Important Message

No Official Addenda to ICD-9-CM Volumes 1 & 2 for 2013

Because the Centers for Medicare and Medicaid Services and the National Center for Health Statistics (NCHS) did not release official ICD-9-CM addenda for volumes 1 & 2 for fiscal 2013, there will be no ICD-9-CM code changes. As a result, the "Summary of Code Changes" and the "ICD-9-CM Code Changes: An Insider's View" (Expert editions only) are not included in this manual. There are no official changes to the Alphabetic Index and Tabular List sections, including instructional notes, title revisions, or other content, though there are changes to other parts of the manual that keep the book up-to-date (see "What is NEW for the 2013 ICD-9-CM Volumes 1 & 2," below).

The Official ICD-9-CM Guidelines for Coding and Reporting included in this manual were effective October 1, 2011. This set of guidelines was approved by the Cooperating Parties and the Editorial Advisory Board for *Coding Clinic for ICD-9-CM*. The Health Insurance Portability and Accountability Act (HIPAA) requires adherence to these guidelines when ICD-9-CM diagnosis codes are being assigned. Since no official ICD-9-CM addendum to the guidelines was released in 2012, the guidelines included in this book stand as the official version effective October 1, 2012, through September 30, 2013. ICD-9-CM is under a "limited update" or "code set freeze" as we prepare for the transition to and implementation of ICD-10-CM on October 1, 2014.

Remember: ICD-9-CM remains the valid code set for reporting until October 1, 2014. Optum is committed to keeping users up-to-date and will continue to update the code books during the code set freeze.

- HIPAA compliance is mandatory—ICD-9-CM is still the valid code set for reporting under HIPAA.
- There is no freeze on the regulatory changes to the payment systems—our hallmark color coding and symbols will be updated.

What is NEW for the 2013 ICD-9-CM Volumes 1 & 2

Your 2013 ICD-9-CM code book includes this new features plus this updated content:

- *New Feature*: ICD-10-CM Coding Proficiency and Documentation Self-Assessment Test with Answers—How ready are you for ICD-10-CM? This is a self-assessment tool for identifying the areas that may require additional coding training or documentation improvement.
- Updated official coding tips
- Updated Medicare Code Edits (color-coding and symbols)
- Updated American Hospital Association's *Coding Clinic for ICD-9-CM* references
- Updated AHA's *Coding Clinic for ICD-9-CM* topic summaries (Expert updateable edition *only*)

- Monthly "Inside Track" eZine: See "Product Alerts and Regulatory Updates" below

ICD-10 Implementation Date Delayed One Year

Due to previous rulemaking, the ICD-10 code set was to be implemented on October 1, 2013, as described in the final rule, "Health Insurance Portability and Accountability Act (HIPAA) Administrative Simplification: Modifications to Medical Data Code Sets Standards to Adopt ICD-10-CM and ICD-10-PCS" (74 FR 3328–3362, January 16, 2009). However, on April 17, 2012, a proposed rule was released (45 CFR Part 162) that would delay for one year implementation of the ICD-10-CM and ICD-10-PCS data sets until October 1, 2014. The Centers for Medicare and Medicaid Services believes this change will give covered entities the additional time needed to synchronize system and business process preparation and to make the necessary changes to accommodate the updated medical data code sets.

In addition, the ICD-10 final rule analyzed the compliance date, emphasizing the interdependency between implementation of ICD-10 and version 5010 of the transaction standards under HIPAA, and the need to balance the benefits of ICD-10 with the need to ensure adequate time for preparation and testing before implementation. The original version 5010 standards compliance date was set for January 1, 2012, but due to a number of issues, the full compliance date was delayed until June 30, 2012. It was recognized that any delay in attaining compliance with version 5010 would negatively impact ICD-10 implementation and compliance. Based on the National Committee on Vital and Health Statistics (NCVHS) recommendations and industry feedback, it was determined that 24 months is the minimum amount of time the industry needs to achieve compliance with ICD-10 once version 5010 has moved into external (level 2) testing.

While considering a number of alternatives for the delay, CMS determined that a one-year delay would provide sufficient time for small providers and small hospitals to become ICD-10 compliant and would be the least financially burdensome to those who had planned to be compliant on October 1, 2013. In its March 2, 2012, letter to the Health and Human Services secretary on a possible delay of the ICD-10 compliance date, the NCVHS urged that any delay should be announced as soon as possible and should not be for more than one year. Among the alternatives ruled out were setting different implementation dates for ICD-10-CM and ICD-10-PCS, moving directly to ICD-11, and implementing a delay of two years. The one-year delay, with a compliance date of October 1, 2014, best meets the objectives for all covered entities.

Effect on Code Set Freeze

A code set freeze is a suspension of updates to ICD-9-CM and ICD-10 code sets. The ICD-9-CM Coordination and Maintenance Committee implemented a partial code set freeze of the ICD-9-CM and ICD-10 codes before the October 1, 2013, ICD-10 compliance deadline. As a result, on October 1, 2012, there will be only limited code updates to both the ICD-9-CM and ICD-10 code sets to capture new technologies and diseases as required by section 503(a) of Pub. L. 108-173. With the one-year delay in the compliance and implementation date, the same limited code set freeze will be in effect for October 1, 2013.

Please note that while the code set freeze limits the number of new codes, it does not limit any necessary corrections or adjustments to the existing classification systems. This means that until ICD-10-CM and PCS are implemented (October 1, 2014), changes may occur to the draft indexes, tabular lists, and coding guidelines. It is essential at this time to stay updated on all the changes to the code sets. Effective training requires using the most current code set version.

Also note that while the ICD-9-CM code set may be under the freeze, regulatory issues continue to evolve that may affect coding guidance and coding edits in the code books.

ICD-10 Readiness Recommendations

Most industry experts recommend that providers and others remain HIPAA compliant by continuing to submit claims using current ICD-9-CM coding resources until the compliance date of October 1, 2014, and to continue to aggressively prepare for the new ICD-10 implementation date by fully assessing the impact of ICD-10, working with software and systems vendors to ensure all systems are fully compliant, and training staff well in advance to help mitigate any loss of productivity or revenue.

Product Alerts and Regulatory Updates

Optum is committed to providing customers with the latest information to code accurately and remain HIPAA compliant. Log on to www.optumcoding.com/productalerts to view, download, and print special reports and announcements regarding official changes to the ICD-9-CM code set or guidelines, as well as regulatory changes affecting coding and reimbursement.

In addition, the purchase of this ICD-9-CM code book automatically entitles the user to receive the complimentary *Inside Track to ICD-10*, a monthly eNewsletter that will help readers stay current on all regulatory changes regarding ICD-9-CM and transition more smoothly to ICD-10-CM.

ICD-9-CM

for Physicians – Volumes 1 & 2

2013 | Expert

International Classification of Diseases
9th Revision
Clinical Modification
Sixth Edition

Edited by:
Anita C. Hart, RHIA, CCS, CCS-P
Melinda S. Stegman, MBA, CCS
Beth Ford, RHIT, CCS

Optum is committed to providing you with the ICD-9-CM code update information you need to code accurately and to be in compliance with HIPAA regulations. In case of adoption of additional ICD-9-CM code changes effective April 1, 2013, Optum will provide these code changes to you at no additional cost! Just check back at www.optumcoding.com/productalerts to review the latest information concerning any new code changes.

Codes Valid October 1, 2012, through September 30, 2013

IPES ISBN 978-1-60151-618-3

Publisher's Notice

Our Commitment to Accuracy

Optum is committed to producing accurate and reliable materials. To report corrections, please visit www.optumcoding.com/accuracy or email accuracy@optum.com. You can also reach customer service by calling 1.800.464.3649, option 1.

Special Reports and Announcements

Purchase of this publication entitles you to Special Reports and announcements via email. Please call customer service at 800-464-3649 or contact your bookstore to take advantage of this exciting free service that will keep you abreast of important code changes and regulatory developments.

Review, download, and print the Special Reports in .pdf format. Log on to www.optumcoding.com/productalerts

Preface

ICD-9-CM for Physicians has been designed with the physician office professional in mind. The most recent official government versions of volumes 1 and 2 have been combined to provide physicians and their office staff with an ICD-9-CM book that is easy to use.

In addition, our technical experts have drawn upon their extensive hands-on experience to enhance the government's official version with valuable features essential to correct coding and reimbursement. With these enhancements, physician office health information professionals will increase the efficiency and timeliness of claim submission for both Medicare and other third-party payers.

As you review the content, you'll find the following:

- All the official ICD-9-CM codes, indexes, notes, footnotes and symbols
- Complete official coding guidelines
- Our exclusive color coding, symbols, and footnotes that alert coders to coding and reimbursement issues. Medicare outpatient code edits, such as invalid fourth or fifth digit for diagnosis codes are identified.
- Illustrations and clinically oriented definitions to aid in correct code assignment
- Coding tips based upon the official coding guidelines and advice found in AHA's *Coding Clinic for ICD-9-CM*
- Symbols identifying new codes and text revisions; pages are dated to indicate when the changes were made
- Exclusive QuickFlip Color Tabs for quick, easy location of terms and codes in the Alphabetic Index and Tabular List

Use of Official Sources

This *ICD-9-CM for Physicians* contains the official U.S. Department of Health and Human Services, ICD-9-CM codes, effective for the current year.

The color coding, footnotes and symbols, which identify coding and reimbursement issues, are derived from official federal government sources, including the Medicare Outpatient Code Editor as well as the knowledge of our technical experts.

The American Hospital Association's (AHA) *Coding Clinic for ICD-9-CM* references are used with permission of the AHA.

Important Information About Your Subscription Service

If you have purchased the updateable *ICD-9-CM for Physicians*, your subscription includes an updating service throughout the year to keep the code book current and accurate. Whenever CMS issues changes or corrections to the ICD-9-CM codes, We will issue an update to the book. In July you will receive a list of all new, revised, and invalid codes for the upcoming year.

Technical Editors

Anita C. Hart, RHIA, CCS, CCS-P, *Product Manager, Optum*
Ms. Hart's experience includes 15 years conducting and publishing research in clinical medicine and human genetics for Yale University, Massachusetts General Hospital, and Massachusetts Institute of Technology. Her research conclusions have been published in several peer-reviewed journals. In addition, Ms. Hart has supervised medical records management, health information management, coding and reimbursement, and workers' compensation issues as the office manager for a physical therapy rehabilitation clinic. Ms. Hart is an expert in physician and facility coding, reimbursement systems, and compliance issues. She is also the author of several Optum publications and has served as subject matter advisor on numerous other publications for hospital and physician practices. Ms. Hart is

the ICD-9-CM and ICD-10-CM/PCS subject matter expert for the Optum, has served as the product manager for that product line for 15 years, and has presented at numerous national conferences. Ms. Hart is a member of the American Academy of Professional Coders (AAPC) and a fully credentialed active member of the American Health Information Management Association (AHIMA). Ms Hart is a current AHIMA Approved ICD-10-CM/PCS Trainer and leads the training initiatives within Optum Coding Solutions business unit.

Melinda S. Stegman, MBA, CCS, *Clinical/Technical Editor, Optum*
Ms. Stegman has more than 25 years of experience in the HIM profession and has been responsible for the update and maintenance of the ICD-9-CM, ICD-10, DRG resources and some cross coder products for Optum. In the past, she also managed the clinical aspects of the HSS/Optum HIM Consulting practice in the Washington, DC area office. Her areas of specialization include training on inpatient and DRG coding, outpatient coding, and Ambulatory Payment Classifications (APCs) for HIM professionals, software developers, and other clients; developing an outpatient billing/coding compliance tool for a major accounting firm; and managing HIM consulting practices. Ms. Stegman is a regular contributing author for *Advance for Health Information Management Professionals* and for the *Journal of Health Care Compliance.* She has performed coding assessments and educational sessions throughout the country. Ms. Stegman is credentialed by the American Health Information Management Association (AHIMA) as a Certified Coding Specialist (CCS), AHIMA-Approved ICD-10-CM/PCS Trainer, and holds a Master of Business Administration degree with a concentration in health care management from the University of New Mexico – Albuquerque.

Beth Ford, RHIT, CCS, *Clinical/Technical Editor, Optum*
Ms. Ford is a clinical/technical editor for Optum. She has more than 25 years experience in both physician and facility ICD-9-CM and CPT/HCPCS coding and compliance. Ms. Ford has extensive experience in a variety of healthcare settings including acute and post-acute facilities, occupational health and ambulatory care. She has provided coding education and consulting services to hospitals and physician practices, and has developed curriculum for medical terminology and ICD-9-CM and CPT coding education for a large healthcare system and multi-specialty physician groups. Formerly, she served as a coding specialist, coding manager, coding trainer/educator, coding consultant, and a health information management director. Her areas of specialization include coding auditing and training for DRG, inpatient, outpatient and physician coding. She is credentialed by the American Health Information Management Association (AHIMA) as a Registered Health Information Technologist (RHIT) and a Certified Coding Specialist (CCS). She is an active member of the AHIMA and is an AHIMA-Approved ICD-10-CM/PCS Trainer.

In addition to the editors, the following people have contributed to this book:

Stacy Perry, *Manager, Desktop Publishing*
Tracy Betzler, *Senior Desktop Publishing Specialist*
Hope M. Dunn, *Senior Desktop Publishing Specialist*
Katie Russell, *Desktop Publishing Specialist*
Kate Holden, *Editor*

What to Do If You Have Questions

If you have any questions call our customer service department toll-free at 800-464-3649, option 1.

If you have comments on the content of this book, please e-mail them to customerservice@ingenix.com or fax to 801-982-4033.

Additional Copies

Contact the customer service order department toll-free at 800-464-3649, option 1.

Introduction

History and Future of ICD-9-CM

The International Classification of Diseases, Ninth Revision, Clinical Modification (ICD-9-CM) is based on the official version of the World Health Organization's Ninth Revision, International Classification of Diseases (ICD-9). ICD-9-CM classifies morbidity and mortality information for statistical purposes, indexing of hospital records by disease and operations, data storage, and retrieval.

This modification of ICD-9 supplants the Eighth Revision International Classification of Diseases, Adapted for Use in the United States (ICDA-8) and the Hospital Adaptation of ICDA (H-ICDA).

The concept of extending the International Classification of Diseases for use in hospital indexing was originally developed in response to a need for a more efficient basis for storage and retrieval of diagnostic data. In 1950, the U.S. Public Health Service and the Veterans Administration began independent tests of the International Classification of Diseases for hospital indexing purposes. The following year, the Columbia Presbyterian Medical Center in New York City adopted the International Classification of Diseases, Sixth Revision, with some modifications for use in its medical record department. A few years later, the Commission on Professional and Hospital Activities (CPHA) in Ann Arbor, Mich., adopted the International Classification of Diseases with similar modifications for use in hospitals participating in the Professional Activity Study.

The problem of adapting ICD for indexing hospital records was addressed by the U.S. National Committee on Vital and Health Statistics through its subcommittee on hospital statistics. The subcommittee reviewed the modifications made by the various users of ICD and proposed that uniform changes be made. This was done by a small working party.

In view of the growing interest in the use of the International Classification of Diseases for hospital indexing, a study was undertaken in 1956 by the American Hospital Association and the American Medical Record Association (then the American Association of Medical Record Librarians) of the relative efficiencies of coding systems for diagnostic indexing. This study indicated the International Classification of Diseases provided a suitable and efficient framework for indexing hospital records. The major users of the International Classification of Diseases for hospital indexing purposes then consolidated their experiences, and an adaptation was first published in December 1959. A revision was issued in 1962 and the first "Classification of Operations and Treatments" was included.

In 1966, the international conference for revising the International Classification of Diseases noted the eighth revision of ICD had been constructed with hospital indexing in mind and considered the revised classification suitable, in itself, for hospital use in some countries. However, it was recognized that the basic classification might provide inadequate detail for diagnostic indexing in other countries. A group of consultants was asked to study the eighth revision of ICD (ICD-8) for applicability to various users in the United States. This group recommended that further detail be provided for coding of hospital and morbidity data. The American Hospital Association was requested to develop the needed adaptation proposals. This was done by an advisory committee (the Advisory Committee to the Central Office on ICDA). In 1968 the United States Public Health Service published the product, Eighth Revision International Classification of Diseases, Adapted for Use in the United States. This became commonly known as ICDA-8, and beginning in 1968 it served as the basis for coding diagnostic data for both official morbidity and mortality statistics in the United States.

In 1968, the CPHA published the Hospital Adaptation of ICDA (H-ICDA) based on both the original ICD-8 and ICDA-8. In 1973, CPHA published a revision of H-ICDA, referred to as H-ICDA-2. Hospitals throughout the United States were divided in their use of these classifications until January 1979, when ICD-9-CM was made the single classification intended primarily for use in the United States, replacing these earlier related, but somewhat dissimilar, classifications.

Physicians have been required by law to submit diagnosis codes for Medicare reimbursement since the passage of the Medicare Catastrophic Coverage Act of 1988. This act requires physician offices to include the appropriate diagnosis codes when billing for services provided to Medicare beneficiaries on or after April 1, 1989. The Centers for Medicare and Medicaid Services (CMS) designated ICD-9-CM as the coding system physicians must use.

The ICD-10-CM classification system was developed by the National Center for Health Statistics (NCHS) as a clinical modification to the ICD-10 system developed by the World Health Organization (WHO), primarily as a unique system for use in the United States for morbidity and mortality reporting. Although ICD-10-CM has not yet been implemented for use in the United States, ICD-10 has been adopted for use in the coding and classification or mortality data from death certificates. ICD-10 replaced ICD-9 for this purpose as of January 1, 1999. The Department of Health and Human Services (HHS) published the final rule regarding the adoption of both ICD-10-CM and ICD-10-PCS in the January 16, 2009 *Federal Register* (45 CFR part 162 [CMS—0013—F]). April 17, 2012, the Department of Health and Human Services released a notice postponing the date by which certain health care entities must comply with diagnosis and procedure codes from the International Classification of Diseases, 10th edition (ICD-10). The compliance date for implementing ICD-10-CM and ICD-10-PCS as a replacement for ICD-9-CM is October 1, 2014.

ICD-9-CM Background

In February 1977, a steering committee was convened by the National Center for Health Statistics to provide advice and counsel in developing a clinical modification of ICD-9. The organizations represented on the steering committee included the following:

- American Association of Health Data Systems
- American Hospital Association
- American Medical Record Association
- Association for Health Records
- Council on Clinical Classifications
- Centers for Medicare and Medicaid Services, Department of Health and Human Services
- WHO Center for Classification of Diseases for North America, sponsored by the National Center for Health Statistics, Department of Health and Human Services

The Council on Clinical Classifications was sponsored by the following:

- American Academy of Pediatrics
- American College of Obstetricians and Gynecologists
- American College of Physicians
- American College of Surgeons
- American Psychiatric Association
- Commission on Professional and Hospital Activities

The steering committee met periodically in 1977. Clinical guidance and technical input were provided by task forces on classification from the Council on Clinical Classification's sponsoring organizations.

ICD-9-CM is a clinical modification of the World Health Organization's ICD-9. The term "clinical" is used to emphasize the modification's intent: to serve as a useful tool to classify morbidity data for indexing medical records, medical care review, and ambulatory and other medical care programs, as well as for basic health statistics. To describe the clinical picture of the patient, the codes must be more precise than those needed only for statistical groupings and trend analysis.

Characteristics of ICD-9-CM

ICD-9-CM far exceeds its predecessors in the number of codes provided. The disease classification has been expanded to include health-related conditions and to provide greater specificity at the fifth-digit level of detail. These fifth digits are not optional; they are intended for use in recording the information substantiated in the clinical record.

Volume I (Tabular List) of ICD-9-CM contains four appendixes:

Appendix A: Morphology of Neoplasms

Appendix B: Deleted effective October 1, 2004

Appendix C: Classification of Drugs by American Hospital Formulary Service List Number and Their ICD-9-CM Equivalents

Appendix D: Classification of Industrial Accidents According to Agency

Appendix E: List of Three-Digit Categories

These appendixes are included as a reference to provide further information about the patient's clinical picture, to further define a diagnostic statement, to aid in classifying new drugs or to reference three-digit categories.

Volume 2 (Alphabetic Index) of ICD-9-CM contains many diagnostic terms that do not appear in volume I since the index includes most diagnostic terms currently in use.

The Disease Classification

ICD-9-CM is totally compatible with its parent system, ICD-9, thus meeting the need for comparability of morbidity and mortality statistics at the international level. A few fourth-digit codes were created in existing three-digit rubrics only when the necessary detail could not be accommodated by the use of a fifth-digit subclassification. To ensure that each rubric of ICD-9-CM collapses back to its ICD-9 counterpart the following specifications governed the ICD-9-CM disease classification:

Specifications for the Tabular List:

1.   Three-digit rubrics and their contents are unchanged from ICD-9.

2.   The sequence of three-digit rubrics is unchanged from ICD-9.

3.   Three-digit rubrics are not added to the main body of the classification.

4.   Unsubdivided three-digit rubrics are subdivided where necessary to

    • add clinical detail

    • isolate terms for clinical accuracy

5.   The modification in ICD-9-CM is accomplished by adding a fifth digit to existing ICD-9 rubrics, except as noted under #7 below.

6.   The optional dual classification in ICD-9 is modified.

    • Duplicate rubrics are deleted:

        – four-digit manifestation categories duplicating etiology entries

        – manifestation inclusion terms duplicating etiology entries[2]

    • Manifestations of disease are identified, to the extent possible, by creating five-digit codes in the etiology rubrics.

    • When the manifestation of a disease cannot be included in the etiology rubrics, provision for its identification is made by retaining the ICD-9 rubrics used for classifying manifestations of disease.

7.   The format of ICD-9-CM is revised from that used in ICD-9.

    • American spelling of medical terms is used.

    • Inclusion terms are indented beneath the titles of codes.

    • Codes not to be used for primary tabulation of disease are printed in italics with the notation, "code first underlying disease."

Specifications for the Alphabetic Index:

1.   The format of the Alphabetic Index follows that of ICD-9.

2.   When two codes are required to indicate etiology and manifestation, the manifestation code appears in brackets (e.g., diabetic cataract 250.5 [366.41]).

The ICD-9-CM Coordination and Maintenance Committee

The ICD-9-CM Coordination and Maintenance Committee, a federal committee, was created as a forum for proposals to update International Classification of Diseases, Ninth Revision, Clinical Modification, Sixth Edition (ICD-9-CM). A representative from the National Center for Health Statistics (NCHS) and one from the Centers for Medicare and Medicaid Services (CMS) co-chair the ICD-9-CM Coordination and Maintenance Committee meetings. Responsibility for maintaining ICD-9-CM is divided between the two agencies, with NCHS classifying diagnoses (volumes 1 and 2) and CMS classifying procedures (volume 3).

Proposals for changes to the ICD-9-CM classification system are submitted and discussed in open forum meetings held in March and September of each year at the headquarters of CMS in Baltimore. Comments received during or after the meetings are then reviewed and evaluated. All final decisions are made by the director of NCHS and the administrator of CMS. The complete official document of changes to the classification system is released as the Addenda for the International Classification of Disease, Ninth Revision, Clinical Modification, Sixth Edition, Volume 1, 2, & 3.

The *ICD-9-CM for Physicians, Volumes 1 & 2,* is based on the official version of the International Classification of Diseases, Ninth Revision, Clinical Modification, Sixth Edition, issued by the U.S. Department of Health and Human Services. Annual code changes are implemented by the government and are effective October 1 and valid through September 30 of the following year. If a convincing case is made that requires a new code to capture new technology or an emerging disease, this new code may be implemented on April 1 of the following year.

How to Use the ICD-9-CM for Physicians (Volumes 1 & 2)

ICD-9-CM for Physicians is based on the official version of the International Classification of Diseases, Ninth Revision, Clinical Modification, Sixth Edition, issued by the U.S. Department of Health and Human Services. Annual code changes are implemented by the government and are effective Oct. 1 and valid through Sept. 30 of the following year.

To accommodate the coder's approach to coding, the Alphabetic Index (Volume 2) has been placed before the Tabular List (Volume 1). This allows the user to locate the term in the index, then confirm the accuracy of the code in the Tabular List.

10 Steps to Correct Coding

To code accurately, it is necessary to have a working knowledge of medical terminology and to understand the characteristics, terminology and conventions of ICD-9-CM. Transforming descriptions of diseases, injuries, conditions and procedures into numerical designations (coding) is a complex activity and should not be undertaken without proper training.

Originally, coding allowed retrieval of medical information by diagnoses and operations for medical research, education and administration. Coding today is used to describe the medical necessity of a procedure and facilitate payment of health services, to evaluate utilization patterns and to study the appropriateness of health care costs. Coding provides the basis for epidemiological studies and research into the quality of health care. Incorrect or inaccurate coding can lead to investigations of fraud and abuse. Therefore, coding must be performed correctly and consistently to produce meaningful statistics to aid in planning for the health needs of the nation.

Follow the steps below to code correctly:

Step 1: Identify the reason for the visit (e.g., sign, symptom, diagnosis, condition to be coded).

Physicians describe the patient's condition using terminology that includes specific diagnoses as well as symptoms, problems or reasons for the encounter. If symptoms are present but a definitive diagnosis has not yet been determined, code the symptoms. Do not code conditions that are referred to as "rule out," "suspected," "probable" or "questionable."

Step 2: Always consult the Alphabetic Index, Volume 2, before turning to the Tabular List.

The most critical rule is to begin a code search in the index. Never turn first to the Tabular List (Volume 1), as this will lead to coding errors and less specificity in code assignments. To prevent coding errors, use both the Alphabetic Index and the Tabular List when locating and assigning a code.

Step 3: Locate the main entry term.

The Alphabetic Index is arranged by condition. Conditions may be expressed as nouns, adjectives and eponyms. Some conditions have multiple entries under their synonyms. Main terms are identified using boldface type.

Step 4: Read and interpret any notes listed with the main term.

Notes are identified using italicized type.

Step 5: Review entries for modifiers.

Nonessential modifiers are in parentheses. These parenthetical terms are supplementary words or explanatory information that may either be present or absent in the diagnostic statement and do not affect code assignment.

Step 6: Interpret abbreviations, cross-references, symbols and brackets.

Cross-references used are "*see*," "*see* category," or "*see* also." The abbreviation NEC may follow main terms or subterms. NEC (not elsewhere classified) indicates that there is no specific code for the condition even though the medical documentation may be very specific. The ☑ box indicates the code requires an additional digit. If the appropriate digits are not found in the index, in a box beneath the main term, you MUST refer to the Tabular List. Italicized brackets [ ], are used to enclose a second code number that must be used with the code immediately preceding it and in that sequence.

Step 7: Choose a tentative code and locate it in the Tabular List.

Be guided by any inclusion or exclusion terms, notes or other instructions, such as "*code first*" and "use additional code," that would direct the use of a different or additional code from that selected in the index for a particular diagnosis, condition or disease.

Step 8: Determine whether the code is at the highest level of specificity.

Assign three-digit codes (category codes) if there are no four-digit codes within the code category. Assign four-digit codes (subcategory codes) if there are no five-digit codes for that category. Assign five-digit codes (fifth-digit subclassification codes) for those categories where they are available.

Step 9: Consult the color coding and reimbursement prompts, including the age and sex edits.

Consult the official ICD-9-CM guidelines for coding and reporting, and refer to the AHA's *Coding Clinic for ICD-9-CM* for coding guidelines governing the use of specific codes.

Step 10: Assign the code.

Organization

Introduction

The introductory material in this book includes the history and future of ICD-9-CM as well as an overview of the classification system

Official ICD-9-CM Conventions

This section provides a full explanation of all the official footnotes, symbols, instructional notes, and conventions found in the official government version

Additional Conventions

Exclusive color-coding, symbols, and notations have been included in the *ICD-9-CM for Physicians, Volumes 1 and 2* to alert coders to important coding and reimbursement issues. This section provides a full explanation of the additional conventions used throughout this book.

ICD-10-CM Coding Proficiency and Documentation Self-Assessment

Use this self-assessment to identify the areas that may require additional coding training or documentation improvement prior to the implementation of ICD-10-CM on October 1, 2014.

Summary of AHA's *Coding Clinic for ICD-9-CM* Topics

This is a brief summary of the official advice concerning coding topics covered in the latest issues of AHA's *Coding Clinic for ICD-9-CM* and is found **ONLY** in the *ICD-9-CM Expert for Physicians* updateable edition.

Coding Guidelines

Included in this book are the official ICD-9-CM coding guidelines as approved by the four cooperating parties of the ICD-9-CM Coordination and Maintenance Committee. Failure to comply with these official coding guidelines may result in denied or delayed claims.

Disease Classification: Alphabetic Index to Diseases

The Alphabetic Index to Diseases is separated by tabs labeled with the letters of the alphabet, contains diagnostic terms for illnesses, injuries and reasons for encounters with health care professionals. Both the Table of Drugs and Chemicals and the Alphabetic Index to External Causes of Injury and Poisoning are easily located with the tabs in this section.

The warning statement at the bottom of every page of the index, ▽ Subterms under main terms may continue to next column or page, is a reminder to always check for additional subterms before making final selection.

Disease Classification: Tabular List of Diseases

The Tabular List of Diseases arranges the ICD-9-CM codes and descriptors numerically. Tabs divide this section into chapters, identified by the code range on the tab.

The Tabular List includes two supplementary classifications:

- V Codes–Supplementary Classification of Factors Influencing Health Status and Contact with Health Services (V01–V91)
- E Codes–Supplementary Classification of External Causes of Injury and Poisoning (E000–E999)

ICD-9-CM includes four official appendixes.

- Appendix A   Morphology of Neoplasms
- Appendix B   Deleted effective October 1, 2004
- Appendix C   Classification of Drugs by AHFS List
- Appendix D   Classification of Industrial Accidents According to Agency
- Appendix E   List of Three-digit Categories

These appendixes are included as a reference to provide further information about the patient's circumstances, help further define a diagnostic statement, maintain a tumor registry and aid in classifying new drugs.

Resources

Listed below are the exclusive resources found **ONLY** in the *ICD-9-CM Expert for Physicians, Volumes 1 & 2.*

10 Steps to Correct Coding

This is a valuable resource that takes the coder step by step through the coding process with detailed explanations accompanied by coding examples that demonstrate the practical application of ICD-9-CM conventions and coding guidelines in 10 steps.

Valid Three-digit Code Table

ICD-9-CM is composed of codes with either 3, 4, or 5 digits. A code is invalid if it has not been coded to the full number of digits required for that code. There are a certain number codes that are valid for reporting as three digit codes. A list of these valid three-digit code is included as a convenient reference when auditing claims.

Code Tables

Exclusive coding tables covering abortion, burns, complications, diabetes, hernia, pregnancy, and others are provided to simplify those complex coding issues.

ICD-9-CM Official Conventions

ICD-9-CM Footnotes, Symbols, Instructional Notes and Conventions

This *ICD-9-CM for Physicians* preserves all the footnotes, symbols, instructional notes and conventions found in the government's official version. Accurate coding depends upon understanding the meaning of these elements.

The following appear in the disease Tabular List, unless otherwise noted.

Official Government Symbols

§   The section mark preceding a code denotes a footnote on the page. This symbol is used in the Tabular List of Diseases.

ICD-9-CM Conventions Used in the Tabular List

In addition to the symbols and footnotes above, the ICD-9-CM disease tabular has certain abbreviations, punctuation, symbols and other conventions. Our *ICD-9-CM for Physicians* preserves these conventions. Proper use of the conventions will lead to efficient and accurate coding.

Abbreviations

NEC   Not elsewhere classifiable
This abbreviation is used when the ICD-9-CM system does not provide a code specific for the patient's condition.

NOS   Not otherwise specified
This abbreviation is the equivalent of "unspecified" and is used only when the coder lacks the information necessary to code to a more specific four-digit subcategory.

[ ]   Brackets enclose synonyms, alternative terminology or explanatory phrases:

> **482.2   Pneumonia due to Hemophilus influenzae [H. influenzae]**

Brackets that appear beneath a code indicate the fifth digits that are considered valid fifth digits for the code. This convention is applied for those instances in ICD-9-CM where not all common fifth digits are considered valid for each subcategory within a category.

> **715.0   Osteoarthrosis, generalized**
> [0,4,9]

Generalized arthrosis can only be assigned in cases for which the degenerative joint disease involves multiple joints. Therefore, this code is considered for arthrosis in the sites described as unspecified, hand (which consists of multiple joints), or multiple sites. Therefore, only fifth digits 0, 4, and 9 are valid with subcategory 715.0.

[ ]   Slanted brackets that appear in the Alphabetic Index indicate mandatory multiple coding. Both codes must be assigned to fully describe the condition and are sequenced in the order listed.

> **Tachycardia**
> ventricular (paroxysmal)
>   psychogenic 316 *[427.1]*

Psychogenic paroxysmal tachycardia is reported using both 316, Psychogenic factors associated with diseases classified elsewhere, and 427.1, Paroxysmal ventricular tachycardia.

( )   Parentheses enclose supplementary words, called nonessential modifiers, that may be present in the narrative description of a disease without affecting the code assignment:

> **198.4   Other parts of nervous system**
> Meninges (cerebral) (spinal)

:   Colons are used in the Tabular List after an incomplete term that needs one or more of the modifiers that follow in order to make it assignable to a given category:

> **021.1   Enteric tularemia**
> Tularemia:
>   cryptogenic
>   intestinal
>   typhoidal

}   Braces enclose a series of terms, each of which is modified by the statement appearing to the right of the brace:

> **560.2   Volvulus**
> Knotting
> Strangulation   } of intestine, bowel, or
> Torsion   colon
> Twist

Other Conventions

Boldface   Boldface type is used for all codes and titles in the Tabular List.

Italicized   Italicized type is used for all exclusion notes and to identify codes that should not be used for describing the primary diagnosis.

General Notes Used in the Tabular List

These notes appear only in the Tabular List of Diseases:

Includes   An includes note further defines or clarifies the content of the chapter, subchapter, category, subcategory or subclassification. The includes note in the example below applies only to category 461.

Excludes   following the word "Excludes" are not classified to the chapter, subchapter, category, subcategory or specific subclassification code under which it is found. The note also may provide the location of the excluded diagnosis. Excludes notes are italicized.

> **461   Acute sinusitis**
> [INCLUDES] abscess
>   empyema   } acute, of sinus
>   infection   (accessory)
>   inflammation (nasal)
>   suppuration
>   *EXCLUDES* *chronic or unspecified sinusitis (473.0-473.9)*

Instructional Notes

The following official instructional notes are critical to correct coding practices. The instructional notes appear in red type in the Tabular List.

Use additional code:
This instruction signals the coder that an additional code should be used if the information is available to provide a more complete picture of that diagnosis.

> **362.13 Changes in vascular appearance**
> Vascular sheathing of retina
> Use additional code for any associated atherosclerosis (440.8)

For emphasis this instructional note appears in red type in the tabular section.

There are coding circumstances outside of the etiology/ manifestation convention when multiple coding for a single condition is required. The "Use additional code" note will be found under the associated condition code in the tabular. In the index, the multiple coding requirement is indicated by the use of the slanted bracket. The two codes are to be sequenced as listed in the index. For example, retinal arteriosclerosis must be coded using two codes sequenced as listed in the index.

> **Arteriosclerosis, arteriosclerotic**
> retinal (vascular) 440.8 *[362.13]*

Code first underlying disease:

The *"Code first underlying"* instructional note found under certain codes is a sequencing rule. Most often this sequencing rule applies to the etiology/manifestation convention and is found under the manifestation code. The manifestation code may never be used alone or as a primary diagnosis (i.e., sequenced first). The instructional note, the code and its descriptor appear in italics in the Tabular List.

> **590.81 *Pyelitis or pyelonephritis in diseases classified elsewhere***
> *Code first underlying disease as:*
>   tuberculosis (016.0)

Not all codes with a "Code first underlying disease" instructional note are part of the etiology/manifestation convention. The `Code first' note will appear, but the title of the code and the instructional note are not in italics. These codes may be reported alone or as the secondary diagnosis. For example, disseminated chorioretinitis may be reported as a principal or first-listed diagnosis. However, if the underlying condition that caused disseminated chorioretinitis is known, such as tuberculous disseminated chorioretinitis, two codes are required and sequenced as listed in the index.

> **363.13 Disseminated choroiditis and chorioretinitis, generalized**
>   Code first underlying disease as:
>   tuberculosis (017.3)

For emphasis this instructional note appears in red type in the tabular section.

Code, if applicable, any causal condition first:

A code with this note indicates that this code may be assigned as a principal diagnosis when the causal condition is unknown or not applicable. If a causal condition is known, then the code for that condition should be sequenced as the principal or first-listed diagnosis.

> **590.0 Chronic pyelonephritis**
>   Chronic pyelitis
>   Chronic pyonephrosis
>   Code, if applicable, any causal condition first

For emphasis this instructional note appears in red type in the tabular section.

Instructional Notes Used in the Index

Omit code:

"Omit code" is used to instruct the coder that no code is to be assigned. When this instruction is found in the Alphabetic Index to Diseases the medical term should not be coded as a diagnosis.

> **Metaplasia**
>   cervix — *omit code*

See Condition:

The "see condition" note found in the Alphabetic Index to Disease instructs the coder to refer to a main term for the condition. This note will follow index terms that are nouns for anatomical sites or adjectival forms of disease term. In the example below, the index terms "Cervix" and "Diffuse" are followed by the — see condition. Coders should search the index using a condition term such as atrophy or prolapse.

> **Cervix** — *see* condition
> **Diffuse** — *see* condition

Morphology Codes:

For each neoplastic disease listed in the index, a morphology code is provided that identifies histological type and behavior.

> *Example:*
>
> **Myelolipoma** (M8870/0) — *see* Neoplasm, by site, benign

The histology is identified by the first four digits and the behavior is identified by the digit following the slash. Appendix A of Volume 1 contains a listing of morphology codes. This appendix is helpful when the pathology report identifies the neoplasm by using an M code. The coder may refer to Appendix A to determine the nomenclature of the neoplasm that will be the main term to search in the Index. The behavior classification is as follows:

0 Benign

1 Uncertain whether benign or malignant
    Borderline malignancy

2 Carcinoma in situ
    Intraepithelial
    Noninfiltrating
    Noninvasive

3 Malignant, primary site

6 Malignant, metastatic site
    Secondary site

9 Malignant, uncertain whether primary or metastatic site

Additional Conventions

Symbols and Notations

New and Revised Text Symbols

●   A bullet at a code or line of text indicates that the entry is new.

▲   A triangle in the Tabular List indicates that the code title is revised. In the Alphabetic Index the triangle indicates that a code has changed.

►◄   These symbols appear at the beginning and at the end of a section of new or revised text.

When these symbols appear on a page there will be a date on the lower outside corner of the page indicating the date of the change, (e.g., October 2011).

Additional Digits Required

☑4ᵗʰ   This symbol indicates that the code requires a fourth digit.

☑5ᵗʰ   This symbol indicates that a code requires a fifth digit.

☑   This symbol found only in the Alphabetic Index sections and the Table of Drugs and Chemicals indicates that an additional digit is required. Referring to the tabular section is essential to locate the appropriate additional digit.

AHA's *Coding Clinic for ICD-9-CM* References

The four cooperating parties have designated the AHA's *Coding Clinic for ICD-9-CM* as the official publication for coding guidelines. The references are identified by the notation **AHA:** followed by the issue, year and page number.

In the example below, AHA's *Coding Clinic for ICD-9-CM*, third quarter 1991, page 15, contains a discussion on code assignment for vitreous hemorrhage:

> **379.23 Vitreous hemorrhage**
> **AHA:** 3Q, '91, 15

The table below explains the abbreviations in the *Coding Clinic* references:

J-F	January/February
M-A	March/April
M-J	May/June
J-A	July/August
S-O	September/October
N-D	November/December
1Q	First quarter
2Q	Second quarter
3Q	Third quarter
4Q	Fourth quarter

AHA's *Coding Clinic for ICD-9-CM* references appear in blue type in the Tabular List.

Age and Sex Edit Symbols

The age edits below address OCE edits and are used to detect inconsistencies between the patient's age and diagnosis. They appear in the Tabular List of Diseases to the right of the code description.

Newborn Age: 0   N

These diagnoses are intended for newborns and neonates and the patient's age must be 0 years.

Pediatric Age: 0-17   P

These diagnoses are intended for children and the patient's age must between 0 and 17 years.

Maternity Age: 12-55   M

These diagnoses are intended for the patients between the age of 12 and 55 years.

Adult Age: 15-124   A

These diagnoses are intended for the patients between the age of 15 and 124 years.

The sex symbols below address OCE edits and are used to detect inconsistencies between the patient's sex and diagnosis. They appear in the Tabular List of Diseases to the right of the code description:

♂   **Male diagnosis only**
This symbol appears to the right of the code description. This reference appears in the disease Tabular List.

♀   **Female diagnosis only**
This symbol appears to the right of the code description. This reference appears in the disease Tabular List.

Color Coding

To alert the coder to Medicare outpatient code edits and other important reimbursement issues, color bars have been added over the code descriptors in the Tabular List. Some codes carry more than one color.

Carriers use the Medicare Outpatient Code Editor (OCE) to examine claims for coding and billing accuracy and completeness. Color codes in this book signify Medicare code edits for manifestation codes not to be reported as a primary diagnosis, and when a more specific diagnosis code should be used.

Manifestation Code

These codes will appear in italic type as well as with a blue color bar over the code title. A manifestation code is not allowed to be reported as a first-listed diagnosis because each describes a manifestation of some other underlying disease, not the disease itself. This is referred to as mandatory multiple coding of etiology and manifestation. Code the underlying disease first. A *Code first underlying disease* instructional note will appear with underlying disease codes identified. In the Alphabetic Index these codes are listed as the secondary code in slanted brackets with the code for the underlying disease listed first.

Other Specified Code

These codes will appear with a gray color bar over the code title. Use these codes when the documentation indicates a specified diagnosis, but the ICD-9-CM system does not have a specific code that describes the diagnosis. These codes are may be stated as "Other" or "Not elsewhere classified (NEC)."

Unspecified Code

These codes will have a yellow color bar over the code title. Use these codes when the neither the diagnostic statement nor the documentation provides enough information to assign a more specified diagnosis code. These codes may be stated as "Unspecified" or "Not otherwise specified (NOS)." Note: Do not assign these codes when a more specific diagnosis has been determined.

Other Notations

DEF: This symbol indicates a definition of disease term. The definition will appear in blue type in the Disease Tabular Lists.

TIPS: This symbol precedes official coding advice found in the official coding guidelines and AHA's *Coding Clinic for ICD-9-CM*. Coding tips appear in blue type in the Tabular List.

I-10   In preparation for the transition to coding using the ICD-10-CM classification system, examples of ICD-10-CM codes have been provided for selected ICD-9-CM diagnosis codes. This symbol indicates that the code provided is an ICD-10-CM code to which the selected ICD-9-CM code is mapped.

Note: Coding professionals should keep in mind the following points when referring to the ICD-10-CM codes provided:

- ICD-10-CM codes are not currently valid for reporting purposes.
- The ICD-10-CM code may represent only one possible coding option. Since mappings between ICD-9-CM and ICD-10-CM are not always straightforward one-to-one correspondences due to the differences in terminology and clinical concepts, the mapping may result in a one-to-many code option. Not all code options for a particular ICD-9-CM

code are provided. For cases in which many code alternatives are possible in ICD-10-CM, only one example is provided.

- The ICD-10-CM code examples are provided only for the most frequently reported ICD-9-CM codes in each chapter.
- The ICD-10-CM codes are examples only and are provided to ease the transition to the new classification system.

PDx

This symbol identifies a V code that generally is for use as a first listed diagnosis only (primary) but may be used as an additional diagnosis if the patient has more than one encounter on one day or there is more than one reason for the encounter.

The instructions for V code use contained in the new official coding guidelines only identify those V codes that can only be used as a PDx. All other V codes may either be SDx or PDx depending upon circumstances of the encounter, by meeting the definition of first-listed or principal diagnosis, and by following any specific V code guidelines in section I.C.18 a-e. With the elimination of the V Code Table, the responsibility of those assigning the V codes as PDx is to make sure the circumstances of the encounter meet the definition of first-listed or principal diagnosis, follow all coding instructions, and follow the V code specific guidelines. Optum does not include the SDx edit since it is no longer based on an official source and the V code use is determined by circumstances of the encounter.

Note: Please note that the symbols indicating the V code designation and the V codes that may be principal or first listed (primary) diagnoses included in the official coding guidelines [Section 1.C.18.e] are consistent with reporting guidelines for health care encounters *excluding acute care inpatient admissions*. These V code edits are often in conflict with the inpatient prospective payment system (IPPS) edits. For example, V22.0 Encounter for supervision of a normal first pregnancy, may be an appropriate primary reason for an outpatient encounter. However, supervision for a normal pregnancy is not an acceptable principal diagnosis for an inpatient admission and will have an unacceptable principal diagnosis edit under IPPS.

Wrong Surgery Edit

When a particular surgical or other invasive procedure is indicated to treat a medical condition and the wrong procedure is performed, the procedure is not considered reasonable and necessary. Assign E codes to report these wrong surgery incidents. A Wrong Surgery edit associated with the E code will be triggered and the claim will be denied and returned to the provider. The wrong surgery E codes are identified with an asterisk (*) and a footnote.

Alphabetic Indexes

▽ **Subterms under main terms may continue to next column/page.**

This warning statement is a reminder to always check for additional subterms and information that may continue on to the next page or column before making a final selection.

ICD-10-CM Coding and Documentation Proficiency Self-Assessment

Introduction

This self-assessment covers ICD-10-CM coding guidance and the required level of detail for clinical documentation of heart disease, diabetes, and pneumonia. These high-volume diagnoses have numerous coding guidelines and documentation requirements. The assessment also covers ICD-10-CM conventions that are new or problematic. Use this self-assessment to identify the areas that may require additional coding training or documentation improvement before ICD-10-CM is implemented on October 1, 2014.

Instructions

Code assignments are based upon the 2012 ICD-10-CM diagnosis code set for all reportable diagnoses, including external causes of morbidity (V00–Y99), as appropriate, according to the instructions in ICD-10-CM conventions and the 2012 *ICD-10-CM Draft Official Guidelines for Coding and Reporting*. Answer each question based on the information provided. Note that for some questions, the codes in the answer are not based upon the information provided, requiring that the provider be queried for specific information because the documentation is insufficient to assign codes correctly.

Self-Assessment Questions

1. In ICD-10-CM what are the two anatomical classifications of pneumonia and the sites of the lung affected by each?

2. The attending physician's final diagnosis on the progress note on the day of discharge: atypical pneumonia. Sputum results: normal flora. Chest x-ray: bilateral lower lobe consolidation.

   A Assign J18.9 Pneumonia, unspecified organism.

   B Documentation does not follow guidelines and/or the physician must be queried to determine the following:

   - Clinical significance of the sputum results
   - Clinical significance of the chest x-ray

3. What is the appropriate diagnosis code assignment(s) for ESRD due to type I diabetes on chronic dialysis via right arm AV shunt and hypertension as documented by the provider?

   Code assignment:_____

4. Attending admission note: Patient is a 42-year-old female who presents with diabetes with hypoglycemia.

   A Assign E11.649 Type II diabetes mellitus with hypoglycemia without coma.

   B Documentation does not follow guidelines and/or the physician must be queried to determine the following:

   - Type of diabetes mellitus
   - Cause of the hypoglycemia

5. Assign the appropriate code(s) for a diagnosis by the provider of ischemic heart disease and coronary artery disease without history of coronary bypass and current smoker.

   Code assignment:_____

6. Assign the appropriate code(s) for a patient diagnosed by the provider with community-acquired pneumonia who presented with hemoptysis, productive cough, fever, and an increased respiratory rate with sputum culture stain showing gram-negative bacilli.

   Code assignment:_____

7. Discharge summary: 1. VAP, with sputum stain identifying *Klebsiella pneumoniae*, sensitivity performed and Keflex administered. 2. Vent-dependent patient.

   A Assign J95.851 Ventilator associated pneumonia, B96.1 Klebsiella pneumoniae [K. pneumoniae] as the cause of diseases classified elsewhere, and Z99.11 Dependence on respirator [ventilator] status.

   B Documentation does not follow guidelines and/or the physician must be queried to determine the following:

   - Clinical significance of the sputum results
   - Pneumonia: present on admission or post admission

8. Assign the appropriate diagnosis code(s) for diabetes II with Charcôt joint, left hallux with ulcer, with dry gangrene and with chronic osteomyelitis. The patient is admitted for amputation due to osteomyelitis documented in the surgeon's admission note.

   Code assignment:_____

9. What is the appropriate code assignment for a diagnosis of ischemic cardiomyopathy and coronary artery disease, as documented by the provider?

   Code assignment:_____

10. Discharge summary: Patient was admitted from the ED for work-up of precordial chest pain, elevated troponin; history of CABG, congestive heart failure, hypertension. Final diagnosis: ASCAD with USA, s/p CABG, CHF. Most recent diagnostic left heart catheterization showed clean vein and mammary grafts with 90% atherosclerotic stenosis of the native LAD portion. Plans are for future coronary angioplasty as an outpatient. Continue Lasix, Norvasc, and Nitrolingual.

    A Assign I25.110 Atherosclerotic heart disease of native coronary artery with unstable angina, I11.9 Hypertensive heart disease without heart failure, I50.9 Heart failure, unspecified, Z95.1 Presence of aortocoronary bypass graft.

    B Documentation does not follow guidelines and/or the physician must be queried to determine the following:

    - Description of relationship between the hypertension and congestive heart failure
    - Type of congestive heart failure

11. What is the appropriate diagnosis code assignment for the postobstructive pneumonia, right middle lobe, due to hilar lung cancer right lobe when the treatment is directed only toward the pneumonia as documented in the admission note by the resident?

    Code assignment:_____

12. **Discharge summary: RSV pneumonia with acute bronchiolitis in one-month-old, high-risk due to being ex-35-week preemie.**

    A   Assign J12.1 Respiratory syncytial virus pneumonia, J21.Ø Acute bronchiolitis due to RSV, PØ7.38 Preterm newborn, gestational age 35 completed weeks.

    B   Documentation does not follow guidelines and/or the physician must be queried to determine the following:

    - Clinical significance of the history of prematurity
    - Identification of the causal organism of the bronchiolitis

13. **Assign the appropriate diagnosis code(s) for a subsequent encounter for a patient on prescribed steroids with steroid-induced diabetes mellitus, requiring insulin regimen, determined to be inadequately controlled due to dietary noncompliance as documented by the provider.**

    Code assignment:_____

14. **What is the appropriate code assignment for a diagnosis of unstable angina in a patient who is a nonsmoker with coronary artery disease due to second-hand smoke, as documented by the provider?**

    Code assignment:_____

15. **Order for outpatient pre-op labs via telephone by office manager of surgeon's office; registrar sends a fax-back form that confirms the order with physician signature. Both office and lab enter note into medical record of phone order. Reason for the surgery and history are furnished by the patient at registration: angioplasty of AV fistula, right arm due to stenosis, end-stage kidney disease, hypertension, on weekly dialysis.**

    A   Assign ZØ1.812 Encounter for preprocedural laboratory examination, T82.858A Stenosis of vascular prosthetic devices, implants and grafts, initial encounter, I12.Ø Hypertensive chronic kidney disease with stage 5 chronic kidney disease or end-stage renal disease, N18.6 End-stage renal disease, and Z99.2 Dependence on renal dialysis.

    B   Documentation does not follow guidelines and/or the physician must be queried to determine the following:

    - Etiology of the end-stage renal failure
    - Hypertension, further qualified

16. **What is the appropriate code assignment for the diagnosis of mixed bacterial pneumonia due to *Streptococcus pneumoniae* and *Hemophilus influenzae* identified on sputum culture stain and confirmed by the attending physician in the discharge summary?**

    Code assignment:_____

17. **Discharge summary: Atypical pneumonia, based on presentation clinical indicators and chest CT showing bronchial wall thickening. Last progress note: Awaiting immunoassay results. Addendum to last progress note by PA: Change antibiotic to Azithromycin. At the time of coding, the immunoassay report is posted to the chart and indicates mycoplasma pneumonia. Upon review of the sensitivity test post discharge, the provider's PA ordered a different antibiotic after consulting the attending by phone.**

    A   Assign J18.9 Pneumonia, unspecified organism.

    B   Documentation does not follow guidelines and/or the physician must be queried to determine the following:

    - Clinical significance of the immunoassay results and treatment re-evaluation
    - Provide an addendum if the type of pneumonia can be further specified

18. **What is the appropriate diagnosis code assignment for physician documentation of a 15-year-old with diabetes on insulin regimen?**

    Code assignment:_____

19. **Discharge summary signed by attending: A diagnosis of borderline diabetes is listed and body of summary notes FPG test of 124 mg/dl and indicates a need for follow-up testing in three months with diabetic counseling on next office visit recommended.**

    Code assignment:_____

20. **What is the appropriate diagnosis code assignment for an admission documented by the resident as due to decompensated congestive heart failure with chronic diastolic heart failure, due to patient not refilling her prescription for Lanoxin because she cannot afford the medication this month?**

    Code assignment:_____

21. **Order for outpatient echocardiogram. Reason: O9Ø.3, with stamped signature of treating physician. Patient presents to testing facility with order. States order is for monitoring since she is being treated for congestive heart failure and is two months post delivery.**

    A   Assign O9Ø.3 Peripartum cardiomyopathy, I5Ø.9 Heart failure.

    B   Documentation does not follow guidelines and/or the physician must be queried to determine the following:

    - Provide signed/dated order
    - Provide a written diagnostic statement

22. **Which code is appropriate for the diagnosis of gram-positive pneumonia: J15.8 Pneumonia due to other specified bacteria, or J15.9 Unspecified bacterial pneumonia?**

    Code assignment:_____

23. **What is the appropriate diagnosis code to reflect physician documentation of an office visit of a 14-year-old female G1PØ for evaluation of diet-controlled gestational diabetes, second trimester at 26 weeks?**

    Code assignment:_____

24. **Progress note: Patient with chronic deep ulcer on right heel. Schedule surgery to debride and consult wound care. Monitor glucose levels for patient's diabetes 2.**

   A   Assign E11.621 Type 2 diabetes mellitus with foot ulcer, and L97.419 Non-pressure chronic ulcer of right heel and midfoot with unspecified severity.

   B   Documentation does not follow guidelines and/or the physician must be queried to determine the following:

   - Etiology of the ulcer
   - Stage or severity of the ulcer

25. **What is the appropriate diagnosis code when the PA documents a history of congestive heart failure and combined diastolic and systolic dysfunction under treatment?**

   Code assignment:_____

26. **Office note by provider: Patient presents today for prenatal visit. Patient is 36-year-old G1P2, at 32 weeks, with history of essential hypertension, currently treated and monitored for signs of pre-eclampsia, asymptomatic mitral valve prolapse, history of smoking that ceased prior to pregnancy.**

   A   Assign O09.523 Supervision of elderly multigravida, third trimester, O10.013 Pre-existing essential hypertension complicating pregnancy, third trimester, I34.1 Nonrheumatic mitral (valve) prolapse, Z3A.32 32 weeks gestation of pregnancy.

   B   Documentation does not follow guidelines and/or the physician must be queried to determine the following:

   - Type of hypertension
   - Significance of patient's age affecting the pregnancy

27. **Which of these two coding conventions means the information is insufficient to assign a more specific code; for example, for the diagnosis of bacterial pneumonia?**

   A   NOS

   B   NEC

28. **Discharge summary: CMV pneumonia right lung, s/p right lung transplant in 2010 for end-stage emphysema. History of smoking. Continue outpatient pulmonary rehab.**

   A   Assign T86.812 Lung transplant infection, B25.0 Cytomegaloviral pneumonitis, J43.9 Emphysema, unspecified.

   B   Documentation does not follow guidelines and/or the physician must be queried to determine the following:

   - Whether the CMV infection of the right lung transplant is a complication of the transplant or unrelated to the transplant
   - Whether the emphysema is a current diagnosis or by history only
   - History of smoking: former history of use or dependence

29. **What is the appropriate diagnosis code for an emergency department visit for an 89-year-old patient with bleeding of a left calf ulcer due to diabetes 2 with diabetic peripheral angiopathy, exacerbated by Coumadin use for chronic atrial fibrillation. The bleeding could not be controlled by pressure at nursing home as documented by the ED physician.**

   Code assignment:_____

30. **Physician office visit note by provider: Weekly obstetric visit. 27-year-old G4P2A1, now at 30 weeks with history of miscarriage, current gestational diabetes, being treated with insulin.**

   A   Assign O09.293 Supervision of pregnancy with other poor reproductive or obstetric history, third trimester, O24.414 Gestational diabetes mellitus in pregnancy, insulin controlled, Z3A.30 30 weeks gestation of pregnancy.

   B   Documentation does not follow guidelines and/or the physician must be queried to determine the following:

   - Insulin as a long-term medication
   - Clinical significance of previous miscarriage

31. **What is the appropriate code assignment for a diagnosis of hypertensive heart disease with congestive heart failure, as documented by the emergency department physician?**

   Code assignment:_____

32. **Observation record final diagnosis by nephrologist: Admitted to observation from emergency department due to fluid overload from missing weekly dialysis, acute renal failure, end-stage renal failure, hypertension, history of congestive heart failure on Lasix (compensated). Treated with dialysis.**

   A   Assign E87.70 Fluid overload unspecified, N17.9 Acute kidney failure, I50.9 heart failure, I12.0 Hypertensive chronic kidney disease with stage 5 chronic kidney disease or end-stage renal disease, N18.6 End-stage renal disease, Z91.15 Patient's noncompliance with renal dialysis.

   B   Documentation does not follow guidelines and/or the physician must be queried to determine the following:

   - End-stage renal failure relationship to hypertension
   - Etiology of the fluid overload

33. **Which of these two coding conventions means the information provides detail for which a specific code does not exist. An example of when the convention is used is for the diagnosis *Moraxella catarrhalis* pneumonia.**

   A   NOS

   B   NEC

34. **Admitting note LTCH: 1. Gram-negative pneumonia, resolving: Admit to continue antibiotics three days more to complete regimen ordered during acute inpatient admission, then repeat chest x-ray to evaluate for presence of previously seen consolidation.**

   A   Assign J15.9 Unspecified bacterial pneumonia.

   B   Documentation does not follow guidelines and/or the physician must be queried to determine the following:

   - Whether the diagnosis of pneumonia is current (acute phase) for this encounter or resolved on admission and sequela of illness is under treatment (specify residual)
   - Clinical significance of the repeat chest x-ray (results)

35. **What are the appropriate diagnosis codes for admission to the ASC, as documented by the procedure physician, for pancreatic transplant biopsy to evaluate ongoing rejection. The patient has diabetes type 1 with severe nonproliferative retinopathy and gastroparesis and is on the transplant list awaiting a second pancreas transplant. The patient has a functioning kidney allograft with CKD stage 1, due to diabetic renal disease.**

   Code assignment:_____

36. Wound care note by wound care nurse: 32-year-old male with diabetes 1 (poly)neuropathic ulcer, 2cmx1cm improvement from last week of 2cmx2xm, right lateral 5th toe, Grade 2 subcutaneous tissue involvement, presented with dry, clean dressing, no drainage present, no odor, granular tissue present, no signs of infection, will continue enzymatic debridement. Note: patient is status post kidney/pancreas transplants, which are functioning.

A   Assign E10.621 Type 1 diabetes mellitus with foot ulcer, E10.42 Type 1 diabetes mellitus with diabetic polyneuropathy, L97.512 Non-pressure chronic ulcer of other part of right foot with fat layer exposed, Z94.0 Kidney transplant status, Z94.83 Pancreas transplant status.

B   Documentation does not follow guidelines and/or the physician must be queried to determine the following:

   • Physician must co-sign wound care note

   • Diabetes current diagnosis

37. What is the appropriate diagnosis code for Hospital B for a transfer for therapeutic intervention due to an acute STEMI inferior wall myocardial infarction where the patient suffered an acute subendocardial myocardial infarction prior to discharge, as the physician documented in the discharge summary?

   Code assignment:_____

38. Script written by PCP for outpatient chest x-ray: Productive cough, increased respiratory rate, crackles on inspiration, fever, rule out pneumonia. Script written by PCP for outpatient urinalysis and culture: Fever, tachypnea, history of recurrent urinary tract infections. Radiologist final reading: Pneumonia, COPD. Lab results: Urinalysis was abnormal, culture showed *E. coli*. Sensitivity test results were also performed.

A   Radiology: Assign J18.9 Pneumonia, unspecified organism. Lab: Assign R50.9 Fever, unspecified, R06.82 Tachypnea, not elsewhere classified, Z87.440 Personal history of urinary (tract) infections.

B   Documentation does not follow guidelines and/or the physician must be queried to determine the following:

   • PCP: Etiology for the presenting symptoms identified

   • PCP: Clinical significance of the finding of COPD

39. What is the appropriate diagnosis code for a patient with diabetes 1, inadequately controlled, with an insulin pump who is admitted as an outpatient to evaluate insulin pump function. Insulin pump was found to be functioning. The insulin dosage and titration were changed, as documented by the procedure physician.

   Code assignment:_____

40. What is the appropriate diagnosis code for an encounter the emergency department physician documents as for cardiac arrest due to ventricular fibrillation with cardiogenic shock?

   Code assignment:_____

41. ED record, signed by ED attending: Cardiac arrest, history of coronary artery disease, s/p CABG in 2011, hypertension, history of myocardial infarction in 2011. Patient admitted in cardiac arrest, CPR and defibrillation in the ED, resuscitation was unsuccessful and patient expired. Labs: CK-MB: 12.6, troponin I: 5.0. EKG: ST segment elevation and ventricular fibrillation.

A   Assign I46.9 Cardiac arrest, cause unspecified, I25.10 Atherosclerotic heart disease of native coronary artery without angina pectoris, I10 Essential (primary) hypertension, Z95.1 Presence of aortocoronary bypass graft, I25.2 Old myocardial infarction.

B   Documentation does not follow guidelines and/or the physician must be queried to determine the following:

   • Etiology of cardiac arrest

   • Clinical significance of the lab results and EKG reading

42. What is the appropriate diagnosis code for the second episode in six months of *Pneumocystis jiroveci* pneumonia in a patient who is noted to be HIV positive, as documented by the provider?

   Code assignment:_____

43. Office visit note: Follow-up for recent pneumonia, course of antibiotics completed last week. Patient without complaint. Repeat chest x-ray is negative.

A   Assign Z09 Encounter for follow-up examination after completed treatment for conditions other than malignant neoplasm, Z87.01 Personal history of pneumonia (recurrent).

B   Documentation does not follow guidelines and/or the physician must be queried to determine the following:

   • Type of pneumonia be further specified

   • Pneumonia current or by history only

44. Emergency department record, signed by ED attending: Fractured nose, right black eye of eyelid/ocular area, due to battery assault by boyfriend during domestic abuse incident; apartment residence. Patient is 20-year-old female, G3P2 at 35 weeks with diabetes 1, on insulin, with poor control due to noncompliance and financial difficulties. Admit to labor and delivery observation.

A   Assign O9A.313 Physical abuse complicating pregnancy, third trimester, S02.2XXA Fracture of nasal bones, initial encounter for closed fracture, S00.11XA Contusion of right eyelid and periocular area, initial encounter, O24.013 Pre-existing diabetes mellitus, type 1, in pregnancy, third trimester, E10.65 Type 1 diabetes mellitus with hyperglycemia, T38.3X6A Underdosing of insulin and oral hypoglycemic [antidiabetic] drugs, initial encounter, Z3A.35 35 weeks gestation of pregnancy, Y04.0XXA Assault by unarmed brawl or fight, Y07.03 Male partner, perpetrator of maltreatment and neglect, Z91.14 Patient's other noncompliance with medication regimen, Z91.120 Patient's intentional underdosing of medication regimen due to financial hardship, Z79.4 Long-term (current) use of insulin, Y92.039 Unspecified place in apartment as the place of occurrence of the external cause.

B   Documentation does not follow guidelines and/or the physician must be queried to determine the following:

   • Medical significance of noncompliance

   • Effects of trauma on pregnancy

45. **Progress note by critical care physician: Code blue called after patient arrived on floor after cardiac catheterization with stent placement for coronary artery disease stenosis, history of recent myocardial infarction, no intraop complications noted. Nurse found patient in cardiac arrest; responding team initiated CPR, defibrillation, endotrachial intubation, epinephrine administered. Patient was resuscitated successfully; admit to inpatient status.**

   A   Assign I46.9 Cardiac arrest cause unspecified.

   B   Documentation does not follow guidelines and/or the physician must be queried to determine the following:

   - Cause of cardiac arrest
   - Whether the cardiac arrest was a complication of the procedure

46. **What is the correct code if the resident documents the diagnosis of pneumonia due to mechanical ventilation and the lab record shows vent cultures growing yeast?**

   Code assignment:_____

47. **What is the appropriate diagnosis code when a surgeon documents that a newborn infant was delivered by cesarean on this encounter with macrosomia and the newborn has a diagnosis of syndrome of infant of a diabetic mother?**

   Code assignment:_____

48. **Visit to endocrinologist: Progress note, signed by provider: diabetes 2; 4 months postpartum who had developed gestational diabetes, now with peripartum diabetes 2, under treatment with metaformin.**

   A   Assign E11.9 Type 2 diabetes mellitus without complications, Z86.32 Personal history of gestational diabetes, and O94 Sequela of complication of pregnancy, childbirth, and the puerperium.

   B   Documentation does not follow guidelines and/or the physician must be queried to determine the following:

   - Risk factors for diabetes
   - Diabetic complications

49. **What is the appropriate diagnosis code assignment as documented by the emergency department physician for an encounter with a woman who had acute chest pain on inspiration while surveying the damage in the yard of her former home, with acute emotional stress reaction due to surviving a tornado and losing her home to it today?**

   Code assignment:_____

50. **Admit note by resident: PMH: h/o cardiac arrest due to acute myocardial infarction in 2010, treated by thrombolysis. Admit note: Found to have coronary artery disease, treated medically until now. Admitted today for CABG due to progressive angina. What past history would be appropriate to assign?**

   A   Assign Z86.74 Personal history of sudden cardiac arrest, and I25.2 Old myocardial infarction.

   B   Documentation does not follow guidelines and/or the physician must be queried to determine the following:

   - Type of angina
   - Significance of history of myocardial infarction treatment

Coding and Documentation Review Answers

1. *Answer:* **Lobar affects an area of a lobe of the lung, Bronch(o)(ial) affects the walls of the bronchioles.**

   Rationale: Under the ICD-10-CM Alphabetic Index entry for pneumonia, the subterms that indicate anatomical areas, such as alveolar, apex, confluent, diffuse, etc., index to *"see"* references. The two *"see"* references are *"see* Pneumonia, lobar" or *"see* Pneumonia, broncho." These two terms are anatomical classifications of pneumonia that indicate the sites in the lung where clinical indicators of consolidation can be seen on radiologic displays. Lobar affects an area of the lung lobe. Bronch(o)(ial)pneumonia or lobular pneumonia affects the walls of the bronchioles with multiple foci of isolated consolidation in one or more basal lobes of the lung.

2. *Answer:* <u>A</u> **Assign J18.9 Pneumonia, unspecified organism.**

   Rationale: The type of pneumonia is identified only as "atypical," and no specific organism is attributable; the Alphabetic Index entry for "Pneumonia, atypical" lists J18.9 Pneumonia, unspecified organism. Normal flora identified in a culture indicates a mixture of bacteria normally found at specific body sites and does not represent pathogens and is not clinically significant. The chest x-ray shows bilateral lower lobe consolidation, which can also be seen in congestive heart failure and empyema, among other causes. OCG.I.C.18.b states that signs or symptoms routinely associated with a disease process should not be identified with additional codes unless the physician instructs otherwise.

3. *Answer:* **E10.22 Type 1 diabetes mellitus with diabetic chronic kidney disease, I12.0 Hypertensive chronic kidney disease with stage 5 chronic kidney disease or end-stage renal disease, N18.6 End-stage renal disease, Z99.2 Dependence on renal dialysis**

   Rationale: The type of diabetes is stated as type I, and the chronic kidney disease is due to the diabetes; therefore, assign a code from category E10. ICD-10-CM assumes a cause-and-effect relationship when both hypertension and chronic kidney disease are present (*Official Coding Guidelines* [OCG], section I.C.9.a.2); consequently a code from category I12 is assigned. The tabular "code also" note indicates that the coder should assign an additional code to identify the stage of chronic kidney disease, in this case, end-stage renal disease, N18.6. An instructional note under code N18.6 instructs the coder to use an additional code to identify dialysis status, which is Z99.2 Dependence on renal dialysis.

4. *Answer:* <u>A</u> **E11.649 Type II diabetes mellitus with hypoglycemia without coma**

   Rationale: ICD-10-CM OCG section I.C.4.a.2 states that E11- Type 2 diabetes mellitus, is assigned as the default when the type is not specified. Guideline section I.A.15 indicates that the word "with" means "due to" in the Alphabetic Index; therefore, the documentation links the diabetes and hypoglycemia. Diabetes mellitus codes are combination codes, and the Alphabetic Index entry for diabetes with hypoglycemia, Type 2, refers to E11.649 Type II diabetes mellitus with hypoglycemia without coma.

5. *Answer:* **I25.10 Atherosclerotic heart disease of native coronary artery without angina pectoris, Z72.0 Tobacco use**

   Rationale: The ICD-10-CM Alphabetic Index main term "Disease, coronary (artery)" directs the coder to *"see"* Disease, heart, ischemic, atherosclerotic. Under "Disease/heart/ischemic/atherosclerotic," the code default is I25.10. Both stated conditions are classified to the single code I25.10 Atherosclerotic heart disease of native coronary artery without angina pectoris. When there is no history or documentation of a previous coronary artery bypass graft (CABG) or heart transplant, a code for atherosclerosis of native artery should be assigned. The Alphabetic Index lists code Z72.0 under "Tobacco, use."

6. *Answer:* **J18.9 Pneumonia, unspecified organism, R04.2 Hemoptysis**

   Rationale: The ICD-10-CM Alphabetic Index does not list the nonessential modifier "hemorrhagic" after the term "pneumonia." Therefore, unless documentation links this symptom to the pneumonia, the hemoptysis would be assigned as an additional code. The provider/documentation does not confirm that the sputum culture stain showing gram-negative bacilli is clinically significant. See OCG 1.C.18.b, "Use of a symptom code with a definitive diagnosis," and OCG III, "Reporting Additional Findings, B. Abnormal findings."

7. *Answer:* <u>A</u> **Assign J95.851 Ventilator associated pneumonia, B96.1 Klebsiella pneumoniae [K. pneumoniae] as the cause of diseases classified elsewhere, Z99.11 Dependence on respirator [ventilator] status.**

   Rationale: The ICD-10-CM OCG section I.C.10.d.1 states that the assignment of a complication code is based on the provider's documentation of the relationship between the pneumonia and the mechanical ventilation. In this case, the documentation describes the pneumonia as due to the ventilator. An additional code is assigned if an identified organism is attributed to the VAP, but not a pneumonia code from J12–J18.

8. *Answer:* **E11.610 Type 2 diabetes mellitus with diabetic neuropathic arthropathy, E11.621 Type 2 diabetes mellitus with foot ulcer, E11.52 Type 2 diabetes mellitus with diabetic peripheral angiopathy with gangrene, L97.524 Non-pressure chronic ulcer of other part of left foot with necrosis of bone**

   Rationale: ICD-10-CM OCG section I.A.15 states that the use of the term "with" is to be interpreted to mean "associated with" or "due to" when it appears in a code title, the Alphabetic Index, or an instructional note in the Tabular List. Therefore, the listed conditions are coded as diabetic complications. Guideline section I.C.4.a states that as many codes within a particular category should be assigned as describe all the complications, with sequencing based on the reason for a particular encounter. E11.610 Type 2 diabetes mellitus with diabetic neuropathic arthropathy is sequenced first since this describes the osteomyelitis.

9. *Answer:* **I25.5 Ischemic cardiomyopathy and I25.10 Atherosclerotic heart disease of native coronary artery without angina pectoris**

   Rationale: Ischemic cardiomyopathy is an extrinsic cardiomyopathy due to reduced blood flow to the heart muscle. The ICD-10-CM Alphabetic Index lists I25.5 Ischemic cardiomyopathy under the term "Cardiomyopathy, ischemic to." The "excludes2" note under I25.5 indicates that coronary atherosclerosis (I25.1-, I25.7-) is not included; therefore, these two conditions can be coded together when documented.

10. *Answer:* <u>B</u> **Documentation does not follow guidelines and/or the physician must be queried to determine the following: description of relationship between the hypertension and congestive heart failure, and specify type of the congestive heart failure.**

    Rationale: The relationship between hypertension and congestive heart failure is not assumed in ICD-10-CM and must be documented. Second, if the type of heart failure can be further specified as diastolic, systolic, or both, a more accurate code can be assigned from category I50 Heart failure. Heart disease without a stated causal relationship to hypertension is coded separately.

11. *Answer:* **J18.9 Pneumonia, unspecified organism, and C34.01 Malignant neoplasm of right main bronchus or lung**

Rationale: There is no specific entry in the Alphabetic Index for postobstructive pneumonia; therefore, only the term "Pneumonia" is listed. When a specified type of pneumonia is not documented, J18.9 Pneumonia, unspecified organism, is the default code and should be assigned. The malignancy is sequenced as an additional code according to OCG section C.2.I.4.

12. *Answer:* **A Assign J12.1 Respiratory syncytial virus pneumonia, J21.0 Acute bronchiolitis due to RSV, P07.38 Preterm newborn, gestational age 35 completed weeks.**

Rationale: The ICD-10-CM Alphabetic Index entry for "Pneumonia, respiratory syncytial virus" lists J12.1. Respiratory syncytial virus is a common community-acquired infection in children. OCG section I.C.16.a.5 states that if a newborn condition is community-acquired, a code from chapter 16, "Certain Conditions Originating in the Perinatal Period," is not assigned. RSV bronchiolitis is also documented and is also assigned. Both are acute conditions, and when the patient is admitted for both and both are equal in work-up, focus, and treatment, either can be sequenced as the principal diagnosis, following OCG section II.B. The additional information that the patient is a former preemie is coded as its clinical significance is documented and OCG section I.C.16.e states that prematurity is coded when it affects the patient's current health status.

13. *Answer:* **E09.65 Drug or chemical induced diabetes mellitus with hyperglycemia, T38.0X5D Adverse effect of glucocorticoids and synthetic analogues subsequent encounter, Z79.4 Long term (current) use of insulin, Z91.11 Patient's noncompliance with dietary regimen**

Rationale: Since the steroid use is prescribed and there is no indication of incorrect usage, this is considered an adverse effect and not a poisoning. The diabetes is drug-induced, and according to OCG section I.C.4.a.6.b, sequencing is to "code first" E09 Drug or chemical induced diabetes mellitus, followed by an additional code for the adverse effect to identify the drug T36–T50 with a fifth/sixth character of 5. ICD-10-CM does not use the terms "uncontrolled," "inadequately controlled," or "out of control, poorly controlled." The index instructs the user to "code Diabetes, by type, with hyperglycemia." Therefore, the first-listed code is E09.65 Drug or chemical induced diabetes mellitus with hyperglycemia. This is followed by T38.0X5- Adverse effect of glucocorticoids and synthetic analogues, which is located in the Table of Drugs and Chemicals under the main term "Steroid" with the appropriate additional character requirement, which in this case is a character for a subsequent encounter (D). The patient is maintained on insulin, Z79.4, which OCG section I.C.4.a.6.a, indicates is coded when documented. The diabetes is inadequately controlled due to dietary noncompliance, Z91.11, which is located in the Alphabetic Index under "Noncompliance, with, dietary regimen."

14. *Answer:* **I25.110 Atherosclerotic heart disease of native coronary artery with unstable angina pectoris, Z77.22 Contact with and (suspected) exposure to environmental tobacco smoke (acute) (chronic)**

Rationale: OCG section I.C.9.b states that ICD-10-CM provides combination codes that link coronary artery disease with angina since the relationship between them is to be assumed unless otherwise documented. No separate code is assigned from category I20 Angina pectoris. Code Z77.22 Contact with and (suspected) exposure to environmental tobacco smoke (acute) (chronic) is assigned as a secondary code when the provider documents that the second-hand smoke is the external cause of the patient's condition. Locate the code in the Alphabetic Index under the term "Exposure, second hand tobacco smoke (acute) (chronic)." When there is no history or documentation of a previous coronary artery bypass graft (CABG) or heart transplant, a code for atherosclerosis of native artery is assigned.

15. *Answer:* **A Assign Z01.812 Encounter for preprocedural laboratory examination, T82.858A Stenosis of vascular prosthetic devices, implants and grafts, initial encounter, I12.0 Hypertensive chronic kidney disease with stage 5 chronic kidney disease or end-stage renal disease, N18.6 End-stage renal disease, and Z99.2 Dependence on renal dialysis.**

Rationale: A telephone call from the treating physician's office to the testing facility to order a diagnostic outpatient service is acceptable if, as required by the Centers for Medicare and Medicaid Services, payer, state, conditions of participation bylaws, Joint Commission and Office of Inspector General requirements, both the treating physician/office and the testing facility document the phone call in their copies of the patient's medical record. This information may be obtained from the patient or the medical record, but the coder should attempt to confirm this information with the physician, and it is recommended to have a "fax-back" policy in place for the registration sites. In the example, the reason for the order is to have pre-op lab testing performed; "Examination, pre-procedural (pre-operative), laboratory" in the Alphabetic Index lists Z01.812 Encounter for preprocedural laboratory examination. OCG section I.C.21.c.16 indicates that category Z01 is a "first-listed" diagnosis and therefore should be sequenced first followed by the reason for the surgery/procedure.

16. *Answer:* **J13 Pneumonia due to Streptococcus pneumoniae, and J14 Pneumonia due to Haemophilus influenzae**

Rationale: Since the attending physician confirmed both identified infective organisms, both individual codes are assigned. If the organisms were not identified, then only pneumonia, bacterial (unspecified organism) would be assigned, not the "bacterial, specified" code, since the terms "mixed bacterial" do not identify specified organisms not elsewhere classified.

17. *Answer:* **B Documentation does not follow guidelines and/or the physician must be queried to determine the following: the clinical significance of the immunoassay results and treatment re-evaluation and provide an addendum if the type of pneumonia can be further specified.**

Rationale: After the documentation is reviewed, a query is warranted to further specify the type of pneumonia. The physician assistant documented a change in treatment based upon the results of the immunoassay test. Although the test results are posted to the chart, the coder should ask about their clinical significance and the reason behind the change in medication. Additionally, the findings on chest x-ray further support a more specific pneumonia as due to the identified organism. Coders are responsible for querying when the clinical documentation as a whole suggests a higher level of specificity.

18. *Answer:* **E11.9 Type 2 diabetes mellitus without complications, and Z79.4 Long-term (current) use of insulin**

Rationale: According to OCG section I.C.4.a.2.3, the type of diabetes mellitus cannot be determined by patient age or the use of insulin. The guideline further states that when the type of diabetes is not documented, the default is diabetes mellitus type 2 and that insulin documented as a maintenance drug is assigned as an additional code.

19. *Answer:* **Assign R73.09 Other abnormal glucose.**

Rationale: Without further documentation of a diagnosis of diabetes, the attending's attestation to the discharge summary confirming the lab findings and the indication of clinical significance, only a code from subcategory "abnormal glucose" can be assigned. This can be found in the Alphabetic Index under the main term "Findings, abnormal, inconclusive, without findings, glucose" or by the documentation of borderline diabetes mellitus or diabetes, latent. Code R73.09 Other abnormal glucose, lists "prediabetes" and "latent diabetes" as inclusion terms.

20. *Answer:* I50.33 Acute on chronic diastolic (congestive) heart failure, T46.ØX6A Underdosing of cardiac-stimulant glycosides and drugs of similar action initial encounter, and Z91.12Ø Patient's intentional underdosing of medication regimen due to financial hardship

Rationale: The code for "chronic on acute (i.e., acute on chronic)" is assigned because the acute exacerbation of a chronic condition is coded as acute on chronic, and when a combination code is available, only a single code is assigned. The exacerbation of the congestive heart failure was due to the lack of Lanoxin and is sequenced before the code for the underdosing, according to OCG section I.C.19.e.5.c. The seventh-character assignment of A, indicating the initial encounter, is required to complete code T46.ØX6. An additional code to represent noncompliance and the reason and intent is assigned: Z91.12Ø Patient's intentional underdosing of medication regimen due to financial hardship. The ICD-10-CM Alphabetic Index and Tabular List now provide the nonessential modifier "congestive" in the descriptor of the diastolic and systolic types of heart failure. Therefore an additional code for "congestive heart failure" is not assigned.

21. *Answer:* **B** Documentation does not follow guidelines and/or the physician must be queried to determine the following: provide signed/dated order and provide a written diagnostic statement.

Rationale: A valid order must follow CMS, payer, state, conditions of participation, bylaws and Joint Commission and OIG requirements. Signatures are required for certain diagnostic tests, and CMS Transmittal 327 states that stamped signatures are not acceptable. The introduction to the OCG states that ICD-10-CM is a morbidity classification for classifying diagnoses and reason for health care visits. Codes are not diagnoses—they may not be used as a substitute for a written diagnostic statement within the medical record.

22. *Answer:* J15.9 Unspecified bacterial pneumonia

Rationale: Since the term "gram-positive" is nonspecific and does not identify a specific organism, assign J15.9 Unspecified bacterial pneumonia. When a specific bacterial organism is identified but has no specific entry in the Alphabetic Index or a corresponding ICD-10-CM diagnosis code, the default is J15.8 Pneumonia due to other specified bacteria. The same applies to viral pneumonia coding.

23. *Answer:* OØ9.612 Supervision of young primigravida, second trimester, O24.41Ø Gestational diabetes mellitus in pregnancy, diet controlled, Z3A.26, 26 weeks gestation of pregnancy

Rationale: OCG section I.C.15.i covers gestational diabetes. Since the patient is 14 years old and this is her first pregnancy (identified by "G1PØ"), the coder would look in the index under "Pregnancy, supervision of, young mother, primigravida." The sixth character "2" specifies second trimester as defined by the note at the introduction to chapter 15. The Alphabetic Index lists the main term "Diabetes" with the subterm "gestational, diet controlled," which references code O24.41Ø. Follow the instructional note for chapter 15 and use an additional code from category Z3A to describe the number of weeks of gestation.

24. *Answer:* **B** Documentation does not follow guidelines and/or the physician must be queried to determine the following: etiology of the ulcer and stage or severity of the ulcer.

Rationale: If the ulcer is of diabetic origin, the link to diabetes must be stated before the ulcer can be coded. The term "deep" does not indicate the tissues involved, and the tissues need to be documented to further classify the stage or level of necrosis for code severity specificity.

25. *Answer:* I50.42 Chronic combined systolic (congestive) and diastolic (congestive) heart failure

Rationale: The ICD-10-CM Alphabetic Index does not have entries for diastolic or systolic under the main term "Dysfunction." Diastolic dysfunction is the decline in performance of one or both ventricles of the

heart during the time phase of diastole; left/systemic/body and right/pulmonary/lungs. Dysfunction has a subterm "ventricular/with congestive heart failure," which references I50.9 Heart failure unspecified. However, when there is diastolic or systolic dysfunction in the presence of heart failure, the relationship is assumed. In this example, the heart failure is specified as combined diastolic and systolic. Code I50.42 is the appropriate code. If diastolic or systolic dysfunction is documented without documentation of heart failure, assign I51.9 Heart disease, unspecified. In this case, however, because of the known history of heart failure, the case is coded as chronic.

26. *Answer:* **A** Assign OØ9.523 Supervision of elderly multigravida, third trimester, O1Ø.Ø13 Pre-existing essential hypertension complicating pregnancy third trimester, I34.1 Nonrheumatic mitral (valve) prolapse, Z3A.32 32 weeks gestation of pregnancy.

Rationale: For this scenario, OCG section I.C.15.b.2 states that the principal diagnosis should be a code from category OØ9 for supervision of a high-risk (elderly) pregnancy. The patient is 36 years old and has delivered once (G1P2). Assign code OØ9.523 as the first-listed diagnosis. The sixth character indicates the third trimester, as defined by the note in the introduction to chapter 15. Code Z3A.32 32 weeks gestation of pregnancy, is assigned according to the instructional note for chapter 15. Code O1Ø.Ø13 Pre-existing essential hypertension complicating pregnancy, third trimester, would be assigned as a secondary diagnosis code. Mitral valve prolapse, although asymptomatic, is coded because it is medically significant during pregnancy.

27. *Answer:* **A** NOS

Rationale: The coding convention NOS, or not otherwise specified, is the equivalent of "unspecified" and is assigned when the documentation does not provide more specific information about the condition. In the example, the term bacterial pneumonia means that the specified bacterial organism causing the pneumonia is unknown, or cannot be determined. What is known is that the causal organism is bacterial as opposed to viral. The Alphabetic Index lists the terms "Pneumonia, bacterial"; therefore, the default is J15.9 Unspecified bacterial pneumonia.

28. *Answer:* **A** Assign T86.812 Lung transplant infection, B25.Ø Cytomegaloviral pneumonitis, J43.9 Emphysema, unspecified.

Rationale: According to OCG section I.C.19.g.3.a, the code for transplant complications is assigned only if the complication affects the function of the transplanted organ. The complication requires two codes, one from category T86 to identify the type of complication and a second to identify the manifestation. Cytomegaloviral pneumonitis, or CMV, is an opportunistic pneumonia. Since the pneumonitis is in the allograft, it is coded as a lung transplant complication, specifically as an infection. The transplant was performed only on the right, so the emphysema is not "cured" and is still present. Therefore, the emphysema is assigned as an additional diagnosis. Only history of tobacco dependence, not history of smoking or tobacco use, has an index entry. Therefore, the history of smoking is not coded.

29. *Answer:* E11.622 Type 2 diabetes mellitus with other skin ulcer, T45.515A Adverse effect of anticoagulants, E11.51 Type 2 diabetes mellitus with diabetic peripheral angiopathy without gangrene, L97.229 Non-pressure chronic ulcer of left calf with unspecified severity, I48.2 Chronic atrial fibrillation

Rationale: As the bleeding from the ulcer is an adverse effect of the prescribed Coumadin, follow the guidelines in OCG section I.C.19.e.5.a and sequence the nature of the adverse effect first, which in this case is also a diabetic complication, E11.622 Type 2 diabetes mellitus with other skin ulcer. This is followed by the code identifying the drug and adverse effect, T45.515A Adverse effect of anticoagulants, found in the Table of Drugs and Chemicals. Code also all other diabetic complications, E11.51 Type 2 diabetes mellitus with diabetic peripheral angiopathy without gangrene. Also list code L97.229 Non-pressure chronic ulcer of left calf with unspecified severity to identify the site and severity of the ulcer per the "use additional code" instruction note under E11.622. Code I48.2 Chronic atrial fibrillation, indicates the condition for which the Coumadin is taken.

30. *Answer:* **A** Assign O09.293 Supervision of pregnancy with other poor reproductive or obstetric history, third trimester, O24.414 Gestational diabetes mellitus in pregnancy, insulin controlled, Z3A.30, 30 weeks gestation of pregnancy.

Rationale: The provider's documentation indicates this is a routine prenatal visit for a high-risk pregnancy due to a history of miscarriage with current gestational diabetes. OCG section I.C.15.b.2 states that a code from category O09 Supervision of high-risk pregnancy, should be assigned as the first-listed diagnosis, followed by any other applicable chapter 15 codes to describe comorbid conditions affecting the pregnancy. The code for gestational diabetes does not indicate trimester, but the fourth character does represent "in pregnancy." From the instructional note "use additional code from category Z3A" for chapter 15, code Z3A.30 30 weeks gestation of pregnancy, is assigned. OCG section I.C.15.i notes that additional code Z79.4 Long-term (current) use of insulin, should not be assigned with codes from subcategory O24.4.

31. *Answer:* I11.0 Hypertensive heart disease with heart failure, I50.9 Heart failure, unspecified

Rationale: According to OCG section I.C.9.1, when a causal relationship between hypertension and heart failure (I50.-) or heart disease (I51.4.-I51.9) is stated (due to) or implied (hypertensive), assign a code from category I11 Hypertensive heart disease. Also the OCG section I.A.15 states that in the Alphabetic Index, the subentry term "with" means "associated with" or "due to." Therefore, a diagnostic statement of "with" provides the link between two conditions. The tabular note instructs the coder to "use additional code to identify type of heart failure I50.-." In the example, the type is not documented; therefore an additional code for heart failure, unspecified is assigned.

32. *Answer:* **A** Assign E87.70 Fluid overload unspecified, N17.9 Acute kidney failure, I50.9 Heart failure, I12.0 Hypertensive chronic kidney disease with stage 5 chronic kidney disease or end-stage renal disease, N18.6 End-stage renal disease, Z91.15 Patient's noncompliance with renal dialysis.

Rationale: The acute conditions necessitating admission were the fluid overload and the acute renal failure. Since the dialysis is treatment for both conditions, according to OCG section II.C either may be sequenced as the principal diagnosis unless one is considered the more significant problem. As long as the admission is clearly documented as to treat the fluid overload and as not related to the history of congestive heart failure, the fluid overload can be coded separately. The congestive heart failure is noted to be "compensated," meaning it is not in acute exacerbation; note that unspecified heart failure I50.9 makes no distinction between acute or decompensated and compensated. If the record indicates that the type of heart failure can be specified further, the coder should query the physician for the type as well as a possible relationship between the heart failure and hypertension. Acute renal failure can be coded in the presence of end-stage kidney disease as there are no excludes or includes notes or instructional notes that indicate otherwise. The cause of the fluid overload was the noncompliance with dialysis, which is in the Alphabetic Index as "Noncompliance, with, dialysis," Z91.15. The dialysis status code is not assigned when the noncompliance is coded, Z91.15, as indicated by the "excludes1" note under Z99.2 Dependence on renal dialysis.

33. *Answer:* **B** NEC

Rationale: The coding convention NEC, or not elsewhere classified, is the equivalent of "specified (other, other specified)" and applies when the

documentation specifies a condition but there is no individual code for that condition. In the example, the type of bacteria causing the pneumonia is identified (specified), but the ICD-10-CM Alphabetic Index does not list an individual code for that particular organism. Therefore, the user would look in the index under "Pneumonia, specified, bacterium NEC," leading to J15.8 Pneumonia due to other specified bacteria.

34. *Answer:* **B** Documentation does not follow guidelines and/or the physician must be queried to determine the following: diagnosis of pneumonia current (acute phase) for this encounter or resolved on admission and sequela of illness is under treatment (specify residual); and clinical significance of the repeat chest x-ray (results).

Rationale: Long-term care hospitals may assign codes for acute unresolved conditions, sequelae, or rehab. The selection of principal diagnosis follows the guidelines in OCG section II. When the patient is admitted for continuation of treatment of an acute condition, OCG section I.B.10 may apply if the acute phase has resolved and it is the sequela that is being treated. This provider must document that the residual condition is being treated and is the reason for admission. If the patient no longer has the clinical indicators of the acute disease, the coder should query the physician for clarification as to whether the acute condition is present or if a sequela is receiving the continuation of care and treatment. As long as an acute condition is the target of treatment, it is coded. For this example, the facility must decide how to address the issue of acute condition versus sequela for "resolving" conditions that may or may not have clinical indicators.

35. *Answer:* T86.890 Other transplanted tissue rejection, E10.349 Type 1 diabetes mellitus with severe nonproliferative diabetic retinopathy without macular edema, E10.43 Type 1 diabetes mellitus with diabetic autonomic (poly)neuropathy (gastroparesis), E10.22 Type 1 diabetes mellitus with diabetic chronic kidney disease, N18.1 Chronic kidney disease, stage 1, Z94.0 Kidney transplant status, and Z76.82 Awaiting organ transplant status

Rationale: Rejection affects the transplanted pancreas and is a complication of the pancreas transplant. As the reason for the encounter, the transplant rejection is sequenced first. The patient has ongoing complications of retinopathy and gastroparesis due to diabetes 1, which must also be coded. The patient is also status post kidney transplant due to diabetic renal disease, and the transplanted kidney is functioning with mild CKD stage 1, which is not documented as a complication but is residual renal disease. OCG section I.C.14.a.2 indicates that the CKD stage with kidney transplant status should be assigned. Also indicate that the patient is awaiting transplant by looking in the index under "Transplant, awaiting organ," code Z76.82.

36. *Answer:* **A** Assign E10.621 Type 1 diabetes mellitus with foot ulcer, E10.42 Type 1 diabetes mellitus with diabetic polyneuropathy, L97.512 Non-pressure chronic ulcer of other part of right foot with fat layer exposed, Z94.0 Kidney transplant status, Z94.83 Pancreas transplant status.

Rationale: The term provider is used throughout the *Official Coding Guidelines* to indicate a physician or any qualified health care practitioner who is legally accountable for establishing the patient's diagnosis. State laws define the scope of practice and, for health care entities, regulatory laws establish who may provide documentation; wound care nursing documentation is recognized as valid. Although the patient has a functioning pancreas transplant, diabetes is coded since there are related complications. The diabetes 1 is linked to the ulcer by its description as diabetes 1 neuropathic ulcer. Because the Wagner non-pressure foot ulcer classification grade 2 is penetration through the subcutaneous tissue, the severity chosen is "with fat layer exposed." The ulcer is sequenced first before the neuropathy because it is the reason for the encounter.

37. *Answer:* I21.19 ST elevation (STEMI) myocardial infarction involving other coronary artery of inferior wall, and I22.2 Subsequent non-ST elevation (NSTEMI) myocardial infarction

Rationale: OCG section I.C.9.e.1 states that a code for the site is assigned for an acute STEMI myocardial infarction for encounters occurring when the MI is equal to or less than four weeks old, including transfers during this timeframe. New for ICD-10-CM, OCG section I.C.9.e.4 states that after an initial myocardial infarction, a subsequent or new acute myocardial infarction during the same four-week timeframe is coded to category I22 Subsequent ST elevation (STEMI) and non-ST elevation (NSTEMI) myocardial infarction. When there are both an initial and subsequent acute myocardial infarction, codes from both I21 and I22 are assigned, sequenced based on the circumstances of the encounter.

38. *Answer:* **A** Radiology: Assign J18.9 Pneumonia, unspecified organism. Lab: Assign R50.9 Fever, unspecified, R06.82 Tachypnea, not elsewhere classified, Z87.440 Personal history of urinary (tract) infections.

Rationale: In the outpatient setting, uncertain diagnoses cannot be assigned (OCG section IV.H). The referring provider should document signs, symptoms, and abnormal findings that prompt the outpatient encounter. If a physician has interpreted a diagnostic test and the results are available, the confirmed or definitive diagnosis is coded; the related or integral signs and symptoms are not coded, according to OCG section IV.K.. The second script lists signs and symptoms and history, but the test results are by lab only. Therefore, the signs and symptoms and history codes are assigned. When possible, the coder should ask the PCP to clarify the lab results. Until the PCP confirms the test results for the scripts, only the codes for the symptoms for which the tests were ordered are assigned.

39. *Answer:* E10.65 Type 1 diabetes mellitus with hyperglycemia and Z46.81 Encounter for fitting and adjustment of insulin pump

Rationale: The ICD-10-CM Alphabetic Index lists the terms inadequately controlled, out of control, and poorly controlled to represent diabetes mellitus uncontrolled, with the instruction to assign diabetes, by type, with hyperglycemia. Therefore, assign E10.65 Type 1 diabetes mellitus with hyperglycemia as the first diagnosis as the diabetes was symptomatic and the reason for the encounter, not just an evaluation of the insulin pump or for titration adjustment. Add Z46.81 Encounter for fitting and adjustment of insulin pump, since titration adjustment was performed. The status code Z96.41 Presence of insulin pump (external) (internal) is not assigned since the reason for encounter code indicates the type of status according to OCG section I.C.21.c.3.

40. *Answer:* I49.01 Ventricular fibrillation, I46.2 Cardiac arrest due to underlying cardiac condition, and R57.0 Cardiogenic shock

Rationale: The ICD-10-CM Alphabetic Index now provides separate codes for cardiac arrest due to underlying cardiac condition, due to (other) specified underlying condition (trauma, overdose, etc.) or unspecified cause. Codes for both the cardiac arrest and the underlying condition should be assigned, when the condition is known. In the example for the ED encounter, the ventricular fibrillation is known and should be sequenced first, followed by the code for the cardiac arrest as instructed by the tabular "code first" note under category I46 Cardiac arrest. If further work-up determines the cause of the ventricular fibrillation, such as cardiac ischemia or coronary artery disease, cardiomyopathy, acute myocardial infarction, trauma, overdose, etc., that condition is the principal diagnosis and the appropriate code from category I46 Cardiac arrest, is secondary, along with I49.01 Ventricular fibrillation. Since the cardiogenic shock is not integral to the ventricular fibrillation or the cardiac arrest, the code for shock is assigned even though it is not a chapter 18 code (OCG section I.C.18.b). Review and apply the guidelines in the OCG section II introduction for the UHDDS definition of principal diagnosis for inpatient, and in OCG section IV.G, IV.k and IV.l for the reason of the outpatient encounter. Keep in mind that, according to OCG section IV.A, the coding conventions and the general

and disease-specific guidelines take precedence over the outpatient guidelines.

41. *Answer:* **A** Assign I46.9 Cardiac arrest, cause unspecified, I25.10 Atherosclerotic heart disease of native coronary artery without angina pectoris, I10 Essential (primary) hypertension, Z95.1 Presence of aortocoronary bypass graft, I25.2 Old myocardial infarction.

Rationale: When an emergency department patient dies before the cause of a cardiac arrest is known, the code for the cardiac arrest is the first-listed diagnosis. When the underlying condition is known, the code for the condition is sequenced first, with the code for cardiac arrest as an additional diagnosis. In ICD-10-CM, cardiac arrest now has three subcategories based on whether the underlying condition is known or not and whether it is cardiac or other specified condition. Since there is no documentation of recent cardiac catheterization, the coronary artery disease post CABG is assumed to be of native vessel without angina pectoris.

42. *Answer:* B20 Human immunodeficiency virus [HIV] disease and B59 Pneumocystosis

Rationale: ICD-10-CM OCG section I.C.1.a.1 instructs that confirmation of HIV status can be made by the provider's statement that the patient has an HIV-related illness. Also, section I.C.1.a.2.f states that cases involving patients with any known prior diagnosis of an HIV-related illness are assigned code B20 Human immunodeficiency virus [HIV] disease. The Centers for Disease Control (CDC) classifies *Pneumocystis jiroveci* pneumonia, an opportunistic pneumonia, as an AIDS-defining condition and one of the clinical criteria for HIV stage 3 or AIDS. Another clinical criterion is an HIV-positive patient having bacterial pneumonia twice within one year.

43. *Answer:* **A** Assign Z09 Encounter for follow-up examination after completed treatment for conditions other than malignant neoplasm, Z87.01 Personal history of pneumonia (recurrent).

Rationale: OCG section I.C.21.c.8 states that follow-up codes are assigned when the encounter is for surveillance following completed treatment and the condition no longer exists. Follow-up codes are not used for sequelae or ongoing care of a condition that is healing or resolving. A history code representing the healed/resolved condition is assigned as a secondary code to fully explain the reason for the encounter. The follow-up code is not assigned if the condition is found to have recurred on the follow-up encounter, and instead the code for the condition is listed first.

44. *Answer:* **A** Assign O9A.313 Physical abuse complicating pregnancy, third trimester, S02.2XXA Fracture of nasal bones, initial encounter for closed fracture, S00.11XA Contusion of right eyelid and periocular area, initial encounter, O24.013 Pre-existing diabetes mellitus, type 1, in pregnancy, third trimester, E10.65 Type 1 diabetes mellitus with hyperglycemia, T38.3X6A Underdosing of insulin and oral hypoglycemic [antidiabetic] drugs, initial encounter, Z3A.35 35 weeks gestation of pregnancy, Y04.0XXA Assault by unarmed brawl or fight, Y07.03 Male partner, perpetrator of maltreatment and neglect, Z91.120 Patient's intentional underdosing of medication regimen due to financial hardship, Z79.4 Long term (current) use of insulin, Y92.039 Unspecified place in apartment as the place of occurrence of the external cause

Rationale: The ED provider documentation that is attested by signature confirms the injuries are due to physical abuse. The *Official Coding Guidelines* section I.C.15.r states that abuse in a pregnant patient is sequenced first and coded to category O9A Physical abuse complicating pregnancy, childbirth, and the puerperium, when suspected or confirmed; associated injuries are coded as additional diagnoses. Pre-existing diabetes 1 with poor control is assigned to category O24

Diabetes mellitus in pregnancy, childbirth, and the puerperium, with an additional code from category E10 Type 1 diabetes mellitus, to further identify manifestation of hyperglycemia, indicated in the Alphabetic Index as poor control. Underdosing of medication is covered in OCG section I.C.19.e.5.c and is assigned from category T38 with the sixth character of 6. Sequencing of multiple codes from chapter 20, "External Causes of Morbidity," is explained in OCG section I.C.20.f.

45. *Answer:* <u>B</u> **Documentation does not follow guidelines and/or the physician must be queried to determine the following: cause of cardiac arrest and whether the cardiac arrest a complication of the procedure.**

    Rationale: When a cardiac arrest occurs during an inpatient hospitalization and the patient is resuscitated, a code from category I46 Cardiac arrest, is assigned as an additional diagnosis. It would be appropriate to ask the physician the cause or contributing cause if it is not stated when there is clinical evidence to support the query. When a cardiac arrest is the reason for an inpatient death (the patient is not resuscitated) and the cause or contributing cause is known, the code for cardiac arrest is not assigned.

46. *Answer:* **J95.851 Ventilator associated pneumonia**

    Rationale: ICD-10-CM OCG section I.C.10.d.1 states that the code for a complication is based on the provider's documentation of the relationship between the complication and the cause, in this case, the pneumonia and the mechanical ventilation. Therefore, code J95.851 Ventilator associated pneumonia, is assigned only when the link is expressly stated and not merely when a patient on a mechanical ventilator has pneumonia. An additional code is assigned if an identified organism is attributed to the VAP, but not a code from J12–J18. In the example, since the yeast cultures are identified only as a lab value and are not documented by the provider as related to the VAP, a code for the yeast organism is not assigned. The coder should ask the provider to state the clinical significance of the lab results; if the results are related to the VAP, B37.9 Candidiasis, unspecified, would be assigned.

47. *Answer:* **Z38.01 Single liveborn infant, delivered by cesarean, P70.1 Syndrome of infant of a diabetic mother**

    Rationale: The code for a newborn delivered by cesarean on this admission is found by looking in the Alphabetic Index under "Newborn, born in hospital, by cesarean," code Z38.01. Macrosomia is not listed in the ICD-10-CM Alphabetic Index but is synonymous with "large for gestational age," or LGA, which the index entry for "Large, baby" indicates is coded with P08.1. This is not assigned, however, because subcategory E08.1 has an "excludes1" note indicating that LGA in "syndrome of diabetic mother" is to be included in P70.1.

48. *Answer:* <u>A</u> **Assign E11.9 Type 2 diabetes mellitus without complications, Z86.32 Personal history of gestational diabetes, and O94 Sequela of complication of pregnancy, childbirth, and the puerperium.**

    Rationale: When diagnosed with gestational diabetes mellitus, patients have a high risk of developing diabetes 2 post delivery, which is why clinical guidelines recommend the patients return for postpartum glucose testing. When the postpartum impaired glucose regulation indicates diabetes, the case is coded as diabetes and no longer abnormal glucose finding. OCG section I.C.15.o.3 states that if the provider documents a condition as related to pregnancy, codes from chapter 15 may be assigned. OCG section I.C.15.p states that when an initial complication of a pregnancy develops a sequela requiring care or treatment, code O94 is assigned and sequenced after the code identifying the sequela condition. The documented personal history of gestational diabetes is also coded.

49. *Answer:* **R07.1 Chest pain on breathing, F43.0 Acute stress reaction, X37.1XXA Tornado, and Y92.017 Garden or yard in a single-family (private) house as the place of occurrence of the external cause**

    Rationale: The ICD-10-CM Alphabetic Index no longer provides a separate code for other acute pain for use with a specified site of pain. Instead, only the pain of the site is coded when stated as acute of a specified site. The index entry for "Pain, acute" shows R52 Pain, unspecified, which has an "excludes1" note instructing the user to code to pain by site for localized pain of unspecified type. The chest pain is described as "on inspiration"; the Alphabetic Index lists "Pain, chest, on breathing or pleurodynia," R07.1. Always review the entire record for a description of the chest pain and assign a code of the highest level of specificity based on physician documentation; query when appropriate. Since the chest pain is not linked to the stress the patient is experiencing, code F43.9 Acute stress reaction is assigned. To describe the situation related to the diagnoses, assign X37.1XXA Tornado, and Y92.017 Garden or yard in a single-family (private) house, as the place of occurrence of the external cause, for this initial encounter, according to OCG section I.C.20.b.

50. *Answer:* <u>A</u> **Assign Z86.74 Personal history of sudden cardiac arrest, and I25.2 Old myocardial infarction.**

    Rationale: The past medical history documents a past cardiac arrest and myocardial infarction. Since the patient presents for CABG due to progressive angina for which the history of cardiac arrest and myocardial infarction would be relevant, assign the personal history code for both. The Alphabetic Index lists "History, personal, cardiac arrest (death) successfully resuscitated," code Z86.74. The index entry for history of myocardial infarction is "History, personal, myocardial infarction (old)," code I25.2. History codes are appropriate for an encounter when facility policy requires them or when the history is significant to the encounter based on medical significance or in relationship to other diagnoses or conditions. OCG section III.A states that previous conditions may be coded as additional diagnoses when they affect current care or treatment.

Official ICD-9-CM Guidelines for Coding and Reporting

Effective October 1, 2011

Note: Since no official ICD-9-CM addendum to the guidelines was released in 2012, the guidelines included in this book stand as the official guidelines effective October 1, 2012 through September 30, 2013.

The Centers for Medicare and Medicaid Services (CMS) and the National Center for Health Statistics (NCHS), two departments within the U.S. Federal Government's Department of Health and Human Services (DHHS) provide the following guidelines for coding and reporting using the International Classification of Diseases, 9th Revision, Clinical Modification (ICD-9-CM). These guidelines should be used as a companion document to the official version of the ICD-9-CM as published on CD-ROM by the U.S. Government Printing Office (GPO).

These guidelines have been approved by the four organizations that make up the Cooperating Parties for the ICD-9-CM: the American Hospital Association (AHA), the American Health Information Management Association (AHIMA), CMS, and NCHS. These guidelines are included on the official government version of the ICD-9-CM, and also appear in *Coding Clinic for ICD-9-CM* published by the AHA.

These guidelines are a set of rules that have been developed to accompany and complement the official conventions and instructions provided within the ICD-9-CM itself. The instructions and conventions of the classification take precedence over guidelines. These guidelines are based on the coding and sequencing instructions in Volumes I, II and III of ICD-9-CM, but provide additional instruction. Adherence to these guidelines when assigning ICD-9-CM diagnosis and procedure codes is required under the Health Insurance Portability and Accountability Act (HIPAA). The diagnosis codes (Volumes 1-2) have been adopted under HIPAA for all healthcare settings. Volume 3 procedure codes have been adopted for inpatient procedures reported by hospitals. A joint effort between the healthcare provider and the coder is essential to achieve complete and accurate documentation, code assignment, and reporting of diagnoses and procedures. These guidelines have been developed to assist both the healthcare provider and the coder in identifying those diagnoses and procedures that are to be reported. The importance of consistent, complete documentation in the medical record cannot be overemphasized. Without such documentation accurate coding cannot be achieved. The entire record should be reviewed to determine the specific reason for the encounter and the conditions treated.

The term encounter is used for all settings, including hospital admissions. In the context of these guidelines, the term provider is used throughout the guidelines to mean physician or any qualified health care practitioner who is legally accountable for establishing the patient's diagnosis. Only this set of guidelines, approved by the Cooperating Parties, is official.

The guidelines are organized into sections. Section I includes the structure and conventions of the classification and general guidelines that apply to the entire classification, and chapter-specific guidelines that correspond to the chapters as they are arranged in the classification. Section II includes guidelines for selection of principal diagnosis for non-outpatient settings. Section III includes guidelines for reporting additional diagnoses in non-outpatient settings. Section IV is for outpatient coding and reporting.

Section I. Conventions, general coding guidelines and chapter specific guidelines

A. Conventions for the ICD-9-CM
1. Format:
2. Abbreviations
   a. Index abbreviations
   b. Tabular abbreviations
3. Punctuation
4. Includes and Excludes Notes and Inclusion terms
5. Other and Unspecified codes
   a. "Other" codes
   b. "Unspecified" codes

6. Etiology/manifestation convention ("code first", "use additional code" and "in diseases classified elsewhere" notes)
7. "And"
8. "With"
9. "See" and "See Also"

B. General Coding Guidelines
1. Use of Both Alphabetic Index and Tabular List
2. Locate each term in the Alphabetic Index
3. Level of Detail in Coding
4. Code or codes from 001.0 through V91.99
5. Selection of codes 001.0 through 999.9
6. Signs and symptoms
7. Conditions that are an integral part of a disease process
8. Conditions that are not an integral part of a disease process
9. Multiple coding for a single condition
10. Acute and Chronic Conditions
11. Combination Code
12. Late Effects
13. Impending or Threatened Condition
14. Reporting Same Diagnosis Code more than Once
15. Admissions/Encounters for Rehabilitation
16. Documentation for BMI and Pressure Ulcer Stages
17. Syndromes
18. Documentation of Complications of Care

C. Chapter-Specific Coding Guidelines
1. Chapter 1: Infectious and Parasitic Diseases (001-139)
   a. Human Immunodeficiency Virus (HIV) Infections
   b. Septicemia, Systemic Inflammatory Response Syndrome (SIRS), Sepsis, Severe Sepsis and Septic Shock
   c. Methicillin Resistant *Staphylococcus aureus* (MRSA) Conditions
2. Chapter 2: Neoplasms (140-239)
   a. Treatment directed at the malignancy
   b. Treatment of secondary site
   c. Coding and sequencing of complications
   d. Primary malignancy previously excised
   e. Admissions/Encounters involving chemotherapy, immunotherapy and radiation therapy
   f. Admission/encounter to determine extent of malignancy
   g. Symptoms, signs, and ill-defined conditions listed in Chapter 16 associated with neoplasms
   h. Admission/encounter for pain control/management
   i. Malignant neoplasm associated with transplanted organ
3. Chapter 3: Endocrine, Nutritional, and Metabolic Diseases and Immunity Disorders (240-279)
   a. Diabetes mellitus
4. Chapter 4: Diseases of Blood and Blood Forming Organs (280-289)
   a. Anemia of chronic disease
5. Chapter 5: Mental Disorders (290-319)
   Reserved for future guideline expansion
6. Chapter 6: Diseases of Nervous System and Sense Organs (320-389)
   a. Pain - Category 338
   b. Glaucoma
7. Chapter 7: Diseases of Circulatory System (390-459)
   a. Hypertension

K.   Code all documented conditions that coexist

L.   Patients receiving diagnostic services only

M.   Patients receiving therapeutic services only

N.   Patients receiving preoperative evaluations only

O.   Ambulatory surgery

P.   Routine outpatient prenatal visits

Appendix I: Present on Admission Reporting Guidelines

Section I. Conventions, general coding guidelines and chapter specific guidelines

The conventions, general guidelines and chapter-specific guidelines are applicable to all health care settings unless otherwise indicated. The conventions and instructions of the classification take precedence over guidelines.

A.   Conventions for the ICD-9-CM

The conventions for the ICD-9-CM are the general rules for use of the classification independent of the guidelines. These conventions are incorporated within the index and tabular of the ICD-9-CM as instructional notes. The conventions are as follows:

1.   Format:

The ICD-9-CM uses an indented format for ease in reference

2.   Abbreviations

a.   Index abbreviations

NEC "Not elsewhere classifiable"

This abbreviation in the index represents "other specified" when a specific code is not available for a condition the index directs the coder to the "other specified" code in the tabular.

b.   Tabular abbreviations

NEC "Not elsewhere classifiable"

This abbreviation in the tabular represents "other specified". When a specific code is not available for a condition the tabular includes an NEC entry under a code to identify the code as the "other specified" code.
(See Section I.A.5.a. "Other" codes").

NOS "Not otherwise specified"

This abbreviation is the equivalent of unspecified.
(See Section I.A.5.b., "Unspecified" codes)

3.   Punctuation

[ ]   Brackets are used in the tabular list to enclose synonyms, alternative wording or explanatory phrases. Brackets are used in the index to identify manifestation codes.
(See Section I.A.6. "Etiology/manifestations")

( )   Parentheses are used in both the index and tabular to enclose supplementary words that may be present or absent in the statement of a disease or procedure without affecting the code number to which it is assigned. The terms within the parentheses are referred to as nonessential modifiers.

:   Colons are used in the Tabular list after an incomplete term which needs one or more of the modifiers following the colon to make it assignable to a given category.

4.   Includes and Excludes Notes and Inclusion terms

Includes: This note appears immediately under a three-digit code title to further define, or give examples of, the content of the category.

Excludes: An excludes note under a code indicates that the terms excluded from the code are to be coded elsewhere. In some cases the codes for the excluded terms should not be used in conjunction with the code from which it is excluded. An example of this is a congenital condition excluded from an acquired form of the same condition. The congenital and acquired codes should not be used together. In other cases, the excluded terms may be used together with an excluded code. An example of this is when fractures of different bones are coded to different codes. Both codes may be used together if both types of fractures are present.

Inclusion terms: List of terms is included under certain four and five digit codes. These terms are the conditions for which that code number is to be used. The terms may be synonyms of the code title, or, in the case of "other specified" codes, the terms are a list of the various conditions assigned to that code. The inclusion terms are not necessarily exhaustive. Additional terms found only in the index may also be assigned to a code.

5.   Other and Unspecified codes

a.   "Other" codes

Codes titled "other" or "other specified" (usually a code with a 4th digit 8 or fifth-digit 9 for diagnosis codes) are for use when the information in the medical record provides detail for which a specific code does not exist. Index entries with NEC in the line designate "other" codes in the tabular. These index entries represent specific disease entities for which no specific code exists so the term is included within an "other" code.

b.   "Unspecified" codes

Codes (usually a code with a 4th digit 9 or 5th digit 0 for diagnosis codes) titled "unspecified" are for use when the information in the medical record is insufficient to assign a more specific code.

6.   Etiology/manifestation convention ("code first", "use additional code" and "in diseases classified elsewhere" notes)

Certain conditions have both an underlying etiology and multiple body system manifestations due to the underlying etiology. For such conditions, the ICD-9-CM has a coding convention that requires the underlying condition be sequenced first followed by the manifestation. Wherever such a combination exists, there is a "use additional code" note at the etiology code, and a "code first" note at the manifestation code. These instructional notes indicate the proper sequencing order of the codes, etiology followed by manifestation.

In most cases the manifestation codes will have in the code title, "in diseases classified elsewhere." Codes with this title are a component of the etiology/ manifestation convention. The code title indicates that it is a manifestation code. "In diseases classified elsewhere" codes are never permitted to be used as first listed or principal diagnosis codes. They must be used in conjunction with an underlying condition code and they must be listed following the underlying condition.

There are manifestation codes that do not have "in diseases classified elsewhere" in the title. For such codes a "use additional code" note will still be present and the rules for sequencing apply.

In addition to the notes in the tabular, these conditions also have a specific index entry structure. In the index both conditions are listed together with the etiology code first followed by the manifestation codes in brackets. The code in brackets is always to be sequenced second.

The most commonly used etiology/manifestation combinations are the codes for Diabetes mellitus, category 250. For each code under category 250 there is a use additional code note for the manifestation that is specific for that particular diabetic manifestation. Should a patient have more than one manifestation of diabetes, more than one code from category 250 may be used with as many manifestation codes as are needed to fully describe the patient's complete diabetic condition. The category 250 diabetes codes should be sequenced first, followed by the manifestation codes.

"Code first" and "Use additional code" notes are also used as sequencing rules in the classification for certain codes that are not part of an etiology/ manifestation combination.
See - Section I.B.9. "Multiple coding for a single condition".

7.   "And"

The word "and" should be interpreted to mean either "and" or "or" when it appears in a title.

8.   "With"

The word "with" should be interpreted to mean "associated with" or "due to" when it appears in a code title, the Alphabetic Index, or an instructional note in the Tabular List.

The word "with" in the alphabetic index is sequenced immediately following the main term, not in alphabetical order.

9. "See" and "See Also"

The "see" instruction following a main term in the index indicates that another term should be referenced. It is necessary to go to the main term referenced with the "see" note to locate the correct code.

A "see also" instruction following a main term in the index instructs that there is another main term that may also be referenced that may provide additional index entries that may be useful. It is not necessary to follow the "see also" note when the original main term provides the necessary code.

B. General Coding Guidelines

1. Use of Both Alphabetic Index and Tabular List

Use both the Alphabetic Index and the Tabular List when locating and assigning a code. Reliance on only the Alphabetic Index or the Tabular List leads to errors in code assignments and less specificity in code selection.

2. Locate each term in the Alphabetic Index

Locate each term in the Alphabetic Index and verify the code selected in the Tabular List. Read and be guided by instructional notations that appear in both the Alphabetic Index and the Tabular List.

3. Level of Detail in Coding

Diagnosis and procedure codes are to be used at their highest number of digits available.

ICD-9-CM diagnosis codes are composed of codes with 3, 4, or 5 digits. Codes with three digits are included in ICD-9-CM as the heading of a category of codes that may be further subdivided by the use of fourth and/or fifth digits, which provide greater detail.

A three-digit code is to be used only if it is not further subdivided. Where fourth-digit subcategories and/or fifth-digit subclassifications are provided, they must be assigned. A code is invalid if it has not been coded to the full number of digits required for that code. For example, Acute myocardial infarction, code 410, has fourth digits that describe the location of the infarction (e.g., 410.2, Of inferolateral wall), and fifth digits that identify the episode of care. It would be incorrect to report a code in category 410 without a fourth and fifth digit.

ICD-9-CM Volume 3 procedure codes are composed of codes with either 3 or 4 digits. Codes with two digits are included in ICD-9-CM as the heading of a category of codes that may be further subdivided by the use of third and/or fourth digits, which provide greater detail.

4. Code or codes from 001.0 through V91.99

The appropriate code or codes from 001.0 through V91.99 must be used to identify diagnoses, symptoms, conditions, problems, complaints or other reason(s) for the encounter/visit.

5. Selection of codes 001.0 through 999.9

The selection of codes 001.0 through 999.9 will frequently be used to describe the reason for the admission/encounter. These codes are from the section of ICD-9-CM for the classification of diseases and injuries (e.g., infectious and parasitic diseases; neoplasms; symptoms, signs, and ill-defined conditions, etc.).

6. Signs and symptoms

Codes that describe symptoms and signs, as opposed to diagnoses, are acceptable for reporting purposes when a related definitive diagnosis has not been established (confirmed) by the provider. Chapter 16 of ICD-9-CM, Symptoms, Signs, and Ill-defined conditions (codes 780.0 - 799.9) contain many, but not all codes for symptoms.

7. Conditions that are an integral part of a disease process

Signs and symptoms that are associated routinely with a disease process should not be assigned as additional codes, unless otherwise instructed by the classification.

8. Conditions that are not an integral part of a disease process

Additional signs and symptoms that may not be associated routinely with a disease process should be coded when present.

9. Multiple coding for a single condition

In addition to the etiology/manifestation convention that requires two codes to fully describe a single condition that affects multiple body systems, there are other single conditions that also require more than one code. "Use additional code" notes are found in the tabular at codes that are not part of an etiology/manifestation pair where a secondary code is useful to fully describe a condition. The sequencing rule is the same as the etiology/manifestation pair - "use additional code" indicates that a secondary code should be added.

For example, for infections that are not included in chapter 1, a secondary code from category 041, Bacterial infection in conditions classified elsewhere and of unspecified site, may be required to identify the bacterial organism causing the infection. A "use additional code" note will normally be found at the infectious disease code, indicating a need for the organism code to be added as a secondary code.

"Code first" notes are also under certain codes that are not specifically manifestation codes but may be due to an underlying cause. When a "code first" note is present and an underlying condition is present the underlying condition should be sequenced first.

"Code, if applicable, any causal condition first", notes indicate that this code may be assigned as a principal diagnosis when the causal condition is unknown or not applicable. If a causal condition is known, then the code for that condition should be sequenced as the principal or first-listed diagnosis.

Multiple codes may be needed for late effects, complication codes and obstetric codes to more fully describe a condition. See the specific guidelines for these conditions for further instruction.

10. Acute and Chronic Conditions

If the same condition is described as both acute (subacute) and chronic, and separate subentries exist in the Alphabetic Index at the same indentation level, code both and sequence the acute (subacute) code first.

11. Combination Code

A combination code is a single code used to classify:

- Two diagnoses, or
- A diagnosis with an associated secondary process (manifestation)
- A diagnosis with an associated complication

Combination codes are identified by referring to subterm entries in the Alphabetic Index and by reading the inclusion and exclusion notes in the Tabular List.

Assign only the combination code when that code fully identifies the diagnostic conditions involved or when the Alphabetic Index so directs. Multiple coding should not be used when the classification provides a combination code that clearly identifies all of the elements documented in the diagnosis. When the combination code lacks necessary specificity in describing the manifestation or complication, an additional code should be used as a secondary code.

12. Late Effects

A late effect is the residual effect (condition produced) after the acute phase of an illness or injury has terminated. There is no time limit on when a late effect code can be used. The residual may be apparent early, such as in cerebrovascular accident cases, or it may occur months or years later, such as that due to a previous injury. Coding of late effects generally requires two codes sequenced in the following order: The condition or nature of the late effect is sequenced first. The late effect code is sequenced second.

Exceptions to the above guidelines are those instances the late effect code has been expanded (at the fourth and fifth-digit levels) to include the manifestation(s) or the classification instructs otherwise. The code for the acute phase of an illness or injury that led to the late effect is never used with a code for the late effect.

13. Impending or Threatened Condition

Code any condition described at the time of discharge as "impending" or "threatened" as follows:

If it did occur, code as confirmed diagnosis.

If it did not occur, reference the Alphabetic Index to determine if the condition has a subentry term for "impending" or "threatened" and also reference main term entries for "Impending" and for "Threatened."

If the subterms are listed, assign the given code.

If the subterms are not listed, code the existing underlying condition(s) and not the condition described as impending or threatened.

14. **Reporting Same Diagnosis Code more than Once**

Each unique ICD-9-CM diagnosis code may be reported only once for an encounter. This applies to bilateral conditions or two different conditions classified to the same ICD-9-CM diagnosis code.

15. **Admissions/Encounters for Rehabilitation**

When the purpose for the admission/encounter is rehabilitation, sequence the appropriate V code from category V57, Care involving use of rehabilitation procedures, as the principal/first-listed diagnosis. The code for the condition for which the service is being performed should be reported as an additional diagnosis.

Only one code from category V57 is required. Code V57.89, Other specified rehabilitation procedures, should be assigned if more than one type of rehabilitation is performed during a single encounter. A procedure code should be reported to identify each type of rehabilitation therapy actually performed.

16. **Documentation for BMI and Pressure Ulcer Stages**

For the Body Mass Index (BMI) and pressure ulcer stage codes, code assignment may be based on medical record documentation from clinicians who are not the patient's provider (i.e., physician or other qualified healthcare practitioner legally accountable for establishing the patient's diagnosis), since this information is typically documented by other clinicians involved in the care of the patient (e.g., a dietitian often documents the BMI and nurses often documents the pressure ulcer stages). However, the associated diagnosis (such as overweight, obesity, or pressure ulcer) must be documented by the patient's provider. If there is conflicting medical record documentation, either from the same clinician or different clinicians, the patient's attending provider should be queried for clarification.

The BMI and pressure ulcer stage codes should only be reported as secondary diagnoses. As with all other secondary diagnosis codes, the BMI and pressure ulcer stage codes should only be assigned when they meet the definition of a reportable additional diagnosis (see Section III, Reporting Additional Diagnoses).

17. **Syndromes**

Follow the Alphabetic Index guidance when coding syndromes. In the absence of index guidance, assign codes for the documented manifestations of the syndrome.

18. **Documentation of complications of care**

Code assignment is based on the provider's documentation of the relationship between the condition and the care or procedure. The guideline extends to any complications of care, regardless of the chapter the code is located in. It is important to note that not all conditions that occur during or following medical care or surgery are classified as complications. There must be a cause-and-effect relationship between the care provided and the condition, and an indication in the documentation that it is a complication. Query the provider for clarification, if the complication is not clearly documented.

C. **Chapter-Specific Coding Guidelines**

In addition to general coding guidelines, there are guidelines for specific diagnoses and/or conditions in the classification. Unless otherwise indicated, these guidelines apply to all health care settings. Please refer to Section II for guidelines on the selection of principal diagnosis.

1. **Chapter 1: Infectious and Parasitic Diseases (001-139)**

   a. **Human Immunodeficiency Virus (HIV) Infections**

      1) **Code only confirmed cases**

         Code only confirmed cases of HIV infection/illness. This is an exception to the hospital inpatient guideline Section II, H.

         In this context, "confirmation" does not require documentation of positive serology or culture for HIV; the provider's diagnostic statement that the patient is HIV positive, or has an HIV-related illness is sufficient.

      2) **Selection and sequencing of HIV codes**

         (a) **Patient admitted for HIV-related condition**

            If a patient is admitted for an HIV-related condition, the principal diagnosis should be 042, followed by additional diagnosis codes for all reported HIV-related conditions.

         (b) **Patient with HIV disease admitted for unrelated condition**

            If a patient with HIV disease is admitted for an unrelated condition (such as a traumatic injury), the code for the unrelated condition (e.g., the nature of injury code) should be the principal diagnosis. Other diagnoses would be 042 followed by additional diagnosis codes for all reported HIV-related conditions.

         (c) **Whether the patient is newly diagnosed**

            Whether the patient is newly diagnosed or has had previous admissions/encounters for HIV conditions is irrelevant to the sequencing decision.

         (d) **Asymptomatic human immunodeficiency virus**

            V08 Asymptomatic human immunodeficiency virus [HIV] infection, is to be applied when the patient without any documentation of symptoms is listed as being "HIV positive," "known HIV," "HIV test positive," or similar terminology. Do not use this code if the term "AIDS" is used or if the patient is treated for any HIV-related illness or is described as having any condition(s) resulting from his/her HIV positive status; use 042 in these cases.

         (e) **Patients with inconclusive HIV serology**

            Patients with inconclusive HIV serology, but no definitive diagnosis or manifestations of the illness, may be assigned code 795.71, Inconclusive serologic test for Human Immunodeficiency Virus [HIV].

         (f) **Previously diagnosed HIV-related illness**

            Patients with any known prior diagnosis of an HIV-related illness should be coded to 042. Once a patient has developed an HIV-related illness, the patient should always be assigned code 042 on every subsequent admission/encounter. Patients previously diagnosed with any HIV illness (042) should never be assigned to 795.71 or V08.

         (g) **HIV Infection in Pregnancy, Childbirth and the Puerperium**

            During pregnancy, childbirth or the puerperium, a patient admitted (or presenting for a health care encounter) because of an HIV-related illness should receive a principal diagnosis code of 647.6x, Other specified infectious and parasitic diseases in the mother classifiable elsewhere, but complicating the pregnancy, childbirth or the puerperium, followed by 042 and the code(s) for the HIV-related illness(es). Codes from Chapter 15 always take sequencing priority.

            Patients with asymptomatic HIV infection status admitted (or presenting for a health care encounter) during pregnancy, childbirth, or the puerperium should receive codes of 647.6x and V08.

(h) Encounters for testing for HIV

If a patient is being seen to determine his/her HIV status, use code V73.89, Screening for other specified viral disease. Use code V69.8, Other problems related to lifestyle, as a secondary code if an asymptomatic patient is in a known high risk group for HIV. Should a patient with signs or symptoms or illness, or a confirmed HIV related diagnosis be tested for HIV, code the signs and symptoms or the diagnosis. An additional counseling code V65.44 may be used if counseling is provided during the encounter for the test.

When a patient returns to be informed of his/her HIV test results use code V65.44, HIV counseling, if the results of the test are negative.

If the results are positive but the patient is asymptomatic use code V08, Asymptomatic HIV infection. If the results are positive and the patient is symptomatic use code 042, HIV infection, with codes for the HIV related symptoms or diagnosis. The HIV counseling code may also be used if counseling is provided for patients with positive test results.

b. **Septicemia, Systemic Inflammatory Response Syndrome (SIRS), Sepsis, Severe Sepsis, and Septic Shock**

1) **SIRS, Septicemia, and Sepsis**

(a) The terms *septicemia* and *sepsis* are often used interchangeably by providers, however they are not considered synonymous terms. The following descriptions are provided for reference but do not preclude querying the provider for clarification about terms used in the documentation:

(i) Septicemia generally refers to a systemic disease associated with the presence of pathological microorganisms or toxins in the blood, which can include bacteria, viruses, fungi or other organisms.

(ii) Systemic inflammatory response syndrome (SIRS) generally refers to the systemic response to infection, trauma/burns, or other insult (such as cancer) with symptoms including fever, tachycardia, tachypnea, and leukocytosis.

(iii) Sepsis generally refers to SIRS due to infection.

(iv) Severe sepsis generally refers to sepsis with associated acute organ dysfunction.

(b) **The Coding of SIRS, sepsis and severe sepsis**

The coding of SIRS, sepsis and severe sepsis requires a minimum of 2 codes: a code for the underlying cause (such as infection or trauma) and a code from subcategory 995.9 Systemic inflammatory response syndrome (SIRS).

(i) The code for the underlying cause (such as infection or trauma) must be sequenced before the code from subcategory 995.9 Systemic inflammatory response syndrome (SIRS).

(ii) Sepsis and severe sepsis require a code for the systemic infection (038.xx, 112.5, etc.) and either code 995.91, Sepsis, or 995.92, Severe sepsis. If the causal organism is not documented, assign code 038.9, Unspecified septicemia.

(iii) Severe sepsis requires additional code(s) for the associated acute organ dysfunction(s).

(iv) If a patient has sepsis with multiple organ dysfunctions, follow the instructions for coding severe sepsis.

(v) Either the term sepsis or SIRS must be documented to assign a code from subcategory 995.9.

(vi) See Section I.C.17.g), Injury and poisoning, for information regarding systemic inflammatory

response syndrome (SIRS) due to trauma/burns and other non-infectious processes.

(c) Due to the complex nature of sepsis and severe sepsis, some cases may require querying the provider prior to assignment of the codes.

2) **Sequencing sepsis and severe sepsis**

(a) **Sepsis and severe sepsis as principal diagnosis**

If sepsis or severe sepsis is present on admission, and meets the definition of principal diagnosis, the systemic infection code (e.g., 038.xx, 112.5, etc) should be assigned as the principal diagnosis, followed by code 995.91, Sepsis, or 995.92, Severe sepsis, as required by the sequencing rules in the Tabular List. Codes from subcategory 995.9 can never be assigned as a principal diagnosis. A code should also be assigned for any localized infection, if present.

If the sepsis or severe sepsis is due to a postprocedural infection, see Section I.C.1.b.10 for guidelines related to sepsis due to postprocedural infection.

(b) **Sepsis and severe sepsis as secondary diagnoses**

When sepsis or severe sepsis develops during the encounter (it was not present on admission), the systemic infection code and code 995.91 or 995.92 should be assigned as secondary diagnoses.

(c) **Documentation unclear as to whether sepsis or severe sepsis is present on admission**

Sepsis or severe sepsis may be present on admission but the diagnosis may not be confirmed until sometime after admission. If the documentation is not clear whether the sepsis or severe sepsis was present on admission, the provider should be queried.

3) **Sepsis/SIRS with Localized Infection**

If the reason for admission is both sepsis, severe sepsis, or SIRS and a localized infection, such as pneumonia or cellulitis, a code for the systemic infection (038.xx, 112.5, etc) should be assigned first, then code 995.91 or 995.92, followed by the code for the localized infection. If the patient is admitted with a localized infection, such as pneumonia, and sepsis/SIRS doesn't develop until after admission, see guideline I.C.1.b.2.b).

If the localized infection is postprocedural, *see Section I.C.1.b.10 for guidelines related to sepsis due to postprocedural infection.*

Note: The term urosepsis is a nonspecific term. If that is the only term documented then only code 599.0 should be assigned based on the default for the term in the ICD-9-CM index, in addition to the code for the causal organism if known.

4) **Bacterial Sepsis and Septicemia**

In most cases, it will be a code from category 038, Septicemia, that will be used in conjunction with a code from subcategory 995.9 such as the following:

(a) **Streptococcal sepsis**

If the documentation in the record states streptococcal sepsis, codes 038.0, Streptococcal septicemia, and code 995.91 should be used, in that sequence.

(b) **Streptococcal septicemia**

If the documentation states streptococcal septicemia, only code 038.0 should be assigned, however, the provider should be queried whether the patient has sepsis, an infection with SIRS.

5) **Acute organ dysfunction that is not clearly associated with the sepsis**

If a patient has sepsis and an acute organ dysfunction, but the medical record documentation indicates that the acute organ dysfunction is related to a medical condition other than the sepsis, do not assign code 995.92, Severe sepsis. An acute organ dysfunction must be associated with the sepsis in order to assign the severe sepsis code. If the documentation is not clear as to whether an acute organ dysfunction is related to the sepsis or another medical condition, query the provider.

6) **Septic shock**

   (a) **Sequencing of septic shock**

   Septic shock generally refers to circulatory failure associated with severe sepsis, and, therefore, it represents a type of acute organ dysfunction.

   For cases of septic shock, the code for the systemic infection should be sequenced first, followed by codes 995.92, Severe sepsis and 785.52, Septic shock or 998.02, Postoperative septic shock. Any additional codes for other acute organ dysfunctions should also be assigned. As noted in the sequencing instructions in the Tabular List, the code for septic shock cannot be assigned as a principal diagnosis.

   (b) **Septic Shock without documentation of severe sepsis**

   Since septic shock indicates the presence of severe sepsis, code 995.92, Severe sepsis, can be assigned with code 785.52, Septic shock, or code 998.02 Postoperative shock, septic, even if the term severe sepsis is not documented in the record.

7) **Sepsis and septic shock complicating abortion and pregnancy**

   Sepsis and septic shock complicating abortion, ectopic pregnancy, and molar pregnancy are classified to category codes in Chapter 11 (630-639).

   See section I.C.11.i.7. for information on the coding of puerperal sepsis.

8) **Negative or inconclusive blood cultures**

   Negative or inconclusive blood cultures do not preclude a diagnosis of septicemia or sepsis in patients with clinical evidence of the condition, however, the provider should be queried.

9) **Newborn sepsis**

   See Section I.C.15.j for information on the coding of newborn sepsis.

10) **Sepsis due to a Postprocedural Infection**

   (a) **Documentation of causal relationship**

   As with all postprocedural complications, code assignment is based on the provider's documentation of the relationship between the infection and the procedure.

   (b) **Sepsis due to postprocedural infection**

   In cases of postprocedural sepsis, the complication code, such as code 998.59, Other postoperative infection, or 674.3x, Other complications of obstetrical surgical wounds should be coded first followed by the appropriate sepsis codes (systemic infection code and either code 995.91 or 995.92). An additional code(s) for any acute organ dysfunction should also be assigned for cases of severe sepsis.

   See Section see Section I.C.1.b.6 if the sepsis or severe sepsis results in postprocedural septic shock.

   (c) **Postprocedural infection and postprocedural septic shock**

   In cases where a postprocedural infection has occurred and has resulted in severe sepsis and postprocedural septic shock, the code for the precipitating complication such as code 998.59, Other postoperative infection, or 674.3x, Other complications of obstetrical surgical wounds should be coded first followed by the

appropriate sepsis codes (systemic infection code and code 995.92). Code 998.02, Postoperative septic shock, should be assigned as an additional code. In cases of severe sepsis, an additional code(s) for any acute organ dysfunction should also be assigned.

11) **External cause of injury codes with SIRS**

   Refer to Section I.C.19.a.7 for instruction on the use of external cause of injury codes with codes for SIRS resulting from trauma.

12) **Sepsis and Severe Sepsis Associated with Non-infectious Process**

   In some cases, a non-infectious process, such as trauma, may lead to an infection which can result in sepsis or severe sepsis. If sepsis or severe sepsis is documented as associated with a non-infectious condition, such as a burn or serious injury, and this condition meets the definition for principal diagnosis, the code for the non-infectious condition should be sequenced first, followed by the code for the systemic infection and either code 995.91, Sepsis, or 995.92, Severe sepsis. Additional codes for any associated acute organ dysfunction(s) should also be assigned for cases of severe sepsis. If the sepsis or severe sepsis meets the definition of principal diagnosis, the systemic infection and sepsis codes should be sequenced before the non-infectious condition. When both the associated non-infectious condition and the sepsis or severe sepsis meet the definition of principal diagnosis, either may be assigned as principal diagnosis.

   See Section I.C.1.b.2.a. for guidelines pertaining to sepsis or severe sepsis as the principal diagnosis.

   Only one code from subcategory 995.9 should be assigned. Therefore, when a non-infectious condition leads to an infection resulting in sepsis or severe sepsis, assign either code 995.91 or 995.92. Do not additionally assign code 995.93, Systemic inflammatory response syndrome due to non-infectious process without acute organ dysfunction, or 995.94, Systemic inflammatory response syndrome with acute organ dysfunction.

   See Section I.C.17.g for information on the coding of SIRS due to trauma/burns or other non-infectious disease processes.

c. **Methicillin Resistant Staphylococcus aureus (MRSA) Conditions**

   1) **Selection and sequencing of MRSA codes**

      (a) **Combination codes for MRSA infection**

      When a patient is diagnosed with an infection that is due to methicillin resistant *Staphylococcus aureus* (MRSA), and that infection has a combination code that includes the causal organism (e.g., septicemia, pneumonia) assign the appropriate code for the condition (e.g., code 038.12, Methicillin resistant Staphylococcus aureus septicemia or code 482.42, Methicillin resistant pneumonia due to Staphylococcus aureus). Do not assign code 041.12, Methicillin resistant Staphylococcus aureus, as an additional code because the code includes the type of infection and the MRSA organism. Do not assign a code from subcategory V09.0, Infection with microorganisms resistant to penicillins, as an additional diagnosis.

      See Section C.1.b.1 for instructions on coding and sequencing of septicemia.

      (b) **Other codes for MRSA infection**

      When there is documentation of a current infection (e.g., wound infection, stitch abscess, urinary tract infection) due to MRSA, and that infection does not have a combination code that includes the causal organism, select the appropriate code to identify the condition along with code 041.12, Methicillin resistant Staphylococcus aureus, for the MRSA infection. Do not assign a code from subcategory V09.0, Infection with microorganisms resistant to penicillins.

(c) Methicillin susceptible Staphylococcus aureus (MSSA) and MRSA colonization

The condition or state of being colonized or carrying MSSA or MRSA is called colonization or carriage, while an individual person is described as being colonized or being a carrier. Colonization means that MSSA or MSRA is present on or in the body without necessarily causing illness. A positive MRSA colonization test might be documented by the provider as "MRSA screen positive" or "MRSA nasal swab positive".

Assign code V02.54, Carrier or suspected carrier, Methicillin resistant Staphylococcus aureus, for patients documented as having MRSA colonization. Assign code V02.53, Carrier or suspected carrier, Methicillin susceptible Staphylococcus aureus, for patient documented as having MSSA colonization. Colonization is not necessarily indicative of a disease process or as the cause of a specific condition the patient may have unless documented as such by the provider.

Code V02.59, Other specified bacterial diseases, should be assigned for other types of staphylococcal colonization (e.g., S. epidermidis, S. saprophyticus). Code V02.59 should not be assigned for colonization with any type of Staphylococcus aureus (MRSA, MSSA).

(d) MRSA colonization and infection

If a patient is documented as having both MRSA colonization and infection during a hospital admission, code V02.54, Carrier or suspected carrier, Methicillin resistant Staphylococcus aureus, and a code for the MRSA infection may both be assigned.

2. Chapter 2: Neoplasms (140-239)

General guidelines

Chapter 2 of the ICD-9-CM contains the codes for most benign and all malignant neoplasms. Certain benign neoplasms, such as prostatic adenomas, may be found in the specific body system chapters. To properly code a neoplasm it is necessary to determine from the record if the neoplasm is benign, in-situ, malignant, or of uncertain histologic behavior. If malignant, any secondary (metastatic) sites should also be determined.

The neoplasm table in the Alphabetic Index should be referenced first. However, if the histological term is documented, that term should be referenced first, rather than going immediately to the Neoplasm Table, in order to determine which column in the Neoplasm Table is appropriate. For example, if the documentation indicates "adenoma," refer to the term in the Alphabetic Index to review the entries under this term and the instructional note to "see also neoplasm, by site, benign." The table provides the proper code based on the type of neoplasm and the site. It is important to select the proper column in the table that corresponds to the type of neoplasm. The tabular should then be referenced to verify that the correct code has been selected from the table and that a more specific site code does not exist.

See Section I. C. 18.d.4. for information regarding V codes for genetic susceptibility to cancer.

a. Treatment directed at the malignancy

If the treatment is directed at the malignancy, designate the malignancy as the principal diagnosis.

The only exception to this guideline is if a patient admission/encounter is solely for the administration of chemotherapy, immunotherapy or radiation therapy, assign the appropriate V58.x code as the first-listed or principal diagnosis, and the diagnosis or problem for which the service is being performed as a secondary diagnosis.

b. Treatment of secondary site

When a patient is admitted because of a primary neoplasm with metastasis and treatment is directed toward the secondary site only, the secondary neoplasm is designated as the principal diagnosis even though the primary malignancy is still present.

c. Coding and sequencing of complications

Coding and sequencing of complications associated with the malignancies or with the therapy thereof are subject to the following guidelines:

1) Anemia associated with malignancy

When admission/encounter is for management of an anemia associated with the malignancy, and the treatment is only for anemia, the appropriate anemia code (such as code 285.22, Anemia in neoplastic disease) is designated as the principal diagnosis and is followed by the appropriate code(s) for the malignancy.

Code 285.22 may also be used as a secondary code if the patient suffers from anemia and is being treated for the malignancy.

If anemia in neoplastic disease and anemia due to antineoplastic chemotherapy are both documented, assign codes for both conditions.

2) Anemia associated with chemotherapy, immunotherapy and radiation therapy

When the admission/encounter is for management of an anemia associated with chemotherapy, immunotherapy or radiotherapy and the only treatment is for the anemia, the anemia is sequenced first. The appropriate neoplasm code should be assigned as an additional code.

3) Management of dehydration due to the malignancy

When the admission/encounter is for management of dehydration due to the malignancy or the therapy, or a combination of both, and only the dehydration is being treated (intravenous rehydration), the dehydration is sequenced first, followed by the code(s) for the malignancy.

4) Treatment of a complication resulting from a surgical procedure

When the admission/encounter is for treatment of a complication resulting from a surgical procedure, designate the complication as the principal or first-listed diagnosis if treatment is directed at resolving the complication.

d. Primary malignancy previously excised

When a primary malignancy has been previously excised or eradicated from its site and there is no further treatment directed to that site and there is no evidence of any existing primary malignancy, a code from category V10, Personal history of malignant neoplasm, should be used to indicate the former site of the malignancy. Any mention of extension, invasion, or metastasis to another site is coded as a secondary malignant neoplasm to that site. The secondary site may be the principal or first-listed with the V10 code used as a secondary code.

e. Admissions/Encounters involving chemotherapy, immunotherapy and radiation therapy

1) Episode of care involves surgical removal of neoplasm

When an episode of care involves the surgical removal of a neoplasm, primary or secondary site, followed by adjunct chemotherapy or radiation treatment during the same episode of care, the neoplasm code should be assigned as principal or first-listed diagnosis, using codes in the 140-198 series or where appropriate in the 200-203 series.

2) Patient admission/encounter solely for administration of chemotherapy, immunotherapy and radiation therapy

If a patient admission/encounter is solely for the administration of chemotherapy, immunotherapy or radiation therapy assign code V58.0, Encounter for radiation therapy, or V58.11, Encounter for antineoplastic chemotherapy, or V58.12, Encounter for antineoplastic immunotherapy as the first-listed or principal diagnosis. If a patient receives more than one of these therapies during the same admission more than one of these codes may be assigned, in any sequence.

The malignancy for which the therapy is being administered should be assigned as a secondary diagnosis.

3) Patient admitted for radiotherapy/chemotherapy and immunotherapy and develops complications

When a patient is admitted for the purpose of radiotherapy, immunotherapy or chemotherapy and develops complications such as uncontrolled nausea and vomiting or dehydration, the principal or first-listed diagnosis is V58.0, Encounter for radiotherapy, or V58.11, Encounter for antineoplastic chemotherapy, or V58.12, Encounter for antineoplastic immunotherapy followed by any codes for the complications.

f. Admission/encounter to determine extent of malignancy

When the reason for admission/encounter is to determine the extent of the malignancy, or for a procedure such as paracentesis or thoracentesis, the primary malignancy or appropriate metastatic site is designated as the principal or first-listed diagnosis, even though chemotherapy or radiotherapy is administered.

g. Symptoms, signs, and ill-defined conditions listed in Chapter 16 associated with neoplasms

Symptoms, signs, and ill-defined conditions listed in Chapter 16 characteristic of, or associated with, an existing primary or secondary site malignancy cannot be used to replace the malignancy as principal or first-listed diagnosis, regardless of the number of admissions or encounters for treatment and care of the neoplasm.

h. Admission/encounter for pain control/management

See Section I.C.6.a.5 for information on coding admission/encounter for pain control/management.

i. Malignant neoplasm associated with transplanted organ

A malignant neoplasm of a transplanted organ should be coded as a transplant complication. Assign first the appropriate code from subcategory 996.8, Complications of transplanted organ, followed by code 199.2, Malignant neoplasm associated with transplanted organ. Use an additional code for the specific malignancy.

3. Chapter 3: Endocrine, Nutritional, and Metabolic Diseases and Immunity Disorders (240-279)

a. Diabetes mellitus

Codes under category 250, Diabetes mellitus, identify complications/manifestations associated with diabetes mellitus. A fifth-digit is required for all category 250 codes to identify the type of diabetes mellitus and whether the diabetes is controlled or uncontrolled.

See I.C.3.a.7 for secondary diabetes

1) Fifth-digits for category 250:

The following are the fifth-digits for the codes under category 250:

0   type II or unspecified type, not stated as uncontrolled

1   type I, [juvenile type], not stated as uncontrolled

2   type II or unspecified type, uncontrolled

3   type I, [juvenile type], uncontrolled

The age of a patient is not the sole determining factor, though most type I diabetics develop the condition before reaching puberty. For this reason type I diabetes mellitus is also referred to as juvenile diabetes.

2) Type of diabetes mellitus not documented

If the type of diabetes mellitus is not documented in the medical record the default is type II.

3) Diabetes mellitus and the use of insulin

All type I diabetics must use insulin to replace what their bodies do not produce. However, the use of insulin does not mean that a patient is a type I diabetic. Some patients with type II diabetes mellitus are unable to control their blood sugar through diet and oral medication alone and do require insulin. If the documentation in a medical record does not indicate the type of diabetes but does indicate that the patient uses insulin, the appropriate fifth-digit for type II must be used. For type II patients who routinely use insulin, code V58.67, Long-term (current) use of insulin, should also be assigned to indicate that the patient uses insulin. Code V58.67 should not be assigned if insulin is given temporarily to bring a type II patient's blood sugar under control during an encounter.

4) Assigning and sequencing diabetes codes and associated conditions

When assigning codes for diabetes and its associated conditions, the code(s) from category 250 must be sequenced before the codes for the associated conditions. The diabetes codes and the secondary codes that correspond to them are paired codes that follow the etiology/manifestation convention of the classification *(See Section I.A.6., Etiology/manifestation convention)*. Assign as many codes from category 250 as needed to identify all of the associated conditions that the patient has. The corresponding secondary codes are listed under each of the diabetes codes.

(a) Diabetic retinopathy/diabetic macular edema

Diabetic macular edema, code 362.07, is only present with diabetic retinopathy. Another code from subcategory 362.0, Diabetic retinopathy, must be used with code 362.07. Codes under subcategory 362.0 are diabetes manifestation codes, so they must be used following the appropriate diabetes code.

5) Diabetes mellitus in pregnancy and gestational diabetes

(a) For diabetes mellitus complicating pregnancy, *see Section I.C.11.f., Diabetes mellitus in pregnancy.*

(b) For gestational diabetes, *see Section I.C.11, g., Gestational diabetes.*

6) Insulin pump malfunction

(a) Underdose of insulin due insulin pump failure

An underdose of insulin due to an insulin pump failure should be assigned 996.57, Mechanical complication due to insulin pump, as the principal or first listed code, followed by the appropriate diabetes mellitus code based on documentation.

(b) Overdose of insulin due to insulin pump failure

The principal or first listed code for an encounter due to an insulin pump malfunction resulting in an overdose of insulin, should also be 996.57, Mechanical complication due to insulin pump, followed by code 962.3, Poisoning by insulins and antidiabetic agents, and the appropriate diabetes mellitus code based on documentation.

7) Secondary Diabetes Mellitus

Codes under category 249, Secondary diabetes mellitus, identify complications/manifestations associated with secondary diabetes mellitus. Secondary diabetes is always caused by another condition or event (e.g., cystic fibrosis, malignant neoplasm of pancreas, pancreatectomy, adverse effect of drug, or poisoning).

(a) Fifth-digits for category 249:

A fifth-digit is required for all category 249 codes to identify whether the diabetes is controlled or uncontrolled.

(b) Secondary diabetes mellitus and the use of insulin

For patients who routinely use insulin, code V58.67, Long-term (current) use of insulin, should also be assigned. Code V58.67 should not be assigned if insulin is given temporarily to bring a patient's blood sugar under control during an encounter.

(c) Assigning and sequencing secondary diabetes codes and associated conditions

When assigning codes for secondary diabetes and its associated conditions (e.g. renal manifestations), the code(s) from category 249 must be sequenced before the codes for the associated conditions. The secondary diabetes codes and the diabetic manifestation codes that correspond to them are paired codes that follow the etiology/manifestation convention of the classification. Assign as many codes from category 249 as needed to identify all of the associated conditions that the patient has. The corresponding codes for the associated conditions are listed under each of the secondary diabetes codes. For example, secondary diabetes with diabetic nephrosis is assigned to code 249.40, followed by 581.81.

(d) Assigning and sequencing secondary diabetes codes and its causes

The sequencing of the secondary diabetes codes in relationship to codes for the cause of the diabetes is based on the reason for the encounter, applicable ICD-9-CM sequencing conventions, and chapter-specific guidelines.

If a patient is seen for treatment of the secondary diabetes or one of its associated conditions, a code from category 249 is sequenced as the principal or first-listed diagnosis, with the cause of the secondary diabetes (e.g. cystic fibrosis) sequenced as an additional diagnosis.

If, however, the patient is seen for the treatment of the condition causing the secondary diabetes (e.g., malignant neoplasm of pancreas), the code for the cause of the secondary diabetes should be sequenced as the principal or first-listed diagnosis followed by a code from category 249.

(i) Secondary diabetes mellitus due to pancreatectomy

For postpancreatectomy diabetes mellitus (lack of insulin due to the surgical removal of all or part of the pancreas), assign code 251.3, Postsurgical hypoinsulinemia. Assign a code from subcategory 249, Secondary diabetes mellitus and a code from subcategory V88.1, Acquired absence of pancreas as additional codes. Code also any diabetic manifestations (e.g. diabetic nephrosis 581.81).

(ii) Secondary diabetes due to drugs

Secondary diabetes may be caused by an adverse effect of correctly administered medications, poisoning or late effect of poisoning.

See section I.C.17.e for coding of adverse effects and poisoning, and section I.C.19 for E code reporting.

4. Chapter 4: Diseases of Blood and Blood Forming Organs (280-289)

a. Anemia of chronic disease

Subcategory 285.2, Anemia in chronic illness, has codes for anemia in chronic kidney disease, code 285.21; anemia in neoplastic disease, code 285.22; and anemia in other chronic illness, code 285.29. These codes can be used as the principal/first listed code if the reason for the encounter is to treat the anemia. They may also be used as secondary codes if treatment of the anemia is a component of an encounter, but not the primary reason for the encounter. When using a code from

subcategory 285 it is also necessary to use the code for the chronic condition causing the anemia.

1) Anemia in chronic kidney disease

When assigning code 285.21, Anemia in chronic kidney disease, it is also necessary to assign a code from category 585, Chronic kidney disease, to indicate the stage of chronic kidney disease.

See I.C.10.a. Chronic kidney disease (CKD).

2) Anemia in neoplastic disease

When assigning code 285.22, Anemia in neoplastic disease, it is also necessary to assign the neoplasm code that is responsible for the anemia. Code 285.22 is for use for anemia that is due to the malignancy, not for anemia due to antineoplastic chemotherapy drugs. Assign the appropriate code for anemia due to antineoplastic chemotherapy.

See I.C.2.c.1 Anemia associated with malignancy.

See I.C.2.c.2 Anemia associated with chemotherapy, immunotherapy and radiation therapy.

5. Chapter 5: Mental Disorders (290-319)

Reserved for future guideline expansion

6. Chapter 6: Diseases of Nervous System and Sense Organs (320-389)

a. Pain - Category 338

1) General coding information

Codes in category 338 may be used in conjunction with codes from other categories and chapters to provide more detail about acute or chronic pain and neoplasm-related pain, unless otherwise indicated below.

If the pain is not specified as acute or chronic, do not assign codes from category 338, except for post-thoracotomy pain, postoperative pain, neoplasm related pain, or central pain syndrome.

A code from subcategories 338.1 and 338.2 should not be assigned if the underlying (definitive) diagnosis is known, unless the reason for the encounter is pain control/management and not management of the underlying condition.

(a) Category 338 Codes as Principal or First-Listed Diagnosis

Category 338 codes are acceptable as principal diagnosis or the first-listed code:

- When pain control or pain management is the reason for the admission/encounter (e.g., a patient with displaced intervertebral disc, nerve impingement and severe back pain presents for injection of steroid into the spinal canal). The underlying cause of the pain should be reported as an additional diagnosis, if known.

- When an admission or encounter is for a procedure aimed at treating the underlying condition (e.g., spinal fusion, kyphoplasty), a code for the underlying condition (e.g., vertebral fracture, spinal stenosis) should be assigned as the principal diagnosis. No code from category 338 should be assigned.

- When a patient is admitted for the insertion of a neurostimulator for pain control, assign the appropriate pain code as the principal or first listed diagnosis. When an admission or encounter is for a procedure aimed at treating the underlying condition and a neurostimulator is inserted for pain control during the same admission/encounter, a code for the underlying condition should be assigned as the principal diagnosis and the appropriate pain code should be assigned as a secondary diagnosis.

(b) **Use of Category 338 Codes in Conjunction with Site Specific Pain Codes**

(i) **Assigning Category 338 Codes and Site-Specific Pain Codes**

Codes from category 338 may be used in conjunction with codes that identify the site of pain (including codes from chapter 16) if the category 338 code provides additional information. For example, if the code describes the site of the pain, but does not fully describe whether the pain is acute or chronic, then both codes should be assigned.

(ii) **Sequencing of Category 338 Codes with Site-Specific Pain Codes**

The sequencing of category 338 codes with site-specific pain codes (including chapter 16 codes), is dependent on the circumstances of the encounter/admission as follows:

- If the encounter is for pain control or pain management, assign the code from category 338 followed by the code identifying the specific site of pain (e.g., encounter for pain management for acute neck pain from trauma is assigned code 338.11, Acute pain due to trauma, followed by code 723.1, Cervicalgia, to identify the site of pain).

- If the encounter is for any other reason except pain control or pain management, and a related definitive diagnosis has not been established (confirmed) by the provider, assign the code for the specific site of pain first, followed by the appropriate code from category 338.

2) **Pain due to devices, implants and grafts**

Pain associated with devices, implants or grafts left in a surgical site (for example painful hip prosthesis) is assigned to the appropriate code(s) found in Chapter 17, Injury and Poisoning. Use additional code(s) from category 338 to identify acute or chronic pain due to presence of the device, implant or graft (338.18-338.19 or 338.28-338.29).

3) **Postoperative Pain**

Post-thoracotomy pain and other postoperative pain are classified to subcategories 338.1 and 338.2, depending on whether the pain is acute or chronic. The default for post-thoracotomy and other postoperative pain not specified as acute or chronic is the code for the acute form.

Routine or expected postoperative pain immediately after surgery should not be coded.

(a) **Postoperative pain not associated with specific postoperative complication**

Postoperative pain not associated with a specific postoperative complication is assigned to the appropriate postoperative pain code in category 338.

(b) **Postoperative pain associated with specific postoperative complication**

Postoperative pain associated with a specific postoperative complication (such as painful wire sutures) is assigned to the appropriate code(s) found in Chapter 17, Injury and Poisoning. If appropriate, use additional code(s) from category 338 to identify acute or chronic pain (338.18 or 338.28). If pain control/management is the reason for the encounter, a code from category 338 should be assigned as the principal or first-listed diagnosis in accordance with *Section I.C.6.a.1.a above.*

(c) **Postoperative pain as principal or first-listed diagnosis**

Postoperative pain may be reported as the principal or first-listed diagnosis when the stated reason for the admission/encounter is documented as postoperative pain control/ management.

(d) **Postoperative pain as secondary diagnosis**

Postoperative pain may be reported as a secondary diagnosis code when a patient presents for outpatient surgery and develops an unusual or inordinate amount of postoperative pain.

The provider's documentation should be used to guide the coding of postoperative pain, as well as *Section III. Reporting Additional Diagnoses and Section IV. Diagnostic Coding and Reporting in the Outpatient Setting.*

See Section II.I.2 for information on sequencing of diagnoses for patients admitted to hospital inpatient care following post-operative observation.

See Section II.J for information on sequencing of diagnoses for patients admitted to hospital inpatient care from outpatient surgery.

See Section IV.A.2 for information on sequencing of diagnoses for patients admitted for observation.

4) **Chronic pain**

Chronic pain is classified to subcategory 338.2. There is no time frame defining when pain becomes chronic pain. The provider's documentation should be used to guide use of these codes.

5) **Neoplasm Related Pain**

Code 338.3 is assigned to pain documented as being related, associated or due to cancer, primary or secondary malignancy, or tumor. This code is assigned regardless of whether the pain is acute or chronic.

This code may be assigned as the principal or first-listed code when the stated reason for the admission/encounter is documented as pain control/pain management. The underlying neoplasm should be reported as an additional diagnosis.

When the reason for the admission/encounter is management of the neoplasm and the pain associated with the neoplasm is also documented, code 338.3 may be assigned as an additional diagnosis.

See Section I.C.2 for instructions on the sequencing of neoplasms for all other stated reasons for the admission/encounter (except for pain control/pain management).

6) **Chronic pain syndrome**

This condition is different than the term "chronic pain," and therefore this code should only be used when the provider has specifically documented this condition.

b. **Glaucoma**

1) **Glaucoma**

For types of glaucoma classified to subcategories 365.1-365.6, an additional code should be assigned from subcategory 365.7, Glaucoma stage, to identify the glaucoma stage. Codes from 365.7, Glaucoma stage, may not be assigned as a principal or first-listed diagnosis.

2) **Bilateral glaucoma with same stage**

When a patient has bilateral glaucoma and both are documented as being the same type and stage, report only the code for the type of glaucoma and one code for the stage.

3) **Bilateral glaucoma stage with different stages**

When a patient has bilateral glaucoma and each eye is documented as having a different stage, assign one code for the type of glaucoma and one code for the highest glaucoma stage.

4) Bilateral glaucoma with different types and different stages

When a patient has bilateral glaucoma and each eye is documented as having a different type and a different stage, assign one code for each type of glaucoma and one code for the highest glaucoma stage.

5) Patient admitted with glaucoma and stage evolves during the admission

If a patient is admitted with glaucoma and the stage progresses during the admission, assign the code for highest stage documented.

6) Indeterminate stage glaucoma

Assignment of code 365.74, Indeterminate stage glaucoma, should be based on the clinical documentation. Code 365.74 is used for glaucoma whose stage cannot be clinically determined. This code should not be confused with code 365.70, Glaucoma stage, unspecified. Code 365.70 should be assigned when there is no documentation regarding the stage of the glaucoma.

7. Chapter 7: Diseases of Circulatory System (390-459)

a. Hypertension

Hypertension Table

The Hypertension Table, found under the main term, "Hypertension", in the Alphabetic Index, contains a complete listing of all conditions due to or associated with hypertension and classifies them according to malignant, benign, and unspecified.

1) Hypertension, Essential, or NOS

Assign hypertension (arterial) (essential) (primary) (systemic) (NOS) to category code 401 with the appropriate fourth digit to indicate malignant (.0), benign (.1), or unspecified (.9). Do not use either .0 malignant or .1 benign unless medical record documentation supports such a designation.

2) Hypertension with Heart Disease

Heart conditions (425.8, 429.0-429.3, 429.8, 429.9) are assigned to a code from category 402 when a causal relationship is stated (due to hypertension) or implied (hypertensive). Use an additional code from category 428 to identify the type of heart failure in those patients with heart failure. More than one code from category 428 may be assigned if the patient has systolic or diastolic failure and congestive heart failure.

The same heart conditions (425.8, 429.0-429.3, 429.8, 429.9) with hypertension, but without a stated causal relationship, are coded separately. Sequence according to the circumstances of the admission/encounter.

3) Hypertensive Chronic Kidney Disease

Assign codes from category 403, Hypertensive chronic kidney disease, when conditions classified to category 585 or code 587 are present with hypertension. Unlike hypertension with heart disease, ICD-9-CM presumes a cause-and-effect relationship and classifies chronic kidney disease (CKD) with hypertension as hypertensive chronic kidney disease.

Fifth digits for category 403 should be assigned as follows:

- 0 with CKD stage I through stage IV, or unspecified.
- 1 with CKD stage V or end stage renal disease.

The appropriate code from category 585, Chronic kidney disease, should be used as a secondary code with a code from category 403 to identify the stage of chronic kidney disease.

See Section I.C.10.a for information on the coding of chronic kidney disease.

4) Hypertensive Heart and Chronic Kidney Disease

Assign codes from combination category 404, Hypertensive heart and chronic kidney disease, when both hypertensive kidney disease and hypertensive heart disease are stated in the diagnosis. Assume a relationship between the hypertension and the chronic kidney disease, whether or not the condition is so designated. Assign an additional code from category 428, to identify the type of heart failure. More than one code from category 428 may be assigned if the patient has systolic or diastolic failure and congestive heart failure.

Fifth digits for category 404 should be assigned as follows:

- 0 without heart failure and with chronic kidney disease (CKD) stage I through stage IV, or unspecified
- 1 with heart failure and with CKD stage I through stage IV, or unspecified
- 2 without heart failure and with CKD stage V or end stage renal disease
- 3 with heart failure and with CKD stage V or end stage renal disease

The appropriate code from category 585, Chronic kidney disease, should be used as a secondary code with a code from category 404 to identify the stage of kidney disease.

See Section I.C.10.a for information on the coding of chronic kidney disease.

5) Hypertensive Cerebrovascular Disease

First assign codes from 430-438, Cerebrovascular disease, then the appropriate hypertension code from categories 401-405.

6) Hypertensive Retinopathy

Two codes are necessary to identify the condition. First assign the code from subcategory 362.11, Hypertensive retinopathy, then the appropriate code from categories 401-405 to indicate the type of hypertension.

7) Hypertension, Secondary

Two codes are required: one to identify the underlying etiology and one from category 405 to identify the hypertension. Sequencing of codes is determined by the reason for admission/encounter.

8) Hypertension, Transient

Assign code 796.2, Elevated blood pressure reading without diagnosis of hypertension, unless patient has an established diagnosis of hypertension. Assign code 642.3x for transient hypertension of pregnancy.

9) Hypertension, Controlled

Assign appropriate code from categories 401-405. This diagnostic statement usually refers to an existing state of hypertension under control by therapy.

10) Hypertension, Uncontrolled

Uncontrolled hypertension may refer to untreated hypertension or hypertension not responding to current therapeutic regimen. In either case, assign the appropriate code from categories 401-405 to designate the stage and type of hypertension. Code to the type of hypertension.

11) Elevated Blood Pressure

For a statement of elevated blood pressure without further specificity, assign code 796.2, Elevated blood pressure reading without diagnosis of hypertension, rather than a code from category 401.

b. Cerebral infarction/stroke/cerebrovascular accident (CVA)

The terms stroke and CVA are often used interchangeably to refer to a cerebral infarction. The terms stroke, CVA, and cerebral infarction NOS are all indexed to the default code 434.91, Cerebral artery occlusion, unspecified, with infarction.

Additional code(s) should be assigned for any neurologic deficits associated with the acute CVA, regardless of whether or not the neurologic deficit resolves prior to discharge.

See Section I.C.18.d.3 for information on coding status post administration of tPA in a different facility within the last 24 hours.

c. Postoperative cerebrovascular accident

A cerebrovascular hemorrhage or infarction that occurs as a result of medical intervention is coded to 997.02, Iatrogenic cerebrovascular infarction or hemorrhage. Medical record documentation should clearly specify the cause- and-effect relationship between the medical intervention and the cerebrovascular accident in order to assign this code. A secondary code from the code range 430-432 or from a code from subcategories 433 or 434 with a fifth digit of "1" should also be used to identify the type of hemorrhage or infarct.

This guideline conforms to the use additional code note instruction at category 997. Code 436, Acute, but ill-defined, cerebrovascular disease, should not be used as a secondary code with code 997.02.

d. Late Effects of Cerebrovascular Disease

1) Category 438, Late Effects of Cerebrovascular disease

Category 438 is used to indicate conditions classifiable to categories 430-437 as the causes of late effects (neurologic deficits), themselves classified elsewhere. These "late effects" include neurologic deficits that persist after initial onset of conditions classifiable to 430-437. The neurologic deficits caused by cerebrovascular disease may be present from the onset or may arise at any time after the onset of the condition classifiable to 430-437.

Codes in category 438 are only for use for late effects of cerebrovascular disease, not for neurologic deficits associated with an acute CVA.

2) Codes from category 438 with codes from 430-437

Codes from category 438 may be assigned on a health care record with codes from 430-437, if the patient has a current cerebrovascular accident (CVA) and deficits from an old CVA.

3) Code V12.54

Assign code V12.54, Transient ischemic attack (TIA), and cerebral infarction without residual deficits (and not a code from category 438) as an additional code for history of cerebrovascular disease when no neurologic deficits are present.

e. Acute myocardial infarction (AMI)

1) ST elevation myocardial infarction (STEMI) and non ST elevation myocardial infarction (NSTEMI)

The ICD-9-CM codes for acute myocardial infarction (AMI) identify the site, such as anterolateral wall or true posterior wall. Subcategories 410.0-410.6 and 410.8 are used for ST elevation myocardial infarction (STEMI). Subcategory 410.7, Subendocardial infarction, is used for non ST elevation myocardial infarction (NSTEMI) and nontransmural MIs.

2) Acute myocardial infarction, unspecified

Subcategory 410.9 is the default for the unspecified term acute myocardial infarction. If only STEMI or transmural MI without the site is documented, query the provider as to the site, or assign a code from subcategory 410.9.

3) AMI documented as nontransmural or subendocardial but site provided

If an AMI is documented as nontransmural or subendocardial, but the site is provided, it is still coded as a subendocardial AMI. If NSTEMI evolves to STEMI, assign the STEMI code. If STEMI converts to NSTEMI due to thrombolytic therapy, it is still coded as STEMI.

See Section I.C.18.d.3 for information on coding status post administration of tPA in a different facility within the last 24 hours.

8. Chapter 8: Diseases of Respiratory System (460-519)

See I.C.17.f. for ventilator-associated pneumonia.

a. Chronic Obstructive Pulmonary Disease [COPD] and Asthma

1) Conditions that comprise COPD and Asthma

The conditions that comprise COPD are obstructive chronic bronchitis, subcategory 491.2, and emphysema, category 492. All asthma codes are under category 493, Asthma. Code 496, Chronic airway obstruction, not elsewhere classified, is a nonspecific code that should only be used when the documentation in a medical record does not specify the type of COPD being treated.

2) Acute exacerbation of chronic obstructive bronchitis and asthma

The codes for chronic obstructive bronchitis and asthma distinguish between uncomplicated cases and those in acute exacerbation. An acute exacerbation is a worsening or a decompensation of a chronic condition. An acute exacerbation is not equivalent to an infection superimposed on a chronic condition, though an exacerbation may be triggered by an infection.

3) Overlapping nature of the conditions that comprise COPD and asthma

Due to the overlapping nature of the conditions that make up COPD and asthma, there are many variations in the way these conditions are documented. Code selection must be based on the terms as documented. When selecting the correct code for the documented type of COPD and asthma, it is essential to first review the index, and then verify the code in the tabular list. There are many instructional notes under the different COPD subcategories and codes. It is important that all such notes be reviewed to assure correct code assignment.

4) Acute exacerbation of asthma and status asthmaticus

An acute exacerbation of asthma is an increased severity of the asthma symptoms, such as wheezing and shortness of breath. Status asthmaticus refers to a patient's failure to respond to therapy administered during an asthmatic episode and is a life threatening complication that requires emergency care. If status asthmaticus is documented by the provider with any type of COPD or with acute bronchitis, the status asthmaticus should be sequenced first. It supersedes any type of COPD including that with acute exacerbation or acute bronchitis. It is inappropriate to assign an asthma code with 5th digit 2, with acute exacerbation, together with an asthma code with 5th digit 1, with status asthmatics. Only the 5th digit 1 should be assigned.

b. Chronic Obstructive Pulmonary Disease [COPD] and Bronchitis

1) Acute bronchitis with COPD

Acute bronchitis, code 466.0, is due to an infectious organism. When acute bronchitis is documented with COPD, code 491.22, Obstructive chronic bronchitis with acute bronchitis, should be assigned. It is not necessary to also assign code 466.0. If a medical record documents acute bronchitis with COPD with acute exacerbation, only code 491.22 should be assigned. The acute bronchitis included in code 491.22 supersedes the acute exacerbation. If a medical record documents COPD with acute exacerbation without mention of acute bronchitis, only code 491.21 should be assigned.

c. Acute Respiratory Failure

1) Acute respiratory failure as principal diagnosis

Code 518.81, Acute respiratory failure, may be assigned as a principal diagnosis when it is the condition established after study to be chiefly responsible for occasioning the admission to the hospital, and the selection is supported by the Alphabetic Index and Tabular List. However, chapter-specific coding guidelines (such as obstetrics, poisoning, HIV, newborn) that provide sequencing direction take precedence.

2) **Acute respiratory failure as secondary diagnosis**

Respiratory failure may be listed as a secondary diagnosis if it occurs after admission, or if it is present on admission, but does not meet the definition of principal diagnosis.

3) **Sequencing of acute respiratory failure and another acute condition**

When a patient is admitted with respiratory failure and another acute condition, (e.g., myocardial infarction, cerebrovascular accident, aspiration pneumonia), the principal diagnosis will not be the same in every situation. This applies whether the other acute condition is a respiratory or nonrespiratory condition. Selection of the principal diagnosis will be dependent on the circumstances of admission. If both the respiratory failure and the other acute condition are equally responsible for occasioning the admission to the hospital, and there are no chapter-specific sequencing rules, the guideline regarding two or more diagnoses that equally meet the definition for principal diagnosis *(Section II, C.)* may be applied in these situations.

If the documentation is not clear as to whether acute respiratory failure and another condition are equally responsible for occasioning the admission, query the provider for clarification.

d. **Influenza due to certain identified viruses**

Code only confirmed cases of avian influenza (codes 488.01-488.02, 488.09, Influenza due to identified avian influenza virus), 2009 H1N1 influenza virus (codes 488.11-488.12, 488.19), or novel influenza A (codes 488.81-488.82, 488.89, Influenza due to identified novel influenza A virus). This is an exception to the hospital inpatient guideline Section II, H. (Uncertain Diagnosis).

In this context, "confirmation" does not require documentation of positive laboratory testing specific for avian, 2009 H1N1 or novel influenza A virus. However, coding should be based on the provider's diagnostic statement that the patient has avian influenza, 2009 H1N1 influenza, or novel influenza A.

If the provider records "suspected" or "possible" or "probable" avian, 2009 H1N1, or novel influenza A, the appropriate influenza code from category 487, Influenza should be assigned. A code from category 488, Influenza due to certain identified influenza viruses, should not be assigned.

9. **Chapter 9: Diseases of Digestive System (520-579)**

Reserved for future guideline expansion

10. **Chapter 10: Diseases of Genitourinary System (580-629)**

a. **Chronic kidney disease**

1) **Stages of chronic kidney disease (CKD)**

The ICD-9-CM classifies CKD based on severity. The severity of CKD is designated by stages I-V. Stage II, code 585.2, equates to mild CKD; stage III, code 585.3, equates to moderate CKD; and stage IV, code 585.4, equates to severe CKD. Code 585.6, End stage renal disease (ESRD), is assigned when the provider has documented end-stage-renal disease (ESRD).

If both a stage of CKD and ESRD are documented, assign code 585.6 only.

2) **Chronic kidney disease and kidney transplant status**

Patients who have undergone kidney transplant may still have some form of CKD, because the kidney transplant may not fully restore kidney function. Therefore, the presence of CKD alone does not constitute a transplant complication. Assign the appropriate 585 code for the patient's stage of CKD and code V42.0. If a transplant complication such as failure or rejection is documented, see section I.C.17.f.2.b for information on coding complications of a kidney transplant. If the documentation is unclear as to whether the patient has a complication of the transplant, query the provider.

3) **Chronic kidney disease with other conditions**

Patients with CKD may also suffer from other serious conditions, most commonly diabetes mellitus and hypertension. The sequencing of the CKD code in relationship to codes for other contributing conditions is based on the conventions in the tabular list.

See I.C.3.a.4 for sequencing instructions for diabetes.

See I.C.4.a.1 for anemia in CKD.

See I.C.7.a.3 for hypertensive chronic kidney disease.

See I.C.17.f.2.b, Kidney transplant complications, for instructions on coding of documented rejection or failure.

11. **Chapter 11: Complications of Pregnancy, Childbirth, and the Puerperium (630-679)**

a. **General Rules for Obstetric Cases**

1) **Codes from chapter 11 and sequencing priority**

Obstetric cases require codes from chapter 11, codes in the range 630-679, Complications of Pregnancy, Childbirth, and the Puerperium. Chapter 11 codes have sequencing priority over codes from other chapters. Additional codes from other chapters may be used in conjunction with chapter 11 codes to further specify conditions. Should the provider document that the pregnancy is incidental to the encounter, then code V22.2 should be used in place of any chapter 11 codes. It is the provider's responsibility to state that the condition being treated is not affecting the pregnancy.

2) **Chapter 11 codes used only on the maternal record**

Chapter 11 codes are to be used only on the maternal record, never on the record of the newborn.

3) **Chapter 11 fifth-digits**

Categories 640-648, 651-676 have required fifth-digits, which indicate whether the encounter is antepartum, postpartum and whether a delivery has also occurred.

4) **Fifth-digits, appropriate for each code**

The fifth-digits, which are appropriate for each code number, are listed in brackets under each code. The fifth-digits on each code should all be consistent with each other. That is, should a delivery occur all of the fifth-digits should indicate the delivery.

b. **Selection of OB Principal or First-listed Diagnosis**

1) **Routine outpatient prenatal visits**

For routine outpatient prenatal visits when no complications are present codes V22.0, Supervision of normal first pregnancy, and V22.1, Supervision of other normal pregnancy, should be used as the first-listed diagnoses. These codes should not be used in conjunction with chapter 11 codes.

2) **Prenatal outpatient visits for high-risk patients**

For routine prenatal outpatient visits for patients with high-risk pregnancies, a code from category V23, Supervision of high-risk pregnancy, should be used as the first-listed diagnosis. Secondary chapter 11 codes may be used in conjunction with these codes if appropriate.

3) **Episodes when no delivery occurs**

In episodes when no delivery occurs, the principal diagnosis should correspond to the principal complication of the pregnancy, which necessitated the encounter. Should more than one complication exist, all of which are treated or monitored, any of the complications codes may be sequenced first.

4) **When a delivery occurs**

When a delivery occurs, the principal diagnosis should correspond to the main circumstances or complication of the delivery. In cases of cesarean delivery, the selection of the principal diagnosis should be the condition established after study that was responsible for the patient's admission. If the patient was admitted with a condition that resulted in the performance of a cesarean procedure, that condition should be selected as the principal diagnosis. If the reason for the admission/encounter was unrelated to the condition resulting in the cesarean delivery, the condition related to the reason for the admission/encounter should be selected as the principal diagnosis, even if a cesarean was performed.

5) Outcome of delivery

An outcome of delivery code, V27.0-V27.9, should be included on every maternal record when a delivery has occurred. These codes are not to be used on subsequent records or on the newborn record.

c. Fetal Conditions Affecting the Management of the Mother

1) Codes from categories 655 and 656

Codes from categories 655, Known or suspected fetal abnormality affecting management of the mother, and 656, Other known or suspected fetal and placental problems affecting the management of the mother, are assigned only when the fetal condition is actually responsible for modifying the management of the mother, i.e., by requiring diagnostic studies, additional observation, special care, or termination of pregnancy. The fact that the fetal condition exists does not justify assigning a code from this series to the mother's record.

See I.C.18.d. for suspected maternal and fetal conditions not found

2) In utero surgery

In cases when surgery is performed on the fetus, a diagnosis code from category 655, Known or suspected fetal abnormalities affecting management of the mother, should be assigned identifying the fetal condition. Procedure code 75.36, Correction of fetal defect, should be assigned on the hospital inpatient record.

No code from Chapter 15, the perinatal codes, should be used on the mother's record to identify fetal conditions. Surgery performed in utero on a fetus is still to be coded as an obstetric encounter.

d. HIV Infection in Pregnancy, Childbirth and the Puerperium

During pregnancy, childbirth or the puerperium, a patient admitted because of an HIV-related illness should receive a principal diagnosis of 647.6x, Other specified infectious and parasitic diseases in the mother classifiable elsewhere, but complicating the pregnancy, childbirth or the puerperium, followed by 042 and the code(s) for the HIV-related illness(es).

Patients with asymptomatic HIV infection status admitted during pregnancy, childbirth, or the puerperium should receive codes of 647.6x and V08.

e. Current Conditions Complicating Pregnancy

Assign a code from subcategory 648.x for patients that have current conditions when the condition affects the management of the pregnancy, childbirth, or the puerperium. Use additional secondary codes from other chapters to identify the conditions, as appropriate.

f. Diabetes mellitus in pregnancy

Diabetes mellitus is a significant complicating factor in pregnancy. Pregnant women who are diabetic should be assigned code 648.0x, Diabetes mellitus complicating pregnancy, and a secondary code from category 250, Diabetes mellitus, or category 249, Secondary diabetes to identify the type of diabetes.

Code V58.67, Long-term (current) use of insulin, should also be assigned if the diabetes mellitus is being treated with insulin.

g. Gestational diabetes

Gestational diabetes can occur during the second and third trimester of pregnancy in women who were not diabetic prior to pregnancy. Gestational diabetes can cause complications in the pregnancy similar to those of pre-existing diabetes mellitus. It also puts the woman at greater risk of developing diabetes after the pregnancy. Gestational diabetes is coded to 648.8x, Abnormal glucose tolerance. Codes 648.0x and 648.8x should never be used together on the same record.

Code V58.67, Long-term (current) use of insulin, should also be assigned if the gestational diabetes is being treated with insulin.

h. Normal Delivery, Code 650

1) Normal delivery

Code 650 is for use in cases when a woman is admitted for a full-term normal delivery and delivers a single, healthy infant without any complications antepartum, during the delivery, or postpartum during the delivery episode. Code 650 is always a principal diagnosis. It is not to be used if any other code from chapter 11 is needed to describe a current complication of the antenatal, delivery, or perinatal period. Additional codes from other chapters may be used with code 650 if they are not related to or are in any way complicating the pregnancy.

2) Normal delivery with resolved antepartum complication

Code 650 may be used if the patient had a complication at some point during her pregnancy, but the complication is not present at the time of the admission for delivery.

3) V27.0, Single liveborn, outcome of delivery

V27.0, Single liveborn, is the only outcome of delivery code appropriate for use with 650.

i. The Postpartum and Peripartum Periods

1) Postpartum and peripartum periods

The postpartum period begins immediately after delivery and continues for six weeks following delivery. The peripartum period is defined as the last month of pregnancy to five months postpartum.

2) Postpartum complication

A postpartum complication is any complication occurring within the six-week period.

3) Pregnancy-related complications after 6 week period

Chapter 11 codes may also be used to describe pregnancy-related complications after the six-week period should the provider document that a condition is pregnancy related.

4) Postpartum complications occurring during the same admission as delivery

Postpartum complications that occur during the same admission as the delivery are identified with a fifth digit of "2." Subsequent admissions/encounters for postpartum complications should be identified with a fifth digit of "4."

5) Admission for routine postpartum care following delivery outside hospital

When the mother delivers outside the hospital prior to admission and is admitted for routine postpartum care and no complications are noted, code V24.0, Postpartum care and examination immediately after delivery, should be assigned as the principal diagnosis.

6) Admission following delivery outside hospital with postpartum conditions

A delivery diagnosis code should not be used for a woman who has delivered prior to admission to the hospital. Any postpartum conditions and/or postpartum procedures should be coded.

7) Puerperal sepsis

Code 670.2x, Puerperal sepsis, should be assigned with a secondary code to identify the causal organism (e.g., for a bacterial infection, assign a code from category 041, Bacterial infections in conditions classified elsewhere and of unspecified site). A code from category 038, Septicemia, should not be used for puerperal sepsis. Do not assign code 995.91, Sepsis, as code 670.2x describes the sepsis. If applicable, use additional codes to identify severe sepsis (995.92) and any associated acute organ dysfunction.

j. Code 677, Late effect of complication of pregnancy

1) Code 677

Code 677, Late effect of complication of pregnancy, childbirth, and the puerperium is for use in those cases when an initial complication of a pregnancy develops a sequelae requiring care or treatment at a future date.

2) After the initial postpartum period

This code may be used at any time after the initial postpartum period.

3) Sequencing of Code 677

This code, like all late effect codes, is to be sequenced following the code describing the sequelae of the complication.

k. Abortions

1) Fifth-digits required for abortion categories

Fifth-digits are required for abortion categories 634-637. Fifth digit assignment is based on the status of the patient at the beginning (or start) of the encounter. Fifth-digit 1, incomplete, indicates that all of the products of conception have not been expelled from the uterus. Fifth-digit 2, complete, indicates that all products of conception have been expelled from the uterus.

2) Code from categories 640-648 and 651-659

A code from categories 640-648 and 651-659 may be used as additional codes with an abortion code to indicate the complication leading to the abortion.

Fifth digit 3 is assigned with codes from these categories when used with an abortion code because the other fifth digits will not apply. Codes from the 660-669 series are not to be used for complications of abortion.

3) Code 639 for complications

Code 639 is to be used for all complications following abortion. Code 639 cannot be assigned with codes from categories 634-638.

4) Abortion with Liveborn Fetus

When an attempted termination of pregnancy results in a liveborn fetus assign code 644.21, Early onset of delivery, with an appropriate code from category V27, Outcome of Delivery. The procedure code for the attempted termination of pregnancy should also be assigned.

5) Retained Products of Conception following an abortion

Subsequent admissions for retained products of conception following a spontaneous or legally induced abortion are assigned the appropriate code from category 634, Spontaneous abortion, or 635 Legally induced abortion, with a fifth digit of "1" (incomplete). This advice is appropriate even when the patient was discharged previously with a discharge diagnosis of complete abortion.

12. Chapter 12: Diseases Skin and Subcutaneous Tissue (680-709)

a. Pressure ulcer stage codes

1) Pressure ulcer stages

Two codes are needed to completely describe a pressure ulcer: A code from subcategory 707.0, Pressure ulcer, to identify the site of the pressure ulcer and a code from subcategory 707.2, Pressure ulcer stages.

The codes in subcategory 707.2, Pressure ulcer stages, are to be used as an additional diagnosis with a code(s) from subcategory 707.0, Pressure Ulcer. Codes from 707.2, Pressure ulcer stages, may not be assigned as a principal or first-listed diagnosis. The pressure ulcer stage codes should

only be used with pressure ulcers and not with other types of ulcers (e.g., stasis ulcer).

The ICD-9-CM classifies pressure ulcer stages based on severity, which is designated by stages I-IV and unstageable.

2) Unstageable pressure ulcers

Assignment of code 707.25, Pressure ulcer, unstageable, should be based on the clinical documentation. Code 707.25 is used for pressure ulcers whose stage cannot be clinically determined (e.g., the ulcer is covered by eschar or has been treated with a skin or muscle graft) and pressure ulcers that are documented as deep tissue injury but not documented as due to trauma. This code should not be confused with code 707.20, Pressure ulcer, stage unspecified. Code 707.20 should be assigned when there is no documentation regarding the stage of the pressure ulcer.

3) Documented pressure ulcer stage

Assignment of the pressure ulcer stage code should be guided by clinical documentation of the stage or documentation of the terms found in the index. For clinical terms describing the stage that are not found in the index, and there is no documentation of the stage, the provider should be queried.

4) Bilateral pressure ulcers with same stage

When a patient has bilateral pressure ulcers (e.g., both buttocks) and both pressure ulcers are documented as being the same stage, only the code for the site and one code for the stage should be reported.

5) Bilateral pressure ulcers with different stages

When a patient has bilateral pressure ulcers at the same site (e.g., both buttocks) and each pressure ulcer is documented as being at a different stage, assign one code for the site and the appropriate codes for the pressure ulcer stage.

6) Multiple pressure ulcers of different sites and stages

When a patient has multiple pressure ulcers at different sites (e.g., buttock, heel, shoulder) and each pressure ulcer is documented as being at different stages (e.g., stage 3 and stage 4), assign the appropriate codes for each different site and a code for each different pressure ulcer stage.

7) Patients admitted with pressure ulcers documented as healed

No code is assigned if the documentation states that the pressure ulcer is completely healed.

8) Patients admitted with pressure ulcers documented as healing

Pressure ulcers described as healing should be assigned the appropriate pressure ulcer stage code based on the documentation in the medical record. If the documentation does not provide information about the stage of the healing pressure ulcer, assign code 707.20, Pressure ulcer stage, unspecified.

If the documentation is unclear as to whether the patient has a current (new) pressure ulcer or if the patient is being treated for a healing pressure ulcer, query the provider.

9) Patient admitted with pressure ulcer evolving into another stage during the admission

If a patient is admitted with a pressure ulcer at one stage and it progresses to a higher stage, assign the code for highest stage reported for that site.

13. Chapter 13: Diseases of Musculoskeletal and Connective Tissue (710-739)

a. Coding of Pathologic Fractures

1) Acute Fractures vs. Aftercare

Pathologic fractures are reported using subcategory 733.1, when the fracture is newly diagnosed. Subcategory 733.1 may be used while the patient is receiving active treatment for the fracture. Examples of active treatment are: surgical treatment, emergency department encounter, evaluation and treatment by a new physician.

Fractures are coded using the aftercare codes (subcategories V54.0, V54.2, V54.8 or V54.9) for encounters after the patient has completed active treatment of the fracture and is receiving routine care for the fracture during the healing or recovery phase. Examples of fracture aftercare are: cast change or removal, removal of external or internal fixation device, medication adjustment, and follow up visits following fracture treatment.

Care for complications of surgical treatment for fracture repairs during the healing or recovery phase should be coded with the appropriate complication codes.

Care of complications of fractures, such as malunion and nonunion, should be reported with the appropriate codes.

See Section I. C. 17.b for information on the coding of traumatic fractures.

14. Chapter 14: Congenital Anomalies (740-759)

a. Codes in categories 740-759, Congenital Anomalies

Assign an appropriate code(s) from categories 740-759, Congenital Anomalies, when an anomaly is documented. A congenital anomaly may be the principal/first listed diagnosis on a record or a secondary diagnosis.

When a congenital anomaly does not have a unique code assignment, assign additional code(s) for any manifestations that may be present.

When the code assignment specifically identifies the congenital anomaly, manifestations that are an inherent component of the anomaly should not be coded separately. Additional codes should be assigned for manifestations that are not an inherent component.

Codes from Chapter 14 may be used throughout the life of the patient. If a congenital anomaly has been corrected, a personal history code should be used to identify the history of the anomaly. Although present at birth, a congenital anomaly may not be identified until later in life. Whenever the condition is diagnosed by the physician, it is appropriate to assign a code from codes 740-759.

For the birth admission, the appropriate code from category V30, Liveborn infants, according to type of birth should be sequenced as the principal diagnosis, followed by any congenital anomaly codes, 740-759.

15. Chapter 15: Newborn (Perinatal) Guidelines (760-779)

For coding and reporting purposes the perinatal period is defined as before birth through the 28th day following birth. The following guidelines are provided for reporting purposes. Hospitals may record other diagnoses as needed for internal data use.

a. General Perinatal Rules

1) Chapter 15 Codes

They are <u>never</u> for use on the maternal record. Codes from Chapter 11, the obstetric chapter, are never permitted on the newborn record. Chapter 15 code may be used throughout the life of the patient if the condition is still present.

2) Sequencing of perinatal codes

Generally, codes from Chapter 15 should be sequenced as the principal/first-listed diagnosis on the newborn record, with the exception of the appropriate V30 code for the birth episode, followed by codes from any other chapter that provide additional detail. The "use additional code" note at the beginning of the chapter supports this guideline. If the index does not provide a specific code for a perinatal condition, assign code 779.89, Other specified conditions originating in the perinatal period, followed by the code from another chapter that specifies the condition. Codes for signs and symptoms may be assigned when a definitive diagnosis has not been established.

3) Birth process or community acquired conditions

If a newborn has a condition that may be either due to the birth process or community acquired and the documentation does not indicate which it is, the default is due to the birth process and the code from Chapter 15 should be used. If the condition is community-acquired, a code from Chapter 15 should not be assigned.

4) Code all clinically significant conditions

All clinically significant conditions noted on routine newborn examination should be coded. A condition is clinically significant if it requires:

- clinical evaluation; or
- therapeutic treatment; or
- diagnostic procedures; or
- extended length of hospital stay; or
- increased nursing care and/or monitoring; or
- has implications for future health care needs

Note: The perinatal guidelines listed above are the same as the general coding guidelines for "additional diagnoses", except for the final point regarding implications for future health care needs. Codes should be assigned for conditions that have been specified by the provider as having implications for future health care needs. Codes from the perinatal chapter should not be assigned unless the provider has established a definitive diagnosis.

b. Use of codes V30-V39

When coding the birth of an infant, assign a code from categories V30-V39, according to the type of birth. A code from this series is assigned as a principal diagnosis, and assigned only once to a newborn at the time of birth.

c. Newborn transfers

If the newborn is transferred to another institution, the V30 series is not used at the receiving hospital.

d. Use of category V29

1) Assigning a code from category V29

Assign a code from category V29, Observation and evaluation of newborns and infants for suspected conditions not found, to identify those instances when a healthy newborn is evaluated for a suspected condition that is determined after study not to be present. Do not use a code from category V29 when the patient has identified signs or symptoms of a suspected problem; in such cases, code the sign or symptom.

A code from category V29 may also be assigned as a principal code for readmissions or encounters when the V30 code no longer applies. Codes from category V29 are for use only for healthy newborns and infants for which no condition after study is found to be present.

2) V29 code on a birth record

A V29 code is to be used as a secondary code after the V30, Outcome of delivery, code.

e. Use of other V codes on perinatal records

V codes other than V30 and V29 may be assigned on a perinatal or newborn record code. The codes may be used as a principal or first-listed diagnosis for specific types of encounters or for readmissions or encounters when the V30 code no longer applies.

See Section I.C.18 for information regarding the assignment of V codes.

f. Maternal Causes of Perinatal Morbidity

Codes from categories 760-763, Maternal causes of perinatal morbidity and mortality, are assigned only when the maternal condition has actually affected the fetus or newborn. The fact that the mother has an associated medical condition or experiences some complication of pregnancy, labor or delivery does not justify the routine assignment of codes from these categories to the newborn record.

g. Congenital Anomalies in Newborns

For the birth admission, the appropriate code from category V30, Liveborn infants according to type of birth, should be used, followed by any congenital anomaly codes, categories 740-759. Use additional secondary codes from other chapters to specify conditions associated with the anomaly, if applicable.

Also, see Section I.C.14 for information on the coding of congenital anomalies.

h. Coding Additional Perinatal Diagnoses

1) Assigning codes for conditions that require treatment

Assign codes for conditions that require treatment or further investigation, prolong the length of stay, or require resource utilization.

2) Codes for conditions specified as having implications for future health care needs

Assign codes for conditions that have been specified by the provider as having implications for future health care needs.

Note: This guideline should not be used for adult patients.

3) Codes for newborn conditions originating in the perinatal period

Assign a code for newborn conditions originating in the perinatal period (categories 760-779), as well as complications arising during the current episode of care classified in other chapters, only if the diagnoses have been documented by the responsible provider at the time of transfer or discharge as having affected the fetus or newborn.

i. Prematurity and Fetal Growth Retardation

Providers utilize different criteria in determining prematurity. A code for prematurity should not be assigned unless it is documented. The 5th digit assignment for codes from category 764 and subcategories 765.0 and 765.1 should be based on the recorded birth weight and estimated gestational age.

A code from subcategory 765.2, Weeks of gestation, should be assigned as an additional code with category 764 and codes from 765.0 and 765.1 to specify weeks of gestation as documented by the provider in the record.

j. Newborn sepsis

Code 771.81, Septicemia [sepsis] of newborn, should be assigned with a secondary code from category 041, Bacterial infections in conditions classified elsewhere and of unspecified site, to identify the organism. A code from category 038, Septicemia, should not be used on a newborn record. Do not assign code 995.91, Sepsis, as code 771.81 describes the sepsis. If applicable, use additional codes to identify severe sepsis (995.92) and any associated acute organ dysfunction.

16. Chapter 16: Signs, Symptoms and Ill-Defined Conditions (780-799)

Reserved for future guideline expansion

17. Chapter 17: Injury and Poisoning (800-999)

a. Coding of Injuries

When coding injuries, assign separate codes for each injury unless a combination code is provided, in which case the combination code is assigned. Multiple injury codes are provided in ICD-9-CM, but should not be assigned unless information for a more specific code is not available. These traumatic injury codes are not to be used for normal, healing surgical wounds or to identify complications of surgical wounds.

The code for the most serious injury, as determined by the provider and the focus of treatment, is sequenced first.

1) Superficial injuries

Superficial injuries such as abrasions or contusions are not coded when associated with more severe injuries of the same site.

2) Primary injury with damage to nerves/blood vessels

When a primary injury results in minor damage to peripheral nerves or blood vessels, the primary injury is sequenced first with additional code(s) from categories 950-957, Injury to nerves and spinal cord, and/or 900-904, Injury to blood vessels. When the primary injury is to the blood vessels or nerves, that injury should be sequenced first.

b. Coding of Traumatic Fractures

The principles of multiple coding of injuries should be followed in coding fractures. Fractures of specified sites are coded individually by site in accordance with both the provisions within categories 800-829 and the level of detail furnished by medical record content. Combination categories for multiple fractures are provided for use when there is insufficient detail in the medical record (such as trauma cases transferred to another hospital), when the reporting form limits the number of codes that can be used in reporting pertinent clinical data, or when there is insufficient specificity at the fourth-digit or fifth-digit level. More specific guidelines are as follows:

1) Acute Fractures vs. Aftercare

Traumatic fractures are coded using the acute fracture codes (800-829) while the patient is receiving active treatment for the fracture. Examples of active treatment are: surgical treatment, emergency department encounter, and evaluation and treatment by a new physician.

Fractures are coded using the aftercare codes (subcategories V54.0, V54.1, V54.8, or V54.9) for encounters after the patient has completed active treatment of the fracture and is receiving routine care for the fracture during the healing or recovery phase. Examples of fracture aftercare are: cast change or removal, removal of external or internal fixation device, medication adjustment, and follow up visits following fracture treatment.

Care for complications of surgical treatment for fracture repairs during the healing or recovery phase should be coded with the appropriate complication codes.

Care of complications of fractures, such as malunion and nonunion, should be reported with the appropriate codes.

Pathologic fractures are not coded in the 800-829 range, but instead are assigned to subcategory 733.1. *See Section I.C.13.a for additional information.*

2) Multiple fractures of same limb

Multiple fractures of same limb classifiable to the same three-digit or four-digit category are coded to that category.

3) Multiple unilateral or bilateral fractures of same bone

Multiple unilateral or bilateral fractures of same bone(s) but classified to different fourth-digit subdivisions (bone part) within the same three-digit category are coded individually by site.

4) Multiple fracture categories 819 and 828

Multiple fracture categories 819 and 828 classify bilateral fractures of both upper limbs (819) and both lower limbs (828), but without any detail at the fourth-digit level other than open and closed type of fractures.

5) Multiple fractures sequencing

Multiple fractures are sequenced in accordance with the severity of the fracture. The provider should be asked to list the fracture diagnoses in the order of severity.

c. Coding of Burns

Current burns (940-948) are classified by depth, extent and by agent (E code). Burns are classified by depth as first degree (erythema), second degree (blistering), and third degree (full-thickness involvement).

1) Sequencing of burn and related condition codes

Sequence first the code that reflects the highest degree of burn when more than one burn is present.

a. When the reason for the admission or encounter is for treatment of external multiple burns, sequence first the code that reflects the burn of the highest degree.

b. When a patient has both internal and external burns, the circumstances of admission govern the selection of the principal diagnosis or first-listed diagnosis.

c. When a patient is admitted for burn injuries and other related conditions such as smoke inhalation and/or respiratory failure, the circumstances of admission govern the selection of the principal or first-listed diagnosis.

2) Burns of the same local site

Classify burns of the same local site (three-digit category level, 940-947) but of different degrees to the subcategory identifying the highest degree recorded in the diagnosis.

3) Non-healing burns

Non-healing burns are coded as acute burns.

Necrosis of burned skin should be coded as a non-healed burn.

4) Code 958.3, Posttraumatic wound infection

Assign code 958.3, Posttraumatic wound infection, not elsewhere classified, as an additional code for any documented infected burn site.

5) Assign separate codes for each burn site

When coding burns, assign separate codes for each burn site. Category 946 Burns of Multiple specified sites, should only be used if the location of the burns are not documented.

Category 949, Burn, unspecified, is extremely vague and should rarely be used.

6) Assign codes from category 948, Burns

Burns classified according to extent of body surface involved, when the site of the burn is not specified or when there is a need for additional data. It is advisable to use category 948 as additional coding when needed to provide data for evaluating burn mortality, such as that needed by burn units. It is also advisable to use category 948 as an additional code for reporting purposes when there is mention of a third-degree burn involving 20 percent or more of the body surface.

In assigning a code from category 948:

Fourth-digit codes are used to identify the percentage of total body surface involved in a burn (all degree).

Fifth-digits are assigned to identify the percentage of body surface involved in third-degree burn.

Fifth-digit zero (0) is assigned when less than 10 percent or when no body surface is involved in a third-degree burn.

Category 948 is based on the classic "rule of nines" in estimating body surface involved: head and neck are assigned nine percent, each arm nine percent, each leg 18 percent, the anterior trunk 18 percent, posterior trunk 18 percent, and genitalia one percent. Providers may change these percentage assignments where necessary to accommodate infants and children who have proportionately larger heads than adults and patients who have large buttocks, thighs, or abdomen that involve burns.

7) Encounters for treatment of late effects of burns

Encounters for the treatment of the late effects of burns (i.e., scars or joint contractures) should be coded to the residual

condition (sequelae) followed by the appropriate late effect code (906.5-906.9). A late effect E code may also be used, if desired.

8) Sequelae with a late effect code and current burn

When appropriate, both a sequelae with a late effect code, and a current burn code may be assigned on the same record (when both a current burn and sequelae of an old burn exist).

d. Coding of Debridement of Wound, Infection, or Burn

Excisional debridement involves surgical removal or cutting away, as opposed to a mechanical (brushing, scrubbing, washing) debridement.

For coding purposes, excisional debridement is assigned to code 86.22.

Nonexcisional debridement is assigned to code 86.28.

e. Adverse Effects, Poisoning and Toxic Effects

The properties of certain drugs, medicinal and biological substances or combinations of such substances, may cause toxic reactions. The occurrence of drug toxicity is classified in ICD-9-CM as follows:

1) Adverse Effect

When the drug was correctly prescribed and properly administered, code the reaction plus the appropriate code from the E930-E949 series. Codes from the E930-E949 series must be used to identify the causative substance for an adverse effect of drug, medicinal and biological substances, correctly prescribed and properly administered. The effect, such as tachycardia, delirium, gastrointestinal hemorrhaging, vomiting, hypokalemia, hepatitis, renal failure, or respiratory failure, is coded and followed by the appropriate code from the E930-E949 series.

Adverse effects of therapeutic substances correctly prescribed and properly administered (toxicity, synergistic reaction, side effect, and idiosyncratic reaction) may be due to (1) differences among patients, such as age, sex, disease, and genetic factors, and (2) drug-related factors, such as type of drug, route of administration, duration of therapy, dosage, and bioavailability.

2) Poisoning

(a) Error was made in drug prescription

Errors made in drug prescription or in the administration of the drug by provider, nurse, patient, or other person, use the appropriate poisoning code from the 960-979 series.

(b) Overdose of a drug intentionally taken

If an overdose of a drug was intentionally taken or administered and resulted in drug toxicity, it would be coded as a poisoning (960-979 series).

(c) Nonprescribed drug taken with correctly prescribed and properly administered drug

If a nonprescribed drug or medicinal agent was taken in combination with a correctly prescribed and properly administered drug, any drug toxicity or other reaction resulting from the interaction of the two drugs would be classified as a poisoning.

(d) Interaction of drug(s) and alcohol

When a reaction results from the interaction of a drug(s) and alcohol, this would be classified as poisoning.

(e) Sequencing of poisoning

When coding a poisoning or reaction to the improper use of a medication (e.g., wrong dose, wrong substance, wrong route of administration) the poisoning code is sequenced first, followed by a code for the manifestation. If there is also a diagnosis of drug abuse or dependence to the substance, the abuse or dependence is coded as an additional code.

See Section I.C.3.a.6.b. if poisoning is the result of insulin pump malfunctions and Section I.C.19 for general use of E-codes.

3) Toxic Effects

(a) Toxic effect codes

When a harmful substance is ingested or comes in contact with a person, this is classified as a toxic effect. The toxic effect codes are in categories 980-989.

(b) Sequencing toxic effect codes

A toxic effect code should be sequenced first, followed by the code(s) that identify the result of the toxic effect.

(c) External cause codes for toxic effects

An external cause code from categories E860-E869 for accidental exposure, codes E950.6 or E950.7 for intentional self-harm, category E962 for assault, or categories E980-E982, for undetermined, should also be assigned to indicate intent.

f. Complications of care

1) Complications of care

(a) Documentation of complications of care

See Section I.B.18. for information on documentation of complications of care.

(b) Use additional code to identify nature of complication

An additional code identifying the complication should be assigned with codes in categories 996-999, Complications of Surgical and Medical Care NEC, when the additional code provides greater specificity as to the nature of the condition. If the complication code fully describes the condition, no additional code is necessary.

2) Transplant complications

(a) Transplant complications other than kidney

Codes under subcategory 996.8, Complications of transplanted organ, are for use for both complications and rejection of transplanted organs. A transplant complication code is only assigned if the complication affects the function of the transplanted organ. Two codes are required to fully describe a transplant complication, the appropriate code from subcategory 996.8 and a secondary code that identifies the complication.

Pre-existing conditions or conditions that develop after the transplant are not coded as complications unless they affect the function of the transplanted organs.

See I.C.18.d.3 for transplant organ removal status

See I.C.2.i for malignant neoplasm associated with transplanted organ.

(b) Chronic kidney disease and kidney transplant complications

Patients who have undergone kidney transplant may still have some form of chronic kidney disease (CKD) because the kidney transplant may not fully restore kidney function. Code 996.81 should be assigned for documented complications of a kidney transplant, such as transplant failure or rejection or other transplant complication. Code 996.81 should not be assigned for post kidney transplant patients who have chronic kidney (CKD) unless a transplant complication such as transplant failure or rejection is documented. If the documentation is unclear as to whether the patient has a complication of the transplant, query the provider.

Conditions that affect the function of the transplanted kidney, other than CKD, should be assigned code

996.81, Complications of transplanted organ, Kidney, and a secondary code that identifies the complication.

For patients with CKD following a kidney transplant, but who do not have a complication such as failure or rejection, *see section I.C.10.a.2, Chronic kidney disease and kidney transplant status.*

3) Ventilator associated pneumonia

(a) Documentation of Ventilator associated Pneumonia

As with all procedural or postprocedural complications, code assignment is based on the provider's documentation of the relationship between the condition and the procedure.

Code 997.31, Ventilator associated pneumonia, should be assigned only when the provider has documented ventilator associated pneumonia (VAP). An additional code to identify the organism (e.g., Pseudomonas aeruginosa, code 041.7) should also be assigned. Do not assign an additional code from categories 480-484 to identify the type of pneumonia.

Code 997.31 should not be assigned for cases where the patient has pneumonia and is on a mechanical ventilator but the provider has not specifically stated that the pneumonia is ventilator-associated pneumonia.

If the documentation is unclear as to whether the patient has a pneumonia that is a complication attributable to the mechanical ventilator, query the provider.

(b) Patient admitted with pneumonia and develops VAP

A patient may be admitted with one type of pneumonia (e.g., code 481, Pneumococcal pneumonia) and subsequently develop VAP. In this instance, the principal diagnosis would be the appropriate code from categories 480-484 for the pneumonia diagnosed at the time of admission. Code 997.31, Ventilator associated pneumonia, would be assigned as an additional diagnosis when the provider has also documented the presence of ventilator associated pneumonia.

g. SIRS due to Non-infectious Process

The systemic inflammatory response syndrome (SIRS) can develop as a result of certain non-infectious disease processes, such as trauma, malignant neoplasm, or pancreatitis. When SIRS is documented with a noninfectious condition, and no subsequent infection is documented, the code for the underlying condition, such as an injury, should be assigned, followed by code 995.93, Systemic inflammatory response syndrome due to noninfectious process without acute organ dysfunction, or 995.94, Systemic inflammatory response syndrome due to non-infectious process with acute organ dysfunction. If an acute organ dysfunction is documented, the appropriate code(s) for the associated acute organ dysfunction(s) should be assigned in addition to code 995.94. If acute organ dysfunction is documented, but it cannot be determined if the acute organ dysfunction is associated with SIRS or due to another condition (e.g., directly due to the trauma), the provider should be queried.

When the non-infectious condition has led to an infection that results in SIRS, *see Section I.C.1.b.12 for the guideline for sepsis and severe sepsis associated with a non-infectious process.*

18. Classification of Factors Influencing Health Status and Contact with Health Service (Supplemental V01-V91)

Note: The chapter specific guidelines provide additional information about the use of V codes for specified encounters.

a. Introduction

ICD-9-CM provides codes to deal with encounters for circumstances other than a disease or injury. The Supplementary Classification of Factors Influencing Health Status and Contact with Health Services (V01.0 - V91.99) is provided to deal with occasions when circumstances other than a disease or injury (codes 001-999) are recorded as a diagnosis or problem.

There are four primary circumstances for the use of V codes:

1) A person who is not currently sick encounters the health services for some specific reason, such as to act as an organ donor, to receive prophylactic care, such as inoculations or health screenings, or to receive counseling on health related issues.

2) A person with a resolving disease or injury, or a chronic, long-term condition requiring continuous care, encounters the health care system for specific aftercare of that disease or injury (e.g., dialysis for renal disease; chemotherapy for malignancy; cast change). A diagnosis/symptom code should be used whenever a current, acute, diagnosis is being treated or a sign or symptom is being studied.

3) Circumstances or problems influence a person's health status but are not in themselves a current illness or injury.

4) Newborns, to indicate birth status

b.   V codes use in any healthcare setting

V codes are for use in any healthcare setting. V codes may be used as either a first listed (principal diagnosis code in the inpatient setting) or secondary code, depending on the circumstances of the encounter. Certain V codes may only be used as first listed, others only as secondary codes.

See Section I.C.18.e, V Codes That May Only Be Principal/First-Listed Diagnosis.

c.   V Codes indicate a reason for an encounter

They are not procedure codes. A corresponding procedure code must accompany a V code to describe the procedure performed.

d.   Categories of V Codes

1)   Contact/Exposure

Category V01 indicates contact with or exposure to communicable diseases. These codes are for patients who do not show any sign or symptom of a disease but have been exposed to it by close personal contact with an infected individual or are in an area where a disease is epidemic. These codes may be used as a first listed code to explain an encounter for testing, or, more commonly, as a secondary code to identify a potential risk.

Codes V15.84 – V15.86 describe contact with or (suspected) exposure to asbestos, potentially hazardous body fluids, and lead.

Subcategories V87.0 – V87.3 describe contact with or (suspected) exposure to hazardous metals, aromatic compounds, other potentially hazardous chemicals, and other potentially hazardous substances.

2)   Inoculations and vaccinations

Categories V03-V06 are for encounters for inoculations and vaccinations. They indicate that a patient is being seen to receive a prophylactic inoculation against a disease. The injection itself must be represented by the appropriate procedure code. A code from V03-V06 may be used as a secondary code if the inoculation is given as a routine part of preventive health care, such as a well-baby visit.

3)   Status

Status codes indicate that a patient is a carrier of a disease, has the sequelae or residual of a past disease or condition, or has another factor influencing a person's health status. This includes such things as the presence of prosthetic or mechanical devices resulting from past treatment. A status code is informative, because the status may affect the course of treatment and its outcome. A status code is distinct from a history code. The history code indicates that the patient no longer has the condition.

A status code should not be used with a diagnosis code from one of the body system chapters, if the diagnosis code

includes the information provided by the status code. For example, code V42.1, Heart transplant status, should not be used with code 996.83, Complications of transplanted heart. The status code does not provide additional information. The complication code indicates that the patient is a heart transplant patient.

The status V codes/categories are:

V02   Carrier or suspected carrier of infectious diseases

Carrier status indicates that a person harbors the specific organisms of a disease without manifest symptoms and is capable of transmitting the infection.

V07.5x   Use of agents affecting estrogen receptors and estrogen level

This code indicates when a patient is receiving a drug that affects estrogen receptors and estrogen levels for prevention of cancer.

V08   Asymptomatic HIV infection status

This code indicates that a patient has tested positive for HIV but has manifested no signs or symptoms of the disease.

V09   Infection with drug-resistant microorganisms

This category indicates that a patient has an infection that is resistant to drug treatment. Sequence the infection code first.

V21   Constitutional states in development

V22.2   Pregnant state, incidental

This code is a secondary code only for use when the pregnancy is in no way complicating the reason for visit. Otherwise, a code from the obstetric chapter is required.

V26.5x   Sterilization status

V42   Organ or tissue replaced by transplant

V43   Organ or tissue replaced by other means

V44   Artificial opening status

V45   Other postsurgical states

Assign code V45.87, Transplant organ removal status, to indicate that a transplanted organ has been previously removed. This code should not be assigned for the encounter in which the transplanted organ is removed. The complication necessitating removal of the transplant organ should be assigned for that encounter.

See section I.C17.f.2. for information on the coding of organ transplant complications.

Assign code V45.88, Status post administration of tPA (rtPA) in a different facility within the last 24 hours prior to admission to the current facility, as a secondary diagnosis when a patient is received by transfer into a facility and documentation indicates they were administered tissue plasminogen activator (tPA) within the last 24 hours prior to admission to the current facility.

This guideline applies even if the patient is still receiving the tPA at the time they are received into the current facility.

The appropriate code for the condition for which the tPA was administered (such as cerebrovascular disease or myocardial infarction) should be assigned first.

Code V45.88 is only applicable to the receiving facility record and not to the transferring facility record.

V46   Other dependence on machines

V49.6   Upper limb amputation status

V49.7   Lower limb amputation status

Note: Categories V42-V46, and subcategories V49.6, V49.7 are for use only if there are no complications or malfunctions of the organ or tissue replaced, the amputation site or the equipment on which the patient is dependent.

V49.81 Asymptomatic postmenopausal status (age-related) (natural)

V49.82 Dental sealant status

V49.83 Awaiting organ transplant status

V49.86 Do not resuscitate status

This code may be used when it is documented by the provider that a patient is on do not resuscitate status at any time during the stay.

V49.87 Physical restraint status

This code may be used when it is documented by the provider that a patient has been put in restraints during the current encounter. Please note that this code should not be reported when it is documented by the provider that a patient is temporarily restrained during a procedure.

V58.6x Long-term (current) drug use

Codes from this subcategory indicate a patient's continuous use of a prescribed drug (including such things as aspirin therapy) for the long-term treatment of a condition or for prophylactic use. It is not for use for patients who have addictions to drugs. This subcategory is not for use of medications for detoxification or maintenance programs to prevent withdrawal symptoms in patients with drug dependence (e.g., methadone maintenance for opiate dependence). Assign the appropriate code for the drug dependence instead.

Assign a code from subcategory V58.6, Long-term (current) drug use, if the patient is receiving a medication for an extended period as a prophylactic measure (such as for the prevention of deep vein thrombosis) or as treatment of a chronic condition (such as arthritis) or a disease requiring a lengthy course of treatment (such as cancer). Do not assign a code from subcategory V58.6 for medication being administered for a brief period of time to treat an acute illness or injury (such as a course of antibiotics to treat acute bronchitis).

V83 Genetic carrier status

Genetic carrier status indicates that a person carries a gene, associated with a particular disease, which may be passed to offspring who may develop that disease. The person does not have the disease and is not at risk of developing the disease.

V84 Genetic susceptibility status

Genetic susceptibility indicates that a person has a gene that increases the risk of that person developing the disease.

Codes from category V84, Genetic susceptibility to disease, should not be used as principal or first-listed codes. If the patient has the condition to which he/she is susceptible, and that condition is the reason for the encounter, the code for the current condition should be sequenced first. If the patient is being seen for follow-up after completed treatment for this condition, and the condition no longer exists, a follow-up code should be sequenced first, followed by the appropriate personal history and genetic susceptibility codes. If the purpose of the encounter is genetic counseling associated with procreative management, a code from subcategory V26.3, Genetic counseling and testing, should be assigned as the first-listed code,

followed by a code from category V84. Additional codes should be assigned for any applicable family or personal history.

See Section I.C. 18.d.14 for information on prophylactic organ removal due to a genetic susceptibility.

V85 Body Mass Index (BMI)

V86 Estrogen receptor status

V88 Acquired absence of other organs and tissue

V90 Retained foreign body

4) **History (of)**

There are two types of history V codes, personal and family. Personal history codes explain a patient's past medical condition that no longer exists and is not receiving any treatment, but that has the potential for recurrence, and therefore may require continued monitoring. The exceptions to this general rule are category V14, Personal history of allergy to medicinal agents, and subcategory V15.0, Allergy, other than to medicinal agents. A person who has had an allergic episode to a substance or food in the past should always be considered allergic to the substance.

Family history codes are for use when a patient has a family member(s) who has had a particular disease that causes the patient to be at higher risk of also contracting the disease.

Personal history codes may be used in conjunction with follow-up codes and family history codes may be used in conjunction with screening codes to explain the need for a test or procedure. History codes are also acceptable on any medical record regardless of the reason for visit. A history of an illness, even if no longer present, is important information that may alter the type of treatment ordered.

The history V code categories are:

V10 Personal history of malignant neoplasm

V12 Personal history of certain other diseases

V13 Personal history of other diseases

Except: V13.4, Personal history of arthritis, and subcategory V13.6, Personal history of congenital (corrected) malformations. These conditions are life-long so are not true history codes.

V14 Personal history of allergy to medicinal agents

V15 Other personal history presenting hazards to health

Except: Codes V15.7, Personal history of contraception; V15.84, Contact with and (suspected) exposure to asbestos; V15.85, Contact with and (suspected) exposure to potentially hazardous body fluids; V15.86, Contact with and (suspected) exposure to lead.

V16 Family history of malignant neoplasm

V17 Family history of certain chronic disabling diseases

V18 Family history of certain other specific diseases

V19 Family history of other conditions

V87 Other specified personal exposures and history presenting hazards to health

Except: Subcategories V87.0, Contact with and (suspected) exposure to hazardous metals; V87.1, Contact with and (suspected) exposure to hazardous aromatic compounds; V87.2, Contact with and (suspected) exposure to other potentially hazardous chemicals; and V87.3, Contact with and (suspected) exposure to other potentially hazardous substances.

5) **Screening**

Screening is the testing for disease or disease precursors in seemingly well individuals so that early detection and treatment can be provided for those who test positive for the disease. Screenings that are recommended for many subgroups in a population include: routine mammograms for women over 40, a fecal occult blood test for everyone over 50, an amniocentesis to rule out a fetal anomaly for pregnant women over 35, because the incidence of breast cancer and colon cancer in these subgroups is higher than in the general population, as is the incidence of Down's syndrome in older mothers.

The testing of a person to rule out or confirm a suspected diagnosis because the patient has some sign or symptom is a diagnostic examination, not a screening. In these cases, the sign or symptom is used to explain the reason for the test.

A screening code may be a first listed code if the reason for the visit is specifically the screening exam. It may also be used as an additional code if the screening is done during an office visit for other health problems. A screening code is not necessary if the screening is inherent to a routine examination, such as a pap smear done during a routine pelvic examination.

Should a condition be discovered during the screening then the code for the condition may be assigned as an additional diagnosis.

The V code indicates that a screening exam is planned. A procedure code is required to confirm that the screening was performed.

The screening V code categories:

V28   Antenatal screening
V73-V82 Special screening examinations

6) Observation

There are three observation V code categories. They are for use in very limited circumstances when a person is being observed for a suspected condition that is ruled out. The observation codes are not for use if an injury or illness or any signs or symptoms related to the suspected condition are present. In such cases the diagnosis/symptom code is used with the corresponding E code to identify any external cause. The observation codes are to be used as principal diagnosis only. The only exception to this is when the principal diagnosis is required to be a code from the V30, Live born infant, category. Then the V29 observation code is sequenced after the V30 code. Additional codes may be used in addition to the observation code but only if they are unrelated to the suspected condition being observed.

Codes from subcategory V89.0, Suspected maternal and fetal conditions not found, may either be used as a first listed or as an additional code assignment depending on the case. They are for use in very limited circumstances on a maternal record when an encounter is for a suspected maternal or fetal condition that is ruled out during that encounter (for example, a maternal or fetal condition may be suspected due to an abnormal test result). These codes should not be used when the condition is confirmed. In those cases, the confirmed condition should be coded. In addition, these codes are not for use if an illness or any signs or symptoms related to the suspected condition or problem are present. In such cases the diagnosis/symptom code is used.

Additional codes may be used in addition to the code from subcategory V89.0, but only if they are unrelated to the suspected condition being evaluated.

Codes from subcategory V89.0 may not be used for encounters for antenatal screening of mother. *See Section I.C.18.d., Screening.*

For encounters for suspected fetal condition that are inconclusive following testing and evaluation, assign the appropriate code from category 655, 656, 657 or 658.

The observation V code categories:

V29   Observation and evaluation of newborns for suspected condition not found

For the birth encounter, a code from category V30 should be sequenced before the V29 code.
V71   Observation and evaluation for suspected condition not found
V89   Suspected maternal and fetal conditions not found

7) Aftercare

Aftercare visit codes cover situations when the initial treatment of a disease or injury has been performed and the patient requires continued care during the healing or recovery phase, or for the long-term consequences of the disease. The aftercare V code should not be used if treatment is directed at a current, acute disease or injury. The diagnosis code is to be used in these cases. Exceptions to this rule are codes V58.0, Radiotherapy, and codes from subcategory V58.1, Encounter for chemotherapy and immunotherapy for neoplastic conditions. These codes are to be first listed, followed by the diagnosis code when a patient's encounter is solely to receive radiation therapy or chemotherapy for the treatment of a neoplasm. Should a patient receive both chemotherapy and radiation therapy during the same encounter code V58.0 and V58.1 may be used together on a record with either one being sequenced first.

The aftercare codes are generally first listed to explain the specific reason for the encounter. An aftercare code may be used as an additional code when some type of aftercare is provided in addition to the reason for admission and no diagnosis code is applicable. An example of this would be the closure of a colostomy during an encounter for treatment of another condition.

Aftercare codes should be used in conjunction with any other aftercare codes or other diagnosis codes to provide better detail on the specifics of an aftercare encounter visit, unless otherwise directed by the classification. The sequencing of multiple aftercare codes is discretionary.

Certain aftercare V code categories need a secondary diagnosis code to describe the resolving condition or sequelae, for others, the condition is inherent in the code title.

Additional V code aftercare category terms include fitting and adjustment, and attention to artificial openings.

Status V codes may be used with aftercare V codes to indicate the nature of the aftercare. For example code V45.81, Aortocoronary bypass status, may be used with code V58.73, Aftercare following surgery of the circulatory system, NEC, to indicate the surgery for which the aftercare is being performed. Also, a transplant status code may be used following code V58.44, Aftercare following organ transplant, to identify the organ transplanted. A status code should not be used when the aftercare code indicates the type of status, such as using V55.0, Attention to tracheostomy with V44.0, Tracheostomy status.

See Section I. B.16 Admissions/Encounter for Rehabilitation

The aftercare V category/codes:

V51.0   Encounter for breast reconstruction following mastectomy
V52   Fitting and adjustment of prosthetic device and implant
V53   Fitting and adjustment of other device
V54   Other orthopedic aftercare
V55   Attention to artificial openings
V56   Encounter for dialysis and dialysis catheter care
V57   Care involving the use of rehabilitation procedures
V58.0   Radiotherapy
V58.11   Encounter for antineoplastic chemotherapy
V58.12   Encounter for antineoplastic immunotherapy
V58.3x   Attention to dressings and sutures

V58.41	Encounter for planned post-operative wound closure
V58.42	Aftercare, surgery, neoplasm
V58.43	Aftercare, surgery, trauma
V58.44	Aftercare involving organ transplant
V58.49	Other specified aftercare following surgery
V58.7x	Aftercare following surgery
V58.81	Fitting and adjustment of vascular catheter
V58.82	Fitting and adjustment of non-vascular catheter
V58.83	Monitoring therapeutic drug
V58.89	Other specified aftercare

8) Follow-up

The follow-up codes are used to explain continuing surveillance following completed treatment of a disease, condition, or injury. They imply that the condition has been fully treated and no longer exists. They should not be confused with aftercare codes that explain current treatment for a healing condition or its sequelae. Follow-up codes may be used in conjunction with history codes to provide the full picture of the healed condition and its treatment. The follow-up code is sequenced first, followed by the history code.

A follow-up code may be used to explain repeated visits. Should a condition be found to have recurred on the follow-up visit, then the diagnosis code should be used in place of the follow-up code.

The follow-up V code categories:

| V24 | Postpartum care and evaluation |
| V67 | Follow-up examination |

9) Donor

Category V59 is the donor codes. They are used for living individuals who are donating blood or other body tissue. These codes are only for individuals donating for others, not for self donations. They are not for use to identify cadaveric donations.

10) Counseling

Counseling V codes are used when a patient or family member receives assistance in the aftermath of an illness or injury, or when support is required in coping with family or social problems. They are not necessary for use in conjunction with a diagnosis code when the counseling component of care is considered integral to standard treatment.

The counseling V categories/codes:

V25.0	General counseling and advice for contraceptive management
V26.3	Genetic counseling
V26.4	General counseling and advice for procreative management
V61.x	Other family circumstances
V65.1	Person consulted on behalf of another person
V65.3	Dietary surveillance and counseling
V65.4	Other counseling, not elsewhere classified

11) Obstetrics and related conditions

See Section I.C.11., the Obstetrics guidelines for further instruction on the use of these codes.

V codes for pregnancy are for use in those circumstances when none of the problems or complications included in the codes from the Obstetrics chapter exist (a routine prenatal visit or postpartum care). Codes V22.0, Supervision of normal first pregnancy, and V22.1, Supervision of other normal pregnancy, are always first listed and are not to be used with any other code from the OB chapter.

The outcome of delivery, category V27, should be included on all maternal delivery records. It is always a secondary code.

V codes for family planning (contraceptive) or procreative management and counseling should be included on an obstetric record either during the pregnancy or the postpartum stage, if applicable.

Obstetrics and related conditions V code categories:

V22	Normal pregnancy
V23	Supervision of high-risk pregnancy
	Except: V23.2, Pregnancy with history of abortion. Code 646.3, Recurrent pregnancy loss, from the OB chapter is required to indicate a history of abortion during a pregnancy.
V24	Postpartum care and evaluation
V25	Encounter for contraceptive management
	Except V25.0x
	(See Section I.C.18.d.11, Counseling)
V26	Procreative management
	Except: V26.5x, Sterilization status, V26.3 and V26.4
	(See Section I.C.18.d.11., Counseling)
V27	Outcome of delivery
V28	Antenatal screening
	(See Section I.C.18.d.6., Screening)
V91	Multiple gestation placenta status

12) Newborn, infant and child

See Section I.C.15, the Newborn guidelines for further instruction on the use of these codes.

Newborn V code categories:

V20	Health supervision of infant or child
V29	Observation and evaluation of newborns for suspected condition not found
	(See Section I.C.18.d.7, Observation)
V30-V39	Liveborn infant according to type of birth

13) Routine and administrative examinations

The V codes allow for the description of encounters for routine examinations, such as, a general check-up, or examinations for administrative purposes, such as a pre-employment physical. The codes are not to be used if the examination is for diagnosis of a suspected condition or for treatment purposes. In such cases the diagnosis code is used. During a routine exam, should a diagnosis or condition be discovered, it should be coded as an additional code. Pre-existing and chronic conditions and history codes may also be included as additional codes as long as the examination is for administrative purposes and not focused on any particular condition.

Pre-operative examination and pre-procedural laboratory examination V codes are for use only in those situations when a patient is being cleared for a procedure or surgery and no treatment is given.

The V codes categories/code for routine and administrative examinations:

V20.2	Routine infant or child health check
	Any injections given should have a corresponding procedure code.
V70	General medical examination
V72	Special investigations and examinations
	Codes V72.5 and V72.62 may be used if the reason for the patient encounter is for routine laboratory/radiology testing in the absence of any signs, symptoms, or associated diagnosis. If routine testing is performed during the same encounter as

a test to evaluate a sign, symptom, or diagnosis, it is appropriate to assign both the V code and the code describing the reason for the non-routine test.

14) Miscellaneous V codes

The miscellaneous V codes capture a number of other health care encounters that do not fall into one of the other categories. Certain of these codes identify the reason for the encounter, others are for use as additional codes that provide useful information on circumstances that may affect a patient's care and treatment.

Prophylactic Organ Removal

For encounters specifically for prophylactic removal of breasts, ovaries, or another organ due to a genetic susceptibility to cancer or a family history of cancer, the principal or first listed code should be a code from subcategory V50.4, Prophylactic organ removal, followed by the appropriate genetic susceptibility code and the appropriate family history code.

If the patient has a malignancy of one site and is having prophylactic removal at another site to prevent either a new primary malignancy or metastatic disease, a code for the malignancy should also be assigned in addition to a code from subcategory V50.4. A V50.4 code should not be assigned if the patient is having organ removal for treatment of a malignancy, such as the removal of the testes for the treatment of prostate cancer.

Miscellaneous V code categories/codes:

V07	Need for isolation and other prophylactic or treatment measures
	Except V07.5X, Use of agents affecting estrogen receptors and estrogen levels
V40.31	Wandering in diseases classified elsewhere
V50	Elective surgery for purposes other than remedying health states
V58.5	Orthodontics
V60	Housing, household, and economic circumstances
V62	Other psychosocial circumstances
V63	Unavailability of other medical facilities for care
V64	Persons encountering health services for specific procedures, not carried out
V66	Convalescence and Palliative Care
V68	Encounters for administrative purposes
V69	Problems related to lifestyle

15) Nonspecific V codes

Certain V codes are so non-specific, or potentially redundant with other codes in the classification, that there can be little justification for their use in the inpatient setting. Their use in the outpatient setting should be limited to those instances when there is no further documentation to permit more precise coding. Otherwise, any sign or symptom or any other reason for visit that is captured in another code should be used.

Nonspecific V code categories/codes:

V11	Personal history of mental disorder
	A code from the mental disorders chapter, with an in remission fifth-digit, should be used.
V13.4	Personal history of arthritis
V13.6	Personal history of congenital malformations
V15.7	Personal history of contraception
V23.2	Pregnancy with history of abortion
V40	Mental and behavioral problems
	Exception: V40.31 Wandering in diseases classified elsewhere
V41	Problems with special senses and other special functions

V47	Other problems with internal organs
V48	Problems with head, neck, and trunk
V49	Problems with limbs and other problems

Exceptions:

V49.6	Upper limb amputation status
V49.7	Lower limb amputation status
V49.81	Asymptomatic postmenopausal status (age-related) (natural)
V49.82	Dental sealant status
V49.83	Awaiting organ transplant status
V49.86	Do not resuscitate status
V49.87	Physical restraints status

V51.8	Other aftercare involving the use of plastic surgery
V58.2	Blood transfusion, without reported diagnosis
V58.9	Unspecified aftercare
	See Section IV.K. and Section IV.L. of the Outpatient guidelines.

e. V Codes That May Only be Principal/First-Listed Diagnosis

The list of V codes/categories below may only be reported as the principal/first-listed diagnosis, except when there are multiple encounters on the same day and the medical records for the encounters are combined or when there is more than one V code that meets the definition of principal diagnosis (e.g., a patient is admitted to home healthcare for both aftercare and rehabilitation and they equally meet the definition of principal diagnosis). These codes should not be reported if they do not meet the definition of principal or first-listed diagnosis.

See Section II and Section IV.A for information on selection of principal and first-listed diagnosis.

See Section II.C for information on two or more diagnoses that equally meet the definition for principal diagnosis.

V20.x	Health supervision of infant or child
V22.0	Supervision of normal first pregnancy
V22.1	Supervision of other normal pregnancy
V24.x	Postpartum care and examination
V26.81	Encounter for assisted reproductive fertility procedure cycle
V26.82	Encounter for fertility preservation procedure
V30.x	Single liveborn
V31.x	Twin, mate liveborn
V32.x	Twin, mate stillborn
V33.x	Twin, unspecified
V34.x	Other multiple, mates all liveborn
V35.x	Other multiple, mates all stillborn
V36.x	Other multiple, mates live- and stillborn
V37.x	Other multiple, unspecified
V39.x	Unspecified
V46.12	Encounter for respirator dependence during power failure
V46.13	Encounter for weaning from respirator [ventilator]
V51.0	Encounter for breast reconstruction following mastectomy
V56.0	Extracorporeal dialysis
V57.x	Care involving use of rehabilitation procedures
V58.0	Radiotherapy
V58.11	Encounter for antineoplastic chemotherapy
V58.12	Encounter for antineoplastic immunotherapy
V59.x	Donors
V66.0	Convalescence and palliative care following surgery V66.1 Convalescence and palliative care following radiotherapy

V66.2	Convalescence and palliative care following chemotherapy
V66.3	Convalescence and palliative care following psychotherapy and other treatment for mental disorder
V66.4	Convalescence and palliative care following treatment of fracture
V66.5	Convalescence and palliative care following other treatment
V66.6	Convalescence and palliative care following combined treatment
V66.9	Unspecified convalescence
V68.x	Encounters for administrative purposes
V70.0	Routine general medical examination at a health care facility
V70.1	General psychiatric examination, requested by the authority
V70.2	General psychiatric examination, other and unspecified
V70.3	Other medical examination for administrative purposes
V70.4	Examination for medicolegal reasons
V70.5	Health examination of defined subpopulations
V70.6	Health examination in population surveys
V70.8	Other specified general medical examinations
V70.9	Unspecified general medical examination
V71.x	Observation and evaluation for suspected conditions not found

19. Supplemental Classification of External Causes of Injury and Poisoning (E-codes, E000-E999)

Introduction: These guidelines are provided for those who are currently collecting E codes in order that there will be standardization in the process. If your institution plans to begin collecting E codes, these guidelines are to be applied. The use of E codes is supplemental to the application of ICD-9-CM diagnosis codes.

External causes of injury and poisoning codes (categories E000 and E800-E999) are intended to provide data for injury research and evaluation of injury prevention strategies. Activity codes (categories E001-E030) are intended to be used to describe the activity of a person seeking care for injuries as well as other health conditions, when the injury or other health condition resulted from an activity or the activity contributed to a condition. E codes capture how the injury, poisoning, or adverse effect happened (cause), the intent (unintentional or accidental; or intentional, such as suicide or assault), the person's status (e.g. civilian, military), the associated activity and the place where the event occurred.

Some major categories of E codes include:

    transport accidents

    poisoning and adverse effects of drugs, medicinal substances and biologicals

    accidental falls

    accidents caused by fire and flames

    accidents due to natural and environmental factors

    late effects of accidents, assaults or self injury

    assaults or purposely inflicted injury

    suicide or self inflicted injury

These guidelines apply for the coding and collection of E codes from records in hospitals, outpatient clinics, emergency departments, other ambulatory care settings and provider offices, and nonacute care settings, except when other specific guidelines apply.

a. General E Code Coding Guidelines

1) Used with any code in the range of 001-V91

An E code from categories E800-E999 may be used with any code in the range of 001-V91, which indicates an injury, poisoning, or adverse effect due to an external cause.

An activity E code (categories E001-E030) may be used with any code in the range of 001-V91 that indicates an injury, or other health condition that resulted from an activity, or the activity contributed to a condition.

2) Assign the appropriate E code for all initial treatments

Assign the appropriate E code for the initial encounter of an injury, poisoning, or adverse effect of drugs, not for subsequent treatment.

External cause of injury codes (E-codes) may be assigned while the acute fracture codes are still applicable.

See Section I.C.17.b.1 for coding of acute fractures.

3) Use the full range of E codes

Use the full range of E codes (E800 – E999) to completely describe the cause, the intent and the place of occurrence, if applicable, for all injuries, poisonings, and adverse effects of drugs.

See a.1.), j.), and k.) in this section for information on the use of status and activity E codes.

4) Assign as many E codes as necessary

Assign as many E codes as necessary to fully explain each cause.

5) The selection of the appropriate E code

The selection of the appropriate E code is guided by the Index to External Causes, which is located after the alphabetical index to diseases and by Inclusion and Exclusion notes in the Tabular List.

6) E code can never be a principal diagnosis

An E code can never be a principal (first listed) diagnosis.

7) External cause code(s) with systemic inflammatory response syndrome (SIRS)

An external cause code is not appropriate with a code from subcategory 995.9, unless the patient also has another condition for which an E code would be appropriate (such as an injury, poisoning, or adverse effect of drugs.

8) Multiple Cause E Code Coding Guidelines

More than one E-code is required to fully describe the external cause of an illness, injury or poisoning. The assignment of E-codes should be sequenced in the following priority:

If two or more events cause separate injuries, an E code should be assigned for each cause. The first listed E code will be selected in the following order:

E codes for child and adult abuse take priority over all other E codes.

See Section I.C.19.e., Child and Adult abuse guidelines.

E codes for terrorism events take priority over all other E codes except child and adult abuse.

E codes for cataclysmic events take priority over all other E codes except child and adult abuse and terrorism.

E codes for transport accidents take priority over all other E codes except cataclysmic events, child and adult abuse and terrorism.

Activity and external cause status codes are assigned following all causal (intent) E codes.

The first-listed E code should correspond to the cause of the most serious diagnosis due to an assault, accident, or self-harm, following the order of hierarchy listed above.

9)   If the reporting format limits the number of E codes

If the reporting format limits the number of E codes that can be used in reporting clinical data, report the code for the cause/intent most related to the principal diagnosis. If the format permits capture of additional E codes, the cause/intent, including medical misadventures, of the additional events should be reported rather than the codes for place, activity or external status.

b.   Place of Occurrence Guideline

Use an additional code from category E849 to indicate the Place of Occurrence. The Place of Occurrence describes the place where the event occurred and not the patient's activity at the time of the event.

Do not use E849.9 if the place of occurrence is not stated.

c.   Adverse Effects of Drugs, Medicinal and Biological Substances Guidelines

1)   Do not code directly from the Table of Drugs

Do not code directly from the Table of Drugs and Chemicals. Always refer back to the Tabular List.

2)   Use as many codes as necessary to describe

Use as many codes as necessary to describe completely all drugs, medicinal or biological substances.

If the reporting format limits the number of E codes, and there are different fourth digit codes in the same three digit category, use the code for "Other specified" of that category of drugs, medicinal or biological substances. If there is no "Other specified" code in that category, use the appropriate "Unspecified" code in that category.

If the reporting format limits the number of E codes, and the codes are in different three digit categories, assign the appropriate E code for other multiple drugs and medicinal substances.

3)   If the same E code would describe the causative agent

If the same E code would describe the causative agent for more than one adverse reaction, assign the code only once.

4)   If two or more drugs, medicinal or biological substances

If two or more drugs, medicinal or biological substances are reported, code each individually unless the combination code is listed in the Table of Drugs and Chemicals. In that case, assign the E code for the combination.

5)   When a reaction results from the interaction of a drug(s)

When a reaction results from the interaction of a drug(s) and alcohol, use poisoning codes and E codes for both.

6)   Codes from the E930-E949 series

Codes from the E930-E949 series must be used to identify the causative substance for an adverse effect of drug, medicinal and biological substances, correctly prescribed and properly administered. The effect, such as tachycardia, delirium, gastrointestinal hemorrhaging, vomiting, hypokalemia, hepatitis, renal failure, or respiratory failure, is coded and followed by the appropriate code from the E930-E949 series.

d.   Child and Adult Abuse Guideline

1)   Intentional injury

When the cause of an injury or neglect is intentional child or adult abuse, the first listed E code should be assigned from categories E960-E968, Homicide and injury purposely inflicted by other persons, (except category E967). An E code from category E967, Child and adult battering and other maltreatment, should be added as an additional code to identify the perpetrator, if known.

2)   Accidental intent

In cases of neglect when the intent is determined to be accidental E code E904.0, Abandonment or neglect of infant and helpless person, should be the first listed E code.

e.   Unknown or Suspected Intent Guideline

1)   If the intent (accident, self-harm, assault) of the cause of an injury or poisoning is unknown

If the intent (accident, self-harm, assault) of the cause of an injury or poisoning is unknown or unspecified, code the intent as undetermined E980-E989.

2)   If the intent (accident, self-harm, assault) of the cause of an injury or poisoning is questionable

If the intent (accident, self-harm, assault) of the cause of an injury or poisoning is questionable, probable or suspected, code the intent as undetermined E980-E989.

f.   Undetermined Cause

When the intent of an injury or poisoning is known, but the cause is unknown, use codes: E928.9, Unspecified accident, E958.9, Suicide and self-inflicted injury by unspecified means, and E968.9, Assault by unspecified means.

These E codes should rarely be used, as the documentation in the medical record, in both the inpatient outpatient and other settings, should normally provide sufficient detail to determine the cause of the injury.

g.   Late Effects of External Cause Guidelines

1)   Late effect E codes

Late effect E codes exist for injuries and poisonings but not for adverse effects of drugs, misadventures and surgical complications.

2)   Late effect E codes (E929, E959, E969, E977, E989, or E999.1)

A late effect E code (E929, E959, E969, E977, E989, or E999.1) should be used with any report of a late effect or sequela resulting from a previous injury or poisoning (905-909).

3)   Late effect E code with a related current injury

A late effect E code should never be used with a related current nature of injury code.

4)   Use of late effect E codes for subsequent visits

Use a late effect E code for subsequent visits when a late effect of the initial injury or poisoning is being treated. There is no late effect E code for adverse effects of drugs.

Do not use a late effect E code for subsequent visits for follow-up care (e.g., to assess healing, to receive rehabilitative therapy) of the injury or poisoning when no late effect of the injury has been documented.

h.   Misadventures and Complications of Care Guidelines

1)   Code range E870-E876

Assign a code in the range of E870-E876 if misadventures are stated by the provider. When applying the E code guidelines pertaining to sequencing, these E codes are considered causal codes.

2)   Code range E878-E879

Assign a code in the range of E878-E879 if the provider attributes an abnormal reaction or later complication to a surgical or medical procedure, but does not mention misadventure at the time of the procedure as the cause of the reaction.

i.   Terrorism Guidelines

1)   Cause of injury identified by the Federal Government (FBI) as terrorism

When the cause of an injury is identified by the Federal Government (FBI) as terrorism, the first-listed E-code should be a code from category E979, Terrorism. The definition of terrorism employed by the FBI is found at the inclusion note at E979. The terrorism E-code is the only E-code that should be assigned. Additional E codes from the assault categories should not be assigned.

2) **Cause of an injury is suspected to be the result of terrorism**

When the cause of an injury is suspected to be the result of terrorism a code from category E979 should not be assigned. Assign a code in the range of E codes based circumstances on the documentation of intent and mechanism.

3) **Code E979.9, Terrorism, secondary effects**

Assign code E979.9, Terrorism, secondary effects, for conditions occurring subsequent to the terrorist event. This code should not be assigned for conditions that are due to the initial terrorist act.

4) **Statistical tabulation of terrorism codes**

For statistical purposes these codes will be tabulated within the category for assault, expanding the current category from E960-E969 to include E979 and E999.1.

j. **Activity Code Guidelines**

Assign a code from category E001-E030 to describe the activity that caused or contributed to the injury or other health condition.

Unlike other E codes, activity E codes may be assigned to indicate a health condition (not just injuries) resulted from an activity, or the activity contributed to the condition.

The activity codes are not applicable to poisonings, adverse effects, misadventures or late effects.

Do not assign E030, Unspecified activity, if the activity is not stated.

k. **External cause status**

A code from category E000, External cause status, should be assigned whenever any other E code is assigned for an encounter, including an Activity E code, except for the events noted below. Assign a code from category E000, External cause status, to indicate the work status of the person at the time the event occurred. The status code indicates whether the event occurred during military activity, whether a non-military person was at work, whether an individual including a student or volunteer was involved in a non-work activity at the time of the causal event.

A code from E000, External cause status, should be assigned, when applicable, with other external cause codes, such as transport accidents and falls. The external cause status codes are not applicable to poisonings, adverse effects, misadventures or late effects.

Do not assign a code from category E000 if no other E codes (cause, activity) are applicable for the encounter.

Do not assign code E000.9, Unspecified external cause status, if the status is not stated.

Section II. Selection of Principal Diagnosis

The circumstances of inpatient admission always govern the selection of principal diagnosis. The principal diagnosis is defined in the Uniform Hospital Discharge Data Set (UHDDS) as "that condition established after study to be chiefly responsible for occasioning the admission of the patient to the hospital for care."

The UHDDS definitions are used by hospitals to report inpatient data elements in a standardized manner. These data elements and their definitions can be found in the July 31, 1985, Federal Register (Vol. 50, No, 147), pp. 31038-40.

Since that time the application of the UHDDS definitions has been expanded to include all non-outpatient settings (acute care, short term, long term care and psychiatric hospitals; home health agencies; rehab facilities; nursing homes, etc).

In determining principal diagnosis the coding conventions in the ICD-9-CM, Volumes I and II take precedence over these official coding guidelines.

(See Section I.A., Conventions for the ICD-9-CM)

The importance of consistent, complete documentation in the medical record cannot be overemphasized. Without such documentation the application of all coding guidelines is a difficult, if not impossible, task.

A. **Codes for symptoms, signs, and ill-defined conditions**

Codes for symptoms, signs, and ill-defined conditions from Chapter 16 are not to be used as principal diagnosis when a related definitive diagnosis has been established.

B. **Two or more interrelated conditions, each potentially meeting the definition for principal diagnosis.**

When there are two or more interrelated conditions (such as diseases in the same ICD-9-CM chapter or manifestations characteristically associated with a certain disease) potentially meeting the definition of principal diagnosis, either condition may be sequenced first, unless the circumstances of the admission, the therapy provided, the Tabular List, or the Alphabetic Index indicate otherwise.

C. **Two or more diagnoses that equally meet the definition for principal diagnosis**

In the unusual instance when two or more diagnoses equally meet the criteria for principal diagnosis as determined by the circumstances of admission, diagnostic workup and/or therapy provided, and the Alphabetic Index, Tabular List, or another coding guidelines does not provide sequencing direction, any one of the diagnoses may be sequenced first.

D. **Two or more comparative or contrasting conditions.**

In those rare instances when two or more contrasting or comparative diagnoses are documented as "either/or" (or similar terminology), they are coded as if the diagnoses were confirmed and the diagnoses are sequenced according to the circumstances of the admission. If no further determination can be made as to which diagnosis should be principal, either diagnosis may be sequenced first.

E. **A symptom(s) followed by contrasting/comparative diagnoses**

When a symptom(s) is followed by contrasting/comparative diagnoses, the symptom code is sequenced first. All the contrasting/comparative diagnoses should be coded as additional diagnoses.

F. **Original treatment plan not carried out**

Sequence as the principal diagnosis the condition, which after study occasioned the admission to the hospital, even though treatment may not have been carried out due to unforeseen circumstances.

G. **Complications of surgery and other medical care**

When the admission is for treatment of a complication resulting from surgery or other medical care, the complication code is sequenced as the principal diagnosis. If the complication is classified to the 996-999 series and the code lacks the necessary specificity in describing the complication, an additional code for the specific complication should be assigned.

H. **Uncertain Diagnosis**

If the diagnosis documented at the time of discharge is qualified as "probable", "suspected", "likely", "questionable", "possible", or "still to be ruled out", or other similar terms indicating uncertainty, code the condition as if it existed or was established. The bases for these guidelines are the diagnostic workup, arrangements for further workup or observation, and initial therapeutic approach that correspond most closely with the established diagnosis.

Note: This guideline is applicable only to inpatient admissions to short-term, acute, long-term care and psychiatric hospitals.

I. **Admission from Observation Unit**

1. **Admission Following Medical Observation**

When a patient is admitted to an observation unit for a medical condition, which either worsens or does not improve, and is subsequently admitted as an inpatient of the same hospital for this same medical condition, the principal diagnosis would be the medical condition which led to the hospital admission.

2. **Admission Following Post-Operative Observation**

When a patient is admitted to an observation unit to monitor a condition (or complication) that develops following outpatient surgery, and then is subsequently admitted as an inpatient of the same hospital, hospitals should apply the Uniform Hospital Discharge Data Set (UHDDS) definition of principal diagnosis as "that condition established after study to be chiefly responsible for occasioning the admission of the patient to the hospital for care."

J. Admission from Outpatient Surgery

When a patient receives surgery in the hospital's outpatient surgery department and is subsequently admitted for continuing inpatient care at the same hospital, the following guidelines should be followed in selecting the principal diagnosis for the inpatient admission:

- If the reason for the inpatient admission is a complication, assign the complication as the principal diagnosis.

- If no complication, or other condition, is documented as the reason for the inpatient admission, assign the reason for the outpatient surgery as the principal diagnosis.

- If the reason for the inpatient admission is another condition unrelated to the surgery, assign the unrelated condition as the principal diagnosis.

Section III. Reporting Additional Diagnoses

GENERAL RULES FOR OTHER (ADDITIONAL) DIAGNOSES

For reporting purposes the definition for "other diagnoses" is interpreted as additional conditions that affect patient care in terms of requiring:

> clinical evaluation; or
>
> therapeutic treatment; or
>
> diagnostic procedures; or
>
> extended length of hospital stay; or
>
> increased nursing care and/or monitoring.

The UHDDS item #11-b defines Other Diagnoses as "all conditions that coexist at the time of admission, that develop subsequently, or that affect the treatment received and/or the length of stay. Diagnoses that relate to an earlier episode which have no bearing on the current hospital stay are to be excluded." UHDDS definitions apply to inpatients in acute care, short-term, long term care and psychiatric hospital setting. The UHDDS definitions are used by acute care short-term hospitals to report inpatient data elements in a standardized manner. These data elements and their definitions can be found in the July 31, 1985, Federal Register (Vol. 50, No, 147), pp. 31038-40.

Since that time the application of the UHDDS definitions has been expanded to include all non-outpatient settings (acute care, short term, long term care and psychiatric hospitals; home health agencies; rehab facilities; nursing homes, etc).

The following guidelines are to be applied in designating "other diagnoses" when neither the Alphabetic Index nor the Tabular List in ICD-9-CM provide direction. The listing of the diagnoses in the patient record is the responsibility of the attending provider.

A. Previous conditions

If the provider has included a diagnosis in the final diagnostic statement, such as the discharge summary or the face sheet, it should ordinarily be coded. Some providers include in the diagnostic statement resolved conditions or diagnoses and status-post procedures from previous admission that have no bearing on the current stay. Such conditions are not to be reported and are coded only if required by hospital policy.

However, history codes (V10-V19) may be used as secondary codes if the historical condition or family history has an impact on current care or influences treatment.

B. Abnormal findings

Abnormal findings (laboratory, x-ray, pathologic, and other diagnostic results) are not coded and reported unless the provider indicates their clinical significance. If the findings are outside the normal range and the attending provider has ordered other tests to evaluate the condition or prescribed treatment, it is appropriate to ask the provider whether the abnormal finding should be added.

Please note: This differs from the coding practices in the outpatient setting for coding encounters for diagnostic tests that have been interpreted by a provider.

C. Uncertain Diagnosis

If the diagnosis documented at the time of discharge is qualified as "probable", "suspected", "likely", "questionable", "possible", or "still to be ruled out" or other similar terms indicating uncertainty, code the condition as if it existed or was established. The bases for these guidelines are the diagnostic workup, arrangements for further workup or observation, and

initial therapeutic approach that correspond most closely with the established diagnosis.

Note: This guideline is applicable only to inpatient admissions to short-term, acute, long-term care and psychiatric hospitals.

Section IV. Diagnostic Coding and Reporting Guidelines for Outpatient Services

These coding guidelines for outpatient diagnoses have been approved for use by hospitals/ providers in coding and reporting hospital-based outpatient services and provider-based office visits.

Information about the use of certain abbreviations, punctuation, symbols, and other conventions used in the ICD-9-CM Tabular List (code numbers and titles), can be found in Section IA of these guidelines, under "Conventions Used in the Tabular List." Information about the correct sequence to use in finding a code is also described in Section I.

The terms encounter and visit are often used interchangeably in describing outpatient service contacts and, therefore, appear together in these guidelines without distinguishing one from the other.

Though the conventions and general guidelines apply to all settings, coding guidelines for outpatient and provider reporting of diagnoses will vary in a number of instances from those for inpatient diagnoses, recognizing that:

> The Uniform Hospital Discharge Data Set (UHDDS) definition of principal diagnosis applies only to inpatients in acute, short-term, long-term care and psychiatric hospitals.
>
> Coding guidelines for inconclusive diagnoses (probable, suspected, rule out, etc.) were developed for inpatient reporting and do not apply to outpatients.

A. Selection of first-listed condition

In the outpatient setting, the term first-listed diagnosis is used in lieu of principal diagnosis.

In determining the first-listed diagnosis the coding conventions of ICD-9-CM, as well as the general and disease specific guidelines take precedence over the outpatient guidelines.

Diagnoses often are not established at the time of the initial encounter/visit. It may take two or more visits before the diagnosis is confirmed.

The most critical rule involves beginning the search for the correct code assignment through the Alphabetic Index. Never begin searching initially in the Tabular List as this will lead to coding errors.

1. Outpatient Surgery

When a patient presents for outpatient surgery, code the reason for the surgery as the first-listed diagnosis (reason for the encounter), even if the surgery is not performed due to a contraindication.

2. Observation Stay

When a patient is admitted for observation for a medical condition, assign a code for the medical condition as the first-listed diagnosis.

When a patient presents for outpatient surgery and develops complications requiring admission to observation, code the reason for the surgery as the first reported diagnosis (reason for the encounter), followed by codes for the complications as secondary diagnoses.

B. Codes from 001.0 through V91.99

The appropriate code or codes from 001.0 through V91.99 must be used to identify diagnoses, symptoms, conditions, problems, complaints, or other reason(s) for the encounter/visit.

C. Accurate reporting of ICD-9-CM diagnosis codes

For accurate reporting of ICD-9-CM diagnosis codes, the documentation should describe the patient's condition, using terminology which includes specific diagnoses as well as symptoms, problems, or reasons for the encounter. There are ICD-9-CM codes to describe all of these.

D. Selection of codes 001.0 through 999.9

The selection of codes 001.0 through 999.9 will frequently be used to describe the reason for the encounter. These codes are from the section of ICD-9-CM for the classification of diseases and injuries (e.g. infectious and parasitic diseases; neoplasms; symptoms, signs, and ill-defined conditions, etc.).

E.   Codes that describe symptoms and signs

Codes that describe symptoms and signs, as opposed to diagnoses, are acceptable for reporting purposes when a diagnosis has not been established (confirmed) by the provider. Chapter 16 of ICD-9-CM, Symptoms, Signs, and Ill-defined conditions (codes 780.0 - 799.9) contain many, but not all codes for symptoms.

F.   Encounters for circumstances other than a disease or injury

ICD-9-CM provides codes to deal with encounters for circumstances other than a disease or injury. The Supplementary Classification of factors Influencing Health Status and Contact with Health Services (V01.0- V91.99) is provided to deal with occasions when circumstances other than a disease or injury are recorded as diagnosis or problems. *See Section I.C. 18 for information on V-codes.*

G.   Level of Detail in Coding

1.   ICD-9-CM codes with 3, 4, or 5 digits

ICD-9-CM is composed of codes with either 3, 4, or 5 digits. Codes with three digits are included in ICD-9-CM as the heading of a category of codes that may be further subdivided by the use of fourth and/or fifth digits, which provide greater specificity.

2.   Use of full number of digits required for a code

A three-digit code is to be used only if it is not further subdivided. Where fourth-digit subcategories and/or fifth-digit subclassifications are provided, they must be assigned. A code is invalid if it has not been coded to the full number of digits required for that code.

See also discussion under Section I.b.3., General Coding Guidelines, Level of Detail in Coding.

H.   ICD-9-CM code for the diagnosis, condition, problem, or other reason for encounter/visit

List first the ICD-9-CM code for the diagnosis, condition, problem, or other reason for encounter/visit shown in the medical record to be chiefly responsible for the services provided. List additional codes that describe any coexisting conditions. In some cases the first-listed diagnosis may be a symptom when a diagnosis has not been established (confirmed) by the physician.

I.   Uncertain diagnosis

Do not code diagnoses documented as "probable", "suspected," "questionable," "rule out," or "working diagnosis" or other similar terms indicating uncertainty. Rather, code the condition(s) to the highest degree of certainty for that encounter/visit, such as symptoms, signs, abnormal test results, or other reason for the visit.

Please note: This differs from the coding practices used by short-term, acute care, long-term care and psychiatric hospitals.

J.   Chronic diseases

Chronic diseases treated on an ongoing basis may be coded and reported as many times as the patient receives treatment and care for the condition(s)

K.   Code all documented conditions that coexist

Code all documented conditions that coexist at the time of the encounter/visit, and require or affect patient care treatment or management. Do not code conditions that were previously treated and no longer exist. However, history codes (V10-V19) may be used as secondary codes if the historical condition or family history has an impact on current care or influences treatment.

L.   Patients receiving diagnostic services only

For patients receiving diagnostic services only during an encounter/visit, sequence first the diagnosis, condition, problem, or other reason for encounter/visit shown in the medical record to be chiefly responsible for the outpatient services provided during the encounter/visit. Codes for other diagnoses (e.g., chronic conditions) may be sequenced as additional diagnoses.

For encounters for routine laboratory/radiology testing in the absence of any signs, symptoms, or associated diagnosis, assign V72.5 and/or a code from subcategory V72.6. If routine testing is performed during the same encounter as a test to evaluate a sign, symptom, or diagnosis, it is appropriate to assign both the V code and the code describing the reason for the non-routine test.

For outpatient encounters for diagnostic tests that have been interpreted by a physician, and the final report is available at the time of coding, code any confirmed or definitive diagnosis(es) documented in the interpretation. Do not code related signs and symptoms as additional diagnoses.

Please note: This differs from the coding practice in the hospital inpatient setting regarding abnormal findings on test results.

M.   Patients receiving therapeutic services only

For patients receiving therapeutic services only during an encounter/visit, sequence first the diagnosis, condition, problem, or other reason for encounter/visit shown in the medical record to be chiefly responsible for the outpatient services provided during the encounter/visit. Codes for other diagnoses (e.g., chronic conditions) may be sequenced as additional diagnoses.

The only exception to this rule is that when the primary reason for the admission/encounter is chemotherapy, radiation therapy, or rehabilitation, the appropriate V code for the service is listed first, and the diagnosis or problem for which the service is being performed listed second.

N.   Patients receiving preoperative evaluations only

For patients receiving preoperative evaluations only, sequence first a code from category V72.8, Other specified examinations, to describe the pre-op consultations. Assign a code for the condition to describe the reason for the surgery as an additional diagnosis. Code also any findings related to the pre-op evaluation.

O.   Ambulatory surgery

For ambulatory surgery, code the diagnosis for which the surgery was performed. If the postoperative diagnosis is known to be different from the preoperative diagnosis at the time the diagnosis is confirmed, select the postoperative diagnosis for coding, since it is the most definitive.

P.   Routine outpatient prenatal visits

For routine outpatient prenatal visits when no complications are present, codes V22.0, Supervision of normal first pregnancy, or V22.1, Supervision of other normal pregnancy, should be used as the principal diagnosis. These codes should not be used in conjunction with chapter 11 codes.

APPENDIX I. PRESENT ON ADMISSION REPORTING GUIDELINES

Introduction

These guidelines are to be used as a supplement to the *ICD-9-CM Official Guidelines for Coding and Reporting* to facilitate the assignment of the Present on Admission (POA) indicator for each diagnosis and external cause of injury code reported on claim forms (UB-04 and 837 Institutional).

These guidelines are not intended to replace any guidelines in the main body of the *ICD-9-CM Official Guidelines for Coding and Reporting*. The POA guidelines are not intended to provide guidance on when a condition should be coded, but rather, how to apply the POA indicator to the final set of diagnosis codes that have been assigned in accordance with Sections I, II, and III of the official coding guidelines. Subsequent to the assignment of the ICD-9-CM codes, the POA indicator should then be assigned to those conditions that have been coded.

As stated in the Introduction to the ICD-9-CM Official Guidelines for Coding and Reporting, a joint effort between the healthcare provider and the coder is essential to achieve complete and accurate documentation, code assignment, and reporting of diagnoses and procedures. The importance of consistent, complete documentation in the medical record cannot be overemphasized. Medical record documentation from any provider involved in the care and treatment of the patient may be used to support the determination of whether a condition was present on admission or not. In the context of the official coding guidelines, the term "provider" means a physician or any qualified healthcare practitioner who is legally accountable for establishing the patient's diagnosis.

These guidelines are not a substitute for the provider's clinical judgment as to the determination of whether a condition was/was not present on admission. The provider should be queried regarding issues related to the linking of signs/symptoms, timing of test results, and the timing of findings.

General Reporting Requirements

All claims involving inpatient admissions to general acute care hospitals or other facilities that are subject to a law or regulation mandating collection of present on admission information.

Present on admission is defined as present at the time the order for inpatient admission occurs -- conditions that develop during an outpatient encounter, including emergency department, observation, or outpatient surgery, are considered as present on admission.

POA indicator is assigned to principal and secondary diagnoses (as defined in Section II of the Official Guidelines for Coding and Reporting) and the external cause of injury codes.

Issues related to inconsistent, missing, conflicting or unclear documentation must still be resolved by the provider.

If a condition would not be coded and reported based on UHDDS definitions and current official coding guidelines, then the POA indicator would not be reported.

Reporting Options

Y - Yes

N - No

U - Unknown

W – Clinically undetermined

Unreported/Not used (or "1" for Medicare usage) – (Exempt from POA reporting)

Reporting Definitions

Y = present at the time of inpatient admission

N = not present at the time of inpatient admission

U = documentation is insufficient to determine if condition is present on admission

W = provider is unable to clinically determine whether condition was present on admission or not

Timeframe for POA Identification and Documentation

There is no required timeframe as to when a provider (per the definition of "provider" used in these guidelines) must identify or document a condition to be present on admission. In some clinical situations, it may not be possible for a provider to make a definitive diagnosis (or a condition may not be recognized or reported by the patient) for a period of time after admission. In some cases it may be several days before the provider arrives at a definitive diagnosis. This does not mean that the condition was not present on admission. Determination of whether the condition was present on admission or not will be based on the applicable POA guideline as identified in this document, or on the provider's best clinical judgment.

If at the time of code assignment the documentation is unclear as to whether a condition was present on admission or not, it is appropriate to query the provider for clarification.

ASSIGNING THE POA INDICATOR

Condition is on the "Exempt from Reporting" list

Leave the "present on admission" field blank if the condition is on the list of ICD-9-CM codes for which this field is not applicable. This is the only circumstance in which the field maybe left blank.

POA explicitly documented

Assign Y for any condition the provider explicitly documents as being present on admission.

Assign N for any condition the provider explicitly documents as not present at the time of admission.

Conditions diagnosed prior to inpatient admission

Assign "Y" for conditions that were diagnosed prior to admission (example: hypertension, diabetes mellitus, asthma)

Conditions diagnosed during the admission but clearly present before admission

Assign "Y" for conditions diagnosed during the admission that were clearly present but not diagnosed until after admission occurred.

Diagnoses subsequently confirmed after admission are considered present on admission if at the time of admission they are documented as suspected, possible, rule out, differential diagnosis, or constitute an underlying cause of a symptom that is present at the time of admission.

Condition develops during outpatient encounter prior to inpatient admission

Assign Y for any condition that develops during an outpatient encounter prior to a written order for inpatient admission.

Documentation does not indicate whether condition was present on admission

Assign "U" when the medical record documentation is unclear as to whether the condition was present on admission. "U" should not be routinely assigned and used only in very limited circumstances. Coders are encouraged to query the providers when the documentation is unclear.

Documentation states that it cannot be determined whether the condition was or was not present on admission

Assign "W" when the medical record documentation indicates that it cannot be clinically determined whether or not the condition was present on admission.

Chronic condition with acute exacerbation during the admission

If the code is a combination code that identifies both the chronic condition and the acute exacerbation, see POA guidelines pertaining to combination codes.

If the combination code only identifies the chronic condition and not the acute exacerbation (e.g., acute exacerbation of chronic leukemia), assign "Y."

Conditions documented as possible, probable, suspected, or rule out at the time of discharge

If the final diagnosis contains a possible, probable, suspected, or rule out diagnosis, and this diagnosis was based on signs, symptoms or clinical findings suspected at the time of inpatient admission, assign "Y."

If the final diagnosis contains a possible, probable, suspected, or rule out diagnosis, and this diagnosis was based on signs, symptoms or clinical findings that were not present on admission, assign "N".

Conditions documented as impending or threatened at the time of discharge

If the final diagnosis contains an impending or threatened diagnosis, and this diagnosis is based on symptoms or clinical findings that were present on admission, assign "Y".

If the final diagnosis contains an impending or threatened diagnosis, and this diagnosis is based on symptoms or clinical findings that were not present on admission, assign "N".

Acute and chronic conditions

Assign "Y" for acute conditions that are present at time of admission and N for acute conditions that are not present at time of admission.

Assign "Y" for chronic conditions, even though the condition may not be diagnosed until after admission.

If a single code identifies both an acute and chronic condition, see the POA guidelines for combination codes.

Combination codes

Assign "N" if any part of the combination code was not present on admission (e.g., obstructive chronic bronchitis with acute exacerbation and the exacerbation was not present on admission; gastric ulcer that does not start bleeding until after admission; asthma patient develops status asthmaticus after admission)

Assign "Y" if all parts of the combination code were present on admission (e.g., patient with diabetic nephropathy is admitted with uncontrolled diabetes).

If the final diagnosis includes comparative or contrasting diagnoses, and both were present, or suspected, at the time of admission, assign "Y".

For infection codes that include the causal organism, assign "Y" if the infection (or signs of the infection) was present on admission, even though the culture results may not be known until after admission (e.g., patient is admitted with pneumonia and the provider documents pseudomonas as the causal organism a few days later).

Same diagnosis code for two or more conditions

When the same ICD-9-CM diagnosis code applies to two or more conditions during the same encounter (e.g. bilateral condition, or two separate conditions classified to the same ICD-9-CM diagnosis code):

Assign "Y" if all conditions represented by the single ICD-9-CM code were present on admission (e.g. bilateral fracture of the same bone, same site, and both fractures were present on admission)

Assign "N" if any of the conditions represented by the single ICD-9-CM code was not present on admission (e.g. dehydration with hyponatremia is assigned to code 276.1, but only one of these conditions was present on admission).

Obstetrical conditions

Whether or not the patient delivers during the current hospitalization does not affect assignment of the POA indicator. The determining factor for POA assignment is whether the pregnancy complication or obstetrical condition described by the code was present at the time of admission or not.

If the pregnancy complication or obstetrical condition was present on admission (e.g., patient admitted in preterm labor), assign "Y".

If the pregnancy complication or obstetrical condition was not present on admission (e.g., 2nd degree laceration during delivery, postpartum hemorrhage that occurred during current hospitalization, fetal distress develops after admission), assign "N".

If the obstetrical code includes more than one diagnosis and any of the diagnoses identified by the code were not present on admission assign "N". (e.g., Code 642.7, Pre-eclampsia or eclampsia superimposed on pre-existing hypertension).

If the obstetrical code includes information that is not a diagnosis, do not consider that information in the POA determination. (e.g. Code 652.1x, Breech or other malpresentation successfully converted to cephalic presentation should be reported as present on admission if the fetus was breech on admission but was converted to cephalic presentation after admission (since the conversion to cephalic presentation does not represent a diagnosis, the fact that the conversion occurred after admission has no bearing on the POA determination).

Perinatal conditions

Newborns are not considered to be admitted until after birth. Therefore, any condition present at birth or that developed in utero is considered present at admission and should be assigned "Y". This includes conditions that occur during delivery (e.g., injury during delivery, meconium aspiration, exposure to streptococcus B in the vaginal canal).

Congenital conditions and anomalies

Assign "Y" for congenital conditions and anomalies, **except for categories 740-759, Congenital anomalies, which are on the exempt list.** Congenital conditions are always considered present on admission.

External cause of injury codes

Assign "Y" for any E code representing an external cause of injury or poisoning that occurred prior to inpatient admission (e.g., patient fell out of bed at home, patient fell out of bed in emergency room prior to admission)

Assign "N" for any E code representing an external cause of injury or poisoning that occurred during inpatient hospitalization (e.g., patient fell out of hospital bed during hospital stay, patient experienced an adverse reaction to a medication administered after inpatient admission)

CATEGORIES AND CODES EXEMPT FROM DIAGNOSIS PRESENT ON ADMISSION REQUIREMENT

Note: *"Diagnosis present on admission" for these code categories are exempt because they represent circumstances regarding the healthcare encounter or factors influencing health status that do not represent a current disease or injury or are always present on admission.*

Categories or subcategories listed are inclusive of all codes within those categories or subcategories, unless otherwise indicated. In order to streamline the POA exempt list and make it easier to read, where all of the codes in a code range are POA exempt, only the code range is shown, rather than listing each of the individual codes in the range.

137-139	Late effects of infectious and parasitic diseases
268.1	Rickets, late effect
326	Late effects of intracranial abscess or pyogenic infection
412	Old myocardial infarction
438	Late effects of cerebrovascular disease
650	Normal delivery
660.7	Failed forceps or vacuum extractor, unspecified
677	Late effect of complication of pregnancy, childbirth, and the puerperium
740-759	Congenital anomalies
905-909	Late effects of injuries, poisonings, toxic effects, and other external causes
V02	Carrier or suspected carrier of infectious diseases
V03	Need for prophylactic vaccination and inoculation against bacterial diseases
V04	Need for prophylactic vaccination and inoculation against certain viral diseases
V05	Need for other prophylactic vaccination and inoculation against single diseases
V06	Need for prophylactic vaccination and inoculation against combinations of diseases
V07	Need for isolation and other prophylactic or treatment measures
V10	Personal history of malignant neoplasm
V11	Personal history of mental disorder
V12	Personal history of certain other diseases
V13	Personal history of other diseases
V14	Personal history of allergy to medicinal agents
V15	Other personal history presenting hazards to health
V16	Family history of malignant neoplasm
V17	Family history of certain chronic disabling diseases
V18	Family history of certain other specific conditions
V19	Family history of other conditions
V20	Health supervision of infant or child
V21	Constitutional states in development
V22	Normal pregnancy
V23	Supervision of high-risk pregnancy
V24	Postpartum care and examination
V25	Encounter for contraceptive management
V26	Procreative management
V27	Outcome of delivery
V28	Antenatal screening
V29	Observation and evaluation of newborns for suspected condition not found
V30-V39	Liveborn infants according to type of birth
V42	Organ or tissue replaced by transplant
V43	Organ or tissue replaced by other means
V44	Artificial opening status
V45	Other postprocedural states
V46	Other dependence on machines and devices
V49.60-V49.77	Upper and lower limb amputation status
V49.81-V49.85	Other specified conditions influencing health status
V50	Elective surgery for purposes other than remedying health states
V51	Aftercare involving the use of plastic surgery
V52	Fitting and adjustment of prosthetic device and implant
V53	Fitting and adjustment of other device
V54	Other orthopedic aftercare
V55	Attention to artificial openings
V56	Encounter for dialysis and dialysis catheter care

V57	Care involving use of rehabilitation procedures	E885.1	Fall from roller skates
V58	Encounter for other and unspecified procedures and aftercare	E885.2	Fall from skateboard
V59	Donors	E885.3	Fall from skis
V60	Housing, household, and economic circumstances	E885.4	Fall from snowboard
V61	Other family circumstances	E886.0	Fall on same level from collision, pushing, or shoving, by or with other person, In sports
V62	Other psychosocial circumstances	E890.0-E890.9	Conflagration in private dwelling
V64	Persons encountering health services for specific procedures, not carried out	E893.0	Accident caused by ignition of clothing, from controlled fire in private dwelling
V65	Other persons seeking consultation	E893.2	Accident caused by ignition of clothing, from controlled fire not in building or structure
V66	Convalescence and palliative care	E894	Ignition of highly inflammable material
V67	Follow-up examination	E895	Accident caused by controlled fire in private dwelling
V68	Encounters for administrative purposes	E897	Accident caused by controlled fire not in building or structure
V69	Problems related to lifestyle	E917.0	Striking against or struck accidentally by objects or persons, in sports without subsequent fall
V70	General medical examination		
V71	Observation and evaluation for suspected condition not found	E917.1	Striking against or struck accidentally by objects or persons, caused by a crowd, by collective fear or panic without subsequent fall
V72	Special investigations and examinations		
V73	Special screening examination for viral and chlamydial diseases	E917.2	Striking against or struck accidentally by objects or persons, in running water without subsequent fall
V74	Special screening examination for bacterial and spirochetal diseases	E917.5	Striking against or struck accidentally by objects or persons, object in sports with subsequent fall
V75	Special screening examination for other infectious diseases	E917.6	Striking against or struck accidentally by objects or persons, caused by a crowd, by collective fear or panic with subsequent fall
V76	Special screening for malignant neoplasms		
V77	Special screening for endocrine, nutritional, metabolic, and immunity disorders		
V78	Special screening for disorders of blood and blood-forming organs	E919	Accident caused by machinery (Except E919.2)
		E921	Accident caused by explosion of pressure vessel
V79	Special screening for mental disorders and developmental handicaps	E922	Accident caused by firearm and air gun missile
		E926.2	Visible and ultraviolet light sources
V80	Special screening for neurological, eye, and ear diseases	E928.0-E928.8	Other and unspecified environmental and accidental causes
V81	Special screening for cardiovascular, respiratory, and genitourinary diseases	E929.0-E929.9	Late effects of accidental injury
		E959	Late effects of self-inflicted injury
V82	Special screening for other conditions	E970-E978	Legal intervention
V83	Genetic carrier status	E979	Terrorism
V84	Genetic susceptibility to disease	E981	Poisoning by gases in domestic use, undetermined whether accidentally or purposely inflicted
V85	Body Mass Index		
V86	Estrogen receptor status	E982	Poisoning by other gases, undetermined whether accidentally or purposely inflicted
V87.32	Contact with and (suspected) exposure to algae bloom		
V87.4	Personal history of drug therapy	E985	Injury by firearms, air guns and explosives, undetermined whether accidentally or purposely inflicted
V88	Acquired absence of other organs and tissue		
V89	Suspected maternal and fetal conditions not found	E987.0	Falling from high place, undetermined whether accidentally or purposely inflicted, residential premises
V90	Retained foreign body		
V91	Multiple gestation placenta status	E987.2	Falling from high place, undetermined whether accidentally or purposely inflicted, natural sites
E000	External cause status		
E001-E030	Activity	E989	Late effects of injury, undetermined whether accidentally or purposely inflicted
E800-E807	Railway accidents		
E810-E819	Motor vehicle traffic accidents	E990-E999	Injury resulting from operations of war
E820-E825	Motor vehicle nontraffic accidents		
E826-E829	Other road vehicle accidents		
E830-E838	Water transport accidents		
E840-E845	Air and space transport accidents		
E846-E848	Vehicle accidents not elsewhere classifiable		
E849	Place of occurrence (Except E849.7)		
E883.1	Accidental fall into well		
E883.2	Accidental fall into storm drain or manhole		
E884.0	Fall from playground equipment		
E884.1	Fall from cliff		
E885.0	Fall from (nonmotorized) scooter		

A

AAT (alpha-1 antitrypsin) deficiency 273.4

AAV (disease) (illness) (infection) — *see* Human immunodeficiency virus (disease) (illness) (infection)

Abactio — *see* Abortion, induced

Abactus venter — *see* Abortion, induced

Abarognosis 781.99

Abasia (-astasia) 307.9
- atactica 781.3
- choreic 781.3
- hysterical 300.11
- paroxysmal trepidant 781.3
- spastic 781.3
- trembling 781.3
- trepidans 781.3

Abderhalden-Kaufmann-Lignac syndrome (cystinosis) 270.0

Abdomen, abdominal — *see also* condition
- accordion 306.4
- acute 789.0 ☑
- angina 557.1
- burst 868.00
- convulsive equivalent (*see also* Epilepsy) 345.5 ☑
- heart 746.87
- muscle deficiency syndrome 756.79
- obstipum 756.79

Abdominalgia 789.0 ☑
- periodic 277.31

Abduction contracture, hip or other joint — *see* Contraction, joint

Abercrombie's syndrome (amyloid degeneration) 277.39

Aberrant (congenital) — *see also* Malposition, congenital
- adrenal gland 759.1
- blood vessel NEC 747.60
  - arteriovenous NEC 747.60
  - cerebrovascular 747.81
  - gastrointestinal 747.61
  - lower limb 747.64
  - renal 747.62
  - spinal 747.82
  - upper limb 747.63
- breast 757.6
- endocrine gland NEC 759.2
- gastrointestinal vessel (peripheral) 747.61
- hepatic duct 751.69
- lower limb vessel (peripheral) 747.64
- pancreas 751.7
- parathyroid gland 759.2
- peripheral vascular vessel NEC 747.60
- pituitary gland (pharyngeal) 759.2
- renal blood vessel 747.62
- sebaceous glands, mucous membrane, mouth 750.26
- spinal vessel 747.82
- spleen 759.0
- testis (descent) 752.51
- thymus gland 759.2
- thyroid gland 759.2
- upper limb vessel (peripheral) 747.63

Aberratio
- lactis 757.6
- testis 752.51

Aberration — *see also* Anomaly
- chromosome — *see* Anomaly, chromosome(s)
- distantial 368.9
- mental (*see also* Disorder, mental, nonpsychotic) 300.9

Abetalipoproteinemia 272.5

Abionarce 780.79

Abiotrophy 799.89

Ablatio
- placentae — *see* Placenta, ablatio
- retinae (*see also* Detachment, retina) 361.9

Ablation
- pituitary (gland) (with hypofunction) 253.7
- placenta — *see* Placenta, ablatio
- uterus 621.8

Ablepharia, ablepharon, ablephary 743.62

Ablepsia — *see* Blindness

Ablepsy — *see* Blindness

Ablutomania 300.3

Abnormal, abnormality, abnormalities — *see also* Anomaly
- acid-base balance 276.4
  - fetus or newborn — *see* Distress, fetal
- adaptation curve, dark 368.63
- alveolar ridge 525.9
- amnion 658.9 ☑
  - affecting fetus or newborn 762.9
- anatomical relationship NEC 759.9
- apertures, congenital, diaphragm 756.6
- auditory perception NEC 388.40
- autosomes NEC 758.5
  - 13 758.1
  - 18 758.2
  - 21 or 22 758.0
  - D₁ 758.1
  - E₃ 758.2
  - G 758.0
- ballistocardiogram 794.39
- basal metabolic rate (BMR) 794.7
- biosynthesis, testicular androgen 257.2
- blood level (of)
  - cobalt 790.6
  - copper 790.6
  - iron 790.6
  - lead 790.6
  - lithium 790.6
  - magnesium 790.6
  - mineral 790.6
  - zinc 790.6
- blood pressure
  - elevated (without diagnosis of hypertension) 796.2
  - low (*see also* Hypotension) 458.9
    - reading (incidental) (isolated) (nonspecific) 796.3
- blood sugar 790.29
- bowel sounds 787.5
- breathing behavior — *see* Respiration
- caloric test 794.19
- cervix (acquired) NEC 622.9
  - congenital 752.40
  - in pregnancy or childbirth 654.6 ☑
    - causing obstructed labor 660.2 ☑
      - affecting fetus or newborn 763.1
- chemistry, blood NEC 790.6
- chest sounds 786.7
- chorion 658.9 ☑
  - affecting fetus or newborn 762.9
- chromosomal NEC 758.89
  - analysis, nonspecific result 795.2
  - autosomes (*see also* Abnormal, autosomes NEC) 758.5
  - fetal, (suspected) affecting management of pregnancy 655.1 ☑
  - sex 758.81
- clinical findings NEC 796.4
- communication — *see* Fistula
- configuration of pupils 379.49
- coronary
  - artery 746.85
  - vein 746.9
- cortisol-binding globulin 255.8
- course, Eustachian tube 744.24
- creatinine clearance 794.4
- dentofacial NEC 524.9
  - functional 524.50
  - specified type NEC 524.89
- development, developmental NEC 759.9
  - bone 756.9
  - central nervous system 742.9
- direction, teeth 524.30
- Dynia (*see also* Defect, coagulation) 286.9
- Ebstein 746.2
- echocardiogram 793.2
- echoencephalogram 794.01
- echogram NEC — *see* Findings, abnormal, structure
- electrocardiogram (ECG) (EKG) 794.31
- electroencephalogram (EEG) 794.02
- electromyogram (EMG) 794.17
  - ocular 794.14
- electro-oculogram (EOG) 794.12
- electroretinogram (ERG) 794.11
- erythrocytes 289.9

Abnormal, abnormality, abnormalities — *see also* Anomaly — *continued*
- erythrocytes — *continued*
  - congenital, with perinatal jaundice 282.9 [774.0]
- Eustachian valve 746.9
- excitability under minor stress 301.9
- fat distribution 782.9
- feces 787.7
- fetal heart rate — *see* Distress, fetal
- fetus NEC
  - affecting management of pregnancy — *see* Pregnancy, management affected by, fetal
  - causing disproportion 653.7 ☑
    - affecting fetus or newborn 763.1
    - causing obstructed labor 660.1 ☑
      - affecting fetus or newborn 763.1
  - findings without manifest disease — *see* Findings, abnormal
- fluid
  - amniotic 792.3
  - cerebrospinal 792.0
  - peritoneal 792.9
  - pleural 792.9
  - synovial 792.9
  - vaginal 792.9
- forces of labor NEC 661.9 ☑
  - affecting fetus or newborn 763.7
- form, teeth 520.2
- function studies
  - auditory 794.15
  - bladder 794.9
  - brain 794.00
  - cardiovascular 794.30
  - endocrine NEC 794.6
  - kidney 794.4
  - liver 794.8
  - nervous system
    - central 794.00
    - peripheral 794.19
  - oculomotor 794.14
  - pancreas 794.9
  - placenta 794.9
  - pulmonary 794.2
  - retina 794.11
  - special senses 794.19
  - spleen 794.9
  - thyroid 794.5
  - vestibular 794.16
- gait 781.2
  - hysterical 300.11
- gastrin secretion 251.5
- globulin
  - cortisol-binding 255.8
  - thyroid-binding 246.8
- glucagon secretion 251.4
- glucose 790.29
  - in pregnancy, childbirth, or puerperium 648.8 ☑
    - fetus or newborn 775.0
  - non-fasting 790.29
- gravitational (G) forces or states 994.9
- hair NEC 704.2
- hard tissue formation in pulp 522.3
- head movement 781.0
- heart
  - rate
    - fetus, affecting liveborn infant
      - before the onset of labor 763.81
      - during labor 763.82
      - unspecified as to time of onset 763.83
    - intrauterine
      - before the onset of labor 763.81
      - during labor 763.82
      - unspecified as to time of onset 763.83
    - newborn
      - before the onset of labor 763.81
      - during labor 763.82
      - unspecified as to time of onset 763.83
  - shadow 793.2
  - sounds NEC 785.3

Abnormal, abnormality, abnormalities — *see also* Anomaly — *continued*
- hemoglobin (*see also* Disease, hemoglobin) 282.7
  - trait — *see* Trait, hemoglobin, abnormal
- hemorrhage, uterus — *see* Hemorrhage, uterus
- histology NEC 795.4
- increase
  - in
    - appetite 783.6
    - development 783.9
- involuntary movement 781.0
- jaw closure 524.51
- karyotype 795.2
- knee jerk 796.1
- labor NEC 661.9 ☑
  - affecting fetus or newborn 763.7
- laboratory findings — *see* Findings, abnormal
- length, organ or site, congenital — *see* Distortion
- liver function test 790.6
- loss of height 781.91
- loss of weight 783.21
- lung shadow 793.19
- mammogram 793.80
  - calcification 793.89
  - calculus 793.89
  - microcalcification 793.81
- Mantoux test 795.51
- membranes (fetal)
  - affecting fetus or newborn 762.9
  - complicating pregnancy 658.8 ☑
- menstruation — *see* Menstruation
- metabolism (*see also* condition) 783.9
- movement 781.0
  - disorder NEC 333.90
    - sleep related, unspecified 780.58
    - specified NEC 333.99
  - head 781.0
  - involuntary 781.0
  - specified type NEC 333.99
- muscle contraction, localized 728.85
- myoglobin (Aberdeen) (Annapolis) 289.9
- narrowness, eyelid 743.62
- optokinetic response 379.57
- organs or tissues of pelvis NEC
  - in pregnancy or childbirth 654.9 ☑
    - affecting fetus or newborn 763.89
    - causing obstructed labor 660.2 ☑
      - affecting fetus or newborn 763.1
  - origin — *see* Malposition, congenital
- palmar creases 757.2
- Papanicolaou (smear)
  - anus 796.70
    - with
      - atypical squamous cells
        - cannot exclude high grade squamous intraepithelial lesion (ASC-H) 796.72
        - of undetermined significance (ASC-US) 796.71
      - cytologic evidence of malignancy 796.76
      - high grade squamous intraepithelial lesion (HGSIL) 796.74
      - low grade squamous intraepithelial lesion (LGSIL) 796.73
    - glandular 796.70
    - specified finding NEC 796.79
  - cervix 795.00
    - with
      - atypical squamous cells
        - cannot exclude high grade squamous intraepithelial lesion (ASC-H) 795.02
        - of undetermined significance (ASC-US) 795.01
      - cytologic evidence of malignancy 795.06
      - high grade squamous intraepithelial lesion (HGSIL) 795.04

☑ **Additional Digit Required — Refer to the Tabular List for Digit Selection**   ▽ **Subterms under main terms may continue to next column or page**

Abnormal, abnormality, abnormalities —
  see also Anomaly — *continued*
    Papanicolaou — *continued*
      cervix — *continued*
        with — *continued*
          low grade squamous intraepithe-
            lial lesion (LGSIL) 795.03
          nonspecific finding NEC 795.09
        other site 796.9
        vagina 795.10
          with
            atypical squamous cells
              cannot exclude high grade
                squamous intraepithe-
                lial lesion (ASC-H)
                795.12
              of undetermined significance
                (ASC-US) 795.11
            cytologic evidence of malignancy
              795.16
            high grade squamous intraepithe-
              lial lesion (HGSIL) 795.14
            low grade squamous intraepithe-
              lial lesion (LGSIL) 795.13
        glandular 795.10
        specified finding NEC 795.19
  parturition
    affecting fetus or newborn 763.9
    mother — *see* Delivery, complicated
  pelvis (bony) — *see* Deformity, pelvis
  percussion, chest 786.7
  periods (grossly) (*see also* Menstruation)
    626.9
  phonocardiogram 794.39
  placenta — *see* Placenta, abnormal
  plantar reflex 796.1
  plasma protein — *see* Deficiency, plasma,
    protein
  pleural folds 748.8
  position (*see also* Malposition)
    gravid uterus 654.4 ☑
      causing obstructed labor 660.2 ☑
        affecting fetus or newborn 763.1
  posture NEC 781.92
  presentation (fetus) — *see* Presentation,
    fetus, abnormal
  product of conception NEC 631.8
  puberty — *see* Puberty
  pulmonary
    artery 747.39
    function, newborn 770.89
    test results 794.2
    ventilation, newborn 770.89
      hyperventilation 786.01
  pulsations in neck 785.1
  pupil reflexes 379.40
  quality of milk 676.8 ☑
  radiological examination 793.99
    abdomen NEC 793.6
    biliary tract 793.3
    breast 793.89
      mammogram NOS 793.80
      mammographic
        calcification 793.89
        calculus 793.89
        microcalcification 793.81
    gastrointestinal tract 793.4
    genitourinary organs 793.5
    head 793.0
    image test inconclusive due to excess
      body fat 793.91
    intrathoracic organ NEC 793.2
    lung (field) 793.19
    musculoskeletal system 793.7
    retroperitoneum 793.6
    skin and subcutaneous tissue 793.99
    skull 793.0
  red blood cells 790.09
    morphology 790.09
    volume 790.09
  reflex NEC 796.1
  renal function test 794.4
  respiration signs — *see* Respiration
  response to nerve stimulation 794.10
  retinal correspondence 368.34
  rhythm, heart (*see also* Arrhythmia)

Abnormal, abnormality, abnormalities —
  see also Anomaly — *continued*
  rhythm, heart (*see also* Arrhythmia) — *con-
    tinued*
    fetus — *see* Distress, fetal
  saliva 792.4
  scan
    brain 794.09
    kidney 794.4
    liver 794.8
    lung 794.2
    thyroid 794.5
  secretion
    gastrin 251.5
    glucagon 251.4
  semen 792.2
  serum level (of)
    acid phosphatase 790.5
    alkaline phosphatase 790.5
    amylase 790.5
    enzymes NEC 790.5
    lipase 790.5
  shape
    cornea 743.41
    gallbladder 751.69
    gravid uterus 654.4 ☑
      affecting fetus or newborn 763.89
      causing obstructed labor 660.2 ☑
        affecting fetus or newborn 763.1
    head (*see also* Anomaly, skull) 756.0
    organ or site, congenital NEC — *see*
      Distortion
  sinus venosus 747.40
  size
    fetus, complicating delivery 653.5 ☑
      causing obstructed labor 660.1 ☑
    gallbladder 751.69
    head (*see also* Anomaly, skull) 756.0
    organ or site, congenital NEC — *see*
      Distortion
    teeth 520.2
  skin and appendages, congenital NEC 757.9
  soft parts of pelvis — *see* Abnormal, organs
    or tissues of pelvis
  spermatozoa 792.2
  sputum (amount) (color) (excessive) (odor)
    (purulent) 786.4
  stool NEC 787.7
    bloody 578.1
      occult 792.1
    bulky 787.7
    color (dark) (light) 792.1
    content (fat) (mucus) (pus) 792.1
    occult blood 792.1
  synchondrosis 756.9
  test results without manifest disease — *see*
    Findings, abnormal
  thebesian valve 746.9
  thermography — *see* Findings, abnormal,
    structure
  threshold, cones or rods (eye) 368.63
  thyroid-binding globulin 246.8
  thyroid product 246.8
  toxicology (findings) NEC 796.0
  tracheal cartilage (congenital) 748.3
  transport protein 273.8
  ultrasound results — *see* Findings, abnor-
    mal, structure
  umbilical cord
    affecting fetus or newborn 762.6
    complicating delivery 663.9 ☑
    specified NEC 663.8 ☑
  union
    cricoid cartilage and thyroid cartilage
      748.3
    larynx and trachea 748.3
    thyroid cartilage and hyoid bone 748.3
  urination NEC 788.69
    psychogenic 306.53
    stream
      intermittent 788.61
      slowing 788.62
      splitting 788.61
      weak 788.62
    urgency 788.63
  urine (constituents) NEC 791.9

Abnormal, abnormality, abnormalities —
  see also Anomaly — *continued*
  uterine hemorrhage (*see also* Hemorrhage,
    uterus) 626.9
    climacteric 627.0
    postmenopausal 627.1
  vagina (acquired) (congenital)
    in pregnancy or childbirth 654.7 ☑
      affecting fetus or newborn 763.89
      causing obstructed labor 660.2 ☑
        affecting fetus or newborn 763.1
  vascular sounds 785.9
  vectorcardiogram 794.39
  visually evoked potential (VEP) 794.13
  vulva (acquired) (congenital)
    in pregnancy or childbirth 654.8 ☑
      affecting fetus or newborn 763.89
      causing obstructed labor 660.2 ☑
        affecting fetus or newborn 763.1
  weight
    gain 783.1
      of pregnancy 646.1 ☑
        with hypertension — *see* Tox-
          emia, of pregnancy
    loss 783.21
  x-ray examination — *see* Abnormal, radio-
    logical examination

Abnormally formed uterus — *see* Anomaly,
  uterus
Abnormity (any organ or part) — *see* Anomaly
ABO
  hemolytic disease 773.1
  incompatibility (due to transfusion of blood
    or blood products)
    with hemolytic transfusion reaction
      (HTR) (not specified as acute or
      delayed) 999.61
      24 hours or more after transfusion
        999.63
      acute 999.62
      delayed 999.63
      less than 24 hours after transfusion
        999.62
      unspecified time after transfusion
        999.61
    reaction 999.60
      specified NEC 999.69
Abocclusion 524.20
Abolition, language 784.69
Aborter, habitual or recurrent NEC
  without current pregnancy 629.81
  current abortion (*see also* Abortion, sponta-
    neous) 634.9 ☑
    affecting fetus or newborn 761.8
  observation in current pregnancy 646.3 ☑
Abortion (complete) (incomplete) (inevitable)
  (with retained products of conception)
  637.9 ☑

Note — Use the following fifth-digit
subclassification with categories
634–637:

0   unspecified

1   incomplete

2   complete

---

  with
    complication(s) (any) following previous
      abortion — *see* category 639 ☑
    damage to pelvic organ (laceration)
      (rupture) (tear) 637.2 ☑
    embolism (air) (amniotic fluid) (blood
      clot) (pulmonary) (pyemic) (sep-
      tic) (soap) 637.6 ☑
    genital tract and pelvic infection
      637.0 ☑
    hemorrhage, delayed or excessive
      637.1 ☑
    metabolic disorder 637.4 ☑
    renal failure (acute) 637.3 ☑
    sepsis (genital tract) (pelvic organ)
      637.0 ☑
      urinary tract 637.7 ☑
    shock (postoperative) (septic) 637.5 ☑
    specified complication NEC 637.7 ☑

Abortion — *continued*
  with — *continued*
    toxemia 637.3 ☑
    unspecified complication(s) 637.8 ☑
    urinary tract infection 637.7 ☑
  accidental — *see* Abortion, spontaneous
  artificial — *see* Abortion, induced
  attempted (failed) — *see* Abortion, failed
  criminal — *see* Abortion, illegal
  early — *see* Abortion, spontaneous
  elective — *see* Abortion, legal
  failed (legal) 638.9
    with
      damage to pelvic organ (laceration)
        (rupture) (tear) 638.2
      embolism (air) (amniotic fluid) (blood
        clot) (pulmonary) (pyemic)
        (septic) (soap) 638.6
      genital tract and pelvic infection
        638.0
      hemorrhage, delayed or excessive
        638.1
      metabolic disorder 638.4
      renal failure (acute) 638.3
      sepsis (genital tract) (pelvic organ)
        638.0
        urinary tract 638.7
      shock (postoperative) (septic) 638.5
      specified complication NEC 638.7
      toxemia 638.3
      unspecified complication(s) 638.8
      urinary tract infection 638.7
  fetal indication — *see* Abortion, legal
  fetus 779.6
  following threatened abortion — *see* Abor-
    tion, by type
  habitual or recurrent (care during pregnan-
    cy) 646.3 ☑
    with current abortion (*see also* Abortion,
      spontaneous) 634.9 ☑
      affecting fetus or newborn 761.8
    without current pregnancy 629.81
  homicidal — *see* Abortion, illegal
  illegal 636.9 ☑
    with
      damage to pelvic organ (laceration)
        (rupture) (tear) 636.2 ☑
      embolism (air) (amniotic fluid) (blood
        clot) (pulmonary) (pyemic)
        (septic) (soap) 636.6 ☑
      genital tract and pelvic infection
        636.0 ☑
      hemorrhage, delayed or excessive
        636.1 ☑
      metabolic disorder 636.4 ☑
      renal failure 636.3 ☑
      sepsis (genital tract) (pelvic organ)
        636.0 ☑
        urinary tract 636.7 ☑
      shock (postoperative) (septic)
        636.5 ☑
      specified complication NEC 636.7 ☑
      toxemia 636.3 ☑
      unspecified complication(s) 636.8 ☑
      urinary tract infection 636.7 ☑
    fetus 779.6
  induced 637.9 ☑
    illegal — *see* Abortion, illegal
    legal indications — *see* Abortion, legal
    medical indications — *see* Abortion, le-
      gal
    therapeutic — *see* Abortion, legal
  late — *see* Abortion, spontaneous
  legal (legal indication) (medical indication)
    (under medical supervision) 635.9 ☑
    with
      damage to pelvic organ (laceration)
        (rupture) (tear) 635.2 ☑
      embolism (air) (amniotic fluid) (blood
        clot) (pulmonary) (pyemic)
        (septic) (soap) 635.6 ☑
      genital tract and pelvic infection
        635.0 ☑
      hemorrhage, delayed or excessive
        635.1 ☑

☑ **Additional Digit Required** — Refer to the Tabular List for Digit Selection   ⩊ **Subterms under main terms may continue to next column or page**

2 — Volume 2   ▶◀ **Revised Text**   ● **New Line**   ▲ **Revised Code**   **2013 ICD-9-CM**

Abortion — *continued*
  legal — *continued*
    with — *continued*
      metabolic disorder 635.4 ☑
      renal failure (acute) 635.3 ☑
      sepsis (genital tract) (pelvic organ) 635.0 ☑
      urinary tract 635.7 ☑
      shock (postoperative) (septic) 635.5 ☑
      specified complication NEC 635.7 ☑
      toxemia 635.3 ☑
      unspecified complication(s) 635.8 ☑
      urinary tract infection 635.7 ☑
    fetus 779.6
  medical indication — *see* Abortion, legal
  mental hygiene problem — *see* Abortion, legal
  missed 632
  operative — *see* Abortion, legal
  psychiatric indication — *see* Abortion, legal
  recurrent — *see* Abortion, spontaneous
  self-induced — *see* Abortion, illegal
  septic — *see* Abortion, by type, with sepsis
  spontaneous 634.9 ☑
    with
      damage to pelvic organ (laceration) (rupture) (tear) 634.2 ☑
      embolism (air) (amniotic fluid) (blood clot) (pulmonary) (pyemic) (septic) (soap) 634.6 ☑
      genital tract and pelvic infection 634.0 ☑
      hemorrhage, delayed or excessive 634.1 ☑
      metabolic disorder 634.4 ☑
      renal failure 634.3 ☑
      sepsis (genital tract) (pelvic organ) 634.0 ☑
        urinary tract 634.7 ☑
      shock (postoperative) (septic) 634.5 ☑
      specified complication NEC 634.7 ☑
      toxemia 634.3 ☑
      unspecified complication(s) 634.8 ☑
      urinary tract infection 634.7 ☑
    fetus 761.8
    threatened 640.0 ☑
      affecting fetus or newborn 762.1
  surgical — *see* Abortion, legal
  therapeutic — *see* Abortion, legal
  threatened 640.0 ☑
    affecting fetus or newborn 762.1
  tubal — *see* Pregnancy, tubal
  voluntary — *see* Abortion, legal
Abortus fever 023.9
Aboulomania 301.6
Abrachia 755.20
Abrachiatism 755.20
Abrachiocephalia 759.89
Abrachiocephalus 759.89
Abrami's disease (acquired hemolytic jaundice) 283.9
Abramov-Fiedler myocarditis (acute isolated myocarditis) 422.91
Abrasion — *see also* Injury, superficial, by site
  cornea 918.1
  dental 521.20
    extending into
      dentine 521.22
      pulp 521.23
    generalized 521.25
    limited to enamel 521.21
    localized 521.24
  teeth, tooth (dentifrice) (habitual) (hard tissues) (occupational) (ritual) (traditional) (wedge defect) (*see also* Abrasion, dental) 521.20
Abrikossov's tumor (M9580/0) — *see also* Neoplasm, connective tissue, benign
  malignant (M9580/3) — *see* Neoplasm, connective tissue, malignant
Abrism 988.8
Abruption, placenta — *see* Placenta, abruptio
Abruptio placentae — *see* Placenta, abruptio

Abscess (acute) (chronic) (infectional) (lymphangitic) (metastatic) (multiple) (pyogenic) (septic) (with lymphangitis) — *see also* Cellulitis 682.9
  abdomen, abdominal
    cavity 567.22
    wall 682.2
  abdominopelvic 567.22
  accessory sinus (chronic) (*see also* Sinusitis) 473.9
  adrenal (capsule) (gland) 255.8
  alveolar 522.5
    with sinus 522.7
  amebic 006.3
    bladder 006.8
    brain (with liver or lung abscess) 006.5
    liver (without mention of brain or lung abscess) 006.3
      with
        brain abscess (and lung abscess) 006.5
        lung abscess 006.4
    lung (with liver abscess) 006.4
      with brain abscess 006.5
    seminal vesicle 006.8
    specified site NEC 006.8
    spleen 006.8
  anaerobic 040.0
  ankle 682.6
  anorectal 566
  antecubital space 682.3
  antrum (chronic) (Highmore) (*see also* Sinusitis, maxillary) 473.0
  anus 566
  apical (tooth) 522.5
    with sinus (alveolar) 522.7
  appendix 540.1
  areola (acute) (chronic) (nonpuerperal) 611.0
    puerperal, postpartum 675.1 ☑
  arm (any part, above wrist) 682.3
  artery (wall) 447.2
  atheromatous 447.2
  auditory canal (external) 380.10
  auricle (ear) (staphylococcal) (streptococcal) 380.10
  axilla, axillary (region) 682.3
    lymph gland or node 683
  back (any part) 682.2
  Bartholin's gland 616.3
    with
      abortion — *see* Abortion, by type, with sepsis
      ectopic pregnancy (*see also* categories 633.0–633.9) 639.0
      molar pregnancy (*see also* categories 630–632) 639.0
    complicating pregnancy or puerperium 646.6 ☑
    following
      abortion 639.0
      ectopic or molar pregnancy 639.0
  bartholinian 616.3
  Bezold's 383.01
  bile, biliary, duct or tract (*see also* Cholecystitis) 576.8
  bilharziasis 120.1
  bladder (wall) 595.89
    amebic 006.8
  bone (subperiosteal) (*see also* Osteomyelitis) 730.0 ☑
    accessory sinus (chronic) (*see also* Sinusitis) 473.9
    acute 730.0 ☑
    chronic or old 730.1 ☑
    jaw (lower) (upper) 526.4
    mastoid — *see* Mastoiditis, acute
    petrous (*see also* Petrositis) 383.20
    spinal (tuberculous) (*see also* Tuberculosis) 015.0 ☑ *[730.88]*
      nontuberculous 730.08
  bowel 569.5
  brain (any part) 324.0
    amebic (with liver or lung abscess) 006.5
    cystic 324.0
    late effect — *see* category 326

Abscess — *see also* Cellulitis — *continued*
  brain — *continued*
    otogenic 324.0
    tuberculous (*see also* Tuberculosis) 013.3 ☑
  breast (acute) (chronic) (nonpuerperal) 611.0
    newborn 771.5
    puerperal, postpartum 675.1 ☑
    tuberculous (*see also* Tuberculosis) 017.9 ☑
  broad ligament (chronic) (*see also* Disease, pelvis, inflammatory) 614.4
    acute 614.3
  Brodie's (chronic) (localized) (*see also* Osteomyelitis) 730.1 ☑
  bronchus 519.19
  buccal cavity 528.3
  bulbourethral gland 597.0
  bursa 727.89
    pharyngeal 478.29
  buttock 682.5
  canaliculus, breast 611.0
  canthus 372.20
  cartilage 733.99
  cecum 569.5
    with appendicitis 540.1
  cerebellum, cerebellar 324.0
    late effect — *see* category 326
  cerebral (embolic) 324.0
    late effect — *see* category 326
  cervical (neck region) 682.1
    lymph gland or node 683
    stump (*see also* Cervicitis) 616.0
  cervix (stump) (uteri) (*see also* Cervicitis) 616.0
  cheek, external 682.0
    inner 528.3
  chest 510.9
    with fistula 510.0
    wall 682.2
  chin 682.0
  choroid 363.00
  ciliary body 364.3
  circumtonsillar 475
  cold (tuberculous) (*see also* Tuberculosis, abscess)
    articular — *see* Tuberculosis, joint
  colon (wall) 569.5
  colostomy or enterostomy 569.61
  conjunctiva 372.00
  connective tissue NEC 682.9
  cornea 370.55
    with ulcer 370.00
  corpus
    cavernosum 607.2
    luteum (*see also* Salpingo-oophoritis) 614.2
  Cowper's gland 597.0
  cranium 324.0
  cul-de-sac (Douglas') (posterior) (*see also* Disease, pelvis, inflammatory) 614.4
    acute 614.3
  dental 522.5
    with sinus (alveolar) 522.7
  dentoalveolar 522.5
    with sinus (alveolar) 522.7
  diaphragm, diaphragmatic 567.22
  digit NEC 681.9
  Douglas' cul-de-sac or pouch (*see also* Disease, pelvis, inflammatory) 614.4
    acute 614.3
  Dubois' 090.5
  ductless gland 259.8
  ear
    acute 382.00
    external 380.10
    inner 386.30
    middle — *see* Otitis media
  elbow 682.3
  endamebic — *see* Abscess, amebic
  entamebic — *see* Abscess, amebic
  enterostomy 569.61
  epididymis 604.0
  epidural 324.9
    brain 324.0

Abscess — *see also* Cellulitis — *continued*
  epidural — *continued*
    late effect — *see* category 326
    spinal cord 324.1
  epiglottis 478.79
  epiploon, epiploic 567.22
  erysipelatous (*see also* Erysipelas) 035
  esophagostomy 530.86
  esophagus 530.19
  ethmoid (bone) (chronic) (sinus) (*see also* Sinusitis, ethmoidal) 473.2
  external auditory canal 380.10
  extradural 324.9
    brain 324.0
    late effect — *see* category 326
    spinal cord 324.1
  extraperitoneal — *see* Abscess, peritoneum
  eye 360.00
  eyelid 373.13
  face (any part, except eye) 682.0
  fallopian tube (*see also* Salpingo-oophoritis) 614.2
  fascia 728.89
  fauces 478.29
  fecal 569.5
  femoral (region) 682.6
  filaria, filarial (*see also* Infestation, filarial) 125.9
  finger (any) (intrathecal) (periosteal) (subcutaneous) (subcuticular) 681.00
  fistulous NEC 682.9
  flank 682.2
  foot (except toe) 682.7
  forearm 682.3
  forehead 682.0
  frontal (sinus) (chronic) (*see also* Sinusitis, frontal) 473.1
  gallbladder (*see also* Cholecystitis, acute) 575.0
  gastric 535.0 ☑
  genital organ or tract NEC
    female 616.9
      with
        abortion — *see* Abortion, by type, with sepsis
        ectopic pregnancy (*see also* categories 633.0–633.9) 639.0
        molar pregnancy (*see also* categories 630–632) 639.0
      following
        abortion 639.0
        ectopic or molar pregnancy 639.0
      puerperal, postpartum, childbirth 670.8 ☑
    male 608.4
  genitourinary system, tuberculous (*see also* Tuberculosis) 016.9 ☑
  gingival 523.30
  gland, glandular (lymph) (acute) NEC 683
  glottis 478.79
  gluteal (region) 682.5
  gonorrheal NEC (*see also* Gonococcus) 098.0
  groin 682.2
  gum 523.30
  hand (except finger or thumb) 682.4
  head (except face) 682.8
  heart 429.89
  heel 682.7
  helminthic (*see also* Infestation, by specific parasite) 128.9
  hepatic 572.0
    amebic (*see also* Abscess, liver, amebic) 006.3
    duct 576.8
  hip 682.6
    tuberculous (active) (*see also* Tuberculosis) 015.1 ☑
  ileocecal 540.1
  ileostomy (bud) 569.61
  iliac (region) 682.2
    fossa 540.1
  iliopsoas 567.31
    nontuberculous 728.89
    tuberculous (*see also* Tuberculosis) 015.0 ☑ *[730.88]*
  infraclavicular (fossa) 682.3

☑ **Additional Digit Required — Refer to the Tabular List for Digit Selection**
▽ **Subterms under main terms may continue to next column or page**

2013 ICD-9-CM   ▶◀ Revised Text   ● New Line   ▲ Revised Code   Volume 2 — 3

Abortion — Abscess

Abscess — *see also* Cellulitis — *continued*
  inguinal (region) 682.2
    lymph gland or node 683
  intersphincteric (anus) 566
  intestine, intestinal 569.5
    rectal 566
  intra-abdominal (*see also* Abscess, peritoneum) 567.22
    postoperative 998.59
  intracranial 324.0
    late effect — *see* category 326
  intramammary — *see* Abscess, breast
  intramastoid (*see also* Mastoiditis, acute) 383.00
  intraorbital 376.01
  intraperitoneal 567.22
  intraspinal 324.1
    late effect — *see* category 326
  intratonsillar 475
  iris 364.3
  ischiorectal 566
  jaw (bone) (lower) (upper) 526.4
    skin 682.0
  joint (*see also* Arthritis, pyogenic) 711.0 ☑
    vertebral (tuberculous) (*see also* Tuberculosis) 015.0 ☑ *[730.88]*
      nontuberculous 724.8
  kidney 590.2
    with
      abortion — *see* Abortion, by type, with urinary tract infection
      calculus 592.0
      ectopic pregnancy (*see also* categories 633.0–633.9) 639.8
      molar pregnancy (*see also* categories 630–632) 639.8
    complicating pregnancy or puerperium 646.6 ☑
      affecting fetus or newborn 760.1
    following
      abortion 639.8
      ectopic or molar pregnancy 639.8
  knee 682.6
    joint 711.06
    tuberculous (active) (*see also* Tuberculosis) 015.2 ☑
  labium (majus) (minus) 616.4
    complicating pregnancy, childbirth, or puerperium 646.6 ☑
  lacrimal (passages) (sac) (*see also* Dacryocystitis) 375.30
    caruncle 375.30
    gland (*see also* Dacryoadenitis) 375.00
  lacunar 597.0
  larynx 478.79
  lateral (alveolar) 522.5
    with sinus 522.7
  leg, except foot 682.6
  lens 360.00
  lid 373.13
  lingual 529.0
    tonsil 475
  lip 528.5
  Littre's gland 597.0
  liver 572.0
    amebic 006.3
      with
        brain abscess (and lung abscess) 006.5
        lung abscess 006.4
      due to Entamoeba histolytica 006.3
    dysenteric (*see also* Abscess, liver, amebic) 006.3
    pyogenic 572.0
    tropical (*see also* Abscess, liver, amebic) 006.3
  loin (region) 682.2
  lumbar (tuberculous) (*see also* Tuberculosis) 015.0 ☑ *[730.88]*
    nontuberculous 682.2
  lung (miliary) (putrid) 513.0
    amebic (with liver abscess) 006.4
      with brain abscess 006.5
  lymphangitic, acute — *see* Cellulitis
  lymph, lymphatic, gland or node (acute) 683
    any site, except mesenteric 683

Abscess — *see also* Cellulitis — *continued*
  lymph, lymphatic, gland or node — *continued*
    mesentery 289.2
  malar 526.4
  mammary gland — *see* Abscess, breast
  marginal (anus) 566
  mastoid (process) (*see also* Mastoiditis, acute) 383.00
    subperiosteal 383.01
  maxilla, maxillary 526.4
    molar (tooth) 522.5
      with sinus 522.7
    premolar 522.5
    sinus (chronic) (*see also* Sinusitis, maxillary) 473.0
  mediastinum 513.1
  meibomian gland 373.12
  meninges (*see also* Meningitis) 320.9
  mesentery, mesenteric 567.22
  mesosalpinx (*see also* Salpingo-oophoritis) 614.2
  milk 675.1 ☑
  Monro's (psoriasis) 696.1
  mons pubis 682.2
  mouth (floor) 528.3
  multiple sites NEC 682.9
  mural 682.2
  muscle 728.89
    psoas 567.31
  myocardium 422.92
  nabothian (follicle) (*see also* Cervicitis) 616.0
  nail (chronic) (with lymphangitis) 681.9
    finger 681.02
    toe 681.11
  nasal (fossa) (septum) 478.19
    sinus (chronic) (*see also* Sinusitis) 473.9
  nasopharyngeal 478.29
  nates 682.5
  navel 682.2
    newborn NEC 771.4
  neck (region) 682.1
    lymph gland or node 683
  nephritic (*see also* Abscess, kidney) 590.2
  nipple 611.0
    puerperal, postpartum 675.0 ☑
  nose (septum) 478.19
    external 682.0
  omentum 567.22
  operative wound 998.59
  orbit, orbital 376.01
  ossifluent — *see* Abscess, bone
  ovary, ovarian (corpus luteum) (*see also* Salpingo-oophoritis) 614.2
  oviduct (*see also* Salpingo-oophoritis) 614.2
  palate (soft) 528.3
    hard 526.4
  palmar (space) 682.4
  pancreas (duct) 577.0
  paradontal 523.30
  parafrenal 607.2
  parametric, parametrium (chronic) (*see also* Disease, pelvis, inflammatory) 614.4
    acute 614.3
  paranephric 590.2
  parapancreatic 577.0
  parapharyngeal 478.22
  pararectal 566
  parasinus (*see also* Sinusitis) 473.9
  parauterine (*see also* Disease, pelvis, inflammatory) 614.4
    acute 614.3
  paravaginal (*see also* Vaginitis) 616.10
  parietal region 682.8
  parodontal 523.30
  parotid (duct) (gland) 527.3
    region 528.3
  parumbilical 682.2
    newborn 771.4
  pectoral (region) 682.2
  pelvirectal 567.22
  pelvis, pelvic
    female (chronic) (*see also* Disease, pelvis, inflammatory) 614.4
      acute 614.3

Abscess — *see also* Cellulitis — *continued*
  pelvis, pelvic — *continued*
    male, peritoneal (cellular tissue) — *see* Abscess, peritoneum
    tuberculous (*see also* Tuberculosis) 016.9 ☑
  penis 607.2
    gonococcal (acute) 098.0
      chronic or duration of 2 months or over 098.2
  perianal 566
  periapical 522.5
    with sinus (alveolar) 522.7
  periappendiceal 540.1
  pericardial 420.99
  pericecal 540.1
  pericemental 523.30
  pericholecystic (*see also* Cholecystitis, acute) 575.0
  pericoronal 523.30
  peridental 523.30
  perigastric 535.0 ☑
  perimetric (*see also* Disease, pelvis, inflammatory) 614.4
    acute 614.3
  perinephric, perinephritic (*see also* Abscess, kidney) 590.2
  perineum, perineal (superficial) 682.2
    deep (with urethral involvement) 597.0
    urethra 597.0
  periodontal (parietal) 523.31
    apical 522.5
  periosteum, periosteal (*see also* Periostitis) 730.3 ☑
    with osteomyelitis (*see also* Osteomyelitis) 730.2 ☑
      acute or subacute 730.0 ☑
      chronic or old 730.1 ☑
  peripleuritic 510.9
    with fistula 510.0
  periproctic 566
  periprostatic 601.2
  perirectal (staphylococcal) 566
  perirenal (tissue) (*see also* Abscess, kidney) 590.2
  perisinuous (nose) (*see also* Sinusitis) 473.9
  peritoneum, peritoneal (perforated) (ruptured) 567.22
    with
      abortion — *see* Abortion, by type, with sepsis
      appendicitis 540.1
      ectopic pregnancy (*see also* categories 633.0–633.9) 639.0
      molar pregnancy (*see also* categories 630–632) 639.0
    following
      abortion 639.0
      ectopic or molar pregnancy 639.0
    pelvic, female (*see also* Disease, pelvis, inflammatory) 614.4
      acute 614.3
    postoperative 998.59
    puerperal, postpartum, childbirth 670.8 ☑
    tuberculous (*see also* Tuberculosis) 014.0 ☑
  peritonsillar 475
  perityphlic 540.1
  periureteral 593.89
  periurethral 597.0
    gonococcal (acute) 098.0
      chronic or duration of 2 months or over 098.2
  periuterine (*see also* Disease, pelvis, inflammatory) 614.4
    acute 614.3
  perivesical 595.89
  pernicious NEC 682.9
  petrous bone — *see* Petrositis
  phagedenic NEC 682.9
    chancroid 099.0
  pharynx, pharyngeal (lateral) 478.29
  phlegmonous NEC 682.9
  pilonidal 685.0
  pituitary (gland) 253.8

Abscess — *see also* Cellulitis — *continued*
  pleura 510.9
    with fistula 510.0
  popliteal 682.6
  postanal 566
  postcecal 540.1
  postlaryngeal 478.79
  postnasal 478.19
  postpharyngeal 478.24
  posttonsillar 475
  posttyphoid 002.0
  Pott's (*see also* Tuberculosis) 015.0 ☑ *[730.88]*
  pouch of Douglas (chronic) (*see also* Disease, pelvis, inflammatory) 614.4
  premammary — *see* Abscess, breast
  prepatellar 682.6
  prostate (*see also* Prostatitis) 601.2
    gonococcal (acute) 098.12
      chronic or duration of 2 months or over 098.32
  psoas 567.31
    nontuberculous 728.89
    tuberculous (*see also* Tuberculosis) 015.0 ☑ *[730.88]*
  pterygopalatine fossa 682.8
  pubis 682.2
  puerperal — *see* Puerperal, abscess, by site
  pulmonary — *see* Abscess, lung
  pulp, pulpal (dental) 522.0
    finger 681.01
    toe 681.10
  pyemic — *see* Septicemia
  pyloric valve 535.0 ☑
  rectovaginal septum 569.5
  rectovesical 595.89
  rectum 566
  regional NEC 682.9
  renal (*see also* Abscess, kidney) 590.2
  retina 363.00
  retrobulbar 376.01
  retrocecal 567.22
  retrolaryngeal 478.79
  retromammary — *see* Abscess, breast
  retroperineal 682.2
  retroperitoneal 567.38
    postprocedural 998.59
  retropharyngeal 478.24
    tuberculous (*see also* Tuberculosis) 012.8 ☑
  retrorectal 566
  retrouterine (*see also* Disease, pelvis, inflammatory) 614.4
    acute 614.3
  retrovesical 595.89
  root, tooth 522.5
    with sinus (alveolar) 522.7
  round ligament (*see also* Disease, pelvis, inflammatory) 614.4
    acute 614.3
  rupture (spontaneous) NEC 682.9
  sacrum (tuberculous) (*see also* Tuberculosis) 015.0 ☑ *[730.88]*
    nontuberculous 730.08
  salivary duct or gland 527.3
  scalp (any part) 682.8
  scapular 730.01
  sclera 379.09
  scrofulous (*see also* Tuberculosis) 017.2 ☑
  scrotum 608.4
  seminal vesicle 608.0
    amebic 006.8
  septal, dental 522.5
    with sinus (alveolar) 522.7
  septum (nasal) 478.19
  serous (*see also* Periostitis) 730.3 ☑
  shoulder 682.3
  side 682.2
  sigmoid 569.5
  sinus (accessory) (chronic) (nasal) (*see also* Sinusitis) 473.9
    intracranial venous (any) 324.0
      late effect — *see* category 326
  Skene's duct or gland 597.0
  skin NEC 682.9

☑ **Additional Digit Required — Refer to the Tabular List for Digit Selection**

🔻 **Subterms under main terms may continue to next column or page**

Abscess — see also Cellulitis — continued
  skin — continued
    tuberculous (primary) (see also Tuberculosis) 017.0 ☑
  sloughing NEC 682.9
  specified site NEC 682.8
    amebic 006.8
  spermatic cord 608.4
  sphenoidal (sinus) (see also Sinusitis, sphenoidal) 473.3
  spinal
    cord (any part) (staphylococcal) 324.1
      tuberculous (see also Tuberculosis) 013.5 ☑
    epidural 324.1
  spine (column) (tuberculous) (see also Tuberculosis) 015.0 ☑ [730.88]
    nontuberculous 730.08
  spleen 289.59
    amebic 006.8
  staphylococcal NEC 682.9
  stitch 998.59
  stomach (wall) 535.0 ☑
  strumous (tuberculous) (see also Tuberculosis) 017.2 ☑
  subarachnoid 324.9
    brain 324.0
    cerebral 324.0
    late effect — see category 326
    spinal cord 324.1
  subareolar (see also Abscess, breast)
    puerperal, postpartum 675.1 ☑
  subcecal 540.1
  subcutaneous NEC 682.9
  subdiaphragmatic 567.22
  subdorsal 682.2
  subdural 324.9
    brain 324.0
    late effect — see category 326
    spinal cord 324.1
  subgaleal 682.8
  subhepatic 567.22
  sublingual 528.3
    gland 527.3
  submammary — see Abscess, breast
  submandibular (region) (space) (triangle) 682.0
    gland 527.3
  submaxillary (region) 682.0
    gland 527.3
  submental (pyogenic) 682.0
    gland 527.3
  subpectoral 682.2
  subperiosteal — see Abscess, bone
  subperitoneal 567.22
  subphrenic (see also Abscess, peritoneum) 567.22
    postoperative 998.59
  subscapular 682.2
  subungual 681.9
  suburethral 597.0
  sudoriparous 705.89
  suppurative NEC 682.9
  supraclavicular (fossa) 682.3
  suprahepatic 567.22
  suprapelvic (see also Disease, pelvis, inflammatory) 614.4
    acute 614.3
  suprapubic 682.2
  suprarenal (capsule) (gland) 255.8
  sweat gland 705.89
  syphilitic 095.8
  teeth, tooth (root) 522.5
    with sinus (alveolar) 522.7
    supporting structures NEC 523.30
  temple 682.0
  temporal region 682.0
  temporosphenoidal 324.0
    late effect — see category 326
  tendon (sheath) 727.89
  testicle — see Orchitis
  thecal 728.89
  thigh (acquired) 682.6
  thorax 510.9
    with fistula 510.0
  throat 478.29

Abscess — see also Cellulitis — continued
  thumb (intrathecal) (periosteal) (subcutaneous) (subcuticular) 681.00
  thymus (gland) 254.1
  thyroid (gland) 245.0
  toe (any) (intrathecal) (periosteal) (subcutaneous) (subcuticular) 681.10
  tongue (staphylococcal) 529.0
  tonsil(s) (lingual) 475
  tonsillopharyngeal 475
  tooth, teeth (root) 522.5
    with sinus (alveolar) 522.7
      supporting structure NEC 523.30
  trachea 478.9
  trunk 682.2
  tubal (see also Salpingo-oophoritis) 614.2
  tuberculous — see Tuberculosis, abscess
  tubo-ovarian (see also Salpingo-oophoritis) 614.2
  tunica vaginalis 608.4
  umbilicus NEC 682.2
    newborn 771.4
  upper arm 682.3
  upper respiratory 478.9
  urachus 682.2
  urethra (gland) 597.0
  urinary 597.0
  uterus, uterine (wall) (see also Endometritis) 615.9
    ligament (see also Disease, pelvis, inflammatory) 614.4
      acute 614.3
    neck (see also Cervicitis) 616.0
  uvula 528.3
  vagina (wall) (see also Vaginitis) 616.10
  vaginorectal (see also Vaginitis) 616.10
  vas deferens 608.4
  vermiform appendix 540.1
  vertebra (column) (tuberculous) (see also Tuberculosis) 015.0 ☑ [730.88]
    nontuberculous 730.0 ☑
  vesical 595.89
  vesicouterine pouch (see also Disease, pelvis, inflammatory) 614.4
  vitreous (humor) (pneumococcal) 360.04
  vocal cord 478.5
  von Bezold's 383.01
  vulva 616.4
    complicating pregnancy, childbirth, or puerperium 646.6 ☑
  vulvovaginal gland (see also Vaginitis) 616.3
  web-space 682.4
  wrist 682.4
Absence (organ or part) (complete or partial)
  acoustic nerve 742.8
  adrenal (gland) (congenital) 759.1
    acquired V45.79
  albumin (blood) 273.8
  alimentary tract (complete) (congenital) (partial) 751.8
    lower 751.5
    upper 750.8
  alpha-fucosidase 271.8
  alveolar process (acquired) 525.8
    congenital 750.26
  anus, anal (canal) (congenital) 751.2
  aorta (congenital) 747.22
  aortic valve (congenital) 746.89
  appendix, congenital 751.2
  arm (acquired) V49.60
    above elbow V49.66
    below elbow V49.65
    congenital (see also Deformity, reduction, upper limb) 755.20
      lower — see Absence, forearm, congenital
      upper (complete) (partial) (with absence of distal elements, incomplete) 755.24
        with
          complete absence of distal elements 755.21
            forearm (incomplete) 755.23
  artery (congenital) (peripheral) NEC (see also Anomaly, peripheral vascular system) 747.60

Absence — continued
  artery (see also Anomaly, peripheral vascular system) — continued
    brain 747.81
    cerebral 747.81
    coronary 746.85
    pulmonary 747.31
    umbilical 747.5
  atrial septum 745.69
  auditory canal (congenital) (external) 744.01
  auricle (ear) (with stenosis or atresia of auditory canal), congenital 744.01
  bile, biliary duct (common) or passage (congenital) 751.61
  bladder (acquired) V45.74
    congenital 753.8
  bone (congenital) NEC 756.9
    marrow 284.9
      acquired (secondary) 284.89
      congenital 284.01
      hereditary 284.09
      idiopathic 284.9
    skull 756.0
  bowel sounds 787.5
  brain 740.0
    specified part 742.2
  breast(s) (acquired) V45.71
    congenital 757.6
  broad ligament (congenital) 752.19
  bronchus (congenital) 748.3
  calvarium, calvaria (skull) 756.0
  canaliculus lacrimalis, congenital 743.65
  carpal(s) (congenital) (complete) (partial) (with absence of distal elements, incomplete) (see also Deformity, reduction, upper limb) 755.28
    with complete absence of distal elements 755.21
  cartilage 756.9
  caudal spine 756.13
  cecum (acquired) (postoperative) (posttraumatic) V45.72
    congenital 751.2
  cementum 520.4
  cerebellum (congenital) (vermis) 742.2
  cervix (acquired) (uteri) V88.01
    with remaining uterus V88.03
      and uterus V88.01
    congenital 752.43
  chin, congenital 744.89
  cilia (congenital) 743.63
    acquired 374.89
  circulatory system, part NEC 747.89
  clavicle 755.51
  clitoris (congenital) 752.49
  coccyx, congenital 756.13
  cold sense (see also Disturbance, sensation) 782.0
  colon (acquired) (postoperative) V45.72
    congenital 751.2
  congenital
    lumen — see Atresia
    organ or site NEC — see Agenesis
    septum — see Imperfect, closure
  corpus callosum (congenital) 742.2
  cricoid cartilage 748.3
  diaphragm (congenital) (with hernia) 756.6
    with obstruction 756.6
  digestive organ(s) or tract, congenital (complete) (partial) 751.8
    acquired V45.79
    lower 751.5
    upper 750.8
  ductus arteriosus 747.89
  duodenum (acquired) (postoperative) V45.72
    congenital 751.1
  ear, congenital 744.09
    acquired V45.79
    auricle 744.01
    external 744.01
    inner 744.05
    lobe, lobule 744.21
    middle, except ossicles 744.03
      ossicles 744.04
    ossicles 744.04

Absence — continued
  ejaculatory duct (congenital) 752.89
  endocrine gland NEC (congenital) 759.2
  epididymis (congenital) 752.89
    acquired V45.77
  epiglottis, congenital 748.3
  epileptic (atonic) (typical) (see also Epilepsy) 345.0 ☑
  erythrocyte 284.9
  erythropoiesis 284.9
    congenital 284.01
  esophagus (congenital) 750.3
  Eustachian tube (congenital) 744.24
  extremity (acquired)
    congenital (see also Deformity, reduction) 755.4
    lower V49.70
    upper V49.60
  extrinsic muscle, eye 743.69
  eye (acquired) V45.78
    adnexa (congenital) 743.69
    congenital 743.00
    muscle (congenital) 743.69
  eyelid (fold), congenital 743.62
    acquired 374.89
  face
    bones NEC 756.0
    specified part NEC 744.89
  fallopian tube(s) (acquired) V45.77
    congenital 752.19
  femur, congenital (complete) (partial) (with absence of distal elements, incomplete) (see also Deformity, reduction, lower limb) 755.34
    with
      complete absence of distal elements 755.31
        tibia and fibula (incomplete) 755.33
  fibrin 790.92
  fibrinogen (congenital) 286.3
    acquired 286.6
  fibula, congenital (complete) (partial) (with absence of distal elements, incomplete) (see also Deformity, reduction, lower limb) 755.37
    with
      complete absence of distal elements 755.31
        tibia 755.35
          with
            complete absence of distal elements 755.31
              femur (incomplete) 755.33
                with complete absence of distal elements 755.31
  finger (acquired) V49.62
    congenital (complete) (partial) (see also Deformity, reduction, upper limb) 755.29
      meaning all fingers (complete) (partial) 755.21
      transverse 755.21
  fissures of lungs (congenital) 748.5
  foot (acquired) V49.73
    congenital (complete) 755.31
  forearm (acquired) V49.65
    congenital (complete) (partial) (with absence of distal elements, incomplete) (see also Deformity, reduction, upper limb) 755.25
      with
        complete absence of distal elements (hand and fingers) 755.21
          humerus (incomplete) 755.23
  fovea centralis 743.55
  fucosidase 271.8
  gallbladder (acquired) V45.79
    congenital 751.69
  gamma globulin (blood) 279.00
  genital organs
    acquired V45.77
    congenital
      female 752.89
        external 752.49

☑ Additional Digit Required — Refer to the Tabular List for Digit Selection   ▽ Subterms under main terms may continue to next column or page

2013 ICD-9-CM   ▶◀ Revised Text   ● New Line   ▲ Revised Code   Volume 2 — 5

Absence — *continued*
  genital organs — *continued*
    congenital — *continued*
      female — *continued*
        internal NEC 752.89
        male 752.89
        penis 752.69
  genitourinary organs, congenital NEC 752.89
  glottis 748.3
  gonadal, congenital NEC 758.6
  hair (congenital) 757.4
    acquired — *see* Alopecia
  hand (acquired) V49.63
    congenital (complete) (*see also* Deformity, reduction, upper limb) 755.21
  heart 759.89
    acquired — *see* Status, organ replacement
  heat sense (*see also* Disturbance, sensation) 782.0
  humerus, congenital (complete) (partial) (with absence of distal elements, incomplete) (*see also* Deformity, reduction, upper limb) 755.24
    with
      complete absence of distal elements 755.21
      radius and ulna (incomplete) 755.23
  hymen (congenital) 752.49
  ileum (acquired) (postoperative) (posttraumatic) V45.72
    congenital 751.1
  immunoglobulin, isolated NEC 279.03
    IgA 279.01
    IgG 279.03
    IgM 279.02
  incus (acquired) 385.24
    congenital 744.04
  internal ear (congenital) 744.05
  intestine (acquired) (small) V45.72
    congenital 751.1
    large 751.2
    large V45.72
      congenital 751.2
  iris (congenital) 743.45
  jaw — *see* Absence, mandible
  jejunum (acquired) V45.72
    congenital 751.1
  joint (acquired) (following prior explantation of joint prosthesis) (with or without presence of antibiotic-impregnated cement spacer) NEC V88.29
    congenital NEC 755.8
    hip V88.21
    knee V88.22
  kidney(s) (acquired) V45.73
    congenital 753.0
  labium (congenital) (majus) (minus) 752.49
  labyrinth, membranous 744.05
  lacrimal apparatus (congenital) 743.65
  larynx (congenital) 748.3
  leg (acquired) V49.70
    above knee V49.76
    below knee V49.75
    congenital (partial) (unilateral) (*see also* Deformity, reduction, lower limb) 755.31
      lower (complete) (partial) (with absence of distal elements, incomplete) 755.35
      with
        complete absence of distal elements (foot and toes) 755.31
        thigh (incomplete) 755.33
          with complete absence of distal elements 755.31
      upper — *see* Absence, femur
  lens (congenital) 743.35
    acquired 379.31
  ligament, broad (congenital) 752.19
  limb (acquired)
    congenital (complete) (partial) (*see also* Deformity, reduction) 755.4
      lower 755.30

Absence — *continued*
  limb — *continued*
    congenital (*see also* Deformity, reduction) — *continued*
      lower — *continued*
        complete 755.31
        incomplete 755.32
        longitudinal — *see* Deficiency, lower limb, longitudinal
        transverse 755.31
      upper 755.20
        complete 755.21
        incomplete 755.22
        longitudinal — *see* Deficiency, upper limb, longitudinal
        transverse 755.21
      lower NEC V49.70
      upper NEC V49.60
  lip 750.26
  liver (congenital) (lobe) 751.69
  lumbar (congenital) (vertebra) 756.13
    isthmus 756.11
    pars articularis 756.11
  lumen — *see* Atresia
  lung (bilateral) (congenital) (fissure) (lobe) (unilateral) 748.5
    acquired (any part) V45.76
  mandible (congenital) 524.09
  maxilla (congenital) 524.09
  menstruation 626.0
  metacarpal(s), congenital (complete) (partial) (with absence of distal elements, incomplete) (*see also* Deformity, reduction, upper limb) 755.28
    with all fingers, complete 755.21
  metatarsal(s), congenital (complete) (partial) (with absence of distal elements, incomplete) (*see also* Deformity, reduction, lower limb) 755.38
    with complete absence of distal elements 755.31
  muscle (congenital) (pectoral) 756.81
    ocular 743.69
  musculoskeletal system (congenital) NEC 756.9
  nail(s) (congenital) 757.5
  neck, part 744.89
  nerve 742.8
  nervous system, part NEC 742.8
  neutrophil 288.00
  nipple (congenital) 757.6
    acquired V45.71
  nose (congenital) 748.1
    acquired 738.0
  nuclear 742.8
  ocular muscle (congenital) 743.69
  organ
    of Corti (congenital) 744.05
    or site
      acquired V45.79
      congenital NEC 759.89
  osseous meatus (ear) 744.03
  ovary (acquired) V45.77
    congenital 752.0
  oviduct (acquired) V45.77
    congenital 752.19
  pancreas (congenital) 751.7
    acquired (postoperative) (posttraumatic) V88.11
    partial V88.12
    total V88.11
  parathyroid gland (congenital) 759.2
  parotid gland(s) (congenital) 750.21
  patella, congenital 755.64
  pelvic girdle (congenital) 755.69
  penis (congenital) 752.69
    acquired V45.77
  pericardium (congenital) 746.89
  perineal body (congenital) 756.81
  phalange(s), congenital 755.4
    lower limb (complete) (intercalary) (partial) (terminal) (*see also* Deformity, reduction, lower limb) 755.39
      meaning all toes (complete) (partial) 755.31

Absence — *continued*
  phalange(s), congenital — *continued*
    lower limb (*see also* Deformity, reduction, lower limb) — *continued*
      transverse 755.31
    upper limb (complete) (intercalary) (partial) (terminal) (*see also* Deformity, reduction, upper limb) 755.29
      meaning all digits (complete) (partial) 755.21
      transverse 755.21
  pituitary gland (congenital) 759.2
  postoperative — *see* Absence, by site, acquired
  prostate (congenital) 752.89
    acquired V45.77
  pulmonary
    artery 747.31
    trunk 747.31
    valve (congenital) 746.01
    vein 747.49
  punctum lacrimale (congenital) 743.65
  radius, congenital (complete) (partial) (with absence of distal elements, incomplete) 755.26
    with
      complete absence of distal elements 755.21
      ulna 755.25
        with
          complete absence of distal elements 755.21
          humerus (incomplete) 755.23
  ray, congenital 755.4
    lower limb (complete) (partial) (*see also* Deformity, reduction, lower limb) 755.38
      meaning all rays 755.31
      transverse 755.31
    upper limb (complete) (partial) (*see also* Deformity, reduction, upper limb) 755.28
      meaning all rays 755.21
      transverse 755.21
  rectum (congenital) 751.2
    acquired V45.79
  red cell 284.9
    acquired (secondary) 284.81
    congenital 284.01
    hereditary 284.01
    idiopathic 284.9
  respiratory organ (congenital) NEC 748.9
  rib (acquired) 738.3
    congenital 756.3
  roof of orbit (congenital) 742.0
  round ligament (congenital) 752.89
  sacrum, congenital 756.13
  salivary gland(s) (congenital) 750.21
  scapula 755.59
  scrotum, congenital 752.89
  seminal tract or duct (congenital) 752.89
    acquired V45.77
  septum (congenital) (*see also* Imperfect, closure, septum)
    atrial 745.69
      and ventricular 745.7
    between aorta and pulmonary artery 745.0
    ventricular 745.3
      and atrial 745.7
  sex chromosomes 758.81
  shoulder girdle, congenital (complete) (partial) 755.59
  skin (congenital) 757.39
  skull bone 756.0
    with
      anencephalus 740.0
      encephalocele 742.0
      hydrocephalus 742.3
        with spina bifida (*see also* Spina bifida) 741.0 ☒
      microcephalus 742.1
  spermatic cord (congenital) 752.89
  spinal cord 742.59
  spine, congenital 756.13

Absence — *continued*
  spleen (congenital) 759.0
    acquired V45.79
  sternum, congenital 756.3
  stomach (acquired) (partial) (postoperative) V45.75
    with postgastric surgery syndrome 564.2
    congenital 750.7
  submaxillary gland(s) (congenital) 750.21
  superior vena cava (congenital) 747.49
  tarsal(s), congenital (complete) (partial) (with absence of distal elements, incomplete) (*see also* Deformity, reduction, lower limb) 755.38
  teeth, tooth (congenital) 520.0
    with abnormal spacing 524.30
    acquired 525.10
      with malocclusion 524.30
      due to
        caries 525.13
        extraction 525.10
        periodontal disease 525.12
        trauma 525.11
  tendon (congenital) 756.81
  testis (congenital) 752.89
    acquired V45.77
  thigh (acquired) 736.89
  thumb (acquired) V49.61
    congenital 755.29
  thymus gland (congenital) 759.2
  thyroid (gland) (surgical) 246.8
    with hypothyroidism 244.0
    cartilage, congenital 748.3
    congenital 243
  tibia, congenital (complete) (partial) (with absence of distal elements, incomplete) (*see also* Deformity, reduction, lower limb) 755.36
    with
      complete absence of distal elements 755.31
      fibula 755.35
        with
          complete absence of distal elements 755.31
          femur (incomplete) 755.33
            with complete absence of distal elements 755.31
  toe (acquired) V49.72
    congenital (complete) (partial) 755.39
      meaning all toes 755.31
      transverse 755.31
    great V49.71
  tongue (congenital) 750.11
  tooth, teeth (congenital) 520.0
    with abnormal spacing 524.30
    acquired 525.10
      with malocclusion 524.30
      due to
        caries 525.13
        extraction 525.10
        periodontal disease 525.12
        trauma 525.11
  trachea (cartilage) (congenital) (rings) 748.3
  transverse aortic arch (congenital) 747.21
  tricuspid valve 746.1
  ulna, congenital (complete) (partial) (with absence of distal elements, incomplete) (*see also* Deformity, reduction, upper limb) 755.27
    with
      complete absence of distal elements 755.21
      radius 755.25
        with
          complete absence of distal elements 755.21
          humerus (incomplete) 755.23
  umbilical artery (congenital) 747.5
  ureter (congenital) 753.4
    acquired V45.74
  urethra, congenital 753.8
    acquired V45.74
  urinary system, part NEC, congenital 753.8
    acquired V45.74

☒ **Additional Digit Required — Refer to the Tabular List for Digit Selection**   ▽ **Subterms under main terms may continue to next column or page**

6 — Volume 2   ▶◀ Revised Text   ● New Line   ▲ Revised Code   **2013 ICD-9-CM**

Absence — *continued*
  uterus (acquired) V88.01
    with remaining cervical stump V88.02
      and cervix V88.01
    congenital 752.31
  uvula (congenital) 750.26
  vagina, congenital 752.45
    acquired V45.77
  vas deferens (congenital) 752.89
    acquired V45.77
  vein (congenital) (peripheral) NEC (*see also*
      Anomaly, peripheral vascular system)
      747.60
    brain 747.81
    great 747.49
    portal 747.49
    pulmonary 747.49
  vena cava (congenital) (inferior) (superior)
      747.49
  ventral horn cell 742.59
  ventricular septum 745.3
  vermis of cerebellum 742.2
  vertebra, congenital 756.13
  vulva, congenital 752.49
Absentia epileptica — *see also* Epilepsy
    345.0 ☑
Absinthemia — *see also* Dependence 304.6 ☑
Absinthism — *see also* Dependence 304.6 ☑
Absorbent system disease 459.89
Absorption
  alcohol, through placenta or breast milk
      760.71
  antibiotics, through placenta or breast milk
      760.74
  anticonvulsants, through placenta or breast
      milk 760.77
  antifungals, through placenta or breast milk
      760.74
  anti-infective, through placenta or breast
      milk 760.74
  antimetabolics, through placenta or breast
      milk 760.78
  chemical NEC 989.9
    specified chemical or substance — *see*
        Table of Drugs and Chemicals
    through placenta or breast milk (fetus
        or newborn) 760.70
      alcohol 760.71
      anticonvulsants 760.77
      antifungals 760.74
      anti-infective agents 760.74
      antimetabolics 760.78
      cocaine 760.75
      "crack" 760.75
      diethylstilbestrol [DES] 760.76
      hallucinogenic agents 760.73
      medicinal agents NEC 760.79
      narcotics 760.72
      obstetric anesthetic or analgesic drug
          763.5
      specified agent NEC 760.79
      suspected, affecting management of
          pregnancy 655.5 ☑
  cocaine, through placenta or breast milk
      760.75
  drug NEC (*see also* Reaction, drug)
    through placenta or breast milk (fetus
        or newborn) 760.70
      alcohol 760.71
      anticonvulsants 760.77
      antifungals 760.74
      anti-infective agents 760.74
      antimetabolics 760.78
      cocaine 760.75
      "crack" 760.75
      diethylstilbestrol [DES] 760.76
      hallucinogenic agents 760.73
      medicinal agents NEC 760.79
      narcotics 760.72
      obstetric anesthetic or analgesic drug
          763.5
      specified agent NEC 760.79
      suspected, affecting management of
          pregnancy 655.5 ☑
  fat, disturbance 579.8

Absorption — *continued*
  hallucinogenic agents, through placenta or
      breast milk 760.73
  immune sera, through placenta or breast
      milk 760.79
  lactose defect 271.3
  medicinal agents NEC, through placenta or
      breast milk 760.79
  narcotics, through placenta or breast milk
      760.72
  noxious substance — *see* Absorption,
      chemical
  protein, disturbance 579.8
  pus or septic, general — *see* Septicemia
  quinine, through placenta or breast milk
      760.74
  toxic substance — *see* Absorption, chemical
  uremic — *see* Uremia
Abstinence symptoms or syndrome
  alcohol 291.81
  drug 292.0
  neonatal 779.5
Abt-Letterer-Siwe syndrome (acute histiocy-
    tosis X) (M9722/3) 202.5 ☑
Abulia 799.89
Abulomania 301.6
Abuse
  adult 995.80
    emotional 995.82
    multiple forms 995.85
    neglect (nutritional) 995.84
    physical 995.81
    psychological 995.82
    sexual 995.83
  alcohol — *see also* Alcoholism 305.0 ☑
    dependent 303.9 ☑
    non-dependent 305.0 ☑
  child 995.50
    counseling
      perpetrator
        non-parent V62.83
        parent V61.22
      victim V61.21
    emotional 995.51
    multiple forms 995.59
    neglect (nutritional) 995.52
    physical 995.54
      shaken infant syndrome 995.55
    psychological 995.51
    sexual 995.53
  drugs, nondependent 305.9 ☑

Note — Use the following fifth-digit
subclassification with the following
codes: 305.0, 305.2–305.9:

  0   unspecified
  1   continuous
  2   episodic
  3   in remission
---

    amphetamine type 305.7 ☑
    antidepressants 305.8 ☑
    anxiolytic 305.4 ☑
    barbiturates 305.4 ☑
    caffeine 305.9 ☑
    cannabis 305.2 ☑
    cocaine type 305.6 ☑
    hallucinogens 305.3 ☑
    hashish 305.2 ☑
    hypnotic 305.4 ☑
    inhalant 305.9 ☑
    LSD 305.3 ☑
    marijuana 305.2 ☑
    mixed 305.9 ☑
    morphine type 305.5 ☑
    opioid type 305.5 ☑
    phencyclidine (PCP) 305.9 ☑
    sedative 305.4 ☑
    specified NEC 305.9 ☑
    tranquilizers 305.4 ☑
  spouse 995.80
  tobacco 305.1
Acalcerosis 275.40
Acalcicosis 275.40
Acalculia 784.69

Acalculia — *continued*
  developmental 315.1
Acanthocheilonemiasis 125.4
Acanthocytosis 272.5
Acanthokeratodermia 701.1
Acantholysis 701.8
  bullosa 757.39
Acanthoma (benign) (M8070/0) — *see also*
    Neoplasm, by site, benign
  malignant (M8070/3) — *see* Neoplasm, by
      site, malignant
Acanthosis (acquired) (nigricans) 701.2
  adult 701.2
  benign (congenital) 757.39
  congenital 757.39
  glycogenic
    esophagus 530.89
  juvenile 701.2
  tongue 529.8
Acanthrocytosis 272.5
Acapnia 276.3
Acarbia 276.2
Acardia 759.89
Acardiacus amorphus 759.89
Acardiotrophia 429.1
Acardius 759.89
Acariasis 133.9
  sarcoptic 133.0
Acaridiasis 133.9
Acarinosis 133.9
Acariosis 133.9
Acarodermatitis 133.9
  urticarioides 133.9
Acarophobia 300.29
Acatalasemia 277.89
Acatalasia 277.89
Acatamathesia 784.69
Acataphasia 784.59
Acathisia 781.0
  due to drugs 333.99
Acceleration, accelerated
  atrioventricular conduction 426.7
  idioventricular rhythm 427.89
Accessory (congenital)
  adrenal gland 759.1
  anus 751.5
  appendix 751.5
  atrioventricular conduction 426.7
  auditory ossicles 744.04
  auricle (ear) 744.1
  autosome(s) NEC 758.5
    21 or 22 758.0
  biliary duct or passage 751.69
  bladder 753.8
  blood vessels (peripheral) (congenital) NEC
      (*see also* Anomaly, peripheral vascu-
      lar system) 747.60
    cerebral 747.81
    coronary 746.85
  bone NEC 756.9
    foot 755.67
  breast tissue, axilla 757.6
  carpal bones 755.56
  cecum 751.5
  cervix 752.44
  chromosome(s) NEC 758.5
    13-15 758.1
    16-18 758.2
    21 or 22 758.0
    autosome(s) NEC 758.5
    D_1 758.1
    E_3 758.2
    G 758.0
    sex 758.81
  coronary artery 746.85
  cusp(s), heart valve NEC 746.89
    pulmonary 746.09
  cystic duct 751.69
  digits 755.00
  ear (auricle) (lobe) 744.1
  endocrine gland NEC 759.2
  external os 752.44
  eyelid 743.62
  eye muscle 743.69
  face bone(s) 756.0
  fallopian tube (fimbria) (ostium) 752.19

Accessory — *continued*
  fingers 755.01
  foreskin 605
  frontonasal process 756.0
  gallbladder 751.69
  genital organ(s)
    female 752.49
      external 752.49
      internal NEC 752.89
    male NEC 752.89
      penis 752.69
  genitourinary organs NEC 752.89
  heart 746.89
    valve NEC 746.89
      pulmonary 746.09
  hepatic ducts 751.69
  hymen 752.49
  intestine (large) (small) 751.5
  kidney 753.3
  lacrimal canal 743.65
  leaflet, heart valve NEC 746.89
    pulmonary 746.09
  ligament, broad 752.19
  liver (duct) 751.69
  lobule (ear) 744.1
  lung (lobe) 748.69
  muscle 756.82
  navicular of carpus 755.56
  nervous system, part NEC 742.8
  nipple 757.6
  nose 748.1
  organ or site NEC — *see* Anomaly, specified
      type NEC
  ovary 752.0
  oviduct 752.19
  pancreas 751.7
  parathyroid gland 759.2
  parotid gland (and duct) 750.22
  pituitary gland 759.2
  placental lobe — *see* Placenta, abnormal
  preauricular appendage 744.1
  prepuce 605
  renal arteries (multiple) 747.62
  rib 756.3
    cervical 756.2
  roots (teeth) 520.2
  salivary gland 750.22
  sesamoids 755.8
  sinus — *see* condition
  skin tags 757.39
  spleen 759.0
  sternum 756.3
  submaxillary gland 750.22
  tarsal bones 755.67
  teeth, tooth 520.1
    causing crowding 524.31
  tendon 756.89
  thumb 755.01
  thymus gland 759.2
  thyroid gland 759.2
  toes 755.02
  tongue 750.13
  tragus 744.1
  ureter 753.4
  urethra 753.8
  urinary organ or tract NEC 753.8
  uterus 752.2
  vagina 752.49
  valve, heart NEC 746.89
    pulmonary 746.09
  vertebra 756.19
  vocal cords 748.3
  vulva 752.49
Accident, accidental — *see also* condition
  birth NEC 767.9
  cardiovascular (*see also* Disease, cardiovas-
      cular) 429.2
  cerebral (*see also* Disease, cerebrovascular,
      acute) 434.91
  cerebrovascular (current) (CVA) (*see also*
      Disease, cerebrovascular, acute)
      434.91
    aborted 434.91
    embolic 434.11
    healed or old V12.54
    hemorrhagic — *see* Hemorrhage, brain

☑ **Additional Digit Required** — Refer to the Tabular List for Digit Selection   ▽ **Subterms under main terms may continue to next column or page**

2013 ICD-9-CM   ▶◀ **Revised Text**   ● **New Line**   ▲ **Revised Code**   Volume 2 — 7

Accident, accidental — *see also* condition — *continued*
  cerebrovascular (*see also* Disease, cerebrovascular, acute) — *continued*
    impending 435.9
    ischemic 434.91
    late effect — *see* Late effect(s) (of) cerebrovascular disease
    postoperative 997.02
    thrombotic 434.01
  coronary (*see also* Infarct, myocardium) 410.9 ☑
  craniovascular (*see also* Disease, cerebrovascular, acute) 436
  during pregnancy, to mother, affecting fetus or newborn 760.5
  heart, cardiac (*see also* Infarct, myocardium) 410.9 ☑
  intrauterine 779.89
  vascular — *see* Disease, cerebrovascular, acute
Accommodation
  disorder of 367.51
    drug-induced 367.89
    toxic 367.89
  insufficiency of 367.4
  paralysis of 367.51
    hysterical 300.11
  spasm of 367.53
Accouchement — *see* Delivery
Accreta placenta (without hemorrhage) 667.0 ☑
  with hemorrhage 666.0 ☑
Accretio cordis (nonrheumatic) 423.1
Accretions on teeth 523.6
Accumulation secretion, prostate 602.8
Acephalia, acephalism, acephaly 740.0
Acephalic 740.0
Acephalobrachia 759.89
Acephalocardia 759.89
Acephalocardius 759.89
Acephalochiria 759.89
Acephalochirus 759.89
Acephalogaster 759.89
Acephalostomus 759.89
Acephalothorax 759.89
Acephalus 740.0
Acetonemia 790.6
  diabetic 250.1 ☑
    due to secondary diabetes 249.1 ☑
Acetonglycosuria 982.8
Acetonuria 791.6
Achalasia 530.0
  cardia 530.0
  digestive organs congenital NEC 751.8
  esophagus 530.0
  pelvirectal 751.3
  psychogenic 306.4
  pylorus 750.5
  sphincteral NEC 564.89
Achard-Thiers syndrome (adrenogenital) 255.2
Ache(s) — *see* Pain
Acheilia 750.26
Acheiria 755.21
Achillobursitis 726.71
Achillodynia 726.71
Achlorhydria, achlorhydric 536.0
  anemia 280.9
  diarrhea 536.0
  neurogenic 536.0
  postvagotomy 564.2
  psychogenic 306.4
  secondary to vagotomy 564.2
Achloroblepsia 368.52
Achloropsia 368.52
Acholia 575.8
Acholuric jaundice (familial) (splenomegalic) — *see also* Spherocytosis 282.0
  acquired 283.9
Achondroplasia 756.4
Achrestic anemia 281.8
Achroacytosis, lacrimal gland 375.00
  tuberculous (*see also* Tuberculosis) 017.3 ☑
Achroma, cutis 709.00
Achromate (congenital) 368.54

Achromatopia 368.54
Achromatopsia (congenital) 368.54
Achromia
  congenital 270.2
  parasitica 111.0
  unguium 703.8
Achylia
  gastrica 536.8
    neurogenic 536.3
    psychogenic 306.4
  pancreatica 577.1
Achylosis 536.8
Acid
  burn (*see also* Burn, by site)
    from swallowing acid — *see* Burn, internal organs
  deficiency
    amide nicotinic 265.2
    amino 270.9
    ascorbic 267
    folic 266.2
    nicotinic (amide) 265.2
    pantothenic 266.2
  intoxication 276.2
  peptic disease 536.8
  stomach 536.8
    psychogenic 306.4
Acidemia 276.2
  arginosuccinic 270.6
  fetal
    affecting management of pregnancy 656.3 ☑
    before onset of labor, in liveborn infant 768.2
    during labor and delivery in liveborn infant 768.3
    intrauterine 656.3 ☑
    unspecified as to time of onset, in liveborn infant 768.4
  newborn 775.81
  pipecolic 270.7
Acidity, gastric (high) (low) 536.8
  psychogenic 306.4
Acidocytopenia 288.59
Acidocytosis 288.3
Acidopenia 288.59
Acidosis 276.2
  diabetic 250.1 ☑
    due to secondary diabetes 249.1 ☑
  fetal, affecting management of pregnancy 656.8 ☑
  fetal, affecting newborn 775.81
  kidney tubular 588.89
    newborn 775.81
  lactic 276.2
  metabolic NEC 276.2
    with respiratory acidosis 276.4
      of newborn 775.81
    late, of newborn 775.7
  newborn 775.81
  renal
    hyperchloremic 588.89
    tubular (distal) (proximal) 588.89
  respiratory 276.2
    complicated by
      metabolic acidosis 276.4
        of newborn 775.81
      metabolic alkalosis 276.4
Aciduria 791.9
  arginosuccinic 270.6
  beta-aminoisobutyric (BAIB) 277.2
  glutaric
    type I 270.7
    type II (type IIA, IIB, IIC) 277.85
    type III 277.86
  glycolic 271.8
  methylmalonic 270.3
    with glycinemia 270.7
  organic 270.9
  orotic (congenital) (hereditary) (pyrimidine deficiency) 281.4
Acladiosis 111.8
  skin 111.8
Aclasis
  diaphyseal 756.4
  tarsoepiphyseal 756.59

Acleistocardia 745.5
Aclusion 524.4
Acmesthesia 782.0
Acne (pustular) (vulgaris) 706.1
  agminata (*see also* Tuberculosis) 017.0 ☑
  artificialis 706.1
  atrophica 706.0
  cachecticorum (Hebra) 706.1
  conglobata 706.1
  conjunctiva 706.1
  cystic 706.1
  decalvans 704.09
  erythematosa 695.3
  eyelid 706.1
  frontalis 706.0
  indurata 706.1
  keloid 706.1
  lupoid 706.0
  necrotic, necrotica 706.0
    miliaris 704.8
  neonatal 706.1
  nodular 706.1
  occupational 706.1
  papulosa 706.1
  rodens 706.0
  rosacea 695.3
  scorbutica 267
  scrofulosorum (Bazin) (*see also* Tuberculosis) 017.0 ☑
  summer 692.72
  tropical 706.1
  varioliformis 706.0
Acneiform drug eruptions 692.3
Acnitis (primary) — *see also* Tuberculosis 017.0 ☑
Acomia 704.00
Acontractile bladder 344.61
Aconuresis — *see also* Incontinence 788.30
Acosta's disease 993.2
Acousma 780.1
Acoustic — *see* condition
Acousticophobia 300.29
Acquired — *see* condition
Acquired immune deficiency syndrome — *see* Human immunodeficiency virus (disease) (illness) (infection)
Acquired immunodeficiency syndrome — *see* Human immunodeficiency virus (disease) (illness) (infection)
Acragnosis 781.99
Acrania 740.0
Acroagnosis 781.99
Acroangiodermatitis 448.9
Acroasphyxia, chronic 443.89
Acrobrachycephaly 756.0
Acrobystiolith 608.89
Acrobystitis 607.2
Acrocephalopolysyndactyly 755.55
Acrocephalosyndactyly 755.55
Acrocephaly 756.0
Acrochondrohyperplasia 759.82
Acrocyanosis 443.89
  newborn 770.83
    meaning transient blue hands and feet — *omit code*
Acrodermatitis 686.8
  atrophicans (chronica) 701.8
  continua (Hallopeau) 696.1
  enteropathica 686.8
  Hallopeau's 696.1
  perstans 696.1
  pustulosa continua 696.1
  recalcitrant pustular 696.1
Acrodynia 985.0
Acrodysplasia 755.55
Acrohyperhidrosis — *see also* Hyperhidrosis 780.8
Acrokeratosis verruciformis 757.39
Acromastitis 611.0
Acromegaly, acromegalia (skin) 253.0
Acromelalgia 443.82
Acromicria, acromikria 756.59
Acronyx 703.0
Acropachyderma 757.39
Acropachy, thyroid — *see also* Thyrotoxicosis 242.9 ☑

Acroparesthesia 443.89
  simple (Schultz's type) 443.89
  vasomotor (Nothnagel's type) 443.89
Acropathy thyroid — *see also* Thyrotoxicosis 242.9 ☑
Acrophobia 300.29
Acroposthitis 607.2
Acroscleriasis — *see also* Scleroderma 710.1
Acroscleroderma — *see also* Scleroderma 710.1
Acrosclerosis — *see also* Scleroderma 710.1
Acrosphacelus 785.4
Acrosphenosyndactylia 755.55
Acrospiroma, eccrine (M8402/0) — *see* Neoplasm, skin, benign
Acrostealgia 732.9
Acrosyndactyly — *see also* Syndactylism 755.10
Acrotrophodynia 991.4
Actinic — *see also* condition
  cheilitis (due to sun) 692.72
    chronic NEC 692.74
    due to radiation, except from sun 692.82
  conjunctivitis 370.24
  dermatitis (due to sun) (*see also* Dermatitis, actinic) 692.70
    due to
      roentgen rays or radioactive substance 692.82
      ultraviolet radiation, except from sun 692.82
      sun NEC 692.70
  elastosis solare 692.74
  granuloma 692.73
  keratitis 370.24
  ophthalmia 370.24
  reticuloid 692.73
Actinobacillosis, general 027.8
Actinobacillus
  lignieresii 027.8
  mallei 024
  muris 026.1
Actinocutitis NEC — *see also* Dermatitis, actinic 692.70
Actinodermatitis NEC — *see also* Dermatitis, actinic 692.70
Actinomyces
  israelii (infection) — *see* Actinomycosis
  muris-ratti (infection) 026.1
Actinomycosis, actinomycotic 039.9
  with
    pneumonia 039.1
  abdominal 039.2
  cervicofacial 039.3
  cutaneous 039.0
  pulmonary 039.1
  specified site NEC 039.8
  thoracic 039.1
Actinoneuritis 357.89
Action, heart
  disorder 427.9
    postoperative 997.1
  irregular 427.9
    postoperative 997.1
    psychogenic 306.2
Active — *see* condition
Activity decrease, functional 780.99
Acute — *see also* condition
  abdomen NEC 789.0 ☑
  gallbladder (*see also* Cholecystitis, acute) 575.0
Acyanoblepsia 368.53
Acyanopsia 368.53
Acystia 753.8
Acystinervia — *see* Neurogenic, bladder
Acystineuria — *see* Neurogenic, bladder
Adactylia, adactyly (congenital) 755.4
  lower limb (complete) (intercalary) (partial) (terminal) (*see also* Deformity, reduction, lower limb) 755.39
    meaning all digits (complete) (partial) 755.31
    transverse (complete) (partial) 755.31
  upper limb (complete) (intercalary) (partial) (terminal) (*see also* Deformity, reduction, upper limb) 755.29

☑ **Additional Digit Required** — Refer to the Tabular List for Digit Selection   🆆 **Subterms under main terms may continue to next column or page**

8 — Volume 2   ▶◀ Revised Text   ● New Line   ▲ Revised Code   **2013 ICD-9-CM**

Adactylia, adactyly — *continued*
> upper limb (*see also* Deformity, reduction, upper limb) — *continued*
>> meaning all digits (complete) (partial) 755.21
>> transverse (complete) (partial) 755.21

Adair-Dighton syndrome (brittle bones and blue sclera, deafness) 756.51

Adamantinoblastoma (M9310/0) — *see* Ameloblastoma

Adamantinoma (M9310/0) — *see* Ameloblastoma

Adamantoblastoma (M9310/0) — *see* Ameloblastoma

Adams-Stokes (-Morgagni) disease or syndrome (syncope with heart block) 426.9

Adaptation reaction — *see also* Reaction, adjustment 309.9

Addiction — *see also* Dependence
> absinthe 304.6 ☑
> alcoholic (ethyl) (methyl) (wood) 303.9 ☑
>> complicating pregnancy, childbirth, or puerperium 648.4 ☑
>>> affecting fetus or newborn 760.71
>>> suspected damage to fetus affecting management of pregnancy 655.4 ☑
> drug (*see also* Dependence) 304.9 ☑
> ethyl alcohol 303.9 ☑
> heroin 304.0 ☑
> hospital 301.51
> methyl alcohol 303.9 ☑
> methylated spirit 303.9 ☑
> morphine (-like substances) 304.0 ☑
> nicotine 305.1
> opium 304.0 ☑
> tobacco 305.1
> wine 303.9 ☑

Addison's
> anemia (pernicious) 281.0
> disease (bronze) (primary adrenal insufficiency) 255.41
>> tuberculous (*see also* Tuberculosis) 017.6 ☑
> keloid (morphea) 701.0
> melanoderma (adrenal cortical hypofunction) 255.41

Addison-Biermer anemia (pernicious) 281.0

Addison-Gull disease — *see* Xanthoma

Addisonian crisis or melanosis (acute adrenocortical insufficiency) 255.41

Additional — *see also* Accessory
> chromosome(s) 758.5
>> 13-15 758.1
>> 16-18 758.2
>> 21 758.0
>> autosome(s) NEC 758.5
>> sex 758.81

Adduction contracture, hip or other joint — *see* Contraction, joint

ADEM (acute disseminated encephalomyelitis) (postinfectious) 136.9 *[323.61]*
> infectious 136.9 *[323.61]*
> noninfectious 323.81

Adenasthenia gastrica 536.0

Aden fever 061

Adenitis — *see also* Lymphadenitis 289.3
> acute, unspecified site 683
>> epidemic infectious 075
> axillary 289.3
>> acute 683
>> chronic or subacute 289.1
> Bartholin's gland 616.89
> bulbourethral gland (*see also* Urethritis) 597.89
> cervical 289.3
>> acute 683
>> chronic or subacute 289.1
> chancroid (Ducrey's bacillus) 099.0
> chronic (any lymph node, except mesenteric) 289.1
>> mesenteric 289.2
> Cowper's gland (*see also* Urethritis) 597.89
> epidemic, acute 075
> gangrenous 683
> gonorrheal NEC 098.89

Adenitis — *see also* Lymphadenitis — *continued*
> groin 289.3
>> acute 683
>> chronic or subacute 289.1
> infectious 075
> inguinal (region) 289.3
>> acute 683
>> chronic or subacute 289.1
> lymph gland or node, except mesenteric 289.3
>> acute 683
>> chronic or subacute 289.1
>> mesenteric (acute) (chronic) (nonspecific) (subacute) 289.2
> mesenteric (acute) (chronic) (nonspecific) (subacute) 289.2
>> due to Pasteurella multocida (P. septica) 027.2
> parotid gland (suppurative) 527.2
> phlegmonous 683
> salivary duct or gland (any) (recurring) (suppurative) 527.2
> scrofulous (*see also* Tuberculosis) 017.2 ☑
> septic 289.3
> Skene's duct or gland (*see also* Urethritis) 597.89
> strumous, tuberculous (*see also* Tuberculosis) 017.2 ☑
> subacute, unspecified site 289.1
> sublingual gland (suppurative) 527.2
> submandibular gland (suppurative) 527.2
> submaxillary gland (suppurative) 527.2
> suppurative 683
> tuberculous — *see* Tuberculosis, lymph gland
> urethral gland (*see also* Urethritis) 597.89
> venereal NEC 099.8
> Wharton's duct (suppurative) 527.2

Adenoacanthoma (M8570/3) — *see* Neoplasm, by site, malignant

Adenoameloblastoma (M9300/0) 213.1
> upper jaw (bone) 213.0

Adenocarcinoma (M8140/3) — *see also* Neoplasm, by site, malignant

> *Note — The list of adjectival modifiers below is not exhaustive. A description of adenocarcinoma that does not appear in this list should be coded in the same manner as carcinoma with that description. Thus, "mixed acidophil-basophil adenocarcinoma," should be coded in the same manner as "mixed acidophil-basophil carcinoma," which appears in the list under "Carcinoma."*
>
> *Except where otherwise indicated, the morphological varieties of adenocarcinoma in the list below should be coded by site as for "Neoplasm, malignant."*

> with
>> apocrine metaplasia (M8573/3)
>> cartilaginous (and osseous) metaplasia (M8571/3)
>> osseous (and cartilaginous) metaplasia (M8571/3)
>> spindle cell metaplasia (M8572/3)
>> squamous metaplasia (M8570/3)
> acidophil (M8280/3)
>> specified site — *see* Neoplasm, by site, malignant
>> unspecified site 194.3
> acinar (M8550/3)
> acinic cell (M8550/3)
> adrenal cortical (M8370/3) 194.0
> alveolar (M8251/3)
>> and
>>> epidermoid carcinoma, mixed (M8560/3)
>>> squamous cell carcinoma, mixed (M8560/3)
> apocrine (M8401/3)
>> breast — *see* Neoplasm, breast, malignant
>> specified site NEC — *see* Neoplasm, skin, malignant

Adenocarcinoma — *see also* Neoplasm, by site, malignant — *continued*
> apocrine — *continued*
>> unspecified site 173.99
> basophil (M8300/3)
>> specified site — *see* Neoplasm, by site, malignant
>> unspecified site 194.3
> bile duct type (M8160/3)
>> liver 155.1
>> specified site NEC — *see* Neoplasm, by site, malignant
>> unspecified site 155.1
> bronchiolar (M8250/3) — *see* Neoplasm, lung, malignant
> ceruminous (M8420/3) 173.29
> chromophobe (M8270/3)
>> specified site — *see* Neoplasm, by site, malignant
>> unspecified site 194.3
> clear cell (mesonephroid type) (M8310/3)
> colloid (M8480/3)
> cylindroid type (M8200/3)
> diffuse type (M8145/3)
>> specified site — *see* Neoplasm, by site, malignant
>> unspecified site 151.9
> duct (infiltrating) (M8500/3)
>> with Paget's disease (M8541/3) — *see* Neoplasm, breast, malignant
>> specified site — *see* Neoplasm, by site, malignant
>> unspecified site 174.9
> embryonal (M9070/3)
> endometrioid (M8380/3) — *see* Neoplasm, by site, malignant
> eosinophil (M8280/3)
>> specified site — *see* Neoplasm, by site, malignant
>> unspecified site 194.3
> follicular (M8330/3)
>> and papillary (M8340/3) 193
>> moderately differentiated type (M8332/3) 193
>> pure follicle type (M8331/3) 193
>> specified site — *see* Neoplasm, by site, malignant
>> trabecular type (M8332/3) 193
>> unspecified type 193
>> well differentiated type (M8331/3) 193
> gelatinous (M8480/3)
> granular cell (M8320/3)
> Hürthle cell (M8290/3) 193
> in
>> adenomatous
>>> polyp (M8210/3)
>>> polyposis coli (M8220/3) 153.9
>> polypoid adenoma (M8210/3)
>> tubular adenoma (M8210/3)
>> villous adenoma (M8261/3)
> infiltrating duct (M8500/3)
>> with Paget's disease (M8541/3) — *see* Neoplasm, breast, malignant
>> specified site — *see* Neoplasm, by site, malignant
>> unspecified site 174.9
> inflammatory (M8530/3)
>> specified site — *see* Neoplasm, by site, malignant
>> unspecified site 174.9
> in situ (M8140/2) — *see* Neoplasm, by site, in situ
> intestinal type (M8144/3)
>> specified site — *see* Neoplasm, by site, malignant
>> unspecified site 151.9
> intraductal (noninfiltrating) (M8500/2)
>> papillary (M8503/2)
>>> specified site — *see* Neoplasm, by site, in situ
>>> unspecified site 233.0
>> specified site — *see* Neoplasm, by site, in situ
>> unspecified site 233.0

Adenocarcinoma — *see also* Neoplasm, by site, malignant — *continued*
> islet cell (M8150/3)
>> and exocrine, mixed (M8154/3)
>>> specified site — *see* Neoplasm, by site, malignant
>>> unspecified site 157.9
>> pancreas 157.4
>> specified site NEC — *see* Neoplasm, by site, malignant
>> unspecified site 157.4
> lobular (M8520/3)
>> specified site — *see* Neoplasm, by site, malignant
>> unspecified site 174.9
> medullary (M8510/3)
> mesonephric (M9110/3)
> mixed cell (M8323/3)
> mucinous (M8480/3)
> mucin-producing (M8481/3)
> mucoid (M8480/3) (*see also* Neoplasm, by site, malignant)
>> cell (M8300/3)
>>> specified site — *see* Neoplasm, by site, malignant
>>> unspecified site 194.3
> nonencapsulated sclerosing (M8350/3) 193
> oncocytic (M8290/3)
> oxyphilic (M8290/3)
> papillary (M8260/3)
>> and follicular (M8340/3) 193
>> intraductal (noninfiltrating) (M8503/2)
>>> specified site — *see* Neoplasm, by site, in situ
>>> unspecified site 233.0
>> serous (M8460/3)
>>> specified site — *see* Neoplasm, by site, malignant
>>> unspecified site 183.0
> papillocystic (M8450/3)
>> specified site — *see* Neoplasm, by site, malignant
>> unspecified site 183.0
> pseudomucinous (M8470/3)
>> specified site — *see* Neoplasm, by site, malignant
>> unspecified site 183.0
> renal cell (M8312/3) 189.0
> sebaceous (M8410/3)
> serous (M8441/3) (*see also* Neoplasm, by site, malignant)
>> papillary
>>> specified site — *see* Neoplasm, by site, malignant
>>> unspecified site 183.0
> signet ring cell (M8490/3)
> superficial spreading (M8143/3)
> sweat gland (M8400/3) — *see* Neoplasm, skin, malignant
> trabecular (M8190/3)
> tubular (M8211/3)
> villous (M8262/3)
> water-clear cell (M8322/3) 194.1

Adenofibroma (M9013/0)
> clear cell (M8313/0) — *see* Neoplasm, by site, benign
> endometrioid (M8381/0) 220
>> borderline malignancy (M8381/1) 236.2
>> malignant (M8381/3) 183.0
> mucinous (M9015/0)
>> specified site — *see* Neoplasm, by site, benign
>> unspecified site 220
> prostate
>> with
>>> other lower urinary tract symptoms (LUTS) 600.21
>>> urinary
>>>> obstruction 600.21
>>>> retention 600.21
> serous (M9014/0)
>> specified site — *see* Neoplasm, by site, benign
>> unspecified site 220
> specified site — *see* Neoplasm, by site, benign

☑ Additional Digit Required — Refer to the Tabular List for Digit Selection   ᵂ Subterms under main terms may continue to next column or page

2013 ICD-9-CM   ►◄ Revised Text   ● New Line   ▲ Revised Code   Volume 2 — 9

Adenofibroma — *continued*
  unspecified site 220
Adenofibrosis
  breast 610.2
  endometrioid 617.0
Adenoiditis 474.01
  acute 463
  chronic 474.01
    with chronic tonsillitis 474.02
Adenoids (congenital) (of nasal fossa) 474.9
  hypertrophy 474.12
  vegetations 474.2
Adenolipomatosis (symmetrical) 272.8
Adenolymphoma (M8561/0)
  specified site — *see* Neoplasm, by site, benign
  unspecified 210.2
Adenomatosis (M8220/0)
  endocrine (multiple) (M8360/1)
    single specified site — *see* Neoplasm, by site, uncertain behavior
    two or more specified sites 237.4
    unspecified site 237.4
  erosive of nipple (M8506/0) 217
  pluriendocrine — *see* Adenomatosis, endocrine
  pulmonary (M8250/1) 235.7
    malignant (M8250/3) — *see* Neoplasm, lung, malignant
  specified site — *see* Neoplasm, by site, benign
  unspecified site 211.3
Adenomatous
  cyst, thyroid (gland) — *see* Goiter, nodular
  goiter (nontoxic) (*see also* Goiter, nodular) 241.9
    toxic or with hyperthyroidism 242.3 ☑
Adenoma (sessile) (M8140/0) — *see also* Neoplasm, by site, benign

Note — Except where otherwise indicated, the morphological varieties of adenoma in the list below should be coded by site as for "Neoplasm, benign."

  acidophil (M8280/0)
    specified site — *see* Neoplasm, by site, benign
    unspecified site 227.3
  acinar (cell) (M8550/0)
  acinic cell (M8550/0)
  adrenal (cortex) (cortical) (functioning) (M8370/0) 227.0
    clear cell type (M8373/0) 227.0
    compact cell type (M8371/0) 227.0
    glomerulosa cell type (M8374/0) 227.0
    heavily pigmented variant (M8372/0) 227.0
    mixed cell type (M8375/0) 227.0
  alpha cell (M8152/0)
    pancreas 211.7
    specified site NEC — *see* Neoplasm, by site, benign
    unspecified site 211.7
  alveolar (M8251/0)
  apocrine (M8401/0)
    breast 217
    specified site NEC — *see* Neoplasm, skin, benign
    unspecified site 216.9
  basal cell (M8147/0)
  basophil (M8300/0)
    specified site — *see* Neoplasm, by site, benign
    unspecified site 227.3
  beta cell (M8151/0)
    pancreas 211.7
    specified site NEC — *see* Neoplasm, by site, benign
    unspecified site 211.7
  bile duct (M8160/0) 211.5
  black (M8372/0) 227.0
  bronchial (M8140/1) 235.7
    carcinoid type (M8240/3) — *see* Neoplasm, lung, malignant
    cylindroid type (M8200/3) — *see* Neoplasm, lung, malignant
  ceruminous (M8420/0) 216.2

Adenoma — *see* also Neoplasm, by site, benign — *continued*
  chief cell (M8321/0) 227.1
  chromophobe (M8270/0)
    specified site — *see* Neoplasm, by site, benign
    unspecified site 227.3
  clear cell (M8310/0)
  colloid (M8334/0)
    specified site — *see* Neoplasm, by site, benign
    unspecified site 226
  cylindroid type, bronchus (M8200/3) — *see* Neoplasm, lung, malignant
  duct (M8503/0)
  embryonal (M8191/0)
  endocrine, multiple (M8360/1)
    single specified site — *see* Neoplasm, by site, uncertain behavior
    two or more specified sites 237.4
    unspecified site 237.4
  endometrioid (M8380/0) (*see also* Neoplasm, by site, benign)
    borderline malignancy (M8380/1) — *see* Neoplasm, by site, uncertain behavior
  eosinophil (M8280/0)
    specified site — *see* Neoplasm, by site, benign
    unspecified site 227.3
  fetal (M8333/0)
    specified site — *see* Neoplasm, by site, benign
    unspecified site 226
  follicular (M8330/0)
    specified site — *see* Neoplasm, by site, benign
    unspecified site 226
  hepatocellular (M8170/0) 211.5
  Hürthle cell (M8290/0) 226
  intracystic papillary (M8504/0)
  islet cell (functioning) (M8150/0)
    pancreas 211.7
    specified site NEC — *see* Neoplasm, by site, benign
    unspecified site 211.7
  liver cell (M8170/0) 211.5
  macrofollicular (M8334/0)
    specified site NEC — *see* Neoplasm, by site, benign
    unspecified site 226
  malignant, malignum (M8140/3) — *see* Neoplasm, by site, malignant
  mesonephric (M9110/0)
  microfollicular (M8333/0)
    specified site — *see* Neoplasm, by site, benign
    unspecified site 226
  mixed cell (M8323/0)
  monomorphic (M8146/0)
  mucinous (M8480/0)
  mucoid cell (M8300/0)
    specified site — *see* Neoplasm, by site, benign
    unspecified site 227.3
  multiple endocrine (M8360/1)
    single specified site — *see* Neoplasm, by site, uncertain behavior
    two or more specified sites 237.4
    unspecified site 237.4
  nipple (M8506/0) 217
  oncocytic (M8290/0)
  oxyphilic (M8290/0)
  papillary (M8260/0) (*see also* Neoplasm, by site, benign)
    intracystic (M8504/0)
  papillotubular (M8263/0)
  Pick's tubular (M8640/0)
    specified site — *see* Neoplasm, by site, benign
    unspecified site
      female 220
      male 222.0
  pleomorphic (M8940/0)
  polypoid (M8210/0)
  prostate (benign) 600.20

Adenoma — *see* also Neoplasm, by site, benign — *continued*
  prostate — *continued*
    with
      other lower urinary tract symptoms (LUTS) 600.21
      urinary
        obstruction 600.21
        retention 600.21
  rete cell 222.0
  sebaceous, sebaceum (gland) (senile) (M8410/0) (*see also* Neoplasm, skin, benign)
    disseminata 759.5
  Sertoli cell (M8640/0)
    specified site — *see* Neoplasm, by site, benign
    unspecified site
      female 220
      male 222.0
  skin appendage (M8390/0) — *see* Neoplasm, skin, benign
  sudoriferous gland (M8400/0) — *see* Neoplasm, skin, benign
  sweat gland or duct (M8400/0) — *see* Neoplasm, skin, benign
  testicular (M8640/0)
    specified site — *see* Neoplasm, by site, benign
    unspecified site
      female 220
      male 222.0
  thyroid 226
  trabecular (M8190/0)
  tubular (M8211/0) (*see also* Neoplasm, by site, benign)
    papillary (M8460/3)
    Pick's (M8640/0)
      specified site — *see* Neoplasm, by site, benign
      unspecified site
        female 220
        male 222.0
  tubulovillous (M8263/0)
  villoglandular (M8263/0)
  villous (M8261/1) — *see* Neoplasm, by site, uncertain behavior
  water-clear cell (M8322/0) 227.1
  wolffian duct (M9110/0)
Adenomyoma (M8932/0) — *see also* Neoplasm, by site, benign
  prostate 600.20
    with
      other lower urinary tract symptoms (LUTS) 600.21
      urinary
        obstruction 600.21
        retention 600.21
Adenomyometritis 617.0
Adenomyosis (uterus) (internal) 617.0
Adenopathy (lymph gland) 785.6
  inguinal 785.6
  mediastinal 785.6
  mesentery 785.6
  syphilitic (secondary) 091.4
  tracheobronchial 785.6
    tuberculous (*see also* Tuberculosis) 012.1 ☑
      primary, progressive 010.8 ☑
  tuberculous (*see also* Tuberculosis, lymph gland) 017.2 ☑
    tracheobronchial 012.1 ☑
      primary, progressive 010.8 ☑
Adenopharyngitis 462
Adenophlegmon 683
Adenosalpingitis 614.1
Adenosarcoma (M8960/3) 189.0
Adenosclerosis 289.3
Adenosis
  breast (sclerosing) 610.2
  vagina, congenital 752.49
Adentia (complete) (partial) — *see also* Absence, teeth 520.0
Adherent
  labium (minus) 624.4
  pericardium (nonrheumatic) 423.1

Adherent — *continued*
  pericardium — *continued*
    rheumatic 393
  placenta 667.0 ☑
    with hemorrhage 666.0 ☑
  prepuce 605
  scar (skin) NEC 709.2
  tendon in scar 709.2
Adhesion(s), adhesive (postinfectional) (postoperative)
  abdominal (wall) (*see also* Adhesions, peritoneum) 568.0
  amnion to fetus 658.8 ☑
    affecting fetus or newborn 762.8
  appendix 543.9
  arachnoiditis — *see* Meningitis
  auditory tube (Eustachian) 381.89
  bands (*see also* Adhesions, peritoneum)
    cervix 622.3
    uterus 621.5
  bile duct (any) 576.8
  bladder (sphincter) 596.89
  bowel (*see also* Adhesions, peritoneum) 568.0
  cardiac 423.1
    rheumatic 398.99
  cecum (*see also* Adhesions, peritoneum) 568.0
  cervicovaginal 622.3
    congenital 752.49
    postpartal 674.8 ☑
      old 622.3
  cervix 622.3
  clitoris 624.4
  colon (*see also* Adhesions, peritoneum) 568.0
  common duct 576.8
  congenital (*see also* Anomaly, specified type NEC)
    fingers (*see also* Syndactylism, fingers) 755.11
    labium (majus) (minus) 752.49
    omental, anomalous 751.4
    ovary 752.0
    peritoneal 751.4
    toes (*see also* Syndactylism, toes) 755.13
    tongue (to gum or roof of mouth) 750.12
  conjunctiva (acquired) (localized) 372.62
    congenital 743.63
    extensive 372.63
  cornea — *see* Opacity, cornea
  cystic duct 575.8
  diaphragm (*see also* Adhesions, peritoneum) 568.0
  due to foreign body — *see* Foreign body
  duodenum (*see also* Adhesions, peritoneum) 568.0
    with obstruction 537.3
  ear, middle — *see* Adhesions, middle ear
  epididymis 608.89
  epidural — *see* Adhesions, meninges
  epiglottis 478.79
  Eustachian tube 381.89
  eyelid 374.46
    postoperative 997.99
    surgically created V45.69
  gallbladder (*see also* Disease, gallbladder) 575.8
  globe 360.89
  heart 423.1
    rheumatic 398.99
  ileocecal (coil) (*see also* Adhesions, peritoneum) 568.0
  ileum (*see also* Adhesions, peritoneum) 568.0
  intestine (postoperative) (*see also* Adhesions, peritoneum) 568.0
    with obstruction 560.81
      with hernia (*see also* Hernia, by site, with obstruction)
        gangrenous — *see* Hernia, by site, with gangrene
  intra-abdominal (*see also* Adhesions, peritoneum) 568.0
  iris 364.70
    to corneal graft 996.79

☑ Additional Digit Required — Refer to the Tabular List for Digit Selection   Ⓦ Subterms under main terms may continue to next column or page

10 — Volume 2   ▶◀ Revised Text   ● New Line   ▲ Revised Code   2013 ICD-9-CM

☑ **Additional Digit Required** — Refer to the Tabular List for Digit Selection   ▽ **Subterms under main terms may continue to next column or page**

2013 ICD-9-CM   ▶◀ **Revised Text**   ● **New Line**   ▲ **Revised Code**   **Volume 2 — 11**

Admission — *continued*
  for — *continued*
    breast — *continued*
      removal
        prophylactic V50.41
        tissue expander without synchronous insertion of permanent implant V52.4
    change of
      cardiac pacemaker (battery) V53.31
      carotid sinus pacemaker V53.39
      catheter in artificial opening — *see* Attention to, artificial, opening
      drains V58.49
      dressing
        wound V58.30
          nonsurgical V58.30
          surgical V58.31
      fixation device
        external V54.89
        internal V54.01
      Kirschner wire V54.89
      neuropacemaker device (brain) (peripheral nerve) (spinal cord) V53.02
      nonsurgical wound dressing V58.30
      pacemaker device
        brain V53.02
        cardiac V53.31
        carotid sinus V53.39
        nervous system V53.02
      plaster cast V54.89
      splint, external V54.89
      Steinmann pin V54.89
      surgical wound dressing V58.31
      traction device V54.89
      wound packing V58.30
        nonsurgical V58.30
        surgical V58.31
    checkup only V70.0
    chemotherapy, (oral) (intravenous) antineoplastic V58.11
    circumcision, ritual or routine (in absence of medical indication) V50.2
    clinical research investigation (control) (normal comparison) (participant) V70.7
    closure of artificial opening — *see* Attention to, artificial, opening
    contraceptive
      counseling V25.09
        emergency V25.03
        postcoital V25.03
      management V25.9
        specified type NEC V25.8
    convalescence following V66.9
      chemotherapy V66.2
      psychotherapy V66.3
      radiotherapy V66.1
      surgery V66.0
      treatment (for) V66.5
        combined V66.6
        fracture V66.4
        mental disorder NEC V66.3
        specified condition NEC V66.5
    cosmetic surgery NEC V50.1
      breast reconstruction following mastectomy V51.0
      following healed injury or operation V51.8
    counseling (*see also* Counseling) V65.40
      without complaint or sickness V65.49
      contraceptive management V25.09
        emergency V25.03
        postcoital V25.03
      dietary V65.3
      exercise V65.41
      fertility preservation (prior to cancer therapy) (prior to surgical removal of gonads) V26.42
      for
        nonattending third party V65.19

Admission — *continued*
  for — *continued*
    counseling (*see also* Counseling) — *continued*
      for — *continued*
        pediatric
          pre-adoption visit for adoptive parent(s) V65.11
          pre-birth visit for expectant parent(s) V65.11
        victim of abuse
          child V61.21
          partner or spouse V61.11
      genetic V26.33
      gonorrhea V65.45
      HIV V65.44
      human immunodeficiency virus V65.44
      injury prevention V65.43
      insulin pump training V65.46
      natural family planning
        procreative V26.41
        to avoid pregnancy V25.04
      procreative management V26.49
        using natural family planning V26.41
      sexually transmitted disease NEC V65.45
        HIV V65.44
      specified reason NEC V65.49
      substance use and abuse V65.42
      syphilis V65.45
      victim of abuse
        child V61.21
        partner or spouse V61.11
    desensitization to allergens V07.1
    dialysis V56.0
      catheter
        fitting and adjustment
          extracorporeal V56.1
          peritoneal V56.2
        removal or replacement
          extracorporeal V56.1
          peritoneal V56.2
      extracorporeal (renal) V56.0
      peritoneal V56.8
      renal V56.0
    dietary surveillance and counseling V65.3
    drug monitoring, therapeutic V58.83
    ear piercing V50.3
    elective surgery V50.9
      breast
        augmentation or reduction V50.1
        reconstruction following mastectomy V51.0
        removal, prophylactic V50.41
      circumcision, ritual or routine (in absence of medical indication) V50.2
      cosmetic NEC V50.1
        breast reconstruction following mastectomy V51.0
        following healed injury or operation V51.8
      ear piercing V50.3
      face-lift V50.1
      hair transplant V50.0
      plastic
        breast reconstruction following mastectomy V51.0
        cosmetic NEC V50.1
        following healed injury or operation V51.8
      prophylactic organ removal V50.49
        breast V50.41
        ovary V50.42
      repair of scarred tissue (following healed injury or operation) V51.8
      specified type NEC V50.8
    end-of-life care V66.7
    examination (*see also* Examination) V70.9
      administrative purpose NEC V70.3
      adoption V70.3

Admission — *continued*
  for — *continued*
    examination (*see also* Examination) — *continued*
      allergy V72.7
      antibody response V72.61
      at health care facility V70.0
      athletic team V70.3
      camp V70.3
      cardiovascular, preoperative V72.81
      clinical research investigation (control) (participant) V70.7
      dental V72.2
      developmental testing (child) (infant) V20.2
      donor (potential) V70.8
      driver's license V70.3
      ear V72.19
      employment V70.5
      eye V72.0
      fertility preservation (prior to cancer therapy) (prior to surgical removal of gonads) V26.82
      follow-up (routine) — *see* Examination, follow-up
      for admission to
        old age home V70.3
        school V70.3
      general V70.9
        specified reason NEC V70.8
      gynecological V72.31
      health supervision
        child (over 28 days old) V20.2
        infant (over 28 days old) V20.2
        newborn
          8 to 28 days old V20.32
          under 8 days old V20.31
      hearing V72.19
        following failed hearing screening V72.11
      immigration V70.3
      infant
        8 to 28 days old V20.32
        over 28 days old, routine V20.2
        under 8 days old V20.31
      insurance certification V70.3
      laboratory V72.60
        ordered as part of a routine general medical examination V72.62
        pre-operative V72.63
        pre-procedural V72.63
        specified NEC V72.69
      marriage license V70.3
      medical (general) (*see also* Examination, medical) V70.9
      medicolegal reasons V70.4
      naturalization V70.3
      pelvic (annual) (periodic) V72.31
      postpartum checkup V24.2
      pregnancy (possible) (unconfirmed) V72.40
        negative result V72.41
        positive result V72.42
      preoperative V72.84
        cardiovascular V72.81
        respiratory V72.82
        specified NEC V72.83
      preprocedural V72.84
        cardiovascular V72.81
        general physical V72.83
        respiratory V72.82
        specified NEC V72.83
      prior to chemotherapy V72.83
      prison V70.3
      psychiatric (general) V70.2
        requested by authority V70.1
      radiological NEC V72.5
      respiratory, preoperative V72.82
      school V70.3
      screening — *see* Screening
      skin hypersensitivity V72.7
      specified type NEC V72.85
      sport competition V70.3
      vision V72.0
      well baby and child care V20.2

Admission — *continued*
  for — *continued*
    exercise therapy V57.1
    face-lift, cosmetic reason V50.1
    fertility preservation (prior to cancer therapy) (prior to surgical removal of gonads) V26.82
    fitting (of)
      artificial
        arm (complete) (partial) V52.0
        eye V52.2
        leg (complete) (partial) V52.1
      biliary drainage tube V58.82
      brain neuropacemaker V53.02
      breast V52.4
        implant V52.4
        prosthesis V52.4
      cardiac pacemaker V53.31
      catheter
        non-vascular V58.82
        vascular V58.81
      cerebral ventricle (communicating) shunt V53.01
      chest tube V58.82
      colostomy belt V55.2
      contact lenses V53.1
      cystostomy device V53.6
      dental prosthesis V52.3
      device, unspecified type V53.90
        abdominal V53.59
        cerebral ventricle (communicating) shunt V53.01
        gastrointestinal NEC V53.59
        insulin pump V53.91
        intestinal V53.50
        intrauterine contraceptive
          insertion V25.11
          removal V25.12
            and reinsertion V25.13
          replacement V25.13
        nervous system V53.09
        orthodontic V53.4
        other device V53.99
        prosthetic V52.9
          breast V52.4
          dental V52.3
          eye V52.2
        special senses V53.09
        substitution
          auditory V53.09
          nervous system V53.09
          visual V53.09
      diaphragm (contraceptive) V25.02
      fistula (sinus tract) drainage tube V58.82
      gastric lap band V53.51
      gastrointestinal appliance and device NEC V53.59
      growth rod V54.02
      hearing aid V53.2
      ileostomy device V55.2
      intestinal appliance and device V53.50
      intrauterine contraceptive device
        insertion V25.11
        removal V25.12
          and reinsertion V25.13
        replacement V25.13
      neuropacemaker (brain) (peripheral nerve) (spinal cord) V53.02
      orthodontic device V53.4
      orthopedic (device) V53.7
        brace V53.7
        cast V53.7
        shoes V53.7
      pacemaker
        brain V53.02
        cardiac V53.31
        carotid sinus V53.39
        spinal cord V53.02
      pleural drainage tube V58.82
      portacath V58.81
      prosthesis V52.9
        arm (complete) (partial) V52.0
        breast V52.4
        dental V52.3

☑ **Additional Digit Required — Refer to the Tabular List for Digit Selection**   � **Subterms under main terms may continue to next column or page**

Admission — *continued*
  for — *continued*
    fitting — *continued*
      prosthesis — *continued*
        eye V52.2
        leg (complete) (partial) V52.1
        specified type NEC V52.8
      spectacles V53.1
      wheelchair V53.8
    follow-up examination (routine) (following) V67.9
      cancer chemotherapy V67.2
      chemotherapy V67.2
      high-risk medication NEC V67.51
      injury NEC V67.59
      psychiatric V67.3
      psychotherapy V67.3
      radiotherapy V67.1
      specified surgery NEC V67.09
      surgery V67.00
        vaginal pap smear V67.01
      treatment (for) V67.9
        combined V67.6
        fracture V67.4
        involving high-risk medication NEC V67.51
        mental disorder V67.3
        specified NEC V67.59
    hair transplant, for cosmetic reason V50.0
    health advice, education, or instruction V65.4 ☑
    hearing conservation and treatment V72.12
    hormone replacement therapy (postmenopausal) V07.4
    hospice care V66.7
    immunizations (childhood) appropriate for age V20.2
    immunotherapy, antineoplastic V58.12
    insertion (of)
      intrauterine contraceptive device V25.11
      subdermal implantable contraceptive V25.5
    insulin pump titration V53.91
    insulin pump training V65.46
    intrauterine device
      insertion V25.11
      management V25.42
      removal V25.12
        and reinsertion V25.13
      replacement V25.13
    investigation to determine further disposition V63.8
    in vitro fertilization cycle V26.81
    isolation V07.0
    issue of
      disability examination certificate V68.01
      medical certificate NEC V68.09
      repeat prescription NEC V68.1
        contraceptive device NEC V25.49
    kidney dialysis V56.0
    lengthening of growth rod V54.02
    mental health evaluation V70.2
      requested by authority V70.1
    natural family planning counseling and advice
      procreative V26.41
      to avoid pregnancy V25.04
    nonmedical reason NEC V68.89
    nursing care evaluation V63.8
    observation (without need for further medical care) (*see also* Observation) V71.9
      accident V71.4
      alleged rape or seduction V71.5
      criminal assault V71.6
      following accident V71.4
        at work V71.3
      foreign body ingestion V71.89
      growth and development variations, childhood V21.0
      inflicted injury NEC V71.6

Admission — *continued*
  for — *continued*
    observation (*see also* Observation) — *continued*
      ingestion of deleterious agent or foreign body V71.89
      injury V71.6
      malignant neoplasm V71.1
      mental disorder V71.09
      newborn — *see* Observation, suspected, condition, newborn
      rape V71.5
      specified NEC V71.89
      suspected
        abuse V71.81
        accident V71.4
          at work V71.3
        benign neoplasm V71.89
        cardiovascular V71.7
        disorder V71.9
        exposure
          anthrax V71.82
          biological agent NEC V71.83
          SARS V71.83
        heart V71.7
        inflicted injury NEC V71.6
        malignant neoplasm V71.1
        maternal and fetal problem not found
          amniotic cavity and membrane V89.01
          cervical shortening V89.05
          fetal anomaly V89.03
          fetal growth V89.04
          oligohydramnios V89.01
          other specified NEC V89.09
          placenta V89.02
          polyhydramnios V89.01
        mental NEC V71.09
        neglect V71.81
        specified condition NEC V71.89
        tuberculosis V71.2
      tuberculosis V71.2
    occupational therapy V57.21
    organ transplant, donor — *see* Donor
    ovary, ovarian removal, prophylactic V50.42
    palliative care V66.7
    Papanicolaou smear
      cervix V76.2
        for suspected malignant neoplasm V76.2
        no disease found V71.1
        routine, as part of gynecological examination V72.31
        to confirm findings of recent normal smear following initial abnormal smear V72.32
      vaginal V76.47
        following hysterectomy for malignant condition V67.01
    passage of sounds or bougie in artificial opening — *see* Attention to, artificial, opening
    paternity testing V70.4
    peritoneal dialysis V56.32
    physical therapy NEC V57.1
    plastic surgery
      breast reconstruction following mastectomy V51.0
      cosmetic NEC V50.1
      following healed injury or operation V51.8
    postmenopausal hormone replacement therapy V07.4
    postpartum observation
      immediately after delivery V24.0
      routine follow-up V24.2
    poststerilization (for restoration) V26.0
    procreative management V26.9
      assisted reproductive fertility procedure cycle V26.81
      in vitro fertilization cycle V26.81
      specified type NEC V26.89

Admission — *continued*
  for — *continued*
    prophylactic
      administration of
        antibiotics, long-term V58.62
          short-term use — *omit code*
        antitoxin, any V07.2
        antivenin V07.2
        chemotherapeutic agent NEC V07.39
        chemotherapy NEC V07.39
        diphtheria antitoxin V07.2
        fluoride V07.31
        gamma globulin V07.2
        immune sera (gamma globulin) V07.2
        RhoGAM V07.2
        tetanus antitoxin V07.2
      breathing exercises V57.0
      chemotherapy NEC V07.39
        fluoride V07.31
      measure V07.9
        specified type NEC V07.8
      organ removal V50.49
        breast V50.41
        ovary V50.42
    psychiatric examination (general) V70.2
      requested by authority V70.1
    radiation management V58.0
    radiotherapy V58.0
    reconstruction following mastectomy V51.0
    reforming of artificial opening — *see* Attention to, artificial, opening
    rehabilitation V57.9
      multiple types V57.89
      occupational V57.21
      orthoptic V57.4
      orthotic V57.81
      physical NEC V57.1
      specified type NEC V57.89
      speech (-language) V57.3
      vocational V57.22
    removal of
      breast tissue expander without synchronous insertion of permanent implant V52.4
      cardiac pacemaker V53.31
      cast (plaster) V54.89
      catheter from artificial opening — *see* Attention to, artificial, opening
      cerebral ventricle (communicating) shunt V53.01
      cystostomy catheter V55.5
      device
        cerebral ventricle (communicating) shunt V53.01
        fixation
          external V54.89
          internal V54.01
        intrauterine contraceptive V25.12
        traction, external V54.89
      drains V58.49
      dressing
        wound V58.30
          nonsurgical V58.30
          surgical V58.31
      fixation device
        external V54.89
        internal V54.01
      intrauterine contraceptive device V25.12
      Kirschner wire V54.89
      neuropacemaker (brain) (peripheral nerve) (spinal cord) V53.02
      nonsurgical wound dressing V58.30
      orthopedic fixation device
        external V54.89
        internal V54.01
      pacemaker device
        brain V53.02
        cardiac V53.31
        carotid sinus V53.39
        nervous system V53.02
      plaster cast V54.89

Admission — *continued*
  for — *continued*
    removal of — *continued*
      plate (fracture) V54.01
      rod V54.01
      screw (fracture) V54.01
      splint, traction V54.89
      staples V58.32
      Steinmann pin V54.89
      subdermal implantable contraceptive V25.43
      surgical wound dressing V58.31
      sutures V58.32
      traction device, external V54.89
      ureteral stent V53.6
      wound packing V58.30
        nonsurgical V58.30
        surgical V58.31
    repair of scarred tissue (following healed injury or operation) V51.8
    replacement of intrauterine contraceptive device V25.13
    reprogramming of cardiac pacemaker V53.31
    respirator [ventilator] dependence during
        mechanical failure V46.14
        power failure V46.12
      for weaning V46.13
    restoration of organ continuity (poststerilization) (tuboplasty) (vasoplasty) V26.0
    Rh typing V72.86
    routine infant and child vision and hearing testing V20.2
    sensitivity test (*see also* Test, skin)
      allergy NEC V72.7
      bacterial disease NEC V74.9
      Dick V74.8
      Kveim V82.89
      Mantoux V74.1
      mycotic infection NEC V75.4
      parasitic disease NEC V75.8
      Schick V74.3
      Schultz-Charlton V74.8
    social service (agency) referral or evaluation V63.8
    speech (-language) therapy V57.3
    sterilization V25.2
    suspected disorder (ruled out) (without need for further care) — *see* Observation
    terminal care V66.7
    tests only — *see* Test
    therapeutic drug monitoring V58.83
    therapy
      blood transfusion, without reported diagnosis V58.2
      breathing exercises V57.0
      chemotherapy, antineoplastic V58.11
        prophylactic NEC V07.39
        fluoride V07.31
      dialysis (intermittent) (treatment)
        extracorporeal V56.0
        peritoneal V56.8
        renal V56.0
        specified type NEC V56.8
      exercise (remedial) NEC V57.1
        breathing V57.0
      immunotherapy, antineoplastic V58.12
      long-term (current) (prophylactic) drug use NEC V58.69
        antibiotics V58.62
          short-term use — *omit code*
        anticoagulants V58.61
        anti-inflammatories, nonsteroidal (NSAID) V58.64
        antiplatelets V58.63
        antithrombotics V58.63
        aspirin V58.66
        bisphosphonates V58.68
        high-risk medications NEC V58.69
        insulin V58.67
        methadone for pain control V58.69

☑ **Additional Digit Required — Refer to the Tabular List for Digit Selection**   ▼ **Subterms under main terms may continue to next column or page**

2013 ICD-9-CM   ▶◀ Revised Text   ● New Line   ▲ Revised Code   **Volume 2 — 13**

Admission — *continued*
  for — *continued*
    therapy — *continued*
      long-term drug use — *continued*
        opiate analgesic V58.69
        steroids V58.65
      occupational V57.21
      orthoptic V57.4
      physical NEC V57.1
      radiation V58.0
      speech (-language) V57.3
      vocational V57.22
    toilet or cleaning
      of artificial opening — *see* Attention to, artificial, opening
      of non-vascular catheter V58.82
      of vascular catheter V58.81
    treatment
      measure V07.9
        specified type NEC V07.8
    tubal ligation V25.2
    tuboplasty for previous sterilization V26.0
    ultrasound, routine fetal V28.3
    vaccination, prophylactic (against)
      arthropod-borne virus, viral NEC V05.1
        disease NEC V05.1
        encephalitis V05.0
      Bacille Calmette Guérin (BCG) V03.2
      BCG V03.2
      chickenpox V05.4
      cholera alone V03.0
        with typhoid-paratyphoid (cholera + TAB) V06.0
      common cold V04.7
      dengue V05.1
      diphtheria alone V03.5
      diphtheria-tetanus-pertussis (DTP) (DTaP) V06.1
        with
          poliomyelitis (DTP + polio) V06.3
          typhoid-paratyphoid (DTP + TAB) V06.2
      diphtheria-tetanus [Td] [DT] without pertussis V06.5
      disease (single) NEC V05.9
        bacterial NEC V03.9
          specified type NEC V03.89
        combinations NEC V06.9
          specified type NEC V06.8
        specified type NEC V05.8
        viral NEC V04.89
      encephalitis, viral, arthropod-borne V05.0
      Hemophilus influenzae, type B [Hib] V03.81
      hepatitis, viral V05.3
      human papillomavirus (HPV) V04.89
      immune sera (gamma globulin) V07.2
      influenza V04.81
        with
          Streptococcus pneumoniae [pneumococcus] V06.6
      Leishmaniasis V05.2
      measles alone V04.2
      measles-mumps-rubella (MMR) V06.4
      mumps alone V04.6
        with measles and rubella (MMR) V06.4
      not done because of contraindication V64.09
      pertussis alone V03.6
      plague V03.3
      pneumonia V03.82
      poliomyelitis V04.0
        with diphtheria-tetanus-pertussis (DTP+ polio) V06.3
      rabies V04.5
      respiratory syncytial virus (RSV) V04.82
      rubella alone V04.3
        with measles and mumps (MMR) V06.4

Admission — *continued*
  for — *continued*
    vaccination, prophylactic — *continued*
      smallpox V04.1
      specified type NEC V05.8
      Streptococcus pneumoniae [pneumococcus] V03.82
        with
          influenza V06.6
      tetanus toxoid alone V03.7
        with diphtheria [Td] [DT] V06.5
          and pertussis (DTP) (DTaP) V06.1
      tuberculosis (BCG) V03.2
      tularemia V03.4
      typhoid alone V03.1
        with diphtheria-tetanus-pertussis (TAB + DTP) V06.2
      typhoid-paratyphoid alone (TAB) V03.1
      typhus V05.8
      varicella (chicken pox) V05.4
      viral encephalitis, arthropod-borne V05.0
      viral hepatitis V05.3
      yellow fever V04.4
    vasectomy V25.2
    vasoplasty for previous sterilization V26.0
    vision examination V72.0
    vocational therapy V57.22
    waiting period for admission to other facility V63.2
      undergoing social agency investigation V63.8
    well baby and child care V20.2
    x-ray of chest
      for suspected tuberculosis V71.2
      routine V72.5
Adnexitis (suppurative) — *see also* Salpingo-oophoritis 614.2
Adolescence NEC V21.2
Adoption
  agency referral V68.89
  examination V70.3
  held for V68.89
Adrenal gland — *see* condition
Adrenalism 255.9
  tuberculous (*see also* Tuberculosis) 017.6 ☑
Adrenalitis, adrenitis 255.8
  meningococcal hemorrhagic 036.3
Adrenarche, precocious 259.1
Adrenocortical syndrome 255.2
Adrenogenital syndrome (acquired) (congenital) 255.2
  iatrogenic, fetus or newborn 760.79
Adrenoleukodystrophy 277.86
  neonatal 277.86
  x-linked 277.86
Adrenomyeloneuropathy 277.86
Adventitious bursa — *see* Bursitis
Adynamia (episodica) (hereditary) (periodic) 359.3
Adynamic
  ileus or intestine (*see also* Ileus) 560.1
  ureter 753.22
Aeration lung, imperfect, newborn 770.5
Aerobullosis 993.3
Aerocele — *see* Embolism, air
Aerodermectasia
  subcutaneous (traumatic) 958.7
    surgical 998.81
  surgical 998.81
Aerodontalgia 993.2
Aeroembolism 993.3
Aerogenes capsulatus infection — *see also* Gangrene, gas 040.0
Aero-otitis media 993.0
Aerophagy, aerophagia 306.4
  psychogenic 306.4
Aerosinusitis 993.1
Aerotitis 993.0
Affection, affections — *see also* Disease
  sacroiliac (joint), old 724.6
  shoulder region NEC 726.2

Afibrinogenemia 286.3
  acquired 286.6
  congenital 286.3
  postpartum 666.3 ☑
African
  sleeping sickness 086.5
  tick fever 087.1
  trypanosomiasis 086.5
    Gambian 086.3
    Rhodesian 086.4
Aftercare V58.9
  amputation stump V54.89
  artificial openings — *see* Attention to, artificial, opening
  blood transfusion without reported diagnosis V58.2
  breathing exercise V57.0
  cardiac device V53.39
    defibrillator, automatic implantable (with synchronous cardiac pacemaker) V53.32
    pacemaker V53.31
      carotid sinus V53.39
  carotid sinus pacemaker V53.39
  cerebral ventricle (communicating) shunt V53.01
  chemotherapy (oral) (intravenous) session (adjunctive) (maintenance) V58.11
  defibrillator, automatic implantable cardiac (with synchronous cardiac pacemaker) V53.32
  exercise (remedial) (therapeutic) V57.1
    breathing V57.0
  extracorporeal dialysis (intermittent) (treatment) V56.0
  following surgery NEC V58.49
    for
      injury V58.43
      neoplasm V58.42
      organ transplant V58.44
      trauma V58.43
    joint
      explantation of prosthesis (staged procedure) V54.82
      replacement V54.81
    of
      circulatory system V58.73
      digestive system V58.75
      genital organs V58.76
      genitourinary system V58.76
      musculoskeletal system V58.78
      nervous system V58.72
      oral cavity V58.75
      respiratory system V58.74
      sense organs V58.71
      skin V58.77
      subcutaneous tissue V58.77
      teeth V58.75
      urinary system V58.76
    spinal — *see* Aftercare, following surgery, of, specified body system
    wound closure, planned V58.41
  fracture V54.9
    healing V54.89
      pathologic
        ankle V54.29
        arm V54.20
          lower V54.22
          upper V54.21
        finger V54.29
        foot V54.29
        hand V54.29
        hip V54.23
        leg V54.24
          lower V54.26
          upper V54.25
        pelvis V54.29
        specified site NEC V54.29
        toe(s) V54.29
        vertebrae V54.27
        wrist V54.29
      traumatic
        ankle V54.19
        arm V54.10
          lower V54.12
          upper V54.11

Aftercare — *continued*
  fracture — *continued*
    healing — *continued*
      traumatic — *continued*
        finger V54.19
        foot V54.19
        hand V54.19
        hip V54.13
        leg V54.14
          lower V54.16
          upper V54.15
        pelvis V54.19
        specified site NEC V54.19
        toe(s) V54.19
        vertebrae V54.17
        wrist V54.19
    removal of
      external fixation device V54.89
      internal fixation device V54.01
    specified care NEC V54.89
  gait training V57.1
    for use of artificial limb(s) V57.81
  internal fixation device V54.09
  involving
    dialysis (intermittent) (treatment)
      extracorporeal V56.0
      peritoneal V56.8
      renal V56.0
    gait training V57.1
      for use of artificial limb(s) V57.81
    growth rod
      adjustment V54.02
      lengthening V54.02
    internal fixation device V54.09
    orthoptic training V57.4
    orthotic training V57.81
    radiotherapy session V58.0
    removal of
      drains V58.49
      dressings
        wound V58.30
          nonsurgical V58.30
          surgical V58.31
      fixation device
        external V54.89
        internal V54.01
      fracture plate V54.01
      nonsurgical wound dressing V58.30
      pins V54.01
      plaster cast V54.89
      rods V54.01
      screws V58.32
      staples V58.32
      surgical wound dressings V58.31
      sutures V58.32
      traction device, external V54.89
      wound packing V58.30
        nonsurgical V58.30
        surgical V58.31
  neuropacemaker (brain) (peripheral nerve) (spinal cord) V53.02
  occupational therapy V57.21
  orthodontic V58.5
  orthopedic V54.9
    change of external fixation or traction device V54.89
    following joint
      explantation of prosthesis (staged procedure) V54.82
      replacement V54.81
    internal fixation device V54.09
    removal of fixation device
      external V54.89
      internal V54.01
    specified care NEC V54.89
  orthoptic training V57.4
  orthotic training V57.81
  pacemaker
    brain V53.02
    cardiac V53.31
    carotid sinus V53.39
    peripheral nerve V53.02
    spinal cord V53.02
  peritoneal dialysis (intermittent) (treatment) V56.8
  physical therapy NEC V57.1

☑ **Additional Digit Required** — Refer to the Tabular List for Digit Selection
◥ **Subterms under main terms may continue to next column or page**
14 — Volume 2
▶◀ Revised Text
● New Line
▲ Revised Code
2013 ICD-9-CM

Aftercare — *continued*
  physical therapy — *continued*
    breathing exercises V57.0
  radiotherapy session V58.0
  rehabilitation procedure V57.9
    breathing exercises V57.0
    multiple types V57.89
    occupational V57.21
    orthoptic V57.4
    orthotic V57.81
    physical therapy NEC V57.1
    remedial exercises V57.1
    specified type NEC V57.89
    speech (-language) V57.3
    therapeutic exercises V57.1
    vocational V57.22
  renal dialysis (intermittent) (treatment) V56.0
  specified type NEC V58.89
    removal of non-vascular catheter V58.82
    removal of vascular catheter V58.81
  speech (-language) therapy V57.3
  stump, amputation V54.89
  vocational rehabilitation V57.22
After-cataract 366.50
  obscuring vision 366.53
  specified type, not obscuring vision 366.52
Agalactia 676.4 ☑
Agammaglobulinemia 279.00
  with lymphopenia 279.2
  acquired (primary) (secondary) 279.06
  Bruton's X-linked 279.04
  infantile sex-linked (Bruton's) (congenital) 279.04
  Swiss-type 279.2
Aganglionosis (bowel) (colon) 751.3
Age (old) — *see also* Senile 797
Agenesis — *see also* Absence, by site, congenital
  acoustic nerve 742.8
  adrenal (gland) 759.1
  alimentary tract (complete) (partial) NEC 751.8
    lower 751.2
    upper 750.8
  anus, anal (canal) 751.2
  aorta 747.22
  appendix 751.2
  arm (complete) (partial) (*see also* Deformity, reduction, upper limb) 755.20
  artery (peripheral) NEC (*see also* Anomaly, peripheral vascular system) 747.60
    brain 747.81
    coronary 746.85
    pulmonary 747.31
    umbilical 747.5
  auditory (canal) (external) 744.01
  auricle (ear) 744.01
  bile, biliary duct or passage 751.61
  bone NEC 756.9
  brain 740.0
    specified part 742.2
  breast 757.6
  bronchus 748.3
  canaliculus lacrimalis 743.65
  carpus NEC (*see also* Deformity, reduction, upper limb) 755.28
  cartilage 756.9
  cecum 751.2
  cerebellum 742.2
  cervix 752.43
  chin 744.89
  cilia 743.63
  circulatory system, part NEC 747.89
  clavicle 755.51
  clitoris 752.49
  coccyx 756.13
  colon 751.2
  corpus callosum 742.2
  cricoid cartilage 748.3
  diaphragm (with hernia) 756.6
  digestive organ(s) or tract (complete) (partial) NEC 751.8
    lower 751.2
    upper 750.8
  ductus arteriosus 747.89

Agenesis — *see also* Absence, by site, congenital — *continued*
  duodenum 751.1
  ear NEC 744.09
    auricle 744.01
    lobe 744.21
  ejaculatory duct 752.89
  endocrine (gland) NEC 759.2
  epiglottis 748.3
  esophagus 750.3
  Eustachian tube 744.24
  extrinsic muscle, eye 743.69
  eye 743.00
    adnexa 743.69
  eyelid (fold) 743.62
  face
    bones NEC 756.0
    specified part NEC 744.89
  fallopian tube 752.19
  femur NEC (*see also* Absence, femur, congenital) 755.34
  fibula NEC (*see also* Absence, fibula, congenital) 755.37
  finger NEC (*see also* Absence, finger, congenital) 755.29
  foot (complete) (*see also* Deformity, reduction, lower limb) 755.31
  gallbladder 751.69
  gastric 750.8
  genitalia, genital (organ)
    female 752.89
     external 752.49
     internal NEC 752.89
    male 752.89
     penis 752.69
  glottis 748.3
  gonadal 758.6
  hair 757.4
  hand (complete) (*see also* Deformity, reduction, upper limb) 755.21
  heart 746.89
    valve NEC 746.89
     aortic 746.89
     mitral 746.89
     pulmonary 746.01
  hepatic 751.69
  humerus NEC (*see also* Absence, humerus, congenital) 755.24
  hymen 752.49
  ileum 751.1
  incus 744.04
  intestine (small) 751.1
    large 751.2
  iris (dilator fibers) 743.45
  jaw 524.09
  jejunum 751.1
  kidney(s) (partial) (unilateral) 753.0
  labium (majus) (minus) 752.49
  labyrinth, membranous 744.05
  lacrimal apparatus (congenital) 743.65
  larynx 748.3
  leg NEC (*see also* Deformity, reduction, lower limb) 755.30
  lens 743.35
  limb (complete) (partial) (*see also* Deformity, reduction) 755.4
    lower NEC 755.30
    upper 755.20
  lip 750.26
  liver 751.69
  lung (bilateral) (fissures) (lobe) (unilateral) 748.5
  mandible 524.09
  maxilla 524.09
  metacarpus NEC 755.28
  metatarsus NEC 755.38
  muscle (any) 756.81
  musculoskeletal system NEC 756.9
  nail(s) 757.5
  neck, part 744.89
  nerve 742.8
  nervous system, part NEC 742.8
  nipple 757.6
  nose 748.1
  nuclear 742.8

Agenesis — *see also* Absence, by site, congenital — *continued*
  organ
    of Corti 744.05
    or site not listed — *see* Anomaly, specified type NEC
  osseous meatus (ear) 744.03
  ovary 752.0
  oviduct 752.19
  pancreas 751.7
  parathyroid (gland) 759.2
  patella 755.64
  pelvic girdle (complete) (partial) 755.69
  penis 752.69
  pericardium 746.89
  perineal body 756.81
  pituitary (gland) 759.2
  prostate 752.89
  pulmonary
    artery 747.31
    trunk 747.31
    vein 747.49
  punctum lacrimale 743.65
  radioulnar NEC (*see also* Absence, forearm, congenital) 755.25
  radius NEC (*see also* Absence, radius, congenital) 755.26
  rectum 751.2
  renal 753.0
  respiratory organ NEC 748.9
  rib 756.3
  roof of orbit 742.0
  round ligament 752.89
  sacrum 756.13
  salivary gland 750.21
  scapula 755.59
  scrotum 752.89
  seminal duct or tract 752.89
  septum
    atrial 745.69
    between aorta and pulmonary artery 745.0
    ventricular 745.3
  shoulder girdle (complete) (partial) 755.59
  skull (bone) 756.0
    with
     anencephalus 740.0
     encephalocele 742.0
     hydrocephalus 742.3
      with spina bifida (*see also* Spina bifida) 741.0 ☑
     microcephalus 742.1
  spermatic cord 752.89
  spinal cord 742.59
  spine 756.13
    lumbar 756.13
     isthmus 756.11
     pars articularis 756.11
  spleen 759.0
  sternum 756.3
  stomach 750.7
  tarsus NEC 755.38
  tendon 756.81
  testicular 752.89
  testis 752.89
  thymus (gland) 759.2
  thyroid (gland) 243
    cartilage 748.3
  tibia NEC (*see also* Absence, tibia, congenital) 755.36
  tibiofibular NEC 755.35
  toe (complete) (partial) (*see also* Absence, toe, congenital) 755.39
  tongue 750.11
  trachea (cartilage) 748.3
  ulna NEC (*see also* Absence, ulna, congenital) 755.27
  ureter 753.4
  urethra 753.8
  urinary tract NEC 753.8
  uterus 752.31
  uvula 750.26
  vagina (total) (partial) 752.45
  vas deferens 752.89
  vein(s) (peripheral) NEC (*see also* Anomaly, peripheral vascular system) 747.60

Agenesis — *see also* Absence, by site, congenital — *continued*
  vein(s) (*see also* Anomaly, peripheral vascular system) — *continued*
    brain 747.81
    great 747.49
    portal 747.49
    pulmonary 747.49
   vena cava (inferior) (superior) 747.49
  vermis of cerebellum 742.2
  vertebra 756.13
    lumbar 756.13
     isthmus 756.11
     pars articularis 756.11
  vulva 752.49
Ageusia — *see also* Disturbance, sensation 781.1
Aggressiveness 301.3
Aggressive outburst — *see also* Disturbance, conduct 312.0 ☑
  in children or adolescents 313.9
Aging skin 701.8
Agitated — *see* condition
Agitation 307.9
  catatonic (*see also* Schizophrenia) 295.2 ☑
Aglossia (congenital) 750.11
Aglycogenosis 271.0
Agnail (finger) (with lymphangitis) 681.02
Agnosia (body image) (tactile) 784.69
  verbal 784.69
    auditory 784.69
     secondary to organic lesion 784.69
    developmental 315.8
    secondary to organic lesion 784.69
  visual 368.16
    object 368.16
Agoraphobia 300.22
  with panic disorder 300.21
Agrammatism 784.69
Agranulocytopenia — *see also* Agranulocytosis 288.09
Agranulocytosis — *see also* Neutropenia 288.09
  chronic 288.09
  cyclical 288.02
  due to infection 288.04
  genetic 288.01
  infantile 288.01
  periodic 288.02
  pernicious 288.09
Agraphia (absolute) 784.69
  with alexia 784.61
  developmental 315.39
Agrypnia — *see also* Insomnia 780.52
Ague — *see also* Malaria 084.6
  brass-founders' 985.8
  dumb 084.6
  tertian 084.1
Agyria 742.2
AHTR (acute hemolytic transfusion reaction) — *see* Complications, transfusion
Ahumada-del Castillo syndrome (nonpuerperal galactorrhea and amenorrhea) 253.1
AIDS 042
AIDS-associated retrovirus (disease) (illness) 042
  infection — *see* Human immunodeficiency virus, infection
AIDS-associated virus (disease) (illness) 042
  infection — *see* Human immunodeficiency virus, infection
AIDS-like disease (illness) (syndrome) 042
AIDS-related complex 042
AIDS-related conditions 042
AIDS-related virus (disease) (illness) 042
  infection — *see* Human immunodeficiency virus, infection
AIDS virus (disease) (illness) 042
  infection — *see* Human immunodeficiency virus, infection
Ailment, heart — *see* Disease, heart
Ailurophobia 300.29
Ainhum (disease) 136.0
AIN I (anal intraepithelial neoplasia I) (histologically confirmed) 569.44

AIN II (anal intraepithelial neoplasia II) (histologically confirmed) 569.44
AIN III (anal intraepithelial neoplasia III) 230.6
 anal canal 230.5
AIPHI (acute idiopathic pulmonary hemorrhage in infants (over 28 days old)) 786.31
Air
 anterior mediastinum 518.1
 compressed, disease 993.3
 embolism (any site) (artery) (cerebral) 958.0
  with
   abortion — *see* Abortion, by type, with embolism
   ectopic pregnancy (*see also* categories 633.0–633.9) 639.6
   molar pregnancy (*see also* categories 630–632) 639.6
  due to implanted device — *see* Complications, due to (presence of) any device, implant, or graft classified to 996.0–996.5 NEC
  following
   abortion 639.6
   ectopic or molar pregnancy 639.6
  infusion, perfusion, or transfusion 999.1
  in pregnancy, childbirth, or puerperium 673.0 ☑
  traumatic 958.0
 hunger 786.09
  psychogenic 306.1
 leak (lung) (pulmonary) (thorax) 512.84
  iatrogenic 512.1
  persistent 512.84
  postoperative 512.2
 rarefied, effects of — *see* Effect, adverse, high altitude
 sickness 994.6
Airplane sickness 994.6
Akathisia, acathisia 781.0
 due to drugs 333.99
 neuroleptic-induced acute 333.99
Akinesia algeria 352.6
Akiyami 100.89
Akureyri disease (epidemic neuromyasthenia) 049.8
Alacrima (congenital) 743.65
Alactasia (hereditary) 271.3
Alagille syndrome 759.89
Alalia 784.3
 developmental 315.31
  receptive-expressive 315.32
 secondary to organic lesion 784.3
Alaninemia 270.8
Alastrim 050.1
Albarrán's disease (colibacilluria) 791.9
Albers-Schönberg's disease (marble bones) 756.52
Albert's disease 726.71
Albinism, albino (choroid) (cutaneous) (eye) (generalized) (isolated) (ocular) (oculocutaneous) (partial) 270.2
Albinismus 270.2
Albright (-Martin) (-Bantam) disease (pseudohypoparathyroidism) 275.49
Albright (-McCune) (-Sternberg) syndrome (osteitis fibrosa disseminata) 756.59
Albuminous — *see* condition
Albuminuria, albuminuric (acute) (chronic) (subacute) 791.0
 Bence-Jones 791.0
 cardiac 785.9
 complicating pregnancy, childbirth, or puerperium 646.2 ☑
  with hypertension — *see* Toxemia, of pregnancy
  affecting fetus or newborn 760.1
 cyclic 593.6
 gestational 646.2 ☑
 gravidarum 646.2 ☑
  with hypertension — *see* Toxemia, of pregnancy
  affecting fetus or newborn 760.1
 heart 785.9
 idiopathic 593.6
 orthostatic 593.6

Albuminuria, albuminuric — *continued*
 postural 593.6
 pre-eclamptic (mild) 642.4 ☑
  affecting fetus or newborn 760.0
  severe 642.5 ☑
   affecting fetus or newborn 760.0
 recurrent physiologic 593.6
 scarlatinal 034.1
Albumosuria 791.0
 Bence-Jones 791.0
 myelopathic (M9730/3) 203.0 ☑
Alcaptonuria 270.2
Alcohol, alcoholic
 abstinence 291.81
 acute intoxication 305.0 ☑
  with dependence 303.0 ☑
 addiction (*see also* Alcoholism) 303.9 ☑
  maternal
   with suspected fetal damage affecting management of pregnancy 655.4 ☑
   affecting fetus or newborn 760.71
 amnestic disorder, persisting 291.1
 anxiety 291.89
 brain syndrome, chronic 291.2
 cardiopathy 425.5
 chronic (*see also* Alcoholism) 303.9 ☑
 cirrhosis (liver) 571.2
 delirium 291.0
  acute 291.0
  chronic 291.1
  tremens 291.0
  withdrawal 291.0
 dementia NEC 291.2
 deterioration 291.2
 drunkenness (simple) 305.0 ☑
 hallucinosis (acute) 291.3
 induced
  circadian rhythm sleep disorder 291.82
  hypersomnia 291.82
  insomnia 291.82
  mental disorder 291.9
   anxiety 291.89
   mood 291.89
   sexual 291.89
   sleep 291.82
   specified type 291.89
  parasomnia 291.82
  persisting
   amnestic disorder 291.1
   dementia 291.2
  psychotic disorder
   with
    delusions 291.5
    hallucinations 291.3
  sleep disorder 291.82
 insanity 291.9
 intoxication (acute) 305.0 ☑
  with dependence 303.0 ☑
  pathological 291.4
 jealousy 291.5
 Korsakoff's, Korsakov's, Korsakow's 291.1
 liver NEC 571.3
  acute 571.1
  chronic 571.2
 mania (acute) (chronic) 291.9
 mood 291.89
 paranoia 291.5
 paranoid (type) psychosis 291.5
 pellagra 265.2
 poisoning, accidental (acute) NEC 980.9
  specified type of alcohol — *see* Table of Drugs and Chemicals
 psychosis (*see also* Psychosis, alcoholic) 291.9
  Korsakoff's, Korsakov's, Korsakow's 291.1
  polyneuritic 291.1
   with
    delusions 291.5
    hallucinations 291.3
 related disorder 291.9
 withdrawal symptoms, syndrome NEC 291.81
  delirium 291.0
  hallucinosis 291.3

Alcoholism 303.9 ☑

Note — Use the following fifth-digit subclassification with category 303:

0 unspecified

1 continuous

2 episodic

3 in remission

 with psychosis (*see also* Psychosis, alcoholic) 291.9
 acute 303.0 ☑
 chronic 303.9 ☑
  with psychosis 291.9
 complicating pregnancy, childbirth, or puerperium 648.4 ☑
  affecting fetus or newborn 760.71
 history V11.3
 Korsakoff's, Korsakov's, Korsakow's 291.1
 suspected damage to fetus affecting management of pregnancy 655.4 ☑
Alder's anomaly or syndrome (leukocyte granulation anomaly) 288.2
Alder-Reilly anomaly (leukocyte granulation) 288.2
Aldosteronism (primary) 255.10
 congenital 255.10
 familial type I 255.11
 glucocorticoid-remediable 255.11
 secondary 255.14
Aldosteronoma (M8370/1) 237.2
Aldrich (-Wiskott) syndrome (eczema-thrombocytopenia) 279.12
Aleppo boil 085.1
Aleukemic — *see* condition
Aleukia
 congenital 288.09
 hemorrhagica 284.9
  acquired (secondary) 284.89
  congenital 284.09
  idiopathic 284.9
 splenica 289.4
Alexia (congenital) (developmental) 315.01
 secondary to organic lesion 784.61
Algoneurodystrophy 733.7
Algophobia 300.29
Alibert-Bazin disease (M9700/3) 202.1 ☑
Alibert's disease (mycosis fungoides) (M9700/3) 202.1 ☑
Alice in Wonderland syndrome 293.89
Alienation, mental — *see also* Psychosis 298.9
Alkalemia 276.3
Alkalosis 276.3
 metabolic 276.3
  with respiratory acidosis 276.4
 respiratory 276.3
Alkaptonuria 270.2
Allen-Masters syndrome 620.6
Allergic bronchopulmonary aspergillosis 518.6
Allergy, allergic (reaction) 995.3
 air-borne substance — *see also* Fever, hay 477.9
  specified allergen NEC 477.8
 alveolitis (extrinsic) 495.9
  due to
   Aspergillus clavatus 495.4
   cryptostroma corticale 495.6
   organisms (fungal, thermophilic actinomycete, other) growing in ventilation (air conditioning systems) 495.7
  specified type NEC 495.8
 anaphylactic reaction or shock 995.0
  due to food — *see* Anaphylactic reaction or shock, due to, food
 angioderma 995.1
 angioneurotic edema 995.1
 animal (cat) (dog) (epidermal) 477.8
  dander 477.2
  hair 477.2
 arthritis (*see also* Arthritis, allergic) 716.2 ☑
 asthma — *see* Asthma
 bee sting (anaphylactic shock) 989.5
 biological — *see* Allergy, drug

Allergy, allergic — *continued*
 bronchial asthma — *see* Asthma
 conjunctivitis (eczematous) 372.14
 dander, animal (cat) (dog) 477.2
 dandruff 477.8
 dermatitis (venenata) — *see* Dermatitis
 diathesis V15.09
 drug, medicinal substance, and biological (any) (correct medicinal substance properly administered) (external) (internal) 995.27
  wrong substance given or taken NEC 977.9
   specified drug or substance — *see* Table of Drugs and Chemicals
 dust (house) (stock) 477.8
 eczema — *see* Eczema
 endophthalmitis 360.19
 epidermal (animal) 477.8
 existing dental restorative material
 feathers 477.8
 food (any) (ingested) 693.1
  atopic 691.8
  in contact with skin 692.5
 gastritis 535.4 ☑
 gastroenteritis 558.3
 gastrointestinal 558.3
 grain 477.0
 grass (pollen) 477.0
  asthma (*see also* Asthma) 493.0 ☑
  hay fever 477.0
 hair, animal (cat) (dog) 477.2
 hay fever (grass) (pollen) (ragweed) (tree) (*see also* Fever, hay) 477.9
 history (of) V15.09
  to
   arachnid bite V15.06
   eggs V15.03
   food additives V15.05
   insect bite V15.06
   latex V15.07
   milk products V15.02
   nuts V15.05
    peanuts V15.01
   radiographic dye V15.08
   seafood V15.04
   specified food NEC V15.05
   spider bite V15.06
 horse serum — *see* Allergy, serum
 inhalant 477.9
  dust 477.8
  pollen 477.0
  specified allergen other than pollen 477.8
 kapok 477.8
 medicine — *see* Allergy, drug
 migraine 339.00
 milk protein 558.3
 pannus 370.62
 pneumonia 518.3
 pollen (any) (hay fever) 477.0
  asthma (*see also* Asthma) 493.0 ☑
 primrose 477.0
 primula 477.0
 purpura 287.0
 ragweed (pollen) (Senecio jacobae) 477.0
  asthma (*see also* Asthma) 493.0 ☑
  hay fever 477.0
 respiratory (*see also* Allergy, inhalant) 477.9
  due to
   drug — *see* Allergy, drug
   food — *see* Allergy, food
 rhinitis (*see also* Fever, hay) 477.9
  due to food 477.1
 rose 477.0
 Senecio jacobae 477.0
 serum (prophylactic) (therapeutic) 999.59
  anaphylactic reaction or shock 999.49
 shock (anaphylactic) (due to adverse effect of correct medicinal substance properly administered) 995.0
  food — *see* Anaphylactic reaction or shock, due to, food
  from
   administration of blood and blood products 999.41

Allergy, allergic — *continued*
  shock — *continued*
    from — *continued*
      immunization 999.42
        serum NEC 999.49
  sinusitis (*see also* Fever, hay) 477.9
  skin reaction 692.9
    specified substance — *see* Dermatitis, due to
  tree (any) (hay fever) (pollen) 477.0
    asthma (*see also* Asthma) 493.0 ☑
  upper respiratory (*see also* Fever, hay) 477.9
  urethritis 597.89
  urticaria 708.0
  vaccine — *see* Allergy, serum
Allescheriosis 117.6
Alligator skin disease (ichthyosis congenita) 757.1
  acquired 701.1
Allocheiria, allochiria — *see also* Disturbance, sensation 782.0
Almeida's disease (Brazilian blastomycosis) 116.1
Alopecia (atrophicans) (pregnancy) (premature) (senile) 704.00
  adnata 757.4
  areata 704.01
  celsi 704.01
  cicatrisata 704.09
  circumscripta 704.01
  congenital, congenitalis 757.4
  disseminata 704.01
  effluvium (telogen) 704.02
  febrile 704.09
  generalisata 704.09
  hereditaria 704.09
  marginalis 704.01
  mucinosa 704.09
  postinfectional 704.09
  seborrheica 704.09
  specific 091.82
  syphilitic (secondary) 091.82
  telogen effluvium 704.02
  totalis 704.09
  toxica 704.09
  universalis 704.09
  x-ray 704.09
Alpers' disease 330.8
Alpha-lipoproteinemia 272.4
Alpha thalassemia 282.43
Alphos 696.1
Alpine sickness 993.2
Alport's syndrome (hereditary hematuri-anephropathy-deafness) 759.89
ALPS (autoimmune lymphoproliferative syndrome) 279.41
ALTE (apparent life threatening event) **in newborn and infant)** 799.82
Alteration (of), altered
  awareness 780.09
    transient 780.02
  consciousness 780.09
    persistent vegetative state 780.03
    transient 780.02
  mental status 780.97
    amnesia (retrograde) 780.93
    memory loss 780.93
Alternaria (infection) 118
Alternating — *see* condition
Altitude, high (effects) — *see* Effect, adverse, high altitude
Aluminosis (of lung) 503
Alvarez syndrome (transient cerebral ischemia) 435.9
Alveolar capillary block syndrome 516.64
Alveolitis
  allergic (extrinsic) 495.9
    due to organisms (fungal, thermophilic actinomycete, other) growing in ventilation (air conditioning systems) 495.7
    specified type NEC 495.8
  due to
    Aspergillus clavatus 495.4
    Cryptostroma corticale 495.6

Alveolitis — *continued*
  fibrosing (chronic) (cryptogenic) (lung) 516.31
  idiopathic 516.30
  rheumatoid 714.81
  jaw 526.5
  sicca dolorosa 526.5
Alveolus, alveolar — *see* condition
Alymphocytosis (pure) 279.2
Alymphoplasia, thymic 279.2
Alzheimer's
  dementia (senile)
    with behavioral disturbance 331.0 *[294.11]*
    without behavioral disturbance 331.0 *[294.10]*
  disease or sclerosis 331.0
    with dementia — *see* Alzheimer's, dementia
Amastia — *see also* Absence, breast 611.89
Amaurosis (acquired) (congenital) — *see also* Blindness 369.00
  fugax 362.34
  hysterical 300.11
  Leber's (congenital) 362.76
  tobacco 377.34
  uremic — *see* Uremia
Amaurotic familial idiocy (infantile) (juvenile) (late) 330.1
Ambisexual 752.7
Amblyopia (acquired) (congenital) (partial) 368.00
  color 368.59
    acquired 368.55
  deprivation 368.02
  ex anopsia 368.00
  hysterical 300.11
  nocturnal 368.60
    vitamin A deficiency 264.5
  refractive 368.03
  strabismic 368.01
  suppression 368.01
  tobacco 377.34
  toxic NEC 377.34
  uremic — *see* Uremia
Ameba, amebic (histolytica) — *see also* Amebiasis
  abscess 006.3
    bladder 006.8
    brain (with liver and lung abscess) 006.5
    liver 006.3
      with
        brain abscess (and lung abscess) 006.5
        lung abscess 006.4
    lung (with liver abscess) 006.4
      with brain abscess 006.5
    seminal vesicle 006.8
    spleen 006.8
  carrier (suspected of) V02.2
  meningoencephalitis
    due to Naegleria (gruberi) 136.29
    primary 136.29
Amebiasis NEC 006.9
  with
    brain abscess (with liver or lung abscess) 006.5
    liver abscess (without mention of brain or lung abscess) 006.3
    lung abscess (with liver abscess) 006.4
      with brain abscess 006.5
  acute 006.0
  bladder 006.8
  chronic 006.1
  cutaneous 006.6
  cutis 006.6
  due to organism other than Entamoeba histolytica 007.8
  hepatic (*see also* Abscess, liver, amebic) 006.3
  nondysenteric 006.2
  seminal vesicle 006.8
  specified
    organism NEC 007.8
    site NEC 006.8
Ameboma 006.8

Amelia 755.4
  lower limb 755.31
  upper limb 755.21
Ameloblastoma (M9310/0) 213.1
  jaw (bone) (lower) 213.1
    upper 213.0
  long bones (M9261/3) — *see* Neoplasm, bone, malignant
  malignant (M9310/3) 170.1
    jaw (bone) (lower) 170.1
      upper 170.0
  mandible 213.1
  tibial (M9261/3) 170.7
Amelogenesis imperfecta 520.5
  nonhereditaria (segmentalis) 520.4
Amenorrhea (primary) (secondary) 626.0
  due to ovarian dysfunction 256.8
  hyperhormonal 256.8
Amentia — *see also* Disability, intellectual 319
  Meynert's (nonalcoholic) 294.0
    alcoholic 291.1
  nevoid 759.6
American
  leishmaniasis 085.5
  mountain tick fever 066.1
  trypanosomiasis — *see* Trypanosomiasis, American
Ametropia — *see also* Disorder, accommodation 367.9
Amianthosis 501
Amimia 784.69
Amino acid
  deficiency 270.9
    anemia 281.4
  metabolic disorder (*see also* Disorder, amino acid) 270.9
Aminoaciduria 270.9
  imidazole 270.5
Amnesia (retrograde) 780.93
  auditory 784.69
    developmental 315.31
    secondary to organic lesion 784.69
  dissociative 300.12
  hysterical or dissociative type 300.12
  psychogenic 300.12
  transient global 437.7
Amnestic (confabulatory) **syndrome** 294.0
  alcohol-induced persisting 291.1
  drug-induced persisting 292.83
  posttraumatic 294.0
Amniocentesis screening (for) V28.2
  alphafetoprotein level, raised V28.1
  chromosomal anomalies V28.0
Amnion, amniotic — *see also* condition
  nodosum 658.8 ☑
Amnionitis (complicating pregnancy) 658.4 ☑
  affecting fetus or newborn 762.7
Amoral trends 301.7
Amotio retinae — *see also* Detachment, retina 361.9
Ampulla
  lower esophagus 530.89
  phrenic 530.89
Amputation
  any part of fetus, to facilitate delivery 763.89
  cervix (supravaginal) (uteri) 622.8
    in pregnancy or childbirth 654.6 ☑
      affecting fetus or newborn 763.89
  clitoris — *see* Wound, open, clitoris
  congenital
    lower limb 755.31
    upper limb 755.21
  neuroma (traumatic) (*see also* Injury, nerve, by site)
    surgical complication (late) 997.61
  penis — *see* Amputation, traumatic, penis
  status (without complication) — *see* Absence, by site, acquired
  stump (surgical) (posttraumatic)
    abnormal, painful, or with complication (late) 997.60
    healed or old NEC (*see also* Absence, by site, acquired)
      lower V49.70
      upper V49.60

Amputation — *continued*
  traumatic (complete) (partial)

Note — "Complicated" includes traumatic amputation with delayed healing, delayed treatment, foreign body, or infection.

    arm 887.4
      at or above elbow 887.2
        complicated 887.3
      below elbow 887.0
        complicated 887.1
      both (bilateral) (any level(s)) 887.6
        complicated 887.7
      complicated 887.5
    finger(s) (one or both hands) 886.0
      with thumb(s) 885.0
        complicated 885.1
      complicated 886.1
    foot (except toe(s) only) 896.0
      and other leg 897.6
        complicated 897.7
      both (bilateral) 896.2
        complicated 896.3
      complicated 896.1
      toe(s) only (one or both feet) 895.0
        complicated 895.1
    genital organ(s) (external) NEC 878.8
      complicated 878.9
    hand (except finger(s) only) 887.0
      and other arm 887.6
        complicated 887.7
      both (bilateral) 887.6
        complicated 887.7
      complicated 887.1
    finger(s) (one or both hands) 886.0
      with thumb(s) 885.0
        complicated 885.1
      complicated 886.1
      thumb(s) (with fingers of either hand) 885.0
        complicated 885.1
    head 874.9
    late effect — *see* Late, effects (of), amputation
    leg 897.4
      and other foot 897.6
        complicated 897.7
      at or above knee 897.2
        complicated 897.3
      below knee 897.0
        complicated 897.1
      both (bilateral) 897.6
        complicated 897.7
      complicated 897.5
    lower limb(s) except toe(s) — *see* Amputation, traumatic, leg
    nose — *see* Wound, open, nose
    penis 878.0
      complicated 878.1
    sites other than limbs — *see* Wound, open, by site
    thumb(s) (with finger(s) of either hand) 885.0
      complicated 885.1
    toe(s) (one or both feet) 895.0
      complicated 895.1
    upper limb(s) — *see* Amputation, traumatic, arm
Amputee (bilateral) (old) — *see also* Absence, by site, acquired V49.70
Amusia 784.69
  developmental 315.39
  secondary to organic lesion 784.69
Amyelencephalus 740.0
Amyelia 742.59
Amygdalitis — *see* Tonsillitis
Amygdalolith 474.8
Amyloid disease or degeneration 277.30
  heart 277.39 *[425.7]*
Amyloidosis (familial) (general) (generalized) (genetic) (primary) 277.30
  with lung involvement 277.39 *[517.8]*
  cardiac, hereditary 277.39
  heart 277.39 *[425.7]*
  nephropathic 277.39 *[583.81]*

☑ Additional Digit Required — Refer to the Tabular List for Digit Selection   Subterms under main terms may continue to next column or page

2013 ICD-9-CM   ▶◀ Revised Text   ● New Line   ▲ Revised Code   Volume 2 — 17

Amyloidosis — continued
neuropathic (Portuguese) (Swiss)
277.39 *[357.4]*
pulmonary 277.39 *[517.8]*
secondary 277.39
systemic, inherited 277.39
Amylopectinosis (brancher enzyme deficiency)
271.0
Amylophagia 307.52
Amyoplasia, congenita 756.89
Amyotonia 728.2
congenita 358.8
Amyotrophia, amyotrophy, amyotrophic
728.2
congenita 756.89
diabetic 250.6 ☑ *[353.5]*
due to secondary diabetes
249.6 ☑ *[353.5]*
lateral sclerosis (syndrome) 335.20
neuralgic 353.5
sclerosis (lateral) 335.20
spinal progressive 335.21
Anacidity, gastric 536.0
psychogenic 306.4
Anaerosis of newborn 770.88
Analbuminemia 273.8
Analgesia — see also Anesthesia 782.0
Analphalipoproteinemia 272.5
Anaphylactic reaction or shock (correct
substance properly administered) 995.0
due to
administration of blood and blood
products 999.41
chemical — see Table of Drugs and
Chemicals
correct medicinal substance properly
administered 995.0
drug or medicinal substance
correct substance properly administered 995.0
overdose or wrong substance given
or taken 977.9
specified drug — see Table of
Drugs and Chemicals
following sting(s) 989.5
food 995.60
additives 995.66
crustaceans 995.62
eggs 995.68
fish 995.65
fruits 995.63
milk products 995.67
nuts (tree) 995.64
peanuts 995.61
seeds 995.64
specified NEC 995.69
tree nuts 995.64
vegetables 995.63
immunization 999.42
overdose or wrong substance given or
taken 977.9
specified drug — see Table of Drugs
and Chemicals
serum NEC 999.49
following sting(s) 989.5
purpura 287.0
serum NEC 999.49
Anaphylactoid reaction or shock — see
Anaphylactic reaction or shock
Anaphylaxis — see Anaphylactic reaction or
shock
Anaplasia, cervix 622.10
Anaplasmosis, human 082.49
Anarthria 784.51
Anarthritic rheumatoid disease 446.5
Anasarca 782.3
cardiac (see also Failure, heart) 428.0
fetus or newborn 778.0
lung 514
nutritional 262
pulmonary 514
renal (see also Nephrosis) 581.9
Anaspadias 752.62
Anastomosis
aneurysmal — see Aneurysm

Anastomosis — continued
arteriovenous, congenital NEC (see also
Anomaly, arteriovenous) 747.60
ruptured, of brain (see also Hemorrhage,
subarachnoid) 430
intestinal 569.89
complicated NEC 997.49
involving urinary tract 997.5
retinal and choroidal vessels 743.58
acquired 362.17
Anatomical narrow angle (glaucoma) 365.02
Ancylostoma (infection) (infestation) 126.9
americanus 126.1
braziliense 126.2
caninum 126.8
ceylanicum 126.3
duodenale 126.0
Necator americanus 126.1
Ancylostomiasis (intestinal) 126.9
ancylostoma
americanus 126.1
caninum 126.8
ceylanicum 126.3
duodenale 126.0
braziliense 126.2
Necator americanus 126.1
Anders' disease or syndrome (adiposis
tuberosa simplex) 272.8
Andersen's glycogen storage disease 271.0
Anderson's disease 272.7
Andes disease 993.2
Andrews' disease (bacterid) 686.8
Androblastoma (M8630/1)
benign (M8630/0)
specified site — see Neoplasm, by site,
benign
unspecified site
female 220
male 222.0
malignant (M8630/3)
specified site — see Neoplasm, by site,
malignant
unspecified site
female 183.0
male 186.9
specified site — see Neoplasm, by site, uncertain behavior
tubular (M8640/0)
with lipid storage (M8641/0)
specified site — see Neoplasm, by
site, benign
unspecified site
female 220
male 222.0
specified site — see Neoplasm, by site,
benign
unspecified site
female 220
male 222.0
unspecified site
female 236.2
male 236.4
Android pelvis 755.69
with disproportion (fetopelvic) 653.3 ☑
affecting fetus or newborn 763.1
causing obstructed labor 660.1 ☑
affecting fetus or newborn 763.1
Anectasis, pulmonary (newborn or fetus)
770.5
Anemia 285.9
with
disorder of
anaerobic glycolysis 282.3
pentose phosphate pathway 282.2
koilonychia 285.9
6-phosphogluconic dehydrogenase deficiency 282.2
achlorhydric 280.9
achrestic 281.8
Addison's (pernicious) 281.0
Addison-Biermer (pernicious) 281.0
agranulocytic 288.09
amino acid deficiency 281.4
antineoplastic chemotherapy induced 285.3
aplastic 284.9
acquired (secondary) 284.89

Anemia — continued
aplastic — continued
congenital 284.01
constitutional 284.01
due to
antineoplastic chemotherapy 284.89
chronic systemic disease 284.89
drugs 284.89
infection 284.89
radiation 284.89
idiopathic 284.9
myxedema 244.9
of or complicating pregnancy 648.2 ☑
red cell (acquired) (adult) (with thymoma) 284.81
congenital 284.01
pure 284.01
specified type NEC 284.89
toxic (paralytic) 284.89
aregenerative 284.9
congenital 284.01
asiderotic 280.9
atypical (primary) 285.9
autohemolysis of Selwyn and Dacie (type I)
282.2
autoimmune hemolytic 283.0
Baghdad Spring 282.2
Balantidium coli 007.0
Biermer's (pernicious) 281.0
blood loss (chronic) 280.0
acute 285.1
bothriocephalus 123.4
brickmakers' (see also Ancylostomiasis)
126.9
cerebral 437.8
childhood 282.9
chlorotic 280.9
chronic 285.9
blood loss 280.0
hemolytic 282.9
idiopathic 283.9
simple 281.9
chronica congenita aregenerativa 284.01
combined system disease NEC 281.0 *[336.2]*
due to dietary deficiency 281.1 *[336.2]*
complicating pregnancy or childbirth
648.2 ☑
congenital (following fetal blood loss) 776.5
aplastic 284.01
due to isoimmunization NEC 773.2
Heinz-body 282.7
hereditary hemolytic NEC 282.9
nonspherocytic
Type I 282.2
Type II 282.3
pernicious 281.0
spherocytic (see also Spherocytosis)
282.0
Cooley's (erythroblastic) 282.44
crescent — see Disease, sickle-cell
cytogenic 281.0
Dacie's (nonspherocytic)
type I 282.2
type II 282.3
Davidson's (refractory) 284.9
deficiency 281.9
2, 3 diphosphoglycurate mutase 282.3
2, 3 PG 282.3
6-PGD 282.2
6-phosphogluronic dehydrogenase
282.2
amino acid 281.4
combined B₁₂ and folate 281.3
enzyme, drug-induced (hemolytic) 282.2
erythrocytic glutathione 282.2
folate 281.2
dietary 281.2
drug-induced 281.2
folic acid 281.2
dietary 281.2
drug-induced 281.2
G-6-PD 282.2
GGS-R 282.2
glucose-6-phosphate dehydrogenase
(G-6-PD) 282.2
glucose-phosphate isomerase 282.3

Anemia — continued
deficiency — continued
glutathione peroxidase 282.2
glutathione reductase 282.2
glyceraldehyde phosphate dehydrogenase 282.3
GPI 282.3
G SH 282.2
hexokinase 282.3
iron (Fe) 280.9
specified NEC 280.8
nutritional 281.9
with
poor iron absorption 280.9
specified deficiency NEC 281.8
due to inadequate dietary iron intake
280.1
specified type NEC 281.8
of or complicating pregnancy 648.2 ☑
pentose phosphate pathway 282.2
PFK 282.3
phosphofructo-aldolase 282.3
phosphofructokinase 282.3
phosphoglycerate kinase 282.3
PK 282.3
protein 281.4
pyruvate kinase (PK) 282.3
TPI 282.3
triosephosphate isomerase 282.3
vitamin B₁₂ NEC 281.1
dietary 281.1
pernicious 281.0
Diamond-Blackfan (congenital hypoplastic)
284.01
dibothriocephalus 123.4
dimorphic 281.9
diphasic 281.8
diphtheritic 032.89
Diphyllobothrium 123.4
drepanocytic (see also Disease, sickle-cell)
282.60
due to
antineoplastic chemotherapy 285.3
blood loss (chronic) 280.0
acute 285.1
chemotherapy, antineoplastic 285.3
defect of Embden-Meyerhof pathway
glycolysis 282.3
disorder of glutathione metabolism
282.2
drug — see Anemia, by type (see also
Table of Drugs and Chemicals)
chemotherapy, antineoplastic 285.3
fetal blood loss 776.5
fish tapeworm (D. latum) infestation
123.4
glutathione metabolism disorder 282.2
hemorrhage (chronic) 280.0
acute 285.1
hexose monophosphate (HMP) shunt
deficiency 282.2
impaired absorption 280.9
loss of blood (chronic) 280.0
acute 285.1
myxedema 244.9
Necator americanus 126.1
prematurity 776.6
selective vitamin B₁₂ malabsorption with
proteinuria 281.1
Dyke-Young type (secondary)
(symptomatic) 283.9
dyserythropoietic (congenital) (types I, II,
III) 285.8
dyshemopoietic (congenital) 285.8
Egypt (see also Ancylostomiasis) 126.9
elliptocytosis (see also Elliptocytosis) 282.1
enzyme deficiency, drug-induced 282.2
epidemic (see also Ancylostomiasis) 126.9
EPO resistant 285.21
erythroblastic
familial 282.44
fetus or newborn (see also Disease,
hemolytic) 773.2
late 773.5
erythrocytic glutathione deficiency 282.2

☑ Additional Digit Required — Refer to the Tabular List for Digit Selection   ⩊ Subterms under main terms may continue to next column or page

18 — Volume 2   ▶◀ Revised Text   ● New Line   ▲ Revised Code   2013 ICD-9-CM

Anemia — *continued*
  erythropoietin-resistant (EPO resistant anemia) 285.21
  essential 285.9
  Faber's (achlorhydric anemia) 280.9
  factitious (self-induced blood letting) 280.0
  familial erythroblastic (microcytic) 282.44
  Fanconi's (congenital pancytopenia) 284.09
  favism 282.2
  fetal 678.0 ☑
    following blood loss, affecting newborn 776.5
  fetus or newborn
    due to
      ABO
        antibodies 773.1
        incompatibility, maternal/fetal 773.1
        isoimmunization 773.1
      Rh
        antibodies 773.0
        incompatibility, maternal/fetal 773.0
        isoimmunization 773.0
    following fetal blood loss 776.5
  fish tapeworm (D. latum) infestation 123.4
  folate (folic acid) deficiency 281.2
    dietary 281.2
    drug-induced 281.2
  folate malabsorption, congenital 281.2
  folic acid deficiency 281.2
    dietary 281.2
    drug-induced 281.2
  G-6-PD 282.2
  general 285.9
  glucose-6-phosphate dehydrogenase deficiency 282.2
  glutathione-reductase deficiency 282.2
  goat's milk 281.2
  granulocytic 288.09
  Heinz-body, congenital 282.7
  hemoglobin deficiency 285.9
  hemolytic 283.9
    acquired 283.9
      with hemoglobinuria NEC 283.2
      autoimmune (cold type) (idiopathic) (primary) (secondary) (symptomatic) (warm type) 283.0
      due to
        cold reactive antibodies 283.0
        drug exposure 283.0
        warm reactive antibodies 283.0
      fragmentation 283.19
      idiopathic (chronic) 283.9
      infectious 283.19
        autoimmune 283.0
        non-autoimmune 283.10
      toxic 283.19
      traumatic cardiac 283.19
    acute 283.9
      due to enzyme deficiency NEC 282.3
      fetus or newborn (*see also* Disease, hemolytic) 773.2
        late 773.5
      Lederer's (acquired infectious hemolytic anemia) 283.19
    autoimmune (acquired) 283.0
    chronic 282.9
      idiopathic 283.9
    cold type (secondary) (symptomatic) 283.0
    congenital (spherocytic) (*see also* Spherocytosis) 282.0
      nonspherocytic — *see* Anemia, hemolytic, nonspherocytic, congenital
    drug-induced 283.0
      enzyme deficiency 282.2
    due to
      cardiac conditions 283.19
      drugs 283.0
      enzyme deficiency NEC 282.3
        drug-induced 282.2
      presence of shunt or other internal prosthetic device 283.19

Anemia — *continued*
  hemolytic — *continued*
    due to — *continued*
      thrombotic thrombocytopenic purpura 446.6
    elliptocytotic (*see also* Elliptocytosis) 282.1
    familial 282.9
    hereditary 282.9
      due to enzyme deficiency NEC 282.3
      specified NEC 282.8
    idiopathic (chronic) 283.9
    infectious (acquired) 283.19
    mechanical 283.19
    microangiopathic 283.19
    non-autoimmune NEC 283.10
    nonspherocytic
      congenital or hereditary NEC 282.3
        glucose-6-phosphate dehydrogenase deficiency 282.2
        pyruvate kinase (PK) deficiency 282.3
        type I 282.2
        type II 282.3
        type I 282.2
        type II 282.3
    of or complicating pregnancy 648.2 ☑
    resulting from presence of shunt or other internal prosthetic device 283.19
    secondary 283.19
      autoimmune 283.0
    sickle-cell — *see* Disease, sickle-cell
    Stransky-Regala type (Hb-E) (*see also* Disease, hemoglobin) 282.7
    symptomatic 283.19
      autoimmune 283.0
    toxic (acquired) 283.19
    uremic (adult) (child) 283.11
    warm type (secondary) (symptomatic) 283.0
  hemorrhagic (chronic) 280.0
    acute 285.1
  HEMPAS 285.8
  hereditary erythroblast multinuclearity-positive acidified serum test 285.8
  Herrick's (hemoglobin S disease) 282.61
  hexokinase deficiency 282.3
  high A$_2$ 282.46
  hookworm (*see also* Ancylostomiasis) 126.9
  hypochromic (idiopathic) (microcytic) (normoblastic) 280.9
    with iron loading 285.0
    due to blood loss (chronic) 280.0
      acute 285.1
    familial sex linked 285.0
    pyridoxine-responsive 285.0
  hypoplasia, red blood cells 284.81
    congenital or familial 284.01
  hypoplastic (idiopathic) 284.9
    congenital 284.01
    familial 284.01
    of childhood 284.09
  idiopathic 285.9
    hemolytic, chronic 283.9
  in (due to) (with)
    chronic illness NEC 285.29
    chronic kidney disease 285.21
    end-stage renal disease 285.21
    neoplastic disease 285.22
  infantile 285.9
  infective, infectional 285.9
  intertropical (*see also* Ancylostomiasis) 126.9
  iron (Fe) deficiency 280.9
    due to blood loss (chronic) 280.0
      acute 285.1
    of or complicating pregnancy 648.2 ☑
    specified NEC 280.8
  Jaksch's (pseudoleukemia infantum) 285.8
  Joseph-Diamond-Blackfan (congenital hypoplastic) 284.01
  labyrinth 386.50
  Lederer's (acquired infectious hemolytic anemia) 283.19
  leptocytosis (hereditary) 282.40
  leukoerythroblastic 284.2

Anemia — *continued*
  macrocytic 281.9
    nutritional 281.2
    of or complicating pregnancy 648.2 ☑
    tropical 281.2
  malabsorption (familial), selective B$_{12}$ with proteinuria 281.1
  malarial (*see also* Malaria) 084.6
  malignant (progressive) 281.0
  malnutrition 281.9
  marsh (*see also* Malaria) 084.6
  Mediterranean 282.40
    with hemoglobinopathy 282.49
  megaloblastic 281.9
    combined B$_{12}$ and folate deficiency 281.3
    nutritional (of infancy) 281.2
    of infancy 281.2
    of or complicating pregnancy 648.2 ☑
    refractory 281.3
    specified NEC 281.3
  megalocytic 281.9
  microangiopathic hemolytic 283.19
  microcytic (hypochromic) 280.9
    due to blood loss (chronic) 280.0
      acute 285.1
    familial 282.49
    hypochromic 280.9
  microdrepanocytosis 282.41
  miners' (*see also* Ancylostomiasis) 126.9
  myelopathic 285.8
  myelophthisic (normocytic) 284.2
  newborn (*see also* Disease, hemolytic) 773.2
    due to isoimmunization (*see also* Disease, hemolytic) 773.2
    late, due to isoimmunization 773.5
    posthemorrhagic 776.5
  nonregenerative 284.9
  nonspherocytic hemolytic — *see* Anemia, hemolytic, nonspherocytic
  normocytic (infectional) (not due to blood loss) 285.9
    due to blood loss (chronic) 280.0
      acute 285.1
    myelophthisic 284.2
  nutritional (deficiency) 281.9
    with
      poor iron absorption 280.9
      specified deficiency NEC 281.8
    due to inadequate dietary iron intake 280.1
    megaloblastic (of infancy) 281.2
  of childhood 282.9
  of chronic
    disease NEC 285.29
    illness NEC 285.29
  of or complicating pregnancy 648.2 ☑
    affecting fetus or newborn 760.8
  of prematurity 776.6
  orotic aciduric (congenital) (hereditary) 281.4
  osteosclerotic 289.89
  ovalocytosis (hereditary) (*see also* Elliptocytosis) 282.1
  paludal (*see also* Malaria) 084.6
  pentose phosphate pathway deficiency 282.2
  pernicious (combined system disease) (congenital) (dorsolateral spinal degeneration) (juvenile) (myelopathy) (neuropathy) (posterior sclerosis) (primary) (progressive) (spleen) 281.0
    of or complicating pregnancy 648.2 ☑
  pleochromic 285.9
    of sprue 281.8
  portal 285.8
  posthemorrhagic (chronic) 280.0
    acute 285.1
    newborn 776.5
  postoperative
    due to (acute) blood loss 285.1
      chronic blood loss 280.0
    other 285.9
  postpartum 648.2 ☑
  pressure 285.9
  primary 285.9

Anemia — *continued*
  profound 285.9
  progressive 285.9
    malignant 281.0
    pernicious 281.0
  protein-deficiency 281.4
  pseudoleukemica infantum 285.8
  puerperal 648.2 ☑
  pure red cell 284.81
    congenital 284.01
  pyridoxine-responsive (hypochromic) 285.0
  pyruvate kinase (PK) deficiency 282.3
  refractoria sideroblastica 238.72
  refractory (primary) 238.72
    with
      excess
        blasts-1 (RAEB-1) 238.72
        blasts-2 (RAEB-2) 238.73
      hemochromatosis 238.72
      ringed sideroblasts (RARS) 238.72
    due to
      drug 285.0
      myelodysplastic syndrome 238.72
      toxin 285.0
    hereditary 285.0
    idiopathic 238.72
    megaloblastic 281.3
    sideroblastic 238.72
      hereditary 285.0
    sideropenic 280.9
  Rietti-Greppi-Micheli (thalassemia minor) 282.46
  scorbutic 281.8
  secondary (to) 285.9
    blood loss (chronic) 280.0
      acute 285.1
    hemorrhage 280.0
      acute 285.1
    inadequate dietary iron intake 280.1
  semiplastic 284.9
  septic 285.9
  sickle-cell (*see also* Disease, sickle-cell) 282.60
  sideroachrestic 285.0
  sideroblastic (acquired) (any type) (congenital) (drug-induced) (due to disease) (hereditary) (primary) (secondary) (sex-linked hypochromic) (vitamin B$_6$ responsive) 285.0
    refractory 238.72
      congenital 285.0
      drug-induced 285.0
      hereditary 285.0
      sex-linked hypochromic 285.0
      vitamin B$_6$-responsive 285.0
  sideropenic (refractory) 280.9
    due to blood loss (chronic) 280.0
      acute 285.1
  simple chronic 281.9
  specified type NEC 285.8
  spherocytic (hereditary) (*see also* Spherocytosis) 282.0
  splenic 285.8
    familial (Gaucher's) 272.7
  splenomegalic 285.8
  stomatocytosis 282.8
  syphilitic 095.8
  target cell (oval) 285.8
    with thalassemia — *see* Thalassemia
  thalassemia 282.40
  thrombocytopenic (*see also* Thrombocytopenia) 287.5
  toxic 284.89
  triosephosphate isomerase deficiency 282.3
  tropical, macrocytic 281.2
  tuberculous (*see also* Tuberculosis) 017.9 ☑
  vegan's 281.1
  vitamin
    B$_6$-responsive 285.0
    B$_{12}$ deficiency (dietary) 281.1
      pernicious 281.0
  von Jaksch's (pseudoleukemia infantum) 285.8
  Witts' (achlorhydric anemia) 280.9

☑ **Additional Digit Required — Refer to the Tabular List for Digit Selection**   ▽ **Subterms under main terms may continue to next column or page**

Anemia — continued
  Zuelzer (-Ogden) (nutritional megaloblastic anemia) 281.2
Anencephalus, anencephaly 740.0
  fetal, affecting management of pregnancy 655.0 ☑
Anergasia — see also Psychosis, organic 294.9
  senile 290.0
Anesthesia, anesthetic 782.0
  complication or reaction NEC 995.22
    due to
      correct substance properly administered 995.22
      overdose or wrong substance given 968.4
        specified anesthetic — see Table of Drugs and Chemicals
  cornea 371.81
  death from
    correct substance properly administered 995.4
    during delivery 668.9 ☑
    overdose or wrong substance given 968.4
    specified anesthetic — see Table of Drugs and Chemicals
  eye 371.81
  functional 300.11
  hyperesthetic, thalamic 338.0
  hysterical 300.11
  local skin lesion 782.0
  olfactory 781.1
  sexual (psychogenic) 302.72
  shock
    due to
      correct substance properly administered 995.4
      overdose or wrong substance given 968.4
      specified anesthetic — see Table of Drugs and Chemicals
  skin 782.0
  tactile 782.0
  testicular 608.9
  thermal 782.0
Anetoderma (maculosum) 701.3
Aneuploidy NEC 758.5
Aneurin deficiency 265.1
Aneurysm (anastomotic) (artery) (cirsoid) (diffuse) (false) (fusiform) (multiple) (ruptured) (saccular) (varicose) 442.9
  abdominal (aorta) 441.4
    ruptured 441.3
    syphilitic 093.0
  aorta, aortic (nonsyphilitic) 441.9
    abdominal 441.4
      dissecting 441.02
      ruptured 441.3
      syphilitic 093.0
    arch 441.2
      ruptured 441.1
    arteriosclerotic NEC 441.9
      ruptured 441.5
    ascending 441.2
      ruptured 441.1
    congenital 747.29
    descending 441.9
      abdominal 441.4
        ruptured 441.3
      ruptured 441.5
      thoracic 441.2
        ruptured 441.1
    dissecting 441.00
      abdominal 441.02
      thoracic 441.01
      thoracoabdominal 441.03
    due to coarctation (aorta) 747.10
    ruptured 441.5
    sinus, right 747.29
    syphilitic 093.0
    thoracoabdominal 441.7
      ruptured 441.6
    thorax, thoracic (arch) (nonsyphilitic) 441.2
      dissecting 441.01
      ruptured 441.1

Aneurysm — continued
  aorta, aortic — continued
    thorax, thoracic — continued
      syphilitic 093.0
      transverse 441.2
      ruptured 441.1
    valve (heart) (see also Endocarditis, aortic) 424.1
  arteriosclerotic NEC 442.9
    cerebral 437.3
      ruptured (see also Hemorrhage, subarachnoid) 430
  arteriovenous (congenital) (peripheral) NEC (see also Anomaly, arteriovenous) 747.60
    acquired NEC 447.0
      brain 437.3
        ruptured (see also Hemorrhage, subarachnoid) 430
      coronary 414.11
      pulmonary 417.0
    brain (cerebral) 747.81
      ruptured (see also Hemorrhage, subarachnoid) 430
    coronary 746.85
    pulmonary 747.32
    retina 743.58
    specified site NEC 747.89
    acquired 447.0
    traumatic (see also Injury, blood vessel, by site) 904.9
  basal — see Aneurysm, brain
  berry (congenital) (ruptured) (see also Hemorrhage, subarachnoid) 430
    nonruptured 437.3
  brain 437.3
    arteriosclerotic 437.3
      ruptured (see also Hemorrhage, subarachnoid) 430
    arteriovenous 747.81
      acquired 437.3
        ruptured (see also Hemorrhage, subarachnoid) 430
      ruptured (see also Hemorrhage, subarachnoid) 430
    berry (congenital) (ruptured) (see also Hemorrhage, subarachnoid) 430
      nonruptured 437.3
    congenital 747.81
      ruptured (see also Hemorrhage, subarachnoid) 430
    meninges 437.3
      ruptured (see also Hemorrhage, subarachnoid) 430
    miliary (congenital) (ruptured) (see also Hemorrhage, subarachnoid) 430
    mycotic 421.0
      ruptured (see also Hemorrhage, subarachnoid) 430
    nonruptured 437.3
    ruptured (see also Hemorrhage, subarachnoid) 430
    syphilitic 094.87
  syphilitic (hemorrhage) 094.87
  traumatic — see Injury, intracranial
  cardiac (false) (see also Aneurysm, heart) 414.10
  carotid artery (common) (external) 442.81
    internal (intracranial portion) 437.3
      extracranial portion 442.81
      ruptured into brain (see also Hemorrhage, subarachnoid) 430
    syphilitic 093.89
      intracranial 094.87
  cavernous sinus (see also Aneurysm, brain) 437.3
    arteriovenous 747.81
      ruptured (see also Hemorrhage, subarachnoid) 430
    congenital 747.81
      ruptured (see also Hemorrhage, subarachnoid) 430
  celiac 442.84
  central nervous system, syphilitic 094.89
  cerebral — see Aneurysm, brain
  chest — see Aneurysm, thorax

Aneurysm — continued
  circle of Willis (see also Aneurysm, brain) 437.3
    congenital 747.81
      ruptured (see also Hemorrhage, subarachnoid) 430
    ruptured (see also Hemorrhage, subarachnoid) 430
  common iliac artery 442.2
  congenital (peripheral) NEC 747.60
    brain 747.81
      ruptured (see also Hemorrhage, subarachnoid) 430
    cerebral — see Aneurysm, brain, congenital
    coronary 746.85
    gastrointestinal 747.61
    lower limb 747.64
    pulmonary 747.32
    renal 747.62
    retina 743.58
    specified site NEC 747.89
    spinal 747.82
    upper limb 747.63
  conjunctiva 372.74
  conus arteriosus (see also Aneurysm, heart) 414.10
  coronary (arteriosclerotic) (artery) (vein) (see also Aneurysm, heart) 414.11
    arteriovenous 746.85
    congenital 746.85
    syphilitic 093.89
  cylindrical 441.9
    ruptured 441.5
    syphilitic 093.9
  dissecting 442.9
    aorta 441.00
      abdominal 441.02
      thoracic 441.01
      thoracoabdominal 441.03
    syphilitic 093.9
  ductus arteriosus 747.0
  embolic — see Embolism, artery
  endocardial, infective (any valve) 421.0
  femoral 442.3
  gastroduodenal 442.84
  gastroepiploic 442.84
  heart (chronic or with a stated duration of over 8 weeks) (infectional) (wall) 414.10
    acute or with a stated duration of 8 weeks or less (see also Infarct, myocardium) 410.9 ☑
    congenital 746.89
    valve — see Endocarditis
  hepatic 442.84
  iliac (common) 442.2
  infective (any valve) 421.0
  innominate (nonsyphilitic) 442.89
    syphilitic 093.89
  interauricular septum (see also Aneurysm, heart) 414.10
  interventricular septum (see also Aneurysm, heart) 414.10
  intracranial — see Aneurysm, brain
  intrathoracic (nonsyphilitic) 441.2
    ruptured 441.1
    syphilitic 093.0
  jugular vein (acute) 453.89
    chronic 453.76
  lower extremity 442.3
  lung (pulmonary artery) 417.1
  malignant 093.9
  mediastinal (nonsyphilitic) 442.89
    syphilitic 093.89
  miliary (congenital) (ruptured) (see also Hemorrhage, subarachnoid) 430
  mitral (heart) (valve) 424.0
  mural (arteriovenous) (heart) (see also Aneurysm, heart) 414.10
  mycotic, any site 421.0
    without endocarditis — see Aneurysm by site
    ruptured, brain (see also Hemorrhage, subarachnoid) 430

Aneurysm — continued
  myocardium (see also Aneurysm, heart) 414.10
  neck 442.81
  pancreaticoduodenal 442.84
  patent ductus arteriosus 747.0
  peripheral NEC 442.89
    congenital NEC (see also Aneurysm, congenital) 747.60
  popliteal 442.3
  pulmonary 417.1
    arteriovenous 747.32
      acquired 417.0
    syphilitic 093.89
    valve (heart) (see also Endocarditis, pulmonary) 424.3
  racemose 442.9
    congenital (peripheral) NEC 747.60
  radial 442.0
  Rasmussen's (see also Tuberculosis) 011.2 ☑
  renal 442.1
  retinal (acquired) 362.17
    congenital 743.58
    diabetic 250.5 ☑ [362.01]
      due to secondary diabetes 249.5 ☑ [362.01]
  sinus, aortic (of Valsalva) 747.29
  specified site NEC 442.89
  spinal (cord) 442.89
    congenital 747.82
    syphilitic (hemorrhage) 094.89
  spleen, splenic 442.83
  subclavian 442.82
    syphilitic 093.89
  superior mesenteric 442.84
  syphilitic 093.9
    aorta 093.0
    central nervous system 094.89
    congenital 090.5
    spine, spinal 094.89
  thoracoabdominal 441.7
    ruptured 441.6
  thorax, thoracic (arch) (nonsyphilitic) 441.2
    dissecting 441.01
    ruptured 441.1
    syphilitic 093.0
  traumatic (complication) (early) — see Injury, blood vessel, by site
  tricuspid (heart) (valve) — see Endocarditis, tricuspid
  ulnar 442.0
  upper extremity 442.0
  valve, valvular — see Endocarditis
  venous 456.8
    congenital NEC (see also Aneurysm, congenital) 747.60
  ventricle (arteriovenous) (see also Aneurysm, heart) 414.10
  visceral artery NEC 442.84
Angiectasis 459.89
Angiectopia 459.9
Angiitis 447.6
  allergic granulomatous 446.4
  hypersensitivity 446.20
    Goodpasture's syndrome 446.21
    specified NEC 446.29
  necrotizing 446.0
  Wegener's (necrotizing respiratory granulomatosis) 446.4
Angina (attack) (cardiac) (chest) (effort) (heart) (pectoris) (syndrome) (vasomotor) 413.9
  abdominal 557.1
  accelerated 411.1
  agranulocytic 288.03
  aphthous 074.0
  catarrhal 462
  crescendo 411.1
  croupous 464.4
  cruris 443.9
    due to atherosclerosis NEC (see also Arteriosclerosis, extremities) 440.20
  decubitus 413.0
  diphtheritic (membranous) 032.0
  equivalent 413.9
  erysipelatous 034.0
  erythematous 462

☑ **Additional Digit Required** — Refer to the Tabular List for Digit Selection   ▼ **Subterms under main terms may continue to next column or page**

20 — Volume 2   ▶◀ Revised Text   ● New Line   ▲ Revised Code   **2013 ICD-9-CM**

Angina — *continued*
exudative, chronic 476.0
faucium 478.29
gangrenous 462
diphtheritic 032.0
infectious 462
initial 411.1
intestinal 557.1
ludovici 528.3
Ludwig's 528.3
malignant 462
diphtheritic 032.0
membranous 464.4
diphtheritic 032.0
mesenteric 557.1
monocytic 075
nocturnal 413.0
phlegmonous 475
diphtheritic 032.0
preinfarctional 411.1
Prinzmetal's 413.1
progressive 411.1
pseudomembranous 101
psychogenic 306.2
pultaceous, diphtheritic 032.0
scarlatinal 034.1
septic 034.0
simple 462
stable NEC 413.9
staphylococcal 462
streptococcal 034.0
stridulous, diphtheritic 032.3
syphilitic 093.9
congenital 090.5
tonsil 475
trachealis 464.4
unstable 411.1
variant 413.1
Vincent's 101
Angioblastoma (M9161/1) — *see* Neoplasm, connective tissue, uncertain behavior
Angiocholecystitis — *see also* Cholecystitis, acute 575.0
Angiocholitis — *see also* Cholecystitis, acute 576.1
Angiodysgensis spinalis 336.1
Angiodysplasia (intestinalis) (intestine) 569.84
with hemorrhage 569.85
duodenum 537.82
with hemorrhage 537.83
stomach 537.82
with hemorrhage 537.83
Angioedema (allergic) (any site) (with urticaria) 995.1
hereditary 277.6
Angioendothelioma (M9130/1) — *see also* Neoplasm, by site, uncertain behavior
benign (M9130/0) (*see also* Hemangioma, by site) 228.00
bone (M9260/3) — *see* Neoplasm, bone, malignant
Ewing's (M9260/3) — *see* Neoplasm, bone, malignant
nervous system (M9130/0) 228.09
Angiofibroma (M9160/0) — *see also* Neoplasm, by site, benign
juvenile (M9160/0) 210.7
specified site — *see* Neoplasm, by site, benign
unspecified site 210.7
Angiohemophilia (A) (B) 286.4
Angioid streaks (choroid) (retina) 363.43
Angiokeratoma (M9141/0) — *see also* Neoplasm, skin, benign
corporis diffusum 272.7
Angiokeratosis
diffuse 272.7
Angioleiomyoma (M8894/0) — *see* Neoplasm, connective tissue, benign
Angioleucitis 683
Angiolipoma (M8861/0) — *see also* Lipoma, by site 214.9
infiltrating (M8861/1) — *see* Neoplasm, connective tissue, uncertain behavior
Angioma (M9120/0) — *see also* Hemangioma, by site 228.00

Angioma — *see also* Hemangioma, by site — *continued*
capillary 448.1
hemorrhagicum hereditaria 448.0
malignant (M9120/3) — *see* Neoplasm, connective tissue, malignant
pigmentosum et atrophicum 757.33
placenta — *see* Placenta, abnormal
plexiform (M9131/0) — *see* Hemangioma, by site
senile 448.1
serpiginosum 709.1
spider 448.1
stellate 448.1
Angiomatosis 757.32
bacillary 083.8
corporis diffusum universale 272.7
cutaneocerebral 759.6
encephalocutaneous 759.6
encephalofacial 759.6
encephalotrigeminal 759.6
hemorrhagic familial 448.0
hereditary familial 448.0
heredofamilial 448.0
meningo-oculofacial 759.6
multiple sites 228.09
neuro-oculocutaneous 759.6
retina (Hippel's disease) 759.6
retinocerebellosa 759.6
retinocerebral 759.6
systemic 228.09
Angiomyolipoma (M8860/0)
specified site — *see* Neoplasm, connective tissue, benign
unspecified site 223.0
Angiomyoliposarcoma (M8860/3) — *see* Neoplasm, connective tissue, malignant
Angiomyoma (M8894/0) — *see* Neoplasm, connective tissue, benign
Angiomyosarcoma (M8894/3) — *see* Neoplasm, connective tissue, malignant
Angioneurosis 306.2
Angioneurotic edema (allergic) (any site) (with urticaria) 995.1
hereditary 277.6
Angiopathia, angiopathy 459.9
diabetic (peripheral) 250.7 ☑ *[443.81]*
due to secondary diabetes 249.7 ☑ *[443.81]*
peripheral 443.9
diabetic 250.7 ☑ *[443.81]*
due to secondary diabetes 249.7 ☑ *[443.81]*
specified type NEC 443.89
retinae syphilitica 093.89
retinalis (juvenilis) 362.18
background 362.10
diabetic 250.5 ☑ *[362.01]*
due to secondary diabetes 249.5 ☑ *[362.01]*
proliferative 362.29
tuberculous (*see also* Tuberculosis) 017.3 ☑ *[362.18]*
Angiosarcoma (M9120/3) — *see* Neoplasm, connective tissue, malignant
Angiosclerosis — *see* Arteriosclerosis
Angioscotoma, enlarged 368.42
Angiospasm 443.9
brachial plexus 353.0
cerebral 435.9
cervical plexus 353.2
nerve
arm 354.9
axillary 353.0
median 354.1
ulnar 354.2
autonomic (*see also* Neuropathy, peripheral, autonomic) 337.9
axillary 353.0
leg 355.8
plantar 355.6
lower extremity — *see* Angiospasm, nerve, leg
median 354.1
peripheral NEC 355.9
spinal NEC 355.9

Angiospasm — *continued*
nerve — *continued*
sympathetic (*see also* Neuropathy, peripheral, autonomic) 337.9
ulnar 354.2
upper extremity — *see* Angiospasm, nerve, arm
peripheral NEC 443.9
traumatic 443.9
foot 443.9
leg 443.9
vessel 443.9
Angiospastic disease or edema 443.9
Angle's
class I 524.21
class II 524.22
class III 524.23
Anguillulosis 127.2
Angulation
cecum (*see also* Obstruction, intestine) 560.9
coccyx (acquired) 738.6
congenital 756.19
femur (acquired) 736.39
congenital 755.69
intestine (large) (small) (*see also* Obstruction, intestine) 560.9
sacrum (acquired) 738.5
congenital 756.19
sigmoid (flexure) (*see also* Obstruction, intestine) 560.9
spine (*see also* Curvature, spine) 737.9
tibia (acquired) 736.89
congenital 755.69
ureter 593.3
wrist (acquired) 736.09
congenital 755.59
Angulus infectiosus 686.8
Anhedonia 780.99
Anhidrosis (lid) (neurogenic) (thermogenic) 705.0
Anhydration 276.51
with
hypernatremia 276.0
hyponatremia 276.1
Anhydremia 276.52
with
hypernatremia 276.0
hyponatremia 276.1
Anidrosis 705.0
Aniridia (congenital) 743.45
Anisakiasis (infection) (infestation) 127.1
Anisakis larva infestation 127.1
Aniseikonia 367.32
Anisocoria (pupil) 379.41
congenital 743.46
Anisocytosis 790.09
Anisometropia (congenital) 367.31
Ankle — *see* condition
Ankyloblepharon (acquired) (eyelid) 374.46
filiforme (adnatum) (congenital) 743.62
total 743.62
Ankylodactly — *see also* Syndactylism 755.10
Ankyloglossia 750.0
Ankylosis (fibrous) (osseous) 718.50
ankle 718.57
any joint, produced by surgical fusion V45.4
cricoarytenoid (cartilage) (joint) (larynx) 478.79
dental 521.6
ear ossicle NEC 385.22
malleus 385.21
elbow 718.52
finger 718.54
hip 718.55
incostapedial joint (infectional) 385.22
joint, produced by surgical fusion NEC V45.4
knee 718.56
lumbosacral (joint) 724.6
malleus 385.21
multiple sites 718.59
postoperative (status) V45.4
sacroiliac (joint) 724.6
shoulder 718.51
specified site NEC 718.58
spine NEC 724.9
surgical V45.4

Ankylosis — *continued*
teeth, tooth (hard tissues) 521.6
temporomandibular joint 524.61
wrist 718.53
Ankylostoma — *see* Ancylostoma
Ankylostomiasis (intestinal) — *see* Ancylostomiasis
Ankylurethria — *see also* Stricture, urethra 598.9
Annular — *see also* condition
detachment, cervix 622.8
organ or site, congenital NEC — *see* Distortion
pancreas (congenital) 751.7
Anodontia (complete) (partial) (vera) 520.0
with abnormal spacing 524.30
acquired 525.10
causing malocclusion 524.30
due to
caries 525.13
extraction 525.10
periodontal disease 525.12
trauma 525.11
Anomaly, anomalous (congenital) (unspecified type) 759.9
abdomen 759.9
abdominal wall 756.70
acoustic nerve 742.9
adrenal (gland) 759.1
Alder (-Reilly) (leukocyte granulation) 288.2
alimentary tract 751.9
lower 751.5
specified type NEC 751.8
upper (any part, except tongue) 750.9
tongue 750.10
specified type NEC 750.19
alveolar 524.70
ridge (process) 525.8
specified NEC 524.79
ankle (joint) 755.69
anus, anal (canal) 751.5
aorta, aortic 747.20
arch 747.21
coarctation (postductal) (preductal) 747.10
cusp or valve NEC 746.9
septum 745.0
specified type NEC 747.29
aorticopulmonary septum 745.0
apertures, diaphragm 756.6
appendix 751.5
aqueduct of Sylvius 742.3
with spina bifida (*see also* Spina bifida) 741.0 ☑
arm 755.50
reduction (*see also* Deformity, reduction, upper limb) 755.20
arteriovenous (congenital) (peripheral) NEC 747.60
brain 747.81
cerebral 747.81
coronary 746.85
gastrointestinal 747.61
acquired — *see* Angiodysplasia
lower limb 747.64
renal 747.62
specified site NEC 747.69
spinal 747.82
upper limb 747.63
artery (*see also* Anomaly, peripheral vascular system) NEC 747.60
brain 747.81
cerebral 747.81
coronary 746.85
eye 743.9
pulmonary 747.39
renal 747.62
retina 743.9
umbilical 747.5
arytenoepiglottic folds 748.3
atrial
bands 746.9
folds 746.9
septa 745.5
atrioventricular
canal 745.69

Anomaly, anomalous — continued
  atrioventricular — continued
    common 745.69
    conduction 426.7
    excitation 426.7
    septum 745.4
  atrium — see Anomaly, atrial
  auditory canal 744.3
    specified type NEC 744.29
      with hearing impairment 744.02
  auricle
    ear 744.3
      causing impairment of hearing
        744.02
    heart 746.9
      septum 745.5
  autosomes, autosomal NEC 758.5
  Axenfeld's 743.44
  back 759.9
  band
    atrial 746.9
    heart 746.9
    ventricular 746.9
  Bartholin's duct 750.9
  biliary duct or passage 751.60
    atresia 751.61
  bladder (neck) (sphincter) (trigone) 753.9
    specified type NEC 753.8
  blood vessel 747.9
    artery — see Anomaly, artery
    peripheral vascular — see Anomaly, pe-
      ripheral vascular system
    vein — see Anomaly, vein
  bone NEC 756.9
    ankle 755.69
    arm 755.50
    chest 756.3
    cranium 756.0
    face 756.0
    finger 755.50
    foot 755.67
    forearm 755.50
    frontal 756.0
    head 756.0
    hip 755.63
    leg 755.60
    lumbosacral 756.10
    nose 748.1
    pelvic girdle 755.60
    rachitic 756.4
    rib 756.3
    shoulder girdle 755.50
    skull 756.0
      with
        anencephalus 740.0
        encephalocele 742.0
        hydrocephalus 742.3
          with spina bifida (see also
            Spina bifida) 741.0 ☑
        microcephalus 742.1
    toe 755.66
  brain 742.9
    multiple 742.4
    reduction 742.2
    specified type NEC 742.4
    vessel 747.81
  branchial cleft NEC 744.49
    cyst 744.42
    fistula 744.41
    persistent 744.41
    sinus (external) (internal) 744.41
  breast 757.6
  broad ligament 752.10
    specified type NEC 752.19
  bronchus 748.3
  bulbar septum 745.0
  bulbus cordis 745.9
    persistent (in left ventricle) 745.8
  bursa 756.9
  canal of Nuck 752.9
  canthus 743.9
  capillary NEC (see also Anomaly, peripheral
    vascular system) 747.60
  cardiac 746.9
    septal closure 745.9
      acquired 429.71

Anomaly, anomalous — continued
  cardiac — continued
    valve NEC 746.9
      pulmonary 746.00
        specified type NEC 746.89
  cardiovascular system 746.9
    complicating pregnancy, childbirth, or
      puerperium 648.5 ☑
  carpus 755.50
  cartilage, trachea 748.3
  cartilaginous 756.9
  caruncle, lacrimal, lachrymal 743.9
  cascade stomach 750.7
  cauda equina 742.59
  cecum 751.5
  cerebral (see also Anomaly, brain vessels)
    747.81
  cerebrovascular system 747.81
  cervix (uterus) 752.40
    with doubling of vagina and uterus
      752.2
    in pregnancy or childbirth 654.6 ☑
      affecting fetus or newborn 763.89
      causing obstructed labor 660.2 ☑
        affecting fetus or newborn 763.1
  Chédiak-Higashi (-Steinbrinck) (congenital
    gigantism of peroxidase granules)
    288.2
  cheek 744.9
  chest (wall) 756.3
  chin 744.9
    specified type NEC 744.89
  chordae tendineae 746.9
  choroid 743.9
    plexus 742.9
  chromosomes, chromosomal 758.9
    13 (13-15) 758.1
    18 (16-18) 758.2
    21 or 22 758.0
    autosomes NEC (see also Abnormal, au-
      tosomes) 758.5
    deletion 758.39
    Christchurch 758.39
    D₁ 758.1
    E₃ 758.2
    G 758.0
    mitochondrial 758.9
    mosaics 758.89
    sex 758.81
      complement, XO 758.6
      complement, XXX 758.81
      complement, XXY 758.7
      complement, XYY 758.81
      gonadal dysgenesis 758.6
      Klinefelter's 758.7
      Turner's 758.6
      trisomy 21 758.0
  cilia 743.9
  circulatory system 747.9
    specified type NEC 747.89
  clavicle 755.51
  clitoris 752.40
  coccyx 756.10
  colon 751.5
  common duct 751.60
  communication
    coronary artery 746.85
    left ventricle with right atrium 745.4
  concha (ear) 744.3
  connection
    renal vessels with kidney 747.62
    total pulmonary venous 747.41
  connective tissue 756.9
    specified type NEC 756.89
  cornea 743.9
    shape 743.41
    size 743.41
    specified type NEC 743.49
  coronary
    artery 746.85
    vein 746.89
  cranium — see Anomaly, skull
  cricoid cartilage 748.3
  cushion, endocardial 745.60
    specified type NEC 745.69
  cystic duct 751.60

Anomaly, anomalous — continued
  dental arch 524.20
    specified NEC 524.29
  dental arch relationship 524.20
    angle's class I 524.21
    angle's class II 524.22
    angle's class III 524.23
    articulation
      anterior 524.27
      posterior 524.27
      reverse 524.27
    disto-occlusion 524.22
      division I 524.22
      division II 524.22
    excessive horizontal overlap 524.26
    interarch distance (excessive) (inade-
      quate) 524.28
    mesio-occlusion 524.23
    neutro-occlusion 524.21
    open
      anterior occlusal relationship 524.24
      posterior occlusal relationship 524.25
    specified NEC 524.29
  dentition 520.6
  dentofacial NEC 524.9
    functional 524.50
    specified type NEC 524.89
  dermatoglyphic 757.2
  Descemet's membrane 743.9
    specified type NEC 743.49
  development
    cervix 752.40
    vagina 752.40
    vulva 752.40
  diaphragm, diaphragmatic (apertures) NEC
    756.6
  digestive organ(s) or system 751.9
    lower 751.5
    specified type NEC 751.8
    upper 750.9
  distribution, coronary artery 746.85
  ductus
    arteriosus 747.0
    Botalli 747.0
  duodenum 751.5
  dura 742.9
    brain 742.4
    spinal cord 742.59
  ear 744.3
    causing impairment of hearing 744.00
      specified type NEC 744.09
    external 744.3
      causing impairment of hearing
        744.02
      specified type NEC 744.29
    inner (causing impairment of hearing)
      744.05
    middle, except ossicles (causing impair-
      ment of hearing) 744.03
      ossicles 744.04
    ossicles 744.04
    prominent auricle 744.29
    specified type NEC 744.29
      with hearing impairment 744.09
  Ebstein's (heart) 746.2
    tricuspid valve 746.2
  ectodermal 757.9
  Eisenmenger's (ventricular septal defect)
    745.4
  ejaculatory duct 752.9
    specified type NEC 752.89
  elbow (joint) 755.50
  endocardial cushion 745.60
    specified type NEC 745.69
  endocrine gland NEC 759.2
  epididymis 752.9
  epiglottis 748.3
  esophagus 750.9
    specified type NEC 750.4
  Eustachian tube 744.3
    specified type NEC 744.24
  eye (any part) 743.9
    adnexa 743.9
      specified type NEC 743.69
    anophthalmos 743.00

Anomaly, anomalous — continued
  eye — continued
    anterior
      chamber and related structures 743.9
        angle 743.9
          specified type NEC 743.44
        specified type NEC 743.44
      segment 743.9
        combined 743.48
        multiple 743.48
        specified type NEC 743.49
    cataract (see also Cataract) 743.30
    glaucoma (see also Buphthalmia) 743.20
    lid 743.9
      specified type NEC 743.63
    microphthalmos (see also Microphthal-
      mos) 743.10
    posterior segment 743.9
      specified type NEC 743.59
      vascular 743.58
      vitreous 743.9
        specified type NEC 743.51
    ptosis (eyelid) 743.61
    retina 743.9
      specified type NEC 743.59
    sclera 743.9
      specified type NEC 743.47
    specified type NEC 743.8
  eyebrow 744.89
  eyelid 743.9
    specified type NEC 743.63
  face (any part) 744.9
    bone(s) 756.0
    specified type NEC 744.89
  fallopian tube 752.10
    specified type NEC 752.19
  fascia 756.9
    specified type NEC 756.89
  femur 755.60
  fibula 755.60
  finger 755.50
    supernumerary 755.01
    webbed (see also Syndactylism, fingers)
      755.11
  fixation, intestine 751.4
  flexion (joint) 755.9
    hip or thigh (see also Dislocation, hip,
      congenital) 754.30
  folds, heart 746.9
  foot 755.67
  foramen
    Botalli 745.5
    ovale 745.5
  forearm 755.50
  forehead (see also Anomaly, skull) 756.0
  form, teeth 520.2
  fovea centralis 743.9
  frontal bone (see also Anomaly, skull) 756.0
  gallbladder 751.60
  Gartner's duct 752.41
  gastrointestinal tract 751.9
    specified type NEC 751.8
    vessel 747.61
  genitalia, genital organ(s) or system
    female 752.9
      external 752.40
        specified type NEC 752.49
      internal NEC 752.9
    male (external and internal) 752.9
      epispadias 752.62
      hidden penis 752.65
      hydrocele, congenital 778.6
      hypospadias 752.61
      micropenis 752.64
      testis, undescended 752.51
        retractile 752.52
    specified type NEC 752.89
  genitourinary NEC 752.9
  Gerbode 745.4
  globe (eye) 743.9
  glottis 748.3
  granulation or granulocyte, genetic 288.2
    constitutional 288.2
    leukocyte 288.2
  gum 750.9
  gyri 742.9

☑ **Additional Digit Required** — Refer to the Tabular List for Digit Selection　　　　　　☜ **Subterms under main terms may continue to next column or page**

22 — Volume 2　　　▶◀ **Revised Text**　　　● **New Line**　　　▲ **Revised Code**　　　**2013 ICD-9-CM**

Anomaly, anomalous — *continued*
- hair 757.9
  - specified type NEC 757.4
- hand 755.50
- hard tissue formation in pulp 522.3
- head (*see also* Anomaly, skull) 756.0
- heart 746.9
  - auricle 746.9
  - bands 746.9
  - fibroelastosis cordis 425.3
  - folds 746.9
  - malposition 746.87
  - maternal, affecting fetus or newborn 760.3
  - obstructive NEC 746.84
  - patent ductus arteriosus (Botalli) 747.0
  - septum 745.9
    - acquired 429.71
    - aortic 745.0
    - aorticopulmonary 745.0
    - atrial 745.5
    - auricular 745.5
    - between aorta and pulmonary artery 745.0
    - endocardial cushion type 745.60
      - specified type NEC 745.69
    - interatrial 745.5
    - interventricular 745.4
      - with pulmonary stenosis or atresia, dextraposition of aorta, and hypertrophy of right ventricle 745.2
      - acquired 429.71
    - specified type NEC 745.8
    - ventricular 745.4
      - with pulmonary stenosis or atresia, dextraposition of aorta, and hypertrophy of right ventricle 745.2
      - acquired 429.71
  - specified type NEC 746.89
  - tetralogy of Fallot 745.2
  - valve NEC 746.9
    - aortic 746.9
      - atresia 746.89
      - bicuspid valve 746.4
      - insufficiency 746.4
      - specified type NEC 746.89
      - stenosis 746.3
        - subaortic 746.81
        - supravalvular 747.22
    - mitral 746.9
      - atresia 746.89
      - insufficiency 746.6
      - specified type NEC 746.89
      - stenosis 746.5
    - pulmonary 746.00
      - atresia 746.01
      - insufficiency 746.09
      - stenosis 746.02
        - infundibular 746.83
        - subvalvular 746.83
    - tricuspid 746.9
      - atresia 746.1
      - stenosis 746.1
  - ventricle 746.9
- heel 755.67
- Hegglin's 288.2
- hemianencephaly 740.0
- hemicephaly 740.0
- hemicrania 740.0
- hepatic duct 751.60
- hip (joint) 755.63
- hourglass
  - bladder 753.8
  - gallbladder 751.69
  - stomach 750.7
- humerus 755.50
- hymen 752.40
- hypersegmentation of neutrophils, hereditary 288.2
- hypophyseal 759.2
- ileocecal (coil) (valve) 751.5
- ileum (intestine) 751.5
- ilium 755.60
- integument 757.9

Anomaly, anomalous — *continued*
- integument — *continued*
  - specified type NEC 757.8
- interarch distance (excessive) (inadequate) 524.28
- intervertebral cartilage or disc 756.10
- intestine (large) (small) 751.5
  - fixational type 751.4
- iris 743.9
  - specified type NEC 743.46
- ischium 755.60
- jaw NEC 524.9
  - closure 524.51
  - size (major) NEC 524.00
  - specified type NEC 524.89
- jaw-cranial base relationship 524.10
  - specified NEC 524.19
- jejunum 751.5
- joint 755.9
  - hip
    - dislocation (*see also* Dislocation, hip, congenital) 754.30
    - predislocation (*see also* Subluxation, congenital, hip) 754.32
    - preluxation (*see also* Subluxation, congenital, hip) 754.32
    - subluxation (*see also* Subluxation, congenital, hip) 754.32
  - lumbosacral 756.10
    - spondylolisthesis 756.12
    - spondylosis 756.11
  - multiple arthrogryposis 754.89
  - sacroiliac 755.69
- Jordan's 288.2
- kidney(s) (calyx) (pelvis) 753.9
  - vessel 747.62
- Klippel-Feil (brevicollis) 756.16
- knee (joint) 755.64
- labium (majus) (minus) 752.40
- labyrinth, membranous (causing impairment of hearing) 744.05
- lacrimal
  - apparatus, duct or passage 743.9
    - specified type NEC 743.65
  - gland 743.9
    - specified type NEC 743.64
- Langdon Down (mongolism) 758.0
- larynx, laryngeal (muscle) 748.3
  - web, webbed 748.2
- leg (lower) (upper) 755.60
  - reduction NEC (*see also* Deformity, reduction, lower limb) 755.30
- lens 743.9
  - shape 743.36
  - specified type NEC 743.39
- leukocytes, genetic 288.2
  - granulation (constitutional) 288.2
- lid (fold) 743.9
- ligament 756.9
  - broad 752.10
  - round 752.9
- limb, except reduction deformity 755.9
  - lower 755.60
    - reduction deformity (*see also* Deformity, reduction, lower limb) 755.30
    - specified type NEC 755.69
  - upper 755.50
    - reduction deformity (*see also* Deformity, reduction, upper limb) 755.20
    - specified type NEC 755.59
- lip 750.9
  - harelip (*see also* Cleft, lip) 749.10
  - specified type NEC 750.26
- liver (duct) 751.60
  - atresia 751.69
- lower extremity 755.60
  - vessel 747.64
- lumbosacral (joint) (region) 756.10
- lung (fissure) (lobe) NEC 748.60
  - agenesis 748.5
  - specified type NEC 748.69
- lymphatic system 759.9
- Madelung's (radius) 755.54
- mandible 524.9

Anomaly, anomalous — *continued*
- mandible — *continued*
  - size NEC 524.00
- maxilla 524.9
  - size NEC 524.00
- May (-Hegglin) 288.2
- meatus urinarius 753.9
  - specified type NEC 753.8
- meningeal bands or folds, constriction of 742.8
- meninges 742.9
  - brain 742.4
  - spinal 742.59
- meningocele (*see also* Spina bifida) 741.9 ☑
  - acquired 349.2
- mesentery 751.9
- metacarpus 755.50
- metatarsus 755.67
- middle ear, except ossicles (causing impairment of hearing) 744.03
  - ossicles 744.04
- mitral (leaflets) (valve) 746.9
  - atresia 746.89
  - insufficiency 746.6
  - specified type NEC 746.89
  - stenosis 746.5
- mouth 750.9
  - specified type NEC 750.26
- multiple NEC 759.7
  - specified type NEC 759.89
- muscle 756.9
  - eye 743.9
    - specified type NEC 743.69
  - specified type NEC 756.89
- musculoskeletal system, except limbs 756.9
  - specified type NEC 756.9
- nail 757.9
  - specified type NEC 757.5
- narrowness, eyelid 743.62
- nasal sinus or septum 748.1
- neck (any part) 744.9
  - specified type NEC 744.89
- nerve 742.9
  - acoustic 742.9
    - specified type NEC 742.8
  - optic 742.9
    - specified type NEC 742.8
- nervous system NEC 742.9
  - brain 742.9
    - specified type NEC 742.4
  - specified type NEC 742.8
- neurological 742.9
- nipple 757.6
- nonteratogenic NEC 754.89
- nose, nasal (bone) (cartilage) (septum) (sinus) 748.1
- ocular muscle 743.9
- omphalomesenteric duct 751.0
- opening, pulmonary veins 747.49
- optic
  - disc 743.9
    - specified type NEC 743.57
  - nerve 742.9
- opticociliary vessels 743.9
- orbit (eye) 743.9
  - specified type NEC 743.66
- organ
  - of Corti (causing impairment of hearing) 744.05
  - or site 759.9
    - specified type NEC 759.89
- origin
  - both great arteries from same ventricle 745.11
  - coronary artery 746.85
  - innominate artery 747.69
  - left coronary artery from pulmonary artery 746.85
  - pulmonary artery 747.39
  - renal vessels 747.62
  - subclavian artery (left) (right) 747.21
- osseous meatus (ear) 744.03
- ovary 752.0
- oviduct 752.10
- palate (hard) (soft) 750.9

Anomaly, anomalous — *continued*
- palate — *continued*
  - cleft (*see also* Cleft, palate) 749.00
- pancreas (duct) 751.7
- papillary muscles 746.9
- parathyroid gland 759.2
- paraurethral ducts 753.9
- parotid (gland) 750.9
- patella 755.64
- Pelger-Huët (hereditary hyposegmentation) 288.2
- pelvic girdle 755.60
  - specified type NEC 755.69
- pelvis (bony) 755.60
  - complicating delivery 653.0 ☑
  - rachitic 268.1
    - fetal 756.4
- penis (glans) 752.69
- pericardium 746.89
- peripheral vascular system NEC 747.60
  - gastrointestinal 747.61
  - lower limb 747.64
  - renal 747.62
  - specified site NEC 747.69
  - spinal 747.82
  - upper limb 747.63
- Peter's 743.44
- pharynx 750.9
  - branchial cleft 744.41
  - specified type NEC 750.29
- Pierre Robin 756.0
- pigmentation 709.00
  - congenital 757.33
  - specified NEC 709.09
- pituitary (gland) 759.2
- pleural folds 748.8
- portal vein 747.40
- position tooth, teeth 524.30
  - crowding 524.31
  - displacement 524.30
    - horizontal 524.33
    - vertical 524.34
  - distance
    - interocclusal
      - excessive 524.37
      - insufficient 524.36
  - excessive spacing 524.32
  - rotation 524.35
  - specified NEC 524.39
- preauricular sinus 744.46
- prepuce 752.9
- prostate 752.9
- pulmonary 748.60
  - artery 747.39
  - circulation 747.39
  - specified type NEC 748.69
  - valve 746.00
    - atresia 746.01
    - insufficiency 746.09
    - specified type NEC 746.09
    - stenosis 746.02
      - infundibular 746.83
      - subvalvular 746.83
  - vein 747.40
  - venous
    - connection 747.49
      - partial 747.42
      - total 747.41
    - return 747.49
      - partial 747.42
      - total (TAPVR) (complete) (subdiaphragmatic) (supradiaphragmatic) 747.41
- pupil 743.9
- pylorus 750.9
  - hypertrophy 750.5
  - stenosis 750.5
- rachitic, fetal 756.4
- radius 755.50
- rectovaginal (septum) 752.40
- rectum 751.5
- refraction 367.9
- renal 753.9
  - vessel 747.62
- respiratory system 748.9
  - specified type NEC 748.8

☑ **Additional Digit Required** — Refer to the Tabular List for Digit Selection   🔅 **Subterms under main terms may continue to next column or page**

2013 ICD-9-CM   ▶◀ Revised Text   ● New Line   ▲ Revised Code   **Volume 2 — 23**

Anomaly, anomalous — *continued*
rib 756.3
  cervical 756.2
Rieger's 743.44
rings, trachea 748.3
rotation (*see also* Malrotation)
  hip or thigh (*see also* Subluxation, con-
    genital, hip) 754.32
round ligament 752.9
sacroiliac (joint) 755.69
sacrum 756.10
saddle
  back 754.2
  nose 754.0
    syphilitic 090.5
salivary gland or duct 750.9
  specified type NEC 750.26
scapula 755.50
sclera 743.9
  specified type NEC 743.47
scrotum 752.9
sebaceous gland 757.9
seminal duct or tract 752.9
sense organs 742.9
  specified type NEC 742.8
septum
  heart — *see* Anomaly, heart, septum
  nasal 748.1
sex chromosomes NEC (*see also* Anomaly,
  chromosomes) 758.81
shoulder (girdle) (joint) 755.50
  specified type NEC 755.59
sigmoid (flexure) 751.5
sinus of Valsalva 747.29
site NEC 759.9
skeleton generalized NEC 756.50
skin (appendage) 757.9
  specified type NEC 757.39
skull (bone) 756.0
  with
    anencephalus 740.0
    encephalocele 742.0
    hydrocephalus 742.3
      with spina bifida (*see also* Spina
       bifida) 741.0 ☑
    microcephalus 742.1
specified type NEC
  adrenal (gland) 759.1
  alimentary tract (complete) (partial)
    751.8
    lower 751.5
    upper 750.8
  ankle 755.69
  anus, anal (canal) 751.5
  aorta, aortic 747.29
    arch 747.21
  appendix 751.5
  arm 755.59
  artery (peripheral) NEC (*see also*
    Anomaly, peripheral vascular
    system) 747.60
    brain 747.81
    coronary 746.85
    eye 743.58
    pulmonary 747.39
    retinal 743.58
    umbilical 747.5
  auditory canal 744.29
    causing impairment of hearing
      744.02
  bile duct or passage 751.69
  bladder 753.8
    neck 753.8
  bone(s) 756.9
    arm 755.59
    face 756.0
    leg 755.69
    pelvic girdle 755.69
    shoulder girdle 755.59
    skull 756.0
      with
        anencephalus 740.0
        encephalocele 742.0
        hydrocephalus 742.3

Anomaly, anomalous — *continued*
specified type — *continued*
  bone(s) — *continued*
    skull — *continued*
      with — *continued*
        hydrocephalus — *contin-*
         ued
          with spina bifida (*see also*
            Spina bifida)
            741.0 ☑
        microcephalus 742.1
  brain 742.4
  breast 757.6
  broad ligament 752.19
  bronchus 748.3
  canal of Nuck 752.89
  cardiac septal closure 745.8
  carpus 755.59
  cartilaginous 756.9
  cecum 751.5
  cervix 752.49
  chest (wall) 756.3
  chin 744.89
  ciliary body 743.46
  circulatory system 747.89
  clavicle 755.51
  clitoris 752.49
  coccyx 756.19
  colon 751.5
  common duct 751.69
  connective tissue 756.89
  cricoid cartilage 748.3
  cystic duct 751.69
  diaphragm 756.6
  digestive organ(s) or tract 751.8
    lower 751.5
    upper 750.8
  duodenum 751.5
  ear 744.29
    auricle 744.29
      causing impairment of hearing
        744.02
    causing impairment of hearing
      744.09
    inner (causing impairment of hear-
      ing) 744.05
    middle, except ossicles 744.03
      ossicles 744.04
  ejaculatory duct 752.89
  endocrine 759.2
  epiglottis 748.3
  esophagus 750.4
  Eustachian tube 744.24
  eye 743.8
    lid 743.63
    muscle 743.69
  face 744.89
    bone(s) 756.0
  fallopian tube 752.19
  fascia 756.89
  femur 755.69
  fibula 755.69
  finger 755.59
  foot 755.67
  fovea centralis 743.55
  gallbladder 751.69
  Gartner's duct 752.89
  gastrointestinal tract 751.8
  genitalia, genital organ(s)
    female 752.89
      external 752.49
      internal NEC 752.89
    male 752.89
      penis 752.69
      scrotal transposition 752.81
  genitourinary tract NEC 752.89
  glottis 748.3
  hair 757.4
  hand 755.59
  heart 746.89
    valve NEC 746.89
      pulmonary 746.09
  hepatic duct 751.69
  hydatid of Morgagni 752.89
  hymen 752.49
  integument 757.8

Anomaly, anomalous — *continued*
specified type — *continued*
  intestine (large) (small) 751.5
    fixational type 751.4
  iris 743.46
  jejunum 751.5
  joint 755.8
  kidney 753.3
  knee 755.64
  labium (majus) (minus) 752.49
  labyrinth, membranous 744.05
  larynx 748.3
  leg 755.69
  lens 743.39
  limb, except reduction deformity 755.8
    lower 755.69
      reduction deformity (*see also* De-
        formity, reduction, lower
        limb) 755.30
    upper 755.59
      reduction deformity (*see also* De-
        formity, reduction, upper
        limb) 755.20
  lip 750.26
  liver 751.69
  lung (fissure) (lobe) 748.69
  meatus urinarius 753.8
  metacarpus 755.59
  mouth 750.26
  Müllerian
    cervix 752.49
    uterus 752.39
    vagina 752.49
  muscle 756.89
    eye 743.69
  musculoskeletal system, except limbs
    756.9
  nail 757.5
  neck 744.89
  nerve 742.8
    acoustic 742.8
    optic 742.8
  nervous system 742.8
  nipple 757.6
  nose 748.1
  organ NEC 759.89
    of Corti 744.05
  osseous meatus (ear) 744.03
  ovary 752.0
  oviduct 752.19
  pancreas 751.7
  parathyroid 759.2
  patella 755.64
  pelvic girdle 755.69
  penis 752.69
  pericardium 746.89
  peripheral vascular system NEC (*see also*
    Anomaly, peripheral vascular
    system) 747.60
  pharynx 750.29
  pituitary 759.2
  prostate 752.89
  radius 755.59
  rectum 751.5
  respiratory system 748.8
  rib 756.3
  round ligament 752.89
  sacrum 756.19
  salivary duct or gland 750.26
  scapula 755.59
  sclera 743.47
  scrotum 752.89
    transposition 752.81
  seminal duct or tract 752.89
  shoulder girdle 755.59
  site NEC 759.89
  skin 757.39
  skull (bone(s)) 756.0
    with
      anencephalus 740.0
      encephalocele 742.0
      hydrocephalus 742.3
        with spina bifida (*see also*
          Spina bifida) 741.0 ☑
      microcephalus 742.1
  specified organ or site NEC 759.89

Anomaly, anomalous — *continued*
specified type — *continued*
  spermatic cord 752.89
  spinal cord 742.59
  spine 756.19
  spleen 759.0
  sternum 756.3
  stomach 750.7
  tarsus 755.67
  tendon 756.89
  testis 752.89
  thorax (wall) 756.3
  thymus 759.2
  thyroid (gland) 759.2
    cartilage 748.3
  tibia 755.69
  toe 755.66
  tongue 750.19
  trachea (cartilage) 748.3
  ulna 755.59
  urachus 753.7
  ureter 753.4
    obstructive 753.29
  urethra 753.8
    obstructive 753.6
  urinary tract 753.8
  uterus (Müllerian) 752.39
  uvula 750.26
  vagina 752.49
  vascular NEC (*see also* Anomaly, periph-
    eral vascular system) 747.60
    brain 747.81
  vas deferens 752.89
  vein(s) (peripheral) NEC (*see also*
    Anomaly, peripheral vascular
    system) 747.60
    brain 747.81
    great 747.49
    portal 747.49
    pulmonary 747.49
  vena cava (inferior) (superior) 747.49
  vertebra 756.19
  vulva 752.49
spermatic cord 752.9
spine, spinal 756.10
  column 756.10
  cord 742.9
    meningocele (*see also* Spina bifida)
      741.9 ☑
    specified type NEC 742.59
    spina bifida (*see also* Spina bifida)
      741.9 ☑
    vessel 747.82
  meninges 742.59
  nerve root 742.9
spleen 759.0
Sprengel's 755.52
sternum 756.3
stomach 750.9
  specified type NEC 750.7
submaxillary gland 750.9
superior vena cava 747.40
talipes — *see* Talipes
tarsus 755.67
  with complete absence of distal ele-
    ments 755.31
teeth, tooth NEC 520.9
  position 524.30
    crowding 524.31
    displacement 524.30
      horizontal 524.33
      vertical 524.34
    distance
      interocclusal
        excessive 524.37
        insufficient 524.36
    excessive spacing 524.32
    rotation 524.35
    specified NEC 524.39
    spacing 524.30
tendon 756.9
  specified type NEC 756.89
termination
  coronary artery 746.85
testis 752.9
thebesian valve 746.9

☑ **Additional Digit Required** — Refer to the Tabular List for Digit Selection   ▽ **Subterms under main terms may continue to next column or page**

24 — Volume 2   ►◄ Revised Text   ● New Line   ▲ Revised Code   **2013 ICD-9-CM**

Anomaly, anomalous — continued
thigh 755.60
flexion (see also Subluxation, congenital, hip) 754.32
thorax (wall) 756.3
throat 750.9
thumb 755.50
supernumerary 755.01
thymus gland 759.2
thyroid (gland) 759.2
cartilage 748.3
tibia 755.60
saber 090.5
toe 755.66
supernumerary 755.02
webbed (see also Syndactylism, toes) 755.13
tongue 750.10
specified type NEC 750.19
trachea, tracheal 748.3
cartilage 748.3
rings 748.3
tragus 744.3
transverse aortic arch 747.21
trichromata 368.59
trichromatopsia 368.59
tricuspid (leaflet) (valve) 746.9
atresia 746.1
Ebstein's 746.2
specified type NEC 746.89
stenosis 746.1
trunk 759.9
Uhl's (hypoplasia of myocardium, right ventricle) 746.84
ulna 755.50
umbilicus 759.9
artery 747.5
union, trachea with larynx 748.3
unspecified site 759.9
upper extremity 755.50
vessel 747.63
urachus 753.7
specified type NEC 753.7
ureter 753.9
obstructive 753.20
specified type NEC 753.4
obstructive 753.29
urethra (valve) 753.9
obstructive 753.6
specified type NEC 753.8
urinary tract or system (any part, except urachus) 753.9
specified type NEC 753.8
urachus 753.7
uterus 752.39
with only one functioning horn 752.33
in pregnancy or childbirth 654.0 ☑
affecting fetus or newborn 763.89
causing obstructed labor 660.2 ☑
affecting fetus or newborn 763.1
uvula 750.9
vagina 752.40
valleculae 748.3
valve (heart) NEC 746.9
formation, ureter 753.29
pulmonary 746.00
specified type NEC 746.89
vascular NEC (see also Anomaly, peripheral vascular system) 747.60
ring 747.21
vas deferens 752.9
vein(s) (peripheral) NEC (see also Anomaly, peripheral vascular system) 747.60
brain 747.81
cerebral 747.81
coronary 746.89
great 747.40
specified type NEC 747.49
portal 747.40
pulmonary 747.40
retina 743.9
vena cava (inferior) (superior) 747.40
venous — see Anomaly, vein
venous return (pulmonary) 747.49
partial 747.42
total 747.41

Anomaly, anomalous — continued
ventricle, ventricular (heart) 746.9
bands 746.9
folds 746.9
septa 745.4
vertebra 756.10
vesicourethral orifice 753.9
vessels NEC (see also Anomaly, peripheral vascular system) 747.60
optic papilla 743.9
vitelline duct 751.0
vitreous humor 743.9
specified type NEC 743.51
vulva 752.40
wrist (joint) 755.50
Anomia 784.69
Anonychia 757.5
acquired 703.8
Anophthalmos, anophthalmus (clinical) (congenital) (globe) 743.00
acquired V45.78
Anopsia (altitudinal) (quadrant) 368.46
Anorchia 752.89
Anorchism, anorchidism 752.89
Anorexia 783.0
hysterical 300.11
nervosa 307.1
Anosmia — see also Disturbance, sensation 781.1
hysterical 300.11
postinfectional 478.9
psychogenic 306.7
traumatic 951.8
Anosognosia 780.99
Anosphrasia 781.1
Anosteoplasia 756.50
Anotia 744.09
Anovulatory cycle 628.0
Anoxemia 799.02
newborn 770.88
Anoxia 799.02
altitude 993.2
cerebral 348.1
with
abortion — see Abortion, by type, with specified complication NEC
ectopic pregnancy (see also categories 633.0–633.9) 639.8
molar pregnancy (see also categories 630–632) 639.8
complicating
delivery (cesarean) (instrumental) 669.4 ☑
ectopic or molar pregnancy 639.8
obstetric anesthesia or sedation 668.2 ☑
during or resulting from a procedure 997.01
following
abortion 639.8
ectopic or molar pregnancy 639.8
newborn (see also Distress, fetal, liveborn infant) 770.88
due to drowning 994.1
fetal, affecting newborn 770.88
heart — see Insufficiency, coronary
high altitude 993.2
intrauterine
fetal death (before onset of labor) 768.0
during labor 768.1
liveborn infant — see Distress, fetal, liveborn infant
myocardial — see Insufficiency, coronary
newborn 768.9
mild or moderate 768.6
severe 768.5
pathological 799.02
Anteflexion — see Anteversion
Antenatal
care, normal pregnancy V22.1
first V22.0
sampling
chorionic villus V28.89
screening of mother (for) V28.9
based on amniocentesis NEC V28.2

Antenatal — continued
screening of mother — continued
based on amniocentesis — continued
chromosomal anomalies V28.0
raised alphafetoprotein levels V28.1
chromosomal anomalies V28.0
fetal growth retardation using ulatrasonics V28.4
genomic V28.89
isoimmunization V28.5
malformations using ulatrasonics V28.3
proteomic V28.89
raised alphafetoprotein levels in amniotic fluid V28.1
risk
pre-term labor V28.82
specified condition NEC V28.89
Streptococcus B V28.6
survey
fetal anatomic V28.81
testing
nuchal translucency V28.89
Antepartum — see condition
Anterior — see also condition
spinal artery compression syndrome 721.1
Antero-occlusion 524.24
Anteversion
cervix — see Anteversion, uterus
femur (neck), congenital 755.63
uterus, uterine (cervix) (postinfectional) (postpartal, old) 621.6
congenital 752.39
in pregnancy or childbirth 654.4 ☑
affecting fetus or newborn 763.89
causing obstructed labor 660.2 ☑
affecting fetus or newborn 763.1
Anthracosilicosis (occupational) 500
Anthracosis (lung) (occupational) 500
lingua 529.3
Anthrax 022.9
with pneumonia 022.1 [484.5]
colitis 022.2
cutaneous 022.0
gastrointestinal 022.2
intestinal 022.2
pulmonary 022.1
respiratory 022.1
septicemia 022.3
specified manifestation NEC 022.8
Anthropoid pelvis 755.69
with disproportion (fetopelvic) 653.2 ☑
affecting fetus or newborn 763.1
causing obstructed labor 660.1 ☑
affecting fetus or newborn 763.1
Anthropophobia 300.29
Antibioma, breast 611.0
Antibodies
maternal (blood group) (see also Incompatibility) 656.2 ☑
anti-D, cord blood 656.1 ☑
fetus or newborn 773.0
Antibody
anticardiolipin 795.79
with
hemorrhagic disorder 286.53
hypercoagulable state 289.81
antiphosphatidylglycerol 795.79
with
hemorrhagic disorder 286.53
hypercoagulable state 289.81
antiphosphatidylinositol 795.79
with
hemorrhagic disorder 286.53
hypercoagulable state 289.81
antiphosphatidylserine 795.79
with
hemorrhagic disorder 286.53
hypercoagulable state 289.81
antiphospholipid 795.79
with
hemorrhagic disorder 286.53
hypercoagulable state 289.81
deficiency syndrome
agammaglobulinemic 279.00
congenital 279.04

Antibody — continued
deficiency syndrome — continued
hypogammaglobulinemic 279.00
Anticoagulant
intrinsic, circulating, causing hemorrhagic disorder (see also Circulating, anticoagulants) 286.59
lupus (LAC) 795.79
with
hemorrhagic disorder 286.53
hypercoagulable state 289.81
Antimongolism syndrome 758.39
Antimonial cholera 985.4
Antisocial personality 301.7
Antithrombinemia — see also Circulating anticoagulants 286.59
Antithromboplastinemia — see also Circulating anticoagulants 286.59
Antithromboplastinogenemia — see also Circulating anticoagulants 286.59
Antitoxin complication or reaction — see Complications, vaccination
Anton (-Babinski) syndrome (hemiasomatognosia) 307.9
Antritis (chronic) 473.0
maxilla 473.0
acute 461.0
stomach 535.4 ☑
Antrum, antral — see condition
Anuria 788.5
with
abortion — see Abortion, by type, with renal failure
ectopic pregnancy (see also categories 633.0–633.9) 639.3
molar pregnancy (see also categories 630–632) 639.3
calculus (impacted) (recurrent) 592.9
kidney 592.0
ureter 592.1
congenital 753.3
due to a procedure 997.5
following
abortion 639.3
ectopic or molar pregnancy 639.3
newborn 753.3
postrenal 593.4
puerperal, postpartum, childbirth 669.3 ☑
specified as due to a procedure 997.5
sulfonamide
correct substance properly administered 788.5
overdose or wrong substance given or taken 961.0
traumatic (following crushing) 958.5
Anus, anal — see also condition
high risk human papillomavirus (HPV) DNA test positive 796.75
low risk human papillomavirus (HPV) DNA test positive 796.79
Anusitis 569.49
Anxiety (neurosis) (reaction) (state) 300.00
alcohol-induced 291.89
depression 300.4
drug-induced 292.89
due to or associated with physical condition 293.84
generalized 300.02
hysteria 300.20
in
acute stress reaction 308.0
transient adjustment reaction 309.24
panic type 300.01
separation, abnormal 309.21
syndrome (organic) (transient) 293.84
Aorta, aortic — see condition
Aortectasia — see also Ectasia, aortic 447.70
with aneurysm 441.9
Aortitis (nonsyphilitic) 447.6
arteriosclerotic 440.0
calcific 447.6
Döhle-Heller 093.1
luetic 093.1
rheumatic (see also Endocarditis, acute, rheumatic) 391.1
rheumatoid — see Arthritis, rheumatoid

☑ Additional Digit Required — Refer to the Tabular List for Digit Selection
🔻 Subterms under main terms may continue to next column or page
2013 ICD-9-CM
▶◀ Revised Text
● New Line
▲ Revised Code
Volume 2 — 25

Anomaly, anomalous — Aortitis

Aortitis — continued
specific 093.1
syphilitic 093.1
congenital 090.5
Apathetic 799.25
thyroid storm (see also Thyrotoxicosis)
242.9 ☑
Apathy 799.25
Apepsia 536.8
achlorhydric 536.0
psychogenic 306.4
Aperistalsis, esophagus 530.0
Apert-Gallais syndrome (adrenogenital) 255.2
Apertognathia 524.20
Apert's syndrome (acrocephalosyndactyly)
755.55
Aphagia 787.20
psychogenic 307.1
Aphakia (acquired) (bilateral) (postoperative)
(unilateral) 379.31
congenital 743.35
Aphalangia (congenital) 755.4
lower limb (complete) (intercalary) (partial)
(terminal) 755.39
meaning all digits (complete) (partial)
755.31
transverse 755.31
upper limb (complete) (intercalary) (partial)
(terminal) 755.29
meaning all digits (complete) (partial)
755.21
transverse 755.21
Aphasia (amnestic) (ataxic) (auditory) (Broca's)
(choreatic) (classic) (expressive) (global)
(ideational) (ideokinetic) (ideomotor)
(jargon) (motor) (nominal) (receptive)
(semantic) (sensory) (syntactic) (verbal)
(visual) (Wernicke's) 784.3
developmental 315.31
syphilis, tertiary 094.89
uremic — see Uremia
Aphemia 784.3
uremic — see Uremia
Aphonia 784.41
clericorum 784.49
hysterical 300.11
organic 784.41
psychogenic 306.1
Aphthae, aphthous — see also condition
Bednar's 528.2
cachectic 529.0
epizootic 078.4
fever 078.4
oral 528.2
stomatitis 528.2
thrush 112.0
ulcer (oral) (recurrent) 528.2
genital organ(s) NEC
female 616.50
male 608.89
larynx 478.79
Apical — see condition
Apical ballooning syndrome 429.83
Aplasia — see also Agenesis
alveolar process (acquired) 525.8
congenital 750.26
aorta (congenital) 747.22
aortic valve (congenital) 746.89
axialis extracorticalis (congenital) 330.0
bone marrow (myeloid) 284.9
acquired (secondary) 284.89
congenital 284.01
idiopathic 284.9
brain 740.0
specified part 742.2
breast 757.6
bronchus 748.3
cementum 520.4
cerebellar 742.2
congenital (pure) red cell 284.01
corpus callosum 742.2
erythrocyte 284.81
congenital 284.01
extracortical axial 330.0
eye (congenital) 743.00
fovea centralis (congenital) 743.55

Aplasia — see also Agenesis — continued
germinal (cell) 606.0
iris 743.45
labyrinth, membranous 744.05
limb (congenital) 755.4
lower NEC 755.30
upper NEC 755.20
lung (bilateral) (congenital) (unilateral)
748.5
nervous system NEC 742.8
nuclear 742.8
ovary 752.0
Pelizaeus-Merzbacher 330.0
prostate (congenital) 752.89
red cell (with thymoma) 284.81
acquired (secondary) 284.81
due to drugs 284.81
adult 284.81
congenital 284.01
hereditary 284.01
of infants 284.01
primary 284.01
pure 284.01
due to drugs 284.81
round ligament (congenital) 752.89
salivary gland 750.21
skin (congenital) 757.39
spinal cord 742.59
spleen 759.0
testis (congenital) 752.89
thymic, with immunodeficiency 279.2
thyroid 243
uterus 752.39
ventral horn cell 742.59
Apleuria 756.3
Apnea, apneic (spells) 786.03
newborn, neonatorum 770.81
essential 770.81
obstructive 770.82
primary 770.81
sleep 770.81
specified NEC 770.82
psychogenic 306.1
sleep, unspecified 780.57
with
hypersomnia, unspecified 780.53
hyposomnia, unspecified 780.51
insomnia, unspecified 780.51
sleep disturbance 780.57
central, in conditions classified elsewhere 327.27
obstructive (adult) (pediatric) 327.23
organic 327.20
other 327.29
primary central 327.21
Apneumatosis newborn 770.4
Apodia 755.31
Aponeurosis 726.90
Apophysitis (bone) — see also Osteochondrosis 732.9
calcaneus 732.5
juvenile 732.6
Apoplectiform convulsions — see also Disease, cerebrovascular, acute 436
Apoplexia, apoplexy, apoplectic — see also
Disease, cerebrovascular, acute 436
abdominal 569.89
adrenal 036.3
attack 436
basilar (see also Disease, cerebrovascular,
acute) 436
brain (see also Disease, cerebrovascular,
acute) 436
bulbar (see also Disease, cerebrovascular,
acute) 436
capillary (see also Disease, cerebrovascular,
acute) 436
cardiac (see also Infarct, myocardium)
410.9 ☑
cerebral (see also Disease, cerebrovascular,
acute) 436
chorea (see also Disease, cerebrovascular,
acute) 436
congestive (see also Disease, cerebrovascular, acute) 436
newborn 767.4

Apoplexia, apoplexy, apoplectic — see also
Disease, cerebrovascular, acute —
continued
embolic (see also Embolism, brain) 434.1 ☑
fetus 767.0
fit (see also Disease, cerebrovascular, acute)
436
healed or old V12.54
heart (auricle) (ventricle) (see also Infarct,
myocardium) 410.9 ☑
heat 992.0
hemiplegia (see also Disease, cerebrovascular, acute) 436
hemorrhagic (stroke) (see also Hemorrhage,
brain) 432.9
ingravescent (see also Disease, cerebrovascular, acute) 436
late effect — see Late effect(s) (of) cerebrovascular disease
lung — see Embolism, pulmonary
meninges, hemorrhagic (see also Hemorrhage, subarachnoid) 430
neonatorum 767.0
newborn 767.0
pancreatitis 577.0
placenta 641.2 ☑
progressive (see also Disease, cerebrovascular, acute) 436
pulmonary (artery) (vein) — see Embolism,
pulmonary
sanguineous (see also Disease, cerebrovascular, acute) 436
seizure (see also Disease, cerebrovascular,
acute) 436
serous (see also Disease, cerebrovascular,
acute) 436
spleen 289.59
stroke (see also Disease, cerebrovascular,
acute) 436
thrombotic (see also Thrombosis, brain)
434.0 ☑
uremic — see Uremia
uteroplacental 641.2 ☑
Appendage
fallopian tube (cyst of Morgagni) 752.11
intestine (epiploic) 751.5
preauricular 744.1
testicular (organ of Morgagni) 752.89
Appendicitis 541
with
perforation, peritonitis (generalized), or
rupture 540.0
with peritoneal abscess 540.1
peritoneal abscess 540.1
acute (catarrhal) (fulminating) (gangrenous)
(inflammatory) (obstructive) (retrocecal) (suppurative) 540.9
with
perforation, peritonitis, or rupture
540.0
with peritoneal abscess 540.1
peritoneal abscess 540.1
amebic 006.8
chronic (recurrent) 542
exacerbation — see Appendicitis, acute
fulminating — see Appendicitis, acute
gangrenous — see Appendicitis, acute
healed (obliterative) 542
interval 542
neurogenic 542
obstructive 542
pneumococcal 541
recurrent 542
relapsing 542
retrocecal 541
subacute (adhesive) 542
subsiding 542
suppurative — see Appendicitis, acute
tuberculous (see also Tuberculosis) 014.8 ☑
Appendiclausis 543.9
Appendicolithiasis 543.9
Appendicopathia oxyurica 127.4
Appendix, appendicular — see also condition
Morgagni (male) 752.89
fallopian tube 752.11

Appetite
depraved 307.52
excessive 783.6
psychogenic 307.51
lack or loss (see also Anorexia) 783.0
nonorganic origin 307.59
perverted 307.52
hysterical 300.11
Apprehension, apprehensiveness (abnormal)
(state) 300.00
specified type NEC 300.09
Approximal wear 521.10
Apraxia (classic) (ideational) (ideokinetic)
(ideomotor) (motor) 784.69
oculomotor, congenital 379.51
verbal 784.69
Aptyalism 527.7
Aqueous misdirection 365.83
Arabicum elephantiasis — see also Infestation, filarial 125.9
Arachnidism 989.5
Arachnitis — see Meningitis
Arachnodactyly 759.82
Arachnoidism 989.5
Arachnoiditis (acute) (adhesive) (basic) (brain)
(cerebrospinal) (chiasmal) (chronic)
(spinal) — see also Meningitis 322.9
meningococcal (chronic) 036.0
syphilitic 094.2
tuberculous (see also Tuberculosis,
meninges) 013.0 ☑
Araneism 989.5
Arboencephalitis, Australian 062.4
Arborization block (heart) 426.6
Arbor virus, arbovirus (infection) NEC 066.9
ARC 042
Arches — see condition
Arcuate uterus 752.36
Arcuatus uterus 752.36
Arcus (cornea)
juvenilis 743.43
interfering with vision 743.42
senilis 371.41
Arc-welders' lung 503
Arc-welders' syndrome (photokeratitis) 370.24
Areflexia 796.1
Areola — see condition
Argentaffinoma (M8241/1) — see also Neo-
plasm, by site, uncertain behavior
benign (M8241/0) — see Neoplasm, by site,
benign
malignant (M8241/3) — see Neoplasm, by
site, malignant
syndrome 259.2
Argentinian hemorrhagic fever 078.7
Arginosuccinicaciduria 270.6
Argonz-Del Castillo syndrome (nonpuerperal
galactorrhea and amenorrhea) 253.1
**Argyll-Robertson phenomenon, pupil, or
syndrome** (syphilitic) 094.89
atypical 379.45
nonluetic 379.45
nonsyphilitic 379.45
reversed 379.45
Argyria, argyriasis NEC 985.8
conjunctiva 372.55
cornea 371.16
from drug or medicinal agent
correct substance properly administered
709.09
overdose or wrong substance given or
taken 961.2
Arhinencephaly 742.2
Arias-Stella phenomenon 621.30
Ariboflavinosis 266.0
Arizona enteritis 008.1
Arm — see condition
Armenian disease 277.31
Arnold-Chiari obstruction or syndrome —
see also Spina bifida 741.0 ☑
type I 348.4
type II (see also Spina bifida) 741.0 ☑
type III 742.0
type IV 742.2
Arousals
confusional 327.41

☑ **Additional Digit Required — Refer to the Tabular List for Digit Selection**

ᵂ **Subterms under main terms may continue to next column or page**

26 — Volume 2

▶◀ Revised Text

● New Line

▲ Revised Code

2013 ICD-9-CM

Arrest, arrested
active phase of labor 661.1 ☑
affecting fetus or newborn 763.7
any plane in pelvis
complicating delivery 660.1 ☑
affecting fetus or newborn 763.1
bone marrow (see also Anemia, aplastic) 284.9
cardiac 427.5
with
abortion — see Abortion, by type, with specified complication NEC
ectopic pregnancy (see also categories 633.0–633.9) 639.8
molar pregnancy (see also categories 630–632) 639.8
complicating
anesthesia
correct substance properly administered 427.5
obstetric 668.1 ☑
overdose or wrong substance given 968.4
specified anesthetic — see Table of Drugs and Chemicals
delivery (cesarean) (instrumental) 669.4 ☑
ectopic or molar pregnancy 639.8
surgery (nontherapeutic) (therapeutic) 997.1
fetus or newborn 779.85
following
abortion 639.8
ectopic or molar pregnancy 639.8
personal history, successfully resuscitated V12.53
postoperative (immediate) 997.1
long-term effect of cardiac surgery 429.4
cardiorespiratory (see also Arrest, cardiac) 427.5
deep transverse 660.3 ☑
affecting fetus or newborn 763.1
development or growth
bone 733.91
child 783.40
fetus 764.9 ☑
affecting management of pregnancy 656.5 ☑
tracheal rings 748.3
epiphyseal 733.91
granulopoiesis 288.09
heart — see Arrest, cardiac
respiratory 799.1
newborn 770.87
sinus 426.6
transverse (deep) 660.3 ☑
affecting fetus or newborn 763.1
Arrhenoblastoma (M8630/1)
benign (M8630/0)
specified site — see Neoplasm, by site, benign
unspecified site
female 220
male 222.0
malignant (M8630/3)
specified site — see Neoplasm, by site, malignant
unspecified site
female 183.0
male 186.9
specified site — see Neoplasm, by site, uncertain behavior
unspecified site
female 236.2
male 236.4
Arrhinencephaly 742.2
due to
trisomy 13 (13-15) 758.1
trisomy 18 (16-18) 758.2
Arrhythmia (auricle) (cardiac) (cordis) (gallop rhythm) (juvenile) (nodal) (reflex) (sinus) (supraventricular) (transitory) (ventricle) 427.9

Arrhythmia — continued
bigeminal rhythm 427.89
block 426.9
bradycardia 427.89
contractions, premature 427.60
coronary sinus 427.89
ectopic 427.89
extrasystolic 427.60
postoperative 997.1
psychogenic 306.2
vagal 780.2
Arrillaga-Ayerza syndrome (pulmonary artery sclerosis with pulmonary hypertension) 416.0
Arsenical
dermatitis 692.4
keratosis 692.4
pigmentation 985.1
from drug or medicinal agent
correct substance properly administered 709.09
overdose or wrong substance given or taken 961.1
Arsenism 985.1
from drug or medicinal agent
correct substance properly administered 692.4
overdose or wrong substance given or taken 961.1
Arterial — see condition
Arteriectasis 447.8
Arteriofibrosis — see Arteriosclerosis
Arteriolar sclerosis — see Arteriosclerosis
Arteriolith — see Arteriosclerosis
Arteriolitis 447.6
necrotizing, kidney 447.5
renal — see Hypertension, kidney
Arteriolosclerosis — see Arteriosclerosis
Arterionephrosclerosis — see also Hypertension, kidney 403.90
Arteriopathy 447.9
Arteriosclerosis, arteriosclerotic (artery) (deformans) (diffuse) (disease) (endarteritis) (general) (obliterans) (obliterative) (occlusive) (senile) (with calcification) 440.9
with
gangrene 440.24
psychosis (see also Psychosis, arteriosclerotic) 290.40
ulceration 440.23
aorta 440.0
arteries of extremities — see Arteriosclerosis, extremities
basilar (artery) (see also Occlusion, artery, basilar) 433.0 ☑
brain 437.0
bypass graft
coronary artery 414.05
autologous artery (gastroepiploic) (internal mammary) 414.04
autologous vein 414.02
nonautologous biological 414.03
of transplanted heart 414.07
extremity 440.30
autologous vein 440.31
nonautologous biological 440.32
cardiac — see Arteriosclerosis, coronary
cardiopathy — see Arteriosclerosis, coronary
cardiorenal (see also Hypertension, cardiorenal) 404.90
cardiovascular (see also Disease, cardiovascular) 429.2
carotid (artery) (common) (internal) (see also Occlusion, artery, carotid) 433.1 ☑
central nervous system 437.0
cerebral 437.0
late effect — see Late effect(s) (of) cerebrovascular disease
cerebrospinal 437.0
cerebrovascular 437.0
coronary (artery) 414.00
due to
calcified coronary lesion (severely) 414.4
lipid rich plaque 414.3

Arteriosclerosis, arteriosclerotic — continued
coronary — continued
graft — see Arteriosclerosis, bypass graft
native artery 414.01
of transplanted heart 414.06
extremities (native artery) NEC 440.20
bypass graft 440.30
autologous vein 440.31
nonautologous biological 440.32
claudication (intermittent) 440.21
and
gangrene 440.24
rest pain 440.22
and
gangrene 440.24
ulceration 440.23
and gangrene 440.24
ulceration 440.23
and gangrene 440.24
gangrene 440.24
rest pain 440.22
and
gangrene 440.24
ulceration 440.23
and gangrene 440.24
specified site NEC 440.29
ulceration 440.23
and gangrene 440.24
heart (disease) (see also Arteriosclerosis, coronary)
valve 424.99
aortic 424.1
mitral 424.0
pulmonary 424.3
tricuspid 424.2
iliac 440.8
kidney (see also Hypertension, kidney) 403.90
labyrinth, labyrinthine 388.00
medial NEC (see also Arteriosclerosis, extremities) 440.20
mesentery (artery) 557.1
Mönckeberg's (see also Arteriosclerosis, extremities) 440.20
myocarditis 429.0
nephrosclerosis (see also Hypertension, kidney) 403.90
peripheral (of extremities) — see Arteriosclerosis, extremities
precerebral 433.9 ☑
specified artery NEC 433.8 ☑
pulmonary (idiopathic) 416.0
renal (see also Hypertension, kidney) 403.90
arterioles (see also Hypertension, kidney) 403.90
artery 440.1
retinal (vascular) 440.8 [362.13]
specified artery NEC 440.8
with gangrene 440.8 [785.4]
spinal (cord) 437.0
vertebral (artery) (see also Occlusion, artery, vertebral) 433.2 ☑
Arteriospasm 443.9
Arteriovenous — see condition
Arteritis 447.6
allergic (see also Angiitis, hypersensitivity) 446.20
aorta (nonsyphilitic) 447.6
syphilitic 093.1
aortic arch 446.7
brachiocephalica 446.7
brain 437.4
syphilitic 094.89
branchial 446.7
cerebral 437.4
late effect — see Late effect(s) (of) cerebrovascular disease
syphilitic 094.89
coronary (artery) (see also Arteriosclerosis, coronary)
rheumatic 391.9
chronic 398.99
syphilitic 093.89
cranial (left) (right) 446.5
deformans — see Arteriosclerosis

Arteritis — continued
giant cell 446.5
necrosing or necrotizing 446.0
nodosa 446.0
obliterans (see also Arteriosclerosis)
subclaviocarotica 446.7
pulmonary 417.8
retina 362.18
rheumatic — see Fever, rheumatic
senile — see Arteriosclerosis
suppurative 447.2
syphilitic (general) 093.89
brain 094.89
coronary 093.89
spinal 094.89
temporal 446.5
young female, syndrome 446.7
Artery, arterial — see condition
Arthralgia — see also Pain, joint 719.4 ☑
allergic (see also Pain, joint) 719.4 ☑
in caisson disease 993.3
psychogenic 307.89
rubella 056.71
Salmonella 003.23
temporomandibular joint 524.62
Arthritis, arthritic (acute) (chronic) (subacute) 716.9 ☑
meaning Osteoarthritis — see Osteoarthrosis

Note — Use the following fifth-digit subclassification with categories 711–712, 715–716:

0   site unspecified

1   shoulder region

2   upper arm

3   forearm

4   hand

5   pelvic region and thigh

6   lower leg

7   ankle and foot

8   other specified sites

9   multiple sites

allergic 716.2 ☑
ankylosing (crippling) (spine) 720.0
sites other than spine 716.9 ☑
atrophic 714.0
spine 720.9
back (see also Arthritis, spine) 721.90
Bechterew's (ankylosing spondylitis) 720.0
blennorrhagic 098.50
cervical, cervicodorsal (see also Spondylosis, cervical) 721.0
Charcôt's 094.0 [713.5]
diabetic 250.6 ☑ [713.5]
due to secondary diabetes 249.6 ☑ [713.5]
syringomyelic 336.0 [713.5]
tabetic 094.0 [713.5]
chylous (see also Filariasis) 125.9 [711.7] ☑
climacteric NEC 716.3 ☑
coccyx 721.8
cricoarytenoid 478.79
crystal (-induced) — see Arthritis, due to crystals
deformans (see also Osteoarthrosis) 715.9 ☑
spine 721.90
with myelopathy 721.91
degenerative (see also Osteoarthrosis) 715.9 ☑
idiopathic 715.09
polyarticular 715.09
spine 721.90
with myelopathy 721.91
dermatoarthritis, lipoid 272.8 [713.0]
due to or associated with
acromegaly 253.0 [713.0]
actinomycosis 039.8 [711.4] ☑
amyloidosis 277.39 [713.7]
bacterial disease NEC 040.89 [711.4] ☑
Behçet's syndrome 136.1 [711.2] ☑

☑ **Additional Digit Required** — Refer to the Tabular List for Digit Selection

Ⓦ **Subterms under main terms may continue to next column or page**

2013 ICD-9-CM

▶◀ Revised Text   ● New Line   ▲ Revised Code

Volume 2 — 27

Arrest, arrested — Arthritis, arthritic

Arthritis, arthritic — continued
due to or associated with — continued
blastomycosis 116.0 [711.6] ☑
brucellosis (see also Brucellosis)
023.9 [711.4] ☑
caisson disease 993.3
coccidioidomycosis 114.3 [711.6] ☑
coliform (Escherichia coli) 711.0 ☑
colitis, ulcerative (see also Colitis, ulcerative) 556.9 [713.1]
cowpox 051.01 [711.5] ☑
crystals (see also Gout)
dicalcium phosphate
275.49 [712.1] ☑
pyrophosphate 275.49 [712.2] ☑
specified NEC 275.49 [712.8] ☑
dermatoarthritis, lipoid 272.8 [713.0]
dermatological disorder NEC
709.9 [713.3]
diabetes 250.6 ☑ [713.5]
due to secondary diabetes
249.6 ☑ [713.5]
diphtheria 032.89 [711.4] ☑
dracontiasis 125.7 [711.7] ☑
dysentery 009.0 [711.3] ☑
endocrine disorder NEC 259.9 [713.0]
enteritis NEC 009.1 [711.3] ☑
infectious (see also Enteritis, infectious) 009.0 [711.3] ☑
specified organism NEC
008.8 [711.3] ☑
regional (see also Enteritis, regional)
555.9 [713.1]
specified organism NEC
008.8 [711.3] ☑
epiphyseal slip, nontraumatic (old)
716.8 ☑
erysipelas 035 [711.4] ☑
erythema
epidemic 026.1
multiforme 695.10 [713.3]
nodosum 695.2 [713.3]
Escherichia coli 711.0 ☑
filariasis NEC 125.9 [711.7] ☑
gastrointestinal condition NEC
569.9 [713.1]
glanders 024 [711.4] ☑
Gonococcus 098.50
gout 274.00
helminthiasis NEC 128.9 [711.7] ☑
hematological disorder NEC 289.9 [713.2]
hemochromatosis 275.03 [713.0]
hemoglobinopathy NEC (see also Disease, hemoglobin) 282.7 [713.2]
hemophilia (see also Hemophilia)
286.0 [713.2]
Hemophilus influenzae (H. influenzae)
711.0 ☑
Henoch (-Schönlein) purpura
287.0 [713.6]
H. influenzae 711.0 ☑
histoplasmosis NEC (see also Histoplasmosis) 115.99 [711.6] ☑
human parvovirus 079.83 [711.5] ☑
hyperparathyroidism 252.00 [713.0]
hypersensitivity reaction NEC
995.3 [713.6]
hypogammaglobulinemia (see also Hypogamma-globulinemia)
279.00 [713.0]
hypothyroidism NEC 244.9 [713.0]
infection (see also Arthritis, infectious)
711.9 ☑
infectious disease NEC 136.9 [711.8] ☑
leprosy (see also Leprosy)
030.9 [711.4] ☑
leukemia NEC (M9800/3) 208.9 [713.2]
lipoid dermatoarthritis 272.8 [713.0]
Lyme disease 088.81 [711.8] ☑
Mediterranean fever, familial
277.31 [713.7]
meningococcal infection 036.82
metabolic disorder NEC 277.9 [713.0]
multiple myelomatosis (M9730/3) 203.0
[713.2]

Arthritis, arthritic — continued
due to or associated with — continued
mumps 072.79 [711.5] ☑
mycobacteria 031.8 [711.4] ☑
mycosis NEC 117.9 [711.6] ☑
neurological disorder NEC 349.9 [713.5]
ochronosis 270.2 [713.0]
O'Nyong Nyong 066.3 [711.5] ☑
parasitic disease NEC 136.9 [711.8] ☑
paratyphoid fever (see also Fever,
paratyphoid) 002.9 [711.3] ☑
parvovirus B19 079.83 [711.5] ☑
Pneumococcus 711.0 ☑
poliomyelitis (see also Poliomyelitis)
045.9 [711.5] ☑
Pseudomonas 711.0 ☑
psoriasis 696.0
pyogenic organism (E. coli) (H. influenzae) (Pseudomonas) (Streptococcus) 711.0 ☑
rat-bite fever 026.1 [711.4] ☑
regional enteritis (see also Enteritis, regional) 555.9 [713.1]
Reiter's disease 099.3 [711.1] ☑
respiratory disorder NEC 519.9 [713.4]
reticulosis, malignant (M9720/3) 202.3
[713.2]
rubella 056.71
salmonellosis 003.23
sarcoidosis 135 [713.7]
serum sickness 999.59 [713.6]
Staphylococcus 711.0 ☑
Streptococcus 711.0 ☑
syphilis (see also Syphilis)
094.0 [711.4] ☑
syringomyelia 336.0 [713.5]
thalassemia (see also Thalassemia)
282.40 [713.2]
tuberculosis (see also Tuberculosis,
arthritis) 015.9 ☑ [711.4] ☑
typhoid fever 002.0 [711.3] ☑
ulcerative colitis (see also Colitis, ulcerative) 556.9 [713.1]
urethritis
nongonococcal (see also Urethritis,
nongonococcal)
099.40 [711.1] ☑
nonspecific (see also Urethritis, nongonococcal) 099.40 [711.1] ☑
Reiter's 099.3
viral disease NEC 079.99 [711.5] ☑
erythema epidemic 026.1
gonococcal 098.50
gouty 274.00
acute 274.01
hypertrophic (see also Osteoarthrosis)
715.9 ☑
spine 721.90
with myelopathy 721.91
idiopathic, blennorrheal 099.3
in caisson disease 993.3 [713.8]
infectious or infective (acute) (chronic)
(subacute) NEC 711.9 ☑
nonpyogenic 711.9 ☑
spine 720.9
inflammatory NEC 714.9
juvenile rheumatoid (chronic) (polyarticular)
714.30
acute 714.31
monoarticular 714.33
pauciarticular 714.32
lumbar (see also Spondylosis, lumbar) 721.3
meningococcal 036.82
menopausal NEC 716.3 ☑
migratory — see Fever, rheumatic
neuropathic (Charcôt's) 094.0 [713.5]
diabetic 250.6 ☑ [713.5]
due to secondary diabetes
249.6 ☑ [713.5]
nonsyphilitic NEC 349.9 [713.5]
syringomyelic 336.0 [713.5]
tabetic 094.0 [713.5]
nodosa (see also Osteoarthrosis) 715.9 ☑
spine 721.90
with myelopathy 721.91

Arthritis, arthritic — continued
nonpyogenic NEC 716.9 ☑
spine 721.90
with myelopathy 721.91
ochronotic 270.2 [713.0]
palindromic (see also Rheumatism, palindromic) 719.3
pneumococcal 711.0 ☑
postdysenteric 009.0 [711.3] ☑
postrheumatic, chronic (Jaccoud's) 714.4
primary progressive 714.0
spine 720.9
proliferative 714.0
spine 720.0
psoriatic 696.0
purulent 711.0 ☑
pyogenic or pyemic 711.0 ☑
reactive 099.3
rheumatic 714.0
acute or subacute — see Fever,
rheumatic
chronic 714.0
spine 720.9
rheumatoid (nodular) 714.0
with
splenoadenomegaly and leukopenia
714.1
visceral or systemic involvement
714.2
aortitis 714.89
carditis 714.2
heart disease 714.2
juvenile (chronic) (polyarticular) 714.30
acute 714.31
monoarticular 714.33
pauciarticular 714.32
spine 720.0
rubella 056.71
sacral, sacroiliac, sacrococcygeal (see also
Spondylosis, sacral) 721.3
scorbutic 267
senile or senescent (see also Osteoarthrosis)
715.9 ☑
spine 721.90
with myelopathy 721.91
septic 711.0 ☑
serum (nontherapeutic) (therapeutic)
999.59 [713.6]
specified form NEC 716.8 ☑
spine 721.90
with myelopathy 721.91
atrophic 720.9
degenerative 721.90
with myelopathy 721.91
hypertrophic (with deformity) 721.90
with myelopathy 721.91
infectious or infective NEC 720.9
Marie-Strümpell 720.0
nonpyogenic 721.90
with myelopathy 721.91
pyogenic 720.9
rheumatoid 720.0
traumatic (old) 721.7
tuberculous (see also Tuberculosis)
015.0 ☑ [720.81]
staphylococcal 711.0 ☑
streptococcal 711.0 ☑
suppurative 711.0 ☑
syphilitic 094.0 [713.5]
congenital 090.49 [713.5]
syphilitica deformans (Charcôt) 094.0 [713.5]
temporomandibular joint 524.69
thoracic (see also Spondylosis, thoracic)
721.2
toxic of menopause 716.3 ☑
transient 716.4 ☑
traumatic (chronic) (old) (post) 716.1 ☑
current injury — see nature of injury
tuberculous (see also Tuberculosis, arthritis)
015.9 ☑ [711.4] ☑
urethritica 099.3 [711.1] ☑
urica, uratic 274.00
venereal 099.3 [711.1] ☑
vertebral (see also Arthritis, spine) 721.90
villous 716.8 ☑
von Bechterew's 720.0

Arthrocele — see also Effusion, joint 719.0 ☑
Arthrochondritis — see Arthritis
Arthrodesis status V45.4
Arthrodynia — see also Pain, joint 719.4 ☑
psychogenic 307.89
Arthrodysplasia 755.9
Arthrofibrosis joint — see also Ankylosis
718.5 ☑
Arthrogryposis 728.3
multiplex, congenita 754.89
Arthrokatadysis 715.35
Arthrolithiasis 274.00
Arthro-onychodysplasia 756.89
Arthro-osteo-onychodysplasia 756.89
Arthropathy — see also Arthritis 716.9 ☑

> Note — Use the following fifth-digit subclassification with categories 711–712, 716:
>
> 0   site unspecified
> 1   shoulder region
> 2   upper arm
> 3   forearm
> 4   hand
> 5   pelvic region and thigh
> 6   lower leg
> 7   ankle and foot
> 8   other specified sites
> 9   multiple sites

Behçet's 136.1 [711.2] ☑
Charcôt's 094.0 [713.5]
diabetic 250.6 ☑ [713.5]
due to secondary diabetes
249.6 ☑ [713.5]
syringomyelic 336.0 [713.5]
tabetic 094.0 [713.5]
crystal (-induced) — see Arthritis, due to
crystals
gouty 274.00
acute 274.01
chronic (without mention of tophus
(tophi)) 274.02
with tophus (tophi) 274.03
neurogenic, neuropathic (Charcôt's) (tabetic) 094.0 [713.5]
diabetic 250.6 ☑ [713.5]
due to secondary diabetes
249.6 ☑ [713.5]
nonsyphilitic NEC 349.9 [713.5]
syringomyelic 336.0 [713.5]
postdysenteric NEC 009.0 [711.3] ☑
postrheumatic, chronic (Jaccoud's) 714.4
psoriatic 696.0
pulmonary 731.2
specified NEC 716.8 ☑
syringomyelia 336.0 [713.5]
tabes dorsalis 094.0 [713.5]
tabetic 094.0 [713.5]
transient 716.4 ☑
traumatic 716.1 ☑
uric acid 274.00
Arthrophyte — see also Loose, body, joint
718.1 ☑
Arthrophytis 719.80
ankle 719.87
elbow 719.82
foot 719.87
hand 719.84
hip 719.85
knee 719.86
multiple sites 719.89
pelvic region 719.85
shoulder (region) 719.81
specified site NEC 719.88
wrist 719.83
Arthropyosis — see also Arthritis, pyogenic
711.0 ☑
**Arthroscopic surgical procedure converted
to open procedure** V64.43
Arthrosis (deformans) (degenerative) — see
also Osteoarthrosis 715.9 ☑

☑ Additional Digit Required — Refer to the Tabular List for Digit Selection   ▽ Subterms under main terms may continue to next column or page

28 — Volume 2   ▶◀ Revised Text   ● New Line   ▲ Revised Code   2013 ICD-9-CM

Arthrosis — see also Osteoarthrosis — continued
  Charcôt's 094.0 [713.5]
  polyarticular 715.09
  spine (see also Spondylosis) 721.90
Arthus phenomenon 995.21
  due to
    correct substance properly administered 995.21
    overdose or wrong substance given or taken 977.9
      specified drug — see Table of Drugs and Chemicals
    serum 999.59
Articular — see also condition
  disc disorder (reducing or non-reducing) 524.63
  spondylolisthesis 756.12
Articulation
  anterior 524.27
  posterior 524.27
  reverse 524.27
Artificial
  device (prosthetic) — see Fitting, device
  insemination V26.1
  menopause (states) (symptoms) (syndrome) 627.4
  opening status (functioning) (without complication) V44.9
    anus (colostomy) V44.3
    colostomy V44.3
    cystostomy V44.50
      appendico-vesicostomy V44.52
      cutaneous-vesicostomy V44.51
      specified type NEC V44.59
    enterostomy V44.4
    gastrostomy V44.1
    ileostomy V44.2
    intestinal tract NEC V44.4
    jejunostomy V44.4
    nephrostomy V44.6
    specified site NEC V44.8
    tracheostomy V44.0
    ureterostomy V44.6
    urethrostomy V44.6
    urinary tract NEC V44.6
    vagina V44.7
  vagina status V44.7
ARV (disease) (illness) (infection) — see Human immunodeficiency virus (disease) (illness) (infection)
Arytenoid — see condition
Asbestosis (occupational) 501
Asboe-Hansen's disease (incontinentia pigmenti) 757.33
Ascariasis (intestinal) (lung) 127.0
Ascaridiasis 127.0
Ascaridosis 127.0
Ascaris 127.0
  lumbricoides (infestation) 127.0
  pneumonia 127.0
Ascending — see condition
ASC-H (atypical squamous cells cannot exclude high grade squamous intraepithelial lesion)
  anus 796.72
  cervix 795.02
  vagina 795.12
Aschoff's bodies — see also Myocarditis, rheumatic 398.0
Ascites 789.59
  abdominal NEC 789.59
  cancerous (M8000/6) 789.51
  cardiac 428.0
  chylous (nonfilarial) 457.8
    filarial (see also Infestation, filarial) 125.9
  congenital 778.0
  due to S. japonicum 120.2
  fetal, causing fetopelvic disproportion 653.7 ☑
  heart 428.0
  joint (see also Effusion, joint) 719.0 ☑
  malignant (M8000/6) 789.51
  pseudochylous 789.59
  syphilitic 095.2
  tuberculous (see also Tuberculosis) 014.0 ☑

Ascorbic acid (vitamin C) **deficiency** (scurvy) 267
ASC-US (atypical squamous cells of undetermined significance)
  anus 796.71
  cervix 795.01
  vagina 795.11
ASCVD (arteriosclerotic cardiovascular disease) 429.2
Aseptic — see condition
Asherman's syndrome 621.5
Asialia 527.7
Asiatic cholera — see also Cholera 001.9
Asocial personality or trends 301.7
Asomatognosia 781.8
Aspergillosis 117.3
  with pneumonia 117.3 [484.6]
  allergic bronchopulmonary 518.6
  nonsyphilitic NEC 117.3
Aspergillus (flavus) (fumigatus) (infection) (terreus) 117.3
Aspermatogenesis 606.0
Aspermia (testis) 606.0
Asphyxia, asphyxiation (by) 799.01
  antenatal — see Distress, fetal
  bedclothes 994.7
  birth (see also Asphyxia, newborn) 768.9
  bunny bag 994.7
  carbon monoxide 986
  caul (see also Asphyxia, newborn) 768.9
  cave-in 994.7
    crushing — see Injury, internal, intrathoracic organs
  constriction 994.7
  crushing — see Injury, internal, intrathoracic organs
  drowning 994.1
  fetal, affecting newborn 768.9
  food or foreign body (in larynx) 933.1
    bronchioles 934.8
    bronchus (main) 934.1
    lung 934.8
    nasopharynx 933.0
    nose, nasal passages 932
    pharynx 933.0
    respiratory tract 934.9
      specified part NEC 934.8
    throat 933.0
    trachea 934.0
  gas, fumes, or vapor NEC 987.9
    specified — see Table of Drugs and Chemicals
  gravitational changes 994.7
  hanging 994.7
  inhalation — see Inhalation
  intrauterine
    fetal death (before onset of labor) 768.0
      during labor 768.1
    liveborn infant — see Distress, fetal, liveborn infant
  local 443.0
  mechanical 994.7
    during birth (see also Distress, fetal) 768.9
  mucus 933.1
    bronchus (main) 934.1
    larynx 933.1
    lung 934.8
    nasal passages 932
    newborn 770.18
    pharynx 933.0
    respiratory tract 934.9
      specified part NEC 934.8
    throat 933.0
    trachea 934.0
    vaginal (fetus or newborn) 770.18
  newborn 768.9
    with neurologic involvement 768.5
    blue 768.6
    livida 768.6
    mild or moderate 768.6
    pallida 768.5
    severe 768.5
    white 768.5
  pathological 799.01
  plastic bag 994.7

Asphyxia, asphyxiation — continued
  postnatal (see also Asphyxia, newborn) 768.9
    mechanical 994.7
  pressure 994.7
  reticularis 782.61
  strangulation 994.7
  submersion 994.1
  traumatic NEC — see Injury, internal, intrathoracic organs
  vomiting, vomitus — see Asphyxia, food or foreign body
Aspiration
  acid pulmonary (syndrome) 997.39
    obstetric 668.0 ☑
  amniotic fluid 770.13
    with respiratory symptoms 770.14
  bronchitis 507.0
  clear amniotic fluid 770.13
    with
      pneumonia 770.14
      pneumonitis 770.14
      respiratory symptoms 770.14
  contents of birth canal 770.17
    with respiratory symptoms 770.18
  fetal 770.10
    blood 770.15
      with
        pneumonia 770.16
        pneumonitis 770.16
    pneumonia 770.18
  food, foreign body, or gasoline (with asphyxiation) — see Asphyxia, food or foreign body
  meconium 770.11
    with
      pneumonia 770.12
      pneumonitis 770.12
      respiratory symptoms 770.12
    below vocal cords 770.11
      with respiratory symptoms 770.12
  mucus 933.1
    into
      bronchus (main) 934.1
      lung 934.8
      respiratory tract 934.9
        specified part NEC 934.8
      trachea 934.0
    newborn 770.17
    vaginal (fetus or newborn) 770.17
  newborn 770.10
    with respiratory symptoms 770.18
    blood 770.15
      with
        pneumonia 770.16
        pneumonitis 770.16
        respiratory symptoms 770.16
  pneumonia 507.0
    fetus or newborn 770.18
      meconium 770.12
  pneumonitis 507.0
    fetus or newborn 770.18
      meconium 770.12
    obstetric 668.0 ☑
  postnatal stomach contents 770.85
    with
      pneumonia 770.86
      pneumonitis 770.86
      respiratory symptoms 770.86
  syndrome of newborn (massive) 770.18
    meconium 770.12
  vernix caseosa 770.12
Asplenia 759.0
  with mesocardia 746.87
Assam fever 085.0
Assimilation, pelvis
  with disproportion 653.2 ☑
    affecting fetus or newborn 763.1
    causing obstructed labor 660.1 ☑
      affecting fetus or newborn 763.1
Assmann's focus — see also Tuberculosis 011.0 ☑
Astasia (-abasia) 307.9
  hysterical 300.11
Asteatosis 706.8
  cutis 706.8
Astereognosis 780.99

Asterixis 781.3
  in liver disease 572.8
Asteroid hyalitis 379.22
Asthenia, asthenic 780.79
  cardiac (see also Failure, heart) 428.9
    psychogenic 306.2
  cardiovascular (see also Failure, heart) 428.9
    psychogenic 306.2
  heart (see also Failure, heart) 428.9
    psychogenic 306.2
  hysterical 300.11
  myocardial (see also Failure, heart) 428.9
    psychogenic 306.2
  nervous 300.5
  neurocirculatory 306.2
  neurotic 300.5
  psychogenic 300.5
  psychoneurotic 300.5
  psychophysiologic 300.5
  reaction, psychoneurotic 300.5
  senile 797
  Stiller's 780.79
  tropical anhidrotic 705.1
Asthenopia 368.13
  accommodative 367.4
  hysterical (muscular) 300.11
  psychogenic 306.7
Asthenospermia 792.2
Asthma, asthmatic (bronchial) (catarrh) (spasmodic) 493.9 ☑

> Note — Use the following fifth-digit subclassification with codes 493.0–493.2, 493.9:
>
> 0   without mention of status asthmaticus or acute exacerbation or unspecified
>
> 1   with status asthmaticus
>
> 2   with acute exacerbation

  with
    chronic obstructive pulmonary disease (COPD) 493.2 ☑
    hay fever 493.0 ☑
    rhinitis, allergic 493.0 ☑
  allergic 493.9 ☑
    stated cause (external allergen) 493.0 ☑
  atopic 493.0 ☑
  cardiac (see also Failure, ventricular, left) 428.1
  cardiobronchial (see also Failure, ventricular, left) 428.1
  cardiorenal (see also Hypertension, cardiorenal) 404.90
  childhood 493.0 ☑
  Colliers' 500
  cough variant 493.82
  croup 493.9 ☑
  detergent 507.8
  due to
    detergent 507.8
    inhalation of fumes 506.3
    internal immunological process 493.0 ☑
  endogenous (intrinsic) 493.1 ☑
  eosinophilic 518.3
  exercise induced bronchospasm 493.81
  exogenous (cosmetics) (dander or dust) (drugs) (dust) (feathers) (food) (hay) (platinum) (pollen) 493.0 ☑
  extrinsic 493.0 ☑
  grinders' 502
  hay 493.0 ☑
  heart (see also Failure, ventricular, left) 428.1
  IgE 493.0 ☑
  infective 493.1 ☑
  intrinsic 493.1 ☑
  Kopp's 254.8
  late-onset 493.1 ☑
  meat-wrappers' 506.9
  Millar's (laryngismus stridulus) 478.75
  millstone makers' 502
  miners' 500
  Monday morning 504
  New Orleans (epidemic) 493.0 ☑
  platinum 493.0 ☑

Arthrosis — Asthma, asthmatic

☑ Additional Digit Required — Refer to the Tabular List for Digit Selection   ⟲ Subterms under main terms may continue to next column or page

2013 ICD-9-CM   ►◄ Revised Text   ● New Line   ▲ Revised Code   Volume 2 — 29

Asthma, asthmatic — *continued*
  pneumoconiotic (occupational) NEC 505
    potters' 502
  psychogenic 316 *[493.9]* ☑
  pulmonary eosinophilic 518.3
  red cedar 495.8
  Rostan's (*see also* Failure, ventricular, left)
    428.1
  sandblasters' 502
  sequoiosis 495.8
  stonemasons' 502
  thymic 254.8
  tuberculous (*see also* Tuberculosis, pulmonary) 011.9 ☑
  Wichmann's (laryngismus stridulus) 478.75
  wood 495.8
Astigmatism (compound) (congenital) 367.20
  irregular 367.22
  regular 367.21
Astroblastoma (M9430/3)
  nose 748.1
  specified site — *see* Neoplasm, by site, malignant
  unspecified site 191.9
Astrocytoma (cystic) (M9400/3)
  anaplastic type (M9401/3)
    specified site — *see* Neoplasm, by site, malignant
    unspecified site 191.9
  fibrillary (M9420/3)
    specified site — *see* Neoplasm, by site, malignant
    unspecified site 191.9
  fibrous (M9420/3)
    specified site — *see* Neoplasm, by site, malignant
    unspecified site 191.9
  gemistocytic (M9411/3)
    specified site — *see* Neoplasm, by site, malignant
    unspecified site 191.9
  juvenile (M9421/3)
    specified site — *see* Neoplasm, by site, malignant
    unspecified site 191.9
  nose 748.1
  pilocytic (M9421/3)
    specified site — *see* Neoplasm, by site, malignant
    unspecified site 191.9
  piloid (M9421/3)
    specified site — *see* Neoplasm, by site, malignant
    unspecified site 191.9
  protoplasmic (M9410/3)
    specified site — *see* Neoplasm, by site, malignant
    unspecified site 191.9
  specified site — *see* Neoplasm, by site, malignant
  subependymal (M9383/1) 237.5
    giant cell (M9384/1) 237.5
  unspecified site 191.9
Astroglioma (M9400/3)
  nose 748.1
  specified site — *see* Neoplasm, by site, malignant
  unspecified site 191.9
Asymbolia 784.60
Asymmetrical breathing 786.09
Asymmetry — *see also* Distortion
  breast, between native and reconstructed
    612.1
  chest 786.9
  face 754.0
  jaw NEC 524.12
    maxillary 524.11
  pelvis with disproportion 653.0 ☑
    affecting fetus or newborn 763.1
    causing obstructed labor 660.1 ☑
      affecting fetus or newborn 763.1
Asynergia 781.3
Asynergy 781.3
  ventricular 429.89
Asystole (heart) — *see also* Arrest, cardiac
  427.5

Ataxia, ataxy, ataxic 781.3
  acute 781.3
  brain 331.89
  cerebellar 334.3
    hereditary (Marie's) 334.2
    in
      alcoholism 303.9 ☑ *[334.4]*
      myxedema (*see also* Myxedema)
        244.9 *[334.4]*
      neoplastic disease NEC 239.9 *[334.4]*
  cerebral 331.89
  family, familial 334.2
    cerebral (Marie's) 334.2
    spinal (Friedreich's) 334.0
  Friedreich's (heredofamilial) (spinal) 334.0
  frontal lobe 781.3
  gait 781.2
    hysterical 300.11
  general 781.3
  hereditary NEC 334.2
    cerebellar 334.2
    spastic 334.1
    spinal 334.0
  heredofamilial (Marie's) 334.2
  hysterical 300.11
  locomotor (progressive) 094.0
    diabetic 250.6 ☑ *[337.1]*
      due to secondary diabetes
        249.6 ☑ *[337.1]*
  Marie's (cerebellar) (heredofamilial) 334.2
  nonorganic origin 307.9
  partial 094.0
  postchickenpox 052.7
  progressive locomotor 094.0
  psychogenic 307.9
  Sanger-Brown's 334.2
  spastic 094.0
    hereditary 334.1
    syphilitic 094.0
  spinal
    hereditary 334.0
    progressive locomotor 094.0
  telangiectasia 334.8
Ataxia-telangiectasia 334.8
Atelectasis (absorption collapse) (complete)
    (compression) (massive) (partial)
    (postinfective) (pressure collapse) (pulmonary) (relaxation) 518.0
  newborn (congenital) (partial) 770.5
    primary 770.4
  primary 770.4
  tuberculous (*see also* Tuberculosis, pulmonary) 011.9 ☑
Ateleiosis, ateliosis 253.3
Atelia — *see* Distortion
Ateliosis 253.3
Atelocardia 746.9
Atelomyelia 742.59
Athelia 757.6
Atheroembolism
  extremity
    lower 445.02
    upper 445.01
  kidney 445.81
  specified site NEC 445.89
Atheroma, atheromatous — *see also* Arteriosclerosis 440.9
  aorta, aortic 440.0
    valve (*see also* Endocarditis, aortic) 424.1
  artery — *see* Arteriosclerosis
  basilar (artery) (*see also* Occlusion, artery, basilar) 433.0 ☑
  carotid (artery) (common) (internal) (*see also* Occlusion, artery, carotid) 433.1 ☑
  cerebral (arteries) 437.0
  coronary (artery) — *see* Arteriosclerosis, coronary
  degeneration — *see* Arteriosclerosis
  heart, cardiac — *see* Arteriosclerosis, coronary
  mitral (valve) 424.0
  myocardium, myocardial — *see* Arteriosclerosis, coronary
  pulmonary valve (heart) (*see also* Endocarditis, pulmonary) 424.3
  skin 706.2

Atheroma, atheromatous — *see also*
    Arteriosclerosis — *continued*
  tricuspid (heart) (valve) 424.2
  valve, valvular — *see* Endocarditis
  vertebral (artery) (*see also* Occlusion, artery, vertebral) 433.2 ☑
Atheromatosis — *see also* Arteriosclerosis
  arterial, congenital 272.8
Atherosclerosis — *see* Arteriosclerosis
Athetosis (acquired) 781.0
  bilateral 333.79
  congenital (bilateral) 333.6
  double 333.71
  unilateral 781.0
Athlete's
  foot 110.4
  heart 429.3
Athletic team examination V70.3
Athrepsia 261
Athyrea (acquired) — *see also* Hypothyroidism
    244.9
  congenital 243
Athyreosis (congenital) 243
  acquired — *see* Hypothyroidism
Athyroidism (acquired) — *see also* Hypothyroidism 244.9
  congenital 243
Atmospheric pyrexia 992.0
Atonia, atony, atonic
  abdominal wall 728.2
  bladder (sphincter) 596.4
    neurogenic NEC 596.54
      with cauda equina syndrome 344.61
  capillary 448.9
  cecum 564.89
    psychogenic 306.4
  colon 564.89
    psychogenic 306.4
  congenital 779.89
  dyspepsia 536.3
    psychogenic 306.4
  intestine 564.89
    psychogenic 306.4
  stomach 536.3
    neurotic or psychogenic 306.4
    psychogenic 306.4
  uterus 661.2 ☑
    with hemorrhage (postpartum) 666.1 ☑
    without hemorrhage
      intrapartum 661.2 ☑
      postpartum 669.8 ☑
  vesical 596.4
Atopy NEC V15.09
Atransferrinemia, congenital 273.8
Atresia, atretic (congenital) 759.89
  alimentary organ or tract NEC 751.8
    lower 751.2
    upper 750.8
  ani, anus, anal (canal) 751.2
  aorta 747.22
    with hypoplasia of ascending aorta and
      defective development of left
      ventricle (with mitral valve atresia) 746.7
    arch 747.11
    ring 747.21
  aortic (orifice) (valve) 746.89
    arch 747.11
  aqueduct of Sylvius 742.3
    with spina bifida (*see also* Spina bifida)
      741.0 ☑
  artery NEC (*see also* Atresia, blood vessel)
    747.60
    cerebral 747.81
    coronary 746.85
    eye 743.58
    pulmonary 747.31
    umbilical 747.5
  auditory canal (external) 744.02
  bile, biliary duct (common) or passage
    751.61
    acquired (*see also* Obstruction, biliary)
      576.2
  bladder (neck) 753.6
  blood vessel (peripheral) NEC 747.60
    cerebral 747.81

Atresia, atretic — *continued*
  blood vessel — *continued*
    gastrointestinal 747.61
    lower limb 747.64
    pulmonary artery 747.31
    renal 747.62
    spinal 747.82
    upper limb 747.63
  bronchus 748.3
  canal, ear 744.02
  cardiac
    valve 746.89
      aortic 746.89
      mitral 746.89
      pulmonary 746.01
      tricuspid 746.1
  cecum 751.2
  cervix (acquired) 622.4
    congenital 752.43
    in pregnancy or childbirth 654.6 ☑
      affecting fetus or newborn 763.89
      causing obstructed labor 660.2 ☑
        affecting fetus or newborn 763.1
  choana 748.0
  colon 751.2
  cystic duct 751.61
    acquired 575.8
      with obstruction (*see also* Obstruction, gallbladder) 575.2
  digestive organs NEC 751.8
  duodenum 751.1
  ear canal 744.02
  ejaculatory duct 752.89
  epiglottis 748.3
  esophagus 750.3
  Eustachian tube 744.24
  fallopian tube (acquired) 628.2
    congenital 752.19
  follicular cyst 620.0
  foramen of
    Luschka 742.3
      with spina bifida (*see also* Spina bifida) 741.0 ☑
    Magendie 742.3
      with spina bifida (*see also* Spina bifida) 741.0 ☑
  gallbladder 751.69
  genital organ
    external
      female 752.49
      male NEC 752.89
        penis 752.69
    internal
      female 752.89
      male 752.89
  glottis 748.3
  gullet 750.3
  heart
    valve NEC 746.89
      aortic 746.89
      mitral 746.89
      pulmonary 746.01
      tricuspid 746.1
  hymen 752.42
    acquired 623.3
    postinfective 623.3
  ileum 751.1
  intestine (small) 751.1
    large 751.2
  iris, filtration angle (*see also* Buphthalmia)
    743.20
  jejunum 751.1
  kidney 753.3
  lacrimal, apparatus 743.65
    acquired — *see* Stenosis, lacrimal
  larynx 748.3
  ligament, broad 752.19
  lung 748.5
  meatus urinarius 753.6
  mitral valve 746.89
    with atresia or hypoplasia of aortic orifice or valve, with hypoplasia of
      ascending aorta and defective
      development of left ventricle
      746.7
  nares (anterior) (posterior) 748.0

☑ **Additional Digit Required** — Refer to the Tabular List for Digit Selection   🗤 **Subterms under main terms may continue to next column or page**

30 — Volume 2   ▶◀ Revised Text   ● New Line   ▲ Revised Code   2013 ICD-9-CM

Atresia, atretic — *continued*
  nasolacrimal duct 743.65
  nasopharynx 748.8
  nose, nostril 748.0
    acquired 738.0
  organ or site NEC — *see* Anomaly, specified
    type NEC
  osseous meatus (ear) 744.03
  oviduct (acquired) 628.2
    congenital 752.19
  parotid duct 750.23
    acquired 527.8
  pulmonary (artery) 747.31
    valve 746.01
    vein 747.49
  pulmonic 746.01
  pupil 743.46
  rectum 751.2
  salivary duct or gland 750.23
    acquired 527.8
  sublingual duct 750.23
    acquired 527.8
  submaxillary duct or gland 750.23
    acquired 527.8
  trachea 748.3
  tricuspid valve 746.1
  ureter 753.29
  ureteropelvic junction 753.21
  ureterovesical orifice 753.22
  urethra (valvular) 753.6
  urinary tract NEC 753.29
  uterus 752.31
    acquired 621.8
  vagina (acquired) 623.2
    congenital (total) (partial) 752.45
    postgonococcal (old) 098.2
    postinfectional 623.2
    senile 623.2
  vascular NEC (*see also* Atresia, blood vessel)
    747.60
    cerebral 747.81
  vas deferens 752.89
  vein NEC (*see also* Atresia, blood vessel)
    747.60
    cardiac 746.89
    great 747.49
    portal 747.49
    pulmonary 747.49
  vena cava (inferior) (superior) 747.49
  vesicourethral orifice 753.6
  vulva 752.49
    acquired 624.8
Atrichia, atrichosis 704.00
  congenital (universal) 757.4
Atrioventricularis commune 745.69
At risk for falling V15.88
Atrophia — *see also* Atrophy
  alba 709.09
  cutis 701.8
    idiopathica progressiva 701.8
    senilis 701.8
  dermatological, diffuse (idiopathic) 701.8
  flava hepatis (acuta) (subacuta) (*see also*
    Necrosis, liver) 570
  gyrata of choroid and retina (central) 363.54
    generalized 363.57
  senilis 797
    dermatological 701.8
  unguium 703.8
    congenita 757.5
Atrophoderma, atrophodermia 701.9
  diffusum (idiopathic) 701.8
  maculatum 701.3
    et striatum 701.3
      due to syphilis 095.8
    syphilitic 091.3
  neuriticum 701.8
  pigmentosum 757.33
  reticulatum symmetricum faciei 701.8
  senile 701.8
  symmetrical 701.8
  vermiculata 701.8
Atrophy, atrophic
  adrenal (autoimmune) (capsule) (cortex)
    (gland) 255.41
    with hypofunction 255.41

Atrophy, atrophic — *continued*
  alveolar process or ridge (edentulous)
    525.20
    mandible 525.20
      minimal 525.21
      moderate 525.22
      severe 525.23
    maxilla 525.20
      minimal 525.24
      moderate 525.25
      severe 525.26
  appendix 543.9
  Aran-Duchenne muscular 335.21
  arm 728.2
  arteriosclerotic — *see* Arteriosclerosis
  arthritis 714.0
    spine 720.9
  bile duct (any) 576.8
  bladder 596.89
  blanche (of Milian) 701.3
  bone (senile) 733.99
    due to
      disuse 733.7
      infection 733.99
      tabes dorsalis (neurogenic) 094.0
    posttraumatic 733.99
  brain (cortex) (progressive) 331.9
    with dementia 290.10
    Alzheimer's 331.0
      with dementia — *see* Alzheimer's,
        dementia
    circumscribed (Pick's) 331.11
      with dementia
        with behavioral disturbance
          331.11 *[294.11]*
        without behavioral disturbance
          331.11 *[294.10]*
    congenital 742.4
    hereditary 331.9
    senile 331.2
  breast 611.4
    puerperal, postpartum 676.3 ☑
  buccal cavity 528.9
  cardiac (brown) (senile) (*see also* Degenera-
    tion, myocardial) 429.1
  cartilage (infectional) (joint) 733.99
  cast, plaster of Paris 728.2
  cerebellar — *see* Atrophy, brain
  cerebral — *see* Atrophy, brain
  cervix (endometrium) (mucosa) (myometri-
    um) (senile) (uteri) 622.8
    menopausal 627.8
  Charcôt-Marie-Tooth 356.1
  choroid 363.40
    diffuse secondary 363.42
    hereditary (*see also* Dystrophy, choroid)
      363.50
    gyrate
      central 363.54
      diffuse 363.57
      generalized 363.57
    senile 363.41
  ciliary body 364.57
  colloid, degenerative 701.3
  conjunctiva (senile) 372.89
  corpus cavernosum 607.89
  cortical (*see also* Atrophy, brain) 331.9
  Cruveilhier's 335.21
  cystic duct 576.8
  dacryosialadenopathy 710.2
  degenerative
    colloid 701.3
    senile 701.3
  Déjérine-Thomas 333.0
  diffuse idiopathic, dermatological 701.8
  disuse
    bone 733.7
    muscle 728.2
    pelvic muscles and anal sphincter 618.83
  Duchenne-Aran 335.21
  ear 388.9
  edentulous alveolar ridge 525.20
    mandible 525.20
      minimal 525.21
      moderate 525.22
      severe 525.23

Atrophy, atrophic — *continued*
  edentulous alveolar ridge — *continued*
    maxilla 525.20
      minimal 525.24
      moderate 525.25
      severe 525.26
  emphysema, lung 492.8
  endometrium (senile) 621.8
    cervix 622.8
  enteric 569.89
  epididymis 608.3
  eyeball, cause unknown 360.41
  eyelid (senile) 374.50
  facial (skin) 701.9
  facioscapulohumeral (Landouzy-Déjérine)
    359.1
  fallopian tube (senile), acquired 620.3
  fatty, thymus (gland) 254.8
  gallbladder 575.8
  gastric 537.89
  gastritis (chronic) 535.1 ☑
  gastrointestinal 569.89
  genital organ, male 608.89
  glandular 289.3
  globe (phthisis bulbi) 360.41
  gum (*see also* Recession, gingival) 523.20
  hair 704.2
  heart (brown) (senile) (*see also* Degenera-
    tion, myocardial) 429.1
  hemifacial 754.0
    Romberg 349.89
  hydronephrosis 591
  infantile 261
    paralysis, acute (*see also* Poliomyelitis,
      with paralysis) 045.1 ☑
  intestine 569.89
  iris (generalized) (postinfectional) (sector
    shaped) 364.59
    essential 364.51
    progressive 364.51
    sphincter 364.54
  kidney (senile) (*see also* Sclerosis, renal) 587
    with hypertension (*see also* Hyperten-
      sion, kidney) 403.90
    congenital 753.0
    hydronephrotic 591
    infantile 753.0
  lacrimal apparatus (primary) 375.13
    secondary 375.14
  Landouzy-Déjérine 359.1
  laryngitis, infection 476.0
  larynx 478.79
  Leber's optic 377.16
  lip 528.5
  liver (acute) (subacute) (*see also* Necrosis,
    liver) 570
    chronic (yellow) 571.8
    yellow (congenital) 570
      with
        abortion — *see* Abortion, by type,
          with specified complica-
          tion NEC
        ectopic pregnancy (*see also* cate-
          gories 633.0–633.9) 639.8
        molar pregnancy (*see also* cate-
          gories 630–632) 639.8
      chronic 571.8
      complicating pregnancy 646.7 ☑
      following
        abortion 639.8
        ectopic or molar pregnancy 639.8
      from injection, inoculation or transfu-
        sion (onset within 8 months
        after administration) — *see*
        Hepatitis, viral
      healed 571.5
      obstetric 646.7 ☑
      postabortal 639.8
      postimmunization — *see* Hepatitis,
        viral
      posttransfusion — *see* Hepatitis, viral
      puerperal, postpartum 674.8 ☑
  lung (senile) 518.89
    congenital 748.69
  macular (dermatological) 701.3
    syphilitic, skin 091.3

Atrophy, atrophic — *continued*
  macular — *continued*
    syphilitic, skin — *continued*
      striated 095.8
  muscle, muscular 728.2
    disuse 728.2
    Duchenne-Aran 335.21
    extremity (lower) (upper) 728.2
    familial spinal 335.11
    general 728.2
    idiopathic 728.2
    infantile spinal 335.0
    myelopathic (progressive) 335.10
    myotonic 359.21
    neuritic 356.1
    neuropathic (peroneal) (progressive)
      356.1
    peroneal 356.1
    primary (idiopathic) 728.2
    progressive (familial) (hereditary) (pure)
      335.21
      adult (spinal) 335.19
      infantile (spinal) 335.0
      juvenile (spinal) 335.11
      spinal 335.10
        adult 335.19
        hereditary or familial 335.11
        infantile 335.0
    pseudohypertrophic 359.1
    spinal (progressive) 335.10
      adult 335.19
      Aran-Duchenne 335.21
      familial 335.11
      hereditary 335.11
      infantile 335.0
      juvenile 335.11
    syphilitic 095.6
  myocardium (*see also* Degeneration, myocar-
    dial) 429.1
  myometrium (senile) 621.8
    cervix 622.8
  myotatic 728.2
  myotonia 359.21
  nail 703.8
    congenital 757.5
  nasopharynx 472.2
  nerve (*see also* Disorder, nerve)
    abducens 378.54
    accessory 352.4
    acoustic or auditory 388.5
    cranial 352.9
      first (olfactory) 352.0
      second (optic) (*see also* Atrophy, op-
        tic nerve) 377.10
      third (oculomotor) (partial) 378.51
        total 378.52
      fourth (trochlear) 378.53
      fifth (trigeminal) 350.8
      sixth (abducens) 378.54
      seventh (facial) 351.8
      eighth (auditory) 388.5
      ninth (glossopharyngeal) 352.2
      tenth (pneumogastric) (vagus) 352.3
      eleventh (accessory) 352.4
      twelfth (hypoglossal) 352.5
    facial 351.8
    glossopharyngeal 352.2
    hypoglossal 352.5
    oculomotor (partial) 378.51
      total 378.52
    olfactory 352.0
    peripheral 355.9
    pneumogastric 352.3
    trigeminal 350.8
    trochlear 378.53
    vagus (pneumogastric) 352.3
  nervous system, congenital 742.8
  neuritic (*see also* Disorder, nerve) 355.9
  neurogenic NEC 355.9
    bone
      tabetic 094.0
  nutritional 261
  old age 797
  olivopontocerebellar 333.0

☑ **Additional Digit Required** — Refer to the Tabular List for Digit Selection   ⒲ **Subterms under main terms may continue to next column or page**

2013 ICD-9-CM   ▶◀ **Revised Text**   ● **New Line**   ▲ **Revised Code**   Volume 2 — 31

Atrophy, atrophic — *continued*
  optic nerve (ascending) (descending) (infectional) (nonfamilial) (papillomacular bundle) (postretinal) (secondary NEC) (simple) 377.10
    associated with retinal dystrophy 377.13
    dominant hereditary 377.16
    glaucomatous 377.14
    hereditary (dominant) (Leber's) 377.16
    Leber's (hereditary) 377.16
    partial 377.15
    postinflammatory 377.12
    primary 377.11
    syphilitic 094.84
      congenital 090.49
      tabes dorsalis 094.0
  orbit 376.45
  ovary (senile), acquired 620.3
  oviduct (senile), acquired 620.3
  palsy, diffuse 335.20
  pancreas (duct) (senile) 577.8
  papillary muscle 429.81
  paralysis 355.9
  parotid gland 527.0
  patches skin 701.3
    senile 701.8
  penis 607.89
  pharyngitis 472.1
  pharynx 478.29
  pluriglandular 258.8
  polyarthritis 714.0
  prostate 602.2
  pseudohypertrophic 359.1
  renal (see also Sclerosis, renal) 587
  reticulata 701.8
  retina (see also Degeneration, retina) 362.60
    hereditary (see also Dystrophy, retina) 362.70
  rhinitis 472.0
  salivary duct or gland 527.0
  scar NEC 709.2
  sclerosis, lobar (of brain) 331.0
    with dementia
      with behavioral disturbance 331.0 [294.11]
      without behavioral disturbance 331.0 [294.10]
  scrotum 608.89
  seminal vesicle 608.89
  senile 797
    degenerative, of skin 701.3
  skin (patches) (senile) 701.8
  spermatic cord 608.89
  spinal (cord) 336.8
    acute 336.8
    muscular (chronic) 335.10
      adult 335.19
      familial 335.11
      juvenile 335.10
    paralysis 335.10
      acute (see also Poliomyelitis, with paralysis) 045.1 ☑
  spine (column) 733.99
  spleen (senile) 289.59
  spots (skin) 701.3
    senile 701.8
  stomach 537.89
  striate and macular 701.3
    syphilitic 095.8
  subcutaneous 701.9
    due to injection 999.9
  sublingual gland 527.0
  submaxillary gland 527.0
  Sudeck's 733.7
  suprarenal (autoimmune) (capsule) (gland) 255.41
    with hypofunction 255.41
  tarso-orbital fascia, congenital 743.66
  testis 608.3
  thenar, partial 354.0
  throat 478.29
  thymus (fat) 254.8
  thyroid (gland) 246.8
    with
      cretinism 243
      myxedema 244.9

Atrophy, atrophic — *continued*
  thyroid — *continued*
    congenital 243
  tongue (senile) 529.8
    papillae 529.4
    smooth 529.4
  trachea 519.19
  tunica vaginalis 608.89
  turbinate 733.99
  tympanic membrane (nonflaccid) 384.82
    flaccid 384.81
  ulcer (see also Ulcer, skin) 707.9
  upper respiratory tract 478.9
  uterus, uterine (acquired) (senile) 621.8
    cervix 622.8
    due to radiation (intended effect) 621.8
  vagina (senile) 627.3
  vascular 459.89
  vas deferens 608.89
  vertebra (senile) 733.99
  vulva (primary) (senile) 624.1
  Werdnig-Hoffmann 335.0
  yellow (acute) (congenital) (liver) (subacute) (see also Necrosis, liver) 570
    chronic 571.8
    resulting from administration of blood, plasma, serum, or other biological substance (within 8 months of administration) — see Hepatitis, viral

Attack
  akinetic (see also Epilepsy) 345.0 ☑
  angina — see Angina
  apoplectic (see also Disease, cerebrovascular, acute) 436
  benign shuddering 333.93
  bilious — see Vomiting
  cataleptic 300.11
  cerebral (see also Disease, cerebrovascular, acute) 436
  coronary (see also Infarct, myocardium) 410.9 ☑
  cyanotic, newborn 770.83
  epileptic (see also Epilepsy) 345.9 ☑
  epileptiform 780.39
  heart (see also Infarct, myocardium) 410.9 ☑
  hemiplegia (see also Disease, cerebrovascular, acute) 436
  hysterical 300.11
  jacksonian (see also Epilepsy) 345.5 ☑
  myocardium, myocardial (see also Infarct, myocardium) 410.9 ☑
  myoclonic (see also Epilepsy) 345.1 ☑
  panic 300.01
  paralysis (see also Disease, cerebrovascular, acute) 436
  paroxysmal 780.39
  psychomotor (see also Epilepsy) 345.4 ☑
  salaam (see also Epilepsy) 345.6 ☑
  schizophreniform (see also Schizophrenia) 295.4 ☑
  sensory and motor 780.39
  syncope 780.2
  toxic, cerebral 780.39
  transient ischemic (TIA) 435.9
  unconsciousness 780.2
    hysterical 300.11
  vasomotor 780.2
  vasovagal (idiopathic) (paroxysmal) 780.2

Attention to — *continued*
  artificial opening (of) V55.9
    digestive tract NEC V55.4
    specified site NEC V55.8
    urinary tract NEC V55.6
    vagina V55.7
  colostomy V55.3
  cystostomy V55.5
  dressing
    wound V58.30
      nonsurgical V58.30
      surgical V58.31
  gastrostomy V55.1
  ileostomy V55.2
  jejunostomy V55.4
  nephrostomy V55.6

Attention to — *continued*
  surgical dressings V58.31
  sutures V58.32
  tracheostomy V55.0
  ureterostomy V55.6
  urethrostomy V55.6
Attrition
  gum (see also Recession, gingival) 523.20
  teeth (hard tissues) 521.10
    excessive 521.10
      extending into
        dentine 521.12
        pulp 521.13
      generalized 521.15
      limited to enamel 521.11
      localized 521.14
Atypical — *see also* condition
  cells
    endocervical 795.00
    endometrial 795.00
    glandular
      anus 796.70
      cervical 795.00
      vaginal 795.10
  distribution, vessel (congenital) (peripheral) NEC 747.60
  endometrium 621.9
  kidney 593.89
Atypism, cervix 622.10
Audible tinnitus — *see also* Tinnitus 388.30
Auditory — *see* condition
Audry's syndrome (acropachyderma) 757.39
Aujeszky's disease 078.89
Aura
  jacksonian (see also Epilepsy) 345.5 ☑
  persistent migraine 346.5 ☑
    with cerebral infarction 346.6 ☑
    without cerebral infarction 346.5 ☑
Aurantiasis, cutis 278.3
Auricle, auricular — *see* condition
Auriculotemporal syndrome 350.8
Australian
  Q fever 083.0
  X disease 062.4
Autism, autistic (child) (infantile) 299.0 ☑
Autodigestion 799.89
Autoerythrocyte sensitization 287.2
Autographism 708.3
Autoimmune
  cold sensitivity 283.0
  disease NEC 279.49
  hemolytic anemia 283.0
  inhibitors to clotting factors 286.52
  lymphoproliferative syndrome (ALPS) 279.41
  thyroiditis 245.2
Autoinfection, septic — *see* Septicemia
Autointoxication 799.89
Automatism 348.89
  with temporal sclerosis 348.81
  epileptic (see also Epilepsy) 345.4 ☑
  paroxysmal, idiopathic (see also Epilepsy) 345.4 ☑
Autonomic, autonomous
  bladder 596.54
    neurogenic 596.54
      with cauda equina 344.61
  dysreflexia 337.3
  faciocephalalgia (see also Neuropathy, peripheral, autonomic) 337.9
  hysterical seizure 300.11
  imbalance (see also Neuropathy, peripheral, autonomic) 337.9
Autophony 388.40
Autosensitivity, erythrocyte 287.2
Autotopagnosia 780.99
Autotoxemia 799.89
Autumn — *see* condition
Avellis' syndrome 344.89
Aversion
  oral 783.3
    newborn 779.31
    nonorganic origin 307.59
Aviators
  disease or sickness (see also Effect, adverse, high altitude) 993.2

Aviators — *continued*
  ear 993.0
  effort syndrome 306.2
Avitaminosis (multiple NEC) — *see also* Deficiency, vitamin 269.2
  A 264.9
  B 266.9
    with
      beriberi 265.0
      pellagra 265.2
  B_1 265.1
  B_2 266.0
  B_6 266.1
  B_{12} 266.2
  C (with scurvy) 267
  D 268.9
    with
      osteomalacia 268.2
      rickets 268.0
  E 269.1
  G 266.0
  H 269.1
  K 269.0
  multiple 269.2
  nicotinic acid 265.2
  P 269.1
Avulsion (traumatic) 879.8
  blood vessel — *see* Injury, blood vessel, by site
  cartilage (see also Dislocation, by site)
    knee, current (see also Tear, meniscus) 836.2
    symphyseal (inner), complicating delivery 665.6 ☑
  complicated 879.9
  diaphragm — *see* Injury, internal, diaphragm
  ear — *see* Wound, open, ear
  epiphysis of bone — *see* Fracture, by site
  external site other than limb — *see* Wound, open, by site
  eye 871.3
  fingernail — *see* Wound, open, finger
  fracture — *see* Fracture, by site
  genital organs, external — *see* Wound, open, genital organs
  head (intracranial) NEC (see also Injury, intracranial, with open intracranial wound)
    complete 874.9
    external site NEC 873.8
      complicated 873.9
  internal organ or site — *see* Injury, internal, by site
  joint (see also Dislocation, by site)
    capsule — *see* Sprain, by site
  ligament — *see* Sprain, by site
  limb (see also Amputation, traumatic, by site)
    skin and subcutaneous tissue — *see* Wound, open, by site
  muscle — *see* Sprain, by site
  nerve (root) — *see* Injury, nerve, by site
  scalp — *see* Wound, open, scalp
  skin and subcutaneous tissue — *see* Wound, open, by site
  symphyseal cartilage (inner), complicating delivery 665.6 ☑
  tendon (see also Sprain, by site)
    with open wound — *see* Wound, open, by site
  toenail — *see* Wound, open, toe(s)
  tooth 873.63
    complicated 873.73
Awaiting organ transplant status V49.83
Awareness of heart beat 785.1
Axe grinders' disease 502
Axenfeld's anomaly or syndrome 743.44
Axilla, axillary — *see also* condition
  breast 757.6
Axonotmesis — *see* Injury, nerve, by site
Ayala's disease 756.89
Ayerza's disease or syndrome (pulmonary artery sclerosis with pulmonary hypertension) 416.0

Azoospermia 606.0
Azorean disease (of the nervous system) 334.8
Azotemia 790.6
    meaning uremia (*see also* Uremia) 586
Aztec ear 744.29
Azygos lobe, lung (fissure) 748.69

B

Baader's syndrome (erythema multiforme exudativum) 695.19
Baastrup's syndrome 721.5
Babesiasis 088.82
Babesiosis 088.82
Babington's disease (familial hemorrhagic telangiectasia) 448.0
Babinski-Fröhlich syndrome (adiposogenital dystrophy) 253.8
Babinski-Nageotte syndrome 344.89
Babinski's syndrome (cardiovascular syphilis) 093.89
Bacillary — *see* condition
Bacilluria 791.9
    asymptomatic, in pregnancy or puerperium 646.5 ☑
    tuberculous (*see also* Tuberculosis) 016.9 ☑
Bacillus — *see also* Infection, bacillus
    abortus infection 023.1
    anthracis infection 022.9
    coli
        infection 041.49
            generalized 038.42
            intestinal 008.00
        pyemia 038.42
        septicemia 038.42
    Flexner's 004.1
    fusiformis infestation 101
    mallei infection 024
    Shiga's 004.0
    suipestifer infection (*see also* Infection, Salmonella) 003.9
Back — *see* condition
Backache (postural) 724.5
    psychogenic 307.89
    sacroiliac 724.6
Backflow (pyelovenous) — *see also* Disease, renal 593.9
Backknee — *see also* Genu, recurvatum 736.5
Bacteremia 790.7
    newborn 771.83
Bacteria
    in blood (*see also* Bacteremia) 790.7
    in urine (*see also* Bacteriuria) 599.0
Bacterial — *see* condition
Bactericholia — *see also* Cholecystitis, acute 575.0
Bacterid, bacteride (Andrews' pustular) 686.8
Bacteriuria, bacteruria 791.9
    with
        urinary tract infection 599.0
    asymptomatic 791.9
        in pregnancy or puerperium 646.5 ☑
            affecting fetus or newborn 760.1
Bad
    breath 784.99
    heart — *see* Disease, heart
    trip (*see also* Abuse, drugs, nondependent) 305.3 ☑
Baehr-Schiffrin disease (thrombotic thrombocytopenic purpura) 446.6
Baelz's disease (cheilitis glandularis apostematosa) 528.5
Baerensprung's disease (eczema marginatum) 110.3
Bagassosis (occupational) 495.1
Baghdad boil 085.1
Bagratuni's syndrome (temporal arteritis) 446.5
Baker's
    cyst (knee) 727.51
        tuberculous (*see also* Tuberculosis) 015.2 ☑
    itch 692.89
Bakwin-Krida syndrome (craniometaphyseal dysplasia) 756.89
Balanitis (circinata) (gangraenosa) (infectious) (vulgaris) 607.1

Balanitis — *continued*
    amebic 006.8
    candidal 112.2
    chlamydial 099.53
    due to Ducrey's bacillus 099.0
    erosiva circinata et gangraenosa 607.1
    gangrenous 607.1
    gonococcal (acute) 098.0
        chronic or duration of 2 months or over 098.2
    nongonococcal 607.1
    phagedenic 607.1
    venereal NEC 099.8
    xerotica obliterans 607.81
Balanoposthitis 607.1
    chlamydial 099.53
    gonococcal (acute) 098.0
        chronic or duration of 2 months or over 098.2
    ulcerative NEC 099.8
Balanorrhagia — *see* Balanitis
Balantidiasis 007.0
Balantidiosis 007.0
Balbuties, balbutio — *see also* Disorder, fluency 315.35
Bald
    patches on scalp 704.00
    tongue 529.4
Baldness — *see also* Alopecia 704.00
Balfour's disease (chloroma) 205.3 ☑
Balint's syndrome (psychic paralysis of visual fixation) 368.16
Balkan grippe 083.0
Ball
    food 938
    hair 938
Ballantyne (-Runge) syndrome (postmaturity) 766.22
Balloon disease — *see also* Effect, adverse, high altitude 993.2
Ballooning posterior leaflet syndrome 424.0
Baló's disease or concentric sclerosis 341.1
Bamberger's disease (hypertrophic pulmonary osteoarthropathy) 731.2
Bamberger-Marie disease (hypertrophic pulmonary osteoarthropathy) 731.2
Bamboo spine 720.0
Bancroft's filariasis 125.0
Band(s)
    adhesive (*see also* Adhesions, peritoneum) 568.0
    amniotic 658.8 ☑
        affecting fetus or newborn 762.8
    anomalous or congenital (*see also* Anomaly, specified type NEC)
        atrial 746.9
        heart 746.9
        intestine 751.4
        omentum 751.4
        ventricular 746.9
    cervix 622.3
    gallbladder (congenital) 751.69
    intestinal (adhesive) (*see also* Adhesions, peritoneum) 568.0
        congenital 751.4
    obstructive (*see also* Obstruction, intestine) 560.81
    periappendiceal (congenital) 751.4
    peritoneal (adhesive) (*see also* Adhesions, peritoneum) 568.0
        with intestinal obstruction 560.81
        congenital 751.4
    uterus 621.5
    vagina 623.2
Bandemia (without diagnosis of specific infection) 288.66
Bandl's ring (contraction)
    complicating delivery 661.4 ☑
        affecting fetus or newborn 763.7
Bang's disease (Brucella abortus) 023.1
Bangkok hemorrhagic fever 065.4
Bannister's disease 995.1
Bantam-Albright-Martin disease (pseudohypoparathyroidism) 275.49

Banti's disease or syndrome (with cirrhosis) (with portal hypertension) — *see* Cirrhosis, liver
Bar
    calcaneocuboid 755.67
    calcaneonavicular 755.67
    cubonavicular 755.67
    prostate 600.90
        with
            other lower urinary tract symptoms (LUTS) 600.91
        urinary
            obstruction 600.91
            retention 600.91
    talocalcaneal 755.67
Baragnosis 780.99
Barasheh, barashek 266.2
Barcoo disease or rot — *see also* Ulcer, skin 707.9
Bard-Pic syndrome (carcinoma, head of pancreas) 157.0
Bärensprung's disease (eczema marginatum) 110.3
Baritosis 503
Barium lung disease 503
Barlow (-Möller) disease or syndrome (meaning infantile scurvy) 267
Barlow's syndrome (meaning mitral valve prolapse) 424.0
Barodontalgia 993.2
Baron Münchausen syndrome 301.51
Barosinusitis 993.1
Barotitis 993.0
Barotrauma 993.2
    odontalgia 993.2
    otitic 993.0
    sinus 993.1
Barraquer's disease or syndrome (progressive lipodystrophy) 272.6
Barré-Guillain syndrome 357.0
Barrel chest 738.3
Barré-Liéou syndrome (posterior cervical sympathetic) 723.2
Barrett's esophagus 530.85
Barrett's syndrome or ulcer (chronic peptic ulcer of esophagus) 530.85
Bársony-Polgár syndrome (corkscrew esophagus) 530.5
Bársony-Teschendorf syndrome (corkscrew esophagus) 530.5
Bartholin's
    adenitis (*see also* Bartholinitis) 616.89
    gland — *see* condition
Bartholinitis (suppurating) 616.89
    gonococcal (acute) 098.0
        chronic or duration of 2 months or over 098.2
Barth syndrome 759.89
Bartonellosis 088.0
Bartter's syndrome (secondary hyperaldosteronism with juxtaglomerular hyperplasia) 255.13
Basal — *see* condition
Basan's (hidrotic) **ectodermal dysplasia** 757.31
Baseball finger 842.13
Basedow's disease or syndrome (exophthalmic goiter) 242.0 ☑
Basic — *see* condition
Basilar — *see* condition
Bason's (hidrotic) **ectodermal dysplasia** 757.31
Basopenia 288.59
Basophilia 288.65
Basophilism (corticoadrenal) (Cushing's) (pituitary) (thymic) 255.0
Bassen-Kornzweig syndrome (abetalipoproteinemia) 272.5
Bat ear 744.29
Bateman's
    disease 078.0
    purpura (senile) 287.2
Bathing cramp 994.1
Bathophobia 300.23
Batten's disease, retina 330.1 *[362.71]*
Batten-Mayou disease 330.1 *[362.71]*

Batten-Steinert syndrome 359.21
Battered
    adult (syndrome) 995.81
    baby or child (syndrome) 995.54
    spouse (syndrome) 995.81
Battey mycobacterium infection 031.0
Battledore placenta — *see* Placenta, abnormal
Battle exhaustion — *see also* Reaction, stress, acute 308.9
Baumgarten-Cruveilhier (cirrhosis) **disease, or syndrome** 571.5
Bauxite
    fibrosis (of lung) 503
    workers' disease 503
Bayle's disease (dementia paralytica) 094.1
Bazin's disease (primary) — *see also* Tuberculosis 017.1 ☑
Beach ear 380.12
Beaded hair (congenital) 757.4
Beals syndrome 759.82
Beard's disease (neurasthenia) 300.5
Bearn-Kunkel (-Slater) syndrome (lupoid hepatitis) 571.49
Beat
    elbow 727.2
    hand 727.2
    knee 727.2
Beats
    ectopic 427.60
    escaped, heart 427.60
        postoperative 997.1
    premature (nodal) 427.60
        atrial 427.61
        auricular 427.61
        postoperative 997.1
        specified type NEC 427.69
        supraventricular 427.61
        ventricular 427.69
Beau's
    disease or syndrome (*see also* Degeneration, myocardial) 429.1
    lines (transverse furrows on fingernails) 703.8
Bechterew's disease (ankylosing spondylitis) 720.0
Bechterew-Strümpell-Marie syndrome (ankylosing spondylitis) 720.0
Becker's
    disease
        idiopathic mural endomyocardial disease 425.2
        myotonia congenita, recessive form 359.22
    dystrophy 359.22
Beck's syndrome (anterior spinal artery occlusion) 433.8 ☑
Beckwith (-Wiedemann) syndrome 759.89
Bedbugs bite(s) — *see* Injury, superficial, by site
Bedclothes, asphyxiation or suffocation by 994.7
Bed confinement status V49.84
Bednar's aphthae 528.2
Bedsore (*see also* Ulcer, pressure) 707.00
    with gangrene 707.00 *[785.4]*
Bedwetting — *see also* Enuresis 788.36
Beer-drinkers' heart (disease) 425.5
Bee sting (with allergic or anaphylactic shock) 989.5
Begbie's disease (exophthalmic goiter) 242.0 ☑
Behavior disorder, disturbance — *see also* Disturbance, conduct
    antisocial, without manifest psychiatric disorder
        adolescent V71.02
        adult V71.01
        child V71.02
    dyssocial, without manifest psychiatric disorder
        adolescent V71.02
        adult V71.01
        child V71.02
    high risk — *see* Problem
Behçet's syndrome 136.1
Behr's disease 362.50

☑ Additional Digit Required — Refer to the Tabular List for Digit Selection   ⬙ Subterms under main terms may continue to next column or page

2013 ICD-9-CM   ▶◀ Revised Text   ● New Line   ▲ Revised Code   **Volume 2 — 33**

Beigel's disease or morbus (white piedra)
111.2
Bejel 104.0
Bekhterev's disease (ankylosing spondylitis)
720.0
Bekhterev-Strümpell-Marie syndrome
(ankylosing spondylitis) 720.0
Belching — *see also* Eructation 787.3
Bell's
disease (*see also* Psychosis, affective)
296.0 ☑
mania (*see also* Psychosis, affective) 296.0 ☑
palsy, paralysis 351.0
infant 767.5
newborn 767.5
syphilitic 094.89
spasm 351.0
**Bence-Jones albuminuria, albuminosuria,
or proteinuria** 791.0
Bends 993.3
Benedikt's syndrome (paralysis) 344.89
Benign — *see also* condition
cellular changes, cervix 795.09
prostate
with
other lower urinary tract symptoms
(LUTS) 600.21
urinary
obstruction 600.21
retention 600.21
hyperplasia 600.20
neoplasm 222.2
Bennett's
disease (leukemia) 208.9 ☑
fracture (closed) 815.01
open 815.11
Benson's disease 379.22
Bent
back (hysterical) 300.11
nose 738.0
congenital 754.0
Bereavement V62.82
as adjustment reaction 309.0
Bergeron's disease (hysteroepilepsy) 300.11
Berger's paresthesia (lower limb) 782.0
Beriberi (acute) (atrophic) (chronic) (dry)
(subacute) (wet) 265.0
with polyneuropathy 265.0 *[357.4]*
heart (disease) 265.0 *[425.7]*
leprosy 030.1
neuritis 265.0 *[357.4]*
Berlin's disease or edema (traumatic) 921.3
Berloque dermatitis 692.72
Bernard-Horner syndrome — *see also* Neuropathy, peripheral, autonomic 337.9
Bernard-Sergent syndrome (acute adrenocortical insufficiency) 255.41
Bernard-Soulier disease or thrombopathy
287.1
Bernhardt's disease or paresthesia 355.1
Bernhardt-Roth disease or syndrome
(paresthesia) 355.1
Bernheim's syndrome — *see also* Failure,
heart 428.0
Bertielliasis 123.8
Bertolotti's syndrome (sacralization of fifth
lumbar vertebra) 756.15
Berylliosis (acute) (chronic) (lung) (occupational) 503
Besnier's
lupus pernio 135
prurigo (atopic dermatitis) (infantile
eczema) 691.8
Besnier-Boeck disease or sarcoid 135
Besnier-Boeck-Schaumann disease (sarcoidosis) 135
Best's disease 362.76
Bestiality 302.1
**Beta-adrenergic hyperdynamic circulatory
state** 429.82
Beta-aminoisobutyric aciduria 277.2
Beta-mercaptolactate-cysteine disulfiduria
270.0
Beta thalassemia (mixed) 282.44
major 282.44
minor 282.46

Beurmann's disease (sporotrichosis) 117.1
Bezoar 938
intestine 936
stomach 935.2
Bezold's abscess — *see also* Mastoiditis 383.01
Bianchi's syndrome (aphasia-apraxia-alexia)
784.69
Bicornuate or bicornis uterus (complete)
(partial) 752.34
in pregnancy or childbirth 654.0 ☑
with obstructed labor 660.2 ☑
affecting fetus or newborn 763.1
affecting fetus or newborn 763.89
Bicuspid aortic valve 746.4
Biedl-Bardet syndrome 759.89
Bielschowsky's disease 330.1
Bielschowsky-Jansky
amaurotic familial idiocy 330.1
disease 330.1
Biemond's syndrome (obesity, polydactyly,
and intellectual disabilities) 759.89
Biermer's anemia or disease (pernicious
anemia) 281.0
Biett's disease 695.4
Bifid (congenital) — *see also* Imperfect, closure
apex, heart 746.89
clitoris 752.49
epiglottis 748.3
kidney 753.3
nose 748.1
patella 755.64
scrotum 752.89
toe 755.66
tongue 750.13
ureter 753.4
uterus 752.34
uvula 749.02
with cleft lip (*see also* Cleft, palate, with
cleft lip) 749.20
Biforis uterus (suprasimplex) 752.34
Bifurcation (congenital) — *see also* Imperfect,
closure
gallbladder 751.69
kidney pelvis 753.3
renal pelvis 753.3
rib 756.3
tongue 750.13
trachea 748.3
ureter 753.4
urethra 753.8
uvula 749.02
with cleft lip (*see also* Cleft, palate, with
cleft lip) 749.20
vertebra 756.19
Bigeminal pulse 427.89
Bigeminy 427.89
Big spleen syndrome 289.4
Bilateral — *see* condition
Bile duct — *see* condition
Bile pigments in urine 791.4
Bilharziasis — *see also* Schistosomiasis 120.9
chyluria 120.0
cutaneous 120.3
galacturia 120.0
hematochyluria 120.0
intestinal 120.1
lipemia 120.9
lipuria 120.0
Oriental 120.2
piarhemia 120.9
pulmonary 120.2
tropical hematuria 120.0
vesical 120.0
Biliary — *see* condition
Bilious (attack) — *see also* Vomiting
fever, hemoglobinuric 084.8
Bilirubinuria 791.4
Biliuria 791.4
Billroth's disease
meningocele (*see also* Spina bifida) 741.9 ☑
Bilobate placenta — *see* Placenta, abnormal
Bilocular
heart 745.7
stomach 536.8
Bing-Horton syndrome (histamine cephalgia)
339.00

Binswanger's disease or dementia 290.12
Biörck (-Thorson) syndrome (malignant carcinoid) 259.2
Biparta, bipartite — *see also* Imperfect, closure
carpal scaphoid 755.59
patella 755.64
placenta — *see* Placenta, abnormal
vagina 752.49
Bird
face 756.0
fanciers' lung or disease 495.2
flu — *see also* Influenza, avian 488.02
Bird's disease (oxaluria) 271.8
Birth
abnormal fetus or newborn 763.9
accident, fetus or newborn — *see* Birth, injury
complications in mother — *see* Delivery,
complicated
compression during NEC 767.9
defect — *see* Anomaly
delayed, fetus 763.9
difficult NEC, affecting fetus or newborn
763.9
dry, affecting fetus or newborn 761.1
forced, NEC, affecting fetus or newborn
763.89
forceps, affecting fetus or newborn 763.2
hematoma of sternomastoid 767.8
immature 765.1 ☑
extremely 765.0 ☑
inattention, after or at 995.52
induced, affecting fetus or newborn 763.89
infant — *see* Newborn
injury NEC 767.9
adrenal gland 767.8
basal ganglia 767.0
brachial plexus (paralysis) 767.6
brain (compression) (pressure) 767.0
cerebellum 767.0
cerebral hemorrhage 767.0
conjunctiva 767.8
eye 767.8
fracture
bone, any except clavicle or spine
767.3
clavicle 767.2
femur 767.3
humerus 767.3
long bone 767.3
radius and ulna 767.3
skeleton NEC 767.3
skull 767.3
spine 767.4
tibia and fibula 767.3
hematoma 767.8
liver (subcapsular) 767.8
mastoid 767.8
skull 767.19
sternomastoid 767.8
testes 767.8
vulva 767.8
intracranial (edema) 767.0
laceration
brain 767.0
by scalpel 767.8
peripheral nerve 767.7
liver 767.8
meninges
brain 767.0
spinal cord 767.4
nerves (cranial, peripheral) 767.7
brachial plexus 767.6
facial 767.5
paralysis 767.7
brachial plexus 767.6
Erb (-Duchenne) 767.6
facial nerve 767.5
Klumpke (-Déjérine) 767.6
radial nerve 767.6
spinal (cord) (hemorrhage) (laceration) (rupture) 767.4
rupture
intracranial 767.0
liver 767.8

Birth — *continued*
injury — *continued*
rupture — *continued*
spinal cord 767.4
spleen 767.8
viscera 767.8
scalp 767.19
scalpel wound 767.8
skeleton NEC 767.3
specified NEC 767.8
spinal cord 767.4
spleen 767.8
subdural hemorrhage 767.0
tentorial, tear 767.0
testes 767.8
vulva 767.8
instrumental, NEC, affecting fetus or newborn 763.2
lack of care, after or at 995.52
multiple
affected by maternal complications of
pregnancy 761.5
healthy liveborn — *see* Newborn, multiple
neglect, after or at 995.52
newborn — *see* Newborn
palsy or paralysis NEC 767.7
precipitate, fetus or newborn 763.6
premature (infant) 765.1 ☑
prolonged, affecting fetus or newborn 763.9
retarded, fetus or newborn 763.9
shock, newborn 779.89
strangulation or suffocation
due to aspiration of clear amniotic fluid
770.13
with respiratory symptoms 770.14
mechanical 767.8
trauma NEC 767.9
triplet
affected by maternal complications of
pregnancy 761.5
healthy liveborn — *see* Newborn, multiple
twin
affected by maternal complications of
pregnancy 761.5
healthy liveborn — *see* Newborn, twin
ventouse, affecting fetus or newborn 763.3
Birthmark 757.32
Birt-Hogg-Dube syndrome 759.89
Bisalbuminemia 273.8
Biskra button 085.1
Bite(s)
with intact skin surface — *see* Contusion
animal — *see* Wound, open, by site
intact skin surface — *see* Contusion
bedbug — *see* Injury, superficial, by site
centipede 989.5
chigger 133.8
fire ant 989.5
flea — *see* Injury, superficial, by site
human (open wound) (*see also* Wound,
open, by site)
intact skin surface — *see* Contusion
insect
nonvenomous — *see* Injury, superficial,
by site
venomous 989.5
mad dog (death from) 071
open
anterior 524.24
posterior 524.25
poisonous 989.5
red bug 133.8
reptile 989.5
nonvenomous — *see* Wound, open, by
site
snake 989.5
nonvenomous — *see* Wound, open, by
site
spider (venomous) 989.5
nonvenomous — *see* Injury, superficial,
by site
venomous 989.5
Biting
cheek or lip 528.9

☑ **Additional Digit Required** — Refer to the Tabular List for Digit Selection

✍ **Subterms under main terms may continue to next column or page**

34 — Volume 2

▶◀ **Revised Text**

● **New Line**

▲ **Revised Code**

2013 ICD-9-CM

Biting — *continued*
  nail 307.9
Black
  death 020.9
  eye NEC 921.0
  hairy tongue 529.3
  heel 924.20
  lung disease 500
  palm 923.20
Blackfan-Diamond anemia or syndrome
  (congenital hypoplastic anemia) 284.01
Blackhead 706.1
Blackout 780.2
Blackwater fever 084.8
Bladder — *see* condition
Blast
  blindness 921.3
  concussion — *see* Blast, injury
  injury 869.0
    with open wound into cavity 869.1
    abdomen or thorax — *see* Injury, internal, by site
    brain (*see also* Concussion, brain) 850.9
      with skull fracture — *see* Fracture, skull
    ear (acoustic nerve trauma) 951.5
      with perforation, tympanic membrane — *see* Wound, open, ear, drum
    lung (*see also* Injury, internal, lung) 861.20
    otitic (explosive) 388.11
Blastomycosis, blastomycotic (chronic) (cutaneous) (disseminated) (lung) (pulmonary) (systemic) 116.0
  Brazilian 116.1
  European 117.5
  keloidal 116.2
  North American 116.0
  primary pulmonary 116.0
  South American 116.1
Bleb(s) 709.8
  emphysematous (bullous) (diffuse) (lung) (ruptured) (solitary) 492.0
  filtering, eye (postglaucoma) (status) V45.69
    with complication 997.99
      postcataract extraction (complication) 997.99
  lung (ruptured) 492.0
    congenital 770.5
  subpleural (emphysematous) 492.0
Bleeder (familial) (hereditary) — *see also* Defect, coagulation 286.9
  nonfamilial 286.9
Bleeding — *see also* Hemorrhage 459.0
  anal 569.3
  anovulatory 628.0
  atonic, following delivery 666.1 ☑
  capillary 448.9
  due to subinvolution 621.1
    puerperal 666.2 ☑
  ear 388.69
  excessive, associated with menopausal onset 627.0
  familial (*see also* Defect, coagulation) 286.9
  following intercourse 626.7
  gastrointestinal 578.9
  gums 523.8
  hemorrhoids — *see* Hemorrhoids, bleeding
  intermenstrual
    irregular 626.6
    regular 626.5
  intraoperative 998.11
  irregular NEC 626.4
  menopausal 627.0
  mouth 528.9
  nipple 611.79
  nose 784.7
  ovulation 626.5
  postclimacteric 627.1
  postcoital 626.7
  postmenopausal 627.1
    following induced menopause 627.4
  postoperative 998.11
  preclimacteric 627.0
  puberty 626.3

Bleeding — *see also* Hemorrhage — *continued*
  puberty — *continued*
    excessive, with onset of menstrual periods 626.3
  rectum, rectal 569.3
  tendencies (*see also* Defect, coagulation) 286.9
  throat 784.8
  umbilical stump 772.3
  umbilicus 789.9
  unrelated to menstrual cycle 626.6
  uterus, uterine 626.9
    climacteric 627.0
    dysfunctional 626.8
    functional 626.8
    unrelated to menstrual cycle 626.6
  vagina, vaginal 623.8
    functional 626.8
  vicarious 625.8
Blennorrhagia, blennorrhagic — *see* Blennorrhea
Blennorrhea (acute) 098.0
  adultorum 098.40
  alveolaris 523.40
  chronic or duration of 2 months or over 098.2
  gonococcal (neonatorum) 098.40
  inclusion (neonatal) (newborn) 771.6
  neonatorum 098.40
Blepharelosis — *see also* Entropion 374.00
Blepharitis (eyelid) 373.00
  angularis 373.01
  ciliaris 373.00
    with ulcer 373.01
  marginal 373.00
    with ulcer 373.01
  scrofulous (*see also* Tuberculosis) 017.3 ☑ [373.00]
  squamous 373.02
  ulcerative 373.01
Blepharochalasis 374.34
  congenital 743.62
Blepharoclonus 333.81
Blepharoconjunctivitis — *see also* Conjunctivitis 372.20
  angular 372.21
  contact 372.22
Blepharophimosis (eyelid) 374.46
  congenital 743.62
Blepharoplegia 374.89
Blepharoptosis 374.30
  congenital 743.61
Blepharopyorrhea 098.49
Blepharospasm 333.81
  due to drugs 333.85
Blessig's cyst 362.62
Blighted ovum 631.8
Blind
  bronchus (congenital) 748.3
  eye (*see also* Blindness)
    hypertensive 360.42
    hypotensive 360.41
  loop syndrome (postoperative) 579.2
  sac, fallopian tube (congenital) 752.19
  spot, enlarged 368.42
  tract or tube (congenital) NEC — *see* Atresia
Blindness (acquired) (congenital) (both eyes) 369.00
  with deafness V49.85
  blast 921.3
    with nerve injury — *see* Injury, nerve, optic
  Bright's — *see* Uremia
  color (congenital) 368.59
    acquired 368.55
    blue 368.53
    green 368.52
    red 368.51
    total 368.54
  concussion 950.9
  cortical 377.75
  day 368.10
    acquired 368.10
    congenital 368.10
    hereditary 368.10

Blindness — *continued*
  day — *continued*
    specified type NEC 368.10
  due to
    injury NEC 950.9
    refractive error — *see* Error, refractive
  eclipse (total) 363.31
  emotional 300.11
  face 368.16
  hysterical 300.11
  legal (both eyes) (USA definition) 369.4
    with impairment of better (less impaired) eye
    near-total 369.02
      with
        lesser eye impairment 369.02
        near-total 369.04
        total 369.03
      profound 369.05
        with
          lesser eye impairment 369.05
          near-total 369.07
          profound 369.08
          total 369.06
      severe 369.21
        with
          lesser eye impairment 369.21
          blind 369.11
          near-total 369.13
          profound 369.14
          severe 369.22
          total 369.12
      total
        with lesser eye impairment
          total 369.01
  mind 784.69
  moderate
    both eyes 369.25
      with impairment of lesser eye (specified as)
        blind, not further specified 369.15
        low vision, not further specified 369.23
        near-total 369.17
        profound 369.18
        severe 369.24
        total 369.16
    one eye 369.74
      with vision of other eye (specified as)
        near-normal 369.75
        normal 369.76
  near-total
    both eyes 369.04
      with impairment of lesser eye (specified as)
        blind, not further specified 369.02
        total 369.03
    one eye 369.64
      with vision of other eye (specified as)
        near-normal 369.65
        normal 369.66
  night 368.60
    acquired 368.62
    congenital (Japanese) 368.61
    hereditary 368.61
    specified type NEC 368.69
    vitamin A deficiency 264.5
  nocturnal — *see* Blindness, night
  one eye 369.60
    with low vision of other eye 369.10
  profound
    both eyes 369.08
      with impairment of lesser eye (specified as)
        blind, not further specified 369.05
        near-total 369.07
        total 369.06
    one eye 369.67
      with vision of other eye (specified as)
        near-normal 369.68
        normal 369.69
  psychic 784.69
  severe
    both eyes 369.22

Blindness — *continued*
  severe — *continued*
    both eyes — *continued*
      with impairment of lesser eye (specified as)
        blind, not further specified 369.11
        low vision, not further specified 369.21
        near-total 369.13
        profound 369.14
        total 369.12
    one eye 369.71
      with vision of other eye (specified as)
        near-normal 369.72
        normal 369.73
  snow 370.24
  sun 363.31
  temporary 368.12
  total
    both eyes 369.01
    one eye 369.61
      with vision of other eye (specified as)
        near-normal 369.62
        normal 369.63
  transient 368.12
  traumatic NEC 950.9
  word (developmental) 315.01
    acquired 784.61
    secondary to organic lesion 784.61
Blister — *see also* Injury, superficial, by site
  beetle dermatitis 692.89
  due to burn — *see* Burn, by site, second degree
  fever 054.9
  fracture — *omit code*
  multiple, skin, nontraumatic 709.8
Bloating 787.3
Bloch-Siemens syndrome (incontinentia pigmenti) 757.33
Bloch-Stauffer dyshormonal dermatosis 757.33
Bloch-Sulzberger disease or syndrome (incontinentia pigmenti) (melanoblastosis) 757.33
Block
  alveolar capillary 516.8
  arborization (heart) 426.6
  arrhythmic 426.9
  atrioventricular (AV) (incomplete) (partial) 426.10
    with
      2:1 atrioventricular response block 426.13
      atrioventricular dissociation 426.0
    first degree (incomplete) 426.11
    second degree (Mobitz type I) 426.13
      Mobitz (type) II 426.12
    third degree 426.0
    complete 426.0
      congenital 746.86
    congenital 746.86
    Mobitz (incomplete)
      type I (Wenckebach's) 426.13
      type II 426.12
    partial 426.13
  auriculoventricular (*see also* Block, atrioventricular) 426.10
    complete 426.0
      congenital 746.86
    congenital 746.86
  bifascicular (cardiac) 426.53
  bundle branch (complete) (false) (incomplete) 426.50
    bilateral 426.53
    left (complete) (main stem) 426.3
      with right bundle branch block 426.53
      anterior fascicular 426.2
        with
          posterior fascicular block 426.3
          right bundle branch block 426.52
      hemiblock 426.2
      incomplete 426.2

Block — *continued*
  bundle branch — *continued*
    left — *continued*
      incomplete — *continued*
        with right bundle branch block 426.53
        posterior fascicular 426.2
          with
            anterior fascicular block 426.3
            right bundle branch block 426.51
      right 426.4
        with
          left bundle branch block (incomplete) (main stem) 426.53
          left fascicular block 426.53
            anterior 426.52
            posterior 426.51
      Wilson's type 426.4
  cardiac 426.9
  conduction 426.9
    complete 426.0
  Eustachian tube (*see also* Obstruction, Eustachian tube) 381.60
  fascicular (left anterior) (left posterior) 426.2
  foramen Magendie (acquired) 331.3
    congenital 742.3
      with spina bifida (*see also* Spina bifida) 741.0 ☑
  heart 426.9
    first degree (atrioventricular) 426.11
    second degree (atrioventricular) 426.13
    third degree (atrioventricular) 426.0
    bundle branch (complete) (false) (incomplete) 426.50
      bilateral 426.53
      left (*see also* Block, bundle branch, left) 426.3
      right (*see also* Block, bundle branch, right) 426.4
    complete (atrioventricular) 426.0
    congenital 746.86
    incomplete 426.13
    intra-atrial 426.6
    intraventricular NEC 426.6
    sinoatrial 426.6
    specified type NEC 426.6
  hepatic vein 453.0
  intraventricular (diffuse) (myofibrillar) 426.6
    bundle branch (complete) (false) (incomplete) 426.50
      bilateral 426.53
      left (*see also* Block, bundle branch, left) 426.3
      right (*see also* Block, bundle branch, right) 426.4
  kidney (*see also* Disease, renal) 593.9
    postcystoscopic 997.5
  myocardial (*see also* Block, heart) 426.9
  nodal 426.10
  optic nerve 377.49
  organ or site (congenital) NEC — *see* Atresia
  parietal 426.6
  peri-infarction 426.6
  portal (vein) 452
  sinoatrial 426.6
  sinoauricular 426.6
  spinal cord 336.9
  trifascicular 426.54
  tubal 628.2
  vein NEC 453.9
Blocq's disease or syndrome (astasia-abasia) 307.9
Blood
  constituents, abnormal NEC 790.6
  disease 289.9
    specified NEC 289.89
  donor V59.01
    other blood components V59.09
    stem cells V59.02
    whole blood V59.01
  dyscrasia 289.9
    with
      abortion — *see* Abortion, by type, with hemorrhage, delayed or excessive

Blood — *continued*
  dyscrasia — *continued*
    with — *continued*
      ectopic pregnancy (*see also* categories 633.0–633.9) 639.1
      molar pregnancy (*see also* categories 630–632) 639.1
    following
      abortion 639.1
      ectopic or molar pregnancy 639.1
    newborn NEC 776.9
    puerperal, postpartum 666.3 ☑
  flukes NEC (*see also* Infestation, Schistosoma) 120.9
  in
    feces (*see also* Melena) 578.1
      occult 792.1
    urine (*see also* Hematuria) 599.70
  mole 631.8
  occult 792.1
  poisoning (*see also* Septicemia) 038.9
  pressure
    decreased, due to shock following injury 958.4
    fluctuating 796.4
    high (*see also* Hypertension) 401.9
      borderline 796.2
      incidental reading (isolated) (nonspecific), without diagnosis of hypertension 796.2
    low (*see also* Hypotension) 458.9
      incidental reading (isolated) (nonspecific), without diagnosis of hypotension 796.3
  spitting (*see also* Hemoptysis) 786.30
  staining cornea 371.12
  transfusion
    without reported diagnosis V58.2
    donor V59.01
      stem cells V59.02
    reaction or complication — *see* Complications, transfusion
  tumor — *see* Hematoma
  vessel rupture — *see* Hemorrhage
  vomiting (*see also* Hematemesis) 578.0
Blood-forming organ disease 289.9
Bloodgood's disease 610.1
Bloodshot eye 379.93
Bloom (-Machacek) (-Torre) syndrome 757.39
Blotch, palpebral 372.55
Blount-Barber syndrome (tibia vara) 732.4
Blount's disease (tibia vara) 732.4
Blue
  baby 746.9
  bloater 491.20
    with
      acute bronchitis 491.22
      exacerbation (acute) 491.21
  diaper syndrome 270.0
  disease 746.9
  dome cyst 610.0
  drum syndrome 381.02
  sclera 743.47
    with fragility of bone and deafness 756.51
  toe syndrome 445.02
Blueness — *see also* Cyanosis 782.5
Blurring, visual 368.8
Blushing (abnormal) (excessive) 782.62
BMI (body mass index)
  adult
    25.0-25.9 V85.21
    26.0-26.9 V85.22
    27.0-27.9 V85.23
    28.0-28.9 V85.24
    29.0-29.9 V85.25
    30.0-30.9 V85.30
    31.0-31.9 V85.31
    32.0-32.9 V85.32
    33.0-33.9 V85.33
    34.0-34.9 V85.34
    35.0-35.9 V85.35
    36.0-36.9 V85.36
    37.0-37.9 V85.37
    38.0-38.9 V85.38
    39.0-39.9 V85.39

BMI — *continued*
  adult — *continued*
    40.0-44.9 V85.41
    45.0-49.9 V85.42
    50.0-59.9 V85.43
    60.0-69.9 V85.44
    70 and over V85.45
    between 19-24 V85.1
    less than 19 V85.0
  pediatric
    5th percentile to less than 85th percentile for age V85.52
    85th percentile to less than 95th percentile for age V85.53
    greater than or equal to 95th percentile for age V85.54
    less than 5th percentile for age V85.51
Boarder, hospital V65.0
  infant V65.0
Bockhart's impetigo (superficial folliculitis) 704.8
Bodechtel-Guttmann disease (subacute sclerosing panencephalitis) 046.2
Boder-Sedgwick syndrome (ataxia-telangiectasia) 334.8
Body, bodies
  Aschoff (*see also* Myocarditis, rheumatic) 398.0
  asteroid, vitreous 379.22
  choroid, colloid (degenerative) 362.57
    hereditary 362.77
  cytoid (retina) 362.82
  drusen (retina) (*see also* Drusen) 362.57
    optic disc 377.21
  fibrin, pleura 511.0
  foreign — *see* Foreign body
  Hassall-Henle 371.41
  loose
    joint (*see also* Loose, body, joint) 718.1 ☑
    knee 717.6
    knee 717.6
    sheath, tendon 727.82
  Mallory's 034.1
  mass index (BMI)
    adult
      25.0-25.9 V85.21
      26.0-26.9 V85.22
      27.0-27.9 V85.23
      28.0-28.9 V85.24
      29.0-29.9 V85.25
      30.0-30.9 V85.30
      31.0-31.9 V85.31
      32.0-32.9 V85.32
      33.0-33.9 V85.33
      34.0-34.9 V85.34
      35.0-35.9 V85.35
      36.0-36.9 V85.36
      37.0-37.9 V85.37
      38.0-38.9 V85.38
      39.0-39.9 V85.39
      40.0-44.9 V85.41
      45.0-49.9 V85.42
      50.0-59.9 V85.43
      60.0-69.9 V85.44
      70 and over V85.45
      between 19-24 V85.1
      less than 19 V85.0
    pediatric
      5th percentile to less than 85th percentile for age V85.52
      85th percentile to less than 95th percentile for age V85.53
      greater than or equal to 95th percentile for age V85.54
      less than 5th percentile for age V85.51
  Mooser 081.0
  Negri 071
  rice (joint) (*see also* Loose, body, joint) 718.1 ☑
    knee 717.6
  rocking 307.3
Boeck's
  disease (sarcoidosis) 135
  lupoid (miliary) 135

Boeck's — *continued*
  sarcoid 135
Boerhaave's syndrome (spontaneous esophageal rupture) 530.4
Boggy
  cervix 622.8
  uterus 621.8
Boil — *see also* Carbuncle 680.9
  abdominal wall 680.2
  Aleppo 085.1
  ankle 680.6
  anus 680.5
  arm (any part, above wrist) 680.3
  auditory canal, external 680.0
  axilla 680.3
  back (any part) 680.2
  Baghdad 085.1
  breast 680.2
  buttock 680.5
  chest wall 680.2
  corpus cavernosum 607.2
  Delhi 085.1
  ear (any part) 680.0
  eyelid 373.13
  face (any part, except eye) 680.0
  finger (any) 680.4
  flank 680.2
  foot (any part) 680.7
  forearm 680.3
  Gafsa 085.1
  genital organ, male 608.4
  gluteal (region) 680.5
  groin 680.2
  hand (any part) 680.4
  head (any part, except face) 680.8
  heel 680.7
  hip 680.6
  knee 680.6
  labia 616.4
  lacrimal (*see also* Dacryocystitis) 375.30
    gland (*see also* Dacryoadenitis) 375.00
    passages (duct) (sac) (*see also* Dacryocystitis) 375.30
  leg, any part, except foot 680.6
  multiple sites 680.9
  natal 085.1
  neck 680.1
  nose (external) (septum) 680.0
  orbit, orbital 376.01
  partes posteriores 680.5
  pectoral region 680.2
  penis 607.2
  perineum 680.2
  pinna 680.0
  scalp (any part) 680.8
  scrotum 608.4
  seminal vesicle 608.0
  shoulder 680.3
  skin NEC 680.9
  specified site NEC 680.8
  spermatic cord 608.4
  temple (region) 680.0
  testis 608.4
  thigh 680.6
  thumb 680.4
  toe (any) 680.7
  tropical 085.1
  trunk 680.2
  tunica vaginalis 608.4
  umbilicus 680.2
  upper arm 680.3
  vas deferens 608.4
  vulva 616.4
  wrist 680.4
Bold hives — *see also* Urticaria 708.9
Bolivian hemorrhagic fever 078.7
Bombé, iris 364.74
Bomford-Rhoads anemia (refractory) 238.72
Bone — *see* condition
Bonnevie-Ullrich syndrome 758.6
Bonnier's syndrome 386.19
Bonvale Dam fever 780.79
Bony block of joint 718.80
  ankle 718.87
  elbow 718.82
  foot 718.87

Bony block of joint — *continued*
  hand 718.84
  hip 718.85
  knee 718.86
  multiple sites 718.89
  pelvic region 718.85
  shoulder (region) 718.81
  specified site NEC 718.88
  wrist 718.83
BOOP (bronchiolitis obliterans organized
    pneumonia) 516.8
Borderline
  diabetes mellitus 790.29
  hypertension 796.2
  intellectual functioning V62.89
  osteopenia 733.90
  pelvis 653.1 ☑
    with obstruction during labor 660.1 ☑
      affecting fetus or newborn 763.1
  psychosis (*see also* Schizophrenia) 295.5 ☑
    of childhood (*see also* Psychosis, child-
      hood) 299.8 ☑
  schizophrenia (*see also* Schizophrenia)
    295.5 ☑
Borna disease 062.9
Bornholm disease (epidemic pleurodynia)
    074.1
Borrelia vincentii (mouth) (pharynx) (tonsils)
    101
Bostock's catarrh — *see also* Fever, hay 477.9
Boston exanthem 048
Botalli, ductus (patent) (persistent) 747.0
Bothriocephalus latus infestation 123.4
Botulism 005.1
  food poisoning 005.1
  infant 040.41
  non-foodborne 040.42
  wound 040.42
Bouba — *see also* Yaws 102.9
Bouffée délirante 298.3
Bouillaud's disease or syndrome (rheumatic
    heart disease) 391.9
Bourneville's disease (tuberous sclerosis)
    759.5
Boutonneuse fever 082.1
Boutonniere
  deformity (finger) 736.21
  hand (intrinsic) 736.21
Bouveret (-Hoffmann) disease or syndrome
    (paroxysmal tachycardia) 427.2
Bovine heart — *see* Hypertrophy, cardiac
Bowel — *see* condition
Bowen's
  dermatosis (precancerous) (M8081/2) —
    see Neoplasm, skin, in situ
  disease (M8081/2) — *see* Neoplasm, skin,
    in situ
  epithelioma (M8081/2) — *see* Neoplasm,
    skin, in situ
  type
    epidermoid carcinoma in situ (M8081/2)
      — *see* Neoplasm, skin, in situ
    intraepidermal squamous cell carcinoma
      (M8081/2) — *see* Neoplasm, skin,
      in situ
Bowing
  femur 736.89
    congenital 754.42
  fibula 736.89
    congenital 754.43
  forearm 736.09
    away from midline (cubitus valgus)
      736.01
    toward midline (cubitus varus) 736.02
  leg(s), long bones, congenital 754.44
  radius 736.09
    away from midline (cubitus valgus)
      736.01
    toward midline (cubitus varus) 736.02
  tibia 736.89
    congenital 754.43
Bowleg(s) 736.42
  congenital 754.44
  rachitic 268.1
Boyd's dysentery 004.2
Brachial — *see* condition

Brachman-de Lange syndrome (Amsterdam
    dwarf, intellectual disabilities, and
    brachycephaly) 759.89
Brachycardia 427.89
Brachycephaly 756.0
Brachymorphism and ectopia lentis 759.89
Bradley's disease (epidemic vomiting) 078.82
Bradycardia 427.89
  chronic (sinus) 427.81
  newborn 779.81
  nodal 427.89
  postoperative 997.1
  reflex 337.09
  sinoatrial 427.89
    with paroxysmal tachyarrhythmia or
      tachycardia 427.81
    chronic 427.81
  sinus 427.89
    with paroxysmal tachyarrhythmia or
      tachycardia 427.81
    chronic 427.81
    persistent 427.81
    severe 427.81
  tachycardia syndrome 427.81
  vagal 427.89
Bradykinesia 781.0
Bradypnea 786.09
Brailsford's disease 732.3
  radial head 732.3
  tarsal scaphoid 732.5
Brailsford-Morquio disease or syndrome
    (mucopolysaccharidosis IV) 277.5
Brain — *see also* condition
  death 348.82
  syndrome (acute) (chronic) (nonpsychotic)
    (organic) (with neurotic reaction)
    (with behavioral reaction) (*see al-*
    so Syndrome, brain) 310.9
    with
      presenile brain disease 290.10
      psychosis, psychotic reaction (*see al-*
        so Psychosis, organic) 294.9
  congenital (*see also* Disability, intellectu-
    al) 319
Branched-chain amino-acid disease 270.3
Branchial — *see* condition
Brandt's syndrome (acrodermatitis enteropath-
    ica) 686.8
Brash (water) 787.1
Brass-founders' ague 985.8
Bravais-Jacksonian epilepsy — *see also*
    Epilepsy 345.5 ☑
Braxton Hicks contractions 644.1 ☑
Braziers' disease 985.8
Brazilian
  blastomycosis 116.1
  leishmaniasis 085.5
BRBPR (bright red blood per rectum) 569.3
Break
  cardiorenal — *see* Hypertension, cardiorenal
  retina (*see also* Defect, retina) 361.30
Breakbone fever 061
Breakdown
  device, implant, or graft — *see* Complica-
    tions, mechanical
  nervous (*see also* Disorder, mental, nonpsy-
    chotic) 300.9
  perineum 674.2 ☑
Breast — *see also* condition
  buds 259.1
    in newborn 779.89
  dense 793.82
  nodule 793.89
Breast feeding difficulties 676.8 ☑
Breath
  foul 784.99
  holder, child 312.81
  holding spells 786.9
  shortness 786.05
Breathing
  asymmetrical 786.09
  bronchial 786.09
  exercises V57.0
  labored 786.09
  mouth 784.99
    causing malocclusion 524.59

Breathing — *continued*
  periodic 786.09
    high altitude 327.22
  tic 307.20
Breathlessness 786.09
Breda's disease — *see also* Yaws 102.9
Breech
  delivery, affecting fetus or newborn 763.0
  extraction, affecting fetus or newborn 763.0
  presentation (buttocks) (complete) (frank)
    652.2 ☑
    with successful version 652.1 ☑
    before labor, affecting fetus or newborn
      761.7
    during labor, affecting fetus or newborn
      763.0
Breisky's disease (kraurosis vulvae) 624.09
Brennemann's syndrome (acute mesenteric
    lymphadenitis) 289.2
Brenner's
  tumor (benign) (M9000/0) 220
    borderline malignancy (M9000/1) 236.2
    malignant (M9000/3) 183.0
    proliferating (M9000/1) 236.2
Bretonneau's disease (diphtheritic malignant
    angina) 032.0
Breus' mole 631.8
Brevicollis 756.16
Bricklayers' itch 692.89
Brickmakers' anemia 126.9
Bridge
  myocardial 746.85
Bright's
  blindness — *see* Uremia
  disease (*see also* Nephritis) 583.9
    arteriosclerotic (*see also* Hypertension,
      kidney) 403.90
Bright red blood per rectum (BRBPR) 569.3
Brill's disease (recrudescent typhus) 081.1
  flea-borne 081.0
  louse-borne 081.1
Brill-Symmers disease (follicular lymphoma)
    (M9690/3) 202.0 ☑
Brill-Zinsser disease (recrudescent typhus)
    081.1
Brinton's disease (linitis plastica) (M8142/3)
    151.9
Brion-Kayser disease — *see also* Fever,
    paratyphoid 002.9
Briquet's disorder or syndrome 300.81
Brissaud's
  infantilism (infantile myxedema) 244.9
  motor-verbal tic 307.23
Brissaud-Meige syndrome (infantile
    myxedema) 244.9
Brittle
  bones (congenital) 756.51
  nails 703.8
    congenital 757.5
Broad — *see also* condition
  beta disease 272.2
  ligament laceration syndrome 620.6
Brock's syndrome (atelectasis due to enlarged
    lymph nodes) 518.0
Brocq's disease 691.8
  atopic (diffuse) neurodermatitis 691.8
  lichen simplex chronicus 698.3
  parakeratosis psoriasiformis 696.2
  parapsoriasis 696.2
Brocq-Duhring disease (dermatitis herpeti-
    formis) 694.0
Brodie's
  abscess (localized) (chronic) (*see also* Os-
    teomyelitis) 730.1 ☑
  disease (joint) (*see also* Osteomyelitis)
    730.1 ☑
Broken
  arches 734
    congenital 755.67
  back — *see* Fracture, vertebra, by site
  bone — *see* Fracture, by site
  compensation — *see* Disease, heart
  heart syndrome 429.83
  implant or internal device — *see* listing un-
    der Complications, mechanical
  neck — *see* Fracture, vertebra, cervical

Broken — *continued*
  nose 802.0
    open 802.1
  tooth, teeth 873.63
    complicated 873.73
Bromhidrosis 705.89
Bromidism, bromism
  acute 967.3
    correct substance properly administered
      349.82
    overdose or wrong substance given or
      taken 967.3
  chronic (*see also* Dependence) 304.1 ☑
Bromidrosiphobia 300.23
Bromidrosis 705.89
Bronchi, bronchial — *see* condition
Bronchiectasis (cylindrical) (diffuse) (fusiform)
    (localized) (moniliform) (postinfectious)
    (recurrent) (saccular) 494.0
  with acute exacerbation 494.1
  congenital 748.61
  tuberculosis (*see also* Tuberculosis) 011.5 ☑
Bronchiolectasis — *see* Bronchiectasis
Bronchiolitis (acute) (infectious) (subacute)
    466.19
  with
    bronchospasm or obstruction 466.19
    influenza, flu, or grippe (*see also* Influen-
      za) 487.1
  catarrhal (acute) (subacute) 466.19
  chemical 506.0
    chronic 506.4
  chronic (obliterative) 491.8
  due to external agent — *see* Bronchitis,
    acute, due to
  fibrosa obliterans 491.8
  influenzal (*see also* Influenza) 487.1
  obliterans 491.8
    with organizing pneumonia (BOOP)
      516.8
    status post lung transplant 996.84
  obliterative (chronic) (diffuse) (subacute)
    491.8
    due to fumes or vapors 506.4
  respiratory syncytial virus 466.11
  vesicular — *see* Pneumonia, broncho-
Bronchitis (diffuse) (hypostatic) (infectious)
    (inflammatory) (simple) 490
  with
    emphysema — *see* Emphysema
    influenza, flu, or grippe (*see also* Influen-
      za) 487.1
    obstruction airway, chronic 491.20
      with
        acute bronchitis 491.22
        exacerbation (acute) 491.21
    tracheitis 490
      acute or subacute 466.0
        with bronchospasm or obstruc-
          tion 466.0
      chronic 491.8
  acute or subacute 466.0
    with
      bronchiectasis 494.1
      bronchospasm 466.0
      obstruction 466.0
      tracheitis 466.0
    chemical (due to fumes or vapors) 506.0
    due to
      fumes or vapors 506.0
      radiation 508.8
  allergic (acute) (*see also* Asthma) 493.9 ☑
  arachidic 934.1
  aspiration 507.0
    due to fumes or vapors 506.0
  asthmatic (acute) 493.90
    with
      acute exacerbation 493.92
      status asthmaticus 493.91
    chronic 493.2 ☑
  capillary 466.19
    with bronchospasm or obstruction
      466.19
    chronic 491.8
  caseous (*see also* Tuberculosis) 011.3 ☑
  Castellani's 104.8

☑ Additional Digit Required — Refer to the Tabular List for Digit Selection   ⓦ **Subterms under main terms may continue to next column or page**

2013 ICD-9-CM   ▶◀ Revised Text   ● New Line   ▲ Revised Code   **Volume 2 — 37**

Bronchitis — continued
  catarrhal 490
    acute — see Bronchitis, acute
    chronic 491.0
  chemical (acute) (subacute) 506.0
    chronic 506.4
    due to fumes or vapors (acute) (subacute) 506.0
      chronic 506.4
  chronic 491.9
    with
      tracheitis (chronic) 491.8
    asthmatic 493.2 ☑
    catarrhal 491.0
    chemical (due to fumes and vapors) 506.4
    due to
      fumes or vapors (chemical) (inhalation) 506.4
      radiation 508.8
      tobacco smoking 491.0
    mucopurulent 491.1
    obstructive 491.20
      with
        acute bronchitis 491.22
        exacerbation (acute) 491.21
      purulent 491.1
      simple 491.0
      specified type NEC 491.8
  croupous 466.0
    with bronchospasm or obstruction 466.0
    due to fumes or vapors 506.0
  emphysematous 491.20
    with
      acute bronchitis 491.22
      exacerbation (acute) 491.21
  exudative 466.0
  fetid (chronic) (recurrent) 491.1
  fibrinous, acute or subacute 466.0
    with bronchospasm or obstruction 466.0
  grippal (see also Influenza) 487.1
  influenzal (see also Influenza) 487.1
  membranous, acute or subacute 466.0
    with bronchospasm or obstruction 466.0
  moulders' 502
  mucopurulent (chronic) (recurrent) 491.1
    acute or subacute 466.0
  obliterans 491.8
  obstructive (chronic) 491.20
    with
      acute bronchitis 491.22
      exacerbation (acute) 491.21
  pituitous 491.1
  plastic (inflammatory) 466.0
  pneumococcal, acute or subacute 466.0
    with bronchospasm or obstruction 466.0
  pseudomembranous 466.0
  purulent (chronic) (recurrent) 491.1
    acute or subacute 466.0
      with bronchospasm or obstruction 466.0
  putrid 491.1
  scrofulous (see also Tuberculosis) 011.3 ☑
  senile 491.9
  septic, acute or subacute 466.0
    with bronchospasm or obstruction 466.0
  smokers' 491.0
  spirochetal 104.8
  suffocative, acute or subacute 466.0
  summer (see also Asthma) 493.9 ☑
  suppurative (chronic) 491.1
    acute or subacute 466.0
  tuberculous (see also Tuberculosis) 011.3 ☑
  ulcerative 491.8
    Vincent's 101
  Vincent's 101
  viral, acute or subacute 466.0
Bronchoalveolitis 485
Bronchoaspergillosis 117.3
Bronchocele
  meaning
    dilatation of bronchus 519.19
    goiter 240.9
Bronchogenic carcinoma 162.9
Bronchohemisporosis 117.9
Broncholithiasis 518.89

Broncholithiasis — continued
  tuberculous (see also Tuberculosis) 011.3 ☑
Bronchomalacia 748.3
Bronchomoniliasis 112.89
Bronchomycosis 112.89
Bronchonocardiosis 039.1
Bronchopleuropneumonia — see Pneumonia, broncho-
Bronchopneumonia — see Pneumonia, broncho-
Bronchopneumonitis — see Pneumonia, broncho-
Bronchopulmonary — see condition
Bronchopulmonitis — see Pneumonia, broncho-
Bronchorrhagia 786.30
  newborn 770.3
  tuberculous (see also Tuberculosis) 011.3 ☑
Bronchorrhea (chronic) (purulent) 491.0
  acute 466.0
Bronchospasm 519.11
  with
    asthma — see Asthma
    bronchiolitis, acute 466.19
      due to respiratory syncytial virus 466.11
    bronchitis — see Bronchitis
    chronic obstructive pulmonary disease (COPD) 496
    emphysema — see Emphysema
      due to external agent — see Condition, respiratory, acute, due to
  acute 519.11
  exercise induced 493.81
Bronchospirochetosis 104.8
Bronchostenosis 519.19
Bronchus — see condition
Bronze, bronzed
  diabetes 275.01
  disease (Addison's) (skin) 255.41
    tuberculous (see also Tuberculosis) 017.6 ☑
Brooke's disease or tumor (M8100/0) — see Neoplasm, skin, benign
Brown enamel of teeth (hereditary) 520.5
Brown-Séquard's paralysis (syndrome) 344.89
Brown's tendon sheath syndrome 378.61
Brow presentation complicating delivery 652.4 ☑
Brucella, brucellosis (infection) 023.9
  abortus 023.1
  canis 023.3
  dermatitis, skin 023.9
  melitensis 023.0
  mixed 023.8
  suis 023.2
Bruck-de Lange disease or syndrome (Amsterdam dwarf, intellectual disabilities, and brachycephaly) 759.89
Bruck's disease 733.99
Brugada syndrome 746.89
Brug's filariasis 125.1
Brugsch's syndrome (acropachyderma) 757.39
Bruhl's disease (splenic anemia with fever) 285.8
Bruise (skin surface intact) — see also Contusion
  with
    fracture — see Fracture, by site
    open wound — see Wound, open, by site
  internal organ (abdomen, chest, or pelvis) — see Injury, internal, by site
  umbilical cord 663.6 ☑
    affecting fetus or newborn 762.6
Bruit 785.9
  arterial (abdominal) (carotid) 785.9
  supraclavicular 785.9
Brushburn — see Injury, superficial, by site
Bruton's X-linked agammaglobulinemia 279.04
Bruxism 306.8
  sleep related 327.53
Bubbly lung syndrome 770.7
Bubo 289.3
  blennorrhagic 098.89

Bubo — continued
  chancroidal 099.0
  climatic 099.1
    due to Hemophilus ducreyi 099.0
  gonococcal 098.89
  indolent NEC 099.8
  inguinal NEC 099.8
    chancroidal 099.0
    climatic 099.1
    due to H. ducreyi 099.0
  scrofulous (see also Tuberculosis) 017.2 ☑
  soft chancre 099.0
  suppurating 683
  syphilitic 091.0
    congenital 090.0
  tropical 099.1
  venereal NEC 099.8
  virulent 099.0
Bubonic plague 020.0
Bubonocele — see Hernia, inguinal
Buccal — see condition
Buchanan's disease (juvenile osteochondrosis of iliac crest) 732.1
Buchem's syndrome (hyperostosis corticalis) 733.3
Buchman's disease (osteochondrosis, juvenile) 732.1
Bucket handle fracture (semilunar cartilage) — see also Tear, meniscus 836.2
Budd-Chiari syndrome (hepatic vein thrombosis) 453.0
Budgerigar-fanciers' disease or lung 495.2
Büdinger-Ludloff-Läwen disease 717.89
Buds
  breast 259.1
  in newborn 779.89
Buerger's disease (thromboangiitis obliterans) 443.1
Bulbar — see condition
Bulbus cordis 745.9
  persistent (in left ventricle) 745.8
Bulging fontanels (congenital) 756.0
Bulimia 783.6
  nervosa 307.51
  nonorganic origin 307.51
Bulky uterus 621.2
Bulla(e) 709.8
  lung (emphysematous) (solitary) 492.0
Bullet wound — see also Wound, open, by site
  fracture — see Fracture, by site, open
  internal organ (abdomen, chest, or pelvis) — see Injury, internal, by site, with open wound
  intracranial — see Laceration, brain, with open wound
Bullis fever 082.8
Bullying — see also Disturbance, conduct 312.0 ☑
Bundle
  branch block (complete) (false) (incomplete) 426.50
    bilateral 426.53
    left (see also Block, bundle branch, left) 426.3
      hemiblock 426.2
    right (see also Block, bundle branch, right) 426.4
  of His — see condition
  of Kent syndrome (anomalous atrioventricular excitation) 426.7
Bungpagga 040.81
Bunion 727.1
Bunionette 727.1
Bunyamwera fever 066.3
Buphthalmia, buphthalmos (congenital) 743.20
  associated with
    keratoglobus, congenital 743.22
    megalocornea 743.22
    ocular anomalies NEC 743.22
  isolated 743.21
  simple 743.21
Bürger-Grütz disease or syndrome (essential familial hyperlipemia) 272.3
Buried roots 525.3

Burke's syndrome 577.8
Burkitt's
  tumor (M9750/3) 200.2 ☑
  type malignant, lymphoma, lymphoblastic, or undifferentiated (M9750/3) 200.2 ☑
Burn (acid) (cathode ray) (caustic) (chemical) (electric heating appliance) (electricity) (fire) (flame) (hot liquid or object) (irradiation) (lime) (radiation) (steam) (thermal) (x-ray) 949.0

Note — Use the following fifth-digit subclassification with category 948 to indicate the percent of body surface with third degree burn:
0	Less than 10% or unspecified
1	10–19%
2	20–29%
3	30–39%
4	40–49%
5	50–59%
6	60–69%
7	70–79%
8	80–89%
9	90% or more of body surface

  with
    blisters — see Burn, by site, second degree
    erythema — see Burn, by site, first degree
    skin loss (epidermal) (see also Burn, by site, second degree)
      full thickness (see also Burn, by site, third degree)
        with necrosis of underlying tissues — see Burn, by site, third degree, deep
  first degree — see Burn, by site, first degree
  second degree — see Burn, by site, second degree
  third degree — see Burn, by site, third degree
    deep — see Burn, by site, third degree, deep
  abdomen, abdominal (muscle) (wall) 942.03
    with
      trunk — see Burn, trunk, multiple sites
    first degree 942.13
    second degree 942.23
    third degree 942.33
      deep 942.43
        with loss of body part 942.53
  ankle 945.03
    with
      lower limb(s) — see Burn, leg, multiple sites
    first degree 945.13
    second degree 945.23
    third degree 945.33
      deep 945.43
        with loss of body part 945.53
  anus — see Burn, trunk, specified site NEC
  arm(s) 943.00
    first degree 943.10
    second degree 943.20
    third degree 943.30
      deep 943.40
        with loss of body part 943.50
    lower — see Burn, forearm(s)
    multiple sites, except hand(s) or wrist(s) 943.09
      first degree 943.19
      second degree 943.29
      third degree 943.39
        deep 943.49
          with loss of body part 943.59
    upper 943.03
      first degree 943.13
      second degree 943.23
      third degree 943.33

☑ Additional Digit Required — Refer to the Tabular List for Digit Selection   Subterms under main terms may continue to next column or page

38 — Volume 2   ▶◀ Revised Text   ● New Line   ▲ Revised Code   2013 ICD-9-CM

Burn — *continued*
　arm(s) — *continued*
　　upper — *continued*
　　　third degree — *continued*
　　　　deep 943.43
　　　　　with loss of body part 943.53
　auditory canal (external) — *see* Burn, ear
　auricle (ear) — *see* Burn, ear
　axilla 943.04
　　with
　　　upper limb(s), except hand(s) or wrist(s) — *see* Burn, arm(s), multiple sites
　　first degree 943.14
　　second degree 943.24
　　third degree 943.34
　　　deep 943.44
　　　　with loss of body part 943.54
　back 942.04
　　with
　　　trunk — *see* Burn, trunk, multiple sites
　　first degree 942.14
　　second degree 942.24
　　third degree 942.34
　　　deep 942.44
　　　　with loss of body part 942.54
　biceps
　　brachii — *see* Burn, arm(s), upper
　　femoris — *see* Burn, thigh
　breast(s) 942.01
　　with
　　　trunk — *see* Burn, trunk, multiple sites
　　first degree 942.11
　　second degree 942.21
　　third degree 942.31
　　　deep 942.41
　　　　with loss of body part 942.51
　brow — *see* Burn, forehead
　buttock(s) — *see* Burn, back
　canthus (eye) 940.1
　　chemical 940.0
　cervix (uteri) 947.4
　cheek (cutaneous) 941.07
　　with
　　　face or head — *see* Burn, head, multiple sites
　　first degree 941.17
　　second degree 941.27
　　third degree 941.37
　　　deep 941.47
　　　　with loss of body part 941.57
　chest wall (anterior) 942.02
　　with
　　　trunk — *see* Burn, trunk, multiple sites
　　first degree 942.12
　　second degree 942.22
　　third degree 942.32
　　　deep 942.42
　　　　with loss of body part 942.52
　chin 941.04
　　with
　　　face or head — *see* Burn, head, multiple sites
　　first degree 941.14
　　second degree 941.24
　　third degree 941.34
　　　deep 941.44
　　　　with loss of body part 941.54
　clitoris — *see* Burn, genitourinary organs, external
　colon 947.3
　conjunctiva (and cornea) 940.4
　　chemical
　　　acid 940.3
　　　alkaline 940.2
　cornea (and conjunctiva) 940.4
　　chemical
　　　acid 940.3
　　　alkaline 940.2
　costal region — *see* Burn, chest wall
　due to ingested chemical agent — *see* Burn, internal organs
　ear (auricle) (canal) (drum) (external) 941.01

Burn — *continued*
　ear — *continued*
　　with
　　　face or head — *see* Burn, head, multiple sites
　　first degree 941.11
　　second degree 941.21
　　third degree 941.31
　　　deep 941.41
　　　　with loss of a body part 941.51
　elbow 943.02
　　with
　　　hand(s) and wrist(s) — *see* Burn, multiple specified sites
　　　upper limb(s), except hand(s) or wrist(s) (*see also* Burn, arm(s), multiple sites)
　　first degree 943.12
　　second degree 943.22
　　third degree 943.32
　　　deep 943.42
　　　　with loss of body part 943.52
　electricity, electric current — *see* Burn, by site
　entire body — *see* Burn, multiple, specified sites
　epididymis — *see* Burn, genitourinary organs, external
　epigastric region — *see* Burn, abdomen
　epiglottis 947.1
　esophagus 947.2
　extent (percent of body surface)
　　less than 10 percent 948.0 ☑
　　10-19 percent 948.1 ☑
　　20-29 percent 948.2 ☑
　　30-39 percent 948.3 ☑
　　40-49 percent 948.4 ☑
　　50-59 percent 948.5 ☑
　　60-69 percent 948.6 ☑
　　70-79 percent 948.7 ☑
　　80-89 percent 948.8 ☑
　　90 percent or more 948.9 ☑
　extremity
　　lower — *see* Burn, leg
　　upper — *see* Burn, arm(s)
　eye(s) (and adnexa) (only) 940.9
　　with
　　　face, head, or neck 941.02
　　　　first degree 941.12
　　　　second degree 941.22
　　　　third degree 941.32
　　　　　deep 941.42
　　　　　　with loss of body part 941.52
　　　other sites (classifiable to more than one category in 940–945) — *see* Burn, multiple, specified sites
　　　resulting rupture and destruction of eyeball 940.5
　　specified part — *see* Burn, by site
　eyeball (*see also* Burn, eye)
　　with resulting rupture and destruction of eyeball 940.5
　eyelid(s) 940.1
　　chemical 940.0
　face — *see* Burn, head
　finger (nail) (subungual) 944.01
　　with
　　　hand(s) — *see* Burn, hand(s), multiple sites
　　　other sites — *see* Burn, multiple, specified sites
　　　thumb 944.04
　　　　first degree 944.14
　　　　second degree 944.24
　　　　third degree 944.34
　　　　　deep 944.44
　　　　　　with loss of body part 944.54
　　first degree 944.11
　　second degree 944.21
　　third degree 944.31
　　　deep 944.41
　　　　with loss of body part 944.51
　　multiple (digits) 944.03

Burn — *continued*
　finger — *continued*
　　multiple — *continued*
　　　with thumb — *see* Burn, finger, with thumb
　　　first degree 944.13
　　　second degree 944.23
　　　third degree 944.33
　　　　deep 944.43
　　　　　with loss of body part 944.53
　flank — *see* Burn, abdomen
　foot 945.02
　　with
　　　lower limb(s) — *see* Burn, leg, multiple sites
　　first degree 945.12
　　second degree 945.22
　　third degree 945.32
　　　deep 945.42
　　　　with loss of body part 945.52
　forearm(s) 943.01
　　with
　　　upper limb(s), except hand(s) or wrist(s) — *see* Burn, arm(s), multiple sites
　　first degree 943.11
　　second degree 943.21
　　third degree 943.31
　　　deep 943.41
　　　　with loss of body part 943.51
　forehead 941.07
　　with
　　　face or head — *see* Burn, head, multiple sites
　　first degree 941.17
　　second degree 941.27
　　third degree 941.37
　　　deep 941.47
　　　　with loss of body part 941.57
　fourth degree — *see* Burn, by site, third degree, deep
　friction — *see* Injury, superficial, by site
　from swallowing caustic or corrosive substance NEC — *see* Burn, internal organs
　full thickness — *see* Burn, by site, third degree
　gastrointestinal tract 947.3
　genitourinary organs
　　external 942.05
　　　with
　　　　trunk — *see* Burn, trunk, multiple sites
　　　first degree 942.15
　　　second degree 942.25
　　　third degree 942.35
　　　　deep 942.45
　　　　　with loss of body part 942.55
　　internal 947.8
　globe (eye) — *see* Burn, eyeball
　groin — *see* Burn, abdomen
　gum 947.0
　hand(s) (phalanges) (and wrist) 944.00
　　first degree 944.10
　　second degree 944.20
　　third degree 944.30
　　　deep 944.40
　　　　with loss of body part 944.50
　　back (dorsal surface) 944.06
　　　first degree 944.16
　　　second degree 944.26
　　　third degree 944.36
　　　　deep 944.46
　　　　　with loss of body part 944.56
　　multiple sites 944.08
　　　first degree 944.18
　　　second degree 944.28
　　　third degree 944.38
　　　　deep 944.48
　　　　　with loss of body part 944.58
　head (and face) 941.00
　　first degree 941.10
　　second degree 941.20
　　third degree 941.30
　　　deep 941.40
　　　　with loss of body part 941.50

Burn — *continued*
　head — *continued*
　　eye(s) only 940.9
　　　specified part — *see* Burn, by site
　　multiple sites 941.09
　　　with eyes — *see* Burn, eyes, with face, head, or neck
　　　first degree 941.19
　　　second degree 941.29
　　　third degree 941.39
　　　　deep 941.49
　　　　　with loss of body part 941.59
　heel — *see* Burn, foot
　hip — *see* Burn, trunk, specified site NEC
　iliac region — *see* Burn, trunk, specified site NEC
　infected 958.3
　inhalation (*see also* Burn, internal organs) 947.9
　internal organs 947.9
　　from caustic or corrosive substance (swallowing) NEC 947.9
　　specified NEC (*see also* Burn, by site) 947.8
　interscapular region — *see* Burn, back
　intestine (large) (small) 947.3
　iris — *see* Burn, eyeball
　knee 945.05
　　with
　　　lower limb(s) — *see* Burn, leg, multiple sites
　　first degree 945.15
　　second degree 945.25
　　third degree 945.35
　　　deep 945.45
　　　　with loss of body part 945.55
　labium (majus) (minus) — *see* Burn, genitourinary organs, external
　lacrimal apparatus, duct, gland, or sac 940.1
　　chemical 940.0
　larynx 947.1
　late effect — *see* Late, effects (of), burn
　leg 945.00
　　first degree 945.10
　　second degree 945.20
　　third degree 945.30
　　　deep 945.40
　　　　with loss of body part 945.50
　　lower 945.04
　　　with other part(s) of lower limb(s) — *see* Burn, leg, multiple sites
　　　first degree 945.14
　　　second degree 945.24
　　　third degree 945.34
　　　　deep 945.44
　　　　　with loss of body part 945.54
　　multiple sites 945.09
　　　first degree 945.19
　　　second degree 945.29
　　　third degree 945.39
　　　　deep 945.49
　　　　　with loss of body part 945.59
　　upper — *see* Burn, thigh
　lightning — *see* Burn, by site
　limb(s)
　　lower (including foot or toe(s)) — *see* Burn, leg
　　upper (except wrist and hand) — *see* Burn, arm(s)
　lip(s) 941.03
　　with
　　　face or head — *see* Burn, head, multiple sites
　　first degree 941.13
　　second degree 941.23
　　third degree 941.33
　　　deep 941.43
　　　　with loss of body part 941.53
　lumbar region — *see* Burn, back
　lung 947.1
　malar region — *see* Burn, cheek
　mastoid region — *see* Burn, scalp
　membrane, tympanic — *see* Burn, ear
　midthoracic region — *see* Burn, chest wall
　mouth 947.0
　multiple (*see also* Burn, unspecified) 949.0

Burn — Burn

☑ **Additional Digit Required — Refer to the Tabular List for Digit Selection**　　　　🔟 **Subterms under main terms may continue to next column or page**

Burn — *continued*
  multiple (*see also* Burn, unspecified) — *continued*
    specified sites classifiable to more than one category in 940-945 ☑, 946.0
      first degree 946.1
      second degree 946.2
      third degree 946.3
        deep 946.4
          with loss of body part 946.5
  muscle, abdominal — *see* Burn, abdomen
  nasal (septum) — *see* Burn, nose
  neck 941.08
    with
      face or head — *see* Burn, head, multiple sites
    first degree 941.18
    second degree 941.28
    third degree 941.38
      deep 941.48
        with loss of body part 941.58
  nose (septum) 941.05
    with
      face or head — *see* Burn, head, multiple sites
    first degree 941.15
    second degree 941.25
    third degree 941.35
      deep 941.45
        with loss of body part 941.55
  occipital region — *see* Burn, scalp
  orbit region 940.1
    chemical 940.0
  oronasopharynx 947.0
  palate 947.0
  palm(s) 944.05
    with
      hand(s) and wrist(s) — *see* Burn, hand(s), multiple sites
    first degree 944.15
    second degree 944.25
    third degree 944.35
      deep 944.45
        with loss of a body part 944.55
  parietal region — *see* Burn, scalp
  penis — *see* Burn, genitourinary organs, external
  perineum — *see* Burn, genitourinary organs, external
  periocular area 940.1
    chemical 940.0
  pharynx 947.0
  pleura 947.1
  popliteal space — *see* Burn, knee
  prepuce — *see* Burn, genitourinary organs, external
  pubic region — *see* Burn, genitourinary organs, external
  pudenda — *see* Burn, genitourinary organs, external
  rectum 947.3
  sac, lacrimal 940.1
    chemical 940.0
  sacral region — *see* Burn, back
  salivary (ducts) (glands) 947.0
  scalp 941.06
    with
      face or neck — *see* Burn, head, multiple sites
    first degree 941.16
    second degree 941.26
    third degree 941.36
      deep 941.46
        with loss of body part 941.56
  scapular region 943.06
    with
      upper limb(s), except hand(s) or wrist(s) — *see* Burn, arm(s), multiple sites
    first degree 943.16
    second degree 943.26
    third degree 943.36
      deep 943.46
        with loss of body part 943.56
  sclera — *see* Burn, eyeball

Burn — *continued*
  scrotum — *see* Burn, genitourinary organs, external
  septum, nasal — *see* Burn, nose
  shoulder(s) 943.05
    with
      hand(s) and wrist(s) — *see* Burn, multiple, specified sites
      upper limb(s), except hand(s) or wrist(s) — *see* Burn, arm(s), multiple sites
    first degree 943.15
    second degree 943.25
    third degree 943.35
      deep 943.45
        with loss of body part 943.55
  skin NEC (*see also* Burn, unspecified) 949.0
  skull — *see* Burn, head
  small intestine 947.3
  sternal region — *see* Burn, chest wall
  stomach 947.3
  subconjunctival — *see* Burn, conjunctiva
  subcutaneous — *see* Burn, by site, third degree
  submaxillary region — *see* Burn, head
  submental region — *see* Burn, chin
  sun — *see* Sunburn
  supraclavicular fossa — *see* Burn, neck
  supraorbital — *see* Burn, forehead
  temple — *see* Burn, scalp
  temporal region — *see* Burn, scalp
  testicle — *see* Burn, genitourinary organs, external
  testis — *see* Burn, genitourinary organs, external
  thigh 945.06
    with
      lower limb(s) — *see* Burn, leg, multiple sites
    first degree 945.16
    second degree 945.26
    third degree 945.36
      deep 945.46
        with loss of body part 945.56
  thorax (external) — *see* Burn, chest wall
  throat 947.0
  thumb(s) (nail) (subungual) 944.02
    with
      finger(s) — *see* Burn, finger, with other sites, thumb
      hand(s) and wrist(s) — *see* Burn, hand(s), multiple sites
    first degree 944.12
    second degree 944.22
    third degree 944.32
      deep 944.42
        with loss of body part 944.52
  toe (nail) (subungual) 945.01
    with
      lower limb(s) — *see* Burn, leg, multiple sites
    first degree 945.11
    second degree 945.21
    third degree 945.31
      deep 945.41
        with loss of body part 945.51
  tongue 947.0
  tonsil 947.0
  trachea 947.1
  trunk 942.00
    first degree 942.10
    second degree 942.20
    third degree 942.30
      deep 942.40
        with loss of body part 942.50
    multiple sites 942.09
      first degree 942.19
      second degree 942.29
      third degree 942.39
        deep 942.49
          with loss of body part 942.59
    specified site NEC 942.09
      first degree 942.19
      second degree 942.29
      third degree 942.39
        deep 942.49

Burn — *continued*
  trunk — *continued*
    specified site — *continued*
      third degree — *continued*
        deep — *continued*
          with loss of body part 942.59
  tunica vaginalis — *see* Burn, genitourinary organs, external
  tympanic membrane — *see* Burn, ear
  tympanum — *see* Burn, ear
  ultraviolet 692.82
  unspecified site (multiple) 949.0
    with extent of body surface involved specified
      less than 10 percent 948.0 ☑
      10-19 percent 948.1 ☑
      20-29 percent 948.2 ☑
      30-39 percent 948.3 ☑
      40-49 percent 948.4 ☑
      50-59 percent 948.5 ☑
      60-69 percent 948.6 ☑
      70-79 percent 948.7 ☑
      80-89 percent 948.8 ☑
      90 percent or more 948.9 ☑
    first degree 949.1
    second degree 949.2
    third degree 949.3
      deep 949.4
        with loss of body part 949.5
  uterus 947.4
  uvula 947.0
  vagina 947.4
  vulva — *see* Burn, genitourinary organs, external
  wrist(s) 944.07
    with
      hand(s) — *see* Burn, hand(s), multiple sites
    first degree 944.17
    second degree 944.27
    third degree 944.37
      deep 944.47
        with loss of body part 944.57

Burnett's syndrome (milk-alkali) 275.42
Burnier's syndrome (hypophyseal dwarfism) 253.3
Burning
  feet syndrome 266.2
  sensation (*see also* Disturbance, sensation) 782.0
  tongue 529.6
Burns' disease (osteochondrosis, lower ulna) 732.3
Bursa — *see also* condition
  pharynx 478.29
Bursitis NEC 727.3
  Achilles tendon 726.71
  adhesive 726.90
    shoulder 726.0
  ankle 726.79
  buttock 726.5
  calcaneal 726.79
  collateral ligament
    fibular 726.63
    tibial 726.62
  Duplay's 726.2
  elbow 726.33
  finger 726.8
  foot 726.79
  gonococcal 098.52
  hand 726.4
  hip 726.5
  infrapatellar 726.69
  ischiogluteal 726.5
  knee 726.60
  occupational NEC 727.2
  olecranon 726.33
  pes anserinus 726.61
  pharyngeal 478.29
  popliteal 727.51
  prepatellar 726.65
  radiohumeral 727.3
  scapulohumeral 726.19
    adhesive 726.0
  shoulder 726.10
    adhesive 726.0

Bursitis — *continued*
  subacromial 726.19
    adhesive 726.0
  subcoracoid 726.19
  subdeltoid 726.19
    adhesive 726.0
  subpatellar 726.69
  syphilitic 095.7
  Thornwaldt's, Tornwaldt's (pharyngeal) 478.29
  toe 726.79
  trochanteric area 726.5
  wrist 726.4
Burst stitches or sutures (complication of surgery) (external) (*see also* Dehiscence) 998.32
  internal 998.31
Buruli ulcer 031.1
Bury's disease (erythema elevatum diutinum) 695.89
Buschke's disease or scleredema (adultorum) 710.1
Busquet's disease (osteoperiostitis) — *see also* Osteomyelitis 730.1 ☑
Busse-Buschke disease (cryptococcosis) 117.5
Buttock — *see* condition
Button
  Biskra 085.1
  Delhi 085.1
  oriental 085.1
Buttonhole hand (intrinsic) 736.21
Bwamba fever (encephalitis) 066.3
Byssinosis (occupational) 504
Bywaters' syndrome 958.5

C

Cacergasia 300.9
Cachexia 799.4
  cancerous (*see also* Neoplasm, by site, malignant) 799.4
  cardiac — *see* Disease, heart
  dehydration 276.51
    with
      hypernatremia 276.0
      hyponatremia 276.1
  due to malnutrition 799.4
  exophthalmic 242.0 ☑
  heart — *see* Disease, heart
  hypophyseal 253.2
  hypopituitary 253.2
  lead 984.9
    specified type of lead — *see* Table of Drugs and Chemicals
  malaria 084.9
  malignant (*see also* Neoplasm, by site, malignant) 799.4
  marsh 084.9
  nervous 300.5
  old age 797
  pachydermic — *see* Hypothyroidism
  paludal 084.9
  pituitary (postpartum) 253.2
  renal (*see also* Disease, renal) 593.9
  saturnine 984.9
    specified type of lead — *see* Table of Drugs and Chemicals
  senile 797
  Simmonds' (pituitary cachexia) 253.2
  splenica 289.59
  strumipriva (*see also* Hypothyroidism) 244.9
  tuberculous NEC (*see also* Tuberculosis) 011.9 ☑
Café au lait spots 709.09
Caffey's disease or syndrome (infantile cortical hyperostosis) 756.59
Caisson disease 993.3
Caked breast (puerperal, postpartum) 676.2 ☑
Cake kidney 753.3
Calabar swelling 125.2
Calcaneal spur 726.73
Calcaneoapophysitis 732.5
Calcaneonavicular bar 755.67
Calcareous — *see* condition
Calcicosis (occupational) 502
Calciferol (vitamin D) **deficiency** 268.9

Calciferol (vitamin D) **deficiency** —
   continued
   with
      osteomalacia 268.2
      rickets (*see also* Rickets) 268.0
Calcification
   adrenal (capsule) (gland) 255.41
      tuberculous (*see also* Tuberculosis)
         017.6 ☑
   aorta 440.0
   artery (annular) — *see* Arteriosclerosis
   auricle (ear) 380.89
   bladder 596.89
      due to S. hematobium 120.0
   brain (cortex) — *see* Calcification, cerebral
   bronchus 519.19
   bursa 727.82
   cardiac (*see also* Degeneration, myocardial)
      429.1
   cartilage (postinfectional) 733.99
   cerebral (cortex) 348.89
      artery 437.0
   cervix (uteri) 622.8
   choroid plexus 349.2
   conjunctiva 372.54
   corpora cavernosa (penis) 607.89
   cortex (brain) — *see* Calcification, cerebral
   dental pulp (nodular) 522.2
   dentinal papilla 520.4
   disc, intervertebral 722.90
      cervical, cervicothoracic 722.91
      lumbar, lumbosacral 722.93
      thoracic, thoracolumbar 722.92
   fallopian tube 620.8
   falx cerebri — *see* Calcification, cerebral
   fascia 728.89
   gallbladder 575.8
   general 275.40
   heart (*see also* Degeneration, myocardial)
      429.1
      valve — *see* Endocarditis
   intervertebral cartilage or disc (postinfection-
      al) 722.90
      cervical, cervicothoracic 722.91
      lumbar, lumbosacral 722.93
      thoracic, thoracolumbar 722.92
   intracranial — *see* Calcification, cerebral
   intraspinal ligament 728.89
   joint 719.80
      ankle 719.87
      elbow 719.82
      foot 719.87
      hand 719.84
      hip 719.85
      knee 719.86
      multiple sites 719.89
      pelvic region 719.85
      shoulder (region) 719.81
      specified site NEC 719.88
      wrist 719.83
   kidney 593.89
      tuberculous (*see also* Tuberculosis)
         016.0 ☑
   larynx (senile) 478.79
   lens 366.8
   ligament 728.89
      intraspinal 728.89
      knee (medial collateral) 717.89
   lung 518.89
      active 518.89
      postinfectional 518.89
      tuberculous (*see also* Tuberculosis, pul-
         monary) 011.9 ☑
   lymph gland or node (postinfectional) 289.3
      tuberculous (*see also* Tuberculosis,
         lymph gland) 017.2 ☑
   mammographic 793.89
   massive (paraplegic) 728.10
   medial NEC (*see also* Arteriosclerosis, extrem-
      ities) 440.20
   meninges (cerebral) 349.2
   metastatic 275.40
   Mönckeberg's — *see* Arteriosclerosis
   muscle 728.10
      heterotopic, postoperative 728.13

Calcification — *continued*
   myocardium, myocardial (*see also* Degener-
      ation, myocardial) 429.1
   ovary 620.8
   pancreas 577.8
   penis 607.89
   periarticular 728.89
   pericardium (*see also* Pericarditis) 423.8
   pineal gland 259.8
   pleura 511.0
      postinfectional 518.89
      tuberculous (*see also* Tuberculosis,
         pleura) 012.0 ☑
   pulp (dental) (nodular) 522.2
   renal 593.89
   Rider's bone 733.99
   sclera 379.16
   semilunar cartilage 717.89
   spleen 289.59
   subcutaneous 709.3
   suprarenal (capsule) (gland) 255.41
   tendon (sheath) 727.82
      with bursitis, synovitis or tenosynovitis
         727.82
   trachea 519.19
   ureter 593.89
   uterus 621.8
   vitreous 379.29
Calcified — *see also* Calcification
   hematoma NEC 959.9
Calcinosis (generalized) (interstitial) (tumoral)
   (universalis) 275.49
   circumscripta 709.3
   cutis 709.3
   intervertebralis 275.49 [722.90]
   Raynaud's phenomenonsclerodactylytelang-
      iectasis (CRST) 710.1
Calciphylaxis — *see also* Calcification, by site
   275.49
Calcium
   blood
      high (*see also* Hypercalcemia) 275.42
      low (*see also* Hypocalcemia) 275.41
   deposits (*see also* Calcification, by site)
      in bursa 727.82
      in tendon (sheath) 727.82
         with bursitis, synovitis or tenosynovi-
            tis 727.82
   salts or soaps in vitreous 379.22
Calciuria 791.9
Calculi — *see* Calculus
Calculosis, intrahepatic — *see* Choledocholithiasis
Calculus, calculi, calculous 592.9
   ampulla of Vater — *see* Choledocholithiasis
   anuria (impacted) (recurrent) 592.0
   appendix 543.9
   bile duct (any) — *see* Choledocholithiasis
   biliary — *see* Cholelithiasis
   bilirubin, multiple — *see* Cholelithiasis
   bladder (encysted) (impacted) (urinary)
      594.1
      diverticulum 594.0
   bronchus 518.89
   calyx (kidney) (renal) 592.0
      congenital 753.3
   cholesterol (pure) (solitary) — *see*
      Cholelithiasis
   common duct (bile) — *see* Choledocholithi-
      asis
   conjunctiva 372.54
   cystic 594.1
      duct — *see* Cholelithiasis
   dental 523.6
      subgingival 523.6
      supragingival 523.6
   epididymis 608.89
   gallbladder (*see also* Cholelithiasis)
      congenital 751.69
   hepatic (duct) — *see* Choledocholithiasis
   intestine (impaction) (obstruction) 560.39
   kidney (impacted) (multiple) (pelvis) (recur-
      rent) (staghorn) 592.0
      congenital 753.3
   lacrimal (passages) 375.57
   liver (impacted) — *see* Choledocholithiasis

Calculus, calculi, calculous — *continued*
   lung 518.89
   mammographic 793.89
   nephritic (impacted) (recurrent) 592.0
   nose 478.19
   pancreas (duct) 577.8
   parotid gland 527.5
   pelvis, encysted 592.0
   prostate 602.0
   pulmonary 518.89
   renal (impacted) (recurrent) 592.0
      congenital 753.3
   salivary (duct) (gland) 527.5
   seminal vesicle 608.89
   staghorn 592.0
   Stensen's duct 527.5
   sublingual duct or gland 527.5
      congenital 750.26
   submaxillary duct, gland, or region 527.5
   suburethral 594.8
   tonsil 474.8
   tooth, teeth 523.6
   tunica vaginalis 608.89
   ureter (impacted) (recurrent) 592.1
   urethra (impacted) 594.2
   urinary (duct) (impacted) (passage) (tract)
      592.9
      lower tract NEC 594.9
         specified site 594.8
   vagina 623.8
   vesical (impacted) 594.1
   Wharton's duct 527.5
Caliectasis 593.89
California
   disease 114.0
   encephalitis 062.5
Caligo cornea 371.03
Callositas, callosity (infected) 700
Callus (infected) 700
   bone 726.91
   excessive, following fracture (*see also* Late,
      effect (of), fracture)
Calvé (-Perthes) disease (osteochondrosis,
   femoral capital) 732.1
Calvities — *see also* Alopecia 704.00
Cameroon fever — *see also* Malaria 084.6
Camptocormia 300.11
Camptodactyly (congenital) 755.59
Camurati-Engelmann disease (diaphyseal
   sclerosis) 756.59
Canal — *see* condition
Canaliculitis (lacrimal) (acute) 375.31
   Actinomyces 039.8
   chronic 375.41
Canavan's disease 330.0
Cancer (M8000/3) — *see also* Neoplasm, by
   site, malignant

> Note — The term "cancer" when modi-
> fied by an adjective or adjectival phrase
> indicating a morphological type should
> be coded in the same manner as "carci-
> noma" with that adjective or phrase.
> Thus, "squamous-cell cancer" should be
> coded in the same manner as "squa-
> mous-cell carcinoma," which appears in
> the list under "Carcinoma."

   bile duct type (M8160/3), liver 155.1
   hepatocellular (M8170/3) 155.0
Cancerous (M8000/3) — *see* Neoplasm, by site,
   malignant
Cancerphobia 300.29
Cancrum oris 528.1
Candidiasis, candidal 112.9
   with pneumonia 112.4
   balanitis 112.2
   congenital 771.7
   disseminated 112.5
   endocarditis 112.81
   esophagus 112.84
   intertrigo 112.3
   intestine 112.85
   lung 112.4
   meningitis 112.83
   mouth 112.0
   nails 112.3
   neonatal 771.7

Candidiasis, candidal — *continued*
   onychia 112.3
   otitis externa 112.82
   otomycosis 112.82
   paronychia 112.3
   perionyxis 112.3
   pneumonia 112.4
   pneumonitis 112.4
   skin 112.3
   specified site NEC 112.89
   systemic 112.5
   urogenital site NEC 112.2
   vagina 112.1
   vulva 112.1
   vulvovaginitis 112.1
Candidiosis — *see* Candidiasis
Candiru infection or infestation 136.8
Canities (premature) 704.3
   congenital 757.4
Canker (mouth) (sore) 528.2
   rash 034.1
Cannabinosis 504
Canton fever 081.9
Cap
   cradle 690.11
Capillariasis 127.5
Capillary — *see* condition
Caplan-Colinet syndrome 714.81
Caplan's syndrome 714.81
Capsule — *see* condition
Capsulitis (joint) 726.90
   adhesive (shoulder) 726.0
   hip 726.5
   knee 726.60
   labyrinthine 387.8
   thyroid 245.9
   wrist 726.4
Caput
   crepitus 756.0
   medusae 456.8
   succedaneum 767.19
Carapata disease 087.1
Carate — *see* Pinta
**Carbohydrate-deficient glycoprotein syn-
   drome** (CGDS) 271.8
Carboxyhemoglobinemia 986
Carbuncle 680.9
   abdominal wall 680.2
   ankle 680.6
   anus 680.5
   arm (any part, above wrist) 680.3
   auditory canal, external 680.0
   axilla 680.3
   back (any part) 680.2
   breast 680.2
   buttock 680.5
   chest wall 680.2
   corpus cavernosum 607.2
   ear (any part) (external) 680.0
   eyelid 373.13
   face (any part, except eye) 680.0
   finger (any) 680.4
   flank 680.2
   foot (any part) 680.7
   forearm 680.3
   genital organ (male) 608.4
   gluteal (region) 680.5
   groin 680.2
   hand (any part) 680.4
   head (any part, except face) 680.8
   heel 680.7
   hip 680.6
   kidney (*see also* Abscess, kidney) 590.2
   knee 680.6
   labia 616.4
   lacrimal
      gland (*see also* Dacryoadenitis) 375.00
      passages (duct) (sac) (*see also* Dacryocys-
         titis) 375.30
   leg, any part except foot 680.6
   lower extremity, any part except foot 680.6
   malignant 022.0
   multiple sites 680.9
   neck 680.1
   nose (external) (septum) 680.0
   orbit, orbital 376.01

☑ **Additional Digit Required** — Refer to the Tabular List for Digit Selection   ▼ **Subterms under main terms may continue to next column or page**

2013 ICD-9-CM   ►◄ **Revised Text**   ● **New Line**   ▲ **Revised Code**   **Volume 2 — 41**

Carbuncle — continued
partes posteriores 680.5
pectoral region 680.2
penis 607.2
perineum 680.2
pinna 680.0
scalp (any part) 680.8
scrotum 608.4
seminal vesicle 608.0
shoulder 680.3
skin NEC 680.9
specified site NEC 680.8
spermatic cord 608.4
temple (region) 680.0
testis 608.4
thigh 680.6
thumb 680.4
toe (any) 680.7
trunk 680.2
tunica vaginalis 608.4
umbilicus 680.2
upper arm 680.3
urethra 597.0
vas deferens 608.4
vulva 616.4
wrist 680.4
Carbunculus — see also Carbuncle 680.9
Carcinoid (tumor) (M8240/1) — see Tumor, carcinoid
Carcinoidosis 259.2
Carcinomaphobia 300.29
Carcinomatosis
peritonei (M8010/6) 197.6
specified site NEC (M8010/3) — see Neoplasm, by site, malignant
unspecified site (M8010/6) 199.0
Carcinoma (M8010/3) — see also Neoplasm, by site, malignant

Note — Except where otherwise indicated, the morphological varieties of carcinoma in the list below should be coded by site as for "Neoplasm, malignant."

with
apocrine metaplasia (M8573/3)
cartilaginous (and osseous) metaplasia (M8571/3)
osseous (and cartilaginous) metaplasia (M8571/3)
productive fibrosis (M8141/3)
spindle cell metaplasia (M8572/3)
squamous metaplasia (M8570/3)
acidophil (M8280/3)
specified site — see Neoplasm, by site, malignant
unspecified site 194.3
acidophil-basophil, mixed (M8281/3)
specified site — see Neoplasm, by site, malignant
unspecified site 194.3
acinar (cell) (M8550/3)
acinic cell (M8550/3)
adenocystic (M8200/3)
adenoid
cystic (M8200/3)
squamous cell (M8075/3)
adenosquamous (M8560/3)
adnexal (skin) (M8390/3) — see Neoplasm, skin, malignant
adrenal cortical (M8370/3) 194.0
alveolar (M8251/3)
cell (M8250/3) — see Neoplasm, lung, malignant
anaplastic type (M8021/3)
apocrine (M8401/3)
breast — see Neoplasm, breast, malignant
specified site NEC — see Neoplasm, skin, malignant
unspecified site 173.99
basal cell (pigmented) (M8090/3) (see also Neoplasm, skin, malignant) 173.91
fibro-epithelial type (M8093/3) — see Neoplasm, skin, malignant
morphea type (M8092/3) — see Neoplasm, skin, malignant

Carcinoma — see also Neoplasm, by site, malignant — continued
basal cell (see also Neoplasm, skin, malignant) — continued
multicentric (M8091/3) — see Neoplasm, skin, malignant
basaloid (M8123/3)
basal-squamous cell, mixed (M8094/3) — see Neoplasm, skin, malignant
basophil (M8300/3)
specified site — see Neoplasm, by site, malignant
unspecified site 194.3
basophil-acidophil, mixed (M8281/3)
specified site — see Neoplasm, by site, malignant
unspecified site 194.3
basosquamous (M8094/3) — see Neoplasm, skin, malignant
bile duct type (M8160/3)
and hepatocellular, mixed (M8180/3) 155.0
liver 155.1
specified site NEC — see Neoplasm, by site, malignant
unspecified site 155.1
branchial or branchiogenic 146.8
bronchial or bronchogenic — see Neoplasm, lung, malignant
bronchiolar (terminal) (M8250/3) — see Neoplasm, lung, malignant
bronchiolo-alveolar (M8250/3) — see Neoplasm, lung, malignant
bronchogenic (epidermoid) 162.9
C cell (M8510/3)
specified site — see Neoplasm, by site, malignant
unspecified site 193
ceruminous (M8420/3) 173.29
chorionic (M9100/3)
specified site — see Neoplasm, by site, malignant
unspecified site
female 181
male 186.9
chromophobe (M8270/3)
specified site — see Neoplasm, by site, malignant
unspecified site 194.3
clear cell (mesonephroid type) (M8310/3)
cloacogenic (M8124/3)
specified site — see Neoplasm, by site, malignant
unspecified site 154.8
colloid (M8480/3)
cribriform (M8201/3)
cylindroid type (M8200/3)
diffuse type (M8145/3)
specified site — see Neoplasm, by site, malignant
unspecified site 151.9
duct (cell) (M8500/3)
with Paget's disease (M8541/3) — see Neoplasm, breast, malignant
infiltrating (M8500/3)
specified site — see Neoplasm, by site, malignant
unspecified site 174.9
ductal (M8500/3)
ductular, infiltrating (M8521/3)
embryonal (M9070/3)
and teratoma, mixed (M9081/3)
combined with choriocarcinoma (M9101/3) — see Neoplasm, by site, malignant
infantile type (M9071/3)
liver 155.0
polyembryonal type (M9072/3)
endometrioid (M8380/3)
eosinophil (M8280/3)
specified site — see Neoplasm, by site, malignant
unspecified site 194.3
epidermoid (M8070/3) (see also Carcinoma, squamous cell)

Carcinoma — see also Neoplasm, by site, malignant — continued
epidermoid (see also Carcinoma, squamous cell) — continued
and adenocarcinoma, mixed (M8560/3)
in situ, Bowen's type (M8081/2) — see Neoplasm, skin, in situ
intradermal — see Neoplasm, skin, in situ
fibroepithelial type basal cell (M8093/3) — see Neoplasm, skin, malignant
follicular (M8330/3)
and papillary (mixed) (M8340/3) 193
moderately differentiated type (M8332/3) 193
pure follicle type (M8331/3) 193
specified site — see Neoplasm, by site, malignant
trabecular type (M8332/3) 193
unspecified site 193
well differentiated type (M8331/3) 193
gelatinous (M8480/3)
giant cell (M8031/3)
and spindle cell (M8030/3)
granular cell (M8320/3)
granulosa cell (M8620/3) 183.0
hepatic cell (M8170/3) 155.0
hepatocellular (M8170/3) 155.0
and bile duct, mixed (M8180/3) 155.0
hepatocholangiolitic (M8180/3) 155.0
Hürthle cell (thyroid) 193
hypernephroid (M8311/3)
in
adenomatous
polyp (M8210/3)
polyposis coli (M8220/3) 153.9
pleomorphic adenoma (M8940/3)
polypoid adenoma (M8210/3)
situ (M8010/3) — see Carcinoma, in situ
tubular adenoma (M8210/3)
villous adenoma (M8261/3)
infiltrating duct (M8500/3)
with Paget's disease (M8541/3) — see Neoplasm, breast, malignant
specified site — see Neoplasm, by site, malignant
unspecified site 174.9
inflammatory (M8530/3)
specified site — see Neoplasm, by site, malignant
unspecified site 174.9
in situ (M8010/2) (see also Neoplasm, by site, in situ)
epidermoid (M8070/2) (see also Neoplasm, by site, in situ)
with questionable stromal invasion (M8076/2)
specified site — see Neoplasm, by site, in situ
unspecified site 233.1
Bowen's type (M8081/2) — see Neoplasm, skin, in situ
intraductal (M8500/2)
specified site — see Neoplasm, by site, in situ
unspecified site 233.0
lobular (M8520/2)
specified site — see Neoplasm, by site, in situ
unspecified site 233.0
papillary (M8050/2) — see Neoplasm, by site, in situ
squamous cell (M8070/2) (see also Neoplasm, by site, in situ)
with questionable stromal invasion (M8076/2)
specified site — see Neoplasm, by site, in situ
unspecified site 233.1
transitional cell (M8120/2) — see Neoplasm, by site, in situ
intestinal type (M8144/3)
specified site — see Neoplasm, by site, malignant
unspecified site 151.9

Carcinoma — see also Neoplasm, by site, malignant — continued
intraductal (noninfiltrating) (M8500/2)
papillary (M8503/2)
specified site — see Neoplasm, by site, in situ
unspecified site 233.0
specified site — see Neoplasm, by site, in situ
unspecified site 233.0
intraepidermal (M8070/2) (see also Neoplasm, skin, in situ)
squamous cell, Bowen's type (M8081/2) — see Neoplasm, skin, in situ
intraepithelial (M8010/2) (see also Neoplasm, by site, in situ)
squamous cell (M8072/2) — see Neoplasm, by site, in situ
intraosseous (M9270/3) 170.1
upper jaw (bone) 170.0
islet cell (M8150/3)
and exocrine, mixed (M8154/3)
specified site — see Neoplasm, by site, malignant
unspecified site 157.9
pancreas 157.4
specified site NEC — see Neoplasm, by site, malignant
unspecified site 157.4
juvenile, breast (M8502/3) — see Neoplasm, breast, malignant
Kulchitsky's cell (carcinoid tumor of intestine) 259.2
large cell (M8012/3)
squamous cell, non-keratinizing type (M8072/3)
Leydig cell (testis) (M8650/3)
specified site — see Neoplasm, by site, malignant
unspecified site 186.9
female 183.0
male 186.9
liver cell (M8170/3) 155.0
lobular (infiltrating) (M8520/3)
non-infiltrating (M8520/3)
specified site — see Neoplasm, by site, in situ
unspecified site 233.0
specified site — see Neoplasm, by site, malignant
unspecified site 174.9
lymphoepithelial (M8082/3)
medullary (M8510/3)
with
amyloid stroma (M8511/3)
specified site — see Neoplasm, by site, malignant
unspecified site 193
lymphoid stroma (M8512/3)
specified site — see Neoplasm, by site, malignant
unspecified site 174.9
Merkel cell 209.36
buttock 209.36
ear 209.31
eyelid, including canthus 209.31
face 209.31
genitals 209.36
lip 209.31
lower limb 209.34
neck 209.32
nodal presentation 209.75
scalp 209.32
secondary (any site) 209.75
specified site NEC 209.36
trunk 209.35
unknown primary site 209.75
upper limb 209.33
visceral metastatic presentation 209.75
mesometanephric (M9110/3)
mesonephric (M9110/3)
metastatic (M8010/6) — see Metastasis, cancer
metatypical (M8095/3) — see Neoplasm, skin, malignant

☑ Additional Digit Required — Refer to the Tabular List for Digit Selection   ⬝ Subterms under main terms may continue to next column or page

42 — Volume 2   ▶◀ Revised Text   ● New Line   ▲ Revised Code   2013 ICD-9-CM

Carcinoma — *see also* Neoplasm, by site, malignant — *continued*
  morphea type basal cell (M8092/3) — *see* Neoplasm, skin, malignant
  mucinous (M8480/3)
  mucin-producing (M8481/3)
  mucin-secreting (M8481/3)
  mucoepidermoid (M8430/3)
  mucoid (M8480/3)
    cell (M8300/3)
      specified site — *see* Neoplasm, by site, malignant
      unspecified site 194.3
  mucous (M8480/3)
  neuroendocrine
    high grade (M8240/3) 209.30
    malignant poorly differentiated (M8240/3) 209.30
  nonencapsulated sclerosing (M8350/3) 193
  noninfiltrating
    intracystic (M8504/2) — *see* Neoplasm, by site, in situ
    intraductal (M8500/2)
      papillary (M8503/2)
        specified site — *see* Neoplasm, by site, in situ
        unspecified site 233.0
      specified site — *see* Neoplasm, by site, in situ
      unspecified site 233.0
    lobular (M8520/2)
      specified site — *see* Neoplasm, by site, in situ
      unspecified site 233.0
  oat cell (M8042/3)
    specified site — *see* Neoplasm, by site, malignant
    unspecified site 162.9
  odontogenic (M9270/3) 170.1
    upper jaw (bone) 170.0
  onocytic (M8290/3)
  oxyphilic (M8290/3)
  papillary (M8050/3)
    and follicular (mixed) (M8340/3) 193
    epidermoid (M8052/3)
    intraductal (noninfiltrating) (M8503/2)
      specified site — *see* Neoplasm, by site, in situ
      unspecified site 233.0
    serous (M8460/3)
      specified site — *see* Neoplasm, by site, malignant
      surface (M8461/3)
        specified site — *see* Neoplasm, by site, malignant
        unspecified site 183.0
      unspecified site 183.0
    squamous cell (M8052/3)
    transitional cell (M8130/3)
  papillocystic (M8450/3)
    specified site — *see* Neoplasm, by site, malignant
    unspecified site 183.0
  parafollicular cell (M8510/3)
    specified site — *see* Neoplasm, by site, malignant
    unspecified site 193
  pleomorphic (M8022/3)
  polygonal cell (M8034/3)
  prickle cell (M8070/3)
  pseudoglandular, squamous cell (M8075/3)
  pseudomucinous (M8470/3)
    specified site — *see* Neoplasm, by site, malignant
    unspecified site 183.0
  pseudosarcomatous (M8033/3)
  regaud type (M8082/3) — *see* Neoplasm, nasopharynx, malignant
  renal cell (M8312/3) 189.0
  reserve cell (M8041/3)
  round cell (M8041/3)
  Schmincke (M8082/3) — *see* Neoplasm, nasopharynx, malignant
  Schneiderian (M8121/3)
    specified site — *see* Neoplasm, by site, malignant

Carcinoma — *see also* Neoplasm, by site, malignant — *continued*
  Schneiderian — *continued*
    unspecified site 160.0
  scirrhous (M8141/3)
  sebaceous (M8410/3) — *see* Neoplasm, skin, malignant
  secondary (M8010/6) — *see* Neoplasm, by site, malignant, secondary
  secretory, breast (M8502/3) — *see* Neoplasm, breast, malignant
  serous (M8441/3)
    papillary (M8460/3)
      specified site — *see* Neoplasm, by site, malignant
      unspecified site 183.0
    surface, papillary (M8461/3)
      specified site — *see* Neoplasm, by site, malignant
      unspecified site 183.0
  Sertoli cell (M8640/3)
    specified site — *see* Neoplasm, by site, malignant
    unspecified site 186.9
  signet ring cell (M8490/3)
    metastatic (M8490/6) — *see* Neoplasm, by site, secondary
  simplex (M8231/3)
  skin appendage (M8390/3) — *see* Neoplasm, skin, malignant
  small cell (M8041/3)
    fusiform cell type (M8043/3)
    squamous cell, non-keratinizing type (M8073/3)
  solid (M8230/3)
    with amyloid stroma (M8511/3)
      specified site — *see* Neoplasm, by site, malignant
      unspecified site 193
  spheroidal cell (M8035/3)
  spindle cell (M8032/3)
    and giant cell (M8030/3)
  spinous cell (M8070/3)
  squamous (cell) (M8070/3)
    adenoid type (M8075/3)
    and adenocarcinoma, mixed (M8560/3)
    intraepidermal, Bowen's type — *see* Neoplasm, skin, in situ
    keratinizing type (large cell) (M8071/3)
    large cell, non-keratinizing type (M8072/3)
    microinvasive (M8076/3)
      specified site — *see* Neoplasm, by site, malignant
      unspecified site 180.9
    non-keratinizing type (M8072/3)
    papillary (M8052/3)
    pseudoglandular (M8075/3)
    skin (*see also* Neoplasm, skin, malignant) 173.92
    small cell, non-keratinizing type (M8073/3)
    spindle cell type (M8074/3)
    verrucous (M8051/3)
  superficial spreading (M8143/3)
  sweat gland (M8400/3) — *see* Neoplasm, skin, malignant
  theca cell (M8600/3) 183.0
  thymic (M8580/3) 164.0
  trabecular (M8190/3)
  transitional (cell) (M8120/3)
    papillary (M8130/3)
    spindle cell type (M8122/3)
  tubular (M8211/3)
  undifferentiated type (M8020/3)
  urothelial (M8120/3)
  ventriculi 151.9
  verrucous (epidermoid) (squamous cell) (M8051/3)
  villous (M8262/3)
  water-clear cell (M8322/3) 194.1
  wolffian duct (M9110/3)
Carcinosarcoma (M8980/3) — *see also* Neoplasm, by site, malignant
  embryonal type (M8981/3) — *see* Neoplasm, by site, malignant

Cardiac — *see also* condition
  death — *see* Disease, heart
  device
    defibrillator, automatic implantable (with synchronous cardiac pacemaker) V45.02
      in situ NEC V45.00
    pacemaker
      cardiac
        fitting or adjustment V53.31
        in situ V45.01
      carotid sinus
        fitting or adjustment V53.39
        in situ V45.09
  pacemaker — *see* Cardiac, device, pacemaker
  tamponade 423.3
Cardia, cardial — *see* condition
Cardialgia — *see also* Pain, precordial 786.51
Cardiectasis — *see* Hypertrophy, cardiac
Cardiochalasia 530.81
Cardiomalacia — *see also* Degeneration, myocardial 429.1
Cardiomegalia glycogenica diffusa 271.0
Cardiomegaly — *see also* Hypertrophy, cardiac 429.3
  congenital 746.89
  glycogen 271.0
  hypertensive (*see also* Hypertension, heart) 402.90
  idiopathic 429.3
Cardiomyoliposis — *see also* Degeneration, myocardial 429.1
Cardiomyopathy (congestive) (constrictive) (familial) (infiltrative) (obstructive) (restrictive) (sporadic) 425.4
  alcoholic 425.5
  amyloid 277.39 *[425.7]*
  beriberi 265.0 *[425.7]*
  cobalt-beer 425.5
  congenital 425.3
  due to
    amyloidosis 277.39 *[425.7]*
    beriberi 265.0 *[425.7]*
    cardiac glycogenosis 271.0 *[425.7]*
    Chagas' disease 086.0
    Friedreich's ataxia 334.0 *[425.8]*
    hypertension — *see* Hypertension, with, heart involvement
    mucopolysaccharidosis 277.5 *[425.7]*
    myotonia atrophica 359.21 *[425.8]*
    progressive muscular dystrophy 359.1 *[425.8]*
    sarcoidosis 135 *[425.8]*
  glycogen storage 271.0 *[425.7]*
  hypertensive — *see* Hypertension, with, heart involvement
  hypertrophic 425.18
    nonobstructive 425.18
    obstructive 425.11
      congenital 746.84
  idiopathic (concentric) 425.4
  in
    Chagas' disease 086.0
    sarcoidosis 135 *[425.8]*
  ischemic 414.8
  metabolic NEC 277.9 *[425.7]*
    amyloid 277.39 *[425.7]*
    thyrotoxic (*see also* Thyrotoxicosis) 242.9 ☑ *[425.7]*
    thyrotoxicosis (*see also* Thyrotoxicosis) 242.9 ☑ *[425.7]*
  newborn 425.4
    congenital 425.3
  nutritional 269.9 *[425.7]*
    beriberi 265.0 *[425.7]*
  obscure of Africa 425.2
  peripartum 674.5 ☑
  postpartum 674.5 ☑
  primary 425.4
  secondary 425.9
  stress inuced 429.83
  takotsubo 429.83
  thyrotoxic (*see also* Thyrotoxicosis) 242.9 ☑ *[425.7]*
  toxic NEC 425.9

Cardiomyopathy — *continued*
  tuberculous (*see also* Tuberculosis) 017.9 ☑ *[425.8]*
Cardionephritis — *see* Hypertension, cardiorenal
Cardionephropathy — *see* Hypertension, cardiorenal
Cardionephrosis — *see* Hypertension, cardiorenal
Cardioneurosis 306.2
Cardiopathia nigra 416.0
Cardiopathy — *see also* Disease, heart 429.9
  hypertensive (*see also* Hypertension, heart) 402.90
  idiopathic 425.4
  mucopolysaccharidosis 277.5 *[425.7]*
Cardiopericarditis — *see also* Pericarditis 423.9
Cardiophobia 300.29
Cardioptosis 746.87
Cardiorenal — *see* condition
Cardiorrhexis — *see also* Infarct, myocardium 410.9 ☑
Cardiosclerosis — *see* Arteriosclerosis, coronary
Cardiosis — *see* Disease, heart
Cardiospasm (esophagus) (reflex) (stomach) 530.0
  congenital 750.7
Cardiostenosis — *see* Disease, heart
Cardiosymphysis 423.1
Cardiothyrotoxicosis — *see* Hyperthyroidism
Cardiovascular — *see* condition
Carditis (acute) (bacterial) (chronic) (subacute) 429.89
  Coxsackie 074.20
  hypertensive (*see also* Hypertension, heart) 402.90
  meningococcal 036.40
  rheumatic — *see* Disease, heart, rheumatic
  rheumatoid 714.2
Care (of)
  child (routine) V20.1
  convalescent following V66.9
    chemotherapy V66.2
    medical NEC V66.5
    psychotherapy V66.3
    radiotherapy V66.1
    surgery V66.0
    surgical NEC V66.0
    treatment (for) V66.5
      combined V66.6
      fracture V66.4
      mental disorder NEC V66.3
      specified type NEC V66.5
  end-of-life V66.7
  family member (handicapped) (sick)
    creating problem for family V61.49
    provided away from home for holiday relief V60.5
    unavailable, due to
      absence (person rendering care) (sufferer) V60.4
      inability (any reason) of person rendering care V60.4
  holiday relief V60.5
  hospice V66.7
  lack of (at or after birth) (infant) (child) 995.52
    adult 995.84
  lactation of mother V24.1
  palliative V66.7
  postpartum
    immediately after delivery V24.0
    routine follow-up V24.2
  prenatal V22.1
    first pregnancy V22.0
    high-risk pregnancy V23.9
      inconclusive fetal viability V23.87
      specified problem NEC V23.89
  terminal V66.7
  unavailable, due to
    absence of person rendering care V60.4
    inability (any reason) of person rendering care V60.4
  well baby V20.1

☑ Additional Digit Required — Refer to the Tabular List for Digit Selection   ᵂ Subterms under main terms may continue to next column or page

2013 ICD-9-CM   ▶◀ Revised Text   ● New Line   ▲ Revised Code   Volume 2 — 43

Carcinoma — Care

Caries (bone) — *see also* Tuberculosis, bone
  015.9 ☑ *[730.8]* ☑
  arrested 521.04
  cementum 521.03
  cerebrospinal (tuberculous)
    015.0 ☑ *[730.88]*
  dental (acute) (chronic) (incipient) (infected)
    521.00
    with pulp exposure 521.03
    extending to
      dentine 521.02
      pulp 521.03
    other specified NEC 521.09
    pit and fissure 521.06
    primary
      pit and fissure origin 521.06
      root surface 521.08
      smooth surface origin 521.07
    root surface 521.08
    smooth surface 521.07
  dentin (acute) (chronic) 521.02
  enamel (acute) (chronic) (incipient) 521.01
  external meatus 380.89
  hip (*see also* Tuberculosis) 015.1 ☑ *[730.85]*
  initial 521.01
  knee 015.2 ☑ *[730.86]*
  labyrinth 386.8
  limb NEC 015.7 ☑ *[730.88]*
  mastoid (chronic) (process) 383.1
  middle ear 385.89
  nose 015.7 ☑ *[730.88]*
  orbit 015.7 ☑ *[730.88]*
  ossicle 385.24
  petrous bone 383.20
  sacrum (tuberculous) 015.0 ☑ *[730.88]*
  spine, spinal (column) (tuberculous)
    015.0 ☑ *[730.88]*
  syphilitic 095.5
    congenital 090.0 *[730.8]* ☑
  teeth (internal) 521.00
    initial 521.01
  vertebra (column) (tuberculous)
    015.0 ☑ *[730.88]*
Carini's syndrome (ichthyosis congenita) 757.1
Carious teeth 521.00
Carneous mole 631.8
Carnosinemia 270.5
Carotid body or sinus syndrome 337.01
Carotidynia 337.01
Carotinemia (dietary) 278.3
Carotinosis (cutis) (skin) 278.3
Carpal tunnel syndrome 354.0
Carpenter's syndrome 759.89
Carpopedal spasm — *see also* Tetany 781.7
Carpoptosis 736.05
Carrier (suspected) **of**
  amebiasis V02.2
  bacterial disease (meningococcal, staphylo-
    coccal) NEC V02.59
  cholera V02.0
  cystic fibrosis gene V83.81
  defective gene V83.89
  diphtheria V02.4
  dysentery (bacillary) V02.3
    amebic V02.2
  Endamoeba histolytica V02.2
  gastrointestinal pathogens NEC V02.3
  genetic defect V83.89
  gonorrhea V02.7
  group B streptococcus V02.51
  HAA (hepatitis Australian-antigen) V02.61
  hemophilia A (asymptomatic) V83.01
    symptomatic V83.02
  hepatitis V02.60
    Australian-antigen (HAA) V02.61
    B V02.61
    C V02.62
    serum V02.61
    specified type NEC V02.69
    viral V02.60
  infective organism NEC V02.9
  malaria V02.9
  paratyphoid V02.3
  Salmonella V02.3
    typhosa V02.1
  serum hepatitis V02.61

Carrier (suspected) **of** — *continued*
  Shigella V02.3
  Staphylococcus NEC V02.59
    methicillin
      resistant Staphylococcus aureus
        V02.54
      susceptible Staphylococcus aureus
        V02.53
  Streptococcus NEC V02.52
    group B V02.51
  typhoid V02.1
  venereal disease NEC V02.8
Carrión's disease (Bartonellosis) 088.0
Car sickness 994.6
Carter's
  relapsing fever (Asiatic) 087.0
Cartilage — *see* condition
Caruncle (inflamed)
  abscess, lacrimal (*see also* Dacryocystitis)
    375.30
  conjunctiva 372.00
    acute 372.00
  eyelid 373.00
  labium (majus) (minus) 616.89
  lacrimal 375.30
  urethra (benign) 599.3
  vagina (wall) 616.89
Cascade stomach 537.6
Caseation lymphatic gland — *see also* Tuberculosis 017.2 ☑
Caseous
  bronchitis — *see* Tuberculosis, pulmonary
  meningitis 013.0 ☑
  pneumonia — *see* Tuberculosis, pulmonary
Cassidy (-Scholte) syndrome (malignant carcinoid) 259.2
Castellani's bronchitis 104.8
Castleman's tumor or lymphoma (mediastinal lymph node hyperplasia) 785.6
Castration, traumatic 878.2
  complicated 878.3
Casts in urine 791.7
Catalepsy 300.11
  catatonic (acute) (*see also* Schizophrenia)
    295.2 ☑
  hysterical 300.11
  schizophrenic (*see also* Schizophrenia)
    295.2 ☑
Cataphasia — *see also* Disorder, fluency 315.35
Cataplexy (idiopathic) — *see* Narcolepsy
Cataract (anterior cortical) (anterior polar)
    (black) (capsular) (central) (cortical) (hy-
    permature) (immature) (incipient) (ma-
    ture) 366.9
  anterior
    and posterior axial embryonal 743.33
    pyramidal 743.31
    subcapsular polar
      infantile, juvenile, or presenile 366.01
      senile 366.13
  associated with
    calcinosis 275.40 *[366.42]*
    craniofacial dysostosis 756.0 *[366.44]*
    galactosemia 271.1 *[366.44]*
    hypoparathyroidism 252.1 *[366.42]*
    myotonic disorders 359.21 *[366.43]*
    neovascularization 366.33
  blue dot 743.39
  cerulean 743.39
  complicated NEC 366.30
  congenital 743.30
    capsular or subcapsular 743.31
    cortical 743.32
    nuclear 743.33
    specified type NEC 743.39
    total or subtotal 743.34
    zonular 743.32
  coronary (congenital) 743.39
    acquired 366.12
  cupuliform 366.14
  diabetic 250.5 ☑ *[366.41]*
    due to secondary diabetes
      249.5 ☑ *[366.41]*
  drug-induced 366.45
  due to
    chalcosis 360.24 *[366.34]*

Cataract — *continued*
  due to — *continued*
    chronic choroiditis (*see also* Choroiditis)
      363.20 *[366.32]*
    degenerative myopia 360.21 *[366.34]*
    glaucoma (*see also* Glaucoma)
      365.9 *[366.31]*
    infection, intraocular NEC 366.32
    inflammatory ocular disorder NEC 366.32
    iridocyclitis, chronic 364.10 *[366.33]*
    pigmentary retinal dystrophy
      362.74 *[366.34]*
    radiation 366.46
  electric 366.46
  glassblowers' 366.46
  heat ray 366.46
  heterochromic 366.33
  in eye disease NEC 366.30
  infantile (*see also* Cataract, juvenile) 366.00
  intumescent 366.12
  irradiational 366.46
  juvenile 366.00
    anterior subcapsular polar 366.01
    combined forms 366.09
    cortical 366.03
    lamellar 366.03
    nuclear 366.04
    posterior subcapsular polar 366.02
    specified NEC 366.09
    zonular 366.03
  lamellar 743.32
    infantile, juvenile, or presenile 366.03
  morgagnian 366.18
  myotonic 359.21 *[366.43]*
  myxedema 244.9 *[366.44]*
  nuclear 366.16
  posterior, polar (capsular) 743.31
    infantile, juvenile, or presenile 366.02
    senile 366.14
  presenile (*see also* Cataract, juvenile) 366.00
  punctate
    acquired 366.12
    congenital 743.39
  secondary (membrane) 366.50
    obscuring vision 366.53
    specified type, not obscuring vision
      366.52
  senile 366.10
    anterior subcapsular polar 366.13
    combined forms 366.19
    cortical 366.15
    hypermature 366.18
    immature 366.12
    incipient 366.12
    mature 366.17
    nuclear 366.16
    posterior subcapsular polar 366.14
    specified NEC 366.19
    total or subtotal 366.17
  snowflake 250.5 ☑ *[366.41]*
    due to secondary diabetes
      249.5 ☑ *[366.41]*
  specified NEC 366.8
  subtotal (senile) 366.17
    congenital 743.34
  sunflower 360.24 *[366.34]*
  tetanic NEC 252.1 *[366.42]*
  total (mature) (senile) 366.17
    congenital 743.34
    localized 366.21
    traumatic 366.22
  toxic 366.45
  traumatic 366.20
    partially resolved 366.23
    total 366.22
  zonular (perinuclear) 743.32
    infantile, juvenile, or presenile 366.03
Cataracta 366.10
  brunescens 366.16
  cerulea 743.39
  complicata 366.30
  congenita 743.30
  coralliformis 743.39
  coronaria (congenital) 743.39
    acquired 366.12
  diabetic 250.5 ☑ *[366.41]*

Cataracta — *continued*
  diabetic — *continued*
    due to secondary diabetes
      249.5 ☑ *[366.41]*
  floriformis 360.24 *[366.34]*
  membranacea
    accreta 366.50
    congenita 743.39
  nigra 366.16
Catarrh, catarrhal (inflammation) — *see also*
  condition 460
  acute 460
  asthma, asthmatic (*see also* Asthma)
    493.9 ☑
  Bostock's (*see also* Fever, hay) 477.9
  bowel — *see* Enteritis
  bronchial 490
    acute 466.0
    chronic 491.0
    subacute 466.0
  cervix, cervical (canal) (uteri) — *see* Cervicitis
  chest (*see also* Bronchitis) 490
  chronic 472.0
  congestion 472.0
  conjunctivitis 372.03
  due to syphilis 095.9
    congenital 090.0
  enteric — *see* Enteritis
  epidemic (*see also* Influenza) 487.1
  Eustachian 381.50
  eye (acute) (vernal) 372.03
  fauces (*see also* Pharyngitis) 462
  febrile 460
  fibrinous acute 466.0
  gastroenteric — *see* Enteritis
  gastrointestinal — *see* Enteritis
  gingivitis 523.00
  hay (*see also* Fever, hay) 477.9
  infectious 460
  intestinal — *see* Enteritis
  larynx (*see also* Laryngitis, chronic) 476.0
  liver 070.1
    with hepatic coma 070.0
  lung (*see also* Bronchitis) 490
    acute 466.0
    chronic 491.0
  middle ear (chronic) — *see* Otitis media,
    chronic
  mouth 528.00
  nasal (chronic) (*see also* Rhinitis) 472.0
    acute 460
  nasobronchial 472.2
  nasopharyngeal (chronic) 472.2
    acute 460
  nose — *see* Catarrh, nasal
  ophthalmia 372.03
  pneumococcal, acute 466.0
  pulmonary (*see also* Bronchitis) 490
    acute 466.0
    chronic 491.0
  spring (eye) 372.13
  suffocating (*see also* Asthma) 493.9 ☑
  summer (hay) (*see also* Fever, hay) 477.9
  throat 472.1
  tracheitis 464.10
    with obstruction 464.11
  tubotympanal 381.4
    acute (*see also* Otitis media, acute, non-
      suppurative) 381.00
    chronic 381.10
  vasomotor (*see also* Fever, hay) 477.9
  vesical (bladder) — *see* Cystitis
Catarrhus aestivus — *see also* Fever, hay 477.9
Catastrophe, cerebral — *see also* Disease,
  cerebrovascular, acute 436
Catatonia, catatonic (acute) 781.99
  with
    affective psychosis — *see* Psychosis, af-
      fective
  agitation 295.2 ☑
  dementia (praecox) 295.2 ☑
  due to or associated with physical condition
    293.89
  excitation 295.2 ☑
  excited type 295.2 ☑
  in conditions classified elsewhere 293.89

Catatonia, catatonic — *continued*
 schizophrenia 295.2 ☑
 stupor 295.2 ☑
Cat's ear 744.29
Cat-scratch — *see also* Injury, superficial
 disease or fever 078.3
Cauda equina — *see also* condition
 syndrome 344.60
Cauliflower ear 738.7
Caul over face 768.9
Causalgia 355.9
 lower limb 355.71
 upper limb 354.4
Cause
 external, general effects NEC 994.9
 not stated 799.9
 unknown 799.9
Caustic burn — *see also* Burn, by site
 from swallowing caustic or corrosive substance — *see* Burn, internal organs
Cavare's disease (familial periodic paralysis) 359.3
Cave-in, injury
 crushing (severe) (*see also* Crush, by site) 869.1
 suffocation 994.7
Cavernitis (penis) 607.2
 lymph vessel — *see* Lymphangioma
Cavernositis 607.2
Cavernous — *see* condition
Cavitation of lung — *see also* Tuberculosis 011.2 ☑
 nontuberculous 518.89
 primary, progressive 010.8 ☑
Cavity
 lung — *see* Cavitation of lung
 optic papilla 743.57
 pulmonary — *see* Cavitation of lung
 teeth 521.00
 vitreous (humor) 379.21
Cavovarus foot, congenital 754.59
Cavus foot (congenital) 754.71
 acquired 736.73
Cazenave's
 disease (pemphigus) NEC 694.4
 lupus (erythematosus) 695.4
CDGS (carbohydrate-deficient glycoprotein syndrome) 271.8
Cecitis — *see* Appendicitis
Cecocele — *see* Hernia
Cecum — *see* condition
Celiac
 artery compression syndrome 447.4
 disease 579.0
 infantilism 579.0
Cell, cellular — *see also* condition
 anterior chamber (eye) (positive aqueous ray) 364.04
Cellulitis (diffuse) (with lymphangitis) — *see also* Abscess 682.9
 abdominal wall 682.2
 anaerobic (*see also* Gas gangrene) 040.0
 ankle 682.6
 anus 566
 areola 611.0
 arm (any part, above wrist) 682.3
 auditory canal (external) 380.10
 axilla 682.3
 back (any part) 682.2
 breast 611.0
  postpartum 675.1 ☑
 broad ligament (*see also* Disease, pelvis, inflammatory) 614.4
  acute 614.3
 buttock 682.5
 cervical (neck region) 682.1
 cervix (uteri) (*see also* Cervicitis) 616.0
 cheek, external 682.0
  internal 528.3
 chest wall 682.2
 chronic NEC 682.9
 colostomy 569.61
 corpus cavernosum 607.2
 digit 681.9

Cellulitis — *see also* Abscess — *continued*
 Douglas' cul-de-sac or pouch (chronic) (*see also* Disease, pelvis, inflammatory) 614.4
  acute 614.3
 drainage site (following operation) 998.59
 ear, external 380.10
 enterostomy 569.61
 erysipelar (*see also* Erysipelas) 035
 esophagostomy 530.86
 eyelid 373.13
 face (any part, except eye) 682.0
 finger (intrathecal) (periosteal) (subcutaneous) (subcuticular) 681.00
 flank 682.2
 foot (except toe) 682.7
 forearm 682.3
 gangrenous (*see also* Gangrene) 785.4
 genital organ NEC
  female — *see* Abscess, genital organ, female
  male 608.4
 glottis 478.71
 gluteal (region) 682.5
 gonococcal NEC 098.0
 groin 682.2
 hand (except finger or thumb) 682.4
 head (except face) NEC 682.8
 heel 682.7
 hip 682.6
 jaw (region) 682.0
 knee 682.6
 labium (majus) (minus) (*see also* Vulvitis) 616.10
 larynx 478.71
 leg, except foot 682.6
 lip 528.5
 mammary gland 611.0
 mouth (floor) 528.3
 multiple sites NEC 682.9
 nasopharynx 478.21
 navel 682.2
  newborn NEC 771.4
 neck (region) 682.1
 nipple 611.0
 nose 478.19
  external 682.0
 orbit, orbital 376.01
 palate (soft) 528.3
 pectoral (region) 682.2
 pelvis, pelvic
  with
   abortion — *see* Abortion, by type, with sepsis
   ectopic pregnancy (*see also* categories 633.0–633.9) 639.0
   molar pregnancy (*see also* categories 630–632) 639.0
  female (*see also* Disease, pelvis, inflammatory) 614.4
   acute 614.3
  following
   abortion 639.0
   ectopic or molar pregnancy 639.0
  male 567.21
  puerperal, postpartum, childbirth 670.8 ☑
 penis 607.2
 perineal, perineum 682.2
 perirectal 566
 peritonsillar 475
 periurethral 597.0
 periuterine (*see also* Disease, pelvis, inflammatory) 614.4
  acute 614.3
 pharynx 478.21
 phlegmonous NEC 682.9
 rectum 566
 retromammary 611.0
 retroperitoneal (*see also* Peritonitis) 567.2 ☑, 567.38
 round ligament (*see also* Disease, pelvis, inflammatory) 614.4
  acute 614.3
 scalp (any part) 682.8
  dissecting 704.8

Cellulitis — *see also* Abscess — *continued*
 scrotum 608.4
 seminal vesicle 608.0
 septic NEC 682.9
 shoulder 682.3
 specified sites NEC 682.8
 spermatic cord 608.4
 submandibular (region) (space) (triangle) 682.0
  gland 527.3
 submaxillary 528.3
  gland 527.3
 submental (pyogenic) 682.0
  gland 527.3
 suppurative NEC 682.9
 testis 608.4
 thigh 682.6
 thumb (intrathecal) (periosteal) (subcutaneous) (subcuticular) 681.00
 toe (intrathecal) (periosteal) (subcutaneous) (subcuticular) 681.10
 tonsil 475
 trunk 682.2
 tuberculous (primary) (*see also* Tuberculosis) 017.0 ☑
 tunica vaginalis 608.4
 umbilical 682.2
  newborn NEC 771.4
 vaccinal 999.39
 vagina — *see* Vaginitis
 vas deferens 608.4
 vocal cords 478.5
 vulva (*see also* Vulvitis) 616.10
 wrist 682.4
Cementoblastoma, benign (M9273/0) 213.1
 upper jaw (bone) 213.0
Cementoma (M9273/0) 213.1
 gigantiform (M9275/0) 213.1
  upper jaw (bone) 213.0
 upper jaw (bone) 213.0
Cementoperiostitis 523.40
 acute 523.33
 apical 523.40
Cephalgia, cephalalgia — *see also* Headache 784.0
 histamine 339.00
 nonorganic origin 307.81
 other trigeminal autonomic (TACS) 339.09
 psychogenic 307.81
 tension 307.81
Cephalhematocele, cephalematocele
 due to birth injury 767.19
 fetus or newborn 767.19
 traumatic (*see also* Contusion, head) 920
Cephalhematoma, cephalematoma (calcified)
 due to birth injury 767.19
 fetus or newborn 767.19
 traumatic (*see also* Contusion, head) 920
Cephalic — *see* condition
Cephalitis — *see* Encephalitis
Cephalocele 742.0
Cephaloma — *see* Neoplasm, by site, malignant
Cephalomenia 625.8
Cephalopelvic — *see* condition
Cercomoniasis 007.3
Cerebellitis — *see* Encephalitis
Cerebellum (cerebellar) — *see* condition
Cerebral — *see* condition
Cerebritis — *see* Encephalitis
Cerebrohepatorenal syndrome 759.89
Cerebromacular degeneration 330.1
Cerebromalacia — *see also* Softening, brain 348.89
 due to cerebrovascular accident 438.89
Cerebrosidosis 272.7
Cerebrospasticity — *see* Palsy, cerebral
Cerebrospinal — *see* condition
Cerebrum — *see* condition
Ceroid storage disease 272.7
Cerumen (accumulation) (impacted) 380.4
Cervical — *see also* condition
 auricle 744.43
 high risk human papillomavirus (HPV) DNA test positive 795.05

Cervical — *see also* condition — *continued*
 intraepithelial glandular neoplasia 233.1
 low risk human papillomavirus (HPV) DNA test positive 795.09
 rib 756.2
 shortening — *see* Short, cervical
Cervicalgia 723.1
Cervicitis (acute) (chronic) (nonvenereal) (subacute) (with erosion or ectropion) 616.0
 with
  abortion — *see* Abortion, by type, with sepsis
  ectopic pregnancy (*see also* categories 633.0–633.9) 639.0
  molar pregnancy (*see also* categories 630–632) 639.0
  ulceration 616.0
 chlamydial 099.53
 complicating pregnancy or puerperium 646.6 ☑
  affecting fetus or newborn 760.8
 following
  abortion 639.0
  ectopic or molar pregnancy 639.0
 gonococcal (acute) 098.15
  chronic or duration of 2 months or more 098.35
 senile (atrophic) 616.0
 syphilitic 095.8
 trichomonal 131.09
 tuberculous (*see also* Tuberculosis) 016.7 ☑
Cervicoaural fistula 744.49
Cervicocolpitis (emphysematosa) — *see also* Cervicitis 616.0
Cervix — *see* condition
Cesarean delivery, operation or section NEC 669.7 ☑
 affecting fetus or newborn 763.4
 (planned) occurring after 37 completed weeks of gestation but before 39 completed weeks gestation due to (spontaneous) onset of labor 649.8 ☑
 post mortem, affecting fetus or newborn 761.6
 previous, affecting management of pregnancy 654.2 ☑
Céstan-Chenais paralysis 344.89
Céstan-Raymond syndrome 433.8 ☑
Céstan's syndrome 344.89
Cestode infestation NEC 123.9
 specified type NEC 123.8
Cestodiasis 123.9
CGF (congenital generalized fibromatosis) 759.89
Chabert's disease 022.9
Chacaleh 266.2
Chafing 709.8
Chagas' disease — *see also* Trypanosomiasis, American 086.2
 with heart involvement 086.0
Chagres fever 084.0
Chalasia (cardiac sphincter) 530.81
Chalazion 373.2
Chalazoderma 757.39
Chalcosis 360.24
 cornea 371.15
 crystalline lens 360.24 [366.34]
 retina 360.24
Chalicosis (occupational) (pulmonum) 502
Chancre (any genital site) (hard) (indurated) (infecting) (primary) (recurrent) 091.0
 congenital 090.0
 conjunctiva 091.2
 Ducrey's 099.0
 extragenital 091.2
 eyelid 091.2
 Hunterian 091.0
 lip (syphilis) 091.2
 mixed 099.8
 nipple 091.2
 Nisbet's 099.0
 of
  carate 103.0
  pinta 103.0

Catatonia, catatonic — Chancre

☑ **Additional Digit Required** — Refer to the Tabular List for Digit Selection   🔻 **Subterms under main terms may continue to next column or page**

Chancre — continued
of — continued
yaws 102.0
palate, soft 091.2
phagedenic 099.0
Ricord's 091.0
Rollet's (syphilitic) 091.0
seronegative 091.0
seropositive 091.0
simple 099.0
soft 099.0
bubo 099.0
urethra 091.0
yaws 102.0
Chancriform syndrome 114.1
Chancroid 099.0
anus 099.0
penis (Ducrey's bacillus) 099.0
perineum 099.0
rectum 099.0
scrotum 099.0
urethra 099.0
vulva 099.0
Chandipura fever 066.8
Chandler's disease (osteochondritis dissecans, hip) 732.7
Change(s) (of) — see also Removal of
arteriosclerotic — see Arteriosclerosis
battery
cardiac pacemaker V53.31
bone 733.90
diabetic 250.8 ☑ [731.8]
due to secondary diabetes 249.8 ☑ [731.8]
in disease, unknown cause 733.90
bowel habits 787.99
cardiorenal (vascular) (see also Hypertension, cardiorenal) 404.90
cardiovascular — see Disease, cardiovascular
circulatory 459.9
cognitive or personality change of other type, nonpsychotic 310.1
color, teeth, tooth
during formation 520.8
extrinsic 523.6
intrinsic posteruptive 521.7
contraceptive device V25.42
cornea, corneal
degenerative NEC 371.40
membrane NEC 371.30
senile 371.41
coronary (see also Ischemia, heart) 414.9
degenerative
chamber angle (anterior) (iris) 364.56
ciliary body 364.57
spine or vertebra (see also Spondylosis) 721.90
dental pulp, regressive 522.2
drains V58.49
dressing
wound V58.30
nonsurgical V58.30
surgical V58.31
fixation device V54.89
external V54.89
internal V54.01
heart (see also Disease, heart)
hip joint 718.95
hyperplastic larynx 478.79
hypertrophic
nasal sinus (see also Sinusitis) 473.9
turbinate, nasal 478.0
upper respiratory tract 478.9
inflammatory — see Inflammation
joint (see also Derangement, joint) 718.90
sacroiliac 724.6
Kirschner wire V54.89
knee 717.9
macular, congenital 743.55

Change(s) — see also Removal of — continued
malignant (M — — /3) (see also Neoplasm, by site, malignant)

Note — for malignant change occurring in a neoplasm, use the appropriate M code with behavior digit /3 e.g., malignant change in uterine fibroid — M8890/3. For malignant change occurring in a nonneoplastic condition (e.g., gastric ulcer) use the M code M8000/3.

mental (status) NEC 780.97
due to or associated with physical condition — see Syndrome, brain
myocardium, myocardial — see Degeneration, myocardial
of life (see also Menopause) 627.2
pacemaker battery (cardiac) V53.31
peripheral nerve 355.9
personality (nonpsychotic) NEC 310.1
plaster cast V54.89
refractive, transient 367.81
regressive, dental pulp 522.2
retina 362.9
myopic (degenerative) (malignant) 360.21
vascular appearance 362.13
sacroiliac joint 724.6
scleral 379.19
degenerative 379.16
senile (see also Senility) 797
sensory (see also Disturbance, sensation) 782.0
skin texture 782.8
spinal cord 336.9
splint, external V54.89
subdermal implantable contraceptive V25.5
suture V58.32
traction device V54.89
trophic 355.9
arm NEC 354.9
leg NEC 355.8
lower extremity NEC 355.8
upper extremity NEC 354.9
vascular 459.9
vasomotor 443.9
voice 784.49
psychogenic 306.1
wound packing V58.30
nonsurgical V58.30
surgical V58.31
Changing sleep-work schedule, affecting sleep 327.36
Changuinola fever 066.0
Chapping skin 709.8
Character
depressive 301.12
Charcôt's
arthropathy 094.0 [713.5]
cirrhosis — see Cirrhosis, biliary
disease 094.0
spinal cord 094.0
fever (biliary) (hepatic) (intermittent) — see Choledocholithiasis
joint (disease) 094.0 [713.5]
diabetic 250.6 ☑ [713.5]
due to secondary diabetes 249.6 ☑ [713.5]
syringomyelic 336.0 [713.5]
syndrome (intermittent claudication) 443.9
due to atherosclerosis 440.21
Charcôt-Marie-Tooth disease, paralysis, or syndrome 356.1
CHARGE association (syndrome) 759.89
Charleyhorse (quadriceps) 843.8
muscle, except quadriceps — see Sprain, by site
Charlouis' disease — see also Yaws 102.9
Chauffeur's fracture — see Fracture, ulna, lower end
Cheadle (-Möller) (-Barlow) disease or syndrome (infantile scurvy) 267
Checking (of)
contraceptive device (intrauterine) V25.42
device
fixation V54.89

Checking — continued
device — continued
fixation — continued
external V54.89
internal V54.09
traction V54.89
Kirschner wire V54.89
plaster cast V54.89
splint, external V54.89
Checkup
following treatment — see Examination
health V70.0
infant (over 28 days old) (not sick) V20.2
newborn, routine
8 to 28 days old V20.32
over 28 days old, routine V20.2
under 8 days old V20.31
weight V20.32
pregnancy (normal) V22.1
first V22.0
high-risk pregnancy V23.9
inconclusive fetal viability V23.87
specified problem NEC V23.89
Chédiak-Higashi (-Steinbrinck) anomaly, disease, or syndrome (congenital gigantism of peroxidase granules) 288.2
Cheek — see also condition
biting 528.9
Cheese itch 133.8
Cheese washers' lung 495.8
Cheilitis 528.5
actinic (due to sun) 692.72
chronic NEC 692.74
due to radiation, except from sun 692.82
due to radiation, except from sun 692.82
acute 528.5
angular 528.5
catarrhal 528.5
chronic 528.5
exfoliative 528.5
gangrenous 528.5
glandularis apostematosa 528.5
granulomatosa 351.8
infectional 528.5
membranous 528.5
Miescher's 351.8
suppurative 528.5
ulcerative 528.5
vesicular 528.5
Cheilodynia 528.5
Cheilopalatoschisis — see also Cleft, palate, with cleft lip 749.20
Cheilophagia 528.9
Cheiloschisis — see also Cleft, lip 749.10
Cheilosis 528.5
with pellagra 265.2
angular 528.5
due to
dietary deficiency 266.0
vitamin deficiency 266.0
Cheiromegaly 729.89
Cheiropompholyx 705.81
Cheloid — see also Keloid 701.4
Chemical burn — see also Burn, by site
from swallowing chemical — see Burn, internal organs
Chemodectoma (M8693/1) — see Paraganglioma, nonchromaffin
Chemoprophylaxis NEC V07.39
Chemosis, conjunctiva 372.73
Chemotherapy
convalescence V66.2
encounter (for) (oral) (intravenous) V58.11
maintenance (oral) (intravenous) V58.11
prophylactic NEC V07.39
fluoride V07.31
Cherubism 526.89
Chest — see condition
Cheyne-Stokes respiration (periodic) 786.04
Chiari's
disease or syndrome (hepatic vein thrombosis) 453.0
malformation
type I 348.4
type II (see also Spina bifida) 741.0 ☑

Chiari's — continued
malformation — continued
type III 742.0
type IV 742.2
network 746.89
Chiari-Frommel syndrome 676.6 ☑
Chicago disease (North American blastomycosis) 116.0
Chickenpox — see also Varicella 052.9
exposure to V01.71
vaccination and inoculation (prophylactic) V05.4
Chiclero ulcer 085.4
Chiggers 133.8
Chignon 111.2
fetus or newborn (from vacuum extraction) 767.19
Chigoe disease 134.1
Chikungunya fever 066.3
Chilaiditi's syndrome (subphrenic displacement, colon) 751.4
Chilblains 991.5
lupus 991.5
Child
behavior causing concern V61.20
adopted child V61.24
biological child V61.23
foster child V61.25
Childbed fever 670.8 ☑
Childbirth — see also Delivery
puerperal complications — see Puerperal
Childhood, period of rapid growth V21.0
Chill(s) 780.64
with fever 780.60
without fever 780.64
congestive 780.99
in malarial regions 084.6
septic — see Septicemia
urethral 599.84
Chilomastigiasis 007.8
Chin — see condition
Chinese dysentery 004.9
Chiropractic dislocation — see also Lesion, nonallopathic, by site 739.9
Chitral fever 066.0
Chlamydia, chlamydial — see condition
Chloasma 709.09
cachecticorum 709.09
eyelid 374.52
congenital 757.33
hyperthyroid 242.0 ☑
gravidarum 646.8 ☑
idiopathic 709.09
skin 709.09
symptomatic 709.09
Chloroma (M9930/3) 205.3 ☑
Chlorosis 280.9
Egyptian (see also Ancylostomiasis) 126.9
miners' (see also Ancylostomiasis) 126.9
Chlorotic anemia 280.9
Chocolate cyst (ovary) 617.1
Choked
disk or disc — see Papilledema
on food, phlegm, or vomitus NEC (see also Asphyxia, food) 933.1
phlegm 933.1
while vomiting NEC (see also Asphyxia, food) 933.1
Chokes (resulting from bends) 993.3
Choking sensation 784.99
Cholangiectasis — see also Disease, gallbladder 575.8
Cholangiocarcinoma (M8160/3)
and hepatocellular carcinoma, combined (M8180/3) 155.0
liver 155.1
specified site NEC — see Neoplasm, by site, malignant
unspecified site 155.1
Cholangiohepatitis 575.8
due to fluke infestation 121.1
Cholangiohepatoma (M8180/3) 155.0
Cholangiolitis (acute) (chronic) (extrahepatic) (gangrenous) 576.1
intrahepatic 575.8

☑ **Additional Digit Required** — Refer to the Tabular List for Digit Selection

▽ **Subterms under main terms may continue to next column or page**

46 — Volume 2
▶◀ **Revised Text**
● **New Line**
▲ **Revised Code**
2013 ICD-9-CM

Cholangiolitis — *continued*
  paratyphoidal (*see also* Fever, paratyphoid)
    002.9
  typhoidal 002.0
Cholangioma (M8160/0) 211.5
  malignant — *see* Cholangiocarcinoma
Cholangitis (acute) (ascending) (catarrhal)
  (chronic) (infective) (malignant) (primary) (recurrent) (sclerosing) (secondary)
  (stenosing) (suppurative) 576.1
  chronic nonsuppurative destructive 571.6
  nonsuppurative destructive (chronic) 571.6
Cholecystdocholithiasis — *see* Choledocholithiasis
Cholecystitis 575.10
  with
    calculus, stones in
      bile duct (common) (hepatic) — *see*
        Choledocholithiasis
      gallbladder — *see* Cholelithiasis
  acute 575.0
  acute and chronic 575.12
  chronic 575.11
  emphysematous (acute) (*see also* Cholecys-
    titis, acute) 575.0
  gangrenous (*see also* Cholecystitis, acute)
    575.0
  paratyphoidal, current (*see also* Fever,
    paratyphoid) 002.9
  suppurative (*see also* Cholecystitis, acute)
    575.0
  typhoidal 002.0
Choledochitis (suppurative) 576.1
Choledocholith — *see* Choledocholithiasis
Choledocholithiasis 574.5 ☑

Note — Use the following fifth-digit
subclassification with category 574:
  0 without mention of obstruction
  1 with obstruction

  with
    cholecystitis 574.4 ☑
      acute 574.3 ☑
      chronic 574.4 ☑
    cholelithiasis 574.9 ☑
      with
        cholecystitis 574.7 ☑
          acute 574.6 ☑
          and chronic 574.8 ☑
        chronic 574.7 ☑
Cholelithiasis (impacted) (multiple) 574.2 ☑

Note — Use the following fifth-digit
subclassification with category 574:
  0 without mention of obstruction
  1 with obstruction

  with
    cholecystitis 574.1 ☑
      acute 574.0 ☑
      chronic 574.1 ☑
    choledocholithiasis 574.9 ☑
      with
        cholecystitis 574.7 ☑
          acute 574.6 ☑
          and chronic 574.8 ☑
        chronic cholecystitis 574.7 ☑
Cholemia — *see also* Jaundice 782.4
  familial 277.4
  Gilbert's (familial nonhemolytic) 277.4
Cholemic gallstone — *see* Cholelithiasis
Choleperitoneum, choleperitonitis — *see
  also* Disease, gallbladder 567.81
Cholera (algid) (Asiatic) (asphyctic) (epidemic)
  (gravis) (Indian) (malignant) (morbus)
  (pestilential) (spasmodic) 001.9
  antimonial 985.4
  carrier (suspected) of V02.0
  classical 001.0
  contact V01.0
  due to
    Vibrio
      cholerae (Inaba, Ogawa, Hikojima
        serotypes) 001.0
      El Tor 001.1

Cholera — *continued*
  El Tor 001.1
    exposure to V01.0
    vaccination, prophylactic (against) V03.0
Cholerine — *see also* Cholera 001.9
Cholestasis 576.8
  due to total parenteral nutrition (TPN) 573.8
Cholesteatoma (ear) 385.30
  attic (primary) 385.31
  diffuse 385.35
  external ear (canal) 380.21
  marginal (middle ear) 385.32
    with involvement of mastoid cavity
      385.33
    secondary (with middle ear involvement)
      385.33
  mastoid cavity 385.30
  middle ear (secondary) 385.32
    with involvement of mastoid cavity
      385.33
  postmastoidectomy cavity (recurrent)
    383.32
  primary 385.31
  recurrent, postmastoidectomy cavity 383.32
  secondary (middle ear) 385.32
    with involvement of mastoid cavity
      385.33
Cholesteatosis (middle ear) — *see also*
  Cholesteatoma 385.30
  diffuse 385.35
Cholesteremia 272.0
Cholesterin
  granuloma, middle ear 385.82
  in vitreous 379.22
Cholesterol
  deposit
    retina 362.82
    vitreous 379.22
  elevated (high) 272.0
    with elevated (high) triglycerides 272.2
  imbibition of gallbladder (*see also* Disease,
    gallbladder) 575.6
Cholesterolemia 272.0
  essential 272.0
  familial 272.0
  hereditary 272.0
Cholesterosis, cholesterolosis (gallbladder)
  575.6
  with
    cholecystitis — *see* Cholecystitis
    cholelithiasis — *see* Cholelithiasis
  middle ear (*see also* Cholesteatoma) 385.30
Cholocolic fistula — *see also* Fistula, gallbladder 575.5
Choluria 791.4
Chondritis (purulent) 733.99
  auricle 380.03
  costal 733.6
    Tietze's 733.6
  patella, posttraumatic 717.7
  pinna 380.03
  posttraumatica patellae 717.7
  tuberculous (active) (*see also* Tuberculosis)
    015.9 ☑
    intervertebral 015.0 ☑ *[730.88]*
Chondroangiopathia calcarea seu punctate
  756.59
Chondroblastoma (M9230/0) — *see also*
  Neoplasm, bone, benign
  malignant (M9230/3) — *see* Neoplasm,
    bone, malignant
Chondrocalcinosis (articular) (crystal deposition) (dihydrate) — *see also* Arthritis, due
  to, crystals 275.49 *[712.3]* ☑
  due to
    calcium pyrophosphate
      275.49 *[712.2]* ☑
    dicalcium phosphate crystals
      275.49 *[712.1]* ☑
    pyrophosphate crystals 275.49 *[712.2]* ☑
Chondrodermatitis nodularis helicis 380.00
Chondrodysplasia 756.4
  angiomatose 756.4
  calcificans congenita 756.59
  epiphysialis punctata 756.59
  hereditary deforming 756.4

Chondrodysplasia — *continued*
  rhizomelic punctata 277.86
Chondrodystrophia (fetalis) 756.4
  calcarea 756.4
  calcificans congenita 756.59
  fetalis hypoplastica 756.59
  hypoplastica calcinosa 756.59
  punctata 756.59
  tarda 277.5
Chondrodystrophy (familial) (hypoplastic)
  756.4
  myotonic (congenital) 359.23
Chondroectodermal dysplasia 756.55
Chondrolysis 733.99
Chondroma (M9220/0) — *see also* Neoplasm
  cartilage, benign
  juxtacortical (M9221/0) — *see* Neoplasm,
    bone, benign
  periosteal (M9221/0) — *see* Neoplasm,
    bone, benign
Chondromalacia 733.92
  epiglottis (congenital) 748.3
  generalized 733.92
  knee 717.7
  larynx (congenital) 748.3
  localized, except patella 733.92
  patella, patellae 717.7
  systemic 733.92
  tibial plateau 733.92
  trachea (congenital) 748.3
Chondromatosis (M9220/1) — *see* Neoplasm,
  cartilage, uncertain behavior
Chondromyxosarcoma (M9220/3) — *see*
  Neoplasm, cartilage, malignant
Chondro-osteodysplasia (Morquio-Brailsford
  type) 277.5
Chondro-osteodystrophy 277.5
Chondro-osteoma (M9210/0) — *see* Neoplasm, bone, benign
Chondropathia tuberosa 733.6
Chondrosarcoma (M9220/3) — *see also* Neoplasm, cartilage, malignant
  juxtacortical (M9221/3) — *see* Neoplasm,
    bone, malignant
  mesenchymal (M9240/3) — *see* Neoplasm,
    connective tissue, malignant
Chordae tendineae rupture (chronic) 429.5
Chordee (nonvenereal) 607.89
  congenital 752.63
  gonococcal 098.2
Chorditis (fibrinous) (nodosa) (tuberosa) 478.5
Chordoma (M9370/3) — *see* Neoplasm, by site,
  malignant
Chorea (gravis) (minor) (spasmodic) 333.5
  with
    heart involvement — *see* Chorea with
      rheumatic heart disease
    rheumatic heart disease (chronic, inac-
      tive, or quiescent) (conditions
      classifiable to 393–398) (*see*
      rheumatic heart condition in-
      volved)
      active or acute (conditions classifi-
        able to 391) 392.0
  acute — *see* Chorea, Sydenham's
  apoplectic (*see also* Disease, cerebrovascu-
    lar, acute) 436
  chronic 333.4
  electric 049.8
  gravidarum — *see* Eclampsia, pregnancy
  habit 307.22
  hereditary 333.4
  Huntington's 333.4
  posthemiplegic 344.89
  pregnancy — *see* Eclampsia, pregnancy
  progressive 333.4
    chronic 333.4
    hereditary 333.4
  rheumatic (chronic) 392.9
    with heart disease or involvement — *see*
      Chorea, with rheumatic heart
      disease
  senile 333.5
  Sydenham's 392.9
    with heart involvement — *see* Chorea,
      with rheumatic heart disease

Chorea — *continued*
  Sydenham's — *continued*
    nonrheumatic 333.5
  variabilis 307.23
Choreoathetosis (paroxysmal) 333.5
Chorioadenoma (destruens) (M9100/1) 236.1
Chorioamnionitis 658.4 ☑
  affecting fetus or newborn 762.7
Chorioangioma (M9120/0) 219.8
Choriocarcinoma (M9100/3)
  combined with
    embryonal carcinoma (M9101/3) — *see*
      Neoplasm, by site, malignant
    teratoma (M9101/3) — *see* Neoplasm,
      by site, malignant
  specified site — *see* Neoplasm, by site, ma-
    lignant
  unspecified site
    female 181
    male 186.9
Chorioencephalitis, lymphocytic (acute)
  (serous) 049.0
Chorioepithelioma (M9100/3) — *see* Choriocarcinoma
Choriomeningitis (acute) (benign) (lymphocytic) (serous) 049.0
Chorionepithelioma (M9100/3) — *see* Choriocarcinoma
Chorionitis — *see also* Scleroderma 710.1
Chorioretinitis 363.20
  disseminated 363.10
    generalized 363.13
    in
      neurosyphilis 094.83
      secondary syphilis 091.51
    peripheral 363.12
    posterior pole 363.11
    tuberculous (*see also* Tuberculosis)
      017.3 ☑ *[363.13]*
  due to
    histoplasmosis (*see also* Histoplasmosis)
      115.92
    toxoplasmosis (acquired) 130.2
      congenital (active) 771.2
  focal 363.00
    juxtapapillary 363.01
    peripheral 363.04
    posterior pole NEC 363.03
  juxtapapillaris, juxtapapillary 363.01
  progressive myopia (degeneration) 360.21
  syphilitic (secondary) 091.51
    congenital (early) 090.0 *[363.13]*
      late 090.5 *[363.13]*
    late 095.8 *[363.13]*
  tuberculous (*see also* Tuberculosis)
    017.3 ☑ *[363.13]*
Choristoma — *see* Neoplasm, by site, benign
Choroid — *see* condition
Choroideremia, choroidermia (initial stage)
  (late stage) (partial or total atrophy)
  363.55
Choroiditis — *see also* Chorioretinitis 363.20
  leprous 030.9 *[363.13]*
  senile guttate 363.41
  sympathetic 360.11
  syphilitic (secondary) 091.51
    congenital (early) 090.0 *[363.13]*
      late 090.5 *[363.13]*
    late 095.8 *[363.13]*
  Tay's 363.41
  tuberculous (*see also* Tuberculosis)
    017.3 ☑ *[363.13]*
Choroidopathy NEC 363.9
  degenerative (*see also* Degeneration,
    choroid) 363.40
  hereditary (*see also* Dystrophy, choroid)
    363.50
  specified type NEC 363.8
Choroidoretinitis — *see* Chorioretinitis
Choroidosis, central serous 362.41
Choroidretinopathy, serous 362.41
Christian's syndrome (chronic histiocytosis X)
  277.89
Christian-Weber disease (nodular nonsuppu-
  rative panniculitis) 729.30
Christmas disease 286.1

☑ Additional Digit Required — Refer to the Tabular List for Digit Selection   Subterms under main terms may continue to next column or page

Chromaffinoma (M8700/0) — *see also* Neoplasm, by site, benign
  malignant (M8700/3) — *see* Neoplasm, by site, malignant
Chromatopsia 368.59
Chromhidrosis, chromidrosis 705.89
Chromoblastomycosis 117.2
Chromomycosis 117.2
Chromophytosis 111.0
Chromotrichomycosis 111.8
Chronic — *see* condition
Churg-Strauss syndrome 446.4
Chyle cyst, mesentery 457.8
Chylocele (nonfilarial) 457.8
  filarial (*see also* Infestation, filarial) 125.9
  tunica vaginalis (nonfilarial) 608.84
    filarial (*see also* Infestation, filarial) 125.9
Chylomicronemia (fasting) (with hyperprebe-talipoproteinemia) 272.3
Chylopericardium (acute) 420.90
Chylothorax (nonfilarial) 457.8
  filarial (*see also* Infestation, filarial) 125.9
Chylous
  ascites 457.8
  cyst of peritoneum 457.8
  hydrocele 603.9
  hydrothorax (nonfilarial) 457.8
    filarial (*see also* Infestation, filarial) 125.9
Chyluria 791.1
  bilharziasis 120.0
  due to
    Brugia (malayi) 125.1
    Wuchereria (bancrofti) 125.0
      malayi 125.1
  filarial (*see also* Infestation, filarial) 125.9
  filariasis (*see also* Infestation, filarial) 125.9
  nonfilarial 791.1
Cicatricial (deformity) — *see* Cicatrix
Cicatrix (adherent) (contracted) (painful) (vicious) 709.2
  adenoid 474.8
  alveolar process 525.8
  anus 569.49
  auricle 380.89
  bile duct (*see also* Disease, biliary) 576.8
  bladder 596.89
  bone 733.99
  brain 348.89
  cervix (postoperative) (postpartal) 622.3
    in pregnancy or childbirth 654.6 ☑
      causing obstructed labor 660.2 ☑
  chorioretinal 363.30
    disseminated 363.35
    macular 363.32
    peripheral 363.34
    posterior pole NEC 363.33
  choroid — *see* Cicatrix, chorioretinal
  common duct (*see also* Disease, biliary) 576.8
  congenital 757.39
  conjunctiva 372.64
  cornea 371.00
    tuberculous (*see also* Tuberculosis) 017.3 ☑ [371.05]
  duodenum (bulb) 537.3
  esophagus 530.3
  eyelid 374.46
    with
      ectropion — *see* Ectropion
      entropion — *see* Entropion
  hypopharynx 478.29
  knee, semilunar cartilage 717.5
  lacrimal
    canaliculi 375.53
    duct
      acquired 375.56
      neonatal 375.55
    punctum 375.52
    sac 375.54
  larynx 478.79
  limbus (cystoid) 372.64
  lung 518.89
  macular 363.32
    disseminated 363.35
    peripheral 363.34
  middle ear 385.89

Cicatrix — *continued*
  mouth 528.9
  muscle 728.89
  nasolacrimal duct
    acquired 375.56
    neonatal 375.55
  nasopharynx 478.29
  palate (soft) 528.9
  penis 607.89
  prostate 602.8
  rectum 569.49
  retina 363.30
    disseminated 363.35
    macular 363.32
    peripheral 363.34
    posterior pole NEC 363.33
  semilunar cartilage — *see* Derangement, meniscus
  seminal vesicle 608.89
  skin 709.2
    infected 686.8
    postinfectional 709.2
    tuberculous (*see also* Tuberculosis) 017.0 ☑
  specified site NEC 709.2
  throat 478.29
  tongue 529.8
  tonsil (and adenoid) 474.8
  trachea 478.9
  tuberculous NEC (*see also* Tuberculosis) 011.9 ☑
  ureter 593.89
  urethra 599.84
  uterus 621.8
  vagina 623.4
    in pregnancy or childbirth 654.7 ☑
      causing obstructed labor 660.2 ☑
  vocal cord 478.5
  wrist, constricting (annular) 709.2
CIDP (chronic inflammatory demyelinating polyneuropathy) 357.81
CIN I (cervical intraepithelial neoplasia I) 622.11
CIN II (cervical intraepithelial neoplasia II) 622.12
CIN III (cervical intraepithelial neoplasia III) 233.1
Cinchonism
  correct substance properly administered 386.9
  overdose or wrong substance given or taken 961.4
Circine herpes 110.5
Circle of Willis — *see* condition
Circular — *see also* condition
  hymen 752.49
Circulating anticoagulants, antibodies, or inhibitors — *see also* Anticoagulants 286.59
  extrinsic 287.8
  following childbirth 666.3 ☑
  intrinsic, causing hemorrhagic disorder 286.59
    with
      acquired hemophilia 286.52
      antiphospholipid antibody 286.53
  postpartum 666.3 ☑
Circulation
  collateral (venous), any site 459.89
  defective 459.9
    congenital 747.9
    lower extremity 459.89
  embryonic 747.9
  failure 799.89
    fetus or newborn 779.89
    peripheral 785.59
  fetal, persistent 747.83
  heart, incomplete 747.9
Circulatory system — *see* condition
Circulus senilis 371.41
Circumcision
  in absence of medical indication V50.2
  ritual V50.2
  routine V50.2
  status (post), female 629.20
Circumscribed — *see* condition

Circumvallata placenta — *see* Placenta, abnormal
Cirrhosis, cirrhotic 571.5
  with alcoholism 571.2
  alcoholic (liver) 571.2
  atrophic (of liver) — *see* Cirrhosis, portal
  Baumgarten-Cruveilhier 571.5
  biliary (cholangiolitic) (cholangitic) (cholestatic) (extrahepatic) (hypertrophic) (intrahepatic) (nonobstructive) (obstructive) (pericholangiolitic) (posthepatic) (primary) (secondary) (xanthomatous) 571.6
    due to
      clonorchiasis 121.1
      flukes 121.3
  brain 331.9
  capsular — *see* Cirrhosis, portal
  cardiac 571.5
    alcoholic 571.2
  central (liver) — *see* Cirrhosis, liver
  Charcôt's 571.6
  cholangiolitic — *see* Cirrhosis, biliary
  cholangitic — *see* Cirrhosis, biliary
  cholestatic — *see* Cirrhosis, biliary
  clitoris (hypertrophic) 624.2
  coarsely nodular 571.5
  congestive (liver) — *see* Cirrhosis, cardiac
  Cruveilhier-Baumgarten 571.5
  cryptogenic (of liver) 571.5
    alcoholic 571.2
  dietary (*see also* Cirrhosis, portal) 571.5
  due to
    bronzed diabetes 275.01
    congestive hepatomegaly — *see* Cirrhosis, cardiac
    cystic fibrosis 277.00
    hemochromatosis (*see also* Hemochromatosis) 275.03
    hepatolenticular degeneration 275.1
    passive congestion (chronic) — *see* Cirrhosis, cardiac
    Wilson's disease 275.1
    xanthomatosis 272.2
  extrahepatic (obstructive) — *see* Cirrhosis, biliary
  fatty 571.8
    alcoholic 571.0
  florid 571.2
  Glisson's — *see* Cirrhosis, portal
  Hanot's (hypertrophic) — *see* Cirrhosis, biliary
  hepatic — *see* Cirrhosis, liver
  hepatolienal — *see* Cirrhosis, liver
  hobnail — *see* Cirrhosis, portal
  hypertrophic (*see also* Cirrhosis, liver)
    biliary — *see* Cirrhosis, biliary
    Hanot's — *see* Cirrhosis, biliary
  infectious NEC — *see* Cirrhosis, portal
  insular — *see* Cirrhosis, portal
  intrahepatic (obstructive) (primary) (secondary) — *see* Cirrhosis, biliary
  juvenile (*see also* Cirrhosis, portal) 571.5
  kidney (*see also* Sclerosis, renal) 587
  Laennec's (of liver) 571.2
    nonalcoholic 571.5
  liver (chronic) (hepatolienal) (hypertrophic) (nodular) (splenomegalic) (unilobar) 571.5
    with alcoholism 571.2
    alcoholic 571.2
    congenital (due to failure of obliteration of umbilical vein) 777.8
    cryptogenic 571.5
      alcoholic 571.2
    fatty 571.8
      alcoholic 571.0
    macronodular 571.5
      alcoholic 571.2
    micronodular 571.5
      alcoholic 571.2
    nodular, diffuse 571.5
      alcoholic 571.2
    pigmentary 275.01
    portal 571.5
      alcoholic 571.2

Cirrhosis, cirrhotic — *continued*
  liver — *continued*
    postnecrotic 571.5
      alcoholic 571.2
    syphilitic 095.3
  lung (chronic) (*see also* Fibrosis, lung) 515
  macronodular (of liver) 571.5
    alcoholic 571.2
  malarial 084.9
  metabolic NEC 571.5
  micronodular (of liver) 571.5
    alcoholic 571.2
  monolobular — *see* Cirrhosis, portal
  multilobular — *see* Cirrhosis, portal
  nephritis (*see also* Sclerosis, renal) 587
  nodular — *see* Cirrhosis, liver
  nutritional (fatty) 571.5
  obstructive (biliary) (extrahepatic) (intrahepatic) — *see* Cirrhosis, biliary
  ovarian 620.8
  paludal 084.9
  pancreas (duct) 577.8
  pericholangiolitic — *see* Cirrhosis, biliary
  periportal — *see* Cirrhosis, portal
  pigment, pigmentary (of liver) 275.01
  portal (of liver) 571.5
    alcoholic 571.2
  posthepatitic (*see also* Cirrhosis, postnecrotic) 571.5
  postnecrotic (of liver) 571.5
    alcoholic 571.2
  primary (intrahepatic) — *see* Cirrhosis, biliary
  pulmonary (*see also* Fibrosis, lung) 515
  renal (*see also* Sclerosis, renal) 587
  septal (*see also* Cirrhosis, postnecrotic) 571.5
  spleen 289.51
  splenomegalic (of liver) — *see* Cirrhosis, liver
  stasis (liver) — *see* Cirrhosis, liver
  stomach 535.4 ☑
  Todd's (*see also* Cirrhosis, biliary) 571.6
  toxic (nodular) — *see* Cirrhosis, postnecrotic
  trabecular — *see* Cirrhosis, postnecrotic
  unilobar — *see* Cirrhosis, liver
  vascular (of liver) — *see* Cirrhosis, liver
  xanthomatous (biliary) (*see also* Cirrhosis, biliary) 571.6
    due to xanthomatosis (familial) (metabolic) (primary) 272.2
Cistern, subarachnoid 793.0
Citrullinemia 270.6
Citrullinuria 270.6
Ciuffini-Pancoast tumor (M8010/3) (carcinoma, pulmonary apex) 162.3
Civatte's disease or poikiloderma 709.09
CJD (Creutzfeldt-Jakob disease) 046.19
  variant (vCJD) 046.11
CLABSI (central line-associated bloodstream infection) 999.32
Clam diggers' itch 120.3
Clap — *see* Gonorrhea
Clarke-Hadfield syndrome (pancreatic infantilism) 577.8
Clark's paralysis 343.9
Clastothrix 704.2
Claude Bernard-Horner syndrome — *see also* Neuropathy, peripheral, autonomic 337.9
Claude's syndrome 352.6
Claudication, intermittent 443.9
  cerebral (artery) (*see also* Ischemia, cerebral, transient) 435.9
  due to atherosclerosis 440.21
  spinal cord (arteriosclerotic) 435.1
    syphilitic 094.89
  spinalis 435.1
  venous (axillary) 453.89
Claudicatio venosa intermittens 453.89
Claustrophobia 300.29
Clavus (infected) 700
Clawfoot (congenital) 754.71
  acquired 736.74
Clawhand (acquired) 736.06
  congenital 755.59
Clawtoe (congenital) 754.71

Clawtoe — continued
acquired 735.5
Clay eating 307.52
Clay shovelers' fracture — see Fracture, vertebra, cervical
Cleansing of artificial opening — see also Attention to artificial opening V55.9
Cleft (congenital) — see also Imperfect, closure
alveolar process 525.8
branchial (persistent) 744.41
cyst 744.42
clitoris 752.49
cricoid cartilage, posterior 748.3
facial (see also Cleft, lip) 749.10
lip 749.10
with cleft palate 749.20
bilateral (lip and palate) 749.24
with unilateral lip or palate 749.25
complete 749.23
incomplete 749.24
unilateral (lip and palate) 749.22
with bilateral lip or palate 749.25
complete 749.21
incomplete 749.22
bilateral 749.14
with cleft palate, unilateral 749.25
complete 749.13
incomplete 749.14
unilateral 749.12
with cleft palate, bilateral 749.25
complete 749.11
incomplete 749.12
nose 748.1
palate 749.00
with cleft lip 749.20
bilateral (lip and palate) 749.24
with unilateral lip or palate 749.25
complete 749.23
incomplete 749.24
unilateral (lip and palate) 749.22
with bilateral lip or palate 749.25
complete 749.21
incomplete 749.22
bilateral 749.04
with cleft lip, unilateral 749.25
complete 749.03
incomplete 749.04
unilateral 749.02
with cleft lip, bilateral 749.25
complete 749.01
incomplete 749.02
penis 752.69
posterior, cricoid cartilage 748.3
scrotum 752.89
sternum (congenital) 756.3
thyroid cartilage (congenital) 748.3
tongue 750.13
uvula 749.02
with cleft lip (see also Cleft, lip, with cleft palate) 749.20
water 366.12
Cleft hand (congenital) 755.58
Cleidocranial dysostosis 755.59
Cleidotomy, fetal 763.89
Cleptomania 312.32
Clérambault's syndrome 297.8
erotomania 302.89
Clergyman's sore throat 784.49
Click, clicking
systolic syndrome 785.2
Clifford's syndrome (postmaturity) 766.22
Climacteric — see also Menopause 627.2
arthritis NEC (see also Arthritis, climacteric) 716.3 ☑
depression (see also Psychosis, affective) 296.2 ☑
disease 627.2
recurrent episode 296.3 ☑
single episode 296.2 ☑
female (symptoms) 627.2
male (symptoms) (syndrome) 608.89
melancholia (see also Psychosis, affective) 296.2 ☑
recurrent episode 296.3 ☑

Climacteric — see also Menopause — continued
melancholia (see also Psychosis, affective) — continued
single episode 296.2 ☑
paranoid state 297.2
paraphrenia 297.2
polyarthritis NEC 716.39
male 608.89
symptoms (female) 627.2
Clinical research investigation (control) (participant) V70.7
Clinodactyly 755.59
Clitoris — see condition
Cloaca, persistent 751.5
Clonorchiasis 121.1
Clonorchiosis 121.1
Clonorchis infection, liver 121.1
Clonus 781.0
Closed bite 524.20
Closed surgical procedure converted to open procedure
arthroscopic V64.43
laparoscopic V64.41
thoracoscopic V64.42
Closure
artificial opening (see also Attention to artificial opening) V55.9
congenital, nose 748.0
cranial sutures, premature 756.0
defective or imperfect NEC — see Imperfect, closure
fistula, delayed — see Fistula
fontanelle, delayed 756.0
foramen ovale, imperfect 745.5
hymen 623.3
interauricular septum, defective 745.5
interventricular septum, defective 745.4
lacrimal duct 375.56
congenital 743.65
neonatal 375.55
nose (congenital) 748.0
acquired 738.0
primary angle without glaucoma damage 365.06
vagina 623.2
valve — see Endocarditis
vulva 624.8
Clot (blood)
artery (obstruction) (occlusion) (see also Embolism) 444.9
atrial appendage 429.89
bladder 596.7
brain (extradural or intradural) (see also Thrombosis, brain) 434.0 ☑
late effect — see Late effect(s) (of) cerebrovascular disease
circulation 444.9
heart (see also Infarct, myocardium) 410.9 ☑
without myocardial infarction 429.89
vein (see also Thrombosis) 453.9
Clotting defect NEC — see also Defect, coagulation 286.9
Clouded state 780.09
epileptic (see also Epilepsy) 345.9 ☑
paroxysmal (idiopathic) (see also Epilepsy) 345.9 ☑
Clouding
corneal graft 996.51
Cloudy
antrum, antra 473.0
dialysis effluent 792.5
Clouston's (hidrotic) ectodermal dysplasia 757.31
Clubbing of fingers 781.5
Clubfinger 736.29
acquired 736.29
congenital 754.89
Clubfoot (congenital) 754.70
acquired 736.71
equinovarus 754.51
paralytic 736.71
Club hand (congenital) 754.89
acquired 736.07
Clubnail (acquired) 703.8

Clubnail — continued
congenital 757.5
Clump kidney 753.3
Clumsiness 781.3
syndrome 315.4
Cluttering — see also Disorder, fluency 315.35
Clutton's joints 090.5
Coagulation, intravascular (diffuse) (disseminated) — see also Fibrinolysis 286.6
newborn 776.2
Coagulopathy — see also Defect, coagulation 286.9
consumption 286.6
intravascular (disseminated) NEC 286.6
newborn 776.2
Coalition
calcaneoscaphoid 755.67
calcaneus 755.67
tarsal 755.67
Coal miners'
elbow 727.2
lung 500
Coal workers' lung or pneumoconiosis 500
Coarctation
aorta (postductal) (preductal) 747.10
pulmonary artery 747.31
Coated tongue 529.3
Coats' disease 362.12
Cocainism — see also Dependence 304.2 ☑
Coccidioidal granuloma 114.3
Coccidioidomycosis 114.9
with pneumonia 114.0
cutaneous (primary) 114.1
disseminated 114.3
extrapulmonary (primary) 114.1
lung 114.5
acute 114.0
chronic 114.4
primary 114.0
meninges 114.2
primary (pulmonary) 114.0
acute 114.0
prostate 114.3
pulmonary 114.5
acute 114.0
chronic 114.4
primary 114.0
specified site NEC 114.3
Coccidioidosis 114.9
lung 114.5
acute 114.0
chronic 114.4
primary 114.0
meninges 114.2
Coccidiosis (colitis) (diarrhea) (dysentery) 007.2
Cocciuria 791.9
Coccus in urine 791.9
Coccydynia 724.79
Coccygodynia 724.79
Coccyx — see condition
Cochin-China
diarrhea 579.1
anguilluliasis 127.2
ulcer 085.1
Cockayne's disease or syndrome (microcephaly and dwarfism) 759.89
Cockayne-Weber syndrome (epidermolysis bullosa) 757.39
Cocked-up toe 735.2
Cock's peculiar tumor 706.2
Codman's tumor (benign chondroblastoma) (M9230/0) — see Neoplasm, bone, benign
Coenurosis 123.8
Coffee workers' lung 495.8
Cogan's syndrome 370.52
congenital oculomotor apraxia 379.51
nonsyphilitic interstitial keratitis 370.52
Coiling, umbilical cord — see Complications, umbilical cord
Coitus, painful (female) 625.0
male 608.89
psychogenic 302.76
Cold 460
with influenza, flu, or grippe (see also Influenza) 487.1

Cold — continued
abscess (see also Tuberculosis, abscess)
articular — see Tuberculosis, joint
agglutinin
disease (chronic) or syndrome 283.0
hemoglobinuria 283.0
paroxysmal (cold) (nocturnal) 283.2
allergic (see also Fever, hay) 477.9
bronchus or chest — see Bronchitis
with grippe or influenza (see also Influenza) 487.1
common (head) 460
vaccination, prophylactic (against) V04.7
deep 464.10
effects of 991.9
specified effect NEC 991.8
excessive 991.9
specified effect NEC 991.8
exhaustion from 991.8
exposure to 991.9
specified effect NEC 991.8
grippy (see also Influenza) 487.1
head 460
injury syndrome (newborn) 778.2
intolerance 780.99
on lung — see Bronchitis
rose 477.0
sensitivity, autoimmune 283.0
virus 460
Coldsore — see also Herpes, simplex 054.9
Colibacillosis 041.49
generalized 038.42
Colibacilluria 791.9
Colic (recurrent) 789.7
abdomen 789.7
psychogenic 307.89
appendicular 543.9
appendix 543.9
bile duct — see Choledocholithiasis
biliary — see Cholelithiasis
bilious — see Cholelithiasis
common duct — see Choledocholithiasis
Devonshire NEC 984.9
specified type of lead — see Table of Drugs and Chemicals
flatulent 787.3
gallbladder or gallstone — see Cholelithiasis
gastric 536.8
hepatic (duct) — see Choledocholithiasis
hysterical 300.11
in
adult 789.0 ☑
child over 12 months old 789.0 ☑
infant 789.7
infantile 789.7
intestinal 789.7
kidney 788.0
lead NEC 984.9
specified type of lead — see Table of Drugs and Chemicals
liver (duct) — see Choledocholithiasis
mucous 564.9
psychogenic 316 [564.9]
nephritic 788.0
painter's NEC 984.9
pancreas 577.8
psychogenic 306.4
renal 788.0
saturnine NEC 984.9
specified type of lead — see Table of Drugs and Chemicals
spasmodic 789.7
ureter 788.0
urethral 599.84
due to calculus 594.2
uterus 625.8
menstrual 625.3
vermicular 543.9
virus 460
worm NEC 128.9
Colicystitis — see also Cystitis 595.9
Colitis (acute) (catarrhal) (croupous) (cystica superficialis) (exudative) (hemorrhagic) (noninfectious) (phlegmonous) (presumed noninfectious) 558.9
adaptive 564.9

☑ Additional Digit Required — Refer to the Tabular List for Digit Selection   ᴺᴱᵂ Subterms under main terms may continue to next column or page

2013 ICD-9-CM   ▶◀ Revised Text   ● New Line   ▲ Revised Code   Volume 2 — 49

Colitis — *continued*
  allergic 558.3
  amebic (*see also* Amebiasis) 006.9
    nondysenteric 006.2
  anthrax 022.2
  bacillary (*see also* Infection, Shigella) 004.9
  balantidial 007.0
  chronic 558.9
    ulcerative (*see also* Colitis, ulcerative) 556.9
  coccidial 007.2
  dietetic 558.9
  due to radiation 558.1
  eosinophilic 558.42
  functional 558.9
  gangrenous 009.0
  giardial 007.1
  granulomatous 555.1
  gravis (*see also* Colitis, ulcerative) 556.9
  infectious (*see also* Enteritis, due to, specific organism) 009.0
    presumed 009.1
  ischemic 557.9
    acute 557.0
    chronic 557.1
      due to mesenteric artery insufficiency 557.1
  membranous 564.9
    psychogenic 316 *[564.9]*
  mucous 564.9
    psychogenic 316 *[564.9]*
  necrotic 009.0
  polyposa (*see also* Colitis, ulcerative) 556.9
  protozoal NEC 007.9
  pseudomembranous 008.45
  pseudomucinous 564.9
  regional 555.1
  segmental 555.1
  septic (*see also* Enteritis, due to, specific organism) 009.0
  spastic 564.9
    psychogenic 316 *[564.9]*
  Staphylococcus 008.41
    food 005.0
  thromboulcerative 557.0
  toxic 558.2
  transmural 555.1
  trichomonal 007.3
  tuberculous (ulcerative) 014.8 ☑
  ulcerative (chronic) (idiopathic) (nonspecific) 556.9
    entero- 556.0
    fulminant 557.0
    ileo- 556.1
    left-sided 556.5
    procto- 556.2
    proctosigmoid 556.3
      psychogenic 316 *[556]* ☑
    specified NEC 556.8
    universal 556.6
Collagen disease NEC 710.9
  nonvascular 710.9
  vascular (allergic) (*see also* Angiitis, hypersensitivity) 446.20
Collagenosis — *see also* Collagen disease 710.9
  cardiovascular 425.4
  mediastinal 519.3
Collapse 780.2
  adrenal 255.8
  cardiorenal (*see also* Hypertension, cardiorenal) 404.90
  cardiorespiratory 785.51
    fetus or newborn 779.85
  cardiovascular (*see also* Disease, heart) 785.51
    fetus or newborn 779.85
  circulatory (peripheral) 785.59
    with
      abortion — *see* Abortion, by type, with shock
      ectopic pregnancy (*see also* categories 633.0–633.9) 639.5
      molar pregnancy (*see also* categories 630–632) 639.5
    during or after labor and delivery 669.1 ☑

Collapse — *continued*
  circulatory — *continued*
    fetus or newborn 779.85
    following
      abortion 639.5
      ectopic or molar pregnancy 639.5
    during or after labor and delivery 669.1 ☑
      fetus or newborn 779.89
    during or resulting from a surgical procedure 998.00
  external ear canal 380.50
    secondary to
      inflammation 380.53
      surgery 380.52
      trauma 380.51
  general 780.2
  heart — *see* Disease, heart
  heat 992.1
  hysterical 300.11
  labyrinth, membranous (congenital) 744.05
  lung (massive) (*see also* Atelectasis) 518.0
    pressure, during labor 668.0 ☑
  myocardial — *see* Disease, heart
  nervous (*see also* Disorder, mental, nonpsychotic) 300.9
  neurocirculatory 306.2
  nose 738.0
  postoperative (cardiovascular) 998.09
  pulmonary (see also Atelectasis) 518.0
    fetus or newborn 770.5
      partial 770.5
      primary 770.4
  thorax 512.89
    iatrogenic 512.1
    postoperative 512.1
  trachea 519.19
  valvular — *see* Endocarditis
  vascular (peripheral) 785.59
    with
      abortion — *see* Abortion, by type, with shock
      ectopic pregnancy (*see also* categories 633.0–633.9) 639.5
      molar pregnancy (*see also* categories 630–632) 639.5
    cerebral (*see also* Disease, cerebrovascular, acute) 436
    during or after labor and delivery 669.1 ☑
    fetus or newborn 779.89
    following
      abortion 639.5
      ectopic or molar pregnancy 639.5
    vasomotor 785.59
    vertebra 733.13
Collateral — *see also* condition
  circulation (venous) 459.89
  dilation, veins 459.89
Colles' fracture (closed) (reversed) (separation) 813.41
  open 813.51
Collet-Sicard syndrome 352.6
Collet's syndrome 352.6
Colliculitis urethralis — *see also* Urethritis 597.89
Colliers'
  asthma 500
  lung 500
  phthisis (*see also* Tuberculosis) 011.4 ☑
Collodion baby (ichthyosis congenita) 757.1
Colloid milium 709.3
Coloboma NEC 743.49
  choroid 743.59
  fundus 743.52
  iris 743.46
  lens 743.36
  lids 743.62
  optic disc (congenital) 743.57
    acquired 377.23
  retina 743.56
  sclera 743.47
Coloenteritis — *see* Enteritis
Colon — *see* condition
Colonization
  MRSA (methicillin resistant Staphylococcus aureus) V02.54

Colonization — *continued*
  MSSA (methicillin susceptible Staphylococcus aureus) V02.53
Coloptosis 569.89
Color
  amblyopia NEC 368.59
    acquired 368.55
  blindness NEC (congenital) 368.59
    acquired 368.55
Colostomy
  attention to V55.3
  fitting or adjustment V55.3
  malfunctioning 569.62
  status V44.3
Colpitis — *see also* Vaginitis 616.10
Colpocele 618.6
Colpocystitis — *see also* Vaginitis 616.10
Colporrhexis 665.4 ☑
Colpospasm 625.1
Column, spinal, vertebral — *see* condition
Coma 780.01
  apoplectic (*see also* Disease, cerebrovascular, acute) 436
  diabetic (with ketoacidosis) 250.3 ☑
    due to secondary diabetes 249.3 ☑
    hyperosmolar 250.2 ☑
      due to secondary diabetes 249.2 ☑
  eclamptic (*see also* Eclampsia) 780.39
  epileptic 345.3
  hepatic 572.2
  hyperglycemic 250.3 ☑
    due to secondary diabetes 249.3 ☑
  hyperosmolar (diabetic) (nonketotic) 250.2 ☑
    due to secondary diabetes 249.2 ☑
  hypoglycemic 251.0
    diabetic 250.3 ☑
      due to secondary diabetes 249.3 ☑
  insulin 250.3 ☑
    due to secondary diabetes 249.3 ☑
    hyperosmolar 250.2 ☑
      due to secondary diabetes 249.2 ☑
    non-diabetic 251.0
    organic hyperinsulinism 251.0
  Kussmaul's (diabetic) 250.3 ☑
    due to secondary diabetes 249.3 ☑
  liver 572.2
  newborn 779.2
  prediabetic 250.2 ☑
    due to secondary diabetes 249.2 ☑
  uremic — *see* Uremia
Combat fatigue — *see also* Reaction, stress, acute 308.9
Combined — *see* condition
Comedo 706.1
Comedocarcinoma (M8501/3) — *see also* Neoplasm, breast, malignant
  noninfiltrating (M8501/2)
    specified site — *see* Neoplasm, by site, in situ
    unspecified site 233.0
Comedomastitis 610.4
Comedones 706.1
  lanugo 757.4
Comma bacillus, carrier (suspected) of V02.3
Comminuted fracture — *see* Fracture, by site
Common
  aortopulmonary trunk 745.0
  atrioventricular canal (defect) 745.69
  atrium 745.69
  cold (head) 460
    vaccination, prophylactic (against) V04.7
  truncus (arteriosus) 745.0
  ventricle 745.3
Commotio (current)
  cerebri (*see also* Concussion, brain) 850.9
    with skull fracture — *see* Fracture, skull, by site
  retinae 921.3
  spinalis — *see* Injury, spinal, by site
Commotion (current)
  brain (without skull fracture) (*see also* Concussion, brain) 850.9
    with skull fracture — *see* Fracture, skull, by site
  spinal cord — *see* Injury, spinal, by site

Communication
  abnormal (*see also* Fistula)
    between
      base of aorta and pulmonary artery 745.0
      left ventricle and right atrium 745.4
      pericardial sac and pleural sac 748.8
      pulmonary artery and pulmonary vein 747.39
    congenital, between uterus and anterior abdominal wall 752.39
      bladder 752.39
      intestine 752.39
      rectum 752.39
    left ventricular — right atrial 745.4
    pulmonary artery-pulmonary vein 747.39
Compartment syndrome — *see* Syndrome, compartment
Compensation
  broken — *see* Failure, heart
  failure — *see* Failure, heart
  neurosis, psychoneurosis 300.11
Complaint — *see also* Disease
  bowel, functional 564.9
    psychogenic 306.4
  intestine, functional 564.9
    psychogenic 306.4
  kidney (*see also* Disease, renal) 593.9
  liver 573.9
  miners' 500
Complete — *see* condition
Complex
  cardiorenal (*see also* Hypertension, cardiorenal) 404.90
  castration 300.9
  Costen's 524.60
  ego-dystonic homosexuality 302.0
  Eisenmenger's (ventricular septal defect) 745.4
  homosexual, ego-dystonic 302.0
  hypersexual 302.89
  inferiority 301.9
  jumped process
    spine — *see* Dislocation, vertebra
  primary, tuberculosis (*see also* Tuberculosis) 010.0 ☑
  regional pain syndrome 355.9
    type I 337.20
      lower limb 337.22
      specified site NEC 337.29
      upper limb 337.21
    type II
      lower limb 355.71
      upper limb 354.4
  Taussig-Bing (transposition, aorta and overriding pulmonary artery) 745.11
Complications
  abortion NEC — *see* categories 634-639 ☑
  accidental puncture or laceration during a procedure 998.2
  amniocentesis, fetal 679.1 ☑
  amputation stump (late) (surgical) 997.60
    traumatic — *see* Amputation, traumatic
  anastomosis (and bypass) (*see also* Complications, due to (presence of) any device, implant, or graft classified to 996.0–996.5 NEC)
    hemorrhage NEC 998.11
    intestinal (internal) NEC 997.49
      involving urinary tract 997.5
    mechanical — *see* Complications, mechanical, graft
    urinary tract (involving intestinal tract) 997.5
  anesthesia, anesthetic NEC (*see also* Anesthesia, complication) 995.22
    in labor and delivery 668.9 ☑
      affecting fetus or newborn 763.5
      cardiac 668.1 ☑
      central nervous system 668.2 ☑
      pulmonary 668.0 ☑
      specified type NEC 668.8 ☑
  aortocoronary (bypass) graft 996.03
    atherosclerosis — *see* Arteriosclerosis, coronary
    embolism 996.72

☑ **Additional Digit Required — Refer to the Tabular List for Digit Selection**   � **Subterms under main terms may continue to next column or page**

Index
Colitis — Complications

Complications — *continued*
  infection and inflammation — *continued*
    due to any device, implant or graft classified to 996.0–996.5 — *continued*
      Hickman catheter — *continued*
        bloodstream 999.32
        localized 999.33
      infusion pump 996.62
      insulin pump 996.69
      intrauterine contraceptive device 996.65
      joint prosthesis, internal 996.66
      ocular lens 996.69
      orbital (implant) 996.69
      orthopedic NEC 996.67
        joint, internal 996.66
      peripherally inserted central catheter (PICC) 999.31
        bloodstream 999.32
        localized 999.33
      portacath (port-a-cath) 999.31
        bloodstream 999.32
        localized 999.33
      specified type NEC 996.69
      triple lumen catheter 999.31
        bloodstream 999.32
        localized 999.33
      umbilical venous catheter 999.31
        bloodstream 999.32
        localized 999.33
      urinary catheter, indwelling 996.64
      ventricular shunt 996.63
  infusion (procedure) 999.88
    blood — *see* Complications, transfusion
    infection NEC 999.39
    sepsis NEC 999.39
  inhalation therapy NEC 999.9
  injection (procedure) 999.9
    drug reaction (*see also* Reaction, drug) 995.27
    infection NEC 999.39
    sepsis NEC 999.39
    serum (prophylactic) (therapeutic) — *see* Complications, vaccination
    vaccine (any) — *see* Complications, vaccination
  inoculation (any) — *see* Complications, vaccination
  insulin pump 996.57
  internal device (catheter) (electronic) (fixation) (prosthetic) (*see also* Complications, due to (presence of) any device, implant, or graft classified to 996.0–996.5 NEC)
    mechanical — *see* Complications, mechanical
  intestinal pouch, specified NEC 569.79
  intestinal transplant (immune or nonimmune cause) 996.87
  intraoperative bleeding or hemorrhage 998.11
  intrauterine contraceptive device (*see also* Complications, contraceptive device) 996.76
    with fetal damage affecting management of pregnancy 655.8 ☑
    infection or inflammation 996.65
  in utero procedure
    fetal 679.1 ☑
    maternal 679.0 ☑
  jejunostomy 569.60
  kidney transplant (immune or nonimmune cause) 996.81
  labor 669.9 ☑
    specified condition NEC 669.8 ☑
  liver transplant (immune or nonimmune cause) 996.82
  lumbar puncture 349.0
  mechanical
    anastomosis — *see* Complications, mechanical, graft
    artificial heart 996.09
    bypass — *see* Complications, mechanical, graft

Complications — *continued*
  mechanical — *continued*
    catheter NEC 996.59
      cardiac 996.09
      cystostomy 596.82
      dialysis (hemodialysis) 996.1
        peritoneal 996.56
      during a procedure 998.2
      urethral, indwelling 996.31
    colostomy 569.62
    device NEC 996.59
      balloon (counterpulsation), intra-aortic 996.1
      cardiac 996.00
        automatic implantable defibrillator 996.04
        long-term effect 429.4
        specified NEC 996.09
      contraceptive, intrauterine 996.32
      counterpulsation, intra-aortic 996.1
      fixation, external, with internal components 996.49
      fixation, internal (nail, rod, plate) 996.40
      genitourinary 996.30
        specified NEC 996.39
      insulin pump 996.57
      nervous system 996.2
      orthopedic, internal 996.40
        prosthetic joint (*see also* Complications, mechanical, device, orthopedic, prosthetic, joint) 996.47
      prosthetic NEC 996.59
        joint 996.47
          articular bearing surface wear 996.46
          aseptic loosening 996.41
          breakage 996.43
          dislocation 996.42
          failure 996.47
          fracture 996.43
            around prosthetic 996.44
            peri-prosthetic 996.44
          instability 996.42
          loosening 996.41
          peri-prosthetic osteolysis 996.45
          subluxation 996.42
          wear 996.46
      umbrella, vena cava 996.1
      vascular 996.1
    dorsal column stimulator 996.2
    electrode NEC 996.59
      brain 996.2
      cardiac 996.01
      spinal column 996.2
    enterostomy 569.62
    esophagostomy 530.87
    fistula, arteriovenous, surgically created 996.1
    gastrostomy 536.42
    graft NEC 996.52
      aortic (bifurcation) 996.1
      aortocoronary bypass 996.03
      blood vessel NEC 996.1
      bone 996.49
      cardiac 996.00
      carotid artery bypass 996.1
      cartilage 996.49
      corneal 996.51
      coronary bypass 996.03
      decellularized allodermis 996.55
      genitourinary 996.30
        specified NEC 996.39
      muscle 996.49
      nervous system 996.2
      organ (immune or nonimmune cause) 996.80
        heart 996.83
        intestines 996.87
        kidney 996.81
        liver 996.82
        lung 996.84
        pancreas 996.86
        specified NEC 996.89

Complications — *continued*
  mechanical — *continued*
    graft — *continued*
      orthopedic, internal 996.49
      peripheral nerve 996.2
      prosthetic NEC 996.59
      skin 996.52
        artificial 996.55
      specified NEC 996.59
      tendon 996.49
      tissue NEC 996.52
      tooth 996.59
      ureter, without mention of resection 996.39
      vascular 996.1
    heart valve prosthesis 996.02
      long-term effect 429.4
    implant NEC 996.59
      cardiac 996.00
        automatic implantable defibrillator 996.04
        long-term effect 429.4
        specified NEC 996.09
      electrode NEC 996.59
        brain 996.2
        cardiac 996.01
        spinal column 996.2
      genitourinary 996.30
      nervous system 996.2
      orthopedic, internal 996.49
      prosthetic NEC 996.59
        in
          bile duct 996.59
          breast 996.54
          chin 996.59
          eye
            ocular lens 996.53
            orbital globe 996.59
      vascular 996.1
    insulin pump 996.57
    nonabsorbable surgical material 996.59
    pacemaker NEC 996.59
      brain 996.2
      cardiac 996.01
      nerve (phrenic) 996.2
    patch — *see* Complications, mechanical, graft
    prosthesis NEC 996.59
      bile duct 996.59
      breast 996.54
      chin 996.59
      ocular lens 996.53
      reconstruction, vas deferens 996.39
    reimplant NEC 996.59
      extremity (*see also* Complications, reattached, extremity) 996.90
      organ (*see also* Complications, transplant, organ, by site) 996.80
    repair — *see* Complications, mechanical, graft
    respirator [ventilator] V46.14
    shunt NEC 996.59
      arteriovenous, surgically created 996.1
      ventricular (communicating) 996.2
    stent NEC 996.59
    tracheostomy 519.02
    vas deferens reconstruction 996.39
    ventilator [respirator] V46.14
  medical care NEC 999.9
    cardiac NEC 997.1
    gastrointestinal NEC 997.49
    nervous system NEC 997.00
    peripheral vascular NEC 997.2
    respiratory NEC 997.39
    urinary NEC 997.5
    vascular
      mesenteric artery 997.71
      other vessels 997.79
      peripheral vessels 997.2
      renal artery 997.72
  nephrostomy 997.5
  nervous system
    device, implant, or graft NEC 349.1
      mechanical 996.2
    postoperative NEC 997.00

Complications — *continued*
  obstetric 669.9 ☑
    procedure (instrumental) (manual) (surgical) 669.4 ☑
    specified NEC 669.8 ☑
    surgical wound 674.3 ☑
  ocular lens implant NEC 996.79
    infection or inflammation 996.69
    mechanical 996.53
  organ transplant — *see* Complications, transplant, organ, by site
  orthopedic device, implant, or graft
    internal (fixation) (nail) (plate) (rod) NEC 996.78
      infection or inflammation 996.67
      joint prosthesis 996.77
        infection or inflammation 996.66
      mechanical 996.40
  pacemaker (cardiac) 996.72
    infection or inflammation 996.61
    mechanical 996.01
  pancreas transplant (immune or nonimmune cause) 996.86
  perfusion NEC 999.9
  perineal repair (obstetrical) 674.3 ☑
    disruption 674.2 ☑
  pessary (uterus) (vagina) — *see* Complications, contraceptive device
  phototherapy 990
  postcystoscopic 997.5
  postmastoidectomy NEC 383.30
  postoperative — *see* Complications, surgical procedures
  pregnancy NEC 646.9 ☑
    affecting fetus or newborn 761.9
  prosthetic device, internal (*see also* Complications, due to (presence of) any device, implant or graft classified to 996.0–996.5 NEC)
    mechanical NEC (*see also* Complications, mechanical) 996.59
  puerperium NEC (*see also* Puerperal) 674.9 ☑
  puncture, spinal 349.0
  pyelogram 997.5
  radiation 990
  radiotherapy 990
  reattached
    body part, except extremity 996.99
    extremity (infection) (rejection) 996.90
      arm(s) 996.94
        digit(s) (hand) 996.93
          foot 996.95
        finger(s) 996.93
        foot 996.95
        forearm 996.91
        hand 996.92
        leg 996.96
        lower NEC 996.96
        toe(s) 996.95
        upper NEC 996.94
  reimplant NEC (*see also* Complications, due to (presence of) any device, implant, or graft classified to 996.0–996.5 NEC)
    bone marrow 996.85
    extremity (*see also* Complications, reattached, extremity) 996.90
      due to infection 996.90
    mechanical — *see* Complications, mechanical, reimplant
    organ (immune or nonimmune cause) (partial) (total) (*see also* Complications, transplant, organ, by site) 996.80
  renal allograft 996.81
  renal dialysis — *see* Complications, dialysis
  respirator [ventilator], mechanical V46.14
  respiratory 519.9
    device, implant or graft NEC 996.79
      infection or inflammation 996.69
      mechanical 996.59
    distress syndrome, adult, following trauma and surgery 518.52
    insufficiency, acute, postoperative 518.52

Complications — *continued*
respiratory — *continued*
postoperative NEC 997.39
therapy NEC 999.9
sedation during labor and delivery 668.9 ☑
affecting fetus or newborn 763.5
cardiac 668.1 ☑
central nervous system 668.2 ☑
pulmonary 668.0 ☑
specified type NEC 668.8 ☑
seroma (intraoperative) (postoperative) (noninfected) 998.13
infected 998.51
shunt (*see also* Complications, due to (presence of) any device, implant, or graft classified to 996.0–996.5 NEC)
mechanical — *see* Complications, mechanical, shunt
specified body system NEC
device, implant, or graft — *see* Complications, due to (presence of) any device, implant, or graft classified to 996.0–996.5 NEC
postoperative NEC 997.99
spinal puncture or tap 349.0
stoma, external
gastrointestinal tract
colostomy 569.60
enterostomy 569.60
esophagostomy 530.87
infection 530.86
mechanical 530.87
gastrostomy 536.40
urinary tract 997.5
stomach banding 539.09
stomach stapling 539.89
surgical procedures 998.9
accidental puncture or laceration 998.2
amputation stump (late) 997.60
anastomosis — *see* Complications, anastomosis
burst stitches or sutures (external) (*see also* Dehiscence) 998.32
internal 998.31
cardiac 997.1
long-term effect following cardiac surgery 429.4
cataract fragments in eye 998.82
catheter device — *see* Complications, catheter device
cecostomy malfunction 569.62
colostomy malfunction 569.62
cystostomy malfunction 596.82
infection 596.81
mechanical 596.82
specified complication NEC 596.83
dehiscence (of incision) (external) (*see also* Dehiscence) 998.32
internal 998.31
dialysis NEC (*see also* Complications, dialysis) 999.9
disruption (*see also* Dehiscence)
anastomosis (internal) — *see* Complications, mechanical, graft
internal suture (line) 998.31
wound (external) 998.32
internal 998.31
dumping syndrome (postgastrectomy) 564.2
elephantiasis or lymphedema 997.99
postmastectomy 457.0
emphysema (surgical) 998.81
enterostomy malfunction 569.62
esophagostomy malfunction 530.87
evisceration 998.32
fistula (persistent postoperative) 998.6
foreign body inadvertently left in wound (sponge) (suture) (swab) 998.4
from nonabsorbable surgical material (Dacron) (mesh) (permanent suture) (reinforcing) (Teflon) — *see* Complications, due to (presence of) any device, implant, or graft classified to 996.0–996.5 NEC
gastrointestinal NEC 997.49
gastrostomy malfunction 536.42

Complications — *continued*
surgical procedures — *continued*
hematoma 998.12
hemorrhage 998.11
ileostomy malfunction 569.62
internal prosthetic device NEC (*see also* Complications, internal device) 996.70
hemolytic anemia 283.19
infection or inflammation 996.60
malfunction — *see* Complications, mechanical
mechanical complication — *see* Complications, mechanical
thrombus 996.70
jejunostomy malfunction 569.62
nervous system NEC 997.00
obstruction, internal anastomosis — *see* Complications, mechanical, graft
other body system NEC 997.99
peripheral vascular NEC 997.2
postcardiotomy syndrome 429.4
postcholecystectomy syndrome 576.0
postcommissurotomy syndrome 429.4
postgastrectomy dumping syndrome 564.2
postmastectomy lymphedema syndrome 457.0
postmastoidectomy 383.30
cholesteatoma, recurrent 383.32
cyst, mucosal 383.31
granulation 383.33
inflammation, chronic 383.33
postvagotomy syndrome 564.2
postvalvulotomy syndrome 429.4
reattached extremity (infection) (rejection) (*see also* Complications, reattached, extremity) 996.90
respiratory NEC 997.39
seroma 998.13
shock (endotoxic) (septic) 998.02
hypovolemic 998.09
shunt, prosthetic (thrombus) (*see also* Complications, due to (presence of) any device, implant, or graft classified to 996.0–996.5 NEC)
hemolytic anemia 283.19
specified complication NEC 596.83
specified complication NEC 998.89
stitch abscess 998.59
transplant — *see* Complications, graft
ureterostomy malfunction 997.5
urethrostomy malfunction 997.5
urinary NEC 997.5
vascular
mesenteric artery 997.71
other vessels 997.79
peripheral vessels 997.2
renal artery 997.72
wound infection 998.59
therapeutic misadventure NEC 999.9
surgical treatment 998.9
tracheostomy 519.00
transfusion (blood) (lymphocytes) (plasma) 999.80
acute lung injury (TRALI) 518.7
atrophy, liver, yellow, subacute (within 8 months of administration) — *see* Hepatitis, viral
bone marrow 996.85
embolism
air 999.1
thrombus 999.2
febrile nonhemolytic reaction (FNHTR) 780.66
hemolysis NEC 999.89
bone marrow 996.85
hemolytic reaction, incompatibility unspecified 999.83
acute 999.84
delayed 999.85
hepatitis (serum) (type B) (within 8 months after administration) — *see* Hepatitis, viral
incompatibility reaction
ABO 999.60

Complications — *continued*
transfusion — *continued*
incompatibility reaction — *continued*
ABO — *continued*
with hemolytic transfusion reaction (HTR) (not specified as acute or delayed) 999.61
acute 999.62
delayed 999.63
specified type NEC 999.69
minor blood group 999.89
non-ABO (minor antigens) (Duffy) (Kell) (Kidd) (Lewis) (M) (N) (P) (S) 999.75
with hemolytic transfusion reaction (HTR) (not specified as acute or delayed) 999.76
acute 999.77
delayed 999.78
specified type NEC 999.79
Rh antigen (C) (c) (D) (E) (e) (factor) 999.70
with hemolytic transfusion reaction (HTR) (not specified as acute or delayed) 999.71
acute 999.72
delayed 999.73
specified type NEC 999.74
infection 999.39
acute 999.34
jaundice (serum) (within 8 months after administration) — *see* Hepatitis, viral
sepsis 999.39
shock or reaction NEC 999.89
bone marrow 996.85
specified reaction NEC 999.89
subacute yellow atrophy of liver (within 8 months after administration) — *see* Hepatitis, viral
thromboembolism 999.2
transplant NEC (*see also* Complications, due to (presence of) any device, implant, or graft classified to 996.0–996.5 NEC)
bone marrow 996.85
organ (immune or nonimmune cause) (partial) (total) 996.80
bone marrow 996.85
heart 996.83
intestines 996.87
kidney 996.81
liver 996.82
lung 996.84
pancreas 996.86
specified NEC 996.89
stem cell(s) 996.88
from
peripheral blood 996.88
umbilical cord 996.88
trauma NEC (early) 958.8
ultrasound therapy NEC 999.9
umbilical cord
affecting fetus or newborn 762.6
complicating delivery 663.9 ☑
affecting fetus or newborn 762.6
specified type NEC 663.8 ☑
urethral catheter NEC 996.76
infection or inflammation 996.64
mechanical 996.31
urinary, postoperative NEC 997.5
vaccination 999.9
anaphylaxis NEC 999.42
cellulitis 999.39
encephalitis or encephalomyelitis 323.51
hepatitis (serum) (type B) (within 8 months after administration) — *see* Hepatitis, viral
infection (general) (local) NEC 999.39
jaundice (serum) (within 8 months after administration) — *see* Hepatitis, viral
meningitis 997.09 [321.8]
myelitis 323.52
protein sickness 999.52

Complications — *continued*
vaccination — *continued*
reaction (allergic) 999.52
serum 999.52
sepsis 999.39
serum intoxication, sickness, rash, or other serum reaction NEC 999.52
shock (allergic) (anaphylactic) 999.49
subacute yellow atrophy of liver (within 8 months after administration) — *see* Hepatitis, viral
vaccinia (generalized) 999.0
localized 999.39
vascular
device, implant, or graft NEC 996.74
infection or inflammation 996.62
mechanical NEC 996.1
cardiac (*see also* Complications, mechanical, by type) 996.00
following infusion, perfusion, or transfusion 999.2
postoperative NEC 997.2
mesenteric artery 997.71
other vessels 997.79
peripheral vessels 997.2
renal artery 997.72
ventilation therapy NEC 999.9
ventilator [respirator], mechanical V46.14

Compound presentation, complicating delivery 652.8 ☑
causing obstructed labor 660.0 ☑
Compressed air disease 993.3
Compression
with injury — *see* specific injury
arm NEC 354.9
artery 447.1
celiac, syndrome 447.4
brachial plexus 353.0
brain (stem) 348.4
due to
contusion, brain — *see* Contusion, brain
injury NEC (*see also* Hemorrhage, brain, traumatic)
birth — *see* Birth, injury, brain
laceration, brain — *see* Laceration, brain
osteopathic 739.0
bronchus 519.19
by cicatrix — *see* Cicatrix
cardiac 423.9
cauda equina 344.60
with neurogenic bladder 344.61
celiac (artery) (axis) 447.4
cerebral — *see* Compression, brain
cervical plexus 353.2
cord (umbilical) — *see* Compression, umbilical cord
cranial nerve 352.9
second 377.49
third (partial) 378.51
total 378.52
fourth 378.53
fifth 350.8
sixth 378.54
seventh 351.8
divers' squeeze 993.3
duodenum (external) (*see also* Obstruction, duodenum) 537.3
during birth 767.9
esophagus 530.3
congenital, external 750.3
Eustachian tube 381.63
facies (congenital) 754.0
fracture — *see* Fracture, by site
heart — *see* Disease, heart
intestine (*see also* Obstruction, intestine) 560.9
with hernia — *see* Hernia, by site, with obstruction
laryngeal nerve, recurrent 478.79
leg NEC 355.8
lower extremity NEC 355.8
lumbosacral plexus 353.1
lung 518.89

Complications — Compression

☑ Additional Digit Required — Refer to the Tabular List for Digit Selection   🔻 Subterms under main terms may continue to next column or page

2013 ICD-9-CM   ▶◀ Revised Text   ● New Line   ▲ Revised Code   Volume 2 — 53

Compression — *continued*
  lymphatic vessel 457.1
  medulla — *see* Compression, brain
  nerve NEC (*see also* Disorder, nerve)
    arm NEC 354.9
    autonomic nervous system (*see also*
      Neuropathy, peripheral, autonom-
      ic) 337.9
    axillary 353.0
    cranial NEC 352.9
    due to displacement of intervertebral
      disc 722.2
      with myelopathy 722.70
      cervical 722.0
        with myelopathy 722.71
      lumbar, lumbosacral 722.10
        with myelopathy 722.73
      thoracic, thoracolumbar 722.11
        with myelopathy 722.72
    iliohypogastric 355.79
    ilioinguinal 355.79
    leg NEC 355.8
    lower extremity NEC 355.8
    median (in carpal tunnel) 354.0
    obturator 355.79
    optic 377.49
    plantar 355.6
    posterior tibial (in tarsal tunnel) 355.5
    root (by scar tissue) NEC 724.9
      cervical NEC 723.4
      lumbar NEC 724.4
      lumbosacral 724.4
      thoracic 724.4
    saphenous 355.79
    sciatic (acute) 355.0
    sympathetic 337.9
    traumatic — *see* Injury, nerve
    ulnar 354.2
    upper extremity NEC 354.9
  peripheral — *see* Compression, nerve
  spinal (cord) (old or nontraumatic) 336.9
    by displacement of intervertebral disc
      — *see* Displacement, interverte-
      bral disc
    nerve
      root NEC 724.9
        postoperative 722.80
          cervical region 722.81
          lumbar region 722.83
          thoracic region 722.82
        traumatic — *see* Injury, nerve,
          spinal
      traumatic — *see* Injury, nerve, spinal
    spondylogenic 721.91
      cervical 721.1
      lumbar, lumbosacral 721.42
      thoracic 721.41
    traumatic (*see also* Injury, spinal, by site)
      with fracture, vertebra — *see* Frac-
        ture, vertebra, by site, with
        spinal cord injury
  spondylogenic — *see* Compression, spinal
    cord, spondylogenic
  subcostal nerve (syndrome) 354.8
  sympathetic nerve NEC 337.9
  syndrome 958.5
  thorax 512.89
    iatrogenic 512.1
    postoperative 512.1
  trachea 519.19
    congenital 748.3
  ulnar nerve (by scar tissue) 354.2
  umbilical cord
    affecting fetus or newborn 762.5
      cord prolapsed 762.4
    complicating delivery 663.2 ☑
      cord around neck 663.1 ☑
      cord prolapsed 663.0 ☑
  upper extremity NEC 354.9
  ureter 593.3
  urethra — *see* Stricture, urethra
  vein 459.2
  vena cava (inferior) (superior) 459.2
  vertebral NEC — *see* Compression, spinal
    (cord)

Compulsion, compulsive
  eating 307.51
  neurosis (obsessive) 300.3
  personality 301.4
  states (mixed) 300.3
  swearing 300.3
    in Gilles de la Tourette's syndrome
      307.23
  tics and spasms 307.22
  water drinking NEC (syndrome) 307.9
Concato's disease (pericardial polyserositis)
  423.2
  peritoneal 568.82
  pleural — *see* Pleurisy
Concavity, chest wall 738.3
Concealed
  hemorrhage NEC 459.0
  penis 752.65
Concentric fading 368.12
Concern (normal) **about sick person in family**
  V61.49
Concrescence (teeth) 520.2
Concretio cordis 423.1
  rheumatic 393
Concretion — *see also* Calculus
  appendicular 543.9
  canaliculus 375.57
  clitoris 624.8
  conjunctiva 372.54
  eyelid 374.56
  intestine (impaction) (obstruction) 560.39
  lacrimal (passages) 375.57
  prepuce (male) 605
    female (clitoris) 624.8
  salivary gland (any) 527.5
  seminal vesicle 608.89
  stomach 537.89
  tonsil 474.8
Concussion (current) 850.9
  with
    loss of consciousness 850.5
      brief (less than one hour)
        30 minutes or less 850.11
        31-59 minutes 850.12
      moderate (1-24 hours) 850.2
      prolonged (more than 24 hours)
        (with complete recovery)
        (with return to pre-existing
        conscious level) 850.3
        without return to pre-existing
        conscious level 850.4
    mental confusion or disorientation
      (without loss of consciousness)
      850.0
      with loss of consciousness — *see*
        Concussion, with, loss of con-
        sciousness
  without loss of consciousness 850.0
  blast (air) (hydraulic) (immersion) (underwa-
    ter) 869.0
    with open wound into cavity 869.1
    abdomen or thorax — *see* Injury, inter-
      nal, by site
    brain — *see* Concussion, brain
    ear (acoustic nerve trauma) 951.5
      with perforation, tympanic mem-
        brane — *see* Wound, open,
        ear drum
    thorax — *see* Injury, internal, intratho-
      racic organs NEC
  brain or cerebral (without skull fracture)
    850.9
    with
      loss of consciousness 850.5
        brief (less than one hour)
          30 minutes or less 850.11
          31-59 minutes 850.12
        moderate (1-24 hours) 850.2
        prolonged (more than 24 hours)
          (with complete recovery)
          (with return to pre-exist-
          ing conscious level) 850.3
        without return to pre-existing
          conscious level 850.4

Concussion — *continued*
  brain or cerebral — *continued*
    with — *continued*
      mental confusion or disorientation
        (without loss of conscious-
        ness) 850.0
      with loss of consciousness — *see*
        Concussion, brain, with,
        loss of consciousness
      skull fracture — *see* Fracture, skull,
        by site
      without loss of consciousness 850.0
  cauda equina 952.4
  cerebral — *see* Concussion, brain
  conus medullaris (spine) 952.4
  hydraulic — *see* Concussion, blast
  internal organs — *see* Injury, internal, by
    site
  labyrinth — *see* Injury, intracranial
  ocular 921.3
  osseous labyrinth — *see* Injury, intracranial
  spinal (cord) (*see also* Injury, spinal, by site)
    due to
      broken
        back — *see* Fracture, vertebra, by
          site, with spinal cord injury
        neck — *see* Fracture, vertebra,
          cervical, with spinal cord
          injury
      fracture, fracture dislocation, or
        compression fracture of spine
        or vertebra — *see* Fracture,
        vertebra, by site, with spinal
        cord injury
  syndrome 310.2
  underwater blast — *see* Concussion, blast
Condition — *see also* Disease
  fetal hematologic 678.0 ☑
  psychiatric 298.9
  respiratory NEC 519.9
    acute or subacute NEC 519.9
      due to
        external agent 508.9
          specified type NEC 508.8
        fumes or vapors (chemical) (in-
          halation) 506.3
        radiation 508.0
    chronic NEC 519.9
      due to
        external agent 508.9
          specified type NEC 508.8
        fumes or vapors (chemical) (in-
          halation) 506.4
        radiation 508.1
    due to
      external agent 508.9
        specified type NEC 508.8
      fumes or vapors (chemical) (inhala-
        tion) 506.9
      smoke inhalation 508.2
Conduct disturbance — *see also* Disturbance,
  conduct 312.9
  adjustment reaction 309.3
  hyperkinetic 314.2
Condyloma NEC 078.11
  acuminatum 078.11
  gonorrheal 098.0
  latum 091.3
  syphilitic 091.3
    congenital 090.0
  venereal, syphilitic 091.3
Confinement — *see* Delivery
Conflagration — *see also* Burn, by site
  asphyxia (by inhalation of gases, fumes, or
    vapors) 987.9
  specified agent — *see* Table of Drugs
    and Chemicals
Conflict
  family V61.9
    specified circumstance NEC V61.8
  interpersonal NEC V62.81
  marital V61.10
    involving
      divorce V61.03
      estrangement V61.09
  parent (guardian)-child V61.20

Conflict — *continued*
  parent-child — *continued*
    adopted child V61.24
    biological child V61.23
    foster child V61.25
  partner V61.10
Confluent — *see* condition
Confusional arousals 327.41
Confusion, confused (mental) (state) — *see*
  also State, confusional 298.9
  acute 293.0
  epileptic 293.0
  postoperative 293.9
  psychogenic 298.2
  reactive (from emotional stress, psycholog-
    ical trauma) 298.2
  subacute 293.1
Congelation 991.9
Congenital — *see also* condition
  aortic septum 747.29
  generalized fibromatosis (CGF) 759.89
  intrinsic factor deficiency 281.0
  malformation — *see* Anomaly
Congestion, congestive
  asphyxia, newborn 768.9
  bladder 596.89
  bowel 569.89
  brain (*see also* Disease, cerebrovascular NEC)
    437.8
    malarial 084.9
  breast 611.79
  bronchi 519.19
  bronchial tube 519.19
  catarrhal 472.0
  cerebral — *see* Congestion, brain
  cerebrospinal — *see* Congestion, brain
  chest 786.9
  chill 780.99
    malarial (*see also* Malaria) 084.6
  circulatory NEC 459.9
  conjunctiva 372.71
  due to disturbance of circulation 459.9
  duodenum 537.3
  enteritis — *see* Enteritis
  eye 372.71
  fibrosis syndrome (pelvic) 625.5
  gastroenteritis — *see* Enteritis
  general 799.89
  glottis 476.0
  heart (*see also* Failure, heart) 428.0
  hepatic 573.0
  hypostatic (lung) 514
  intestine 569.89
  intracranial — *see* Congestion, brain
  kidney 593.89
  labyrinth 386.50
  larynx 476.0
  liver 573.0
  lung 786.9
    active or acute (*see also* Pneumonia) 486
      congenital 770.0
    chronic 514
    hypostatic 514
    idiopathic, acute 518.52
    passive 514
  malaria, malarial (brain) (fever) (*see also*
    Malaria) 084.6
  medulla — *see* Congestion, brain
  nasal 478.19
  nose 478.19
  orbit, orbital 376.33
    inflammatory (chronic) 376.10
      acute 376.00
  ovary 620.8
  pancreas 577.8
  pelvic, female 625.5
  pleural 511.0
  prostate (active) 602.1
  pulmonary — *see* Congestion, lung
  renal 593.89
  retina 362.89
  seminal vesicle 608.89
  spinal cord 336.1
  spleen 289.51
    chronic 289.51
  stomach 537.89

☑ **Additional Digit Required — Refer to the Tabular List for Digit Selection**   ⱽᵂ **Subterms under main terms may continue to next column or page**

Congestion, congestive — continued
  trachea 464.11
  urethra 599.84
  uterus 625.5
    with subinvolution 621.1
  viscera 799.89
Congestive — see Congestion
Conical
  cervix 622.6
  cornea 371.60
  teeth 520.2
Conjoined twins 759.4
  causing disproportion (fetopelvic) 678.1 ☑
  fetal 678.1 ☑
Conjugal maladjustment V61.10
  involving
    divorce V61.03
    estrangement V61.09
Conjunctiva — see condition
Conjunctivitis (exposure) (infectious)
  (nondiphtheritic) (pneumococcal) (pustular) (staphylococcal) (streptococcal)
  NEC 372.30
  actinic 370.24
  acute 372.00
    atopic 372.05
    chemical 372.06
    contagious 372.03
    follicular 372.02
    hemorrhagic (viral) 077.4
    toxic 372.06
  adenoviral (acute) 077.3
  allergic (chronic) 372.14
    with hay fever 372.05
  anaphylactic 372.05
  angular 372.03
  Apollo (viral) 077.4
  atopic 372.05
  blennorrhagic (neonatorum) 098.40
  catarrhal 372.03
  chemical 372.06
    allergic 372.05
    meaning corrosion — see Burn, conjunc-
    tiva
  chlamydial 077.98
    due to
      Chlamydia trachomatis — see Tra-
      choma
      paratrachoma 077.0
  chronic 372.10
    allergic 372.14
    follicular 372.12
    simple 372.11
    specified type NEC 372.14
    vernal 372.13
  diphtheritic 032.81
  due to
    dust 372.05
    enterovirus type 70 077.4
    erythema multiforme 695.10 [372.33]
    filariasis (see also Filariasis) 125.9 [372.15]
    mucocutaneous
      disease NEC 372.33
      leishmaniasis 085.5 [372.15]
    Reiter's disease 099.3 [372.33]
    syphilis 095.8 [372.10]
    toxoplasmosis (acquired) 130.1
      congenital (active) 771.2
    trachoma — see Trachoma
  dust 372.05
  eczematous 370.31
  epidemic 077.1
    hemorrhagic 077.4
  follicular (acute) 372.02
    adenoviral (acute) 077.3
    chronic 372.12
  glare 370.24
  gonococcal (neonatorum) 098.40
  granular (trachomatous) 076.1
    late effect 139.1
  hemorrhagic (acute) (epidemic) 077.4
  herpetic (simplex) 054.43
    zoster 053.21
  inclusion 077.0
  infantile 771.6
  influenzal 372.03

Conjunctivitis — continued
  Koch-Weeks 372.03
  light 372.05
  medicamentosa 372.05
  membranous 372.04
  meningococcic 036.89
  Morax-Axenfeld 372.02
  mucopurulent NEC 372.03
  neonatal 771.6
    gonococcal 098.40
  Newcastle's 077.8
  nodosa 360.14
  of Beal 077.3
  parasitic 372.15
    filariasis (see also Filariasis) 125.9 [372.15]
    mucocutaneous leishmaniasis
      085.5 [372.15]
  Parinaud's 372.02
  petrificans 372.39
  phlyctenular 370.31
  pseudomembranous 372.04
    diphtheritic 032.81
  purulent 372.03
  Reiter's 099.3 [372.33]
  rosacea 695.3 [372.31]
  serous 372.01
    viral 077.99
  simple chronic 372.11
  specified NEC 372.39
  sunlamp 372.04
  swimming pool 077.0
  toxic 372.06
  trachomatous (follicular) 076.1
    acute 076.0
    late effect 139.1
  traumatic NEC 372.39
  tuberculous (see also Tuberculosis)
    017.3 ☑ [370.31]
  tularemic 021.3
  tularensis 021.3
  vernal 372.13
    limbar 372.13 [370.32]
  viral 077.99
    acute hemorrhagic 077.4
    specified NEC 077.8
Conjunctivochalasis 372.81
Conjunctoblepharitis — see Conjunctivitis
Connective tissue — see condition
Conn (-Louis) syndrome (primary aldosteronism) 255.12
Conradi (-Hünermann) syndrome or disease
  (chondrodysplasia calcificans congenita)
  756.59
Consanguinity V19.7
Consecutive — see condition
Consolidated lung (base) — see Pneumonia,
  lobar
Constipation 564.00
  atonic 564.09
  drug induced
    correct substance properly administered
      564.09
    overdose or wrong substance given or
      taken 977.9
      specified drug — see Table of Drugs
      and Chemicals
  neurogenic 564.09
  other specified NEC 564.09
  outlet dysfunction 564.02
  psychogenic 306.4
  simple 564.00
  slow transit 564.01
  spastic 564.09
Constitutional — see also condition
  arterial hypotension (see also Hypotension)
    458.9
  obesity 278.00
    morbid 278.01
  psychopathic state 301.9
  short stature in childhood 783.43
  state, developmental V21.9
    specified development NEC V21.8
  substandard 301.6
Constitutionally substandard 301.6
Constriction
  anomalous, meningeal bands or folds 742.8

Constriction — continued
  aortic arch (congenital) 747.10
  asphyxiation or suffocation by 994.7
  bronchus 519.19
  canal, ear (see also Stricture, ear canal, ac-
    quired) 380.50
  duodenum 537.3
  gallbladder (see also Obstruction, gallblad-
    der) 575.2
    congenital 751.69
  intestine (see also Obstruction, intestine)
    560.9
  larynx 478.74
    congenital 748.3
  meningeal bands or folds, anomalous 742.8
  organ or site, congenital NEC — see Atresia
  prepuce (congenital) 605
  pylorus 537.0
    adult hypertrophic 537.0
    congenital or infantile 750.5
    newborn 750.5
  ring (uterus) 661.4 ☑
    affecting fetus or newborn 763.7
  spastic (see also Spasm)
    ureter 593.3
    urethra — see Stricture, urethra
  stomach 537.89
  ureter 593.3
  urethra — see Stricture, urethra
  visual field (functional) (peripheral) 368.45
Constrictive — see condition
Consultation
  without complaint or sickness V65.9
    feared complaint unfounded V65.5
    specified reason NEC V65.8
  medical (see also Counseling, medical)
  specified reason NEC V65.8
Consumption — see Tuberculosis
Contact — see also Exposure (suspected)
  with
    AIDS virus V01.79
    anthrax V01.81
    asbestos V15.84
    cholera V01.0
    communicable disease V01.9
      specified type NEC V01.89
      viral NEC V01.79
    Escherichia coli (E. coli) V01.83
    German measles V01.4
    gonorrhea V01.6
    HIV V01.79
    human immunodeficiency virus V01.79
    lead V15.86
    meningococcus V01.84
    parasitic disease NEC V01.89
    poliomyelitis V01.2
    potentially hazardous body fluids V15.85
    rabies V01.5
    rubella V01.4
    SARS-associated coronavirus V01.82
    smallpox V01.3
    syphilis V01.6
    tuberculosis V01.1
    varicella V01.71
    venereal disease V01.6
    viral disease NEC V01.79
  dermatitis — see Dermatitis
Contamination, food — see also Poisoning,
  food 005.9
Contraception, contraceptive
  advice NEC V25.09
    family planning V25.09
    fitting of diaphragm V25.02
    prescribing or use of
      oral contraceptive agent V25.01
      specified agent NEC V25.02
  counseling NEC V25.09
    emergency V25.03
    family planning V25.09
    fitting of diaphragm V25.02
    prescribing or use of
      oral contraceptive agent V25.01
      emergency V25.03
      postcoital V25.03
      specified agent NEC V25.02
  device (in situ) V45.59

Contraception, contraceptive —
  continued
  device — continued
    causing menorrhagia 996.76
    checking V25.42
    complications 996.32
    insertion V25.11
    intrauterine V45.51
    reinsertion V25.13
    removal V25.12
      and reinsertion V25.13
    replacement V25.13
    subdermal V45.52
  fitting of diaphragm V25.02
  insertion
    intrauterine contraceptive device V25.11
    subdermal implantable V25.5
  maintenance V25.40
    examination V25.40
      oral contraceptive V25.41
      specified method NEC V25.49
      subdermal implantable V25.43
        intrauterine device V25.42
    intrauterine device V25.42
    oral contraceptive V25.41
    specified method NEC V25.49
    subdermal implantable V25.43
  management NEC V25.49
  prescription
    oral contraceptive agent V25.01
      emergency V25.03
      postcoital V25.03
      repeat V25.41
    specified agent NEC V25.02
      repeat V25.49
  sterilization V25.2
  surveillance V25.40
    intrauterine device V25.42
    oral contraceptive agent V25.41
      subdermal implantable V25.43
    specified method NEC V25.49
Contraction, contracture, contracted
  Achilles tendon (see also Short, tendon,
    Achilles) 727.81
  anus 564.89
  axilla 729.90
  bile duct (see also Disease, biliary) 576.8
  bladder 596.89
    neck or sphincter 596.0
  bowel (see also Obstruction, intestine) 560.9
  Braxton Hicks 644.1 ☑
  breast implant, capsular 611.83
  bronchus 519.19
  burn (old) — see Cicatrix
  capsular, of breast implant 611.83
  cecum (see also Obstruction, intestine) 560.9
  cervix (see also Stricture, cervix) 622.4
    congenital 752.49
  cicatricial — see Cicatrix
  colon (see also Obstruction, intestine) 560.9
  conjunctiva trachomatous, active 076.1
    late effect 139.1
  Dupuytren's 728.6
  eyelid 374.41
  eye socket (after enucleation) 372.64
  face 729.90
  fascia (lata) (postural) 728.89
    Dupuytren's 728.6
    palmar 728.6
    plantar 728.71
  finger NEC 736.29
    congenital 755.59
    joint (see also Contraction, joint) 718.44
  flaccid, paralytic
    joint (see also Contraction, joint)
      718.4 ☑
    muscle 728.85
    ocular 378.50
  gallbladder (see also Obstruction, gallblad-
    der) 575.2
  hamstring 728.89
    tendon 727.81
  heart valve — see Endocarditis
  Hicks' 644.1 ☑
  hip (see also Contraction, joint) 718.4 ☑

☑ Additional Digit Required — Refer to the Tabular List for Digit Selection   Ⱳ Subterms under main terms may continue to next column or page

Contraction, contracture, contracted — *continued*
hourglass
  bladder 596.89
    congenital 753.8
  gallbladder (*see also* Obstruction, gallbladder) 575.2
    congenital 751.69
  stomach 536.8
    congenital 750.7
    psychogenic 306.4
  uterus 661.4 ☑
    affecting fetus or newborn 763.7
hysterical 300.11
infantile (*see also* Epilepsy) 345.6 ☑
internal os (*see also* Stricture, cervix) 622.4
intestine (*see also* Obstruction, intestine) 560.9
joint (abduction) (acquired) (adduction) (flexion) (rotation) 718.40
  ankle 718.47
  congenital NEC 755.8
    generalized or multiple 754.89
      lower limb joints 754.89
    hip (*see also* Subluxation, congenital, hip) 754.32
    lower limb (including pelvic girdle) not involving hip 754.89
    upper limb (including shoulder girdle) 755.59
  elbow 718.42
  foot 718.47
  hand 718.44
  hip 718.45
  hysterical 300.11
  knee 718.46
  multiple sites 718.49
  pelvic region 718.45
  shoulder (region) 718.41
  specified site NEC 718.48
  wrist 718.43
kidney (granular) (secondary) (*see also* Sclerosis, renal) 587
  congenital 753.3
  hydronephritic 591
  pyelonephritic (*see also* Pyelitis, chronic) 590.00
  tuberculous (*see also* Tuberculosis) 016.0 ☑
ligament 728.89
  congenital 756.89
liver — *see* Cirrhosis, liver
muscle (postinfectional) (postural) NEC 728.85
  congenital 756.89
    sternocleidomastoid 754.1
  extraocular 378.60
  eye (extrinsic) (*see also* Strabismus) 378.9
    paralytic (*see also* Strabismus, paralytic) 378.50
  flaccid 728.85
  hysterical 300.11
  ischemic (Volkmann's) 958.6
  paralytic 728.85
  posttraumatic 958.6
  psychogenic 306.0
    specified as conversion reaction 300.11
  myotonic 728.85
  neck (*see also* Torticollis) 723.5
    congenital 754.1
    psychogenic 306.0
  ocular muscle (*see also* Strabismus) 378.9
    paralytic (*see also* Strabismus, paralytic) 378.50
organ or site, congenital NEC — *see* Atresia
outlet (pelvis) — *see* Contraction, pelvis
palmar fascia 728.6
paralytic
  joint (*see also* Contraction, joint) 718.4 ☑
  muscle 728.85
    ocular (*see also* Strabismus, paralytic) 378.50
pelvis (acquired) (general) 738.6
  affecting fetus or newborn 763.1

Contraction, contracture, contracted — *continued*
pelvis — *continued*
  complicating delivery 653.1 ☑
    causing obstructed labor 660.1 ☑
    generally contracted 653.1 ☑
      causing obstructed labor 660.1 ☑
    inlet 653.2 ☑
      causing obstructed labor 660.1 ☑
    midpelvic 653.8 ☑
      causing obstructed labor 660.1 ☑
    midplane 653.8 ☑
      causing obstructed labor 660.1 ☑
    outlet 653.3 ☑
      causing obstructed labor 660.1 ☑
plantar fascia 728.71
premature
  atrial 427.61
  auricular 427.61
  auriculoventricular 427.61
  heart (junctional) (nodal) 427.60
  supraventricular 427.61
  ventricular 427.69
prostate 602.8
pylorus (*see also* Pylorospasm) 537.81
rectosigmoid (*see also* Obstruction, intestine) 560.9
rectum, rectal (sphincter) 564.89
  psychogenic 306.4
ring (Bandl's) 661.4 ☑
  affecting fetus or newborn 763.7
scar — *see* Cicatrix
sigmoid (*see also* Obstruction, intestine) 560.9
socket, eye 372.64
spine (*see also* Curvature, spine) 737.9
stomach 536.8
  hourglass 536.8
    congenital 750.7
  psychogenic 306.4
tendon (sheath) (*see also* Short, tendon) 727.81
toe 735.8
ureterovesical orifice (postinfectional) 593.3
urethra 599.84
uterus 621.8
  abnormal 661.9 ☑
    affecting fetus or newborn 763.7
  clonic, hourglass or tetanic 661.4 ☑
    affecting fetus or newborn 763.7
  dyscoordinate 661.4 ☑
    affecting fetus or newborn 763.7
  hourglass 661.4 ☑
    affecting fetus or newborn 763.7
  hypotonic NEC 661.2 ☑
    affecting fetus or newborn 763.7
  incoordinate 661.4 ☑
    affecting fetus or newborn 763.7
  inefficient or poor 661.2 ☑
    affecting fetus or newborn 763.7
  irregular 661.2 ☑
    affecting fetus or newborn 763.7
  tetanic 661.4 ☑
    affecting fetus or newborn 763.7
vagina (outlet) 623.2
vesical 596.89
  neck or urethral orifice 596.0
visual field, generalized 368.45
Volkmann's (ischemic) 958.6
Contusion (skin surface intact) 924.9
with
  crush injury — *see* Crush
  dislocation — *see* Dislocation, by site
  fracture — *see* Fracture, by site
  internal injury (*see also* Injury, internal, by site)
    heart — *see* Contusion, cardiac
    kidney — *see* Contusion, kidney
    liver — *see* Contusion, liver
    lung — *see* Contusion, lung
    spleen — *see* Contusion, spleen

Contusion — *continued*
with — *continued*
  intracranial injury — *see* Injury, intracranial
  nerve injury — *see* Injury, nerve
  open wound — *see* Wound, open, by site
abdomen, abdominal (muscle) (wall) 922.2
  organ(s) NEC 868.00
adnexa, eye NEC 921.9
ankle 924.21
  with other parts of foot 924.20
arm 923.9
  lower (with elbow) 923.10
  upper 923.03
    with shoulder or axillary region 923.09
auditory canal (external) (meatus) (and other part(s) of neck, scalp, or face, except eye) 920
auricle, ear (and other part(s) of neck, scalp, or face except eye) 920
axilla 923.02
  with shoulder or upper arm 923.09
back 922.31
bone NEC 924.9
brain (cerebral) (membrane) (with hemorrhage) 851.8 ☑

Note — *Use the following fifth-digit subclassification with categories 851–854:*

0   *unspecified state of consciousness*

1   *with no loss of consciousness*

2   *with brief [less than one hour] loss of consciousness*

3   *with moderate [1–24 hours] loss of consciousness*

4   *with prolonged [more than 24 hours] loss of consciousness and return to pre-existing conscious level*

5   *with prolonged [more than 24 hours] loss of consciousness, without return to pre-existing conscious level*

Use fifth-digit 5 to designate when a patient is unconscious and dies before regaining consciousness, regardless of the duration of the loss of consciousness

6   *with loss of consciousness of unspecified duration*

9   *with concussion, unspecified*

with
  open intracranial wound 851.9 ☑
  skull fracture — *see* Fracture, skull, by site
cerebellum 851.4 ☑
  with open intracranial wound 851.5 ☑
cortex 851.0 ☑
  with open intracranial wound 851.1 ☑
occipital lobe 851.4 ☑
  with open intracranial wound 851.5 ☑
stem 851.4 ☑
  with open intracranial wound 851.5 ☑
breast 922.0
brow (and other part(s) of neck, scalp, or face, except eye) 920
buttock 922.32
canthus 921.1
cardiac 861.01
  with open wound into thorax 861.11
cauda equina (spine) 952.4
cerebellum — *see* Contusion, brain, cerebellum
cerebral — *see* Contusion, brain
cheek(s) (and other part(s) of neck, scalp, or face, except eye) 920

Contusion — *continued*
chest (wall) 922.1
chin (and other part(s) of neck, scalp, or face, except eye) 920
clitoris 922.4
conjunctiva 921.1
conus medullaris (spine) 952.4
cornea 921.3
corpus cavernosum 922.4
cortex (brain) (cerebral) — *see* Contusion, brain, cortex
costal region 922.1
ear (and other part(s) of neck, scalp, or face except eye) 920
elbow 923.11
  with forearm 923.10
epididymis 922.4
epigastric region 922.2
eye NEC 921.9
eyeball 921.3
eyelid(s) (and periocular area) 921.1
face (and neck, or scalp, any part, except eye) 920
femoral triangle 922.2
fetus or newborn 772.6
finger(s) (nail) (subungual) 923.3
flank 922.2
foot (with ankle) (excluding toe(s)) 924.20
forearm (and elbow) 923.10
forehead (and other part(s) of neck, scalp, or face, except eye) 920
genital organs, external 922.4
globe (eye) 921.3
groin 922.2
gum(s) (and other part(s) of neck, scalp, or face, except eye) 920
hand(s) (except fingers alone) 923.20
head (any part, except eye) (and face) (and neck) 920
heart — *see* Contusion, cardiac
heel 924.20
hip 924.01
  with thigh 924.00
iliac region 922.2
inguinal region 922.2
internal organs (abdomen, chest, or pelvis) NEC — *see* Injury, internal, by site
interscapular region 922.33
iris (eye) 921.3
kidney 866.01
  with open wound into cavity 866.11
knee 924.11
  with lower leg 924.10
labium (majus) (minus) 922.4
lacrimal apparatus, gland, or sac 921.1
larynx (and other part(s) of neck, scalp, or face, except eye) 920
late effect — *see* Late, effects (of), contusion
leg 924.5
  lower (with knee) 924.10
lens 921.3
lingual (and other part(s) of neck, scalp, or face, except eye) 920
lip(s) (and other part(s) of neck, scalp, or face, except eye) 920
liver 864.01
  with
    laceration — *see* Laceration, liver
    open wound into cavity 864.11
lower extremity 924.5
  multiple sites 924.4
lumbar region 922.31
lung 861.21
  with open wound into thorax 861.31
malar region (and other part(s) of neck, scalp, or face, except eye) 920
mandibular joint (and other part(s) of neck, scalp, or face, except eye) 920
mastoid region (and other part(s) of neck, scalp, or face, except eye) 920
membrane, brain — *see* Contusion, brain
midthoracic region 922.1
mouth (and other part(s) of neck, scalp, or face, except eye) 920
multiple sites (not classifiable to same three-digit category) 924.8

Contusion — *continued*
  multiple sites — *continued*
    lower limb 924.4
    trunk 922.8
    upper limb 923.8
  muscle NEC 924.9
  myocardium — *see* Contusion, cardiac
  nasal (septum) (and other part(s) of neck, scalp, or face, except eye) 920
  neck (and scalp or face, any part, except eye) 920
  nerve — *see* Injury, nerve, by site
  nose (and other part(s) of neck, scalp, or face, except eye) 920
  occipital region (scalp) (and neck or face, except eye) 920
    lobe — *see* Contusion, brain, occipital lobe
  orbit (region) (tissues) 921.2
  palate (soft) (and other part(s) of neck, scalp, or face, except eye) 920
  parietal region (scalp) (and neck, or face, except eye) 920
    lobe — *see* Contusion, brain
  penis 922.4
  pericardium — *see* Contusion, cardiac
  perineum 922.4
  periocular area 921.1
  pharynx (and other part(s) of neck, scalp, or face, except eye) 920
  popliteal space (*see also* Contusion, knee) 924.11
  prepuce 922.4
  pubic region 922.4
  pudenda 922.4
  pulmonary — *see* Contusion, lung
  quadriceps femoralis 924.00
  rib cage 922.1
  sacral region 922.32
  salivary ducts or glands (and other part(s) of neck, scalp, or face, except eye) 920
  scalp (and neck, or face any part, except eye) 920
  scapular region 923.01
    with shoulder or upper arm 923.09
  sclera (eye) 921.3
  scrotum 922.4
  shoulder 923.00
    with upper arm or axillar regions 923.09
  skin NEC 924.9
  skull 920
  spermatic cord 922.4
  spinal cord (*see also* Injury, spinal, by site)
    cauda equina 952.4
    conus medullaris 952.4
  spleen 865.01
    with open wound into cavity 865.11
  sternal region 922.1
  stomach — *see* Injury, internal, stomach
  subconjunctival 921.1
  subcutaneous NEC 924.9
  submaxillary region (and other part(s) of neck, scalp, or face, except eye) 920
  submental region (and other part(s) of neck, scalp, or face, except eye) 920
  subperiosteal NEC 924.9
  supraclavicular fossa (and other part(s) of neck, scalp, or face, except eye) 920
  supraorbital (and other part(s) of neck, scalp, or face, except eye) 920
  temple (region) (and other part(s) of neck, scalp, or face, except eye) 920
  testis 922.4
  thigh (and hip) 924.00
  thorax 922.1
    organ — *see* Injury, internal, intrathoracic
  throat (and other part(s) of neck, scalp, or face, except eye) 920
  thumb(s) (nail) (subungual) 923.3
  toe(s) (nail) (subungual) 924.3
  tongue (and other part(s) of neck, scalp, or face, except eye) 920
  trunk 922.9
    multiple sites 922.8

Contusion — *continued*
  trunk — *continued*
    specified site — *see* Contusion, by site
  tunica vaginalis 922.4
  tympanum (membrane) (and other part(s) of neck, scalp, or face, except eye) 920
  upper extremity 923.9
    multiple sites 923.8
  uvula (and other part(s) of neck, scalp, or face, except eye) 920
  vagina 922.4
  vocal cord(s) (and other part(s) of neck, scalp, or face, except eye) 920
  vulva 922.4
  wrist 923.21
    with hand(s), except finger(s) alone 923.20
Conus (any type) (congenital) 743.57
  acquired 371.60
  medullaris syndrome 336.8
Convalescence (following) V66.9
  chemotherapy V66.2
  medical NEC V66.5
  psychotherapy V66.3
  radiotherapy V66.1
  surgery NEC V66.0
  treatment (for) NEC V66.5
    combined V66.6
    fracture V66.4
    mental disorder NEC V66.3
    specified disorder NEC V66.5
Conversion
  closed surgical procedure to open procedure
    arthroscopic V64.43
    laparoscopic V64.41
    thoracoscopic V64.42
  hysteria, hysterical, any type 300.11
  neurosis, any 300.11
  reaction, any 300.11
Converter, tuberculosis (test reaction) 795.51
Convulsions (idiopathic) 780.39
  apoplectiform (*see also* Disease, cerebrovascular, acute) 436
  brain 780.39
  cerebral 780.39
  cerebrospinal 780.39
  due to trauma NEC — *see* Injury, intracranial
  eclamptic (*see also* Eclampsia) 780.39
  epileptic (*see also* Epilepsy) 345.9 ☑
  epileptiform (*see also* Seizure, epileptiform) 780.39
  epileptoid (*see also* Seizure, epileptiform) 780.39
  ether
    anesthetic
      correct substance properly administered 780.39
      overdose or wrong substance given 968.2
    other specified type — *see* Table of Drugs and Chemicals
  febrile (simple) 780.31
    complex 780.32
  generalized 780.39
  hysterical 300.11
  infantile 780.39
    epilepsy — *see* Epilepsy
  internal 780.39
  jacksonian (*see also* Epilepsy) 345.5 ☑
  myoclonic 333.2
  newborn 779.0
  paretic 094.1
  pregnancy (nephritic) (uremic) — *see* Eclampsia, pregnancy
  psychomotor (*see also* Epilepsy) 345.4 ☑
  puerperal, postpartum — *see* Eclampsia, pregnancy
  recurrent 780.39
    epileptic — *see* Epilepsy
  reflex 781.0
  repetitive 780.39
    epileptic — *see* Epilepsy
  salaam (*see also* Epilepsy) 345.6 ☑
  scarlatinal 034.1

Convulsions — *continued*
  spasmodic 780.39
  tetanus, tetanic (*see also* Tetanus) 037
  thymic 254.8
  uncinate 780.39
  uremic 586
Convulsive — *see also* Convulsions
  disorder or state 780.39
    epileptic — *see* Epilepsy
  equivalent, abdominal (*see also* Epilepsy) 345.5 ☑
Cooke-Apert-Gallais syndrome (adrenogenital) 255.2
Cooley's anemia (erythroblastic) 282.44
Coolie itch 126.9
Cooper's
  disease 610.1
  hernia — *see* Hernia, Cooper's
Coordination disturbance 781.3
Copper wire arteries, retina 362.13
Copra itch 133.8
Coprolith 560.39
Coprophilia 302.89
Coproporphyria, hereditary 277.1
Coprostasis 560.32
  with hernia (*see also* Hernia, by site, with obstruction)
    gangrenous — *see* Hernia, by site, with gangrene
Cor
  biloculare 745.7
  bovinum — *see* Hypertrophy, cardiac
  bovis (*see also* Hypertrophy, cardiac)
  pulmonale (chronic) 416.9
    acute 415.0
  triatriatum, triatrium 746.82
  triloculare 745.8
    biatriatum 745.3
    biventriculare 745.69
Corbus' disease 607.1
Cord — *see also* condition
  around neck (tightly) (with compression)
    affecting fetus or newborn 762.5
    complicating delivery 663.1 ☑
      without compression 663.3 ☑
        affecting fetus or newborn 762.6
  bladder NEC 344.61
    tabetic 094.0
  prolapse
    affecting fetus or newborn 762.4
    complicating delivery 663.0 ☑
Cord's angiopathy — *see also* Tuberculosis 017.3 ☑ *[362.18]*
Cordis ectopia 746.87
Corditis (spermatic) 608.4
Corectopia 743.46
Cori type glycogen storage disease — *see* Disease, glycogen storage
Cork-handlers' disease or lung 495.3
Corkscrew esophagus 530.5
Corlett's pyosis (impetigo) 684
Corn (infected) 700
Cornea — *see also* condition
  donor V59.5
  guttata (dystrophy) 371.57
  plana 743.41
Cornelia de Lange's syndrome (Amsterdam dwarf, intellectual disabilities, and brachycephaly) 759.89
Cornual gestation or pregnancy — *see* Pregnancy, cornual
Cornu cutaneum 702.8
Coronary (artery) — *see also* condition
  arising from aorta or pulmonary trunk 746.85
Corpora — *see also* condition
  amylacea (prostate) 602.8
  cavernosa — *see* condition
Corpulence — *see* Obesity
Corpus — *see* condition
Corrigan's disease — *see* Insufficiency, aortic
Corrosive burn — *see* Burn, by site
Corsican fever — *see also* Malaria 084.6
Cortical — *see also* condition
  blindness 377.75
  necrosis, kidney (bilateral) 583.6

Corticoadrenal — *see* condition
Corticosexual syndrome 255.2
Coryza (acute) 460
  with grippe or influenza (*see also* Influenza) 487.1
  syphilitic 095.8
    congenital (chronic) 090.0
Costen's syndrome or complex 524.60
Costiveness — *see also* Constipation 564.00
Costochondritis 733.6
Cotard's syndrome (paranoia) 297.1
Cot death 798.0
Cotia virus 059.8
Cotungo's disease 724.3
Cough 786.2
  with hemorrhage (*see also* Hemoptysis) 786.39
  affected 786.2
  bronchial 786.2
    with grippe or influenza (*see also* Influenza) 487.1
  chronic 786.2
  epidemic 786.2
  functional 306.1
  hemorrhagic 786.39
  hysterical 300.11
  laryngeal, spasmodic 786.2
  nervous 786.2
  psychogenic 306.1
  smokers' 491.0
  tea tasters' 112.89
Counseling NEC V65.40
  without complaint or sickness V65.49
  abuse victim NEC V62.89
    child V61.21
    partner V61.11
    spouse V61.11
  child abuse, maltreatment, or neglect V61.21
  contraceptive NEC V25.09
    device (intrauterine) V25.02
      maintenance V25.40
        intrauterine contraceptive device V25.42
        oral contraceptive (pill) V25.41
        specified type NEC V25.49
        subdermal implantable V25.43
      management NEC V25.9
      oral contraceptive (pill) V25.01
        emergency V25.03
        postcoital V25.03
      prescription NEC V25.02
        oral contraceptive (pill) V25.01
          emergency V25.03
          postcoital V25.03
        repeat prescription V25.41
      repeat prescription V25.40
      subdermal implantable V25.43
      surveillance NEC V25.40
  dietary V65.3
  exercise V65.41
  expectant parent(s)
    pediatric pre-adoption visit V65.11
    pediatric pre-birth visit V65.11
  explanation of
    investigation finding NEC V65.49
    medication NEC V65.49
  family planning V25.09
    natural
      procreative V26.41
      to avoid pregnancy V25.04
  for nonattending third party V65.19
  genetic V26.33
  gonorrhea V65.45
  health (advice) (education) (instruction) NEC V65.49
  HIV V65.44
  human immunodeficiency virus V65.44
  injury prevention V65.43
  insulin pump training V65.46
  marital V61.10
  medical (for) V65.9
    boarding school resident V60.6
    condition not demonstrated V65.5
    feared complaint and no disease found V65.5

☑ **Additional Digit Required — Refer to the Tabular List for Digit Selection**   ▽ **Subterms under main terms may continue to next column or page**

Index

Counseling — Crush, crushed, crushing

Counseling — *continued*
　medical — *continued*
　　institutional resident V60.6
　　on behalf of another V65.19
　　person living alone V60.3
　natural family planning
　　procreative V26.41
　　to avoid pregnancy V25.04
　parent (guardian)-child conflict V61.20
　　adopted child V61.24
　　biological child V61.23
　　foster child V61.25
　　specified problem NEC V61.29
　partner abuse
　　perpetrator V61.12
　　victim V61.11
　pediatric
　　pre-adoption visit for adoptive parent(s)
　　　V65.11
　　pre-birth visit for expectant parents
　　　V65.11
　perpetrator of
　　child abuse V62.83
　　　parental V61.22
　　partner abuse V61.12
　　spouse abuse V61.12
　procreative V65.49
　sex NEC V65.49
　　transmitted disease NEC V65.45
　　　HIV V65.44
　specified reason NEC V65.49
　spousal abuse
　　perpetrator V61.12
　　victim V61.11
　substance use and abuse V65.42
　syphilis V65.45
　victim (of)
　　abuse NEC V62.89
　　child abuse V61.21
　　partner abuse V61.11
　　spousal abuse V61.11
Coupled rhythm 427.89
Couvelaire uterus (complicating delivery) —
　see Placenta, separation
Cowper's gland — *see* condition
Cowperitis — *see also* Urethritis 597.89
　gonorrheal (acute) 098.0
　　chronic or duration of 2 months or over
　　　098.2
Cowpox (abortive) 051.01
　due to vaccination 999.0
　eyelid 051.01 [373.5]
　　postvaccination 999.0 [373.5]
Coxa
　plana 732.1
　valga (acquired) 736.31
　　congenital 755.61
　　late effect of rickets 268.1
　vara (acquired) 736.32
　　congenital 755.62
　　late effect of rickets 268.1
Coxae malum senilis 715.25
Coxalgia (nontuberculous) 719.45
　tuberculous (*see also* Tuberculosis)
　　015.1 ☑ [730.85]
Coxalgic pelvis 736.30
Coxitis 716.65
Coxsackie (infection) (virus) 079.2
　central nervous system NEC 048
　endocarditis 074.22
　enteritis 008.67
　meningitis (aseptic) 047.0
　myocarditis 074.23
　pericarditis 074.21
　pharyngitis 074.0
　pleurodynia 074.1
　specific disease NEC 074.8
Crabs, meaning pubic lice 132.2
Crack baby 760.75
Cracked
　nipple 611.2
　　puerperal, postpartum 676.1 ☑
　tooth 521.81
Cradle cap 690.11
Craft neurosis 300.89
Craigiasis 007.8

Cramp(s) 729.82
　abdominal 789.0 ☑
　bathing 994.1
　colic 789.7
　　infantile 789.7
　　psychogenic 306.4
　due to immersion 994.1
　extremity (lower) (upper) NEC 729.82
　fireman 992.2
　heat 992.2
　hysterical 300.11
　immersion 994.1
　intestinal 789.0 ☑
　　psychogenic 306.4
　linotypist's 300.89
　　organic 333.84
　muscle (extremity) (general) 729.82
　　due to immersion 994.1
　　hysterical 300.11
　occupational (hand) 300.89
　　organic 333.84
　psychogenic 307.89
　salt depletion 276.1
　sleep related leg 327.52
　stoker 992.2
　stomach 789.0 ☑
　telegraphers' 300.89
　　organic 333.84
　typists' 300.89
　　organic 333.84
　uterus 625.8
　　menstrual 625.3
　writers' 333.84
　　organic 333.84
　　psychogenic 300.89
Cranial — *see* condition
Cranioclasis, fetal 763.89
Craniocleidodysostosis 755.59
Craniofenestria (skull) 756.0
Craniolacunia (skull) 756.0
Craniopagus 759.4
Craniopathy, metabolic 733.3
Craniopharyngeal — *see* condition
Craniopharyngioma (M9350/1) 237.0
Craniorachischisis (totalis) 740.1
Cranioschisis 756.0
Craniostenosis 756.0
Craniosynostosis 756.0
Craniotabes (cause unknown) 733.3
　rachitic 268.1
　syphilitic 090.5
Craniotomy, fetal 763.89
Cranium — *see* condition
Craw-craw 125.3
CRBSI (catheter-related bloodstream infection)
　999.31
Creaking joint 719.60
　ankle 719.67
　elbow 719.62
　foot 719.67
　hand 719.64
　hip 719.65
　knee 719.66
　multiple sites 719.69
　pelvic region 719.65
　shoulder (region) 719.61
　specified site NEC 719.68
　wrist 719.63
Creeping
　eruption 126.9
　palsy 335.21
　paralysis 335.21
Crenated tongue 529.8
Creotoxism 005.9
Crepitus
　caput 756.0
　joint 719.60
　　ankle 719.67
　　elbow 719.62
　　foot 719.67
　　hand 719.64
　　hip 719.65
　　knee 719.66
　　multiple sites 719.69
　　pelvic region 719.65
　　shoulder (region) 719.61

Crepitus — *continued*
　joint — *continued*
　　specified site NEC 719.68
　　wrist 719.63
Crescent or conus choroid, congenital 743.57
Cretin, cretinism (athyrotic) (congenital) (en-
　demic) (metabolic) (nongoitrous) (spo-
　radic) 243
　goitrous (sporadic) 246.1
　pelvis (dwarf type) (male type) 243
　　with disproportion (fetopelvic) 653.1 ☑
　　　affecting fetus or newborn 763.1
　　　causing obstructed labor 660.1 ☑
　　　　affecting fetus or newborn 763.1
　pituitary 253.3
Cretinoid degeneration 243
Creutzfeldt-Jakob disease (CJD) (syndrome)
　046.19
　with dementia
　　with behavioral disturbance
　　　046.19 [294.11]
　　without behavioral disturbance
　　　046.19 [294.10]
　familial 046.19
　iatrogenic 046.19
　specified NEC 046.19
　sporadic 046.19
　variant (vCJD) 046.11
　　with dementia
　　　with behavioral disturbance
　　　　046.11 [294.11]
　　　without behavioral disturbance
　　　　046.11 [294.10]
Crib death 798.0
Cribriform hymen 752.49
Cri-du-chat syndrome 758.31
Crigler-Najjar disease or syndrome (congen-
　ital hyperbilirubinemia) 277.4
Crimean hemorrhagic fever 065.0
Criminalism 301.7
Crisis
　abdomen 789.0 ☑
　addisonian (acute adrenocortical insufficien-
　　cy) 255.41
　adrenal (cortical) 255.41
　asthmatic — *see* Asthma
　brain, cerebral (*see also* Disease, cerebrovas-
　　cular, acute) 436
　celiac 579.0
　Dietl's 593.4
　emotional NEC 309.29
　　acute reaction to stress 308.0
　　adjustment reaction 309.9
　　specific to childhood or adolescence
　　　313.9
　gastric (tabetic) 094.0
　glaucomatocyclitic 364.22
　heart (*see also* Failure, heart) 428.9
　hypertensive — *see* Hypertension
　nitritoid
　　correct substance properly administered
　　　458.29
　　overdose or wrong substance given or
　　　taken 961.1
　oculogyric 378.87
　　psychogenic 306.7
　Pel's 094.0
　psychosexual identity 302.6
　rectum 094.0
　renal 593.81
　sickle cell 282.62
　stomach (tabetic) 094.0
　tabetic 094.0
　thyroid (*see also* Thyrotoxicosis) 242.9 ☑
　thyrotoxic (*see also* Thyrotoxicosis) 242.9 ☑
　vascular — *see* Disease, cerebrovascular,
　　acute
Crocq's disease (acrocyanosis) 443.89
Crohn's disease — *see also* Enteritis, regional
　555.9
Cronkhite-Canada syndrome 211.3
Crooked septum, nasal 470
Cross
　birth (of fetus) complicating delivery
　　652.3 ☑
　　with successful version 652.1 ☑

Cross — *continued*
　birth complicating delivery — *continued*
　　causing obstructed labor 660.0 ☑
　bite, anterior or posterior 524.27
　eye (*see also* Esotropia) 378.00
Crossed ectopia of kidney 753.3
Crossfoot 754.50
Croup, croupous (acute) (angina) (catarrhal)
　(infective) (inflammatory) (laryngeal)
　(membranous) (nondiphtheritic) (pseu-
　domembranous) 464.4
　asthmatic (*see also* Asthma) 493.9 ☑
　bronchial 466.0
　diphtheritic (membranous) 032.3
　false 478.75
　spasmodic 478.75
　　diphtheritic 032.3
　stridulous 478.75
　　diphtheritic 032.3
Crouzon's disease (craniofacial dysostosis)
　756.0
Crowding, teeth 524.31
CRST syndrome (cutaneous systemic sclerosis)
　710.1
Cruchet's disease (encephalitis lethargica)
　049.8
Cruelty in children — *see also* Disturbance,
　conduct 312.9
Crural ulcer — *see also* Ulcer, lower extremity
　707.10
Crush, crushed, crushing (injury) 929.9
　abdomen 926.19
　　internal — *see* Injury, internal, abdomen
　ankle 928.21
　　with other parts of foot 928.20
　arm 927.9
　　lower (and elbow) 927.10
　　upper 927.03
　　　with shoulder or axillary region
　　　　927.09
　axilla 927.02
　　with shoulder or upper arm 927.09
　back 926.11
　breast 926.19
　buttock 926.12
　cheek 925.1
　chest — *see* Injury, internal, chest
　ear 925.1
　elbow 927.11
　　with forearm 927.10
　face 925.1
　finger(s) 927.3
　　with hand(s) 927.20
　　　and wrist(s) 927.21
　flank 926.19
　foot, excluding toe(s) alone (with ankle)
　　928.20
　forearm (and elbow) 927.10
　genitalia, external (female) (male) 926.0
　　internal — *see* Injury, internal, genital
　　　organ NEC
　hand, except finger(s) alone (and wrist)
　　927.20
　head — *see* Fracture, skull, by site
　heel 928.20
　hip 928.01
　　with thigh 928.00
　internal organ (abdomen, chest, or pelvis)
　　— *see* Injury, internal, by site
　knee 928.11
　　with leg, lower 928.10
　labium (majus) (minus) 926.0
　larynx 925.2
　late effect — *see* Late, effects (of), crushing
　leg 928.9
　　lower 928.10
　　　and knee 928.11
　　upper 928.00
　limb
　　lower 928.9
　　　multiple sites 928.8
　　upper 927.9
　　　multiple sites 927.8
　multiple sites NEC 929.0
　neck 925.2
　nerve — *see* Injury, nerve, by site

☑ **Additional Digit Required** — Refer to the Tabular List for Digit Selection　　　　　　　🔻 **Subterms under main terms may continue to next column or page**

58 — Volume 2　　　　▶◀ **Revised Text**　　　● **New Line**　　　▲ **Revised Code**　　　**2013 ICD-9-CM**

Crush, crushed, crushing — *continued*
　　nose 802.0
　　　　open 802.1
　　penis 926.0
　　pharynx 925.2
　　scalp 925.1
　　scapular region 927.01
　　　　with shoulder or upper arm 927.09
　　scrotum 926.0
　　shoulder 927.00
　　　　with upper arm or axillary region 927.09
　　skull or cranium — *see* Fracture, skull, by
　　　　　site
　　spinal cord — *see* Injury, spinal, by site
　　syndrome (complication of trauma) 958.5
　　testis 926.0
　　thigh (with hip) 928.00
　　throat 925.2
　　thumb(s) (and fingers) 927.3
　　toe(s) 928.3
　　　　with foot 928.20
　　　　　　and ankle 928.21
　　tonsil 925.2
　　trunk 926.9
　　　　chest — *see* Injury, internal, intrathoracic
　　　　　　organs NEC
　　　　internal organ — *see* Injury, internal, by
　　　　　　site
　　　　multiple sites 926.8
　　　　specified site NEC 926.19
　　vulva 926.0
　　wrist 927.21
　　　　with hand(s), except fingers alone 927.20
Crusta lactea 690.11
Crusts 782.8
Crutch paralysis 953.4
Cruveilhier-Baumgarten cirrhosis, disease,
　　or syndrome 571.5
Cruveilhier's disease 335.21
Cruz-Chagas disease — *see also* Trypanosomi-
　　asis 086.2
Crying
　　constant, continuous
　　　　adolescent 780.95
　　　　adult 780.95
　　　　baby 780.92
　　　　child 780.95
　　　　infant 780.92
　　　　newborn 780.92
　　excessive
　　　　adolescent 780.95
　　　　adult 780.95
　　　　baby 780.92
　　　　child 780.95
　　　　infant 780.92
　　　　newborn 780.92
Cryofibrinogenemia 273.2
Cryoglobulinemia (mixed) 273.2
Crypt (anal) (rectal) 569.49
Cryptitis (anal) (rectal) 569.49
Cryptococcosis (European) (pulmonary) (sys-
　　temic) 117.5
Cryptococcus 117.5
　　epidermicus 117.5
　　neoformans, infection by 117.5
Cryptopapillitis (anus) 569.49
Cryptophthalmos (eyelid) 743.06
Cryptorchid, cryptorchism, cryptorchidism
　　752.51
Cryptosporidiosis 007.4
　　hepatobiliary 136.8
　　respiratory 136.8
Cryptotia 744.29
Crystallopathy
　　calcium pyrophosphate (*see also* Arthritis)
　　　　275.49 *[712.2]* ☑
　　dicalcium phosphate (*see also* Arthritis)
　　　　275.49 *[712.1]* ☑
　　gouty 274.00
　　pyrophosphate NEC (*see also* Arthritis)
　　　　275.49 *[712.2]* ☑
　　uric acid 274.00
Crystalluria 791.9
Csillag's disease (lichen sclerosis et atrophicus)
　　701.0
Cuban itch 050.1

Cubitus
　　valgus (acquired) 736.01
　　　　congenital 755.59
　　　　late effect of rickets 268.1
　　varus (acquired) 736.02
　　　　congenital 755.59
　　　　late effect of rickets 268.1
Cultural deprivation V62.4
Cupping of optic disc 377.14
Curling esophagus 530.5
Curling's ulcer — *see* Ulcer, duodenum
Curschmann (-Batten) (-Steinert) disease or
　　syndrome 359.21
Curvature
　　organ or site, congenital NEC — *see* Distor-
　　　　tion
　　penis (lateral) 752.69
　　Pott's (spinal) (*see also* Tuberculosis)
　　　　015.0 ☑ *[737.43]*
　　radius, idiopathic, progressive (congenital)
　　　　755.54
　　spine (acquired) (angular) (idiopathic) (incor-
　　　　rect) (postural) 737.9
　　　　congenital 754.2
　　　　due to or associated with
　　　　　　Charcôt-Marie-Tooth disease
　　　　　　　　356.1 *[737.40]*
　　　　　　mucopolysaccharidosis
　　　　　　　　277.5 *[737.40]*
　　　　　　neurofibromatosis 237.71 *[737.40]*
　　　　　　osteitis
　　　　　　　　deformans 731.0 *[737.40]*
　　　　　　　　fibrosa cystica 252.01 *[737.40]*
　　　　　　osteoporosis (*see also* Osteoporosis)
　　　　　　　　733.00 *[737.40]*
　　　　　　poliomyelitis (*see also* Poliomyelitis)
　　　　　　　　138 *[737.40]*
　　　　　　tuberculosis (Pott's curvature) (*see*
　　　　　　　　also Tuberculosis)
　　　　　　　　015.0 ☑ *[737.43]*
　　　　kyphoscoliotic (*see also* Kyphoscoliosis)
　　　　　　737.30
　　　　kyphotic (*see also* Kyphosis) 737.10
　　　　late effect of rickets 268.1 *[737.40]*
　　　　Pott's 015.0 ☑ *[737.40]*
　　　　scoliotic (*see also* Scoliosis) 737.30
　　　　specified NEC 737.8
　　　　tuberculous 015.0 ☑ *[737.40]*
Cushing's
　　basophilism, disease, or syndrome (iatro-
　　　　genic) (idiopathic) (pituitary ba-
　　　　sophilism) (pituitary dependent)
　　　　255.0
　　ulcer — *see* Ulcer, peptic
Cushingoid due to steroid therapy
　　correct substance properly administered
　　　　255.0
　　overdose or wrong substance given or taken
　　　　962.0
Cut (external) — *see* Wound, open, by site
Cutaneous — *see also* condition
　　hemorrhage 782.7
　　horn (cheek) (eyelid) (mouth) 702.8
　　larva migrans 126.9
Cutis — *see also* condition
　　hyperelastic 756.83
　　　　acquired 701.8
　　laxa 756.83
　　　　senilis 701.8
　　marmorata 782.61
　　osteosis 709.3
　　pendula 756.83
　　　　acquired 701.8
　　rhomboidalis nuchae 701.8
　　verticis gyrata 757.39
　　　　acquired 701.8
Cyanopathy, newborn 770.83
Cyanosis 782.5
　　autotoxic 289.7
　　common atrioventricular canal 745.69
　　congenital 770.83
　　conjunctiva 372.71
　　due to
　　　　endocardial cushion defect 745.60
　　　　nonclosure, foramen botalli 745.5
　　　　patent foramen botalli 745.5

Cyanosis — *continued*
　　due to — *continued*
　　　　persistent foramen ovale 745.5
　　enterogenous 289.7
　　fetus or newborn 770.83
　　ostium primum defect 745.61
　　paroxysmal digital 443.0
　　retina, retinal 362.10
Cycle
　　anovulatory 628.0
　　menstrual, irregular 626.4
Cyclencephaly 759.89
Cyclical vomiting 536.2
　　associated with migraine 346.2 ☑
　　psychogenic 306.4
Cyclitic membrane 364.74
Cyclitis — *see also* Iridocyclitis 364.3
　　acute 364.00
　　　　primary 364.01
　　　　recurrent 364.02
　　chronic 364.10
　　　　in
　　　　　　sarcoidosis 135 *[364.11]*
　　　　　　tuberculosis (*see also* Tuberculosis)
　　　　　　　　017.3 ☑ *[364.11]*
　　Fuchs' heterochromic 364.21
　　granulomatous 364.10
　　lens induced 364.23
　　nongranulomatous 364.00
　　posterior 363.21
　　primary 364.01
　　recurrent 364.02
　　secondary (noninfectious) 364.04
　　　　infectious 364.03
　　subacute 364.00
　　　　primary 364.01
　　　　recurrent 364.02
Cyclokeratitis — *see* Keratitis
Cyclophoria 378.44
Cyclopia, cyclops 759.89
Cycloplegia 367.51
Cyclospasm 367.53
Cyclosporiasis 007.5
Cyclothymia 301.13
Cyclothymic personality 301.13
Cyclotropia 378.33
Cyesis — *see* Pregnancy
Cylindroma (M8200/3) — *see also* Neoplasm,
　　by site, malignant
　　eccrine dermal (M8200/0) — *see* Neoplasm,
　　　　skin, benign
　　skin (M8200/0) — *see* Neoplasm, skin, be-
　　　　nign
Cylindruria 791.7
Cyllosoma 759.89
Cynanche
　　diphtheritic 032.3
　　tonsillaris 475
Cynorexia 783.6
Cyphosis — *see* Kyphosis
Cyprus fever — *see also* Brucellosis 023.9
Cyriax's syndrome (slipping rib) 733.99
Cyst (mucus) (retention) (serous) (simple)

Note — *In general, cysts are not neoplastic and are classified to the appropriate category for disease of the specified anatomical site. This generalization
does not apply to certain types of cysts
which are neoplastic in nature, for example, dermoid, nor does it apply to
cysts of certain structures, for example,
branchial cleft, which are classified as
developmental anomalies.*

*The following listing includes some of
the most frequently reported sites of
cysts as well as qualifiers which indicate
the type of cyst. The latter qualifiers
usually are not repeated under the
anatomical sites. Since the code assignment for a given site may vary depending upon the type of cyst, the coder
should refer to the listings under the
specified type of cyst before considera-
tion is given to the site.*

　　accessory, fallopian tube 752.11

Cyst — *continued*
　　adenoid (infected) 474.8
　　adrenal gland 255.8
　　　　congenital 759.1
　　air, lung 518.89
　　allantoic 753.7
　　alveolar process (jaw bone) 526.2
　　amnion, amniotic 658.8 ☑
　　anterior chamber (eye) 364.60
　　　　exudative 364.62
　　　　implantation (surgical) (traumatic)
　　　　　　364.61
　　　　parasitic 360.13
　　anterior nasopalatine 526.1
　　antrum 478.19
　　anus 569.49
　　apical (periodontal) (tooth) 522.8
　　appendix 543.9
　　arachnoid, brain 348.0
　　arytenoid 478.79
　　auricle 706.2
　　Baker's (knee) 727.51
　　　　tuberculous (*see also* Tuberculosis)
　　　　　　015.2 ☑
　　Bartholin's gland or duct 616.2
　　bile duct (*see also* Disease, biliary) 576.8
　　bladder (multiple) (trigone) 596.89
　　Blessig's 362.62
　　blood, endocardial (*see also* Endocarditis)
　　　　424.90
　　blue dome 610.0
　　bone (local) 733.20
　　　　aneurysmal 733.22
　　　　jaw 526.2
　　　　　　developmental (odontogenic) 526.0
　　　　　　fissural 526.1
　　　　　　latent 526.89
　　　　solitary 733.21
　　　　unicameral 733.21
　　brain 348.0
　　　　congenital 742.4
　　　　hydatid (*see also* Echinococcus) 122.9
　　　　third ventricle (colloid) 742.4
　　branchial (cleft) 744.42
　　branchiogenic 744.42
　　breast (benign) (blue dome) (pedunculated)
　　　　(solitary) (traumatic) 610.0
　　　　involution 610.4
　　　　sebaceous 610.8
　　broad ligament (benign) 620.8
　　　　embryonic 752.11
　　bronchogenic (mediastinal) (sequestration)
　　　　518.89
　　　　congenital 748.4
　　buccal 528.4
　　bulbourethral gland (Cowper's) 599.89
　　bursa, bursal 727.49
　　　　pharyngeal 478.26
　　calcifying odontogenic (M9301/0) 213.1
　　　　upper jaw (bone) 213.0
　　canal of Nuck (acquired) (serous) 629.1
　　　　congenital 752.41
　　canthus 372.75
　　carcinomatous (M8010/3) — *see* Neoplasm,
　　　　by site, malignant
　　cartilage (joint) — *see* Derangement, joint
　　cauda equina 336.8
　　cavum septi pellucidi NEC 348.0
　　celomic (pericardium) 746.89
　　cerebellopontine (angle) — *see* Cyst, brain
　　cerebellum — *see* Cyst, brain
　　cerebral — *see* Cyst, brain
　　cervical lateral 744.42
　　cervix 622.8
　　　　embryonal 752.41
　　　　nabothian (gland) 616.0
　　chamber, anterior (eye) 364.60
　　　　exudative 364.62
　　　　implantation (surgical) (traumatic)
　　　　　　364.61
　　　　parasitic 360.13
　　chiasmal, optic NEC (*see also* Lesion, chias-
　　　　mal) 377.54
　　chocolate (ovary) 617.1
　　choledochal (congenital) 751.69
　　　　acquired 576.8

☑ **Additional Digit Required — Refer to the Tabular List for Digit Selection**　　　　　　　　　　　　　　👁 **Subterms under main terms may continue to next column or page**

2013 ICD-9-CM　　　　　▶◀ **Revised Text**　　　　　● **New Line**　　　▲ **Revised Code**　　　　　　　　　　**Volume 2 — 59**

Crush, crushed, crushing — Cyst

Cyst — continued
choledochus 751.69
chorion 658.8 ☑
choroid plexus 348.0
chyle, mesentery 457.8
ciliary body 364.60
   exudative 364.64
   implantation 364.61
   primary 364.63
clitoris 624.8
coccyx (see also Cyst, bone) 733.20
colloid
   third ventricle (brain) 742.4
   thyroid gland — see Goiter
colon 569.89
common (bile) duct (see also Disease, biliary) 576.8
congenital NEC 759.89
   adrenal glands 759.1
   epiglottis 748.3
   esophagus 750.4
   fallopian tube 752.11
   kidney 753.10
      multiple 753.19
      single 753.11
   larynx 748.3
   liver 751.62
   lung 748.4
   mediastinum 748.8
   ovary 752.0
   oviduct 752.11
   pancreas 751.7
   periurethral (tissue) 753.8
   prepuce NEC 752.69
      penis 752.69
   sublingual 750.26
   submaxillary gland 750.26
   thymus (gland) 759.2
   tongue 750.19
   ureterovesical orifice 753.4
   vulva 752.41
conjunctiva 372.75
cornea 371.23
corpora quadrigemina 348.0
corpus
   albicans (ovary) 620.2
   luteum (ruptured) 620.1
Cowper's gland (benign) (infected) 599.89
cranial meninges 348.0
craniobuccal pouch 253.8
craniopharyngeal pouch 253.8
cystic duct (see also Disease, gallbladder) 575.8
Cysticercus (any site) 123.1
Dandy-Walker 742.3
   with spina bifida (see also Spina bifida) 741.0 ☑
dental 522.8
   developmental 526.0
   eruption 526.0
   lateral periodontal 526.0
   primordial (keratocyst) 526.0
   root 522.8
dentigerous 526.0
   mandible 526.0
   maxilla 526.0
dermoid (M9084/0) (see also Neoplasm, by site, benign)
   with malignant transformation (M9084/3) 183.0
   implantation
      external area or site (skin) NEC 709.8
      iris 364.61
      skin 709.8
      vagina 623.8
      vulva 624.8
   mouth 528.4
   oral soft tissue 528.4
   sacrococcygeal 685.1
      with abscess 685.0
   developmental of ovary, ovarian 752.0
dura (cerebral) 348.0
   spinal 349.2
ear (external) 706.2
echinococcal (see also Echinococcus) 122.9

Cyst — continued
embryonal
   cervix uteri 752.41
   genitalia, female external 752.41
   uterus 752.39
   vagina 752.41
endometrial 621.8
   ectopic 617.9
endometrium (uterus) 621.8
   ectopic — see Endometriosis
enteric 751.5
enterogenous 751.5
epidermal (inclusion) (see also Cyst, skin) 706.2
epidermoid (inclusion) (see also Cyst, skin) 706.2
   mouth 528.4
   not of skin — see Cyst, by site
   oral soft tissue 528.4
epididymis 608.89
epiglottis 478.79
epiphysis cerebri 259.8
epithelial (inclusion) (see also Cyst, skin) 706.2
epoophoron 752.11
eruption 526.0
esophagus 530.89
ethmoid sinus 478.19
eye (retention) 379.8
   congenital 743.03
   posterior segment, congenital 743.54
eyebrow 706.2
eyelid (sebaceous) 374.84
   infected 373.13
   sweat glands or ducts 374.84
falciform ligament (inflammatory) 573.8
fallopian tube 620.8
   congenital 752.11
female genital organs NEC 629.89
fimbrial (congenital) 752.11
fissural (oral region) 526.1
follicle (atretic) (graafian) (ovarian) 620.0
   nabothian (gland) 616.0
follicular (atretic) (ovarian) 620.0
   dentigerous 526.0
frontal sinus 478.19
gallbladder or duct 575.8
ganglion 727.43
Gartner's duct 752.41
gas, of mesentery 568.89
gingiva 523.8
gland of moll 374.84
globulomaxillary 526.1
graafian follicle 620.0
granulosal lutein 620.2
hemangiomatous (M9121/0) (see also Hemangioma) 228.00
hydatid (see also Echinococcus) 122.9
   fallopian tube (Morgagni) 752.11
   liver NEC 122.8
   lung NEC 122.9
   Morgagni 752.89
      fallopian tube 752.11
   specified site NEC 122.9
hymen 623.8
   embryonal 752.41
hypopharynx 478.26
hypophysis, hypophyseal (duct) (recurrent) 253.8
   cerebri 253.8
implantation (dermoid)
   anterior chamber (eye) 364.61
   external area or site (skin) NEC 709.8
   iris 364.61
   vagina 623.8
   vulva 624.8
incisor, incisive canal 526.1
inclusion (epidermal) (epithelial) (epidermoid) (mucous) (squamous) (see also Cyst, skin) 706.2
   not of skin — see Neoplasm, by site, benign
intestine (large) (small) 569.89
intracranial — see Cyst, brain
intraligamentous 728.89
   knee 717.89

Cyst — continued
intrasellar 253.8
iris (idiopathic) 364.60
   exudative 364.62
   implantation (surgical) (traumatic) 364.61
   miotic pupillary 364.55
   parasitic 360.13
Iwanoff's 362.62
jaw (bone) (aneurysmal) (extravasation) (hemorrhagic) (traumatic) 526.2
   developmental (odontogenic) 526.0
   fissural 526.1
keratin 706.2
kidney (congenital) 753.10
   acquired 593.2
   calyceal (see also Hydronephrosis) 591
   multiple 753.19
   pyelogenic (see also Hydronephrosis) 591
   simple 593.2
   single 753.11
   solitary (not congenital) 593.2
labium (majus) (minus) 624.8
   sebaceous 624.8
lacrimal
   apparatus 375.43
   gland or sac 375.12
larynx 478.79
lens 379.39
   congenital 743.39
lip (gland) 528.5
liver 573.8
   congenital 751.62
   hydatid (see also Echinococcus) 122.8
      granulosis 122.0
      multilocularis 122.5
lung 518.89
   congenital 748.4
   giant bullous 492.0
lutein 620.1
lymphangiomatous (M9173/0) 228.1
lymphoepithelial
   mouth 528.4
   oral soft tissue 528.4
macula 362.54
malignant (M8000/3) — see Neoplasm, by site, malignant
mammary gland (sweat gland) (see also Cyst, breast) 610.0
mandible 526.2
   dentigerous 526.0
   radicular 522.8
maxilla 526.2
   dentigerous 526.0
   radicular 522.8
median
   anterior maxillary 526.1
   palatal 526.1
mediastinum (congenital) 748.8
meibomian (gland) (retention) 373.2
   infected 373.12
membrane, brain 348.0
meninges (cerebral) 348.0
   spinal 349.2
meniscus knee 717.5
mesentery, mesenteric (gas) 568.89
   chyle 457.8
   gas 568.89
mesonephric duct 752.89
mesothelial
   peritoneum 568.89
   pleura (peritoneal) 568.89
milk 611.5
miotic pupillary (iris) 364.55
Morgagni (hydatid) 752.89
   fallopian tube 752.11
mouth 528.4
Müllerian duct 752.89
   appendix testis 608.89
   cervix (embryonal) 752.41
   fallopian tube 752.11
   prostatic utricle 599.89
   vagina (embryonal) 752.41
multilocular (ovary) (M8000/1) 239.5
myometrium 621.8

Cyst — continued
nabothian (follicle) (ruptured) 616.0
nasal sinus 478.19
nasoalveolar 528.4
nasolabial 528.4
nasopalatine (duct) 526.1
   anterior 526.1
nasopharynx 478.26
neoplastic (M8000/1) (see also Neoplasm, by site, unspecified nature)
   benign (M8000/0) — see Neoplasm, by site, benign
   uterus 621.8
nervous system — see Cyst, brain
neuroenteric 742.59
neuroepithelial ventricle 348.0
nipple 610.0
nose 478.19
   skin of 706.2
odontogenic, developmental 526.0
omentum (lesser) 568.89
   congenital 751.8
oral soft tissue (dermoid) (epidermoid) (lymphoepithelial) 528.4
ora serrata 361.19
orbit 376.81
ovary, ovarian (twisted) 620.2
   adherent 620.2
   chocolate 617.1
   corpus
      albicans 620.2
      luteum 620.1
   dermoid (M9084/0) 220
   developmental 752.0
   due to failure of involution NEC 620.2
   endometrial 617.1
   follicular (atretic) (graafian) (hemorrhagic) 620.0
   hemorrhagic 620.2
   in pregnancy or childbirth 654.4 ☑
      affecting fetus or newborn 763.89
      causing obstructed labor 660.2 ☑
         affecting fetus or newborn 763.1
   multilocular (M8000/1) 239.5
   pseudomucinous (M8470/0) 220
   retention 620.2
   serous 620.2
   theca lutein 620.2
   tuberculous (see also Tuberculosis) 016.6 ☑
   unspecified 620.2
oviduct 620.8
palatal papilla (jaw) 526.1
palate 526.1
   fissural 526.1
   median (fissural) 526.1
palatine, of papilla 526.1
pancreas, pancreatic 577.2
   congenital 751.7
   false 577.2
   hemorrhagic 577.2
   true 577.2
paralabral
   hip 718.85
   shoulder 840.7
paramesonephric duct — see Cyst, Müllerian duct
paranephric 593.2
para ovarian 752.11
paraphysis, cerebri 742.4
parasitic NEC 136.9
parathyroid (gland) 252.8
paratubal (fallopian) 620.8
paraurethral duct 599.89
paroophoron 752.11
parotid gland 527.6
   mucous extravasation or retention 527.6
parovarian 752.11
pars planus 364.60
   exudative 364.64
   primary 364.63
pelvis, female
   in pregnancy or childbirth 654.4 ☑
      affecting fetus or newborn 763.89
      causing obstructed labor 660.2 ☑
         affecting fetus or newborn 763.1

☑ Additional Digit Required — Refer to the Tabular List for Digit Selection   ᵂ Subterms under main terms may continue to next column or page

Cyst — *continued*
  penis (sebaceous) 607.89
  periapical 522.8
  pericardial (congenital) 746.89
    acquired (secondary) 423.8
  pericoronal 526.0
  perineural (Tarlov's) 355.9
  periodontal 522.8
    lateral 526.0
  peripancreatic 577.2
  peripelvic (lymphatic) 593.2
  peritoneum 568.89
    chylous 457.8
  pharynx (wall) 478.26
  pilar 704.41
  pilonidal (infected) (rectum) 685.1
    with abscess 685.0
    malignant (M9084/3) 173.59
  pituitary (duct) (gland) 253.8
  placenta (amniotic) — *see* Placenta, abnormal
  pleura 519.8
  popliteal 727.51
  porencephalic 742.4
    acquired 348.0
  postanal (infected) 685.1
    with abscess 685.0
  posterior segment of eye, congenital 743.54
  postmastoidectomy cavity 383.31
  preauricular 744.47
  prepuce 607.89
    congenital 752.69
  primordial (jaw) 526.0
  prostate 600.3
  pseudomucinous (ovary) (M8470/0) 220
  pudenda (sweat glands) 624.8
  pupillary, miotic 364.55
    sebaceous 624.8
  radicular (residual) 522.8
  radiculodental 522.8
  ranular 527.6
  Rathke's pouch 253.8
  rectum (epithelium) (mucous) 569.49
  renal — *see* Cyst, kidney
  residual (radicular) 522.8
  retention (ovary) 620.2
  retina 361.19
    macular 362.54
    parasitic 360.13
    primary 361.13
    secondary 361.14
  retroperitoneal 568.89
  sacrococcygeal (dermoid) 685.1
    with abscess 685.0
  salivary gland or duct 527.6
    mucous extravasation or retention 527.6
  Sampson's 617.1
  sclera 379.19
  scrotum (sebaceous) 706.2
    sweat glands 706.2
  sebaceous (duct) (gland) 706.2
    breast 610.8
    eyelid 374.84
    genital organ NEC
      female 629.89
      male 608.89
    scrotum 706.2
  semilunar cartilage (knee) (multiple) 717.5
  seminal vesicle 608.89
  serous (ovary) 620.2
  sinus (antral) (ethmoidal) (frontal) (maxillary) (nasal) (sphenoidal) 478.19
  Skene's gland 599.89
  skin (epidermal) (epidermoid, inclusion) (epithelial) (inclusion) (retention) (sebaceous) 706.2
    breast 610.8
    eyelid 374.84
    genital organ NEC
      female 629.89
      male 608.89
    neoplastic 216.3
    scrotum 706.2
    sweat gland or duct 705.89
  solitary
    bone 733.21

Cyst — *continued*
  solitary — *continued*
    kidney 593.2
  spermatic cord 608.89
  sphenoid sinus 478.19
  spinal meninges 349.2
  spine (*see also* Cyst, bone) 733.20
  spleen NEC 289.59
    congenital 759.0
    hydatid (*see also* Echinococcus) 122.9
  spring water (pericardium) 746.89
  subarachnoid 348.0
    intrasellar 793.0
  subdural (cerebral) 348.0
    spinal cord 349.2
  sublingual gland 527.6
    mucous extravasation or retention 527.6
  submaxillary gland 527.6
    mucous extravasation or retention 527.6
  suburethral 599.89
  suprarenal gland 255.8
  suprasellar — *see* Cyst, brain
  sweat gland or duct 705.89
  sympathetic nervous system 337.9
  synovial 727.40
    popliteal space 727.51
  Tarlov's 355.9
  tarsal 373.2
  tendon (sheath) 727.42
  testis 608.89
  theca-lutein (ovary) 620.2
  Thornwaldt's, Tornwaldt's 478.26
  thymus (gland) 254.8
  thyroglossal (duct) (infected) (persistent) 759.2
  thyroid 246.2
    adenomatous — *see* Goiter, nodular
    colloid (*see also* Goiter) 240.9
  thyrolingual duct (infected) (persistent) 759.2
  tongue (mucous) 529.8
  tonsil 474.8
  tooth (dental root) 522.8
  trichilemmal (proliferating) 704.42
  tubo-ovarian 620.8
    inflammatory 614.1
  tunica vaginalis 608.89
  turbinate (nose) (*see also* Cyst, bone) 733.20
  Tyson's gland (benign) (infected) 607.89
  umbilicus 759.89
  urachus 753.7
  ureter 593.89
  ureterovesical orifice 593.89
    congenital 753.4
  urethra 599.84
  urethral gland (Cowper's) 599.89
  uterine
    ligament 620.8
      embryonic 752.11
    tube 620.8
  uterus (body) (corpus) (recurrent) 621.8
    embryonal 752.39
  utricle (ear) 386.8
    prostatic 599.89
  utriculus masculinus 599.89
  vagina, vaginal (squamous cell) (wall) 623.8
    embryonal 752.41
    implantation 623.8
    inclusion 623.8
  vallecula, vallecular 478.79
  ventricle, neuroepithelial 348.0
  verumontanum 599.89
  vesical (orifice) 596.89
  vitreous humor 379.29
  vulva (sweat glands) 624.8
    congenital 752.41
    implantation 624.8
    inclusion 624.8
    sebaceous gland 624.8
  vulvovaginal gland 624.8
  wolffian 752.89
Cystadenocarcinoma (M8440/3) — *see also* Neoplasm, by site, malignant
  bile duct type (M8161/3) 155.1
  endometrioid (M8380/3) — *see* Neoplasm, by site, malignant

Cystadenocarcinoma — *see also* Neoplasm, by site, malignant — *continued*
  mucinous (M8470/3)
    papillary (M8471/3)
      specified site — *see* Neoplasm, by site, malignant
      unspecified site 183.0
    specified site — *see* Neoplasm, by site, malignant
    unspecified site 183.0
  papillary (M8450/3)
    mucinous (M8471/3)
      specified site — *see* Neoplasm, by site, malignant
      unspecified site 183.0
    pseudomucinous (M8471/3)
      specified site — *see* Neoplasm, by site, malignant
      unspecified site 183.0
    serous (M8460/3)
      specified site — *see* Neoplasm, by site, malignant
      unspecified site 183.0
    specified site — *see* Neoplasm, by site, malignant
    unspecified 183.0
  pseudomucinous (M8470/3)
    papillary (M8471/3)
      specified site — *see* Neoplasm, by site, malignant
      unspecified site 183.0
    specified site — *see* Neoplasm, by site, malignant
    unspecified site 183.0
  serous (M8441/3)
    papillary (M8460/3)
      specified site — *see* Neoplasm, by site, malignant
      unspecified site 183.0
    specified site — *see* Neoplasm, by site, malignant
    unspecified site 183.0
Cystadenofibroma (M9013/0)
  clear cell (M8313/0) — *see* Neoplasm, by site, benign
  endometrioid (M8381/0) 220
    borderline malignancy (M8381/1) 236.2
    malignant (M8381/3) 183.0
  mucinous (M9015/0)
    specified site — *see* Neoplasm, by site, benign
    unspecified site 220
  serous (M9014/0)
    specified site — *see* Neoplasm, by site, benign
    unspecified site 220
  specified site — *see* Neoplasm, by site, benign
  unspecified site 220
Cystadenoma (M8440/0) — *see also* Neoplasm, by site, benign
  bile duct (M8161/0) 211.5
  endometrioid (M8380/0) (*see also* Neoplasm, by site, benign)
    borderline malignancy (M8380/1) — *see* Neoplasm, by site, uncertain behavior
  malignant (M8440/3) — *see* Neoplasm, by site, malignant
  mucinous (M8470/0)
    borderline malignancy (M8470/1)
      specified site — *see* Neoplasm, uncertain behavior
      unspecified site 236.2
    papillary (M8471/0)
      borderline malignancy (M8471/1)
        specified site — *see* Neoplasm, by site, uncertain behavior
        unspecified site 236.2
      specified site — *see* Neoplasm, by site, benign
      unspecified site 220
    specified site — *see* Neoplasm, by site, benign
    unspecified site 220

Cystadenoma — *see also* Neoplasm, by site, benign — *continued*
  papillary (M8450/0)
    borderline malignancy (M8450/1)
      specified site — *see* Neoplasm, by site, uncertain behavior
      unspecified site 236.2
    lymphomatosum (M8561/0) 210.2
    mucinous (M8471/0)
      borderline malignancy (M8471/1)
        specified site — *see* Neoplasm, by site, uncertain behavior
        unspecified site 236.2
      specified site — *see* Neoplasm, by site, benign
      unspecified site 220
    pseudomucinous (M8471/0)
      borderline malignancy (M8471/1)
        specified site — *see* Neoplasm, by site, uncertain behavior
        unspecified site 236.2
      specified site — *see* Neoplasm, by site, benign
      unspecified site 220
    serous (M8460/0)
      borderline malignancy (M8460/1)
        specified site — *see* Neoplasm, by site, uncertain behavior
        unspecified site 236.2
      specified site — *see* Neoplasm, by site, benign
      unspecified site 220
    specified site — *see* Neoplasm, by site, benign
    unspecified site 220
  pseudomucinous (M8470/0)
    borderline malignancy (M8470/1)
      specified site — *see* Neoplasm, by site, uncertain behavior
      unspecified site 236.2
    papillary (M8471/0)
      borderline malignancy (M8471/1)
        specified site — *see* Neoplasm, by site, uncertain behavior
        unspecified site 236.2
      specified site — *see* Neoplasm, by site, benign
      unspecified site 220
    specified site — *see* Neoplasm, by site, benign
    unspecified site 220
  serous (M8441/0)
    borderline malignancy (M8441/1)
      specified site — *see* Neoplasm, by site, uncertain behavior
      unspecified site 236.2
    papillary (M8460/0)
      borderline malignancy (M8460/1)
        specified site — *see* Neoplasm, by site, uncertain behavior
        unspecified site 236.2
      specified site — *see* Neoplasm, by site, benign
      unspecified site 220
    specified site — *see* Neoplasm, by site, benign
    unspecified site 220
  thyroid 226
Cystathioninemia 270.4
Cystathioninuria 270.4
Cystic — *see also* condition
  breast, chronic 610.1
  corpora lutea 620.1
  degeneration, congenital
    brain 742.4
    kidney (*see also* Cystic, disease, kidney) 753.10
  disease
    breast, chronic 610.1
    kidney, congenital 753.10
      medullary 753.16
      multiple 753.19
      polycystic — *see* Polycystic, kidney
      single 753.11
      specified NEC 753.19
    liver, congenital 751.62

Cyst — Cystic

☑ **Additional Digit Required** — Refer to the Tabular List for Digit Selection   ▽ **Subterms under main terms may continue to next column or page**

2013 ICD-9-CM   ▶◀ Revised Text   ● New Line   ▲ Revised Code   **Volume 2 — 61**

Index

Cystic — see also condition — continued
　disease — continued
　　lung 518.89
　　　congenital 748.4
　　pancreas, congenital 751.7
　　semilunar cartilage 717.5
　duct — see condition
　eyeball, congenital 743.03
　fibrosis (pancreas) 277.00
　　with
　　　manifestations
　　　　gastrointestinal 277.03
　　　　pulmonary 277.02
　　　　specified NEC 277.09
　　　meconium ileus 277.01
　　　pulmonary exacerbation 277.02
　hygroma (M9173/0) 228.1
　kidney, congenital 753.10
　　medullary 753.16
　　multiple 753.19
　　polycystic — see Polycystic, kidney
　　single 753.11
　　specified NEC 753.19
　liver, congenital 751.62
　lung 518.89
　　congenital 748.4
　mass — see Cyst
　mastitis, chronic 610.1
　ovary 620.2
　pancreas, congenital 751.7
Cysticerciasis 123.1
Cysticercosis (mammary) (subretinal) 123.1
Cysticercus 123.1
　cellulosae infestation 123.1
Cystinosis (malignant) 270.0
Cystinuria 270.0
Cystitis (bacillary) (colli) (diffuse) (exudative)
　(hemorrhagic) (purulent) (recurrent)
　(septic) (suppurative) (ulcerative) 595.9
　with
　　abortion — see Abortion, by type, with
　　　urinary tract infection
　　ectopic pregnancy (see also categories
　　　633.0–633.9) 639.8

Cystitis — continued
　with — continued
　　fibrosis 595.1
　　leukoplakia 595.1
　　malakoplakia 595.1
　　metaplasia 595.1
　　molar pregnancy (see also categories
　　　630–632) 639.8
　actinomycotic 039.8 [595.4]
　acute 595.0
　　of trigone 595.3
　allergic 595.89
　amebic 006.8 [595.4]
　bilharzial 120.9 [595.4]
　blennorrhagic (acute) 098.11
　　chronic or duration of 2 months or more
　　　098.31
　bullous 595.89
　calculous 594.1
　chlamydial 099.53
　chronic 595.2
　　interstitial 595.1
　　of trigone 595.3
　complicating pregnancy, childbirth, or
　　puerperium 646.6 ☑
　　affecting fetus or newborn 760.1
　cystic(a) 595.81
　diphtheritic 032.84
　echinococcal
　　granulosus 122.3 [595.4]
　　multilocularis 122.6 [595.4]
　emphysematous 595.89
　encysted 595.81
　follicular 595.3
　following
　　abortion 639.8
　　ectopic or molar pregnancy 639.8
　gangrenous 595.89
　glandularis 595.89
　gonococcal (acute) 098.11
　　chronic or duration of 2 months or more
　　　098.31
　incrusted 595.89
　interstitial 595.1

Cystitis — continued
　irradiation 595.82
　irritation 595.89
　malignant 595.89
　monilial 112.2
　of trigone 595.3
　panmural 595.1
　polyposa 595.89
　prostatic 601.3
　radiation 595.82
　Reiter's (abacterial) 099.3
　specified NEC 595.89
　subacute 595.2
　submucous 595.1
　syphilitic 095.8
　trichomoniasis 131.09
　tuberculous (see also Tuberculosis) 016.1 ☑
　ulcerative 595.1
Cystocele
　female (without uterine prolapse) 618.01
　　with uterine prolapse 618.4
　　　complete 618.3
　　　incomplete 618.2
　　lateral 618.02
　　midline 618.01
　　paravaginal 618.02
　in pregnancy or childbirth 654.4 ☑
　　affecting fetus or newborn 763.89
　　causing obstructed labor 660.2 ☑
　　　affecting fetus or newborn 763.1
　male 596.89
Cystoid
　cicatrix limbus 372.64
　degeneration macula 362.53
Cystolithiasis 594.1
Cystoma (M8440/0) — see also Neoplasm, by
　site, benign
　endometrial, ovary 617.1
　mucinous (M8470/0)
　　specified site — see Neoplasm, by site,
　　　benign
　　unspecified site 220

Cystoma — see also Neoplasm, by site, benign
　— continued
　serous (M8441/0)
　　specified site — see Neoplasm, by site,
　　　benign
　　unspecified site 220
　simple (ovary) 620.2
Cystoplegia 596.53
Cystoptosis 596.89
Cystopyelitis — see also Pyelitis 590.80
Cystorrhagia 596.89
Cystosarcoma phyllodes (M9020/1) 238.3
　benign (M9020/0) 217
　malignant (M9020/3) — see Neoplasm,
　　breast, malignant
Cystostomy status V44.50
　with complication 596.83
　　infection 596.81
　　mechanical 596.82
　　specified complication NEC 596.83
　appendico-vesicostomy V44.52
　cutaneous-vesicostomy V44.51
　specified type NEC V44.59
Cystourethritis — see also Urethritis 597.89
Cystourethrocele — see also Cystocele
　female (without uterine prolapse) 618.09
　　with uterine prolapse 618.4
　　　complete 618.3
　　　incomplete 618.2
　male 596.89
Cytomegalic inclusion disease 078.5
　congenital 771.1
Cytomycosis, reticuloendothelial — see also
　Histoplasmosis, American 115.00
Cytopenia 289.9
　refractory
　　with
　　　multilineage dysplasia (RCMD)
　　　　238.72
　　　and ringed sideroblasts (RCMD-
　　　　RS) 238.72

☑ Additional Digit Required — Refer to the Tabular List for Digit Selection　　　　　　　　　　　　　🔲 Subterms under main terms may continue to next column or page

　　　　▶◀ Revised Text　　　　● New Line　　　　▲ Revised Code　　　　**2013 ICD-9-CM**

D

Daae (-Finsen) disease (epidemic pleurodynia) 074.1
Dabney's grip 074.1
Da Costa's syndrome (neurocirculatory asthenia) 306.2
Dacryoadenitis, dacryadenitis 375.00
  acute 375.01
  chronic 375.02
Dacryocystitis 375.30
  acute 375.32
  chronic 375.42
  neonatal 771.6
  phlegmonous 375.33
  syphilitic 095.8
    congenital 090.0
  trachomatous, active 076.1
    late effect 139.1
  tuberculous (see also Tuberculosis) 017.3 ☑
Dacryocystoblenorrhea 375.42
Dacryocystocele 375.43
Dacryolith, dacryolithiasis 375.57
Dacryoma 375.43
Dacryopericystitis (acute) (subacute) 375.32
  chronic 375.42
Dacryops 375.11
Dacryosialadenopathy, atrophic 710.2
Dacryostenosis 375.56
  congenital 743.65
Dactylitis
  bone (see also Osteomyelitis) 730.2 ☑
  sickle-cell 282.62
    Hb-C 282.64
    Hb-SS 282.62
    specified NEC 282.69
  syphilitic 095.5
  tuberculous (see also Tuberculosis) 015.5 ☑
Dactylolysis spontanea 136.0
Dactylosymphysis — see also Syndactylism 755.10
Damage
  arteriosclerotic — see Arteriosclerosis
  brain 348.9
    anoxic, hypoxic 348.1
      during or resulting from a procedure 997.01
      ischemic, in newborn 768.70
        mild 768.71
        moderate 768.72
        severe 768.73
    child NEC 343.9
    due to birth injury 767.0
    minimal (child) (see also Hyperkinesia) 314.9
    newborn 767.0
  cardiac (see also Disease, heart)
  cardiorenal (vascular) (see also Hypertension, cardiorenal) 404.90
  central nervous system — see Damage, brain
  cerebral NEC — see Damage, brain
  coccyx, complicating delivery 665.6 ☑
  coronary (see also Ischemia, heart) 414.9
  eye, birth injury 767.8
  heart (see also Disease, heart)
    valve — see Endocarditis
  hypothalamus NEC 348.9
  liver 571.9
    alcoholic 571.3
  medication 995.20
  myocardium (see also Degeneration, myocardial) 429.1
  pelvic
    joint or ligament, during delivery 665.6 ☑
    organ NEC
      with
        abortion — see Abortion, by type, with damage to pelvic organs
        ectopic pregnancy (see also categories 633.0–633.9) 639.2
        molar pregnancy (see also categories 630–632) 639.2
      during delivery 665.5 ☑

Damage — continued
  pelvic — continued
    organ — continued
      following
        abortion 639.2
        ectopic or molar pregnancy 639.2
  renal (see also Disease, renal) 593.9
  skin, solar 692.79
    acute 692.72
    chronic 692.74
  subendocardium, subendocardial (see also Degeneration, myocardial) 429.1
  vascular 459.9
Dameshek's syndrome (erythroblastic anemia) 282.49
Dana-Putnam syndrome (subacute combined sclerosis with pernicious anemia) 281.0 [336.2]
Danbolt (-Closs) syndrome (acrodermatitis enteropathica) 686.8
Dandruff 690.18
Dandy fever 061
Dandy-Walker deformity or syndrome (atresia, foramen of Magendie) 742.3
  with spina bifida (see also Spina bifida) 741.0 ☑
Dangle foot 736.79
Danielssen's disease (anesthetic leprosy) 030.1
Danlos' syndrome 756.83
Darier's disease (congenital) (keratosis follicularis) 757.39
  due to vitamin A deficiency 264.8
  meaning erythema annulare centrifugum 695.0
Darier-Roussy sarcoid 135
Dark area on retina 239.81
Darling's
  disease (see also Histoplasmosis, American) 115.00
  histoplasmosis (see also Histoplasmosis, American) 115.00
Dartre 054.9
Darwin's tubercle 744.29
Davidson's anemia (refractory) 284.9
Davies-Colley syndrome (slipping rib) 733.99
Davies' disease 425.0
Dawson's encephalitis 046.2
Day blindness — see also Blindness, day 368.60
Dead
  fetus
    retained (in utero) 656.4 ☑
      early pregnancy (death before 22 completed weeks gestation) 632
      late (death after 22 completed weeks gestation) 656.4 ☑
    syndrome 641.3 ☑
  labyrinth 386.50
  ovum, retained 631.8
Deaf and dumb NEC 389.7
Deaf mutism (acquired) (congenital) NEC 389.7
  endemic 243
  hysterical 300.11
  syphilitic, congenital 090.0
Deafness (acquired) (complete) (congenital) (hereditary) (middle ear) (partial) 389.9
  with
    blindness V49.85
    blue sclera and fragility of bone 756.51
  auditory fatigue 389.9
  aviation 993.0
    nerve injury 951.5
  boilermakers' 951.5
  central 389.14
    with conductive hearing loss 389.20
      bilateral 389.22
      unilateral 389.21
  conductive (air) 389.00
    with sensorineural hearing loss 389.20
      bilateral 389.22
      unilateral 389.21
    bilateral 389.06
    combined types 389.08
    external ear 389.01

Deafness — continued
  conductive — continued
    inner ear 389.04
    middle ear 389.03
    multiple types 389.08
    tympanic membrane 389.02
    unilateral 389.05
  emotional (complete) 300.11
  functional (complete) 300.11
  high frequency 389.8
  hysterical (complete) 300.11
  injury 951.5
  low frequency 389.8
  mental 784.69
  mixed conductive and sensorineural 389.20
    bilateral 389.22
    unilateral 389.21
  nerve
    with conductive hearing loss 389.20
      bilateral 389.22
      unilateral 389.21
    bilateral 389.12
    unilateral 389.13
  neural
    with conductive hearing loss 389.20
      bilateral 389.22
      unilateral 389.21
    bilateral 389.12
    unilateral 389.13
  noise-induced 388.12
    nerve injury 951.5
  nonspeaking 389.7
  perceptive 389.10
    with conductive hearing loss 389.20
      bilateral 389.22
      unilateral 389.21
    central 389.14
    neural
      bilateral 389.12
      unilateral 389.13
    sensorineural 389.10
      asymmetrical 389.16
      bilateral 389.18
      unilateral 389.15
    sensory
      bilateral 389.11
      unilateral 389.17
  psychogenic (complete) 306.7
  sensorineural (see also Deafness, perceptive) 389.10
    asymmetrical 389.16
    bilateral 389.18
    unilateral 389.15
  sensory
    with conductive hearing loss 389.20
      bilateral 389.22
      unilateral 389.21
    bilateral 389.11
    unilateral 389.17
  specified type NEC 389.8
  sudden NEC 388.2
  syphilitic 094.89
  transient ischemic 388.02
  transmission — see Deafness, conductive
  traumatic 951.5
  word (secondary to organic lesion) 784.69
    developmental 315.31
Death
  after delivery (cause not stated) (sudden) 674.9 ☑
  anesthetic
    due to
      correct substance properly administered 995.4
      overdose or wrong substance given 968.4
        specified anesthetic — see Table of Drugs and Chemicals
    during delivery 668.9 ☑
  brain 348.82
  cardiac (sudden) (SCD) — code to underlying condition
    family history of V17.41
    personal history of, successfully resuscitated V12.53
  cause unknown 798.2

Death — continued
  cot (infant) 798.0
  crib (infant) 798.0
  fetus, fetal (cause not stated) (intrauterine) 779.9
    early, with retention (before 22 completed weeks gestation) 632
    from asphyxia or anoxia (before labor) 768.0
      during labor 768.1
    late, affecting management of pregnancy (after 22 completed weeks gestation) 656.4 ☑
  from pregnancy NEC 646.9 ☑
  instantaneous 798.1
  intrauterine (see also Death, fetus) 779.9
    complicating pregnancy 656.4 ☑
  maternal, affecting fetus or newborn 761.6
  neonatal NEC 779.9
  sudden (cause unknown) 798.1
    cardiac (SCD)
      family history of V17.41
      personal history of, successfully resuscitated V12.53
    during delivery 669.9 ☑
      under anesthesia NEC 668.9 ☑
    infant, syndrome (SIDS) 798.0
    puerperal, during puerperium 674.9 ☑
  unattended (cause unknown) 798.9
  under anesthesia NEC
    due to
      correct substance properly administered 995.4
      overdose or wrong substance given 968.4
        specified anesthetic — see Table of Drugs and Chemicals
    during delivery 668.9 ☑
  violent 798.1
de Beurmann-Gougerot disease (sporotrichosis) 117.1
Debility (general) (infantile) (postinfectional) 799.3
  with nutritional difficulty 269.9
  congenital or neonatal NEC 779.9
  nervous 300.5
  old age 797
  senile 797
Débove's disease (splenomegaly) 789.2
Decalcification
  bone (see also Osteoporosis) 733.00
  teeth 521.89
Decapitation 874.9
  fetal (to facilitate delivery) 763.89
Decapsulation, kidney 593.89
Decay
  dental 521.00
  senile 797
  tooth, teeth 521.00
Decensus, uterus — see Prolapse, uterus
Deciduitis (acute)
  with
    abortion — see Abortion, by type, with sepsis
    ectopic pregnancy (see also categories 633.0–633.9) 639.0
    molar pregnancy (see also categories 630–632) 639.0
  affecting fetus or newborn 760.8
  following
    abortion 639.0
    ectopic or molar pregnancy 639.0
  in pregnancy 646.6 ☑
  puerperal, postpartum 670.1 ☑
Deciduoma malignum (M9100/3) 181
Deciduous tooth (retained) 520.6
Decline (general) — see also Debility 799.3
Decompensation
  cardiac (acute) (chronic) (see also Disease, heart) 429.9
    failure — see Failure, heart
  cardiorenal (see also Hypertension, cardiorenal) 404.90
  cardiovascular (see also Disease, cardiovascular) 429.2
  heart (see also Disease, heart) 429.9

☑ Additional Digit Required — Refer to the Tabular List for Digit Selection   ⚐ Subterms under main terms may continue to next column or page

2013 ICD-9-CM   ▶◀ Revised Text   ● New Line   ▲ Revised Code   Volume 2 — 63

Decompensation — continued
  heart (see also Disease, heart) (contin-
      ued
    failure — see Failure, heart
  hepatic 572.2
  myocardial (acute) (chronic) (see also Dis-
      ease, heart) 429.9
    failure — see Failure, heart
  respiratory 519.9
Decompression sickness 993.3
Decrease, decreased
  blood
    platelets (see also Thrombocytopenia)
        287.5
    pressure 796.3
      due to shock following
          injury 958.4
          operation 998.00
    white cell count 288.50
      specified NEC 288.59
  cardiac reserve — see Disease, heart
  estrogen 256.39
    postablative 256.2
  fetal movements 655.7 ☑
  fragility of erythrocytes 289.89
  function
    adrenal (cortex) 255.41
      medulla 255.5
    ovary in hypopituitarism 253.4
    parenchyma of pancreas 577.8
    pituitary (gland) (lobe) (anterior) 253.2
      posterior (lobe) 253.8
  functional activity 780.99
  glucose 790.29
  haptoglobin (serum) NEC 273.8
  leukocytes 288.50
  libido 799.81
  lymphocytes 288.51
  platelets (see also Thrombocytopenia) 287.5
  pulse pressure 785.9
  respiration due to shock following injury
      958.4
  sexual desire 799.81
  tear secretion NEC 375.15
  tolerance
    fat 579.8
    salt and water 276.9
  vision NEC 369.9
  white blood cell count 288.50
Decubital gangrene — see also Ulcer, pressure
    707.00 [785.4]
Decubiti — see also Ulcer, pressure 707.00
Decubitus (ulcer) — see also Ulcer, pressure
    707.00
  with gangrene 707.00 [785.4]
  ankle 707.06
  back
    lower 707.03
    upper 707.02
  buttock 707.05
  coccyx 707.03
  elbow 707.01
  head 707.09
  heel 707.07
  hip 707.04
  other site 707.09
  sacrum 707.03
  shoulder blades 707.02
Deepening acetabulum 718.85
Defect, defective 759.9
  3-beta-hydroxysteroid dehydrogenase 255.2
  11-hydroxylase 255.2
  21-hydroxylase 255.2
  abdominal wall, congenital 756.70
  aorticopulmonary septum 745.0
  aortic septal 745.0
  atrial septal (ostium secundum type) 745.5
    acquired 429.71
    ostium primum type 745.61
    sinus venosus 745.8
  atrioventricular
    canal 745.69
    septum 745.4
      acquired 429.71
  atrium secundum 745.5
    acquired 429.71

Defect, defective — continued
  auricular septal 745.5
    acquired 429.71
  bilirubin excretion 277.4
  biosynthesis, testicular androgen 257.2
  bridge 525.60
  bulbar septum 745.0
  butanol-insoluble iodide 246.1
  chromosome — see Anomaly, chromosome
  circulation (acquired) 459.9
    congenital 747.9
    newborn 747.9
  clotting NEC (see also Defect, coagulation)
      286.9
  coagulation (factor) (see also Deficiency,
      coagulation factor) 286.9
    with
      abortion — see Abortion, by type,
          with hemorrhage
      ectopic pregnancy (see also cate-
          gories 634–638) 639.1
      molar pregnancy (see also categories
          630–632) 639.1
    acquired (any) 286.7
    antepartum or intrapartum 641.3 ☑
      affecting fetus or newborn 762.1
    causing hemorrhage of pregnancy or
        delivery 641.3 ☑
    complicating pregnancy, childbirth, or
        puerperium 649.3 ☑
    due to
      liver disease 286.7
      vitamin K deficiency 286.7
    newborn, transient 776.3
    postpartum 666.3 ☑
    specified type NEC 286.9
  conduction (heart) 426.9
  bone (see also Deafness, conductive)
      389.00
  congenital, organ or site NEC (see also
      Anomaly)
    circulation 747.9
    Descemet's membrane 743.9
      specified type NEC 743.49
    diaphragm 756.6
    ectodermal 757.9
    esophagus 750.9
    pulmonic cusps — see Anomaly, heart
        valve
    respiratory system 748.9
      specified type NEC 748.8
  crown 525.60
  cushion endocardial 745.60
  dental restoration 525.60
  dentin (hereditary) 520.5
  Descemet's membrane (congenital) 743.9
    acquired 371.30
    specific type NEC 743.49
  deutan 368.52
  developmental (see also Anomaly, by site)
    cauda equina 742.59
    left ventricle 746.9
      with atresia or hypoplasia of aortic
          orifice or valve, with hypopla-
          sia of ascending aorta 746.7
      in hypoplastic left heart syndrome
          746.7
    testis 752.9
    vessel 747.9
  diaphragm
    with elevation, eventration, or hernia —
        see Hernia, diaphragm
    congenital 756.6
      with elevation, eventration, or hernia
          756.6
      gross (with elevation, eventration, or
          hernia) 756.6
  ectodermal, congenital 757.9
  Eisenmenger's (ventricular septal defect)
      745.4
  endocardial cushion 745.60
    specified type NEC 745.69
  esophagus, congenital 750.9
  extensor retinaculum 728.9
  fibrin polymerization (see also Defect, coag-
      ulation) 286.3

Defect, defective — continued
  filling
    biliary tract 793.3
    bladder 793.5
    dental 525.60
    gallbladder 793.3
    kidney 793.5
    stomach 793.4
    ureter 793.5
  fossa ovalis 745.5
  gene, carrier (suspected) of V83.89
  Gerbode 745.4
  glaucomatous, without elevated tension
      365.89
  Hageman (factor) (see also Defect, coagula-
      tion) 286.3
  hearing (see also Deafness) 389.9
  high grade 317
  homogentisic acid 270.2
  interatrial septal 745.5
    acquired 429.71
  interauricular septal 745.5
    acquired 429.71
  interventricular septal 745.4
    with pulmonary stenosis or atresia, dex-
        traposition of aorta, and hypertro-
        phy of right ventricle 745.2
    acquired 429.71
    in tetralogy of Fallot 745.2
  iodide trapping 246.1
  iodotyrosine dehalogenase 246.1
  kynureninase 270.2
  learning, specific 315.2
  major osseous 731.3
  mental (see also Disability, intellectual) 319
  osseous, major 731.3
  osteochondral NEC 738.8
  ostium
    primum 745.61
    secundum 745.5
  pericardium 746.89
  peroxidase-binding 246.1
  placental blood supply — see Placenta, in-
      sufficiency
  platelet (qualitative) 287.1
    constitutional 286.4
  postural, spine 737.9
  protan 368.51
  pulmonic cusps, congenital 746.00
  renal pelvis 753.9
    obstructive 753.29
    specified type NEC 753.3
  respiratory system, congenital 748.9
    specified type NEC 748.8
  retina, retinal 361.30
    with detachment (see also Detachment,
        retina, with retinal defect) 361.00
    multiple 361.33
      with detachment 361.02
    nerve fiber bundle 362.85
    single 361.30
      with detachment 361.01
  septal (closure) (heart) NEC 745.9
    acquired 429.71
    atrial 745.5
    specified type NEC 745.8
  speech NEC 784.59
    developmental 315.39
    late effect of cerebrovascular disease —
        see Late effect(s) (of) cerebrovas-
        cular disease, speech and lan-
        guage deficit
    secondary to organic lesion 784.59
  Taussig-Bing (transposition, aorta and
      overriding pulmonary artery) 745.11
  teeth, wedge 521.20
  thyroid hormone synthesis 246.1
  tritan 368.53
  ureter 753.9
    obstructive 753.29
  vascular (acquired) (local) 459.9
    congenital (peripheral) NEC 747.60
      gastrointestinal 747.61
      lower limb 747.64
      renal 747.62
      specified NEC 747.69

Defect, defective — continued
  vascular — continued
    congenital — continued
      spinal 747.82
      upper limb 747.63
  ventricular septal 745.4
    with pulmonary stenosis or atresia, dex-
        traposition of aorta, and hypertro-
        phy of right ventricle 745.2
    acquired 429.71
    atrioventricular canal type 745.69
    between infundibulum and anterior
        portion 745.4
    in tetralogy of Fallot 745.2
    isolated anterior 745.4
  vision NEC 369.9
  visual field 368.40
    arcuate 368.43
    heteronymous, bilateral 368.47
    homonymous, bilateral 368.46
    localized NEC 368.44
    nasal step 368.44
    peripheral 368.44
    sector 368.43
  voice and resonance 784.40
  wedge, teeth (abrasion) 521.20
Defeminization syndrome 255.2
Deferentitis 608.4
  gonorrheal (acute) 098.14
    chronic or duration of 2 months or over
        098.34
Defibrination syndrome — see also Fibrinoly-
    sis 286.6
Deficiency, deficient
  3-beta-hydroxysteroid dehydrogenase 255.2
  6-phosphogluconic dehydrogenase (ane-
      mia) 282.2
  11-beta-hydroxylase 255.2
  17-alpha-hydroxylase 255.2
  18-hydroxysteroid dehydrogenase 255.2
  20-alpha-hydroxylase 255.2
  21-hydroxylase 255.2
  AAT (alpha-1 antitrypsin) 273.4
  abdominal muscle syndrome 756.79
  accelerator globulin (Ac G) (blood) (see also
      Defect, coagulation) 286.3
  AC globulin (congenital) (see also Defect,
      coagulation) 286.3
    acquired 286.7
  activating factor (blood) (see also Defect,
      coagulation) 286.3
  adenohypophyseal 253.2
  adenosine deaminase 277.2
  aldolase (hereditary) 271.2
  alpha-1-antitrypsin 273.4
  alpha-1-trypsin inhibitor 273.4
  alpha-fucosidase 271.8
  alpha-lipoprotein 272.5
  alpha-mannosidase 271.8
  amino acid 270.9
  anemia — see Anemia, deficiency
  aneurin 265.1
    with beriberi 265.0
  antibody NEC 279.00
  antidiuretic hormone 253.5
  antihemophilic
    factor (A) 286.0
      B 286.1
      C 286.2
    globulin (AHG) NEC 286.0
  antithrombin III 289.81
  antitrypsin 273.4
  argininosuccinate synthetase or lyase 270.6
  ascorbic acid (with scurvy) 267
  autoprothrombin
    I (see also Defect, coagulation) 286.3
    II 286.1
    C (see also Defect, coagulation) 286.3
  bile salt 579.8
  biotin 266.2
  biotinidase 277.6
  bradykinase-1 277.6
  brancher enzyme (amylopectinosis) 271.0
  calciferol 268.9
    with
      osteomalacia 268.2

☑ **Additional Digit Required** — Refer to the Tabular List for Digit Selection   Subterms under main terms may continue to next column or page

64 — Volume 2   ▶◀ Revised Text   ● New Line   ▲ Revised Code   2013 ICD-9-CM

Deficiency, deficient — *continued*
calciferol — *continued*
  with — *continued*
    rickets (*see also* Rickets) 268.0
calcium 275.40
  dietary 269.3
calorie, severe 261
carbamyl phosphate synthetase 270.6
cardiac (*see also* Insufficiency, myocardial) 428.0
carnitine 277.81
  due to
    hemodialysis 277.83
    inborn errors of metabolism 277.82
    valproic acid therapy 277.83
  iatrogenic 277.83
  palmitoyltransferase (CPT1, CPT2) 277.85
  palmityl transferase (CPT1, CPT2) 277.85
  primary 277.81
  secondary 277.84
carotene 264.9
Carr factor (*see also* Defect, coagulation) 286.9
central nervous system 349.9
ceruloplasmin 275.1
cevitamic acid (with scurvy) 267
choline 266.2
Christmas factor 286.1
chromium 269.3
citrin 269.1
clotting (blood) (*see also* Defect, coagulation) 286.9
coagulation factor NEC 286.9
  with
    abortion — *see* Abortion, by type, with hemorrhage
    ectopic pregnancy (*see also* categories 634–638) 639.1
    molar pregnancy (*see also* categories 630–632) 639.1
  acquired (any) 286.7
  antepartum or intrapartum 641.3 ☑
    affecting fetus or newborn 762.1
  complicating pregnancy, childbirth, or puerperium 649.3 ☑
  due to
    liver disease 286.7
    vitamin K deficiency 286.7
  newborn, transient 776.3
  postpartum 666.3 ☑
  specified type NEC 286.3
color vision (congenital) 368.59
  acquired 368.55
combined glucocorticoid and mineralocorticoid 255.41
combined, two or more coagulation factors (*see also* Defect, coagulation) 286.9
complement factor NEC 279.8
contact factor (*see also* Defect, coagulation) 286.3
copper NEC 275.1
corticoadrenal 255.41
craniofacial axis 756.0
cyanocobalamin (vitamin B₁₂) 266.2
debrancher enzyme (limit dextrinosis) 271.0
desmolase 255.2
diet 269.9
dihydrofolate reductase 281.2
dihydropteridine reductase 270.1
dihydropyrimidine dehydrogenase (DPD) 277.6
disaccharidase (intestinal) 271.3
disease NEC 269.9
ear(s) V48.8
edema 262
endocrine 259.9
enzymes, circulating NEC (*see also* Deficiency, by specific enzyme) 277.6
ergosterol 268.9
  with
    osteomalacia 268.2
    rickets (*see also* Rickets) 268.0
erythrocytic glutathione (anemia) 282.2
eyelid(s) V48.8
factor (*see also* Defect, coagulation) 286.9
  I (congenital) (fibrinogen) 286.3

Deficiency, deficient — *continued*
factor (*see also* Defect, coagulation) — *continued*
  I — *continued*
    antepartum or intrapartum 641.3 ☑
      affecting fetus or newborn 762.1
    newborn, transient 776.3
    postpartum 666.3 ☑
  II (congenital) (prothrombin) 286.3
  V (congenital) (labile) 286.3
  VII (congenital) (stable) 286.3
  VIII (congenital) (functional) 286.0
    with
      functional defect 286.0
      vascular defect 286.4
  IX (Christmas) (congenital) (functional) 286.1
  X (congenital) (Stuart-Prower) 286.3
  XI (congenital) (plasma thromboplastin antecedent) 286.2
  XII (congenital) (Hageman) 286.3
  XIII (congenital) (fibrin stabilizing) 286.3
  Hageman 286.3
  multiple (congenital) 286.9
    acquired 286.7
fibrinase (*see also* Defect, coagulation) 286.3
fibrinogen (congenital) (*see also* Defect, coagulation) 286.3
  acquired 286.6
fibrin-stabilizing factor (congenital) (*see also* Defect, coagulation) 286.3
finger — *see* Absence, finger
fletcher factor (*see also* Defect, coagulation) 286.9
fluorine 269.3
folate, anemia 281.2
folic acid (vitamin Bc) 266.2
  anemia 281.2
follicle-stimulating hormone (FSH) 253.4
fructokinase 271.2
fructose-1, 6-diphosphate 271.2
fructose-1-phosphate aldolase 271.2
FSH (follicle-stimulating hormone) 253.4
fucosidase 271.8
galactokinase 271.1
galactose-1-phosphate uridyl transferase 271.1
gamma globulin in blood 279.00
glass factor (*see also* Defect, coagulation) 286.3
glucocorticoid 255.41
glucose-6-phosphatase 271.0
glucose-6-phosphate dehydrogenase anemia 282.2
glucuronyl transferase 277.4
glutathione-reductase (anemia) 282.2
glycogen synthetase 271.0
growth hormone 253.3
Hageman factor (congenital) (*see also* Defect, coagulation) 286.3
head V48.0
hemoglobin (*see also* Anemia) 285.9
hepatophosphorylase 271.0
hexose monophosphate (HMP) shunt 282.2
HGH (human growth hormone) 253.3
HG-PRT 277.2
homogentisic acid oxidase 270.2
hormone (*see also* Deficiency, by specific hormone)
  anterior pituitary (isolated) (partial) NEC 253.4
  growth (human) 253.3
  follicle-stimulating 253.4
  growth (human) (isolated) 253.3
  human growth 253.3
  interstitial cell-stimulating 253.4
  luteinizing 253.4
  melanocyte-stimulating 253.4
  testicular 257.2
human growth hormone 253.3
humoral 279.00
  with
    hyper-IgM 279.05
      autosomal recessive 279.05
      X-linked 279.05
    increased IgM 279.05

Deficiency, deficient — *continued*
humoral — *continued*
  congenital hypogammaglobulinemia 279.04
  non-sex-linked 279.06
  selective immunoglobulin NEC 279.03
    IgA 279.01
    IgG 279.03
    IgM 279.02
      increased 279.05
  specified NEC 279.09
hydroxylase 255.2
hypoxanthine-guanine phosphoribosyltransferase (HG-PRT) 277.2
ICSH (interstitial cell-stimulating hormone) 253.4
immunity NEC 279.3
  cell-mediated 279.10
    with
      hyperimmunoglobulinemia 279.2
      thrombocytopenia and eczema 279.12
    specified NEC 279.19
  combined (severe) 279.2
    syndrome 279.2
  common variable 279.06
  humoral NEC 279.00
    IgA (secretory) 279.01
    IgG 279.03
    IgM 279.02
  immunoglobulin, selective NEC 279.03
    IgA 279.01
    IgG 279.03
    IgM 279.02
inositol (B complex) 266.2
interferon 279.49
internal organ V47.0
interstitial cell-stimulating hormone (ICSH) 253.4
intrinsic factor (Castle's) (congenital) 281.0
intrinsic (urethral) sphincter (ISD) 599.82
invertase 271.3
iodine 269.3
iron, anemia 280.9
labile factor (congenital) (*see also* Defect, coagulation) 286.3
  acquired 286.7
lacrimal fluid (acquired) 375.15
  congenital 743.64
lactase 271.3
Laki-Lorand factor (*see also* Defect, coagulation) 286.3
lecithin-cholesterol acyltranferase 272.5
LH (luteinizing hormone) 253.4
limb V49.0
  lower V49.0
    congenital (*see also* Deficiency, lower limb, congenital) 755.30
  upper V49.0
    congenital (*see also* Deficiency, upper limb, congenital) 755.20
lipocaic 577.8
lipoid (high-density) 272.5
lipoprotein (familial) (high density) 272.5
liver phosphorylase 271.0
long chain 3-hydroxyacyl CoA dehydrogenase (LCHAD) 277.85
long chain/very long chain acyl CoA dehydrogenase (LCAD, VLCAD) 277.85
lower limb V49.0
  congenital 755.30
    with complete absence of distal elements 755.31
    longitudinal (complete) (partial) (with distal deficiencies, incomplete) 755.32
      with complete absence of distal elements 755.31
      combined femoral, tibial, fibular (incomplete) 755.33
      femoral 755.34
      fibular 755.37
      metatarsal(s) 755.38
      phalange(s) 755.39
        meaning all digits 755.31
      tarsal(s) 755.38

Deficiency, deficient — *continued*
lower limb — *continued*
  congenital — *continued*
    longitudinal — *continued*
      tibia 755.36
      tibiofibular 755.35
      transverse 755.31
luteinizing hormone (LH) 253.4
lysosomal alpha-1, 4 glucosidase 271.0
magnesium 275.2
mannosidase 271.8
medium chain acyl CoA dehydrogenase (MCAD) 277.85
melanocyte-stimulating hormone (MSH) 253.4
menadione (vitamin K) 269.0
  newborn 776.0
mental (familial) (hereditary) (*see also* Disability, intellectual) 319
methylenetetrahydrofolate reductase (MTHFR) 270.4
mineral NEC 269.3
mineralocorticoid 255.42
molybdenum 269.3
moral 301.7
multiple, syndrome 260
myocardial (*see also* Insufficiency, myocardial) 428.0
myophosphorylase 271.0
NADH-diaphorase or reductase (congenital) 289.7
NADH (DPNH)-methemoglobin-reductase (congenital) 289.7
neck V48.1
niacin (amide) (-tryptophan) 265.2
nicotinamide 265.2
nicotinic acid (amide) 265.2
nose V48.8
number of teeth (*see also* Anodontia) 520.0
nutrition, nutritional 269.9
  specified NEC 269.8
ornithine transcarbamylase 270.6
ovarian 256.39
oxygen (*see also* Anoxia) 799.02
pantothenic acid 266.2
parathyroid (gland) 252.1
phenylalanine hydroxylase 270.1
phosphoenolpyruvate carboxykinase 271.8
phosphofructokinase 271.2
phosphoglucomutase 271.0
phosphohexoisomerase 271.0
phosphomannomutase 271.8
phosphomannose isomerase 271.8
phosphomannosyl mutase 271.8
phosphorylase kinase, liver 271.0
pituitary (anterior) 253.2
  posterior 253.5
placenta — *see* Placenta, insufficiency
plasma
  cell 279.00
  protein (paraproteinemia) (pyroglobulinemia) 273.8
  gamma globulin 279.00
  thromboplastin
    antecedent (PTA) 286.2
    component (PTC) 286.1
platelet NEC 287.1
  constitutional 286.4
polyglandular 258.9
potassium (K) 276.8
proaccelerin (congenital) (*see also* Defect, congenital) 286.3
  acquired 286.7
proconvertin factor (congenital) (*see also* Defect, coagulation) 286.3
  acquired 286.7
prolactin 253.4
protein 260
  anemia 281.4
  C 289.81
  plasma — *see* Deficiency, plasma, protein
  S 289.81
prothrombin (congenital) (*see also* Defect, coagulation) 286.3
  acquired 286.7

☑ **Additional Digit Required — Refer to the Tabular List for Digit Selection**   ▽ **Subterms under main terms may continue to next column or page**

2013 ICD-9-CM   ▶◀ **Revised Text**   ● **New Line**   ▲ **Revised Code**   **Volume 2 — 65**

Deficiency, deficient — Deficiency, deficient

Deficiency, deficient — *continued*
Prower factor (*see also* Defect, coagulation) 286.3
PRT 277.2
pseudocholinesterase 289.89
psychobiological 301.6
PTA 286.2
PTC 286.1
purine nucleoside phosphorylase 277.2
pyracin (alpha) (beta) 266.1
pyridoxal 266.1
pyridoxamine 266.1
pyridoxine (derivatives) 266.1
pyruvate carboxylase 271.8
pyruvate dehydrogenase 271.8
pyruvate kinase (PK) 282.3
riboflavin (vitamin B_2) 266.0
saccadic eye movements 379.57
salivation 527.7
salt 276.1
secretion
  ovary 256.39
  salivary gland (any) 527.7
  urine 788.5
selenium 269.3
serum
  antitrypsin, familial 273.4
  protein (congenital) 273.8
short chain acyl CoA dehydrogenase (SCAD) 277.85
short stature homeobox gene (SHOX)
  with
    dyschondrosteosis 756.89
    short stature (idiopathic) 783.43
    Turner's syndrome 758.6
smooth pursuit movements (eye) 379.58
sodium (Na) 276.1
SPCA (*see also* Defect, coagulation) 286.3
specified NEC 269.8
stable factor (congenital) (*see also* Defect, coagulation) 286.3
  acquired 286.7
Stuart (-Prower) factor (*see also* Defect, coagulation) 286.3
sucrase 271.3
sucrase-isomaltase 271.3
sulfite oxidase 270.0
syndrome, multiple 260
thiamine, thiaminic (chloride) 265.1
thrombokinase (*see also* Defect, coagulation) 286.3
  newborn 776.0
thrombopoieten 287.39
thymolymphatic 279.2
thyroid (gland) 244.9
tocopherol 269.1
toe — *see* Absence, toe
tooth bud (*see also* Anodontia) 520.0
trunk V48.1
UDPG-glycogen transferase 271.0
upper limb V49.0
  congenital 755.20
    with complete absence of distal elements 755.21
    longitudinal (complete) (partial) (with distal deficiencies, incomplete) 755.22
      carpal(s) 755.28
      combined humeral, radial, ulnar (incomplete) 755.23
      humeral 755.24
      metacarpal(s) 755.28
      phalange(s) 755.29
        meaning all digits 755.21
      radial 755.26
      radioulnar 755.25
      ulnar 755.27
    transverse (complete) (partial) 755.21
vascular 459.9
vasopressin 253.5
viosterol (*see also* Deficiency, calciferol) 268.9
vitamin (multiple) NEC 269.2
  A 264.9
    with
      Bitôt's spot 264.1

Deficiency, deficient — *continued*
vitamin — *continued*
  A — *continued*
    with — *continued*
      Bitôt's spot — *continued*
        corneal 264.2
          with corneal ulceration 264.3
      keratomalacia 264.4
      keratosis, follicular 264.8
      night blindness 264.5
      scar of cornea, xerophthalmic 264.6
      specified manifestation NEC 264.8
        ocular 264.7
      xeroderma 264.8
      xerophthalmia 264.7
      xerosis
        conjunctival 264.0
          with Bitôt's spot 264.1
        corneal 264.2
          with corneal ulceration 264.3
  B (complex) NEC 266.9
    with
      beriberi 265.0
      pellagra 265.2
    specified type NEC 266.2
  B_1 NEC 265.1
    beriberi 265.0
  B_2 266.0
  B_6 266.1
  B_{12} 266.2
  B_c (folic acid) 266.2
  C (ascorbic acid) (with scurvy) 267
  D (calciferol) (ergosterol) 268.9
    with
      osteomalacia 268.2
      rickets (*see also* Rickets) 268.0
  E 269.1
  folic acid 266.2
  G 266.0
  H 266.2
  K 269.0
    of newborn 776.0
  nicotinic acid 265.2
  P 269.1
  PP 265.2
  specified NEC 269.1
  zinc 269.3
Deficient — *see also* Deficiency
blink reflex 374.45
craniofacial axis 756.0
number of teeth (*see also* Anodontia) 520.0
secretion of urine 788.5
Deficit
attention 799.51
cognitive communication 799.52
concentration 799.51
executive function 799.55
frontal lobe 799.55
neurologic NEC 781.99
  due to
    cerebrovascular lesion (*see also* Disease, cerebrovascular, acute) 436
      late effect — *see* Late effect(s) (of) cerebrovascular disease
    transient ischemic attack 435.9
  ischemic
    reversible (RIND) 434.91
      history of (personal) V12.54
      prolonged (PRIND) 434.91
        history of (personal) V12.54
oxygen 799.02
psychomotor 799.54
visuospatial 799.53
Deflection
radius 736.09
septum (acquired) (nasal) (nose) 470
spine — *see* Curvature, spine
turbinate (nose) 470
Defluvium
capillorum (*see also* Alopecia) 704.00
ciliorum 374.55

Defluvium — *continued*
unguium 703.8
Deformity 738.9
abdomen, congenital 759.9
abdominal wall
  acquired 738.8
  congenital 756.70
  muscle deficiency syndrome 756.79
acquired (unspecified site) 738.9
  specified site NEC 738.8
adrenal gland (congenital) 759.1
alimentary tract, congenital 751.9
  lower 751.5
  specified type NEC 751.8
  upper (any part, except tongue) 750.9
    specified type NEC 750.8
    tongue 750.10
      specified type NEC 750.19
ankle (joint) (acquired) 736.70
  abduction 718.47
  congenital 755.69
  contraction 718.47
  specified NEC 736.79
anus (congenital) 751.5
  acquired 569.49
aorta (congenital) 747.20
  acquired 447.8
  arch 747.21
    acquired 447.8
  coarctation 747.10
aortic
  arch 747.21
    acquired 447.8
  cusp or valve (congenital) 746.9
    acquired (*see also* Endocarditis, aortic) 424.1
  ring 747.21
appendix 751.5
arm (acquired) 736.89
  congenital 755.50
arteriovenous (congenital) (peripheral) NEC 747.60
  gastrointestinal 747.61
  lower limb 747.64
  renal 747.62
  specified NEC 747.69
  spinal 747.82
  upper limb 747.63
artery (congenital) (peripheral) NEC (*see also* Deformity, vascular) 747.60
  acquired 447.8
  cerebral 747.81
  coronary (congenital) 746.85
    acquired (*see also* Ischemia, heart) 414.9
  retinal 743.9
  umbilical 747.5
atrial septal (congenital) (heart) 745.5
auditory canal (congenital) (external) (*see also* Deformity, ear) 744.3
  acquired 380.50
auricle
  ear (congenital) (*see also* Deformity, ear) 744.3
    acquired 380.32
  heart (congenital) 746.9
back (acquired) — *see* Deformity, spine
Bartholin's duct (congenital) 750.9
bile duct (congenital) 751.60
  acquired 576.8
    with calculus, choledocholithiasis, or stones — *see* Choledocholithiasis
biliary duct or passage (congenital) 751.60
  acquired 576.8
    with calculus, choledocholithiasis, or stones — *see* Choledocholithiasis
bladder (neck) (sphincter) (trigone) (acquired) 596.89
  congenital 753.9
bone (acquired) NEC 738.9
  congenital 756.9
  turbinate 738.0
boutonniere (finger) 736.21
brain (congenital) 742.9

Deformity — *continued*
brain — *continued*
  acquired 348.89
  multiple 742.4
  reduction 742.2
  vessel (congenital) 747.81
breast (acquired) 611.89
  congenital 757.6
  reconstructed 612.0
bronchus (congenital) 748.3
  acquired 519.19
bursa, congenital 756.9
canal of Nuck 752.9
canthus (congenital) 743.9
  acquired 374.89
capillary (acquired) 448.9
  congenital NEC (*see also* Deformity, vascular) 747.60
cardiac — *see* Deformity, heart
cardiovascular system (congenital) 746.9
caruncle, lacrimal (congenital) 743.9
  acquired 375.69
cascade, stomach 537.6
cecum (congenital) 751.5
  acquired 569.89
cerebral (congenital) 742.9
  acquired 348.89
cervix (acquired) (uterus) 622.8
  congenital 752.40
cheek (acquired) 738.19
  congenital 744.9
chest (wall) (acquired) 738.3
  congenital 754.89
  late effect of rickets 268.1
chin (acquired) 738.19
  congenital 744.9
choroid (congenital) 743.9
  acquired 363.8
  plexus (congenital) 742.9
    acquired 349.2
cicatricial — *see* Cicatrix
cilia (congenital) 743.9
  acquired 374.89
circulatory system (congenital) 747.9
clavicle (acquired) 738.8
  congenital 755.51
clitoris (congenital) 752.40
  acquired 624.8
clubfoot — *see* Clubfoot
coccyx (acquired) 738.6
  congenital 756.10
colon (congenital) 751.5
  acquired 569.89
concha (ear) (congenital) (*see also* Deformity, ear) 744.3
  acquired 380.32
congenital, organ or site not listed (*see also* Anomaly) 759.9
cornea (congenital) 743.9
  acquired 371.70
coronary artery (congenital) 746.85
  acquired (*see also* Ischemia, heart) 414.9
cranium (acquired) 738.19
  congenital (*see also* Deformity, skull, congenital) 756.0
cricoid cartilage (congenital) 748.3
  acquired 478.79
cystic duct (congenital) 751.60
  acquired 575.8
Dandy-Walker 742.3
  with spina bifida (*see also* Spina bifida) 741.0 ☑
diaphragm (congenital) 756.6
  acquired 738.8
digestive organ(s) or system (congenital) NEC 751.9
  specified type NEC 751.8
ductus arteriosus 747.0
duodenal bulb 537.89
duodenum (congenital) 751.5
  acquired 537.89
dura (congenital) 742.9
  brain 742.4
    acquired 349.2
  spinal 742.59
    acquired 349.2

☑ **Additional Digit Required** — Refer to the Tabular List for Digit Selection   ᵂ **Subterms under main terms may continue to next column or page**

66 — Volume 2   ▶◀ **Revised Text**   ● **New Line**   ▲ **Revised Code**   2013 ICD-9-CM

Deformity — *continued*
- ear (congenital) 744.3
  - acquired 380.32
  - auricle 744.3
    - causing impairment of hearing 744.02
  - causing impairment of hearing 744.00
  - external 744.3
    - causing impairment of hearing 744.02
  - internal 744.05
  - lobule 744.3
  - middle 744.03
    - ossicles 744.04
  - ossicles 744.04
- ectodermal (congenital) NEC 757.9
  - specified type NEC 757.8
- ejaculatory duct (congenital) 752.9
  - acquired 608.89
- elbow (joint) (acquired) 736.00
  - congenital 755.50
  - contraction 718.42
- endocrine gland NEC 759.2
- epididymis (congenital) 752.9
  - acquired 608.89
  - torsion 608.24
- epiglottis (congenital) 748.3
  - acquired 478.79
- esophagus (congenital) 750.9
  - acquired 530.89
- Eustachian tube (congenital) NEC 744.3
  - specified type NEC 744.24
- extremity (acquired) 736.9
  - congenital, except reduction deformity 755.9
    - lower 755.60
    - upper 755.50
  - reduction — *see* Deformity, reduction
- eye (congenital) 743.9
  - acquired 379.8
  - muscle 743.9
- eyebrow (congenital) 744.89
- eyelid (congenital) 743.9
  - acquired 374.89
  - specified type NEC 743.62
- face (acquired) 738.19
  - congenital (any part) 744.9
    - due to intrauterine malposition and pressure 754.0
- fallopian tube (congenital) 752.10
  - acquired 620.8
- femur (acquired) 736.89
  - congenital 755.60
- fetal
  - with fetopelvic disproportion 653.7 ☑
    - affecting fetus or newborn 763.1
  - causing obstructed labor 660.1 ☑
    - affecting fetus or newborn 763.1
  - known or suspected, affecting management of pregnancy 655.9 ☑
- finger (acquired) 736.20
  - boutonniere type 736.21
  - congenital 755.50
  - flexion contracture 718.44
  - swan neck 736.22
- flexion (joint) (acquired) 736.9
  - congenital NEC 755.9
  - hip or thigh (acquired) 736.39
    - congenital (*see also* Subluxation, congenital, hip) 754.32
- foot (acquired) 736.70
  - cavovarus 736.75
    - congenital 754.59
  - congenital NEC 754.70
    - specified type NEC 754.79
  - valgus (acquired) 736.79
    - congenital 754.60
      - specified type NEC 754.69
  - varus (acquired) 736.79
    - congenital 754.50
      - specified type NEC 754.59
- forearm (acquired) 736.00
  - congenital 755.50
- forehead (acquired) 738.19
  - congenital (*see also* Deformity, skull, congenital) 756.0

Deformity — *continued*
- frontal bone (acquired) 738.19
  - congenital (*see also* Deformity, skull, congenital) 756.0
- gallbladder (congenital) 751.60
  - acquired 575.8
- gastrointestinal tract (congenital) NEC 751.9
  - acquired 569.89
  - specified type NEC 751.8
- genitalia, genital organ(s) or system NEC
  - congenital 752.9
  - female (congenital) 752.9
    - acquired 629.89
    - external 752.40
    - internal 752.9
  - male (congenital) 752.9
    - acquired 608.89
- globe (eye) (congenital) 743.9
  - acquired 360.89
- gum (congenital) 750.9
  - acquired 523.9
- gunstock 736.02
- hand (acquired) 736.00
  - claw 736.06
  - congenital 755.50
  - minus (and plus) (intrinsic) 736.09
  - pill roller (intrinsic) 736.09
  - plus (and minus) (intrinsic) 736.09
  - swan neck (intrinsic) 736.09
- head (acquired) 738.10
  - congenital (*see also* Deformity, skull congenital) 756.0
  - specified NEC 738.19
- heart (congenital) 746.9
  - auricle (congenital) 746.9
  - septum 745.9
    - auricular 745.5
    - specified type NEC 745.8
    - ventricular 745.4
  - valve (congenital) NEC 746.9
    - acquired — *see* Endocarditis
    - pulmonary (congenital) 746.00
    - specified type NEC 746.89
  - ventricle (congenital) 746.9
- heel (acquired) 736.76
  - congenital 755.67
- hepatic duct (congenital) 751.60
  - acquired 576.8
    - with calculus, choledocholithiasis, or stones — *see* Choledocholithiasis
- hip (joint) (acquired) 736.30
  - congenital NEC 755.63
  - flexion 718.45
    - congenital (*see also* Subluxation, congenital, hip) 754.32
- hourglass — *see* Contraction, hourglass
- humerus (acquired) 736.89
  - congenital 755.50
- hymen (congenital) 752.40
- hypophyseal (congenital) 759.2
- ileocecal (coil) (valve) (congenital) 751.5
  - acquired 569.89
- ileum (intestine) (congenital) 751.5
  - acquired 569.89
- ilium (acquired) 738.6
  - congenital 755.60
- integument (congenital) 757.9
- intervertebral cartilage or disc (acquired) (*see also* Displacement, intervertebral disc)
  - congenital 756.10
- intestine (large) (small) (congenital) 751.5
  - acquired 569.89
- iris (acquired) 364.75
  - congenital 743.9
  - prolapse 364.89
- ischium (acquired) 738.6
  - congenital 755.60
- jaw (acquired) (congenital) NEC 524.9
  - due to intrauterine malposition and pressure 754.0
- joint (acquired) NEC 738.8
  - congenital 755.9

Deformity — *continued*
- joint — *continued*
  - contraction (abduction) (adduction) (extension) (flexion) — *see* Contraction, joint
  - kidney(s) (calyx) (pelvis) (congenital) 753.9
    - acquired 593.89
    - vessel 747.62
      - acquired 459.9
  - Klippel-Feil (brevicollis) 756.16
  - knee (acquired) NEC 736.6
    - congenital 755.64
  - labium (majus) (minus) (congenital) 752.40
    - acquired 624.8
  - lacrimal apparatus or duct (congenital) 743.9
    - acquired 375.69
  - larynx (muscle) (congenital) 748.3
    - acquired 478.79
    - web (glottic) (subglottic) 748.2
  - leg (lower) (upper) (acquired) NEC 736.89
    - congenital 755.60
      - reduction — *see* Deformity, reduction, lower limb
  - lens (congenital) 743.9
    - acquired 379.39
  - lid (fold) (congenital) 743.9
    - acquired 374.89
  - ligament (acquired) 728.9
    - congenital 756.9
  - limb (acquired) 736.9
    - congenital, except reduction deformity 755.9
      - lower 755.60
        - reduction (*see also* Deformity, reduction, lower limb) 755.30
      - upper 755.50
        - reduction (*see also* Deformity, reduction, upper limb) 755.20
    - specified NEC 736.89
  - lip (congenital) NEC 750.9
    - acquired 528.5
    - specified type NEC 750.26
  - liver (congenital) 751.60
    - acquired 573.8
    - duct (congenital) 751.60
      - acquired 576.8
        - with calculus, choledocholithiasis, or stones — *see* Choledocholithiasis
  - lower extremity — *see* Deformity, leg
  - lumbosacral (joint) (region) (congenital) 756.10
    - acquired 738.5
  - lung (congenital) 748.60
    - acquired 518.89
    - specified type NEC 748.69
  - lymphatic system, congenital 759.9
  - Madelung's (radius) 755.54
  - maxilla (acquired) (congenital) 524.9
  - meninges or membrane (congenital) 742.9
    - brain 742.4
      - acquired 349.2
    - spinal (cord) 742.59
      - acquired 349.2
  - mesentery (congenital) 751.9
    - acquired 568.89
  - metacarpus (acquired) 736.00
    - congenital 755.50
  - metatarsus (acquired) 736.70
    - congenital 754.70
  - middle ear, except ossicles (congenital) 744.03
    - ossicles 744.04
  - mitral (leaflets) (valve) (congenital) 746.9
    - acquired — *see* Endocarditis, mitral
    - Ebstein's 746.89
    - parachute 746.5
    - specified type NEC 746.89
    - stenosis, congenital 746.5
  - mouth (acquired) 528.9
    - congenital NEC 750.9
      - specified type NEC 750.26
  - multiple, congenital NEC 759.7

Deformity — *continued*
- multiple, congenital — *continued*
  - specified type NEC 759.89
- muscle (acquired) 728.9
  - congenital 756.9
    - specified type NEC 756.89
    - sternocleidomastoid (due to intrauterine malposition and pressure) 754.1
- musculoskeletal system, congenital NEC 756.9
  - specified type NEC 756.9
- nail (acquired) 703.9
  - congenital 757.9
- nasal — *see* Deformity, nose
- neck (acquired) NEC 738.2
  - congenital (any part) 744.9
    - sternocleidomastoid 754.1
- nervous system (congenital) 742.9
- nipple (congenital) 757.6
  - acquired 611.89
- nose, nasal (cartilage) (acquired) 738.0
  - bone (turbinate) 738.0
  - congenital 748.1
    - bent 754.0
    - squashed 754.0
  - saddle 738.0
    - syphilitic 090.5
  - septum 470
    - congenital 748.1
  - sinus (wall) (congenital) 748.1
    - acquired 738.0
  - syphilitic (congenital) 090.5
    - late 095.8
- ocular muscle (congenital) 743.9
  - acquired 378.60
- opticociliary vessels (congenital) 743.9
- orbit (congenital) (eye) 743.9
  - acquired NEC 376.40
    - associated with craniofacial deformities 376.44
    - due to
      - bone disease 376.43
      - surgery 376.47
      - trauma 376.47
- organ of Corti (congenital) 744.05
- ovary (congenital) 752.0
  - acquired 620.8
- oviduct (congenital) 752.10
  - acquired 620.8
- palate (congenital) 750.9
  - acquired 526.89
  - cleft (congenital) (*see also* Cleft, palate) 749.00
  - hard, acquired 526.89
  - soft, acquired 528.9
- pancreas (congenital) 751.7
  - acquired 577.8
- parachute, mitral valve 746.5
- parathyroid (gland) 759.2
- parotid (gland) (congenital) 750.9
  - acquired 527.8
- patella (acquired) 736.6
  - congenital 755.64
- pelvis, pelvic (acquired) (bony) 738.6
  - with disproportion (fetopelvic) 653.0 ☑
    - affecting fetus or newborn 763.1
    - causing obstructed labor 660.1 ☑
      - affecting fetus or newborn 763.1
  - congenital 755.60
  - rachitic (late effect) 268.1
- penis (glans) (congenital) 752.9
  - acquired 607.89
- pericardium (congenital) 746.9
  - acquired — *see* Pericarditis
- pharynx (congenital) 750.9
  - acquired 478.29
- Pierre Robin (congenital) 756.0
- pinna (acquired) 380.32
  - congenital 744.3
- pituitary (congenital) 759.2
- pleural folds (congenital) 748.8
- portal vein (congenital) 747.40
- posture — *see* Curvature, spine
- prepuce (congenital) 752.9
  - acquired 607.89

☑ **Additional Digit Required — Refer to the Tabular List for Digit Selection**   ▽ **Subterms under main terms may continue to next column or page**

2013 ICD-9-CM   ▶◀ **Revised Text**   ● **New Line**   ▲ **Revised Code**   **Volume 2 — 67**

Index — Deformity — Degeneration, degenerative

Degeneration, degenerative — continued
cervix 622.8
due to radiation (intended effect) 622.8
adverse effect or misadventure 622.8
changes, spine or vertebra (see also
Spondylosis) 721.90
chitinous 277.39
chorioretinal 363.40
congenital 743.53
hereditary 363.50
choroid (colloid) (drusen) 363.40
hereditary 363.50
senile 363.41
diffuse secondary 363.42
cochlear 386.8
collateral ligament (knee) (medial) 717.82
lateral 717.81
combined (spinal cord) (subacute)
266.2 [336.2]
with anemia (pernicious) 281.0 [336.2]
due to dietary deficiency
281.1 [336.2]
due to vitamin B$_{12}$ deficiency anemia
(dietary) 281.1 [336.2]
conjunctiva 372.50
amyloid 277.39 [372.50]
cornea 371.40
calcerous 371.44
familial (hereditary) (see also Dystrophy,
cornea) 371.50
macular 371.55
reticular 371.54
hyaline (of old scars) 371.41
marginal (Terrien's) 371.48
mosaic (shagreen) 371.41
nodular 371.46
peripheral 371.48
senile 371.41
cortical (cerebellar) (parenchymatous) 334.2
alcoholic 303.9 ☑ [334.4]
diffuse, due to arteriopathy 437.0
corticobasal 331.6
corticostriatal-spinal 334.8
cretinoid 243
cruciate ligament (knee) (posterior) 717.84
anterior 717.83
cutis 709.3
amyloid 277.39
dental pulp 522.2
disc disease — see Degeneration, intervertebral disc
dorsolateral (spinal cord) — see Degeneration, combined
endocardial 424.90
extrapyramidal NEC 333.90
eye NEC 360.40
macular (see also Degeneration, macula)
362.50
congenital 362.75
hereditary 362.76
fatty (diffuse) (general) 272.8
liver 571.8
alcoholic 571.0
localized site — see Degeneration, by
site, fatty
placenta — see Placenta, abnormal
globe (eye) NEC 360.40
macular — see Degeneration, macula
grey matter 330.8
heart (brown) (calcareous) (fatty) (fibrous)
(hyaline) (mural) (muscular) (pigmentary) (senile) (with arteriosclerosis)
(see also Degeneration, myocardial)
429.1
amyloid 277.39 [425.7]
atheromatous — see Arteriosclerosis,
coronary
gouty 274.82
hypertensive (see also Hypertension,
heart) 402.90
ischemic 414.9
valve, valvular — see Endocarditis
hepatolenticular (Wilson's) 275.1
hepatorenal 572.4
heredofamilial
brain NEC 331.89

Degeneration, degenerative — continued
heredofamilial — continued
spinal cord NEC 336.8
hyaline (diffuse) (generalized) 728.9
localized (see also Degeneration, by site)
cornea 371.41
keratitis 371.41
hypertensive vascular — see Hypertension
infrapatellar fat pad 729.31
internal semilunar cartilage 717.3
intervertebral disc 722.6
with myelopathy 722.70
cervical, cervicothoracic 722.4
with myelopathy 722.71
lumbar, lumbosacral 722.52
with myelopathy 722.73
thoracic, thoracolumbar 722.51
with myelopathy 722.72
intestine 569.89
amyloid 277.39
lardaceous 277.39
iris (generalized) (see also Atrophy, iris)
364.59
pigmentary 364.53
pupillary margin 364.54
ischemic — see Ischemia
joint disease (see also Osteoarthrosis)
715.9 ☑
multiple sites 715.09
spine (see also Spondylosis) 721.90
kidney (see also Sclerosis, renal) 587
amyloid 277.39 [583.81]
cyst, cystic (multiple) (solitary) 593.2
congenital (see also Cystic, disease,
kidney) 753.10
fatty 593.89
fibrocystic (congenital) 753.19
lardaceous 277.39 [583.81]
polycystic (congenital) 753.12
adult type (APKD) 753.13
autosomal dominant 753.13
autosomal recessive 753.14
childhood type (CPKD) 753.14
infantile type 753.14
waxy 277.39 [583.81]
Kuhnt-Junius (retina) 362.52
labyrinth, osseous 386.8
lacrimal passages, cystic 375.12
lardaceous (any site) 277.39
lateral column (posterior), spinal cord (see
also Degeneration, combined)
266.2 [336.2]
lattice 362.63
lens 366.9
infantile, juvenile, or presenile 366.00
senile 366.10
lenticular (familial) (progressive) (Wilson's)
(with cirrhosis of liver) 275.1
striate artery 437.0
lethal ball, prosthetic heart valve 996.02
ligament
collateral (knee) (medial) 717.82
lateral 717.81
cruciate (knee) (posterior) 717.84
anterior 717.83
liver (diffuse) 572.8
amyloid 277.39
congenital (cystic) 751.62
cystic 572.8
congenital 751.62
fatty 571.8
alcoholic 571.0
hypertrophic 572.8
lardaceous 277.39
parenchymatous, acute or subacute (see
also Necrosis, liver) 570
pigmentary 572.8
toxic (acute) 573.8
waxy 277.39
lung 518.89
lymph gland 289.3
hyaline 289.3
lardaceous 277.39
macula (acquired) (senile) 362.50
atrophic 362.51
Best's 362.76

Degeneration, degenerative — continued
macula — continued
congenital 362.75
cystic 362.54
cystoid 362.53
disciform 362.52
dry 362.51
exudative 362.52
familial pseudoinflammatory 362.77
hereditary 362.76
hole 362.54
juvenile (Stargardt's) 362.75
nonexudative 362.51
pseudohole 362.54
wet 362.52
medullary — see Degeneration, brain
membranous labyrinth, congenital (causing
impairment of hearing) 744.05
meniscus — see Derangement, joint
microcystoid 362.62
mitral — see Insufficiency, mitral
Mönckeberg's (see also Arteriosclerosis, extremities) 440.20
moral 301.7
motor centers, senile 331.2
mural (see also Degeneration, myocardial)
429.1
heart, cardiac (see also Degeneration,
myocardial) 429.1
myocardium, myocardial (see also Degeneration, myocardial) 429.1
muscle 728.9
fatty 728.9
fibrous 728.9
heart (see also Degeneration, myocardial) 429.1
hyaline 728.9
muscular progressive 728.2
myelin, central nervous system NEC 341.9
myocardium, myocardial (brown) (calcareous) (fatty) (fibrous) (hyaline) (mural)
(muscular) (pigmentary) (senile)
(with arteriosclerosis) 429.1
with rheumatic fever (conditions classifiable to 390) 398.0
active, acute, or subacute 391.2
with chorea 392.0
inactive or quiescent (with chorea)
398.0
amyloid 277.39 [425.7]
congenital 746.89
fetus or newborn 779.89
gouty 274.82
hypertensive (see also Hypertension,
heart) 402.90
ischemic 414.8
rheumatic (see also Degeneration, myocardium, with rheumatic fever)
398.0
syphilitic 093.82
nasal sinus (mucosa) (see also Sinusitis)
473.9
frontal 473.1
maxillary 473.0
nerve — see Disorder, nerve
nervous system 349.89
amyloid 277.39 [357.4]
autonomic (see also Neuropathy, peripheral, autonomic) 337.9
fatty 349.89
peripheral autonomic NEC (see also
Neuropathy, peripheral, autonomic) 337.9
nipple 611.9
nose 478.19
oculoacousticocerebral, congenital (progressive) 743.8
olivopontocerebellar (familial) (hereditary)
333.0
osseous labyrinth 386.8
ovary 620.8
cystic 620.2
microcystic 620.2
pallidal, pigmentary (progressive) 333.0
pancreas 577.8

Degeneration, degenerative — continued
pancreas — continued
tuberculous (see also Tuberculosis)
017.9 ☑
papillary muscle 429.81
paving stone 362.61
penis 607.89
peritoneum 568.89
pigmentary (diffuse) (general)
localized — see Degeneration, by site
pallidal (progressive) 333.0
secondary 362.65
pineal gland 259.8
pituitary (gland) 253.8
placenta (fatty) (fibrinoid) (fibroid) — see
Placenta, abnormal
popliteal fat pad 729.31
posterolateral (spinal cord) (see also Degeneration, combined) 266.2 [336.2]
pulmonary valve (heart) (see also Endocarditis, pulmonary) 424.3
pulp (tooth) 522.2
pupillary margin 364.54
renal (see also Sclerosis, renal) 587
fibrocystic 753.19
polycystic 753.12
adult type (APKD) 753.13
autosomal dominant 753.13
autosomal recessive 753.14
childhood type (CPKD) 753.14
infantile type 753.14
reticuloendothelial system 289.89
retina (peripheral) 362.60
with retinal defect (see also Detachment,
retina, with retinal defect) 361.00
cystic (senile) 362.50
cystoid 362.53
hereditary (see also Dystrophy, retina)
362.70
cerebroretinal 362.71
congenital 362.75
juvenile (Stargardt's) 362.75
macula 362.76
Kuhnt-Junius 362.52
lattice 362.63
macular (see also Degeneration, macula)
362.50
microcystoid 362.62
palisade 362.63
paving stone 362.61
pigmentary (primary) 362.74
secondary 362.65
posterior pole (see also Degeneration,
macula) 362.50
secondary 362.66
senile 362.60
cystic 362.53
reticular 362.64
saccule, congenital (causing impairment of
hearing) 744.05
sacculocochlear 386.8
senile 797
brain 331.2
cardiac, heart, or myocardium (see also
Degeneration, myocardial) 429.1
motor centers 331.2
reticule 362.64
retina, cystic 362.50
vascular — see Arteriosclerosis
silicone rubber poppet (prosthetic valve)
996.02
sinus (cystic) (see also Sinusitis) 473.9
polypoid 471.1
skin 709.3
amyloid 277.39
colloid 709.3
spinal (cord) 336.8
amyloid 277.39
column 733.90
combined (subacute) (see also Degeneration, combined) 266.2 [336.2]
with anemia (pernicious)
281.0 [336.2]
dorsolateral (see also Degeneration,
combined) 266.2 [336.2]
familial NEC 336.8

Degeneration, degenerative — continued
  spinal — continued
    fatty 336.8
    funicular (see also Degeneration, combined) 266.2 [336.2]
    heredofamilial NEC 336.8
    posterolateral (see also Degeneration, combined) 266.2 [336.2]
    subacute combined — see Degeneration, combined
    tuberculous (see also Tuberculosis) 013.8 ☑
  spine 733.90
  spleen 289.59
    amyloid 277.39
    lardaceous 277.39
  stomach 537.89
    lardaceous 277.39
  strionigral 333.0
  sudoriparous (cystic) 705.89
  suprarenal (capsule) (gland) 255.8
    with hypofunction 255.41
  sweat gland 705.89
  synovial membrane (pulpy) 727.9
  tapetoretinal 362.74
    adult or presenile form 362.50
  testis (postinfectional) 608.89
  thymus (gland) 254.8
    fatty 254.8
    lardaceous 277.39
  thyroid (gland) 246.8
  tricuspid (heart) (valve) — see Endocarditis, tricuspid
  tuberculous NEC (see also Tuberculosis) 011.9 ☑
  turbinate 733.90
  uterus 621.8
    cystic 621.8
  vascular (senile) (see also Arteriosclerosis)
    hypertensive — see Hypertension
  vitreoretinal (primary) 362.73
    secondary 362.66
  vitreous humor (with infiltration) 379.21
  wallerian NEC — see Disorder, nerve
  waxy (any site) 277.39
  Wilson's hepatolenticular 275.1
Deglutition
  paralysis 784.99
    hysterical 300.11
  pneumonia 507.0
Degos' disease or syndrome 447.8
Degradation disorder, branched-chain amino acid 270.3
Dehiscence
  anastomosis — see Complications, anastomosis
  cesarean wound 674.1 ☑
  closure of
    cornea 998.32
    fascia, superficial or muscular 998.31
    internal organ 998.31
    mucosa 998.32
    muscle or muscle flap 998.31
    ribs or rib cage 998.31
    skin 998.32
    skull or craniotomy 998.31
    sternum or sternotomy 998.31
    subcutaneous tissue 998.32
    tendon or ligament 998.31
    traumatic laceration (external) (internal) 998.33
  episiotomy 674.2 ☑
  operation wound 998.32
    deep 998.31
    external 998.32
    internal 998.31
    superficial 998.32
  perineal wound (postpartum) 674.2 ☑
  postoperative 998.32
    abdomen 998.32
      internal 998.31
    internal 998.31
  traumatic injury wound repair 998.33
  uterine wound 674.1 ☑
Dehydration (cachexia) 276.51

Dehydration — continued
  with
    hypernatremia 276.0
    hyponatremia 276.1
  newborn 775.5
Deiters' nucleus syndrome 386.19
Déjérine's disease 356.0
Déjérine-Klumpke paralysis 767.6
Déjérine-Roussy syndrome 338.0
Déjérine-Sottas disease or neuropathy (hypertrophic) 356.0
Déjérine-Thomas atrophy or syndrome 333.0
de Lange's syndrome (Amsterdam dwarf, intellectual disabilities, and brachycephaly) 759.89
Delay, delayed
  adaptation, cones or rods 368.63
  any plane in pelvis
    affecting fetus or newborn 763.1
    complicating delivery 660.1 ☑
  birth or delivery NEC 662.1 ☑
    affecting fetus or newborn 763.89
    second twin, triplet, or multiple mate 662.3 ☑
  closure (see also Fistula)
    cranial suture 756.0
    fontanel 756.0
  coagulation NEC 790.92
  conduction (cardiac) (ventricular) 426.9
  delivery NEC 662.1 ☑
    second twin, triplet, etc. 662.3 ☑
      affecting fetus or newborn 763.89
  development
    in childhood 783.40
      physiological 783.40
    intellectual NEC 315.9
    learning NEC 315.2
    reading 315.00
    sexual 259.0
    speech 315.39
      and language due to hearing loss 315.34
      associated with hyperkinesis 314.1
    spelling 315.09
  gastric emptying 536.8
  menarche 256.39
    due to pituitary hypofunction 253.4
  menstruation (cause unknown) 626.8
  milestone in childhood 783.42
  motility — see Hypomotility
  passage of meconium (newborn) 777.1
  primary respiration 768.9
  puberty 259.0
  separation of umbilical cord 779.83
  sexual maturation, female 259.0
  vaccination V64.00
Del Castillo's syndrome (germinal aplasia) 606.0
Déleage's disease 359.89
Deletion syndrome
  5p 758.31
  22q11.2 758.32
  autosomal NEC 758.39
  constitutional 5q deletion 758.39
Delhi (boil) (button) (sore) 085.1
Delinquency (juvenile) 312.9
  group (see also Disturbance, conduct) 312.2
  neurotic 312.4
Delirium, delirious 780.09
  acute 780.09
    due to conditions classified elsewhere 293.0
  alcoholic 291.0
    acute 291.0
    chronic 291.1
  alcoholicum 291.0
  chronic (see also Psychosis) 293.89
    due to or associated with physical condition — see Psychosis, organic
  drug-induced 292.81
  due to conditions classified elsewhere 293.0
  eclamptic (see also Eclampsia) 780.39
  exhaustion (see also Reaction, stress, acute) 308.9
  hysterical 300.11

Delirium, delirious — continued
  in
    presenile dementia 290.11
    senile dementia 290.3
  induced by drug 292.81
  manic, maniacal (acute) (see also Psychosis, affective) 296.0
    recurrent episode 296.1 ☑
    single episode 296.0 ☑
  puerperal 293.9
  senile 290.3
  subacute (psychotic) 293.1
  thyroid (see also Thyrotoxicosis) 242.9 ☑
  traumatic (see also Injury, intracranial)
    with
      lesion, spinal cord — see Injury, spinal, by site
      shock, spinal — see Injury, spinal, by site
  tremens (impending) 291.0
  uremic — see Uremia
  withdrawal
    alcoholic (acute) 291.0
      chronic 291.1
    drug 292.0
Delivery

> Note — Use the following fifth-digit subclassification with categories 640–649, 651–676:
>
> 0   unspecified as to episode of care
>
> 1   delivered, with or without mention of antepartum condition
>
> 2   delivered, with mention of postpartum complication
>
> 3   antepartum condition or complication
>
> 4   postpartum condition or complication

  breech (assisted) (buttocks) (complete) (frank) (spontaneous) 652.2 ☑
    affecting fetus or newborn 763.0
    extraction NEC 669.6 ☑
  cesarean (for) 669.7 ☑
    abnormal
      cervix 654.6 ☑
      pelvic organs or tissues 654.9 ☑
      pelvis (bony) (major) NEC 653.0 ☑
      presentation or position 652.9 ☑
        in multiple gestation 652.6 ☑
      size, fetus 653.5 ☑
      soft parts (of pelvis) 654.9 ☑
      uterus, congenital 654.0 ☑
      vagina 654.7 ☑
      vulva 654.8 ☑
    abruptio placentae 641.2 ☑
    acromion presentation 652.8 ☑
    affecting fetus or newborn 763.4
    anteversion, cervix or uterus 654.4 ☑
    atony, uterus 661.2 ☑
      with hemorrhage 666.1 ☑
    bicornis or bicornuate uterus 654.0 ☑
    breech presentation (buttocks) (complete) (frank) 652.2 ☑
    brow presentation 652.4 ☑
    cephalopelvic disproportion (normally formed fetus) 653.4 ☑
    chin presentation 652.4 ☑
    cicatrix of cervix 654.6 ☑
    contracted pelvis (general) 653.1 ☑
      inlet 653.2 ☑
      outlet 653.3 ☑
    cord presentation or prolapse 663.0 ☑
    cystocele 654.4 ☑
    deformity (acquired) (congenital)
      pelvic organs or tissues NEC 654.9 ☑
      pelvis (bony) NEC 653.0 ☑
    displacement, uterus NEC 654.4 ☑
    disproportion NEC 653.9 ☑
    distress
      fetal 656.8 ☑
      maternal 669.0 ☑
    eclampsia 642.6 ☑

Delivery — continued
  cesarean — continued
    face presentation 652.4 ☑
    failed
      forceps 660.7 ☑
      trial of labor NEC 660.6 ☑
      vacuum extraction 660.7 ☑
      ventouse 660.7 ☑
    fetal deformity 653.7 ☑
    fetal-maternal hemorrhage 656.0 ☑
    fetus, fetal
      distress 656.8 ☑
      prematurity 656.8 ☑
    fibroid (tumor) (uterus) 654.1 ☑
    footling 652.8 ☑
      with successful version 652.1 ☑
    hemorrhage (antepartum) (intrapartum) NEC 641.9 ☑
    hydrocephalic fetus 653.6 ☑
    incarceration of uterus 654.3 ☑
    incoordinate uterine action 661.4 ☑
    inertia, uterus 661.2 ☑
      primary 661.0 ☑
      secondary 661.1 ☑
    lateroversion, uterus or cervix 654.4 ☑
    mal lie 652.9 ☑
    malposition
      fetus 652.9 ☑
        in multiple gestation 652.6 ☑
      pelvic organs or tissues NEC 654.9 ☑
      uterus NEC or cervix 654.4 ☑
    malpresentation NEC 652.9 ☑
      in multiple gestation 652.6 ☑
    maternal
      diabetes mellitus (conditions classifiable to 249 and 250) 648.0 ☑
      heart disease NEC 648.6 ☑
    meconium in liquor 656.8 ☑
      staining only 792.3
    oblique presentation 652.3 ☑
    oversize fetus 653.5 ☑
    pelvic tumor NEC 654.9 ☑
    placental insufficiency 656.5 ☑
    placenta previa 641.0 ☑
      with hemorrhage 641.1 ☑
    (planned) occurring after 37 completed weeks of gestation but before 39 completed weeks gestation due to (spontaneous) onset of labor 649.8 ☑
    poor dilation, cervix 661.0 ☑
    pre-eclampsia 642.4 ☑
      severe 642.5 ☑
    previous
      cesarean delivery, section 654.2 ☑
      surgery (to)
        cervix 654.6 ☑
        gynecological NEC 654.9 ☑
        rectum 654.8 ☑
        uterus NEC 654.9 ☑
          previous cesarean delivery, section 654.2 ☑
        vagina 654.7 ☑
    prolapse
      arm or hand 652.7 ☑
      uterus 654.4 ☑
    prolonged labor 662.1 ☑
    rectocele 654.4 ☑
    retroversion, uterus or cervix 654.3 ☑
    rigid
      cervix 654.6 ☑
      pelvic floor 654.4 ☑
      perineum 654.8 ☑
      vagina 654.7 ☑
      vulva 654.8 ☑
    sacculation, pregnant uterus 654.4 ☑
    scar(s)
      cervix 654.6 ☑
      cesarean delivery, section 654.2 ☑
      uterus NEC 654.9 ☑
        due to previous cesarean delivery, section 654.2 ☑
    Shirodkar suture in situ 654.5 ☑
    shoulder presentation 652.8 ☑

☑ Additional Digit Required — Refer to the Tabular List for Digit Selection

Subterms under main terms may continue to next column or page

▶◀ Revised Text   ● New Line   ▲ Revised Code

Delivery — *continued*
  cesarean — *continued*
    stenosis or stricture, cervix 654.6 ☑
    transverse presentation or lie 652.3 ☑
    tumor, pelvic organs or tissues NEC 654.4 ☑
    umbilical cord presentation or prolapse 663.0 ☑
  completely normal case — *see* category 650
  complicated (by) NEC 669.9 ☑
    abdominal tumor, fetal 653.7 ☑
      causing obstructed labor 660.1 ☑
    abnormal, abnormality of
      cervix 654.6 ☑
        causing obstructed labor 660.2 ☑
      forces of labor 661.9 ☑
      formation of uterus 654.0 ☑
      pelvic organs or tissues 654.9 ☑
        causing obstructed labor 660.2 ☑
      pelvis (bony) (major) NEC 653.0 ☑
        causing obstructed labor 660.1 ☑
      presentation or position NEC 652.9 ☑
        causing obstructed labor 660.0 ☑
      size, fetus 653.5 ☑
        causing obstructed labor 660.1 ☑
      soft parts (of pelvis) 654.9 ☑
        causing obstructed labor 660.2 ☑
      uterine contractions NEC 661.9 ☑
      uterus (formation) 654.0 ☑
        causing obstructed labor 660.2 ☑
      vagina 654.7 ☑
        causing obstructed labor 660.2 ☑
    abnormally formed uterus (any type) (congenital) 654.0 ☑
      causing obstructed labor 660.2 ☑
    acromion presentation 652.8 ☑
      causing obstructed labor 660.0 ☑
    adherent placenta 667.0 ☑
      with hemorrhage 666.0 ☑
    adhesions, uterus (to abdominal wall) 654.4 ☑
    advanced maternal age NEC 659.6 ☑
      multigravida 659.6 ☑
      primigravida 659.5 ☑
    air embolism 673.0 ☑
    amnionitis 658.4 ☑
    amniotic fluid embolism 673.1 ☑
    anesthetic death 668.9 ☑
    annular detachment, cervix 665.3 ☑
    antepartum hemorrhage — *see* Delivery, complicated, hemorrhage
    anteversion, cervix or uterus 654.4 ☑
      causing obstructed labor 660.2 ☑
    apoplexy 674.0 ☑
      placenta 641.2 ☑
    arrested active phase 661.1 ☑
    asymmetrical pelvis bone 653.0 ☑
      causing obstructed labor 660.1 ☑
    atony, uterus with hemorrhage (hypotonic) (inertia) 666.1 ☑
      hypertonic 661.4 ☑
    Bandl's ring 661.4 ☑
    battledore placenta — *see* Placenta, abnormal
    bicornis or bicornuate uterus 654.0 ☑
      causing obstructed labor 660.2 ☑
    birth injury to mother NEC 665.9 ☑
    bleeding (*see also* Delivery, complicated, hemorrhage) 641.9 ☑
    breech presentation (assisted) (buttocks) (complete) (frank) (spontaneous) 652.2 ☑
      with successful version 652.1 ☑
    brow presentation 652.4 ☑

Delivery — *continued*
  complicated — *continued*
    cephalopelvic disproportion (normally formed fetus) 653.4 ☑
      causing obstructed labor 660.1 ☑
    cerebral hemorrhage 674.0 ☑
    cervical dystocia 661.2 ☑
    chin presentation 652.4 ☑
      causing obstructed labor 660.0 ☑
    cicatrix
      cervix 654.6 ☑
        causing obstructed labor 660.2 ☑
      vagina 654.7 ☑
        causing obstructed labor 660.2 ☑
    coagulation defect 649.3 ☑
    colporrhexis 665.4 ☑
      with perineal laceration 664.0 ☑
    compound presentation 652.8 ☑
      causing obstructed labor 660.0 ☑
    compression of cord (umbilical) 663.2 ☑
      around neck 663.1 ☑
      cord prolapsed 663.0 ☑
    contraction, contracted pelvis 653.1 ☑
      causing obstructed labor 660.1 ☑
      general 653.1 ☑
        causing obstructed labor 660.1 ☑
      inlet 653.2 ☑
        causing obstructed labor 660.1 ☑
      midpelvic 653.8 ☑
        causing obstructed labor 660.1 ☑
      midplane 653.8 ☑
        causing obstructed labor 660.1 ☑
      outlet 653.3 ☑
        causing obstructed labor 660.1 ☑
    contraction ring 661.4 ☑
    cord (umbilical) 663.9 ☑
      around neck, tightly or with compression 663.1 ☑
        without compression 663.3 ☑
      bruising 663.6 ☑
      complication NEC 663.9 ☑
        specified type NEC 663.8 ☑
      compression NEC 663.2 ☑
      entanglement NEC 663.3 ☑
        with compression 663.2 ☑
      forelying 663.0 ☑
      hematoma 663.6 ☑
      marginal attachment 663.8 ☑
      presentation 663.0 ☑
      prolapse (complete) (occult) (partial) 663.0 ☑
      short 663.4 ☑
      specified complication NEC 663.8 ☑
      thrombosis (vessels) 663.6 ☑
      vascular lesion 663.6 ☑
      velamentous insertion 663.8 ☑
    Couvelaire uterus 641.2 ☑
    cretin pelvis (dwarf type) (male type) 653.1 ☑
      causing obstructed labor 660.1 ☑
    crossbirth 652.3 ☑
      with successful version 652.1 ☑
      causing obstructed labor 660.0 ☑
    cyst (Gartner's duct) 654.7 ☑
    cystocele 654.4 ☑
      causing obstructed labor 660.2 ☑
    death of fetus (near term) 656.4 ☑
      early (before 22 completed weeks gestation) 632
    deformity (acquired) (congenital) fetus 653.7 ☑
      causing obstructed labor 660.1 ☑
      pelvic organs or tissues NEC 654.9 ☑
        causing obstructed labor 660.2 ☑
      pelvis (bony) NEC 653.0 ☑

Delivery — *continued*
  complicated — *continued*
    deformity — *continued*
      pelvis — *continued*
        causing obstructed labor 660.1 ☑
    delay, delayed
      delivery in multiple pregnancy 662.3 ☑
      due to locked mates 660.5 ☑
      following rupture of membranes (spontaneous) 658.2 ☑
        artificial 658.3 ☑
    depressed fetal heart tones 659.7 ☑
    diastasis recti 665.8 ☑
    dilatation
      bladder 654.4 ☑
        causing obstructed labor 660.2 ☑
      cervix, incomplete, poor or slow 661.0 ☑
    diseased placenta 656.7 ☑
    displacement uterus NEC 654.4 ☑
      causing obstructed labor 660.2 ☑
    disproportion NEC 653.9 ☑
      causing obstructed labor 660.1 ☑
    disruptio uteri — *see* Delivery, complicated, rupture, uterus
    distress
      fetal 656.8 ☑
      maternal 669.0 ☑
    double uterus (congenital) 654.0 ☑
      causing obstructed labor 660.2 ☑
    dropsy amnion 657.0 ☑
    dysfunction, uterus 661.9 ☑
      hypertonic 661.4 ☑
      hypotonic 661.2 ☑
        primary 661.0 ☑
        secondary 661.1 ☑
      incoordinate 661.4 ☑
    dystocia
      cervical 661.2 ☑
      fetal — *see* Delivery, complicated, abnormal, presentation
      maternal — *see* Delivery, complicated, prolonged labor
      pelvic — *see* Delivery, complicated, contraction pelvis
      positional 652.8 ☑
      shoulder girdle 660.4 ☑
    eclampsia 642.6 ☑
    ectopic kidney 654.4 ☑
      causing obstructed labor 660.2 ☑
    edema, cervix 654.6 ☑
      causing obstructed labor 660.2 ☑
    effusion, amniotic fluid 658.1 ☑
    elderly multigravida 659.6 ☑
    elderly primigravida 659.5 ☑
    embolism (pulmonary) 673.2 ☑
      air 673.0 ☑
      amniotic fluid 673.1 ☑
      blood clot 673.2 ☑
      cerebral 674.0 ☑
      fat 673.8 ☑
      pyemic 673.3 ☑
      septic 673.3 ☑
    entanglement, umbilical cord 663.3 ☑
      with compression 663.2 ☑
      around neck (with compression) 663.1 ☑
    eversion, cervix or uterus 665.2 ☑
    excessive
      fetal growth 653.5 ☑
        causing obstructed labor 660.1 ☑
      size of fetus 653.5 ☑
        causing obstructed labor 660.1 ☑
    face presentation 652.4 ☑
      causing obstructed labor 660.0 ☑
      to pubes 660.3 ☑
    failure, fetal head to enter pelvic brim 652.5 ☑
      causing obstructed labor 660.0 ☑

Delivery — *continued*
  complicated — *continued*
    female genital mutilation 660.8 ☑
    fetal
      acid-base balance 656.8 ☑
      death (near term) NEC 656.4 ☑
        early (before 22 completed weeks gestation) 632
      deformity 653.7 ☑
        causing obstructed labor 660.1 ☑
      distress 656.8 ☑
      heart rate or rhythm 659.7 ☑
      reduction of multiple fetuses reduced to single fetus 651.7 ☑
    fetopelvic disproportion 653.4 ☑
      causing obstructed labor 660.1 ☑
    fever during labor 659.2 ☑
    fibroid (tumor) (uterus) 654.1 ☑
      causing obstructed labor 660.2 ☑
    fibromyomata 654.1 ☑
      causing obstructed labor 660.2 ☑
    forelying umbilical cord 663.0 ☑
    fracture of coccyx 665.6 ☑
    hematoma 664.5 ☑
      broad ligament 665.7 ☑
      ischial spine 665.7 ☑
      pelvic 665.7 ☑
      perineum 664.5 ☑
      soft tissues 665.7 ☑
      subdural 674.0 ☑
      umbilical cord 663.6 ☑
      vagina 665.7 ☑
      vulva or perineum 664.5 ☑
    hemorrhage (uterine) (antepartum) (intrapartum) (pregnancy) 641.9 ☑
      accidental 641.2 ☑
      associated with
        afibrinogenemia 641.3 ☑
        coagulation defect 641.3 ☑
          hyperfibrinolysis 641.3 ☑
          hypofibrinogenemia 641.3 ☑
      cerebral 674.0 ☑
      due to
        low-lying placenta 641.1 ☑
        placenta previa 641.1 ☑
        premature separation of placenta (normally implanted) 641.2 ☑
        retained placenta 666.0 ☑
        trauma 641.8 ☑
        uterine leiomyoma 641.8 ☑
      marginal sinus rupture 641.2 ☑
      placenta NEC 641.9 ☑
      postpartum (atonic) (immediate) (within 24 hours) 666.1 ☑
        with retained or trapped placenta 666.0 ☑
        delayed 666.2 ☑
        secondary 666.2 ☑
        third stage 666.0 ☑
    hourglass contraction, uterus 661.4 ☑
    hydramnios 657.0 ☑
    hydrocephalic fetus 653.6 ☑
      causing obstructed labor 660.1 ☑
    hydrops fetalis 653.7 ☑
      causing obstructed labor 660.1 ☑
    hypertension — *see* Hypertension, complicating pregnancy
    hypertonic uterine dysfunction 661.4 ☑
    hypotonic uterine dysfunction 661.2 ☑
    impacted shoulders 660.4 ☑
    incarceration, uterus 654.3 ☑
      causing obstructed labor 660.2 ☑
    incomplete dilation (cervix) 661.0 ☑
    incoordinate uterus 661.4 ☑
    indication NEC 659.9 ☑
      specified type NEC 659.8 ☑
    inertia, uterus 661.2 ☑
      hypertonic 661.4 ☑
      hypotonic 661.2 ☑
        primary 661.0 ☑
        secondary 661.1 ☑

☑ Additional Digit Required — Refer to the Tabular List for Digit Selection   ⏳ Subterms under main terms may continue to next column or page

2013 ICD-9-CM   ▶◀ Revised Text   ● New Line   ▲ Revised Code   Volume 2 — 71

Delivery — *continued*
  complicated — *continued*
    infantile
      genitalia 654.4 ☑
        causing obstructed labor
          660.2 ☑
      uterus (os) 654.4 ☑
        causing obstructed labor
          660.2 ☑
    injury (to mother) NEC 665.9 ☑
    intrauterine fetal death (near term) NEC
      656.4 ☑
      early (before 22 completed weeks
        gestation) 632
    inversion, uterus 665.2 ☑
    kidney, ectopic 654.4 ☑
      causing obstructed labor 660.2 ☑
    knot (true), umbilical cord 663.2 ☑
    labor
      onset (spontaneous) after 37 complet-
        ed weeks of gestation but be-
        fore 39 completed weeks
        gestation with delivery by
        (planned) cesarean section
        649.8 ☑
      premature (before 37 completed
        weeks gestation) 644.2 ☑
    laceration 664.9 ☑
      anus (sphincter) (healed) (old)
        654.8 ☑
        with mucosa 664.3 ☑
        not associated with third-degree
          perineal laceration
          664.6 ☑
      bladder (urinary) 665.5 ☑
      bowel 665.5 ☑
      central 664.4 ☑
      cervix (uteri) 665.3 ☑
      fourchette 664.0 ☑
      hymen 664.0 ☑
      labia (majora) (minora) 664.0 ☑
      pelvic
        floor 664.1 ☑
        organ NEC 665.5 ☑
      perineum, perineal 664.4 ☑
        first degree 664.0 ☑
        second degree 664.1 ☑
        third degree 664.2 ☑
        fourth degree 664.3 ☑
        central 664.4 ☑
        extensive NEC 664.4 ☑
        muscles 664.1 ☑
        skin 664.0 ☑
        slight 664.0 ☑
      peritoneum (pelvic) 665.5 ☑
      periurethral tissue 664.8 ☑
      rectovaginal (septum) (without per-
        ineal laceration) 665.4 ☑
        with perineum 664.2 ☑
          with anal or rectal mucosa
          664.3 ☑
      skin (perineum) 664.0 ☑
      specified site or type NEC 664.8 ☑
      sphincter ani (healed) (old) 654.8 ☑
        with mucosa 664.3 ☑
        not associated with third-degree
          perineal laceration
          664.6 ☑
      urethra 665.5 ☑
      uterus 665.1 ☑
        before labor 665.0 ☑
      vagina, vaginal (deep) (high) (sulcus)
        (wall) (without perineal lacer-
        ation) 665.4 ☑
        with perineum 664.0 ☑
        muscles, with perineum 664.1 ☑
      vulva 664.0 ☑
    lateroversion, uterus or cervix 654.4 ☑
      causing obstructed labor 660.2 ☑
    locked mates 660.5 ☑
    low implantation of placenta — *see* De-
      livery, complicated, placenta,
      previa
    mal lie 652.9 ☑

Delivery — *continued*
  complicated — *continued*
    malposition
      fetus NEC 652.9 ☑
        causing obstructed labor
          660.0 ☑
      pelvic organs or tissues NEC 654.9 ☑
        causing obstructed labor
          660.2 ☑
      placenta 641.1 ☑
        without hemorrhage 641.0 ☑
      uterus NEC or cervix 654.4 ☑
        causing obstructed labor
          660.2 ☑
    malpresentation 652.9 ☑
      causing obstructed labor 660.0 ☑
    marginal sinus (bleeding) (rupture)
      641.2 ☑
    maternal hypotension syndrome
      669.2 ☑
    meconium in liquor 656.8 ☑
    membranes, retained — *see* Delivery,
      complicated, placenta, retained
    mentum presentation 652.4 ☑
      causing obstructed labor 660.0 ☑
    metrorrhagia (myopathia) — *see* Deliv-
      ery, complicated, hemorrhage
    metrorrhexis — *see* Delivery, complicat-
      ed, rupture, uterus
    multiparity (grand) 659.4 ☑
    myelomeningocele, fetus 653.7 ☑
      causing obstructed labor 660.1 ☑
    Nägele's pelvis 653.0 ☑
      causing obstructed labor 660.1 ☑
    nonengagement, fetal head 652.5 ☑
      causing obstructed labor 660.0 ☑
    oblique presentation 652.3 ☑
      causing obstructed labor 660.0 ☑
    obstetric
      shock 669.1 ☑
      trauma NEC 665.9 ☑
    obstructed labor 660.9 ☑
      due to
        abnormality of pelvic organs or
          tissues (conditions classifi-
          able to 654.0–654.9)
          660.2 ☑
        deep transverse arrest 660.3 ☑
        impacted shoulders 660.4 ☑
        locked twins 660.5 ☑
        malposition and malpresentation
          of fetus (conditions classi-
          fiable to 652.0–652.9)
          660.0 ☑
        persistent occipitoposterior
          660.3 ☑
        shoulder dystocia 660.4 ☑
    occult prolapse of umbilical cord
      663.0 ☑
    oversize fetus 653.5 ☑
      causing obstructed labor 660.1 ☑
    pathological retraction ring, uterus
      661.4 ☑
    pelvic
      arrest (deep) (high) (of fetal head)
        (transverse) 660.3 ☑
      deformity (bone) (*see also* Deformity,
        pelvis, with disproportion)
      soft tissue 654.9 ☑
        causing obstructed labor
          660.2 ☑
      tumor NEC 654.9 ☑
        causing obstructed labor
          660.2 ☑
    penetration, pregnant uterus by instru-
      ment 665.1 ☑
    perforation — *see* Delivery, complicated,
      laceration
    persistent
      hymen 654.8 ☑
        causing obstructed labor
          660.2 ☑
      occipitoposterior 660.3 ☑

Delivery — *continued*
  complicated — *continued*
    placenta, placental
      ablatio 641.2 ☑
      abnormality 656.7 ☑
        with hemorrhage 641.2 ☑
      abruptio 641.2 ☑
      accreta 667.0 ☑
        with hemorrhage 666.0 ☑
      adherent (without hemorrhage)
        667.0 ☑
        with hemorrhage 666.0 ☑
      apoplexy 641.2 ☑
      battledore placenta — *see* Placenta,
        abnormal
      detachment (premature) 641.2 ☑
      disease 656.7 ☑
      hemorrhage NEC 641.9 ☑
      increta (without hemorrhage)
        667.0 ☑
        with hemorrhage 666.0 ☑
      low (implantation) 641.1 ☑
        without hemorrhage 641.0 ☑
      malformation 656.7 ☑
        with hemorrhage 641.2 ☑
      malposition 641.1 ☑
        without hemorrhage 641.0 ☑
      marginal sinus rupture 641.2 ☑
      percreta 667.0 ☑
        with hemorrhage 666.0 ☑
      premature separation 641.2 ☑
      previa (central) (lateral) (marginal)
        (partial) 641.1 ☑
        without hemorrhage 641.0 ☑
      retained (with hemorrhage) 666.0 ☑
        without hemorrhage 667.0 ☑
      rupture of marginal sinus 641.2 ☑
      separation (premature) 641.2 ☑
      trapped 666.0 ☑
        without hemorrhage 667.0 ☑
      vicious insertion 641.1 ☑
    polyhydramnios 657.0 ☑
    polyp, cervix 654.6 ☑
      causing obstructed labor 660.2 ☑
    precipitate labor 661.3 ☑
    premature
      labor (before 37 completed weeks
        gestation) 644.2 ☑
      rupture, membranes 658.1 ☑
        delayed delivery following
          658.2 ☑
    presenting umbilical cord 663.0 ☑
    previous
      cesarean delivery, section 654.2 ☑
      surgery
        cervix 654.6 ☑
          causing obstructed labor
            660.2 ☑
        gynecological NEC 654.9 ☑
          causing obstructed labor
            660.2 ☑
        perineum 654.8 ☑
        rectum 654.8 ☑
        uterus NEC 654.9 ☑
          due to previous cesarean de-
            livery, section 654.2 ☑
        vagina 654.7 ☑
          causing obstructed labor
            660.2 ☑
        vulva 654.8 ☑
    primary uterine inertia 661.0 ☑
    primipara, elderly or old 659.5 ☑
    prolapse
      arm or hand 652.7 ☑
        causing obstructed labor
          660.0 ☑
      cord (umbilical) 663.0 ☑
      fetal extremity 652.8 ☑
      foot or leg 652.8 ☑
        causing obstructed labor
          660.0 ☑
      umbilical cord (complete) (occult)
        (partial) 663.0 ☑
      uterus 654.4 ☑

Delivery — *continued*
  complicated — *continued*
    prolapse — *continued*
      uterus — *continued*
        causing obstructed labor
          660.2 ☑
    prolonged labor 662.1 ☑
      first stage 662.0 ☑
      second stage 662.2 ☑
      active phase 661.2 ☑
      due to
        cervical dystocia 661.2 ☑
        contraction ring 661.4 ☑
        tetanic uterus 661.4 ☑
        uterine inertia 661.2 ☑
          primary 661.0 ☑
          secondary 661.1 ☑
      latent phase 661.0 ☑
    pyrexia during labor 659.2 ☑
    rachitic pelvis 653.2 ☑
      causing obstructed labor 660.1 ☑
    rectocele 654.4 ☑
      causing obstructed labor 660.2 ☑
    retained membranes or portions of pla-
      centa 666.2 ☑
      without hemorrhage 667.1 ☑
    retarded (prolonged) birth 662.1 ☑
    retention secundines (with hemorrhage)
      666.2 ☑
      without hemorrhage 667.1 ☑
    retroversion, uterus or cervix 654.3 ☑
      causing obstructed labor 660.2 ☑
    rigid
      cervix 654.6 ☑
        causing obstructed labor
          660.2 ☑
      pelvic floor 654.4 ☑
        causing obstructed labor
          660.2 ☑
      perineum or vulva 654.8 ☑
        causing obstructed labor
          660.2 ☑
      vagina 654.7 ☑
        causing obstructed labor
          660.2 ☑
    Robert's pelvis 653.0 ☑
      causing obstructed labor 660.1 ☑
    rupture (*see also* Delivery, complicated,
      laceration)
      bladder (urinary) 665.5 ☑
      cervix 665.3 ☑
      marginal sinus 641.2 ☑
      membranes, premature 658.1 ☑
      pelvic organ NEC 665.5 ☑
      perineum (without mention of other
        laceration) — *see* Delivery,
        complicated, laceration, per-
        ineum
      peritoneum (pelvic) 665.5 ☑
      urethra 665.5 ☑
      uterus (during labor) 665.1 ☑
        before labor 665.0 ☑
    sacculation, pregnant uterus 654.4 ☑
    sacral teratomas, fetal 653.7 ☑
      causing obstructed labor 660.1 ☑
    scar(s)
      cervix 654.6 ☑
        causing obstructed labor
          660.2 ☑
      cesarean delivery, section 654.2 ☑
        causing obstructed labor
          660.2 ☑
      perineum 654.8 ☑
        causing obstructed labor
          660.2 ☑
      uterus NEC 654.9 ☑
        causing obstructed labor
          660.2 ☑
        due to previous cesarean delivery,
          section 654.2 ☑
      vagina 654.7 ☑
        causing obstructed labor
          660.2 ☑
      vulva 654.8 ☑

Delivery — continued
  complicated — continued
    scar(s) — continued
      vulva — continued
        causing obstructed labor
          660.2 ☑
    scoliotic pelvis 653.0 ☑
      causing obstructed labor 660.1 ☑
    secondary uterine inertia 661.1 ☑
    secundines, retained — see Delivery,
      complicated, placenta, retained
    separation
      placenta (premature) 641.2 ☑
      pubic bone 665.6 ☑
      symphysis pubis 665.6 ☑
    septate vagina 654.7 ☑
      causing obstructed labor 660.2 ☑
    shock (birth) (obstetric) (puerperal)
      669.1 ☑
    short cord syndrome 663.4 ☑
    shoulder
      girdle dystocia 660.4 ☑
      presentation 652.8 ☑
        causing obstructed labor
          660.0 ☑
    Siamese twins 678.1 ☑
    slow slope active phase 661.2 ☑
    spasm
      cervix 661.4 ☑
      uterus 661.4 ☑
    spondylolisthesis, pelvis 653.3 ☑
      causing obstructed labor 660.1 ☑
    spondylolysis (lumbosacral) 653.3 ☑
      causing obstructed labor 660.1 ☑
    spondylosis 653.0 ☑
      causing obstructed labor 660.1 ☑
    stenosis or stricture
      cervix 654.6 ☑
        causing obstructed labor
          660.2 ☑
      vagina 654.7 ☑
        causing obstructed labor
          660.2 ☑
    sudden death, unknown cause 669.9 ☑
    tear (pelvic organ) (see also Delivery,
      complicated, laceration) 664.9 ☑
      anal sphincter (healed) (old) 654.8 ☑
        not associated with third-degree
          perineal laceration
          664.6 ☑
    teratomas, sacral, fetal 653.7 ☑
      causing obstructed labor 660.1 ☑
    tetanic uterus 661.4 ☑
    tipping pelvis 653.0 ☑
      causing obstructed labor 660.1 ☑
    transverse
      arrest (deep) 660.3 ☑
      presentation or lie 652.3 ☑
        with successful version 652.1 ☑
        causing obstructed labor
          660.0 ☑
    trauma (obstetrical) NEC 665.9 ☑
      periurethral 664.8 ☑
    tumor
      abdominal, fetal 653.7 ☑
        causing obstructed labor
          660.1 ☑
      pelvic organs or tissues NEC 654.9 ☑
        causing obstructed labor
          660.2 ☑
    umbilical cord (see also Delivery, compli-
      cated, cord) 663.9 ☑
      around neck tightly, or with compres-
        sion 663.1 ☑
      entanglement NEC 663.3 ☑
        with compression 663.2 ☑
      prolapse (complete) (occult) (partial)
        663.0 ☑
    unstable lie 652.0 ☑
      causing obstructed labor 660.0 ☑
    uterine
      inertia (see also Delivery, complicat-
        ed, inertia, uterus) 661.2 ☑
      spasm 661.4 ☑

Delivery — continued
  complicated — continued
    vasa previa 663.5 ☑
    velamentous insertion of cord 663.8 ☑
    young maternal age 659.8 ☑
  delayed NEC 662.1 ☑
    following rupture of membranes (spon-
      taneous) 658.2 ☑
    artificial 658.3 ☑
    second twin, triplet, etc. 662.3 ☑
  difficult NEC 669.9 ☑
    previous, affecting management of
      pregnancy or childbirth V23.49
    specified type NEC 669.8 ☑
  early onset (spontaneous) 644.2 ☑
  footling 652.8 ☑
    with successful version 652.1 ☑
  forceps NEC 669.5 ☑
    affecting fetus or newborn 763.2
  missed (at or near term) 656.4 ☑
  multiple gestation NEC 651.9 ☑
    with fetal loss and retention of one or
      more fetus(es) 651.6 ☑
    following (elective) fetal reduction
      651.7 ☑
    specified type NEC 651.8 ☑
      with fetal loss and retention of one
        or more fetus(es) 651.6 ☑
      following (elective) fetal reduction
        651.7 ☑
  nonviable infant 656.4 ☑
  normal — see category 650
  precipitate 661.3 ☑
    affecting fetus or newborn 763.6
  premature NEC (before 37 completed weeks
    gestation) 644.2 ☑
    previous, affecting management of
      pregnancy V23.41
  quadruplet NEC 651.2 ☑
    with fetal loss and retention of one or
      more fetus(es) 651.5 ☑
    following (elective) fetal reduction
      651.7 ☑
  quintuplet NEC 651.8 ☑
    with fetal loss and retention of one or
      more fetus(es) 651.6 ☑
    following (elective) fetal reduction
      651.7 ☑
  sextuplet NEC 651.8 ☑
    with fetal loss and retention of one or
      more fetus(es) 651.6 ☑
    following (elective) fetal reduction
      651.7 ☑
  specified complication NEC 669.8 ☑
  stillbirth (near term) NEC 656.4 ☑
    early (before 22 completed weeks gesta-
      tion) 632
  term pregnancy (live birth) NEC — see cate-
    gory 650
    stillbirth NEC 656.4 ☑
  threatened premature 644.2 ☑
  triplets NEC 651.1 ☑
    with fetal loss and retention of one or
      more fetus(es) 651.4 ☑
    delayed delivery (one or more mates)
      662.3 ☑
    following (elective) fetal reduction
      651.7 ☑
    locked mates 660.5 ☑
  twins NEC 651.0 ☑
    with fetal loss and retention of one fetus
      651.3 ☑
    delayed delivery (one or more mates)
      662.3 ☑
    following (elective) fetal reduction
      651.7 ☑
    locked mates 660.5 ☑
  uncomplicated — see category 650
  vacuum extractor NEC 669.5 ☑
    affecting fetus or newborn 763.3
  ventouse NEC 669.5 ☑
    affecting fetus or newborn 763.3
Dellen, cornea 371.41
Delusions (paranoid) 297.9

Delusions — continued
  grandiose 297.1
  parasitosis 300.29
  systematized 297.1
Dementia 294.20
  with behavioral disturbance (aggressive)
    (combative) (violent) 294.21
  alcohol-induced persisting (see also Psy-
    chosis, alcoholic) 291.2
  Alzheimer's — see Alzheimer's, dementia
  arteriosclerotic (simple type) (uncomplicat-
    ed) 290.40
    with
      acute confusional state 290.41
      delirium 290.41
      delusions 290.42
      depressed mood 290.43
    depressed type 290.43
    paranoid type 290.42
  Binswanger's 290.12
  catatonic (acute) (see also Schizophrenia)
    295.2 ☑
  congenital (see also Disability, intellectual)
    319
  degenerative 290.9
    presenile-onset — see Dementia, prese-
      nile
    senile-onset — see Dementia, senile
  developmental (see also Schizophrenia)
    295.9 ☑
  dialysis 294.8
    transient 293.9
  drug-induced persisting (see also Psychosis,
    drug) 292.82
  due to or associated with condition(s) clas-
    sified elsewhere
    Alzheimer's
      with behavioral disturbance
        331.0 [294.11]
      without behavioral disturbance
        331.0 [294.10]
    cerebral lipidoses
      with behavioral disturbance
        330.1 [294.11]
      without behavioral disturbance
        330.1 [294.10]
    epilepsy
      with behavioral disturbance
        345.9 ☑ [294.11]
      without behavioral disturbance
        345.9 ☑ [294.10]
    hepatolenticular degeneration
      with behavioral disturbance
        275.1 [294.11]
      without behavioral disturbance
        275.1 [294.10]
    HIV
      with behavioral disturbance
        042 [294.11]
      without behavioral disturbance
        042 [294.10]
    Huntington's chorea
      with behavioral disturbance
        333.4 [294.11]
      without behavioral disturbance
        333.4 [294.10]
    Jakob-Creutzfeldt disease (CJD)
      with behavioral disturbance
        046.19 [294.11]
      without behavioral disturbance
        046.19 [294.10]
      variant (vCJD) 046.11
        with dementia
          with behavioral disturbance
            046.11 [294.11]
          without behavioral disbur-
            bance 046.11 [294.10]
    Lewy bodies
      with behavioral disturbance
        331.82 [294.11]
      without behavioral disturbance
        331.82 [294.10]
    multiple sclerosis
      with behavioral disturbance
        340 [294.11]

Dementia — continued
  due to or associated with condition(s) classi-
    fied elsewhere — continued
    multiple sclerosis — continued
      without behavioral disturbance
        340 [294.10]
    neurosyphilis
      with behavioral disturbance
        094.9 [294.11]
      without behavioral disturbance
        094.9 [294.10]
    Parkinsonism
      with behavioral disturbance
        331.82 [294.11]
      without behavioral disturbance
        331.82 [294.10]
    Parkinson's disease
      with behavioral disturbance
        332.0 [294.11]
      without behavioral disturbance
        332.0 [294.10]
    Pelizaeus-Merzbacher disease
      with behavioral disturbance
        333.0 [294.11]
      without behavioral disturbance
        333.0 [294.10]
    Pick's disease
      with behavioral disturbance
        331.11 [294.11]
      without behavioral disturbance
        331.11 [294.10]
    polyarteritis nodosa
      with behavioral disturbance
        446.0 [294.11]
      without behavioral disturbance
        446.0 [294.10]
    syphilis
      with behavioral disturbance
        094.1 [294.11]
      without behavioral disturbance
        094.1 [294.10]
    Wilson's disease
      with behavioral disturbance
        275.1 [294.11]
      without behavioral disturbance
        275.1 [294.10]
  frontal 331.19
    with behavioral disturbance
      331.19 [294.11]
    without behavioral disturbance
      331.19 [294.10]
  frontotemporal 331.19
    with behavioral disturbance
      331.19 [294.11]
    without behavioral disturbance
      331.19 [294.10]
  hebephrenic (acute) 295.1 ☑
  Heller's (infantile psychosis) (see also Psy-
    chosis, childhood) 299.1 ☑
  idiopathic 290.9
    presenile-onset — see Dementia, prese-
      nile
    senile-onset — see Dementia, senile
  in
    arteriosclerotic brain disease 290.40
    senility 290.0
  induced by drug 292.82
  infantile, infantilia (see also Psychosis,
    childhood) 299.0 ☑
  Lewy body 331.82
    with behavioral disturbance
      331.82 [294.11]
    without behavioral disturbance
      331.82 [294.10]
  multi-infarct (cerebrovascular) (see also De-
    mentia, arteriosclerotic) 290.40
  old age 290.0
  paralytica, paralytic 094.1
    juvenilis 090.40
    syphilitic 094.1
      congenital 090.40
    tabetic form 094.1
  paranoid (see also Schizophrenia) 295.3 ☑
  paraphrenic (see also Schizophrenia)
    295.3 ☑
  paretic 094.1

Dementia — continued
  praecox (see also Schizophrenia) 295.9 ☑
  presenile 290.10
    with
      acute confusional state 290.11
      delirium 290.11
      delusional features 290.12
      depressive features 290.13
    depressed type 290.13
    paranoid type 290.12
    simple type 290.10
    uncomplicated 290.10
  primary (acute) (see also Schizophrenia)
      295.0 ☑
  progressive, syphilitic 094.1
  puerperal — see Psychosis, puerperal
  schizophrenic (see also Schizophrenia)
      295.9 ☑
  senile 290.0
    with
      acute confusional state 290.3
      delirium 290.3
      delusional features 290.20
      depressive features 290.21
    depressed type 290.21
    exhaustion 290.0
    paranoid type 290.20
  simple type (acute) (see also Schizophrenia)
      295.0 ☑
  simplex (acute) (see also Schizophrenia)
      295.0 ☑
  syphilitic 094.1
  uremic — see Uremia
  vascular 290.40
    with
      delirium 290.41
      delusions 290.42
      depressed mood 290.43
Demerol dependence — see also Dependence
      304.0 ☑
Demineralization, ankle — see also Osteo-
      porosis 733.00
Demodex folliculorum (infestation) 133.8
Demoralization 799.25
de Morgan's spots (senile angiomas) 448.1
Demyelinating
  polyneuritis, chronic inflammatory 357.81
Demyelination, demyelinization
  central nervous system 341.9
      specified NEC 341.8
  corpus callosum (central) 341.8
  global 340
Dengue (fever) 061
  sandfly 061
  vaccination, prophylactic (against) V05.1
  virus hemorrhagic fever 065.4
Dens
  evaginatus 520.2
  in dente 520.2
  invaginatus 520.2
Dense
  breast(s) 793.82
Density
  increased, bone (disseminated) (general-
      ized) (spotted) 733.99
  lung (nodular) 518.89
Dental — see also condition
  examination only V72.2
Dentia praecox 520.6
Denticles (in pulp) 522.2
Dentigerous cyst 526.0
Dentin
  irregular (in pulp) 522.3
  opalescent 520.5
  secondary (in pulp) 522.3
  sensitive 521.89
Dentinogenesis imperfecta 520.5
Dentinoma (M9271/0) 213.1
  upper jaw (bone) 213.0
Dentition 520.7
  abnormal 520.6
  anomaly 520.6
  delayed 520.6
  difficult 520.7
  disorder of 520.6
  precocious 520.6

Dentition — continued
  retarded 520.6
Denture sore (mouth) 528.9
Dependence

Note — Use the following fifth-digit
subclassification with category 304:

0   unspecified
1   continuous
2   episodic
3   in remission

  with
    withdrawal symptoms
      alcohol 291.81
      drug 292.0
  14-hydroxy-dihydromorphinone 304.0 ☑
  absinthe 304.6 ☑
  acemorphan 304.0 ☑
  acetanilid(e) 304.6 ☑
  acetophenetidin 304.6 ☑
  acetorphine 304.0 ☑
  acetyldihydrocodeine 304.0 ☑
  acetyldihydrocodeinone 304.0 ☑
  Adalin 304.1 ☑
  Afghanistan black 304.3 ☑
  agrypnal 304.1 ☑
  alcohol, alcoholic (ethyl) (methyl) (wood)
      303.9 ☑
    maternal, with suspected fetal damage
        affecting management of preg-
        nancy 655.4 ☑
  allobarbitone 304.1 ☑
  allonal 304.1 ☑
  allylisopropylacetylurea 304.1 ☑
  alphaprodine (hydrochloride) 304.0 ☑
  Alurate 304.1 ☑
  Alvodine 304.0 ☑
  amethocaine 304.6 ☑
  amidone 304.0 ☑
  amidopyrine 304.6 ☑
  aminopyrine 304.6 ☑
  amobarbital 304.1 ☑
  amphetamine(s) (type) (drugs classifiable
      to 969.7) 304.4 ☑
  amylene hydrate 304.6 ☑
  amylobarbitone 304.1 ☑
  amylocaine 304.6 ☑
  Amytal (sodium) 304.1 ☑
  analgesic (drug) NEC 304.6 ☑
    synthetic with morphine-like effect
        304.0 ☑
  anesthetic (agent) (drug) (gas) (general)
      (local) NEC 304.6 ☑
  Angel dust 304.6 ☑
  anileridine 304.0 ☑
  antipyrine 304.6 ☑
  anxiolytic 304.1 ☑
  aprobarbital 304.1 ☑
  aprobarbitone 304.1 ☑
  atropine 304.0 ☑
  Avertin (bromide) 304.6 ☑
  barbenyl 304.1 ☑
  barbital(s) 304.1 ☑
  barbitone 304.1 ☑
  barbiturate(s) (compounds) (drugs classifi-
      able to 967.0) 304.1 ☑
  barbituric acid (and compounds) 304.1 ☑
  benzedrine 304.4 ☑
  benzylmorphine 304.0 ☑
  Beta-chlor 304.1 ☑
  bhang 304.3 ☑
  blue velvet 304.0 ☑
  Brevital 304.1 ☑
  bromal (hydrate) 304.1 ☑
  bromide(s) NEC 304.1 ☑
  bromine compounds NEC 304.1 ☑
  bromisovalum 304.1 ☑
  bromoform 304.1 ☑
  Bromo-seltzer 304.1 ☑
  bromural 304.1 ☑
  butabarbital (sodium) 304.1 ☑
  butabarpal 304.1 ☑

Dependence — continued
  butallylonal 304.1 ☑
  butethal 304.1 ☑
  buthalitone (sodium) 304.1 ☑
  Butisol 304.1 ☑
  butobarbitone 304.1 ☑
  butyl chloral (hydrate) 304.1 ☑
  caffeine 304.4 ☑
  cannabis (indica) (sativa) (resin) (derivatives)
      (type) 304.3 ☑
  carbamazepine 304.6 ☑
  Carbrital 304.1 ☑
  carbromal 304.1 ☑
  carisoprodol 304.6 ☑
  Catha (edulis) 304.4 ☑
  chloral (betaine) (hydrate) 304.1 ☑
  chloralamide 304.1 ☑
  chloralformamide 304.1 ☑
  chloralose 304.1 ☑
  chlordiazepoxide 304.1 ☑
  Chloretone 304.1 ☑
  chlorobutanol 304.1 ☑
  chlorodyne 304.1 ☑
  chloroform 304.6 ☑
  Cliradon 304.0 ☑
  coca (leaf) and derivatives 304.2 ☑
  cocaine 304.2 ☑
    hydrochloride 304.2 ☑
    salt (any) 304.2 ☑
  codeine 304.0 ☑
  combination of drugs (excluding morphine
      or opioid type drug) NEC 304.8 ☑
    morphine or opioid type drug with any
        other drug 304.7 ☑
  croton-chloral 304.1 ☑
  cyclobarbital 304.1 ☑
  cyclobarbitone 304.1 ☑
  dagga 304.3 ☑
  Delvinal 304.1 ☑
  Demerol 304.0 ☑
  desocodeine 304.0 ☑
  desomorphine 304.0 ☑
  desoxyephedrine 304.4 ☑
  DET 304.5 ☑
  dexamphetamine 304.4 ☑
  dexedrine 304.4 ☑
  dextromethorphan 304.0 ☑
  dextromoramide 304.0 ☑
  dextronorpseudoephedrine 304.4 ☑
  dextrorphan 304.0 ☑
  diacetylmorphine 304.0 ☑
  Dial 304.1 ☑
  diallylbarbituric acid 304.1 ☑
  diamorphine 304.0 ☑
  diazepam 304.1 ☑
  dibucaine 304.6 ☑
  dichloroethane 304.6 ☑
  diethyl barbituric acid 304.1 ☑
  diethylsulfone-diethylmethane 304.1 ☑
  difencloxazine 304.0 ☑
  dihydrocodeine 304.0 ☑
  dihydrocodeinone 304.0 ☑
  dihydrohydroxycodeinone 304.0 ☑
  dihydroisocodeine 304.0 ☑
  dihydromorphine 304.0 ☑
  dihydromorphinone 304.0 ☑
  dihydroxycodeinone 304.0 ☑
  Dilaudid 304.0 ☑
  dimenhydrinate 304.6 ☑
  dimethylmeperidine 304.0 ☑
  dimethyltriptamine 304.5 ☑
  Dionin 304.0 ☑
  diphenoxylate 304.6 ☑
  dipipanone 304.0 ☑
  d-lysergic acid diethylamide 304.5 ☑
  DMT 304.5 ☑
  Dolophine 304.0 ☑
  DOM 304.2 ☑
  Doriden 304.1 ☑
  dormiral 304.1 ☑
  Dormison 304.1 ☑
  Dromoran 304.0 ☑
  drug NEC 304.9 ☑

Dependence — continued
  drug — continued
    analgesic NEC 304.6 ☑
    combination (excluding morphine or
        opioid type drug) NEC 304.8 ☑
      morphine or opioid type drug with
          any other drug 304.7 ☑
    complicating pregnancy, childbirth, or
        puerperium 648.3 ☑
      affecting fetus or newborn 779.5
    hallucinogenic 304.5 ☑
    hypnotic NEC 304.1 ☑
    narcotic NEC 304.9 ☑
    psychostimulant NEC 304.4 ☑
    sedative 304.1 ☑
    soporific NEC 304.1 ☑
    specified type NEC 304.6 ☑
    suspected damage to fetus affecting
        management of pregnancy
        655.5 ☑
    synthetic, with morphine-like effect
        304.0 ☑
    tranquilizing 304.1 ☑
  duboisine 304.6 ☑
  ectylurea 304.1 ☑
  Endocaine 304.6 ☑
  Equanil 304.1 ☑
  Eskabarb 304.1 ☑
  ethchlorvynol 304.1 ☑
  ether (ethyl) (liquid) (vapor) (vinyl) 304.6 ☑
  ethidene 304.6 ☑
  ethinamate 304.1 ☑
  ethoheptazine 304.6 ☑
  ethyl
    alcohol 303.9 ☑
    bromide 304.6 ☑
    carbamate 304.6 ☑
    chloride 304.6 ☑
    morphine 304.0 ☑
  ethylene (gas) 304.6 ☑
    dichloride 304.6 ☑
  ethylidene chloride 304.6 ☑
  etilfen 304.1 ☑
  etorphine 304.0 ☑
  etoval 304.1 ☑
  eucodal 304.0 ☑
  euneryl 304.1 ☑
  Evipal 304.1 ☑
  Evipan 304.1 ☑
  fentanyl 304.0 ☑
  ganja 304.3 ☑
  gardenal 304.1 ☑
  gardenpanyl 304.1 ☑
  gelsemine 304.6 ☑
  Gelsemium 304.6 ☑
  Gemonil 304.1 ☑
  glucochloral 304.1 ☑
  glue (airplane) (sniffing) 304.6 ☑
  glutethimide 304.1 ☑
  hallucinogenics 304.5 ☑
  hashish 304.3 ☑
  headache powder NEC 304.6 ☑
  Heavenly Blue 304.5 ☑
  hedonal 304.1 ☑
  hemp 304.3 ☑
  heptabarbital 304.1 ☑
  Heptalgin 304.0 ☑
  heptobarbitone 304.1 ☑
  heroin 304.0 ☑
    salt (any) 304.0 ☑
  hexethal (sodium) 304.1 ☑
  hexobarbital 304.1 ☑
  Hycodan 304.0 ☑
  hydrocodone 304.0 ☑
  hydromorphinol 304.0 ☑
  hydromorphinone 304.0 ☑
  hydromorphone 304.0 ☑
  hydroxycodeine 304.0 ☑
  hypnotic NEC 304.1 ☑
  Indian hemp 304.3 ☑
  inhalant 304.6 ☑
  intranarcon 304.1 ☑
  Kemithal 304.1 ☑

☑ Additional Digit Required — Refer to the Tabular List for Digit Selection   ⅏ Subterms under main terms may continue to next column or page

74 — Volume 2   ▶◀ Revised Text   ● New Line   ▲ Revised Code   2013 ICD-9-CM

Dependence — *continued*
- ketobemidone 304.0 ☑
- khat 304.4 ☑
- kif 304.3 ☑
- Lactuca (virosa) extract 304.1 ☑
- lactucarium 304.1 ☑
- laudanum 304.0 ☑
- Lebanese red 304.3 ☑
- Leritine 304.0 ☑
- lettuce opium 304.1 ☑
- Levanil 304.1 ☑
- Levo-Dromoran 304.0 ☑
- levo-iso-methadone 304.0 ☑
- levorphanol 304.0 ☑
- Librium 304.1 ☑
- Lomotil 304.6 ☑
- Lotusate 304.1 ☑
- LSD (-25) (and derivatives) 304.5 ☑
- Luminal 304.1 ☑
- lysergic acid 304.5 ☑
  - amide 304.5 ☑
- maconha 304.3 ☑
- magic mushroom 304.5 ☑
- marihuana 304.3 ☑
- MDA (methylene dioxyamphetamine) 304.4 ☑
- Mebaral 304.1 ☑
- Medinal 304.1 ☑
- Medomin 304.1 ☑
- megahallucinogenics 304.5 ☑
- meperidine 304.0 ☑
- mephobarbital 304.1 ☑
- meprobamate 304.1 ☑
- mescaline 304.5 ☑
- methadone 304.0 ☑
- methamphetamine(s) 304.4 ☑
- methaqualone 304.1 ☑
- metharbital 304.1 ☑
- methitural 304.1 ☑
- methobarbitone 304.1 ☑
- methohexital 304.1 ☑
- methopholine 304.6 ☑
- methyl
  - alcohol 303.9 ☑
  - bromide 304.6 ☑
  - morphine 304.0 ☑
  - sulfonal 304.1 ☑
- methylaparafynol 304.1 ☑
- methylated spirit 303.9 ☑
- methylbutinol 304.6 ☑
- methyldihydromorphinone 304.0 ☑
- methylene
  - chloride 304.6 ☑
  - dichloride 304.6 ☑
  - dioxyamphetamine (MDA) 304.4 ☑
- methylphenidate 304.4 ☑
- methyprylone 304.1 ☑
- metopon 304.0 ☑
- Miltown 304.1 ☑
- morning glory seeds 304.5 ☑
- morphinan(s) 304.0 ☑
- morphine (sulfate) (sulfite) (type) (drugs classifiable to 965.00–965.09) 304.0 ☑
- morphine or opioid type drug (drugs classifiable to 965.00–965.09) with any other drug 304.7 ☑
- morphinol(s) 304.0 ☑
- morphinon 304.0 ☑
- morpholinylethylmorphine 304.0 ☑
- mylomide 304.1 ☑
- myristicin 304.5 ☑
- narcotic (drug) NEC 304.9 ☑
- nealbarbital 304.1 ☑
- nealbarbitone 304.1 ☑
- Nembutal 304.1 ☑
- Neonal 304.1 ☑
- Neraval 304.1 ☑
- Neravan 304.1 ☑
- neurobarb 304.1 ☑
- nicotine 305.1
- Nisentil 304.0 ☑
- nitrous oxide 304.6 ☑

Dependence — *continued*
- Noctec 304.1 ☑
- Noludar 304.1 ☑
- nonbarbiturate sedatives and tranquilizers with similar effect 304.1 ☑
- noptil 304.1 ☑
- normorphine 304.0 ☑
- noscapine 304.0 ☑
- Novocaine 304.6 ☑
- Numorphan 304.0 ☑
- nunol 304.1 ☑
- Nupercaine 304.6 ☑
- Oblivon 304.1 ☑
- on
  - aspirator V46.0
  - hemodialysis V45.11
  - hyperbaric chamber V46.8
  - iron lung V46.11
  - machine (enabling) V46.9
    - specified type NEC V46.8
  - peritoneal dialysis V45.11
  - Possum (Patient-Operated-Selector-Mechanism) V46.8
  - renal dialysis machine V45.11
  - respirator [ventilator] V46.11
    - encounter
      - during
        - mechanical failure V46.14
        - power failure V46.12
      - for weaning V46.13
  - supplemental oxygen V46.2
  - wheelchair V46.3
- opiate 304.0 ☑
- opioids 304.0 ☑
- opioid type drug 304.0 ☑
  - with any other drug 304.7 ☑
- opium (alkaloids) (derivatives) (tincture) 304.0 ☑
- ortal 304.1 ☑
- Oxazepam 304.1 ☑
- oxycodone 304.0 ☑
- oxymorphone 304.0 ☑
- Palfium 304.0 ☑
- Panadol 304.6 ☑
- pantopium 304.0 ☑
- pantopon 304.0 ☑
- papaverine 304.0 ☑
- paracetamol 304.6 ☑
- paracodin 304.0 ☑
- paraldehyde 304.1 ☑
- paregoric 304.0 ☑
- Parzone 304.0 ☑
- PCP (phencyclidine) 304.6 ☑
- Pearly Gates 304.5 ☑
- pentazocine 304.0 ☑
- pentobarbital 304.1 ☑
- pentobarbitone (sodium) 304.1 ☑
- Pentothal 304.1 ☑
- Percaine 304.6 ☑
- Percodan 304.0 ☑
- Perichlor 304.1 ☑
- Pernocton 304.1 ☑
- Pernoston 304.1 ☑
- peronine 304.0 ☑
- pethidine (hydrochloride) 304.0 ☑
- petrichloral 304.1 ☑
- peyote 304.5 ☑
- Phanodron 304.1 ☑
- phenacetin 304.6 ☑
- phenadoxone 304.0 ☑
- phenaglycodol 304.1 ☑
- phenazocine 304.0 ☑
- phencyclidine 304.6 ☑
- phenmetrazine 304.4 ☑
- phenobal 304.1 ☑
- phenobarbital 304.1 ☑
- phenobarbitone 304.1 ☑
- phenomorphan 304.0 ☑
- phenonyl 304.1 ☑
- phenoperidine 304.0 ☑
- pholcodine 304.0 ☑
- piminodine 304.0 ☑
- Pipadone 304.0 ☑
- Pitkin's solution 304.6 ☑

Dependence — *continued*
- Placidyl 304.1 ☑
- polysubstance 304.8 ☑
- Pontocaine 304.6 ☑
- pot 304.3 ☑
- potassium bromide 304.1 ☑
- Preludin 304.4 ☑
- Prinadol 304.0 ☑
- probarbital 304.1 ☑
- procaine 304.6 ☑
- propanal 304.1 ☑
- propoxyphene 304.6 ☑
- psilocibin 304.5 ☑
- psilocin 304.5 ☑
- psilocybin 304.5 ☑
- psilocyline 304.5 ☑
- psilocyn 304.5 ☑
- psychedelic agents 304.5 ☑
- psychostimulant NEC 304.4 ☑
- psychotomimetic agents 304.5 ☑
- pyrahexyl 304.3 ☑
- Pyramidon 304.6 ☑
- quinalbarbitone 304.1 ☑
- racemoramide 304.0 ☑
- racemorphan 304.0 ☑
- Rela 304.6 ☑
- scopolamine 304.6 ☑
- secobarbital 304.1 ☑
- Seconal 304.1 ☑
- sedative NEC 304.1 ☑
  - nonbarbiturate with barbiturate effect 304.1 ☑
- Sedormid 304.1 ☑
- sernyl 304.1 ☑
- sodium bromide 304.1 ☑
- Soma 304.6 ☑
- Somnal 304.1 ☑
- Somnos 304.1 ☑
- Soneryl 304.1 ☑
- soporific (drug) NEC 304.1 ☑
- specified drug NEC 304.6 ☑
- speed 304.4 ☑
- spinocaine 304.6 ☑
- Stovaine 304.6 ☑
- STP 304.5 ☑
- stramonium 304.6 ☑
- Sulfonal 304.1 ☑
- sulfonethylmethane 304.1 ☑
- sulfonmethane 304.1 ☑
- Surital 304.1 ☑
- synthetic drug with morphine-like effect 304.0 ☑
- talbutal 304.1 ☑
- tetracaine 304.6 ☑
- tetrahydrocannabinol 304.3 ☑
- tetronal 304.1 ☑
- THC 304.3 ☑
- thebacon 304.0 ☑
- thebaine 304.0 ☑
- thiamil 304.1 ☑
- thiamylal 304.1 ☑
- thiopental 304.1 ☑
- tobacco 305.1
- toluene, toluol 304.6 ☑
- tranquilizer NEC 304.1 ☑
  - nonbarbiturate with barbiturate effect 304.1 ☑
- tribromacetaldehyde 304.6 ☑
- tribromethanol 304.6 ☑
- tribromomethane 304.6 ☑
- trichloroethanol 304.6 ☑
- trichoroethyl phosphate 304.1 ☑
- triclofos 304.1 ☑
- Trional 304.1 ☑
- Tuinal 304.1 ☑
- Turkish Green 304.3 ☑
- urethan(e) 304.6 ☑
- Valium 304.1 ☑
- Valmid 304.1 ☑
- veganin 304.0 ☑
- veramon 304.1 ☑
- Veronal 304.1 ☑
- versidyne 304.6 ☑

Dependence — *continued*
- vinbarbital 304.1 ☑
- vinbarbitone 304.1 ☑
- vinyl bitone 304.1 ☑
- vitamin B₆ 266.1
- wine 303.9 ☑
- Zactane 304.6 ☑

Dependency
- passive 301.6
- reactions 301.6

Depersonalization (episode, in neurotic state) (neurotic) (syndrome) 300.6

Depletion
- carbohydrates 271.9
- complement factor 279.8
- extracellular fluid 276.52
- plasma 276.52
- potassium 276.8
  - nephropathy 588.89
- salt or sodium 276.1
  - causing heat exhaustion or prostration 992.4
  - nephropathy 593.9
- volume 276.50
  - extracellular fluid 276.52
  - plasma 276.52

Deployment (military)
- personal history of V62.22
- returned from V62.22
- status V62.21

Deposit
- argentous, cornea 371.16
- bone, in Boeck's sarcoid 135
- calcareous, calcium — *see* Calcification
- cholesterol
  - retina 362.82
  - skin 709.3
  - vitreous (humor) 379.22
- conjunctival 372.56
- cornea, corneal NEC 371.10
  - argentous 371.16
  - in
    - cystinosis 270.0 *[371.15]*
    - mucopolysaccharidosis 277.5 *[371.15]*
- crystalline, vitreous (humor) 379.22
- hemosiderin, in old scars of cornea 371.11
- metallic, in lens 366.45
- skin 709.3
- teeth, tooth (betel) (black) (green) (materia alba) (orange) (soft) (tobacco) 523.6
- urate, in kidney (*see also* Disease, renal) 593.9

Depraved appetite 307.52

Depression 311
- acute (*see also* Psychosis, affective) 296.2 ☑
  - recurrent episode 296.3 ☑
  - single episode 296.2 ☑
- agitated (*see also* Psychosis, affective) 296.2 ☑
  - recurrent episode 296.3 ☑
  - single episode 296.2 ☑
- anaclitic 309.21
- anxiety 300.4
- arches 734
  - congenital 754.61
- autogenous (*see also* Psychosis, affective) 296.2 ☑
  - recurrent episode 296.3 ☑
  - single episode 296.2 ☑
- basal metabolic rate (BMR) 794.7
- bone marrow 289.9
- central nervous system 799.1
  - newborn 779.2
- cerebral 331.9
  - newborn 779.2
- cerebrovascular 437.8
  - newborn 779.2
- chest wall 738.3
- endogenous (*see also* Psychosis, affective) 296.2 ☑
  - recurrent episode 296.3 ☑
  - single episode 296.2 ☑
- functional activity 780.99
- hysterical 300.11

☑ **Additional Digit Required — Refer to the Tabular List for Digit Selection**   ▽ **Subterms under main terms may continue to next column or page**

2013 ICD-9-CM   ▶◀ Revised Text   ● New Line   ▲ Revised Code   **Volume 2 — 75**

Depression — *continued*
  involutional, climacteric, or menopausal (*see also* Psychosis, affective) 296.2 ☑
    recurrent episode 296.3 ☑
    single episode 296.2 ☑
  major 296.2 ☑
    recurrent episode 296.3 ☑
    single episode 296.2 ☑
  manic (*see also* Psychosis, affective) 296.80
  medullary 348.89
    newborn 779.2
  mental 300.4
  metatarsal heads — *see* Depression, arches
  metatarsus — *see* Depression, arches
  monopolar (*see also* Psychosis, affective) 296.2 ☑
    recurrent episode 296.3 ☑
    single episode 296.2 ☑
  nervous 300.4
  neurotic 300.4
  nose 738.0
  postpartum 648.4 ☑
  psychogenic 300.4
    reactive 298.0
  psychoneurotic 300.4
  psychotic (*see also* Psychosis, affective) 296.2 ☑
    reactive 298.0
    recurrent episode 296.3 ☑
    single episode 296.2 ☑
  reactive 300.4
    neurotic 300.4
    psychogenic 298.0
    psychoneurotic 300.4
    psychotic 298.0
  recurrent 296.3 ☑
  respiratory center 348.89
    newborn 770.89
  scapula 736.89
  senile 290.21
  situational (acute) (brief) 309.0
    prolonged 309.1
  skull 754.0
  sternum 738.3
  visual field 368.40
Depressive reaction — *see also* Reaction, depressive
  acute (transient) 309.0
    with anxiety 309.28
  prolonged 309.1
  situational (acute) 309.0
    prolonged 309.1
Deprivation
  cultural V62.4
  emotional V62.89
    affecting
      adult 995.82
      infant or child 995.51
  food 994.2
    specific substance NEC 269.8
  protein (familial) (kwashiorkor) 260
  sleep V69.4
  social V62.4
    affecting
      adult 995.82
      infant or child 995.51
  symptoms, syndrome
    alcohol 291.81
    drug 292.0
  vitamins (*see also* Deficiency, vitamin) 269.2
  water 994.3
de Quervain's
  disease (tendon sheath) 727.04
  syndrome 259.51
  thyroiditis (subacute granulomatous thyroiditis) 245.1
Derangement
  ankle (internal) 718.97
    current injury (*see also* Dislocation, ankle) 837.0
    recurrent 718.37
  cartilage (articular) NEC (*see also* Disorder, cartilage, articular) 718.0 ☑
    knee 717.9
      recurrent 718.36
    recurrent 718.3 ☑

Derangement — *continued*
  collateral ligament (knee) (medial) (tibial) 717.82
    current injury 844.1
      lateral (fibular) 844.0
    lateral (fibular) 717.81
      current injury 844.0
  cruciate ligament (knee) (posterior) 717.84
    anterior 717.83
      current injury 844.2
    current injury 844.2
  elbow (internal) 718.92
    current injury (*see also* Dislocation, elbow) 832.00
    recurrent 718.32
  gastrointestinal 536.9
  heart — *see* Disease, heart
  hip (joint) (internal) (old) 718.95
    current injury (*see also* Dislocation, hip) 835.00
    recurrent 718.35
  intervertebral disc — *see* Displacement, intervertebral disc
  joint (internal) 718.90
    ankle 718.97
    current injury (*see also* Dislocation, by site)
      knee, meniscus or cartilage (*see also* Tear, meniscus) 836.2
    elbow 718.92
    foot 718.97
    hand 718.94
    hip 718.95
    knee 717.9
    multiple sites 718.99
    pelvic region 718.95
    recurrent 718.30
      ankle 718.37
      elbow 718.32
      foot 718.37
      hand 718.34
      hip 718.35
      knee 718.36
      multiple sites 718.39
      pelvic region 718.35
      shoulder (region) 718.31
      specified site NEC 718.38
      temporomandibular (old) 524.69
      wrist 718.33
    shoulder (region) 718.91
    specified site NEC 718.98
    spine NEC 724.9
    temporomandibular 524.69
    wrist 718.93
  knee (cartilage) (internal) 717.9
    current injury (*see also* Tear, meniscus) 836.2
    ligament 717.89
      capsular 717.85
      collateral — *see* Derangement, collateral ligament
      cruciate — *see* Derangement, cruciate ligament
      specified NEC 717.85
    recurrent 718.36
  low back NEC 724.9
  meniscus NEC (knee) 717.5
    current injury (*see also* Tear, meniscus) 836.2
    lateral 717.40
      anterior horn 717.42
      posterior horn 717.43
      specified NEC 717.49
    medial 717.3
      anterior horn 717.1
      posterior horn 717.2
    recurrent 718.3 ☑
    site other than knee — *see* Disorder, cartilage, articular
  mental (*see also* Psychosis) 298.9
  rotator cuff (recurrent) (tear) 726.10
    current 840.4
  sacroiliac (old) 724.6
    current — *see* Dislocation, sacroiliac
  semilunar cartilage (knee) 717.5
    current injury 836.2

Derangement — *continued*
  semilunar cartilage — *continued*
    current injury — *continued*
      lateral 836.1
      medial 836.0
    recurrent 718.3 ☑
  shoulder (internal) 718.91
    current injury (*see also* Dislocation, shoulder) 831.00
    recurrent 718.31
  spine (recurrent) NEC 724.9
    current — *see* Dislocation, spine
  temporomandibular (internal) (joint) (old) 524.69
    current — *see* Dislocation, jaw
Dercum's disease or syndrome (adiposis dolorosa) 272.8
Derealization (neurotic) 300.6
Dermal — *see* condition
Dermaphytid — *see* Dermatophytosis
Dermatergosis — *see* Dermatitis
Dermatitis (allergic) (contact) (occupational) (venenata) 692.9
  ab igne 692.82
  acneiform 692.9
  actinic (due to sun) 692.70
    acute 692.72
    chronic NEC 692.74
    other than from sun NEC 692.82
  ambustionis
    due to
      burn or scald — *see* Burn, by site
      sunburn (*see also* Sunburn) 692.71
  amebic 006.6
  ammonia 691.0
  anaphylactoid NEC 692.9
  arsenical 692.4
  artefacta 698.4
    psychogenic 316 [698.4]
  asthmatic 691.8
  atopic (allergic) (intrinsic) 691.8
    psychogenic 316 [691.8]
  atrophicans 701.8
    diffusa 701.8
    maculosa 701.3
  autoimmune progesterone 279.49
  berlock, berloque 692.72
  blastomycetic 116.0
  blister beetle 692.89
  Brucella NEC 023.9
  bullosa 694.9
    striata pratensis 692.6
  bullous 694.9
    mucosynechial, atrophic 694.60
      with ocular involvement 694.61
    seasonal 694.8
  calorica
    due to
      burn or scald — *see* Burn, by site
      cold 692.89
      sunburn (*see also* Sunburn) 692.71
  caterpillar 692.89
  cercarial 120.3
  combustionis
    due to
      burn or scald — *see* Burn, by site
      sunburn (*see also* Sunburn) 692.71
  congelationis 991.5
  contusiformis 695.2
  diabetic 250.8 ☑
  diaper 691.0
  diphtheritica 032.85
  due to
    acetone 692.2
    acids 692.4
    adhesive plaster 692.4
    alcohol (skin contact) (substances classifiable to 980.0–980.9) 692.4
      taken internally 693.8
    alkalis 692.4
    allergy NEC 692.9
    ammonia (household) (liquid) 692.4
    animal
      dander (cat) (dog) 692.84
      hair (cat) (dog) 692.84
    arnica 692.3

Dermatitis — *continued*
  due to — *continued*
    arsenic 692.4
      taken internally 693.8
    blister beetle 692.89
    cantharides 692.3
    carbon disulphide 692.2
    caterpillar 692.89
    caustics 692.4
    cereal (ingested) 693.1
      contact with skin 692.5
    chemical(s) NEC 692.4
      internal 693.8
      irritant NEC 692.4
      taken internally 693.8
    chlorocompounds 692.2
    coffee (ingested) 693.1
      contact with skin 692.5
    cold weather 692.89
    cosmetics 692.81
    cyclohexanes 692.2
    dander, animal (cat) (dog) 692.84
    deodorant 692.81
    detergents 692.0
    dichromate 692.4
    drugs and medicinals (correct substance properly administered) (internal use) 693.0
      external (in contact with skin) 692.3
      wrong substance given or taken 976.9
        specified substance — *see* Table of Drugs and Chemicals
      wrong substance given or taken 977.9
        specified substance — *see* Table of Drugs and Chemicals
    dyes 692.89
      hair 692.89
    epidermophytosis — *see* Dermatophytosis
    esters 692.2
    external irritant NEC 692.9
      specified agent NEC 692.89
    eye shadow 692.81
    fish (ingested) 693.1
      contact with skin 692.5
    flour (ingested) 693.1
      contact with skin 692.5
    food (ingested) 693.1
      in contact with skin 692.5
    fruit (ingested) 693.1
      contact with skin 692.5
    fungicides 692.3
    furs 692.84
    glycols 692.2
    greases NEC 692.1
    hair, animal (cat) (dog) 692.84
    hair dyes 692.89
    hot
      objects and materials — *see* Burn, by site
      weather or places 692.89
    hydrocarbons 692.2
    infrared rays, except from sun 692.82
      solar NEC (*see also* Dermatitis, due to, sun) 692.70
    ingested substance 693.9
      drugs and medicinals (*see also* Dermatitis, due to, drugs and medicinals) 693.0
      food 693.1
      specified substance NEC 693.8
    ingestion or injection of chemical 693.8
      drug (correct substance properly administered) 693.0
        wrong substance given or taken 977.9
          specified substance — *see* Table of Drugs and Chemicals
    insecticides 692.4
    internal agent 693.9
      drugs and medicinals (*see also* Dermatitis, due to, drugs and medicinals) 693.0

☑ **Additional Digit Required — Refer to the Tabular List for Digit Selection**   ᵀᴱᴺ **Subterms under main terms may continue to next column or page**

76 — Volume 2   ▶◀ Revised Text   ● New Line   ▲ Revised Code   2013 ICD-9-CM

Dermatitis — *continued*
due to — *continued*
  internal agent — *continued*
    food (ingested) 693.1
      in contact with skin 692.5
      specified agent NEC 693.8
    iodine 692.3
    iodoform 692.3
    irradiation 692.82
    jewelry 692.83
    keratolytics 692.3
    ketones 692.2
    lacquer tree (Rhus verniciflua) 692.6
    light (sun) NEC (*see also* Dermatitis, due
      to, sun) 692.70
      other 692.82
    low temperature 692.89
    mascara 692.81
    meat (ingested) 693.1
      contact with skin 692.5
    mercury, mercurials 692.3
    metals 692.83
    milk (ingested) 693.1
      contact with skin 692.5
    Neomycin 692.3
    nylon 692.4
    oils NEC 692.1
    paint solvent 692.2
    pediculocides 692.3
    petroleum products (substances classifi-
      able to 981) 692.4
    phenol 692.3
    photosensitiveness, photosensitivity
      (sun) 692.72
      other light 692.82
    plants NEC 692.6
    plasters, medicated (any) 692.3
    plastic 692.4
    poison
      ivy (Rhus toxicodendron) 692.6
      oak (Rhus diversiloba) 692.6
      plant or vine 692.6
      sumac (Rhus venenata) 692.6
      vine (Rhus radicans) 692.6
    preservatives 692.89
    primrose (primula) 692.6
    primula 692.6
    radiation 692.82
      sun NEC (*see also* Dermatitis, due to,
        sun) 692.70
      tanning bed 692.82
    radioactive substance 692.82
    radium 692.82
    ragweed (Senecio jacobae) 692.6
    Rhus (diversiloba) (radicans) (toxicoden-
      dron) (venenata) (verniciflua)
      692.6
    rubber 692.4
    scabicides 692.3
    Senecio jacobae 692.6
    solar radiation — *see* Dermatitis, due to,
      sun
    solvents (any) (substances classifiable to
      982.0–982.8) 692.2
      chlorocompound group 692.2
      cyclohexane group 692.2
      ester group 692.2
      glycol group 692.2
      hydrocarbon group 692.2
      ketone group 692.2
      paint 692.2
    specified agent NEC 692.89
    sun 692.70
      acute 692.72
      chronic NEC 692.74
      specified NEC 692.79
    sunburn (*see also* Sunburn) 692.71
    sunshine NEC (*see also* Dermatitis, due
      to, sun) 692.70
    tanning bed 692.82
    tetrachlorethylene 692.2
    toluene 692.2
    topical medications 692.3
    turpentine 692.2
    ultraviolet rays, except from sun 692.82

Dermatitis — *continued*
due to — *continued*
  ultraviolet rays, except from sun — *con-*
    tinued
    sun NEC (*see also* Dermatitis, due to,
      sun) 692.70
  vaccine or vaccination (correct substance
    properly administered) 693.0
    wrong substance given or taken
      bacterial vaccine 978.8
        specified — *see* Table of
          Drugs and Chemicals
      other vaccines NEC 979.9
        specified — *see* Table of
          Drugs and Chemicals
  varicose veins (*see also* Varicose, vein,
    inflamed or infected) 454.1
  x-rays 692.82
dyshydrotic 705.81
dysmenorrheica 625.8
eczematoid NEC 692.9
  infectious 690.8
eczematous NEC 692.9
epidemica 695.89
erysipelatosa 695.81
escharotica — *see* Burn, by site
exfoliativa, exfoliative 695.89
  generalized 695.89
  infantum 695.81
  neonatorum 695.81
eyelid 373.31
  allergic 373.32
  contact 373.32
  eczematous 373.31
  herpes (zoster) 053.20
    simplex 054.41
  infective 373.5
    due to
      actinomycosis 039.3 *[373.5]*
      herpes
        simplex 054.41
        zoster 053.20
      impetigo 684 *[373.5]*
      leprosy (*see also* Leprosy)
        030.0 *[373.4]*
      lupus vulgaris (tuberculous) (*see*
        also Tuberculosis)
        017.0 ☑ *[373.4]*
      mycotic dermatitis (*see also* Der-
        matomycosis)
        111.9 *[373.5]*
      vaccinia 051.02 *[373.5]*
        postvaccination 999.0 *[373.5]*
      yaws (*see also* Yaws) 102.9 *[373.4]*
facta, factitia 698.4
  psychogenic 316 *[698.4]*
ficta 698.4
  psychogenic 316 *[698.4]*
flexural 691.8
follicularis 704.8
friction 709.8
fungus 111.9
  specified type NEC 111.8
gangrenosa, gangrenous (infantum) (*see*
  also Gangrene) 785.4
gestationis 646.8 ☑
gonococcal 098.89
gouty 274.89
harvest mite 133.8
heat 692.89
herpetiformis (bullous) (erythematous)
  (pustular) (vesicular) 694.0
  juvenile 694.2
  senile 694.5
hiemalis 692.89
hypostatic, hypostatica 454.1
  with ulcer 454.2
impetiginous 684
infantile (acute) (chronic) (intertriginous)
  (intrinsic) (seborrheic) 690.12
infectiosa eczematoides 690.8
infectious (staphylococcal) (streptococcal)
  686.9
  eczematoid 690.8
infective eczematoid 690.8
Jacquet's (diaper dermatitis) 691.0

Dermatitis — *continued*
due to — *continued*
  leptus 133.8
lichenified NEC 692.9
lichenoid, chronic 701.0
lichenoides purpurica pigmentosa 709.1
meadow 692.6
medicamentosa (correct substance properly
  administered) (internal use) (*see also*
  Dermatitis, due to, drugs or medicinals) 693.0
  due to contact with skin 692.3
mite 133.8
multiformis 694.0
  juvenile 694.2
  senile 694.5
napkin 691.0
neuro 698.3
neurotica 694.0
nummular NEC 692.9
osteatosis, osteatotic 706.8
papillaris capillitii 706.1
pellagrous 265.2
perioral 695.3
perstans 696.1
photosensitivity (sun) 692.72
  other light 692.82
pigmented purpuric lichenoid 709.1
polymorpha dolorosa 694.0
primary irritant 692.9
pruriginosa 694.0
pruritic NEC 692.9
psoriasiform nodularis 696.2
psychogenic 316
purulent 686.00
pustular contagious 051.2
pyococcal 686.00
pyocyaneus 686.09
pyogenica 686.00
radiation 692.82
repens 696.1
Ritter's (exfoliativa) 695.81
Schamberg's (progressive pigmentary dermatosis) 709.09
schistosome 120.3
seasonal bullous 694.8
seborrheic 690.10
  infantile 690.12
sensitization NEC 692.9
septic (*see also* Septicemia) 686.00
  gonococcal 098.89
solar, solare NEC (*see also* Dermatitis, due
  to, sun) 692.70
stasis 454.1
  due to
    postphlebitic syndrome 459.12
      with ulcer 459.13
    varicose veins — *see* Varicose
    ulcerated or with ulcer (varicose) 454.2
sunburn (*see also* Sunburn) 692.71
suppurative 686.00
traumatic NEC 709.8
trophoneurotica 694.0
ultraviolet, except from sun 692.82
  due to sun NEC (*see also* Dermatitis, due
    to, sun) 692.82
varicose 454.1
  with ulcer 454.2
vegetans 686.8
verrucosa 117.2
xerotic 706.8
Dermatoarthritis, lipoid 272.8 *[713.0]*
Dermatochalasia, dermatochalasis 374.87
Dermatofibroma (lenticulare) (M8832/0) —
  see also Neoplasm, skin, benign
  protuberans (M8832/1) — *see* Neoplasm,
    skin, uncertain behavior
Dermatofibrosarcoma (protuberans)
  (M8832/3) — *see* Neoplasm, skin, malignant
Dermatographia 708.3
Dermatolysis (congenital) (exfoliativa) 757.39
  acquired 701.8
  eyelids 374.34
  palpebrarum 374.34
  senile 701.8
Dermatomegaly NEC 701.8

Dermatomucomyositis 710.3
Dermatomycosis 111.9
  furfuracea 111.0
  specified type NEC 111.8
Dermatomyositis (acute) (chronic) 710.3
Dermatoneuritis of children 985.0
Dermatophiliasis 134.1
Dermatophytide — *see* Dermatophytosis
Dermatophytosis (Epidermophyton) (infection) (microsporum) (tinea) (Trichophyton) 110.9
  beard 110.0
  body 110.5
  deep seated 110.6
  fingernails 110.1
  foot 110.4
  groin 110.3
  hand 110.2
  nail 110.1
  perianal (area) 110.3
  scalp 110.0
  scrotal 110.8
  specified site NEC 110.8
  toenails 110.1
  vulva 110.8
Dermatopolyneuritis 985.0
Dermatorrhexis 756.83
  acquired 701.8
Dermatosclerosis — *see also* Scleroderma
  710.1
  localized 701.0
Dermatosis 709.9
  Andrews' 686.8
  atopic 691.8
  Bowen's (M8081/2) — *see* Neoplasm, skin,
    in situ
  bullous 694.9
    specified type NEC 694.8
  erythematosquamous 690.8
  exfoliativa 695.89
  factitial 698.4
  gonococcal 098.89
  herpetiformis 694.0
    juvenile 694.2
    senile 694.5
  hysterical 300.11
  linear IgA 694.8
  menstrual NEC 709.8
  neutrophilic, acute febrile 695.89
  occupational (*see also* Dermatitis) 692.9
  papulosa nigra 709.8
  pigmentary NEC 709.00
    progressive 709.09
      Schamberg's 709.09
      Siemens-Bloch 757.33
  progressive pigmentary 709.09
  psychogenic 316
  pustular subcorneal 694.1
  Schamberg's (progressive pigmentary)
    709.09
  senile NEC 709.3
  specified NEC 702.8
  Unna's (seborrheic dermatitis) 690.10
Dermographia 708.3
Dermographism 708.3
Dermoid (cyst) (M9084/0) — *see also* Neoplasm, by site, benign
  with malignant transformation (M9084/3)
    183.0
Dermopathy
  infiltrative, with thyrotoxicosis 242.0 ☑
  nephrogenic fibrosing 701.8
  senile NEC 709.3
Dermophytosis — *see* Dermatophytosis
Descemet's membrane — *see* condition
Descemetocele 371.72
Descending — *see* condition
Descensus uteri (complete) (incomplete)
  (partial) (without vaginal wall prolapse)
  618.1
  with mention of vaginal wall prolapse —
    see Prolapse, uterovaginal
Desensitization to allergens V07.1
Desert
  rheumatism 114.0
  sore (*see also* Ulcer, skin) 707.9

☑ **Additional Digit Required — Refer to the Tabular List for Digit Selection**

🔺 **Subterms under main terms may continue to next column or page**

Desertion (child) (newborn) 995.52
  adult 995.84
Desmoid (extra-abdominal) (tumor) (M8821/1) — *see also* Neoplasm, connective tissue, uncertain behavior
  abdominal (M8822/1) — *see* Neoplasm, connective tissue, uncertain behavior
Despondency 300.4
Desquamative dermatitis NEC 695.89
Destruction
  articular facet (*see also* Derangement, joint) 718.9 ☑
    vertebra 724.9
  bone 733.90
    syphilitic 095.5
  joint (*see also* Derangement, joint) 718.9 ☑
    sacroiliac 724.6
  kidney 593.89
  live fetus to facilitate birth NEC 763.89
  ossicles (ear) 385.24
  rectal sphincter 569.49
  septum (nasal) 478.19
  tuberculous NEC (*see also* Tuberculosis) 011.9 ☑
  tympanic membrane 384.82
  tympanum 385.89
  vertebral disc — *see* Degeneration, intervertebral disc
Destructiveness — *see also* Disturbance, conduct 312.9
  adjustment reaction 309.3
Detachment
  cartilage (*see also* Sprain, by site)
    knee — *see* Tear, meniscus
  cervix, annular 622.8
    complicating delivery 665.3 ☑
  choroid (old) (postinfectional) (simple) (spontaneous) 363.70
    hemorrhagic 363.72
    serous 363.71
  knee, medial meniscus (old) 717.3
    current injury 836.0
  ligament — *see* Sprain, by site
  placenta (premature) — *see* Placenta, separation
  retina (recent) 361.9
    with retinal defect (rhegmatogenous) 361.00
      giant tear 361.03
      multiple 361.02
      partial
        with
          giant tear 361.03
          multiple defects 361.02
          retinal dialysis (juvenile) 361.04
          single defect 361.01
      retinal dialysis (juvenile) 361.04
      single 361.01
      subtotal 361.05
      total 361.05
    delimited (old) (partial) 361.06
    old
      delimited 361.06
      partial 361.06
      total or subtotal 361.07
    pigment epithelium (RPE) (serous) 362.42
      exudative 362.42
      hemorrhagic 362.43
    rhegmatogenous (*see also* Detachment, retina, with retinal defect) 361.00
    serous (without retinal defect) 361.2
    specified type NEC 361.89
    traction (with vitreoretinal organization) 361.81
  vitreous humor 379.21
Detergent asthma 507.8
Deterioration
  epileptic
    with behavioral disturbance 345.9 ☑ *[294.11]*
    without behavioral disturbance 345.9 ☑ *[294.10]*
  heart, cardiac (*see also* Degeneration, myocardial) 429.1

Deterioration — *continued*
  mental (*see also* Psychosis) 298.9
  myocardium, myocardial (*see also* Degeneration, myocardial) 429.1
  senile (simple) 797
  transplanted organ — *see* Complications, transplant, organ, by site
de Toni-Fanconi syndrome (cystinosis) 270.0
Deuteranomaly 368.52
Deuteranopia (anomalous trichromat) (complete) (incomplete) 368.52
Deutschländer's disease — *see* Fracture, foot
Development
  abnormal, bone 756.9
  arrested 783.40
    bone 733.91
    child 783.40
      due to malnutrition (protein-calorie) 263.2
    fetus or newborn 764.9 ☑
    tracheal rings (congenital) 748.3
  defective, congenital (*see also* Anomaly)
    cauda equina 742.59
    left ventricle 746.9
      with atresia or hypoplasia of aortic orifice or valve with hypoplasia of ascending aorta 746.7
      in hypoplastic left heart syndrome 746.7
  delayed (*see also* Delay, development) 783.40
    arithmetical skills 315.1
    language (skills) 315.31
      and speech due to hearing loss 315.34
      expressive 315.31
      mixed receptive-expressive 315.32
    learning skill, specified NEC 315.2
    mixed skills 315.5
    motor coordination 315.4
    reading 315.00
    specified
      learning skill NEC 315.2
      type NEC, except learning 315.8
    speech 315.39
      and language due to hearing loss 315.34
      associated with hyperkinesia 314.1
      phonological 315.39
    spelling 315.09
    written expression 315.2
  imperfect, congenital (*see also* Anomaly)
    heart 746.9
    lungs 748.60
  improper (fetus or newborn) 764.9 ☑
  incomplete (fetus or newborn) 764.9 ☑
    affecting management of pregnancy 656.5 ☑
    bronchial tree 748.3
    organ or site not listed — *see* Hypoplasia
    respiratory system 748.9
  sexual, precocious NEC 259.1
  tardy, mental (*see also* Disability, intellectual) 319
Developmental — *see* condition
Devergie's disease (pityriasis rubra pilaris) 696.4
Deviation
  conjugate (eye) 378.87
    palsy 378.81
    spasm, spastic 378.82
  esophagus 530.89
  eye, skew 378.87
  mandible, opening and closing 524.53
  midline (jaw) (teeth) 524.29
    specified site NEC — *see* Malposition
  occlusal plane 524.76
  organ or site, congenital NEC — *see* Malposition, congenital
  septum (acquired) (nasal) 470
    congenital 754.0
  sexual 302.9
    bestiality 302.1
    coprophilia 302.89
    ego-dystonic
      homosexuality 302.0

Deviation — *continued*
  sexual — *continued*
    ego-dystonic — *continued*
      lesbianism 302.0
    erotomania 302.89
      Clérambault's 297.8
    exhibitionism (sexual) 302.4
    fetishism 302.81
      transvestic 302.3
    frotteurism 302.89
    homosexuality, ego-dystonic 302.0
      pedophilic 302.2
    lesbianism, ego-dystonic 302.0
    masochism 302.83
    narcissism 302.89
    necrophilia 302.89
    nymphomania 302.89
    pederosis 302.2
    pedophilia 302.2
    sadism 302.84
    sadomasochism 302.84
    satyriasis 302.89
    specified type NEC 302.89
    transvestic fetishism 302.3
    transvestism 302.3
    voyeurism 302.82
    zoophilia (erotica) 302.1
  teeth, midline 524.29
  trachea 519.19
  ureter (congenital) 753.4
Devic's disease 341.0
Device
  cerebral ventricle (communicating) in situ V45.2
  contraceptive — *see* Contraceptive, device
  drainage, cerebrospinal fluid V45.2
Devil's
  grip 074.1
  pinches (purpura simplex) 287.2
Devitalized tooth 522.9
Devonshire colic 984.9
  specified type of lead — *see* Table of Drugs and Chemicals
Dextraposition, aorta 747.21
  with ventricular septal defect, pulmonary stenosis or atresia, and hypertrophy of right ventricle 745.2
  in tetralogy of Fallot 745.2
Dextratransposition, aorta 745.11
Dextrinosis, limit (debrancher enzyme deficiency) 271.0
Dextrocardia (corrected) (false) (isolated) (secondary) (true) 746.87
  with
    complete transposition of viscera 759.3
    situs inversus 759.3
Dextroversion, kidney (left) 753.3
Dhobie itch 110.3
DHTR (delayed hemolytic transfusion reaction) — *see* Complications, transfusion
Diabetes, diabetic (brittle) (congenital) (familial) (mellitus) (severe) (slight) (without complication) 250.0 ☑

> *Note* — Use the following fifth-digit subclassification with category 250:
>
> 0 type II or unspecified type, not stated as uncontrolled
>
> Fifth-digit 0 is for use for type II patients, even if the patient requires insulin
>
> 1 type I [juvenile type], not stated as uncontrolled
>
> 2 type II or unspecified type, uncontrolled
>
> Fifth-digit 2 is for use for type II patients, even if the patient requires insulin
>
> 3 type I [juvenile type], uncontrolled

  with
    coma (with ketoacidosis) 250.3 ☑
      due to secondary diabetes 249.3 ☑
      hyperosmolar (nonketotic) 250.2 ☑
        due to secondary diabetes 249.2 ☑

Diabetes, diabetic — *continued*
  with — *continued*
    complication NEC 250.9 ☑
      due to secondary diabetes 249.9 ☑
      specified NEC 250.8 ☑
        due to secondary diabetes 249.8 ☑
    gangrene 250.7 ☑ *[785.4]*
      due to secondary diabetes 249.7 ☑ *[785.4]*
    hyperglycemia — code to Diabetes, by type, with 5th digit for not stated as uncontrolled
    hyperosmolarity 250.2 ☑
      due to secondary diabetes 249.2 ☑
    ketosis, ketoacidosis 250.1 ☑
      due to secondary diabetes 249.1 ☑
    loss of protective sensation (LOPS) — *see* Diabetes, neuropathy
    osteomyelitis 250.8 ☑ *[731.8]*
      due to secondary diabetes 249.8 ☑ *[731.8]*
    specified manisfestations NEC 250.8 ☑
      due to secondary diabetes 249.8 ☑
  acetonemia 250.1 ☑
    due to secondary diabetes 249.1 ☑
  acidosis 250.1 ☑
    due to secondary diabetes 249.1 ☑
  amyotrophy 250.6 ☑ *[353.5]*
    due to secondary diabetes 249.6 ☑ *[353.5]*
  angiopathy, peripheral 250.7 ☑ *[443.81]*
    due to secondary diabetes 249.7 ☑ *[443.81]*
  asymptomatic 790.29
  autonomic neuropathy (peripheral) 250.6 ☑ *[337.1]*
    due to secondary diabetes 249.6 ☑ *[337.1]*
  bone change 250.8 ☑ *[731.8]*
    due to secondary diabetes 249.8 ☑ *[731.8]*
  borderline 790.29
  bronze, bronzed 275.01
  cataract 250.5 ☑ *[366.41]*
    due to secondary diabetes 249.5 ☑ *[366.41]*
  chemical induced — *see* Diabetes, secondary
  complicating pregnancy, childbirth, or puerperium 648.0 ☑
  coma (with ketoacidosis) 250.3 ☑
    due to secondary diabetes 249.3 ☑
    hyperglycemic 250.3 ☑
      due to secondary diabetes 249.3 ☑
    hyperosmolar (nonketotic) 250.2 ☑
      due to secondary diabetes 249.2 ☑
    hypoglycemic 250.3 ☑
      due to secondary diabetes 249.3 ☑
    insulin 250.3 ☑
      due to secondary diabetes 249.3 ☑
  complicating pregnancy, childbirth, or puerperium (maternal) (conditions classifiable to 249 and 250) 648.0 ☑
    affecting fetus or newborn 775.0
  complication NEC 250.9 ☑
    due to secondary diabetes 249.9 ☑
    specified NEC 250.8 ☑
      due to secondary diabetes 249.8 ☑
  dorsal sclerosis 250.6 ☑ *[340]*
    due to secondary diabetes 249.6 ☑ *[340]*
  drug-induced — *see also* Diabetes, secondary
    overdose or wrong substance given or taken — *see* Table of Drugs and Chemicals
  due to
    cystic fibrosis — *see* Diabetes, secondary
    infection — *see* Diabetes, secondary
  dwarfism-obesity syndrome 258.1
  gangrene 250.7 ☑ *[785.4]*
    due to secondary diabetes 249.7 ☑ *[785.4]*

Diabetes, diabetic — *continued*
gastroparesis 250.6 ☑ *[536.3]*
  due to secondary diabetes
    249.6 ☑ *[536.3]*
gestational 648.8 ☑
  complicating pregnancy, childbirth, or
    puerperium 648.8 ☑
glaucoma 250.5 ☑ *[365.44]*
  due to secondary diabetes
    249.5 ☑ *[365.44]*
glomerulosclerosis (intercapillary)
  250.4 ☑ *[581.81]*
  due to secondary diabetes
    249.4 ☑ *[581.81]*
glycogenosis, secondary 250.8 ☑ *[259.8]*
  due to secondary diabetes
    249.8 ☑ *[259.8]*
hemochromatosis (*see also* Hemochromatosis) 275.03
hyperosmolar coma 250.2 ☑
  due to secondary diabetes 249.2 ☑
hyperosmolarity 250.2 ☑
  due to secondary diabetes 249.2 ☑
hypertension-nephrosis syndrome
  250.4 ☑ *[581.81]*
  due to secondary diabetes
    249.4 ☑ *[581.81]*
hypoglycemia 250.8 ☑
  due to secondary diabetes 249.8 ☑
hypoglycemic shock 250.8 ☑
  due to secondary diabetes 249.8 ☑
inadequately controlled — code to Diabetes, by type, with 5th digit for not stated as uncontrolled
insipidus 253.5
  nephrogenic 588.1
  pituitary 253.5
  vasopressin-resistant 588.1
intercapillary glomerulosclerosis
  250.4 ☑ *[581.81]*
  due to secondary diabetes
    249.4 ☑ *[581.81]*
iritis 250.5 ☑ *[364.42]*
  due to secondary diabetes
    249.5 ☑ *[364.42]*
ketosis, ketoacidosis 250.1 ☑
  due to secondary diabetes 249.1 ☑
Kimmelstiel (-Wilson) disease or syndrome (intercapillary glomerulosclerosis)
  250.4 ☑ *[581.81]*
  due to secondary diabetes
    249.4 ☑ *[581.81]*
Lancereaux's (diabetes mellitus with marked emaciation) 250.8 ☑ *[261]*
  due to secondary diabetes
    249.8 ☑ *[261]*
latent (chemical) — *see* Diabetes, secondary
complicating pregnancy, childbirth, or puerperium 648.0 ☑
lipoidosis 250.8 ☑ *[272.7]*
  due to secondary diabetes
    249.8 ☑ *[272.7]*
macular edema 250.5 ☑ *[362.07]*
  due to secondary diabetes
    249.5 ☑ *[362.07]*
maternal
  with manifest disease in the infant 775.1
  affecting fetus or newborn 775.0
microaneurysms, retinal 250.5 ☑ *[362.01]*
  due to secondary diabetes
    249.5 ☑ *[362.01]*
mononeuropathy 250.6 ☑ *[355.9]*
  due to secondary diabetes
    249.6 ☑ *[355.9]*
neonatal, transient 775.1
nephropathy 250.4 ☑ *[583.81]*
  due to secondary diabetes
    249.4 ☑ *[583.81]*
nephrosis (syndrome) 250.4 ☑ *[581.81]*
  due to secondary diabetes
    249.4 ☑ *[581.81]*
neuralgia 250.6 ☑ *[357.2]*
  due to secondary diabetes
    249.6 ☑ *[357.2]*

Diabetes, diabetic — *continued*
neuritis 250.6 ☑ *[357.2]*
  due to secondary diabetes
    249.6 ☑ *[357.2]*
neurogenic arthropathy 250.6 ☑ *[713.5]*
  due to secondary diabetes
    249.6 ☑ *[713.5]*
neuropathy 250.6 ☑ *[357.2]*
  autonomic (peripheral) 250.6 ☑ *[337.1]*
    due to secondary diabetes
      249.6 ☑ *[337.1]*
  due to secondary diabetes
    249.6 ☑ *[357.2]*
nonclinical 790.29
osteomyelitis 250.8 ☑ *[731.8]*
  due to secondary diabetes
    249.8 ☑ *[731.8]*
out of control — code to Diabetes, by type, with 5th digit for uncontrolled
peripheral autonomic neuropathy
  250.6 ☑ *[337.1]*
  due to secondary diabetes
    249.6 ☑ *[337.1]*
phosphate 275.3
polyneuropathy 250.6 ☑ *[357.2]*
  due to secondary diabetes
    249.6 ☑ *[357.2]*
poorly controlled — code to Diabetes, by type, with 5th digit for not stated as uncontrolled
renal (true) 271.4
retinal
  edema 250.5 ☑ *[362.07]*
    due to secondary diabetes
      249.5 ☑ *[362.07]*
  hemorrhage 250.5 ☑ *[362.01]*
    due to secondary diabetes
      249.5 ☑ *[362.01]*
  microaneurysms 250.5 ☑ *[362.01]*
    due to secondary diabetes
      249.5 ☑ *[362.01]*
  retinitis 250.5 ☑ *[362.01]*
    due to secondary diabetes
      249.5 ☑ *[362.01]*
  retinopathy 250.5 ☑ *[362.01]*
    background 250.5 ☑ *[362.01]*
      due to secondary diabetes
        249.5 ☑ *[362.01]*
    due to secondary diabetes
      249.5 ☑ *[362.01]*
    nonproliferative 250.5 ☑ *[362.03]*
      due to secondary diabetes
        249.5 ☑ *[362.03]*
    mild 250.5 ☑ *[362.04]*
      due to secondary diabetes
        249.5 ☑ *[362.04]*
    moderate 250.5 ☑ *[362.05]*
      due to secondary diabetes
        249.5 ☑ *[362.05]*
    severe 250.5 ☑ *[362.06]*
      due to secondary diabetes
        249.5 ☑ *[362.06]*
    proliferative 250.5 ☑ *[362.02]*
      due to secondary diabetes
        249.5 ☑ *[362.02]*
secondary (chemical-induced) (due to chronic condition) (due to infection) (drug-induced) 249.0 ☑
  with
    coma (with ketoacidosis) 249.3 ☑
      hyperosmolar (nonketotic)
        249.2 ☑
    complication NEC 249.9 ☑
      specified NEC 249.8 ☑
    gangrene 249.7 ☑ *[785.4]*
    hyperosmolarity 249.2 ☑
    ketosis, ketoacidosis 249.1 ☑
    osteomyelitis 249.8 ☑ *[731.8]*
    specified manifestations NEC
      249.8 ☑
  acetonemia 249.1 ☑
  acidosis 249.1 ☑
  amyotrophy 249.6 ☑ *[353.5]*
  angiopathy, peripheral 249.7 ☑ *[443.81]*

Diabetes, diabetic — *continued*
secondary — *continued*
  autonomic neuropathy (peripheral)
    249.6 ☑ *[337.1]*
  bone change 249.8 ☑ *[731.8]*
  cataract 249.5 ☑ *[366.41]*
  coma (with ketoacidosis) 249.3 ☑
    hyperglycemic 249.3 ☑
    hyperosmolar (nonketotic) 249.2 ☑
    hypoglycemic 249.3 ☑
    insulin 249.3 ☑
  complicating pregnancy, childbirth, or puerperium (maternal) 648.0 ☑
    affecting fetus or newborn 775.0
  complication NEC 249.9 ☑
    specified NEC 249.8 ☑
  dorsal sclerosis 249.6 ☑ *[340]*
  due to overdose or wrong substance given or taken — *see* Table of Drugs and Chemicals
  gangrene 249.7 ☑ *[785.4]*
  gastroparesis 249.6 ☑ *[536.3]*
  glaucoma 249.5 ☑ *[365.44]*
  glomerulosclerosis (intercapillary)
    249.4 ☑ *[581.81]*
  glycogenosis, secondary 249.8 ☑ *[259.8]*
  hyperosmolar coma 249.2 ☑
  hyperosmolarity 249.2 ☑
  hypertension-nephrosis syndrome
    249.4 ☑ *[581.81]*
  hypoglycemia 249.8 ☑
  hypoglycemic shock 249.8 ☑
  intercapillary glomerulosclerosis
    249.4 ☑ *[581.81]*
  iritis 249.5 ☑ *[364.42]*
  ketosis, ketoacidosis 249.1 ☑
  Kimmelstiel (-Wilson) disease or syndrome (intercapillary glomerulosclerosis) 249.4 ☑ *[581.81]*
  Lancereaux's (diabetes mellitus with marked emaciation)
    249.8 ☑ *[261]*
  lipoidosis 249.8 ☑ *[272.7]*
  macular edema 249.5 ☑ *[362.07]*
  maternal
    with manifest disease in the infant 775.1
    affecting fetus or newborn 775.0
  microaneurysms, retinal
    249.5 ☑ *[362.01]*
  mononeuropathy 249.6 ☑ *[355.9]*
  nephropathy 249.4 ☑ *[583.81]*
  nephrosis (syndrome) 249.4 ☑ *[581.81]*
  neuralgia 249.6 ☑ *[357.2]*
  neuritis 249.6 ☑ *[357.2]*
  neurogenic arthropathy 249.6 ☑ *[713.5]*
  neuropathy 249.6 ☑ *[357.2]*
    autonomic (peripheral)
      249.6 ☑ *[337.1]*
  osteomyelitis 249.8 ☑ *[731.8]*
  peripheral autonomic neuropathy
    249.6 ☑ *[337.1]*
  polyneuropathy 249.6 ☑ *[357.2]*
  retinal
    edema 249.5 ☑ *[362.07]*
    hemorrhage 249.5 ☑ *[362.01]*
    microaneurysms 249.5 ☑ *[362.01]*
    retinitis 249.5 ☑ *[362.01]*
    retinopathy 249.5 ☑ *[362.01]*
      background 249.5 ☑ *[362.01]*
      nonproliferative 249.5 ☑ *[362.03]*
        mild 249.5 ☑ *[362.04]*
        moderate 249.5 ☑ *[362.05]*
        severe 249.5 ☑ *[362.06]*
      proliferative 249.5 ☑ *[362.02]*
  ulcer (skin) 249.8 ☑ *[707.9]*
    lower extemity 249.8 ☑ *[707.10]*
      ankle 249.8 ☑ *[707.13]*
      calf 249.8 ☑ *[707.12]*
      foot 249.8 ☑ *[707.15]*
      heel 249.8 ☑ *[707.14]*
      knee 249.8 ☑ *[707.19]*
      specified site NEC
        249.8 ☑ *[707.19]*

Diabetes, diabetic — *continued*
secondary — *continued*
  ulcer — *continued*
    lower extemity — *continued*
      thigh 249.8 ☑ *[707.11]*
      toes 249.8 ☑ *[707.15]*
    specified site NEC 249.8 ☑ *[707.8]*
    xanthoma 249.8 ☑ *[272.2]*
  steroid induced — *see also* Diabetes, secondary
    overdose or wrong substance given or taken 962.0
  stress 790.29
  subclinical 790.29
  subliminal 790.29
  sugar 250.0 ☑
  ulcer (skin) 250.8 ☑ *[707.9]*
    due to secondary diabetes
      249.8 ☑ *[707.9]*
    lower extremity 250.8 ☑ *[707.10]*
      ankle 250.8 ☑ *[707.13]*
        due to secondary diabetes
          249.8 ☑ *[707.13]*
      calf 250.8 ☑ *[707.12]*
        due to secondary diabetes
          249.8 ☑ *[707.12]*
      due to secondary diabetes
        249.8 ☑ *[707.10]*
      foot 250.8 ☑ *[707.15]*
        due to secondary diabetes
          249.8 ☑ *[707.15]*
      heel 250.8 ☑ *[707.14]*
        due to secondary diabetes
          249.8 ☑ *[707.14]*
      knee 250.8 ☑ *[707.19]*
        due to secondary diabetes
          249.8 ☑ *[707.19]*
      specified site NEC 250.8 ☑ *[707.19]*
        due to secondary diabetes
          249.8 ☑ *[707.19]*
      thigh 250.8 ☑ *[707.11]*
        due to secondary diabetes
          249.8 ☑ *[707.11]*
      toes 250.8 ☑ *[707.15]*
        due to secondary diabetes
          249.8 ☑ *[707.15]*
    specified site NEC 250.8 ☑ *[707.8]*
      due to secondary diabetes
        249.8 ☑ *[707.8]*
  xanthoma 250.8 ☑ *[272.2]*
    due to secondary diabetes
      249.8 ☑ *[272.2]*
Diacyclothrombopathia 287.1
Diagnosis deferred 799.9
Dialysis (intermittent) (treatment)
  anterior retinal (juvenile) (with detachment) 361.04
  extracorporeal V56.0
  hemodialysis V56.0
    status only V45.11
  peritoneal V56.8
    status only V45.11
  renal V56.0
    status only V45.11
  specified type NEC V56.8
Diamond-Blackfan anemia or syndrome (congenital hypoplastic anemia) 284.01
Diamond-Gardener syndrome (autoerythrocyte sensitization) 287.2
Diaper rash 691.0
Diaphoresis (excessive) NEC — *see also* Hyperhidrosis) 780.8
Diaphragm — *see* condition
Diaphragmalgia 786.52
Diaphragmitis 519.4
Diaphyseal aclasis 756.4
Diaphysitis 733.99
Diarrhea, diarrheal (acute) (autumn) (bilious) (bloody) (catarrhal) (choleraic) (chronic) (gravis) (green) (infantile) (lienteric) (noninfectious) (presumed noninfectious) (putrefactive) (secondary) (sporadic) (summer) (symptomatic) (thermic) 787.91
  achlorhydric 536.0

☑ Additional Digit Required — Refer to the Tabular List for Digit Selection   ▽ Subterms under main terms may continue to next column or page

2013 ICD-9-CM   ▶◀ Revised Text   ● New Line   ▲ Revised Code   Volume 2 — 79

Diarrhea, diarrheal — *continued*
  allergic 558.3
  amebic (*see also* Amebiasis) 006.9
    with abscess — *see* Abscess, amebic
    acute 006.0
    chronic 006.1
    nondysenteric 006.2
  bacillary — *see* Dysentery, bacillary
  bacterial NEC 008.5
  balantidial 007.0
  bile salt-induced 579.8
  cachectic NEC 787.91
  chilomastix 007.8
  choleriformis 001.1
  coccidial 007.2
  Cochin-China 579.1
    anguilluliasis 127.2
    psilosis 579.1
  Dientamoeba 007.8
  dietetic 787.91
  due to
    achylia gastrica 536.8
    Aerobacter aerogenes 008.2
    Bacillus coli — *see* Enteritis, E. coli
    bacteria NEC 008.5
    bile salts 579.8
    Capillaria
      hepatica 128.8
      philippinensis 127.5
    Clostridium perfringens (C) (F) 008.46
    Enterobacter aerogenes 008.2
    enterococci 008.49
    Escherichia coli — *see* Enteritis, E. coli
    Giardia lamblia 007.1
    Heterophyes heterophyes 121.6
    irritating foods 787.91
    Metagonimus yokogawai 121.5
    Necator americanus 126.1
    Paracolobactrum arizonae 008.1
    Paracolon bacillus NEC 008.47
      Arizona 008.1
    Proteus (bacillus) (mirabilis) (Morganii)
      008.3
    Pseudomonas aeruginosa 008.42
    S. japonicum 120.2
    specified organism NEC 008.8
      bacterial 008.49
      viral NEC 008.69
    Staphylococcus 008.41
    Streptococcus 008.49
      anaerobic 008.46
    Strongyloides stercoralis 127.2
    Trichuris trichiura 127.3
    virus NEC (*see also* Enteritis, viral) 008.69
  dysenteric 009.2
    due to specified organism NEC 008.8
  dyspeptic 787.91
  endemic 009.3
    due to specified organism NEC 008.8
  epidemic 009.2
    due to specified organism NEC 008.8
  fermentative 787.91
  flagellate 007.9
  Flexner's (ulcerative) 004.1
  functional 564.5
    following gastrointestinal surgery 564.4
    psychogenic 306.4
  giardial 007.1
  Giardia lamblia 007.1
  hill 579.1
  hyperperistalsis (nervous) 306.4
  infectious 009.2
    due to specified organism NEC 008.8
    presumed 009.3
  inflammatory 787.91
    due to specified organism NEC 008.8
  malarial (*see also* Malaria) 084.6
  mite 133.8
  mycotic 117.9
  nervous 306.4
  neurogenic 564.5
  parenteral NEC 009.2
  postgastrectomy 564.4
  postvagotomy 564.4
  prostaglandin induced 579.8
  protozoal NEC 007.9

Diarrhea, diarrheal — *continued*
  psychogenic 306.4
  septic 009.2
    due to specified organism NEC 008.8
  specified organism NEC 008.8
    bacterial 008.49
    viral NEC 008.69
  Staphylococcus 008.41
  Streptococcus 008.49
    anaerobic 008.46
  toxic 558.2
  travelers' 009.2
    due to specified organism NEC 008.8
  trichomonal 007.3
  tropical 579.1
  tuberculous 014.8 ☑
  ulcerative (chronic) (*see also* Colitis, ulcerative) 556.9
  viral (*see also* Enteritis, viral) 008.8
  zymotic NEC 009.2
Diastasis
  cranial bones 733.99
    congenital 756.0
  joint (traumatic) — *see* Dislocation, by site
  muscle 728.84
    congenital 756.89
  recti (abdomen) 728.84
    complicating delivery 665.8 ☑
    congenital 756.79
Diastema, teeth, tooth 524.30
Diastematomyelia 742.51
Diataxia, cerebral, infantile 343.0
Diathesis
  allergic V15.09
  bleeding (familial) 287.9
  cystine (familial) 270.0
  gouty 274.9
  hemorrhagic (familial) 287.9
    newborn NEC 776.0
  oxalic 271.8
  scrofulous (*see also* Tuberculosis) 017.2 ☑
  spasmophilic (*see also* Tetany) 781.7
  ulcer 536.9
  uric acid 274.9
Diaz's disease or osteochondrosis 732.5
Dibothriocephaliasis 123.4
  larval 123.5
Dibothriocephalus (infection) (infestation)
    (latus) 123.4
  larval 123.5
Dicephalus 759.4
Dichotomy, teeth 520.2
Dichromat, dichromata (congenital) 368.59
Dichromatopsia (congenital) 368.59
Dichuchwa 104.0
Dicroceliasis 121.8
Didelphys, didelphic — *see also* Double uterus
    752.2
Didymitis — *see also* Epididymitis 604.90
Died — *see also* Death
  without
    medical attention (cause unknown)
      798.9
    sign of disease 798.2
Dientamoeba diarrhea 007.8
Dietary
  inadequacy or deficiency 269.9
  surveillance and counseling V65.3
Dietl's crisis 593.4
Dieulafoy lesion (hemorrhagic)
  of
    duodenum 537.84
    esophagus 530.82
    intestine 569.86
    stomach 537.84
Difficult
  birth, affecting fetus or newborn 763.9
  delivery NEC 669.9 ☑
Difficulty
  feeding 783.3
    adult 783.3
    breast 676.8 ☑
    child 783.3
    elderly 783.3
    infant 783.3
    newborn 779.31

Difficulty — *continued*
  feeding — *continued*
    nonorganic (infant) NEC 307.59
  mechanical, gastroduodenal stoma 537.89
  reading 315.00
  specific, spelling 315.09
  swallowing (*see also* Dysphagia) 787.20
  walking 719.7
Diffuse — *see* condition
Diffused ganglion 727.42
Di George's syndrome (thymic hypoplasia)
    279.11
Digestive — *see* condition
Di Guglielmo's disease or syndrome
    (M9841/3) 207.0 ☑
Dihydropyrimidine dehydrogenase disease
    (DPD) 277.6
Diktyoma (M9051/3) — *see* Neoplasm, by site,
    malignant
Dilaceration, tooth 520.4
Dilatation
  anus 564.89
    venule — *see* Hemorrhoids
  aorta (focal) (general) (*see also* Ectasia, aortic) 447.70
    with aneurysm 441.9
    congenital 747.29
    infectional 093.0
    ruptured 441.5
    syphilitic 093.0
  appendix (cystic) 543.9
  artery 447.8
  bile duct (common) (congenital) 751.69
    acquired 576.8
  bladder (sphincter) 596.89
    congenital 753.8
    in pregnancy or childbirth 654.4 ☑
      causing obstructed labor 660.2 ☑
      affecting fetus or newborn 763.1
  blood vessel 459.89
  bronchus, bronchi 494.0
    with acute exacerbation 494.1
  calyx (due to obstruction) 593.89
  capillaries 448.9
  cardiac (acute) (chronic) (*see also* Hypertrophy, cardiac) 429.3
    congenital 746.89
      valve NEC 746.89
      pulmonary 746.09
    hypertensive (*see also* Hypertension,
      heart) 402.90
  cavum septi pellucidi 742.4
  cecum 564.89
    psychogenic 306.4
  cervix (uteri) (*see also* Incompetency, cervix)
    incomplete, poor, slow
      affecting fetus or newborn 763.7
      complicating delivery 661.0 ☑
      affecting fetus or newborn 763.7
  colon 564.7
    congenital 751.3
    due to mechanical obstruction 560.89
    psychogenic 306.4
  common bile duct (congenital) 751.69
    acquired 576.8
      with calculus, choledocholithiasis, or
        stones — *see* Choledocholithiasis
  cystic duct 751.69
    acquired (any bile duct) 575.8
  duct, mammary 610.4
  duodenum 564.89
  esophagus 530.89
    congenital 750.4
    due to
      achalasia 530.0
      cardiospasm 530.0
  Eustachian tube, congenital 744.24
  fontanel 756.0
  gallbladder 575.8
    congenital 751.69
  gastric 536.8
    acute 536.1
    psychogenic 306.4
  heart (acute) (chronic) (*see also* Hypertrophy, cardiac) 429.3

Dilatation — *continued*
  heart (*see also* Hypertrophy, cardiac) —
    continued
    congenital 746.89
    hypertensive (*see also* Hypertension,
      heart) 402.90
    valve (*see also* Endocarditis)
      congenital 746.89
  ileum 564.89
    psychogenic 306.4
  inguinal rings — *see* Hernia, inguinal
  jejunum 564.89
    psychogenic 306.4
  kidney (calyx) (collecting structures) (cystic)
    (parenchyma) (pelvis) 593.89
  lacrimal passages 375.69
  lymphatic vessel 457.1
  mammary duct 610.4
  Meckel's diverticulum (congenital) 751.0
  meningeal vessels, congenital 742.8
  myocardium (acute) (chronic) (*see also* Hypertrophy, cardiac) 429.3
  organ or site, congenital NEC — *see* Distortion
  pancreatic duct 577.8
  pelvis, kidney 593.89
  pericardium — *see* Pericarditis
  pharynx 478.29
  prostate 602.8
  pulmonary
    artery (idiopathic) 417.8
      congenital 747.39
    valve, congenital 746.09
  pupil 379.43
  rectum 564.89
  renal 593.89
  saccule vestibularis, congenital 744.05
  salivary gland (duct) 527.8
  sphincter ani 564.89
  stomach 536.8
    acute 536.1
    psychogenic 306.4
  submaxillary duct 527.8
  trachea, congenital 748.3
  ureter (idiopathic) 593.89
    congenital 753.20
    due to obstruction 593.5
  urethra (acquired) 599.84
  vasomotor 443.9
  vein 459.89
  ventricular, ventricle (acute) (chronic) (*see
    also* Hypertrophy, cardiac) 429.3
    cerebral, congenital 742.4
    hypertensive (*see also* Hypertension,
      heart) 402.90
  venule 459.89
    anus — *see* Hemorrhoids
  vesical orifice 596.89
Dilated, dilation — *see* Dilatation
Diminished
  hearing (acuity) (*see also* Deafness) 389.9
  pulse pressure 785.9
  vision NEC 369.9
  vital capacity 794.2
Diminuta taenia 123.6
Diminution, sense or sensation (cold) (heat)
    (tactile) (vibratory) — *see also* Disturbance, sensation 782.0
Dimitri-Sturge-Weber disease (encephalocutaneous angiomatosis) 759.6
Dimple
  parasacral 685.1
    with abscess 685.0
  pilonidal 685.1
    with abscess 685.0
  postanal 685.1
    with abscess 685.0
Dioctophyma renale (infection) (infestation)
    128.8
Dipetalonemiasis 125.4
Diphallus 752.69
Diphtheria, diphtheritic (gangrenous) (hemorrhagic) 032.9
  carrier (suspected) of V02.4
  cutaneous 032.85
  cystitis 032.84

☑ **Additional Digit Required** — Refer to the Tabular List for Digit Selection

ᵂ **Subterms under main terms may continue to next column or page**

Diphtheria, diphtheritic — *continued*
  faucial 032.0
  infection of wound 032.85
  inoculation (anti) (not sick) V03.5
  laryngeal 032.3
  myocarditis 032.82
  nasal anterior 032.2
  nasopharyngeal 032.1
  neurological complication 032.89
  peritonitis 032.83
  specified site NEC 032.89
Diphyllobothriasis (intestine) 123.4
  larval 123.5
Diplacusis 388.41
Diplegia (upper limbs) 344.2
  brain or cerebral 437.8
  congenital 343.0
  facial 351.0
    congenital 352.6
  infantile or congenital (cerebral) (spastic) (spinal) 343.0
  lower limbs 344.1
  syphilitic, congenital 090.49
Diplococcus, diplococcal — *see* condition
Diplomyelia 742.59
Diplopia 368.2
  refractive 368.15
Dipsomania — *see also* Alcoholism 303.9 ☑
  with psychosis (*see also* Psychosis, alcoholic) 291.9
Dipylidiasis 123.8
  intestine 123.8
Direction, teeth, abnormal 524.30
Dirt-eating child 307.52
Disability, disabilities
  heart — *see* Disease, heart
  intellectual 319
    borderline V62.89
    mild, IQ 50-70 317
    moderate, IQ 35-49 318.0
    profound, IQ under 20 318.2
    severe, IQ 20-34 318.1
  learning NEC 315.2
  special spelling 315.09
Disarticulation — *see also* Derangement, joint 718.9 ☑
  meaning
    amputation
      status — *see* Absence, by site
      traumatic — *see* Amputation, traumatic
    dislocation, traumatic or congenital — *see* Dislocation
Disaster, cerebrovascular — *see also* Disease, cerebrovascular, acute 436
Discharge
  anal NEC 787.99
  breast (female) (male) 611.79
  conjunctiva 372.89
  continued locomotor idiopathic (*see also* Epilepsy) 345.5 ☑
  diencephalic autonomic idiopathic (*see also* Epilepsy) 345.5 ☑
  ear 388.60
    blood 388.69
    cerebrospinal fluid 388.61
  excessive urine 788.42
  eye 379.93
  nasal 478.19
  nipple 611.79
  patterned motor idiopathic (*see also* Epilepsy) 345.5 ☑
  penile 788.7
  postnasal — *see* Sinusitis
  sinus, from mediastinum 510.0
  umbilicus 789.9
  urethral 788.7
    bloody 599.84
  vaginal 623.5
Discitis 722.90
  cervical, cervicothoracic 722.91
  lumbar, lumbosacral 722.93
  thoracic, thoracolumbar 722.92
Discogenic syndrome — *see* Displacement, intervertebral disc

Discoid
  kidney 753.3
  meniscus, congenital 717.5
  semilunar cartilage 717.5
Discoloration
  mouth 528.9
  nails 703.8
  teeth 521.7
    due to
      drugs 521.7
      metals (copper) (silver) 521.7
      pulpal bleeding 521.7
    during formation 520.8
    extrinsic 523.6
    intrinsic posteruptive 521.7
Discomfort
  chest 786.59
  visual 368.13
Discomycosis — *see* Actinomycosis
Discontinuity, ossicles, ossicular chain 385.23
Discrepancy
  centric occlusion
    maximum intercuspation 524.55
    of teeth 524.55
  leg length (acquired) 736.81
    congenital 755.30
  uterine size-date 649.6 ☑
Discrimination
  political V62.4
  racial V62.4
  religious V62.4
  sex V62.4
Disease, diseased — *see also* Syndrome
  Abrami's (acquired hemolytic jaundice) 283.9
  absorbent system 459.89
  accumulation — *see* Thesaurismosis
  acid-peptic 536.8
  Acosta's 993.2
  Adams-Stokes (-Morgagni) (syncope with heart block) 426.9
  Addison's (bronze) (primary adrenal insufficiency) 255.41
    anemia (pernicious) 281.0
    tuberculous (*see also* Tuberculosis) 017.6 ☑
  Addison-Gull — *see* Xanthoma
  adenoids (and tonsils) (chronic) 474.9
  adrenal (gland) (capsule) (cortex) 255.9
    hyperfunction 255.3
    hypofunction 255.41
    specified type NEC 255.8
  ainhum (dactylolysis spontanea) 136.0
  akamushi (scrub typhus) 081.2
  Akureyri (epidemic neuromyasthenia) 049.8
  Albarrán's (colibacilluria) 791.9
  Albers-Schönberg's (marble bones) 756.52
  Albert's 726.71
  Albright (-Martin) (-Bantam) 275.49
  Alibert's (mycosis fungoides) (M9700/3) 202.1 ☑
  Alibert-Bazin (M9700/3) 202.1 ☑
  alimentary canal 569.9
  alligator skin (ichthyosis congenita) 757.1
    acquired 701.1
  Almeida's (Brazilian blastomycosis) 116.1
  Alpers' 330.8
  alpine 993.2
  altitude 993.2
  alveoli, teeth 525.9
  Alzheimer's — *see* Alzheimer's
  amyloid (any site) 277.30
  anarthritic rheumatoid 446.5
  Anders' (adiposis tuberosa simplex) 272.8
  Andersen's (glycogenosis IV) 271.0
  Anderson's (angiokeratoma corporis diffusum) 272.7
  Andes 993.2
  Andrews' (bacterid) 686.8
  angiospastic, angiospasmodic 443.9
    cerebral 435.9
      with transient neurologic deficit 435.9
    vein 459.89

Disease, diseased — *see also* Syndrome — *continued*
  anterior
    chamber 364.9
    horn cell 335.9
      specified type NEC 335.8
  antral (chronic) 473.0
    acute 461.0
  anus NEC 569.49
  aorta (nonsyphilitic) 447.9
    syphilitic NEC 093.89
  aortic (heart) (valve) (*see also* Endocarditis, aortic) 424.1
  apollo 077.4
  aponeurosis 726.90
  appendix 543.9
  aqueous (chamber) 364.9
  arc-welders' lung 503
  Armenian 277.31
  Arnold-Chiari (*see also* Spina bifida) 741.0 ☑
  arterial 447.9
    occlusive (*see also* Occlusion, by site) 444.22
      with embolus or thrombus — *see* Occlusion, by site
      due to stricture or stenosis 447.1
    specified type NEC 447.8
  arteriocardiorenal (*see also* Hypertension, cardiorenal) 404.90
  arteriolar (generalized) (obliterative) 447.9
    specified type NEC 447.8
  arteriorenal — *see* Hypertension, kidney
  arteriosclerotic (*see also* Arteriosclerosis)
    cardiovascular 429.2
    coronary — *see* Arteriosclerosis, coronary
    heart — *see* Arteriosclerosis, coronary
    vascular — *see* Arteriosclerosis
  artery 447.9
    cerebral 437.9
    coronary — *see* Arteriosclerosis, coronary
    specified type NEC 447.8
  arthropod-borne NEC 088.9
    specified type NEC 088.89
  Asboe-Hansen's (incontinentia pigmenti) 757.33
  atticoantral, chronic (with posterior or superior marginal perforation of ear drum) 382.2
  auditory canal, ear 380.9
  Aujeszky's 078.89
  auricle, ear NEC 380.30
  Australian X 062.4
  autoimmune NEC 279.49
    hemolytic (cold type) (warm type) 283.0
    parathyroid 252.1
    thyroid 245.2
  aviators' (*see also* Effect, adverse, high altitude) 993.2
  ax(e)-grinders' 502
  Ayala's 756.89
  Ayerza's (pulmonary artery sclerosis with pulmonary hypertension) 416.0
  Azorean (of the nervous system) 334.8
  Babington's (familial hemorrhagic telangiectasia) 448.0
  back bone NEC 733.90
  bacterial NEC 040.89
    zoonotic NEC 027.9
      specified type NEC 027.8
  Baehr-Schiffrin (thrombotic thrombocytopenic purpura) 446.6
  Baelz's (cheilitis glandularis apostematosa) 528.5
  Baerensprung's (eczema marginatum) 110.3
  Balfour's (chloroma) 205.3 ☑
  balloon (*see also* Effect, adverse, high altitude) 993.2
  Baló's 341.1
  Bamberger (-Marie) (hypertrophic pulmonary osteoarthropathy) 731.2
  Bang's (Brucella abortus) 023.1
  Bannister's 995.1
  Banti's (with cirrhosis) (with portal hypertension) — *see* Cirrhosis, liver

Disease, diseased — *see also* Syndrome — *continued*
  Barcoo (*see also* Ulcer, skin) 707.9
  barium lung 503
  Barlow (-Möller) (infantile scurvy) 267
  barometer makers' 985.0
  Barraquer (-Simons) (progressive lipodystrophy) 272.6
  basal ganglia 333.90
    degenerative NEC 333.0
    specified NEC 333.89
  Basedow's (exophthalmic goiter) 242.0 ☑
  basement membrane NEC 583.89
    with
      pulmonary hemorrhage (Goodpasture's syndrome) 446.21 [583.81]
  Bateman's 078.0
    purpura (senile) 287.2
  Batten's 330.1 [362.71]
  Batten-Mayou (retina) 330.1 [362.71]
  Batten-Steinert 359.21
  Battey 031.0
  Baumgarten-Cruveilhier (cirrhosis of liver) 571.5
  bauxite-workers' 503
  Bayle's (dementia paralytica) 094.1
  Bazin's (primary) (*see also* Tuberculosis) 017.1 ☑
  Beard's (neurasthenia) 300.5
  Beau's (*see also* Degeneration, myocardial) 429.1
  Bechterew's (ankylosing spondylitis) 720.0
  Becker's
    idiopathic mural endomyocardial disease 425.2
    myotonia congenita, recessive form 359.22
  Begbie's (exophthalmic goiter) 242.0 ☑
  Behr's 362.50
  Beigel's (white piedra) 111.2
  Bekhterev's (ankylosing spondylitis) 720.0
  Bell's (*see also* Psychosis, affective) 296.0 ☑
  Bennett's (leukemia) 208.9 ☑
  Benson's 379.22
  Bergeron's (hysteroepilepsy) 300.11
  Berlin's 921.3
  Bernard-Soulier (thrombopathy) 287.1
  Bernhardt (-Roth) 355.1
  beryllium 503
  Besnier-Boeck (-Schaumann) (sarcoidosis) 135
  Best's 362.76
  Beurmann's (sporotrichosis) 117.1
  Bielschowsky (-Jansky) 330.1
  Biermer's (pernicious anemia) 281.0
  Biett's (discoid lupus erythematosus) 695.4
  bile duct (*see also* Disease, biliary) 576.9
  biliary (duct) (tract) 576.9
    with calculus, choledocholithiasis, or stones — *see* Choledocholithiasis
  Billroth's (meningocele) (*see also* Spina bifida) 741.9 ☑
  Binswanger's 290.12
  Bird's (oxaluria) 271.8
  bird fanciers' 495.2
  black lung 500
  bladder 596.9
    specified NEC 596.89
  bleeder's 286.0
  Bloch-Sulzberger (incontinentia pigmenti) 757.33
  Blocq's (astasia-abasia) 307.9
  blood (-forming organs) 289.9
    specified NEC 289.89
    vessel 459.9
  Bloodgood's 610.1
  Blount's (tibia vara) 732.4
  blue 746.9
  Bodechtel-Guttmann (subacute sclerosing panencephalitis) 046.2
  Boeck's (sarcoidosis) 135
  bone 733.90
    fibrocystic NEC 733.29
      jaw 526.2
    marrow 289.9

☑ Additional Digit Required — Refer to the Tabular List for Digit Selection   ᵂ Subterms under main terms may continue to next column or page

2013 ICD-9-CM   ▶◀ Revised Text   ● New Line   ▲ Revised Code   Volume 2 — 81

Diphtheria, diphtheritic — Disease, diseased

Disease, diseased — *see also* Syndrome — *continued*

bone — *continued*
Paget's (osteitis deformans) 731.0
specified type NEC 733.99
von Recklinghausen's (osteitis fibrosa cystica) 252.01
Bonfils' — *see* Disease, Hodgkin's
Borna 062.9
Bornholm (epidemic pleurodynia) 074.1
Bostock's (*see also* Fever, hay) 477.9
Bouchard's (myopathic dilatation of the stomach) 536.1
Bouillaud's (rheumatic heart disease) 391.9
Bourneville (-Brissaud) (tuberous sclerosis) 759.5
Bouveret (-Hoffmann) (paroxysmal tachycardia) 427.2
bowel 569.9
functional 564.9
psychogenic 306.4
Bowen's (M8081/2) — *see* Neoplasm, skin, in situ
Bozzolo's (multiple myeloma) (M9730/3) 203.0 ☑
Bradley's (epidemic vomiting) 078.82
Brailsford's 732.3
radius, head 732.3
tarsal, scaphoid 732.5
Brailsford-Morquio (mucopolysaccharidosis IV) 277.5
brain 348.9
Alzheimer's 331.0
with dementia — *see* Alzheimer's, dementia
arterial, artery 437.9
arteriosclerotic 437.0
congenital 742.9
degenerative — *see* Degeneration, brain
inflammatory (*see also* Encephalitis)
late effect — *see* category 326
organic 348.9
arteriosclerotic 437.0
parasitic NEC 123.9
Pick's 331.11
with dementia
with behavioral disturbance 331.11 [294.11]
without behavioral disturbance 331.11 [294.10]
senile 331.2
braziers' 985.8
breast 611.9
cystic (chronic) 610.1
fibrocystic 610.1
inflammatory 611.0
Paget's (M8540/3) 174.0
puerperal, postpartum NEC 676.3 ☑
specified NEC 611.89
Breda's (*see also* Yaws) 102.9
Breisky's (kraurosis vulvae) 624.09
Bretonneau's (diphtheritic malignant angina) 032.0
Bright's (*see also* Nephritis) 583.9
arteriosclerotic (*see also* Hypertension, kidney) 403.90
Brill's (recrudescent typhus) 081.1
flea-borne 081.0
louse-borne 081.1
Brill-Symmers (follicular lymphoma) (M9690/3) 202.0 ☑
Brill-Zinsser (recrudescent typhus) 081.1
Brinton's (leather bottle stomach) (M8142/3) 151.9
Brion-Kayser (*see also* Fever, paratyphoid) 002.9
broad
beta 272.2
ligament, noninflammatory 620.9
specified NEC 620.8
Brocq's 691.8
meaning
atopic (diffuse) neurodermatitis 691.8
dermatitis herpetiformis 694.0
lichen simplex chronicus 698.3

Disease, diseased — *see also* Syndrome — *continued*

Brocq's — *continued*
meaning — *continued*
parapsoriasis 696.2
prurigo 698.2
Brocq-Duhring (dermatitis herpetiformis) 694.0
Brodie's (joint) (*see also* Osteomyelitis) 730.1 ☑
bronchi 519.19
bronchopulmonary 519.19
bronze (Addison's) 255.41
tuberculous (*see also* Tuberculosis) 017.6 ☑
Brown-Séquard 344.89
Bruck's 733.99
Bruck-de Lange (Amsterdam dwarf, intellectual disabilities, and brachycephaly) 759.89
Bruhl's (splenic anemia with fever) 285.8
Bruton's (X-linked agammaglobulinemia) 279.04
buccal cavity 528.9
Buchanan's (juvenile osteochondrosis, iliac crest) 732.1
Buchman's (osteochondrosis juvenile) 732.1
Budgerigar-Fanciers' 495.2
Büdinger-Ludloff-Läwen 717.89
Buerger's (thromboangiitis obliterans) 443.1
Bürger-Grütz (essential familial hyperlipemia) 272.3
Burns' (lower ulna) 732.3
bursa 727.9
Bury's (erythema elevatum diutinum) 695.89
Buschke's 710.1
Busquet's (*see also* Osteomyelitis) 730.1 ☑
Busse-Buschke (cryptococcosis) 117.5
C₂ (*see also* Alcoholism) 303.9 ☑
Caffey's (infantile cortical hyperostosis) 756.59
caisson 993.3
calculous 592.9
California 114.0
Calvé (-Perthes) (osteochondrosis, femoral capital) 732.1
Camurati-Engelmann (diaphyseal sclerosis) 756.59
Canavan's 330.0
capillaries 448.9
Carapata 087.1
cardiac — *see* Disease, heart
cardiopulmonary, chronic 416.9
cardiorenal (arteriosclerotic) (hepatic) (hypertensive) (vascular) (*see also* Hypertension, cardiorenal) 404.90
cardiovascular (arteriosclerotic) 429.2
congenital 746.9
hypertensive (*see also* Hypertension, heart) 402.90
benign 402.10
malignant 402.00
renal (*see also* Hypertension, cardiorenal) 404.90
syphilitic (asymptomatic) 093.9
carotid gland 259.8
Carrión's (Bartonellosis) 088.0
cartilage NEC 733.90
specified NEC 733.99
Castellani's 104.8
cat-scratch 078.3
Cavare's (familial periodic paralysis) 359.3
Cazenave's (pemphigus) 694.4
cecum 569.9
celiac (adult) 579.0
infantile 579.0
cellular tissue NEC 709.9
central core 359.0
cerebellar, cerebellum — *see* Disease, brain
cerebral (*see also* Disease, brain) 348.9
arterial, artery 437.9
degenerative — *see* Degeneration, brain
cerebrospinal 349.9
cerebrovascular NEC 437.9
acute 436
embolic — *see* Embolism, brain

Disease, diseased — *see also* Syndrome — *continued*

cerebrovascular — *continued*
acute — *continued*
late effect — *see* Late effect(s) (of) cerebrovascular disease
puerperal, postpartum, childbirth 674.0 ☑
thrombotic — *see* Thrombosis, brain
arteriosclerotic 437.0
embolic — *see* Embolism, brain
ischemic, generalized NEC 437.1
late effect — *see* Late effect(s) (of) cerebrovascular disease
occlusive 437.1
puerperal, postpartum, childbirth 674.0 ☑
specified type NEC 437.8
thrombotic — *see* Thrombosis, brain
ceroid storage 272.7
cervix (uteri)
inflammatory 616.0
noninflammatory 622.9
specified NEC 622.8
Chabert's 022.9
Chagas' (*see also* Trypanosomiasis, American) 086.2
Chandler's (osteochondritis dissecans, hip) 732.7
Charcôt-Marie-Tooth 356.1
Charcôt's (joint) 094.0 [713.5]
spinal cord 094.0
Charlouis' (*see also* Yaws) 102.9
Cheadle (-Möller) (-Barlow) (infantile scurvy) 267
Chédiak-Steinbrinck (-Higashi) (congenital gigantism of peroxidase granules) 288.2
cheek, inner 528.9
chest 519.9
Chiari's (hepatic vein thrombosis) 453.0
Chicago (North American blastomycosis) 116.0
chignon (white piedra) 111.2
chigoe, chigo (jigger) 134.1
childhood granulomatous 288.1
Chinese liver fluke 121.1
chlamydial NEC 078.88
cholecystic (*see also* Disease, gallbladder) 575.9
choroid 363.9
degenerative (*see also* Degeneration, choroid) 363.40
hereditary (*see also* Dystrophy, choroid) 363.50
specified type NEC 363.8
Christian's (chronic histiocytosis X) 277.89
Christian-Weber (nodular nonsuppurative panniculitis) 729.30
Christmas 286.1
ciliary body 364.9
specified NEC 364.89
circulatory (system) NEC 459.9
chronic, maternal, affecting fetus or newborn 760.3
specified NEC 459.89
syphilitic 093.9
congenital 090.5
Civatte's (poikiloderma) 709.09
climacteric 627.2
male 608.89
coagulation factor deficiency (congenital) (*see also* Defect, coagulation) 286.9
Coats' 362.12
coccidioidal pulmonary 114.5
acute 114.0
chronic 114.4
primary 114.0
residual 114.4
Cockayne's (microcephaly and dwarfism) 759.89
Cogan's 370.52
cold
agglutinin 283.0
or hemoglobinuria 283.0

Disease, diseased — *see also* Syndrome — *continued*

cold — *continued*
agglutinin — *continued*
or hemoglobinuria — *continued*
paroxysmal (cold) (nocturnal) 283.2
hemagglutinin (chronic) 283.0
collagen NEC 710.9
nonvascular 710.9
specified NEC 710.8
vascular (allergic) (*see also* Angiitis, hypersensitivity) 446.20
colon 569.9
functional 564.9
congenital 751.3
ischemic 557.0
combined system (of spinal cord) 266.2 [336.2]
with anemia (pernicious) 281.0 [336.2]
compressed air 993.3
Concato's (pericardial polyserositis) 423.2
peritoneal 568.82
pleural — *see* Pleurisy
congenital NEC 799.89
conjunctiva 372.9
chlamydial 077.98
specified NEC 077.8
specified type NEC 372.89
viral 077.99
specified NEC 077.8
connective tissue, diffuse (*see also* Disease, collagen) 710.9
Conor and Bruch's (boutonneuse fever) 082.1
Conradi (-Hünermann) 756.59
Cooley's (erythroblastic anemia) 282.44
Cooper's 610.1
Corbus' 607.1
cork-handlers' 495.3
cornea (*see also* Keratopathy) 371.9
coronary (*see also* Ischemia, heart) 414.9
congenital 746.85
ostial, syphilitic 093.20
aortic 093.22
mitral 093.21
pulmonary 093.24
tricuspid 093.23
Corrigan's — *see* Insufficiency, aortic
Cotugno's 724.3
Coxsackie (virus) NEC 074.8
cranial nerve NEC 352.9
Creutzfeldt-Jakob (CJD) 046.19
with dementia
with behavioral disturbance 046.19 [294.11]
without behavioral disturbance 046.19 [294.10]
familial 046.19
iatrogenic 046.19
specified NEC 046.19
sporadic 046.19
variant (vCJD) 046.11
with dementia
with behavioral disturbance 046.11 [294.11]
without behavioral disturbance 046.11 [294.10]
Crigler-Najjar (congenital hyperbilirubinemia) 277.4
Crocq's (acrocyanosis) 443.89
Crohn's (intestine) (*see also* Enteritis, regional) 555.9
Crouzon's (craniofacial dysostosis) 756.0
Cruchet's (encephalitis lethargica) 049.8
Cruveilhier's 335.21
Cruz-Chagas (*see also* Trypanosomiasis, American) 086.2
crystal deposition (*see also* Arthritis, due to, crystals) 712.9 ☑
Csillag's (lichen sclerosus et atrophicus) 701.0
Curschmann's 359.21
Cushing's (pituitary basophilism) 255.0
cystic
breast (chronic) 610.1

Disease, diseased — *see also* Syndrome — *continued*

cystic — *continued*

kidney, congenital (*see also* Cystic, disease, kidney) 753.10

liver, congenital 751.62

lung 518.89

congenital 748.4

pancreas 577.2

congenital 751.7

renal, congenital (*see also* Cystic, disease, kidney) 753.10

semilunar cartilage 717.5

cysticercus 123.1

cystine storage (with renal sclerosis) 270.0

cytomegalic inclusion (generalized) 078.5

with

pneumonia 078.5 [484.1]

congenital 771.1

Daae (-Finsen) (epidemic pleurodynia) 074.1

dancing 297.8

Danielssen's (anesthetic leprosy) 030.1

Darier's (congenital) (keratosis follicularis) 757.39

erythema annulare centrifugum 695.0

vitamin A deficiency 264.8

Darling's (histoplasmosis) (*see also* Histoplasmosis, American) 115.00

Davies' 425.0

de Beurmann-Gougerot (sporotrichosis) 117.1

Débove's (splenomegaly) 789.2

deer fly (*see also* Tularemia) 021.9

deficiency 269.9

degenerative (*see also* Degeneration)

disc — *see* Degeneration, intervertebral disc

Degos' 447.8

Déjérine (-Sottas) 356.0

Déleage's 359.89

demyelinating, demyelinizating (brain stem) (central nervous system) 341.9

multiple sclerosis 340

specified NEC 341.8

de Quervain's (tendon sheath) 727.04

thyroid (subacute granulomatous thyroiditis) 245.1

Dercum's (adiposis dolorosa) 272.8

Deutschländer's — *see* Fracture, foot

Devergie's (pityriasis rubra pilaris) 696.4

Devic's 341.0

diaphorase deficiency 289.7

diaphragm 519.4

diarrheal, infectious 009.2

diatomaceous earth 502

Diaz's (osteochondrosis astragalus) 732.5

digestive system 569.9

Di Guglielmo's (erythemic myelosis) (M9841/3) 207.0 ☑

Dimitri-Sturge-Weber (encephalocutaneous angiomatosis) 759.6

disc, degenerative — *see* Degeneration, intervertebral disc

discogenic (*see also* Disease, intervertebral disc) 722.90

diverticular — *see* Diverticula

Down's (mongolism) 758.0

Dubini's (electric chorea) 049.8

Dubois' (thymus gland) 090.5

Duchenne's 094.0

locomotor ataxia 094.0

muscular dystrophy 359.1

paralysis 335.22

pseudohypertrophy, muscles 359.1

Duchenne-Griesinger 359.1

ductless glands 259.9

Duhring's (dermatitis herpetiformis) 694.0

Dukes (-Filatov) 057.8

duodenum NEC 537.9

specified NEC 537.89

Duplay's 726.2

Dupré's (meningism) 781.6

Dupuytren's (muscle contracture) 728.6

Durand-Nicolas-Favre (climatic bubo) 099.1

Duroziez's (congenital mitral stenosis) 746.5

Dutton's (trypanosomiasis) 086.9

Disease, diseased — *see also* Syndrome — *continued*

Eales' 362.18

ear (chronic) (inner) NEC 388.9

middle 385.9

adhesive (*see also* Adhesions, middle ear) 385.10

specified NEC 385.89

Eberth's (typhoid fever) 002.0

Ebstein's

heart 746.2

meaning diabetes 250.4 ☑ [581.81]

due to secondary diabetes 249.4 ☑ [581.81]

Echinococcus (*see also* Echinococcus) 122.9

ECHO virus NEC 078.89

Economo's (encephalitis lethargica) 049.8

Eddowes' (brittle bones and blue sclera) 756.51

Edsall's 992.2

Eichstedt's (pityriasis versicolor) 111.0

Ellis-van Creveld (chondroectodermal dysplasia) 756.55

endocardium — *see* Endocarditis

endocrine glands or system NEC 259.9

specified NEC 259.8

endomyocardial, idiopathic mural 425.2

Engelmann's (diaphyseal sclerosis) 756.59

Engel-von Recklinghausen (osteitis fibrosa cystica) 252.01

English (rickets) 268.0

Engman's (infectious eczematoid dermatitis) 690.8

enteroviral, enterovirus NEC 078.89

central nervous system NEC 048

epidemic NEC 136.9

epididymis 608.9

epigastric, functional 536.9

psychogenic 306.4

Erb (-Landouzy) 359.1

Erb-Goldflam 358.00

Erdheim-Chester (ECD) 277.89

Erichsen's (railway spine) 300.16

esophagus 530.9

functional 530.5

psychogenic 306.4

Eulenburg's (congenital paramyotonia) 359.29

Eustachian tube 381.9

Evans' (thrombocytopenic purpura) 287.32

external auditory canal 380.9

extrapyramidal NEC 333.90

eye 379.90

anterior chamber 364.9

inflammatory NEC 364.3

muscle 378.9

eyeball 360.9

eyelid 374.9

eyeworm of Africa 125.2

Fabry's (angiokeratoma corporis diffusum) 272.7

facial nerve (seventh) 351.9

newborn 767.5

Fahr-Volhard (malignant nephrosclerosis) 403.00

fallopian tube, noninflammatory 620.9

specified NEC 620.8

familial periodic 277.31

paralysis 359.3

Fanconi's (congenital pancytopenia) 284.09

Farber's (disseminated lipogranulomatosis) 272.8

fascia 728.9

inflammatory 728.9

Fauchard's (periodontitis) 523.40

Favre-Durand-Nicolas (climatic bubo) 099.1

Favre-Racouchot (elastoidosis cutanea nodularis) 701.8

Fede's 529.0

Feer's 985.0

Felix's (juvenile osteochondrosis, hip) 732.1

Fenwick's (gastric atrophy) 537.89

Fernels' (aortic aneurysm) 441.9

fibrocaseous, of lung (*see also* Tuberculosis, pulmonary) 011.9 ☑

fibrocystic (*see also* Fibrocystic, disease)

Disease, diseased — *see also* Syndrome — *continued*

fibrocystic (*see also* Fibrocystic, disease) — *continued*

newborn 277.01

Fiedler's (leptospiral jaundice) 100.0

fifth 057.0

Filatoff's (infectious mononucleosis) 075

Filatov's (infectious mononucleosis) 075

file-cutters' 984.9

specified type of lead — *see* Table of Drugs and Chemicals

filterable virus NEC 078.89

fish skin 757.1

acquired 701.1

Flajani (-Basedow) (exophthalmic goiter) 242.0 ☑

Flatau-Schilder 341.1

flax-dressers' 504

Fleischner's 732.3

flint 502

fluke — *see* Infestation, fluke

Følling's (phenylketonuria) 270.1

foot and mouth 078.4

foot process 581.3

Forbes' (glycogenosis III) 271.0

Fordyce's (ectopic sebaceous glands) (mouth) 750.26

Fordyce-Fox (apocrine miliaria) 705.82

Fothergill's

meaning scarlatina anginosa 034.1

neuralgia (*see also* Neuralgia, trigeminal) 350.1

Fournier's 608.83

female 616.89

fourth 057.8

Fox (-Fordyce) (apocrine miliaria) 705.82

Francis' (*see also* Tularemia) 021.9

Franklin's (heavy chain) 273.2

Frei's (climatic bubo) 099.1

Freiberg's (flattening metatarsal) 732.5

Friedländer's (endarteritis obliterans) — *see* Arteriosclerosis

Friedreich's

combined systemic or ataxia 334.0

facial hemihypertrophy 756.0

myoclonia 333.2

Fröhlich's (adiposogenital dystrophy) 253.8

Frommel's 676.6 ☑

frontal sinus (chronic) 473.1

acute 461.1

Fuller's earth 502

fungus, fungous NEC 117.9

Gaisböck's (polycythemia hypertonica) 289.0

gallbladder 575.9

congenital 751.60

Gamna's (siderotic splenomegaly) 289.51

Gamstorp's (adynamia episodica hereditaria) 359.3

Gandy-Nanta (siderotic splenomegaly) 289.51

Gannister (occupational) 502

Garré's (*see also* Osteomyelitis) 730.1 ☑

gastric (*see also* Disease, stomach) 537.9

gastroesophageal reflux (GERD) 530.81

gastrointestinal (tract) 569.9

amyloid 277.39

functional 536.9

psychogenic 306.4

Gaucher's (adult) (cerebroside lipidosis) (infantile) 272.7

Gayet's (superior hemorrhagic polioencephalitis) 265.1

Gee (-Herter) (-Heubner) (-Thaysen) (nontropical sprue) 579.0

generalized neoplastic (M8000/6) 199.0

genital organs NEC

female 629.9

specified NEC 629.89

male 608.9

Gerhardt's (erythromelalgia) 443.82

Gerlier's (epidemic vertigo) 078.81

Gibert's (pityriasis rosea) 696.3

Gibney's (perispondylitis) 720.9

Gierke's (glycogenosis I) 271.0

Disease, diseased — *see also* Syndrome — *continued*

Gilbert's (familial nonhemolytic jaundice) 277.4

Gilchrist's (North American blastomycosis) 116.0

Gilford (-Hutchinson) (progeria) 259.8

Gilles de la Tourette's (motor-verbal tic) 307.23

Giovannini's 117.9

gland (lymph) 289.9

Glanzmann's (hereditary hemorrhagic thrombasthenia) 287.1

glassblowers' 527.1

Glénard's (enteroptosis) 569.89

Glisson's (*see also* Rickets) 268.0

glomerular

membranous, idiopathic 581.1

minimal change 581.3

glycogen storage (Andersen's) (Cori types 1-7) (Forbes') (McArdle-Schmid-Pearson) (Pompe's) (types I-VII) 271.0

cardiac 271.0 [425.7]

generalized 271.0

glucose–6–phosphatase deficiency 271.0

heart 271.0 [425.7]

hepatorenal 271.0

liver and kidneys 271.0

myocardium 271.0 [425.7]

von Gierke's (glycogenosis I) 271.0

Goldflam-Erb 358.00

Goldscheider's (epidermolysis bullosa) 757.39

Goldstein's (familial hemorrhagic telangiectasia) 448.0

gonococcal NEC 098.0

Goodall's (epidemic vomiting) 078.82

Gordon's (exudative enteropathy) 579.8

Gougerot's (trisymptomatic) 709.1

Gougerot-Carteaud (confluent reticulate papillomatosis) 701.8

Gougerot-Hailey-Hailey (benign familial chronic pemphigus) 757.39

graft-versus-host 279.50

acute 279.51

on chronic 279.53

chronic 279.52

grain-handlers' 495.8

Grancher's (splenopneumonia) — *see* Pneumonia

granulomatous (childhood) (chronic) 288.1

graphite lung 503

Graves' (exophthalmic goiter) 242.0 ☑

Greenfield's 330.0

green monkey 078.89

Griesinger's (*see also* Ancylostomiasis) 126.9

grinders' 502

Grisel's 723.5

Gruby's (tinea tonsurans) 110.0

Guertin's (electric chorea) 049.8

Guillain-Barré 357.0

Guinon's (motor-verbal tic) 307.23

Gull's (thyroid atrophy with myxedema) 244.8

Gull and Sutton's — *see* Hypertension, kidney

gum NEC 523.9

Günther's (congenital erythropoietic porphyria) 277.1

gynecological 629.9

specified NEC 629.89

H 270.0

Haas' 732.3

Habermann's (acute parapsoriasis varioliformis) 696.2

Haff 985.1

Hageman (congenital factor XII deficiency) (*see also* Defect, congenital) 286.3

Haglund's (osteochondrosis os tibiale externum) 732.5

Hagner's (hypertrophic pulmonary osteoarthropathy) 731.2

Hailey-Hailey (benign familial chronic pemphigus) 757.39

hair (follicles) NEC 704.9

Disease, diseased — *see also* Syndrome — *continued*
  hair — *continued*
    specified type NEC 704.8
  Hallervorden-Spatz 333.0
  Hallopeau's (lichen sclerosus et atrophicus) 701.0
  Hamman's (spontaneous mediastinal emphysema) 518.1
  hand, foot, and mouth 074.3
  Hand-Schüller-Christian (chronic histiocytosis X) 277.89
  Hanot's — *see* Cirrhosis, biliary
  Hansen's (leprosy) 030.9
    benign form 030.1
    malignant form 030.0
  Harada's 363.22
  Harley's (intermittent hemoglobinuria) 283.2
  Hartnup (pellagra-cerebellar ataxia-renal aminoaciduria) 270.0
  Hart's (pellagra-cerebellar ataxia-renal aminoaciduria) 270.0
  Hashimoto's (struma lymphomatosa) 245.2
  Hb — *see* Disease, hemoglobin
  heart (organic) 429.9
    with
      acute pulmonary edema (*see also* Failure, ventricular, left) 428.1
      hypertensive 402.91
        with renal failure 404.93
        benign 402.11
          with renal failure 404.13
        malignant 402.01
          with renal failure 404.03
      kidney disease — *see* Hypertension, cardiorenal
      rheumatic fever (conditions classifiable to 390)
        active 391.9
          with chorea 392.0
        inactive or quiescent (with chorea) 398.90
    amyloid 277.39 *[425.7]*
    aortic (valve) (*see also* Endocarditis, aortic) 424.1
    arteriosclerotic or sclerotic (minimal) (senile) — *see* Arteriosclerosis, coronary
    artery, arterial — *see* Arteriosclerosis, coronary
    atherosclerotic — *see* Arteriosclerosis, coronary
    beer drinkers' 425.5
    beriberi 265.0 *[425.7]*
    black 416.0
    congenital NEC 746.9
      cyanotic 746.9
      maternal, affecting fetus or newborn 760.3
      specified type NEC 746.89
    congestive (*see also* Failure, heart) 428.0
    coronary 414.9
    cryptogenic 429.9
    due to
      amyloidosis 277.39 *[425.7]*
      beriberi 265.0 *[425.7]*
      cardiac glycogenosis 271.0 *[425.7]*
      Friedreich's ataxia 334.0 *[425.8]*
      gout 274.82
      mucopolysaccharidosis 277.5 *[425.7]*
      myotonia atrophica 359.21 *[425.8]*
      progressive muscular dystrophy 359.1 *[425.8]*
      sarcoidosis 135 *[425.8]*
    fetal 746.9
      inflammatory 746.89
    fibroid (*see also* Myocarditis) 429.0
    functional 427.9
      postoperative 997.1
      psychogenic 306.2
    glycogen storage 271.0 *[425.7]*
    gonococcal NEC 098.85
    gouty 274.82
    hypertensive (*see also* Hypertension, heart) 402.90

Disease, diseased — *see also* Syndrome — *continued*
  heart — *continued*
    hypertensive (*see also* Hypertension, heart) — *continued*
      benign 402.10
      malignant 402.00
    hyperthyroid (*see also* Hyperthyroidism) 242.9 ☑ *[425.7]*
    incompletely diagnosed — *see* Disease, heart
    ischemic (chronic) (*see also* Ischemia, heart) 414.9
      acute (*see also* Infarct, myocardium) 410.9 ☑
        without myocardial infarction 411.89
          with coronary (artery) occlusion 411.81
      asymptomatic 412
      diagnosed on ECG or other special investigation but currently presenting no symptoms 412
    kyphoscoliotic 416.1
    mitral (*see also* Endocarditis, mitral) 394.9
    muscular (*see also* Degeneration, myocardial) 429.1
    postpartum 674.8 ☑
    psychogenic (functional) 306.2
    pulmonary (chronic) 416.9
      acute 415.0
      specified NEC 416.8
    rheumatic (chronic) (inactive) (old) (quiescent) (with chorea) 398.90
      active or acute 391.9
        with chorea (active) (rheumatic) (Sydenham's) 392.0
        specified type NEC 391.8
      maternal, affecting fetus or newborn 760.3
    rheumatoid — *see* Arthritis, rheumatoid
    sclerotic — *see* Arteriosclerosis, coronary
    senile (*see also* Myocarditis) 429.0
    specified type NEC 429.89
    syphilitic 093.89
      aortic 093.1
        aneurysm 093.0
      asymptomatic 093.89
      congenital 090.5
    thyroid (gland) (*see also* Hyper-thyroidism) 242.9 ☑ *[425.7]*
    thyrotoxic (*see also* Thyrotoxicosis) 242.9 ☑ *[425.7]*
    tuberculous (*see also* Tuberculosis) 017.9 ☑ *[425.8]*
    valve, valvular (obstructive) (regurgitant) (*see also* Endocarditis)
      congenital NEC (*see also* Anomaly, heart, valve) 746.9
      pulmonary 746.00
        specified type NEC 746.89
    vascular — *see* Disease, cardiovascular
  heavy-chain (gamma G) 273.2
  Heberden's 715.04
  Hebra's
    dermatitis exfoliativa 695.89
    erythema multiforme exudativum 695.19
    pityriasis
      maculata et circinata 696.3
      rubra 695.89
        pilaris 696.4
    prurigo 698.2
  Heerfordt's (uveoparotitis) 135
  Heidenhain's 290.10
    with dementia 290.10
  Heilmeyer-Schöner (M9842/3) 207.1 ☑
  Heine-Medin (*see also* Poliomyelitis) 045.9 ☑
  Heller's (*see also* Psychosis, childhood) 299.1 ☑
  Heller-Döhle (syphilitic aortitis) 093.1
  hematopoietic organs 289.9
  hemoglobin (Hb) 282.7
    with thalassemia 282.49

Disease, diseased — *see also* Syndrome — *continued*
  hemoglobin — *continued*
    abnormal (mixed) NEC 282.7
      with thalassemia 282.49
    AS genotype 282.5
    Bart's 282.43
    C (Hb-C) 282.7
      with other abnormal hemoglobin NEC 282.7
      elliptocytosis 282.7
      Hb-S (without crisis) 282.63
        with
          crisis 282.64
          vaso-occlusive pain 282.64
      sickle-cell (without crisis) 282.63
        with
          crisis 282.64
          vaso-occlusive pain 282.64
      thalassemia 282.49
    constant spring 282.7
    D (Hb-D) 282.7
      with other abnormal hemoglobin NEC 282.7
      Hb-S (without crisis) 282.68
        with crisis 282.69
      sickle-cell (without crisis) 282.68
        with crisis 282.69
      thalassemia 282.49
    E (Hb-E) 282.7
      with other abnormal hemoglobin NEC 282.7
      Hb-S (without crisis) 282.68
        with crisis 282.69
      sickle-cell (without crisis) 282.68
        with crisis 282.69
      thalassemia 282.47
    elliptocytosis 282.7
    F (Hb-F) 282.7
    G (Hb-G) 282.7
    H (Hb-H) 282.43
    hereditary persistence, fetal (HPFH) ("Swiss variety") 282.7
    high fetal gene 282.7
    I thalassemia 282.49
    M 289.7
    S (*see also* Disease, sickle-cell, Hb-S)
      thalassemia (without crisis) 282.41
        with
          crisis 282.42
          vaso-occlusive pain 282.42
    spherocytosis 282.7
    unstable, hemolytic 282.7
    Zurich (Hb-Zurich) 282.7
  hemolytic (fetus) (newborn) 773.2
    autoimmune (cold type) (warm type) 283.0
    due to or with
      incompatibility
        ABO (blood group) 773.1
        blood (group) (Duffy) (Kell) (Kidd) (Lewis) (M) (S) NEC 773.2
        Rh (blood group) (factor) 773.0
      Rh negative mother 773.0
    unstable hemoglobin 282.7
  hemorrhagic 287.9
    newborn 776.0
  Henoch (-Schönlein) (purpura nervosa) 287.0
  hepatic — *see* Disease, liver
  hepatolenticular 275.1
  heredodegenerative NEC
    brain 331.89
    spinal cord 336.8
  Hers' (glycogenosis VI) 271.0
  Herter (-Gee) (-Heubner) (nontropical sprue) 579.0
  Herxheimer's (diffuse idiopathic cutaneous atrophy) 701.8
  Heubner's 094.89
  Heubner-Herter (nontropical sprue) 579.0
  high fetal gene or hemoglobin thalassemia (*see also* Thalassemia) 282.40
  Hildenbrand's (typhus) 081.9
  hip (joint) NEC 719.95
    congenital 755.63

Disease, diseased — *see also* Syndrome — *continued*
  hip — *continued*
    suppurative 711.05
    tuberculous (*see also* Tuberculosis) 015.1 ☑ *[730.85]*
  Hippel's (retinocerebral angiomatosis) 759.6
  Hirschfeld's (acute diabetes mellitus) (*see also* Diabetes) 250.0 ☑
    due to secondary diabetes 249.0 ☑
  Hirschsprung's (congenital megacolon) 751.3
  His (-Werner) (trench fever) 083.1
  HIV 042
  Hodgkin's (M9650/3) 201.9 ☑

> **Note** — *Use the following fifth-digit subclassification with category 201:*
>
> 0   *unspecified site*
>
> 1   *lymph nodes of head, face, and neck*
>
> 2   *intrathoracic lymph nodes*
>
> 3   *intra-abdominal lymph nodes*
>
> 4   *lymph nodes of axilla and upper limb*
>
> 5   *lymph nodes of inguinal region and lower limb*
>
> 6   *intrapelvic lymph nodes*
>
> 7   *spleen*
>
> 8   *lymph nodes of multiple sites*

    lymphocytic
      depletion (M9653/3) 201.7 ☑
        diffuse fibrosis (M9654/3) 201.7 ☑
        reticular type (M9655/3) 201.7 ☑
      predominance (M9651/3) 201.4 ☑
    lymphocytic-histiocytic predominance (M9651/3) 201.4 ☑
    mixed cellularity (M9652/3) 201.6 ☑
    nodular sclerosis (M9656/3) 201.5 ☑
      cellular phase (M9657/3) 201.5 ☑
  Hodgson's 441.9
    ruptured 441.5
  Hoffa (-Kastert) (liposynovitis prepatellaris) 272.8
  Holla (*see also* Spherocytosis) 282.0
  homozygous-Hb-S 282.61
  hoof and mouth 078.4
  hookworm (*see also* Ancylostomiasis) 126.9
  Horton's (temporal arteritis) 446.5
  host-versus-graft (immune or nonimmune cause) 279.50
  HPFH (hereditary persistence of fetal hemoglobin) ("Swiss variety") 282.7
  Huchard's disease (continued arterial hypertension) 401.9
  Huguier's (uterine fibroma) 218.9
  human immunodeficiency (virus) 042
  hunger 251.1
  Hunt's
    dyssynergia cerebellaris myoclonica 334.2
    herpetic geniculate ganglionitis 053.11
  Huntington's 333.4
  Huppert's (multiple myeloma) (M9730/3) 203.0 ☑
  Hurler's (mucopolysaccharidosis I) 277.5
  Hutchinson-Boeck (sarcoidosis) 135
  Hutchinson-Gilford (progeria) 259.8
  Hutchinson's, meaning
    angioma serpiginosum 709.1
    cheiropompholyx 705.81
    prurigo estivalis 692.72
  hyaline (diffuse) (generalized) 728.9
    membrane (lung) (newborn) 769
  hydatid (*see also* Echinococcus) 122.9
  Hyde's (prurigo nodularis) 698.3
  hyperkinetic (*see also* Hyperkinesia) 314.9
    heart 429.82
  hypertensive (*see also* Hypertension) 401.9
  hypophysis 253.9
    hyperfunction 253.1

☑ **Additional Digit Required — Refer to the Tabular List for Digit Selection**   ⬙ **Subterms under main terms may continue to next column or page**

84 — Volume 2   ▶◀ Revised Text   ● New Line   ▲ Revised Code   2013 ICD-9-CM

Disease, diseased — *see also* Syndrome — *continued*

hypophysis — *continued*
   hypofunction 253.2
Iceland (epidemic neuromyasthenia) 049.8
I cell 272.7
ill-defined 799.89
immunologic NEC 279.9
immunoproliferative 203.8 ☑
inclusion 078.5
   salivary gland 078.5
infancy, early NEC 779.9
infective NEC 136.9
inguinal gland 289.9
internal semilunar cartilage, cystic 717.5
intervertebral disc 722.90
   with myelopathy 722.70
   cervical, cervicothoracic 722.91
      with myelopathy 722.71
   lumbar, lumbosacral 722.93
      with myelopathy 722.73
   thoracic, thoracolumbar 722.92
      with myelopathy 722.72
intestine 569.9
   functional 564.9
      congenital 751.3
      psychogenic 306.4
   lardaceous 277.39
   organic 569.9
   protozoal NEC 007.9
iris 364.9
   specified NEC 364.89
iron
   metabolism (*see also* Hemochromatosis) 275.09
   storage (*see also* Hemochromatosis) 275.03
Isambert's (*see also* Tuberculosis, larynx) 012.3 ☑
Iselin's (osteochondrosis, fifth metatarsal) 732.5
island (scrub typhus) 081.2
itai-itai 985.5
Jadassohn's (maculopapular erythroderma) 696.2
Jadassohn-Pellizari's (anetoderma) 701.3
Jakob-Creutzfeldt (CJD) 046.19
   with dementia
      with behavioral disturbance 046.19 *[294.11]*
      without behavioral disturbance 046.19 *[294.10]*
   familial 046.19
   iatrogenic 046.19
   specified NEC 046.19
   sporadic 046.19
   variant (vCJD) 046.11
      with dementia
         with behavioral disturbance 046.11 *[294.11]*
         without behavioral disturbance 046.11 *[294.10]*
Jaksch (-Luzet) (pseudoleukemia infantum) 285.8
Janet's 300.89
Jansky-Bielschowsky 330.1
jaw NEC 526.9
   fibrocystic 526.2
Jensen's 363.05
Jeune's (asphyxiating thoracic dystrophy) 756.4
jigger 134.1
Johnson-Stevens (erythema multiforme exudativum) 695.13
joint NEC 719.9 ☑
   ankle 719.97
   Charcôt 094.0 *[713.5]*
   degenerative (*see also* Osteoarthrosis) 715.9 ☑
      multiple 715.09
      spine (*see also* Spondylosis) 721.90
   elbow 719.92
   foot 719.97
   hand 719.94
   hip 719.95

Disease, diseased — *see also* Syndrome — *continued*

joint — *continued*
   hypertrophic (chronic) (degenerative) (*see also* Osteoarthrosis) 715.9 ☑
      spine (*see also* Spondylosis) 721.90
   knee 719.96
   Luschka 721.90
   multiple sites 719.99
   pelvic region 719.95
   sacroiliac 724.6
   shoulder (region) 719.91
   specified site NEC 719.98
   spine NEC 724.9
      pseudarthrosis following fusion 733.82
      sacroiliac 724.6
   wrist 719.93
Jourdain's (acute gingivitis) 523.00
Jüngling's (sarcoidosis) 135
Kahler (-Bozzolo) (multiple myeloma) (M9730/3) 203.0 ☑
Kalischer's 759.6
Kaposi's 757.33
   lichen ruber 697.8
      acuminatus 696.4
      moniliformis 697.8
   xeroderma pigmentosum 757.33
Kaschin-Beck (endemic polyarthritis) 716.00
   ankle 716.07
   arm 716.02
      lower (and wrist) 716.03
      upper (and elbow) 716.02
   foot (and ankle) 716.07
   forearm (and wrist) 716.03
   hand 716.04
   leg 716.06
      lower 716.06
      upper 716.05
   multiple sites 716.09
   pelvic region (hip) (thigh) 716.05
   shoulder region 716.01
   specified site NEC 716.08
Katayama 120.2
Kawasaki 446.1
Kedani (scrub typhus) 081.2
kidney (functional) (pelvis) (*see also* Disease, renal) 593.9
   chronic 585.9
      requiring chronic dialysis 585.6
      stage
         I 585.1
         II (mild) 585.2
         III (moderate) 585.3
         IV (severe) 585.4
         V 585.5
   cystic (congenital) 753.10
      multiple 753.19
      single 753.11
      specified NEC 753.19
   fibrocystic (congenital) 753.19
   in gout 274.10
   polycystic (congenital) 753.12
      adult type (APKD) 753.13
      autosomal dominant 753.13
      autosomal recessive 753.14
      childhood type (CPKD) 753.14
      infantile type 753.14
Kienböck's (carpal lunate) (wrist) 732.3
Kimmelstiel (-Wilson) (intercapillary glomerulosclerosis) 250.4 ☑ *[581.81]*
   due to secondary diabetes 249.4 ☑ *[581.81]*
Kinnier Wilson's (hepatolenticular degeneration) 275.1
kissing 075
Kleb's (*see also* Nephritis) 583.9
Klinger's 446.4
Klippel's 723.8
Klippel-Feil (brevicollis) 756.16
knight's 911.1
Köbner's (epidermolysis bullosa) 757.39
Koenig-Wichmann (pemphigus) 694.4
Köhler's
   first (osteoarthrosis juvenilis) 732.5

Disease, diseased — *see also* Syndrome — *continued*

Köhler's — *continued*
   second (Freiberg's infraction, metatarsal head) 732.5
   patellar 732.4
   tarsal navicular (bone) (osteoarthrosis juvenilis) 732.5
Köhler-Freiberg (infraction, metatarsal head) 732.5
Köhler-Mouchet (osteoarthrosis juvenilis) 732.5
Köhler-Pellegrini-Stieda (calcification, knee joint) 726.62
Kok 759.89
König's (osteochondritis dissecans) 732.7
Korsakoff's (nonalcoholic) 294.0
   alcoholic 291.1
Kostmann's (infantile genetic agranulocytosis) 288.01
Krabbe's 330.0
Kraepelin-Morel (*see also* Schizophrenia) 295.9 ☑
Kraft-Weber-Dimitri 759.6
Kufs' 330.1
Kugelberg-Welander 335.11
Kuhnt-Junius 362.52
Kümmell's (-Verneuil) (spondylitis) 721.7
Kundrat's (lymphosarcoma) 200.1 ☑
kuru 046.0
Kussmaul (-Meier) (polyarteritis nodosa) 446.0
Kyasanur Forest 065.2
Kyrle's (hyperkeratosis follicularis in cutem penetrans) 701.1
labia
   inflammatory 616.10
   noninflammatory 624.9
      specified NEC 624.8
labyrinth, ear 386.8
lacrimal system (apparatus) (passages) 375.9
   gland 375.00
      specified NEC 375.89
Lafora's 333.2
Lagleyze-von Hippel (retinocerebral angiomatosis) 759.6
Lancereaux-Mathieu (leptospiral jaundice) 100.0
Landry's 357.0
Lane's 569.89
lardaceous (any site) 277.39
Larrey-Weil (leptospiral jaundice) 100.0
Larsen (-Johansson) (juvenile osteopathia patellae) 732.4
larynx 478.70
Lasègue's (persecution mania) 297.9
Leber's 377.16
Lederer's (acquired infectious hemolytic anemia) 283.19
Legg's (capital femoral osteochondrosis) 732.1
Legg-Calvé-Perthes (capital femoral osteochondrosis) 732.1
Legg-Calvé-Waldenström (femoral capital osteochondrosis) 732.1
Legg-Perthes (femoral capital osteochrondosis) 732.1
Legionnaires' 482.84
Leigh's 330.8
Leiner's (exfoliative dermatitis) 695.89
Leloir's (lupus erythematosus) 695.4
Lenegre's 426.0
lens (eye) 379.39
Leriche's (osteoporosis, posttraumatic) 733.7
Letterer-Siwe (acute histiocytosis X) (M9722/3) 202.5 ☑
Lev's (acquired complete heart block) 426.0
Lewandowski's (*see also* Tuberculosis) 017.0 ☑
Lewandowski-Lutz (epidermodysplasia verruciformis) 078.19
Lewy body 331.82
   with dementia
      with behavioral disturbance 331.82 *[294.11]*

Disease, diseased — *see also* Syndrome — *continued*

Lewy body — *continued*
   with dementia — *continued*
      without behavioral disturbance 331.82 *[294.10]*
Leyden's (periodic vomiting) 536.2
Libman-Sacks (verrucous endocarditis) 710.0 *[424.91]*
Lichtheim's (subacute combined sclerosis with pernicious anemia) 281.0 *[336.2]*
ligament 728.9
light chain 203.0 ☑
Lightwood's (renal tubular acidosis) 588.89
Lignac's (cystinosis) 270.0
Lindau's (retinocerebral angiomatosis) 759.6
Lindau-von Hippel (angiomatosis retinocerebellosa) 759.6
lip NEC 528.5
lipidosis 272.7
lipoid storage NEC 272.7
Lipschütz's 616.50
Little's — *see* Palsy, cerebral
liver 573.9
   alcoholic 571.3
      acute 571.1
      chronic 571.3
   chronic 571.9
      alcoholic 571.3
   cystic, congenital 751.62
   drug-induced 573.3
   due to
      chemicals 573.3
      fluorinated agents 573.3
      hypersensitivity drugs 573.3
      isoniazids 573.3
   end stage NEC 572.8
      due to hepatitis — *see* Hepatitis
   fibrocystic (congenital) 751.62
   glycogen storage 271.0
   organic 573.9
   polycystic (congenital) 751.62
Lobo's (keloid blastomycosis) 116.2
Lobstein's (brittle bones and blue sclera) 756.51
locomotor system 334.9
Lorain's (pituitary dwarfism) 253.3
Lou Gehrig's 335.20
Lucas-Championnière (fibrinous bronchitis) 466.0
Ludwig's (submaxillary cellulitis) 528.3
luetic — *see* Syphilis
lumbosacral region 724.6
lung NEC 518.89
   black 500
   congenital 748.60
   cystic 518.89
      congenital 748.4
   fibroid (chronic) (*see also* Fibrosis, lung) 515
   fluke 121.2
      oriental 121.2
   in
      amyloidosis 277.39 *[517.8]*
      polymyositis 710.4 *[517.8]*
      sarcoidosis 135 *[517.8]*
      Sjögren's syndrome 710.2 *[517.8]*
      syphilis 095.1
      systemic lupus erythematosus 710.0 *[517.8]*
      systemic sclerosis 710.1 *[517.2]*
   interstitial (chronic) 515
      acute 136.3
      respiratory bronchiolitis 516.34
   nonspecific, chronic 496
   obstructive (chronic) (COPD) 496
      with
         acute
            bronchitis 491.22
            exacerbation NEC 491.21
         alveolitis, allergic (*see also* Alveolitis, allergic) 495.9
         asthma (chronic) (obstructive) 493.2 ☑
         bronchiectasis 494.0
            with acute exacerbation 494.1

☑ Additional Digit Required — Refer to the Tabular List for Digit Selection   ▽ Subterms under main terms may continue to next column or page

2013 ICD-9-CM   ▶◀ Revised Text   ● New Line   ▲ Revised Code   Volume 2 — 85

Disease, diseased — *see also* Syndrome — *continued*

lung — *continued*
 obstructive — *continued*
  with — *continued*
   bronchitis (chronic) 491.20
    with
     acute bronchitis 491.22
     exacerbation (acute) 491.21
    decompensated 491.21
     with exacerbation 491.21
    emphysema NEC 492.8
  diffuse (with fibrosis) 496
  of childhood, specific NEC 516.69
  polycystic 518.89
   asthma (chronic) (obstructive) 493.2 ☑
   congenital 748.4
   purulent (cavitary) 513.0
  restrictive 518.89
  rheumatoid 714.81
   diffuse interstitial 714.81
  specified NEC 518.89
Lutembacher's (atrial septal defect with mitral stenosis) 745.5
Lutz-Miescher (elastosis perforans serpiginosa) 701.1
Lutz-Splendore-de Almeida (Brazilian blastomycosis) 116.1
Lyell's (toxic epidermal necrolysis) 695.15
 due to drug
  correct substance properly administered 695.15
  overdose or wrong substance given or taken 977.9
  specific drug — *see* Table of Drugs and Chemicals
Lyme 088.81
lymphatic (gland) (system) 289.9
 channel (noninfective) 457.9
 vessel (noninfective) 457.9
 specified NEC 457.8
lymphoproliferative (chronic) (M9970/1) 238.79
 X linked 759.89
Machado-Joseph 334.8
Madelung's (lipomatosis) 272.8
Madura (actinomycotic) 039.9
 mycotic 117.4
Magitot's 526.4
Majocchi's (purpura annularis telangiectodes) 709.1
malarial (*see also* Malaria) 084.6
Malassez's (cystic) 608.89
Malibu 919.8
 infected 919.9
malignant (M8000/3) (*see also* Neoplasm, by site, malignant)
 previous, affecting management of pregnancy V23.89
Manson's 120.1
maple bark 495.6
maple syrup (urine) 270.3
Marburg (virus) 078.89
Marchiafava (-Bignami) 341.8
Marfan's 090.49
 congenital syphilis 090.49
 meaning Marfan's syndrome 759.82
Marie-Bamberger (hypertrophic pulmonary osteoarthropathy) (secondary) 731.2
 primary or idiopathic (acropachyderma) 757.39
 pulmonary (hypertrophic osteoarthropathy) 731.2
Marie-Strümpell (ankylosing spondylitis) 720.0
Marion's (bladder neck obstruction) 596.0
Marsh's (exophthalmic goiter) 242.0 ☑
Martin's 715.27
mast cell 757.33
 systemic (M9741/3) 202.6 ☑
mastoid (*see also* Mastoiditis) 383.9
 process 385.9
maternal, unrelated to pregnancy NEC, affecting fetus or newborn 760.9

Disease, diseased — *see also* Syndrome — *continued*

Mathieu's (leptospiral jaundice) 100.0
Mauclaire's 732.3
Mauriac's (erythema nodosum syphiliticum) 091.3
Maxcy's 081.0
McArdle (-Schmid-Pearson) (glycogenosis V) 271.0
mediastinum NEC 519.3
Medin's (*see also* Poliomyelitis) 045.9 ☑
Mediterranean 282.40
 with hemoglobinopathy 282.49
medullary center (idiopathic) (respiratory) 348.89
Meige's (chronic hereditary edema) 757.0
Meleda 757.39
Ménétrier's (hypertrophic gastritis) 535.2 ☑
Ménière's (active) 386.00
 cochlear 386.02
 cochleovestibular 386.01
 inactive 386.04
 in remission 386.04
 vestibular 386.03
meningeal — *see* Meningitis
mental (*see also* Psychosis) 298.9
Merzbacher-Pelizaeus 330.0
mesenchymal 710.9
mesenteric embolic 557.0
metabolic NEC 277.9
metal polishers' 502
metastatic — *see* Metastasis
Mibelli's 757.39
microdrepanocytic 282.41
microvascular — code to condition
microvillus
 atrophy 751.5
 inclusion (MVD) 751.5
Miescher's 709.3
Mikulicz's (dryness of mouth, absent or decreased lacrimation) 527.1
Milkman (-Looser) (osteomalacia with pseudofractures) 268.2
Miller's (osteomalacia) 268.2
Mills' 335.29
Milroy's (chronic hereditary edema) 757.0
Minamata 985.0
Minor's 336.1
Minot's (hemorrhagic disease, newborn) 776.0
Minot-von Willebrand-Jürgens (angiohemophilia) 286.4
Mitchell's (erythromelalgia) 443.82
mitral — *see* Endocarditis, mitral
Mljet (mal de Meleda) 757.39
Möbius', Moebius' 346.2 ☑
Moeller's 267
Möller (-Barlow) (infantile scurvy) 267
Mönckeberg's (*see also* Arteriosclerosis, extremities) 440.20
Mondor's (thrombophlebitis of breast) 451.89
Monge's 993.2
Morel-Kraepelin (*see also* Schizophrenia) 295.9 ☑
Morgagni's (syndrome) (hyperostosis frontalis interna) 733.3
Morgagni-Adams-Stokes (syncope with heart block) 426.9
Morquio (-Brailsford) (-Ullrich) (mucopolysaccharidosis IV) 277.5
Morton's (with metatarsalgia) 355.6
Morvan's 336.0
motor neuron (bulbar) (mixed type) 335.20
Mouchet's (juvenile osteochondrosis, foot) 732.5
mouth 528.9
Moyamoya 437.5
Mucha's (acute parapsoriasis varioliformis) 696.2
mu-chain 273.2
mucolipidosis (I) (II) (III) 272.7
Münchmeyer's (exostosis luxurians) 728.11
Murri's (intermittent hemoglobinuria) 283.2
muscle 359.9
 inflammatory 728.9

Disease, diseased — *see also* Syndrome — *continued*

muscle — *continued*
 ocular 378.9
musculoskeletal system 729.90
mushroom workers' 495.5
Myà's (congenital dilation, colon) 751.3
mycotic 117.9
myeloproliferative (chronic) (M9960/1) 238.79
myocardium, myocardial (*see also* Degeneration, myocardial) 429.1
 hypertensive (*see also* Hypertension, heart 402.90
 primary (idiopathic) 425.4
myoneural 358.9
Naegeli's 287.1
nail 703.9
 specified type NEC 703.8
Nairobi sheep 066.1
nasal 478.9
 cavity NEC 478.19
 sinus (chronic) — *see* Sinusitis
navel (newborn) NEC 779.89
 delayed separation of umbilical cord 779.83
nemaline body 359.0
neoplastic, generalized (M8000/6) 199.0
nerve — *see* Disorder, nerve
nervous system (central) 349.9
 autonomic, peripheral (*see also* Neuropathy, peripheral, autonomic) 337.9
 congenital 742.9
 inflammatory — *see* Encephalitis
 parasympathetic (*see also* Neuropathy, peripheral, autonomic) 337.9
 peripheral NEC 355.9
 prion NEC 046.79
 specified NEC 349.89
 sympathetic (*see also* Neuropathy, peripheral, autonomic) 337.9
 vegetative (*see also* Neuropathy, peripheral, autonomic) 337.9
Nettleship's (urticaria pigmentosa) 757.33
Neumann's (pemphigus vegetans) 694.4
neurologic (central) NEC (*see also* Disease, nervous system) 349.9
 peripheral NEC 355.9
neuromuscular system NEC 358.9
Newcastle 077.8
Nicolas (-Durand) — Favre (climatic bubo) 099.1
Niemann-Pick (lipid histiocytosis) 272.7
nipple 611.9
 Paget's (M8540/3) 174.0
Nishimoto (-Takeuchi) 437.5
nonarthropod-borne NEC 078.89
 central nervous system NEC 049.9
 enterovirus NEC 078.89
nonautoimmune hemolytic NEC 283.10
Nonne-Milroy-Meige (chronic hereditary edema) 757.0
Norrie's (congenital progressive oculoacousticocerebral degeneration) 743.8
nose 478.19
nucleus pulposus — *see* Disease, intervertebral disc
nutritional 269.9
 maternal, affecting fetus or newborn 760.4
oasthouse, urine 270.2
obliterative vascular 447.1
Odelberg's (juvenile osteochondrosis) 732.1
Oguchi's (retina) 368.61
Ohara's (*see also* Tularemia) 021.9
Ollier's (chondrodysplasia) 756.4
Opitz's (congestive splenomegaly) 289.51
Oppenheim's 358.8
Oppenheim-Urbach (necrobiosis lipoidica diabeticorum) 250.8 ☑ [709.3]
 due to secondary diabetes 249.8 ☑ [709.3]
optic nerve NEC 377.49
orbit 376.9
 specified NEC 376.89
Oriental liver fluke 121.1

Disease, diseased — *see also* Syndrome — *continued*

Oriental lung fluke 121.2
Ormond's 593.4
Osgood-Schlatter 732.4
Osgood's tibia (tubercle) 732.4
Osler (-Vaquez) (polycythemia vera) (M9950/1) 238.4
Osler-Rendu (familial hemorrhagic telangiectasia) 448.0
osteofibrocystic 252.01
Otto's 715.35
outer ear 380.9
ovary (noninflammatory) NEC 620.9
 cystic 620.2
 polycystic 256.4
 specified NEC 620.8
Owren's (congenital) (*see also* Defect, coagulation) 286.3
Paas' 756.59
Paget's (osteitis deformans) 731.0
 with infiltrating duct carcinoma of the breast (M8541/3) — *see* Neoplasm, breast, malignant
 bone 731.0
  osteosarcoma in (M9184/3) — *see* Neoplasm, bone, malignant
 breast (M8540/3) 174.0
 extramammary (M8542/3) (*see also* Neoplasm, skin, malignant)
  anus 154.3
  skin 173.59
 malignant (M8540/3)
  breast 174.0
  specified site NEC (M8542/3) — *see* Neoplasm, skin, malignant
  unspecified site 174.0
 mammary (M8540/3) 174.0
 nipple (M8540/3) 174.0
palate (soft) 528.9
Paltauf-Sternberg 201.9 ☑
pancreas 577.9
 cystic 577.2
  congenital 751.7
 fibrocystic 277.00
Panner's 732.3
 capitellum humeri 732.3
 head of humerus 732.3
 tarsal navicular (bone) (osteochondrosis) 732.5
panvalvular — *see* Endocarditis, mitral
parametrium 629.9
parasitic NEC 136.9
 cerebral NEC 123.9
 intestinal NEC 129
 mouth 112.0
 skin NEC 134.9
 specified type — *see* Infestation
 tongue 112.0
parathyroid (gland) 252.9
 specified NEC 252.8
Parkinson's 332.0
parodontal 523.9
Parrot's (syphilitic osteochondritis) 090.0
Parry's (exophthalmic goiter) 242.0 ☑
Parson's (exophthalmic goiter) 242.0 ☑
Pavy's 593.6
Paxton's (white piedra) 111.2
Payr's (splenic flexure syndrome) 569.89
pearl-workers' (chronic osteomyelitis) (*see also* Osteomyelitis) 730.1 ☑
Pel-Ebstein — *see* Disease, Hodgkin's
Pelizaeus-Merzbacher 330.0
 with dementia
  with behavioral disturbance 330.0 [294.11]
  without behavioral disturbance 330.0 [294.10]
Pellegrini-Stieda (calcification, knee joint) 726.62
pelvis, pelvic
 female NEC 629.9
  specified NEC 629.89
 gonococcal (acute) 098.19
  chronic or duration of 2 months or over 098.39

☑ **Additional Digit Required — Refer to the Tabular List for Digit Selection**

▼ **Subterms under main terms may continue to next column or page**

Disease, diseased — *see also* Syndrome — *continued*

pelvis, pelvic — *continued*
infection (*see also* Disease, pelvis, inflammatory) 614.9
inflammatory (female) (PID) 614.9
with
abortion — *see* Abortion, by type, with sepsis
ectopic pregnancy (*see also* categories 633.0–633.9) 639.0
molar pregnancy (*see also* categories 630–632) 639.0
acute 614.3
chronic 614.4
complicating pregnancy 646.6 ☑
affecting fetus or newborn 760.8
following
abortion 639.0
ectopic or molar pregnancy 639.0
peritonitis (acute) 614.5
chronic NEC 614.7
puerperal, postpartum, childbirth 670.8 ☑
specified NEC 614.8
organ, female NEC 629.9
specified NEC 629.89
peritoneum, female NEC 629.9
specified NEC 629.89
penis 607.9
inflammatory 607.2
peptic NEC 536.9
acid 536.8
periapical tissues NEC 522.9
pericardium 423.9
specified type NEC 423.8
perineum
female
inflammatory 616.9
specified NEC 616.89
noninflammatory 624.9
specified NEC 624.8
male (inflammatory) 682.2
periodic (familial) (Reimann's) NEC 277.31
paralysis 359.3
periodontal NEC 523.9
specified NEC 523.8
periosteum 733.90
peripheral
arterial 443.9
autonomic nervous system (*see also* Neuropathy, autonomic) 337.9
nerve NEC (*see also* Neuropathy) 356.9
multiple — *see* Polyneuropathy
vascular 443.9
specified type NEC 443.89
peritoneum 568.9
pelvic, female 629.9
specified NEC 629.89
Perrin-Ferraton (snapping hip) 719.65
persistent mucosal (middle ear) (with posterior or superior marginal perforation of ear drum) 382.2
Perthes' (capital femoral osteochondrosis) 732.1
Petit's (*see also* Hernia, lumbar) 553.8
Peutz-Jeghers 759.6
Peyronie's 607.85
Pfeiffer's (infectious mononucleosis) 075
pharynx 478.20
Phocas' 610.1
photochromogenic (acid-fast bacilli) (pulmonary) 031.0
nonpulmonary 031.9
Pick's
brain 331.11
with dementia
with behavioral disturbance 331.11 [294.11]
without behavioral disturbance 331.11 [294.10]
cerebral atrophy 331.11
with dementia
with behavioral disturbance 331.11 [294.11]

Disease, diseased — *see also* Syndrome — *continued*

Pick's — *continued*
cerebral atrophy — *continued*
with dementia — *continued*
without behavioral disturbance 331.11 [294.10]
lipid histiocytosis 272.7
liver (pericardial pseudocirrhosis of liver) 423.2
pericardium (pericardial pseudocirrhosis of liver) 423.2
polyserositis (pericardial pseudocirrhosis of liver) 423.2
Pierson's (osteochondrosis) 732.1
pigeon fanciers' or breeders' 495.2
pineal gland 259.8
pink 985.0
Pinkus' (lichen nitidus) 697.1
pinworm 127.4
pituitary (gland) 253.9
hyperfunction 253.1
hypofunction 253.2
pituitary snuff-takers' 495.8
placenta
affecting fetus or newborn 762.2
complicating pregnancy or childbirth 656.7 ☑
pleura (cavity) (*see also* Pleurisy) 511.0
Plummer's (toxic nodular goiter) 242.3 ☑
pneumatic
drill 994.9
hammer 994.9
policeman's 729.2
Pollitzer's (hidradenitis suppurativa) 705.83
polycystic (congenital) 759.89
congenital 748.4
kidney or renal 753.12
adult type (APKD) 753.13
autosomal dominant 753.13
autosomal recessive 753.14
childhood type (CPKD) 753.14
infantile type 753.14
liver or hepatic 751.62
lung or pulmonary 518.89
ovary, ovaries 256.4
spleen 759.0
polyethylene 996.45
Pompe's (glycogenosis II) 271.0
Poncet's (tuberculous rheumatism) (*see also* Tuberculosis) 015.9 ☑
Posada-Wernicke 114.9
Potain's (pulmonary edema) 514
Pott's (*see also* Tuberculosis)
015.0 ☑ [730.88]
osteomyelitis 015.0 ☑ [730.88]
paraplegia 015.0 ☑ [730.88]
spinal curvature 015.0 ☑ [737.43]
spondylitis 015.0 ☑ [720.81]
Potter's 753.0
Poulet's 714.2
pregnancy NEC (*see also* Pregnancy) 646.9 ☑
Preiser's (osteoporosis) 733.09
Pringle's (tuberous sclerosis) 759.5
Profichet's 729.90
prostate 602.9
specified type NEC 602.8
protozoal NEC 136.8
intestine, intestinal NEC 007.9
pseudo-Hurler's (mucolipidosis III) 272.7
psychiatric (*see also* Psychosis) 298.9
psychotic (*see also* Psychosis) 298.9
Puente's (simple glandular cheilitis) 528.5
puerperal NEC (*see also* Puerperal) 674.9 ☑
pulmonary (*see also* Disease, lung)
amyloid 277.39 [517.8]
artery 417.9
circulation, circulatory 417.9
specified NEC 417.8
diffuse obstructive (chronic) 496
with
acute bronchitis 491.22
asthma (chronic) (obstructive) 493.2 ☑
exacerbation NEC (acute) 491.21

Disease, diseased — *see also* Syndrome — *continued*

pulmonary (*see also* Disease, lung) — *continued*
heart (chronic) 416.9
specified NEC 416.8
hypertensive (vascular) 416.0
cardiovascular 416.0
obstructive diffuse (chronic) 496
with
acute bronchitis 491.22
asthma (chronic) (obstructive) 493.2 ☑
bronchitis (chronic) 491.20
with
exacerbation (acute) 491.21
acute 491.22
exacerbation NEC (acute) 491.21
decompensated 491.21
with exacerbation 491.21
valve (*see also* Endocarditis, pulmonary) 424.3
pulp (dental) NEC 522.9
pulseless 446.7
Putnam's (subacute combined sclerosis with pernicious anemia) 281.0 [336.2]
Pyle (-Cohn) (craniometaphyseal dysplasia) 756.89
pyramidal tract 333.90
Quervain's
tendon sheath 727.04
thyroid (subacute granulomatous thyroiditis) 245.1
Quincke's — *see* Edema, angioneurotic
Quinquaud (acne decalvans) 704.09
rag sorters' 022.1
Raynaud's (paroxysmal digital cyanosis) 443.0
reactive airway — *see* Asthma
Recklinghausen's (M9540/1) 237.71
bone (osteitis fibrosa cystica) 252.01
Recklinghausen-Applebaum (hemochromatosis) (*see also* Hemochromatosis) 275.03
Reclus' (cystic) 610.1
rectum NEC 569.49
Refsum's (heredopathia atactica polyneuritiformis) 356.3
Reichmann's (gastrosuccorrhea) 536.8
Reimann's (periodic) 277.31
Reiter's 099.3
renal (functional) (pelvis) (*see also* Disease, kidney) 593.9
with
edema (*see also* Nephrosis) 581.9
exudative nephritis 583.89
lesion of interstitial nephritis 583.89
stated generalized cause — *see* Nephritis
acute 593.9
basement membrane NEC 583.89
with
pulmonary hemorrhage (Goodpasture's syndrome) 446.21 [583.81]
chronic (*see also* Disease, kidney, chronic) 585.9
complicating pregnancy or puerperium NEC 646.2 ☑
with hypertension — *see* Toxemia, of pregnancy
affecting fetus or newborn 760.1
cystic, congenital (*see also* Cystic, disease, kidney) 753.10
diabetic 250.4 ☑ [583.81]
due to secondary diabetes 249.4 ☑ [581.81]
due to
amyloidosis 277.39 [583.81]
diabetes mellitus 250.4 ☑ [583.81]
due to secondary diabetes 249.4 ☑ [581.81]
systemic lupus erythematosis 710.0 [583.81]

Disease, diseased — *see also* Syndrome — *continued*

renal (*see also* Disease, kidney) — *continued*
end-stage 585.6
exudative 583.89
fibrocystic (congenital) 753.19
gonococcal 098.19 [583.81]
gouty 274.10
hypertensive (*see also* Hypertension, kidney) 403.90
immune complex NEC 583.89
interstitial (diffuse) (focal) 583.89
lupus 710.0 [583.81]
maternal, affecting fetus or newborn 760.1
hypertensive 760.0
phosphate-losing (tubular) 588.0
polycystic (congenital) 753.12
adult type (APKD) 753.13
autosomal dominant 753.13
autosomal recessive 753.14
childhood type (CPKD) 753.14
infantile type 753.14
specified lesion or cause NEC (*see also* Glomerulonephritis) 583.89
subacute 581.9
syphilitic 095.4
tuberculous (*see also* Tuberculosis) 016.0 ☑ [583.81]
tubular (*see also* Nephrosis, tubular) 584.5
Rendu-Osler-Weber (familial hemorrhagic telangiectasia) 448.0
renovascular (arteriosclerotic) (*see also* Hypertension, kidney) 403.90
respiratory (tract) 519.9
acute or subacute (upper) NEC 465.9
due to fumes or vapors 506.3
multiple sites NEC 465.8
noninfectious 478.9
streptococcal 034.0
chronic 519.9
arising in the perinatal period 770.7
due to fumes or vapors 506.4
due to
aspiration of liquids or solids 508.9
external agents 508.9
specified NEC 508.8
fumes or vapors 506.9
acute or subacute NEC 506.3
chronic 506.4
fetus or newborn NEC 770.9
obstructive 496
smoke inhalation 508.2
specified type NEC 519.8
upper (acute) (infectious) NEC 465.9
multiple sites NEC 465.8
noninfectious NEC 478.9
streptococcal 034.0
retina, retinal NEC 362.9
Batten's or Batten-Mayou 330.1 [362.71]
degeneration 362.89
vascular lesion 362.17
rheumatic (*see also* Arthritis) 716.8 ☑
heart — *see* Disease, heart, rheumatic
rheumatoid (heart) — *see* Arthritis, rheumatoid
rickettsial NEC 083.9
specified type NEC 083.8
Riedel's (ligneous thyroiditis) 245.3
Riga (-Fede) (cachectic aphthae) 529.0
Riggs' (compound periodontitis) 523.40
Ritter's 695.81
Rivalta's (cervicofacial actinomycosis) 039.3
Robles' (onchocerciasis) 125.3 [360.13]
Roger's (congenital interventricular septal defect) 745.4
Rokitansky's (*see also* Necrosis, liver) 570
Romberg's 349.89
Rosenthal's (factor XI deficiency) 286.2
Rossbach's (hyperchlorhydria) 536.8
psychogenic 306.4
Roth (-Bernhardt) 355.1
Runeberg's (progressive pernicious anemia) 281.0

☑ **Additional Digit Required — Refer to the Tabular List for Digit Selection**   ᵂ **Subterms under main terms may continue to next column or page**

2013 ICD-9-CM   ▶◀ **Revised Text**   ● **New Line**   ▲ **Revised Code**   **Volume 2 — 87**

Disease, diseased — *see also* Syndrome — *continued*

Rust's (tuberculous spondylitis) (*see also* Tuberculosis) 015.0 ☑ *[720.81]*
Rustitskii's (multiple myeloma) (M9730/3) 203.0 ☑
Ruysch's (Hirschsprung's disease) 751.3
Sachs (-Tay) 330.1
sacroiliac NEC 724.6
salivary gland or duct NEC 527.9
  inclusion 078.5
    streptococcal 034.0
  virus 078.5
Sander's (paranoia) 297.1
Sandhoff's 330.1
sandworm 126.9
Savill's (epidemic exfoliative dermatitis) 695.89
Schamberg's (progressive pigmentary dermatosis) 709.09
Schaumann's (sarcoidosis) 135
Schenck's (sporotrichosis) 117.1
Scheuermann's (osteochondrosis) 732.0
Schilder (-Flatau) 341.1
Schimmelbusch's 610.1
Schlatter-Osgood 732.4
Schlatter's tibia (tubercle) 732.4
Schmorl's 722.30
  cervical 722.39
  lumbar, lumbosacral 722.32
  specified region NEC 722.39
  thoracic, thoracolumbar 722.31
Scholz's 330.0
Schönlein (-Henoch) (purpura rheumatica) 287.0
Schottmüller's (*see also* Fever, paratyphoid) 002.9
Schüller-Christian (chronic histiocytosis X) 277.89
Schultz's (agranulocytosis) 288.09
Schwalbe-Ziehen-Oppenheimer 333.6
Schwartz-Jampel 359.23
Schweninger-Buzzi (macular atrophy) 701.3
sclera 379.19
scrofulous (*see also* Tuberculosis) 017.2 ☑
scrotum 608.9
sebaceous glands NEC 706.9
Secretan's (posttraumatic edema) 782.3
semilunar cartilage, cystic 717.5
seminal vesicle 608.9
Senear-Usher (pemphigus erythematosus) 694.4
serum NEC 999.59
Sever's (osteochondrosis calcaneum) 732.5
sexually transmitted — *see* Disease, venereal
Sézary's (reticulosis) (M9701/3) 202.2 ☑
Shaver's (bauxite pneumoconiosis) 503
Sheehan's (postpartum pituitary necrosis) 253.2
shimamushi (scrub typhus) 081.2
shipyard 077.1
sickle cell 282.60
  with
    crisis 282.62
      Hb-S disease 282.61
    other abnormal hemoglobin (Hb-D) (Hb-E) (Hb-G) (Hb-J) (Hb-K) (Hb-O) (Hb-P) (high fetal gene) (without crisis) 282.68
      with crisis 282.69
  elliptocytosis 282.60
  Hb-C (without crisis) 282.63
    with
      crisis 282.64
      vaso-occlusive pain 282.64
  Hb-S 282.61
    with
      crisis 282.62
      Hb-C (without crisis) 282.63
        with
          crisis 282.64
          vaso-occlusive pain 282.64

Disease, diseased — *see also* Syndrome — *continued*

sickle cell — *continued*
  Hb-S — *continued*
    with — *continued*
      other abnormal hemoglobin (Hb-D) (Hb-E) (Hb-G) (Hb-J) (Hb-K) (Hb-O) (Hb-P) (high fetal gene) (without crisis) 282.68
        with crisis 282.69
  spherocytosis 282.60
  thalassemia (without crisis) 282.41
    with
      crisis 282.42
      vaso-occlusive pain 282.42
Siegal-Cattan-Mamou (periodic) 277.31
silo fillers' 506.9
Simian B 054.3
Simmonds' (pituitary cachexia) 253.2
Simons' (progressive lipodystrophy) 272.6
Sinding-Larsen (juvenile osteopathia patellae) 732.4
sinus (*see also* Sinusitis)
  brain 437.9
  specified NEC 478.19
Sirkari's 085.0
sixth (*see also* Exanthem subitum) 058.10
Sjögren (-Gougerot) 710.2
  with lung involvement 710.2 *[517.8]*
Skevas-Zerfus 989.5
skin NEC 709.9
  due to metabolic disorder 277.9
  specified type NEC 709.8
sleeping (*see also* Narcolepsy) 347.00
  meaning sleeping sickness (*see also* Trypanosomiasis) 086.5
small vessel 443.9
Smith-Strang (oasthouse urine) 270.2
Sneddon-Wilkinson (subcorneal pustular dermatosis) 694.1
South African creeping 133.8
Spencer's (epidemic vomiting) 078.82
Spielmeyer-Stock 330.1
Spielmeyer-Vogt 330.1
spine, spinal 733.90
  combined system (*see also* Degeneration, combined) 266.2 *[336.2]*
    with pernicious anemia 281.0 *[336.2]*
  cord NEC 336.9
    congenital 742.9
    demyelinating NEC 341.8
  joint (*see also* Disease, joint, spine) 724.9
    tuberculous 015.0 ☑ *[730.8]* ☑
spinocerebellar 334.9
  specified NEC 334.8
spleen (organic) (postinfectional) 289.50
  amyloid 277.39
  lardaceous 277.39
  polycystic 759.0
  specified NEC 289.59
sponge divers' 989.5
Stanton's (melioidosis) 025
Stargardt's 362.75
Startle 759.89
Steinert's 359.21
Sternberg's — *see* Disease, Hodgkin's
Stevens-Johnson (erythema multiforme exudativum) 695.13
Sticker's (erythema infectiosum) 057.0
Stieda's (calcification, knee joint) 726.62
Still's (juvenile rheumatoid arthritis) 714.30
  adult onset 714.2
Stiller's (asthenia) 780.79
Stokes' (exophthalmic goiter) 242.0 ☑
Stokes-Adams (syncope with heart block) 426.9
Stokvis (-Talma) (enterogenous cyanosis) 289.7
stomach NEC (organic) 537.9
  functional 536.9
    psychogenic 306.4
  lardaceous 277.39
stonemasons' 502

Disease, diseased — *see also* Syndrome — *continued*

storage
  glycogen (*see also* Disease, glycogen storage) 271.0
  lipid 272.7
  mucopolysaccharide 277.5
striatopallidal system 333.90
  specified NEC 333.89
Strümpell-Marie (ankylosing spondylitis) 720.0
Stuart's (congenital factor X deficiency) (*see also* Defect, coagulation) 286.3
Stuart-Prower (congenital factor X deficiency) (*see also* Defect, coagulation) 286.3
Sturge (-Weber) (-Dimitri) (encephalocutaneous angiomatosis) 759.6
Stuttgart 100.89
Sudeck's 733.7
supporting structures of teeth NEC 525.9
suprarenal (gland) (capsule) 255.9
  hyperfunction 255.3
  hypofunction 255.41
Sutton's 709.09
Sutton and Gull's — *see* Hypertension, kidney
sweat glands NEC 705.9
  specified type NEC 705.89
sweating 078.2
Sweeley-Klionsky 272.7
Swift (-Feer) 985.0
swimming pool (bacillus) 031.1
swineherd's 100.89
Sylvest's (epidemic pleurodynia) 074.1
Symmers (follicular lymphoma) (M9690/3) 202.0 ☑
sympathetic nervous system (*see also* Neuropathy, peripheral, autonomic) 337.9
synovium 727.9
syphilitic — *see* Syphilis
systemic tissue mast cell (M9741/3) 202.6 ☑
Taenzer's 757.4
Takayasu's (pulseless) 446.7
Talma's 728.85
Tangier (familial high-density lipoprotein deficiency) 272.5
Tarral-Besnier (pityriasis rubra pilaris) 696.4
Taylor's 701.8
Tay-Sachs 330.1
tear duct 375.69
teeth, tooth 525.9
  hard tissues 521.9
    specified NEC 521.89
  pulp NEC 522.9
tendon 727.9
  inflammatory NEC 727.9
terminal vessel 443.9
testis 608.9
Thaysen-Gee (nontropical sprue) 579.0
Thomsen's 359.22
Thomson's (congenital poikiloderma) 757.33
Thornwaldt's, Tornwaldt's (pharyngeal bursitis) 478.29
throat 478.20
  septic 034.0
thromboembolic (*see also* Embolism) 444.9
thymus (gland) 254.9
  specified NEC 254.8
thyroid (gland) NEC 246.9
  heart (*see also* Hyperthyroidism) 242.9 ☑ *[425.7]*
  lardaceous 277.39
  specified NEC 246.8
Tietze's 733.6
Tommaselli's
  correct substance properly administered 599.70
  overdose or wrong substance given or taken 961.4
tongue 529.9
tonsils, tonsillar (and adenoids) (chronic) 474.9
  specified NEC 474.8
tooth, teeth 525.9

Disease, diseased — *see also* Syndrome — *continued*

tooth, teeth — *continued*
  hard tissues 521.9
    specified NEC 521.89
  pulp NEC 522.9
Tornwaldt's (pharyngeal bursitis) 478.29
Tourette's 307.23
trachea 519.19
tricuspid — *see* Endocarditis, tricuspid
triglyceride-storage, type I, II, III 272.7
triple vessel (coronary arteries) — *see* Arteriosclerosis, coronary
trisymptomatic, Gougerot's 709.1
trophoblastic (*see also* Hydatidiform mole) 630
  previous, affecting management of pregnancy V23.1
tsutsugamushi (scrub typhus) 081.2
tube (fallopian), noninflammatory 620.9
  specified NEC 620.8
tuberculous NEC (*see also* Tuberculosis) 011.9 ☑
tubo-ovarian
  inflammatory (*see also* Salpingo-oophoritis) 614.2
  noninflammatory 620.9
    specified NEC 620.8
tubotympanic, chronic (with anterior perforation of ear drum) 382.1
tympanum 385.9
Uhl's 746.84
umbilicus (newborn) NEC 779.89
  delayed separation 779.83
Underwood's (sclerema neonatorum) 778.1
undiagnosed 799.9
Unna's (seborrheic dermatitis) 690.18
unstable hemoglobin hemolytic 282.7
Unverricht (-Lundborg) 345.1 ☑
Urbach-Oppenheim (necrobiosis lipoidica diabeticorum) 250.8 ☑ *[709.3]*
  due to secondary diabetes 249.8 ☑ *[709.3]*
Urbach-Wiethe (lipoid proteinosis) 272.8
ureter 593.9
urethra 599.9
  specified type NEC 599.84
urinary (tract) 599.9
  bladder 596.9
    specified NEC 596.89
  maternal, affecting fetus or newborn 760.1
Usher-Senear (pemphigus erythematosus) 694.4
uterus (organic) 621.9
  infective (*see also* Endometritis) 615.9
  inflammatory (*see also* Endometritis) 615.9
  noninflammatory 621.9
    specified type NEC 621.8
uveal tract
  anterior 364.9
  posterior 363.9
vagabonds' 132.1
vagina, vaginal
  inflammatory 616.10
  noninflammatory 623.9
    specified NEC 623.8
Valsuani's (progressive pernicious anemia, puerperal) 648.2 ☑
  complicating pregnancy or puerperium 648.2 ☑
valve, valvular — *see also* Endocarditis
  congenital NEC (*see also* Anomaly, heart, valve) 746.9
  pulmonary 746.00
  specified type NEC 746.89
van Bogaert-Nijssen (-Peiffer) 330.0
van Creveld-von Gierke (glycogenosis I) 271.0
van den Bergh's (enterogenous cyanosis) 289.7
van Neck's (juvenile osteochondrosis) 732.1
Vaquez (-Osler) (polycythemia vera) (M9950/1) 238.4
vascular 459.9

☑ **Additional Digit Required** — Refer to the Tabular List for Digit Selection   ▼ **Subterms under main terms may continue to next column or page**

88 — Volume 2   ▶◀ Revised Text   ● New Line   ▲ Revised Code   2013 ICD-9-CM

Disease, diseased — *see also* Syndrome — *continued*

vascular — *continued*
arteriosclerotic — *see* Arteriosclerosis
hypertensive — *see* Hypertension
obliterative 447.1
peripheral 443.9
occlusive 459.9
peripheral (occlusive) 443.9
in (due to) (with) diabetes mellitus 250.7 ☑ [443.81]
in (due to) (with) secondary diabetes 249.7 ☑ [443.81]
specified type NEC 443.89
vas deferens 608.9
vasomotor 443.9
vasospastic 443.9
vein 459.9
venereal 099.9
chlamydial NEC 099.50
anus 099.52
bladder 099.53
cervix 099.53
epididymis 099.54
genitourinary NEC 099.55
lower 099.53
specified NEC 099.54
pelvic inflammatory disease 099.54
perihepatic 099.56
peritoneum 099.56
pharynx 099.51
rectum 099.52
specified site NEC 099.59
testis 099.54
vagina 099.53
vulva 099.53
complicating pregnancy, childbirth, or puerperium 647.2 ☑
fifth 099.1
sixth 099.1
specified nature or type NEC 099.8
chlamydial — *see* Disease, venereal, chlamydial
Verneuil's (syphilitic bursitis) 095.7
Verse's (calcinosis intervertebralis) 275.49 [722.90]
vertebra, vertebral NEC 733.90
disc — *see* Disease, Intervertebral disc
vibration NEC 994.9
Vidal's (lichen simplex chronicus) 698.3
Vincent's (trench mouth) 101
Virchow's 733.99
virus (filterable) NEC 078.89
arbovirus NEC 066.9
arthropod-borne NEC 066.9
central nervous system NEC 049.9
specified type NEC 049.8
complicating pregnancy, childbirth, or puerperium 647.6 ☑
contact (with) V01.79
varicella V01.71
exposure to V01.79
varicella V01.71
Marburg 078.89
maternal
with fetal damage affecting management of pregnancy 655.3 ☑
nonarthropod-borne NEC 078.89
central nervous system NEC 049.9
specified NEC 049.8
vaccination, prophylactic (against) V04.89
vitreous 379.29
vocal cords NEC 478.5
Vogt's (Cecile) 333.71
Vogt-Spielmeyer 330.1
Volhard-Fahr (malignant nephrosclerosis) 403.00
Volkmann's
acquired 958.6
von Bechterew's (ankylosing spondylitis) 720.0
von Economo's (encephalitis lethargica) 049.8
von Eulenburg's (congenital paramyotonia) 359.29

Disease, diseased — *see also* Syndrome — *continued*

von Gierke's (glycogenosis I) 271.0
von Graefe's 378.72
von Hippel's (retinocerebral angiomatosis) 759.6
von Hippel-Lindau (angiomatosis retinocerebellosa) 759.6
von Jaksch's (pseudoleukemia infantum) 285.8
von Recklinghausen's (M9540/1) 237.71
bone (osteitis fibrosa cystica) 252.01
von Recklinghausen-Applebaum (hemochromatosis) (*see also* Hemochromatosis) 275.03
von Willebrand (-Jürgens) (angiohemophilia) 286.4
von Zambusch's (lichen sclerosus et atrophicus) 701.0
Voorhoeve's (dyschondroplasia) 756.4
Vrolik's (osteogenesis imperfecta) 756.51
vulva
inflammatory 616.10
noninflammatory 624.9
specified NEC 624.8
Wagner's (colloid milium) 709.3
Waldenström's (osteochondrosis capital femoral) 732.1
Wallgren's (obstruction of splenic vein with collateral circulation) 459.89
Wardrop's (with lymphangitis) 681.9
finger 681.02
toe 681.11
Wassilieff's (leptospiral jaundice) 100.0
wasting NEC 799.4
due to malnutrition 261
paralysis 335.21
Waterhouse-Friderichsen 036.3
waxy (any site) 277.39
Weber-Christian (nodular nonsuppurative panniculitis) 729.30
Wegner's (syphilitic osteochondritis) 090.0
Weil's (leptospiral jaundice) 100.0
of lung 100.0
Weir Mitchell's (erythromelalgia) 443.82
Werdnig-Hoffmann 335.0
Werlhof's (*see also* Purpura, thrombocytopenic) 287.39
Wermer's 258.01
Werner's (progeria adultorum) 259.8
Werner-His (trench fever) 083.1
Werner-Schultz (agranulocytosis) 288.09
Wernicke's (superior hemorrhagic polioencephalitis) 265.1
Wernicke-Posadas 114.9
Whipple's (intestinal lipodystrophy) 040.2
whipworm 127.3
White's (congenital) (keratosis follicularis) 757.39
white
blood cell 288.9
specified NEC 288.8
spot 701.0
Whitmore's (melioidosis) 025
Widal-Abrami (acquired hemolytic jaundice) 283.9
Wilkie's 557.1
Wilkinson-Sneddon (subcorneal pustular dermatosis) 694.1
Willis' (diabetes mellitus) (*see also* Diabetes) 250.0 ☑
due to secondary diabetes 249.0 ☑
Wilson's (hepatolenticular degeneration) 275.1
Wilson-Brocq (dermatitis exfoliativa) 695.89
winter vomiting 078.82
Wise's 696.2
Wohlfart-Kugelberg-Welander 335.11
Woillez's (acute idiopathic pulmonary congestion) 518.52
Wolman's (primary familial xanthomatosis) 272.7
wool-sorters' 022.1
Zagari's (xerostomia) 527.7
Zahorsky's (exanthem subitum) 058.10
Ziehen-Oppenheim 333.6

Disease, diseased — *see also* Syndrome — *continued*

zoonotic, bacterial NEC 027.9
specified type NEC 027.8
Disfigurement (due to scar) 709.2
head V48.6
limb V49.4
neck V48.7
trunk V48.7
Disgerminoma — *see* Dysgerminoma
Disinsertion, retina 361.04
Disintegration, complete, of the body 799.89
traumatic 869.1
Disk kidney 753.3
Dislocatable hip, congenital — *see also* Dislocation, hip, congenital 754.30
Dislocation (articulation) (closed) (displacement) (simple) (subluxation) 839.8

Note — "Closed" includes simple, complete, partial, uncomplicated, and unspecified dislocation.

"Open" includes dislocation specified as infected or compound and dislocation with foreign body.

"Chronic," "habitual," "old," or "recurrent" dislocations should be coded as indicated under the entry "Dislocation, recurrent," and "pathological" as indicated under the entry "Dislocation, pathological."

For late effect of dislocation see Late, effect, dislocation.

with fracture — *see* Fracture, by site
acromioclavicular (joint) (closed) 831.04
open 831.14
anatomical site (closed)
specified NEC 839.69
open 839.79
unspecified or ill-defined 839.8
open 839.9
ankle (scaphoid bone) (closed) 837.0
open 837.1
arm (closed) 839.8
open 839.9
astragalus (closed) 837.0
open 837.1
atlanto-axial (closed) 839.01
open 839.11
atlas (closed) 839.01
open 839.11
axis (closed) 839.02
open 839.12
back (closed) 839.8
open 839.9
Bell-Daly 723.8
breast bone (closed) 839.61
open 839.71
capsule, joint — *see* Dislocation, by site
carpal (bone) — *see* Dislocation, wrist
carpometacarpal (joint) (closed) 833.04
open 833.14
cartilage (joint) (*see also* Dislocation, by site)
knee — *see* Tear, meniscus
cervical, cervicodorsal, or cervicothoracic (spine) (vertebra) — *see* Dislocation, vertebra, cervical
chiropractic (*see also* Lesion, nonallopathic) 739.9
chondrocostal — *see* Dislocation, costochondral
chronic — *see* Dislocation, recurrent
clavicle (closed) 831.04
open 831.14
coccyx (closed) 839.41
open 839.51
collar bone (closed) 831.04
open 831.14
compound (open) NEC 839.9
congenital NEC 755.8
hip (*see also* Dislocation, hip, congenital) 754.30
lens 743.37
rib 756.3
sacroiliac 755.69

Dislocation — *continued*

congenital — *continued*
spine NEC 756.19
vertebra 756.19
coracoid (closed) 831.09
open 831.19
costal cartilage (closed) 839.69
open 839.79
costochondral (closed) 839.69
open 839.79
cricoarytenoid articulation (closed) 839.69
open 839.79
cricothyroid (cartilage) articulation (closed) 839.69
open 839.79
dorsal vertebrae (closed) 839.21
open 839.31
ear ossicle 385.23
elbow (closed) 832.00
anterior (closed) 832.01
open 832.11
congenital 754.89
divergent (closed) 832.09
open 832.19
lateral (closed) 832.04
open 832.14
medial (closed) 832.03
open 832.13
posterior (closed) 832.02
open 832.12
recurrent 718.32
specified type NEC 832.09
open 832.19
eye 360.81
lateral 376.36
eyeball 360.81
lateral 376.36
femur
distal end (closed) 836.50
anterior 836.52
open 836.62
lateral 836.54
open 836.64
medial 836.53
open 836.63
open 836.60
posterior 836.51
open 836.61
proximal end (closed) 835.00
anterior (pubic) 835.03
open 835.13
obturator 835.02
open 835.12
open 835.10
posterior 835.01
open 835.11
fibula
distal end (closed) 837.0
open 837.1
proximal end (closed) 836.59
open 836.69
finger(s) (phalanx) (thumb) (closed) 834.00
interphalangeal (joint) 834.02
open 834.12
metacarpal (bone), distal end 834.01
open 834.11
metacarpophalangeal (joint) 834.01
open 834.11
open 834.10
recurrent 718.34
foot (closed) 838.00
open 838.10
recurrent 718.37
forearm (closed) 839.8
open 839.9
fracture — *see* Fracture, by site
glenoid (closed) 831.09
open 831.19
habitual — *see* Dislocation, recurrent
hand (closed) 839.8
open 839.9
hip (closed) 835.00
anterior 835.03
obturator 835.02
open 835.12

☑ Additional Digit Required — Refer to the Tabular List for Digit Selection   ▽ Subterms under main terms may continue to next column or page

2013 ICD-9-CM   ▶◀ Revised Text   ● New Line   ▲ Revised Code   Volume 2 — 89

Disease, diseased — Dislocation

☑ **Additional Digit Required — Refer to the Tabular List for Digit Selection**   🔽 **Subterms under main terms may continue to next column or page**

90 — Volume 2   ▶◀ Revised Text   ● New Line   ▲ Revised Code   2013 ICD-9-CM

Dislocation — *continued*
  wrist — *continued*
    metacarpal bone, proximal end 833.05
      open 833.15
    midcarpal (joint) 833.03
      open 833.13
    open 833.10
    radiocarpal (joint) 833.02
      open 833.12
    radioulnar (joint) 833.01
      open 833.11
    recurrent 718.33
    specified site NEC 833.09
      open 833.19
  xiphoid cartilage (closed) 839.61
    open 839.71
Dislodgement
  artificial skin graft 996.55
  decellularized allodermis graft 996.55
Disobedience, hostile (covert) (overt) — *see also* Disturbance, conduct 312.0 ☑
Disorder — *see also* Disease
  academic underachievement, childhood and adolescence 313.83
  accommodation 367.51
    drug-induced 367.89
    toxic 367.89
  adjustment (*see also* Reaction, adjustment) 309.9
    with
      anxiety 309.24
      anxiety and depressed mood 309.28
      depressed mood 309.0
      disturbance of conduct 309.3
      disturbance of emotions and conduct 309.4
  adrenal (capsule) (cortex) (gland) 255.9
    specified type NEC 255.8
  adrenogenital 255.2
  affective (*see also* Psychosis, affective) 296.90
    atypical 296.81
  aggressive, unsocialized (*see also* Disturbance, conduct) 312.0 ☑
  alcohol, alcoholic (*see also* Alcohol) 291.9
    induced mood 291.89
  allergic — *see* Allergy
  amino acid (metabolic) (*see also* Disturbance, metabolism, amino acid) 270.9
    albinism 270.2
    alkaptonuria 270.2
    argininosuccinicaciduria 270.6
    beta-amino-isobutyricaciduria 277.2
    cystathioninuria 270.4
    cystinosis 270.0
    cystinuria 270.0
    glycinuria 270.0
    homocystinuria 270.4
    imidazole 270.5
    maple syrup (urine) disease 270.3
    neonatal, transitory 775.89
    oasthouse urine disease 270.2
    ochronosis 270.2
    phenylketonuria 270.1
    phenylpyruvic oligophrenia 270.1
    purine NEC 277.2
    pyrimidine NEC 277.2
    renal transport NEC 270.0
    specified type NEC 270.8
    transport NEC 270.0
      renal 270.0
    xanthinuria 277.2
  amnestic (*see also* Amnestic syndrome) 294.8
    alcohol-induced persisting 291.1
    drug-induced persisting 292.83
    in conditions classified elsewhere 294.0
  anaerobic glycolysis with anemia 282.3
  anxiety (*see also* Anxiety) 300.00
    due to or associated with physical condition 293.84
  arteriole 447.9
    specified type NEC 447.8
  artery 447.9
    specified type NEC 447.8

Disorder — *see also* Disease — *continued*
  articulation — *see* Disorder, joint
  Asperger's 299.8 ☑
  attachment of infancy or early childhood 313.89
  attention deficit 314.00
    with hyperactivity 314.01
    predominantly
      combined hyperactive/inattentive 314.01
      hyperactive/impulsive 314.01
      inattentive 314.00
    residual type 314.8
  auditory processing disorder 388.45
    acquired 388.45
    developmental 315.32
  autistic 299.0 ☑
  autoimmune NEC 279.49
    hemolytic (cold type) (warm type) 283.0
    parathyroid 252.1
    thyroid 245.2
  avoidant, childhood or adolescence 313.21
  balance
    acid-base 276.9
      mixed (with hypercapnia) 276.4
    electrolyte 276.9
    fluid 276.9
  behavior NEC (*see also* Disturbance, conduct) 312.9
    disruptive 312.9
  bilirubin excretion 277.4
  bipolar (affective) (alternating) 296.80

Note — Use the following fifth-digit subclassification with categories 296.0–296.6:

0   unspecifed

1   mild

2   moderate

3   severe, without mention of psychotic behavior

4   severe, specified as with psychotic behavior

5   in partial or unspecified remission

6   in full remission

---

    atypical 296.7
    currently
      depressed 296.5 ☑
      hypomanic 296.4 ☑
      manic 296.4 ☑
    mixed 296.6 ☑
    specified type NEC 296.89
    type I 296.7
      most recent episode (or current)
        depressed 296.5 ☑
        hypomanic 296.4 ☑
        manic 296.4 ☑
        mixed 296.6 ☑
        unspecified 296.7
      single manic episode 296.0 ☑
    type II (recurrent major depressive episodes with hypomania) 296.89
  bladder 596.9
    functional NEC 596.59
    specified NEC 596.89
  bleeding 286.9
  bone NEC 733.90
    specified NEC 733.99
  brachial plexus 353.0
  branched-chain amino-acid degradation 270.3
  breast 611.9
    puerperal, postpartum 676.3 ☑
    specified NEC 611.89
  Briquet's 300.81
  bursa 727.9
    shoulder region 726.10
  carbohydrate metabolism, congenital 271.9
  cardiac, functional 427.9
    postoperative 997.1
    psychogenic 306.2
  cardiovascular, psychogenic 306.2
  cartilage NEC 733.90

Disorder — *see also* Disease — *continued*
  cartilage — *continued*
    articular 718.9
      ankle 718.07
      elbow 718.02
      foot 718.07
      hand 718.04
      hip 718.05
      knee 717.9
      multiple sites 718.09
      pelvic region 718.05
      shoulder region 718.01
      specified
        site NEC 718.08
        type NEC 733.99
      wrist 718.03
  catatonic — *see* Catatonia
  central auditory processing 315.32
    acquired 388.45
    developmental 315.32
  cervical region NEC 723.9
  cervical root (nerve) NEC 353.2
  character NEC (*see also* Disorder, personality) 301.9
  ciliary body 364.9
    specified NEC 364.89
  coagulation (factor) (*see also* Defect, coagulation) 286.9
    factor VIII (congenital) (functional) 286.0
    factor IX (congenital) (functional) 286.1
    neonatal, transitory 776.3
  coccyx 724.70
    specified NEC 724.79
  cognitive 294.9
  colon 569.9
    functional 564.9
      congenital 751.3
  communication 307.9
  conduct (*see also* Disturbance, conduct) 312.9
    adjustment reaction 309.3
    adolescent onset type 312.82
    childhood onset type 312.81
    compulsive 312.30
      specified type NEC 312.39
    hyperkinetic 314.2
    onset unspecified 312.89
    socialized (type) 312.20
      aggressive 312.23
      unaggressive 312.21
    specified NEC 312.89
  conduction, heart 426.9
    specified NEC 426.89
  conflict
    sexual orientation 302.0
  congenital
    glycosylation (CDG) 271.8
  convulsive (secondary) (*see also* Convulsions) 780.39
    due to injury at birth 767.0
    idiopathic 780.39
  coordination 781.3
  cornea NEC 371.89
    due to contact lens 371.82
  corticosteroid metabolism NEC 255.2
  cranial nerve — *see* Disorder, nerve, cranial
  cyclothymic 301.13
  degradation, branched-chain amino acid 270.3
  delusional 297.1
  dentition 520.6
  depersonalization 300.6
  depressive NEC 311
    atypical 296.82
    major (*see also* Psychosis, affective) 296.2 ☑
      recurrent episode 296.3 ☑
      single episode 296.2 ☑
  development, specific 315.9
    associated with hyperkinesia 314.1
    coordination 315.4
    language 315.31
      and speech due to hearing loss 315.34
    learning 315.2
      arithmetical 315.1

Disorder — *see also* Disease — *continued*
  development, specific — *continued*
    learning — *continued*
      reading 315.00
    mixed 315.5
    motor coordination 315.4
    specified type NEC 315.8
    speech 315.39
      and language due to hearing loss 315.34
  diaphragm 519.4
  digestive 536.9
    fetus or newborn 777.9
      specified NEC 777.8
    psychogenic 306.4
  disintegrative, childhood 299.1 ☑
  dissociative 300.15
    identity 300.14
    nocturnal 307.47
  drug-related 292.9
  dysmorphic body 300.7
  dysthymic 300.4
  ear 388.9
    degenerative NEC 388.00
    external 380.9
      specified 380.89
    pinna 380.30
    specified type NEC 388.8
    vascular NEC 388.00
  eating NEC 307.50
  electrolyte NEC 276.9
    with
      abortion — *see* Abortion, by type, with metabolic disorder
      ectopic pregnancy (*see also* categories 633.0–633.9) 639.4
      molar pregnancy (*see also* categories 630–632) 639.4
    acidosis 276.2
      metabolic 276.2
      respiratory 276.2
    alkalosis 276.3
      metabolic 276.3
      respiratory 276.3
    following
      abortion 639.4
      ectopic or molar pregnancy 639.4
    neonatal, transitory NEC 775.5
  emancipation as adjustment reaction 309.22
  emotional (*see also* Disorder, mental, nonpsychotic) V40.9
  endocrine 259.9
    specified type NEC 259.8
  esophagus 530.9
    functional 530.5
    psychogenic 306.4
  explosive
    intermittent 312.34
    isolated 312.35
  expressive language 315.31
  eye 379.90
    globe — *see* Disorder, globe
    ill-defined NEC 379.99
    limited duction NEC 378.63
    specified NEC 379.8
  eyelid 374.9
    degenerative 374.50
    sensory 374.44
    specified type NEC 374.89
    vascular 374.85
  factitious (with combined psychological and physical signs and symptoms) (with predominantly physical signs and symptoms) 300.19
    with predominantly psychological signs and symptoms 300.16
  factor, coagulation (*see also* Defect, coagulation) 286.9
    IX (congenital) (funcitonal) 286.1
    VIII (congenital) (functional) 286.0
  fascia 728.9
  fatty acid oxidation 277.85
  feeding — *see* Feeding
  female sexual arousal 302.72
  fluency 315.35
    adult onset 307.0

☑ Additional Digit Required — Refer to the Tabular List for Digit Selection   ᴿᴱⱽ Subterms under main terms may continue to next column or page

2013 ICD-9-CM   ▶◀ Revised Text   ● New Line   ▲ Revised Code   Volume 2 — 91

Disorder — see also Disease — continued

fluency — continued
  childhood onset 315.35
  due to late effect of cerebrovascular accident 438.14
  in conditions classified elsewhere 784.52
fluid NEC 276.9
gastric (functional) 536.9
  motility 536.8
  psychogenic 306.4
  secretion 536.8
gastrointestinal (functional) NEC 536.9
  newborn (neonatal) 777.9
    specified NEC 777.8
  psychogenic 306.4
gender (child) 302.6
  adult 302.85
gender identity (childhood) 302.6
  adolescents 302.85
  adults (-life) 302.85
genitourinary system, psychogenic 306.50
globe 360.9
  degenerative 360.20
    specified NEC 360.29
  specified type NEC 360.89
hearing (see also Deafness)
  conductive type (air) (see also Deafness, conductive) 389.00
  mixed conductive and sensorineural 389.20
    bilateral 389.22
    unilateral 389.21
  nerve
    bilateral 389.12
    unilateral 389.13
  perceptive (see also Deafness, perceptive) 389.10
  sensorineural type NEC (see also Deafness, sensorineural 389.10
heart action 427.9
  postoperative 997.1
hematological, transient neonatal 776.9
  specified type NEC 776.8
hematopoietic organs 289.9
hemorrhagic NEC 287.9
  due to intrinsic circulating anticoagulants, antibodies, or inhibitors 286.59
    with
      acquired hemophilia 286.52
      antiphospholipid antibody 286.53
  specified type NEC 287.8
hemostasis (see also Defect, coagulation) 286.9
homosexual conflict 302.0
hypomanic (chronic) 301.11
identity
  childhood and adolescence 313.82
    gender 302.6
immune mechanism (immunity) 279.9
  single complement (C1-C9) 279.8
  specified type NEC 279.8
impulse control (see also Disturbance, conduct, compulsive) 312.30
infant sialic acid storage 271.8
integument, fetus or newborn 778.9
  specified type NEC 778.8
interactional psychotic (childhood) (see also Psychosis, childhood) 299.1 ☑
intermittent explosive 312.34
intervertebral disc 722.90
  cervical, cervicothoracic 722.91
  lumbar, lumbosacral 722.93
  thoracic, thoracolumbar 722.92
intestinal 569.9
  functional NEC 564.9
    congenital 751.3
    postoperative 564.4
  psychogenic 306.4
introverted, of childhood and adolescence 313.22
involuntary emotional expression (IEED) 310.81
iris 364.9
  specified NEC 364.89
iron, metabolism 275.09

Disorder — see also Disease — continued

iron, metabolism — continued
  specified type NEC 275.09
isolated explosive 312.35
joint NEC 719.90
  ankle 719.97
  elbow 719.92
  foot 719.97
  hand 719.94
  hip 719.95
  knee 719.96
  multiple sites 719.99
  pelvic region 719.95
  psychogenic 306.0
  shoulder (region) 719.91
  specified site NEC 719.98
  temporomandibular 524.60
    sounds on opening or closing 524.64
    specified NEC 524.69
  wrist 719.93
kidney 593.9
  functional 588.9
    specified NEC 588.89
labyrinth, labyrinthine 386.9
  specified type NEC 386.8
lactation 676.9 ☑
language (developmental) (expressive) 315.31
  mixed receptive-expressive 315.32
learning 315.9
ligament 728.9
ligamentous attachments, peripheral (see also Enthesopathy)
  spine 720.1
limb NEC 729.90
  psychogenic 306.0
lipid
  metabolism, congenital 272.9
  storage 272.7
lipoprotein deficiency (familial) 272.5
low back NEC 724.9
  psychogenic 306.0
lumbosacral
  plexus 353.1
  root (nerve) NEC 353.4
lymphoproliferative (chronic) NEC (M9970/1) 238.79
  post-transplant (PTLD) 238.77
major depressive (see also Psychosis, affective) 296.2 ☑
  recurrent episode 296.3 ☑
  single episode 296.2 ☑
male erectile 607.84
  nonorganic origin 302.72
manic (see also Psychosis, affective) 296.0 ☑
  atypical 296.81
mathematics 315.1
meniscus NEC (see also Disorder, cartilage, articular) 718.0 ☑
menopausal 627.9
  specified NEC 627.8
menstrual 626.9
  psychogenic 306.52
  specified NEC 626.8
mental (nonpsychotic) 300.9
  affecting management of pregnancy, childbirth, or puerperium 648.4 ☑
  drug-induced 292.9
    hallucinogen persisting perception 292.89
    specified type NEC 292.89
  due to or associated with
    alcoholism 291.9
    drug consumption NEC 292.9
      specified type NEC 292.89
    physical condition NEC 293.9
  induced by drug 292.9
    specified type NEC 292.89
  neurotic (see also Neurosis) 300.9
  of infancy, childhood or adolescence 313.9
  persistent
    other
      due to conditions classified elsewhere 294.8

Disorder — see also Disease — continued

mental — continued
  persistent — continued
    unspecified
      due to conditions classified elsewhere 294.9
  presenile 310.1
    psychotic NEC 290.10
  previous, affecting management of pregnancy V23.89
  psychoneurotic (see also Neurosis) 300.9
  psychotic (see also Psychosis) 298.9
    brief 298.8
    senile 290.20
  specific, following organic brain damage 310.9
    cognitive or personality change of other type 310.1
    frontal lobe syndrome 310.0
    postconcussional syndrome 310.2
    specified type NEC 310.89
  transient
    in conditions classified elsewhere 293.9
metabolism NEC 277.9
  with
    abortion — see Abortion, by type, with metabolic disorder
    ectopic pregnancy (see also categories 633.0–633.9) 639.4
    molar pregnancy (see also categories 630–632) 639.4
  alkaptonuria 270.2
  amino acid (see also Disorder, amino acid) 270.9
    specified type NEC 270.8
  ammonia 270.6
  arginine 270.6
  argininosuccinic acid 270.6
  basal 794.7
  bilirubin 277.4
  calcium 275.40
  carbohydrate 271.9
    specified type NEC 271.8
  cholesterol 272.9
  citrulline 270.6
  copper 275.1
  corticosteroid 255.2
  cystine storage 270.0
  cystinuria 270.0
  fat 272.9
  fatty acid oxidation 277.85
  following
    abortion 639.4
    ectopic or molar pregnancy 639.4
  fructosemia 271.2
  fructosuria 271.2
  fucosidosis 271.8
  galactose-1-phosphate uridyl transferase 271.1
  glutamine 270.7
  glycine 270.7
  glycogen storage NEC 271.0
    hepatorenal 271.0
  hemochromatosis (see also Hemochromatosis) 275.03
  in labor and delivery 669.0 ☑
  iron 275.09
  lactose 271.3
  lipid 272.9
    specified type NEC 272.8
    storage 272.7
  lipoprotein (see also Hyperlipemia deficiency (familial)) 272.5
  lysine 270.7
  magnesium 275.2
  mannosidosis 271.8
  mineral 275.9
    specified type NEC 275.8
  mitochondrial 277.87
  mucopolysaccharide 277.5
  nitrogen 270.9
  ornithine 270.6
  oxalosis 271.8
  pentosuria 271.8
  phenylketonuria 270.1

Disorder — see also Disease — continued

metabolism — continued
  phosphate 275.3
  phosphorous 275.3
  plasma protein 273.9
    specified type NEC 273.8
  porphyrin 277.1
  purine 277.2
  pyrimidine 277.2
  serine 270.7
  sodium 276.9
  specified type NEC 277.89
  steroid 255.2
  threonine 270.7
  urea cycle 270.6
  xylose 271.8
micturition NEC 788.69
  psychogenic 306.53
misery and unhappiness, of childhood and adolescence 313.1
mitochondrial metabolism 277.87
mitral valve 424.0
mood (see also Disorder, bipolar) 296.90
  alcohol-induced 291.89
  episodic 296.90
    specified NEC 296.99
  in conditions classified elsewhere 293.83
motor tic 307.20
  chronic 307.22
  transient (childhood) 307.21
movement NEC 333.90
  hysterical 300.11
  medication-induced 333.90
  periodic limb 327.51
  sleep related, unspecified 780.58
    other organic 327.59
  specified type NEC 333.99
  stereotypic 307.3
mucopolysaccharide 277.5
muscle 728.9
  psychogenic 306.0
  specified type NEC 728.3
muscular attachments, peripheral (see also Enthesopathy)
  spine 720.1
musculoskeletal system NEC 729.90
  psychogenic 306.0
myeloproliferative (chronic) NEC (M9960/1) 238.79
myoneural 358.9
  due to lead 358.2
  specified type NEC 358.8
  toxic 358.2
myotonic 359.29
neck region NEC 723.9
nerve 349.9
  abducens NEC 378.54
  accessory 352.4
  acoustic 388.5
  auditory 388.5
  auriculotemporal 350.8
  axillary 353.0
  cerebral — see Disorder, nerve, cranial
  cranial 352.9
    first 352.0
    second 377.49
    third
      partial 378.51
      total 378.52
    fourth 378.53
    fifth 350.9
    sixth 378.54
    seventh NEC 351.9
    eighth 388.5
    ninth 352.2
    tenth 352.3
    eleventh 352.4
    twelfth 352.5
    multiple 352.6
  entrapment — see Neuropathy, entrapment
  facial 351.9
    specified NEC 351.8
  femoral 355.2
  glossopharyngeal NEC 352.2
  hypoglossal 352.5

Disorder — see also Disease — continued

nerve — continued
iliohypogastric 355.79
ilioinguinal 355.79
intercostal 353.8
lateral
cutaneous of thigh 355.1
popliteal 355.3
lower limb NEC 355.8
medial, popliteal 355.4
median NEC 354.1
obturator 355.79
oculomotor
partial 378.51
total 378.52
olfactory 352.0
optic 377.49
hypoplasia 377.43
ischemic 377.41
nutritional 377.33
toxic 377.34
peroneal 355.3
phrenic 354.8
plantar 355.6
pneumogastric 352.3
posterior tibial 355.5
radial 354.3
recurrent laryngeal 352.3
root 353.9
specified NEC 353.8
saphenous 355.79
sciatic NEC 355.0
specified NEC 355.9
lower limb 355.79
upper limb 354.8
spinal 355.9
sympathetic NEC 337.9
trigeminal 350.9
specified NEC 350.8
trochlear 378.53
ulnar 354.2
upper limb NEC 354.9
vagus 352.3
nervous system NEC 349.9
autonomic (peripheral) (see also Neuropathy, peripheral, autonomic) 337.9
cranial 352.9
parasympathetic (see also Neuropathy, peripheral, autonomic) 337.9
specified type NEC 349.89
sympathetic (see also Neuropathy, peripheral, autonomic) 337.9
vegetative (see also Neuropathy, peripheral, autonomic) 337.9
neurohypophysis NEC 253.6
neurological NEC 781.99
peripheral NEC 355.9
neuromuscular NEC 358.9
hereditary NEC 359.1
specified NEC 358.8
toxic 358.2
neurotic 300.9
specified type NEC 300.89
neutrophil, polymorphonuclear (functional) 288.1
nightmare 307.47
night terror 307.46
obsessive-compulsive 300.3
oppositional defiant, childhood and adolescence 313.81
optic
chiasm 377.54
associated with
inflammatory disorders 377.54
neoplasm NEC 377.52
pituitary 377.51
pituitary disorders 377.51
vascular disorders 377.53
nerve 377.49
radiations 377.63
tracts 377.63
orbit 376.9
specified NEC 376.89
orgasmic
female 302.73
male 302.74

Disorder — see also Disease — continued

overanxious, of childhood and adolescence 313.0
oxidation, fatty acid 277.85
pancreas, internal secretion (other than diabetes mellitus) 251.9
specified type NEC 251.8
panic 300.01
with agoraphobia 300.21
papillary muscle NEC 429.81
paranoid 297.9
induced 297.3
shared 297.3
parathyroid 252.9
specified type NEC 252.8
paroxysmal, mixed 780.39
pentose phosphate pathway with anemia 282.2
periodic limb movement 327.51
peroxisomal 277.86
personality 301.9
affective 301.10
aggressive 301.3
amoral 301.7
anancastic, anankastic 301.4
antisocial 301.7
asocial 301.7
asthenic 301.6
avoidant 301.82
borderline 301.83
compulsive 301.4
cyclothymic 301.13
dependent-passive 301.6
dyssocial 301.7
emotional instability 301.59
epileptoid 301.3
explosive 301.3
following organic brain damage 310.1
histrionic 301.50
hyperthymic 301.11
hypomanic (chronic) 301.11
hypothymic 301.12
hysterical 301.50
immature 301.89
inadequate 301.6
introverted 301.21
labile 301.59
moral deficiency 301.7
narcissistic 301.81
obsessional 301.4
obsessive-compulsive 301.4
overconscientious 301.4
paranoid 301.0
passive (-dependent) 301.6
passive-aggressive 301.84
pathological NEC 301.9
pseudosocial 301.7
psychopathic 301.9
schizoid 301.20
introverted 301.21
schizotypal 301.22
schizotypal 301.22
seductive 301.59
type A 301.4
unstable 301.59
pervasive developmental 299.9 ☑
childhood-onset 299.8 ☑
specified NEC 299.8 ☑
phonological 315.39
pigmentation, choroid (congenital) 743.53
pinna 380.30
specified type NEC 380.39
pituitary, thalamic 253.9
anterior NEC 253.4
iatrogenic 253.7
postablative 253.7
specified NEC 253.8
pityriasis-like NEC 696.8
platelets (blood) 287.1
polymorphonuclear neutrophils (functional) 288.1
porphyrin metabolism 277.1
postmenopausal 627.9
specified type NEC 627.8
post-transplant lymphoproliferative (PTLD) 238.77

Disorder — see also Disease — continued

posttraumatic stress 309.81
post-traumatic stress (PTSD) 309.81
acute 309.81
brief 309.81
chronic 309.81
premenstrual dysphoric (PMDD) 625.4
psoriatic-like NEC 696.8
psychic, with diseases classified elsewhere 316
psychogenic NEC (see also condition) 300.9
allergic NEC
respiratory 306.1
anxiety 300.00
atypical 300.00
generalized 300.02
appetite 307.59
articulation, joint 306.0
asthenic 300.5
blood 306.8
cardiovascular (system) 306.2
compulsive 300.3
cutaneous 306.3
depressive 300.4
digestive (system) 306.4
dysmenorrheic 306.52
dyspneic 306.1
eczematous 306.3
endocrine (system) 306.6
eye 306.7
feeding 307.59
functional NEC 306.9
gastric 306.4
gastrointestinal (system) 306.4
genitourinary (system) 306.50
heart (function) (rhythm) 306.2
hemic 306.8
hyperventilatory 306.1
hypochondriacal 300.7
hysterical 300.10
intestinal 306.4
joint 306.0
learning 315.2
limb 306.0
lymphatic (system) 306.8
menstrual 306.52
micturition 306.53
monoplegic NEC 306.0
motor 307.9
muscle 306.0
musculoskeletal 306.0
neurocirculatory 306.2
obsessive 300.3
occupational 300.89
organ or part of body NEC 306.9
organs of special sense 306.7
paralytic NEC 306.0
phobic 300.20
physical NEC 306.9
pruritic 306.3
rectal 306.4
respiratory (system) 306.1
rheumatic 306.0
sexual (function) 302.70
specified type NEC 302.79
sexual orientation conflict 302.0
skin (allergic) (eczematous) (pruritic) 306.3
sleep 307.40
initiation or maintenance 307.41
persistent 307.42
transient 307.41
movement 780.58
sleep terror 307.46
specified type NEC 307.49
specified part of body NEC 306.8
stomach 306.4
psychomotor NEC 307.9
hysterical 300.11
psychoneurotic (see also Neurosis) 300.9
mixed NEC 300.89
psychophysiologic (see also Disorder, psychosomatic) 306.9
psychosexual identity (childhood) 302.6
adult-life 302.85
psychosomatic NEC 306.9

Disorder — see also Disease — continued

psychosomatic — continued
allergic NEC
respiratory 306.1
articulation, joint 306.0
cardiovascular (system) 306.2
cutaneous 306.3
digestive (system) 306.4
dysmenorrheic 306.52
dyspneic 306.1
endocrine (system) 306.6
eye 306.7
gastric 306.4
gastrointestinal (system) 306.4
genitourinary (system) 306.50
heart (functional) (rhythm) 306.2
hyperventilatory 306.1
intestinal 306.4
joint 306.0
limb 306.0
lymphatic (system) 306.8
menstrual 306.52
micturition 306.53
monoplegic NEC 306.0
muscle 306.0
musculoskeletal 306.0
neurocirculatory 306.2
organs of special sense 306.7
paralytic NEC 306.0
pruritic 306.3
rectal 306.4
respiratory (system) 306.1
rheumatic 306.0
sexual (function) 302.70
skin 306.3
specified part of body NEC 306.8
specified type NEC 302.79
stomach 306.4
psychotic (see also Psychosis) 298.9
brief 298.8
purine metabolism NEC 277.2
pyrimidine metabolism NEC 277.2
reactive attachment of infancy or early childhood 313.89
reading, developmental 315.00
reflex 796.1
REM sleep behavior 327.42
renal function, impaired 588.9
specified type NEC 588.89
renal transport NEC 588.89
respiration, respiratory NEC 519.9
due to
aspiration of liquids or solids 508.9
inhalation of fumes or vapors 506.9
smoke inhalation 508.2
psychogenic 306.1
retina 362.9
specified type NEC 362.89
rumination 307.53
sacroiliac joint NEC 724.6
sacrum 724.6
schizo-affective (see also Schizophrenia) 295.7 ☑
schizoid, childhood or adolescence 313.22
schizophreniform 295.4 ☑
schizotypal personality 301.22
secretion, thyrocalcitonin 246.0
seizure 345.9 ☑
recurrent 345.9 ☑
epileptic — see Epilepsy
semantic pragmatic 315.39
with autism 299.0 ☑
sense of smell 781.1
psychogenic 306.7
separation anxiety 309.21
sexual (see also Deviation, sexual) 302.9
aversion 302.79
desire, hypoactive 302.71
function, psychogenic 302.70
shyness, of childhood and adolescence 313.21
single complement (C1-C9) 279.8
skin NEC 709.9
fetus or newborn 778.9
specified type 778.8

☑ **Additional Digit Required — Refer to the Tabular List for Digit Selection**   🔻 **Subterms under main terms may continue to next column or page**

2013 ICD-9-CM   ▶◀ **Revised Text**   ● **New Line**   ▲ **Revised Code**   **Volume 2 — 93**

Disorder — see also Disease — continued

skin — continued

  psychogenic (allergic) (eczematous) (pruritic) 306.3

  specified type NEC 709.8

  vascular 709.1

sleep 780.50

  with apnea — see Apnea, sleep

  alcohol induced 291.82

  arousal 307.46

    confusional 327.41

  circadian rhythm 327.30

    advanced sleep phase type 327.32

    alcohol induced 291.82

    delayed sleep phase type 327.31

    drug induced 292.85

    free running type 327.34

    in conditions classified elsewhere 327.37

    irregular sleep-wake type 327.33

    jet lag type 327.35

    other 327.39

    shift work type 327.36

  drug induced 292.85

  initiation or maintenance (see also Insomnia) 780.52

    nonorganic origin (transient) 307.41

      persistent 307.42

  nonorganic origin 307.40

    specified type NEC 307.49

  organic specified type NEC 327.8

  periodic limb movement 327.51

  specified NEC 780.59

  wake

    cycle — see Disorder, sleep, circadian rhythm

    schedule — see Disorer, sleep, circadian rhythm

social, of childhood and adolescence 313.22

soft tissue 729.90

  specified type NEC 729.99

somatization 300.81

somatoform (atypical) (undifferentiated) 300.82

  severe 300.81

  specified type NEC 300.89

speech NEC 784.59

  nonorganic origin 307.9

spine NEC 724.9

  ligamentous or muscular attachments, peripheral 720.1

steroid metabolism NEC 255.2

stomach (functional) (see also Disorder, gastric) 536.9

  psychogenic 306.4

storage, iron 275.09

stress (see also Reaction, stress, acute) 308.3

  posttraumatic

    acute 309.81

    brief 309.81

    chronic 309.81

substitution 300.11

suspected — see Observation

synovium 727.9

temperature regulation, fetus or newborn 778.4

temporomandibular joint NEC 524.60

  sounds on opening or closing 524.64

  specified NEC 524.69

tendon 727.9

  shoulder region 726.10

thoracic root (nerve) NEC 353.3

thyrocalcitonin secretion 246.0

thyroid (gland) NEC 246.9

  specified type NEC 246.8

tic 307.20

  chronic (motor or vocal) 307.22

  motor-verbal 307.23

  organic origin 333.1

  transient (of childhood) 307.21

tooth NEC 525.9

  development NEC 520.9

    specified type NEC 520.8

  eruption 520.6

  specified type NEC 525.8

Tourette's 307.23

Disorder — see also Disease — continued

transport, carbohydrate 271.9

  specified type NEC 271.8

tubular, phosphate-losing 588.0

tympanic membrane 384.9

unaggressive, unsocialized (see also Disturbance, conduct) 312.1 ☑

undersocialized, unsocialized (see also Disturbance, conduct)

  aggressive (type) 312.0 ☑

  unaggressive (type) 312.1 ☑

vision, visual NEC 368.9

  binocular NEC 368.30

  cortex 377.73

    associated with

      inflammatory disorders 377.73

      neoplasms 377.71

      vascular disorders 377.72

  pathway NEC 377.63

    associated with

      inflammatory disorders 377.63

      neoplasms 377.61

      vascular disorders 377.62

vocal tic

  chronic 307.22

wakefulness (see also Hypersomnia) 780.54

  nonorganic origin (transient) 307.43

    persistent 307.44

written expression 315.2

Disorganized globe 360.29

Displacement, displaced

Note — For acquired displacement of bones, cartilage, joints, tendons, due to injury, see also Dislocation.

Displacements at ages under one year should be considered congenital, provided there is no indication the condition was acquired after birth.

acquired traumatic of bone, cartilage, joint, tendon NEC (without fracture) (see also Dislocation) 839.8

  with fracture — see Fracture, by site

adrenal gland (congenital) 759.1

alveolus and teeth, vertical 524.75

appendix, retrocecal (congenital) 751.5

auricle (congenital) **744.29**

bladder (acquired) 596.**89**

  congenital 753.8

brachial plexus (congenital) 742.8

brain stem, caudal 742.4

canaliculus lacrimalis 743.65

cardia, through esophageal hiatus 750.6

cerebellum, caudal 742.4

cervix — see Displacement, uterus

colon (congenital) 751.4

device, implant, or graft — see Complications, mechanical

epithelium

  columnar of cervix 622.10

  cuboidal, beyond limits of external os (uterus) 752.49

esophageal mucosa into cardia of stomach, congenital 750.4

esophagus (acquired) 530.89

  congenital 750.4

eyeball (acquired) (old) 376.36

  congenital 743.8

  current injury 871.3

  lateral 376.36

fallopian tube (acquired) 620.4

  congenital 752.19

  opening (congenital) 752.19

gallbladder (congenital) 751.69

gastric mucosa 750.7

  into

    duodenum 750.7

    esophagus 750.7

    Meckel's diverticulum, congenital 750.7

globe (acquired) (lateral) (old) 376.36

  current injury 871.3

graft

  artificial skin graft 996.55

  decellularized allodermis graft 996.55

heart (congenital) 746.87

Displacement, displaced — continued

heart — continued

  acquired 429.89

hymen (congenital) (upward) 752.49

internal prosthesis NEC — see Complications, mechanical

intervertebral disc (with neuritis, radiculitis, sciatica, or other pain) 722.2

  with myelopathy 722.70

  cervical, cervicodorsal, cervicothoracic 722.0

    with myelopathy 722.71

    due to major trauma — see Dislocation, vertebra, cervical

  due to trauma — see Dislocation, vertebra

  lumbar, lumbosacral 722.10

    with myelopathy 722.73

    due to major trauma — see Dislocation, vertebra, lumbar

  thoracic, thoracolumbar 722.11

    with myelopathy 722.72

    due to major trauma — see Dislocation, vertebra, thoracic

intrauterine device 996.32

kidney (acquired) 593.0

  congenital 753.3

lacrimal apparatus or duct (congenital) 743.65

macula (congenital) 743.55

Meckel's diverticulum (congenital) 751.0

nail (congenital) 757.5

  acquired 703.8

opening of Wharton's duct in mouth 750.26

organ or site, congenital NEC — see Malposition, congenital

ovary (acquired) 620.4

  congenital 752.0

  free in peritoneal cavity (congenital) 752.0

  into hernial sac 620.4

oviduct (acquired) 620.4

  congenital 752.19

parathyroid (gland) 252.8

parotid gland (congenital) 750.26

punctum lacrimale (congenital) 743.65

sacroiliac (congenital) (joint) 755.69

  current injury — see Dislocation, sacroiliac

  old 724.6

spine (congenital) 756.19

spleen, congenital 759.0

stomach (congenital) 750.7

  acquired 537.89

subglenoid (closed) 831.01

sublingual duct (congenital) 750.26

teeth, tooth 524.30

  horizontal 524.33

  vertical 524.34

tongue (congenital) (downward) 750.19

trachea (congenital) 748.3

ureter or ureteric opening or orifice (congenital) 753.4

uterine opening of oviducts or fallopian tubes 752.19

uterus, uterine (see also Malposition, uterus) 621.6

  congenital 752.39

ventricular septum 746.89

  with rudimentary ventricle 746.89

xyphoid bone (process) 738.3

Disproportion 653.9 ☑

affecting fetus or newborn 763.1

breast, reconstructed 612.1

  between native and reconstructed 612.1

caused by

  conjoined twins 678.1 ☑

  contraction, pelvis (general) 653.1 ☑

    inlet 653.2 ☑

    midpelvic 653.8 ☑

    midplane 653.8 ☑

    outlet 653.3 ☑

  fetal

    ascites 653.7 ☑

    hydrocephalus 653.6 ☑

    hydrops 653.7 ☑

Disproportion — continued

caused by — continued

  fetal — continued

    meningomyelocele 653.7 ☑

    sacral teratoma 653.7 ☑

    tumor 653.7 ☑

    hydrocephalic fetus 653.6 ☑

    pelvis, pelvic, abnormality (bony) NEC 653.0 ☑

    unusually large fetus 653.5 ☑

  causing obstructed labor 660.1 ☑

cephalopelvic, normally formed fetus 653.4 ☑

  causing obstructed labor 660.1 ☑

fetal NEC 653.5 ☑

  causing obstructed labor 660.1 ☑

fetopelvic, normally formed fetus 653.4 ☑

  causing obstructed labor 660.1 ☑

mixed maternal and fetal origin, normally formed fetus 653.4 ☑

pelvis, pelvic (bony) NEC 653.1 ☑

  causing obstructed labor 660.1 ☑

specified type NEC 653.8 ☑

Disruption

cesarean wound 674.1 ☑

family V61.09

  due to

    child in

      care of non-parental family member V61.06

      foster care V61.06

      welfare custody V61.05

    death of family member V61.07

    divorce V61.03

    estrangement V61.09

      parent-child V61.04

    extended absence of family member NEC V61.08

    family member

      on military deployment V61.01

      return from military deployment V61.02

    legal separation V61.03

gastrointestinal anastomosis 997.49

ligament(s) (see also Sprain)

  knee

    current injury — see Dislocation, knee

    old 717.89

      capsular 717.85

      collateral (medial) 717.82

        lateral 717.81

      cruciate (posterior) 717.84

        anterior 717.83

      specified site NEC 717.85

marital V61.10

  involving

    divorce V61.03

    estrangement V61.09

operation wound (external) (see also Dehiscence) 998.32

  internal 998.31

organ transplant, anastomosis site — see Complications, transplant, organ, by site

ossicles, ossicular chain 385.23

  traumatic — see Fracture, skull, base

parenchyma

  liver (hepatic) — see Laceration, liver, major

  spleen — see Laceration, spleen, parenchyma, massive

phase-shift, of 24-hour sleep-wake cycle, unspecified 780.55

  nonorganic origin 307.45

sleep-wake cycle (24-hour), unspecified 780.55

  circadian rhythm 327.33

  nonorganic origin 307.45

suture line (external) (see also Dehiscence) 998.32

  internal 998.31

wound 998.30

  cesarean operation 674.1 ☑

  episiotomy 674.2 ☑

  operation (surgical) 998.32

☑ Additional Digit Required — Refer to the Tabular List for Digit Selection   ᵂ Subterms under main terms may continue to next column or page

94 — Volume 2   ▶◀ Revised Text   ● New Line   ▲ Revised Code   2013 ICD-9-CM

Disruption — *continued*
 wound — *continued*
  operation — *continued*
   cesarean 674.1 ☑
   internal 998.31
   perineal (obstetric) 674.2 ☑
   uterine 674.1 ☑
Disruptio uteri — *see also* Rupture, uterus
 complicating delivery — *see* Delivery, complicated, rupture, uterus
Dissatisfaction with
 employment V62.29
 school environment V62.3
Dissecting — *see* condition
Dissection
 aorta 441.00
  abdominal 441.02
  thoracic 441.01
  thoracoabdominal 441.03
 artery, arterial
  carotid 443.21
  coronary 414.12
  iliac 443.22
  renal 443.23
  specified NEC 443.29
  vertebral 443.24
 vascular 459.9
 wound — *see* Wound, open, by site
Disseminated — *see* condition
Dissociated personality NEC 300.15
Dissociation
 auriculoventricular or atrioventricular (any degree) (AV) 426.89
  with heart block 426.0
 interference 426.89
 isorhythmic 426.89
 rhythm
  atrioventricular (AV) 426.89
  interference 426.89
Dissociative
 identity disorder 300.14
 reaction NEC 300.15
Dissolution, vertebra — *see also* Osteoporosis 733.00
Distention
 abdomen (gaseous) 787.3
 bladder 596.89
 cecum 569.89
 colon 569.89
 gallbladder 575.8
 gaseous (abdomen) 787.3
 intestine 569.89
 kidney 593.89
 liver 573.9
 seminal vesicle 608.89
 stomach 536.8
  acute 536.1
  psychogenic 306.4
 ureter 593.5
 uterus 621.8
Distichia, distichiasis (eyelid) 743.63
Distoma hepaticum infestation 121.3
Distomiasis 121.9
 bile passages 121.3
  due to Clonorchis sinensis 121.1
 hemic 120.9
 hepatic (liver) 121.3
  due to Clonorchis sinensis (clonorchiasis) 121.1
 intestinal 121.4
 liver 121.3
  due to Clonorchis sinensis 121.1
 lung 121.2
 pulmonary 121.2
Distomolar (fourth molar) 520.1
 causing crowding 524.31
Disto-occlusion (division I) (division II) 524.22
Distortion (congenital)
 adrenal (gland) 759.1
 ankle (joint) 755.69
 anus 751.5
 aorta 747.29
 appendix 751.5
 arm 755.59
 artery (peripheral) NEC (*see also* Distortion, peripheral vascular system) 747.60

Distortion — *continued*
 artery (*see also* Distortion, peripheral vascular system) — *continued*
  cerebral 747.81
  coronary 746.85
  pulmonary 747.39
  retinal 743.58
  umbilical 747.5
 auditory canal 744.29
  causing impairment of hearing 744.02
 bile duct or passage 751.69
 bladder 753.8
 brain 742.4
 bronchus 748.3
 cecum 751.5
 cervix (uteri) 752.49
 chest (wall) 756.3
 clavicle 755.51
 clitoris 752.49
 coccyx 756.19
 colon 751.5
 common duct 751.69
 cornea 743.41
 cricoid cartilage 748.3
 cystic duct 751.69
 duodenum 751.5
 ear 744.29
  auricle 744.29
   causing impairment of hearing 744.02
  causing impairment of hearing 744.09
  external 744.29
   causing impairment of hearing 744.02
  inner 744.05
  middle, except ossicles 744.03
   ossicles 744.04
  ossicles 744.04
 endocrine (gland) NEC 759.2
 epiglottis 748.3
 Eustachian tube 744.24
 eye 743.8
  adnexa 743.69
 face bone(s) 756.0
 fallopian tube 752.19
 femur 755.69
 fibula 755.69
 finger(s) 755.59
 foot 755.67
 gallbladder 751.69
 genitalia, genital organ(s)
  female 752.89
   external 752.49
   internal NEC 752.89
  male 752.89
   penis 752.69
 glottis 748.3
 gyri 742.4
 hand bone(s) 755.59
 heart (auricle) (ventricle) 746.89
  valve (cusp) 746.89
 hepatic duct 751.69
 humerus 755.59
 hymen 752.49
 ileum 751.5
 intestine (large) (small) 751.5
  with anomalous adhesions, fixation or malrotation 751.4
 jaw NEC 524.89
 jejunum 751.5
 kidney 753.3
 knee (joint) 755.64
 labium (majus) (minus) 752.49
 larynx 748.3
 leg 755.69
 lens 743.36
 liver 751.69
 lumbar spine 756.19
  with disproportion (fetopelvic) 653.0 ☑
   affecting fetus or newborn 763.1
   causing obstructed labor 660.1 ☑
 lumbosacral (joint) (region) 756.19
 lung (fissures) (lobe) 748.69
 nerve 742.8
 nose 748.1

Distortion — *continued*
 organ
  of Corti 744.05
  of site not listed — *see* Anomaly, specified type NEC
 ossicles, ear 744.04
 ovary 752.0
 oviduct 752.19
 pancreas 751.7
 parathyroid (gland) 759.2
 patella 755.64
 peripheral vascular system NEC 747.60
  gastrointestinal 747.61
  lower limb 747.64
  renal 747.62
  spinal 747.82
  upper limb 747.63
 pituitary (gland) 759.2
 radius 755.59
 rectum 751.5
 rib 756.3
 sacroiliac joint 755.69
 sacrum 756.19
 scapula 755.59
 shoulder girdle 755.59
 site not listed — *see* Anomaly, specified type NEC
 skull bone(s) 756.0
  with
   anencephalus 740.0
   encephalocele 742.0
   hydrocephalus 742.3
    with spina bifida (*see also* Spina bifida) 741.0 ☑
   microcephalus 742.1
 spinal cord 742.59
 spine 756.19
 spleen 759.0
 sternum 756.3
 thorax (wall) 756.3
 thymus (gland) 759.2
 thyroid (gland) 759.2
  cartilage 748.3
 tibia 755.69
 toe(s) 755.66
 tongue 750.19
 trachea (cartilage) 748.3
 ulna 755.59
 ureter 753.4
  causing obstruction 753.20
 urethra 753.8
  causing obstruction 753.6
 uterus 752.39
 vagina 752.49
 vein (peripheral) NEC (*see also* Distortion, peripheral vascular system) 747.60
  great 747.49
  portal 747.49
  pulmonary 747.49
 vena cava (inferior) (superior) 747.49
 vertebra 756.19
 visual NEC 368.15
  shape or size 368.14
 vulva 752.49
 wrist (bones) (joint) 755.59
Distress
 abdomen 789.0 ☑
 colon 564.9
 emotional V40.9
 epigastric 789.0 ☑
 fetal (syndrome) 768.4
  affecting management of pregnancy or childbirth 656.8 ☑
  liveborn infant 768.4
   first noted
    before onset of labor 768.2
    during labor and delivery 768.3
  stillborn infant (death before onset of labor) 768.0
  death during labor 768.1
 gastrointestinal (functional) 536.9
  psychogenic 306.4
 intestinal (functional) NEC 564.9
  psychogenic 306.4
 intrauterine — *see* Distress, fetal
 leg 729.5

Distress — *continued*
 maternal 669.0 ☑
 mental V40.9
 respiratory 786.09
  acute (adult) 518.82
   adult syndrome (following trauma and surgery) 518.52
   specified NEC 518.82
  fetus or newborn 770.89
  syndrome (idiopathic) (newborn) 769
 stomach 536.9
  psychogenic 306.4
Distribution vessel, atypical NEC 747.60
 coronary artery 746.85
 spinal 747.82
Districhiasis 704.2
Disturbance — *see also* Disease
 absorption NEC 579.9
  calcium 269.3
  carbohydrate 579.8
  fat 579.8
  protein 579.8
  specified type NEC 579.8
  vitamin (*see also* Deficiency, vitamin) 269.2
 acid-base equilibrium 276.9
 activity and attention, simple, with hyperkinesis 314.01
 amino acid (metabolic) (*see also* Disorder, amino acid) 270.9
  imidazole 270.5
  maple syrup (urine) disease 270.3
  transport 270.0
 assimilation, food 579.9
 attention, simple 314.00
  with hyperactivity 314.01
 auditory, nerve, except deafness 388.5
 behavior (*see also* Disturbance, conduct) 312.9
 blood clotting (hypoproteinemia) (mechanism) (*see also* Defect, coagulation) 286.9
 central nervous system NEC 349.9
 cerebral nerve NEC 352.9
 circulatory 459.9
 conduct 312.9

Note — Use the following fifth-digit subclassification with categories 312.0–312.2:

0 *unspecified*

1 *mild*

2 *moderate*

3 *severe*

---

 adjustment reaction 309.3
 adolescent onset type 312.82
 childhood onset type 312.81
 compulsive 312.30
  intermittent explosive disorder 312.34
  isolated explosive disorder 312.35
  kleptomania 312.32
  pathological gambling 312.31
  pyromania 312.33
 hyperkinetic 314.2
 intermittent explosive 312.34
 isolated explosive 312.35
 mixed with emotions 312.4
 socialized (type) 312.20
  aggressive 312.23
  unaggressive 312.21
 specified type NEC 312.89
 undersocialized, unsocialized
  aggressive (type) 312.0 ☑
  unaggressive (type) 312.1 ☑
 coordination 781.3
 cranial nerve NEC 352.9
 deep sensibility — *see* Disturbance, sensation
 digestive 536.9
  psychogenic 306.4
 electrolyte — *see* Imbalance, electrolyte
 emotions specific to childhood or adolescence 313.9

☑ **Additional Digit Required** — **Refer to the Tabular List for Digit Selection**   ᵂ **Subterms under main terms may continue to next column or page**

2013 ICD-9-CM   ▶◀ **Revised Text**   ● **New Line**   ▲ **Revised Code**   **Volume 2 — 95**

Disruption — Disturbance

Disturbance — see also Disease —
  continued
  emotions specific to childhood or adoles-
    cence — continued
    with
      academic underachievement 313.83
      anxiety and fearfulness 313.0
      elective mutism 313.23
      identity disorder 313.82
      jealousy 313.3
      misery and unhappiness 313.1
      oppositional defiant disorder 313.81
      overanxiousness 313.0
      sensitivity 313.21
      shyness 313.21
      social withdrawal 313.22
      withdrawal reaction 313.22
    involving relationship problems 313.3
    mixed 313.89
    specified type NEC 313.89
  endocrine (gland) 259.9
    neonatal, transitory 775.9
      specified NEC 775.89
  equilibrium 780.4
  feeding (elderly) (infant) 783.3
    newborn 779.31
    nonorganic origin NEC 307.59
    psychogenic NEC 307.59
  fructose metabolism 271.2
  gait 781.2
    hysterical 300.11
  gastric (functional) 536.9
    motility 536.8
    psychogenic 306.4
    secretion 536.8
  gastrointestinal (functional) 536.9
    psychogenic 306.4
  habit, child 307.9
  hearing, except deafness 388.40
  heart, functional (conditions classifiable to
    426, 427, 428)
    due to presence of (cardiac) prosthesis
      429.4
    postoperative (immediate) 997.1
      long-term effect of cardiac surgery
        429.4
    psychogenic 306.2
  hormone 259.9
  innervation uterus, sympathetic, parasym-
    pathetic 621.8
  keratinization NEC
    gingiva 523.10
    lip 528.5
    oral (mucosa) (soft tissue) 528.79
      residual ridge mucosa
        excessive 528.72
        minimal 528.71
      tongue 528.79
  labyrinth, labyrinthine (vestibule) 386.9
  learning, specific NEC 315.2
  memory (see also Amnesia) 780.93
    mild, following organic brain damage
      310.89
  mental (see also Disorder, mental) 300.9
    associated with diseases classified else-
      where 316
  metabolism (acquired) (congenital) (see also
    Disorder, metabolism) 277.9
    with
      abortion — see Abortion, by type,
        with metabolic disorder
      ectopic pregnancy (see also cate-
        gories 633.0–633.9) 639.4
      molar pregnancy (see also categories
        630–632) 639.4
    amino acid (see also Disorder, amino
      acid) 270.9
      aromatic NEC 270.2
      branched-chain 270.3
      specified type NEC 270.8
      straight-chain NEC 270.7
      sulfur-bearing 270.4
      transport 270.0
    ammonia 270.6
    arginine 270.6
    argininosuccinic acid 270.6

Disturbance — see also Disease —
  continued
  metabolism (see also Disorder, metabolism)
    — continued
    carbohydrate NEC 271.9
    cholesterol 272.9
    citrulline 270.6
    cystathionine 270.4
    fat 272.9
    following
      abortion 639.4
      ectopic or molar pregnancy 639.4
    general 277.9
      carbohydrate 271.9
      iron 275.09
      phosphate 275.3
      sodium 276.9
    glutamine 270.7
    glycine 270.7
    histidine 270.5
    homocystine 270.4
    in labor or delivery 669.0 ☑
    iron 275.09
    isoleucine 270.3
    leucine 270.3
    lipoid 272.9
      specified type NEC 272.8
    lysine 270.7
    methionine 270.4
    neonatal, transitory 775.9
      specified type NEC 775.89
    nitrogen 788.99
    ornithine 270.6
    phosphate 275.3
    phosphatides 272.7
    serine 270.7
    sodium NEC 276.9
    threonine 270.7
    tryptophan 270.2
    tyrosine 270.2
    urea cycle 270.6
    valine 270.3
  motor 796.1
  nervous functional 799.21
  neuromuscular mechanism (eye) due to
    syphilis 094.84
  nutritional 269.9
    nail 703.8
  ocular motion 378.87
    psychogenic 306.7
  oculogyric 378.87
    psychogenic 306.7
  oculomotor NEC 378.87
    psychogenic 306.7
  olfactory nerve 781.1
  optic nerve NEC 377.49
  oral epithelium, including tongue 528.79
    residual ridge mucosa
      excessive 528.72
      minimal 528.71
  personality (pattern) (trait) (see also Disor-
    der, personality) 301.9
    following organic brain damage 310.1
  polyglandular 258.9
  psychomotor 307.9
  pupillary 379.49
  reflex 796.1
  rhythm, heart 427.9
    postoperative (immediate) 997.1
      long-term effect of cardiac surgery
        429.4
    psychogenic 306.2
  salivary secretion 527.7
  sensation (cold) (heat) (localization) (tactile
    discrimination localization) (texture)
    (vibratory) NEC 782.0
    hysterical 300.11
    skin 782.0
    smell 781.1
    taste 781.1
  sensory (see also Disturbance, sensation)
    782.0
    innervation 782.0
  situational (transient) (see also Reaction,
    adjustment) 309.9
    acute 308.3

Disturbance — see also Disease —
  continued
  sleep 780.50
    with apnea — see Apnea, sleep
    initiation or maintenance (see also Insom-
      nia) 780.52
      nonorganic origin 307.41
    nonorganic origin 307.40
      specified type NEC 307.49
    specified NEC 780.59
      nonorganic origin 307.49
    wakefulness (see also Hypersomnia)
      780.54
      nonorganic origin 307.43
  sociopathic 301.7
  speech NEC 784.59
    developmental 315.39
      associated with hyperkinesis 314.1
    secondary to organic lesion 784.59
  stomach (functional) (see also Disturbance,
    gastric) 536.9
  sympathetic (nerve) (see also Neuropathy,
    peripheral, autonomic) 337.9
  temperature sense 782.0
    hysterical 300.11
  tooth
    eruption 520.6
    formation 520.4
    structure, hereditary NEC 520.5
  touch (see also Disturbance, sensation) 782.0
  vascular 459.9
    arteriosclerotic — see Arteriosclerosis
  vasomotor 443.9
  vasospastic 443.9
  vestibular labyrinth 386.9
  vision, visual NEC 368.9
    psychophysical 368.16
    specified NEC 368.8
    subjective 368.10
  voice and resonance 784.40
  wakefulness (initiation or maintenance) (see
    also Hypersomnia) 780.54
    nonorganic origin 307.43
Disulfiduria, beta-mercaptolactate-cysteine
  270.0
Disuse atrophy, bone 733.7
Ditthomska syndrome 307.81
Diuresis 788.42
Divers'
  palsy or paralysis 993.3
  squeeze 993.3
Diverticula, diverticulosis, diverticulum
  (acute) (multiple) (perforated) (ruptured)
    562.10
  with diverticulitis 562.11
  aorta (Kommerell's) 747.21
  appendix (noninflammatory) 543.9
  bladder (acquired) (sphincter) 596.3
    congenital 753.8
  broad ligament 620.8
  bronchus (congenital) 748.3
    acquired 494.0
      with acute exacerbation 494.1
  calyx, calyceal (kidney) 593.89
  cardia (stomach) 537.1
  cecum 562.10
    with
      diverticulitis 562.11
        with hemorrhage 562.13
      hemorrhage 562.12
    congenital 751.5
  colon (acquired) 562.10
    with
      diverticulitis 562.11
        with hemorrhage 562.13
      hemorrhage 562.12
    congenital 751.5
  duodenum 562.00
    with
      diverticulitis 562.01
        with hemorrhage 562.03
      hemorrhage 562.02
    congenital 751.5
  epiphrenic (esophagus) 530.6
  esophagus (congenital) 750.4
    acquired 530.6

Diverticula, diverticulosis, diverticulum —
  continued
  esophagus — continued
    epiphrenic 530.6
    pulsion 530.6
    traction 530.6
    Zenker's 530.6
  Eustachian tube 381.89
  fallopian tube 620.8
  gallbladder (congenital) 751.69
  gastric 537.1
  heart (congenital) 746.89
  ileum 562.00
    with
      diverticulitis 562.01
        with hemorrhage 562.03
      hemorrhage 562.02
  intestine (large) 562.10
    with
      diverticulitis 562.11
        with hemorrhage 562.13
      hemorrhage 562.12
    congenital 751.5
    small 562.00
      with
        diverticulitis 562.01
          with hemorrhage 562.03
        hemorrhage 562.02
      congenital 751.5
  jejunum 562.00
    with
      diverticulitis 562.01
        with hemorrhage 562.03
      hemorrhage 562.02
  kidney (calyx) (pelvis) 593.89
    with calculus 592.0
  Kommerell's 747.21
  laryngeal ventricle (congenital) 748.3
  Meckel's (displaced) (hypertrophic) 751.0
  midthoracic 530.6
  organ or site, congenital NEC — see Distor-
    tion
  pericardium (conginital) (cyst) 746.89
    acquired (true) 423.8
  pharyngoesophageal (pulsion) 530.6
  pharynx (congenital) 750.27
  pulsion (esophagus) 530.6
  rectosigmoid 562.10
    with
      diverticulitis 562.11
        with hemorrhage 562.13
      hemorrhage 562.12
    congenital 751.5
  rectum 562.10
    with
      diverticulitis 562.11
        with hemorrhage 562.13
      hemorrhage 562.12
  renal (calyces) (pelvis) 593.89
    with calculus 592.0
  Rokitansky's 530.6
  seminal vesicle 608.0
  sigmoid 562.10
    with
      diverticulitis 562.11
        with hemorrhage 562.13
      hemorrhage 562.12
    congenital 751.5
  small intestine 562.00
    with
      diverticulitis 562.01
        with hemorrhage 562.03
      hemorrhage 562.02
  stomach (cardia) (juxtacardia) (juxtapyloric)
    (acquired) 537.1
    congenital 750.7
  subdiaphragmatic 530.6
  trachea (congenital) 748.3
    acquired 519.19
  traction (esophagus) 530.6
  ureter (acquired) 593.89
    congenital 753.4
  ureterovesical orifice 593.89
  urethra (acquired) 599.2
    congenital 753.8
  ventricle, left (congenital) 746.89

☑ **Additional Digit Required — Refer to the Tabular List for Digit Selection**   ▽ **Subterms under main terms may continue to next column or page**

2013 ICD-9-CM   ▶◀ **Revised Text**   ● **New Line**   ▲ **Revised Code**   **Volume 2 — 97**

☑ **Additional Digit Required — Refer to the Tabular List for Digit Selection**
                                                       🔟 **Subterms under main terms may continue to next column or page**
98 — Volume 2   ▶◀ **Revised Text**   ● **New Line**   ▲ **Revised Code**   **2013 ICD-9-CM**

Dysfunction — continued
  senile 797
  sexual 302.70
  sinoatrial node 427.81
  somatic 739.9
    abdomen 739.9
    acromioclavicular 739.7
    cervical 739.1
    cervicothoracic 739.1
    costochondral 739.8
    costovertebral 739.8
    extremities
      lower 739.6
      upper 739.7
    head 739.0
    hip 739.5
    lumbar, lumbosacral 739.3
    occipitocervical 739.0
    pelvic 739.5
    pubic 739.5
    rib cage 739.8
    sacral 739.4
    sacrococcygeal 739.4
    sacroiliac 739.4
    specified site NEC 739.9
    sternochondral 739.8
    sternoclavicular 739.7
    temporomandibular 739.0
    thoracic, thoracolumbar 739.2
  stomach 536.9
    psychogenic 306.4
  suprarenal 255.9
    hyperfunction 255.3
    hypofunction 255.41
  symbolic NEC 784.60
    specified type NEC 784.69
  systolic 429.9
    with heart failure — see Failure, heart
  temporomandibular (joint) (joint-pain-syndrome) NEC 524.60
    sounds on opening or closing 524.64
    specified NEC 524.69
  testicular 257.9
    hyperfunction 257.0
    hypofunction 257.2
    specified type NEC 257.8
  thymus 254.9
  thyroid 246.9
    complicating pregnancy, childbirth, or puerperium 648.1 ☑
    hyperfunction — see Hyperthyroidism
    hypofunction — see Hypothyroidism
  uterus, complicating delivery 661.9 ☑
    affecting fetus or newborn 763.7
    hypertonic 661.4 ☑
    hypotonic 661.2 ☑
      primary 661.0 ☑
      secondary 661.1 ☑
  velopharyngeal (acquired) 528.9
    congenital 750.29
  ventricular 429.9
    with congestive heart failure (see also Failure, heart) 428.0
    due to
      cardiomyopathy — see Cardiomyopathy
      hypertension — see Hypertension, heart
    left, reversible following sudden emotional stress 429.83
  vesicourethral NEC 596.59
  vestibular 386.50
    specified type NEC 386.58
Dysgammaglobulinemia 279.06
Dysgenesis
  gonadal (due to chromosomal anomaly) 758.6
    pure 752.7
  kidney(s) 753.0
  ovarian 758.6
  renal 753.0
  reticular 279.2
  seminiferous tubules 758.6
  tidal platelet 287.31

Dysgerminoma (M9060/3)
  specified site — see Neoplasm, by site, malignant
  unspecified site
    female 183.0
    male 186.9
Dysgeusia 781.1
Dysgraphia 781.3
Dyshidrosis 705.81
Dysidrosis 705.81
Dysinsulinism 251.8
Dyskaryotic cervical smear 795.09
Dyskeratosis — see also Keratosis 701.1
  bullosa hereditaria 757.39
  cervix 622.10
  congenital 757.39
  follicularis 757.39
    vitamin A deficiency 264.8
  gingiva 523.8
  oral soft tissue NEC 528.79
  tongue 528.79
  uterus NEC 621.8
Dyskinesia 781.3
  biliary 575.8
  esophagus 530.5
  hysterical 300.11
  intestinal 564.89
  neuroleptic-induced tardive 333.85
  nonorganic origin 307.9
  orofacial 333.82
    due to drugs 333.85
  psychogenic 307.9
  subacute, due to drugs 333.85
  tardive (oral) 333.85
Dyslalia 784.59
  developmental 315.39
Dyslexia 784.61
  developmental 315.02
  secondary to organic lesion 784.61
Dyslipidemia 272.4
Dysmaturity — see also Immaturity 765.1 ☑
  lung 770.4
  pulmonary 770.4
Dysmenorrhea (essential) (exfoliative) (functional) (intrinsic) (membranous) (primary) (secondary) 625.3
  psychogenic 306.52
Dysmetabolic syndrome X 277.7
Dysmetria 781.3
Dysmorodystrophia mesodermalis congenita 759.82
Dysnomia 784.3
Dysorexia 783.0
  hysterical 300.11
Dysostosis
  cleidocranial, cleidocranialis 755.59
  craniofacial 756.0
  Fairbank's (idiopathic familial generalized osteophytosis) 756.50
  mandibularis 756.0
  mandibulofacial, incomplete 756.0
  multiplex 277.5
  orodigitofacial 759.89
Dyspareunia (female) 625.0
  male 608.89
  psychogenic 302.76
Dyspepsia (allergic) (congenital) (fermentative) (flatulent) (functional) (gastric) (gastrointestinal) (neurogenic) (occupational) (reflex) 536.8
  acid 536.8
  atonic 536.3
    psychogenic 306.4
  diarrhea 787.91
    psychogenic 306.4
  intestinal 564.89
    psychogenic 306.4
  nervous 306.4
  neurotic 306.4
  psychogenic 306.4
Dysphagia 787.20
  cervical 787.29
  functional 300.11
  hysterical 300.11
  nervous 300.11
  neurogenic 787.29

Dysphagia — continued
  oral phase 787.21
  oropharyngeal phase 787.22
  pharyngeal phase 787.23
  pharyngoesophageal phase 787.24
  psychogenic 306.4
  sideropenic 280.8
  spastica 530.5
  specified NEC 787.29
Dysphagocytosis, congenital 288.1
Dysphasia 784.59
Dysphonia 784.42
  clericorum 784.49
  functional 300.11
  hysterical 300.11
  psychogenic 306.1
  spastica 478.79
Dyspigmentation — see also Pigmentation
  eyelid (acquired) 374.52
Dyspituitarism 253.9
  hyperfunction 253.1
  hypofunction 253.2
  posterior lobe 253.6
Dysplasia — see also Anomaly
  alveolar capillary, with vein misalignment 516.64
  anus 569.44
    intraepithelial neoplasia I (AIN I) (histologically confirmed) 569.44
    intraepithelial neoplasia II (AIN II) (histologically confirmed) 569.44
    intraepithelial neoplasia III (AIN III) 230.6
      anal canal 230.5
    mild (histologically confirmed) 569.44
    moderate (histologically confirmed) 569.44
    severe 230.6
      anal canal 230.5
  artery
    fibromuscular NEC 447.8
      carotid 447.8
      renal 447.3
  bladder 596.89
  bone (fibrous) NEC 733.29
    diaphyseal, progressive 756.59
    jaw 526.89
    monostotic 733.29
    polyostotic 756.54
    solitary 733.29
  brain 742.9
  bronchopulmonary, fetus or newborn 770.7
  cervix (uteri) 622.10
    cervical intraepithelial neoplasia I (CIN I) 622.11
    cervical intraepithelial neoplasia II (CIN II) 622.12
    cervical intraepithelial neoplasia III (CIN III) 233.1
    CIN I 622.11
    CIN II 622.12
    CIN III 233.1
    mild 622.11
    moderate 622.12
    severe 233.1
  chondroectodermal 756.55
  chondromatose 756.4
  colon 211.3
  craniocarpotarsal 759.89
  craniometaphyseal 756.89
  dentinal 520.5
  diaphyseal, progressive 756.59
  ectodermal (anhidrotic) (Bason) (Clouston's) (congenital) (Feinmesser) (hereditary) (hidrotic) (Marshall) (Robinson's) 757.31
  epiphysealis 756.9
    multiplex 756.56
    punctata 756.59
  epiphysis 756.9
    multiple 756.56
  epithelial
    epiglottis 478.79
    uterine cervix 622.10
  erythroid NEC 289.89
  eye (see also Microphthalmos) 743.10
  familial metaphyseal 756.89

Dysplasia — see also Anomaly — continued
  fibromuscular, artery NEC 447.8
    carotid 447.8
    renal 447.3
  fibrous
    bone NEC 733.29
      diaphyseal, progressive 756.59
      jaw 526.89
      monostotic 733.29
      polyostotic 756.54
      solitary 733.29
  high-grade, focal — see Neoplasm, by site, benign
  hip (congenital) 755.63
    with dislocation (see also Dislocation, hip, congenital) 754.30
  hypohidrotic ectodermal 757.31
  joint 755.8
  kidney 753.15
  leg 755.69
  linguofacialis 759.89
  lung 748.5
  macular 743.55
  mammary (benign) (gland) 610.9
    cystic 610.1
    specified type NEC 610.8
  metaphyseal 756.9
    familial 756.89
  monostotic fibrous 733.29
  muscle 756.89
  myeloid NEC 289.89
  nervous system (general) 742.9
  neuroectodermal 759.6
  oculoauriculovertebral 756.0
  oculodentodigital 759.89
  olfactogenital 253.4
  osteo-onycho-arthro (hereditary) 756.89
  periosteum 733.99
  polyostotic fibrous 756.54
  progressive diaphyseal 756.59
  prostate 602.3
    intraepithelial neoplasia I [PIN I] 602.3
    intraepithelial neoplasia II [PIN II] 602.3
    intraepithelial neoplasia III [PIN III] 233.4
  renal 753.15
  renofacialis 753.0
  retinal NEC 743.56
  retrolental (see also Retinopathy of prematurity) 362.21
  skin 709.8
  spinal cord 742.9
  thymic, with immunodeficiency 279.2
  vagina 623.0
    mild 623.0
    moderate 623.0
    severe 233.31
  vocal cord 478.5
  vulva 624.8
    intraepithelial neoplasia I (VIN I) 624.01
    intraepithelial neoplasia II (VIN II) 624.02
    intraepithelial neoplasia III (VIN III) 233.32
    mild 624.01
    moderate 624.02
    severe 233.32
    VIN I 624.01
    VIN II 624.02
    VIN III 233.32
Dyspnea (nocturnal) (paroxysmal) 786.09
  asthmatic (bronchial) (see also Asthma) 493.9 ☑
    with bronchitis (see also Asthma) 493.9 ☑
      chronic 493.2 ☑
    cardiac (see also Failure, ventricular, left) 428.1
  cardiac (see also Failure, ventricular, left) 428.1
  functional 300.11
  hyperventilation 786.01
  hysterical 300.11
  Monday morning 504
  newborn 770.89
  psychogenic 306.1
  uremic — see Uremia

☑ **Additional Digit Required — Refer to the Tabular List for Digit Selection**   ▽ **Subterms under main terms may continue to next column or page**

2013 ICD-9-CM   ▶◀ Revised Text   ● New Line   ▲ Revised Code   **Volume 2 — 99**

Dyspraxia — Ectopic, ectopia

Dyspraxia 781.3
  syndrome 315.4
Dysproteinemia 273.8
  transient with copper deficiency 281.4
Dysprothrombinemia (constitutional) — see
    also Defect, coagulation 286.3
Dysreflexia, autonomic 337.3
Dysrhythmia
  cardiac 427.9
    postoperative (immediate) 997.1
      long-term effect of cardiac surgery
        429.4
    specified type NEC 427.89
  cerebral or cortical 348.30
Dyssecretosis, mucoserous 710.2
**Dyssocial reaction, without manifest psychi-
    atric disorder**
  adolescent V71.02
  adult V71.01
  child V71.02
Dyssomnia NEC 780.56
  nonorganic origin 307.47
Dyssplenism 289.4
Dyssynergia
  biliary (see also Disease, biliary) 576.8
  cerebellaris myoclonica 334.2
  detrusor sphincter (bladder) 596.55
  ventricular 429.89
Dystasia, hereditary areflexic 334.3
Dysthymia 300.4
Dysthymic disorder 300.4
Dysthyroidism 246.9
Dystocia 660.9 ☑
  affecting fetus or newborn 763.1
  cervical 661.2 ☑
    affecting fetus or newborn 763.7
  contraction ring 661.4 ☑
    affecting fetus or newborn 763.7
  fetal 660.9 ☑
    abnormal size 653.5 ☑
      affecting fetus or newborn 763.1
    deformity 653.7 ☑
      affecting fetus or newborn 763.1
  maternal 660.9 ☑
    affecting fetus or newborn 763.1
  positional 660.0 ☑
    affecting fetus or newborn 763.1
  shoulder (girdle) 660.4 ☑
    affecting fetus or newborn 763.1
  uterine NEC 661.4 ☑
    affecting fetus or newborn 763.7
Dystonia
  acute
    due to drugs 333.72
      neuroleptic-induced acute 333.72
  deformans progressiva 333.6
  lenticularis 333.6
  musculorum deformans 333.6
  torsion (idiopathic) 333.6
    acquired 333.79
    fragments (of) 333.89
    genetic 333.6
    symptomatic 333.79
Dystonic
  movements 781.0
Dystopia kidney 753.3
Dystrophia myotonica 359.2 ☑
Dystrophy, dystrophia 783.9
  adiposogenital 253.8
  asphyxiating thoracic 756.4
  Becker's type 359.22
  brevicollis 756.16
  Bruch's membrane 362.77
  cervical (sympathetic) NEC 337.09
  chondro-osseous with punctate epiphyseal
    dysplasia 756.59
  choroid (hereditary) 363.50
    central (areolar) (partial) 363.53
      total (gyrate) 363.54
    circinate 363.53
    circumpapillary (partial) 363.51
      total 363.52
    diffuse
      partial 363.56
      total 363.57
    generalized
      partial 363.56

Dystrophy, dystrophia — continued
  choroid — continued
    generalized — continued
      total 363.57
    gyrate
      central 363.54
      generalized 363.57
    helicoid 363.52
    peripapillary — see Dystrophy, choroid,
      circumpapillary
    serpiginous 363.54
  cornea (hereditary) 371.50
    anterior NEC 371.52
    Cogan's 371.52
    combined 371.57
    crystalline 371.56
    endothelial (Fuchs') 371.57
    epithelial 371.50
      juvenile 371.51
      microscopic cystic 371.52
    granular 371.53
    lattice 371.54
    macular 371.55
    marginal (Terrien's) 371.48
    Meesman's 371.51
    microscopic cystic (epithelial) 371.52
    nodular, Salzmann's 371.46
    polymorphous 371.58
    posterior NEC 371.58
    ring-like 371.52
    Salzmann's nodular 371.46
    stromal NEC 371.56
  dermatochondrocorneal 371.50
  Duchenne's 359.1
  due to malnutrition 263.9
  Erb's 359.1
  familial
    hyperplastic periosteal 756.59
    osseous 277.5
  foveal 362.77
  Fuchs', cornea 371.57
  Gowers' muscular 359.1
  hair 704.2
  hereditary, progressive muscular 359.1
  hypogenital, with diabetic tendency 759.81
  Landouzy-Déjérine 359.1
  Leyden-Möbius 359.1
  mesodermalis congenita 759.82
  muscular 359.1
    congenital (hereditary) 359.0
      myotonic 359.22
    distal 359.1
    Duchenne's 359.1
    Erb's 359.1
    fascioscapulohumeral 359.1
    Gowers' 359.1
    hereditary (progressive) 359.1
    Landouzy-Déjérine 359.1
    limb-girdle 359.1
    myotonic 359.21
    progressive (hereditary) 359.1
      Charcôt-Marie-Tooth 356.1
    pseudohypertrophic (infantile) 359.1
  myocardium, myocardial (see also Degener-
    ation, myocardial) 429.1
  myotonic 359.21
  myotonica 359.21
  nail 703.8
    congenital 757.5
  neurovascular (traumatic) (see also Neuropa-
    thy, peripheral, autonomic) 337.9
  nutritional 263.9
  ocular 359.1
  oculocerebrorenal 270.8
  oculopharyngeal 359.1
  ovarian 620.8
  papillary (and pigmentary) 701.1
  pelvicrural atrophic 359.1
  pigmentary (see also Acanthosis) 701.2
  pituitary (gland) 253.8
  polyglandular 258.8
  posttraumatic sympathetic — see Dystro-
    phy, sympathetic
  progressive ophthalmoplegic 359.1
  reflex neuromuscular — see Dystrophy,
    sympathetic

Dystrophy, dystrophia — continued
  retina, retinal (hereditary) 362.70
    albipunctate 362.74
    Bruch's membrane 362.77
    cone, progressive 362.75
    hyaline 362.77
    in
      Bassen-Kornzweig syndrome
        272.5 [362.72]
      cerebroretinal lipidosis 330.1 [362.71]
      Refsum's disease 356.3 [362.72]
      systemic lipidosis 272.7 [362.71]
    juvenile (Stargardt's) 362.75
    pigmentary 362.74
    pigment epithelium 362.76
    progressive cone (-rod) 362.75
    pseudoinflammatory foveal 362.77
    rod, progressive 362.75
    sensory 362.75
    vitelliform 362.76
  Salzmann's nodular 371.46
  scapuloperoneal 359.1
  skin NEC 709.9
  sympathetic (posttraumatic) (reflex) 337.20
    lower limb 337.22
    specified site NEC 337.29
    upper limb 337.21
  tapetoretinal NEC 362.74
  thoracic asphyxiating 756.4
  unguium 703.8
    congenital 757.5
  vitreoretinal (primary) 362.73
    secondary 362.66
  vulva 624.09
Dysuria 788.1
  psychogenic 306.53

E

Eagle-Barrett syndrome 756.71
Eales' disease (syndrome) 362.18
Ear — see also condition
  ache 388.70
    otogenic 388.71
    referred 388.72
  lop 744.29
  piercing V50.3
  swimmers' acute 380.12
  tank 380.12
  tropical 111.8 [380.15]
  wax 380.4
Earache 388.70
  otogenic 388.71
  referred 388.72
Early satiety 780.94
Eaton-Lambert syndrome — see also Syn-
    drome, Lambert-Eaton) 358.30
Eberth's disease (typhoid fever) 002.0
Ebstein's
  anomaly or syndrome (downward displace-
    ment, tricuspid valve into right ven-
    tricle) 746.2
  disease (diabetes) 250.4 ☑ [581.81]
    due to secondary diabetes
      249.4 ☑ [581.81]
Eccentro-osteochondrodysplasia 277.5
Ecchondroma (M9210/0) — see Neoplasm,
    bone, benign
Ecchondrosis (M9210/1) 238.0
Ecchordosis physaliphora 756.0
Ecchymosis (multiple) 459.89
  conjunctiva 372.72
  eye (traumatic) 921.0
  eyelids (traumatic) 921.1
  newborn 772.6
  spontaneous 782.7
  traumatic — see Contusion
ECD (Erdheim-Chester disease) 277.89
Echinococciasis — see Echinococcus
Echinococcosis — see Echinococcus
Echinococcus (infection) 122.9
  granulosus 122.4
    liver 122.0
    lung 122.1
    orbit 122.3 [376.13]
    specified site NEC 122.3
    thyroid 122.2

Echinococcus — continued
  liver NEC 122.8
    granulosus 122.0
    multilocularis 122.5
  lung NEC 122.9
    granulosus 122.1
    multilocularis 122.6
  multilocularis 122.7
    liver 122.5
    specified site NEC 122.6
  orbit 122.9 [376.13]
    granulosus 122.3 [376.13]
    multilocularis 122.6 [376.13]
  specified site NEC 122.9
    granulosus 122.3
    multilocularis 122.6 [376.13]
  thyroid NEC 122.9
    granulosus 122.2
    multilocularis 122.6
Echinorhynchiasis 127.7
Echinostomiasis 121.8
Echolalia 784.69
ECHO virus infection NEC 079.1
Eclampsia, eclamptic (coma) (convulsions)
    (delirium) 780.39
  female, child-bearing age NEC — see
    Eclampsia, pregnancy
  gravidarum — see Eclampsia, pregnancy
  male 780.39
  not associated with pregnancy or childbirth
    780.39
  pregnancy, childbirth, or puerperium
    642.6 ☑
    with pre-existing hypertension 642.7 ☑
    affecting fetus or newborn 760.0
  uremic 586
Eclipse blindness (total) 363.31
Economic circumstance affecting care V60.9
  specified type NEC V60.89
Economo's disease (encephalitis lethargica)
    049.8
Ectasia, ectasis
  annuloaortic 424.1
  aorta (see also Ectasia, aortic) 447.70
    with aneurysm 441.9
    ruptured 441.5
  aortic 447.70
    with aneurysm 441.9
    abdominal 447.72
    thoracic 447.71
    thoracoabdominal 447.73
  breast 610.4
  capillary 448.9
  cornea (marginal) (postinfectional) 371.71
  duct (mammary) 610.4
  gastric antral vascular (GAVE) 537.82
    with hemorrhage 537.83
    without hemorrhage 537.82
  kidney 593.89
  mammary duct (gland) 610.4
  papillary 448.9
  renal 593.89
  salivary gland (duct) 527.8
  scar, cornea 371.71
  sclera 379.11
Ecthyma 686.8
  contagiosum 051.2
  gangrenosum 686.09
  infectiosum 051.2
Ectocardia 746.87
Ectodermal dysplasia, congenital 757.31
Ectodermosis erosiva pluriorificialis 695.19
Ectopic, ectopia (congenital) 759.89
  abdominal viscera 751.8
    due to defect in anterior abdominal wall
      756.79
  ACTH syndrome 255.0
  adrenal gland 759.1
  anus 751.5
  auricular beats 427.61
  beats 427.60
  bladder 753.5
  bone and cartilage in lung 748.69
  brain 742.4
  breast tissue 757.6
  cardiac 746.87

☑ **Additional Digit Required** — Refer to the Tabular List for Digit Selection   ᵂ **Subterms under main terms may continue to next column or page**

100 — Volume 2   ▶◀ Revised Text   ● New Line   ▲ Revised Code   **2013 ICD-9-CM**

Ectopic, ectopia — *continued*
cerebral 742.4
cordis 746.87
endometrium 617.9
gallbladder 751.69
gastric mucosa 750.7
gestation — *see* Pregnancy, ectopic
heart 746.87
hormone secretion NEC 259.3
hyperparathyroidism 259.3
kidney (crossed) (intrathoracic) (pelvis)
753.3
in pregnancy or childbirth 654.4 ☑
causing obstructed labor 660.2 ☑
lens 743.37
lentis 743.37
mole — *see* Pregnancy, ectopic
organ or site NEC — *see* Malposition, congenital
ovary 752.0
pancreas, pancreatic tissue 751.7
pregnancy — *see* Pregnancy, ectopic
pupil 364.75
renal 753.3
sebaceous glands of mouth 750.26
secretion
ACTH 255.0
adrenal hormone 259.3
adrenalin 259.3
adrenocorticotropin 255.0
antidiuretic hormone (ADH) 259.3
epinephrine 259.3
hormone NEC 259.3
norepinephrine 259.3
pituitary (posterior) 259.3
spleen 759.0
testis 752.51
thyroid 759.2
ureter 753.4
ventricular beats 427.69
vesicae 753.5
Ectrodactyly 755.4
finger (*see also* Absence, finger, congenital)
755.29
toe (*see also* Absence, toe, congenital)
755.39
Ectromelia 755.4
lower limb 755.30
upper limb 755.20
Ectropion 374.10
anus 569.49
cervix 622.0
with mention of cervicitis 616.0
cicatricial 374.14
congenital 743.62
eyelid 374.10
cicatricial 374.14
congenital 743.62
mechanical 374.12
paralytic 374.12
senile 374.11
spastic 374.13
iris (pigment epithelium) 364.54
lip (congenital) 750.26
acquired 528.5
mechanical 374.12
paralytic 374.12
rectum 569.49
senile 374.11
spastic 374.13
urethra 599.84
uvea 364.54
Eczema (acute) (allergic) (chronic) (erythematous) (fissum) (occupational) (rubrum)
(squamous) 692.9
asteatotic 706.8
atopic 691.8
contact NEC 692.9
dermatitis NEC 692.9
due to specified cause — *see* Dermatitis,
due to
dyshidrotic 705.81
external ear 380.22
flexural 691.8
gouty 274.89
herpeticum 054.0

Eczema — *continued*
hypertrophicum 701.8
hypostatic — *see* Varicose, vein
impetiginous 684
infantile (acute) (chronic) (due to any substance) (intertriginous) (seborrheic)
690.12
intertriginous NEC 692.9
infantile 690.12
intrinsic 691.8
lichenified NEC 692.9
marginatum 110.3
nummular 692.9
pustular 686.8
seborrheic 690.18
infantile 690.12
solare 692.72
stasis (lower extremity) 454.1
ulcerated 454.2
vaccination, vaccinatum 999.0
varicose (lower extremity) — *see* Varicose,
vein
verrucosum callosum 698.3
Eczematoid, exudative 691.8
Eddowes' syndrome (brittle bones and blue
sclera) 756.51
Edema, edematous 782.3
with nephritis (*see also* Nephrosis) 581.9
allergic 995.1
angioneurotic (allergic) (any site) (with urticaria) 995.1
hereditary 277.6
angiospastic 443.9
Berlin's (traumatic) 921.3
brain (cytotoxic) (vasogenic) 348.5
due to birth injury 767.8
fetus or newborn 767.8
cardiac (*see also* Failure, heart) 428.0
cardiovascular (*see also* Failure, heart) 428.0
cerebral — *see* Edema, brain
cerebrospinal vessel — *see* Edema, brain
cervix (acute) (uteri) 622.8
puerperal, postpartum 674.8 ☑
chronic hereditary 757.0
circumscribed, acute 995.1
hereditary 277.6
complicating pregnancy (gestational)
646.1 ☑
with hypertension — *see* Toxemia, of
pregnancy
conjunctiva 372.73
connective tissue 782.3
cornea 371.20
due to contact lenses 371.24
idiopathic 371.21
secondary 371.22
cystoid macular 362.53
due to
lymphatic obstruction — *see* Edema,
lymphatic
salt retention 276.0
epiglottis — *see* Edema, glottis
essential, acute 995.1
hereditary 277.6
extremities, lower — *see* Edema, legs
eyelid NEC 374.82
familial, hereditary (legs) 757.0
famine 262
fetus or newborn 778.5
genital organs
female 629.89
male 608.86
gestational 646.1 ☑
with hypertension — *see* Toxemia, of
pregnancy
glottis, glottic, glottides (obstructive) (passive) 478.6
allergic 995.1
hereditary 277.6
due to external agent — *see* Condition,
respiratory, acute, due to specified agent
heart (*see also* Failure, heart) 428.0
newborn 779.89
heat 992.7
hereditary (legs) 757.0

Edema, edematous — *continued*
inanition 262
infectious 782.3
intracranial 348.5
due to injury at birth 767.8
iris 364.89
joint (*see also* Effusion, joint) 719.0 ☑
larynx (*see also* Edema, glottis) 478.6
legs 782.3
due to venous obstruction 459.2
hereditary 757.0
localized 782.3
due to venous obstruction 459.2
lower extremity 459.2
lower extremities — *see* Edema, legs
lung 514
acute 518.4
with heart disease or failure (*see also*
Failure, ventricular, left) 428.1
congestive 428.0
chemical (due to fumes or vapors)
506.1
due to
external agent(s) NEC 508.9
specified NEC 508.8
fumes and vapors (chemical) (inhalation) 506.1
radiation 508.0
chemical (acute) 506.1
chronic 506.4
chronic 514
chemical (due to fumes or vapors)
506.4
due to
external agent(s) NEC 508.9
specified NEC 508.8
fumes or vapors (chemical) (inhalation) 506.4
radiation 508.1
due to
external agent 508.9
specified NEC 508.8
high altitude 993.2
near drowning 994.1
postoperative 518.4
terminal 514
lymphatic 457.1
due to mastectomy operation 457.0
macula 362.83
cystoid 362.53
diabetic 250.5 ☑ [362.07]
due to secondary diabetes
249.5 ☑ [362.07]
malignant (*see also* Gangrene, gas) 040.0
Milroy's 757.0
nasopharynx 478.25
neonatorum 778.5
nutritional (newborn) 262
with dyspigmentation, skin and hair 260
optic disc or nerve — *see* Papilledema
orbit 376.33
circulatory 459.89
palate (soft) (hard) 528.9
pancreas 577.8
penis 607.83
periodic 995.1
hereditary 277.6
pharynx 478.25
pitting 782.3
pulmonary — *see* Edema, lung
Quincke's 995.1
hereditary 277.6
renal (*see also* Nephrosis) 581.9
retina (localized) (macular) (peripheral)
362.83
cystoid 362.53
diabetic 250.5 ☑ [362.07]
due to secondary diabetes
249.5 ☑ [362.07]
salt 276.0
scrotum 608.86
seminal vesicle 608.86
spermatic cord 608.86
spinal cord 336.1
starvation 262
stasis (*see also* Hypertension, venous) 459.30

Edema, edematous — *continued*
subconjunctival 372.73
subglottic (*see also* Edema, glottis) 478.6
supraglottic (*see also* Edema, glottis) 478.6
testis 608.86
toxic NEC 782.3
traumatic NEC 782.3
tunica vaginalis 608.86
vas deferens 608.86
vocal cord — *see* Edema, glottis
vulva (acute) 624.8
Edentia (complete) (partial) — *see also* Absence, tooth 520.0
acquired (*see also* Edentulism) 525.40
due to
caries 525.13
extraction 525.10
periodontal disease 525.12
specified NEC 525.19
trauma 525.11
causing malocclusion 524.30
congenital (deficiency of tooth buds) 520.0
Edentulism 525.40
complete 525.40
class I 525.41
class II 525.42
class III 525.43
class IV 525.44
partial 525.50
class I 525.51
class II 525.52
class III 525.53
class IV 525.54
Edsall's disease 992.2
Educational handicap V62.3
Edwards' syndrome 758.2
Effect, adverse NEC
abnormal gravitational (G) forces or states
994.9
air pressure — *see* Effect, adverse, atmospheric pressure
altitude (high) — *see* Effect, adverse, high
altitude
anesthetic
in labor and delivery NEC 668.9 ☑
affecting fetus or newborn 763.5
antitoxin — *see* Complications, vaccination
atmospheric pressure 993.9
due to explosion 993.4
high 993.3
low — *see* Effect, adverse, high altitude
specified effect NEC 993.8
biological, correct substance properly administered (*see also* Effect, adverse, drug)
995.20
blood (derivatives) (serum) (transfusion) —
see Complications, transfusion
chemical substance NEC 989.9
specified — *see* Table of Drugs and
Chemicals
cobalt, radioactive (*see also* Effect, adverse,
radioactive substance) 990
cold (temperature) (weather) 991.9
chilblains 991.5
frostbite — *see* Frostbite
specified effect NEC 991.8
drugs and medicinals 995.20
correct substance properly administered
995.20
overdose or wrong substance given or
taken 977.9
specified drug — *see* Table of Drugs
and Chemicals
electric current (shock) 994.8
burn — *see* Burn, by site
electricity (electrocution) (shock) 994.8
burn — *see* Burn, by site
exertion (excessive) 994.5
exposure 994.9
exhaustion 994.4
external cause NEC 994.9
fallout (radioactive) NEC 990
fluoroscopy NEC 990

☑ Additional Digit Required — Refer to the Tabular List for Digit Selection
2013 ICD-9-CM ▶◀ Revised Text ● New Line ▲ Revised Code
Subterms under main terms may continue to next column or page
Volume 2 — 101

Effect, adverse — Elongation, elongated

Effect, adverse — *continued*
foodstuffs
anaphylactic reaction or shock due to food NEC — *see* Anaphylactic reaction or shock, due to food
noxious 988.9
specified type NEC (*see also* Poisoning, by name of noxious foodstuff) 988.8
gases, fumes, or vapors — *see* Table of Drugs and Chemicals
glue (airplane) sniffing 304.6 ☑
heat — *see* Heat
high altitude NEC 993.2
anoxia 993.2
on
ears 993.0
sinuses 993.1
polycythemia 289.0
hot weather — *see* Heat
hunger 994.2
immersion, foot 991.4
immunization — *see* Complications, vaccination
immunological agents — *see* Complications, vaccination
implantation (removable) of isotope or radium NEC 990
infrared (radiation) (rays) NEC 990
burn — *see* Burn, by site
dermatitis or eczema 692.82
infusion — *see* Complications, infusion
ingestion or injection of isotope (therapeutic) NEC 990
irradiation NEC (*see also* Effect, adverse, radiation) 990
isotope (radioactive) NEC 990
lack of care (child) (infant) (newborn) 995.52
adult 995.84
lightning 994.0
burn — *see* Burn, by site
Lirugin — *see* Complications, vaccination
medicinal substance, correct, properly administered (*see also* Effect, adverse, drugs) 995.20
mesothorium NEC 990
motion 994.6
noise, inner ear 388.10
other drug, medicinal and biological substance 995.29
overheated places — *see* Heat
polonium NEC 990
psychosocial, of work environment V62.1
radiation (diagnostic) (fallout) (infrared) (natural source) (therapeutic) (tracer) (ultraviolet) (x-ray) NEC 990
with pulmonary manifestations
acute 508.0
chronic 508.1
dermatitis or eczema 692.82
due to sun NEC (*see also* Dermatitis, due to, sun) 692.70
fibrosis of lungs 508.1
maternal with suspected damage to fetus affecting management of pregnancy 655.6 ☑
pneumonitis 508.0
radioactive substance NEC 990
dermatitis or eczema 692.82
radioactivity NEC 990
radiotherapy NEC 990
dermatitis or eczema 692.82
radium NEC 990
reduced temperature 991.9
frostbite — *see* Frostbite
immersion, foot (hand) 991.4
specified effect NEC 991.8
roentgenography NEC 990
roentgenoscopy NEC 990
roentgen rays NEC 990
serum (prophylactic) (therapeutic) NEC 999.59
specified NEC 995.89
external cause NEC 994.9
strangulation 994.7
submersion 994.1

Effect, adverse — *continued*
teletherapy NEC 990
thirst 994.3
transfusion — *see* Complications, transfusion
ultraviolet (radiation) (rays) NEC 990
burn (*see also* Burn, by site)
from sun (*see also* Sunburn) 692.71
dermatitis or eczema 692.82
due to sun NEC (*see also* Dermatitis, due to, sun) 692.70
uranium NEC 990
vaccine (any) — *see* Complications, vaccination
weightlessness 994.9
whole blood (*see also* Complications, transfusion)
overdose or wrong substance given (*see also* Table of Drugs and Chemicals) 964.7
working environment V62.1
x-rays NEC 990
dermatitis or eczema 692.82
Effect, remote
of cancer — *see* condition
Effects, late — *see* Late, effect (of)
Effluvium, telogen 704.02
Effort
intolerance 306.2
syndrome (aviators) (psychogenic) 306.2
Effusion
amniotic fluid (*see also* Rupture, membranes, premature) 658.1 ☑
brain (serous) 348.5
bronchial (*see also* Bronchitis) 490
cerebral 348.5
cerebrospinal (*see also* Meningitis) 322.9
vessel 348.5
chest — *see* Effusion, pleura
intracranial 348.5
joint 719.00
ankle 719.07
elbow 719.02
foot 719.07
hand 719.04
hip 719.05
knee 719.06
multiple sites 719.09
pelvic region 719.05
shoulder (region) 719.01
specified site NEC 719.08
wrist 719.03
meninges (*see also* Meningitis) 322.9
pericardium, pericardial (*see also* Pericarditis) 423.9
acute 420.90
peritoneal (chronic) 568.82
pleura, pleurisy, pleuritic, pleuropericardial 511.9
bacterial, nontuberculous 511.1
fetus or newborn 511.9
malignant 511.81
nontuberculous 511.9
bacterial 511.1
pneumococcal 511.1
staphylococcal 511.1
streptococcal 511.1
traumatic 862.29
with open wound 862.39
tuberculous (*see also* Tuberculosis, pleura) 012.0 ☑
primary progressive 010.1 ☑
pulmonary — *see* Effusion, pleura
spinal (*see also* Meningitis) 322.9
thorax, thoracic — *see* Effusion, pleura
Egg (oocyte) (ovum)
donor V59.70
over age 35 V59.73
anonymous recipient V59.73
designated recipient V59.74
under age 35 V59.71
anonymous recipient V59.71
designated recipient V59.72
Eggshell nails 703.8
congenital 757.5

Ego-dystonic
homosexuality 302.0
lesbianism 302.0
sexual orientation 302.0
Egyptian splenomegaly 120.1
Ehlers-Danlos syndrome 756.83
Ehrlichiosis 082.40
chaffeensis 082.41
specified type NEC 082.49
Eichstedt's disease (pityriasis versicolor) 111.0
EIN (endometrial intraepithelial neoplasia) 621.35
Eisenmenger's complex or syndrome (ventricular septal defect) 745.4
Ejaculation, semen
painful 608.89
psychogenic 306.59
premature 302.75
retrograde 608.87
Ekbom syndrome (restless legs) 333.94
Ekman's syndrome (brittle bones and blue sclera) 756.51
Elastic skin 756.83
acquired 701.8
Elastofibroma (M8820/0) — *see* Neoplasm, connective tissue, benign
Elastoidosis
cutanea nodularis 701.8
cutis cystica et comedonica 701.8
Elastoma 757.39
juvenile 757.39
Miescher's (elastosis perforans serpiginosa) 701.1
Elastomyofibrosis 425.3
Elastosis 701.8
atrophicans 701.8
perforans serpiginosa 701.1
reactive perforating 701.1
senilis 701.8
solar (actinic) 692.74
Elbow — *see* condition
Electric
current, electricity, effects (concussion) (fatal) (nonfatal) (shock) 994.8
burn — *see* Burn, by site
feet (foot) syndrome 266.2
shock from electroshock gun (taser) 994.8
Electrocution 994.8
Electrolyte imbalance 276.9
with
abortion — *see* Abortion, by type, with metabolic disorder
ectopic pregnancy (*see also* categories 633.0–633.9) 639.4
hyperemesis gravidarum (before 22 completed weeks gestation) 643.1 ☑
molar pregnancy (*see also* categories 630–632) 639.4
following
abortion 639.4
ectopic or molar pregnancy 639.4
Elephantiasis (nonfilarial) 457.1
arabicum (*see also* Infestation, filarial) 125.9
congenita hereditaria 757.0
congenital (any site) 757.0
due to
Brugia (malayi) 125.1
mastectomy operation 457.0
Wuchereria (bancrofti) 125.0
malayi 125.1
eyelid 374.83
filarial (*see also* Infestation, filarial) 125.9
filariensis (*see also* Infestation, filarial) 125.9
gingival 523.8
glandular 457.1
graecorum 030.9
lymphangiectatic 457.1
lymphatic vessel 457.1
due to mastectomy operation 457.0
neuromatosa 237.71
postmastectomy 457.0
scrotum 457.1
streptococcal 457.1
surgical 997.99
postmastectomy 457.0

Elephantiasis — *continued*
telangiectodes 457.1
vulva (nonfilarial) 624.8
Elephant man syndrome 237.71
Elevated — *see* Elevation
findings on laboratory examination — *see* Findings, abnormal, without diagnosis (examination) (laboratory test)
GFR (glomerular filtration rate) — *see* Findings, abnormal, without diagnosis (examination) (laboratory test)
Elevation
17-ketosteroids 791.9
acid phosphatase 790.5
alkaline phosphatase 790.5
amylase 790.5
antibody titers 795.79
basal metabolic rate (BMR) 794.7
blood pressure (*see also* Hypertension) 401.9
reading (incidental) (isolated) (nonspecific), no diagnosis of hypertension 796.2
blood sugar 790.29
body temperature (of unknown origin) (*see also* Pyrexia) 780.60
cancer antigen 125 [CA 125] 795.82
carcinoembryonic antigen [CEA] 795.81
cholesterol 272.0
with high triglycerides 272.2
conjugate, eye 378.81
C-reactive protein (CRP) 790.95
CRP (C-reactive protein) 790.95
diaphragm, congenital 756.6
GFR (glomerular filtration rate) — *see* Findings, abnormal, without diagnosis (examination) (laboratory test)
glucose
fasting 790.21
tolerance test 790.22
immunoglobulin level 795.79
indolacetic acid 791.9
lactic acid dehydrogenase (LDH) level 790.4
leukocytes 288.60
lipase 790.5
lipoprotein a level 272.8
liver function test (LFT) 790.6
alkaline phosphatase 790.5
aminotransferase 790.4
bilirubin 782.4
hepatic enzyme NEC 790.5
lactate dehydrogenase 790.4
lymphocytes 288.61
prostate specific antigen (PSA) 790.93
renin 790.99
in hypertension (*see also* Hypertension, renovascular) 405.91
Rh titer (*see also* Complications, transfusion) 999.70
scapula, congenital 755.52
sedimentation rate 790.1
SGOT 790.4
SGPT 790.4
transaminase 790.4
triglycerides 272.1
with high cholesterol 272.2
vanillylmandelic acid 791.9
venous pressure 459.89
VMA 791.9
white blood cell count 288.60
specified NEC 288.69
Elliptocytosis (congenital) (hereditary) 282.1
Hb-C (disease) 282.7
hemoglobin disease 282.7
sickle-cell (disease) 282.60
trait 282.5
Ellison-Zollinger syndrome (gastric hypersecretion with pancreatic islet cell tumor) 251.5
Ellis-van Creveld disease or syndrome (chondroectodermal dysplasia) 756.55
Elongation, elongated (congenital) — *see also* Distortion
bone 756.9
cervix (uteri) 752.49
acquired 622.6
hypertrophic 622.6

☑ **Additional Digit Required** — Refer to the Tabular List for Digit Selection   ▽ **Subterms under main terms may continue to next column or page**

102 — Volume 2   ▶◀ Revised Text   ● New Line   ▲ Revised Code   2013 ICD-9-CM

Elongation, elongated — see also Distortion
  — continued
  colon 751.5
  common bile duct 751.69
  cystic duct 751.69
  frenulum, penis 752.69
  labia minora, acquired 624.8
  ligamentum patellae 756.89
  petiolus (epiglottidis) 748.3
  styloid bone (process) 733.99
  tooth, teeth 520.2
  uvula 750.26
    acquired 528.9
Elschnig bodies or pearls 366.51
El Tor cholera 001.1
Emaciation (due to malnutrition) 261
Emancipation disorder 309.22
Embadomoniasis 007.8
Embarrassment heart, cardiac — see Disease,
    heart
Embedded
  fragment (status) — see Foreign body, re-
    tained
  splinter (status) — see Foreign body, re-
    tained
  tooth, teeth 520.6
    root only 525.3
Embolic — see condition
Embolism 444.9
  with
    abortion — see Abortion, by type, with
      embolism
    ectopic pregnancy (see also categories
      633.0–633.9) 639.6
    molar pregnancy (see also categories
      630–632) 639.6
  air (any site) 958.0
    with
      abortion — see Abortion, by type,
        with embolism
      ectopic pregnancy (see also cate-
        gories 633.0–633.9) 639.6
      molar pregnancy (see also categories
        630–632) 639.6
    due to implanted device — see Compli-
      cations, due to (presence of) any
      device, implant, or graft classified
      to 996.0–996.5 NEC
    following
      abortion 639.6
      ectopic or molar pregnancy 639.6
      infusion, perfusion, or transfusion
        999.1
    in pregnancy, childbirth, or puerperium
      673.0 ☑
    traumatic 958.0
  amniotic fluid (pulmonary) 673.1 ☑
    with
      abortion — see Abortion, by type,
        with embolism
      ectopic pregnancy (see also cate-
        gories 633.0–633.9) 639.6
      molar pregnancy (see also categories
        630–632) 639.6
    following
      abortion 639.6
      ectopic or molar pregnancy 639.6
  aorta, aortic 444.1
    abdominal 444.09
      saddle 444.01
    bifurcation 444.09
    saddle 444.01
    thoracic 444.1
  artery 444.9
    auditory, internal 433.8 ☑
    basilar (see also Occlusion, artery, basilar)
      433.0 ☑
    bladder 444.89
    carotid (common) (internal) (see also
      Occlusion, artery, carotid)
      433.1 ☑
    cerebellar (anterior inferior) (posterior
      inferior) (superior) 433.8 ☑
    cerebral (see also Embolism, brain)
      434.1 ☑
    choroidal (anterior) 433.8 ☑

Embolism — continued
  artery — continued
    communicating posterior 433.8 ☑
    coronary (see also Infarct, myocardium)
      410.9 ☑
      without myocardial infarction 411.81
    extremity 444.22
      lower 444.22
      upper 444.21
    hypophyseal 433.8 ☑
    mesenteric (with gangrene) 557.0
    ophthalmic (see also Occlusion, retina)
      362.30
    peripheral 444.22
    pontine 433.8 ☑
    precerebral NEC — see Occlusion, artery,
      precerebral
    pulmonary — see Embolism, pulmonary
    pyemic 449
      pulmonary 415.12
    renal 593.81
    retinal (see also Occlusion, retina) 362.30
    septic 449
      pulmonary 415.12
    specified site NEC 444.89
    vertebral (see also Occlusion, artery, ver-
      tebral) 433.2 ☑
  auditory, internal 433.8 ☑
  basilar (artery) (see also Occlusion, artery,
    basilar) 433.0 ☑
  birth, mother — see Embolism, obstetrical
  blood-clot
    with
      abortion — see Abortion, by type,
        with embolism
      ectopic pregnancy (see also cate-
        gories 633.0–633.9) 639.6
      molar pregnancy (see also categories
        630–632) 639.6
    following
      abortion 639.6
      ectopic or molar pregnancy 639.6
    in pregnancy, childbirth, or puerperium
      673.2 ☑
  brain 434.1 ☑
    with
      abortion — see Abortion, by type,
        with embolism
      ectopic pregnancy (see also cate-
        gories 633.0–633.9) 639.6
      molar pregnancy (see also categories
        630–632) 639.6
    following
      abortion 639.6
      ectopic or molar pregnancy 639.6
    late effect — see Late effect(s) (of) cere-
      brovascular disease
    puerperal, postpartum, childbirth
      674.0 ☑
  capillary 448.9
  cardiac (see also Infarct, myocardium)
    410.9 ☑
  carotid (artery) (common) (internal) (see also
    Occlusion, artery, carotid) 433.1 ☑
  cavernous sinus (venous) — see Embolism,
    intracranial venous sinus
  cerebral (see also Embolism, brain) 434.1 ☑
  cholesterol — see Atheroembolism
  choroidal (anterior) (artery) 433.8 ☑
  coronary (artery or vein) (systemic) (see also
    Infarct, myocardium) 410.9 ☑
    without myocardial infarction 411.81
  due to (presence of) any device, implant, or
    graft classifiable to 996.0–996.5 —
    see Complications, due to (presence
    of) any device, implant, or graft clas-
    sified to 996.0–996.5 NEC
  encephalomalacia (see also Embolism, brain)
    434.1 ☑
  extremities 444.22
    lower 444.22
    upper 444.21
  eye 362.30
  fat (cerebral) (pulmonary) (systemic) 958.1

Embolism — continued
  fat — continued
    with
      abortion — see Abortion, by type,
        with embolism
      ectopic pregnancy (see also cate-
        gories 633.0–633.9) 639.6
      molar pregnancy (see also categories
        630–632) 639.6
    complicating delivery or puerperium
      673.8 ☑
    following
      abortion 639.6
      ectopic or molar pregnancy 639.6
    in pregnancy, childbirth, or the puerperi-
      um 673.8 ☑
  femoral (artery) 444.22
    vein 453.6
      deep 453.41
  following
    abortion 639.6
    ectopic or molar pregnancy 639.6
    infusion, perfusion, or transfusion
      air 999.1
      thrombus 999.2
  heart (fatty) (see also Infarct, myocardium)
    410.9 ☑
  hepatic (vein) 453.0
  iliac (artery) 444.81
  iliofemoral 444.81
  in pregnancy, childbirth, or puerperium
    (pulmonary) — see Embolism, obstet-
    rical
  intestine (artery) (vein) (with gangrene)
    557.0
  intracranial (see also Embolism, brain)
    434.1 ☑
    venous sinus (any) 325
      late effect — see category 326
      nonpyogenic 437.6
        in pregnancy or puerperium
          671.5 ☑
  kidney (artery) 593.81
  lateral sinus (venous) — see Embolism, in-
    tracranial venous sinus
  longitudinal sinus (venous) — see Em-
    bolism, intracranial venous sinus
  lower extremity 444.22
  lung (massive) — see Embolism, pulmonary
  meninges (see also Embolism, brain)
    434.1 ☑
  mesenteric (artery) (with gangrene) 557.0
  multiple NEC 444.9
  obstetrical (pulmonary) 673.2 ☑
    air 673.0 ☑
    amniotic fluid (pulmonary) 673.1 ☑
    blood-clot 673.2 ☑
    cardiac 674.8 ☑
    fat 673.8 ☑
    heart 674.8 ☑
    pyemic 673.3 ☑
    septic 673.3 ☑
    specified NEC 674.8 ☑
  ophthalmic (see also Occlusion, retina)
    362.30
  paradoxical NEC 444.9
  penis 607.82
  peripheral arteries NEC 444.22
    lower 444.22
    upper 444.21
  pituitary 253.8
  popliteal (artery) 444.22
  portal (vein) 452
  postoperative NEC 997.2
    cerebral 997.02
    mesenteric artery 997.71
    other vessels 997.79
    peripheral vascular 997.2
    pulmonary 415.11
      septic 415.11
    renal artery 997.72
  precerebral artery (see also Occlusion, artery,
    precerebral) 433.9 ☑
  puerperal — see Embolism, obstetrical
  pulmonary (acute) (artery) (vein) 415.19

Embolism — continued
  pulmonary — continued
    with
      abortion — see Abortion, by type,
        with embolism
      ectopic pregnancy (see also cate-
        gories 633.0–633.9) 639.6
      molar pregnancy (see also categories
        630–632) 639.6
    chronic 416.2
    following
      abortion 639.6
      ectopic or molar pregnancy 639.6
    healed or old V12.55
    iatrogenic 415.11
    in pregnancy, childbirth, or puerperium
      — see Embolism, obstetrical
    personal history of V12.55
    postoperative 415.11
    septic 415.12
  pyemic (multiple) (see also Septicemia)
    415.12
    with
      abortion — see Abortion, by type,
        with embolism
      ectopic pregnancy (see also cate-
        gories 633.0–633.9) 639.6
      molar pregnancy (see also categories
        630–632) 639.6
    Aerobacter aerogenes 415.12
    enteric gram-negative bacilli 415.12
    Enterobacter aerogenes 415.12
    Escherichia coli 415.12
    following
      abortion 639.6
      ectopic or molar pregnancy 639.6
    Hemophilus influenzae 415.12
    pneumococcal 415.12
    Proteus vulgaris 415.12
    Pseudomonas (aeruginosa) 415.12
    puerperal, postpartum, childbirth (any
      organism) 673.3 ☑
    Serratia 415.12
    specified organism NEC 415.12
    staphylococcal 415.12
      aureus 415.12
      specified organism NEC 415.12
    streptococcal 415.12
  renal (artery) 593.81
    vein 453.3
  retina, retinal (see also Occlusion, retina)
    362.30
  saddle
    abdominal aorta 444.01
    pulmonary artery 415.13
  septic 415.12
    arterial 449
  septicemic — see Embolism, pyemic
  sinus — see Embolism, intracranial venous
    sinus
  soap
    with
      abortion — see Abortion, by type,
        with embolism
      ectopic pregnancy (see also cate-
        gories 633.0–633.9) 639.6
      molar pregnancy (see also categories
        630–632) 639.6
    following
      abortion 639.6
      ectopic or molar pregnancy 639.6
  spinal cord (nonpyogenic) 336.1
    in pregnancy or puerperium 671.5 ☑
    pyogenic origin 324.1
    late effect — see category 326
  spleen, splenic (artery) 444.89
  thrombus (thromboembolism) following
    infusion, perfusion, or transfusion
    999.2
  upper extremity 444.21
  vein 453.9
    with inflammation or phlebitis — see
      Thrombophlebitis
    antecubital (acute) 453.81
      chronic 453.71
    axillary (acute) 453.84

☑ Additional Digit Required — Refer to the Tabular List for Digit Selection   ⬛ Subterms under main terms may continue to next column or page

2013 ICD-9-CM   ▶◀ Revised Text   ● New Line   ▲ Revised Code   Volume 2 — 103

Embolism — continued
vein — continued
axillary — continued
chronic 453.74
basilic (acute) 453.81
chronic 453.71
brachial (acute) 453.82
chronic 453.72
brachiocephalic (acute) (innominate) 453.87
chronic 453.77
cephalic (acute) 453.81
chronic 453.71
cerebral (see also Embolism, brain) 434.1 ☑
coronary (see also Infarct, myocardium) 410.9 ☑
without myocardial infarction 411.81
hepatic 453.0
internal jugular (acute) 453.86
chronic 453.76
lower extremity (superficial) 453.6
deep 453.40
acute 453.40
calf 453.42
distal (lower leg) 453.42
femoral 453.41
iliac 453.41
lower leg 453.42
peroneal 453.42
popliteal 453.41
proximal (upper leg) 453.41
thigh 453.41
tibial 453.42
chronic 453.50
calf 453.52
disal (lower leg) 453.52
femoral 453.51
iliac 453.51
lower leg 453.52
peroneal 453.52
popliteal 453.51
proximal (upper leg) 453.51
thigh 453.51
tibial 453.52
saphenous (greater) (lesser) 453.6
superficial 453.6
mesenteric (with gangrene) 557.0
portal 452
pulmonary — see Embolism, pulmonary
radial (acute) 453.82
chronic 453.72
renal 453.3
saphenous (greater) (lesser) 453.6
specified NEC (acute) 453.89
with inflammation or phlebitis — see Thrombophlebitis
chronic 453.79
subclavian (acute) 453.85
chronic 453.75
superior vena cava (acute) 453.87
chronic 453.77
thoracic (acute) 453.87
chronic 453.77
ulnar (acute) 453.82
chronic 453.72
upper extremity (acute) 453.83
chronic 453.73
deep 453.72
superficial 453.71
deep 453.82
superficial 453.81
vena cava
inferior 453.2
superior (acute) 453.87
chronic 453.77
vessels of brain (see also Embolism, brain) 434.1 ☑
Embolization — see Embolism
Embolus — see Embolism
Embryoma (M9080/1) — see also Neoplasm, by site, uncertain behavior
benign (M9080/0) — see Neoplasm, by site, benign
kidney (M8960/3) 189.0
liver (M8970/3) 155.0

Embryoma (M9080/1) — see also Neoplasm, by site, uncertain behavior — continued
malignant (M9080/3) (see also Neoplasm, by site, malignant)
kidney (M8960/3) 189.0
liver (M8970/3) 155.0
testis (M9070/3) 186.9
undescended 186.0
testis (M9070/3) 186.9
undescended 186.0
Embryonic
circulation 747.9
heart 747.9
vas deferens 752.89
Embryopathia NEC 759.9
Embryotomy, fetal 763.89
Embryotoxon 743.43
interfering with vision 743.42
Emesis — see also Vomiting
bilious 787.04
gravidarum — see Hyperemesis, gravidarum
Emissions, nocturnal (semen) 608.89
Emotional
crisis — see Crisis, emotional
disorder (see also Disorder, mental) 300.9
instability (excessive) 301.3
lability 799.24
overlay — see Reaction, adjustment
upset 300.9
Emotionality, pathological 301.3
Emotogenic disease — see also Disorder, psychogenic 306.9
Emphysema (atrophic) (centriacinar) (centrilobular) (chronic) (diffuse) (essential) (hypertrophic) (interlobular) (lung) (obstructive) (panlobular) (paracicatricial) (paracinar) (postural) (pulmonary) (senile) (subpleural) (traction) (unilateral) (unilobular) (vesicular) 492.8
with bronchitis
chronic 491.20
with
acute bronchitis 491.22
exacerbation (acute) 491.21
bullous (giant) 492.0
cellular tissue 958.7
surgical 998.81
compensatory 518.2
congenital 770.2
conjunctiva 372.89
connective tissue 958.7
surgical 998.81
due to fumes or vapors 506.4
eye 376.89
eyelid 374.85
surgical 998.81
traumatic 958.7
fetus or newborn (interstitial) (mediastinal) (unilobular) 770.2
heart 416.9
interstitial 518.1
congenital 770.2
fetus or newborn 770.2
laminated tissue 958.7
surgical 998.81
mediastinal 518.1
fetus or newborn 770.2
newborn (interstitial) (mediastinal) (unilobular) 770.2
obstructive diffuse with fibrosis 492.8
orbit 376.89
subcutaneous 958.7
due to trauma 958.7
nontraumatic 518.1
surgical 998.81
surgical 998.81
thymus (gland) (congenital) 254.8
traumatic 958.7
tuberculous (see also Tuberculosis, pulmonary) 011.9 ☑
Employment examination (certification) V70.5
Empty sella (turcica) syndrome 253.8

Empyema (chest) (diaphragmatic) (double) (encapsulated) (general) (interlobar) (lung) (medial) (necessitatis) (perforating chest wall) (pleura) (pneumococcal) (residual) (sacculated) (streptococcal) (supradiaphragmatic) 510.9
with fistula 510.0
accessory sinus (chronic) (see also Sinusitis) 473.9
acute 510.9
with fistula 510.0
antrum (chronic) (see also Sinusitis, maxillary) 473.0
brain (any part) (see also Abscess, brain) 324.0
ethmoidal (sinus) (chronic) (see also Sinusitis, ethmoidal) 473.2
extradural (see also Abscess, extradural) 324.9
frontal (sinus) (chronic) (see also Sinusitis, frontal) 473.1
gallbladder (see also Cholecystitis, acute) 575.0
mastoid (process) (acute) (see also Mastoiditis, acute) 383.00
maxilla, maxillary 526.4
sinus (chronic) (see also Sinusitis, maxillary) 473.0
nasal sinus (chronic) (see also Sinusitis) 473.9
sinus (accessory) (nasal) (see also Sinusitis) 473.9
sphenoidal (chronic) (sinus) (see also Sinusitis, sphenoidal) 473.3
subarachnoid (see also Abscess, extradural) 324.9
subdural (see also Abscess, extradural) 324.9
tuberculous (see also Tuberculosis, pleura) 012.0 ☑
ureter (see also Ureteritis) 593.89
ventricular (see also Abscess, brain) 324.0
Enameloma 520.2
Encephalitis (bacterial) (chronic) (hemorrhagic) (idiopathic) (nonepidemic) (spurious) (subacute) 323.9
acute (see also Encephalitis, viral)
disseminated (postinfectious) NEC 136.9 [323.61]
postimmunization or postvaccination 323.51
inclusional 049.8
inclusion body 049.8
necrotizing 049.8
arboviral, arbovirus NEC 064
arthropod-borne (see also Encephalitis, viral, arthropod-borne) 064
Australian X 062.4
Bwamba fever 066.3
California (virus) 062.5
Central European 063.2
Czechoslovakian 063.2
Dawson's (inclusion body) 046.2
diffuse sclerosing 046.2
due to
actinomycosis 039.8 [323.41]
cat-scratch disease 078.3 [323.01]
human herpesvirus NEC 058.29
human herpesvirus 6 058.21
human herpesvirus 7 058.29
human immunodeficiency virus (HIV) disease 042 [323.01]
infectious mononucleosis 075 [323.01]
malaria (see also Malaria) 084.6 [323.2]
Negishi virus 064
ornithosis 073.7 [323.01]
other infection classified elsewhere 136.9 [323.41]
prophylactic inoculation against smallpox 323.51
rickettsiosis (see also Rickettsiosis) 083.9 [323.1]
rubella 056.01
toxoplasmosis (acquired) 130.0
congenital (active) 771.2 [323.41]
typhus (fever) (see also Typhus) 081.9 [323.1]
vaccination (smallpox) 323.51

Encephalitis — continued
Eastern equine 062.2
endemic 049.8
epidemic 049.8
equine (acute) (infectious) (viral) 062.9
Eastern 062.2
Venezuelan 066.2
Western 062.1
Far Eastern 063.0
following vaccination or other immunization procedure 323.51
herpes 054.3
human herpesvirus NEC 058.29
human herpesvirus 6 058.21
human herpesvirus 7 058.29
Ilheus (virus) 062.8
inclusion body 046.2
infectious (acute) (virus) NEC 049.8
influenzal (see also Influenza) 487.8 [323.41]
lethargic 049.8
Japanese (B type) 062.0
La Crosse 062.5
Langat 063.8
late effect — see Late, effect, encephalitis
lead 984.9 [323.71]
lethargic (acute) (infectious) (influenzal) 049.8
lethargica 049.8
louping ill 063.1
lupus 710.0 [323.81]
lymphatica 049.0
Mengo 049.8
meningococcal 036.1
mumps 072.2
Murray Valley 062.4
myoclonic 049.8
Negishi virus 064
otitic NEC 382.4 [323.41]
parasitic NEC 123.9 [323.41]
periaxialis (concentrica) (diffusa) 341.1
postchickenpox 052.0
postexanthematous NEC 057.9 [323.62]
postimmunization 323.51
postinfectious NEC 136.9 [323.62]
postmeasles 055.0
posttraumatic 323.81
postvaccinal (smallpox) 323.51
postvaricella 052.0
postviral NEC 079.99 [323.62]
postexanthematous 057.9 [323.62]
specified NEC 057.8 [323.62]
Powassan 063.8
progressive subcortical (Binswanger's) 290.12
Rasmussen 323.81
Rio Bravo 049.8
rubella 056.01
Russian
autumnal 062.0
spring-summer type (taiga) 063.0
saturnine 984.9 [323.71]
Semliki Forest 062.8
serous 048
slow-acting virus NEC 046.8
specified cause NEC 323.81
St. Louis type 062.3
subacute sclerosing 046.2
subcorticalis chronica 290.12
summer 062.0
suppurative 324.0
syphilitic 094.81
congenital 090.41
tick-borne 063.9
torula, torular 117.5 [323.41]
toxic NEC 989.9 [323.71]
toxoplasmic (acquired) 130.0
congenital (active) 771.2 [323.41]
trichinosis 124 [323.41]
Trypanosomiasis (see also Trypanosomiasis) 086.9 [323.2]
tuberculous (see also Tuberculosis) 013.6 ☑
type B (Japanese) 062.0
type C 062.3
van Bogaert's 046.2
Venezuelan 066.2
Vienna type 049.8

☑ Additional Digit Required — Refer to the Tabular List for Digit Selection   Ⓦ Subterms under main terms may continue to next column or page

104 — Volume 2   ▶◀ Revised Text   ● New Line   ▲ Revised Code   2013 ICD-9-CM

Encephalitis — *continued*
  viral, virus 049.9
    arthropod-borne NEC 064
      mosquito-borne 062.9
        Australian X disease 062.4
        California virus 062.5
        Eastern equine 062.2
        Ilheus virus 062.8
        Japanese (B type) 062.0
        Murray Valley 062.4
        specified type NEC 062.8
        St. Louis 062.3
        type B 062.0
        type C 062.3
        Western equine 062.1
      tick-borne 063.9
        biundulant 063.2
        Central European 063.2
        Czechoslovakian 063.2
        diphasic meningoencephalitis 063.2
        Far Eastern 063.0
        Langat 063.8
        louping ill 063.1
        Powassan 063.8
        Russian spring-summer (taiga) 063.0
        specified type NEC 063.8
      vector unknown 064
      Western equine 062.1
    slow acting NEC 046.8
    specified type NEC 049.8
    vaccination, prophylactic (against) V05.0
    von Economo's 049.8
    Western equine 062.1
    West Nile type 066.41
Encephalocele 742.0
  orbit 376.81
Encephalocystocele 742.0
Encephaloduroarteriomyosynangiosis
    (EDAMS) 437.5
Encephalomalacia (brain) (cerebellar) (cere-
    bral) (cerebrospinal) — *see also* Soften-
    ing, brain 348.89
  due to
    hemorrhage (*see also* Hemorrhage,
      brain) 431
    recurrent spasm of artery 435.9
  embolic (cerebral) (*see also* Embolism, brain)
      434.1 ☑
  subcorticalis chronicus arteriosclerotica
      290.12
  thrombotic (*see also* Thrombosis, brain)
      434.0 ☑
Encephalomeningitis — *see* Meningoen-
    cephalitis
Encephalomeningocele 742.0
Encephalomeningomyelitis — *see* Menin-
    goencephalitis
Encephalomeningopathy — *see also* Menin-
    goencephalitis 349.9
Encephalomyelitis (chronic) (granulomatous)
    (myalgic, benign) — *see also* Encephalitis
    323.9
  abortive disseminated 049.8
  acute disseminated (ADEM) (postinfectious)
      136.9 [323.61]
    infectious 136.9 [323.61]
    noninfectious 323.81
    postimmunization 323.51
  due to
    cat-scratch disease 078.3 [323.01]
    infectious mononucleosis 075 [323.01]
    ornithosis 073.7 [323.01]
    vaccination (any) 323.51
  equine (acute) (infectious) 062.9
    Eastern 062.2
    Venezuelan 066.2
    Western 062.1
  funicularis infectiosa 049.8
  late effect — *see* Late, effect, encephalitis
  Munch-Peterson's 049.8
  postchickenpox 052.0
  postimmunization 323.51
  postmeasles 055.0
  postvaccinal (smallpox) 323.51

Encephalomyelitis — *see also* Encephalitis —
    continued
  rubella 056.01
  specified cause NEC 323.81
  syphilitic 094.81
  West Nile 066.41
Encephalomyelocele 742.0
Encephalomyelomeningitis — *see* Menin-
    goencephalitis
Encephalomyeloneuropathy 349.9
Encephalomyelopathy 349.9
  subacute necrotizing (infantile) 330.8
Encephalomyeloradiculitis (acute) 357.0
Encephalomyeloradiculoneuritis (acute)
    357.0
Encephalomyeloradiculopathy 349.9
Encephalomyocarditis 074.23
Encephalopathia hyperbilirubinemica,
    newborn 774.7
  due to isoimmunization (conditions classifi-
    able to 773.0–773.2) 773.4
Encephalopathy (acute) 348.30
  alcoholic 291.2
  anoxic — *see* Damage, brain, anoxic
  arteriosclerotic 437.0
    late effect — *see* Late effect(s) (of) cere-
      brovascular disease
  bilirubin, newborn 774.7
    due to isoimmunization 773.4
  congenital 742.9
  demyelinating (callosal) 341.8
  due to
    birth injury (intracranial) 767.8
    dialysis 294.8
      transient 293.9
    drugs — (*see also* Table of Drugs and
      Chemicals) 349.82
    hyperinsulinism — *see* Hyperinsulinism
    influenza (virus) (*see also* Influenza)
      487.8
      identified
        avian 488.09
        (novel) 2009 H1N1 488.19
    lack of vitamin (*see also* Deficiency, vita-
      min) 269.2
    nicotinic acid deficiency 291.2
    serum (nontherapeutic) (therapeutic)
      999.59
    syphilis 094.81
    trauma (postconcussional) 310.2
      current (*see also* Concussion, brain)
        850.9
        with skull fracture — *see* Fracture,
          skull, by site, with intracra-
          nial injury
    vaccination 323.51
  hepatic 572.2
  hyperbilirubinemic, newborn 774.7
    due to isoimmunization (conditions
      classifiable to 773.0–773.2) 773.4
  hypertensive 437.2
  hypoglycemic 251.2
  hypoxic (*see also* Damage, brain, anoxic)
    ischemic (HIE) 768.70
      mild 768.71
      moderate 768.72
      severe 768.73
  infantile cystic necrotizing (congenital)
    341.8
  lead 984.9 [323.71]
  leukopolio 330.0
  metabolic (*see also* Delirium) 348.31
    drug induced 349.82
    toxic 349.82
  necrotizing
    hemorrhagic (acute) 323.61
    subacute 330.8
  other specified type NEC 348.39
  pellagrous 265.2
  portal-systemic 572.2
  postcontusional 310.2
  posttraumatic 310.2
  saturnine 984.9 [323.71]
  septic 348.31
  spongioform, subacute (viral) 046.19

Encephalopathy — *continued*
  subacute
    necrotizing 330.8
    spongiform 046.19
    viral, spongiform 046.19
  subcortical progressive (Schilder) 341.1
    chronic (Binswanger's) 290.12
  toxic 349.82
    metabolic 349.82
  traumatic (postconcussional) 310.2
    current (*see also* Concussion, brain) 850.9
      with skull fracture — *see* Fracture,
        skull, by site, with intracranial
        injury
  vitamin B deficiency NEC 266.9
  Wernicke's (superior hemorrhagic polioen-
    cephalitis) 265.1
Encephalorrhagia — *see also* Hemorrhage,
    brain 432.9
  healed or old V12.54
  late effect — *see* Late effect(s) (of) cere-
    brovascular disease
Encephalosis, posttraumatic 310.2
Enchondroma (M9220/0) — *see also* Neo-
    plasm, bone, benign
  multiple, congenital 756.4
Enchondromatosis (cartilaginous) (congenital)
    (multiple) 756.4
Enchondroses, multiple (cartilaginous) (con-
    genital) 756.4
Encopresis — *see also* Incontinence, feces
    787.60
  nonorganic origin 307.7
Encounter for — *see also* Admission for
  administrative purpose only V68.9
    referral of patient without examination
      or treatment V68.81
    specified purpose NEC V68.89
  chemotherapy, (oral) (intravenous), antineo-
    plastic V58.11
  determination of fetal viability of pregnancy
    V23.87
  dialysis
    extracorporeal (renal) V56.0
    peritoneal V56.8
  disability examination V68.01
  end-of-life care V66.7
  hospice care V66.7
  immunizations (childhood) appropriate for
    age V20.2
  immunotherapy, antineoplastic V58.12
  joint prosthesis insertion following prior
    explantation of joint prosthesis
    V54.82
  palliative care V66.7
  paternity testing V70.4
  radiotherapy V58.0
  respirator [ventilator] dependence
    during
      mechanical failure V46.14
      power failure V46.12
    for weaning V46.13
  routine infant and child vision and hearing
    testing V20.2
  school examination V70.3
    following surgery V67.09
  screening mammogram NEC V76.12
    for high-risk patient V76.11
  terminal care V66.7
  weaning from respirator [ventilator] V46.13
Encystment — *see* Cyst
Endamebiasis — *see* Amebiasis
Endamoeba — *see* Amebiasis
Endarteritis (bacterial, subacute) (infective)
    (septic) 447.6
  brain, cerebral or cerebrospinal 437.4
    late effect — *see* Late effect(s) (of) cere-
      brovascular disease
  coronary (artery) — *see* Arteriosclerosis,
    coronary
  deformans — *see* Arteriosclerosis
  embolic (*see also* Embolism) 444.9
  obliterans (*see also* Arteriosclerosis)
    pulmonary 417.8
  pulmonary 417.8
  retina 362.18

Endarteritis — *continued*
  senile — *see* Arteriosclerosis
  syphilitic 093.89
    brain or cerebral 094.89
    congenital 090.5
    spinal 094.89
  tuberculous (*see also* Tuberculosis) 017.9 ☑
Endemic — *see* condition
Endocarditis (chronic) (indeterminate) (inter-
    stitial) (marantic) (nonbacterial throm-
    botic) (residual) (sclerotic) (sclerous)
    (senile) (valvular) 424.90
  with
    rheumatic fever (conditions classifiable
      to 390)
      active — *see* Endocarditis, acute,
        rheumatic
      inactive or quiescent (with chorea)
        397.9
  acute or subacute 421.9
    rheumatic (aortic) (mitral) (pulmonary)
      (tricuspid) 391.1
      with chorea (acute) (rheumatic)
        (Sydenham's) 392.0
  aortic (heart) (nonrheumatic) (valve) 424.1
    with
      mitral (valve) disease 396.9
        active or acute 391.1
          with chorea (acute)
            (rheumatic) (Syden-
            ham's) 392.0
      bacterial 421.0
      rheumatic fever (conditions classifi-
        able to 390)
        active — *see* Endocarditis, acute,
          rheumatic
        inactive or quiescent (with
          chorea) 395.9
          with mitral disease 396.9
  acute or subacute 421.9
  arteriosclerotic 424.1
  congenital 746.89
  hypertensive 424.1
  rheumatic (chronic) (inactive) 395.9
    with mitral (valve) disease 396.9
      active or acute 391.1
        with chorea (acute)
          (rheumatic) (Syden-
          ham's) 392.0
      active or acute 391.1
        with chorea (acute) (rheumatic)
          (Sydenham's) 392.0
  specified cause, except rheumatic 424.1
  syphilitic 093.22
  arteriosclerotic or due to arteriosclerosis
    424.99
  atypical verrucous (Libman-Sacks)
    710.0 [424.91]
  bacterial (acute) (any valve) (chronic) (suba-
    cute) 421.0
  blastomycotic 116.0 [421.1]
  candidal 112.81
  congenital 425.3
  constrictive 421.0
  Coxsackie 074.22
  due to
    blastomycosis 116.0 [421.1]
    candidiasis 112.81
    Coxsackie (virus) 074.22
    disseminated lupus erythematosus
      710.0 [424.91]
    histoplasmosis (*see also* Histoplasmosis)
      115.94
    hypertension (benign) 424.99
    moniliasis 112.81
    prosthetic cardiac valve 996.61
    Q fever 083.0 [421.1]
    serratia marcescens 421.0
    typhoid (fever) 002.0 [421.1]
  fetal 425.3
  gonococcal 098.84
  hypertensive 424.99
  infectious or infective (acute) (any valve)
    (chronic) (subacute) 421.0
  lenta (acute) (any valve) (chronic) (subacute)
    421.0

☑ **Additional Digit Required — Refer to the Tabular List for Digit Selection**   ▿ **Subterms under main terms may continue to next column or page**

2013 ICD-9-CM   ▶◀ **Revised Text**   ● **New Line**   ▲ **Revised Code**   **Volume 2 — 105**

Enteritis — *continued*
  chronic — *continued*
    ulcerative (*see also* Colitis, ulcerative)
        556.9
    cicatrizing (chronic) 555.0
  Clostridium
    botulinum 005.1
    difficile 008.45
    haemolyticum 008.46
    novyi 008.46
    perfringens (C) (F) 008.46
    specified type NEC 008.46
  coccidial 007.2
  dietetic 558.9
  due to
    achylia gastrica 536.8
    adenovirus 008.62
    Aerobacter aerogenes 008.2
    anaerobes (*see also* Enteritis, anaerobic)
        008.46
    Arizona (bacillus) 008.1
    astrovirus 008.66
    Bacillus coli — *see* Enteritis, E. coli
    bacteria NEC 008.5
      specified NEC 008.49
    Bacteroides (*see also* Enteritis, Bacteroides) 008.46
    Butyrivibrio (fibriosolvens) 008.46
    calicivirus 008.65
    Camplyobacter 008.43
    Clostridium — *see* Enteritis, Clostridium
    Cockle agent 008.64
    Coxsackie (virus) 008.67
    Ditchling agent 008.64
    ECHO virus 008.67
    Enterobacter aerogenes 008.2
    enterococci 008.49
    enterovirus NEC 008.67
    Escherichia coli — *see* Enteritis, E. coli
    Eubacterium 008.46
    Fusobacterium (nucleatum) 008.46
    gram-negative bacteria NEC 008.47
      anaerobic NEC 008.46
    Hawaii agent 008.63
    irritating foods 558.9
    Klebsiella aerogenes 008.47
    Marin County agent 008.66
    Montgomery County agent 008.63
    norovirus 008.63
    Norwalk-like agent 008.63
    Norwalk virus 008.63
    Otofuke agent 008.63
    Paracolobactrum arizonae 008.1
    paracolon bacillus NEC 008.47
      Arizona 008.1
    Paramatta agent 008.64
    Peptococcus 008.46
    Peptostreptococcus 008.46
    Proteus (bacillus) (mirabilis) (morganii)
        008.3
    Pseudomonas aeruginosa 008.42
    Rotavirus 008.61
    Sapporo agent 008.63
    small round virus (SRV) NEC 008.64
      featureless NEC 008.63
      structured NEC 008.63
    Snow Mountain (SM) agent 008.63
    specified
      bacteria NEC 008.49
      organism, nonbacterial NEC 008.8
      virus NEC 008.69
    Staphylococcus 008.41
    Streptococcus 008.49
      anaerobic 008.46
    Taunton agent 008.63
    Torovirus 008.69
    Treponema 008.46
    Veillonella 008.46
    virus 008.8
      specified type NEC 008.69
    Wollan (W) agent 008.64
    Yersinia enterocolitica 008.44
  dysentery — *see* Dysentery
  E. coli 008.00
    enterohemorrhagic 008.04

Enteritis — *continued*
  E. coli — *continued*
    enteroinvasive 008.03
    enteropathogenic 008.01
    enterotoxigenic 008.02
    specified type NEC 008.09
  el tor 001.1
  embadomonial 007.8
  eosinophilic 558.41
  epidemic 009.0
  Eubacterium 008.46
  fermentative 558.9
  fulminant 557.0
  Fusobacterium (nucleatum) 008.46
  gangrenous (*see also* Enteritis, due to, by
      organism) 009.0
  giardial 007.1
  gram-negative bacteria NEC 008.47
    anaerobic NEC 008.46
  infectious NEC (*see also* Enteritis, due to, by
      organism) 009.0
    presumed 009.1
  influenzal (*see also* Influenza) 487.8
  ischemic 557.9
    acute 557.0
    chronic 557.1
    due to mesenteric artery insufficiency
        557.1
  membranous 564.9
  mucous 564.9
  myxomembranous 564.9
  necrotic (*see also* Enteritis, due to, by organism) 009.0
  necroticans 005.2
  necrotizing of fetus or newborn (*see also*
      Enterocolitis, necrotizing, newborn)
      777.50
  neurogenic 564.9
  newborn 777.8
    necrotizing (*see also* Enterocolitis,
        necrotizing, newborn) 777.50
  parasitic NEC 129
  paratyphoid (fever) (*see also* Fever, paratyphoid) 002.9
  Peptococcus 008.46
  Peptostreptococcus 008.46
  Proprionibacterium 008.46
  protozoal NEC 007.9
  radiation 558.1
  regional (of) 555.9
    intestine
      large (bowel, colon, or rectum) 555.1
        with small intestine 555.2
      small (duodenum, ileum, or jejunum)
          555.0
        with large intestine 555.2
  Salmonella infection 003.0
  salmonellosis 003.0
  segmental (*see also* Enteritis, regional) 555.9
  septic (*see also* Enteritis, due to, by organism) 009.0
  Shigella 004.9
  simple 558.9
  spasmodic 564.9
  spastic 564.9
  staphylococcal 008.41
    due to food 005.0
  streptococcal 008.49
    anaerobic 008.46
  toxic 558.2
  Treponema (denticola) (macrodentium)
      008.46
  trichomonal 007.3
  tuberculous (*see also* Tuberculosis) 014.8 ☑
  typhosa 002.0
  ulcerative (chronic) (*see also* Colitis, ulcerative) 556.9
  Veillonella 008.46
  viral 008.8
    adenovirus 008.62
    enterovirus 008.67
    specified virus NEC 008.69
  Yersinia enterocolitica 008.44
  zymotic 009.0
Enteroarticular syndrome 099.3
Enterobiasis 127.4

Enterobius vermicularis 127.4
Enterocele — *see also* Hernia 553.9
  pelvis, pelvic (acquired) (congenital) 618.6
  vagina, vaginal (acquired) (congenital) 618.6
Enterocolitis — *see also* Enteritis
  fetus or newborn (*see also* Enterocolitis,
      necrotizing, newborn) 777.8
    necrotizing 777.50
  fulminant 557.0
  granulomatous 555.2
  hemorrhagic (acute) 557.0
    chronic 557.1
  necrotizing (acute) (membranous) 557.0
    newborn 777.50
      with
        perforation 777.53
        pneumatosis and perforation
            777.53
        pneumatosis without perforation
            777.52
        without pneumatosis, without perforation 777.51
      stage I 777.51
      stage II 777.52
      stage III 777.53
    primary necrotizing (*see also* Enterocolitis,
        necrotizing, newborn) 777.50
  pseudomembranous 008.45
    newborn 008.45
  radiation 558.1
    newborn (*see also* Enterocolitis, necrotizing, newborn) 777.50
  ulcerative 556.0
Enterocystoma 751.5
Enterogastritis — *see* Enteritis
Enterogenous cyanosis 289.7
Enterolith, enterolithiasis (impaction) 560.39
  with hernia (*see also* Hernia, by site, with
      obstruction)
    gangrenous — *see* Hernia, by site, with
        gangrene
Enteropathy 569.9
  exudative (of Gordon) 579.8
  gluten 579.0
  hemorrhagic, terminal 557.0
  protein-losing 579.8
Enteroperitonitis — *see also* Peritonitis 567.9
Enteroptosis 569.89
Enterorrhagia 578.9
Enterospasm 564.9
  psychogenic 306.4
Enterostenosis — *see also* Obstruction, intestine 560.9
Enterostomy status V44.4
  with complication 569.60
Enthesopathy 726.90
  ankle and tarsus 726.70
  elbow region 726.30
    specified NEC 726.39
  hip 726.5
  knee 726.60
  peripheral NEC 726.8
  shoulder region 726.10
    adhesive 726.0
  spinal 720.1
  wrist and carpus 726.4
Entrance, air into vein — *see* Embolism, air
Entrapment, nerve — *see* Neuropathy, entrapment
Entropion (eyelid) 374.00
  cicatricial 374.04
  congenital 743.62
  late effect of trachoma (healed) 139.1
  mechanical 374.02
  paralytic 374.02
  senile 374.01
  spastic 374.03
Enucleation of eye (current) (traumatic) 871.3
Enuresis 788.30
  habit disturbance 307.6
  nocturnal 788.36
    psychogenic 307.6
  nonorganic origin 307.6
  psychogenic 307.6
Enzymopathy 277.9
Eosinopenia 288.59

Eosinophilia 288.3
  with
    angiolymphoid hyperplasia (ALHE)
        228.01
  allergic 288.3
  hereditary 288.3
  idiopathic 288.3
  infiltrative 518.3
  Loeffler's 518.3
  myalgia syndrome 710.5
  pulmonary (tropical) 518.3
  secondary 288.3
  tropical 518.3
Eosinophilic — *see also* condition
  fasciitis 728.89
  granuloma (bone) 277.89
  infiltration lung 518.3
Ependymitis (acute) (cerebral) (chronic)
    (granular) — *see also* Meningitis 322.9
Ependymoblastoma (M9392/3)
  specified site — *see* Neoplasm, by site, malignant
  unspecified site 191.9
Ependymoma (epithelial) (malignant)
    (M9391/3)
  anaplastic type (M9392/3)
    specified site — *see* Neoplasm, by site,
        malignant
    unspecified site 191.9
  benign (M9391/0)
    specified site — *see* Neoplasm, by site,
        benign
    unspecified site 225.0
  myxopapillary (M9394/1) 237.5
  papillary (M9393/1) 237.5
  specified site — *see* Neoplasm, by site, malignant
  unspecified site 191.9
Ependymopathy 349.2
  spinal cord 349.2
Ephelides, ephelis 709.09
Ephemeral fever — *see also* Pyrexia 780.60
Epiblepharon (congenital) 743.62
Epicanthus, epicanthic fold (congenital)
    (eyelid) 743.63
Epicondylitis (elbow) (lateral) 726.32
  medial 726.31
Epicystitis — *see also* Cystitis 595.9
Epidemic — *see* condition
Epidermidalization, cervix — *see* condition
Epidermidization, cervix — *see* condition
Epidermis, epidermal — *see* condition
Epidermization, cervix — *see* condition
Epidermodysplasia verruciformis 078.19
Epidermoid
  cholesteatoma — *see* Cholesteatoma
  inclusion (*see also* Cyst, skin) 706.2
Epidermolysis
  acuta (combustiformis) (toxica) 695.15
  bullosa 757.39
  necroticans combustiformis 695.15
  due to drug
    correct substance properly administered 695.15
    overdose or wrong substance given
        or taken 977.9
    specified drug — *see* Table of
        Drugs and Chemicals
Epidermophytid — *see* Dermatophytosis
Epidermophytosis (infected) — *see* Dermatophytosis
Epidermosis, ear (middle) — *see also*
    Cholesteatoma 385.30
Epididymis — *see* condition
Epididymitis (nonvenereal) 604.90
  with abscess 604.0
  acute 604.99
  blennorrhagic (acute) 098.0
    chronic or duration of 2 months or over
        098.2
  caseous (*see also* Tuberculosis) 016.4 ☑
  chlamydial 099.54
  diphtheritic 032.89 [604.91]
  filarial 125.9 [604.91]
  gonococcal (acute) 098.0

☑ Additional Digit Required — Refer to the Tabular List for Digit Selection   ⟱ Subterms under main terms may continue to next column or page

2013 ICD-9-CM   ▶◀ Revised Text   ● New Line   ▲ Revised Code   Volume 2 — 107

Index

Epididymitis — Error

Epididymitis — continued
  gonococcal — continued
    chronic or duration of 2 months or over 098.2
    recurrent 604.99
    residual 604.99
    syphilitic 095.8 [604.91]
    tuberculous (see also Tuberculosis) 016.4 ☑
Epididymo-orchitis — see also Epididymitis 604.90
  with abscess 604.0
  chlamydial 099.54
  gonococcal (acute) 098.13
    chronic or duration of 2 months or over 098.33
Epidural — see condition
Epigastritis — see also Gastritis 535.5 ☑
Epigastrium, epigastric — see condition
Epigastrocele — see also Hernia, epigastric 553.29
Epiglottiditis (acute) 464.30
  with obstruction 464.31
  chronic 476.1
  viral 464.30
    with obstruction 464.31
Epiglottis — see condition
Epiglottitis (acute) 464.30
  with obstruction 464.31
  chronic 476.1
  viral 464.30
    with obstruction 464.31
Epignathus 759.4
Epilepsia
  partialis continua (see also Epilepsy) 345.7 ☑
  procursiva (see also Epilepsy) 345.8 ☑
Epilepsy, epileptic (idiopathic) 345.9 ☑

Note — use the following fifth-digit subclassification with categories 345.0, 345.1, 345.4–345.9:
0 without mention of intractable epilepsy
1 with intractable epilepsy
    pharmacoresistant (pharmacologically resistant)
    poorly controlled
    refractory (medically)
    treatment resistant

  abdominal 345.5 ☑
  absence (attack) 345.0 ☑
  akinetic 345.0 ☑
    psychomotor 345.4 ☑
  automatism 345.4 ☑
  autonomic diencephalic 345.5 ☑
  brain 345.9 ☑
  Bravais-Jacksonian 345.5 ☑
  cerebral 345.9 ☑
  climacteric 345.9 ☑
  clonic 345.1 ☑
  clouded state 345.9 ☑
  coma 345.3
  communicating 345.4 ☑
  complicating pregnancy, childbirth, or the puerperium 649.4 ☑
  congenital 345.9 ☑
  convulsions 345.9 ☑
  cortical (focal) (motor) 345.5 ☑
  cursive (running) 345.8 ☑
  cysticercosis 123.1
  deterioration
    with behavioral disturbance 345.9 ☑ [294.11]
    without behavioral disturbance 345.9 ☑ [294.10]
  due to syphilis 094.89
  equivalent 345.5 ☑
  fit 345.9 ☑
  focal (motor) 345.5 ☑
  gelastic 345.8 ☑
  generalized 345.9 ☑
    convulsive 345.1 ☑

Epilepsy, epileptic — continued
  generalized — continued
    flexion 345.1 ☑
    nonconvulsive 345.0 ☑
  grand mal (idiopathic) 345.1 ☑
  Jacksonian (motor) (sensory) 345.5 ☑
  Kojevnikoff's, Kojevnikov's, Kojewnikoff's 345.7 ☑
  laryngeal 786.2
  limbic system 345.4 ☑
  localization related (focal) (partial) and epileptic syndromes
    with
      complex partial seizures 345.4 ☑
      simple partial seizures 345.5 ☑
  major (motor) 345.1 ☑
  minor 345.0 ☑
  mixed (type) 345.9 ☑
  motor partial 345.5 ☑
  musicogenic 345.1 ☑
  myoclonus, myoclonic 345.1 ☑
    progressive (familial) 345.1 ☑
  nonconvulsive, generalized 345.0 ☑
  parasitic NEC 123.9
  partial (focalized) 345.5 ☑
    with
      impairment of consciousness 345.4 ☑
      memory and ideational disturbances 345.4 ☑
      without impairment of consciousness 345.5 ☑
    abdominal type 345.5 ☑
    motor type 345.5 ☑
    psychomotor type 345.4 ☑
    psychosensory type 345.4 ☑
    secondarily generalized 345.4 ☑
    sensory type 345.5 ☑
    somatomotor type 345.5 ☑
    somatosensory type 345.5 ☑
    temporal lobe type 345.4 ☑
    visceral type 345.5 ☑
    visual type 345.5 ☑
  peripheral 345.9 ☑
  petit mal 345.0 ☑
  photokinetic 345.8 ☑
  progressive myoclonic (familial) 345.1 ☑
  psychic equivalent 345.5 ☑
  psychomotor 345.4 ☑
  psychosensory 345.4 ☑
  reflex 345.1 ☑
  seizure 345.9 ☑
  senile 345.9 ☑
  sensory-induced 345.5 ☑
  sleep (see also Narcolepsy) 347.00
  somatomotor 345.5 ☑
  somatosensory 345.5 ☑
  specified type NEC 345.8 ☑
  status (grand mal) 345.3
    focal motor 345.7 ☑
    petit mal 345.2
    psychomotor 345.7 ☑
    temporal lobe 345.7 ☑
  symptomatic 345.9 ☑
  temporal lobe 345.4 ☑
  tonic (-clonic) 345.1 ☑
  traumatic (injury unspecified) 907.0
    injury specified — see Late, effect (of) specified injury
  twilight 293.0
  uncinate (gyrus) 345.4 ☑
  Unverricht (-Lundborg) (familial myoclonic) 345.1 ☑
  visceral 345.5 ☑
  visual 345.5 ☑
Epileptiform
  convulsions 780.39
  seizure 780.39
Epiloia 759.5
Epimenorrhea 626.2
Epipharyngitis — see also Nasopharyngitis 460
Epiphora 375.20

Epiphora — continued
  due to
    excess lacrimation 375.21
    insufficient drainage 375.22
Epiphyseal arrest 733.91
  femoral head 732.2
Epiphyseolysis, epiphysiolysis — see also Osteochondrosis 732.9
Epiphysitis — see also Osteochondrosis 732.9
  juvenile 732.6
  marginal (Scheuermann's) 732.0
  os calcis 732.5
  syphilitic (congenital) 090.0
  vertebral (Scheuermann's) 732.0
Epiplocele — see also Hernia 553.9
Epiploitis — see also Peritonitis 567.9
Epiplosarcomphalocele — see also Hernia, umbilicus 553.1
Episcleritis 379.00
  gouty 274.89 [379.09]
  nodular 379.02
  periodica fugax 379.01
    angioneurotic — see Edema, angioneurotic
  specified NEC 379.09
  staphylococcal 379.00
  suppurative 379.00
  syphilitic 095.0
  tuberculous (see also Tuberculosis) 017.3 ☑ [379.09]
Episode
  brain (see also Disease, cerebrovascular, acute) 436
  cerebral (see also Disease, cerebrovascular, acute) 436
  depersonalization (in neurotic state) 300.6
  hyporesponsive 780.09
  psychotic (see also Psychosis) 298.9
    organic, transient 293.9
  schizophrenic (acute) NEC (see also Schizophrenia) 295.4 ☑
Epispadias
  female 753.8
  male 752.62
Episplenitis 289.59
Epistaxis (multiple) 784.7
  hereditary 448.0
  vicarious menstruation 625.8
Epithelioma (malignant) (M8011/3) — see also Neoplasm, by site, malignant
  adenoides cysticum (M8100/0) — see Neoplasm, skin, benign
  basal cell (M8090/3) — see Neoplasm, skin, malignant
  benign (M8011/0) — see Neoplasm, by site, benign
  Bowen's (M8081/2) — see Neoplasm, skin, in situ
  calcifying (benign) (Malherbe's) (M8110/0) — see Neoplasm, skin, benign
  external site — see Neoplasm, skin, malignant
  intraepidermal, Jadassohn (M8096/0) — see Neoplasm, skin, benign
  squamous cell (M8070/3) — see Neoplasm, by site, malignant
Epitheliopathy
  pigment, retina 363.15
  posterior multifocal placoid (acute) 363.15
Epithelium, epithelial — see condition
Epituberculosis (allergic) (with atelectasis) — see also Tuberculosis 010.8 ☑
Eponychia 757.5
Epstein's
  nephrosis or syndrome (see also Nephrosis) 581.9
  pearl (mouth) 528.4
Epstein-Barr infection (viral) 075
  chronic 780.79 [139.8]
Epulis (giant cell) (gingiva) 523.8
Equinia 024
Equinovarus (congenital) 754.51
  acquired 736.71
Equivalent
  angina 413.9

Equivalent — continued
  convulsive (abdominal) (see also Epilepsy) 345.5 ☑
  epileptic (psychic) (see also Epilepsy) 345.5 ☑
Erb's
  disease 359.1
  palsy, paralysis (birth) (brachial) (newborn) 767.6
    spinal (spastic) syphilitic 094.89
  pseudohypertrophic muscular dystrophy 359.1
Erb-Goldflam disease or syndrome 358.00
Erb (-Duchenne) paralysis (birth injury) (newborn) 767.6
Erdheim-Chester disease (ECD) 277.89
Erdheim's syndrome (acromegalic macrospondylitis) 253.0
Erection, painful (persistent) 607.3
Ergosterol deficiency (vitamin D) 268.9
  with
    osteomalacia 268.2
    rickets (see also Rickets) 268.0
Ergotism (ergotized grain) 988.2
  from ergot used as drug (migraine therapy)
    correct substance properly administered 349.82
    overdose or wrong substance given or taken 975.0
Erichsen's disease (railway spine) 300.16
Erlacher-Blount syndrome (tibia vara) 732.4
Erosio interdigitalis blastomycetica 112.3
Erosion
  arteriosclerotic plaque — see Arteriosclerosis, by site
  artery NEC 447.2
    without rupture 447.8
  bone 733.99
  bronchus 519.19
  cartilage (joint) 733.99
  cervix (uteri) (acquired) (chronic) (congenital) 622.0
    with mention of cervicitis 616.0
  cornea (recurrent) (see also Keratitis) 371.42
    traumatic 918.1
  dental (idiopathic) (occupational) 521.30
    extending into
      dentine 521.32
      pulp 521.33
    generalized 521.35
    limited to enamel 521.31
    localized 521.34
  duodenum, postpyloric — see Ulcer, duodenum
  esophagus 530.89
  gastric 535.4 ☑
  implanted vaginal mesh
    in, into
      pelvic floor muscles 629.31
      surrounding organ(s) or tissue 629.31
  intestine 569.89
  lymphatic vessel 457.8
  pylorus, pyloric (ulcer) 535.4 ☑
  sclera 379.16
  spine, aneurysmal 094.89
  spleen 289.59
  stomach 535.4 ☑
  teeth (idiopathic) (occupational) (see also Erosion, dental) 521.30
    due to
      medicine 521.30
      persistent vomiting 521.30
  urethra 599.84
  uterus 621.8
  vaginal prosthetic materials NEC
    in, into
      pelvic floor muscles 629.31
      surrounding organ(s) or tissue 629.31
  vertebra 733.99
Erotomania 302.89
  Clérambault's 297.8
Error
  in diet 269.9
  refractive 367.9
    astigmatism (see also Astigmatism) 367.20

Error — continued
  refractive — continued
    drug-induced 367.89
    hypermetropia 367.0
    hyperopia 367.0
    myopia 367.1
    presbyopia 367.4
    toxic 367.89
Eructation 787.3
  nervous 306.4
  psychogenic 306.4
Eruption
  creeping 126.9
  drug — see Dermatitis, due to, drug
  Hutchinson, summer 692.72
  Kaposi's varicelliform 054.0
  napkin (psoriasiform) 691.0
  polymorphous
    light (sun) 692.72
    other source 692.82
  psoriasiform, napkin 691.0
  recalcitrant pustular 694.8
  ringed 695.89
  skin (see also Dermatitis) 782.1
    creeping (meaning hookworm) 126.9
    due to
      chemical(s) NEC 692.4
        internal use 693.8
      drug — see Dermatitis, due to, drug
      prophylactic inoculation or vaccina-
        tion against disease — see
        Dermatitis, due to, vaccine
      smallpox vaccination NEC — see
        Dermatitis, due to, vaccine
    erysipeloid 027.1
    feigned 698.4
    Hutchinson, summer 692.72
    Kaposi's, varicelliform 054.0
      vaccinia 999.0
    lichenoid, axilla 698.3
    polymorphous, due to light 692.72
    toxic NEC 695.0
    vesicular 709.8
  teeth, tooth
    accelerated 520.6
    delayed 520.6
    difficult 520.6
    disturbance of 520.6
    in abnormal sequence 520.6
    incomplete 520.6
    late 520.6
    natal 520.6
    neonatal 520.6
    obstructed 520.6
    partial 520.6
    persistent primary 520.6
    premature 520.6
    prenatal 520.6
  vesicular 709.8
Erysipelas (gangrenous) (infantile) (newborn)
    (phlegmonous) (suppurative) 035
  external ear 035 [380.13]
  puerperal, postpartum, childbirth 670.8 ☑
Erysipelatoid (Rosenbach's) 027.1
Erysipeloid (Rosenbach's) 027.1
Erythema, erythematous (generalized) 695.9
  ab igne — see Burn, by site, first degree
  annulare (centrifugum) (rheumaticum)
    695.0
  arthriticum epidemicum 026.1
  brucellum (see also Brucellosis) 023.9
  bullosum 695.19
  caloricum — see Burn, by site, first degree
  chronicum migrans 088.81
  circinatum 695.19
  diaper 691.0
  due to
    chemical (contact) NEC 692.4
      internal 693.8
    drug (internal use) 693.0
      contact 692.3
  elevatum diutinum 695.89
  endemic 265.2
  epidemic, arthritic 026.1
  figuratum perstans 695.0
  gluteal 691.0

Erythema, erythematous — continued
  gyratum (perstans) (repens) 695.19
  heat — see Burn, by site, first degree
  ichthyosiforme congenitum 757.1
  induratum (primary) (scrofulosorum) (see
    also Tuberculosis) 017.1 ☑
    nontuberculous 695.2
  infantum febrile 057.8
  infectional NEC 695.9
  infectiosum 057.0
  inflammation NEC 695.9
  intertrigo 695.89
  iris 695.10
  lupus (discoid) (localized) (see also Lupus,
    erythematosus) 695.4
  marginatum 695.0
    rheumaticum — see Fever, rheumatic
  medicamentosum — see Dermatitis, due
    to, drug
  migrans 529.1
    chronicum 088.81
  multiforme 695.10
    bullosum 695.19
    conjunctiva 695.19
    exudativum (Hebra) 695.19
    major 695.12
    minor 695.11
    pemphigoides 694.5
  napkin 691.0
  neonatorum 778.8
  nodosum 695.2
    tuberculous (see also Tuberculosis)
      017.1 ☑
  nummular, nummulare 695.19
  palmar 695.0
  palmaris hereditarium 695.0
  pernio 991.5
  perstans solare 692.72
  rash, newborn 778.8
  scarlatiniform (exfoliative) (recurrent) 695.0
  simplex marginatum 057.8
  solare (see also Sunburn) 692.71
  streptogenes 696.5
  toxic, toxicum NEC 695.0
    newborn 778.8
  tuberculous (primary) (see also Tuberculosis)
      017.0 ☑
  venenatum 695.0
Erythematosus — see condition
Erythematous — see condition
Erythermalgia (primary) 443.82
Erythralgia 443.82
Erythrasma 039.0
Erythredema 985.0
  polyneuritica 985.0
  polyneuropathy 985.0
Erythremia (acute) (M9841/3) 207.0 ☑
  chronic (M9842/3) 207.1 ☑
  secondary 289.0
Erythroblastopenia (acquired) 284.89
  congenital 284.01
Erythroblastophthisis 284.01
Erythroblastosis (fetalis) (newborn) 773.2
  due to
    ABO
      antibodies 773.1
      incompatibility, maternal/fetal 773.1
      isoimmunization 773.1
    Rh
      antibodies 773.0
      incompatibility, maternal/fetal 773.0
      isoimmunization 773.0
Erythrocyanosis (crurum) 443.89
Erythrocythemia — see Erythremia
Erythrocytopenia 285.9
Erythrocytosis (megalosplenic)
  familial 289.6
  oval, hereditary (see also Elliptocytosis)
    282.1
  secondary 289.0
  stress 289.0
Erythroderma — see also Erythema 695.9
  desquamativa (in infants) 695.89
  exfoliative 695.89
  ichthyosiform, congenital 757.1
  infantum 695.89

Erythroderma — see also Erythema —
    continued
  maculopapular 696.2
  neonatorum 778.8
  psoriaticum 696.1
  secondary 695.9
Erythrodysesthesia, palmar plantar (PPE)
    693.0
Erythrogenesis imperfecta 284.09
Erythroleukemia (M9840/3) 207.0 ☑
Erythromelalgia 443.82
Erythromelia 701.8
Erythropenia 285.9
Erythrophagocytosis 289.9
Erythrophobia 300.23
Erythroplakia
  oral mucosa 528.79
  tongue 528.79
Erythroplasia (Queyrat) (M8080/2)
  specified site — see Neoplasm, skin, in situ
  unspecified site 233.5
Erythropoiesis, idiopathic ineffective 285.0
Escaped beats, heart 427.60
  postoperative 997.1
Escherichia coli (E. coli) — see Infection, Es-
    cherichia coli
Esoenteritis — see Enteritis
Esophagalgia 530.89
Esophagectasis 530.89
  due to cardiospasm 530.0
Esophagismus 530.5
Esophagitis (alkaline) (chemical) (chronic) (in-
    fectional) (necrotic) (peptic) (postopera-
    tive) (regurgitant) 530.10
  acute 530.12
  candidal 112.84
  eosinophilic 530.13
  reflux 530.11
  specified NEC 530.19
  tuberculous (see also Tuberculosis) 017.8 ☑
  ulcerative 530.19
Esophagocele 530.6
Esophagodynia 530.89
Esophagomalacia 530.89
Esophagoptosis 530.89
Esophagospasm 530.5
Esophagostenosis 530.3
Esophagostomiasis 127.7
Esophagostomy
  complication 530.87
    infection 530.86
    malfunctioning 530.87
    mechanical 530.87
Esophagotracheal — see condition
Esophagus — see condition
Esophoria 378.41
  convergence, excess 378.84
  divergence, insufficiency 378.85
Esotropia (nonaccommodative) 378.00
  accommodative 378.35
  alternating 378.05
    with
      A pattern 378.06
      specified noncomitancy NEC 378.08
      V pattern 378.07
      X pattern 378.08
      Y pattern 378.08
    intermittent 378.22
  intermittent 378.20
    alternating 378.22
    monocular 378.21
  monocular 378.01
    with
      A pattern 378.02
      specified noncomitancy NEC 378.04
      V pattern 378.03
      X pattern 378.04
      Y pattern 378.04
    intermittent 378.21
Espundia 085.5
Essential — see condition
Esterapenia 289.89
Esthesioneuroblastoma (M9522/3) 160.0
Esthesioneurocytoma (M9521/3) 160.0
Esthesioneuroepithelioma (M9523/3) 160.0
Esthiomene 099.1

Estivo-autumnal
  fever 084.0
  malaria 084.0
Estrangement V61.09
Estriasis 134.0
Ethanolaminuria 270.8
Ethanolism — see also Alcoholism 303.9 ☑
Ether dependence, dependency — see also
    Dependence 304.6 ☑
Etherism — see also Dependence 304.6 ☑
Ethmoid, ethmoidal — see condition
Ethmoiditis (chronic) (nonpurulent) (purulent)
    — see also Sinusitis, ethmoidal 473.2
  influenzal (see also Influenza) 487.1
  Woakes' 471.1
Ethylism — see also Alcoholism 303.9 ☑
Eulenburg's disease (congenital paramyoto-
    nia) 359.29
Eunuchism 257.2
Eunuchoidism 257.2
  hypogonadotropic 257.2
European blastomycosis 117.5
Eustachian — see condition
Euthyroidism 244.9
Euthyroid sick syndrome 790.94
Evaluation
  fetal lung maturity 659.8 ☑
  for suspected condition (see also Observa-
    tion) V71.9
    abuse V71.81
    exposure
      anthrax V71.82
      biologic agent NEC V71.83
      SARS V71.83
    neglect V71.81
    newborn — see Observation, suspected,
      condition, newborn
    specified condition NEC V71.89
  mental health V70.2
    requested by authority V70.1
  nursing care V63.8
  social service V63.8
Evans' syndrome (thrombocytopenic purpura)
    287.32
Event, apparent life threatening in newborn
    and infant (ALTE) 799.82
Eventration
  colon into chest — see Hernia, diaphragm
  diaphragm (congenital) 756.6
Eversion
  bladder 596.89
  cervix (uteri) 622.0
    with mention of cervicitis 616.0
  foot NEC 736.79
    congenital 755.67
  lacrimal punctum 375.51
  punctum lacrimale (postinfectional) (senile)
    375.51
  ureter (meatus) 593.89
  urethra (meatus) 599.84
  uterus 618.1
    complicating delivery 665.2 ☑
      affecting fetus or newborn 763.89
    puerperal, postpartum 674.8 ☑
Evidence
  of malignancy
    cytologic
      without histologic confirmation
        anus 796.76
        cervix 795.06
        vagina 795.16
Evisceration
  birth injury 767.8
  bowel (congenital) — see Hernia, ventral
  congenital (see also Hernia, ventral) 553.29
  operative wound 998.32
  traumatic NEC 869.1
    eye 871.3
Evulsion — see Avulsion
Ewing's
  angioendothelioma (M9260/3) — see Neo-
    plasm, bone, malignant
  sarcoma (M9260/3) — see Neoplasm, bone,
    malignant
  tumor (M9260/3) — see Neoplasm, bone,
    malignant

Error — Ewing's

☑ **Additional Digit Required — Refer to the Tabular List for Digit Selection**   ▽ **Subterms under main terms may continue to next column or page**

2013 ICD-9-CM   ▶◀ **Revised Text**   ● **New Line**   ▲ **Revised Code**   **Volume 2 — 109**

Exaggerated lumbosacral angle (with imping-
ing spine) 756.12
Examination (general) (routine) (of) (for) V70.9
allergy V72.7
annual V70.0
cardiovascular preoperative V72.81
cervical Papanicolaou smear V76.2
as a part of routine gynecological examination V72.31
to confirm findings of recent normal
smear following initial abnormal
smear V72.32
child care (routine) V20.2
clinical research investigation (normal control patient) (participant) V70.7
dental V72.2
developmental testing (child) (infant) V20.2
donor (potential) V70.8
ear V72.19
eye V72.0
following
accident (motor vehicle) V71.4
alleged rape or seduction (victim or culprit) V71.5
inflicted injury (victim or culprit) NEC
V71.6
rape or seduction, alleged (victim or
culprit) V71.5
treatment (for) V67.9
combined V67.6
fracture V67.4
involving high-risk medication NEC
V67.51
mental disorder V67.3
specified condition NEC V67.59
follow-up (routine) (following) V67.9
cancer chemotherapy V67.2
chemotherapy V67.2
disease NEC V67.59
high-risk medication NEC V67.51
injury NEC V67.59
population survey V70.6
postpartum V24.2
psychiatric V67.3
psychotherapy V67.3
radiotherapy V67.1
specified surgery NEC V67.09
surgery V67.00
vaginal pap smear V67.01
gynecological V72.31
for contraceptive maintenance V25.40
intrauterine device V25.42
pill V25.41
specified method NEC V25.49
health (of)
armed forces personnel V70.5
checkup V70.0
child, routine V20.2
defined subpopulation NEC V70.5
inhabitants of institutions V70.5
occupational V70.5
pre-employment screening V70.5
preschool children V70.5
for admission to school V70.3
prisoners V70.5
for entrance into prison V70.3
prostitutes V70.5
refugees V70.5
school children V70.5
students V70.5
hearing V72.19
following failed hearing screening
V72.11
infant
8 to 28 days old V20.32
over 28 days old, routine V20.2
under 8 days old V20.31
laboratory V72.60
ordered as part of a routine general
medical examination V72.62
pre-operative V72.63
pre-procedural V72.63
specified NEC V72.69
lactating mother V24.1
medical (for) (of) V70.9
administrative purpose NEC V70.3

Examination — continued
medical — continued
admission to
old age home V70.3
prison V70.3
school V70.3
adoption V70.3
armed forces personnel V70.5
at health care facility V70.0
camp V70.3
child, routine V20.2
clinical research (control) (normal comparison) (participant) V70.7
defined subpopulation NEC V70.5
donor (potential) V70.8
driving license V70.3
general V70.9
routine V70.0
specified reason NEC V70.8
immigration V70.3
inhabitants of institutions V70.5
insurance certification V70.3
marriage V70.3
medicolegal reasons V70.4
naturalization V70.3
occupational V70.5
population survey V70.6
pre-employment V70.5
preschool children V70.5
for admission to school V70.3
prison V70.3
prisoners V70.5
for entrance into prison V70.3
prostitutes V70.5
refugees V70.5
school children V70.5
specified reason NEC V70.8
sport competition V70.3
students V70.5
medicolegal reason V70.4
pelvic (annual) (periodic) V72.31
periodic (annual) (routine) V70.0
postpartum
immediately after delivery V24.0
routine follow-up V24.2
pregnancy (unconfirmed) (possible) V72.40
negative result V72.41
positive result V72.42
prenatal V22.1
first pregnancy V22.0
high-risk pregnancy V23.9
specified problem NEC V23.89
to determine fetal viability V23.87
preoperative V72.84
cardiovascular V72.81
respiratory V72.82
specified NEC V72.83
preprocedural V72.84
cardiovascular V72.81
general physical V72.83
respiratory V72.82
specified NEC V72.83
prior to chemotherapy V72.83
psychiatric V70.2
follow-up not needing further care V67.3
requested by authority V70.1
radiological NEC V72.5
respiratory preoperative V72.82
screening — see Screening
sensitization V72.7
skin V72.7
hypersensitivity V72.7
special V72.9
specified type or reason NEC V72.85
preoperative V72.83
specified NEC V72.83
teeth V72.2
vaginal Papanicolaou smear V76.47
following hysterectomy for malignant
condition V67.01
victim or culprit following
alleged rape or seduction V71.5
inflicted injury NEC V71.6
vision V72.0
well baby V20.2
Exanthem, exanthema — see also Rash 782.1

Exanthem, exanthema — see also Rash —
continued
Boston 048
epidemic, with meningitis 048
lichenoid psoriasiform 696.2
subitum 058.10
due to
human herpesvirus 6 058.11
human herpesvirus 7 058.12
viral, virus NEC 057.9
specified type NEC 057.8
Excess, excessive, excessively
alcohol level in blood 790.3
carbohydrate tissue, localized 278.1
carotene (dietary) 278.3
cold 991.9
specified effect NEC 991.8
convergence 378.84
crying 780.95
of
adolescent 780.95
adult 780.95
baby 780.92
child 780.95
infant (baby) 780.92
newborn 780.92
development, breast 611.1
diaphoresis (see also Hyperhidrosis) 780.8
distance, interarch 524.28
divergence 378.85
drinking (alcohol) NEC (see also Abuse,
drugs, nondependent) 305.0 ☑
continual (see also Alcoholism) 303.9 ☑
habitual (see also Alcoholism) 303.9 ☑
eating 783.6
eyelid fold (congenital) 743.62
fat 278.02
in heart (see also Degeneration, myocardial) 429.1
tissue, localized 278.1
foreskin 605
gas 787.3
gastrin 251.5
glucagon 251.4
heat (see also Heat) 992.9
horizontal
overjet 524.26
overlap 524.26
interarch distance 524.28
intermaxillary vertical dimension 524.37
interocclusal distance of teeth 524.37
large
colon 564.7
congenital 751.3
fetus or infant 766.0
with obstructed labor 660.1 ☑
affecting management of pregnancy
656.6 ☑
causing disproportion 653.5 ☑
newborn (weight of 4500 grams or
more) 766.0
organ or site, congenital NEC — see
Anomaly, specified type NEC
lid fold (congenital) 743.62
long
colon 751.5
organ or site, congenital NEC — see
Anomaly, specified type NEC
umbilical cord (entangled)
affecting fetus or newborn 762.5 ☑
in pregnancy or childbirth 663.3 ☑
with compression 663.2 ☑
menstruation 626.2
number of teeth 520.1
causing crowding 524.31
nutrients (dietary) NEC 783.6
potassium (K) 276.7
salivation (see also Ptyalism) 527.7
secretion (see also Hypersecretion)
milk 676.6 ☑
sputum 786.4
sweat (see also Hyperhidrosis) 780.8
short
organ or site, congenital NEC — see
Anomaly, specified type NEC

Excess, excessive, excessively —
continued
short — continued
umbilical cord
affecting fetus or newborn 762.6
in pregnancy or childbirth 663.4 ☑
skin NEC 701.9
eyelid 743.62
acquired 374.30
sodium (Na) 276.0
spacing of teeth 524.32
sputum 786.4
sweating (see also Hyperhidrosis) 780.8
tearing (ducts) (eye) (see also Epiphora)
375.20
thirst 783.5
due to deprivation of water 994.3
tissue in reconstructed breast 612.0
tuberosity 524.07
vitamin
A (dietary) 278.2
administered as drug (chronic) (prolonged excessive intake) 278.2
reaction to sudden overdose
963.5
D (dietary) 278.4
administered as drug (chronic) (prolonged excessive intake) 278.4
reaction to sudden overdose
963.5
weight 278.02
gain 783.1
of pregnancy 646.1 ☑
loss 783.21
Excitability, abnormal, under minor stress
309.29
Excitation
catatonic (see also Schizophrenia) 295.2 ☑
psychogenic 298.1
reactive (from emotional stress, psychological trauma) 298.1
Excitement
manic (see also Psychosis, affective) 296.0 ☑
recurrent episode 296.1 ☑
single episode 296.0 ☑
mental, reactive (from emotional stress,
psychological trauma) 298.1
state, reactive (from emotional stress, psychological trauma) 298.1
Excluded pupils 364.76
Excoriation (traumatic) — see also Injury, superficial, by site 919.8
neurotic 698.4
Excyclophoria 378.44
Excyclotropia 378.33
Exencephalus, exencephaly 742.0
Exercise
breathing V57.0
remedial NEC V57.1
therapeutic NEC V57.1
Exfoliation
skin
due to erythematous condition 695.50
involving (percent of body surface)
less than 10 percent 695.50
10-19 percent 695.51
20-29 percent 695.52
30-39 percent 695.53
40-49 percent 695.54
50-59 percent 695.55
60-69 percent 695.56
70-79 percent 695.57
80-89 percent 695.58
90 percent or more 695.59
teeth
due to systemic causes 525.0
Exfoliative — see also condition
dermatitis 695.89
Exhaustion, exhaustive (physical NEC) 780.79
battle (see also Reaction, stress, acute) 308.9
cardiac (see also Failure, heart) 428.9
delirium (see also Reaction, stress, acute)
308.9
due to
cold 991.8
excessive exertion 994.5

Exhaustion, exhaustive — continued
  due to — continued
    exposure 994.4
    overexertion 994.5
  fetus or newborn 779.89
  heart (see also Failure, heart) 428.9
  heat 992.5
    due to
      salt depletion 992.4
      water depletion 992.3
  manic (see also Psychosis, affective) 296.0 ☑
    recurrent episode 296.1 ☑
    single episode 296.0 ☑
  maternal, complicating delivery 669.8 ☑
    affecting fetus or newborn 763.89
  mental 300.5
  myocardium, myocardial (see also Failure, heart) 428.9
  nervous 300.5
  old age 797
  postinfectional NEC 780.79
  psychogenic 300.5
  psychosis (see also Reaction, stress, acute) 308.9
  senile 797
    dementia 290.0
Exhibitionism (sexual) 302.4
Exomphalos 756.72
Exophoria 378.42
  convergence, insufficiency 378.83
  divergence, excess 378.85
Exophthalmic
  cachexia 242.0 ☑
  goiter 242.0 ☑
  ophthalmoplegia 242.0 ☑ [376.22]
Exophthalmos 376.30
  congenital 743.66
  constant 376.31
  endocrine NEC 259.9 [376.22]
  hyperthyroidism 242.0 ☑ [376.21]
  intermittent NEC 376.34
  malignant 242.0 ☑ [376.21]
  pulsating 376.35
    endocrine NEC 259.9 [376.22]
  thyrotoxic 242.0 ☑ [376.21]
Exostosis 726.91
  cartilaginous (M9210/0) — see Neoplasm, bone, benign
  congenital 756.4
  ear canal, external 380.81
  gonococcal 098.89
  hip 726.5
  intracranial 733.3
  jaw (bone) 526.81
  luxurians 728.11
  multiple (cancellous) (congenital) (hereditary) 756.4
  nasal bones 726.91
  orbit, orbital 376.42
  osteocartilaginous (M9210/0) — see Neoplasm, bone, benign
  spine 721.8
    with spondylosis — see Spondylosis
  syphilitic 095.5
  wrist 726.4
Exotropia 378.10
  alternating 378.15
    with
      A pattern 378.16
      specified noncomitancy NEC 378.18
      V pattern 378.17
      X pattern 378.18
      Y pattern 378.18
    intermittent 378.24
  intermittent 378.20
    alternating 378.24
    monocular 378.23
  monocular 378.11
    with
      A pattern 378.12
      specified noncomitancy NEC 378.14
      V pattern 378.13
      X pattern 378.14
      Y pattern 378.14
    intermittent 378.23

Explanation of
  investigation finding V65.4 ☑
  medication V65.4 ☑
Exposure (suspected) 994.9
  algae bloom V87.32
  cold 991.9
    specified effect NEC 991.8
  effects of 994.9
  exhaustion due to 994.4
  implanted vaginal mesh
    into vagina 629.32
    through vaginal wall 629.32
  to
    AIDS virus V01.79
    anthrax V01.81
    aromatic
      amines V87.11
      dyes V87.19
    arsenic V87.01
    asbestos V15.84
    benzene V87.12
    body fluids (hazardous) V15.85
    cholera V01.0
    chromium compounds V87.09
    communicable disease V01.9
      specified type NEC V01.89
    dyes V87.2
      aromatic V87.19
    Escherichia coli (E. coli) V01.83
    German measles V01.4
    gonorrhea V01.6
    hazardous
      aromatic compounds NEC V87.19
      body fluids V15.85
      chemicals NEC V87.2
      metals V87.09
      substances V87.39
    HIV V01.79
    human immunodeficiency virus V01.79
    lead V15.86
    meningococcus V01.84
    mold V87.31
    nickel dust V87.09
    parasitic disease V01.89
    poliomyelitis V01.2
    polycyclic aromatic hydrocarbons V87.19
    potentially hazardous body fluids V15.85
    rabies V01.5
    rubella V01.4
    SARS-associated coronavirus V01.82
    smallpox V01.3
    syphilis V01.6
    tuberculosis V01.1
    uranium V87.02
    varicella V01.71
    venereal disease V01.6
    viral disease NEC V01.79
      varicella V01.71
  vaginal prosthetic materials NEC
    into vagina 629.32
    through vaginal wall 629.32
Exsanguination, fetal 772.0
Exstrophy
  abdominal content 751.8
  bladder (urinary) 753.5
Extensive — see condition
Extra — see also Accessory
  rib 756.3
    cervical 756.2
Extraction
  with hook 763.89
  breech NEC 669.6 ☑
    affecting fetus or newborn 763.0
  cataract postsurgical V45.61
  manual NEC 669.8 ☑
    affecting fetus or newborn 763.89
Extrasystole 427.60
  atrial 427.61
  postoperative 997.1
  ventricular 427.69
Extrauterine gestation or pregnancy — see Pregnancy, ectopic
Extravasation
  blood 459.0
    lower extremity 459.0
  chemotherapy, vesicant 999.81

Extravasation — continued
  chyle into mesentery 457.8
  pelvicalyceal 593.4
  pyelosinus 593.4
  urine 788.8
    from ureter 788.8
  vesicant
    agent NEC 999.82
    chemotherapy 999.81
Extremity — see condition
Extrophy — see Exstrophy
Extroversion
  bladder 753.5
  uterus 618.1
    complicating delivery 665.2 ☑
      affecting fetus or newborn 763.89
    postpartal (old) 618.1
Extruded tooth 524.34
Extrusion
  alveolus and teeth 524.75
  breast implant (prosthetic) 996.54
  device, implant, or graft — see Complications, mechanical
  eye implant (ball) (globe) 996.59
  intervertebral disc — see Displacement, intervertebral disc
  lacrimal gland 375.43
  mesh (reinforcing) 996.59
  ocular lens implant 996.53
  prosthetic device NEC — see Complications, mechanical
  vitreous 379.26
Exudate, pleura — see Effusion, pleura
Exudates, retina 362.82
Exudative — see condition
Eye, eyeball, eyelid — see condition
Eyestrain 368.13
Eyeworm disease of Africa 125.2

F

Faber's anemia or syndrome (achlorhydric anemia) 280.9
Fabry's disease (angiokeratoma corporis diffusum) 272.7
Face, facial — see condition
Facet of cornea 371.44
Faciocephalalgia, autonomic — see also Neuropathy, peripheral, autonomic 337.9
Facioscapulohumeral myopathy 359.1
Factitious disorder, illness — see Illness, factitious
Factor
  deficiency — see Deficiency, factor
  psychic, associated with diseases classified elsewhere 316
  risk — see Problem
  V Leiden mutation 289.81
Fahr-Volhard disease (malignant nephrosclerosis) 403.00
Failure, failed
  adenohypophyseal 253.2
  attempted abortion (legal) (see also Abortion, failed) 638.9
  bone marrow (anemia) 284.9
    acquired (secondary) 284.89
    congenital 284.09
    idiopathic 284.9
  cardiac (see also Failure, heart) 428.9
    newborn 779.89
  cardiorenal (chronic) 428.9
    hypertensive (see also Hypertension, cardiorenal) 404.93
  cardiorespiratory 799.1
    specified during or due to a procedure 997.1
    long-term effect of cardiac surgery 429.4
  cardiovascular (chronic) 428.9
  cerebrovascular 437.8
  cervical dilatation in labor 661.0 ☑
    affecting fetus or newborn 763.7
  circulation, circulatory 799.89
    fetus or newborn 779.89
    peripheral 785.50
    postoperative 998.00

Failure, failed — continued
  compensation — see Disease, heart
  congestive (see also Failure, heart) 428.0
  conscious sedation, during procedure 995.24
  coronary (see also Insufficiency, coronary) 411.89
  dental implant 525.79
    due to
      infection 525.71
      lack of attached gingiva 525.72
      occlusal trauma (caused by poor prosthetic design) 525.72
      parafunctional habits 525.72
      periodontal infection (peri-implantitis) 525.72
      poor oral hygiene 525.72
      unintentional loading 525.71
    endosseous NEC 525.79
    mechanical 525.73
    osseointegration 525.71
      due to
        complications of systemic disease 525.71
        poor bone quality 525.71
        premature loading 525.71
      iatrogenic 525.71
      prior to intentional prosthetic loading 525.71
    post-osseointegration
      biological 525.72
      iatrogenic 525.72
      due to complications of systemic disease 525.72
      mechanical 525.73
    pre-integration 525.71
    pre-osseointegration 525.71
  dental prosthesis causing loss of dental implant 525.73
  dental restoration
    marginal integrity 525.61
    periodontal anatomical integrity 525.65
  descent of head (at term) 652.5 ☑
    affecting fetus or newborn 763.1
    in labor 660.0 ☑
      affecting fetus or newborn 763.1
  device, implant, or graft — see Complications, mechanical
  engagement of head NEC 652.5 ☑
    in labor 660.0 ☑
  extrarenal 788.99
  fetal head to enter pelvic brim 652.5 ☑
    affecting fetus or newborn 763.1
    in labor 660.0 ☑
      affecting fetus or newborn 763.1
  forceps NEC 660.7 ☑
    affecting fetus or newborn 763.1
  fusion (joint) (spinal) 996.49
  growth in childhood 783.43
  heart (acute) (sudden) 428.9
    with
      abortion — see Abortion, by type, with specified complication NEC
      acute pulmonary edema (see also Failure, ventricular, left) 428.1
      with congestion (see also Failure, heart) 428.0
      decompensation (see also Failure, heart) 428.0
      dilation — see Disease, heart
      ectopic pregnancy (see also categories 633.0–633.9) 639.8
      molar pregnancy (see also categories 630–632) 639.8
    arteriosclerotic 440.9
    combined left-right sided 428.0
    combined systolic and diastolic 428.40
      acute 428.41
      acute on chronic 428.43
      chronic 428.42
    compensated (see also Failure, heart) 428.0

☑ **Additional Digit Required** — Refer to the Tabular List for Digit Selection

⬛ **Subterms under main terms may continue to next column or page**

2013 ICD-9-CM

▶◀ **Revised Text**

● **New Line**

▲ **Revised Code**

Volume 2 — 111

Failure, failed — *continued*
  heart — *continued*
    complicating
      abortion — *see* Abortion, by type, with specified complication NEC
      delivery (cesarean) (instrumental) 669.4 ☑
      ectopic pregnancy (*see also* categories 633.0–633.9) 639.8
      molar pregnancy (*see also* categories 630–632) 639.8
      obstetric anesthesia or sedation 668.1 ☑
      surgery 997.1
    congestive (compensated) (decompensated) (*see also* Failure, heart) 428.0
      with rheumatic fever (conditions classifiable to 390)
        active 391.8
        inactive or quiescent (with chorea) 398.91
      fetus or newborn 779.89
      hypertensive (*see also* Hypertension, heart) 402.91
        with renal disease (*see also* Hypertension, cardiorenal) 404.91
          with renal failure 404.93
        benign 402.11
        malignant 402.01
      rheumatic (chronic) (inactive) (with chorea) 398.91
        active or acute 391.8
          with chorea (Sydenham's) 392.0
    decompensated (*see also* Failure, heart) 428.0
    degenerative (*see also* Degeneration, myocardial) 429.1
    diastolic 428.30
      acute 428.31
      acute on chronic 428.33
      chronic 428.32
    due to presence of (cardiac) prosthesis 429.4
    fetus or newborn 779.89
    following
      abortion 639.8
      cardiac surgery 429.4
      ectopic or molar pregnancy 639.8
    high output NEC 428.9
    hypertensive (*see also* Hypertension, heart) 402.91
      with renal disease (*see also* Hypertension, cardiorenal) 404.91
        with renal failure 404.93
      benign 402.11
      malignant 402.01
    left (ventricular) (*see also* Failure, ventricular, left) 428.1
      with right-sided failure (see also Failure, heart) 428.0
    low output (syndrome) NEC 428.9
    organic — *see* Disease, heart
    postoperative (immediate) 997.1
      long term effect of cardiac surgery 429.4
    rheumatic (chronic) (congestive) (inactive) 398.91
    right (secondary to left heart failure, conditions classifiable to 428.1) (ventricular) (*see also* Failure, heart) 428.0
    senile 797
    specified during or due to a procedure 997.1
      long-term effect of cardiac surgery 429.4
    systolic 428.20
      acute 428.21
      acute on chronic 428.23
      chronic 428.22
    thyrotoxic (*see also* Thyrotoxicosis) 242.9 ☑ *[425.7]*

Failure, failed — *continued*
  heart — *continued*
    valvular — *see* Endocarditis
  hepatic 572.8
    acute 570
    due to a procedure 997.49
  hepatorenal 572.4
  hypertensive heart (*see also* Hypertension, heart) 402.91
    benign 402.11
    malignant 402.01
  induction (of labor) 659.1 ☑
    abortion (legal) (*see also* Abortion, failed) 638.9
    affecting fetus or newborn 763.89
    by oxytocic drugs 659.1 ☑
    instrumental 659.0 ☑
    mechanical 659.0 ☑
    medical 659.1 ☑
    surgical 659.0 ☑
  initial alveolar expansion, newborn 770.4
  involution, thymus (gland) 254.8
  kidney — *see* Failure, renal
  lactation 676.4 ☑
  Leydig's cell, adult 257.2
  liver 572.8
    acute 570
  medullary 799.89
  mitral — *see* Endocarditis, mitral
  moderate sedation, during procedure 995.24
  myocardium, myocardial (*see also* Failure, heart) 428.9
    chronic (*see also* Failure, heart) 428.0
    congestive (*see also* Failure, heart) 428.0
  ovarian (primary) 256.39
    iatrogenic 256.2
    postablative 256.2
    postirradiation 256.2
    postsurgical 256.2
  ovulation 628.0
  prerenal 788.99
  renal (kidney) 586
    with
      abortion — *see* Abortion, by type, with renal failure
      ectopic pregnancy (*see also* categories 633.0–633.9) 639.3
      edema (*see also* Nephrosis) 581.9
      hypertension (*see also* Hypertension, kidney) 403.91
      hypertensive heart disease (conditions classifiable to 402) 404.92
        with heart failure 404.93
        benign 404.12
          with heart failure 404.13
        malignant 404.02
          with heart failure 404.03
      molar pregnancy (*see also* categories 630–632) 639.3
      tubular necrosis (acute) 584.5
    acute 584.9
      with lesion of
        necrosis
          cortical (renal) 584.6
          medullary (renal) (papillary) 584.7
          tubular 584.5
        specified pathology NEC 584.8
    chronic 585.9
      hypertensive or with hypertension (*see also* Hypertension, kidney) 403.91
    due to a procedure 997.5
    following
      abortion 639.3
      crushing 958.5
      ectopic or molar pregnancy 639.3
      labor and delivery (acute) 669.3 ☑
    hypertensive (*see also* Hypertension, kidney) 403.91
    puerperal, postpartum 669.3 ☑
  respiration, respiratory 518.81
    acute 518.81
      following trauma and surgery 518.51

Failure, failed — *continued*
  respiration, respiratory — *continued*
    acute and chronic 518.84
      following trauma and surgery 518.53
    center 348.89
      newborn 770.84
    chronic 518.83
      following trauma and surgery or shock 518.51
      newborn 770.84
  rotation
    cecum 751.4
    colon 751.4
    intestine 751.4
    kidney 753.3
  sedation, during procedure
    conscious 995.24
    moderate 995.24
  segmentation (*see also* Fusion)
    fingers (*see also* Syndactylism, fingers) 755.11
    toes (*see also* Syndactylism, toes) 755.13
  seminiferous tubule, adult 257.2
  senile (general) 797
    with psychosis 290.20
  testis, primary (seminal) 257.2
  to progress 661.2 ☑
  to thrive
    adult 783.7
    child 783.41
    newborn 779.34
  transplant 996.80
    bone marrow 996.85
    organ (immune or nonimmune cause) 996.80
      bone marrow 996.85
      heart 996.83
      intestines 996.87
      kidney 996.81
      liver 996.82
      lung 996.84
      pancreas 996.86
      specified NEC 996.89
    skin 996.52
      artificial 996.55
      decellularized allodermis 996.55
      temporary allograft or pigskin graft — omit code
    stem cell(s) 996.88
      from
        peripheral blood 996.88
        umbilical cord 996.88
  trial of labor NEC 660.6 ☑
    affecting fetus or newborn 763.1
  tubal ligation 998.89
  urinary 586
  vacuum extraction
    abortion — *see* Abortion, failed
    delivery NEC 660.7 ☑
      affecting fetus or newborn 763.1
  vasectomy 998.89
  ventouse NEC 660.7 ☑
    affecting fetus or newborn 763.1
  ventricular (*see also* Failure, heart) 428.9
    left 428.1
      with rheumatic fever (conditions classifiable to 390)
        active 391.8
          with chorea 392.0
        inactive or quiescent (with chorea) 398.91
      hypertensive (*see also* Hypertension, heart) 402.91
        benign 402.11
        malignant 402.01
      rheumatic (chronic) (inactive) (with chorea) 398.91
        active or acute 391.8
          with chorea 392.0
    right (*see also* Failure, heart) 428.0
  vital centers, fetus or newborn 779.89
  weight gain in childhood 783.41
Fainting (fit) (spell) 780.2
Falciform hymen 752.49
Fallen arches 734
Falling, any organ or part — *see* Prolapse

Fall, maternal, affecting fetus or newborn 760.5
Fallopian
  insufflation
    fertility testing V26.21
    following sterilization reversal V26.22
  tube — *see* condition
Fallot's
  pentalogy 745.2
  tetrad or tetralogy 745.2
  triad or trilogy 746.09
Fallout, radioactive (adverse effect) NEC 990
False — *see also* condition
  bundle branch block 426.50
  bursa 727.89
  croup 478.75
  joint 733.82
  labor (pains) 644.1 ☑
  opening, urinary, male 752.69
  passage, urethra (prostatic) 599.4
  positive
    serological test for syphilis 795.6
    Wassermann reaction 795.6
  pregnancy 300.11
Family, familial — *see also* condition
  affected by
    family member
      currently on deployment (military) V61.01
      returned from deployment (military) (current or past conflict) V61.02
  disruption (*see also* Disruption, family) V61.09
  estrangement V61.09
  hemophagocytic
    lymphohistiocytosis 288.4
    reticulosis 288.4
  Li-Fraumeni (syndrome) V84.01
  planning advice V25.09
    natural
      procreative V26.41
      to avoid pregnancy V25.04
  problem V61.9
    specified circumstance NEC V61.8
  retinoblastoma (syndrome) 190.5
Famine 994.2
  edema 262
Fanconi's anemia (congenital pancytopenia) 284.09
Fanconi (-de Toni) (-Debré) syndrome (cystinosis) 270.0
Farber (-Uzman) syndrome or disease (disseminated lipogranulomatosis) 272.8
Farcin 024
Farcy 024
Farmers'
  lung 495.0
  skin 692.74
Farsightedness 367.0
Fascia — *see* condition
Fasciculation 781.0
Fasciculitis optica 377.32
Fasciitis 729.4
  eosinophilic 728.89
  necrotizing 728.86
  nodular 728.79
  perirenal 593.4
  plantar 728.71
  pseudosarcomatous 728.79
  traumatic (old) NEC 728.79
    current — *see* Sprain, by site
Fasciola hepatica infestation 121.3
Fascioliasis 121.3
Fasciolopsiasis (small intestine) 121.4
Fasciolopsis (small intestine) 121.4
Fast pulse 785.0
Fat
  embolism (cerebral) (pulmonary) (systemic) 958.1
    with
      abortion — *see* Abortion, by type, with embolism
      ectopic pregnancy (*see also* categories 633.0–633.9) 639.6

☑ **Additional Digit Required** — Refer to the Tabular List for Digit Selection
🔻 **Subterms under main terms may continue to next column or page**

112 — Volume 2   ▶◀ Revised Text   ● New Line   ▲ Revised Code   2013 ICD-9-CM

Fat — *continued*
embolism — *continued*
with — *continued*
molar pregnancy (*see also* categories 630–632) 639.6
complicating delivery or puerperium 673.8 ☑
following
abortion 639.6
ectopic or molar pregnancy 639.6
in pregnancy, childbirth, or the puerperium 673.8 ☑
excessive 278.02
in heart (*see also* Degeneration, myocardial) 429.1
general 278.02
hernia, herniation 729.30
eyelid 374.34
knee 729.31
orbit 374.34
retro-orbital 374.34
retropatellar 729.31
specified site NEC 729.39
indigestion 579.8
in stool 792.1
localized (pad) 278.1
heart (*see also* Degeneration, myocardial) 429.1
knee 729.31
retropatellar 729.31
necrosis (*see also* Fatty, degeneration)
breast (aseptic) (segmental) 611.3
mesentery 567.82
omentum 567.82
peritoneum 567.82
pad 278.1
Fatal familial insomnia (FFI) 046.72
Fatal syncope 798.1
Fatigue 780.79
auditory deafness (*see also* Deafness) 389.9
chronic, syndrome 780.71
combat (*see also* Reaction, stress, acute) 308.9
during pregnancy 646.8 ☑
general 780.79
psychogenic 300.5
heat (transient) 992.6
muscle 729.89
myocardium (*see also* Failure, heart) 428.9
nervous 300.5
neurosis 300.5
operational 300.89
postural 729.89
posture 729.89
psychogenic (general) 300.5
senile 797
syndrome NEC 300.5
chronic 780.71
undue 780.79
voice 784.49
Fatness 278.02
Fatty — *see also* condition
apron 278.1
degeneration (diffuse) (general) NEC 272.8
localized — *see* Degeneration, by site, fatty
placenta — *see* Placenta, abnormal
heart (enlarged) (*see also* Degeneration, myocardial) 429.1
infiltration (diffuse) (general) (*see also* Degeneration, by site, fatty) 272.8
heart (enlarged) (*see also* Degeneration, myocardial) 429.1
liver 571.8
alcoholic 571.0
necrosis — *see* Degeneration, fatty
phanerosis 272.8
Fauces — *see* condition
Fauchard's disease (periodontitis) 523.40
Faucitis 478.29
Faulty — *see also* condition
position of teeth 524.30
Favism (anemia) 282.2
Favre-Racouchot disease (elastoidosis cutanea nodularis) 701.8
Favus 110.9

Favus — *continued*
beard 110.0
capitis 110.0
corporis 110.5
eyelid 110.8
foot 110.4
hand 110.2
scalp 110.0
specified site NEC 110.8
Feared complaint unfounded V65.5
Fear, fearfulness (complex) (reaction) 300.20
child 313.0
of
animals 300.29
closed spaces 300.29
crowds 300.29
eating in public 300.23
heights 300.29
open spaces 300.22
with panic attacks 300.21
public speaking 300.23
streets 300.22
with panic attacks 300.21
travel 300.22
with panic attacks 300.21
washing in public 300.23
transient 308.0
Febricula (continued) (simple) — *see also* Pyrexia 780.60
Febrile — *see also* Pyrexia 780.60
convulsion (simple) 780.31
complex 780.32
nonhemolytic transfusion reaction (FNHTR) 780.66
seizure (simple) 780.31
atypical 780.32
complex 780.32
complicated 780.32
Febris — *see also* Fever 780.60
aestiva (*see also* Fever, hay) 477.9
flava (*see also* Fever, yellow) 060.9
melitensis 023.0
pestis (*see also* Plague) 020.9
puerperalis 672.0 ☑
recurrens (*see also* Fever, relapsing) 087.9
pediculo vestimenti 087.0
rubra 034.1
typhoidea 002.0
typhosa 002.0
Fecal — *see* condition
Fecalith (impaction) 560.32
with hernia (*see also* Hernia, by site, with obstruction)
gangrenous — *see* Hernia, by site, with gangrene
appendix 543.9
congenital 777.1
Fede's disease 529.0
Feeble-minded 317
Feeble rapid pulse due to shock following injury 958.4
Feeding
faulty (elderly) (infant) 783.3
newborn 779.31
formula check V20.2
improper (elderly) (infant) 783.3
newborn 779.31
problem (elderly) (infant) 783.3
newborn 779.31
nonorganic origin 307.59
Feeling of foreign body in throat 784.99
Feer's disease 985.0
Feet — *see* condition
Feigned illness V65.2
Feil-Klippel syndrome (brevicollis) 756.16
Feinmesser's (hidrotic) **ectodermal dysplasia** 757.31
Felix's disease (juvenile osteochondrosis, hip) 732.1
Felon (any digit) (with lymphangitis) 681.01
herpetic 054.6
Felty's syndrome (rheumatoid arthritis with splenomegaly and leukopenia) 714.1
Feminism in boys 302.6
Feminization, testicular 259.51
with pseudohermaphroditism, male 259.51

Femoral hernia — *see* Hernia, femoral
Femora vara 736.32
Femur, femoral — *see* condition
Fenestrata placenta — *see* Placenta, abnormal
Fenestration, fenestrated — *see also* Imperfect, closure
aorta-pulmonary 745.0
aorticopulmonary 745.0
aortopulmonary 745.0
cusps, heart valve NEC 746.89
pulmonary 746.09
hymen 752.49
pulmonic cusps 746.09
Fenwick's disease 537.89
Fermentation (gastric) (gastrointestinal) (stomach) 536.8
intestine 564.89
psychogenic 306.4
psychogenic 306.4
Fernell's disease (aortic aneurysm) 441.9
Fertile eunuch syndrome 257.2
Fertility, meaning multiparity — *see* Multiparity
Fetal
alcohol syndrome 760.71
anemia 678.0 ☑
thrombocytopenia 678.0 ☑
twin to twin transfusion 678.0 ☑
Fetalis uterus 752.39
Fetid
breath 784.99
sweat 705.89
Fetishism 302.81
transvestic 302.3
Fetomaternal hemorrhage
affecting management of pregnancy 656.0 ☑
fetus or newborn 772.0
Fetus, fetal — *see also* condition
papyraceous 779.89
type lung tissue 770.4
Fever 780.60
with chills 780.60
in malarial regions (*see also* Malaria) 084.6
abortus NEC 023.9
aden 061
African tick-borne 087.1
American
mountain tick 066.1
spotted 082.0
and ague (*see also* Malaria) 084.6
aphthous 078.4
arbovirus hemorrhagic 065.9
Assam 085.0
Australian A or Q 083.0
Bangkok hemorrhagic 065.4
biliary, Charcôt's intermittent — *see* Choledocholithiasis
bilious, hemoglobinuric 084.8
blackwater 084.8
blister 054.9
Bonvale Dam 780.79
boutonneuse 082.1
brain 323.9
late effect — *see* category 326
breakbone 061
Bullis 082.8
Bunyamwera 066.3
Burdwan 085.0
Bwamba (encephalitis) 066.3
Cameroon (*see also* Malaria) 084.6
Canton 081.9
catarrhal (acute) 460
chronic 472.0
cat-scratch 078.3
cerebral 323.9
late effect — *see* category 326
cerebrospinal (meningococcal) (*see also* Meningitis, cerebrospinal) 036.0
Chagres 084.0
Chandipura 066.8
changuinola 066.0
Charcôt's (biliary) (hepatic) (intermittent) — *see* Choledocholithiasis
Chikungunya (viral) 066.3

Fever — *continued*
Chikungunya — *continued*
hemorrhagic 065.4
childbed 670.8 ☑
Chitral 066.0
Colombo (*see also* Fever, paratyphoid) 002.9
Colorado tick (virus) 066.1
congestive
malarial (*see also* Malaria) 084.6
remittent (*see also* Malaria) 084.6
Congo virus 065.0
continued 780.60
malarial 084.0
Corsican (*see also* Malaria) 084.6
Crimean hemorrhagic 065.0
Cyprus (*see also* Brucellosis) 023.9
dandy 061
deer fly (*see also* Tularemia) 021.9
dehydration, newborn 778.4
dengue (virus) 061
hemorrhagic 065.4
desert 114.0
due to heat 992.0
Dumdum 085.0
enteric 002.0
ephemeral (of unknown origin) (*see also* Pyrexia) 780.60
epidemic, hemorrhagic of the Far East 065.0
erysipelatous (*see also* Erysipelas) 035
estivo-autumnal (malarial) 084.0
etiocholanolone 277.31
famine (*see also* Fever, relapsing)
meaning typhus — *see* Typhus
Far Eastern hemorrhagic 065.0
five day 083.1
Fort Bragg 100.89
gastroenteric 002.0
gastromalarial (*see also* Malaria) 084.6
Gibraltar (*see also* Brucellosis) 023.9
glandular 075
Guama (viral) 066.3
Haverhill 026.1
hay (allergic) (with rhinitis) 477.9
with
asthma (bronchial) (*see also* Asthma) 493.0 ☑
due to
dander, animal (cat) (dog) 477.2
dust 477.8
fowl 477.8
hair, animal (cat) (dog) 477.2
pollen, any plant or tree 477.0
specified allergen other than pollen 477.8
heat (effects) 992.0
hematuric, bilious 084.8
hemoglobinuric (malarial) 084.8
bilious 084.8
hemorrhagic (arthropod-borne) NEC 065.9
with renal syndrome 078.6
arenaviral 078.7
Argentine 078.7
Bangkok 065.4
Bolivian 078.7
Central Asian 065.0
chikungunya 065.4
Crimean 065.0
dengue (virus) 065.4
Ebola 065.8
epidemic 078.6
of Far East 065.0
Far Eastern 065.0
Junin virus 078.7
Korean 078.6
Kyasanur forest 065.2
Machupo virus 078.7
mite-borne NEC 065.8
mosquito-borne 065.4
Omsk 065.1
Philippine 065.4
Russian (Yaroslav) 078.6
Singapore 065.4
Southeast Asia 065.4
Thailand 065.4
tick-borne NEC 065.3
hepatic (*see also* Cholecystitis) 575.8

☑ **Additional Digit Required — Refer to the Tabular List for Digit Selection**

ⓦ **Subterms under main terms may continue to next column or page**

Fever — *continued*
  hepatic (*see also* Cholecystitis) — *continued*
    intermittent (Charcôt's) — *see* Choledocholithiasis
  herpetic (*see also* Herpes) 054.9
  Hyalomma tick 065.0
  icterohemorrhagic 100.0
  inanition 780.60
    newborn 778.4
  in conditions classified elsewhere 780.61
  infective NEC 136.9
  intermittent (bilious) (*see also* Malaria) 084.6
    hepatic (Charcôt) — *see* Choledocholithiasis
    of unknown origin (*see also* Pyrexia) 780.60
    pernicious 084.0
  iodide
    correct substance properly administered 780.60
    overdose or wrong substance given or taken 975.5
  Japanese river 081.2
  jungle yellow 060.0
  Junin virus, hemorrhagic 078.7
  Katayama 120.2
  Kedani 081.2
  Kenya 082.1
  Korean hemorrhagic 078.6
  Lassa 078.89
  Lone Star 082.8
  lung — *see* Pneumonia
  Machupo virus, hemorrhagic 078.7
  malaria, malarial (*see also* Malaria) 084.6
  Malta (*see also* Brucellosis) 023.9
  Marseilles 082.1
  marsh (*see also* Malaria) 084.6
  Mayaro (viral) 066.3
  Mediterranean (*see also* Brucellosis) 023.9
    familial 277.31
    tick 082.1
  meningeal — *see* Meningitis
  metal fumes NEC 985.8
  Meuse 083.1
  Mexican — *see* Typhus, Mexican
  Mianeh 087.1
  miasmatic (*see also* Malaria) 084.6
  miliary 078.2
  milk, female 672.0 ☑
  mill 504
  mite-borne hemorrhagic 065.8
  Monday 504
  mosquito-borne NEC 066.3
    hemorrhagic NEC 065.4
  mountain 066.1
    meaning
      Rocky Mountain spotted 082.0
      undulant fever (*see also* Brucellosis) 023.9
    tick (American) 066.1
  Mucambo (viral) 066.3
  mud 100.89
  Neapolitan (*see also* Brucellosis) 023.9
  neutropenic 288.00
  newborn (environmentally-induced) 778.4
  nine-mile 083.0
  nonexanthematous tick 066.1
  North Asian tick-borne typhus 082.2
  Omsk hemorrhagic 065.1
  O'nyong-nyong (viral) 066.3
  Oropouche (viral) 066.3
  Oroya 088.0
  paludal (*see also* Malaria) 084.6
  Panama 084.0
  pappataci 066.0
  paratyphoid 002.9
    A 002.1
    B (Schottmüller's) 002.2
    C (Hirschfeld) 002.3
  parrot 073.9
  periodic 277.31
  pernicious, acute 084.0
  persistent (of unknown origin) (*see also* Pyrexia) 780.60
  petechial 036.0

Fever — *continued*
  pharyngoconjunctival 077.2
    adenoviral type 3 077.2
  Philippine hemorrhagic 065.4
  phlebotomus 066.0
  Piry 066.8
  Pixuna (viral) 066.3
  Plasmodium ovale 084.3
  pleural (*see also* Pleurisy) 511.0
  pneumonic — *see* Pneumonia
  polymer fume 987.8
  postimmunization 780.63
  postoperative 780.62
    due to infection 998.59
  posttransfusion 780.66
  postvaccination 780.63
  pretibial 100.89
  puerperal, postpartum 672.0 ☑
  putrid — *see* Septicemia
  pyemic — *see* Septicemia
  Q 083.0
    with pneumonia 083.0 *[484.8]*
  quadrilateral 083.0
  quartan (malaria) 084.2
  Queensland (coastal) 083.0
    seven-day 100.89
  Quintan (A) 083.1
  quotidian 084.0
  rabbit (*see also* Tularemia) 021.9
  rat-bite 026.9
    due to
      Spirillum minor or minus 026.0
      Spirochaeta morsus muris 026.0
      Streptobacillus moniliformis 026.1
  recurrent — *see* Fever, relapsing
  relapsing 087.9
    Carter's (Asiatic) 087.0
    Dutton's (West African) 087.1
    Koch's 087.9
    louse-borne (epidemic) 087.0
    Novy's (American) 087.1
    Obermeyer's (European) 087.0
    spirillum NEC 087.9
    tick-borne (endemic) 087.1
  remittent (bilious) (congestive) (gastric) (*see also* Malaria) 084.6
  rheumatic (active) (acute) (chronic) (subacute) 390
    with heart involvement 391.9
      carditis 391.9
      endocarditis (aortic) (mitral) (pulmonary) (tricuspid) 391.1
      multiple sites 391.8
      myocarditis 391.2
      pancarditis, acute 391.8
      pericarditis 391.0
      specified type NEC 391.8
      valvulitis 391.1
    cardiac hypertrophy 398.99
    inactive or quiescent
      with cardiac hypertrophy 398.99
      carditis 398.90
      endocarditis 397.9
        aortic (valve) 395.9
          with mitral (valve) disease 396.9
        mitral (valve) 394.9
          with aortic (valve) disease 396.9
        pulmonary (valve) 397.1
        tricuspid (valve) 397.0
      heart conditions (classifiable to 429.3, 429.6, 429.9) 398.99
      failure (congestive) (conditions classifiable to 428.0, 428.9) 398.91
      left ventricular failure (conditions classifiable to 428.1) 398.91
      myocardial degeneration (conditions classifiable to 429.1) 398.0
      myocarditis (conditions classifiable to 429.0) 398.0
      pancarditis 398.99
      pericarditis 393
  Rift Valley (viral) 066.3
  Rocky Mountain spotted 082.0

Fever — *continued*
  rose 477.0
  Ross river (viral) 066.3
  Russian hemorrhagic 078.6
  sandfly 066.0
  San Joaquin (valley) 114.0
  São Paulo 082.0
  scarlet 034.1
  septic — *see* Septicemia
  seven-day 061
    Japan 100.89
    Queensland 100.89
  shin bone 083.1
  Singapore hemorrhagic 065.4
  solar 061
  sore 054.9
  South African tick-bite 087.1
  Southeast Asia hemorrhagic 065.4
  spinal — *see* Meningitis
  spirillary 026.0
  splenic (*see also* Anthrax) 022.9
  spotted (Rocky Mountain) 082.0
    American 082.0
    Brazilian 082.0
    Colombian 082.0
    meaning
      cerebrospinal meningitis 036.0
      typhus 082.9
  spring 309.23
  steroid
    correct substance properly administered 780.60
    overdose or wrong substance given or taken 962.0
  streptobacillary 026.1
  subtertian 084.0
  Sumatran mite 081.2
  sun 061
  swamp 100.89
  sweating 078.2
  swine 003.8
  sylvatic yellow 060.0
  Tahyna 062.5
  tertian — *see* Malaria, tertian
  Thailand hemorrhagic 065.4
  thermic 992.0
  three day 066.0
    with Coxsackie exanthem 074.8
  tick
    American mountain 066.1
    Colorado 066.1
    Kemerovo 066.1
    Mediterranean 082.1
    mountain 066.1
    nonexanthematous 066.1
    Quaranfil 066.1
  tick-bite NEC 066.1
  tick-borne NEC 066.1
    hemorrhagic NEC 065.3
  transitory of newborn 778.4
  trench 083.1
  tsutsugamushi 081.2
  typhogastric 002.0
  typhoid (abortive) (ambulant) (any site) (hemorrhagic) (infection) (intermittent) (malignant) (rheumatic) 002.0
  typhomalarial (*see also* Malaria) 084.6
  typhus — *see* Typhus
  undulant (*see also* Brucellosis) 023.9
  unknown origin (*see also* Pyrexia) 780.60
  uremic — *see* Uremia
  uveoparotid 135
  valley (Coccidioidomycosis) 114.0
  Venezuelan equine 066.2
  Volhynian 083.1
  Wesselsbron (viral) 066.3
  West
    African 084.8
    Nile (viral) 066.40
      with
        cranial nerve disorders 066.42
        encephalitis 066.41
        optic neuritis 066.42
        other complications 066.49
        other neurologic manifestations 066.42

Fever — *continued*
  West — *continued*
    Nile — *continued*
      with — *continued*
        polyradiculitis 066.42
  Whitmore's 025
  Wolhynian 083.1
  worm 128.9
  Yaroslav hemorrhagic 078.6
  yellow 060.9
    jungle 060.0
    sylvatic 060.0
    urban 060.1
    vaccination, prophylactic (against) V04.4
  Zika (viral) 066.3
Fibrillation
  atrial (established) (paroxysmal) 427.31
  auricular (atrial) (established) 427.31
  cardiac (ventricular) 427.41
  coronary (*see also* Infarct, myocardium) 410.9 ☑
  heart (ventricular) 427.41
  muscular 728.9
  postoperative 997.1
  ventricular 427.41
Fibrin
  ball or bodies, pleural (sac) 511.0
  chamber, anterior (eye) (gelatinous exudate) 364.04
Fibrinogenolysis (hemorrhagic) — *see* Fibrinolysis
Fibrinogenopenia (congenital) (hereditary) — *see also* Defect, coagulation 286.3
  acquired 286.6
Fibrinolysis (acquired) (hemorrhagic) (pathologic) 286.6
  with
    abortion — *see* Abortion, by type, with hemorrhage, delayed or excessive
    ectopic pregnancy (*see also* categories 633.0–633.9) 639.1
    molar pregnancy (*see also* categories 630–632) 639.1
  antepartum or intrapartum 641.3 ☑
    affecting fetus or newborn 762.1
  following
    abortion 639.1
    ectopic or molar pregnancy 639.1
  newborn, transient 776.2
  postpartum 666.3 ☑
Fibrinopenia (hereditary) — *see also* Defect, coagulation 286.3
  acquired 286.6
Fibrinopurulent — *see* condition
Fibrinous — *see* condition
Fibroadenoma (M9010/0)
  cellular intracanalicular (M9020/0) 217
  giant (intracanalicular) (M9020/0) 217
  intracanalicular (M9011/0)
    cellular (M9020/0) 217
    giant (M9020/0) 217
    specified site — *see* Neoplasm, by site, benign
    unspecified site 217
  juvenile (M9030/0) 217
  pericanicular (M9012/0)
    specified site — *see* Neoplasm, by site, benign
    unspecified site 217
  phyllodes (M9020/0) 217
  prostate 600.20
    with
      other lower urinary tract symptoms (LUTS) 600.21
      urinary
        obstruction 600.21
        retention 600.21
  specified site — *see* Neoplasm, by site, benign
  unspecified site 217
Fibroadenosis, breast (chronic) (cystic) (diffuse) (periodic) (segmental) 610.2
Fibroangioma (M9160/0) — *see also* Neoplasm, by site, benign

Fibroangioma — see also Neoplasm, by site, benign — continued
  juvenile (M9160/0)
    specified site — see Neoplasm, by site, benign
    unspecified site 210.7
Fibrocellulitis progressiva ossificans 728.11
Fibrochondrosarcoma (M9220/3) — see Neoplasm, cartilage, malignant
Fibrocystic
  disease 277.00
    bone NEC 733.29
    breast 610.1
    jaw 526.2
    kidney (congenital) 753.19
    liver 751.62
    lung 518.89
      congenital 748.4
    pancreas 277.00
  kidney (congenital) 753.19
Fibrodysplasia ossificans multiplex (progressiva) 728.11
Fibroelastosis (cordis) (endocardial) (endomyocardial) 425.3
Fibroid (tumor) (M8890/0) — see also Neoplasm, connective tissue, benign
  disease, lung (chronic) (see also Fibrosis, lung) 515
  heart (disease) (see also Myocarditis) 429.0
  induration, lung (chronic) (see also Fibrosis, lung) 515
  in pregnancy or childbirth 654.1 ☑
    affecting fetus or newborn 763.89
    causing obstructed labor 660.2 ☑
      affecting fetus or newborn 763.1
  liver — see Cirrhosis, liver
  lung (see also Fibrosis, lung) 515
  pneumonia (chronic) (see also Fibrosis, lung) 515
  uterus (M8890/0) (see also Leiomyoma, uterus) 218.9
Fibrolipoma (M8851/0) — see also Lipoma, by site 214.9
Fibroliposarcoma (M8850/3) — see Neoplasm, connective tissue, malignant
Fibroma (M8810/0) — see also Neoplasm, connective tissue, benign
  ameloblastic (M9330/0) 213.1
    upper jaw (bone) 213.0
  bone (nonossifying) 733.99
    ossifying (M9262/0) — see Neoplasm, bone, benign
  cementifying (M9274/0) — see Neoplasm, bone, benign
  chondromyxoid (M9241/0) — see Neoplasm, bone, benign
  desmoplastic (M8823/1) — see Neoplasm, connective tissue, uncertain behavior
  facial (M8813/0) — see Neoplasm, connective tissue, benign
  invasive (M8821/1) — see Neoplasm, connective tissue, uncertain behavior
  molle (M8851/0) — see Lipoma, by site) 214.9
  myxoid (M8811/0) — see Neoplasm, connective tissue, benign
  nasopharynx, nasopharyngeal (juvenile) (M9160/0) 210.7
  nonosteogenic (nonossifying) — see Dysplasia, fibrous
  odontogenic (M9321/0) 213.1
    upper jaw (bone) 213.0
  ossifying (M9262/0) — see Neoplasm, bone, benign
  periosteal (M8812/0) — see Neoplasm, bone, benign
  prostate 600.20
    with
      other lower urinary tract symptoms (LUTS) 600.21
      urinary
        obstruction 600.21
        retention 600.21
  soft (M8851/0) (see also Lipoma, by site) 214.9
Fibromatosis 728.79

Fibromatosis — continued
  abdominal (M8822/1) — see Neoplasm, connective tissue, uncertain behavior
  aggressive (M8821/1) — see Neoplasm, connective tissue, uncertain behavior
  congenital generalized (CGF) 759.89
  Dupuytren's 728.6
  gingival 523.8
  plantar fascia 728.71
  proliferative 728.79
  pseudosarcomatous (proliferative) (subcutaneous) 728.79
  subcutaneous pseudosarcomatous (proliferative) 728.79
Fibromyalgia 729.1
Fibromyoma (M8890/0) — see also Neoplasm, connective tissue, benign
  uterus (corpus) (see also Leiomyoma, uterus) 218.9
    in pregnancy or childbirth 654.1 ☑
      affecting fetus or newborn 763.89
      causing obstructed labor 660.2 ☑
        affecting fetus or newborn 763.1
Fibromyositis — see also Myositis 729.1
  scapulohumeral 726.2
Fibromyxolipoma (M8852/0) — see also Lipoma, by site 214.9
Fibromyxoma (M8811/0) — see Neoplasm, connective tissue, benign
Fibromyxosarcoma (M8811/3) — see Neoplasm, connective tissue, malignant
Fibro-odontoma, ameloblastic (M9290/0) 213.1
  upper jaw (bone) 213.0
Fibro-osteoma (M9262/0) — see Neoplasm, bone, benign
Fibroplasia, retrolental (see also Retinopathy of prematurity) 362.21
Fibropurulent — see condition
Fibrosarcoma (M8810/3) — see also Neoplasm, connective tissue, malignant
  ameloblastic (M9330/3) 170.1
    upper jaw (bone) 170.0
  congenital (M8814/3) — see Neoplasm, connective tissue, malignant
  fascial (M8813/3) — see Neoplasm, connective tissue, malignant
  infantile (M8814/3) — see Neoplasm, connective tissue, malignant
  odontogenic (M9330/3) 170.1
    upper jaw (bone) 170.0
  periosteal (M8812/3) — see Neoplasm, bone, malignant
Fibrosclerosis
  breast 610.3
  corpora cavernosa (penis) 607.89
  familial multifocal NEC 710.8
  multifocal (idiopathic) NEC 710.8
  penis (corpora cavernosa) 607.89
Fibrosis, fibrotic
  adrenal (gland) 255.8
  alveolar (diffuse) 516.31
  amnion 658.8 ☑
  anal papillae 569.49
  anus 569.49
  appendix, appendiceal, noninflammatory 543.9
  arteriocapillary — see Arteriosclerosis
  bauxite (of lung) 503
  biliary 576.8
    due to Clonorchis sinensis 121.1
  bladder 596.89
    interstitial 595.1
    localized submucosal 595.1
    panmural 595.1
  bone, diffuse 756.59
  breast 610.3
  capillary (see also Arteriosclerosis)
    lung (chronic) (see also Fibrosis, lung) 515
  cardiac (see also Myocarditis) 429.0
  cervix 622.8
  chorion 658.8 ☑
  corpus cavernosum 607.89
  cystic (of pancreas) 277.00

Fibrosis, fibrotic — continued
  cystic — continued
    with
      manifestations
        gastrointestinal 277.03
        pulmonary 277.02
        specified NEC 277.09
      meconium ileus 277.01
      pulmonary exacerbation 277.02
  due to (presence of) any device, implant, or graft — see Complications, due to (presence of) any device, implant, or graft classified to 996.0–996.5 NEC
  ejaculatory duct 608.89
  endocardium (see also Endocarditis) 424.90
  endomyocardial (African) 425.0
  epididymis 608.89
  eye muscle 378.62
  graphite (of lung) 503
  heart (see also Myocarditis) 429.0
  hepatic (see also Cirrhosis, liver)
    due to Clonorchis sinensis 121.1
  hepatolienal — see Cirrhosis, liver
  hepatosplenic — see Cirrhosis, liver
  infrapatellar fat pad 729.31
  interstitial pulmonary, newborn 770.7
  intrascrotal 608.89
  kidney (see also Sclerosis, renal) 587
  liver — see Cirrhosis, liver
  lung (atrophic) (capillary) (chronic) (confluent) (massive) (perialveolar) (peribronchial) 515
    with
      anthracosilicosis (occupational) 500
      anthracosis (occupational) 500
      asbestosis (occupational) 501
      bagassosis (occupational) 495.1
      bauxite 503
      berylliosis (occupational) 503
      byssinosis (occupational) 504
      calcicosis (occupational) 502
      chalicosis (occupational) 502
      dust reticulation (occupational) 504
      farmers' lung 495.0
      gannister disease (occupational) 502
      graphite 503
      pneumoconiosis (occupational) 505
      pneumosiderosis (occupational) 503
      siderosis (occupational) 503
      silicosis (occupational) 502
      tuberculosis (see also Tuberculosis) 011.4 ☑
    diffuse (idiopathic) (interstitial) 516.31
    due to
      bauxite 503
      fumes or vapors (chemical) (inhalation) 506.4
      graphite 503
    following radiation 508.1
    postinflammatory 515
    silicotic (massive) (occupational) 502
    tuberculous (see also Tuberculosis) 011.4 ☑
  lymphatic gland 289.3
  median bar 600.90
    with
      other lower urinary tract symptoms (LUTS) 600.91
      urinary
        obstruction 600.91
        retention 600.91
  mediastinum (idiopathic) 519.3
  meninges 349.2
  muscle NEC 728.2
    iatrogenic (from injection) 999.9
  myocardium, myocardial (see also Myocarditis) 429.0
  oral submucous 528.8
  ovary 620.8
  oviduct 620.8
  pancreas 577.8
    cystic 277.00
      with
        manifestations
          gastrointestinal 277.03

Fibrosis, fibrotic — continued
  pancreas — continued
    cystic — continued
      with — continued
        manifestations — continued
          pulmonary 277.02
          specified NEC 277.09
        meconium ileus 277.01
        pulmonary exacerbation 277.02
  penis 607.89
  periappendiceal 543.9
  periarticular (see also Ankylosis) 718.5 ☑
  pericardium 423.1
  perineum, in pregnancy or childbirth 654.8 ☑
    affecting fetus or newborn 763.89
    causing obstructed labor 660.2 ☑
      affecting fetus or newborn 763.1
  perineural NEC 355.9
    foot 355.6
  periureteral 593.89
  placenta — see Placenta, abnormal
  pleura 511.0
  popliteal fat pad 729.31
  preretinal 362.56
  prostate (chronic) 600.90
    with
      other lower urinary tract symptoms (LUTS) 600.91
      urinary
        obstruction 600.91
        retention 600.91
  pulmonary (chronic) (see also Fibrosis, lung) 515
    alveolar capillary block 516.8
    idiopathic 516.31
    interstitial
      diffuse (idiopathic) 516.31
      newborn 770.7
  radiation — see Effect, adverse, radiation
  rectal sphincter 569.49
  retroperitoneal, idiopathic 593.4
  sclerosing mesenteric (idiopathic) 567.82
  scrotum 608.89
  seminal vesicle 608.89
  senile 797
  skin NEC 709.2
  spermatic cord 608.89
  spleen 289.59
    bilharzial (see also Schistosomiasis) 120.9
  subepidermal nodular (M8832/0) — see Neoplasm, skin, benign
  submucous NEC 709.2
    oral 528.8
    tongue 528.8
  syncytium — see Placenta, abnormal
  testis 608.89
    chronic, due to syphilis 095.8
  thymus (gland) 254.8
  tunica vaginalis 608.89
  ureter 593.89
  urethra 599.84
  uterus (nonneoplastic) 621.8
    bilharzial (see also Schistosomiasis) 120.9
    neoplastic (see also Leiomyoma, uterus) 218.9
  vagina 623.8
  valve, heart (see also Endocarditis) 424.90
  vas deferens 608.89
  vein 459.89
    lower extremities 459.89
  vesical 595.1
Fibrositis (periarticular) (rheumatoid) 729.0
  humeroscapular region 726.2
  nodular, chronic
    Jaccoud's 714.4
    rheumatoid 714.4
  ossificans 728.11
  scapulohumeral 726.2
Fibrothorax 511.0
Fibrotic — see Fibrosis
Fibrous — see condition
Fibroxanthoma (M8831/0) — see also Neoplasm, connective tissue, benign
  atypical (M8831/1) — see Neoplasm, connective tissue, uncertain behavior

☑ **Additional Digit Required** — Refer to the Tabular List for Digit Selection   ▽ **Subterms under main terms may continue to next column or page**

2013 ICD-9-CM   ▶◀ Revised Text   ● New Line   ▲ Revised Code   **Volume 2 — 115**

Fibroxanthoma — see also Neoplasm, connective tissue, benign — continued
  malignant (M8831/3) — see Neoplasm, connective tissue, malignant
Fibroxanthosarcoma (M8831/3) — see Neoplasm, connective tissue, malignant
Fiedler's
  disease (leptospiral jaundice) 100.0
  myocarditis or syndrome (acute isolated myocarditis) 422.91
Fiessinger-Leroy (-Reiter) syndrome 099.3
Fiessinger-Rendu syndrome (erythema muliforme exudativum) 695.19
Fifth disease (eruptive) 057.0
  venereal 099.1
Filaria, filarial — see Infestation, filarial
Filariasis — see also Infestation, filarial 125.9
  bancroftian 125.0
  Brug's 125.1
  due to
    bancrofti 125.0
    Brugia (Wuchereria) (malayi) 125.1
    Loa loa 125.2
    malayi 125.1
    organism NEC 125.6
    Wuchereria (bancrofti) 125.0
      malayi 125.1
  Malayan 125.1
  ozzardi 125.5
  specified type NEC 125.6
Filatoff's, Filatov's, Filatow's disease (infectious mononucleosis) 075
File-cutters' disease 984.9
  specified type of lead — see Table of Drugs and Chemicals
Filling defect
  biliary tract 793.3
  bladder 793.5
  duodenum 793.4
  gallbladder 793.3
  gastrointestinal tract 793.4
  intestine 793.4
  kidney 793.5
  stomach 793.4
  ureter 793.5
Filtering bleb, eye (postglaucoma) (status) V45.69
  with complication or rupture 997.99
  postcataract extraction (complication) 997.99
Fimbrial cyst (congenital) 752.11
Fimbriated hymen 752.49
Financial problem affecting care V60.2
Findings, (abnormal), without diagnosis (examination) (laboratory test) 796.4
  17-ketosteroids, elevated 791.9
  acetonuria 791.6
  acid phosphatase 790.5
  albumin-globulin ratio 790.99
  albuminuria 791.0
  alcohol in blood 790.3
  alkaline phosphatase 790.5
  amniotic fluid 792.3
  amylase 790.5
  anisocytosis 790.09
  antenatal screening 796.5
  anthrax, positive 795.31
  antibody titers, elevated 795.79
  anticardiolipin antibody 795.79
  antigen-antibody reaction 795.79
  antiphosphatidylglycerol antibody 795.79
  antiphosphatidylinositol antibody 795.79
  antiphosphatidylserine antibody 795.79
  antiphospholipid antibody 795.79
  bacteriuria 791.9
  ballistocardiogram 794.39
  bicarbonate 276.9
  bile in urine 791.4
  bilirubin 277.4
  bleeding time (prolonged) 790.92
  blood culture, positive 790.7
  blood gas level (arterial) 790.91
  blood sugar level 790.29
    high 790.29
      fasting glucose 790.21

Findings, (abnormal), without diagnosis — continued
  blood sugar level — continued
    high — continued
      glucose tolerance test 790.22
    low 251.2
  calcium 275.40
  cancer antigen 125 [CA 125] 795.82
  carbonate 276.9
  carcinoembryonic antigen [CEA] 795.81
  casts, urine 791.7
  catecholamines 791.9
  cells, urine 791.7
  cerebrospinal fluid (color) (content) (pressure) 792.0
  cervical
    high risk human papillomavirus (HPV) DNA test positive 795.05
    low risk human papillomavirus (HPV) DNA test positive 795.09
    non-atypical endometrial cells 795.09
  chloride 276.9
  cholesterol 272.9
    high 272.0
      with high triglycerides 272.2
  chromosome analysis 795.2
  chyluria 791.1
  circulation time 794.39
  cloudy dialysis effluent 792.5
  cloudy urine 791.9
  coagulation study 790.92
  cobalt, blood 790.6
  color of urine (unusual) NEC 791.9
  copper, blood 790.6
  C-reactive protein (CRP) 790.95
  creatinine clearance 794.4
  crystals, urine 791.9
  culture, positive NEC 795.39
    blood 790.7
    HIV V08
    human immunodeficiency virus V08
    nose 795.39
      Staphylococcus — see Carrier (suspected) of, Staphylococcus
    skin lesion NEC 795.39
    spinal fluid 792.0
    sputum 795.39
    stool 792.1
    throat 795.39
    urine 791.9
    viral
      human immunodeficiency V08
    wound 795.39
  cytology specified site NEC 796.9
  echocardiogram 793.2
  echoencephalogram 794.01
  echogram NEC — see Findings, abnormal, structure
  electrocardiogram (ECG) (EKG) 794.31
  electroencephalogram (EEG) 794.02
  electrolyte level, urinary 791.9
  electromyogram (EMG) 794.17
    ocular 794.14
  electro-oculogram (EOG) 794.12
  electroretinogram (ERG) 794.11
  enzymes, serum NEC 790.5
  fibrinogen titer coagulation study 790.92
  filling defect — see Filling defect
  function study NEC 794.9
    auditory 794.15
    bladder 794.9
    brain 794.00
    cardiac 794.30
    endocrine NEC 794.6
      thyroid 794.5
    kidney 794.4
    liver 794.8
    nervous system
      central 794.00
      peripheral 794.19
    oculomotor 794.14
    pancreas 794.9
    placenta 794.9
    pulmonary 794.2
    retina 794.11
    special senses 794.19

Findings, (abnormal), without diagnosis — continued
  function study — continued
    spleen 794.9
    vestibular 794.16
  gallbladder, nonvisualization 793.3
  glucose 790.29
    elevated
      fasting 790.21
      tolerance test 790.22
  glycosuria 791.5
  heart
    shadow 793.2
    sounds 785.3
  hematinuria 791.2
  hematocrit
    drop (precipitous) 790.01
    elevated 282.7
    low 285.9
  hematologic NEC 790.99
  hematuria 599.70
  hemoglobin
    drop 790.01
    elevated 282.7
    low 285.9
  hemoglobinuria 791.2
  histological NEC 795.4
  hormones 259.9
  immunoglobulins, elevated 795.79
  indolacetic acid, elevated 791.9
  iron 790.6
  karyotype 795.2
  ketonuria 791.6
  lactic acid dehydrogenase (LDH) 790.4
  lead 790.6
  lipase 790.5
  lipids NEC 272.9
  lithium, blood 790.6
  liver function test 790.6
  lung field (shadow) 793.19
    coin lesion 793.11
  magnesium, blood 790.6
  mammogram 793.80
    calcification 793.89
    calculus 793.89
    dense breasts 793.82
    inconclusive 793.82
      due to dense breasts 793.82
    microcalcification 793.81
  mediastinal shift 793.2
  melanin, urine 791.9
  microbiologic NEC 795.39
  mineral, blood NEC 790.6
  myoglobinuria 791.3
  nasal swab, anthrax 795.31
  neonatal screening 796.6
  nitrogen derivatives, blood 790.6
  nonvisualization of gallbladder 793.3
  nose culture, positive 795.39
  odor of urine (unusual) NEC 791.9
  oxygen saturation 790.91
  Papanicolaou (smear) 796.9
    anus 796.70
      with
        atypical squamous cells
          cannot exclude high grade squamous intraepithelial lesion (ASC-H) 796.72
          of undetermined significance (ASC-US) 796.71
        cytologic evidence of malignancy 796.76
        high grade squamous intraepithelial lesion (HGSIL) 796.74
        low grade squamous intraepithelial lesion (LGSIL) 796.73
      glandular 796.70
      specified finding NEC 796.79
    cervix 795.00
      with
        atypical squamous cells
          cannot exclude high grade squamous intraepithelial lesion (ASC-H) 795.02

Findings, (abnormal), without diagnosis — continued
  Papanicolaou — continued
    cervix — continued
      with — continued
        atypical squamous cells — continued
          of undetermined significance (ASC-US) 795.01
        cytologic evidence of malignancy 795.06
        high grade squamous intraepithelial lesion (HGSIL) 795.04
        low grade squamous intraepithelial lesion (LGSIL) 795.03
        non-atypical endometrial cells 795.09
      dyskaryotic 795.09
      non-atypical endometrial cells 795.09
      nonspecific finding NEC 795.09
    other site 796.9
    vagina 795.10
      with
        atypical squamous cells
          cannot exclude high grade squamous intraepithelial lesion (ASC-H) 795.12
          of undetermined significance (ASC-US) 795.11
        cytologic evidence of malignancy 795.16
        high grade squamous intraepithelial lesion (HGSIL) 795.14
        low grade squamous intraepithelial lesion (LGSIL) 795.13
      glandular 795.10
      specified NEC 795.19
  peritoneal fluid 792.9
  phonocardiogram 794.39
  phosphorus 275.3
  pleural fluid 792.9
  pneumoencephalogram 793.0
  PO2-oxygen ratio 790.91
  poikilocytosis 790.09
  potassium
    deficiency 276.8
    excess 276.7
  PPD 795.51
  prostate specific antigen (PSA) 790.93
  protein, serum NEC 790.99
  proteinuria 791.0
  prothrombin time (partial) (prolonged) (PT) (PTT) 790.92
  pyuria 791.9
  radiologic (x-ray) 793.99
    abdomen 793.6
    biliary tract 793.3
    breast 793.89
      abnormal mammogram NOS 793.80
      mammographic
        calcification 793.89
        calculus 793.89
        microcalcification 793.81
    gastrointestinal tract 793.4
    genitourinary organs 793.5
    head 793.0
    image test inconclusive due to excess body fat 793.91
    intrathoracic organs NEC 793.2
    lung 793.19
    musculoskeletal 793.7
    placenta 793.99
    retroperitoneum 793.6
    skin 793.99
    skull 793.0
    subcutaneous tissue 793.99
  red blood cell 790.09
    count 790.09
    morphology 790.09
    sickling 790.09
    volume 790.09
  saliva 792.4
  scan NEC 794.9
    bladder 794.9
    bone 794.9

☑ **Additional Digit Required** — Refer to the Tabular List for Digit Selection   ⩗ **Subterms under main terms may continue to next column or page**

116 — Volume 2   ▶◀ Revised Text   ● New Line   ▲ Revised Code   2013 ICD-9-CM

Findings, (abnormal), without diagnosis —
continued
  scan — *continued*
    brain 794.09
    kidney 794.4
    liver 794.8
    lung 794.2
    pancreas 794.9
    placental 794.9
    spleen 794.9
    thyroid 794.5
  sedimentation rate, elevated 790.1
  semen 792.2
  serological (for)
    human immunodeficiency virus (HIV)
      inconclusive 795.71
      positive V08
    syphilis — *see* Findings, serology for
      syphilis
  serology for syphilis
    false positive 795.6
    positive 097.1
      false 795.6
      follow-up of latent syphilis — *see*
        Syphilis, latent
      only finding — *see* Syphilis, latent
  serum 790.99
    blood NEC 790.99
    enzymes NEC 790.5
    proteins 790.99
  SGOT 790.4
  SGPT 790.4
  sickling of red blood cells 790.09
  skin test, positive 795.79
    tuberculin (without active tuberculosis)
      795.51
  sodium 790.6
    deficiency 276.1
    excess 276.0
  specified NEC 796.9
  spermatozoa 792.2
  spinal fluid 792.0
    culture, positive 792.0
  sputum culture, positive 795.39
    for acid-fast bacilli 795.39
  stool NEC 792.1
    bloody 578.1
      occult 792.1
    color 792.1
    culture, positive 792.1
    occult blood 792.1
  stress test 794.39
  structure, body (echogram) (thermogram)
    (ultrasound) (x-ray) NEC 793.99
    abdomen 793.6
    breast 793.89
      abnormal mammogram 793.80
      mammographic
        calcification 793.89
        calculus 793.89
        microcalcification 793.81
    gastrointestinal tract 793.4
    genitourinary organs 793.5
    head 793.0
      echogram (ultrasound) 794.01
    intrathoracic organs NEC 793.2
    lung 793.19
    musculoskeletal 793.7
    placenta 793.99
    retroperitoneum 793.6
    skin 793.99
    subcutaneous tissue NEC 793.99
  synovial fluid 792.9
  thermogram — *see* Findings, abnormal,
    structure
  throat culture, positive 795.39
  thyroid (function) 794.5
    metabolism (rate) 794.5
    scan 794.5
    uptake 794.5
  total proteins 790.99
  toxicology (drugs) (heavy metals) 796.0
  transaminase (level) 790.4
  triglycerides 272.9
    high 272.1
      with high cholesterol 272.2

Findings, (abnormal), without diagnosis —
continued
  tuberculin skin test (without active tuberculosis) 795.51
  tumor markers NEC 795.89
  ultrasound (*see also* Findings, abnormal,
    structure)
    cardiogram 793.2
  uric acid, blood 790.6
  urine, urinary constituents 791.9
    acetone 791.6
    albumin 791.0
    bacteria 791.9
    bile 791.4
    blood 599.70
    casts or cells 791.7
    chyle 791.1
    culture, positive 791.9
    glucose 791.5
    hemoglobin 791.2
    ketone 791.6
    protein 791.0
    pus 791.9
    sugar 791.5
  vaginal
    fluid 792.9
    high risk human papillomavirus (HPV)
      DNA test positive 795.15
    low risk human papillomavirus (HPV)
      DNA test positive 795.19
  vanillylmandelic acid, elevated 791.9
  vectorcardiogram (VCG) 794.39
  ventriculogram (cerebral) 793.0
  VMA, elevated 791.9
  Wassermann reaction
    false positive 795.6
    positive 097.1
      follow-up of latent syphilis — *see*
        Syphilis, latent
      only finding — *see* Syphilis, latent
  white blood cell 288.9
    count 288.9
      elevated 288.60
      low 288.50
    differential 288.9
    morphology 288.9
  wound culture 795.39
  xerography 793.89
  zinc, blood 790.6
Finger — *see* condition
Finnish type nephrosis (congenital) 759.89
Fire, St. Anthony's — *see also* Erysipelas 035
Fish
  hook stomach 537.89
  meal workers' lung 495.8
Fisher's syndrome 357.0
Fissure, fissured
  abdominal wall (congenital) 756.79
  anus, anal 565.0
    congenital 751.5
  buccal cavity 528.9
  clitoris (congenital) 752.49
  ear, lobule (congenital) 744.29
  epiglottis (congenital) 748.3
  larynx 478.79
    congenital 748.3
  lip 528.5
    congenital (*see also* Cleft, lip) 749.10
  nipple 611.2
    puerperal, postpartum 676.1 ☑
  palate (congenital) (*see also* Cleft, palate)
    749.00
  postanal 565.0
  rectum 565.0
  skin 709.8
    streptococcal 686.9
  spine (congenital) (*see also* Spina bifida)
    741.9 ☑
  sternum (congenital) 756.3
  tongue (acquired) 529.5
    congenital 750.13
Fistula (sinus) 686.9
  abdomen (wall) 569.81
    bladder 596.2
    intestine 569.81
    ureter 593.82

Fistula — *continued*
  abdomen — *continued*
    uterus 619.2
  abdominorectal 569.81
  abdominosigmoidal 569.81
  abdominothoracic 510.0
  abdominouterine 619.2
    congenital 752.39
  abdominovesical 596.2
  accessory sinuses (*see also* Sinusitis) 473.9
  actinomycotic — *see* Actinomycosis
  alveolar
    antrum (*see also* Sinusitis, maxillary)
      473.0
    process 522.7
  anorectal 565.1
  antrobuccal (*see also* Sinusitis, maxillary)
    473.0
  antrum (*see also* Sinusitis, maxillary) 473.0
  anus, anal (infectional) (recurrent) 565.1
    congenital 751.5
    tuberculous (*see also* Tuberculosis)
      014.8 ☑
  aortic sinus 747.29
  aortoduodenal 447.2
  appendix, appendicular 543.9
  arteriovenous (acquired) 447.0
    brain 437.3
      congenital 747.81
        ruptured (*see also* Hemorrhage,
          subarachnoid) 430
      ruptured (*see also* Hemorrhage, sub-
        arachnoid) 430
    cerebral 437.3
      congenital 747.81
    congenital (peripheral) 747.60
      brain — *see* Fistula, arteriovenous,
        brain, congenital
      coronary 746.85
      gastrointestinal 747.61
      lower limb 747.64
      pulmonary 747.39
      renal 747.62
      specified site NEC 747.69
      upper limb 747.63
    coronary 414.19
      congenital 746.85
    heart 414.19
    pulmonary (vessels) 417.0
      congenital 747.39
    surgically created (for dialysis) V45.11
      complication NEC 996.73
        atherosclerosis — *see* Arteriosclerosis, extremities
        embolism 996.74
        infection or inflammation 996.62
        mechanical 996.1
        occlusion NEC 996.74
        thrombus 996.74
    traumatic — *see* Injury, blood vessel, by
      site
  artery 447.2
  aural 383.81
    congenital 744.49
  auricle 383.81
    congenital 744.49
  Bartholin's gland 619.8
  bile duct (*see also* Fistula, biliary) 576.4
  biliary (duct) (tract) 576.4
    congenital 751.69
  bladder (neck) (sphincter) 596.2
    into seminal vesicle 596.2
  bone 733.99
  brain 348.89
    arteriovenous — *see* Fistula, arteriovenous, brain
  branchial (cleft) 744.41
  branchiogenous 744.41
  breast 611.0
    puerperal, postpartum 675.1 ☑
  bronchial 510.0
  bronchocutaneous, bronchomediastinal,
    bronchopleural, bronchopleuromediastinal (infective) 510.0
    tuberculous (*see also* Tuberculosis)
      011.3 ☑

Fistula — *continued*
  bronchoesophageal 530.89
    congenital 750.3
  buccal cavity (infective) 528.3
  canal, ear 380.89
  carotid-cavernous
    congenital 747.81
      with hemorrhage 430
    traumatic 900.82
      with hemorrhage (*see also* Hemorrhage, brain, traumatic)
        853.0 ☑
      late effect 908.3
  cecosigmoidal 569.81
  cecum 569.81
  cerebrospinal (fluid) 349.81
  cervical, lateral (congenital) 744.41
  cervicoaural (congenital) 744.49
  cervicosigmoidal 619.1
  cervicovesical 619.0
  cervix 619.8
  chest (wall) 510.0
  cholecystocolic (*see also* Fistula, gallbladder)
    575.5
  cholecystocolonic (*see also* Fistula, gallbladder) 575.5
  cholecystoduodenal (*see also* Fistula, gallbladder) 575.5
  cholecystoenteric (*see also* Fistula, gallbladder) 575.5
  cholecystogastric (*see also* Fistula, gallbladder) 575.5
  cholecystointestinal (*see also* Fistula, gallbladder) 575.5
  choledochoduodenal 576.4
  cholocolic (*see also* Fistula, gallbladder)
    575.5
  coccyx 685.1
    with abscess 685.0
  colon 569.81
  colostomy 569.69
  colovaginal (acquired) 619.1
  common duct (bile duct) 576.4
  congenital, NEC — *see* Anomaly, specified type NEC
  cornea, causing hypotony 360.32
  coronary, arteriovenous 414.19
    congenital 746.85
  costal region 510.0
  cul-de-sac, Douglas' 619.8
  cutaneous 686.9
  cystic duct (*see also* Fistula, gallbladder)
    575.5
    congenital 751.69
  cystostomy 596.83
  dental 522.7
  diaphragm 510.0
    bronchovisceral 510.0
    pleuroperitoneal 510.0
    pulmonoperitoneal 510.0
  duodenum 537.4
  ear (canal) (external) 380.89
  enterocolic 569.81
  enterocutaneous 569.81
  enteroenteric 569.81
  entero-uterine 619.1
    congenital 752.39
  enterovaginal 619.1
    congenital 752.49
  enterovesical 596.1
  epididymis 608.89
    tuberculous (*see also* Tuberculosis)
      016.4 ☑
  esophagobronchial 530.89
    congenital 750.3
  esophagocutaneous 530.89
  esophagopleurocutaneous 530.89
  esophagotracheal 530.84
    congenital 750.3
  esophagus 530.89
    congenital 750.4
  ethmoid (*see also* Sinusitis, ethmoidal) 473.2
  eyeball (cornea) (sclera) 360.32
  eyelid 373.11
  fallopian tube (external) 619.2
  fecal 569.81

☑ **Additional Digit Required — Refer to the Tabular List for Digit Selection**   ⬃ **Subterms under main terms may continue to next column or page**

2013 ICD-9-CM   ▶◀ Revised Text   ● New Line   ▲ Revised Code   **Volume 2 — 117**

Fistula — *continued*
fecal — *continued*
congenital 751.5
from periapical lesion 522.7
frontal sinus (*see also* Sinusitis, frontal) 473.1
gallbladder 575.5
with calculus, cholelithiasis, stones (*see also* Cholelithiasis) 574.2 ☑
congenital 751.69
gastric 537.4
gastrocolic 537.4
congenital 750.7
tuberculous (*see also* Tuberculosis) 014.8 ☑
gastroenterocolic 537.4
gastroesophageal 537.4
gastrojejunal 537.4
gastrojejunocolic 537.4
genital
organs
female 619.9
specified site NEC 619.8
male 608.89
tract-skin (female) 619.2
hepatopleural 510.0
hepatopulmonary 510.0
horseshoe 565.1
ileorectal 569.81
ileosigmoidal 569.81
ileostomy 569.69
ileovesical 596.1
ileum 569.81
in ano 565.1
tuberculous (*see also* Tuberculosis) 014.8 ☑
inner ear (*see also* Fistula, labyrinth) 386.40
intestine 569.81
intestinocolonic (abdominal) 569.81
intestinoureteral 593.82
intestinouterine 619.1
intestinovaginal 619.1
congenital 752.49
intestinovesical 596.1
involving female genital tract 619.9
digestive-genital 619.1
genital tract-skin 619.2
specified site NEC 619.8
urinary-genital 619.0
ischiorectal (fossa) 566
jejunostomy 569.69
jejunum 569.81
joint 719.80
ankle 719.87
elbow 719.82
foot 719.87
hand 719.84
hip 719.85
knee 719.86
multiple sites 719.89
pelvic region 719.85
shoulder (region) 719.81
specified site NEC 719.88
tuberculous — *see* Tuberculosis, joint
wrist 719.83
kidney 593.89
labium (majus) (minus) 619.8
labyrinth, labyrinthine NEC 386.40
combined sites 386.48
multiple sites 386.48
oval window 386.42
round window 386.41
semicircular canal 386.43
lacrimal, lachrymal (duct) (gland) (sac) 375.61
lacrimonasal duct 375.61
laryngotracheal 748.3
larynx 478.79
lip 528.5
congenital 750.25
lumbar, tuberculous (*see also* Tuberculosis) 015.0 ☑ *[730.8]* ☑
lung 510.0
lymphatic (node) (vessel) 457.8
mamillary 611.0
mammary (gland) 611.0
puerperal, postpartum 675.1 ☑

Fistula — *continued*
mastoid (process) (region) 383.1
maxillary (*see also* Sinusitis, maxillary) 473.0
mediastinal 510.0
mediastinobronchial 510.0
mediastinocutaneous 510.0
middle ear 385.89
mouth 528.3
nasal 478.19
sinus (*see also* Sinusitis) 473.9
nasopharynx 478.29
nipple — *see* Fistula, breast
nose 478.19
oral (cutaneous) 528.3
maxillary (*see also* Sinusitis, maxillary) 473.0
nasal (with cleft palate) (*see also* Cleft, palate) 749.00
orbit, orbital 376.10
oro-antral (*see also* Sinusitis, maxillary) 473.0
oval window (internal ear) 386.42
oviduct (external) 619.2
palate (hard) 526.89
soft 528.9
pancreatic 577.8
pancreaticoduodenal 577.8
parotid (gland) 527.4
region 528.3
pelvoabdominointestinal 569.81
penis 607.89
perianal 565.1
pericardium (pleura) (sac) (*see also* Pericarditis) 423.8
pericecal 569.81
perineal — *see* Fistula, perineum
perineorectal 569.81
perineosigmoidal 569.81
perineo-urethroscrotal 608.89
perineum, perineal (with urethral involvement) NEC 599.1
tuberculous (*see also* Tuberculosis) 017.9 ☑
ureter 593.82
perirectal 565.1
tuberculous (*see also* Tuberculosis) 014.8 ☑
peritoneum (*see also* Peritonitis) 567.22
periurethral 599.1
pharyngo-esophageal 478.29
pharynx 478.29
branchial cleft (congenital) 744.41
pilonidal (infected) (rectum) 685.1
with abscess 685.0
pleura, pleural, pleurocutaneous, pleuroperitoneal 510.0
stomach 510.0
tuberculous (*see also* Tuberculosis) 012.0 ☑
pleuropericardial 423.8
postauricular 383.81
postoperative, persistent 998.6
preauricular (congenital) 744.46
prostate 602.8
pulmonary 510.0
arteriovenous 417.0
congenital 747.39
tuberculous (*see also* Tuberculosis, pulmonary) 011.9 ☑
pulmonoperitoneal 510.0
rectolabial 619.1
rectosigmoid (intercommunicating) 569.81
rectoureteral 593.82
rectourethral 599.1
congenital 753.8
rectouterine 619.1
congenital 752.39
rectovaginal 619.1
congenital 752.49
old, postpartal 619.1
tuberculous (*see also* Tuberculosis) 014.8 ☑
rectovesical 596.1
congenital 753.8
rectovesicovaginal 619.1
rectovulvar 619.1
congenital 752.49

Fistula — *continued*
rectum (to skin) 565.1
tuberculous (*see also* Tuberculosis) 014.8 ☑
renal 593.89
retroauricular 383.81
round window (internal ear) 386.41
salivary duct or gland 527.4
congenital 750.24
sclera 360.32
scrotum (urinary) 608.89
tuberculous (*see also* Tuberculosis) 016.5 ☑
semicircular canals (internal ear) 386.43
sigmoid 569.81
vesicoabdominal 596.1
sigmoidovaginal 619.1
congenital 752.49
skin 686.9
ureter 593.82
vagina 619.2
sphenoidal sinus (*see also* Sinusitis, sphenoidal) 473.3
splenocolic 289.59
stercoral 569.81
stomach 537.4
sublingual gland 527.4
congenital 750.24
submaxillary
gland 527.4
congenital 750.24
region 528.3
thoracic 510.0
duct 457.8
thoracoabdominal 510.0
thoracogastric 510.0
thoracicointestinal 510.0
thoracoabdominal 510.0
thoracogastric 510.0
thorax 510.0
thyroglossal duct 759.2
thyroid 246.8
trachea (congenital) (external) (internal) 748.3
tracheoesophageal 530.84
congenital 750.3
following tracheostomy 519.09
traumatic
arteriovenous (*see also* Injury, blood vessel, by site) 904.9
brain — *see* Injury, intracranial
tuberculous — *see* Tuberculosis, by site
typhoid 002.0
umbilical 759.89
umbilico-urinary 753.8
urachal, urachus 753.7
ureter (persistent) 593.82
ureteroabdominal 593.82
ureterocervical 593.82
ureterorectal 593.82
ureterosigmoido-abdominal 593.82
ureterovaginal 619.0
ureterovesical 596.2
urethra 599.1
congenital 753.8
tuberculous (*see also* Tuberculosis) 016.3 ☑
urethroperineal 599.1
urethroperineovesical 596.2
urethrorectal 599.1
congenital 753.8
urethroscrotal 608.89
urethrovaginal 619.0
urethrovesical 596.2
urethrovesicovaginal 619.0
urinary (persistent) (recurrent) 599.1
uteroabdominal (anterior wall) 619.2
congenital 752.39
uteroenteric 619.1
uterofecal 619.1
uterointestinal 619.1
congenital 752.39
uterorectal 619.1
congenital 752.39
uteroureteric 619.0
uterovaginal 619.8

Fistula — *continued*
uterovesical 619.0
congenital 752.39
uterus 619.8
vagina (wall) 619.8
postpartal, old 619.8
vaginocutaneous (postpartal) 619.2
vaginoileal (acquired) 619.1
vaginoperineal 619.2
vesical NEC 596.2
vesicoabdominal 596.2
vesicocervicovaginal 619.0
vesicocolic 596.1
vesicocutaneous 596.2
vesicoenteric 596.1
vesicointestinal 596.1
vesicometrorectal 619.1
vesicoperineal 596.2
vesicorectal 596.1
congenital 753.8
vesicosigmoidal 596.1
vesicosigmoidovaginal 619.1
vesicoureteral 596.2
vesicoureterovaginal 619.0
vesicourethral 596.2
vesicourethrorectal 596.1
vesicouterine 619.0
congenital 752.39
vesicovaginal 619.0
vulvorectal 619.1
congenital 752.49
Fit 780.39
apoplectic (*see also* Disease, cerebrovascular, acute) 436
late effect — *see* Late effect(s) (of) cerebrovascular disease
epileptic (*see also* Epilepsy) 345.9 ☑
fainting 780.2
hysterical 300.11
newborn 779.0
Fitting (of)
artificial
arm (complete) (partial) V52.0
breast V52.4
implant exchange (different material) (different size) V52.4
eye(s) V52.2
leg(s) (complete) (partial) V52.1
brain neuropacemaker V53.02
cardiac pacemaker V53.31
carotid sinus pacemaker V53.39
cerebral ventricle (communicating) shunt V53.01
colostomy belt V53.5 ☑
contact lenses V53.1
cystostomy device V53.6
defibrillator, automatic implantable cardiac (with synchronous cardiac pacemaker) V53.32
dentures V52.3
device, unspecified type V53.90
abdominal V53.59
cardiac
defibrillator, automatic implantable (with synchronous cardiac pacemaker) V53.32
pacemaker V53.31
specified NEC V53.39
cerebral ventricle (communicating) shunt V53.01
gastrointestinal NEC V53.59
insulin pump V53.91
intestinal V53.50
intrauterine contraceptive
insertion V25.11
removal V25.12
and reinsertion V25.13
replacement V25.13
nervous system V53.09
orthodontic V53.4
orthoptic V53.1
other device V53.99
prosthetic V52.9
breast V52.4
dental V52.3
eye V52.2

☑ **Additional Digit Required** — Refer to the Tabular List for Digit Selection   ▽ **Subterms under main terms may continue to next column or page**

118 — Volume 2   ▶◀ Revised Text   ● New Line   ▲ Revised Code   2013 ICD-9-CM

Fitting — *continued*
  device, unspecified type — *continued*
    prosthetic — *continued*
      specified type NEC V52.8
    special senses V53.09
    substitution
      auditory V53.09
      nervous system V53.09
      visual V53.09
    urinary V53.6
  diaphragm (contraceptive) V25.02
  gastric lap band V53.51
  gastrointestinal appliance and device NEC V53.59
  glasses (reading) V53.1
  growth rod V54.02
  hearing aid V53.2
  ileostomy device V53.5 ☑
  intestinal appliance and device V53.50
  intestinal appliance or device NEC V53.5 ☑
  intrauterine contraceptive device
    insertion V25.11
    removal V25.12
      and reinsertion V25.13
    replacement V25.13
  neuropacemaker (brain) (peripheral nerve) (spinal cord) V53.02
  orthodontic device V53.4
  orthopedic (device) V53.7
    brace V53.7
    cast V53.7
    corset V53.7
    shoes V53.7
  pacemaker (cardiac) V53.31
    brain V53.02
    carotid sinus V53.39
    peripheral nerve V53.02
    spinal cord V53.02
  prosthesis V52.9
    arm (complete) (partial) V52.0
    breast V52.4
      implant exchange (different material) (different size) V52.4
    dental V52.3
    eye V52.2
    leg (complete) (partial) V52.1
    specified type NEC V52.8
  spectacles V53.1
  wheelchair V53.8
Fitz-Hugh and Curtis syndrome 098.86
  due to
    Chlamydia trachomatis 099.56
    Neisseria gonorrhoeae (gonococcal peritonitis) 098.86
Fitz's syndrome (acute hemorrhagic pancreatitis) 577.0
Fixation
  joint — *see* Ankylosis
  larynx 478.79
  pupil 364.76
  stapes 385.22
    deafness (*see also* Deafness, conductive) 389.04
  uterus (acquired) — *see* Malposition, uterus
  vocal cord 478.5
Flaccid — *see also* condition
  foot 736.79
  forearm 736.09
  palate, congenital 750.26
Flail
  chest 807.4
    newborn 767.3
  joint (paralytic) 718.80
    ankle 718.87
    elbow 718.82
    foot 718.87
    hand 718.84
    hip 718.85
    knee 718.86
    multiple sites 718.89
    pelvic region 718.85
    shoulder (region) 718.81
    specified site NEC 718.88
    wrist 718.83
Flajani (-Basedow) syndrome or disease (exophthalmic goiter) 242.0 ☑

Flap, liver 572.8
Flare, anterior chamber (aqueous) (eye) 364.04
Flashback phenomena (drug) (hallucinogenic) 292.89
Flat
  chamber (anterior) (eye) 360.34
  chest, congenital 754.89
  electroencephalogram (EEG) 348.89
  foot (acquired) (fixed type) (painful) (postural) (spastic) 734
    congenital 754.61
      rocker bottom 754.61
      vertical talus 754.61
    rachitic 268.1
    rocker bottom (congenital) 754.61
    vertical talus, congenital 754.61
  organ or site, congenital NEC — *see* Anomaly, specified type NEC
  pelvis 738.6
    with disproportion (fetopelvic) 653.2 ☑
      affecting fetus or newborn 763.1
      causing obstructed labor 660.1 ☑
        affecting fetus or newborn 763.1
    congenital 755.69
Flatau-Schilder disease 341.1
Flattening
  head, femur 736.39
  hip 736.39
  lip (congenital) 744.89
  nose (congenital) 754.0
    acquired 738.0
Flatulence 787.3
Flatus 787.3
  vaginalis 629.89
Flax dressers' disease 504
Flea bite — *see* Injury, superficial, by site
Fleischer (-Kayser) ring (corneal pigmentation) 275.1 *[371.14]*
Fleischner's disease 732.3
Fleshy mole 631.8
Flexibilitas cerea — *see also* Catalepsy 300.11
Flexion
  cervix — *see* Flexion, uterus
  contracture, joint (*see also* Contraction, joint) 718.4 ☑
  deformity, joint (*see also* Contraction, joint) 736.9
    hip, congenital (*see also* Subluxation, congenital, hip) 754.32
  uterus (*see also* Malposition, uterus) 621.6
Flexner's
  bacillus 004.1
  diarrhea (ulcerative) 004.1
  dysentery 004.1
Flexner-Boyd dysentery 004.2
Flexure — *see* condition
Floater, vitreous 379.24
Floating
  cartilage (joint) (*see also* Disorder, cartilage, articular) 718.0 ☑
    knee 717.6
  gallbladder (congenital) 751.69
  kidney 593.0
    congenital 753.3
  liver (congenital) 751.69
  rib 756.3
  spleen 289.59
Flooding 626.2
Floor — *see* condition
Floppy
  infant NEC 781.99
  iris syndrome 364.81
  valve syndrome (mitral) 424.0
Flu — *see also* Influenza
  bird (*see also* Influenza, avian) 488.02
  gastric NEC 008.8
  swine — *see* Influenza (novel) 2009 H1N1
Fluctuating blood pressure 796.4
Fluid
  abdomen 789.59
  chest (*see also* Pleurisy, with effusion) 511.9
  heart (*see also* Failure, heart) 428.0
  joint (*see also* Effusion, joint) 719.0 ☑
  loss (acute) 276.50

Fluid — *continued*
  loss — *continued*
    with
      hypernatremia 276.0
      hyponatremia 276.1
  lung (*see also* Edema, lung)
    encysted 511.89
  peritoneal cavity 789.59
    malignant 789.51
  pleural cavity (*see also* Pleurisy, with effusion) 511.9
  retention 276.69
Flukes NEC — *see also* Infestation, fluke 121.9
  blood NEC (*see also* Infestation, Schistosoma) 120.9
  liver 121.3
Fluor (albus) (vaginalis) 623.5
  trichomonal (Trichomonas vaginalis) 131.00
Fluorosis (dental) (chronic) 520.3
Flushing 782.62
  menopausal 627.2
Flush syndrome 259.2
Flutter
  atrial or auricular 427.32
  heart (ventricular) 427.42
    atrial 427.32
    impure 427.32
    postoperative 997.1
    ventricular 427.42
Flux (bloody) (serosanguineous) 009.0
FNHTR (febrile nonhemolytic transfusion reaction) 780.66
Focal — *see* condition
Fochier's abscess — *see* Abscess, by site
Focus, Assmann's — *see also* Tuberculosis 011.0 ☑
Fogo selvagem 694.4
Foix-Alajouanine syndrome 336.1
Folds, anomalous — *see also* Anomaly, specified type NEC
  Bowman's membrane 371.31
  Descemet's membrane 371.32
  epicanthic 743.63
  heart 746.89
  posterior segment of eye, congenital 743.54
Folie à deux 297.3
Follicle
  cervix (nabothian) (ruptured) 616.0
  graafian, ruptured, with hemorrhage 620.0
  nabothian 616.0
Folliclis (primary) — *see also* Tuberculosis 017.0 ☑
Follicular — *see also* condition
  cyst (atretic) 620.0
Folliculitis 704.8
  abscedens et suffodiens 704.8
  decalvans 704.09
  gonorrheal (acute) 098.0
    chronic or duration of 2 months or more 098.2
  keloid, keloidalis 706.1
  pustular 704.8
  ulerythematosa reticulata 701.8
Folliculosis, conjunctival 372.02
Følling's disease (phenylketonuria) 270.1
Follow-up (examination) (routine) (following) V67.9
  cancer chemotherapy V67.2
  chemotherapy V67.2
  fracture V67.4
  high-risk medication V67.51
  injury NEC V67.59
  postpartum
    immediately after delivery V24.0
    routine V24.2
  psychiatric V67.3
  psychotherapy V67.3
  radiotherapy V67.1
  specified condition NEC V67.59
  specified surgery NEC V67.09
  surgery V67.00
    vaginal pap smear V67.01
  treatment V67.9
    combined NEC V67.6
    fracture V67.4

Follow-up — *continued*
  treatment — *continued*
    involving high-risk medication NEC V67.51
    mental disorder V67.3
    specified NEC V67.59
Fong's syndrome (hereditary osteoonychodysplasia) 756.89
Food
  allergy 693.1
  anaphylactic reaction or shock due to food 995.60
  asphyxia (from aspiration or inhalation) (*see also* Asphyxia, food) 933.1
  choked on (*see also* Asphyxia, food) 933.1
  deprivation 994.2
    specified kind of food NEC 269.8
  intoxication (*see also* Poisoning, food) 005.9
  lack of 994.2
  poisoning (*see also* Poisoning, food) 005.9
  refusal or rejection NEC 307.59
  strangulation or suffocation (*see also* Asphyxia, food) 933.1
  toxemia (*see also* Poisoning, food) 005.9
Foot — *see also* condition
  and mouth disease 078.4
  process disease 581.3
Foramen ovale (nonclosure) (patent) (persistent) 745.5
Forbes-Albright syndrome (nonpuerperal amenorrhea and lactation associated with pituitary tumor) 253.1
Forbes'(glycogen storage) disease 271.0
Forced birth or delivery NEC 669.8 ☑
  affecting fetus or newborn NEC 763.89
Forceps
  delivery NEC 669.5 ☑
    affecting fetus or newborn 763.2
Fordyce's disease (ectopic sebaceous glands) (mouth) 750.26
Fordyce-Fox disease (apocrine miliaria) 705.82
Forearm — *see* condition
Foreign body

> *Note* — *For foreign body with open wound, or other injury, see Wound, open, or the type of injury specified.*

  accidentally left during a procedure 998.4
  anterior chamber (eye) 871.6
    magnetic 871.5
      retained or old 360.51
    retained or old 360.61
  ciliary body (eye) 871.6
    magnetic 871.5
      retained or old 360.52
    retained or old 360.62
  entering through orifice (current) (old)
    accessory sinus 932
    air passage (upper) 933.0
      lower 934.8
    alimentary canal 938
    alveolar process 935.0
    antrum (Highmore) 932
    anus 937
    appendix 936
    asphyxia due to (*see also* Asphyxia, food) 933.1
    auditory canal 931
    auricle 931
    bladder 939.0
    bronchioles 934.8
    bronchus (main) 934.1
    buccal cavity 935.0
    canthus (inner) 930.1
    cecum 936
    cervix (canal) uterine 939.1
    coil, ileocecal 936
    colon 936
    conjunctiva 930.1
    conjunctival sac 930.1
    cornea 930.0
    digestive organ or tract NEC 938
    duodenum 936
    ear (external) 931
    esophagus 935.1
    eye (external) 930.9
      combined sites 930.8

☑ **Additional Digit Required** — Refer to the Tabular List for Digit Selection   ▽ **Subterms under main terms may continue to next column or page**

Foreign body — *continued*
  entering through orifice — *continued*
    eye — *continued*
      intraocular — *see* Foreign body, by site
      specified site NEC 930.8
    eyeball 930.8
      intraocular — *see* Foreign body, intraocular
    eyelid 930.1
      retained or old 374.86
    frontal sinus 932
    gastrointestinal tract 938
    genitourinary tract 939.9
    globe 930.8
      penetrating 871.6
        magnetic 871.5
          retained or old 360.50
        retained or old 360.60
    gum 935.0
    Highmore's antrum 932
    hypopharynx 933.0
    ileocecal coil 936
    ileum 936
    inspiration (of) 933.1
    intestine (large) (small) 936
    lacrimal apparatus, duct, gland, or sac 930.2
    larynx 933.1
    lung 934.8
    maxillary sinus 932
    mouth 935.0
    nasal sinus 932
    nasopharynx 933.0
    nose (passage) 932
    nostril 932
    oral cavity 935.0
    palate 935.0
    penis 939.3
    pharynx 933.0
    pyriform sinus 933.0
    rectosigmoid 937
      junction 937
    rectum 937
    respiratory tract 934.9
      specified part NEC 934.8
    sclera 930.1
    sinus 932
      accessory 932
      frontal 932
      maxillary 932
      nasal 932
      pyriform 933.0
    small intestine 936
    stomach (hairball) 935.2
    suffocation by (*see also* Asphyxia, food) 933.1
    swallowed 938
      tongue 933.0
    tear ducts or glands 930.2
    throat 933.0
    tongue 935.0
      swallowed 933.0
    tonsil, tonsillar 933.0
      fossa 933.0
    trachea 934.0
    ureter 939.0
    urethra 939.0
    uterus (any part) 939.1
    vagina 939.2
    vulva 939.2
    wind pipe 934.0
  feeling of, in throat 784.99
  granuloma (old) 728.82
    bone 733.99
    in operative wound (inadvertently left) 998.4
      due to surgical material intentionally left — *see* Complications, due to (presence of) any device, implant, or graft classified to 996.0–996.5 NEC
    muscle 728.82
    skin 709.4
    soft tissue 709.4
    subcutaneous tissue 709.4

Foreign body — *continued*
  in
    bone (residual) 733.99
    open wound — *see* Wound, open, by site complicated
    soft tissue (residual) 729.6
  inadvertently left in operation wound (causing adhesions, obstruction, or perforation) 998.4
  ingestion, ingested NEC 938
  inhalation or inspiration (*see also* Asphyxia, food) 933.1
  internal organ, not entering through an orifice — *see* Injury, internal, by site, with open wound
  intraocular (nonmagnetic) 871.6
    combined sites 871.6
      magnetic 871.5
        retained or old 360.59
      retained or old 360.69
    magnetic 871.5
      retained or old 360.50
    retained or old 360.60
    specified site NEC 871.6
      magnetic 871.5
        retained or old 360.59
      retained or old 360.69
    iris (nonmagnetic) 871.6
      magnetic 871.5
        retained or old 360.52
      retained or old 360.62
    lens (nonmagnetic) 871.6
      magnetic 871.5
        retained or old 360.53
      retained or old 360.63
    lid, eye 930.1
    ocular muscle 870.4
      retained or old 376.6
    old or residual
      bone 733.99
      eyelid 374.86
      middle ear 385.83
      muscle 729.6
        ocular 376.6
      retrobulbar 376.6
      skin 729.6
        with granuloma 709.4
      soft tissue 729.6
        with granuloma 709.4
      subcutaneous tissue 729.6
        with granuloma 709.4
    operation wound, left accidentally 998.4
    orbit 870.4
      retained or old 376.6
    posterior wall, eye 871.6
      magnetic 871.5
        retained or old 360.55
      retained or old 360.65
    respiratory tree 934.9
      specified site NEC 934.8
    retained (old) (nonmagnetic) (in) V90.9
      anterior chamber (eye) 360.61
        magnetic 360.51
      ciliary body 360.62
        magnetic 360.52
      eyelid 374.86
      fragment(s)
        acrylics V90.2
        animal quills V90.31
        animal spines V90.31
        cement V90.83
        concrete V90.83
        crystalline V90.83
        depleted
          isotope V90.09
          uranium V90.01
        diethylhexylphthalates V90.2
        glass V90.81
        isocyanate V90.2
        metal V90.10
          magnetic V90.11
          nonmagnetic V90.12
        organic NEC V90.39
        plastic V90.2
        radioactive
          nontherapeutic V90.09

Foreign body — *continued*
  retained — *continued*
    fragment(s) — *continued*
      radioactive — *continued*
        specified NEC V90.09
      stone V90.83
      tooth V90.32
      wood V90.33
    globe 360.60
      magnetic 360.50
    intraocular 360.60
      magnetic 360.50
      specified site NEC 360.69
        magnetic 360.59
    iris 360.62
      magnetic 360.52
    lens 360.63
      magnetic 360.53
    muscle 729.6
    orbit 376.6
    posterior wall of globe 360.65
      magnetic 360.55
    retina 360.65
      magnetic 360.55
    retrobulbar 376.6
    skin 729.6
      with granuloma 709.4
    soft tissue 729.6
      with granuloma 709.4
    specified NEC V90.89
    subcutaneous tissue 729.6
      with granuloma 709.4
    vitreous 360.64
      magnetic 360.54
  retina 871.6
    magnetic 871.5
      retained or old 360.55
    retained or old 360.65
  superficial, without major open wound (*see also* Injury, superficial, by site) 919.6
  swallowed NEC 938
  throat, feeling of 784.99
  vitreous (humor) 871.6
    magnetic 871.5
      retained or old 360.54
    retained or old 360.64

Forking, aqueduct of Sylvius 742.3
  with spina bifida (*see also* Spina bifida) 741.0 ☑
Formation
  bone in scar tissue (skin) 709.3
  connective tissue in vitreous 379.25
  Elschnig pearls (postcataract extraction) 366.51
  hyaline in cornea 371.49
  sequestrum in bone (due to infection) (*see also* Osteomyelitis) 730.1 ☑
  valve
    colon, congenital 751.5
    ureter (congenital) 753.29
Formication 782.0
Fort Bragg fever 100.89
Fossa — *see also* condition
  pyriform — *see* condition
Foster care (status) V60.81
Foster-Kennedy syndrome 377.04
Fothergill's
  disease, meaning scarlatina anginosa 034.1
  neuralgia (*see also* Neuralgia, trigeminal) 350.1
Foul breath 784.99
Found dead (cause unknown) 798.9
Foundling V20.0
Fournier's disease (idiopathic gangrene) 608.83
  female 616.89
Fourth
  cranial nerve — *see* condition
  disease 057.8
  molar 520.1
Foville's syndrome 344.89
Fox's
  disease (apocrine miliaria) 705.82
  impetigo (contagiosa) 684
Fox-Fordyce disease (apocrine miliaria) 705.82

Fracture (abduction) (adduction) (avulsion) (compression) (crush) (dislocation) (oblique) (separation) (closed) 829.0

Note — For fracture of any of the following sites with fracture of other bones — see Fracture, multiple.

"Closed" includes the following descriptions of fractures, with or without delayed healing, unless they are specified as open or compound:

comminuted	linear
depressed	simple
elevated	slipped epiphysis
fissured	spiral
greenstick	unspecified
impacted	

"Open" includes the following descriptions of fractures, with or without delayed healing:

compound	puncture
infected	with foreign body
missile	

For late effect of fracture, see Late, effect, fracture, by site.

  with
    internal injuries in same region (conditions classifiable to 860–869) (*see also* Injury, internal, by site)
    pelvic region — *see* Fracture, pelvis
  acetabulum (with visceral injury) (closed) 808.0
    open 808.1
  acromion (process) (closed) 811.01
    open 811.11
  alveolus (closed) 802.8
    open 802.9
  ankle (malleolus) (closed) 824.8
    bimalleolar (Dupuytren's) (Pott's) 824.4
      open 824.5
    bone 825.21
      open 825.31
    lateral malleolus only (fibular) 824.2
      open 824.3
    medial malleolus only (tibial) 824.0
      open 824.1
    open 824.9
    pathologic 733.16
    talus 825.21
      open 825.31
    trimalleolar 824.6
      open 824.7
  antrum — *see* Fracture, skull, base
  arm (closed) 818.0
    and leg(s) (any bones) 828.0
      open 828.1
    both (any bones) (with rib(s)) (with sternum) 819.0
      open 819.1
    lower 813.80
      open 813.90
    open 818.1
    upper — *see* Fracture, humerus
  astragalus (closed) 825.21
    open 825.31
  atlas — *see* Fracture, vertebra, cervical, first
  axis — *see* Fracture, vertebra, cervical, second
  back — *see* Fracture, vertebra, by site
  Barton's — *see* Fracture, radius, lower end
  basal (skull) — *see* Fracture, skull, base
  Bennett's (closed) 815.01
    open 815.11
  bimalleolar (closed) 824.4
    open 824.5
  bone (closed) NEC 829.0
    birth injury NEC 767.3
    open 829.1
    pathologic NEC (*see also* Fracture, pathologic) 733.10

☑ Additional Digit Required — Refer to the Tabular List for Digit Selection   ▽ Subterms under main terms may continue to next column or page

120 — Volume 2   ▶◀ Revised Text   ● New Line   ▲ Revised Code   2013 ICD-9-CM

Fracture — continued
　bone — continued
　　stress NEC (see also Fracture, stress)
　　　733.95
　boot top — see Fracture, fibula
　boxers' — see Fracture, metacarpal bone(s)
　breast bone — see Fracture, sternum
　bucket handle (semilunar cartilage) — see
　　　Tear, meniscus
　buckle — see Fracture, torus
　burst — see Fracture, traumatic, by site
　bursting — see Fracture, phalanx, hand,
　　　distal
　calcaneus (closed) 825.0
　　open 825.1
　capitate (bone) (closed) 814.07
　　open 814.17
　capitellum (humerus) (closed) 812.49
　　open 812.59
　carpal bone(s) (wrist NEC) (closed) 814.00
　　open 814.10
　　specified site NEC 814.09
　　　open 814.19
　cartilage, knee (semilunar) — see Tear,
　　　meniscus
　cervical — see Fracture, vertebra, cervical
　chauffeur's — see Fracture, ulna, lower end
　chisel — see Fracture, radius, upper end
　chronic — see Fracture, pathologic
　clavicle (interligamentous part) (closed)
　　　810.00
　　acromial end 810.03
　　　open 810.13
　　due to birth trauma 767.2
　　open 810.10
　　shaft (middle third) 810.02
　　　open 810.12
　　sternal end 810.01
　　　open 810.11
　clayshovelers' — see Fracture, vertebra,
　　　cervical
　coccyx (see also Fracture, vertebra, coccyx)
　　complicating delivery 665.6 ☑
　collar bone — see Fracture, clavicle
　Colles' (reversed) (closed) 813.41
　　open 813.51
　comminuted — see Fracture, by site
　compression (see also Fracture, by site)
　　nontraumatic — see Fracture, pathologic
　congenital 756.9
　coracoid process (closed) 811.02
　　open 811.12
　coronoid process (ulna) (closed) 813.02
　　mandible (closed) 802.23
　　　open 802.33
　　open 813.12
　corpus cavernosum penis 959.13
　costochondral junction — see Fracture, rib
　costosternal junction — see Fracture, rib
　cranium — see Fracture, skull, by site
　cricoid cartilage (closed) 807.5
　　open 807.6
　cuboid (ankle) (closed) 825.23
　　open 825.33
　cuneiform
　　foot (closed) 825.24
　　　open 825.34
　　wrist (closed) 814.03
　　　open 814.13
　dental implant 525.73
　dental restorative material
　　with loss of material 525.64
　　without loss of material 525.63
　due to
　　birth injury — see Birth injury, fracture
　　gunshot — see Fracture, by site, open
　　neoplasm — see Fracture, pathologic
　　osteoporosis — see Fracture, pathologic
　Dupuytren's (ankle) (fibula) (closed) 824.4
　　open 824.5
　　radius 813.42
　　　open 813.52
　Duverney's — see Fracture, ilium
　elbow (see also Fracture, humerus, lower
　　　end)
　　olecranon (process) (closed) 813.01

Fracture — continued
　elbow (see also Fracture, humerus, lower
　　　end) — continued
　　olecranon — continued
　　　open 813.11
　　supracondylar (closed) 812.41
　　　open 812.51
　ethmoid (bone) (sinus) — see Fracture, skull,
　　　base
　face bone(s) (closed) NEC 802.8
　　with
　　　other bone(s) — see Fracture, multi-
　　　　ple, skull
　　　skull (see also Fracture, skull)
　　　　involving other bones — see
　　　　　Fracture, multiple, skull
　　open 802.9
　fatigue — see Fracture, march
　femur, femoral (closed) 821.00
　　cervicotrochanteric 820.03
　　　open 820.13
　　condyles, epicondyles 821.21
　　　open 821.31
　　distal end — see Fracture, femur, lower
　　　　end
　　epiphysis (separation)
　　　capital 820.01
　　　　open 820.11
　　　head 820.01
　　　　open 820.11
　　　lower 821.22
　　　　open 821.32
　　　trochanteric 820.01
　　　　open 820.11
　　　upper 820.01
　　　　open 820.11
　　head 820.09
　　　open 820.19
　　lower end or extremity (distal end)
　　　　(closed) 821.20
　　　condyles, epicondyles 821.21
　　　　open 821.31
　　　epiphysis (separation) 821.22
　　　　open 821.32
　　　multiple sites 821.29
　　　　open 821.39
　　　open 821.30
　　　specified site NEC 821.29
　　　　open 821.39
　　　supracondylar 821.23
　　　　open 821.33
　　　T-shaped 821.21
　　　　open 821.31
　　neck (closed) 820.8
　　　base (cervicotrochanteric) 820.03
　　　　open 820.13
　　　extracapsular 820.20
　　　　open 820.30
　　　intertrochanteric (section) 820.21
　　　　open 820.31
　　　intracapsular 820.00
　　　　open 820.10
　　　intratrochanteric 820.21
　　　　open 820.31
　　　midcervical 820.02
　　　　open 820.12
　　　open 820.9
　　　pathologic 733.14
　　　　specified part NEC 733.15
　　　specified site NEC 820.09
　　　　open 820.19
　　　stress 733.96
　　　transcervical 820.02
　　　　open 820.12
　　　transtrochanteric 820.20
　　　　open 820.30
　　　open 821.10
　　pathologic 733.14
　　　specified part NEC 733.15
　　peritrochanteric (section) 820.20
　　　open 820.30
　　shaft (lower third) (middle third) (upper
　　　　third) 821.01
　　　open 821.11
　　　stress 733.97
　　subcapital 820.09

Fracture — continued
　femur, femoral — continued
　　subcapital — continued
　　　open 820.19
　　subtrochanteric (region) (section) 820.22
　　　open 820.32
　　supracondylar 821.23
　　　open 821.33
　　transepiphyseal 820.01
　　　open 820.11
　　trochanter (greater) (lesser) (see also
　　　　Fracture, femur, neck, by site)
　　　　820.20
　　　open 820.30
　　T-shaped, into knee joint 821.21
　　　open 821.31
　　upper end 820.8
　　　open 820.9
　fibula (closed) 823.81
　　with tibia 823.82
　　　open 823.92
　　distal end 824.8
　　　open 824.9
　　epiphysis
　　　lower 824.8
　　　　open 824.9
　　　upper — see Fracture, fibula, upper
　　　　end
　　head — see Fracture, fibula, upper end
　　involving ankle 824.2
　　　open 824.3
　　lower end or extremity 824.8
　　　open 824.9
　　malleolus (external) (lateral) 824.2
　　　open 824.3
　　open NEC 823.91
　　pathologic 733.16
　　proximal end — see Fracture, fibula,
　　　　upper end
　　shaft 823.21
　　　with tibia 823.22
　　　　open 823.32
　　　open 823.31
　　stress 733.93
　　torus 823.41
　　　with tibia 823.42
　　upper end or extremity (epiphysis)
　　　　(head) (proximal end) (styloid)
　　　　823.01
　　　with tibia 823.02
　　　　open 823.12
　　　open 823.11
　finger(s), of one hand (closed) (see also
　　　Fracture, phalanx, hand) 816.00
　　with
　　　metacarpal bone(s), of same hand
　　　　817.0
　　　　open 817.1
　　　thumb of same hand 816.03
　　　　open 816.13
　　open 816.10
　foot, except toe(s) alone (closed) 825.20
　　open 825.30
　forearm (closed) NEC 813.80
　　lower end (distal end) (lower epiphysis)
　　　　813.40
　　　open 813.50
　　open 813.90
　　shaft 813.20
　　　open 813.30
　　upper end (proximal end) (upper epiph-
　　　　ysis) 813.00
　　　open 813.10
　fossa, anterior, middle, or posterior — see
　　　Fracture, skull, base
　Fracture (abduction) (adduction) (avulsion)
　　　(compression) (crush) (dislocation)
　　　(oblique) (separation) (closed) 829.0
　frontal (bone) (see also Fracture, skull, vault)
　　sinus — see Fracture, skull, base
　Galeazzi's — see Fracture, radius, lower end
　glenoid (cavity) (fossa) (scapula) (closed)
　　　811.03
　　open 811.13
　Gosselin's — see Fracture, ankle
　greenstick — see Fracture, by site

Fracture — continued
　grenade-throwers' — see Fracture, humerus,
　　　shaft
　gutter — see Fracture, skull, vault
　hamate (closed) 814.08
　　open 814.18
　hand, one (closed) 815.00
　　carpals 814.00
　　　open 814.10
　　　specified site NEC 814.09
　　　　open 814.19
　　metacarpals 815.00
　　　open 815.10
　　multiple, bones of one hand 817.0
　　　open 817.1
　　open 815.10
　　phalanges (see also Fracture, phalanx,
　　　　hand) 816.00
　　　open 816.10
　healing
　　aftercare (see also Aftercare, fracture)
　　　　V54.89
　　change of cast V54.89
　　complications — see condition
　　convalescence V66.4
　　removal of
　　　cast V54.89
　　　fixation device
　　　　external V54.89
　　　　internal V54.01
　heel bone (closed) 825.0
　　open 825.1
　Hill-Sachs 812.09
　hip (closed) (see also Fracture, femur, neck)
　　　820.8
　　open 820.9
　　pathologic 733.14
　humerus (closed) 812.20
　　anatomical neck 812.02
　　　open 812.12
　　articular process (see also Fracture
　　　　humerus, condyle(s)) 812.44
　　　open 812.54
　　capitellum 812.49
　　　open 812.59
　　condyle(s) 812.44
　　　lateral (external) 812.42
　　　　open 812.52
　　　medial (internal epicondyle) 812.43
　　　　open 812.53
　　　open 812.54
　　distal end — see Fracture, humerus,
　　　　lower end
　　epiphysis
　　　lower (see also Fracture, humerus,
　　　　condyle(s)) 812.44
　　　　open 812.54
　　　upper 812.09
　　　　open 812.19
　　external condyle 812.42
　　　open 812.52
　　great tuberosity 812.03
　　　open 812.13
　　head 812.09
　　　open 812.19
　　internal epicondyle 812.43
　　　open 812.53
　　lesser tuberosity 812.09
　　　open 812.19
　　lower end or extremity (distal end) (see
　　　　also Fracture, humerus, by site)
　　　　812.40
　　　multiple sites NEC 812.49
　　　　open 812.59
　　　open 812.50
　　　specified site NEC 812.49
　　　　open 812.59
　　neck 812.01
　　　open 812.11
　　open 812.30
　　pathologic 733.11
　　proximal end — see Fracture, humerus,
　　　　upper end
　　shaft 812.21
　　　open 812.31
　　supracondylar 812.41

☑ Additional Digit Required — Refer to the Tabular List for Digit Selection　　　　　　　　　🔳 Subterms under main terms may continue to next column or page

2013 ICD-9-CM　　　　　　　▶◀ Revised Text　　　　　● New Line　　　▲ Revised Code　　　　　　　　　Volume 2 — 121

Fracture — *continued*
  humerus — *continued*
    supracondylar — *continued*
      open 812.51
    surgical neck 812.01
      open 812.11
    trochlea 812.49
      open 812.59
    T-shaped 812.44
      open 812.54
    tuberosity — *see* Fracture, humerus, upper end
    upper end or extremity (proximal end) (*see also* Fracture, humerus, by site) 812.00
      open 812.10
      specified site NEC 812.09
        open 812.19
  hyoid bone (closed) 807.5
    open 807.6
  hyperextension — *see* Fracture, radius, lower end
  ilium (with visceral injury) (closed) 808.41
    open 808.51
  impaction, impacted — *see* Fracture, by site
  incus — *see* Fracture, skull, base
  innominate bone (with visceral injury) (closed) 808.49
    open 808.59
  instep, of one foot (closed) 825.20
    with toe(s) of same foot 827.0
      open 827.1
    open 825.30
  insufficiency — *see* Fracture, pathologic, by site
  internal
    ear — *see* Fracture, skull, base
    semilunar cartilage, knee — *see* Tear, meniscus, medial
  intertrochanteric — *see* Fracture, femur, neck, intertrochanteric
  ischium (with visceral injury) (closed) 808.42
    open 808.52
  jaw (bone) (lower) (closed) (*see also* Fracture, mandible) 802.20
    angle 802.25
      open 802.35
    open 802.30
    upper — *see* Fracture, maxilla
  knee
    cap (closed) 822.0
      open 822.1
    cartilage (semilunar) — *see* Tear, meniscus
  labyrinth (osseous) — *see* Fracture, skull, base
  larynx (closed) 807.5
    open 807.6
  late effect — *see* Late, effects (of), fracture
  Le Fort's — *see* Fracture, maxilla
  leg (closed) 827.0
    with rib(s) or sternum 828.0
      open 828.1
    both (any bones) 828.0
      open 828.1
    lower — *see* Fracture, tibia
      open 827.1
    upper — *see* Fracture, femur
  limb
    lower (multiple) (closed) NEC 827.0
      open 827.1
    upper (multiple) (closed) NEC 818.0
      open 818.1
  long bones, due to birth trauma — *see* Birth injury, fracture
  lower end or extremity (anterior lip) (posterior) 824.8
    open 824.9
  lumbar — *see* Fracture, vertebra, lumbar
  lunate bone (closed) 814.02
    open 814.12
  malar bone (closed) 802.4
    open 802.5
  Malgaigne's (closed) 808.43
    open 808.53
  malleolus (closed) 824.8

Fracture — *continued*
  malleolus — *continued*
    bimalleolar 824.4
      open 824.5
    lateral 824.2
      and medial (*see also* Fracture, malleolus, bimalleolar)
        with lip of tibia — *see* Fracture, malleolus, trimalleolar
        open 824.3
    medial (closed) 824.0
      and lateral (*see also* Fracture, malleolus, bimalleolar)
        with lip of tibia — *see* Fracture, malleolus, trimalleolar
        open 824.1
    open 824.9
    trimalleolar (closed) 824.6
      open 824.7
  malleus — *see* Fracture, skull, base
  malunion 733.81
  mandible (closed) 802.20
    angle 802.25
      open 802.35
    body 802.28
      alveolar border 802.27
        open 802.37
      open 802.38
      symphysis 802.26
        open 802.36
    condylar process 802.21
      open 802.31
    coronoid process 802.23
      open 802.33
    multiple sites 802.29
      open 802.39
    open 802.30
    ramus NEC 802.24
      open 802.34
    subcondylar 802.22
      open 802.32
  manubrium — *see* Fracture, sternum
  march 733.95
    femoral neck 733.96
    fibula 733.93
    metatarsals 733.94
    pelvis 733.98
    shaft of femur 733.97
    tibia 733.93
  maxilla, maxillary (superior) (upper jaw) (closed) 802.4
    inferior — *see* Fracture, mandible
    open 802.5
  meniscus, knee — *see* Tear, meniscus
  metacarpus, metacarpal (bone(s)), of one hand (closed) 815.00
    with phalanx, phalanges, hand (finger(s)) (thumb) of same hand 817.0
      open 817.1
    base 815.02
      first metacarpal 815.01
        open 815.11
      open 815.12
      thumb 815.01
        open 815.11
    multiple sites 815.09
      open 815.19
    neck 815.04
      open 815.14
    open 815.10
    shaft 815.03
      open 815.13
  metatarsus, metatarsal (bone(s)), of one foot (closed) 825.25
    with tarsal bone(s) 825.29
      open 825.39
    open 825.35
  Monteggia's (closed) 813.03
    open 813.13
  Moore's — *see* Fracture, radius, lower end
  multangular bone (closed)
    larger 814.05
      open 814.15
    smaller 814.06
      open 814.16

Fracture — *continued*
  multiple (closed) 829.0

Note — Multiple fractures of sites classifiable to the same three- or four-digit category are coded to that category, except for sites classifiable to 810–818 or 820–827 in different limbs.

Multiple fractures of sites classifiable to different fourth-digit subdivisions within the same three–digit category should be dealt with according to coding rules.

Multiple fractures of sites classifiable to different three–digit categories (identifiable from the listing under "Fracture"), and of sites classifiable to 810–818 or 820–827 in different limbs should be coded according to the following list, which should be referred to in the following priority order: skull or face bones, pelvis or vertebral column, legs, arms.

  arm (multiple bones in same arm except in hand alone) (sites classifiable to 810–817 with sites classifiable to a different three–digit category in 810–817 in same arm) (closed) 818.0
    open 818.1
  arms, both or arm(s) with rib(s) or sternum (sites classifiable to 810–818 with sites classifiable to same range of categories in other limb or to 807) (closed) 819.0
    open 819.1
  bones of trunk NEC (closed) 809.0
    open 809.1
  hand, metacarpal bone(s) with phalanx or phalanges of same hand (sites classifiable to 815 with sites classifiable to 816 in same hand) (closed) 817.0
    open 817.1
  leg (multiple bones in same leg) (sites classifiable to 820–826 with sites classifiable to a different three–digit category in that range in same leg) (closed) 827.0
    open 827.1
  legs, both or leg(s) with arm(s), rib(s), or sternum (sites classifiable to 820–827 with sites classifiable to same range of categories in other leg or to 807 or 810–819) (closed) 828.0
    open 828.1
  open 829.1
  pelvis with other bones except skull or face bones (sites classifiable to 808 with sites classifiable to 805–807 or 810–829) (closed) 809.0
    open 809.1

Fracture — *continued*
  multiple — *continued*
    skull, specified or unspecified bones, or face bone(s) with any other bone(s) (sites classifiable to 800–803 with sites classifiable to 805–829) (closed) 804.0 ☑

Note — Use the following fifth-digit subclassification with categories 800, 801, 803, and 804:

0   *unspecified state of consciousness*

1   *with no loss of consciousness*

2   *with brief [less than one hour] loss of consciousness*

3   *with moderate [1–24 hours] loss of consciousness*

4   *with prolonged [more than 24 hours] loss of consciousness and return to pre–existing conscious level*

5   *with prolonged [more than 24 hours] loss of consciousness, without return to pre–existing conscious level*

Use fifth-digit 5 to designate when a patient is unconscious and dies before regaining consciousness, regardless of the duration of the loss of consciousness

6   *with loss of consciousness of unspecified duration*

9   *with concussion, unspecified*

    with
      contusion, cerebral 804.1 ☑
      epidural hemorrhage 804.2 ☑
      extradural hemorrhage 804.2 ☑
      hemorrhage (intracranial) NEC 804.3 ☑
      intracranial injury NEC 804.4 ☑
      laceration, cerebral 804.1 ☑
      subarachnoid hemorrhage 804.2 ☑
      subdural hemorrhage 804.2 ☑
      open 804.5 ☑
        with
          contusion, cerebral 804.6 ☑
          epidural hemorrhage 804.7 ☑
          extradural hemorrhage 804.7 ☑
          hemorrhage (intracranial) NEC 804.8 ☑
          intracranial injury NEC 804.9 ☑
          laceration, cerebral 804.6 ☑
          subarachnoid hemorrhage 804.7 ☑
          subdural hemorrhage 804.7 ☑
      vertebral column with other bones, except skull or face bones (sites classifiable to 805 or 806 with sites classifiable to 807–808 or 810–829) (closed) 809.0
        open 809.1
  nasal (bone(s)) (closed) 802.0
    open 802.1
    sinus — *see* Fracture, skull, base
  navicular
    carpal (wrist) (closed) 814.01
      open 814.11
    tarsal (ankle) (closed) 825.22
      open 825.32
  neck — *see* Fracture, vertebra, cervical
  neural arch — *see* Fracture, vertebra, by site
  nonunion 733.82
  nose, nasal, (bone) (septum) (closed) 802.0
    open 802.1
  occiput — *see* Fracture, skull, base
  odontoid process — *see* Fracture, vertebra, cervical
  olecranon (process) (ulna) (closed) 813.01

☑ **Additional Digit Required** — Refer to the Tabular List for Digit Selection

⬚ **Subterms under main terms may continue to next column or page**

Fracture — *continued*
  olecranon — *continued*
    open 813.11
   open 829.1
  orbit, orbital (bone) (region) (closed) 802.8
    floor (blow-out) 802.6
      open 802.7
    open 802.9
    roof — *see* Fracture, skull, base
    specified part NEC 802.8
      open 802.9
  os
    calcis (closed) 825.0
      open 825.1
    magnum (closed) 814.07
      open 814.17
    pubis (with visceral injury) (closed) 808.2
      open 808.3
    triquetrum (closed) 814.03
      open 814.13
  osseous
    auditory meatus — *see* Fracture, skull, base
    labyrinth — *see* Fracture, skull, base
  ossicles, auditory (incus) (malleus) (stapes) — *see* Fracture, skull, base
  osteoporotic — *see* Fracture, pathologic
  palate (closed) 802.8
    open 802.9
  paratrooper — *see* Fracture, tibia, lower end
  parietal bone — *see* Fracture, skull, vault
  parry — *see* Fracture, Monteggia's
  patella (closed) 822.0
    open 822.1
  pathologic (cause unknown) 733.10
    ankle 733.16
    femur (neck) 733.14
      specified NEC 733.15
    fibula 733.16
    hip 733.14
    humerus 733.11
    radius (distal) 733.12
    specified site NEC 733.19
    tibia 733.16
    ulna 733.12
    vertebrae (collapse) 733.13
    wrist 733.12
  pedicle (of vertebral arch) — *see* Fracture, vertebra, by site
  pelvis, pelvic (bone(s)) (with visceral injury) (closed) 808.8
    multiple
      with
        disruption of pelvic circle 808.43
          open 808.53
        disruption of pelvic ring 808.43
          open 808.53
      without
        disruption of pelvic circle 808.44
          open 808.54
        disruption of pelvic ring 808.44
          open 808.54
    open 808.9
    rim (closed) 808.49
      open 808.59
    stress 733.98
  peritrochanteric (closed) 820.20
    open 820.30
  phalanx, phalanges, of one
    foot (closed) 826.0
      with bone(s) of same lower limb 827.0
        open 827.1
      open 826.1
    hand (closed) 816.00
      with metacarpal bone(s) of same hand 817.0
        open 817.1
      distal 816.02
        open 816.12
      middle 816.01
        open 816.11
      multiple sites NEC 816.03
        open 816.13
      open 816.10
      proximal 816.01

Fracture — *continued*
  phalanx, phalanges, of one — *continued*
    hand — *continued*
      proximal — *continued*
        open 816.11
  pisiform (closed) 814.04
    open 814.14
  pond — *see* Fracture, skull, vault
  Pott's (closed) 824.4
    open 824.5
  prosthetic device, internal — *see* Complications, mechanical
  pubis (with visceral injury) (closed) 808.2
    open 808.3
  Quervain's (closed) 814.01
    open 814.11
  radius (alone) (closed) 813.81
    with ulna NEC 813.83
      open 813.93
    distal end — *see* Fracture, radius, lower end
    epiphysis
      lower — *see* Fracture, radius, lower end
      upper — *see* Fracture, radius, upper end
    head — *see* Fracture, radius, upper end
    lower end or extremity (distal end) (lower epiphysis) 813.42
      with ulna (lower end) 813.44
        open 813.54
      open 813.52
      torus 813.45
        with ulna 813.47
    neck — *see* Fracture, radius, upper end
    open NEC 813.91
    pathologic 733.12
    proximal end — *see* Fracture, radius, upper end
    shaft (closed) 813.21
      with ulna (shaft) 813.23
        open 813.33
      open 813.31
    upper end 813.07
      with ulna (upper end) 813.08
        open 813.18
      epiphysis 813.05
        open 813.15
      head 813.05
        open 813.15
      multiple sites 813.07
        open 813.17
      neck 813.06
        open 813.16
      open 813.17
      specified site NEC 813.07
        open 813.17
  ramus
    inferior or superior (with visceral injury) (closed) 808.2
      open 808.3
    ischium — *see* Fracture, ischium
    mandible 802.24
      open 802.34
  rib(s) (closed) 807.0 ☑

> *Note* — Use the following fifth-digit subclassification with categories 807.0–807.1:
>
> 0   rib(s), unspecified
>
> 1   one rib
>
> 2   two ribs
>
> 3   three ribs
>
> 4   four ribs
>
> 5   five ribs
>
> 6   six ribs
>
> 7   seven ribs
>
> 8   eight or more ribs
>
> 9   multiple ribs, unspecified

    with flail chest (open) 807.4
    open 807.1 ☑
  root, tooth 873.63

Fracture — *continued*
  root, tooth — *continued*
    complicated 873.73
  sacrum — *see* Fracture, vertebra, sacrum
  scaphoid
    ankle (closed) 825.22
      open 825.32
    wrist (closed) 814.01
      open 814.11
  scapula (closed) 811.00
    acromial, acromion (process) 811.01
      open 811.11
    body 811.09
      open 811.19
    coracoid process 811.02
      open 811.12
    glenoid (cavity) (fossa) 811.03
      open 811.13
    neck 811.03
      open 811.13
    open 811.10
  semilunar
    bone, wrist (closed) 814.02
      open 814.12
    cartilage (interior) (knee) — *see* Tear, meniscus
  sesamoid bone — *see* Fracture, by site
  Shepherd's (closed) 825.21
    open 825.31
  shoulder (*see also* Fracture, humerus, upper end)
    blade — *see* Fracture, scapula
  silverfork — *see* Fracture, radius, lower end
  sinus (ethmoid) (frontal) (maxillary) (nasal) (sphenoidal) — *see* Fracture, skull, base
  Skillern's — *see* Fracture, radius, shaft
  skull (multiple NEC) (with face bones) (closed) 803.0 ☑

> *Note* — Use the following fifth-digit subclassification with categories 800, 801, 803, and 804:
>
> 0   unspecified state of consciousness
>
> 1   with no loss of consciousness
>
> 2   with brief [less than one hour] loss of consciousness
>
> 3   with moderate [1-24 hours] loss of consciousness
>
> 4   with prolonged [more than 24 hours] loss of consciousness and return to pre-existing conscious level
>
> 5   with prolonged [more than 24 hours] loss of consciousness, without return to pre-existing conscious level
>
> Use fifth-digit 5 to designate when a patient is unconscious and dies before regaining consciousness, regardless of the duration of the loss of consciousness
>
> 6   with loss of consciousness of unspecified duration
>
> 9   with concussion, unspecified

    with
      contusion, cerebral 803.1 ☑
      epidural hemorrhage 803.2 ☑
      extradural hemorrhage 803.2 ☑
      hemorrhage (intracranial) NEC 803.3 ☑
      intracranial injury NEC 803.4 ☑
      laceration, cerebral 803.1 ☑
      other bones — *see* Fracture, multiple, skull
      subarachnoid hemorrhage 803.2 ☑
      subdural hemorrhage 803.2 ☑
    base (antrum) (ethmoid bone) (fossa) (internal ear) (nasal sinus) (occiput) (sphenoid) (temporal bone) (closed) 801.0 ☑

Fracture — *continued*
  skull — *continued*
    base — *continued*
      with
        contusion, cerebral 801.1 ☑
        epidural hemorrhage 801.2 ☑
        extradural hemorrhage 801.2 ☑
        hemorrhage (intracranial) NEC 801.3 ☑
        intracranial injury NEC 801.4 ☑
        laceration, cerebral 801.1 ☑
        subarachnoid hemorrhage 801.2 ☑
        subdural hemorrhage 801.2 ☑
      open 801.5 ☑
        with
          contusion, cerebral 801.6 ☑
          epidural hemorrhage 801.7 ☑
          extradural hemorrhage 801.7 ☑
          hemorrhage (intracranial) NEC 801.8 ☑
          intracranial injury NEC 801.9 ☑
          laceration, cerebral 801.6 ☑
          subarachnoid hemorrhage 801.7 ☑
          subdural hemorrhage 801.7 ☑
    birth injury 767.3
    face bones — *see* Fracture, face bones
    open 803.5 ☑
      with
        contusion, cerebral 803.6 ☑
        epidural hemorrhage 803.7 ☑
        extradural hemorrhage 803.7 ☑
        hemorrhage (intracranial) NEC 803.8 ☑
        intracranial injury NEC 803.9 ☑
        laceration, cerebral 803.6 ☑
        subarachnoid hemorrhage 803.7 ☑
        subdural hemorrhage 803.7 ☑
    vault (frontal bone) (parietal bone) (vertex) (closed) 800.0 ☑
      with
        contusion, cerebral 800.1 ☑
        epidural hemorrhage 800.2 ☑
        extradural hemorrhage 800.2 ☑
        hemorrhage (intracranial) NEC 800.3 ☑
        intracranial injury NEC 800.4 ☑
        laceration, cerebral 800.1 ☑
        subarachnoid hemorrhage 800.2 ☑
        subdural hemorrhage 800.2 ☑
      open 800.5 ☑
        with
          contusion, cerebral 800.6 ☑
          epidural hemorrhage 800.7 ☑
          extradural hemorrhage 800.7 ☑
          hemorrhage (intracranial) NEC 800.8 ☑
          intracranial injury NEC 800.9 ☑
          laceration, cerebral 800.6 ☑

☑ Additional Digit Required — Refer to the Tabular List for Digit Selection   ᐁ Subterms under main terms may continue to next column or page

2013 ICD-9-CM   ▶◀ Revised Text   ● New Line   ▲ Revised Code   Volume 2 — 123

☑ Additional Digit Required — Refer to the Tabular List for Digit Selection   ᵂ Subterms under main terms may continue to next column or page

124 — Volume 2   ▶◀ Revised Text   ● New Line   ▲ Revised Code   2013 ICD-9-CM

Fracture — Fragilitas

Fragilitas — *continued*
  ossium — *continued*
    with blue sclera 756.51
    unguium 703.8
      congenital 757.5
Fragility
  bone 756.51
    with deafness and blue sclera 756.51
  capillary (hereditary) 287.8
  hair 704.2
  nails 703.8
Fragmentation — *see* Fracture, by site
Frailty 797
Frambesia, frambesial (tropica) — *see also*
    Yaws 102.9
  initial lesion or ulcer 102.0
  primary 102.0
Frambeside
  gummatous 102.4
  of early yaws 102.2
Frambesioma 102.1
Franceschetti's syndrome (mandibulofacial
    dysostosis) 756.0
Francis' disease — *see also* Tularemia 021.9
Franklin's disease (heavy chain) 273.2
Frank's essential thrombocytopenia — *see*
    also Purpura, thrombocytopenic 287.39
Fraser's syndrome 759.89
Freckle 709.09
  malignant melanoma in (M8742/3) — *see*
    Melanoma
  melanotic (of Hutchinson) (M8742/2) — *see*
    Neoplasm, skin, in situ
  retinal 239.81
Freeman-Sheldon syndrome 759.89
Freezing 991.9
  specified effect NEC 991.8
Freiberg's
  disease (osteochondrosis, second
    metatarsal) 732.5
  infraction of metatarsal head 732.5
  osteochondrosis 732.5
Frei's disease (climatic bubo) 099.1
Fremitus, friction, cardiac 785.3
Frenulum linguae 750.0
Frenum
  external os 752.44
  tongue 750.0
Frequency (urinary) NEC 788.41
  micturition 788.41
  nocturnal 788.43
  polyuria 788.42
  psychogenic 306.53
Frey's syndrome (auriculotemporal syndrome)
    705.22
Friction
  burn (*see also* Injury, superficial, by site)
    919.0
  fremitus, cardiac 785.3
  precordial 785.3
  sounds, chest 786.7
Friderichsen-Waterhouse syndrome or disease 036.3
Friedländer's
  B (bacillus) NEC (*see also* condition) 041.3
  sepsis or septicemia 038.49
  disease (endarteritis obliterans) — *see* Arteriosclerosis
Friedreich's
  ataxia 334.0
  combined systemic disease 334.0
  disease 333.2
    combined systemic 334.0
  myoclonia 333.2

Friedreich's — *continued*
  sclerosis (spinal cord) 334.0
Friedrich-Erb-Arnold syndrome (acropachyderma) 757.39
Frigidity 302.72
  psychic or psychogenic 302.72
Fröhlich's disease or syndrome (adiposogenital dystrophy) 253.8
Froin's syndrome 336.8
Frommel-Chiari syndrome 676.6 ☑
Frommel's disease 676.6 ☑
Frontal — *see also* condition
  lobe syndrome 310.0
Frostbite 991.3
  face 991.0
  foot 991.2
  hand 991.1
  specified site NEC 991.3
Frotteurism 302.89
Frozen 991.9
  pelvis 620.8
  shoulder 726.0
Fructosemia 271.2
Fructosuria (benign) (essential) 271.2
Fuchs'
  black spot (myopic) 360.21
  corneal dystrophy (endothelial) 371.57
  heterochromic cyclitis 364.21
Fucosidosis 271.8
Fugue 780.99
  dissociative 300.13
  hysterical (dissociative) 300.13
  reaction to exceptional stress (transient)
    308.1
Fukuhara syndrome 277.87
Fuller Albright's syndrome (osteitis fibrosa
    disseminata) 756.59
Fuller's earth disease 502
Fulminant, fulminating — *see* condition
Functional — *see* condition
Functioning
  borderline intellectual V62.89
Fundus — *see also* condition
  flavimaculatus 362.76
Fungemia 117.9
Fungus, fungous
  cerebral 348.89
  disease NEC 117.9
  infection — *see* Infection, fungus
  testis (*see also* Tuberculosis)
    016.5 ☑ [608.81]
Funiculitis (acute) 608.4
  chronic 608.4
  endemic 608.4
  gonococcal (acute) 098.14
    chronic or duration of 2 months or over
      098.34
  tuberculous (*see also* Tuberculosis) 016.5 ☑
Funnel
  breast (acquired) 738.3
    congenital 754.81
    late effect of rickets 268.1
  chest (acquired) 738.3
    congenital 754.81
    late effect of rickets 268.1
  pelvis (acquired) 738.6
    with disproportion (fetopelvic) 653.3 ☑
      affecting fetus or newborn 763.1
      causing obstructed labor 660.1 ☑
        affecting fetus or newborn 763.1
    congenital 755.69
    tuberculous (*see also* Tuberculosis)
      016.9 ☑

FUO — *see also* Pyrexia 780.60
Furfur 690.18
  microsporon 111.0
Furor, paroxysmal (idiopathic) — *see also*
    Epilepsy 345.8 ☑
Furriers' lung 495.8
Furrowed tongue 529.5
  congenital 750.13
Furrowing nail(s) (transverse) 703.8
  congenital 757.5
Furuncle 680.9
  abdominal wall 680.2
  ankle 680.6
  anus 680.5
  arm (any part, above wrist) 680.3
  auditory canal, external 680.0
  axilla 680.3
  back (any part) 680.2
  breast 680.2
  buttock 680.5
  chest wall 680.2
  corpus cavernosum 607.2
  ear (any part) 680.0
  eyelid 373.13
  face (any part, except eye) 680.0
  finger (any) 680.4
  flank 680.2
  foot (any part) 680.7
  forearm 680.3
  gluteal (region) 680.5
  groin 680.2
  hand (any part) 680.4
  head (any part, except face) 680.8
  heel 680.7
  hip 680.6
  kidney (*see also* Abscess, kidney) 590.2
  knee 680.6
  labium (majus) (minus) 616.4
  lacrimal
    gland (*see also* Dacryoadenitis) 375.00
    passages (duct) (sac) (*see also* Dacryocystitis) 375.30
  leg, any part except foot 680.6
  malignant 022.0
  multiple sites 680.9
  neck 680.1
  nose (external) (septum) 680.0
  orbit 376.01
  partes posteriores 680.5
  pectoral region 680.2
  penis 607.2
  perineum 680.2
  pinna 680.0
  scalp (any part) 680.8
  scrotum 608.4
  seminal vesicle 608.0
  shoulder 680.3
  skin NEC 680.9
  specified site NEC 680.8
  spermatic cord 608.4
  temple (region) 680.0
  testis 604.90
  thigh 680.6
  thumb 680.4
  toe (any) 680.7
  trunk 680.2
  tunica vaginalis 608.4
  umbilicus 680.2
  upper arm 680.3
  vas deferens 608.4
  vulva 616.4
  wrist 680.4
Furunculosis — *see also* Furuncle 680.9
  external auditory meatus 680.0 *[380.13]*

Fusarium (infection) 118
Fusion, fused (congenital)
  anal (with urogenital canal) 751.5
  aorta and pulmonary artery 745.0
  astragaloscaphoid 755.67
  atria 745.5
  atrium and ventricle 745.69
  auditory canal 744.02
  auricles, heart 745.5
  binocular, with defective stereopsis 368.33
  bone 756.9
  cervical spine — *see* Fusion, spine
  choanal 748.0
  commissure, mitral valve 746.5
  cranial sutures, premature 756.0
  cusps, heart valve NEC 746.89
    mitral 746.5
    tricuspid 746.89
  ear ossicles 744.04
  fingers (*see also* Syndactylism, fingers)
    755.11
  hymen 752.42
  hymeno-urethral 599.89
    causing obstructed labor 660.1 ☑
      affecting fetus or newborn 763.1
  joint (acquired) (*see also* Ankylosis)
    congenital 755.8
  kidneys (incomplete) 753.3
  labium (majus) (minus) 752.49
  larynx and trachea 748.3
  limb 755.8
    lower 755.69
    upper 755.59
  lobe, lung 748.5
  lumbosacral (acquired) 724.6
    congenital 756.15
    surgical V45.4
  nares (anterior) (posterior) 748.0
  nose, nasal 748.0
  nostril(s) 748.0
  organ or site NEC — *see* Anomaly, specified
    type NEC
  ossicles 756.9
    auditory 744.04
  pulmonary valve segment 746.02
  pulmonic cusps 746.02
  ribs 756.3
  sacroiliac (acquired) (joint) 724.6
    congenital 755.69
    surgical V45.4
  skull, imperfect 756.0
  spine (acquired) 724.9
    arthrodesis status V45.4
    congenital (vertebra) 756.15
    postoperative status V45.4
  sublingual duct with submaxillary duct at
    opening in mouth 750.26
  talonavicular (bar) 755.67
  teeth, tooth 520.2
  testes 752.89
  toes (*see also* Syndactylism, toes) 755.13
  trachea and esophagus 750.3
  twins 759.4
  urethral-hymenal 599.89
  vagina 752.49
  valve cusps — *see* Fusion, cusps, heart valve
  ventricles, heart 745.4
  vertebra (arch) — *see* Fusion, spine
  vulva 752.49
Fusospirillosis (mouth) (tongue) (tonsil) 101
Fussy infant (baby) 780.91

☑ Additional Digit Required — Refer to the Tabular List for Digit Selection   🔻 Subterms under main terms may continue to next column or page

2013 ICD-9-CM   ▶◀ Revised Text   ● New Line   ▲ Revised Code   Volume 2 — 125

G

Gafsa boil 085.1
Gain, weight (abnormal) (excessive) — *see also*
Weight, gain 783.1
Gaisböck's disease or syndrome (polycythemia hypertonica) 289.0
Gait
abnormality 781.2
hysterical 300.11
ataxic 781.2
hysterical 300.11
disturbance 781.2
hysterical 300.11
paralytic 781.2
scissor 781.2
spastic 781.2
staggering 781.2
hysterical 300.11
Galactocele (breast) (infected) 611.5
puerperal, postpartum 676.8 ☑
Galactophoritis 611.0
puerperal, postpartum 675.2 ☑
Galactorrhea 676.6 ☑
not associated with childbirth 611.6
Galactosemia (classic) (congenital) 271.1
Galactosuria 271.1
Galacturia 791.1
bilharziasis 120.0
Galen's vein — *see* condition
Gallbladder — *see also* condition
acute (*see also* Disease, gallbladder) 575.0
Gall duct — *see* condition
Gallop rhythm 427.89
Gallstone (cholemic) (colic) (impacted) — *see also* Cholelithiasis
causing intestinal obstruction 560.31
Gambling, pathological 312.31
Gammaloidosis 277.39
Gammopathy 273.9
macroglobulinemia 273.3
monoclonal (benign) (essential) (idiopathic) (with lymphoplasmacytic dyscrasia) 273.1
Gamna's disease (siderotic splenomegaly) 289.51
Gampsodactylia (congenital) 754.71
Gamstorp's disease (adynamia episodica hereditaria) 359.3
Gandy-Nanta disease (siderotic splenomegaly) 289.51
Gang activity, without manifest psychiatric disorder V71.09
adolescent V71.02
adult V71.01
child V71.02
Gangliocytoma (M9490/0) — *see* Neoplasm, connective tissue, benign
Ganglioglioma (M9505/1) — *see* Neoplasm, by site, uncertain behavior
Ganglion 727.43
joint 727.41
of yaws (early) (late) 102.6
periosteal (*see also* Periostitis) 730.3 ☑
tendon sheath (compound) (diffuse) 727.42
tuberculous (*see also* Tuberculosis) 015.9 ☑
Ganglioneuroblastoma (M9490/3) — *see* Neoplasm, connective tissue, malignant
Ganglioneuroma (M9490/0) — *see also* Neoplasm, connective tissue, benign
malignant (M9490/3) — *see* Neoplasm, connective tissue, malignant
Ganglioneuromatosis (M9491/0) — *see* Neoplasm, connective tissue, benign
Ganglionitis
fifth nerve (*see also* Neuralgia, trigeminal) 350.1
gasserian 350.1
geniculate 351.1
herpetic 053.11
newborn 767.5
herpes zoster 053.11
herpetic geniculate (Hunt's syndrome) 053.11
Gangliosidosis 330.1
Gangosa 102.5

Gangrene, gangrenous (anemia) (artery) (cellulitis) (dermatitis) (dry) (infective) (moist) (pemphigus) (septic) (skin) (stasis) (ulcer) 785.4
with
arteriosclerosis (native artery) 440.24
bypass graft 440.30
autologous vein 440.31
nonautologous biological 440.32
diabetes (mellitus) 250.7 ☑ *[785.4]*
due to secondary diabetes 249.7 ☑ *[785.4]*
abdomen (wall) 785.4
adenitis 683
alveolar 526.5
angina 462
diphtheritic 032.0
anus 569.49
appendices epiploicae — *see* Gangrene, mesentery
appendix — *see* Appendicitis, acute
arteriosclerotic — *see* Arteriosclerosis, with, gangrene
auricle 785.4
Bacillus welchii (*see also* Gangrene, gas) 040.0
bile duct (*see also* Cholangitis) 576.8
bladder 595.89
bowel — *see* Gangrene, intestine
cecum — *see* Gangrene, intestine
Clostridium perfringens or welchii (*see also* Gangrene, gas) 040.0
colon — *see* Gangrene, intestine
connective tissue 785.4
cornea 371.40
corpora cavernosa (infective) 607.2
noninfective 607.89
cutaneous, spreading 785.4
decubital (*see also* Ulcer, pressure) 707.00 *[785.4]*
diabetic (any site) 250.7 ☑ *[785.4]*
due to secondary diabetes 249.7 ☑ *[785.4]*
dropsical 785.4
emphysematous (*see also* Gangrene, gas) 040.0
epidemic (ergotized grain) 988.2
epididymis (infectional) (*see also* Epididymitis) 604.99
erysipelas (*see also* Erysipelas) 035
extremity (lower) (upper) 785.4
gallbladder or duct (*see also* Cholecystitis, acute) 575.0
gas (bacillus) 040.0
with
abortion — *see* Abortion, by type, with sepsis
ectopic pregnancy (*see also* categories 633.0–633.9) 639.0
molar pregnancy (*see also* categories 630–632) 639.0
following
abortion 639.0
ectopic or molar pregnancy 639.0
puerperal, postpartum, childbirth 670.8 ☑
glossitis 529.0
gum 523.8
hernia — *see* Hernia, by site, with gangrene
hospital noma 528.1
intestine, intestinal (acute) (hemorrhagic) (massive) 557.0
with
hernia — *see* Hernia, by site, with gangrene
mesenteric embolism or infarction 557.0
obstruction (*see also* Obstruction, intestine) 560.9
laryngitis 464.00
with obstruction 464.01
liver 573.8
lung 513.0
spirochetal 104.8
lymphangitis 457.2
Meleney's (cutaneous) 686.09

Gangrene, gangrenous — *continued*
mesentery 557.0
with
embolism or infarction 557.0
intestinal obstruction (*see also* Obstruction, intestine) 560.9
mouth 528.1
noma 528.1
orchitis 604.90
ovary (*see also* Salpingo-oophoritis) 614.2
pancreas 577.0
penis (infectional) 607.2
noninfective 607.89
perineum 785.4
pharynx 462
pneumonia 513.0
Pott's 440.24
presenile 443.1
pulmonary 513.0
pulp, tooth 522.1
quinsy 475
Raynaud's (symmetric gangrene) 443.0 *[785.4]*
rectum 569.49
retropharyngeal 478.24
rupture — *see* Hernia, by site, with gangrene
scrotum 608.4
noninfective 608.83
senile 440.24
septic 034.0
septic 034.0
sore throat 462
spermatic cord 608.4
noninfective 608.89
spine 785.4
spirochetal NEC 104.8
spreading cutaneous 785.4
stomach 537.89
stomatitis 528.1
symmetrical 443.0 *[785.4]*
testis (infectional) (*see also* Orchitis) 604.99
noninfective 608.89
throat 462
diphtheritic 032.0
thyroid (gland) 246.8
tonsillitis (acute) 463
tooth (pulp) 522.1
tuberculous NEC (*see also* Tuberculosis) 011.9 ☑
tunica vaginalis 608.4
noninfective 608.89
umbilicus 785.4
uterus (*see also* Endometritis) 615.9
uvulitis 528.3
vas deferens 608.4
noninfective 608.89
vulva (*see also* Vulvitis) 616.10
Gannister disease (occupational) 502
with tuberculosis — *see* Tuberculosis, pulmonary
Ganser's syndrome, hysterical 300.16
Gardner-Diamond syndrome (autoerythrocyte sensitization) 287.2
Gargoylism 277.5
Garré's
disease (*see also* Osteomyelitis) 730.1 ☑
osteitis (sclerosing) (*see also* Osteomyelitis) 730.1 ☑
osteomyelitis (*see also* Osteomyelitis) 730.1 ☑
Garrod's pads, knuckle 728.79
Gartner's duct
cyst 752.41
persistent 752.41
Gas 787.3
asphyxia, asphyxiation, inhalation, poisoning, suffocation NEC 987.9
specified gas — *see* Table of Drugs and Chemicals
bacillus gangrene or infection — *see* Gas, gangrene
cyst, mesentery 568.89
excessive 787.3
gangrene 040.0

Gas — *continued*
gangrene — *continued*
with
abortion — *see* Abortion, by type, with sepsis
ectopic pregnancy (*see also* categories 633.0–633.9) 639.0
molar pregnancy (*see also* categories 630–632) 639.0
following
abortion 639.0
ectopic or molar pregnancy 639.0
puerperal, postpartum, childbirth 670.8 ☑
on stomach 787.3
pains 787.3
Gastradenitis 535.0 ☑
Gastralgia 536.8
psychogenic 307.89
Gastrectasis, gastrectasia 536.1
psychogenic 306.4
Gastric — *see* condition
Gastrinoma (M8153/1)
malignant (M8153/3)
pancreas 157.4
specified site NEC — *see* Neoplasm, by site, malignant
unspecified site 157.4
specified site — *see* Neoplasm, by site, uncertain behavior
unspecified site 235.5
Gastritis 535.5 ☑

Note — Use the following fifth-digit subclassification for category 535:
0   without mention of hemorrhage
1   with hemorrhage

acute 535.0 ☑
alcoholic 535.3 ☑
allergic 535.4 ☑
antral 535.4 ☑
atrophic 535.1 ☑
atrophic-hyperplastic 535.1 ☑
bile-induced 535.4 ☑
catarrhal 535.0 ☑
chronic (atrophic) 535.1 ☑
cirrhotic 535.4 ☑
corrosive (acute) 535.4 ☑
dietetic 535.4 ☑
due to diet deficiency 269.9 *[535.4]* ☑
eosinophilic 535.7 ☑
erosive 535.4 ☑
follicular 535.4 ☑
chronic 535.1 ☑
giant hypertrophic 535.2 ☑
glandular 535.4 ☑
chronic 535.1 ☑
hypertrophic (mucosa) 535.2 ☑
chronic giant 211.1
irritant 535.4 ☑
nervous 306.4
phlegmonous 535.0 ☑
psychogenic 306.4
sclerotic 535.4 ☑
spastic 536.8
subacute 535.0 ☑
superficial 535.4 ☑
suppurative 535.0 ☑
toxic 535.4 ☑
tuberculous (*see also* Tuberculosis) 017.9 ☑
Gastrocarcinoma (M8010/3) 151.9
Gastrocolic — *see* condition
Gastrocolitis — *see* Enteritis
Gastrodisciasis 121.8
Gastroduodenitis — *see also* Gastritis 535.5 ☑
catarrhal 535.0 ☑
infectional 535.0 ☑
virus, viral 008.8
specified type NEC 008.69
Gastrodynia 536.8
Gastroenteritis (acute) (catarrhal) (congestive) (hemorrhagic) (noninfectious) — *see also* Enteritis 558.9
aertrycke infection 003.0

Gastroenteritis — *see also* Enteritis — *continued*
  allergic 558.3
  chronic 558.9
    ulcerative (*see also* Colitis, ulcerative) 556.9
  dietetic 558.9
  due to
    antineoplastic chemotherapy 558.9
    food poisoning (*see also* Poisoning, food) 005.9
    radiation 558.1
  eosinophilic 558.41
  epidemic 009.0
  functional 558.9
  infectious (*see also* Enteritis, due to, by organism) 009.0
    presumed 009.1
  salmonella 003.0
  septic (*see also* Enteritis, due to, by organism) 009.0
  toxic 558.2
  tuberculous (*see also* Tuberculosis) 014.8 ☑
  ulcerative (*see also* Colitis, ulcerative) 556.9
  viral NEC 008.8
    specified type NEC 008.69
  zymotic 009.0
Gastroenterocolitis — *see* Enteritis
Gastroenteropathy, protein-losing 579.8
Gastroenteroptosis 569.89
Gastroesophageal laceration-hemorrhage syndrome 530.7
Gastroesophagitis 530.19
Gastrohepatitis — *see also* Gastritis 535.5 ☑
Gastrointestinal — *see* condition
Gastrojejunal — *see* condition
Gastrojejunitis — *see also* Gastritis 535.5 ☑
Gastrojejunocolic — *see* condition
Gastroliths 537.89
Gastromalacia 537.89
Gastroparalysis 536.3
  diabetic 250.6 ☑ *[536.3]*
    due to secondary diabetes 249.6 ☑ *[536.3]*
Gastroparesis 536.3
  diabetic 250.6 ☑ *[536.3]*
    due to secondary diabetes 249.6 ☑ *[536.3]*
Gastropathy 537.9
  congestive portal 537.89
  erythematous 535.5 ☑
  exudative 579.8
  portal hypertensive 537.89
Gastroptosis 537.5
Gastrorrhagia 578.0
Gastrorrhea 536.8
  psychogenic 306.4
Gastroschisis (congenital) 756.73
  acquired 569.89
Gastrospasm (neurogenic) (reflex) 536.8
  neurotic 306.4
  psychogenic 306.4
Gastrostaxis 578.0
Gastrostenosis 537.89
Gastrostomy
  attention to V55.1
  complication 536.40
    specified type 536.49
  infection 536.41
  malfunctioning 536.42
  status V44.1
Gastrosuccorrhea (continuous) (intermittent) 536.8
  neurotic 306.4
  psychogenic 306.4
Gaucher's
  disease (adult) (cerebroside lipidosis) (infantile) 272.7
  hepatomegaly 272.7
  splenomegaly (cerebroside lipidosis) 272.7
GAVE (gastric antral vascular ectasia) 537.82
  with hemorrhage 537.83
  without hemorrhage 537.82
Gayet's disease (superior hemorrhagic polioencephalitis) 265.1

Gayet-Wernicke's syndrome (superior hemorrhagic polioencephalitis) 265.1
Gee (-Herter) (-Heubner) (-Thaysen) disease or syndrome (nontropical sprue) 579.0
Gélineau's syndrome — *see also* Narcolepsy 347.00
Gemination, teeth 520.2
Gemistocytoma (M9411/3)
  specified site — *see* Neoplasm, by site, malignant
  unspecified site 191.9
General, generalized — *see* condtion
Genetic
  susceptibility to
    MEN (multiple endocrine neoplasia) V84.81
    neoplasia
      multiple endocrine (MEN) V84.81
    neoplasm
      malignant, of
        breast V84.01
        endometrium V84.04
        other V84.09
        ovary V84.02
        prostate V84.03
    specified disease NEC V84.89
Genital — *see* condition
  warts 078.11
Genito-anorectal syndrome 099.1
Genitourinary system — *see* condition
Genu
  congenital 755.64
  extrorsum (acquired) 736.42
    congenital 755.64
    late effects of rickets 268.1
  introrsum (acquired) 736.41
    congenital 755.64
    late effects of rickets 268.1
  rachitic (old) 268.1
  recurvatum (acquired) 736.5
    congenital 754.40
      with dislocation of knee 754.41
    late effects of rickets 268.1
  valgum (acquired) (knock-knee) 736.41
    congenital 755.64
    late effects of rickets 268.1
  varum (acquired) (bowleg) 736.42
    congenital 755.64
    late effect of rickets 268.1
Geographic tongue 529.1
Geophagia 307.52
Geotrichosis 117.9
  intestine 117.9
  lung 117.9
  mouth 117.9
Gephyrophobia 300.29
Gerbode defect 745.4
GERD (gastroesophageal reflux disease) 530.81
Gerhardt's
  disease (erythromelalgia) 443.82
  syndrome (vocal cord paralysis) 478.30
Gerlier's disease (epidemic vertigo) 078.81
German measles 056.9
  exposure to V01.4
Germinoblastoma (diffuse) (M9614/3) 202.8 ☑
  follicular (M9692/3) 202.0 ☑
Germinoma (M9064/3) — *see* Neoplasm, by site, malignant
Gerontoxon 371.41
Gerstmann-Sträussler-Scheinker syndrome (GSS) 046.71
Gerstmann's syndrome (finger agnosia) 784.69
Gestation (period) — *see also* Pregnancy
  ectopic NEC (*see also* Pregnancy, ectopic) 633.90
    with intrauterine pregnancy 633.91
  multiple
    placenta status
      quadruplet
        two or more monoamniotic fetuses V91.22
        two or more monochorionic fetuses V91.21

Gestation — *see also* Pregnancy — *continued*
  multiple — *continued*
    placenta status — *continued*
      quadruplet — *continued*
        unable to determine number of placenta and number of amniotic sacs V91.29
        unspecified number of placenta and unspecified number of amniotic sacs V91.20
      specified (greater than quadruplets) NEC
        two or more monoamniotic fetuses V91.92
        two or more monochorionic fetuses V91.91
        unable to determine number of placenta and number of amniotic sacs V91.99
        unspecified number of placenta and unspecified number of amniotic sacs V91.90
      triplet
        two or more monoamniotic fetuses V91.12
        two or more monochorionic fetuses V91.11
        unable to determine number of placenta and number of amniotic sacs V91.19
        unspecified number of placenta, unspecified number of amniotic sacs V91.10
      twin
        dichorionic/diamniotic (two placentae, two amniotic sacs) V91.03
        monochorionic/diamniotic (one placenta, two amniotic sacs) V91.02
        monochorionic/monoamniotic (one placenta, one amniotic sac) V91.01
        unable to determine number of placenta and number of amniotic sacs V91.09
        unspecified number of placenta, unspecified number of amniotic sacs V91.00
Gestational proteinuria 646.2 ☑
  with hypertension — *see* Toxemia, of pregnancy
Ghon tubercle primary infection — *see also* Tuberculosis 010.0 ☑
Ghost
  teeth 520.4
  vessels, cornea 370.64
Ghoul hand 102.3
Gianotti Crosti syndrome 057.8
  due to known virus — *see* Infection, virus
  due to unknown virus 057.8
Giant
  cell
    epulis 523.8
    peripheral (gingiva) 523.8
    tumor, tendon sheath 727.02
  colon (congenital) 751.3
  esophagus (congenital) 750.4
  kidney 753.3
  urticaria 995.1
    hereditary 277.6
Giardia lamblia infestation 007.1
Giardiasis 007.1
Gibert's disease (pityriasis rosea) 696.3
Gibraltar fever — *see* Brucellosis
Giddiness 780.4
  hysterical 300.11
  psychogenic 306.9
Gierke's disease (glycogenosis I) 271.0
Gigantism (cerebral) (hypophyseal) (pituitary) 253.0
Gilbert's disease or cholemia (familial nonhemolytic jaundice) 277.4
Gilchrist's disease (North American blastomycosis) 116.0

Gilford (-Hutchinson) disease or syndrome (progeria) 259.8
Gilles de la Tourette's disease (motor-verbal tic) 307.23
Gillespie's syndrome (dysplasia oculodentodigitalis) 759.89
Gingivitis 523.10
  acute 523.00
    necrotizing 101
    non-plaque induced 523.01
    plaque induced 523.00
  catarrhal 523.10
  chronic 523.10
    non-plaque induced 523.11
  desquamative 523.10
  expulsiva 523.40
  hyperplastic 523.10
  marginal, simple 523.10
  necrotizing, acute 101
  non-plaque induced 523.11
  pellagrous 265.2
  plaque induced 523.10
  ulcerative 523.10
    acute necrotizing 101
  Vincent's 101
Gingivoglossitis 529.0
Gingivopericementitis 523.40
Gingivosis 523.10
Gingivostomatitis 523.10
  herpetic 054.2
Giovannini's disease 117.9
GISA (glycopeptide intermediate staphylococcus aureus) V09.8 ☑
Glanders 024
Gland, glandular — *see* condition
Glanzmann (-Naegeli) disease or thrombasthenia 287.1
Glassblowers' disease 527.1
Glaucoma (capsular) (inflammatory) (noninflammatory) (primary) 365.9
  with increased episcleral venous pressure 365.82
  absolute 360.42
  acute 365.22
    narrow angle 365.22
    secondary 365.60
  angle closure 365.20
    acute 365.22
    attack 365.22
    chronic 365.23
    crisis 365.22
    intermittent 365.21
    interval 365.21
    primary 365.20
      chronic 365.23
    residual stage 365.24
    subacute 365.21
  angle recession 365.65
  borderline 365.00
  chronic 365.11
    noncongestive 365.11
    open angle 365.11
    simple 365.11
  closed angle — *see* Glaucoma, angle closure
  congenital 743.20
    associated with other eye anomalies 743.22
    simple 743.21
  congestive — *see* Glaucoma, narrow angle
  corticosteroid-induced (glaucomatous stage) 365.31
    residual stage 365.32
  exfoliation 365.52
  hemorrhagic 365.60
  hypersecretion 365.81
  infantile 365.14
    congenital 743.20
      associated with other eye anomalies 743.22
      simple 743.21
  inflammatory 365.62
  in or with
    aniridia 365.42
    Axenfeld's anomaly 365.41
    congenital syndromes NEC 759.89 *[365.44]*

Glaucoma — *continued*
  in or with — *continued*
    disorder of lens NEC 365.59
    inflammation, ocular 365.62
    iris
      anomalies NEC 365.42
      atrophy, essential 365.42
      bombé 365.61
    microcornea 365.43
    neurofibromatosis 237.71 [365.44]
    ocular
      cysts NEC 365.64
      disorders NEC 365.60
      trauma 365.65
      tumors NEC 365.64
    pupillary block or seclusion 365.61
    Rieger's anomaly or syndrome 365.41
    seclusion of pupil 365.61
    Sturge-Weber (-Dimitri) syndrome
      759.6 [365.44]
    systemic syndrome NEC 365.44
    tumor of globe 365.64
    vascular disorders NEC 365.63
  juvenile 365.14
  low tension 365.12
  malignant 365.83
  narrow angle (primary) 365.20
    acute 365.22
    chronic 365.23
    intermittent 365.21
    interval 365.21
    residual stage 365.24
    subacute 365.21
  neovascular 365.63
  newborn 743.20
    associated with other eye anomalies
      743.22
    simple 743.21
  noncongestive (chronic) 365.11
  nonobstructive (chronic) 365.11
  normal tension 365.12
  obstructive 365.60
    due to lens changes 365.59
  open angle 365.10
    with
      abnormal optic disc appearance or
        asymmetry 365.01
      borderline findings
        high risk 365.05
        intraocular pressure 365.01
        low risk 365.01
      cupping of optic discs 365.01
      thin central corneal thickness
        (pachymetry) 365.01
    high risk 365.05
    low risk 365.01
    primary 365.11
    residual stage 365.15
  phacoanaphylactic 365.59
  phacolytic 365.51
  phacomorphic
    acute 365.22
    borderline 365.06
  pigmentary 365.13
  pigment dispersion 365.13
  postinfectious 365.60
  pseudoexfoliation 365.52
  secondary NEC 365.60
    due to
      steroids 365.31
      surgery 365.60
  simple (chronic) 365.11
  simplex 365.11
  stage
    advanced 365.73
    early 365.71
    end-stage 365.73
    indeterminate 365.74
    mild 365.71
    moderate 365.72
    severe 365.73
    unspecified 365.70
  steroid
    induced 365.31
    responders 365.03
  suspect 365.00

Glaucoma — *continued*
  suspect — *continued*
    primary angle closure 365.02
  syphilitic 095.8
  traumatic NEC 365.65
    newborn 767.8
  uveitic 365.62
  wide angle (*see also* Glaucoma, open angle)
    365.10
Glaucomatous flecks (subcapsular) 366.31
Glazed tongue 529.4
Gleet 098.2
Glénard's disease or syndrome (enteroptosis)
  569.89
Glinski-Simmonds syndrome (pituitary
  cachexia) 253.2
Glioblastoma (multiforme) (M9440/3)
  with sarcomatous component (M9442/3)
    specified site — *see* Neoplasm, by site,
      malignant
    unspecified site 191.9
  giant cell (M9441/3)
    specified site — *see* Neoplasm, by site,
      malignant
    unspecified site 191.9
  specified site — *see* Neoplasm, by site, ma-
    lignant
  unspecified site 191.9
Glioma (malignant) (M9380/3)
  astrocytic (M9400/3)
    specified site — *see* Neoplasm, by site,
      malignant
    unspecified site 191.9
  mixed (M9382/3)
    specified site — *see* Neoplasm, by site,
      malignant
    unspecified site 191.9
  nose 748.1
  specified site NEC — *see* Neoplasm, by site,
    malignant
  subependymal (M9383/1) 237.5
  unspecified site 191.9
Gliomatosis cerebri (M9381/3) 191.0
Glioneuroma (M9505/1) — *see* Neoplasm, by
  site, uncertain behavior
Gliosarcoma (M9380/3)
  specified site — *see* Neoplasm, by site, ma-
    lignant
  unspecified site 191.9
Gliosis (cerebral) 349.89
  spinal 336.0
Glisson's
  cirrhosis — *see* Cirrhosis, portal
  disease (*see also* Rickets) 268.0
Glissonitis 573.3
Globinuria 791.2
Globus 306.4
  hystericus 300.11
Glomangioma (M8712/0) — *see also* Heman-
  gioma 228.00
Glomangiosarcoma (M8710/3) — *see* Neoplasm, connective tissue, malignant
Glomerular nephritis — *see also* Nephritis
  583.9
Glomerulitis — *see also* Nephritis 583.9
Glomerulonephritis — *see also* Nephritis 583.9
  with
    edema (*see also* Nephrosis) 581.9
    lesion of
      exudative nephritis 583.89
      interstitial nephritis (diffuse) (focal)
        583.89
      necrotizing glomerulitis 583.4
        acute 580.4
        chronic 582.4
      renal necrosis 583.9
        cortical 583.6
        medullary 583.7
      specified pathology NEC 583.89
        acute 580.89
        chronic 582.89
    necrosis, renal 583.9
      cortical 583.6
      medullary (papillary) 583.7
    specified pathology or lesion NEC 583.89
  acute 580.9

Glomerulonephritis — *see also* Nephritis —
  continued
  acute — *continued*
    with
      exudative nephritis 580.89
      interstitial nephritis (diffuse) (focal)
        580.89
      necrotizing glomerulitis 580.4
      extracapillary with epithelial crescents
        580.4
      poststreptococcal 580.0
      proliferative (diffuse) 580.0
      rapidly progressive 580.4
      specified pathology NEC 580.89
  arteriolar (*see also* Hypertension, kidney)
    403.90
  arteriosclerotic (*see also* Hypertension, kid-
    ney) 403.90
  ascending (*see also* Pyelitis) 590.80
  basement membrane NEC 583.89
    with
      pulmonary hemorrhage (Goodpas-
        ture's syndrome)
        446.21 [583.81]
  chronic 582.9
    with
      exudative nephritis 582.89
      interstitial nephritis (diffuse) (focal)
        582.89
      necrotizing glomerulitis 582.4
      specified pathology or lesion NEC
        582.89
    endothelial 582.2
    extracapillary with epithelial crescents
      582.4
    hypocomplementemic persistent 582.2
    lobular 582.2
    membranoproliferative 582.2
    membranous 582.1
      and proliferative (mixed) 582.2
      sclerosing 582.1
    mesangiocapillary 582.2
    mixed membranous and proliferative
      582.2
    proliferative (diffuse) 582.0
    rapidly progressive 582.4
    sclerosing 582.1
  cirrhotic — *see* Sclerosis, renal
  desquamative — *see* Nephrosis
  due to or associated with
    amyloidosis 277.39 [583.81]
      with nephrotic syndrome
        277.39 [581.81]
      chronic 277.39 [582.81]
    diabetes mellitus 250.4 ☑ [583.81]
      with nephrotic syndrome
        250.4 ☑ [581.81]
        due to secondary diabetes
          249.4 ☑ [581.81]
      due to secondary diabetes
        249.4 ☑ [581.81]
    diphtheria 032.89 [580.81]
    gonococcal infection (acute)
      098.19 [583.81]
      chronic or duration of 2 months or
        over 098.39 [583.81]
    infectious hepatitis 070.9 [580.81]
    malaria (with nephrotic syndrome)
      084.9 [581.81]
    mumps 072.79 [580.81]
    polyarteritis (nodosa) (with nephrotic
      syndrome) 446.0 [581.81]
    specified pathology NEC 583.89
      acute 580.89
      chronic 582.89
    streptotrichosis 039.8 [583.81]
    subacute bacterial endocarditis
      421.0 [580.81]
    syphilis (late) 095.4
      congenital 090.5 [583.81]
      early 091.69 [583.81]
    systemic lupus erythematosus
      710.0 [583.81]
      with nephrotic syndrome
        710.0 [581.81]
      chronic 710.0 [582.81]

Glomerulonephritis — *see also* Nephritis —
  continued
  due to or associated with — *continued*
    tuberculosis (*see also* Tuberculosis)
      016.0 ☑ [583.81]
      typhoid fever 002.0 [580.81]
  extracapillary with epithelial crescents 583.4
    acute 580.4
    chronic 582.4
  exudative 583.89
    acute 580.89
    chronic 582.89
  focal (*see also* Nephritis) 583.9
    embolic 580.4
  granular 582.89
  granulomatous 582.89
  hydremic (*see also* Nephrosis) 581.9
  hypocomplementemic persistent 583.2
    with nephrotic syndrome 581.2
    chronic 582.2
  immune complex NEC 583.89
  infective (*see also* Pyelitis) 590.80
  interstitial (diffuse) (focal) 583.89
    with nephrotic syndrome 581.89
    acute 580.89
    chronic 582.89
  latent or quiescent 582.9
  lobular 583.2
    with nephrotic syndrome 581.2
    chronic 582.2
  membranoproliferative 583.2
    with nephrotic syndrome 581.2
    chronic 582.2
  membranous 583.1
    with nephrotic syndrome 581.1
    and proliferative (mixed) 583.2
      with nephrotic syndrome 581.2
      chronic 582.2
    chronic 582.1
    sclerosing 582.1
      with nephrotic syndrome 581.1
  mesangiocapillary 583.2
    with nephrotic syndrome 581.2
    chronic 582.2
  minimal change 581.3
  mixed membranous and proliferative 583.2
    with nephrotic syndrome 581.2
    chronic 582.2
  necrotizing 583.4
    acute 580.4
    chronic 582.4
  nephrotic (*see also* Nephrosis) 581.9
  old — *see* Glomerulonephritis, chronic
  parenchymatous 581.89
  poststreptococcal 580.0
  proliferative (diffuse) 583.0
    with nephrotic syndrome 581.0
    acute 580.0
    chronic 582.0
  purulent (*see also* Pyelitis) 590.80
  quiescent — *see* Nephritis, chronic
  rapidly progressive 583.4
    acute 580.4
    chronic 582.4
  sclerosing membranous (chronic) 582.1
    with nephrotic syndrome 581.1
  septic (*see also* Pyelitis) 590.80
  specified pathology or lesion NEC 583.89
    with nephrotic syndrome 581.89
    acute 580.89
    chronic 582.89
  suppurative (acute) (disseminated) (*see also*
    Pyelitis) 590.80
  toxic — *see* Nephritis, acute
  tubal, tubular — *see* Nephrosis, tubular
  type II (Ellis) — *see* Nephrosis
  vascular — *see* Hypertension, kidney
Glomerulosclerosis — *see also* Sclerosis, renal
  587
  focal 582.1
    with nephrotic syndrome 581.1
  intercapillary (nodular) (with diabetes)
    250.4 ☑ [581.81]
    due to secondary diabetes
      249.4 ☑ [581.81]
Glossagra 529.6

☑ **Additional Digit Required — Refer to the Tabular List for Digit Selection**   ᴺᴱᵂ **Subterms under main terms may continue to next column or page**

2013 ICD-9-CM   ▶◀ **Revised Text**   ● **New Line**   ▲ **Revised Code**   **Volume 2 — 129**

Glossalgia 529.6
Glossitis 529.0
  areata exfoliativa 529.1
  atrophic 529.4
  benign migratory 529.1
  gangrenous 529.0
  Hunter's 529.4
  median rhomboid 529.2
  Moeller's 529.4
  pellagrous 265.2
Glossocele 529.8
Glossodynia 529.6
  exfoliativa 529.4
Glossoncus 529.8
Glossophytia 529.3
Glossoplegia 529.8
Glossoptosis 529.8
Glossopyrosis 529.6
Glossotrichia 529.3
Glossy skin 701.9
Glottis — see condition
Glottitis — see Glossitis
Glucagonoma (M8152/0)
  malignant (M8152/3)
    pancreas 157.4
    specified site NEC — see Neoplasm, by
      site, malignant
    unspecified site 157.4
  pancreas 211.7
  specified site NEC — see Neoplasm, by site,
    benign
  unspecified site 211.7
Glucoglycinuria 270.7
Glue ear syndrome 381.20
Glue sniffing (airplane glue) — see also Depen-
    dence 304.6 ☑
Glycinemia (with methylmalonic acidemia)
    270.7
Glycinuria (renal) (with ketosis) 270.0
Glycogen
  infiltration (see also Disease, glycogen stor-
    age) 271.0
  storage disease (see also Disease, glycogen
    storage) 271.0
Glycogenosis — see also Disease, glycogen
    storage 271.0
  cardiac 271.0 [425.7]
  Cori, types I-VII 271.0
  diabetic, secondary 250.8 ☑ [259.8]
    due to secondary diabetes
      249.8 ☑ [259.8]
  diffuse (with hepatic cirrhosis) 271.0
  generalized 271.0
  glucose-6-phosphatase deficiency 271.0
  hepatophosphorylase deficiency 271.0
  hepatorenal 271.0
  myophosphorylase deficiency 271.0
  pulmonary interstitial 516.62
Glycopenia 251.2
Glycopeptide
  intermediate staphylococcus aureus (GISA)
    V09.8 ☑
  resistant
    enterococcus V09.8 ☑
    staphylococcus aureus (GRSA) V09.8 ☑
Glycoprolinuria 270.8
Glycosuria 791.5
  renal 271.4
Gnathostoma (spinigerum) (infection) (infes-
    tation) 128.1
  wandering swellings from 128.1
Gnathostomiasis 128.1
Goiter (adolescent) (colloid) (diffuse) (dipping)
    (due to iodine deficiency) (endemic)
    (euthyroid) (heart) (hyperplastic) (inter-
    nal) (intrathoracic) (juvenile) (mixed
    type) (nonendemic) (parenchymatous)
    (plunging) (sporadic) (subclavicular)
    (substernal) 240.9
  with
    hyperthyroidism (recurrent) (see also
      Goiter, toxic) 242.0 ☑
    thyrotoxicosis (see also Goiter, toxic)
      242.0 ☑
  adenomatous (see also Goiter, nodular)
    241.9

Goiter — continued
  cancerous (M8000/3) 193
  complicating pregnancy, childbirth, or
    puerperium 648.1 ☑
  congenital 246.1
  cystic (see also Goiter, nodular) 241.9
  due to enzyme defect in synthesis of thyroid
    hormone (butane-insoluble iodine)
    (coupling) (deiodinase) (iodide trap-
    ping or organification) (iodotyrosine
    dehalogenase) (peroxidase) 246.1
  dyshormonogenic 246.1
  exophthalmic (see also Goiter, toxic)
    242.0 ☑
  familial (with deaf-mutism) 243
  fibrous 245.3
  lingual 759.2
  lymphadenoid 245.2
  malignant (M8000/3) 193
  multinodular (nontoxic) 241.1
    toxic or with hyperthyroidism (see also
      Goiter, toxic) 242.2 ☑
  nodular (nontoxic) 241.9
    with
      hyperthyroidism (see also Goiter,
        toxic) 242.3 ☑
      thyrotoxicosis (see also Goiter, toxic)
        242.3 ☑
    endemic 241.9
    exophthalmic (diffuse) (see also Goiter,
      toxic) 242.0 ☑
    multinodular (nontoxic) 241.1
    sporadic 241.9
    toxic (see also Goiter, toxic) 242.3 ☑
    uninodular (nontoxic) 241.0
  nontoxic (nodular) 241.9
    multinodular 241.1
    uninodular 241.0
  pulsating (see also Goiter, toxic) 242.0 ☑
  simple 240.0
  toxic 242.0 ☑

  Note — Use the following fifth-digit
  subclassification with category 242:

  0   without mention of thyrotoxic
      crisis or storm

  1   with mention of thyrotoxic crisis
      or storm

    adenomatous 242.3 ☑
      multinodular 242.2 ☑
      uninodular 242.1 ☑
    multinodular 242.2 ☑
    nodular 242.3 ☑
      multinodular 242.2 ☑
      uninodular 242.1 ☑
    uninodular 242.1 ☑
  uninodular (nontoxic) 241.0
    toxic or with hyperthyroidism (see also
      Goiter, toxic) 242.1 ☑
Goldberg (-Maxwell) (-Morris) syndrome
    (testicular feminization) 259.51
Goldblatt's
  hypertension 440.1
  kidney 440.1
Goldenhar's syndrome (oculoauriculoverte-
    bral dysplasia) 756.0
Goldflam-Erb disease or syndrome 358.00
Goldscheider's disease (epidermolysis bullosa)
    757.39
Goldstein's disease (familial hemorrhagic
    telangiectasia) 448.0
Golfer's elbow 726.32
Goltz-Gorlin syndrome (dermal hypoplasia)
    757.39
Gonadoblastoma (M9073/1)
  specified site — see Neoplasm, by site un-
    certain behavior
  unspecified site
    female 236.2
    male 236.4
Gonecystitis — see also Vesiculitis 608.0
Gongylonemiasis 125.6
  mouth 125.6
Goniosynechiae 364.73
Gonococcemia 098.89

Gonococcus, gonococcal (disease) (infection)
    — see also condition 098.0
  anus 098.7
  bursa 098.52
  chronic NEC 098.2
  complicating pregnancy, childbirth, or
    puerperium 647.1 ☑
    affecting fetus or newborn 760.2
  conjunctiva, conjunctivitis (neonatorum)
    098.40
  dermatosis 098.89
  endocardium 098.84
  epididymo-orchitis 098.13
    chronic or duration of 2 months or over
      098.33
  eye (newborn) 098.40
  fallopian tube (chronic) 098.37
    acute 098.17
  genitourinary (acute) (organ) (system) (tract)
    (see also Gonorrhea) 098.0
    lower 098.0
      chronic 098.2
    upper 098.10
      chronic 098.30
  heart NEC 098.85
  joint 098.50
  keratoderma 098.81
  keratosis (blennorrhagica) 098.81
  lymphatic (gland) (node) 098.89
  meninges 098.82
  orchitis (acute) 098.13
    chronic or duration of 2 months or over
      098.33
  pelvis (acute) 098.19
    chronic or duration of 2 months or over
      098.39
  pericarditis 098.83
  peritonitis 098.86
  pharyngitis 098.6
  pharynx 098.6
  proctitis 098.7
  pyosalpinx (chronic) 098.37
    acute 098.17
  rectum 098.7
  septicemia 098.89
  skin 098.89
  specified site NEC 098.89
  synovitis 098.51
  tendon sheath 098.51
  throat 098.6
  urethra (acute) 098.0
    chronic or duration of 2 months or over
      098.2
  vulva (acute) 098.0
    chronic or duration of 2 months or over
      098.2
Gonocytoma (M9073/1)
  specified site — see Neoplasm, by site, un-
    certain behavior
  unspecified site
    female 236.2
    male 236.4
Gonorrhea 098.0
  acute 098.0
  Bartholin's gland (acute) 098.0
    chronic or duration of 2 months or over
      098.2
  bladder (acute) 098.11
    chronic or duration of 2 months or over
      098.31
  carrier (suspected of) V02.7
  cervix (acute) 098.15
    chronic or duration of 2 months or over
      098.35
  chronic 098.2
  complicating pregnancy, childbirth, or
    puerperium 647.1 ☑
    affecting fetus or newborn 760.2
  conjunctiva, conjunctivitis (neonatorum)
    098.40
  contact V01.6
  Cowper's gland (acute) 098.0
    chronic or duration of 2 months or over
      098.2
  duration of two months or over 098.2
  exposure to V01.6

Gonorrhea — continued
  fallopian tube (chronic) 098.37
    acute 098.17
  genitourinary (acute) (organ) (system) (tract)
    098.0
    chronic 098.2
    duration of two months or over 098.2
  kidney (acute) 098.19
    chronic or duration of 2 months or over
      098.39
  ovary (acute) 098.19
    chronic or duration of 2 months or over
      098.39
  pelvis (acute) 098.19
    chronic or duration of 2 months or over
      098.39
  penis (acute) 098.0
    chronic or duration of 2 months or over
      098.2
  prostate (acute) 098.12
    chronic or duration of 2 months or over
      098.32
  seminal vesicle (acute) 098.14
    chronic or duration of 2 months or over
      098.34
  specified site NEC — see Gonococcus
  spermatic cord (acute) 098.14
    chronic or duration of 2 months or over
      098.34
  urethra (acute) 098.0
    chronic or duration of 2 months or over
      098.2
  vagina (acute) 098.0
    chronic or duration of 2 months or over
      098.2
  vas deferens (acute) 098.14
    chronic or duration of 2 months or over
      098.34
  vulva (acute) 098.0
    chronic or duration of 2 months or over
      098.2
Goodpasture's syndrome (pneumorenal)
    446.21
Good's syndrome 279.06
Gopalan's syndrome (burning feet) 266.2
Gordon's disease (exudative enteropathy)
    579.8
Gorlin-Chaudhry-Moss syndrome 759.89
Gougerot-Blum syndrome (pigmented pur-
    puric lichenoid dermatitis) 709.1
Gougerot-Carteaud disease or syndrome
    (confluent reticulate papillomatosis)
    701.8
Gougerot-Hailey-Hailey disease (benign fa-
    milial chronic pemphigus) 757.39
Gougerot (-Houwer) -Sjögren syndrome
    (keratoconjunctivitis sicca) 710.2
Gougerot's syndrome (trisymptomatic) 709.1
Gouley's syndrome (constrictive pericarditis)
    423.2
Goundou 102.6
Gout, gouty 274.9
  with
    specified manifestations NEC 274.89
    tophi (tophus) 274.03
  acute 274.01
  arthritis 274.00
    acute 274.01
  arthropathy 274.00
    acute 274.01
    chronic (without mention of tophus
      (tophi)) 274.02
      with tophus (tophi) 274.03
  attack 274.01
  chronic 274.02
    tophaceous 274.03
  degeneration, heart 274.82
  diathesis 274.9
  eczema 274.89
  episcleritis 274.89 [379.09]
  external ear (tophus) 274.81
  flare 274.01
  glomerulonephritis 274.10
  iritis 274.89 [364.11]
  joint 274.00
  kidney 274.10

Gout, gouty — *continued*
lead 984.9
  specified type of lead — *see* Table of Drugs and Chemicals
nephritis 274.10
neuritis 274.89 *[357.4]*
phlebitis 274.89 *[451.9]*
rheumatic 714.0
saturnine 984.9
  specified type of lead — *see* Table of Drugs and Chemicals
spondylitis 274.00
synovitis 274.00
syphilitic 095.8
tophi 274.03
  ear 274.81
  heart 274.82
  specified site NEC 274.82
Gowers'
muscular dystrophy 359.1
syndrome (vasovagal attack) 780.2
Gowers-Paton-Kennedy syndrome 377.04
Gradenigo's syndrome 383.02
Graft-versus-host disease 279.50
due to organ transplant NEC — *see* Complications, transplant, organ
Graham Steell's murmur (pulmonic regurgitation) — *see also* Endocarditis, pulmonary 424.3
Grain-handlers' disease or lung 495.8
Grain mite (itch) 133.8
Grand
mal (idiopathic) (*see also* Epilepsy) 345.1 ✓
  hysteria of Charcôt 300.11
  nonrecurrent or isolated 780.39
multipara
  affecting management of labor and delivery 659.4 ✓
  status only (not pregnant) V61.5
Granite workers' lung 502
Granular — *see also* condition
inflammation, pharynx 472.1
kidney (contracting) (*see also* Sclerosis, renal) 587
liver — *see* Cirrhosis, liver
nephritis — *see* Nephritis
Granulation tissue, abnormal — *see also* Granuloma
abnormal or excessive 701.5
postmastoidectomy cavity 383.33
postoperative 701.5
skin 701.5
Granulocytopenia, granulocytopenic (primary) 288.00
malignant 288.09
Granuloma NEC 686.1
abdomen (wall) 568.89
  skin (pyogenicum) 686.1
    from residual foreign body 709.4
annulare 695.89
anus 569.49
apical 522.6
appendix 543.9
aural 380.23
beryllium (skin) 709.4
  lung 503
bone (*see also* Osteomyelitis) 730.1 ✓
  eosinophilic 277.89
  from residual foreign body 733.99
canaliculus lacrimalis 375.81
cerebral 348.89
cholesterin, middle ear 385.82
coccidioidal (progressive) 114.3
  lung 114.4
  meninges 114.2
  primary (lung) 114.0
colon 569.89
conjunctiva 372.61
dental 522.6
ear, middle (cholesterin) 385.82
  with otitis media — *see* Otitis media
eosinophilic 277.89
  bone 277.89
  lung 277.89
  oral mucosa 528.9
exuberant 701.5

Granuloma — *continued*
eyelid 374.89
facial
  lethal midline 446.3
  malignant 446.3
faciale 701.8
fissuratum (gum) 523.8
foot NEC 686.1
foreign body (in soft tissue) NEC 728.82
  bone 733.99
  in operative wound 998.4
  muscle 728.82
  skin 709.4
  subcutaneous tissue 709.4
fungoides 202.1 ✓
gangraenescens 446.3
giant cell (central) (jaw) (reparative) 526.3
  gingiva 523.8
  peripheral (gingiva) 523.8
gland (lymph) 289.3
Hodgkin's (M9661/3) 201.1 ✓
ileum 569.89
infectious NEC 136.9
inguinale (Donovan) 099.2
  venereal 099.2
intestine 569.89
iridocyclitis 364.10
jaw (bone) 526.3
  reparative giant cell 526.3
kidney (*see also* Infection, kidney) 590.9
lacrimal sac 375.81
larynx 478.79
lethal midline 446.3
lipid 277.89
lipoid 277.89
liver 572.8
lung (infectious) (*see also* Fibrosis, lung) 515
  coccidioidal 114.4
  eosinophilic 277.89
lymph gland 289.3
Majocchi's 110.6
malignant, face 446.3
mandible 526.3
mediastinum 519.3
midline 446.3
monilial 112.3
muscle 728.82
  from residual foreign body 728.82
nasal sinus (*see also* Sinusitis) 473.9
operation wound 998.59
  foreign body 998.4
  stitch (external) 998.89
    internal wound 998.89
  talc 998.7
oral mucosa, eosinophilic or pyogenic 528.9
orbit, orbital 376.11
paracoccidioidal 116.1
penis, venereal 099.2
periapical 522.6
peritoneum 568.89
  due to ova of helminths NEC (*see also* Helminthiasis) 128.9
postmastoidectomy cavity 383.33
postoperative — *see* Granuloma, operation wound
prostate 601.8
pudendi (ulcerating) 099.2
pudendorum (ulcerative) 099.2
pulp, internal (tooth) 521.49
pyogenic, pyogenicum (skin) 686.1
  maxillary alveolar ridge 522.6
  oral mucosa 528.9
rectum 569.49
reticulohistiocytic 277.89
rubrum nasi 705.89
sarcoid 135
Schistosoma 120.9
septic (skin) 686.1
silica (skin) 709.4
sinus (accessory) (infectional) (nasal) (*see also* Sinusitis) 473.9
skin (pyogenicum) 686.1
  from foreign body or material 709.4
sperm 608.89
spine
  syphilitic (epidural) 094.89

Granuloma — *continued*
spine — *continued*
  tuberculous (*see also* Tuberculosis) 015.0 ✓ *[730.88]*
stitch (postoperative) 998.89
  internal wound 998.89
suppurative (skin) 686.1
suture (postoperative) 998.89
  internal wound 998.89
swimming pool 031.1
talc 728.82
  in operation wound 998.7
telangiectaticum (skin) 686.1
tracheostomy 519.09
trichophyticum 110.6
tropicum 102.4
umbilicus 686.1
  newborn 771.4
urethra 599.84
uveitis 364.10
vagina 099.2
venereum 099.2
vocal cords 478.5
Wegener's (necrotizing respiratory granulomatosis) 446.4
Granulomatosis NEC 686.1
disciformis chronica et progressiva 709.3
infantiseptica 771.2
lipoid 277.89
lipophagic, intestinal 040.2
miliary 027.0
necrotizing, respiratory 446.4
progressive, septic 288.1
Wegener's (necrotizing respiratory) 446.4
Granulomatous tissue — *see* Granuloma
Granulosis rubra nasi 705.89
Graphite fibrosis (of lung) 503
Graphospasm 300.89
organic 333.84
Grating scapula 733.99
Gravel (urinary) — *see also* Calculus 592.9
Graves' disease (exophthalmic goiter) — *see also* Goiter, toxic 242.0 ✓
Gravis — *see* condition
Grawitz's tumor (hypernephroma) (M8312/3) 189.0
Grayness, hair (premature) 704.3
congenital 757.4
Gray or grey syndrome (chloramphenicol) (newborn) 779.4
Greenfield's disease 330.0
Green sickness 280.9
Greenstick fracture — *see* Fracture, by site
Greig's syndrome (hypertelorism) 756.0
Grief 309.0
Griesinger's disease — *see also* Ancylostomiasis 126.9
Grinders'
asthma 502
lung 502
phthisis (*see also* Tuberculosis) 011.4 ✓
Grinding, teeth 306.8
Grip
Dabney's 074.1
devil's 074.1
Grippe, grippal — *see also* Influenza
Balkan 083.0
intestinal (*see also* Influenza) 487.8
summer 074.8
Grippy cold — *see also* Influenza 487.1
Grisel's disease 723.5
Groin — *see* condition
Grooved
nails (transverse) 703.8
tongue 529.5
  congenital 750.13
Ground itch 126.9
Growing pains, children 781.99
Growth (fungoid) (neoplastic) (new) (M8000/1) — *see also* Neoplasm, by site, unspecified nature
adenoid (vegetative) 474.12
benign (M8000/0) — *see* Neoplasm, by site, benign
fetal, poor 764.9 ✓

Growth — *see also* Neoplasm, by site, unspecified nature — *continued*
fetal, poor — *continued*
  affecting management of pregnancy 656.5 ✓
malignant (M8000/3) — *see* Neoplasm, by site, malignant
rapid, childhood V21.0
secondary (M8000/6) — *see* Neoplasm, by site, malignant, secondary
GRSA (glycopeptide resistant staphylococcus aureus) V09.8 ✓
Gruber's hernia — *see* Hernia, Gruber's
Gruby's disease (tinea tonsurans) 110.0
GSS (Gerstmann-Sträussler-Scheinker syndrome) 046.71
G-trisomy 758.0
Guama fever 066.3
Gubler (-Millard) paralysis or syndrome 344.89
Guérin-Stern syndrome (arthrogryposis multiplex congenita) 754.89
Guertin's disease (electric chorea) 049.8
Guillain-Barré disease or syndrome 357.0
Guinea worms (infection) (infestation) 125.7
Guinon's disease (motor-verbal tic) 307.23
Gull and Sutton's disease — *see* Hypertension, kidney
Gull's disease (thyroid atrophy with myxedema) 244.8
Gum — *see* condition
Gumboil 522.7
Gumma (syphilitic) 095.9
artery 093.89
  cerebral or spinal 094.89
bone 095.5
  of yaws (late) 102.6
brain 094.89
cauda equina 094.89
central nervous system NEC 094.9
ciliary body 095.8 *[364.11]*
congenital 090.5
  testis 090.5
eyelid 095.8 *[373.5]*
heart 093.89
intracranial 094.89
iris 095.8 *[364.11]*
kidney 095.4
larynx 095.8
leptomeninges 094.2
liver 095.3
meninges 094.2
myocardium 093.82
nasopharynx 095.8
neurosyphilitic 094.9
nose 095.8
orbit 095.8
palate (soft) 095.8
penis 095.8
pericardium 093.81
pharynx 095.8
pituitary 095.8
scrofulous (*see also* Tuberculosis) 017.0 ✓
skin 095.8
specified site NEC 095.8
spinal cord 094.89
tongue 095.8
tonsil 095.8
trachea 095.8
tuberculous (*see also* Tuberculosis) 017.0 ✓
ulcerative due to yaws 102.4
ureter 095.8
yaws 102.4
  bone 102.6
Gunn's syndrome (jaw-winking syndrome) 742.8
Gunshot wound — *see also* Wound, open, by site
fracture — *see* Fracture, by site, open
internal organs (abdomen, chest, or pelvis) — *see* Injury, internal, by site, with open wound
intracranial — *see* Laceration, brain, with open intracranial wound
Günther's disease or syndrome (congenital erythropoietic porphyria) 277.1

Index

Gustatory hallucination — Heidenhain's disease

Gustatory hallucination 780.1
Gynandrism 752.7
Gynandroblastoma (M8632/1)
  specified site — *see* Neoplasm, by site, uncertain behavior
  unspecified site
    female 236.2
    male 236.4
Gynandromorphism 752.7
Gynatresia (congenital) 752.49
Gynecoid pelvis, male 738.6
Gynecological examination V72.31
  for contraceptive maintenance V25.40
Gynecomastia 611.1
Gynephobia 300.29
Gyrate scalp 757.39

H

Haas' disease (osteochondrosis head of humerus) 732.3
Habermann's disease (acute parapsoriasis varioliformis) 696.2
Habit, habituation
  chorea 307.22
  disturbance, child 307.9
  drug (*see also* Dependence) 304.9 ☑
  laxative (*see also* Abuse, drugs, nondependent) 305.9 ☑
  spasm 307.20
    chronic 307.22
    transient (of childhood) 307.21
  tic 307.20
    chronic 307.22
    transient (of childhood) 307.21
  use of
    nonprescribed drugs (*see also* Abuse, drugs, nondependent) 305.9 ☑
    patent medicines (*see also* Abuse, drugs, nondependent) 305.9 ☑
  vomiting 536.2
Hadfield-Clarke syndrome (pancreatic infantilism) 577.8
Haff disease 985.1
Hageman factor defect, deficiency, or disease — *see also* Defect, coagulation 286.3
Haglund's disease (osteochondrosis os tibiale externum) 732.5
Haglund-Läwen-Fründ syndrome 717.89
Hagner's disease (hypertrophic pulmonary osteoarthropathy) 731.2
Hag teeth, tooth 524.39
Hailey-Hailey disease (benign familial chronic pemphigus) 757.39
Hair — *see also* condition
  plucking 307.9
Hairball in stomach 935.2
Hairy black tongue 529.3
Half vertebra 756.14
Halitosis 784.99
Hallermann-Streiff syndrome 756.0
Hallervorden-Spatz disease or syndrome 333.0
Hallopeau's
  acrodermatitis (continua) 696.1
  disease (lichen sclerosis et atrophicus) 701.0
Hallucination (auditory) (gustatory) (olfactory) (tactile) 780.1
  alcohol-induced 291.3
  drug-induced 292.12
  visual 368.16
Hallucinosis 298.9
  alcohol-induced (acute) 291.3
  drug-induced 292.12
Hallus — *see* Hallux
Hallux 735.9
  limitus 735.8
  malleus (acquired) 735.3
  rigidus (acquired) 735.2
    congenital 755.66
    late effects of rickets 268.1
  valgus (acquired) 735.0
    congenital 755.66
  varus (acquired) 735.1
    congenital 755.66
Halo, visual 368.15

Hamartoblastoma 759.6
Hamartoma 759.6
  epithelial (gingival), odontogenic, central, or peripheral (M9321/0) 213.1
    upper jaw (bone) 213.0
  vascular 757.32
Hamartosis, hamartoses NEC 759.6
Hamman's disease or syndrome (spontaneous mediastinal emphysema) 518.1
Hamman-Rich syndrome (diffuse interstitial pulmonary fibrosis) 516.33
Hammer toe (acquired) 735.4
  congenital 755.66
  late effects of rickets 268.1
Hand — *see* condition
Hand-foot syndrome 693.0
Hand-Schüller-Christian disease or syndrome (chronic histiocytosis x) 277.89
Hanging (asphyxia) (strangulation) (suffocation) 994.7
Hangnail (finger) (with lymphangitis) 681.02
Hangover (alcohol) — *see also* Abuse, drugs, nondependent 305.0 ☑
Hanot-Chauffard (-Troisier) syndrome (bronze diabetes) 275.01
Hanot's cirrhosis or disease — *see* Cirrhosis, biliary
Hansen's disease (leprosy) 030.9
  benign form 030.1
  malignant form 030.0
Harada's disease or syndrome 363.22
Hard chancre 091.0
Hardening
  artery — *see* Arteriosclerosis
  brain 348.89
  liver 571.8
Hard firm prostate 600.10
  with
    urinary
      obstruction 600.11
      retention 600.11
Harelip — *see also* Cleft, lip 749.10
Hare's syndrome (M8010/3) (carcinoma, pulmonary apex) 162.3
Harkavy's syndrome 446.0
Harlequin (fetus) 757.1
  color change syndrome 779.89
Harley's disease (intermittent hemoglobinuria) 283.2
Harris'
  lines 733.91
  syndrome (organic hyperinsulinism) 251.1
Hart's disease or syndrome (pellagra-cerebellar ataxia-renal aminoaciduria) 270.0
Hartmann's pouch (abnormal sacculation of gallbladder neck) 575.8
  of intestine V44.3
    attention to V55.3
Hartnup disease (pellagra-cerebellar ataxia-renal aminoaciduria) 270.0
Harvester lung 495.0
Hashimoto's disease or struma (struma lymphomatosa) 245.2
Hassall-Henle bodies (corneal warts) 371.41
Haut mal — *see also* Epilepsy 345.1 ☑
Haverhill fever 026.1
Hawaiian wood rose dependence 304.5 ☑
Hawkins' keloid 701.4
Hay
  asthma (*see also* Asthma) 493.0 ☑
  fever (allergic) (with rhinitis) 477.9
    with asthma (bronchial) (*see also* Asthma) 493.0 ☑
    allergic, due to grass, pollen, ragweed, or tree 477.0
    conjunctivitis 372.05
    due to
      dander, animal (cat) (dog) 477.2
      dust 477.8
      fowl 477.8
      hair, animal (cat) (dog) 477.2
      pollen 477.0
      specified allergen other than pollen 477.8
Hayem-Faber syndrome (achlorhydric anemia) 280.9

Hayem-Widal syndrome (acquired hemolytic jaundice) 283.9
Haygarth's nodosities 715.04
Hazard-Crile tumor (M8350/3) 193
Hb (abnormal)
  disease — *see* Disease, hemoglobin
  trait — *see* Trait
H disease 270.0
Head — *see also* condition
  banging 307.3
Headache 784.0
  allergic 339.00
  associated with sexual activity 339.82
  cluster 339.00
    chronic 339.02
    episodic 339.01
  daily
    chronic 784.0
    new persistent (NPDH) 339.42
  drug induced 339.3
  due to
    loss, spinal fluid 349.0
    lumbar puncture 349.0
    saddle block 349.0
  emotional 307.81
  histamine 339.00
  hypnic 339.81
  lumbar puncture 349.0
  medication overuse 339.3
  menopausal 627.2
  menstrual 346.4 ☑
  migraine 346.9 ☑
  nasal septum 784.0
  nonorganic origin 307.81
  orgasmic 339.82
  postspinal 349.0
  post-traumatic 339.20
    acute 339.21
    chronic 339.22
  premenstrual 346.4 ☑
  preorgasmic 339.82
  primary
    cough 339.83
    exertional 339.84
    stabbing 339.85
    thunderclap 339.43
  psychogenic 307.81
  psychophysiologic 307.81
  rebound 339.3
  short lasting unilateral neuralgiform with conjunctival injection and tearing (SUNCT) 339.05
  sick 346.9 ☑
  spinal 349.0
    complicating labor and delivery 668.8 ☑
    postpartum 668.8 ☑
  spinal fluid loss 349.0
  syndrome
    cluster 339.00
    complicated NEC 339.44
    periodic in child or adolescent 346.2 ☑
    specified NEC 339.89
  tension 307.81
    type 339.10
      chronic 339.12
      episodic 339.11
  vascular 784.0
    migraine type 346.9 ☑
  vasomotor 346.9 ☑
Health
  advice V65.4 ☑
  audit V70.0
  checkup V70.0
  education V65.4 ☑
  hazard (*see also* History of) V15.9
    falling V15.88
    specified cause NEC V15.89
  instruction V65.4 ☑
  services provided because (of)
    boarding school residence V60.6
    holiday relief for person providing home care V60.5
    inadequate
      housing V60.1
      resources V60.2
    lack of housing V60.0

Health — *continued*
  services provided because — *continued*
    no care available in home V60.4
    person living alone V60.3
    poverty V60.3
    residence in institution V60.6
    specified cause NEC V60.89
    vacation relief for person providing home care V60.5
Healthy
  donor (*see also* Donor) V59.9
  infant or child
    accompanying sick mother V65.0
    receiving care V20.1
  person
    accompanying sick relative V65.0
    admitted for sterilization V25.2
    receiving prophylactic inoculation or vaccination (*see also* Vaccination, prophylactic) V05.9
Hearing
  conservation and treatment V72.12
  examination V72.19
    following failed hearing screening V72.11
Heart — *see* condition
Heartburn 787.1
  psychogenic 306.4
Heat (effects) 992.9
  apoplexy 992.0
  burn (*see also* Burn, by site)
    from sun (*see also* Sunburn) 692.71
  collapse 992.1
  cramps 992.2
  dermatitis or eczema 692.89
  edema 992.7
  erythema — *see* Burn, by site
  excessive 992.9
    specified effect NEC 992.8
  exhaustion 992.5
    anhydrotic 992.3
    due to
      salt (and water) depletion 992.4
      water depletion 992.3
  fatigue (transient) 992.6
  fever 992.0
  hyperpyrexia 992.0
  prickly 705.1
  prostration — *see* Heat, exhaustion
  pyrexia 992.0
  rash 705.1
  specified effect NEC 992.8
  stroke 992.0
  sunburn (*see also* Sunburn) 692.71
  syncope 992.1
Heavy-chain disease 273.2
Heavy-for-dates (fetus or infant) 766.1
  4500 grams or more 766.0
  exceptionally 766.0
Hebephrenia, hebephrenic (acute) — *see also* Schizophrenia 295.1 ☑
  dementia (praecox) (*see also* Schizophrenia) 295.1 ☑
  schizophrenia (*see also* Schizophrenia) 295.1 ☑
Heberden's
  disease or nodes 715.04
  syndrome (angina pectoris) 413.9
Hebra's disease
  dermatitis exfoliativa 695.89
  erythema multiforme exudativum 695.19
  pityriasis 695.89
    maculata et circinata 696.3
    rubra 695.89
      pilaris 696.4
  prurigo 698.2
Hebra, nose 040.1
Hedinger's syndrome (malignant carcinoid) 259.2
Heel — *see* condition
Heerfordt's disease or syndrome (uveoparotitis) 135
Hegglin's anomaly or syndrome 288.2
Heidenhain's disease 290.10
  with dementia 290.10

Heilmeyer-Schöner disease (M9842/3) 207.1 ☑

Heine-Medin disease — see also Poliomyelitis 045.9 ☑

Heinz-body anemia, congenital 282.7

Heller's disease or syndrome (infantile psychosis) — see also Psychosis, childhood 299.1 ☑

H.E.L.L.P 642.5 ☑

Helminthiasis — see also Infestation, by specific parasite 128.9

Ancylostoma (see also Ancylostoma) 126.9

intestinal 127.9

mixed types (types classifiable to more than one of the categories 120.0–127.7) 127.8

specified type 127.7

mixed types (intestinal) (types classifiable to more than one of the categories 120.0–127.7) 127.8

Necator americanus 126.1

specified type NEC 128.8

Trichinella 124

Heloma 700

Hemangioblastoma (M9161/1) — see also Neoplasm, connective tissue, uncertain behavior

malignant (M9161/3) — see Neoplasm, connective tissue, malignant

Hemangioblastomatosis, cerebelloretinal 759.6

Hemangioendothelioma (M9130/1) — see also Neoplasm, by site, uncertain behavior

benign (M9130/0) 228.00

bone (diffuse) (M9130/3) — see Neoplasm, bone, malignant

malignant (M9130/3) — see Neoplasm, connective tissue, malignant

nervous system (M9130/0) 228.09

Hemangioendotheliosarcoma (M9130/3) — see Neoplasm, connective tissue, malignant

Hemangiofibroma (M9160/0) — see Neoplasm, by site, benign

Hemangiolipoma (M8861/0) — see Lipoma

Hemangioma (M9120/0) 228.00

arteriovenous (M9123/0) — see Hemangioma, by site

brain 228.02

capillary (M9131/0) — see Hemangioma, by site

cavernous (M9121/0) — see Hemangioma, by site

central nervous system NEC 228.09

choroid 228.09

heart 228.09

infantile (M9131/0) — see Hemangioma, by site

intra-abdominal structures 228.04

intracranial structures 228.02

intramuscular (M9132/0) — see Hemangioma, by site

iris 228.09

juvenile (M9131/0) — see Hemangioma, by site

malignant (M9120/3) — see Neoplasm, connective tissue, malignant

meninges 228.09

brain 228.02

spinal cord 228.09

peritoneum 228.04

placenta — see Placenta, abnormal

plexiform (M9131/0) — see Hemangioma, by site

racemose (M9123/0) — see Hemangioma, by site

retina 228.03

retroperitoneal tissue 228.04

sclerosing (M8832/0) — see Neoplasm, skin, benign

simplex (M9131/0) — see Hemangioma, by site

skin and subcutaneous tissue 228.01

specified site NEC 228.09

spinal cord 228.09

Hemangioma — continued

venous (M9122/0) — see Hemangioma, by site

verrucous keratotic (M9142/0) — see Hemangioma, by site

Hemangiomatosis (systemic) 757.32

involving single site — see Hemangioma

Hemangiopericytoma (M9150/1) — see also Neoplasm, connective tissue, uncertain behavior

benign (M9150/0) — see Neoplasm, connective tissue, benign

malignant (M9150/3) — see Neoplasm, connective tissue, malignant

Hemangiosarcoma (M9120/3) — see Neoplasm, connective tissue, malignant

Hemarthrosis (nontraumatic) 719.10

ankle 719.17

elbow 719.12

foot 719.17

hand 719.14

hip 719.15

knee 719.16

multiple sites 719.19

pelvic region 719.15

shoulder (region) 719.11

specified site NEC 719.18

traumatic — see Sprain, by site

wrist 719.13

Hematemesis 578.0

with ulcer — see Ulcer, by site, with hemorrhage

due to S. japonicum 120.2

Goldstein's (familial hemorrhagic telangiectasia) 448.0

newborn 772.4

due to swallowed maternal blood 777.3

Hematidrosis 705.89

Hematinuria — see also Hemoglobinuria 791.2

malarial 084.8

paroxysmal 283.2

Hematite miners' lung 503

Hematobilia 576.8

Hematocele (congenital) (diffuse) (idiopathic) 608.83

broad ligament 620.7

canal of Nuck 629.0

cord, male 608.83

fallopian tube 620.8

female NEC 629.0

ischiorectal 569.89

male NEC 608.83

ovary 629.0

pelvis, pelvic

female 629.0

with ectopic pregnancy (see also Pregnancy, ectopic) 633.90

with intrauterine pregnancy 633.91

male 608.83

periuterine 629.0

retrouterine 629.0

scrotum 608.83

spermatic cord (diffuse) 608.83

testis 608.84

traumatic — see Injury, internal, pelvis

tunica vaginalis 608.83

uterine ligament 629.0

uterus 621.4

vagina 623.6

vulva 624.5

Hematocephalus 742.4

Hematochezia — see also Melena 578.1

Hematochyluria — see also Infestation, filarial 125.9

Hematocolpos 626.8

Hematocornea 371.12

Hematogenous — see condition

Hematoma (skin surface intact) (traumatic) — see also Contusion

Note — Hematomas are coded according to origin and the nature and site of the hematoma or the accompanying injury. Hematomas of unspecified origin are coded as injuries of the sites involved, except:

(a) hematomas of genital organs which are coded as diseases of the organ involved unless they complicate pregnancy or delivery

(b) hematomas of the eye which are coded as diseases of the eye.

For late effect of hematoma classifiable to 920–924 see Late, effect, contusion

with

crush injury — see Crush

fracture — see Fracture, by site

injury of internal organs (see also Injury, internal, by site)

kidney — see Hematoma, kidney, traumatic

liver — see Hematoma, liver, traumatic

spleen — see Hematoma, spleen

nerve injury — see Injury, nerve

open wound — see Wound, open, by site

skin surface intact — see Contusion

abdomen (wall) — see Contusion, abdomen

amnion 658.8 ☑

aorta, dissecting 441.00

abdominal 441.02

thoracic 441.01

thoracoabdominal 441.03

aortic intramural — see Dissection, aorta

arterial (complicating trauma) 904.9

specified site — see Injury, blood vessel, by site

auricle (ear) 380.31

birth injury 767.8

skull 767.19

brain (traumatic) 853.0 ☑

Note — Use the following fifth-digit subclassification with categories 851–854:

0 unspecified state of consciousness

1 with no loss of consciousness

2 with brief [less than one hour] loss of consciousness

3 with moderate [1–24 hours] loss of consciousness

4 with prolonged [more than 24 hours] loss of consciousness and return to pre–existing conscious level

5 with prolonged [more than 24 hours] loss of consciousness, without return to pre–existing conscious level

Use fifth-digit 5 to designate when a patient is unconscious and dies before regaining consciousness, regardless of the duration of the loss of consciousness

6 with loss of consciousness of unspecified duration

9 with concussion, unspecified

with

cerebral

contusion — see Contusion, brain

laceration — see Laceration, brain

open intracranial wound 853.1 ☑

skull fracture — see Fracture, skull, by site

extradural or epidural 852.4 ☑

with open intracranial wound 852.5 ☑

fetus or newborn 767.0

Hematoma — see also Contusion — continued

brain — continued

extradural or epidural — continued

nontraumatic 432.0

fetus or newborn NEC 767.0

nontraumatic (see also Hemorrhage, brain) 431

epidural or extradural 432.0

newborn NEC 772.8

subarachnoid, arachnoid, or meningeal (see also Hemorrhage, subarachnoid) 430

subdural (see also Hemorrhage, subdural) 432.1

subarachnoid, arachnoid, or meningeal 852.0 ☑

with open intracranial wound 852.1 ☑

fetus or newborn 772.2

nontraumatic (see also Hemorrhage, subarachnoid) 430

subdural 852.2 ☑

with open intracranial wound 852.3 ☑

fetus or newborn (localized) 767.0

nontraumatic (see also Hemorrhage, subdural) 432.1

breast (nontraumatic) 611.89

broad ligament (nontraumatic) 620.7

complicating delivery 665.7 ☑

traumatic — see Injury, internal, broad ligament

calcified NEC 959.9

capitis 920

due to birth injury 767.19

newborn 767.19

cerebral — see Hematoma, brain

cesarean section wound 674.3 ☑

chorion — see Placenta, abnormal

complicating delivery (perineum) (vulva) 664.5 ☑

pelvic 665.7 ☑

vagina 665.7 ☑

corpus

cavernosum (nontraumatic) 607.82

luteum (nontraumatic) (ruptured) 620.1

dura (mater) — see Hematoma, brain, subdural

epididymis (nontraumatic) 608.83

epidural (traumatic) (see also Hematoma, brain, extradural)

spinal — see Injury, spinal, by site

episiotomy 674.3 ☑

external ear 380.31

extradural (see also Hematoma, brain, extradural)

fetus or newborn 767.0

nontraumatic 432.0

fetus or newborn 767.0

fallopian tube 620.8

genital organ (nontraumatic)

female NEC 629.89

male NEC 608.83

traumatic (external site) 922.4

internal — see Injury, internal, genital organ

graafian follicle (ruptured) 620.0

internal organs (abdomen, chest, or pelvis) (see also Injury, internal, by site)

kidney — see Hematoma, kidney, traumatic

liver — see Hematoma, liver, traumatic

spleen — see Hematoma, spleen

intracranial — see Hematoma, brain

kidney, cystic 593.81

traumatic 866.01

with open wound into cavity 866.11

labia (nontraumatic) 624.5

lingual (and other parts of neck, scalp, or face, except eye) 920

liver (subcapsular) 573.8

birth injury 767.8

fetus or newborn 767.8

traumatic NEC 864.01

Hematoma — *see also* Contusion — *continued*
  liver — *continued*
    traumatic — *continued*
      with
        laceration — *see* Laceration, liver
        open wound into cavity 864.11
  mediastinum — *see* Injury, internal, mediastinum
  meninges, meningeal (brain) (*see also* Hematoma, brain, subarachnoid)
    spinal — *see* Injury, spinal, by site
  mesosalpinx (nontraumatic) 620.8
    traumatic — *see* Injury, internal, pelvis
  muscle (traumatic) — *see* Contusion, by site
    nontraumatic 729.92
  nasal (septum) (and other part(s) of neck, scalp, or face, except eye) 920
  obstetrical surgical wound 674.3 ☑
  orbit, orbital (nontraumatic) 376.32
    traumatic 921.2
  ovary (corpus luteum) (nontraumatic) 620.1
    traumatic — *see* Injury, internal, ovary
  pelvis (female) (nontraumatic) 629.89
    complicating delivery 665.7 ☑
    male 608.83
    traumatic (*see also* Injury, internal, pelvis)
      specified organ NEC (*see also* Injury, internal, pelvis) 867.6
  penis (nontraumatic) 607.82
  pericranial (and neck, or face any part, except eye) 920
    due to injury at birth 767.19
  perineal wound (obstetrical) 674.3 ☑
    complicating delivery 664.5 ☑
  perirenal, cystic 593.81
  pinna 380.31
  placenta — *see* Placenta, abnormal
  postoperative 998.12
  retroperitoneal (nontraumatic) 568.81
    traumatic — *see* Injury, internal, retroperitoneum
  retropubic, male 568.81
  scalp (and neck, or face any part, except eye) 920
    fetus or newborn 767.19
  scrotum (nontraumatic) 608.83
    traumatic 922.4
  seminal vesicle (nontraumatic) 608.83
    traumatic — *see* Injury, internal, seminal, vesicle
  soft tissue 729.92
  spermatic cord (*see also* Injury, internal, spermatic cord)
    nontraumatic 608.83
  spinal (cord) (meninges) (*see also* Injury, spinal, by site)
    fetus or newborn 767.4
    nontraumatic 336.1
  spleen 865.01
    with
      laceration — *see* Laceration, spleen
      open wound into cavity 865.11
  sternocleidomastoid, birth injury 767.8
  sternomastoid, birth injury 767.8
  subarachnoid (*see also* Hematoma, brain, subarachnoid)
    fetus or newborn 772.2
    nontraumatic (*see also* Hemorrhage, subarachnoid) 430
    newborn 772.2
  subdural (*see also* Hematoma, brain, subdural)
    fetus or newborn (localized) 767.0
    nontraumatic (*see also* Hemorrhage, subdural) 432.1
  subperiosteal (syndrome) 267
    traumatic — *see* Hematoma, by site
  superficial, fetus or newborn 772.6
  syncytium — *see* Placenta, abnormal
  testis (nontraumatic) 608.83
    birth injury 767.8
    traumatic 922.4
  tunica vaginalis (nontraumatic) 608.83
  umbilical cord 663.6 ☑
    affecting fetus or newborn 762.6

Hematoma — *see also* Contusion — *continued*
  uterine ligament (nontraumatic) 620.7
    traumatic — *see* Injury, internal, pelvis
  uterus 621.4
    traumatic — *see* Injury, internal, pelvis
  vagina (nontraumatic) (ruptured) 623.6
    complicating delivery 665.7 ☑
    traumatic 922.4
  vas deferens (nontraumatic) 608.83
    traumatic — *see* Injury, internal, vas deferens
  vitreous 379.23
  vocal cord 920
  vulva (nontraumatic) 624.5
    complicating delivery 664.5 ☑
    fetus or newborn 767.8
    traumatic 922.4
Hematometra 621.4
Hematomyelia 336.1
  with fracture of vertebra (*see also* Fracture, vertebra, by site, with spinal cord injury) 806.8
  fetus or newborn 767.4
Hematomyelitis 323.9
  late effect — *see* category 326
Hematoperitoneum — *see also* Hemoperitoneum 568.81
Hematopneumothorax — *see also* Hemothorax 511.89
Hematopoiesis, cyclic 288.02
Hematoporphyria (acquired) (congenital) 277.1
Hematoporphyrinuria (acquired) (congenital) 277.1
Hematorachis, hematorrhachis 336.1
  fetus or newborn 767.4
Hematosalpinx 620.8
  with
    ectopic pregnancy (*see also* categories 633.0–633.9) 639.2
    infectional (*see also* Salpingo-oophoritis) 614.2
    molar pregnancy (*see also* categories 630–632) 639.2
Hematospermia 608.82
Hematothorax — *see also* Hemothorax 511.89
Hematotympanum 381.03
Hematuria (benign) (essential) (idiopathic) 599.70
  due to S. hematobium 120.0
  endemic 120.0
  gross 599.71
  intermittent 599.70
  malarial 084.8
  microscopic 599.72
  paroxysmal 599.70
  sulfonamide
    correct substance properly administered 599.70
    overdose or wrong substance given or taken 961.0
  tropical (bilharziasis) 120.0
  tuberculous (*see also* Tuberculosis) 016.9 ☑
Hematuric bilious fever 084.8
Hemeralopia 368.10
Hemiabiotrophy 799.89
Hemi-akinesia 781.8
Hemianalgesia — *see also* Disturbance, sensation 782.0
Hemianencephaly 740.0
Hemianesthesia — *see also* Disturbance, sensation 782.0
Hemianopia, hemianopsia (altitudinal) (homonymous) 368.46
  binasal 368.47
  bitemporal 368.47
  heteronymous 368.47
  syphilitic 095.8
Hemiasomatognosia 307.9
Hemiathetosis 781.0
Hemiatrophy 799.89
  cerebellar 334.8
  face 349.89
    progressive 349.89
  fascia 728.9

Hemiatrophy — *continued*
  leg 728.2
  tongue 529.8
Hemiballism (us) 333.5
Hemiblock (cardiac) (heart) (left) 426.2
Hemicardia 746.89
Hemicephalus, hemicephaly 740.0
Hemichorea 333.5
Hemicrania 346.9 ☑
  congenital malformation 740.0
  continua 339.41
  paroxysmal 339.03
    chronic 339.04
    episodic 339.03
Hemidystrophy — *see* Hemiatrophy
Hemiectromelia 755.4
Hemihypalgesia — *see also* Disturbance, sensation 782.0
Hemihypertrophy (congenital) 759.89
  cranial 756.0
Hemihypesthesia — *see also* Disturbance, sensation 782.0
Hemi-inattention 781.8
Hemimelia 755.4
  lower limb 755.30
    paraxial (complete) (incomplete) (intercalary) (terminal) 755.32
      fibula 755.37
      tibia 755.36
    transverse (complete) (partial) 755.31
  upper limb 755.20
    paraxial (complete) (incomplete) (intercalary) (terminal) 755.22
      radial 755.26
      ulnar 755.27
    transverse (complete) (partial) 755.21
Hemiparalysis — *see also* Hemiplegia 342.9 ☑
Hemiparesis — *see also* Hemiplegia 342.9 ☑
Hemiparesthesia — *see also* Disturbance, sensation 782.0
Hemiplegia 342.9 ☑
  acute (*see also* Disease, cerebrovascular, acute) 436
  alternans facialis 344.89
  apoplectic (*see also* Disease, cerebrovascular, acute) 436
    late effect or residual
      affecting
        dominant side 438.21
        nondominant side 438.22
        unspecified side 438.20
  arteriosclerotic 437.0
    late effect or residual
      affecting
        dominant side 438.21
        nondominant side 438.22
        unspecified side 438.20
  ascending (spinal) NEC 344.89
  attack (*see also* Disease, cerebrovascular, acute) 436
  brain, cerebral (current episode) 437.8
    congenital 343.1
  cerebral — *see* Hemiplegia, brain
  congenital (cerebral) (spastic) (spinal) 343.1
  conversion neurosis (hysterical) 300.11
  cortical — *see* Hemiplegia, brain
  due to
    arteriosclerosis 437.0
      late effect or residual
        affecting
          dominant side 438.21
          nondominant side 438.22
          unspecified side 438.20
    cerebrovascular lesion (*see also* Disease, cerebrovascular, acute) 436
      late effect
        affecting
          dominant side 438.21
          nondominant side 438.22
          unspecified side 438.20
  embolic (current) (*see also* Embolism, brain) 434.1 ☑
    late effect
      affecting
        dominant side 438.21
        nondominant side 438.22

Hemiplegia — *continued*
  embolic (*see also* Embolism, brain) — *continued*
    late effect — *continued*
      affecting — *continued*
        unspecified side 438.20
  flaccid 342.0 ☑
  hypertensive (current episode) 437.8
  infantile (postnatal) 343.4
  late effect
    birth injury, intracranial or spinal 343.4
    cerebrovascular lesion — *see* Late effect(s) (of) cerebrovascular disease
    viral encephalitis 139.0
  middle alternating NEC 344.89
  newborn NEC 767.0
  seizure (current episode) (*see also* Disease, cerebrovascular, acute) 436
  spastic 342.1 ☑
    congenital or infantile 343.1
  specified NEC 342.8 ☑
  thrombotic (current) (*see also* Thrombosis, brain) 434.0 ☑
    late effect — *see* Late effect(s) (of) cerebrovascular disease
Hemisection, spinal cord — *see* Fracture, vertebra, by site, with spinal cord injury
Hemispasm 781.0
  facial 781.0
Hemispatial neglect 781.8
Hemisporosis 117.9
Hemitremor 781.0
Hemivertebra 756.14
Hemobilia 576.8
Hemocholecyst 575.8
Hemochromatosis (acquired) (liver) (myocardium) (secondary) 275.03
  with refractory anemia 238.72
  diabetic 275.03
  due to repeated red blood cell transfusions 275.02
  hereditary 275.01
  primary idiopathic 275.01
  specified NEC 275.03
  transfusion associated (red blood cell) 275.02
Hemodialysis V56.0
Hemoglobin — *see also* condition
  abnormal (disease) — *see* Disease, hemoglobin
  AS genotype 282.5
  fetal, hereditary persistence 282.7
  H Constant Spring 282.43
  H disease 282.43
  high-oxygen-affinity 289.0
  low NEC 285.9
  S (Hb-S), heterozygous 282.5
Hemoglobinemia 283.2
  due to blood transfusion NEC 999.89
    bone marrow 996.85
  paroxysmal 283.2
Hemoglobinopathy (mixed) — *see also* Disease, hemoglobin 282.7
  with thalassemia 282.49
  sickle-cell 282.60
    with thalassemia (without crisis) 282.41
    with
      crisis 282.42
      vaso-occlusive pain 282.42
Hemoglobinuria, hemoglobinuric 791.2
  with anemia, hemolytic, acquired (chronic) NEC 283.2
  cold (agglutinin) (paroxysmal) (with Raynaud's syndrome) 283.2
  due to
    exertion 283.2
    hemolysis (from external causes) NEC 283.2
  exercise 283.2
  fever (malaria) 084.8
  infantile 791.2
  intermittent 283.2
  malarial 084.8
  march 283.2
  nocturnal (paroxysmal) 283.2

☑ **Additional Digit Required** — Refer to the Tabular List for Digit Selection   Subterms under main terms may continue to next column or page

134 — Volume 2   ▶◀ Revised Text   ● New Line   ▲ Revised Code   2013 ICD-9-CM

Hemoglobinuria, hemoglobinuric —
continued
  paroxysmal (cold) (nocturnal) 283.2
Hemolymphangioma (M9175/0) 228.1
Hemolysis
  fetal — *see* Jaundice, fetus or newborn
  intravascular (disseminated) NEC 286.6
    with
      abortion — *see* Abortion, by type,
        with hemorrhage, delayed or
        excessive
      ectopic pregnancy (*see also* cate-
        gories 633.0–633.9) 639.1
      hemorrhage of pregnancy 641.3 ☑
        affecting fetus or newborn 762.1
      molar pregnancy (*see also* categories
        630–632) 639.1
    acute 283.2
    following
      abortion 639.1
      ectopic or molar pregnancy 639.1
    neonatal — *see* Jaundice, fetus or newborn
    transfusion NEC 999.89
  bone marrow 996.85
Hemolytic — *see also* condition
  anemia — *see* Anemia, hemolytic
  uremic syndrome 283.11
Hemometra 621.4
Hemopericardium (with effusion) 423.0
  newborn 772.8
  traumatic (*see also* Hemothorax, traumatic)
    860.2
    with open wound into thorax 860.3
Hemoperitoneum 568.81
  infectional (*see also* Peritonitis) 567.29
  traumatic — *see* Injury, internal, peritoneum
Hemophagocytic syndrome 288.4
  infection-associated 288.4
Hemophilia (familial) (hereditary) 286.0
  A 286.0
    carrier (asymptomatic) V83.01
      symptomatic V83.02
  acquired 286.52
  autoimmune 286.52
  B (Leyden) 286.1
  C 286.2
  calcipriva (*see also* Fibrinolysis) 286.7
  classical 286.0
  nonfamilial 286.7
  secondary 286.52
  vascular 286.4
Hemophilus influenzae NEC 041.5
  arachnoiditis (basic) (brain) (spinal) 320.0
    late effect — *see* category 326
  bronchopneumonia 482.2
  cerebral ventriculitis 320.0
    late effect — *see* category 326
  cerebrospinal inflammation 320.0
    late effect — *see* category 326
  infection NEC 041.5
  leptomeningitis 320.0
    late effect — *see* category 326
  meningitis (cerebral) (cerebrospinal) (spinal)
    320.0
    late effect — *see* category 326
  meningomyelitis 320.0
    late effect — *see* category 326
  pachymeningitis (adhesive) (fibrous) (hem-
    orrhagic) (hypertrophic) (spinal)
    320.0
    late effect — *see* category 326
  pneumonia (broncho-) 482.2
Hemophthalmos 360.43
Hemopneumothorax — *see also* Hemothorax
  511.89
  traumatic 860.4
    with open wound into thorax 860.5
Hemoptysis 786.30
  due to Paragonimus (westermani) 121.2
  newborn 770.3
  specified NEC 786.39
  tuberculous (*see also* Tuberculosis, pul-
    monary) 011.9 ☑
Hemorrhage, hemorrhagic (nontraumatic)
  459.0
  abdomen 459.0

Hemorrhage, hemorrhagic — *continued*
  accidental (antepartum) 641.2 ☑
    affecting fetus or newborn 762.1
  adenoid 474.8
  adrenal (capsule) (gland) (medulla) 255.41
    newborn 772.5
  after labor — *see* Hemorrhage, postpartum
  alveolar
    lung, newborn 770.3
    process 525.8
  alveolus 525.8
  amputation stump (surgical) 998.11
    secondary, delayed 997.69
  anemia (chronic) 280.0
    acute 285.1
  antepartum — *see* Hemorrhage, pregnancy
  anus (sphincter) 569.3
  apoplexy (stroke) 432.9
  arachnoid — *see* Hemorrhage, subarach-
    noid
  artery NEC 459.0
    brain (*see also* Hemorrhage, brain) 431
    middle meningeal — *see* Hemorrhage,
      subarachnoid
  basilar (ganglion) (*see also* Hemorrhage,
    brain) 431
  bladder 596.89
  blood dyscrasia 289.9
  bowel 578.9
    newborn 772.4
  brain (miliary) (nontraumatic) 431
    with
      birth injury 767.0
    arachnoid — *see* Hemorrhage, subarach-
      noid
    due to
      birth injury 767.0
      rupture of aneurysm (congenital) (*see
        also* Hemorrhage, subarach-
        noid) 430
      mycotic 431
      syphilis 094.89
    epidural or extradural — *see* Hemor-
      rhage, extradural
    fetus or newborn (anoxic) (hypoxic) (due
      to birth trauma) (nontraumatic)
      767.0
      intraventricular 772.10
        grade I 772.11
        grade II 772.12
        grade III 772.13
        grade IV 772.14
    iatrogenic 997.02
    postoperative 997.02
    puerperal, postpartum, childbirth
      674.0 ☑
    stem 431
    subarachnoid, arachnoid, or meningeal
      — *see* Hemorrhage, subarach-
      noid
    subdural — *see* Hemorrhage, subdural

Hemorrhage, hemorrhagic — *continued*
  brain — *continued*
    traumatic NEC 853.0 ☑

> *Note* — *Use the following fifth-digit
> subclassification with categories
> 851–854:*
>
> 0 *unspecified state of consciousness*
>
> 1 *with no loss of consciousness*
>
> 2 *with brief [less than one hour]
> loss of consciousness*
>
> 3 *with moderate [1–24 hours] loss
> of consciousness*
>
> 4 *with prolonged [more than 24
> hours] loss of consciousness and
> return to pre–existing conscious
> level*
>
> 5 *with prolonged [more than 24
> hours] loss of consciousness,
> without return to pre–existing
> conscious level*
>
> *Use fifth-digit 5 to designate when a
> patient is unconscious and dies before
> regaining consciousness, regardless of
> the duration of the loss of consciousness*
>
> 6 *with loss of consciousness of un-
> specified duration*
>
> 9 *with concussion, unspecified*

      with
        cerebral
          contusion — *see* Contusion,
            brain
          laceration — *see* Laceration,
            brain
        open intracranial wound 853.1 ☑
        skull fracture — *see* Fracture,
          skull, by site
      extradural or epidural 852.4 ☑
        with open intracranial wound
          852.5 ☑
      subarachnoid 852.0 ☑
        with open intracranial wound
          852.1 ☑
      subdural 852.2 ☑
        with open intracranial wound
          852.3 ☑
  breast 611.79
  bronchial tube — *see* Hemorrhage, lung
  bronchopulmonary — *see* Hemorrhage,
    lung
  bronchus (cause unknown) (*see also* Hemor-
    rhage, lung) 786.30
  bulbar (*see also* Hemorrhage, brain) 431
  bursa 727.89
  capillary 448.9
    primary 287.8
  capsular — *see* Hemorrhage, brain
  cardiovascular 429.89
  cecum 578.9
  cephalic (*see also* Hemorrhage, brain) 431
  cerebellar (*see also* Hemorrhage, brain) 431
  cerebellum (*see also* Hemorrhage, brain) 431
  cerebral (*see also* Hemorrhage, brain) 431
    fetus or newborn (anoxic) (traumatic)
      767.0
  cerebromeningeal (*see also* Hemorrhage,
    brain) 431
  cerebrospinal (*see also* Hemorrhage, brain)
    431
  cerebrovascular accident — *see* Hemor-
    rhage, brain
  cerebrum (*see also* Hemorrhage, brain) 431
  cervix (stump) (uteri) 622.8
  cesarean section wound 674.3 ☑
  chamber, anterior (eye) 364.41
  childbirth — *see* Hemorrhage, complicating,
    delivery
  choroid 363.61
    expulsive 363.62
  ciliary body 364.41
  cochlea 386.8
  colon — *see* Hemorrhage, intestine

Hemorrhage, hemorrhagic — *continued*
  complicating
    delivery 641.9 ☑
      affecting fetus or newborn 762.1
      associated with
        afibrinogenemia 641.3 ☑
          affecting fetus or newborn
            763.89
        coagulation defect 641.3 ☑
          affecting fetus or newborn
            763.89
        hyperfibrinolysis 641.3 ☑
          affecting fetus or newborn
            763.89
        hypofibrinogenemia 641.3 ☑
          affecting fetus or newborn
            763.89
      due to
        low-lying placenta 641.1 ☑
          affecting fetus or newborn
            762.0
        placenta previa 641.1 ☑
          affecting fetus or newborn
            762.0
        premature separation of placenta
          641.2 ☑
          affecting fetus or newborn
            762.1
      retained
        placenta 666.0 ☑
        secundines 666.2 ☑
      trauma 641.8 ☑
        affecting fetus or newborn
          763.89
      uterine leiomyoma 641.8 ☑
        affecting fetus or newborn
          763.89
    surgical procedure 998.11
  complication(s)
    of dental implant placement 525.71
  concealed NEC 459.0
  congenital 772.9
  conjunctiva 372.72
    newborn 772.8
  cord, newborn 772.0
    slipped ligature 772.3
    stump 772.3
  corpus luteum (ruptured) 620.1
  cortical (*see also* Hemorrhage, brain) 431
  cranial 432.9
  cutaneous 782.7
    newborn 772.6
  cystitis — *see* Cystitis
  cyst, pancreas 577.2
  delayed
    with
      abortion — *see* Abortion, by type,
        with hemorrhage, delayed or
        excessive
      ectopic pregnancy (*see also* cate-
        gories 633.0–633.9) 639.1
      molar pregnancy (*see also* categories
        630–632) 639.1
    following
      abortion 639.1
      ectopic or molar pregnancy 639.1
    postpartum 666.2 ☑
  diathesis (familial) 287.9
    newborn 776.0
  disease 287.9
    newborn 776.0
    specified type NEC 287.8
  disorder 287.9
    due to intrinsic circulating anticoagu-
      lants, antibodies, or inhibitors
      286.59
      with
        acquired hemophilia 286.52
        antiphospholipid antibody 286.53
    specified type NEC 287.8
  due to
    any device, implant or graft (presence
      of) classifiable to 996.0–996.5 —
      see Complications, due to (pres-
      ence of) any device, implant, or
      graft classified to 996.0–996.5NEC

☑ **Additional Digit Required — Refer to the Tabular List for Digit Selection**   ☝ **Subterms under main terms may continue to next column or page**

2013 ICD-9-CM   ▶◀ **Revised Text**   ● **New Line**   ▲ **Revised Code**   **Volume 2 — 135**

Index — Hemorrhage, hemorrhagic — Hemorrhage, hemorrhagic

Hemorrhage, hemorrhagic — *continued*
due to — *continued*
intrinsic circulating anticoagulant, antibodies, or inhibitors 286.59
with
acquired hemophilia 286.52
antiphospholipid antibody 286.53
duodenum, duodenal 537.89
ulcer — *see* Ulcer, duodenum, with hemorrhage
dura mater — *see* Hemorrhage, subdural
endotracheal — *see* Hemorrhage, lung
epicranial subaponeurotic (massive) 767.11
epidural — *see* Hemorrhage, extradural
episiotomy 674.3 ☑
esophagus 530.82
varix (*see also* Varix, esophagus, bleeding) 456.0
excessive
with
abortion — *see* Abortion, by type, with hemorrhage, delayed or excessive
ectopic pregnancy (*see also* categories 633.0–633.9) 639.1
molar pregnancy (*see also* categories 630–632) 639.1
following
abortion 639.1
ectopic or molar pregnancy 639.1
external 459.0
extradural (traumatic) (*see also* Hemorrhage, brain, traumatic, extradural)
birth injury 767.0
fetus or newborn (anoxic) (traumatic) 767.0
nontraumatic 432.0
eye 360.43
chamber (anterior) (aqueous) 364.41
fundus 362.81
eyelid 374.81
fallopian tube 620.8
fetomaternal 772.0
affecting management of pregnancy or puerperium 656.0 ☑
fetus, fetal, affecting newborn 772.0
from
cut end of co-twin's cord 772.0
placenta 772.0
ruptured cord 772.0
vasa previa 772.0
into
co-twin 772.0
mother's circulation 772.0
affecting management of pregnancy or puerperium 656.0 ☑
fever (*see also* Fever, hemorrhagic) 065.9
with renal syndrome 078.6
arthropod-borne NEC 065.9
Bangkok 065.4
Crimean 065.0
dengue virus 065.4
epidemic 078.6
Junin virus 078.7
Korean 078.6
Machupo virus 078.7
mite-borne 065.8
mosquito-borne 065.4
Philippine 065.4
Russian (Yaroslav) 078.6
Singapore 065.4
southeast Asia 065.4
Thailand 065.4
tick-borne NEC 065.3
fibrinogenolysis (*see also* Fibrinolysis) 286.6
fibrinolytic (acquired) (*see also* Fibrinolysis) 286.6
fontanel 767.19
from tracheostomy stoma 519.09
fundus, eye 362.81
funis
affecting fetus or newborn 772.0
complicating delivery 663.8 ☑
gastric (*see also* Hemorrhage, stomach) 578.9

Hemorrhage, hemorrhagic — *continued*
gastroenteric 578.9
newborn 772.4
gastrointestinal (tract) 578.9
newborn 772.4
genitourinary (tract) NEC 599.89
gingiva 523.8
globe 360.43
gravidarum — *see* Hemorrhage, pregnancy
gum 523.8
heart 429.89
hypopharyngeal (throat) 784.8
intermenstrual 626.6
irregular 626.6
regular 626.5
internal (organs) 459.0
capsule (*see also* Hemorrhage, brain) 431
ear 386.8
newborn 772.8
intestine 578.9
congenital 772.4
newborn 772.4
into
bladder wall 596.7
bursa 727.89
corpus luysii (*see also* Hemorrhage, brain) 431
intra-abdominal 459.0
during or following surgery 998.11
intra-alveolar, newborn (lung) 770.3
intracerebral (*see also* Hemorrhage, brain) 431
intracranial NEC 432.9
puerperal, postpartum, childbirth 674.0 ☑
traumatic — *see* Hemorrhage, brain, traumatic
intramedullary NEC 336.1
intraocular 360.43
intraoperative 998.11
intrapartum — *see* Hemorrhage, complicating, delivery
intrapelvic
female 629.89
male 459.0
intraperitoneal 459.0
intrapontine (*see also* Hemorrhage, brain) 431
intrauterine 621.4
complicating delivery — *see* Hemorrhage, complicating, delivery
in pregnancy or childbirth — *see* Hemorrhage, pregnancy
postpartum (*see also* Hemorrhage, postpartum) 666.1 ☑
intraventricular (*see also* Hemorrhage, brain) 431
fetus or newborn (anoxic) (traumatic) 772.10
grade I 772.11
grade II 772.12
grade III 772.13
grade IV 772.14
intravesical 596.7
iris (postinfectional) (postinflammatory) (toxic) 364.41
joint (nontraumatic) 719.10
ankle 719.17
elbow 719.12
foot 719.17
forearm 719.13
hand 719.14
hip 719.15
knee 719.16
lower leg 719.16
multiple sites 719.19
pelvic region 719.15
shoulder (region) 719.11
specified site NEC 719.18
thigh 719.15
upper arm 719.12
wrist 719.13
kidney 593.81
knee (joint) 719.16
labyrinth 386.8
leg NEC 459.0

Hemorrhage, hemorrhagic — *continued*
lenticular striate artery (*see also* Hemorrhage, brain) 431
ligature, vessel 998.11
liver 573.8
lower extremity NEC 459.0
lung 786.30
newborn 770.3
tuberculous (*see also* Tuberculosis, pulmonary) 011.9 ☑
malaria 084.8
marginal sinus 641.2 ☑
massive subaponeurotic, birth injury 767.11
maternal, affecting fetus or newborn 762.1
mediastinum 786.30
medulla (*see also* Hemorrhage, brain) 431
membrane (brain) (*see also* Hemorrhage, subarachnoid) 430
spinal cord — *see* Hemorrhage, spinal cord
meninges, meningeal (brain) (middle) (*see also* Hemorrhage, subarachnoid) 430
spinal cord — *see* Hemorrhage, spinal cord
mesentery 568.81
metritis 626.8
midbrain (*see also* Hemorrhage, brain) 431
mole 631.8
mouth 528.9
mucous membrane NEC 459.0
newborn 772.8
muscle 728.89
nail (subungual) 703.8
nasal turbinate 784.7
newborn 772.8
nasopharynx 478.29
navel, newborn 772.3
newborn 772.9
adrenal 772.5
alveolar (lung) 770.3
brain (anoxic) (hypoxic) (due to birth trauma) 767.0
cerebral (anoxic) (hypoxic) (due to birth trauma) 767.0
conjunctiva 772.8
cutaneous 772.6
diathesis 776.0
due to vitamin K deficiency 776.0
epicranial subaponeurotic (massive) 767.11
gastrointestinal 772.4
internal (organs) 772.8
intestines 772.4
intra-alveolar (lung) 770.3
intracranial (from any perinatal cause) 767.0
intraventricular (from any perinatal cause) 772.10
grade I 772.11
grade II 772.12
grade III 772.13
grade IV 772.14
lung 770.3
pulmonary (massive) 770.3
spinal cord, traumatic 767.4
stomach 772.4
subaponeurotic (massive) 767.11
subarachnoid (from any perinatal cause) 772.2
subconjunctival 772.8
subgaleal 767.11
umbilicus 772.0
slipped ligature 772.3
vasa previa 772.0
nipple 611.79
nose 784.7
newborn 772.8
obstetrical surgical wound 674.3 ☑
omentum 568.89
newborn 772.4
optic nerve (sheath) 377.42
orbit 376.32
ovary 620.1
oviduct 620.8
pancreas 577.8
parathyroid (gland) (spontaneous) 252.8

Hemorrhage, hemorrhagic — *continued*
parturition — *see* Hemorrhage, complicating, delivery
penis 607.82
pericardium, pericarditis 423.0
perineal wound (obstetrical) 674.3 ☑
peritoneum, peritoneal 459.0
peritonsillar tissue 474.8
after operation on tonsils 998.11
due to infection 475
petechial 782.7
pituitary (gland) 253.8
placenta NEC 641.9 ☑
affecting fetus or newborn 762.1
from surgical or instrumental damage 641.8 ☑
affecting fetus or newborn 762.1
previa 641.1 ☑
affecting fetus or newborn 762.0
pleura — *see* Hemorrhage, lung
polioencephalitis, superior 265.1
polymyositis — *see* Polymyositis
pons (*see also* Hemorrhage, brain) 431
pontine (*see also* Hemorrhage, brain) 431
popliteal 459.0
postcoital 626.7
postextraction (dental) 998.11
postmenopausal 627.1
postnasal 784.7
postoperative 998.11
postpartum (atonic) (following delivery of placenta) 666.1 ☑
delayed or secondary (after 24 hours) 666.2 ☑
retained placenta 666.0 ☑
third stage 666.0 ☑
pregnancy (concealed) 641.9 ☑
accidental 641.2 ☑
affecting fetus or newborn 762.1
before 22 completed weeks gestation 640.9 ☑
affecting fetus or newborn 762.1
due to
abruptio placenta 641.2 ☑
affecting fetus or newborn 762.1
afibrinogenemia or other coagulation defect (conditions classifiable to 286.0–286.9) 641.3 ☑
affecting fetus or newborn 762.1
coagulation defect 641.3 ☑
affecting fetus or newborn 762.1
hyperfibrinolysis 641.3 ☑
affecting fetus or newborn 762.1
hypofibrinogenemia 641.3 ☑
affecting fetus or newborn 762.1
leiomyoma, uterus 641.8 ☑
affecting fetus or newborn 762.1
low-lying placenta 641.1 ☑
affecting fetus or newborn 762.1
marginal sinus (rupture) 641.2 ☑
affecting fetus or newborn 762.1
placenta previa 641.1 ☑
affecting fetus or newborn 762.0
premature separation of placenta (normally implanted) 641.2 ☑
affecting fetus or newborn 762.1
threatened abortion 640.0 ☑
affecting fetus or newborn 762.1
trauma 641.8 ☑
affecting fetus or newborn 762.1
early (before 22 completed weeks gestation) 640.9 ☑
affecting fetus or newborn 762.1
previous, affecting management of pregnancy or childbirth V23.49
unavoidable — *see* Hemorrhage, pregnancy, due to placenta previa
prepartum (mother) — *see* Hemorrhage, pregnancy
preretinal, cause unspecified 362.81
prostate 602.1
puerperal (*see also* Hemorrhage, postpartum) 666.1 ☑

Hemorrhage, hemorrhagic — *continued*
  pulmonary (*see also* Hemorrhage, lung)
    786.30
      acute idiopathic in infants (AIPHI) (over
        28 days old) 786.31
      newborn (massive) 770.3
      renal syndrome 446.21
  purpura (primary) (*see also* Purpura, throm-
    bocytopenic) 287.39
  rectum (sphincter) 569.3
  recurring, following initial hemorrhage at
    time of injury 958.2
  renal 593.81
    pulmonary syndrome 446.21
  respiratory tract (*see also* Hemorrhage, lung)
    786.30
  retina, retinal (deep) (superficial) (vessels)
    362.81
    diabetic 250.5 ☑ *[362.01]*
      due to secondary diabetes
        249.5 ☑ *[362.01]*
    due to birth injury 772.8
  retrobulbar 376.89
  retroperitoneal 459.0
  retroplacental (*see also* Placenta, separation)
    641.2 ☑
  scalp 459.0
    due to injury at birth 767.19
  scrotum 608.83
  secondary (nontraumatic) 459.0
    following initial hemorrhage at time of
      injury 958.2
  seminal vesicle 608.83
  skin 782.7
    newborn 772.6
  spermatic cord 608.83
  spinal (cord) 336.1
    aneurysm (ruptured) 336.1
      syphilitic 094.89
    due to birth injury 767.4
    fetus or newborn 767.4
  spleen 289.59
  spontaneous NEC 459.0
    petechial 782.7
  stomach 578.9
    newborn 772.4
    ulcer — *see* Ulcer, stomach, with hemor-
      rhage
  subaponeurotic, newborn 767.11
    massive (birth injury) 767.11
  subarachnoid (nontraumatic) 430
    fetus or newborn (anoxic) (traumatic)
      772.2
    puerperal, postpartum, childbirth
      674.0 ☑
    traumatic — *see* Hemorrhage, brain,
      traumatic, subarachnoid
  subconjunctival 372.72
    due to birth injury 772.8
    newborn 772.8
  subcortical (*see also* Hemorrhage, brain) 431
  subcutaneous 782.7
  subdiaphragmatic 459.0
  subdural (nontraumatic) 432.1
    due to birth injury 767.0
    fetus or newborn (anoxic) (hypoxic) (due
      to birth trauma) 767.0
    puerperal, postpartum, childbirth
      674.0 ☑
    spinal 336.1
    traumatic — *see* Hemorrhage, brain,
      traumatic, subdural
  subgaleal 767.11
  subhyaloid 362.81
  subperiosteal 733.99
  subretinal 362.81
  subtentorial (*see also* Hemorrhage, subdu-
    ral) 432.1
  subungual 703.8
    due to blood dyscrasia 287.8
  suprarenal (capsule) (gland) 255.41
    fetus or newborn 772.5
  tentorium (traumatic) (*see also* Hemorrhage,
    brain, traumatic)
    fetus or newborn 767.0

Hemorrhage, hemorrhagic — *continued*
  tentorium (*see also* Hemorrhage, brain,
    traumatic) — *continued*
    nontraumatic — *see* Hemorrhage, sub-
      dural
  testis 608.83
  thigh 459.0
  third stage 666.0 ☑
  thorax — *see* Hemorrhage, lung
  throat 784.8
  thrombocythemia 238.71
  thymus (gland) 254.8
  thyroid (gland) 246.3
    cyst 246.3
  tongue 529.8
  tonsil 474.8
    postoperative 998.11
  tooth socket (postextraction) 998.11
  trachea — *see* Hemorrhage, lung
  traumatic (*see also* nature of injury)
    brain — *see* Hemorrhage, brain, traumat-
      ic
    recurring or secondary (following initial
      hemorrhage at time of injury)
      958.2
  tuberculous NEC (*see also* Tuberculosis,
    pulmonary) 011.9 ☑
  tunica vaginalis 608.83
  ulcer — *see* Ulcer, by site, with hemorrhage
  umbilicus, umbilical cord 772.0
    after birth, newborn 772.3
    complicating delivery 663.8 ☑
      affecting fetus or newborn 772.0
    slipped ligature 772.3
    stump 772.3
  unavoidable (due to placenta previa)
    641.1 ☑
    affecting fetus or newborn 762.0
  upper extremity 459.0
  urethra (idiopathic) 599.84
  uterus, uterine (abnormal) 626.9
    climacteric 627.0
    complicating delivery — *see* Hemor-
      rhage, complicating, delivery
    due to
      intrauterine contraceptive device
        996.76
      perforating uterus 996.32
    functional or dysfunctional 626.8
    in pregnancy — *see* Hemorrhage, preg-
      nancy
    intermenstrual 626.6
      irregular 626.6
      regular 626.5
    postmenopausal 627.1
    postpartum (*see also* Hemorrhage,
      postpartum) 666.1 ☑
    prepubertal 626.8
    pubertal 626.3
    puerperal (immediate) 666.1 ☑
  vagina 623.8
  vasa previa 663.5 ☑
    affecting fetus or newborn 772.0
  vas deferens 608.83
  ventricular (*see also* Hemorrhage, brain) 431
  vesical 596.89
  viscera 459.0
    newborn 772.8
  vitreous (humor) (intraocular) 379.23
  vocal cord 478.5
  vulva 624.8
Hemorrhoids (anus) (rectum) (without complication) 455.6
  bleeding, prolapsed, strangulated, or ulcer-
    ated NEC 455.8
    external 455.5
    internal 455.2
  complicated NEC 455.8
  complicating pregnancy and puerperium
    671.8 ☑
  external 455.3
    with complication NEC 455.5
      bleeding, prolapsed, strangulated, or
        ulcerated 455.5
      thrombosed 455.4
  internal 455.0

Hemorrhoids — *continued*
  internal — *continued*
    with complication NEC 455.2
      bleeding, prolapsed, strangulated, or
        ulcerated 455.2
      thrombosed 455.1
    residual skin tag 455.9
    sentinel pile 455.9
    thrombosed NEC 455.7
      external 455.4
      internal 455.1
Hemosalpinx 620.8
Hemosiderosis 275.09
  dietary 275.09
  pulmonary (idiopathic) 275.09 *[516.1]*
  transfusion NEC 275.02
    bone marrow 996.85
Hemospermia 608.82
Hemothorax 511.89
  bacterial, nontuberculous 511.1
  newborn 772.8
  nontuberculous 511.89
    bacterial 511.1
  pneumococcal 511.1
  postoperative 998.11
  staphylococcal 511.1
  streptococcal 511.1
  traumatic 860.2
    with
      open wound into thorax 860.3
      pneumothorax 860.4
        with open wound into thorax
          860.5
  tuberculous (*see also* Tuberculosis, pleura)
    012.0 ☑
Hemotympanum 385.89
Hench-Rosenberg syndrome (palindromic
  arthritis) — *see also* Rheumatism, palindromic 719.3 ☑
Henle's warts 371.41
Henoch (-Schönlein)
  disease or syndrome (allergic purpura) 287.0
  purpura (allergic) 287.0
Henpue, henpuye 102.6
Heparin-induced thrombocytopenia (HIT)
  289.84
Heparitinuria 277.5
Hepar lobatum 095.3
Hepatalgia 573.8
Hepatic — *see also* condition
  flexure syndrome 569.89
Hepatitis 573.3
  acute (*see also* Necrosis, liver) 570
    alcoholic 571.1
    infective 070.1
      with hepatic coma 070.0
  alcoholic 571.1
  amebic — *see* Abscess, liver, amebic
  anicteric (acute) — *see* Hepatitis, viral
  antigen-associated (HAA) — *see* Hepatitis,
    viral, type B
  Australian antigen (positive) — *see* Hepati-
    tis, viral, type B
  autoimmune 571.42
  catarrhal (acute) 070.1
    with hepatic coma 070.0
    chronic 571.40
    newborn 070.1
      with hepatic coma 070.0
  chemical 573.3
  cholangiolitic 573.8
  cholestatic 573.8
  chronic 571.40
    active 571.49
      viral — *see* Hepatitis, viral
    aggressive 571.49
    persistent 571.41
    viral — *see* Hepatitis, viral
  cytomegalic inclusion virus 078.5 *[573.1]*
  diffuse 573.3
  "dirty needle" — *see* Hepatitis, viral
  drug-induced 573.3
  due to
    Coxsackie 074.8 *[573.1]*
    cytomegalic inclusion virus 078.5 *[573.1]*
    infectious mononucleosis 075 *[573.1]*

Hepatitis — *continued*
  due to — *continued*
    malaria 084.9 *[573.2]*
    mumps 072.71
    secondary syphilis 091.62
    toxoplasmosis (acquired) 130.5
      congenital (active) 771.2
  epidemic — *see* Hepatitis, viral, type A
  fetus or newborn 774.4
  fibrous (chronic) 571.49
    acute 570
  from injection, inoculation, or transfusion
    (blood) (other substance) (plasma)
    (serum) (onset within 8 months after
    administration) — *see* Hepatitis, viral
  fulminant (viral) (*see also* Hepatitis, viral)
    070.9
    with hepatic coma 070.6
    type A 070.1
      with hepatic coma 070.0
    type B — *see* Hepatitis, viral, type B
  giant cell (neonatal) 774.4
  hemorrhagic 573.8
  history of
    B V12.09
    C V12.09
  homologous serum — *see* Hepatitis, viral
  hypertrophic (chronic) 571.49
    acute 570
  infectious, infective (acute) (chronic) (suba-
    cute) 070.1
    with hepatic coma 070.0
  inoculation — *see* Hepatitis, viral
  interstitial (chronic) 571.49
    acute 570
  lupoid 571.49
  malarial 084.9 *[573.2]*
  malignant (*see also* Necrosis, liver) 570
  neonatal (toxic) 774.4
  newborn 774.4
  parenchymatous (acute) (*see also* Necrosis,
    liver) 570
  peliosis 573.3
  persistent, chronic 571.41
  plasma cell 571.49
  postimmunization — *see* Hepatitis, viral
  postnecrotic 571.49
  posttransfusion — *see* Hepatitis, viral
  recurrent 571.49
  septic 573.3
  serum — *see* Hepatitis, viral
    carrier (suspected of) V02.61
  subacute (*see also* Necrosis, liver) 570
  suppurative (diffuse) 572.0
  syphilitic (late) 095.3
    congenital (early) 090.0 *[573.2]*
      late 090.5 *[573.2]*
    secondary 091.62
  toxic (noninfectious) 573.3
    fetus or newborn 774.4
  tuberculous (*see also* Tuberculosis) 017.9 ☑
  viral (acute) (anicteric) (cholangiolitic)
    (cholestatic) (chronic) (subacute)
    070.9
    with hepatic coma 070.6
    AU-SH type virus — *see* Hepatitis, viral,
      type B
    Australian antigen — *see* Hepatitis, viral,
      type B
    B-antigen — *see* Hepatitis, viral, type B
    Coxsackie 074.8 *[573.1]*
    cytomegalic inclusion 078.5 *[573.1]*
    IH (virus) — *see* Hepatitis, viral, type A
    infectious hepatitis virus — *see* Hepati-
      tis, viral, type A
    serum hepatitis virus — *see* Hepatitis,
      viral, type B
    SH — *see* Hepatitis, viral, type B
    specified type NEC 070.59
      with hepatic coma 070.49
    type A 070.1
      with hepatic coma 070.0
    type B (acute) 070.30
      with
        hepatic coma 070.20
          with hepatitis delta 070.21

☑ **Additional Digit Required — Refer to the Tabular List for Digit Selection**   〽 **Subterms under main terms may continue to next column or page**

2013 ICD-9-CM   ▶◀ Revised Text   ● New Line   ▲ Revised Code   Volume 2 — 137

Hepatitis — continued
  viral — continued
    type B — continued
      with — continued
        hepatitis delta 070.31
          with hepatic coma 070.21
      carrier status V02.61
      chronic 070.32
        with
          hepatic coma 070.22
            with hepatitis delta 070.23
          hepatitis delta 070.33
            with hepatic coma 070.23
    type C
      acute 070.51
        with hepatic coma 070.41
      carrier status V02.62
      chronic 070.54
        with hepatic coma 070.44
      in remission 070.54
      unspecified 070.70
        with hepatic coma 070.71
    type delta (with hepatitis B carrier state)
      070.52
      with
        active hepatitis B disease — see
          Hepatitis, viral, type B
        hepatic coma 070.42
    type E 070.53
      with hepatic coma 070.43
    vaccination and inoculation (prophylactic) V05.3
  Waldenström's (lupoid hepatitis) 571.49
Hepatization, lung (acute) — see also Pneumonia, lobar
  chronic (see also Fibrosis, lung) 515
Hepatoblastoma (M8970/3) 155.0
Hepatocarcinoma (M8170/3) 155.0
Hepatocholangiocarcinoma (M8180/3) 155.0
Hepatocholangioma, benign (M8180/0) 211.5
Hepatocholangitis 573.8
Hepatocystitis — see also Cholecystitis 575.10
Hepatodystrophy 570
Hepatolenticular degeneration 275.1
Hepatolithiasis — see Choledocholithiasis
Hepatoma (malignant) (M8170/3) 155.0
  benign (M8170/0) 211.5
  congenital (M8970/3) 155.0
  embryonal (M8970/3) 155.0
Hepatomegalia glycogenica diffusa 271.0
Hepatomegaly — see also Hypertrophy, liver
  789.1
  congenital 751.69
    syphilitic 090.0
  due to Clonorchis sinensis 121.1
  Gaucher's 272.7
  syphilitic (congenital) 090.0
Hepatoptosis 573.8
Hepatorrhexis 573.8
Hepatosis, toxic 573.8
Hepatosplenomegaly 571.8
  due to S. japonicum 120.2
  hyperlipemic (Bürger-Grutz type) 272.3
Herald patch 696.3
Hereditary — see condition
Heredodegeneration 330.9
  macular 362.70
Heredopathia atactica polyneuritiformis
  356.3
Heredosyphilis — see also Syphilis, congenital
  090.9
Hermaphroditism (true) 752.7
  with specified chromosomal anomaly —
    see Anomaly, chromosomes, sex
Hernia, hernial (acquired) (recurrent) 553.9
  with
    gangrene (obstructed) NEC 551.9
    obstruction NEC 552.9
      and gangrene 551.9
  abdomen (wall) — see Hernia, ventral
  abdominal, specified site NEC 553.8
    with
      gangrene (obstructed) 551.8
      obstruction 552.8
        and gangrene 551.8
  appendix 553.8

Hernia, hernial — continued
  appendix — continued
    with
      gangrene (obstructed) 551.8
      obstruction 552.8
        and gangrene 551.8
  bilateral (inguinal) — see Hernia, inguinal
  bladder (sphincter)
    congenital (female) (male) 756.71
    female (see also Cystocele, female)
      618.01
    male 596.89
  brain 348.4
    congenital 742.0
  broad ligament 553.8
  cartilage, vertebral — see Displacement,
    intervertebral disc
  cerebral 348.4
    congenital 742.0
    endaural 742.0
  ciliary body 364.89
    traumatic 871.1
  colic 553.9
    with
      gangrene (obstructed) 551.9
      obstruction 552.9
        and gangrene 551.9
  colon 553.9
    with
      gangrene (obstructed) 551.9
      obstruction 552.9
        and gangrene 551.9
  colostomy (stoma) 569.69
  Cooper's (retroperitoneal) 553.8
    with
      gangrene (obstructed) 551.8
      obstruction 552.8
        and gangrene 551.8
  crural — see Hernia, femoral
  cystostomy 596.83
  diaphragm, diaphragmatic 553.3
    with
      gangrene (obstructed) 551.3
      obstruction 552.3
        and gangrene 551.3
    congenital 756.6
    due to gross defect of diaphragm 756.6
    traumatic 862.0
      with open wound into cavity 862.1
  direct (inguinal) — see Hernia, inguinal
  disc, intervertebral — see Displacement,
    intervertebral disc
  diverticulum, intestine 553.9
    with
      gangrene (obstructed) 551.9
      obstruction 552.9
        and gangrene 551.9
  double (inguinal) — see Hernia, inguinal
  due to adhesion with obstruction 552.9
  duodenojejunal 553.8
    with
      gangrene (obstructed) 551.8
      obstruction 552.8
        and gangrene 551.8
  en glissade — see Hernia, inguinal
  enterostomy (stoma) 569.69
  epigastric 553.29
    with
      gangrene (obstruction) 551.29
      obstruction 552.29
        and gangrene 551.29
    recurrent 553.21
      with
        gangrene (obstructed) 551.21
        obstruction 552.21
          and gangrene 551.21
  esophageal hiatus (sliding) 553.3
    with
      gangrene (obstructed) 551.3
      obstruction 552.3
        and gangrene 551.3
    congenital 750.6
  external (inguinal) — see Hernia, inguinal
  fallopian tube 620.4
  fascia 728.89
  fat 729.30

Hernia, hernial — continued
  fat — continued
    eyelid 374.34
    orbital 374.34
    pad 729.30
      eye, eyelid 374.34
      knee 729.31
      orbit 374.34
      popliteal (space) 729.31
      specified site NEC 729.39
  femoral (unilateral) 553.00
    with
      gangrene (obstructed) 551.00
      obstruction 552.00
        with gangrene 551.00
    bilateral 553.02
      gangrenous (obstructed) 551.02
      obstructed 552.02
        with gangrene 551.02
      recurrent 553.03
        gangrenous (obstructed) 551.03
        obstructed 552.03
          with gangrene 551.03
    recurrent (unilateral) 553.01
      bilateral 553.03
        gangrenous (obstructed) 551.03
        obstructed 552.03
          with gangrene 551.01
      gangrenous (obstructed) 551.01
      obstructed 552.01
        with gangrene 551.01
  foramen
    Bochdalek 553.3
      with
        gangrene (obstructed) 551.3
        obstruction 552.3
          and gangrene 551.3
      congenital 756.6
    magnum 348.4
    Morgagni, Morgagnian 553.3
      with
        gangrene 551.3
        obstruction 552.3
          and gangrene 551.3
      congenital 756.6
  funicular (umbilical) 553.1
    with
      gangrene (obstructed) 551.1
      obstruction 552.1
        and gangrene 551.1
    spermatic cord — see Hernia, inguinal
  gangrenous — see Hernia, by site, with
    gangrene
  gastrointestinal tract 553.9
    with
      gangrene (obstructed) 551.9
      obstruction 552.9
        and gangrene 551.9
  gluteal — see Hernia, femoral
  Gruber's (internal mesogastric) 553.8
    with
      gangrene (obstructed) 551.8
      obstruction 552.8
        and gangrene 551.8
  Hesselbach's 553.8
    with
      gangrene (obstructed) 551.8
      obstruction 552.8
        and gangrene 551.8
  hiatal (esophageal) (sliding) 553.3
    with
      gangrene (obstructed) 551.3
      obstruction 552.3
        and gangrene 551.3
    congenital 750.6
  incarcerated (see also Hernia, by site, with
    obstruction) 552.9
    gangrenous (see also Hernia, by site, with
      gangrene) 551.9
  incisional 553.21
    with
      gangrene (obstructed) 551.21
      obstruction 552.21
        and gangrene 551.21
    lumbar — see Hernia, lumbar
    recurrent 553.21

Hernia, hernial — continued
  incisional — continued
    recurrent — continued
      with
        gangrene (obstructed) 551.21
        obstruction 552.21
          and gangrene 551.21
  indirect (inguinal) — see Hernia, inguinal
  infantile — see Hernia, inguinal
  infrapatellar fat pad 729.31
  inguinal (direct) (double) (encysted) (external) (funicular) (indirect) (infantile)
    (internal) (interstitial) (oblique)
    (scrotal) (sliding) 550.9 ☑

> Note — Use the following fifth-digit
> subclassification with category 550:
>
> 0 unilateral or unspecified (not
>   specified as recurrent)
>
> 1 unilateral or unspecified, recurrent
>
> 2 bilateral (not specified as recurrent)
>
> 3 bilateral, recurrent

    with
      gangrene (obstructed) 550.0 ☑
      obstruction 550.1 ☑
        and gangrene 550.0 ☑
  internal 553.8
    with
      gangrene (obstructed) 551.8
      obstruction 552.8
        and gangrene 551.8
    inguinal — see Hernia, inguinal
  interstitial 553.9
    with
      gangrene (obstructed) 551.9
      obstruction 552.9
        and gangrene 551.9
    inguinal — see Hernia, inguinal
  intervertebral cartilage or disc — see Displacement, intervertebral disc
  intestine, intestinal 553.9
    with
      gangrene (obstructed) 551.9
      obstruction 552.9
        and gangrene 551.9
  intra-abdominal 553.9
    with
      gangrene (obstructed) 551.9
      obstruction 552.9
        and gangrene 551.9
  intraparietal 553.9
    with
      gangrene (obstructed) 551.9
      obstruction 552.9
        and gangrene 551.9
  iris 364.89
    traumatic 871.1
  irreducible (see also Hernia, by site, with
    obstruction) 552.9
    gangrenous (with obstruction) (see also
      Hernia, by site, with gangrene)
      551.9
  ischiatic 553.8
    with
      gangrene (obstructed) 551.8
      obstruction 552.8
        and gangrene 551.8
  ischiorectal 553.8
    with
      gangrene (obstructed) 551.8
      obstruction 552.8
        and gangrene 551.8
  lens 379.32
    traumatic 871.1
  linea
    alba — see Hernia, epigastric
    semilunaris — see Hernia, spigelian
  Littre's (diverticular) 553.9
    with
      gangrene (obstructed) 551.9
      obstruction 552.9
        and gangrene 551.9
  lumbar 553.8

☑ **Additional Digit Required — Refer to the Tabular List for Digit Selection**

🔻 **Subterms under main terms may continue to next column or page**

Hidradenoma — see also Neoplasm, skin, benign — continued
   papillary (M8405/0) — see Neoplasm, skin, benign
Hidrocystoma (M8404/0) — see Neoplasm, skin, benign
HIE (hypoxic-ischemic encephalopathy) 768.70
   mild 768.71
   moderate 768.72
   severe 768.73
High
   A₂ anemia 282.46

   A_2 anemia 282.46
   altitude effects 993.2
      anoxia 993.2
      on
         ears 993.0
         sinuses 993.1
      polycythemia 289.0
   arch
      foot 755.67
      palate 750.26
   artery (arterial) tension (see also Hypertension) 401.9
      without diagnosis of hypertension 796.2
   basal metabolic rate (BMR) 794.7
   blood pressure (see also Hypertension) 401.9
      borderline 796.2
      incidental reading (isolated) (nonspecific), no diagnosis of hypertension 796.2
   cholesterol 272.0
      with high triglycerides 272.2
   compliance bladder 596.4
   diaphragm (congenital) 756.6
   frequency deafness (congenital) (regional) 389.8
   head at term 652.5 ☑
      affecting fetus or newborn 763.1
   output failure (cardiac) (see also Failure, heart) 428.9
   oxygen-affinity hemoglobin 289.0
   palate 750.26
   risk
      behavior — see Problem
      family situation V61.9
         specified circumstance NEC V61.8
      human papillomavirus (HPV) DNA test positive
         anal 796.75
         cervical 795.05
         vaginal 795.15
      individual NEC V62.89
      infant NEC V20.1
      patient taking drugs (prescribed) V67.51
         nonprescribed (see also Abuse, drugs, nondependent) 305.9 ☑
      pregnancy V23.9
         inadequate prenatal care V23.7
         inconclusive fetal viability V23.87
         specified problem NEC V23.89
   temperature (of unknown origin) (see also Pyrexia) 780.60
   thoracic rib 756.3
   triglycerides 272.1
      with high cholesterol 272.2
Hildenbrand's disease (typhus) 081.9
Hilger's syndrome 337.09
Hill diarrhea 579.1
Hilliard's lupus — see also Tuberculosis 017.0 ☑
Hilum — see condition
Hip — see condition
Hippel's disease (retinocerebral angiomatosis) 759.6
Hippus 379.49
Hirschfeld's disease (acute diabetes mellitus) — see also Diabetes 250.0 ☑
   due to secondary diabetes 249.0 ☑
Hirschsprung's disease or megacolon (congenital) 751.3
Hirsuties — see also Hypertrichosis 704.1
Hirsutism — see also Hypertrichosis 704.1
Hirudiniasis (external) (internal) 134.2
Hiss-Russell dysentery 004.1
Histamine cephalgia 339.00
Histidinemia 270.5

Histidinuria 270.5
Histiocytic syndromes 288.4
Histiocytoma (M8832/0) — see also Neoplasm, skin, benign
   fibrous (M8830/0) (see also Neoplasm, skin, benign)
      atypical (M8830/1) — see Neoplasm, connective tissue, uncertain behavior
      malignant (M8830/3) — see Neoplasm, connective tissue, malignant
Histiocytosis (acute) (chronic) (subacute) 277.89
   acute differentiated progressive (M9722/3) 202.5 ☑
   adult pulmonary Langerhans cell (PLCH) 516.5
   cholesterol 277.89
   essential 277.89
   lipid, lipoid (essential) 272.7
   lipochrome (familial) 288.1
   malignant (M9720/3) 202.3 ☑
   non-Langerhans cell 277.89
   polyostotic sclerosing 277.89
   X (chronic) 277.89
      acute (progressive) (M9722/3) 202.5 ☑
Histoplasmosis 115.90
   with
      endocarditis 115.94
      meningitis 115.91
      pericarditis 115.93
      pneumonia 115.95
      retinitis 115.92
      specified manifestation NEC 115.99
   African (due to Histoplasma duboisii) 115.10
   with
      endocarditis 115.14
      meningitis 115.11
      pericarditis 115.13
      pneumonia 115.15
      retinitis 115.12
      specified manifestation NEC 115.19
   American (due to Histoplasma capsulatum) 115.00
   with
      endocarditis 115.04
      meningitis 115.01
      pericarditis 115.03
      pneumonia 115.05
      retinitis 115.02
      specified manifestation NEC 115.09
   Darling's — see Histoplasmosis, American
   large form (see also Histoplasmosis, African) 115.10
   lung 115.05
   small form (see also Histoplasmosis, American) 115.00
History (personal) of
   abuse
      emotional V15.42
      neglect V15.42
      physical V15.41
      sexual V15.41
   affective psychosis V11.1
   alcoholism V11.3
      specified as drinking problem (see also Abuse, drugs, nondependent) 305.0 ☑
   allergy to V15.09
      analgesic agent NEC V14.6
      anesthetic NEC V14.4
      antibiotic agent NEC V14.1
         penicillin V14.0
      anti-infective agent NEC V14.3
      arachnid bite V15.06
      diathesis V15.09
      drug V14.9
         specified type NEC V14.8
      eggs V15.03
      food additives V15.05
      insect bite V15.06
      latex V15.07
      medicinal agents V14.9
         specified type NEC V14.8
      milk products V15.02
      narcotic agent NEC V14.5

History of — continued
   allergy to — continued
      nuts V15.05
         peanuts V15.01
      penicillin V14.0
      radiographic dye V15.08
      seafood V15.04
      serum V14.7
      specified food NEC V15.05
      specified nonmedicinal agents NEC V15.09
      spider bite V15.06
      sulfa V14.2
      sulfonamides V14.2
      therapeutic agent NEC V15.09
      vaccine V14.7
   anaphylactic reaction or shock V13.81
   anaphylaxis V13.81
   anemia V12.3
   arrest, sudden cardiac V12.53
   arthritis V13.4
   attack, transient ischemic (TIA) V12.54
   benign neoplasm of brain V12.41
   blood disease V12.3
   calculi, urinary V13.01
   cardiovascular disease V12.50
      myocardial infarction 412
   chemotherapy, antineoplastic V87.41
   child abuse V15.41
   cigarette smoking V15.82
   circulatory system disease V12.50
      myocardial infarction 412
   cleft lip and palate, corrected V13.64
   combat and operational stress reaction V11.4
   congenital malformation (corrected)
      circulatory system V13.65
      digestive system V13.67
      ear V13.64
      eye V13.64
      face V13.64
      genitourinary system V13.62
      heart V13.65
      integument V13.68
      limbs V13.68
      musculoskeletal V13.68
      neck V13.64
      nervous system V13.63
      respiratory system V13.66
      specified type NEC V13.69
   contraception V15.7
   death, sudden, successfully resuscitated V12.53
   deficit
      prolonged reversible ischemic neurologic (PRIND) V12.54
      reversible ischemic neurologic (RIND) V12.54
   diathesis, allergic V15.09
   digestive system disease V12.70
      peptic ulcer V12.71
      polyps, colonic V12.72
      specified NEC V12.79
   disease (of) V13.9
      blood V12.3
      blood-forming organs V12.3
      cardiovascular system V12.50
      circulatory system V12.50
         specified NEC V12.59
      digestive system V12.70
         peptic ulcer V12.71
         polyps, colonic V12.72
         specified NEC V12.79
      infectious V12.00
         malaria V12.03
         methicillin resistant Staphylococcus aureus (MRSA) V12.04
         MRSA (methicillin resistant Staphylococcus aureus) V12.04
         poliomyelitis V12.02
         specified NEC V12.09
         tuberculosis V12.01
      parasitic V12.00
         specified NEC V12.09
      respiratory system V12.60
         pneumonia V12.61

History of — continued
   disease — continued
      respiratory system — continued
         specified NEC V12.69
      skin V13.3
      specified site NEC V13.89
      subcutaneous tissue V13.3
      trophoblastic V13.1
         affecting management of pregnancy V23.1
   disorder (of) V13.9
      endocrine V12.29
         gestational diabetes V12.21
      genital system V13.29
      hematological V12.3
      immunity V12.29
      mental V11.9
         affective type V11.1
         manic-depressive V11.1
         neurosis V11.2
         schizophrenia V11.0
         specified type NEC V11.8
      metabolic V12.29
      musculoskeletal NEC V13.59
      nervous system V12.40
         specified type NEC V12.49
      obstetric V13.29
         affecting management of current pregnancy V23.49
         ectopic pregnancy V23.42
         pre-term labor V23.41
         pre-term labor V13.21
      sense organs V12.40
         specified type NEC V12.49
      specified site NEC V13.89
      urinary system V13.00
         calculi V13.01
         infection V13.02
         nephrotic syndrome V13.03
         specified NEC V13.09
   drug use
      nonprescribed (see also Abuse, drugs, nondependent) 305.9 ☑
      patent (see also Abuse, drugs, nondependent) 305.9 ☑
   dysplasia
      cervical (conditions classifiable to 622.10-622.12) V13.22
      vaginal (conditions classifiable to 623.0) V13.23
      vulvar (conditions classifiable to 624.01-624.02) V13.24
   effect NEC of external cause V15.89
   embolism V12.51
      pulmonary V12.55
   emotional abuse V15.42
   encephalitis V12.42
   endocrine disorder V12.29
      gestational diabetes V12.21
   estrogen therapy V87.43
   extracorporeal membrane oxygenation (ECMO) V15.87
   failed
      conscious sedation V15.80
      moderate sedation V15.80
   falling V15.88
   family
      allergy V19.6
      anemia V18.2
      arteriosclerosis V17.49
      arthritis V17.7
      asthma V17.5
      blindness V19.0
      blood disorder NEC V18.3
      cardiovascular disease V17.49
      carrier, genetic disease V18.9
      cerebrovascular disease V17.1
      chronic respiratory condition NEC V17.6
      colonic polyps V18.51
      congenital anomalies V19.5
      consanguinity V19.7
      coronary artery disease V17.3
      cystic fibrosis V18.19
      deafness V19.2
      diabetes mellitus V18.0
      digestive disorders V18.59

☑ Additional Digit Required — Refer to the Tabular List for Digit Selection   ▼ Subterms under main terms may continue to next column or page

140 — Volume 2   ▶◀ Revised Text   ● New Line   ▲ Revised Code   2013 ICD-9-CM

History of — *continued*
family — *continued*
disabilities, intellectual V18.4
disease or disorder (of)
allergic V19.6
blood NEC V18.3
cardiovascular NEC V17.49
cerebrovascular V17.1
colonic polyps V18.51
coronary artery V17.3
death, sudden cardiac (SCD) V17.41
digestive V18.59
ear NEC V19.3
endocrine V18.19
multiple neoplasia (MEN) syndrome V18.11
eye NEC V19.19
glaucoma V19.11
genitourinary NEC V18.7
glaucoma V19.11
hypertensive V17.49
infectious V18.8
ischemic heart V17.3
kidney V18.69
polycystic V18.61
mental V17.0
metabolic V18.19
musculoskeletal NEC V17.89
osteoporosis V17.81
neurological NEC V17.2
parasitic V18.8
psychiatric condition V17.0
skin condition V19.4
ear disorder NEC V19.3
endocrine disease V18.19
multiple neoplasia (MEN) syndrome V18.11
epilepsy V17.2
eye disorder NEC V19.19
glaucoma V19.11
genetic disease carrier V18.9
genitourinary disease NEC V18.7
glaucoma V19.11
glomerulonephritis V18.69
gout V18.19
hay fever V17.6
hearing loss V19.2
hematopoietic neoplasia V16.7
Hodgkin's disease V16.7
Huntington's chorea V17.2
hydrocephalus V19.5
hypertension V17.49
infarction, myocardial V17.3
infectious disease V18.8
intellectual disabilities V18.4
ischemic heart disease V17.3
kidney disease V18.69
polycystic V18.61
leukemia V16.6
lymphatic malignant neoplasia NEC V16.7
malignant neoplasm (of) NEC V16.9
anorectal V16.0
anus V16.0
appendix V16.0
bladder V16.52
bone V16.8
brain V16.8
breast V16.3
male V16.8
bronchus V16.1
cecum V16.0
cervix V16.49
colon V16.0
duodenum V16.0
esophagus V16.0
eye V16.8
gallbladder V16.0
gastrointestinal tract V16.0
genital organs V16.40
hemopoietic NEC V16.7
ileum V16.0
ilium V16.8
intestine V16.0
intrathoracic organs NEC V16.2
kidney V16.51

History of — *continued*
family — *continued*
malignant neoplasm — *continued*
larynx V16.2
liver V16.0
lung V16.1
lymphatic NEC V16.7
ovary V16.41
oviduct V16.41
pancreas V16.0
penis V16.49
prostate V16.42
rectum V16.0
respiratory organs NEC V16.2
skin V16.8
specified site NEC V16.8
stomach V16.0
testis V16.43
trachea V16.1
ureter V16.59
urethra V16.59
urinary organs V16.59
uterus V16.49
vagina V16.49
vulva V16.49
MEN (multiple endocrine neoplasia syndrome) V18.11
mental retardation — *see* History, family, intellectual disabilities
metabolic disease NEC V18.19
mongolism V19.5
multiple
endocrine neoplasia (MEN) syndrome V18.11
myeloma V16.7
musculoskeletal disease NEC V17.89
osteoporosis V17.81
myocardial infarction V17.3
nephritis V18.69
nephrosis V18.69
osteoporosis V17.81
parasitic disease V18.8
polycystic kidney disease V18.61
psychiatric disorder V17.0
psychosis V17.0
retinitis pigmentosa V19.19
schizophrenia V17.0
skin conditions V19.4
specified condition NEC V19.8
stroke (cerebrovascular) V17.1
sudden cardiac death (SCD) V17.41
visual loss V19.0
foreign body fully removed V15.53
fracture, healed
pathologic V13.51
stress V13.52
traumatic V15.51
genital system disorder V13.29
pre-term labor V13.21
gestational diabetes V12.21
health hazard V15.9
falling V15.88
specified cause NEC V15.89
hepatitis
B V12.09
C V12.09
Hodgkin's disease V10.72
hypospadias (corrected) V13.61
immunity disorder V12.29
immunosuppression therapy V87.46
infarction, cerebral, without residual deficits V12.54
infection
central nervous system V12.42
urinary (tract) V13.02
infectious disease V12.00
malaria V12.03
methicillin resistant Staphylococcus aureus (MRSA) V12.04
MRSA (methicillin resistant Staphylococcus aureus) V12.04
poliomyelitis V12.02
specified NEC V12.09
tuberculosis V12.01
injury NEC V15.59
traumatic brain V15.52

History of — *continued*
insufficient prenatal care V23.7
in utero procedure
during pregnancy V15.21
while a fetus V15.22
irradiation V15.3
leukemia V10.60
lymphoid V10.61
monocytic V10.63
myeloid V10.62
specified type NEC V10.69
little or no prenatal care V23.7
low birth weight (*see also* Status, low birth weight) V21.30
lymphosarcoma V10.71
malaria V12.03
malignant carcinoid tumor V10.91
malignant neoplasm (of) V10.90
accessory sinus V10.22
adrenal V10.88
anus V10.06
bile duct V10.09
bladder V10.51
bone V10.81
brain V10.85
breast V10.3
bronchus V10.11
cervix uteri V10.41
colon V10.05
connective tissue NEC V10.89
corpus uteri V10.42
digestive system V10.00
specified part NEC V10.09
duodenum V10.09
endocrine gland NEC V10.88
epididymis V10.48
esophagus V10.03
eye V10.84
fallopian tube V10.44
female genital organ V10.40
specified site NEC V10.44
gallbladder V10.09
gastrointestinal tract V10.00
gum V10.02
hematopoietic NEC V10.79
hypopharynx V10.02
ileum V10.09
intrathoracic organs NEC V10.20
jejunum V10.09
kidney V10.52
large intestine V10.05
larynx V10.21
lip V10.02
liver V10.07
lung V10.11
lymphatic NEC V10.79
lymph glands or nodes NEC V10.79
male genital organ V10.45
specified site NEC V10.49
mediastinum V10.29
melanoma (of skin) V10.82
middle ear V10.22
mouth V10.02
specified part NEC V10.02
nasal cavities V10.22
nasopharynx V10.02
nervous system NEC V10.86
nose V10.22
oropharynx V10.02
ovary V10.43
pancreas V10.09
parathyroid V10.88
penis V10.49
pharynx V10.02
pineal V10.88
pituitary V10.88
placenta V10.44
pleura V10.29
prostate V10.46
rectosigmoid junction V10.06
rectum V10.06
renal pelvis V10.53
respiratory organs NEC V10.20
salivary gland V10.02
skin V10.83
melanoma V10.82

History of — *continued*
malignant neoplasm — *continued*
small intestine NEC V10.09
soft tissue NEC V10.89
specified site NEC V10.89
stomach V10.04
testis V10.47
thymus V10.29
thyroid V10.87
tongue V10.01
trachea V10.12
ureter V10.59
urethra V10.59
urinary organ V10.50
uterine adnexa V10.44
uterus V10.42
vagina V10.44
vulva V10.44
malignant neuroendocrine tumor V10.91
manic-depressive psychosis V11.1
meningitis V12.42
mental disorder V11.9
affective type V11.1
manic-depressive V11.1
neurosis V11.2
schizophrenia V11.0
specified type NEC V11.8
Merkel cell carcinoma V10.91
metabolic disorder V12.29
methicillin resistant Staphylococcus aureus (MRSA) V12.04
MRSA (methicillin resistant Staphylococcus aureus) V12.04
musculoskeletal disorder NEC V13.59
myocardial infarction 412
neglect (emotional) V15.42
nephrotic syndrome V13.03
nervous system disorder V12.40
specified type NEC V12.49
neurosis V11.2
noncompliance with medical treatment V15.81
nutritional deficiency V12.1
obstetric disorder V13.29
affecting management of current pregnancy V23.49
ectopic pregnancy V23.42
pre-term labor V23.41
pre-term labor V13.21
parasitic disease V12.00
specified NEC V12.09
perinatal problems V13.7
low birth weight (*see also* Status, low birth weight) V21.30
physical abuse V15.41
poisoning V15.6
poliomyelitis V12.02
polyps, colonic V12.72
poor obstetric V13.29
affecting management of current pregnancy V23.49
ectopic pregnancy V23.42
pre-term labor V23.41
pre-term labor V13.21
prolonged reversible ischemic neurologic deficit (PRIND) V12.54
psychiatric disorder V11.9
affective type V11.1
manic-depressive V11.1
neurosis V11.2
schizophrenia V11.0
specified type NEC V11.8
psychological trauma V15.49
emotional abuse V15.42
neglect V15.42
physical abuse V15.41
rape V15.41
psychoneurosis V11.2
radiation therapy V15.3
rape V15.41
respiratory system disease V12.60
pneumonia V12.61
specified NEC V12.69
reticulosarcoma V10.71
return from military deployment V62.22

✓ Additional Digit Required — Refer to the Tabular List for Digit Selection   Subterms under main terms may continue to next column or page

2013 ICD-9-CM   ▶◀ Revised Text   ● New Line   ▲ Revised Code   Volume 2 — 141

History of — *continued*
  reversible ischemic neurologic deficit (RIND) V12.54
  schizophrenia V11.0
  skin disease V13.3
  smoking (tobacco) V15.82
  steroid therapy V87.45
    inhaled V87.44
    systemic V87.45
  stroke without residual deficits V12.54
  subcutaneous tissue disease V13.3
  sudden
    cardiac
      arrest V12.53
      death (successfully resuscitated) V12.53
  surgery to
    great vessels V15.1
    heart V15.1
    in utero
      during pregnancy V15.21
      while a fetus V15.22
    organs NEC V15.29
  syndrome, nephrotic V13.03
  therapy
    antineoplastic drug V87.41
    drug NEC V87.49
    estrogen V87.43
    immunosuppression V87.46
    monoclonal drug V87.42
    steroid V87.45
      inhaled V87.44
      systemic V87.45
  thrombophlebitis V12.52
  thrombosis V12.51
    pulmonary V12.55
  tobacco use V15.82
  trophoblastic disease V13.1
    affecting management of pregnancy V23.1
  tuberculosis V12.01
  ulcer, peptic V12.71
  urinary system disorder V13.00
    calculi V13.01
    infection V13.02
    nephrotic syndrome V13.03
    specified NEC V13.09
His-Werner disease (trench fever) 083.1
HIT (heparin-induced thrombocytopenia) 289.84
Hives (bold) — *see also* Urticaria 708.9
HIV infection (disease) (illness) — *see* Human immunodeficiency virus (disease) (illness) (infection)
Hoarseness 784.42
Hobnail liver — *see* Cirrhosis, portal
Hobo, hoboism V60.0
Hodgkin's
  disease (M9650/3) 201.9 ☑
  lymphocytic
    depletion (M9653/3) 201.7 ☑
      diffuse fibrosis (M9654/3) 201.7 ☑
      reticular type (M9655/3) 201.7 ☑
    predominance (M9651/3) 201.4 ☑
  lymphocytic-histiocytic predominance (M9651/3) 201.4 ☑
  mixed cellularity (M9652/3) 201.6 ☑
  nodular sclerosis (M9656/3) 201.5 ☑
    cellular phase (M9657/3) 201.5 ☑
  granuloma (M9661/3) 201.1 ☑
  lymphogranulomatosis (M9650/3) 201.9 ☑
  lymphoma (M9650/3) 201.9 ☑
  lymphosarcoma (M9650/3) 201.9 ☑
  paragranuloma (M9660/3) 201.0 ☑
  sarcoma (M9662/3) 201.2 ☑
Hodgson's disease (aneurysmal dilatation of aorta) 441.9
  ruptured 441.5
Hodi-potsy 111.0
Hoffa (-Kastert) disease or syndrome (liposynovitis prepatellaris) 272.8
Hoffmann-Bouveret syndrome (paroxysmal tachycardia) 427.2
Hoffman's syndrome 244.9 *[359.5]*

Hole
  macula 362.54
  optic disc, crater-like 377.22
  retina (macula) 362.54
    round 361.31
      with detachment 361.01
Holla disease — *see also* Spherocytosis 282.0
Holländer-Simons syndrome (progressive lipodystrophy) 272.6
Hollow foot (congenital) 754.71
  acquired 736.73
Holmes' syndrome (visual disorientation) 368.16
Holoprosencephaly 742.2
  due to
    trisomy 13 758.1
    trisomy 18 758.2
Holthouse's hernia — *see* Hernia, inguinal
Homesickness 309.89
Homicidal ideation V62.85
Homocystinemia 270.4
Homocystinuria 270.4
Homologous serum jaundice (prophylactic) (therapeutic) — *see* Hepatitis, viral
Homosexuality — omit code
  ego-dystonic 302.0
  pedophilic 302.2
  problems with 302.0
Homozygous Hb-S disease 282.61
Honeycomb lung 518.89
  congenital 748.4
Hong Kong ear 117.3
HOOD (hereditary osteo-onychodysplasia) 756.89
Hooded
  clitoris 752.49
  penis 752.69
Hookworm (anemia) (disease) (infestation) — *see* Ancylostomiasis
Hoppe-Goldflam syndrome 358.00
Hordeolum (external) (eyelid) 373.11
  internal 373.12
Horn
  cutaneous 702.8
    cheek 702.8
    eyelid 702.8
    penis 702.8
    iliac 756.89
    nail 703.8
      congenital 757.5
  papillary 700
Horner's
  syndrome (*see also* Neuropathy, peripheral, autonomic) 337.9
    traumatic 954.0
  teeth 520.4
Horseshoe kidney (congenital) 753.3
Horton's
  disease (temporal arteritis) 446.5
  headache or neuralgia 339.00
Hospice care V66.7
Hospitalism (in children) NEC 309.83
Hourglass contraction, contracture
  bladder 596.89
  gallbladder 575.2
    congenital 751.69
  stomach 536.8
    congenital 750.7
    psychogenic 306.4
  uterus 661.4 ☑
    affecting fetus or newborn 763.7
Household circumstance affecting care V60.9
  specified type NEC V60.89
Housemaid's knee 727.2
Housing circumstance affecting care V60.9
  specified type NEC V60.89
HTLV-I infection 079.51
HTLV-II infection 079.52
HTLV-III/LAV (disease) (illness) (infection) — *see* Human immunodeficiency virus (disease) (illness) (infection)
HTLV-III (disease) (illness) (infection) — *see* Human immunodeficiency virus (disease) (illness) (infection)

HTR (hemolytic transfusion reaction)
  due to or resulting from
    incompatibility
      ABO 999.61
        acute 999.62
        delayed 999.63
      non-ABO antigen (minor) (Duffy) (Kell) (Kidd) (Lewis) (M) (N) (P) (S) 999.76
        acute 999.77
        delayed 999.78
      Rh antigen (C) (c) (D) (E) (e) 999.71
        acute 999.72
        delayed 999.73
Huchard's disease (continued arterial hypertension) 401.9
Hudson-Stähli lines 371.11
Huguier's disease (uterine fibroma) 218.9
Human bite (open wound) — *see also* Wound, open, by site
  intact skin surface — *see* Contusion
Human immunodeficiency virus (disease) (illness) 042
  infection V08
    with symptoms, symptomatic 042
Human immunodeficiency virus-2 infection 079.53
Human immunovirus (disease) (illness) (infection) — *see* Human immunodeficiency virus (disease) (illness) (infection)
Human papillomavirus 079.4
  high risk, DNA test positive
    anal 796.75
    cervical 795.05
    vaginal 795.15
  low risk, DNA test positive
    anal 796.79
    cervical 795.09
    vaginal 795.19
Human parvovirus 079.83
Human T-cell lymphotrophic virus-I infection 079.51
Human T-cell lymphotrophic virus-II infection 079.52
Human T-cell lymphotrophic virus-III (disease) (illness) (infection) — *see* Human immunodeficiency virus (disease) (illness) (infection)
Humpback (acquired) 737.9
  congenital 756.19
Hum, venous — omit code
Hunchback (acquired) 737.9
  congenital 756.19
Hunger 994.2
  air, psychogenic 306.1
  disease 251.1
Hungry bone syndrome 275.5
Hunner's ulcer — *see also* Cystitis 595.1
Hunt's
  neuralgia 053.11
  syndrome (herpetic geniculate ganglionitis) 053.11
    dyssynergia cerebellaris myoclonica 334.2
Hunter's glossitis 529.4
Hunterian chancre 091.0
Hunter (-Hurler) syndrome (mucopolysaccharidosis II) 277.5
Huntington's
  chorea 333.4
  disease 333.4
Huppert's disease (multiple myeloma) (M9730/3) 203.0 ☑
Hurler (-Hunter) disease or syndrome (mucopolysaccharidosis II) 277.5
Hürthle cell
  adenocarcinoma (M8290/3) 193
  adenoma (M8290/0) 226
  carcinoma (M8290/3) 193
  tumor (M8290/0) 226
Hutchinson's
  disease meaning
    angioma serpiginosum 709.1
    cheiropompholyx 705.81
    prurigo estivalis 692.72

Hutchinson's — *continued*
  disease meaning — *continued*
    summer eruption, or summer prurigo 692.72
  incisors 090.5
  melanotic freckle (M8742/2) (*see also* Neoplasm, skin, in situ)
    malignant melanoma in (M8742/3) — *see* Melanoma
  teeth or incisors (congenital syphilis) 090.5
Hutchinson-Boeck disease or syndrome (sarcoidosis) 135
Hutchinson-Gilford disease or syndrome (progeria) 259.8
Hyaline
  degeneration (diffuse) (generalized) 728.9
    localized — *see* Degeneration, by site
  membrane (disease) (lung) (newborn) 769
Hyalinosis cutis et mucosae 272.8
Hyalin plaque, sclera, senile 379.16
Hyalitis (asteroid) 379.22
  syphilitic 095.8
Hydatid
  cyst or tumor (*see also* Echinococcus)
    fallopian tube 752.11
  mole — *see* Hydatidiform mole
  Morgagni (congenital) 752.89
    fallopian tube 752.11
Hydatidiform mole (benign) (complicating pregnancy) (delivered) (undelivered) 630
  invasive (M9100/1) 236.1
  malignant (M9100/1) 236.1
  previous, affecting management of pregnancy V23.1
Hydatidosis — *see* Echinococcus
Hyde's disease (prurigo nodularis) 698.3
Hydradenitis 705.83
Hydradenoma (M8400/0) — *see* Hidradenoma
Hydralazine lupus or syndrome
  correct substance properly administered 695.4
  overdose or wrong substance given or taken 972.6
Hydramnios 657.0 ☑
  affecting fetus or newborn 761.3
Hydrancephaly 742.3
  with spina bifida (*see also* Spina bifida) 741.0 ☑
Hydranencephaly 742.3
  with spina bifida (*see also* Spina bifida) 741.0 ☑
Hydrargyrism NEC 985.0
Hydrarthrosis — *see also* Effusion, joint 719.0 ☑
  gonococcal 098.50
  intermittent (*see also* Rheumatism, palindromic) 719.3 ☑
  of yaws (early) (late) 102.6
  syphilitic 095.8
    congenital 090.5
Hydremia 285.9
Hydrencephalocele (congenital) 742.0
Hydrencephalomeningocele (congenital) 742.0
Hydroa 694.0
  aestivale 692.72
  gestationis 646.8 ☑
  herpetiformis 694.0
  pruriginosa 694.0
  vacciniforme 692.72
Hydroadenitis 705.83
Hydrocalycosis — *see also* Hydronephrosis 591
  congenital 753.29
Hydrocalyx — *see also* Hydronephrosis 591
Hydrocele (calcified) (chylous) (idiopathic) (infantile) (inguinal canal) (recurrent) (senile) (spermatic cord) (testis) (tunica vaginalis) 603.9
  canal of Nuck (female) 629.1
    male 603.9
  congenital 778.6
  encysted 603.0
    congenital 778.6
  female NEC 629.89
  infected 603.1
  round ligament 629.89

☑ **Additional Digit Required** — Refer to the Tabular List for Digit Selection   👑 **Subterms under main terms may continue to next column or page**

142 — Volume 2   ▶◀ Revised Text   ● New Line   ▲ Revised Code   **2013 ICD-9-CM**

Hydrocele — *continued*
 specified type NEC 603.8
  congenital 778.6
 spinalis (*see also* Spina bifida) 741.9 ☑
 vulva 624.8
Hydrocephalic fetus
 affecting management or pregnancy
  655.0 ☑
 causing disproportion 653.6 ☑
  with obstructed labor 660.1 ☑
   affecting fetus or newborn 763.1
Hydrocephalus (acquired) (external) (internal)
 (malignant) (noncommunicating) (obstructive) (recurrent) 331.4
 aqueduct of Sylvius stricture 742.3
  with spina bifida (*see also* Spina bifida)
   741.0 ☑
 chronic 742.3
  with spina bifida (*see also* Spina bifida)
   741.0 ☑
 communicating 331.3
 congenital (external) (internal) 742.3
  with spina bifida (*see also* Spina bifida)
   741.0 ☑
 due to
  stricture of aqueduct of Sylvius 742.3
   with spina bifida (*see also* Spina bifi-
    da) 741.0 ☑
  toxoplasmosis (congenital) 771.2
 fetal affecting management of pregnancy
  655.0 ☑
 foramen Magendie block (acquired) 331.3
  congenital 742.3
   with spina bifida (*see also* Spina bifi-
    da) 741.0 ☑
 newborn 742.3
  with spina bifida (*see also* Spina bifida)
   741.0 ☑
 normal pressure 331.5
  idiopathic (INPH) 331.5
  secondary 331.3
 otitic 348.2
 syphilitic, congenital 090.49
 tuberculous (*see also* Tuberculosis) 013.8 ☑
Hydrocolpos (congenital) 623.8
Hydrocystoma (M8404/0) — *see* Neoplasm,
 skin, benign
Hydroencephalocele (congenital) 742.0
Hydroencephalomeningocele (congenital)
 742.0
Hydrohematopneumothorax — *see also*
 Hemothorax 511.89
Hydromeningitis — *see* Meningitis
Hydromeningocele (spinal) — *see also* Spina
 bifida 741.9 ☑
 cranial 742.0
Hydrometra 621.8
Hydrometrocolpos 623.8
Hydromicrocephaly 742.1
Hydromphalus (congenital) (since birth)
 757.39
Hydromyelia 742.53
Hydromyelocele — *see also* Spina bifida
 741.9 ☑
Hydronephrosis 591
 atrophic 591
 congenital 753.29
 due to S. hematobium 120.0
 early 591
 functionless (infected) 591
 infected 591
 intermittent 591
 primary 591
 secondary 591
 tuberculous (*see also* Tuberculosis) 016.0 ☑
Hydropericarditis — *see also* Pericarditis 423.9
Hydropericardium — *see also* Pericarditis
 423.9
Hydroperitoneum 789.59
Hydrophobia 071
Hydrophthalmos — *see also* Buphthalmia
 743.20
Hydropneumohemothorax — *see also*
 Hemothorax 511.89
Hydropneumopericarditis — *see also* Pericarditis 423.9

Hydropneumopericardium — *see also* Pericarditis 423.9
Hydropneumothorax 511.89
 nontuberculous 511.89
  bacterial 511.1
  pneumococcal 511.1
  staphylococcal 511.1
  streptococcal 511.1
 traumatic 860.0
  with open wound into thorax 860.1
 tuberculous (*see also* Tuberculosis, pleura)
  012.0 ☑
Hydrops 782.3
 abdominis 789.59
 amnii (complicating pregnancy) (*see also*
  Hydramnios) 657.0 ☑
 articulorum intermittens (*see also* Rheumatism, palindromic) 719.3 ☑
 cardiac (*see also* Failure, heart) 428.0
 congenital — *see* Hydrops, fetalis
 endolymphatic (*see also* Disease, Ménière's)
  386.00
 fetal, fetalis or newborn 778.0
  due to
   alpha thalassemia 282.43
   isoimmunization 773.3
  not due to isoimmunization 778.0
 gallbladder 575.3
 idiopathic (fetus or newborn) 778.0
 joint (*see also* Effusion, joint) 719.0 ☑
 labyrinth (*see also* Disease, Ménière's) 386.00
 meningeal NEC 331.4
 nutritional 262
 pericardium — *see* Pericarditis
 pleura (*see also* Hydrothorax) 511.89
 renal (*see also* Nephrosis) 581.9
 spermatic cord (*see also* Hydrocele) 603.9
Hydropyonephrosis — *see also* Pyelitis 590.80
 chronic 590.00
Hydrorachis 742.53
Hydrorrhea (nasal) 478.19
 gravidarum 658.1 ☑
 pregnancy 658.1 ☑
Hydrosadenitis 705.83
Hydrosalpinx (fallopian tube) (follicularis)
 614.1
Hydrothorax (double) (pleural) 511.89
 chylous (nonfilarial) 457.8
  filaria (*see also* Infestation, filarial) 125.9
 nontuberculous 511.89
  bacterial 511.1
  pneumococcal 511.1
  staphylococcal 511.1
  streptococcal 511.1
 traumatic 862.29
  with open wound into thorax 862.39
 tuberculous (*see also* Tuberculosis, pleura)
  012.0 ☑
Hydroureter 593.5
 congenital 753.22
Hydroureteronephrosis — *see also* Hydronephrosis 591
Hydrourethra 599.84
Hydroxykynureninuria 270.2
Hydroxyprolinemia 270.8
Hydroxyprolinuria 270.8
Hygroma (congenital) (cystic) (M9173/0) 228.1
 prepatellar 727.3
 subdural — *see* Hematoma, subdural
Hymen — *see* condition
Hymenolepiasis (diminuta) (infection) (infestation) (nana) 123.6
Hymenolepsis (diminuta) (infection) (infestation) (nana) 123.6
Hypalgesia — *see also* Disturbance, sensation
 782.0
Hyperabduction syndrome 447.8
Hyperacidity, gastric 536.8
 psychogenic 306.4
Hyperactive, hyperactivity 314.01
 basal cell, uterine cervix 622.10
 bladder 596.51
 bowel (syndrome) 564.9
  sounds 787.5
 cervix epithelial (basal) 622.10
 child 314.01

Hyperactive, hyperactivity — *continued*
 colon 564.9
 gastrointestinal 536.8
  psychogenic 306.4
 intestine 564.9
 labyrinth (unilateral) 386.51
  with loss of labyrinthine reactivity 386.58
   bilateral 386.52
 nasal mucous membrane 478.19
 stomach 536.8
 thyroid (gland) (*see also* Thyrotoxicosis)
  242.9 ☑
Hyperacusis 388.42
Hyperadrenalism (cortical) 255.3
 medullary 255.6
Hyperadrenocorticism 255.3
 congenital 255.2
 iatrogenic
  correct substance properly administered
   255.3
  overdose or wrong substance given or
   taken 962.0
Hyperaffectivity 301.11
Hyperaldosteronism (atypical) (hyperplastic)
 (normoaldosteronal) (normotensive)
 (primary) 255.10
 secondary 255.14
Hyperalgesia — *see also* Disturbance, sensation 782.0
Hyperalimentation 783.6
 carotene 278.3
 specified NEC 278.8
 vitamin A 278.2
 vitamin D 278.4
Hyperaminoaciduria 270.9
 arginine 270.6
 citrulline 270.6
 cystine 270.0
 glycine 270.0
 lysine 270.7
 ornithine 270.6
 renal (types I, II, III) 270.0
Hyperammonemia (congenital) 270.6
Hyperamnesia 780.99
Hyperamylasemia 790.5
Hyperaphia 782.0
Hyperazotemia 791.9
Hyperbetalipoproteinemia (acquired) (essential) (familial) (hereditary) (primary)
 (secondary) 272.0
 with prebetalipoproteinemia 272.2
Hyperbilirubinemia 782.4
 congenital 277.4
 constitutional 277.4
 neonatal (transient) (*see also* Jaundice, fetus
  or newborn) 774.6
  of prematurity 774.2
**Hyperbilirubinemica encephalopathia,
 newborn** 774.7
 due to isoimmunization 773.4
Hypercalcemia, hypercalcemic (idiopathic)
 275.42
 nephropathy 588.89
Hypercalcinuria 275.40
Hypercapnia 786.09
 with mixed acid-based disorder 276.4
 fetal, affecting newborn 770.89
Hypercarotinemia 278.3
Hypercementosis 521.5
Hyperchloremia 276.9
Hyperchlorhydria 536.8
 neurotic 306.4
 psychogenic 306.4
Hypercholesterinemia — *see* Hypercholesterolemia
Hypercholesterolemia 272.0
 with hyperglyceridemia, endogenous 272.2
 essential 272.0
 familial 272.0
 hereditary 272.0
 primary 272.0
 pure 272.0
Hypercholesterolosis 272.0
Hyperchylia gastrica 536.8
 psychogenic 306.4

Hyperchylomicronemia (familial) (with hyperbetalipoproteinemia) 272.3
Hypercoagulation syndrome (primary) 289.81
 secondary 289.82
Hypercorticosteronism
 correct substance properly administered
  255.3
 overdose or wrong substance given or taken
  962.0
Hypercortisonism
 correct substance properly administered
  255.3
 overdose or wrong substance given or taken
  962.0
**Hyperdynamic beta-adrenergic state or
 syndrome** (circulatory) 429.82
Hyperekplexia 759.89
Hyperelectrolytemia 276.9
Hyperemesis 536.2
 arising during pregnancy — *see* Hyperemesis, gravidarum
 gravidarum (mild) (before 22 completed
  weeks gestation) 643.0 ☑
  with
   carbohydrate depletion 643.1 ☑
   dehydration 643.1 ☑
   electrolyte imbalance 643.1 ☑
   metabolic disturbance 643.1 ☑
  affecting fetus or newborn 761.8
  severe (with metabolic disturbance)
   643.1 ☑
 psychogenic 306.4
Hyperemia (acute) 780.99
 anal mucosa 569.49
 bladder 596.7
 cerebral 437.8
 conjunctiva 372.71
 ear, internal, acute 386.30
 enteric 564.89
 eye 372.71
 eyelid (active) (passive) 374.82
 intestine 564.89
 iris 364.41
 kidney 593.81
 labyrinth 386.30
 liver (active) (passive) 573.8
 lung 514
 ovary 620.8
 passive 780.99
 pulmonary 514
 renal 593.81
 retina 362.89
 spleen 289.59
 stomach 537.89
Hyperesthesia (body surface) — *see also* Disturbance, sensation 782.0
 larynx (reflex) 478.79
  hysterical 300.11
 pharynx (reflex) 478.29
Hyperestrinism 256.0
Hyperestrogenism 256.0
Hyperestrogenosis 256.0
Hyperexplexia 759.89
Hyperextension, joint 718.80
 ankle 718.87
 elbow 718.82
 foot 718.87
 hand 718.84
 hip 718.85
 knee 718.86
 multiple sites 718.89
 pelvic region 718.85
 shoulder (region) 718.81
 specified site NEC 718.88
 wrist 718.83
Hyperfibrinolysis — *see* Fibrinolysis
Hyperfolliculinism 256.0
Hyperfructosemia 271.2
Hyperfunction
 adrenal (cortex) 255.3
  androgenic, acquired benign 255.3
  medulla 255.6
  virilism 255.2
 corticoadrenal NEC 255.3
 labyrinth — *see* Hyperactive, labyrinth
 medulloadrenal 255.6

☑ Additional Digit Required — Refer to the Tabular List for Digit Selection   ▧ Subterms under main terms may continue to next column or page

2013 ICD-9-CM   ▶◀ Revised Text   ● New Line   ▲ Revised Code   Volume 2 — 143

Hyperfunction — *continued*
- ovary 256.1
  - estrogen 256.0
- pancreas 577.8
- parathyroid (gland) 252.00
- pituitary (anterior) (gland) (lobe) 253.1
- testicular 257.0

Hypergammaglobulinemia 289.89
- monoclonal, benign (BMH) 273.1
- polyclonal 273.0
- Waldenström's 273.0

Hyperglobulinemia 273.8

Hyperglycemia 790.29
- maternal
  - affecting fetus or newborn 775.0
  - manifest diabetes in infant 775.1
- postpancreatectomy (complete) (partial) 251.3

Hyperglyceridemia 272.1
- endogenous 272.1
- essential 272.1
- familial 272.1
- hereditary 272.1
- mixed 272.3
- pure 272.1

Hyperglycinemia 270.7

Hypergonadism
- ovarian 256.1
- testicular (infantile) (primary) 257.0

Hyperheparinemia — *see also* Circulating, intrinsic anticoagulants 287.5

Hyperhidrosis, hyperidrosis 705.21
- axilla 705.21
- face 705.21
- focal (localized) 705.21
  - primary 705.21
    - axilla 705.21
    - face 705.21
    - palms 705.21
    - soles 705.21
  - secondary 705.22
    - axilla 705.22
    - face 705.22
    - palms 705.22
    - soles 705.22
- generalized 780.8
- palms 705.21
- psychogenic 306.3
- secondary 780.8
- soles 705.21

Hyperhistidinemia 270.5

Hyperinsulinism (ectopic) (functional) (organic) NEC 251.1
- iatrogenic 251.0
- reactive 251.2
- spontaneous 251.2
- therapeutic misadventure (from administration of insulin) 962.3

Hyperiodemia 276.9

Hyperirritability (cerebral), in newborn 779.1

Hyperkalemia 276.7

Hyperkeratosis — *see also* Keratosis 701.1
- cervix 622.2
- congenital 757.39
- cornea 371.89
- due to yaws (early) (late) (palmar or plantar) 102.3
- eccentrica 757.39
- figurata centrifuga atrophica 757.39
- follicularis 757.39
  - in cutem penetrans 701.1
- limbic (cornea) 371.89
- palmoplantaris climacterica 701.1
- pinta (carate) 103.1
- senile (with pruritus) 702.0
- tongue 528.79
- universalis congenita 757.1
- vagina 623.1
- vocal cord 478.5
- vulva 624.09

Hyperkinesia, hyperkinetic (disease) (reaction) (syndrome) 314.9
- with
  - attention deficit — *see* Disorder, attention deficit
  - conduct disorder 314.2

Hyperkinesia, hyperkinetic — *continued*
- with — *continued*
  - developmental delay 314.1
  - simple disturbance of activity and attention 314.01
  - specified manifestation NEC 314.8
- heart (disease) 429.82
- of childhood or adolescence NEC 314.9

Hyperlacrimation — *see also* Epiphora 375.20

Hyperlipemia — *see also* Hyperlipidemia 272.4

Hyperlipidemia 272.4
- carbohydrate-induced 272.1
- combined 272.2
- endogenous 272.1
- exogenous 272.3
- fat-induced 272.3
- group
  - A 272.0
  - B 272.1
  - C 272.2
  - D 272.3
- mixed 272.2
- specified type NEC 272.4

Hyperlipidosis 272.7
- hereditary 272.7

Hyperlipoproteinemia (acquired) (essential) (familial) (hereditary) (primary) (secondary) 272.4
- Fredrickson type
  - I 272.3
  - IIa 272.0
  - IIb 272.2
  - III 272.2
  - IV 272.1
  - V 272.3
- low-density-lipoid-type (LDL) 272.0
- very-low-density-lipoid-type (VLDL) 272.1

Hyperlucent lung, unilateral 492.8

Hyperluteinization 256.1

Hyperlysinemia 270.7

Hypermagnesemia 275.2
- neonatal 775.5

Hypermaturity (fetus or newborn)
- post-term infant 766.21
- prolonged gestation infant 766.22

Hypermenorrhea 626.2

Hypermetabolism 794.7

Hypermethioninemia 270.4

Hypermetropia (congenital) 367.0

Hypermobility
- cecum 564.9
- coccyx 724.71
- colon 564.9
  - psychogenic 306.4
- ileum 564.89
- joint (acquired) 718.80
  - ankle 718.87
  - elbow 718.82
  - foot 718.87
  - hand 718.84
  - hip 718.85
  - knee 718.86
  - multiple sites 718.89
  - pelvic region 718.85
  - shoulder (region) 718.81
  - specified site NEC 718.88
  - wrist 718.83
- kidney, congenital 753.3
- meniscus (knee) 717.5
- scapula 718.81
- stomach 536.8
  - psychogenic 306.4
- syndrome 728.5
- testis, congenital 752.52
- urethral 599.81

Hypermotility
- gastrointestinal 536.8
- intestine 564.9
  - psychogenic 306.4
- stomach 536.8

Hypernasality 784.43

Hypernatremia 276.0
- with water depletion 276.0

Hypernephroma (M8312/3) 189.0

Hyperopia 367.0

Hyperorexia 783.6

Hyperornithinemia 270.6

Hyperosmia — *see also* Disturbance, sensation 781.1

Hyperosmolality 276.0

Hyperosteogenesis 733.99

Hyperostosis 733.99
- calvarial 733.3
- cortical 733.3
  - infantile 756.59
- frontal, internal of skull 733.3
- interna frontalis 733.3
- monomelic 733.99
- skull 733.3
  - congenital 756.0
- vertebral 721.8
  - with spondylosis — *see* Spondylosis
  - ankylosing 721.6

Hyperovarianism 256.1

Hyperovarism, hyperovaria 256.1

Hyperoxaluria (primary) 271.8

Hyperoxia 987.8

Hyperparathyroidism 252.00
- ectopic 259.3
- other 252.08
- primary 252.01
- secondary (of renal origin) 588.81
  - non-renal 252.02
- tertiary 252.08

Hyperpathia — *see also* Disturbance, sensation 782.0
- psychogenic 307.80

Hyperperistalsis 787.4
- psychogenic 306.4

Hyperpermeability, capillary 448.9

Hyperphagia 783.6

Hyperphenylalaninemia 270.1

Hyperphoria 378.40
- alternating 378.45

Hyperphosphatemia 275.3

Hyperpiesia — *see also* Hypertension 401.9

Hyperpiesis — *see also* Hypertension 401.9

Hyperpigmentation — *see* Pigmentation

Hyperpinealism 259.8

Hyperpipecolatemia 270.7

Hyperpituitarism 253.1

Hyperplasia, hyperplastic
- adenoids (lymphoid tissue) 474.12
  - and tonsils 474.10
- adrenal (capsule) (cortex) (gland) 255.8
  - with
    - sexual precocity (male) 255.2
    - virilism, adrenal 255.2
    - virilization (female) 255.2
  - congenital 255.2
  - due to excess ACTH (ectopic) (pituitary) 255.0
  - medulla 255.8
- alpha cells (pancreatic)
  - with
    - gastrin excess 251.5
    - glucagon excess 251.4
- angiolymphoid, with eosinophilia (ALHE) 228.01
- appendix (lymphoid) 543.0
- artery, fibromuscular NEC 447.8
  - carotid 447.8
  - renal 447.3
- bone 733.99
  - marrow 289.9
- breast (*see also* Hypertrophy, breast) 611.1
  - ductal 610.8
    - atypical 610.8
- carotid artery 447.8
- cementation, cementum (teeth) (tooth) 521.5
- cervical gland 785.6
- cervix (uteri) 622.10
  - basal cell 622.10
  - congenital 752.49
  - endometrium 622.10
  - polypoid 622.10
- chin 524.05
- clitoris, congenital 752.49
- dentin 521.5
- endocervicitis 616.0

Hyperplasia, hyperplastic — *continued*
- endometrium, endometrial (adenomatous) (atypical) (cystic) (glandular) (polypoid) (uterus) 621.30
  - with atypia 621.33
  - without atypia
    - complex 621.32
    - simple 621.31
  - benign 621.34
  - cervix 622.10
- epithelial 709.8
  - focal, oral, including tongue 528.79
  - mouth (focal) 528.79
  - nipple 611.89
  - skin 709.8
  - tongue (focal) 528.79
  - vaginal wall 623.0
- erythroid 289.9
- fascialis ossificans (progressiva) 728.11
- fibromuscular, artery NEC 447.8
  - carotid 447.8
  - renal 447.3
- genital
  - female 629.89
  - male 608.89
- gingiva 523.8
- glandularis
  - cystica uteri 621.30
  - endometrium (uterus) 621.30
  - interstitialis uteri 621.30
- granulocytic 288.69
- gum 523.8
- hymen, congenital 752.49
- islands of Langerhans 251.1
- islet cell (pancreatic) 251.9
  - alpha cells
    - with excess
      - gastrin 251.5
      - glucagon 251.4
  - beta cells 251.1
- juxtaglomerular (complex) (kidney) 593.89
- kidney (congenital) 753.3
- liver (congenital) 751.69
- lymph node (gland) 785.6
- lymphoid (diffuse) (nodular) 785.6
  - appendix 543.0
  - intestine 569.89
- mandibular 524.02
  - alveolar 524.72
  - unilateral condylar 526.89
- Marchand multiple nodular (liver) — *see* Cirrhosis, postnecrotic
- maxillary 524.01
  - alveolar 524.71
- medulla, adrenal 255.8
- myometrium, myometrial 621.2
- neuroendocrine cell, of infancy 516.61
- nose (lymphoid) (polypoid) 478.19
- oral soft tissue (inflammatory) (irritative) (mucosa) NEC 528.9
  - gingiva 523.8
  - tongue 528.9
- organ or site, congenital NEC — *see* Anomaly, specified type NEC
- ovary 620.8
- palate, papillary 528.9
- pancreatic islet cells 251.9
  - alpha
    - with excess
      - gastrin 251.5
      - glucagon 251.4
  - beta 251.1
- parathyroid (gland) 252.01
- persistent, vitreous (primary) 743.51
- pharynx (lymphoid) 478.29
- prostate 600.90
  - with
    - other lower urinary tract symptoms (LUTS) 600.91
    - urinary
      - obstruction 600.91
      - retention 600.91
  - adenofibromatous 600.20
    - with
      - other lower urinary tract symptoms (LUTS) 600.21

Hyperplasia, hyperplastic — *continued*
  prostate — *continued*
    adenofibromatous — *continued*
      with — *continued*
        urinary
          obstruction 600.21
          retention 600.21
      nodular 600.10
        with
          urinary
            obstruction 600.11
            retention 600.11
  renal artery (fibromuscular) 447.3
  reticuloendothelial (cell) 289.9
  salivary gland (any) 527.1
  Schimmelbusch's 610.1
  suprarenal (capsule) (gland) 255.8
  thymus (gland) (persistent) 254.0
  thyroid (*see also* Goiter) 240.9
    primary 242.0 ☑
    secondary 242.2 ☑
  tonsil (lymphoid tissue) 474.11
    and adenoids 474.10
  urethrovaginal 599.89
  uterus, uterine (myometrium) 621.2
    endometrium (*see also* Hyperplasia, en-
      dometrium) 621.30
  vitreous (humor), primary persistent 743.51
  vulva 624.3
  zygoma 738.11
Hyperpnea — *see also* Hyperventilation 786.01
Hyperpotassemia 276.7
Hyperprebetalipoproteinemia 272.1
  with chylomicronemia 272.3
  familial 272.1

Hyperprolactinemia 253.1
Hyperprolinemia 270.8
Hyperproteinemia 273.8
Hyperprothrombinemia 289.89
Hyperpselaphesia 782.0
Hyperpyrexia 780.60
  heat (effects of) 992.0
  malarial (*see also* Malaria) 084.6
  malignant, due to anesthetic 995.86
  rheumatic — *see* Fever, rheumatic
  unknown origin (*see also* Pyrexia) 780.60
Hyperreactor, vascular 780.2
Hyperreflexia 796.1
  bladder, autonomic 596.54
    with cauda equina 344.61
  detrusor 344.61
Hypersalivation — *see also* Ptyalism 527.7
Hypersarcosinemia 270.8
Hypersecretion
  ACTH 255.3
  androgens (ovarian) 256.1
  calcitonin 246.0
  corticoadrenal 255.3
  cortisol 255.3
  estrogen 256.0
  gastric 536.8
    psychogenic 306.4
  gastrin 251.5
  glucagon 251.4
  hormone
    ACTH 255.3
    anterior pituitary 253.1
    growth NEC 253.0
    ovarian androgen 256.1
    testicular 257.0

Hypersecretion — *continued*
  hormone — *continued*
    thyroid stimulating 242.8 ☑
  insulin — *see* Hyperinsulinism
  lacrimal glands (*see also* Epiphora) 375.20
  medulloadrenal 255.6
  milk 676.6 ☑
  ovarian androgens 256.1
  pituitary (anterior) 253.1
  salivary gland (any) 527.7
  testicular hormones 257.0
  thyrocalcitonin 246.0
  upper respiratory 478.9
Hypersegmentation, hereditary 288.2
  eosinophils 288.2
  neutrophil nuclei 288.2
Hypersensitive, hypersensitiveness, hyper-
   sensitivity — *see also* Allergy
  angiitis 446.20
    specified NEC 446.29
  carotid sinus 337.01
  colon 564.9
    psychogenic 306.4
  DNA (deoxyribonucleic acid) NEC 287.2
  drug (*see also* Allergy, drug) 995.27
  due to correct medical substance properly
    administered 995.27
  esophagus 530.89
  insect bites — *see* Injury, superficial, by site
  labyrinth 386.58
  pain (*see also* Disturbance, sensation) 782.0
  pneumonitis NEC 495.9
  reaction (*see also* Allergy) 995.3
    upper respiratory tract NEC 478.8
  stomach (allergic) (nonallergic) 536.8

Hypersensitive, hypersensitiveness,
   hypersensitivity — *see also* Allergy —
   continued
  stomach — *continued*
    psychogenic 306.4
Hypersomatotropism (classic) 253.0
Hypersomnia, unspecified 780.54
  with sleep apnea, unspecified 780.53
  alcohol induced 291.82
  drug induced 292.85
  due to
    medical condition classified elsewhere
      327.14
    mental disorder 327.15
  idiopathic
    with long sleep time 327.11
    without long sleep time 327.12
  menstrual related 327.13
  nonorganic origin 307.43
    persistent (primary) 307.44
    transient 307.43
  organic 327.10
    other 327.19
  primary 307.44
  recurrent 327.13
Hypersplenia 289.4
Hypersplenism 289.4
Hypersteatosis 706.3
Hyperstimulation, ovarian 256.1
Hypersuprarenalism 255.3
Hypersusceptibility — *see* Allergy
Hyper-TBG-nemia 246.8
Hypertelorism 756.0
  orbit, orbital 376.41

☑ **Additional Digit Required — Refer to the Tabular List for Digit Selection**   ⬇ **Subterms under main terms may continue to next column or page**

	Malignant	Benign	Unspecified
Hypertension, hypertensive (arterial) (arteriolar) (crisis) (degeneration) (disease) (essential) (fluctuating) (idiopathic) (intermittent) (labile) (low renin) (orthostatic) (paroxysmal) (primary) (systemic) (uncontrolled) (vascular)	401.0	401.1	401.9
with			
chronic kidney disease			
stage I through stage IV, or unspecified	403.00	403.10	403.90
stage V or end stage renal disese	403.01	403.11	403.91
heart involvement (conditions classifiable to 429.0–429.3, 429.8, 429.9 due to hypertension) (see also Hypertension, heart)	402.00	402.10	402.90
with kidney involvement — see Hypertension, cardiorenal			
renal (kidney) involvement (only conditions classifiable to 585, 587) (excludes conditions classifiable to 584) (see also Hypertension, kidney)	403.00	403.10	403.90
with heart involvement — see Hypertension, cardiorenal			
failure (and sclerosis) (see also Hypertension, kidney)	403.01	403.11	403.91
sclerosis without failure (see also Hypertension, kidney)	403.00	403.10	403.90
accelerated (see also Hypertension, by type, malignant))	401.0	—	—
antepartum — see Hypertension, complicating pregnancy, childbirth, or the puerperium			
borderline	—	—	796.2
cardiorenal (disease)	404.00	404.10	404.90
with			
chronic kidney disease			
stage I through stage IV, or unspecified	404.00	404.10	404.90
and heart failure	404.01	404.11	404.91
stage V or end stage renal disease	404.02	404.12	404.92
and heart failure	404.03	404.13	404.93
heart failure	404.01	404.11	404.91
and chronic kidney disease	404.01	404.11	404.91
stage I through stage IV or unspecified	404.01	404.11	404.91
stave V or end stage renal disease	404.03	404.13	404.93
cardiovascular disease (arteriosclerotic) (sclerotic)	402.00	402.10	402.90
with			
heart failure	402.01	402.11	402.91
renal involvement (conditions classifiable to 403) (see also Hypertension, cardiorenal)	404.00	404.10	404.90
cardiovascular-renal (disease) (sclerosis) (see also Hypertension, cardiorenal)	404.00	404.10	404.90
cerebrovascular disease NEC	437.2	—	—
complicating pregnancy, childbirth, or the puerperium	642.2	642.0	642.9
with			
albuminuria (and edema) (mild)	—	—	642.4
severe	—	—	642.5
chronic kidney disesae	642.2	—	—
and heart disease	642.2	—	—
edema (mild)	—	—	642.4
severe	—	—	642.5
heart disease	642.2	—	—
and chronic kidney disease	642.2	—	—
renal disease	642.2	—	—
and heart disease	642.2	—	—
chronic	642.2	642.0	—
with pre-eclampsia or eclampsia	642.7	—	—
fetus or newborn	760.0	—	—
essential	—	642.0	—
with pre-eclampsia or eclampsia	—	642.7	—
fetus or newborn	760.0	—	—
fetus or newborn	760.0	—	—
gestational	—	—	642.3
pre-existing	642.2	642.0	—
with pre-eclampsia or eclampsia	642.7	—	—
fetus or newborn	760.0	—	—
secondary to renal disease	642.1	—	—
with pre-eclampsia or eclampsia	642.7	—	—
fetus or newborn	760.0	—	—
transient	—	—	642.3
due to			
aldosteronism, primary	405.09	405.19	405.99
brain tumor	405.09	405.19	405.99
bulbar poliomyelitis	405.09	405.19	405.99
calculus			
kidney	405.09	405.19	405.99

	Malignant	Benign	Unspecified
Hypertension, hypertensive — continued			
due to — continued			
calculus — continued			
ureter	405.09	405.19	405.99
coarctation, aorta	405.09	405.19	405.99
Cushing's disease	405.09	405.19	405.99
glomerulosclerosis (see also Hypertension, kidney)	403.00	403.10	403.90
periarteritis nodosa	405.09	405.19	405.99
pheochromocytoma	405.09	405.19	405.99
polycystic kidney(s)	405.09	405.19	405.99
polycythemia	405.09	405.19	405.99
porphyria	405.09	405.19	405.99
pyelonephritis	405.09	405.19	405.99
renal (artery)			
aneurysm	405.01	405.11	405.91
anomaly	405.01	405.11	405.91
embolism	405.01	405.11	405.91
fibromuscular hyperplasia	405.01	405.11	405.91
occlusion	405.01	405.11	405.91
stenosis	405.01	405.11	405.91
thrombosis	405.01	405.11	405.91
encephalopathy	437.2	—	—
gestational (transient) NEC	—	—	642.3
Goldblatt's	440.1	—	—
heart (disease) (conditions classifiable to 429.0–429.3, 429.8, 429.9 due to hypertension)	402.00	402.10	402.90
with heart failure	402.01	402.11	402.91
hypertensive kidney disease (conditions classifiable to 403) (see also Hypertension, cardiorenal)	404.00	404.10	404.90
renal sclerosis (see also Hypertension, cardiorenal)	404.00	404.10	404.90
intracranial, benign	—	348.2	—
intraocular	—	—	365.04
kidney	403.00	403.10	403.90
with			
chronic kidney disease			
stage I through stage IV, or unspecified	403.00	403.10	403.90
stage V or end stage renal disese	403.01	403.11	403.91
heart involvement (conditions classifiable to 429.0–429.3, 429.8, 429.9 due to hypertension) (see also Hypertension, cardiorenal)	404.00	404.10	404.90
hypertensive heart (disease) (conditions classifiable to 402) (see also Hypertension, cardiorenal)	404.00	404.10	404.90
lesser circulation	—	—	416.0
necrotizing	401.0	—	—
ocular	—	—	365.04
pancreatic duct — code to underlying condition			
with			
chronic pancreatitis	—	—	577.1
portal (due to chronic liver disease)	—	—	572.3
postoperative	—	—	997.91
psychogenic	—	—	306.2
puerperal, postpartum — see Hypertension, complicating pregnancy, childbirth, or the puerperium			
pulmonary (artery) (secondary)	—	—	416.8
with			
cor pulmonale (chronic)	—	—	416.8
acute	—	—	415.0
right heart ventricular strain/failure	—	—	416.8
acute	—	—	415.0
idiopathic	—	—	416.0
primary	—	—	416.0
of newborn	—	—	747.83
secondary	—	—	416.8
renal (disease) (see also Hypertension, kidney)	403.00	403.10	403.90
renovascular NEC	405.01	405.11	405.91
secondary NEC	405.09	405.19	405.99
due to			
aldosteronism, primary	405.09	405.19	405.99
brain tumor	405.09	405.19	405.99
bulbar poliomyelitis	405.09	405.19	405.99
calculus			
kidney	405.09	405.19	405.99
ureter	405.09	405.19	405.99
coarctation, aorta	405.09	405.19	405.99
Cushing's disease	405.09	405.19	405.99
glomerulosclerosis (see also Hypertension, kidney)	403.00	403.10	403.90

☑ **Additional Digit Required — Refer to the Tabular List for Digit Selection**   ▽ **Subterms under main terms may continue to next column or page**

	Malignant	Benign	Unspecified
Hypertension, hypertensive — *continued*			
secondary — *continued*			
due to — *continued*			
periarteritis nodosa	405.09	405.19	405.99
pheochromocytoma	405.09	405.19	405.99
polycystic kidney(s)	405.09	405.19	405.99
polycythemia	405.09	405.19	405.99
porphyria	405.09	405.19	405.99
pyelonephritis	405.09	405.19	405.99
renal (artery)			
aneurysm	405.01	405.11	405.91
anomaly	405.01	405.11	405.91
embolism	405.01	405.11	405.91
fibromuscular hyperplasia	405.01	405.11	405.91
occlusion	405.01	405.11	405.91
stenosis	405.01	405.11	405.91
thrombosis	405.01	405.11	405.91
transient	—	—	796.2
of pregnancy	—	—	642.3
vascular degeneration	401.0	401.1	401.9
venous, chronic (asymptomatic) (idiopathic)	—	—	459.30
with			
complication, NEC	—	—	459.39
inflammation	—	—	459.32
with ulcer	—	—	459.33
ulcer	—	—	459.31
with inflammation	—	—	459.33
due to			
deep vein thrombosis (*see also* Syndrome, postphlebetic)	—	—	459.10

☑ **Additional Digit Required** — **Refer to the Tabular List for Digit Selection**   ⓦ **Subterms under main terms may continue to next column or page**

2013 ICD-9-CM   ▶◀ **Revised Text**   ● **New Line**   ▲ **Revised Code**   **Volume 2 — 147**

Hypertensive urgency — *see* Hypertension
Hyperthecosis, ovary 256.8
Hyperthermia (of unknown origin) — *see also* Pyrexia 780.60
   malignant (due to anesthesia) 995.86
   newborn 778.4
Hyperthymergasia — *see also* Psychosis, affective 296.0 ☑
   reactive (from emotional stress, psychological trauma) 298.1
   recurrent episode 296.1 ☑
   single episode 296.0 ☑
Hyperthymism 254.8
Hyperthyroid (recurrent) — *see* Hyperthyroidism
Hyperthyroidism (latent) (preadult) (recurrent) (without goiter) 242.9 ☑

> *Note — Use the following fifth-digit subclassification with category 242:*
>
> 0   *without mention of thyrotoxic crisis or storm*
>
> 1   *with mention of thyrotoxic crisis or storm*

   with
      goiter (diffuse) 242.0 ☑
         adenomatous 242.3 ☑
            multinodular 242.2 ☑
            uninodular 242.1 ☑
         nodular 242.3 ☑
            multinodular 242.2 ☑
            uninodular 242.1 ☑
         thyroid nodule 242.1 ☑
      complicating pregnancy, childbirth, or puerperium 648.1 ☑
      neonatal (transient) 775.3
Hypertonia — *see* Hypertonicity
Hypertonicity
   bladder 596.51
   fetus or newborn 779.89
   gastrointestinal (tract) 536.8
   infancy 779.89
      due to electrolyte imbalance 779.89
   muscle 728.85
   stomach 536.8
      psychogenic 306.4
   uterus, uterine (contractions) 661.4 ☑
      affecting fetus or newborn 763.7
Hypertony — *see* Hypertonicity
Hypertransaminemia 790.4
Hypertrichosis 704.1
   congenital 757.4
   eyelid 374.54
   lanuginosa 757.4
      acquired 704.1
Hypertriglyceridemia, essential 272.1
Hypertrophy, hypertrophic
   adenoids (infectional) 474.12
      and tonsils (faucial) (infective) (lingual) (lymphoid) 474.10
   adrenal 255.8
   alveolar process or ridge 525.8
   anal papillae 569.49
   apocrine gland 705.82
   artery NEC 447.8
      carotid 447.8
      congenital (peripheral) NEC 747.60
         gastrointestinal 747.61
         lower limb 747.64
         renal 747.62
         specified NEC 747.69
         spinal 747.82
         upper limb 747.63
      renal 447.3
   arthritis (chronic) (*see also* Osteoarthrosis) 715.9 ☑
      spine (*see also* Spondylosis) 721.90
   arytenoid 478.79
   asymmetrical (heart) 429.9
   auricular — *see* Hypertrophy, cardiac
   Bartholin's gland 624.8
   bile duct 576.8
   bladder (sphincter) (trigone) 596.89
   blind spot, visual field 368.42
   bone 733.99

Hypertrophy, hypertrophic — *continued*
   brain 348.89
   breast 611.1
      cystic 610.1
      fetus or newborn 778.7
      fibrocystic 610.1
      massive pubertal 611.1
      puerperal, postpartum 676.3 ☑
      senile (parenchymatous) 611.1
   cardiac (chronic) (idiopathic) 429.3
      with
         rheumatic fever (conditions classifiable to 390)
            active 391.8
               with chorea 392.0
            inactive or quiescent (with chorea) 398.99
      congenital NEC 746.89
      fatty (*see also* Degeneration, myocardial) 429.1
      hypertensive (*see also* Hypertension, heart) 402.90
      rheumatic (with chorea) 398.99
         active or acute 391.8
            with chorea 392.0
      valve (*see also* Endocarditis) 424.90
         congenital NEC 746.89
   cartilage 733.99
   cecum 569.89
   cervix (uteri) 622.6
      congenital 752.49
      elongation 622.6
   clitoris (cirrhotic) 624.2
      congenital 752.49
   colon 569.89
      congenital 751.3
   conjunctiva, lymphoid 372.73
   cornea 371.89
   corpora cavernosa 607.89
   duodenum 537.89
   endometrium (uterus) (*see also* Hyperplasia, endometrium) 621.30
      cervix 622.6
   epididymis 608.89
   esophageal hiatus (congenital) 756.6
      with hernia — *see* Hernia, diaphragm
   eyelid 374.30
   falx, skull 733.99
   fat pad 729.30
      infrapatellar 729.31
      knee 729.31
      orbital 374.34
      popliteal 729.31
      prepatellar 729.31
      retropatellar 729.31
      specified site NEC 729.39
   foot (congenital) 755.67
   frenum, frenulum (tongue) 529.8
      linguae 529.8
      lip 528.5
   gallbladder or cystic duct 575.8
   gastric mucosa 535.2 ☑
   gingiva 523.8
   gland, glandular (general) NEC 785.6
   gum (mucous membrane) 523.8
   heart (idiopathic) (*see also* Hypertrophy, cardiac)
      valve (*see also* Endocarditis)
         congenital NEC 746.89
   hemifacial 754.0
   hepatic — *see* Hypertrophy, liver
   hiatus (esophageal) 756.6
   hilus gland 785.6
   hymen, congenital 752.49
   ileum 569.89
   infrapatellar fat pad 729.31
   intestine 569.89
   jejunum 569.89
   kidney (compensatory) 593.1
      congenital 753.3
   labial frenulum 528.5
   labium (majus) (minus) 624.3
   lacrimal gland, chronic 375.03
   ligament 728.9
      spinal 724.8
   linguae frenulum 529.8

Hypertrophy, hypertrophic — *continued*
   lingual tonsil (infectional) 474.11
   lip (frenum) 528.5
      congenital 744.81
   liver 789.1
      acute 573.8
      cirrhotic — *see* Cirrhosis, liver
      congenital 751.69
      fatty — *see* Fatty, liver
   lymph gland 785.6
      tubercuious — *see* Tuberculosis, lymph gland
   mammary gland — *see* Hypertrophy, breast
   maxillary frenulum 528.5
   Meckel's diverticulum (congenital) 751.0
   medial meniscus, acquired 717.3
   median bar 600.90
      with
         other lower urinary tract symptoms (LUTS) 600.91
         urinary
            obstruction 600.91
            retention 600.91
   mediastinum 519.3
   meibomian gland 373.2
   meniscus, knee, congenital 755.64
   metatarsal head 733.99
   metatarsus 733.99
   mouth 528.9
   mucous membrane
      alveolar process 523.8
      nose 478.19
      turbinate (nasal) 478.0
   muscle 728.9
   muscular coat, artery NEC 447.8
      carotid 447.8
      renal 447.3
   myocardium (*see also* Hypertrophy, cardiac) 429.3
      idiopathic 425.18
   myometrium 621.2
   nail 703.8
      congenital 757.5
   nasal 478.19
      alae 478.19
      bone 738.0
      cartilage 478.19
      mucous membrane (septum) 478.19
      sinus (*see also* Sinusitis) 473.9
      turbinate 478.0
   nasopharynx, lymphoid (infectional) (tissue) (wall) 478.29
   neck, uterus 622.6
   nipple 611.1
   normal aperture diaphragm (congenital) 756.6
   nose (*see also* Hypertrophy, nasal) 478.19
   orbit 376.46
   organ or site, congenital NEC — *see* Anomaly, specified type NEC
   osteoarthropathy (pulmonary) 731.2
   ovary 620.8
   palate (hard) 526.89
      soft 528.9
   pancreas (congenital) 751.7
   papillae
      anal 569.49
      tongue 529.3
   parathyroid (gland) 252.01
   parotid gland 527.1
   penis 607.89
   phallus 607.89
      female (clitoris) 624.2
   pharyngeal tonsil 474.12
   pharyngitis 472.1
   pharynx 478.29
      lymphoid (infectional) (tissue) (wall) 478.29
   pituitary (fossa) (gland) 253.8
   popliteal fat pad 729.31
   preauricular (lymph) gland (Hampstead) 785.6
   prepuce (congenital) 605
      female 624.2
   prostate (asymptomatic) (early) (recurrent) 600.90

Hypertrophy, hypertrophic — *continued*
   prostate — *continued*
      with
         other lower urinary tract symptoms (LUTS) 600.91
         urinary
            obstruction 600.91
            retention 600.91
      adenofibromatous 600.20
         with
            other lower urinary tract symptoms (LUTS) 600.21
            urinary
               obstruction 600.21
               retention 600.21
      benign 600.00
         with
            other lower urinary tract symptoms (LUTS) 600.01
            urinary
               obstruction 600.01
               retention 600.01
      congenital 752.89
   pseudoedematous hypodermal 757.0
   pseudomuscular 359.1
   pylorus (muscle) (sphincter) 537.0
      congenital 750.5
      infantile 750.5
   rectal sphincter 569.49
   rectum 569.49
   renal 593.1
   rhinitis (turbinate) 472.0
   salivary duct or gland 527.1
      congenital 750.26
   scaphoid (tarsal) 733.99
   scar 701.4
   scrotum 608.89
   sella turcica 253.8
   seminal vesicle 608.89
   sigmoid 569.89
   skin condition NEC 701.9
   spermatic cord 608.89
   spinal ligament 724.8
   spleen — *see* Splenomegaly
   spondylitis (spine) (*see also* Spondylosis) 721.90
   stomach 537.89
   subaortic stenosis (idiopathic) 425.11
   sublingual gland 527.1
      congenital 750.26
   submaxillary gland 527.1
   suprarenal (gland) 255.8
   tendon 727.9
   testis 608.89
      congenital 752.89
   thymic, thymus (congenital) (gland) 254.0
   thyroid (gland) (*see also* Goiter) 240.9
      primary 242.0 ☑
      secondary 242.2 ☑
   toe (congenital) 755.65
      acquired 735.8
   tongue 529.8
      congenital 750.15
      frenum 529.8
      papillae (foliate) 529.3
   tonsil (faucial) (infective) (lingual) (lymphoid) 474.11
      with
         adenoiditis 474.01
         tonsillitis 474.00
            and adenoiditis 474.02
      and adenoids 474.10
   tunica vaginalis 608.89
   turbinate (mucous membrane) 478.0
   ureter 593.89
   urethra 599.84
   uterus 621.2
      puerperal, postpartum 674.8 ☑
   uvula 528.9
   vagina 623.8
   vas deferens 608.89
   vein 459.89
   ventricle, ventricular (heart) (left) (right) (*see also* Hypertrophy, cardiac)
      congenital 746.89

☑ **Additional Digit Required — Refer to the Tabular List for Digit Selection**   ▽ **Subterms under main terms may continue to next column or page**

148 — Volume 2   ▶◀ Revised Text   ● New Line   ▲ Revised Code   **2013 ICD-9-CM**

Hypertrophy, hypertrophic — continued
 ventricle, ventricular (see also Hypertrophy, cardiac) — continued
  due to hypertension (left) (right) (see also Hypertension, heart) 402.90
   benign 402.10
   malignant 402.00
  right with ventricular septal defect, pulmonary stenosis or atresia, and dextraposition of aorta 745.2
 verumontanum 599.89
 vesical 596.89
 vocal cord 478.5
 vulva 624.3
  stasis (nonfilarial) 624.3
Hypertropia (intermittent) (periodic) 378.31
Hypertyrosinemia 270.2
Hyperuricemia 790.6
Hypervalinemia 270.3
Hyperventilation (tetany) 786.01
 hysterical 300.11
 psychogenic 306.1
 syndrome 306.1
Hyperviscidosis 277.00
Hyperviscosity (of serum) (syndrome) NEC 273.3
 polycythemic 289.0
 sclerocythemic 282.8
Hypervitaminosis (dietary) NEC 278.8
 A (dietary) 278.2
 D (dietary) 278.4
 from excessive administration or use of vitamin preparations (chronic) 278.8
  reaction to sudden overdose 963.5
 vitamin A 278.2
  reaction to sudden overdose 963.5
 vitamin D 278.4
  reaction to sudden overdose 963.5
 vitamin K
  correct substance properly administered 278.8
  overdose or wrong substance given or taken 964.3
Hypervolemia 276.69
Hypesthesia — see also Disturbance, sensation 782.0
 cornea 371.81
Hyphema (anterior chamber) (ciliary body) (iris) 364.41
 traumatic 921.3
Hyphemia — see Hyphema
Hypoacidity, gastric 536.8
 psychogenic 306.4
Hypoactive labyrinth (function) — see Hypofunction, labyrinth
Hypoadrenalism 255.41
 tuberculous (see also Tuberculosis) 017.6 ☑
Hypoadrenocorticism 255.41
 pituitary 253.4
Hypoalbuminemia 273.8
Hypoaldosteronism 255.42
Hypoalphalipoproteinemia 272.5
Hypobarism 993.2
Hypobaropathy 993.2
Hypobetalipoproteinemia (familial) 272.5
Hypocalcemia 275.41
 cow's milk 775.4
 dietary 269.3
 neonatal 775.4
 phosphate-loading 775.4
Hypocalcification, teeth 520.4
Hypochloremia 276.9
Hypochlorhydria 536.8
 neurotic 306.4
 psychogenic 306.4
Hypocholesteremia 272.5
Hypochondria (reaction) 300.7
Hypochondriac 300.7
Hypochondriasis 300.7
Hypochromasia blood cells 280.9
Hypochromic anemia 280.9
 due to blood loss (chronic) 280.0
  acute 285.1
 microcytic 280.9
Hypocoagulability — see also Defect, coagulation 286.9

Hypocomplementemia 279.8
Hypocythemia (progressive) 284.9
Hypodontia — see also Anodontia 520.0
Hypoeosinophilia 288.59
Hypoesthesia — see also Disturbance, sensation 782.0
 cornea 371.81
 tactile 782.0
Hypoestrinism 256.39
Hypoestrogenism 256.39
Hypoferremia 280.9
 due to blood loss (chronic) 280.0
Hypofertility
 female 628.9
 male 606.1
Hypofibrinogenemia 286.3
 acquired 286.6
 congenital 286.3
Hypofunction
 adrenal (gland) 255.41
  cortex 255.41
  medulla 255.5
  specified NEC 255.5
 cerebral 331.9
 corticoadrenal NEC 255.41
 intestinal 564.89
 labyrinth (unilateral) 386.53
  with loss of labyrinthine reactivity 386.55
  bilateral 386.54
   with loss of labyrinthine reactivity 386.56
 Leydig cell 257.2
 ovary 256.39
  postablative 256.2
 pituitary (anterior) (gland) (lobe) 253.2
  posterior 253.5
 testicular 257.2
  iatrogenic 257.1
  postablative 257.1
  postirradiation 257.1
  postsurgical 257.1
Hypogammaglobulinemia 279.00
 acquired primary 279.06
 non-sex-linked, congenital 279.06
 sporadic 279.06
 transient of infancy 279.09
Hypogenitalism (congenital) (female) (male) 752.89
 penis 752.69
Hypoglycemia (spontaneous) 251.2
 coma 251.0
  diabetic 250.3 ☑
   due to secondary diabetes 249.3 ☑
 diabetic 250.8 ☑
  due to secondary diabetes 249.8 ☑
 due to insulin 251.0
  therapeutic misadventure 962.3
 familial (idiopathic) 251.2
 following gastrointestinal surgery 579.3
 infantile (idiopathic) 251.2
 in infant of diabetic mother 775.0
 leucine-induced 270.3
 neonatal 775.6
 reactive 251.2
 specified NEC 251.1
Hypoglycemic shock 251.0
 diabetic 250.8 ☑
  due to secondary diabetes 249.8 ☑
 due to insulin 251.0
 functional (syndrome) 251.1
Hypogonadism
 female 256.39
 gonadotrophic (isolated) 253.4
 hypogonadotropic (isolated) (with anosmia) 253.4
 isolated 253.4
 male 257.2
  hereditary familial (Reifenstein's syndrome) 259.52
 ovarian (primary) 256.39
 pituitary (secondary) 253.4
 testicular (primary) (secondary) 257.2
Hypohidrosis 705.0
Hypohidrotic ectodermal dysplasia 757.31
Hypoidrosis 705.0
Hypoinsulinemia, postsurgical 251.3

Hypoinsulinemia, postsurgical — continued
 postpancreatectomy (complete) (partial) 251.3
Hypokalemia 276.8
Hypokinesia 780.99
Hypoleukia splenica 289.4
Hypoleukocytosis 288.50
Hypolipidemia 272.5
Hypolipoproteinemia 272.5
Hypomagnesemia 275.2
 neonatal 775.4
Hypomania, hypomanic reaction — see also Psychosis, affective 296.0 ☑
 recurrent episode 296.1 ☑
 single episode 296.0 ☑
Hypomastia (congenital) 611.82
Hypomenorrhea 626.1
Hypometabolism 783.9
Hypomotility
 gastrointestinal tract 536.8
  psychogenic 306.4
 intestine 564.89
  psychogenic 306.4
 stomach 536.8
  psychogenic 306.4
Hyponasality 784.44
Hyponatremia 276.1
Hypo-ovarianism 256.39
Hypo-ovarism 256.39
Hypoparathyroidism (idiopathic) (surgically induced) 252.1
 neonatal 775.4
Hypoperfusion (in)
 newborn 779.89
Hypopharyngitis 462
Hypophoria 378.40
Hypophosphatasia 275.3
Hypophosphatemia (acquired) (congenital) (familial) 275.3
 renal 275.3
Hypophyseal, hypophysis — see also condition
 dwarfism 253.3
 gigantism 253.0
 syndrome 253.8
Hypophyseothalamic syndrome 253.8
Hypopiesis — see Hypotension
Hypopigmentation 709.00
 eyelid 374.53
Hypopinealism 259.8
Hypopituitarism (juvenile) (syndrome) 253.2
 due to
  hormone therapy 253.7
  hypophysectomy 253.7
  radiotherapy 253.7
 postablative 253.7
 postpartum hemorrhage 253.2
Hypoplasia, hypoplasis 759.89
 adrenal (gland) 759.1
 alimentary tract 751.8
  lower 751.2
  upper 750.8
 angiolymphoid, with eosinophilia (ALHE) 228.01
 anus, anal (canal) 751.2
 aorta 747.22
 aortic
  arch (tubular) 747.10
  orifice or valve with hypoplasia of ascending aorta and defective development of left ventricle (with mitral valve atresia) 746.7
 appendix 751.2
 areola 757.6
 arm (see also Absence, arm, congenital) 755.20
 artery (congenital) (peripheral) 747.60
  brain 747.81
  cerebral 747.81
  coronary 746.85
  gastrointestinal 747.61
  lower limb 747.64
  pulmonary 747.31
  renal 747.62
  retinal 743.58

Hypoplasia, hypoplasis — continued
 artery — continued
  specified NEC 747.69
  spinal 747.82
  umbilical 747.5
  upper limb 747.63
 auditory canal 744.29
  causing impairment of hearing 744.02
 biliary duct (common) or passage 751.61
 bladder 753.8
 bone NEC 756.9
  face 756.0
  malar 756.0
  mandible 524.04
   alveolar 524.74
  marrow 284.9
   acquired (secondary) 284.89
   congenital 284.09
   idiopathic 284.9
  maxilla 524.03
   alveolar 524.73
  skull (see also Hypoplasia, skull) 756.0
 brain 742.1
  gyri 742.2
  specified part 742.2
 breast (areola) 611.82
 bronchus (tree) 748.3
 cardiac 746.89
  valve — see Hypoplasia, heart, valve
  vein 746.89
 carpus (see also Absence, carpal, congenital) 755.28
 cartilaginous 756.9
 cecum 751.2
 cementum 520.4
  hereditary 520.5
 cephalic 742.1
 cerebellum 742.2
 cervix (uteri) 752.43
 chin 524.06
 clavicle 755.51
 coccyx 756.19
 colon 751.2
 corpus callosum 742.2
 cricoid cartilage 748.3
 dermal, focal (Goltz) 757.39
 digestive organ(s) or tract NEC 751.8
  lower 751.2
  upper 750.8
 ear 744.29
  auricle 744.23
  lobe 744.29
  middle, except ossicles 744.03
   ossicles 744.04
  ossicles 744.04
 enamel of teeth (neonatal) (postnatal) (prenatal) 520.4
  hereditary 520.5
 endocrine (gland) NEC 759.2
 endometrium 621.8
 epididymis 752.89
 epiglottis 748.3
 erythroid, congenital 284.01
 erythropoietic, chronic acquired 284.81
 esophagus 750.3
 Eustachian tube 744.24
 eye (see also Microphthalmos) 743.10
  lid 743.62
 face 744.89
  bone(s) 756.0
 fallopian tube 752.19
 femur (see also Absence, femur, congenital) 755.34
 fibula (see also Absence, fibula, congenital) 755.37
 finger (see also Absence, finger, congenital) 755.29
 focal dermal 757.39
 foot 755.31
 gallbladder 751.69
 genitalia, genital organ(s)
  female 752.89
   external 752.49
   internal NEC 752.89
   in adiposogenital dystrophy 253.8
  male 752.89

☑ Additional Digit Required — Refer to the Tabular List for Digit Selection   Subterms under main terms may continue to next column or page

2013 ICD-9-CM   ►◄ Revised Text   ● New Line   ▲ Revised Code   Volume 2 — 149

Hypoplasia, hypoplasis — *continued*
  genitalia, genital organ(s) — *continued*
    male — *continued*
      penis 752.69
  glottis 748.3
  hair 757.4
  hand 755.21
  heart 746.89
    left (complex) (syndrome) 746.7
    valve NEC 746.89
      pulmonary 746.01
  humerus (*see also* Absence, humerus, congenital) 755.24
  hymen 752.49
  intestine (small) 751.1
    large 751.2
  iris 743.46
  jaw 524.09
  kidney(s) 753.0
  labium (majus) (minus) 752.49
  labyrinth, membranous 744.05
  lacrimal duct (apparatus) 743.65
  larynx 748.3
  leg (*see also* Absence, limb, congenital, lower) 755.30
  limb 755.4
    lower (*see also* Absence, limb, congenital, lower) 755.30
    upper (*see also* Absence, limb, congenital, upper) 755.20
  liver 751.69
  lung (lobe) 748.5
  mammary (areolar) 611.82
  mandibular 524.04
    alveolar 524.74
    unilateral condylar 526.89
  maxillary 524.03
    alveolar 524.73
  medullary 284.9
  megakaryocytic 287.30
  metacarpus (*see also* Absence, metacarpal, congenital) 755.28
  metatarsus (*see also* Absence, metatarsal, congenital) 755.38
  muscle 756.89
    eye 743.69
  myocardium (congenital) (Uhl's anomaly) 746.84
  nail(s) 757.5
  nasolacrimal duct 743.65
  nervous system NEC 742.8
  neural 742.8
  nose, nasal 748.1
  ophthalmic (*see also* Microphthalmos) 743.10
  optic nerve 377.43
  organ
    of Corti 744.05
    or site NEC — *see* Anomaly, by site
  osseous meatus (ear) 744.03
  ovary 752.0
  oviduct 752.19
  pancreas 751.7
  parathyroid (gland) 759.2
  parotid gland 750.26
  patella 755.64
  pelvis, pelvic girdle 755.69
  penis 752.69
  peripheral vascular system (congenital) NEC 747.60
    gastrointestinal 747.61
    lower limb 747.64
    renal 747.62
    specified NEC 747.69
    spinal 747.82
    upper limb 747.63
  pituitary (gland) 759.2
  pulmonary 748.5

Hypoplasia, hypoplasis — *continued*
  pulmonary — *continued*
    arteriovenous 747.32
    artery 747.31
    valve 746.01
  punctum lacrimale 743.65
  radioulnar (*see also* Absence, radius, congenital, with ulna) 755.25
  radius (*see also* Absence, radius, congenital) 755.26
  rectum 751.2
  respiratory system NEC 748.9
  rib 756.3
  sacrum 756.19
  scapula 755.59
  shoulder girdle 755.59
  skin 757.39
  skull (bone) 756.0
    with
      anencephalus 740.0
      encephalocele 742.0
      hydrocephalus 742.3
        with spina bifida (*see also* Spina bifida) 741.0 ☑
      microcephalus 742.1
  spinal (cord) (ventral horn cell) 742.59
    vessel 747.82
  spine 756.19
  spleen 759.0
  sternum 756.3
  tarsus (*see also* Absence, tarsal, congenital) 755.38
  testis, testicle 752.89
  thymus (gland) 279.11
  thyroid (gland) 243
    cartilage 748.3
  tibiofibular (*see also* Absence, tibia, congenital, with fibula) 755.35
  toe (*see also* Absence, toe, congenital) 755.39
  tongue 750.16
  trachea (cartilage) (rings) 748.3
  Turner's (tooth) 520.4
  ulna (*see also* Absence, ulna, congenital) 755.27
  umbilical artery 747.5
  ureter 753.29
  uterus 752.32
  vagina 752.45
  vascular (peripheral) NEC (*see also* Hypoplasia, peripheral vascular system) 747.60
    brain 747.81
  vein(s) (peripheral) NEC (*see also* Hypoplasia, peripheral vascular system) 747.60
    brain 747.81
    cardiac 746.89
    great 747.49
    portal 747.49
    pulmonary 747.49
    vena cava (inferior) (superior) 747.49
  vertebra 756.19
  vulva 752.49
  zonule (ciliary) 743.39
  zygoma 738.12
Hypopotassemia 276.8
Hypoproaccelerinemia — *see* Defect, coagulation 286.3
Hypoproconvertinemia (congenital) — *see also* Defect, coagulation 286.3
Hypoproteinemia (essential) (hypermetabolic) (idiopathic) 273.8
Hypoproteinosis 260
Hypoprothrombinemia (congenital) (hereditary) (idiopathic) — *see also* Defect, coagulation 286.3
  acquired 286.7
  newborn 776.3

Hypopselaphesia 782.0
Hypopyon (anterior chamber) (eye) 364.05
  iritis 364.05
  ulcer (cornea) 370.04
Hypopyrexia 780.99
Hyporeflex 796.1
Hyporeninemia, extreme 790.99
  in primary aldosteronism 255.10
Hyporesponsive episode 780.09
Hyposecretion
  ACTH 253.4
  ovary 256.39
    postablative 256.2
  salivary gland (any) 527.7
Hyposegmentation of neutrophils, hereditary 288.2
Hyposiderinemia 280.9
Hyposmolality 276.1
  syndrome 276.1
Hyposomatotropism 253.3
Hyposomnia, unspecified — *see also* Insomnia 780.52
  with sleep apnea, unspecified 780.51
Hypospadias (male) 752.61
  female 753.8
Hypospermatogenesis 606.1
Hyposphagma 372.72
Hyposplenism 289.59
Hypostasis, pulmonary 514
Hypostatic — *see* condition
Hyposthenuria 593.89
Hyposuprarenalism 255.41
Hypo-TBG-nemia 246.8
Hypotension (arterial) (constitutional) 458.9
  chronic 458.1
  iatrogenic 458.29
  maternal, syndrome (following labor and delivery) 669.2 ☑
  of hemodialysis 458.21
  orthostatic (chronic) 458.0
    dysautonomic-dyskinetic syndrome 333.0
  permanent idiopathic 458.1
  postoperative 458.29
  postural 458.0
  specified type NEC 458.8
  transient 796.3
Hypothermia (accidental) 991.6
  anesthetic 995.89
  associated with low environmental temperature 991.6
  newborn NEC 778.3
  not associated with low environmental temperature 780.65
Hypothymergasia — *see also* Psychosis, affective 296.2 ☑
  recurrent episode 296.3 ☑
  single episode 296.2 ☑
Hypothyroidism (acquired) 244.9
  complicating pregnancy, childbirth, or puerperium 648.1 ☑
  congenital 243
  due to
    ablation 244.1
      radioactive iodine 244.1
      surgical 244.0
    iodine (administration) (ingestion) 244.2
      radioactive 244.1
    irradiation therapy 244.1
    p-aminosalicylic acid (PAS) 244.3
    phenylbutazone 244.3
    resorcinol 244.3
    specified cause NEC 244.8
    surgery 244.0
  goitrous (sporadic) 246.1
  iatrogenic NEC 244.3
  iodine 244.2

Hypothyroidism — *continued*
  pituitary 244.8
  postablative NEC 244.1
  postsurgical 244.0
  primary 244.9
  secondary NEC 244.8
  specified cause NEC 244.8
  sporadic goitrous 246.1
Hypotonia, hypotonicity, hypotony 781.3
  benign congenital 358.8
  bladder 596.4
  congenital 779.89
    benign 358.8
  eye 360.30
    due to
      fistula 360.32
      ocular disorder NEC 360.33
      following loss of aqueous or vitreous 360.33
    primary 360.31
  infantile muscular (benign) 359.0
  muscle 728.9
  uterus, uterine (contractions) — *see* Inertia, uterus
Hypotrichosis 704.09
  congenital 757.4
  lid (congenital) 757.4
    acquired 374.55
  postinfectional NEC 704.09
Hypotropia 378.32
Hypoventilation 786.09
  congenital central alveolar syndrome 327.25
  idiopathic sleep related nonobstructive alveolar 327.24
  obesity 278.03
  sleep related, in conditions classifiable elsewhere 327.26
Hypovitaminosis — *see also* Deficiency, vitamin 269.2
Hypovolemia 276.52
  surgical shock 998.09
  traumatic (shock) 958.4
Hypoxemia — *see also* Anoxia 799.02
  sleep related, in conditions classifiable elsewhere 327.26
Hypoxia — *see also* Anoxia 799.02
  cerebral 348.1
    during or resulting from a procedure 997.01
    newborn 770.88
      mild or moderate 768.6
      severe 768.5
  fetal, affecting newborn 770.88
  intrauterine — *see* Distress, fetal
  myocardial (*see also* Insufficiency, coronary) 411.89
    arteriosclerotic — *see* Arteriosclerosis, coronary
  newborn 770.88
  sleep related 327.24
Hypoxic-ischemic encephalopathy (HIE) 768.70
  mild 768.71
  moderate 768.72
  severe 768.73
Hypsarrhythmia — *see also* Epilepsy 345.6 ☑
Hysteralgia, pregnant uterus 646.8 ☑
Hysteria, hysterical 300.10
  anxiety 300.20
  Charcôt's gland 300.11
  conversion (any manifestation) 300.11
  dissociative type NEC 300.15
  psychosis, acute 298.1
Hysteroepilepsy 300.11
Hysterotomy, affecting fetus or newborn 763.89

☑ Additional Digit Required — Refer to the Tabular List for Digit Selection   ▽ Subterms under main terms may continue to next column or page

150 — Volume 2   ▶◀ Revised Text   ● New Line   ▲ Revised Code   2013 ICD-9-CM

I

Iatrogenic syndrome of excess cortisol 255.0
IBM (inclusion body myositis) 359.71
Iceland disease (epidemic neuromyasthenia) 049.8
Ichthyosis (congenita) 757.1
  acquired 701.1
  fetalis gravior 757.1
  follicularis 757.1
  hystrix 757.39
  lamellar 757.1
  lingual 528.6
  palmaris and plantaris 757.39
  simplex 757.1
  vera 757.1
  vulgaris 757.1
Ichthyotoxism 988.0
  bacterial (see also Poisoning, food) 005.9
Icteroanemia, hemolytic (acquired) 283.9
  congenital (see also Spherocytosis) 282.0
Icterus — see also Jaundice 782.4
  catarrhal — see Icterus, infectious
  conjunctiva 782.4
    newborn 774.6
  epidemic — see Icterus, infectious
  febrilis — see Icterus, infectious
  fetus or newborn — see Jaundice, fetus or newborn
  gravis (see also Necrosis, liver) 570
    complicating pregnancy 646.7 ☑
      affecting fetus or newborn 760.8
    fetus or newborn NEC 773.0
    obstetrical 646.7 ☑
      affecting fetus or newborn 760.8
  hematogenous (acquired) 283.9
  hemolytic (acquired) 283.9
    congenital (see also Spherocytosis) 282.0
  hemorrhagic (acute) 100.0
    leptospiral 100.0
    newborn 776.0
    spirochetal 100.0
  infectious 070.1
    with hepatic coma 070.0
    leptospiral 100.0
    spirochetal 100.0
  intermittens juvenilis 277.4
  malignant (see also Necrosis, liver) 570
  neonatorum (see also Jaundice, fetus or newborn) 774.6
  pernicious (see also Necrosis, liver) 570
  spirochetal 100.0
Ictus solaris, solis 992.0
Ideation
  homicidal V62.85
  suicidal V62.84
Identity disorder 313.82
  dissociative 300.14
  gender role (child) 302.6
    adult 302.85
  psychosexual (child) 302.6
    adult 302.85
Idioglossia 307.9
Idiopathic — see condition
Idiosyncrasy — see also Allergy 995.3
  drug, medicinal substance, and biological — see Allergy, drug
Idiot, idiocy (congenital) 318.2
  amaurotic (Bielschowsky) (-Jansky) (family) (infantile) (late) (juvenile) (late) (Vogt-Spielmeyer) 330.1
  microcephalic 742.1
  Mongolian 758.0
  oxycephalic 756.0
Id reaction (due to bacteria) 692.89
IEED (involuntary emotional expression disorder) 310.81
IFIS (intraoperative floppy iris syndrome) 364.81
IgE asthma 493.0 ☑
Ileitis (chronic) — see also Enteritis 558.9
  infectious 009.0
  noninfectious 558.9
  regional (ulcerative) 555.0
    with large intestine 555.2
  segmental 555.0

Ileitis — see also Enteritis — continued
  segmental — continued
    with large intestine 555.2
  terminal (ulcerative) 555.0
    with large intestine 555.2
Ileocolitis — see also Enteritis 558.9
  infectious 009.0
  regional 555.2
  ulcerative 556.1
Ileostomy status V44.2
  with complication 569.60
Ileotyphus 002.0
Ileum — see condition
Ileus (adynamic) (bowel) (colon) (inhibitory) (intestine) (neurogenic) (paralytic) 560.1
  arteriomesenteric duodenal 537.2
  due to gallstone (in intestine) 560.31
  duodenal, chronic 537.2
  following gastrointestinal surgery 997.49
  gallstone 560.31
  mechanical (see also Obstruction, intestine) 560.9
  meconium 777.1
    due to cystic fibrosis 277.01
  myxedema 564.89
  postoperative 997.49
  transitory, newborn 777.4
Iliac — see condition
Iliotibial band friction syndrome 728.89
Illegitimacy V61.6
Ill, louping 063.1
Illness — see also Disease
  factitious 300.19
    with
      combined psychological and physical signs and symptoms 300.19
      predominantly
        physical signs and symptoms 300.19
        psychological symptoms 300.16
    chronic (with physical symptoms) 301.51
  heart — see Disease, heart
  manic-depressive (see also Psychosis, affective) 296.80
  mental (see also Disorder, mental) 300.9
Imbalance 781.2
  autonomic (see also Neuropathy, peripheral, autonomic) 337.9
  electrolyte 276.9
    with
      abortion — see Abortion, by type, with metabolic disorder
      ectopic pregnancy (see also categories 633.0–633.9) 639.4
      hyperemesis gravidarum (before 22 completed weeks gestation) 643.1 ☑
      molar pregnancy (see also categories 630–632) 639.4
    following
      abortion 639.4
      ectopic or molar pregnancy 639.4
    neonatal, transitory NEC 775.5
  endocrine 259.9
  eye muscle NEC 378.9
    heterophoria — see Heterophoria
  glomerulotubular NEC 593.89
  hormone 259.9
  hysterical (see also Hysteria) 300.10
  labyrinth NEC 386.50
  posture 729.90
  sympathetic (see also Neuropathy, peripheral, autonomic) 337.9
Imbecile, imbecility 318.0
  moral 301.7
  old age 290.9
  senile 290.9
  specified IQ — see IQ
  unspecified IQ 318.0
Imbedding, intrauterine device 996.32
Imbibition, cholesterol (gallbladder) 575.6
Imerslund (-Gräsbeck) syndrome (anemia due to familial selective vitamin B_{12} malabsorption) 281.1
Iminoacidopathy 270.8
Iminoglycinuria, familial 270.8

Immature — see also Immaturity
  personality 301.89
Immaturity 765.1 ☑
  extreme 765.0 ☑
  fetus or infant light-for-dates — see Light-for-dates
  lung, fetus or newborn 770.4
  organ or site NEC — see Hypoplasia
  pulmonary, fetus or newborn 770.4
  reaction 301.89
  sexual (female) (male) 259.0
Immersion 994.1
  foot 991.4
  hand 991.4
Immobile, immobility
  complete
    due to severe physical disability or frailty 780.72
  intestine 560.89
  joint — see Ankylosis
  syndrome (paraplegic) 728.3
Immunization
  ABO
    affecting management of pregnancy 656.2 ☑
    fetus or newborn 773.1
  complication — see Complications, vaccination
  Rh factor
    affecting management of pregnancy 656.1 ☑
    fetus or newborn 773.0
    from transfusion (see also Complications, transfusion) 999.70
Immunodeficiency 279.3
  with
    adenosine-deaminase deficiency 279.2
    defect, predominant
      B-cell 279.00
      T-cell 279.10
    hyperimmunoglobulinemia 279.2
    lymphopenia, hereditary 279.2
    thrombocytopenia and eczema 279.12
    thymic
      aplasia 279.2
      dysplasia 279.2
  autosomal recessive, Swiss-type 279.2
  common variable 279.06
  severe combined (SCID) 279.2
  to Rh factor
    affecting management of pregnancy 656.1 ☑
    fetus or newborn 773.0
  X-linked, with increased IgM 279.05
Immunotherapy, prophylactic V07.2
  antineoplastic V58.12
Impaction, impacted
  bowel, colon, rectum 560.30
    with hernia (see also Hernia, by site, with obstruction)
      gangrenous — see Hernia, by site, with gangrene
    by
      calculus 560.32
      gallstone 560.31
      fecal 560.32
      specified type NEC 560.32
  calculus — see Calculus
  cerumen (ear) (external) 380.4
  cuspid 520.6
  dental 520.6
  fecal, feces 560.32
    with hernia (see also Hernia, by site, with obstruction)
      gangrenous — see Hernia, by site, with gangrene
  fracture — see Fracture, by site
  gallbladder — see Cholelithiasis
  gallstone(s) — see Cholelithiasis
    in intestine (any part) 560.31
  intestine(s) 560.30
    with hernia (see also Hernia, by site, with obstruction)
      gangrenous — see Hernia, by site, with gangrene

Impaction, impacted — continued
  intestine(s) — continued
    by
      calculus 560.32
      gallstone 560.31
      fecal 560.32
      specified type NEC 560.32
  intrauterine device (IUD) 996.32
  molar 520.6
  shoulder 660.4 ☑
    affecting fetus or newborn 763.1
  tooth, teeth 520.6
  turbinate 733.99
Impaired, impairment (function)
  arm V49.1
    movement, involving
      musculoskeletal system V49.1
      nervous system V49.2
  auditory discrimination 388.43
  back V48.3
  body (entire) V49.89
  cognitive, mild, so stated 331.83
  combined visual hearing V49.85
  dual sensory V49.85
  glucose
    fasting 790.21
    tolerance test (oral) 790.22
  hearing (see also Deafness) 389.9
    combined with visual impairment V49.85
  heart — see Disease, heart
  kidney (see also Disease, renal) 593.9
    disorder resulting from 588.9
      specified NEC 588.89
  leg V49.1
    movement, involving
      musculoskeletal system V49.1
      nervous system V49.2
  limb V49.1
    movement, involving
      musculoskeletal system V49.1
      nervous system V49.2
  liver 573.8
  mastication 524.9
  mild cognitive, so stated 331.83
  mobility
    ear ossicles NEC 385.22
    incostapedial joint 385.22
    malleus 385.21
  myocardium, myocardial (see also Insufficiency, myocardial) 428.0
  neuromusculoskeletal NEC V49.89
    back V48.3
    head V48.2
    limb V49.2
    neck V48.3
    spine V48.3
    trunk V48.3
  rectal sphincter 787.99
  renal (see also Disease, renal) 593.9
    disorder resulting from 588.9
      specified NEC 588.89
  spine V48.3
  vision NEC 369.9
    both eyes NEC 369.3
    combined with hearing impairment V49.85
    moderate 369.74
      both eyes 369.25
        with impairment of lesser eye (specified as)
          blind, not further specified 369.15
          low vision, not further specified 369.23
          near-total 369.17
          profound 369.18
          severe 369.24
          total 369.16
    one eye 369.74
      with vision of other eye (specified as)
        near-normal 369.75
        normal 369.76
    near-total 369.64
      both eyes 369.04

☑ **Additional Digit Required — Refer to the Tabular List for Digit Selection**   ▽ **Subterms under main terms may continue to next column or page**

2013 ICD-9-CM   ▶◀ Revised Text   ● New Line   ▲ Revised Code   Volume 2 — 151

Impaired, impairment — *continued*
  vision — *continued*
    near-total — *continued*
      both eyes — *continued*
        with impairment of lesser eye
          (specified as)
            blind, not further specified
              369.02
            total 369.03
        one eye 369.64
          with vision of other eye (specified
            as)
            near normal 369.65
            normal 369.66
    one eye 369.60
      with low vision of other eye 369.10
    profound 369.67
      both eyes 369.08
        with impairment of lesser eye
          (specified as)
            blind, not further specified
              369.05
            near-total 369.07
            total 369.06
      one eye 369.67
        with vision of other eye (specified
          as)
            near-normal 369.68
            normal 369.69
    severe 369.71
      both eyes 369.22
        with impairment of lesser eye
          (specified as)
            blind, not further specified
              369.11
           low vision, not further speci-
             fied 369.21
           near-total 369.13
           profound 369.14
           total 369.12
      one eye 369.71
        with vision of other eye (specified
          as)
            near-normal 369.72
            normal 369.73
    total
      both eyes 369.01
      one eye 369.61
        with vision of other eye (specified
          as)
            near-normal 369.62
            normal 369.63
Impaludism — *see* Malaria
Impediment, speech NEC 784.59
  psychogenic 307.9
  secondary to organic lesion 784.59
Impending
  cerebrovascular accident or attack 435.9
  coronary syndrome 411.1
  delirium tremens 291.0
  myocardial infarction 411.1
Imperception, auditory (acquired) (congenital) 389.9
Imperfect
  aeration, lung (newborn) 770.5
  closure (congenital)
    alimentary tract NEC 751.8
      lower 751.5
      upper 750.8
    atrioventricular ostium 745.69
    atrium (secundum) 745.5
      primum 745.61
    branchial cleft or sinus 744.41
    choroid 743.59
    cricoid cartilage 748.3
    cusps, heart valve NEC 746.89
      pulmonary 746.09
    ductus
      arteriosus 747.0
      Botalli 747.0
    ear drum 744.29
      causing impairment of hearing
        744.03
    endocardial cushion 745.60
    epiglottis 748.3

Imperfect — *continued*
  closure — *continued*
    esophagus with communication to
      bronchus or trachea 750.3
    Eustachian valve 746.89
    eyelid 743.62
    face, facial (*see also* Cleft, lip) 749.10
    foramen
      Botalli 745.5
      ovale 745.5
    genitalia, genital organ(s) or system
      female 752.89
        external 752.49
        internal NEC 752.89
        uterus 752.39
      male 752.89
        penis 752.69
    glottis 748.3
    heart valve (cusps) NEC 746.89
    interatrial ostium or septum 745.5
    interauricular ostium or septum 745.5
    interventricular ostium or septum 745.4
    iris 743.46
    kidney 753.3
    larynx 748.3
    lens 743.36
    lip (*see also* Cleft, lip) 749.10
    nasal septum or sinus 748.1
    nose 748.1
    omphalomesenteric duct 751.0
    optic nerve entry 743.57
    organ or site NEC — *see* Anomaly, spec-
      ified type, by site
    ostium
      interatrial 745.5
      interauricular 745.5
      interventricular 745.4
    palate (*see also* Cleft, palate) 749.00
    preauricular sinus 744.46
    retina 743.56
    roof of orbit 742.0
    sclera 743.47
    septum
      aortic 745.0
      aorticopulmonary 745.0
      atrial (secundum) 745.5
        primum 745.61
      between aorta and pulmonary artery
        745.0
      heart 745.9
      interatrial (secundum) 745.5
        primum 745.61
      interauricular (secundum) 745.5
        primum 745.61
      interventricular 745.4
        with pulmonary stenosis or atre-
          sia, dextraposition of aor-
          ta, and hypertrophy of
          right ventricle 745.2
        in tetralogy of Fallot 745.2
      nasal 748.1
      ventricular 745.4
        with pulmonary stenosis or atre-
          sia, dextraposition of aor-
          ta, and hypertrophy of
          right ventricle 745.2
        in tetralogy of Fallot 745.2
    skull 756.0
      with
        anencephalus 740.0
        encephalocele 742.0
        hydrocephalus 742.3
          with spina bifida (*see also*
            Spina bifida) 741.0 ☑
        microcephalus 742.1
    spine (with meningocele) (*see also* Spina
      bifida) 741.90
    thyroid cartilage 748.3
    trachea 748.3
    tympanic membrane 744.29
      causing impairment of hearing
        744.03
    uterus (with communication to bladder,
      intestine, or rectum) 752.39
    uvula 749.02

Imperfect — *continued*
  closure — *continued*
    uvula — *continued*
      with cleft lip (*see also* Cleft, palate,
        with cleft lip) 749.20
      vitelline duct 751.0
  development — *see* Anomaly, by site
  erection 607.84
  fusion — *see* Imperfect, closure
  inflation lung (newborn) 770.5
  intestinal canal 751.5
  poise 729.90
  rotation — *see* Malrotation
  septum, ventricular 745.4
Imperfectly descended testis 752.51
Imperforate (congenital) — *see also* Atresia
  anus 751.2
  bile duct 751.61
  cervix (uteri) 752.49
  esophagus 750.3
  hymen 752.42
  intestine (small) 751.1
    large 751.2
  jejunum 751.1
  pharynx 750.29
  rectum 751.2
  salivary duct 750.23
  urethra 753.6
  urinary meatus 753.6
  vagina 752.49
Impervious (congenital) — *see also* Atresia
  anus 751.2
  bile duct 751.61
  esophagus 750.3
  intestine (small) 751.1
    large 751.2
  rectum 751.2
  urethra 753.6
Impetiginization of other dermatoses 684
Impetigo (any organism) (any site) (bullous)
  (circinate) (contagiosa) (neonatorum)
  (simplex) 684
  Bockhart's (superficial folliculitis) 704.8
  external ear 684 [380.13]
  eyelid 684 [373.5]
  Fox's (contagiosa) 684
  furfuracea 696.5
  herpetiformis 694.3
    nonobstetrical 694.3
  staphylococcal infection 684
  ulcerative 686.8
  vulgaris 684
Impingement, soft tissue between teeth
  524.89
  anterior 524.81
  posterior 524.82
Implantation
  anomalous (*see also* Anomaly, specified
    type, by site)
    ureter 753.4
  cyst
    external area or site (skin) NEC 709.8
    iris 364.61
    vagina 623.8
    vulva 624.8
  dermoid (cyst)
    external area or site (skin) NEC 709.8
    iris 364.61
    vagina 623.8
    vulva 624.8
  placenta, low or marginal — *see* Placenta
    previa
Implant, endometrial 617.9
Impotence (sexual) 607.84
  organic origin NEC 607.84
  psychogenic 302.72
Impoverished blood 285.9
Impression, basilar 756.0
Imprisonment V62.5
Improper
  development, infant 764.9 ☑
Improperly tied umbilical cord (causing
  hemorrhage) 772.3
Impulses, obsessional 300.3
Impulsive 799.23
  neurosis 300.3

Impulsiveness 799.23
Inaction, kidney — *see also* Disease, renal
  593.9
Inactive — *see* condition
Inadequate, inadequacy
  aesthetics of dental restoration 525.67
  biologic 301.6
  cardiac and renal — *see* Hypertension, car-
    diorenal
  constitutional 301.6
  development
    child 783.40
    fetus 764.9 ☑
      affecting management of pregnancy
        656.5 ☑
    genitalia
      after puberty NEC 259.0
      congenital — *see* Hypoplasia, geni-
        talia
    lungs 748.5
    organ or site NEC — *see* Hypoplasia, by
      site
  dietary 269.9
  distance, interarch 524.28
  education V62.3
  environment
    economic problem V60.2
    household condition NEC V60.1
    poverty V60.2
    unemployment V62.0
  functional 301.6
  household care, due to
    family member
      handicapped or ill V60.4
      temporarily away from home V60.4
        on vacation V60.5
    technical defects in home V60.1
    temporary absence from home of person
      rendering care V60.4
  housing (heating) (space) V60.1
  interarch distance 524.28
  material resources V60.2
  mental (*see also* Disability, intellectual) 319
  nervous system 799.29
  personality 301.6
  prenatal care in current pregnancy V23.7
  pulmonary
    function 786.09
    newborn 770.89
    ventilation, newborn 770.89
  respiration 786.09
    newborn 770.89
  sample
    cytology
      anal 796.78
      cervical 795.08
      vaginal 795.18
  social 301.6
Inanition 263.9
  with edema 262
  due to
    deprivation of food 994.2
    malnutrition 263.9
  fever 780.60
Inappropriate
  change in quantitative human chorionic
    gonadotropin (hCG) in early pregnan-
    cy 631.0
  level of quantitative human chorionic go-
    nadotropin (hCG) for gestational age
    in early pregnancy 631.0
  secretion
    ACTH 255.0
    antidiuretic hormone (ADH) (excessive)
      253.6
      deficiency 253.5
    ectopic hormone NEC 259.3
    pituitary (posterior) 253.6
Inattention after or at birth 995.52
Inborn errors of metabolism — *see* Disorder,
  metabolism
Incarceration, incarcerated
  bubonocele (*see also* Hernia, inguinal, with
    obstruction)
    gangrenous — *see* Hernia, inguinal, with
      gangrene

☑ Additional Digit Required — Refer to the Tabular List for Digit Selection   Subterms under main terms may continue to next column or page

152 — Volume 2   ▶◀ Revised Text   ● New Line   ▲ Revised Code   2013 ICD-9-CM

Incarceration, incarcerated — continued
colon (by hernia) (see also Hernia, by site with obstruction)
  gangrenous — see Hernia, by site, with gangrene
enterocele 552.9
  gangrenous 551.9
epigastrocele 552.29
  gangrenous 551.29
epiplocele 552.9
  gangrenous 551.9
exomphalos 552.1
  gangrenous 551.1
fallopian tube 620.8
hernia (see also Hernia, by site, with obstruction)
  gangrenous — see Hernia, by site, with gangrene
iris, in wound 871.1
lens, in wound 871.1
merocele (see also Hernia, femoral, with obstruction) 552.00
omentum (by hernia) (see also Hernia, by site, with obstruction)
  gangrenous — see Hernia, by site, with gangrene
omphalocele 756.72
rupture (meaning hernia) (see also Hernia, by site, with obstruction) 552.9
  gangrenous (see also Hernia, by site, with gangrene) 551.9
sarcoepiplocele 552.9
  gangrenous 551.9
sarcoepiplomphalocele 552.1
  with gangrene 551.1
uterus 621.8
  gravid 654.3 ☑
    causing obstructed labor 660.2 ☑
    affecting fetus or newborn 763.1

Incident, cerebrovascular — see also Disease, cerebrovascular, acute 436

Incineration (entire body) (from fire, conflagration, electricity, or lightning) — see Burn, multiple, specified sites

Incised wound
external — see Wound, open, by site
internal organs (abdomen, chest, or pelvis) — see Injury, internal, by site, with open wound

Incision, incisional
hernia — see Hernia, incisional
surgical, complication — see Complications, surgical procedures
traumatic
  external — see Wound, open, by site
  internal organs (abdomen, chest, or pelvis) — see Injury, internal, by site, with open wound

Inclusion
azurophilic leukocytic 288.2
blennorrhea (neonatal) (newborn) 771.6
cyst — see Cyst, skin
gallbladder in liver (congenital) 751.69

Incompatibility
ABO
  affecting management of pregnancy 656.2 ☑
  fetus or newborn 773.1
  infusion or transfusion reaction (see also Complications, transfusion) 999.60
blood (group) (Duffy) (E) (K(ell)) (Kidd) (Lewis) (M) (N) (P) (S) NEC
  affecting management of pregnancy 656.2 ☑
  fetus or newborn 773.2
  infusion or transfusion reaction (see also Complications, transfusion) 999.75
contour of existing restoration of tooth with oral health 525.65
marital V61.10
  involving
    divorce V61.03
    estrangement V61.09

Incompatibility — continued
non-ABO (see also Complications, transfusion) 999.75
Rh (antigen) (C) (c) (D) (E) (e) (blood group) (factor)
  affecting management of pregnancy 656.1 ☑
  fetus or newborn 773.0
  infusion or transfusion reaction (see also Complications, transfusion) 999.70
Rhesus — see Incompatibility, Rh

Incompetency, incompetence, incompetent
annular
  aortic (valve) (see also Insufficiency, aortic) 424.1
  mitral (valve) (see also Insufficiency, mitral) 424.0
  pulmonary valve (heart) (see also Endocarditis, pulmonary) 424.3
aortic (valve) (see also Insufficiency, aortic) 424.1
  syphilitic 093.22
cardiac (orifice) 530.0
  valve — see Endocarditis
cervix, cervical (os) 622.5
  in pregnancy 654.5 ☑
    affecting fetus or newborn 761.0
chronotropic 426.89
  with
    autonomic dysfunction 337.9
    ischemic heart disease 414.9
    left ventricular dysfunction 429.89
    sinus node dysfunction 427.81
esophagogastric (junction) (sphincter) 530.0
heart valve, congenital 746.89
mitral (valve) — see Insufficiency, mitral
papillary muscle (heart) 429.81
pelvic
  pubocervical tissue 618.81
  rectovaginal tissue 618.82
pulmonary valve (heart) (see also Endocarditis, pulmonary) 424.3
  congenital 746.09
tricuspid (annular) (rheumatic) (valve) (see also Endocarditis, tricuspid) 397.0
valvular — see Endocarditis
vein, venous (saphenous) (varicose) (see also Varicose, vein) 454.9
velopharyngeal (closure)
  acquired 528.9
  congenital 750.29

Incomplete — see also condition
bladder emptying 788.21
defecation 787.61
expansion lungs (newborn) 770.5
gestation (liveborn) — see Immaturity
rotation — see Malrotation

Inconclusive
image test due to excess body fat 793.91
mammogram, mammography 793.82
  due to dense breasts 793.82

Incontinence 788.30
without sensory awareness 788.34
anal sphincter 787.60
continuous leakage 788.37
feces, fecal 787.60
  due to hysteria 300.11
  nonorganic origin 307.7
hysterical 300.11
mixed (male) (female) (urge and stress) 788.33
overflow 788.38
paradoxical 788.39
rectal 787.60
specified NEC 788.39
stress (female) 625.6
  male NEC 788.32
urethral sphincter 599.84
urge 788.31
  and stress (male) (female) 788.33
urine 788.30
  active 788.30
  due to
    cognitive impairment 788.91
    immobility 788.91

Incontinence — continued
urine — continued
  due to — continued
    severe physical disability 788.91
  functional 788.91
  male 788.30
    stress 788.32
    and urge 788.33
  neurogenic 788.39
  nonorganic origin 307.6
  stress (female) 625.6
    male NEC 788.32
  urge 788.31
  and stress 788.33

Incontinentia pigmenti 757.33

Incoordinate
uterus (action) (contractions) 661.4 ☑
  affecting fetus or newborn 763.7

Incoordination
esophageal-pharyngeal (newborn) 787.24
muscular 781.3
papillary muscle 429.81

Increase, increased
abnormal, in development 783.9
androgens (ovarian) 256.1
anticoagulants (antithrombin) (anti-II) (anti-VIIIa) (anti-IXa) (anti-XIa) (prothrombin) (see also Anticoagulants 286.59
  anti-IIa 287.8
  anti-Xa 287.8
  extrinsic 287.8
  postpartum 666.3 ☑
cold sense (see also Disturbance, sensation) 782.0
estrogen 256.0
function
  adrenal (cortex) 255.3
    medulla 255.6
  pituitary (anterior) (gland) (lobe) 253.1
    posterior 253.6
heat sense (see also Disturbance, sensation) 782.0
intracranial pressure 781.99
  injury at birth 767.8
light reflex of retina 362.13
permeability, capillary 448.9
pressure
  intracranial 781.99
    injury at birth 767.8
  intraocular 365.00
pulsations 785.9
pulse pressure 785.9
sphericity, lens 743.36
splenic activity 289.4
venous pressure 459.89
  portal 572.3

Incrustation, cornea, lead or zinc 930.0

Incyclophoria 378.44

Incyclotropia 378.33

Indeterminate sex 752.7

India rubber skin 756.83

Indicanuria 270.2

Indigestion (bilious) (functional) 536.8
acid 536.8
catarrhal 536.8
due to decomposed food NEC 005.9
fat 579.8
nervous 306.4
psychogenic 306.4

Indirect — see condition

Indolent bubo NEC 099.8

Induced
abortion — see Abortion, induced
birth, affecting fetus or newborn 763.89
delivery — see Delivery
labor — see Delivery

Induration, indurated
brain 348.89
breast (fibrous) 611.79
  puerperal, postpartum 676.3 ☑
broad ligament 620.8
chancre 091.0
  anus 091.1
  congenital 090.0
  extragenital NEC 091.2
corpora cavernosa (penis) (plastic) 607.89

Induration, indurated — continued
liver (chronic) 573.8
  acute 573.8
lung (black) (brown) (chronic) (fibroid) (see also Fibrosis, lung) 515
  essential brown 275.09 [516.1]
penile 607.89
phlebitic — see Phlebitis
skin 782.8
stomach 537.89

Induratio penis plastica 607.89

Industrial — see condition

Inebriety — see also Abuse, drugs, nondependent 305.0 ☑

Inefficiency
kidney (see also Disease, renal) 593.9
thyroid (acquired) (gland) 244.9

Inelasticity, skin 782.8

Inequality, leg (acquired) (length) 736.81
congenital 755.30

Inertia
bladder 596.4
  neurogenic 596.54
    with cauda equina syndrome 344.61
stomach 536.8
  psychogenic 306.4
uterus, uterine 661.2 ☑
  affecting fetus or newborn 763.7
  primary 661.0 ☑
  secondary 661.1 ☑
vesical 596.4
  neurogenic 596.54
    with cauda equina 344.61

Infant — see also condition
excessive crying of 780.92
fussy (baby) 780.91
held for adoption V68.89
newborn — see Newborn
post-term (gestation period over 40 completed weeks to 42 completed weeks) 766.21
prolonged gestation of (period over 42 completed weeks) 766.22
syndrome of diabetic mother 775.0

"Infant Hercules" syndrome 255.2

Infantile — see also condition
genitalia, genitals 259.0
  in pregnancy or childbirth NEC 654.4 ☑
    affecting fetus or newborn 763.89
    causing obstructed labor 660.2 ☑
      affecting fetus or newborn 763.1
heart 746.9
kidney 753.3
lack of care 995.52
macula degeneration 362.75
melanodontia 521.05
os, uterus (see also Infantile, genitalia) 259.0
pelvis 738.6
  with disproportion (fetopelvic) 653.1 ☑
    affecting fetus or newborn 763.1
    causing obstructed labor 660.1 ☑
      affecting fetus or newborn 763.1
penis 259.0
testis 257.2
uterus (see also Infantile, genitalia) 259.0
vulva 752.49

Infantilism 259.9
with dwarfism (hypophyseal) 253.3
Brissaud's (infantile myxedema) 244.9
celiac 579.0
Herter's (nontropical sprue) 579.0
hypophyseal 253.3
hypothalamic (with obesity) 253.8
idiopathic 259.9
intestinal 579.0
pancreatic 577.8
pituitary 253.3
renal 588.0
sexual (with obesity) 259.0

Infants, healthy liveborn — see Newborn

Infarct, infarction
adrenal (capsule) (gland) 255.41
amnion 658.8 ☑
anterior (with contiguous portion of intraventricular septum) NEC (see also Infarct, myocardium) 410.1 ☑

Infarct, infarction — *continued*
  appendices epiploicae 557.0
  bowel 557.0
  brain (stem) 434.91
    embolic (*see also* Embolism, brain) 434.11
    healed or old without residuals V12.54
    iatrogenic 997.02
    lacunar 434.91
    late effect — *see* Late effect(s) (of) cerebrovascular disease
    postoperative 997.02
    puerperal, postpartum, childbirth 674.0 ☑
    thrombotic (*see also* Thrombosis, brain) 434.01
  breast 611.89
  Brewer's (kidney) 593.81
  cardiac (*see also* Infarct, myocardium) 410.9 ☑
  cerebellar (*see also* Infarct, brain) 434.91
    embolic (*see also* Embolism, brain) 434.11
  cerebral (*see also* Infarct, brain) 434.91
    aborted 434.91
    embolic (*see also* Embolism, brain) 434.11
    thrombotic (*see also* Infarct, brain) 434.01
  chorion 658.8 ☑
  colon (acute) (agnogenic) (embolic) (hemorrhagic) (nonocclusive) (nonthrombotic) (occlusive) (segmental) (thrombotic) (with gangrene) 557.0
  coronary artery (*see also* Infarct, myocardium) 410.9 ☑
  cortical 434.91
  embolic (*see also* Embolism) 444.9
  fallopian tube 620.8
  gallbladder 575.8
  heart (*see also* Infarct, myocardium) 410.9 ☑
  hepatic 573.4
  hypophysis (anterior lobe) 253.8
  impending (myocardium) 411.1
  intestine (acute) (agnogenic) (embolic) (hemorrhagic) (nonocclusive) (nonthrombotic) (occlusive) (thrombotic) (with gangrene) 557.0
  kidney 593.81
  lacunar 434.91
  liver 573.4
  lung (embolic) (thrombotic) 415.19
    with
      abortion — *see* Abortion, by type, with, embolism
      ectopic pregnancy (*see also* categories 633.0–633.9) 639.6
      molar pregnancy (*see also* categories 630–632) 639.6
    following
      abortion 639.6
      ectopic or molar pregnancy 639.6
    iatrogenic 415.11
    in pregnancy, childbirth, or puerperium — *see* Embolism, obstetrical
    postoperative 415.11
    septic 415.12
  lymph node or vessel 457.8
  medullary (brain) — *see* Infarct, brain
  meibomian gland (eyelid) 374.85
  mesentery, mesenteric (embolic) (thrombotic) (with gangrene) 557.0
  midbrain — *see* Infarct, brain
  myocardium, myocardial (acute or with a stated duration of 8 weeks or less) (with hypertension) 410.9 ☑

Note — Use the following fifth-digit subclassification with category 410:

0   episode unspecified

1   initial episode

2   subsequent episode without recurrence

Infarct, infarction — *continued*
  myocardium, myocardial — *continued*
    with symptoms after 8 weeks from date of infarction 414.8
    anterior (wall) (with contiguous portion of intraventricular septum) NEC 410.1 ☑
    anteroapical (with contiguous portion of intraventricular septum) 410.1 ☑
    anterolateral (wall) 410.0 ☑
    anteroseptal (with contiguous portion of intraventricular septum) 410.1 ☑
    apical-lateral 410.5 ☑
    atrial 410.8 ☑
    basal-lateral 410.5 ☑
    chronic (with symptoms after 8 weeks from date of infarction) 414.8
    diagnosed on ECG, but presenting no symptoms 412
    diaphragmatic wall (with contiguous portion of intraventricular septum) 410.4 ☑
    healed or old, currently presenting no symptoms 412
    high lateral 410.5 ☑
    impending 411.1
    inferior (wall) (with contiguous portion of intraventricular septum) 410.4 ☑
    inferolateral (wall) 410.2 ☑
    inferoposterior wall 410.3 ☑
    intraoperative 997.1
    lateral wall 410.5 ☑
    non-Q wave 410.7 ☑
    non-ST elevation (NSTEMI) 410.7 ☑
    nontransmural 410.7 ☑
    papillary muscle 410.8 ☑
    past (diagnosed on ECG or other special investigation, but currently presenting no symptoms) 412
      with symptoms NEC 414.8
    posterior (strictly) (true) (wall) 410.6 ☑
    posterobasal 410.6 ☑
    posteroinferior 410.3 ☑
    posterolateral 410.5 ☑
    postprocedural 997.1
    previous, currently presenting no symptoms 412
    Q wave (*see also* Infarct, myo-cardium, by site) 410.9 ☑
    septal 410.8 ☑
    specified site NEC 410.8 ☑
    ST elevation (STEMI) 410.9 ☑
      anterior (wall) 410.1 ☑
      anterolateral (wall) 410.0 ☑
      inferior (wall) 410.4 ☑
      inferolateral (wall) 410.2 ☑
      inferoposterior wall 410.3 ☑
      lateral wall 410.5 ☑
      posterior (strictly) (true) (wall) 410.6 ☑
      specified site NEC 410.8 ☑
    subendocardial 410.7 ☑
    syphilitic 093.82
    non-ST elevation myocardial infarction (NSTEMI) 410.7 ☑
  nontransmural 410.7 ☑
  omentum 557.0
  ovary 620.8
  pancreas 577.8
  papillary muscle (*see also* Infarct, myocardium) 410.8 ☑
  parathyroid gland 252.8
  pituitary (gland) 253.8
  placenta (complicating pregnancy) 656.7 ☑
    affecting fetus or newborn 762.2
  pontine — *see* Infarct, brain
  posterior NEC (*see also* Infarct, myocardium) 410.6 ☑
  prostate 602.8
  pulmonary (artery) (hemorrhagic) (vein) 415.19

Infarct, infarction — *continued*
  pulmonary — *continued*
    with
      abortion — *see* Abortion, by type, with embolism
      ectopic pregnancy (*see also* categories 633.0–633.9) 639.6
      molar pregnancy (*see also* categories 630–632) 639.6
    following
      abortion 639.6
      ectopic or molar pregnancy 639.6
    iatrogenic 415.11
    in pregnancy, childbirth, or puerperium — *see* Embolism, obstetrical
    postoperative 415.11
    septic 415.12
  renal 593.81
    embolic or thrombotic 593.81
  retina, retinal 362.84
    with occlusion — *see* Occlusion, retina
  spinal (acute) (cord) (embolic) (nonembolic) 336.1
  spleen 289.59
    embolic or thrombotic 444.89
  subchorionic — *see* Infarct, placenta
  subendocardial (*see also* Infarct, myocardium) 410.7 ☑
  suprarenal (capsule) (gland) 255.41
  syncytium — *see* Infarct, placenta
  testis 608.83
  thrombotic (*see also* Thrombosis) 453.9
    artery, arterial — *see* Embolism
  thyroid (gland) 246.3
  ventricle (heart) (*see also* Infarct, myocardium) 410.9 ☑
Infecting — *see* condition
Infection, infected, infective (opportunistic) 136.9
  with
    influenza viruses occurring in pigs or other animals — *see* Influenza, due to identified, novel influenza A virus
    lymphangitis — *see* Lymphangitis
  abortion — *see* Abortion, by type, with, sepsis
  abscess (skin) — *see* Abscess, by site
  Absidia 117.7
  acanthamoeba 136.21
  Acanthocheilonema (perstans) 125.4
    streptocerca 125.6
  accessory sinus (chronic) (*see also* Sinusitis) 473.9
  Achorion — *see* Dermatophytosis
  Acremonium falciforme 117.4
  acromioclavicular (joint) 711.91
  actinobacillus
    lignieresii 027.8
    mallei 024
    muris 026.1
  actinomadura — *see* Actinomycosis
  Actinomyces (israelii) (*see also* Actinomycosis)
    muris-ratti 026.1
  Actinomycetales (actinomadura) (Actinomyces) (Nocardia) (Streptomyces) — *see* Actinomycosis
  actinomycotic NEC (*see also* Actinomycosis) 039.9
  adenoid (chronic) 474.01
    acute 463
    and tonsil (chronic) 474.02
      acute or subacute 463
  adenovirus NEC 079.0
    in diseases classified elsewhere — *see* category 079 ☑
    unspecified nature or site 079.0
  Aerobacter aerogenes NEC 041.85
    enteritis 008.2
  aerogenes capsulatus (*see also* Gangrene, gas) 040.0
  aertrycke (*see also* Infection, Salmonella) 003.9
  ajellomyces dermatitidis 116.0

Infection, infected, infective — *continued*
  alimentary canal NEC (*see also* Enteritis, due to, by organism) 009.0
  Allescheria boydii 117.6
  Alternaria 118
  alveolus, alveolar (process) (pulpal origin) 522.4
  ameba, amebic (histolytica) (*see also* Amebiasis) 006.9
    acute 006.0
    chronic 006.1
    free-living 136.29
    hartmanni 007.8
    specified
      site NEC 006.8
      type NEC 007.8
  amniotic fluid or cavity 658.4 ☑
    affecting fetus or newborn 762.7
  anaerobes (cocci) (gram-negative) (gram-positive) (mixed) NEC 041.84
  anal canal 569.49
  Ancylostoma braziliense 126.2
  Angiostrongylus cantonensis 128.8
  anisakiasis 127.1
  Anisakis larva 127.1
  anthrax (*see also* Anthrax) 022.9
  antrum (chronic) (*see also* Sinusitis, maxillary) 473.0
  anus (papillae) (sphincter) 569.49
  arbor virus NEC 066.9
  arbovirus NEC 066.9
  argentophil-rod 027.0
  Ascaris lumbricoides 127.0
  ascomycetes 117.4
  Aspergillus (flavus) (fumigatus) (terreus) 117.3
  atypical
    acid-fast (bacilli) (*see also* Mycobacterium, atypical) 031.9
    mycobacteria (*see also* Mycobacterium, atypical) 031.9
  auditory meatus (circumscribed) (diffuse) (external) (*see also* Otitis, externa) 380.10
  auricle (ear) (*see also* Otitis, externa) 380.10
  axillary gland 683
  Babesiasis 088.82
  Babesiosis 088.82
  Bacillus NEC 041.89
    abortus 023.1
    anthracis (*see also* Anthrax) 022.9
    cereus (food poisoning) 005.89
    coli — *see* Infection, Escherichia coli
    coliform NEC 041.85
    Ducrey's (any location) 099.0
    Flexner's 004.1
    Friedländer's NEC 041.3
    fusiformis 101
    gas (gangrene) (*see also* Gangrene, gas) 040.0
    mallei 024
    melitensis 023.0
    paratyphoid, paratyphosus 002.9
      A 002.1
      B 002.2
      C 002.3
    Schmorl's 040.3
    Shiga 004.0
    suipestifer (*see also* Infection, Salmonella) 003.9
    swimming pool 031.1
    typhosa 002.0
    welchii (*see also* Gangrene, gas) 040.0
    Whitmore's 025
  bacterial NEC 041.9
    specified NEC 041.89
      anaerobic NEC 041.84
      gram-negative NEC 041.85
        anaerobic NEC 041.84
  Bacterium
    paratyphosum 002.9
      A 002.1
      B 002.2
      C 002.3
    typhosum 002.0

☑ Additional Digit Required — Refer to the Tabular List for Digit Selection   ⬇ Subterms under main terms may continue to next column or page

154 — Volume 2   ▶◀ Revised Text   ● New Line   ▲ Revised Code   2013 ICD-9-CM

Infection, infected, infective — *continued*
  Bacteroides (fragilis) (melaninogenicus) (oralis) NEC 041.82
  balantidium coli 007.0
  Bartholin's gland 616.89
  Basidiobolus 117.7
  Bedsonia 079.98
    specified NEC 079.88
  bile duct 576.1
  bladder (*see also* Cystitis) 595.9
  Blastomyces, blastomycotic 116.0
    brasiliensis 116.1
    dermatitidis 116.0
    European 117.5
    loboi 116.2
    North American 116.0
    South American 116.1
  bleb
    postprocedural 379.60
      stage 1 379.61
      stage 2 379.62
      stage 3 379.63
  blood stream — *see also* Septicemia
    catheter-related (CRBSI) 999.31
    central line-associated (CLABSI) 999.32
    due to central venous catheter 999.32
  bone 730.9 ☑
    specified — *see* Osteomyelitis
  Bordetella 033.9
    bronchiseptica 033.8
    parapertussis 033.1
    pertussis 033.0
  Borrelia
    bergdorfi 088.81
    vincentii (mouth) (pharynx) (tonsil) 101
  bovine stomatitis 059.11
  brain (*see also* Encephalitis) 323.9
    late effect — *see* category 326
    membranes (*see also* Meningitis) 322.9
    septic 324.0
      late effect — *see* category 326
      meninges (*see also* Meningitis) 320.9
  branchial cyst 744.42
  breast 611.0
    puerperal, postpartum 675.2 ☑
      with nipple 675.9 ☑
        specified type NEC 675.8 ☑
      nonpurulent 675.2 ☑
      purulent 675.1 ☑
  bronchus (*see also* Bronchitis) 490
    fungus NEC 117.9
  Brucella 023.9
    abortus 023.1
    canis 023.3
    melitensis 023.0
    mixed 023.8
    suis 023.2
  Brugia (Wuchereria) malayi 125.1
  bursa — *see* Bursitis
  buttocks (skin) 686.9
  Candida (albicans) (tropicalis) (*see also* Candidiasis) 112.9
    congenital 771.7
  Candiru 136.8
  Capillaria
    hepatica 128.8
    philippinensis 127.5
  cartilage 733.99
  catheter-related bloodstream (CRBSI) 999.31
  cat liver fluke 121.0
  cellulitis — *see* Cellulitis, by site
  central line-associated 999.31
    bloodstream 999.32
  Cephalosporum falciforme 117.4
  Cercomonas hominis (intestinal) 007.3
  cerebrospinal (*see also* Meningitis) 322.9
    late effect — *see* category 326
  cervical gland 683
  cervix (*see also* Cervicitis) 616.0
  cesarean section wound 674.3 ☑
  Chilomastix (intestinal) 007.8
  Chlamydia 079.98
    specified NEC 079.88
  cholera (*see also* Cholera) 001.9
  chorionic plate 658.8 ☑

Infection, infected, infective — *continued*
  Cladosporium
    bantianum 117.8
    carrionii 117.2
    mansoni 111.1
    trichoides 117.8
    wernecki 111.1
  Clonorchis (sinensis) (liver) 121.1
  Clostridium (haemolyticum) (novyi) NEC 041.84
    botulinum 005.1
    histolyticum (*see also* Gangrene, gas) 040.0
    oedematiens (*see also* Gangrene, gas) 040.0
    perfringens 041.83
      due to food 005.2
    septicum (*see also* Gangrene, gas) 040.0
    sordellii (*see also* Gangrene, gas) 040.0
    welchii (*see also* Gangrene, gas) 040.0
      due to food 005.2
  Coccidioides (immitis) (*see also* Coccidioidomycosis) 114.9
  coccus NEC 041.89
  colon (*see also* Enteritis, due to, by organism) 009.0
    bacillus — *see* Infection, Escherichia coli
  colostomy or enterostomy 569.61
  common duct 576.1
  complicating pregnancy, childbirth, or puerperium NEC 647.9 ☑
    affecting fetus or newborn 760.2
  Condiobolus 117.7
  congenital NEC 771.89
    Candida albicans 771.7
    chronic 771.2
    cytomegalovirus 771.1
    hepatitis, viral 771.2
    herpes simplex 771.2
    listeriosis 771.2
    malaria 771.2
    poliomyelitis 771.2
    rubella 771.0
    toxoplasmosis 771.2
    tuberculosis 771.2
    urinary (tract) 771.82
    vaccinia 771.2
  coronavirus 079.89
    SARS-associated 079.82
  corpus luteum (*see also* Salpingo-oophoritis) 614.2
  Corynebacterium diphtheriae — *see* Diphtheria
  cotia virus 059.8
  Coxsackie (*see also* Coxsackie) 079.2
    endocardium 074.22
    heart NEC 074.20
    in diseases classified elsewhere — *see* category 079 ☑
    meninges 047.0
    myocardium 074.23
    pericardium 074.21
    pharynx 074.0
    specified disease NEC 074.8
    unspecified nature or site 079.2
  Cryptococcus neoformans 117.5
  Cryptosporidia 007.4
  Cunninghamella 117.7
  cyst — *see* Cyst
  Cysticercus cellulosae 123.1
  cystostomy 596.83
  cytomegalovirus 078.5
    congenital 771.1
  dental (pulpal origin) 522.4
  deuteromycetes 117.4
  Dicrocoelium dendriticum 121.8
  Dipetalonema (perstans) 125.4
    streptocerca 125.6
  diptherial — *see* Diphtheria
  Diphyllobothrium (adult) (latum) (pacificum) 123.4
    larval 123.5
  Diplogonoporus (grandis) 123.8
  Dipylidium (caninum) 123.8
  Dirofilaria 125.6
  dog tapeworm 123.8

Infection, infected, infective — *continued*
  Dracunculus medinensis 125.7
  Dreschlera 118
    hawaiiensis 117.8
  Ducrey's bacillus (any site) 099.0
  due to or resulting from
    central venous catheter (*see also* Complications, due to, catheter, central venous) 999.31
      bloodstream 999.32
      localized 999.33
    device, implant, or graft (any) (presence of) — *see* Complications, infection and inflammation, due to (presence of) any device, implant, or graft classified to 996.0–996.5 NEC
    injection, inoculation, infusion, transfusion, or vaccination (prophylactic) (therapeutic) 999.39
      blood and blood products
        acute 999.34
    injury NEC — *see* Wound, open, by site, complicated
    surgery 998.59
  duodenum 535.6 ☑
  ear (*see also* Otitis)
    external (*see also* Otitis, externa) 380.10
    inner (*see also* Labyrinthitis) 386.30
    middle — *see* Otitis, media
  Eaton's agent NEC 041.81
  Eberthella typhosa 002.0
  Ebola 078.89
  echinococcosis 122.9
  Echinococcus (*see also* Echinococcus) 122.9
  Echinostoma 121.8
  ECHO virus 079.1
    in diseases classified elsewhere — *see* category 079 ☑
    unspecified nature or site 079.1
  Ehrlichiosis 082.40
    chaffeensis 082.41
    specified type NEC 082.49
  Endamoeba — *see* Infection, ameba
  endocardium (*see also* Endocarditis) 421.0
  endocervix (*see also* Cervicitis) 616.0
  Entamoeba — *see* Infection, ameba
  enteric (*see also* Enteritis, due to, by organism) 009.0
  Enterobacter aerogenes NEC 041.85
  Enterobacter sakazakii 041.85
  Enterobius vermicularis 127.4
  enterococcus NEC 041.04
  enterovirus NEC 079.89
    central nervous system NEC 048
    enteritis 008.67
    meningitis 047.9
  Entomophthora 117.7
  Epidermophyton — *see* Dermatophytosis
  epidermophytosis — *see* Dermatophytosis
  episiotomy 674.3 ☑
  Epstein-Barr virus 075
    chronic 780.79 [139.8]
  erysipeloid 027.1
  Erysipelothrix (insidiosa) (rhusiopathiae) 027.1
  erythema infectiosum 057.0
  Escherichia coli (E. coli) 041.49
    enteritis — *see* Enteritis, E. coli
    generalized 038.42
    intestinal — *see* Enteritis, E. coli
    non-Shiga toxin-producing 041.49
    Shiga toxin-producing (STEC) 041.43
      with
        unspecified O group 041.43
        non-O157 (with known O group) 041.43
        O157 (with confirmation of Shiga toxin when H antigen is unknown, or is not H7) 041.41
        O157:H7 with or without confirmation of Shiga toxin-production 041.41
        O157H:- (nonmotile) with confirmation of Shiga toxin 041.41
    specified NEC 041.42

Infection, infected, infective — *continued*
  esophagostomy 530.86
  ethmoidal (chronic) (sinus) (*see also* Sinusitis, ethmoidal) 473.2
  Eubacterium 041.84
  Eustachian tube (ear) 381.50
    acute 381.51
    chronic 381.52
  exanthema subitum (*see also* Exanthem subitum) 058.10
  exit site 999.33
  external auditory canal (meatus) (*see also* Otitis, externa) 380.10
  eye NEC 360.00
  eyelid 373.9
    specified NEC 373.8
  fallopian tube (*see also* Salpingo-oophoritis) 614.2
  fascia 728.89
  Fasciola
    gigantica 121.3
    hepatica 121.3
  Fasciolopsis (buski) 121.4
  fetus (intra-amniotic) — *see* Infection, congenital
  filarial — *see* Infestation, filarial
  finger (skin) 686.9
    abscess (with lymphangitis) 681.00
      pulp 681.01
    cellulitis (with lymphangitis) 681.00
    distal closed space (with lymphangitis) 681.00
    nail 681.02
      fungus 110.1
  fish tapeworm 123.4
    larval 123.5
  flagellate, intestinal 007.9
  fluke — *see* Infestation, fluke
  focal
    teeth (pulpal origin) 522.4
    tonsils 474.00
      and adenoids 474.02
  Fonsecaea
    compactum 117.2
    pedrosoi 117.2
  food (*see also* Poisoning, food) 005.9
  foot (skin) 686.9
    fungus 110.4
  Francisella tularensis (*see also* Tularemia) 021.9
  frontal sinus (chronic) (*see also* Sinusitis, frontal) 473.1
  fungus NEC 117.9
    beard 110.0
    body 110.5
    dermatiacious NEC 117.8
    foot 110.4
    groin 110.3
    hand 110.2
    nail 110.1
    pathogenic to compromised host only 118
    perianal (area) 110.3
    scalp 110.0
    scrotum 110.8
    skin 111.9
      foot 110.4
      hand 110.2
      toenails 110.1
    trachea 117.9
  Fusarium 118
  Fusobacterium 041.84
  gallbladder (*see also* Cholecystitis, acute) 575.0
  Gardnerella vaginalis 041.89
  gas bacillus (*see also* Gas, gangrene) 040.0
  gastric (*see also* Gastritis) 535.5 ☑
  Gastrodiscoides hominis 121.8
  gastroenteric (*see also* Enteritis, due to, by organism) 009.0
  gastrointestinal (*see also* Enteritis, due to, by organism) 009.0
  gastrostomy 536.41
  generalized NEC (*see also* Septicemia) 038.9
  genital organ or tract NEC
    female 614.9

☑ **Additional Digit Required** — Refer to the Tabular List for Digit Selection   ▽ **Subterms under main terms may continue to next column or page**

2013 ICD-9-CM   ▶◀ **Revised Text**   ● **New Line**   ▲ **Revised Code**   **Volume 2 — 155**

Infection, infected, infective — *continued*
  genital organ or tract — *continued*
    female — *continued*
      with
        abortion — *see* Abortion, by type,
          with sepsis
        ectopic pregnancy (*see also* cate-
          gories 633.0–633.9) 639.0
        molar pregnancy (*see also* cate-
          gories 630–632) 639.0
        complicating pregnancy 646.6 ☑
          affecting fetus or newborn 760.8
        following
          abortion 639.0
          ectopic or molar pregnancy 639.0
        puerperal, postpartum, childbirth
          670.8 ☑
        minor or localized 646.6 ☑
          affecting fetus or newborn
            760.8
    male 608.4
  genitourinary tract NEC 599.0
  Ghon tubercle, primary (*see also* Tuberculo-
    sis) 010.0 ☑
  Giardia lamblia 007.1
  gingival (chronic) 523.10
    acute 523.00
    Vincent's 101
  glanders 024
  Glenosporopsis amazonica 116.2
  Gnathostoma spinigerum 128.1
  Gongylonema 125.6
  gonococcal NEC (*see also* Gonococcus) 098.0
  gram-negative bacilli NEC 041.85
    anaerobic 041.84
  guinea worm 125.7
  gum (*see also* Infection, gingival) 523.10
  Hantavirus 079.81
  heart 429.89
  Helicobacter pylori [H. pylori] 041.86
  helminths NEC 128.9
    intestinal 127.9
      mixed (types classifiable to more
        than one category in
        120.0–127.7) 127.8
      specified type NEC 127.7
    specified type NEC 128.8
  Hemophilus influenzae NEC 041.5
    generalized 038.41
  herpes (simplex) (*see also* Herpes, simplex)
    054.9
    congenital 771.2
    zoster (*see also* Herpes, zoster) 053.9
      eye NEC 053.29
  Heterophyes heterophyes 121.6
  Histoplasma (*see also* Histoplasmosis) 115.90
    capsulatum (*see also* Histoplasmosis,
      American) 115.00
    duboisii (*see also* Histoplasmosis, African)
      115.10
  HIV V08
    with symptoms, symptomatic 042
  hookworm (*see also* Ancylostomiasis) 126.9
  human herpesvirus NEC 058.89
  human herpesvirus 6 058.81
  human herpesvirus 7 058.82
  human herpesvirus 8 058.89
  human immunodeficiency virus V08
    with symptoms, symptomatic 042
  human papillomavirus 079.4
  hydrocele 603.1
  hydronephrosis 591
  Hymenolepis 123.6
  hypopharynx 478.29
  inguinal glands 683
    due to soft chancre 099.0
  insertion site 999.33
  intestine, intestinal (*see also* Enteritis, due
    to, by organism) 009.0
  intrauterine (*see also* Endometritis) 615.9
    complicating delivery 646.6 ☑
  isospora belli or hominis 007.2
  Japanese B encephalitis 062.0
  jaw (bone) (acute) (chronic) (lower) (suba-
    cute) (upper) 526.4
  joint — *see* Arthritis, infectious or infective

Infection, infected, infective — *continued*
  Kaposi's sarcoma-associated herpesvirus
    058.89
  kidney (cortex) (hematogenous) 590.9
    with
      abortion — *see* Abortion, by type,
        with urinary tract infection
      calculus 592.0
      ectopic pregnancy (*see also* cate-
        gories 633.0–633.9) 639.8
      molar pregnancy (*see also* categories
        630–632) 639.8
      complicating pregnancy or puerperium
        646.6 ☑
        affecting fetus or newborn 760.1
      following
        abortion 639.8
        ectopic or molar pregnancy 639.8
      pelvis and ureter 590.3
  Klebsiella pneumoniae NEC 041.3
  knee (skin) NEC 686.9
    joint — *see* Arthritis, infectious
  Koch's (*see also* Tuberculosis, pulmonary)
    011.9 ☑
  labia (majora) (minora) (*see also* Vulvitis)
    616.10
  lacrimal
    gland (*see also* Dacryoadenitis) 375.00
    passages (duct) (sac) (*see also* Dacryocys-
      titis) 375.30
  larynx NEC 478.79
  leg (skin) NEC 686.9
  Leishmania (*see also* Leishmaniasis) 085.9
    braziliensis 085.5
    donovani 085.0
    ethiopica 085.3
    furunculosa 085.1
    infantum 085.0
    mexicana 085.4
    tropica (minor) 085.1
    major 085.2
  Leptosphaeria senegalensis 117.4
  leptospira (*see also* Leptospirosis) 100.9
    Australis 100.89
    Bataviae 100.89
    pyrogenes 100.89
    specified type NEC 100.89
  leptospirochetal NEC (*see also* Leptospirosis)
    100.9
  Leptothrix — *see* Actinomycosis
  Listeria monocytogenes (listeriosis) 027.0
    congenital 771.2
  liver fluke — *see* Infestation, fluke, liver
  Loa loa 125.2
    eyelid 125.2 *[373.6]*
  Loboa loboi 116.2
  local, skin (staphylococcal) (streptococcal)
    NEC 686.9
    abscess — *see* Abscess, by site
    cellulitis — *see* Cellulitis, by site
    ulcer (*see also* Ulcer, skin) 707.9
  Loefflerella
    mallei 024
    whitmori 025
  lung 518.89
    atypical Mycobacterium 031.0
      tuberculous (*see also* Tuberculosis,
        pulmonary) 011.9 ☑
    basilar 518.89
    chronic 518.89
    fungus NEC 117.9
    spirochetal 104.8
    virus — *see* Pneumonia, virus
  lymph gland (axillary) (cervical) (inguinal)
    683
    mesenteric 289.2
  lymphoid tissue, base of tongue or posterior
    pharynx, NEC 474.00
  madurella
    grisea 117.4
    mycetomii 117.4
  major
    with
      abortion — *see* Abortion, by type,
        with sepsis

Infection, infected, infective — *continued*
  major — *continued*
    with — *continued*
      ectopic pregnancy (*see also* cate-
        gories 633.0–633.9) 639.0
      molar pregnancy (*see also* categories
        630–632) 639.0
    following
      abortion 639.0
      ectopic or molar pregnancy 639.0
    puerperal, postpartum, childbirth
      670.0 ☑
  Malassezia furfur 111.0
  Malleomyces
    mallei 024
    pseudomallei 025
  mammary gland 611.0
    puerperal, postpartum 675.2 ☑
  Mansonella (ozzardi) 125.5
  mastoid (suppurative) — *see* Mastoiditis
  maxilla, maxillary 526.4
    sinus (chronic) (*see also* Sinusitis, maxil-
      lary) 473.0
  mediastinum 519.2
  medina 125.7
  meibomian
    cyst 373.12
    gland 373.12
  melioidosis 025
  meninges (*see also* Meningitis) 320.9
  meningococcal (*see also* condition) 036.9
    brain 036.1
    cerebrospinal 036.0
    endocardium 036.42
    generalized 036.2
    meninges 036.0
    meningococcemia 036.2
    specified site NEC 036.89
  mesenteric lymph nodes or glands NEC
    289.2
  Metagonimus 121.5
  metatarsophalangeal 711.97
  methicillin
    resistant Staphylococcus aureus (MRSA)
      041.12
    susceptible Staphylococcus aureus
      (MSSA) 041.11
  microorganism resistant to drugs — *see*
    Resistance (to), drugs by microorgan-
    isms
  Microsporidia 136.8
  microsporum, microsporic — *see* Dermato-
    phytosis
  Mima polymorpha NEC 041.85
  mixed flora NEC 041.89
  Monilia (*see also* Candidiasis) 112.9
    neonatal 771.7
  monkeypox 059.01
  Monosporium apiospermum 117.6
  mouth (focus) NEC 528.9
    parasitic 136.9
  MRSA (methicillin resistant Staphylococcus
    aureus) 041.12
  MSSA (methicillin susceptible Staphylococ-
    cus aureus) 041.11
  Mucor 117.7
  muscle NEC 728.89
  mycelium NEC 117.9
  mycetoma
    actinomycotic NEC (*see also* Actinomyco-
      sis) 039.9
    mycotic NEC 117.4
  Mycobacterium, mycobacterial (*see also*
    Mycobacterium) 031.9
  Mycoplasma NEC 041.81
  mycotic NEC 117.9
    pathogenic to compromised host only
      118
    skin NEC 111.9
    systemic 117.9
  myocardium NEC 422.90
  nail (chronic) (with lymphangitis) 681.9
    finger 681.02
      fungus 110.1
    ingrowing 703.0
    toe 681.11

Infection, infected, infective — *continued*
  nail — *continued*
    toe — *continued*
      fungus 110.1
  nasal sinus (chronic) (*see also* Sinusitis) 473.9
  nasopharynx (chronic) 478.29
    acute 460
  navel 686.9
    newborn 771.4
  Neisserian — *see* Gonococcus
  Neotestudina rosatii 117.4
  newborn, generalized 771.89
  nipple 611.0
    puerperal, postpartum 675.0 ☑
      with breast 675.9 ☑
        specified type NEC 675.8 ☑
  Nocardia — *see* Actinomycosis
  nose 478.19
  nostril 478.19
  obstetrical surgical wound 674.3 ☑
  Oesophagostomum (apiostomum) 127.7
  Oestrus ovis 134.0
  Oidium albicans (*see also* Candidiasis) 112.9
  Onchocerca (volvulus) 125.3
    eye 125.3 *[360.13]*
    eyelid 125.3 *[373.6]*
  operation wound 998.59
  Opisthorchis (felineus) (tenuicollis) (viverri-
    ni) 121.0
  orbit 376.00
    chronic 376.10
  orthopoxvirus 059.00
    specified NEC 059.09
  ovary (*see also* Salpingo-oophoritis) 614.2
  Oxyuris vermicularis 127.4
  pancreas 577.0
  Paracoccidioides brasiliensis 116.1
  Paragonimus (westermani) 121.2
  parainfluenza virus 079.89
  parameningococcus NEC 036.9
    with meningitis 036.0
  parapoxvirus 059.10
    specified NEC 059.19
  parasitic NEC 136.9
  paratyphoid 002.9
    type A 002.1
    type B 002.2
    type C 002.3
  paraurethral ducts 597.89
  parotid gland 527.2
  Pasteurella NEC 027.2
    multocida (cat-bite) (dog-bite) 027.2
    pestis (*see also* Plague) 020.9
    pseudotuberculosis 027.2
    septica (cat-bite) (dog-bite) 027.2
    tularensis (*see also* Tularemia) 021.9
  pelvic, female (*see also* Disease, pelvis, in-
    flammatory) 614.9
  penis (glans) (retention) NEC 607.2
    herpetic 054.13
  Peptococcus 041.84
  Peptostreptococcus 041.84
  periapical (pulpal origin) 522.4
  peridental 523.30
  perineal wound (obstetrical) 674.3 ☑
  periodontal 523.31
  periorbital 376.00
    chronic 376.10
  perirectal 569.49
  perirenal (*see also* Infection, kidney) 590.9
  peritoneal (*see also* Peritonitis) 567.9
  periureteral 593.89
  periurethral 597.89
  Petriellidium boydii 117.6
  pharynx 478.29
    Coxsackie virus 074.0
    phlegmonous 462
    posterior, lymphoid 474.00
  Phialophora
    gougerotii 117.8
    jeanselmei 117.8
    verrucosa 117.2
  Piedraia hortai 111.3
  pinna, acute 380.11
  pinta 103.9
    intermediate 103.1

☑ **Additional Digit Required** — Refer to the Tabular List for Digit Selection   ⩘ **Subterms under main terms may continue to next column or page**

156 — Volume 2   ▶◀ **Revised Text**   ● **New Line**   ▲ **Revised Code**   2013 ICD-9-CM

☑ Additional Digit Required — Refer to the Tabular List for Digit Selection   ▼ Subterms under main terms may continue to next column or page

2013 ICD-9-CM   ▶◀ Revised Text   ● New Line   ▲ Revised Code   Volume 2 — 157

Infection, infected, infective — Infection, infected, infective

Infection, infected, infective — continued
typhus 081.9
  flea-borne (endemic) 081.0
  louse-borne (epidemic) 080
  mite-borne 081.2
  recrudescent 081.1
  tick-borne 082.9
   African 082.1
   North Asian 082.2
umbilicus (septic) 686.9
  newborn NEC 771.4
ureter 593.89
urethra (see also Urethritis) 597.80
urinary (tract) NEC 599.0
  with
   abortion — see Abortion, by type, with urinary tract infection
   ectopic pregnancy (see also categories 633.0–633.9) 639.8
   molar pregnancy (see also categories 630–632) 639.8
  candidal 112.2
  complicating pregnancy, childbirth, or puerperium 646.6 ☑
   affecting fetus or newborn 760.1
   asymptomatic 646.5 ☑
    affecting fetus or newborn 760.1
  diplococcal (acute) 098.0
   chronic 098.2
  due to Trichomonas (vaginalis) 131.00
  following
   abortion 639.8
   ectopic or molar pregnancy 639.8
  gonococcal (acute) 098.0
   chronic or duration of 2 months or over 098.2
  newborn 771.82
  trichomonal 131.00
  tuberculous (see also Tuberculosis) 016.3 ☑
uterus, uterine (see also Endometritis) 615.9
utriculus masculinus NEC 597.89
vaccination 999.39
vagina (granulation tissue) (wall) (see also Vaginitis) 616.10
varicella 052.9
varicose veins — see Varicose, veins
variola 050.9
  major 050.0
  minor 050.1
vas deferens NEC 608.4
Veillonella 041.84
verumontanum 597.89
vesical (see also Cystitis) 595.9
Vibrio
  cholerae 001.0
   El Tor 001.1
  parahaemolyticus (food poisoning) 005.4
  vulnificus 041.85
Vincent's (gums) (mouth) (tonsil) 101
vaccination 999.39
virus, viral 079.99
  adenovirus
   in diseases classified elsewhere — see category 079 ☑
   unspecified nature or site 079.0
  central nervous system NEC 049.9
   enterovirus 048
    meningitis 047.9
     specified type NEC 047.8
   slow virus 046.9
   specified condition NEC 046.8
  chest 519.8
  conjunctivitis 077.99
   specified type NEC 077.8
  coronavirus 079.89
   SARS-associated 079.82
  Coxsackie (see also Infection, Coxsackie) 079.2
  Ebola 065.8
  ECHO
   in diseases classified elsewhere — see category 079 ☑
   unspecified nature or site 079.1

Infection, infected, infective — continued
virus, viral — continued
  encephalitis 049.9
   arthropod-borne NEC 064
   tick-borne 063.9
    specified type NEC 063.8
  enteritis NEC (see also Enteritis, viral) 008.8
  exanthem NEC 057.9
  Hantavirus 079.81
  human papilloma 079.4
  in diseases classified elsewhere — see category 079 ☑
  intestine (see also Enteritis, viral) 008.8
  lung — see Pneumonia, viral
  respiratory syncytial (RSV) 079.6
  retrovirus 079.50
  rhinovirus
   in diseases classified elsewhere — see category 079 ☑
   unspecified nature or site 079.3
  salivary gland disease 078.5
  slow 046.9
   specified condition NEC 046.8
  specified type NEC 079.89
   in diseases classified elsewhere — see category 079 ☑
  unspecified nature or site 079.99
  warts 078.10
   specified NEC 078.19
  yaba monkey tumor 059.22
  vulva (see also Vulvitis) 616.10
whipworm 127.3
Whitmore's bacillus 025
wound (local) (posttraumatic) NEC 958.3
  with
   dislocation — see Dislocation, by site, open
   fracture — see Fracture, by site, open
   open wound — see Wound, open, by site, complicated
  postoperative 998.59
  surgical 998.59
Wuchereria 125.0
  bancrofti 125.0
  malayi 125.1
yaba monkey tumor virus 059.22
yatapoxvirus 059.20
yaws — see Yaws
yeast (see also Candidiasis) 112.9
yellow fever (see also Fever, yellow) 060.9
Yersinia pestis (see also Plague) 020.9
Zeis' gland 373.12
zoonotic bacterial NEC 027.9
Zopfia senegalensis 117.4
Infective, infectious — see condition
Inferiority complex 301.9
  constitutional psychopathic 301.9
Infertility
female 628.9
  age related 628.8
  associated with
   adhesions, peritubal 614.6 [628.2]
   anomaly
    cervical mucus 628.4
    congenital
     cervix 628.4
     fallopian tube 628.2
     uterus 628.3
     vagina 628.4
   anovulation 628.0
   dysmucorrhea 628.4
   endometritis, tuberculous (see also Tuberculosis) 016.7 ☑ [628.3]
   Stein-Leventhal syndrome 256.4 [628.0]
  due to
   adiposogenital dystrophy 253.8 [628.1]
   anterior pituitary disorder NEC 253.4 [628.1]
    hyperfunction 253.1 [628.1]
   cervical anomaly 628.4
   fallopian tube anomaly 628.2
   ovarian failure 256.39 [628.0]

Infertility — continued
female — continued
  due to — continued
   Stein-Leventhal syndrome 256.4 [628.0]
   uterine anomaly 628.3
   vaginal anomaly 628.4
  nonimplantation 628.3
  origin
   cervical 628.4
   pituitary-hypothalamus NEC 253.8 [628.1]
    anterior pituitary NEC 253.4 [628.1]
     hyperfunction NEC 253.1 [628.1]
    dwarfism 253.3 [628.1]
    panhypopituitarism 253.2 [628.1]
   specified NEC 628.8
   tubal (block) (occlusion) (stenosis) 628.2
    adhesions 614.6 [628.2]
   uterine 628.3
   vaginal 628.4
  previous, requiring supervision of pregnancy V23.0
male 606.9
  absolute 606.0
  due to
   azoospermia 606.0
   drug therapy 606.8
   extratesticular cause NEC 606.8
   germinal cell
    aplasia 606.0
    desquamation 606.1
   hypospermatogenesis 606.1
   infection 606.8
   obstruction, afferent ducts 606.8
   oligospermia 606.1
   radiation 606.8
   spermatogenic arrest (complete) 606.0
    incomplete 606.1
   systemic disease 606.8
Infestation 134.9
Acanthocheilonema (perstans) 125.4
  streptocerca 125.6
Acariasis 133.9
  demodex folliculorum 133.8
  Sarcoptes scabiei 133.0
  trombiculae 133.8
Agamofilaria streptocerca 125.6
Ancylostoma, Ankylostoma 126.9
  americanum 126.1
  braziliense 126.2
  canium 126.8
  ceylanicum 126.3
  duodenale 126.0
  new world 126.1
  old world 126.0
Angiostrongylus cantonensis 128.8
anisakiasis 127.1
Anisakis larva 127.1
arthropod NEC 134.1
Ascaris lumbricoides 127.0
Bacillus fusiformis 101
Balantidium coli 007.0
beef tapeworm 123.2
Bothriocephalus (latus) 123.4
  larval 123.5
broad tapeworm 123.4
  larval 123.5
Brugia malayi 125.1
Candiru 136.8
Capillaria
  hepatica 128.8
  philippinensis 127.5
cat liver fluke 121.0
Cercomonas hominis (intestinal) 007.3
cestodes 123.9
  specified type NEC 123.8
chigger 133.8
chigoe 134.1
Chilomastix 007.8
Clonorchis (sinensis) (liver) 121.1
coccidia 007.2

Infestation — continued
complicating pregnancy, childbirth, or puerperium 647.9 ☑
  affecting fetus or newborn 760.8
Cysticercus cellulosae 123.1
Demodex folliculorum 133.8
Dermatobia (hominis) 134.0
Dibothriocephalus (latus) 123.4
  larval 123.5
Dicrocoelium dendriticum 121.8
Diphyllobothrium (adult) (intestinal) (latum) (pacificum) 123.4
  larval 123.5
Diplogonoporus (grandis) 123.8
Dipylidium (caninum) 123.8
Distoma hepaticum 121.3
dog tapeworm 123.8
Dracunculus medinensis 125.7
dragon worm 125.7
dwarf tapeworm 123.6
Echinococcus (see also Echinococcus) 122.9
Echinostoma ilocanum 121.8
Embadomonas 007.8
Endamoeba (histolytica) — see Infection, ameba
Entamoeba (histolytica) — see Infection, ameba
Enterobius vermicularis 127.4
Epidermophyton — see Dermatophytosis
eyeworm 125.2
Fasciola
  gigantica 121.3
  hepatica 121.3
Fasciolopsis (buski) (small intestine) 121.4
  blood NEC (see also Schistosomiasis) 120.9
  cat liver 121.0
  filarial 125.9
   due to
    Acanthocheilonema (perstans) 125.4
     streptocerca 125.6
    Brugia (Wuchereria) malayi 125.1
    Dracunculus medinensis 125.7
    guinea worms 125.7
    Mansonella (ozzardi) 125.5
    Onchocerca volvulus 125.3
     eye 125.3 [360.13]
     eyelid 125.3 [373.6]
    Wuchereria (bancrofti) 125.0
     malayi 125.1
   specified type NEC 125.6
  fish tapeworm 123.4
   larval 123.5
  fluke 121.9
  intestinal (giant) 121.4
  liver (sheep) 121.3
   cat 121.0
   Chinese 121.1
   clonorchiasis 121.1
   fascioliasis 121.3
   Oriental 121.1
  lung (oriental) 121.2
  sheep liver 121.3
fly larva 134.0
Gasterophilus (intestinalis) 134.0
Gastrodiscoides hominis 121.8
Giardia lamblia 007.1
Gnathostoma (spinigerum) 128.1
Gongylonema 125.6
guinea worm 125.7
helminth NEC 128.9
  intestinal 127.9
   mixed (types classifiable to more than one category in 120.0–127.7) 127.8
   specified type NEC 127.7
  specified type NEC 128.8
Heterophyes heterophyes (small intestine) 121.6
hookworm (see also Infestation, ancylostoma) 126.9
Hymenolepis (diminuta) (nana) 123.6
intestinal NEC 129
leeches (aquatic) (land) 134.2
Leishmania — see Leishmaniasis

Infestation — *continued*
- lice (*see also* Infestation, pediculus) 132.9
- Linguatulidae, linguatula (pentastoma) (serrata) 134.1
- Loa loa 125.2
  - eyelid 125.2 *[373.6]*
- louse (*see also* Infestation, pediculus) 132.9
  - body 132.1
  - head 132.0
  - pubic 132.2
- maggots 134.0
- Mansonella (ozzardi) 125.5
- medina 125.7
- Metagonimus yokogawai (small intestine) 121.5
- Microfilaria streptocerca 125.3
  - eye 125.3 *[360.13]*
  - eyelid 125.3 *[373.6]*
- Microsporon furfur 111.0
- microsporum — *see* Dermatophytosis
- mites 133.9
  - scabic 133.0
  - specified type NEC 133.8
- monilia (albicans) (*see also* Candidiasis) 112.9
  - vagina 112.1
  - vulva 112.1
- mouth 112.0
- Necator americanus 126.1
- nematode (intestinal) 127.9
  - Ancylostoma (*see also* Ancylostoma) 126.9
  - Ascaris lumbricoides 127.0
  - conjunctiva NEC 128.9
  - Dioctophyma 128.8
  - Enterobius vermicularis 127.4
  - Gnathostoma spinigerum 128.1
  - Oesophagostomum (apiostomum) 127.7
  - Physaloptera 127.4
  - specified type NEC 127.7
  - Strongyloides stercoralis 127.2
  - Ternidens diminutus 127.7
  - Trichinella spiralis 124
  - Trichostrongylus 127.6
  - Trichuris (trichiuria) 127.3
- Oesophagostomum (apiostomum) 127.7
- Oestrus ovis 134.0
- Onchocerca (volvulus) 125.3
  - eye 125.3 *[360.13]*
  - eyelid 125.3 *[373.6]*
- Opisthorchis (felineus) (tenuicollis) (viverrini) 121.0
- Oxyuris vermicularis 127.4
- Paragonimus (westermani) 121.2
- parasite, parasitic NEC 136.9
  - eyelid 134.9 *[373.6]*
  - intestinal 129
  - mouth 112.0
  - orbit 376.13
  - skin 134.9
  - tongue 112.0
- pediculus 132.9
  - capitis (humanus) (any site) 132.0
  - corporis (humanus) (any site) 132.1
  - eyelid 132.0 *[373.6]*
  - mixed (classifiable to more than one category in 132.0–132.2) 132.3
  - pubis (any site) 132.2
- phthirus (pubis) (any site) 132.2
  - with any infestation classifiable to 132.0, 132.1 and 132.3
- pinworm 127.4
- pork tapeworm (adult) 123.0
- protozoal NEC 136.8
- pubic louse 132.2
- rat tapeworm 123.6
- red bug 133.8
- roundworm (large) NEC 127.0
- sand flea 134.1
- saprophytic NEC 136.8
- Sarcoptes scabiei 133.0
- scabies 133.0
- Schistosoma 120.9
  - bovis 120.8
  - cercariae 120.3
  - hematobium 120.0

Infestation — *continued*
- Schistosoma — *continued*
  - intercalatum 120.8
  - japonicum 120.2
  - mansoni 120.1
  - mattheii 120.8
  - specified
    - site — *see* Schistosomiasis
    - type NEC 120.8
  - spindale 120.8
- screw worms 134.0
- skin NEC 134.9
- Sparganum (mansoni) (proliferum) 123.5
  - larval 123.5
- specified type NEC 134.8
- Spirometra larvae 123.5
- Sporozoa NEC 136.8
- Stellantchasmus falcatus 121.6
- Strongyloides 127.2
- Strongylus (gibsoni) 127.7
- Taenia 123.3
  - diminuta 123.6
  - Echinococcus (*see also* Echinococcus) 122.9
  - mediocanellata 123.2
  - nana 123.6
  - saginata (mediocanellata) 123.2
  - solium (intestinal form) 123.0
    - larval form 123.1
- Taeniarhynchus saginatus 123.2
- tapeworm 123.9
  - beef 123.2
  - broad 123.4
    - larval 123.5
  - dog 123.8
  - dwarf 123.6
  - fish 123.4
    - larval 123.5
  - pork 123.0
  - rat 123.6
- Ternidens diminutus 127.7
- Tetranychus molestissimus 133.8
- threadworm 127.4
- tongue 112.0
- Toxocara (cani) (cati) (felis) 128.0
- trematode(s) NEC 121.9
- Trichina spiralis 124
- Trichinella spiralis 124
- Trichocephalus 127.3
- Trichomonas 131.9
  - bladder 131.09
  - cervix 131.09
  - intestine 007.3
  - prostate 131.03
  - specified site NEC 131.8
  - urethra (female) (male) 131.02
  - urogenital 131.00
  - vagina 131.01
  - vulva 131.01
- Trichophyton — *see* Dermatophytosis
- Trichostrongylus instabilis 127.6
- Trichuris (trichiuria) 127.3
- Trombicula (irritans) 133.8
- Trypanosoma — *see* Trypanosomiasis
- Tunga penetrans 134.1
- Uncinaria americana 126.1
- whipworm 127.3
- worms NEC 128.9
  - intestinal 127.9
- Wuchereria 125.0
  - bancrofti 125.0
  - malayi 125.1

Infiltrate, infiltration
- with an iron compound 275.09
- amyloid (any site) (generalized) 277.39
- calcareous (muscle) NEC 275.49
  - localized — *see* Degeneration, by site
- calcium salt (muscle) 275.49
- chemotherapy, vesicant 999.81
- corneal (*see also* Edema, cornea) 371.20
- eyelid 373.9
- fatty (diffuse) (generalized) 272.8
  - localized — *see* Degeneration, by site, fatty
- glycogen, glycogenic (*see also* Disease, glycogen storage) 271.0

Infiltrate, infiltration — *continued*
- heart, cardiac
  - fatty (*see also* Degeneration, myocardial) 429.1
  - glycogenic 271.0 *[425.7]*
- inflammatory in vitreous 379.29
- kidney (*see also* Disease, renal) 593.9
- leukemic (M9800/3) — *see* Leukemia
- liver 573.8
  - fatty — *see* Fatty, liver
  - glycogen (*see also* Disease, glycogen storage) 271.0
- lung (*see also* Infiltrate, pulmonary) 793.19
  - eosinophilic 518.3
  - x-ray finding only 793.19
- lymphatic (*see also* Leukemia, lymphatic) 204.9 ☑
  - gland, pigmentary 289.3
- muscle, fatty 728.9
- myelogenous (*see also* Leukemia, myeloid) 205.9 ☑
- myocardium, myocardial
  - fatty (*see also* Degeneration, myocardial) 429.1
  - glycogenic 271.0 *[425.7]*
- pulmonary 793.19
  - with
    - eosinophilia 518.3
    - pneumonia — *see* Pneumonia, by type
  - x-ray finding only 793.19
  - Ranke's primary (*see also* Tuberculosis) 010.0 ☑
- skin, lymphocytic (benign) 709.8
- thymus (gland) (fatty) 254.8
- urine 788.8
- vesicant
  - agent NEC 999.82
  - chemotherapy 999.81
- vitreous humor 379.29

Infirmity 799.89
- senile 797

Inflammation, inflamed, inflammatory (with exudation)
- abducens (nerve) 378.54
- accessory sinus (chronic) (*see also* Sinusitis) 473.9
- adrenal (gland) 255.8
- alimentary canal — *see* Enteritis
- alveoli (teeth) 526.5
  - scorbutic 267
- amnion — *see* Amnionitis
- anal canal 569.49
- antrum (chronic) (*see also* Sinusitis, maxillary) 473.0
- anus 569.49
- appendix (*see also* Appendicitis) 541
- arachnoid — *see* Meningitis
- areola 611.0
  - puerperal, postpartum 675.0 ☑
- areolar tissue NEC 686.9
- artery — *see* Arteritis
- auditory meatus (external) (*see also* Otitis, externa) 380.10
- Bartholin's gland 616.89
- bile duct or passage 576.1
- bladder (*see also* Cystitis) 595.9
- bleb
  - postprocedural 379.60
    - stage 1 379.61
    - stage 2 379.62
    - stage 3 379.63
- bone — *see* Osteomyelitis
- bowel (*see also* Enteritis) 558.9
- brain (*see also* Encephalitis) 323.9
  - late effect — *see* category 326
  - membrane — *see* Meningitis
- breast 611.0
  - puerperal, postpartum 675.2 ☑
- broad ligament (*see also* Disease, pelvis, inflammatory) 614.4
  - acute 614.3
- bronchus — *see* Bronchitis
- bursa — *see* Bursitis
- capsule
  - liver 573.3

Inflammation, inflamed, inflammatory — *continued*
- capsule — *continued*
  - spleen 289.59
- catarrhal (*see also* Catarrh) 460
  - vagina 616.10
- cecum (*see also* Appendicitis) 541
- cerebral (*see also* Encephalitis) 323.9
  - late effect — *see* category 326
  - membrane — *see* Meningitis
- cerebrospinal (*see also* Meningitis) 322.9
  - late effect — *see* category 326
  - meningococcal 036.0
  - tuberculous (*see also* Tuberculosis) 013.6 ☑
- cervix (uteri) (*see also* Cervicitis) 616.0
- chest 519.9
- choroid NEC (*see also* Choroiditis) 363.20
- cicatrix (tissue) — *see* Cicatrix
- colon (*see also* Enteritis) 558.9
  - granulomatous 555.1
  - newborn 558.9
- connective tissue (diffuse) NEC 728.9
- cornea (*see also* Keratitis) 370.9
  - with ulcer (*see also* Ulcer, cornea) 370.00
- corpora cavernosa (penis) 607.2
- cranial nerve — *see* Disorder, nerve, cranial
- diarrhea — *see* Diarrhea
- disc (intervertebral) (space) 722.90
  - cervical, cervicothoracic 722.91
  - lumbar, lumbosacral 722.93
  - thoracic, thoracolumbar 722.92
- Douglas' cul-de-sac or pouch (chronic) (*see also* Disease, pelvis, inflammatory) 614.4
  - acute 614.3
- due to (presence of) any device, implant, or graft classifiable to 996.0–996.5 — *see* Complications, infection and inflammation, due to (presence of) any device, implant, or graft classified to 996.0–996.5 NEC
- duodenum 535.6 ☑
- dura mater — *see* Meningitis
- ear (*see also* Otitis)
  - external (*see also* Otitis, externa) 380.10
  - inner (*see also* Labyrinthitis) 386.30
  - middle — *see* Otitis media
- esophagus 530.10
- ethmoidal (chronic) (sinus) (*see also* Sinusitis, ethmoidal) 473.2
- Eustachian tube (catarrhal) 381.50
  - acute 381.51
  - chronic 381.52
- extrarectal 569.49
- eye 379.99
- eyelid 373.9
  - specified NEC 373.8
- fallopian tube (*see also* Salpingo-oophoritis) 614.2
- fascia 728.9
- fetal membranes (acute) 658.4 ☑
  - affecting fetus or newborn 762.7
- follicular, pharynx 472.1
- frontal (chronic) (sinus) (*see also* Sinusitis, frontal) 473.1
- gallbladder (*see also* Cholecystitis, acute) 575.0
- gall duct (*see also* Cholecystitis) 575.10
- gastrointestinal (*see also* Enteritis) 558.9
- genital organ (diffuse) (internal)
  - female 614.9
    - with
      - abortion — *see* Abortion, by type, with sepsis
      - ectopic pregnancy (*see also* categories 633.0–633.9) 639.0
      - molar pregnancy (*see also* categories 630–632) 639.0
    - complicating pregnancy, childbirth, or puerperium 646.6 ☑
      - affecting fetus or newborn 760.8
    - following
      - abortion 639.0
      - ectopic or molar pregnancy 639.0
  - male 608.4

☑ **Additional Digit Required** — Refer to the Tabular List for Digit Selection   ▽ **Subterms under main terms may continue to next column or page**

2013 ICD-9-CM   ▶◀ **Revised Text**   ● **New Line**   ▲ **Revised Code**   **Volume 2 — 159**

Inflammation, inflamed, inflammatory — *continued*
gland (lymph) (*see also* Lymphadenitis) 289.3
glottis (*see also* Laryngitis) 464.00
  with obstruction 464.01
granular, pharynx 472.1
gum 523.10
heart (*see also* Carditis) 429.89
hepatic duct 576.8
hernial sac — *see* Hernia, by site
ileum (*see also* Enteritis) 558.9
  terminal or regional 555.0
    with large intestine 555.2
intervertebral disc 722.90
  cervical, cervicothoracic 722.91
  lumbar, lumbosacral 722.93
  thoracic, thoracolumbar 722.92
intestine (*see also* Enteritis) 558.9
jaw (acute) (bone) (chronic) (lower) (suppurative) (upper) 526.4
jejunum — *see* Enteritis
joint NEC (*see also* Arthritis) 716.9 ☑
  sacroiliac 720.2
kidney (*see also* Nephritis) 583.9
knee (joint) 716.66
  tuberculous (active) (*see also* Tuberculosis) 015.2 ☑
labium (majus) (minus) (*see also* Vulvitis) 616.10
lacrimal
  gland (*see also* Dacryoadenitis) 375.00
  passages (duct) (sac) (*see also* Dacryocystitis) 375.30
larynx (*see also* Laryngitis) 464.00
  with obstruction 464.01
  diphtheritic 032.3
leg NEC 686.9
lip 528.5
liver (capsule) (*see also* Hepatitis) 573.3
  acute 570
  chronic 571.40
  suppurative 572.0
lung (acute) (*see also* Pneumonia) 486
  chronic (interstitial) 518.89
lymphatic vessel (*see also* Lymphangitis) 457.2
lymph node or gland (*see also* Lymphadenitis) 289.3
mammary gland 611.0
  puerperal, postpartum 675.2 ☑
maxilla, maxillary 526.4
  sinus (chronic) (*see also* Sinusitis, maxillary) 473.0
membranes of brain or spinal cord — *see* Meningitis
meninges — *see* Meningitis
mouth 528.00
muscle 728.9
myocardium (*see also* Myocarditis) 429.0
nasal sinus (chronic) (*see also* Sinusitis) 473.9
nasopharynx — *see* Nasopharyngitis
navel 686.9
  newborn NEC 771.4
nerve NEC 729.2
nipple 611.0
  puerperal, postpartum 675.0 ☑
nose 478.19
  suppurative 472.0
oculomotor nerve 378.51
optic nerve 377.30
orbit (chronic) 376.10
  acute 376.00
  chronic 376.10
ovary (*see also* Salpingo-oophoritis) 614.2
oviduct (*see also* Salpingo-oophoritis) 614.2
pancreas — *see* Pancreatitis
parametrium (chronic) (*see also* Disease, pelvis, inflammatory) 614.4
  acute 614.3
parotid region 686.9
  gland 527.2
pelvis, female (*see also* Disease, pelvis, inflammatory) 614.9
penis (corpora cavernosa) 607.2
perianal 569.49

Inflammation, inflamed, inflammatory — *continued*
pericardium (*see also* Pericarditis) 423.9
perineum (female) (male) 686.9
perirectal 569.49
peritoneum (*see also* Peritonitis) 567.9
periuterine (*see also* Disease, pelvis, inflammatory) 614.9
perivesical (*see also* Cystitis) 595.9
petrous bone (*see also* Petrositis) 383.20
pharynx (*see also* Pharyngitis) 462
  follicular 472.1
  granular 472.1
pia mater — *see* Meningitis
pleura — *see* Pleurisy
postmastoidectomy cavity 383.30
  chronic 383.33
pouch, internal ileoanal 569.71
prostate (*see also* Prostatitis) 601.9
rectosigmoid — *see* Rectosigmoiditis
rectum (*see also* Proctitis) 569.49
respiratory, upper (*see also* Infection, respiratory, upper) 465.9
  chronic, due to external agent — *see* Condition, respiratory, chronic, due to, external agent
  due to
    fumes or vapors (chemical) (inhalation) 506.2
    radiation 508.1
retina (*see also* Retinitis) 363.20
retrocecal (*see also* Appendicitis) 541
retroperitoneal (*see also* Peritonitis) 567.9
salivary duct or gland (any) (suppurative) 527.2
scorbutic, alveoli, teeth 267
scrotum 608.4
sigmoid — *see* Enteritis
sinus (*see also* Sinusitis) 473.9
Skene's duct or gland (*see also* Urethritis) 597.89
skin 686.9
spermatic cord 608.4
sphenoidal (sinus) (*see also* Sinusitis, sphenoidal) 473.3
spinal
  cord (*see also* Encephalitis) 323.9
    late effect — *see* category 326
  membrane — *see* Meningitis
  nerve — *see* Disorder, nerve
spine (*see also* Spondylitis) 720.9
spleen (capsule) 289.59
stomach — *see* Gastritis
stricture, rectum 569.49
subcutaneous tissue NEC 686.9
suprarenal (gland) 255.8
synovial (fringe) (membrane) — *see* Bursitis
tendon (sheath) NEC 726.90
testis (*see also* Orchitis) 604.90
thigh 686.9
throat (*see also* Sore throat) 462
thymus (gland) 254.8
thyroid (gland) (*see also* Thyroiditis) 245.9
tongue 529.0
tonsil — *see* Tonsillitis
trachea — *see* Tracheitis
trochlear nerve 378.53
tubal (*see also* Salpingo-oophoritis) 614.2
tuberculous NEC (*see also* Tuberculosis) 011.9 ☑
tubo-ovarian (*see also* Salpingo-oophoritis) 614.2
tunica vaginalis 608.4
tympanic membrane — *see* Myringitis
umbilicus, umbilical 686.9
  newborn NEC 771.4
uterine ligament (*see also* Disease, pelvis, inflammatory) 614.4
  acute 614.3
uterus (catarrhal) (*see also* Endometritis) 615.9
uveal tract (anterior) (*see also* Iridocyclitis) 364.3
  posterior — *see* Chorioretinitis
  sympathetic 360.11
vagina (*see also* Vaginitis) 616.10

Inflammation, inflamed, inflammatory — *continued*
vas deferens 608.4
vein (*see also* Phlebitis) 451.9
  thrombotic 451.9
    cerebral (*see also* Thrombosis, brain) 434.0 ☑
  leg 451.2
    deep (vessels) NEC 451.19
    superficial (vessels) 451.0
  lower extremity 451.2
    deep (vessels) NEC 451.19
    superficial (vessels) 451.0
vocal cord 478.5
vulva (*see also* Vulvitis) 616.10
Inflation, lung imperfect (newborn) 770.5
Influenza, influenzal 487.1
  with
    bronchitis 487.1
    bronchopneumonia 487.0
    cold (any type) 487.1
    digestive manifestations 487.8
    hemoptysis 487.1
    involvement of
      gastrointestinal tract 487.8
      nervous system 487.8
    laryngitis 487.1
    manifestations NEC 487.8
      respiratory 487.1
        pneumonia 487.0
    pharyngitis 487.1
    pneumonia (any form classifiable to 480-483, 485–486) 487.0
    respiratory manifestations NEC 487.1
    sinusitis 487.1
    sore throat 487.1
    tonsillitis 487.1
    tracheitis 487.1
    upper respiratory infection (acute) 487.1
  abdominal 487.8
  A/H5N1 (*see also* Influenza, avian) 488.02
  Asian 487.1
  avian 488.02
    with involvement of gastrointestinal tract 488.09
    bronchopneumonia 488.01
    laryngitis 488.02
    manifestations NEC 488.09
      respiratory 488.02
    pharyngitis 488.02
    pneumonia (any form classifiable to 480-483, 485-486) 488.01
    respiratory infection (acute) (upper) 488.02
  bronchial 487.1
  bronchopneumonia 487.0
  catarrhal 487.1
  due to identified
    animal origin influenza virus — *see* Influenza, due to identified, novel influenza A virus
    avian influenza virus 488.02
      with
        manifestations NEC 488.09
          respiratory 488.02
        pneumonia (any form classifiable to 480-483, 485-486) 488.01
    (novel 2009) H1N1 influenza virus 488.12
      with
        manifestations NEC 488.19
          respiratory 488.12
        pneumonia 488.11
    novel influenza A virus 488.82
      with
        encephalopathy 488.89
        involvement of gastrointestinal tract 488.89
        laryngitis 488.82
        manifestations NEC 488.89
          respiratory (acute) (upper) 488.82
        pharyngitis 488.82
        pneumonia 488.81
  epidemic 487.1
  gastric 487.8

Influenza, influenzal — *continued*
  intestinal 487.8
  laryngitis 487.1
  maternal affecting fetus or newborn 760.2
    manifest influenza in infant 771.2
  (novel) 2009 H1N1 488.12
    with involvement of gastrointestinal tract 488.19
    bronchopneumonia 488.11
    laryngitis 488.12
    manifestations NEC 488.19
      respiratory 488.12
    pharyngitis 488.12
    pneumonia (any form classifiable to 480-483, 485-486) 488.11
    respiratory infection (acute) (upper) 488.12
  novel A/H1N1 (*see also* Influenza, (novel) 2009 H1N1) 488.12
  novel influenza A viruses not previously found in humans — *see* Influenza, due to identified, novel influenza A virus
  pharyngitis 487.1
  pneumonia (any form) 487.0
  respiratory (upper) 487.1
  specified NEC 487.1
  stomach 487.8
  vaccination, prophylactic (against) V04.81
Influenza-like disease — *see also* Influenza 487.1
Infraction, Freiberg's (metatarsal head) 732.5
Infraeruption, teeth 524.34
Infusion complication, misadventure, or reaction — *see* Complication, infusion
Ingestion
  chemical — *see* Table of Drugs and Chemicals
  drug or medicinal substance
    overdose or wrong substance given or taken 977.9
      specified drug — *see* Table of Drugs and Chemicals
  foreign body NEC (*see also* Foreign body) 938
Ingrowing
  hair 704.8
  nail (finger) (toe) (infected) 703.0
Inguinal — *see also* condition
  testis 752.51
Inhalation
  carbon monoxide 986
  flame
    lung 947.1
    mouth 947.0
  food or foreign body (*see also* Asphyxia, food or foreign body) 933.1
  gas, fumes, or vapor (noxious) 987.9
    specified agent — *see* Table of Drugs and Chemicals
  liquid or vomitus (*see also* Asphyxia, food or foreign body) 933.1
  lower respiratory tract NEC 934.9
  meconium (fetus or newborn) 770.11
    with respiratory symptoms 770.12
  mucus (*see also* Asphyxia, mucus) 933.1
  oil (causing suffocation) (*see also* Asphyxia, food or foreign body) 933.1
  pneumonia — *see* Pneumonia, aspiration
  smoke 508.2
  steam 987.9
  stomach contents or secretions (*see also* Asphyxia, food or foreign body) 933.1
    in labor and delivery 668.0 ☑
Inhibition, inhibited
  academic as adjustment reaction 309.23
  orgasm
    female 302.73
    male 302.74
  sexual
    desire 302.71
    excitement 302.72
  work as adjustment reaction 309.23
Inhibitor
  autoimmune, to clotting factors 286.52

☑ Additional Digit Required — Refer to the Tabular List for Digit Selection   ▧ Subterms under main terms may continue to next column or page

Inhibitor — *continued*
  systemic lupus erythematosus (presence of) 795.79
    with
      hemorrhagic disorder 286.53
      hypercoagulable state 289.81
Iniencephalus, iniencephaly 740.2
Injected eye 372.74
Injury 959.9

> *Note* — *For abrasion, insect bite (non-venomous), blister, or scratch, see Injury, superficial.*
>
> *For laceration, traumatic rupture, tear, or penetrating wound of internal organs, such as heart, lung, liver, kidney, pelvic organs, whether or not accompanied by open wound in the same region, see Injury, internal.*
>
> *For nerve injury, see Injury, nerve.*
>
> *For late effect of injuries classifiable to 850–854, 860–869, 900–919, 950–959, see Late, effect, injury, by type.*

  abdomen, abdominal (viscera) (*see also* Injury, internal, abdomen)
    muscle or wall 959.12
  acoustic, resulting in deafness 951.5
  adenoid 959.09
  adrenal (gland) — *see* Injury, internal, adrenal
  alveolar (process) 959.09
  ankle (and foot) (and knee) (and leg, except thigh) 959.7
  anterior chamber, eye 921.3
  anus 959.19
  aorta (thoracic) 901.0
    abdominal 902.0
  appendix — *see* Injury, internal, appendix
  arm, upper (and shoulder) 959.2
  artery (complicating trauma) (*see also* Injury, blood vessel, by site) 904.9
    cerebral or meningeal (*see also* Hemorrhage, brain, traumatic, subarachnoid) 852.0 ☑
  auditory canal (external) (meatus) 959.09
  auricle, auris, ear 959.09
  axilla 959.2
  back 959.19
  bile duct — *see* Injury, internal, bile duct
  birth (*see also* Birth, injury)
    canal NEC, complicating delivery 665.9 ☑
  bladder (sphincter) — *see* Injury, internal, bladder
  blast (air) (hydraulic) (immersion) (underwater) NEC 869.0
    with open wound into cavity NEC 869.1
    abdomen or thorax — *see* Injury, internal, by site
    brain — *see* Concussion, brain
    ear (acoustic nerve trauma) 951.5
      with perforation of tympanic membrane — *see* Wound, open, ear, drum
  blood vessel NEC 904.9
    abdomen 902.9
      multiple 902.87
      specified NEC 902.89
    aorta (thoracic) 901.0
      abdominal 902.0
    arm NEC 903.9
    axillary 903.00
      artery 903.01
      vein 903.02
    azygos vein 901.89
    basilic vein 903.1
    brachial (artery) (vein) 903.1
    bronchial 901.89
    carotid artery 900.00
      common 900.01
      external 900.02
      internal 900.03
    celiac artery 902.20
      specified branch NEC 902.24
    cephalic vein (arm) 903.1

Injury — *continued*
  blood vessel — *continued*
    colica dextra 902.26
    cystic
      artery 902.24
      vein 902.39
    deep plantar 904.6
    digital (artery) (vein) 903.5
    due to accidental puncture or laceration during procedure 998.2
    extremity
      lower 904.8
        multiple 904.7
        specified NEC 904.7
      upper 903.9
        multiple 903.8
        specified NEC 903.8
    femoral
      artery (superficial) 904.1
        above profunda origin 904.0
        common 904.0
      vein 904.2
    gastric
      artery 902.21
      vein 902.39
    head 900.9
      intracranial — *see* Injury, intracranial
      multiple 900.82
      specified NEC 900.89
    hemiazygos vein 901.89
    hepatic
      artery 902.22
      vein 902.11
    hypogastric 902.59
      artery 902.51
      vein 902.52
    ileocolic
      artery 902.26
      vein 902.31
    iliac 902.50
      artery 902.53
      specified branch NEC 902.59
      vein 902.54
    innominate
      artery 901.1
      vein 901.3
    intercostal (artery) (vein) 901.81
    jugular vein (external) 900.81
      internal 900.1
    leg NEC 904.8
    mammary (artery) (vein) 901.82
    mesenteric
      artery 902.20
        inferior 902.27
        specified branch NEC 902.29
        superior (trunk) 902.25
          branches, primary 902.26
      vein 902.39
        inferior 902.32
        superior (and primary subdivisions) 902.31
    neck 900.9
      multiple 900.82
      specified NEC 900.89
    ovarian 902.89
      artery 902.81
      vein 902.82
    palmar artery 903.4
    pelvis 902.9
      multiple 902.87
      specified NEC 902.89
    plantar (deep) (artery) (vein) 904.6
    popliteal 904.40
      artery 904.41
      vein 904.42
    portal 902.33
    pulmonary 901.40
      artery 901.41
      vein 901.42
    radial (artery) (vein) 903.2
    renal 902.40
      artery 902.41
      specified NEC 902.49
      vein 902.42
    saphenous
      artery 904.7

Injury — *continued*
  blood vessel — *continued*
    saphenous — *continued*
      vein (greater) (lesser) 904.3
    splenic
      artery 902.23
      vein 902.34
    subclavian
      artery 901.1
      vein 901.3
    suprarenal 902.49
    thoracic 901.9
      multiple 901.83
      specified NEC 901.89
    tibial 904.50
      artery 904.50
        anterior 904.51
        posterior 904.53
      vein 904.50
        anterior 904.52
        posterior 904.54
    ulnar (artery) (vein) 903.3
    uterine 902.59
      artery 902.55
      vein 902.56
    vena cava
      inferior 902.10
        specified branches NEC 902.19
      superior 901.2
  brachial plexus 953.4
    newborn 767.6
  brain (traumatic) NEC (*see also* Injury, intracranial) 854.0 ☑
    due to fracture of skull — *see* Fracture, skull, by site
  breast 959.19
  broad ligament — *see* Injury, internal, broad ligament
  bronchus, bronchi — *see* Injury, internal, bronchus
  brow 959.09
  buttock 959.19
  canthus, eye 921.1
  cathode ray 990
  cauda equina 952.4
    with fracture, vertebra — *see* Fracture, vertebra, sacrum
  cavernous sinus (*see also* Injury, intracranial) 854.0 ☑
  cecum — *see* Injury, internal, cecum
  celiac ganglion or plexus 954.1
  cerebellum (*see also* Injury, intracranial) 854.0 ☑
  cervix (uteri) — *see* Injury, internal, cervix
  cheek 959.09
  chest (*see also* Injury, internal, chest)
    wall 959.11
  childbirth (*see also* Birth, injury)
    maternal NEC 665.9 ☑
  chin 959.09
  choroid (eye) 921.3
  clitoris 959.14
  coccyx 959.19
    complicating delivery 665.6 ☑
  colon — *see* Injury, internal, colon
  common duct — *see* Injury, internal, common duct
  conjunctiva 921.1
    superficial 918.2
  cord
    spermatic — *see* Injury, internal, spermatic cord
    spinal — *see* Injury, spinal, by site
  cornea 921.3
    abrasion 918.1
      due to contact lens 371.82
    penetrating — *see* Injury, eyeball, penetrating
    superficial 918.1
      due to contact lens 371.82
  cortex (cerebral) (*see also* Injury, intracranial) 854.0 ☑
    visual 950.3
  costal region 959.11
  costochondral 959.11

Injury — *continued*
  cranial
    bones — *see* Fracture, skull, by site
    cavity (*see also* Injury, intracranial) 854.0 ☑
    nerve — *see* Injury, nerve, cranial
  crushing — *see* Crush
  cutaneous sensory nerve
    lower limb 956.4
    upper limb 955.5
  deep tissue — *see* Contusion, by site
    meaning pressure ulcer 707.25
  delivery (*see also* Birth, injury)
    maternal NEC 665.9 ☑
  Descemet's membrane — *see* Injury, eyeball, penetrating
  diaphragm — *see* Injury, internal, diaphragm
  diffuse axonal — *see* Injury, intracranial
  duodenum — *see* Injury, internal, duodenum
  ear (auricle) (canal) (drum) (external) 959.09
  elbow (and forearm) (and wrist) 959.3
  epididymis 959.14
  epigastric region 959.12
  epiglottis 959.09
  epiphyseal, current — *see* Fracture, by site
  esophagus — *see* Injury, internal, esophagus
  Eustachian tube 959.09
  extremity (lower) (upper) NEC 959.8
  eye 921.9
    penetrating eyeball — *see* Injury, eyeball, penetrating
    superficial 918.9
  eyeball 921.3
    penetrating 871.7
      with
        partial loss (of intraocular tissue) 871.2
        prolapse or exposure (of intraocular tissue) 871.1
        without prolapse 871.0
        foreign body (nonmagnetic) 871.6
          magnetic 871.5
    superficial 918.9
  eyebrow 959.09
  eyelid(s) 921.1
    laceration — *see* Laceration, eyelid
    superficial 918.0
  face (and neck) 959.09
  fallopian tube — *see* Injury, internal, fallopian tube
  finger(s) (nail) 959.5
  flank 959.19
  foot (and ankle) (and knee) (and leg, except thigh) 959.7
  forceps NEC 767.9
    scalp 767.19
  forearm (and elbow) (and wrist) 959.3
  forehead 959.09
  gallbladder — *see* Injury, internal, gallbladder
  gasserian ganglion 951.2
  gastrointestinal tract — *see* Injury, internal, gastrointestinal tract
  genital organ(s)
    with
      abortion — *see* Abortion, by type, with damage to pelvic organs
      ectopic pregnancy (*see also* categories 633.0–633.9) 639.2
      molar pregnancy (*see also* categories 630–632) 639.2
    external 959.14
      fracture of corpus cavernosum penis 959.13
    following
      abortion 639.2
      ectopic or molar pregnancy 639.2
    internal — *see* Injury, internal, genital organs
    obstetrical trauma NEC 665.9 ☑
      affecting fetus or newborn 763.89
  gland
    lacrimal 921.1

☑ **Additional Digit Required** — Refer to the Tabular List for Digit Selection   ⏭ **Subterms under main terms may continue to next column or page**

2013 ICD-9-CM   ▶◀ **Revised Text**   ● **New Line**   ▲ **Revised Code**   **Volume 2 — 161**

Injury — continued
  gland — continued
    lacrimal — continued
      laceration 870.8
    parathyroid 959.09
    salivary 959.09
    thyroid 959.09
  globe (eye) (see also Injury, eyeball) 921.3
  grease gun — see Wound, open, by site, complicated
  groin 959.19
  gum 959.09
  hand(s) (except fingers) 959.4
  head NEC 959.01
    with
      loss of consciousness 850.5
      skull fracture — see Fracture, skull, by site
  heart — see Injury, internal, heart
  heel 959.7
  hip (and thigh) 959.6
  hymen 959.14
  hyperextension (cervical) (vertebra) 847.0
  ileum — see Injury, internal, ileum
  iliac region 959.19
  infrared rays NEC 990
  instrumental (during surgery) 998.2
    birth injury — see Birth, injury
    nonsurgical (see also Injury, by site) 959.9
    obstetrical 665.9 ☑
      affecting fetus or newborn 763.89
      bladder 665.5 ☑
      cervix 665.3 ☑
      high vaginal 665.4 ☑
      perineal NEC 664.9 ☑
      urethra 665.5 ☑
      uterus 665.5 ☑
  internal 869.0

> Note — For injury of internal organ(s) by foreign body entering through a natural orifice (e.g., inhaled, ingested, or swallowed) — see Foreign body, entering through orifice.
>
> For internal injury of any of the following sites with internal injury of any other of the sites — see Injury, internal, multiple.

    with
      fracture
        pelvis — see Fracture, pelvis
        specified site, except pelvis — see Injury, internal, by site
      open wound into cavity 869.1
    abdomen, abdominal (viscera) NEC 868.00
      with
        fracture, pelvis — see Fracture, pelvis
        open wound into cavity 868.10
        specified site NEC 868.09
          with open wound into cavity 868.19
    adrenal (gland) 868.01
      with open wound into cavity 868.11
    aorta (thoracic) 901.0
      abdominal 902.0
    appendix 863.85
      with open wound into cavity 863.95
    bile duct 868.02
      with open wound into cavity 868.12
    bladder (sphincter) 867.0
      with
        abortion — see Abortion, by type, with damage to pelvic organs
        ectopic pregnancy (see also categories 633.0–633.9) 639.2
        molar pregnancy (see also categories 630–632) 639.2
        open wound into cavity 867.1
      following
        abortion 639.2
        ectopic or molar pregnancy 639.2
      obstetrical trauma 665.5 ☑

Injury — continued
  internal — continued
    bladder — continued
      obstetrical trauma — continued
        affecting fetus or newborn 763.89
    blood vessel — see Injury, blood vessel, by site
    broad ligament 867.6
      with open wound into cavity 867.7
    bronchus, bronchi 862.21
      with open wound into cavity 862.31
    cecum 863.89
      with open wound into cavity 863.99
    cervix (uteri) 867.4
      with
        abortion — see Abortion, by type, with damage to pelvic organs
        ectopic pregnancy (see also categories 633.0–633.9) 639.2
        molar pregnancy (see also categories 630–632) 639.2
        open wound into cavity 867.5
      following
        abortion 639.2
        ectopic or molar pregnancy 639.2
      obstetrical trauma 665.3 ☑
        affecting fetus or newborn 763.89
    chest (see also Injury, internal, intrathoracic organs) 862.8
      with open wound into cavity 862.9
    colon 863.40
      with
        open wound into cavity 863.50
        rectum 863.46
          with open wound into cavity 863.56
      ascending (right) 863.41
        with open wound into cavity 863.51
      descending (left) 863.43
        with open wound into cavity 863.53
      multiple sites 863.46
        with open wound into cavity 863.56
      sigmoid 863.44
        with open wound into cavity 863.54
      specified site NEC 863.49
        with open wound into cavity 863.59
      transverse 863.42
        with open wound into cavity 863.52
    common duct 868.02
      with open wound into cavity 868.12
    complicating delivery 665.9 ☑
      affecting fetus or newborn 763.89
    diaphragm 862.0
      with open wound into cavity 862.1
    duodenum 863.21
      with open wound into cavity 863.31
    esophagus (intrathoracic) 862.22
      with open wound into cavity 862.32
      cervical region 874.4
        complicated 874.5
    fallopian tube 867.6
      with open wound into cavity 867.7
    gallbladder 868.02
      with open wound into cavity 868.12
    gastrointestinal tract NEC 863.80
      with open wound into cavity 863.90
    genital organ NEC 867.6
      with open wound into cavity 867.7
    heart 861.00
      with open wound into thorax 861.10
    ileum 863.29
      with open wound into cavity 863.39
    intestine NEC 863.89
      with open wound into cavity 863.99
      large NEC 863.40
        with open wound into cavity 863.50
      small NEC 863.20

Injury — continued
  internal — continued
    intestine — continued
      small — continued
        with open wound into cavity 863.30
    intra-abdominal (organ) 868.00
      with open wound into cavity 868.10
      multiple sites 868.09
        with open wound into cavity 868.19
      specified site NEC 868.09
        with open wound into cavity 868.19
    intrathoracic organs (multiple) 862.8
      with open wound into cavity 862.9
      diaphragm (only) — see Injury, internal, diaphragm
      heart (only) — see Injury, internal, heart
      lung (only) — see Injury, internal, lung
      specified site NEC 862.29
        with open wound into cavity 862.39
    intrauterine (see also Injury, internal, uterus) 867.4
      with open wound into cavity 867.5
    jejunum 863.29
      with open wound into cavity 863.39
    kidney (subcapsular) 866.00
      with
        disruption of parenchyma (complete) 866.03
          with open wound into cavity 866.13
        hematoma (without rupture of capsule) 866.01
          with open wound into cavity 866.11
        laceration 866.02
          with open wound into cavity 866.12
        open wound into cavity 866.10
    liver 864.00
      with
        contusion 864.01
          with open wound into cavity 864.11
        hematoma 864.01
          with open wound into cavity 864.11
        laceration 864.05
          with open wound into cavity 864.15
        major (disruption of hepatic parenchyma) 864.04
          with open wound into cavity 864.14
        minor (capsule only) 864.02
          with open wound into cavity 864.12
        moderate (involving parenchyma) 864.03
          with open wound into cavity 864.13
        multiple 864.04
        stellate 864.04
          with open wound into cavity 864.14
        open wound into cavity 864.10
    lung 861.20
      with open wound into thorax 861.30
      aspiration 507.0
      hemopneumothorax — see Hemopneumothorax, traumatic
      hemothorax — see Hemothorax, traumatic
      pneumohemothorax — see Pneumohemothorax, traumatic
      pneumothorax — see Pneumothorax, traumatic
      transfusion related, acute (TRALI) 518.7
    mediastinum 862.29
      with open wound into cavity 862.39

Injury — continued
  internal — continued
    mesentery 863.89
      with open wound into cavity 863.99
    mesosalpinx 867.6
      with open wound into cavity 867.7
    multiple 869.0

> Note — Multiple internal injuries of sites classifiable to the same three- or four-digit category should be classified to that category.
>
> Multiple injuries classifiable to different fourth-digit subdivisions of 861 (heart and lung injuries) should be dealt with according to coding rules.

      internal
        with open wound into cavity 869.1
      intra-abdominal organ (sites classifiable to 863–868)
        with
          intrathoracic organ(s) (sites classifiable to 861–862) 869.0
            with open wound into cavity 869.1
          other intra-abdominal organ(s) (sites classifiable to 863–868, except where classifiable to the same three-digit category) 868.09
            with open wound into cavity 868.19
      intrathoracic organ (sites classifiable to 861–862)
        with
          intra-abdominal organ(s) (sites classifiable to 863–868) 869.0
            with open wound into cavity 869.1
          other intrathoracic organ(s) (sites classifiable to 861–862, except where classifiable to the same three-digit category) 862.8
            with open wound into cavity 862.9
    myocardium — see Injury, internal, heart
    ovary 867.6
      with open wound into cavity 867.7
    pancreas (multiple sites) 863.84
      with open wound into cavity 863.94
      body 863.82
        with open wound into cavity 863.92
      head 863.81
        with open wound into cavity 863.91
      tail 863.83
        with open wound into cavity 863.93
    pelvis, pelvic (organs) (viscera) 867.8
      with
        fracture, pelvis — see Fracture, pelvis
        open wound into cavity 867.9
      specified site NEC 867.6
        with open wound into cavity 867.7
    peritoneum 868.03
      with open wound into cavity 868.13
    pleura 862.29
      with open wound into cavity 862.39
    prostate 867.6
      with open wound into cavity 867.7
    rectum 863.45
      with
        colon 863.46
          with open wound into cavity 863.56
        open wound into cavity 863.55
    retroperitoneum 868.04

☑ Additional Digit Required — Refer to the Tabular List for Digit Selection   ▽ Subterms under main terms may continue to next column or page

162 — Volume 2   ▶◀ Revised Text   ● New Line   ▲ Revised Code   2013 ICD-9-CM

Injury — continued
  internal — continued
    retroperitoneum — continued
      with open wound into cavity 868.14
    round ligament 867.6
      with open wound into cavity 867.7
    seminal vesicle 867.6
      with open wound into cavity 867.7
    spermatic cord 867.6
      with open wound into cavity 867.7
      scrotal — see Wound, open, spermatic cord
    spleen 865.00
      with
        disruption of parenchyma (massive) 865.04
          with open wound into cavity 865.14
        hematoma (without rupture of capsule) 865.01
          with open wound into cavity 865.11
        open wound into cavity 865.10
        tear, capsular 865.02
          with open wound into cavity 865.12
        extending into parenchyma 865.03
          with open wound into cavity 865.13
    stomach 863.0
      with open wound into cavity 863.1
    suprarenal gland (multiple) 868.01
      with open wound into cavity 868.11
    thorax, thoracic (cavity) (organs) (multiple) (see also Injury, internal, intrathoracic organs) 862.8
      with open wound into cavity 862.9
    thymus (gland) 862.29
      with open wound into cavity 862.39
    trachea (intrathoracic) 862.29
      with open wound into cavity 862.39
      cervical region (see also Wound, open, trachea) 874.02
    ureter 867.2
      with open wound into cavity 867.3
    urethra (sphincter) 867.0
      with
        abortion — see Abortion, by type, with damage to pelvic organs
        ectopic pregnancy (see also categories 633.0–633.9) 639.2
        molar pregnancy (see also categories 630–632) 639.2
        open wound into cavity 867.1
      following
        abortion 639.2
        ectopic or molar pregnancy 639.2
      obstetrical trauma 665.5 ☑
        affecting fetus or newborn 763.89
    uterus 867.4
      with
        abortion — see Abortion, by type, with damage to pelvic organs
        ectopic pregnancy (see also categories 633.0–633.9) 639.2
        molar pregnancy (see also categories 630–632) 639.2
        open wound into cavity 867.5
      following
        abortion 639.2
        ectopic or molar pregnancy 639.2
      obstetrical trauma NEC 665.5 ☑
        affecting fetus or newborn 763.89
    vas deferens 867.6
      with open wound into cavity 867.7
    vesical (sphincter) 867.0
      with open wound into cavity 867.1
    viscera (abdominal) (see also Injury, internal, multiple) 868.00
      with
        fracture, pelvis — see Fracture, pelvis
        open wound into cavity 868.10

Injury — continued
  internal — continued
    viscera (see also Injury, internal, multiple) — continued
      thoracic NEC (see also Injury, internal, intrathoracic organs) 862.8
        with open wound into cavity 862.9
    interscapular region 959.19
    intervertebral disc 959.19
    intestine — see Injury, internal, intestine
    intra-abdominal (organs) NEC — see Injury, internal, intra-abdominal
    intracranial (traumatic) 854.0 ☑

> Note — Use the following fifth-digit subclassification with categories 851–854:
>
> 0   unspecified state of consciousness
>
> 1   with no loss of consciousness
>
> 2   with brief [less than one hour] loss of consciousness
>
> 3   with moderate [1–24 hours] loss of consciousness
>
> 4   with prolonged [more than 24 hours] loss of consciousness and return to pre–existing conscious level
>
> 5   with prolonged [more than 24 hours] loss of consciousness, without return to pre–existing conscious level
>
> Use fifth-digit 5 to designate when a patient is unconscious and dies before regaining consciousness, regardless of the duration of the loss of consciousness
>
> 6   with loss of consciousness of unspecified duration
>
> 9   with concussion, unspecified

      with
        open intracranial wound 854.1 ☑
        skull fracture — see Fracture, skull, by site
      contusion 851.8 ☑
        with open intracranial wound 851.9 ☑
        brain stem 851.4 ☑
          with open intracranial wound 851.5 ☑
        cerebellum 851.4 ☑
          with open intracranial wound 851.5 ☑
        cortex (cerebral) 851.0 ☑
          with open intracranial wound 851.2 ☑
      hematoma — see Injury, intracranial, hemorrhage
      hemorrhage 853.0 ☑
        with
          laceration — see Injury, intracranial, laceration
          open intracranial wound 853.1 ☑
        extradural 852.4 ☑
          with open intracranial wound 852.5 ☑
        subarachnoid 852.0 ☑
          with open intracranial wound 852.1 ☑
        subdural 852.2 ☑
          with open intracranial wound 852.3 ☑
      laceration 851.8 ☑
        with open intracranial wound 851.9 ☑
        brain stem 851.6 ☑
          with open intracranial wound 851.7 ☑
        cerebellum 851.6 ☑
          with open intracranial wound 851.7 ☑
        cortex (cerebral) 851.2 ☑

Injury — continued
  intracranial — continued
    laceration — continued
      cortex — continued
        with open intracranial wound 851.3 ☑
    intraocular — see Injury, eyeball, penetrating
    intrathoracic organs (multiple) — see Injury, internal, intrathoracic organs
    intrauterine — see Injury, internal, intrauterine
    iris 921.3
      penetrating — see Injury, eyeball, penetrating
    jaw 959.09
    jejunum — see Injury, internal, jejunum
    joint NEC 959.9
      old or residual 718.80
        ankle 718.87
        elbow 718.82
        foot 718.87
        hand 718.84
        hip 718.85
        knee 718.86
        multiple sites 718.89
        pelvic region 718.85
        shoulder (region) 718.81
        specified site NEC 718.88
        wrist 718.83
    kidney — see Injury, internal, kidney
      acute (nontraumatic) 584.9
    knee (and ankle) (and foot) (and leg, except thigh) 959.7
    labium (majus) (minus) 959.14
    labyrinth, ear 959.09
    lacrimal apparatus, gland, or sac 921.1
      laceration 870.8
    larynx 959.09
    late effect — see Late, effects (of), injury
    leg, except thigh (and ankle) (and foot) (and knee) 959.7
      upper or thigh 959.6
    lens, eye 921.3
      penetrating — see Injury, eyeball, penetrating
    lid, eye — see Injury, eyelid
    lip 959.09
    liver — see Injury, internal, liver
    lobe, parietal — see Injury, intracranial
    lumbar (region) 959.19
      plexus 953.5
    lumbosacral (region) 959.19
      plexus 953.5
    lung — see Injury, internal, lung
    malar region 959.09
    mastoid region 959.09
    maternal, during pregnancy, affecting fetus or newborn 760.5
    maxilla 959.09
    mediastinum — see Injury, internal, mediastinum
    membrane
      brain (see also Injury, intracranial) 854.0 ☑
      tympanic 959.09
    meningeal artery — see Hemorrhage, brain, traumatic, subarachnoid
    meninges (cerebral) — see Injury, intracranial
    mesenteric
      artery — see Injury, blood vessel, mesenteric, artery
      plexus, inferior 954.1
      vein — see Injury, blood vessel, mesenteric, vein
    mesentery — see Injury, internal, mesentery
    mesosalpinx — see Injury, internal, mesosalpinx
    middle ear 959.09
    midthoracic region 959.11
    mouth 959.09
    multiple (sites not classifiable to the same four–digit category in 959.0–959.7) 959.8
      internal 869.0

Injury — continued
  multiple — continued
    internal — continued
      with open wound into cavity 869.1
  musculocutaneous nerve 955.4
  nail
    finger 959.5
    toe 959.7
  nasal (septum) (sinus) 959.09
  nasopharynx 959.09
  neck (and face) 959.09
  nerve 957.9
    abducens 951.3
    abducent 951.3
    accessory 951.6
    acoustic 951.5
    ankle and foot 956.9
    anterior crural, femoral 956.1
    arm (see also Injury, nerve, upper limb) 955.9
    auditory 951.5
    axillary 955.0
    brachial plexus 953.4
    cervical sympathetic 954.0
    cranial 951.9
      first or olfactory 951.8
      second or optic 950.0
      third or oculomotor 951.0
      fourth or trochlear 951.1
      fifth or trigeminal 951.2
      sixth or abducens 951.3
      seventh or facial 951.4
      eighth, acoustic, or auditory 951.5
      ninth or glossopharyngeal 951.8
      tenth, pneumogastric, or vagus 951.8
      eleventh or accessory 951.6
      twelfth or hypoglossal 951.7
      newborn 767.7
    cutaneous sensory
      lower limb 956.4
      upper limb 955.5
    digital (finger) 955.6
      toe 956.5
    facial 951.4
      newborn 767.5
    femoral 956.1
    finger 955.9
    foot and ankle 956.9
    forearm 955.9
    glossopharyngeal 951.8
    hand and wrist 955.9
    head and neck, superficial 957.0
    hypoglossal 951.7
    involving several parts of body 957.8
    leg (see also Injury, nerve, lower limb) 956.9
    lower limb 956.9
      multiple 956.8
      specified site NEC 956.5
    lumbar plexus 953.5
    lumbosacral plexus 953.5
    median 955.1
      forearm 955.1
      wrist and hand 955.1
    multiple (in several parts of body) (sites not classifiable to the same three-digit category) 957.8
    musculocutaneous 955.4
    musculospiral 955.3
      upper arm 955.3
    oculomotor 951.0
    olfactory 951.8
    optic 950.0
    pelvic girdle 956.9
      multiple sites 956.8
      specified site NEC 956.5
    peripheral 957.9
      multiple (in several regions) (sites not classifiable to the same three-digit category) 957.8
      specified site NEC 957.1
    peroneal 956.3
      ankle and foot 956.3
      lower leg 956.3
    plantar 956.5
    plexus 957.9

☑ Additional Digit Required — Refer to the Tabular List for Digit Selection   ▽ Subterms under main terms may continue to next column or page

2013 ICD-9-CM   ▶◀ Revised Text   ● New Line   ▲ Revised Code   Volume 2 — 163

Injury — Injury

Injury — *continued*
　nerve — *continued*
　　plexus — *continued*
　　　celiac 954.1
　　　mesenteric, inferior 954.1
　　　spinal 953.9
　　　　brachial 953.4
　　　　lumbosacral 953.5
　　　　multiple sites 953.8
　　　sympathetic NEC 954.1
　　pneumogastric 951.8
　　radial 955.3
　　　wrist and hand 955.3
　　sacral plexus 953.5
　　sciatic 956.0
　　　thigh 956.0
　　shoulder girdle 955.9
　　　multiple 955.8
　　　specified site NEC 955.7
　　specified site NEC 957.1
　　spinal 953.9
　　　plexus — *see* Injury, nerve, plexus, spinal
　　　root 953.9
　　　　cervical 953.0
　　　　dorsal 953.1
　　　　lumbar 953.2
　　　　multiple sites 953.8
　　　　sacral 953.3
　　splanchnic 954.1
　　sympathetic NEC 954.1
　　　cervical 954.0
　　thigh 956.9
　　tibial 956.5
　　　ankle and foot 956.2
　　　lower leg 956.5
　　　posterior 956.2
　　toe 956.9
　　trigeminal 951.2
　　trochlear 951.1
　　trunk, excluding shoulder and pelvic girdles 954.9
　　　specified site NEC 954.8
　　　sympathetic NEC 954.1
　　ulnar 955.2
　　　forearm 955.2
　　　wrist (and hand) 955.2
　　upper limb 955.9
　　　multiple 955.8
　　　specified site NEC 955.7
　　vagus 951.8
　　wrist and hand 955.9
　nervous system, diffuse 957.8
　nose (septum) 959.09
　obstetrical NEC 665.9 ☑
　　affecting fetus or newborn 763.89
　occipital (region) (scalp) 959.09
　　lobe (*see also* Injury, intracranial) 854.0 ☑
　optic 950.9
　　chiasm 950.1
　　cortex 950.3
　　nerve 950.0
　　pathways 950.2
　orbit, orbital (region) 921.2
　　penetrating 870.3
　　　with foreign body 870.4
　ovary — *see* Injury, internal, ovary
　paint-gun — *see* Wound, open, by site, complicated
　palate (soft) 959.09
　pancreas — *see* Injury, internal, pancreas
　parathyroid (gland) 959.09
　parietal (region) (scalp) 959.09
　　lobe — *see* Injury, intracranial
　pelvic
　　floor 959.19
　　　complicating delivery 664.1 ☑
　　　　affecting fetus or newborn 763.89
　　joint or ligament, complicating delivery 665.6 ☑
　　　affecting fetus or newborn 763.89
　　organs (*see also* Injury, internal, pelvis)

Injury — *continued*
　pelvic — *continued*
　　organs (*see also* Injury, internal, pelvis) — *continued*
　　　with
　　　　abortion — *see* Abortion, by type, with damage to pelvic organs
　　　　ectopic pregnancy (*see also* categories 633.0–633.9) 639.2
　　　　molar pregnancy (*see also* categories 633.0–633.9) 639.2
　　　following
　　　　abortion 639.2
　　　　ectopic or molar pregnancy 639.2
　　　obstetrical trauma 665.5 ☑
　　　　affecting fetus or newborn 763.89
　pelvis 959.19
　penis 959.14
　　fracture of corpus cavernosum 959.13
　perineum 959.14
　peritoneum — *see* Injury, internal, peritoneum
　periurethral tissue
　　with
　　　abortion — *see* Abortion, by type, with damage to pelvic organs
　　　ectopic pregnancy (*see also* categories 633.0–633.9) 639.2
　　　molar pregnancy (*see also* categories 630–632) 639.2
　　complicating delivery 664.8 ☑
　　　affecting fetus or newborn 763.89
　　following
　　　abortion 639.2
　　　ectopic or molar pregnancy 639.2
　phalanges
　　foot 959.7
　　hand 959.5
　pharynx 959.09
　pleura — *see* Injury, internal, pleura
　popliteal space 959.7
　post-cardiac surgery (syndrome) 429.4
　prepuce 959.14
　prostate — *see* Injury, internal, prostate
　pubic region 959.19
　pudenda 959.14
　radiation NEC 990
　radioactive substance or radium NEC 990
　rectovaginal septum 959.14
　rectum — *see* Injury, internal, rectum
　retina 921.3
　　penetrating — *see* Injury, eyeball, penetrating
　retroperitoneal — *see* Injury, internal, retroperitoneum
　roentgen rays NEC 990
　round ligament — *see* Injury, internal, round ligament
　sacral (region) 959.19
　　plexus 953.5
　sacroiliac ligament NEC 959.19
　sacrum 959.19
　salivary ducts or glands 959.09
　scalp 959.09
　　due to birth trauma 767.19
　　fetus or newborn 767.19
　scapular region 959.2
　sclera 921.3
　　penetrating — *see* Injury, eyeball, penetrating
　　superficial 918.2
　scrotum 959.14
　seminal vesicle — *see* Injury, internal, seminal vesicle
　shoulder (and upper arm) 959.2
　sinus
　　cavernous (*see also* Injury, intracranial) 854.0 ☑
　　nasal 959.09
　skeleton NEC, birth injury 767.3
　skin NEC 959.9
　skull — *see* Fracture, skull, by site
　soft tissue (of external sites) (severe) — *see* Wound, open, by site
　specified site NEC 959.8

Injury — *continued*
　spermatic cord — *see* Injury, internal, spermatic cord
　spinal (cord) 952.9
　　with fracture, vertebra — *see* Fracture, vertebra, by site, with spinal cord injury
　　cervical (C₁-C₄) 952.00
　　　with
　　　　anterior cord syndrome 952.02
　　　　central cord syndrome 952.03
　　　　complete lesion of cord 952.01
　　　　incomplete lesion NEC 952.04
　　　　posterior cord syndrome 952.04
　　　C₅-C₇ level 952.05
　　　　with
　　　　　anterior cord syndrome 952.07
　　　　　central cord syndrome 952.08
　　　　　complete lesion of cord 952.06
　　　　　incomplete lesion NEC 952.09
　　　　　posterior cord syndrome 952.09
　　　　specified type NEC 952.09
　　　specified type NEC 952.04
　　dorsal (D₁-D₆) (T₁-T₆) (thoracic) 952.10
　　　with
　　　　anterior cord syndrome 952.12
　　　　central cord syndrome 952.13
　　　　complete lesion of cord 952.11
　　　　incomplete lesion NEC 952.14
　　　　posterior cord syndrome 952.14
　　　D₇-D₁₂ level (T₇-T₁₂) 952.15
　　　　with
　　　　　anterior cord syndrome 952.17
　　　　　central cord syndrome 952.18
　　　　　complete lesion of cord 952.16
　　　　　incomplete lesion NEC 952.19
　　　　　posterior cord syndrome 952.19
　　　　specified type NEC 952.19
　　　specified type NEC 952.14
　　lumbar 952.2
　　multiple sites 952.8
　　nerve (root) NEC — *see* Injury, nerve, spinal, root
　　plexus 953.9
　　　brachial 953.4
　　　lumbosacral 953.5
　　　multiple sites 953.8
　　sacral 952.3
　　thoracic (*see also* Injury, spinal, dorsal) 952.10
　spleen — *see* Injury, internal, spleen
　stellate ganglion 954.1
　sternal region 959.11
　stomach — *see* Injury, internal, stomach
　subconjunctival 921.1
　subcutaneous 959.9
　subdural — *see* Injury, intracranial
　submaxillary region 959.09
　submental region 959.09
　subungual
　　fingers 959.5
　　toes 959.7

Injury — *continued*
　superficial 919 ☑

> *Note* — Use the following fourth-digit subdivisions with categories 910–919:
>
> 0　Abrasion or friction burn without mention of infection
> 1　Abrasion or friction burn, infected
> 2　Blister without mention of infection
> 3　Blister, infected
> 4　Insect bite, nonvenomous, without mention of infection
> 5　Insect bite, nonvenomous, infected
> 6　Superficial foreign body (splinter) without major open wound and without mention of infection
> 7　Superficial foreign body (splinter) without major open wound, infected
> 8　Other and unspecified superficial injury without mention of infection
> 9　Other and unspecified superficial injury, infected
>
> For late effects of superficial injury, see category 906.2.

　　abdomen, abdominal (muscle) (wall) (and other part(s) of trunk) 911 ☑
　　ankle (and hip, knee, leg, or thigh) 916 ☑
　　anus (and other part(s) of trunk) 911 ☑
　　arm 913 ☑
　　　upper (and shoulder) 912 ☑
　　auditory canal (external) (meatus) (and other part(s) of face, neck, or scalp, except eye) 910 ☑
　　axilla (and upper arm) 912 ☑
　　back (and other part(s) of trunk) 911 ☑
　　breast (and other part(s) of trunk) 911 ☑
　　brow (and other part(s) of face, neck, or scalp, except eye) 910 ☑
　　buttock (and other part(s) of trunk) 911 ☑
　　canthus, eye 918.0
　　cheek(s) (and other part(s) of face, neck, or scalp, except eye) 910 ☑
　　chest wall (and other part(s) of trunk) 911 ☑
　　chin (and other part(s) of face, neck, or scalp, except eye) 910 ☑
　　clitoris (and other part(s) of trunk) 911 ☑
　　conjunctiva 918.2
　　cornea 918.1
　　　due to contact lens 371.82
　　costal region (and other part(s) of trunk) 911 ☑
　　ear(s) (auricle) (canal) (drum) (external) (and other part(s) of face, neck, or scalp, except eye) 910 ☑
　　elbow (and forearm) (and wrist) 913 ☑
　　epididymis (and other part(s) of trunk) 911 ☑
　　epigastric region (and other part(s) of trunk) 911 ☑
　　epiglottis (and other part(s) of face, neck, or scalp, except eye) 910 ☑
　　eye(s) (and adnexa) NEC 918.9
　　eyelid(s) (and periocular area) 918.0
　　face (any part(s), except eye) (and neck or scalp) 910 ☑
　　finger(s) (nail) (any) 915 ☑
　　flank (and other part(s) of trunk) 911 ☑
　　foot (phalanges) (and toe(s)) 917 ☑
　　forearm (and elbow) (and wrist) 913 ☑
　　forehead (and other part(s) of face, neck, or scalp, except eye) 910 ☑
　　globe (eye) 918.9

☑ Additional Digit Required — Refer to the Tabular List for Digit Selection　　　　　　🔁 Subterms under main terms may continue to next column or page

164 — Volume 2　　　　▶◀ Revised Text　　　● New Line　　　▲ Revised Code　　　　2013 ICD-9-CM

Injury — *continued*
  superficial — *continued*
    groin (and other part(s) of trunk) 911 ☑
    gum(s) (and other part(s) of face, neck, or scalp, except eye) 910 ☑
    hand(s) (except fingers alone) 914 ☑
    head (and other part(s) of face, neck, or scalp, except eye) 910 ☑
    heel (and foot or toe) 917 ☑
    hip (and ankle, knee, leg, or thigh) 916 ☑
    iliac region (and other part(s) of trunk) 911 ☑
    interscapular region (and other part(s) of trunk) 911 ☑
    iris 918.9
    knee (and ankle, hip, leg, or thigh) 916 ☑
    labium (majus) (minus) (and other part(s) of trunk) 911 ☑
    lacrimal (apparatus) (gland) (sac) 918.0
    leg (lower) (upper) (and ankle, hip, knee, or thigh) 916 ☑
    lip(s) (and other part(s) of face, neck, or scalp, except eye) 910 ☑
    lower extremity (except foot) 916 ☑
    lumbar region (and other part(s) of trunk) 911 ☑
    malar region (and other part(s) of face, neck, or scalp, except eye) 910 ☑
    mastoid region (and other part(s) of face, neck, or scalp, except eye) 910 ☑
    midthoracic region (and other part(s) of trunk) 911 ☑
    mouth (and other part(s) of face, neck, or scalp, except eye) 910 ☑
    multiple sites (not classifiable to the same three-digit category) 919 ☑
    nasal (septum) (and other part(s) of face, neck, or scalp, except eye) 910 ☑
    neck (and face or scalp, any part(s), except eye) 910 ☑
    nose (septum) (and other part(s) of face, neck, or scalp, except eye) 910 ☑
    occipital region (and other part(s) of face, neck, or scalp, except eye) 910 ☑
    orbital region 918.0
    palate (soft) (and other part(s) of face, neck, or scalp, except eye) 910 ☑
    parietal region (and other part(s) of face, neck, or scalp, except eye) 910 ☑
    penis (and other part(s) of trunk) 911 ☑
    perineum (and other part(s) of trunk) 911 ☑
    periocular area 918.0
    pharynx (and other part(s) of face, neck, or scalp, except eye) 910 ☑
    popliteal space (and ankle, hip, leg, or thigh) 916 ☑
    prepuce (and other part(s) of trunk) 911 ☑
    pubic region (and other part(s) of trunk) 911 ☑
    pudenda (and other part(s) of trunk) 911 ☑
    sacral region (and other part(s) of trunk) 911 ☑
    salivary (ducts) (glands) (and other part(s) of face, neck, or scalp, except eye) 910 ☑
    scalp (and other part(s) of face or neck, except eye) 910 ☑
    scapular region (and upper arm) 912 ☑
    sclera 918.2
    scrotum (and other part(s) of trunk) 911 ☑
    shoulder (and upper arm) 912 ☑
    skin NEC 919 ☑
    specified site(s) NEC 919 ☑
    sternal region (and other part(s) of trunk) 911 ☑
    subconjunctival 918.2
    subcutaneous NEC 919 ☑

Injury — *continued*
  superficial — *continued*
    submaxillary region (and other part(s) of face, neck, or scalp, except eye) 910 ☑
    submental region (and other part(s) of face, neck, or scalp, except eye) 910 ☑
    supraclavicular fossa (and other part(s) of face, neck, or scalp, except eye) 910 ☑
    supraorbital 918.0
    temple (and other part(s) of face, neck, or scalp, except eye) 910 ☑
    temporal region (and other part(s) of face, neck, or scalp, except eye) 910 ☑
    testis (and other part(s) of trunk) 911 ☑
    thigh (and ankle, hip, knee, or leg) 916 ☑
    thorax, thoracic (external) (and other part(s) of trunk) 911 ☑
    throat (and other part(s) of face, neck, or scalp, except eye) 910 ☑
    thumb(s) (nail) 915 ☑
    toe(s) (nail) (subungual) (and foot) 917 ☑
    tongue (and other part(s) of face, neck, or scalp, except eye) 910 ☑
    tooth, teeth (*see also* Abrasion, dental) 521.20
    trunk (any part(s)) 911 ☑
    tunica vaginalis 959.14
    tympanum, tympanic membrane (and other part(s) of face, neck, or scalp, except eye) 910 ☑
    upper extremity NEC 913 ☑
    uvula (and other part(s) of face, neck, or scalp, except eye) 910 ☑
    vagina (and other part(s) of trunk) 911 ☑
    vulva (and other part(s) of trunk) 911 ☑
    wrist (and elbow) (and forearm) 913 ☑
  supraclavicular fossa 959.19
  supraorbital 959.09
  surgical complication (external or internal site) 998.2
  symphysis pubis 959.19
    complicating delivery 665.6 ☑
      affecting fetus or newborn 763.89
  temple 959.09
  temporal region 959.09
  testis 959.14
  thigh (and hip) 959.6
  thorax, thoracic (external) 959.11
    cavity — *see* Injury, internal, thorax
    internal — *see* Injury, internal, intrathoracic organs
  throat 959.09
  thumb(s) (nail) 959.5
  thymus — *see* Injury, internal, thymus
  thyroid (gland) 959.09
  toe (nail) (any) 959.7
  tongue 959.09
  tonsil 959.09
  tooth NEC 873.63
    complicated 873.73
  trachea — *see* Injury, internal, trachea
  trunk 959.19
  tunica vaginalis 959.14
  tympanum, tympanic membrane 959.09
  ultraviolet rays NEC 990
  ureter — *see* Injury, internal, ureter
  urethra (sphincter) — *see* Injury, internal, urethra
  uterus — *see* Injury, internal, uterus
  uvula 959.09
  vagina 959.14
  vascular — *see* Injury, blood vessel
  vas deferens — *see* Injury, internal, vas deferens
  vein (*see also* Injury, blood vessel, by site) 904.9
  vena cava
    inferior 902.10
    superior 901.2

Injury — *continued*
  vesical (sphincter) — *see* Injury, internal, vesical
  viscera (abdominal) — *see* Injury, internal, viscera
    with fracture, pelvis — *see* Fracture, pelvis
  visual 950.9
    cortex 950.3
  vitreous (humor) 871.2
  vulva 959.14
  whiplash (cervical spine) 847.0
  wringer — *see* Crush, by site
  wrist (and elbow) (and forearm) 959.3
  x-ray NEC 990
Inoculation — *see also* Vaccination
  complication or reaction — *see* Complication, vaccination
INPH (idiopathic normal pressure hydrocephalus) 331.5
Insanity, insane — *see also* Psychosis 298.9
  adolescent (*see also* Schizophrenia) 295.9 ☑
  alternating (*see also* Psychosis, affective, circular) 296.7
  confusional 298.9
    acute 293.0
    subacute 293.1
  delusional 298.9
  paralysis, general 094.1
    progressive 094.1
  paresis, general 094.1
  senile 290.20
Insect
  bite — *see* Injury, superficial, by site
  venomous, poisoning by 989.5
Insemination, artificial V26.1
Insensitivity
  adrenocorticotropin hormone (ACTH) 255.41
  androgen 259.50
    complete 259.51
    partial 259.52
Insertion
  cord (umbilical) lateral or velamentous 663.8 ☑
    affecting fetus or newborn 762.6
  intrauterine contraceptive device V25.11
  placenta, vicious — *see* Placenta, previa
  subdermal implantable contraceptive V25.5
  velamentous, umbilical cord 663.8 ☑
    affecting fetus or newborn 762.6
Insolation 992.0
  meaning sunstroke 992.0
Insomnia, unspecified 780.52
  with sleep apnea, unspecified 780.51
  adjustment 307.41
  alcohol induced 291.82
  behavioral, of childhood V69.5
  drug induced 292.85
  due to
    medical condition classified elsewhere 327.01
    mental disorder 327.02
  fatal familial (FFI) 046.72
  idiopathic 307.42
  nonorganic origin 307.41
    persistent (primary) 307.42
    transient 307.41
  organic 327.00
    other 327.09
  paradoxical 307.42
  primary 307.42
  psychophysiological 307.42
  subjective complaint 307.49
Inspiration
  food or foreign body (*see also* Asphyxia, food or foreign body) 933.1
  mucus (*see also* Asphyxia, mucus) 933.1
Inspissated bile syndrome, newborn 774.4
Instability
  detrusor 596.59
  emotional (excessive) 301.3
  joint (posttraumatic) 718.80
    ankle 718.87
    elbow 718.82
    foot 718.87

Instability — *continued*
  joint — *continued*
    hand 718.84
    hip 718.85
    knee 718.86
    lumbosacral 724.6
    multiple sites 718.89
    pelvic region 718.85
    sacroiliac 724.6
    shoulder (region) 718.81
    specified site NEC 718.88
    wrist 718.83
  lumbosacral 724.6
  nervous 301.89
  personality (emotional) 301.59
  thyroid, paroxysmal 242.9 ☑
  urethral 599.83
  vasomotor 780.2
Insufficiency, insufficient
  accommodation 367.4
  adrenal (gland) (acute) (chronic) 255.41
    medulla 255.5
    primary 255.41
    specified site NEC 255.5
  adrenocortical 255.41
  anterior (occlusal) guidance 524.54
  anus 569.49
  aortic (valve) 424.1
    with
      mitral (valve) disease 396.1
        insufficiency, incompetence, or regurgitation 396.3
        stenosis or obstruction 396.1
      stenosis or obstruction 424.1
        with mitral (valve) disease 396.8
    congenital 746.4
    rheumatic 395.1
      with
        mitral (valve) disease 396.1
          insufficiency, incompetence, or regurgitation 396.3
          stenosis or obstruction 396.1
        stenosis or obstruction 395.2
          with mitral (valve) disease 396.8
    specified cause NEC 424.1
    syphilitic 093.22
  arterial 447.1
    basilar artery 435.0
    carotid artery 435.8
    cerebral 437.1
    coronary (acute or subacute) 411.89
    mesenteric 557.1
    peripheral 443.9
    precerebral 435.9
    vertebral artery 435.1
    vertebrobasilar 435.3
  arteriovenous 459.9
  basilar artery 435.0
  biliary 575.8
  cardiac (*see also* Insufficiency, myocardial) 428.0
    complicating surgery 997.1
    due to presence of (cardiac) prosthesis 429.4
    postoperative 997.1
      long-term effect of cardiac surgery 429.4
    specified during or due to a procedure 997.1
      long-term effect of cardiac surgery 429.4
  cardiorenal (*see also* Hypertension, cardiorenal) 404.90
  cardiovascular (*see also* Disease, cardiovascular) 429.2
    renal (*see also* Hypertension, cardiorenal) 404.90
  carotid artery 435.8
  cerebral (vascular) 437.9
  cerebrovascular 437.9
    with transient focal neurological signs and symptoms 435.9
    acute 437.1
      with transient focal neurological signs and symptoms 435.9

☑ **Additional Digit Required** — Refer to the Tabular List for Digit Selection   ▽ **Subterms under main terms may continue to next column or page**

Insufficiency, insufficient — *continued*
circulatory NEC 459.9
fetus or newborn 779.89
convergence 378.83
coronary (acute or subacute) 411.89
chronic or with a stated duration of over 8 weeks 414.8
corticoadrenal 255.41
dietary 269.9
divergence 378.85
food 994.2
gastroesophageal 530.89
gonadal
ovary 256.39
testis 257.2
gonadotropic hormone secretion 253.4
heart (*see also* Insufficiency, myocardial)
fetus or newborn 779.89
valve (*see also* Endocarditis) 424.90
congenital NEC 746.89
hepatic 573.8
idiopathic autonomic 333.0
interocclusal distance of teeth (ridge) 524.36
kidney
acute 593.9
chronic 585.9
labyrinth, labyrinthine (function) 386.53
bilateral 386.54
unilateral 386.53
lacrimal 375.15
liver 573.8
lung (acute) (*see also* Insufficiency, pulmonary) 518.82
following trauma and surgery 518.52
newborn 770.89
mental (congenital) (*see also* Disability, intellectual) 319
mesenteric 557.1
mitral (valve) 424.0
with
aortic (valve) disease 396.3
insufficiency, incompetence, or regurgitation 396.3
stenosis or obstruction 396.2
obstruction or stenosis 394.2
with aortic valve disease 396.8
congenital 746.6
rheumatic 394.1
with
aortic (valve) disease 396.3
insufficiency, incompetence, or regurgitation 396.3
stenosis or obstruction 396.2
obstruction or stenosis 394.2
with aortic valve disease 396.8
active or acute 391.1
with chorea, rheumatic (Sydenham's) 392.0
specified cause, except rheumatic 424.0
muscle
heart — *see* Insufficiency, myocardial
ocular (*see also* Strabismus) 378.9
myocardial, myocardium (with arteriosclerosis) 428.0
with rheumatic fever (conditions classifiable to 390)
active, acute, or subacute 391.2
with chorea 392.0
inactive or quiescent (with chorea) 398.0
congenital 746.89
due to presence of (cardiac) prosthesis 429.4
fetus or newborn 779.89
following cardiac surgery 429.4
hypertensive (*see also* Hypertension, heart) 402.91
benign 402.11
malignant 402.01
postoperative 997.1
long-term effect of cardiac surgery 429.4
rheumatic 398.0
active, acute, or subacute 391.2
with chorea (Sydenham's) 392.0
syphilitic 093.82

Insufficiency, insufficient — *continued*
nourishment 994.2
organic 799.89
ovary 256.39
postablative 256.2
pancreatic 577.8
parathyroid (gland) 252.1
peripheral vascular (arterial) 443.9
pituitary (anterior) 253.2
posterior 253.5
placental — *see* Placenta, insufficiency
platelets 287.5
prenatal care in current pregnancy V23.7
progressive pluriglandular 258.9
pseudocholinesterase 289.89
pulmonary (acute) 518.82
following
shock 518.52
surgery 518.52
trauma 518.52
newborn 770.89
valve (*see also* Endocarditis, pulmonary) 424.3
congenital 746.09
pyloric 537.0
renal 593.9
acute 593.9
chronic 585.9
due to a procedure 997.5
respiratory 786.09
acute 518.82
following trauma and surgery 518.52
newborn 770.89
rotation — *see* Malrotation
suprarenal 255.41
medulla 255.5
tarso-orbital fascia, congenital 743.66
tear film 375.15
testis 257.2
thyroid (gland) (acquired) (*see also* Hypothyroidism)
congenital 243
tricuspid (*see also* Endocarditis, tricuspid) 397.0
congenital 746.89
syphilitic 093.23
urethral sphincter 599.84
valve, valvular (heart) (*see also* Endocarditis) 424.90
vascular 459.9
intestine NEC 557.9
mesenteric 557.1
peripheral 443.9
renal (*see also* Hypertension, kidney) 403.90
velopharyngeal
acquired 528.9
congenital 750.29
venous (peripheral) 459.81
ventricular — *see* Insufficiency, myocardial
vertebral artery 435.1
vertebrobasilar artery 435.3
weight gain during pregnancy 646.8 ☑
zinc 269.3
Insufflation
fallopian
fertility testing V26.21
following sterilization reversal V26.22
meconium 770.11
with respiratory symptoms 770.12
Insular — *see* condition
Insulinoma (M8151/0)
malignant (M8151/3)
pancreas 157.4
specified site — *see* Neoplasm, by site, malignant
unspecified site 157.4
pancreas 211.7
specified site — *see* Neoplasm, by site, benign
unspecified site 211.7
Insuloma — *see* Insulinoma
Insult
brain 437.9
acute 436
cerebral 437.9

Insult — *continued*
cerebral — *continued*
acute 436
cerebrovascular 437.9
acute 436
vascular NEC 437.9
acute 436
Insurance examination (certification) V70.3
Intemperance — *see also* Alcoholism 303.9 ☑
Interception of pregnancy (menstrual extraction) V25.3
Interference
balancing side 524.56
non-working side 524.56
Intermenstrual
bleeding 626.6
irregular 626.6
regular 626.5
hemorrhage 626.6
irregular 626.6
regular 626.5
pain(s) 625.2
Intermittent — *see* condition
Internal — *see* condition
Interproximal wear 521.10
Interrogation
cardiac defibrillator (automatic) (implantable) V53.32
cardiac pacemaker V53.31
cardiac (event) (loop) recorder V53.39
infusion pump (implanted) (intrathecal) V53.09
neurostimulator V53.02
Interruption
aortic arch 747.11
bundle of His 426.50
fallopian tube (for sterilization) V25.2
phase-shift, sleep cycle 307.45
repeated REM-sleep 307.48
sleep
due to perceived environmental disturbances 307.48
phase-shift, of 24-hour sleep-wake cycle 307.45
repeated REM-sleep type 307.48
vas deferens (for sterilization) V25.2
Intersexuality 752.7
Interstitial — *see* condition
Intertrigo 695.89
labialis 528.5
Intervertebral disc — *see* condition
Intestine, intestinal — *see also* condition
flu 487.8
Intolerance
carbohydrate NEC 579.8
cardiovascular exercise, with pain (at rest) (with less than ordinary activity) (with ordinary activity) V47.2
cold 780.99
dissacharide (hereditary) 271.3
drug
correct substance properly administered 995.27
wrong substance given or taken in error 977.9
specified drug — *see* Table of Drugs and Chemicals
effort 306.2
fat NEC 579.8
foods NEC 579.8
fructose (hereditary) 271.2
glucose (-galactose) (congenital) 271.3
gluten 579.0
lactose (hereditary) (infantile) 271.3
lysine (congenital) 270.7
milk NEC 579.8
protein (familial) 270.7
starch NEC 579.8
sucrose (-isomaltose) (congenital) 271.3
Intoxicated NEC — *see also* Alcoholism 305.0 ☑
Intoxication
acid 276.2
acute
alcoholic 305.0 ☑
with alcoholism 303.0 ☑

Intoxication — *continued*
acute — *continued*
alcoholic — *continued*
hangover effects 305.0 ☑
caffeine 305.9 ☑
hallucinogenic (*see also* Abuse, drugs, nondependent) 305.3 ☑
alcohol (acute) 305.0 ☑
with alcoholism 303.0 ☑
hangover effects 305.0 ☑
idiosyncratic 291.4
pathological 291.4
alimentary canal 558.2
ammonia (hepatic) 572.2
caffeine 305.9 ☑
chemical (*see also* Table of Drugs and Chemicals)
via placenta or breast milk 760.70
alcohol 760.71
anticonvulsants
antifungals
anti-infective agents 760.74
antimetabolics
cocaine 760.75
"crack" 760.75
hallucinogenic agents NEC 760.73
medicinal agents NEC 760.79
narcotics 760.72
obstetric anesthetic or analgesic drug 763.5
specified agent NEC 760.79
suspected, affecting management of pregnancy 655.5 ☑
cocaine, through placenta or breast milk 760.75
delirium
alcohol 291.0
drug 292.81
drug 292.89
with delirium 292.81
correct substance properly administered (*see also* Allergy, drug) 995.27
newborn 779.4
obstetric anesthetic or sedation 668.9 ☑
affecting fetus or newborn 763.5
overdose or wrong substance given or taken — *see* Table of Drugs and Chemicals
pathologic 292.2
specific to newborn 779.4
via placenta or breast milk 760.70
alcohol 760.71
anticonvulsants 760.77
antifungals 760.74
anti-infective agents 760.74
antimetabolics 760.78
cocaine 760.75
"crack" 760.75
hallucinogenic agents 760.73
medicinal agents NEC 760.79
narcotics 760.72
obstetric anesthetic or analgesic drug 763.5
specified agent NEC 760.79
suspected, affecting management of pregnancy 655.5 ☑
enteric — *see* Intoxication, intestinal
fetus or newborn, via placenta or breast milk 760.70
alcohol 760.71
anticonvulsants 760.77
antifungals 760.74
anti-infective agents 760.74
antimetabolics 760.78
cocaine 760.75
"crack" 760.75
hallucinogenic agents 760.73
medicinal agents NEC 760.79
narcotics 760.72
obstetric anesthetic or analgesic drug 763.5
specified agent NEC 760.79
suspected, affecting management of pregnancy 655.5 ☑
food — *see* Poisoning, food
gastrointestinal 558.2

☑ Additional Digit Required — Refer to the Tabular List for Digit Selection   ▽ Subterms under main terms may continue to next column or page

Intoxication — *continued*
  hallucinogenic (acute) 305.3 ☑
  hepatocerebral 572.2
  idiosyncratic alcohol 291.4
  intestinal 569.89
    due to putrefaction of food 005.9
  methyl alcohol (*see also* Alcoholism)
      305.0 ☑
    with alcoholism 303.0 ☑
  non-foodborne due to toxins of Clostridium
      botulinum [C. botulinum] — *see* Botulism
  pathologic 291.4
    drug 292.2
  potassium (K) 276.7
  septic
    with
      abortion — *see* Abortion, by type,
          with sepsis
      ectopic pregnancy (*see also* categories 633.0–633.9) 639.0
      molar pregnancy (*see also* categories 630–632) 639.0
    during labor 659.3 ☑
    following
      abortion 639.0
      ectopic or molar pregnancy 639.0
    generalized — *see* Septicemia
    puerperal, postpartum, childbirth 670.2 ☑
  serum (prophylactic) (therapeutic) 999.59
  uremic — *see* Uremia
  water 276.69
Intracranial — *see* condition
Intrahepatic gallbladder 751.69
Intraligamentous — *see also* condition
  pregnancy — *see* Pregnancy, cornual
Intraocular — *see also* condition
  sepsis 360.00
Intrathoracic — *see also* condition
  kidney 753.3
  stomach — *see* Hernia, diaphragm
Intrauterine contraceptive device
  checking V25.42
  insertion V25.11
  in situ V45.51
  management V25.42
  prescription V25.02
    repeat V25.42
  reinsertion V25.13
  removal V25.12
    and reinsertion V25.13
  replacement V25.13
Intraventricular — *see* condition
Intrinsic deformity — *see* Deformity
Intruded tooth 524.34
Intrusion, repetitive, of sleep (due to environmental disturbances) (with atypical polysomnographic features) 307.48
Intumescent, lens (eye) NEC 366.9
  senile 366.12
Intussusception (colon) (enteric) (intestine) (rectum) 560.0
  appendix 543.9
  congenital 751.5
  fallopian tube 620.8
  ileocecal 560.0
  ileocolic 560.0
  ureter (with obstruction) 593.4
Invagination
  basilar 756.0
  colon or intestine 560.0
Invalid (since birth) 799.89
Invalidism (chronic) 799.89
Inversion
  albumin-globulin (A-G) ratio 273.8
  bladder 596.89
  cecum (*see also* Intussusception) 560.0
  cervix 622.8
  nipple 611.79
    congenital 757.6
    puerperal, postpartum 676.3 ☑
  optic papilla 743.57
  organ or site, congenital NEC — *see* Anomaly, specified type NEC
  sleep rhythm 327.39

Inversion — *continued*
  sleep rhythm — *continued*
    nonorganic origin 307.45
  testis (congenital) 752.51
  uterus (postinfectional) (postpartal, old) 621.7
    chronic 621.7
    complicating delivery 665.2 ☑
      affecting fetus or newborn 763.89
  vagina — *see* Prolapse, vagina
Investigation
  allergens V72.7
  clinical research (control) (normal comparison) (participant) V70.7
Inviability — *see* Immaturity
Involuntary movement, abnormal 781.0
Involution, involutional — *see also* condition
  breast, cystic or fibrocystic 610.1
  depression (*see also* Psychosis, affective) 296.2 ☑
    recurrent episode 296.3 ☑
    single episode 296.2 ☑
  melancholia (*see also* Psychosis, affective) 296.2 ☑
    recurrent episode 296.3 ☑
    single episode 296.2 ☑
  ovary, senile 620.3
  paranoid state (reaction) 297.2
  paraphrenia (climacteric) (menopause) 297.2
  psychosis 298.8
  thymus failure 254.8
IQ
  under 20 318.2
  20-34 318.1
  35-49 318.0
  50-70 317
IRDS 769
Irideremia 743.45
Iridis rubeosis 364.42
  diabetic 250.5 ☑ [364.42]
    due to secondary diabetes 249.5 ☑ [364.42]
Iridochoroiditis (panuveitis) 360.12
Iridocyclitis NEC 364.3
  acute 364.00
    primary 364.01
    recurrent 364.02
  chronic 364.10
    in
      lepromatous leprosy 030.0 [364.11]
      sarcoidosis 135 [364.11]
      tuberculosis (*see also* Tuberculosis) 017.3 ☑ [364.11]
  due to allergy 364.04
  endogenous 364.01
  gonococcal 098.41
  granulomatous 364.10
  herpetic (simplex) 054.44
    zoster 053.22
  hypopyon 364.05
  lens induced 364.23
  nongranulomatous 364.00
  primary 364.01
  recurrent 364.02
  rheumatic 364.10
  secondary 364.04
    infectious 364.03
    noninfectious 364.04
  subacute 364.00
    primary 364.01
    recurrent 364.02
  sympathetic 360.11
  syphilitic (secondary) 091.52
  tuberculous (chronic) (*see also* Tuberculosis) 017.3 ☑ [364.11]
Iridocyclochoroiditis (panuveitis) 360.12
Iridodialysis 364.76
Iridodonesis 364.89
Iridoplegia (complete) (partial) (reflex) 379.49
Iridoschisis 364.52
IRIS (Immune Reconstitution Inflammatory Syndrome) 995.90
Iris — *see* condition
Iritis 364.3
  acute 364.00

Iritis — *continued*
  acute — *continued*
    primary 364.01
    recurrent 364.02
  chronic 364.10
    in
      sarcoidosis 135 [364.11]
      tuberculosis (*see also* Tuberculosis) 017.3 ☑ [364.11]
  diabetic 250.5 ☑ [364.42]
    due to secondary diabetes 249.5 ☑ [364.42]
  due to
    allergy 364.04
    herpes simplex 054.44
    leprosy 030.0 [364.11]
  endogenous 364.01
  gonococcal 098.41
  gouty 274.89 [364.11]
  granulomatous 364.10
  hypopyon 364.05
  lens induced 364.23
  nongranulomatous 364.00
  papulosa 095.8 [364.11]
  primary 364.01
  recurrent 364.02
  rheumatic 364.10
  secondary 364.04
    infectious 364.03
    noninfectious 364.04
  subacute 364.00
    primary 364.01
    recurrent 364.02
  sympathetic 360.11
  syphilitic (secondary) 091.52
    congenital 090.0 [364.11]
    late 095.8 [364.11]
  tuberculous (*see also* Tuberculosis) 017.3 ☑ [364.11]
  uratic 274.89 [364.11]
Iron
  deficiency anemia 280.9
  metabolism disease 275.09
  storage disease 275.09
Iron-miners' lung 503
Irradiated enamel (tooth, teeth) 521.89
Irradiation
  burn — *see* Burn, by site
  effects, adverse 990
Irreducible, irreducibility — *see* condition
Irregular, irregularity
  action, heart 427.9
  alveolar process 525.8
  bleeding NEC 626.4
  breathing 786.09
  colon 569.89
  contour
    acquired 371.70
    of cornea 743.41
      acquired 371.70
    reconstructed breast 612.0
  dentin in pulp 522.3
  eye movements NEC 379.59
  menstruation (cause unknown) 626.4
  periods 626.4
  prostate 602.9
  pupil 364.75
  respiratory 786.09
  septum (nasal) 470
  shape, organ or site, congenital NEC — *see* Distortion
  sleep-wake rhythm (non-24-hour) 327.39
    nonorganic origin 307.45
  vertebra 733.99
Irritability 799.22
  bladder 596.89
    neurogenic 596.54
      with cauda equina syndrome 344.61
  bowel (syndrome) 564.1
  bronchial (*see also* Bronchitis) 490
  cerebral, newborn 779.1
  colon 564.1
    psychogenic 306.4
  duodenum 564.89
  heart (psychogenic) 306.2
  ileum 564.89

Irritability — *continued*
  jejunum 564.89
  myocardium 306.2
  nervousness 799.21
  rectum 564.89
  stomach 536.9
    psychogenic 306.4
  sympathetic (nervous system) (*see also* Neuropathy, peripheral, autonomic) 337.9
  urethra 599.84
  ventricular (heart) (psychogenic) 306.2
Irritable — *see also* Irritability 799.22
Irritation
  anus 569.49
  axillary nerve 353.0
  bladder 596.89
  brachial plexus 353.0
  brain (traumatic) (*see also* Injury, intracranial) 854.0 ☑
    nontraumatic — *see* Encephalitis
  bronchial (*see also* Bronchitis) 490
  cerebral (traumatic) (*see also* Injury, intracranial) 854.0 ☑
    nontraumatic — *see* Encephalitis
  cervical plexus 353.2
  cervix (*see also* Cervicitis) 616.0
  choroid, sympathetic 360.11
  cranial nerve — *see* Disorder, nerve, cranial
  digestive tract 536.9
    psychogenic 306.4
  gastric 536.9
    psychogenic 306.4
  gastrointestinal (tract) 536.9
    functional 536.9
    psychogenic 306.4
  globe, sympathetic 360.11
  intestinal (bowel) 564.9
  labyrinth 386.50
  lumbosacral plexus 353.1
  meninges (traumatic) (*see also* Injury, intracranial) 854.0 ☑
    nontraumatic — *see* Meningitis
  myocardium 306.2
  nerve — *see* Disorder, nerve
  nervous 799.21
  nose 478.19
  penis 607.89
  perineum 709.9
  peripheral
    autonomic nervous system (*see also* Neuropathy, peripheral, autonomic) 337.9
    nerve — *see* Disorder, nerve
  peritoneum (*see also* Peritonitis) 567.9
  pharynx 478.29
  plantar nerve 355.6
  spinal (cord) (traumatic) (*see also* Injury, spinal, by site)
    nerve (*see also* Disorder, nerve)
      root NEC 724.9
      traumatic — *see* Injury, nerve, spinal
    nontraumatic — *see* Myelitis
  stomach 536.9
    psychogenic 306.4
  sympathetic nerve NEC (*see also* Neuropathy, peripheral, autonomic) 337.9
  ulnar nerve 354.2
  vagina 623.9
Isambert's disease 012.3 ☑
Ischemia, ischemic 459.9
  basilar artery (with transient neurologic deficit) 435.0
  bone NEC 733.40
  bowel (transient) 557.9
    acute 557.0
    chronic 557.1
    due to mesenteric artery insufficiency 557.1
  brain (*see also* Ischemia, cerebral)
    recurrent focal 435.9
  cardiac (*see also* Ischemia, heart) 414.9
  cardiomyopathy 414.8
  carotid artery (with transient neurologic deficit) 435.8
  cerebral (chronic) (generalized) 437.1

Ischemia, ischemic — *continued*
  cerebral — *continued*
    arteriosclerotic 437.0
      intermittent (with transient neurologic
          deficit) 435.9
      newborn 779.2
      puerperal, postpartum, childbirth
          674.0 ☑
      recurrent focal (with transient neurologic
          deficit) 435.9
      transient (with transient neurologic
          deficit) 435.9
  colon 557.9
    acute 557.0
    chronic 557.1
    due to mesenteric artery insufficiency
        557.1
  coronary (chronic) (*see also* Ischemia, heart)
      414.9
  demand 411.89
  heart (chronic or with a stated duration of
      over 8 weeks) 414.9
    acute or with a stated duration of 8
        weeks or less (*see also* Infarct,
        myocardium) 410.9 ☑
      without myocardial infarction 411.89
        with coronary (artery) occlusion
            411.81
    subacute 411.89
  intestine (transient) 557.9
    acute 557.0
    chronic 557.1
    due to mesenteric artery insufficiency
        557.1
  kidney 593.81
  labyrinth 386.50

Ischemia, ischemic — *continued*
  muscles, leg 728.89
  myocardium, myocardial (chronic or with a
      stated duration of over 8 weeks)
      414.8
    acute (*see also* Infarct, myocardium)
        410.9 ☑
      without myocardial infarction 411.89
        with coronary (artery) occlusion
            411.81
  renal 593.81
  retina, retinal 362.84
  small bowel 557.9
    acute 557.0
    chronic 557.1
    due to mesenteric artery insufficiency
        557.1
  spinal cord 336.1
  subendocardial (*see also* Insufficiency,
      coronary) 411.89
  supply (*see also* Angina) 414.9
  vertebral artery (with transient neurologic
      deficit) 435.1
Ischialgia — *see also* Sciatica 724.3
Ischiopagus 759.4
Ischium, ischial — *see* condition
Ischomenia 626.8
Ischuria 788.5
Iselin's disease or osteochondrosis 732.5
Islands of
  parotid tissue in
    lymph nodes 750.26
    neck structures 750.26
  submaxillary glands in
    fascia 750.26
    lymph nodes 750.26

Islands of — *continued*
  submaxillary glands in — *continued*
    neck muscles 750.26
Islet cell tumor, pancreas (M8150/0) 211.7
Isoimmunization NEC — *see also* Incompati-
      bility 656.2 ☑
  anti-E 656.2 ☑
  fetus or newborn 773.2
    ABO blood groups 773.1
    Rhesus (Rh) factor 773.0
Isolation V07.0
  social V62.4
Isosporosis 007.2
Issue
  medical certificate NEC V68.09
    cause of death V68.09
    disability examination V68.01
    fitness V68.09
    incapacity V68.09
  repeat prescription NEC V68.1
    appliance V68.1
    contraceptive V25.40
      device NEC V25.49
        intrauterine V25.42
        specified type NEC V25.49
      pill V25.41
    glasses V68.1
    medicinal substance V68.1
Itch — *see also* Pruritus 698.9
  bakers' 692.89
  barbers' 110.0
  bricklayers' 692.89
  cheese 133.8
  clam diggers' 120.3
  coolie 126.9
  copra 133.8

Itch — *see also* Pruritus — *continued*
  Cuban 050.1
  dew 126.9
  dhobie 110.3
  eye 379.99
  filarial (*see also* Infestation, filarial) 125.9
  grain 133.8
  grocers' 133.8
  ground 126.9
  harvest 133.8
  jock 110.3
  Malabar 110.9
    beard 110.0
    foot 110.4
    scalp 110.0
  meaning scabies 133.0
  Norwegian 133.0
  perianal 698.0
  poultrymen's 133.8
  sarcoptic 133.0
  scrub 134.1
  seven year V61.10
    meaning scabies 133.0
  straw 133.8
  swimmers' 120.3
  washerwoman's 692.4
  water 120.3
  winter 698.8
Itsenko-Cushing syndrome (pituitary ba-
      sophilism) 255.0
Ivemark's syndrome (asplenia with congenital
      heart disease) 759.0
Ivory bones 756.52
Ixodes 134.8
Ixodiasis 134.8

☑ **Additional Digit Required — Refer to the Tabular List for Digit Selection**   ⩊ **Subterms under main terms may continue to next column or page**

J

Jaccoud's nodular fibrositis, chronic (Jaccoud's syndrome) 714.4
Jackson's
  membrane 751.4
  paralysis or syndrome 344.89
  veil 751.4
Jacksonian
  epilepsy (*see also* Epilepsy) 345.5 ☑
  seizures (focal) (*see also* Epilepsy) 345.5 ☑
Jacob's ulcer (M8090/3) — *see* Neoplasm, skin, malignant, by site
Jacquet's dermatitis (diaper dermatitis) 691.0
Jadassohn's
  blue nevus (M8780/0) — *see* Neoplasm, skin, benign
  disease (maculopapular erythroderma) 696.2
  intraepidermal epithelioma (M8096/0) — *see* Neoplasm, skin, benign
Jadassohn-Lewandowski syndrome (pachyonychia congenita) 757.5
Jadassohn-Pellizari's disease (anetoderma) 701.3
Jadassohn-Tièche nevus (M8780/0) — *see* Neoplasm, skin, benign
Jaffe-Lichtenstein (-Uehlinger) syndrome 252.01
Jahnke's syndrome (encephalocutaneous angiomatosis) 759.6
Jakob-Creutzfeldt disease (CJD) (syndrome) 046.19
  with dementia
    with behavioral disturbance 046.19 [294.11]
    without behavioral disturbance 046.19 [294.10]
  familial 046.19
  iatrogenic 046.19
  specified NEC 046.19
  sporadic 046.19
  variant (vCJD) 046.11
    with dementia
      with behavioral disturbance 046.11 [294.11]
      without behavioral disturbance 046.11 [294.10]
Jaksch (-Luzet) disease or syndrome (pseudoleukemia infantum) 285.8
Jamaican
  neuropathy 349.82
  paraplegic tropical ataxic-spastic syndrome 349.82
Janet's disease (psychasthenia) 300.89
Janiceps 759.4
Jansky-Bielschowsky amaurotic familial idiocy 330.1
Japanese
  B type encephalitis 062.0
  river fever 081.2
  seven-day fever 100.89
Jaundice (yellow) 782.4
  acholuric (familial) (splenomegalic) (*see also* Spherocytosis) 282.0
    acquired 283.9
  breast milk 774.39
  catarrhal (acute) 070.1
    with hepatic coma 070.0
    chronic 571.9
    epidemic — *see* Jaundice, epidemic
  cholestatic (benign) 782.4
  chronic idiopathic 277.4
  epidemic (catarrhal) 070.1
    with hepatic coma 070.0
    leptospiral 100.0
    spirochetal 100.0
  febrile (acute) 070.1
    with hepatic coma 070.0
    leptospiral 100.0
    spirochetal 100.0
  fetus or newborn 774.6
    due to or associated with
      ABO
        absence or deficiency of enzyme system for bilirubin conjugation (congenital) 774.39

Jaundice — *continued*
  fetus or newborn — *continued*
    due to or associated with — *continued*
      antibodies 773.1
      blood group incompatibility NEC 773.2
      breast milk inhibitors to conjugation 774.39
        associated with preterm delivery 774.2
      bruising 774.1
      Crigler-Najjar syndrome 277.4 [774.31]
      delayed conjugation 774.30
        associated with preterm delivery 774.2
      development 774.39
      drugs or toxins transmitted from mother 774.1
      G-6-PD deficiency 282.2 [774.0]
      galactosemia 271.1 [774.5]
      Gilbert's syndrome 277.4 [774.31]
      hepatocellular damage 774.4
      hereditary hemolytic anemia (*see also* Anemia, hemolytic) 282.9 [774.0]
      hypothyroidism, congenital 243 [774.31]
      incompatibility, maternal/fetal NEC 773.2
      incompatibility, maternal/fetal 773.2
      infection 774.1
      inspissated bile syndrome 774.4
      isoimmunization NEC 773.2
      isoimmunization 773.1
      mucoviscidosis 277.01 [774.5]
      obliteration of bile duct, congenital 751.61 [774.5]
      polycythemia 774.1
      preterm delivery 774.2
      red cell defect 282.9 [774.0]
      Rh
        antibodies 773.0
        incompatibility, maternal/fetal 773.0
        isoimmunization 773.0
      spherocytosis (congenital) 282.0 [774.0]
      swallowed maternal blood 774.1
    physiological NEC 774.6
  from injection, inoculation, infusion, or transfusion (blood) (plasma) (serum) (other substance) (onset within 8 months after administration) — *see* Hepatitis, viral
  Gilbert's (familial nonhemolytic) 277.4
  hematogenous 283.9
  hemolytic (acquired) 283.9
    congenital (*see also* Spherocytosis) 282.0
  hemorrhagic (acute) 100.0
    leptospiral 100.0
    newborn 776.0
    spirochetal 100.0
  hepatocellular 573.8
  homologous (serum) — *see* Hepatitis, viral
  idiopathic, chronic 277.4
  infectious (acute) (subacute) 070.1
    with hepatic coma 070.0
    leptospiral 100.0
    spirochetal 100.0
  leptospiral 100.0
  malignant (*see also* Necrosis, liver) 570
  newborn (physiological) (*see also* Jaundice, fetus or newborn) 774.6
  nonhemolytic, congenital familial (Gilbert's) 277.4
  nuclear, newborn (*see also* Kernicterus of newborn) 774.7
  obstructive NEC (*see also* Obstruction, biliary) 576.8
  postimmunization — *see* Hepatitis, viral
  posttransfusion — *see* Hepatitis, viral
  regurgitation (*see also* Obstruction, biliary) 576.8

Jaundice — *continued*
  serum (homologous) (prophylactic) (therapeutic) — *see* Hepatitis, viral
  spirochetal (hemorrhagic) 100.0
  symptomatic 782.4
    newborn 774.6
Jaw — *see* condition
Jaw-blinking 374.43
  congenital 742.8
Jaw-winking phenomenon or syndrome 742.8
Jealousy
  alcoholic 291.5
  childhood 313.3
  sibling 313.3
Jejunitis — *see also* Enteritis 558.9
Jejunostomy status V44.4
Jejunum, jejunal — *see* condition
Jensen's disease 363.05
Jericho boil 085.1
Jerks, myoclonic 333.2
Jervell-Lange-Nielsen syndrome 426.82
Jeune's disease or syndrome (asphyxiating thoracic dystrophy) 756.4
Jigger disease 134.1
Job's syndrome (chronic granulomatous disease) 288.1
Jod-Basedow phenomenon 242.8 ☑
Johnson-Stevens disease (erythema multiforme exudativum) 695.13
Joint — *see also* condition
  Charcôt's 094.0 [713.5]
  false 733.82
  flail — *see* Flail, joint
  mice — *see* Loose, body, joint, by site
  sinus to bone 730.9 ☑
  von Gies' 095.8
Jordan's anomaly or syndrome 288.2
Josephs-Diamond-Blackfan anemia (congenital hypoplastic) 284.01
Joubert syndrome 759.89
Jumpers' knee 727.2
Jungle yellow fever 060.0
Jüngling's disease (sarcoidosis) 135
Junin virus hemorrhagic fever 078.7
Juvenile — *see also* condition
  delinquent 312.9
    group (*see also* Disturbance, conduct) 312.2 ☑
    neurotic 312.4

K

Kabuki syndrome 759.89
Kahler (-Bozzolo) disease (multiple myeloma) (M9730/3) 203.0 ☑
Kakergasia 300.9
Kakke 265.0
Kala-azar (Indian) (infantile) (Mediterranean) (Sudanese) 085.0
Kalischer's syndrome (encephalocutaneous angiomatosis) 759.6
Kallmann's syndrome (hypogonadotropic hypogonadism with anosmia) 253.4
Kanner's syndrome (autism) — *see also* Psychosis, childhood 299.0 ☑
Kaolinosis 502
Kaposi's
  disease 757.33
    lichen ruber 696.4
      acuminatus 696.4
      moniliformis 697.8
    xeroderma pigmentosum 757.33
  sarcoma (M9140/3) 176.9
    adipose tissue 176.1
    aponeurosis 176.1
    artery 176.1
    associated herpesvirus infection 058.89
    blood vessel 176.1
    bursa 176.1
    connective tissue 176.1
    external genitalia 176.8
    fascia 176.1
    fatty tissue 176.1
    fibrous tissue 176.1
    gastrointestinal tract NEC 176.3
    ligament 176.1

Kaposi's — *continued*
  sarcoma — *continued*
    lung 176.4
    lymph
      gland(s) 176.5
      node(s) 176.5
    lymphatic(s) NEC 176.1
    muscle (skeletal) 176.1
    oral cavity NEC 176.8
    palate 176.2
    scrotum 176.8
    skin 176.0
    soft tissue 176.1
    specified site NEC 176.8
    subcutaneous tissue 176.1
    synovia 176.1
    tendon (sheath) 176.1
    vein 176.1
    vessel 176.1
    viscera NEC 176.9
    vulva 176.8
  varicelliform eruption 054.0
    vaccinia 999.0
Kartagener's syndrome or triad (sinusitis, bronchiectasis, situs inversus) 759.3
Kasabach-Merritt syndrome (capillary hemangioma associated with thrombocytopenic purpura) 287.39
Kaschin-Beck disease (endemic polyarthritis) — *see* Disease, Kaschin-Beck
Kast's syndrome (dyschondroplasia with hemangiomas) 756.4
Katatonia — *see* Catatonia
Katayama disease or fever 120.2
Kathisophobia 781.0
Kawasaki disease 446.1
Kayser-Fleischer ring (cornea) (pseudosclerosis) 275.1 [371.14]
Kaznelson's syndrome (congenital hypoplastic anemia) 284.01
Kearns-Sayre syndrome 277.87
Kedani fever 081.2
Kelis 701.4
Kelly (-Patterson) syndrome (sideropenic dysphagia) 280.8
Keloid, cheloid 701.4
  Addison's (morphea) 701.0
  cornea 371.00
  Hawkins' 701.4
  scar 701.4
Keloma 701.4
Kenya fever 082.1
Keratectasia 371.71
  congenital 743.41
Keratinization NEC
  alveolar ridge mucosa
    excessive 528.72
    minimal 528.71
Keratitis (nodular) (nonulcerative) (simple) (zonular) NEC 370.9
  with ulceration (*see also* Ulcer, cornea) 370.00
  actinic 370.24
  arborescens 054.42
  areolar 370.22
  bullosa 370.8
  deep — *see* Keratitis, interstitial
  dendritic(a) 054.42
  desiccation 370.34
  diffuse interstitial 370.52
  disciform(is) 054.43
    varicella 052.7 [370.44]
  epithelialis vernalis 372.13 [370.32]
  exposure 370.34
  filamentary 370.23
  gonococcal (congenital) (prenatal) 098.43
  herpes, herpetic (simplex) NEC 054.43
    zoster 053.21
  hypopyon 370.04
  in
    chickenpox 052.7 [370.44]
    exanthema (*see also* Exanthem) 057.9 [370.44]
    paravaccinia (*see also* Paravaccinia) 051.9 [370.44]

☑ Additional Digit Required — Refer to the Tabular List for Digit Selection   🔖 Subterms under main terms may continue to next column or page

2013 ICD-9-CM   ►◄ Revised Text   ● New Line   ▲ Revised Code   Volume 2 — 169

Keratitis — *continued*
  in — *continued*
    smallpox (*see also* Smallpox)
      050.9 *[370.44]*
      vernal conjunctivitis 372.13 *[370.32]*
    interstitial (nonsyphilitic) 370.50
      with ulcer (*see also* Ulcer, cornea) 370.00
      diffuse 370.52
      herpes, herpetic (simplex) 054.43
        zoster 053.21
      syphilitic (congenital) (hereditary) 090.3
      tuberculous (*see also* Tuberculosis)
        017.3 ☑ *[370.59]*
    lagophthalmic 370.34
    macular 370.22
    neuroparalytic 370.35
    neurotrophic 370.35
    nummular 370.22
    oyster-shuckers' 370.8
    parenchymatous — *see* Keratitis, interstitial
    petrificans 370.8
    phlyctenular 370.31
    postmeasles 055.71
    punctata, punctate 370.21
      leprosa 030.0 *[370.21]*
      profunda 090.3
      superficial (Thygeson's) 370.21
    purulent 370.8
    pustuliformis profunda 090.3
    rosacea 695.3 *[370.49]*
    sclerosing 370.54
    specified type NEC 370.8
    stellate 370.22
    striate 370.22
    superficial 370.20
      with conjunctivitis (*see also* Keratoconjunctivitis) 370.40
      punctate (Thygeson's) 370.21
    suppurative 370.8
    syphilitic (congenital) (prenatal) 090.3
    trachomatous 076.1
      late effect 139.1
    tuberculous (phlyctenular) (*see also* Tuberculosis) 017.3 ☑ *[370.31]*
    ulcerated (*see also* Ulcer, cornea) 370.00
    vesicular 370.8
    welders' 370.24
    xerotic (*see also* Keratomalacia) 371.45
      vitamin A deficiency 264.4
Keratoacanthoma 238.2
Keratocele 371.72
Keratoconjunctivitis — *see also* Keratitis 370.40
  adenovirus type 8 077.1
  epidemic 077.1
  exposure 370.34
  gonococcal 098.43
  herpetic (simplex) 054.43
    zoster 053.21
  in
    chickenpox 052.7 *[370.44]*
    exanthema (*see also* Exanthem) 057.9 *[370.44]*
    paravaccinia (*see also* Paravaccinia) 051.9 *[370.44]*
    smallpox (*see also* Smallpox) 050.9 *[370.44]*
  infectious 077.1
  neurotrophic 370.35
  phlyctenular 370.31
  postmeasles 055.71
  shipyard 077.1
  sicca (Sjögren's syndrome) 710.2
    not in Sjögren's syndrome 370.33
  specified type NEC 370.49
  tuberculous (phlyctenular) (*see also* Tuberculosis) 017.3 ☑ *[370.31]*
Keratoconus 371.60
  acute hydrops 371.62
  congenital 743.41
  stable 371.61
Keratocyst (dental) 526.0
Keratoderma, keratodermia (congenital) (palmaris et plantaris) (symmetrical) 757.39
  acquired 701.1

Keratoderma, keratodermia — *continued*
  blennorrhagica 701.1
    gonococcal 098.81
  climacterium 701.1
  eccentrica 757.39
  gonorrheal 098.81
  punctata 701.1
  tylodes, progressive 701.1
Keratodermatocele 371.72
Keratoglobus 371.70
  congenital 743.41
    associated with buphthalmos 743.22
Keratohemia 371.12
Keratoiritis — *see also* Iridocyclitis 364.3
  syphilitic 090.3
  tuberculous (*see also* Tuberculosis) 017.3 ☑ *[364.11]*
Keratolysis exfoliativa (congenital) 757.39
  acquired 695.89
  neonatorum 757.39
Keratoma 701.1
  congenital 757.39
  malignum congenitale 757.1
  palmaris et plantaris hereditarium 757.39
  senile 702.0
Keratomalacia 371.45
  vitamin A deficiency 264.4
Keratomegaly 743.41
Keratomycosis 111.1
  nigricans (palmaris) 111.1
Keratopathy 371.40
  band (*see also* Keratitis) 371.43
  bullous (*see also* Keratitis) 371.23
  degenerative (*see also* Degeneration, cornea) 371.40
    hereditary (*see also* Dystrophy, cornea) 371.50
  discrete colliquative 371.49
Keratoscleritis, tuberculous — *see also* Tuberculosis 017.3 ☑ *[370.31]*
Keratosis 701.1
  actinic 702.0
  arsenical 692.4
  blennorrhagica 701.1
    gonococcal 098.81
  congenital (any type) 757.39
  ear (middle) (*see also* Cholesteatoma) 385.30
  female genital (external) 629.89
  follicularis 757.39
    acquired 701.1
    congenital (acneiformis) (Siemens') 757.39
    spinulosa (decalvans) 757.39
    vitamin A deficiency 264.8
  follicular, vitamin A deficiency 264.8
  gonococcal 098.81
  larynx, laryngeal 478.79
  male genital (external) 608.89
  middle ear (*see also* Cholesteatoma) 385.30
  nigricans 701.2
    congenital 757.39
  obturans 380.21
  oral epithelium
    residual ridge mucosa
      excessive 528.72
      minimal 528.71
  palmaris et plantaris (symmetrical) 757.39
  penile 607.89
  pharyngeus 478.29
  pilaris 757.39
    acquired 701.1
    punctata (palmaris et plantaris) 701.1
  scrotal 608.89
  seborrheic 702.19
    inflamed 702.11
  senilis 702.0
  solar 702.0
  suprafollicularis 757.39
  tonsillaris 478.29
  vagina 623.1
  vegetans 757.39
  vitamin A deficiency 264.8
Kerato-uveitis — *see also* Iridocyclitis 364.3
Keraunoparalysis 994.0
Kerion (celsi) 110.0

Kernicterus of newborn (not due to isoimmunization) 774.7
  due to isoimmunization (conditions classifiable to 773.0–773.2) 773.4
Ketoacidosis 276.2
  diabetic 250.1 ☑
    due to secondary diabetes 249.1 ☑
Ketonuria 791.6
  branched-chain, intermittent 270.3
Ketosis 276.2
  diabetic 250.1 ☑
    due to secondary diabetes 249.1 ☑
Kidney — *see* condition
Kienböck's
  disease 732.3
    adult 732.8
  osteochondrosis 732.3
Kimmelstiel (-Wilson) disease or syndrome (intercapillary glomerulosclerosis) 250.4 ☑ *[581.81]*
  due to secondary diabetes 249.4 ☑ *[581.81]*
Kink, kinking
  appendix 543.9
  artery 447.1
  cystic duct, congenital 751.61
  hair (acquired) 704.2
  ileum or intestine (*see also* Obstruction, intestine) 560.9
  Lane's (*see also* Obstruction, intestine) 560.9
  organ or site, congenital NEC — *see* Anomaly, specified type NEC, by site
  ureter (pelvic junction) 593.3
    congenital 753.20
  vein(s) 459.2
    caval 459.2
    peripheral 459.2
Kinnier Wilson's disease (hepatolenticular degeneration) 275.1
Kissing
  osteophytes 721.5
  spine 721.5
  vertebra 721.5
Klauder's syndrome (erythema multiforme, exudativum) 695.19
Klebs' disease — *see also* Nephritis 583.9
Kleine-Levin syndrome 327.13
Klein-Waardenburg syndrome (ptosisepicanthus) 270.2
Kleptomania 312.32
Klinefelter's syndrome 758.7
Klinger's disease 446.4
Klippel's disease 723.8
Klippel-Feil disease or syndrome (brevicollis) 756.16
Klippel-Trenaunay syndrome 759.89
Klumpke (-Déjérine) palsy, paralysis (birth) (newborn) 767.6
Klüver-Bucy (-Terzian) syndrome 310.0
Knee — *see* condition
Knifegrinders' rot — *see also* Tuberculosis 011.4 ☑
Knock-knee (acquired) 736.41
  congenital 755.64
Knot
  intestinal, syndrome (volvulus) 560.2
  umbilical cord (true) 663.2 ☑
    affecting fetus or newborn 762.5
Knots, surfer 919.8
  infected 919.9
Knotting (of)
  hair 704.2
  intestine 560.2
Knuckle pads (Garrod's) 728.79
Köbner's disease (epidermolysis bullosa) 757.39
Koch's
  infection (*see also* Tuberculosis, pulmonary) 011.9 ☑
  relapsing fever 087.9
Koch-Weeks conjunctivitis 372.03
Koenig-Wichman disease (pemphigus) 694.4
Köhler's disease (osteochondrosis) 732.5
  first (osteochondrosis juvenilis) 732.5
  second (Freiburg's infarction, metatarsal head) 732.5
  patellar 732.4

Köhler's disease — *continued*
  tarsal navicular (bone) (osteoarthrosis juvenilis) 732.5
Köhler-Mouchet disease (osteoarthrosis juvenilis) 732.5
Köhler-Pellegrini-Stieda disease or syndrome (calcification, knee joint) 726.62
Koilonychia 703.8
  congenital 757.5
Kojevnikov's, Kojewnikoff's epilepsy — *see also* Epilepsy 345.7 ☑
König's
  disease (osteochondritis dissecans) 732.7
  syndrome 564.89
Koniophthisis — *see also* Tuberculosis 011.4 ☑
Koplik's spots 055.9
Kopp's asthma 254.8
Korean hemorrhagic fever 078.6
Korsakoff (-Wernicke) disease, psychosis, or syndrome (nonalcoholic) 294.0
  alcoholic 291.1
Korsakov's disease — *see* Korsakoff's disease
Korsakow's disease — *see* Korsakoff's disease
Kostmann's disease or syndrome (infantile genetic agranulocytosis) 288.01
Krabbe's
  disease (leukodystrophy) 330.0
  syndrome
    congenital muscle hypoplasia 756.89
    cutaneocerebral angioma 759.6
Kraepelin-Morel disease — *see also* Schizophrenia 295.9 ☑
Kraft-Weber-Dimitri disease 759.6
Kraurosis
  ani 569.49
  penis 607.0
  vagina 623.8
  vulva 624.09
Kreotoxism 005.9
Krukenberg's
  spindle 371.13
  tumor (M8490/6) 198.6
Kufs' disease 330.1
Kugelberg-Welander disease 335.11
Kuhnt-Junius degeneration or disease 362.52
Kulchitsky's cell carcinoma (carcinoid tumor of intestine) 259.2
Kümmell's disease or spondylitis 721.7
Kundrat's disease (lymphosarcoma) 200.1 ☑
Kunekune — *see* Dermatophytosis
Kunkel syndrome (lupoid hepatitis) 571.49
Kupffer cell sarcoma (M9124/3) 155.0
Kuru 046.0
Kussmaul's
  coma (diabetic) 250.3 ☑
    due to secondary diabetes 249.3 ☑
  disease (polyarteritis nodosa) 446.0
  respiration (air hunger) 786.09
Kwashiorkor (marasmus type) 260
Kyasanur Forest disease 065.2
Kyphoscoliosis, kyphoscoliotic (acquired) — *see also* Scoliosis 737.30
  congenital 756.19
  due to radiation 737.33
  heart (disease) 416.1
  idiopathic 737.30
  infantile
    progressive 737.32
    resolving 737.31
  late effect of rickets 268.1 *[737.43]*
  specified NEC 737.39
  thoracogenic 737.34
  tuberculous (*see also* Tuberculosis) 015.0 ☑ *[737.43]*
Kyphosis, kyphotic (acquired) (postural) 737.10
  adolescent postural 737.0
  congenital 756.19
  dorsalis juvenilis 732.0
  due to or associated with
    Charcôt-Marie-Tooth disease 356.1 *[737.41]*
    mucopolysaccharidosis 277.5 *[737.41]*
    neurofibromatosis 237.71 *[737.41]*

☑ Additional Digit Required — Refer to the Tabular List for Digit Selection · Subterms under main terms may continue to next column or page

170 — Volume 2 · ►◄ Revised Text · ● New Line · ▲ Revised Code · 2013 ICD-9-CM

Kyphosis, kyphotic — *continued*
due to or associated with — *continued*
osteitis
deformans 731.0 [737.41]
fibrosa cystica 252.01 [737.41]
osteoporosis (*see also* Osteoporosis)
733.0 ✓ [737.41]
poliomyelitis (*see also* Poliomyelitis)
138 [737.41]
radiation 737.11
tuberculosis (*see also* Tuberculosis)
015.0 ✓ [737.41]
Kümmell's 721.7
late effect of rickets 268.1 [737.41]
Morquio-Brailsford type (spinal)
277.5 [737.41]
pelvis 738.6
postlaminectomy 737.12
specified cause NEC 737.19
syphilitic, congenital 090.5 [737.41]
tuberculous (*see also* Tuberculous)
015.0 ✓ [737.41]
Kyrle's disease (hyperkeratosis follicularis in cutem penetrans) 701.1

L

Labia, labium — *see* condition
Labiated hymen 752.49
Labile
blood pressure 796.2
emotions, emotionality 301.3
vasomotor system 443.9
Lability, emotional 799.24
Labioglossal paralysis 335.22
Labium leporinum — *see also* Cleft, lip 749.10
Labor — *see also* Delivery
with complications — *see* Delivery, complicated
abnormal NEC 661.9 ✓
affecting fetus or newborn 763.7
arrested active phase 661.1 ✓
affecting fetus or newborn 763.7
desultory 661.2 ✓
affecting fetus or newborn 763.7
dyscoordinate 661.4 ✓
affecting fetus or newborn 763.7
early onset (22-36 weeks gestation)
644.2 ✓
failed
induction 659.1 ✓
mechanical 659.0 ✓
medical 659.1 ✓
surgical 659.0 ✓
trial (vaginal delivery) 660.6 ✓
false 644.1 ✓
forced or induced, affecting fetus or newborn 763.89
hypertonic 661.4 ✓
affecting fetus or newborn 763.7
hypotonic 661.2 ✓
affecting fetus or newborn 763.7
primary 661.0 ✓
affecting fetus or newborn 763.7
secondary 661.1 ✓
affecting fetus or newborn 763.7
incoordinate 661.4 ✓
affecting fetus or newborn 763.7
irregular 661.2 ✓
affecting fetus or newborn 763.7
long — *see* Labor, prolonged
missed (at or near term) 656.4 ✓
obstructed NEC 660.9 ✓
affecting fetus or newborn 763.1
due to female genital mutilation
660.8 ✓
specified cause NEC 660.8 ✓
affecting fetus or newborn 763.1
pains, spurious 644.1 ✓
precipitate 661.3 ✓
affecting fetus or newborn 763.6
premature 644.2 ✓
threatened 644.0 ✓
prolonged or protracted 662.1 ✓
first stage 662.0 ✓
affecting fetus or newborn 763.89

Labor — *see also* Delivery — *continued*
prolonged or protracted — *continued*
second stage 662.2 ✓
affecting fetus or newborn 763.89
affecting fetus or newborn 763.89
threatened NEC 644.1 ✓
undelivered 644.1 ✓
Labored breathing — *see also* Hyperventilation 786.09
Labyrinthitis (inner ear) (destructive) (latent)
386.30
circumscribed 386.32
diffuse 386.31
focal 386.32
purulent 386.33
serous 386.31
suppurative 386.33
syphilitic 095.8
toxic 386.34
viral 386.35
Laceration — *see also* Wound, open, by site
accidental, complicating surgery 998.2
Achilles tendon 845.09
with open wound 892.2
anus (sphincter) 879.6
with
abortion — *see* Abortion, by type, with damage to pelvic organs
ectopic pregnancy (*see also* categories 633.0–633.9) 639.2
molar pregnancy (*see also* categories 630–632) 639.2
complicated 879.7
complicating delivery (healed) (old)
654.8 ✓
with laceration of anal or rectal mucosa 664.3 ✓
not associated with third-degree perineal laceration 664.6 ✓
following
abortion 639.2
ectopic or molar pregnancy 639.2
nontraumatic, nonpuerperal (healed)
(old) 569.43
bladder (urinary)
with
abortion — *see* Abortion, by type, with damage to pelvic organs
ectopic pregnancy (*see also* categories 633.0–633.9) 639.2
molar pregnancy (*see also* categories 630–632) 639.2
following
abortion 639.2
ectopic or molar pregnancy 639.2
obstetrical trauma 665.5 ✓
blood vessel — *see* Injury, blood vessel, by site
bowel
with
abortion — *see* Abortion, by type, with damage to pelvic organs
ectopic pregnancy (*see also* categories 633.0–633.9) 639.2
molar pregnancy (*see also* categories 630–632) 639.2
following
abortion 639.2
ectopic or molar pregnancy 639.2
obstetrical trauma 665.5 ✓

Laceration — *see also* Wound, open, by site — *continued*
brain (cerebral) (membrane) (with hemorrhage) 851.8 ✓

Note — Use the following fifth-digit subclassification with categories 851–854:

0   unspecified state of consciousness

1   with no loss of consciousness

2   with brief [less than one hour] loss of consciousness

3   with moderate [1–24 hours] loss of consciousness

4   with prolonged [more than 24 hours] loss of consciousness and return to pre–existing conscious level

5   with prolonged [more than 24 hours] loss of consciousness, without return to pre–existing conscious level

Use fifth-digit 5 to designate when a patient is unconscious and dies before regaining consciousness, regardless of the duration of the loss of consciousness

6   with loss of consciousness of unspecified duration

9   with concussion, unspecified

with
open intracranial wound 851.9 ✓
skull fracture — *see* Fracture, skull, by site
cerebellum 851.6 ✓
with open intracranial wound
851.7 ✓
cortex 851.2 ✓
with open intracranial wound
851.3 ✓
during birth 767.0
stem 851.6 ✓
with open intracranial wound
851.7 ✓
broad ligament
with
abortion — *see* Abortion, by type, with damage to pelvic organs
ectopic pregnancy (*see also* categories 633.0–633.9) 639.2
molar pregnancy (*see also* categories 630–632) 639.2
following
abortion 639.2
ectopic or molar pregnancy 639.2
nontraumatic 620.6
obstetrical trauma 665.6 ✓
syndrome (nontraumatic) 620.6
capsule, joint — *see* Sprain, by site
cardiac — *see* Laceration, heart
causing eversion of cervix uteri (old) 622.0
central, complicating delivery 664.4 ✓
cerebellum — *see* Laceration, brain, cerebellum
cerebral (*see also* Laceration, brain)
during birth 767.0
cervix (uteri)
with
abortion — *see* Abortion, by type, with damage to pelvic organs
ectopic pregnancy (*see also* categories 633.0–633.9) 639.2
molar pregnancy (*see also* categories 630–632) 639.2
following
abortion 639.2
ectopic or molar pregnancy 639.2
nonpuerperal, nontraumatic 622.3
obstetrical trauma (current) 665.3 ✓
old (postpartal) 622.3
traumatic — *see* Injury, internal, cervix
chordae heart 429.5
complicated 879.9

Laceration — *see also* Wound, open, by site — *continued*
cornea — *see* Laceration, eyeball
superficial 918.1
cortex (cerebral) — *see* Laceration, brain, cortex
esophagus 530.89
eye(s) — *see* Laceration, ocular
eyeball NEC 871.4
with prolapse or exposure of intraocular tissue 871.1
penetrating — *see* Penetrating wound, eyeball
specified as without prolapse of intraocular tissue 871.0
eyelid NEC 870.8
full thickness 870.1
involving lacrimal passages 870.2
skin (and periocular area) 870.0
penetrating — *see* Penetrating wound, orbit
fourchette
with
abortion — *see* Abortion, by type, with damage to pelvic organs
ectopic pregnancy (*see also* categories 633.0–633.9) 639.2
molar pregnancy (*see also* categories 630–632) 639.2
complicating delivery 664.0 ✓
following
abortion 639.2
ectopic or molar pregnancy 639.2
heart (without penetration of heart chambers) 861.02
with
open wound into thorax 861.12
penetration of heart chambers
861.03
with open wound into thorax
861.13
hernial sac — *see* Hernia, by site
internal organ (abdomen) (chest) (pelvis)
NEC — *see* Injury, internal, by site
NEC — *see* Injury, internal, by site
kidney (parenchyma) 866.02
with
complete disruption of parenchyma
(rupture) 866.03
with open wound into cavity
866.13
open wound into cavity 866.12
labia
complicating delivery 664.0 ✓
ligament (*see also* Sprain, by site)
with open wound — *see* Wound, open, by site
liver 864.05
with open wound into cavity 864.15
major (disruption of hepatic parenchyma) 864.04
with open wound into cavity 864.14
minor (capsule only) 864.02
with open wound into cavity 864.12
moderate (involving parenchyma without major disruption) 864.03
with open wound into cavity 864.13
multiple 864.04
with open wound into cavity
864.14
stellate 864.04
with open wound into cavity 864.14
lung 861.22
with open wound into thorax 861.32
meninges — *see* Laceration, brain
meniscus (knee) (*see also* Tear, meniscus)
836.2
old 717.5
site other than knee (*see also* Sprain, by site)
old NEC (*see also* Disorder, cartilage, articular) 718.0 ✓
muscle (*see also* Sprain, by site)
with open wound — *see* Wound, open, by site
myocardium — *see* Laceration, heart

Laceration — see also Wound, open, by site — continued
nerve — see Injury, nerve, by site
ocular NEC (see also Laceration, eyeball) 871.4
  adnexa NEC 870.8
    penetrating 870.3
      with foreign body 870.4
  orbit (eye) 870.8
    penetrating 870.3
      with foreign body 870.4
pelvic
  floor (muscles)
    with
      abortion — see Abortion, by type, with damage to pelvic organs
      ectopic pregnancy (see also categories 633.0–633.9) 639.2
      molar pregnancy (see also categories 630–632) 639.2
    complicating delivery 664.1 ☑
    following
      abortion 639.2
      ectopic or molar pregnancy 639.2
    nonpuerperal 618.7
    old (postpartal) 618.7
  organ NEC
    with
      abortion — see Abortion, by type, with damage to pelvic organs
      ectopic pregnancy (see also categories 633.0–633.9) 639.2
      molar pregnancy (see also categories 630–632) 639.2
    complicating delivery 665.5 ☑
      affecting fetus or newborn 763.89
    following
      abortion 639.2
      ectopic or molar pregnancy 639.2
    obstetrical trauma 665.5 ☑
perineum, perineal (old) (postpartal) 618.7
  with
    abortion — see Abortion, by type, with damage to pelvic floor
    ectopic pregnancy (see also categories 633.0–633.9) 639.2
    molar pregnancy (see also categories 630–632) 639.2
  complicating delivery 664.4 ☑
    first degree 664.0 ☑
    second degree 664.1 ☑
    third degree 664.2 ☑
    fourth degree 664.3 ☑
    anal sphincter (healed) (old) 654.8 ☑
      not associated with third-degree perineal laceration 664.6 ☑
      sphincter (anal) (healed) (old) 654.8 ☑
        not associated with third-degree perineal laceration 664.6 ☑
    central 664.4 ☑
    involving
      anal sphincter 664.2 ☑
      fourchette 664.0 ☑
      hymen 664.0 ☑
      labia 664.0 ☑
      pelvic floor 664.1 ☑
      perineal muscles 664.1 ☑
      rectovaginal septum 664.2 ☑
        with anal mucosa 664.3 ☑
      skin 664.0 ☑
      sphincter (anal) 664.2 ☑
        with anal mucosa 664.3 ☑
      vagina 664.0 ☑
      vaginal muscles 664.1 ☑
      vulva 664.0 ☑
    secondary 674.2 ☑
  following
    abortion 639.2
    ectopic or molar pregnancy 639.2
  male 879.6

Laceration — see also Wound, open, by site — continued
perineum, perineal — continued
  male — continued
    complicated 879.7
    muscles, complicating delivery 664.1 ☑
    nonpuerperal, current injury 879.6
      complicated 879.7
    secondary (postpartal) 674.2 ☑
peritoneum
  with
    abortion — see Abortion, by type, with damage to pelvic organs
    ectopic pregnancy (see also categories 633.0–633.9) 639.2
    molar pregnancy (see also categories 630–632) 639.2
  following
    abortion 639.2
    ectopic or molar pregnancy 639.2
  obstetrical trauma 665.5 ☑
periurethral tissue
  with
    abortion — see Abortion, by type, with damage to pelvic organs
    ectopic pregnancy (see also categories 633.0–633.9) 639.2
    molar pregnancy (see also categories 630–632) 639.2
  following
    abortion 639.2
    ectopic or molar pregnancy 639.2
  obstetrical trauma 664.8 ☑
rectovaginal (septum)
  with
    abortion — see Abortion, by type, with damage to pelvic organs
    ectopic pregnancy (see also categories 633.0–633.9) 639.2
    molar pregnancy (see also categories 630–632) 639.2
  complicating delivery 665.4 ☑
    with perineum 665.4 ☑
      involving anal or rectal mucosa 664.3 ☑
  following
    abortion 639.2
    ectopic or molar pregnancy 639.2
  nonpuerperal 623.4
  old (postpartal) 623.4
spinal cord (meninges) (see also Injury, spinal, by site)
  due to injury at birth 767.4
  fetus or newborn 767.4
spleen 865.09
  with
    disruption of parenchyma (massive) 865.04
      with open wound into cavity 865.14
    open wound into cavity 865.19
  capsule (without disruption of parenchyma) 865.02
    with open wound into cavity 865.12
  parenchyma 865.03
    with open wound into cavity 865.13
    massive disruption (rupture) 865.04
      with open wound into cavity 865.14
tendon 848.9
  with open wound — see Wound, open, by site
  Achilles 845.09
    with open wound 892.2
  lower limb NEC 844.9
    with open wound NEC 894.2
  upper limb NEC 840.9
    with open wound NEC 884.2
tentorium cerebelli — see Laceration, brain, cerebellum
tongue 873.64
  complicated 873.74
urethra
  with
    abortion — see Abortion, by type, with damage to pelvic organs

Laceration — see also Wound, open, by site — continued
urethra — continued
  with — continued
    ectopic pregnancy (see also categories 633.0–633.9) 639.2
    molar pregnancy (see also categories 630–632) 639.2
  following
    abortion 639.2
    ectopic or molar pregnancy 639.2
  nonpuerperal, nontraumatic 599.84
  obstetrical trauma 665.5 ☑
uterus
  with
    abortion — see Abortion, by type, with damage to pelvic organs
    ectopic pregnancy (see also categories 633.0–633.9) 639.2
    molar pregnancy (see also categories 630–632) 639.2
  following
    abortion 639.2
    ectopic or molar pregnancy 639.2
  nonpuerperal, nontraumatic 621.8
  obstetrical trauma NEC 665.5 ☑
  old (postpartal) 621.8
vagina
  with
    abortion — see Abortion, by type, with damage to pelvic organs
    ectopic pregnancy (see also categories 633.0–633.9) 639.2
    molar pregnancy (see also categories 630–632) 639.2
    perineal involvement, complicating delivery 664.0 ☑
  complicating delivery 665.4 ☑
    first degree 664.0 ☑
    second degree 664.1 ☑
    third degree 664.2 ☑
    fourth degree 664.3 ☑
    high 665.4 ☑
    muscles 664.1 ☑
    sulcus 665.4 ☑
    wall 665.4 ☑
  following
    abortion 639.2
    ectopic or molar pregnancy 639.2
  nonpuerperal, nontraumatic 623.4
  old (postpartal) 623.4
valve, heart — see Endocarditis
vulva
  with
    abortion — see Abortion, by type, with damage to pelvic organs
    ectopic pregnancy (see also categories 633.0–633.9) 639.2
    molar pregnancy (see also categories 630–632) 639.2
  complicating delivery 664.0 ☑
  following
    abortion 639.2
    ectopic or molar pregnancy 639.2
  nonpuerperal, nontraumatic 624.4
  old (postpartal) 624.4
Lachrymal — see condition
Lachrymonasal duct — see condition
Lack of
  adequate intermaxillary vertical dimension 524.36
  appetite (see also Anorexia) 783.0
  care
    in home V60.4
    of adult 995.84
    of infant (at or after birth) 995.52
  coordination 781.3
  development (see also Hypoplasia)
    physiological in childhood 783.40
  education V62.3
  energy 780.79
  financial resources V60.2
  food 994.2
    in environment V60.89
  growth in childhood 783.43
  heating V60.1

Lack of — continued
  housing (permanent) (temporary) V60.0
    adequate V60.1
  material resources V60.2
  medical attention 799.89
  memory (see also Amnesia) 780.93
    mild, following organic brain damage 310.89
  ovulation 628.0
  person able to render necessary care V60.4
  physical exercise V69.0
  physiologic development in childhood 783.40
  posterior occlusal support 524.57
  prenatal care in current pregnancy V23.7
  shelter V60.0
  sleep V69.4
  water 994.3
Lacrimal — see condition
Lacrimation, abnormal — see also Epiphora 375.20
Lacrimonasal duct — see condition
Lactation, lactating (breast) (puerperal) (postpartum)
  defective 676.4 ☑
  disorder 676.9 ☑
    specified type NEC 676.8 ☑
  excessive 676.6 ☑
  failed 676.4 ☑
  mastitis NEC 675.2 ☑
  mother (care and/or examination) V24.1
  nonpuerperal 611.6
  suppressed 676.5 ☑
Lacticemia 271.3
  excessive 276.2
Lactosuria 271.3
Lacunar skull 756.0
Laennec's cirrhosis (alcoholic) 571.2
  nonalcoholic 571.5
Lafora's disease 333.2
Lagleyze-von Hippel disease (retinocerebral angiomatosis) 759.6
Lag, lid (nervous) 374.41
Lagophthalmos (eyelid) (nervous) 374.20
  cicatricial 374.23
  keratitis (see also Keratitis) 370.34
  mechanical 374.22
  paralytic 374.21
La grippe — see Influenza
Lahore sore 085.1
Lakes, venous (cerebral) 437.8
Laki-Lorand factor deficiency — see also Defect, coagulation 286.3
Lalling 307.9
Lambliasis 007.1
Lame back 724.5
Lancereaux's diabetes (diabetes mellitus with marked emaciation) 250.8 ☑ [261]
  due to secondary diabetes 249.8 ☑ [261]
Landau-Kleffner syndrome 345.8 ☑
Landouzy-Déjérine dystrophy (fascioscapulohumeral atrophy) 359.1
Landry's disease or paralysis 357.0
Landry-Guillain-Barré syndrome 357.0
Lane's
  band 751.4
  disease 569.89
  kink (see also Obstruction, intestine) 560.9
Langdon Down's syndrome (mongolism) 758.0
Language abolition 784.69
Lanugo (persistent) 757.4
Laparoscopic surgical procedure converted to open procedure V64.41
Lardaceous
  degeneration (any site) 277.39
  disease 277.39
  kidney 277.39 [583.81]
  liver 277.39
Large
  baby (regardless of gestational age) 766.1
    exceptionally (weight of 4500 grams or more) 766.0
    of diabetic mother 775.0
  ear 744.22
  fetus (see also Oversize, fetus)

☑ **Additional Digit Required** — Refer to the Tabular List for Digit Selection   ☝ **Subterms under main terms may continue to next column or page**

172 — Volume 2   ►◄ Revised Text   ● New Line   ▲ Revised Code   2013 ICD-9-CM

Large — *continued*
fetus (*see also* Oversize, fetus) — *continued*
causing disproportion 653.5 ☑
with obstructed labor 660.1 ☑
for dates
fetus or newborn (regardless of gestational age) 766.1
affecting management of pregnancy 656.6 ☑
exceptionally (weight of 4500 grams or more) 766.0
physiological cup 743.57
stature 783.9
waxy liver 277.39
white kidney — *see* Nephrosis
Larsen-Johansson disease (juvenile osteopathia patellae) 732.4
Larsen's syndrome (flattened facies and multiple congenital dislocations) 755.8
Larva migrans
cutaneous NEC 126.9
ancylostoma 126.9
of Diptera in vitreous 128.0
visceral NEC 128.0
Laryngeal — *see also* condition 786.2
syncope 786.2
Laryngismus (acute) (infectious) (stridulous) 478.75
congenital 748.3
diphtheritic 032.3
Laryngitis (acute) (edematous) (fibrinous) (gangrenous) (infective) (infiltrative) (malignant) (membranous) (phlegmonous) (pneumococcal) (pseudomembranous) (septic) (subglottic) (suppurative) (ulcerative) (viral) 464.00
with
influenza, flu, or grippe (*see also* Influenza) 487.1
obstruction 464.01
tracheitis (*see also* Laryngotracheitis) 464.20
with obstruction 464.21
acute 464.20
with obstruction 464.21
chronic 476.1
atrophic 476.0
Borrelia vincentii 101
catarrhal 476.0
chronic 476.0
with tracheitis (chronic) 476.1
due to external agent — *see* Condition, respiratory, chronic, due to
diphtheritic (membranous) 032.3
due to external agent — *see* Inflammation, respiratory, upper, due to
Hemophilus influenza 464.00
with obstruction 464.01
H. influenzae 464.00
with obstruction 464.01
hypertrophic 476.0
influenzal (*see also* Influenza) 487.1
pachydermic 478.79
sicca 476.0
spasmodic 478.75
acute 464.00
with obstruction 464.01
streptococcal 034.0
stridulous 478.75
syphilitic 095.8
congenital 090.5
tuberculous (*see also* Tuberculosis, larynx) 012.3 ☑
Vincent's 101
Laryngocele (congenital) (ventricular) 748.3
Laryngofissure 478.79
congenital 748.3
Laryngomalacia (congenital) 748.3
Laryngopharyngitis (acute) 465.0
chronic 478.9
due to external agent — *see* Condition, respiratory, chronic, due to
due to external agent — *see* Inflammation, respiratory, upper, due to
septic 034.0

Laryngoplegia — *see also* Paralysis, vocal cord 478.30
Laryngoptosis 478.79
Laryngospasm 478.75
due to external agent — *see* Condition, respiratory, acute, due to
Laryngostenosis 478.74
congenital 748.3
Laryngotracheitis (acute) (infectional) (viral) — *see also* Laryngitis 464.20
with obstruction 464.21
atrophic 476.1
Borrelia vincenti 101
catarrhal 476.1
chronic 476.1
due to external agent — *see* Condition, respiratory, chronic, due to
diphtheritic (membranous) 032.3
due to external agent — *see* Inflammation, respiratory, upper, due to
H. influenzae 464.20
with obstruction 464.21
hypertrophic 476.1
influenzal (*see also* Influenza) 487.1
pachydermic 478.75
sicca 476.1
spasmodic 478.75
acute 464.20
with obstruction 464.21
streptococcal 034.0
stridulous 478.75
syphilitic 095.8
congenital 090.5
tuberculous (*see also* Tuberculosis, larynx) 012.3 ☑
Vincent's 101
Laryngotracheobronchitis — *see also* Bronchitis 490
acute 466.0
chronic 491.8
viral 466.0
Laryngotracheobronchopneumonitis — *see* Pneumonia, broncho-
Larynx, laryngeal — *see* condition
Lasègue's disease (persecution mania) 297.9
Lassa fever 078.89
Lassitude — *see also* Weakness 780.79
Late — *see also* condition
effect(s) (of) (*see also* condition)
abscess
intracranial or intraspinal (conditions classifiable to 324) — *see* category 326
adverse effect of drug, medicinal or biological substance 909.5
allergic reaction 909.9
amputation
postoperative (late) 997.60
traumatic (injury classifiable to 885–887 and 895–897) 905.9
burn (injury classifiable to 948–949) 906.9
extremities NEC (injury classifiable to 943 or 945) 906.7
hand or wrist (injury classifiable to 944) 906.6
eye (injury classifiable to 940) 906.5
face, head, and neck (injury classifiable to 941) 906.5
specified site NEC (injury classifiable to 942 and 946–947) 906.8
cerebrovascular disease (conditions classifiable to 430–437) 438.9
with
alterations of sensations 438.6
aphasia 438.11
apraxia 438.81
ataxia 438.84
cognitive deficits 438.0
disturbances of vision 438.7
dysarthria 438.13
dysphagia 438.82
dysphasia 438.12
facial droop 438.83
facial weakness 438.83
fluency disorder 438.14

Late — *see also* condition — *continued*
effect(s) (*see also* condition) — *continued*
cerebrovascular disease — *continued*
with — *continued*
hemiplegia/hemiparesis
affecting
dominant side 438.21
nondominant side 438.22
unspecified side 438.20
monoplegia of lower limb
affecting
dominant side 438.41
nondominant side 438.42
unspecified side 438.40
monoplegia of upper limb
affecting
dominant side 438.31
nondominant side 438.32
unspecified side 438.30
paralytic syndrome NEC
affecting
bilateral 438.53
dominant side 438.51
nondominant side 438.52
unspecified side 438.50
speech and language deficit 438.10
specified type NEC 438.19
stuttering 438.14
vertigo 438.85
specified type NEC 438.89
childbirth complication(s) 677
complication(s) of
childbirth 677
delivery 677
pregnancy 677
puerperium 677
surgical and medical care (conditions classifiable to 996–999) 909.3
trauma (conditions classifiable to 958) 908.6
contusion (injury classifiable to 920–924) 906.3
crushing (injury classifiable to 925–929) 906.4
delivery complication(s) 677
dislocation (injury classifiable to 830–839) 905.6
encephalitis or encephalomyelitis (conditions classifiable to 323) — *see* category 326
in infectious diseases 139.8
viral (conditions classifiable to 049.8, 049.9, 062–064) 139.0
external cause NEC (conditions classifiable to 995) 909.9
certain conditions classifiable to categories 991-994 909.4
foreign body in orifice (injury classifiable to 930–939) 908.5
fracture (multiple) (injury classifiable to 828–829) 905.5
extremity
lower (injury classifiable to 821–827) 905.4
neck of femur (injury classifiable to 820) 905.3
upper (injury classifiable to 810–819) 905.2
face and skull (injury classifiable to 800–804) 905.0
skull and face (injury classifiable to 800–804) 905.0
spine and trunk (injury classifiable to 805 and 807–809) 905.1
with spinal cord lesion (injury classifiable to 806) 907.2
infection
pyogenic, intracranial — *see* category 326
infectious diseases (conditions classifiable to 001–136) NEC 139.8
injury (injury classifiable to 959) 908.9

Late — *see also* condition — *continued*
effect(s) (*see also* condition) — *continued*
injury — *continued*
blood vessel 908.3
abdomen and pelvis (injury classifiable to 902) 908.4
extremity (injury classifiable to 903–904) 908.3
head and neck (injury classifiable to 900) 908.3
intracranial (injury classifiable to 850–854) 907.0
with skull fracture 905.0
thorax (injury classifiable to 901) 908.4
internal organ NEC (injury classifiable to 867 and 869) 908.2
abdomen (injury classifiable to 863–866 and 868) 908.1
thorax (injury classifiable to 860–862) 908.0
intracranial (injury classifiable to 850–854) 907.0
with skull fracture (injury classifiable to 800–801 and 803–804) 905.0
nerve NEC (injury classifiable to 957) 907.9
cranial (injury classifiable to 950–951) 907.1
peripheral NEC (injury classifiable to 957) 907.9
lower limb and pelvic girdle (injury classifiable to 956) 907.5
upper limb and shoulder girdle (injury classifiable to 955) 907.4
roots and plexus(es), spinal (injury classifiable to 953) 907.3
trunk (injury classifiable to 954) 907.3
spinal
cord (injury classifiable to 806 and 952) 907.2
nerve root(s) and plexus(es) (injury classifiable to 953) 907.3
superficial (injury classifiable to 910–919) 906.2
tendon (tendon injury classifiable to 840–848, 880–884 with .2, and 890–894 with .2) 905.8
meningitis
bacterial (conditions classifiable to 320) — *see* category 326
unspecified cause (conditions classifiable to 322) — *see* category 326
myelitis (*see also* Late, effect(s) (of), encephalitis) — *see* category 326
parasitic diseases (conditions classifiable to 001–136 NEC) 139.8
phlebitis or thrombophlebitis of intracranial venous sinuses (conditions classifiable to 325) — *see* category 326
poisoning due to drug, medicinal or biological substance (conditions classifiable to 960–979) 909.0
poliomyelitis, acute (conditions classifiable to 045) 138
pregnancy complication(s) 677
puerperal complication(s) 677
radiation (conditions classifiable to 990) 909.2
rickets 268.1
sprain and strain without mention of tendon injury (injury classifiable to 840–848, except tendon injury) 905.7
tendon involvement 905.8

☑ Additional Digit Required — Refer to the Tabular List for Digit Selection   ▽ Subterms under main terms may continue to next column or page
2013 ICD-9-CM   ▶◀ Revised Text   ● New Line   ▲ Revised Code   Volume 2 — 173

Large — Late

Late — see also condition — continued
  effect(s) (see also condition) — contin-
    ued
    toxic effect of
      drug, medicinal or biological sub-
        stance (conditions classifiable
        to 960–979) 909.0
      nonmedical substance (conditions
        classifiable to 980–989) 909.1
      trachoma (conditions classifiable to 076)
        139.1
    tuberculosis 137.0
      bones and joints (conditions classifi-
        able to 015) 137.3
      central nervous system (conditions
        classifiable to 013) 137.1
      genitourinary (conditions classifiable
        to 016) 137.2
      pulmonary (conditions classifiable to
        010–012) 137.0
      specified organs NEC (conditions
        classifiable to 014, 017–018)
        137.4
    viral encephalitis (conditions classifiable
      to 049.8, 049.9, 062–064) 139.0
    wound, open
      extremity (injury classifiable to
        880–884 and 890–894, except
        .2) 906.1
      tendon (injury classifiable to
        880–884 with .2 and
        890–894 with .2) 905.8
      head, neck, and trunk (injury classifi-
        able to 870–879) 906.0
  infant
    post-term (gestation period over 40
      completed weeks to 42 complet-
      ed weeks) 766.21
    prolonged gestation (period over 42
      completed weeks) 766.22
Latent — see condition
Lateral — see condition
Laterocession — see Lateroversion
Lateroflexion — see Lateroversion
Lateroversion
  cervix — see Lateroversion, uterus
  uterus, uterine (cervix) (postinfectional)
    (postpartal, old) 621.6
    congenital 752.39
    in pregnancy or childbirth 654.4 ☑
      affecting fetus or newborn 763.89
Lathyrism 988.2
Launois-Bensaude's lipomatosis 272.8
Launois-Cléret syndrome (adiposogenital
  dystrophy) 253.8
Launois' syndrome (pituitary gigantism) 253.0
Laurence-Moon-Biedl syndrome (obesity,
  polydactyly, and intellectual disabilities)
  759.89
LAV (disease) (illness) (infection) — see Human
  immunodeficiency virus (disease) (illness) (infection)
LAV/HTLV-III (disease) (illness) (infection) —
  see Human immunodeficiency virus
  (disease) (illness) (infection)
Lawford's syndrome (encephalocutaneous
  angiomatosis) 759.6
Laxative habit — see also Abuse, drugs, nondependent 305.9 ☑
Lax, laxity — see also Relaxation
  ligament 728.4
  skin (acquired) 701.8
    congenital 756.83
Lazy leukocyte syndrome 288.09
LCAD (long chain/very long chain acyl CoA dehydrogenase deficiency, VLCAD) 277.85
LCHAD (long chain 3-hydroxyacyl CoA dehydrogenase deficiency) 277.85
Lead — see also condition
  exposure (suspected) to V15.86
  incrustation of cornea 371.15
  poisoning 984.9
    specified type of lead — see Table of
      Drugs and Chemicals
Lead miners' lung 503

Leakage
  amniotic fluid 658.1 ☑
    with delayed delivery 658.2 ☑
    affecting fetus or newborn 761.1
  bile from drainage tube (T tube) 997.49
  blood (microscopic), fetal, into maternal
    circulation 656.0 ☑
    affecting management of pregnancy or
      puerperium 656.0 ☑
  device, implant, or graft — see Complica-
    tions, mechanical
  spinal fluid at lumbar puncture site 997.09
  urine, continuous 788.37
Leaky heart — see Endocarditis
Learning defect, specific NEC (strephosymbolia) 315.2
Leather bottle stomach (M8142/3) 151.9
Leber's
  congenital amaurosis 362.76
  optic atrophy (hereditary) 377.16
Lederer's anemia or disease (acquired infec-
  tious hemolytic anemia) 283.19
Lederer-Brill syndrome (acquired infectious
  hemolytic anemia) 283.19
Leeches (aquatic) (land) 134.2
Left-sided neglect 781.8
Leg — see condition
Legal investigation V62.5
Legg (-Calvé) -Perthes disease or syndrome
  (osteochondrosis, femoral capital) 732.1
Legionnaires' disease 482.84
Leigh's disease 330.8
Leiner's disease (exfoliative dermatitis) 695.89
Leiofibromyoma (M8890/0) — see also
  Leiomyoma
  uterus (cervix) (corpus) (see also Leiomyoma,
    uterus) 218.9
Leiomyoblastoma (M8891/1) — see Neo-
  plasm, connective tissue, uncertain be-
  havior
Leiomyofibroma (M8890/0) — see also Neoplasm, connective tissue, benign
  uterus (cervix) (corpus) (see also Leiomyoma,
    uterus) 218.9
Leiomyoma (M8890/0) — see also Neoplasm,
  connective tissue, benign
  bizarre (M8893/0) — see Neoplasm, connec-
    tive tissue, benign
  cellular (M8892/1) — see Neoplasm, connec-
    tive tissue, uncertain behavior
  epithelioid (M8891/1) — see Neoplasm,
    connective tissue, uncertain behavior
  prostate (polypoid) 600.20
    with
      other lower urinary tract symptoms
        (LUTS) 600.21
      urinary
        obstruction 600.21
        retention 600.21
  uterus (cervix) (corpus) 218.9
    interstitial 218.1
    intramural 218.1
    submucous 218.0
    subperitoneal 218.2
    subserous 218.2
  vascular (M8894/0) — see Neoplasm, con-
    nective tissue, benign
Leiomyomatosis (intravascular) (M8890/1) —
  see Neoplasm, connective tissue, uncertain behavior
Leiomyosarcoma (M8890/3) — see also Neoplasm, connective tissue, malignant
  epithelioid (M8891/3) — see Neoplasm,
    connective tissue, malignant
Leishmaniasis 085.9
  American 085.5
    cutaneous 085.4
    mucocutaneous 085.5
  Asian desert 085.2
  Brazilian 085.5
  cutaneous 085.9
    acute necrotizing 085.2
    American 085.4
    Asian desert 085.2
    diffuse 085.3
    dry form 085.1

Leishmaniasis — continued
  cutaneous — continued
    Ethiopian 085.3
    eyelid 085.5 [373.6]
    late 085.1
    lepromatous 085.3
    recurrent 085.1
    rural 085.2
    ulcerating 085.1
    urban 085.1
    wet form 085.2
    zoonotic form 085.2
  dermal (see also Leishmaniasis, cutaneous)
    post kala-azar 085.0
  eyelid 085.5 [373.6]
  infantile 085.0
  Mediterranean 085.0
  mucocutaneous (American) 085.5
  naso-oral 085.5
  nasopharyngeal 085.5
  Old World 085.1
  tegumentaria diffusa 085.4
  vaccination, prophylactic (against) V05.2
  visceral (Indian) 085.0
Leishmanoid, dermal — see also Leishmaniasis, cutaneous
  post kala-azar 085.0
Leloir's disease 695.4
Lemiere syndrome 451.89
Lenegre's disease 426.0
Lengthening, leg 736.81
Lennox-Gastaut syndrome 345.0 ☑
  with tonic seizures 345.1 ☑
Lennox's syndrome — see also Epilepsy
  345.0 ☑
Lens — see condition
Lenticonus (anterior) (posterior) (congenital)
  743.36
Lenticular degeneration, progressive 275.1
Lentiglobus (posterior) (congenital) 743.36
Lentigo (congenital) 709.09
  juvenile 709.09
  Maligna (M8742/2) (see also Neoplasm, skin,
    in situ)
    melanoma (M8742/3) — see Melanoma
  senile 709.09
Leonine leprosy 030.0
Leontiasis
  ossium 733.3
  syphilitic 095.8
    congenital 090.5
Léopold-Lévi's syndrome (paroxysmal thyroid
  instability) 242.9 ☑
Lepore hemoglobin syndrome 282.45
Lepothrix 039.0
Lepra 030.9
  Willan's 696.1
Leprechaunism 259.8
Lepromatous leprosy 030.0
Leprosy 030.9
  anesthetic 030.1
  beriberi 030.1
  borderline (group B) (infiltrated) (neuritic)
    030.3
  cornea (see also Leprosy, by type)
    030.9 [371.89]
  dimorphous (group B) (infiltrated) (leproma-
    tous) (neuritic) (tuberculoid) 030.3
  eyelid 030.0 [373.4]
  indeterminate (group I) (macular) (neuritic)
    (uncharacteristic) 030.2
  leonine 030.0
  lepromatous (diffuse) (infiltrated) (macular)
    (neuritic) (nodular) (type L) 030.0
  macular (early) (neuritic) (simple) 030.2
  maculoanesthetic 030.1
  mixed 030.0
  neuro 030.1
  nodular 030.0
  primary neuritic 030.3
  specified type or group NEC 030.8
  tubercular 030.1
  tuberculoid (macular) (maculoanesthetic)
    (major) (minor) (neuritic) (type T)
    030.1
Leptocytosis, hereditary 282.40

Leptomeningitis (chronic) (circumscribed)
  (hemorrhagic) (nonsuppurative) — see
  also Meningitis 322.9
  aseptic 047.9
    adenovirus 049.1
    Coxsackie virus 047.0
    ECHO virus 047.1
    enterovirus 047.9
    lymphocytic choriomeningitis 049.0
  epidemic 036.0
  late effect — see category 326
  meningococcal 036.0
  pneumococcal 320.1
  syphilitic 094.2
  tuberculous (see also Tuberculosis,
    meninges) 013.0 ☑
Leptomeningopathy — see also Meningitis
  322.9
Leptospiral — see condition
Leptospirochetal — see condition
Leptospirosis 100.9
  autumnalis 100.89
  canicula 100.89
  grippotyphosa 100.89
  hebdomidis 100.89
  icterohemorrhagica 100.0
  nanukayami 100.89
  pomona 100.89
  Weil's disease 100.0
Leptothricosis — see Actinomycosis
Leptothrix infestation — see Actinomycosis
Leptotricosis — see Actinomycosis
Leptus dermatitis 133.8
Leriche's syndrome (aortic bifurcation occlusion) 444.09
Léris pleonosteosis 756.89
Léri-Weill syndrome 756.59
Lermoyez's syndrome — see also Disease,
  Ménière's 386.00
Lesbianism — omit code
  ego-dystonic 302.0
  problems with 302.0
Lesch-Nyhan syndrome (hypoxanthinegua-
  nine-phosphoribosyltransferase deficiency) 277.2
Lesion(s)
  abducens nerve 378.54
  alveolar process 525.8
  anorectal 569.49
  aortic (valve) — see Endocarditis, aortic
  auditory nerve 388.5
  basal ganglion 333.90
  bile duct (see also Disease, biliary) 576.8
  bladder 596.9
  bone 733.90
  brachial plexus 353.0
  brain 348.89
    congenital 742.9
    vascular (see also Lesion, cerebrovascu-
      lar) 437.9
      degenerative 437.1
      healed or old without residuals
        V12.54
      hypertensive 437.2
      late effect — see Late effect(s) (of)
        cerebrovascular disease
  buccal 528.9
  calcified — see Calcification
  canthus 373.9
  carate — see Pinta, lesions
  cardia 537.89
  cardiac — see also Disease, heart
    congenital 746.9
    valvular — see Endocarditis
  cauda equina 344.60
    with neurogenic bladder 344.61
  cecum 569.89
  cerebral — see Lesion, brain
  cerebrovascular (see also Disease, cere-
    brovascular NEC) 437.9
    degenerative 437.1
      healed or old without residuals
        V12.54
    hypertensive 437.2
    specified type NEC 437.8
  cervical root (nerve) NEC 353.2

Lesion(s) — *continued*
- chiasmal 377.54
  - associated with
    - inflammatory disorders 377.54
    - neoplasm NEC 377.52
      - pituitary 377.51
    - pituitary disorders 377.51
    - vascular disorders 377.53
- chorda tympani 351.8
- coin, lung 793.11
- colon 569.89
- congenital — *see* Anomaly
- conjunctiva 372.9
- coronary artery (*see also* Ischemia, heart) 414.9
- cranial nerve 352.9
  - first 352.0
  - second 377.49
  - third
    - partial 378.51
    - total 378.52
  - fourth 378.53
  - fifth 350.9
  - sixth 378.54
  - seventh 351.9
  - eighth 388.5
  - ninth 352.2
  - tenth 352.3
  - eleventh 352.4
  - twelfth 352.5
- cystic — *see* Cyst
- degenerative — *see* Degeneration
- dermal (skin) 709.9
- Dieulafoy (hemorrhagic)
  - of
    - duodenum 537.84
    - intestine 569.86
    - stomach 537.84
- duodenum 537.89
  - with obstruction 537.3
- eyelid 373.9
- gasserian ganglion 350.8
- gastric 537.89
- gastroduodenal 537.89
- gastrointestinal 569.89
- glossopharyngeal nerve 352.2
- heart (organic) (*see also* Disease, heart)
  - vascular — *see* Disease, cardiovascular
- helix (ear) 709.9
- high grade myelodysplastic syndrome 238.73
- hyperchromic, due to pinta (carate) 103.1
- hyperkeratotic (*see also* Hyperkeratosis) 701.1
- hypoglossal nerve 352.5
- hypopharynx 478.29
- hypothalamic 253.9
- ileocecal coil 569.89
- ileum 569.89
- iliohypogastric nerve 355.79
- ilioinguinal nerve 355.79
- in continuity — *see* Injury, nerve, by site
- inflammatory — *see* Inflammation
- intestine 569.89
- intracerebral — *see* Lesion, brain
- intrachiasmal (optic) (*see also* Lesion, chiasmal) 377.54
- intracranial, space-occupying NEC 784.2
- joint 719.90
  - ankle 719.97
  - elbow 719.92
  - foot 719.97
  - hand 719.94
  - hip 719.95
  - knee 719.96
  - multiple sites 719.99
  - pelvic region 719.95
  - sacroiliac (old) 724.6
  - shoulder (region) 719.91
  - specified site NEC 719.98
  - wrist 719.93
- keratotic (*see also* Keratosis) 701.1
- kidney (*see also* Disease, renal) 593.9
- laryngeal nerve (recurrent) 352.3
- leonine 030.0
- lip 528.5

Lesion(s) — *continued*
- liver 573.8
- low grade myelodysplastic syndrome 238.72
- lumbosacral
  - plexus 353.1
  - root (nerve) NEC 353.4
- lung 518.89
  - coin 793.11
- maxillary sinus 473.0
- mitral — *see* Endocarditis, mitral
- Morel Lavallée — *see* Hematoma, by site
- motor cortex 348.89
- nerve (*see also* Disorder, nerve) 355.9
- nervous system 349.9
  - congenital 742.9
- nonallopathic NEC 739.9
  - in region (of)
    - abdomen 739.9
    - acromioclavicular 739.7
    - cervical, cervicothoracic 739.1
    - costochondral 739.8
    - costovertebral 739.8
    - extremity
      - lower 739.6
      - upper 739.7
    - head 739.0
    - hip 739.5
    - lower extremity 739.6
    - lumbar, lumbosacral 739.3
    - occipitocervical 739.0
    - pelvic 739.5
    - pubic 739.5
    - rib cage 739.8
    - sacral, sacrococcygeal, sacroiliac 739.4
    - sternochondral 739.8
    - sternoclavicular 739.7
    - thoracic, thoracolumbar 739.2
    - upper extremity 739.7
- nose (internal) 478.19
- obstructive — *see* Obstruction
- obturator nerve 355.79
- occlusive
  - artery — *see* Embolism, artery
- organ or site NEC — *see* Disease, by site
- osteolytic 733.90
- paramacular, of retina 363.32
- peptic 537.89
- periodontal, due to traumatic occlusion 523.8
- perirectal 569.49
- peritoneum (granulomatous) 568.89
- pigmented (skin) 709.00
- pinta — *see* Pinta, lesions
- polypoid — *see* Polyp
- prechiasmal (optic) (*see also* Lesion, chiasmal) 377.54
- primary (*see also* Syphilis, primary)
  - carate 103.0
  - pinta 103.0
  - yaws 102.0
- pulmonary 518.89
  - valve (*see also* Endocarditis, pulmonary) 424.3
- pylorus 537.89
- radiation NEC 990
- radium NEC 990
- rectosigmoid 569.89
- retina, retinal (*see also* Retinopathy)
  - vascular 362.17
- retroperitoneal 568.89
- romanus 720.1
- sacroiliac (joint) 724.6
- salivary gland 527.8
  - benign lymphoepithelial 527.8
- saphenous nerve 355.79
- secondary — *see* Syphilis, secondary
- sigmoid 569.89
- sinus (accessory) (nasal) (*see also* Sinusitis) 473.9
- skin 709.9
  - suppurative 686.00
- SLAP (superior glenoid labrum) 840.7
- space-occupying, intracranial NEC 784.2
- spinal cord 336.9
  - congenital 742.9

Lesion(s) — *continued*
- spinal cord — *continued*
  - traumatic (complete) (incomplete) (transverse) (*see also* Injury, spinal, by site)
    - with
      - broken
        - back — *see* Fracture, vertebra, by site, with spinal cord injury
        - neck — *see* Fracture, vertebra, cervical, with spinal cord injury
      - fracture, vertebra — *see* Fracture, vertebra, by site, with spinal cord injury
- spleen 289.50
- stomach 537.89
- superior glenoid labrum (SLAP) 840.7
- syphilitic — *see* Syphilis
- tertiary — *see* Syphilis, tertiary
- thoracic root (nerve) 353.3
- tonsillar fossa 474.9
- tooth, teeth 525.8
  - white spot 521.01
- traumatic NEC (*see also* nature and site of injury) 959.9
- tricuspid (valve) — *see* Endocarditis, tricuspid
- trigeminal nerve 350.9
- ulcerated or ulcerative — *see* Ulcer
- uterus NEC 621.9
- vagina 623.8
- vagus nerve 352.3
- valvular — *see* Endocarditis
- vascular 459.9
  - affecting central nervous system (*see also* Lesion, cerebrovascular) 437.9
  - following trauma (*see also* Injury, blood vessel, by site) 904.9
  - retina 362.17
  - traumatic — *see* Injury, blood vessel, by site
  - umbilical cord 663.6 ☑
    - affecting fetus or newborn 762.6
- visual
  - cortex NEC (*see also* Disorder, visual, cortex) 377.73
  - pathway NEC (*see also* Disorder, visual, pathway) 377.63
- warty — *see* Verruca
- white spot, on teeth 521.01
- x-ray NEC 990

Lethargic — *see* condition
Lethargy 780.79
Letterer-Siwe disease (acute histiocytosis X) (M9722/3) 202.5 ☑
Leucinosis 270.3
Leucocoria 360.44
Leucosarcoma (M9850/3) 207.8 ☑
Leukasmus 270.2
Leukemia, leukemic (congenital) (M9800/3) 208.9 ☑

> *Note* – Use the following fifth-digit subclassification for categories 203–208:
>
> 0   *without mention of having achieved remission*
>
>   *failed remission*
>
> 1   *with remission*
>
> 2   *in relapse*

- acute NEC (M9801/3) 208.0 ☑
- aleukemic NEC (M9804/3) 208.8 ☑
  - granulocytic (M9864/3) 205.8 ☑
- basophilic (M9870/3) 205.1 ☑
- blast (cell) (M9801/3) 208.0 ☑
- blastic (M9801/3) 208.0 ☑
  - granulocytic (M9861/3) 205.0 ☑
- chronic NEC (M9803/3) 208.1 ☑
- compound (M9810/3) 207.8 ☑
- eosinophilic (M9880/3) 205.1 ☑
- giant cell (M9910/3) 207.2 ☑
- granulocytic (M9860/3) 205.9 ☑
  - acute (M9861/3) 205.0 ☑

Leukemia, leukemic — *continued*
- granulocytic — *continued*
  - aleukemic (M9864/3) 205.8 ☑
  - blastic (M9861/3) 205.0 ☑
  - chronic (M9863/3) 205.1 ☑
  - subacute (M9862/3) 205.2 ☑
  - subleukemic (M9864/3) 205.8 ☑
- hairy cell (M9940/3) 202.4 ☑
- hemoblastic (M9801/3) 208.0 ☑
- histiocytic (M9890/3) 206.9 ☑
- lymphatic (M9820/3) 204.9 ☑
  - acute (M9821/3) 204.0 ☑
  - aleukemic (M9824/3) 204.8 ☑
  - chronic (M9823/3) 204.1 ☑
  - subacute (M9822/3) 204.2 ☑
  - subleukemic (M9824/3) 204.8 ☑
- lymphoblastic (M9821/3) 204.0 ☑
- lymphocytic (M9820/3) 204.9 ☑
  - acute (M9821/3) 204.0 ☑
  - aleukemic (M9824/3) 204.8 ☑
  - chronic (M9823/3) 204.1 ☑
  - granular
    - large T-cell 204.8 ☑
  - subacute (M9822/3) 204.2 ☑
  - subleukemic (M9824/3) 204.8 ☑
- lymphogenous (M9820/3) — *see* Leukemia, lymphoid
- lymphoid (M9820/3) 204.9 ☑
  - acute (M9821/3) 204.0 ☑
  - aleukemic (M9824/3) 204.8 ☑
  - blastic (M9821/3) 204.0 ☑
  - chronic (M9823/3) 204.1 ☑
  - subacute (M9822/3) 204.2 ☑
  - subleukemic (M9824/3) 204.8 ☑
- lymphosarcoma cell (M9850/3) 207.8 ☑
- mast cell (M9900/3) 207.8 ☑
- megakaryocytic (M9910/3) 207.2 ☑
- megakaryocytoid (M9910/3) 207.2 ☑
- mixed (cell) (M9810/3) 207.8 ☑
- monoblastic (M9891/3) 206.0 ☑
- monocytic (Schilling-type) (M9890/3) 206.9 ☑
  - acute (M9891/3) 206.0 ☑
  - aleukemic (M9894/3) 206.8 ☑
  - chronic (M9893/3) 206.1 ☑
  - Naegeli-type (M9863/3) 205.1 ☑
  - subacute (M9892/3) 206.2 ☑
  - subleukemic (M9894/3) 206.8 ☑
- monocytoid (M9890/3) 206.9 ☑
  - acute (M9891/3) 206.0 ☑
  - aleukemic (M9894/3) 206.8 ☑
  - chronic (M9893/3) 206.1 ☑
  - myelogenous (M9863/3) 205.1 ☑
  - subacute (M9892/3) 206.2 ☑
  - subleukemic (M9894/3) 206.8 ☑
- monomyelocytic (M9860/3) — *see* Leukemia, myelomonocytic
- myeloblastic (M9861/3) 205.0 ☑
- myelocytic (M9863/3) 205.1 ☑
  - acute (M9861/3) 205.0 ☑
- myelogenous (M9860/3) 205.9 ☑
  - acute (M9861/3) 205.0 ☑
  - aleukemic (M9864/3) 205.8 ☑
  - chronic (M9863/3) 205.1 ☑
  - monocytoid (M9863/3) 205.1 ☑
  - subacute (M9862/3) 205.2 ☑
  - subleukemic (M9864) 205.8 ☑
- myeloid (M9860/3) 205.9 ☑
  - acute (M9861/3) 205.0 ☑
  - aleukemic (M9864/3) 205.8 ☑
  - chronic (M9863/3) 205.1 ☑
  - subacute (M9862/3) 205.2 ☑
  - subleukemic (M9864/3) 205.8 ☑
- myelomonocytic (M9860/3) 205.9 ☑
  - acute (M9861/3) 205.0 ☑
  - chronic (M9863/3) 205.1 ☑
- Naegeli-type monocytic (M9863/3) 205.1 ☑
- neutrophilic (M9865/3) 205.1 ☑
- plasma cell (M9830/3) 203.1 ☑
- plasmacytic (M9830/3) 203.1 ☑
- prolymphocytic (M9825/3) — *see* Leukemia, lymphoid
- promyelocytic, acute (M9866/3) 205.0 ☑

☑ **Additional Digit Required — Refer to the Tabular List for Digit Selection**   ▽ **Subterms under main terms may continue to next column or page**

2013 ICD-9-CM   ▶◀ **Revised Text**   ● **New Line**   ▲ **Revised Code**   **Volume 2 — 175**

Lesion(s) — Leukemia, leukemic

Index

Leukemia, leukemic — Lipomatosis

Leukemia, leukemic — *continued*
  Schilling-type monocytic (M9890/3) — *see* Leukemia, monocytic
  stem cell (M9801/3) 208.0 ☑
  subacute NEC (M9802/3) 208.2 ☑
  subleukemic NEC (M9804/3) 208.8 ☑
  thrombocytic (M9910/3) 207.2 ☑
  undifferentiated (M9801/3) 208.0 ☑
Leukemoid reaction (basophilic) (lymphocytic) (monocytic) (myelocytic) (neutrophilic) 288.62
Leukoaraiosis (hypertensive) 437.1
Leukoariosis — *see* Leukoaraiosis
Leukoclastic vasculitis 446.29
Leukocoria 360.44
Leukocythemia — *see* Leukemia
Leukocytopenia 288.50
Leukocytosis 288.60
  basophilic 288.8
  eosinophilic 288.3
  lymphocytic 288.8
  monocytic 288.8
  neutrophilic 288.8
Leukoderma 709.09
  syphilitic 091.3
    late 095.8
Leukodermia — *see also* Leukoderma 709.09
Leukodystrophy (cerebral) (globoid cell) (metachromatic) (progressive) (sudanophilic) 330.0
Leukoedema, mouth or tongue 528.79
Leukoencephalitis
  acute hemorrhagic (postinfectious) NEC 136.9 [323.61]
    postimmunization or postvaccinal 323.51
  subacute sclerosing 046.2
  van Bogaert's 046.2
  van Bogaert's (sclerosing) 046.2
Leukoencephalopathy — *see also* Encephalitis 323.9
  acute necrotizing hemorrhagic (postinfectious) 136.9 [323.61]
    postimmunization or postvaccinal 323.51
  arteriosclerotic 437.0
  Binswanger's 290.12
  metachromatic 330.0
  multifocal (progressive) 046.3
  progressive multifocal 046.3
  reversible, posterior 348.5
Leukoerythroblastosis 289.9
Leukoerythrosis 289.0
Leukokeratosis — *see also* Leukoplakia 702.8
  mouth 528.6
  nicotina palati 528.79
  tongue 528.6
Leukokoria 360.44
Leukokraurosis vulva, vulvae 624.09
Leukolymphosarcoma (M9850/3) 207.8 ☑
Leukoma (cornea) (interfering with central vision) 371.03
  adherent 371.04
Leukomalacia, periventricular 779.7
Leukomelanopathy, hereditary 288.2
Leukonychia (punctata) (striata) 703.8
  congenital 757.5
Leukopathia
  unguium 703.8
    congenital 757.5
Leukopenia 288.50
  basophilic 288.59
  cyclic 288.02
  eosinophilic 288.59
  familial 288.59
  malignant (*see also* Agranulocytosis) 288.09
  periodic 288.02
  transitory neonatal 776.7
Leukopenic — *see* condition
Leukoplakia 702.8
  anus 569.49
  bladder (postinfectional) 596.89
  buccal 528.6
  cervix (uteri) 622.2
  esophagus 530.83
  gingiva 528.6

Leukoplakia — *continued*
  kidney (pelvis) 593.89
  larynx 478.79
  lip 528.6
  mouth 528.6
  oral soft tissue (including tongue) (mucosa) 528.6
  palate 528.6
  pelvis (kidney) 593.89
  penis (infectional) 607.0
  rectum 569.49
  syphilitic 095.8
  tongue 528.6
  tonsil 478.29
  ureter (postinfectional) 593.89
  urethra (postinfectional) 599.84
  uterus 621.8
  vagina 623.1
  vesical 596.89
  vocal cords 478.5
  vulva 624.09
Leukopolioencephalopathy 330.0
Leukorrhea (vagina) 623.5
  due to trichomonas (vaginalis) 131.00
  trichomonal (Trichomonas vaginalis) 131.00
Leukosarcoma (M9850/3) 207.8 ☑
Leukosis (M9800/3) — *see* Leukemia
Lev's disease or syndrome (acquired complete heart block) 426.0
Levi's syndrome (pituitary dwarfism) 253.3
Levocardia (isolated) 746.87
  with situs inversus 759.3
Levulosuria 271.2
Lewandowski's disease (primary) — *see also* Tuberculosis 017.0 ☑
Lewandowski-Lutz disease (epidermodysplasia verruciformis) 078.19
Lewy body dementia 331.82
Lewy body disease 331.82
Leyden's disease (periodic vomiting) 536.2
Leyden-Möbius dystrophy 359.1
Leydig cell
  carcinoma (M8650/3)
    specified site — *see* Neoplasm, by site, malignant
    unspecified site
      female 183.0
      male 186.9
  tumor (M8650/1)
    benign (M8650/0)
      specified site — *see* Neoplasm, by site, benign
      unspecified site
        female 220
        male 222.0
    malignant (M8650/3)
      specified site — *see* Neoplasm, by site, malignant
      unspecified site
        female 183.0
        male 186.9
    specified site — *see* Neoplasm, by site, uncertain behavior
    unspecified site
      female 236.2
      male 236.4
Leydig-Sertoli cell tumor (M8631/0)
  specified site — *see* Neoplasm, by site, benign
  unspecified site
    female 220
    male 222.0
LGSIL (low grade squamous intraepithelial lesion)
  anus 796.73
  cervix 795.03
  vagina 795.13
Liar, pathologic 301.7
Libman-Sacks disease or syndrome 710.0 [424.91]
Lice (infestation) 132.9
  body (pediculus corporis) 132.1
  crab 132.2
  head (pediculus capitis) 132.0
  mixed (classifiable to more than one of the categories 132.0–132.2) 132.3

Lice — *continued*
  pubic (pediculus pubis) 132.2
Lichen 697.9
  albus 701.0
  annularis 695.89
  atrophicus 701.0
  corneus obtusus 698.3
  myxedematous 701.8
  nitidus 697.1
  pilaris 757.39
    acquired 701.1
  planopilaris 697.0
  planus (acute) (chronicus) (hypertrophic) (verrucous) 697.0
    morphoeicus 701.0
    sclerosus (et atrophicus) 701.0
  ruber 696.4
    acuminatus 696.4
    moniliformis 697.8
    obtusus corneus 698.3
    of Wilson 697.0
    planus 697.0
  sclerosus (et atrophicus) 701.0
  scrofulosus (primary) (*see also* Tuberculosis) 017.0 ☑
  simplex (Vidal's) 698.3
    chronicus 698.3
    circumscriptus 698.3
  spinulosus 757.39
    mycotic 117.9
  striata 697.8
  urticatus 698.2
Lichenification 698.3
  nodular 698.3
Lichenoides tuberculosis (primary) — *see also* Tuberculosis 017.0 ☑
Lichtheim's disease or syndrome (subacute combined sclerosis with pernicious anemia) 281.0 [336.2]
Lien migrans 289.59
Lientery — *see also* Diarrhea 787.91
  infectious 009.2
Life circumstance problem NEC V62.89
Li-Fraumeni cancer syndrome V84.01
Ligament — *see* condition
Light-for-dates (infant) 764.0 ☑
  with signs of fetal malnutrition 764.1 ☑
  affecting management of pregnancy 656.5 ☑
Light-headedness 780.4
Lightning (effects) (shock) (stroke) (struck by) 994.0
  burn — *see* Burn, by site
  foot 266.2
Lightwood's disease or syndrome (renal tubular acidosis) 588.89
Lignac's disease (cystinosis) 270.0
Lignac (-Fanconi) syndrome (cystinosis) 270.0
Lignac (-de Toni) (-Fanconi) (-Debré) syndrome (cystinosis) 270.0
Ligneous thyroiditis 245.3
Likoff's syndrome (angina in menopausal women) 413.9
Limb — *see* condition
Limitation of joint motion — *see also* Stiffness, joint 719.5 ☑
  sacroiliac 724.6
Limit dextrinosis 271.0
Limited
  cardiac reserve — *see* Disease, heart
  duction, eye NEC 378.63
  mandibular range of motion 524.52
Lindau (-von Hippel) disease (angiomatosis retinocerebellosa) 759.6
Lindau's disease (retinocerebral angiomatosis) 759.6
Linea corneae senilis 371.41
Lines
  Beau's (transverse furrows on fingernails) 703.8
  Harris' 733.91
  Hudson-Stähli 371.11
  Stähli's 371.11
Lingua
  geographical 529.1
  nigra (villosa) 529.3

Lingua — *continued*
  plicata 529.5
    congenital 750.13
  tylosis 528.6
Lingual (tongue) — *see also* condition
  thyroid 759.2
Linitis (gastric) 535.4 ☑
  plastica (M8142/3) 151.9
Lioderma essentialis (cum melanosis et telangiectasia) 757.33
Lip — *see also* condition
  biting 528.9
Lipalgia 272.8
Lipedema — *see* Edema
Lipemia — *see also* Hyperlipidemia 272.4
  retina, retinalis 272.3
Lipidosis 272.7
  cephalin 272.7
  cerebral (infantile) (juvenile) (late) 330.1
  cerebroretinal 330.1 [362.71]
  cerebroside 272.7
  cerebrospinal 272.7
  chemically-induced 272.7
  cholesterol 272.7
  diabetic 250.8 ☑ [272.7]
    due to secondary diabetes 249.8 ☑ [272.7]
  dystopic (hereditary) 272.7
  glycolipid 272.7
  hepatosplenomegalic 272.3
  hereditary, dystopic 272.7
  sulfatide 330.0
Lipoadenoma (M8324/0) — *see* Neoplasm, by site, benign
Lipoblastoma (M8881/0) — *see* Lipoma, by site
Lipoblastomatosis (M8881/0) — *see* Lipoma, by site
Lipochondrodystrophy 277.5
Lipochrome histiocytosis (familial) 288.1
Lipodermatosclerosis 729.39
Lipodystrophia progressiva 272.6
Lipodystrophy (progressive) 272.6
  insulin 272.6
  intestinal 040.2
  mesenteric 567.82
Lipofibroma (M8851/0) — *see* Lipoma, by site
Lipoglycoproteinosis 272.8
Lipogranuloma, sclerosing 709.8
Lipogranulomatosis (disseminated) 272.8
  kidney 272.8
Lipoid — *see also* condition
  histiocytosis 272.7
    essential 272.7
  nephrosis (*see also* Nephrosis) 581.3
  proteinosis of Urbach 272.8
Lipoidemia — *see also* Hyperlipidemia 272.4
Lipoidosis — *see also* Lipidosis 272.7
Lipoma (M8850/0) 214.9
  breast (skin) 214.1
  face 214.0
  fetal (M8881/0) (*see also* Lipoma, by site)
    fat cell (M8880/0) — *see* Lipoma, by site
  infiltrating (M8856/0) — *see* Lipoma, by site
  intra-abdominal 214.3
  intramuscular (M8856/0) — *see* Lipoma, by site
  intrathoracic 214.2
  kidney 214.3
  mediastinum 214.2
  muscle 214.8
  peritoneum 214.3
  retroperitoneum 214.3
  skin 214.1
    face 214.0
  spermatic cord 214.4
  spindle cell (M8857/0) — *see* Lipoma, by site
  stomach 214.3
  subcutaneous tissue 214.1
    face 214.0
  thymus 214.2
  thyroid gland 214.2
Lipomatosis (dolorosa) 272.8
  epidural 214.8
  fetal (M8881/0) — *see* Lipoma, by site

☑ **Additional Digit Required** — Refer to the Tabular List for Digit Selection   ▽ **Subterms under main terms may continue to next column or page**

176 — Volume 2   ▶◀ Revised Text   ● New Line   ▲ Revised Code   **2013 ICD-9-CM**

Lipomatosis — *continued*
- Launois-Bensaude's 272.8

Lipomyohemangioma (M8860/0)
- specified site — *see* Neoplasm, connective tissue, benign
- unspecified site 223.0

Lipomyoma (M8860/0)
- specified site — *see* Neoplasm, connective tissue, benign
- unspecified site 223.0

Lipomyxoma (M8852/0) — *see* Lipoma, by site
Lipomyxosarcoma (M8852/3) — *see* Neoplasm, connective tissue, malignant
Lipophagocytosis 289.89
Lipoproteinemia (alpha) 272.4
- broad-beta 272.2
- floating-beta 272.2
- hyper-pre-beta 272.1

Lipoproteinosis (Rössle-Urbach-Wiethe) 272.8
Liposarcoma (M8850/3) — *see also* Neoplasm, connective tissue, malignant
- differentiated type (M8851/3) — *see* Neoplasm, connective tissue, malignant
- embryonal (M8852/3) — *see* Neoplasm, connective tissue, malignant
- mixed type (M8855/3) — *see* Neoplasm, connective tissue, malignant
- myxoid (M8852/3) — *see* Neoplasm, connective tissue, malignant
- pleomorphic (M8854/3) — *see* Neoplasm, connective tissue, malignant
- round cell (M8853/3) — *see* Neoplasm, connective tissue, malignant
- well differentiated type (M8851/3) — *see* Neoplasm, connective tissue, malignant

Liposynovitis prepatellaris 272.8
Lipping
- cervix 622.0
- spine (*see also* Spondylosis) 721.90
- vertebra (*see also* Spondylosis) 721.90

Lip pits (mucus), congenital 750.25
Lipschütz disease or ulcer 616.50
Lipuria 791.1
- bilharziasis 120.0

Liquefaction, vitreous humor 379.21
Lisping 307.9
Lissauer's paralysis 094.1
Lissencephalia, lissencephaly 742.2
Listerellose 027.0
Listeriose 027.0
Listeriosis 027.0
- congenital 771.2
- fetal 771.2
- suspected fetal damage affecting management of pregnancy 655.4 ☑

Listlessness 780.79
Lithemia 790.6
Lithiasis — *see also* Calculus
- hepatic (duct) — *see* Choledocholithiasis
- urinary 592.9

Lithopedion 779.9
- affecting management of pregnancy 656.8 ☑

Lithosis (occupational) 502
- with tuberculosis — *see* Tuberculosis, pulmonary

Lithuria 791.9
Litigation V62.5
Little
- league elbow 718.82
- stroke syndrome 435.9

Little's disease — *see* Palsy, cerebral
Littre's
- gland — *see* condition
- hernia — *see* Hernia, Littre's

Littritis — *see also* Urethritis 597.89
Livedo 782.61
- annularis 782.61
- racemose 782.61
- reticularis 782.61

Live flesh 781.0
Liver — *see also* condition
- donor V59.6

Livida, asphyxia
- newborn 768.6

Living
- alone V60.3
- with handicapped person V60.4

Lloyd's syndrome 258.1
Loa loa 125.2
Loasis 125.2
Lobe, lobar — *see* condition
Lobo's disease or blastomycosis 116.2
Lobomycosis 116.2
Lobotomy syndrome 310.0
Lobstein's disease (brittle bones and blue sclera) 756.51
Lobster-claw hand 755.58
Lobulation (congenital) — *see also* Anomaly, specified type NEC, by site
- kidney, fetal 753.3
- liver, abnormal 751.69
- spleen 759.0

Lobule, lobular — *see* condition
Local, localized — *see* condition
Locked bowel or intestine — *see also* Obstruction, intestine 560.9
Locked-in state 344.81
Locked twins 660.5 ☑
- affecting fetus or newborn 763.1

Locking
- joint (*see also* Derangement, joint) 718.90
- knee 717.9

Lockjaw — *see also* Tetanus 037
Locomotor ataxia (progressive) 094.0
Löffler's
- endocarditis 421.0
- eosinophilia or syndrome 518.3
- pneumonia 518.3
- syndrome (eosinophilic pneumonitis) 518.3

Löfgren's syndrome (sarcoidosis) 135
Loiasis 125.2
- eyelid 125.2 [373.6]

Loneliness V62.89
Lone star fever 082.8
Longitudinal stripes or grooves, nails 703.8
- congenital 757.5

Long labor 662.1 ☑
- affecting fetus or newborn 763.89
- first stage 662.0 ☑
- second stage 662.2 ☑

Long-term (current) (prophylactic) **drug use** V58.69
- antibiotics V58.62
- anticoagulants V58.61
- anti-inflammatories, non-steroidal (NSAID) V58.64
- antiplatelets/antithrombotics V58.63
- aspirin V58.66
- bisphosphonates V58.68
- high-risk medications NEC V58.69
- insulin V58.67
- methadone for pain control V58.69
- opiate analgesic V58.69
- pain killers V58.69
  - anti-inflammatories, non-steroidal (NSAID) V58.64
  - aspirin V58.66
- steroids V58.65
- tamoxifen V07.51

Loop
- intestine (*see also* Volvulus) 560.2
- intrascleral nerve 379.29
- vascular on papilla (optic) 743.57

Loose — *see also* condition
- body
  - in tendon sheath 727.82
  - joint 718.10
    - ankle 718.17
    - elbow 718.12
    - foot 718.17
    - hand 718.14
    - hip 718.15
    - knee 717.6
    - multiple sites 718.19
    - pelvic region 718.15
    - prosthetic implant — *see* Complications, mechanical
    - shoulder (region) 718.11
    - specified site NEC 718.18
    - wrist 718.13

Loose — *see also* condition — *continued*
- cartilage (joint) (*see also* Loose, body, joint) 718.1 ☑
  - knee 717.6
- facet (vertebral) 724.9
- prosthetic implant — *see* Complications, mechanical
- sesamoid, joint (*see also* Loose, body, joint) 718.1 ☑
- tooth, teeth 525.8

Loosening epiphysis 732.9
Looser (-Debray)-Milkman syndrome (osteomalacia with pseudofractures) 268.2
Lop ear (deformity) 744.29
Lorain's disease or syndrome (pituitary dwarfism) 253.3
Lorain-Levi syndrome (pituitary dwarfism) 253.3
Lordosis (acquired) (postural) 737.20
- congenital 754.2
- due to or associated with
  - Charcôt-Marie-Tooth disease 356.1 [737.42]
  - mucopolysaccharidosis 277.5 [737.42]
  - neurofibromatosis 237.71 [737.42]
  - osteitis
    - deformans 731.0 [737.42]
    - fibrosa cystica 252.01 [737.42]
  - osteoporosis (*see also* Osteoporosis) 733.00 [737.42]
  - poliomyelitis (*see also* Poliomyelitis) 138 [737.42]
  - tuberculosis (*see also* Tuberculosis) 015.0 ☑ [737.42]
- late effect of rickets 268.1 [737.42]
- postlaminectomy 737.21
- postsurgical NEC 737.22
- rachitic 268.1 [737.42]
- specified NEC 737.29
- tuberculous (*see also* Tuberculosis) 015.0 ☑ [737.42]

Loss
- appetite 783.0
  - hysterical 300.11
  - nonorganic origin 307.59
  - psychogenic 307.59
- blood — *see* Hemorrhage
- central vision 368.41
- consciousness 780.09
  - transient 780.2
- control, sphincter, rectum 787.60
  - nonorganic origin 307.7
- ear ossicle, partial 385.24
- elasticity, skin 782.8
- extremity or member, traumatic, current — *see* Amputation, traumatic
- fluid (acute) 276.50
  - with
    - hypernatremia 276.0
    - hyponatremia 276.1
  - fetus or newborn 775.5
- hair 704.00
- hearing (*see also* Deafness)
  - central 389.14
  - conductive (air) 389.00
    - with sensorineural hearing loss 389.20
      - bilateral 389.22
      - unilateral 389.21
    - bilateral 389.06
    - combined types 389.08
    - external ear 389.01
    - inner ear 389.04
    - middle ear 389.03
    - multiple types 389.08
    - tympanic membrane 389.02
    - unilateral 389.05
  - mixed conductive and sensorineural 389.20
    - bilateral 389.22
    - unilateral 389.21
  - mixed type 389.20
    - bilateral 389.22
    - unilateral 389.21
  - nerve
    - bilateral 389.12

Loss — *continued*
- hearing (*see also* Deafness) — *continued*
  - nerve — *continued*
    - unilateral 389.13
  - neural
    - bilateral 389.12
    - unilateral 389.13
  - noise-induced 388.12
  - perceptive NEC (*see also* Loss, hearing, sensorineural) 389.10
  - sensorineural 389.10
    - with conductive hearing loss 389.20
      - bilateral 389.22
      - unilateral 389.21
    - asymmetrical 389.16
      - bilateral 389.18
    - central 389.14
    - neural 389.12
      - bilateral 389.12
      - unilateral 389.13
    - sensory
      - bilateral 389.11
      - unilateral 389.17
    - unilateral 389.15
  - sensory
    - bilateral 389.11
    - unilateral 389.17
  - specified type NEC 389.8
  - sudden NEC 388.2
- height 781.91
- labyrinthine reactivity (unilateral) 386.55
  - bilateral 386.56
- memory (*see also* Amnesia) 780.93
  - mild, following organic brain damage 310.89
- mind (*see also* Psychosis) 298.9
- occlusal vertical dimension 524.37
- organ or part — *see* Absence, by site, acquired
- recurrent pregnancy — *see* Pregnancy, management affected by, abortion, habitual
- sensation 782.0
- sense of
  - smell (*see also* Disturbance, sensation) 781.1
  - taste (*see also* Disturbance, sensation) 781.1
  - touch (*see also* Disturbance, sensation) 781.1
- sight (acquired) (complete) (congenital) — *see* Blindness
- spinal fluid
  - headache 349.0
- substance of
  - bone (*see also* Osteoporosis) 733.00
  - cartilage 733.99
  - ear 380.32
  - vitreous (humor) 379.26
- tooth, teeth
  - acquired 525.10
    - due to
      - caries 525.13
      - extraction 525.10
      - periodontal disease 525.12
      - specified NEC 525.19
      - trauma 525.11
- vision, visual (*see also* Blindness) 369.9
  - both eyes (*see also* Blindness, both eyes) 369.3
  - complete (*see also* Blindness, both eyes) 369.00
  - one eye 369.8
  - sudden 368.11
  - transient 368.12
- vitreous 379.26
- voice (*see also* Aphonia) 784.41
- weight (cause unknown) 783.21

Lou Gehrig's disease 335.20
Louis-Bar syndrome (ataxia-telangiectasia) 334.8
Louping ill 063.1
Lousiness — *see* Lice
Low
- back syndrome 724.2
- basal metabolic rate (BMR) 794.7

☑ **Additional Digit Required** — Refer to the Tabular List for Digit Selection   🆆 **Subterms under main terms may continue to next column or page**

2013 ICD-9-CM   ▶◀ **Revised Text**   ● **New Line**   ▲ **Revised Code**   **Volume 2 — 177**

Lymphohistiocytosis, familial hemophago-cytic 288.4
Lymphoid — *see* condition
Lympholeukoblastoma (M9850/3) 207.8 ☑
Lympholeukosarcoma (M9850/3) 207.8 ☑
Lymphoma (malignant) (M9590/3) 202.8 ☑

> *Note* — *Use the following fifth-digit subclassification with categories 200–202:*
>
> 0 *unspecified site, extranodal and solid organ sites*
> 1 *lymph nodes of head, face, and neck*
> 2 *intrathoracic lymph nodes*
> 3 *intra–abdominal lymph nodes*
> 4 *lymph nodes of axilla and upper limb*
> 5 *lymph nodes of inguinal region and lower limb*
> 6 *intrapelvic lymph nodes*
> 7 *spleen*
> 8 *lymph nodes of multiple sites*

   benign (M9590/0) — *see* Neoplasm, by site, benign
   Burkitt's type (lymphoblastic) (undifferenti-ated) (M9750/3) 200.2 ☑
   Castleman's (mediastinal lymph node hyper-plasia) 785.6
   centroblastic-centrocytic
      diffuse (M9614/3) 202.8 ☑
      follicular (M9692/3) 202.0 ☑
   centroblastic type (diffuse) (M9632/3) 202.8 ☑
      follicular (M9697/3) 202.0 ☑
   centrocytic (M9622/3) 202.8 ☑
   compound (M9613/3) 200.8 ☑
   convoluted cell type (lymphoblastic) (M9602/3) 202.8 ☑
   diffuse NEC (M9590/3) 202.8 ☑
      large B cell 202.8 ☑
   follicular (giant) (M9690/3) 202.0 ☑
      center cell (diffuse) (M9615/3) 202.8 ☑
         cleaved (diffuse) (M9623/3) 202.8 ☑
            follicular (M9695/3) 202.0 ☑
         non-cleaved (diffuse) (M9633/3) 202.8 ☑
            follicular (M9698/3) 202.0 ☑
      centroblastic-centrocytic (M9692/3) 202.0 ☑
      centroblastic type (M9697/3) 202.0 ☑
      large cell 202.0 ☑
      lymphocytic
         intermediate differentiation (M9694/3) 202.0 ☑
         poorly differentiated (M9696/3) 202.0 ☑
      mixed (cell type) (lymphocytic-histiocyt-ic) (small cell and large cell) (M9691/3) 202.0 ☑
      germinocytic (M9622/3) 202.8 ☑
   giant, follicular or follicle (M9690/3) 202.0 ☑
   histiocytic (diffuse) (M9640/3) 200.0 ☑
      nodular (M9642/3) 200.0 ☑
      pleomorphic cell type (M9641/3) 200.0 ☑
   Hodgkin's (M9650/3) (*see also* Disease, Hodgkin's) 201.9 ☑
   immunoblastic (type) (M9612/3) 200.8 ☑
   large cell (M9640/3) 200.7 ☑
      anaplastic 200.6 ☑
      nodular (M9642/3) 202.0 ☑
      pleomorphic cell type (M9641/3) 200.0 ☑
   lymphoblastic (diffuse) (M9630/3) 200.1 ☑
      Burkitt's type (M9750/3) 200.2 ☑
      convoluted cell type (M9602/3) 202.8 ☑
   lymphocytic (cell type) (diffuse) (M9620/3) 200.1 ☑

Lymphoma — *continued*
   lymphocytic — *continued*
      with plasmacytoid differentiation, dif-fuse (M9611/3) 200.8 ☑
      intermediate differentiation (diffuse) (M9621/3) 200.1 ☑
         follicular (M9694/3) 202.0 ☑
         nodular (M9694/3) 202.0 ☑
      nodular (M9690/3) 202.0 ☑
      poorly differentiated (diffuse) (M9630/3) 200.1 ☑
         follicular (M9696/3) 202.0 ☑
         nodular (M9696/3) 202.0 ☑
      well differentiated (diffuse) (M9620/3) 200.1 ☑
         follicular (M9693/3) 202.0 ☑
         nodular (M9693/3) 202.0 ☑
   lymphocytic-histiocytic, mixed (diffuse) (M9613/3) 200.8 ☑
      follicular (M9691/3) 202.0 ☑
      nodular (M9691/3) 202.0 ☑
   lymphoplasmacytoid type (M9611/3) 200.8 ☑
   lymphosarcoma type (M9610/3) 200.1 ☑
   macrofollicular (M9690/3) 202.0 ☑
   mantle cell 200.4 ☑
   marginal zone 200.3 ☑
      extranodal B-cell 200.3 ☑
      nodal B-cell 200.3 ☑
      splenic B-cell 200.3 ☑
   mixed cell type (diffuse) (M9613/3) 200.8 ☑
      follicular (M9691/3) 202.0 ☑
      nodular (M9691/3) 202.0 ☑
   nodular (M9690/3) 202.0 ☑
      histiocytic (M9642/3) 200.0 ☑
      lymphocytic (M9690/3) 202.0 ☑
         intermediate differentiation (M9694/3) 202.0 ☑
         poorly differentiated (M9696/3) 202.0 ☑
      mixed (cell type) (lymphocytic-histiocyt-ic) (small cell and large cell) (M9691/3) 202.0 ☑
   non-Hodgkin's type NEC (M9591/3) 202.8 ☑
   peripheral T-cell 202.7 ☑
   primary central nervous system 200.5 ☑
   reticulum cell (type) (M9640/3) 200.0 ☑
   small cell and large cell, mixed (diffuse) (M9613/3) 200.8 ☑
      follicular (M9691/3) 202.0 ☑
      nodular (M9691/3) 202.0 ☑
   stem cell (type) (M9601/3) 202.8 ☑
   T-cell 202.1 ☑
      peripheral 202.7 ☑
   undifferentiated (cell type) (non-Burkitt's) (M9600/3) 202.8 ☑
      Burkitt's type (M9750/3) 200.2 ☑
Lymphomatosis (M9590/3) — *see also* Lym-phoma
   granulomatous 099.1
Lymphopathia
   venereum 099.1
   veneris 099.1
Lymphopenia 288.51
   familial 279.2
Lymphoreticulosis, benign (of inoculation) 078.3
Lymphorrhea 457.8
Lymphosarcoma (M9610/3) 200.1 ☑
   diffuse (M9610/3) 200.1 ☑
      with plasmacytoid differentiation (M9611/3) 200.8 ☑
      lymphoplasmacytic (M9611/3) 200.8 ☑
   follicular (giant) (M9690/3) 202.0 ☑
      lymphoblastic (M9696/3) 202.0 ☑
      lymphocytic, intermediate differentia-tion (M9694/3) 202.0 ☑
      mixed cell type (M9691/3) 202.0 ☑
   giant follicular (M9690/3) 202.0 ☑
   Hodgkin's (M9650/3) 201.9 ☑
   immunoblastic (M9612/3) 200.8 ☑
   lymphoblastic (diffuse) (M9630/3) 200.1 ☑
      follicular (M9696/3) 202.0 ☑
      nodular (M9696/3) 202.0 ☑

Lymphosarcoma — *continued*
   lymphocytic (diffuse) (M9620/3) 200.1 ☑
      intermediate differentiation (diffuse) (M9621/3) 200.1 ☑
         follicular (M9694/3) 202.0 ☑
         nodular (M9694/3) 202.0 ☑
   mixed cell type (diffuse) (M9613/3) 200.8 ☑
      follicular (M9691/3) 202.0 ☑
      nodular (M9691/3) 202.0 ☑
   nodular (M9690/3) 202.0 ☑
      lymphoblastic (M9696/3) 202.0 ☑
      lymphocytic, intermediate differentia-tion (M9694/3) 202.0 ☑
      mixed cell type (M9691/3) 202.0 ☑
   prolymphocytic (M9631/3) 200.1 ☑
   reticulum cell (M9640/3) 200.0 ☑
Lymphostasis 457.8
Lypemania — *see also* Melancholia 296.2 ☑
Lyssa 071

<h2 align="center">M</h2>

Macacus ear 744.29
Maceration
   fetus (cause not stated) 779.9
   wet feet, tropical (syndrome) 991.4
Machado-Joseph disease 334.8
Machupo virus hemorrhagic fever 078.7
Macleod's syndrome (abnormal transradiancy, one lung) 492.8
Macrocephalia, macrocephaly 756.0
Macrocheilia (congenital) 744.81
Macrochilia (congenital) 744.81
Macrocolon (congenital) 751.3
Macrocornea 743.41
   associated with buphthalmos 743.22
Macrocytic — *see* condition
Macrocytosis 289.89
Macrodactylia, macrodactylism (fingers) (thumbs) 755.57
   toes 755.65
Macrodontia 520.2
Macroencephaly 742.4
Macrogenia 524.05
Macrogenitosomia (female) (male) (praecox) 255.2
Macrogingivae 523.8
Macroglobulinemia (essential) (idiopathic) (monoclonal) (primary) (syndrome) (Waldenström's) 273.3
Macroglossia (congenital) 750.15
   acquired 529.8
Macrognathia, macrognathism (congenital) 524.00
   mandibular 524.02
      alveolar 524.72
   maxillary 524.01
      alveolar 524.71
Macrogyria (congenital) 742.4
Macrohydrocephalus — *see also* Hydro-cephalus 331.4
Macromastia — *see also* Hypertrophy, breast 611.1
Macrophage activation syndrome 288.4
Macropsia 368.14
Macrosigmoid 564.7
   congenital 751.3
Macrospondylitis, acromegalic 253.0
Macrostomia (congenital) 744.83
Macrotia (external ear) (congenital) 744.22
Macula
   cornea, corneal
      congenital 743.43
         interfering with vision 743.42
      interfering with central vision 371.03
      not interfering with central vision 371.02
   degeneration (*see also* Degeneration, mac-ula) 362.50
      hereditary (*see also* Dystrophy, retina) 362.70
   edema, cystoid 362.53
Maculae ceruleae 132.1
Macules and papules 709.8
Maculopathy, toxic 362.55
Madarosis 374.55

Madelung's
   deformity (radius) 755.54
   disease (lipomatosis) 272.8
   lipomatosis 272.8
Madness — *see also* Psychosis 298.9
   myxedema (acute) 293.0
   subacute 293.1
Madura
   disease (actinomycotic) 039.9
      mycotic 117.4
   foot (actinomycotic) 039.4
      mycotic 117.4
Maduromycosis (actinomycotic) 039.9
   mycotic 117.4
Maffucci's syndrome (dyschondroplasia with hemangiomas) 756.4
Magenblase syndrome 306.4
Main en griffe (acquired) 736.06
   congenital 755.59
Maintenance
   chemotherapy regimen or treatment V58.11
   dialysis regimen or treatment
      extracorporeal (renal) V56.0
      peritoneal V56.8
      renal V56.0
   drug therapy or regimen
      chemotherapy, antineoplastic V58.11
      immunotherapy, antineoplastic V58.12
   external fixation NEC V54.89
   methadone 304.00
   radiotherapy V58.0
   traction NEC V54.89
Majocchi's
   disease (purpura annularis telangiectodes) 709.1
   granuloma 110.6
Major — *see* condition
Mal
   cerebral (idiopathic) (*see also* Epilepsy) 345.9 ☑
   comital (*see also* Epilepsy) 345.9 ☑
   de los pintos (*see also* Pinta) 103.9
   de Meleda 757.39
   de mer 994.6
   lie — *see* Presentation, fetal
   perforant (*see also* Ulcer, lower extremity) 707.15
Malabar itch 110.9
   beard 110.0
   foot 110.4
   scalp 110.0
Malabsorption 579.9
   calcium 579.8
   carbohydrate 579.8
   disaccharide 271.3
   drug-induced 579.8
   due to bacterial overgrowth 579.8
   fat 579.8
   folate, congenital 281.2
   galactose 271.1
   glucose-galactose (congenital) 271.3
   intestinal 579.9
   isomaltose 271.3
   lactose (hereditary) 271.3
   methionine 270.4
   monosaccharide 271.8
   postgastrectomy 579.3
   postsurgical 579.3
   protein 579.8
   sucrose (-isomaltose) (congenital) 271.3
   syndrome 579.9
      postgastrectomy 579.3
      postsurgical 579.3
Malacia, bone 268.2
   juvenile (*see also* Rickets) 268.0
   Kienböck's (juvenile) (lunate) (wrist) 732.3
      adult 732.8
Malacoplakia
   bladder 596.89
   colon 569.89
   pelvis (kidney) 593.89
   ureter 593.89
   urethra 599.84
Malacosteon 268.2
   juvenile (*see also* Rickets) 268.0
Maladaptation — *see* Maladjustment

Maladie de Roger 745.4
Maladjustment
conjugal V61.10
  involving
    divorce V61.03
    estrangement V61.09
educational V62.3
family V61.9
  specified circumstance NEC V61.8
marital V61.10
  involving
    divorce V61.03
    estrangement V61.09
occupational V62.29
  current military deployment status
    V62.21
simple, adult (see also Reaction, adjustment)
  309.9
situational acute (see also Reaction, adjustment) 309.9
social V62.4
Malaise 780.79
Malakoplakia — see Malacoplakia
Malaria, malarial (fever) 084.6
algid 084.9
any type, with
  algid malaria 084.9
  blackwater fever 084.8
  fever
    blackwater 084.8
    hemoglobinuric (bilious) 084.8
  hemoglobinuria, malarial 084.8
  hepatitis 084.9 [573.2]
  nephrosis 084.9 [581.81]
  pernicious complication NEC 084.9
    cardiac 084.9
    cerebral 084.9
cardiac 084.9
carrier (suspected) of V02.9
cerebral 084.9
complicating pregnancy, childbirth, or
  puerperium 647.4 ☑
congenital 771.2
congestion, congestive 084.6
  brain 084.9
continued 084.0
estivo-autumnal 084.0
falciparum (malignant tertian) 084.0
hematinuria 084.8
hematuria 084.8
hemoglobinuria 084.8
hemorrhagic 084.6
induced (therapeutically) 084.7
  accidental — see Malaria, by type
liver 084.9 [573.2]
malariae (quartan) 084.2
malignant (tertian) 084.0
mixed infections 084.5
monkey 084.4
ovale 084.3
pernicious, acute 084.0
Plasmodium, P.
  falciparum 084.0
  malariae 084.2
  ovale 084.3
  vivax 084.1
quartan 084.2
quotidian 084.0
recurrent 084.6
  induced (therapeutically) 084.7
    accidental — see Malaria, by type
remittent 084.6
specified types NEC 084.4
spleen 084.6
subtertian 084.0
tertian (benign) 084.1
  malignant 084.0
tropical 084.0
typhoid 084.6
vivax (benign tertian) 084.1
Malassez's disease (testicular cyst) 608.89
Malassimilation 579.9
Maldescent, testis 752.51
Maldevelopment — see also Anomaly, by site
brain 742.9
colon 751.5

Maldevelopment — see also Anomaly, by site
  — continued
hip (joint) 755.63
  congenital dislocation (see also Disloca-
    tion, hip, congenital) 754.30
mastoid process 756.0
middle ear, except ossicles 744.03
  ossicles 744.04
newborn (not malformation) 764.9 ☑
ossicles, ear 744.04
spine 756.10
toe 755.66
Male type pelvis 755.69
with disproportion (fetopelvic) 653.2 ☑
  affecting fetus or newborn 763.1
  causing obstructed labor 660.1 ☑
    affecting fetus or newborn 763.1
Malformation (congenital) — see also
  Anomaly
arteriovenous
  pulmonary 747.32
bone 756.9
bursa 756.9
Chiari
  type I 348.4
  type II (see also Spina bifida) 741.0 ☑
  type III 742.0
  type IV 742.2
circulatory system NEC 747.9
  specified type NEC 747.89
cochlea 744.05
digestive system NEC 751.9
  lower 751.5
  specified type NEC 751.8
  upper 750.9
eye 743.9
gum 750.9
heart NEC 746.9
  specified type NEC 746.89
  valve 746.9
internal ear 744.05
joint NEC 755.9
  specified type NEC 755.8
Mondini's (congenital) (malformation,
  cochlea) 744.05
muscle 756.9
nervous system (central) 742.9
pelvic organs or tissues
  in pregnancy or childbirth 654.9 ☑
    affecting fetus or newborn 763.89
    causing obstructed labor 660.2 ☑
      affecting fetus or newborn 763.1
placenta (see also Placenta, abnormal)
  656.7 ☑
respiratory organs 748.9
  specified type NEC 748.8
Rieger's 743.44
sense organs NEC 742.9
  specified type NEC 742.8
skin 757.9
  specified type NEC 757.8
spinal cord 742.9
teeth, tooth NEC 520.9
tendon 756.9
throat 750.9
umbilical cord (complicating delivery)
  663.9 ☑
  affecting fetus or newborn 762.6
umbilicus 759.9
urinary system NEC 753.9
  specified type NEC 753.8
venous — see Anomaly, vein
Malfunction — see also Dysfunction
arterial graft 996.1
cardiac pacemaker 996.01
catheter device — see Complications, mechanical, catheter
colostomy 569.62
  valve 569.62
cystostomy 596.82
  infection 596.81
  mechanical 596.82
  specified complication NEC 596.83
device, implant, or graft NEC — see Complications, mechanical
enteric stoma 569.62

Malfunction — see also Dysfunction —
  continued
enterostomy 569.62
esophagostomy 530.87
gastroenteric 536.8
gastrostomy 536.42
ileostomy
  valve 569.62
nephrostomy 997.5
pacemaker — see Complications, mechanical, pacemaker
prosthetic device, internal — see Complications, mechanical
tracheostomy 519.02
valve
  colostomy 569.62
  ileostomy 569.62
vascular graft or shunt 996.1
Malgaigne's fracture (closed) 808.43
open 808.53
Malherbe's
calcifying epithelioma (M8110/0) — see
  Neoplasm, skin, benign
tumor (M8110/0) — see Neoplasm, skin,
  benign
Malibu disease 919.8
infected 919.9
Malignancy (M8000/3) — see Neoplasm, by
  site, malignant
Malignant — see condition
Malingerer, malingering V65.2
Mallet, finger (acquired) 736.1
congenital 755.59
late effect of rickets 268.1
Malleus 024
Mallory's bodies 034.1
Mallory-Weiss syndrome 530.7
Malnutrition (calorie) 263.9
complicating pregnancy 648.9 ☑
degree
  first 263.1
  second 263.0
  third 262
  mild (protein) 263.1
  moderate (protein) 263.0
  severe 261
    protein-calorie 262
fetus 764.2 ☑
  "light-for-dates" 764.1 ☑
following gastrointestinal surgery 579.3
intrauterine or fetal 764.2 ☑
  fetus or infant "light-for-dates" 764.1 ☑
lack of care, or neglect (child) (infant) 995.52
  adult 995.84
malignant 260
mild (protein) 263.1
moderate (protein) 263.0
protein 260
protein-calorie 263.9
  mild 263.1
  moderate 263.0
  severe 262
  specified type NEC 263.8
severe 261
  protein-calorie NEC 262
Malocclusion (teeth) 524.4
angle's class I 524.21
angle's class II 524.22
angle's class III 524.23
due to
  abnormal swallowing 524.59
  accessory teeth (causing crowding)
    524.31
  dentofacial abnormality NEC 524.89
  impacted teeth (causing crowding) 520.6
  missing teeth 524.30
  mouth breathing 524.59
  sleep postures 524.59
  supernumerary teeth (causing crowding)
    524.31
  thumb sucking 524.59
  tongue, lip, or finger habits 524.59
  temporomandibular (joint) 524.69
Malposition
cardiac apex (congenital) 746.87
cervix — see Malposition, uterus

Malposition — continued
congenital
  adrenal (gland) 759.1
  alimentary tract 751.8
    lower 751.5
    upper 750.8
  aorta 747.21
  appendix 751.5
  arterial trunk 747.29
  artery (peripheral) NEC (see also Malposi-
    tion, congenital, peripheral vascu-
    lar system) 747.60
    coronary 746.85
    pulmonary 747.39
  auditory canal 744.29
    causing impairment of hearing
      744.02
  auricle (ear) 744.29
    causing impairment of hearing
      744.02
  cervical 744.43
  biliary duct or passage 751.69
  bladder (mucosa) 753.8
    exteriorized or extroverted 753.5
  brachial plexus 742.8
  brain tissue 742.4
  breast 757.6
  bronchus 748.3
  cardiac apex 746.87
  cecum 751.5
  clavicle 755.51
  colon 751.5
  digestive organ or tract NEC 751.8
    lower 751.5
    upper 750.8
  ear (auricle) (external) 744.29
    ossicles 744.04
  endocrine (gland) NEC 759.2
  epiglottis 748.3
  Eustachian tube 744.24
  eye 743.8
  facial features 744.89
  fallopian tube 752.19
  finger(s) 755.59
    supernumerary 755.01
  foot 755.67
  gallbladder 751.69
  gastrointestinal tract 751.8
  genitalia, genital organ(s) or tract
    female 752.89
      external 752.49
      internal NEC 752.89
    male 752.89
      penis 752.69
      scrotal transposition 752.81
  glottis 748.3
  hand 755.59
  heart 746.87
    dextrocardia 746.87
      with complete transposition of
        viscera 759.3
  hepatic duct 751.69
  hip (joint) (see also Dislocation, hip,
    congenital) 754.30
  intestine (large) (small) 751.5
    with anomalous adhesions, fixation,
      or malrotation 751.4
  joint NEC 755.8
  kidney 753.3
  larynx 748.3
  limb 755.8
    lower 755.69
    upper 755.59
  liver 751.69
  lung (lobe) 748.69
  nail(s) 757.5
  nerve 742.8
  nervous system NEC 742.8
  nose, nasal (septum) 748.1
  organ or site NEC — see Anomaly, spec-
    ified type NEC, by site
  ovary 752.0
  pancreas 751.7
  parathyroid (gland) 759.2
  patella 755.64
  peripheral vascular system 747.60

☑ **Additional Digit Required** — Refer to the Tabular List for Digit Selection ⓦ **Subterms under main terms may continue to next column or page**

180 — Volume 2 ▶◄ Revised Text ● New Line ▲ Revised Code 2013 ICD-9-CM

Malposition — *continued*
  congenital — *continued*
    peripheral vascular system — *continued*
      gastrointestinal 747.61
      lower limb 747.64
      renal 747.62
      specified NEC 747.69
      spinal 747.82
      upper limb 747.63
    pituitary (gland) 759.2
    respiratory organ or system NEC 748.9
    rib (cage) 756.3
      supernumerary in cervical region 756.2
    scapula 755.59
    shoulder 755.59
    spinal cord 742.59
    spine 756.19
    spleen 759.0
    sternum 756.3
    stomach 750.7
    symphysis pubis 755.69
    testis (undescended) 752.51
    thymus (gland) 759.2
    thyroid (gland) (tissue) 759.2
      cartilage 748.3
    toe(s) 755.66
      supernumerary 755.02
    tongue 750.19
    trachea 748.3
    uterus 752.39
    vein(s) (peripheral) NEC (*see also* Malposition, congenital, peripheral vascular system) 747.60
      great 747.49
      portal 747.49
      pulmonary 747.49
      vena cava (inferior) (superior) 747.49
  device, implant, or graft — *see* Complications, mechanical
  fetus NEC (*see also* Presentation, fetal) 652.9 ☑
    with successful version 652.1 ☑
    affecting fetus or newborn 763.1
    before labor, affecting fetus or newborn 761.7
    causing obstructed labor 660.0 ☑
    in multiple gestation (one fetus or more) 652.6 ☑
      with locking 660.5 ☑
      causing obstructed labor 660.0 ☑
  gallbladder (*see also* Disease, gallbladder) 575.8
  gastrointestinal tract 569.89
    congenital 751.8
  heart (*see also* Malposition, congenital, heart) 746.87
  intestine 569.89
    congenital 751.5
  pelvic organs or tissues
    in pregnancy or childbirth 654.4 ☑
      affecting fetus or newborn 763.89
      causing obstructed labor 660.2 ☑
        affecting fetus or newborn 763.1
  placenta — *see* Placenta, previa
  stomach 537.89
    congenital 750.7
  tooth, teeth 524.30
    with impaction 520.6
  uterus (acquired) (acute) (adherent) (any degree) (asymptomatic) (postinfectional) (postpartal, old) 621.6
    anteflexion or anteversion (*see also* Anteversion, uterus) 621.6
    congenital 752.39
    flexion 621.6
      lateral (*see also* Lateroversion, uterus) 621.6
    in pregnancy or childbirth 654.4 ☑
      affecting fetus or newborn 763.89
      causing obstructed labor 660.2 ☑
        affecting fetus or newborn 763.1
    inversion 621.6
    lateral (flexion) (version) (*see also* Lateroversion, uterus)

Malposition — *continued*
  uterus — *continued*
    lateroflexion (*see also* Lateroversion, uterus) 621.6
    lateroversion (*see also* Lateroversion, uterus) 621.6
    retroflexion or retroversion (*see also* Retroversion, uterus) 621.6
Malposture 729.90
Malpresentation, fetus — *see also* Presentation, fetal 652.9 ☑
Malrotation
  cecum 751.4
  colon 751.4
  intestine 751.4
  kidney 753.3
MALT (mucosa associated lymphoid tissue) 200.3 ☑
Malta fever — *see also* Brucellosis 023.9
Maltosuria 271.3
Maltreatment (of)
  adult 995.80
    emotional 995.82
    multiple forms 995.85
    neglect (nutritional) 995.84
    physical 995.81
    psychological 995.82
    sexual 995.83
  child 995.50
    emotional 995.51
    multiple forms 995.59
    neglect (nutritional) 995.52
    physical 995.54
      shaken infant syndrome 995.55
    psychological 995.51
    sexual 995.53
  spouse (*see also* Maltreatment, adult) 995.80
Malt workers' lung 495.4
Malum coxae senilis 715.25
Malunion, fracture 733.81
Mammillitis — *see also* Mastitis 611.0
  puerperal, postpartum 675.2 ☑
Mammitis — *see also* Mastitis 611.0
  puerperal, postpartum 675.2 ☑
Mammographic
  calcification 793.89
  calculus 793.89
  microcalcification 793.81
Mammoplasia 611.1
Management
  contraceptive V25.9
    specified type NEC V25.8
  procreative V26.9
    specified type NEC V26.89
Mangled NEC — *see also* nature and site of injury 959.9
Mania (monopolar) — *see also* Psychosis, affective 296.0 ☑
  alcoholic (acute) (chronic) 291.9
  Bell's — *see* Mania, chronic
  chronic 296.0 ☑
    recurrent episode 296.1 ☑
    single episode 296.0 ☑
  compulsive 300.3
  delirious (acute) 296.0 ☑
    recurrent episode 296.1 ☑
    single episode 296.0 ☑
  epileptic (*see also* Epilepsy) 345.4 ☑
  hysterical 300.10
  inhibited 296.89
  puerperal (after delivery) 296.0 ☑
    recurrent episode 296.1 ☑
    single episode 296.0 ☑
  recurrent episode 296.1 ☑
  senile 290.8
  single episode 296.0 ☑
  stupor 296.89
  stuporous 296.89
  unproductive 296.89
Manic-depressive insanity, psychosis, reaction, or syndrome — *see also* Psychosis, affective 296.80
  circular (alternating) 296.7
    currently
      depressed 296.5 ☑
      episode unspecified 296.7

Manic-depressive insanity, psychosis, reaction, or syndrome — *see also* Psychosis, affective — *continued*
  circular — *continued*
    currently — *continued*
      hypomanic, previously depressed 296.4 ☑
      manic 296.4 ☑
    mixed 296.6 ☑
  depressed (type), depressive 296.2 ☑
    atypical 296.82
    recurrent episode 296.3 ☑
    single episode 296.2 ☑
  hypomanic 296.0 ☑
    recurrent episode 296.1 ☑
    single episode 296.0 ☑
  manic 296.0 ☑
    atypical 296.81
    recurrent episode 296.1 ☑
    single episode 296.0 ☑
  mixed NEC 296.89
  perplexed 296.89
  stuporous 296.89
Manifestations, rheumatoid
  lungs 714.81
  pannus — *see* Arthritis, rheumatoid
  subcutaneous nodules — *see* Arthritis, rheumatoid
Mankowsky's syndrome (familial dysplastic osteopathy) 731.2
Mannoheptulosuria 271.8
Mannosidosis 271.8
Manson's
  disease (schistosomiasis) 120.1
  pyosis (pemphigus contagiosus) 684
  schistosomiasis 120.1
Mansonellosis 125.5
Manual — *see* condition
Maple bark disease 495.6
Maple bark-strippers' lung 495.6
Maple syrup (urine) disease or syndrome 270.3
Marable's syndrome (celiac artery compression) 447.4
Marasmus 261
  brain 331.9
  due to malnutrition 261
  intestinal 569.89
  nutritional 261
  senile 797
  tuberculous NEC (*see also* Tuberculosis) 011.9 ☑
Marble
  bones 756.52
  skin 782.61
Marburg disease (virus) 078.89
March
  foot 733.94
  hemoglobinuria 283.2
Marchand multiple nodular hyperplasia (liver) 571.5
Marchesani (-Weill) syndrome (brachymorphism and ectopia lentis) 759.89
Marchiafava (-Bignami) disease or syndrome 341.8
Marchiafava-Micheli syndrome (paroxysmal nocturnal hemoglobinuria) 283.2
Marcus Gunn's syndrome (jaw-winking syndrome) 742.8
Marfan's
  congenital syphilis 090.49
  disease 090.49
  syndrome (arachnodactyly) 759.82
    meaning congenital syphilis 090.49
    with luxation of lens 090.49 [379.32]
Marginal
  implantation, placenta — *see* Placenta, previa
  placenta — *see* Placenta, previa
  sinus (hemorrhage) (rupture) 641.2 ☑
    affecting fetus or newborn 762.1
Marie's
  cerebellar ataxia 334.2
  syndrome (acromegaly) 253.0

Marie-Bamberger disease or syndrome (hypertrophic) (pulmonary) (secondary) 731.2
  idiopathic (acropachyderma) 757.39
  primary (acropachyderma) 757.39
Marie-Charcôt-Tooth neuropathic atrophy, muscle 356.1
Marie-Strümpell arthritis or disease (ankylosing spondylitis) 720.0
Marihuana, marijuana
  abuse (*see also* Abuse, drugs, nondependent) 305.2 ☑
  dependence (*see also* Dependence) 304.3 ☑
Marion's disease (bladder neck obstruction) 596.0
Marital conflict V61.10
Mark
  port wine 757.32
  raspberry 757.32
  strawberry 757.32
  stretch 701.3
  tattoo 709.09
Maroteaux-Lamy syndrome (mucopolysaccharidosis VI) 277.5
Marriage license examination V70.3
Marrow (bone)
  arrest 284.9
  megakaryocytic 287.30
  poor function 289.9
Marseilles fever 082.1
Marshall's (hidrotic) **ectodermal dysplasia** 757.31
Marsh's disease (exophthalmic goiter) 242.0 ☑
Marsh fever — *see also* Malaria 084.6
Martin-Albright syndrome (pseudohypoparathyroidism) 275.49
Martin's disease 715.27
Martorell-Fabre syndrome (pulseless disease) 446.7
Masculinization, female, with adrenal hyperplasia 255.2
Masculinovoblastoma (M8670/0) 220
Masochism 302.83
Masons' lung 502
Mass
  abdominal 789.3 ☑
  anus 787.99
  bone 733.90
  breast 611.72
  cheek 784.2
  chest 786.6
  cystic — *see* Cyst
  ear 388.8
  epigastric 789.3 ☑
  eye 379.92
  female genital organ 625.8
  gum 784.2
  head 784.2
  intracranial 784.2
  joint 719.60
    ankle 719.67
    elbow 719.62
    foot 719.67
    hand 719.64
    hip 719.65
    knee 719.66
    multiple sites 719.69
    pelvic region 719.65
    shoulder (region) 719.61
    specified site NEC 719.68
    wrist 719.63
  kidney (*see also* Disease, kidney) 593.9
  lung 786.6
  lymph node 785.6
  malignant (M8000/3) — *see* Neoplasm, by site, malignant
  mediastinal 786.6
  mouth 784.2
  muscle (limb) 729.89
  neck 784.2
  nose or sinus 784.2
  palate 784.2
  pelvis, pelvic 789.3 ☑
  penis 607.89
  perineum 625.8

☑ Additional Digit Required — Refer to the Tabular List for Digit Selection   ⩔ Subterms under main terms may continue to next column or page

2013 ICD-9-CM   ▶◀ Revised Text   ● New Line   ▲ Revised Code   Volume 2 — 181

Mass — *continued*
rectum 787.99
scrotum 608.89
skin 782.2
specified organ NEC — *see* Disease of specified organ or site
splenic 789.2
substernal 786.6
thyroid (*see also* Goiter) 240.9
superficial (localized) 782.2
testes 608.89
throat 784.2
tongue 784.2
umbilicus 789.3 ☑
uterus 625.8
vagina 625.8
vulva 625.8
Massive — *see* condition
Mastalgia 611.71
psychogenic 307.89
Mast cell
disease 757.33
systemic (M9741/3) 202.6 ☑
leukemia (M9900/3) 207.8 ☑
sarcoma (M9740/3 202.6 ☑
tumor (M9740/1) 238.5
malignant (M9740/3) 202.6 ☑
Masters-Allen syndrome 620.6
Mastitis (acute) (adolescent) (diffuse) (interstitial) (lobular) (nonpuerperal) (nonsuppurative) (parenchymatous) (phlegmonous) (simple) (subacute) (suppurative) 611.0
chronic (cystic) (fibrocystic) 610.1
cystic 610.1
Schimmelbusch's type 610.1
fibrocystic 610.1
infective 611.0
lactational 675.2 ☑
lymphangitis 611.0
neonatal (noninfective) 778.7
infective 771.5
periductal 610.4
plasma cell 610.4
puerperalis 675.2 ☑
puerperal, postpartum, (interstitial) (nonpurulent) (parenchymatous) 675.2 ☑
purulent 675.1 ☑
stagnation 676.2 ☑
retromammary 611.0
puerperal, postpartum 675.1 ☑
submammary 611.0
puerperal, postpartum 675.1 ☑
Mastocytoma (M9740/1) 238.5
malignant (M9740/3) 202.6 ☑
Mastocytosis 757.33
malignant (M9741/3) 202.6 ☑
systemic (M9741/3) 202.6 ☑
Mastodynia 611.71
psychogenic 307.89
Mastoid — *see* condition
Mastoidalgia — *see also* Otalgia 388.70
Mastoiditis (coalescent) (hemorrhagic) (pneumococcal) (streptococcal) (suppurative) 383.9
acute or subacute 383.00
with
Gradenigo's syndrome 383.02
petrositis 383.02
specified complication NEC 383.02
subperiosteal abscess 383.01
chronic (necrotic) (recurrent) 383.1
tuberculous (*see also* Tuberculosis) 015.6 ☑
Mastopathy, mastopathia 611.9
chronica cystica 610.1
diffuse cystic 610.1
estrogenic 611.89
ovarian origin 611.89
Mastoplasia 611.1
Masturbation 307.9
Maternal condition, affecting fetus or newborn
acute yellow atrophy of liver 760.8
albuminuria 760.1
anesthesia or analgesia 763.5
blood loss 762.1

Maternal condition, affecting fetus or newborn — *continued*
chorioamnionitis 762.7
circulatory disease, chronic (conditions classifiable to 390–459, 745–747) 760.3
congenital heart disease (conditions classifiable to 745–746) 760.3
cortical necrosis of kidney 760.1
death 761.6
diabetes mellitus 775.0
manifest diabetes in the infant 775.1
disease NEC 760.9
circulatory system, chronic (conditions classifiable to 390–459, 745–747) 760.3
genitourinary system (conditions classifiable to 580–599) 760.1
respiratory (conditions classifiable to 490–519, 748) 760.3
eclampsia 760.0
hemorrhage NEC 762.1
hepatitis acute, malignant, or subacute 760.8
hyperemesis (gravidarum) 761.8
hypertension (arising during pregnancy) (conditions classifiable to 642) 760.0
infection
disease classifiable to 001–136 ☑, 760.2
genital tract NEC 760.8
urinary tract 760.1
influenza 760.2
manifest influenza in the infant 771.2
injury (conditions classifiable to 800–996) 760.5
malaria 760.2
manifest malaria in infant or fetus 771.2
malnutrition 760.4
necrosis of liver 760.8
nephritis (conditions classifiable to 580–583) 760.1
nephrosis (conditions classifiable to 581) 760.1
noxious substance transmitted via breast milk or placenta 760.70
alcohol 760.71
anticonvulsants 760.77
antifungals 760.74
anti-infective agents 760.74
antimetabolics 760.78
cocaine 760.75
"crack" 760.75
diethylstilbestrol [DES] 760.76
hallucinogenic agents 760.73
medicinal agents NEC 760.79
narcotics 760.72
obstetric anesthetic or analgesic drug 760.72
specified agent NEC 760.79
nutritional disorder (conditions classifiable to 260–269) 760.4
operation unrelated to current delivery (*see also* Newborn, affected by) 760.64
pre-eclampsia 760.0
pyelitis or pyelonephritis, arising during pregnancy (conditions classifiable to 590) 760.1
renal disease or failure 760.1
respiratory disease, chronic (conditions classifiable to 490–519, 748) 760.3
rheumatic heart disease (chronic) (conditions classifiable to 393–398) 760.3
rubella (conditions classifiable to 056) 760.2
manifest rubella in the infant or fetus 771.0
surgery unrelated to current delivery (*see also* Newborn, affected by) 760.64
to uterus or pelvic organs 760.64
syphilis (conditions classifiable to 090–097) 760.2
manifest syphilis in the infant or fetus 090.0
thrombophlebitis 760.3
toxemia (of pregnancy) 760.0
pre-eclamptic 760.0

Maternal condition, affecting fetus or newborn — *continued*
toxoplasmosis (conditions classifiable to 130) 760.2
manifest toxoplasmosis in the infant or fetus 771.2
transmission of chemical substance through the placenta 760.70
alcohol 760.71
anticonvulsants 760.77
antifungals 760.74
anti-infective 760.74
antimetabolics 760.78
cocaine 760.75
"crack" 760.75
diethylstilbestrol [DES] 760.76
hallucinogenic agents 760.73
narcotics 760.72
specified substance NEC 760.79
uremia 760.1
urinary tract conditions (conditions classifiable to 580–599) 760.1
vomiting (pernicious) (persistent) (vicious) 761.8
Maternity — *see* Delivery
Matheiu's disease (leptospiral jaundice) 100.0
Mauclaire's disease or osteochondrosis 732.3
Maxcy's disease 081.0
Maxilla, maxillary — *see* condition
May (-Hegglin) anomaly or syndrome 288.2
Mayaro fever 066.3
Mazoplasia 610.8
MBD (minimal brain dysfunction), child — *see also* Hyperkinesia 314.9
MCAD (medium chain acyl CoA dehydrogenase deficiency) 277.85
McArdle (-Schmid-Pearson) disease or syndrome (glycogenosis V) 271.0
McCune-Albright syndrome (osteitis fibrosa disseminata) 756.59
MCLS (mucocutaneous lymph node syndrome) 446.1
McQuarrie's syndrome (idiopathic familial hypoglycemia) 251.2
Measles (black) (hemorrhagic) (suppressed) 055.9
with
encephalitis 055.0
keratitis 055.71
keratoconjunctivitis 055.71
otitis media 055.2
pneumonia 055.1
complication 055.8
specified type NEC 055.79
encephalitis 055.0
French 056.9
German 056.9
keratitis 055.71
keratoconjunctivitis 055.71
liberty 056.9
otitis media 055.2
pneumonia 055.1
specified complications NEC 055.79
vaccination, prophylactic (against) V04.2
Meatitis, urethral — *see also* Urethritis 597.89
Meat poisoning — *see* Poisoning, food
Meatus, meatal — *see* condition
Meat-wrappers' asthma 506.9
Meckel's
diverticulitis 751.0
diverticulum (displaced) (hypertrophic) 751.0
Meconium
aspiration 770.11
with
pneumonia 770.12
pneumonitis 770.12
respiratory symptoms 770.12
below vocal cords 770.11
with respiratory symptoms 770.12
syndrome 770.12
delayed passage in newborn 777.1
ileus 777.1
due to cystic fibrosis 277.01
in liquor 792.3
noted during delivery 656.8 ☑

Meconium — *continued*
insufflation 770.11
with respiratory symptoms 770.12
obstruction
fetus or newborn 777.1
in mucoviscidosis 277.01
passage of 792.3
noted during delivery 763.84
peritonitis 777.6
plug syndrome (newborn) NEC 777.1
staining 779.84
Median — *see also* condition
arcuate ligament syndrome 447.4
bar (prostate) 600.90
with
other lower urinary tract symptoms (LUTS) 600.91
urinary
obstruction 600.91
retention 600.91
rhomboid glossitis 529.2
vesical orifice 600.90
with
other lower urinary tract symptoms (LUTS) 600.91
urinary
obstruction 600.91
retention 600.91
Mediastinal shift 793.2
Mediastinitis (acute) (chronic) 519.2
actinomycotic 039.8
syphilitic 095.8
tuberculous (*see also* Tuberculosis) 012.8 ☑
Mediastinopericarditis — *see also* Pericarditis 423.9
acute 420.90
chronic 423.8
rheumatic 393
rheumatic, chronic 393
Mediastinum, mediastinal — *see* condition
Medical services provided for — *see* Health, services provided because (of)
Medicine poisoning (by overdose) (wrong substance given or taken in error) 977.9
specified drug or substance — *see* Table of Drugs and Chemicals
Medin's disease (poliomyelitis) 045.9 ☑
Mediterranean
anemia 282.40
with other hemoglobinopathy 282.49
disease or syndrome (hemopathic) 282.40
with other hemoglobinopathy 282.49
fever (*see also* Brucellosis) 023.9
familial 277.31
kala-azar 085.0
leishmaniasis 085.0
tick fever 082.1
Medulla — *see* condition
Medullary
cystic kidney 753.16
sponge kidney 753.17
Medullated fibers
optic (nerve) 743.57
retina 362.85
Medulloblastoma (M9470/3)
desmoplastic (M9471/3) 191.6
specified site — *see* Neoplasm, by site, malignant
unspecified site 191.6
Medulloepithelioma (M9501/3) — *see also* Neoplasm, by site, malignant
teratoid (M9502/3) — *see* Neoplasm, by site, malignant
Medullomyoblastoma (M9472/3)
specified site — *see* Neoplasm, by site, malignant
unspecified site 191.6
Meekeren-Ehlers-Danlos syndrome 756.83
Megacaryocytic — *see* condition
Megacolon (acquired) (functional) (not Hirschsprung's disease) 564.7
aganglionic 751.3
congenital, congenitum 751.3
Hirschsprung's (disease) 751.3
psychogenic 306.4
toxic (*see also* Colitis, ulcerative) 556.9

☑ **Additional Digit Required** — Refer to the Tabular List for Digit Selection   🅦 **Subterms under main terms may continue to next column or page**

182 — Volume 2   ▶◀ Revised Text   ● New Line   ▲ Revised Code   2013 ICD-9-CM

Megaduodenum 537.3
Megaesophagus (functional) 530.0
  congenital 750.4
Megakaryocytic — *see* condition
Megalencephaly 742.4
Megalerythema (epidermicum) (infectiosum) 057.0
Megalia, cutis et ossium 757.39
Megaloappendix 751.5
Megalocephalus, megalocephaly NEC 756.0
Megalocornea 743.41
  associated with buphthalmos 743.22
Megalocytic anemia 281.9
Megalodactylia (fingers) (thumbs) 755.57
  toes 755.65
Megaloduodenum 751.5
Megaloesophagus (functional) 530.0
  congenital 750.4
Megalogastria (congenital) 750.7
Megalomania 307.9
Megalophthalmos 743.8
Megalopsia 368.14
Megalosplenia — *see also* Splenomegaly 789.2
Megaloureter 593.89
  congenital 753.22
Megarectum 569.49
Megasigmoid 564.7
  congenital 751.3
Megaureter 593.89
  congenital 753.22
Megrim 346.9 ☑
Meibomian
  cyst 373.2
    infected 373.12
  gland — *see* condition
  infarct (eyelid) 374.85
  stye 373.11
Meibomitis 373.12
Meige
  -Milroy disease (chronic hereditary edema) 757.0
  syndrome (blepharospasm-oromandibular dystonia) 333.82
Melalgia, nutritional 266.2
Melancholia — *see also* Psychosis, affective 296.90
  climacteric 296.2 ☑
    recurrent episode 296.3 ☑
    single episode 296.2 ☑
  hypochondriac 300.7
  intermittent 296.2 ☑
    recurrent episode 296.3 ☑
    single episode 296.2 ☑
  involutional 296.2 ☑
    recurrent episode 296.3 ☑
    single episode 296.2 ☑
  menopausal 296.2 ☑
    recurrent episode 296.3 ☑
    single episode 296.2 ☑
  puerperal 296.2 ☑
  reactive (from emotional stress, psychological trauma) 298.0
  recurrent 296.3 ☑
  senile 290.21
  stuporous 296.2 ☑
    recurrent episode 296.3 ☑
    single episode 296.2 ☑
Melanemia 275.09
Melanoameloblastoma (M9363/0) — *see* Neoplasm, bone, benign
Melanoblastoma (M8720/3) — *see* Melanoma
Melanoblastosis
  Block-Sulzberger 757.33
  cutis linearis sive systematisata 757.33
Melanocarcinoma (M8720/3) — *see* Melanoma
Melanocytoma, eyeball (M8726/0) 224.0
Melanocytosis, neurocutaneous 757.33
Melanoderma, melanodermia 709.09
  Addison's (primary adrenal insufficiency) 255.41
Melanodontia, infantile 521.05
Melanodontoclasia 521.05
Melanoepithelioma (M8720/3) — *see* Melanoma

Melanoma (malignant) (M8720/3) 172.9

> *Note* — Except where otherwise indicated, the morphological varieties of melanoma in the list below should be coded by site as for "Melanoma (malignant)". Internal sites should be coded to malignant neoplasm of those sites.

  abdominal wall 172.5
  ala nasi 172.3
  amelanotic (M8730/3) — *see* Melanoma, by site
  ankle 172.7
  anus, anal 154.3
    canal 154.2
  arm 172.6
  auditory canal (external) 172.2
  auricle (ear) 172.2
  auricular canal (external) 172.2
  axilla 172.5
  axillary fold 172.5
  back 172.5
  balloon cell (M8722/3) — *see* Melanoma, by site
  benign (M8720/0) — *see* Neoplasm, skin, benign
  breast (female) (male) 172.5
  brow 172.3
  buttock 172.5
  canthus (eye) 172.1
  cheek (external) 172.3
  chest wall 172.5
  chin 172.3
  choroid 190.6
  conjunctiva 190.3
  ear (external) 172.2
  epithelioid cell (M8771/3) (*see also* Melanoma, by site)
    and spindle cell, mixed (M8775/3) — *see* Melanoma, by site
  external meatus (ear) 172.2
  eye 190.9
  eyebrow 172.3
  eyelid (lower) (upper) 172.1
  face NEC 172.3
  female genital organ (external) NEC 184.4
  finger 172.6
  flank 172.5
  foot 172.7
  forearm 172.6
  forehead 172.3
  foreskin 187.1
  gluteal region 172.5
  groin 172.5
  hand 172.6
  heel 172.7
  helix 172.2
  hip 172.7
  in
    giant pigmented nevus (M8761/3) — *see* Melanoma, by site
    Hutchinson's melanotic freckle (M8742/3) — *see* Melanoma, by site
    junctional nevus (M8740/3) — *see* Melanoma, by site
    precancerous melanosis (M8741/3) — *see* Melanoma, by site
  in situ — *see* Melanoma, by site
    skin 172.9
  interscapular region 172.5
  iris 190.0
  jaw 172.3
  juvenile (M8770/0) — *see* Neoplasm, skin, benign
  knee 172.7
  labium
    majus 184.1
    minus 184.2
  lacrimal gland 190.2
  leg 172.7
  lip (lower) (upper) 172.0
  liver 197.7
  lower limb NEC 172.7
  male genital organ (external) NEC 187.9
  meatus, acoustic (external) 172.2
  meibomian gland 172.1

Melanoma — *continued*
  metastatic
    of or from specified site — *see* Melanoma, by site
    site not of skin — *see* Neoplasm, by site, malignant, secondary
    to specified site — *see* Neoplasm, by site, malignant, secondary
    unspecified site 172.9
  nail 172.9
    finger 172.6
    toe 172.7
  neck 172.4
  nodular (M8721/3) — *see* Melanoma, by site
  nose, external 172.3
  orbit 190.1
  penis 187.4
  perianal skin 172.5
  perineum 172.5
  pinna 172.2
  popliteal (fossa) (space) 172.7
  prepuce 187.1
  pubes 172.5
  pudendum 184.4
  retina 190.5
  scalp 172.4
  scrotum 187.7
  septum nasal (skin) 172.3
  shoulder 172.6
  skin NEC 172.8
    in situ 172.9
  spindle cell (M8772/3) (*see also* Melanoma, by site)
    type A (M8773/3) 190.0
    type B (M8774/3) 190.0
  submammary fold 172.5
  superficial spreading (M8743/3) — *see* Melanoma, by site
  temple 172.3
  thigh 172.7
  toe 172.7
  trunk NEC 172.5
  umbilicus 172.5
  upper limb NEC 172.6
  vagina vault 184.0
  vulva 184.4
Melanoplakia 528.9
Melanosarcoma (M8720/3) — *see also* Melanoma
  epithelioid cell (M8771/3) — *see* Melanoma
Melanosis 709.09
  addisonian (primary adrenal insufficiency) 255.41
    tuberculous (*see also* Tuberculosis) 017.6 ☑
  adrenal 255.41
  colon 569.89
  conjunctiva 372.55
    congenital 743.49
  corii degenerativa 757.33
  cornea (presenile) (senile) 371.12
    congenital 743.43
      interfering with vision 743.42
  eye 372.55
    congenital 743.49
  jute spinners' 709.09
  lenticularis progressiva 757.33
  liver 573.8
  precancerous (M8741/2) (*see also* Neoplasm, skin, in situ)
    malignant melanoma in (M8741/3) — *see* Melanoma
  prenatal 743.43
    interfering with vision 743.42
  Riehl's 709.09
  sclera 379.19
    congenital 743.47
  suprarenal 255.41
  tar 709.09
  toxic 709.09
Melanuria 791.9
Melasma 709.09
  adrenal (gland) 255.41
  suprarenal (gland) 255.41

MELAS syndrome (mitochondrial encephalopathy, lactic acidosis and stroke-like episodes) 277.87
Melena 578.1
  due to
    swallowed maternal blood 777.3
    ulcer — *see* Ulcer, by site, with hemorrhage
  newborn 772.4
    due to swallowed maternal blood 777.3
Meleney's
  gangrene (cutaneous) 686.09
  ulcer (chronic undermining) 686.09
Melioidosis 025
Melitensis, febris 023.0
Melitococcosis 023.0
Melkersson (-Rosenthal) syndrome 351.8
Mellitus, diabetes — *see* Diabetes
Melorheostosis (bone) (leri) 733.99
Meloschisis 744.83
Melotia 744.29
Membrana
  capsularis lentis posterior 743.39
  epipapillaris 743.57
Membranacea placenta — *see* Placenta, abnormal
Membranaceous uterus 621.8
Membrane, membranous — *see also* condition
  folds, congenital — *see* Web
  Jackson's 751.4
  over face (causing asphyxia), fetus or newborn 768.9
  premature rupture — *see* Rupture, membranes, premature
  pupillary 364.74
    persistent 743.46
  retained (complicating delivery) (with hemorrhage) 666.2 ☑
    without hemorrhage 667.1 ☑
  secondary (eye) 366.50
  unruptured (causing asphyxia) 768.9
  vitreous humor 379.25
Membranitis, fetal 658.4 ☑
  affecting fetus or newborn 762.7
Memory disturbance, loss or lack — *see also* Amnesia 780.93
  mild, following organic brain damage 310.89
MEN (multiple endocrine neoplasia) (syndromes)
  type I 258.01
  type IIA 258.02
  type IIB 258.03
Menadione (vitamin K) **deficiency** 269.0
Menarche, precocious 259.1
Mendacity, pathologic 301.7
Mendelson's syndrome (resulting from a procedure) 997.32
  obstetric 668.0 ☑
Mende's syndrome (ptosis-epicanthus) 270.2
Ménétrier's disease or syndrome (hypertrophic gastritis) 535.2 ☑
Ménière's disease, syndrome, or vertigo 386.00
  cochlear 386.02
  cochleovestibular 386.01
  inactive 386.04
  in remission 386.04
  vestibular 386.03
Meninges, meningeal — *see* condition
Meningioma (M9530/0) — *see also* Neoplasm, meninges, benign
  angioblastic (M9535/0) — *see* Neoplasm, meninges, benign
  angiomatous (M9534/0) — *see* Neoplasm, meninges, benign
  endotheliomatous (M9531/0) — *see* Neoplasm, meninges, benign
  fibroblastic (M9532/0) — *see* Neoplasm, meninges, benign
  fibrous (M9532/0) — *see* Neoplasm, meninges, benign
  hemangioblastic (M9535/0) — *see* Neoplasm, meninges, benign

---

☑ **Additional Digit Required** — Refer to the Tabular List for Digit Selection   ⩔ **Subterms under main terms may continue to next column or page**

Meningioma — see also Neoplasm, meninges, benign — continued
 hemangiopericytic (M9536/0) — see Neoplasm, meninges, benign
 malignant (M9530/3) — see Neoplasm, meninges, malignant
 meningiothelial (M9531/0) — see Neoplasm, meninges, benign
 meningotheliomatous (M9531/0) — see Neoplasm, meninges, benign
 mixed (M9537/0) — see Neoplasm, meninges, benign
 multiple (M9530/1) 237.6
 papillary (M9538/1) 237.6
 psammomatous (M9533/0) — see Neoplasm, meninges, benign
 syncytial (M9531/0) — see Neoplasm, meninges, benign
 transitional (M9537/0) — see Neoplasm, meninges, benign
Meningiomatosis (diffuse) (M9530/1) 237.6
Meningism — see also Meningismus 781.6
Meningismus (infectional) (pneumococcal) 781.6
 due to serum or vaccine 997.09 [321.8]
 influenzal NEC (see also Influenza) 487.8
Meningitis (basal) (basic) (basilar) (brain) (cerebral) (cervical) (congestive) (diffuse) (hemorrhagic) (infantile) (membranous) (metastatic) (nonspecific) (pontine) (progressive) (simple) (spinal) (subacute) (sympathetica) (toxic) 322.9
 abacterial NEC (see also Meningitis, aseptic) 047.9
 actinomycotic 039.8 [320.7]
 adenoviral 049.1
 Aerobacter aerogenes 320.82
 anaerobes (cocci) (gram-negative) (gram-positive) (mixed) (NEC) 320.81
 arbovirus NEC 066.9 [321.2]
 specified type NEC 066.8 [321.2]
 aseptic (acute) NEC 047.9
 adenovirus 049.1
 Coxsackie virus 047.0
 due to
 adenovirus 049.1
 Coxsackie virus 047.0
 ECHO virus 047.1
 enterovirus 047.9
 mumps 072.1
 poliovirus (see also Poliomyelitis) 045.2 ☑ [321.2]
 ECHO virus 047.1
 herpes (simplex) virus 054.72
 zoster 053.0
 leptospiral 100.81
 lymphocytic choriomeningitis 049.0
 noninfective 322.0
 Bacillus pyocyaneus 320.89
 bacterial NEC 320.9
 anaerobic 320.81
 gram-negative 320.82
 anaerobic 320.81
 Bacteroides (fragilis) (oralis) (melaninogenicus) 320.81
 cancerous (M8000/6) 198.4
 candidal 112.83
 carcinomatous (M8010/6) 198.4
 caseous (see also Tuberculosis, meninges) 013.0 ☑
 cerebrospinal (acute) (chronic) (diplococcal) (endemic) (epidemic) (fulminant) (infectious) (malignant) (meningococcal) (sporadic) 036.0
 carrier (suspected) of V02.59
 chronic NEC 322.2
 clear cerebrospinal fluid NEC 322.0
 Clostridium (haemolyticum) (novyi) NEC 320.81
 coccidioidomycosis 114.2
 Coxsackie virus 047.0
 cryptococcal 117.5 [321.0]
 diplococcal 036.0
 gram-negative 036.0
 gram-positive 320.1

Meningitis — continued
 Diplococcus pneumoniae 320.1
 due to
 actinomycosis 039.8 [320.7]
 adenovirus 049.1
 coccidiomycosis 114.2
 enterovirus 047.9
 specified NEC 047.8
 histoplasmosis (see also Histoplasmosis) 115.91
 Listerosis 027.0 [320.7]
 Lyme disease 088.81 [320.7]
 moniliasis 112.83
 mumps 072.1
 neurosyphilis 094.2
 nonbacterial organisms NEC 321.8
 oidiomycosis 112.83
 poliovirus (see also Poliomyelitis) 045.2 ☑ [321.2]
 preventive immunization, inoculation, or vaccination 997.09 [321.8]
 sarcoidosis 135 [321.4]
 sporotrichosis 117.1 [321.1]
 syphilis 094.2
 acute 091.81
 congenital 090.42
 secondary 091.81
 trypanosomiasis (see also Trypanosomiasis) 086.9 [321.3]
 whooping cough 033.9 [320.7]
 ECHO virus 047.1
 E. coli 320.82
 endothelial-leukocytic, benign, recurrent 047.9
 Enterobacter aerogenes 320.82
 enteroviral 047.9
 specified type NEC 047.8
 enterovirus 047.9
 specified NEC 047.8
 eosinophilic 322.1
 epidemic NEC 036.0
 Escherichia coli (E. coli) 320.82
 Eubacterium 320.81
 fibrinopurulent NEC 320.9
 specified type NEC 320.89
 Friedländer (bacillus) 320.82
 fungal NEC 117.9 [321.1]
 Fusobacterium 320.81
 gonococcal 098.82
 gram-negative bacteria NEC 320.82
 anaerobic 320.81
 cocci 036.0
 specified NEC 320.82
 gram-negative cocci NEC 036.0
 specified NEC 320.82
 gram-positive cocci NEC 320.9
 herpes (simplex) virus 054.72
 zoster 053.0
 H. influenzae 320.0
 infectious NEC 320.9
 influenzal 320.0
 Klebsiella pneumoniae 320.82
 late effect — see Late, effect, meningitis
 leptospiral (aseptic) 100.81
 Listerella (monocytogenes) 027.0 [320.7]
 Listeria monocytogenes 027.0 [320.7]
 lymphocytic (acute) (benign) (serous) 049.0
 choriomeningitis virus 049.0
 meningococcal (chronic) 036.0
 Mima polymorpha 320.82
 Mollaret's 047.9
 monilial 112.83
 mumps (virus) 072.1
 mycotic NEC 117.9 [321.1]
 Neisseria 036.0
 neurosyphilis 094.2
 nonbacterial NEC (see also Meningitis, aseptic) 047.9
 nonpyogenic NEC 322.0
 oidiomycosis 112.83
 ossificans 349.2
 Peptococcus 320.81
 Peptostreptococcus 320.81
 pneumococcal 320.1
 poliovirus (see also Poliomyelitis) 045.2 ☑ [321.2]

Meningitis — continued
 Proprionibacterium 320.81
 Proteus morganii 320.82
 Pseudomonas (aeruginosa) (pyocyaneus) 320.82
 purulent NEC 320.9
 specified organism NEC 320.89
 pyogenic NEC 320.9
 specified organism NEC 320.89
 Salmonella 003.21
 septic NEC 320.9
 specified organism NEC 320.89
 serosa circumscripta NEC 322.0
 serous NEC (see also Meningitis, aseptic) 047.9
 lymphocytic 049.0
 syndrome 348.2
 Serratia (marcescens) 320.82
 specified organism NEC 320.89
 sporadic cerebrospinal 036.0
 sporotrichosis 117.1 [321.1]
 staphylococcal 320.3
 sterile 997.09
 streptococcal (acute) 320.2
 suppurative 320.9
 specified organism NEC 320.89
 syphilitic 094.2
 acute 091.81
 congenital 090.42
 secondary 091.81
 torula 117.5 [321.0]
 traumatic (complication of injury) 958.8
 Treponema (denticola) (macrodenticum) 320.81
 trypanosomiasis 086.1 [321.3]
 tuberculous (see also Tuberculosis, meninges) 013.0 ☑
 typhoid 002.0 [320.7]
 Veillonella 320.81
 Vibrio vulnificus 320.82
 viral, virus NEC (see also Meningitis, aseptic) 047.9
 Wallgren's (see also Meningitis, aseptic) 047.9
Meningocele (congenital) (spinal) — see also Spina bifida 741.9 ☑
 acquired (traumatic) 349.2
 cerebral 742.0
 cranial 742.0
Meningocerebritis — see Meningoencephalitis
Meningococcemia (acute) (chronic) 036.2
Meningococcus, meningococcal — see also condition 036.9
 adrenalitis, hemorrhagic 036.3
 carditis 036.40
 carrier (suspected) of V02.59
 cerebrospinal fever 036.0
 encephalitis 036.1
 endocarditis 036.42
 exposure to V01.84
 infection NEC 036.9
 meningitis (cerebrospinal) 036.0
 myocarditis 036.43
 optic neuritis 036.81
 pericarditis 036.41
 septicemia (chronic) 036.2
Meningoencephalitis — see also Encephalitis 323.9
 acute NEC 048
 bacterial, purulent, pyogenic, or septic — see Meningitis
 chronic NEC 094.1
 diffuse NEC 094.1
 diphasic 063.2
 due to
 actinomycosis 039.8 [320.7]
 blastomycosis NEC (see also Blastomycosis) 116.0 [323.41]
 free-living amebae 136.29
 Listeria monocytogenes 027.0 [320.7]
 Lyme disease 088.81 [320.7]
 mumps 072.2
 Naegleria (amebae) (gruberi) (organisms) 136.29
 rubella 056.01

Meningoencephalitis — see also Encephalitis — continued
 due to — continued
 sporotrichosis 117.1 [321.1]
 toxoplasmosis (acquired) 130.0
 congenital (active) 771.2 [323.41]
 Trypanosoma 086.1 [323.2]
 epidemic 036.0
 herpes 054.3
 herpetic 054.3
 H. influenzae 320.0
 infectious (acute) 048
 influenzal 320.0
 late effect — see category 326
 Listeria monocytogenes 027.0 [320.7]
 lymphocytic (serous) 049.0
 mumps 072.2
 parasitic NEC 123.9 [323.41]
 pneumococcal 320.1
 primary amebic 136.29
 rubella 056.01
 serous 048
 lymphocytic 049.0
 specific 094.2
 staphylococcal 320.3
 streptococcal 320.2
 syphilitic 094.2
 toxic NEC 989.9 [323.71]
 due to
 carbon tetrachloride (vapor) 987.8 [323.71]
 hydroxyquinoline derivatives poisoning 961.3 [323.71]
 lead 984.9 [323.71]
 mercury 985.0 [323.71]
 thallium 985.8 [323.71]
 toxoplasmosis (acquired) 130.0
 trypanosomic 086.1 [323.2]
 tuberculous (see also Tuberculosis, meninges) 013.0 ☑
 virus NEC 048
Meningoencephalocele 742.0
 syphilitic 094.89
 congenital 090.49
Meningoencephalomyelitis — see also Meningoencephalitis 323.9
 acute NEC 048
 disseminated (postinfectious) 136.9 [323.61]
 postimmunization or postvaccination 323.51
 due to
 actinomycosis 039.8 [320.7]
 torula 117.5 [323.41]
 toxoplasma or toxoplasmosis (acquired) 130.0
 congenital (active) 771.2 [323.41]
 late effect — see category 326
Meningoencephalomyelopathy — see also Meningoencephalomyelitis 349.9
Meningoencephalopathy — see also Meningoencephalitis 348.39
Meningoencephalopoliomyelitis — see also Poliomyelitis, bulbar 045.0 ☑
 late effect 138
Meningomyelitis — see also Meningoencephalitis 323.9
 blastomycotic NEC (see also Blastomycosis) 116.0 [323.41]
 due to
 actinomycosis 039.8 [320.7]
 blastomycosis (see also Blastomycosis) 116.0 [323.41]
 Meningococcus 036.0
 sporotrichosis 117.1 [323.41]
 torula 117.5 [323.41]
 late effect — see category 326
 lethargic 049.8
 meningococcal 036.0
 syphilitic 094.2
 tuberculous (see also Tuberculosis, meninges) 013.0 ☑
Meningomyelocele — see also Spina bifida 741.9 ☑
 syphilitic 094.89

☑ Additional Digit Required — Refer to the Tabular List for Digit Selection   ⩊ Subterms under main terms may continue to next column or page

Meningomyeloneuritis — *see* Meningoencephalitis
Meningoradiculitis — *see* Meningitis
Meningovascular — *see* condition
Meniscocytosis 282.60
Menkes' syndrome — *see* Syndrome, Menkes'
Menolipsis 626.0
Menometrorrhagia 626.2
Menopause, menopausal (symptoms) (syndrome) 627.2
  arthritis (any site) NEC 716.3 ☑
  artificial 627.4
  bleeding 627.0
  crisis 627.2
  depression (*see also* Psychosis, affective)
    296.2 ☑
    agitated 296.2 ☑
      recurrent episode 296.3 ☑
      single episode 296.2 ☑
    psychotic 296.2 ☑
      recurrent episode 296.3 ☑
      single episode 296.2 ☑
    recurrent episode 296.3 ☑
    single episode 296.2 ☑
    melancholia (*see also* Psychosis, affective)
      296.2 ☑
      recurrent episode 296.3 ☑
      single episode 296.2 ☑
  paranoid state 297.2
  paraphrenia 297.2
  postsurgical 627.4
  premature 256.31
    postirradiation 256.2
    postsurgical 256.2
  psychoneurosis 627.2
  psychosis NEC 298.8
  surgical 627.4
  toxic polyarthritis NEC 716.39
Menorrhagia (primary) 626.2
  climacteric 627.0
  menopausal 627.0
  postclimacteric 627.1
  postmenopausal 627.1
  preclimacteric 627.0
  premenopausal 627.0
  puberty (menses retained) 626.3
Menorrhalgia 625.3
Menoschesis 626.8
Menostaxis 626.2
Menses, retention 626.8
Menstrual — *see also* Menstruation
  cycle, irregular 626.4
  disorders NEC 626.9
  extraction V25.3
  fluid, retained 626.8
  molimen 625.4
  period, normal V65.5
  regulation V25.3
Menstruation
  absent 626.0
  anovulatory 628.0
  delayed 626.8
  difficult 625.3
  disorder 626.9
    psychogenic 306.52
    specified NEC 626.8
  during pregnancy 640.8 ☑
  excessive 626.2
  frequent 626.2
  infrequent 626.1
  irregular 626.4
  latent 626.8
  membranous 626.8
  painful (primary) (secondary) 625.3
    psychogenic 306.52
  passage of clots 626.2
  precocious 259.1
  protracted 626.8
  retained 626.8
  retrograde 626.8
  scanty 626.1
  suppression 626.8
  vicarious (nasal) 625.8
Mentagra — *see also* Sycosis 704.8
Mental — *see also* condition

Mental — *see also* condition — *continued*
  deficiency (*see also* Disability, intellectual)
    319
  deterioration (*see also* Psychosis) 298.9
  disorder (*see also* Disorder, mental) 300.9
  exhaustion 300.5
  insufficiency (congenital) (*see also* Disability,
    intellectual) 319
  observation without need for further medi-
    cal care NEC V71.09
  retardation —*see* Disability, intellectual
  subnormality (*see also* Disability, intellectu-
    al) 319
    mild 317
    moderate 318.0
    profound 318.2
    severe 318.1
  upset (*see also* Disorder, mental) 300.9
Meralgia paresthetica 355.1
Mercurial — *see* condition
Mercurialism NEC 985.0
Merergasia 300.9
Merkel cell tumor — *see* Carcinoma, Merkel
cell
Merocele — *see also* Hernia, femoral 553.00
Meromelia 755.4
  lower limb 755.30
    intercalary 755.32
      femur 755.34
        tibiofibular (complete) (incom-
          plete) 755.33
      fibula 755.37
      metatarsal(s) 755.38
      tarsal(s) 755.38
      tibia 755.36
      tibiofibular 755.35
    terminal (complete) (partial) (transverse)
      755.31
      longitudinal 755.32
        metatarsal(s) 755.38
        phalange(s) 755.39
        tarsal(s) 755.38
      transverse 755.31
  upper limb 755.20
    intercalary 755.22
      carpal(s) 755.28
      humeral 755.24
        radioulnar (complete) (incom-
          plete) 755.23
      metacarpal(s) 755.28
      phalange(s) 755.29
      radial 755.26
      radioulnar 755.25
      ulnar 755.27
    terminal (complete) (partial) (transverse)
      755.21
      longitudinal 755.22
        carpal(s) 755.28
        metacarpal(s) 755.28
        phalange(s) 755.29
      transverse 755.21
Merosmia 781.1
MERRF syndrome (myoclonus with epilepsy
and with ragged red fibers) 277.87
Merycism — *see also* Vomiting
  psychogenic 307.53
Merzbacher-Pelizaeus disease 330.0
Mesaortitis — *see* Aortitis
Mesarteritis — *see* Arteritis
Mesencephalitis — *see also* Encephalitis 323.9
  late effect — *see* category 326
Mesenchymoma (M8990/1) — *see also* Neo-
plasm, connective tissue, uncertain be-
havior
  benign (M8990/0) — *see* Neoplasm, connec-
tive tissue, benign
  malignant (M8990/3) — *see* Neoplasm,
connective tissue, malignant
Mesenteritis
  retractile 567.82
  sclerosing 567.82
Mesentery, mesenteric — *see* condition
Mesiodens, mesiodentes 520.1
  causing crowding 524.31
Mesio-occlusion 524.23
Mesocardia (with asplenia) 746.87

Mesocolon — *see* condition
Mesonephroma (malignant) (M9110/3) — *see*
also Neoplasm, by site, malignant
  benign (M9110/0) — *see* Neoplasm, by site,
benign
Mesophlebitis — *see* Phlebitis
Mesostromal dysgenesis 743.51
Mesothelioma (malignant) (M9050/3) — *see*
also Neoplasm, by site, malignant
  benign (M9050/0) — *see* Neoplasm, by site,
benign
  biphasic type (M9053/3) (*see also* Neoplasm,
by site, malignant)
    benign (M9053/0) — *see* Neoplasm, by
site, benign
  epithelioid (M9052/3) (*see also* Neoplasm,
by site, malignant)
    benign (M9052/0) — *see* Neoplasm, by
site, benign
  fibrous (M9051/3) (*see also* Neoplasm, by
site, malignant)
    benign (M9051/0) — *see* Neoplasm, by
site, benign
Metabolic syndrome 277.7
Metabolism disorder 277.9
  specified type NEC 277.89
Metagonimiasis 121.5
Metagonimus infestation (small intestine)
121.5
Metal
  pigmentation (skin) 709.00
  polishers' disease 502
Metalliferous miners' lung 503
Metamorphopsia 368.14
Metaplasia
  bone, in skin 709.3
  breast 611.89
  cervix — *omit code*
  endometrium (squamous) 621.8
  esophagus 530.85
  intestinal, of gastric mucosa 537.89
  kidney (pelvis) (squamous) (*see also* Disease,
renal) 593.89
  myelogenous 289.89
  myeloid 289.89
    agnogenic 238.76
    megakaryocytic 238.76
  spleen 289.59
  squamous cell
    amnion 658.8 ☑
    bladder 596.89
    cervix — *see* condition
    trachea 519.19
    tracheobronchial tree 519.19
    uterus 621.8
      cervix — *see* condition
Metastasis, metastatic
  abscess — *see* Abscess
  calcification 275.40
  cancer, neoplasm, or disease
    from specified site (M8000/3) — *see*
Neoplasm, by site, malignant
    to specified site (M8000/6) — *see* Neo-
plasm, by site, secondary
  deposits (in) (M8000/6) — *see* Neoplasm,
by site, secondary
  mesentery, of neuroendocrine tumor 209.74
  pneumonia 038.8 *[484.8]*
  spread (to) (M8000/6) — *see* Neoplasm, by
site, secondary
Metatarsalgia 726.70
  anterior 355.6
  due to Freiberg's disease 732.5
  Morton's 355.6
Metatarsus, metatarsal — *see also* condition
  abductus valgus (congenital) 754.60
  adductus varus (congenital) 754.53
  primus varus 754.52
  valgus (adductus) (congenital) 754.60
  varus (abductus) (congenital) 754.53
    primus 754.52
Methadone use 304.00
Methemoglobinemia 289.7
  acquired (with sulfhemoglobinemia) 289.7
  congenital 289.7
  enzymatic 289.7

Methemoglobinemia — *continued*
  Hb-M disease 289.7
  hereditary 289.7
  toxic 289.7
Methemoglobinuria — *see also*
Hemoglobinuria 791.2
Methicillin
  resistant staphyloccocus aureus (MRSA)
041.12
    colonization V02.54
    personal history of V12.04
  susceptible staphylococcus aureus (MSSA)
041.11
    colonization V02.53
Methioninemia 270.4
Metritis (catarrhal) (septic) (suppurative) —
see also Endometritis 615.9
  blennorrhagic 098.16
    chronic or duration of 2 months or over
098.36
  cervical (*see also* Cervicitis) 616.0
  gonococcal 098.16
    chronic or duration of 2 months or over
098.36
  hemorrhagic 626.8
  puerperal, postpartum, childbirth 670.1 ☑
    septic 670.2 ☑
  tuberculous (*see also* Tuberculosis) 016.7 ☑
Metropathia hemorrhagica 626.8
Metroperitonitis — *see also* Peritonitis, pelvic,
female 614.5
Metrorrhagia 626.6
  arising during pregnancy — *see* Hemorrhage, pregnancy
  postpartum NEC 666.2 ☑
  primary 626.6
  psychogenic 306.59
  puerperal 666.2 ☑
Metrorrhexis — *see* Rupture, uterus
Metrosalpingitis — *see also* Salpingo-
oophoritis 614.2
Metrostaxis 626.6
Metrovaginitis — *see also* Endometritis 615.9
  gonococcal (acute) 098.16
    chronic or duration of 2 months or over
098.36
Mexican fever — *see* Typhus, Mexican
Meyenburg-Altherr-Uehlinger syndrome
733.99
Meyer-Schwickerath and Weyers syndrome
(dysplasia oculodentodigitalis) 759.89
Meynert's amentia (nonalcoholic) 294.0
  alcoholic 291.1
Mibelli's disease 757.39
Mice, joint — *see also* Loose, body, joint
718.1 ☑
  knee 717.6
Micheli-Rietti syndrome (thalassemia minor)
282.46
Michotte's syndrome 721.5
Micrencephalon, micrencephaly 742.1
Microalbuminuria 791.0
Microaneurysm, retina 362.14
  diabetic 250.5 ☑ *[362.01]*
    due to secondary diabetes
249.5 ☑ *[362.01]*
Microangiopathy 443.9
  diabetic (peripheral) 250.7 ☑ *[443.81]*
    due to secondary diabetes
249.7 ☑ *[443.81]*
    retinal 250.5 ☑ *[362.01]*
      due to secondary diabetes
249.5 ☑ *[362.01]*
  peripheral 443.9
    diabetic 250.7 ☑ *[443.81]*
      due to secondary diabetes
249.7 ☑ *[443.81]*
  retinal 362.18
    diabetic 250.5 ☑ *[362.01]*
      due to secondary diabetes
249.5 ☑ *[362.01]*
  thrombotic 446.6
    Moschcowitz's (thrombotic thrombocy-
topenic purpura) 446.6
Microcalcification, mammographic 793.81

☑ **Additional Digit Required — Refer to the Tabular List for Digit Selection**   ⬛ **Subterms under main terms may continue to next column or page**

2013 ICD-9-CM   ▶◀ **Revised Text**   ● **New Line**   ▲ **Revised Code**   **Volume 2 — 185**

Microcephalus, microcephalic, microcephaly 742.1
  due to toxoplasmosis (congenital) 771.2
Microcheilia 744.82
Microcolon (congenital) 751.5
Microcornea (congenital) 743.41
Microcytic — see condition
Microdeletions NEC 758.33
Microdontia 520.2
Microdrepanocytosis (thalassemia-Hb-S disease) 282.41
  with sickle cell crisis 282.42
Microembolism
  atherothrombotic — see Atheroembolism
  retina 362.33
Microencephalon 742.1
Microfilaria streptocerca infestation 125.3
Microgastria (congenital) 750.7
Microgenia 524.06
Microgenitalia (congenital) 752.89
  penis 752.64
Microglioma (M9710/3)
  specified site — see Neoplasm, by site, malignant
  unspecified site 191.9
Microglossia (congenital) 750.16
Micrognathia, micrognathism (congenital) 524.00
  mandibular 524.04
    alveolar 524.74
  maxillary 524.03
    alveolar 524.73
Microgyria (congenital) 742.2
Microinfarct, heart — see also Insufficiency, coronary 411.89
Microlithiasis, alveolar, pulmonary 516.2
Micromastia 611.82
Micromyelia (congenital) 742.59
Micropenis 752.64
Microphakia (congenital) 743.36
Microphthalmia (congenital) — see also Microphthalmos 743.10
Microphthalmos (congenital) 743.10
  associated with eye and adnexal anomalies NEC 743.12
  due to toxoplasmosis (congenital) 771.2
  isolated 743.11
  simple 743.11
  syndrome 759.89
Micropsia 368.14
Microsporidiosis 136.8
Microsporon furfur infestation 111.0
Microsporosis — see also Dermatophytosis 110.9
  nigra 111.1
Microstomia (congenital) 744.84
Microthelia 757.6
Microthromboembolism — see Embolism
Microtia (congenital) (external ear) 744.23
Microtropia 378.34
Microvillus inclusion disease (MVD) 751.5
Micturition
  disorder NEC 788.69
    psychogenic 306.53
  frequency 788.41
    psychogenic 306.53
  nocturnal 788.43
  painful 788.1
    psychogenic 306.53
Middle
  ear — see condition
  lobe (right) syndrome 518.0
Midplane — see condition
Miescher's disease 709.3
  cheilitis 351.8
  granulomatosis disciformis 709.3
Miescher-Leder syndrome or granulomatosis 709.3
Mieten's syndrome 759.89

Migraine (idiopathic) 346.9 ☑

Note — The following fifth digit subclassification is for use with category 346:

0   without mention of intractable migraine without mention of status migrainosus

       without mention of refractory migraine without mention of status migrainosus

1   with intractable migraine, so stated, without mention of status migrainosus

       with refractory migraine, so stated, without mention of status migrainosus

2   without mention of intractable migraine with status migrainosus

       without mention of refractory migraine with status migrainosus

3   with intractable migraine, so stated, with status migrainosus

       with refractory migraine, so stated, with status migrainosus

  with aura (acute-onset) (without headache) (prolonged) (typical) 346.0 ☑
  without aura 346.1 ☑
    chronic 346.7 ☑
    transformed 346.7 ☑
  abdominal (syndrome) 346.2 ☑
  allergic (histamine) 346.2 ☑
  atypical 346.8 ☑
  basilar 346.0 ☑
  chronic without aura 346.7 ☑
  classic(al) 346.0 ☑
  common 346.1 ☑
  complicated 346.0 ☑
  hemiplegic 346.3 ☑
    familial 346.3 ☑
    sporadic 346.3 ☑
  lower-half 339.00
  menstrual 346.4 ☑
  menstrually related 346.4 ☑
  ophthalmic 346.8 ☑
  ophthalmoplegic 346.2 ☑
  premenstrual 346.4 ☑
  pure menstrual 346.4 ☑
  retinal 346.0 ☑
  specified form NEC 346.8 ☑
  transformed without aura 346.7 ☑
  variant 346.2 ☑
Migrant, social V60.0
Migratory, migrating — see also condition
  person V60.0
  testis, congenital 752.52
Mikulicz's disease or syndrome (dryness of mouth, absent or decreased lacrimation) 527.1
Milian atrophia blanche 701.3
Miliaria (crystallina) (rubra) (tropicalis) 705.1
  apocrine 705.82
Miliary — see condition
Milium — see also Cyst, sebaceous 706.2
  colloid 709.3
  eyelid 374.84
Milk
  crust 690.11
  excess secretion 676.6 ☑
  fever, female 672.0 ☑
  poisoning 988.8
  retention 676.2 ☑
  sickness 988.8
  spots 423.1
Milkers' nodes 051.1
Milk-leg (deep vessels) 671.4 ☑
  complicating pregnancy 671.3 ☑
  nonpuerperal 451.19
  puerperal, postpartum, childbirth 671.4 ☑
Milkman (-Looser) disease or syndrome (osteomalacia with pseudofractures) 268.2

Milky urine — see also Chyluria 791.1
Millar's asthma (laryngismus stridulus) 478.75
Millard-Gubler-Foville paralysis 344.89
Millard-Gubler paralysis or syndrome 344.89
Miller-Dieker syndrome 758.33
Miller's disease (osteomalacia) 268.2
Miller Fisher's syndrome 357.0
Milles' syndrome (encephalocutaneous angiomatosis) 759.6
Mills' disease 335.29
Millstone makers' asthma or lung 502
Milroy's disease (chronic hereditary edema) 757.0
Miners' — see also condition
  asthma 500
  elbow 727.2
  knee 727.2
  lung 500
  nystagmus 300.89
  phthisis (see also Tuberculosis) 011.4 ☑
  tuberculosis (see also Tuberculosis) 011.4 ☑
Minkowski-Chauffard syndrome — see also Spherocytosis 282.0
Minor — see condition
Minor's disease 336.1
Minot's disease (hemorrhagic disease, newborn) 776.0
Minot-von Willebrand (-Jürgens) disease or syndrome (angiohemophilia) 286.4
Minus (and plus) hand (intrinsic) 736.09
Miosis (persistent) (pupil) 379.42
Mirizzi's syndrome (hepatic duct stenosis) — see also Obstruction, biliary 576.2
  with calculus, cholelithiasis, or stones — see Choledocholithiasis
Mirror writing 315.09
  secondary to organic lesion 784.69
Misadventure (prophylactic) (therapeutic) — see also Complications 999.9
  administration of insulin 962.3
  infusion — see Complications, infusion
  local applications (of fomentations, plasters, etc.) 999.9
    burn or scald — see Burn, by site
  medical care (early) (late) NEC 999.9
    adverse effect of drugs or chemicals — see Table of Drugs and Chemicals
    burn or scald — see Burn, by site
  radiation NEC 990
  radiotherapy NEC 990
  surgical procedure (early) (late) — see Complications, surgical procedure
  transfusion — see Complications, transfusion
  vaccination or other immunological procedure — see Complications, vaccination
Misanthropy 301.7
Miscarriage — see Abortion, spontaneous
Mischief, malicious, child — see also Disturbance, conduct 312.0 ☑
Misdirection
  aqueous 365.83
Mismanagement, feeding 783.3
Misplaced, misplacement
  kidney (see also Disease, renal) 593.0
    congenital 753.3
  organ or site, congenital NEC — see Malposition, congenital
Missed
  abortion 632
  delivery (at or near term) 656.4 ☑
  labor (at or near term) 656.4 ☑
Misshapen reconstructed breast 612.0
Missing — see also Absence
  teeth (acquired) 525.10
    congenital (see also Anodontia) 520.0
    due to
      caries 525.13
      extraction 525.10
      periodontal disease 525.12
      specified NEC 525.19
      trauma 525.11
  vertebrae (congenital) 756.13
Misuse of drugs NEC — see also Abuse, drug, nondependent 305.9 ☑

Mitchell's disease (erythromelalgia) 443.82
Mite(s)
  diarrhea 133.8
  grain (itch) 133.8
  hair follicle (itch) 133.8
  in sputum 133.8
Mitochondrial encephalopathy, lactic acidosis and stroke-like episodes (MELAS syndrome) 277.87
Mitochondrial neurogastrointestinal encephalopathy syndrome (MNGIE) 277.87
Mitral — see condition
Mittelschmerz 625.2
Mixed — see condition
Mljet disease (mal de Meleda) 757.39
Mobile, mobility
  cecum 751.4
  coccyx 733.99
  excessive — see Hypermobility
  gallbladder 751.69
  kidney 593.0
    congenital 753.3
  organ or site, congenital NEC — see Malposition, congenital
  spleen 289.59
Mobitz heart block (atrioventricular) 426.10
  type I (Wenckebach's) 426.13
  type II 426.12
Möbius'
  disease 346.2 ☑
  syndrome
    congenital oculofacial paralysis 352.6
    ophthalmoplegic migraine 346.2 ☑
Moeller(-Barlow) disease (infantile scurvy) 267
  glossitis 529.4
Mohr's syndrome (types I and II) 759.89
Mola destruens (M9100/1) 236.1
Molarization, premolars 520.2
Molar pregnancy 631.8
  hydatidiform (delivered) (undelivered) 630
Molding, head (during birth) — omit code
Mold(s) in vitreous 117.9
Mole (pigmented) (M8720/0) — see also Neoplasm, skin, benign
  blood 631.8
  Breus' 631.8
  cancerous (M8720/3) — see Melanoma
  carneous 631.8
  destructive (M9100/1) 236.1
  ectopic — see Pregnancy, ectopic
  fleshy 631.8
  hemorrhagic 631.8
  hydatid, hydatidiform (benign) (complicating pregnancy) (delivered) (undelivered) (see also Hydatidiform mole) 630
    invasive (M9100/1) 236.1
    malignant (M9100/1) 236.1
    previous, affecting management of pregnancy V23.1
  invasive (hydatidiform) (M9100/1) 236.1
  malignant
    meaning
      malignant hydatidiform mole (M9100/1) 236.1
      melanoma (M8720/3) — see Melanoma
  nonpigmented (M8730/0) — see Neoplasm, skin, benign
  pregnancy NEC 631.8
  skin (M8720/0) — see Neoplasm, skin, benign
  stone 631.8
  tubal — see Pregnancy, tubal
  vesicular (see also Hydatidiform mole) 630
Molimen, molimina (menstrual) 625.4
Mollaret's meningitis 047.9
Mollities (cerebellar) (cerebral) 437.8
  ossium 268.2
Molluscum
  contagiosum 078.0
  epitheliale 078.0
  fibrosum (M8851/0) — see Lipoma, by site
  pendulum (M8851/0) — see Lipoma, by site

☑ Additional Digit Required — Refer to the Tabular List for Digit Selection   ᵂ Subterms under main terms may continue to next column or page

186 — Volume 2   ▶◀ Revised Text   ● New Line   ▲ Revised Code   2013 ICD-9-CM

Mönckeberg's arteriosclerosis, degeneration, disease, or sclerosis — see also
    Arteriosclerosis, extremities 440.20
Monday fever 504
Monday morning dyspnea or asthma 504
Mondini's malformation (cochlea) 744.05
Mondor's disease (thrombophlebitis of breast) 451.89
Mongolian, mongolianism, mongolism, mongoloid 758.0
    spot 757.33
Monilethrix (congenital) 757.4
Monilia infestation — see Candidiasis
Moniliasis — see also Candidiasis
    neonatal 771.7
    vulvovaginitis 112.1
Monkeypox 059.01
Monoarthritis 716.60
    ankle 716.67
    arm 716.62
        lower (and wrist) 716.63
        upper (and elbow) 716.62
    foot (and ankle) 716.67
    forearm (and wrist) 716.63
    hand 716.64
    leg 716.66
        lower 716.66
        upper 716.65
    pelvic region (hip) (thigh) 716.65
    shoulder (region) 716.61
    specified site NEC 716.68
Monoblastic — see condition
Monochromatism (cone) (rod) 368.54
Monocytic — see condition
Monocytopenia 288.59
Monocytosis (symptomatic) 288.63
Monofixation syndrome 378.34
Monomania — see also Psychosis 298.9
Mononeuritis 355.9
    cranial nerve — see Disorder, nerve, cranial
    femoral nerve 355.2
    lateral
        cutaneous nerve of thigh 355.1
        popliteal nerve 355.3
    lower limb 355.8
        specified nerve NEC 355.79
    medial popliteal nerve 355.4
    median nerve 354.1
    multiplex 354.5
    plantar nerve 355.6
    posterior tibial nerve 355.5
    radial nerve 354.3
    sciatic nerve 355.0
    ulnar nerve 354.2
    upper limb 354.9
        specified nerve NEC 354.8
    vestibular 388.5
Mononeuropathy — see also Mononeuritis 355.9
    diabetic NEC 250.6 ☑ [355.9]
        due to secondary diabetes 249.6 ☑ [355.9]
        lower limb 250.6 ☑ [355.8]
            due to secondary diabetes 249.6 ☑ [355.8]
        upper limb 250.6 ☑ [354.9]
            due to secondary diabetes 249.6 ☑ [354.9]
    iliohypogastric nerve 355.79
    ilioinguinal nerve 355.79
    obturator nerve 355.79
    saphenous nerve 355.79
Mononucleosis, infectious 075
    with hepatitis 075 [573.1]
Monoplegia 344.5
    brain (current episode) (see also Paralysis, brain) 437.8
        fetus or newborn 767.8
    cerebral (current episode) (see also Paralysis, brain) 437.8
    congenital or infantile (cerebral) (spastic) (spinal) 343.3
    embolic (current) (see also Embolism, brain) 434.1 ☑
        late effect — see Late effect(s) (of) cerebrovascular disease

Monoplegia — continued
    infantile (cerebral) (spastic) (spinal) 343.3
    lower limb 344.30
        affecting
            dominant side 344.31
            nondominant side 344.32
        due to late effect of cerebrovascular accident — see Late effect(s) (of) cerebrovascular accident
    newborn 767.8
    psychogenic 306.0
        specified as conversion reaction 300.11
    thrombotic (current) (see also Thrombosis, brain) 434.0 ☑
        late effect — see Late effect(s) (of) cerebrovascular disease
    transient 781.4
    upper limb 344.40
        affecting
            dominant side 344.41
            nondominant side 344.42
        due to late effect of cerebrovascular accident — see Late effect(s) (of) cerebrovascular accident
Monorchism, monorchidism 752.89
Monteggia's fracture (closed) 813.03
    open 813.13
Mood swings
    brief compensatory 296.99
    rebound 296.99
Mooren's ulcer (cornea) 370.07
Moore's syndrome — see also Epilepsy 345.5 ☑
Mooser bodies 081.0
Mooser-Neill reaction 081.0
Moral
    deficiency 301.7
    imbecility 301.7
Morax-Axenfeld conjunctivitis 372.03
Morbilli — see also Measles 055.9
Morbus
    anglicus, anglorum 268.0
    Beigel 111.2
    caducus (see also Epilepsy) 345.9 ☑
    caeruleus 746.89
    celiacus 579.0
    comitialis (see also Epilepsy) 345.9 ☑
    cordis (see also Disease, heart)
        valvulorum — see Endocarditis
    coxae 719.95
        tuberculous (see also Tuberculosis) 015.1 ☑
    hemorrhagicus neonatorum 776.0
    maculosus neonatorum 772.6
    renum 593.0
    senilis (see also Osteoarthrosis) 715.9 ☑
Morel-Kraepelin disease — see also Schizophrenia 295.9 ☑
Morel-Moore syndrome (hyperostosis frontalis interna) 733.3
Morel-Morgagni syndrome (hyperostosis frontalis interna) 733.3
Morgagni
    cyst, organ, hydatid, or appendage 752.89
        fallopian tube 752.11
    disease or syndrome (hyperostosis frontalis interna) 733.3
Morgagni-Adams-Stokes syndrome (syncope with heart block) 426.9
Morgagni-Stewart-Morel syndrome (hyperostosis frontalis interna) 733.3
Moria — see also Psychosis 298.9
Morning sickness 643.0 ☑
Moron 317
Morphea (guttate) (linear) 701.0
Morphine dependence — see also Dependence 304.0 ☑
Morphinism — see also Dependence 304.0 ☑
Morphinomania — see also Dependence 304.0 ☑
Morphoea 701.0
Morquio (-Brailsford) (-Ullrich) disease or syndrome (mucopolysaccharidosis IV) 277.5
    kyphosis 277.5

Morris syndrome (testicular feminization) 259.51
Morsus humanus (open wound) — see also Wound, open, by site
    skin surface intact — see Contusion
Mortification (dry) (moist) — see also Gangrene 785.4
Morton's
    disease 355.6
    foot 355.6
    metatarsalgia (syndrome) 355.6
    neuralgia 355.6
    neuroma 355.6
    syndrome (metatarsalgia) (neuralgia) 355.6
    toe 355.6
Morvan's disease 336.0
Mosaicism, mosaic (chromosomal) 758.9
    autosomal 758.5
    sex 758.81
Moschcowitz's syndrome (thrombotic thrombocytopenic purpura) 446.6
Mother yaw 102.0
Motion sickness (from travel, any vehicle) (from roundabouts or swings) 994.6
Mottled teeth (enamel) (endemic) (nonendemic) 520.3
Mottling enamel (endemic) (nonendemic) (teeth) 520.3
Mouchet's disease 732.5
Mould(s) (in vitreous) 117.9
Moulders'
    bronchitis 502
    tuberculosis (see also Tuberculosis) 011.4 ☑
Mounier-Kuhn syndrome 748.3
    with
        acute exacerbation 494.1
        bronchiectasis 494.0
            with (acute) exacerbation 494.1
    acquired 519.19
        with bronchiectasis 494.0
            with (acute) exacerbation 494.1
Mountain
    fever — see Fever, mountain
    sickness 993.2
        with polycythemia, acquired 289.0
        acute 289.0
    tick fever 066.1
Mouse, joint — see also Loose, body, joint 718.1 ☑
    knee 717.6
Mouth — see condition
Movable
    coccyx 724.71
    kidney (see also Disease, renal) 593.0
        congenital 753.3
    organ or site, congenital NEC — see Malposition, congenital
    spleen 289.59
Movement
    abnormal (dystonic) (involuntary) 781.0
    decreased fetal 655.7 ☑
    paradoxical facial 374.43
Moya Moya disease 437.5
Mozart's ear 744.29
MRSA (methicillin-resistant staphylococcus aureus) 041.12
    colonization V02.54
    personal history of V12.04
MSSA (methicillin susceptible staphylococcus aureus) 041.11
    colonization V02.53
Mucha's disease (acute parapsoriasis varioliformis) 696.2
Mucha-Haberman syndrome (acute parapsoriasis varioliformis) 696.2
Mu-chain disease 273.2
Mucinosis (cutaneous) (papular) 701.8
Mucocele
    appendix 543.9
    buccal cavity 528.9
    gallbladder (see also Disease, gallbladder) 575.3
    lacrimal sac 375.43
    orbit (eye) 376.81
    salivary gland (any) 527.6
    sinus (accessory) (nasal) 478.19

Mucocele — continued
    turbinate (bone) (middle) (nasal) 478.19
    uterus 621.8
Mucocutaneous lymph node syndrome (acute) (febrile) (infantile) 446.1
Mucoenteritis 564.9
Mucolipidosis I, II, III 272.7
Mucopolysaccharidosis (types 1-6) 277.5
    cardiopathy 277.5 [425.7]
Mucormycosis (lung) 117.7
Mucosa associated lymphoid tissue (MALT) 200.3 ☑
Mucositis — see also Inflammation, by site 528.00
    cervix (ulcerative) 616.81
    due to
        antineoplastic therapy (ulcerative) 528.01
        other drugs (ulcerative) 528.02
        specified NEC 528.09
    gastrointestinal (ulcerative) 538
    nasal (ulcerative) 478.11
    necroticans agranulocytica (see also Agranulocytosis) 288.09
    ulcerative 528.00
    vagina (ulcerative) 616.81
    vulva (ulcerative) 616.81
Mucous — see also condition
    patches (syphilitic) 091.3
        congenital 090.0
Mucoviscidosis 277.00
    with meconium obstruction 277.01
Mucus
    asphyxia or suffocation (see also Asphyxia, mucus) 933.1
        newborn 770.18
    in stool 792.1
    plug (see also Asphyxia, mucus) 933.1
        aspiration, of newborn 770.17
        tracheobronchial 519.19
            newborn 770.18
Muguet 112.0
Mulberry molars 090.5
Müllerian mixed tumor (M8950/3) — see Neoplasm, by site, malignant
Multicystic kidney 753.19
Multilobed placenta — see Placenta, abnormal
Multinodular prostate 600.10
    with
        urinary
            obstruction 600.11
            retention 600.11
Multiparity V61.5
    affecting
        fetus or newborn 763.89
        management of
            labor and delivery 659.4 ☑
            pregnancy V23.3
    requiring contraceptive management (see also Contraception) V25.9
Multipartita placenta — see Placenta, abnormal
Multiple, multiplex — see also condition
    birth
        affecting fetus or newborn 761.5
        healthy liveborn — see Newborn, multiple
    digits (congenital) 755.00
        fingers 755.01
        toes 755.02
    organ or site NEC — see Accessory
    personality 300.14
    renal arteries 747.62
Mumps 072.9
    with complication 072.8
        specified type NEC 072.79
    encephalitis 072.2
    hepatitis 072.71
    meningitis (aseptic) 072.1
    meningoencephalitis 072.2
    oophoritis 072.79
    orchitis 072.0
    pancreatitis 072.3
    polyneuropathy 072.72
    vaccination, prophylactic (against) V04.6

☑ **Additional Digit Required — Refer to the Tabular List for Digit Selection**					▽ **Subterms under main terms may continue to next column or page**

2013 ICD-9-CM					▶◀ Revised Text					● New Line					▲ Revised Code					Volume 2 — 187

Mumu — *see also* Infestation, filarial 125.9
Münchausen syndrome 301.51
Münchmeyer's disease or syndrome (exostosis luxurians) 728.11
Mural — *see* condition
Murmur (cardiac) (heart) (nonorganic) (organic) 785.2
  abdominal 787.5
  aortic (valve) (*see also* Endocarditis, aortic) 424.1
  benign — *omit code*
  cardiorespiratory 785.2
  diastolic — *see* condition
  Flint (*see also* Endocarditis, aortic) 424.1
  functional — *omit code*
  Graham Steell (pulmonic regurgitation) (*see also* Endocarditis, pulmonary) 424.3
  innocent — *omit code*
  insignificant — *omit code*
  midsystolic 785.2
  mitral (valve) — *see* Stenosis, mitral
  physiologic — *see* condition
  presystolic, mitral — *see* Insufficiency, mitral
  pulmonic (valve) (*see also* Endocarditis, pulmonary) 424.3
  Still's (vibratory) — *omit code*
  systolic (valvular) — *see* condition
  tricuspid (valve) — *see* Endocarditis, tricuspid
  undiagnosed 785.2
  valvular — *see* condition
  vibratory — *omit code*
Murri's disease (intermittent hemoglobinuria) 283.2
Muscae volitantes 379.24
Muscle, muscular — *see* condition
Musculoneuralgia 729.1
Mushrooming hip 718.95
Mushroom workers' (pickers') lung 495.5
Mutation(s)
  factor V Leiden 289.81
  prothrombin gene 289.81
  surfactant, of lung 516.63
Mutism — *see also* Aphasia 784.3
  akinetic 784.3
  deaf (acquired) (congenital) 389.7
  hysterical 300.11
  selective (elective) 313.23
    adjustment reaction 309.83
MVD (microvillus inclusion disease) 751.5
MVID (microvillus inclusion disease) 751.5
Myà's disease (congenital dilation, colon) 751.3
Myalgia (intercostal) 729.1
  eosinophilia syndrome 710.5
  epidemic 074.1
    cervical 078.89
  psychogenic 307.89
  traumatic NEC 959.9
Myasthenia 358.00
  cordis — *see* Failure, heart
  gravis 358.00
    with exacerbation (acute) 358.01
    in crisis 358.01
    neonatal 775.2
    pseudoparalytica 358.00
  stomach 536.8
    psychogenic 306.4
  syndrome
    in
      botulism 005.1 *[358.1]*
      diabetes mellitus 250.6 ☑ *[358.1]*
        due to secondary diabetes 249.6 ☑ *[358.1]*
      hypothyroidism (*see also* Hypothyroidism) 244.9 *[358.1]*
      malignant neoplasm NEC 199.1 *[358.1]*
      pernicious anemia 281.0 *[358.1]*
      thyrotoxicosis (*see also* Thyrotoxicosis) 242.9 ☑ *[358.1]*
Myasthenic 728.87
Mycelium infection NEC 117.9
Mycetismus 988.1
Mycetoma (actinomycotic) 039.9
  bone 039.8

Mycetoma — *continued*
  bone — *continued*
    mycotic 117.4
  foot 039.4
    mycotic 117.4
  madurae 039.9
    mycotic 117.4
  maduromycotic 039.9
    mycotic 117.4
  mycotic 117.4
  nocardial 039.9
Mycobacteriosis — *see* Mycobacterium
Mycobacterium, mycobacterial (infection) 031.9
  acid-fast (bacilli) 031.9
  anonymous (*see also* Mycobacterium, atypical) 031.9
  atypical (acid-fast bacilli) 031.9
    cutaneous 031.1
    pulmonary 031.0
      tuberculous (*see also* Tuberculosis, pulmonary) 011.9 ☑
    specified site NEC 031.8
  avium 031.0
    intracellulare complex bacteremia (MAC) 031.2
  balnei 031.1
  Battey 031.0
  cutaneous 031.1
  disseminated 031.2
    avium-intracellulare complex (DMAC) 031.2
  fortuitum 031.0
  intracellulare (battey bacillus) 031.0
  kakerifu 031.8
  kansasii 031.0
  kasongo 031.8
  leprae — *see* Leprosy
  luciflavum 031.0
  marinum 031.1
  pulmonary 031.0
    tuberculous (*see also* Tuberculosis, pulmonary) 011.9 ☑
  scrofulaceum 031.1
  tuberculosis (human, bovine) (*see also* Tuberculosis)
    avian type 031.0
  ulcerans 031.1
  xenopi 031.0
Mycosis, mycotic 117.9
  cutaneous NEC 111.9
  ear 111.8 *[380.15]*
  fungoides (M9700/3) 202.1 ☑
  mouth 112.0
  pharynx 117.9
  skin NEC 111.9
  stomatitis 112.0
  systemic NEC 117.9
  tonsil 117.9
  vagina, vaginitis 112.1
Mydriasis (persistent) (pupil) 379.43
Myelatelia 742.59
Myelinoclasis, perivascular, acute (postinfectious) NEC 136.9 *[323.61]*
  postimmunization or postvaccinal 323.51
Myelinosis, central pontine 341.8
Myelitis (ascending) (cerebellar) (childhood) (chronic) (descending) (diffuse) (disseminated) (pressure) (progressive) (spinal cord) (subacute) — *see also* Encephalitis 323.9
  acute (transverse) 341.20
    idiopathic 341.22
    in conditions classified elsewhere 341.21
  due to
    other infection classified elsewhere 136.9 *[323.42]*
    specified cause NEC 323.82
    vaccination (any) 323.52
    viral diseases classified elsewhere 323.02
  herpes simplex 054.74
  herpes zoster 053.14
  late effect — *see* category 326
  optic neuritis in 341.0
  postchickenpox 052.2
  postimmunization 323.52

Myelitis — *see also* Encephalitis — *continued*
  postinfectious 136.9 *[323.63]*
  postvaccinal 323.52
  postvaricella 052.2
  syphilitic (transverse) 094.89
  toxic 989.9 *[323.72]*
  transverse 323.82
    acute 341.20
      idiopathic 341.22
      in conditions classified elsewhere 341.21
    idiopathic 341.22
  tuberculous (*see also* Tuberculosis) 013.6 ☑
  virus 049.9
Myeloblastic — *see* condition
Myelocele — *see also* Spina bifida 741.9 ☑
  with hydrocephalus 741.0 ☑
Myelocystocele — *see also* Spina bifida 741.9 ☑
Myelocytic — *see* condition
Myelocytoma 205.1 ☑
Myelodysplasia (spinal cord) 742.59
  meaning myelodysplastic syndrome — *see* Syndrome, myelodysplastic
Myeloencephalitis — *see* Encephalitis
Myelofibrosis 289.83
  with myeloid metaplasia 238.76
  idiopathic (chronic) 238.76
  megakaryocytic 238.79
  primary 238.76
  secondary 289.83
Myelogenous — *see* condition
Myeloid — *see* condition
Myelokathexis 288.09
Myeloleukodystrophy 330.0
Myelolipoma (M8870/0) — *see* Neoplasm, by site, benign
Myeloma (multiple) (plasma cell) (plasmacytic) (M9730/3) 203.0 ☑
  monostotic (M9731/1) 238.6
  solitary (M9731/1) 238.6
Myelomalacia 336.8
Myelomata, multiple (M9730/3) 203.0 ☑
Myelomatosis (M9730/3) 203.0 ☑
Myelomeningitis — *see* Meningoencephalitis
Myelomeningocele (spinal cord) — *see also* Spina bifida 741.9 ☑
  fetal, causing fetopelvic disproportion 653.7 ☑
Myelo-osteo-musculodysplasia hereditaria 756.89
Myelopathic — *see* condition
Myelopathy (spinal cord) 336.9
  cervical 721.1
  diabetic 250.6 ☑ *[336.3]*
    due to secondary diabetes 249.6 ☑ *[336.3]*
  drug-induced 336.8
  due to or with
    carbon tetrachloride 987.8 *[323.72]*
    degeneration or displacement, intervertebral disc 722.70
      cervical, cervicothoracic 722.71
      lumbar, lumbosacral 722.73
      thoracic, thoracolumbar 722.72
    hydroxyquinoline derivatives 961.3 *[323.72]*
    infection — *see* Encephalitis
    intervertebral disc disorder 722.70
      cervical, cervicothoracic 722.71
      lumbar, lumbosacral 722.73
      thoracic, thoracolumbar 722.72
    lead 984.9 *[323.72]*
    mercury 985.0 *[323.72]*
    neoplastic disease (*see also* Neoplasm, by site) 239.9 *[336.3]*
    pernicious anemia 281.0 *[336.3]*
    spondylosis 721.91
      cervical 721.1
      lumbar, lumbosacral 721.42
      thoracic 721.41
    thallium 985.8 *[323.72]*
  lumbar, lumbosacral 721.42
  necrotic (subacute) 336.1
  radiation-induced 336.8

Myelopathy — *continued*
  spondylogenic NEC 721.91
    cervical 721.1
    lumbar, lumbosacral 721.42
    thoracic 721.41
  thoracic 721.41
  toxic NEC 989.9 *[323.72]*
  transverse (*see also* Myelitis) 323.82
  vascular 336.1
Myelophthisis 284.2
Myeloproliferative disease (M9960/1) 238.79
Myeloradiculitis — *see also* Polyneuropathy 357.0
Myeloradiculodysplasia (spinal) 742.59
Myelosarcoma (M9930/3) 205.3 ☑
Myelosclerosis 289.89
  with myeloid metaplasia (M9961/1) 238.76
  disseminated, of nervous system 340
  megakaryocytic (M9961/1) 238.79
Myelosis (M9860/3) — *see also* Leukemia, myeloid 205.9 ☑
  acute (M9861/3) 205.0 ☑
  aleukemic (M9864/3) 205.8 ☑
  chronic (M9863/3) 205.1 ☑
  erythremic (M9840/3) 207.0 ☑
    acute (M9841/3) 207.0 ☑
  megakaryocytic (M9920/3) 207.2 ☑
  nonleukemic (chronic) 288.8
  subacute (M9862/3) 205.2 ☑
Myesthenia — *see* Myasthenia
Myiasis (cavernous) 134.0
  orbit 134.0 *[376.13]*
Myoadenoma, prostate 600.20
  with
    other lower urinary tract symptoms (LUTS) 600.21
    urinary
      obstruction 600.21
      retention 600.21
Myoblastoma
  granular cell (M9580/0) (*see also* Neoplasm, connective tissue, benign)
    malignant (M9580/3) — *see* Neoplasm, connective tissue, malignant
  tongue (M9580/0) 210.1
Myocardial — *see* condition
Myocardiopathy (congestive) (constrictive) (familial) (idiopathic) (infiltrative) (obstructive) (primary) (restrictive) (sporadic) 425.4
  alcoholic 425.5
  amyloid 277.39 *[425.7]*
  beriberi 265.0 *[425.7]*
  cobalt-beer 425.5
  due to
    amyloidosis 277.39 *[425.7]*
    beriberi 265.0 *[425.7]*
    cardiac glycogenosis 271.0 *[425.7]*
    Chagas' disease 086.0
    Friedreich's ataxia 334.0 *[425.8]*
    influenza (*see also* Influenza) 487.8 *[425.8]*
    mucopolysaccharidosis 277.5 *[425.7]*
    myotonia atrophica 359.21 *[425.8]*
    progressive muscular dystrophy 359.1 *[425.8]*
    sarcoidosis 135 *[425.8]*
  glycogen storage 271.0 *[425.7]*
  hypertrophic 425.18
    nonobstructive 425.18
    obstructive 425.11
  metabolic NEC 277.9 *[425.7]*
  nutritional 269.9 *[425.7]*
  obscure (African) 425.2
  peripartum 674.5 ☑
  postpartum 674.5 ☑
  secondary 425.9
  thyrotoxic (*see also* Thyrotoxicosis) 242.9 ☑ *[425.7]*
  toxic NEC 425.9
Myocarditis (fibroid) (interstitial) (old) (progressive) (senile) (with arteriosclerosis) 429.0
  with
    rheumatic fever (conditions classifiable to 390) 398.0

Myocarditis — *continued*
  with — *continued*
    rheumatic fever — *continued*
      active (*see also* Myocarditis, acute, rheumatic) 391.2
      inactive or quiescent (with chorea) 398.0
  active (nonrheumatic) 422.90
    rheumatic 391.2
      with chorea (acute) (rheumatic) (Sydenham's) 392.0
  acute or subacute (interstitial) 422.90
    due to Streptococcus (beta-hemolytic) 391.2
    idiopathic 422.91
    rheumatic 391.2
      with chorea (acute) (rheumatic) (Sydenham's) 392.0
    specified type NEC 422.99
  aseptic of newborn 074.23
  bacterial (acute) 422.92
  chagasic 086.0
  chronic (interstitial) 429.0
  congenital 746.89
  constrictive 425.4
  Coxsackie (virus) 074.23
  diphtheritic 032.82
  due to or in
    Coxsackie (virus) 074.23
    diphtheria 032.82
    epidemic louse-borne typhus 080 [422.0]
    influenza (*see also* Influenza) 487.8 [422.0]
    Lyme disease 088.81 [422.0]
    scarlet fever 034.1 [422.0]
    toxoplasmosis (acquired) 130.3
    tuberculosis (*see also* Tuberculosis) 017.9 ☑ [422.0]
    typhoid 002.0 [422.0]
    typhus NEC 081.9 [422.0]
  eosinophilic 422.91
  epidemic of newborn 074.23
  Fiedler's (acute) (isolated) (subacute) 422.91
  giant cell (acute) (subacute) 422.91
  gonococcal 098.85
  granulomatous (idiopathic) (isolated) (nonspecific) 422.91
  hypertensive (*see also* Hypertension, heart) 402.90
  idiopathic 422.91
    granulomatous 422.91
  infective 422.92
  influenzal (*see also* Influenza) 487.8 [422.0]
  isolated (diffuse) (granulomatous) 422.91
  malignant 422.99
  meningococcal 036.43
  nonrheumatic, active 422.90
  parenchymatous 422.90
  pneumococcal (acute) (subacute) 422.92
  rheumatic (chronic) (inactive) (with chorea) 398.0
    active or acute 391.2
      with chorea (acute) (rheumatic) (Sydenham's) 392.0
  septic 422.92
  specific (giant cell) (productive) 422.91
  staphylococcal (acute) (subacute) 422.92
  suppurative 422.92
  syphilitic (chronic) 093.82
  toxic 422.93
    rheumatic (*see also* Myocarditis, acute rheumatic) 391.2
  tuberculous (*see also* Tuberculosis) 017.9 ☑ [422.0]
  typhoid 002.0 [422.0]
  valvular — *see* Endocarditis
  viral, except Coxsackie 422.91
    Coxsackie 074.23
    of newborn (Coxsackie) 074.23
Myocardium, myocardial — *see* condition
Myocardosis — *see also* Cardiomyopathy 425.4
Myoclonia (essential) 333.2
  epileptica 345.1 ☑
  Friedrich's 333.2
  massive 333.2

Myoclonic
  epilepsy, familial (progressive) 345.1 ☑
  jerks 333.2
Myoclonus (familial essential) (multifocal) (simplex) 333.2
  with epilepsy and with ragged red fibers (MERRF syndrome) 277.87
  facial 351.8
  massive (infantile) 333.2
  palatal 333.2
  pharyngeal 333.2
Myocytolysis 429.1
Myodiastasis 728.84
Myoendocarditis — *see also* Endocarditis
  acute or subacute 421.9
Myoepithelioma (M8982/0) — *see* Neoplasm, by site, benign
Myofascitis (acute) 729.1
  low back 724.2
Myofibroma (M8890/0) — *see also* Neoplasm, connective tissue, benign
  uterus (cervix) (corpus) (*see also* Leiomyoma) 218.9
Myofibromatosis
  infantile 759.89
Myofibrosis 728.2
  heart (*see also* Myocarditis) 429.0
  humeroscapular region 726.2
  scapulohumeral 726.2
Myofibrositis — *see also* Myositis 729.1
  scapulohumeral 726.2
Myogelosis (occupational) 728.89
Myoglobinuria 791.3
Myoglobulinuria, primary 791.3
Myokymia — *see also* Myoclonus
  facial 351.8
Myolipoma (M8860/0)
  specified site — *see* Neoplasm, connective tissue, benign
  unspecified site 223.0
Myoma (M8895/0) — *see also* Neoplasm, connective tissue, benign
  cervix (stump) (uterus) (*see also* Leiomyoma) 218.9
  malignant (M8895/3) — *see* Neoplasm, connective tissue, malignant
  prostate 600.20
    with
      other lower urinary tract symptoms (LUTS) 600.21
      urinary
        obstruction 600.21
        retention 600.21
  uterus (cervix) (corpus) (*see also* Leiomyoma) 218.9
    in pregnancy or childbirth 654.1 ☑
      affecting fetus or newborn 763.89
      causing obstructed labor 660.2 ☑
        affecting fetus or newborn 763.1
Myomalacia 728.9
  cordis, heart (*see also* Degeneration, myocardial) 429.1
Myometritis — *see also* Endometritis 615.9
Myometrium — *see* condition
Myonecrosis, clostridial 040.0
Myopathy 359.9
  alcoholic 359.4
  amyloid 277.39 [359.6]
  benign, congenital 359.0
  central core 359.0
  centronuclear 359.0
  congenital (benign) 359.0
  critical illness 359.81
  distal 359.1
  due to drugs 359.4
  endocrine 259.9 [359.5]
    specified type NEC 259.8 [359.5]
  extraocular muscles 376.82
  facioscapulohumeral 359.1
  in
    Addison's disease 255.41 [359.5]
    amyloidosis 277.39 [359.6]
    cretinism 243 [359.5]
    Cushing's syndrome 255.0 [359.5]
    disseminated lupus erythematosus 710.0 [359.6]

Myopathy — *continued*
  in — *continued*
    giant cell arteritis 446.5 [359.6]
    hyperadrenocorticism NEC 255.3 [359.5]
    hyperparathyroidism 252.01 [359.5]
    hypopituitarism 253.2 [359.5]
    hypothyroidism (*see also* Hypothyroidism) 244.9 [359.5]
    malignant neoplasm NEC (M8000/3) 199.1 [359.6]
    myxedema (*see also* Myxedema) 244.9 [359.5]
    polyarteritis nodosa 446.0 [359.6]
    rheumatoid arthritis 714.0 [359.6]
    sarcoidosis 135 [359.6]
    scleroderma 710.1 [359.6]
    Sjögren's disease 710.2 [359.6]
    thyrotoxicosis (*see also* Thyrotoxicosis) 242.9 ☑ [359.5]
  inflammatory 359.79
    immune NEC 359.79
    specified NEC 359.79
  intensive care (ICU) 359.81
  limb-girdle 359.1
  myotubular 359.0
  necrotizing, acute 359.81
  nemaline 359.0
  ocular 359.1
  oculopharyngeal 359.1
  of critical illness 359.81
  primary 359.89
  progressive NEC 359.89
  proximal myotonic (PROMM) 359.21
  quadriplegic, acute 359.81
  rod body 359.0
  scapulohumeral 359.1
  specified type NEC 359.89
  toxic 359.4
Myopericarditis — *see also* Pericarditis 423.9
Myopia (axial) (congenital) (increased curvature or refraction, nucleus of lens) 367.1
  degenerative, malignant 360.21
  malignant 360.21
  progressive high (degenerative) 360.21
Myosarcoma (M8895/3) — *see* Neoplasm, connective tissue, malignant
Myosis (persistent) 379.42
  stromal (endolymphatic) (M8931/1) 236.0
Myositis 729.1
  clostridial 040.0
  due to posture 729.1
  epidemic 074.1
  fibrosa or fibrous (chronic) 728.2
    Volkmann's (complicating trauma) 958.6
  inclusion body (IBM) 359.71
  infective 728.0
  interstitial 728.81
  multiple — *see* Polymyositis
  occupational 729.1
  orbital, chronic 376.12
  ossificans 728.12
    circumscribed 728.12
    progressive 728.11
    traumatic 728.12
  progressive fibrosing 728.11
  purulent 728.0
  rheumatic 729.1
  rheumatoid 729.1
  suppurative 728.0
  syphilitic 095.6
  traumatic (old) 729.1
Myospasia impulsiva 307.23
Myotonia (acquisita) (intermittens) 728.85
  atrophica 359.21
  congenita 359.22
    acetazolamide responsive 359.22
    dominant form 359.22
    recessive form 359.22
  drug-induced 359.24
  dystrophica 359.21
  fluctuans 359.29
  levior 359.22
  permanens 359.29
Myotonic pupil 379.46
Myriapodiasis 134.1

Myringitis
  with otitis media — *see* Otitis media
  acute 384.00
    specified type NEC 384.09
  bullosa hemorrhagica 384.01
  bullous 384.01
  chronic 384.1
Mysophobia 300.29
Mytilotoxism 988.0
Myxadenitis labialis 528.5
Myxedema (adult) (idiocy) (infantile) (juvenile) (thyroid gland) — *see also* Hypothyroidism 244.9
  circumscribed 242.9 ☑
  congenital 243
  cutis 701.8
  localized (pretibial) 242.9 ☑
  madness (acute) 293.0
    subacute 293.1
  papular 701.8
  pituitary 244.8
  postpartum 674.8 ☑
  pretibial 242.9 ☑
  primary 244.9
Myxochondrosarcoma (M9220/3) — *see* Neoplasm, cartilage, malignant
Myxofibroma (M8811/0) — *see also* Neoplasm, connective tissue, benign
  odontogenic (M9320/0) 213.1
    upper jaw (bone) 213.0
Myxofibrosarcoma (M8811/3) — *see* Neoplasm, connective tissue, malignant
Myxolipoma (M8852/0) — *see also* Lipoma, by site 214.9
Myxoliposarcoma (M8852/3) — *see* Neoplasm, connective tissue, malignant
Myxoma (M8840/0) — *see also* Neoplasm, connective tissue, benign
  odontogenic (M9320/0) 213.1
    upper jaw (bone) 213.0
Myxosarcoma (M8840/3) — *see* Neoplasm, connective tissue, malignant

N

Naegeli's
  disease (hereditary hemorrhagic thrombasthenia) 287.1
  leukemia, monocytic (M9863/3) 205.1 ☑
  syndrome (incontinentia pigmenti) 757.33
Naffziger's syndrome 353.0
Naga sore — *see also* Ulcer, skin 707.9
Nägele's pelvis 738.6
  with disproportion (fetopelvic) 653.0 ☑
    affecting fetus or newborn 763.1
    causing obstructed labor 660.1 ☑
      affecting fetus or newborn 763.1
Nager-de Reynier syndrome (dysostosis mandibularis) 756.0
Nail — *see also* condition
  biting 307.9
  patella syndrome (hereditary osteoonychodysplasia) 756.89
Nanism, nanosomia — *see also* Dwarfism 259.4
  hypophyseal 253.3
  pituitary 253.3
  renis, renalis 588.0
Nanukayami 100.89
Napkin rash 691.0
Narcissism 301.81
Narcolepsy 347.00
  with cataplexy 347.01
  in conditions classified elsewhere 347.10
    with cataplexy 347.11
Narcosis
  carbon dioxide (respiratory) 786.09
  due to drug
    correct substance properly administered 780.09
    overdose or wrong substance given or taken 977.9
      specified drug — *see* Table of Drugs and Chemicals
Narcotism (chronic) — *see also* Dependence 304.9 ☑

☑ **Additional Digit Required — Refer to the Tabular List for Digit Selection**   ⤵ **Subterms under main terms may continue to next column or page**

2013 ICD-9-CM   ▶◀ Revised Text   ● New Line   ▲ Revised Code   Volume 2 — 189

Myocarditis — Narcotism (chronic)

Narcotism (chronic) — *see also* Dependence
— *continued*
  acute
    correct substance properly administered
      349.82
    overdose or wrong substance given or
      taken 967.8
      specified drug — *see* Table of Drugs
        and Chemicals
NARP (ataxia and retinitis pigmentosa) 277.87
Narrow
  anterior chamber angle 365.02
  pelvis (inlet) (outlet) — *see* Contraction,
    pelvis
Narrowing
  artery NEC 447.1
    auditory, internal 433.8 ☑
    basilar 433.0 ☑
      with other precerebral artery
        433.3 ☑
      bilateral 433.3 ☑
    carotid 433.1 ☑
      with other precerebral artery
        433.3 ☑
      bilateral 433.3 ☑
    cerebellar 433.8 ☑
    choroidal 433.8 ☑
    communicating posterior 433.8 ☑
    coronary (*see also* Arteriosclerosis, coro-
      nary)
      congenital 746.85
      due to syphilis 090.5
    hypophyseal 433.8 ☑
    pontine 433.8 ☑
    precerebral NEC 433.9 ☑
      multiple or bilateral 433.3 ☑
      specified NEC 433.8 ☑
    vertebral 433.2 ☑
      with other precerebral artery
        433.3 ☑
      bilateral 433.3 ☑
  auditory canal (external) (*see also* Stricture,
    ear canal, acquired) 380.50
  cerebral arteries 437.0
  cicatricial — *see* Cicatrix
  congenital — *see* Anomaly, congenital
  coronary artery — *see* Narrowing, artery,
    coronary
  ear, middle 385.22
  Eustachian tube (*see also* Obstruction, Eu-
    stachian tube) 381.60
  eyelid 374.46
    congenital 743.62
  intervertebral disc or space NEC — *see* De-
    generation, intervertebral disc
  joint space, hip 719.85
  larynx 478.74
  lids 374.46
    congenital 743.62
  mesenteric artery (with gangrene) 557.0
  palate 524.89
  palpebral fissure 374.46
  retinal artery 362.13
  ureter 593.3
  urethra (*see also* Stricture, urethra) 598.9
Narrowness, abnormal, eyelid 743.62
Nasal — *see* condition
Nasolacrimal — *see* condition
Nasopharyngeal — *see also* condition
  bursa 478.29
  pituitary gland 759.2
  torticollis 723.5
Nasopharyngitis (acute) (infective) (subacute)
  460
  chronic 472.2
    due to external agent — *see* Condition,
      respiratory, chronic, due to
  due to external agent — *see* Condition,
    respiratory, due to
  septic 034.0
  streptococcal 034.0
  suppurative (chronic) 472.2
  ulcerative (chronic) 472.2
Nasopharynx, nasopharyngeal — *see* condition
Natal tooth, teeth 520.6

Nausea — *see also* Vomiting 787.02
  with vomiting 787.01
  epidemic 078.82
  gravidarum — *see* Hyperemesis, gravidarum
  marina 994.6
Navel — *see* condition
Neapolitan fever — *see also* Brucellosis 023.9
Near drowning 994.1
Nearsightedness 367.1
Near-syncope 780.2
Nebécourt's syndrome 253.3
Nebula, cornea (eye) 371.01
  congenital 743.43
    interfering with vision 743.42
Necator americanus infestation 126.1
Necatoriasis 126.1
Neck — *see* condition
Necrencephalus — *see also* Softening, brain
  437.8
Necrobacillosis 040.3
Necrobiosis 799.89
  brain or cerebral (*see also* Softening, brain)
    437.8
  lipoidica 709.3
    diabeticorum 250.8 ☑ *[709.3]*
      due to secondary diabetes
        249.8 ☑ *[709.3]*
Necrodermolysis 695.15
Necrolysis, toxic epidermal 695.15
  due to drug
    correct substance properly administered
      695.15
    overdose or wrong substance given or
      taken 977.9
      specified drug — *see* Table of Drugs
        and Chemicals
  Stevens-Johnson syndrome overlap (SJS-
    TEN overlap syndrome) 695.14
Necrophilia 302.89
Necrosis, necrotic
  adrenal (capsule) (gland) 255.8
  antrum, nasal sinus 478.19
  aorta (hyaline) (*see also* Aneurysm, aorta)
    441.9
    cystic medial 441.00
      abdominal 441.02
      thoracic 441.01
      thoracoabdominal 441.03
    ruptured 441.5
  arteritis 446.0
  artery 447.5
  aseptic, bone 733.40
    femur (head) (neck) 733.42
      medial condyle 733.43
    humoral head 733.41
    jaw 733.45
    medial femoral condyle 733.43
    specific site NEC 733.49
    talus 733.44
  avascular, bone NEC (*see also* Necrosis,
    aseptic, bone) 733.40
  bladder (aseptic) (sphincter) 596.89
  bone (*see also* Osteomyelitis) 730.1 ☑
    acute 730.0 ☑
    aseptic or avascular 733.40
      femur (head) (neck) 733.42
        medial condyle 733.43
      humoral head 733.41
      jaw 733.45
      medial femoral condyle 733.43
      specified site NEC 733.49
      talus 733.44
    ethmoid 478.19
    ischemic 733.40
    jaw 526.4
      aseptic 733.45
    marrow 289.89
    Paget's (osteitis deformans) 731.0
    tuberculous — *see* Tuberculosis, bone
  brain (softening) (*see also* Softening, brain)
    437.8
  breast (aseptic) (fat) (segmental) 611.3
  bronchus, bronchi 519.19
  central nervous system NEC (*see also* Soften-
    ing, brain) 437.8
  cerebellar (*see also* Softening, brain) 437.8

Necrosis, necrotic — *continued*
  cerebral (softening) (*see also* Softening,
    brain) 437.8
  cerebrospinal (softening) (*see also* Soften-
    ing, brain) 437.8
  colon 557.0
  cornea (*see also* Keratitis) 371.40
  cortical, kidney 583.6
  cystic medial (aorta) 441.00
    abdominal 441.02
    thoracic 441.01
    thoracoabdominal 441.03
  dental 521.09
    pulp 522.1
  due to swallowing corrosive substance —
    see Burn, by site
  ear (ossicle) 385.24
  esophagus 530.89
  ethmoid (bone) 478.19
  eyelid 374.50
  fat, fatty (generalized) (*see also* Degenera-
    tion, fatty) 272.8
    abdominal wall 567.82
    breast (aseptic) (segmental) 611.3
    intestine 569.89
    localized — *see* Degeneration, by site,
      fatty
    mesentery 567.82
    omentum 567.82
    pancreas 577.8
    peritoneum 567.82
    skin (subcutaneous) 709.3
      newborn 778.1
  femur (aseptic) (avascular) 733.42
    head 733.42
    medial condyle 733.43
    neck 733.42
  gallbladder (*see also* Cholecystitis, acute)
    575.0
  gangrenous 785.4
  gastric 537.89
  glottis 478.79
  heart (myocardium) — *see* Infarct, myocardi-
    um
  hepatic (*see also* Necrosis, liver) 570
  hip (aseptic) (avascular) 733.42
  intestine (acute) (hemorrhagic) (massive)
    557.0
  ischemic 785.4
  jaw 526.4
    asceptic 733.45
  kidney (bilateral) 583.9
    acute 584.9
    cortical 583.6
      acute 584.6
        with
          abortion — *see* Abortion, by
            type, with renal failure
          ectopic pregnancy (*see also*
            categories
            633.0–633.9) 639.3
          molar pregnancy (*see also*
            categories 630–632)
            639.3
        complicating pregnancy 646.2 ☑
          affecting fetus or newborn
            760.1
        following labor and delivery
          669.3 ☑
    medullary (papillary) (*see also* Pyelitis)
      590.80
    in
      acute renal failure 584.7
      nephritis, nephropathy 583.7
    papillary (*see also* Pyelitis) 590.80
    in
      acute renal failure 584.7
      nephritis, nephropathy 583.7
    tubular 584.5
      with
        abortion — *see* Abortion, by type,
          with renal failure
        ectopic pregnancy (*see also* cate-
          gories 633.0–633.9) 639.3
        molar pregnancy (*see also* cate-
          gories 630–632) 639.3

Necrosis, necrotic — *continued*
  kidney — *continued*
    tubular — *continued*
      complicating
        abortion 639.3
        ectopic or molar pregnancy 639.3
        pregnancy 646.2 ☑
          affecting fetus or newborn
            760.1
        following labor and delivery 669.3 ☑
      traumatic 958.5
  larynx 478.79
  liver (acute) (congenital) (diffuse) (massive)
    (subacute) 570
    with
      abortion — *see* Abortion, by type,
        with specified complication
        NEC
      ectopic pregnancy (*see also* cate-
        gories 633.0–633.9) 639.8
      molar pregnancy (*see also* categories
        630–632) 639.8
    complicating pregnancy 646.7 ☑
      affecting fetus or newborn 760.8
    following
      abortion 639.8
      ectopic or molar pregnancy 639.8
    obstetrical 646.7 ☑
    postabortal 639.8
    puerperal, postpartum 674.8 ☑
    toxic 573.3
  lung 513.0
  lymphatic gland 683
  mammary gland 611.3
  mastoid (chronic) 383.1
  mesentery 557.0
    fat 567.82
  mitral valve — *see* Insufficiency, mitral
  myocardium, myocardial — *see* Infarct,
    myocardium
  nose (septum) 478.19
  omentum 557.0
    with mesenteric infarction 557.0
    fat 567.82
  orbit, orbital 376.10
  ossicles, ear (aseptic) 385.24
  ovary (*see also* Salpingo-oophoritis) 614.2
  pancreas (aseptic) (duct) (fat) 577.8
    acute 577.0
    infective 577.0
  papillary, kidney (*see also* Pyelitis) 590.80
  perineum 624.8
  peritoneum 557.0
    with mesenteric infarction 557.0
    fat 567.82
  pharynx 462
    in granulocytopenia 288.09
  phosphorus 983.9
  pituitary (gland) (postpartum) (Sheehan)
    253.2
  placenta (*see also* Placenta, abnormal)
    656.7 ☑
  pneumonia 513.0
  pulmonary 513.0
  pulp (dental) 522.1
  pylorus 537.89
  radiation — *see* Necrosis, by site
  radium — *see* Necrosis, by site
  renal — *see* Necrosis, kidney
  sclera 379.19
  scrotum 608.89
  skin or subcutaneous tissue 709.8
    due to burn — *see* Burn, by site
    gangrenous 785.4
  spine, spinal (column) 730.18
    acute 730.18
    cord 336.1
  spleen 289.59
  stomach 537.89
  stomatitis 528.1
  subcutaneous fat 709.3
    fetus or newborn 778.1
  subendocardial — *see* Infarct, myocardium
  suprarenal (capsule) (gland) 255.8
  teeth, tooth 521.09
  testis 608.89

Necrosis, necrotic — *continued*
  thymus (gland) 254.8
  tonsil 474.8
  trachea 519.19
  tuberculous NEC — *see* Tuberculosis
  tubular (acute) (anoxic) (toxic) 584.5
    due to a procedure 997.5
  umbilical cord, affecting fetus or newborn
      762.6
  vagina 623.8
  vertebra (lumbar) 730.18
    acute 730.18
    tuberculous (*see also* Tuberculosis)
        015.0 ☑ *[730.8]* ☑
  vesical (aseptic) (bladder) 596.89
  vulva 624.8

Necrosis, necrotic — *continued*
  x-ray — *see* Necrosis, by site
Necrospermia 606.0
Necrotizing angiitis 446.0
Negativism 301.7
Neglect (child) (newborn) NEC 995.52
  adult 995.84
  after or at birth 995.52
  hemispatial 781.8
  left-sided 781.8
  sensory 781.8
  visuospatial 781.8
Negri bodies 071
Neill-Dingwall syndrome (microcephaly and
      dwarfism) 759.89
Neisserian infection NEC — *see* Gonococcus

Nematodiasis NEC — *see also* Infestation, Ne-
      matode 127.9
  ancylostoma (*see also* Ancylostomiasis)
      126.9
Neoformans cryptococcus infection 117.5
Neonatal — *see also* condition
  abstinence syndrome 779.5
  adrenoleukodystrophy 277.86
  teeth, tooth 520.6
Neonatorum — *see* condition
Neoplasia
  anal intraepithelial I (AIN I) (histologically
      confirmed) 569.44
  anal intraepithelial II (AIN II) (histologically
      confirmed) 569.44
  anal intraepithelial III (AIN III) 230.6

Neoplasia — *continued*
  anal intraepithelial III — *continued*
    anal canal 230.5
  endometrial intraepithelial (EIN) 621.35
  multiple endocrine (MEN)
    type I 258.01
    type IIA 258.02
    type IIB 258.03
  vaginal intraepithelial I (VAIN I) 623.0
  vaginal intraepithelial II (VAIN II) 623.0
  vaginal intraepithelial III (VAIN III) 233.31
  vulvular intraepithelial I (VIN I) 624.01
  vulvular intraepithelial II (VIN II) 624.02
  vulvular intraepithelial III (VIN III) 233.32

☑ **Additional Digit Required — Refer to the Tabular List for Digit Selection**   ▽ **Subterms under main terms may continue to next column or page**

2013 ICD-9-CM   ▶◀ **Revised Text**   ● **New Line**   ▲ **Revised Code**   **Volume 2 — 191**

	Malignant					
	Primary	Secondary	Ca in situ	Benign	Uncertain Behavior	Unspecified
Neoplasm, neoplastic	199.1	—	234.9	229.9	238.9	239.9

Notes — 1. The list below gives the code numbers for neoplasms by anatomical site. For each site there are six possible code numbers according to whether the neoplasm in question is malignant, benign, in situ, of uncertain behavior, or of unspecified nature. The description of the neoplasm will often indicate which of the six columns is appropriate; e.g., malignant melanoma of skin, benign fibroadenoma of breast, carcinoma in situ of cervix uteri.

Where such descriptors are not present, the remainder of the Index should be consulted where guidance is given to the appropriate column for each morphological (histological) variety listed; e.g., Mesonephroma — see Neoplasm, malignant; Embryoma — see also Neoplasm, uncertain behavior; Disease, Bowen's — see Neoplasm, skin, in situ. However, the guidance in the Index can be overridden if one of the descriptors mentioned above is present; e.g., malignant adenoma of colon is coded to 153.9 and not to 211.3 as the adjective "malignant" overrides the Index entry "Adenoma — see also Neoplasm, benign."

2. Sites marked with the sign * (e.g., face NEC*) should be classified to malignant neoplasm of skin of these sites if the variety of neoplasm is a squamous cell carcinoma or an epidermoid carcinoma, and to benign neoplasm of skin of these sites if the variety of neoplasm is a papilloma (any type).

	Malignant					
	Primary	Secondary	Ca in situ	Benign	Uncertain Behavior	Unspecified
abdomen, abdominal	195.2	198.89	234.8	229.8	238.8	239.89
cavity	195.2	198.89	234.8	229.8	238.8	239.89
organ	195.2	198.89	234.8	229.8	238.8	239.89
viscera	195.2	198.89	234.8	229.8	238.8	239.89
wall	173.50	198.2	232.5	216.5	238.2	239.2
basal cell carcinoma	173.51	—	—	—	—	—
connective tissue	171.5	198.89	—	215.5	238.1	239.2
specified type NEC	173.59	—	—	—	—	—
squamous cell carcinoma	173.52	—	—	—	—	—
abdominopelvic	195.8	198.89	234.8	229.8	238.8	239.89
accessory sinus — see Neoplasm, sinus						
acoustic nerve	192.0	198.4		225.1	237.9	239.7
acromion (process)	170.4	198.5		213.4	238.0	239.2
adenoid (pharynx) (tissue)	147.1	198.89	230.0	210.7	235.1	239.0
adipose tissue (see also Neoplasm, connective tissue)	171.9	198.89	—	215.9	238.1	239.2
adnexa (uterine)	183.9	198.82	233.39	221.8	236.3	239.5
adrenal (cortex) (gland) (medulla)	194.0	198.7	234.8	227.0	237.2	239.7
ala nasi (external)	173.30	198.2	232.3	216.3	238.2	239.2
alimentary canal or tract NEC	159.9	197.8	230.9	211.9	235.5	239.0
alveolar	143.9	198.89	230.0	210.4	235.1	239.0
mucosa	143.9	198.89	230.0	210.4	235.1	239.0
lower	143.1	198.89	230.0	210.4	235.1	239.0
upper	143.0	198.89	230.0	210.4	235.1	239.0
ridge or process	170.1	198.5	—	213.1	238.0	239.2
carcinoma	143.9	—	—	—	—	—
lower	143.1	—	—	—	—	—
upper	143.0	—	—	—	—	—
lower	170.1	198.5	—	213.1	238.0	239.2
mucosa	143.9	198.89	230.0	210.4	235.1	239.0
lower	143.1	198.89	230.0	210.4	235.1	239.0
upper	143.0	198.89	230.0	210.4	235.1	239.0
upper	170.0	198.5	—	213.0	238.0	239.2
sulcus	145.1	198.89	230.0	210.4	235.1	239.0
alveolus	143.9	198.89	230.0	210.4	235.1	239.0
lower	143.1	198.89	230.0	210.4	235.1	239.0
upper	143.0	198.89	230.0	210.4	235.1	239.0
ampulla of Vater	156.2	197.8	230.8	211.5	235.3	239.0
ankle NEC*	195.5	198.89	232.7	229.8	238.8	239.89
anorectum, anorectal (junction)	154.8	197.5	230.7	211.4	235.2	239.0
antecubital fossa or space*	195.4	198.89	232.6	229.8	238.8	239.89

	Malignant					
	Primary	Secondary	Ca in situ	Benign	Uncertain Behavior	Unspecified
Neoplasm, neoplastic — continued						
antrum (Highmore) (maxillary)	160.2	197.3	231.8	212.0	235.9	239.1
pyloric	151.2	197.8	230.2	211.1	235.2	239.0
tympanicum	160.1	197.3	231.8	212.0	235.9	239.1
anus, anal	154.3	197.5	230.6	211.4	235.5	239.0
canal	154.2	197.5	230.5	211.4	235.5	239.0
contiguous sites with rectosigmoid junction or rectum	154.8	—	—	—	—	—
margin (see also Neoplasm, anus, skin)	173.50	198.2	232.5	216.6	238.2	239.2
skin	173.50	198.2	232.5	216.5	238.2	239.2
basal cell carcinoma	173.51					
specified type NEC	173.59	—	—	—	—	—
squamous cell carcinoma	173.52	—	—	—	—	—
sphincter	154.2	197.5	230.5	211.4	235.5	239.0
aorta (thoracic)	171.4	198.89	—	215.4	238.1	239.2
abdominal	171.5	198.89	—	215.5	238.1	239.2
aortic body	194.6	198.89	—	227.6	237.3	239.7
aponeurosis	171.9	198.89	—	215.9	238.1	239.2
palmar	171.2	198.89	—	215.2	238.1	239.2
plantar	171.3	198.89	—	215.3	238.1	239.2
appendix	153.5	197.5	230.3	211.3	235.2	239.0
arachnoid (cerebral)	192.1	198.4		225.2	237.6	239.7
spinal	192.3	198.4		225.4	237.6	239.7
areola (female)	174.0	198.81	233.0	217	238.3	239.3
male	175.0	198.81	233.0	217	238.3	239.3
arm NEC*	195.4	198.89	232.6	229.8	238.8	239.89
artery — see Neoplasm, connective tissue						
aryepiglottic fold	148.2	198.89	230.0	210.8	235.1	239.0
hypopharyngeal aspect	148.2	198.89	230.0	210.8	235.1	239.0
laryngeal aspect	161.1	197.3	231.0	212.1	235.6	239.1
marginal zone	148.2	198.89	230.0	210.8	235.1	239.0
arytenoid (cartilage)	161.3	197.3	231.0	212.1	235.6	239.1
fold — see Neoplasm, aryepiglottic						
associated with transplanted organ	199.2	—		—	—	—
atlas	170.2	198.5	—	213.2	238.0	239.2
atrium, cardiac	164.1	198.89		212.7	238.8	239.89
auditory canal (external) (skin) (see also Neoplasm, skin, ear)	173.20	198.2	232.2	216.2	238.2	239.2
internal	160.1	197.3	231.8	212.0	235.9	239.1
nerve	192.0	198.4	—	225.1	237.9	239.7
tube	160.1	197.3	231.8	212.0	235.9	239.1
Eustachian	160.1	197.3	231.8	212.0	235.9	239.1
opening	147.2	198.89	230.0	210.7	235.1	239.0
auricle, ear see also Neoplasm, skin, ear)	173.20	198.2	232.2	216.2	238.2	239.2
cartilage	171.0	198.89	—	215.0	238.1	239.2
auricular canal (external) (see also Neoplasm, skin, ear)	173.20	198.2	232.2	216.2	238.2	239.2
internal	160.1	197.3	231.8	212.0	235.9	239.1
autonomic nerve or nervous system NEC	171.9	198.89	—	215.9	238.1	239.2
axilla, axillary	195.1	198.89	234.8	229.8	238.8	239.89
fold (see also Neoplasm, skin, trunk)	173.50	198.2	232.5	216.5	238.2	239.2

Neoplasm, neoplastic — continued

	Malignant					
	Primary	Secondary	Ca in situ	Benign	Uncertain Behavior	Unspecified
back NEC*	195.8	198.89	232.5	229.8	238.8	239.89
Bartholin's gland	184.1	198.82	233.32	221.2	236.3	239.5
basal ganglia	191.0	198.3	—	225.0	237.5	239.6
basis pedunculi	191.7	198.3	—	225.0	237.5	239.6
bile or biliary (tract)	156.9	197.8	230.8	211.5	235.3	239.0
canaliculi (biliferi) (intrahepatic)	155.1	197.8	230.8	211.5	235.3	239.0
canals, interlobular	155.1	197.8	230.8	211.5	235.3	239.0
contiguous sites	156.8	—	—	—	—	—
duct or passage (common) (cystic) (extrahepatic)	156.1	197.8	230.8	211.5	235.3	239.0
contiguous sites with gallbladder	156.8	—	—	—	—	—
interlobular	155.1	197.8	230.8	211.5	235.3	239.0
intrahepatic	155.1	197.8	230.8	211.5	235.3	239.0
and extrahepatic	156.9	197.8	230.8	211.5	235.3	239.0
bladder (urinary)	188.9	198.1	233.7	223.3	236.7	239.4
contiguous sites	188.8	—	—	—	—	—
dome	188.1	198.1	233.7	223.3	236.7	239.4
neck	188.5	198.1	233.7	223.3	236.7	239.4
orifice	188.9	198.1	233.7	223.3	236.7	239.4
ureteric	188.6	198.1	233.7	223.3	236.7	239.4
urethral	188.5	198.1	233.7	223.3	236.7	239.4
sphincter	188.8	198.1	233.7	223.3	236.7	239.4
trigone	188.0	198.1	233.7	223.3	236.7	239.4
urachus	188.7	—	233.7	223.3	236.7	239.4
wall	188.9	198.1	233.7	223.3	236.7	239.4
anterior	188.3	198.1	233.7	223.3	236.7	239.4
lateral	188.2	198.1	233.7	223.3	236.7	239.4
posterior	188.4	198.1	233.7	223.3	236.7	239.4
blood vessel — *see* Neoplasm, connective tissue						
bone (periosteum)	170.9	198.5	—	213.9	238.0	239.2

Note — Carcinomas and adenocarcinomas, of any type other than intraosseous or odontogenic, of the sites listed under "Neoplasm, bone" should be considered as constituting metastatic spread from an unspecified primary site and coded to 198.5 for morbidity coding.

	Malignant					
	Primary	Secondary	Ca in situ	Benign	Uncertain Behavior	Unspecified
acetabulum	170.6	198.5	—	213.6	238.0	239.2
acromion (process)	170.4	198.5	—	213.4	238.0	239.2
ankle	170.8	198.5	—	213.8	238.0	239.2
arm NEC	170.4	198.5	—	213.4	238.0	239.2
astragalus	170.8	198.5	—	213.8	238.0	239.2
atlas	170.2	198.5	—	213.2	238.0	239.2
axis	170.2	198.5	—	213.2	238.0	239.2
back NEC	170.2	198.5	—	213.2	238.0	239.2
calcaneus	170.8	198.5	—	213.8	238.0	239.2
calvarium	170.0	198.5	—	213.0	238.0	239.2
carpus (any)	170.5	198.5	—	213.5	238.0	239.2
cartilage NEC	170.9	198.5	—	213.9	238.0	239.2
clavicle	170.3	198.5	—	213.3	238.0	239.2
clivus	170.0	198.5	—	213.0	238.0	239.2
coccygeal vertebra	170.6	198.5	—	213.6	238.0	239.2
coccyx	170.6	198.5	—	213.6	238.0	239.2
costal cartilage	170.3	198.5	—	213.3	238.0	239.2
costovertebral joint	170.3	198.5	—	213.3	238.0	239.2
cranial	170.0	198.5	—	213.0	238.0	239.2
cuboid	170.8	198.5	—	213.8	238.0	239.2
cuneiform	170.9	198.5	—	213.9	238.0	239.2
ankle	170.8	198.5	—	213.8	238.0	239.2
wrist	170.5	198.5	—	213.5	238.0	239.2
digital	170.9	198.5	—	213.9	238.0	239.2
finger	170.5	198.5	—	213.5	238.0	239.2
toe	170.8	198.5	—	213.8	238.0	239.2

Neoplasm, neoplastic — continued
bone — continued

	Malignant					
	Primary	Secondary	Ca in situ	Benign	Uncertain Behavior	Unspecified
elbow	170.4	198.5	—	213.4	238.0	239.2
ethmoid (labyrinth)	170.0	198.5	—	213.0	238.0	239.2
face	170.0	198.5	—	213.0	238.0	239.2
lower jaw	170.1	198.5	—	213.1	238.0	239.2
femur (any part)	170.7	198.5	—	213.7	238.0	239.2
fibula (any part)	170.7	198.5	—	213.7	238.0	239.2
finger (any)	170.5	198.5	—	213.5	238.0	239.2
foot	170.8	198.5	—	213.8	238.0	239.2
forearm	170.4	198.5	—	213.4	238.0	239.2
frontal	170.0	198.5	—	213.0	238.0	239.2
hand	170.5	198.5	—	213.5	238.0	239.2
heel	170.8	198.5	—	213.8	238.0	239.2
hip	170.6	198.5	—	213.6	238.0	239.2
humerus (any part)	170.4	198.5	—	213.4	238.0	239.2
hyoid	170.0	198.5	—	213.0	238.0	239.2
ilium	170.6	198.5	—	213.6	238.0	239.2
innominate	170.6	198.5	—	213.6	238.0	239.2
intervertebral cartilage or disc	170.2	198.5	—	213.2	238.0	239.2
ischium	170.6	198.5	—	213.6	238.0	239.2
jaw (lower)	170.1	198.5	—	213.1	238.0	239.2
upper	170.0	198.5	—	213.0	238.0	239.2
knee	170.7	198.5	—	213.7	238.0	239.2
leg NEC	170.7	198.5	—	213.7	238.0	239.2
limb NEC	170.9	198.5	—	213.9	238.0	239.2
lower (long bones)	170.7	198.5	—	213.7	238.0	239.2
short bones	170.8	198.5	—	213.8	238.0	239.2
upper (long bones)	170.4	198.5	—	213.4	238.0	239.2
short bones	170.5	198.5	—	213.5	238.0	239.2
long	170.9	198.5	—	213.9	238.0	239.2
lower limbs NEC	170.7	198.5	—	213.7	238.0	239.2
upper limbs NEC	170.4	198.5	—	213.4	238.0	239.2
malar	170.0	198.5	—	213.0	238.0	239.2
mandible	170.1	198.5	—	213.1	238.0	239.2
marrow NEC	202.9	198.5	—	—	—	238.79
mastoid	170.0	198.5	—	213.0	238.0	239.2
maxilla, maxillary (superior)	170.0	198.5	—	213.0	238.0	239.2
inferior	170.1	198.5	—	213.1	238.0	239.2
metacarpus (any)	170.5	198.5	—	213.5	238.0	239.2
metatarsus (any)	170.8	198.5	—	213.8	238.0	239.2
navicular (ankle)	170.8	198.5	—	213.8	238.0	239.2
hand	170.5	198.5	—	213.5	238.0	239.2
nose, nasal	170.0	198.5	—	213.0	238.0	239.2
occipital	170.0	198.5	—	213.0	238.0	239.2
orbit	170.0	198.5	—	213.0	238.0	239.2
parietal	170.0	198.5	—	213.0	238.0	239.2
patella	170.8	198.5	—	213.8	238.0	239.2
pelvic	170.6	198.5	—	213.6	238.0	239.2
phalanges	170.9	198.5	—	213.9	238.0	239.2
foot	170.8	198.5	—	213.8	238.0	239.2
hand	170.5	198.5	—	213.5	238.0	239.2
pubic	170.6	198.5	—	213.6	238.0	239.2
radius (any part)	170.4	198.5	—	213.4	238.0	239.2
rib	170.3	198.5	—	213.3	238.0	239.2
sacral vertebra	170.6	198.5	—	213.6	238.0	239.2
sacrum	170.6	198.5	—	213.6	238.0	239.2
scaphoid (of hand)	170.5	198.5	—	213.5	238.0	239.2
of ankle	170.8	198.5	—	213.8	238.0	239.2
scapula (any part)	170.4	198.5	—	213.4	238.0	239.2
sella turcica	170.0	198.5	—	213.0	238.0	239.2
short	170.9	198.5	—	213.9	238.0	239.2
lower limb	170.8	198.5	—	213.8	238.0	239.2

Neoplasm, neoplastic — continued	Primary	Secondary	Ca in situ	Benign	Uncertain Behavior	Unspecified
bone — continued						
short — continued						
upper limb	170.5	198.5	—	213.5	238.0	239.2
shoulder	170.4	198.5	—	213.4	238.0	239.2
skeleton, skeletal NEC	170.9	198.5	—	213.9	238.0	239.2
skull	170.0	198.5	—	213.0	238.0	239.2
sphenoid	170.0	198.5	—	213.0	238.0	239.2
spine, spinal (column)	170.2	198.5	—	213.2	238.0	239.2
coccyx	170.6	198.5	—	213.6	238.0	239.2
sacrum	170.6	198.5	—	213.6	238.0	239.2
sternum	170.3	198.5	—	213.3	238.0	239.2
tarsus (any)	170.8	198.5	—	213.8	238.0	239.2
temporal	170.0	198.5	—	213.0	238.0	239.2
thumb	170.5	198.5	—	213.5	238.0	239.2
tibia (any part)	170.7	198.5	—	213.7	238.0	239.2
toe (any)	170.8	198.5	—	213.8	238.0	239.2
trapezium	170.5	198.5	—	213.5	238.0	239.2
trapezoid	170.5	198.5	—	213.5	238.0	239.2
turbinate	170.0	198.5	—	213.0	238.0	239.2
ulna (any part)	170.4	198.5	—	213.4	238.0	239.2
unciform	170.5	198.5	—	213.5	238.0	239.2
vertebra (column)	170.2	198.5	—	213.2	238.0	239.2
coccyx	170.6	198.5	—	213.6	238.0	239.2
sacrum	170.6	198.5	—	213.6	238.0	239.2
vomer	170.0	198.5	—	213.0	238.0	239.2
wrist	170.5	198.5	—	213.5	238.0	239.2
xiphoid process	170.3	198.5	—	213.3	238.0	239.2
zygomatic	170.0	198.5	—	213.0	238.0	239.2
book-leaf (mouth)	145.8	198.89	230.0	210.4	235.1	239.0
bowel — see Neoplasm, intestine						
brachial plexus	171.2	198.89	—	215.2	238.1	239.2
brain NEC	191.9	198.3	—	225.0	237.5	239.6
basal ganglia	191.0	198.3	—	225.0	237.5	239.6
cerebellopontine angle	191.6	198.3	—	225.0	237.5	239.6
cerebellum NOS	191.6	198.3	—	225.0	237.5	239.6
cerebrum	191.0	198.3	—	225.0	237.5	239.6
choroid plexus	191.5	198.3	—	225.0	237.5	239.6
contiguous sites	191.8	—	—	—	—	—
corpus callosum	191.8	198.3	—	225.0	237.5	239.6
corpus striatum	191.0	198.3	—	225.0	237.5	239.6
cortex (cerebral)	191.0	198.3	—	225.0	237.5	239.6
frontal lobe	191.1	198.3	—	225.0	237.5	239.6
globus pallidus	191.0	198.3	—	225.0	237.5	239.6
hippocampus	191.2	198.3	—	225.0	237.5	239.6
hypothalamus	191.0	198.3	—	225.0	237.5	239.6
internal capsule	191.0	198.3	—	225.0	237.5	239.6
medulla oblongata	191.7	198.3	—	225.0	237.5	239.6
meninges	192.1	198.4	—	225.2	237.6	239.7
midbrain	191.7	198.3	—	225.0	237.5	239.6
occipital lobe	191.4	198.3	—	225.0	237.5	239.6
parietal lobe	191.3	198.3	—	225.0	237.5	239.6
peduncle	191.7	198.3	—	225.0	237.5	239.6
pons	191.7	198.3	—	225.0	237.5	239.6
stem	191.7	198.3	—	225.0	237.5	239.6
tapetum	191.8	198.3	—	225.0	237.5	239.6
temporal lobe	191.2	198.3	—	225.0	237.5	239.6
thalamus	191.0	198.3	—	225.0	237.5	239.6
uncus	191.2	198.3	—	225.0	237.5	239.6
ventricle (floor)	191.5	198.3	—	225.0	237.5	239.6
branchial (cleft) (vestiges)	146.8	198.89	230.0	210.6	235.1	239.0
breast (connective tissue) (female) (glandular tissue) (soft parts)	174.9	198.81	233.0	217	238.3	239.3
areola	174.0	198.81	233.0	217	238.3	239.3
male	175.0	198.81	233.0	217	238.3	239.3
axillary tail	174.6	198.81	233.0	217	238.3	239.3

Neoplasm, neoplastic — continued	Primary	Secondary	Ca in situ	Benign	Uncertain Behavior	Unspecified
breast — continued						
central portion	174.1	198.81	233.0	217	238.3	239.3
contiguous sites	174.8	—	—	—	—	—
ectopic sites	174.8	198.81	233.0	217	238.3	239.3
inner	174.8	198.81	233.0	217	238.3	239.3
lower	174.8	198.81	233.0	217	238.3	239.3
lower-inner quadrant	174.3	198.81	233.0	217	238.3	239.3
lower-outer quadrant	174.5	198.81	233.0	217	238.3	239.3
male	175.9	198.81	233.0	217	238.3	239.3
areola	175.0	198.81	233.0	217	238.3	239.3
ectopic tissue	175.9	198.81	233.0	217	238.3	239.3
nipple	175.0	198.81	233.0	217	238.3	239.3
mastectomy site (skin) (see also Neoplasm, mastectomy site)	173.50	198.2	—	—	—	—
specified as breast tissue	174.8	198.81	—	—	—	—
midline	174.8	198.81	233.0	217	238.3	239.3
nipple	174.0	198.81	233.0	217	238.3	239.3
male	175.0	198.81	233.0	217	238.3	239.3
outer	174.8	198.81	233.0	217	238.3	239.3
skin (see also Neoplasm, mastectomy site)	173.50	198.2	232.5	216.5	238.2	239.2
tail (axillary)	174.6	198.81	233.0	217	238.3	239.3
upper	174.8	198.81	233.0	217	238.3	239.3
upper-inner quadrant	174.2	198.81	233.0	217	238.3	239.3
upper-outer quadrant	174.4	198.81	233.0	217	238.3	239.3
broad ligament	183.3	198.82	233.39	221.0	236.3	239.5
bronchiogenic, bronchogenic (lung)	162.9	197.0	231.2	212.3	235.7	239.1
bronchiole	162.9	197.0	231.2	212.3	235.7	239.1
bronchus	162.9	197.0	231.2	212.3	235.7	239.1
carina	162.2	197.0	231.2	212.3	235.7	239.1
contiguous sites with lung or trachea	162.8	—	—	—	—	—
lower lobe of lung	162.5	197.0	231.2	212.3	235.7	239.1
main	162.2	197.0	231.2	212.3	235.7	239.1
middle lobe of lung	162.4	197.0	231.2	212.3	235.7	239.1
upper lobe of lung	162.3	197.0	231.2	212.3	235.7	239.1
brow	173.30	198.2	232.3	216.3	238.2	239.2
basal cell carcinoma	173.31	—	—	—	—	—
specified type NEC	173.39	—	—	—	—	—
squamous cell carcinoma	173.32	—	—	—	—	—
buccal (cavity)	145.9	198.89	230.0	210.4	235.1	239.0
commissure	145.0	198.89	230.0	210.4	235.1	239.0
groove (lower) (upper)	145.1	198.89	230.0	210.4	235.1	239.0
mucosa	145.0	198.89	230.0	210.4	235.1	239.0
sulcus (lower) (upper)	145.1	198.89	230.0	210.4	235.1	239.0
bulbourethral gland	189.3	198.1	233.9	223.81	236.99	239.5
bursa — see Neoplasm, connective tissue						
buttock NEC*	195.3	198.89	232.5	229.8	238.8	239.89
calf*	195.5	198.89	232.7	229.8	238.8	239.89
calvarium	170.0	198.5	—	213.0	238.0	239.2
calyx, renal	189.1	198.0	233.9	223.1	236.91	239.5
canal anal	154.2	197.5	230.5	211.4	235.5	239.0

☑ **Additional Digit Required — Refer to the Tabular List for Digit Selection**

ᴺᵉʷ **Subterms under main terms may continue to next column or page**

Neoplasm, neoplastic — continued

	Malignant					
	Primary	Secondary	Ca in situ	Benign	Uncertain Behavior	Unspecified
canal — *continued*						
auditory (external) (*see also* Neoplasm, skin, ear)	173.20	198.2	232.2	216.2	238.2	239.2
auricular (external) (*see also* Neoplasm, skin, ear)	173.20	198.2	232.2	216.2	238.2	239.2
canaliculi, biliary (biliferi) (intrahepatic)	155.1	197.8	230.8	211.5	235.3	239.0
canthus (eye) (inner) (outer)	173.10	198.2	232.1	216.1	238.2	239.2
basal cell carcinoma	173.11	—	—	—	—	—
specified type NEC	173.19	—	—	—	—	—
squamous cell carcinoma	173.12	—	—	—	—	—
capillary — *see* Neoplasm, connective tissue						
caput coli	153.4	197.5	230.3	211.3	235.2	239.0
cardia (gastric)	151.0	197.8	230.2	211.1	235.2	239.0
cardiac orifice (stomach)	151.0	197.8	230.2	211.1	235.2	239.0
cardio-esophageal junction	151.0	197.8	230.2	211.1	235.2	239.0
cardio-esophagus	151.0	197.8	230.2	211.1	235.2	239.0
carina (bronchus)	162.2	197.0	231.2	212.3	235.7	239.1
carotid (artery)	171.0	198.89	—	215.0	238.1	239.2
body	194.5	198.89	—	227.5	237.3	239.7
carpus (any bone)	170.5	198.5	—	213.5	238.0	239.2
cartilage (articular) (joint) NEC (*see also* Neoplasm, bone)	170.9	198.5	—	213.9	238.0	239.2
arytenoid	161.3	197.3	231.0	212.1	235.6	239.1
auricular	171.0	198.89	—	215.0	238.1	239.2
bronchi	162.2	197.3	—	212.3	235.7	239.1
connective tissue — *see* Neoplasm, connective tissue						
costal	170.3	198.5	—	213.3	238.0	239.2
cricoid	161.3	197.3	231.0	212.1	235.6	239.1
cuneiform	161.3	197.3	231.0	212.1	235.6	239.1
ear (external)	171.0	198.89	—	215.0	238.1	239.2
ensiform	170.3	198.5	—	213.3	238.0	239.2
epiglottis	161.1	197.3	231.0	212.1	235.6	239.1
anterior surface	146.4	198.89	230.0	210.6	235.1	239.0
eyelid	171.0	198.89	—	215.0	238.1	239.2
intervertebral	170.2	198.5	—	213.2	238.0	239.2
larynx, laryngeal	161.3	197.3	231.0	212.1	235.6	239.1
nose, nasal	160.0	197.3	231.8	212.0	235.9	239.1
pinna	171.0	198.89	—	215.0	238.1	239.2
rib	170.3	198.5	—	213.3	238.0	239.2
semilunar (knee)	170.7	198.5	—	213.7	238.0	239.2
thyroid	161.3	197.3	231.0	212.1	235.6	239.1
trachea	162.0	197.3	231.1	212.2	235.7	239.1
cauda equina	192.2	198.3	—	225.3	237.5	239.7
cavity						
buccal	145.9	198.89	230.0	210.4	235.1	239.0
nasal	160.0	197.3	231.8	212.0	235.9	239.1
oral	145.9	198.89	230.0	210.4	235.1	239.0
peritoneal	158.9	197.6	—	211.8	235.4	239.0
tympanic	160.1	197.3	231.8	212.0	235.9	239.1
cecum	153.4	197.5	230.3	211.3	235.2	239.0
central						
nervous system — *see* Neoplasm, nervous system						
white matter	191.0	198.3	—	225.0	237.5	239.6

Neoplasm, neoplastic — continued

	Malignant					
	Primary	Secondary	Ca in situ	Benign	Uncertain Behavior	Unspecified
cerebellopontine (angle)	191.6	198.3	—	225.0	237.5	239.6
cerebellum, cerebellar	191.6	198.3	—	225.0	237.5	239.6
cerebrum, cerebral (cortex) (hemisphere) (white matter)	191.0	198.3	—	225.0	237.5	239.6
meninges	192.1	198.4	—	225.2	237.6	239.7
peduncle	191.7	198.3	—	225.0	237.5	239.6
ventricle (any)	191.5	198.3	—	225.0	237.5	239.6
cervical region	195.0	198.89	234.8	229.8	238.8	239.89
cervix (cervical) (uteri) (uterus)	180.9	198.82	233.1	219.0	236.0	239.5
canal	180.0	198.82	233.1	219.0	236.0	239.5
contiguous sites	180.8	—	—	—	—	—
endocervix (canal) (gland)	180.0	198.82	233.1	219.0	236.0	239.5
exocervix	180.1	198.82	233.1	219.0	236.0	239.5
external os	180.1	198.82	233.1	219.0	236.0	239.5
internal os	180.0	198.82	233.1	219.0	236.0	239.5
nabothian gland	180.0	198.82	233.1	219.0	236.0	239.5
squamocolumnar junction	180.8	198.82	233.1	219.0	236.0	239.5
stump	180.8	198.82	233.1	219.0	236.0	239.5
cheek	195.0	198.89	234.8	229.8	238.8	239.89
external	173.30	198.2	232.3	216.3	238.2	239.2
basal cell carcinoma	173.31	—	—	—	—	—
specified type NEC	173.39	—	—	—	—	—
squamous cell carcinoma	173.32	—	—	—	—	—
inner aspect	145.0	198.89	230.0	210.4	235.1	239.0
internal	145.0	198.89	230.0	210.4	235.1	239.0
mucosa	145.0	198.89	230.0	210.4	235.1	239.0
chest (wall) NEC	195.1	198.89	234.8	229.8	238.8	239.89
chiasma opticum	192.0	198.4	—	225.1	237.9	239.7
chin	173.30	198.2	232.3	216.3	238.2	239.2
basal cell carcinoma	173.31	—	—	—	—	—
specified type NEC	173.39	—	—	—	—	—
squamous cell carcinoma	173.32	—	—	—	—	—
choana	147.3	198.89	230.0	210.7	235.1	239.0
cholangiole	155.1	197.8	230.8	211.5	235.3	239.0
choledochal duct	156.1	197.8	230.8	211.5	235.3	239.0
choroid	190.6	198.4	234.0	224.6	238.8	239.81
plexus	191.5	198.3	—	225.0	237.5	239.6
ciliary body	190.0	198.4	234.0	224.0	238.8	239.89
clavicle	170.3	198.5	—	213.3	238.0	239.2
clitoris	184.3	198.82	233.32	221.2	236.3	239.5
clivus	170.0	198.5	—	213.0	238.0	239.2
cloacogenic zone	154.8	197.5	230.7	211.4	235.5	239.0
coccygeal						
body or glomus	194.6	198.89	—	227.6	237.3	239.7
vertebra	170.6	198.5	—	213.6	238.0	239.2
coccyx	170.6	198.5	—	213.6	238.0	239.2
colon — *see also* Neoplasm, intestine, large	153.9	197.5	230.3	211.3	235.2	239.0
with rectum	154.0	197.5	230.4	211.4	235.2	239.0
columnella (*see also* Neoplasm, skin, face)	173.30	198.2	232.3	216.3	238.2	239.2
column, spinal — *see* Neoplasm, spine						
commissure						
labial, lip	140.6	198.89	230.0	210.4	235.1	239.0
laryngeal	161.0	197.3	231.0	212.1	235.6	239.1
common (bile) duct	156.1	197.8	230.8	211.5	235.3	239.0

☑ **Additional Digit Required** — Refer to the Tabular List for Digit Selection

▽ Subterms under main terms may continue to next column or page

Neoplasm, neoplastic — continued

	Malignant					
	Primary	Secondary	Ca in situ	Benign	Uncertain Behavior	Unspecified
concha (see also Neoplasm, skin, ear)	173.20	198.2	232.2	216.2	238.2	239.2
nose	160.0	197.3	231.8	212.0	235.9	239.1
conjunctiva	190.3	198.4	234.0	224.3	238.8	239.89
connective tissue NEC	171.9	198.89	—	215.9	238.1	239.2

Note — For neoplasms of connective tissue (blood vessel, bursa, fascia, ligament, muscle, peripheral nerves, sympathetic and parasympathetic nerves and ganglia, synovia, tendon, etc.) or of morphological types that indicate connective tissue, code according to the list under "Neoplasm, connective tissue"; for sites that do not appear in this list, code to neoplasm of that site; e.g.,

liposarcoma, shoulder 171.2

leiomyosarcoma, stomach 151.9

neurofibroma, chest wall 215.4

Morphological types that indicate connective tissue appear in the proper place in the alphabetic index with the instruction "see Neoplasm, connective tissue..."

	Primary	Secondary	Ca in situ	Benign	Uncertain Behavior	Unspecified
abdomen	171.5	198.89	—	215.5	238.1	239.2
abdominal wall	171.5	198.89	—	215.5	238.1	239.2
ankle	171.3	198.89	—	215.3	238.1	239.2
antecubital fossa or space	171.2	198.89	—	215.2	238.1	239.2
arm	171.2	198.89	—	215.2	238.1	239.2
auricle (ear)	171.0	198.89	—	215.0	238.1	239.2
axilla	171.4	198.89	—	215.4	238.1	239.2
back	171.7	198.89	—	215.7	238.1	239.2
breast (female) (see also Neoplasm, breast)	174.9	198.81	233.0	217	238.3	239.3
male	175.9	198.81	233.0	217	238.3	239.3
buttock	171.6	198.89	—	215.6	238.1	239.2
calf	171.3	198.89	—	215.3	238.1	239.2
cervical region	171.0	198.89	—	215.0	238.1	239.2
cheek	171.0	198.89	—	215.0	238.1	239.2
chest (wall)	171.4	198.89	—	215.4	238.1	239.2
chin	171.0	198.89	—	215.0	238.1	239.2
contiguous sites	171.8	—	—	—	—	—
diaphragm	171.4	198.89	—	215.4	238.1	239.2
ear (external)	171.0	198.89	—	215.0	238.1	239.2
elbow	171.2	198.89	—	215.2	238.1	239.2
extrarectal	171.6	198.89	—	215.6	238.1	239.2
extremity	171.8	198.89	—	215.8	238.1	239.2
lower	171.3	198.89	—	215.3	238.1	239.2
upper	171.2	198.89	—	215.2	238.1	239.2
eyelid	171.0	198.89	—	215.0	238.1	239.2
face	171.0	198.89	—	215.0	238.1	239.2
finger	171.2	198.89	—	215.2	238.1	239.2
flank	171.7	198.89	—	215.7	238.1	239.2
foot	171.3	198.89	—	215.3	238.1	239.2
forearm	171.2	198.89	—	215.2	238.1	239.2
forehead	171.0	198.89	—	215.0	238.1	239.2
gastric	171.5	198.89	—	215.5	238.1	—
gastrointestinal	171.5	198.89	—	215.5	238.1	—
gluteal region	171.6	198.89	—	215.6	238.1	239.2
great vessels NEC	171.4	198.89	—	215.4	238.1	239.2
groin	171.6	198.89	—	215.6	238.1	239.2
hand	171.2	198.89	—	215.2	238.1	239.2
head	171.0	198.89	—	215.0	238.1	239.2
heel	171.3	198.89	—	215.3	238.1	239.2
hip	171.3	198.89	—	215.3	238.1	239.2
hypochondrium	171.5	198.89	—	215.5	238.1	239.2
iliopsoas muscle	171.6	198.89	—	215.5	238.1	239.2
infraclavicular region	171.4	198.89	—	215.4	238.1	239.2
inguinal (canal) (region)	171.6	198.89	—	215.6	238.1	239.2
intestine	171.5	198.89	—	215.5	238.1	—
intrathoracic	171.4	198.89	—	215.4	238.1	239.2
ischiorectal fossa	171.6	198.89	—	215.6	238.1	239.2
jaw	143.9	198.89	230.0	210.4	235.1	239.0

Neoplasm, neoplastic — continued
connective tissue — continued

	Primary	Secondary	Ca in situ	Benign	Uncertain Behavior	Unspecified
knee	171.3	198.89	—	215.3	238.1	239.2
leg	171.3	198.89	—	215.3	238.1	239.2
limb NEC	171.9	198.89	—	215.8	238.1	239.2
lower	171.3	198.89	—	215.3	238.1	239.2
upper	171.2	198.89	—	215.2	238.1	239.2
nates	171.6	198.89	—	215.6	238.1	239.2
neck	171.0	198.89	—	215.0	238.1	239.2
orbit	190.1	198.4	234.0	224.1	238.8	239.89
pararectal	171.6	198.89	—	215.6	238.1	239.2
para-urethral	171.6	198.89	—	215.6	238.1	239.2
paravaginal	171.6	198.89	—	215.6	238.1	239.2
pelvis (floor)	171.6	198.89	—	215.6	238.1	239.2
pelvo-abdominal	171.8	198.89	—	215.8	238.1	239.2
perineum	171.6	198.89	—	215.6	238.1	239.2
perirectal (tissue)	171.6	198.89	—	215.6	238.1	239.2
periurethral (tissue)	171.6	198.89	—	215.6	238.1	239.2
popliteal fossa or space	171.3	198.89	—	215.3	238.1	239.2
presacral	171.6	198.89	—	215.6	238.1	239.2
psoas muscle	171.5	198.89	—	215.5	238.1	239.2
pterygoid fossa	171.0	198.89	—	215.0	238.1	239.2
rectovaginal septum or wall	171.6	198.89	—	215.6	238.1	239.2
rectovesical	171.6	198.89	—	215.6	238.1	239.2
retroperitoneum	158.0	197.6	—	211.8	235.4	239.0
sacrococcygeal region	171.6	198.89	—	215.6	238.1	239.2
scalp	171.0	198.89	—	215.0	238.1	239.2
scapular region	171.4	198.89	—	215.4	238.1	239.2
shoulder	171.2	198.89	—	215.2	238.1	239.2
skin (dermis) NEC	173.90	198.2	232.9	216.9	238.2	239.2
stomach	171.5	198.89	—	215.5	238.1	—
submental	171.0	198.89	—	215.0	238.1	239.2
supraclavicular region	171.0	198.89	—	215.0	238.1	239.2
temple	171.0	198.89	—	215.0	238.1	239.2
temporal region	171.0	198.89	—	215.0	238.1	239.2
thigh	171.3	198.89	—	215.3	238.1	239.2
thoracic (duct) (wall)	171.4	198.89	—	215.4	238.1	239.2
thorax	171.4	198.89	—	215.4	238.1	239.2
thumb	171.2	198.89	—	215.2	238.1	239.2
toe	171.3	198.89	—	215.3	238.1	239.2
trunk	171.7	198.89	—	215.7	238.1	239.2
umbilicus	171.5	198.89	—	215.5	238.1	239.2
vesicorectal	171.6	198.89	—	215.6	238.1	239.2
wrist	171.2	198.89	—	215.2	238.1	239.2
conus medullaris	192.2	198.3	—	225.3	237.5	239.7
cord (true) (vocal)	161.0	197.3	231.0	212.1	235.6	239.1
false	161.1	197.3	231.0	212.1	235.6	239.1
spermatic	187.6	198.82	233.6	222.8	236.6	239.5
spinal (cervical) (lumbar) (thoracic)	192.2	198.3	—	225.3	237.5	239.7
cornea (limbus)	190.4	198.4	234.0	224.4	238.8	239.89
corpus						
albicans	183.0	198.6	233.39	220	236.2	239.5
callosum, brain	191.8	198.3	—	225.0	237.5	239.6
cavernosum	187.3	198.82	233.5	222.1	236.6	239.5
gastric	151.4	197.8	230.2	211.1	235.2	239.0
penis	187.3	198.82	233.5	222.1	236.6	239.5
striatum, cerebrum	191.0	198.3	—	225.0	237.5	239.6
uteri	182.0	198.82	233.2	219.1	236.0	239.5
isthmus	182.1	198.82	233.2	219.1	236.0	239.5
cortex						
adrenal	194.0	198.7	234.8	227.0	237.2	239.7
cerebral	191.0	198.3	—	225.0	237.5	239.6
costal cartilage	170.3	198.5	—	213.3	238.0	239.2

Left column table:

	Malignant			Benign	Uncertain Behavior	Unspecified
	Primary	Secondary	Ca in situ			
Neoplasm, neoplastic — *continued*						
costovertebral joint	170.3	198.5	—	213.3	238.0	239.2
Cowper's gland	189.3	198.1	233.9	223.81	236.99	239.5
cranial (fossa, any)	191.9	198.3	—	225.0	237.5	239.6
meninges	192.1	198.4	—	225.2	237.6	239.7
nerve (any)	192.0	198.4	—	225.1	237.9	239.7
craniobuccal pouch	194.3	198.89	234.8	227.3	237.0	239.7
craniopharyngeal (duct) (pouch)	194.3	198.89	234.8	227.3	237.0	239.7
cricoid	148.0	198.89	230.0	210.8	235.1	239.0
cartilage	161.3	197.3	231.0	212.1	235.6	239.1
cricopharynx	148.0	198.89	230.0	210.8	235.1	239.0
crypt of Morgagni	154.8	197.5	230.7	211.4	235.2	239.0
crystalline lens	190.0	198.4	234.0	224.0	238.8	239.89
cul-de-sac (Douglas')	158.8	197.6	—	211.8	235.4	239.0
cuneiform cartilage	161.3	197.3	231.0	212.1	235.6	239.1
cutaneous — *see* Neoplasm, skin						
cutis — *see* Neoplasm, skin						
cystic (bile) duct (common)	156.1	197.8	230.8	211.5	235.3	239.0
dermis — *see* Neoplasm, skin						
diaphragm	171.4	198.89	—	215.4	238.1	239.2
digestive organs, system, tube, or tract NEC	159.9	197.8	230.9	211.9	235.5	239.0
contiguous sites with peritoneum	159.8	—	—	—	—	—
disc, intervertebral	170.2	198.5	—	213.2	238.0	239.2
disease, generalized	199.0	—	234.9	229.9	238.9	—
disseminated	199.0	—	234.9	229.9	238.9	—
Douglas' cul-de-sac or pouch	158.8	197.6	—	211.8	235.4	239.0
duodenojejunal junction	152.8	197.4	230.7	211.2	235.2	239.0
duodenum	152.0	197.4	230.7	211.2	235.2	239.0
dura (cranial) (mater)	192.1	198.4	—	225.2	237.6	239.7
cerebral	192.1	198.4	—	225.2	237.6	239.7
spinal	192.3	198.4	—	225.4	237.6	239.7
ear (external) (*see also* Neoplasm, ear, skin)	173.20	198.2	232.2	216.2	238.2	239.2
auricle or auris (*see also* Neoplasm, ear, skin)	173.20	198.2	232.2	216.2	238.2	239.2
canal, external (*see also* Neoplasm, ear, skin)	173.20	198.2	232.2	216.2	238.2	239.2
cartilage	171.0	198.89	—	215.0	238.1	239.2
external meatus (*see also* Neoplasm, ear, skin)	173.20	198.2	232.2	216.2	238.2	239.2
inner	160.1	197.3	231.8	212.0	235.9	239.89
lobule (*see also* Neoplasm, ear, skin)	173.20	198.2	232.2	216.2	238.2	239.2
middle	160.1	197.3	231.8	212.0	235.9	239.89
contiguous sites with accessory sinuses or nasal cavities	160.8	—	—	—	—	—
skin	173.20	198.2	232.2	216.2	238.2	239.2
basal cell carcinoma	173.21	—	—	—	—	—
specified type NEC	173.29	—	—	—	—	—
squamous cell carcinoma	173.22	—	—	—	—	—
earlobe	173.20	198.2	232.2	216.2	238.2	239.2

Right column table:

	Malignant			Benign	Uncertain Behavior	Unspecified
	Primary	Secondary	Ca in situ			
Neoplasm, neoplastic — *continued*						
earlobe — *continued*						
basal cell carcinoma	173.21	—	—	—	—	—
specified type NEC	173.29	—	—	—	—	—
squamous cell carcinoma	173.22	—	—	—	—	—
ejaculatory duct	187.8	198.82	233.6	222.8	236.6	239.5
elbow NEC*	195.4	198.89	232.6	229.8	238.8	239.89
endocardium	164.1	198.89	—	212.7	238.8	239.89
endocervix (canal) (gland)	180.0	198.82	233.1	219.0	236.0	239.5
endocrine gland NEC	194.9	198.89	—	227.9	237.4	239.7
pluriglandular NEC	194.8	198.89	234.8	227.8	237.4	239.7
endometrium (gland) (stroma)	182.0	198.82	233.2	219.1	236.0	239.5
ensiform cartilage	170.3	198.5	—	213.3	238.0	239.2
enteric — *see* Neoplasm, intestine						
ependyma (brain)	191.5	198.3	—	225.0	237.5	239.6
epicardium	164.1	198.89	—	212.7	238.8	239.89
epididymis	187.5	198.82	233.6	222.3	236.6	239.5
epidural	192.9	198.4	—	225.9	237.9	239.7
epiglottis	161.1	197.3	231.0	212.1	235.6	239.1
anterior aspect or surface	146.4	198.89	230.0	210.6	235.1	239.0
cartilage	161.3	197.3	231.0	212.1	235.6	239.1
free border (margin)	146.4	198.89	230.0	210.6	235.1	239.0
junctional region	146.5	198.89	230.0	210.6	235.1	239.0
posterior (laryngeal) surface	161.1	197.3	231.0	212.1	235.6	239.1
suprahyoid portion	161.1	197.3	231.0	212.1	235.6	239.1
esophagogastric junction	151.0	197.8	230.2	211.1	235.2	239.0
esophagus	150.9	197.8	230.1	211.0	235.5	239.0
abdominal	150.2	197.8	230.1	211.0	235.5	239.0
cervical	150.0	197.8	230.1	211.0	235.5	239.0
contiguous sites	150.8	—	—	—	—	—
distal (third)	150.5	197.8	230.1	211.0	235.5	239.0
lower (third)	150.5	197.8	230.1	211.0	235.5	239.0
middle (third)	150.4	197.8	230.1	211.0	235.5	239.0
proximal (third)	150.3	197.8	230.1	211.0	235.5	239.0
specified part NEC	150.8	197.8	230.1	211.0	235.5	239.0
thoracic	150.1	197.8	230.1	211.0	235.5	239.0
upper (third)	150.3	197.8	230.1	211.0	235.5	239.0
ethmoid (sinus)	160.3	197.3	231.8	212.0	235.9	239.1
bone or labyrinth	170.0	198.5	—	213.0	238.0	239.2
Eustachian tube	160.1	197.3	231.8	212.0	235.9	239.1
exocervix	180.1	198.82	233.1	219.0	236.0	239.5
external meatus (ear) (*see also* Neoplasm, skin, ear)	173.20	198.2	232.2	216.2	238.2	239.2
os, cervix uteri	180.1	198.82	233.1	219.0	236.0	239.5
extradural	192.9	198.4	—	225.9	237.9	239.7
extrahepatic (bile) duct	156.1	197.8	230.8	211.5	235.3	239.0
contiguous sites with gallbladder	156.8	—	—	—	—	—
extraocular muscle	190.1	198.4	234.0	224.1	238.8	239.89
extrarectal	195.3	198.89	234.8	229.8	238.8	239.89
extremity*	195.8	198.89	232.8	229.8	238.8	239.89
lower*	195.5	198.89	232.7	229.8	238.8	239.89
upper*	195.4	198.89	232.6	229.8	238.8	239.89
eye NEC	190.9	198.4	234.0	224.9	238.8	239.89
contiguous sites	190.8	—	—	—	—	—

☑ **Additional Digit Required — Refer to the Tabular List for Digit Selection**

Ⓦ **Subterms under main terms may continue to next column or page**

	Malignant			Benign	Uncertain Behavior	Unspecified
	Primary	Secondary	Ca in situ			
Neoplasm, neoplastic — *continued*						
eye — *continued*						
specified sites NEC	190.8	198.4	234.0	224.8	238.8	239.89
eyeball	190.0	198.4	234.0	224.0	238.8	239.89
eyebrow	173.30	198.2	232.3	216.3	238.2	239.2
basal cell carcinoma	173.31	—	—	—	—	—
specified type NEC	173.39	—	—	—	—	—
squamous cell carcinoma	173.32	—	—	—	—	—
eyelid (lower) (skin) (upper)	173.10	198.2	232.1	216.1	238.2	239.2
basal cell carcinoma	173.11	—	—	—	—	—
cartilage	171.0	198.89	—	215.0	238.1	239.2
specified type NEC	173.19	—	—	—	—	—
squamous cell carcinoma	173.12	—	—	—	—	—
face NEC*	195.0	198.89	232.3	229.8	238.8	239.89
fallopian tube (accessory)	183.2	198.82	233.39	221.0	236.3	239.5
falx (cerebelli) (cerebri)	192.1	198.4		225.2	237.6	239.7
fascia (*see also* Neoplasm, connective tissue)						
palmar	171.2	198.89	—	215.2	238.1	239.2
plantar	171.3	198.89	—	215.3	238.1	239.2
fatty tissue — *see* Neoplasm, connective tissue						
fauces, faucial NEC	146.9	198.89	230.0	210.6	235.1	239.0
pillars	146.2	198.89	230.0	210.6	235.1	239.0
tonsil	146.0	198.89	230.0	210.5	235.1	239.0
femur (any part)	170.7	198.5	—	213.7	238.0	239.2
fetal membrane	181	198.82	233.2	219.8	236.1	239.5
fibrous tissue — *see* Neoplasm, connective tissue						
fibula (any part)	170.7	198.5	—	213.7	238.0	239.2
filum terminale	192.2	198.3	—	225.3	237.5	239.7
finger NEC*	195.4	198.89	232.6	229.8	238.8	239.89
flank NEC*	195.8	198.89	232.5	229.8	238.8	239.89
follicle, nabothian	180.0	198.82	233.1	219.0	236.0	239.5
foot NEC*	195.5	198.89	232.7	229.8	238.8	239.89
forearm NEC*	195.4	198.89	232.6	229.8	238.8	239.89
forehead (skin)	173.30	198.2	232.3	216.3	238.2	239.2
basal cell carcinoma	173.31	—	—	—	—	—
specified type NEC	173.39	—	—	—	—	—
squamous cell carcinoma	173.32	—	—	—	—	—
foreskin	187.1	198.82	233.5	222.1	236.6	239.5
fornix						
pharyngeal	147.3	198.89	230.0	210.7	235.1	239.0
vagina	184.0	198.82	233.31	221.1	236.3	239.5
fossa (of)						
anterior (cranial)	191.9	198.3	—	225.0	237.5	239.6
cranial	191.9	198.3	—	225.0	237.5	239.6
ischiorectal	195.3	198.89	234.8	229.8	238.8	239.89
middle (cranial)	191.9	198.3	—	225.0	237.5	239.6
pituitary	194.3	198.89	234.8	227.3	237.0	239.7
posterior (cranial)	191.9	198.3	—	225.0	237.5	239.6
pterygoid	171.0	198.89	—	215.0	238.1	239.2
pyriform	148.1	198.89	230.0	210.8	235.1	239.0
Rosenmüller	147.2	198.89	230.0	210.7	235.1	239.0
tonsillar	146.1	198.89	230.0	210.6	235.1	239.0
fourchette	184.4	198.82	233.32	221.2	236.3	239.5
frenulum						
labii — *see* Neoplasm, lip, internal						

	Malignant			Benign	Uncertain Behavior	Unspecified
	Primary	Secondary	Ca in situ			
Neoplasm, neoplastic — *continued*						
frenulum — *continued*						
linguae	141.3	198.89	230.0	210.1	235.1	239.0
frontal						
bone	170.0	198.5	—	213.0	238.0	239.2
lobe, brain	191.1	198.3	—	225.0	237.5	239.6
meninges	192.1	198.4	—	225.2	237.6	239.7
pole	191.1	198.3	—	225.0	237.5	239.6
sinus	160.4	197.3	231.8	212.0	235.9	239.1
fundus						
stomach	151.3	197.8	230.2	211.1	235.2	239.0
uterus	182.0	198.82	233.2	219.1	236.0	239.5
gallbladder	156.0	197.8	230.8	211.5	235.3	239.0
contiguous sites with extrahepatic bile ducts	156.8	—	—	—	—	—
gall duct (extrahepatic)	156.1	197.8	230.8	211.5	235.3	239.0
intrahepatic	155.1	197.8	230.8	211.5	235.3	239.0
ganglia (*see also* Neoplasm, connective tissue)	171.9	198.89	—	215.9	238.1	239.2
basal	191.0	198.3	—	225.0	237.5	239.6
ganglion (*see also* Neoplasm, connective tissue)	171.9	198.89	—	215.9	238.1	239.2
cranial nerve	192.0	198.4	—	225.1	237.9	239.7
Gartner's duct	184.0	198.82	233.31	221.1	236.3	239.5
gastric — *see* Neoplasm, stomach						
gastrocolic	159.8	197.8	230.9	211.9	235.5	239.0
gastroesophageal junction	151.0	197.8	230.2	211.1	235.2	239.0
gastrointestinal (tract) NEC	159.9	197.8	230.9	211.9	235.5	239.0
generalized	199.0	—	234.9	229.9	238.9	—
genital organ or tract						
female NEC	184.9	198.82	233.39	221.9	236.3	239.5
contiguous sites	184.8	—	—	—	—	—
specified site NEC	184.8	198.82	233.39	221.8	236.3	239.5
male NEC	187.9	198.82	233.6	222.9	236.6	239.5
contiguous sites	187.8	—	—	—	—	—
specified site NEC	187.8	198.82	233.6	222.8	236.6	239.5
genitourinary tract						
female	184.9	198.82	233.39	221.9	236.3	239.5
male	187.9	198.82	233.6	222.9	236.6	239.5
gingiva (alveolar) (marginal)	143.9	198.89	230.0	210.4	235.1	239.0
lower	143.1	198.89	230.0	210.4	235.1	239.0
mandibular	143.1	198.89	230.0	210.4	235.1	239.0
maxillary	143.0	198.89	230.0	210.4	235.1	239.0
upper	143.0	198.89	230.0	210.4	235.1	239.0
gland, glandular (lymphatic) (system) (*see also* Neoplasm, lymph gland)						
endocrine NEC	194.9	198.89	—	227.9	237.4	239.7
salivary — *see* Neoplasm, salivary, gland						
glans penis	187.2	198.82	233.5	222.1	236.6	239.5
globus pallidus	191.0	198.3	—	225.0	237.5	239.6
glomus						
coccygeal	194.6	198.89	—	227.6	237.3	239.7
jugularis	194.6	198.89		227.6	237.3	239.7
glosso-epiglottic fold(s)	146.4	198.89	230.0	210.6	235.1	239.0
glossopalatine fold	146.2	198.89	230.0	210.6	235.1	239.0
glossopharyngeal sulcus	146.1	198.89	230.0	210.6	235.1	239.0

☑ Additional Digit Required — Refer to the Tabular List for Digit Selection ▽ Subterms under main terms may continue to next column or page

198 — Volume 2 ►◄ Revised Text ● New Line ▲ Revised Code 2013 ICD-9-CM

Neoplasm, neoplastic— continued	Primary	Secondary	Ca in situ	Benign	Uncertain Behavior	Unspecified
glottis	161.0	197.3	231.0	212.1	235.6	239.1
gluteal region*	195.3	198.89	232.5	229.8	238.8	239.89
great vessels NEC	171.4	198.89	—	215.4	238.1	239.2
groin NEC	195.3	198.89	232.5	229.8	238.8	239.89
gum	143.9	198.89	230.0	210.4	235.1	239.0
contiguous sites	143.8	—	—	—	—	—
lower	143.1	198.89	230.0	210.4	235.1	239.0
upper	143.0	198.89	230.0	210.4	235.1	239.0
hand NEC*	195.4	198.89	232.6	229.8	238.8	239.89
head NEC*	195.0	198.89	232.4	229.8	238.8	239.89
heart	164.1	198.89	—	212.7	238.8	239.89
contiguous sites with mediastinum or thymus	164.8	—	—	—	—	—
heel NEC*	195.5	198.89	232.7	229.8	238.8	239.89
helix (see also Neoplasm, skin, ear)	173.20	198.2	232.2	216.2	238.2	239.2
hematopoietic, hemopoietic tissue NEC	202.8	198.89	—	—	—	238.79
hemisphere, cerebral	191.0	198.3	—	225.0	237.5	239.6
hemorrhoidal zone	154.2	197.5	230.5	211.4	235.5	239.0
hepatic	155.2	197.7	230.8	211.5	235.3	239.0
duct (bile)	156.1	197.8	230.8	211.5	235.3	239.0
flexure (colon)	153.0	197.5	230.3	211.3	235.2	239.0
primary	155.0	—	—	—	—	—
hilus of lung	162.2	197.0	231.2	212.3	235.7	239.1
hip NEC*	195.5	198.89	232.7	229.8	238.8	239.89
hippocampus, brain	191.2	198.3	—	225.0	237.5	239.6
humerus (any part)	170.4	198.5	—	213.4	238.0	239.2
hymen	184.0	198.82	233.31	221.1	236.3	239.5
hypopharynx, hypopharyngeal NEC	148.9	198.89	230.0	210.8	235.1	239.0
contiguous sites	148.8	—	—	—	—	—
postcricoid region	148.0	198.89	230.0	210.8	235.1	239.0
posterior wall	148.3	198.89	230.0	210.8	235.1	239.0
pyriform fossa (sinus)	148.1	198.89	230.0	210.8	235.1	239.0
specified site NEC	148.8	198.89	230.0	210.8	235.1	239.0
wall	148.9	198.89	230.0	210.8	235.1	239.0
posterior	148.3	198.89	230.0	210.8	235.1	239.0
hypophysis	194.3	198.89	234.8	227.3	237.0	239.7
hypothalamus	191.0	198.3	—	225.0	237.5	239.6
ileocecum, ileocecal (coil) (junction) (valve)	153.4	197.5	230.3	211.3	235.2	239.0
ileum	152.2	197.4	230.7	211.2	235.2	239.0
ilium	170.6	198.5	—	213.6	238.0	239.2
immunoproliferative NEC	203.8	—	—	—	—	—
infraclavicular (region)*	195.1	198.89	232.5	229.8	238.8	239.89
inguinal (region)*	195.3	198.89	232.5	229.8	238.8	239.89
insula	191.0	198.3	—	225.0	237.5	239.6
insular tissue (pancreas)	157.4	197.8	230.9	211.7	235.5	239.0
brain	191.0	198.3	—	225.0	237.5	239.6
interarytenoid fold	148.2	198.89	230.0	210.8	235.1	239.0
hypopharyngeal aspect	148.2	198.89	230.0	210.8	235.1	239.0
laryngeal aspect	161.1	197.3	231.0	212.1	235.6	239.1
marginal zone	148.2	198.89	230.0	210.8	235.1	239.0
interdental papillae	143.9	198.89	230.0	210.4	235.1	239.0
lower	143.1	198.89	230.0	210.4	235.1	239.0
upper	143.0	198.89	230.0	210.4	235.1	239.0
internal capsule	191.0	198.3	—	225.0	237.5	239.6
os (cervix)	180.0	198.82	233.1	219.0	236.0	239.5

Neoplasm, neoplastic— continued	Primary	Secondary	Ca in situ	Benign	Uncertain Behavior	Unspecified
intervertebral cartilage or disc	170.2	198.5	—	213.2	238.0	239.2
intestine, intestinal	159.0	197.8	230.7	211.9	235.2	239.0
large	153.9	197.5	230.3	211.3	235.2	239.0
appendix	153.5	197.5	230.3	211.3	235.2	239.0
caput coli	153.4	197.5	230.3	211.3	235.2	239.0
cecum	153.4	197.5	230.3	211.3	235.2	239.0
colon	153.9	197.5	230.3	211.3	235.2	239.0
and rectum*	154.0	197.5	230.4	211.4	235.2	239.0
ascending	153.6	197.5	230.3	211.3	235.2	239.0
caput	153.4	197.5	230.3	211.3	235.2	239.0
contiguous sites	153.8	—	—	—	—	—
descending	153.2	197.5	230.3	211.3	235.2	239.0
distal	153.2	197.5	230.3	211.3	235.2	239.0
left	153.2	197.5	230.3	211.3	235.2	239.0
pelvic	153.3	197.5	230.3	211.3	235.2	239.0
right	153.6	197.5	230.3	211.3	235.2	239.0
sigmoid (flexure)	153.3	197.5	230.3	211.3	235.2	239.0
transverse	153.1	197.5	230.3	211.3	235.2	239.0
contiguous sites	153.8	—	—	—	—	—
hepatic flexure	153.0	197.5	230.3	211.3	235.2	239.0
ileocecum, ileocecal (coil) (valve)	153.4	197.5	230.3	211.3	235.2	239.0
sigmoid flexure (lower) (upper)	153.3	197.5	230.3	211.3	235.2	239.0
splenic flexure	153.7	197.5	230.3	211.3	235.2	239.0
small	152.9	197.4	230.7	211.2	235.2	239.0
contiguous sites	152.8	—	—	—	—	—
duodenum	152.0	197.4	230.7	211.2	235.2	239.0
ileum	152.2	197.4	230.7	211.2	235.2	239.0
jejunum	152.1	197.4	230.7	211.2	235.2	239.0
tract NEC	159.0	197.8	230.7	211.9	235.2	239.0
intra-abdominal	195.2	198.89	234.8	229.8	238.8	239.89
intracranial NEC	191.9	198.3	—	225.0	237.5	239.6
intrahepatic (bile) duct	155.1	197.8	230.8	211.5	235.3	239.0
intraocular	190.0	198.4	234.0	224.0	238.8	239.89
intraorbital	190.1	198.4	234.0	224.1	238.8	239.89
intrasellar	194.3	198.89	234.8	227.3	237.0	239.7
intrathoracic (cavity) (organs NEC)	195.1	198.89	234.8	229.8	238.8	239.89
contiguous sites with respiratory organs	165.8	—	—	—	—	—
iris	190.0	198.4	234.0	224.0	238.8	239.89
ischiorectal (fossa)	195.3	198.89	234.8	229.8	238.8	239.89
ischium	170.6	198.5	—	213.6	238.0	239.2
island of Reil	191.0	198.3	—	225.0	237.5	239.6
islands or islets of Langerhans	157.4	197.8	230.9	211.7	235.5	239.0
isthmus uteri	182.1	198.82	233.2	219.1	236.0	239.5
jaw	195.0	198.89	234.8	229.8	238.8	239.89
bone	170.1	198.5	—	213.1	238.0	239.2
carcinoma	143.9	—	—	—	—	—
lower	143.1	—	—	—	—	—
upper	143.0	—	—	—	—	—
lower	170.1	198.5	—	213.1	238.0	239.2
upper	170.0	198.5	—	213.0	238.0	239.2
carcinoma (any type) (lower) (upper)	195.0	—	—	—	—	—
skin (see also Neoplasm, skin, face)	173.30	198.2	232.3	216.3	238.2	239.2
soft tissues	143.9	198.89	230.0	210.4	235.1	239.0
lower	143.1	198.89	230.0	210.4	235.1	239.0
upper	143.0	198.89	230.0	210.4	235.1	239.0
jejunum	152.1	197.4	230.7	211.2	235.2	239.0

☑ Additional Digit Required — Refer to the Tabular List for Digit Selection

Subterms under main terms may continue to next column or page

	Malignant					
	Primary	Secondary	Ca in situ	Benign	Uncertain Behavior	Unspecified
Neoplasm, neoplastic— continued						
joint NEC (see also Neoplasm, bone)						
bone)	170.9	198.5	—	213.9	238.0	239.2
acromioclavicular	170.4	198.5	—	213.4	238.0	239.2
bursa or synovial membrane — see Neoplasm, connective tissue						
costovertebral	170.3	198.5	—	213.3	238.0	239.2
sternocostal	170.3	198.5	—	213.3	238.0	239.2
temporomandibular	170.1	198.5	—	213.1	238.0	239.2
junction						
anorectal	154.8	197.5	230.7	211.4	235.5	239.0
cardioesophageal	151.0	197.8	230.2	211.1	235.2	239.0
esophagogastric	151.0	197.8	230.2	211.1	235.2	239.0
gastroesophageal	151.0	197.8	230.2	211.1	235.2	239.0
hard and soft palate	145.5	198.89	230.0	210.4	235.1	239.0
ileocecal	153.4	197.5	230.3	211.3	235.2	239.0
pelvirectal	154.0	197.5	230.4	211.4	235.2	239.0
pelviureteric	189.1	198.0	233.9	223.1	236.91	239.5
rectosigmoid	154.0	197.5	230.4	211.4	235.2	239.0
squamocolumnar, of cervix	180.8	198.82	233.1	219.0	236.0	239.5
kidney (parenchyma)	189.0	198.0	233.9	223.0	236.91	239.5
calyx	189.1	198.0	233.9	223.1	236.91	239.5
hilus	189.1	198.0	233.9	223.1	236.91	239.5
pelvis	189.1	198.0	233.9	223.1	236.91	239.5
knee NEC*	195.5	198.89	232.7	229.8	238.8	239.89
labia (skin)	184.4	198.82	233.32	221.2	236.3	239.5
majora	184.1	198.82	233.32	221.2	236.3	239.5
minora	184.2	198.82	233.32	221.2	236.3	239.5
labial (see also Neoplasm, lip) sulcus (lower) (upper)	145.1	198.89	230.0	210.4	235.1	239.0
labium (skin)	184.4	198.82	233.32	221.2	236.3	239.5
majus	184.1	198.82	233.32	221.2	236.3	239.5
minus	184.2	198.82	233.32	221.2	236.3	239.5
lacrimal						
canaliculi	190.7	198.4	234.0	224.7	238.8	239.89
duct (nasal)	190.7	198.4	234.0	224.7	238.8	239.89
gland	190.2	198.4	234.0	224.2	238.8	239.89
punctum	190.7	198.4	234.0	224.7	238.8	239.89
sac	190.7	198.4	234.0	224.7	238.8	239.89
Langerhans, islands or islets	157.4	197.8	230.9	211.7	235.5	239.0
laryngopharynx	148.9	198.89	230.0	210.8	235.1	239.0
larynx, laryngeal NEC	161.9	197.3	231.0	212.1	235.6	239.1
aryepiglottic fold	161.1	197.3	231.0	212.1	235.6	239.1
cartilage (arytenoid) (cricoid) (cuneiform) (thyroid)	161.3	197.3	231.0	212.1	235.6	239.1
commissure (anterior) (posterior)	161.0	197.3	231.0	212.1	235.6	239.1
contiguous sites	161.8	—	—	—	—	—
extrinsic NEC	161.1	197.3	231.0	212.1	235.6	239.1
meaning hypopharynx	148.9	198.89	230.0	210.8	235.1	239.0
interarytenoid fold	161.1	197.3	231.0	212.1	235.6	239.1
intrinsic	161.0	197.3	231.0	212.1	235.6	239.1
ventricular band	161.1	197.3	231.0	212.1	235.6	239.1
leg NEC*	195.5	198.89	232.7	229.8	238.8	239.89
lens, crystalline	190.0	198.4	234.0	224.0	238.8	239.89
lid (lower) (upper)	173.10	198.2	232.1	216.1	238.2	239.2
basal cell carcinoma	173.11	—	—	—	—	—
specified type NEC	173.19	—	—	—	—	—
squamous cell carcinoma	173.12	—	—	—	—	—
Neoplasm, neoplastic— continued						
ligament (see also Neoplasm, connective tissue)						
broad	183.3	198.82	233.39	221.0	236.3	239.5
Mackenrodt's	183.8	198.82	233.39	221.8	236.3	239.5
non-uterine — see Neoplasm, connective tissue						
round	183.5	198.82	—	221.0	236.3	239.5
sacro-uterine	183.4	198.82	—	221.0	236.3	239.5
uterine	183.4	198.82	—	221.0	236.3	239.5
utero-ovarian	183.8	198.82	233.39	221.8	236.3	239.5
uterosacral	183.4	198.82	—	221.0	236.3	239.5
limb*	195.8	198.89	232.8	229.8	238.8	239.89
lower*	195.5	198.89	232.7	229.8	238.8	239.89
upper*	195.4	198.89	232.6	229.8	238.8	239.89
limbus of cornea	190.4	198.4	234.0	224.4	238.8	239.89
lingual NEC (see also Neoplasm, tongue)	141.9	198.89	230.0	210.1	235.1	239.0
lingula, lung	162.3	197.0	231.2	212.3	235.7	239.1
lip (external) (lipstick area) (vermillion border)	140.9	198.89	230.0	210.0	235.1	239.0
buccal aspect — see Neoplasm, lip, internal						
commissure	140.6	198.89	230.0	210.4	235.1	239.0
contiguous sites	140.8	—	—	—	—	—
with oral cavity or pharynx	149.8	—	—	—	—	—
frenulum — see Neoplasm, lip, internal						
inner aspect — see Neoplasm, lip, internal						
internal (buccal) (frenulum) (mucosa) (oral)	140.5	198.89	230.0	210.0	235.1	239.0
lower	140.4	198.89	230.0	210.0	235.1	239.0
upper	140.3	198.89	230.0	210.0	235.1	239.0
lower	140.1	198.89	230.0	210.0	235.1	239.0
internal (buccal) (frenulum) (mucosa) (oral)	140.4	198.89	230.0	210.0	235.1	239.0
mucosa — see Neoplasm, lip, internal						
oral aspect — see Neoplasm, lip, internal						
skin (commissure) (lower) (upper)	173.00	198.2	232.0	216.0	238.2	239.2
basal cell carcinoma	173.01	—	—	—	—	—
specified type NEC	173.09	—	—	—	—	—
squamous cell carcinoma	173.02	—	—	—	—	—
upper	140.0	198.89	230.0	210.0	235.1	239.0
internal (buccal) (frenulum) (mucosa) (oral)	140.3	198.89	230.0	210.0	235.1	239.0
liver	155.2	197.7	230.8	211.5	235.3	239.0
primary	155.0	—	—	—	—	—
lobe						
azygos	162.3	197.0	231.2	212.3	235.7	239.1
frontal	191.1	198.3	—	225.0	237.5	239.6
lower	162.5	197.0	231.2	212.3	235.7	239.1
middle	162.4	197.0	231.2	212.3	235.7	239.1
occipital	191.4	198.3	—	225.0	237.5	239.6

☑ **Additional Digit Required — Refer to the Tabular List for Digit Selection**

Ⓦ **Subterms under main terms may continue to next column or page**

	Malignant			Benign	Uncertain Behavior	Unspecified
	Primary	Secondary	Ca in situ			

Neoplasm, neoplastic — continued						
lobe — continued						
parietal	191.3	198.3	—	225.0	237.5	239.6
temporal	191.2	198.3	—	225.0	237.5	239.6
upper	162.3	197.0	231.2	212.3	235.7	239.1
lumbosacral plexus	171.6	198.4	—	215.6	238.1	239.2
lung	162.9	197.0	231.2	212.3	235.7	239.1
azygos lobe	162.3	197.0	231.2	212.3	235.7	239.1
carina	162.2	197.0	231.2	212.3	235.7	239.1
contiguous sites with bronchus or trachea	162.8	—	—	—	—	—
hilus	162.2	197.0	231.2	212.3	235.7	239.1
lingula	162.3	197.0	231.2	212.3	235.7	239.1
lobe NEC	162.9	197.0	231.2	212.3	235.7	239.1
lower lobe	162.5	197.0	231.2	212.3	235.7	239.1
main bronchus	162.2	197.0	231.2	212.3	235.7	239.1
middle lobe	162.4	197.0	231.2	212.3	235.7	239.1
upper lobe	162.3	197.0	231.2	212.3	235.7	239.1
lymph, lymphatic channel NEC (see also Neoplasm, connective tissue)	171.9	198.89	—	215.9	238.1	239.2
gland (secondary)	—	196.9	—	229.0	238.8	239.89
abdominal	—	196.2	—	229.0	238.8	239.89
aortic	—	196.2	—	229.0	238.8	239.89
arm	—	196.3	—	229.0	238.8	239.89
auricular (anterior) (posterior)	—	196.0	—	229.0	238.8	239.89
axilla, axillary	—	196.3	—	229.0	238.8	239.89
brachial	—	196.3	—	229.0	238.8	239.89
bronchial	—	196.1	—	229.0	238.8	239.89
bronchopulmonary	—	196.1	—	229.0	238.8	239.89
celiac	—	196.2	—	229.0	238.8	239.89
cervical	—	196.0	—	229.0	238.8	239.89
cervicofacial	—	196.0	—	229.0	238.8	239.89
Cloquet	—	196.5	—	229.0	238.8	239.89
colic	—	196.2	—	229.0	238.8	239.89
common duct	—	196.2	—	229.0	238.8	239.89
cubital	—	196.3	—	229.0	238.8	239.89
diaphragmatic	—	196.1	—	229.0	238.8	239.89
epigastric, inferior	—	196.6	—	229.0	238.8	239.89
epitrochlear	—	196.3	—	229.0	238.8	239.89
esophageal	—	196.1	—	229.0	238.8	239.89
face	—	196.0	—	229.0	238.8	239.89
femoral	—	196.5	—	229.0	238.8	239.89
gastric	—	196.2	—	229.0	238.8	239.89
groin	—	196.5	—	229.0	238.8	239.89
head	—	196.0	—	229.0	238.8	239.89
hepatic	—	196.2	—	229.0	238.8	239.89
hilar (pulmonary)	—	196.1	—	229.0	238.8	239.89
splenic	—	196.2	—	229.0	238.8	239.89
hypogastric	—	196.6	—	229.0	238.8	239.89
ileocolic	—	196.2	—	229.0	238.8	239.89
iliac	—	196.6	—	229.0	238.8	239.89
infraclavicular	—	196.3	—	229.0	238.8	239.89
inguina, inguinal	—	196.5	—	229.0	238.8	239.89
innominate	—	196.1	—	229.0	238.8	239.89
intercostal	—	196.1	—	229.0	238.8	239.89
intestinal	—	196.2	—	229.0	238.8	239.89
intra-abdominal	—	196.2	—	229.0	238.8	239.89
intrapelvic	—	196.6	—	229.0	238.8	239.89
intrathoracic	—	196.1	—	229.0	238.8	239.9
jugular	—	196.0	—	229.0	238.8	239.89
leg	—	196.5	—	229.0	238.8	239.89
limb lower	—	196.5	—	229.0	238.8	239.9
upper	—	196.3	—	229.0	238.8	239.89
lower limb	—	196.5	—	229.0	238.8	239.9
lumbar	—	196.2	—	229.0	238.8	239.89

	Malignant			Benign	Uncertain Behavior	Unspecified
	Primary	Secondary	Ca in situ			

Neoplasm, neoplastic — continued						
lymph, lymphatic — continued						
gland — continued						
mandibular	—	196.0	—	229.0	238.8	239.89
mediastinal	—	196.1	—	229.0	238.8	239.89
mesenteric (inferior) (superior)	—	196.2	—	229.0	238.8	239.89
midcolic	—	196.2	—	229.0	238.8	239.89
multiple sites in categories 196.0–196.6	—	196.8	—	229.0	238.8	239.89
neck	—	196.0	—	229.0	238.8	239.89
obturator	—	196.6	—	229.0	238.8	239.89
occipital	—	196.0	—	229.0	238.8	239.89
pancreatic	—	196.2	—	229.0	238.8	239.89
para-aortic	—	196.2	—	229.0	238.8	239.89
paracervical	—	196.6	—	229.0	238.8	239.89
parametrial	—	196.6	—	229.0	238.8	239.89
parasternal	—	196.1	—	229.0	238.8	239.89
parotid	—	196.0	—	229.0	238.8	239.89
pectoral	—	196.3	—	229.0	238.8	239.89
pelvic	—	196.6	—	229.0	238.8	239.89
peri-aortic	—	196.2	—	229.0	238.8	239.89
peripancreatic	—	196.2	—	229.0	238.8	239.89
popliteal	—	196.5	—	229.0	238.8	239.89
porta hepatis	—	196.2	—	229.0	238.8	239.89
portal	—	196.2	—	229.0	238.8	239.89
preauricular	—	196.0	—	229.0	238.8	239.89
prelaryngeal	—	196.0	—	229.0	238.8	239.89
presymphysial	—	196.6	—	229.0	238.8	239.89
pretracheal	—	196.0	—	229.0	238.8	239.89
primary (any site) NEC	202.9	—	—	—	—	—
pulmonary (hiler)	—	196.1	—	229.0	238.8	239.89
pyloric	—	196.2	—	229.0	238.8	239.89
retroperitoneal	—	196.2	—	229.0	238.8	239.89
retropharyngeal	—	196.0	—	229.0	238.8	239.89
Rosenmüller's	—	196.5	—	229.0	238.8	239.89
sacral	—	196.6	—	229.0	238.8	239.89
scalene	—	196.0	—	229.0	238.8	239.89
site NEC	—	196.9	—	229.0	238.8	239.89
splenic (hilar)	—	196.2	—	229.0	238.8	239.89
subclavicular	—	196.3	—	229.0	238.8	239.89
subinguinal	—	196.5	—	229.0	238.8	239.89
sublingual	—	196.0	—	229.0	238.8	239.89
submandibular	—	196.0	—	229.0	238.8	239.89
submaxillary	—	196.0	—	229.0	238.8	239.89
submental	—	196.0	—	229.0	238.8	239.89
subscapular	—	196.3	—	229.0	238.8	239.89
supraclavicular	—	196.0	—	229.0	238.8	239.89
thoracic	—	196.1	—	229.0	238.8	239.89
tibial	—	196.5	—	229.0	238.8	239.89
tracheal	—	196.1	—	229.0	238.8	239.89
tracheobronchial	—	196.1	—	229.0	238.8	239.89
upper limb	—	196.3	—	229.0	238.8	239.89
Virchow's	—	196.0	—	229.0	238.8	239.89
node (see also Neoplasm, lymph gland) primary NEC	202.9	—	—	—	—	—
vessel (see also Neoplasm, connective tissue)	171.9	198.89	—	215.9	238.1	239.2
Mackenrodt's ligament	183.8	198.82	233.39	221.8	236.3	239.5
malar	170.0	198.5	—	213.0	238.0	239.2
region — see Neoplasm, cheek						
mammary gland — see Neoplasm, breast						
mandible	170.1	198.5	—	213.1	238.0	239.2
alveolar						

Neoplasm, neoplastic—	Malignant			Benign	Uncertain Behavior	Unspecified
	Primary	Secondary	Ca in situ			
continued						
mandible — *continued*						
alveolar — *continued*						
mucosa	143.1	198.89	230.0	210.4	235.1	239.0
mucose	143.1	198.89	230.0	210.4	235.1	239.0
ridge or process	170.1	198.5	—	213.1	238.0	239.2
carcinoma	143.1	—	—	—	—	—
carcinoma	143.1	—	—	—	—	—
marrow (bone) NEC	202.9	198.5	—	—	—	238.79
mastectomy site (skin)	173.50	198.2				
basal cell carcinoma	173.51	—	—	—	—	—
specified as breast tissue	174.8	198.81				
specified type NEC	173.59	—	—	—	—	—
squamous cell carcinoma	173.52	—	—	—	—	—
mastoid (air cells) (antrum) (cavity)	160.1	197.3	231.8	212.0	235.9	239.1
bone or process	170.0	198.5	—	213.0	238.0	239.2
maxilla, maxillary (superior)	170.0	198.5	—	213.0	238.0	239.2
alveolar mucosa	143.0	198.89	230.0	210.4	235.1	239.0
ridge or process	170.0	198.5	—	213.0	238.0	239.2
carcinoma	143.0	—	—	—	—	—
antrum	160.2	197.3	231.8	212.0	235.9	239.1
carcinoma	143.0	—	—	—	—	—
inferior — *see* Neoplasm, mandible						
sinus	160.2	197.3	231.8	212.0	235.9	239.1
meatus external (ear) (*see also* Neoplasm, skin, ear)	173.20	198.2	232.2	216.2	238.2	239.2
Meckel's diverticulum	152.3	197.4	230.7	211.2	235.2	239.0
mediastinum, mediastinal	164.9	197.1	—	212.5	235.8	239.89
anterior	164.2	197.1	—	212.5	235.8	239.89
contiguous sites with heart and thymus	164.8	—	—	—	—	—
posterior	164.3	197.1	—	212.5	235.8	239.89
medulla adrenal	194.0	198.7	234.8	227.0	237.2	239.7
oblongata	191.7	198.3	—	225.0	237.5	239.6
meibomian gland	173.10	198.2	232.1	216.1	238.2	239.2
basal cell carcinoma	173.11	—	—	—	—	—
specified type NEC	173.19	—	—	—	—	—
squamous cell carcinoma	173.12	—	—	—	—	—
meninges (brain) (cerebral) (cranial) (intracranial)	192.1	198.4	—	225.2	237.6	239.7
spinal (cord)	192.3	198.4	—	225.4	237.6	239.7
meniscus, knee joint (lateral) (medial)	170.7	198.5	—	213.7	238.0	239.2
mesentery, mesenteric	158.8	197.6	—	211.8	235.4	239.0
mesoappendix	158.8	197.6	—	211.8	235.4	239.0
mesocolon	158.8	197.6	—	211.8	235.4	239.0
mesopharynx — *see* Neoplasm, oropharynx						
mesosalpinx	183.3	198.82	233.39	221.0	236.3	239.5
mesovarium	183.3	198.82	233.39	221.0	236.3	239.5

Neoplasm, neoplastic—	Malignant			Benign	Uncertain Behavior	Unspecified
	Primary	Secondary	Ca in situ			
continued						
metacarpus (any bone)	170.5	198.5	—	213.5	238.0	239.2
metastatic NEC (*see also* Neoplasm, by site, secondary)	—	199.1	—	—	—	—
metatarsus (any bone)	170.8	198.5	—	213.8	238.0	239.2
midbrain	191.7	198.3	—	225.0	237.5	239.6
milk duct — *see* Neoplasm, breast						
mons pubis	184.4	198.82	233.32	221.2	236.3	239.5
veneris	184.4	198.82	233.32	221.2	236.3	239.5
motor tract	192.9	198.4	—	225.9	237.9	239.7
brain	191.9	198.3	—	225.0	237.5	239.6
spinal	192.2	198.3	—	225.3	237.5	239.7
mouth	145.9	198.89	230.0	210.4	235.1	239.0
contiguous sites	145.8	—	—	—	—	—
floor	144.9	198.89	230.0	210.3	235.1	239.0
anterior portion	144.0	198.89	230.0	210.3	235.1	239.0
contiguous sites	144.8	—	—	—	—	—
lateral portion	144.1	198.89	230.0	210.3	235.1	239.0
roof	145.5	198.89	230.0	210.4	235.1	239.0
specified part NEC	145.8	198.89	230.0	210.4	235.1	239.0
vestibule	145.1	198.89	230.0	210.4	235.1	239.0
mucosa alveolar (ridge or process)	143.9	198.89	230.0	210.4	235.1	239.0
lower	143.1	198.89	230.0	210.4	235.1	239.0
upper	143.0	198.89	230.0	210.4	235.1	239.0
buccal	145.0	198.89	230.0	210.4	235.1	239.0
cheek	145.0	198.89	230.0	210.4	235.1	239.0
lip — *see* Neoplasm, lip, internal						
nasal	160.0	197.3	231.8	212.0	235.9	239.1
oral	145.0	198.89	230.0	210.4	235.1	239.0
Müllerian duct female	184.8	198.82	233.39	221.8	236.3	239.5
male	187.8	198.82	233.6	222.8	236.6	239.5
multiple sites NEC	199.0	—	234.9	229.9	238.9	—
muscle (*see also* Neoplasm, connective tissue) extraocular	190.1	198.4	234.0	224.1	238.8	239.89
myocardium	164.1	198.89	—	212.7	238.8	239.89
myometrium	182.0	198.82	233.2	219.1	236.0	239.5
myopericardium	164.1	198.89	—	212.7	238.8	239.89
nabothian gland (follicle)	180.0	198.82	233.1	219.0	236.0	239.5
nail	173.90	198.2	232.9	216.9	238.2	239.2
finger (*see also* Neoplasm, skin, limb, upper)	173.60	198.2	232.6	216.6	238.2	239.2
toe (*see also* Neoplasm, skin, limb, lower)	173.70	198.2	232.7	216.7	238.2	239.2
nares, naris (anterior) (posterior)	160.0	197.3	231.8	212.0	235.9	239.1
nasal — *see* Neoplasm, nose						
nasolabial groove (*see also* Neoplasm, skin, face)	173.30	198.2	232.3	216.3	238.2	239.2
nasolacrimal duct	190.7	198.4	234.0	224.7	238.8	239.89
nasopharynx, nasopharyngeal	147.9	198.89	230.0	210.7	235.1	239.0
contiguous sites	147.8	—	—	—	—	—
floor	147.3	198.89	230.0	210.7	235.1	239.0
roof	147.0	198.89	230.0	210.7	235.1	239.0
specified site NEC	147.8	198.89	230.0	210.7	235.1	239.0
wall	147.9	198.89	230.0	210.7	235.1	239.0

☑ **Additional Digit Required — Refer to the Tabular List for Digit Selection**　　　　　　　　　　〰 **Subterms under main terms may continue to next column or page**

Neoplasm, neoplastic—	Malignant			Benign	Uncertain Behavior	Unspecified
	Primary	Secondary	Ca in situ			
continued						
nasopharynx,						
nasopharyngeal —						
continued						
wall — *continued*						
anterior	147.3	198.89	230.0	210.7	235.1	239.0
lateral	147.2	198.89	230.0	210.7	235.1	239.0
posterior	147.1	198.89	230.0	210.7	235.1	239.0
superior	147.0	198.89	230.0	210.7	235.1	239.0
nates (*see also*						
Neoplasm, skin,						
trunk)	173.50	198.2	232.5	216.5	238.2	239.2
neck NEC*	195.0	198.89	234.8	229.8	238.8	239.89
skin	173.40	198.2	232.4	216.4	238.2	239.2
basal cell						
carcinoma	173.41	—	—	—	—	—
specified type						
NEC	173.49	—	—	—	—	—
squamous cell						
carcinoma	173.42	—	—	—	—	—
nerve (autonomic)						
(ganglion)						
(parasympathetic)						
(peripheral)						
(sympathetic) (*see*						
also Neoplasm,						
connective tissue)						
abducens	192.0	198.4	—	225.1	237.9	239.7
accessory						
(spinal)	192.0	198.4	—	225.1	237.9	239.7
acoustic	192.0	198.4	—	225.1	237.9	239.7
auditory	192.0	198.4	—	225.1	237.9	239.7
brachial	171.2	198.89	—	215.2	238.1	239.2
cranial (any)	192.0	198.4	—	225.1	237.9	239.7
facial	192.0	198.4	—	225.1	237.9	239.7
femoral	171.3	198.89	—	215.3	238.1	239.2
glossopharyngeal	192.0	198.4	—	225.1	237.9	239.7
hypoglossal	192.0	198.4	—	225.1	237.9	239.7
intercostal	171.4	198.89	—	215.4	238.1	239.2
lumbar	171.7	198.89	—	215.7	238.1	239.2
median	171.2	198.89	—	215.2	238.1	239.2
obturator	171.3	198.89	—	215.3	238.1	239.2
oculomotor	192.0	198.4	—	225.1	237.9	239.7
olfactory	192.0	198.4	—	225.1	237.9	239.7
optic	192.0	198.4	—	225.1	237.9	239.7
peripheral NEC	171.9	198.89	—	215.9	238.1	239.2
radial	171.2	198.89	—	215.2	238.1	239.2
sacral	171.6	198.89	—	215.6	238.1	239.2
sciatic	171.3	198.89	—	215.3	238.1	239.2
spinal NEC	171.9	198.89	—	215.9	238.1	239.2
trigeminal	192.0	198.4	—	225.1	237.9	239.7
trochlear	192.0	198.4	—	225.1	237.9	239.7
ulnar	171.2	198.89	—	215.2	238.1	239.2
vagus	192.0	198.4	—	225.1	237.9	239.7
nervous system						
(central) NEC	192.9	198.4	—	225.9	237.9	239.7
autonomic NEC	171.9	198.89	—	215.9	238.1	239.2
brain (*see also*						
Neoplasm, brain)						
membrane or						
meninges	192.1	198.4	—	225.2	237.6	239.7
contiguous sites	192.8	—	—	—	—	—
parasympathetic						
NEC	171.9	198.89	—	215.9	238.1	239.2
sympathetic NEC	171.9	198.89	—	215.9	238.1	239.2
nipple (female)	174.0	198.81	233.0	217	238.3	239.3
male	175.0	198.81	233.0	217	238.3	239.3
nose, nasal	195.0	198.89	234.8	229.8	238.8	239.89
ala (external) (*see also*						
Neoplasm, nose,						
skin)	173.30	198.2	232.3	216.3	238.2	239.2
bone	170.0	198.5	—	213.0	238.0	239.2
cartilage	160.0	197.3	231.8	212.0	235.9	239.1
cavity	160.0	197.3	231.8	212.0	235.9	239.1
contiguous sites						
with accessory	160.8	—	—	—	—	—

Neoplasm, neoplastic—	Malignant			Benign	Uncertain Behavior	Unspecified
	Primary	Secondary	Ca in situ			
continued						
nose, nasal — *continued*						
cavity — *continued*						
contiguous sites						
with accessory						
sinuses or						
middle ear —						
continued						
sinuses or						
middle ear						
choana	147.3	198.89	230.0	210.7	235.1	239.0
external (skin) (*see*						
also Neoplasm,						
nose, skin)	173.30	198.2	232.3	216.3	238.2	239.2
fossa	160.0	197.3	231.8	212.0	235.9	239.1
internal	160.0	197.3	231.8	212.0	235.9	239.1
mucosa	160.0	197.3	231.8	212.0	235.9	239.1
septum	160.0	197.3	231.8	212.0	235.9	239.1
posterior						
margin	147.3	198.89	230.0	210.7	235.1	239.0
sinus — *see*						
Neoplasm, sinus						
skin	173.30	198.2	232.3	216.3	238.2	239.2
basal cell						
carcinoma	173.31	—	—	—	—	—
specified type						
NEC	173.39	—	—	—	—	—
squamous cell						
carcinoma	173.32	—	—	—	—	—
turbinate						
(mucosa)	160.0	197.3	231.8	212.0	235.9	239.1
bone	170.0	198.5	—	213.0	238.0	239.2
vestibule	160.0	197.3	231.8	212.0	235.9	239.1
nostril	160.0	197.3	231.8	212.0	235.9	239.1
nucleus pulposus	170.2	198.5	—	213.2	238.0	239.2
occipital						
bone	170.0	198.5	—	213.0	238.0	239.2
lobe or pole,						
brain	191.4	198.3	—	225.0	237.5	239.6
odontogenic — *see*						
Neoplasm, jaw						
bone						
oesophagus — *see*						
Neoplasm,						
esophagus						
olfactory nerve or						
bulb	192.0	198.4	—	225.1	237.9	239.7
olive (brain)	191.7	198.3	—	225.0	237.5	239.6
omentum	158.8	197.6	—	211.8	235.4	239.0
operculum (brain)	191.0	198.3	—	225.0	237.5	239.6
optic nerve, chiasm, or						
tract	192.0	198.4	—	225.1	237.9	239.7
oral (cavity)	145.9	198.89	230.0	210.4	235.1	239.0
contiguous sites with						
lip or						
pharynx	149.8	—	—	—	—	—
ill-defined	149.9	198.89	230.0	210.4	235.1	239.0
mucosa	145.9	198.89	230.0	210.4	235.1	239.0
orbit	190.1	198.4	234.0	224.1	238.8	239.89
bone	170.0	198.5	—	213.0	238.0	239.2
eye	190.1	198.4	234.0	224.1	238.8	239.89
soft parts	190.1	198.4	234.0	224.1	238.8	239.89
organ of						
Zuckerkandl	194.6	198.89	—	227.6	237.3	239.7
oropharynx	146.9	198.89	230.0	210.6	235.1	239.0
branchial cleft						
(vestige)	146.8	198.89	230.0	210.6	235.1	239.0
contiguous sites	146.8	—	—	—	—	—
junctional region	146.5	198.89	230.0	210.6	235.1	239.0
lateral wall	146.6	198.89	230.0	210.6	235.1	239.0
pillars of fauces	146.2	198.89	230.0	210.6	235.1	239.0
posterior wall	146.7	198.89	230.0	210.6	235.1	239.0
specified part						
NEC	146.8	198.89	230.0	210.6	235.1	239.0
vallecula	146.3	198.89	230.0	210.6	235.1	239.0
os						
external	180.1	198.82	233.1	219.0	236.0	239.5

☑ Additional Digit Required — Refer to the Tabular List for Digit Selection   ▽ Subterms under main terms may continue to next column or page

2013 ICD-9-CM   ►◄ Revised Text   ● New Line   ▲ Revised Code   Volume 2 — 203

Neoplasm, neoplastic — continued	Malignant Primary	Malignant Secondary	Malignant Ca in situ	Benign	Uncertain Behavior	Unspecified
os — continued						
internal	180.0	198.82	233.1	219.0	236.0	239.5
ovary	183.0	198.6	233.39	220	236.2	239.5
oviduct	183.2	198.82	233.39	221.0	236.3	239.5
palate	145.5	198.89	230.0	210.4	235.1	239.0
hard	145.2	198.89	230.0	210.4	235.1	239.0
junction of hard and soft palate	145.5	198.89	230.0	210.4	235.1	239.0
soft	145.3	198.89	230.0	210.4	235.1	239.0
nasopharyngeal surface	147.3	198.89	230.0	210.7	235.1	239.0
posterior surface	147.3	198.89	230.0	210.7	235.1	239.0
superior surface	147.3	198.89	230.0	210.7	235.1	239.0
palatoglossal arch	146.2	198.89	230.0	210.6	235.1	239.0
palatopharyngeal arch	146.2	198.89	230.0	210.6	235.1	239.0
pallium	191.0	198.3	—	225.0	237.5	239.6
palpebra	173.10	198.2	232.1	216.1	238.2	239.2
basal cell carcinoma	173.11	—	—	—	—	—
specified type NEC	173.19	—	—	—	—	—
squamous cell carcinoma	173.12	—	—	—	—	—
pancreas	157.9	197.8	230.9	211.6	235.5	239.0
body	157.1	197.8	230.9	211.6	235.5	239.0
contiguous sites	157.8	—	—	—	—	—
duct (of Santorini) (of Wirsung)	157.3	197.8	230.9	211.6	235.5	239.0
ectopic tissue	157.8	197.8	230.9	211.6	235.5	239.0
head	157.0	197.8	230.9	211.6	235.5	239.0
islet cells	157.4	197.8	230.9	211.7	235.5	239.0
neck	157.8	197.8	230.9	211.6	235.5	239.0
tail	157.2	197.8	230.9	211.6	235.5	239.0
para-aortic body	194.6	198.89	—	227.6	237.3	239.7
paraganglion NEC	194.6	198.89	—	227.6	237.3	239.7
parametrium	183.4	198.82	—	221.0	236.3	239.5
paranephric	158.0	197.6	—	211.8	235.4	239.0
pararectal	195.3	198.89	—	229.8	238.8	239.89
parasagittal (region)	195.0	198.89	234.8	229.8	238.8	239.89
parasellar	192.9	198.4	—	225.9	237.9	239.7
parathyroid (gland)	194.1	198.89	234.8	227.1	237.4	239.7
paraurethral	195.3	198.89	—	229.8	238.8	239.89
gland	189.4	198.1	233.9	223.89	236.99	239.5
paravaginal	195.3	198.89	—	229.8	238.8	239.89
parenchyma, kidney	189.0	198.0	233.9	223.0	236.91	239.5
parietal						
bone	170.0	198.5	—	213.0	238.0	239.2
lobe, brain	191.3	198.3	—	225.0	237.5	239.6
paroophoron	183.3	198.82	233.39	221.0	236.3	239.5
parotid (duct) (gland)	142.0	198.89	230.0	210.2	235.0	239.0
parovarium	183.3	198.82	233.39	221.0	236.3	239.5
patella	170.8	198.5	—	213.8	238.0	239.2
peduncle, cerebral	191.7	198.3	—	225.0	237.5	239.6
pelvirectal junction	154.0	197.5	230.4	211.4	235.2	239.0
pelvis, pelvic	195.3	198.89	234.8	229.8	238.8	239.89
bone	170.6	198.5	—	213.6	238.0	239.2
floor	195.3	198.89	234.8	229.8	238.8	239.89
renal	189.1	198.0	233.9	223.1	236.91	239.5
viscera	195.3	198.89	234.8	229.8	238.8	239.89
wall	195.3	198.89	234.8	229.8	238.8	239.89
pelvo-abdominal	195.8	198.89	234.8	229.8	238.8	239.89
penis	187.4	198.82	233.5	222.1	236.6	239.5
body	187.3	198.82	233.5	222.1	236.6	239.5
corpus (cavernosum)	187.3	198.82	233.5	222.1	236.6	239.5
glans	187.2	198.82	233.5	222.1	236.6	239.5
skin NEC	187.4	198.82	233.5	222.1	236.6	239.5
periadrenal (tissue)	158.0	197.6	—	211.8	235.4	239.0
perianal (skin) (see also Neoplasm, skin, anus)	173.50	198.2	232.5	216.5	238.2	239.2
pericardium	164.1	198.89	—	212.7	238.8	239.89
perinephric	158.0	197.6	—	211.8	235.4	239.0
perineum	195.3	198.89	234.8	229.8	238.8	239.89
periodontal tissue NEC	143.9	198.89	230.0	210.4	235.1	239.0
periosteum — see Neoplasm, bone						
peripancreatic	158.0	197.6	—	211.8	235.4	239.0
peripheral nerve NEC	171.9	198.89	—	215.9	238.1	239.2
perirectal (tissue)	195.3	198.89	—	229.8	238.8	239.89
perirenal (tissue)	158.0	197.6	—	211.8	235.4	239.0
peritoneum, peritoneal (cavity)	158.9	197.6	—	211.8	235.4	239.0
contiguous sites	158.8	—	—	—	—	—
with digestive organs	159.8	—	—	—	—	—
parietal	158.8	197.6	—	211.8	235.4	239.0
pelvic	158.8	197.6	—	211.8	235.4	239.0
specified part NEC	158.8	197.6	—	211.8	235.4	239.0
peritonsillar (tissue)	195.0	198.89	234.8	229.8	238.8	239.89
periurethral tissue	195.3	198.89	—	229.8	238.8	239.89
phalanges	170.9	198.5	—	213.9	238.0	239.2
foot	170.8	198.5	—	213.8	238.0	239.2
hand	170.5	198.5	—	213.5	238.0	239.2
pharynx, pharyngeal	149.0	198.89	230.0	210.9	235.1	239.0
bursa	147.1	198.89	230.0	210.7	235.1	239.0
fornix	147.3	198.89	230.0	210.7	235.1	239.0
recess	147.2	198.89	230.0	210.7	235.1	239.0
region	149.0	198.89	230.0	210.9	235.1	239.0
tonsil	147.1	198.89	230.0	210.7	235.1	239.0
wall (lateral) (posterior)	149.0	198.89	230.0	210.9	235.1	239.0
pia mater (cerebral) (cranial)	192.1	198.4	—	225.2	237.6	239.7
spinal	192.3	198.4	—	225.4	237.6	239.7
pillars of fauces	146.2	198.89	230.0	210.6	235.1	239.0
pineal (body) (gland)	194.4	198.89	234.8	227.4	237.1	239.7
pinna (ear) NEC (see also Neoplasm, skin, ear)	173.20	198.2	232.2	216.2	238.2	239.2
cartilage	171.0	198.89	—	215.0	238.1	239.2
piriform fossa or sinus	148.1	198.89	230.0	210.8	235.1	239.0
pituitary (body) (fossa) (gland) (lobe)	194.3	198.89	234.8	227.3	237.0	239.7
placenta	181	198.82	233.2	219.8	236.1	239.5
pleura, pleural (cavity)	163.9	197.2	—	212.4	235.8	239.1
contiguous sites	163.8	—	—	—	—	—
parietal	163.0	197.2	—	212.4	235.8	239.1
visceral	163.1	197.2	—	212.4	235.8	239.1
plexus						
brachial	171.2	198.89	—	215.2	238.1	239.2
cervical	171.0	198.89	—	215.0	238.1	239.2
choroid	191.5	198.3	—	225.0	237.5	239.6
lumbosacral	171.6	198.89	—	215.6	238.1	239.2
sacral	171.6	198.89	—	215.6	238.1	239.2
pluri-endocrine	194.8	198.89	234.8	227.8	237.4	239.7
pole						
frontal	191.1	198.3	—	225.0	237.5	239.6
occipital	191.4	198.3	—	225.0	237.5	239.6
pons (varolii)	191.7	198.3	—	225.0	237.5	239.6
popliteal fossa or space*	195.5	198.89	234.8	229.8	238.8	239.89
postcricoid (region)	148.0	198.89	230.0	210.8	235.1	239.0

☑ Additional Digit Required — Refer to the Tabular List for Digit Selection   ▼ Subterms under main terms may continue to next column or page

204 — Volume 2   ►◄ Revised Text   ● New Line   ▲ Revised Code   2013 ICD-9-CM

Neoplasm, neoplastic— *continued*

	Malignant					
	Primary	Secondary	Ca in situ	Benign	Uncertain Behavior	Unspecified
posterior fossa (cranial)	191.9	198.3	—	225.0	237.5	239.6
postnasal space	147.9	198.89	230	210.7	235.1	239.0
prepuce	187.1	198.82	233.5	222.1	236.6	239.5
prepylorus	151.1	197.8	230.2	211.1	235.2	239.0
presacral (region)	195.3	198.89	—	229.8	238.8	239.89
prostate (gland)	185	198.82	233.4	222.2	236.5	239.5
utricle	189.3	198.1	233.9	223.81	236.99	239.5
pterygoid fossa	171.0	198.89	—	215.0	238.1	239.2
pubic bone	170.6	198.5	—	213.6	238.0	239.2
pudenda, pudendum (female)	184.4	198.82	233.32	221.2	236.3	239.5
pulmonary	162.9	197.0	231.2	212.3	235.7	239.1
putamen	191.0	198.3	—	225.0	237.5	239.6
pyloric antrum	151.2	197.8	230.2	211.1	235.2	239.0
canal	151.1	197.8	230.2	211.1	235.2	239.0
pylorus	151.1	197.8	230.2	211.1	235.2	239.0
pyramid (brain)	191.7	198.3	—	225.0	237.5	239.6
pyriform fossa or sinus	148.1	198.89	230.0	210.8	235.1	239.0
radius (any part)	170.4	198.5	—	213.4	238.0	239.2
Rathke's pouch	194.3	198.89	234.8	227.3	237.0	239.7
rectosigmoid (colon) (junction)	154.0	197.5	230.4	211.4	235.2	239.0
contiguous sites with anus or rectum	154.8	—	—	—	—	—
rectouterine pouch	158.8	197.6	—	211.8	235.4	239.0
rectovaginal septum or wall	195.3	198.89	234.8	229.8	238.8	239.89
rectovesical septum	195.3	198.89	234.8	229.8	238.8	239.89
rectum (ampulla)	154.1	197.5	230.4	211.4	235.2	239.0
and colon	154.0	197.5	230.4	211.4	235.2	239.0
contiguous sites with anus or rectosigmoid junction	154.8	—	—	—	—	—
renal	189.0	198.0	233.9	223.0	236.91	239.5
calyx	189.1	198.0	233.9	223.1	236.91	239.5
hilus	189.1	198.0	233.9	223.1	236.91	239.5
parenchyma	189.0	198.0	233.9	223.0	236.91	239.5
pelvis	189.1	198.0	233.9	223.1	236.91	239.5
respiratory organs or system NEC	165.9	197.3	231.9	212.9	235.9	239.1
contiguous sites with intrathoracic organs	165.8	—	—	—	—	—
specified sites NEC	165.8	197.3	231.8	212.8	235.9	239.1
tract NEC	165.9	197.3	231.9	212.9	235.9	239.1
upper	165.0	197.3	231.9	212.9	235.9	239.1
retina	190.5	198.4	234.0	224.5	238.8	239.81
retrobulbar	190.1	198.4	—	224.1	238.8	239.89
retrocecal	158.0	197.6	—	211.8	235.4	239.0
retromolar (area) (triangle) (trigone)	145.6	198.89	230.0	210.4	235.1	239.0
retro-orbital	195.0	198.89	234.8	229.8	238.8	239.89
retroperitoneal (space) (tissue)	158.0	197.6	—	211.8	235.4	239.0
contiguous sites	158.8	—	—	—	—	—
retroperitoneum	158.0	197.6	—	211.8	235.4	239.0
contiguous sites	158.8	—	—	—	—	—
retropharyngeal	149.0	198.89	230.0	210.9	235.1	239.0
retrovesical (septum)	195.3	198.89	234.8	229.8	238.8	239.89
rhinencephalon	191.0	198.3	—	225.0	237.5	239.6
rib	170.3	198.5	—	213.3	238.0	239.2
Rosenmüller's fossa	147.2	198.89	230.0	210.7	235.1	239.0
round ligament	183.5	198.82	—	221.0	236.3	239.5

Neoplasm, neoplastic— *continued*

	Malignant					
	Primary	Secondary	Ca in situ	Benign	Uncertain Behavior	Unspecified
sacrococcyx, sacrococcygeal	170.6	198.5	—	213.6	238.0	239.2
region	195.3	198.89	234.8	229.8	238.8	239.89
sacrouterine ligament	183.4	198.82	—	221.0	236.3	239.5
sacrum, sacral (vertebra)	170.6	198.5	—	213.6	238.0	239.2
salivary gland or duct (major)	142.9	198.89	230.0	210.2	235.0	239.0
contiguous sites	142.8	—	—	—	—	—
minor NEC	145.9	198.89	230.0	210.4	235.1	239.0
parotid	142.0	198.89	230.0	210.2	235.0	239.0
pluriglandular	142.8	198.89	—	210.2	235.0	239.0
sublingual	142.2	198.89	230.0	210.2	235.0	239.0
submandibular	142.1	198.89	230.0	210.2	235.0	239.0
submaxillary	142.1	198.89	230.0	210.2	235.0	239.0
salpinx (uterine)	183.2	198.82	233.39	221.0	236.3	239.5
Santorini's duct	157.3	197.8	230.9	211.6	235.5	239.0
scalp	173.40	198.2	232.4	216.4	238.2	239.2
basal cell carcinoma	173.41	—	—	—	—	—
specified type NEC	173.49	—	—	—	—	—
squamous cell carcinoma	173.42	—	—	—	—	—
scapula (any part)	170.4	198.5	—	213.4	238.0	239.2
scapular region	195.1	198.89	234.8	229.8	238.8	239.89
scar NEC (*see also* Neoplasm, skin)	173.90	198.2	232.9	216.9	238.2	239.2
sciatic nerve	171.3	198.89	—	215.3	238.1	239.2
sclera	190.0	198.4	234.0	224.0	238.8	239.89
scrotum (skin)	187.7	198.82	—	222.4	236.6	239.5
sebaceous gland — *see* Neoplasm, skin						
sella turcica	194.3	198.89	234.8	227.3	237.0	239.7
bone	170.0	198.5	—	213.0	238.0	239.2
semilunar cartilage (knee)	170.7	198.5	—	213.7	238.0	239.2
seminal vesicle	187.8	198.82	233.6	222.8	236.6	239.5
septum nasal	160.0	197.3	231.8	212.0	235.9	239.1
posterior margin	147.3	198.89	230.0	210.7	235.1	239.0
rectovaginal	195.3	198.89	234.8	229.8	238.8	239.89
rectovesical	195.3	198.89	234.8	229.8	238.8	239.89
urethrovaginal	184.9	198.82	233.39	221.9	236.3	239.5
vesicovaginal	184.9	198.82	233.39	221.9	236.3	239.5
shoulder NEC*	195.4	198.89	232.6	229.8	238.8	239.89
sigmoid flexure (lower) (upper)	153.3	197.5	230.3	211.3	235.2	239.0
sinus (accessory)	160.9	197.3	231.8	212.0	235.9	239.1
bone (any)	170.0	198.5	—	213.0	238.0	239.2
contiguous sites with middle ear or nasal cavities	160.8	—	—	—	—	—
ethmoidal	160.3	197.3	231.8	212.0	235.9	239.1
frontal	160.4	197.3	231.8	212.0	235.9	239.1
maxillary	160.2	197.3	231.8	212.0	235.9	239.1
nasal, paranasal NEC	160.9	197.3	231.8	212.0	235.9	239.1
pyriform	148.1	198.89	230.0	210.8	235.1	239.0
sphenoidal	160.5	197.3	231.8	212.0	235.9	239.1
skeleton, skeletal NEC	170.9	198.5	—	213.9	238.0	239.2
Skene's gland	189.4	198.1	233.9	223.89	236.99	239.5
skin NOS	173.90	198.2	232.9	216.9	238.2	239.2
abdominal wall	173.50	198.2	232.5	216.5	238.2	239.2
basal cell carcinoma	173.51	—	—	—	—	—
specified type NEC	173.59	—	—	—	—	—
squamous cell carcinoma	173.52	—	—	—	—	—

☑ Additional Digit Required — Refer to the Tabular List for Digit Selection   ▽ Subterms under main terms may continue to next column or page

2013 ICD-9-CM   ▶◀ Revised Text   ● New Line   ▲ Revised Code   Volume 2 — 205

Neoplasm, neoplastic —	Malignant			Benign	Uncertain Behavior	Unspecified
	Primary	Secondary	Ca in situ			
continued						
skin — continued						
ala nasi (*see also* Neoplasm, skin, face)	173.30	198.2	232.3	216.3	238.2	239.2
ankle (*see also* Neoplasm, skin, limb, lower)	173.70	198.2	232.7	216.7	238.2	239.2
antecubital space (*see also* Neoplasm, skin, limb, upper)	173.60	198.2	232.6	216.6	238.2	239.2
anus	173.50	198.2	232.5	216.5	238.2	239.2
basal cell carcinoma	173.51	—	—	—	—	—
specified type NEC	173.59	—	—	—	—	—
squamous cell carcinoma	173.52	—	—	—	—	—
arm (*see also* Neoplasm, skin, limb, upper)	173.60	198.2	232.6	216.6	238.2	239.2
auditory canal (external) (*see also* Neoplasm, skin, ear)	173.20	198.2	232.2	216.2	238.2	239.2
auricle (ear) (*see also* Neoplasm, skin, ear)	173.20	198.2	232.2	216.2	238.2	239.2
auricular canal (external) (*see also* Neoplasm, skin, ear)	173.20	198.2	232.2	216.2	238.2	239.2
axilla, axillary fold (*see also* Neoplasm, skin, trunk)	173.50	198.2	232.5	216.5	238.2	239.2
back	173.50	198.2	232.5	216.5	238.2	239.2
basal cell carcinoma	173.51	—	—	—	—	—
specified type NEC	173.59	—	—	—	—	—
squamous cell carcinoma	173.52	—	—	—	—	—
basal cell carcinoma, unspecified site	173.91	—	—	—	—	—
breast (*see also* Neoplasm, skin, trunk)	173.50	198.2	232.5	216.5	238.2	239.2
brow (*see also* Neoplasm, skin, face)	173.30	198.2	232.3	216.3	238.2	239.2
buttock (*see also* Neoplasm, skin, trunk)	173.50	198.2	232.5	216.5	238.2	239.2
calf (*see also* Neoplasm, skin, limb, lower)	173.70	198.2	232.7	216.7	238.2	239.2
canthus (eye) (inner) (outer)	173.10	198.2	232.1	216.1	238.2	239.2
basal cell carcinoma	173.11	—	—	—	—	—
specified type NEC	173.19	—	—	—	—	—
squamous cell carcinoma	173.12	—	—	—	—	—
cervical region (*see also* Neoplasm, skin, neck)	173.40	198.2	232.4	216.4	238.2	239.2
cheek (external) (*see also* Neoplasm, skin, face)	173.30	198.2	232.3	216.3	238.2	239.2
chest (wall) (*see also* Neoplasm, skin, trunk)	173.50	198.2	232.5	216.5	238.2	239.2
chin (*see also* Neoplasm, skin, face)	173.30	198.2	232.3	216.3	238.2	239.2
Neoplasm, neoplastic — continued						
skin — continued						
clavicular area (*see also* Neoplasm, skin, trunk)	173.50	198.2	232.5	216.5	238.2	239.2
clitoris	—	198.82	233.32	221.2	236.3	239.5
columnella (*see also* Neoplasm, skin, face)	173.30	198.2	232.3	216.3	238.2	239.2
concha (*see also* Neoplasm, skin, ear)	173.20	198.2	232.2	216.2	238.2	239.2
contiguous sites	173.80	—	—	—	—	—
basal cell carcinoma	173.81	—	—	—	—	—
specified type NEC	173.89	—	—	—	—	—
squamous cell carcinoma	173.82	—	—	—	—	—
ear (external)	173.20	198.2	232.2	216.2	238.2	239.2
basal cell carcinoma	173.21	—	—	—	—	—
specified type NEC	173.29	—	—	—	—	—
squamous cell carcinoma	173.22	—	—	—	—	—
elbow (*see also* Neoplasm, skin, limb, upper)	173.60	198.2	232.6	216.6	238.2	239.2
eyebrow (*see also* Neoplasm, skin, face)	173.30	198.2	232.3	216.3	238.2	239.2
eyelid	173.10	198.2	232.1	—	238.2	239.2
basal cell carcinoma	173.11	—	—	—	—	—
specified type NEC	173.19	—	—	—	—	—
squamous cell carcinoma	173.12	—	—	—	—	—
face NEC	173.30	198.2	232.3	216.3	238.2	239.2
basal cell carcinoma	173.31	—	—	—	—	—
specified type NEC	173.39	—	—	—	—	—
squamous cell carcinoma	173.32	—	—	—	—	—
female genital organs (external)	184.4	198.82	233.30	221.2	236.3	239.5
clitoris	184.3	198.82	233.32	221.2	236.3	239.5
labium NEC	184.4	198.82	233.32	221.2	236.3	239.5
majus	184.1	198.82	233.32	221.2	236.3	239.5
minus	184.2	198.82	233.32	221.2	236.3	239.5
pudendum	184.4	198.82	233.32	221.2	236.3	239.5
vulva	184.4	198.82	233.32	221.2	236.3	239.5
finger (*see also* Neoplasm, skin, limb, upper)	173.60	198.2	232.6	216.6	238.2	239.2
flank (*see also* Neoplasm, skin, trunk)	173.50	198.2	232.5	216.5	238.2	239.2
foot (*see also* Neoplasm, skin, limb, lower)	173.70	198.2	232.7	216.7	238.2	239.2
forearm (*see also* Neoplasm, skin, limb, upper)	173.60	198.2	232.6	216.6	238.2	239.2
forehead (*see also* Neoplasm, skin, face)	173.30	198.2	232.3	216.3	238.2	239.2
glabella (*see also* Neoplasm, skin, face)	173.30	198.2	232.3	216.3	238.2	239.2
gluteal region (*see also* Neoplasm, skin, trunk)	173.50	198.2	232.5	216.5	238.2	239.2
groin (*see also* Neoplasm, skin, trunk)	173.50	198.2	232.5	216.5	238.2	239.2

☑ Additional Digit Required — Refer to the Tabular List for Digit Selection

▽ Subterms under main terms may continue to next column or page

Neoplasm, neoplastic — continued skin — continued	Malignant			Benign	Uncertain Behavior	Unspecified
	Primary	Secondary	Ca in situ			
hand (see also Neoplasm, skin, limb, upper)	173.60	198.2	232.6	216.6	238.2	239.2
head NEC (see also Neoplasm, skin, scalp)	173.40	198.2	232.4	216.4	238.2	239.2
heel (see also Neoplasm, skin, limb, lower)	173.70	198.2	232.7	216.7	238.2	239.2
helix (see also Neoplasm, skin, ear)	173.20	198.2	—	216.2	238.2	239.2
hip	173.70	198.2	232.7	216.7	238.2	239.2
basal cell carcinoma	173.71	—	—	—	—	—
specified type NEC	173.79	—	—	—	—	—
squamous cell carcinoma	173.72	—	—	—	—	—
infraclavicular region (see also Neoplasm, skin, trunk)	173.50	198.2	232.5	216.5	238.2	239.2
inguinal region (see also Neoplasm, skin, trunk)	173.50	198.2	232.5	216.5	238.2	239.2
jaw (see also Neoplasm, skin, face)	173.30	198.2	232.3	216.3	238.2	239.2
knee (see also Neoplasm, skin, limb, lower)	173.70	198.2	232.7	216.7	238.2	239.2
labia						
majora	184.1	198.82	233.32	221.2	236.3	239.5
minora	184.2	198.82	233.32	221.2	236.3	239.5
leg (see also Neoplasm, skin, limb, lower)	173.70	198.2	232.7	216.7	238.2	239.2
lid (lower) (upper)	173.10	198.2	232.1	216.1	238.2	239.2
basal cell carcinoma	173.11	—	—	—	—	—
specified type NEC	173.19	—	—	—	—	—
squamous cell carcinoma	173.12	—	—	—	—	—
limb NEC	173.90	198.2	232.9	216.9	238.2	239.5
lower	173.70	198.2	232.7	216.7	238.2	239.2
basal cell carcinoma	173.71	—	—	—	—	—
specified type NEC	173.79	—	—	—	—	—
squamous cell carcinoma	173.72	—	—	—	—	—
upper	173.60	198.2	232.6	216.6	238.2	239.2
basal cell carcinoma	173.61	—	—	—	—	—
specified type NEC	173.69	—	—	—	—	—
squamous cell carcinoma	173.62	—	—	—	—	—
lip (lower) (upper)	173.00	198.2	232.0	216.0	238.2	239.2
basal cell carcinoma	173.01	—	—	—	—	—
specified type NEC	173.09	—	—	—	—	—
squamous cell carcinoma	173.02	—	—	—	—	—
male genital organs	187.9	198.82	233.6	222.9	236.6	239.5
penis	187.4	198.82	233.5	222.1	236.6	239.5
prepuce	187.1	198.82	233.5	222.1	236.6	239.5
scrotum	187.7	198.82	233.6	222.4	236.6	239.5
mastectomy site (see also Neoplasm, skin, trunk)	173.50	198.2	—	—	—	—
specified as breast tissue	174.8	198.81	—	—	—	—
meatus, acoustic (external) (see also Neoplasm, skin, ear)	173.20	198.2	232.2	216.2	238.2	239.2
nates (see also Neoplasm, skin, trunk)	173.50	198.2	232.5	216.5	238.2	239.0
neck	173.40	198.2	232.4	216.4	238.2	239.2
basal cell carcinoma	173.41	—	—	—	—	—
specified type NEC	173.49	—	—	—	—	—
squamous cell carcinoma	173.42	—	—	—	—	—
nose (external) (see also Neoplasm, skin, face)	173.30	198.2	232.3	216.3	238.2	239.2
palm (see also Neoplasm, skin, limb, upper)	173.60	198.2	232.6	216.6	238.2	239.2
palpebra	173.10	198.2	232.1	216.1	238.2	239.2
basal cell carcinoma	173.11	—	—	—	—	—
specified type NEC	173.19	—	—	—	—	—
squamous cell carcinoma	173.12	—	—	—	—	—
penis NEC	187.4	198.82	233.5	222.1	236.6	239.5
perianal (see also Neoplasm, skin, anus)	173.50	198.2	232.5	216.5	238.2	239.2
perineum (see also Neoplasm, skin, anus)	173.50	198.2	232.5	216.5	238.2	239.2
pinna (see also Neoplasm, skin, ear)	173.20	198.2	232.2	216.2	238.2	239.2
plantar (see also Neoplasm, skin, limb, lower)	173.70	198.2	232.7	216.7	238.2	239.2
popliteal fossa or space (see also Neoplasm, skin, limb, lower)	173.70	198.2	232.7	216.7	238.2	239.2
prepuce	187.1	198.82	233.5	222.1	236.6	239.5
pubes (see also Neoplasm, skin, trunk)	173.50	198.2	232.5	216.5	238.2	239.2
sacrococcygeal region (see also Neoplasm, skin, trunk)	173.50	198.2	232.5	216.5	238.2	239.2
scalp	173.40	198.2	232.4	216.4	238.2	239.2
basal cell carcinoma	173.41	—	—	—	—	—
specified type NEC	173.49	—	—	—	—	—
squamous cell carcinoma	173.42	—	—	—	—	—
scapular region (see also Neoplasm, skin, trunk)	173.50	198.2	232.5	216.5	238.2	239.2
scrotum	187.7	198.82	233.6	222.4	236.6	239.5
shoulder	173.60	198.2	232.6	216.6	238.2	239.2
basal cell carcinoma	173.61	—	—	—	—	—
specified type NEC	173.69	—	—	—	—	—
squamous cell carcinoma	173.62	—	—	—	—	—

	Malignant					
	Primary	Secondary	Ca in situ	Benign	Uncertain Behavior	Unspecified
Neoplasm, neoplastic— continued						
skin — continued						
sole (foot) (see also Neoplasm, skin, limb, lower)	173.70	198.2	232.7	216.7	238.2	239.2
specified sites NEC	173.80	198.2	232.8	216.8	—	239.2
basal cell carcinoma	173.81	—	—	—	—	—
specified type NEC	173.89	—	—	—	—	—
squamous cell carcinoma	173.82	—	—	—	—	—
specified type NEC, unspecified site	173.99	—	—	—	—	—
squamous cell carcinoma, unspecified site	173.92	—	—	—	—	—
submammary fold (see also Neoplasm, skin, trunk)	173.50	198.2	232.5	216.5	238.2	239.2
supraclavicular region (see also Neoplasm, skin, neck)	173.40	198.2	232.4	216.4	238.2	239.2
temple (see also Neoplasm, skin, face)	173.30	198.2	232.3	216.3	238.2	239.2
thigh (see also Neoplasm, skin, limb, lower)	173.70	198.2	232.7	216.7	238.2	239.2
thoracic wall (see also Neoplasm, skin, trunk)	173.50	198.2	232.5	216.5	238.2	239.2
thumb (see also Neoplasm, skin, limb, upper)	173.60	198.2	232.6	216.6	238.2	239.2
toe (see also Neoplasm, skin, limb, lower)	173.70	198.2	232.7	216.7	238.2	239.2
tragus (see also Neoplasm, skin, ear)	173.20	198.2	232.2	216.2	238.2	239.2
trunk	173.50	198.2	232.5	216.5	238.2	239.2
basal cell carcinoma	173.51	—	—	—	—	—
specified type NEC	173.59	—	—	—	—	—
squamous cell carcinoma	173.52	—	—	—	—	—
umbilicus (see also Neoplasm, skin, trunk)	173.50	198.2	232.5	216.5	238.2	239.2
vulva	184.4	198.82	233.32	221.2	236.3	239.5
wrist (see also Neoplasm, skin, limb, upper)	173.60	198.2	232.6	216.6	238.2	239.2
skull	170.0	198.5	—	213.0	238.0	239.2
soft parts or tissues — see Neoplasm, connective tissue						
specified site NEC	195.8	198.89	234.8	229.8	238.8	239.89
specified site — see Neoplasm, skin						
spermatic cord	187.6	198.82	233.6	222.8	236.6	239.5
sphenoid	160.5	197.3	231.8	212.0	235.9	239.1
bone	170.0	198.5	—	213.0	238.0	239.2
sinus	160.5	197.3	231.8	212.0	235.9	239.1
sphincter						
anal	154.2	197.5	230.5	211.4	235.5	239.0
of Oddi	156.1	197.8	230.8	211.5	235.3	239.0
spine, spinal (column)	170.2	198.5	—	213.2	238.0	239.2
bulb	191.7	198.3	—	225.0	237.5	239.6
coccyx	170.6	198.5	—	213.6	238.0	239.2

	Malignant					
	Primary	Secondary	Ca in situ	Benign	Uncertain Behavior	Unspecified
Neoplasm, neoplastic— continued						
spine, spinal — continued						
cord (cervical) (lumbar) (sacral) (thoracic)	192.2	198.3	—	225.3	237.5	239.7
dura mater	192.3	198.4	—	225.4	237.6	239.7
lumbosacral	170.2	198.5	—	213.2	238.0	239.2
membrane	192.3	198.4	—	225.4	237.6	239.7
meninges	192.3	198.4	—	225.4	237.6	239.7
nerve (root)	171.9	198.89	—	215.9	238.1	239.2
pia mater	192.3	198.4	—	225.4	237.6	239.7
root	171.9	198.89	—	215.9	238.1	239.2
sacrum	170.6	198.5	—	213.6	238.0	239.2
spleen, splenic NEC	159.1	197.8	230.9	211.9	235.5	239.0
flexure (colon)	153.7	197.5	230.3	211.3	235.2	239.0
stem, brain	191.7	198.3	—	225.0	237.5	239.6
Stensen's duct	142.0	198.89	230.0	210.2	235.0	239.0
sternum	170.3	198.5	—	213.3	238.0	239.2
stomach	151.9	197.8	230.2	211.1	235.2	239.0
antrum (pyloric)	151.2	197.8	230.2	211.1	235.2	239.0
body	151.4	197.8	230.2	211.1	235.2	239.0
cardia	151.0	197.8	230.2	211.1	235.2	239.0
cardiac orifice	151.0	197.8	230.2	211.1	235.2	239.0
contiguous sites	151.8	—	—	—	—	—
corpus	151.4	197.8	230.2	211.1	235.2	239.0
fundus	151.3	197.8	230.2	211.1	235.2	239.0
greater curvature NEC	151.6	197.8	230.2	211.1	235.2	239.0
lesser curvature NEC	151.5	197.8	230.2	211.1	235.2	239.0
prepylorus	151.1	197.8	230.2	211.1	235.2	239.0
pylorus	151.1	197.8	230.2	211.1	235.2	239.0
wall NEC	151.9	197.8	230.2	211.1	235.2	239.0
anterior NEC	151.8	197.8	230.2	211.1	235.2	239.0
posterior NEC	151.8	197.8	230.2	211.1	235.2	239.0
stroma, endometrial	182.0	198.82	233.2	219.1	236.0	239.5
stump, cervical	180.8	198.82	233.1	219.0	236.0	239.5
subcutaneous (nodule) (tissue) NEC — see Neoplasm, connective tissue						
subdural	192.1	198.4	—	225.2	237.6	239.7
subglottis, subglottic	161.2	197.3	231.0	212.1	235.6	239.1
sublingual	144.9	198.89	230.0	210.3	235.1	239.0
gland or duct	142.2	198.89	230.0	210.2	235.0	239.0
submandibular gland	142.1	198.89	230.0	210.2	235.0	239.0
submaxillary gland or duct	142.1	198.89	230.0	210.2	235.0	239.0
submental	195.0	198.89	234.8	229.8	238.8	239.89
subpleural	162.9	197.0	—	212.3	235.7	239.1
substernal	164.2	197.1	—	212.5	235.8	239.89
sudoriferous, sudoriparous gland, site unspecified	173.90	198.2	232.9	216.9	238.2	239.2
specified site — see Neoplasm, skin						
supraclavicular region	195.0	198.89	234.8	229.8	238.8	239.89
supraglottis	161.1	197.3	231.0	212.1	235.6	239.1
suprarenal (capsule) (cortex) (gland) (medulla)	194.0	198.7	234.8	227.0	237.2	239.7
suprasellar (region)	191.9	198.3	—	225.0	237.5	239.6
sweat gland (apocrine) (eccrine), site unspecified	173.90	198.2	232.9	216.9	238.2	239.2
sympathetic nerve or nervous system NEC	171.9	198.89	—	215.9	238.1	239.2

☑ Additional Digit Required — Refer to the Tabular List for Digit Selection　　　　　　　　▽ Subterms under main terms may continue to next column or page

208 — Volume 2　　　　▶◀ Revised Text　　　　● New Line　　　▲ Revised Code　　　　2013 ICD-9-CM

	Malignant					
	Primary	Secondary	Ca in situ	Benign	Uncertain Behavior	Unspecified
Neoplasm, neoplastic — continued						
symphysis pubis	170.6	198.5	—	213.6	238.0	239.2
synovial membrane — see Neoplasm, connective tissue						
tapetum, brain	191.8	198.3	—	225.0	237.5	239.6
tarsus (any bone)	170.8	198.5	—	213.8	238.0	239.2
temple (skin) (see also Neoplasm, skin, face)	173.30	198.2	232.3	216.3	238.2	239.2
temporal						
bone	170.0	198.5	—	213.0	238.0	239.2
lobe or pole	191.2	198.3	—	225.0	237.5	239.6
region	195.0	198.89	234.8	229.8	238.8	239.89
skin (see also Neoplasm, skin, face)	173.30	198.2	232.3	216.3	238.2	239.2
tendon (sheath) — see Neoplasm, connective tissue						
tentorium (cerebelli)	192.1	198.4	—	225.2	237.6	239.7
testis, testes (descended) (scrotal)	186.9	198.82	233.6	222.0	236.4	239.5
ectopic	186.0	198.82	233.6	222.0	236.4	239.5
retained	186.0	198.82	233.6	222.0	236.4	239.5
undescended	186.0	198.82	233.6	222.0	236.4	239.5
thalamus	191.0	198.3	—	225.0	237.5	239.6
thigh NEC*	195.5	198.89	234.8	229.8	238.8	239.89
thorax, thoracic (cavity) (organs NEC)	195.1	198.89	234.8	229.8	238.8	239.89
duct	171.4	198.89	—	215.4	238.1	239.2
wall NEC	195.1	198.89	234.8	229.8	238.8	239.89
throat	149.0	198.89	230.0	210.9	235.1	239.0
thumb NEC*	195.4	198.89	232.6	229.8	238.8	239.89
thymus (gland)	164.0	198.89	—	212.6	235.8	239.89
contiguous sites with heart and mediastinum	164.8	—	—	—	—	—
thyroglossal duct	193	198.89	234.8	226	237.4	239.7
thyroid (gland)	193	198.89	234.8	226	237.4	239.7
cartilage	161.3	197.3	231.0	212.1	235.6	239.1
tibia (any part)	170.7	198.5	—	213.7	238.0	239.2
toe NEC*	195.5	198.89	232.7	229.8	238.8	239.89
tongue	141.9	198.89	230.0	210.1	235.1	239.0
anterior (two-thirds) NEC	141.4	198.89	230.0	210.1	235.1	239.0
dorsal surface	141.1	198.89	230.0	210.1	235.1	239.0
ventral surface	141.3	198.89	230.0	210.1	235.1	239.0
base (dorsal surface)	141.0	198.89	230.0	210.1	235.1	239.0
border (lateral)	141.2	198.89	230.0	210.1	235.1	239.0
contiguous sites	141.8	—	—	—	—	—
dorsal surface NEC	141.1	198.89	230.0	210.1	235.1	239.0
fixed part NEC	141.0	198.89	230.0	210.1	235.1	239.0
foreamen cecum	141.1	198.89	230.0	210.1	235.1	239.0
frenulum linguae	141.3	198.89	230.0	210.1	235.1	239.0
junctional zone	141.5	198.89	230.0	210.1	235.1	239.0
margin (lateral)	141.2	198.89	230.0	210.1	235.1	239.0
midline NEC	141.1	198.89	230.0	210.1	235.1	239.0
mobile part NEC	141.4	198.89	230.0	210.1	235.1	239.0
posterior (third)	141.0	198.89	230.0	210.1	235.1	239.0
root	141.0	198.89	230.0	210.1	235.1	239.0
surface (dorsal)	141.1	198.89	230.0	210.1	235.1	239.0
base	141.0	198.89	230.0	210.1	235.1	239.0
ventral	141.3	198.89	230.0	210.1	235.1	239.0
tip	141.2	198.89	230.0	210.1	235.1	239.0
tonsil	141.6	198.89	230.0	210.1	235.1	239.0
tonsil	146.0	198.89	230.0	210.5	235.1	239.0
fauces, faucial	146.0	198.89	230.0	210.5	235.1	239.0
lingual	141.6	198.89	230.0	210.1	235.1	239.0
palatine	146.0	198.89	230.0	210.5	235.1	239.0
pharyngeal	147.1	198.89	230.0	210.7	235.1	239.0

	Malignant					
	Primary	Secondary	Ca in situ	Benign	Uncertain Behavior	Unspecified
Neoplasm, neoplastic — continued						
tonsil — continued						
pillar (anterior) (posterior)	146.2	198.89	230.0	210.6	235.1	239.0
tonsillar fossa	146.1	198.89	230.0	210.6	235.1	239.0
tooth socket NEC	143.9	198.89	230.0	210.4	235.1	239.0
trachea (cartilage) (mucosa)	162.0	197.3	231.1	212.2	235.7	239.1
contiguous sites with bronchus or lung	162.8	—	—	—	—	—
tracheobronchial	162.8	197.3	231.1	212.2	235.7	239.1
contiguous sites with lung	162.8	—	—	—	—	—
tragus (see also Neoplasm, skin, ear)	173.20	198.2	232.2	216.2	238.2	239.2
trunk NEC*	195.8	198.89	232.5	229.8	238.8	239.89
tubo-ovarian	183.8	198.82	233.39	221.8	236.3	239.5
tunica vaginalis	187.8	198.82	233.6	222.8	236.6	239.5
turbinate (bone)	170.0	198.5	—	213.0	238.0	239.2
nasal	160.0	197.3	231.8	212.0	235.9	239.1
tympanic cavity	160.1	197.3	231.8	212.0	235.9	239.1
ulna (any part)	170.4	198.5	—	213.4	238.0	239.2
umbilicus, umbilical (see also Neoplasm, skin, trunk)	173.50	198.2	232.5	216.5	238.2	239.2
uncus, brain	191.2	198.3	—	225.0	237.5	239.6
unknown site or unspecified	199.1	199.1	234.9	229.9	238.9	239.9
urachus	188.7	198.1	233.7	223.3	236.7	239.4
ureter-bladder (junction)	188.6	198.1	233.7	223.3	236.7	239.4
ureter, ureteral	189.2	198.1	233.9	223.2	236.91	239.5
orifice (bladder)	188.6	198.1	233.7	223.3	236.7	239.4
urethra, urethral (gland)	189.3	198.1	233.9	223.81	236.99	239.5
orifice, internal	188.5	198.1	233.7	223.3	236.7	239.4
urethrovaginal (septum)	184.9	198.82	233.39	221.9	236.3	239.5
urinary organ or system NEC	189.9	198.1	233.9	223.9	236.99	239.5
bladder — see Neoplasm, bladder						
contiguous sites	189.8	—	—	—	—	—
specified sites NEC	189.8	198.1	233.9	223.89	236.99	239.5
utero-ovarian	183.8	198.82	233.39	221.8	236.3	239.5
ligament	183.3	198.82	—	221.0	236.3	239.5
uterosacral ligament	183.4	198.82	—	221.0	236.3	239.5
uterus, uteri, uterine	179	198.82	233.2	219.9	236.0	239.5
adnexa NEC	183.9	198.82	233.39	221.8	236.3	239.5
contiguous sites	183.8	—	—	—	—	—
body	182.0	198.82	233.2	219.1	236.0	239.5
contiguous sites	182.8	—	—	—	—	—
cervix	180.9	198.82	233.1	219.0	236.0	239.5
cornu	182.0	198.82	233.2	219.1	236.0	239.5
corpus	182.0	198.82	233.2	219.1	236.0	239.5
endocervix (canal) (gland)	180.0	198.82	233.1	219.0	236.0	239.5
endometrium	182.0	198.82	233.2	219.1	236.0	239.5
exocervix	180.1	198.82	233.1	219.0	236.0	239.5
external os	180.1	198.82	233.1	219.0	236.0	239.5
fundus	182.0	198.82	233.2	219.1	236.0	239.5
internal os	180.0	198.82	233.1	219.0	236.0	239.5
isthmus	182.1	198.82	233.2	219.1	236.0	239.5
ligament	183.4	198.82	—	221.0	236.3	239.5
broad	183.3	198.82	233.39	221.0	236.3	239.5
round	183.5	198.82	—	221.0	236.3	239.5
lower segment	182.1	198.82	233.2	219.1	236.0	239.5
myometrium	182.0	198.82	233.2	219.1	236.0	239.5

☑ Additional Digit Required — Refer to the Tabular List for Digit Selection   Subterms under main terms may continue to next column or page

2013 ICD-9-CM   ►◄ Revised Text   ● New Line   ▲ Revised Code   Volume 2 — 209

Neoplasm, neoplastic — continued	Malignant			Benign	Uncertain Behavior	Unspecified
	Primary	Secondary	Ca in situ			
uterus, uteri, uterine — *continued*						
squamocolumnar junction	180.8	198.82	233.1	219.0	236.0	239.5
tube	183.2	198.82	233.39	221.0	236.3	239.5
utricle, prostatic	189.3	198.1	233.9	223.81	236.99	239.5
uveal tract	190.0	198.4	234.0	224.0	238.8	239.89
uvula	145.4	198.89	230.0	210.4	235.1	239.0
vagina, vaginal (fornix) (vault) (wall)	184.0	198.82	233.31	221.1	236.3	239.5
vaginovesical	184.9	198.82	233.39	221.9	236.3	239.5
septum	184.9	198.82	233.39	221.9	236.3	239.5
vallecula (epiglottis)	146.3	198.89	230.0	210.6	235.1	239.0
vascular — *see* Neoplasm, connective tissue						
vas deferens	187.6	198.82	233.6	222.8	236.6	239.5
Vater's ampulla	156.2	197.8	230.8	211.5	235.3	239.0
vein, venous — *see* Neoplasm, connective tissue						
vena cava (abdominal) (inferior)	171.5	198.89	—	215.5	238.1	239.2
superior	171.4	198.89	—	215.4	238.1	239.2
ventricle (cerebral) (floor) (fourth) (lateral) (third)	191.5	198.3	—	225.0	237.5	239.6
cardiac (left) (right)	164.1	198.89	—	212.7	238.8	239.89
ventricular band of larynx	161.1	197.3	231.0	212.1	235.6	239.1
ventriculus — see Neoplasm, stomach						
vermillion border — *see* Neoplasm, lip						
vermis, cerebellum	191.6	198.3	—	225.0	237.5	239.6
vertebra (column)	170.2	198.5	—	213.2	238.0	239.2
coccyx	170.6	198.5	—	213.6	238.0	239.2
sacrum	170.6	198.5	—	213.6	238.0	239.2
vesical — *see* Neoplasm, bladder						
vesicle, seminal	187.8	198.82	233.6	222.8	236.6	239.5
vesicocervical tissue	184.9	198.82	233.39	221.9	236.3	239.5
vesicorectal	195.3	198.89	234.8	229.8	238.8	239.89
vesicovaginal	184.9	198.82	233.39	221.9	236.3	239.5
septum	184.9	198.82	233.39	221.9	236.3	239.5
vessel (blood) — *see* Neoplasm, connective tissue						
vestibular gland, greater	184.1	198.82	233.32	221.2	236.3	239.5
vestibule						
mouth	145.1	198.89	230.0	210.4	235.1	239.0
nose	160.0	197.3	231.8	212.0	235.9	239.1
Virchow's gland	—	196.0	—	229.0	238.8	239.89
viscera NEC	195.8	198.89	234.8	229.8	238.8	239.89
vocal cords (true)	161.0	197.3	231.0	212.1	235.6	239.1
false	161.1	197.3	231.0	212.1	235.6	239.1
vomer	170.0	198.5	—	213.0	238.0	239.2
vulva	184.4	198.82	233.32	221.2	236.3	239.5
vulvovaginal gland	184.4	198.82	233.32	221.2	236.3	239.5
Waldeyer's ring	149.1	198.89	230.0	210.9	235.1	239.0
Wharton's duct	142.1	198.89	230.0	210.2	235.0	239.0
white matter (central) (cerebral)	191.0	198.3	—	225.0	237.5	239.6
windpipe	162.0	197.3	231.1	212.2	235.7	239.1
Wirsung's duct	157.3	197.8	230.9	211.6	235.5	239.0
wolffian (body) (duct) female	184.8	198.82	233.39	221.8	236.3	239.5
male	187.8	198.82	233.6	222.8	236.6	239.5
womb — *see* Neoplasm, uterus						

Neoplasm, neoplastic — continued	Malignant			Benign	Uncertain Behavior	Unspecified
	Primary	Secondary	Ca in situ			
wrist NEC*	195.4	198.89	232.6	229.8	238.8	239.89
xiphoid process	170.3	198.5	—	213.3	238.0	239.2
Zuckerkandl's organ	194.6	198.89	—	227.6	237.3	239.7

☑ **Additional Digit Required — Refer to the Tabular List for Digit Selection**   ▽ **Subterms under main terms may continue to next column or page**

210 — Volume 2   ▶◀ **Revised Text**   ● **New Line**   ▲ **Revised Code**   2013 ICD-9-CM

Neovascularization
  choroid 362.16
  ciliary body 364.42
  cornea 370.60
    deep 370.63
    localized 370.61
  iris 364.42
  retina 362.16
  subretinal 362.16
Nephralgia 788.0
Nephritis, nephritic (albuminuric) (azotemic) (congenital) (degenerative) (diffuse) (disseminated) (epithelial) (familial) (focal) (granulomatous) (hemorrhagic) (infantile) (nonsuppurative, excretory) (uremic) 583.9
  with
    edema — see Nephrosis
    lesion of
      glomerulonephritis
        hypocomplementemic persistent 583.2
          with nephrotic syndrome 581.2
          chronic 582.2
        lobular 583.2
          with nephrotic syndrome 581.2
          chronic 582.2
        membranoproliferative 583.2
          with nephrotic syndrome 581.2
          chronic 582.2
        membranous 583.1
          with nephrotic syndrome 581.1
          chronic 582.1
        mesangiocapillary 583.2
          with nephrotic syndrome 581.2
          chronic 582.2
        mixed membranous and proliferative 583.2
          with nephrotic syndrome 581.2
          chronic 582.2
        proliferative (diffuse) 583.0
          with nephrotic syndrome 581.0
          acute 580.0
          chronic 582.0
        rapidly progressive 583.4
          acute 580.4
          chronic 582.4
      interstitial nephritis (diffuse) (focal) 583.89
        with nephrotic syndrome 581.89
        acute 580.89
        chronic 582.89
      necrotizing glomerulitis 583.4
        acute 580.4
        chronic 582.4
      renal necrosis 583.9
        cortical 583.6
        medullary 583.7
      specified pathology NEC 583.89
        with nephrotic syndrome 581.89
        acute 580.89
        chronic 582.89
    necrosis, renal 583.9
      cortical 583.6
      medullary (papillary) 583.7
    nephrotic syndrome (see also Nephrosis) 581.9
    papillary necrosis 583.7
    specified pathology NEC 583.89
  acute 580.9
    extracapillary with epithelial crescents 580.4
    hypertensive (see also Hypertension, kidney) 403.90
    necrotizing 580.4
    poststreptococcal 580.0
    proliferative (diffuse) 580.0
    rapidly progressive 580.4
    specified pathology NEC 580.89

Nephritis, nephritic — continued
  amyloid 277.39 [583.81]
    chronic 277.39 [582.81]
  arteriolar (see also Hypertension, kidney) 403.90
  arteriosclerotic (see also Hypertension, kidney) 403.90
  ascending (see also Pyelitis) 590.80
  atrophic 582.9
  basement membrane NEC 583.89
    with
      pulmonary hemorrhage (Goodpasture's syndrome) 446.21 [583.81]
  calculous, calculus 592.0
  cardiac (see also Hypertension, kidney) 403.90
  cardiovascular (see also Hypertension, kidney) 403.90
  chronic 582.9
    arteriosclerotic (see also Hypertension, kidney) 403.90
    hypertensive (see also Hypertension, kidney) 403.90
  cirrhotic (see also Sclerosis, renal) 587
  complicating pregnancy, childbirth, or puerperium 646.2 ✓
    with hypertension 642.1 ✓
      affecting fetus or newborn 760.0
    affecting fetus or newborn 760.1
  croupous 580.9
  desquamative — see Nephrosis
  due to
    amyloidosis 277.39 [583.81]
      chronic 277.39 [582.81]
    arteriosclerosis (see also Hypertension, kidney) 403.90
    diabetes mellitus 250.4 ✓ [583.81]
      with nephrotic syndrome 250.4 ✓ [581.81]
      due to secondary diabetes 249.4 ✓ [583.81]
    due to secondary diabetes 249.4 ✓ [583.81]
    diphtheria 032.89 [580.81]
    gonococcal infection (acute) 098.19 [583.81]
      chronic or duration of 2 months or over 098.39 [583.81]
    gout 274.10
    infectious hepatitis 070.9 [580.81]
    mumps 072.79 [580.81]
    specified kidney pathology NEC 583.89
      acute 580.89
      chronic 582.89
    streptotrichosis 039.8 [583.81]
    subacute bacterial endocarditis 421.0 [580.81]
    systemic lupus erythematosus 710.0 [583.81]
      chronic 710.0 [582.81]
    typhoid fever 002.0 [580.81]
  endothelial 582.2
  end stage (chronic) (terminal) NEC 585.6
  epimembranous 581.1
  exudative 583.89
    with nephrotic syndrome 581.89
    acute 580.89
    chronic 582.89
  gonococcal (acute) 098.19 [583.81]
    chronic or duration of 2 months or over 098.39 [583.81]
  gouty 274.10
  hereditary (Alport's syndrome) 759.89
  hydremic — see Nephrosis
  hypertensive (see also Hypertension, kidney) 403.90
  hypocomplementemic persistent 583.2
    with nephrotic syndrome 581.2
    chronic 582.2
  immune complex NEC 583.89
  infective (see also Pyelitis) 590.80
  interstitial (diffuse) (focal) 583.89
    with nephrotic syndrome 581.89
    acute 580.89
    chronic 582.89

Nephritis, nephritic — continued
  latent or quiescent — see Nephritis, chronic
  lead 984.9
    specified type of lead — see Table of Drugs and Chemicals
  lobular 583.2
    with nephrotic syndrome 581.2
    chronic 582.2
  lupus 710.0 [583.81]
    acute 710.0 [580.81]
    chronic 710.0 [582.81]
  membranoproliferative 583.2
    with nephrotic syndrome 581.2
    chronic 582.2
  membranous 583.1
    with nephrotic syndrome 581.1
    chronic 582.1
  mesangiocapillary 583.2
    with nephrotic syndrome 581.2
    chronic 582.2
  minimal change 581.3
  mixed membranous and proliferative 583.2
    with nephrotic syndrome 581.2
    chronic 582.2
  necrotic, necrotizing 583.4
    acute 580.4
    chronic 582.4
  nephrotic — see Nephrosis
  old — see Nephritis, chronic
  parenchymatous 581.89
  polycystic 753.12
    adult type (APKD) 753.13
    autosomal dominant 753.13
    autosomal recessive 753.14
    childhood type (CPKD) 753.14
    infantile type 753.14
  poststreptococcal 580.0
  pregnancy — see Nephritis, complicating pregnancy
  proliferative 583.0
    with nephrotic syndrome 581.0
    acute 580.0
    chronic 582.0
  purulent (see also Pyelitis) 590.80
  rapidly progressive 583.4
    acute 580.4
    chronic 582.4
  salt-losing or salt-wasting (see also Disease, renal) 593.9
  saturnine 584.9
    specified type of lead — see Table of Drugs and Chemicals
  septic (see also Pyelitis) 590.80
  specified pathology NEC 583.89
    acute 580.89
    chronic 582.89
  staphylococcal (see also Pyelitis) 590.80
  streptotrichosis 039.8 [583.81]
  subacute (see also Nephrosis) 581.9
  suppurative (see also Pyelitis) 590.80
  syphilitic (late) 095.4
    congenital 090.5 [583.81]
    early 091.69 [583.81]
  terminal (chronic) (end-stage) NEC 585.6
  toxic — see Nephritis, acute
  tubal, tubular — see Nephrosis, tubular
  tuberculous (see also Tuberculosis) 016.0 ✓ [583.81]
  type II (Ellis) — see Nephrosis
  vascular — see Hypertension, kidney
  war 583.9
Nephroblastoma (M8960/3) 189.0
  epithelial (M8961/3) 189.0
  mesenchymal (M8962/3) 189.0
Nephrocalcinosis 275.49
Nephrocystitis, pustular — see also Pyelitis 590.80
Nephrolithiasis (congenital) (pelvis) (recurrent) 592.0
  uric acid 274.11
Nephroma (M8960/3) 189.0
  mesoblastic (M8960/1) 236.9 ✓
Nephronephritis — see also Nephrosis 581.9
Nephronopthisis 753.16
Nephropathy — see also Nephritis 583.9

Nephropathy — see also Nephritis — continued
  with
    exudative nephritis 583.89
    interstitial nephritis (diffuse) (focal) 583.89
    medullary necrosis 583.7
    necrosis 583.9
      cortical 583.6
      medullary or papillary 583.7
    papillary necrosis 583.7
    specified lesion or cause NEC 583.89
  analgesic 583.89
    with medullary necrosis, acute 584.7
  arteriolar (see also Hypertension, kidney) 403.90
  arteriosclerotic (see also Hypertension, kidney) 403.90
  complicating pregnancy 646.2 ✓
  diabetic 250.4 ✓ [583.81]
    due to secondary diabetes 249.4 ✓ [583.81]
  gouty 274.10
    specified type NEC 274.19
  hereditary amyloid 277.31
  hypercalcemic 588.89
  hypertensive (see also Hypertension, kidney) 403.90
  hypokalemic (vacuolar) 588.89
  IgA 583.9
  obstructive 593.89
    congenital 753.20
  phenacetin 584.7
  phosphate-losing 588.0
  potassium depletion 588.89
  proliferative (see also Nephritis, proliferative) 583.0
  protein-losing 588.89
  salt-losing or salt-wasting (see also Disease, renal) 593.9
  sickle-cell (see also Disease, sickle-cell) 282.60 [583.81]
  toxic 584.5
  vasomotor 584.5
  water-losing 588.89
Nephroptosis — see also Disease, renal 593.9
  congenital (displaced) 753.3
Nephropyosis — see also Abscess, kidney 590.2
Nephrorrhagia 593.81
Nephrosclerosis (arteriolar) (arteriosclerotic) (chronic) (hyaline) — see also Hypertension, kidney 403.90
  gouty 274.10
  hyperplastic (arteriolar) (see also Hypertension, kidney) 403.90
  senile (see also Sclerosis, renal) 587
Nephrosis, nephrotic (Epstein's) (syndrome) 581.9
  with
    lesion of
      focal glomerulosclerosis 581.1
      glomerulonephritis
        endothelial 581.2
        hypocomplementemic persistent 581.2
        lobular 581.2
        membranoproliferative 581.2
        membranous 581.1
        mesangiocapillary 581.2
        minimal change 581.3
        mixed membranous and proliferative 581.2
        proliferative 581.0
      segmental hyalinosis 581.1
      specified pathology NEC 581.89
  acute — see Nephrosis, tubular
  anoxic — see Nephrosis, tubular
  arteriosclerotic (see also Hypertension, kidney) 403.90
  chemical — see Nephrosis, tubular
  cholemic 572.4
  complicating pregnancy, childbirth, or puerperium — see Nephritis, complicating pregnancy
  diabetic 250.4 ✓ [581.81]

✓ **Additional Digit Required** — Refer to the Tabular List for Digit Selection   ▽ **Subterms under main terms may continue to next column or page**

2013 ICD-9-CM   ▶◀ **Revised Text**   ● **New Line**   ▲ **Revised Code**   **Volume 2 — 211**

Nephrosis, nephrotic — continued
- diabetic — continued
  - due to secondary diabetes 249.4 ☑ [581.81]
  - Finnish type (congenital) 759.89
  - hemoglobinuric — see Nephrosis, tubular
- in
  - amyloidosis 277.39 [581.81]
  - diabetes mellitus 250.4 ☑ [581.81]
    - due to secondary diabetes 249.4 ☑ [581.81]
  - epidemic hemorrhagic fever 078.6
  - malaria 084.9 [581.81]
  - polyarteritis 446.0 [581.81]
  - systemic lupus erythematosus 710.0 [581.81]
- ischemic — see Nephrosis, tubular
- lipoid 581.3
- lower nephron — see Nephrosis, tubular
- lupoid 710.0 [581.81]
- lupus 710.0 [581.81]
- malarial 084.9 [581.81]
- minimal change 581.3
- necrotizing — see Nephrosis, tubular
- osmotic (sucrose) 588.89
- polyarteritic 446.0 [581.81]
- radiation 581.9
- specified lesion or cause NEC 581.89
- syphilitic 095.4
- toxic — see Nephrosis, tubular
- tubular (acute) 584.5
  - due to a procedure 997.5
  - radiation 581.9

Nephrosonephritis hemorrhagic (endemic) 078.6

Nephrostomy status V44.6
- with complication 997.5

Nerve — see condition

Nerves 799.21

Nervous — see also condition 799.21
- breakdown 300.9
- heart 306.2
- stomach 306.4
- tension 799.21

Nervousness 799.21

Nesidioblastoma (M8150/0)
- pancreas 211.7
- specified site NEC — see Neoplasm, by site, benign
- unspecified site 211.7

Netherton's syndrome (ichthyosiform erythroderma) 757.1

Nettle rash 708.8

Nettleship's disease (urticaria pigmentosa) 757.33

Neumann's disease (pemphigus vegetans) 694.4

Neuralgia, neuralgic (acute) — see also Neuritis 729.2
- accessory (nerve) 352.4
- acoustic (nerve) 388.5
- ankle 355.8
- anterior crural 355.8
- anus 787.99
- arm 723.4
- auditory (nerve) 388.5
- axilla 353.0
- bladder 788.1
- brachial 723.4
- brain — see Disorder, nerve, cranial
- broad ligament 625.9
- cerebral — see Disorder, nerve, cranial
- ciliary 339.00
- cranial nerve (see also Disorder, nerve, cranial)
  - fifth or trigeminal (see also Neuralgia, trigeminal) 350.1
- ear 388.71
  - middle 352.1
- facial 351.8
- finger 354.9
- flank 355.8
- foot 355.8
- forearm 354.9
- Fothergill's (see also Neuralgia, trigeminal) 350.1

Neuralgia, neuralgic — see also Neuritis — continued
- Fothergill's (see also Neuralgia, trigeminal) — continued
  - postherpetic 053.12
- glossopharyngeal (nerve) 352.1
- groin 355.8
- hand 354.9
- heel 355.8
- Horton's 339.00
- Hunt's 053.11
- hypoglossal (nerve) 352.5
- iliac region 355.8
- infraorbital (see also Neuralgia, trigeminal) 350.1
- inguinal 355.8
- intercostal (nerve) 353.8
  - postherpetic 053.19
- jaw 352.1
- kidney 788.0
- knee 355.8
- loin 355.8
- malarial (see also Malaria) 084.6
- mastoid 385.89
- maxilla 352.1
- median thenar 354.1
- metatarsal 355.6
- middle ear 352.1
- migrainous 339.00
- Morton's 355.6
- nerve, cranial — see Disorder, nerve, cranial
- nose 352.0
- occipital 723.8
- olfactory (nerve) 352.0
- ophthalmic 377.30
  - postherpetic 053.19
- optic (nerve) 377.30
- penis 607.9
- perineum 355.8
- pleura 511.0
- postherpetic NEC 053.19
  - geniculate ganglion 053.11
  - ophthalmic 053.19
  - trifacial 053.12
  - trigeminal 053.12
- pubic region 355.8
- radial (nerve) 723.4
- rectum 787.99
- sacroiliac joint 724.3
- sciatic (nerve) 724.3
- scrotum 608.9
- seminal vesicle 608.9
- shoulder 354.9
- Sluder's 337.09
- specified nerve NEC — see Disorder, nerve
- spermatic cord 608.9
- sphenopalatine (ganglion) 337.09
- subscapular (nerve) 723.4
- suprascapular (nerve) 723.4
- testis 608.89
- thenar (median) 354.1
- thigh 355.8
- tongue 352.5
- trifacial (nerve) (see also Neuralgia, trigeminal) 350.1
- trigeminal (nerve) 350.1
  - postherpetic 053.12
- tympanic plexus 388.71
- ulnar (nerve) 723.4
- vagus (nerve) 352.3
- wrist 354.9
- writers' 300.89
  - organic 333.84

Neurapraxia — see Injury, nerve, by site

Neurasthenia 300.5
- cardiac 306.2
- gastric 306.4
- heart 306.2
- postfebrile 780.79
- postviral 780.79

Neurilemmoma (M9560/0) — see also Neoplasm, connective tissue, benign
- acoustic (nerve) 225.1
- malignant (M9560/3) (see also Neoplasm, connective tissue, malignant)
  - acoustic (nerve) 192.0

Neurilemmosarcoma (M9560/3) — see Neoplasm, connective tissue, malignant

Neurilemoma — see Neurilemmoma

Neurinoma (M9560/0) — see Neurilemmoma

Neurinomatosis (M9560/1) — see also Neoplasm, connective tissue, uncertain behavior
- centralis 759.5

Neuritis — see also Neuralgia 729.2
- abducens (nerve) 378.54
- accessory (nerve) 352.4
- acoustic (nerve) 388.5
  - syphilitic 094.86
- alcoholic 357.5
  - with psychosis 291.1
- amyloid, any site 277.39 [357.4]
- anterior crural 355.8
- arising during pregnancy 646.4 ☑
- arm 723.4
- ascending 355.2
- auditory (nerve) 388.5
- brachial (nerve) NEC 723.4
  - due to displacement, intervertebral disc 722.0
- cervical 723.4
- chest (wall) 353.8
- costal region 353.8
- cranial nerve (see also Disorder, nerve, cranial)
  - first or olfactory 352.0
  - second or optic 377.30
  - third or oculomotor 378.52
  - fourth or trochlear 378.53
  - fifth or trigeminal (see also Neuralgia, trigeminal) 350.1
  - sixth or abducens 378.54
  - seventh or facial 351.8
    - newborn 767.5
  - eighth or acoustic 388.5
  - ninth or glossopharyngeal 352.1
  - tenth or vagus 352.3
  - eleventh or accessory 352.4
  - twelfth or hypoglossal 352.5
- Déjérine-Sottas 356.0
- diabetic 250.6 ☑ [357.2]
  - due to secondary diabetes 249.6 ☑ [357.2]
- diphtheritic 032.89 [357.4]
- due to
  - beriberi 265.0 [357.4]
  - displacement, prolapse, protrusion, or rupture of intervertebral disc 722.2
    - cervical 722.0
    - lumbar, lumbosacral 722.10
    - thoracic, thoracolumbar 722.11
  - herniation, nucleus pulposus 722.2
    - cervical 722.0
    - lumbar, lumbosacral 722.10
    - thoracic, thoracolumbar 722.11
- endemic 265.0 [357.4]
- facial (nerve) 351.8
  - newborn 767.5
- general — see Polyneuropathy
- geniculate ganglion 351.1
  - due to herpes 053.11
- glossopharyngeal (nerve) 352.1
- gouty 274.89 [357.4]
- hypoglossal (nerve) 352.5
- ilioinguinal (nerve) 355.8
- in diseases classified elsewhere — see Polyneuropathy, in
- infectious (multiple) 357.0
- intercostal (nerve) 353.8
- interstitial hypertrophic progressive NEC 356.9
- leg 355.8
- lumbosacral NEC 724.4
- median (nerve) 354.1
  - thenar 354.1
- multiple (acute) (infective) 356.9
  - endemic 265.0 [357.4]
- multiplex endemica 265.0 [357.4]
- nerve root (see also Radiculitis) 729.2
- oculomotor (nerve) 378.52
- olfactory (nerve) 352.0

Neuritis — see also Neuralgia — continued
- optic (nerve) 377.30
  - in myelitis 341.0
  - meningococcal 036.81
- pelvic 355.8
- peripheral (nerve) (see also Neuropathy, peripheral)
  - complicating pregnancy or puerperium 646.4 ☑
  - specified nerve NEC — see Mononeuritis
- pneumogastric (nerve) 352.3
- postchickenpox 052.7
- postherpetic 053.7
- progressive hypertrophic interstitial NEC 356.9
- puerperal, postpartum 646.4 ☑
- radial (nerve) 723.4
- retrobulbar 377.32
  - syphilitic 094.85
- rheumatic (chronic) 729.2
- sacral region 355.8
- sciatic (nerve) 724.3
  - due to displacement of intervertebral disc 722.10
- serum 999.59
- specified nerve NEC — see Disorder, nerve
- spinal (nerve) 355.9
  - root (see also Radiculitis) 729.2
- subscapular (nerve) 723.4
- suprascapular (nerve) 723.4
- syphilitic 095.8
- thenar (median) 354.1
- thoracic NEC 724.4
- toxic NEC 357.7
- trochlear (nerve) 378.53
- ulnar (nerve) 723.4
- vagus (nerve) 352.3

Neuroangiomatosis, encephalofacial 759.6

Neuroastrocytoma (M9505/1) — see Neoplasm, by site, uncertain behavior

Neuro-avitaminosis 269.2

Neuroblastoma (M9500/3)
- olfactory (M9522/3) 160.0
- specified site — see Neoplasm, by site, malignant
- unspecified site 194.0

Neurochorioretinitis — see also Chorioretinitis 363.20

Neurocirculatory asthenia 306.2

Neurocytoma (M9506/0) — see Neoplasm, by site, benign

Neurodermatitis (circumscribed) (circumscripta) (local) 698.3
- atopic 691.8
- diffuse (Brocq) 691.8
- disseminated 691.8
- nodulosa 698.3

Neuroencephalomyelopathy, optic 341.0

Neuroendocrine tumor — see Tumor, neuroendocrine

Neuroepithelioma (M9503/3) — see also Neoplasm, by site, malignant
- olfactory (M9521/3) 160.0

Neurofibroma (M9540/0) — see also Neoplasm, connective tissue, benign
- melanotic (M9541/0) — see Neoplasm, connective tissue, benign
- multiple (M9540/1) 237.70
  - type 1 237.71
  - type 2 237.72
- plexiform (M9550/0) — see Neoplasm, connective tissue, benign

Neurofibromatosis (multiple) (M9540/1) 237.70
- acoustic 237.72
- malignant (M9540/3) — see Neoplasm, connective tissue, malignant
- Schwannomatosis 237.73
- specified type NEC 237.79
- type 1 237.71
- type 2 237.72
- von Recklinghausen's 237.71

Neurofibrosarcoma (M9540/3) — see Neoplasm, connective tissue, malignant

Neurogenic — see also condition

☑ Additional Digit Required — Refer to the Tabular List for Digit Selection   ▽ Subterms under main terms may continue to next column or page

212 — Volume 2   ▶◀ Revised Text   ● New Line   ▲ Revised Code   2013 ICD-9-CM

Neurogenic — *see also* condition —
   continued
  bladder (atonic) (automatic) (autonomic)
   (flaccid) (hypertonic) (hypotonic)
   (inertia) (infranuclear) (irritable)
   (motor) (nonreflex) (nuclear) (paralysis) (reflex) (sensory) (spastic)
   (supranuclear) (uninhibited) 596.54
    with cauda equina syndrome 344.61
  bowel 564.81
  heart 306.2
Neuroglioma (M9505/1) — *see* Neoplasm,
  by site, uncertain behavior
Neurolabyrinthitis (of Dix and Hallpike) 386.12
Neurolathyrism 988.2
Neuroleprosy 030.1
Neuroleptic malignant syndrome 333.92
Neurolipomatosis 272.8
Neuroma (M9570/0) — *see also* Neoplasm,
  connective tissue, benign
  acoustic (nerve) (M9560/0) 225.1
  amputation (traumatic) (*see also* Injury,
   nerve, by site)
    surgical complication (late) 997.61
  appendix 211.3
  auditory nerve 225.1
  digital 355.6
   toe 355.6
  interdigital (toe) 355.6
  intermetatarsal 355.6
  Morton's 355.6
  multiple 237.70
   type 1 237.71
   type 2 237.72
  nonneoplastic 355.9
   arm NEC 354.9
   leg NEC 355.8
   lower extremity NEC 355.8
   specified site NEC — *see* Mononeuritis,
    by site
   upper extremity NEC 354.9
  optic (nerve) 225.1
  plantar 355.6
  plexiform (M9550/0) — *see* Neoplasm,
   connective tissue, benign
  surgical (nonneoplastic) 355.9
   arm NEC 354.9
   leg NEC 355.8
   lower extremity NEC 355.8
   upper extremity NEC 354.9
  traumatic (*see also* Injury, nerve, by site)
   old — *see* Neuroma, nonneoplastic
Neuromyalgia 729.1
Neuromyasthenia (epidemic) 049.8
Neuromyelitis 341.8
  ascending 357.0
  optica 341.0
Neuromyopathy NEC 358.9
Neuromyositis 729.1
Neuronevus (M8725/0) — *see* Neoplasm, skin,
  benign
Neuronitis 357.0
  ascending (acute) 355.2
  vestibular 386.12
Neuroparalytic — *see* condition
Neuropathy, neuropathic — *see also* Disorder,
  nerve 355.9
  acute motor 357.82
  alcoholic 357.5
   with psychosis 291.1
  arm NEC 354.9
  ataxia and retinitis pigmentosa (NARP syndrome) 277.87
  autonomic (peripheral) — *see* Neuropathy,
   peripheral, autonomic
  axillary nerve 353.0
  brachial plexus 353.0
  cervical plexus 353.2
  chronic
   progressive segmentally demyelinating
    357.89
   relapsing demyelinating 357.89
  congenital sensory 356.2
  Déjérine-Sottas 356.0
  diabetic 250.6 ☑ *[357.2]*
   autonomic (peripheral) 250.6 ☑ *[337.1]*

Neuropathy, neuropathic — *see also* Disorder,
  nerve — *continued*
  diabetic — *continued*
   due to secondary diabetes
    249.6 ☑ *[357.2]*
    autonomic (peripheral)
     249.6 ☑ *[337.1]*
  entrapment 355.9
   iliohypogastric nerve 355.79
   ilioinguinal nerve 355.79
   lateral cutaneous nerve of thigh 355.1
   median nerve 354.0
   obturator nerve 355.79
   peroneal nerve 355.3
   posterior tibial nerve 355.5
   saphenous nerve 355.79
   ulnar nerve 354.2
  facial nerve 351.9
  hereditary 356.9
   peripheral 356.0
   sensory (radicular) 356.2
  hypertrophic
   Charcôt-Marie-Tooth 356.1
   Déjérine-Sottas 356.0
   interstitial 356.9
   Refsum 356.3
  intercostal nerve 354.8
  ischemic — *see* Disorder, nerve
  Jamaican (ginger) 357.7
  leg NEC 355.8
  lower extremity NEC 355.8
  lumbar plexus 353.1
  median nerve 354.1
  motor
   acute 357.82
  multiple (acute) (chronic) (*see also*
   Polyneuropathy) 356.9
  optic 377.39
   ischemic 377.41
   nutritional 377.33
   toxic 377.34
  peripheral (nerve) (*see also* Polyneuropathy)
   356.9
   arm NEC 354.9
   autonomic 337.9
    amyloid 277.39 *[337.1]*
    idiopathic 337.00
    in
     amyloidosis 277.39 *[337.1]*
     diabetes (mellitus)
      250.6 ☑ *[337.1]*
      due to secondary diabetes
       249.6 ☑ *[337.1]*
     diseases classified elsewhere
      337.1
     gout 274.89 *[337.1]*
     hyperthyroidism 242.9 ☑ *[337.1]*
   due to
    antitetanus serum 357.6
    arsenic 357.7
    drugs 357.6
    lead 357.7
    organophosphate compounds 357.7
    toxic agent NEC 357.7
   hereditary 356.0
   idiopathic 356.9
    progressive 356.4
    specified type NEC 356.8
   in diseases classified elsewhere — *see*
    Polyneuropathy, in
   leg NEC 355.8
   lower extremity NEC 355.8
   upper extremity NEC 354.9
  plantar nerves 355.6
  progressive
   hypertrophic interstitial 356.9
   inflammatory 357.89
  radicular NEC 729.2
   brachial 723.4
   cervical NEC 723.4
   hereditary sensory 356.2
   lumbar 724.4
   lumbosacral 724.4
   thoracic NEC 724.4
  sacral plexus 353.1
  sciatic 355.0

Neuropathy, neuropathic — *see also* Disorder,
  nerve — *continued*
  spinal nerve NEC 355.9
   root (*see also* Radiculitis) 729.2
  toxic 357.7
  trigeminal sensory 350.8
  ulnar nerve 354.2
  upper extremity NEC 354.9
  uremic 585.9 *[357.4]*
  vitamin B$_{12}$ 266.2 *[357.4]*
   with anemia (pernicious) 281.0 *[357.4]*
    due to dietary deficiency
     281.1 *[357.4]*
Neurophthisis — *see also* Disorder, nerve
  diabetic 250.6 ☑ *[357.2]*
   due to secondary diabetes
    249.6 ☑ *[357.2]*
  peripheral 356.9
Neuropraxia — *see* Injury, nerve
Neuroretinitis 363.05
  syphilitic 094.85
Neurosarcoma (M9540/3) — *see* Neoplasm,
  connective tissue, malignant
Neurosclerosis — *see* Disorder, nerve
Neurosis, neurotic 300.9
  accident 300.16
  anancastic, anankastic 300.3
  anxiety (state) 300.00
   generalized 300.02
   panic type 300.01
  asthenic 300.5
  bladder 306.53
  cardiac (reflex) 306.2
  cardiovascular 306.2
  climacteric, unspecified type 627.2
  colon 306.4
  compensation 300.16
  compulsive, compulsion 300.3
  conversion 300.11
  craft 300.89
  cutaneous 306.3
  depersonalization 300.6
  depressive (reaction) (type) 300.4
  endocrine 306.6
  environmental 300.89
  fatigue 300.5
  functional (*see also* Disorder, psychosomatic) 306.9
  gastric 306.4
  gastrointestinal 306.4
  genitourinary 306.50
  heart 306.2
  hypochondriacal 300.7
  hysterical 300.10
   conversion type 300.11
   dissociative type 300.15
  impulsive 300.3
  incoordination 306.0
   larynx 306.1
   vocal cord 306.1
  intestine 306.4
  larynx 306.1
   hysterical 300.11
   sensory 306.1
  menopause, unspecified type 627.2
  mixed NEC 300.89
  musculoskeletal 306.0
  obsessional 300.3
   phobia 300.3
  obsessive-compulsive 300.3
  occupational 300.89
  ocular 306.7
  oral (*see also* Disorder, fluency) 315.35
  organ (*see also* Disorder, psychosomatic)
   306.9
  pharynx 306.1
  phobic 300.20
  posttraumatic (acute) (situational) 309.81
   chronic 309.81
  psychasthenic (type) 300.89
  railroad 300.16
  rectum 306.4
  respiratory 306.1
  rumination 306.4
  senile 300.89
  sexual 302.70

Neurosis, neurotic — *continued*
  situational 300.89
  specified type NEC 300.89
  state 300.9
   with depersonalization episode 300.6
  stomach 306.4
  vasomotor 306.2
  visceral 306.4
  war 300.16
Neurospongioblastosis diffusa 759.5
Neurosyphilis (arrested) (early) (inactive) (late)
  (latent) (recurrent) 094.9
  with ataxia (cerebellar) (locomotor) (spastic)
   (spinal) 094.0
  acute meningitis 094.2
  aneurysm 094.89
  arachnoid (adhesive) 094.2
  arteritis (any artery) 094.89
  asymptomatic 094.3
  congenital 090.40
  dura (mater) 094.89
  general paresis 094.1
  gumma 094.9
  hemorrhagic 094.9
  juvenile (asymptomatic) (meningeal) 090.40
  leptomeninges (aseptic) 094.2
  meningeal 094.2
  meninges (adhesive) 094.2
  meningovascular (diffuse) 094.2
  optic atrophy 094.84
  parenchymatous (degenerative) 094.1
  paresis (*see also* Paresis, general) 094.1
  paretic (*see also* Paresis, general) 094.1
  relapse 094.9
  remission in (sustained) 094.9
  serological 094.3
  specified nature or site NEC 094.89
  tabes (dorsalis) 094.0
   juvenile 090.40
  tabetic 094.0
   juvenile 090.40
  taboparesis 094.1
   juvenile 090.40
  thrombosis 094.89
  vascular 094.89
Neurotic — *see also* Neurosis 300.9
  excoriation 698.4
   psychogenic 306.3
Neurotmesis — *see* Injury, nerve, by site
Neurotoxemia — *see* Toxemia
Neutro-occlusion 524.21
Neutropenia, neutropenic (idiopathic) (pernicious) (primary) 288.00
  chronic 288.09
   hypoplastic 288.09
  congenital (nontransient) 288.01
  cyclic 288.02
  drug induced 288.03
  due to infection 288.04
  fever 288.00
  genetic 288.01
  immune 288.09
  infantile 288.01
  malignant 288.09
  neonatal, transitory (isoimmune) (maternal
   transfer) 776.7
  periodic 288.02
  splenic 289.53
  splenomegaly 289.53
  toxic 288.09
Neutrophilia, hereditary giant 288.2
Nevocarcinoma (M8720/3) — *see* Melanoma
Nevus (M8720/0) — *see also* Neoplasm, skin,
  benign

> *Note* — *Except where otherwise indicat-
> ed, varieties of nevus in the list below
> that are followed by a morphology code
> number (M----/0) should be coded by
> site as for "Neoplasm, skin, benign."*

  acanthotic 702.8
  achromic (M8730/0)
  amelanotic (M8730/0)
  anemic, anemicus 709.09
  angiomatous (M9120/0) (*see also* Hemangioma) 228.00
  araneus 448.1

☑ **Additional Digit Required** — Refer to the Tabular List for Digit Selection   🔺 **Subterms under main terms may continue to next column or page**

2013 ICD-9-CM   ▶◀ **Revised Text**   ● **New Line**   ▲ **Revised Code**   **Volume 2 — 213**

Nevus — see also Neoplasm, skin, benign — continued
avasculosus 709.09
balloon cell (M8722/0)
bathing trunk (M8761/1) 238.2
blue (M8780/0)
cellular (M8790/0)
giant (M8790/0)
Jadassohn's (M8780/0)
malignant (M8780/3) — see Melanoma
capillary (M9131/0) (see also Hemangioma) 228.00
cavernous (M9121/0) (see also Hemangioma) 228.00
cellular (M8720/0)
blue (M8790/0)
comedonicus 757.33
compound (M8760/0)
conjunctiva (M8720/0) 224.3
dermal (M8750/0)
and epidermal (M8760/0)
epithelioid cell (and spindle cell) (M8770/0)
flammeus 757.32
osteohypertrophic 759.89
hairy (M8720/0)
halo (M8723/0)
hemangiomatous (M9120/0) (see also Hemangioma) 228.00
intradermal (M8750/0)
intraepidermal (M8740/0)
involuting (M8724/0)
Jadassohn's (blue) (M8780/0)
junction, junctional (M8740/0)
malignant melanoma in (M8740/3) — see Melanoma
juvenile (M8770/0)
lymphatic (M9170/0) 228.1
magnocellular (M8726/0)
specified site — see Neoplasm, by site, benign
unspecified site 224.0
malignant (M8720/3) — see Melanoma
meaning hemangioma (M9120/0) (see also Hemangioma) 228.00
melanotic (pigmented) (M8720/0)
multiplex 759.5
nonneoplastic 448.1
nonpigmented (M8730/0)
nonvascular (M8720/0)
oral mucosa, white sponge 750.26
osteohypertrophic, flammeus 759.89
papillaris (M8720/0)
papillomatosus (M8720/0)
pigmented (M8720/0)
giant (M8761/1) (see also Neoplasm, skin, uncertain behavior)
malignant melanoma in (M8761/3) — see Melanoma
systematicus 757.33
pilosus (M8720/0)
port wine 757.32
sanguineous 757.32
sebaceous (senile) 702.8
senile 448.1
spider 448.1
spindle cell (and epithelioid cell) (M8770/0)
stellar 448.1
strawberry 757.32
syringocystadenomatous papilliferous (M8406/0)
unius lateris 757.33
Unna's 757.32
vascular 757.32
verrucous 757.33
white sponge (oral mucosa) 750.26
Newborn (infant) (liveborn)
abstinence syndrome 779.5
affected by
amniocentesis 760.61
maternal abuse of drugs (gestational) (via placenta) (via breast milk) (see also Noxious, substances transmitted through placenta or breast milk (affecting fetus or newborn)) 760.70
methamphetamine(s) 760.72

Newborn — continued
affected by — continued
procedure
amniocentesis 760.61
in utero NEC 760.62
surgical on mother
during pregnancy NEC 760.63
previous not associated with pregnancy 760.64
apnea 770.81
obstructive 770.82
specified NEC 770.82
breast buds 779.89
cardiomyopathy 425.4
congenital 425.3
convulsion 779.0
electrolyte imbalance NEC (transitory) 775.5
fever (environmentally-induced) 778.4
gestation
24 completed weeks 765.22
25-26 completed weeks 765.23
27-28 completed weeks 765.24
29-30 completed weeks 765.25
31-32 completed weeks 765.26
33-34 completed weeks 765.27
35-36 completed weeks 765.28
37 or more completed weeks 765.29
less than 24 completed weeks 765.21
unspecified completed weeks 765.20
infection 771.89
candida 771.7
mastitis 771.5
specified NEC 771.89
urinary tract 771.82
mastitis 771.5
multiple NEC
born in hospital (without mention of cesarean delivery or section) V37.00
with cesarean delivery or section V37.01
born outside hospital
hospitalized V37.1
not hospitalized V37.2
mates all liveborn
born in hospital (without mention of cesarean delivery or section) V34.00
with cesarean delivery or section V34.01
born outside hospital
hospitalized V34.1
not hospitalized V34.2
mates all stillborn
born in hospital (without mention of cesarean delivery or section) V35.00
with cesarean delivery or section V35.01
born outside hospital
hospitalized V35.1
not hospitalized V35.2
mates liveborn and stillborn
born in hospital (without mention of cesarean delivery or section) V36.00
with cesarean delivery or section V36.01
born outside hospital
hospitalized V36.1
not hospitalized V36.2
omphalitis 771.4
seizure 779.0
sepsis 771.81
single
born in hospital (without mention of cesarean delivery or section) V30.00
with cesarean delivery or section V30.01
born outside hospital
hospitalized V30.1
not hospitalized V30.2
specified condition NEC 779.89

Newborn — continued
twin NEC
born in hospital (without mention of cesarean delivery or section) V33.00
with cesarean delivery or section V33.01
born outside hospital
hospitalized V33.1
not hospitalized V33.2
mate liveborn
born in hospital V31.0 ☑
born outside hospital
hospitalized V31.1
not hospitalized V31.2
mate stillborn
born in hospital V32.0 ☑
born outside hospital
hospitalized V32.1
not hospitalized V32.2
unspecified as to single or multiple birth
born in hospital (without mention of cesarean delivery or section) V39.00
with cesarean delivery or section V39.01
born outside hospital
hospitalized V39.1
not hospitalized V39.2
weight check V20.32
Newcastle's conjunctivitis or disease 077.8
Nezelof's syndrome (pure alymphocytosis) 279.13
Niacin (amide) **deficiency** 265.2
Nicolas-Durand-Favre disease (climatic bubo) 099.1
Nicolas-Favre disease (climatic bubo) 099.1
Nicotinic acid (amide) **deficiency** 265.2
Niemann-Pick disease (lipid histiocytosis) (splenomegaly) 272.7
Night
blindness (see also Blindness, night) 368.60
congenital 368.61
vitamin A deficiency 264.5
cramps 729.82
sweats 780.8
terrors, child 307.46
Nightmare 307.47
REM-sleep type 307.47
Nipple — see condition
Nisbet's chancre 099.0
Nishimoto (-Takeuchi) disease 437.5
Nitritoid crisis or reaction — see Crisis, nitritoid
Nitrogen retention, extrarenal 788.99
Nitrosohemoglobinemia 289.89
Njovera 104.0
No
diagnosis 799.9
disease (found) V71.9
room at the inn V65.0
Nocardiasis — see Nocardiosis
Nocardiosis 039.9
with pneumonia 039.1
lung 039.1
specified type NEC 039.8
Nocturia 788.43
psychogenic 306.53
Nocturnal — see also condition
dyspnea (paroxysmal) 786.09
emissions 608.89
enuresis 788.36
psychogenic 307.6
frequency (micturition) 788.43
psychogenic 306.53
Nodal rhythm disorder 427.89
Nodding of head 781.0
Node(s) — see also Nodule(s)
Heberden's 715.04
larynx 478.79
lymph — see condition
milkers' 051.1
Osler's 421.0
rheumatic 729.89
Schmorl's 722.30
lumbar, lumbosacral 722.32

Node(s) — see also Nodule(s) — continued
Schmorl's — continued
specified region NEC 722.39
thoracic, thoracolumbar 722.31
singers' 478.5
skin NEC 782.2
tuberculous — see Tuberculosis, lymph gland
vocal cords 478.5
Nodosities, Haygarth's 715.04
Nodule(s), nodular
actinomycotic (see also Actinomycosis) 039.9
arthritic — see Arthritis, nodosa
breast 793.89
cutaneous 782.2
Haygarth's 715.04
inflammatory — see Inflammation
juxta-articular 102.7
syphilitic 095.7
yaws 102.7
larynx 478.79
lung
emphysematous 492.8
solitary 793.11
milkers' 051.1
prostate 600.10
with
urinary
obstruction 600.11
retention 600.11
pulmonary, solitary (subsegmental branch of the bronchial tree) 793.11
multiple 793.19
retrocardiac 785.9
rheumatic 729.89
rheumatoid — see Arthritis, rheumatoid
scrotum (inflammatory) 608.4
singers' 478.5
skin NEC 782.2
solitary, lung 793.11
emphysematous 492.8
subcutaneous 782.2
thyroid (gland) (nontoxic) (uninodular) 241.0
with
hyperthyroidism 242.1 ☑
thyrotoxicosis 242.1 ☑
toxic or with hyperthyroidism 242.1 ☑
vocal cords 478.5
Noma (gangrenous) (hospital) (infective) 528.1
auricle (see also Gangrene) 785.4
mouth 528.1
pudendi (see also Vulvitis) 616.10
vulvae (see also Vulvitis) 616.10
Nomadism V60.0
Non-adherence
artificial skin graft 996.55
decellularized allodermis graft 996.55
Non-autoimmune hemolytic anemia NEC 283.10
Nonclosure — see also Imperfect, closure
ductus
arteriosus 747.0
Botalli 747.0
Eustachian valve 746.89
foramen
Botalli 745.5
ovale 745.5
Noncompliance with medical treatment V15.81
renal dialysis V45.12
Nondescent (congenital) — see also Malposition, congenital
cecum 751.4
colon 751.4
testis 752.51
Nondevelopment
brain 742.1
specified part 742.2
heart 746.89
organ or site, congenital NEC — see Hypoplasia
Nonengagement
head NEC 652.5 ☑
in labor 660.1 ☑
affecting fetus or newborn 763.1

Nonexanthematous tick fever 066.1
Nonexpansion, lung (newborn) NEC 770.4
Nonfunctioning
    cystic duct (*see also* Disease, gallbladder)
        575.8
    gallbladder (*see also* Disease, gallbladder)
        575.8
    kidney (*see also* Disease, renal) 593.9
    labyrinth 386.58
Nonhealing
    stump (surgical) 997.69
    wound, surgical 998.83
Nonimplantation of ovum, causing infertili-
    ty 628.3
Noninsufflation, fallopian tube 628.2
Nonne-Milroy-Meige syndrome (chronic
    hereditary edema) 757.0
Nonovulation 628.0
Nonpatent fallopian tube 628.2
Nonpneumatization, lung NEC 770.4
Nonreflex bladder 596.54
    with cauda equina 344.61
Nonretention of food — *see* Vomiting
Nonrotation — *see* Malrotation
Nonsecretion, urine — *see also* Anuria 788.5
    newborn 753.3
Nonunion
    fracture 733.82
    organ or site, congenital NEC — *see* Imper-
        fect, closure
    symphysis pubis, congenital 755.69
    top sacrum, congenital 756.19
Nonviability 765.0 ☑
Nonvisualization, gallbladder 793.3
Nonvitalized tooth 522.9
Non-working side interference 524.56
Normal
    delivery — *see* category 650
    menses V65.5
    state (feared complaint unfounded) V65.5
Normoblastosis 289.89

Normocytic anemia (infectional) 285.9
    due to blood loss (chronic) 280.0
        acute 285.1
Norrie's disease (congenital) (progressive
    oculoacousticocerebral degeneration)
    743.8
North American blastomycosis 116.0
Norwegian itch 133.0
Nosebleed 784.7
Nose, nasal — *see* condition
Nosomania 298.9
Nosophobia 300.29
Nostalgia 309.89
Notched lip, congenital — *see also* Cleft, lip
    749.10
Notching nose, congenital (tip) 748.1
Notch of iris 743.46
Nothnagel's
    syndrome 378.52
    vasomotor acroparesthesia 443.89
Novy's relapsing fever (American) 087.1
Noxious
    foodstuffs, poisoning by
        fish 988.0
        fungi 988.1
        mushrooms 988.1
        plants (food) 988.2
        shellfish 988.0
        specified type NEC 988.8
        toadstool 988.1
    substances transmitted through placenta
        or breast milk (affecting fetus or
        newborn) 760.70
        acetretin 760.78
        alcohol 760.71
        aminopterin 760.78
        antiandrogens 760.79
        anticonvulsant 760.77
        antifungal 760.74
        anti-infective agents 760.74
        antimetabolic 760.78

Noxious — *continued*
    substances transmitted through placenta or
        breast milk — *continued*
        atorvastatin 760.78
        carbamazepine 760.77
        cocaine 760.75
        "crack" 760.75
        diethylstilbestrol (DES) 760.76
        divalproex sodium 760.77
        endocrine disrupting chemicals 760.79
        estrogens 760.79
        etretinate 760.78
        fluconazole 760.74
        fluvastatin 760.78
        hallucinogenic agents NEC 760.73
        hormones 760.79
        lithium 760.79
        lovastatin 760.78
        medicinal agents NEC 760.79
        methotrexate 760.78
        misoprostil 760.79
        narcotics 760.72
        obstetric anesthetic or analgesic 763.5
        phenobarbital 760.77
        phenytoin 760.77
        pravastatin 760.78
        progestins 760.79
        retinoic acid 760.78
        simvastatin 760.78
        solvents 760.79
        specified agent NEC 760.79
        statins 760.78
        suspected, affecting management of
            pregnancy 655.5 ☑
        tetracycline 760.74
        thalidomide 760.79
        trimethadione 760.77
        valproate 760.77
        valproic acid 760.77
        vitamin A 760.78
NPDH (new persistent daily headache) 339.42

Nuchal hitch (arm) 652.8 ☑
Nucleus pulposus — *see* condition
Numbness 782.0
Nuns' knee 727.2
Nursemaid's
    elbow 832.2
    shoulder 831.0 ☑
Nutmeg liver 573.8
Nutrition, deficient or insufficient (particular
    kind of food) 269.9
    due to
        insufficient food 994.2
        lack of
            care (child) (infant) 995.52
                adult 995.84
            food 994.2
Nyctalopia — *see also* Blindness, night 368.60
    vitamin A deficiency 264.5
Nycturia 788.43
    psychogenic 306.53
Nymphomania 302.89
Nystagmus 379.50
    associated with vestibular system disorders
        379.54
    benign paroxysmal positional 386.11
    central positional 386.2
    congenital 379.51
    deprivation 379.53
    dissociated 379.55
    latent 379.52
    miners' 300.89
    positional
        benign paroxysmal 386.11
        central 386.2
    specified NEC 379.56
    vestibular 379.54
    visual deprivation 379.53

☑ **Additional Digit Required** — Refer to the Tabular List for Digit Selection   ▽ **Subterms under main terms may continue to next column or page**

2013 ICD-9-CM   ▶◀ **Revised Text**   ● **New Line**   ▲ **Revised Code**   **Volume 2 — 215**

O

Oasthouse urine disease 270.2
Obermeyer's relapsing fever (European) 087.0
Obesity (constitutional) (exogenous) (familial) (nutritional) (simple) 278.00
  adrenal 255.8
  complicating pregnancy, childbirth, or puerperium 649.1 ☑
  due to hyperalimentation 278.00
  endocrine NEC 259.9
  endogenous 259.9
  Fröhlich's (adiposogenital dystrophy) 253.8
  glandular NEC 259.9
  hypothyroid (see also Hypothyroidism) 244.9
  hypoventilation syndrome 278.03
  morbid 278.01
  of pregnancy 649.1 ☑
  pituitary 253.8
  severe 278.01
  thyroid (see also Hypothyroidism) 244.9
Oblique — see also condition
  lie before labor, affecting fetus or newborn 761.7
Obliquity, pelvis 738.6
Obliteration
  abdominal aorta 446.7
  appendix (lumen) 543.9
  artery 447.1
  ascending aorta 446.7
  bile ducts 576.8
    with calculus, choledocholithiasis, or stones — see Choledocholithiasis
    congenital 751.61
      jaundice from 751.61 [774.5]
  common duct 576.8
    with calculus, choledocholithiasis, or stones — see Choledocholithiasis
    congenital 751.61
  cystic duct 575.8
    with calculus, choledocholithiasis, or stones — see Choledocholithiasis
  disease, arteriolar 447.1
  endometrium 621.8
  eye, anterior chamber 360.34
  fallopian tube 628.2
  lymphatic vessel 457.1
    postmastectomy 457.0
  organ or site, congenital NEC — see Atresia
  placental blood vessels — see Placenta, abnormal
  supra-aortic branches 446.7
  ureter 593.89
  urethra 599.84
  vein 459.9
  vestibule (oral) 525.8
Observation (for) V71.9
  without need for further medical care V71.9
  accident NEC V71.4
    at work V71.3
  criminal assault V71.6
  deleterious agent ingestion V71.89
  disease V71.9
    cardiovascular V71.7
    heart V71.7
    mental V71.09
    specified condition NEC V71.89
  foreign body ingestion V71.89
  growth and development variations V21.8
  injuries (accidental) V71.4
    inflicted NEC V71.6
      during alleged rape or seduction V71.5
  malignant neoplasm, suspected V71.1
  postpartum
    immediately after delivery V24.0
    routine follow-up V24.2
  pregnancy
    high-risk V23.9
      inconclusive fetal viability V23.87
      specified problem NEC V23.89
    normal (without complication) V22.1
      with nonobstetric complication V22.2
      first V22.0
  rape or seduction, alleged V71.5
    injury during V71.5

Observation — continued
  suicide attempt, alleged V71.89
  suspected (undiagnosed) (unproven)
    abuse V71.81
    cardiovascular disease V71.7
    child or wife battering victim V71.6
    concussion (cerebral) V71.6
    condition NEC V71.89
      infant — see Observation, suspected, condition, newborn
      maternal and fetal
        amniotic cavity and membrane problem V89.01
        cervical shortening V89.05
        fetal anomaly V89.03
        fetal growth problem V89.04
        oligohydramnios V89.01
        other specified problem NEC V89.09
        placental problem V89.02
        polyhydramnios V89.01
      newborn V29.9
        cardiovascular disease V29.8
        congenital anomaly V29.8
        genetic V29.3
        infectious V29.0
        ingestion foreign object V29.8
        injury V29.8
        metabolic V29.3
        neoplasm V29.8
        neurological V29.1
        poison, poisoning V29.8
        respiratory V29.2
        specified NEC V29.8
    exposure
      anthrax V71.82
      biologic agent NEC V71.83
      SARS V71.83
    infectious disease not requiring isolation V71.89
    malignant neoplasm V71.1
    mental disorder V71.09
    neglect V71.81
    neoplasm
      benign V71.89
      malignant V71.1
    specified condition NEC V71.89
    tuberculosis V71.2
  tuberculosis, suspected V71.2
Obsession, obsessional 300.3
  ideas and mental images 300.3
  impulses 300.3
  neurosis 300.3
  phobia 300.3
  psychasthenia 300.3
  ruminations 300.3
  state 300.3
  syndrome 300.3
Obsessive-compulsive 300.3
  neurosis 300.3
  personality 301.4
  reaction 300.3
Obstetrical trauma NEC (complicating delivery) 665.9 ☑
  with
    abortion — see Abortion, by type, with damage to pelvic organs
    ectopic pregnancy (see also categories 633.0–633.9) 639.2
    molar pregnancy (see also categories 630–632) 639.2
  affecting fetus or newborn 763.89
  following
    abortion 639.2
    ectopic or molar pregnancy 639.2
Obstipation — see also Constipation 564.00
  psychogenic 306.4
Obstruction, obstructed, obstructive
  airway NEC 519.8
    with
      allergic alveolitis NEC 495.9
      asthma NEC (see also Asthma) 493.9 ☑
      bronchiectasis 494.0
        with acute exacerbation 494.1

Obstruction, obstructed, obstructive — continued
  airway — continued
    with — continued
      bronchitis (chronic) (see also Bronchitis, with, obstruction) 491.20
      emphysema NEC 492.8
    chronic 496
      with
        allergic alveolitis NEC 495.5
        asthma NEC (see also Asthma) 493.2 ☑
        bronchiectasis 494.0
          with acute exacerbation 494.1
        bronchitis (chronic) (see also Bronchitis, with, obstruction) 491.20
        emphysema NEC 492.8
    due to
      bronchospasm 519.11
      foreign body 934.9
      inhalation of fumes or vapors 506.9
      laryngospasm 478.75
  alimentary canal (see also Obstruction, intestine) 560.9
  ampulla of Vater 576.2
    with calculus, cholelithiasis, or stones — see Choledocholithiasis
  aortic (heart) (valve) (see also Stenosis, aortic) 424.1
    rheumatic (see also Stenosis, aortic, rheumatic) 395.0
  aortoiliac 444.09
  aqueduct of Sylvius 331.4
    congenital 742.3
      with spina bifida (see also Spina bifida) 741.0 ☑
  Arnold-Chiari (see also Spina bifida) 741.0 ☑
  artery (see also Embolism, artery) 444.9
    basilar (complete) (partial) (see also Occlusion, artery, basilar) 433.0 ☑
    carotid (complete) (partial) (see also Occlusion, artery, carotid) 433.1 ☑
    precerebral — see Occlusion, artery, precerebral NEC
    retinal (central) (see also Occlusion, retina) 362.30
    vertebral (complete) (partial) (see also Occlusion, artery, vertebral) 433.2 ☑
  asthma (chronic) (with obstructive pulmonary disease) 493.2 ☑
  band (intestinal) 560.81
  bile duct or passage (see also Obstruction, biliary) 576.2
    congenital 751.61
      jaundice from 751.61 [774.5]
  biliary (duct) (tract) 576.2
    with calculus 574.51
      with cholecystitis (chronic) 574.41
        acute 574.31
    congenital 751.61
      jaundice from 751.61 [774.5]
    gallbladder 575.2
      with calculus 574.21
        with cholecystitis (chronic) 574.11
          acute 574.01
  bladder neck (acquired) 596.0
    congenital 753.6
  bowel (see also Obstruction, intestine) 560.9
  bronchus 519.19
  canal, ear (see also Stricture, ear canal, acquired) 380.50
  cardia 537.89
  caval veins (inferior) (superior) 459.2
  cecum (see also Obstruction, intestine) 560.9
  circulatory 459.9
  colon (see also Obstruction, intestine) 560.9
    sympathicotonic 560.89
  common duct (see also Obstruction, biliary) 576.2
    congenital 751.61
  coronary (artery) (heart) (see also Arteriosclerosis, coronary)
    acute (see also Infarct, myocardium) 410.9 ☑

Obstruction, obstructed, obstructive — continued
  coronary (see also Arteriosclerosis, coronary) — continued
    acute (see also Infarct, myocardium) — continued
      without myocardial infarction 411.81
  cystic duct (see also Obstruction, gallbladder) 575.2
    congenital 751.61
  device, implant, or graft — see Complications, due to (presence of) any device, implant, or graft classified to 996.0–996.5 NEC
  due to foreign body accidentally left in operation wound 998.4
  duodenum 537.3
    congenital 751.1
    due to
      compression NEC 537.3
      cyst 537.3
      intrinsic lesion or disease NEC 537.3
      scarring 537.3
      torsion 537.3
      ulcer 532.91
      volvulus 537.3
  ejaculatory duct 608.89
  endocardium 424.90
    arteriosclerotic 424.99
    specified cause, except rheumatic 424.99
  esophagus 530.3
  eustachian tube (complete) (partial) 381.60
    cartilaginous
      extrinsic 381.63
      intrinsic 381.62
    due to
      cholesteatoma 381.61
      osseous lesion NEC 381.61
      polyp 381.61
    osseous 381.61
  fallopian tube (bilateral) 628.2
  fecal 560.32
    with hernia (see also Hernia, by site, with obstruction)
      gangrenous — see Hernia, by site, with gangrene
  foramen of Monro (congenital) 742.3
    with spina bifida (see also Spina bifida) 741.0 ☑
  foreign body — see Foreign body
  gallbladder 575.2
    with calculus, cholelithiasis, or stones 574.21
      with cholecystitis (chronic) 574.11
        acute 574.01
    congenital 751.69
      jaundice from 751.69 [774.5]
  gastric outlet 537.0
  gastrointestinal (see also Obstruction, intestine) 560.9
  glottis 478.79
  hepatic 573.8
    duct (see also Obstruction, biliary) 576.2
      congenital 751.61
    icterus (see also Obstruction, biliary) 576.8
      congenital 751.61
  ileocecal coil (see also Obstruction, intestine) 560.9
  ileum (see also Obstruction, intestine) 560.9
  iliofemoral (artery) 444.81
  internal anastomosis — see Complications, mechanical, graft
  intestine (mechanical) (neurogenic) (paroxysmal) (postinfectional) (reflex) 560.9
    with
      adhesions (intestinal) (peritoneal) 560.81
      hernia (see also Hernia, by site, with obstruction)
        gangrenous — see Hernia, by site, with gangrene
    adynamic (see also Ileus) 560.1
    by gallstone 560.31
    congenital or infantile (small) 751.1
      large 751.2

☑ Additional Digit Required — Refer to the Tabular List for Digit Selection

🖝 Subterms under main terms may continue to next column or page

2013 ICD-9-CM

▶◀ Revised Text   ● New Line   ▲ Revised Code

Volume 2 — 217

Oasthouse urine disease — Obstruction, obstructed, obstructive

Obstruction, obstructed, obstructive — *continued*
- intestine — *continued*
  - due to
    - Ascaris lumbricoides 127.0
    - mural thickening 560.89
    - procedure 997.49
      - involving urinary tract 997.5
  - impaction 560.32
  - infantile — *see* Obstruction, intestine, congenital
  - newborn
    - due to
      - fecaliths 777.1
      - inspissated milk 777.2
      - meconium (plug) 777.1
        - in mucoviscidosis 277.01
      - transitory 777.4
  - specified cause NEC 560.89
  - transitory, newborn 777.4
  - volvulus 560.2
- intracardiac ball valve prosthesis 996.02
- jaundice (*see also* Obstruction, biliary) 576.8
  - congenital 751.61
- jejunum (*see also* Obstruction, intestine) 560.9
- kidney 593.89
- labor 660.9 ☑
  - affecting fetus or newborn 763.1
  - by
    - bony pelvis (conditions classifiable to 653.0–653.9) 660.1 ☑
    - deep transverse arrest 660.3 ☑
    - impacted shoulder 660.4 ☑
    - locked twins 660.5 ☑
    - malposition (fetus) (conditions classifiable to 652.0–652.9) 660.0 ☑
      - head during labor 660.3 ☑
    - persistent occipitoposterior position 660.3 ☑
    - soft tissue, pelvic (conditions classifiable to 654.0–654.9) 660.2 ☑
- lacrimal
  - canaliculi 375.53
    - congenital 743.65
  - punctum 375.52
  - sac 375.54
- lacrimonasal duct 375.56
  - congenital 743.65
  - neonatal 375.55
- lacteal, with steatorrhea 579.2
- laryngitis (*see also* Laryngitis) 464.01
- larynx 478.79
  - congenital 748.3
- liver 573.8
  - cirrhotic (*see also* Cirrhosis, liver) 571.5
- lung 518.89
  - with
    - asthma — *see* Asthma
    - bronchitis (chronic) 491.20
    - emphysema NEC 492.8
  - airway, chronic 496
  - chronic NEC 496
    - with
      - asthma (chronic) (obstructive) 493.2 ☑
  - disease, chronic 496
    - with
      - asthma (chronic) (obstructive) 493.2 ☑
  - emphysematous 492.8
- lymphatic 457.1
- meconium
  - fetus or newborn 777.1
    - in mucoviscidosis 277.01
  - newborn due to fecaliths 777.1
- mediastinum 519.3
- mitral (rheumatic) — *see* Stenosis, mitral
- nasal 478.19
  - duct 375.56
    - neonatal 375.55
  - sinus — *see* Sinusitis
- nasolacrimal duct 375.56
  - congenital 743.65
  - neonatal 375.55

Obstruction, obstructed, obstructive — *continued*
- nasopharynx 478.29
- nose 478.19
- organ or site, congenital NEC — *see* Atresia
- pancreatic duct 577.8
- parotid gland 527.8
- pelviureteral junction (*see also* Obstruction, ureter) 593.4
- pharynx 478.29
- portal (circulation) (vein) 452
- prostate 600.90
  - with
    - other lower urinary tract symptoms (LUTS) 600.91
  - urinary
    - obstruction 600.91
    - retention 600.91
  - valve (urinary) 596.0
- pulmonary
  - valve (heart) (*see also* Endocarditis, pulmonary) 424.3
  - vein, isolated 747.49
- pyemic — *see* Septicemia
- pylorus (acquired) 537.0
  - congenital 750.5
  - infantile 750.5
- rectosigmoid (*see also* Obstruction, intestine) 560.9
- rectum 569.49
- renal 593.89
- respiratory 519.8
  - chronic 496
- retinal (artery) (vein) (central) (*see also* Occlusion, retina) 362.30
- salivary duct (any) 527.8
  - with calculus 527.5
- sigmoid (*see also* Obstruction, intestine) 560.9
- sinus (accessory) (nasal) (*see also* Sinusitis) 473.9
- Stensen's duct 527.8
- stomach 537.89
  - acute 536.1
  - congenital 750.7
- submaxillary gland 527.8
  - with calculus 527.5
- thoracic duct 457.1
- thrombotic — *see* Thrombosis
- tooth eruption 520.6
- trachea 519.19
- tracheostomy airway 519.09
- tricuspid — *see* Endocarditis, tricuspid
- upper respiratory, congenital 748.8
- ureter (functional) 593.4
  - congenital 753.20
  - due to calculus 592.1
- ureteropelvic junction, congenital 753.21
- ureterovesical junction, congenital 753.22
- urethra 599.60
  - congenital 753.6
- urinary (moderate) 599.60
  - organ or tract (lower) 599.60
    - due to
      - benign prostatic hypertrophy (BPH) - see category 600
    - specified NEC 599.69
    - due to
      - benign prostatic hypertrophy (BPH) — see category 600
  - prostatic valve 596.0
- uropathy 599.60
- uterus 621.8
- vagina 623.2
- valvular — *see* Endocarditis
- vascular graft or shunt 996.1
  - atherosclerosis — *see* Arteriosclerosis, coronary
  - embolism 996.74
  - occlusion NEC 996.74
  - thrombus 996.74
- vein, venous 459.2
  - caval (inferior) (superior) 459.2
  - thrombotic — *see* Thrombosis
- vena cava (inferior) (superior) 459.2

Obstruction, obstructed, obstructive — *continued*
- ventricular shunt 996.2
- vesical 596.0
- vesicourethral orifice 596.0
- vessel NEC 459.9

Obturator — *see* condition

Occlusal
- plane deviation 524.76
- wear, teeth 521.10

Occlusion
- anus 569.49
  - congenital 751.2
  - infantile 751.2
- aortoiliac (chronic) 444.09
- aqueduct of Sylvius 331.4
  - congenital 742.3
    - with spina bifida (*see also* Spina bifida) 741.0 ☑
- arteries of extremities, lower 444.22
  - without thrombus or embolus (*see also* Arteriosclerosis, extremities) 440.20
  - due to stricture or stenosis 447.1
  - upper 444.21
    - without thrombus or embolus (*see also* Arteriosclerosis, extremities) 440.20
    - due to stricture or stenosis 447.1
- artery NEC (*see also* Embolism, artery) 444.9
  - auditory, internal 433.8 ☑
  - basilar 433.0 ☑
    - with other precerebral artery 433.3 ☑
    - bilateral 433.3 ☑
  - brain or cerebral (*see also* Infarct, brain) 434.9 ☑
  - carotid 433.1 ☑
    - with other precerebral artery 433.3 ☑
    - bilateral 433.3 ☑
  - cerebellar (anterior inferior) (posterior inferior) (superior) 433.8 ☑
  - cerebral (*see also* Infarct, brain) 434.9 ☑
  - choroidal (anterior) 433.8 ☑
  - chronic total
    - coronary 414.2
    - extremity(ies) 440.4
  - communicating posterior 433.8 ☑
  - complete
    - coronary 414.2
    - extremity(ies) 440.4
  - coronary (thrombotic) (*see also* Infarct, myocardium) 410.9 ☑
    - acute 410.9 ☑
      - without myocardial infarction 411.81
    - chronic total 414.2
    - complete 414.2
    - healed or old 412
    - total 414.2
  - extremity(ies)
    - chronic total 440.4
    - complete 440.4
    - total 440.4
  - hypophyseal 433.8 ☑
  - iliac (artery) 444.81
  - mesenteric (embolic) (thrombotic) (with gangrene) 557.0
  - pontine 433.8 ☑
  - precerebral NEC 433.9 ☑
    - late effect — *see* Late effect(s) (of) cerebrovascular disease
    - multiple or bilateral 433.3 ☑
    - puerperal, postpartum, childbirth 674.0 ☑
    - specified NEC 433.8 ☑
  - renal 593.81
  - retinal — *see* Occlusion, retina, artery
  - spinal 433.8 ☑
  - vertebral 433.2 ☑
    - with other precerebral artery 433.3 ☑
    - bilateral 433.3 ☑

Occlusion — *continued*
- basilar (artery) — *see* Occlusion, artery, basilar
- bile duct (any) (*see also* Obstruction, biliary) 576.2
- bowel (*see also* Obstruction, intestine) 560.9
- brain (artery) (vascular) (*see also* Infarct, brain) 434.9 ☑
- breast (duct) 611.89
- carotid (artery) (common) (internal) — *see* Occlusion, artery, carotid
- cerebellar (anterior inferior) (artery) (posterior inferior) (superior) 433.8 ☑
- cerebral (artery) (*see also* Infarct, brain) 434.9 ☑
- cerebrovascular (*see also* Infarct, brain) 434.9 ☑
  - diffuse 437.0
- cervical canal (*see also* Stricture, cervix) 622.4
  - by falciparum malaria 084.0
- cervix (uteri) (*see also* Stricture, cervix) 622.4
- choanal 748.0
- choroidal (artery) 433.8 ☑
- colon (*see also* Obstruction, intestine) 560.9
- communicating posterior artery 433.8 ☑
- coronary (artery) (thrombotic) (*see also* Infarct, myocardium) 410.9 ☑
  - without myocardial infarction 411.81
  - acute 410.9 ☑
    - without myocardial infarction 411.81
  - healed or old 412
- cystic duct (*see also* Obstruction, gallbladder) 575.2
  - congenital 751.69
- disto
  - division I 524.22
  - division II 524.22
- embolic — *see* Embolism
- fallopian tube 628.2
  - congenital 752.19
- gallbladder (*see also* Obstruction, gallbladder) 575.2
  - congenital 751.69
    - jaundice from 751.69 [774.5]
- gingiva, traumatic 523.8
- hymen 623.3
  - congenital 752.42
- hypophyseal (artery) 433.8 ☑
- iliac artery 444.81
- intestine (*see also* Obstruction, intestine) 560.9
- kidney 593.89
- lacrimal apparatus — *see* Stenosis, lacrimal
- lung 518.89
- lymph or lymphatic channel 457.1
- mammary duct 611.89
- mesenteric artery (embolic) (thrombotic) (with gangrene) 557.0
- nose 478.1 ☑
  - congenital 748.0
- organ or site, congenital NEC — *see* Atresia
- oviduct 628.2
  - congenital 752.19
- periodontal, traumatic 523.8
- peripheral arteries (lower extremity) 444.22
  - without thrombus or embolus (*see also* Arteriosclerosis, extremities) 440.20
  - due to stricture or stenosis 447.1
  - upper extremity 444.21
    - without thrombus or embolus (*see also* Arteriosclerosis, extremities) 440.20
    - due to stricture or stenosis 447.1
- pontine (artery) 433.8 ☑
- posterior lingual, of mandibular teeth 524.29
- precerebral artery — *see* Occlusion, artery, precerebral NEC
- puncta lacrimalia 375.52
- pupil 364.74
- pylorus (*see also* Stricture, pylorus) 537.0
- renal artery 593.81
- retina, retinal (vascular) 362.30
  - artery, arterial 362.30

Occlusion — *continued*
  retina, retinal — *continued*
    artery, arterial — *continued*
      branch 362.32
      central (total) 362.31
      partial 362.33
      transient 362.34
      tributary 362.32
    vein 362.30
      branch 362.36
      central (total) 362.35
      incipient 362.37
      partial 362.37
      tributary 362.36
  spinal artery 433.8 ☑
  stent
    coronary 996.72
  teeth (mandibular) (posterior lingual) 524.29
  thoracic duct 457.1
  tubal 628.2
  ureter (complete) (partial) 593.4
    congenital 753.29
  urethra (*see also* Stricture, urethra) 598.9
    congenital 753.6
  uterus 621.8
  vagina 623.2
  vascular NEC 459.9
  vein — *see* Thrombosis
  vena cava
    inferior 453.2
    superior (acute) 453.87
      chronic 453.77
  ventricle (brain) NEC 331.4
  vertebral (artery) — *see* Occlusion, artery, vertebral
  vessel (blood) NEC 459.9
  vulva 624.8
Occlusio pupillae 364.74
Occupational
  problems NEC V62.29
  therapy V57.21
Ochlophobia 300.29
Ochronosis (alkaptonuric) (congenital) (endogenous) 270.2
  with chloasma of eyelid 270.2
Ocular muscle — *see also* condition
  myopathy 359.1
  torticollis 781.93
Oculoauriculovertebral dysplasia 756.0
Oculogyric
  crisis or disturbance 378.87
    psychogenic 306.7
Oculomotor syndrome 378.81
Oddi's sphincter spasm 576.5
Odelberg's disease (juvenile osteochondrosis) 732.1
Odontalgia 525.9
Odontoameloblastoma (M9311/0) 213.1
  upper jaw (bone) 213.0
Odontoclasia 521.05
Odontoclasis 873.63
  complicated 873.73
Odontodysplasia, regional 520.4
Odontogenesis imperfecta 520.5
Odontoma (M9280/0) 213.1
  ameloblastic (M9311/0) 213.1
    upper jaw (bone) 213.0
  calcified (M9280/0) 213.1
    upper jaw (bone) 213.0
  complex (M9282/0) 213.1
    upper jaw (bone) 213.0
  compound (M9281/0) 213.1
    upper jaw (bone) 213.0
  fibroameloblastic (M9290/0) 213.1
    upper jaw (bone) 213.0
  follicular 526.0
  upper jaw (bone) 213.0
Odontomyelitis (closed) (open) 522.0
Odontonecrosis 521.09
Odontorrhagia 525.8
Odontosarcoma, ameloblastic (M9290/3) 170.1
  upper jaw (bone) 170.0
Odynophagia 787.20
Oesophagostomiasis 127.7
Oesophagostomum infestation 127.7

Oestriasis 134.0
Ogilvie's syndrome (sympathicotonic colon obstruction) 560.89
Oguchi's disease (retina) 368.61
Ohara's disease — *see also* Tularemia 021.9
Oidiomycosis — *see also* Candidiasis 112.9
Oidiomycotic meningitis 112.83
Oidium albicans infection — *see also* Candidiasis 112.9
Old age 797
  dementia (of) 290.0
Olfactory — *see* condition
Oligemia 285.9
Oligergasia — *see also* Disability, intellectual 319
Oligoamnios 658.0 ☑
  affecting fetus or newborn 761.2
Oligoastrocytoma, mixed (M9382/3)
  specified site — *see* Neoplasm, by site, malignant
  unspecified site 191.9
Oligocythemia 285.9
Oligodendroblastoma (M9460/3)
  specified site — *see* Neoplasm, by site, malignant
  unspecified site 191.9
Oligodendroglioma (M9450/3)
  anaplastic type (M9451/3)
    specified site — *see* Neoplasm, by site, malignant
    unspecified site 191.9
  specified site — *see* Neoplasm, by site, malignant
  unspecified site 191.9
Oligodendroma — *see* Oligodendroglioma
Oligodontia — *see also* Anodontia 520.0
Oligoencephalon 742.1
Oligohydramnios 658.0 ☑
  affecting fetus or newborn 761.2
  due to premature rupture of membranes 658.1 ☑
  affecting fetus or newborn 761.2
Oligohydrosis 705.0
Oligomenorrhea 626.1
Oligophrenia — *see also* Disability, intellectual 319
  phenylpyruvic 270.1
Oligospermia 606.1
Oligotrichia 704.09
  congenita 757.4
Oliguria 788.5
  with
    abortion — *see* Abortion, by type, with renal failure
    ectopic pregnancy (*see also* categories 633.0–633.9) 639.3
    molar pregnancy (*see also* categories 630–632) 639.3
  complicating
    abortion 639.3
    ectopic or molar pregnancy 639.3
    pregnancy 646.2 ☑
      with hypertension — *see* Toxemia, of pregnancy
    due to a procedure 997.5
    following labor and delivery 669.3 ☑
    heart or cardiac — *see* Failure, heart
    puerperal, postpartum 669.3 ☑
    specified due to a procedure 997.5
Ollier's disease (chondrodysplasia) 756.4
Omentitis — *see also* Peritonitis 567.9
Omentocele — *see also* Hernia, omental 553.8
Omentum, omental — *see* condition
Omphalitis (congenital) (newborn) 771.4
  not of newborn 686.9
  tetanus 771.3
Omphalocele 756.72
Omphalomesenteric duct, persistent 751.0
Omphalorrhagia, newborn 772.3
Omsk hemorrhagic fever 065.1
Onanism 307.9
Onchocerciasis 125.3
  eye 125.3 *[360.13]*
Onchocercosis 125.3
Oncocytoma (M8290/0) — *see* Neoplasm, by site, benign

Ondine's curse 348.89
Oneirophrenia — *see also* Schizophrenia 295.4 ☑
Onychauxis 703.8
  congenital 757.5
Onychia (with lymphangitis) 681.9
  dermatophytic 110.1
  finger 681.02
  toe 681.11
Onychitis (with lymphangitis) 681.9
  finger 681.02
  toe 681.11
Onychocryptosis 703.0
Onychodystrophy 703.8
  congenital 757.5
Onychogryphosis 703.8
Onychogryposis 703.8
Onycholysis 703.8
Onychomadesis 703.8
Onychomalacia 703.8
Onychomycosis 110.1
  finger 110.1
  toe 110.1
Onycho-osteodysplasia 756.89
Onychophagy 307.9
Onychoptosis 703.8
Onychorrhexis 703.8
  congenital 757.5
Onychoschizia 703.8
Onychotrophia — *see also* Atrophy, nail 703.8
O'nyong-nyong fever 066.3
Onyxis (finger) (toe) 703.0
Onyxitis (with lymphangitis) 681.9
  finger 681.02
  toe 681.11
Oocyte (egg) (ovum)
  donor V59.70
    over age 35 V59.73
      anonymous recipient V59.73
      designated recipient V59.74
    under age 35 V59.71
      anonymous recipient V59.71
      designated recipient V59.72
Oophoritis (cystic) (infectional) (interstitial) — *see also* Salpingo-oophoritis 614.2
  complicating pregnancy 646.6 ☑
  fetal (acute) 752.0
  gonococcal (acute) 098.19
    chronic or duration of 2 months or over 098.39
  tuberculous (*see also* Tuberculosis) 016.6 ☑
Opacity, opacities
  cornea 371.00
    central 371.03
    congenital 743.43
      interfering with vision 743.42
    degenerative (*see also* Degeneration, cornea) 371.40
    hereditary (*see also* Dystrophy, cornea) 371.50
    inflammatory (*see also* Keratitis) 370.9
    late effect of trachoma (healed) 139.1
    minor 371.01
    peripheral 371.02
  enamel (fluoride) (nonfluoride) (teeth) 520.3
  lens (*see also* Cataract) 366.9
  snowball 379.22
  vitreous (humor) 379.24
    congenital 743.51
Opalescent dentin (hereditary) 520.5
Open, opening
  abnormal, organ or site, congenital — *see* Imperfect, closure
  angle
    with
      borderline findings
        high risk 365.05
        intraocular pressure 365.01
        low risk 365.01
      cupping of discs 365.01
    high risk 365.05
    low risk 365.01
  bite
    anterior 524.24
    posterior 524.25
  false — *see* Imperfect, closure

Open, opening — *continued*
  margin on tooth restoration 525.61
  restoration margins 525.61
  wound — *see* Wound, open, by site
Operation
  causing mutilation of fetus 763.89
  destructive, on live fetus, to facilitate birth 763.89
  for delivery, fetus or newborn 763.89
  maternal, unrelated to current delivery, affecting fetus or newborn (*see also* Newborn, affected by) 760.64
Operational fatigue 300.89
Operative — *see* condition
Operculitis (chronic) 523.40
  acute 523.30
Operculum, retina 361.32
  with detachment 361.01
Ophiasis 704.01
Ophthalmia — *see also* Conjunctivitis 372.30
  actinic rays 370.24
  allergic (acute) 372.05
    chronic 372.14
  blennorrhagic (neonatorum) 098.40
  catarrhal 372.03
  diphtheritic 032.81
  Egyptian 076.1
  electric, electrica 370.24
  gonococcal (neonatorum) 098.40
  metastatic 360.11
  migraine 346.8 ☑
  neonatorum, newborn 771.6
    gonococcal 098.40
  nodosa 360.14
  phlyctenular 370.31
    with ulcer (*see also* Ulcer, cornea) 370.00
  sympathetic 360.11
Ophthalmitis — *see* Ophthalmia
Ophthalmocele (congenital) 743.66
Ophthalmoneuromyelitis 341.0
Ophthalmopathy, infiltrative with thyrotoxicosis 242.0 ☑
Ophthalmoplegia — *see also* Strabismus 378.9
  anterior internuclear 378.86
  ataxia-areflexia syndrome 357.0
  bilateral 378.9
  diabetic 250.5 ☑ *[378.86]*
    due to secondary diabetes 249.5 ☑ *[378.86]*
  exophthalmic 242.0 ☑ *[376.22]*
  external 378.55
    progressive 378.72
    total 378.56
  internal (complete) (total) 367.52
  internuclear 378.86
  migraine 346.2 ☑
  painful 378.55
  Parinaud's 378.81
  progressive external 378.72
  supranuclear, progressive 333.0
  total (external) 378.56
    internal 367.52
  unilateral 378.9
Opisthognathism 524.00
Opisthorchiasis (felineus) (tenuicollis) (viverrini) 121.0
Opisthotonos, opisthotonus 781.0
Opitz's disease (congestive splenomegaly) 289.51
Opiumism — *see also* Dependence 304.0 ☑
Oppenheim's disease 358.8
Oppenheim-Urbach disease or syndrome (necrobiosis lipoidica diabeticorum) 250.8 ☑ *[709.3]*
  due to secondary diabetes 249.8 ☑ *[709.3]*
Opsoclonia 379.59
Optic nerve — *see* condition
Orbit — *see* condition
Orchioblastoma (M9071/3) 186.9
Orchitis (nonspecific) (septic) 604.90
  with abscess 604.0
  blennorrhagic (acute) 098.13
    chronic or duration of 2 months or over 098.33
  diphtheritic 032.89 *[604.91]*
  filarial 125.9 *[604.91]*

☑ **Additional Digit Required** — Refer to the Tabular List for Digit Selection   ▼ **Subterms under main terms may continue to next column or page**

Orchitis — *continued*
  gangrenous 604.99
  gonococcal (acute) 098.13
    chronic or duration of 2 months or over 098.33
  mumps 072.0
  parotidea 072.0
  suppurative 604.99
  syphilitic 095.8 *[604.91]*
  tuberculous (*see also* Tuberculosis) 016.5 ☑ *[608.81]*
Orf 051.2
Organic — *see also* condition
  heart — *see* Disease, heart
  insufficiency 799.89
Oriental
  bilharziasis 120.2
  schistosomiasis 120.2
  sore 085.1
Orientation
  ego-dystonic sexual 302.0
Orifice — *see* condition
Origin, both great vessels from right ventricle 745.11
Ormond's disease or syndrome 593.4
Ornithosis 073.9
  with
    complication 073.8
      specified NEC 073.7
    pneumonia 073.0
    pneumonitis (lobular) 073.0
Orodigitofacial dysostosis 759.89
Oropouche fever 066.3
Orotaciduria, oroticaciduria (congenital) (hereditary) (pyrimidine deficiency) 281.4
Oroya fever 088.0
Orthodontics V58.5
  adjustment V53.4
  aftercare V58.5
  fitting V53.4
Orthopnea 786.02
Orthoptic training V57.4
Osgood-Schlatter
  disease 732.4
  osteochondrosis 732.4
Osler's
  disease (M9950/1) (polycythemia vera) 238.4
  nodes 421.0
Osler-Rendu disease (familial hemorrhagic telangiectasia) 448.0
Osler-Vaquez disease (M9950/1) (polycythemia vera) 238.4
Osler-Weber-Rendu syndrome (familial hemorrhagic telangiectasia) 448.0
Osmidrosis 705.89
Osseous — *see* condition
Ossification
  artery — *see* Arteriosclerosis
  auricle (ear) 380.39
  bronchus 519.19
  cardiac (*see also* Degeneration, myocardial) 429.1
  cartilage (senile) 733.99
  coronary (artery) — *see* Arteriosclerosis, coronary
  diaphragm 728.10
  ear 380.39
    middle (*see also* Otosclerosis) 387.9
  falx cerebri 349.2
  fascia 728.10
  fontanel
    defective or delayed 756.0
    premature 756.0
  heart (*see also* Degeneration, myocardial) 429.1
    valve — *see* Endocarditis
  larynx 478.79
  ligament
    posterior longitudinal 724.8
      cervical 723.7
  meninges (cerebral) 349.2
    spinal 336.8
  multiple, eccentric centers 733.99
  muscle 728.10

Ossification — *continued*
  muscle — *continued*
    heterotopic, postoperative 728.13
  myocardium, myocardial (*see also* Degeneration, myocardial) 429.1
  penis 607.81
  periarticular 728.89
  sclera 379.16
  tendon 727.82
  trachea 519.19
  tympanic membrane (*see also* Tympanosclerosis) 385.00
  vitreous (humor) 360.44
Osteitis — *see also* Osteomyelitis 730.2 ☑
  acute 730.0 ☑
  alveolar 526.5
  chronic 730.1 ☑
  condensans (ilii) 733.5
  deformans (Paget's) 731.0
    due to or associated with malignant neoplasm (*see also* Neoplasm, bone, malignant) 170.9 *[731.1]*
  due to yaws 102.6
  fibrosa NEC 733.29
    cystica (generalisata) 252.01
    disseminata 756.59
    osteoplastica 252.01
  fragilitans 756.51
  Garré's (sclerosing) 730.1 ☑
  infectious (acute) (subacute) 730.0 ☑
    chronic or old 730.1 ☑
  jaw (acute) (chronic) (lower) (neonatal) (suppurative) (upper) 526.4
  parathyroid 252.01
  petrous bone (*see also* Petrositis) 383.20
  pubis 733.5
  sclerotic, nonsuppurative 730.1 ☑
  syphilitic 095.5
  tuberculosa
    cystica (of Jüngling) 135
    multiplex cystoides 135
Osteoarthritica spondylitis (spine) — *see also* Spondylosis 721.90
Osteoarthritis — *see also* Osteoarthrosis 715.9 ☑
  distal interphalangeal 715.9 ☑
  hyperplastic 731.2
  interspinalis (*see also* Spondylosis) 721.90
  spine, spinal NEC (*see also* Spondylosis) 721.90
Osteoarthropathy — *see also* Osteoarthrosis 715.9 ☑
  chronic idiopathic hypertrophic 757.39
  familial idiopathic 757.39
  hypertrophic pulmonary 731.2
    secondary 731.2
  idiopathic hypertrophic 757.39
  primary hypertrophic 731.2
  pulmonary hypertrophic 731.2
  secondary hypertrophic 731.2
Osteoarthrosis (degenerative) (hypertrophic) (rheumatoid) 715.9 ☑

> *Note — Use the following fifth-digit subclassification with category 715:*
>
> *0   site unspecified*
> *1   shoulder region*
> *2   upper arm*
> *3   forearm*
> *4   hand*
> *5   pelvic region and thigh*
> *6   lower leg*
> *7   ankle and foot*
> *8   other specified sites except spine*
> *9   multiple sites*

  Deformans alkaptonurica 270.2
  generalized 715.09
  juvenilis (Köhler's) 732.5
  localized 715.3 ☑
    idiopathic 715.1 ☑
    primary 715.1 ☑

Osteoarthrosis — *continued*
  localized — *continued*
    secondary 715.2 ☑
  multiple sites, not specified as generalized 715.89
  polyarticular 715.09
  spine (*see also* Spondylosis) 721.90
  temporomandibular joint 524.69
Osteoblastoma (M9200/0) — *see* Neoplasm, bone, benign
Osteochondritis — *see also* Osteochondrosis 732.9
  dissecans 732.7
    hip 732.7
  ischiopubica 732.1
  multiple 756.59
  syphilitic (congenital) 090.0
Osteochondrodermodysplasia 756.59
Osteochondrodystrophy 277.5
  deformans 277.5
  familial 277.5
  fetalis 756.4
Osteochondrolysis 732.7
Osteochondroma (M9210/0) — *see also* Neoplasm, bone, benign
  multiple, congenital 756.4
Osteochondromatosis (M9210/1) 238.0
  synovial 727.82
Osteochondromyxosarcoma (M9180/3) — *see* Neoplasm, bone, malignant
Osteochondropathy NEC 732.9
Osteochondrosarcoma (M9180/3) — *see* Neoplasm, bone, malignant
Osteochondrosis 732.9
  acetabulum 732.1
  adult spine 732.8
  astragalus 732.5
  Blount's 732.4
  Buchanan's (juvenile osteochondrosis of iliac crest) 732.1
  Buchman's (juvenile osteochondrosis) 732.1
  Burns' 732.3
  calcaneus 732.5
  capitular epiphysis (femur) 732.1
  carpal
    lunate (wrist) 732.3
    scaphoid 732.3
  coxae juvenilis 732.1
  deformans juvenilis (coxae) (hip) 732.1
    Scheuermann's 732.0
    spine 732.0
    tibia 732.4
    vertebra 732.0
  Diaz's (astragalus) 732.5
  dissecans (knee) (shoulder) 732.7
  femoral capital epiphysis 732.1
  femur (head) (juvenile) 732.1
  foot (juvenile) 732.5
  Freiberg's (disease) (second metatarsal) 732.5
  Haas' 732.3
  Haglund's (os tibiale externum) 732.5
  hand (juvenile) 732.3
  head of
    femur 732.1
    humerus (juvenile) 732.3
  hip (juvenile) 732.1
  humerus (juvenile) 732.3
  iliac crest (juvenile) 732.1
  ilium (juvenile) 732.1
  ischiopubic synchondrosis 732.1
  Iselin's (osteochondrosis fifth metatarsal) 732.5
  juvenile, juvenilis 732.6
    arm 732.3
    capital femoral epiphysis 732.1
    capitellum humeri 732.3
    capitular epiphysis 732.1
    carpal scaphoid 732.3
    clavicle, sternal epiphysis 732.6
    coxae 732.1
    deformans 732.1
    foot 732.5
    hand 732.3
    hip and pelvis 732.1
    lower extremity, except foot 732.4

Osteochondrosis — *continued*
  juvenile, juvenilis — *continued*
    lunate, wrist 732.3
    medial cuneiform bone 732.5
    metatarsal (head) 732.5
    metatarsophalangeal 732.5
    navicular, ankle 732.5
    patella 732.4
    primary patellar center (of Köhler) 732.4
    specified site NEC 732.6
    spine 732.0
    tarsal scaphoid 732.5
    tibia (epiphysis) (tuberosity) 732.4
    upper extremity 732.3
    vertebra (body) (Calvé) 732.0
      epiphyseal plates (of Scheuermann) 732.0
  Kienböck's (disease) 732.3
  Köhler's (disease) (navicular, ankle) 732.5
    patellar 732.4
    tarsal navicular 732.5
  Legg-Calvé-Perthes (disease) 732.1
  lower extremity (juvenile) 732.4
  lunate bone 732.3
  Mauclaire's 732.3
  metacarpal heads (of Mauclaire) 732.3
  metatarsal (fifth) (head) (second) 732.5
  navicular, ankle 732.5
  os calcis 732.5
  Osgood-Schlatter 732.4
  os tibiale externum 732.5
  Panner's 732.3
  patella (juvenile) 732.4
  patellar center
    primary (of Köhler) 732.4
    secondary (of Sinding-Larsen) 732.4
  pelvis (juvenile) 732.1
  Pierson's 732.1
  radial head (juvenile) 732.3
  Scheuermann's 732.0
  Sever's (calcaneum) 732.5
  Sinding-Larsen (secondary patellar center) 732.4
  spine (juvenile) 732.0
    adult 732.8
  symphysis pubis (of Pierson) (juvenile) 732.1
  syphilitic (congenital) 090.0
  tarsal (navicular) (scaphoid) 732.5
  tibia (proximal) (tubercle) 732.4
  tuberculous — *see* Tuberculosis, bone
  ulna 732.3
  upper extremity (juvenile) 732.3
  van Neck's (juvenile osteochondrosis) 732.1
  vertebral (juvenile) 732.0
    adult 732.8
Osteoclastoma (M9250/1) 238.0
  malignant (M9250/3) — *see* Neoplasm, bone, malignant
Osteocopic pain 733.90
Osteodynia 733.90
Osteodystrophy
  azotemic 588.0
  chronica deformans hypertrophica 731.0
  congenital 756.50
    specified type NEC 756.59
  deformans 731.0
  fibrosa localisata 731.0
  parathyroid 252.01
  renal 588.0
Osteofibroma (M9262/0) — *see* Neoplasm, bone, benign
Osteofibrosarcoma (M9182/3) — *see* Neoplasm, bone, malignant
Osteogenesis imperfecta 756.51
Osteogenic — *see* condition
Osteoma (M9180/0) — *see also* Neoplasm, bone, benign
  osteoid (M9191/0) (*see also* Neoplasm, bone, benign)
    giant (M9200/0) — *see* Neoplasm, bone, benign
Osteomalacia 268.2
  chronica deformans hypertrophica 731.0
  due to vitamin D deficiency 268.2
  infantile (*see also* Rickets) 268.0
  juvenile (*see also* Rickets) 268.0

Osteomalacia — *continued*
oncogenic 275.8
pelvis 268.2
vitamin D-resistant 275.3
Osteomalacic bone 268.2
Osteomalacosis 268.2
Osteomyelitis (general) (infective) (localized) (neonatal) (purulent) (pyogenic) (septic) (staphylococcal) (streptococcal) (suppurative) (with periostitis) 730.2 ☑

	Note — Use the following fifth-digit subclassification with category 730:
0	site unspecified
1	shoulder region
2	upper arm
3	forearm
4	hand
5	pelvic region and thigh
6	lower leg
7	ankle and foot
8	other specified sites
9	multiple sites

acute or subacute 730.0 ☑
chronic or old 730.1 ☑
due to or associated with
diabetes mellitus 250.8 ☑ [731.8]
due to secondary diabetes 249.8 ☑ [731.8]
tuberculosis (see also Tuberculosis, bone) 015.9 ☑ [730.8] ☑
limb bones 015.5 ☑ [730.8] ☑
specified bones NEC 015.7 ☑ [730.8] ☑
spine 015.0 ☑ [730.8] ☑
typhoid 002.0 [730.8] ☑
Garré's 730.1 ☑
jaw (acute) (chronic) (lower) (neonatal) (suppurative) (upper) 526.4
nonsuppurating 730.1 ☑
orbital 376.03
petrous bone (see also Petrositis) 383.20
Salmonella 003.24
sclerosing, nonsuppurative 730.1 ☑
sicca 730.1 ☑
syphilitic 095.5
congenital 090.0 [730.8] ☑
tuberculous — see Tuberculosis, bone
typhoid 002.0 [730.8] ☑
Osteomyelofibrosis 289.89
Osteomyelosclerosis 289.89
Osteonecrosis 733.40
meaning osteomyelitis 730.1 ☑
Osteo-onycho-arthro dysplasia 756.89
Osteo-onychodysplasia, hereditary 756.89
Osteopathia
condensans disseminata 756.53
hyperostotica multiplex infantilis 756.59
hypertrophica toxica 731.2
striata 756.4
Osteopathy resulting from poliomyelitis — see also Poliomyelitis 045.9 ☑ [730.7] ☑
familial dysplastic 731.2
Osteopecilia 756.53
Osteopenia 733.90
borderline 733.90
Osteoperiostitis — see also Osteomyelitis 730.2 ☑
ossificans toxica 731.2
toxica ossificans 731.2
Osteopetrosis (familial) 756.52
Osteophyte — see Exostosis
Osteophytosis — see Exostosis
Osteopoikilosis 756.53
Osteoporosis (generalized) 733.00
circumscripta 731.0
disuse 733.03
drug-induced 733.09
idiopathic 733.02
postmenopausal 733.01
posttraumatic 733.7

Osteoporosis — *continued*
screening V82.81
senile 733.01
specified type NEC 733.09
Osteoporosis-osteomalacia syndrome 268.2
Osteopsathyrosis 756.51
Osteoradionecrosis, jaw 526.89
Osteosarcoma (M9180/3) — see also Neoplasm, bone, malignant
chondroblastic (M9181/3) — see Neoplasm, bone, malignant
fibroblastic (M9182/3) — see Neoplasm, bone, malignant
in Paget's disease of bone (M9184/3) — see Neoplasm, bone, malignant
juxtacortical (M9190/3) — see Neoplasm, bone, malignant
parosteal (M9190/3) — see Neoplasm, bone, malignant
telangiectatic (M9183/3) — see Neoplasm, bone, malignant
Osteosclerosis 756.52
fragilis (generalisata) 756.52
Osteosclerotic anemia 289.89
Osteosis
acromegaloid 757.39
cutis 709.3
parathyroid 252.01
renal fibrocystic 588.0
Österreicher-Turner syndrome 756.89
Ostium
atrioventriculare commune 745.69
primum (arteriosum) (defect) (persistent) 745.61
secundum (arteriosum) (defect) (patent) (persistent) 745.5
Ostrum-Furst syndrome 756.59
Os, uterus — see condition
Otalgia 388.70
otogenic 388.71
referred 388.72
Othematoma 380.31
Otitic hydrocephalus 348.2
Otitis 382.9
with effusion 381.4
purulent 382.4
secretory 381.4
serous 381.4
suppurative 382.4
acute 382.9
adhesive (see also Adhesions, middle ear) 385.10
chronic 382.9
with effusion 381.3
mucoid, mucous (simple) 381.20
purulent 382.3
secretory 381.3
serous 381.10
suppurative 382.3
diffuse parasitic 136.8
externa (acute) (diffuse) (hemorrhagica) 380.10
actinic 380.22
candidal 112.82
chemical 380.22
chronic 380.23
mycotic — see Otitis, externa, mycotic
specified type NEC 380.23
circumscribed 380.10
contact 380.22
due to
erysipelas 035 [380.13]
impetigo 684 [380.13]
seborrheic dermatitis 690.10 [380.13]
eczematoid 380.22
furuncular 680.0 [380.13]
infective 380.10
chronic 380.16
malignant 380.14
mycotic (chronic) 380.15
due to
aspergillosis 117.3 [380.15]
moniliasis 112.82
otomycosis 111.8 [380.15]
reactive 380.22

Otitis — *continued*
externa — *continued*
specified type NEC 380.22
tropical 111.8 [380.15]
insidiosa (see also Otosclerosis) 387.9
interna (see also Labyrinthitis) 386.30
media (hemorrhagic) (staphylococcal) (streptococcal) 382.9
acute 382.9
with effusion 381.00
allergic 381.04
mucoid 381.05
sanguineous 381.06
serous 381.04
catarrhal 381.00
exudative 381.00
mucoid 381.02
allergic 381.05
necrotizing 382.00
with spontaneous rupture of ear drum 382.01
in
influenza (see also Influenza) 487.8 [382.02]
measles 055.2
scarlet fever 034.1 [382.02]
nonsuppurative 381.00
purulent 382.00
with spontaneous rupture of ear drum 382.01
sanguineous 381.03
allergic 381.06
secretory 381.01
seromucinous 381.02
serous 381.01
allergic 381.04
suppurative 382.00
with spontaneous rupture of ear drum 382.01
due to
influenza (see also Influenza) 487.8 [382.02]
scarlet fever 034.1 [382.02]
transudative 381.00
adhesive (see also Adhesions, middle ear) 385.10
allergic 381.4
acute 381.04
mucoid 381.05
sanguineous 381.06
serous 381.04
chronic 381.3
catarrhal 381.4
acute 381.00
chronic (simple) 381.10
chronic 382.9
with effusion 381.3
adhesive (see also Adhesions, middle ear) 385.10
allergic 381.3
atticoantral, suppurative (with posterior or superior marginal perforation of ear drum) 382.2
benign suppurative (with anterior perforation of ear drum) 382.1
catarrhal 381.10
exudative 381.3
mucinous 381.20
mucoid, mucous (simple) 381.20
mucosanguineous 381.29
nonsuppurative 381.3
purulent 382.3
secretory 381.3
seromucinous 381.3
serosanguineous 381.19
serous (simple) 381.10
suppurative 382.3
atticoantral (with posterior or superior marginal perforation of ear drum) 382.2
benign (with anterior perforation of ear drum) 382.1
tuberculous (see also Tuberculosis) 017.4 ☑
tubotympanic 382.1
transudative 381.3

Otitis — *continued*
media — *continued*
exudative 381.4
acute 381.00
chronic 381.3
fibrotic (see also Adhesions, middle ear) 385.10
mucoid, mucous 381.4
acute 381.02
chronic (simple) 381.20
mucosanguineous, chronic 381.29
nonsuppurative 381.4
acute 381.00
chronic 381.3
postmeasles 055.2
purulent 382.4
acute 382.00
with spontaneous rupture of ear drum 382.01
chronic 382.3
sanguineous, acute 381.03
allergic 381.06
secretory 381.4
acute or subacute 381.01
chronic 381.3
seromucinous 381.4
acute or subacute 381.02
chronic 381.3
serosanguineous, chronic 381.19
serous 381.4
acute or subacute 381.01
chronic (simple) 381.10
subacute — see Otitis, media, acute
suppurative 382.4
acute 382.00
with spontaneous rupture of ear drum 382.01
chronic 382.3
atticoantral 382.2
benign 382.1
tuberculous (see also Tuberculosis) 017.4 ☑
tubotympanic 382.1
transudative 381.4
acute 381.00
chronic 381.3
tuberculous (see also Tuberculosis) 017.4 ☑
postmeasles 055.2
Otoconia 386.8
Otolith syndrome 386.19
Otomycosis 111.8 [380.15]
in
aspergillosis 117.3 [380.15]
moniliasis 112.82
Otopathy 388.9
Otoporosis — see also Otosclerosis 387.9
Otorrhagia 388.69
traumatic — see nature of injury
Otorrhea 388.60
blood 388.69
cerebrospinal (fluid) 388.61
Otosclerosis (general) 387.9
cochlear (endosteal) 387.2
involving
otic capsule 387.2
oval window
nonobliterative 387.0
obliterative 387.1
round window 387.2
nonobliterative 387.0
obliterative 387.1
specified type NEC 387.8
Otospongiosis — see also Otosclerosis 387.9
Otto's disease or pelvis 715.35
Outburst, aggressive — see also Disturbance, conduct 312.0 ☑
in children or adolescents 313.9
Outcome of delivery
multiple birth NEC V27.9
all liveborn V27.5
all stillborn V27.7
some liveborn V27.6
unspecified V27.9
single V27.9
liveborn V27.0

Outcome of delivery — *continued*
single — *continued*
stillborn V27.1
twins V27.9
both liveborn V27.2
both stillborn V27.4
one liveborn, one stillborn V27.3
Outlet — *see also* condition
syndrome (thoracic) 353.0
Outstanding ears (bilateral) 744.29
Ovalocytosis (congenital) (hereditary) — *see also* Elliptocytosis 282.1
Ovarian — *see also* condition
pregnancy — *see* Pregnancy, ovarian
remnant syndrome 620.8
vein syndrome 593.4
Ovaritis (cystic) — *see also* Salpingo-oophoritis 614.2
Ovary, ovarian — *see* condition
Overactive — *see also* Hyperfunction
bladder 596.51
eye muscle (*see also* Strabismus) 378.9
hypothalamus 253.8
thyroid (*see also* Thyrotoxicosis) 242.9 ☑
Overactivity, child 314.01
Overbite (deep) (excessive) (horizontal) (vertical) 524.29
Overbreathing — *see also* Hyperventilation 786.01
Overconscientious personality 301.4
Overdevelopment — *see also* Hypertrophy
breast (female) (male) 611.1
nasal bones 738.0
prostate, congenital 752.89
Overdistention — *see* Distention
Overdose overdosage (drug) 977.9
specified drug or substance — *see* Table of Drugs and Chemicals
Overeating 783.6
nonorganic origin 307.51
Overexertion (effects) (exhaustion) 994.5
Overexposure (effects) 994.9
exhaustion 994.4
Overfeeding — *see also* Overeating 783.6
Overfill, endodontic 526.62
Overgrowth, bone NEC 733.99
Overhanging
tooth restoration 525.62
unrepairable, dental restorative materials 525.62
Overheated (effects) (places) — *see* Heat
Overinhibited child 313.0
Overjet 524.29
excessive horizontal 524.26
Overlaid, overlying (suffocation) 994.7
Overlap
excessive horizontal 524.26
Overlapping toe (acquired) 735.8
congenital (fifth toe) 755.66
Overload
fluid 276.69
due to transfusion (blood) (blood components) 276.61
iron, due to repeated red blood cell transfusions 275.02
potassium (K) 276.7
sodium (Na) 276.0
transfusion associated circulatory (TACO) 276.61
Overnutrition — *see also* Hyperalimentation 783.6
Overproduction — *see also* Hypersecretion
ACTH 255.3
cortisol 255.0
growth hormone 253.0
thyroid-stimulating hormone (TSH) 242.8 ☑
Overriding
aorta 747.21
finger (acquired) 736.29
congenital 755.59
toe (acquired) 735.8
congenital 755.66
Oversize
fetus (weight of 4500 grams or more) 766.0
affecting management of pregnancy 656.6 ☑

Oversize — *continued*
fetus — *continued*
causing disproportion 653.5 ☑
with obstructed labor 660.1 ☑
affecting fetus or newborn 763.1
Overstimulation, ovarian 256.1
Overstrained 780.79
heart — *see* Hypertrophy, cardiac
Overweight — *see also* Obesity 278.02
Overwork 780.79
Oviduct — *see* condition
Ovotestis 752.7
Ovulation (cycle)
failure or lack of 628.0
pain 625.2
Ovum
blighted 631.8
donor V59.70
over age 35 V59.73
anonymous recipient V59.73
designated recipient V59.74
under age 35 V59.71
anonymous recipient V59.71
designated recipient V59.72
dropsical 631.8
pathologic 631.8
Owren's disease or syndrome (parahemophilia) — *see also* Defect, coagulation 286.3
Oxalosis 271.8
Oxaluria 271.8
Ox heart — *see* Hypertrophy, cardiac
OX syndrome 758.6
Oxycephaly, oxycephalic 756.0
syphilitic, congenital 090.0
Oxyuriasis 127.4
Oxyuris vermicularis (infestation) 127.4
Ozena 472.0

P

Pacemaker syndrome 429.4
Pachyderma, pachydermia 701.8
laryngis 478.5
laryngitis 478.79
larynx (verrucosa) 478.79
Pachydermatitis 701.8
Pachydermatocele (congenital) 757.39
acquired 701.8
Pachydermatosis 701.8
Pachydermoperiostitis
secondary 731.2
Pachydermoperiostosis
primary idiopathic 757.39
secondary 731.2
Pachymeningitis (adhesive) (basal) (brain) (cerebral) (cervical) (chronic) (circumscribed) (external) (fibrous) (hemorrhagic) (hypertrophic) (internal) (purulent) (spinal) (suppurative) — *see also* Meningitis 322.9
gonococcal 098.82
Pachyonychia (congenital) 757.5
acquired 703.8
Pachyperiosteodermia
primary or idiopathic 757.39
secondary 731.2
Pachyperiostosis
primary or idiopathic 757.39
secondary 731.2
Pacinian tumor (M9507/0) — *see* Neoplasm, skin, benign
Pads, knuckle or Garrod's 728.79
Paget's disease (osteitis deformans) 731.0
with infiltrating duct carcinoma of the breast (M8541/3) — *see* Neoplasm, breast, malignant
bone 731.0
osteosarcoma in (M9184/3) — *see* Neoplasm, bone, malignant
breast (M8540/3) 174.0
extramammary (M8542/3) (*see also* Neoplasm, skin, malignant)
anus 154.3
skin 173.59
malignant (M8540/3)
breast 174.0

Paget's disease — *continued*
malignant — *continued*
specified site NEC (M8542/3) — *see* Neoplasm, skin, malignant
unspecified site 174.0
mammary (M8540/3) 174.0
necrosis of bone 731.0
nipple (M8540/3) 174.0
osteitis deformans 731.0
Paget-Schroetter syndrome (intermittent venous claudication) 453.89
Pain(s) (*see also* Painful) 780.96
abdominal 789.0 ☑
acute 338.19
due to trauma 338.11
postoperative 338.18
post-thoracotomy 338.12
adnexa (uteri) 625.9
alimentary, due to vascular insufficiency 557.9
anginoid (*see also* Pain, precordial) 786.51
anus 569.42
arch 729.5
arm 729.5
axillary 729.5
back (postural) 724.5
low 724.2
psychogenic 307.89
bile duct 576.9
bladder 788.99
bone 733.90
breast 611.71
psychogenic 307.89
broad ligament 625.9
cancer associated 338.3
cartilage NEC 733.90
cecum 789.0 ☑
cervicobrachial 723.3
chest (central) 786.50
atypical 786.59
midsternal 786.51
musculoskeletal 786.59
noncardiac 786.59
substernal 786.51
wall (anterior) 786.52
chronic 338.29
associated with significant psychosocial dysfunction 338.4
due to trauma 338.21
postoperative 338.28
post-thoracotomy 338.22
syndrome 338.4
coccyx 724.79
colon 789.0 ☑
common duct 576.9
coronary — *see* Angina
costochondral 786.52
diaphragm 786.52
due to (presence of) any device, implant, or graft classifiable to 996.0–996.5 — *see* Complications, due to (presence of) any device, implant, or graft classified to 996.0–996.5 NEC
malignancy (primary) (secondary) 338.3
ear (*see also* Otalgia) 388.70
epigastric, epigastrium 789.06
extremity (lower) (upper) 729.5
eye 379.91
face, facial 784.0
atypical 350.2
nerve 351.8
false (labor) 644.1 ☑
female genital organ NEC 625.9
psychogenic 307.89
finger 729.5
flank 789.0 ☑
foot 729.5
gallbladder 575.9
gas (intestinal) 787.3
gastric 536.8
generalized 780.96
genital organ
female 625.9
male 608.9
psychogenic 307.89
groin 789.0 ☑

Pain(s) (*see also* Painful) — *continued*
growing 781.99
hand 729.5
head (*see also* Headache) 784.0
heart (see also Pain, precordial) 786.51
infraorbital (*see also* Neuralgia, trigeminal) 350.1
intermenstrual 625.2
jaw 784.92
joint 719.40
ankle 719.47
elbow 719.42
foot 719.47
hand 719.44
hip 719.45
knee 719.46
multiple sites 719.49
pelvic region 719.45
psychogenic 307.89
shoulder (region) 719.41
specified site NEC 719.48
wrist 719.43
kidney 788.0
labor, false or spurious 644.1 ☑
laryngeal 784.1
leg 729.5
limb 729.5
low back 724.2
lumbar region 724.2
mandible, mandibular 784.92
mastoid (*see also* Otalgia) 388.70
maxilla 784.92
menstrual 625.3
metacarpophalangeal (joint) 719.44
metatarsophalangeal (joint) 719.47
mouth 528.9
muscle 729.1
intercostal 786.59
musculoskeletal (see also Pain, by site) 729.1
nasal 478.19
nasopharynx 478.29
neck NEC 723.1
psychogenic 307.89
neoplasm related (acute) (chronic) 338.3
nerve NEC 729.2
neuromuscular 729.1
nose 478.19
ocular 379.91
ophthalmic 379.91
orbital region 379.91
osteocopic 733.90
ovary 625.9
psychogenic 307.89
over heart (*see also* Pain, precordial) 786.51
ovulation 625.2
pelvic (female) 625.9
male NEC 789.0 ☑
psychogenic 307.89
psychogenic 307.89
penis 607.9
psychogenic 307.89
pericardial (*see also* Pain, precordial) 786.51
perineum
female 625.9
male 608.9
pharynx 478.29
pleura, pleural, pleuritic 786.52
postoperative 338.18
acute 338.18
chronic 338.28
post-thoracotomy 338.12
acute 338.12
chronic 338.22
preauricular 388.70
precordial (region) 786.51
psychogenic 307.89
premenstrual 625.4
psychogenic 307.80
cardiovascular system 307.89
gastrointestinal system 307.89
genitourinary system 307.89
heart 307.89
musculoskeletal system 307.89
respiratory system 307.89
skin 306.3
radicular (spinal) (*see also* Radiculitis) 729.2

Pain(s) (see also Painful) — continued
rectum 569.42
respiration 786.52
retrosternal 786.51
rheumatic NEC 729.0
muscular 729.1
rib 786.50
root (spinal) (see also Radiculitis) 729.2
round ligament (stretch) 625.9
sacroiliac 724.6
sciatic 724.3
scrotum 608.9
psychogenic 307.89
seminal vesicle 608.9
sinus 478.19
skin 782.0
spermatic cord 608.9
spinal root (see also Radiculitis) 729.2
stomach 536.8
psychogenic 307.89
substernal 786.51
testis 608.9
psychogenic 307.89
thoracic spine 724.1
with radicular and visceral pain 724.4
throat 784.1
tibia 733.90
toe 729.5
tongue 529.6
tooth 525.9
total hip replacement 996.77
total knee replacement 996.77
trigeminal (see also Neuralgia, trigeminal) 350.1
tumor associated 338.3
umbilicus 789.05
ureter 788.0
urinary (organ) (system) 788.0
uterus 625.9
psychogenic 307.89
vagina 625.9
vertebrogenic (syndrome) 724.5
vesical 788.99
vulva 625.9
xiphoid 733.90
Painful — see also Pain
arc syndrome 726.19
coitus
female 625.0
male 608.89
psychogenic 302.76
ejaculation (semen) 608.89
psychogenic 302.79
erection 607.3
feet syndrome 266.2
menstruation 625.3
psychogenic 306.52
micturition 788.1
ophthalmoplegia 378.55
respiration 786.52
scar NEC 709.2
urination 788.1
wire sutures 998.89
Painters' colic 984.9
specified type of lead — see Table of Drugs and Chemicals
Palate — see condition
Palatoplegia 528.9
Palatoschisis — see also Cleft, palate 749.00
Palilalia 784.69
Palindromic arthritis — see also Rheumatism, palindromic 719.3 ☑
Palliative care V66.7
Pallor 782.61
temporal, optic disc 377.15
Palmar — see also condition
fascia — see condition
Palpable
cecum 569.89
kidney 593.89
liver 573.9
lymph nodes 785.6
ovary 620.8
prostate 602.9
spleen (see also Splenomegaly) 789.2
uterus 625.8

Palpitation (heart) 785.1
psychogenic 306.2
Palsy — see also Paralysis 344.9
atrophic diffuse 335.20
Bell's 351.0
newborn 767.5
birth 767.7
brachial plexus 353.0
fetus or newborn 767.6
brain (see also Palsy, cerebral)
noncongenital or noninfantile 344.89
late effect — see Late effect(s) (of) cerebrovascular disease
syphilitic 094.89
congenital 090.49
bulbar (chronic) (progressive) 335.22
pseudo NEC 335.23
supranuclear NEC 344.8 ☑
cerebral (congenital) (infantile) (spastic) 343.9
athetoid 333.71
diplegic 343.0
late effect — see Late effect(s) (of) cerebrovascular disease
hemiplegic 343.1
monoplegic 343.3
noncongenital or noninfantile 437.8
late effect — see Late effect(s) (of) cerebrovascular disease
paraplegic 343.0
quadriplegic 343.2
spastic, not congenital or infantile 344.89
syphilitic 094.89
congenital 090.49
tetraplegic 343.2
cranial nerve (see also Disorder, nerve, cranial)
multiple 352.6
creeping 335.21
divers' 993.3
Erb's (birth injury) 767.6
facial 351.0
newborn 767.5
glossopharyngeal 352.2
Klumpke (-Déjérine) 767.6
lead 984.9
specified type of lead — see Table of Drugs and Chemicals
median nerve (tardy) 354.0
peroneal nerve (acute) (tardy) 355.3
progressive supranuclear 333.0
pseudobulbar NEC 335.23
radial nerve (acute) 354.3
seventh nerve 351.0
newborn 767.5
shaking (see also Parkinsonism) 332.0
spastic (cerebral) (spinal) 343.9
hemiplegic 343.1
specified nerve NEC — see Disorder, nerve
supranuclear NEC 356.8
progressive 333.0
ulnar nerve (tardy) 354.2
wasting 335.21
Paltauf-Sternberg disease 201.9 ☑
Paludism — see Malaria
Panama fever 084.0
Panaris (with lymphangitis) 681.9
finger 681.02
toe 681.11
Panaritium (with lymphangitis) 681.9
finger 681.02
toe 681.11
Panarteritis (nodosa) 446.0
brain or cerebral 437.4
Pancake heart 793.2
with cor pulmonale (chronic) 416.9
Pancarditis (acute) (chronic) 429.89
with
rheumatic
fever (active) (acute) (chronic) (subacute) 391.8
inactive or quiescent 398.99
rheumatic, acute 391.8
chronic or inactive 398.99

Pancoast's syndrome or tumor (carcinoma, pulmonary apex) (M8010/3) 162.3
Pancoast-Tobias syndrome (M8010/3) (carcinoma, pulmonary apex) 162.3
Pancolitis 556.6
Pancreas, pancreatic — see condition
Pancreatitis 577.0
acute (edematous) (hemorrhagic) (recurrent) 577.0
annular 577.0
apoplectic 577.0
calcerceous 577.0
chronic (infectious) 577.1
recurrent 577.1
cystic 577.2
fibrous 577.8
gangrenous 577.0
hemorrhagic (acute) 577.0
interstitial (chronic) 577.1
acute 577.0
malignant 577.0
mumps 072.3
painless 577.1
recurrent 577.1
relapsing 577.1
subacute 577.0
suppurative 577.0
syphilitic 095.8
Pancreatolithiasis 577.8
Pancytolysis 289.9
Pancytopenia (acquired) 284.19
with
malformations 284.09
myelodysplastic syndrome — see Syndrome, myelodysplastic
congenital 284.09
due to
antineoplastic chemotherapy 284.11
drug, specified NEC 284.12
specified NEC 284.19
Panencephalitis — see also Encephalitis
subacute, sclerosing 046.2
Panhematopenia 284.81
congenital 284.09
constitutional 284.09
splenic, primary 289.4
Panhemocytopenia 284.81
congenital 284.09
constitutional 284.09
Panhypogonadism 257.2
Panhypopituitarism 253.2
prepubertal 253.3
Panic (attack) (state) 300.01
reaction to exceptional stress (transient) 308.0
Panmyelopathy, familial constitutional 284.09
Panmyelophthisis 284.2
acquired (secondary) 284.81
congenital 284.2
idiopathic 284.9
Panmyelosis (acute) (M9951/1) 238.79
Panner's disease 732.3
capitellum humeri 732.3
head of humerus 732.3
tarsal navicular (bone) (osteochondrosis) 732.5
Panneuritis endemica 265.0 [357.4]
Panniculitis 729.30
back 724.8
knee 729.31
mesenteric 567.82
neck 723.6
nodular, nonsuppurative 729.30
sacral 724.8
specified site NEC 729.39
Panniculus adiposus (abdominal) 278.1
Pannus (corneal) 370.62
abdominal (symptomatic) 278.1
allergic eczematous 370.62
degenerativus 370.62
keratic 370.62
rheumatoid — see Arthritis, rheumatoid
trachomatosus, trachomatous (active) 076.1 [370.62]
late effect 139.1

Panophthalmitis 360.02
Panotitis — see Otitis media
Pansinusitis (chronic) (hyperplastic) (nonpurulent) (purulent) 473.8
acute 461.8
due to fungus NEC 117.9
tuberculous (see also Tuberculosis) 012.8 ☑
Panuveitis 360.12
sympathetic 360.11
Panvalvular disease — see Endocarditis, mitral
Papageienkrankheit 073.9
Papanicolaou smear
anus 796.70
with
atypical squamous cells
cannot exclude high grade squamous intraepithelial lesion (ASC-H) 796.72
of undetermined significance (ASC-US) 796.71
cytologic evidence of malignancy 796.76
high grade squamous intraepithelial lesion (HGSIL) 796.74
low grade squamous intraepithelial lesion (LGSIL) 796.73
glandular 796.70
specified finding NEC 796.79
unsatisfactory cytology 796.78
cervix (screening test) V76.2
as part of gynecological examination V72.31
for suspected malignant neoplasm V76.2
no disease found V71.1
inadequate cytology sample 795.08
nonspecific abnormal finding 795.00
with
atypical squamous cells
cannot exclude high grade squamous intraepithelial lesion (ASC-H) 795.02
of undetermined significance (ASC-US) 795.01
cytologic evidence of malignancy 795.06
high grade squamous intraepithelial lesion (HGSIL) 795.04
low grade squamous intraepithelial lesion (LGSIL) 795.03
nonspecific finding NEC 795.09
to confirm findings of recent normal smear following initial abnormal smear V72.32
satisfactory smear but lacking transformation zone 795.07
unsatisfactory cervical cytology 795.08
other specified site (see also Screening, malignant neoplasm)
for suspected malignant neoplasm (see also Screening, malignant neoplasm)
no disease found V71.1
nonspecific abnormal finding 796.9
vagina V76.47
with
atypical squamous cells
cannot exclude high grade squamous intraepithelial lesion (ASC-H) 795.12
of undetermined significance (ASC-US) 795.11
cytologic evidence of malignancy 795.16
high grade squamous intraepithelial lesion (HGSIL) 795.14
low grade squamous intraepithelial lesion (LGSIL) 795.13
abnormal NEC 795.19
following hysterectomy for malignant condition V67.01
inadequate cytology sample 795.18
unsatisfactory cytology 795.18
Papilledema 377.00
associated with
decreased ocular pressure 377.02

☑ **Additional Digit Required** — Refer to the Tabular List for Digit Selection

🔽 **Subterms under main terms may continue to next column or page**

Papilledema — continued
  associated with — continued
    increased intracranial pressure 377.01
    retinal disorder 377.03
  choked disc 377.00
  infectional 377.00
Papillitis 377.31
  anus 569.49
  chronic lingual 529.4
  necrotizing, kidney 584.7
  optic 377.31
  rectum 569.49
  renal, necrotizing 584.7
  tongue 529.0
Papilloma (M8050/0) — see also Neoplasm, by site, benign

> Note — Except where otherwise indicated, the morphological varieties of papilloma in the list below should be coded by site as for "Neoplasm, benign."

  acuminatum (female) (male) 078.11
  bladder (urinary) (transitional cell) (M8120/1) 236.7
    benign (M8120/0) 223.3
  choroid plexus (M9390/0) 225.0
    anaplastic type (M9390/3) 191.5
    malignant (M9390/3) 191.5
  ductal (M8503/0)
  dyskeratotic (M8052/0)
  epidermoid (M8052/0)
  hyperkeratotic (M8052/0)
  intracystic (M8504/0)
  intraductal (M8503/0)
  inverted (M8053/0)
  keratotic (M8052/0)
  parakeratotic (M8052/0)
  pinta (primary) 103.0
  renal pelvis (transitional cell) (M8120/1) 236.99
    benign (M8120/0) 223.1
  Schneiderian (M8121/0)
    specified site — see Neoplasm, by site, benign
    unspecified site 212.0
  serous surface (M8461/0)
    borderline malignancy (M8461/1)
      specified site — see Neoplasm, by site, uncertain behavior
      unspecified site 236.2
    specified site — see Neoplasm, by site, benign
    unspecified site 220
  squamous (cell) (M8052/0)
  transitional (cell) (M8120/0)
    bladder (urinary) (M8120/1) 236.7
    inverted type (M8121/1) — see Neoplasm, by site, uncertain behavior
    renal pelvis (M8120/1) 236.91
    ureter (M8120/1) 236.91
  ureter (transitional cell) (M8120/1) 236.91
    benign (M8120/0) 223.2
  urothelial (M8120/1) — see Neoplasm, by site, uncertain behavior
  verrucous (M8051/0)
  villous (M8261/1) — see Neoplasm, by site, uncertain behavior
  yaws, plantar or palmar 102.1
Papillomata, multiple, of yaws 102.1
Papillomatosis (M8060/0) — see also Neoplasm, by site, benign
  confluent and reticulate 701.8
  cutaneous 701.8
  ductal, breast 610.1
  Gougerot-Carteaud (confluent reticulate) 701.8
  intraductal (diffuse) (M8505/0) — see Neoplasm, by site, benign
  subareolar duct (M8506/0) 217
Papillon-Léage and Psaume syndrome (orodigitofacial dysostosis) 759.89
Papule 709.8
  carate (primary) 103.0
  fibrous, of nose (M8724/0) 216.3
  pinta (primary) 103.0
Papulosis
  lymphomatoid 709.8

Papulosis — continued
  malignant 447.8
Papyraceous fetus 779.89
  complicating pregnancy 646.0 ☑
Paracephalus 759.7
Parachute mitral valve 746.5
Paracoccidioidomycosis 116.1
  mucocutaneous-lymphangitic 116.1
  pulmonary 116.1
  visceral 116.1
Paracoccidiomycosis — see Paracoccidioidomycosis
Paracusis 388.40
Paradentosis 523.5
Paradoxical facial movements 374.43
Paraffinoma 999.9
Paraganglioma (M8680/1)
  adrenal (M8700/0) 227.0
    malignant (M8700/3) 194.0
  aortic body (M8691/1) 237.3
    malignant (M8691/3) 194.6
  carotid body (M8692/1) 237.3
    malignant (M8692/3) 194.5
  chromaffin (M8700/0) (see also Neoplasm, by site, benign)
    malignant (M8700/3) — see Neoplasm, by site, malignant
  extra-adrenal (M8693/1)
    malignant (M8693/3)
      specified site — see Neoplasm, by site, malignant
      unspecified site 194.6
    specified site — see Neoplasm, by site, uncertain behavior
    unspecified site 237.3
  glomus jugulare (M8690/1) 237.3
    malignant (M8690/3) 194.6
  jugular (M8690/1) 237.3
    malignant (M8680/3)
      specified site — see Neoplasm, by site, malignant
      unspecified site 194.6
  nonchromaffin (M8693/1)
    malignant (M8693/3)
      specified site — see Neoplasm, by site, malignant
      unspecified site 194.6
    specified site — see Neoplasm, by site, uncertain behavior
    unspecified site 237.3
  parasympathetic (M8682/1)
    specified site — see Neoplasm, by site, uncertain behavior
    unspecified site 237.3
  specified site — see Neoplasm, by site, uncertain behavior
  sympathetic (M8681/1)
    specified site — see Neoplasm, by site, uncertain behavior
    unspecified site 237.3
  unspecified site 237.3
Parageusia 781.1
  psychogenic 306.7
Paragonimiasis 121.2
Paragranuloma, Hodgkin's (M9660/3) 201.0 ☑
Parahemophilia — see also Defect, coagulation 286.3
Parakeratosis 690.8
  psoriasiformis 696.2
  variegata 696.2
Paralysis, paralytic (complete) (incomplete) 344.9
  with
    broken
      back — see Fracture, vertebra, by site, with spinal cord injury
      neck — see Fracture, vertebra, cervical, with spinal cord injury
    fracture, vertebra — see Fracture, vertebra, by site, with spinal cord injury
  syphilis 094.89
  abdomen and back muscles 355.9
  abdominal muscles 355.9
  abducens (nerve) 378.54

Paralysis, paralytic — continued
  abductor 355.9
    lower extremity 355.8
    upper extremity 354.9
  accessory nerve 352.4
  accommodation 367.51
    hysterical 300.11
  acoustic nerve 388.5
  agitans 332.0
    arteriosclerotic 332.0
  alternating 344.89
    oculomotor 344.89
  amyotrophic 335.20
  ankle 355.8
  anterior serratus 355.9
  anus (sphincter) 569.49
  apoplectic (current episode) (see also Disease, cerebrovascular, acute) 436
    late effect — see Late effect(s) (of) cerebrovascular disease
  arm 344.40
    affecting
      dominant side 344.41
      nondominant side 344.42
    both 344.2
    hysterical 300.11
    late effect — see Late effect(s) (of) cerebrovascular disease
    psychogenic 306.0
    transient 781.4
    traumatic NEC (see also Injury, nerve, upper limb) 955.9
  arteriosclerotic (current episode) 437.0
    late effect — see Late effect(s) (of) cerebrovascular disease
  ascending (spinal), acute 357.0
  associated, nuclear 344.89
  asthenic bulbar 358.00
  ataxic NEC 334.9
    general 094.1
  athetoid 333.71
  atrophic 356.9
    infantile, acute (see also Poliomyelitis, with paralysis) 045.1 ☑
    muscle NEC 355.9
    progressive 335.21
    spinal (acute) (see also Poliomyelitis, with paralysis) 045.1 ☑
  attack (see also Disease, cerebrovascular, acute) 436
  axillary 353.0
  Babinski-Nageotte's 344.89
  Bell's 351.0
    newborn 767.5
  Benedikt's 344.89
  birth (injury) 767.7
    brain 767.0
    intracranial 767.0
    spinal cord 767.4
  bladder (sphincter) 596.53
    neurogenic 596.54
      with cauda equina syndrome 344.61
    puerperal, postpartum, childbirth 665.5 ☑
    sensory 596.54
      with cauda equina 344.61
    spastic 596.54
      with cauda equina 344.61
  bowel, colon, or intestine (see also Ileus) 560.1
  brachial plexus 353.0
    due to birth injury 767.6
    newborn 767.6
  brain
    congenital — see Palsy, cerebral
    current episode 437.8
    diplegia 344.2
    hemiplegia 342.9 ☑
      late effect — see Late effect(s) (of) cerebrovascular disease
    infantile — see Palsy, cerebral
    late effect — see Late effect(s) (of) cerebrovascular disease
    monoplegia (see also Monoplegia)
      late effect — see Late effect(s) (of) cerebrovascular disease

Paralysis, paralytic — continued
  brain — continued
    paraplegia 344.1
    quadriplegia — see Quadriplegia
    syphilitic, congenital 090.49
    triplegia 344.89
  bronchi 519.19
  Brown-Séquard's 344.89
  bulbar (chronic) (progressive) 335.22
    infantile (see also Poliomyelitis, bulbar) 045.0 ☑
    poliomyelitic (see also Poliomyelitis, bulbar) 045.0 ☑
    pseudo 335.23
    supranuclear 344.89
  bulbospinal 358.00
  cardiac (see also Failure, heart) 428.9
  cerebral
    current episode 437.8
    spastic, infantile — see Palsy, cerebral
  cerebrocerebellar 437.8
    diplegic infantile 343.0
  cervical
    plexus 353.2
    sympathetic NEC 337.09
  Céstan-Chenais 344.89
  Charcôt-Marie-Tooth type 356.1
  childhood — see Palsy, cerebral
  Clark's 343.9
  colon (see also Ileus) 560.1
  compressed air 993.3
  compression
    arm NEC 354.9
    cerebral — see Paralysis, brain
    leg NEC 355.8
    lower extremity NEC 355.8
    upper extremity NEC 354.9
  congenital (cerebral) (spastic) (spinal) — see Palsy, cerebral
  conjugate movement (of eye) 378.81
    cortical (nuclear) (supranuclear) 378.81
  convergence 378.83
  cordis (see also Failure, heart) 428.9
  cortical (see also Paralysis, brain) 437.8
  cranial or cerebral nerve (see also Disorder, nerve, cranial) 352.9
  creeping 335.21
  crossed leg 344.89
  crutch 953.4
  deglutition 784.99
    hysterical 300.11
  dementia 094.1
  descending (spinal) NEC 335.9
  diaphragm (flaccid) 519.4
    due to accidental section of phrenic nerve during procedure 998.2
  digestive organs NEC 564.89
  diplegic — see Diplegia
  divergence (nuclear) 378.85
  divers' 993.3
  Duchenne's 335.22
  due to intracranial or spinal birth injury — see Palsy, cerebral
  embolic (current episode) (see also Embolism, brain) 434.1 ☑
    late effect — see Late effect(s) (of) cerebrovascular disease
  enteric (see also Ileus) 560.1
    with hernia — see Hernia, by site, with obstruction
  Erb (-Duchenne) (birth) (newborn) 767.6
  Erb's syphilitic spastic spinal 094.89
  esophagus 530.89
  essential, infancy (see also Poliomyelitis) 045.9 ☑
  extremity
    lower — see Paralysis, leg
    spastic (hereditary) 343.3
      noncongenital or noninfantile 344.1
    transient (cause unknown) 781.4
    upper — see Paralysis, arm
  eye muscle (extrinsic) 378.55
    intrinsic 367.51
  facial (nerve) 351.0
    birth injury 767.5
    congenital 767.5

☑ Additional Digit Required — Refer to the Tabular List for Digit Selection   �om Subterms under main terms may continue to next column or page

224 — Volume 2   ▶◀ Revised Text   ● New Line   ▲ Revised Code   2013 ICD-9-CM

Paralysis, paralytic — *continued*
facial — *continued*
following operation NEC 998.2
newborn 767.5
familial 359.3
periodic 359.3
spastic 334.1
fauces 478.29
finger NEC 354.9
foot NEC 355.8
gait 781.2
gastric nerve 352.3
gaze 378.81
general 094.1
ataxic 094.1
insane 094.1
juvenile 090.40
progressive 094.1
tabetic 094.1
glossopharyngeal (nerve) 352.2
glottis (*see also* Paralysis, vocal cord) 478.30
gluteal 353.4
Gubler (-Millard) 344.89
hand 354.9
hysterical 300.11
psychogenic 306.0
heart (*see also* Failure, heart) 428.9
hemifacial, progressive 349.89
hemiplegic — *see* Hemiplegia
hyperkalemic periodic (familial) 359.3
hypertensive (current episode) 437.8
hypoglossal (nerve) 352.5
hypokalemic periodic 359.3
Hyrtl's sphincter (rectum) 569.49
hysterical 300.11
ileus (*see also* Ileus) 560.1
infantile (*see also* Poliomyelitis) 045.9 ☑
atrophic acute 045.1 ☑
bulbar 045.0 ☑
cerebral — *see* Palsy, cerebral
paralytic 045.1 ☑
progressive acute 045.9 ☑
spastic — *see* Palsy, cerebral
spinal 045.9 ☑
infective (*see also* Poliomyelitis) 045.9 ☑
inferior nuclear 344.89
insane, general or progressive 094.1
internuclear 378.86
interosseous 355.9
intestine (*see also* Ileus) 560.1
intracranial (current episode) (*see also* Paralysis, brain) 437.8
due to birth injury 767.0
iris 379.49
due to diphtheria (toxin) 032.81 [379.49]
ischemic, Volkmann's (complicating trauma) 958.6
isolated sleep, recurrent
Jackson's 344.89
jake 357.7
Jamaica ginger (jake) 357.7
juvenile general 090.40
Klumpke (-Déjérine) (birth) (newborn) 767.6
labioglossal (laryngeal) (pharyngeal) 335.22
Landry's 357.0
laryngeal nerve (recurrent) (superior) (*see also* Paralysis, vocal cord) 478.30
larynx (*see also* Paralysis, vocal cord) 478.30
due to diphtheria (toxin) 032.3
late effect
due to
birth injury, brain or spinal (cord) — *see* Palsy, cerebral
edema, brain or cerebral — *see* Paralysis, brain
lesion
late effect — *see* Late effect(s) (of) cerebrovascular disease
spinal (cord) — *see* Paralysis, spinal
lateral 335.24
lead 984.9
specified type of lead — *see* Table of Drugs and Chemicals
left side — *see* Hemiplegia
leg 344.30

Paralysis, paralytic — *continued*
leg — *continued*
affecting
dominant side 344.31
nondominant side 344.32
both (*see also* Paraplegia) 344.1
crossed 344.89
hysterical 300.11
psychogenic 306.0
transient or transitory 781.4
traumatic NEC (*see also* Injury, nerve, lower limb) 956.9
levator palpebrae superioris 374.31
limb NEC 344.5
all four — *see* Quadriplegia
quadriplegia — *see* Quadriplegia
lip 528.5
Lissauer's 094.1
local 355.9
lower limb (*see also* Paralysis, leg)
both (*see also* Paraplegia) 344.1
lung 518.89
newborn 770.89
median nerve 354.1
medullary (tegmental) 344.89
mesencephalic NEC 344.89
tegmental 344.89
middle alternating 344.89
Millard-Gubler-Foville 344.89
monoplegic — *see* Monoplegia
motor NEC 344.9
cerebral — *see* Paralysis, brain
spinal — *see* Paralysis, spinal
multiple
cerebral — *see* Paralysis, brain
spinal — *see* Paralysis, spinal
muscle (flaccid) 359.9
due to nerve lesion NEC 355.9
eye (extrinsic) 378.55
intrinsic 367.51
oblique 378.51
iris sphincter 364.89
ischemic (complicating trauma) (Volkmann's) 958.6
pseudohypertrophic 359.1
muscular (atrophic) 359.9
progressive 335.21
musculocutaneous nerve 354.9
musculospiral 354.9
nerve (*see also* Disorder, nerve)
third or oculomotor (partial) 378.51
total 378.52
fourth or trochlear 378.53
sixth or abducens 378.54
seventh or facial 351.0
birth injury 767.5
due to
injection NEC 999.9
operation NEC 997.09
newborn 767.5
accessory 352.4
auditory 388.5
birth injury 767.7
cranial or cerebral (*see also* Disorder, nerve, cranial) 352.9
facial 351.0
birth injury 767.5
newborn 767.5
laryngeal (*see also* Paralysis, vocal cord) 478.30
newborn 767.7
phrenic 354.8
newborn 767.7
radial 354.3
birth injury 767.6
newborn 767.6
syphilitic 094.89
traumatic NEC (*see also* Injury, nerve, by site) 957.9
trigeminal 350.9
ulnar 354.2
newborn NEC 767.0
normokalemic periodic 359.3
obstetrical, newborn 767.7
ocular 378.9
oculofacial, congenital 352.6

Paralysis, paralytic — *continued*
oculomotor (nerve) (partial) 378.51
alternating 344.89
external bilateral 378.55
total 378.52
olfactory nerve 352.0
palate 528.9
palatopharyngolaryngeal 352.6
paratrigeminal 350.9
periodic (familial) (hyperkalemic) (hypokalemic) (normokalemic) (potassium sensitive) (secondary) 359.3
peripheral
autonomic nervous system — *see* Neuropathy, peripheral, autonomic
nerve NEC 355.9
peroneal (nerve) 355.3
pharynx 478.29
phrenic nerve 354.8
plantar nerves 355.6
pneumogastric nerve 352.3
poliomyelitis (current) (*see also* Poliomyelitis, with paralysis) 045.1 ☑
bulbar 045.0 ☑
popliteal nerve 355.3
pressure (*see also* Neuropathy, entrapment) 355.9
progressive 335.21
atrophic 335.21
bulbar 335.22
general 094.1
hemifacial 349.89
infantile, acute (*see also* Poliomyelitis) 045.9 ☑
multiple 335.20
pseudobulbar 335.23
pseudohypertrophic 359.1
muscle 359.1
psychogenic 306.0
pupil, pupillary 379.49
quadriceps 355.8
quadriplegic (*see also* Quadriplegia) 344.0 ☑
radial nerve 354.3
birth injury 767.6
rectum (sphincter) 569.49
rectus muscle (eye) 378.55
recurrent
isolated sleep 327.43
laryngeal nerve (*see also* Paralysis, vocal cord) 478.30
respiratory (muscle) (system) (tract) 786.09
center NEC 344.89
fetus or newborn 770.87
congenital 768.9
newborn 768.9
right side — *see* Hemiplegia
Saturday night 354.3
saturnine 984.9
specified type of lead — *see* Table of Drugs and Chemicals
sciatic nerve 355.0
secondary — *see* Paralysis, late effect
seizure (cerebral) (current episode) (*see also* Disease, cerebrovascular, acute) 436
late effect — *see* Late effect(s) (of) cerebrovascular disease
senile NEC 344.9
serratus magnus 355.9
shaking (*see also* Parkinsonism) 332.0
shock (*see also* Disease, cerebrovascular, acute) 436
late effect — *see* Late effect(s) (of) cerebrovascular disease
shoulder 354.9
soft palate 528.9
spasmodic — *see* Paralysis, spastic
spastic 344.9
cerebral infantile — *see* Palsy, cerebral
congenital (cerebral) — *see* Palsy, cerebral
familial 334.1
hereditary 334.1
infantile 343.9
noncongenital or noninfantile, cerebral 344.9

Paralysis, paralytic — *continued*
spastic — *continued*
syphilitic 094.0
spinal 094.89
sphincter, bladder (*see also* Paralysis, bladder) 596.53
spinal (cord) NEC 344.1
accessory nerve 352.4
acute (*see also* Poliomyelitis) 045.9 ☑
ascending acute 357.0
atrophic (acute) (*see also* Poliomyelitis, with paralysis) 045.1 ☑
spastic, syphilitic 094.89
congenital NEC 343.9
hemiplegic — *see* Hemiplegia
hereditary 336.8
infantile (*see also* Poliomyelitis) 045.9 ☑
late effect NEC 344.89
monoplegic — *see* Monoplegia
nerve 355.9
progressive 335.10
quadriplegic — *see* Quadriplegia
spastic NEC 343.9
traumatic — *see* Injury, spinal, by site
sternomastoid 352.4
stomach 536.3
diabetic 250.6 ☑ [536.3]
due to secondary diabetes 249.6 ☑ [536.3]
nerve (nondiabetic) 352.3
stroke (current episode) — *see* Infarct, brain
late effect — *see* Late effect(s) (of) cerebrovascular disease
subscapularis 354.8
superior nuclear NEC 334.9
supranuclear 356.8
sympathetic
cervical NEC 337.09
nerve NEC (*see also* Neuropathy, peripheral, autonomic) 337.9
nervous system — *see* Neuropathy, peripheral, autonomic
syndrome 344.9
specified NEC 344.89
syphilitic spastic spinal (Erb's) 094.89
tabetic general 094.1
thigh 355.8
throat 478.29
diphtheritic 032.0
muscle 478.29
thrombotic (current episode) (*see also* Thrombosis, brain) 434.0 ☑
late effect — *see* Late effect(s) (of) cerebrovascular disease
thumb NEC 354.9
tick (-bite) 989.5
Todd's (postepileptic transitory paralysis) 344.89
toe 355.6
tongue 529.8
transient
arm or leg NEC 781.4
traumatic NEC (*see also* Injury, nerve, by site) 957.9
trapezius 352.4
traumatic, transient NEC (*see also* Injury, nerve, by site) 957.9
trembling (*see also* Parkinsonism) 332.0
triceps brachii 354.9
trigeminal nerve 350.9
trochlear nerve 378.53
ulnar nerve 354.2
upper limb (*see also* Paralysis, arm)
both (*see also* Diplegia) 344.2
uremic — *see* Uremia
uveoparotitic 135
uvula 528.9
hysterical 300.11
postdiphtheritic 032.0
vagus nerve 352.3
vasomotor NEC 337.9
velum palati 528.9
vesical (*see also* Paralysis, bladder) 596.53
vestibular nerve 388.5
visual field, psychic 368.16
vocal cord 478.30

☑ Additional Digit Required — Refer to the Tabular List for Digit Selection
🖉 Subterms under main terms may continue to next column or page
2013 ICD-9-CM ▶◀ Revised Text ● New Line ▲ Revised Code Volume 2 — 225

Index

Paralysis, paralytic — Pathologic, pathological

Paralysis, paralytic — *continued*
   vocal cord — *continued*
      bilateral (partial) 478.33
         complete 478.34
      complete (bilateral) 478.34
      unilateral (partial) 478.31
         complete 478.32
      Volkmann's (complicating trauma) 958.6
      wasting 335.21
      Weber's 344.89
      wrist NEC 354.9
Paramedial orifice, urethrovesical 753.8
Paramenia 626.9
Parametritis (chronic) — *see also* Disease,
      pelvis, inflammatory 614.4
   acute 614.3
   puerperal, postpartum, childbirth 670.8 ☑
Parametrium, parametric — *see* condition
Paramnesia — *see also* Amnesia 780.93
Paramolar 520.1
   causing crowding 524.31
Paramyloidosis 277.30
Paramyoclonus multiplex 333.2
Paramyotonia 359.29
   congenita (of von Eulenburg) 359.29
Paraneoplastic syndrome — *see* condition
Parangi — *see also* Yaws 102.9
Paranoia 297.1
   alcoholic 291.5
   querulans 297.8
   senile 290.20
Paranoid
   dementia (*see also* Schizophrenia) 295.3 ☑
      praecox (acute) 295.3 ☑
      senile 290.20
   personality 301.0
   psychosis 297.9
      alcoholic 291.5
      climacteric 297.2
      drug-induced 292.11
      involutional 297.2
      menopausal 297.2
      protracted reactive 298.4
      psychogenic 298.4
         acute 298.3
      senile 290.20
   reaction (chronic) 297.9
      acute 298.3
   schizophrenia (acute) (*see also* Schizophre-
      nia) 295.3 ☑
   state 297.9
      alcohol-induced 291.5
      climacteric 297.2
      drug-induced 292.11
      due to or associated with
         arteriosclerosis (cerebrovascular)
            290.42
         presenile brain disease 290.12
         senile brain disease 290.20
      involutional 297.2
      menopausal 297.2
      senile 290.20
      simple 297.0
      specified type NEC 297.8
   tendencies 301.0
   traits 301.0
   trends 301.0
   type, psychopathic personality 301.0
Paraparesis — *see also* Paraplegia 344.1
Paraphasia 784.3
Paraphilia — *see also* Deviation, sexual 302.9
Paraphimosis (congenital) 605
   chancroidal 099.0
Paraphrenia, paraphrenic (late) 297.2
   climacteric 297.2
   dementia (*see also* Schizophrenia) 295.3 ☑
   involutional 297.2
   menopausal 297.2
   schizophrenia (acute) (*see also* Schizophre-
      nia) 295.3 ☑
Paraplegia 344.1
   with
      broken back — *see* Fracture, vertebra,
         by site, with spinal cord injury

Paraplegia — *continued*
   with — *continued*
      fracture, vertebra — *see* Fracture, verte-
         bra, by site, with spinal cord in-
         jury
   ataxic — *see* Degeneration, combined,
      spinal cord
   brain (current episode) (*see also* Paralysis,
      brain) 437.8
   cerebral (current episode) (*see also* Paralysis,
      brain) 437.8
   congenital or infantile (cerebral) (spastic)
      (spinal) 343.0
   cortical — *see* Paralysis, brain
   familial spastic 334.1
   functional (hysterical) 300.11
   hysterical 300.11
   infantile 343.0
   late effect 344.1
   Pott's (*see also* Tuberculosis)
      015.0 ☑ *[730.88]*
   psychogenic 306.0
   spastic
      Erb's spinal 094.89
      hereditary 334.1
      not infantile or congenital 344.1
   spinal (cord)
      traumatic NEC — *see* Injury, spinal, by
         site
   syphilitic (spastic) 094.89
   traumatic NEC — *see* Injury, spinal, by site
Paraproteinemia 273.2
   benign (familial) 273.1
   monoclonal 273.1
   secondary to malignant or inflammatory
      disease 273.1
Parapsoriasis 696.2
   en plaques 696.2
   guttata 696.2
   lichenoides chronica 696.2
   retiformis 696.2
   varioliformis (acuta) 696.2
Parascarlatina 057.8
Parasitic — *see also* condition
   disease NEC (*see also* Infestation, parasitic)
      136.9
      contact V01.89
      exposure to V01.89
   intestinal NEC 129
   skin NEC 134.9
   stomatitis 112.0
   sycosis 110.0
      beard 110.0
      scalp 110.0
   twin 759.4
Parasitism NEC 136.9
   intestinal NEC 129
   skin NEC 134.9
   specified — *see* Infestation
Parasitophobia 300.29
Parasomnia 307.47
   alcohol induced 291.82
   drug induced 292.85
   nonorganic origin 307.47
   organic 327.40
      in conditions classified elsewhere 327.44
      other 327.49
Paraspadias 752.69
Paraspasm facialis 351.8
Parathyroid gland — *see* condition
Parathyroiditis (autoimmune) 252.1
Parathyroprival tetany 252.1
Paratrachoma 077.0
Paratyphilitis — *see also* Appendicitis 541
Paratyphoid (fever) — *see* Fever, paratyphoid
Paratyphus — *see* Fever, paratyphoid
Paraurethral duct 753.8
Para-urethritis 597.89
   gonococcal (acute) 098.0
      chronic or duration of 2 months or over
         098.2
Paravaccinia NEC 051.9
   milkers' node 051.1
Paravaginitis — *see also* Vaginitis 616.10
Parencephalitis — *see also* Encephalitis 323.9
   late effect — *see* category 326

Parergasia 298.9
Paresis — *see also* Paralysis 344.9
   accommodation 367.51
   bladder (spastic) (sphincter) (*see also* Paral-
      ysis, bladder) 596.53
      tabetic 094.0
   bowel, colon, or intestine (*see also* Ileus)
      560.1
   brain or cerebral — *see* Paralysis, brain
   extrinsic muscle, eye 378.55
   general 094.1
      arrested 094.1
      brain 094.1
      cerebral 094.1
      insane 094.1
      juvenile 090.40
         remission 090.49
      progressive 094.1
      remission (sustained) 094.1
      tabetic 094.1
   heart (*see also* Failure, heart) 428.9
   infantile (*see also* Poliomyelitis) 045.9 ☑
   insane 094.1
   juvenile 090.40
   late effect — *see* Paralysis, late effect
   luetic (general) 094.1
   peripheral progressive 356.9
   pseudohypertrophic 359.1
   senile NEC 344.9
   stomach 536.3
      diabetic 250.6 ☑ *[536.3]*
         due to secondary diabetes
            249.6 ☑ *[536.3]*
   syphilitic (general) 094.1
      congenital 090.40
   transient, limb 781.4
   vesical (sphincter) NEC 596.53
Paresthesia — *see also* Disturbance, sensation
   782.0
   Berger's (paresthesia of lower limb) 782.0
   Bernhardt 355.1
   Magnan's 782.0
Paretic — *see* condition
Parinaud's
   conjunctivitis 372.02
   oculoglandular syndrome 372.02
   ophthalmoplegia 378.81
   syndrome (paralysis of conjugate upward
      gaze) 378.81
Parkes Weber and Dimitri syndrome (en-
      cephalocutaneous angiomatosis) 759.6
Parkinson's disease, syndrome, or tremor
      — *see* Parkinsonism
Parkinsonism (arteriosclerotic) (idiopathic)
      (primary) 332.0
   associated with orthostatic hypotension
      (idiopathic) (symptomatic) 333.0
   due to drugs 332.1
   neuroleptic-induced 332.1
   secondary 332.1
   syphilitic 094.82
Parodontitis 523.40
Parodontosis 523.5
Paronychia (with lymphangitis) 681.9
   candidal (chronic) 112.3
   chronic 681.9
      candidal 112.3
      finger 681.02
      toe 681.11
   finger 681.02
   toe 681.11
   tuberculous (primary) (*see also* Tuberculosis)
      017.0 ☑
Parorexia NEC 307.52
   hysterical 300.11
Parosmia 781.1
   psychogenic 306.7
Parotid gland — *see* condition
Parotiditis — *see also* Parotitis 527.2
   epidemic 072.9
   infectious 072.9
Parotitis 527.2
   allergic 527.2
   chronic 527.2
   epidemic (*see also* Mumps) 072.9
   infectious (*see also* Mumps) 072.9

Parotitis — *continued*
   noninfectious 527.2
   nonspecific toxic 527.2
   not mumps 527.2
   postoperative 527.2
   purulent 527.2
   septic 527.2
   suppurative (acute) 527.2
   surgical 527.2
   toxic 527.2
Paroxysmal — *see also* condition
   dyspnea (nocturnal) 786.09
Parrot's disease (syphilitic osteochondritis)
      090.0
Parrot fever 073.9
Parry's disease or syndrome (exophthalmic
      goiter) 242.0 ☑
Parry-Romberg syndrome 349.89
Parsonage-Aldren-Turner syndrome 353.5
Parsonage-Turner syndrome 353.5
Parson's disease (exophthalmic goiter)
      242.0 ☑
Pars planitis 363.21
Particolored infant 757.39
Parturition — *see* Delivery
Parvovirus 079.83
   B19 079.83
   human 079.83
Passage
   false, urethra 599.4
   meconium noted during delivery 763.84
   of sounds or bougies (*see also* Attention to
      artificial opening) V55.9
Passive — *see* condition
Pasteurella septica 027.2
Pasteurellosis — *see also* Infection, Pasteurella
      027.2
PAT (paroxysmal atrial tachycardia) 427.0
Patau's syndrome (trisomy D1) 758.1
Patch
   herald 696.3
Patches
   mucous (syphilitic) 091.3
      congenital 090.0
   smokers' (mouth) 528.6
Patellar — *see* condition
Patellofemoral syndrome 719.46
Patent — *see also* Imperfect closure
   atrioventricular ostium 745.69
   canal of Nuck 752.41
   cervix 622.5
      complicating pregnancy 654.5 ☑
         affecting fetus or newborn 761.0
   ductus arteriosus or Botalli 747.0
   Eustachian
      tube 381.7
      valve 746.89
   foramen
      Botalli 745.5
      ovale 745.5
   interauricular septum 745.5
   interventricular septum 745.4
   omphalomesenteric duct 751.0
   os (uteri) — *see* Patent, cervix
   ostium secundum 745.5
   urachus 753.7
   vitelline duct 751.0
Paternity testing V70.4
Paterson-Kelly syndrome or web (sideropenic
      dysphagia) 280.8
Paterson (-Brown) (-Kelly) syndrome
      (sideropenic dysphagia) 280.8
Paterson's syndrome (sideropenic dysphagia)
      280.8
Pathologic, pathological — *see also* condition
   asphyxia 799.01
   drunkenness 291.4
   emotionality 301.3
   fracture — *see* Fracture, pathologic
   liar 301.7
   personality 301.9
   resorption, tooth 521.40
      external 521.42
      internal 521.41
      specified NEC 521.49
   sexuality (*see also* Deviation, sexual) 302.9

☑ Additional Digit Required — Refer to the Tabular List for Digit Selection   🔄 Subterms under main terms may continue to next column or page

226 — Volume 2   ▶◀ Revised Text   ● New Line   ▲ Revised Code   2013 ICD-9-CM

Pathology (of) — *see also* Disease
  periradicular, associated with previous endodontic treatment 526.69
Patterned motor discharge, idiopathic — *see also* Epilepsy 345.5 ☑
Patulous — *see also* Patent
  anus 569.49
  Eustachian tube 381.7
Pause, sinoatrial 427.81
Pavor nocturnus 307.46
Pavy's disease 593.6
Paxton's disease (white piedra) 111.2
Payr's disease or syndrome (splenic flexure syndrome) 569.89
PBA (pseudobulbar affect) 310.81
Pearls
  Elschnig 366.51
  enamel 520.2
Pearl-workers' disease (chronic osteomyelitis) — *see also* Osteomyelitis 730.1 ☑
Pectenitis 569.49
Pectenosis 569.49
Pectoral — *see* condition
Pectus
  carinatum (congenital) 754.82
    acquired 738.3
    rachitic (*see also* Rickets) 268.0
  excavatum (congenital) 754.81
    acquired 738.3
    rachitic (*see also* Rickets) 268.0
  recurvatum (congenital) 754.81
    acquired 738.3
Pedatrophia 261
Pederosis 302.2
Peg-shaped teeth 520.2
Pelade 704.01
Pel's crisis 094.0
Pel-Ebstein disease — *see* Disease, Hodgkin's
Pelger-Huët anomaly or syndrome (hereditary hyposegmentation) 288.2
Peliosis (rheumatica) 287.0
Pelizaeus-Merzbacher
  disease 330.0
  sclerosis, diffuse cerebral 330.0
Pellagra (alcoholic or with alcoholism) 265.2
  with polyneuropathy 265.2 *[357.4]*
Pellagra-cerebellar-ataxia-renal aminoaciduria syndrome 270.0
Pellegrini's disease (calcification, knee joint) 726.62
Pellegrini (-Stieda) disease or syndrome (calcification, knee joint) 726.62
Pellizzi's syndrome (pineal) 259.8
Pelvic — *see also* condition
  congestion-fibrosis syndrome 625.5
  kidney 753.3
Pelvioectasis 591
Pelviolithiasis 592.0
Pelviperitonitis
  female (*see also* Peritonitis, pelvic, female) 614.5
  male (*see also* Peritonitis) 567.21
Pelvis, pelvic — *see also* condition or type
  infantile 738.6
  Nägele's 738.6
  obliquity 738.6
  Robert's 755.69
Pemphigoid 694.5
  benign, mucous membrane 694.60
    with ocular involvement 694.61
  bullous 694.5
  cicatricial 694.60
    with ocular involvement 694.61
  juvenile 694.2
Pemphigus 694.4

Pemphigus — *continued*
  benign 694.5
    chronic familial 757.39
  Brazilian 694.4
  circinatus 694.0
  congenital, traumatic 757.39
  conjunctiva 694.61
  contagiosus 684
  erythematodes 694.4
  erythematosus 694.4
  foliaceus 694.4
  frambesiodes 694.4
  gangrenous (*see also* Gangrene) 785.4
  malignant 694.4
  neonatorum, newborn 684
  ocular 694.61
  papillaris 694.4
  seborrheic 694.4
  South American 694.4
  syphilitic (congenital) 090.0
  vegetans 694.4
  vulgaris 694.4
  wildfire 694.4
Pendred's syndrome (familial goiter with deafmutism) 243
Pendulous
  abdomen 701.9
    in pregnancy or childbirth 654.4 ☑
      affecting fetus or newborn 763.89
  breast 611.89
Penetrating wound — *see also* Wound, open, by site
  with internal injury — *see* Injury, internal, by site, with open wound
  eyeball 871.7
    with foreign body (nonmagnetic) 871.6
      magnetic 871.5
  ocular (*see also* Penetrating wound, eyeball) 871.7
    adnexa 870.3
      with foreign body 870.4
  orbit 870.3
    with foreign body 870.4
Penetration, pregnant uterus by instrument
  with
    abortion — *see* Abortion, by type, with damage to pelvic organs
    ectopic pregnancy (*see also* categories 633.0–633.9) 639.2
    molar pregnancy (*see also* categories 630–632) 639.2
  complication of delivery 665.1 ☑
    affecting fetus or newborn 763.89
  following
    abortion 639.2
    ectopic or molar pregnancy 639.2
Penfield's syndrome — *see also* Epilepsy 345.5 ☑
Penicilliosis of lung 117.3
Penis — *see* condition
Penitis 607.2
Pentalogy (of Fallot) 745.2
Penta X syndrome 758.81
Pentosuria (benign) (essential) 271.8
Peptic acid disease 536.8
Peregrinating patient V65.2
Perforated — *see* Perforation
Perforation, perforative (nontraumatic)
  antrum (*see also* Sinusitis, maxillary) 473.0
  appendix 540.0
    with peritoneal abscess 540.1
  atrial septum, multiple 745.5
  attic, ear 384.22
    healed 384.81
  bile duct, except cystic (*see also* Disease, biliary) 576.3
    cystic 575.4
  bladder (urinary) 596.6
    with
      abortion — *see* Abortion, by type, with damage to pelvic organs
      ectopic pregnancy (*see also* categories 633.0–633.9) 639.2
      molar pregnancy (*see also* categories 630–632) 639.2

Perforation, perforative — *continued*
  bladder — *continued*
    following
      abortion 639.2
      ectopic or molar pregnancy 639.2
    obstetrical trauma 665.5 ☑
  bowel 569.83
    with
      abortion — *see* Abortion, by type, with damage to pelvic organs
      ectopic pregnancy (*see also* categories 633.0–633.9) 639.2
      molar pregnancy (*see also* categories 630–632) 639.2
    fetus or newborn 777.6
    following
      abortion 639.2
      ectopic or molar pregnancy 639.2
    obstetrical trauma 665.5 ☑
  broad ligament
    with
      abortion — *see* Abortion, by type, with damage to pelvic organs
      ectopic pregnancy (*see also* categories 633.0–633.9) 639.2
      molar pregnancy (*see also* categories 630–632) 639.2
    following
      abortion 639.2
      ectopic or molar pregnancy 639.2
    obstetrical trauma 665.6 ☑
  by
    device, implant, or graft — *see* Complications, mechanical
    foreign body left accidentally in operation wound 998.4
    instrument (any) during a procedure, accidental 998.2
  cecum 540.0
    with peritoneal abscess 540.1
  cervix (uteri) (*see also* Injury, internal, cervix)
    with
      abortion — *see* Abortion, by type, with damage to pelvic organs
      ectopic pregnancy (*see also* categories 633.0–633.9) 639.2
      molar pregnancy (*see also* categories 630–632) 639.2
    following
      abortion 639.2
      ectopic or molar pregnancy 639.2
    obstetrical trauma 665.3 ☑
  colon 569.83
  common duct (bile) 576.3
  cornea (*see also* Ulcer, cornea) 370.00
    due to ulceration 370.06
  cystic duct 575.4
  diverticulum (*see also* Diverticula) 562.10
    small intestine 562.00
  duodenum, duodenal (ulcer) — *see* Ulcer, duodenum, with perforation
  ear drum — *see* Perforation, tympanum
  enteritis — *see* Enteritis
  esophagus 530.4
  ethmoidal sinus (*see also* Sinusitis, ethmoidal) 473.2
  foreign body (external site) (*see also* Wound, open, by site, complicated)
    internal site, by ingested object — *see* Foreign body
  frontal sinus (*see also* Sinusitis, frontal) 473.1
  gallbladder or duct (*see also* Disease, gallbladder) 575.4
  gastric (ulcer) — *see* Ulcer, stomach, with perforation
  heart valve — *see* Endocarditis
  ileum (*see also* Perforation, intestine) 569.83
  instrumental
    external — *see* Wound, open, by site
    pregnant uterus, complicating delivery 665.9 ☑
    surgical (accidental) (blood vessel) (nerve) (organ) 998.2
  intestine 569.83

Perforation, perforative — *continued*
  intestine — *continued*
    with
      abortion — *see* Abortion, by type, with damage to pelvic organs
      ectopic pregnancy (*see also* categories 633.0–633.9) 639.2
      molar pregnancy (*see also* categories 630–632) 639.2
    fetus or newborn 777.6
    obstetrical trauma 665.5 ☑
    ulcerative NEC 569.83
  jejunum, jejunal 569.83
    ulcer — *see* Ulcer, gastrojejunal, with perforation
  mastoid (antrum) (cell) 383.89
  maxillary sinus (*see also* Sinusitis, maxillary) 473.0
  membrana tympani — *see* Perforation, tympanum
  nasal
    septum 478.19
      congenital 748.1
      syphilitic 095.8
    sinus (*see also* Sinusitis) 473.9
      congenital 748.1
  palate (hard) 526.89
    soft 528.9
      syphilitic 095.8
      syphilitic 095.8
  palatine vault 526.89
    syphilitic 095.8
      congenital 090.5
  pelvic
    floor
      with
        abortion — *see* Abortion, by type, with damage to pelvic organs
        ectopic pregnancy (*see also* categories 633.0–633.9) 639.2
        molar pregnancy (*see also* categories 630–632) 639.2
      obstetrical trauma 664.1 ☑
    organ
      with
        abortion — *see* Abortion, by type, with damage to pelvic organs
        ectopic pregnancy (*see also* categories 633.0–633.9) 639.2
        molar pregnancy (*see also* categories 630–632) 639.2
      following
        abortion 639.2
        ectopic or molar pregnancy 639.2
      obstetrical trauma 665.5 ☑
  perineum — *see* Laceration, perineum
  periurethral tissue
    with
      abortion — *see* Abortion, by type, with damage to pelvic organs
      ectopic pregnancy (*see also* categories 630–632) 639.2
      molar pregnancy (*see also* categories 630–632) 639.2
  pharynx 478.29
  pylorus, pyloric (ulcer) — *see* Ulcer, stomach, with perforation
  rectum 569.49
  root canal space 526.61
  sigmoid 569.83
  sinus (accessory) (chronic) (nasal) (*see also* Sinusitis) 473.9
  sphenoidal sinus (*see also* Sinusitis, sphenoidal) 473.3
  stomach (due to ulcer) — *see* Ulcer, stomach, with perforation
  surgical (accidental) (by instrument) (blood vessel) (nerve) (organ) 998.2
  traumatic
    external — *see* Wound, open, by site
    eye (*see also* Penetrating wound, ocular) 871.7
    internal organ — *see* Injury, internal, by site

☑ **Additional Digit Required — Refer to the Tabular List for Digit Selection**   ▽ **Subterms under main terms may continue to next column or page**

Perforation, perforative — *continued*
  tympanum (membrane) (persistent posttrau-
    matic) (postinflammatory) 384.20
    with
      otitis media — *see* Otitis media
    attic 384.22
    central 384.21
    healed 384.81
    marginal NEC 384.23
    multiple 384.24
    pars flaccida 384.22
    total 384.25
    traumatic — *see* Wound, open, ear,
      drum
  typhoid, gastrointestinal 002.0
  ulcer — *see* Ulcer, by site, with perforation
  ureter 593.89
  urethra
    with
      abortion — *see* Abortion, by type,
        with damage to pelvic organs
      ectopic pregnancy (*see also* cate-
        gories 633.0–633.9) 639.2
      molar pregnancy (*see also* categories
        630–632) 639.2
    following
      abortion 639.2
      ectopic or molar pregnancy 639.2
    obstetrical trauma 665.5 ☑
  uterus (*see also* Injury, internal, uterus)
    with
      abortion — *see* Abortion, by type,
        with damage to pelvic organs
      ectopic pregnancy (*see also* cate-
        gories 633.0–633.9) 639.2
      molar pregnancy (*see also* categories
        630–632) 639.2
    by intrauterine contraceptive device
      996.32
    following
      abortion 639.2
      ectopic or molar pregnancy 639.2
    obstetrical trauma — *see* Injury, internal,
      uterus, obstetrical trauma
  uvula 528.9
    syphilitic 095.8
  vagina — *see* Laceration, vagina
  viscus NEC 799.89
    traumatic 868.00
      with open wound into cavity 868.10
Periadenitis mucosa necrotica recurrens
  528.2
Periangiitis 446.0
Periantritis 535.4 ☑
Periappendicitis (acute) — *see also* Appendicitis 541
Periarteritis (disseminated) (infectious)
  (necrotizing) (nodosa) 446.0
Periarthritis (joint) 726.90
  Duplay's 726.2
  gonococcal 098.50
  humeroscapularis 726.2
  scapulohumeral 726.2
  shoulder 726.2
  wrist 726.4
Periarthrosis (angioneural) — *see* Periarthritis
Peribronchitis 491.9
  tuberculous (*see also* Tuberculosis) 011.3 ☑
Pericapsulitis, adhesive (shoulder) 726.0
Pericarditis (granular) (with decompensation)
  (with effusion) 423.9
  with
    rheumatic fever (conditions classifiable
      to 390)
      active (*see also* Pericarditis,
        rheumatic) 391.0
      inactive or quiescent 393
  actinomycotic 039.8 *[420.0]*
  acute (nonrheumatic) 420.90
    with chorea (acute) (rheumatic) (Syden-
      ham's) 392.0
    bacterial 420.99
    benign 420.91
    hemorrhagic 420.90
    idiopathic 420.91
    infective 420.90

Pericarditis — *continued*
  acute — *continued*
    nonspecific 420.91
    rheumatic 391.0
      with chorea (acute) (rheumatic)
        (Sydenham's) 392.0
    sicca 420.90
    viral 420.91
  adhesive or adherent (external) (internal)
    423.1
    acute — *see* Pericarditis, acute
    rheumatic (external) (internal) 393
  amebic 006.8 *[420.0]*
  bacterial (acute) (subacute) (with serous or
    seropurulent effusion) 420.99
  calcareous 423.2
  cholesterol (chronic) 423.8
    acute 420.90
  chronic (nonrheumatic) 423.8
    rheumatic 393
  constrictive 423.2
  Coxsackie 074.21
  due to
    actinomycosis 039.8 *[420.0]*
    amebiasis 006.8 *[420.0]*
    Coxsackie (virus) 074.21
    histoplasmosis (*see also* Histoplasmosis)
      115.93
    nocardiosis 039.8 *[420.0]*
    tuberculosis (*see also* Tuberculosis)
      017.9 ☑ *[420.0]*
  fibrinocaseous (*see also* Tuberculosis)
    017.9 ☑ *[420.0]*
  fibrinopurulent 420.99
  fibrinous — *see* Pericarditis, rheumatic
  fibropurulent 420.99
  fibrous 423.1
  gonococcal 098.83
  hemorrhagic 423.0
  idiopathic (acute) 420.91
  infective (acute) 420.90
  meningococcal 036.41
  neoplastic (chronic) 423.8
    acute 420.90
  nonspecific 420.91
  obliterans, obliterating 423.1
  plastic 423.1
  pneumococcal (acute) 420.99
  postinfarction 411.0
  purulent (acute) 420.99
  rheumatic (active) (acute) (with effusion)
    (with pneumonia) 391.0
    with chorea (acute) (rheumatic) (Syden-
      ham's) 392.0
    chronic or inactive (with chorea) 393
  septic (acute) 420.99
  serofibrinous — *see* Pericarditis, rheumatic
  staphylococcal (acute) 420.99
  streptococcal (acute) 420.99
  suppurative (acute) 420.99
  syphilitic 093.81
  tuberculous (acute) (chronic) (*see also* Tuber-
    culosis) 017.9 ☑ *[420.0]*
  uremic 585.9 *[420.0]*
  viral (acute) 420.91
Pericardium, pericardial — *see* condition
Pericellulitis — *see also* Cellulitis 682.9
Pericementitis 523.40
  acute 523.30
  chronic (suppurative) 523.40
Pericholecystitis — *see also* Cholecystitis
  575.10
Perichondritis
  auricle 380.00
    acute 380.01
    chronic 380.02
  bronchus 491.9
  ear (external) 380.00
    acute 380.01
    chronic 380.02
  larynx 478.71
    syphilitic 095.8
    typhoid 002.0 *[478.71]*
  nose 478.19
  pinna 380.00
    acute 380.01

Perichondritis — *continued*
  pinna — *continued*
    chronic 380.02
  trachea 478.9
Periclasia 523.5
Pericolitis 569.89
Pericoronitis (chronic) 523.40
  acute 523.33
Pericystitis — *see also* Cystitis 595.9
Pericytoma (M9150/1) — *see also* Neoplasm,
  connective tissue, uncertain behavior
  benign (M9150/0) — *see* Neoplasm, connec-
    tive tissue, benign
  malignant (M9150/3) — *see* Neoplasm,
    connective tissue, malignant
Peridacryocystitis, acute 375.32
Peridiverticulitis — *see also* Diverticulitis
  562.11
Periduodenitis 535.6 ☑
Periendocarditis — *see also* Endocarditis
  424.90
  acute or subacute 421.9
Periepididymitis — *see also* Epididymitis
  604.90
Perifolliculitis (abscedens) 704.8
  capitis, abscedens et suffodiens 704.8
  dissecting, scalp 704.8
  scalp 704.8
  superficial pustular 704.8
Perigastritis (acute) 535.0 ☑
Perigastrojejunitis (acute) 535.0 ☑
Perihepatitis (acute) 573.3
  chlamydial 099.56
  gonococcal 098.86
Peri-ileitis (subacute) 569.89
Perilabyrinthitis (acute) — *see* Labyrinthitis
Perimeningitis — *see* Meningitis
Perimetritis — *see also* Endometritis 615.9
Perimetrosalpingitis — *see also* Salpingo-
  oophoritis 614.2
Perineocele 618.05
Perinephric — *see* condition
Perinephritic — *see* condition
Perinephritis — *see also* Infection, kidney
  590.9
  purulent (*see also* Abscess, kidney) 590.2
Perineum, perineal — *see* condition
Perineuritis NEC 729.2
Periodic — *see also* condition
  disease (familial) 277.31
  edema 995.1
    hereditary 277.6
  fever 277.31
  headache syndromes in child or adolescent
    346.2 ☑
  limb movement disorder 327.51
  paralysis (familial) 359.3
  peritonitis 277.31
  polyserositis 277.31
  somnolence (*see also* Narcolepsy) 347.00
Periodontal
  cyst 522.8
  pocket 523.8
Periodontitis (chronic) (complex) (compound)
  (simplex) 523.40
  acute 523.33
  aggressive 523.30
    generalized 523.32
    localized 523.31
  apical 522.6
    acute (pulpal origin) 522.4
  generalized 523.42
  localized 523.41
Periodontoclasia 523.5
Periodontosis 523.5
Periods — *see also* Menstruation
  heavy 626.2
  irregular 626.4
Perionychia (with lymphangitis) 681.9
  finger 681.02
  toe 681.11
Perioophoritis — *see also* Salpingo-oophoritis
  614.2
Periorchitis — *see also* Orchitis 604.90
Periosteum, periosteal — *see* condition

Periostitis (circumscribed) (diffuse) (infective)
  730.3 ☑

Note — *Use the following fifth-digit*
subclassification with category 730:

0	*site unspecified*
1	*shoulder region*
2	*upper arm*
3	*forearm*
4	*hand*
5	*pelvic region and thigh*
6	*lower leg*
7	*ankle and foot*
8	*other specified sites*
9	*multiple sites*

  with osteomyelitis (*see also* Osteomyelitis)
    730.2 ☑
    acute or subacute 730.0 ☑
    chronic or old 730.1 ☑
  albuminosa, albuminosus 730.3 ☑
  alveolar 526.5
  alveolodental 526.5
  dental 526.5
  gonorrheal 098.89
  hyperplastica, generalized 731.2
  jaw (lower) (upper) 526.4
  monomelic 733.99
  orbital 376.02
  syphilitic 095.5
    congenital 090.0 *[730.8]* ☑
    secondary 091.61
  tuberculous (*see also* Tuberculosis, bone)
    015.9 ☑ *[730.8]* ☑
  yaws (early) (hypertrophic) (late) 102.6
Periostosis — *see also* Periostitis 730.3 ☑
  with osteomyelitis (*see also* Osteomyelitis)
    730.2 ☑
    acute or subacute 730.0 ☑
    chronic or old 730.1 ☑
  hyperplastic 756.59
Peripartum cardiomyopathy 674.5 ☑
Periphlebitis — *see also* Phlebitis 451.9
  lower extremity 451.2
    deep (vessels) 451.19
    superficial (vessels) 451.0
  portal 572.1
  retina 362.18
  superficial (vessels) 451.0
  tuberculous (*see also* Tuberculosis) 017.9 ☑
    retina 017.3 ☑ *[362.18]*
Peripneumonia — *see* Pneumonia
Periproctitis 569.49
Periprostatitis — *see also* Prostatitis 601.9
Perirectal — *see* condition
Perirenal — *see* condition
Perisalpingitis — *see also* Salpingo-oophoritis
  614.2
Perisigmoiditis 569.89
Perisplenitis (infectional) 289.59
Perispondylitis — *see* Spondylitis
Peristalsis reversed or visible 787.4
Peritendinitis — *see also* Tenosynovitis 726.90
  adhesive (shoulder) 726.0
Perithelioma (M9150/1) — *see* Pericytoma
Peritoneum, peritoneal — *see also* condition
  equilibration test V56.32
Peritonitis (acute) (adhesive) (fibrinous)
  (hemorrhagic) (idiopathic) (localized)
  (perforative) (primary) (with adhesions)
  (with effusion) 567.9
  with or following
    abortion — *see* Abortion, by type, with
      sepsis
    abscess 567.21
    appendicitis 540.0
      with peritoneal abscess 540.1
    ectopic pregnancy (*see also* categories
      633.0–633.9) 639.0
    molar pregnancy (*see also* categories
      630–632) 639.0
  aseptic 998.7

Peritonitis — *continued*
- bacterial 567.29
  - spontaneous 567.23
- bile, biliary 567.81
- chemical 998.7
- chlamydial 099.56
- chronic proliferative 567.89
- congenital NEC 777.6
- diaphragmatic 567.22
- diffuse NEC 567.29
- diphtheritic 032.83
- disseminated NEC 567.29
- due to
  - bile 567.81
  - foreign
    - body or object accidentally left during a procedure (instrument) (sponge) (swab) 998.4
    - substance accidentally left during a procedure (chemical) (powder) (talc) 998.7
  - talc 998.7
  - urine 567.89
- fibrinopurulent 567.29
- fibrinous 567.29
- fibrocaseous (*see also* Tuberculosis) 014.0 ☑
- fibropurulent 567.29
- general, generalized (acute) 567.21
- gonococcal 098.86
- in infective disease NEC 136.9 *[567.0]*
- meconium (newborn) 777.6
- pancreatic 577.8
- paroxysmal, benign 277.31
- pelvic
  - female (acute) 614.5
    - chronic NEC 614.7
      - with adhesions 614.6
    - puerperal, postpartum, childbirth 670.8 ☑
  - male (acute) 567.21
- periodic (familial) 277.31
- phlegmonous 567.29
- pneumococcal 567.1
- postabortal 639.0
- proliferative, chronic 567.89
- puerperal, postpartum, childbirth 670.8 ☑
- purulent 567.29
- septic 567.29
- spontaneous bacterial 567.23
- staphylococcal 567.29
- streptococcal 567.29
- subdiaphragmatic 567.29
- subphrenic 567.29
- suppurative 567.29
- syphilitic 095.2
  - congenital 090.0 *[567.0]*
- talc 998.7
- tuberculous (*see also* Tuberculosis) 014.0 ☑
- urine 567.89

Peritonsillar — *see* condition
Peritonsillitis 475
Perityphlitis — *see also* Appendicitis 541
Periureteritis 593.89
Periurethral — *see* condition
Periurethritis (gangrenous) 597.89
Periuterine — *see* condition
Perivaginitis — *see also* Vaginitis 616.10
Perivasculitis, retinal 362.18
Perivasitis (chronic) 608.4
Periventricular leukomalacia 779.7
Perivesiculitis (seminal) — *see also* Vesiculitis 608.0
Perlèche 686.8
- due to
  - moniliasis 112.0
  - riboflavin deficiency 266.0
Pernicious — *see* condition
Pernio, perniosis 991.5
Persecution
- delusion 297.9
- social V62.4
Perseveration (tonic) 784.69
Persistence, persistent (congenital) 759.89
- anal membrane 751.2
- arteria stapedia 744.04
- atrioventricular canal 745.69

Persistence, persistent — *continued*
- bloody ejaculate 792.2
- branchial cleft 744.41
- bulbus cordis in left ventricle 745.8
- canal of Cloquet 743.51
- capsule (opaque) 743.51
- cilioretinal artery or vein 743.51
- cloaca 751.5
- communication — *see* Fistula, congenital
- convolutions
  - aortic arch 747.21
  - fallopian tube 752.19
  - oviduct 752.19
  - uterine tube 752.19
- double aortic arch 747.21
- ductus
  - arteriosus 747.0
  - Botalli 747.0
- fetal
  - circulation 747.83
  - form of cervix (uteri) 752.49
  - hemoglobin (hereditary) ("Swiss variety") 282.7
  - pulmonary hypertension 747.83
- foramen
  - Botalli 745.5
  - ovale 745.5
- Gartner's duct 752.41
- hemoglobin, fetal (hereditary) (HPFH) 282.7
- hyaloid
  - artery (generally incomplete) 743.51
  - system 743.51
- hymen (tag)
  - in pregnancy or childbirth 654.8 ☑
    - causing obstructed labor 660.2 ☑
- lanugo 757.4
- left
  - posterior cardinal vein 747.49
  - root with right arch of aorta 747.21
  - superior vena cava 747.49
- Meckel's diverticulum 751.0
- mesonephric duct 752.89
  - fallopian tube 752.11
- mucosal disease (middle ear) (with posterior or superior marginal perforation of ear drum) 382.2
- nail(s), anomalous 757.5
- occiput, anterior or posterior 660.3 ☑
  - fetus or newborn 763.1
- omphalomesenteric duct 751.0
- organ or site NEC — *see* Anomaly, specified type NEC
- ostium
  - atrioventriculare commune 745.69
  - primum 745.61
  - secundum 745.5
- ovarian rests in fallopian tube 752.19
- pancreatic tissue in intestinal tract 751.5
- primary (deciduous)
  - teeth 520.6
  - vitreous hyperplasia 743.51
- pulmonary hypertension 747.83
- pupillary membrane 743.46
  - iris 743.46
- Rhesus (Rh) titer (*see also* Complications, transfusion) 999.70
- right aortic arch 747.21
- sinus
  - urogenitalis 752.89
  - venosus with imperfect incorporation in right auricle 747.49
- thymus (gland) 254.8
  - hyperplasia 254.0
- thyroglossal duct 759.2
- thyrolingual duct 759.2
- truncus arteriosus or communis 745.0
- tunica vasculosa lentis 743.39
- umbilical sinus 753.7
- urachus 753.7
- vegetative state 780.03
- vitelline duct 751.0
- wolffian duct 752.89
Person (with)
- admitted for clinical research, as participant or control subject V70.7

Person — *continued*
- affected by
  - family member
    - currently on deployment (military) V61.01
    - returned from deployment (military) (current or past conflict) V61.02
- awaiting admission to adequate facility elsewhere V63.2
- undergoing social agency investigation V63.8
- concern (normal) about sick person in family V61.49
- consulting on behalf of another V65.19
  - pediatric
    - pre-adoption visit for adoptive parents V65.11
    - pre-birth visit for expectant parents V65.11
- currently deployed in theater or in support of military war, peacekeeping and humanitarian operations V62.21
- feared
  - complaint in whom no diagnosis was made V65.5
  - condition not demonstrated V65.5
- feigning illness V65.2
- healthy, accompanying sick person V65.0
- history of military war, peacekeeping and humanitarian deployment (current or past conflict) V62.22
- living (in)
  - without
    - adequate
      - financial resources V60.2
      - housing (heating) (space) V60.1
    - housing (permanent) (temporary) V60.0
    - material resources V60.2
    - person able to render necessary care V60.4
    - shelter V60.0
  - alone V60.3
  - boarding school V60.6
  - residence remote from hospital or medical care facility V63.0
  - residential institution V60.6
- medical services in home not available V63.1
- on waiting list V63.2
  - undergoing social agency investigation V63.8
- sick or handicapped in family V61.49
- "worried well" V65.5
Personality
- affective 301.10
- aggressive 301.3
- amoral 301.7
- anancastic, anankastic 301.4
- antisocial 301.7
- asocial 301.7
- asthenic 301.6
- avoidant 301.82
- borderline 301.83
- change 310.1
- compulsive 301.4
- cycloid 301.13
- cyclothymic 301.13
- dependent 301.6
- depressive (chronic) 301.12
- disorder, disturbance NEC 301.9
  - with
    - antisocial disturbance 301.7
    - pattern disturbance NEC 301.9
    - sociopathic disturbance 301.7
    - trait disturbance 301.9
- dual 300.14
- dyssocial 301.7
- eccentric 301.89
  - "haltlose" type 301.89
- emotionally unstable 301.59
- epileptoid 301.3
- explosive 301.3
- fanatic 301.0
- histrionic 301.50
- hyperthymic 301.11

Personality — *continued*
- hypomanic 301.11
- hypothymic 301.12
- hysterical 301.50
- immature 301.89
- inadequate 301.6
- labile 301.59
- masochistic 301.89
- morally defective 301.7
- multiple 300.14
- narcissistic 301.81
- obsessional 301.4
- obsessive-compulsive 301.4
- overconscientious 301.4
- paranoid 301.0
- passive (-dependent) 301.6
- passive-aggressive 301.84
- pathologic NEC 301.9
- pattern defect or disturbance 301.9
- pseudosocial 301.7
- psychoinfantile 301.59
- psychoneurotic NEC 301.89
- psychopathic 301.9
  - with
    - amoral trend 301.7
    - antisocial trend 301.7
    - asocial trend 301.7
    - pathologic sexuality (*see also* Deviation, sexual) 302.9
  - mixed types 301.9
- schizoid 301.20
- type A 301.4
- unstable (emotional) 301.59
Perthes' disease (capital femoral osteochondrosis) 732.1
Pertussis — *see also* Whooping cough 033.9
- vaccination, prophylactic (against) V03.6
Peruvian wart 088.0
Perversion, perverted
- appetite 307.52
  - hysterical 300.11
- function
  - pineal gland 259.8
  - pituitary gland 253.9
    - anterior lobe
      - deficient 253.2
      - excessive 253.1
    - posterior lobe 253.6
  - placenta — *see* Placenta, abnormal
- sense of smell or taste 781.1
  - psychogenic 306.7
- sexual (*see also* Deviation, sexual) 302.9
Pervious, congenital — *see also* Imperfect, closure
- ductus arteriosus 747.0
Pes (congenital) — *see also* Talipes 754.70
- abductus (congenital) 754.60
  - acquired 736.79
- acquired NEC 736.79
  - planus 734
- adductus (congenital) 754.79
  - acquired 736.79
- cavus 754.71
  - acquired 736.73
- planovalgus (congenital) 754.69
  - acquired 736.79
- planus (acquired) (any degree) 734
  - congenital 754.61
  - rachitic 268.1
- valgus (congenital) 754.61
  - acquired 736.79
- varus (congenital) 754.50
  - acquired 736.79
Pest — *see also* Plague 020.9
Pestis — *see also* Plague 020.9
- bubonica 020.0
- fulminans 020.0
- minor 020.8
- pneumonica — *see* Plague, pneumonic
Petechial
- fever 036.0
- typhus 081.9
Petechia, petechiae 782.7
- fetus or newborn 772.6
Petges-Cléjat or Petges-Clégat syndrome (poikilodermatomyositis) 710.3

☑ Additional Digit Required — Refer to the Tabular List for Digit Selection   🔻 Subterms under main terms may continue to next column or page

2013 ICD-9-CM   ▶◀ Revised Text   ● New Line   ▲ Revised Code   Volume 2 — 229

Petit's
disease (see also Hernia, lumbar) 553.8
Petit mal (idiopathic) — see also Epilepsy
345.0 ☑
status 345.2
Petrellidosis 117.6
Petrositis 383.20
acute 383.21
chronic 383.22
Peutz-Jeghers disease or syndrome 759.6
Peyronie's disease 607.85
Pfeiffer's disease 075
Phacentocele 379.32
traumatic 921.3
Phacoanaphylaxis 360.19
Phacocele (old) 379.32
traumatic 921.3
Phaehyphomycosis 117.8
Phagedena (dry) (moist) — see also Gangrene
785.4
arteriosclerotic 440.24
geometric 686.09
penis 607.89
senile 440.2 ☑ [785.4]
sloughing 785.4
tropical (see also Ulcer, skin) 707.9
vulva 616.50
Phagedenic — see also condition
abscess (see also Abscess)
chancroid 099.0
bubo NEC 099.8
chancre 099.0
ulcer (tropical) (see also Ulcer, skin) 707.9
Phagomania 307.52
Phakoma 362.89
Phantom limb (syndrome) 353.6
Pharyngeal — see also condition
arch remnant 744.41
pouch syndrome 279.11
Pharyngitis (acute) (catarrhal) (gangrenous)
(infective) (malignant) (membranous)
(phlegmonous) (pneumococcal) (pseudomembranous) (simple) (staphylococcal) (subacute) (suppurative) (ulcerative)
(viral) 462
with influenza, flu, or grippe (see also Influenza) 487.1
aphthous 074.0
atrophic 472.1
chlamydial 099.51
chronic 472.1
Coxsackie virus 074.0
diphtheritic (membranous) 032.0
follicular 472.1
fusospirochetal 101
gonococcal 098.6
granular (chronic) 472.1
herpetic 054.79
hypertrophic 472.1
infectional, chronic 472.1
influenzal (see also Influenza) 487.1
lymphonodular, acute 074.8
septic 034.0
streptococcal 034.0
tuberculous (see also Tuberculosis) 012.8 ☑
vesicular 074.0
Pharyngoconjunctival fever 077.2
Pharyngoconjunctivitis, viral 077.2
Pharyngolaryngitis (acute) 465.0
chronic 478.9
septic 034.0
Pharyngoplegia 478.29
Pharyngotonsillitis 465.8
tuberculous 012.8 ☑
Pharyngotracheitis (acute) 465.8
chronic 478.9
Pharynx, pharyngeal — see condition
Phase of life problem NEC V62.89
Phenomenon
Arthus' 995.21
flashback (drug) 292.89
jaw-winking 742.8
Jod-Basedow 242.8 ☑
L. E. cell 710.0
lupus erythematosus cell 710.0

Phenomenon — continued
Pelger-Huët (hereditary hyposegmentation)
288.2
Raynaud's (paroxysmal digital cyanosis)
(secondary) 443.0
Reilly's (see also Neuropathy, peripheral,
autonomic) 337.9
vasomotor 780.2
vasospastic 443.9
vasovagal 780.2
Wenckebach's, heart block (second degree)
426.13
Phenylketonuria (PKU) 270.1
Phenylpyruvicaciduria 270.1
Pheochromoblastoma (M8700/3)
specified site — see Neoplasm, by site, malignant
unspecified site 194.0
Pheochromocytoma (M8700/0)
malignant (M8700/3)
specified site — see Neoplasm, by site,
malignant
unspecified site 194.0
specified site — see Neoplasm, by site, benign
unspecified site 227.0
Phimosis (congenital) 605
chancroidal 099.0
due to infection 605
Phlebectasia — see also Varicose, vein 454.9
congenital NEC 747.60
esophagus (see also Varix, esophagus) 456.1
with hemorrhage (see also Varix, esophagus, bleeding) 456.0
Phlebitis (infective) (pyemic) (septic) (suppurative) 451.9
antecubital vein 451.82
arm NEC 451.84
axillary vein 451.89
basilic vein 451.82
deep 451.83
superficial 451.82
axillary vein 451.89
basilic vein 451.82
blue 451.9
brachial vein 451.83
breast, superficial 451.89
cavernous (venous) sinus — see Phlebitis,
intracranial sinus
cephalic vein 451.82
cerebral (venous) sinus — see Phlebitis, intracranial sinus
chest wall, superficial 451.89
complicating pregnancy or puerperium
671.2 ☑
affecting fetus or newborn 760.3
cranial (venous) sinus — see Phlebitis, intracranial sinus
deep (vessels) 451.19
femoral vein 451.11
specified vessel NEC 451.19
due to implanted device — see Complications, due to (presence of) any device, implant, or graft classified to
996.0–996.5 NEC
during or resulting from a procedure 997.2
femoral vein (deep) (superficial) 451.11
femoropopliteal 451.19
following infusion, perfusion, or transfusion
999.2
gouty 274.89 [451.9]
hepatic veins 451.89
iliac vein 451.81
iliofemoral 451.11
intracranial sinus (any) (venous) 325
late effect — see category 326
nonpyogenic 437.6
in pregnancy or puerperium 671.5 ☑
jugular vein 451.89
lateral (venous) sinus — see Phlebitis, intracranial sinus
leg 451.2
deep (vessels) 451.19
femoral vein 451.11
specified vessel NEC 451.19
superficial (vessels) 451.0

Phlebitis — continued
leg — continued
superficial — continued
femoral vein 451.11
longitudinal sinus — see Phlebitis, intracranial sinus
lower extremity 451.2
deep (vessels) 451.19
femoral vein 451.11
specified vessel NEC 451.19
migrans, migrating (superficial) 453.1
superficial (vessels) 451.0
femoral vein 451.11
pelvic
with
abortion — see Abortion, by type,
with sepsis
ectopic pregnancy (see also categories 633.0–633.9) 639.0
molar pregnancy (see also categories
630–632) 639.0
following
abortion 639.0
ectopic or molar pregnancy 639.0
puerperal, postpartum 671.4 ☑
popliteal vein 451.19
portal (vein) 572.1
postoperative 997.2
pregnancy 671.2 ☑
deep 671.3 ☑
specified type NEC 671.5 ☑
superficial 671.2 ☑
puerperal, postpartum, childbirth 671.2 ☑
deep 671.4 ☑
lower extremities 671.2 ☑
pelvis 671.4 ☑
specified site NEC 671.5 ☑
superficial 671.2 ☑
radial vein 451.83
retina 362.18
saphenous (great) (long) 451.0
accessory or small 451.0
sinus (meninges) — see Phlebitis, intracranial sinus
specified site NEC 451.89
subclavian vein 451.89
syphilitic 093.89
tibial vein 451.19
ulcer, ulcerative 451.9
leg 451.2
deep (vessels) 451.19
femoral vein 451.11
specified vessel NEC 451.19
superficial (vessels) 451.0
femoral vein 451.11
lower extremity 451.2
deep (vessels) 451.19
femoral vein 451.11
specified vessel NEC 451.19
superficial (vessels) 451.0
ulnar vein 451.83
umbilicus 451.89
upper extremity (see also Phlebitis, arm)
deep (veins) 451.83
brachial vein 451.83
radial vein 451.83
ulnar vein 451.83
superficial (veins) 451.82
antecubital vein 451.82
basilica vein 451.82
cephalic vein 451.82
uterus (septic) (see also Endometritis) 615.9
varicose (leg) (lower extremity) (see also
Varicose, vein) 454.1
Phlebofibrosis 459.89
Phleboliths 459.89
Phlebosclerosis 459.89
Phlebothrombosis — see Thrombosis
Phlebotomus fever 066.0
Phlegmasia
alba dolens (deep vessels) 451.19
complicating pregnancy 671.3 ☑
nonpuerperal 451.19
puerperal, postpartum, childbirth
671.4 ☑
cerulea dolens 451.19

Phlegm, choked on 933.1
Phlegmon — see also Abscess 682.9
erysipelatous (see also Erysipelas) 035
iliac 682.2
fossa 540.1
throat 478.29
Phlegmonous — see condition
Phlyctenulosis (allergic) (keratoconjunctivitis)
(nontuberculous) 370.31
cornea 370.31
with ulcer (see also Ulcer, cornea) 370.00
tuberculous (see also Tuberculosis)
017.3 ☑ [370.31]
Phobia, phobic (reaction) 300.20
animal 300.29
isolated NEC 300.29
obsessional 300.3
simple NEC 300.29
social 300.23
specified NEC 300.29
state 300.20
Phocas' disease 610.1
Phocomelia 755.4
lower limb 755.32
complete 755.33
distal 755.35
proximal 755.34
upper limb 755.22
complete 755.23
distal 755.25
proximal 755.24
Phoria — see also Heterophoria 378.40
Phosphate-losing tubular disorder 588.0
Phosphatemia 275.3
Phosphaturia 275.3
Photoallergic response 692.72
Photocoproporphyria 277.1
Photodermatitis (sun) 692.72
light other than sun 692.82
Photokeratitis 370.24
Photo-ophthalmia 370.24
Photophobia 368.13
Photopsia 368.15
Photoretinitis 363.31
Photoretinopathy 363.31
Photosensitiveness (sun) 692.72
light other than sun 692.82
Photosensitization (skin) (sun) 692.72
light other than sun 692.82
Phototoxic response 692.72
Phrenitis 323.9
Phrynoderma 264.8
Phthiriasis (pubis) (any site) 132.2
with any infestation classifiable to
132.0, 132.1, 132.3
Phthirus infestation — see Phthiriasis
Phthisis — see also Tuberculosis 011.9 ☑
bulbi (infectional) 360.41
colliers' 011.4 ☑
cornea 371.05
eyeball (due to infection) 360.41
millstone makers' 011.4 ☑
miners' 011.4 ☑
potters' 011.4 ☑
sandblasters' 011.4 ☑
stonemasons' 011.4 ☑
Phycomycosis 117.7
Physalopteriasis 127.7
Physical therapy NEC V57.1
breathing exercises V57.0
Physiological cup, optic papilla
borderline, glaucoma suspect 365.00
enlarged 377.14
glaucomatous 377.14
Phytobezoar 938
intestine 936
stomach 935.2
Pian — see also Yaws 102.9
Pianoma 102.1
Piarhemia, piarrhemia — see also Hyperlipemia 272.4
bilharziasis 120.9
Pica 307.52
hysterical 300.11
Pick's
cerebral atrophy 331.11

☑ Additional Digit Required — Refer to the Tabular List for Digit Selection   ⬃ Subterms under main terms may continue to next column or page

230 — Volume 2   ▶◀ Revised Text   ● New Line   ▲ Revised Code   2013 ICD-9-CM

Pick's — continued
  cerebral atrophy — continued
    with dementia
      with behavioral disturbance
        331.11 [294.11]
      without behavioral disturbance
        331.11 [294.10]
  disease
    brain 331.11
      dementia in
        with behavioral disturbance
          331.11 [294.11]
        without behavioral disturbance
          331.11 [294.10]
    lipid histiocytosis 272.7
    liver (pericardial pseudocirrhosis of liver) 423.2
    pericardium (pericardial pseudocirrhosis of liver) 423.2
    polyserositis (pericardial pseudocirrhosis of liver) 423.2
    syndrome
      heart (pericardial pseudocirrhosis of liver) 423.2
      liver (pericardial pseudocirrhosis of liver) 423.2
  tubular adenoma (M8640/0)
    specified site — see Neoplasm, by site, benign
    unspecified site
      female 220
      male 222.0
Pick-Herxheimer syndrome (diffuse idiopathic cutaneous atrophy) 701.8
Pick-Niemann disease (lipid histiocytosis) 272.7
Pickwickian syndrome (cardiopulmonary obesity) 278.03
Piebaldism, classic 709.09
Piedra 111.2
  beard 111.2
    black 111.3
    white 111.2
  black 111.3
  scalp 111.3
    black 111.3
    white 111.2
  white 111.2
Pierre Marie-Bamberger syndrome (hypertrophic pulmonary osteoarthropathy) 731.2
Pierre Marie's syndrome (pulmonary hypertrophic osteoarthropathy) 731.2
Pierre Mauriac's syndrome (diabetes-dwarfism-obesity) 258.1
Pierre Robin deformity or syndrome (congenital) 756.0
Pierson's disease or osteochondrosis 732.1
Pigeon
  breast or chest (acquired) 738.3
    congenital 754.82
    rachitic (see also Rickets) 268.0
  breeders' disease or lung 495.2
  fanciers' disease or lung 495.2
  toe 735.8
Pigmentation (abnormal) 709.00
  anomaly 709.00
    congenital 757.33
    specified NEC 709.09
  conjunctiva 372.55
  cornea 371.10
    anterior 371.11
    posterior 371.13
    stromal 371.12
  lids (congenital) 757.33
    acquired 374.52
  limbus corneae 371.10
  metals 709.00
  optic papilla, congenital 743.57
  retina (congenital) (grouped) (nevoid) 743.53
    acquired 362.74
  scrotum, congenital 757.33
Piles — see Hemorrhoids
Pili
  annulati or torti (congenital) 757.4

Pili — continued
  incarnati 704.8
Pill roller hand (intrinsic) 736.09
Pilomatrixoma (M8110/0) — see Neoplasm, skin, benign
Pilonidal — see condition
Pimple 709.8
PIN I (prostatic intraepithelial neoplasia I) 602.3
PIN II (prostatic intraepithelial neoplasia II) 602.3
PIN III (prostatic intraepithelial neoplasia III) 233.4
Pinched nerve — see Neuropathy, entrapment
Pineal body or gland — see condition
Pinealoblastoma (M9362/3) 194.4
Pinealoma (M9360/1) 237.1
  malignant (M9360/3) 194.4
Pineoblastoma (M9362/3) 194.4
Pineocytoma (M9361/1) 237.1
Pinguecula 372.51
Pingueculitis 372.34
Pinhole meatus — see also Stricture, urethra 598.9
Pink
  disease 985.0
  eye 372.03
  puffer 492.8
Pinkus' disease (lichen nitidus) 697.1
Pinpoint
  meatus (see also Stricture, urethra) 598.9
  os uteri (see also Stricture, cervix) 622.4
Pinselhaare (congenital) 757.4
Pinta 103.9
  cardiovascular lesions 103.2
  chancre (primary) 103.0
  erythematous plaques 103.1
  hyperchrome lesions 103.1
  hyperkeratosis 103.1
  lesions 103.9
    cardiovascular 103.2
    hyperchromic 103.1
    intermediate 103.1
    late 103.2
    mixed 103.3
    primary 103.0
    skin (achromic) (cicatricial) (dyschromic) 103.2
      hyperchromic 103.1
      mixed (achromic and hyperchromic) 103.3
  papule (primary) 103.0
  skin lesions (achromic) (cicatricial) (dyschromic) 103.2
    hyperchromic 103.1
    mixed (achromic and hyperchromic) 103.3
  vitiligo 103.2
Pintid 103.0
Pinworms (disease) (infection) (infestation) 127.4
Piry fever 066.8
Pistol wound — see Gunshot wound
Pitchers' elbow 718.82
Pithecoid pelvis 755.69
  with disproportion (fetopelvic) 653.2 ☑
    affecting fetus or newborn 763.1
    causing obstructed labor 660.1 ☑
Pithiatism 300.11
Pit, lip (mucus), **congenital** 750.25
Pitted — see also Pitting
  teeth 520.4
Pitting (edema) — see also Edema 782.3
  lip 782.3
  nail 703.8
    congenital 757.5
Pituitary gland — see condition
Pituitary snuff-takers' disease 495.8
Pityriasis 696.5
  alba 696.5
  capitis 690.11
  circinata (et maculata) 696.3
  Hebra's (exfoliative dermatitis) 695.89
  lichenoides et varioliformis 696.2
  maculata (et circinata) 696.3
  nigra 111.1
  pilaris 757.39

Pityriasis — continued
  pilaris — continued
    acquired 701.1
    Hebra's 696.4
  rosea 696.3
  rotunda 696.3
  rubra (Hebra) 695.89
    pilaris 696.4
  sicca 690.18
  simplex 690.18
  specified type NEC 696.5
  streptogenes 696.5
  versicolor 111.0
    scrotal 111.0
Placenta, placental
  ablatio 641.2 ☑
    affecting fetus or newborn 762.1
  abnormal, abnormality 656.7 ☑
    with hemorrhage 641.8 ☑
      affecting fetus or newborn 762.1
    affecting fetus or newborn 762.2
  abruptio 641.2 ☑
    affecting fetus or newborn 762.1
  accessory lobe — see Placenta, abnormal
  accreta (without hemorrhage) 667.0 ☑
    with hemorrhage 666.0 ☑
  adherent (without hemorrhage) 667.0 ☑
    with hemorrhage 666.0 ☑
  apoplexy — see Placenta, separation
  battledore — see Placenta, abnormal
  bilobate — see Placenta, abnormal
  bipartita — see Placenta, abnormal
  carneous mole 631.8
  centralis — see Placenta, previa
  circumvallata — see Placenta, abnormal
  cyst (amniotic) — see Placenta, abnormal
  deficiency — see Placenta, insufficiency
  degeneration — see Placenta, insufficiency
  detachment (partial) (premature) (with hemorrhage) 641.2 ☑
    affecting fetus or newborn 762.1
  dimidiata — see Placenta, abnormal
  disease 656.7 ☑
    affecting fetus or newborn 762.2
  duplex — see Placenta, abnormal
  dysfunction — see Placenta, insufficiency
  fenestrata — see Placenta, abnormal
  fibrosis — see Placenta, abnormal
  fleshy mole 631.8
  hematoma — see Placenta, abnormal
  hemorrhage NEC — see Placenta, separation
  hormone disturbance or malfunction — see Placenta, abnormal
  hyperplasia — see Placenta, abnormal
  increta (without hemorrhage) 667.0 ☑
    with hemorrhage 666.0 ☑
  infarction 656.7 ☑
    affecting fetus or newborn 762.2
  insertion, vicious — see Placenta, previa
  insufficiency
    affecting
      fetus or newborn 762.2
      management of pregnancy 656.5 ☑
  lateral — see Placenta, previa
  low implantation or insertion — see Placenta, previa
  low-lying — see Placenta, previa
  malformation — see Placenta, abnormal
  malposition — see Placenta, previa
  marginalis, marginata — see Placenta, previa
  marginal sinus (hemorrhage) (rupture) 641.2 ☑
    affecting fetus or newborn 762.1
  membranacea — see Placenta, abnormal
  multilobed — see Placenta, abnormal
  multipartita — see Placenta, abnormal
  necrosis — see Placenta, abnormal
  percreta (without hemorrhage) 667.0 ☑
    with hemorrhage 666.0 ☑
  polyp 674.4 ☑
  previa (central) (centralis) (complete) (lateral) (marginal) (marginalis) (partial) (partialis) (total) (with hemorrhage) 641.1 ☑

Placenta, placental — continued
  previa — continued
    without hemorrhage (before labor and delivery) (during pregnancy) 641.0 ☑
    affecting fetus or newborn 762.0
    noted
      before labor, without hemorrhage (with cesarean delivery) 641.0 ☑
      during pregnancy (without hemorrhage) 641.0 ☑
  retention (with hemorrhage) 666.0 ☑
    without hemorrhage 667.0 ☑
    fragments, complicating puerperium (delayed hemorrhage) 666.2 ☑
      without hemorrhage 667.1 ☑
    postpartum, puerperal 666.2 ☑
  separation (normally implanted) (partial) (premature) (with hemorrhage) 641.2 ☑
    affecting fetus or newborn 762.1
  septuplex — see Placenta, abnormal
  small — see Placenta, insufficiency
  softening (premature) — see Placenta, abnormal
  spuria — see Placenta, abnormal
  succenturiata — see Placenta, abnormal
  syphilitic 095.8
  transfusion syndromes 762.3
  transmission of chemical substance — see Absorption, chemical, through placenta
  trapped (with hemorrhage) 666.0 ☑
    without hemorrhage 667.0 ☑
  trilobate — see Placenta, abnormal
  tripartita — see Placenta, abnormal
  triplex — see Placenta, abnormal
  varicose vessel — see Placenta, abnormal
  vicious insertion — see Placenta, previa
Placentitis
  affecting fetus or newborn 762.7
  complicating pregnancy 658.4 ☑
Plagiocephaly (skull) 754.0
Plague 020.9
  abortive 020.8
  ambulatory 020.8
  bubonic 020.0
  cellulocutaneous 020.1
  lymphatic gland 020.0
  pneumonic 020.5
    primary 020.3
    secondary 020.4
  pulmonary — see Plague, pneumonic
  pulmonic — see Plague, pneumonic
  septicemic 020.2
  tonsillar 020.9
    septicemic 020.2
  vaccination, prophylactic (against) V03.3
Planning, family V25.09
  contraception V25.9
  natural
    procreative V26.41
    to avoid pregnancy V25.04
  procreation V26.49
    natural V26.41
Plaque
  artery, arterial — see Arteriosclerosis
  calcareous — see Calcification
  Hollenhorst's (retinal) 362.33
  tongue 528.6
Plasma cell myeloma 203.0 ☑
Plasmacytoma, plasmacytoma (solitary) (M9731/1) 238.6
  benign (M9731/0) — see Neoplasm, by site, benign
  malignant (M9731/3) 203.8 ☑
Plasmacytopenia 288.59
Plasmacytosis 288.64
Plaster ulcer — see also Ulcer, pressure 707.00
Plateau iris syndrome (without glaucoma) 364.82
  with glaucoma 365.23
Platybasia 756.0
Platyonychia (congenital) 757.5
  acquired 703.8

☑ **Additional Digit Required** — Refer to the Tabular List for Digit Selection   ™ **Subterms under main terms may continue to next column or page**

2013 ICD-9-CM   ▶◀ Revised Text   ● New Line   ▲ Revised Code   Volume 2 — 231

Platypelloid pelvis 738.6
  with disproportion (fetopelvic) 653.2 ☑
    affecting fetus or newborn 763.1
    causing obstructed labor 660.1 ☑
      affecting fetus or newborn 763.1
  congenital 755.69
Platyspondylia 756.19
Plethora 782.62
  newborn 776.4
Pleuralgia 786.52
Pleura, pleural — see condition
Pleurisy (acute) (adhesive) (chronic) (costal)
    (diaphragmatic) (double) (dry) (fetid)
    (fibrinous) (fibrous) (interlobar) (latent)
    (lung) (old) (plastic) (primary) (residual)
    (sicca) (sterile) (subacute) (unresolved)
    (with adherent pleura) 511.0
  with
    effusion (without mention of cause)
        511.9
      bacterial, nontuberculous 511.1
      nontuberculous NEC 511.9
        bacterial 511.1
        pneumococcal 511.1
        specified type NEC 511.89
        staphylococcal 511.1
        streptococcal 511.1
        tuberculous (see also Tuberculosis,
            pleura) 012.0 ☑
          primary, progressive 010.1 ☑
    influenza, flu, or grippe (see also Influen-
        za) 487.1
    tuberculosis — see Pleurisy, tuberculous
  encysted 511.89
  exudative (see also Pleurisy, with effusion)
      511.9
    bacterial, nontuberculous 511.1
  fibrinopurulent 510.9
    with fistula 510.0
  fibropurulent 510.9
    with fistula 510.0
  hemorrhagic 511.89
  influenzal (see also Influenza) 487.1
  pneumococcal 511.0
    with effusion 511.1
  purulent 510.9
    with fistula 510.0
  septic 510.9
    with fistula 510.0
  serofibrinous (see also Pleurisy, with effu-
      sion) 511.9
    bacterial, nontuberculous 511.1
  seropurulent 510.9
    with fistula 510.0
  serous (see also Pleurisy, with effusion) 511.9
    bacterial, nontuberculous 511.1
  staphylococcal 511.0
    with effusion 511.1
  streptococcal 511.0
    with effusion 511.1
  suppurative 510.9
    with fistula 510.0
  traumatic (post) (current) 862.29
    with open wound into cavity 862.39
  tuberculous (with effusion) (see also Tuber-
      culosis, pleura) 012.0 ☑
    primary, progressive 010.1 ☑
Pleuritis sicca — see Pleurisy
Pleurobronchopneumonia — see also Pneu-
    monia, broncho- 485
Pleurodynia 786.52
  epidemic 074.1
  viral 074.1
Pleurohepatitis 573.8
Pleuropericarditis — see also Pericarditis 423.9
  acute 420.90
Pleuropneumonia (acute) (bilateral) (double)
    (septic) — see also Pneumonia 486
  chronic (see also Fibrosis, lung) 515
Pleurorrhea — see also Hydrothorax 511.89
Plexitis, brachial 353.0
Plica
  knee 727.83
  polonica 132.0
  syndrome 727.83
  tonsil 474.8

Plicae dysphonia ventricularis 784.49
Plicated tongue 529.5
  congenital 750.13
Plug
  bronchus NEC 519.19
  meconium (newborn) NEC 777.1
  mucus — see Mucus, plug
Plumbism 984.9
  specified type of lead — see Table of Drugs
      and Chemicals
Plummer's disease (toxic nodular goiter)
    242.3 ☑
Plummer-Vinson syndrome (sideropenic
    dysphagia) 280.8
Pluricarential syndrome of infancy 260
Plurideficiency syndrome of infancy 260
Plus (and minus) hand (intrinsic) 736.09
PMDD (premenstrual dysphoric disorder) 625.4
PMS 625.4
Pneumathemia — see Air, embolism, by
    type
Pneumatic drill or hammer disease 994.9
Pneumatocele (lung) 518.89
  intracranial 348.89
  tension 492.0
Pneumatosis
  cystoides intestinalis 569.89
  peritonei 568.89
  pulmonum 492.8
Pneumaturia 599.84
Pneumoblastoma (M8981/3) — see Neoplasm,
    lung, malignant
Pneumocephalus 348.89
Pneumococcemia 038.2
Pneumococcus, pneumococcal — see condi-
    tion
Pneumoconiosis (due to) (inhalation of) 505
  aluminum 503
  asbestos 501
  bagasse 495.1
  bauxite 503
  beryllium 503
  carbon electrode makers' 503
  coal
    miners' (simple) 500
    workers' (simple) 500
  cotton dust 504
  diatomite fibrosis 502
  dust NEC 504
    inorganic 503
    lime 502
    marble 502
    organic NEC 504
  fumes or vapors (from silo) 506.9
  graphite 503
  hard metal 503
  mica 502
  moldy hay 495.0
  rheumatoid 714.81
  silica NEC 502
    and carbon 500
  silicate NEC 502
  talc 502
Pneumocystis carinii pneumonia 136.3
Pneumocystis jiroveci pneumonia 136.3
Pneumocystosis 136.3
  with pneumonia 136.3
Pneumoenteritis 025
Pneumohemopericardium — see also Peri-
    carditis 423.9
Pneumohemothorax — see also Hemothorax
    511.89
  traumatic 860.4
    with open wound into thorax 860.5
Pneumohydropericardium — see also Peri-
    carditis 423.9
Pneumohydrothorax — see also Hydrothorax
    511.89
Pneumomediastinum 518.1
  congenital 770.2
  fetus or newborn 770.2
Pneumomycosis 117.9

Pneumonia (acute) (Alpenstich) (benign) (bi-
    lateral) (brain) (cerebral) (circumscribed)
    (congestive) (creeping) (delayed resolu-
    tion) (double) (epidemic) (fever) (flash)
    (fulminant) (fungoid) (granulomatous)
    (hemorrhagic) (incipient) (infantile) (in-
    fectious) (infiltration) (insular) (intermit-
    tent) (latent) (lobe) (migratory) (new-
    born) (organized) (overwhelming) (pri-
    mary) (progressive) (pseudolobar) (puru-
    lent) (resolved) (secondary) (senile)
    (septic) (suppurative) (terminal) (true)
    (unresolved) (vesicular) 486
  with influenza, flu, or grippe 487.0
    due to
      identified (virus)
        avian 488.01
        (novel) 2009 H1N1 488.11
        novel influenza A 488.81
  adenoviral 480.0
  adynamic 514
  alba 090.0
  allergic 518.3
  alveolar — see Pneumonia, lobar
  anaerobes 482.81
  anthrax 022.1 [484.5]
  apex, apical — see Pneumonia, lobar
  ascaris 127.0 [484.8]
  aspiration 507.0
    due to
      aspiration of microorganisms
        bacterial 482.9
          specified type NEC 482.89
        specified organism NEC 483.8
          bacterial NEC 482.89
        viral 480.9
          specified type NEC 480.8
      food (regurgitated) 507.0
      gastric secretions 507.0
      milk 507.0
      oils, essences 507.1
      solids, liquids NEC 507.8
      vomitus 507.0
    fetal 770.18
      due to
        blood 770.16
        clear amniotic fluid 770.14
        meconium 770.12
        postnatal stomach contents
            770.86
    newborn 770.18
      due to
        blood 770.16
        clear amniotic fluid 770.14
        meconium 770.12
        postnatal stomach contents
            770.86
  asthenic 514
  atypical (disseminated) (focal) (primary) 486
    with influenza (see also Influenza) 487.0
  bacillus 482.9
    specified type NEC 482.89
  bacterial 482.9
    specified type NEC 482.89
  Bacteroides (fragilis) (oralis) (melaninogeni-
      cus) 482.81
  basal, basic, basilar — see Pneumonia, by
      type
  bronchiolitis obliterans organized (BOOP)
      516.8
  broncho-, bronchial (confluent) (croupous)
      (diffuse) (disseminated) (hemorrhag-
      ic) (involving lobes) (lobar) (terminal)
      485
    with influenza 487.0
      due to
        identified (virus)
          avian 488.01
          (novel) 2009 H1N1 488.11
          novel influenza A 488.81
    allergic 518.3
    aspiration (see also Pneumonia, aspira-
        tion) 507.0
    bacterial 482.9
      specified type NEC 482.89
    capillary 466.19

Pneumonia — continued
  broncho-, bronchial — continued
    capillary — continued
      with bronchospasm or obstruction
          466.19
    chronic (see also Fibrosis, lung) 515
    congenital (infective) 770.0
    diplococcal 481
    Eaton's agent 483.0
    Escherichia coli (E. coli) 482.82
    Friedländer's bacillus 482.0
    Hemophilus influenzae 482.2
    hiberno-vernal 083.0 [484.8]
    hypostatic 514
    influenzal (see also Influenza) 487.0
    inhalation (see also Pneumonia, aspira-
        tion) 507.0
      due to fumes or vapors (chemical)
          506.0
    Klebsiella 482.0
    lipid 507.1
      endogenous 516.8
    Mycoplasma (pneumoniae) 483.0
    ornithosis 073.0
    pleuropneumonia-like organisms (PPLO)
        483.0
    pneumococcal 481
    Proteus 482.83
    Pseudomonas 482.1
    specified organism NEC 483.8
      bacterial NEC 482.89
    staphylococcal 482.40
      aureus 482.41
        methicillin
          resistant (MRSA) 482.42
          susceptible (MSSA) 482.41
      specified type NEC 482.49
    streptococcal — see Pneumonia, strep-
        tococcal
    typhoid 002.0 [484.8]
    viral, virus (see also Pneumonia, viral)
        480.9
  Butyrivibrio (fibriosolvens) 482.81
  Candida 112.4
  capillary 466.19
    with bronchospasm or obstruction
        466.19
  caseous (see also Tuberculosis) 011.6 ☑
  catarrhal — see Pneumonia, broncho-
  central — see Pneumonia, lobar
  Chlamydia, chlamydial 483.1
    pneumoniae 483.1
    psittaci 073.0
    specified type NEC 483.1
    trachomatis 483.1
  cholesterol 516.8
  chronic (see also Fibrosis, lung) 515
  cirrhotic (chronic) (see also Fibrosis, lung)
      515
  Clostridium (haemolyticum) (novyi) NEC
      482.81
  confluent — see Pneumonia, broncho-
  congenital (infective) 770.0
    aspiration 770.18
  croupous — see Pneumonia, lobar
  cryptogenic organizing 516.36
  cytomegalic inclusion 078.5 [484.1]
  deglutition (see also Pneumonia, aspiration)
      507.0
  desquamative interstitial 516.37
  diffuse — see Pneumonia, broncho-
  diplococcal, diplococcus (broncho-) (lobar)
      481
  disseminated (focal) — see Pneumonia,
      broncho-
  due to
    adenovirus 480.0
    anaerobes 482.81
    Bacterium anitratum 482.83
    Chlamydia, chlamydial 483.1
      pneumoniae 483.1
      psittaci 073.0
      specified type NEC 483.1
      trachomatis 483.1
    coccidioidomycosis 114.0
    Diplococcus (pneumoniae) 481

☑ Additional Digit Required — Refer to the Tabular List for Digit Selection   ⚐ Subterms under main terms may continue to next column or page

232 — Volume 2   ▶◀ Revised Text   ● New Line   ▲ Revised Code   2013 ICD-9-CM

Pneumonia — continued
  due to — continued
    Eaton's agent 483.0
    Escherichia coli (E. coli) 482.82
    Friedländer's bacillus 482.0
    fumes or vapors (chemical) (inhalation) 506.0
    fungus NEC 117.9 [484.7]
      coccidioidomycosis 114.0
    Hemophilus influenzae (H. influenzae) 482.2
    Herellea 482.83
    influenza (see also Influenza) 487.0
    Klebsiella pneumoniae 482.0
    Mycoplasma (pneumoniae) 483.0
    parainfluenza virus 480.2
    pleuropneumonia-like organism (PPLO) 483.0
    Pneumococcus 481
    Pneumocystis carinii 136.3
    Pneumocystis jiroveci 136.3
    Proteus 482.83
    Pseudomonas 482.1
    respiratory syncytial virus 480.1
    rickettsia 083.9 [484.8]
    SARS-associated coronavirus 480.3
    specified
      bacteria NEC 482.89
      organism NEC 483.8
      virus NEC 480.8
    Staphylococcus 482.40
      aureus 482.41
        methicillin
          resistant (MRSA) 482.42
          susceptible (MSSA) 482.41
      specified type NEC 482.49
    Streptococcus (see also Pneumonia, streptococcal)
      pneumoniae 481
    virus (see also Pneumonia, viral) 480.9
      SARS-associated coronavirus 480.3
  Eaton's agent 483.0
  embolic, embolism — (see Embolism, pulmonary
  eosinophilic 518.3
  Escherichia coli (E. coli) 482.82
  Eubacterium 482.81
  fibrinous — see Pneumonia, lobar
  fibroid (chronic) (see also Fibrosis, lung) 515
  fibrous (see also Fibrosis, lung) 515
  Friedländer's bacillus 482.0
  Fusobacterium (nucleatum) 482.81
  gangrenous 513.0
  giant cell (see also Pneumonia, viral) 480.9
  gram-negative bacteria NEC 482.83
    anaerobic 482.81
  grippal (see also Influenza) 487.0
  Hemophilus influenzae (bronchial) (lobar) 482.2
  hypostatic (broncho-) (lobar) 514
  in
    actinomycosis 039.1
    anthrax 022.1 [484.5]
    aspergillosis 117.3 [484.6]
    candidiasis 112.4
    coccidioidomycosis 114.0
    cytomegalic inclusion disease 078.5 [484.1]
    histoplasmosis (see also Histoplasmosis) 115.95
    infectious disease NEC 136.9 [484.8]
    measles 055.1
    mycosis, systemic NEC 117.9 [484.7]
    nocardiasis, nocardiosis 039.1
    ornithosis 073.0
    pneumocystosis 136.3
    psittacosis 073.0
    Q fever 083.0 [484.8]
    salmonellosis 003.22
    toxoplasmosis 130.4
    tularemia 021.2
    typhoid (fever) 002.0 [484.8]
    varicella 052.1
    whooping cough (see also Whooping cough) 033.9 [484.3]
  infective, acquired prenatally 770.0

Pneumonia — continued
  influenzal (broncho) (lobar) (virus) (see also Influenza) 487.0
  inhalation (see also Pneumonia, aspiration) 507.0
    fumes or vapors (chemical) 506.0
  interstitial 516.8
    with influenzal (see also Influenza) 487.0
    acute
      due to Pneumocystis (carinii) (jiroveci) 136.3
      meaning:
        acute interstitial pneumonitis 516.33
        atypical pneumonia — see Pneumonia, atypical
        bacterial pneumonia — see Pneumonia, bacterial
    chronic (see also Fibrosis, lung) 515
    desquamative 516.37
    hypostatic 514
    idiopathic 516.30
      lymphoid 516.35
    lipid 507.1
    lymphoid (due to known underlying cause) 516.8
    non-specific (due to known underlying cause) 516.8
    organizing (due to known underlying cause) 516.8
    plasma cell 136.3
    Pseudomonas 482.1
  intrauterine (infective) 770.0
    aspiration 770.18
      blood 770.16
      clear amniotic fluid 770.14
      meconium 770.12
      postnatal stomach contents 770.86
  Klebsiella pneumoniae 482.0
  Legionnaires' 482.84
  lipid, lipoid (exogenous) (interstitial) 507.1
    endogenous 516.8
  lobar (diplococcal) (disseminated) (double) (interstitial) (pneumococcal, any type) 481
    with influenza (see also Influenza) 487.0
    bacterial 482.9
      specified type NEC 482.89
    chronic (see also Fibrosis, lung) 515
    Escherichia coli (E. coli) 482.82
    Friedländer's bacillus 482.0
    Hemophilus influenzae (H. influenzae) 482.2
    hypostatic 514
    influenzal (see also Influenza) 487.0
    Klebsiella 482.0
    ornithosis 073.0
    Proteus 482.83
    Pseudomonas 482.1
    psittacosis 073.0
    specified organism NEC 483.8
      bacterial NEC 482.89
    staphylococcal 482.40
      aureus 482.41
        methicillin
          resistant (MRSA) 482.42
          susceptible (MSSA) 482.41
        specified type NEC 482.49
    streptococcal — see Pneumonia, streptococcal
    viral, virus (see also Pneumonia, viral) 480.9
  lobular (confluent) — see Pneumonia, broncho-
  Löffler's 518.3
  massive — see Pneumonia, lobar
  meconium aspiration 770.12
  metastatic NEC 038.8 [484.8]
  methicillin resistant Staphylococcus aureus (MRSA) 482.42
  methicillin susceptible Staphylococcus aureus (MSSA) 482.41
  MRSA (methicillin resistant Staphylococcus aureus) 482.42
  MSSA (methicillin susceptible Staphylococcus aureus) 482.41

Pneumonia — continued
  multilobar — see Pneumonia, by type
  Mycoplasma (pneumoniae) 483.0
  necrotic 513.0
  nitrogen dioxide 506.9
  orthostatic 514
  parainfluenza virus 480.2
  parenchymatous (see also Fibrosis, lung) 515
  passive 514
  patchy — see Pneumonia, broncho-
  Peptococcus 482.81
  Peptostreptococcus 482.81
  plasma cell 136.3
  pleurolobar — see Pneumonia, lobar
  pleuropneumonia-like organism (PPLO) 483.0
  pneumococcal (broncho) (lobar) 481
  Pneumocystis (carinii) (jiroveci) 136.3
  postinfectional NEC 136.9 [484.8]
  postmeasles 055.1
  postoperative 997.39
    aspiration 997.32
  primary atypical 486
  Proprionibacterium 482.81
  Proteus 482.83
  Pseudomonas 482.1
  psittacosis 073.0
  radiation 508.0
  respiratory syncytial virus 480.1
  resulting from a procedure 997.39
    aspiration 997.32
  rheumatic 390 [517.1]
  Salmonella 003.22
  SARS-associated coronavirus 480.3
  segmented, segmental — see Pneumonia, broncho-
  Serratia (marcescens) 482.83
  specified
    bacteria NEC 482.89
    organism NEC 483.8
    virus NEC 480.8
  spirochetal 104.8 [484.8]
  staphylococcal (broncho) (lobar) 482.40
    aureus 482.41
      methicillin
        resistant 482.42
        susceptible (MSSA) 482.41
      specified type NEC 482.49
  static, stasis 514
  streptococcal (broncho) (lobar) NEC 482.30
    Group
      A 482.31
      B 482.32
      specified NEC 482.39
    pneumoniae 481
    specified type NEC 482.39
  Streptococcus pneumoniae 481
  traumatic (complication) (early) (secondary) 958.8
  tuberculous (any) (see also Tuberculosis) 011.6 ☑
  tularemic 021.2
  TWAR agent 483.1
  varicella 052.1
  Veillonella 482.81
  ventilator associated 997.31
  viral, virus (broncho) (interstitial) (lobar) 480.9
    with influenza, flu, or grippe (see also Influenza) 487.0
    adenoviral 480.0
    parainfluenza 480.2
    respiratory syncytial 480.1
    SARS-associated coronavirus 480.3
    specified type NEC 480.8
  white (congenital) 090.0
Pneumonic — see condition
Pneumonitis (acute) (primary) — see also Pneumonia 486
  allergic 495.9
    specified type NEC 495.8
  aspiration 507.0
    due to fumes or gases 506.0
    fetal 770.18
      due to
        blood 770.16

Pneumonitis — see also Pneumonia — continued
  aspiration — continued
    fetal — continued
      due to — continued
        clear amniotic fluid 770.14
        meconium 770.12
        postnatal stomach contents 770.86
    newborn 770.18
      due to
        blood 770.16
        clear amniotic fluid 770.14
        meconium 770.12
        postnatal stomach contents 770.86
    obstetric 668.0 ☑
  chemical 506.0
    due to fumes or gases 506.0
    resulting from a procedure 997.32
  cholesterol 516.8
  chronic (see also Fibrosis, lung) 515
  congenital rubella 771.0
  crack 506.0
  due to
    crack (cocaine) 506.0
    fumes or vapors 506.0
    inhalation
      food (regurgitated), milk, vomitus 507.0
      oils, essences 507.1
      saliva 507.0
      solids, liquids NEC 507.8
    toxoplasmosis (acquired) 130.4
      congenital (active) 771.2 [484.8]
  eosinophilic 518.3
  fetal aspiration 770.18
    due to
      blood 770.16
      clear amniotic fluid 770.14
      meconium 770.12
      postnatal stomach contents 770.86
  hypersensitivity 495.9
  interstitial (chronic) (see also Fibrosis, lung) 515
    acute 516.33
    idiopathic
      lymphocytic 516.35
      non-specific 516.32
    lymphoid 516.8
  lymphoid, interstitial 516.8
  meconium aspiration 770.12
  postanesthetic
    correct substance properly administered 507.0
    obstetric 668.0 ☑
    overdose or wrong substance given 968.4
      specified anesthetic — see Table of Drugs and Chemicals
  postoperative 997.3 ☑
    aspiration 997.32
    obstetric 668.0 ☑
  radiation 508.0
  rubella, congenital 771.0
  "ventilation" 495.7
  ventilator associated 997.31
  wood-dust 495.8
Pneumonoconiosis — see Pneumoconiosis
Pneumoparotid 527.8
Pneumopathy NEC 518.89
  alveolar 516.9
    specified NEC 516.8
  due to dust NEC 504
  parietoalveolar 516.9
    specified condition NEC 516.8
Pneumopericarditis — see also Pericarditis 423.9
  acute 420.90
Pneumopericardium — see also Pericarditis
  congenital 770.2
  fetus or newborn 770.2
  traumatic (post) (see also Pneumothorax, traumatic) 860.0
    with open wound into thorax 860.1
Pneumoperitoneum 568.89

☑ Additional Digit Required — Refer to the Tabular List for Digit Selection
🔻 Subterms under main terms may continue to next column or page

Pneumoperitoneum — *continued*
  fetus or newborn 770.2
Pneumophagia (psychogenic) 306.4
Pneumopleurisy, pneumopleuritis — *see also* Pneumonia 486
Pneumopyopericardium 420.99
Pneumopyothorax — *see also* Pyopneumothorax 510.9
  with fistula 510.0
Pneumorrhagia 786.30
  newborn 770.3
  tuberculous (*see also* Tuberculosis, pulmonary) 011.9 ☑
Pneumosiderosis (occupational) 503
Pneumothorax 512.89
  acute 512.89
  chronic 512.83
  congenital 770.2
  due to operative injury of chest wall or lung 512.1
    accidental puncture or laceration 512.1
  fetus or newborn 770.2
  iatrogenic 512.1
  postoperative 512.1
  specified type NEC 512.89
  spontaneous 512.89
    fetus or newborn 770.2
    primary 512.81
    secondary 512.82
    tension 512.0
  sucking 512.89
    iatrogenic 512.1
    postoperative 512.1
  tense valvular, infectional 512.0
  tension 512.0
    iatrogenic 512.1
    postoperative 512.1
    spontaneous 512.0
  traumatic 860.0
    with
      hemothorax 860.4
        with open wound into thorax 860.5
      open wound into thorax 860.1
  tuberculous (*see also* Tuberculosis) 011.7 ☑
Pocket(s)
  endocardial (*see also* Endocarditis) 424.90
  periodontal 523.8
Podagra 274.01
Podencephalus 759.89
Poikilocytosis 790.09
Poikiloderma 709.09
  Civatte's 709.09
  congenital 757.33
  vasculare atrophicans 696.2
Poikilodermatomyositis 710.3
Pointed ear 744.29
Poise imperfect 729.90
Poisoned — *see* Poisoning
Poisoning (acute) — *see also* Table of Drugs and Chemicals
  Bacillus, B.
    aertrycke (*see also* Infection, Salmonella) 003.9
    botulinus 005.1
    cholerae (suis) (*see also* Infection, Salmonella) 003.9
    paratyphosus (*see also* infection, Salmonella) 003.9
    suipestifer (*see also* Infection, Salmonella) 003.9
  bacterial toxins NEC 005.9
  berries, noxious 988.2
  blood (general) — *see* Septicemia
  botulism 005.1
  bread, moldy, mouldy — *see* Poisoning, food
  Ciguatera 988.0
  damaged meat — *see* Poisoning, food
  death-cap (Amanita phalloides) (Amanita verna) 988.1
  decomposed food — *see* Poisoning, food
  diseased food — *see* Poisoning, food
  drug — *see* Table of Drugs and Chemicals
  epidemic, fish, meat, or other food — *see* Poisoning, food

Poisoning — *see also* Table of Drugs and Chemicals — *continued*
  fava bean 282.2
  fish (bacterial) (*see also* Poisoning, food) noxious 988.0
  food (acute) (bacterial) (diseased) (infected) NEC 005.9
  due to
    bacillus
      aertrycke (*see also* Poisoning, food, due to Salmonella) 003.9
      botulinus 005.1
      cereus 005.89
      choleraesuis (*see also* Poisoning, food, due to Salmonella) 003.9
      paratyphosus (*see also* Poisoning, food, due to Salmonella) 003.9
      suipestifer (*see also* Poisoning, food, due to Salmonella) 003.9
    Clostridium 005.3
      botulinum 005.1
      perfringens 005.2
      welchii 005.2
    Salmonella (aertrycke) (callinarum) (choleraesuis) (enteritidis) (paratyphi) (suipestifer) 003.9
      with
        gastroenteritis 003.0
        localized infection(s) (*see also* Infection, Salmonella) 003.20
        septicemia 003.1
        specified manifestation NEC 003.8
    specified bacterium NEC 005.89
    Staphylococcus 005.0
    Streptococcus 005.89
    Vibrio parahaemolyticus 005.4
    Vibrio vulnificus 005.81
  noxious or naturally toxic 988.0
    berries 988.2
    fish 988.0
    mushroom 988.1
    plants NEC 988.2
  ice cream — *see* Poisoning, food
  ichthyotoxism (bacterial) 005.9
  kreotoxism, food 005.9
  malarial — *see* Malaria
  meat — *see* Poisoning, food
  mushroom (noxious) 988.1
  mussel (*see also* Poisoning, food) noxious 988.0
  noxious foodstuffs (*see also* Poisoning, food, noxious) 988.9
    specified type NEC 988.8
  plants, noxious 988.2
  pork (*see also* Poisoning, food)
    specified NEC 988.8
    Trichinosis 124
  ptomaine — *see* Poisoning, food
  putrefaction, food — *see* Poisoning, food
  radiation 508.0
  Salmonella (*see also* Infection, Salmonella) 003.9
  sausage (*see also* Poisoning, food)
    Trichinosis 124
  saxitoxin 988.0
  shellfish (*see also* Poisoning, food)
    noxious (amnesic) (azaspiracid) (diarrheic) (neurotoxic) (paralytic) 988.0
  Staphylococcus, food 005.0
  toxic, from disease NEC 799.89
  truffles — *see* Poisoning, food
  uremic — *see* Uremia
  uric acid 274.9
  water 276.69
Poison ivy, oak, sumac or other plant dermatitis 692.6
Poker spine 720.0
Policeman's disease 729.2
Polioencephalitis (acute) (bulbar) — *see also* Poliomyelitis, bulbar 045.0 ☑

Polioencephalitis — *see also* Poliomyelitis, bulbar — *continued*
  inferior 335.22
  influenzal (*see also* Influenza) 487.8
  superior hemorrhagic (acute) (Wernicke's) 265.1
  Wernicke's (superior hemorrhagic) 265.1
Polioencephalomyelitis (acute) (anterior) (bulbar) — *see also* Polioencephalitis 045.0 ☑
Polioencephalopathy, superior hemorrhagic 265.1
  with
    beriberi 265.0
    pellagra 265.2
Poliomeningoencephalitis — *see* Meningoencephalitis
Poliomyelitis (acute) (anterior) (epidemic) 045.9 ☑

> *Note* — Use the following fifth-digit subclassification with category 045:
>
> 0 poliovirus, unspecified type
> 1 poliovirus, type I
> 2 poliovirus, type II
> 3 poliovirus, type III

  with
    paralysis 045.1 ☑
      bulbar 045.0 ☑
  abortive 045.2 ☑
  ascending 045.9 ☑
    progressive 045.9 ☑
  bulbar 045.0 ☑
  cerebral 045.0 ☑
  chronic 335.21
  congenital 771.2
  contact V01.2
  deformities 138
  exposure to V01.2
  late effect 138
  nonepidemic 045.9 ☑
  nonparalytic 045.2 ☑
  old with deformity 138
  posterior, acute 053.19
  residual 138
  sequelae 138
  spinal, acute 045.9 ☑
  syphilitic (chronic) 094.89
  vaccination, prophylactic (against) V04.0
Poliosis (eyebrow) (eyelashes) 704.3
  circumscripta (congenital) 757.4
    acquired 704.3
  congenital 757.4
Pollakiuria 788.41
  psychogenic 306.53
Pollinosis 477.0
Pollitzer's disease (hidradenitis suppurativa) 705.83
Polyadenitis — *see also* Adenitis 289.3
  malignant 020.0
Polyalgia 729.99
Polyangiitis (essential) 446.0
Polyarteritis (nodosa) (renal) 446.0
Polyarthralgia 719.49
  psychogenic 306.0
Polyarthritis, polyarthropathy NEC 716.59
  due to or associated with other specified conditions — *see* Arthritis, due to or associated with
  endemic (*see also* Disease, Kaschin-Beck) 716.0 ☑
  inflammatory 714.9
    specified type NEC 714.89
  juvenile (chronic) 714.30
    acute 714.31
  migratory — *see* Fever, rheumatic
  rheumatic 714.0
    fever (acute) — *see* Fever, rheumatic
Polycarential syndrome of infancy 260
Polychondritis (atrophic) (chronic) (relapsing) 733.99
Polycoria 743.46
Polycystic (congenital) (disease) 759.89

Polycystic — *continued*
  degeneration, kidney — *see* Polycystic, kidney
  kidney (congenital) 753.12
    adult type (APKD) 753.13
    autosomal dominant 753.13
    autosomal recessive 753.14
    childhood type (CPKD) 753.14
    infantile type 753.14
  liver 751.62
  lung 518.89
    congenital 748.4
  ovary, ovaries 256.4
  spleen 759.0
Polycythemia (primary) (rubra) (vera) (M9950/1) 238.4
  acquired 289.0
  benign 289.0
    familial 289.6
  due to
    donor twin 776.4
    fall in plasma volume 289.0
    high altitude 289.0
    maternal-fetal transfusion 776.4
    stress 289.0
  emotional 289.0
  erythropoietin 289.0
  familial (benign) 289.6
  Gaisböck's (hypertonica) 289.0
  high altitude 289.0
  hypertonica 289.0
  hypoxemic 289.0
  neonatorum 776.4
  nephrogenous 289.0
  relative 289.0
  secondary 289.0
  spurious 289.0
  stress 289.0
Polycytosis cryptogenica 289.0
Polydactylism, polydactyly 755.00
  fingers 755.01
  toes 755.02
Polydipsia 783.5
Polydystrophic oligophrenia 277.5
Polyembryoma (M9072/3) — *see* Neoplasm, by site, malignant
Polygalactia 676.6 ☑
Polyglandular
  deficiency 258.9
  dyscrasia 258.9
  dysfunction 258.9
  syndrome 258.8
Polyhydramnios — *see also* Hydramnios 657.0 ☑
Polymastia 757.6
Polymenorrhea 626.2
Polymicrogyria 742.2
Polymyalgia 725
  arteritica 446.5
  rheumatica 725
Polymyositis (acute) (chronic) (hemorrhagic) 710.4
  with involvement of
    lung 710.4 *[517.8]*
    skin 710.3
  ossificans (generalisata) (progressiva) 728.19
  Wagner's (dermatomyositis) 710.3
Polyneuritis, polyneuritic — *see also* Polyneuropathy 356.9
  alcoholic 357.5
    with psychosis 291.1
  cranialis 352.6
  demyelinating, chronic inflammatory (CIDP) 357.81
  diabetic 250.6 ☑ *[357.2]*
    due to secondary diabetes 249.6 ☑ *[357.2]*
  due to lack of vitamin NEC 269.2 *[357.4]*
  endemic 265.0 *[357.4]*
  erythredema 985.0
  febrile 357.0
  hereditary ataxic 356.3
  idiopathic, acute 357.0
  infective (acute) 357.0
  nutritional 269.9 *[357.4]*
  postinfectious 357.0

Polyneuropathy (peripheral) 356.9
    alcoholic 357.5
    amyloid 277.39 *[357.4]*
    arsenical 357.7
    critical illness 357.82
    demyelinating, chronic inflammatory (CIDP) 357.81
    diabetic 250.6 ☑ *[357.2]*
        due to secondary diabetes 249.6 ☑ *[357.2]*
    due to
        antitetanus serum 357.6
        arsenic 357.7
        drug or medicinal substance 357.6
            correct substance properly administered 357.6
            overdose or wrong substance given or taken 977.9
                specified drug — *see* Table of Drugs and Chemicals
        lack of vitamin NEC 269.2 *[357.4]*
        lead 357.7
        organophosphate compounds 357.7
        pellagra 265.2 *[357.4]*
        porphyria 277.1 *[357.4]*
        serum 357.6
        toxic agent NEC 357.7
    hereditary 356.0
    idiopathic 356.9
        progressive 356.4
    in
        amyloidosis 277.39 *[357.4]*
        avitaminosis 269.2 *[357.4]*
            specified NEC 269.1 *[357.4]*
        beriberi 265.0 *[357.4]*
        collagen vascular disease NEC 710.9 *[357.1]*
        deficiency
            B-complex NEC 266.2 *[357.4]*
            vitamin B 266.1 *[357.4]*
            vitamin B6 266.9 *[357.4]*
        diabetes 250.6 ☑ *[357.2]*
            due to secondary diabetes 249.6 ☑ *[357.2]*
        diphtheria (*see also* Diphtheria) 032.89 *[357.4]*
        disseminated lupus erythematosus 710.0 *[357.1]*
        herpes zoster 053.13
        hypoglycemia 251.2 *[357.4]*
        malignant neoplasm (M8000/3) NEC 199.1 *[357.3]*
        mumps 072.72
        pellagra 265.2 *[357.4]*
        polyarteritis nodosa 446.0 *[357.1]*
        porphyria 277.1 *[357.4]*
        rheumatoid arthritis 714.0 *[357.1]*
        sarcoidosis 135 *[357.4]*
        uremia 585.9 *[357.4]*
    lead 357.7
    nutritional 269.9 *[357.4]*
        specified NEC 269.8 *[357.4]*
    postherpetic 053.13
    progressive 356.4
    sensory (hereditary) 356.2
    specified NEC 356.8
Polyonychia 757.5
Polyopia 368.2
    refractive 368.15
Polyorchism, polyorchidism (three testes) 752.89
Polyorrhymenitis (peritoneal) — *see also* Polyserositis 568.82
    pericardial 423.2
Polyostotic fibrous dysplasia 756.54
Polyotia 744.1
Polyphagia 783.6
Polypoid — *see* condition
Polyposis — *see also* Polyp
    coli (adenomatous) (M8220/0) 211.3
        adenocarcinoma in (M8220/3) 153.9
        carcinoma in (M8220/3) 153.9
    familial (M8220/0) 211.3
    intestinal (adenomatous) (M8220/0) 211.3
    multiple (M8221/0) — *see* Neoplasm, by site, benign

Polyp, polypus

Note — Polyps of organs or sites that do not appear in the list below should be coded to the residual category for diseases of the organ or site concerned.

    accessory sinus 471.8
    adenoid tissue 471.0
    adenomatous (M8210/0) (*see also* Neoplasm, by site, benign)
        adenocarcinoma in (M8210/3) — *see* Neoplasm, by site, malignant
        carcinoma in (M8210/3) — *see* Neoplasm, by site, malignant
        multiple (M8221/0) — *see* Neoplasm, by site, benign
    antrum 471.8
    anus, anal (canal) (nonadenomatous) 569.0
        adenomatous 211.4
    Bartholin's gland 624.6
    bladder (M8120/1) 236.7
    broad ligament 620.8
    cervix (uteri) 622.7
        adenomatous 219.0
        in pregnancy or childbirth 654.6 ☑
            affecting fetus or newborn 763.89
            causing obstructed labor 660.2 ☑
        mucous 622.7
        nonneoplastic 622.7
    choanal 471.0
    cholesterol 575.6
    clitoris 624.6
    colon (M8210/0) (*see also* Polyp, adenomatous) 211.3
    corpus uteri 621.0
    dental 522.0
    ear (middle) 385.30
    endometrium 621.0
    ethmoidal (sinus) 471.8
    fallopian tube 620.8
    female genital organs NEC 624.8
    frontal (sinus) 471.8
    gallbladder 575.6
    gingiva 523.8
    gum 523.8
    labia 624.6
    larynx (mucous) 478.4
    malignant (M8000/3) — *see* Neoplasm, by site, malignant
    maxillary (sinus) 471.8
    middle ear 385.30
    myometrium 621.0
    nares
        anterior 471.9
        posterior 471.0
    nasal (mucous) 471.9
        cavity 471.0
        septum 471.9
    nasopharyngeal 471.0
    neoplastic (M8210/0) — *see* Neoplasm, by site, benign
    nose (mucous) 471.9
    oviduct 620.8
    paratubal 620.8
    pharynx 478.29
        congenital 750.29
    placenta, placental 674.4 ☑
    prostate 600.20
        with
            other lower urinary tract symptoms (LUTS) 600.21
            urinary
                obstruction 600.21
                retention 600.21
    pudenda 624.6
    pulp (dental) 522.0
    rectosigmoid 211.4
    rectum (nonadenomatous) 569.0
        adenomatous 211.4
    septum (nasal) 471.9
    sinus (accessory) (ethmoidal) (frontal) (maxillary) (sphenoidal) 471.8
    sphenoidal (sinus) 471.8
    stomach (M8210/0) 211.1
    tube, fallopian 620.8
    turbinate, mucous membrane 471.8
    ureter 593.89

Polyp, polypus — *continued*
    urethra 599.3
    uterine
        ligament 620.8
        tube 620.8
    uterus (body) (corpus) (mucous) 621.0
        in pregnancy or childbirth 654.1 ☑
            affecting fetus or newborn 763.89
            causing obstructed labor 660.2 ☑
    vagina 623.7
    vocal cord (mucous) 478.4
    vulva 624.6
Polyradiculitis (acute) 357.0
Polyradiculoneuropathy (acute) (segmentally demyelinating) 357.0
Polysarcia 278.00
Polyserositis (peritoneal) 568.82
    due to pericarditis 423.2
    paroxysmal (familial) 277.31
    pericardial 423.2
    periodic (familial) 277.31
    pleural — *see* Pleurisy
    recurrent 277.31
    tuberculous (*see also* Tuberculosis, polyserositis) 018.9 ☑
Polysialia 527.7
Polysplenia syndrome 759.0
Polythelia 757.6
Polytrichia — *see also* Hypertrichosis 704.1
Polyunguia (congenital) 757.5
    acquired 703.8
Polyuria 788.42
Pompe's disease (glycogenosis II) 271.0
Pompholyx 705.81
Poncet's disease (tuberculous rheumatism) — *see also* Tuberculosis 015.9 ☑
Pond fracture — *see* Fracture, skull, vault
Ponos 085.0
Pons, pontine — *see* condition
Poor
    aesthetics of existing restoration of tooth 525.67
    contractions, labor 661.2 ☑
        affecting fetus or newborn 763.7
    fetal growth NEC 764.9 ☑
        affecting management of pregnancy 656.5 ☑
    incorporation
        artificial skin graft 996.55
        decellularized allodermis graft 996.55
    obstetrical history V13.29
        affecting management of current pregnancy V23.49
            ectopic pregnancy V23.42
            pre-term labor V23.41
        pre-term labor V13.21
    sucking reflex (newborn) 796.1
    vision NEC 369.9
Poradenitis, nostras 099.1
Porencephaly (congenital) (developmental) (true) 742.4
    acquired 348.0
    nondevelopmental 348.0
    traumatic (post) 310.2
Porocephaliasis 134.1
Porokeratosis 757.39
    disseminated superficial actinic (DSAP) 692.75
Poroma, eccrine (M8402/0) — *see* Neoplasm, skin, benign
Porphyria (acute) (congenital) (constitutional) (erythropoietic) (familial) (hepatica) (idiopathic) (idiosyncratic) (intermittent) (latent) (mixed hepatic) (photosensitive) (South African genetic) (Swedish) 277.1
    acquired 277.1
    cutaneatarda
        hereditaria 277.1
        symptomatica 277.1
    due to drugs
        correct substance properly administered 277.1
        overdose or wrong substance given or taken 977.9
            specified drug — *see* Table of Drugs and Chemicals

Porphyria — *continued*
    secondary 277.1
    toxic NEC 277.1
    variegata 277.1
Porphyrinuria (acquired) (congenital) (secondary) 277.1
Porphyruria (acquired) (congenital) 277.1
Portal — *see* condition
Port wine nevus or mark 757.32
Posadas-Wernicke disease 114.9
Position
    fetus, abnormal (*see also* Presentation, fetal) 652.9 ☑
    teeth, faulty (*see also* Anomaly, position tooth) 524.30
Positive
    culture (nonspecific) 795.39
        AIDS virus V08
        blood 790.7
        HIV V08
        human immunodeficiency virus V08
        nose 795.39
            Staphylococcus — *see* Carrier (suspected) of, Staphylococcus
        skin lesion NEC 795.39
        spinal fluid 792.0
        sputum 795.39
        stool 792.1
        throat 795.39
        urine 791.9
        wound 795.39
    findings, anthrax 795.31
    HIV V08
    human immunodeficiency virus (HIV) V08
    PPD 795.51
    serology
        AIDS virus V08
            inconclusive 795.71
        HIV V08
            inconclusive 795.71
        human immunodeficiency virus (HIV) V08
            inconclusive 795.71
        syphilis 097.1
            with signs or symptoms — *see* Syphilis, by site and stage
            false 795.6
    skin test 795.7 ☑
        tuberculin (without active tuberculosis) 795.51
    VDRL 097.1
        with signs or symptoms — *see* Syphilis, by site and stage
        false 795.6
    Wassermann reaction 097.1
        false 795.6
Postcardiotomy syndrome 429.4
Postcaval ureter 753.4
Postcholecystectomy syndrome 576.0
Postclimacteric bleeding 627.1
Postcommissurotomy syndrome 429.4
Postconcussional syndrome 310.2
Postcontusional syndrome 310.2
Postcricoid region — *see* condition
Post-dates (pregnancy) — *see* Pregnancy
Postencephalitic — *see also* condition
    syndrome 310.89
Posterior — *see* condition
Posterolateral sclerosis (spinal cord) — *see* Degeneration, combined
Postexanthematous — *see* condition
Postfebrile — *see* condition
Postgastrectomy dumping syndrome 564.2
Posthemiplegic chorea 344.89
Posthemorrhagic anemia (chronic) 280.0
    acute 285.1
    newborn 776.5
Posthepatitis syndrome 780.79
Postherpetic neuralgia (intercostal) (syndrome) (zoster) 053.19
    geniculate ganglion 053.11
    ophthalmica 053.19
    trigeminal 053.12
Posthitis 607.1
Postimmunization complication or reaction
    — *see* Complications, vaccination

☑ **Additional Digit Required — Refer to the Tabular List for Digit Selection**   ⷮ **Subterms under main terms may continue to next column or page**

2013 ICD-9-CM   ▶◀ Revised Text   ● New Line   ▲ Revised Code   **Volume 2 — 235**

Postinfectious — *see* condition
Postinfluenzal syndrome 780.79
Postlaminectomy syndrome 722.80
  cervical, cervicothoracic 722.81
  kyphosis 737.12
  lumbar, lumbosacral 722.83
  thoracic, thoracolumbar 722.82
Postleukotomy syndrome 310.0
Postlobectomy syndrome 310.0
Postmastectomy lymphedema (syndrome) 457.0
Postmaturity, postmature (fetus or newborn) (gestation period over 42 completed weeks) 766.22
  affecting management of pregnancy
    post-term pregnancy 645.1 ☑
    prolonged pregnancy 645.2 ☑
  syndrome 766.22
Postmeasles — *see also* condition
  complication 055.8
    specified NEC 055.79
Postmenopausal
  endometrium (atrophic) 627.8
    suppurative (see also Endometritis) 615.9
  hormone replacement therapy V07.4
  status (age related) (natural) V49.81
Postnasal drip 784.91
Postnatal — *see* condition
Postoperative — *see also* condition
  confusion state 293.9
  psychosis 293.9
  status NEC (*see also* Status (post)) V45.89
Postpancreatectomy hyperglycemia 251.3
Postpartum — *see also* condition
  anemia 648.2 ☑
  cardiomyopathy 674.5 ☑
  observation
    immediately after delivery V24.0
    routine follow-up V24.2
Postperfusion syndrome NEC 999.89
  bone marrow 996.85
Postpoliomyelitic — *see* condition
Postsurgery status NEC — *see also* Status (post V45.89
Post-term (pregnancy) 645.1 ☑
  infant (gestation period over 40 completed weeks to 42 completed weeks) 766.21
Post-transplant lymphoproliferative disorder (PTLD) 238.77
Posttraumatic — *see* condition
Posttraumatic brain syndrome, nonpsychotic 310.2
Post-traumatic stress disorder (PTSD) 309.81
Post-typhoid abscess 002.0
Postures, hysterical 300.11
Postvaccinal reaction or complication — *see* Complications, vaccination
Postvagotomy syndrome 564.2
Postvalvulotomy syndrome 429.4
Postvasectomy sperm count V25.8
Potain's disease (pulmonary edema) 514
Potain's syndrome (gastrectasis with dyspepsia) 536.1
Pott's
  curvature (spinal) (*see also* Tuberculosis) 015.0 ☑ *[737.43]*
  disease or paraplegia (*see also* Tuberculosis) 015.0 ☑ *[730.88]*
  fracture (closed) 824.4
    open 824.5
  gangrene 440.24
  osteomyelitis (*see also* Tuberculosis) 015.0 ☑ *[730.88]*
  spinal curvature (*see also* Tuberculosis) 015.0 ☑ *[737.43]*
  tumor, puffy (*see also* Osteomyelitis) 730.2 ☑
Potter's
  asthma 502
  disease 753.0
  facies 754.0
  lung 502
  syndrome (with renal agenesis) 753.0

Pouch
  bronchus 748.3
  Douglas' — *see* condition
  esophagus, esophageal (congenital) 750.4
    acquired 530.6
  gastric 537.1
  Hartmann's (abnormal sacculation of gallbladder neck) 575.8
    of intestine V44.3
      attention to V55.3
  pharynx, pharyngeal (congenital) 750.27
Pouchitis 569.71
Poulet's disease 714.2
Poultrymen's itch 133.8
Poverty V60.2
PPE (palmar plantar erythrodysesthesia) 693.0
Prader-Labhart-Willi-Fanconi syndrome (hypogenital dystrophy with diabetic tendency) 759.81
Prader-Willi syndrome (hypogenital dystrophy with diabetic tendency) 759.81
Preachers' voice 784.49
Pre-AIDS — *see* Human immunodeficiency virus (disease) (illness) (infection)
Preauricular appendage 744.1
Prebetalipoproteinemia (acquired) (essential) (familial) (hereditary) (primary) (secondary) 272.1
  with chylomicronemia 272.3
Precipitate labor 661.3 ☑
  affecting fetus or newborn 763.6
Preclimacteric bleeding 627.0
  menorrhagia 627.0
Precocious
  adrenarche 259.1
  menarche 259.1
  menstruation 259.1
  pubarche 259.1
  puberty NEC 259.1
  sexual development NEC 259.1
  thelarche 259.1
Precocity, sexual (constitutional) (cryptogenic) (female) (idiopathic) (male) NEC 259.1
  with adrenal hyperplasia 255.2
Precordial pain 786.51
  psychogenic 307.89
Predeciduous teeth 520.2
Prediabetes, prediabetic 790.29
  complicating pregnancy, childbirth, or puerperium 648.8 ☑
  fetus or newborn 775.89
Predislocation status of hip, at birth — *see also* Subluxation, congenital, hip 754.32
Preeclampsia (mild) 642.4 ☑
  with pre-existing hypertension 642.7 ☑
  affecting fetus or newborn 760.0
  severe 642.5 ☑
  superimposed on pre-existing hypertensive disease 642.7 ☑
Preeruptive color change, teeth, tooth 520.8
Preexcitation 426.7
  atrioventricular conduction 426.7
  ventricular 426.7
Preglaucoma 365.00
Pregnancy (single) (uterine) (without sickness) V22.2

> *Note — Use the following fifth-digit subclassification with categories 640–649, 651–679:*
>
> *0   unspecified as to episode of care*
>
> *1   delivered, with or without mention of antepartum condition*
>
> *2   delivered, with mention of postpartum complication*
>
> *3   antepartum condition or complication*
>
> *4   postpartum condition or complication*

  abdominal (ectopic) 633.00
    with intrauterine pregnancy 633.01
    affecting fetus or newborn 761.4
  abnormal NEC 646.9 ☑
  ampullar — *see* Pregnancy, tubal

Pregnancy — *continued*
  biochemical 631.0
  broad ligament — *see* Pregnancy, cornual
  cervical — *see* Pregnancy, cornual
  chemical 631.0
  combined (extrauterine and intrauterine) — *see* Pregnancy, cornual
  complicated (by) 646.9 ☑
    abnormal, abnormality NEC 646.9 ☑
      cervix 654.6 ☑
      cord (umbilical) 663.9 ☑
      glucose tolerance (conditions classifiable to 790.21–790.29) 648.8 ☑
      pelvic organs or tissues NEC 654.9 ☑
      pelvis (bony) 653.0 ☑
      perineum or vulva 654.8 ☑
      placenta, placental (vessel) 656.7 ☑
      position
        cervix 654.4 ☑
        placenta 641.1 ☑
          without hemorrhage 641.0 ☑
        uterus 654.4 ☑
      size, fetus 653.5 ☑
      uterus (congenital) 654.0 ☑
    abscess or cellulitis
      bladder 646.6 ☑
      genitourinary tract (conditions classifiable to 590, 595, 597, 599.0, 614.0–614.5, 614.7–614.9, 615) 646.6 ☑
      kidney 646.6 ☑
      urinary tract NEC 646.6 ☑
    adhesion, pelvic peritoneal 648.9 ☑
    air embolism 673.0 ☑
    albuminuria 646.2 ☑
      with hypertension — *see* Toxemia, of pregnancy
    amnionitis 658.4 ☑
    amniotic fluid embolism 673.1 ☑
    anemia (conditions classifiable to 280–285) 648.2 ☑
    appendicitis 648.9 ☑
    atrophy, yellow (acute) (liver) (subacute) 646.7 ☑
    bacilluria, asymptomatic 646.5 ☑
    bacteriuria, asymptomatic 646.5 ☑
    bariatric surgery status 649.2 ☑
    bicornis or bicornuate uterus 654.0 ☑
    biliary problems 646.7 ☑
    bone and joint disorders (conditions classifiable to 720–724 or conditions affecting lower limbs classifiable to 711–719, 725–738) 648.7 ☑
    breech presentation (buttocks) (complete) (frank) 652.2 ☑
      with successful version 652.1 ☑
    cardiovascular disease (conditions classifiable to 390–398, 410–429) 648.6 ☑
      congenital (conditions classifiable to 745–747) 648.5 ☑
    cerebrovascular disorders (conditions classifiable to 430–434, 436–437) 674.0 ☑
    cervicitis (conditions classifiable to 616.0) 646.6 ☑
    chloasma (gravidarum) 646.8 ☑
    cholelithiasis 646.8 ☑
    cholestasis 646.7 ☑
    chorea (gravidarum) — *see* Eclampsia, pregnancy
    coagulation defect 649.3 ☑
    conjoined twins 678.1 ☑
    contraction, pelvis (general) 653.1 ☑
      inlet 653.2 ☑
      outlet 653.3 ☑
    convulsions (eclamptic) (uremic) 642.6 ☑
      with pre-existing hypertension 642.7 ☑

Pregnancy — *continued*
  complicated — *continued*
    current disease or condition (nonobstetric)
      abnormal glucose tolerance 648.8 ☑
      anemia 648.2 ☑
      biliary tract 646.7 ☑
      bone and joint (lower limb) 648.7 ☑
      cardiovascular 648.6 ☑
        congenital 648.5 ☑
      cerebrovascular 674.0 ☑
      diabetes (conditions classifiable to 249 and 250) 648.0 ☑
      drug dependence 648.3 ☑
      female genital mutilation 648.9 ☑
      genital organ or tract 646.6 ☑
      gonorrheal 647.1 ☑
      hypertensive 642.2 ☑
        chronic kidney 642.2 ☑
        renal 642.1 ☑
      infectious 647.9 ☑
        specified type NEC 647.8 ☑
      liver 646.7 ☑
      malarial 647.4 ☑
      nutritional deficiency 648.9 ☑
      parasitic NEC 647.8 ☑
      periodontal disease 648.9 ☑
      renal 646.2 ☑
        hypertensive 642.1 ☑
      rubella 647.5 ☑
      specified condition NEC 648.9 ☑
      syphilitic 647.0 ☑
      thyroid 648.1 ☑
      tuberculous 647.3 ☑
      urinary 646.6 ☑
      venereal 647.2 ☑
      viral NEC 647.6 ☑
    cystitis 646.6 ☑
    cystocele 654.4 ☑
    death of fetus (near term) 656.4 ☑
      early pregnancy (before 22 completed weeks gestation) 632
    deciduitis 646.6 ☑
    decreased fetal movements 655.7 ☑
    diabetes (mellitus) (conditions classifiable to 249 and 250) 648.0 ☑
    disorders of liver and biliary tract 646.7 ☑
    displacement, uterus NEC 654.4 ☑
    disproportion — *see* Disproportion
    double uterus 654.0 ☑
    drug dependence (conditions classifiable to 304) 648.3 ☑
    dysplasia, cervix 654.6 ☑
    early onset of delivery (spontaneous) 644.2 ☑
    eclampsia, eclamptic (coma) (convulsions) (delirium) (nephritis) (uremia) 642.6 ☑
      with pre-existing hypertension 642.7 ☑
    edema 646.1 ☑
      with hypertension — *see* Toxemia, of pregnancy
    effusion, amniotic fluid 658.1 ☑
      delayed delivery following 658.2 ☑
    embolism
      air 673.0 ☑
      amniotic fluid 673.1 ☑
      blood-clot 673.2 ☑
      cerebral 674.0 ☑
      pulmonary NEC 673.2 ☑
      pyemic 673.3 ☑
      septic 673.3 ☑
    emesis (gravidarum) — *see* Pregnancy, complicated, vomiting
    endometritis (conditions classifiable to 615.0–615.9) 670.1 ☑
      decidual 646.6 ☑
    epilepsy 649.4 ☑
    excessive weight gain NEC 646.1 ☑
    face presentation 652.4 ☑
    failure, fetal head to enter pelvic brim 652.5 ☑

☑ **Additional Digit Required** 7 — **Refer to the Tabular List for Digit Selection**   ⌐ **Subterms under main terms may continue to next column or page**

236 — Volume 2   ▶◀ Revised Text   ● New Line   ▲ Revised Code   **2013 ICD-9-CM**

Pregnancy — *continued*
  complicated — *continued*
    false labor (pains) 644.1 ☑
    fatigue 646.8 ☑
    fatty metamorphosis of liver 646.7 ☑
    female genital mutilation 648.9 ☑
    fetal
      anemia 678.0 ☑
      complications from in utero proce-
        dure 679.1 ☑
      conjoined twins 678.1 ☑
      death (near term) 656.4 ☑
        early (before 22 completed weeks
          gestation) 632
      deformity 653.7 ☑
      distress 656.8 ☑
      hematologic conditions 678.0 ☑
      reduction of multiple fetuses reduced
        to single fetus 651.7 ☑
      thrombocytopenia 678.0 ☑
      twin to twin transfusion 678.0 ☑
    fibroid (tumor) (uterus) 654.1 ☑
    footling presentation 652.8 ☑
      with successful version 652.1 ☑
    gallbladder disease 646.8 ☑
    gastric banding status 649.2 ☑
    gastric bypass status for obesity
    genital herpes (asymptomatic) (history
      of) (inactive) 647.6 ☑
    goiter 648.1 ☑
    gonococcal infection (conditions classifi-
      able to 098) 647.1 ☑
    gonorrhea (conditions classifiable to
      098) 647.1 ☑
    hemorrhage 641.9 ☑
      accidental 641.2 ☑
      before 22 completed weeks gesta-
        tion NEC 640.9 ☑
      cerebrovascular 674.0 ☑
      due to
        afibrinogenemia or other coagu-
          lation defect (conditions
          classifiable to 286.0–286.9)
          641.3 ☑
        leiomyoma, uterine 641.8 ☑
        marginal sinus (rupture) 641.2 ☑
        premature separation, placenta
          641.2 ☑
        trauma 641.8 ☑
      early (before 22 completed weeks
        gestation) 640.9 ☑
      threatened abortion 640.0 ☑
      unavoidable 641.1 ☑
    hepatitis (acute) (malignant) (subacute)
      646.7 ☑
      viral 647.6 ☑
    herniation of uterus 654.4 ☑
    high head at term 652.5 ☑
    hydatidiform mole (delivered) (undeliv-
      ered) 630
    hydramnios 657.0 ☑
    hydrocephalic fetus 653.6 ☑
    hydrops amnii 657.0 ☑
    hydrorrhea 658.1 ☑
    hyperemesis (gravidarum) — *see* Hyper-
      emesis, gravidarum
    hypertension — *see* Hypertension,
      complicating pregnancy
    hypertensive
      chronic kidney disease 642.2 ☑
      heart and chronic kidney disease
        642.2 ☑
      heart and renal disease 642.2 ☑
      heart disease 642.2 ☑
      renal disease 642.2 ☑
    hypertensive heart and chronic kidney
      disease 642.2 ☑
    hyperthyroidism 648.1 ☑
    hypothyroidism 648.1 ☑
    hysteralgia 646.8 ☑
    incarceration, uterus 654.3 ☑
    incompetent cervix (os) 654.5 ☑
    infection 647.9 ☑

Pregnancy — *continued*
  complicated — *continued*
    infection — *continued*
      amniotic fluid 658.4 ☑
      bladder 646.6 ☑
      genital organ (conditions classifiable
        to 614.0–614.5, 614.7–614.9,
        615) 646.6 ☑
      kidney (conditions classifiable to
        590.0–590.9) 646.6 ☑
      urinary (tract) 646.6 ☑
        asymptomatic 646.5 ☑
    infective and parasitic diseases NEC
      647.8 ☑
    inflammation
      bladder 646.6 ☑
      genital organ (conditions classifiable
        to 614.0–614.5, 614.7–614.9,
        615) 646.6 ☑
      urinary tract NEC 646.6 ☑
    insufficient weight gain 646.8 ☑
    insulin resistance 648.8 ☑
    intrauterine fetal death (near term) NEC
      656.4 ☑
      early (before 22 completed weeks'
        gestation) 632
    malaria (conditions classifiable to 084)
      647.4 ☑
    malformation, uterus (congenital)
      654.0 ☑
    malnutrition (conditions classifiable to
      260–269) 648.9 ☑
    malposition
      fetus — *see* Pregnancy, complicated,
        malpresentation
      uterus or cervix 654.4 ☑
    malpresentation 652.9 ☑
      with successful version 652.1 ☑
      in multiple gestation 652.6 ☑
      specified type NEC 652.8 ☑
    marginal sinus hemorrhage or rupture
      641.2 ☑
    maternal complications from in utero
      procedure 679.0 ☑
    maternal drug abuse 648.4 ☑
    maternal obesity syndrome 646.1 ☑
    menstruation 640.8 ☑
    mental disorders (conditions classifiable
      to 290–303, 305.0, 305.2–305.9,
      306–316, 317–319) 648.4 ☑
    mentum presentation 652.4 ☑
    missed
      abortion 632
      delivery (at or near term) 656.4 ☑
      labor (at or near term) 656.4 ☑
    necrosis
      genital organ or tract (conditions
        classifiable to 614.0–614.5,
        614.7–614.9, 615) 646.6 ☑
      liver (conditions classifiable to 570)
        646.7 ☑
      renal, cortical 646.2 ☑
    nephritis or nephrosis (conditions classi-
      fiable to 580–589) 646.2 ☑
      with hypertension 642.1 ☑
    nephropathy NEC 646.2 ☑
    neuritis (peripheral) 646.4 ☑
    nutritional deficiency (conditions classi-
      fiable to 260–269) 648.9 ☑
    obesity 649.1 ☑
      surgery status 649.2 ☑
    oblique lie or presentation 652.3 ☑
      with successful version 652.1 ☑
    obstetrical trauma NEC 665.9 ☑
    oligohydramnios NEC 658.0 ☑
    onset of contractions before 37 weeks
      644.0 ☑
    oversize fetus 653.5 ☑
    papyraceous fetus 646.0 ☑
    patent cervix 654.5 ☑
    pelvic inflammatory disease (conditions
      classifiable to 614.0–614.5,
      614.7–614.9, 615) 646.6 ☑
    pelvic peritoneal adhesion 648.9 ☑

Pregnancy — *continued*
  complicated — *continued*
    placenta, placental
      abnormality 656.7 ☑
      abruptio or ablatio 641.2 ☑
      detachment 641.2 ☑
      disease 656.7 ☑
      infarct 656.7 ☑
      low implantation 641.1 ☑
        without hemorrhage 641.0 ☑
      malformation 656.7 ☑
      malposition 641.1 ☑
        without hemorrhage 641.0 ☑
      marginal sinus hemorrhage 641.2 ☑
      previa 641.1 ☑
        without hemorrhage 641.0 ☑
      separation (premature) (undelivered)
        641.2 ☑
    placentitis 658.4 ☑
    pneumonia 648.9 ☑
    polyhydramnios 657.0 ☑
    postmaturity
      post-term 645.1 ☑
      prolonged 645.2 ☑
    prediabetes 648.8 ☑
    pre-eclampsia (mild) 642.4 ☑
      severe 642.5 ☑
      superimposed on pre-existing hyper-
        tensive disease 642.7 ☑
    premature rupture of membranes
      658.1 ☑
      with delayed delivery 658.2 ☑
    previous
      ectopic pregnancy V23.42
      infertility V23.0
      in utero procedure during previous
        pregnancy V23.86
      nonobstetric condition V23.89
      poor obstetrical history V23.49
      premature delivery V23.41
      trophoblastic disease (conditions
        classifiable to 630) V23.1
    prolapse, uterus 654.4 ☑
    proteinuria (gestational) 646.2 ☑
      with hypertension — *see* Toxemia,
        of pregnancy
    pruritus (neurogenic) 646.8 ☑
    psychosis or psychoneurosis 648.4 ☑
    ptyalism 646.8 ☑
    pyelitis (conditions classifiable to
      590.0–590.9) 646.6 ☑
    renal disease or failure NEC 646.2 ☑
      with secondary hypertension
        642.1 ☑
      hypertensive 642.2 ☑
    retention, retained dead ovum 631.8
    retroversion, uterus 654.3 ☑
    Rh immunization, incompatibility, or
      sensitization 656.1 ☑
    rubella (conditions classifiable to 056)
      647.5 ☑
    rupture
      amnion (premature) 658.1 ☑
        with delayed delivery 658.2 ☑
      marginal sinus (hemorrhage)
        641.2 ☑
      membranes (premature) 658.1 ☑
        with delayed delivery 658.2 ☑
      uterus (before onset of labor)
        665.0 ☑
    salivation (excessive) 646.8 ☑
    salpingo–oophoritis (conditions classifi-
      able to 614.0–614.2) 646.6 ☑
    septicemia (conditions classifiable to
      038.0–038.9) 647.8 ☑
      postpartum 670.2 ☑
      puerperal 670.2 ☑
    smoking 649.0 ☑
    spasms, uterus (abnormal) 646.8 ☑
    specified condition NEC 646.8 ☑
    spotting 649.5 ☑
    spurious labor pains 644.1 ☑
    status post
      bariatric surgery 649.2 ☑

Pregnancy — *continued*
  complicated — *continued*
    status post — *continued*
      gastric banding 649.2 ☑
      gastric bypass for obesity 649.2 ☑
      obesity surgery 649.2 ☑
    superfecundation 651.9 ☑
    superfetation 651.9 ☑
    syphilis (conditions classifiable to
      090–097) 647.0 ☑
    threatened
      abortion 640.0 ☑
      premature delivery 644.2 ☑
      premature labor 644.0 ☑
    thrombophlebitis (superficial) 671.2 ☑
      deep 671.3 ☑
      septic 670.3 ☑
    thrombosis 671.2 ☑
      venous (superficial) 671.2 ☑
        deep 671.3 ☑
    thyroid dysfunction (conditions classifi-
      able to 240–246) 648.1 ☑
    thyroiditis 648.1 ☑
    thyrotoxicosis 648.1 ☑
    tobacco use disorder 649.0 ☑
    torsion of uterus 654.4 ☑
    toxemia — *see* Toxemia, of pregnancy
    transverse lie or presentation 652.3 ☑
      with successful version 652.1 ☑
    trauma 648.9 ☑
      obstetrical 665.9 ☑
    tuberculosis (conditions classifiable to
      010–018) 647.3 ☑
    tumor
      cervix 654.6 ☑
      ovary 654.4 ☑
      pelvic organs or tissue NEC 654.4 ☑
      uterus (body) 654.1 ☑
        cervix 654.6 ☑
      vagina 654.7 ☑
      vulva 654.8 ☑
    unstable lie 652.0 ☑
    uremia — *see* Pregnancy, complicated,
      renal disease
    urethritis 646.6 ☑
    vaginitis or vulvitis (conditions classifi-
      able to 616.1) 646.6 ☑
    varicose
      placental vessels 656.7 ☑
      veins (legs) 671.0 ☑
        perineum 671.1 ☑
        vulva 671.1 ☑
    varicosity, labia or vulva 671.1 ☑
    venereal disease NEC (conditions classi-
      fiable to 099) 647.2 ☑
    venous complication 671.9 ☑
    viral disease NEC (conditions classifiable
      to 042, 050–055, 057–079,
      795.05, 795.15, 796.75) 647.6 ☑
    vomiting (incoercible) (pernicious) (per-
      sistent) (uncontrollable) (vicious)
      643.9 ☑
      due to organic disease or other cause
        643.8 ☑
      early — *see* Hyperemesis, gravi-
        darum
      late (after 22 completed weeks gesta-
        tion) 643.2 ☑
    young maternal age 659.8 ☑
  complications NEC 646.9 ☑
  cornual 633.80
    with intrauterine pregnancy 633.81
    affecting fetus or newborn 761.4
  death, maternal NEC 646.9 ☑
  delivered — *see* Delivery
  ectopic (ruptured) NEC 633.90
    with intrauterine pregnancy 633.91
    abdominal — *see* Pregnancy, abdominal
    affecting fetus or newborn 761.4
    combined (extrauterine and intrauter-
      ine) — *see* Pregnancy, cornual
    ovarian — *see* Pregnancy, ovarian
    specified type NEC 633.80
      with intrauterine pregnancy 633.81

☑ **Additional Digit Required** — **Refer to the Tabular List for Digit Selection**   ▿ **Subterms under main terms may continue to next column or page**

Pregnancy — continued
  ectopic — continued
    specified type — continued
      affecting fetus or newborn 761.4
    tubal — see Pregnancy, tubal
  examination, pregnancy
    negative result V72.41
    not confirmed V72.40
    positive result V72.42
  extrauterine — see Pregnancy, ectopic
  fallopian — see Pregnancy, tubal
  false 300.11
    labor (pains) 644.1 ☑
  fatigue 646.8 ☑
  illegitimate V61.6
  incidental finding V22.2
  in double uterus 654.0 ☑
  interstitial — see Pregnancy, cornual
  intraligamentous — see Pregnancy, cornual
  intramural — see Pregnancy, cornual
  intraperitoneal — see Pregnancy, abdominal
  isthmian — see Pregnancy, tubal
  management affected by
    abnormal, abnormality
      fetus (suspected) 655.9 ☑
        specified NEC 655.8 ☑
      placenta 656.7 ☑
    advanced maternal age NEC 659.6 ☑
      multigravida 659.6 ☑
      primigravida 659.5 ☑
    antibodies (maternal)
      anti-c 656.1 ☑
      anti-d 656.1 ☑
      anti-e 656.1 ☑
      blood group (ABO) 656.2 ☑
        Rh(esus) 656.1 ☑
    appendicitis 648.9 ☑
    bariatric surgery status 649.2 ☑
    coagulation defect 649.3 ☑
    elderly multigravida 659.6 ☑
    elderly primigravida 659.5 ☑
    epilepsy 649.4 ☑
    fetal (suspected)
      abnormality 655.9 ☑
        abdominal 655.8 ☑
        acid-base balance 656.8 ☑
        cardiovascular 655.8 ☑
        facial 655.8 ☑
        gastrointestinal 655.8 ☑
        gentourinary 655.8 ☑
        heart rate or rhythm 659.7 ☑
        limb 655.8 ☑
        specified NEC 655.8 ☑
      acidemia 656.3 ☑
      anencephaly 655.0 ☑
      aneuploidy 655.1 ☑
      bradycardia 659.7 ☑
      central nervous system malformation 655.0 ☑
      chromosomal abnormalities (conditions classifiable to 758.0–758.9) 655.1 ☑
      damage from
        drugs 655.5 ☑
          obstetric, anesthetic, or sedative 655.5 ☑
        environmental toxins 655.8 ☑
        intrauterine contraceptive device 655.8 ☑
        maternal
          alcohol addiction 655.4 ☑
          disease NEC 655.4 ☑
          drug use 655.5 ☑
          listeriosis 655.4 ☑
          rubella 655.3 ☑
          toxoplasmosis 655.4 ☑
          viral infection 655.3 ☑
        radiation 655.6 ☑
      death (near term) 656.4 ☑
        early (before 22 completed weeks' gestation) 632
      distress 656.8 ☑
      excessive growth 656.6 ☑

Pregnancy — continued
  management affected by — continued
    fetal — continued
      fetal-maternal hemorrhage 656.0 ☑
      growth retardation 656.5 ☑
      hereditary disease 655.2 ☑
      hereditary disease in family (possibly) affecting fetus 655.2 ☑
      hydrocephalus 655.0 ☑
      incompatibility, blood groups (ABO) 656.2 ☑
      intrauterine death 656.4 ☑
      poor growth 656.5 ☑
      Rh(esus) 656.1 ☑
      spina bifida (with myelomeningocele) 655.0 ☑
    gastric banding status 649.2 ☑
    gastric bypass status for obesity 649.2 ☑
    insufficient prenatal care V23.7
    insulin resistance 648.8 ☑
    intrauterine death 656.4 ☑
    isoimmunization (ABO) 656.2 ☑
      Rh(esus) 656.1 ☑
    large-for-dates fetus 656.6 ☑
    light-for-dates fetus 656.5 ☑
    meconium in liquor 656.8 ☑
    mental disorder (conditions classifiable to 290–303, 305.0, 305.2–305.9, 306–316, 317–319) 648.4 ☑
    multiparity (grand) 659.4 ☑
    obesity 649.1 ☑
      surgery status 649.2 ☑
    poor obstetric history V23.49
      pre-term labor V23.41
    postmaturity
      post-term 645.1 ☑
      prolonged 645.2 ☑
    post-term pregnancy 645.1 ☑
    previous
      abortion V23.2
        habitual 646.3 ☑
      cesarean delivery 654.2 ☑
      difficult delivery V23.49
      ectopic pregnancy V23.42
      forceps delivery V23.49
      habitual abortions 646.3 ☑
      hemorrhage, antepartum or postpartum V23.49
      hydatidiform mole V23.1
      infertility V23.0
      in utero procedure during previous pregnancy V23.86
      malignancy NEC V23.89
      nonobstetrical conditions V23.8 ☑
      premature delivery V23.41
      recurrent pregnancy loss 646.3 ☑
      trophoblastic disease (conditions in 630) V23.1
      vesicular mole V23.1
    prolonged pregnancy 645.2 ☑
    recurrent pregnancy loss 646.3 ☑
    small-for-dates fetus 656.5 ☑
    smoking 649.0 ☑
    spotting 649.5 ☑
    suspected conditions not found
      amniotic cavity and membrane problem V89.01
      cervical shortening V89.05
      fetal anomaly V89.03
      fetal growth problem V89.04
      oligohydramnios V89.01
      other specified problem NEC V89.09
      placental problem V89.02
      polyhydramnios V89.01
    tobacco use disorder 649.0 ☑
    venous complication 671.9 ☑
    young maternal age 659.8 ☑
  maternal death NEC 646.9 ☑
  mesometric (mural) — see Pregnancy, cornual
  molar 631.8
    hydatidiform (see also Hydatidiform mole) 630
      previous, affecting management of pregnancy V23.1

Pregnancy — continued
  molar — continued
    previous, affecting management of pregnancy V23.49
  multiple NEC 651.9 ☑
    with fetal loss and retention of one or more fetus(es) 651.6 ☑
    affecting fetus or newborn 761.5
    following (elective) fetal reduction 651.7 ☑
    specified type NEC 651.8 ☑
      with fetal loss and retention of one or more fetus(es) 651.6 ☑
      following (elective) fetal reduction 651.7 ☑
  mural — see Pregnancy, cornual
  observation NEC V22.1
    first pregnancy V22.0
    high-risk V23.9
      inconclusive fetal viability V23.87
      specified problem NEC V23.89
  ovarian 633.20
    with intrauterine pregnancy 633.21
    affecting fetus or newborn 761.4
  possible, not (yet) confirmed V72.40
  postmature
    post-term 645.1 ☑
    prolonged 645.2 ☑
  post-term 645.1 ☑
  prenatal care only V22.1
    first pregnancy V22.0
    high-risk V23.9
      inconclusive fetal viability V23.87
      specified problem NEC V23.89
  prolonged 645.2 ☑
  quadruplet NEC 651.2 ☑
    with fetal loss and retention of one or more fetus(es) 651.5 ☑
    affecting fetus or newborn 761.5
    following (elective) fetal reduction 651.7 ☑
  quintuplet NEC 651.8 ☑
    with fetal loss and retention of one or more fetus(es) 651.6 ☑
    affecting fetus or newborn 761.5
    following (elective) fetal reduction 651.7 ☑
  resulting from
    assisted reproductive technology V23.85
    in vitro fertilization V23.85
  sextuplet NEC 651.8 ☑
    with fetal loss and retention of one or more fetus(es) 651.6 ☑
    affecting fetus or newborn 761.5
    following (elective) fetal reduction 651.7 ☑
  spurious 300.11
  superfecundation NEC 651.9 ☑
    with fetal loss and retention of one or more fetus(es) 651.6 ☑
    following (elective) fetal reduction 651.7 ☑
  superfetation NEC 651.9 ☑
    with fetal loss and retention of one or more fetus(es) 651.6 ☑
    following (elective) fetal reduction 651.7 ☑
  supervision (of) (for) (see also Pregnancy, management affected by)
    elderly
      multigravida V23.82
      primigravida V23.81
    high-risk V23.9
      inconclusive fetal viability V23.87
      insufficient prenatal care V23.7
      specified problem NEC V23.89
    inconclusive fetal viability V23.87
    multiparity V23.3
    normal NEC V22.1
      first V22.0
    poor
      obstetric history V23.49
        ectopic pregnancy V23.42
        pre-term labor V23.41
      reproductive history V23.5

Pregnancy — continued
  supervision (see also Pregnancy, management affected by) — continued
    previous
      abortion V23.2
      hydatidiform mole V23.1
      infertility V23.0
      neonatal death V23.5
      stillbirth V23.5
      trophoblastic disease V23.1
      vesicular mole V23.1
    specified problem NEC V23.89
    young
      multigravida V23.84
      primigravida V23.83
  triplet NEC 651.1 ☑
    with fetal loss and retention of one or more fetus(es) 651.4 ☑
    affecting fetus or newborn 761.5
    following (elective) fetal reduction 651.7 ☑
  tubal (with rupture) 633.10
    with intrauterine pregnancy 633.11
    affecting fetus or newborn 761.4
  twin NEC 651.0 ☑
    with fetal loss and retention of one fetus 651.3 ☑
    affecting fetus or newborn 761.5
    conjoined 678.1 ☑
    following (elective) fetal reduction 651.7 ☑
  unconfirmed V72.40
  undelivered (no other diagnosis) V22.2
    with false labor 644.1 ☑
    high-risk V23.9
      specified problem NEC V23.89
  unwanted NEC V61.7
Pregnant uterus — see condition
Preiser's disease (osteoporosis) 733.09
Prekwashiorkor 260
Preleukemia 238.75
Preluxation of hip, congenital — see also Subluxation, congenital, hip 754.32
Premature — see also condition
  beats (nodal) 427.60
    atrial 427.61
    auricular 427.61
    postoperative 997.1
    specified type NEC 427.69
    supraventricular 427.61
    ventricular 427.69
  birth NEC 765.1 ☑
  closure
    cranial suture 756.0
    fontanel 756.0
    foramen ovale 745.8
  contractions 427.60
    atrial 427.61
    auricular 427.61
    auriculoventricular 427.61
    heart (extrasystole) 427.60
    junctional 427.60
    nodal 427.60
    postoperative 997.1
    ventricular 427.69
  ejaculation 302.75
  infant NEC 765.1 ☑
    excessive 765.0 ☑
    light-for-dates — see Light-for-dates
  labor 644.2 ☑
    threatened 644.0 ☑
  lungs 770.4
  menopause 256.31
  puberty 259.1
  rupture of membranes or amnion 658.1 ☑
    affecting fetus or newborn 761.1
    delayed delivery following 658.2 ☑
  senility (syndrome) 259.8
  separation, placenta (partial) — see Placenta, separation
  ventricular systole 427.69
Prematurity NEC 765.1 ☑
  extreme 765.0 ☑
Premenstrual syndrome 625.4
Premenstrual tension 625.4
Premolarization, cuspids 520.2

☑ Additional Digit Required — Refer to the Tabular List for Digit Selection   ▽ Subterms under main terms may continue to next column or page

238 — Volume 2   ►◄ Revised Text   ● New Line   ▲ Revised Code   2013 ICD-9-CM

Premyeloma 273.1
Prenatal
  care, normal pregnancy V22.1
    first V22.0
  death, cause unknown — see Death, fetus
  screening — see Antenatal, screening
  teeth 520.6
Prepartum — see condition
Preponderance, left or right ventricular
  429.3
Prepuce — see condition
PRES (posterior reversible encephalopathy
  syndrome) 348.39
Presbycardia 797
  hypertensive (see also Hypertension, heart)
  402.90
Presbycusis 388.01
Presbyesophagus 530.89
Presbyophrenia 310.1
Presbyopia 367.4
Prescription of contraceptives NEC V25.02
  diaphragm V25.02
  oral (pill) V25.01
    emergency V25.03
    postcoital V25.03
    repeat V25.41
  repeat V25.40
    oral (pill) V25.41
Presenile — see also condition
  aging 259.8
  dementia (see also Dementia, presenile)
    290.10
Presenility 259.8
Presentation, fetal
  abnormal 652.9 ☑
    with successful version 652.1 ☑
    before labor, affecting fetus or newborn
      761.7
    causing obstructed labor 660.0 ☑
      affecting fetus or newborn, any, ex-
        cept breech 763.1
    in multiple gestation (one or more)
      652.6 ☑
    specified NEC 652.8 ☑
  arm 652.7 ☑
    causing obstructed labor 660.0 ☑
  breech (buttocks) (complete) (frank)
    652.2 ☑
    with successful version 652.1 ☑
      before labor, affecting fetus or new-
        born 761.7
    before labor, affecting fetus or newborn
      761.7
  brow 652.4 ☑
    causing obstructed labor 660.0 ☑
  buttocks 652.2 ☑
  chin 652.4 ☑
  complete 652.2 ☑
  compound 652.8 ☑
  cord 663.0 ☑
  extended head 652.4 ☑
  face 652.4 ☑
    to pubes 652.8 ☑
  footling 652.8 ☑
  frank 652.2 ☑
  hand, leg, or foot NEC 652.8 ☑
  incomplete 652.8 ☑
  mentum 652.4 ☑
  multiple gestation (one fetus or more)
    652.6 ☑
  oblique 652.3 ☑
    with successful version 652.1 ☑
  shoulder 652.8 ☑
    affecting fetus or newborn 763.1
  transverse 652.3 ☑
    with successful version 652.1 ☑
  umbilical cord 663.0 ☑
  unstable 652.0 ☑
Prespondylolisthesis (congenital) (lumbosacral) 756.11
Pressure
  area, skin ulcer (see also Ulcer, pressure)
    707.00
  atrophy, spine 733.99
  birth, fetus or newborn NEC 767.9

Pressure — continued
  brachial plexus 353.0
  brain 348.4
    injury at birth 767.0
  cerebral — see Pressure, brain
  chest 786.59
  cone, tentorial 348.4
    injury at birth 767.0
  funis — see Compression, umbilical cord
  hyposystolic (see also Hypotension) 458.9
  increased
    intracranial 781.99
      due to
        benign intracranial hypertension
          348.2
        hydrocephalus — see hydro-
          cephalus
        injury at birth 767.8
    intraocular 365.00
  lumbosacral plexus 353.1
  mediastinum 519.3
  necrosis (chronic) (skin) (see also Decubitus)
    707.00
  nerve — see Compression, nerve
  paralysis (see also Neuropathy, entrapment)
    355.9
  pre-ulcer skin changes limited to persistent
    focal erythema (see also Ulcer, pres-
    sure) 707.21
  sore (chronic) (see also Ulcer, pressure)
    707.00
  spinal cord 336.9
  ulcer (chronic) (see also Ulcer, pressure)
    707.00
  umbilical cord — see Compression, umbili-
    cal cord
  venous, increased 459.89
Pre-syncope 780.2
Preterm infant NEC 765.1 ☑
  extreme 765.0 ☑
Priapism (penis) 607.3
Prickling sensation — see also Disturbance,
  sensation 782.0
Prickly heat 705.1
Primary — see also condition
  angle closure suspect 365.02
Primigravida, elderly
  affecting
    fetus or newborn 763.89
    management of pregnancy, labor, and
      delivery 659.5 ☑
Primipara, old
  affecting
    fetus or newborn 763.89
    management of pregnancy, labor, and
      delivery 659.5 ☑
Primula dermatitis 692.6
Primus varus (bilateral) (metatarsus) 754.52
PRIND (prolonged reversible ischemic neurologic deficit) 434.91
  history of (personal) V12.54
Pringle's disease (tuberous sclerosis) 759.5
Prinzmetal's angina 413.1
Prinzmetal-Massumi syndrome (anterior
  chest wall) 786.52
Prizefighter ear 738.7
Problem (with) V49.9
  academic V62.3
  acculturation V62.4
  adopted child V61.24
  aged
    in-law V61.3
    parent V61.3
    person NEC V61.8
  alcoholism in family V61.41
  anger reaction (see also Disturbance, con-
    duct) 312.0 ☑
  behavioral V40.9
    specified NEC V40.39
  behavior, child 312.9
  betting V69.3
  biological child V61.23
  cardiorespiratory NEC V47.2
  career choice V62.29
  care of sick or handicapped person in family
    or household V61.49

Problem — continued
  communication V40.1
  conscience regarding medical care V62.6
  delinquency (juvenile) 312.9
  diet, inappropriate V69.1
  digestive NEC V47.3
  ear NEC V41.3
  eating habits, inappropriate V69.1
  economic V60.2
    affecting care V60.9
      specified type NEC V60.89
  educational V62.3
  enuresis, child 307.6
  exercise, lack of V69.0
  eye NEC V41.1
  family V61.9
    specified circumstance NEC V61.8
  fear reaction, child 313.0
  feeding (elderly) (infant) 783.3
    newborn 779.31
    nonorganic 307.59
  fetal, affecting management of pregnancy
    656.9 ☑
    specified type NEC 656.8 ☑
  financial V60.2
  foster child V61.25
  functional V41.9
    specified type NEC V41.8
  gambling V69.3
  genital NEC V47.5
  head V48.9
    deficiency V48.0
    disfigurement V48.6
    mechanical V48.2
    motor V48.2
    movement of V48.2
    sensory V48.4
    specified condition NEC V48.8
  hearing V41.2
  high-risk sexual behavior V69.2
  identity 313.82
  influencing health status NEC V49.89
  internal organ NEC V47.9
    deficiency V47.0
    mechanical or motor V47.1
  interpersonal NEC V62.81
  jealousy, child 313.3
  learning V40.0
  legal V62.5
  life circumstance NEC V62.89
  lifestyle V69.9
    specified NEC V69.8
  limb V49.9
    deficiency V49.0
    disfigurement V49.4
    mechanical V49.1
    motor V49.2
    movement, involving
      musculoskeletal system V49.1
      nervous system V49.2
    sensory V49.3
    specified condition NEC V49.5
  litigation V62.5
  living alone V60.3
  loneliness NEC V62.89
  marital V61.10
    involving
      divorce V61.03
      estrangement V61.09
      psychosexual disorder 302.9
      sexual function V41.7
    relationship V61.10
  mastication V41.6
  medical care, within family V61.49
  mental V40.9
    specified NEC V40.2
  mental hygiene, adult V40.9
  multiparity V61.5
  nail biting, child 307.9
  neck V48.9
    deficiency V48.1
    disfigurement V48.7
    mechanical V48.3
    motor V48.3
    movement V48.3
    sensory V48.5

Problem — continued
  neck — continued
    specified condition NEC V48.8
  neurological NEC 781.99
  none (feared complaint unfounded) V65.5
  occupational V62.29
  parent-child V61.20
    adopted child V61.24
    biological child V61.23
    foster child V61.25
    relationship V61.20
  partner V61.10
    relationship V61.10
  personal NEC V62.89
    interpersonal conflict NEC V62.81
  personality (see also Disorder, personality)
    301.9
  phase of life V62.89
  placenta, affecting management of pregnan-
    cy 656.9 ☑
    specified type NEC 656.8 ☑
  poverty V60.2
  presence of sick or handicapped person in
    family or household V61.49
  psychiatric 300.9
  psychosocial V62.9
    specified type NEC V62.89
  relational NEC V62.81
  relationship, childhood 313.3
  religious or spiritual belief
    other than medical care V62.89
    regarding medical care V62.6
  self-damaging behavior V69.8
  sexual
    behavior, high-risk V69.2
    function NEC V41.7
  sibling
    relational V61.8
    relationship V61.8
  sight V41.0
  sleep disorder, child 307.40
  sleep, lack of V69.4
  smell V41.5
  speech V40.1
  spite reaction, child (see also Disturbance,
    conduct) 312.0 ☑
  spoiled child reaction (see also Disturbance,
    conduct) 312.1 ☑
  substance abuse in family V61.42
  swallowing V41.6
  tantrum, child (see also Disturbance, con-
    duct) 312.1 ☑
  taste V41.5
  thumb sucking, child 307.9
  tic (child) 307.21
  trunk V48.9
    deficiency V48.1
    disfigurement V48.7
    mechanical V48.3
    motor V48.3
    movement V48.3
    sensory V48.5
    specified condition NEC V48.8
  unemployment V62.0
  urinary NEC V47.4
  voice production V41.4
Procedure (surgical) **not done** NEC V64.3
  because of
    contraindication V64.1
    patient's decision V64.2
      for reasons of conscience or religion
        V62.6
    specified reason NEC V64.3
Procidentia
  anus (sphincter) 569.1
  rectum (sphincter) 569.1
  stomach 537.89
  uteri 618.1
Proctalgia 569.42
  fugax 564.6
  spasmodic 564.6
    psychogenic 307.89
Proctitis 569.49
  amebic 006.8
  chlamydial 099.52
  gonococcal 098.7

☑ **Additional Digit Required** — Refer to the Tabular List for Digit Selection   ▽ **Subterms under main terms may continue to next column or page**

2013 ICD-9-CM   ▶◀ **Revised Text**   ● **New Line**   ▲ **Revised Code**   **Volume 2 — 239**

Proctitis — continued
  granulomatous 555.1
  idiopathic 556.2
    with ulcerative sigmoiditis 556.3
  tuberculous (see also Tuberculosis) 014.8 ☑
  ulcerative (chronic) (nonspecific) 556.2
    with ulcerative sigmoiditis 556.3
Proctocele
  female (without uterine prolapse) 618.04
    with uterine prolapse 618.4
      complete 618.3
      incomplete 618.2
  male 569.49
Proctocolitis, idiopathic 556.2
  with ulcerative sigmoiditis 556.3
Proctoptosis 569.1
Proctosigmoiditis 569.89
  ulcerative (chronic) 556.3
Proctospasm 564.6
  psychogenic 306.4
Prodromal-AIDS — see Human immunodefi-
    ciency virus (disease) (illness) (infection)
Profichet's disease or syndrome 729.90
Progeria (adultorum) (syndrome) 259.8
Prognathism (mandibular) (maxillary) 524.10
Progonoma (melanotic) (M9363/0) — see
    Neoplasm, by site, benign
Progressive — see condition
Prolapse, prolapsed
  anus, anal (canal) (sphincter) 569.1
  arm or hand, complicating delivery 652.7 ☑
    causing obstructed labor 660.0 ☑
      affecting fetus or newborn 763.1
    fetus or newborn 763.1
  bladder (acquired) (mucosa) (sphincter)
    congenital (female) (male) 756.71
    female (see also Cystocele, female)
      618.01
    male 596.89
  breast implant (prosthetic) 996.54
  cecostomy 569.69
  cecum 569.89
  cervix, cervical (hypertrophied) 618.1
    anterior lip, obstructing labor 660.2 ☑
      affecting fetus or newborn 763.1
    congenital 752.49
    postpartal (old) 618.1
    stump 618.84
  ciliary body 871.1
  colon (pedunculated) 569.89
  colostomy 569.69
  conjunctiva 372.73
  cord — see Prolapse, umbilical cord
  cystostomy 596.83
  disc (intervertebral) — see Displacement,
    intervertebral disc
  duodenum 537.89
  eye implant (orbital) 996.59
    lens (ocular) 996.53
  fallopian tube 620.4
  fetal extremity, complicating delivery
    652.8 ☑
    causing obstructed labor 660.0 ☑
    fetus or newborn 763.1
  funis — see Prolapse, umbilical cord
  gastric (mucosa) 537.89
  genital, female 618.9
    specified NEC 618.89
  globe 360.81
  ileostomy bud 569.69
  intervertebral disc — see Displacement, in-
    tervertebral disc
  intestine (small) 569.89
  iris 364.89
    traumatic 871.1
  kidney (see also Disease, renal) 593.0
    congenital 753.3
  laryngeal muscles or ventricle 478.79
  leg, complicating delivery 652.8 ☑
    causing obstructed labor 660.0 ☑
    fetus or newborn 763.1
  liver 573.8
  meatus urinarius 599.5
  mitral valve 424.0
  ocular lens implant 996.53

Prolapse, prolapsed — continued
  organ or site, congenital NEC — see Malpo-
    sition, congenital
  ovary 620.4
  pelvic (floor), female 618.89
  perineum, female 618.89
  pregnant uterus 654.4 ☑
  rectum (mucosa) (sphincter) 569.1
    due to Trichuris trichiuria 127.3
  spleen 289.59
  stomach 537.89
  umbilical cord
    affecting fetus or newborn 762.4
    complicating delivery 663.0 ☑
  ureter 593.89
    with obstruction 593.4
  ureterovesical orifice 593.89
  urethra (acquired) (infected) (mucosa) 599.5
    congenital 753.8
  uterovaginal 618.4
    complete 618.3
    incomplete 618.2
    specified NEC 618.89
  uterus (first degree) (second degree) (third
    degree) (complete) (without vaginal
    wall prolapse) 618.1
    with mention of vaginal wall prolapse
      — see Prolapse, uterovaginal
    congenital 752.39
    in pregnancy or childbirth 654.4 ☑
      affecting fetus or newborn 763.1
      causing obstructed labor 660.2 ☑
        affecting fetus or newborn 763.1
    postpartal (old) 618.1
  uveal 871.1
  vagina (anterior) (posterior) (vault) (wall)
    (without uterine prolapse) 618.00
    with uterine prolapse 618.4
      complete 618.3
      incomplete 618.2
    paravaginal 618.02
    posthysterectomy 618.5
    specified NEC 618.09
  vitreous (humor) 379.26
    traumatic 871.1
  womb — see Prolapse, uterus
Prolapsus, female 618.9
Proliferative — see condition
Prolinemia 270.8
Prolinuria 270.8
Prolonged, prolongation
  bleeding time (see also Defect, coagulation)
    790.92
    "idiopathic" (in von Willebrand's disease)
      286.4
  coagulation time (see also Defect, coagula-
    tion) 790.92
  gestation syndrome 766.22
  labor 662.1 ☑
    affecting fetus or newborn 763.89
    first stage 662.0 ☑
    second stage 662.2 ☑
  pregnancy 645.2 ☑
  PR interval 426.11
  prothrombin time (see also Defect, coagula-
    tion) 790.92
  QT interval 794.31
    syndrome 426.82
  rupture of membranes (24 hours or more
    prior to onset of labor) 658.2 ☑
  uterine contractions in labor 661.4 ☑
    affecting fetus or newborn 763.7
Prominauris 744.29
Prominence
  auricle (ear) (congenital) 744.29
    acquired 380.32
  ischial spine or sacral promontory
    with disproportion (fetopelvic) 653.3 ☑
      affecting fetus or newborn 763.1
      causing obstructed labor 660.1 ☑
        affecting fetus or newborn 763.1
  nose (congenital) 748.1
    acquired 738.0
PROMM (proximal myotonic myotonia) 359.21
Pronation
  ankle 736.79

Pronation — continued
  foot 736.79
    congenital 755.67
Prophylactic
  administration of
    antibiotics, long-term V58.62
      short-term — omit code
    antitoxin, any V07.2
    antivenin V07.2
    chemotherapeutic agent NEC V07.39
      fluoride V07.31
    diphtheria antitoxin V07.2
    drug V07.39
    exemestar (Aromasin) V07.52
    gamma globulin V07.2
    immune sera (gamma globulin) V07.2
    RhoGAM V07.2
    tetanus antitoxin V07.2
  chemotherapy NEC V07.39
    fluoride V07.31
  hormone replacement (postmenopausal)
    V07.4
  immunotherapy V07.2
  measure V07.9
    specified type NEC V07.8
  medication V07.39
  postmenopausal hormone replacement
    V07.4
  sterilization V25.2
Proptosis (ocular) — see also Exophthalmos
    376.30
  thyroid 242.0 ☑
Propulsion
  eyeball 360.81
Prosecution, anxiety concerning V62.5
Prosopagnosia 368.16
Prostate, prostatic — see condition
Prostatism 600.90
  with
    other lower urinary tract symptoms
      (LUTS) 600.91
    urinary
      obstruction 600.91
      retention 600.91
Prostatitis (congestive) (suppurative) 601.9
  acute 601.0
  cavitary 601.8
  chlamydial 099.54
  chronic 601.1
  diverticular 601.8
  due to Trichomonas (vaginalis) 131.03
  fibrous 600.90
    with
      other lower urinary tract symptoms
        (LUTS) 600.91
      urinary
        obstruction 600.91
        retention 600.91
  gonococcal (acute) 098.12
    chronic or duration of 2 months or over
      098.32
  granulomatous 601.8
  hypertrophic 600.00
    with
      other lower urinary tract symptoms
        (LUTS) 600.01
      urinary
        obstruction 600.01
        retention 600.01
  specified type NEC 601.8
  subacute 601.1
  trichomonal 131.03
  tuberculous (see also Tuberculosis)
    016.5 ☑ [601.4]
Prostatocystitis 601.3
Prostatorrhea 602.8
Prostatoseminovesiculitis, trichomonal
    131.03
Prostration 780.79
  heat 992.5
    anhydrotic 992.3
    due to
      salt (and water) depletion 992.4
      water depletion 992.3
  nervous 300.5
  newborn 779.89

Prostration — continued
  senile 797
Protanomaly 368.51
Protanopia (anomalous trichromat) (complete)
    (incomplete) 368.51
Protection (against) (from) — see Prophylactic
Protein
  deficiency 260
  malnutrition 260
  sickness (prophylactic) (therapeutic) 999.59
Proteinemia 790.99
Proteinosis
  alveolar, lung or pulmonary 516.0
  lipid 272.8
  lipoid (of Urbach) 272.8
Proteinuria — see also Albuminuria 791.0
  Bence-Jones NEC 791.0
  gestational 646.2 ☑
    with hypertension — see Toxemia, of
      pregnancy
  orthostatic 593.6
  postural 593.6
Proteolysis, pathologic 286.6
Protocoproporphyria 277.1
Protoporphyria (erythrohepatic) (erythropoi-
    etic) 277.1
Protrusio acetabuli 718.65
Protrusion
  acetabulum (into pelvis) 718.65
  device, implant, or graft — see Complica-
    tions, mechanical
  ear, congenital 744.29
  intervertebral disc — see Displacement, in-
    tervertebral disc
  nucleus pulposus — see Displacement, in-
    tervertebral disc
Proud flesh 701.5
Prune belly (syndrome) 756.71
Prurigo (ferox) (gravis) (Hebra's) (hebrae) (mi-
    tis) (simplex) 698.2
  agria 698.3
  asthma syndrome 691.8
  Besnier's (atopic dermatitis) (infantile
    eczema) 691.8
  eczematodes allergicum 691.8
  estivalis (Hutchinson's) 692.72
  Hutchinson's 692.72
  nodularis 698.3
  psychogenic 306.3
Pruritus, pruritic 698.9
  ani 698.0
    psychogenic 306.3
  conditions NEC 698.9
    psychogenic 306.3
  due to Onchocerca volvulus 125.3
  ear 698.9
  essential 698.9
  genital organ(s) 698.1
    psychogenic 306.3
  gravidarum 646.8 ☑
  hiemalis 698.8
  neurogenic (any site) 306.3
  perianal 698.0
  psychogenic (any site) 306.3
  scrotum 698.1
    psychogenic 306.3
  senile, senilis 698.8
  Trichomonas 131.9
  vulva, vulvae 698.1
    psychogenic 306.3
Psammocarcinoma (M8140/3) — see Neo-
    plasm, by site, malignant
Pseudarthrosis, pseudoarthrosis (bone)
    733.82
  joint following fusion V45.4
Pseudoacanthosis
  nigricans 701.8
Pseudoaneurysm — see Aneurysm
Pseudoangina (pectoris) — see Angina
Pseudoangioma 452
Pseudo-Argyll-Robertson pupil 379.45
Pseudoarteriosus 747.89
Pseudoarthrosis — see Pseudarthrosis
Pseudoataxia 799.89
Pseudobulbar affect (PBA) 310.81
Pseudobursa 727.89

☑ Additional Digit Required — Refer to the Tabular List for Digit Selection   ▼ Subterms under main terms may continue to next column or page

Pseudocholera 025
Pseudochromidrosis 705.89
Pseudocirrhosis, liver, pericardial 423.2
Pseudocoarctation 747.21
Pseudocowpox 051.1
Pseudocoxalgia 732.1
Pseudocroup 478.75
Pseudocyesis 300.11
Pseudocyst
  lung 518.89
  pancreas 577.2
  retina 361.19
Pseudodementia 300.16
Pseudoelephantiasis neuroarthritica 757.0
Pseudoemphysema 518.89
Pseudoencephalitis
  superior (acute) hemorrhagic 265.1
Pseudoerosion cervix, congenital 752.49
Pseudoexfoliation, lens capsule 366.11
Pseudofracture (idiopathic) (multiple) (spontaneous) (symmetrical) 268.2
Pseudoglanders 025
Pseudoglioma 360.44
Pseudogout — *see* Chondrocalcinosis
Pseudohallucination 780.1
Pseudohemianesthesia 782.0
Pseudohemophilia (Bernuth's) (hereditary) (typeB) 286.4
  type A 287.8
  vascular 287.8
Pseudohermaphroditism 752.7
  with chromosomal anomaly — *see* Anomaly, chromosomal
  adrenal 255.2
  female (without adrenocortical disorder) 752.7
    with adrenocortical disorder 255.2
    adrenal 255.2
  male (without gonadal disorder) 752.7
    with
      adrenocortical disorder 255.2
      cleft scrotum 752.7
      feminizing testis 259.51
      gonadal disorder 257.9
      adrenal 255.2
Pseudohole, macula 362.54
Pseudo-Hurler's disease (mucolipidosis III) 272.7
Pseudohydrocephalus 348.2
Pseudohypertrophic muscular dystrophy (Erb's) 359.1
Pseudohypertrophy, muscle 359.1
Pseudohypoparathyroidism 275.49
Pseudoinfluenza — *see also* Influenza 487.1
Pseudoinsomnia 307.49
Pseudoleukemia 288.8
  infantile 285.8
Pseudomembranous — *see* condition
Pseudomeningocele (cerebral) (infective) 349.2
  postprocedural 997.01
  spinal 349.2
Pseudomenstruation 626.8
Pseudomucinous
  cyst (ovary) (M8470/0) 220
  peritoneum 568.89
Pseudomyeloma 273.1
Pseudomyxoma peritonei (M8480/6) 197.6
Pseudoneuritis optic (nerve) 377.24
  papilla 377.24
  congenital 743.57
Pseudoneuroma — *see* Injury, nerve, by site
Pseudo-obstruction
  intestine (chronic) (idiopathic) (intermittent secondary) (primary) 564.89
  acute 560.89
Pseudopapilledema 377.24
Pseudoparalysis
  arm or leg 781.4
  atonic, congenital 358.8
Pseudopelade 704.09
Pseudophakia V43.1
Pseudopolycythemia 289.0
Pseudopolyposis, colon 556.4
Pseudoporencephaly 348.0
Pseudopseudohypoparathyroidism 275.49

Pseudopsychosis 300.16
Pseudopterygium 372.52
Pseudoptosis (eyelid) 374.34
Pseudorabies 078.89
Pseudoretinitis, pigmentosa 362.65
Pseudorickets 588.0
  senile (Pozzi's) 731.0
Pseudorubella 057.8
Pseudoscarlatina 057.8
Pseudosclerema 778.1
Pseudosclerosis (brain)
  Jakob's 046.19
  of Westphal (-Strümpell) (hepatolenticular degeneration) 275.1
  spastic 046.19
    with dementia
      with behavioral disturbance 046.19 *[294.11]*
      without behavioral disturbance 046.19 *[294.10]*
Pseudoseizure 780.39
  non-psychiatric 780.39
  psychiatric 300.11
Pseudotabes 799.89
  diabetic 250.6 ☑ *[337.1]*
    due to secondary diabetes 249.6 ☑ *[337.1]*
Pseudotetanus — *see also* Convulsions 780.39
Pseudotetany 781.7
  hysterical 300.11
Pseudothalassemia 285.0
Pseudotrichinosis 710.3
Pseudotruncus arteriosus 747.29
Pseudotuberculosis, pasteurella (infection) 027.2
Pseudotumor
  cerebri 348.2
  orbit (inflammatory) 376.11
Pseudo-Turner's syndrome 759.89
Pseudoxanthoma elasticum 757.39
Psilosis (sprue) (tropical) 579.1
  Monilia 112.89
  nontropical 579.0
  not sprue 704.00
Psittacosis 073.9
Psoitis 728.89
Psora NEC 696.1
Psoriasis 696.1
  any type, except arthropathic 696.1
  arthritic, arthropathic 696.0
  buccal 528.6
  flexural 696.1
  follicularis 696.1
  guttate 696.1
  inverse 696.1
  mouth 528.6
  nummularis 696.1
  psychogenic 316 *[696.1]*
  punctata 696.1
  pustular 696.1
  rupioides 696.1
  vulgaris 696.1
Psorospermiasis 136.4
Psorospermosis 136.4
  follicularis (vegetans) 757.39
Psychalgia 307.80
Psychasthenia 300.89
  compulsive 300.3
  mixed compulsive states 300.3
  obsession 300.3
Psychiatric disorder or problem NEC 300.9
Psychogenic — *see also* condition
  factors associated with physical conditions 316
Psychoneurosis, psychoneurotic — *see also* Neurosis 300.9
  anxiety (state) 300.00
  climacteric 627.2
  compensation 300.16
  compulsion 300.3
  conversion hysteria 300.11
  depersonalization 300.6
  depressive type 300.4
  dissociative hysteria 300.15
  hypochondriacal 300.7
  hysteria 300.10

Psychoneurosis, psychoneurotic — *see also* Neurosis — *continued*
  hysteria — *continued*
    conversion type 300.11
    dissociative type 300.15
  mixed NEC 300.89
  neurasthenic 300.5
  obsessional 300.3
  obsessive-compulsive 300.3
  occupational 300.89
  personality NEC 301.89
  phobia 300.20
  senile NEC 300.89
Psychopathic — *see also* condition
  constitution, posttraumatic 310.2
    with psychosis 293.9
  personality 301.9
    amoral trends 301.7
    antisocial trends 301.7
    asocial trends 301.7
    mixed types 301.7
  state 301.9
Psychopathy, sexual — *see also* Deviation, sexual 302.9
Psychophysiologic, psychophysiological condition — *see* Reaction, psychophysiologic
Psychose passionelle 297.8
Psychosexual identity disorder 302.6
  adult-life 302.85
  childhood 302.6
Psychosis 298.9
  acute hysterical 298.1
  affecting management of pregnancy, childbirth, or puerperium 648.4 ☑
  affective (*see also* Disorder, mood) 296.90

> *Note* — Use the following fifth-digit subclassification with categories 296.0–296.6:
>
> 0   unspecified
>
> 1   mild
>
> 2   moderate
>
> 3   severe, without mention of psychotic behavior
>
> 4   severe, specified as with psychotic behavior
>
> 5   in partial or unspecified remission
>
> 6   in full remission

    drug-induced 292.84
    due to or associated with physical condition 293.83
    involutional 293.83
      recurrent episode 296.3 ☑
      single episode 296.2 ☑
    manic-depressive 296.80
      circular (alternating) 296.7
        currently depressed 296.5 ☑
        currently manic 296.4 ☑
      depressed type 296.2 ☑
        atypical 296.82
        recurrent episode 296.3 ☑
        single episode 296.2 ☑
      manic 296.0 ☑
        atypical 296.81
        recurrent episode 296.1 ☑
        single episode 296.0 ☑
      mixed type NEC 296.89
      specified type NEC 296.89
    senile 290.21
    specified type NEC 296.99
  alcoholic 291.9
    with
      anxiety 291.89
      delirium tremens 291.0
      delusions 291.5
      dementia 291.2
      hallucinosis 291.3
      jealousy 291.5
      mood disturbance 291.89
      paranoia 291.5
      persisting amnesia 291.1
      sexual dysfunction 291.89

Psychosis — *continued*
  alcoholic — *continued*
    with — *continued*
      sleep disturbance 291.89
    amnestic confabulatory 291.1
    delirium tremens 291.0
    hallucinosis 291.3
    Korsakoff's, Korsakov's, Korsakow's 291.1
    paranoid type 291.5
    pathological intoxication 291.4
    polyneuritic 291.1
    specified type NEC 291.89
  alternating (*see also* Psychosis, manic-depressive, circular) 296.7
  anergastic (*see also* Psychosis, organic) 294.9
  arteriosclerotic 290.40
    with
      acute confusional state 290.41
      delirium 290.41
      delusions 290.42
      depressed mood 290.43
    depressed type 290.43
    paranoid type 290.42
    simple type 290.40
    uncomplicated 290.40
  atypical 298.9
    depressive 296.82
    manic 296.81
  borderline (schizophrenia) (*see also* Schizophrenia) 295.5 ☑
    of childhood (*see also* Psychosis, childhood) 299.8 ☑
    prepubertal 299.8 ☑
  brief reactive 298.8
  childhood, with origin specific to 299.9 ☑

> *Note* — Use the following fifth-digit subclassification with category 299:
>
> 0   current or active state
>
> 1   residual state

    atypical 299.8 ☑
    specified type NEC 299.8 ☑
  circular (*see also* Psychosis, manic-depressive, circular) 296.7
  climacteric (*see also* Psychosis, involutional) 298.8
  confusional 298.9
    acute 293.0
    reactive 298.2
    subacute 293.1
  depressive (*see also* Psychosis, affective) 296.2 ☑
    atypical 296.82
    involutional 296.2 ☑
      with hypomania (bipolar II) 296.89
      recurrent episode 296.3 ☑
      single episode 296.2 ☑
    psychogenic 298.0
    reactive (emotional stress) (psychological trauma) 298.0
    recurrent episode 296.3 ☑
      with hypomania (bipolar II) 296.89
    single episode 296.2 ☑
  disintegrative, childhood (*see also* Psychosis, childhood) 299.1 ☑
  drug 292.9
    with
      affective syndrome 292.84
      amnestic syndrome 292.83
      anxiety 292.89
      delirium 292.81
        withdrawal 292.0
      delusions 292.11
      dementia 292.82
      depressive state 292.84
      hallucinations 292.12
      hallucinosis 292.12
      mood disorder 292.84
      mood disturbance 292.84
      organic personality syndrome NEC 292.89
      sexual dysfunction 292.89
      sleep disturbance 292.89
      withdrawal syndrome (and delirium) 292.0

☑ **Additional Digit Required** — Refer to the Tabular List for Digit Selection   ▽ **Subterms under main terms may continue to next column or page**

2013 ICD-9-CM   ▶◀ **Revised Text**   ● **New Line**   ▲ **Revised Code**   **Volume 2 — 241**

Psychosis — *continued*
- drug — *continued*
  - affective syndrome 292.84
  - delusions 292.11
  - hallucinatory state 292.12
  - hallucinosis 292.12
  - paranoid state 292.11
  - specified type NEC 292.89
  - withdrawal syndrome (and delirium) 292.0
  - due to or associated with physical condition (*see also* Psychosis, organic) 293.9
- epileptic NEC 293.9
- excitation (psychogenic) (reactive) 298.1
- exhaustive (*see also* Reaction, stress, acute) 308.9
- hypomanic (*see also* Psychosis, affective) 296.0 ☑
  - recurrent episode 296.1 ☑
  - single episode 296.0 ☑
- hysterical 298.8
  - acute 298.1
- in
  - conditions classified elsewhere
    - with
      - delusions 293.81
      - hallucinations 293.82
    - pregnancy, childbirth, or puerperium 648.4 ☑
- incipient 298.8
  - schizophrenic (*see also* Schizophrenia) 295.5 ☑
- induced 297.3
- infantile (*see also* Psychosis, childhood) 299.0 ☑
- infective 293.9
  - acute 293.0
  - subacute 293.1
- interactional (childhood) (*see also* Psychosis, childhood) 299.1 ☑
- involutional 298.8
  - depressive (*see also* Psychosis, affective) 296.2 ☑
    - recurrent episode 296.3 ☑
    - single episode 296.2 ☑
  - melancholic 296.2 ☑
    - recurrent episode 296.3 ☑
    - single episode 296.2 ☑
  - paranoid state 297.2
  - paraphrenia 297.2
- Korsakoff's, Korakov's, Korsakow's (nonalcoholic) 294.0
  - alcoholic 291.1
- mania (phase) (*see also* Psychosis, affective) 296.0 ☑
  - recurrent episode 296.1 ☑
  - single episode 296.0 ☑
- manic (*see also* Psychosis, affective) 296.0 ☑
  - atypical 296.81
  - recurrent episode 296.1 ☑
  - single episode 296.0 ☑
- manic-depressive 296.80
  - circular 296.7
    - currently
      - depressed 296.5 ☑
      - manic 296.4 ☑
    - mixed 296.6 ☑
  - depressive 296.2 ☑
    - recurrent episode 296.3 ☑
      - with hypomania (bipolar II) 296.89
    - single episode 296.2 ☑
  - hypomanic 296.0 ☑
    - recurrent episode 296.1 ☑
    - single episode 296.0 ☑
  - manic 296.0 ☑
    - atypical 296.81
    - recurrent episode 296.1 ☑
    - single episode 296.0 ☑
  - mixed NEC 296.89
  - perplexed 296.89
  - stuporous 296.89
- menopausal (*see also* Psychosis, involutional) 298.8

Psychosis — *continued*
- mixed schizophrenic and affective (*see also* Schizophrenia) 295.7 ☑
- multi-infarct (cerebrovascular) (*see also* Psychosis, arteriosclerotic) 290.40
- organic NEC 294.9
  - due to or associated with
    - addiction
      - alcohol (*see also* Psychosis, alcoholic) 291.9
      - drug (*see also* Psychosis, drug) 292.9
    - alcohol intoxication, acute (*see also* Psychosis, alcoholic) 291.9
    - alcoholism (*see also* Psychosis, alcoholic) 291.9
    - arteriosclerosis (cerebral) (*see also* Psychosis, arteriosclerotic) 290.40
    - cerebrovascular disease
      - acute (psychosis) 293.0
      - arteriosclerotic (*see also* Psychosis, arteriosclerotic) 290.40
    - childbirth — *see* Psychosis, puerperal
    - dependence
      - alcohol (*see also* Psychosis, alcoholic) 291.9
      - drug 292.9
    - disease
      - alcoholic liver (*see also* Psychosis, alcoholic) 291.9
      - brain
        - arteriosclerotic (*see also* Psychosis, arteriosclerotic) 290.40
        - cerebrovascular
          - acute (psychosis) 293.0
          - arteriosclerotic (*see also* Psychosis, arteriosclerotic) 290.40
        - endocrine or metabolic 293.9
          - acute (psychosis) 293.0
          - subacute (psychosis) 293.1
        - Jakob-Creutzfeldt 046.19
          - with behavioral disturbance 046.19 *[294.11]*
          - without behavioral disturbance 046.19 *[294.10]*
          - familial 046.19
          - iatrogenic 046.19
          - specified NEC 046.19
          - sporadic 046.19
          - variant 046.11
            - with dementia
              - with behavioral disturbance 046.11 *[294.11]*
              - without behavioral disturbance 046.11 *[294.10]*
        - liver, alcoholic (*see also* Psychosis, alcoholic) 291.9
      - disorder
        - cerebrovascular
          - acute (psychosis) 293.0
        - endocrine or metabolic 293.9
          - acute (psychosis) 293.0
          - subacute (psychosis) 293.1
      - epilepsy
        - with behavioral disturbance 345.9 ☑ *[294.11]*
        - without behavioral disturbance 345.9 ☑ *[294.10]*
        - transient (acute) 293.0
      - Huntington's chorea
        - with behavioral disturbance 333.4 *[294.11]*
        - without behavioral disturbance 333.4 *[294.10]*
      - infection
        - brain 293.9
          - acute (psychosis) 293.0
          - chronic 294.8
          - subacute (psychosis) 293.1
        - intracranial NEC 293.9

Psychosis — *continued*
- organic — *continued*
  - due to or associated with — *continued*
    - infection — *continued*
      - intracranial — *continued*
        - acute (psychosis) 293.0
        - chronic 294.8
        - subacute (psychosis) 293.1
    - intoxication
      - alcoholic (acute) (*see also* Psychosis, alcoholic) 291.9
      - pathological 291.4
      - drug (*see also* Psychosis, drug) 292.9
    - ischemia
      - cerebrovascular (generalized) (*see also* Psychosis, arteriosclerotic) 290.40
    - Jakob-Creutzfeldt disease (syndrome) 046.19
      - with behavioral disturbance 046.19 *[294.11]*
      - without behavioral disturbance 046.19 *[294.10]*
      - variant 046.11
        - with dementia
          - with behavioral disturbance 046.11 *[294.11]*
          - without behavioral disturbance 046.11 *[294.10]*
    - multiple sclerosis
      - with behavioral disturbance 340 *[294.11]*
      - without behavioral disturbance 340 *[294.10]*
    - physical condition NEC 293.9
      - with
        - delusions 293.81
        - hallucinations 293.82
    - presenility 290.10
    - puerperium — *see* Psychosis, puerperal
    - sclerosis, multiple
      - with behavioral disturbance 340 *[294.11]*
      - without behavioral disturbance 340 *[294.10]*
    - senility 290.20
    - status epilepticus
      - with behavioral disturbance 345.3 *[294.11]*
      - without behavioral disturbance 345.3 *[294.10]*
    - trauma
      - brain (birth) (from electrical current) (surgical) 293.9
        - acute (psychosis) 293.0
        - chronic 294.8
        - subacute (psychosis) 293.1
        - unspecified physical condition 293.9
          - with
            - delusion 293.81
            - hallucinations 293.82
  - infective 293.9
    - acute (psychosis) 293.0
    - subacute 293.1
  - posttraumatic 293.9
    - acute 293.0
    - subacute 293.1
  - specified type NEC 294.8
  - transient 293.9
    - with
      - anxiety 293.84
      - delusions 293.81
      - depression 293.83
      - hallucinations 293.82
    - depressive type 293.83
    - hallucinatory type 293.82
    - paranoid type 293.81
    - specified type NEC 293.89
  - paranoic 297.1
  - paranoid (chronic) 297.9

Psychosis — *continued*
- paranoid — *continued*
  - alcoholic 291.5
  - chronic 297.1
  - climacteric 297.2
  - involutional 297.2
  - menopausal 297.2
  - protracted reactive 298.4
  - psychogenic 298.4
    - acute 298.3
  - schizophrenic (*see also* Schizophrenia) 295.3 ☑
  - senile 290.20
- paroxysmal 298.9
  - senile 290.20
- polyneuritic, alcoholic 291.1
- postoperative 293.9
- postpartum — *see* Psychosis, puerperal
- prepsychotic (*see also* Schizophrenia) 295.5 ☑
- presbyophrenic (type) 290.8
- presenile (*see also* Dementia, presenile) 290.10
- prison 300.16
- psychogenic 298.8
  - depressive 298.0
  - paranoid 298.4
    - acute 298.3
- puerperal
  - specified type — *see* categories 295-298 ☑
  - unspecified type 293.89
    - acute 293.0
    - chronic 293.89
    - subacute 293.1
- reactive (emotional stress) (psychological trauma) 298.8
  - brief 298.8
  - confusion 298.2
  - depressive 298.0
  - excitation 298.1
- schizo-affective (depressed) (excited) (*see also* Schizophrenia) 295.7 ☑
- schizophrenia, schizophrenic (*see also* Schizophrenia) 295.9 ☑
  - borderline type 295.5 ☑
    - of childhood (*see also* Psychosis, childhood) 299.8 ☑
  - catatonic (excited) (withdrawn) 295.2 ☑
  - childhood type (*see also* Psychosis, childhood) 299.9 ☑
  - hebephrenic 295.1 ☑
  - incipient 295.5 ☑
  - latent 295.5 ☑
  - paranoid 295.3 ☑
  - prepsychotic 295.5 ☑
  - prodromal 295.5 ☑
  - pseudoneurotic 295.5 ☑
  - pseudopsychopathic 295.5 ☑
  - schizophreniform 295.4 ☑
  - simple 295.0 ☑
  - undifferentiated type 295.9 ☑
- schizophreniform 295.4 ☑
- senile NEC 290.20
  - with
    - delusional features 290.20
    - depressive features 290.21
  - depressed type 290.21
  - paranoid type 290.20
  - simple deterioration 290.20
  - specified type — *see* categories 295-298 ☑
- shared 297.3
- situational (reactive) 298.8
- symbiotic (childhood) (*see also* Psychosis, childhood) 299.1 ☑
- toxic (acute) 293.9

Psychotic — *see also* condition 298.9
- episode 298.9
  - due to or associated with physical conditions (*see also* Psychosis, organic) 293.9

Pterygium (eye) 372.40
- central 372.43
- colli 744.5

☑ **Additional Digit Required — Refer to the Tabular List for Digit Selection**   ⓦ **Subterms under main terms may continue to next column or page**

242 — Volume 2   ▶◀ **Revised Text**   ● **New Line**   ▲ **Revised Code**   2013 ICD-9-CM

Pterygium — continued
double 372.44
peripheral (stationary) 372.41
progressive 372.42
recurrent 372.45
Ptilosis 374.55
PTLD (post-transplant lymphoproliferative disorder) 238.77
Ptomaine (poisoning) — see also Poisoning, food 005.9
Ptosis (adiposa) 374.30
breast 611.81
cecum 569.89
colon 569.89
congenital (eyelid) 743.61
specified site NEC — see Anomaly, specified type NEC
epicanthus syndrome 270.2
eyelid 374.30
congenital 743.61
mechanical 374.33
myogenic 374.32
paralytic 374.31
gastric 537.5
intestine 569.89
kidney (see also Disease, renal) 593.0
congenital 753.3
liver 573.8
renal (see also Disease, renal) 593.0
congenital 753.3
splanchnic 569.89
spleen 289.59
stomach 537.5
viscera 569.89
PTP (posttransfusion purpura) 287.41
PTSD (Post-traumatic stress disorder) 309.81
Ptyalism 527.7
hysterical 300.11
periodic 527.2
pregnancy 646.8 ☑
psychogenic 306.4
Ptyalolithiasis 527.5
Pubalgia 848.8
Pubarche, precocious 259.1
Pubertas praecox 259.1
Puberty V21.1
abnormal 259.9
bleeding 626.3
delayed 259.0
precocious (constitutional) (cryptogenic) (idiopathic) NEC 259.1
due to
adrenal
cortical hyperfunction 255.2
hyperplasia 255.2
cortical hyperfunction 255.2
ovarian hyperfunction 256.1
estrogen 256.0
pineal tumor 259.8
testicular hyperfunction 257.0
premature 259.1
due to
adrenal cortical hyperfunction 255.2
pineal tumor 259.8
pituitary (anterior) hyperfunction 253.1
Puckering, macula 362.56
Pudenda, pudendum — see condition
Puente's disease (simple glandular cheilitis) 528.5
Puerperal
abscess
areola 675.1 ☑
Bartholin's gland 646.6 ☑
breast 675.1 ☑
cervix (uteri) 670.8 ☑
fallopian tube 670.8 ☑
genital organ 670.8 ☑
kidney 646.6 ☑
mammary 675.1 ☑
mesosalpinx 670.8 ☑
nabothian 646.6 ☑
nipple 675.0 ☑
ovary, ovarian 670.8 ☑
oviduct 670.8 ☑
parametric 670.8 ☑

Puerperal — continued
abscess — continued
para-uterine 670.8 ☑
pelvic 670.8 ☑
perimetric 670.8 ☑
periuterine 670.8 ☑
retro-uterine 670.8 ☑
subareolar 675.1 ☑
suprapelvic 670.8 ☑
tubal (ruptured) 670.8 ☑
tubo-ovarian 670.8 ☑
urinary tract NEC 646.6 ☑
uterine, uterus 670.8 ☑
vagina (wall) 646.6 ☑
vaginorectal 646.6 ☑
vulvovaginal gland 646.6 ☑
accident 674.9 ☑
adnexitis 670.8 ☑
afibrinogenemia, or other coagulation defect 666.3 ☑
albuminuria (acute) (subacute) 646.2 ☑
pre-eclamptic 642.4 ☑
anemia (conditions classifiable to 280–285) 648.2 ☑
anuria 669.3 ☑
apoplexy 674.0 ☑
asymptomatic bacteriuria 646.5 ☑
atrophy, breast 676.3 ☑
blood dyscrasia 666.3 ☑
caked breast 676.2 ☑
cardiomyopathy 674.5 ☑
cellulitis — see Puerperal, abscess
cerebrovascular disorder (conditions classifiable to 430–434, 436–437) 674.0 ☑
cervicitis (conditions classifiable to 616.0) 646.6 ☑
coagulopathy (any) 666.3 ☑
complications 674.9 ☑
specified type NEC 674.8 ☑
convulsions (eclamptic) (uremic) 642.6 ☑
with pre-existing hypertension 642.7 ☑
cracked nipple 676.1 ☑
cystitis 646.6 ☑
cystopyelitis 646.6 ☑
deciduitis (acute) 670.8 ☑
delirium NEC 293.9
diabetes (mellitus) (conditions classifiable to 249 and 250) 648.0 ☑
disease 674.9 ☑
breast NEC 676.3 ☑
cerebrovascular (acute) 674.0 ☑
nonobstetric NEC (see also Pregnancy, complicated, current disease or condition) 648.9 ☑
pelvis inflammatory 670.8 ☑
renal NEC 646.2 ☑
tubo-ovarian 670.8 ☑
Valsuani's (progressive pernicious anemia) 648.2 ☑
disorder
lactation 676.9 ☑
specified type NEC 676.8 ☑
nonobstetric NEC (see also Pregnancy, complicated, current disease or condition) 648.9 ☑
disruption
cesarean wound 674.1 ☑
episiotomy wound 674.2 ☑
perineal laceration wound 674.2 ☑
drug dependence (conditions classifiable to 304) 648.3 ☑
eclampsia 642.6 ☑
with pre-existing hypertension 642.7 ☑
embolism (pulmonary) 673.2 ☑
air 673.0 ☑
amniotic fluid 673.1 ☑
blood-clot 673.2 ☑
brain or cerebral 674.0 ☑
cardiac 674.8 ☑
fat 673.8 ☑
intracranial sinus (venous) 671.5 ☑
pyemic 673.3 ☑
septic 673.3 ☑
spinal cord 671.5 ☑

Puerperal — continued
endometritis (conditions classifiable to 615.0–615.9) 670.1 ☑
endophlebitis — see Puerperal, phlebitis
endotrachelitis 646.6 ☑
engorgement, breasts 676.2 ☑
erysipelas 670.8 ☑
failure
lactation 676.4 ☑
renal, acute 669.3 ☑
fever 672 ☑
meaning pyrexia (of unknown origin) 672.0 ☑
meaning sepsis 670.2 ☑
fissure, nipple 676.1 ☑
fistula
breast 675.1 ☑
mammary gland 675.1 ☑
nipple 675.0 ☑
galactophoritis 675.2 ☑
galactorrhea 676.6 ☑
gangrene
gas 670.8 ☑
with sepsis 670.2 ☑
uterus 670.8 ☑
gonorrhea (conditions classifiable to 098) 647.1 ☑
hematoma, subdural 674.0 ☑
hematosalpinx, infectional 670.8 ☑
hemiplegia, cerebral 674.0 ☑
hemorrhage 666.1 ☑
brain 674.0 ☑
bulbar 674.0 ☑
cerebellar 674.0 ☑
cerebral 674.0 ☑
cortical 674.0 ☑
delayed (after 24 hours) (uterine) 666.2 ☑
extradural 674.0 ☑
internal capsule 674.0 ☑
intracranial 674.0 ☑
intrapontine 674.0 ☑
meningeal 674.0 ☑
pontine 674.0 ☑
subarachnoid 674.0 ☑
subcortical 674.0 ☑
subdural 674.0 ☑
uterine, delayed 666.2 ☑
ventricular 674.0 ☑
hemorrhoids 671.8 ☑
hepatorenal syndrome 674.8 ☑
hypertrophy
breast 676.3 ☑
mammary gland 676.3 ☑
induration breast (fibrous) 676.3 ☑
infarction
lung — see Puerperal, embolism
pulmonary — see Puerperal, embolism
infection
Bartholin's gland 646.6 ☑
breast 675.2 ☑
with nipple 675.9 ☑
specified type NEC 675.8 ☑
cervix 646.6 ☑
endocervix 646.6 ☑
fallopian tube 670.8 ☑
generalized 670.0 ☑
genital tract (major) 670.0 ☑
minor or localized 646.6 ☑
kidney (bacillus coli) 646.6 ☑
mammary gland 675.2 ☑
with nipple 675.9 ☑
specified type NEC 675.8 ☑
nipple 675.0 ☑
with breast 675.9 ☑
specified type NEC 675.8 ☑
ovary 670.8 ☑
pelvic 670.8 ☑
peritoneum 670.8 ☑
renal 646.6 ☑
tubo-ovarian 670.8 ☑
urinary (tract) NEC 646.6 ☑
asymptomatic 646.5 ☑

Puerperal — continued
infection — continued
uterus, uterine 670.8 ☑
vagina 646.6 ☑
inflammation (see also Puerperal, infection)
areola 675.1 ☑
Bartholin's gland 646.6 ☑
breast 675.2 ☑
broad ligament 670.8 ☑
cervix (uteri) 646.6 ☑
fallopian tube 670.8 ☑
genital organs 670.8 ☑
localized 646.6 ☑
mammary gland 675.2 ☑
nipple 675.0 ☑
ovary 670.8 ☑
oviduct 670.8 ☑
pelvis 670.8 ☑
periuterine 670.8 ☑
tubal 670.8 ☑
vagina 646.6 ☑
vein — see Puerperal, phlebitis
inversion, nipple 676.3 ☑
ischemia, cerebral 674.0 ☑
lymphangitis 670.8 ☑
breast 675.2 ☑
malaria (conditions classifiable to 084) 647.4 ☑
malnutrition 648.9 ☑
mammillitis 675.0 ☑
mammitis 675.2 ☑
mania 296.0 ☑
recurrent episode 296.1 ☑
single episode 296.0 ☑
mastitis 675.2 ☑
purulent 675.1 ☑
retromammary 675.1 ☑
submammary 675.1 ☑
melancholia 296.2 ☑
recurrent episode 296.3 ☑
single episode 296.2 ☑
mental disorder (conditions classifiable to 290–303, 305.0, 305.2–305.9, 306–316, 317–319) 648.4 ☑
metritis (suppurative) 670.1 ☑
septic 670.2 ☑
metroperitonitis 670.8 ☑
metrorrhagia 666.2 ☑
metrosalpingitis 670.8 ☑
metrovaginitis 670.8 ☑
milk leg 671.4 ☑
monoplegia, cerebral 674.0 ☑
necrosis
kidney, tubular 669.3 ☑
liver (acute) (subacute) (conditions classifiable to 570) 674.8 ☑
ovary 670.8 ☑
renal cortex 669.3 ☑
nephritis or nephrosis (conditions classifiable to 580–589) 646.2 ☑
with hypertension 642.1 ☑
nutritional deficiency (conditions classifiable to 260–269) 648.9 ☑
occlusion, precerebral artery 674.0 ☑
oliguria 669.3 ☑
oophoritis 670.8 ☑
ovaritis 670.8 ☑
paralysis
bladder (sphincter) 665.5 ☑
cerebral 674.0 ☑
paralytic stroke 674.0 ☑
parametritis 670.8 ☑
paravaginitis 646.6 ☑
pelviperitonitis 670.8 ☑
perimetritis 670.8 ☑
perimetrosalpingitis 670.8 ☑
perinephritis 646.6 ☑
perioophoritis 670.8 ☑
periphlebitis — see Puerperal, phlebitis
perisalpingitis 670.8 ☑
peritoneal infection 670.8 ☑
peritonitis (pelvic) 670.8 ☑
perivaginitis 646.6 ☑

☑ **Additional Digit Required** — Refer to the Tabular List for Digit Selection   🏥 **Subterms under main terms may continue to next column or page**

2013 ICD-9-CM   ▶◀ **Revised Text**   ● **New Line**   ▲ **Revised Code**   **Volume 2 — 243**

Puerperal — *continued*
  phlebitis 671.2 ☑
    deep 671.4 ☑
    intracranial sinus (venous) 671.5 ☑
    pelvic 671.4 ☑
    specified site NEC 671.5 ☑
    superficial 671.2 ☑
  phlegmasia alba dolens 671.4 ☑
  placental polyp 674.4 ☑
  pneumonia, embolic — *see* Puerperal, embolism
  prediabetes 648.8 ☑
  pre-eclampsia (mild) 642.4 ☑
    with pre-existing hypertension 642.7 ☑
    severe 642.5 ☑
  psychosis, unspecified (*see also* Psychosis, puerperal) 293.89
  pyelitis 646.6 ☑
  pyelocystitis 646.6 ☑
  pyelohydronephrosis 646.6 ☑
  pyelonephritis 646.6 ☑
  pyelonephrosis 646.6 ☑
  pyemia 670.2 ☑
  pyocystitis 646.6 ☑
  pyohemia 670.2 ☑
  pyometra 670.8 ☑
  pyonephritis 646.6 ☑
  pyonephrosis 646.6 ☑
  pyo-oophoritis 670.8 ☑
  pyosalpingitis 670.8 ☑
  pyosalpinx 670.8 ☑
  pyrexia (of unknown origin) 672.0 ☑
  renal
    disease NEC 646.2 ☑
    failure, acute 669.3 ☑
  retention
    decidua (fragments) (with delayed hemorrhage) 666.2 ☑
      without hemorrhage 667.1 ☑
    placenta (fragments) (with delayed hemorrhage) 666.2 ☑
      without hemorrhage 667.1 ☑
    secundines (fragments) (with delayed hemorrhage) 666.2 ☑
      without hemorrhage 667.1 ☑
  retracted nipple 676.0 ☑
  rubella (conditions classifiable to 056) 647.5 ☑
  salpingitis 670.8 ☑
  salpingo-oophoritis 670.8 ☑
  salpingo-ovaritis 670.8 ☑
  salpingoperitonitis 670.8 ☑
  sapremia 670.2 ☑
  secondary perineal tear 674.2 ☑
  sepsis (pelvic) 670.2 ☑
  septicemia 670.2 ☑
  subinvolution (uterus) 674.8 ☑
  sudden death (cause unknown) 674.9 ☑
  suppuration — *see* Puerperal, abscess
  syphilis (conditions classifiable to 090–097) 647.0 ☑
  tetanus 670.8 ☑
  thelitis 675.0 ☑
  thrombocytopenia 666.3 ☑
  thrombophlebitis (superficial) 671.2 ☑
    deep 671.4 ☑
    pelvic 671.4 ☑
    septic 670.3 ☑
    specified site NEC 671.5 ☑
  thrombosis (venous) — *see* Thrombosis, puerperal
  thyroid dysfunction (conditions classifiable to 240–246) 648.1 ☑
  toxemia (*see also* Toxemia, of pregnancy) 642.4 ☑
    eclamptic 642.6 ☑
      with pre-existing hypertension 642.7 ☑
    pre-eclamptic (mild) 642.4 ☑
      with
        convulsions 642.6 ☑
        pre-existing hypertension 642.7 ☑
      severe 642.5 ☑

Puerperal — *continued*
  tuberculosis (conditions classifiable to 010–018) 647.3 ☑
  uremia 669.3 ☑
  vaginitis (conditions classifiable to 616.1) 646.6 ☑
  varicose veins (legs) 671.0 ☑
    vulva or perineum 671.1 ☑
  venous complication 671.9 ☑
  vulvitis (conditions classifiable to 616.1) 646.6 ☑
  vulvovaginitis (conditions classifiable to 616.1) 646.6 ☑
  white leg 671.4 ☑
Pulled muscle — *see* Sprain, by site
Pulmolithiasis 518.89
Pulmonary — *see* condition
Pulmonitis (unknown etiology) 486
Pulpitis (acute) (anachoretic) (chronic) (hyperplastic) (putrescent) (suppurative) (ulcerative) 522.0
Pulpless tooth 522.9
Pulse
  alternating 427.89
    psychogenic 306.2
  bigeminal 427.89
  fast 785.0
  feeble, rapid, due to shock following injury 958.4
  rapid 785.0
  slow 427.89
  strong 785.9
  trigeminal 427.89
  water-hammer (*see also* Insufficiency, aortic) 424.1
  weak 785.9
Pulseless disease 446.7
Pulsus
  alternans or trigemini 427.89
    psychogenic 306.2
Punch drunk 310.2
Puncta lacrimalia occlusion 375.52
Punctiform hymen 752.49
Puncture (traumatic) — *see also* Wound, open, by site
  accidental, complicating surgery 998.2
  bladder, nontraumatic 596.6
  by
    device, implant, or graft — *see* Complications, mechanical
    foreign body
      internal organs (*see also* Injury, internal, by site)
        by ingested object — *see* Foreign body
      left accidentally in operation wound 998.4
    instrument (any) during a procedure, accidental 998.2
  internal organs, abdomen, chest, or pelvis — *see* Injury, internal, by site
  kidney, nontraumatic 593.89
Pupil — *see* condition
Pupillary membrane 364.74
  persistent 743.46
Pupillotonia 379.46
  pseudotabetic 379.46
Purpura 287.2
  abdominal 287.0
  allergic 287.0
  anaphylactoid 287.0
  annularis telangiectodes 709.1
  arthritic 287.0
  autoerythrocyte sensitization 287.2
  autoimmune 287.0
  bacterial 287.0
  Bateman's (senile) 287.2
  capillary fragility (hereditary) (idiopathic) 287.8
  cryoglobulinemic 273.2
  devil's pinches 287.2
  fibrinolytic (*see also* Fibrinolysis) 286.6
  fulminans, fulminous 286.6
  gangrenous 287.0
  hemorrhagic (*see also* Purpura, thrombocytopenic) 287.39

Purpura — *continued*
  hemorrhagic (*see also* Purpura, thrombocytopenic) — *continued*
    nodular 272.7
    nonthrombocytopenic 287.0
    thrombocytopenic 287.39
  Henoch's (purpura nervosa) 287.0
  Henoch-Schönlein (allergic) 287.0
  hypergammaglobulinemic (benign primary) (Waldenström's) 273.0
  idiopathic 287.31
    nonthrombocytopenic 287.0
    thrombocytopenic 287.31
  immune thrombocytopenic 287.31
  infectious 287.0
  malignant 287.0
  neonatorum 772.6
  nervosa 287.0
  newborn NEC 772.6
  nonthrombocytopenic 287.2
    hemorrhagic 287.0
    idiopathic 287.0
  nonthrombopenic 287.2
  peliosis rheumatica 287.0
  pigmentaria, progressiva 709.09
  posttransfusion (PTP) 287.41
    from whole blood (fresh) or blood products 287.41
  primary 287.0
  primitive 287.0
  red cell membrane sensitivity 287.2
  rheumatica 287.0
  Schönlein (-Henoch) (allergic) 287.0
  scorbutic 267
  senile 287.2
  simplex 287.2
  symptomatica 287.0
  telangiectasia annularis 709.1
  thrombocytopenic (*see also* Thrombocytopenia) 287.30
    congenital 287.33
    essential 287.30
    hereditary 287.31
    idiopathic 287.31
    immune 287.31
    neonatal, transitory (*see also* Thrombocytopenia, neonatal transitory) 776.1
    primary 287.30
    puerperal, postpartum 666.3 ☑
    thrombotic 446.6
  thrombohemolytic (*see also* Fibrinolysis) 286.6
  thrombopenic (*see also* Thrombocytopenia) 287.30
    congenital 287.33
    essential 287.30
    thrombotic 446.6
      thrombocytic 446.6
      thrombocytopenic 446.6
  toxic 287.0
  variolosa 050.0
  vascular 287.0
  visceral symptoms 287.0
  Werlhof's (*see also* Purpura, thrombocytopenic) 287.39
Purpuric spots 782.7
Purulent — *see* condition
Pus
  absorption, general — *see* Septicemia
  in
    stool 792.1
    urine 791.9
  tube (rupture) (*see also* Salpingo-oophoritis) 614.2
Pustular rash 782.1
Pustule 686.9
  malignant 022.0
  nonmalignant 686.9
Putnam-Dana syndrome (subacute combined sclerosis with pernicious anemia) 281.0 [336.2]
Putnam's disease (subacute combined sclerosis with pernicious anemia) 281.0 [336.2]
Putrefaction, intestinal 569.89
Putrescent pulp (dental) 522.1

Pyarthritis — *see* Pyarthrosis
Pyarthrosis — *see also* Arthritis, pyogenic 711.0 ☑
  tuberculous — *see* Tuberculosis, joint
Pycnoepilepsy, pycnolepsy (idiopathic) — *see also* Epilepsy 345.0 ☑
Pyelectasia 593.89
Pyelectasis 593.89
Pyelitis (congenital) (uremic) 590.80
  with
    abortion — *see* Abortion, by type, with specified complication NEC
    contracted kidney 590.00
    ectopic pregnancy (*see also* categories 633.0–633.9) 639.8
    molar pregnancy (*see also* categories 630–632) 639.8
  acute 590.10
    with renal medullary necrosis 590.11
  chronic 590.00
    with
      renal medullary necrosis 590.01
  complicating pregnancy, childbirth, or puerperium 646.6 ☑
    affecting fetus or newborn 760.1
  cystica 590.3
    following
      abortion 639.8
      ectopic or molar pregnancy 639.8
  gonococcal 098.19
    chronic or duration of 2 months or over 098.39
  tuberculous (*see also* Tuberculosis) 016.0 ☑ [590.81]
Pyelocaliectasis 593.89
Pyelocystitis — *see also* Pyelitis 590.80
Pyelohydronephrosis 591
Pyelonephritis — *see also* Pyelitis 590.80
  acute 590.10
    with renal medullary necrosis 590.11
  chronic 590.00
  syphilitic (late) 095.4
  tuberculous (*see also* Tuberculosis) 016.0 ☑ [590.81]
Pyelonephrosis — *see also* Pyelitis 590.80
  chronic 590.00
Pyelophlebitis 451.89
Pyelo-ureteritis cystica 590.3
Pyemia, pyemic (purulent) — *see also* Septicemia 038.9
  abscess — *see* Abscess
  arthritis (*see also* Arthritis, pyogenic) 711.0 ☑
  Bacillus coli 038.42
  embolism (*see also* Septicemia) 415.12
  fever 038.9
  infection 038.9
  joint (*see also* Arthritis, pyogenic) 711.0 ☑
  liver 572.1
  meningococcal 036.2
  newborn 771.81
  phlebitis — *see* Phlebitis
  pneumococcal 038.2
  portal 572.1
  postvaccinal 999.39
  puerperal 670.2 ☑
  specified organism NEC 038.8
  staphylococcal 038.10
    aureus 038.11
      methicillin
        resistant 038.12
        susceptible 038.11
    specified organism NEC 038.19
  streptococcal 038.0
  tuberculous — *see* Tuberculosis, miliary
Pygopagus 759.4
Pykno-epilepsy, pyknolepsy (idiopathic) — *see also* Epilepsy 345.0 ☑
Pyle (-Cohn) disease (craniometaphyseal dysplasia) 756.89
Pylephlebitis (suppurative) 572.1
Pylethrombophlebitis 572.1
Pylethrombosis 572.1
Pyloritis — *see also* Gastritis 535.5 ☑
Pylorospasm (reflex) 537.81
  congenital or infantile 750.5

☑ Additional Digit Required — Refer to the Tabular List for Digit Selection
                                              ▽ Subterms under main terms may continue to next column or page

Pylorospasm — *continued*
  neurotic 306.4
  newborn 750.5
  psychogenic 306.4
Pylorus, pyloric — *see* condition
Pyoarthrosis — *see* Pyarthrosis
Pyocele
  mastoid 383.00
  sinus (accessory) (nasal) (*see also* Sinusitis)
    473.9
  turbinate (bone) 473.9
  urethra (*see also* Urethritis) 597.0
Pyococcal dermatitis 686.00
Pyococcide, skin 686.00
Pyocolpos — *see also* Vaginitis 616.10
Pyocyaneus dermatitis 686.09
Pyocystitis — *see* Cystitis 595.9
Pyoderma, pyodermia 686.00
  gangrenosum 686.01
  specified type NEC 686.09
  vegetans 686.8
Pyodermatitis 686.00
  vegetans 686.8
Pyogenic — *see* condition
Pyohemia — *see* Septicemia
Pyohydronephrosis — *see also* Pyelitis 590.80
Pyometra 615.9
Pyometritis — *see also* Endometritis 615.9
Pyometrium — *see also* Endometritis 615.9
Pyomyositis 728.0
  ossificans 728.19
  tropical (bungpagga) 040.81
Pyonephritis — *see also* Pyelitis 590.80
  chronic 590.00
Pyonephrosis (congenital) — *see also* Pyelitis
  590.80
  acute 590.10
Pyo-oophoritis — *see also* Salpingo-oophoritis
  614.2
Pyo-ovarium — *see also* Salpingo-oophoritis
  614.2
Pyopericarditis 420.99
Pyopericardium 420.99
Pyophlebitis — *see* Phlebitis
Pyopneumopericardium 420.99
Pyopneumothorax (infectional) 510.9
  with fistula 510.0
  subdiaphragmatic (*see also* Peritonitis)
    567.29
  subphrenic (*see also* Peritonitis) 567.29
  tuberculous (*see also* Tuberculosis, pleura)
    012.0 ☑
Pyorrhea (alveolar) (alveolaris) 523.40
  degenerative 523.5
Pyosalpingitis — *see also* Salpingo-oophoritis
  614.2
Pyosalpinx — *see also* Salpingo-oophoritis
  614.2
Pyosepticemia — *see* Septicemia
Pyosis
  Corlett's (impetigo) 684
  Manson's (pemphigus contagiosus) 684
Pyothorax 510.9
  with fistula 510.0
  tuberculous (*see also* Tuberculosis, pleura)
    012.0 ☑
Pyoureter 593.89
  tuberculous (*see also* Tuberculosis) 016.2 ☑
Pyramidopallidonigral syndrome 332.0
Pyrexia (of unknown origin) (P.U.O.) 780.60
  atmospheric 992.0
  during labor 659.2 ☑
  environmentally-induced newborn 778.4
  heat 992.0
  newborn, environmentally-induced 778.4
  puerperal 672.0 ☑
Pyroglobulinemia 273.8
Pyromania 312.33
Pyrosis 787.1
Pyrroloporphyria 277.1
Pyuria (bacterial) 791.9

Q

Q fever 083.0
  with pneumonia 083.0 [484.8]
Quadricuspid aortic valve 746.89

Quadrilateral fever 083.0
Quadriparesis — *see* Quadriplegia
  meaning muscle weakness 728.87
Quadriplegia 344.00
  with fracture, vertebra (process) — *see*
    Fracture, vertebra, cervical, with
    spinal cord injury
  brain (current episode) 437.8
  C1-C4
    complete 344.01
    incomplete 344.02
  C5-C7
    complete 344.03
    incomplete 344.04
  cerebral (current episode) 437.8
  congenital or infantile (cerebral) (spastic)
    (spinal) 343.2
  cortical 437.8
  embolic (current episode) (*see also* Em-
    bolism, brain) 434.1 ☑
  functional 780.72
  infantile (cerebral) (spastic) (spinal) 343.2
  newborn NEC 767.0
  specified NEC 344.09
  thrombotic (current episode) (*see also*
    Thrombosis, brain) 434.0 ☑
  traumatic — *see* Injury, spinal, cervical
Quadruplet
  affected by maternal complications of
    pregnancy 761.5
  healthy liveborn — *see* Newborn, multiple
  pregnancy (complicating delivery) NEC
    651.8 ☑
    with fetal loss and retention of one or
      more fetus(es) 651.5 ☑
    following (elective) fetal reduction
      651.7 ☑
Quarrelsomeness 301.3
Quartan
  fever 084.2
  malaria (fever) 084.2
Queensland fever 083.0
  coastal 083.0
  seven-day 100.89
Quervain's disease 727.04
  thyroid (subacute granulomatous thyroidi-
    tis) 245.1
Queyrat's erythroplasia (M8080/2)
  specified site — *see* Neoplasm, skin, in situ
  unspecified site 233.5
Quincke's disease or edema — *see* Edema,
  angioneurotic
Quinquaud's disease (acne decalvans) 704.09
Quinsy (gangrenous) 475
Quintan fever 083.1
Quintuplet
  affected by maternal complications of
    pregnancy 761.5
  healthy liveborn — *see* Newborn, multiple
  pregnancy (complicating delivery) NEC
    651.2 ☑
    with fetal loss and retention of one or
      more fetus(es) 651.6 ☑
    following (elective) fetal reduction
      651.7 ☑
Quotidian
  fever 084.0
  malaria (fever) 084.0

R

Rabbia 071
Rabbit fever — *see also* Tularemia 021.9
Rabies 071
  contact V01.5
  exposure to V01.5
  inoculation V04.5
    reaction — *see* Complications, vaccina-
      tion
  vaccination, prophylactic (against) V04.5
Rachischisis — *see also* Spina bifida 741.9 ☑
Rachitic — *see also* condition
  deformities of spine 268.1
  pelvis 268.1
    with disproportion (fetopelvic) 653.2 ☑
      affecting fetus or newborn 763.1

Rachitic — *see also* condition — *continued*
  pelvis — *continued*
    with disproportion — *continued*
      causing obstructed labor 660.1 ☑
        affecting fetus or newborn 763.1
Rachitis, rachitism — *see also* Rickets
  acute 268.0
  fetalis 756.4
  renalis 588.0
  tarda 268.0
Racket nail 757.5
Radial nerve — *see* condition
Radiation effects or sickness — *see also* Effect, adverse, radiation
  cataract 366.46
  dermatitis 692.82
    sunburn (*see also* Sunburn) 692.71
Radiculitis (pressure) (vertebrogenic) 729.2
  accessory nerve 723.4
  anterior crural 724.4
  arm 723.4
  brachial 723.4
  cervical NEC 723.4
  due to displacement of intervertebral disc
    — *see* Neuritis, due to, displacement
    intervertebral disc
  leg 724.4
  lumbar NEC 724.4
  lumbosacral 724.4
  rheumatic 729.2
  syphilitic 094.89
  thoracic (with visceral pain) 724.4
Radiculomyelitis 357.0
  toxic, due to
    Clostridium tetani 037
    Corynebacterium diphtheriae 032.89
Radiculopathy — *see also* Radiculitis 729.2
Radioactive substances, adverse effect —
  see Effect, adverse, radioactive substance
Radiodermal burns (acute) (chronic) (occupa-
  tional) — *see* Burn, by site
Radiodermatitis 692.82
Radionecrosis — *see* Effect, adverse, radiation
Radiotherapy session V58.0
Radium, adverse effect — *see* Effect, adverse,
  radioactive substance
Raeder-Harbitz syndrome (pulseless disease)
  446.7
Rage — *see also* Disturbance, conduct 312.0 ☑
  meaning rabies 071
Rag sorters' disease 022.1
Raillietiniasis 123.8
Railroad neurosis 300.16
Railway spine 300.16
Raised — *see* Elevation
Raiva 071
Rake teeth, tooth 524.39
Rales 786.7
Ramifying renal pelvis 753.3
Ramsay Hunt syndrome (herpetic geniculate
  ganglionitis) 053.11
  meaning dyssynergia cerebellaris myocloni-
    ca 334.2
Ranke's primary infiltration — *see also* Tuberculosis 010.0 ☑
Ranula 527.6
  congenital 750.26
Rape
  adult 995.83
  alleged, observation or examination V71.5
  child 995.53
Rapid
  feeble pulse, due to shock, following injury
    958.4
  heart (beat) 785.0
    psychogenic 306.2
  respiration 786.06
    psychogenic 306.1
  second stage (delivery) 661.3 ☑
    affecting fetus or newborn 763.6
  time-zone change syndrome 327.35
Rarefaction, bone 733.99
Rash 782.1
  canker 034.1
  diaper 691.0
  drug (internal use) 693.0

Rash — *continued*
  drug — *continued*
    contact 692.3
  ECHO 9 virus 078.89
  enema 692.89
  food (*see also* Allergy, food) 693.1
  heat 705.1
  napkin 691.0
  nettle 708.8
  pustular 782.1
  rose 782.1
    epidemic 056.9
    of infants 057.8
  scarlet 034.1
  serum (prophylactic) (therapeutic) 999.59
  toxic 782.1
  wandering tongue 529.1
Rasmussen's aneurysm — *see also* Tuberculosis 011.2 ☑
Rat-bite fever 026.9
  due to Streptobacillus moniliformis 026.1
  spirochetal (morsus muris) 026.0
Rathke's pouch tumor (M9350/1) 237.0
Raymond (-Céstan) syndrome 433.8 ☑
Raynaud's
  disease or syndrome (paroxysmal digital
    cyanosis) 443.0
  gangrene (symmetric) 443.0 [785.4]
  phenomenon (paroxysmal digital cyanosis)
    (secondary) 443.0
RDS 769
Reaction
  acute situational maladjustment (*see also*
    Reaction, adjustment) 309.9
  adaptation (*see also* Reaction, adjustment)
    309.9
  adjustment 309.9
    with
      anxious mood 309.24
        with depressed mood 309.28
      conduct disturbance 309.3
        combined with disturbance of
          emotions 309.4
      depressed mood 309.0
        brief 309.0
          with anxious mood 309.28
        prolonged 309.1
      elective mutism 309.83
      mixed emotions and conduct 309.4
      mutism, elective 309.83
      physical symptoms 309.82
      predominant disturbance (of)
        conduct 309.3
        emotions NEC 309.29
          mixed 309.28
          mixed, emotions and conduct
            309.4
        specified type NEC 309.89
      specific academic or work inhibition
        309.23
      withdrawal 309.83
    depressive 309.0
      with conduct disturbance 309.4
      brief 309.0
      prolonged 309.1
    specified type NEC 309.89
  adverse food NEC 995.7
  affective (*see also* Psychosis, affective)
    296.90
    specified type NEC 296.99
  aggressive 301.3
    unsocialized (*see also* Disturbance, con-
      duct) 312.0 ☑
  allergic (*see also* Allergy) 995.3
    drug, medicinal substance, and biologi-
      cal — *see* Allergy, drug
    due to correct medical substance prop-
      erly administered 995.27
    food — *see* Allergy, food
    serum 999.59
  anaphylactic — *see* Anaphylactic reaction
  anesthesia — *see* Anesthesia, complication
  anger 312.0 ☑
  antisocial 301.7
  antitoxin (prophylactic) (therapeutic) — *see*
    Complications, vaccination

☑ Additional Digit Required — Refer to the Tabular List for Digit Selection   Subterms under main terms may continue to next column or page

Reaction — *continued*
    anxiety 300.00
    Arthus 995.21
    asthenic 300.5
    compulsive 300.3
    conversion (anesthetic) (autonomic) (hyperkinetic) (mixed paralytic) (paresthetic) 300.11
    deoxyribonuclease (DNA) (DNase) hypersensitivity NEC 287.2
    depressive 300.4
        acute 309.0
        affective (*see also* Psychosis, affective) 296.2 ☑
            recurrent episode 296.3 ☑
            single episode 296.2 ☑
        brief 309.0
        manic (*see also* Psychosis, affective) 296.80
        neurotic 300.4
        psychoneurotic 300.4
        psychotic 298.0
    dissociative 300.15
    drug NEC (*see also* Table of Drugs and Chemicals) 995.20
        allergic (*see also* Allergy, drug) 995.27
        correct substance properly administered 995.20
        obstetric anesthetic or analgesic NEC 668.9 ☑
            affecting fetus or newborn 763.5
            specified drug — *see* Table of Drugs and Chemicals
        overdose or poisoning 977.9
            specified drug — *see* Table of Drugs and Chemicals
        specific to newborn 779.4
        transmitted via placenta or breast milk — *see* Absorption, drug, through placenta
        withdrawal NEC 292.0
            infant of dependent mother 779.5
        wrong substance given or taken in error 977.9
            specified drug — *see* Table of Drugs and Chemicals
    dyssocial 301.7
    dystonic, acute, due to drugs 333.72
    erysipeloid 027.1
    fear 300.20
        child 313.0
    fluid loss, cerebrospinal 349.0
    food (*see also* Allergy, food)
        adverse NEC 995.7
        anaphylactic shock — *see* Anaphylactic reaction or shock, due to, food
    foreign
        body NEC 728.82
            in operative wound (inadvertently left) 998.4
            due to surgical material intentionally left — *see* Complications, due to (presence of) any device, implant, or graft classified to 996.0–996.5 NEC
        substance accidentally left during a procedure (chemical) (powder) (talc) 998.7
        body or object (instrument) (sponge) (swab) 998.4
    graft-versus-host (GVH) 279.50
    grief (acute) (brief) 309.0
        prolonged 309.1
    gross stress (*see also* Reaction, stress, acute) 308.9
    group delinquent (*see also* Disturbance, conduct) 312.2 ☑
    Herxheimer's 995.91
    hyperkinetic (*see also* Hyperkinesia) 314.9
    hypochondriacal 300.7
    hypoglycemic, due to insulin 251.0
        therapeutic misadventure 962.3
    hypomanic (*see also* Psychosis, affective) 296.0 ☑
        recurrent episode 296.1 ☑

Reaction — *continued*
    hypomanic (*see also* Psychosis, affective) — *continued*
        single episode 296.0 ☑
    hysterical 300.10
        conversion type 300.11
        dissociative 300.15
    id (bacterial cause) 692.89
    immaturity NEC 301.89
        aggressive 301.3
        emotional instability 301.59
    immunization — *see* Complications, vaccination
    incompatibility
        blood group (*see also* Complications, transfusion) 999.80
            ABO (due to transfusion of blood or blood products) (*see also* Complications, transfusion) 999.60
            minor blood group 999.89
            non-ABO — *see* Complications, transfusion 999.75
            Rh antigen (C) (c) (D) (E) (e) (factor) (infusion) (transfusion) (*see also* Complications, transfusion) 999.70
    inflammatory — *see* Infection
    infusion — *see* Complications, infusion
    inoculation (immune serum) — *see* Complications, vaccination
    insulin 995.23
    involutional
        paranoid 297.2
        psychotic (*see also* Psychosis, affective, depressive) 296.2 ☑
    leukemoid (basophilic) (lymphocytic) (monocytic) (myelocytic) (neutrophilic) 288.62
    LSD (*see also* Abuse, drugs, nondependent) 305.3 ☑
    lumbar puncture 349.0
    manic-depressive (*see also* Psychosis, affective) 296.80
        depressed 296.2 ☑
            recurrent episode 296.3 ☑
            single episode 296.2 ☑
        hypomanic 296.0 ☑
    neurasthenic 300.5
    neurogenic (*see also* Neurosis) 300.9
    neurotic NEC 300.9
    neurotic-depressive 300.4
    nitritoid — *see* Crisis, nitritoid
    nonspecific
        to
            cell mediated immunity measurement of gamma interferon antigen response without active tuberculosis 795.52
            QuantiFERON-TB test (QFT) without active tuberculosis 795.52
            tuberculin test (*see also* Reaction, tuberculin skin test) 795.51
    obsessive compulsive 300.3
    organic 293.9
        acute 293.0
        subacute 293.1
    overanxious, child or adolescent 313.0
    paranoid (chronic) 297.9
        acute 298.3
        climacteric 297.2
        involutional 297.2
        menopausal 297.2
        senile 290.20
        simple 297.0
    passive
        aggressive 301.84
        dependency 301.6
    personality (*see also* Disorder, personality) 301.9
    phobic 300.20
    postradiation — *see* Effect, adverse, radiation
    psychogenic NEC 300.9
    psychoneurotic (*see also* Neurosis) 300.9
        anxiety 300.00
        compulsive 300.3

Reaction — *continued*
    psychoneurotic (*see also* Neurosis) — *continued*
        conversion 300.11
        depersonalization 300.6
        depressive 300.4
        dissociative 300.15
        hypochondriacal 300.7
        hysterical 300.10
            conversion type 300.11
            dissociative type 300.15
        neurasthenic 300.5
        obsessive 300.3
        obsessive-compulsive 300.3
        phobic 300.20
        tension state 300.9
    psychophysiologic NEC (*see also* Disorder, psychosomatic) 306.9
        cardiovascular 306.2
        digestive 306.4
        endocrine 306.6
        gastrointestinal 306.4
        genitourinary 306.50
        heart 306.2
        hemic 306.8
        intestinal (large) (small) 306.4
        laryngeal 306.1
        lymphatic 306.8
        musculoskeletal 306.0
        pharyngeal 306.1
        respiratory 306.1
        skin 306.3
        special sense organs 306.7
    psychosomatic (*see also* Disorder, psychosomatic) 306.9
    psychotic (*see also* Psychosis) 298.9
        depressive 298.0
        due to or associated with physical condition (*see also* Psychosis, organic) 293.9
        involutional (*see also* Psychosis, affective) 296.2 ☑
            recurrent episode 296.3 ☑
            single episode 296.2 ☑
    pupillary (myotonic) (tonic) 379.46
    radiation — *see* Effect, adverse, radiation
    runaway (*see also* Disturbance, conduct)
        socialized 312.2 ☑
        undersocialized, unsocialized 312.1 ☑
    scarlet fever toxin — *see* Complications, vaccination
    schizophrenic (*see also* Schizophrenia) 295.9 ☑
        latent 295.5 ☑
    serological for syphilis — *see* Serology for syphilis
    serum (prophylactic) (therapeutic) 999.59
        anaphylactic 999.49
        due to
            administration of blood and blood products 999.51
                anaphylactic 999.41
            vaccination 999.52
                anaphylactic 999.41
        immediate 999.49
    situational (*see also* Reaction, adjustment) 309.9
        acute, to stress 308.3
        adjustment (*see also* Reaction, adjustment) 309.9
    somatization (*see also* Disorder, psychosomatic) 306.9
    spinal puncture 349.0
    spite, child (*see also* Disturbance, conduct) 312.0 ☑
    stress, acute 308.9
        with predominant disturbance (of)
            consciousness 308.1
            emotions 308.0
            mixed 308.4
            psychomotor 308.2
            specified type NEC 308.3
        bone or cartilage — *see* Fracture, stress
    surgical procedure — *see* Complications, surgical procedure

Reaction — *continued*
    tetanus antitoxin — *see* Complications, vaccination
    toxin-antitoxin — *see* Complications, vaccination
    transfusion (blood) (bone marrow) (lymphocytes) (allergic) (*see also* Complications, transfusion) 999.80
    tuberculin skin test, nonspecific (without active tuberculosis) 795.51
        positive (without active tuberculosis) 795.51
    ultraviolet — *see* Effect, adverse, ultraviolet
    undersocialized, unsocialized (*see also* Disturbance, conduct)
        aggressive (type) 312.0 ☑
        unaggressive (type) 312.1 ☑
    vaccination (any) — *see* Complications, vaccination
    white graft (skin) 996.52
    withdrawing, child or adolescent 313.22
    x-ray — *see* Effect, adverse, x-rays
Reactive depression — *see also* Reaction, depressive 300.4
    neurotic 300.4
    psychoneurotic 300.4
    psychotic 298.0
Rebound tenderness 789.6 ☑
Recalcitrant patient V15.81
Recanalization, thrombus — *see* Thrombosis
Recession, receding
    chamber angle (eye) 364.77
    chin 524.06
    gingival (postinfective) (postoperative) 523.20
        generalized 523.25
        localized 523.24
        minimal 523.21
        moderate 523.22
        severe 523.23
Recklinghausen-Applebaum disease (hemochromatosis) 275.03
Recklinghausen's disease (M9540/1) 237.71
    bones (osteitis fibrosa cystica) 252.01
Reclus' disease (cystic) 610.1
Recrudescent typhus (fever) 081.1
Recruitment, auditory 388.44
Rectalgia 569.42
Rectitis 569.49
Rectocele
    female (without uterine prolapse) 618.04
        with uterine prolapse 618.4
            complete 618.3
            incomplete 618.2
        in pregnancy or childbirth 654.4 ☑
            causing obstructed labor 660.2 ☑
                affecting fetus or newborn 763.1
    male 569.49
    vagina, vaginal (outlet) 618.04
Rectosigmoiditis 569.89
    ulcerative (chronic) 556.3
Rectosigmoid junction — *see* condition
Rectourethral — *see* condition
Rectovaginal — *see* condition
Rectovesical — *see* condition
Rectum, rectal — *see* condition
Recurrent — *see* condition
    pregnancy loss — *see* Pregnancy, management affected by, abortion, habitual
Red bugs 133.8
Red cedar asthma 495.8
Redness
    conjunctiva 379.93
    eye 379.93
    nose 478.19
Reduced ventilatory or vital capacity 794.2
Reduction
    function
        kidney (*see also* Disease, renal) 593.9
        liver 573.8
    ventilatory capacity 794.2
    vital capacity 794.2
Redundant, redundancy
    abdomen 701.9
    anus 751.5
    cardia 537.89

☑ **Additional Digit Required** — Refer to the Tabular List for Digit Selection   ▽ **Subterms under main terms may continue to next column or page**

246 — Volume 2   ▶◀ **Revised Text**   ● **New Line**   ▲ **Revised Code**   2013 ICD-9-CM

Redundant, redundancy — *continued*
  clitoris 624.2
  colon (congenital) 751.5
  foreskin (congenital) 605
  intestine 751.5
  labia 624.3
  organ or site, congenital NEC — *see* Accessory
  panniculus (abdominal) 278.1
  prepuce (congenital) 605
  pylorus 537.89
  rectum 751.5
  scrotum 608.89
  sigmoid 751.5
  skin (of face) 701.9
    eyelids 374.30
  stomach 537.89
  uvula 528.9
  vagina 623.8
Reduplication — *see* Duplication
Referral
  adoption (agency) V68.89
  nursing care V63.8
  patient without examination or treatment V68.81
  social services V63.8
Reflex — *see also* condition
  blink, deficient 374.45
  hyperactive gag 478.29
  neurogenic bladder NEC 596.54
    atonic 596.54
      with cauda equina syndrome 344.61
  vasoconstriction 443.9
  vasovagal 780.2
Reflux 530.81
  acid 530.81
  esophageal 530.81
    with esophagitis 530.11
  esophagitis 530.11
  gastroesophageal 530.81
  mitral — *see* Insufficiency, mitral
  ureteral — *see* Reflux, vesicoureteral
  vesicoureteral 593.70
    with
      reflux nephropathy 593.73
        bilateral 593.72
        unilateral 593.71
Reformed gallbladder 576.0
Reforming, artificial openings — *see also* Attention to, artificial, opening V55.9
Refractive error — *see also* Error, refractive 367.9
Refsum's disease or syndrome (heredopathia atactica polyneuritiformis) 356.3
Refusal of
  food 307.59
    hysterical 300.11
  treatment because of, due to
    patient's decision NEC V64.2
    reason of conscience or religion V62.6
Regaud
  tumor (M8082/3) — *see* Neoplasm, nasopharynx, malignant
  type carcinoma (M8082/3) — *see* Neoplasm, nasopharynx, malignant
Regional — *see* condition
Regulation feeding (elderly) (infant) 783.3
  newborn 779.31
Regurgitated
  food, choked on 933.1
  stomach contents, choked on 933.1
Regurgitation 787.03
  aortic (valve) (*see also* Insufficiency, aortic) 424.1
    congenital 746.4
    syphilitic 093.22
  food (*see also* Vomiting)
    with reswallowing — *see* Rumination
    newborn 779.33
  gastric contents — *see* Vomiting
  heart — *see* Endocarditis
  mitral (valve) (*see also* Insufficiency, mitral)
    congenital 746.6
  myocardial — *see* Endocarditis
  pulmonary (heart) (valve) (*see also* Endocarditis, pulmonary) 424.3

Regurgitation — *continued*
  stomach — *see* Vomiting
  tricuspid — *see* Endocarditis, tricuspid
  valve, valvular — *see* Endocarditis
  vesicoureteral — *see* Reflux, vesicoureteral
Rehabilitation V57.9
  multiple types V57.89
  occupational V57.21
  specified type NEC V57.89
  speech (-language) V57.3
  vocational V57.22
Reichmann's disease or syndrome (gastrosuccorrhea) 536.8
Reifenstein's syndrome (hereditary familial hypogonadism, male) 259.52
Reilly's syndrome or phenomenon — *see also* Neuropathy, peripheral, autonomic 337.9
Reimann's periodic disease 277.31
Reinsertion, contraceptive device V25.42
  intrauterine V25.13
Reiter's disease, syndrome, or urethritis 099.3 *[711.1]* ☑
Rejection
  food, hysterical 300.11
  transplant 996.80
    bone marrow 996.85
    corneal 996.51
    organ (immune or nonimmune cause) 996.80
      bone marrow 996.85
      heart 996.83
      intestines 996.87
      kidney 996.81
      liver 996.82
      lung 996.84
      pancreas 996.86
      specified NEC 996.89
    skin 996.52
      artificial 996.55
      decellularized allodermis 996.55
    stem cells(s) 996.88
      from
        peripheral blood 996.88
        umbilical cord 996.88
Relapsing fever 087.9
  Carter's (Asiatic) 087.0
  Dutton's (West African) 087.1
  Koch's 087.9
  louse-borne (epidemic) 087.0
  Novy's (American) 087.1
  Obermeyer's (European) 087.0
  Spirillum 087.9
  tick-borne (endemic) 087.1
Relaxation
  anus (sphincter) 569.49
    due to hysteria 300.11
  arch (foot) 734
    congenital 754.61
  back ligaments 728.4
  bladder (sphincter) 596.59
  cardio-esophageal 530.89
  cervix (*see also* Incompetency, cervix) 622.5
  diaphragm 519.4
  inguinal rings — *see* Hernia, inguinal
  joint (capsule) (ligament) (paralytic) (*see also* Derangement, joint) 718.90
    congenital 755.8
  lumbosacral joint 724.6
  pelvic floor 618.89
  pelvis 618.89
  perineum 618.89
  posture 729.90
  rectum (sphincter) 569.49
  sacroiliac (joint) 724.6
  scrotum 608.89
  urethra (sphincter) 599.84
  uterus (outlet) 618.89
  vagina (outlet) 618.89
  vesical 596.59
Remains
  canal of Cloquet 743.51
  capsule (opaque) 743.51
Remittent fever (malarial) 084.6
Remnant
  canal of Cloquet 743.51

Remnant — *continued*
  capsule (opaque) 743.51
  cervix, cervical stump (acquired) (postoperative) 622.8
  cystic duct, postcholecystectomy 576.0
  fingernail 703.8
    congenital 757.5
  meniscus, knee 717.5
  thyroglossal duct 759.2
  tonsil 474.8
    infected 474.00
  urachus 753.7
Remote effect of cancer — *see* condition
Removal (of)
  catheter (urinary) (indwelling) V53.6
    from artificial opening — *see* Attention to, artificial, opening
    non-vascular V58.82
    vascular V58.81
  cerebral ventricle (communicating) shunt V53.01
  device (*see also* Fitting (of))
    contraceptive V25.12
      with reinsertion V25.13
    fixation
      external V54.89
      internal V54.01
    traction V54.89
  drains V58.49
  dressing
    wound V58.30
      nonsurgical V58.30
      surgical V58.31
  ileostomy V55.2
  Kirschner wire V54.89
  nonvascular catheter V58.82
  pin V54.01
  plaster cast V54.89
  plate (fracture) V54.01
  rod V54.01
  screw V54.01
  splint, external V54.89
  staples V58.32
  subdermal implantable contraceptive V25.43
  sutures V58.32
  traction device, external V54.89
  vascular catheter V58.81
  wound packing V58.30
    nonsurgical V58.30
    surgical V58.31
Ren
  arcuatus 753.3
  mobile, mobilis (*see also* Disease, renal) 593.0
    congenital 753.3
  unguliformis 753.3
Renal — *see also* condition
  glomerulohyalinosis-diabetic syndrome 250.4 ☑ *[581.81]*
    due to secondary diabetes 249.4 ☑ *[581.81]*
Rendu-Osler-Weber disease or syndrome (familial hemorrhagic telangiectasia) 448.0
Reninoma (M8361/1) 236.91
Rénon-Delille syndrome 253.8
Repair
  pelvic floor, previous, in pregnancy or childbirth 654.4 ☑
    affecting fetus or newborn 763.89
  scarred tissue V51.8
Replacement by artificial or mechanical device or prosthesis of — *see also* Fitting (of
  artificial skin V43.83
  bladder V43.5
  blood vessel V43.4
  breast V43.82
  eye globe V43.0
  heart
    with
      assist device V43.21
      fully implantable artificial heart V43.22
    valve V43.3

Replacement by artificial or mechanical device or prosthesis of — *see also* Fitting (of — *continued*
    intestine V43.89
    joint V43.60
      ankle V43.66
      elbow V43.62
      finger V43.69
      hip (partial) (total) V43.64
      knee V43.65
      shoulder V43.61
      specified NEC V43.69
      wrist V43.63
    kidney V43.89
    larynx V43.81
    lens V43.1
    limb(s) V43.7
    liver V43.89
    lung V43.89
    organ NEC V43.89
    pancreas V43.89
    skin (artificial) V43.83
    tissue NEC V43.89
Reprogramming
  cardiac pacemaker V53.31
Request for expert evidence V68.2
Reserve, decreased or low
  cardiac — *see* Disease, heart
  kidney (*see also* Disease, renal) 593.9
Residual — *see also* condition
  bladder 596.89
  foreign body — *see* Retention, foreign body
  state, schizophrenic (*see also* Schizophrenia) 295.6 ☑
  urine 788.69
Resistance, resistant (to)
  activated protein C 289.81

Note — *use the following subclassification for categories V09.5, V09.7, V09.8, V09.9:*

0 *without mention of resistance to multiple drugs*

1 *with resistance to multiple drugs*

      V09.5 *quinolones and fluoroquinolones*

      V09.7 *antimycobacterial agents*

      V09.8 *specified drugs NEC*

      V09.9 *unspecified drugs*

  drugs by microorganisms V09.9 ☑
    Amikacin V09.4
    aminoglycosides V09.4
    Amodiaquine V09.5 ☑
    Amoxicillin V09.0
    Ampicillin V09.0
    antimycobacterial agents V09.7 ☑
    Azithromycin V09.2
    Azlocillin V09.0
    Aztreonam V09.1
    Bacampicillin V09.0
    Bacitracin V09.8 ☑
    Benznidazole V09.8 ☑
    B-lactam antibiotics V09.1
    Capreomycin V09.7 ☑
    Carbenicillin V09.0
    Cefaclor V09.1
    Cefadroxil V09.1
    Cefamandole V09.1
    Cefatetan V09.1
    Cefazolin V09.1
    Cefixime V09.1
    Cefonicid V09.1
    Cefoperazone V09.1
    Ceforanide V09.1
    Cefotaxime V09.1
    Cefoxitin V09.1
    Ceftazidime V09.1
    Ceftizoxime V09.1
    Ceftriaxone V09.1
    Cefuroxime V09.1
    Cephalexin V09.1
    Cephaloglycin V09.1
    Cephaloridine V09.1

☑ **Additional Digit Required** — Refer to the Tabular List for Digit Selection   ▽ **Subterms under main terms may continue to next column or page**

Resistance, resistant — continued
  drugs by microorganisms — continued
    Cephalosporins V09.1
    Cephalothin V09.1
    Cephapirin V09.1
    Cephradine V09.1
    Chloramphenicol V09.8 ☑
    Chloroquine V09.5 ☑
    Chlorguanide V09.8 ☑
    Chlorproguanil V09.8 ☑
    Chlortetracycline V09.3
    Cinoxacin V09.5 ☑
    Ciprofloxacin V09.5 ☑
    Clarithromycin V09.2
    Clindamycin V09.8 ☑
    Clioquinol V09.5 ☑
    Clofazimine V09.7 ☑
    Cloxacillin V09.0
    Cyclacillin V09.0
    Cycloserine V09.7 ☑
    Dapsone [DZ] V09.7 ☑
    Demeclocycline V09.3
    Dicloxacillin V09.0
    Doxycycline V09.3
    Enoxacin V09.5 ☑
    Erythromycin V09.2
    Ethambutol [EMB] V09.7 ☑
    Ethionamide [ETA] V09.7 ☑
    fluoroquinolones V09.5 ☑
    Gentamicin V09.4
    Halofantrine V09.8 ☑
    Imipenem V09.1
    Iodoquinol V09.5 ☑
    Isoniazid [INH] V09.7 ☑
    Kanamycin V09.4
    macrolides V09.2
    Mafenide V09.6
    MDRO (multiple drug resistant organisms) NOS V09.91
    Mefloquine V09.8 ☑
    Melasoprol V09.8 ☑
    Methacycline V09.3
    Methenamine V09.8 ☑
    Methicillin — see Infection, Methicillin V09.0
    Metronidazole V09.8 ☑
    Mezlocillin V09.0
    Minocycline V09.3
    multiple drug resistant organisms NOS V09.91
    Nafcillin V09.0
    Nalidixic acid V09.5 ☑
    Natamycin V09.2
    Neomycin V09.4
    Netilmicin V09.4
    Nimorazole V09.8 ☑
    Nitrofurantoin V09.8 ☑
    Nitrofurtimox V09.8 ☑
    Norfloxacin V09.5 ☑
    Nystatin V09.2
    Ofloxacin V09.5 ☑
    Oleandomycin V09.2
    Oxacillin V09.0
    Oxytetracycline V09.3
    Para-amino salicylic acid [PAS] V09.7 ☑
    Paromomycin V09.4
    Penicillin (G) (V) (VK) V09.0
    penicillins V09.0
    Pentamidine V09.8 ☑
    Piperacillin V09.0
    Primaquine V09.5 ☑
    Proguanil V09.8 ☑
    Pyrazinamide [PZA] V09.7 ☑
    Pyrimethamine/Sulfalene V09.8 ☑
    Pyrimethamine/Sulfodoxine V09.8 ☑
    Quinacrine V09.5 ☑
    Quinidine V09.8 ☑
    Quinine V09.8 ☑
    quinolones V09.5 ☑
    Rifabutin V09.7 ☑
    Rifampin [RIF] V09.7 ☑
    Rifamycin V09.7 ☑
    Roliletracycline V09.3
    specified drugs NEC V09.8 ☑
    Spectinomycin V09.8 ☑

Resistance, resistant — continued
  drugs by microorganisms — continued
    Spiramycin V09.2
    Streptomycin [SM] V09.4
    Sulfacetamide V09.6
    Sulfacytine V09.6
    Sulfadiazine V09.6
    Sulfadoxine V09.6
    Sulfamethoxazole V09.6
    Sulfapyridine V09.6
    Sulfasalizine V09.6
    Sulfasoxazole V09.6
    sulfonamides V09.6
    Sulfoxone V09.7 ☑
    tetracycline V09.3
    tetracyclines V09.3
    Thiamphenicol V09.8 ☑
    Ticarcillin V09.0
    Tinidazole V09.8 ☑
    Tobramycin V09.4
    Triamphenicol V09.8 ☑
    Trimethoprim V09.8 ☑
    Vancomycin V09.8 ☑
  insulin 277.7
    complicating pregnancy 648.8 ☑
  thyroid hormone 246.8
Resorption
  biliary 576.8
    purulent or putrid (see also Cholecystitis) 576.8
  dental (roots) 521.40
    alveoli 525.8
    pathological
      external 521.42
      internal 521.41
      specified NEC 521.49
  septic — see Septicemia
  teeth (roots) 521.40
    pathological
      external 521.42
      internal 521.41
      specified NEC 521.49
Respiration
  asymmetrical 786.09
  bronchial 786.09
  Cheyne-Stokes (periodic respiration) 786.04
  decreased, due to shock following injury 958.4
  disorder of 786.00
    psychogenic 306.1
    specified NEC 786.09
  failure 518.81
    acute 518.81
      following trauma and surgery 518.51
    acute and chronic 518.84
      following trauma and surgery 518.53
    chronic 518.83
    following trauma and surgery 518.51
    newborn 770.84
  insufficiency 786.09
    acute 518.82
    newborn NEC 770.89
  Kussmaul (air hunger) 786.09
  painful 786.52
  periodic 786.09
    high altitude 327.22
  poor 786.09
    newborn NEC 770.89
  sighing 786.7
    psychogenic 306.1
  wheezing 786.07
Respiratory — see also condition
  distress 786.09
    acute 518.82
    fetus or newborn NEC 770.89
    syndrome (newborn) 769
      adult (following trauma and surgery) 518.52
        specified NEC 518.82
  failure 518.81
    acute 518.81
      following trauma and surgery 518.51
    acute and chronic 518.84
      following trauma and surgery 518.53
    chronic 518.83
    following trauma and surgery 518.51

Respiratory syncytial virus (RSV) 079.6
  bronchiolitis 466.11
  pneumonia 480.1
  vaccination, prophylactic (against) V04.82
Response
  photoallergic 692.72
  phototoxic 692.72
Restless legs syndrome (RLS) 333.94
Restlessness 799.29
Restoration of organ continuity from previous sterilization (tuboplasty) (vasoplasty) V26.0
Rest, rests
  mesonephric duct 752.89
    fallopian tube 752.11
  ovarian, in fallopian tubes 752.19
  wolffian duct 752.89
Restriction of housing space V60.1
Restzustand, schizophrenic — see also
    Schizophrenia 295.6 ☑
Retained — see Retention
Retardation
  development, developmental, specific (see also Disorder, development, specific) 315.9
    learning, specific 315.2
      arithmetical 315.1
      language (skills) 315.31
        expressive 315.31
        mixed receptive-expressive 315.32
      mathematics 315.1
      reading 315.00
        phonological 315.39
        written expression 315.2
      motor 315.4
  endochondral bone growth 733.91
  growth (physical) in childhood 783.43
    due to malnutrition 263.2
    fetal (intrauterine) 764.9 ☑
      affecting management of pregnancy 656.5 ☑
  intrauterine growth 764.9 ☑
    affecting management of pregnancy 656.5 ☑
  mental — see Disability, intellectual
  motor, specific 315.4
  physical 783.43
    child 783.43
    due to malnutrition 263.2
    fetus (intrauterine) 764.9 ☑
      affecting management of pregnancy 656.5 ☑
  psychomotor NEC 307.9
  reading 315.00
Retching — see Vomiting
Retention, retained
  bladder (see also Retention, urine) 788.20
    psychogenic 306.53
  carbon dioxide 276.2
  cholelithiasis, following cholecystectomy 997.41
  cyst — see Cyst
  dead
    fetus (after 22 completed weeks gestation) 656.4 ☑
      early fetal death (before 22 completed weeks gestation) 632
    ovum 631.8
  decidua (following delivery) (fragments) (with hemorrhage) 666.2 ☑
    without hemorrhage 667.1 ☑
  deciduous tooth 520.6
  dental root 525.3
  fecal (see also Constipation) 564.00
  fluid 276.69
  foreign body (see also Foreign body, retained)
    bone 733.99
    current trauma — see Foreign body, by site or type
    middle ear 385.83
    muscle 729.6
    soft tissue NEC 729.6
  gallstones, following cholecystectomy 997.41

Retention, retained — continued
  gastric 536.8
  membranes (following delivery) (with hemorrhage) 666.2 ☑
    with abortion — see Abortion, by type
    without hemorrhage 667.1 ☑
  menses 626.8
  milk (puerperal) 676.2 ☑
  nitrogen, extrarenal 788.99
  placenta (total) (with hemorrhage) 666.0 ☑
    with abortion — see Abortion, by type
    without hemorrhage 667.0 ☑
    portions or fragments 666.2 ☑
      without hemorrhage 667.1 ☑
  products of conception
    early pregnancy (fetal death before 22 completed weeks gestation) 632
    following
      abortion — see Abortion, by type
      delivery 666.2 ☑
        with hemorrhage 666.2 ☑
        without hemorrhage 667.1 ☑
  secundines (following delivery) (with hemorrhage) 666.2 ☑
    with abortion — see Abortion, by type
    without hemorrhage 667.1 ☑
    complicating puerperium (delayed hemorrhage) 666.2 ☑
  smegma, clitoris 624.8
  urine NEC 788.20
    bladder, incomplete emptying 788.21
    due to
      benign prostatic hypertrophy (BPH) — see category 600
    due to
      benign prostatic hypertrophy (BPH) — see category 600
    psychogenic 306.53
    specified NEC 788.29
  water (in tissue) (see also Edema) 782.3
Reticulation, dust (occupational) 504
Reticulocytosis NEC 790.99
Reticuloendotheliosis
  acute infantile (M9722/3) 202.5 ☑
  leukemic (M9940/3) 202.4 ☑
  malignant (M9720/3) 202.3 ☑
  nonlipid (M9722/3) 202.5 ☑
Reticulohistiocytoma (giant cell) 277.89
Reticulohistiocytosis, multicentric 272.8
Reticulolymphosarcoma (diffuse) (M9613/3) 200.8 ☑
  follicular (M9691/3) 202.0 ☑
  nodular (M9691/3) 202.0 ☑
Reticulosarcoma (M9640/3) 200.0 ☑
  nodular (M9642/3) 200.0 ☑
  pleomorphic cell type (M9641/3) 200.0 ☑
Reticulosis (skin)
  acute of infancy (M9722/3) 202.5 ☑
  familial hemophagocytic 288.4
  histiocytic medullary (M9721/3) 202.3 ☑
  lipomelanotic 695.89
  malignant (M9720/3) 202.3 ☑
  Sézary's (M9701/3) 202.2 ☑
Retina, retinal — see condition
Retinitis — see also Chorioretinitis 363.20
  albuminurica 585.9 [363.10]
  arteriosclerotic 440.8 [362.13]
  central angiospastic 362.41
  Coat's 362.12
  diabetic 250.5 ☑ [362.01]
    due to secondary diabetes 249.5 ☑ [362.01]
  disciformis 362.52
  disseminated 363.10
    metastatic 363.14
    neurosyphilitic 094.83
    pigment epitheliopathy 363.15
  exudative 362.12
  focal 363.00
    in histoplasmosis 115.92
      capsulatum 115.02
      duboisii 115.12
    juxtapapillary 363.05
    macular 363.06
    paramacular 363.06

Retinitis — see also Chorioretinitis — continued
  focal — continued
    peripheral 363.08
    posterior pole NEC 363.07
  gravidarum 646.8 ☑
  hemorrhagica externa 362.12
  juxtapapillary (Jensen's) 363.05
  luetic — see Retinitis, syphilitic
  metastatic 363.14
  pigmentosa 362.74
  proliferans 362.29
  proliferating 362.29
  punctata albescens 362.76
  renal 585.9 [363.13]
  syphilitic (secondary) 091.51
    congenital 090.0 [363.13]
    early 091.51
    late 095.8 [363.13]
  syphilitica, central, recurrent 095.8 [363.13]
  tuberculous (see also Tuberculous)
    017.3 ☑ [363.13]
Retinoblastoma (M9510/3) 190.5
  differentiated type (M9511/3) 190.5
  undifferentiated type (M9512/3) 190.5
Retinochoroiditis — see also Chorioretinitis
  363.20
  central angiospastic 362.41
  disseminated 363.10
    metastatic 363.14
    neurosyphilitic 094.83
    pigment epitheliopathy 363.15
    syphilitic 094.83
  due to toxoplasmosis (acquired) (focal)
    130.2
  focal 363.00
    in histoplasmosis 115.92
      capsulatum 115.02
      duboisii 115.12
    juxtapapillary (Jensen's) 363.05
    macular 363.06
    paramacular 363.06
    peripheral 363.08
    posterior pole NEC 363.07
  juxtapapillaris 363.05
  syphilitic (disseminated) 094.83
Retinopathy (background) 362.10
  arteriosclerotic 440.8 [362.13]
  atherosclerotic 440.8 [362.13]
  central serous 362.41
  circinate 362.10
  Coat's 362.12
  diabetic 250.5 ☑ [362.01]
    due to secondary diabetes
      249.5 ☑ [362.01]
    nonproliferative 250.5 ☑ [362.03]
      due to secondary diabetes
        249.5 ☑ [362.03]
      mild 250.5 ☑ [362.04]
        due to secondary diabetes
          249.5 ☑ [362.04]
      moderate 250.5 ☑ [362.05]
        due to secondary diabetes
          249.5 ☑ [362.05]
      severe 250.5 ☑ [362.06]
        due to secondary diabetes
          249.5 ☑ [362.06]
    proliferative 250.5 ☑ [362.02]
      due to secondary diabetes
        249.5 ☑ [362.02]
  exudative 362.12
  hypertensive 362.11
  nonproliferative
    diabetic 250.5 ☑ [362.03]
      due to secondary diabetes
        249.5 ☑ [362.03]
      mild 250.5 ☑ [362.04]
        due to secondary diabetes
          249.5 ☑ [362.04]
      moderate 250.5 ☑ [362.05]
        due to secondary diabetes
          249.5 ☑ [362.05]
      severe 250.5 ☑ [362.06]
        due to secondary diabetes
          249.5 ☑ [362.06]
  of prematurity 362.20

Retinopathy — continued
  of prematurity — continued
    cicatricial 362.21
    stage
      0 362.22
      1 362.23
      2 362.24
      3 362.25
      4 362.26
      5 362.27
  pigmentary, congenital 362.74
  proliferative 362.29
    diabetic 250.5 ☑ [362.02]
      due to secondary diabetes
        249.5 ☑ [362.02]
    sickle-cell 282.60 [362.29]
  solar 363.31
Retinoschisis 361.10
  bullous 361.12
  congenital 743.56
  flat 361.11
  juvenile 362.73
Retractile testis 752.52
Retraction
  cervix — see Retraction, uterus
  drum (membrane) 384.82
  eyelid 374.41
  finger 736.29
  head 781.0
  lid 374.41
  lung 518.89
  mediastinum 519.3
  nipple 611.79
    congenital 757.6
    puerperal, postpartum 676.0 ☑
  palmar fascia 728.6
  pleura (see also Pleurisy) 511.0
  ring, uterus (Bandl's) (pathological) 661.4 ☑
    affecting fetus or newborn 763.7
  sternum (congenital) 756.3
    acquired 738.3
    during respiration 786.9
  substernal 738.3
  supraclavicular 738.8
  syndrome (Duane's) 378.71
  uterus 621.6
  valve (heart) — see Endocarditis
Retrobulbar — see condition
Retrocaval ureter 753.4
Retrocecal — see also condition
  appendix (congenital) 751.5
Retrocession — see Retroversion
Retrodisplacement — see Retroversion
Retroflection, retroflexion — see Retroversion
Retrognathia, retrognathism (mandibular)
  (maxillary) 524.10
Retrograde
  ejaculation 608.87
  menstruation 626.8
Retroiliac ureter 753.4
Retroperineal — see condition
Retroperitoneal — see condition
Retroperitonitis 567.39
Retropharyngeal — see condition
Retroplacental — see condition
Retroposition — see Retroversion
Retroprosthetic membrane 996.51
Retrosternal thyroid (congenital) 759.2
Retroversion, retroverted
  cervix — see Retroversion, uterus
  female NEC (see also Retroversion, uterus)
    621.6
  iris 364.70
  testis (congenital) 752.51
  uterus, uterine (acquired) (acute) (adherent)
    (any degree) (asymptomatic) (cervix)
    (postinfectional) (postpartal, old)
    621.6
    congenital 752.39
    in pregnancy or childbirth 654.3 ☑
      affecting fetus or newborn 763.89
      causing obstructed labor 660.2 ☑
        affecting fetus or newborn 763.1
Retrusion, premaxilla (developmental) 524.04
Rett's syndrome 330.8

Reverse, reversed
  peristalsis 787.4
Reye-Sheehan syndrome (postpartum pituitary necrosis) 253.2
Reye's syndrome 331.81
Rhabdomyolysis (idiopathic) 728.88
Rhabdomyoma (M8900/0) — see also Neoplasm, connective tissue, benign
  adult (M8904/0) — see Neoplasm, connective tissue, benign
  fetal (M8903/0) — see Neoplasm, connective tissue, benign
  glycogenic (M8904/0) — see Neoplasm, connective tissue, benign
Rhabdomyosarcoma (M8900/3) — see also Neoplasm, connective tissue, malignant
  alveolar (M8920/3) — see Neoplasm, connective tissue, malignant
  embryonal (M8910/3) — see Neoplasm, connective tissue, malignant
  mixed type (M8902/3) — see Neoplasm, connective tissue, malignant
  pleomorphic (M8901/3) — see Neoplasm, connective tissue, malignant
Rhabdosarcoma (M8900/3) — see Rhabdomyosarcoma
Rh antigen (C) (c) (D) (E) (e) (factor)
  hemolytic disease 773.0
  incompatibility, immunization, or sensitization
    affecting management of pregnancy
      656.1 ☑
    fetus or newborn 773.0
    transfusion reaction (see also Complications, transfusion) 999.70
  negative mother, affecting fetus or newborn 773.0
  titer elevated (see also Complications, transfusion) 999.70
  transfusion reaction (see also Complications, transfusion) 999.70
Rhesus (factor) (Rh) incompatibility — see Rh, incompatibility
Rheumaticosis — see Rheumatism
Rheumatism, rheumatic (acute NEC) 729.0
  adherent pericardium 393
  arthritis
    acute or subacute — see Fever, rheumatic
    chronic 714.0
      spine 720.0
  articular (chronic) NEC (see also Arthritis) 716.9 ☑
    acute or subacute — see Fever, rheumatic
  back 724.9
  blennorrhagic 098.59
  carditis — see Disease, heart, rheumatic
  cerebral — see Fever, rheumatic
  chorea (acute) — see Chorea, rheumatic
  chronic NEC 729.0
  coronary arteritis 391.9
    chronic 398.99
  degeneration, myocardium (see also Degeneration, myocardium, with rheumatic fever) 398.0
  desert 114.0
  febrile — see Fever, rheumatic
  fever — see Fever, rheumatic
  gonococcal 098.59
  gout 714.0
  heart
    disease (see also Disease, heart, rheumatic) 398.90
    failure (chronic) (congestive) (inactive) 398.91
  hemopericardium — see Rheumatic, pericarditis
  hydropericardium — see Rheumatic, pericarditis
  inflammatory (acute) (chronic) (subacute) — see Fever, rheumatic
  intercostal 729.0
    meaning Tietze's disease 733.6
  joint (chronic) NEC (see also Arthritis) 716.9 ☑

Rheumatism, rheumatic — continued
  joint (see also Arthritis) — continued
    acute — see Fever, rheumatic
  mediastinopericarditis — see Rheumatic, pericarditis
  muscular 729.0
  myocardial degeneration (see also Degeneration, myocardium, with rheumatic fever) 398.0
  myocarditis (chronic) (inactive) (with chorea) 398.0
    active or acute 391.2
      with chorea (acute) (rheumatic) (Sydenham's) 392.0
  myositis 729.1
  neck 724.9
  neuralgic 729.0
  neuritis (acute) (chronic) 729.2
  neuromuscular 729.0
  nodose — see Arthritis, nodosa
  nonarticular 729.0
  palindromic 719.30
    ankle 719.37
    elbow 719.32
    foot 719.37
    hand 719.34
    hip 719.35
    knee 719.36
    multiple sites 719.39
    pelvic region 719.35
    shoulder (region) 719.31
    specified site NEC 719.38
    wrist 719.33
  pancarditis, acute 391.8
    with chorea (acute) (rheumatic) (Sydenham's) 392.0
    chronic or inactive 398.99
  pericarditis (active) (acute) (with effusion) (with pneumonia) 391.0
    with chorea (acute) (rheumatic) (Sydenham's) 392.0
    chronic or inactive 393
  pericardium — see Rheumatic, pericarditis
  pleuropericarditis — see Rheumatic, pericarditis
  pneumonia 390 [517.1]
  pneumonitis 390 [517.1]
  pneumopericarditis — see Rheumatic, pericarditis
  polyarthritis
    acute or subacute — see Fever, rheumatic
    chronic 714.0
  polyarticular NEC (see also Arthritis) 716.9 ☑
  psychogenic 306.0
  radiculitis 729.2
  sciatic 724.3
  septic — see Fever, rheumatic
  spine 724.9
  subacute NEC 729.0
  torticollis 723.5
  tuberculous NEC (see also Tuberculosis) 015.9 ☑
  typhoid fever 002.0
Rheumatoid — see also condition
  lungs 714.81
Rhinitis (atrophic) (catarrhal) (chronic) (croupous) (fibrinous) (hyperplastic) (hypertrophic) (membranous) (purulent) (suppurative) (ulcerative) 472.0
  with
    hay fever (see also Fever, hay) 477.9
      with asthma (bronchial) 493.0 ☑
    sore throat — see Nasopharyngitis
  acute 460
  allergic (nonseasonal) (seasonal) (see also Fever, hay) 477.9
    with asthma (see also Asthma) 493.0 ☑
    due to food 477.1
  granulomatous 472.0
  infective 460
  obstructive 472.0
  pneumococcal 460
  syphilitic 095.8
    congenital 090.0
  tuberculous (see also Tuberculosis) 012.8 ☑

☑ **Additional Digit Required** — Refer to the Tabular List for Digit Selection   ▽ **Subterms under main terms may continue to next column or page**

2013 ICD-9-CM   ▶◀ Revised Text   ● New Line   ▲ Revised Code   **Volume 2 — 249**

Retinitis — Rhinitis

Rhinitis — *continued*
vasomotor (*see also* Fever, hay) 477.9
Rhinoantritis (chronic) 473.0
acute 461.0
Rhinodacryolith 375.57
Rhinolalia (aperta) (clausa) (open) 784.43
Rhinolith 478.19
nasal sinus (*see also* Sinusitis) 473.9
Rhinomegaly 478.19
Rhinopharyngitis (acute) (subacute) — *see also* Nasopharyngitis 460
chronic 472.2
destructive ulcerating 102.5
mutilans 102.5
Rhinophyma 695.3
Rhinorrhea 478.19
cerebrospinal (fluid) 349.81
paroxysmal (*see also* Fever, hay) 477.9
spasmodic (*see also* Fever, hay) 477.9
Rhinosalpingitis 381.50
acute 381.51
chronic 381.52
Rhinoscleroma 040.1
Rhinosporidiosis 117.0
Rhinovirus infection 079.3
Rhizomelic chrondrodysplasia punctata 277.86
Rhizomelique, pseudopolyarthritic 446.5
Rhoads and Bomford anemia (refractory) 238.72
Rhus
diversiloba dermatitis 692.6
radicans dermatitis 692.6
toxicodendron dermatitis 692.6
venenata dermatitis 692.6
verniciflua dermatitis 692.6
Rhythm
atrioventricular nodal 427.89
disorder 427.9
coronary sinus 427.89
ectopic 427.89
nodal 427.89
escape 427.89
heart, abnormal 427.9
fetus or newborn — *see* Abnormal, heart rate
idioventricular 426.89
accelerated 427.89
nodal 427.89
sleep, inversion 327.39
nonorganic origin 307.45
Rhytidosis facialis 701.8
Rib — *see also* condition
cervical 756.2
Riboflavin deficiency 266.0
Rice bodies — *see also* Loose, body, joint 718.1 ☑
knee 717.6
Richter's hernia — *see* Hernia, Richter's
Ricinism 988.2
Rickets (active) (acute) (adolescent) (adult) (chest wall) (congenital) (current) (infantile) (intestinal) 268.0
celiac 579.0
fetal 756.4
hemorrhagic 267
hypophosphatemic with nephrotic-glycosuric dwarfism 270.0
kidney 588.0
late effect 268.1
renal 588.0
scurvy 267
vitamin D-resistant 275.3
Rickettsial disease 083.9
specified type NEC 083.8
Rickettsialpox 083.2
Rickettsiosis NEC 083.9
specified type NEC 083.8
tick-borne 082.9
specified type NEC 082.8
vesicular 083.2
Ricord's chancre 091.0
Riddoch's syndrome (visual disorientation) 368.16
Rider's
bone 733.99

Rider's — *continued*
chancre 091.0
Ridge, alveolus — *see also* condition
edentulous
atrophy 525.20
mandible 525.20
minimal 525.21
moderate 525.22
severe 525.23
maxilla 525.20
minimal 525.24
moderate 525.25
severe 525.26
flabby 525.20
Ridged ear 744.29
Riedel's
disease (ligneous thyroiditis) 245.3
lobe, liver 751.69
struma (ligneous thyroiditis) 245.3
thyroiditis (ligneous) 245.3
Rieger's anomaly or syndrome (mesodermal dysgenesis, anterior ocular segment) 743.44
Riehl's melanosis 709.09
Rietti-Greppi-Micheli anemia or syndrome 282.46
Rieux's hernia — *see* Hernia, Rieux's
Rift Valley fever 066.3
Riga's disease (cachectic aphthae) 529.0
Riga-Fede disease (cachectic aphthae) 529.0
Riggs' disease (compound periodontitis) 523.40
Right middle lobe syndrome 518.0
Rigid, rigidity — *see also* condition
abdominal 789.4 ☑
articular, multiple congenital 754.89
back 724.8
cervix uteri
in pregnancy or childbirth 654.6 ☑
affecting fetus or newborn 763.89
causing obstructed labor 660.2 ☑
affecting fetus or newborn 763.1
hymen (acquired) (congenital) 623.3
nuchal 781.6
pelvic floor
in pregnancy or childbirth 654.4 ☑
affecting fetus or newborn 763.89
causing obstructed labor 660.2 ☑
affecting fetus or newborn 763.1
perineum or vulva
in pregnancy or childbirth 654.8 ☑
affecting fetus or newborn 763.89
causing obstructed labor 660.2 ☑
affecting fetus or newborn 763.1
spine 724.8
vagina
in pregnancy or childbirth 654.7 ☑
affecting fetus or newborn 763.89
causing obstructed labor 660.2 ☑
affecting fetus or newborn 763.1
Rigors 780.99
Riley-Day syndrome (familial dysautonomia) 742.8
RIND (reversible ischemic neurological deficit) 434.91
history of (personal) V12.54
Ring(s)
aorta 747.21
Bandl's, complicating delivery 661.4 ☑
affecting fetus or newborn 763.7
contraction, complicating delivery 661.4 ☑
affecting fetus or newborn 763.7
esophageal (congenital) 750.3
Fleischer (-Kayser) (cornea) 275.1 *[371.14]*
hymenal, tight (acquired) (congenital) 623.3
Kayser-Fleischer (cornea) 275.1 *[371.14]*
retraction, uterus, pathological 661.4 ☑
affecting fetus or newborn 763.7
Schatzki's (esophagus) (congenital) (lower) 750.3
acquired 530.3
Soemmering's 366.51
trachea, abnormal 748.3
vascular (congenital) 747.21
Vossius' 921.3
late effect 366.21

Ringed hair (congenital) 757.4
Ringing in the ear — *see also* Tinnitus 388.30
Ringworm 110.9
beard 110.0
body 110.5
Burmese 110.9
corporeal 110.5
foot 110.4
groin 110.3
hand 110.2
honeycomb 110.0
nails 110.1
perianal (area) 110.3
scalp 110.0
specified site NEC 110.8
Tokelau 110.5
Rise, venous pressure 459.89
Risk
factor — *see* Problem
falling V15.88
suicidal 300.9
Ritter's disease (dermatitis exfoliativa neonatorum) 695.81
Rivalry, sibling 313.3
Rivalta's disease (cervicofacial actinomycosis) 039.3
River blindness 125.3 *[360.13]*
Robert's pelvis 755.69
with disproportion (fetopelvic) 653.0 ☑
affecting fetus or newborn 763.1
causing obstructed labor 660.1 ☑
affecting fetus or newborn 763.1
Robinson's (hidrotic) **ectodermal dysplasia** 757.31
Robin's syndrome 756.0
Robles' disease (onchocerciasis) 125.3 *[360.13]*
Rochalimea — *see* Rickettsial disease
Rocky Mountain fever (spotted) 082.0
Rodent ulcer (M8090/3) — *see also* Neoplasm, skin, malignant
cornea 370.07
Roentgen ray, adverse effect — *see* Effect, adverse, x-ray
Roetheln 056.9
Roger's disease (congenital interventricular septal defect) 745.4
Rokitansky's
disease (*see also* Necrosis, liver) 570
tumor 620.2
Rokitansky-Aschoff sinuses (mucosal outpouching of gallbladder) — *see also* Disease, gallbladder 575.8
Rokitansky-Kuster-Hauser syndrome (congenital absence vagina) 752.45
Rollet's chancre (syphilitic) 091.0
Rolling of head 781.0
Romano-Ward syndrome (prolonged QT interval syndrome) 426.82
Romanus lesion 720.1
Romberg's disease or syndrome 349.89
Roof, mouth — *see* condition
Rosacea 695.3
acne 695.3
keratitis 695.3 *[370.49]*
Rosary, rachitic 268.0
Rose
cold 477.0
fever 477.0
rash 782.1
epidemic 056.9
of infants 057.8
Rosenbach's erysipelatoid or erysipeloid 027.1
Rosen-Castleman-Liebow syndrome (pulmonary proteinosis) 516.0
Rosenthal's disease (factor XI deficiency) 286.2
Roseola 057.8
infantum, infantilis (*see also* Exanthem subitum) 058.10
Rossbach's disease (hyperchlorhydria) 536.8
psychogenic 306.4
Rössle-Urbach-Wiethe lipoproteinosis 272.8
Ross river fever 066.3
Rostan's asthma (cardiac) — *see also* Failure, ventricular, left 428.1

Rot
Barcoo (*see also* Ulcer, skin) 707.9
knife-grinders' (*see also* Tuberculosis) 011.4 ☑
Rotation
anomalous, incomplete or insufficient — *see* Malrotation
cecum (congenital) 751.4
colon (congenital) 751.4
manual, affecting fetus or newborn 763.89
spine, incomplete or insufficient 737.8
tooth, teeth 524.35
vertebra, incomplete or insufficient 737.8
Rot-Bernhardt disease 355.1
Röteln 056.9
Roth-Bernhardt disease or syndrome 355.1
Roth's disease or meralgia 355.1
Rothmund (-Thomson) syndrome 757.33
Rotor's disease or syndrome (idiopathic hyperbilirubinemia) 277.4
Rotundum ulcus — *see* Ulcer, stomach
Round
back (with wedging of vertebrae) 737.10
late effect of rickets 268.1
hole, retina 361.31
with detachment 361.01
ulcer (stomach) — *see* Ulcer, stomach
worms (infestation) (large) NEC 127.0
Roussy-Lévy syndrome 334.3
Routine postpartum follow-up V24.2
Roy (-Jutras) syndrome (acropachyderma) 757.39
Rubella (German measles) 056.9
complicating pregnancy, childbirth, or puerperium 647.5 ☑
complication 056.8
neurological 056.00
encephalomyelitis 056.01
specified type NEC 056.09
specified type NEC 056.79
congenital 771.0
contact V01.4
exposure to V01.4
maternal
with suspected fetal damage affecting management of pregnancy 655.3 ☑
affecting fetus or newborn 760.2
manifest rubella in infant 771.0
specified complications NEC 056.79
vaccination, prophylactic (against) V04.3
Rubeola (measles) — *see also* Measles 055.9
complicated 055.8
meaning rubella (*see also* Rubella) 056.9
scarlatinosis 057.8
Rubeosis iridis 364.42
diabetica 250.5 ☑ *[364.42]*
due to secondary diabetes 249.5 ☑ *[364.42]*
Rubinstein-Taybi's syndrome (brachydactylia, short stature and intellectual disabilities 759.89
Rudimentary (congenital) — *see also* Agenesis
arm 755.22
bone 756.9
cervix uteri 752.43
eye (*see also* Microphthalmos) 743.10
fallopian tube 752.19
leg 755.32
lobule of ear 744.21
patella 755.64
respiratory organs in thoracopagus 759.4
tracheal bronchus 748.3
uterine horn 752.39
uterus 752.39
in male 752.7
solid or with cavity 752.39
vagina 752.45
Rud's syndrome (mental deficiency, epilepsy, and infantilism) 759.89
Ruiter-Pompen (-Wyers) syndrome (angiokeratoma corporis diffusum) 272.7
Ruled out condition — *see also* Observation, suspected V71.9
Rumination — *see also* Vomiting
disorder 307.53

☑ Additional Digit Required — Refer to the Tabular List for Digit Selection   👁 Subterms under main terms may continue to next column or page

250 — Volume 2   ▶◀ Revised Text   ● New Line   ▲ Revised Code   2013 ICD-9-CM

Rumination — *see also* Vomiting — *continued*
  neurotic 300.3
  obsessional 300.3
  psychogenic 307.53
Runaway reaction — *see also* Disturbance, conduct
  socialized 312.2 ☑
  undersocialized, unsocialized 312.1 ☑
Runeberg's disease (progressive pernicious anemia) 281.0
Runge's syndrome (postmaturity) 766.22
Runny nose 784.99
Rupia 091.3
  congenital 090.0
  tertiary 095.9
Rupture, ruptured 553.9
  abdominal viscera NEC 799.89
    obstetrical trauma 665.5 ☑
  abscess (spontaneous) — *see* Abscess, by site
  amnion — *see* Rupture, membranes
  aneurysm — *see* Aneurysm
  anus (sphincter) — *see* Laceration, anus
  aorta, aortic 441.5
    abdominal 441.3
    arch 441.1
    ascending 441.1
    descending 441.5
      abdominal 441.3
      thoracic 441.1
    syphilitic 093.0
    thoracoabdominal 441.6
    thorax, thoracic 441.1
    transverse 441.1
    traumatic (thoracic) 901.0
      abdominal 902.0
    valve or cusp (*see also* Endocarditis, aortic) 424.1
  appendix (with peritonitis) 540.0
    with peritoneal abscess 540.1
    traumatic — *see* Injury, internal, gastrointestinal tract
  arteriovenous fistula, brain (congenital) 430
  artery 447.2
    brain (*see also* Hemorrhage, brain) 431
    coronary (*see also* Infarct, myocardium) 410.9 ☑
    heart (*see also* Infarct, myocardium) 410.9 ☑
    pulmonary 417.8
    traumatic (complication) (*see also* Injury, blood vessel, by site) 904.9
  bile duct, except cystic (*see also* Disease, biliary) 576.3
    cystic 575.4
    traumatic — *see* Injury, internal, intra-abdominal
  bladder (sphincter) 596.6
    with
      abortion — *see* Abortion, by type, with damage to pelvic organs
      ectopic pregnancy (*see also* categories 633.0–633.9) 639.2
      molar pregnancy (*see also* categories 630–632) 639.2
    following
      abortion 639.2
      ectopic or molar pregnancy 639.2
    nontraumatic 596.6
    obstetrical trauma 665.5 ☑
    spontaneous 596.6
    traumatic — *see* Injury, internal, bladder
  blood vessel (*see also* Hemorrhage) 459.0
    brain (*see also* Hemorrhage, brain) 431
    heart (*see also* Infarct, myocardium) 410.9 ☑
    traumatic (complication) (*see also* Injury, blood vessel, by site) 904.9
  bone — *see* Fracture, by site
  bowel 569.89
    traumatic — *see* Injury, internal, intestine
  Bowman's membrane 371.31

Rupture, ruptured — *continued*
  brain
    aneurysm (congenital) (*see also* Hemorrhage, subarachnoid) 430
      late effect — *see* Late effect(s) (of) cerebrovascular disease
      syphilitic 094.87
    hemorrhagic (*see also* Hemorrhage, brain) 431
    injury at birth 767.0
    syphilitic 094.89
  capillaries 448.9
  cardiac (*see also* Infarct, myocardium) 410.9 ☑
  cartilage (articular) (current) (*see also* Sprain, by site)
    knee — *see* Tear, meniscus
    semilunar — *see* Tear, meniscus
  cecum (with peritonitis) 540.0
    with peritoneal abscess 540.1
    traumatic 863.89
      with open wound into cavity 863.99
  cerebral aneurysm (congenital) (*see also* Hemorrhage, subarachnoid) 430
    late effect — *see* Late effect(s) (of) cerebrovascular disease
  cervix (uteri)
    with
      abortion — *see* Abortion, by type, with damage to pelvic organs
      ectopic pregnancy (*see also* categories 633.0–633.9) 639.2
      molar pregnancy (*see also* categories 630–632) 639.2
    following
      abortion 639.2
      ectopic or molar pregnancy 639.2
    obstetrical trauma 665.3 ☑
    traumatic — *see* Injury, internal, cervix
  chordae tendineae 429.5
  choroid (direct) (indirect) (traumatic) 363.63
  circle of Willis (*see also* Hemorrhage, subarachnoid) 430
    late effect — *see* Late effect(s) (of) cerebrovascular disease
  colon 569.89
    traumatic — *see* Injury, internal, colon
  cornea (traumatic) (*see also* Rupture, eye)
    due to ulcer 370.00
  coronary (artery) (thrombotic) (*see also* Infarct, myocardium) 410.9 ☑
  corpus luteum (infected) (ovary) 620.1
  cyst — *see* Cyst
  cystic duct (*see also* Disease, gallbladder) 575.4
  Descemet's membrane 371.33
    traumatic — *see* Rupture, eye
  diaphragm (*see also* Hernia, diaphragm)
    traumatic — *see* Injury, internal, diaphragm
  diverticulum
    bladder 596.3
    intestine (large) (*see also* Diverticula) 562.10
      small 562.00
  duodenal stump 537.89
  duodenum (ulcer) — *see* Ulcer, duodenum, with perforation
  ear drum (*see also* Perforation, tympanum) 384.20
    with otitis media — *see* Otitis media
    traumatic — *see* Wound, open, ear
  esophagus 530.4
    traumatic 862.22
      with open wound into cavity 862.32
      cervical region — *see* Wound, open, esophagus
  eye (without prolapse of intraocular tissue) 871.0
    with
      exposure of intraocular tissue 871.1
      partial loss of intraocular tissue 871.2
      prolapse of intraocular tissue 871.1
    due to burn 940.5
  fallopian tube 620.8

Rupture, ruptured — *continued*
  fallopian tube — *continued*
    due to pregnancy — *see* Pregnancy, tubal
    traumatic — *see* Injury, internal, fallopian tube
  fontanel 767.3
  free wall (ventricle) (*see also* Infarct, myocardium) 410.9 ☑
  gallbladder or duct (*see also* Disease, gallbladder) 575.4
    traumatic — *see* Injury, internal, gallbladder
  gastric (*see also* Rupture, stomach) 537.89
    vessel 459.0
  globe (eye) (traumatic) — *see* Rupture, eye
  graafian follicle (hematoma) 620.0
  heart (auricle) (ventricle) (*see also* Infarct, myocardium) 410.9 ☑
    infectional 422.90
    traumatic — *see* Rupture, myocardium, traumatic
  hymen 623.8
  internal
    organ, traumatic (*see also* Injury, internal, by site)
      heart — *see* Rupture, myocardium, traumatic
      kidney — *see* Rupture, kidney
      liver — *see* Rupture, liver
      spleen — *see* Rupture, spleen, traumatic
    semilunar cartilage — *see* Tear, meniscus
  intervertebral disc — *see* Displacement, intervertebral disc
    traumatic (current) — *see* Dislocation, vertebra
  intestine 569.89
    traumatic — *see* Injury, internal, intestine
  intracranial, birth injury 767.0
  iris 364.76
    traumatic — *see* Rupture, eye
  joint capsule — *see* Sprain, by site
  kidney (traumatic) 866.03
    with open wound into cavity 866.13
    due to birth injury 767.8
    nontraumatic 593.89
  lacrimal apparatus (traumatic) 870.2
  lens (traumatic) 366.20
  ligament (*see also* Sprain, by site)
    with open wound — *see* Wound, open, by site
    old (*see also* Disorder, cartilage, articular) 718.0 ☑
  liver (traumatic) 864.04
    with open wound into cavity 864.14
    due to birth injury 767.8
    nontraumatic 573.8
  lymphatic (node) (vessel) 457.8
  marginal sinus (placental) (with hemorrhage) 641.2 ☑
    affecting fetus or newborn 762.1
  meaning hernia — *see* Hernia
  membrana tympani (*see also* Perforation, tympanum) 384.20
    with otitis media — *see* Otitis media
    traumatic — *see* Wound, open, ear
  membranes (spontaneous)
    artificial
      delayed delivery following 658.3 ☑
        affecting fetus or newborn 761.1
      fetus or newborn 761.1
    delayed delivery following 658.2 ☑
      affecting fetus or newborn 761.1
    premature (less than 24 hours prior to onset of labor) 658.1 ☑
      affecting fetus or newborn 761.1
      delayed delivery following 658.2 ☑
        affecting fetus or newborn 761.1
  meningeal artery (*see also* Hemorrhage, subarachnoid) 430
    late effect — *see* Late effect(s) (of) cerebrovascular disease
  meniscus (knee) (*see also* Tear, meniscus)

Rupture, ruptured — *continued*
  meniscus (*see also* Tear, meniscus) — *continued*
    old (*see also* Derangement, meniscus) 717.5
    site other than knee — *see* Disorder, cartilage, articular
    site other than knee — *see* Sprain, by site
  mesentery 568.89
    traumatic — *see* Injury, internal, mesentery
  mitral — *see* Insufficiency, mitral
  muscle (traumatic) NEC (*see also* Sprain, by site)
    with open wound — *see* Wound, open, by site
    nontraumatic 728.83
  musculotendinous cuff (nontraumatic) (shoulder) 840.4
  mycotic aneurysm, causing cerebral hemorrhage (*see also* Hemorrhage, subarachnoid) 430
    late effect — *see* Late effect(s) (of) cerebrovascular disease
  myocardium, myocardial (*see also* Infarct, myocardium) 410.9 ☑
    traumatic 861.03
      with open wound into thorax 861.13
  nontraumatic (meaning hernia) (*see also* Hernia, by site) 553.9
  obstructed (*see also* Hernia, by site, with obstruction) 552.9
    gangrenous (*see also* Hernia, by site, with gangrene) 551.9
  operation wound (*see also* Dehiscence) 998.32
    internal 998.31
  ovary, ovarian 620.8
    corpus luteum 620.1
    follicle (graafian) 620.0
  oviduct 620.8
    due to pregnancy — *see* Pregnancy, tubal
  pancreas 577.8
    traumatic — *see* Injury, internal, pancreas
  papillary muscle (ventricular) 429.6
  pelvic
    floor, complicating delivery 664.1 ☑
    organ NEC — *see* Injury, pelvic, organs
  penis (traumatic) — *see* Wound, open, penis
  perineum 624.8
    during delivery (*see also* Laceration, perineum, complicating delivery) 664.4 ☑
  pharynx (nontraumatic) (spontaneous) 478.29
  pregnant uterus (before onset of labor) 665.0 ☑
  prostate (traumatic) — *see* Injury, internal, prostate
  pulmonary
    artery 417.8
    valve (heart) (*see also* Endocarditis, pulmonary) 424.3
    vein 417.8
    vessel 417.8
  pupil, sphincter 364.75
  pus tube (*see also* Salpingo-oophoritis) 614.2
  pyosalpinx (*see also* Salpingo-oophoritis) 614.2
  rectum 569.49
    traumatic — *see* Injury, internal, rectum
  retina, retinal (traumatic) (without detachment) 361.30
    with detachment (*see also* Detachment, retina, with retinal defect) 361.00
  rotator cuff (capsule) (traumatic) 840.4
    nontraumatic (complete) 727.61
      partial 726.13
  sclera 871.0
  semilunar cartilage, knee (*see also* Tear, meniscus) 836.2

☑ Additional Digit Required — Refer to the Tabular List for Digit Selection   Subterms under main terms may continue to next column or page

2013 ICD-9-CM   ▶◀ Revised Text   ● New Line   ▲ Revised Code   Volume 2 — 251

Rumination — Rupture, ruptured

Rupture, ruptured — *continued*
    semilunar cartilage, knee (*see also* Tear,
        meniscus) — *continued*
        old (*see also* Derangement, meniscus)
            717.5
    septum (cardiac) 410.8 ☑
    sigmoid 569.89
        traumatic — *see* Injury, internal, colon,
            sigmoid
    sinus of Valsalva 747.29
    spinal cord (*see also* Injury, spinal, by site)
        due to injury at birth 767.4
        fetus or newborn 767.4
        syphilitic 094.89
        traumatic (*see also* Injury, spinal, by site)
           with fracture — *see* Fracture, verte-
               bra, by site, with spinal cord
               injury
    spleen 289.59
        congenital 767.8
        due to injury at birth 767.8
        malarial 084.9
        nontraumatic 289.59
        spontaneous 289.59
        traumatic 865.04
           with open wound into cavity 865.14
    splenic vein 459.0
    stomach 537.89
        due to injury at birth 767.8
        traumatic — *see* Injury, internal, stom-
            ach
        ulcer — *see* Ulcer, stomach, with perfo-
            ration
    synovium 727.50
        specified site NEC 727.59
    tendon (traumatic) (*see also* Sprain, by site)
        with open wound — *see* Wound, open,
            by site
        Achilles 845.09
           nontraumatic 727.67
        ankle 845.09
           nontraumatic 727.68
        biceps (long bead) 840.8
           nontraumatic 727.62
        foot 845.10
           interphalangeal (joint) 845.13

Rupture, ruptured — *continued*
    tendon (*see also* Sprain, by site) — *contin-*
      ued
        foot — *continued*
           metatarsophalangeal (joint) 845.12
           nontraumatic 727.68
           specified site NEC 845.19
           tarsometatarsal (joint) 845.11
        hand 842.10
           carpometacarpal (joint) 842.11
           interphalangeal (joint) 842.13
           metacarpophalangeal (joint) 842.12
           nontraumatic 727.63
               extensors 727.63
               flexors 727.64
           specified site NEC 842.19
        nontraumatic 727.60
           specified site NEC 727.69
        patellar 844.8
           nontraumatic 727.66
        quadriceps 844.8
           nontraumatic 727.65
        rotator cuff (capsule) 840.4
           nontraumatic (complete) 727.61
               partial 726.13
        wrist 842.00
           carpal (joint) 842.01
           nontraumatic 727.63
               extensors 727.63
               flexors 727.64
           radiocarpal (joint) (ligament) 842.02
           radioulnar (joint), distal 842.09
           specified site NEC 842.09
    testis (traumatic) 878.2
        complicated 878.3
        due to syphilis 095.8
    thoracic duct 457.8
    tonsil 474.8
    traumatic
        with open wound — *see* Wound, open,
            by site
        aorta — *see* Rupture, aorta, traumatic
        ear drum — *see* Wound, open, ear, drum
        external site — *see* Wound, open, by site
        eye 871.2
        globe (eye) — *see* Wound, open, eyeball

Rupture, ruptured — *continued*
    traumatic — *continued*
        internal organ (abdomen, chest, or
            pelvis) (*see also* Injury, internal,
            by site)
           heart — *see* Rupture, myocardium,
              traumatic
           kidney — *see* Rupture, kidney
           liver — *see* Rupture, liver
           spleen — *see* Rupture, spleen, trau-
              matic
        ligament, muscle, or tendon (*see also*
            Sprain, by site)
           with open wound — *see* Wound,
              open, by site
        meaning hernia — *see* Hernia
    tricuspid (heart) (valve) — *see* Endocarditis,
        tricuspid
    tube, tubal 620.8
        abscess (*see also* Salpingo-oophoritis)
           614.2
        due to pregnancy — *see* Pregnancy,
           tubal
    tympanum, tympanic (membrane) (*see also*
        Perforation, tympanum) 384.20
        with otitis media — *see* Otitis media
        traumatic — *see* Wound, open, ear,
           drum
    umbilical cord 663.8 ☑
        fetus or newborn 772.0
    ureter (traumatic) (*see also* Injury, internal,
        ureter) 867.2
        nontraumatic 593.89
    urethra 599.84
        with
           abortion — *see* Abortion, by type,
               with damage to pelvic organs
           ectopic pregnancy (*see also* cate-
               gories 633.0–633.9) 639.2
           molar pregnancy (*see also* categories
               630–632) 639.2
        following
           abortion 639.2
           ectopic or molar pregnancy 639.2
        obstetrical trauma 665.5 ☑
        traumatic — *see* Injury, internal urethra

Rupture, ruptured — *continued*
    uterosacral ligament 620.8
    uterus (traumatic) (*see also* Injury, internal
        uterus)
        affecting fetus or newborn 763.89
        during labor 665.1 ☑
        nonpuerperal, nontraumatic 621.8
        nontraumatic 621.8
        pregnant (during labor) 665.1 ☑
           before labor 665.0 ☑
    vagina 878.6
        complicated 878.7
        complicating delivery — *see* Laceration,
           vagina, complicating delivery
    valve, valvular (heart) — *see* Endocarditis
    varicose vein — *see* Varicose, vein
    varix — *see* Varix
    vena cava 459.0
    ventricle (free wall) (left) (*see also* Infarct,
        myocardium) 410.9 ☑
    vesical (urinary) 596.6
        traumatic — *see* Injury, internal, bladder
    vessel (blood) 459.0
        pulmonary 417.8
    viscus 799.89
    vulva 878.4
        complicated 878.5
        complicating delivery 664.0 ☑
Russell's dwarf (uterine dwarfism and cranio-
    facial dysostosis) 759.89
Russell's dysentery 004.8
Russell (-Silver) syndrome (congenital
    hemihypertrophy and short stature)
    759.89
Russian spring-summer type encephalitis
    063.0
Rust's disease (tuberculous spondylitis)
    015.0 ☑ *[720.81]*
Rustitskii's disease (multiple myeloma)
    (M9730/3) 203.0 ☑
Ruysch's disease (Hirschsprung's disease)
    751.3
Rytand-Lipsitch syndrome (complete atrioven-
    tricular block) 426.0

☑ Additional Digit Required — Refer to the Tabular List for Digit Selection   🔻 Subterms under main terms may continue to next column or page

252 — Volume 2   ▶◀ Revised Text   ● New Line   ▲ Revised Code   2013 ICD-9-CM

S

Saber
shin 090.5
tibia 090.5
Saccharomyces infection — *see also* Candidiasis 112.9
Saccharopinuria 270.7
Saccular — *see* condition
Sacculation
aorta (nonsyphilitic) (*see also* Aneurysm, aorta) 441.9
ruptured 441.5
syphilitic 093.0
bladder 596.3
colon 569.89
intralaryngeal (congenital) (ventricular) 748.3
larynx (congenital) (ventricular) 748.3
organ or site, congenital — *see* Distortion
pregnant uterus, complicating delivery 654.4 ☑
affecting fetus or newborn 763.1
causing obstructed labor 660.2 ☑
affecting fetus or newborn 763.1
rectosigmoid 569.89
sigmoid 569.89
ureter 593.89
urethra 599.2
vesical 596.3
Sachs (-Tay) disease (amaurotic familial idiocy) 330.1
Sacks-Libman disease 710.0 [424.91]
Sac, lacrimal — *see* condition
Sacralgia 724.6
Sacralization
fifth lumbar vertebra 756.15
incomplete (vertebra) 756.15
Sacrodynia 724.6
NULL
Sacroiliac joint — *see* condition
Sacroiliitis NEC 720.2
Sacrum — *see* condition
Saddle
back 737.8
embolus
abdominal aorta 444.01
pulmonary artery 415.13
injury — code to condition
nose 738.0
congenital 754.0
due to syphilis 090.5
Sadism (sexual) 302.84
Saemisch's ulcer 370.04
Saenger's syndrome 379.46
Sago spleen 277.39
Sailors' skin 692.74
Saint
Anthony's fire (*see also* Erysipelas) 035
Guy's dance — *see* Chorea
Louis-type encephalitis 062.3
triad (*see also* Hernia, diaphragm) 553.3
Vitus' dance — *see* Chorea
Salicylism
correct substance properly administered 535.4 ☑
overdose or wrong substance given or taken 965.1
Salivary duct or gland — *see also* condition
virus disease 078.5
Salivation (excessive) — *see also* Ptyalism 527.7
Salmonella (aertrycke) (choleraesuis) (enteritidis) (gallinarum) (suipestifer) (typhimurium) — *see also* Infection, Salmonella 003.9
arthritis 003.23
carrier (suspected) of V02.3
meningitis 003.21
osteomyelitis 003.24
pneumonia 003.22
septicemia 003.1
typhosa 002.0
carrier (suspected) of V02.1
Salmonellosis 003.0
with pneumonia 003.22

Salpingitis (catarrhal) (fallopian tube) (nodular) (pseudofollicular) (purulent) (septic) — *see also* Salpingo-oophoritis 614.2
ear 381.50
acute 381.51
chronic 381.52
Eustachian (tube) 381.50
acute 381.51
chronic 381.52
follicularis 614.1
gonococcal (chronic) 098.37
acute 098.17
interstitial, chronic 614.1
isthmica nodosa 614.1
old — *see* Salpingo-oophoritis, chronic
puerperal, postpartum, childbirth 670.8 ☑
specific (chronic) 098.37
acute 098.17
tuberculous (acute) (chronic) (*see also* Tuberculosis) 016.6 ☑
venereal (chronic) 098.37
acute 098.17
Salpingocele 620.4
Salpingo-oophoritis (catarrhal) (purulent) (ruptured) (septic) (suppurative) 614.2
acute 614.0
with
abortion — *see* Abortion, by type, with sepsis
ectopic pregnancy (*see also* categories 633.0–633.9) 639.0
molar pregnancy (*see also* categories 630–632) 639.0
following
abortion 639.0
ectopic or molar pregnancy 639.0
gonococcal 098.17
puerperal, postpartum, childbirth 670.8 ☑
tuberculous (*see also* Tuberculosis) 016.6 ☑
chronic 614.1
gonococcal 098.37
tuberculous (see also Tuberculosis) 016.6 ☑
complicating pregnancy 646.6 ☑
affecting fetus or newborn 760.8
gonococcal (chronic) 098.37
acute 098.17
old — *see* Salpingo-oophoritis, chronic
puerperal 670.8 ☑
specific — *see* Salpingo-oophoritis, gonococcal
subacute (*see also* Salpingo-oophoritis, acute) 614.0
tuberculous (acute) (chronic) (*see also* Tuberculosis) 016.6 ☑
venereal — *see* Salpingo-oophoritis, gonococcal
Salpingo-ovaritis — *see also* Salpingo-oophoritis 614.2
Salpingoperitonitis — *see also* Salpingo-oophoritis 614.2
Salt-losing
nephritis (*see also* Disease, renal) 593.9
syndrome (*see also* Disease, renal) 593.9
Salt-rheum — *see also* Eczema 692.9
Salzmann's nodular dystrophy 371.46
Sampling
chorionic villus V28.89
Sampson's cyst or tumor 617.1
Sandblasters'
asthma 502
lung 502
Sander's disease (paranoia) 297.1
Sandfly fever 066.0
Sandhoff's disease 330.1
Sanfilippo's syndrome (mucopolysaccharidosis III) 277.5
Sanger-Brown's ataxia 334.2
San Joaquin Valley fever 114.0
Sao Paulo fever or typhus 082.0
Saponification, mesenteric 567.89
Sapremia — *see* Septicemia
Sarcocele (benign)
syphilitic 095.8

Sarcocele — *continued*
syphilitic — *continued*
congenital 090.5
Sarcoepiplocele — *see also* Hernia 553.9
Sarcoepiplomphalocele — *see also* Hernia, umbilicus 553.1
Sarcoid (any site) 135
with lung involvement 135 [517.8]
Boeck's 135
Darier-Roussy 135
Spiegler-Fendt 686.8
Sarcoidosis 135
cardiac 135 [425.8]
lung 135 [517.8]
Sarcoma (M8800/3) — *see also* Neoplasm, connective tissue, malignant
alveolar soft part (M9581/3) — *see* Neoplasm, connective tissue, malignant
ameloblastic (M9330/3) 170.1
upper jaw (bone) 170.0
botryoid (M8910/3) — *see* Neoplasm, connective tissue, malignant
botryoides (M8910/3) — *see* Neoplasm, connective tissue, malignant
cerebellar (M9480/3) 191.6
circumscribed (arachnoidal) (M9471/3) 191.6
circumscribed (arachnoidal) cerebellar (M9471/3) 191.6
clear cell, of tendons and aponeuroses (M9044/3) — *see* Neoplasm, connective tissue, malignant
embryonal (M8991/3) — *see* Neoplasm, connective tissue, malignant
endometrial (stromal) (M8930/3) 182.0
isthmus 182.1
endothelial (M9130/3) (*see also* Neoplasm, connective tissue, malignant)
bone (M9260/3) — *see* Neoplasm, bone, malignant
epithelioid cell (M8804/3) — *see* Neoplasm, connective tissue, malignant
Ewing's (M9260/3) — *see* Neoplasm, bone, malignant
follicular dendritic cell 202.9 ☑
germinoblastic (diffuse) (M9632/3) 202.8 ☑
follicular (M9697/3) 202.0 ☑
giant cell (M8802/3) (*see also* Neoplasm, connective tissue, malignant)
bone (M9250/3) — *see* Neoplasm, bone, malignant
glomoid (M8710/3) — *see* Neoplasm, connective tissue, malignant
granulocytic (M9930/3) 205.3 ☑
hemangioendothelial (M9130/3) — *see* Neoplasm, connective tissue, malignant
hemorrhagic, multiple (M9140/3) — *see* Kaposi's, sarcoma
Hodgkin's (M9662/3) 201.2 ☑
immunoblastic (M9612/3) 200.8 ☑
interdigitating dendritic cell 202.9 ☑
Kaposi's (M9140/3) — *see* Kaposi's, sarcoma
Kupffer cell (M9124/3) 155.0
Langerhans cell 202.9 ☑
leptomeningeal (M9530/3) — *see* Neoplasm, meninges, malignant
lymphangioendothelial (M9170/3) — *see* Neoplasm, connective tissue, malignant
lymphoblastic (M9630/3) 200.1 ☑
lymphocytic (M9620/3) 200.1 ☑
mast cell (M9740/3) 202.6 ☑
melanotic (M8720/3) — *see* Melanoma
meningeal (M9530/3) — *see* Neoplasm, meninges, malignant
meningothelial (M9530/3) — *see* Neoplasm, meninges, malignant
mesenchymal (M8800/3) (*see also* Neoplasm, connective tissue, malignant)
mixed (M8990/3) — *see* Neoplasm, connective tissue, malignant
mesothelial (M9050/3) — *see* Neoplasm, by site, malignant

Sarcoma — *see also* Neoplasm, connective tissue, malignant — *continued*
monstrocellular (M9481/3)
specified site — *see* Neoplasm, by site, malignant
unspecified site 191.9
myeloid (M9930/3) 205.3 ☑
neurogenic (M9540/3) — *see* Neoplasm, connective tissue, malignant
odontogenic (M9270/3) 170.1
upper jaw (bone) 170.0
osteoblastic (M9180/3) — *see* Neoplasm, bone, malignant
osteogenic (M9180/3) (*see also* Neoplasm, bone, malignant)
juxtacortical (M9190/3) — *see* Neoplasm, bone, malignant
periosteal (M9190/3) — *see* Neoplasm, bone, malignant
periosteal (M8812/3) (*see also* Neoplasm, bone, malignant)
osteogenic (M9190/3) — *see* Neoplasm, bone, malignant
plasma cell (M9731/3) 203.8 ☑
pleomorphic cell (M8802/3) — *see* Neoplasm, connective tissue, malignant
reticuloendothelial (M9720/3) 202.3 ☑
reticulum cell (M9640/3) 200.0 ☑
nodular (M9642/3) 200.0 ☑
pleomorphic cell type (M9641/3) 200.0 ☑
round cell (M8803/3) — *see* Neoplasm, connective tissue, malignant
small cell (M8803/3) — *see* Neoplasm, connective tissue, malignant
spindle cell (M8801/3) — *see* Neoplasm, connective tissue, malignant
stromal (endometrial) (M8930/3) 182.0
isthmus 182.1
synovial (M9040/3) (*see also* Neoplasm, connective tissue, malignant)
biphasic type (M9043/3) — *see* Neoplasm, connective tissue, malignant
epithelioid cell type (M9042/3) — *see* Neoplasm, connective tissue, malignant
spindle cell type (M9041/3) — *see* Neoplasm, connective tissue, malignant
Sarcomatosis
meningeal (M9539/3) — *see* Neoplasm, meninges, malignant
specified site NEC (M8800/3) — *see* Neoplasm, connective tissue, malignant
unspecified site (M8800/6) 171.9
Sarcosinemia 270.8
Sarcosporidiosis 136.5
Satiety, early 780.94
Satisfactory smear but lacking transformation zone
anal 796.77
cervical 795.07
Saturnine — *see* condition
Saturnism 984.9
specified type of lead — *see* Table of Drugs and Chemicals
Satyriasis 302.89
Sauriasis — *see* Ichthyosis
Sauriderma 757.39
Sauriosis — *see* Ichthyosis
Savill's disease (epidemic exfoliative dermatitis) 695.89
SBE (subacute bacterial endocarditis) 421.0
Scabies (any site) 133.0
Scabs 782.8
Scaglietti-Dagnini syndrome (acromegalic macrospondylitis) 253.0
Scald, scalded — *see also* Burn, by site
skin syndrome 695.81
Scalenus anticus (anterior) syndrome 353.0
Scales 782.8
Scalp — *see* condition
Scaphocephaly 756.0
Scaphoiditis, tarsal 732.5
Scapulalgia 733.90

☑ **Additional Digit Required** — Refer to the Tabular List for Digit Selection

⬮ **Subterms under main terms may continue to next column or page**

Scapulohumeral myopathy 359.1
Scarabiasis 134.1
Scarlatina 034.1
  anginosa 034.1
  maligna 034.1
  myocarditis, acute 034.1 *[422.0]*
    old (*see also* Myocarditis) 429.0
  otitis media 034.1 *[382.02]*
  ulcerosa 034.1
Scarlatinella 057.8
Scarlet fever (albuminuria) (angina) (convulsions) (lesions of lid) (rash) 034.1
Scar, scarring — *see also* Cicatrix 709.2
  adherent 709.2
  atrophic 709.2
  cervix
    in pregnancy or childbirth 654.6 ☑
      affecting fetus or newborn 763.89
      causing obstructed labor 660.2 ☑
        affecting fetus or newborn 763.1
  cheloid 701.4
  chorioretinal 363.30
    disseminated 363.35
    macular 363.32
    peripheral 363.34
    posterior pole NEC 363.33
  choroid (*see also* Scar, chorioretinal) 363.30
  compression, pericardial 423.9
  congenital 757.39
  conjunctiva 372.64
  cornea 371.00
    xerophthalmic 264.6
  due to previous cesarean delivery, complicating pregnancy or childbirth 654.2 ☑
    affecting fetus or newborn 763.89
  duodenal (bulb) (cap) 537.3
  hypertrophic 701.4
  keloid 701.4
  labia 624.4
  lung (base) 518.89
  macula 363.32
    disseminated 363.35
    peripheral 363.34
  muscle 728.89
  myocardium, myocardial 412
  painful 709.2
  papillary muscle 429.81
  posterior pole NEC 363.33
    macular — *see* Scar, macula
  postnecrotic (hepatic) (liver) 571.9
  psychic V15.49
  retina (*see also* Scar, chorioretinal) 363.30
  trachea 478.9
  uterus 621.8
    in pregnancy or childbirth NEC 654.9 ☑
      affecting fetus or newborn 763.89
      due to previous cesarean delivery 654.2 ☑
  vulva 624.4
Schamberg's disease, dermatitis, or dermatosis (progressive pigmentary dermatosis) 709.09
Schatzki's ring (esophagus) (lower) (congenital) 750.3
  acquired 530.3
Schaufenster krankheit 413.9
Schaumann's
  benign lymphogranulomatosis 135
  disease (sarcoidosis) 135
  syndrome (sarcoidosis) 135
Scheie's syndrome (mucopolysaccharidosis IS) 277.5
Schenck's disease (sporotrichosis) 117.1
Scheuermann's disease or osteochondrosis 732.0
Scheuthauer-Marie-Sainton syndrome (cleidocranialis dysostosis) 755.59
Schilder (-Flatau) disease 341.1
Schilling-type monocytic leukemia (M9890/3) 206.9 ☑
Schimmelbusch's disease, cystic mastitis, or hyperplasia 610.1
Schirmer's syndrome (encephalocutaneous angiomatosis) 759.6
Schistocelia 756.79

Schistoglossia 750.13
Schistosoma infestation — *see* Infestation, Schistosoma
Schistosomiasis 120.9
  Asiatic 120.2
  bladder 120.0
  chestermani 120.8
  colon 120.1
  cutaneous 120.3
  due to
    S. hematobium 120.0
    S. japonicum 120.2
    S. mansoni 120.1
    S. mattheii 120.8
  eastern 120.2
  genitourinary tract 120.0
  intestinal 120.1
  lung 120.2
  Manson's (intestinal) 120.1
  Oriental 120.2
  pulmonary 120.2
  specified type NEC 120.8
  vesical 120.0
Schizencephaly 742.4
Schizo-affective psychosis — *see also* Schizophrenia 295.7 ☑
Schizodontia 520.2
Schizoid personality 301.20
  introverted 301.21
  schizotypal 301.22
Schizophrenia, schizophrenic (reaction) 295.9 ☑

Note — *Use the following fifth-digit subclassification with category 295:*

0   unspecified

1   subchronic

2   chronic

3   subchronic with acute exacerbation

4   chronic with acute exacerbation

5   in remission

  acute (attack) NEC 295.8 ☑
    episode 295.4 ☑
  atypical form 295.8 ☑
  borderline 295.5 ☑
  catalepsy 295.2 ☑
  catatonic (type) (acute) (excited) (withdrawn) 295.2 ☑
  childhood (type) (*see also* Psychosis, childhood) 299.9 ☑
  chronic NEC 295.6 ☑
  coenesthesiopathic 295.8 ☑
  cyclic (type) 295.7 ☑
  disorganized (type) 295.1 ☑
  flexibilitas cerea 295.2 ☑
  hebephrenic (type) (acute) 295.1 ☑
  incipient 295.5 ☑
  latent 295.5 ☑
  paranoid (type) (acute) 295.3 ☑
  paraphrenic (acute) 295.3 ☑
  prepsychotic 295.5 ☑
  primary (acute) 295.0 ☑
  prodromal 295.5 ☑
  pseudoneurotic 295.5 ☑
  pseudopsychopathic 295.5 ☑
  reaction 295.9 ☑
  residual type (state) 295.6 ☑
  restzustand 295.6 ☑
  schizo-affective (type) (depressed) (excited) 295.7 ☑
  schizophreniform type 295.4 ☑
  simple (type) (acute) 295.0 ☑
  simplex (acute) 295.0 ☑
  specified type NEC 295.8 ☑
  syndrome of childhood NEC (*see also* Psychosis, childhood) 299.9 ☑
  undifferentiated type 295.9 ☑
    acute 295.8 ☑
    chronic 295.6 ☑
Schizothymia 301.20
  introverted 301.21

Schizothymia — *continued*
  schizotypal 301.22
Schlafkrankheit 086.5
Schlatter-Osgood disease (osteochondrosis, tibial tubercle) 732.4
Schlatter's tibia (osteochondrosis) 732.4
Schloffer's tumor — *see also* Peritonitis 567.29
Schmidt's syndrome
  sphallo-pharyngo-laryngeal hemiplegia 352.6
  thyroid-adrenocortical insufficiency 258.1
  vagoaccessory 352.6
Schmincke
  carcinoma (M8082/3) — *see* Neoplasm, nasopharynx, malignant
  tumor (M8082/3) — *see* Neoplasm, nasopharynx, malignant
Schmitz (-Stutzer) dysentery 004.0
Schmorl's disease or nodes 722.30
  lumbar, lumbosacral 722.32
  specified region NEC 722.39
  thoracic, thoracolumbar 722.31
Schneiderian
  carcinoma (M8121/3)
    specified site — *see* Neoplasm, by site, malignant
    unspecified site 160.0
  papilloma (M8121/0)
    specified site — *see* Neoplasm, by site, benign
    unspecified site 212.0
Schneider's syndrome 047.9
Schnitzler syndrome 273.1
Schoffer's tumor — *see also* Peritonitis 567.29
Scholte's syndrome (malignant carcinoid) 259.2
Scholz's disease 330.0
Scholz (-Bielschowsky-Henneberg) syndrome 330.0
Schönlein (-Henoch) disease (primary) (purpura) (rheumatic) 287.0
School examination V70.3
  following surgery V67.09
Schottmüller's disease — *see also* Fever, paratyphoid 002.9
Schroeder's syndrome (endocrine-hypertensive) 255.3
Schüller-Christian disease or syndrome (chronic histiocytosis X) 277.89
Schultz's disease or syndrome (agranulocytosis) 288.09
Schultze's acroparesthesia, simple 443.89
Schwalbe-Ziehen-Oppenheimer disease 333.6
Schwannoma (M9560/0) — *see also* Neoplasm, connective tissue, benign
  malignant (M9560/3) — *see* Neoplasm, connective tissue, malignant
Schwannomatosis 237.73
Schwartz-Bartter syndrome (inappropriate secretion of antidiuretic hormone) 253.6
Schwartz (-Jampel) syndrome 359.23
Schweninger-Buzzi disease (macular atrophy) 701.3
Sciatic — *see* condition
Sciatica (infectional) 724.3
  due to
    displacement of intervertebral disc 722.10
    herniation, nucleus pulposus 722.10
  wallet 724.3
Scimitar syndrome (anomalous venous drainage, right lung to inferior vena cava) 747.49
Sclera — *see* condition
Sclerectasia 379.11
Scleredema
  adultorum 710.1
  Buschke's 710.1
  newborn 778.1
Sclerema
  adiposum (newborn) 778.1
  adultorum 710.1
  edematosum (newborn) 778.1
  neonatorum 778.1
  newborn 778.1

Scleriasis — *see* Scleroderma
Scleritis 379.00
  with corneal involvement 379.05
  anterior (annular) (localized) 379.03
  brawny 379.06
  granulomatous 379.09
  posterior 379.07
  specified NEC 379.09
  suppurative 379.09
  syphilitic 095.0
  tuberculous (nodular) (*see also* Tuberculosis) 017.3 ☑ *[379.09]*
Sclerochoroiditis — *see also* Scleritis 379.00
Scleroconjunctivitis — *see also* Scleritis 379.00
Sclerocystic ovary (syndrome) 256.4
Sclerodactylia 701.0
Scleroderma, sclerodermia (acrosclerotic) (diffuse) (generalized) (progressive) (pulmonary) 710.1
  circumscribed 701.0
  linear 701.0
  localized (linear) 701.0
  newborn 778.1
Sclerokeratitis 379.05
  meaning sclerosing keratitis 370.54
  tuberculous (*see also* Tuberculosis) 017.3 ☑ *[379.09]*
Scleromalacia
  multiple 731.0
  perforans 379.04
Scleroma, trachea 040.1
Scleromyxedema 701.8
Scleroperikeratitis 379.05
Sclerose en plaques 340
Sclerosis, sclerotic
  adrenal (gland) 255.8
  Alzheimer's 331.0
    with dementia — *see* Alzheimer's, dementia
  amyotrophic (lateral) 335.20
  annularis fibrosi
    aortic 424.1
    mitral 424.0
  aorta, aortic 440.0
    valve (*see also* Endocarditis, aortic) 424.1
  artery, arterial, arteriolar, arteriovascular — *see* Arteriosclerosis
  ascending multiple 340
  Baló's (concentric) 341.1
  basilar — *see* Sclerosis, brain
  bone (localized) NEC 733.99
  brain (general) (lobular) 348.89
    Alzheimer's — *see* Alzheimer's, dementia
    artery, arterial 437.0
    atrophic lobar 331.0
      with dementia
        with behavioral disturbance 331.0 *[294.11]*
        without behavioral disturbance 331.0 *[294.10]*
    diffuse 341.1
      familial (chronic) (infantile) 330.0
      infantile (chronic) (familial) 330.0
      Pelizaeus-Merzbacher type 330.0
    disseminated 340
    hereditary 334.2
    hippocampal 348.81
    infantile (degenerative) (diffuse) 330.0
    insular 340
    Krabbe's 330.0
    mesial temporal 348.81
    miliary 340
    multiple 340
    Pelizaeus-Merzbacher 330.0
    progressive familial 330.0
    senile 437.0
    temporal 348.81
      mesial 348.81
    tuberous 759.5
  bulbar, progressive 340
  bundle of His 426.50
    left 426.3
    right 426.4
  cardiac — *see* Arteriosclerosis, coronary

Sclerosis, sclerotic — *continued*
cardiorenal (*see also* Hypertension, cardiorenal) 404.90
cardiovascular (*see also* Disease, cardiovascular) 429.2
renal (*see also* Hypertension, cardiorenal) 404.90
centrolobar, familial 330.0
cerebellar — *see* Sclerosis, brain
cerebral — *see* Sclerosis, brain
cerebrospinal 340
disseminated 340
multiple 340
cerebrovascular 437.0
choroid 363.40
diffuse 363.56
combined (spinal cord) (*see also* Degeneration, combined)
multiple 340
concentric, Baló's 341.1
cornea 370.54
coronary (artery) — *see* Arteriosclerosis, coronary
corpus cavernosum
female 624.8
male 607.89
Dewitzky's
aortic 424.1
mitral 424.0
diffuse NEC 341.1
disease, heart — *see* Arteriosclerosis, coronary
disseminated 340
dorsal 340
dorsolateral (spinal cord) — *see* Degeneration, combined
endometrium 621.8
extrapyramidal 333.90
eye, nuclear (senile) 366.16
Friedreich's (spinal cord) 334.0
funicular (spermatic cord) 608.89
gastritis 535.4 ☑
general (vascular) — *see* Arteriosclerosis
gland (lymphatic) 457.8
hepatic 571.9
hereditary
cerebellar 334.2
spinal 334.0
hippocampal 348.81
idiopathic cortical (Garré's) (*see also* Osteomyelitis) 730.1 ☑
ilium, piriform 733.5
insular 340
pancreas 251.8
Islands of Langerhans 251.8
kidney — *see* Sclerosis, renal
larynx 478.79
lateral 335.24
amyotrophic 335.20
descending 335.24
primary 335.24
spinal 335.24
liver 571.9
lobar, atrophic (of brain) 331.0
with dementia
with behavioral disturbance 331.0 [294.11]
without behavioral disturbance 331.0 [294.10]
lung (*see also* Fibrosis, lung) 515
mastoid 383.1
mesial temporal 348.81
mitral — *see* Endocarditis, mitral
Mönckeberg's (medial) (*see also* Arteriosclerosis, extremities) 440.20
multiple (brain stem) (cerebral) (generalized) (spinal cord) 340
myocardium, myocardial — *see* Arteriosclerosis, coronary
nuclear (senile), eye 366.16
ovary 620.8
pancreas 577.8
penis 607.89
peripheral arteries (*see also* Arteriosclerosis, extremities) 440.20
plaques 340

Sclerosis, sclerotic — *continued*
pluriglandular 258.8
polyglandular 258.8
posterior (spinal cord) (syphilitic) 094.0
posterolateral (spinal cord) — *see* Degeneration, combined
prepuce 607.89
primary lateral 335.24
progressive systemic 710.1
pulmonary (*see also* Fibrosis, lung) 515
artery 416.0
valve (heart) (*see also* Endocarditis, pulmonary) 424.3
renal 587
with
cystine storage disease 270.0
hypertension (*see also* Hypertension, kidney) 403.90
hypertensive heart disease (conditions classifiable to 402) (*see also* Hypertension, cardiorenal) 404.90
arteriolar (hyaline) (*see also* Hypertension, kidney) 403.90
hyperplastic (*see also* Hypertension, kidney) 403.90
retina (senile) (vascular) 362.17
rheumatic
aortic valve 395.9
mitral valve 394.9
Schilder's 341.1
senile — *see* Arteriosclerosis
spinal (cord) (general) (progressive) (transverse) 336.8
ascending 357.0
combined (*see also* Degeneration, combined)
multiple 340
syphilitic 094.89
disseminated 340
dorsolateral — *see* Degeneration, combined
hereditary (Friedreich's) (mixed form) 334.0
lateral (amyotrophic) 335.24
multiple 340
posterior (syphilitic) 094.0
stomach 537.89
subendocardial, congenital 425.3
systemic (progressive) 710.1
with lung involvement 710.1 [517.2]
temporal 348.81
mesial 348.81
tricuspid (heart) (valve) — *see* Endocarditis, tricuspid
tuberous (brain) 759.5
tympanic membrane (*see also* Tympanosclerosis) 385.00
valve, valvular (heart) — *see* Endocarditis
vascular — *see* Arteriosclerosis
vein 459.89
Sclerotenonitis 379.07
Sclerotitis — *see also* Scleritis 379.00
syphilitic 095.0
tuberculous (*see also* Tuberculosis) 017.3 ☑ [379.09]
Scoliosis (acquired) (postural) 737.30
congenital 754.2
due to or associated with
Charcôt-Marie-Tooth disease 356.1 [737.43]
mucopolysaccharidosis 277.5 [737.43]
neurofibromatosis 237.71 [737.43]
osteitis
deformans 731.0 [737.43]
fibrosa cystica 252.01 [737.43]
osteoporosis (*see also* Osteoporosis) 733.00 [737.43]
poliomyelitis 138 [737.43]
radiation 737.33
tuberculosis (*see also* Tuberculosis) 015.0 ☑ [737.43]
idiopathic 737.30
infantile
progressive 737.32
resolving 737.31

Scoliosis — *continued*
paralytic 737.39
rachitic 268.1
sciatic 724.3
specified NEC 737.39
thoracogenic 737.34
tuberculous (*see also* Tuberculosis) 015.0 ☑ [737.43]
Scoliotic pelvis 738.6
with disproportion (fetopelvic) 653.0 ☑
affecting fetus or newborn 763.1
causing obstructed labor 660.1 ☑
affecting fetus or newborn 763.1
Scorbutus, scorbutic 267
anemia 281.8
Scotoma (ring) 368.44
arcuate 368.43
Bjerrum 368.43
blind spot area 368.42
central 368.41
centrocecal 368.41
paracecal 368.42
paracentral 368.41
scintillating 368.12
Seidel 368.43
Scratch — *see* Injury, superficial, by site
Scratchy throat 784.99
Screening (for) V82.9
alcoholism V79.1
anemia, deficiency NEC V78.1
iron V78.0
anomaly, congenital V82.89
antenatal, of mother V28.9
alphafetoprotein levels, raised V28.1
based on amniocentesis V28.2
chromosomal anomalies V28.0
raised alphafetoprotein levels V28.1
fetal growth retardation using ultrasonics V28.4
ultrasonics V28.4
genomic V28.89
isoimmunization V28.5
malformations using ultrasonics V28.3
proteomic V28.89
raised alphafetoprotein levels V28.1
risk
pre-term labor V28.82
specified condition NEC V28.89
Streptococcus B V28.6
arterial hypertension V81.1
arthropod-borne viral disease NEC V73.5
asymptomatic bacteriuria V81.5
bacterial
and spirochetal sexually transmitted diseases V74.5
conjunctivitis V74.4
disease V74.9
sexually transmitted V74.5
specified condition NEC V74.8
bacteriuria, asymptomatic V81.5
blood disorder NEC V78.9
specified type NEC V78.8
bronchitis, chronic V81.3
brucellosis V74.8
cancer — *see* Screening, malignant neoplasm
cardiovascular disease NEC V81.2
cataract V80.2
Chagas' disease V75.3
chemical poisoning V82.5
cholera V74.0
cholesterol level V77.91
chromosomal
anomalies
by amniocentesis, antenatal V28.0
maternal postnatal V82.4
athletes V70.3
colonoscopy V76.51
condition
cardiovascular NEC V81.2
eye NEC V80.2
genitourinary NEC V81.6
neurological NEC V80.09
respiratory NEC V81.4
skin V82.0
specified NEC V82.89

Screening — *continued*
congenital
anomaly V82.89
eye V80.2
dislocation of hip V82.3
eye condition or disease V80.2
conjunctivitis, bacterial V74.4
contamination NEC (*see also* Poisoning) V82.5
coronary artery disease V81.0
cystic fibrosis V77.6
deficiency anemia NEC V78.1
iron V78.0
dengue fever V73.5
depression V79.0
developmental handicap V79.9
in early childhood V79.3
specified type NEC V79.8
diabetes mellitus V77.1
diphtheria V74.3
disease or disorder V82.9
bacterial V74.9
specified NEC V74.8
blood V78.9
specified type NEC V78.8
blood-forming organ V78.9
specified type NEC V78.8
cardiovascular NEC V81.2
hypertensive V81.1
ischemic V81.0
Chagas' V75.3
chlamydial V73.98
specified NEC V73.88
ear NEC V80.3
endocrine NEC V77.99
eye NEC V80.2
genitourinary NEC V81.6
heart NEC V81.2
hypertensive V81.1
ischemic V81.0
HPV (human papillomavirus) V73.81
human papillomavirus V73.81
immunity NEC V77.99
infectious NEC V75.9
lipoid NEC V77.91
mental V79.9
specified type NEC V79.8
metabolic NEC V77.99
inborn NEC V77.7
neurological NEC V80.09
nutritional NEC V77.99
rheumatic NEC V82.2
rickettsial V75.0
sexually transmitted V74.5
bacterial V74.5
spirochetal V74.5
sickle-cell V78.2
trait V78.2
specified type NEC V82.89
thyroid V77.0
vascular NEC V81.2
ischemic V81.0
venereal V74.5
viral V73.99
arthropod-borne NEC V73.5
specified type NEC V73.89
dislocation of hip, congenital V82.3
drugs in athletes V70.3
elevated titer V82.9
emphysema (chronic) V81.3
encephalitis, viral (mosquito or tick borne) V73.5
endocrine disorder NEC V77.99
eye disorder NEC V80.2
congenital V80.2
fever
dengue V73.5
hemorrhagic V73.5
yellow V73.4
filariasis V75.6
galactosemia V77.4
genetic V82.79
disease carrier status V82.71
genitourinary condition NEC V81.6
glaucoma V80.1
gonorrhea V74.5

☑ **Additional Digit Required** — Refer to the Tabular List for Digit Selection   ⱽ **Subterms under main terms may continue to next column or page**

Screening — *continued*
- gout V77.5
- Hansen's disease V74.2
- heart disease NEC V81.2
  - hypertensive V81.1
  - ischemic V81.0
- heavy metal poisoning V82.5
- helminthiasis, intestinal V75.7
- hematopoietic malignancy V76.89
- hemoglobinopathies NEC V78.3
- hemorrhagic fever V73.5
- Hodgkin's disease V76.89
- hormones in athletes V70.3
- HPV (human papillomavirus) V73.81
- human papillomavirus (HPV) V73.81
- hypercholesterolemia V77.91
- hyperlipidemia V77.91
- hypertension V81.1
- immunity disorder NEC V77.99
- inborn errors of metabolism NEC V77.7
- infection
  - bacterial V74.9
    - specified type NEC V74.8
  - mycotic V75.4
  - parasitic NEC V75.8
- infectious disease V75.9
  - specified type NEC V75.8
- ingestion of radioactive substance V82.5
- intellectual disabilities V79.2
- intestinal helminthiasis V75.7
- iron deficiency anemia V78.0
- ischemic heart disease V81.0
- lead poisoning V82.5
- leishmaniasis V75.2
- leprosy V74.2
- leptospirosis V74.8
- leukemia V76.89
- lipoid disorder NEC V77.91
- lymphoma V76.89
- malaria V75.1
- malignant neoplasm (of) V76.9
  - bladder V76.3
  - blood V76.89
  - breast V76.10
    - mammogram NEC V76.12
      - for high-risk patient V76.11
    - specified type NEC V76.19
  - cervix V76.2
  - colon V76.51
  - colorectal V76.51
  - hematopoietic system V76.89
  - intestine V76.50
    - colon V76.51
    - small V76.52
  - lung V76.0
  - lymph (glands) V76.89
  - nervous system V76.81
  - oral cavity V76.42
  - other specified neoplasm NEC V76.89
  - ovary V76.46
  - prostate V76.44
  - rectum V76.41
  - respiratory organs V76.0
  - skin V76.43
  - specified sites NEC V76.49
  - testis V76.45
  - vagina V76.47
    - following hysterectomy for malignant condition V67.01
- malnutrition V77.2
- mammogram NEC V76.12
  - for high-risk patient V76.11
- maternal postnatal chromosomal anomalies V82.4
- measles V73.2
- mental
  - disorder V79.9
    - specified type NEC V79.8
  - retardation — *see* Screening, intellectual disabilities
- metabolic disorder NEC V77.99
- metabolic errors, inborn V77.7
- mucoviscidosis V77.6
- multiphasic V82.6
- mycosis V75.4
- mycotic infection V75.4

Screening — *continued*
- nephropathy V81.5
- neurological condition NEC V80.09
- nutritional disorder V77.99
- obesity V77.8
- osteoporosis V82.81
- parasitic infection NEC V75.8
- phenylketonuria V77.3
- plague V74.8
- poisoning
  - chemical NEC V82.5
    - contaminated water supply V82.5
      - heavy metal V82.5
- poliomyelitis V73.0
- postnatal chromosomal anomalies, maternal V82.4
- prenatal — *see* Screening, antenatal
- pulmonary tuberculosis V74.1
- radiation exposure V82.5
- renal disease V81.5
- respiratory condition NEC V81.4
- rheumatic disorder NEC V82.2
- rheumatoid arthritis V82.1
- rickettsial disease V75.0
- rubella V73.3
- schistosomiasis V75.5
- senile macular lesions of eye V80.2
- sexually transmitted diseases V74.5
  - bacterial V74.5
  - spirochetal V74.5
- sickle-cell anemia, disease, or trait V78.2
- skin condition V82.0
- sleeping sickness V75.3
- smallpox V73.1
- special V82.9
  - specified condition NEC V82.89
- specified type NEC V82.89
- spirochetal disease V74.9
  - sexually transmitted V74.5
  - specified type NEC V74.8
- stimulants in athletes V70.3
- syphilis V74.5
- tetanus V74.8
- thyroid disorder V77.0
- trachoma V73.6
- traumatic brain injury V80.01
- trypanosomiasis V75.3
- tuberculosis, pulmonary V74.1
- venereal disease V74.5
- viral encephalitis
  - mosquito-borne V73.5
  - tick-borne V73.5
- whooping cough V74.8
- worms, intestinal V75.7
- yaws V74.6
- yellow fever V73.4

Scrofula — *see also* Tuberculosis 017.2 ☑
Scrofulide (primary) — *see also* Tuberculosis 017.0 ☑
Scrofuloderma, scrofulodermia (any site) (primary) — *see also* Tuberculosis 017.0 ☑
Scrofulosis (universal) — *see also* Tuberculosis 017.2 ☑
Scrofulosis lichen (primary) — *see also* Tuberculosis 017.0 ☑
Scrofulous — *see* condition
Scrotal tongue 529.5
- congenital 750.13
Scrotum — *see* condition
Scurvy (gum) (infantile) (rickets) (scorbutic) 267
Sea-blue histiocyte syndrome 272.7
Seabright-Bantam syndrome (pseudohypoparathyroidism) 275.49
Sealpox 059.12
Seasickness 994.6
Seatworm 127.4
Sebaceous
- cyst (*see also* Cyst, sebaceous) 706.2
- gland disease NEC 706.9
Sebocystomatosis 706.2
Seborrhea, seborrheic 706.3
- adiposa 706.3
- capitis 690.11
- congestiva 695.4
- corporis 706.3

Seborrhea, seborrheic — *continued*
- dermatitis 690.10
  - infantile 690.12
- diathesis in infants 695.89
- eczema 690.18
  - infantile 690.12
- keratosis 702.19
  - inflamed 702.11
- nigricans 705.89
- sicca 690.18
- wart 702.19
  - inflamed 702.11
Seckel's syndrome 759.89
Seclusion pupil 364.74
Seclusiveness, child 313.22
Secondary — *see also* condition
- neoplasm — *see* Neoplasm, by site, malignant, secondary
Secretan's disease or syndrome (posttraumatic edema) 782.3
Secretion
- antidiuretic hormone, inappropriate (syndrome) 253.6
- catecholamine, by pheochromocytoma 255.6
- hormone
  - antidiuretic, inappropriate (syndrome) 253.6
  - by
    - carcinoid tumor 259.2
    - pheochromocytoma 255.6
  - ectopic NEC 259.3
- urinary
  - excessive 788.42
  - suppression 788.5
Section
- cesarean
  - affecting fetus or newborn 763.4
  - post mortem, affecting fetus or newborn 761.6
  - previous, in pregnancy or childbirth 654.2 ☑
    - affecting fetus or newborn 763.89
- nerve, traumatic — *see* Injury, nerve, by site
Seeligmann's syndrome (ichthyosis congenita) 757.1
Segmentation, incomplete (congenital) — *see also* Fusion
- bone NEC 756.9
- lumbosacral (joint) 756.15
- vertebra 756.15
  - lumbosacral 756.15
Seizure(s) 780.39
- akinetic (idiopathic) (*see also* Epilepsy) 345.0 ☑
  - psychomotor 345.4 ☑
- apoplexy, apoplectic (*see also* Disease, cerebrovascular, acute) 436
- atonic (*see also* Epilepsy) 345.0 ☑
- autonomic 300.11
- brain or cerebral (*see also* Disease, cerebrovascular, acute) 436
- convulsive (*see also* Convulsions) 780.39
- cortical (focal) (motor) (*see also* Epilepsy) 345.5 ☑
- disorder (*see also* Epilepsy) 345.9 ☑
  - due to stroke 438.89
- epilepsy, epileptic (cryptogenic) (*see also* Epilepsy) 345.9 ☑
- epileptiform, epileptoid 780.39
  - focal (*see also* Epilepsy) 345.5 ☑
- febrile (simple) 780.31
  - with status epilepticus 345.3
  - atypical 780.32
  - complex 780.32
  - complicated 780.32
- heart — *see* Disease, heart
- hysterical 300.11
- Jacksonian (focal) (*see also* Epilepsy) 345.5 ☑
  - motor type 345.5 ☑
  - sensory type 345.5 ☑
- migraine triggered 346.0 ☑
- newborn 779.0
- paralysis (*see also* Disease, cerebrovascular, acute) 436

Seizure(s) — *continued*
- posttraumatic 780.33
- recurrent 345.8 ☑
  - epileptic — *see* Epilepsy
- repetitive 780.39
  - epileptic — *see* Epilepsy
- salaam (*see also* Epilepsy) 345.6 ☑
- uncinate (*see also* Epilepsy) 345.4 ☑
Self-mutilation 300.9
Semicoma 780.09
Semiconsciousness 780.09
Seminal
- vesicle — *see* condition
- vesiculitis (*see also* Vesiculitis) 608.0
Seminoma (M9061/3)
- anaplastic type (M9062/3)
  - specified site — *see* Neoplasm, by site, malignant
  - unspecified site 186.9
- specified site — *see* Neoplasm, by site, malignant
- spermatocytic (M9063/3)
  - specified site — *see* Neoplasm, by site, malignant
  - unspecified site 186.9
- unspecified site 186.9
Semliki Forest encephalitis 062.8
Senear-Usher disease or syndrome (pemphigus erythematosus) 694.4
Senecio jacobae dermatitis 692.6
Senectus 797
Senescence 797
Senile — *see also* condition 797
- cervix (atrophic) 622.8
- degenerative atrophy, skin 701.3
- endometrium (atrophic) 621.8
- fallopian tube (atrophic) 620.3
- heart (failure) 797
- lung 492.8
- ovary (atrophic) 620.3
- syndrome 259.8
- vagina, vaginitis (atrophic) 627.3
- wart 702.0
Senility 797
- with
  - acute confusional state 290.3
  - delirium 290.3
  - mental changes 290.9
  - psychosis NEC (*see also* Psychosis, senile) 290.20
  - premature (syndrome) 259.8
Sensation
- burning (*see also* Disturbance, sensation) 782.0
  - tongue 529.6
- choking 784.99
- loss of (*see also* Disturbance, sensation) 782.0
- prickling (*see also* Disturbance, sensation) 782.0
- tingling (*see also* Disturbance, sensation) 782.0
Sense loss (touch) — *see also* Disturbance, sensation 782.0
- smell 781.1
- taste 781.1
Sensibility disturbance NEC (cortical) (deep) (vibratory) — *see also* Disturbance, sensation 782.0
Sensitive dentine 521.89
Sensitiver Beziehungswahn 297.8
Sensitivity, sensitization — *see also* Allergy
- autoerythrocyte 287.2
- carotid sinus 337.01
- child (excessive) 313.21
- cold, autoimmune 283.0
- methemoglobin 289.7
- suxamethonium 289.89
- tuberculin, without clinical or radiological symptoms 795.51
Sensory
- extinction 781.8
- neglect 781.8
Separation
- acromioclavicular — *see* Dislocation, acromioclavicular

☑ **Additional Digit Required** — Refer to the Tabular List for Digit Selection   ▽ **Subterms under main terms may continue to next column or page**

256 — Volume 2   ▶◀ Revised Text   ● New Line   ▲ Revised Code   2013 ICD-9-CM

Separation — *continued*
anxiety, abnormal 309.21
apophysis, traumatic — *see* Fracture, by site
choroid 363.70
hemorrhagic 363.72
serous 363.71
costochondral (simple) (traumatic) — *see* Dislocation, costochondral
delayed
umbilical cord 779.83
epiphysis, epiphyseal
nontraumatic 732.9
upper femoral 732.2
traumatic — *see* Fracture, by site
fracture — *see* Fracture, by site
infundibulum cardiac from right ventricle by a partition 746.83
joint (current) (traumatic) — *see* Dislocation, by site
placenta (normally implanted) — *see* Placenta, separation
pubic bone, obstetrical trauma 665.6 ☑
retina, retinal (*see also* Detachment, retina) 361.9
layers 362.40
sensory (*see also* Retinoschisis) 361.10
pigment epithelium (exudative) 362.42
hemorrhagic 362.43
sternoclavicular (traumatic) — *see* Dislocation, sternoclavicular
symphysis pubis, obstetrical trauma 665.6 ☑
tracheal ring, incomplete (congenital) 748.3
Sepsis (generalized) 995.91
with
abortion — *see* Abortion, by type, with sepsis
acute organ dysfunction 995.92
ectopic pregnancy (*see also* categories 633.0–633.9) 639.0
molar pregnancy (*see also* categories 630–632) 639.0
multiple organ dysfunction (MOD) 995.92
buccal 528.3
complicating labor 659.3 ☑
dental (pulpal origin) 522.4
female genital organ NEC 614.9
fetus (intrauterine) 771.81
following
abortion 639.0
ectopic or molar pregnancy 639.0
infusion, perfusion, or transfusion 999.39
Friedländer's 038.49
intra-abdominal 567.22
intraocular 360.00
localized — code to specific localized infection
in operation wound 998.59
skin (*see also* Abscess) 682.9
malleus 024
nadir 038.9
newborn (organism unspecified) NEC 771.81
oral 528.3
puerperal, postpartum, childbirth (pelvic) 670.2 ☑
resulting from infusion, injection, transfusion, or vaccination 999.39
severe 995.92
skin, localized (*see also* Abscess) 682.9
umbilical (newborn) (organism unspecified) 771.89
tetanus 771.3
urinary 599.0
meaning sepsis 995.91
meaning urinary tract infection 599.0
Septate — *see also* Septum
Septic — *see also* condition
adenoids 474.01
and tonsils 474.02
arm (with lymphangitis) 682.3
embolus — *see* Embolism
finger (with lymphangitis) 681.00
foot (with lymphangitis) 682.7
gallbladder (*see also* Cholecystitis) 575.8

Septic — *see also* condition — *continued*
hand (with lymphangitis) 682.4
joint (*see also* Arthritis, septic) 711.0 ☑
kidney (*see also* Infection, kidney) 590.9
leg (with lymphangitis) 682.6
mouth 528.3
nail 681.9
finger 681.02
toe 681.11
shock (endotoxic) 785.52
postoperative 998.02
sore (*see also* Abscess) 682.9
throat 034.0
milk-borne 034.0
streptococcal 034.0
spleen (acute) 289.59
teeth (pulpal origin) 522.4
throat 034.0
thrombus — *see* Thrombosis
toe (with lymphangitis) 681.10
tonsils 474.00
and adenoids 474.02
umbilical cord (newborn) (organism unspecified) 771.89
uterus (*see also* Endometritis) 615.9
Septicemia, septicemic (generalized) (suppurative) 038.9
with
abortion — *see* Abortion, by type, with sepsis
ectopic pregnancy (*see also* categories 633.0–633.9) 639.0
molar pregnancy (*see also* categories 630–632) 639.0
Aerobacter aerogenes 038.49
anaerobic 038.3
anthrax 022.3
Bacillus coli 038.42
Bacteroides 038.3
Clostridium 038.3
complicating labor 659.3 ☑
cryptogenic 038.9
enteric gram-negative bacilli 038.40
Enterobacter aerogenes 038.49
Erysipelothrix (insidiosa) (rhusiopathiae) 027.1
Escherichia coli 038.42
following
abortion 639.0
ectopic or molar pregnancy 639.0
infusion, injection, transfusion, or vaccination 999.39
Friedländer's (bacillus) 038.49
gangrenous 038.9
gonococcal 098.89
gram-negative (organism) 038.40
anaerobic 038.3
Hemophilus influenzae 038.41
herpes (simplex) 054.5
herpetic 054.5
Listeria monocytogenes 027.0
meningeal — *see* Meningitis
meningococcal (chronic) (fulminating) 036.2
methicillin
resistant Staphylococcus aureus (MRSA) 038.12
susceptible Staphylococcus aureus (MSSA) 038.11
MRSA (methicillin resistant Staphylococcus aureus) 038.12
MSSA (methicillin susceptible Staphylococcus aureus) 038.11
navel, newborn (organism unspecified) 771.89
newborn (organism unspecified) 771.81
plague 020.2
pneumococcal 038.2
postabortal 639.0
postoperative 998.59
Proteus vulgaris 038.49
Pseudomonas (aeruginosa) 038.43
puerperal, postpartum 670.2 ☑
Salmonella (aertrycke) (callinarum) (choleraesuis) (enteritidis) (suipestifer) 003.1
Serratia 038.44
Shigella (*see also* Dysentery, bacillary) 004.9

Septicemia, septicemic — *continued*
specified organism NEC 038.8
staphylococcal 038.10
aureus 038.11
methicillin
resistant (MRSA) 038.12
susceptible (MSSA) 038.11
specified organism NEC 038.19
streptococcal (anaerobic) 038.0
Streptococcus pneumoniae 038.2
suipestifer 003.1
umbilicus, newborn (organism unspecified) 771.89
viral 079.99
Yersinia enterocolitica 038.49
Septum, septate (congenital) — *see also* Anomaly, specified type NEC
anal 751.2
aqueduct of Sylvius 742.3
with spina bifida (*see also* Spina bifida) 741.0 ☑
hymen 752.49
uterus (complete) (partial) 752.35
vagina
in pregnancy or childbirth 654.7 ☑
affecting fetus or newborn 763.89
causing obstructed labor 660.2 ☑
affecting fetus or newborn 763.1
longitudinal (with or without obstruction) 752.47
transverse 752.46
Sequestration
lung (congenital) (extralobar) (intralobar) 748.5
orbit 376.10
pulmonary artery (congenital) 747.39
splenic 289.52
Sequestrum
bone (*see also* Osteomyelitis) 730.1 ☑
jaw 526.4
dental 525.8
jaw bone 526.4
sinus (accessory) (nasal) (*see also* Sinusitis) 473.9
maxillary 473.0
Sequoiosis asthma 495.8
Serology for syphilis
doubtful
with signs or symptoms — *see* Syphilis, by site and stage
follow-up of latent syphilis — *see* Syphilis, latent
false positive 795.6
negative, with signs or symptoms — *see* Syphilis, by site and stage
positive 097.1
with signs or symptoms — *see* Syphilis, by site and stage
false 795.6
follow-up of latent syphilis — *see* Syphilis, latent
only finding — *see* Syphilis, latent
reactivated 097.1
Seroma (postoperative) (non-infected) 998.13
infected 998.51
post-traumatic 729.91
Seropurulent — *see* condition
Serositis, multiple 569.89
pericardial 423.2
peritoneal 568.82
pleural — *see* Pleurisy
Serotonin syndrome 333.99
Serous — *see* condition
Sertoli cell
adenoma (M8640/0)
specified site — *see* Neoplasm, by site, benign
unspecified site
female 220
male 222.0
carcinoma (M8640/3)
specified site — *see* Neoplasm, by site, malignant
unspecified site 186.9
syndrome (germinal aplasia) 606.0

Sertoli cell — *continued*
tumor (M8640/0)
with lipid storage (M8641/0)
specified site — *see* Neoplasm, by site, benign
unspecified site
female 220
male 222.0
specified site — *see* Neoplasm, by site, benign
unspecified site
female 220
male 222.0
Sertoli-Leydig cell tumor (M8631/0)
specified site — *see* Neoplasm, by site, benign
unspecified site
female 220
male 222.0
Serum
allergy, allergic reaction 999.59
shock 999.49
arthritis 999.59 *[713.6]*
complication or reaction NEC 999.59
disease NEC 999.59
hepatitis 070.3 ☑
intoxication 999.59
jaundice (homologous) — *see* Hepatitis, viral, type B
neuritis 999.59
poisoning NEC 999.59
rash NEC 999.59
reaction NEC 999.59
sickness NEC 999.59
Sesamoiditis 733.99
Seven-day fever 061
of
Japan 100.89
Queensland 100.89
Sever's disease or osteochondrosis (calcaneum) 732.5
Sex chromosome mosaics 758.81
Sex reassignment surgery status (*see also* Trans-sexualism) 302.50
Sextuplet
affected by maternal complications of pregnancy 761.5
healthy liveborn — *see* Newborn, multiple pregnancy (complicating delivery) NEC 651.8 ☑
with fetal loss and retention of one or more fetus(es) 651.6 ☑
following (elective) fetal reduction 651.7 ☑
Sexual
anesthesia 302.72
deviation (*see also* Deviation, sexual) 302.9
disorder (*see also* Deviation, sexual) 302.9
frigidity (female) 302.72
function, disorder of (psychogenic) 302.70
specified type NEC 302.79
immaturity (female) (male) 259.0
impotence 607.84
organic origin NEC 607.84
psychogenic 302.72
precocity (constitutional) (cryptogenic) (female) (idiopathic) (male) NEC 259.1
with adrenal hyperplasia 255.2
sadism 302.84
Sexuality, pathological — *see also* Deviation, sexual 302.9
Sézary's disease, reticulosis, or syndrome (M9701/3) 202.2 ☑
Shadow, lung 793.19
Shaken infant syndrome 995.55
Shaking
head (tremor) 781.0
palsy or paralysis (*see also* Parkinsonism) 332.0
Shallowness, acetabulum 736.39
Shaver's disease or syndrome (bauxite pneumoconiosis) 503
Shearing
artificial skin graft 996.55
decellularized allodermis graft 996.55
Sheath (tendon) — *see* condition

☑ **Additional Digit Required** — Refer to the Tabular List for Digit Selection   ▽ **Subterms under main terms may continue to next column or page**

Shedding
nail 703.8
teeth, premature, primary (deciduous) 520.6
Sheehan's disease or syndrome (postpartum pituitary necrosis) 253.2
Shelf, rectal 569.49
Shell
shock (current) (see also Reaction, stress, acute) 308.9
lasting state 300.16
teeth 520.5
Shield kidney 753.3
Shifting
pacemaker 427.89
sleep-work schedule (affecting sleep) 327.36
Shift, mediastinal 793.2
Shiga's
bacillus 004.0
dysentery 004.0
Shigella (dysentery) — see also Dysentery, bacillary 004.9
carrier (suspected) of V02.3
Shigellosis — see also Dysentery, bacillary 004.9
Shingles — see also Herpes, zoster 053.9
eye NEC 053.29
Shin splints 844.9
Shipyard eye or disease 077.1
Shirodkar suture, in pregnancy 654.5 ☑
Shock 785.50
with
abortion — see Abortion, by type, with shock
ectopic pregnancy (see also categories 633.0–633.9) 639.5
molar pregnancy (see also categories 630–632) 639.5
allergic — see Anaphylactic reaction or shock
anaclitic 309.21
anaphylactic — see also Anaphylactic reaction or shock
due to administration of blood and blood products 999.41
anaphylactoid — see Anaphylactic reaction or shock
anesthetic
correct substance properly administered 995.4
overdose or wrong substance given 968.4
specified anesthetic — see Table of Drugs and Chemicals
birth, fetus or newborn NEC 779.89
cardiogenic 785.51
chemical substance — see Table of Drugs and Chemicals
circulatory 785.59
complicating
abortion — see Abortion, by type, with shock
ectopic pregnancy (see also categories 633.0–633.9) 639.5
labor and delivery 669.1 ☑
molar pregnancy (see also categories 630–632) 639.5
culture 309.29
due to
drug 995.0
correct substance properly administered 995.0
overdose or wrong substance given or taken 977.9
specified drug — see Table of Drugs and Chemicals
food — see Anaphylactic shock, due to, food
during labor and delivery 669.1 ☑
electric 994.8
from electroshock gun (taser) 994.8
endotoxic 785.52
due to surgical procedure 998.02
postoperative 998.02
following
abortion 639.5
ectopic or molar pregnancy 639.5

Shock — continued
following — continued
injury (immediate) (delayed) 958.4
labor and delivery 669.1 ☑
gram-negative 785.52
postoperative 998.02
hematogenic 785.59
hemorrhagic
due to
disease 785.59
surgery (intraoperative) (postoperative) 998.09
trauma 958.4
hypovolemic NEC 785.59
surgical 998.09
traumatic 958.4
insulin 251.0
therapeutic misadventure 962.3
kidney 584.5
traumatic (following crushing) 958.5
lightning 994.0
lung 518.82
related to trauma and surgery 518.52
nervous (see also Reaction, stress, acute) 308.9
obstetric 669.1 ☑
with
abortion — see Abortion, by type, with shock
ectopic pregnancy (see also categories 633.0–633.9) 639.5
molar pregnancy (see also categories 630–632) 639.5
following
abortion 639.5
ectopic or molar pregnancy 639.5
paralysis, paralytic (see also Disease, cerebrovascular, acute) 436
late effect — see Late effect(s) (of) cerebrovascular disease
pleural (surgical) 998.09
due to trauma 958.4
postoperative 998.00
with
abortion — see Abortion, by type, with shock
ectopic pregnancy (see also categories 633.0–633.9) 639.5
molar pregnancy (see also categories 630–632) 639.5
cardiogenic 998.01
following
abortion 639.5
ectopic or molar pregnancy 639.5
hypovolemic 998.09
septic (endotoxic) (gram-negative) 998.02
specified NEC 998.09
psychic (see also Reaction, stress, acute) 308.9
past history (of) V15.49
psychogenic (see also Reaction, stress, acute) 308.9
septic 785.52
with
abortion — see Abortion, by type, with shock
ectopic pregnancy (see also categories 633.0–633.9) 639.5
molar pregnancy (see also categories 630–632) 639.5
due to
surgical procedure 998.02
transfusion NEC 999.89
bone marrow 996.85
following
abortion 639.5
ectopic or molar pregnancy 639.5
surgical procedure 998.02
transfusion NEC 999.89
bone marrow 996.85
postoperative 998.02
spinal (see also Injury, spinal, by site)
with spinal bone injury — see Fracture, vertebra, by site, with spinal cord injury

Shock — continued
surgical 998.00
therapeutic misadventure NEC (see also Complications) 998.89
thyroxin 962.7
toxic 040.82
transfusion — see Complications, transfusion
traumatic (immediate) (delayed) 958.4
Shoemakers' chest 738.3
Short, shortening, shortness
Achilles tendon (acquired) 727.81
arm 736.89
congenital 755.20
back 737.9
bowel syndrome 579.3
breath 786.05
cervical, cervix 649.7 ☑
gravid uterus 649.7 ☑
non-gravid uterus 622.5
acquired 622.5
congenital 752.49
chain acyl CoA dehydrogenase deficiency (SCAD) 277.85
common bile duct, congenital 751.69
cord (umbilical) 663.4 ☑
affecting fetus or newborn 762.6
cystic duct, congenital 751.69
esophagus (congenital) 750.4
femur (acquired) 736.81
congenital 755.34
frenulum linguae 750.0
frenum, lingual 750.0
hamstrings 727.81
hip (acquired) 736.39
congenital 755.63
leg (acquired) 736.81
congenital 755.30
metatarsus (congenital) 754.79
acquired 736.79
organ or site, congenital NEC — see Distortion
palate (congenital) 750.26
P-R interval syndrome 426.81
radius (acquired) 736.09
congenital 755.26
round ligament 629.89
sleeper 307.49
stature, constitutional (hereditary) (idiopathic) 783.43
tendon 727.81
Achilles (acquired) 727.81
congenital 754.79
congenital 756.89
thigh (acquired) 736.81
congenital 755.34
tibialis anticus 727.81
umbilical cord 663.4 ☑
affecting fetus or newborn 762.6
urethra 599.84
uvula (congenital) 750.26
vagina 623.8
Shortsightedness 367.1
Shoshin (acute fulminating beriberi) 265.0
Shoulder — see condition
Shovel-shaped incisors 520.2
Shower, thromboembolic — see Embolism
Shunt (status)
aortocoronary bypass V45.81
arterial-venous (dialysis) V45.11
arteriovenous, pulmonary (acquired) 417.0
congenital 747.39
traumatic (complication) 901.40
cerebral ventricle (communicating) in situ V45.2
coronary artery bypass V45.81
surgical, prosthetic, with complications — see Complications, shunt
vascular NEC V45.89
Shutdown
renal 586
with
abortion — see Abortion, by type, with renal failure
ectopic pregnancy (see also categories 633.0–633.9) 639.3

Shutdown — continued
renal — continued
with — continued
molar pregnancy (see also categories 630–632) 639.3
complicating
abortion 639.3
ectopic or molar pregnancy 639.3
following labor and delivery 669.3 ☑
Shwachman's syndrome 288.02
Shy-Drager syndrome (orthostatic hypotension with multisystem degeneration) 333.0
Sialadenitis (any gland) (chronic) (suppurative) 527.2
epidemic — see Mumps
Sialadenosis, periodic 527.2
Sialaporia 527.7
Sialectasia 527.8
Sialitis 527.2
Sialoadenitis — see also Sialadenitis 527.2
Sialoangitis 527.2
Sialodochitis (fibrinosa) 527.2
Sialodocholithiasis 527.5
Sialolithiasis 527.5
Sialorrhea — see also Ptyalism 527.7
periodic 527.2
Sialosis 527.8
rheumatic 710.2
Siamese twin 759.4
complicating pregnancy 678.1 ☑
Sicard's syndrome 352.6
Sicca syndrome (keratoconjunctivitis) 710.2
Sick 799.9
cilia syndrome 759.89
or handicapped person in family V61.49
Sickle-cell
anemia (see also Disease, sickle-cell) 282.60
disease (see also Disease, sickle-cell) 282.60
hemoglobin
C disease (without crisis) 282.63
with
crisis 282.64
vaso-occlusive pain 282.64
D disease (without crisis) 282.68
with crisis 282.69
E disease (without crisis) 282.68
with crisis 282.69
thalassemia (without crisis) 282.41
with
crisis 282.42
vaso-occlusive pain 282.42
trait 282.5
Sicklemia — see also Disease, sickle-cell 282.60
trait 282.5
Sickness
air (travel) 994.6
airplane 994.6
alpine 993.2
altitude 993.2
Andes 993.2
aviators' 993.2
balloon 993.2
car 994.6
compressed air 993.3
decompression 993.3
green 280.9
harvest 100.89
milk 988.8
morning 643.0 ☑
motion 994.6
mountain 993.2
acute 289.0
protein (see also Complications, vaccination) 999.59
radiation NEC 990
roundabout (motion) 994.6
sea 994.6
serum NEC 999.59
sleeping (African) 086.5
by Trypanosoma 086.5
gambiense 086.3
rhodesiense 086.4
Gambian 086.3
late effect 139.8
Rhodesian 086.4

☑ Additional Digit Required — Refer to the Tabular List for Digit Selection ▽ Subterms under main terms may continue to next column or page

258 — Volume 2 ▶◀ Revised Text ● New Line ▲ Revised Code 2013 ICD-9-CM

Sickness — *continued*
  sweating 078.2
  swing (motion) 994.6
  train (railway) (travel) 994.6
  travel (any vehicle) 994.6
Sick sinus syndrome 427.81
Sideropenia — *see also* Anemia, iron deficiency 280.9
Siderosis (lung) (occupational) 503
  central nervous system (CNS) 437.8
  cornea 371.15
  eye (bulbi) (vitreous) 360.23
  lens 360.23
Siegal-Cattan-Mamou disease (periodic) 277.31
Siemens' syndrome
  ectodermal dysplasia 757.31
  keratosis follicularis spinulosa (decalvans) 757.39
Sighing respiration 786.7
Sigmoid
  flexure — *see* condition
  kidney 753.3
Sigmoiditis — *see* Enteritis
Silfverskiöld's syndrome 756.50
Silicosis, silicotic (complicated) (occupational) (simple) 502
  fibrosis, lung (confluent) (massive) (occupational) 502
  non-nodular 503
  pulmonum 502
Silicotuberculosis — *see also* Tuberculosis 011.4 ☑
Silo fillers' disease 506.9
Silver's syndrome (congenital hemihypertrophy and short stature) 759.89
Silver wire arteries, retina 362.13
Silvestroni-Bianco syndrome (thalassemia minima) 282.49
Simian crease 757.2
Simmonds' cachexia or disease (pituitary cachexia) 253.2
Simons' disease or syndrome (progressive lipodystrophy) 272.6
Simple, simplex — *see* condition
Sinding-Larsen disease (juvenile osteopathia patellae) 732.4
Singapore hemorrhagic fever 065.4
Singers' node or nodule 478.5
Single
  atrium 745.69
  coronary artery 746.85
  umbilical artery 747.5
  ventricle 745.3
Singultus 786.8
  epidemicus 078.89
Sinus — *see also* Fistula
  abdominal 569.81
  arrest 426.6
  arrhythmia 427.89
  bradycardia 427.89
    chronic 427.81
  branchial cleft (external) (internal) 744.41
  coccygeal (infected) 685.1
    with abscess 685.0
  dental 522.7
  dermal (congenital) 685.1
    with abscess 685.0
  draining — *see* Fistula
  infected, skin NEC 686.9
  marginal, ruptured or bleeding 641.2 ☑
    affecting fetus or newborn 762.1
  pause 426.6
  pericranii 742.0
  pilonidal (infected) (rectum) 685.1
    with abscess 685.0
  preauricular 744.46
  rectovaginal 619.1
  sacrococcygeal (dermoid) (infected) 685.1
    with abscess 685.0
  skin
    infected NEC 686.9
    noninfected — *see* Ulcer, skin
  tachycardia 427.89
  tarsi syndrome 726.79
  testis 608.89

Sinus — *see also* Fistula — *continued*
  tract (postinfectional) — *see* Fistula
  urachus 753.7
Sinuses, Rokitansky-Aschoff — *see also* Disease, gallbladder 575.8
Sinusitis (accessory) (nasal) (hyperplastic) (nonpurulent) (purulent) (chronic) 473.9
  with influenza, flu, or grippe (*see also* Influenza) 487.1
  acute 461.9
    ethmoidal 461.2
    frontal 461.1
    maxillary 461.0
    specified type NEC 461.8
    sphenoidal 461.3
  allergic (*see also* Fever, hay) 477.9
  antrum — *see* Sinusitis, maxillary
  due to
    fungus, any sinus 117.9
    high altitude 993.1
  ethmoidal 473.2
    acute 461.2
  frontal 473.1
    acute 461.1
  influenzal (*see also* Influenza) 487.1
  maxillary 473.0
    acute 461.0
  specified site NEC 473.8
  sphenoidal 473.3
    acute 461.3
  syphilitic, any sinus 095.8
  tuberculous, any sinus (*see also* Tuberculosis) 012.8 ☑
Sinusitis-bronchiectasis-situs inversus (syndrome) (triad) 759.3
Sioloangitis 527.2
Sipple's syndrome (medullary thyroid carcinoma-pheochromocytoma) 258.02
Sirenomelia 759.89
Siriasis 992.0
Sirkari's disease 085.0
SIRS (systemic inflammatory response syndrome) 995.90
  due to
    infectious process 995.91
      with acute organ dysfunction 995.92
    non-infectious process 995.93
      with acute organ dysfunction 995.94
Siti 104.0
Sitophobia 300.29
Situational
  disturbance (transient) (*see also* Reaction, adjustment) 309.9
    acute 308.3
  maladjustment, acute (*see also* Reaction, adjustment) 309.9
  reaction (*see also* Reaction, adjustment) 309.9
    acute 308.3
Situation, psychiatric 300.9
Situs inversus or transversus 759.3
  abdominalis 759.3
  thoracis 759.3
Sixth disease
  due to
    human herpesvirus 6 058.11
    human herpesvirus 7 058.12
Sjögren-Larsson syndrome (ichthyosis congenita) 757.1
Sjögren (-Gougerot) syndrome or disease (keratoconjunctivitis sicca) 710.2
  with lung involvement 710.2 [517.8]
SJS-TEN (Stevens-Johnson syndrome - toxic epidermal necrolysis overlap syndrome) 695.14
Skeletal — *see* condition
Skene's gland — *see* condition
Skenitis — *see also* Urethritis 597.89
  gonorrheal (acute) 098.0
    chronic or duration of 2 months or over 098.2
Skerljevo 104.0
Skevas-Zerfus disease 989.5
Skin — *see also* condition
  donor V59.1
  hidebound 710.9

SLAP lesion (superior glenoid labrum) 840.7
Slate-dressers' lung 502
Slate-miners' lung 502
Sleep
  deprivation V69.4
  disorder 780.50
    with apnea — *see* Apnea, sleep
    child 307.40
    movement, unspecified 780.58
    nonorganic origin 307.40
      specified type NEC 307.49
  disturbance 780.50
    with apnea — *see* Apnea, sleep
    nonorganic origin 307.40
      specified type NEC 307.49
  drunkenness 307.47
  movement disorder, unspecified 780.58
  paroxysmal (*see also* Narcolepsy) 347.00
  related movement disorder, unspecified 780.58
  rhythm inversion 327.39
    nonorganic origin 307.45
  walking 307.46
    hysterical 300.13
Sleeping sickness 086.5
  late effect 139.8
Sleeplessness — *see also* Insomnia 780.52
  menopausal 627.2
  nonorganic origin 307.41
Slipped, slipping
  epiphysis (postinfectional) 732.9
    traumatic (old) 732.9
      current — *see* Fracture, by site
    upper femoral (nontraumatic) 732.2
  intervertebral disc — *see* Displacement, intervertebral disc
  ligature, umbilical 772.3
  patella 717.89
  rib 733.99
  sacroiliac joint 724.6
  tendon 727.9
  ulnar nerve, nontraumatic 354.2
  vertebra NEC (*see also* Spondylolisthesis) 756.12
Slocumb's syndrome 255.3
Sloughing (multiple) (skin) 686.9
  abscess — *see* Abscess, by site
  appendix 543.9
  bladder 596.89
  fascia 728.9
  graft — *see* Complications, graft
  phagedena (*see also* Gangrene) 785.4
  reattached extremity (*see also* Complications, reattached extremity) 996.90
  rectum 569.49
  scrotum 608.89
  tendon 727.9
  transplanted organ (*see also* Rejection, transplant, organ, by site) 996.80
  ulcer (*see also* Ulcer, skin) 707.9
Slow
  feeding newborn 779.31
  fetal, growth NEC 764.9 ☑
    affecting management of pregnancy 656.5 ☑
Slowing
  heart 427.89
  urinary stream 788.62
Sluder's neuralgia or syndrome 337.09
Slurred, slurring, speech 784.59
Small-for-dates — *see also* Light-for-dates 764.0 ☑
  affecting management of pregnancy 656.5 ☑
Smallpox 050.9
  contact V01.3
  exposure to V01.3
  hemorrhagic (pustular) 050.0
  malignant 050.0
  modified 050.2
  vaccination
    complications — *see* Complications, vaccination
    prophylactic (against) V04.1
Small, smallness
  cardiac reserve — *see* Disease, heart

Small, smallness — *continued*
  for dates
    fetus or newborn 764.0 ☑
      with malnutrition 764.1 ☑
        affecting management of pregnancy 656.5 ☑
    infant, term 764.0 ☑
      with malnutrition 764.1 ☑
        affecting management of pregnancy 656.5 ☑
  introitus, vagina 623.3
  kidney, unknown cause 589.9
    bilateral 589.1
    unilateral 589.0
  ovary 620.8
  pelvis
    with disproportion (fetopelvic) 653.1 ☑
      affecting fetus or newborn 763.1
    causing obstructed labor 660.1 ☑
      affecting fetus or newborn 763.1
  placenta — *see* Placenta, insufficiency
  uterus 621.8
  white kidney 582.9
Smearing, fecal 787.62
Smith's fracture (separation) (closed) 813.41
  open 813.51
Smith-Lemli Opitz syndrome (cerebrohepatorenal syndrome) 759.89
Smith-Magenis syndrome 758.33
Smith-Strang disease (oasthouse urine) 270.2
Smokers'
  bronchitis 491.0
  cough 491.0
  syndrome (*see also* Abuse, drugs, nondependent) 305.1
  throat 472.1
  tongue 528.6
Smoking complicating pregnancy, childbirth, or the puerperium 649.0 ☑
Smothering spells 786.09
Snaggle teeth, tooth 524.39
Snapping
  finger 727.05
  hip 719.65
  jaw 524.69
    temporomandibular joint sounds on opening or closing 524.64
  knee 717.9
  thumb 727.05
Sneddon-Wilkinson disease or syndrome (subcorneal pustular dermatosis) 694.1
Sneezing 784.99
  intractable 478.19
Sniffing
  cocaine (*see also* Dependence) 304.2 ☑
  ether (*see also* Dependence) 304.6 ☑
  glue (airplane) (*see also* Dependence) 304.6 ☑
Snoring 786.09
Snow blindness 370.24
Snuffles (nonsyphilitic) 460
  syphilitic (infant) 090.0
Social migrant V60.0
Sodoku 026.0
Soemmering's ring 366.51
Soft — *see also* condition
  enlarged prostate 600.00
    with
      other lower urinary tract symptoms (LUTS) 600.01
      urinary
        obstruction 600.01
        retention 600.01
  nails 703.8
Softening
  bone 268.2
  brain (necrotic) (progressive) 348.89
    arteriosclerotic 437.0
    congenital 742.4
    due to cerebrovascular accident 438.89
    embolic (*see also* Embolism, brain) 434.1 ☑
    hemorrhagic (*see also* Hemorrhage, brain) 431
    occlusive 434.9 ☑

☑ Additional Digit Required — Refer to the Tabular List for Digit Selection   ▽ Subterms under main terms may continue to next column or page

2013 ICD-9-CM   ▶◀ Revised Text   ● New Line   ▲ Revised Code   **Volume 2 — 259**

☑ **Additional Digit Required** — Refer to the Tabular List for Digit Selection   ⬇ **Subterms under main terms may continue to next column or page**

260 — Volume 2   ▶◀ Revised Text   ● New Line   ▲ Revised Code   2013 ICD-9-CM

Splenomegaly 789.2
  Bengal 789.2
  cirrhotic 289.51
  congenital 759.0
  congestive, chronic 289.51
  cryptogenic 789.2
  Egyptian 120.1
  Gaucher's (cerebroside lipidosis) 272.7
  idiopathic 789.2
  malarial (see also Malaria) 084.6
  neutropenic 289.53
  Niemann-Pick (lipid histiocytosis) 272.7
  siderotic 289.51
  syphilitic 095.8
    congenital 090.0
  tropical (Bengal) (idiopathic) 789.2
Splenopathy 289.50
Splenopneumonia — see Pneumonia
Splenoptosis 289.59
Splinter — see Injury, superficial, by site
Split, splitting
  heart sounds 427.89
  lip, congenital (see also Cleft, lip) 749.10
  nails 703.8
  urinary stream 788.61
Spoiled child reaction — see also Disturbance, conduct 312.1 ☑
Spondylarthritis — see also Spondylosis 721.90
Spondylarthrosis — see also Spondylosis 721.90
Spondylitis 720.9
  ankylopoietica 720.0
  ankylosing (chronic) 720.0
  atrophic 720.9
    ligamentous 720.9
  chronic (traumatic) (see also Spondylosis) 721.90
  deformans (chronic) (see also Spondylosis) 721.90
  gonococcal 098.53
  gouty 274.00
  hypertrophic (see also Spondylosis) 721.90
  infectious NEC 720.9
  juvenile (adolescent) 720.0
  Kümmell's 721.7
  Marie-Strümpell (ankylosing) 720.0
  muscularis 720.9
  ossificans ligamentosa 721.6
  osteoarthritica (see also Spondylosis) 721.90
  posttraumatic 721.7
  proliferative 720.0
  rheumatoid 720.0
  rhizomelica 720.0
  sacroiliac NEC 720.2
  senescent (see also Spondylosis) 721.90
  senile (see also Spondylosis) 721.90
  static (see also Spondylosis) 721.90
  traumatic (chronic) (see also Spondylosis) 721.90
  tuberculous (see also Tuberculosis) 015.0 ☑ [720.81]
  typhosa 002.0 [720.81]
Spondyloarthrosis — see also Spondylosis 721.90
Spondylolisthesis (congenital) (lumbosacral) 756.12
  with disproportion (fetopelvic) 653.3 ☑
    affecting fetus or newborn 763.1
    causing obstructed labor 660.1 ☑
      affecting fetus or newborn 763.1
  acquired 738.4
  degenerative 738.4
  traumatic 738.4
    acute (lumbar) — see Fracture, vertebra, lumbar
    site other than lumbosacral — see Fracture, vertebra, by site
Spondylolysis (congenital) 756.11
  acquired 738.4
  cervical 756.19
  lumbosacral region 756.11
    with disproportion (fetopelvic) 653.3 ☑
      affecting fetus or newborn 763.1
      causing obstructed labor 660.1 ☑
        affecting fetus or newborn 763.1

Spondylopathy
  inflammatory 720.9
    specified type NEC 720.89
  traumatic 721.7
Spondylose rhizomelique 720.0
Spondylosis 721.90
  with
    disproportion 653.3 ☑
      affecting fetus or newborn 763.1
      causing obstructed labor 660.1 ☑
        affecting fetus or newborn 763.1
    myelopathy NEC 721.91
  cervical, cervicodorsal 721.0
    with myelopathy 721.1
  inflammatory 720.9
  lumbar, lumbosacral 721.3
    with myelopathy 721.42
  sacral 721.3
    with myelopathy 721.42
  thoracic 721.2
    with myelopathy 721.41
  traumatic 721.7
Sponge
  divers' disease 989.5
  inadvertently left in operation wound 998.4
  kidney (medullary) 753.17
Spongioblastoma (M9422/3)
  multiforme (M9440/3)
    specified site — see Neoplasm, by site, malignant
    unspecified site 191.9
  polare (M9423/3)
    specified site — see Neoplasm, by site, malignant
    unspecified site 191.9
  primitive polar (M9443/3)
    specified site — see Neoplasm, by site, malignant
    unspecified site 191.9
  specified site — see Neoplasm, by site, malignant
  unspecified site 191.9
Spongiocytoma (M9400/3)
  specified site — see Neoplasm, by site, malignant
  unspecified site 191.9
Spongioneuroblastoma (M9504/3) — see Neoplasm, by site, malignant
Spontaneous — see also condition
  fracture — see Fracture, pathologic
Spoon nail 703.8
  congenital 757.5
Sporadic — see condition
Sporotrichosis (bones) (cutaneous) (disseminated) (epidermal) (lymphatic) (lymphocutaneous) (mucous membranes) (pulmonary) (skeletal) (visceral) 117.1
Sporotrichum schenckii infection 117.1
Spots, spotting
  atrophic (skin) 701.3
  Bitôt's (in the young child) 264.1
  café au lait 709.09
  cayenne pepper 448.1
  complicating pregnancy 649.5 ☑
  cotton wool (retina) 362.83
  de Morgan's (senile angiomas) 448.1
  Fúchs' black (myopic) 360.21
  intermenstrual
    irregular 626.6
    regular 626.5
  interpalpebral 372.53
  Koplik's 055.9
  liver 709.09
  Mongolian (pigmented) 757.33
  of pregnancy 649.5 ☑
  purpuric 782.7
  ruby 448.1
Spotted fever — see Fever, spotted
Sprain, strain (joint) (ligament) (muscle) (tendon) 848.9
  abdominal wall (muscle) 848.8
  Achilles tendon 845.09
  acromioclavicular 840.0
  ankle 845.00
    and foot 845.00
  anterior longitudinal, cervical 847.0

Sprain, strain — continued
  arm 840.9
    upper 840.9
      and shoulder 840.9
  astragalus 845.00
  atlanto-axial 847.0
  atlanto-occipital 847.0
  atlas 847.0
  axis 847.0
  back (see also Sprain, spine) 847.9
  breast bone 848.40
  broad ligament — see Injury, internal, broad ligament
  calcaneofibular 845.02
  carpal 842.01
  carpometacarpal 842.11
  cartilage
    costal, without mention of injury to sternum 848.3
    involving sternum 848.42
  ear 848.8
  knee 844.9
    with current tear (see also Tear, meniscus) 836.2
  semilunar (knee) 844.8
    with current tear (see also Tear, meniscus) 836.2
  septal, nose 848.0
  thyroid region 848.2
  xiphoid 848.49
  cervical, cervicodorsal, cervicothoracic 847.0
  chondrocostal, without mention of injury to sternum 848.3
    involving sternum 848.42
  chondrosternal 848.42
  chronic (joint) — see Derangement, joint
  clavicle 840.9
  coccyx 847.4
  collar bone 840.9
  collateral, knee (medial) (tibial) 844.1
    lateral (fibular) 844.0
      recurrent or old 717.89
        lateral 717.81
        medial 717.82
  coracoacromial 840.8
  coracoclavicular 840.1
  coracohumeral 840.2
  coracoid (process) 840.9
  coronary, knee 844.8
  costal cartilage, without mention of injury to sternum 848.3
    involving sternum 848.42
  cricoarytenoid articulation 848.2
  cricothyroid articulation 848.2
  cruciate
    knee 844.2
    old 717.89
      anterior 717.83
      posterior 717.84
  deltoid
    ankle 845.01
    shoulder 840.8
  dorsal (spine) 847.1
  ear cartilage 848.8
  elbow 841.9
    and forearm 841.9
    specified site NEC 841.8
  femur (proximal end) 843.9
    distal end 844.9
  fibula (proximal end) 844.9
    distal end 845.00
  fibulocalcaneal 845.02
  finger(s) 842.10
  foot 845.10
    and ankle 845.00
  forearm 841.9
    and elbow 841.9
    specified site NEC 841.8
  glenoid (shoulder) (see also SLAP lesion) 840.8
  hand 842.10
  hip 843.9
    and thigh 843.9
  humerus (proximal end) 840.9
    distal end 841.9
  iliofemoral 843.0

Sprain, strain — continued
  infraspinatus 840.3
  innominate
    acetabulum 843.9
    pubic junction 848.5
    sacral junction 846.1
  internal
    collateral, ankle 845.01
    semilunar cartilage 844.8
      with current tear (see also Tear, meniscus) 836.2
      old 717.5
  interphalangeal
    finger 842.13
    toe 845.13
  ischiocapsular 843.1
  jaw (cartilage) (meniscus) 848.1
    old 524.69
  knee 844.9
    and leg 844.9
    old 717.5
    collateral
      lateral 717.81
      medial 717.82
    cruciate
      anterior 717.83
      posterior 717.84
  late effect — see Late, effects (of), sprain
  lateral collateral, knee 844.0
    old 717.81
  leg 844.9
    and knee 844.9
  ligamentum teres femoris 843.8
  low back 846.9
  lumbar (spine) 847.2
  lumbosacral 846.0
    chronic or old 724.6
  mandible 848.1
    old 524.69
  maxilla 848.1
  medial collateral, knee 844.1
    old 717.82
  meniscus
    jaw 848.1
      old 524.69
    knee 844.8
      with current tear (see also Tear, meniscus) 836.2
      old 717.5
    mandible 848.1
      old 524.69
    specified site NEC 848.8
  metacarpal 842.10
    distal 842.12
    proximal 842.11
  metacarpophalangeal 842.12
  metatarsal 845.10
  metatarsophalangeal 845.12
  midcarpal 842.19
  midtarsal 845.19
  multiple sites, except fingers alone or toes alone 848.8
  neck 847.0
  nose (septal cartilage) 848.0
  occiput from atlas 847.0
  old — see Derangement, joint
  orbicular, hip 843.8
  patella(r) 844.8
    old 717.89
  pelvis 848.5
  phalanx
    finger 842.10
    toe 845.10
  radiocarpal 842.02
  radiohumeral 841.2
  radioulnar 841.9
    distal 842.09
  radius, radial (proximal end) 841.9
    and ulna 841.9
      distal 842.09
    collateral 841.0
      distal end 842.00
  recurrent — see Sprain, by site
  rib (cage), without mention of injury to sternum 848.3
    involving sternum 848.42

☑ Additional Digit Required — Refer to the Tabular List for Digit Selection   ⏷ Subterms under main terms may continue to next column or page

2013 ICD-9-CM   ▶◀ Revised Text   ● New Line   ▲ Revised Code   Volume 2 — 261

Sprain, strain — *continued*
 rotator cuff (capsule) 840.4
 round ligament (*see also* Injury, internal, round ligament)
  femur 843.8
 sacral (spine) 847.3
 sacrococcygeal 847.3
 sacroiliac (region) 846.9
  chronic or old 724.6
  ligament 846.1
  specified site NEC 846.8
 sacrospinatus 846.2
 sacrospinous 846.2
 sacrotuberous 846.3
 scaphoid bone, ankle 845.00
 scapula(r) 840.9
 semilunar cartilage (knee) 844.8
  with current tear (*see also* Tear, meniscus) 836.2
  old 717.5
 septal cartilage (nose) 848.0
 shoulder 840.9
  and arm, upper 840.9
  blade 840.9
 specified site NEC 848.8
 spine 847.9
  cervical 847.0
  coccyx 847.4
  dorsal 847.1
  lumbar 847.2
  lumbosacral 846.0
   chronic or old 724.6
  sacral 847.3
  sacroiliac (*see also* Sprain, sacroiliac) 846.9
   chronic or old 724.6
  thoracic 847.1
 sternoclavicular 848.41
 sternum 848.40
 subglenoid (*see also* SLAP lesion) 840.8
 subscapularis 840.5
 supraspinatus 840.6
 symphysis
  jaw 848.1
   old 524.69
  mandibular 848.1
   old 524.69
  pubis 848.5
 talofibular 845.09
 tarsal 845.10
 tarsometatarsal 845.11
 temporomandibular 848.1
  old 524.69
 teres
  ligamentum femoris 843.8
  major or minor 840.8
 thigh (proximal end) 843.9
  and hip 843.9
  distal end 844.9
 thoracic (spine) 847.1
 thorax 848.8
 thumb 842.10
 thyroid cartilage or region 848.2
 tibia (proximal end) 844.9
  distal end 845.00
 tibiofibular
  distal 845.03
  superior 844.3
 toe(s) 845.10
 trachea 848.8
 trapezoid 840.8
 ulna, ulnar (proximal end) 841.9
  collateral 841.1
  distal end 842.00
 ulnohumeral 841.3
 vertebrae (*see also* Sprain, spine) 847.9
  cervical, cervicodorsal, cervicothoracic 847.0
 wrist (cuneiform) (scaphoid) (semilunar) 842.00
 xiphoid cartilage 848.49
Sprengel's deformity (congenital) 755.52
Spring fever 309.23
Sprue 579.1
 celiac 579.0
 idiopathic 579.0

Sprue — *continued*
 meaning thrush 112.0
 nontropical 579.0
 tropical 579.1
Spur — *see also* Exostosis
 bone 726.91
  calcaneal 726.73
 calcaneal 726.73
 iliac crest 726.5
 nose (septum) 478.19
  bone 726.91
 septal 478.19
Spuria placenta — *see* Placenta, abnormal
Spurway's syndrome (brittle bones and blue sclera) 756.51
Sputum, abnormal (amount) (color) (excessive) (odor) (purulent) 786.4
 bloody 786.30
Squamous — *see also* condition
 cell metaplasia
  bladder 596.89
  cervix — *see* condition
 epithelium in
  cervical canal (congenital) 752.49
  uterine mucosa (congenital) 752.39
 metaplasia
  bladder 596.89
  cervix — *see* condition
Squashed nose 738.0
 congenital 754.0
Squeeze, divers' 993.3
Squint — *see also* Strabismus 378.9
 accommodative (*see also* Esotropia) 378.00
 concomitant (*see also* Heterotropia) 378.30
Stab — *see also* Wound, open, by site
 internal organs — *see* Injury, internal, by site, with open wound
Staggering gait 781.2
 hysterical 300.11
Staghorn calculus 592.0
Stain, staining
 meconium 779.84
 port wine 757.32
 tooth, teeth (hard tissues) 521.7
  due to
   accretions 523.6
   deposits (betel) (black) (green) (materia alba) (orange) (tobacco) 523.6
   metals (copper) (silver) 521.7
   nicotine 523.6
   pulpal bleeding 521.7
   tobacco 523.6
Stälh's
 ear 744.29
 pigment line (cornea) 371.11
Stälhi's pigment lines (cornea) 371.11
Stammering — *see also* Disorder, fluency 315.35
Standstill
 atrial 426.6
 auricular 426.6
 cardiac (*see also* Arrest, cardiac) 427.5
 sinoatrial 426.6
 sinus 426.6
 ventricular (*see also* Arrest, cardiac) 427.5
Stannosis 503
Stanton's disease (melioidosis) 025
Staphylitis (acute) (catarrhal) (chronic) (gangrenous) (membranous) (suppurative) (ulcerative) 528.3
Staphylococcemia 038.10
 aureus 038.11
 specified organism NEC 038.19
Staphylococcus, staphylococcal — *see* condition
Staphyloderma (skin) 686.00
Staphyloma 379.11
 anterior, localized 379.14
 ciliary 379.11
 cornea 371.73
 equatorial 379.13
 posterior 379.12
 posticum 379.12
 ring 379.15
 sclera NEC 379.11

Starch eating 307.52
Stargardt's disease 362.75
Starvation (inanition) (due to lack of food) 994.2
 edema 262
 voluntary NEC 307.1
Stasis
 bile (duct) (*see also* Disease, biliary) 576.8
 bronchus (*see also* Bronchitis) 490
 cardiac (*see also* Failure, heart) 428.0
 cecum 564.89
 colon 564.89
 dermatitis (*see also* Varix, with stasis dermatitis) 454.1
 duodenal 536.8
 eczema (*see also* Varix, with stasis dermatitis) 454.1
 edema (*see also* Hypertension, venous) 459.30
 foot 991.4
 gastric 536.3
 ileocecal coil 564.89
 ileum 564.89
 intestinal 564.89
 jejunum 564.89
 kidney 586
 liver 571.9
  cirrhotic — *see* Cirrhosis, liver
 lymphatic 457.8
 pneumonia 514
 portal 571.9
 pulmonary 514
 rectal 564.89
 renal 586
  tubular 584.5
 stomach 536.3
 ulcer
  with varicose veins 454.0
  without varicose veins 459.81
 urine NEC (*see also* Retention, urine) 788.20
 venous 459.81
State
 affective and paranoid, mixed, organic psychotic 294.8
 agitated 307.9
  acute reaction to stress 308.2
 anxiety (neurotic) (*see also* Anxiety) 300.00
  specified type NEC 300.09
 apprehension (*see also* Anxiety) 300.00
  specified type NEC 300.09
 climacteric, female 627.2
  following induced menopause 627.4
 clouded
  epileptic (*see also* Epilepsy) 345.9 ☑
  paroxysmal (idiopathic) (*see also* Epilepsy) 345.9 ☑
 compulsive (mixed) (with obsession) 300.3
 confusional 298.9
  acute 293.0
   with
    arteriosclerotic dementia 290.41
    presenile brain disease 290.11
    senility 290.3
   alcoholic 291.0
   drug-induced 292.81
  epileptic 293.0
  postoperative 293.9
  reactive (emotional stress) (psychological trauma) 298.2
  subacute 293.1
 constitutional psychopathic 301.9
 convulsive (*see also* Convulsions) 780.39
 depressive NEC 311
  induced by drug 292.84
  neurotic 300.4
 dissociative 300.15
 hallucinatory 780.1
  induced by drug 292.12
 hypercoagulable (primary) 289.81
  secondary 289.82
 hyperdynamic beta-adrenergic circulatory 429.82
 locked-in 344.81
 menopausal 627.2
  artificial 627.4
  following induced menopause 627.4

State — *continued*
 neurotic NEC 300.9
  with depersonalization episode 300.6
 obsessional 300.3
 oneiroid (*see also* Schizophrenia) 295.4 ☑
 panic 300.01
 paranoid 297.9
  alcohol-induced 291.5
  arteriosclerotic 290.42
  climacteric 297.2
  drug-induced 292.11
  in
   presenile brain disease 290.12
   senile brain disease 290.20
  involutional 297.2
  menopausal 297.2
  senile 290.20
  simple 297.0
 postleukotomy 310.0
 pregnant (*see also* Pregnancy) V22.2
 psychogenic, twilight 298.2
 psychotic, organic (*see also* Psychosis, organic) 294.9
  mixed paranoid and affective 294.8
  senile or presenile NEC 290.9
  transient NEC 293.9
   with
    anxiety 293.84
    delusions 293.81
    depression 293.83
    hallucinations 293.82
 residual schizophrenic (*see also* Schizophrenia) 295.6 ☑
 tension (*see also* Anxiety) 300.9
 transient organic psychotic 293.9
  anxiety type 293.84
  depressive type 293.83
  hallucinatory type 293.83
  paranoid type 293.81
  specified type NEC 293.89
 twilight
  epileptic 293.0
  psychogenic 298.2
 vegetative (persistent) 780.03
Status (post)
 absence
  epileptic (*see also* Epilepsy) 345.2
  of organ, acquired (postsurgical) — *see* Absence, by site, acquired
 administration of tPA(rtPA) in a different institution within the last 24 hours prior to admission to facility V45.88
 anastomosis of intestine (for bypass) V45.3
 anginosus 413.9
 angioplasty, percutaneous transluminal coronary V45.82
 ankle prosthesis V43.66
 aortocoronary bypass or shunt V45.81
 arthrodesis V45.4
 artificially induced condition NEC V45.89
 artificial opening (of) V44.9
  gastrointestinal tract NEC V44.4
  specified site NEC V44.8
  urinary tract NEC V44.6
  vagina V44.7
 aspirator V46.0
 asthmaticus (*see also* Asthma) 493.9 ☑
 awaiting organ transplant V49.83
 bariatric surgery V45.86
  complicating pregnancy, childbirth, or the puerperium 649.2 ☑
 bed confinement V49.84
 breast
  correction V43.82
  implant removal V45.83
  reconstruction V43.82
 cardiac
  device (in situ) V45.00
   carotid sinus V45.09
    fitting or adjustment V53.39
   defibrillator, automatic implantable (with synchronous cardiac pacemaker) V45.02
   pacemaker V45.01
    fitting or adjustment V53.31
 carotid sinus stimulator V45.09

☑ **Additional Digit Required** — Refer to the Tabular List for Digit Selection   ⬇ **Subterms under main terms may continue to next column or page**

262 — Volume 2   ▶◀ **Revised Text**   ● **New Line**   ▲ **Revised Code**   2013 ICD-9-CM

Status — continued
  cataract extraction V45.61
  chemotherapy V66.2
    current V58.69
  circumcision, female 629.20
  clitorectomy (female genital mutilation type
      I) 629.21
    with excision of labia minora (female
        genital mutilation type II) 629.22
  colonization — see Carrier (suspected) of
  colostomy V44.3
  contraceptive device V45.59
    intrauterine V45.51
    subdermal V45.52
  convulsivus idiopathicus (see also Epilepsy)
      345.3
  coronary artery bypass or shunt V45.81
  cutting
    female genital 629.20
      specified NEC 629.29
      type I 629.21
      type II 629.22
      type III 629.23
      type IV 629.29
  cystostomy V44.50
    appendico-vesicostomy V44.52
    cutaneous-vesicostomy V44.51
    specified type NEC V44.59
  defibrillator, automatic implantable cardiac
      (with synchronous cardiac pacemak-
      er) V45.02
  delinquent immunization V15.83
  dental crowns V45.84
  dental fillings V45.84
  dental restoration V45.84
  dental sealant V49.82
  dialysis (hemo) (peritoneal) V45.11
  donor V59.9
  do not resuscitate V49.86
  drug therapy or regimen V67.59
    high-risk medication NEC V67.51
  elbow prosthesis V43.62
  embedded
    fragment — see Foreign body, retained
    splinter — see Foreign body, retained
  enterostomy V44.4
  epileptic, epilepticus (absence) (grand mal)
      (see also Epilepsy) 345.3
    focal motor 345.7 ☑
    partial 345.7 ☑
    petit mal 345.2
    psychomotor 345.7 ☑
    temporal lobe 345.7 ☑
  estrogen receptor
    negative [ER-] V86.1
    positive [ER+] V86.0
  explantation of joint prosthesis NEC V88.29
    hip V88.21
    knee V88.22
  eye (adnexa) surgery V45.69
  female genital
    cutting 629.20
      specified NEC 629.29
      type I 629.21
      type II 629.22
      type III 629.23
      type IV 629.29
    mutilation 629.20
      type I 629.21
      type II 629.22
      type III 629.23
      type IV 629.29
  filtering bleb (eye) (postglaucoma) V45.69
    with rupture or complication 997.99
    postcataract extraction (complication)
        997.99
  finger joint prosthesis V43.69
  foster care V60.81
  gastric
    banding V45.86
      complicating pregnancy, childbirth,
          or the puerperium 649.2 ☑
    bypass for obesity V45.86
      complicating pregnancy, childbirth,
          or the puerperium 649.2 ☑
  gastrostomy V44.1

Status — continued
  grand mal 345.3
  heart valve prosthesis V43.3
  hemodialysis V45.11
  hip prosthesis (joint) (partial) (total) V43.64
    explantation V88.21
  hysterectomy V88.01
    partial with remaining cervical stump
        V88.02
    total V88.01
  ileostomy V44.2
  infibulation (female genital mutilation type
      III) 629.23
  insulin pump V45.85
  intestinal bypass V45.3
  intrauterine contraceptive device V45.51
  jejunostomy V44.4
  joint prosthesis NEC V43.69
    explantation V88.29
  knee joint prosthesis V43.65
    explantation V88.22
  lacunaris 437.8
  lacunosis 437.8
  lapsed immunization schedule V15.83
  low birth weight V21.30
    less than 500 grams V21.31
    1000–1499 grams V21.33
    1500–1999 grams V21.34
    2000–2500 grams V21.35
    500–999 grams V21.32
  lymphaticus 254.8
  malignant neoplasm, ablated or excised —
      see History, malignant neoplasm
  marmoratus 333.79
  military deployment V62.22
  mutilation, female 629.20
    type I 629.21
    type II 629.22
    type III 629.23
    type IV 629.29
  nephrostomy V44.6
  neuropacemaker NEC V45.89
    brain V45.89
    carotid sinus V45.09
    neurologic NEC V45.89
  obesity surgery V45.86
    complicating pregnancy, childbirth, or
        the puerperium 649.2 ☑
  organ replacement
    by artificial or mechanical device or
        prosthesis of
      artery V43.4
      artificial skin V43.83
      bladder V43.5
      blood vessel V43.4
      breast V43.82
      eye globe V43.0
      heart
        assist device V43.21
        fully implantable artificial heart
            V43.22
        valve V43.3
      intestine V43.89
      joint V43.60
        ankle V43.66
        elbow V43.62
        finger V43.69
        hip (partial) (total) V43.64
        knee V43.65
        shoulder V43.61
        specified NEC V43.69
        wrist V43.63
      kidney V43.89
      larynx V43.81
      lens V43.1
      limb(s) V43.7
      liver V43.89
      lung V43.89
      organ NEC V43.89
      pancreas V43.89
      skin (artificial) V43.83
      tissue NEC V43.89
      vein V43.4
    by organ transplant (heterologous) (ho-
        mologous) — see Status, trans-
        plant

Status — continued
  pacemaker
    brain V45.89
    cardiac V45.01
    carotid sinus V45.09
    neurologic NEC V45.89
    specified site NEC V45.89
  percutaneous transluminal coronary angio-
      plasty V45.82
  peritoneal dialysis V45.11
  petit mal 345.2
  physical restraints V49.87
  postcommotio cerebri 310.2
  postmenopausal (age related) (natural)
      V49.81
  postoperative NEC V45.89
  postpartum NEC V24.2
    care immediately following delivery
        V24.0
    routine follow-up V24.2
  postsurgical NEC V45.89
  renal dialysis V45.11
    noncompliance V45.12
  respirator [ventilator] V46.11
    encounter
      during
        mechanical failure V46.14
        power failure V46.12
      for weaning V46.13
  retained foreign body — see Foreign body,
      retained
  reversed jejunal transposition (for bypass)
      V45.3
  sex reassignment surgery (see also Trans-
      sexualism) 302.50
  shoulder prosthesis V43.61
  shunt
    aortocoronary bypass V45.81
    arteriovenous (for dialysis) V45.11
    cerebrospinal fluid V45.2
    vascular NEC V45.89
      aortocoronary (bypass) V45.81
    ventricular (communicating) (for
        drainage) V45.2
  sterilization
    tubal ligation V26.51
    vasectomy V26.52
  subdermal contraceptive device V45.52
  thymicolymphaticus 254.8
  thymicus 254.8
  thymolymphaticus 254.8
  tooth extraction 525.10
  tracheostomy V44.0
  transplant
    blood vessel V42.89
    bone V42.4
      marrow V42.81
    cornea V42.5
    heart V42.1
      valve V42.2
    intestine V42.84
    kidney V42.0
    liver V42.7
    lung V42.6
    organ V42.9
      removal (due to complication, failure,
          rejection or infection) V45.87
      specified site NEC V42.89
    pancreas V42.83
    peripheral stem cells V42.82
    skin V42.3
    stem cells, peripheral V42.82
    tissue V42.9
      specified type NEC V42.89
    vessel, blood V42.89
  tubal ligation V26.51
  ureterostomy V44.6
  urethrostomy V44.6
  vagina, artificial V44.7
  vascular shunt NEC V45.89
    aortocoronary (bypass) V45.81
  vasectomy V26.52
  ventilator [respirator] V46.11

Status — continued
  ventilator [respirator] — continued
    encounter
      during
        mechanical failure V46.14
        power failure V46.12
      for weaning V46.13
  wheelchair confinement V46.3
  wrist prosthesis V43.63
Stave fracture — see Fracture, metacarpus,
    metacarpal bone(s)
Steal
  subclavian artery 435.2
  vertebral artery 435.1
Stealing, solitary, child problem — see also
    Disturbance, conduct 312.1 ☑
Steam burn — see Burn, by site
Steatocystoma multiplex 706.2
Steatoma (infected) 706.2
  eyelid (cystic) 374.84
    infected 373.13
Steatorrhea (chronic) 579.8
  with lacteal obstruction 579.2
  idiopathic 579.0
    adult 579.0
    infantile 579.0
  pancreatic 579.4
  primary 579.0
  secondary 579.8
  specified cause NEC 579.8
  tropical 579.1
Steatosis 272.8
  heart (see also Degeneration, myocardial)
      429.1
  kidney 593.89
  liver 571.8
Steele-Richardson (-Olszewski) Syndrome
    333.0
Steinbrocker's syndrome — see also Neuropa-
    thy, peripheral, autonomic 337.9
Steinert's disease 359.21
Stein-Leventhal syndrome (polycystic ovary)
    256.4
Stein's syndrome (polycystic ovary) 256.4
STEMI (ST elevation myocardial infarction) —
    see also — Infarct, myocardium, ST ele-
    vation 410.9 ☑
Stenocardia — see also Angina 413.9
Stenocephaly 756.0
Stenosis (cicatricial) — see also Stricture
  ampulla of Vater 576.2
    with calculus, cholelithiasis, or stones —
        see Choledocholithiasis
  anus, anal (canal) (sphincter) 569.2
    congenital 751.2
  aorta (ascending) 747.22
    arch 747.10
    arteriosclerotic 440.0
    calcified 440.0
  aortic (valve) 424.1
    with
      mitral (valve)
        insufficiency or incompetence
            396.2
        stenosis or obstruction 396.0
    atypical 396.0
    congenital 746.3
    rheumatic 395.0
      with
        insufficiency, incompetency or
            regurgitation 395.2
          with mitral (valve) disease
              396.8
        mitral (valve)
          disease (stenosis) 396.0
          insufficiency or incompetence
              396.2
          stenosis or obstruction 396.0
    specified cause, except rheumatic 424.1
    syphilitic 093.22
  aqueduct of Sylvius (congenital) 742.3
    with spina bifida (see also Spina bifida)
        741.0 ☑
    acquired 331.4
  artery NEC (see also Arteriosclerosis) 447.1
    basilar — see Narrowing, artery, basilar

Status — Stenosis

☑ Additional Digit Required — Refer to the Tabular List for Digit Selection   ▼ Subterms under main terms may continue to next column or page

2013 ICD-9-CM   ▶◀ Revised Text   ● New Line   ▲ Revised Code   Volume 2 — 263

Stomatitis — *continued*
  angular — *continued*
    due to dietary or vitamin deficiency 266.0
  aphthous 528.2
  bovine 059.11
  candidal 112.0
  catarrhal 528.00
  denture 528.9
  diphtheritic (membranous) 032.0
  due to
    dietary deficiency 266.0
    thrush 112.0
    vitamin deficiency 266.0
  epidemic 078.4
  epizootic 078.4
  follicular 528.00
  gangrenous 528.1
  herpetic 054.2
  herpetiformis 528.2
  malignant 528.00
  membranous acute 528.00
  monilial 112.0
  mycotic 112.0
  necrotic 528.1
    ulcerative 101
  necrotizing ulcerative 101
  parasitic 112.0
  septic 528.00
  specified NEC 528.09
  spirochetal 101
  suppurative (acute) 528.00
  ulcerative 528.00
    necrotizing 101
  ulceromembranous 101
  vesicular 528.00
    with exanthem 074.3
  Vincent's 101
Stomatocytosis 282.8
Stomatomycosis 112.0
Stomatorrhagia 528.9
Stone(s) — *see also* Calculus
  bladder 594.1
    diverticulum 594.0
  cystine 270.0
  heart syndrome (*see also* Failure, ventricular, left) 428.1
  kidney 592.0
  prostate 602.0
  pulp (dental) 522.2
  renal 592.0
  salivary duct or gland (any) 527.5
  ureter 592.1
  urethra (impacted) 594.2
  urinary (duct) (impacted) (passage) 592.9
    bladder 594.1
      diverticulum 594.0
    lower tract NEC 594.9
    specified site 594.8
  xanthine 277.2
Stonecutters' lung 502
  tuberculous (*see also* Tuberculosis) 011.4 ☑
Stonemasons'
  asthma, disease, or lung 502
    tuberculous (*see also* Tuberculosis) 011.4 ☑
  phthisis (*see also* Tuberculosis) 011.4 ☑
Stoppage
  bowel (*see also* Obstruction, intestine) 560.9
  heart (*see also* Arrest, cardiac) 427.5
  intestine (*see also* Obstruction, intestine) 560.9
  urine NEC (*see also* Retention, urine) 788.20
Storm, thyroid (apathetic) — *see also* Thyrotoxicosis 242.9 ☑
Strabismus (alternating) (congenital) (nonparalytic) 378.9
  concomitant (*see also* Heterotropia) 378.30
    convergent (*see also* Esotropia) 378.00
    divergent (*see also* Exotropia) 378.10
  convergent (*see also* Esotropia) 378.00
  divergent (*see also* Exotropia) 378.10
  due to adhesions, scars — *see* Strabismus, mechanical
  in neuromuscular disorder NEC 378.73
    intermittent 378.20

Strabismus — *continued*
  in neuromuscular disorder — *continued*
    intermittent — *continued*
      vertical 378.31
  latent 378.40
    convergent (esophoria) 378.41
    divergent (exophoria) 378.42
    vertical 378.43
  mechanical 378.60
    due to
      Brown's tendon sheath syndrome 378.61
      specified musculofascial disorder NEC 378.62
  paralytic 378.50
    third or oculomotor nerve (partial) 378.51
      total 378.52
    fourth or trochlear nerve 378.53
    sixth or abducens nerve 378.54
  specified type NEC 378.73
  vertical (hypertropia) 378.31
Strain — *see also* Sprain, by site
  eye NEC 368.13
  heart — *see* Disease, heart
  meaning gonorrhea — *see* Gonorrhea
  on urination 788.65
  physical NEC V62.89
  postural 729.90
  psychological NEC V62.89
Strands
  conjunctiva 372.62
  vitreous humor 379.25
Strangulation, strangulated 994.7
  appendix 543.9
  asphyxiation or suffocation by 994.7
  bladder neck 596.0
  bowel — *see* Strangulation, intestine
  colon — *see* Strangulation, intestine
  cord (umbilical) — *see* Compression, umbilical cord
  due to birth injury 767.8
  food or foreign body (*see also* Asphyxia, food) 933.1
  hemorrhoids 455.8
    external 455.5
    internal 455.2
  hernia (*see also* Hernia, by site, with obstruction)
    gangrenous — *see* Hernia, by site, with gangrene
  intestine (large) (small) 560.2
    with hernia (*see also* Hernia, by site, with obstruction)
      gangrenous — *see* Hernia, by site, with gangrene
    congenital (small) 751.1
      large 751.2
  mesentery 560.2
  mucus (*see also* Asphyxia, mucus) 933.1
    newborn 770.18
  omentum 560.2
  organ or site, congenital NEC — *see* Atresia
  ovary 620.8
    due to hernia 620.4
  penis 607.89
    foreign body 939.3
  rupture (*see also* Hernia, by site, with obstruction) 552.9
    gangrenous (*see also* Hernia, by site, with gangrene) 551.9
  stomach, due to hernia (*see also* Hernia, by site, with obstruction) 552.9
    with gangrene (*see also* Hernia, by site, with gangrene) 551.9
  umbilical cord — *see* Compression, umbilical cord
  vesicourethral orifice 596.0
Strangury 788.1
Strawberry
  gallbladder (*see also* Disease, gallbladder) 575.6
  mark 757.32
  tongue (red) (white) 529.3
Straw itch 133.8
Streak, ovarian 752.0

Strephosymbolia 315.01
  secondary to organic lesion 784.69
Streptobacillary fever 026.1
Streptobacillus moniliformis 026.1
Streptococcemia 038.0
Streptococcicosis — *see* Infection, streptococcal
Streptococcus, streptococcal — *see* condition
Streptoderma 686.00
Streptomycosis — *see* Actinomycosis
Streptothricosis — *see* Actinomycosis
Streptothrix — *see* Actinomycosis
Streptotrichosis — *see* Actinomycosis
Stress 308.9
  fracture — *see* Fracture, stress
  polycythemia 289.0
  reaction (gross) (*see also* Reaction, stress, acute) 308.9
Stretching, nerve — *see* Injury, nerve, by site
Striae (albicantes) (atrophicae) (cutis distensae) (distensae) 701.3
Striations of nails 703.8
Stricture — *see also* Stenosis 799.89
  ampulla of Vater 576.2
    with calculus, cholelithiasis, or stones — *see* Choledocholithiasis
  anus (sphincter) 569.2
    congenital 751.2
    infantile 751.2
  aorta (ascending) 747.22
    arch 747.10
    arteriosclerotic 440.0
    calcified 440.0
  aortic (valve) (*see also* Stenosis, aortic) 424.1
    congenital 746.3
  aqueduct of Sylvius (congenital) 742.3
    with spina bifida (*see also* Spina bifida) 741.0 ☑
    acquired 331.4
  artery 447.1
    basilar — *see* Narrowing, artery, basilar
    carotid (common) (internal) — *see* Narrowing, artery, carotid
    celiac 447.4
    cerebral 437.0
      congenital 747.81
      due to
        embolism (*see also* Embolism, brain) 434.1 ☑
        thrombus (*see also* Thrombosis, brain) 434.0 ☑
    congenital (peripheral) 747.60
      cerebral 747.81
      coronary 746.85
      gastrointestinal 747.61
      lower limb 747.64
      renal 747.62
      retinal 743.58
      specified NEC 747.69
      spinal 747.82
      umbilical 747.5
      upper limb 747.63
    coronary — *see* Arteriosclerosis, coronary
      congenital 746.85
    precerebral — *see* Narrowing, artery, precerebral NEC
    pulmonary (congenital) 747.31
      acquired 417.8
    renal 440.1
    vertebral — *see* Narrowing, artery, vertebral
  auditory canal (congenital) (external) 744.02
    acquired (*see also* Stricture, ear canal, acquired) 380.50
  bile duct or passage (any) (postoperative) (*see also* Obstruction, biliary) 576.2
    congenital 751.61
  bladder 596.89
    congenital 753.6
    neck 596.0
      congenital 753.6
  bowel (*see also* Obstruction, intestine) 560.9
  brain 348.89
  bronchus 519.19
    syphilitic 095.8

Stricture — *see also* Stenosis — *continued*
  cardia (stomach) 537.89
    congenital 750.7
  cardiac (*see also* Disease, heart)
    orifice (stomach) 537.89
  cardiovascular (*see also* Disease, cardiovascular) 429.2
  carotid artery — *see* Narrowing, artery, carotid
  cecum (*see also* Obstruction, intestine) 560.9
  cervix, cervical (canal) 622.4
    congenital 752.49
    in pregnancy or childbirth 654.6 ☑
      affecting fetus or newborn 763.89
      causing obstructed labor 660.2 ☑
        affecting fetus or newborn 763.1
  colon (*see also* Obstruction, intestine) 560.9
    congenital 751.2
  colostomy 569.62
  common bile duct (*see also* Obstruction, biliary) 576.2
    congenital 751.61
  coronary (artery) — *see* Arteriosclerosis, coronary
    congenital 746.85
  cystic duct (*see also* Obstruction, gallbladder) 575.2
    congenital 751.61
  cystostomy 596.83
  digestive organs NEC, congenital 751.8
  duodenum 537.3
    congenital 751.1
  ear canal (external) (congenital) 744.02
    acquired 380.50
      secondary to
        inflammation 380.53
        surgery 380.52
        trauma 380.51
  ejaculatory duct 608.85
  enterostomy 569.62
  esophagostomy 530.87
  esophagus (corrosive) (peptic) 530.3
    congenital 750.3
    syphilitic 095.8
      congenital 090.5
  eustachian tube (*see also* Obstruction, Eustachian tube) 381.60
    congenital 744.24
  fallopian tube 628.2
    gonococcal (chronic) 098.37
      acute 098.17
    tuberculous (*see also* Tuberculosis) 016.6 ☑
  gallbladder (*see also* Obstruction, gallbladder) 575.2
    congenital 751.69
  glottis 478.74
  heart (*see also* Disease, heart)
    congenital NEC 746.89
    valve (*see also* Endocarditis)
      congenital NEC 746.89
        aortic 746.3
        mitral 746.5
        pulmonary 746.02
        tricuspid 746.1
  hepatic duct (*see also* Obstruction, biliary) 576.2
  hourglass, of stomach 537.6
  hymen 623.3
  hypopharynx 478.29
  intestine (*see also* Obstruction, intestine) 560.9
    congenital (small) 751.1
      large 751.2
    ischemic 557.1
  lacrimal
    canaliculi 375.53
      congenital 743.65
    punctum 375.52
      congenital 743.65
    sac 375.54
      congenital 743.65
  lacrimonasal duct 375.56
    congenital 743.65
    neonatal 375.55
  larynx 478.79

☑ Additional Digit Required — Refer to the Tabular List for Digit Selection   ▒ Subterms under main terms may continue to next column or page

2013 ICD-9-CM   ▶◀ Revised Text   ● New Line   ▲ Revised Code   Volume 2 — 265

Index

Stricture — Subtentorial

Stricture — see also Stenosis — continued
  larynx — continued
    congenital 748.3
    syphilitic 095.8
      congenital 090.5
  lung 518.89
  meatus
    ear (congenital) 744.02
      acquired (see also Stricture, ear canal, acquired) 380.50
      osseous (congenital) (ear) 744.03
        acquired (see also Stricture, ear canal, acquired) 380.50
    urinarius (see also Stricture, urethra) 598.9
      congenital 753.6
  mitral (valve) (see also Stenosis, mitral) 394.0
    congenital 746.5
    specified cause, except rheumatic 424.0
  myocardium, myocardial (see also Degeneration, myocardial) 429.1
    hypertrophic subaortic (idiopathic) 425.11
  nares (anterior) (posterior) 478.19
    congenital 748.0
  nasal duct 375.56
    congenital 743.65
    neonatal 375.55
  nasolacrimal duct 375.56
    congenital 743.65
    neonatal 375.55
  nasopharynx 478.29
    syphilitic 095.8
  nephrostomy 997.5
  nose 478.19
    congenital 748.0
  nostril (anterior) (posterior) 478.19
    congenital 748.0
  organ or site, congenital NEC — see Atresia
  osseous meatus (congenital) (ear) 744.03
    acquired (see also Stricture, ear canal, acquired) 380.50
  os uteri (see also Stricture, cervix) 622.4
  oviduct — see Stricture, fallopian tube
  pelviureteric junction 593.3
  pharynx (dilation) 478.29
  prostate 602.8
  pulmonary, pulmonic
    artery (congenital) 747.31
      acquired 417.8
      noncongenital 417.8
    infundibulum (congenital) 746.83
    valve (see also Endocarditis, pulmonary) 424.3
      congenital 746.02
    vein (congenital) 747.49
      acquired 417.8
    vessel NEC 417.8
  punctum lacrimale 375.52
    congenital 743.65
  pylorus (hypertrophic) 537.0
    adult 537.0
    congenital 750.5
    infantile 750.5
  rectosigmoid 569.89
  rectum (sphincter) 569.2
    congenital 751.2
    due to
      chemical burn 947.3
      irradiation 569.2
      lymphogranuloma venereum 099.1
    gonococcal 098.7
    inflammatory 099.1
    syphilitic 095.8
    tuberculous (see also Tuberculosis) 014.8 ☑
  renal artery 440.1
  salivary duct or gland (any) 527.8
  sigmoid (flexure) (see also Obstruction, intestine) 560.9
  spermatic cord 608.85
  stoma (following) (of)
    colostomy 569.62
    cystostomy 596.83
    enterostomy 569.62
    esophagostomy 530.87

Stricture — see also Stenosis — continued
  stoma — continued
    gastrostomy 536.42
    ileostomy 569.62
    nephrostomy 997.5
    tracheostomy 519.02
    ureterostomy 997.5
  stomach 537.89
    congenital 750.7
    hourglass 537.6
  subaortic 746.81
    hypertrophic (acquired) (idiopathic) 425.11
  subglottic 478.74
  syphilitic NEC 095.8
  tendon (sheath) 727.81
  trachea 519.19
    congenital 748.3
    syphilitic 095.8
    tuberculous (see also Tuberculosis) 012.8 ☑
  tracheostomy 519.02
  tricuspid (valve) (see also Endocarditis, tricuspid) 397.0
    congenital 746.1
    nonrheumatic 424.2
  tunica vaginalis 608.85
  ureter (postoperative) 593.3
    congenital 753.29
    tuberculous (see also Tuberculosis) 016.2 ☑
  ureteropelvic junction 593.3
    congenital 753.21
  ureterovesical orifice 593.3
    congenital 753.22
  urethra (anterior) (meatal) (organic) (posterior) (spasmodic) 598.9
    associated with schistosomiasis (see also Schistosomiasis) 120.9 [598.01]
    congenital (valvular) 753.6
    due to
      infection 598.00
        syphilis 095.8 [598.01]
      trauma 598.1
    gonococcal 098.2 [598.01]
    gonorrheal 098.2 [598.01]
    infective 598.00
    late effect of injury 598.1
    postcatheterization 598.2
    postobstetric 598.1
    postoperative 598.2
    specified cause NEC 598.8
    syphilitic 095.8 [598.01]
    traumatic 598.1
    valvular, congenital 753.6
  urinary meatus (see also Stricture, urethra) 598.9
    congenital 753.6
  uterus, uterine 621.5
    os (external) (internal) — see Stricture, cervix
  vagina (outlet) 623.2
    congenital 752.49
  valve (cardiac) (heart) (see also Endocarditis) 424.90
    congenital (cardiac) (heart) NEC 746.89
      aortic 746.3
      mitral 746.5
      pulmonary 746.02
      tricuspid 746.1
      urethra 753.6
  valvular (see also Endocarditis) 424.90
  vascular graft or shunt 996.1
    atherosclerosis — see Arteriosclerosis, extremities
    embolism 996.74
    occlusion NEC 996.74
    thrombus 996.74
  vas deferens 608.85
    congenital 752.89
  vein 459.2
  vena cava (inferior) (superior) NEC 459.2
    congenital 747.49
  ventricular shunt 996.2
  vesicourethral orifice 596.0
    congenital 753.6

Stricture — see also Stenosis — continued
  vulva (acquired) 624.8
Stridor 786.1
  congenital (larynx) 748.3
Stridulous — see condition
Strippling of nails 703.8
Stroke 434.91
  apoplectic (see also Disease, cerebrovascular, acute) 436
  brain — see Infarct, brain
  embolic 434.11
  epileptic — see Epilepsy
  healed or old V12.54
  heart — see Disease, heart
  heat 992.0
  hemorrhagic — see Hemorrhage, brain
  iatrogenic 997.02
  in evolution 434.91
  ischemic 434.91
  late effect — see Late effect(s) (of) cerebrovascular disease
  lightning 994.0
  paralytic — see Infarct, brain
  postoperative 997.02
  progressive 435.9
  thrombotic 434.01
Stromatosis, endometrial (M8931/1) 236.0
Strong pulse 785.9
Strongyloides stercoralis infestation 127.2
Strongyloidiasis 127.2
Strongyloidosis 127.2
Strongylus (gibsoni) infestation 127.7
Strophulus (newborn) 779.89
  pruriginosus 698.2
Struck by lightning 994.0
Struma — see also Goiter 240.9
  fibrosa 245.3
  Hashimoto (struma lymphomatosa) 245.2
  lymphomatosa 245.2
  nodosa (simplex) 241.9
    endemic 241.9
    multinodular 241.1
    sporadic 241.9
    toxic or with hyperthyroidism 242.3 ☑
      multinodular 242.2 ☑
      uninodular 242.1 ☑
    toxicosa 242.3 ☑
      multinodular 242.2 ☑
      uninodular 242.1 ☑
    uninodular 241.0
  ovarii (M9090/0) 220
    and carcinoid (M9091/1) 236.2
    malignant (M9090/3) 183.0
  Riedel's (ligneous thyroiditis) 245.3
  scrofulous (see also Tuberculosis) 017.2 ☑
  tuberculous (see also Tuberculosis) 017.2 ☑
    abscess 017.2 ☑
    adenitis 017.2 ☑
    lymphangitis 017.2 ☑
    ulcer 017.2 ☑
Strumipriva cachexia — see also Hypothyroidism 244.9
Strümpell-Marie disease or spine (ankylosing spondylitis) 720.0
Strümpell-Westphal pseudosclerosis (hepatolenticular degeneration) 275.1
Stuart's disease (congenital factor X deficiency) — see also Defect, coagulation 286.3
Stuart-Prower factor deficiency (congenital factor X deficiency) — see also Defect, coagulation 286.3
Students' elbow 727.2
Stuffy nose 478.19
Stump — see also Amputation
  cervix, cervical (healed) 622.8
Stupor 780.09
  catatonic (see also Schizophrenia) 295.2 ☑
  circular (see also Psychosis, manic-depressive, circular) 296.7
  manic 296.89
  manic-depressive (see also Psychosis, affective) 296.89
  mental (anergic) (delusional) 298.9
  psychogenic 298.8
  reaction to exceptional stress (transient) 308.2

Stupor — continued
  traumatic NEC (see also Injury, intracranial)
    with spinal (cord)
      lesion — see Injury, spinal, by site
      shock — see Injury, spinal, by site
Sturge (-Weber) (-Dimitri) disease or syndrome (encephalocutaneous angiomatosis) 759.6
Sturge-Kalischer-Weber syndrome (encephalocutaneous angiomatosis) 759.6
Stuttering 315.35
  adult onset 307.0
  childhood onset 315.35
  due to late effect of cerebrovascular disease (see also Late effect(s) (of) cerebrovascular disease) 438.14
  in conditions classified elsewhere 784.52
Sty, stye 373.11
  external 373.11
  internal 373.12
  meibomian 373.12
Subacidity, gastric 536.8
  psychogenic 306.4
Subacute — see condition
Subarachnoid — see condition
Subclavian steal syndrome 435.2
Subcortical — see condition
Subcostal syndrome 098.86
  nerve compression 354.8
Subcutaneous, subcuticular — see condition
Subdelirium 293.1
Subdural — see condition
Subendocardium — see condition
Subependymoma (M9383/1) 237.5
Suberosis 495.3
Subglossitis — see Glossitis
Subhemophilia 286.0
Subinvolution (uterus) 621.1
  breast (postlactational) (postpartum) 611.89
  chronic 621.1
  puerperal, postpartum 674.8 ☑
Sublingual — see condition
Sublinguitis 527.2
Subluxation — see also Dislocation, by site
  congenital NEC (see also Malposition, congenital)
    hip (unilateral) 754.32
      with dislocation of other hip 754.35
      bilateral 754.33
    joint
      lower limb 755.69
      shoulder 755.59
      upper limb 755.59
  lower limb (joint) 755.69
  shoulder (joint) 755.59
  upper limb (joint) 755.59
  lens 379.32
    anterior 379.33
    posterior 379.34
  radial head 832.2
  rotary, cervical region of spine — see Fracture, vertebra, cervical
Submaxillary — see condition
Submersion (fatal) (nonfatal) 994.1
Submissiveness (undue), in child 313.0
Submucous — see condition
Subnormal, subnormality
  accommodation (see also Disorder, accommodation) 367.9
  mental (see also Disability, intellectual) 319
    mild 317
    moderate 318.0
    profound 318.2
    severe 318.1
  temperature (accidental) 991.6
    not associated with low environmental temperature 780.99
Subphrenic — see condition
Subscapular nerve — see condition
Subseptus uterus 752.35
Subsiding appendicitis 542
Substance abuse in family V61.42
Substernal thyroid — see also Goiter 240.9
  congenital 759.2
Substitution disorder 300.11
Subtentorial — see condition

Subtertian
  fever 084.0
  malaria (fever) 084.0
Subthyroidism (acquired) — *see also* Hypothyroidism 244.9
  congenital 243
Succenturiata placenta — *see* Placenta, abnormal
Succussion sounds, chest 786.7
Sucking thumb, child 307.9
Sudamen 705.1
Sudamina 705.1
Sudanese kala-azar 085.0
Sudden
  death, cause unknown (less than 24 hours) 798.1
    cardiac (SCD)
      family history of V17.41
      personal history of, successfully resuscitated V12.53
    during childbirth 669.9 ☑
    infant 798.0
    puerperal, postpartum 674.9 ☑
  hearing loss NEC 388.2
  heart failure (*see also* Failure, heart) 428.9
  infant death syndrome 798.0
Sudeck's atrophy, disease, or syndrome 733.7
SUDS (sudden unexplained death) 798.2
Suffocation — *see also* Asphyxia 799.01
  by
    bed clothes 994.7
    bunny bag 994.7
    cave-in 994.7
    constriction 994.7
    drowning 994.1
    inhalation
      food or foreign body (*see also* Asphyxia, food or foreign body) 933.1
      oil or gasoline (*see also* Asphyxia, food or foreign body) 933.1
    overlying 994.7
    plastic bag 994.7
    pressure 994.7
    strangulation 994.7
  during birth 768.1
  mechanical 994.7
Sugar
  blood
    high 790.29
    low 251.2
  in urine 791.5
Suicide, suicidal (attempted)
  by poisoning — *see* Table of Drugs and Chemicals
  ideation V62.84
  risk 300.9
  tendencies 300.9
  trauma NEC (*see also* nature and site of injury) 959.9
Suipestifer infection — *see also* Infection, Salmonella 003.9
Sulfatidosis 330.0
Sulfhemoglobinemia, sulphemoglobinemia (acquired) (congenital) 289.7
Sumatran mite fever 081.2
Summer — *see* condition
Sunburn 692.71
  first degree 692.71
  second degree 692.76
  third degree 692.77
  dermatitis 692.71
  due to
    other ultraviolet radiation 692.82
    tanning bed 692.82
SUNCT (short lasting unilateral neuralgiform headache with conjunctival injection and tearing) 339.05
Sunken
  acetabulum 718.85
  fontanels 756.0
Sunstroke 992.0
Superfecundation 651.9 ☑
  with fetal loss and retention of one or more fetus(es) 651.6 ☑
  following (elective) fetal reduction 651.7 ☑

Superfetation 651.9 ☑
  with fetal loss and retention of one or more fetus(es) 651.6 ☑
  following (elective) fetal reduction 651.7 ☑
Superinvolution uterus 621.8
Supernumerary (congenital)
  aortic cusps 746.89
  auditory ossicles 744.04
  bone 756.9
  breast 757.6
  carpal bones 755.56
  cusps, heart valve NEC 746.89
    mitral 746.5
    pulmonary 746.09
  digit(s) 755.00
    finger 755.01
    toe 755.02
  ear (lobule) 744.1
  fallopian tube 752.19
  finger 755.01
  hymen 752.49
  kidney 753.3
  lacrimal glands 743.64
  lacrimonasal duct 743.65
  lobule (ear) 744.1
  mitral cusps 746.5
  muscle 756.82
  nipples 757.6
  organ or site NEC — *see* Accessory
  ossicles, auditory 744.04
  ovary 752.0
  oviduct 752.19
  pulmonic cusps 746.09
  rib 756.3
    cervical or first 756.2
      syndrome 756.2
  roots (of teeth) 520.2
  spinal vertebra 756.19
  spleen 759.0
  tarsal bones 755.67
  teeth 520.1
    causing crowding 524.31
  testis 752.89
  thumb 755.01
  toe 755.02
  uterus 752.2
  vagina 752.49
  vertebra 756.19
Supervision (of)
  contraceptive method previously prescribed V25.40
    intrauterine device V25.42
    oral contraceptive (pill) V25.41
    specified type NEC V25.49
    subdermal implantable contraceptive V25.43
  dietary (for) V65.3
    allergy (food) V65.3
    colitis V65.3
    diabetes mellitus V65.3
    food allergy intolerance V65.3
    gastritis V65.3
    hypercholesterolemia V65.3
    hypoglycemia V65.3
    intolerance (food) V65.3
    obesity V65.3
    specified NEC V65.3
  lactation V24.1
  newborn health
    8 to 28 days old V20.32
    under 8 days old V20.31
  pregnancy — *see* Pregnancy, supervision of
Supplemental teeth 520.1
  causing crowding 524.31
Suppression
  binocular vision 368.31
  lactation 676.5 ☑
  menstruation 626.8
  ovarian secretion 256.39
  renal 586
  urinary secretion 788.5
  urine 788.5
Suppuration, suppurative — *see also* condition

Suppuration, suppurative — *see also* condition — *continued*
  accessory sinus (chronic) (*see also* Sinusitis) 473.9
  adrenal gland 255.8
  antrum (chronic) (*see also* Sinusitis, maxillary) 473.0
  bladder (*see also* Cystitis) 595.89
  bowel 569.89
  brain 324.0
    late effect 326
  breast 611.0
    puerperal, postpartum 675.1 ☑
  dental periosteum 526.5
  diffuse (skin) 686.00
  ear (middle) (*see also* Otitis media) 382.4
    external (*see also* Otitis, externa) 380.10
    internal 386.33
  ethmoidal (sinus) (chronic) (*see also* Sinusitis, ethmoidal) 473.2
  fallopian tube (*see also* Salpingo-oophoritis) 614.2
  frontal (sinus) (chronic) (*see also* Sinusitis, frontal) 473.1
  gallbladder (*see also* Cholecystitis, acute) 575.0
  gum 523.30
  hernial sac — *see* Hernia, by site
  intestine 569.89
  joint (*see also* Arthritis, suppurative) 711.0 ☑
  labyrinthine 386.33
  lung 513.0
  mammary gland 611.0
    puerperal, postpartum 675.1 ☑
  maxilla, maxillary 526.4
    sinus (chronic) (*see also* Sinusitis, maxillary) 473.0
  muscle 728.0
  nasal sinus (chronic) (*see also* Sinusitis) 473.9
  pancreas 577.0
  parotid gland 527.2
  pelvis, pelvic
    female (*see also* Disease, pelvis, inflammatory) 614.4
      acute 614.3
    male (*see also* Peritonitis) 567.21
  pericranial (*see also* Osteomyelitis) 730.2 ☑
  salivary duct or gland (any) 527.2
  sinus (nasal) (*see also* Sinusitis) 473.9
  sphenoidal (sinus) (chronic) (*see also* Sinusitis, sphenoidal) 473.3
  thymus (gland) 254.1
  thyroid (gland) 245.0
  tonsil 474.8
  uterus (*see also* Endometritis) 615.9
  vagina 616.10
  wound (*see also* Wound, open, by site, complicated)
    dislocation — *see* Dislocation, by site, compound
    fracture — *see* Fracture, by site, open
    scratch or other superficial injury — *see* Injury, superficial, by site
Supraeruption, teeth 524.34
Supraglottitis 464.50
  with obstruction 464.51
Suprapubic drainage 596.89
Suprarenal (gland) — *see* condition
Suprascapular nerve — *see* condition
Suprasellar — *see* condition
Supraspinatus syndrome 726.10
Surfer knots 919.8
  infected 919.9
Surgery
  cosmetic NEC V50.1
    breast reconstruction following mastectomy V51.0
    following healed injury or operation V51.8
    hair transplant V50.0
  elective V50.9
    breast
      augmentation or reduction V50.1
      reconstruction following mastectomy V51.0

Surgery — *continued*
  elective — *continued*
    circumcision, ritual or routine (in absence of medical indication) V50.2
    cosmetic NEC V50.1
    ear piercing V50.3
    face-lift V50.1
    following healed injury or operation V51.8
    hair transplant V50.0
  not done because of
    contraindication V64.1
    patient's decision V64.2
    specified reason NEC V64.3
  plastic
    breast
      augmentation or reduction V50.1
      reconstruction following mastectomy V51.0
    cosmetic V50.1
    face-lift V50.1
    following healed injury or operation V51.8
    repair of scarred tissue (following healed injury or operation) V51.8
    specified type NEC V50.8
  previous, in pregnancy or childbirth
    cervix 654.6 ☑
      affecting fetus or newborn (*see also* Newborn, affected by) 760.63
      causing obstructed labor 660.2 ☑
        affecting fetus or newborn 763.1
    pelvic soft tissues NEC 654.9 ☑
      affecting fetus or newborn (*see also* Newborn, affected by) 760.63
      causing obstructed labor 660.2 ☑
        affecting fetus or newborn 763.1
    perineum or vulva 654.8 ☑
    uterus NEC 654.9 ☑
      affecting fetus or newborn (*see also* Newborn, affected by) 760.63
      causing obstructed labor 660.2 ☑
        affecting fetus or newborn 763.1
      due to previous cesarean delivery 654.2 ☑
    vagina 654.7 ☑
Surgical
  abortion — *see* Abortion, legal
  emphysema 998.81
  kidney (*see also* Pyelitis) 590.80
  operation NEC 799.9
  procedures, complication or misadventure — *see* Complications, surgical procedure
  shock 998.00
Survey
  fetal anatomic V28.81
Susceptibility
  genetic
    to
      MEN (multiple endocrine neoplasia) V84.81
      neoplasia
        multiple endocrine (MEN) V84.81
      neoplasm
        malignant, of
          breast V84.01
          endometrium V84.04
          other V84.09
          ovary V84.02
          prostate V84.03
        specified disease V84.89
Suspected condition, ruled out — *see also* Observation, suspected V71.9
  specified condition NEC V71.89
Suspended uterus, in pregnancy or childbirth 654.4 ☑
  affecting fetus or newborn 763.89
  causing obstructed labor 660.2 ☑
    affecting fetus or newborn 763.1
Sutton and Gull's disease (arteriolar nephrosclerosis) — *see also* Hypertension, kidney 403.90
Sutton's disease 709.09

☑ Additional Digit Required — Refer to the Tabular List for Digit Selection   ▽ Subterms under main terms may continue to next column or page

2013 ICD-9-CM   ►◄ Revised Text   ● New Line   ▲ Revised Code   Volume 2 — 267

Subtertian — Sutton's disease

Suture
burst (in external operation wound) (see also Dehiscence) 998.32
internal 998.31
inadvertently left in operation wound 998.4
removal V58.32
Shirodkar, in pregnancy (with or without cervical incompetence) 654.5 ☑

Swab inadvertently left in operation wound 998.4

Swallowed, swallowing
difficulty (see also Dysphagia) 787.20
foreign body NEC (see also Foreign body) 938

Swamp fever 100.89
Swan neck hand (intrinsic) 736.09
Sweat(s), sweating
disease or sickness 078.2
excessive (see also Hyperhidrosis) 780.8
fetid 705.89
fever 078.2
gland disease 705.9
specified type NEC 705.89
miliary 078.2
night 780.8

Sweeley-Klionsky disease (angiokeratoma corporis diffusum) 272.7
Sweet's syndrome (acute febrile neutrophilic dermatosis) 695.89
Swelling 782.3
abdominal (not referable to specific organ) 789.3 ☑
adrenal gland, cloudy 255.8
ankle 719.07
anus 787.99
arm 729.81
breast 611.72
Calabar 125.2
cervical gland 785.6
cheek 784.2
chest 786.6
ear 388.8
epigastric 789.3 ☑
extremity (lower) (upper) 729.81
eye 379.92
female genital organ 625.8
finger 729.81
foot 729.81
glands 785.6
gum 784.2
hand 729.81
head 784.2
inflammatory — see Inflammation
joint (see also Effusion, joint) 719.0 ☑
tuberculous — see Tuberculosis, joint
kidney, cloudy 593.89
leg 729.81
limb 729.81
liver 573.8
lung 786.6
lymph nodes 785.6
mediastinal 786.6
mouth 784.2
muscle (limb) 729.81
neck 784.2
nose or sinus 784.2
palate 784.2
pelvis 789.3 ☑
penis 607.83
perineum 625.8
rectum 787.99
scrotum 608.86
skin 782.2
splenic (see also Splenomegaly) 789.2
substernal 786.6
superficial, localized (skin) 782.2
testicle 608.86
throat 784.2
toe 729.81
tongue 784.2
tubular (see also Disease, renal) 593.9
umbilicus 789.3 ☑
uterus 625.8
vagina 625.8
vulva 625.8

Swelling — continued
wandering, due to Gnathostoma (spinigerum) 128.1
white — see Tuberculosis, arthritis
Swift's disease 985.0
Swimmers'
ear (acute) 380.12
itch 120.3
Swimming in the head 780.4
Swollen — see also Swelling
glands 785.6
Swyer-James syndrome (unilateral hyperlucent lung) 492.8
Swyer's syndrome (XY pure gonadal dysgenesis) 752.7
Sycosis 704.8
barbae (not parasitic) 704.8
contagiosa 110.0
lupoid 704.8
mycotic 110.0
parasitic 110.0
vulgaris 704.8
Sydenham's chorea — see Chorea, Sydenham's
Sylvatic yellow fever 060.0
Sylvest's disease (epidemic pleurodynia) 074.1
Symblepharon 372.63
congenital 743.62
Symonds' syndrome 348.2
Sympathetic — see condition
Sympatheticotonia — see also Neuropathy, peripheral, autonomic 337.9
Sympathicoblastoma (M9500/3)
specified site — see Neoplasm, by site, malignant
unspecified site 194.0
Sympathicogonioma (M9500/3) — see Sympathicoblastoma
Sympathoblastoma (M9500/3) — see Sympathicoblastoma
Sympathogonioma (M9500/3) — see Sympathicoblastoma
Symphalangy — see also Syndactylism 755.10
Symptoms, specified (general) NEC 780.99
abdomen NEC 789.9
bone NEC 733.90
breast NEC 611.79
cardiac NEC 785.9
cardiovascular NEC 785.9
chest NEC 786.9
cognition 799.59
development NEC 783.9
digestive system NEC 787.99
emotional state NEC 799.29
eye NEC 379.99
gastrointestinal tract NEC 787.99
genital organs NEC
female 625.9
male 608.9
head and neck NEC 784.99
heart NEC 785.9
jaw 784.92
joint NEC 719.60
ankle 719.67
elbow 719.62
foot 719.67
hand 719.64
hip 719.65
knee 719.66
multiple sites 719.69
pelvic region 719.65
shoulder (region) 719.61
specified site NEC 719.68
temporomandibular 524.69
wrist 719.63
larynx NEC 784.99
limbs NEC 729.89
lymphatic system NEC 785.9
maxilla 784.92
menopausal 627.2
metabolism NEC 783.9
mouth NEC 528.9
muscle NEC 728.9
musculoskeletal NEC 781.99
limbs NEC 729.89
nervous system NEC 781.99

Symptoms, specified — continued
neurotic NEC 300.9
nutrition, metabolism, and development NEC 783.9
pelvis NEC 789.9
female 625.9
peritoneum NEC 789.9
respiratory system NEC 786.9
skin and integument NEC 782.9
subcutaneous tissue NEC 782.9
throat NEC 784.99
tonsil NEC 784.99
urinary system NEC 788.99
vascular NEC 785.9
Sympus 759.89
Synarthrosis 719.80
ankle 719.87
elbow 719.82
foot 719.87
hand 719.84
hip 719.85
knee 719.86
multiple sites 719.89
pelvic region 719.85
shoulder (region) 719.81
specified site NEC 719.88
wrist 719.83
Syncephalus 759.4
Synchondrosis 756.9
abnormal (congenital) 756.9
ischiopubic (van Neck's) 732.1
Synchysis (senile) (vitreous humor) 379.21
scintillans 379.22
Syncope (near) (pre-) 780.2
anginosa 413.9
bradycardia 427.89
cardiac 780.2
carotid sinus 337.01
complicating delivery 669.2 ☑
due to lumbar puncture 349.0
fatal 798.1
heart 780.2
heat 992.1
laryngeal 786.2
tussive 786.2
vasoconstriction 780.2
vasodepressor 780.2
vasomotor 780.2
vasovagal 780.2
Syncytial infarct — see Placenta, abnormal
Syndactylism, syndactyly (multiple sites) 755.10
fingers (without fusion of bone) 755.11
with fusion of bone 755.12
toes (without fusion of bone) 755.13
with fusion of bone 755.14
Syndrome — see also Disease
with 5q deletion 238.74
5q minus 238.74
abdominal
acute 789.0 ☑
migraine 346.2 ☑
muscle deficiency 756.79
Abercrombie's (amyloid degeneration) 277.39
abnormal innervation 374.43
abstinence
alcohol 291.81
drug 292.0
neonatal 779.5
Abt-Letterer-Siwe (acute histiocytosis X) (M9722/3) 202.5 ☑
Achard-Thiers (adrenogenital) 255.2
acid pulmonary aspiration 997.39
obstetric (Mendelson's) 668.0 ☑
acquired immune deficiency 042
acquired immunodeficiency 042
acrocephalosyndactylism 755.55
acute abdominal 789.0 ☑
acute chest 517.3
acute coronary 411.1
Adair-Dighton (brittle bones and blue sclera, deafness) 756.51
Adams-Stokes (-Morgagni) (syncope with heart block) 426.9
Addisonian 255.41

Syndrome — see also Disease — continued
Adie (-Holmes) (pupil) 379.46
adiposogenital 253.8
adrenal
hemorrhage 036.3
meningococcic 036.3
adrenocortical 255.3
adrenogenital (acquired) (congenital) 255.2
feminizing 255.2
iatrogenic 760.79
virilism (acquired) (congenital) 255.2
affective organic NEC 293.89
drug-induced 292.84
afferent loop NEC 537.89
African macroglobulinemia 273.3
Ahumada-Del Castillo (nonpuerperal galactorrhea and amenorrhea) 253.1
air blast concussion — see Injury, internal, by site
Alagille 759.89
Albright (-Martin) (pseudohypoparathyroidism) 275.49
Albright-McCune-Sternberg (osteitis fibrosa disseminata) 756.59
alcohol withdrawal 291.81
Alder's (leukocyte granulation anomaly) 288.2
Aldrich (-Wiskott) (eczema-thrombocytopenia) 279.12
Alibert-Bazin (mycosis fungoides) (M9700/3) 202.1 ☑
Alice in Wonderland 293.89
alien hand 781.8
Allen-Masters 620.6
Alligator baby (ichthyosis congenita) 757.1
Alport's (hereditary hematuria-nephropathy-deafness) 759.89
Alvarez (transient cerebral ischemia) 435.9
alveolar capillary block 516.8
Alzheimer's 331.0
with dementia — see Alzheimer's, dementia
amnestic (confabulatory) 294.0
alcohol-induced persisting 291.1
drug-induced 292.83
posttraumatic 294.0
amotivational 292.89
amyostatic 275.1
amyotrophic lateral sclerosis 335.20
androgen insensitivity 259.51
partial 259.52
Angelman 759.89
angina (see also Angina) 413.9
ankyloglossia superior 750.0
anterior
chest wall 786.52
compartment (tibial) 958.8
spinal artery 433.8 ☑
compression 721.1
tibial (compartment) 958.8
antibody deficiency 279.00
agammaglobulinemic 279.00
congenital 279.04
hypogammaglobulinemic 279.00
anticardiolipin antibody 289.81
antimongolism 758.39
antiphospholipid antibody 289.81
Anton (-Babinski) (hemiasomatognosia) 307.9
anxiety (see also Anxiety) 300.00
organic 293.84
aortic
arch 446.7
bifurcation (occlusion) 444.09
ring 747.21
Apert's (acrocephalosyndactyly) 755.55
Apert-Gallais (adrenogenital) 255.2
aphasia-apraxia-alexia 784.69
apical ballooning 429.83
"approximate answers" 300.16
arcuate ligament (-celiac axis) 447.4
arcus aortae 446.7
arc welders' 370.24
argentaffin, argintaffinoma 259.2
Argonz-Del Castillo (nonpuerperal galactorrhea and amenorrhea) 253.1

☑ Additional Digit Required — Refer to the Tabular List for Digit Selection   ⏷ Subterms under main terms may continue to next column or page

268 — Volume 2   ▶◀ Revised Text   ● New Line   ▲ Revised Code   2013 ICD-9-CM

Syndrome — *see also* Disease — *continued*
  Argyll Robertson's (syphilitic) 094.89
    nonsyphilitic 379.45
  Armenian 277.31
  arm-shoulder (*see also* Neuropathy, periph-
    eral, autonomic) 337.9
  Arnold-Chiari (*see also* Spina bifida) 741.0 ☑
    type I 348.4
    type II 741.0 ☑
    type III 742.0
    type IV 742.2
  Arrillaga-Ayerza (pulmonary artery sclerosis
    with pulmonary hypertension) 416.0
  arteriomesenteric duodenum occlusion
    537.89
  arteriovenous steal 996.73
  arteritis, young female (obliterative brachio-
    cephalic) 446.7
  aseptic meningitis — *see* Meningitis, aseptic
  Asherman's 621.5
  Asperger's 299.8 ☑
  asphyctic (*see also* Anxiety) 300.00
  aspiration, of newborn (massive) 770.18
    meconium 770.12
  ataxia-telangiectasia 334.8
  Audry's (acropachyderma) 757.39
  auriculotemporal 350.8
  autoimmune lymphoproliferative (ALPS)
    279.41
  autosomal (*see also* Abnormal, autosomes
    NEC)
    deletion 758.39
      5p 758.31
      22q11.2 758.32
  Avellis' 344.89
  Axenfeld's 743.44
  Ayerza (-Arrillaga) (pulmonary artery sclero-
    sis with pulmonary hypertension)
    416.0
  Baader's (erythema multiforme exudativum)
    695.19
  Baastrup's 721.5
  Babinski (-Vaquez) (cardiovascular syphilis)
    093.89
  Babinski-Fröhlich (adiposogenital dystro-
    phy) 253.8
  Babinski-Nageotte 344.89
  Bagratuni's (temporal arteritis) 446.5
  Bakwin-Krida (craniometaphyseal dysplasia)
    756.89
  Balint's (psychic paralysis of visual disorien-
    tation) 368.16
  Ballantyne (-Runge) (postmaturity) 766.22
  ballooning posterior leaflet 424.0
  Banti's — *see* Cirrhosis, liver
  Bardet-Biedl (obesity, polydactyly, and intel-
    lectual disabiilties) 759.89
  Bard-Pic's (carcinoma, head of pancreas)
    157.0
  Barlow (-Möller) (infantile scurvy) 267
  Barlow's (mitral valve prolapse) 424.0
  Baron Munchausen's 301.51
  Barré-Guillain 357.0
  Barré-Liéou (posterior cervical sympathetic)
    723.2
  Barrett's (chronic peptic ulcer of esophagus)
    530.85
  Bársony-Polgár (corkscrew esophagus)
    530.5
  Bársony-Teschendorf (corkscrew esophagus)
    530.5
  Barth 759.89
  Bartter's (secondary hyperaldosteronism
    with juxtaglomerular hyperplasia)
    255.13
  basal cell nevus 759.89
  Basedow's (exophthalmic goiter) 242.0 ☑
  basilar artery 435.0
  basofrontal 377.04
  Bassen-Kornzweig (abetalipoproteinemia)
    272.5
  Batten-Steinert 359.21
  battered
    adult 995.81
    baby or child 995.54
    spouse 995.81

Syndrome — *see also* Disease — *continued*
  Baumgarten-Cruveilhier (cirrhosis of liver)
    571.5
  Beals 759.82
  Bearn-Kunkel (-Slater) (lupoid hepatitis)
    571.49
  Beau's (*see also* Degeneration, myocardial)
    429.1
  Bechterew-Strümpell-Marie (ankylosing
    spondylitis) 720.0
  Beck's (anterior spinal artery occlusion)
    433.8 ☑
  Beckwith (-Wiedemann) 759.89
  Behçet's 136.1
  Bekhterev-Strümpell-Marie (ankylosing
    spondylitis) 720.0
  Benedikt's 344.89
  Béquez César (-Steinbrinck-Chédiak-Higashi)
    (congenital gigantism of peroxidase
    granules) 288.2
  Bernard-Horner (*see also* Neuropathy, periph-
    eral, autonomic) 337.9
  Bernard-Sergent (acute adrenocortical insuf-
    ficiency) 255.41
  Bernhardt-Roth 355.1
  Bernheim's (*see also* Failure, heart) 428.0
  Bertolotti's (sacralization of fifth lumbar
    vertebra) 756.15
  Besnier-Boeck-Schaumann (sarcoidosis) 135
  Bianchi's (aphasia-apraxia-alexia syndrome)
    784.69
  Biedl-Bardet (obesity, polydactyly, and intel-
    lectual disabilities) 759.89
  Biemond's (obesity, polydactyly, and intel-
    lectual disabilities) 759.89
  big spleen 289.4
  bilateral polycystic ovarian 256.4
  Bing-Horton's 339.00
  Biörck (-Thorson) (malignant carcinoid)
    259.2
  Birt-Hogg-Dube 759.89
  Blackfan-Diamond (congenital hypoplastic
    anemia) 284.01
  black lung 500
  black widow spider bite 989.5
  bladder neck (*see also* Incontinence, urine)
    788.30
  blast (concussion) — *see* Blast, injury
  blind loop (postoperative) 579.2
  Bloch-Siemens (incontinentia pigmenti)
    757.33
  Bloch-Sulzberger (incontinentia pigmenti)
    757.33
  Bloom (-Machacek) (-Torre) 757.39
  Blount-Barber (tibia vara) 732.4
  blue
    bloater 491.20
      with
        acute bronchitis 491.22
        exacerbation (acute) 491.21
    diaper 270.0
    drum 381.02
    sclera 756.51
    toe 445.02
  Boder-Sedgwick (ataxia-telangiectasia)
    334.8
  Boerhaave's (spontaneous esophageal rup-
    ture) 530.4
  Bonnevie-Ullrich 758.6
  Bonnier's 386.19
  Borjeson-Forssman-Lehmann 759.89
  Bouillaud's (rheumatic heart disease) 391.9
  Bourneville (-Pringle) (tuberous sclerosis)
    759.5
  Bouveret (-Hoffmann) (paroxysmal tachycar-
    dia) 427.2
  brachial plexus 353.0
  Brachman-de Lange (Amsterdam dwarf, in-
    tellectual disabilities, and brachy-
    cephaly) 759.89
  bradycardia-tachycardia 427.81
  Brailsford-Morquio (dystrophy) (mu-
    copolysaccharidosis IV) 277.5
  brain (acute) (chronic) (nonpsychotic) (or-
    ganic) (with behavioral reaction)
    (with neurotic reaction) 310.9

Syndrome — *see also* Disease — *continued*
  brain — *continued*
    with
      presenile brain disease (*see also* De-
        mentia, presenile) 290.10
      psychosis, psychotic reaction (*see al-
        so* Psychosis, organic) 294.9
    chronic alcoholic 291.2
    congenital (*see also* Disability, intellectu-
      al) 319
    postcontusional 310.2
    posttraumatic
      nonpsychotic 310.2
      psychotic 293.9
        acute 293.0
        chronic (*see also* Psychosis, organ-
          ic) 294.8
        subacute 293.1
    psycho-organic (*see also* Syndrome,
      psycho-organic) 310.9
    psychotic (*see also* Psychosis, organic)
      294.9
    senile (*see also* Dementia, senile) 290.0
  branchial arch 744.41
  Brandt's (acrodermatitis enteropathica)
    686.8
  Brennemann's 289.2
  Briquet's 300.81
  Brissaud-Meige (infantile myxedema) 244.9
  broad ligament laceration 620.6
  Brock's (atelectasis due to enlarged lymph
    nodes) 518.0
  broken heart 429.83
  Brown-Séquard 344.89
  brown spot 756.59
  Brown's tendon sheath 378.61
  Brugada 746.89
  Brugsch's (acropachyderma) 757.39
  bubbly lung 770.7
  Buchem's (hyperostosis corticalis) 733.3
  Budd-Chiari (hepatic vein thrombosis) 453.0
  Büdinger-Ludloff-Läwen 717.89
  bulbar 335.22
    lateral (*see also* Disease, cerebrovascular,
      acute) 436
  Bullis fever 082.8
  bundle of Kent (anomalous atrioventricular
    excitation) 426.7
  Bürger-Grütz (essential familial hyper-
    lipemia) 272.3
  Burke's (pancreatic insufficiency and
    chronic neutropenia) 577.8
  Burnett's (milk-alkali) 275.42
  Burnier's (hypophyseal dwarfism) 253.3
  burning feet 266.2
  Bywaters' 958.5
  Caffey's (infantile cortical hyperostosis)
    756.59
  Calvé-Legg-Perthes (osteochondrosis,
    femoral capital) 732.1
  Caplan (-Colinet) syndrome 714.81
  capsular thrombosis (*see also* Thrombosis,
    brain) 434.0 ☑
  carbohydrate-deficient glycoprotein (CDGS)
    271.8
  carcinogenic thrombophlebitis 453.1
  carcinoid 259.2
  cardiac asthma (*see also* Failure, ventricular,
    left) 428.1
  cardiacos negros 416.0
  cardiofaciocutaneous 759.89
  cardiopulmonary obesity 278.03
  cardiorenal (*see also* Hypertension, cardiore-
    nal) 404.90
  cardiorespiratory distress (idiopathic),
    newborn 769
  cardiovascular renal (*see also* Hypertension,
    cardiorenal) 404.90
  cardiovasorenal 272.7
  Carini's (ichthyosis congenita) 757.1
  carotid
    artery (internal) 435.8
    body or sinus 337.01
  carpal tunnel 354.0
  Carpenter's 759.89

Syndrome — *see also* Disease — *continued*
  Cassidy (-Scholte) (malignant carcinoid)
    259.2
  cat-cry 758.31
  cauda equina 344.60
  causalgia 355.9
    lower limb 355.71
    upper limb 354.4
  cavernous sinus 437.6
  celiac 579.0
    artery compression 447.4
    axis 447.4
  central pain 338.0
  cerebellomedullary malformation (*see also*
    Spina bifida) 741.0 ☑
  cerebral gigantism 253.0
  cerebrohepatorenal 759.89
  cervical (root) (spine) NEC 723.8
    disc 722.71
    posterior, sympathetic 723.2
    rib 353.0
    sympathetic paralysis 337.09
    traumatic (acute) NEC 847.0
  cervicobrachial (diffuse) 723.3
  cervicocranial 723.2
  cervicodorsal outlet 353.2
  Céstan (-Raymond) 433.8 ☑
  Céstan's 344.89
  Céstan-Chenais 344.89
  chancriform 114.1
  Charcôt's (intermittent claudication) 443.9
    angina cruris 443.9
    due to atherosclerosis 440.21
  Charcôt-Marie-Tooth 356.1
  Charcôt-Weiss-Baker 337.01
  CHARGE association 759.89
  Cheadle (-Möller) (-Barlow) (infantile scurvy)
    267
  Chédiak-Higashi (-Steinbrinck) (congenital
    gigantism of peroxidase granules)
    288.2
  chest wall 786.52
  Chiari's (hepatic vein thrombosis) 453.0
  Chiari-Frommel 676.6 ☑
  chiasmatic 368.41
  Chilaiditi's (subphrenic displacement, colon)
    751.4
  chondroectodermal dysplasia 756.55
  chorea-athetosis-agitans 275.1
  Christian's (chronic histiocytosis X) 277.89
  chromosome 4 short arm deletion 758.39
  chronic pain 338.4
  Churg-Strauss 446.4
  Clarke-Hadfield (pancreatic infantilism)
    577.8
  Claude's 352.6
  Claude Bernard-Horner (*see also* Neuropa-
    thy, peripheral, autonomic) 337.9
  Clérambault's
    automatism 348.89
    erotomania 297.8
  Clifford's (postmaturity) 766.22
  climacteric 627.2
  Clouston's (hidrotic ectodermal dysplasia)
    757.31
  clumsiness 315.4
  Cockayne's (microencephaly and dwarfism)
    759.89
  Cockayne-Weber (epidermolysis bullosa)
    757.39
  Coffin-Lowry 759.89
  Cogan's (nonsyphilitic interstitial keratitis)
    370.52
  cold injury (newborn) 778.2
  Collet (-Sicard) 352.6
  combined immunity deficiency 279.2
  compartment(al) (anterior) (deep) (posteri-
    or) 958.8
    nontraumatic
      abdomen 729.73
      arm 729.71
      buttock 729.72
      fingers 729.71
      foot 729.72
      forearm 729.71
      hand 729.71

☑ Additional Digit Required — Refer to the Tabular List for Digit Selection   ⊽ Subterms under main terms may continue to next column or page

2013 ICD-9-CM   ▶◀ Revised Text   ● New Line   ▲ Revised Code   Volume 2 — 269

☑ Additional Digit Required — Refer to the Tabular List for Digit Selection

Ⓦ Subterms under main terms may continue to next column or page

270 — Volume 2

▶◀ Revised Text

● New Line

▲ Revised Code

2013 ICD-9-CM

Syndrome — *see also* Disease — *continued*

Gaisböck's (polycythemia hypertonica) 289.0
ganglion (basal, brain) 333.90
  geniculi 351.1
Ganser's, hysterical 300.16
Gardner-Diamond (autoerythrocyte sensitization) 287.2
gastroesophageal junction 530.0
gastroesophageal laceration-hemorrhage 530.7
gastrojejunal loop obstruction 537.89
Gayet-Wernicke's (superior hemorrhagic polioencephalitis) 265.1
Gee-Herter-Heubner (nontropical sprue) 579.0
Gélineau's (*see also* Narcolepsy) 347.00
genito-anorectal 099.1
Gerhardt's (vocal cord paralysis) 478.30
Gerstmann's (finger agnosia) 784.69
Gerstmann-Sträussler-Scheinker (GSS) 046.71
Gianotti Crosti 057.8
  due to known virus — *see* Infection, virus
  due to unknown virus 057.8
Gilbert's 277.4
Gilford (-Hutchinson) (progeria) 259.8
Gilles de la Tourette's 307.23
Gillespie's (dysplasia oculodentodigitalis) 759.89
Glénard's (enteroptosis) 569.89
Glinski-Simmonds (pituitary cachexia) 253.2
glucuronyl transferase 277.4
glue ear 381.20
Goldberg (-Maxwell) (-Morris) (testicular feminization) 259.51
Goldenhar's (oculoauriculovertebral dysplasia) 756.0
Goldflam-Erb 358.00
Goltz-Gorlin (dermal hypoplasia) 757.39
Good's 279.06
Goodpasture's (pneumorenal) 446.21
Gopalan's (burning feet) 266.2
Gorlin's 759.89
Gorlin-Chaudhry-Moss 759.89
Gougerot-Blum (pigmented purpuric lichenoid dermatitis) 709.1
Gougerot-Carteaud (confluent reticulate papillomatosis) 701.8
Gougerot (-Houwer)-Sjögren (keratoconjunctivitis sicca) 710.2
Gouley's (constrictive pericarditis) 423.2
Gowers' (vasovagal attack) 780.2
Gowers-Paton-Kennedy 377.04
Gradenigo's 383.02
gray or grey (chloramphenicol) (newborn) 779.4
Greig's (hypertelorism) 756.0
GSS (Gerstmann-Sträussler-Scheinker) 046.71
Gubler-Millard 344.89
Guérin-Stern (arthrogryposis multiplex congenita) 754.89
Guillain-Barré (-Strohl) 357.0
Gunn's (jaw-winking syndrome) 742.8
Günther's (congenital erythropoietic porphyria) 277.1
gustatory sweating 350.8
H₃O 759.81
Hadfield-Clarke (pancreatic infantilism) 577.8
Haglund-Läwen-Fründ 717.89
hairless women 257.8
hair tourniquet (*see also* Injury, superficial, by site)
  finger 915.8
    infected 915.9
  penis 911.8
    infected 911.9
  toe 917.8
    infected 917.9
Hallermann-Streiff 756.0
Hallervorden-Spatz 333.0
Hamman's (spontaneous mediastinal emphysema) 518.1

Syndrome — *see also* Disease — *continued*

Hamman-Rich (diffuse interstitial pulmonary fibrosis) 516.33
hand-foot 693.0
Hand-Schüller-Christian (chronic histiocytosis X) 277.89
Hanot-Chauffard (-Troisier) (bronze diabetes) 275.01
Harada's 363.22
Hare's (M8010/3) (carcinoma, pulmonary apex) 162.3
Harkavy's 446.0
Harris' (organic hyperinsulinism) 251.1
Hart's (pellagra-cerebellar ataxia-renal aminoaciduria) 270.0
Hayem-Faber (achlorhydric anemia) 280.9
Hayem-Widal (acquired hemolytic jaundice) 283.9
headache — *see* Headache, syndrome
Heberden's (angina pectoris) 413.9
Hedinger's (malignant carcinoid) 259.2
Hegglin's 288.2
Heller's (infantile psychosis) (*see also* Psychosis, childhood) 299.1 ☑
H.E.L.L.P 642.5 ☑
hemolytic-uremic (adult) (child) 283.11
hemophagocytic 288.4
  infection-associated 288.4
Hench-Rosenberg (palindromic arthritis) (*see also* Rheumatism, palindromic) 719.3 ☑
Henoch-Schönlein (allergic purpura) 287.0
hepatic flexure 569.89
hepatopulmonary 573.5
hepatorenal 572.4
  due to a procedure 997.49
  following delivery 674.8 ☑
hepatourologic 572.4
Herrick's (hemoglobin S disease) 282.61
Herter (-Gee) (nontropical sprue) 579.0
Heubner-Herter (nontropical sprue) 579.0
Heyd's (hepatorenal) 572.4
HHHO 759.81
high grade myelodysplastic 238.73
  with 5q deletion 238.73
Hilger's 337.09
histiocytic 288.4
Hoffa (-Kastert) (liposynovitis prepatellaris) 272.8
Hoffmann's 244.9 *[359.5]*
Hoffmann-Bouveret (paroxysmal tachycardia) 427.2
Hoffmann-Werdnig 335.0
Holländer-Simons (progressive lipodystrophy) 272.6
Holmes' (visual disorientation) 368.16
Holmes-Adie 379.46
Hoppe-Goldflam 358.00
Horner's (*see also* Neuropathy, peripheral, autonomic) 337.9
  traumatic — *see* Injury, nerve, cervical sympathetic
hospital addiction 301.51
hungry bone 275.5
Hunt's (herpetic geniculate ganglionitis) 053.11
  dyssynergia cerebellaris myoclonica 334.2
Hunter (-Hurler) (mucopolysaccharidosis II) 277.5
hunterian glossitis 529.4
Hurler (-Hunter) (mucopolysaccharidosis II) 277.5
Hutchinson-Boeck (sarcoidosis) 135
Hutchinson-Gilford (progeria) 259.8
Hutchinson's incisors or teeth 090.5
hydralazine
  correct substance properly administered 695.4
  overdose or wrong substance given or taken 972.6
hydraulic concussion (abdomen) (*see also* Injury, internal, abdomen) 868.00
hyperabduction 447.8
hyperactive bowel 564.9

Syndrome — *see also* Disease — *continued*

hyperaldosteronism with hypokalemic alkalosis (Bartter's) 255.13
hypercalcemic 275.42
hypercoagulation NEC 289.89
hypereosinophilic (idiopathic) 288.3
hyperkalemic 276.7
hyperkinetic (*see also* Hyperkinesia)
  heart 429.82
hyperlipemia-hemolytic anemia-icterus 571.1
hypermobility 728.5
hypernatremia 276.0
hyperosmolarity 276.0
hyperperfusion 997.01
hypersomnia-bulimia 349.89
hypersplenic 289.4
hypersympathetic (*see also* Neuropathy, peripheral, autonomic) 337.9
hypertransfusion, newborn 776.4
hyperventilation, psychogenic 306.1
hyperviscosity (of serum) NEC 273.3
  polycythemic 289.0
  sclerothymic 282.8
hypoglycemic (familial) (neonatal) 251.2
  functional 251.1
hypokalemic 276.8
hypophyseal 253.8
hypophyseothalamic 253.8
hypopituitarism 253.2
hypoplastic left heart 746.7
hypopotassemia 276.8
hyposmolality 276.1
hypotension, maternal 669.2 ☑
hypothenar hammer 443.89
hypotonia-hypomentia-hypogonadism-obesity 759.81
ICF (intravascular coagulation-fibrinolysis) (*see also* Fibrinolysis) 286.6
idiopathic cardiorespiratory distress, newborn 769
idiopathic nephrotic (infantile) 581.9
iliotibial band 728.89
Imerslund (-Gräsbeck) (anemia due to familial selective vitamin B₁₂ malabsorption) 281.1
immobility (paraplegic) 728.3
immune reconstitution inflammatory (IRIS) 995.90
immunity deficiency, combined 279.2
impending coronary 411.1
impingement
  shoulder 726.2
  vertebral bodies 724.4
inappropriate secretion of antidiuretic hormone (ADH) 253.6
incomplete
  mandibulofacial 756.0
infant
  death, sudden (SIDS) 798.0
  Hercules 255.2
  of diabetic mother 775.0
  shaken 995.55
infantilism 253.3
inferior vena cava 459.2
influenza-like (*see also* Influenza) 487.1
inspissated bile, newborn 774.4
insufficient sleep 307.44
intermediate coronary (artery) 411.1
internal carotid artery (*see also* Occlusion, artery, carotid) 433.1 ☑
interspinous ligament 724.8
intestinal
  carcinoid 259.2
  gas 787.3
  knot 560.2
intraoperative floppy iris (IFIS) 364.81
intravascular
  coagulation-fibrinolysis (ICF) (*see also* Fibrinolysis) 286.6
  coagulopathy (*see also* Fibrinolysis) 286.6
inverted Marfan's 759.89
IRDS (idiopathic respiratory distress, newborn) 769
irritable
  bowel 564.1

Syndrome — *see also* Disease — *continued*

irritable — *continued*
  heart 306.2
  weakness 300.5
ischemic bowel (transient) 557.9
  chronic 557.1
  due to mesenteric artery insufficiency 557.1
Itsenko-Cushing (pituitary basophilism) 255.0
IVC (intravascular coagulopathy) (*see also* Fibrinolysis) 286.6
Ivemark's (asplenia with congenital heart disease) 759.0
Jaccoud's 714.4
Jackson's 344.89
Jadassohn-Lewandowski (pachyonchia congenita) 757.5
Jaffe-Lichtenstein (-Uehlinger) 252.01
Jahnke's (encephalocutaneous angiomatosis) 759.6
Jakob-Creutzfeldt 046.19
  with dementia
    with behavioral disturbance 046.19 *[294.11]*
    without behavioral disturbance 046.19 *[294.10]*
  variant 046.11
    with dementia
      with behavioral disturbance 046.11 *[294.11]*
      without behavioral disturbance 046.11 *[294.10]*
Jaksch's (pseudoleukemia infantum) 285.8
Jaksch-Hayem (-Luzet) (pseudoleukemia infantum) 285.8
jaw-winking 742.8
jejunal 564.2
Jervell-Lange-Nielsen 426.82
jet lag 327.35
Jeune's (asphyxiating thoracic dystrophy of newborn) 756.4
Job's (chronic granulomatous disease) 288.1
Jordan's 288.2
Joseph-Diamond-Blackfan (congenital hypoplastic anemia) 284.01
Joubert 759.89
jugular foramen 352.6
Kabuki 759.89
Kahler's (multiple myeloma) (M9730/3) 203.0 ☑
Kalischer's (encephalocutaneous angiomatosis) 759.6
Kallmann's (hypogonadotropic hypogonadism with anosmia) 253.4
Kanner's (autism) (*see also* Psychosis, childhood) 299.0 ☑
Kartagener's (sinusitis, bronchiectasis, situs inversus) 759.3
Kasabach-Merritt (capillary hemangioma associated with thrombocytopenic purpura) 287.39
Kast's (dyschondroplasia with hemangiomas) 756.4
Kaznelson's (congenital hypoplastic anemia) 284.01
Kearns-Sayre 277.87
Kelly's (sideropenic dysphagia) 280.8
Kimmelstiel-Wilson (intercapillary glomerulosclerosis) 250.4 ☑ *[581.81]*
  due to secondary diabetes 249.4 ☑ *[581.81]*
Klauder's (erythema multiforme exudativum) 695.19
Kleine-Levin 327.13
Klein-Waardenburg (ptosis-epicanthus) 270.2
Klinefelter's 758.7
Klippel-Feil (brevicollis) 756.16
Klippel-Trenaunay 759.89
Klumpke (-Déjérine) (injury to brachial plexus at birth) 767.6
Klüver-Bucy (-Terzian) 310.0
Köhler-Pellegrini-Stieda (calcification, knee joint) 726.62
König's 564.89

☑ **Additional Digit Required** — Refer to the Tabular List for Digit Selection   ⩗ **Subterms under main terms may continue to next column or page**

2013 ICD-9-CM   ▶◀ **Revised Text**   ● **New Line**   ▲ **Revised Code**   **Volume 2 — 271**

Syndrome — *see also* Disease — *continued*
Korsakoff (-Wernicke) (nonalcoholic) 294.0
Korsakoff's (nonalcoholic) 294.0
    alcoholic 291.1
    alcoholic 291.1
Kostmann's (infantile genetic agranulocytosis) 288.01
Krabbe's
    congenital muscle hypoplasia 756.89
    cutaneocerebral angioma 759.6
Kunkel (lupoid hepatitis) 571.49
labyrinthine 386.50
laceration, broad ligament 620.6
Lambert-Eaton 358.30
    in
        diseases classified elsewhere 358.39
        neoplastic disease 358.31
Landau-Kieffner 345.8 ☑
Langdon Down (mongolism) 758.0
Larsen's (flattened facies and multiple congenital dislocations) 755.8
lateral
    cutaneous nerve of thigh 355.1
    medullary (*see also* Disease, cerebrovascular acute) 436
Launois' (pituitary gigantism) 253.0
Launois-Cléret (adiposogenital dystrophy) 253.8
Laurence-Moon (-Bardet)-Biedl (obesity, polydactyly, and intellectual disabilities) 759.89
Lawford's (encephalocutaneous angiomatosis) 759.6
lazy
    leukocyte 288.09
    posture 728.3
Lederer-Brill (acquired infectious hemolytic anemia) 283.19
Legg-Calvé-Perthes (osteochondrosis capital femoral) 732.1
Lemiere 451.89
Lennox's (*see also* Epilepsy) 345.0 ☑
Lennox-Gastaut syndrome 345.0 ☑
    with tonic seizures 345.1 ☑
lenticular 275.1
Léopold-Lévi's (paroxysmal thyroid instability) 242.9 ☑
Lepore hemoglobin 282.45
Leriche's (aortic bifurcation occlusion) 444.09
Léri-Weill 756.59
Lermoyez's (*see also* Disease, Ménière's) 386.00
Lesch-Nyhan (hypoxanthine-guanine-phosphoribosyltransferase deficiency) 277.2
leukoencephalopathy, reversible, posterior 348.5
Lev's (acquired complete heart block) 426.0
Levi's (pituitary dwarfism) 253.3
Lévy-Roussy 334.3
Lichtheim's (subacute combined sclerosis with pernicious anemia) 281.0 *[336.2]*
Li-Fraumeni V84.01
Lightwood's (renal tubular acidosis) 588.89
Lignac (-de Toni) (-Fanconi) (-Debré) (cystinosis) 270.0
Likoff's (angina in menopausal women) 413.9
liver-kidney 572.4
Lloyd's 258.1
lobotomy 310.0
Löffler's (eosinophilic pneumonitis) 518.3
Löfgren's (sarcoidosis) 135
long arm 18 or 21 deletion 758.39
Looser (-Debray)-Milkman (osteomalacia with pseudofractures) 268.2
Lorain-Levi (pituitary dwarfism) 253.3
Louis-Bar (ataxia-telangiectasia) 334.8
low
    atmospheric pressure 993.2
    back 724.2
        psychogenic 306.0
    output (cardiac) (*see also* Failure, heart) 428.9
Lowe's (oculocerebrorenal dystrophy) 270.8

Syndrome — *see also* Disease — *continued*
lower radicular, newborn 767.4
Lowe-Terrey-MacLachlan (oculocerebrorenal dystrophy) 270.8
Lown (-Ganong)-Levine (short P-R interval, normal QRS complex, and supraventricular tachycardia) 426.81
Lucey-Driscoll (jaundice due to delayed conjugation) 774.30
Luetscher's (dehydration) 276.51
lumbar vertebral 724.4
Lutembacher's (atrial septal defect with mitral stenosis) 745.5
Lyell's (toxic epidermal necrolysis) 695.15
    due to drug
        correct substance properly administered 695.15
        overdose or wrong substance given or taken 977.9
            specified drug — *see* Table of Drugs and Chemicals
MacLeod's 492.8
macrogenitosomia praecox 259.8
macroglobulinemia 273.3
macrophage activation 288.4
Maffucci's (dyschondroplasia with hemangiomas) 756.4
Magenblase 306.4
magnesium-deficiency 781.7
malabsorption 579.9
    postsurgical 579.3
    spinal fluid 331.3
Mal de Debarquement 780.4
malignant carcinoid 259.2
Mallory-Weiss 530.7
mandibulofacial dysostosis 756.0
manic-depressive (*see also* Psychosis, affective) 296.80
Mankowsky's (familial dysplastic osteopathy) 731.2
maple syrup (urine) 270.3
Marable's (celiac artery compression) 447.4
Marchesani (-Weill) (brachymorphism and ectopia lentis) 759.89
Marchiafava-Bignami 341.8
Marchiafava-Micheli (paroxysmal nocturnal hemoglobinuria) 283.2
Marcus Gunn's (jaw-winking syndrome) 742.8
Marfan's (arachnodactyly) 759.82
    meaning congenital syphilis 090.49
        with luxation of lens 090.49 *[379.32]*
Marie's (acromegaly) 253.0
    primary or idiopathic (acropachyderma) 757.39
    secondary (hypertrophic pulmonary osteoarthropathy) 731.2
Markus-Adie 379.46
Maroteaux-Lamy (mucopolysaccharidosis VI) 277.5
Martin's 715.27
Martin-Albright (pseudohypoparathyroidism) 275.49
Martorell-Fabré (pulseless disease) 446.7
massive aspiration of newborn 770.18
Masters-Allen 620.6
mastocytosis 757.33
maternal hypotension 669.2 ☑
maternal obesity 646.1 ☑
May (-Hegglin) 288.2
McArdle (-Schmid) (-Pearson) (glycogenosis V) 271.0
McCune-Albright (osteitis fibrosa disseminata) 756.59
McQuarrie's (idiopathic familial hypoglycemia) 251.2
meconium
    aspiration 770.12
    plug (newborn) NEC 777.1
median arcuate ligament 447.4
mediastinal fibrosis 519.3
Meekeren-Ehlers-Danlos 756.83
Meige (blepharospasm-oromandibular dystonia) 333.82
    -Milroy (chronic hereditary edema) 757.0

Syndrome — *see also* Disease — *continued*
MELAS (mitochondrial encephalopathy, lactic acidosis and stroke-like episodes) 277.87
Melkersson (-Rosenthal) 351.8
MEN (multiple endocrine neoplasia)
    type I 258.01
    type IIA 258.02
    type IIB 258.03
Mende's (ptosis-epicanthus) 270.2
Mendelson's (resulting from a procedure) 997.32
    during labor 668.0 ☑
    obstetric 668.0 ☑
Ménétrier's (hypertrophic gastritis) 535.2 ☑
Ménière's (*see also* Disease, Ménière's) 386.00
meningo-eruptive 047.1
Menkes' 759.89
    glutamic acid 759.89
    maple syrup (urine) disease 270.3
menopause 627.2
    postartificial 627.4
menstruation 625.4
MERRF (myoclonus with epilepsy and with ragged red fibers) 277.87
mesenteric
    artery, superior 557.1
    vascular insufficiency (with gangrene) 557.1
metabolic 277.7
metastatic carcinoid 259.2
Meyenburg-Altherr-Uehlinger 733.99
Meyer-Schwickerath and Weyers (dysplasia oculodentodigitalis) 759.89
Micheli-Rietti (thalassemia minor) 282.46
Michotte's 721.5
micrognathia-glossoptosis 756.0
microphthalmos (congenital) 759.89
midbrain 348.89
middle
    lobe (lung) (right) 518.0
    radicular 353.0
Miescher's
    familial acanthosis nigricans 701.2
    granulomatosis disciformis 709.3
Mieten's 759.89
migraine 346.0 ☑
Mikity-Wilson (pulmonary dysmaturity) 770.7
Mikulicz's (dryness of mouth, absent or decreased lacrimation) 527.1
milk alkali (milk drinkers') 275.42
Milkman (-Looser) (osteomalacia with pseudofractures) 268.2
Millard-Gubler 344.89
Miller-Dieker 758.33
Miller Fisher's 357.0
Milles' (encephalocutaneous angiomatosis) 759.6
Minkowski-Chauffard (*see also* Spherocytosis) 282.0
Mirizzi's (hepatic duct stenosis) 576.2
    with calculus, cholelithiasis, or stones — *see* Choledocholithiasis
mitochondrial neurogastrointestinal encephalopathy (MNGIE) 277.87
mitral
    click (-murmur) 785.2
    valve prolapse 424.0
MNGIE (mitochondrial neurogastrointestinal encephalopathy) 277.87
Möbius'
    congenital oculofacial paralysis 352.6
    ophthalmoplegic migraine 346.2 ☑
Mohr's (types I and II) 759.89
monofixation 378.34
Moore's (*see also* Epilepsy) 345.5 ☑
Morel-Moore (hyperostosis frontalis interna) 733.3
Morel-Morgagni (hyperostosis frontalis interna) 733.3
Morgagni (-Stewart-Morel) (hyperostosis frontalis interna) 733.3
Morgagni-Adams-Stokes (syncope with heart block) 426.9

Syndrome — *see also* Disease — *continued*
Morquio (-Brailsford) (-Ullrich) (mucopolysaccharidosis IV) 277.5
Morris (testicular feminization) 259.51
Morton's (foot) (metatarsalgia) (metatarsal neuralgia) (neuralgia) (neuroma) (toe) 355.6
Moschcowitz (-Singer-Symmers) (thrombotic thrombocytopenic purpura) 446.6
Mounier-Kuhn 748.3
    with
        acute exacerbation 494.1
        bronchiectasis 494.0
            with (acute) exacerbation 494.1
    acquired 519.19
        with bronchiectasis 494.0
            with (acute) exacerbation 494.1
Mucha-Haberman (acute parapsoriasis varioliformis) 696.2
mucocutaneous lymph node (acute) (febrile) (infantile) (MCLS) 446.1
multiple
    deficiency 260
    endocrine neoplasia (MEN)
        type I 258.01
        type IIA 258.02
        type IIB 258.03
    operations 301.51
Munchausen's 301.51
Münchmeyer's (exostosis luxurians) 728.11
Murchison-Sanderson — *see* Disease, Hodgkin's
myasthenic — *see* Myasthenia, syndrome
myelodysplastic 238.75
    with 5q deletion 238.74
    high grade with 5q deletion 238.73
    lesions, low grade 238.72
    therapy-related 289.83
myeloproliferative (chronic) (M9960/1) 238.79
myofascial pain NEC 729.1
Naffziger's 353.0
Nager-de Reynier (dysostosis mandibularis) 756.0
nail-patella (hereditary osteo-onychodysplasia) 756.89
NARP (neuropathy, ataxia and retinitis pigmentosa) 277.87
Nebécourt's 253.3
Neill-Dingwall (microencephaly and dwarfism) 759.89
nephrotic (*see also* Nephrosis) 581.9
    diabetic 250.4 ☑ *[581.81]*
        due to secondary diabetes 249.4 ☑ *[581.81]*
Netherton's (ichthyosiform erythroderma) 757.1
neurocutaneous 759.6
neuroleptic malignant 333.92
Nezelof's (pure alymphocytosis) 279.13
Niemann-Pick (lipid histiocytosis) 272.7
Nonne-Milroy-Meige (chronic hereditary edema) 757.0
nonsense 300.16
Noonan's 759.89
Nothnagel's
    ophthalmoplegia-cerebellar ataxia 378.52
    vasomotor acroparesthesia 443.89
nucleus ambiguous-hypoglossal 352.6
OAV (oculoauriculovertebral dysplasia) 756.0
obesity hypoventilation 278.03
obsessional 300.3
oculocutaneous 364.24
oculomotor 378.81
oculourethroarticular 099.3
Ogilvie's (sympathicotonic colon obstruction) 560.89
ophthalmoplegia-cerebellar ataxia 378.52
Oppenheim-Urbach (necrobiosis lipoidica diabeticorum) 250.8 ☑ *[709.3]*
    due to secondary diabetes 249.8 ☑ *[709.3]*
oral-facial-digital 759.89

☑ Additional Digit Required — Refer to the Tabular List for Digit Selection   Subterms under main terms may continue to next column or page

272 — Volume 2   ▶◀ Revised Text   ● New Line   ▲ Revised Code   2013 ICD-9-CM

Syndrome — *see also* Disease — *continued*
organic
  affective NEC 293.83
    drug-induced 292.84
  anxiety 293.84
  delusional 293.81
    alcohol-induced 291.5
    drug-induced 292.11
    due to or associated with
      arteriosclerosis 290.42
      presenile brain disease 290.12
      senility 290.20
  depressive 293.83
    drug-induced 292.84
    due to or associated with
      arteriosclerosis 290.43
      presenile brain disease 290.13
      senile brain disease 290.21
  hallucinosis 293.82
    drug-induced 292.84
organic affective 293.83
  induced by drug 292.84
organic personality 310.1
  induced by drug 292.89
Ormond's 593.4
orodigitofacial 759.89
orthostatic hypotensive-dysautonomic
  dyskinetic 333.0
Osler-Weber-Rendu (familial hemorrhagic
  telangiectasia) 448.0
osteodermopathic hyperostosis 757.39
osteoporosis-osteomalacia 268.2
Österreicher-Turner (hereditary osteo-onychodysplasia) 756.89
os trigonum 755.69
Ostrum-Furst 756.59
otolith 386.19
otopalatodigital 759.89
outlet (thoracic) 353.0
ovarian remnant 620.8
Owren's (*see also* Defect, coagulation) 286.3
OX 758.6
pacemaker 429.4
Paget-Schroetter (intermittent venous
  claudication) 453.89
pain (*see also* Pain)
  central 338.0
  chronic 338.4
  complex regional 355.9
    type I 337.20
      lower limb 337.22
      specified site NEC 337.29
      upper limb 337.21
    type II
      lower limb 355.71
      upper limb 354.4
  myelopathic 338.0
  thalamic (hyperesthetic) 338.0
painful
  apicocostal vertebral (M8010/3) 162.3
  arc 726.19
  bruising 287.2
  feet 266.2
Pancoast's (carcinoma, pulmonary apex)
  (M8010/3) 162.3
panhypopituitary (postpartum) 253.2
papillary muscle 429.81
  with myocardial infarction 410.8 ☑
Papillon-Léage and Psaume (orodigitofacial
  dysostosis) 759.89
parabiotic (transfusion)
  donor (twin) 772.0
  recipient (twin) 776.4
paralysis agitans 332.0
paralytic 344.9
  specified type NEC 344.89
paraneoplastic — *see* condition
Parinaud's (paralysis of conjugate upward
  gaze) 378.81
  oculoglandular 372.02
Parkes Weber and Dimitri (encephalocutaneous angiomatosis) 759.6
Parkinson's (*see also* Parkinsonism) 332.0
parkinsonian (*see also* Parkinsonism) 332.0
Parry's (exophthalmic goiter) 242.0 ☑
Parry-Romberg 349.89

Syndrome — *see also* Disease — *continued*
Parsonage-Aldren-Turner 353.5
Parsonage-Turner 353.5
Patau's (trisomy D1) 758.1
patella clunk 719.66
patellofemoral 719.46
Paterson (-Brown) (-Kelly) (sideropenic dysphagia) 280.8
Payr's (splenic flexure syndrome) 569.89
pectoral girdle 447.8
pectoralis minor 447.8
Pelger-Huët (hereditary hyposegmentation)
  288.2
pellagra-cerebellar ataxia-renal
  aminoaciduria 270.0
pellagroid 265.2
Pellegrini-Stieda 726.62
Pellizzi's (pineal) 259.8
pelvic congestion (-fibrosis) 625.5
Pendred's (familial goiter with deaf-mutism)
  243
Penfield's (*see also* Epilepsy) 345.5 ☑
Penta X 758.81
peptic ulcer — *see* Ulcer, peptic 533.9 ☑
perabduction 447.8
periodic 277.31
periurethral fibrosis 593.4
persistent fetal circulation 747.83
Petges-Cléjat (poikilodermatomyositis)
  710.3
Peutz-Jeghers 759.6
Pfeiffer (acrocephalosyndactyly) 755.55
phantom limb 353.6
pharyngeal pouch 279.11
Pick's (pericardial pseudocirrhosis of liver)
  423.2
  heart 423.2
  liver 423.2
Pick-Herxheimer (diffuse idiopathic cutaneous atrophy) 701.8
Pickwickian (cardiopulmonary obesity)
  278.03
PIE (pulmonary infiltration with eosinophilia) 518.3
Pierre Marie-Bamberger (hypertrophic pulmonary osteoarthropathy) 731.2
Pierre Mauriac's (diabetes-dwarfism-obesity)
  258.1
Pierre Robin 756.0
pigment dispersion, iris 364.53
pineal 259.8
pink puffer 492.8
pituitary 253.0
placental
  dysfunction 762.2
  insufficiency 762.2
  transfusion 762.3
plantar fascia 728.71
plateau iris (without glaucoma) 364.82
  with glaucoma 365.23
plica knee 727.83
Plummer-Vinson (sideropenic dysphagia)
  280.8
pluricarential of infancy 260
plurideficiency of infancy 260
pluriglandular (compensatory) 258.8
Poland 756.81
polycarential of infancy 260
polyglandular 258.8
polysplenia 759.0
pontine 433.8 ☑
popliteal
  artery entrapment 447.8
  web 756.89
postartificial menopause 627.4
postcardiac injury
  postcardiotomy 429.4
  postmyocardial infarction 411.0
postcardiotomy 429.4
post chemoembolization — code to associated conditions
postcholecystectomy 576.0
postcommissurotomy 429.4
postconcussional 310.2
postcontusional 310.2
postencephalitic 310.89

Syndrome — *see also* Disease — *continued*
posterior
  cervical sympathetic 723.2
  fossa compression 348.4
  inferior cerebellar artery (*see also* Dis-
    ease, cerebrovascular, acute) 436
  reversible encephalopathy (PRES) 348.39
postgastrectomy (dumping) 564.2
post-gastric surgery 564.2
posthepatitis 780.79
postherpetic (neuralgia) (zoster) 053.19
  geniculate ganglion 053.11
  ophthalmica 053.19
postimmunization — *see* Complications,
  vaccination
postinfarction 411.0
postinfluenza (asthenia) 780.79
postirradiation 990
postlaminectomy 722.80
  cervical, cervicothoracic 722.81
  lumbar, lumbosacral 722.83
  thoracic, thoracolumbar 722.82
postleukotomy 310.0
postlobotomy 310.0
postmastectomy lymphedema 457.0
postmature (of newborn) 766.22
postmyocardial infarction 411.0
postoperative NEC 998.9
  blind loop 579.2
postpartum panhypopituitary 253.2
postperfusion NEC 999.89
  bone marrow 996.85
postpericardiotomy 429.4
postphlebitic (asymptomatic) 459.10
  with
    complications NEC 459.19
    inflammation 459.12
      and ulcer 459.13
    stasis dermatitis 459.12
      with ulcer 459.13
    ulcer 459.11
      with inflammation 459.13
postpolio (myelitis) 138
postvagotomy 564.2
postvalvulotomy 429.4
postviral (asthenia) NEC 780.79
Potain's (gastrectasis with dyspepsia) 536.1
potassium intoxication 276.7
Potter's 753.0
Prader (-Labhart) -Willi (-Fanconi) 759.81
preinfarction 411.1
preleukemic 238.75
premature senility 259.8
premenstrual 625.4
premenstrual tension 625.4
pre ulcer 536.9
Prinzmetal-Massumi (anterior chest wall
  syndrome) 786.52
Profichet's 729.90
progeria 259.8
progressive pallidal degeneration 333.0
prolonged gestation 766.22
Proteus (dermal hypoplasia) 757.39
prune belly 756.71
prurigo-asthma 691.8
pseudocarpal tunnel (sublimis) 354.0
pseudohermaphroditism-virilism-hirsutism
  255.2
pseudoparalytica 358.00
pseudo-Turner's 759.89
psycho-organic 293.9
  acute 293.0
  anxiety type 293.84
  depressive type 293.83
  hallucinatory type 293.82
  nonpsychotic severity 310.1
    specified focal (partial) NEC 310.89
  paranoid type 293.81
  specified type NEC 293.89
  subacute 293.1
pterygolymphangiectasia 758.6
ptosis-epicanthus 270.2
pulmonary
  arteriosclerosis 416.0
  hypoperfusion (idiopathic) 769
  renal (hemorrhagic) 446.21

Syndrome — *see also* Disease — *continued*
pulseless 446.7
Putnam-Dana (subacute combined sclerosis
  with pernicious anemia) 281.0 *[336.2]*
pyloroduodenal 537.89
pyramidopallidonigral 332.0
pyriformis 355.0
QT interval prolongation 426.82
radicular NEC 729.2
  lower limbs 724.4
  upper limbs 723.4
    newborn 767.4
Raeder-Harbitz (pulseless disease) 446.7
Ramsay Hunt's
  dyssynergia cerebellaris myoclonica
    334.2
  herpetic geniculate ganglionitis 053.11
rapid time-zone change 327.35
Raymond (-Céstan) 433.8 ☑
Raynaud's (paroxysmal digital cyanosis)
  443.0
RDS (respiratory distress syndrome, newborn) 769
Refsum's (heredopathia atactica polyneuritiformis) 356.3
Reichmann's (gastrosuccorrhea) 536.8
Reifenstein's (hereditary familial hypogonadism, male) 259.52
Reilly's (*see also* Neuropathy, peripheral,
  autonomic) 337.9
Reiter's 099.3
renal glomerulohyalinosis-diabetic
  250.4 ☑ *[581.81]*
  due to secondary diabetes
    249.4 ☑ *[581.81]*
Rendu-Osler-Weber (familial hemorrhagic
  telangiectasia) 448.0
renofacial (congenital biliary fibroan-
  giomatosis) 753.0
Rénon-Delille 253.8
respiratory distress (idiopathic) (newborn)
  769
  adult (following trauma and surgery)
    518.52
    specified NEC 518.82
  type II 770.6
restless legs (RLS) 333.94
retinoblastoma (familial) 190.5
retraction (Duane's) 378.71
retroperitoneal fibrosis 593.4
retroviral seroconversion (acute) V08
Rett's 330.8
Reye's 331.81
Reye-Sheehan (postpartum pituitary
  necrosis) 253.2
Riddoch's (visual disorientation) 368.16
Ridley's (*see also* Failure, ventricular, left)
  428.1
Rieger's (mesodermal dysgenesis, anterior
  ocular segment) 743.44
Rietti-Greppi-Micheli (thalassemia minor)
  282.46
right ventricular obstruction — *see* Failure,
  heart
Riley-Day (familial dysautonomia) 742.8
Robin's 756.0
Rokitansky-Kuster-Hauser (congenital ab-
  sence, vagina) 752.45
Romano-Ward (prolonged QT interval syn-
  drome) 426.82
Romberg's 349.89
Rosen-Castleman-Liebow (pulmonary pro-
  teinosis) 516.0
rotator cuff, shoulder 726.10
Roth's 355.1
Rothmund's (congenital poikiloderma)
  757.33
Rotor's (idiopathic hyperbilirubinemia)
  277.4
Roussy-Lévy 334.3
Roy (-Jutras) (acropachyderma) 757.39
rubella (congenital) 771.0
Rubinstein-Taybi's (brachydactylia, short
  stature, and intellectual disabilities)
  759.89

☑ **Additional Digit Required — Refer to the Tabular List for Digit Selection**   ᵂᴱᴮ **Subterms under main terms may continue to next column or page**

2013 ICD-9-CM   ▶◀ **Revised Text**   ● **New Line**   ▲ **Revised Code**   **Volume 2 — 273**

Syndrome — see also Disease — continued
- Rud's (mental deficiency, epilepsy, and infantilism) 759.89
- Ruiter-Pompen (-Wyers) (angiokeratoma corporis diffusum) 272.7
- Runge's (postmaturity) 766.22
- Russell (-Silver) (congenital hemihypertrophy and short stature) 759.89
- Rytand-Lipsitch (complete atrioventricular block) 426.0
- sacralization-scoliosis-sciatica 756.15
- sacroiliac 724.6
- Saenger's 379.46
- salt
  - depletion (see also Disease, renal) 593.9
    - due to heat NEC 992.8
      - causing heat exhaustion or prostration 992.4
    - low (see also Disease, renal) 593.9
- salt-losing (see also Disease, renal) 593.9
- Sanfilippo's (mucopolysaccharidosis III) 277.5
- Scaglietti-Dagnini (acromegalic macrospondylitis) 253.0
- scalded skin 695.81
- scalenus anticus (anterior) 353.0
- scapulocostal 354.8
- scapuloperoneal 359.1
- scapulovertebral 723.4
- Schaumann's (sarcoidosis) 135
- Scheie's (mucopolysaccharidosis IS) 277.5
- Scheuthauer-Marie-Sainton (cleidocranialis dysostosis) 755.59
- Schirmer's (encephalocutaneous angiomatosis) 759.6
- schizophrenic, of childhood NEC (see also Psychosis, childhood) 299.9 ☑
- Schmidt's
  - sphallo-pharyngo-laryngeal hemiplegia 352.6
  - thyroid-adrenocortical insufficiency 258.1
  - vagoaccessory 352.6
- Schneider's 047.9
- Schnitzler 273.1
- Scholte's (malignant carcinoid) 259.2
- Scholz (-Bielschowsky-Henneberg) 330.0
- Schroeder's (endocrine-hypertensive) 255.3
- Schüller-Christian (chronic histiocytosis X) 277.89
- Schultz's (agranulocytosis) 288.09
- Schwartz (-Jampel) 359.23
- Schwartz-Bartter (inappropriate secretion of antidiuretic hormone) 253.6
- Scimitar (anomalous venous drainage, right lung to inferior vena cava) 747.49
- sclerocystic ovary 256.4
- sea-blue histiocyte 272.7
- Seabright-Bantam (pseudohypoparathyroidism) 275.49
- Seckel's 759.89
- Secretan's (posttraumatic edema) 782.3
- secretoinhibitor (keratoconjunctivitis sicca) 710.2
- Seeligmann's (ichthyosis congenita) 757.1
- Senear-Usher (pemphigus erythematosus) 694.4
- senilism 259.8
- seroconversion, retroviral (acute) V08
- serotonin 333.99
- serous meningitis 348.2
- Sertoli cell (germinal aplasia) 606.0
- sex chromosome mosaic 758.81
- Sézary's (reticulosis) (M9701/3) 202.2 ☑
- shaken infant 995.55
- Shaver's (bauxite pneumoconiosis) 503
- Sheehan's (postpartum pituitary necrosis) 253.2
- shock (traumatic) 958.4
  - kidney 584.5
    - following crush injury 958.5
  - lung 518.82
    - related to trauma and surgery 518.52
  - neurogenic 308.9
  - psychic 308.9
- Shone's 746.84

Syndrome — see also Disease — continued
- short
  - bowel 579.3
  - P-R interval 426.81
- shoulder-arm (see also Neuropathy, peripheral, autonomic) 337.9
- shoulder-girdle 723.4
- shoulder-hand (see also Neuropathy, peripheral, autonomic) 337.9
- Shwachman's 288.02
- Shy-Drager (orthostatic hypotension with multisystem degeneration) 333.0
- Sicard's 352.6
- sicca (keratoconjunctivitis) 710.2
- sick
  - cell 276.1
  - cilia 759.89
  - sinus 427.81
- sideropenic 280.8
- Siemens'
  - ectodermal dysplasia 757.31
  - keratosis follicularis spinulosa (decalvans) 757.39
- Silfverskiöld's (osteochondrodystrophy, extremities) 756.50
- Silver's (congenital hemihypertrophy and short stature) 759.89
- Silvestroni-Bianco (thalassemia minima) 282.46
- Simons' (progressive lipodystrophy) 272.6
- sinusitis-bronchiectasis-situs inversus 759.3
- sinus tarsi 726.79
- Sipple's (medullary thyroid carcinoma-pheochromocytoma) 258.02
- Sjögren (-Gougerot) (keratoconjunctivitis sicca) 710.2
  - with lung involvement 710.2 [517.8]
- Sjögren-Larsson (ichthyosis congenita) 757.1
- SJS-TEN (Stevens-Johnson syndrome - toxic epidermal necrolysis overlap) 695.14
- Slocumb's 255.3
- Sluder's 337.09
- Smith-Lemli-Opitz (cerebrohepatorenal syndrome) 759.89
- Smith-Magenis 758.33
- smokers' 305.1
- Sneddon-Wilkinson (subcorneal pustular dermatosis) 694.1
- Sotos' (cerebral gigantism) 253.0
- South African cardiomyopathy 425.2
- spasmodic
  - upward movement, eye(s) 378.82
  - winking 307.20
- Spens' (syncope with heart block) 426.9
- spherophakia-brachymorphia 759.89
- spinal cord injury (see also Injury, spinal, by site)
  - with fracture, vertebra — see Fracture, vertebra, by site, with spinal cord injury
  - cervical — see Injury, spinal, cervical
  - fluid malabsorption (acquired) 331.3
- splenic
  - agenesis 759.0
  - flexure 569.89
  - neutropenia 289.53
  - sequestration 289.52
- Spurway's (brittle bones and blue sclera) 756.51
- staphylococcal scalded skin 695.81
- Stein's (polycystic ovary) 256.4
- Steinbrocker's (see also Neuropathy, peripheral, autonomic) 337.9
- Stein-Leventhal (polycystic ovary) 256.4
- Stevens-Johnson (erythema multiforme exudativum) 695.13
  - toxic epidermal necrolysis overlap (SJS-TEN overlap syndrome) 695.14
- Stewart-Morel (hyperostosis frontalis interna) 733.3
- Stickler 759.89
- stiff-baby 759.89
- stiff-man 333.91
- Still's (juvenile rheumatoid arthritis) 714.30

Syndrome — see also Disease — continued
- Still-Felty (rheumatoid arthritis with splenomegaly and leukopenia) 714.1
- Stilling-Türk-Duane (ocular retraction syndrome) 378.71
- Stojano's (subcostal) 098.86
- Stokes (-Adams) (syncope with heart block) 426.9
- Stokvis-Talma (enterogenous cyanosis) 289.7
- stone heart (see also Failure, ventricular, left) 428.1
- straight-back 756.19
- stroke (see also Disease, cerebrovascular, acute) 436
  - little 435.9
- Sturge-Kalischer-Weber (encephalotrigeminal angiomatosis) 759.6
- Sturge-Weber (-Dimitri) (encephalocutaneous angiomatosis) 759.6
- subclavian-carotid obstruction (chronic) 446.7
- subclavian steal 435.2
- subcoracoid-pectoralis minor 447.8
- subcostal 098.86
  - nerve compression 354.8
- subperiosteal hematoma 267
- subphrenic interposition 751.4
- sudden infant death (SIDS) 798.0
- Sudeck's 733.7
- Sudeck-Leriche 733.7
- superior
  - cerebellar artery (see also Disease, cerebrovascular, acute) 436
  - mesenteric artery 557.1
  - pulmonary sulcus (tumor) (M8010/3) 162.3
  - semi-circular canal dehiscence 386.8
  - vena cava 459.2
- suprarenal cortical 255.3
- supraspinatus 726.10
- Susac 348.39
- swallowed blood 777.3
- sweat retention 705.1
- Sweet's (acute febrile neutrophilic dermatosis) 695.89
- Swyer's (XY pure gonadal dysgenesis) 752.7
- Swyer-James (unilateral hyperlucent lung) 492.8
- Symonds' 348.2
- sympathetic
  - cervical paralysis 337.09
  - pelvic 625.5
- syndactylic oxycephaly 755.55
- syphilitic-cardiovascular 093.89
- systemic
  - fibrosclerosing 710.8
  - inflammatory response (SIRS) 995.90
    - due to
      - infectious process 995.91
        - with acute organ dysfunction 995.92
      - non-infectious process 995.93
        - with acute organ dysfunction 995.94
- systolic click (-murmur) 785.2
- Tabagism 305.1
- tachycardia-bradycardia 427.81
- Takayasu (-Onishi) (pulseless disease) 446.7
- Takotsubo 429.83
- Tapia's 352.6
- tarsal tunnel 355.5
- Taussig-Bing (transposition, aorta and overriding pulmonary artery) 745.11
- Taybi's (otopalatodigital) 759.89
- Taylor's 625.5
- teething 520.7
- tegmental 344.89
- telangiectasis-pigmentation-cataract 757.33
- temporal 383.02
  - lobectomy behavior 310.0
- temporomandibular joint-pain-dysfunction [TMJ] NEC 524.60
  - specified NEC 524.69
- Terry's (see also Retinopathy of prematurity) 362.21

Syndrome — see also Disease — continued
- testicular feminization 259.51
- testis, nonvirilizing 257.8
- tethered (spinal) cord 742.59
- thalamic 338.0
- Thibierge-Weissenbach (cutaneous systemic sclerosis) 710.1
- Thiele 724.6
- thoracic outlet (compression) 353.0
- thoracogenous rheumatic (hypertrophic pulmonary osteoarthropathy) 731.2
- Thorn's (see also Disease, renal) 593.9
- Thorson-Biörck (malignant carcinoid) 259.2
- thrombopenia-hemangioma 287.39
- thyroid-adrenocortical insufficiency 258.1
- Tietze's 733.6
- time-zone (rapid) 327.35
- Tobias' (carcinoma, pulmonary apex) (M8010/3) 162.3
- toilet seat 926.0
- Tolosa-Hunt 378.55
- Toni-Fanconi (cystinosis) 270.0
- Touraine's (hereditary osteo-onychodysplasia) 756.89
- Touraine-Solente-Golé (acropachyderma) 757.39
- toxic
  - oil 710.5
  - shock 040.82
- transfusion
  - fetal-maternal 772.0
  - twin
    - donor (infant) 772.0
    - recipient (infant) 776.4
- transient left ventricular apical ballooning 429.83
- Treacher Collins' (incomplete mandibulofacial dysostosis) 756.0
- trigeminal plate 259.8
- triple X female 758.81
- trisomy NEC 758.5
  - 13 or D₁ 758.1
  - 16-18 or E 758.2
  - 18 or E₃ 758.2
  - 20 758.5
  - 21 or G (mongolism) 758.0
  - 22 or G (mongolism) 758.0
  - G 758.0
- Troisier-Hanot-Chauffard (bronze diabetes) 275.01
- tropical wet feet 991.4
- Trousseau's (thrombophlebitis migrans visceral cancer) 453.1
- tumor lysis (following antineoplastic drug therapy) (spontaneous) 277.88
- Türk's (ocular retraction syndrome) 378.71
- Turner's 758.6
- Turner-Varny 758.6
- Twiddler's (due to)
  - automatic implantable defibrillator 996.04
  - pacemaker 996.01
- twin-to-twin transfusion 762.3
  - recipient twin 776.4
- Uehlinger's (acropachyderma) 757.39
- Ullrich (-Bonnevie) (-Turner) 758.6
- Ullrich-Feichtiger 759.89
- underwater blast injury (abdominal) (see also Injury, internal, abdomen) 868.00
- universal joint, cervix 620.6
- Unverricht (-Lundborg) 345.1 ☑
- Unverricht-Wagner (dermatomyositis) 710.3
- upward gaze 378.81
- Urbach-Oppenheim (necrobiosis lipoidica diabeticorum) 250.8 ☑ [709.3]
  - due to secondary diabetes 249.8 ☑ [709.3]
- Urbach-Wiethe (lipoid proteinosis) 272.8
- uremia, chronic 585.9
- urethral 597.81
- urethro-oculoarticular 099.3
- urethro-oculosynovial 099.3
- urohepatic 572.4
- uveocutaneous 364.24
- uveomeningeal, uveomeningitis 363.22

☑ Additional Digit Required — Refer to the Tabular List for Digit Selection   ⱳ Subterms under main terms may continue to next column or page

274 — Volume 2   ▶◀ Revised Text   ● New Line   ▲ Revised Code   2013 ICD-9-CM

Syndrome — *see also* Disease — *continued*
vagohypoglossal 352.6
vagovagal 780.2
van Buchem's (hyperostosis corticalis) 733.3
van der Hoeve's (brittle bones and blue sclera, deafness) 756.51
van der Hoeve-Halbertsma-Waardenburg (ptosis-epicanthus) 270.2
van der Hoeve-Waardenburg-Gualdi (ptosis-epicanthus) 270.2
vanishing twin 651.33
van Neck-Odelberg (juvenile osteochondrosis) 732.1
vascular splanchnic 557.0
vasomotor 443.9
vasovagal 780.2
VATER 759.89
Velo-cardio-facial 758.32
vena cava (inferior) (superior) (obstruction) 459.2
Verbiest's (claudicatio intermittens spinalis) 435.1
Vernet's 352.6
vertebral
artery 435.1
compression 721.1
lumbar 724.4
steal 435.1
vertebrogenic (pain) 724.5
vertiginous NEC 386.9
video display tube 723.8
Villaret's 352.6
Vinson-Plummer (sideropenic dysphagia) 280.8
virilizing adrenocortical hyperplasia, congenital 255.2
virus, viral 079.99
visceral larval migrans 128.0
visual disorientation 368.16
vitamin B$_6$ deficiency 266.1
vitreous touch 997.99
Vogt's (corpus striatum) 333.71
Vogt-Koyanagi 364.24
Volkmann's 958.6
von Bechterew-Strümpell (ankylosing spondylitis) 720.0
von Graefe's 378.72
von Hippel-Lindau (angiomatosis retinocerebellosa) 759.6
von Schroetter's (intermittent venous claudication) 453.89
von Willebrand (-Jürgens) (angiohemophilia) 286.4
Waardenburg-Klein (ptosis epicanthus) 270.2
Wagner (-Unverricht) (dermatomyositis) 710.3
Waldenström's (macroglobulinemia) 273.3
Waldenström-Kjellberg (sideropenic dysphagia) 280.8
Wallenberg's (posterior inferior cerebellar artery) (*see also* Disease, cerebrovascular, acute) 436
Waterhouse (-Friderichsen) 036.3
water retention 276.69
Weber's 344.89
Weber-Christian (nodular nonsuppurative panniculitis) 729.30
Weber-Cockayne (epidermolysis bullosa) 757.39
Weber-Dimitri (encephalocutaneous angiomatosis) 759.6
Weber-Gubler 344.89
Weber-Leyden 344.89
Weber-Osler (familial hemorrhagic telangiectasia) 448.0
Wegener's (necrotizing respiratory granulomatosis) 446.4
Weill-Marchesani (brachymorphism and ectopia lentis) 759.89
Weingarten's (tropical eosinophilia) 518.3
Weiss-Baker (carotid sinus syncope) 337.01
Weissenbach-Thiberge (cutaneous systemic sclerosis) 710.1
Werdnig-Hoffmann 335.0

Syndrome — *see also* Disease — *continued*
Werlhof-Wichmann (*see also* Purpura, thrombocytopenic) 287.39
Wermer's (polyendocrine adenomatosis) 258.01
Werner's (progeria adultorum) 259.8
Wernicke's (nonalcoholic) (superior hemorrhagic polioencephalitis) 265.1
Wernicke-Korsakoff (nonalcoholic) 294.0
alcoholic 291.1
Westphal-Strümpell (hepatolenticular degeneration) 275.1
wet
brain (alcoholic) 303.9 ☑
feet (maceration) (tropical) 991.4
lung
adult 518.52
newborn 770.6
whiplash 847.0
Whipple's (intestinal lipodystrophy) 040.2
"whistling face" (craniocarpotarsal dystrophy) 759.89
Widal (-Abrami) (acquired hemolytic jaundice) 283.9
Wilkie's 557.1
Wilkinson-Sneddon (subcorneal pustular dermatosis) 694.1
Willan-Plumbe (psoriasis) 696.1
Willebrand (-Jürgens) (angiohemophilia) 286.4
Willi-Prader (hypogenital dystrophy with diabetic tendency) 759.81
Wilson's (hepatolenticular degeneration) 275.1
Wilson-Mikity 770.7
Wiskott-Aldrich (eczema-thrombocytopenia) 279.12
withdrawal
alcohol 291.81
drug 292.0
infant of dependent mother 779.5
Woakes' (ethmoiditis) 471.1
Wolff-Parkinson-White (anomalous atrioventricular excitation) 426.7
Wright's (hyperabduction) 447.8
X
cardiac 413.9
dysmetabolic 277.7
xiphoidalgia 733.99
XO 758.6
XXX 758.81
XXXXY 758.81
XXY 758.7
yellow vernix (placental dysfunction) 762.2
Zahorsky's 074.0
Zellweger 277.86
Zieve's (jaundice, hyperlipemia and hemolytic anemia) 571.1
Zollinger-Ellison (gastric hypersecretion with pancreatic islet cell tumor) 251.5
Zuelzer-Ogden (nutritional megaloblastic anemia) 281.2
Synechia (iris) (pupil) 364.70
anterior 364.72
peripheral 364.73
intrauterine (traumatic) 621.5
posterior 364.71
vulvae, congenital 752.49
Synesthesia — *see also* Disturbance, sensation 782.0
Synodontia 520.2
Synophthalmus 759.89
Synorchidism 752.89
Synorchism 752.89
Synostosis (congenital) 756.59
astragaloscaphoid 755.67
radioulnar 755.53
talonavicular (bar) 755.67
tarsal 755.67
Synovial — *see* condition
Synovioma (M9040/3) — *see also* Neoplasm, connective tissue, malignant
benign (M9040/0) — *see* Neoplasm, connective tissue, benign
Synoviosarcoma (M9040/3) — *see* Neoplasm, connective tissue, malignant

Synovitis (*see also* Tenosynovitis) 727.00
chronic crepitant, wrist 727.2
due to crystals — *see* Arthritis, due to crystals
gonococcal 098.51
gouty 274.00
specified NEC 727.09
syphilitic 095.7
congenital 090.0
traumatic, current — *see* Sprain, by site
tuberculous — *see* Tuberculosis, synovitis
villonodular 719.20
ankle 719.27
elbow 719.22
foot 719.27
hand 719.24
hip 719.25
knee 719.26
multiple sites 719.29
pelvic region 719.25
shoulder (region) 719.21
specified site NEC 719.28
wrist 719.23
Syphilide 091.3
congenital 090.0
newborn 090.0
tubercular 095.8
congenital 090.0
Syphilis, syphilitic (acquired) 097.9
with lung involvement 095.1
abdomen (late) 095.2
acoustic nerve 094.86
adenopathy (secondary) 091.4
adrenal (gland) 095.8
with cortical hypofunction 095.8
age under 2 years NEC (*see also* Syphilis, congenital) 090.9
acquired 097.9
alopecia (secondary) 091.82
anemia 095.8
aneurysm (artery) (ruptured) 093.89
aorta 093.0
central nervous system 094.89
congenital 090.5
anus 095.8
primary 091.1
secondary 091.3
aorta, aortic (arch) (abdominal) (insufficiency) (pulmonary) (regurgitation) (stenosis) (thoracic) 093.89
aneurysm 093.0
arachnoid (adhesive) 094.2
artery 093.89
cerebral 094.89
spinal 094.89
arthropathy (neurogenic) (tabetic) 094.0 *[713.5]*
asymptomatic — *see* Syphilis, latent
ataxia, locomotor (progressive) 094.0
atrophoderma maculatum 091.3
auricular fibrillation 093.89
Bell's palsy 094.89
bladder 095.8
bone 095.5
secondary 091.61
brain 094.89
breast 095.8
bronchus 095.8
bubo 091.0
bulbar palsy 094.89
bursa (late) 095.7
cardiac decompensation 093.89
cardiovascular (early) (late) (primary) (secondary) (tertiary) 093.9
specified type and site NEC 093.89
causing death under 2 years of age (*see also* Syphilis, congenital) 090.9
stated to be acquired NEC 097.9
central nervous system (any site) (early) (late) (latent) (primary) (recurrent) (relapse) (secondary) (tertiary) 094.9
with
ataxia 094.0
paralysis, general 094.1
juvenile 090.40
paresis (general) 094.1

Syphilis, syphilitic — *continued*
central nervous system — *continued*
with — *continued*
paresis — *continued*
juvenile 090.40
tabes (dorsalis) 094.0
juvenile 090.40
taboparesis 094.1
juvenile 090.40
aneurysm (ruptured) 094.87
congenital 090.40
juvenile 090.40
remission in (sustained) 094.9
serology doubtful, negative, or positive 094.9
specified nature or site NEC 094.89
vascular 094.89
cerebral 094.89
meningovascular 094.2
nerves 094.89
sclerosis 094.89
thrombosis 094.89
cerebrospinal 094.89
tabetic 094.0
cerebrovascular 094.89
cervix 095.8
chancre (multiple) 091.0
extragenital 091.2
Rollet's 091.2
Charcôt's joint 094.0 *[713.5]*
choked disc 094.89 *[377.00]*
chorioretinitis 091.51
congenital 090.0 *[363.13]*
late 094.83
choroiditis 091.51
congenital 090.0 *[363.13]*
late 094.83
prenatal 090.0 *[363.13]*
choroidoretinitis (secondary) 091.51
congenital 090.0 *[363.13]*
late 094.83
ciliary body (secondary) 091.52
late 095.8 *[364.11]*
colon (late) 095.8
combined sclerosis 094.89
complicating pregnancy, childbirth or puerperium 647.0 ☑
affecting fetus or newborn 760.2
condyloma (latum) 091.3
congenital 090.9
with
encephalitis 090.41
paresis (general) 090.40
tabes (dorsalis) 090.40
taboparesis 090.40
chorioretinitis, choroiditis 090.0 *[363.13]*
early or less than 2 years after birth NEC 090.2
with manifestations 090.0
latent (without manifestations) 090.1
negative spinal fluid test 090.1
serology, positive 090.1
symptomatic 090.0
interstitial keratitis 090.3
juvenile neurosyphilis 090.40
late or 2 years or more after birth NEC 090.7
chorioretinitis, choroiditis 090.5 *[363.13]*
interstitial keratitis 090.3
juvenile neurosyphilis NEC 090.40
latent (without manifestations) 090.6
negative spinal fluid test 090.6
serology, positive 090.6
symptomatic or with manifestations NEC 090.5
interstitial keratitis 090.3
conjugal 097.9
tabes 097.0
conjunctiva 095.8 *[372.10]*
contact V01.6
cord, bladder 094.0
cornea, late 095.8 *[370.59]*
coronary (artery) 093.89
sclerosis 093.89
coryza 095.8

☑ **Additional Digit Required** — Refer to the Tabular List for Digit Selection   ▽ **Subterms under main terms may continue to next column or page**

2013 ICD-9-CM   ▶◀ **Revised Text**   ● **New Line**   ▲ **Revised Code**   **Volume 2 — 275**

Syphilis, syphilitic — *continued*
  coryza — *continued*
    congenital 090.0
  cranial nerve 094.89
  cutaneous — *see* Syphilis, skin
  dacryocystitis 095.8
  degeneration, spinal cord 094.89
  d'emblée 095.8
  dementia 094.1
    paralytica 094.1
      juvenilis 090.40
  destruction of bone 095.5
  dilatation, aorta 093.0
  due to blood transfusion 097.9
  dura mater 094.89
  ear 095.8
    inner 095.8
      nerve (eighth) 094.86
      neurorecurrence 094.86
  early NEC 091.0
    cardiovascular 093.9
    central nervous system 094.9
      paresis 094.1
      tabes 094.0
    latent (without manifestations) (less than 2 years after infection) 092.9
      negative spinal fluid test 092.9
      serological relapse following treatment 092.0
      serology positive 092.9
    paresis 094.1
    relapse (treated, untreated) 091.7
    skin 091.3
    symptomatic NEC 091.89
      extragenital chancre 091.2
      primary, except extragenital chancre 091.0
      secondary (*see also* Syphilis, secondary) 091.3
        relapse (treated, untreated) 091.7
    tabes 094.0
    ulcer 091.3
  eighth nerve 094.86
  endemic, nonvenereal 104.0
  endocarditis 093.20
    aortic 093.22
    mitral 093.21
    pulmonary 093.24
    tricuspid 093.23
  epididymis (late) 095.8
  epiglottis 095.8
  epiphysitis (congenital) 090.0
  esophagus 095.8
  Eustachian tube 095.8
  exposure to V01.6
  eye 095.8 *[363.13]*
    neuromuscular mechanism 094.85
  eyelid 095.8 *[373.5]*
    with gumma 095.8 *[373.5]*
    ptosis 094.89
  fallopian tube 095.8
  fracture 095.5
  gallbladder (late) 095.8
  gastric 095.8
    crisis 094.0
    polyposis 095.8
  general 097.9
    paralysis 094.1
      juvenile 090.40
  genital (primary) 091.0
  glaucoma 095.8
  gumma (late) NEC 095.9
    cardiovascular system 093.9
    central nervous system 094.9
    congenital 090.5
    heart or artery 093.89
  heart 093.89
    block 093.89
    decompensation 093.89
    disease 093.89
    failure 093.89
    valve (*see also* Syphilis, endocarditis) 093.20
  hemianesthesia 094.89
  hemianopsia 095.8
  hemiparesis 094.89

Syphilis, syphilitic — *continued*
  hemiplegia 094.89
  hepatic artery 093.89
  hepatitis 095.3
  hepatomegaly 095.3
    congenital 090.0
  hereditaria tarda (*see also* Syphilis, congenital, late) 090.7
  hereditary (*see also* Syphilis, congenital) 090.9
    interstitial keratitis 090.3
  Hutchinson's teeth 090.5
  hyalitis 095.8
  inactive — *see* Syphilis, latent
  infantum NEC (*see also* Syphilis, congenital) 090.9
  inherited — *see* Syphilis, congenital
  internal ear 095.8
  intestine (late) 095.8
  iris, iritis (secondary) 091.52
    late 095.8 *[364.11]*
  joint (late) 095.8
  keratitis (congenital) (early) (interstitial) (late) (parenchymatous) (punctata profunda) 090.3
  kidney 095.4
  lacrimal apparatus 095.8
  laryngeal paralysis 095.8
  larynx 095.8
  late 097.0
    cardiovascular 093.9
    central nervous system 094.9
    latent or 2 years or more after infection (without manifestations) 096
      negative spinal fluid test 096
      serology positive 096
    paresis 094.1
    specified site NEC 095.8
    symptomatic or with symptoms 095.9
    tabes 094.0
  latent 097.1
    central nervous system 094.9
    date of infection unspecified 097.1
    early or less than 2 years after infection 092.9
    late or 2 years or more after infection 096
    serology
      doubtful
        follow-up of latent syphilis 097.1
        central nervous system 094.9
        date of infection unspecified 097.1
        early or less than 2 years after infection 092.9
        late or 2 years or more after infection 096
      positive, only finding 097.1
        date of infection unspecified 097.1
        early or less than 2 years after infection 097.1
        late or 2 years or more after infection 097.1
  lens 095.8
  leukoderma 091.3
    late 095.8
  lienis 095.8
  lip 091.3
    chancre 091.2
    late 095.8
    primary 091.2
  Lissauer's paralysis 094.1
  liver 095.3
    secondary 091.62
  locomotor ataxia 094.0
  lung 095.1
  lymphadenitis (secondary) 091.4
  lymph gland (early) (secondary) 091.4
    late 095.8
  macular atrophy of skin 091.3
    striated 095.8
  maternal, affecting fetus or newborn 760.2
    manifest syphilis in newborn — *see* Syphilis, congenital
  mediastinum (late) 095.8

Syphilis, syphilitic — *continued*
  meninges (adhesive) (basilar) (brain) (spinal cord) 094.2
  meningitis 094.2
    acute 091.81
    congenital 090.42
  meningoencephalitis 094.2
  meningovascular 094.2
    congenital 090.49
  mesarteritis 093.89
    brain 094.89
    spine 094.89
  middle ear 095.8
  mitral stenosis 093.21
  monoplegia 094.89
  mouth (secondary) 091.3
    late 095.8
  mucocutaneous 091.3
    late 095.8
  mucous
    membrane 091.3
      late 095.8
    patches 091.3
      congenital 090.0
  mulberry molars 090.5
  muscle 095.6
  myocardium 093.82
  myositis 095.6
  nasal sinus 095.8
  neonatorum NEC (*see also* Syphilis, congenital) 090.9
  nerve palsy (any cranial nerve) 094.89
  nervous system, central 094.9
  neuritis 095.8
    acoustic nerve 094.86
  neurorecidive of retina 094.83
  neuroretinitis 094.85
  newborn (*see also* Syphilis, congenital) 090.9
  nodular superficial 095.8
  nonvenereal, endemic 104.0
  nose 095.8
    saddle back deformity 090.5
    septum 095.8
      perforated 095.8
  occlusive arterial disease 093.89
  ophthalmic 095.8 *[363.13]*
  ophthalmoplegia 094.89
  optic nerve (atrophy) (neuritis) (papilla) 094.84
  orbit (late) 095.8
  orchitis 095.8
  organic 097.9
  osseous (late) 095.5
  osteochondritis (congenital) 090.0
  osteoporosis 095.5
  ovary 095.8
  oviduct 095.8
  palate 095.8
    gumma 095.8
    perforated 090.5
  pancreas (late) 095.8
  pancreatitis 095.8
  paralysis 094.89
    general 094.1
    juvenile 090.40
  paraplegia 094.89
  paresis (general) 094.1
    juvenile 090.40
  paresthesia 094.89
  Parkinson's disease or syndrome 094.82
  paroxysmal tachycardia 093.89
  pemphigus (congenital) 090.0
  penis 091.0
    chancre 091.0
    late 095.8
  pericardium 093.81
  perichondritis, larynx 095.8
  periosteum 095.5
    congenital 090.0
    early 091.61
    secondary 091.61
  peripheral nerve 095.8
  petrous bone (late) 095.5
  pharynx 095.8
    secondary 091.3
  pituitary (gland) 095.8

Syphilis, syphilitic — *continued*
  placenta 095.8
  pleura (late) 095.8
  pneumonia, white 090.0
  pontine (lesion) 094.89
  portal vein 093.89
  primary NEC 091.2
    anal 091.1
    and secondary (*see also* Syphilis, secondary) 091.9
    cardiovascular 093.9
    central nervous system 094.9
    extragenital chancre NEC 091.2
    fingers 091.2
    genital 091.0
    lip 091.2
    specified site NEC 091.2
    tonsils 091.2
  prostate 095.8
  psychosis (intracranial gumma) 094.89
  ptosis (eyelid) 094.89
  pulmonary (late) 095.1
    artery 093.89
  pulmonum 095.1
  pyelonephritis 095.4
  recently acquired, symptomatic NEC 091.89
  rectum 095.8
  respiratory tract 095.8
  retina
    late 094.83
    neurorecidive 094.83
  retrobulbar neuritis 094.85
  salpingitis 095.8
  sclera (late) 095.0
  sclerosis
    cerebral 094.89
    coronary 093.89
    multiple 094.89
    subacute 094.89
  scotoma (central) 095.8
  scrotum 095.8
  secondary (and primary) 091.9
    adenopathy 091.4
    anus 091.3
    bone 091.61
    cardiovascular 093.9
    central nervous system 094.9
    chorioretinitis, choroiditis 091.51
    hepatitis 091.62
    liver 091.62
    lymphadenitis 091.4
    meningitis, acute 091.81
    mouth 091.3
    mucous membranes 091.3
    periosteum 091.61
    periostitis 091.61
    pharynx 091.3
    relapse (treated) (untreated) 091.7
    skin 091.3
    specified form NEC 091.89
    tonsil 091.3
    ulcer 091.3
    viscera 091.69
    vulva 091.3
  seminal vesicle (late) 095.8
  seronegative
    with signs or symptoms — *see* Syphilis, by site or stage
  seropositive
    with signs or symptoms — *see* Syphilis, by site and stage
    follow-up of latent syphilis — *see* Syphilis, latent
    only finding — *see* Syphilis, latent
  seventh nerve (paralysis) 094.89
  sinus 095.8
  sinusitis 095.8
  skeletal system 095.5
  skin (early) (secondary) (with ulceration) 091.3
    late or tertiary 095.8
  small intestine 095.8
  spastic spinal paralysis 094.0
  spermatic cord (late) 095.8
  spinal (cord) 094.89

☑ **Additional Digit Required** — Refer to the Tabular List for Digit Selection   ▽ **Subterms under main terms may continue to next column or page**

276 — Volume 2   ▶◀ Revised Text   ● New Line   ▲ Revised Code   2013 ICD-9-CM

Syphilis, syphilitic — *continued*
  spinal — *continued*
    with
      paresis 094.1
      tabes 094.0
  spleen 095.8
  splenomegaly 095.8
  spondylitis 095.5
  staphyloma 095.8
  stigmata (congenital) 090.5
  stomach 095.8
  synovium (late) 095.7
  tabes dorsalis (early) (late) 094.0
    juvenile 090.40
  tabetic type 094.0
    juvenile 090.40
  taboparesis 094.1
    juvenile 090.40
  tachycardia 093.89
  tendon (late) 095.7
  tertiary 097.0
    with symptoms 095.8
    cardiovascular 093.9
    central nervous system 094.9
    multiple NEC 095.8
    specified site NEC 095.8
  testis 095.8
  thorax 095.8
  throat 095.8
  thymus (gland) 095.8
  thyroid (late) 095.8
  tongue 095.8
  tonsil (lingual) 095.8
    primary 091.2
    secondary 091.3
  trachea 095.8
  tricuspid valve 093.23
  tumor, brain 094.89
  tunica vaginalis (late) 095.8
  ulcer (any site) (early) (secondary) 091.3
    late 095.9
    perforating 095.9
      foot 094.0
  urethra (stricture) 095.8
  urogenital 095.8
  uterus 095.8
  uveal tract (secondary) 091.50
    late 095.8 [363.13]
  uveitis (secondary) 091.50
    late 095.8 [363.13]
  uvula (late) 095.8
    perforated 095.8
  vagina 091.0
    late 095.8
  valvulitis NEC 093.20
  vascular 093.89
    brain or cerebral 094.89
  vein 093.89
    cerebral 094.89
  ventriculi 095.8
  vesicae urinariae 095.8
  viscera (abdominal) 095.2
    secondary 091.69
  vitreous (hemorrhage) (opacities) 095.8
  vulva 091.0
    late 095.8
    secondary 091.3
Syphiloma 095.9
  cardiovascular system 093.9
  central nervous system 094.9
  circulatory system 093.9
  congenital 090.5
Syphilophobia 300.29
Syringadenoma (M8400/0) — *see also* Neoplasm, skin, benign
  papillary (M8406/0) — *see* Neoplasm, skin, benign
Syringobulbia 336.0
Syringocarcinoma (M8400/3) — *see* Neoplasm, skin, malignant
Syringocystadenoma (M8400/0) — *see also* Neoplasm, skin, benign
  papillary (M8406/0) — *see* Neoplasm, skin, benign
Syringocystoma (M8407/0) — *see* Neoplasm, skin, benign

Syringoma (M8407/0) — *see also* Neoplasm, skin, benign
  chondroid (M8940/0) — *see* Neoplasm, by site, benign
Syringomyelia 336.0
Syringomyelitis 323.9
  late effect — *see* category 326
Syringomyelocele — *see also* Spina bifida 741.9 ☑
Syringopontia 336.0
System, systemic — *see also* condition
  disease, combined — *see* Degeneration, combined
  fibrosclerosing syndrome 710.8
  inflammatory response syndrome (SIRS) 995.90
    due to
      infectious process 995.91
        with acute organ dysfunction 995.92
      non-infectious process 995.93
        with acute organ dysfunction 995.94
  lupus erythematosus 710.0
    inhibitor 795.79

T

Tab — *see* Tag
Tabacism 989.84
Tabacosis 989.84
Tabardillo 080
  flea-borne 081.0
  louse-borne 080
Tabes, tabetic
  with
    central nervous system syphilis 094.0
    Charcôt's joint 094.0 [713.5]
    cord bladder 094.0
    crisis, viscera (any) 094.0
    paralysis, general 094.1
    paresis (general) 094.1
    perforating ulcer 094.0
  arthropathy 094.0 [713.5]
  bladder 094.0
  bone 094.0
  cerebrospinal 094.0
  congenital 090.40
  conjugal 094.0
  dorsalis 094.0
    neurosyphilis 094.0
  early 094.0
  juvenile 090.40
  latent 094.0
  mesenterica (*see also* Tuberculosis) 014.8 ☑
  paralysis insane, general 094.1
  peripheral (nonsyphilitic) 799.89
  spasmodic 094.0
    not dorsal or dorsalis 343.9
  syphilis (cerebrospinal) 094.0
Taboparalysis 094.1
Taboparesis (remission) 094.1
  with
    Charcôt's joint 094.1 [713.5]
    cord bladder 094.1
    perforating ulcer 094.1
  juvenile 090.40
Tache noir 923.20
Tachyalimentation 579.3
Tachyarrhythmia, tachyrhythmia — *see also* Tachycardia
  paroxysmal with sinus bradycardia 427.81
Tachycardia 785.0
  atrial 427.89
  auricular 427.89
  AV nodal re-entry (re-entrant) 427.89
  junctional ectopic 427.0
  newborn 779.82
  nodal 427.89
    nonparoxysmal atrioventricular 426.89
  nonparoxysmal atrioventricular (nodal) 426.89
  nonsustained 427.2
  paroxysmal 427.2
    with sinus bradycardia 427.81
    atrial (PAT) 427.0
      psychogenic 316 [427.0]

Tachycardia — *continued*
  paroxysmal — *continued*
    atrioventricular (AV) 427.0
      psychogenic 316 [427.0]
    essential 427.2
    junctional 427.0
    nodal 427.0
    psychogenic 316 [427.2]
      atrial 316 [427.0]
      supraventricular 316 [427.0]
      ventricular 316 [427.1]
    supraventricular 427.0
      psychogenic 316 [427.0]
    ventricular 427.1
      psychogenic 316 [427.1]
  postoperative 997.1
  psychogenic 306.2
  sick sinus 427.81
  sinoauricular 427.89
  sinus 427.89
  supraventricular 427.89
  sustained 427.2
    supraventricular 427.0
    ventricular 427.1
  ventricular (paroxysmal) 427.1
    psychogenic 316 [427.1]
Tachygastria 536.8
Tachypnea 786.06
  hysterical 300.11
  newborn (idiopathic) (transitory) 770.6
  psychogenic 306.1
  transitory, of newborn 770.6
TACO (transfusion associated circulatory overload) 276.61
Taenia (infection) (infestation) — *see also* Infestation, taenia 123.3
  diminuta 123.6
  echinococcal infestation (*see also* Echinococcus) 122.9
  nana 123.6
  saginata infestation 123.2
  solium (intestinal form) 123.0
    larval form 123.1
Taeniasis (intestine) — *see also* Infestation, taenia 123.3
  saginata 123.2
  solium 123.0
Taenzer's disease 757.4
Tag (hypertrophied skin) (infected) 701.9
  adenoid 474.8
  anus 455.9
  endocardial (*see also* Endocarditis) 424.90
  hemorrhoidal 455.9
  hymen 623.8
  perineal 624.8
  preauricular 744.1
  rectum 455.9
  sentinel 455.9
  skin 701.9
    accessory 757.39
    anus 455.9
    congenital 757.39
    preauricular 744.1
    rectum 455.9
  tonsil 474.8
  urethra, urethral 599.84
  vulva 624.8
Tahyna fever 062.5
Takayasu (-Onishi) disease or syndrome (pulseless disease) 446.7
Takotsubo syndrome 429.83
Talc granuloma 728.82
  in operation wound 998.7
Talcosis 502
Talipes (congenital) 754.70
  acquired NEC 736.79
    planus 734
  asymmetric 754.79
    acquired 736.79
  calcaneovalgus 754.62
    acquired 736.76
  calcaneovarus 754.59
    acquired 736.76
  calcaneus 754.79
    acquired 736.76
  cavovarus 754.59

Talipes — *continued*
  cavovarus — *continued*
    acquired 736.75
  cavus 754.71
    acquired 736.73
  equinovalgus 754.69
    acquired 736.72
  equinovarus 754.51
    acquired 736.71
  equinus 754.79
    acquired, NEC 736.72
  percavus 754.71
    acquired 736.73
  planovalgus 754.69
    acquired 736.79
  planus (acquired) (any degree) 734
    congenital 754.61
    due to rickets 268.1
  valgus 754.60
    acquired 736.79
  varus 754.50
    acquired 736.79
Talma's disease 728.85
Talon noir 924.20
  hand 923.20
  heel 924.20
  toe 924.3
Tamponade heart (Rose's) — *see also* Pericarditis 423.3
Tanapox 059.21
Tangier disease (familial high-density lipoprotein deficiency) 272.5
Tank ear 380.12
Tantrum (childhood) — *see also* Disturbance, conduct 312.1 ☑
Tapeworm (infection) (infestation) — *see also* Infestation, tapeworm 123.9
Tapia's syndrome 352.6
Tarantism 297.8
Target-oval cell anemia 285.8
  with thalassemia — *see* Thalassemia
Tarlov's cyst 355.9
Tarral-Besnier disease (pityriasis rubra pilaris) 696.4
Tarsalgia 729.2
Tarsal tunnel syndrome 355.5
Tarsitis (eyelid) 373.00
  syphilitic 095.8 [373.00]
  tuberculous (*see also* Tuberculosis) 017.0 ☑ [373.4]
Tartar (teeth) 523.6
Tattoo (mark) 709.09
Taurodontism 520.2
Taussig-Bing defect, heart, or syndrome (transposition, aorta and overriding pulmonary artery) 745.11
Taybi's syndrome (otopalatodigital) 759.89
Tay's choroiditis 363.41
Taylor's
  disease (diffuse idiopathic cutaneous atrophy) 701.8
  syndrome 625.5
Tay-Sachs
  amaurotic familial idiocy 330.1
  disease 330.1
TBI (traumatic brain injury) — *see also* Injury, intracranial 854.0 ☑
  with skull fracture — *see* Fracture, skull, by site
Tear stone 375.57
Tear, torn (traumatic) — *see also* Wound, open, by site
  annular fibrosis 722.51
  anus, anal (sphincter) 863.89
    with open wound in cavity 863.99
    complicating delivery (healed) (old) 654.8 ☑
      with mucosa 664.3 ☑
      not associated with third-degree perineal laceration 664.6 ☑
    nontraumatic, nonpuerperal (healed) (old) 569.43
  articular cartilage, old (*see also* Disorder, cartilage, articular) 718.0 ☑

☑ Additional Digit Required — Refer to the Tabular List for Digit Selection

Subterms under main terms may continue to next column or page

2013 ICD-9-CM

►◄ Revised Text   ● New Line   ▲ Revised Code

Volume 2 — 277

Syphilis, syphilitic — Tear, torn

☑ **Additional Digit Required — Refer to the Tabular List for Digit Selection**   ▼ **Subterms under main terms may continue to next column or page**

Teratoma — *see also* Neoplasm, by site, uncertain behavior — *continued*
  malignant (*see also* Neoplasm, by site, malignant) — *continued*
    trophoblastic (M9102/3)
      specified site — *see* Neoplasm, by site, malignant
      unspecified site 186.9
    undifferentiated type (M9082/3) — *see* Neoplasm, by site, malignant
  mature (M9080/0) — *see* Neoplasm, by site, benign
  malignant (M9080/3) — *see* Neoplasm, by site, malignant
  ovary (M9080/0) 220
    embryonal, immature, or malignant (M9080/3) 183.0
  suprasellar (M9080/3) — *see* Neoplasm, by site, malignant
  testis (M9080/3) 186.9
    adult, benign, cystic, differentiated type or mature (M9080/0) 222.0
    undescended 186.0
Terminal care V66.7
Termination
  anomalous (*see also* Malposition, congenital)
    portal vein 747.49
    right pulmonary vein 747.42
  pregnancy (legal) (therapeutic) — *see* Abortion, legal 635.9 ☑
    fetus NEC 779.6
    illegal (*see also* Abortion, illegal) 636.9 ☑
Ternidens diminutus infestation 127.7
Terrors, night (child) 307.46
Terry's syndrome (*see also* Retinopathy of prematurity) 362.21
Tertiary — *see* condition
Tessellated fundus, retina (tigroid) 362.89
Test(s)
  adequacy
    hemodialysis V56.31
    peritoneal dialysis V56.32
  AIDS virus V72.69
  allergen V72.7
  bacterial disease NEC (*see also* Screening, by name of disease) V74.9
  basal metabolic rate V72.69
  blood
    alcohol V70.4
    drug V70.4
      for therapeutic drug monitoring V58.83
      for routine general physical examination V72.62
      prior to treatment or procedure V72.63
    typing V72.86
      Rh typing V72.86
  developmental, infant or child V20.2
  Dick V74.8
  fertility V26.21
  genetic
    female V26.32
    for genetic disease carrier status
      female V26.31
      male V26.34
    male V26.39
  hearing V72.19
    following failed hearing screening V72.11
    routine, for infant and child V20.2
  HIV V72.69
  human immunodeficiency virus V72.69
  immunity status V72.61
  Kveim V82.89
  laboratory V72.60
    for medicolegal reason V70.4
    ordered as part of a routine general medical examination V72.62
    pre-operative V72.63
    pre-procedural V72.63
    specified NEC V72.69
  male partner of female with recurrent pregnancy loss V26.35
  Mantoux (for tuberculosis) V74.1

Test(s) — *continued*
  mycotic organism V75.4
  nuchal translucency V28.89
  parasitic agent NEC V75.8
  paternity V70.4
  peritoneal equilibration V56.32
  pregnancy
    negative result V72.41
    positive result V72.42
      first pregnancy V72.42
    unconfirmed V72.40
  preoperative V72.84
    cardiovascular V72.81
    respiratory V72.82
    specified NEC V72.83
  procreative management NEC V26.29
    genetic disease carrier status
      female V26.31
      male V26.34
  Rh typing V72.86
  sarcoidosis V82.89
  Schick V74.3
  Schultz-Charlton V74.8
  skin, diagnostic
    allergy V72.7
    bacterial agent NEC (*see also* Screening, by name of disease) V74.9
    Dick V74.8
    hypersensitivity V72.7
    Kveim V82.89
    Mantoux V74.1
    mycotic organism V75.4
    parasitic agent NEC V75.8
    sarcoidosis V82.89
    Schick V74.3
    Schultz-Charlton V74.8
    tuberculin V74.1
  specified type NEC V72.85
  tuberculin V74.1
  vision V72.0
    routine, for infant and child V20.2
  Wassermann
    positive (*see also* Serology for syphilis, positive) 097.1
    false 795.6
Testicle, testicular, testis — *see also* condition
  feminization (syndrome) 259.51
Tetanus, tetanic (cephalic) (convulsions) 037
  with
    abortion — *see* Abortion, by type, with sepsis
    ectopic pregnancy (*see also* categories 633.0–633.9) 639.0
    molar pregnancy — *see* categories 630–632 639.0
  following
    abortion 639.0
    ectopic or molar pregnancy 639.0
  inoculation V03.7
    reaction (due to serum) — *see* Complications, vaccination
  neonatorum 771.3
  puerperal, postpartum, childbirth 670.8 ☑
Tetany, tetanic 781.7
  alkalosis 276.3
  associated with rickets 268.0
  convulsions 781.7
    hysterical 300.11
  functional (hysterical) 300.11
  hyperkinetic 781.7
    hysterical 300.11
  hyperpnea 786.01
    hysterical 300.11
    psychogenic 306.1
  hyperventilation 786.01
    hysterical 300.11
    psychogenic 306.1
  hypocalcemic, neonatal 775.4
  hysterical 300.11
  neonatal 775.4
  parathyroid (gland) 252.1
  parathyroprival 252.1
  postoperative 252.1
  postthyroidectomy 252.1
  pseudotetany 781.7
    hysterical 300.11

Tetany, tetanic — *continued*
  psychogenic 306.1
    specified as conversion reaction 300.11
Tetralogy of Fallot 745.2
Tetraplegia — *see* Quadriplegia
Thailand hemorrhagic fever 065.4
Thalassanemia 282.40
Thalassemia (disease) 282.40
  with other hemoglobinopathy 282.49
  alpha (major) (severe) (triple gene defect) 282.43
    silent carrier 282.46
  beta (homozygous) (major) (severe) 282.44
  delta-beta (homozygous) 282.45
  dominant 282.49
  Hb-S (without crisis) 282.41
    with
      crisis 282.42
      vaso-occlusive pain 282.42
  hemoglobin
    C (Hb-C) 282.49
    D (Hb-D) 282.49
    E (Hb-E) 282.49
    E-beta 282.47
    H (Hb-H) 282.49
    I (Hb-I) 282.49
  high fetal gene (*see also* Thalassemia) 282.40
  high fetal hemoglobin (*see also* Thalassemia) 282.40
  intermedia 282.44
  major 282.44
  minor (alpha) (beta) 282.46
  mixed 282.49
  sickle-cell (without crisis) 282.41
    with
      crisis 282.42
      vaso-occlusive pain 282.42
  specified NEC 282.49
  trait (alpha) (beta) (delta-beta) 282.46
Thalassemic variants 282.49
Thaysen-Gee disease (nontropical sprue) 579.0
Thecoma (M8600/0) 220
  malignant (M8600/3) 183.0
Thelarche, precocious 259.1
Thelitis 611.0
  puerperal, postpartum 675.0 ☑
Therapeutic — *see* condition
Therapy V57.9
  blood transfusion, without reported diagnosis V58.2
  breathing V57.0
  chemotherapy, antineoplastic V58.11
    fluoride V07.31
    prophylactic NEC V07.39
  dialysis (intermittent) (treatment)
    extracorporeal V56.0
    peritoneal V56.8
    renal V56.0
    specified type NEC V56.8
  exercise NEC V57.1
    breathing V57.0
  extracorporeal dialysis (renal) V56.0
  fluoride prophylaxis V07.31
  hemodialysis V56.0
  hormone replacement (postmenopausal) V07.4
  immunotherapy antineoplastic V58.12
  long term oxygen therapy V46.2
  occupational V57.21
  orthoptic V57.4
  orthotic V57.81
  peritoneal dialysis V56.8
  physical NEC V57.1
  postmenopausal hormone replacement V07.4
  radiation V58.0
  speech (-language) V57.3
  vocational V57.22
Thermalgesia 782.0
Thermalgia 782.0
Thermanalgesia 782.0
Thermanesthesia 782.0
Thermic — *see* condition
Thermography (abnormal) 793.99
  breast 793.89

Thermoplegia 992.0
Thesaurismosis
  amyloid 277.39
  bilirubin 277.4
  calcium 275.40
  cystine 270.0
  glycogen (*see also* Disease, glycogen storage) 271.0
  kerasin 272.7
  lipoid 272.7
  melanin 255.41
  phosphatide 272.7
  urate 274.9
Thiaminic deficiency 265.1
  with beriberi 265.0
Thibierge-Weissenbach syndrome (cutaneous systemic sclerosis) 710.1
Thickened endometrium 793.5
Thickening
  bone 733.99
    extremity 733.99
  breast 611.79
  hymen 623.3
  larynx 478.79
  nail 703.8
    congenital 757.5
  periosteal 733.99
  pleura (*see also* Pleurisy) 511.0
  skin 782.8
  subepiglottic 478.79
  tongue 529.8
  valve, heart — *see* Endocarditis
Thiele syndrome 724.6
Thigh — *see* condition
Thinning vertebra — *see also* Osteoporosis 733.00
Thirst, excessive 783.5
  due to deprivation of water 994.3
Thomsen's disease 359.22
Thomson's disease (congenital poikiloderma) 757.33
Thoracic — *see also* condition
  kidney 753.3
  outlet syndrome 353.0
  stomach — *see* Hernia, diaphragm
Thoracogastroschisis (congenital) 759.89
Thoracopagus 759.4
Thoracoschisis 756.3
Thoracoscopic surgical procedure converted to open procedure V64.42
Thorax — *see* condition
Thorn's syndrome — *see also* Disease, renal 593.9
Thornwaldt's, Tornwaldt's
  bursitis (pharyngeal) 478.29
  cyst 478.26
  disease (pharyngeal bursitis) 478.29
Thorson-Biörck syndrome (malignant carcinoid) 259.2
Threadworm (infection) (infestation) 127.4
Threatened
  abortion or miscarriage 640.0 ☑
    with subsequent abortion (*see also* Abortion, spontaneous) 634.9 ☑
    affecting fetus 762.1
  labor 644.1 ☑
    affecting fetus or newborn 761.8
    premature 644.0 ☑
  miscarriage 640.0 ☑
    affecting fetus 762.1
  premature
    delivery 644.2 ☑
      affecting fetus or newborn 761.8
    labor 644.0 ☑
      before 22 completed weeks gestation 640.0 ☑
Three-day fever 066.0
Threshers' lung 495.0
Thrix annulata (congenital) 757.4
Throat — *see* condition
Thrombasthenia (Glanzmann's) (hemorrhagic) (hereditary) 287.1
Thromboangiitis 443.1
  obliterans (general) 443.1
    cerebral 437.1

☑ **Additional Digit Required** — Refer to the Tabular List for Digit Selection   ▽ **Subterms under main terms may continue to next column or page**

Thrombosis, thrombotic — *continued*
  lower extremity — *continued*
    deep vessels — *continued*
      acute — *continued*
        femoral 453.41
        iliac 453.41
        lower leg 453.42
        peroneal 453.42
        popliteal 453.41
        proximal (upper leg) 453.41
        thigh 453.41
        tibial 453.42
      chronic 453.50
        calf 453.52
        distal (lower leg) 453.52
        femoral 453.51
        iliac 453.51
        lower leg 453.52
        peroneal 453.52
        popliteal 453.51
        proximal (upper leg) 453.51
        thigh 453.51
        tibial 453.52
    personal history of V12.51
    saphenous (greater) (lesser) 453.6
    superficial 453.6
  lung 415.19
    iatrogenic 415.11
    personal history of V12.55
    postoperative 415.11
    septic 415.12
  marantic, dural sinus 437.6
  meninges (brain) (*see also* Thrombosis, brain) 434.0 ☑
  mesenteric (artery) (with gangrene) 557.0
    vein (inferior) (superior) 557.0
  mitral — *see* Insufficiency, mitral
  mural (heart chamber) (*see also* Infarct, myocardium) 410.9 ☑
    without
      cardiac condition 429.89
      coronary artery disease 429.89
      myocardial infarction 429.89
    due to syphilis 093.89
    following myocardial infarction 429.79
    healed or specified as old 412
  omentum (with gangrene) 557.0
  ophthalmic (artery) (*see also* Occlusion, retina) 362.30
  pampiniform plexus (male) 608.83
    female 620.8
  parietal (*see also* Infarct, myocardium) 410.9 ☑
  penis, penile 607.82
  peripheral arteries 444.22
    lower 444.22
    upper 444.21
  platelet 446.6
  portal 452
    due to syphilis 093.89
    infectional or septic 572.1
  precerebral artery (*see also* Occlusion, artery, precerebral NEC)
  pregnancy 671.2 ☑
    deep (vein) 671.3 ☑
    superficial (vein) 671.2 ☑
  puerperal, postpartum, childbirth 671.2 ☑
    brain (artery) 674.0 ☑
      venous 671.5 ☑
    cardiac 674.8 ☑
    cerebral (artery) 674.0 ☑
      venous 671.5 ☑
    deep (vein) 671.4 ☑
    intracranial sinus (nonpyogenic) (venous) 671.5 ☑
    pelvic 671.4 ☑
    pulmonary (artery) 673.2 ☑
    specified site NEC 671.5 ☑
    superficial 671.2 ☑
  pulmonary (artery) (vein) 415.19
    iatrogenic 415.11
    personal history of V12.55
    postoperative 415.11
    septic 415.12
  renal (artery) 593.81
    vein 453.3

Thrombosis, thrombotic — *continued*
  resulting from presence of shunt or other internal prosthetic device — *see* Complications, due to (presence of) any device, implant, or graft classified to 996.0–996.5 NEC
  retina, retinal (artery) 362.30
    arterial branch 362.32
    central 362.31
    partial 362.33
    vein
      central 362.35
      tributary (branch) 362.36
  saphenous vein (greater) (lesser) 453.6
  scrotum 608.83
  seminal vesicle 608.83
  sigmoid (venous) sinus — *see* Thrombosis, intracranial venous sinus 325
  silent NEC 453.9
  sinus, intracranial (venous) (any) (*see also* Thrombosis, intracranial venous sinus) 325
  softening, brain (*see also* Thrombosis, brain) 434.0 ☑
  specified site NEC (acute) 453.89
    chronic 453.79
  spermatic cord 608.83
  spinal cord 336.1
    due to syphilis 094.89
    in pregnancy or puerperium 671.5 ☑
    pyogenic origin 324.1
      late effect — *see* category 326
  spleen, splenic 289.59
    artery 444.89
  testis 608.83
  traumatic (complication) (early) (*see also* Injury, blood vessel, by site) 904.9
  tricuspid — *see* Endocarditis, tricuspid
  tumor — *see* Neoplasm, by site
  tunica vaginalis 608.83
  umbilical cord (vessels) 663.6 ☑
    affecting fetus or newborn 762.6
  upper extremity (acute) 453.83
    chronic 453.73
      deep 453.72
      superficial 453.71
    deep 453.82
    superficial 453.81
  vas deferens 608.83
  vein
    antecubital (acute) 453.81
      chronic 453.71
    axillary (acute) 453.84
      chronic 453.74
    basilic (acute) 453.81
      chronic 453.71
    brachial (acute) 453.82
      chronic 453.72
    brachiocephalic (innominate) (acute) 453.87
      chronic 453.77
    cephalic (acute) 453.81
      chronic 453.71
    deep 453.40
      personal history of V12.51
    internal jugular (acute) 453.86
      chronic 453.76
    lower extremity — *see* Thrombosis, lower extremity
    personal history of V12.51
    radial (acute) 453.82
      chronic 453.72
    saphenous (greater) (lesser) 453.6
    specified site NEC (acute) 453.89
      chronic 453.79
    subclavian (acute) 453.85
      chronic 453.75
    superior vena cava (acute) 453.87
      chronic 453.77
    thoracic (acute) 453.87
      chronic 453.77
    ulnar (acute) 453.82
      chronic 453.72
    upper extremity — *see* Thrombosis, upper extremity

Thrombosis, thrombotic — *continued*
  vena cava
    inferior 453.2
    personal history of V12.51
    superior (acute) 453.87
      chronic 453.77
Thrombus — *see* Thrombosis
Thrush 112.0
  newborn 771.7
Thumb — *see also* condition
  gamekeeper's 842.12
  sucking (child problem) 307.9
Thygeson's superficial punctate keratitis 370.21
Thymergasia — *see also* Psychosis, affective 296.80
Thymitis 254.8
Thymoma (benign) (M8580/0) 212.6
  malignant (M8580/3) 164.0
Thymus, thymic (gland) — *see* condition
Thyrocele — *see also* Goiter 240.9
Thyroglossal — *see also* condition
  cyst 759.2
  duct, persistent 759.2
Thyroid (body) (gland) — *see also* condition
  hormone resistance 246.8
  lingual 759.2
Thyroiditis 245.9
  acute (pyogenic) (suppurative) 245.0
    nonsuppurative 245.0
  autoimmune 245.2
  chronic (nonspecific) (sclerosing) 245.8
    fibrous 245.3
    lymphadenoid 245.2
    lymphocytic 245.2
    lymphoid 245.2
  complicating pregnancy, childbirth, or puerperium 648.1 ☑
  de Quervain's (subacute granulomatous) 245.1
  fibrous (chronic) 245.3
  giant (cell) (follicular) 245.1
  granulomatous (de Quervain's) (subacute) 245.1
  Hashimoto's (struma lymphomatosa) 245.2
  iatrogenic 245.4
  invasive (fibrous) 245.3
  ligneous 245.3
  lymphocytic (chronic) 245.2
  lymphoid 245.2
  lymphomatous 245.2
  pseudotuberculous 245.1
  pyogenic 245.0
  radiation 245.4
  Riedel's (ligneous) 245.3
  subacute 245.1
  suppurative 245.0
  tuberculous (*see also* Tuberculosis) 017.5 ☑
  viral 245.1
  woody 245.3
Thyrolingual duct, persistent 759.2
Thyromegaly 240.9
Thyrotoxic
  crisis or storm (*see also* Thyrotoxicosis) 242.9 ☑
  heart failure (*see also* Thyrotoxicosis) 242.9 ☑ [425.7]
Thyrotoxicosis 242.9 ☑

> *Note* — Use the following fifth-digit subclassification with category 242:
>
> 0   without mention of thyrotoxic crisis or storm
>
> 1   with mention of thyrotoxic crisis or storm

  with
    goiter (diffuse) 242.0 ☑
      adenomatous 242.3 ☑
        multinodular 242.2 ☑
        uninodular 242.1 ☑
      nodular 242.3 ☑
        multinodular 242.2 ☑
        uninodular 242.1 ☑
    infiltrative
      dermopathy 242.0 ☑

Thyrotoxicosis — *continued*
  with — *continued*
    infiltrative — *continued*
      ophthalmopathy 242.0 ☑
      thyroid acropachy 242.0 ☑
    complicating pregnancy, childbirth, or puerperium 648.1 ☑
    due to
      ectopic thyroid nodule 242.4 ☑
      ingestion of (excessive) thyroid material 242.8 ☑
      specified cause NEC 242.8 ☑
    factitia 242.8 ☑
    heart 242.9 ☑ [425.7]
    neonatal (transient) 775.3
TIA (transient ischemic attack) 435.9
  with transient neurologic deficit 435.9
  late effect — *see* Late effect(s) (of) cerebrovascular disease
Tibia vara 732.4
Tic 307.20
  breathing 307.20
  child problem 307.21
  compulsive 307.22
  convulsive 307.20
  degenerative (generalized) (localized) 333.3
    facial 351.8
  douloureux (*see also* Neuralgia, trigeminal) 350.1
    atypical 350.2
  habit 307.20
    chronic (motor or vocal) 307.22
    transient (of childhood) 307.21
  lid 307.20
    transient (of childhood) 307.21
  motor-verbal 307.23
  occupational 300.89
  orbicularis 307.20
    transient (of childhood) 307.21
  organic origin 333.3
  postchoreic — *see* Chorea
  psychogenic 307.20
    compulsive 307.22
  salaam 781.0
  spasm 307.20
    chronic (motor or vocal) 307.22
    transient (of childhood) 307.21
Tick-bite fever NEC 066.1
  African 087.1
  Colorado (virus) 066.1
  Rocky Mountain 082.0
Tick (-borne) fever NEC 066.1
  American mountain 066.1
  Colorado 066.1
  hemorrhagic NEC 065.3
    Crimean 065.0
    Kyasanur Forest 065.2
    Omsk 065.1
  mountain 066.1
  nonexanthematous 066.1
Tick paralysis 989.5
Tics and spasms, compulsive 307.22
Tietze's disease or syndrome 733.6
Tight, tightness
  anus 564.89
  chest 786.59
  fascia (lata) 728.9
  foreskin (congenital) 605
  hymen 623.3
  introitus (acquired) (congenital) 623.3
  rectal sphincter 564.89
  tendon 727.81
    Achilles (heel) 727.81
  urethral sphincter 598.9
Tilting vertebra 737.9
Timidity, child 313.21
Tinea (intersecta) (tarsi) 110.9
  amiantacea 110.0
  asbestina 110.0
  barbae 110.0
  beard 110.0
  black dot 110.0
  blanca 111.2
  capitis 110.0
  corporis 110.5
  cruris 110.3

☑ **Additional Digit Required — Refer to the Tabular List for Digit Selection**   ▽ **Subterms under main terms may continue to next column or page**

2013 ICD-9-CM   ▶◀ Revised Text   ● New Line   ▲ Revised Code   Volume 2 — 281

Tinea — *continued*
　decalvans 704.09
　flava 111.0
　foot 110.4
　furfuracea 111.0
　imbricata (Tokelau) 110.5
　lepothrix 039.0
　manuum 110.2
　microsporic (*see also* Dermatophytosis)
　　110.9
　nigra 111.1
　nodosa 111.2
　pedis 110.4
　scalp 110.0
　specified site NEC 110.8
　sycosis 110.0
　tonsurans 110.0
　trichophytic (*see also* Dermatophytosis)
　　110.9
　unguium 110.1
　versicolor 111.0
Tingling sensation — *see also* Disturbance,
　sensation 782.0
Tin-miners' lung 503
Tinnitus (aurium) 388.30
　audible 388.32
　objective 388.32
　subjective 388.31
Tipped, teeth 524.33
Tipping
　pelvis 738.6
　　with disproportion (fetopelvic) 653.0 ☑
　　　affecting fetus or newborn 763.1
　　　causing obstructed labor 660.1 ☑
　　　　affecting fetus or newborn 763.1
　teeth 524.33
Tiredness 780.79
Tissue — *see* condition
Tobacco
　abuse (affecting health) NEC (*see also* Abuse,
　　drugs, nondependent) 305.1
　heart 989.84
　use disorder complicating pregnancy,
　　childbirth, or the puerperium
　　649.0 ☑
Tobias' syndrome (carcinoma, pulmonary
　apex) (M8010/3) 162.3
Tocopherol deficiency 269.1
Todd's
　cirrhosis — *see* Cirrhosis, biliary
　paralysis (postepileptic transitory paralysis)
　　344.89
Toe — *see* condition
Toilet, artificial opening — *see also* Attention
　to, artificial, opening V55.9
Tokelau ringworm 110.5
Tollwut 071
Tolosa-Hunt syndrome 378.55
Tommaselli's disease
　correct substance properly administered
　　599.70
　overdose or wrong substance given or taken
　　961.4
Tongue — *see also* condition
　worms 134.1
Tongue tie 750.0
Tonic pupil 379.46
Toni-Fanconi syndrome (cystinosis) 270.0
Tonsil — *see* condition
Tonsillitis (acute) (catarrhal) (croupous) (follic-
　ular) (gangrenous) (infective) (lacunar)
　(lingual) (malignant) (membranous)
　(phlegmonous) (pneumococcal) (pseu-
　domembranous) (purulent) (septic)
　(staphylococcal) (subacute) (suppura-
　tive) (toxic) (ulcerative) (vesicular) (viral)
　463
　with influenza, flu, or grippe (*see also* Influen-
　　za) 487.1
　chronic 474.00
　diphtheritic (membranous) 032.0
　hypertrophic 474.00
　influenzal (*see also* Influenza) 487.1
　parenchymatous 475
　streptococcal 034.0
　tuberculous (*see also* Tuberculosis) 012.8 ☑

Tonsillitis — *continued*
　Vincent's 101
Tonsillopharyngitis 465.8
Toothache 525.9
Tooth, teeth — *see* condition
Topagnosis 782.0
Tophi (gouty) 274.03
　ear 274.81
　heart 274.82
　specified site NEC 274.82
TORCH infection — *see also* Infection, congen-
　ital 760.2
Torn — *see* Tear, torn
Tornwaldt's bursitis (disease) (pharyngeal
　bursitis) 478.29
　cyst 478.26
Torpid liver 573.9
Torsion
　accessory tube 620.5
　adnexa (female) 620.5
　aorta (congenital) 747.29
　　acquired 447.1
　appendix
　　epididymis 608.24
　　testis 608.23
　bile duct 576.8
　　with calculus, choledocholithiasis or
　　　stones — *see* Choledocholithiasis
　　congenital 751.69
　bowel, colon, or intestine 560.2
　cervix — *see* Malposition, uterus
　duodenum 537.3
　dystonia — *see* Dystonia, torsion
　epididymis 608.24
　　appendix 608.24
　fallopian tube 620.5
　gallbladder (*see also* Disease, gallbladder)
　　575.8
　　congenital 751.69
　gastric 537.89
　hydatid of Morgagni (female) 620.5
　kidney (pedicle) 593.89
　Meckel's diverticulum (congenital) 751.0
　mesentery 560.2
　omentum 560.2
　organ or site, congenital NEC — *see*
　　Anomaly, specified type NEC
　ovary (pedicle) 620.5
　　congenital 752.0
　oviduct 620.5
　penis 607.89
　　congenital 752.69
　renal 593.89
　spasm — *see* Dystonia, torsion
　spermatic cord 608.22
　　extravaginal 608.21
　　intravaginal 608.22
　spleen 289.59
　testicle, testis 608.20
　　appendix 608.23
　tibia 736.89
　umbilical cord — *see* Compression, umbili-
　　cal cord
　uterus (*see also* Malposition, uterus) 621.6
Torticollis (intermittent) (spastic) 723.5
　congenital 754.1
　　sternomastoid 754.1
　due to birth injury 767.8
　hysterical 300.11
　ocular 781.93
　psychogenic 306.0
　　specified as conversion reaction 300.11
　rheumatic 723.5
　rheumatoid 714.0
　spasmodic 333.83
　traumatic, current NEC 847.0
Tortuous
　artery 447.1
　fallopian tube 752.19
　organ or site, congenital NEC — *see* Distor-
　　tion
　renal vessel (congenital) 747.62
　retina vessel (congenital) 743.58
　　acquired 362.17
　ureter 593.4
　urethra 599.84

Tortuous — *continued*
　vein — *see* Varicose, vein
Torula, torular (infection) 117.5
　histolytica 117.5
　lung 117.5
Torulosis 117.5
Torus
　fracture
　　fibula 823.41
　　　with tibia 823.42
　　humerus 812.49
　　radius (alone) 813.45
　　　with ulna 813.47
　　tibia 823.40
　　　with fibula 823.42
　　ulna (alone) 813.46
　　　with radius 813.47
　mandibularis 526.81
　palatinus 526.81
Touch, vitreous 997.99
Touraine-Solente-Golé syndrome
　(acropachyderma) 757.39
Touraine's syndrome (hereditary osteo-ony-
　chodysplasia) 756.89
Tourette's disease (motor-verbal tic) 307.23
Tower skull 756.0
　with exophthalmos 756.0
Toxemia 799.89
　with
　　abortion — *see* Abortion, by type, with
　　　toxemia
　bacterial — *see* Septicemia
　biliary (*see also* Disease, biliary) 576.8
　burn — *see* Burn, by site
　congenital NEC 779.89
　eclamptic 642.6 ☑
　　with pre-existing hypertension 642.7 ☑
　erysipelatous (*see also* Erysipelas) 035
　fatigue 799.89
　fetus or newborn NEC 779.89
　food (*see also* Poisoning, food) 005.9
　gastric 537.89
　gastrointestinal 558.2
　intestinal 558.2
　kidney (*see also* Disease, renal) 593.9
　lung 518.89
　malarial NEC (*see also* Malaria) 084.6
　maternal (of pregnancy), affecting fetus or
　　newborn 760.0
　myocardial — *see* Myocarditis, toxic
　of pregnancy (mild) (pre-eclamptic)
　　642.4 ☑
　　with
　　　convulsions 642.6 ☑
　　　pre-existing hypertension 642.7 ☑
　　affecting fetus or newborn 760.0
　　severe 642.5 ☑
　pre-eclamptic — *see* Toxemia, of pregnancy
　puerperal, postpartum — *see* Toxemia, of
　　pregnancy
　pulmonary 518.89
　renal (*see also* Disease, renal) 593.9
　septic (*see also* Septicemia) 038.9
　small intestine 558.2
　staphylococcal 038.10
　　aureus 038.11
　　due to food 005.0
　　specified organism NEC 038.19
　stasis 799.89
　stomach 537.89
　uremic (*see also* Uremia) 586
　urinary 586
Toxemica cerebropathia psychica (nonalco-
　holic) 294.0
　alcoholic 291.1
Toxic (poisoning) — *see also* condition
　from drug or poison — *see* Table of Drugs
　　and Chemicals
　oil syndrome 710.5
　shock syndrome 040.82
　thyroid (gland) (*see also* Thyrotoxicosis)
　　242.9 ☑
Toxicemia — *see* Toxemia
Toxicity
　dilantin
　　asymptomatic 796.0

Toxicity — *continued*
　dilantin — *continued*
　　symptomatic — *see* Table of Drugs and
　　　Chemicals
　drug
　　asymptomatic 796.0
　　symptomatic — *see* Table of Drugs and
　　　Chemicals
　fava bean 282.2
　from drug or poison
　　asymptomatic 796.0
　　symptomatic — *see* Table of Drugs and
　　　Chemicals
Toxicosis — *see also* Toxemia 799.89
　capillary, hemorrhagic 287.0
Toxinfection 799.89
　gastrointestinal 558.2
Toxocariasis 128.0
Toxoplasma infection, generalized 130.9
Toxoplasmosis (acquired) 130.9
　with pneumonia 130.4
　congenital, active 771.2
　disseminated (multisystemic) 130.8
　maternal
　　with suspected damage to fetus affect-
　　　ing management of pregnancy
　　　655.4 ☑
　　affecting fetus or newborn 760.2
　　　manifest toxoplasmosis in fetus or
　　　　newborn 771.2
　multiple sites 130.8
　multisystemic disseminated 130.8
　specified site NEC 130.7
Trabeculation, bladder 596.89
Trachea — *see* condition
Tracheitis (acute) (catarrhal) (infantile) (mem-
　branous) (plastic) (pneumococcal) (sep-
　tic) (suppurative) (viral) 464.10
　with
　　bronchitis 490
　　　acute or subacute 466.0
　　　chronic 491.8
　　　tuberculosis — *see* Tuberculosis,
　　　　pulmonary
　　laryngitis (acute) 464.20
　　　with obstruction 464.21
　　　chronic 476.1
　　　tuberculous (*see also* Tuberculosis,
　　　　larynx) 012.3 ☑
　　obstruction 464.11
　chronic 491.8
　　with
　　　bronchitis (chronic) 491.8
　　　laryngitis (chronic) 476.1
　　due to external agent — *see* Condition,
　　　respiratory, chronic, due to
　diphtheritic (membranous) 032.3
　due to external agent — *see* Inflamma-
　　tion, respiratory, upper, due to
　edematous 464.11
　influenzal (*see also* Influenza) 487.1
　streptococcal 034.0
　syphilitic 095.8
　tuberculous (*see also* Tuberculosis) 012.8 ☑
Trachelitis (nonvenereal) — *see also* Cervicitis
　616.0
　trichomonal 131.09
Tracheobronchial — *see* condition
Tracheobronchitis — *see also* Bronchitis 490
　acute or subacute 466.0
　　with bronchospasm or obstruction 466.0
　chronic 491.8
　influenzal (*see also* Influenza) 487.1
　senile 491.8
Tracheobronchomegaly (congenital) 748.3
　with bronchiectasis 494.0
　　with (acute) exacerbation 494.1
　acquired 519.19
　　with bronchiectasis 494.0
　　　with (acute) exacerbation 494.1
Tracheobronchopneumonitis — *see* Pneumo-
　nia, broncho
Tracheocele (external) (internal) 519.19
　congenital 748.3
Tracheomalacia 519.19
　congenital 748.3

☑ **Additional Digit Required** — **Refer to the Tabular List for Digit Selection**　　　　　　　　　　(NEW) **Subterms under main terms may continue to next column or page**

Tracheopharyngitis (acute) 465.8
  chronic 478.9
    due to external agent — *see* Condition, respiratory, chronic, due to
    due to external agent — *see* Inflammation, respiratory, upper, due to
Tracheostenosis 519.19
  congenital 748.3
Tracheostomy
  attention to V55.0
  complication 519.00
  granuloma 519.09
  hemorrhage 519.09
  infection 519.01
  malfunctioning 519.02
  obstruction 519.09
  sepsis 519.01
  status V44.0
  stenosis 519.02
Trachoma, trachomatous 076.9
  active (stage) 076.1
  contraction of conjunctiva 076.1
  dubium 076.0
  healed or late effect 139.1
  initial (stage) 076.0
  Türck's (chronic catarrhal laryngitis) 476.0
Trachyphonia 784.49
Traction, vitreomacular 379.27
Training
  insulin pump V65.46
  orthoptic V57.4
  orthotic V57.81
Train sickness 994.6
Trait
  hemoglobin
    abnormal NEC 282.7
      with thalassemia 282.46
    C (*see also* Disease, hemoglobin, C) 282.7
      with elliptocytosis 282.7
    S (Hb-S) 282.5
    Lepore 282.49
    with other abnormal hemoglobin NEC 282.49
  paranoid 301.0
  sickle-cell 282.5
    with
      elliptocytosis 282.5
      spherocytosis 282.5
      thalassemia (alpha) (beta) (delta-beta) 282.46
Traits, paranoid 301.0
Tramp V60.0
Trance 780.09
  hysterical 300.13
Transaminasemia 790.4
Transfusion, blood
  without reported diagnosis V58.2
  donor V59.01
    stem cells V59.02
  fetal twin to twin 678.0 ☑
  incompatible (*see also* Complications, transfusion) 999.80
    ABO (*see also* Complications, transfusion) 999.60
    minor blood group 999.89
    non-ABO (*see also* Complications, transfusion) 999.75
    Rh (antigen) (C) (c) (D) (E) (e) (*see also* Complications, transfusion) 999.70
  reaction or complication — *see* Complications, transfusion
  related acute lung injury (TRALI) 518.7
  syndrome
    fetomaternal 772.0
    twin-to-twin
      blood loss (donor twin) 772.0
      recipient twin 776.4
  twin to twin fetal 678.0 ☑
Transient — *see also* condition
  alteration of awareness 780.02
  blindness 368.12
  deafness (ischemic) 388.02
  global amnesia 437.7
  hyperglycemia (post-procedural) 790.29
  hypoglycemia (post-procedural) 251.2

Transient — *see also* condition — *continued*
  person (homeless) NEC V60.0
Transitional, lumbosacral joint of vertebra 756.19
Translocation
  autosomes NEC 758.5
    13-15 758.1
    16-18 758.2
    21 or 22 758.0
    balanced in normal individual 758.4
    D₁ 758.1
    E₃ 758.2
    G 758.0
  balanced autosomal in normal individual 758.4
  chromosomes NEC 758.89
  Down's syndrome 758.0
Translucency, iris 364.53
Transmission of chemical substances through the placenta (affecting fetus or newborn) 760.70
  alcohol 760.71
  anticonvulsants 760.77
  antifungals 760.74
  anti-infective agents 760.74
  antimetabolics 760.78
  cocaine 760.75
  "crack" 760.75
  diethylstilbestrol [DES] 760.76
  hallucinogenic agents 760.73
  medicinal agents NEC 760.79
  narcotics 760.72
  obstetric anesthetic or analgesic drug 763.5
  specified agent NEC 760.79
  suspected, affecting management of pregnancy 655.5 ☑
Transplant(ed)
  bone V42.4
    marrow V42.81
  complication (*see also* Complications, due to (presence of) any device, implant, or graft classified to 996.0–996.5 NEC)
    bone marrow 996.85
    corneal graft NEC 996.79
      infection or inflammation 996.69
      reaction 996.51
      rejection 996.51
    organ (failure) (immune or nonimmune cause) (infection) (rejection) 996.80
      bone marrow 996.85
      heart 996.83
      intestines 996.87
      kidney 996.81
      liver 996.82
      lung 996.84
      pancreas 996.86
      specified NEC 996.89
    previously removed due to complication, failure, rejection or infection V45.87
    removal status V45.87
    skin NEC 996.79
      infection or inflammation 996.69
      rejection 996.52
        artificial 996.55
        decellularized allodermis 996.55
    stem cell(s) 996.88
      from
        peripheral blood 996.88
        umbilical cord 996.88
  cornea V42.5
  hair V50.0
  heart V42.1
    valve V42.2
  intestine V42.84
  kidney V42.0
  liver V42.7
  lung V42.6
  organ V42.9
    specified NEC V42.89
  pancreas V42.83
  peripheral stem cells V42.82
  skin V42.3

Transplant(ed) — *continued*
  stem cells, peripheral V42.82
  tissue V42.9
    specified NEC V42.89
Transplants, ovarian, endometrial 617.1
Transposed — *see* Transposition
Transposition (congenital) — *see also* Malposition, congenital
  abdominal viscera 759.3
  aorta (dextra) 745.11
  appendix 751.5
  arterial trunk 745.10
  colon 751.5
  great vessels (complete) 745.10
    both originating from right ventricle 745.11
    corrected 745.12
    double outlet right ventricle 745.11
    incomplete 745.11
    partial 745.11
    specified type NEC 745.19
  heart 746.87
    with complete transposition of viscera 759.3
  intestine (large) (small) 751.5
  pulmonary veins 747.49
  reversed jejunal (for bypass) (status) V45.3
  scrotal 752.81
  stomach 750.7
    with general transposition of viscera 759.3
  teeth, tooth 524.30
  vessels (complete) 745.10
    partial 745.11
  viscera (abdominal) (thoracic) 759.3
Trans-sexualism 302.50
  with
    asexual history 302.51
    heterosexual history 302.53
    homosexual history 302.52
Transverse — *see also* condition
  arrest (deep), in labor 660.3 ☑
    affecting fetus or newborn 763.1
  lie 652.3 ☑
    before labor, affecting fetus or newborn 761.7
    causing obstructed labor 660.0 ☑
      affecting fetus or newborn 763.1
    during labor, affecting fetus or newborn 763.1
Transvestism, transvestitism (transvestic fetishism) 302.3
Trapped placenta (with hemorrhage) 666.0 ☑
  without hemorrhage 667.0 ☑
Traumatic — *see also* condition
  brain injury (TBI) (*see also* Injury, intracranial) 854.0 ☑
    with skull fracture — *see* Fracture, skull, by site
Trauma, traumatism — *see also* Injury, by site 959.9
  birth — *see* Birth, injury NEC
  causing hemorrhage of pregnancy or delivery 641.8 ☑
  complicating
    abortion — *see* Abortion, by type, with damage to pelvic organs
    ectopic pregnancy (*see also* categories 633.0–633.9) 639.2
    molar pregnancy (*see also* categories 630–632) 639.2
  during delivery NEC 665.9 ☑
  following
    abortion 639.2
    ectopic or molar pregnancy 639.2
  maternal, during pregnancy, affecting fetus or newborn 760.5
  neuroma — *see* Injury, nerve, by site
  previous major, affecting management of pregnancy, childbirth, or puerperium V23.89
  psychic (current) (*see also* Reaction, adjustment)
    previous (history) V15.49
  psychologic, previous (affecting health) V15.49

Trauma, traumatism — *see also* Injury, by site — *continued*
  transient paralysis — *see* Injury, nerve, by site
Treacher Collins' syndrome (incomplete facial dysostosis) 756.0
Treitz's hernia — *see* Hernia, Treitz's
Trematode infestation NEC 121.9
Trematodiasis NEC 121.9
Trembles 988.8
Trembling paralysis — *see also* Parkinsonism 332.0
Tremor 781.0
  essential (benign) 333.1
  familial 333.1
  flapping (liver) 572.8
  hereditary 333.1
  hysterical 300.11
  intention 333.1
  medication-induced postural 333.1
  mercurial 985.0
  muscle 728.85
  Parkinson's (*see also* Parkinsonism) 332.0
  psychogenic 306.0
    specified as conversion reaction 300.11
  senilis 797
  specified type NEC 333.1
Trench
  fever 083.1
  foot 991.4
  mouth 101
  nephritis — *see* Nephritis, acute
Treponema pallidum infection — *see also* Syphilis 097.9
Treponematosis 102.9
  due to
    T. pallidum — *see* Syphilis
    T. pertenue (yaws) (*see also* Yaws) 102.9
Triad
  Kartagener's 759.3
  Reiter's (complete) (incomplete) 099.3
  Saint's (*see also* Hernia, diaphragm) 553.3
Trichiasis 704.2
  cicatricial 704.2
  eyelid 374.05
    with entropion (*see also* Entropion) 374.00
Trichinella spiralis (infection) (infestation) 124
Trichinelliasis 124
Trichinellosis 124
Trichiniasis 124
Trichinosis 124
Trichobezoar 938
  intestine 936
  stomach 935.2
Trichocephaliasis 127.3
Trichocephalosis 127.3
Trichocephalus infestation 127.3
Trichoclasis 704.2
Trichoepithelioma (M8100/0) — *see also* Neoplasm, skin, benign
  breast 217
  genital organ NEC — *see* Neoplasm, by site, benign
  malignant (M8100/3) — *see* Neoplasm, skin, malignant
Trichofolliculoma (M8101/0) — *see* Neoplasm, skin, benign
Tricholemmoma (M8102/0) — *see* Neoplasm, skin, benign
Trichomatosis 704.2
Trichomoniasis 131.9
  bladder 131.09
  cervix 131.09
  intestinal 007.3
  prostate 131.03
  seminal vesicle 131.09
  specified site NEC 131.8
  urethra 131.02
  urogenitalis 131.00
  vagina 131.01
  vulva 131.01
  vulvovaginal 131.01
Trichomycosis 039.0
  axillaris 039.0
  nodosa 111.2

Tracheopharyngitis — Trichomycosis

☑ **Additional Digit Required** — Refer to the Tabular List for Digit Selection   ▽ **Subterms under main terms may continue to next column or page**

2013 ICD-9-CM   ▶◀ **Revised Text**   ● **New Line**   ▲ **Revised Code**   **Volume 2 — 283**

Trichomycosis — *continued*
nodularis 111.2
rubra 039.0
Trichonocardiosis (axillaris) (palmellina) 039.0
Trichonodosis 704.2
Trichophytide — *see* Dermatophytosis
Trichophytid, trichophyton infection — *see also* Dermatophytosis 110.9
Trichophytobezoar 938
intestine 936
stomach 935.2
Trichophytosis — *see* Dermatophytosis
Trichoptilosis 704.2
Trichorrhexis (nodosa) 704.2
Trichosporosis nodosa 111.2
Trichostasis spinulosa (congenital) 757.4
Trichostrongyliasis (small intestine) 127.6
Trichostrongylosis 127.6
Trichostrongylus (instabilis) infection 127.6
Trichotillomania 312.39
Trichromat, anomalous (congenital) 368.59
Trichromatopsia, anomalous (congenital) 368.59
Trichuriasis 127.3
Trichuris trichiuria (any site) (infection) (infestation) 127.3
Tricuspid (valve) — *see* condition
Trifid — *see also* Accessory
kidney (pelvis) 753.3
tongue 750.13
Trigeminal neuralgia — *see also* Neuralgia, trigeminal 350.1
Trigeminoencephaloangiomatosis 759.6
Trigeminy 427.89
postoperative 997.1
Trigger finger (acquired) 727.03
congenital 756.89
Trigonitis (bladder) (chronic) (pseudomembranous) 595.3
tuberculous (*see also* Tuberculosis) 016.1 ☑
Trigonocephaly 756.0
Trihexosidosis 272.7
Trilobate placenta — *see* Placenta, abnormal
Trilocular heart 745.8
Trimethylaminuria 270.8
Tripartita placenta — *see* Placenta, abnormal
Triple — *see also* Accessory
kidneys 753.3
uteri 752.2
X female 758.81
Triplegia 344.89
congenital or infantile 343.8
Triplet
affected by maternal complications of pregnancy 761.5
healthy liveborn — *see* Newborn, multiple
pregnancy (complicating delivery) NEC 651.1 ☑
with fetal loss and retention of one or more fetus(es) 651.4 ☑
following (elective) fetal reduction 651.7 ☑
Triplex placenta — *see* Placenta, abnormal
Triplication — *see* Accessory
Trismus 781.0
neonatorum 771.3
newborn 771.3
Trisomy (syndrome) NEC 758.5
13 (partial) 758.1
16-18 758.2
18 (partial) 758.2
21 (partial) 758.0
22 758.0
autosomes NEC 758.5
D_1 758.1
E_3 758.2
G (group) 758.0
group D_1 758.1
group E 758.2
group G 758.0
Tritanomaly 368.53
Tritanopia 368.53
Troisier-Hanot-Chauffard syndrome (bronze diabetes) 275.01
Trombidiosis 133.8
Trophedema (hereditary) 757.0

Trophedema — *continued*
congenital 757.0
Trophoblastic disease — *see also* Hydatidiform mole 630
previous, affecting management of pregnancy V23.1
Tropholymphedema 757.0
Trophoneurosis NEC 356.9
arm NEC 354.9
disseminated 710.1
facial 349.89
leg NEC 355.8
lower extremity NEC 355.8
upper extremity NEC 354.9
Tropical — *see also* condition
maceration feet (syndrome) 991.4
wet foot (syndrome) 991.4
Trouble — *see also* Disease
bowel 569.9
heart — *see* Disease, heart
intestine 569.9
kidney (*see also* Disease, renal) 593.9
nervous 799.21
sinus (*see also* Sinusitis) 473.9
Trousseau's syndrome (thrombophlebitis migrans) 453.1
Truancy, childhood — *see also* Disturbance, conduct
socialized 312.2 ☑
undersocialized, unsocialized 312.1 ☑
Truncus
arteriosus (persistent) 745.0
common 745.0
communis 745.0
Trunk — *see* condition
Trychophytide — *see* Dermatophytosis
Trypanosoma infestation — *see* Trypanosomiasis
Trypanosomiasis 086.9
with meningoencephalitis 086.9 [323.2]
African 086.5
due to Trypanosoma 086.5
gambiense 086.3
rhodesiense 086.4
American 086.2
with
heart involvement 086.0
other organ involvement 086.1
without mention of organ involvement 086.2
Brazilian — *see* Trypanosomiasis, American
Chagas' — *see* Trypanosomiasis, American
due to Trypanosoma
cruzi — *see* Trypanosomiasis, American
gambiense 086.3
rhodesiense 086.4
gambiensis, Gambian 086.3
North American — *see* Trypanosomiasis, American
rhodesiensis, Rhodesian 086.4
South American — *see* Trypanosomiasis, American
T-shaped incisors 520.2
Tsutsugamushi fever 081.2
Tubercle — *see also* Tuberculosis
brain, solitary 013.2 ☑
Darwin's 744.29
epithelioid noncaseating 135
Ghon, primary infection 010.0 ☑
Tuberculid, tuberculide (indurating) (lichenoid) (miliary) (papulonecrotic) (primary) (skin) (subcutaneous) — *see also* Tuberculosis 017.0 ☑
Tuberculoma — *see also* Tuberculosis
brain (any part) 013.2 ☑
meninges (cerebral) (spinal) 013.1 ☑
spinal cord 013.4 ☑

Tuberculosis, tubercular, tuberculous (calcification) (calcified) (caseous) (chromogenic acid-fast bacilli) (congenital) (degeneration) (disease) (fibrocaseous) (fistula) (gangrene) (interstitial) (isolated circumscribed lesions) (necrosis) (parenchymatous) (ulcerative) 011.9 ☑

> *Note* — *Use the following fifth-digit subclassification with categories 010–018:*
>
> *0   unspecified*
>
> *1   bacteriological or histological examination not done*
>
> *2   bacteriological or histological examination unknown (at present)*
>
> *3   tubercle bacilli found (in sputum) by microscopy*
>
> *4   tubercle bacilli not found (in sputum) by microscopy, but found by bacterial culture*
>
> *5   tubercle bacilli not found by bacteriological examination, but tuberculosis confirmed histologically*
>
> *6   tubercle bacilli not found by bacteriological or histological examination, but tuberculosis confirmed by other methods [inoculation of animals]*
>
> *For tuberculous conditions specified as late effects or sequelae, see category 137.*

abdomen 014.8 ☑
lymph gland 014.8 ☑
abscess 011.9 ☑
arm 017.9 ☑
bone (*see also* Osteomyelitis, due to, tuberculosis) 015.9 ☑ [730.8]
hip 015.1 ☑ [730.85]
knee 015.2 ☑ [730.86]
sacrum 015.0 ☑ [730.88]
specified site NEC 015.7 ☑ [730.88]
spinal 015.0 ☑ [730.88]
vertebra 015.0 ☑ [730.88]
brain 013.3 ☑
breast 017.9 ☑
Cowper's gland 016.5 ☑
dura (mater) 013.8 ☑
brain 013.3 ☑
spinal cord 013.5 ☑
epidural 013.8 ☑
brain 013.3 ☑
spinal cord 013.5 ☑
frontal sinus — *see* Tuberculosis, sinus
genital organs NEC 016.9 ☑
female 016.7 ☑
male 016.5 ☑
genitourinary NEC 016.9 ☑
gland (lymphatic) — *see* Tuberculosis, lymph gland
hip 015.1 ☑
iliopsoas 015.0 ☑ [730.88]
intestine 014.8 ☑
ischiorectal 014.8 ☑
joint 015.9 ☑
hip 015.1 ☑
knee 015.2 ☑
specified joint NEC 015.8 ☑
vertebral 015.0 ☑ [730.88]
kidney 016.0 ☑ [590.81]
knee 015.2 ☑
lumbar 015.0 ☑ [730.88]
lung 011.2 ☑
primary, progressive 010.8 ☑
meninges (cerebral) (spinal) 013.0 ☑
pelvic 016.9 ☑
female 016.7 ☑
male 016.5 ☑
perianal 014.8 ☑
fistula 014.8 ☑
perinephritic 016.0 ☑ [590.81]

Tuberculosis, tubercular, tuberculous — *continued*
abscess — *continued*
perineum 017.9 ☑
perirectal 014.8 ☑
psoas 015.0 ☑ [730.88]
rectum 014.8 ☑
retropharyngeal 012.8 ☑
sacrum 015.0 ☑ [730.88]
scrofulous 017.2 ☑
scrotum 016.5 ☑
skin 017.0 ☑
primary 017.0 ☑
spinal cord 013.5 ☑
spine or vertebra (column) 015.0 ☑ [730.88]
strumous 017.2 ☑
subdiaphragmatic 014.8 ☑
testis 016.5 ☑
thigh 017.9 ☑
urinary 016.3 ☑
kidney 016.0 ☑ [590.81]
uterus 016.7 ☑
accessory sinus — *see* Tuberculosis, sinus
Addison's disease 017.6 ☑
adenitis (*see also* Tuberculosis, lymph gland) 017.2 ☑
adenoids 012.8 ☑
adenopathy (*see also* Tuberculosis, lymph gland) 017.2 ☑
tracheobronchial 012.1 ☑
primary progressive 010.8 ☑
adherent pericardium 017.9 ☑ [420.0]
adnexa (uteri) 016.7 ☑
adrenal (capsule) (gland) 017.6 ☑
air passage NEC 012.8 ☑
alimentary canal 014.8 ☑
anemia 017.9 ☑
ankle (joint) 015.8 ☑
bone 015.5 ☑ [730.87]
anus 014.8 ☑
apex (*see also* Tuberculosis, pulmonary) 011.9 ☑
apical (*see also* Tuberculosis, pulmonary) 011.9 ☑
appendicitis 014.8 ☑
appendix 014.8 ☑
arachnoid 013.0 ☑
artery 017.9 ☑
arthritis (chronic) (synovial) 015.9 ☑ [711.40]
ankle 015.8 ☑ [730.87]
hip 015.1 ☑ [711.45]
knee 015.2 ☑ [711.46]
specified site NEC 015.8 ☑ [711.48]
spine or vertebra (column) 015.0 ☑ [720.81]
wrist 015.8 ☑ [730.83]
articular — *see* Tuberculosis, joint
ascites 014.0 ☑
asthma (*see also* Tuberculosis, pulmonary) 011.9 ☑
axilla, axillary 017.2 ☑
gland 017.2 ☑
bilateral (*see also* Tuberculosis, pulmonary) 011.9 ☑
bladder 016.1 ☑
bone (*see also* Osteomyelitis, due to, tuberculosis) 015.9 ☑ [730.8]
hip 015.1 ☑ [730.85]
knee 015.2 ☑ [730.86]
limb NEC 015.5 ☑ [730.88]
sacrum 015.0 ☑ [730.88]
specified site NEC 015.7 ☑ [730.88]
spinal or vertebral column 015.0 ☑ [730.88]
bowel 014.8 ☑
miliary 018.9 ☑
brain 013.2 ☑
breast 017.9 ☑
broad ligament 016.7 ☑
bronchi, bronchial, bronchus 011.3 ☑
ectasia, ectasis 011.5 ☑
fistula 011.3 ☑

☑ **Additional Digit Required** — Refer to the Tabular List for Digit Selection   🔍 **Subterms under main terms may continue to next column or page**

284 — Volume 2   ▶◀ Revised Text   ● New Line   ▲ Revised Code   **2013 ICD-9-CM**

Tuberculosis, tubercular, tuberculous — continued

bronchi, bronchial, bronchus — continued
  fistula — continued
    primary, progressive 010.8 ☑
  gland 012.1 ☑
    primary, progressive 010.8 ☑
  isolated 012.2 ☑
  lymph gland or node 012.1 ☑
    primary, progressive 010.8 ☑
bronchiectasis 011.5 ☑
bronchitis 011.3 ☑
bronchopleural 012.0 ☑
bronchopneumonia, bronchopneumonic 011.6 ☑
bronchorrhagia 011.3 ☑
bronchotracheal 011.3 ☑
  isolated 012.2 ☑
bronchus — see Tuberculosis, bronchi
bronze disease (Addison's) 017.6 ☑
buccal cavity 017.9 ☑
bulbourethral gland 016.5 ☑
bursa (see also Tuberculosis, joint) 015.9 ☑
cachexia NEC (see also Tuberculosis, pulmonary) 011.9 ☑
cardiomyopathy 017.9 [425.8]
caries (see also Tuberculosis, bone) 015.9 ☑ [730.8]
cartilage (see also Tuberculosis, bone) 015.9 ☑ [730.8]
  intervertebral 015.0 ☑ [730.88]
catarrhal (see also Tuberculosis, pulmonary) 011.9 ☑
cecum 014.8 ☑
cellular tissue (primary) 017.0 ☑
cellulitis (primary) 017.0 ☑
central nervous system 013.9 ☑
  specified site NEC 013.8 ☑
cerebellum (current) 013.2 ☑
cerebral (current) 013.2 ☑
  meninges 013.0 ☑
cerebrospinal 013.6 ☑
  meninges 013.0 ☑
cerebrum (current) 013.2 ☑
cervical 017.2 ☑
  gland 017.2 ☑
  lymph nodes 017.2 ☑
cervicitis (uteri) 016.7 ☑
cervix 016.7 ☑
chest (see also Tuberculosis, pulmonary) 011.9 ☑
childhood type or first infection 010.0 ☑
choroid 017.3 ☑ [363.13]
choroiditis 017.3 ☑ [363.13]
ciliary body 017.3 ☑ [364.11]
colitis 014.8 ☑
colliers' 011.4 ☑
colliquativa (primary) 017.0 ☑
colon 014.8 ☑
  ulceration 014.8 ☑
complex, primary 010.0 ☑
complicating pregnancy, childbirth, or puerperium 647.3 ☑
  affecting fetus or newborn 760.2
congenital 771.2
conjunctiva 017.3 ☑ [370.31]
connective tissue 017.9 ☑
  bone — see Tuberculosis, bone
contact V01.1
converter (tuberculin skin test) (without disease) 795.51
cornea (ulcer) 017.3 ☑ [370.31]
Cowper's gland 016.5 ☑
coxae 015.1 ☑ [730.85]
coxalgia 015.1 ☑ [730.85]
cul-de-sac of Douglas 014.8 ☑
curvature, spine 015.0 ☑ [737.40]
cutis (colliquativa) (primary) 017.0 ☑
cystitis 016.1 ☑
cyst, ovary 016.6 ☑
dacryocystitis 017.3 ☑ [375.32]
dactylitis 015.5 ☑
diarrhea 014.8 ☑

Tuberculosis, tubercular, tuberculous — continued

diffuse (see also Tuberculosis, miliary) 018.9 ☑
  lung — see Tuberculosis, pulmonary
  meninges 013.0 ☑
digestive tract 014.8 ☑
disseminated (see also Tuberculosis, miliary) 018.9 ☑
  meninges 013.0 ☑
duodenum 014.8 ☑
dura (mater) 013.9 ☑
  abscess 013.8 ☑
    cerebral 013.3 ☑
    spinal 013.5 ☑
dysentery 014.8 ☑
ear (inner) (middle) 017.4 ☑
  bone 015.6 ☑
  external (primary) 017.0 ☑
  skin (primary) 017.0 ☑
elbow 015.8 ☑
emphysema — see Tuberculosis, pulmonary
empyema 012.0 ☑
encephalitis 013.6 ☑
endarteritis 017.9 ☑
endocarditis (any valve) 017.9 ☑ [424.91]
endocardium (any valve) 017.9 ☑ [424.91]
endocrine glands NEC 017.9 ☑
endometrium 016.7 ☑
enteric, enterica 014.8 ☑
enteritis 014.8 ☑
enterocolitis 014.8 ☑
epididymis 016.4 ☑
epididymitis 016.4 ☑
epidural abscess 013.8 ☑
  brain 013.3 ☑
  spinal cord 013.5 ☑
epiglottis 012.3 ☑
episcleritis 017.3 ☑ [379.00]
erythema (induratum) (nodosum) (primary) 017.1 ☑
esophagus 017.8 ☑
Eustachian tube 017.4 ☑
exposure to V01.1
exudative 012.0 ☑
  primary, progressive 010.1 ☑
eye 017.3 ☑
eyelid (primary) 017.0 ☑
  lupus 017.0 ☑ [373.4]
fallopian tube 016.6 ☑
fascia 017.9 ☑
fauces 012.8 ☑
finger 017.9 ☑
first infection 010.0 ☑
fistula, perirectal 014.8 ☑
Florida 011.6 ☑
foot 017.9 ☑
funnel pelvis 137.3
gallbladder 017.9 ☑
galloping (see also Tuberculosis, pulmonary) 011.9 ☑
ganglionic 015.9 ☑
gastritis 017.9 ☑
gastrocolic fistula 014.8 ☑
gastroenteritis 014.8 ☑
gastrointestinal tract 014.8 ☑
general, generalized 018.9 ☑
  acute 018.0 ☑
  chronic 018.8 ☑
genital organs NEC 016.9 ☑
  female 016.7 ☑
  male 016.5 ☑
genitourinary NEC 016.9 ☑
genu 015.2 ☑
glandulae suprarenalis 017.6 ☑
glandular, general 017.2 ☑
glottis 012.3 ☑
grinders' 011.4 ☑
groin 017.2 ☑
gum 017.9 ☑
hand 017.9 ☑
heart 017.9 ☑ [425.8]
hematogenous — see Tuberculosis, miliary

Tuberculosis, tubercular, tuberculous — continued

hemoptysis (see also Tuberculosis, pulmonary) 011.9 ☑
hemorrhage NEC (see also Tuberculosis, pulmonary) 011.9 ☑
hemothorax 012.0 ☑
hepatitis 017.9 ☑
hilar lymph nodes 012.1 ☑
  primary, progressive 010.8 ☑
hip (disease) (joint) 015.1 ☑
  bone 015.1 ☑ [730.85]
hydrocephalus 013.8 ☑
hydropneumothorax 012.0 ☑
hydrothorax 012.0 ☑
hypoadrenalism 017.6 ☑
hypopharynx 012.8 ☑
ileocecal (hyperplastic) 014.8 ☑
ileocolitis 014.8 ☑
ileum 014.8 ☑
iliac spine (superior) 015.0 ☑ [730.88]
incipient NEC (see also Tuberculosis, pulmonary) 011.9 ☑
indurativa (primary) 017.1 ☑
infantile 010.0 ☑
infection NEC 011.9 ☑
  without clinical manifestation 010.0 ☑
infraclavicular gland 017.2 ☑
inguinal gland 017.2 ☑
inguinalis 017.2 ☑
intestine (any part) 014.8 ☑
iris 017.3 ☑ [364.11]
iritis 017.3 ☑ [364.11]
ischiorectal 014.8 ☑
jaw 015.7 ☑ [730.88]
jejunum 014.8 ☑
joint 015.9 ☑
  hip 015.1 ☑
  knee 015.2 ☑
  specified site NEC 015.8 ☑
  vertebral 015.0 ☑ [730.88]
keratitis 017.3 ☑ [370.31]
  interstitial 017.3 ☑ [370.59]
keratoconjunctivitis 017.3 ☑ [370.31]
kidney 016.0 ☑
knee (joint) 015.2 ☑
kyphoscoliosis 015.0 ☑ [737.43]
kyphosis 015.0 ☑ [737.41]
lacrimal apparatus, gland 017.3 ☑
laryngitis 012.3 ☑
larynx 012.3 ☑
latent 795.51
leptomeninges, leptomeningitis (cerebral) (spinal) 013.0 ☑
lichenoides (primary) 017.0 ☑
linguae 017.9 ☑
lip 017.9 ☑
liver 017.9 ☑
lordosis 015.0 ☑ [737.42]
lung — see Tuberculosis, pulmonary
luposa 017.0 ☑
  eyelid 017.0 ☑ [373.4]
lymphadenitis — see Tuberculosis, lymph gland
lymphangitis — see Tuberculosis, lymph gland
lymphatic (gland) (vessel) — see Tuberculosis, lymph gland
lymph gland or node (peripheral) 017.2 ☑
  abdomen 014.8 ☑
  bronchial 012.1 ☑
    primary, progressive 010.8 ☑
  cervical 017.2 ☑
  hilar 012.1 ☑
    primary, progressive 010.8 ☑
  intrathoracic 012.1 ☑
    primary, progressive 010.8 ☑
  mediastinal 012.1 ☑
    primary, progressive 010.8 ☑
  mesenteric 014.8 ☑
  peripheral 017.2 ☑
  retroperitoneal 014.8 ☑
  tracheobronchial 012.1 ☑

Tuberculosis, tubercular, tuberculous — continued

lymph gland or node — continued
  tracheobronchial — continued
    primary, progressive 010.8 ☑
malignant NEC (see also Tuberculosis, pulmonary) 011.9 ☑
mammary gland 017.9 ☑
marasmus NEC (see also Tuberculosis, pulmonary) 011.9 ☑
mastoiditis 015.6 ☑
maternal, affecting fetus or newborn 760.2
mediastinal (lymph) gland or node 012.1 ☑
  primary, progressive 010.8 ☑
mediastinitis 012.8 ☑
  primary, progressive 010.8 ☑
mediastinopericarditis 017.9 ☑ [420.0]
mediastinum 012.8 ☑
  primary, progressive 010.8 ☑
medulla 013.9 ☑
  brain 013.2 ☑
  spinal cord 013.4 ☑
melanosis, Addisonian 017.6 ☑
membrane, brain 013.0 ☑
meninges (cerebral) (spinal) 013.0 ☑
meningitis (basilar) (brain) (cerebral) (cerebrospinal) (spinal) 013.0 ☑
meningoencephalitis 013.0 ☑
mesentery, mesenteric 014.8 ☑
  lymph gland or node 014.8 ☑
miliary (any site) 018.9 ☑
  acute 018.0 ☑
  chronic 018.8 ☑
  specified type NEC 018.8 ☑
millstone makers' 011.4 ☑
miners' 011.4 ☑
moulders' 011.4 ☑
mouth 017.9 ☑
multiple 018.9 ☑
  acute 018.0 ☑
  chronic 018.8 ☑
muscle 017.9 ☑
myelitis 013.6 ☑
myocarditis 017.9 ☑ [422.0]
myocardium 017.9 ☑ [422.0]
nasal (passage) (sinus) 012.8 ☑
nasopharynx 012.8 ☑
neck gland 017.2 ☑
nephritis 016.0 ☑ [583.81]
nerve 017.9 ☑
nose (septum) 012.8 ☑
ocular 017.3 ☑
old NEC 137.0
  without residuals V12.01
omentum 014.8 ☑
oophoritis (acute) (chronic) 016.6 ☑
optic 017.3 ☑ [377.39]
  nerve trunk 017.3 ☑ [377.39]
  papilla, papillae 017.3 ☑ [377.39]
orbit 017.3 ☑
orchitis 016.5 ☑ [608.81]
organ, specified NEC 017.9 ☑
orificialis (primary) 017.0 ☑
osseous (see also Tuberculosis, bone) 015.9 ☑ [730.8]
osteitis (see also Tuberculosis, bone) 015.9 ☑ [730.8]
osteomyelitis (see also Tuberculosis, bone) 015.9 ☑ [730.8]
otitis (media) 017.4 ☑
ovaritis (acute) (chronic) 016.6 ☑
ovary (acute) (chronic) 016.6 ☑
oviducts (acute) (chronic) 016.6 ☑
pachymeningitis 013.0 ☑
palate (soft) 017.9 ☑
pancreas 017.9 ☑
papulonecrotic (primary) 017.0 ☑
parathyroid glands 017.9 ☑
paronychia (primary) 017.0 ☑
parotid gland or region 017.9 ☑
pelvic organ NEC 016.9 ☑
  female 016.7 ☑
  male 016.5 ☑

☑ Additional Digit Required — Refer to the Tabular List for Digit Selection   ▽ Subterms under main terms may continue to next column or page

Tuberculosis, tubercular, tuberculous —
continued
pelvis (bony) 015.7 ✓ [730.85]
penis 016.5 ✓
peribronchitis 011.3 ✓
pericarditis 017.9 ✓ [420.0]
pericardium 017.9 ✓ [420.0]
perichondritis, larynx 012.3 ✓
perineum 017.9 ✓
periostitis (see also Tuberculosis, bone)
    015.9 ✓ [730.8] ✓
periphlebitis 017.9 ✓
    eye vessel 017.3 ✓ [362.18]
    retina 017.3 ✓ [362.18]
perirectal fistula 014.8 ✓
peritoneal gland 014.8 ✓
peritoneum 014.0 ✓
peritonitis 014.0 ✓
pernicious NEC (see also Tuberculosis, pul-
    monary) 011.9 ✓
pharyngitis 012.8 ✓
pharynx 012.8 ✓
phlyctenulosis (conjunctiva)
    017.3 ✓ [370.31]
phthisis NEC (see also Tuberculosis, pul-
    monary) 011.9 ✓
pituitary gland 017.9 ✓
placenta 016.7 ✓
pleura, pleural, pleurisy, pleuritis (fibrinous)
    (obliterative) (purulent) (simple
    plastic) (with effusion) 012.0 ✓
    primary, progressive 010.1 ✓
pneumonia, pneumonic 011.6 ✓
pneumothorax 011.7 ✓
polyserositis 018.9 ✓
    acute 018.0 ✓
    chronic 018.8 ✓
potters' 011.4 ✓
prepuce 016.5 ✓
primary 010.9 ✓
    complex 010.0 ✓
    complicated 010.8 ✓
        with pleurisy or effusion 010.1 ✓
    progressive 010.8 ✓
        with pleurisy or effusion 010.1 ✓
    skin 017.0 ✓
proctitis 014.8 ✓
prostate 016.5 ✓ [601.4]
prostatitis 016.5 ✓ [601.4]
pulmonaris (see also Tuberculosis, pul-
    monary) 011.9 ✓
pulmonary (artery) (incipient) (malignant)
    (multiple round foci) (pernicious)
    (reinfection stage) 011.9 ✓
    cavitated or with cavitation 011.2 ✓
        primary, progressive 010.8 ✓
    childhood type or first infection 010.0 ✓
    chromogenic acid-fast bacilli 795.39
    fibrosis or fibrotic 011.4 ✓
    infiltrative 011.0 ✓
        primary, progressive 010.9 ✓
    nodular 011.1 ✓
    specified NEC 011.8 ✓
    sputum positive only 795.39
    status following surgical collapse of lung
        NEC 011.9 ✓
pyelitis 016.0 ✓ [590.81]
pyelonephritis 016.0 ✓ [590.81]
pyemia — see Tuberculosis, miliary
pyonephrosis 016.0 ✓
pyopneumothorax 012.0 ✓
pyothorax 012.0 ✓
rectum (with abscess) 014.8 ✓
    fistula 014.8 ✓
reinfection stage (see also Tuberculosis,
    pulmonary) 011.9 ✓
renal 016.0 ✓
renis 016.0 ✓
reproductive organ 016.7 ✓
respiratory NEC (see also Tuberculosis, pul-
    monary) 011.9 ✓
    specified site NEC 012.8 ✓
retina 017.3 ✓ [363.13]

Tuberculosis, tubercular, tuberculous —
continued
retroperitoneal (lymph gland or node)
    014.8 ✓
    gland 014.8 ✓
retropharyngeal abscess 012.8 ✓
rheumatism 015.9 ✓
rhinitis 012.8 ✓
sacroiliac (joint) 015.8 ✓
sacrum 015.0 ✓ [730.88]
salivary gland 017.9 ✓
salpingitis (acute) (chronic) 016.6 ✓
sandblasters' 011.4 ✓
sclera 017.3 ✓ [379.09]
scoliosis 015.0 ✓ [737.43]
scrofulous 017.2 ✓
scrotum 016.5 ✓
seminal tract or vesicle 016.5 ✓ [608.81]
senile NEC (see also Tuberculosis, pul-
    monary) 011.9 ✓
septic NEC (see also Tuberculosis, miliary)
    018.9 ✓
shoulder 015.8 ✓
    blade 015.7 ✓ [730.8]
sigmoid 014.8 ✓
sinus (accessory) (nasal) 012.8 ✓
    bone 015.7 ✓ [730.88]
    epididymis 016.4 ✓
skeletal NEC (see also Osteomyelitis, due to
    tuberculosis) 015.9 ✓ [730.8] ✓
skin (any site) (primary) 017.0 ✓
small intestine 014.8 ✓
soft palate 017.9 ✓
spermatic cord 016.5 ✓
spinal
    column 015.0 ✓ [730.88]
    cord 013.4 ✓
    disease 015.0 ✓ [730.88]
    medulla 013.4 ✓
    membrane 013.0 ✓
    meninges 013.0 ✓
spine 015.0 ✓ [730.88]
spleen 017.7 ✓
splenitis 017.7 ✓
spondylitis 015.0 ✓ [720.81]
spontaneous pneumothorax — see Tuber-
    culosis, pulmonary
sternoclavicular joint 015.8 ✓
stomach 017.9 ✓
stonemasons' 011.4 ✓
struma 017.2 ✓
subcutaneous tissue (cellular) (primary)
    017.0 ✓
subcutis (primary) 017.0 ✓
subdeltoid bursa 017.9 ✓
submaxillary 017.9 ✓
    region 017.9 ✓
supraclavicular gland 017.2 ✓
suprarenal (capsule) (gland) 017.6 ✓
swelling, joint (see also Tuberculosis, joint)
    015.9 ✓
symphysis pubis 015.7 ✓ [730.88]
synovitis 015.9 ✓ [727.01]
    hip 015.1 ✓ [727.01]
    knee 015.2 ✓ [727.01]
    specified site NEC 015.8 ✓ [727.01]
    spine or vertebra 015.0 ✓ [727.01]
systemic — see Tuberculosis, miliary
tarsitis (eyelid) 017.0 ✓ [373.4]
    ankle (bone) 015.5 ✓ [730.87]
tendon (sheath) — see Tuberculosis,
    tenosynovitis
tenosynovitis 015.9 ✓ [727.01]
    hip 015.1 ✓ [727.01]
    knee 015.2 ✓ [727.01]
    specified site NEC 015.8 ✓ [727.01]
    spine or vertebra 015.0 ✓ [727.01]
testis 016.5 ✓ [608.81]
throat 012.8 ✓
thymus gland 017.9 ✓
thyroid gland 017.5 ✓
toe 017.9 ✓
tongue 017.9 ✓

Tuberculosis, tubercular, tuberculous —
continued
tonsil (lingual) 012.8 ✓
tonsillitis 012.8 ✓
trachea, tracheal 012.8 ✓
    gland 012.1 ✓
        primary, progressive 010.8 ✓
    isolated 012.2 ✓
tracheobronchial 011.3 ✓
    glandular 012.1 ✓
        primary, progressive 010.8 ✓
    isolated 012.2 ✓
    lymph gland or node 012.1 ✓
        primary, progressive 010.8 ✓
tubal 016.6 ✓
tunica vaginalis 016.5 ✓
typhlitis 014.8 ✓
ulcer (primary) (skin) 017.0 ✓
    bowel or intestine 014.8 ✓
    specified site NEC — see Tuberculosis,
        by site
    unspecified site — see Tuberculosis, pul-
        monary
ureter 016.2 ✓
urethra, urethral 016.3 ✓
urinary organ or tract 016.3 ✓
    kidney 016.0 ✓
uterus 016.7 ✓
uveal tract 017.3 ✓ [363.13]
uvula 017.9 ✓
vaccination, prophylactic (against) V03.2
vagina 016.7 ✓
vas deferens 016.5 ✓
vein 017.9 ✓
verruca (primary) 017.0 ✓
verrucosa (cutis) (primary) 017.0 ✓
vertebra (column) 015.0 ✓ [730.88]
vesiculitis 016.5 ✓ [608.81]
viscera NEC 014.8 ✓
vulva 016.7 ✓ [616.51]
wrist (joint) 015.8 ✓
    bone 015.5 ✓ [730.83]
Tuberculum
auriculae 744.29
occlusal 520.2
paramolare 520.2
Tuberosity
jaw, excessive 524.07
maxillary, entire 524.07
Tuberous sclerosis (brain) 759.5
Tube, tubal, tubular — see also condition
    ligation, admission for V25.2
Tubo-ovarian — see condition
Tuboplasty, after previous sterilization V26.0
Tubotympanitis 381.10
Tularemia 021.9
    with
        conjunctivitis 021.3
        pneumonia 021.2
    bronchopneumonic 021.2
    conjunctivitis 021.3
    cryptogenic 021.1
    disseminated 021.8
    enteric 021.1
    generalized 021.8
    glandular 021.8
    intestinal 021.1
    oculoglandular 021.3
    ophthalmic 021.3
    pneumonia 021.2
    pulmonary 021.2
    specified NEC 021.8
    typhoidal 021.1
    ulceroglandular 021.0
    vaccination, prophylactic (against) V03.4
Tularensis conjunctivitis 021.3
Tumefaction — see also Swelling
    liver (see also Hypertrophy, liver) 789.1
Tumor (M8000/1) — see also Neoplasm, by site,
    unspecified nature
    Abrikossov's (M9580/0) (see also Neoplasm,
        connective tissue, benign)
        malignant (M9580/3) — see Neoplasm,
            connective tissue, malignant

Tumor — see also Neoplasm, by site,
    unspecified nature — *continued*
    acinar cell (M8550/1) — see Neoplasm, by
        site, uncertain behavior
    acinic cell (M8550/1) — see Neoplasm, by
        site, uncertain behavior
    adenomatoid (M9054/0) (see also Neoplasm,
        by site, benign)
        odontogenic (M9300/0) 213.1
        upper jaw (bone) 213.0
    adnexal (skin) (M8390/0) — see Neoplasm,
        skin, benign
    adrenal
        cortical (benign) (M8370/0) 227.0
            malignant (M8370/3) 194.0
        rest (M8671/0) — see Neoplasm, by site,
            benign
    alpha cell (M8152/0)
        malignant (M8152/3)
            pancreas 157.4
            specified site NEC — see Neoplasm,
                by site, malignant
            unspecified site 157.4
        pancreas 211.7
        specified site NEC — see Neoplasm, by
            site, benign
        unspecified site 211.7
    aneurysmal (see also Aneurysm) 442.9
    aortic body (M8691/1) 237.3
        malignant (M8691/3) 194.6
    argentaffin (M8241/1) — see Neoplasm, by
        site, uncertain behavior
    basal cell (M8090/1) (see also Neoplasm,
        skin, uncertain behavior)
    benign (M8000/0) — see Neoplasm, by site,
        benign
    beta cell (M8151/0)
        malignant (M8151/3)
            pancreas 157.4
            specified site — see Neoplasm, by
                site, malignant
            unspecified site 157.4
        pancreas 211.7
        specified site NEC — see Neoplasm, by
            site, benign
        unspecified site 211.7
    blood — see Hematoma
    Brenner (M9000/0) 220
        borderline malignancy (M9000/1) 236.2
        malignant (M9000/3) 183.0
        proliferating (M9000/1) 236.2
    Brooke's (M8100/0) — see Neoplasm, skin,
        benign
    brown fat (M8880/0) — see Lipoma, by site
    Burkitt's (M9750/3) 200.2 ✓
    calcifying epithelial odontogenic (M9340/0)
        213.1
        upper jaw (bone) 213.0
    carcinoid (M8240/1) 209.60
        benign 209.60
            appendix 209.51
            ascending colon 209.53
            bronchus 209.61
            cecum 209.52
            colon 209.50
            descending colon 209.55
            duodenum 209.41
            foregut 209.65
            hindgut 209.67
            ileum 209.43
            jejunum 209.42
            kidney 209.64
            large intestine 209.50
            lung 209.61
            midgut 209.66
            rectum 209.57
            sigmoid colon 209.56
            small intestine 209.40
            specified NEC 209.69
            stomach 209.63
            thymus 209.62
            transverse colon 209.54
        malignant (of) 209.20
            appendix 209.11
            ascending colon 209.13
            bronchus 209.21

✓ **Additional Digit Required** — Refer to the Tabular List for Digit Selection

▽ **Subterms under main terms may continue to next column or page**

Tumor — *see also* Neoplasm, by site, unspecified nature — *continued*
carcinoid — *continued*
  malignant — *continued*
    cecum 209.12
    colon 209.10
    descending colon 209.15
    duodenum 209.01
    foregut 209.25
    hindgut 209.27
    ileum 209.03
    jejunum 209.02
    kidney 209.24
    large intestine 209.10
    lung 209.21
    midgut 209.26
    rectum 209.17
    sigmoid colon 209.16
    small intestine 209.00
    specified NEC 209.29
    stomach 209.23
    thymus 209.22
    transverse colon 209.14
  secondary — *see* Tumor, neuroendocrine, secondary
carotid body (M8692/1) 237.3
  malignant (M8692/3) 194.5
Castleman's (mediastinal lymph node hyperplasia) 785.6
cells (M8001/1) (*see also* Neoplasm, by site, unspecified nature)
  benign (M8001/0) — *see* Neoplasm, by site, benign
  malignant (M8001/3) — *see* Neoplasm, by site, malignant
  uncertain whether benign or malignant (M8001/1) — *see* Neoplasm, by site, uncertain nature
cervix
  in pregnancy or childbirth 654.6 ☑
    affecting fetus or newborn 763.89
    causing obstructed labor 660.2 ☑
      affecting fetus or newborn 763.1
chondromatous giant cell (M9230/0) — *see* Neoplasm, bone, benign
chromaffin (M8700/0) (*see also* Neoplasm, by site, benign)
  malignant (M8700/3) — *see* Neoplasm, by site, malignant
Cock's peculiar 706.2
Codman's (benign chondroblastoma) (M9230/0) — *see* Neoplasm, bone, benign
dentigerous, mixed (M9282/0) 213.1
  upper jaw (bone) 213.0
dermoid (M9084/0) — *see* Neoplasm, by site, benign
  with malignant transformation (M9084/3) 183.0
desmoid (extra-abdominal) (M8821/1) (*see also* Neoplasm, connective tissue, uncertain behavior)
  abdominal (M8822/1) — *see* Neoplasm, connective tissue, uncertain behavior
embryonal (mixed) (M9080/1) (*see also* Neoplasm, by site, uncertain behavior)
  liver (M9080/3) 155.0
endodermal sinus (M9071/3)
  specified site — *see* Neoplasm, by site, malignant
  unspecified site
    female 183.0
    male 186.9
epithelial
  benign (M8010/0) — *see* Neoplasm, by site, benign
  malignant (M8010/3) — *see* Neoplasm, by site, malignant
Ewing's (M9260/3) — *see* Neoplasm, bone, malignant
fatty — *see* Lipoma
fetal, causing disproportion 653.7 ☑
  causing obstructed labor 660.1 ☑
fibroid (M8890/0) — *see* Leiomyoma
	Tumor — *see also* Neoplasm, by site, unspecified nature — *continued*
	G cell (M8153/1)
	  malignant (M8153/3)
	    pancreas 157.4
	    specified site NEC — *see* Neoplasm, by site, malignant
	    unspecified site 157.4
	  specified site — *see* Neoplasm, by site, uncertain behavior
	  unspecified site 235.5
	giant cell (type) (M8003/1) (*see also* Neoplasm, by site, unspecified nature)
	  bone (M9250/1) 238.0
	    malignant (M9250/3) — *see* Neoplasm, bone, malignant
	  chondromatous (M9230/0) — *see* Neoplasm, bone, benign
	  malignant (M8003/3) — *see* Neoplasm, by site, malignant
	  peripheral (gingiva) 523.8
	  soft parts (M9251/1) (*see also* Neoplasm, connective tissue, uncertain behavior)
	    malignant (M9251/3) — *see* Neoplasm, connective tissue, malignant
	  tendon sheath 727.02
	glomus (M8711/0) (*see also* Hemangioma, by site)
	  jugulare (M8690/1) 237.3
	    malignant (M8690/3) 194.6
	gonadal stromal (M8590/1) — *see* Neoplasm, by site, uncertain behavior
	granular cell (M9580/0) (*see also* Neoplasm, connective tissue, benign)
	  malignant (M9580/3) — *see* Neoplasm, connective tissue, malignant
	granulosa cell (M8620/1) 236.2
	  malignant (M8620/3) 183.0
	granulosa cell-theca cell (M8621/1) 236.2
	  malignant (M8621/3) 183.0
	Grawitz's (hypernephroma) (M8312/3) 189.0
	hazard-crile (M8350/3) 193
	hemorrhoidal — *see* Hemorrhoids
	hilar cell (M8660/0) 220
	Hürthle cell (benign) (M8290/0) 226
	  malignant (M8290/3) 193
	hydatid (*see also* Echinococcus) 122.9
	hypernephroid (M8311/1) (*see also* Neoplasm, by site, uncertain behavior)
	interstitial cell (M8650/1) (*see also* Neoplasm, by site, uncertain behavior)
	  benign (M8650/0) — *see* Neoplasm, by site, benign
	  malignant (M8650/3) — *see* Neoplasm, by site, malignant
	islet cell (M8150/0)
	  malignant (M8150/3)
	    pancreas 157.4
	    specified site — *see* Neoplasm, by site, malignant
	    unspecified site 157.4
	  pancreas 211.7
	  specified site NEC — *see* Neoplasm, by site, benign
	  unspecified site 211.7
	juxtaglomerular (M8361/1) 236.91
	Krukenberg's (M8490/6) 198.6
	Leydig cell (M8650/1)
	  benign (M8650/0)
	    specified site — *see* Neoplasm, by site, benign
	    unspecified site
	      female 220
	      male 222.0
	  malignant (M8650/3)
	    specified site — *see* Neoplasm, by site, malignant
	    unspecified site
	      female 183.0
	      male 186.9
	  specified site — *see* Neoplasm, by site, uncertain behavior
	  unspecified site
	    female 236.2
		Tumor — *see also* Neoplasm, by site, unspecified nature — *continued*
		Leydig cell — *continued*
		  unspecified site — *continued*
		    male 236.4
		lipid cell, ovary (M8670/0) 220
		lipoid cell, ovary (M8670/0) 220
		lymphomatous, benign (M9590/0) (*see also* Neoplasm, by site, benign)
		lysis syndrome (following antineoplastic drug therapy) (spontaneous) 277.88
		Malherbe's (M8110/0) — *see* Neoplasm, skin, benign
		malignant (M8000/3) (*see also* Neoplasm, by site, malignant)
		  fusiform cell (type) (M8004/3) — *see* Neoplasm, by site, malignant
		  giant cell (type) (M8003/3) — *see* Neoplasm, by site, malignant
		  mixed NEC (M8940/3) — *see* Neoplasm, by site, malignant
		  small cell (type) (M8002/3) — *see* Neoplasm, by site, malignant
		  spindle cell (type) (M8004/3) — *see* Neoplasm, by site, malignant
		mast cell (M9740/1) 238.5
		  malignant (M9740/3) 202.6 ☑
		melanotic, neuroectodermal (M9363/0) — *see* Neoplasm, by site, benign
		Merkel cell — *see* Carcinoma, Merkel cell
		mesenchymal
		  malignant (M8800/3) — *see* Neoplasm, connective tissue, malignant
		  mixed (M8990/1) — *see* Neoplasm, connective tissue, uncertain behavior
		mesodermal, mixed (M8951/3) (*see also* Neoplasm, by site, malignant)
		  liver 155.0
		mesonephric (M9110/1) (*see also* Neoplasm, by site, uncertain behavior)
		  malignant (M9110/3) — *see* Neoplasm, by site, malignant
		metastatic
		  from specified site (M8000/3) — *see* Neoplasm, by site, malignant
		  to specified site (M8000/6) — *see* Neoplasm, by site, malignant, secondary
		mixed NEC (M8940/0) (*see also* Neoplasm, by site, benign)
		  malignant (M8940/3) — *see* Neoplasm, by site, malignant
		mucocarcinoid, malignant (M8243/3) — *see* Neoplasm, by site, malignant
		mucoepidermoid (M8430/1) — *see* Neoplasm, by site, uncertain behavior
		Müllerian, mixed (M8950/3) — *see* Neoplasm, by site, malignant
		myoepithelial (M8982/0) — *see* Neoplasm, by site, benign
		neuroendocrine 209.60
		  malignant poorly differentiated 209.30
		  secondary 209.70
		    bone 209.73
		    distant lymph nodes 209.71
		    liver 209.72
		    peritoneum 209.74
		    site specified NEC 209.79
		neurogenic olfactory (M9520/3) 160.0
		nonencapsulated sclerosing (M8350/3) 193
		odontogenic (M9270/1) 238.0
		  adenomatoid (M9300/0) 213.1
		    upper jaw (bone) 213.0
		  benign (M9270/0) 213.1
		    upper jaw (bone) 213.0
		  calcifying epithelial (M9340/0) 213.1
		    upper jaw (bone) 213.0
		  malignant (M9270/3) 170.1
		    upper jaw (bone) 170.0
		  squamous (M9312/0) 213.1
		    upper jaw (bone) 213.0
		ovarian stromal (M8590/1) 236.2
		ovary
		  in pregnancy or childbirth 654.4 ☑
		    affecting fetus or newborn 763.89
			Tumor — *see also* Neoplasm, by site, unspecified nature — *continued*
			ovary — *continued*
			  in pregnancy or childbirth — *continued*
			    causing obstructed labor 660.2 ☑
			      affecting fetus or newborn 763.1
			pacinian (M9507/0) — *see* Neoplasm, skin, benign
			Pancoast's (M8010/3) 162.3
			papillary — *see* Papilloma
			pelvic, in pregnancy or childbirth 654.9 ☑
			  affecting fetus or newborn 763.89
			  causing obstructed labor 660.2 ☑
			    affecting fetus or newborn 763.1
			phantom 300.11
			plasma cell (M9731/1) 238.6
			  benign (M9731/0) — *see* Neoplasm, by site, benign
			  malignant (M9731/3) 203.8 ☑
			polyvesicular vitelline (M9071/3)
			  specified site — *see* Neoplasm, by site, malignant
			  unspecified site
			    female 183.0
			    male 186.9
			Pott's puffy (*see also* Osteomyelitis) 730.2 ☑
			Rathke's pouch (M9350/1) 237.0
			regaud's (M8082/3) — *see* Neoplasm, nasopharynx, malignant
			rete cell (M8140/0) 222.0
			retinal anlage (M9363/0) — *see* Neoplasm, by site, benign
			Rokitansky's 620.2
			salivary gland type, mixed (M8940/0) (*see also* Neoplasm, by site, benign)
			  malignant (M8940/3) — *see* Neoplasm, by site, malignant
			Sampson's 617.1
			Schloffer's (*see also* Peritonitis) 567.29
			Schmincke (M8082/3) — *see* Neoplasm, nasopharynx, malignant
			sebaceous (*see also* Cyst, sebaceous) 706.2
			secondary (M8000/6) — *see* Neoplasm, by site, secondary
			  carcinoid — *see* Tumor, neuroendocrine, secondary
			  neuroendocrine — *see* Tumor, neuroendocrine, secondary
			Sertoli cell (M8640/0)
			  with lipid storage (M8641/0)
			    specified site — *see* Neoplasm, by site, benign
			    unspecified site
			      female 220
			      male 222.0
			  specified site — *see* Neoplasm, by site, benign
			  unspecified site
			    female 220
			    male 222.0
			Sertoli-Leydig cell (M8631/0)
			  specified site — *see* Neoplasm, by site, benign
			  unspecified site
			    female 220
			    male 222.0
			sex cord (-stromal) (M8590/1) — *see* Neoplasm, by site, uncertain behavior
			skin appendage (M8390/0) — *see* Neoplasm, skin, benign
			soft tissue
			  benign (M8800/0) — *see* Neoplasm, connective tissue, benign
			  malignant (M8800/3) — *see* Neoplasm, connective tissue, malignant
			sternomastoid 754.1
			stromal
			  abdomen
			    benign 215.5
			    malignant NEC 171.5
			    uncertain behavior 238.1
			  digestive system 238.1
			    benign 215.5
			    malignant NEC 171.5
			    uncertain behavior 238.1

Tumor — Tumor

Tumor — see also Neoplasm, by site, unspecified nature — continued
  stromal — continued
    endometrium (endometrial) 236.0
    gastric 238.1
      benign 215.5
      malignant 151.9
      uncertain behavior 238.1
    gastrointestinal 238.1
      benign 215.5
      malignant NEC 171.5
      uncertain behavior 238.1
    intestine (small) 238.1
      benign 215.5
      malignant 152.9
      uncertain behavior 238.1
    stomach 238.1
      benign 215.5
      malignant 151.9
      uncertain behavior 238.1
  superior sulcus (lung) (pulmonary) (syndrome) (M8010/3) 162.3
  suprasulcus (M8010/3) 162.3
  sweat gland (M8400/1) (see also Neoplasm, skin, uncertain behavior)
    benign (M8400/0) — see Neoplasm, skin, benign
    malignant (M8400/3) — see Neoplasm, skin, malignant
  syphilitic brain 094.89
    congenital 090.49
  testicular stromal (M8590/1) 236.4
  theca cell (M8600/0) 220
  theca cell-granulosa cell (M8621/1) 236.2
  theca-lutein (M8610/0) 220
  turban (M8200/0) 216.4
  uterus
    in pregnancy or childbirth 654.1 ☑
      affecting fetus or newborn 763.89
      causing obstructed labor 660.2 ☑
        affecting fetus or newborn 763.1
  vagina
    in pregnancy or childbirth 654.7 ☑
      affecting fetus or newborn 763.89
      causing obstructed labor 660.2 ☑
        affecting fetus or newborn 763.1
  varicose (see also Varicose, vein) 454.9
  von Recklinghausen's (M9540/1) 237.71
  vulva
    in pregnancy or childbirth 654.8 ☑
      affecting fetus or newborn 763.89
      causing obstructed labor 660.2 ☑
        affecting fetus or newborn 763.1
  Warthin's (salivary gland) (M8561/0) 210.2
  white (see also Tuberculosis, arthritis)
  White-Darier 757.39
  Wilms' (nephroblastoma) (M8960/3) 189.0
  yolk sac (M9071/3)
    specified site — see Neoplasm, by site, malignant
    unspecified site
      female 183.0
      male 186.9
Tumorlet (M8040/1) — see Neoplasm, by site, uncertain behavior
Tungiasis 134.1
Tunica vasculosa lentis 743.39
Tunnel vision 368.45
Turban tumor (M8200/0) 216.4
Türck's trachoma (chronic catarrhal laryngitis) 476.0
Türk's syndrome (ocular retraction syndrome) 378.71
Turner's
  hypoplasia (tooth) 520.4
  syndrome 758.6
  tooth 520.4
Turner-Kieser syndrome (hereditary osteoonychodysplasia) 756.89
Turner-Varny syndrome 758.6
Turricephaly 756.0
Tussis convulsiva — see also Whooping cough 033.9
Twiddler's syndrome (due to)
  automatic implantable defibrillator 996.04
  pacemaker 996.01

Twin
  affected by maternal complications of pregnancy 761.5
  conjoined 759.4
    fetal 678.1 ☑
  healthy liveborn — see Newborn, twin
  pregnancy (complicating delivery) NEC 651.0 ☑
    with fetal loss and retention of one fetus 651.3 ☑
    conjoined 678.1 ☑
    following (elective) fetal reduction 651.7 ☑
Twinning, teeth 520.2
Twist, twisted
  bowel, colon, or intestine 560.2
  hair (congenital) 757.4
  mesentery 560.2
  omentum 560.2
  organ or site, congenital NEC — see Anomaly, specified type NEC
  ovarian pedicle 620.5
    congenital 752.0
  umbilical cord — see Compression, umbilical cord
Twitch 781.0
Tylosis 700
  buccalis 528.6
  gingiva 523.8
  linguae 528.6
  palmaris et plantaris 757.39
Tympanism 787.3
Tympanites (abdominal) (intestine) 787.3
Tympanitis — see Myringitis
Tympanosclerosis 385.00
  involving
    combined sites NEC 385.09
      with tympanic membrane 385.03
    tympanic membrane 385.01
      with ossicles 385.02
        and middle ear 385.03
Tympanum — see condition
Tympany
  abdomen 787.3
  chest 786.7
Typhlitis — see also Appendicitis 541
Typhoenteritis 002.0
Typhogastric fever 002.0
Typhoid (abortive) (ambulant) (any site) (fever) (hemorrhagic) (infection) (intermittent) (malignant) (rheumatic) 002.0
  with pneumonia 002.0 [484.8]
  abdominal 002.0
  carrier (suspected) of V02.1
  cholecystitis (current) 002.0
  clinical (Widal and blood test negative) 002.0
  endocarditis 002.0 [421.1]
  inoculation reaction — see Complications, vaccination
  meningitis 002.0 [320.7]
  mesenteric lymph nodes 002.0
  myocarditis 002.0 [422.0]
  osteomyelitis (see also Osteomyelitis, due to, typhoid) 002.0 [730.8] ☑
  perichondritis, larynx 002.0 [478.71]
  pneumonia 002.0 [484.8]
  spine 002.0 [720.81]
  ulcer (perforating) 002.0
  vaccination, prophylactic (against) V03.1
  Widal negative 002.0
Typhomalaria (fever) — see also Malaria 084.6
Typhomania 002.0
Typhoperitonitis 002.0
Typhus (fever) 081.9
  abdominal, abdominalis 002.0
  African tick 082.1
  amarillic (see also Fever, Yellow) 060.9
  brain 081.9
  cerebral 081.9
  classical 080
  endemic (flea-borne) 081.0
  epidemic (louse-borne) 080
  exanthematic NEC 080
  exanthematicus SAI 080
    brillii SAI 081.1

Typhus — continued
  exanthematicus SAI — continued
    Mexicanus SAI 081.0
    pediculo vestimenti causa 080
    typhus murinus 081.0
  flea-borne 081.0
  Indian tick 082.1
  Kenya tick 082.1
  louse-borne 080
  Mexican 081.0
    flea-borne 081.0
    louse-borne 080
    tabardillo 080
  mite-borne 081.2
  murine 081.0
  North Asian tick-borne 082.2
  petechial 081.9
  Queensland tick 082.3
  rat 081.0
  recrudescent 081.1
  recurrent (see also Fever, relapsing) 087.9
  São Paulo 082.0
  scrub (China) (India) (Malaya) (New Guinea) 081.2
  shop (of Malaya) 081.0
  Siberian tick 082.2
  tick-borne NEC 082.9
  tropical 081.2
  vaccination, prophylactic (against) V05.8
Tyrosinemia 270.2
  neonatal 775.89
Tyrosinosis (Medes) (Sakai) 270.2
Tyrosinuria 270.2
Tyrosyluria 270.2

U

Uehlinger's syndrome (acropachyderma) 757.39
Uhl's anomaly or disease (hypoplasia of myocardium, right ventricle) 746.84
Ulcerosa scarlatina 034.1
Ulcer, ulcerated, ulcerating, ulceration, ulcerative 707.9
  with gangrene 707.9 [785.4]
  abdomen (wall) (see also Ulcer, skin) 707.8
  ala, nose 478.19
  alveolar process 526.5
  amebic (intestine) 006.9
    skin 006.6
  anastomotic — see Ulcer, gastrojejunal
  anorectal 569.41
  antral — see Ulcer, stomach
  anus (sphincter) (solitary) 569.41
    varicose — see Varicose, ulcer, anus
  aorta — see Aneuysm
  aphthous (oral) (recurrent) 528.2
    genital organ(s)
      female 616.50
      male 608.89
    mouth 528.2
  arm (see also Ulcer, skin) 707.8
  arteriosclerotic plaque — see Arteriosclerosis, by site
  artery NEC 447.2
    without rupture 447.8
  atrophic NEC — see Ulcer, skin
  Barrett's (chronic peptic ulcer of esophagus) 530.85
  bile duct 576.8
  bladder (solitary) (sphincter) 596.89
    bilharzial (see also Schistosomiasis) 120.9 [595.4]
    submucosal (see also Cystitis) 595.1
    tuberculous (see also Tuberculosis) 016.1 ☑
  bleeding NEC — see Ulcer, peptic, with hemorrhage
  bone 730.9 ☑
  bowel (see also Ulcer, intestine) 569.82
  breast 611.0
  bronchitis 491.8
  bronchus 519.19
  buccal (cavity) (traumatic) 528.9
  burn (acute) — see Ulcer, duodenum
  Buruli 031.1
  buttock (see also Ulcer, skin) 707.8

Ulcer, ulcerated, ulcerating, ulceration, ulcerative — continued
  buttock (see also Ulcer, skin) — continued
    decubitus (see also Ulcer, pressure) 707.00
  cancerous (M8000/3) — see Neoplasm, by site, malignant
  cardia — see Ulcer, stomach
  cardio-esophageal (peptic) 530.20
    with bleeding 530.21
  cecum (see also Ulcer, intestine) 569.82
  cervix (uteri) (trophic) 622.0
    with mention of cervicitis 616.0
  chancroidal 099.0
  chest (wall) (see also Ulcer, skin) 707.8
  Chiclero 085.4
  chin (pyogenic) (see also Ulcer, skin) 707.8
  chronic (cause unknown) (see also Ulcer, skin)
    penis 607.89
  Cochin-China 085.1
  colitis — see Colitis, ulcerative
  colon (see also Ulcer, intestine) 569.82
  conjunctiva (acute) (postinfectional) 372.00
  cornea (infectional) 370.00
    with perforation 370.06
    annular 370.02
    catarrhal 370.01
    central 370.03
    dendritic 054.42
    marginal 370.01
    mycotic 370.05
    phlyctenular, tuberculous (see also Tuberculosis) 017.3 ☑ [370.31]
    ring 370.02
    rodent 370.07
    serpent, serpiginous 370.04
    superficial marginal 370.01
    tuberculous (see also Tuberculosis) 017.3 ☑ [370.31]
  corpus cavernosum (chronic) 607.89
  crural — see Ulcer, lower extremity
  Curling's — see Ulcer, duodenum
  Cushing's — see Ulcer, peptic
  cystitis (interstitial) 595.1
  decubitus (unspecified site) (see also Ulcer, pressure) 707.00
    with gangrene 707.00 [785.4]
    ankle 707.06
    back
      lower 707.03
      upper 707.02
    buttock 707.05
    coccyx 707.03
    elbow 707.01
    head 707.09
    heel 707.07
    hip 707.04
    other site 707.09
    sacrum 707.03
    shoulder blades 707.02
  dendritic 054.42
  diabetes, diabetic (mellitus) 250.8 ☑ [707.9]
    due to secondary diabetes 249.8 ☑ [707.9]
    lower limb 250.8 ☑ [707.10]
      ankle 250.8 ☑ [707.13]
        due to secondary diabetes 249.8 ☑ [707.13]
      calf 250.8 ☑ [707.12]
        due to secondary diabetes 249.8 ☑ [707.12]
      foot 250.8 ☑ [707.15]
        due to secondary diabetes 249.8 ☑ [707.15]
      heel 250.8 ☑ [707.14]
        due to secondary diabetes 249.8 ☑ [707.14]
      knee 250.8 ☑ [707.19]
        due to secondary diabetes 249.8 ☑ [707.19]
    specified site NEC 250.8 ☑ [707.19]

☑ Additional Digit Required — Refer to the Tabular List for Digit Selection   ▽ Subterms under main terms may continue to next column or page

288 — Volume 2   ▶◀ Revised Text   ● New Line   ▲ Revised Code   2013 ICD-9-CM

Ulcer, ulcerated, ulcerating, ulceration, ulcerative — *continued*

diabetes, diabetic — *continued*
  lower limb — *continued*
    specified site — *continued*
      due to secondary diabetes
        249.8 ☑ *[707.19]*
      thigh 250.8 ☑ *[707.11]*
        due to secondary diabetes
        249.8 ☑ *[707.11]*
      toes 250.8 ☑ *[707.15]*
        due to secondary diabetes
        249.8 ☑ *[707.15]*
    specified site NEC 250.8 ☑ *[707.8]*
      due to secondary diabetes
        249.8 *[707.8]*
Dieulafoy — *see* Lesion, Dieulafoy
due to
  infection NEC — *see* Ulcer, skin
  radiation, radium — *see* Ulcer, by site
  trophic disturbance (any region) — *see*
    Ulcer, skin
  x-ray — *see* Ulcer, by site
duodenum, duodenal (eroded) (peptic)
  532.9 ☑

Note — *Use the following fifth-digit subclassification with categories 531–534:*

0   *without mention of obstruction*

1   *with obstruction*

  with
    hemorrhage (chronic) 532.4 ☑
      and perforation 532.6 ☑
    perforation (chronic) 532.5 ☑
      and hemorrhage 532.6 ☑
  acute 532.3 ☑
    with
      hemorrhage 532.0 ☑
        and perforation 532.2 ☑
      perforation 532.1 ☑
        and hemorrhage 532.2 ☑
  bleeding (recurrent) — *see* Ulcer, duodenum, with hemorrhage
  chronic 532.7 ☑
    with
      hemorrhage 532.4 ☑
        and perforation 532.6 ☑
      perforation 532.5 ☑
        and hemorrhage 532.6 ☑
  penetrating — *see* Ulcer, duodenum, with perforation
  perforating — *see* Ulcer, duodenum, with perforation
dysenteric NEC 009.0
elusive 595.1
endocarditis (any valve) (acute) (chronic) (subacute) 421.0
enteritis — *see* Colitis, ulcerative
enterocolitis 556.0
epiglottis 478.79
esophagus (peptic) 530.20
  with bleeding 530.21
  due to ingestion
    aspirin 530.20
    chemicals 530.20
    medicinal agents 530.20
  fungal 530.20
  infectional 530.20
  varicose (*see also* Varix, esophagus) 456.1
    bleeding (*see also* Varix, esophagus, bleeding) 456.0
eye NEC 360.00
  dendritic 054.42
eyelid (region) 373.01
face (*see also* Ulcer, skin) 707.8
fauces 478.29
Fenwick (-Hunner) (solitary) (*see also* Cystitis) 595.1
fistulous NEC — *see* Ulcer, skin
foot (indolent) (*see also* Ulcer, lower extremity) 707.15
  perforating 707.15
    leprous 030.1
    syphilitic 094.0

Ulcer, ulcerated, ulcerating, ulceration, ulcerative — *continued*

foot (*see also* Ulcer, lower extremity) — *continued*
  trophic 707.15
  varicose 454.0
    inflamed or infected 454.2
frambesial, initial or primary 102.0
gallbladder or duct 575.8
gall duct 576.8
gangrenous (*see also* Gangrene) 785.4
gastric — *see* Ulcer, stomach
gastrocolic — *see* Ulcer, gastrojejunal
gastroduodenal — *see* Ulcer, peptic
gastroesophageal — *see* Ulcer, stomach
gastrohepatic — *see* Ulcer, stomach
gastrointestinal — *see* Ulcer, gastrojejunal
gastrojejunal (eroded) (peptic) 534.9 ☑

Note — *Use the following fifth-digit subclassification with categories 531–534:*

0   *without mention of obstruction*

1   *with obstruction*

  with
    hemorrhage (chronic) 534.4 ☑
      and perforation 534.6 ☑
    perforation 534.5 ☑
      and hemorrhage 534.6 ☑
  acute 534.3 ☑
    with
      hemorrhage 534.0 ☑
        and perforation 534.2 ☑
      perforation 534.1 ☑
        and hemorrhage 534.2 ☑
  bleeding (recurrent) — *see* Ulcer, gastrojejunal, with hemorrhage
  chronic 534.7 ☑
    with
      hemorrhage 534.4 ☑
        and perforation 534.6 ☑
      perforation 534.5 ☑
        and hemorrhage 534.6 ☑
  penetrating — *see* Ulcer, gastrojejunal, with perforation
  perforating — *see* Ulcer, gastrojejunal, with perforation
gastrojejunocolic — *see* Ulcer, gastrojejunal
genital organ
  female 629.89
  male 608.89
gingiva 523.8
gingivitis 523.10
glottis 478.79
granuloma of pudenda 099.2
groin (*see also* Ulcer, skin) 707.8
gum 523.8
gumma, due to yaws 102.4
hand (*see also* Ulcer, skin) 707.8
hard palate 528.9
heel (*see also* Ulcer, lower extremity) 707.14
  decubitus (*see also* Ulcer, pressure) 707.07
hemorrhoids 455.8
  external 455.5
  internal 455.2
hip (*see also* Ulcer, skin) 707.8
  decubitus (*see also* Ulcer, pressure) 707.04
Hunner's 595.1
hypopharynx 478.29
hypopyon (chronic) (subacute) 370.04
hypostaticum — *see* Ulcer, varicose
ileocolitis 556.1
ileum (*see also* Ulcer, intestine) 569.82
intestine, intestinal 569.82
  with perforation 569.83
  amebic 006.9
  duodenal — *see* Ulcer, duodenum
  granulocytopenic (with hemorrhage) 288.09
  marginal 569.82
  perforating 569.83
  small, primary 569.82
  stercoraceous 569.82

Ulcer, ulcerated, ulcerating, ulceration, ulcerative — *continued*

intestine, intestinal — *continued*
  stercoral 569.82
  tuberculous (*see also* Tuberculosis) 014.8 ☑
  typhoid (fever) 002.0
  varicose 456.8
ischemic 707.9
  lower extremity (*see also* Ulcer, lower extremity) 707.10
    ankle 707.13
    calf 707.12
    foot 707.15
    heel 707.14
    knee 707.19
    specified site NEC 707.19
    thigh 707.11
    toes 707.15
jejunum, jejunal — *see* Ulcer, gastrojejunal
keratitis (*see also* Ulcer, cornea) 370.00
knee — *see* Ulcer, lower extremity
labium (majus) (minus) 616.50
laryngitis (*see also* Laryngitis) 464.00
  with obstruction 464.01
larynx (aphthous) (contact) 478.79
  diphtheritic 032.3
leg — *see* Ulcer, lower extremity
lip 528.5
Lipschütz's 616.50
lower extremity (atrophic) (chronic) (neurogenic) (perforating) (pyogenic) (trophic) (tropical) 707.10
  with gangrene (*see also* Ulcer, lower extremity) 707.10 *[785.4]*
    arteriosclerotic 440.24
  ankle 707.13
  arteriosclerotic 440.23
    with gangrene 440.24
  calf 707.12
  decubitus (*see also* Ulcer, pressure) 707.00
    with gangrene 707.00 *[785.4]*
    ankle 707.06
    buttock 707.05
    heel 707.07
    hip 707.04
  foot 707.15
  heel 707.14
  knee 707.19
  specified site NEC 707.19
  thigh 707.11
  toes 707.15
  varicose 454.0
    inflamed or infected 454.2
luetic — *see* Ulcer, syphilitic
lung 518.89
  tuberculous (*see also* Tuberculosis) 011.2 ☑
malignant (M8000/3) — *see* Neoplasm, by site, malignant
marginal NEC — *see* Ulcer, gastrojejunal
meatus (urinarius) 597.89
Meckel's diverticulum 751.0
Meleney's (chronic undermining) 686.09
Mooren's (cornea) 370.07
mouth (traumatic) 528.9
mycobacterial (skin) 031.1
nasopharynx 478.29
navel cord (newborn) 771.4
neck (*see also* Ulcer, skin) 707.8
  uterus 622.0
neurogenic NEC — *see* Ulcer, skin
nose, nasal (infectional) (passage) 478.19
  septum 478.19
    varicose 456.8
  skin — *see* Ulcer, skin
  spirochetal NEC 104.8
oral mucosa (traumatic) 528.9
palate (soft) 528.9
penetrating NEC — *see* Ulcer, peptic, with perforation
penis (chronic) 607.89

Ulcer, ulcerated, ulcerating, ulceration, ulcerative — *continued*

peptic (site unspecified) 533.9 ☑

Note — *Use the following fifth-digit subclassification with categories 531–534:*

0   *without mention of obstruction*

1   *with obstruction*

  with
    hemorrhage 533.4 ☑
      and perforation 533.6 ☑
    perforation (chronic) 533.5 ☑
      and hemorrhage 533.6 ☑
  acute 533.3 ☑
    with
      hemorrhage 533.0 ☑
        and perforation 533.2 ☑
      perforation 533.1 ☑
        and hemorrhage 533.2 ☑
  bleeding (recurrent) — *see* Ulcer, peptic, with hemorrhage
  chronic 533.7 ☑
    with
      hemorrhage 533.4 ☑
        and perforation 533.6 ☑
      perforation 533.5 ☑
        and hemorrhage 533.6 ☑
  penetrating — *see* Ulcer, peptic, with perforation
  perforating NEC (*see also* Ulcer, peptic, with perforation) 533.5 ☑
skin 707.9
perineum (*see also* Ulcer, skin) 707.8
peritonsillar 474.8
phagedenic (tropical) NEC — *see* Ulcer, skin
pharynx 478.29
phlebitis — *see* Phlebitis
plaster (*see also* Ulcer, pressure) 707.00
popliteal space — *see* Ulcer, lower extremity
postpyloric — *see* Ulcer, duodenum
prepuce 607.89
prepyloric — *see* Ulcer, stomach
pressure 707.00
  with
    abrasion, blister, partial thickness skin loss involving epidermis and/or dermis 707.22
    full thickness skin loss involving damage or necrosis of subcutaneous tissue 707.23
    gangrene 707.00 *[785.4]*
    necrosis of soft tissue through to underlying muscle, tendon, or bone 707.24
  ankle 707.06
  back
    lower 707.03
    upper 707.02
  buttock 707.05
  coccyx 707.03
  elbow 707.01
  head 707.09
  healed — omit code
  healing — code to Ulcer, pressure, by stage
  heel 707.07
  hip 707.04
  other site 707.09
  sacrum 707.03
  shoulder blades 707.02
  stage
    I (healing) 707.21
    II (healing) 707.22
    III (healing) 707.23
    IV (healing) 707.24
    unspecified (healing) 707.20
  unstageable 707.25
primary of intestine 569.82
  with perforation 569.83
proctitis 556.2
  with ulcerative sigmoiditis 556.3
prostate 601.8
pseudopeptic — *see* Ulcer, peptic
pyloric — *see* Ulcer, stomach

☑ **Additional Digit Required** — Refer to the Tabular List for Digit Selection   ⩫ **Subterms under main terms may continue to next column or page**

Ulcer, ulcerated, ulcerating, ulceration, ulcerative — *continued*
rectosigmoid 569.82
  with perforation 569.83
rectum (sphincter) (solitary) 569.41
  stercoraceous, stercoral 569.41
  varicose — *see* Varicose, ulcer, anus
retina (*see also* Chorioretinitis) 363.20
rodent (M8090/3) (*see also* Neoplasm, skin, malignant)
  cornea 370.07
round — *see* Ulcer, stomach
sacrum (region) (*see also* Ulcer, skin) 707.8
Saemisch's 370.04
scalp (*see also* Ulcer, skin) 707.8
sclera 379.09
scrofulous (*see also* Tuberculosis) 017.2 ☑
scrotum 608.89
  tuberculous (*see also* Tuberculosis) 016.5 ☑
  varicose 456.4
seminal vesicle 608.89
sigmoid 569.82
  with perforation 569.83
skin (atrophic) (chronic) (neurogenic) (non-healing) (perforating) (pyogenic) (trophic) 707.9
  with gangrene 707.9 [785.4]
  amebic 006.6
  decubitus (*see also* Ulcer, pressure) 707.00
    with gangrene 707.00 [785.4]
    in granulocytopenia 288.09
  lower extremity (*see also* Ulcer, lower extremity) 707.10
    with gangrene 707.10 [785.4]
    arteriosclerotic 440.24
    ankle 707.13
    arteriosclerotic 440.23
      with gangrene 440.24
    calf 707.12
    foot 707.15
    heel 707.14
    knee 707.19
    specified site NEC 707.19
    thigh 707.11
    toes 707.15
  mycobacterial 031.1
  syphilitic (early) (secondary) 091.3
  tuberculous (primary) (*see also* Tuberculosis) 017.0 ☑
  varicose — *see* Ulcer, varicose
sloughing NEC — *see* Ulcer, skin
soft palate 528.9
solitary, anus or rectum (sphincter) 569.41
sore throat 462
  streptococcal 034.0
spermatic cord 608.89
spine (tuberculous) 015.0 ☑ [730.88]
stasis (leg) (venous) 454.0
  with varicose veins 454.0
  without varicose veins 459.81
  inflamed or infected 454.2
stercoral, stercoraceous 569.82
  with perforation 569.83
  anus or rectum 569.41
stoma, stomal — *see* Ulcer, gastrojejunal
stomach (eroded) (peptic) (round) 531.9 ☑

Note — *Use the following fifth-digit subclassification with categories 531–534:*
0 *without mention of obstruction*
1 *with obstruction*

  with
    hemorrhage 531.4 ☑
      and perforation 531.6 ☑
    perforation (chronic) 531.5 ☑
      and hemorrhage 531.6 ☑
  acute 531.3 ☑
    with
      hemorrhage 531.0 ☑
        and perforation 531.2 ☑
      perforation 531.1 ☑
        and hemorrhage 531.2 ☑

Ulcer, ulcerated, ulcerating, ulceration, ulcerative — *continued*
stomach — *continued*
  bleeding (recurrent) — *see* Ulcer, stomach, with hemorrhage
  chronic 531.7 ☑
    with
      hemorrhage 531.4 ☑
        and perforation 531.6 ☑
      perforation 531.5 ☑
        and hemorrhage 531.6 ☑
  penetrating — *see* Ulcer, stomach, with perforation
  perforating — *see* Ulcer, stomach, with perforation
stomatitis 528.00
stress — *see* Ulcer, peptic
strumous (tuberculous) (*see also* Tuberculosis) 017.2 ☑
submental (*see also* Ulcer, skin) 707.8
submucosal, bladder 595.1
syphilitic (any site) (early) (secondary) 091.3
  late 095.9
  perforating 095.9
    foot 094.0
testis 608.89
thigh — *see* Ulcer, lower extremity
throat 478.29
  diphtheritic 032.0
toe — *see* Ulcer, lower extremity
tongue (traumatic) 529.0
tonsil 474.8
  diphtheritic 032.0
trachea 519.19
trophic — *see* Ulcer, skin
tropical NEC (*see also* Ulcer, skin) 707.9
tuberculous — *see* Tuberculosis, ulcer
tunica vaginalis 608.89
turbinate 730.9 ☑
typhoid (fever) 002.0
  perforating 002.0
umbilicus (newborn) 771.4
unspecified site NEC — *see* Ulcer, skin
urethra (meatus) (*see also* Urethritis) 597.89
uterus 621.8
  cervix 622.0
    with mention of cervicitis 616.0
  neck 622.0
    with mention of cervicitis 616.0
vagina 616.89
valve, heart 421.0
varicose (lower extremity, any part) 454.0
  anus — *see* Varicose, ulcer, anus
  broad ligament 456.5
  esophagus (*see also* Varix, esophagus) 456.1
    bleeding (*see also* Varix, esophagus, bleeding) 456.0
  inflamed or infected 454.2
  nasal septum 456.8
  perineum 456.6
  rectum — *see* Varicose, ulcer, anus
  scrotum 456.4
  specified site NEC 456.8
  sublingual 456.3
  vulva 456.6
vas deferens 608.89
vesical (*see also* Ulcer, bladder) 596.89
vulva (acute) (infectional) 616.50
  Behçet's syndrome 136.1 [616.51]
  herpetic 054.12
  tuberculous 016.7 [616.51]
vulvobuccal, recurring 616.50
x-ray — *see* Ulcer, by site
yaws 102.4
Ulcus — *see also* Ulcer
cutis tuberculosum (*see also* Tuberculosis) 017.0 ☑
duodeni — *see* Ulcer, duodenum
durum 091.0
  extragenital 091.2
gastrojejunale — *see* Ulcer, gastrojejunal
hypostaticum — *see* Ulcer, varicose
molle (cutis) (skin) 099.0
serpens corneae (pneumococcal) 370.04
ventriculi — *see* Ulcer, stomach

Ulegyria 742.4
Ulerythema
  acneiforma 701.8
  centrifugum 695.4
  ophryogenes 757.4
Ullrich-Feichtiger syndrome 759.89
Ullrich (-Bonnevie) (-Turner) syndrome 758.6
Ulnar — *see* condition
Ulorrhagia 523.8
Ulorrhea 523.8
Umbilicus, umbilical — *see also* condition
  cord necrosis, affecting fetus or newborn 762.6
Unacceptable
  existing dental restoration
    contours 525.65
    morphology 525.65
Unavailability of medical facilities (at) V63.9
  due to
    investigation by social service agency V63.8
    lack of services at home V63.1
    remoteness from facility V63.0
    waiting list V63.2
  home V63.1
  outpatient clinic V63.0
  specified reason NEC V63.8
Uncinaria americana infestation 126.1
Uncinariasis (*see also* Ancylostomiasis) 126.9
Unconscious, unconsciousness 780.09
Underdevelopment — *see also* Undeveloped
  sexual 259.0
Underfill, endodontic 526.63
Undernourishment 269.9
Undernutrition 269.9
Under observation — *see* Observation
Underweight 783.22
  for gestational age — *see* Light-for-dates
Underwood's disease (sclerema neonatorum) 778.1
Undescended — *see also* Malposition, congenital
  cecum 751.4
  colon 751.4
  testis 752.51
Undetermined diagnosis or cause 799.9
Undeveloped, undevelopment — *see also* Hypoplasia
  brain (congenital) 742.1
  cerebral (congenital) 742.1
  fetus or newborn 764.9 ☑
  heart 746.89
  lung 748.5
  testis 257.2
  uterus 259.0
Undiagnosed (disease) 799.9
Undulant fever — *see also* Brucellosis 023.9
Unemployment, anxiety concerning V62.0
Unequal leg (acquired) (length) 736.81
  congenital 755.30
Unerupted teeth, tooth 520.6
Unextracted dental root 525.3
Unguis incarnatus 703.0
Unicornis uterus 752.33
Unicornuate uterus (with or without a separate uterine horn) 752.33
Unicorporeus uterus 752.39
Uniformis uterus 752.39
Unilateral — *see also* condition
  development, breast 611.89
  organ or site, congenital NEC — *see* Agenesis
  vagina 752.49
Unilateralis uterus 752.39
Unilocular heart 745.8
Uninhibited bladder 596.54
  with cauda equina syndrome 344.61
  neurogenic — *see also* Neurogenic, bladder 596.54
Union, abnormal — *see also* Fusion
  divided tendon 727.89
  larynx and trachea 748.3
Universal
  joint, cervix 620.6
  mesentery 751.4

Unknown
  cause of death 799.9
  diagnosis 799.9
Unna's disease (seborrheic dermatitis) 690.10
Unresponsiveness, adrenocorticotropin (ACTH) 255.41
Unsatisfactory
  cytology smear
    anal 796.78
    cervical 795.08
    vaginal 795.18
  restoration, tooth (existing) 525.60
    specified NEC 525.69
Unsoundness of mind — *see also* Psychosis 298.9
Unspecified cause of death 799.9
Unstable
  back NEC 724.9
  colon 569.89
  joint — *see* Instability, joint
  lie 652.0 ☑
    affecting fetus or newborn (before labor) 761.7
    causing obstructed labor 660.0 ☑
      affecting fetus or newborn 763.1
  lumbosacral joint (congenital) 756.19
    acquired 724.6
  sacroiliac 724.6
  spine NEC 724.9
Untruthfulness, child problem — *see also* Disturbance, conduct 312.0 ☑
Unverricht (-Lundborg) disease, syndrome, or epilepsy 345.1 ☑
Unverricht-Wagner syndrome (dermatomyositis) 710.3
Upper respiratory — *see* condition
Upset
  gastric 536.8
    psychogenic 306.4
  gastrointestinal 536.8
    psychogenic 306.4
    virus (*see also* Enteritis, viral) 008.8
  intestinal (large) (small) 564.9
    psychogenic 306.4
  menstruation 626.9
  mental 300.9
  stomach 536.8
    psychogenic 306.4
Urachus — *see also* condition
  patent 753.7
  persistent 753.7
Uratic arthritis 274.00
Urbach's lipoid proteinosis 272.8
Urbach-Oppenheim disease or syndrome (necrobiosis lipoidica diabeticorum) 250.8 ☑ [709.3]
  due to secondary diabetes 249.8 ☑ [709.3]
Urbach-Wiethe disease or syndrome (lipoid proteinosis) 272.8
Urban yellow fever 060.1
Urea, blood, high — *see* Uremia
Uremia, uremic (absorption) (amaurosis) (amblyopia) (aphasia) (apoplexy) (coma) (delirium) (dementia) (dropsy) (dyspnea) (fever) (intoxication) (mania) (paralysis) (poisoning) (toxemia) (vomiting) 586
  with
    abortion — *see* Abortion, by type, with renal failure
    ectopic pregnancy (*see also* categories 633.0–633.9) 639.3
    hypertension (*see also* Hypertension, kidney) 403.91
    molar pregnancy (*see also* categories 630–632) 639.3
  chronic 585.9
  complicating
    abortion 639.3
    ectopic or molar pregnancy 639.3
    hypertension (*see also* Hypertension, kidney) 403.91
    labor and delivery 669.3 ☑
  congenital 779.89
  extrarenal 788.99
  hypertensive (chronic) (*see also* Hypertension, kidney) 403.91

☑ **Additional Digit Required** — Refer to the Tabular List for Digit Selection   **Subterms under main terms may continue to next column or page**

290 — Volume 2   ▶◀ Revised Text   ● New Line   ▲ Revised Code   2013 ICD-9-CM

Uremia, uremic — *continued*
   maternal NEC, affecting fetus or newborn 760.1
   neuropathy 585.9 *[357.4]*
   pericarditis 585.9 *[420.0]*
   prerenal 788.99
   pyeletic (*see also* Pyelitis) 590.80
Ureteralgia 788.0
Ureterectasis 593.89
Ureteritis 593.89
   cystica 590.3
   due to calculus 592.1
   gonococcal (acute) 098.19
      chronic or duration of 2 months or over 098.39
   nonspecific 593.89
Ureterocele (acquired) 593.89
   congenital 753.23
Ureterolith 592.1
Ureterolithiasis 592.1
Ureterostomy status V44.6
   with complication 997.5
Ureter, ureteral — *see* condition
Urethralgia 788.99
Urethra, urethral — *see* condition
Urethritis (abacterial) (acute) (allergic) (anterior) (chronic) (nonvenereal) (posterior) (recurrent) (simple) (subacute) (ulcerative) (undifferentiated) 597.80
   diplococcal (acute) 098.0
      chronic or duration of 2 months or over 098.2
   due to Trichomonas (vaginalis) 131.02
   gonococcal (acute) 098.0
      chronic or duration of 2 months or over 098.2
   nongonococcal (sexually transmitted) 099.40
      Chlamydia trachomatis 099.41
      Reiter's 099.3
      specified organism NEC 099.49
   nonspecific (sexually transmitted) (*see also* Urethritis, nongonococcal) 099.40
   not sexually transmitted 597.80
   Reiter's 099.3
   trichomonal or due to Trichomonas (vaginalis) 131.02
   tuberculous (*see also* Tuberculosis) 016.3 ☑
   venereal NEC (*see also* Urethritis, nongonococcal) 099.40
Urethrocele
   female 618.03
      with uterine prolapse 618.4
         complete 618.3
         incomplete 618.2
   male 599.5
Urethrolithiasis 594.2
Urethro-oculoarticular syndrome 099.3
Urethro-oculosynovial syndrome 099.3
Urethrorectal — *see* condition
Urethrorrhagia 599.84
Urethrorrhea 788.7
Urethrostomy status V44.6
   with complication 997.5

Urethrotrigonitis 595.3
Urethrovaginal — *see* condition
Urgency
   fecal 787.63
   hypertensive — *see* Hypertension
Urhidrosis, uridrosis 705.89
Uric acid
   diathesis 274.9
   in blood 790.6
Uricacidemia 790.6
Uricemia 790.6
Uricosuria 791.9
Urination
   frequent 788.41
   painful 788.1
   urgency 788.63
Urinemia — *see* Uremia
Urine, urinary — *see also* condition
   abnormality NEC 788.69
   blood in (*see also* Hematuria) 599.70
   discharge, excessive 788.42
   enuresis 788.30
      nonorganic origin 307.6
   extravasation 788.8
   frequency 788.41
   hesitancy 788.64
   incontinence 788.30
      active 788.30
      female 788.30
         stress 625.6
            and urge 788.33
      male 788.30
         stress 788.32
            and urge 788.33
      mixed (stress and urge) 788.33
      neurogenic 788.39
      nonorganic origin 307.6
      overflow 788.38
      stress (female) 625.6
         male NEC 788.32
   intermittent stream 788.61
   pus in 791.9
   retention or stasis NEC 788.20
      bladder, incomplete emptying 788.21
      psychogenic 306.53
      specified NEC 788.29
   secretion
      deficient 788.5
      excessive 788.42
      frequency 788.41
   strain 788.65
   stream
      intermittent 788.61
      slowing 788.62
      splitting 788.61
      weak 788.62
   urgency 788.63
Urinoma NEC 599.9
   bladder 596.89
   kidney 593.89
   renal 593.89
   ureter 593.89
   urethra 599.84
Uroarthritis, infectious 099.3

Urodialysis 788.5
Urolithiasis 592.9
Uronephrosis 593.89
Uropathy 599.9
   obstructive 599.60
Urosepsis 599.0
   meaning sepsis 995.91
   meaning urinary tract infection 599.0
Urticaria 708.9
   with angioneurotic edema 995.1
      hereditary 277.6
   allergic 708.0
   cholinergic 708.5
   chronic 708.8
   cold, familial 708.2
   dermatographic 708.3
   due to
      cold or heat 708.2
      drugs 708.0
      food 708.0
      inhalants 708.0
      plants 708.8
      serum 999.59
   factitial 708.3
   giant 995.1
      hereditary 277.6
   gigantea 995.1
      hereditary 277.6
   idiopathic 708.1
   larynx 995.1
      hereditary 277.6
   neonatorum 778.8
   nonallergic 708.1
   papulosa (Hebra) 698.2
   perstans hemorrhagica 757.39
   pigmentosa 757.33
   recurrent periodic 708.8
   serum 999.59
   solare 692.72
   specified type NEC 708.8
   thermal (cold) (heat) 708.2
   vibratory 708.4
Urticarioides acarodermatitis 133.9
Use of
   agents affecting estrogen receptors and estrogen levels NEC V07.59
   anastrozole (Arimidex) V07.52
   aromatase inhibitors V07.52
   estrogen receptor downregulators V07.59
   exemestane (Aromasin) V07.52
   fulvestrant (Faslodex) V07.59
   gonadotropin-releasing hormone (GnRH) agonist V07.59
   goserelin acetate (Zoladex) V07.59
   letrozole (Femara) V07.52
   leuprolide acetate (leuprorelin) (Lupron) V07.59
   megestrol acetate (Megace) V07.59
   methadone 304.00
   nonprescribed drugs (*see also* Abuse, drugs, nondependent) 305.9 ☑
   patent medicines (*see also* Abuse, drugs, nondependent) 305.9 ☑
   raloxifene (Evista) V07.51

Use of — *continued*
   selective estrogen receptor modulators (SERMs) V07.51
   tamoxifen (Nolvadex) V07.51
   toremifene (Fareston) V07.51
Usher-Senear disease (pemphigus erythematosus) 694.4
Uta 085.5
Uterine size-date discrepancy 649.6 ☑
Uteromegaly 621.2
Uterovaginal — *see* condition
Uterovesical — *see* condition
Uterus — *see also* condition
   with only one functioning horn 752.33
Utriculitis (utriculus prostaticus) 597.89
Uveal — *see* condition
Uveitis (anterior) — *see also* Iridocyclitis 364.3
   acute or subacute 364.00
      due to or associated with
         gonococcal infection 098.41
         herpes (simplex) 054.44
            zoster 053.22
      primary 364.01
      recurrent 364.02
      secondary (noninfectious) 364.04
         infectious 364.03
   allergic 360.11
   chronic 364.10
      due to or associated with
         sarcoidosis 135 *[364.11]*
         tuberculosis (*see also* Tuberculosis) 017.3 ☑ *[364.11]*
   due to
      operation 360.11
      toxoplasmosis (acquired) 130.2
         congenital (active) 771.2
   granulomatous 364.10
   heterochromic 364.21
   lens-induced 364.23
   nongranulomatous 364.00
   posterior 363.20
      disseminated — *see* Chorioretinitis, disseminated
      focal — *see* Chorioretinitis, focal
   recurrent 364.02
   sympathetic 360.11
   syphilitic (secondary) 091.50
      congenital 090.0 *[363.13]*
      late 095.8 *[363.13]*
   tuberculous (*see also* Tuberculosis) 017.3 ☑ *[364.11]*
Uveoencephalitis 363.22
Uveokeratitis — *see also* Iridocyclitis 364.3
Uveoparotid fever 135
Uveoparotitis 135
Uvula — *see* condition
Uvulitis (acute) (catarrhal) (chronic) (gangrenous) (membranous) (suppurative) (ulcerative) 528.3

☑ **Additional Digit Required** — Refer to the Tabular List for Digit Selection   ᵀᴱᴸ **Subterms under main terms may continue to next column or page**

2013 ICD-9-CM   ▶◀ Revised Text   ● New Line   ▲ Revised Code   **Volume 2 — 291**

Uremia, uremic — Uvulitis

V

Vaccination
complication or reaction — *see* Complications, vaccination
delayed V64.00
not carried out V64.00
  because of
    acute illness V64.01
    allergy to vaccine or component V64.04
    caregiver refusal V64.05
    chronic illness V64.02
    guardian refusal V64.05
    immune compromised state V64.03
    parent refusal V64.05
    patient had disease being vaccinated against V64.08
    patient refusal V64.06
    reason NEC V64.09
    religious reasons V64.07
prophylactic (against) V05.9
  arthropod-borne viral
    disease NEC V05.1
    encephalitis V05.0
  chickenpox V05.4
  cholera (alone) V03.0
    with typhoid-paratyphoid (cholera + TAB) V06.0
  common cold V04.7
  diphtheria (alone) V03.5
    with
      poliomyelitis (DTP+ polio) V06.3
      tetanus V06.5
        pertussis combined (DTP) (DTaP) V06.1
        typhoid-paratyphoid (DTP + TAB) V06.2
  disease (single) NEC V05.9
    bacterial NEC V03.9
      specified type NEC V03.89
    combination NEC V06.9
      specified type NEC V06.8
    specified type NEC V05.8
  encephalitis, viral, arthropod-borne V05.0
  Hemophilus influenzae, type B [Hib] V03.81
  hepatitis, viral V05.3
  influenza V04.81
    with
      Streptococcus pneumoniae [pneumococcus] V06.6
  leishmaniasis V05.2
  measles (alone) V04.2
    with mumps-rubella (MMR) V06.4
  mumps (alone) V04.6
    with measles and rubella (MMR) V06.4
  pertussis alone V03.6
  plague V03.3
  poliomyelitis V04.0
    with diphtheria-tetanus-pertussis (DTP + polio) V06.3
  rabies V04.5
  respiratory syncytial virus (RSV) V04.82
  rubella (alone) V04.3
    with measles and mumps (MMR) V06.4
  smallpox V04.1
  Streptococcus pneumoniae [pneumococcus] V03.82
    with
      influenza V06.6
  tetanus toxoid (alone) V03.7
    with diphtheria [Td] [DT] V06.5
      with
        pertussis (DTP) (DTaP) V06.1
          with poliomyelitis (DTP+polio) V06.3
  tuberculosis (BCG) V03.2
  tularemia V03.4
  typhoid-paratyphoid (TAB) (alone) V03.1
    with diphtheria-tetanus-pertussis (TAB + DTP) V06.2
  varicella V05.4

Vaccination — *continued*
  prophylactic — *continued*
    viral
      disease NEC V04.89
      encephalitis, arthropod-borne V05.0
      hepatitis V05.3
      yellow fever V04.4
Vaccinia (generalized) 999.0
  without vaccination 051.02
  congenital 771.2
  conjunctiva 999.39
  eyelids 999.0 *[373.5]*
  localized 999.39
  nose 999.39
  not from vaccination 051.02
    eyelid 051.02 *[373.5]*
  sine vaccinatione 051.02
Vacuum
  extraction of fetus or newborn 763.3
  in sinus (accessory) (nasal) (*see also* Sinusitis) 473.9
Vagabond V60.0
Vagabondage V60.0
Vagabonds' disease 132.1
Vaginalitis (tunica) 608.4
Vagina, vaginal — *see also* condition
  high risk human papillomavirus (HPV) DNA test positive 795.15
  low risk human papillomavirus (HPV) DNA test positive 795.19
Vaginismus (reflex) 625.1
  functional 306.51
  hysterical 300.11
  psychogenic 306.51
Vaginitis (acute) (chronic) (circumscribed) (diffuse) (emphysematous) (Hemophilus vaginalis) (nonspecific) (nonvenereal) (ulcerative) 616.10
  with
    abortion — *see* Abortion, by type, with sepsis
    ectopic pregnancy (*see also* categories 633.0–633.9) 639.0
    molar pregnancy (*see also* categories 630–632) 639.0
  adhesive, congenital 752.49
  atrophic, postmenopausal 627.3
  bacterial 616.10
  blennorrhagic (acute) 098.0
    chronic or duration of 2 months or over 098.2
  candidal 112.1
  chlamydial 099.53
  complicating pregnancy or puerperium 646.6 ☑
    affecting fetus or newborn 760.8
  congenital (adhesive) 752.49
  due to
    C. albicans 112.1
    Trichomonas (vaginalis) 131.01
  following
    abortion 639.0
    ectopic or molar pregnancy 639.0
  gonococcal (acute) 098.0
    chronic or duration of 2 months or over 098.2
  granuloma 099.2
  Monilia 112.1
  mycotic 112.1
  pinworm 127.4 *[616.11]*
  postirradiation 616.10
  postmenopausal atrophic 627.3
  senile (atrophic) 627.3
  syphilitic (early) 091.0
    late 095.8
  trichomonal 131.01
  tuberculous (*see also* Tuberculosis) 016.7 ☑
  venereal NEC 099.8
Vaginosis — *see* Vaginitis
Vagotonia 352.3
Vagrancy V60.0
VAIN I (vaginal intraepithelial neoplasia I) 623.0
VAIN II (vaginal intraepithelial neoplasia II) 623.0
VAIN III (vaginal intraepithelial neoplasia III) 233.31

Vallecula — *see* condition
Valley fever 114.0
Valsuani's disease (progressive pernicious anemia, puerperal) 648.2 ☑
Valve, valvular (formation) — *see also* condition
  cerebral ventricle (communicating) in situ V45.2
  cervix, internal os 752.49
  colon 751.5
  congenital NEC — *see* Atresia
  formation, congenital NEC — *see* Atresia
  heart defect — *see* Anomaly, heart, valve
  ureter 753.29
    pelvic junction 753.21
    vesical orifice 753.22
  urethra 753.6
Valvulitis (chronic) — *see also* Endocarditis 424.90
  rheumatic (chronic) (inactive) (with chorea) 397.9
    active or acute (aortic) (mitral) (pulmonary) (tricuspid) 391.1
  syphilitic NEC 093.20
    aortic 093.22
    mitral 093.21
    pulmonary 093.24
    tricuspid 093.23
Valvulopathy — *see* Endocarditis
van Bogaert-Nijssen (-Peiffer) disease 330.0
van Bogaert's leukoencephalitis (sclerosing) (subacute) 046.2
van Buchem's syndrome (hyperostosis corticalis) 733.3
Vancomycin (glycopeptide)
  intermediate staphylococcus aureus (VISA/GISA) V09.8 ☑
  resistant
    enterococcus (VRE) V09.8 ☑
    staphylococcus aureus (VRSA/GRSA) V09.8 ☑
van Creveld-von Gierke disease (glycogenosis I) 271.0
van den Bergh's disease (enterogenous cyanosis) 289.7
van der Hoeve-Halbertsma-Waardenburg syndrome (ptosis-epicanthus) 270.2
van der Hoeve-Waardenburg-Gualdi syndrome (ptosis epicanthus) 270.2
van der Hoeve's syndrome (brittle bones and blue sclera, deafness) 756.51
Vanillism 692.89
Vanishing lung 492.0
Vanishing twin 651.33
van Neck (-Odelberg) disease or syndrome (juvenile osteochondrosis) 732.1
Vapor asphyxia or suffocation NEC 987.9
  specified agent — *see* Table of Drugs and Chemicals
Vaquez's disease (M9950/1) 238.4
Vaquez-Osler disease (polycythemia vera) (M9950/1) 238.4
Variance, lethal ball, prosthetic heart valve 996.02
Variants, thalassemic 282.49
Variations in hair color 704.3
Varicella 052.9
  with
    complication 052.8
      specified NEC 052.7
    pneumonia 052.1
    vaccination and inoculation (prophylactic) V05.4
  exposure to V01.71
  vaccination and inoculation (against) (prophylactic) V05.4
Varices — *see* Varix
Varicocele (scrotum) (thrombosed) 456.4
  ovary 456.5
  perineum 456.6
  spermatic cord (ulcerated) 456.4
Varicose
  aneurysm (ruptured) (*see also* Aneurysm) 442.9
  dermatitis (lower extremity) — *see* Varicose, vein, inflamed or infected

Varicose — *continued*
  eczema — *see* Varicose, vein
  phlebitis — *see* Varicose, vein, inflamed or infected
  placental vessel — *see* Placenta, abnormal
  tumor — *see* Varicose, vein
  ulcer (lower extremity, any part) 454.0
    anus 455.8
      external 455.5
      internal 455.2
    esophagus (*see also* Varix, esophagus) 456.1
      bleeding (*see also* Varix, esophagus, bleeding) 456.0
    inflamed or infected 454.2
    nasal septum 456.8
    perineum 456.6
    rectum — *see* Varicose, ulcer, anus
    scrotum 456.4
    specified site NEC 456.8
  vein (lower extremity) (ruptured) (*see also* Varix) 454.9
    with
      complications NEC 454.8
      edema 454.8
      inflammation or infection 454.1
        ulcerated 454.2
      pain 454.8
      stasis dermatitis 454.1
        with ulcer 454.2
      swelling 454.8
      ulcer 454.0
        inflamed or infected 454.2
    anus — *see* Hemorrhoids
    broad ligament 456.5
    congenital (peripheral) 747.60
      gastrointestinal 747.61
      lower limb 747.64
      renal 747.62
      specified NEC 747.69
      upper limb 747.63
    esophagus (ulcerated) (*see also* Varix, esophagus) 456.1
      bleeding (*see also* Varix, esophagus, bleeding) 456.0
    inflamed or infected 454.1
      with ulcer 454.2
    in pregnancy or puerperium 671.0 ☑
      vulva or perineum 671.1 ☑
    nasal septum (with ulcer) 456.8
    pelvis 456.5
    perineum 456.6
      in pregnancy, childbirth, or puerperium 671.1 ☑
    rectum — *see* Hemorrhoids
    scrotum (ulcerated) 456.4
    specified site NEC 456.8
    sublingual 456.3
    ulcerated 454.0
      inflamed or infected 454.2
    umbilical cord, affecting fetus or newborn 762.6
    urethra 456.8
    vulva 456.6
      in pregnancy, childbirth, or puerperium 671.1 ☑
  vessel (*see also* Varix)
    placenta — *see* Placenta, abnormal
Varicosis, varicosities, varicosity — *see also* Varix 454.9
Variola 050.9
  hemorrhagic (pustular) 050.0
  major 050.0
  minor 050.1
  modified 050.2
Varioloid 050.2
Variolosa, purpura 050.0
Varix (lower extremity) (ruptured) 454.9
  with
    complications NEC 454.8
    edema 454.8
    inflammation or infection 454.1
      with ulcer 454.2
    pain 454.8
    stasis dermatitis 454.1
      with ulcer 454.2

☑ **Additional Digit Required** — Refer to the Tabular List for Digit Selection   ᴺᴱᶜ **Subterms under main terms may continue to next column or page**

2013 ICD-9-CM   ▶◄ Revised Text   ● New Line   ▲ Revised Code   Volume 2 — 293

Vaccination — Varix

Varix — *continued*
  with — *continued*
    swelling 454.8
    ulcer 454.0
      with inflammation or infection 454.2
  aneurysmal (*see also* Aneurysm) 442.9
  anus — *see* Hemorrhoids
  arteriovenous (congenital) (peripheral) NEC
    747.60
      gastrointestinal 747.61
      lower limb 747.64
      renal 747.62
      specified NEC 747.69
      spinal 747.82
      upper limb 747.63
  bladder 456.5
  broad ligament 456.5
  congenital (peripheral) 747.60
  esophagus (ulcerated) 456.1
    bleeding 456.0
      in
        cirrhosis of liver 571.5 *[456.20]*
        portal hypertension
          572.3 *[456.20]*
    congenital 747.69
      in
        cirrhosis of liver 571.5 *[456.21]*
          with bleeding 571.5 *[456.20]*
        portal hypertension
          572.3 *[456.21]*
          with bleeding 572.3 *[456.20]*
  gastric 456.8
  inflamed or infected 454.1
    ulcerated 454.2
  in pregnancy or puerperium 671.0 ☑
    perineum 671.1 ☑
    vulva 671.1 ☑
  labia (majora) 456.6
  orbit 456.8
    congenital 747.69
  ovary 456.5
  papillary 448.1
  pelvis 456.5
  perineum 456.6
    in pregnancy or puerperium 671.1 ☑
  pharynx 456.8
  placenta — *see* Placenta, abnormal
  prostate 456.8
  rectum — *see* Hemorrhoids
  renal papilla 456.8
  retina 362.17
  scrotum (ulcerated) 456.4
  sigmoid colon 456.8
  specified site NEC 456.8
  spinal (cord) (vessels) 456.8
  spleen, splenic (vein) (with phlebolith) 456.8
  sublingual 456.3
  ulcerated 454.0
    inflamed or infected 454.2
  umbilical cord, affecting fetus or newborn
    762.6
  uterine ligament 456.5
  vocal cord 456.8
  vulva 456.6
    in pregnancy, childbirth, or puerperium
      671.1 ☑
Vasa previa 663.5 ☑
  affecting fetus or newborn 762.6
  hemorrhage from, affecting fetus or new-
    born 772.0
Vascular — *see also* condition
  loop on papilla (optic) 743.57
  sheathing, retina 362.13
  spasm 443.9
  spider 448.1
Vascularity, pulmonary, congenital 747.39
Vascularization
  choroid 362.16
  cornea 370.60
    deep 370.63
    localized 370.61
  retina 362.16
  subretinal 362.16
Vasculitis 447.6
  allergic 287.0
  cryoglobulinemic 273.2

Vasculitis — *continued*
  disseminated 447.6
  kidney 447.8
  leukocytoclastic 446.29
  nodular 695.2
  retinal 362.18
  rheumatic — *see* Fever, rheumatic
Vasculopathy
  cardiac allograft 996.83
Vas deferens — *see* condition
Vas deferentitis 608.4
Vasectomy, admission for V25.2
Vasitis 608.4
  nodosa 608.4
  scrotum 608.4
  spermatic cord 608.4
  testis 608.4
  tuberculous (*see also* Tuberculosis) 016.5 ☑
  tunica vaginalis 608.4
  vas deferens 608.4
Vasodilation 443.9
Vasomotor — *see* condition
Vasoplasty, after previous sterilization V26.0
Vasoplegia, splanchnic — *see also* Neuropathy, peripheral, autonomic 337.9
Vasospasm 443.9
  cerebral (artery) 435.9
    with transient neurologic deficit 435.9
  coronary 413.1
  nerve
    arm NEC 354.9
    autonomic 337.9
    brachial plexus 353.0
    cervical plexus 353.2
    leg NEC 355.8
    lower extremity NEC 355.8
    peripheral NEC 355.9
    spinal NEC 355.9
    sympathetic 337.9
    upper extremity NEC 354.9
  peripheral NEC 443.9
  retina (artery) (*see also* Occlusion, retinal,
    artery) 362.30
Vasospastic — *see* condition
Vasovagal attack (paroxysmal) 780.2
  psychogenic 306.2
Vater's ampulla — *see* condition
VATER syndrome 759.89
vCJD (variant Creutzfeldt-Jakob disease) 046.11
Vegetation, vegetative
  adenoid (nasal fossa) 474.2
  consciousness (persistent) 780.03
  endocarditis (acute) (any valve) (chronic)
    (subacute) 421.0
  heart (mycotic) (valve) 421.0
  state (persistent) 780.03
Veil
  Jackson's 751.4
  over face (causing asphyxia) 768.9
Vein, venous — *see* condition
Veldt sore — *see also* Ulcer, skin 707.9
Velo-cardio-facial syndrome 758.32
Velpeau's hernia — *see* Hernia, femoral
Venereal
  balanitis NEC 099.8
  bubo 099.1
  disease 099.9
    specified nature or type NEC 099.8
  granuloma inguinale 099.2
  lymphogranuloma (Durand-Nicolas-Favre),
    any site 099.1
  salpingitis 098.37
  urethritis (*see also* Urethritis, nongonococ-
    cal) 099.40
  vaginitis NEC 099.8
  warts 078.11
Vengefulness, in child — *see also* Disturbance,
  conduct 312.0 ☑
Venofibrosis 459.89
Venom, venomous
  bite or sting (animal or insect) 989.5
  poisoning 989.5
Venous — *see* condition
Ventouse delivery NEC 669.5 ☑
  affecting fetus or newborn 763.3
Ventral — *see* condition

Ventricle, ventricular — *see also* condition
  escape 427.69
  standstill (*see also* Arrest, cardiac) 427.5
Ventriculitis, cerebral — *see also* Meningitis
  322.9
Ventriculostomy status V45.2
Verbiest's syndrome (claudicatio intermittens
  spinalis) 435.1
Vernet's syndrome 352.6
Verneuil's disease (syphilitic bursitis) 095.7
Verruca (filiformis) 078.10
  acuminata (any site) 078.11
  necrogenica (primary) (*see also* Tuberculosis)
    017.0 ☑
  peruana 088.0
  peruviana 088.0
  plana (juvenilis) 078.19
  plantaris 078.12
  seborrheica 702.19
    inflamed 702.11
  senilis 702.0
  tuberculosa (primary) (*see also* Tuberculosis)
    017.0 ☑
  venereal 078.11
  viral 078.10
    specified NEC 078.19
  vulgaris 078.10
Verrucosities — *see also* Verruca 078.10
Verrucous endocarditis (acute) (any valve)
  (chronic) (subacute) 710.0 *[424.91]*
  nonbacterial 710.0 *[424.91]*
Verruga
  peruana 088.0
  peruviana 088.0
Verse's disease (calcinosis intervertebralis)
  275.49 *[722.90]*
Version
  before labor, affecting fetus or newborn
    761.7
  cephalic (correcting previous malposition)
    652.1 ☑
    affecting fetus or newborn 763.1
  cervix — *see* Version, uterus
  uterus (postinfectional) (postpartal, old) (*see
    also* Malposition, uterus) 621.6
    forward — *see* Anteversion, uterus
    lateral — *see* Lateroversion, uterus
Vertebra, vertebral — *see* condition
Vertigo 780.4
  auditory 386.19
  aural 386.19
  benign paroxysmal positional 386.11
  central origin 386.2
  cerebral 386.2
  Dix and Hallpike (epidemic) 386.12
  endemic paralytic 078.81
  epidemic 078.81
    Dix and Hallpike 386.12
    Gerlier's 078.81
    Pedersen's 386.12
    vestibular neuronitis 386.12
  epileptic — *see* Epilepsy
  Gerlier's (epidemic) 078.81
  hysterical 300.11
  labyrinthine 386.10
  laryngeal 786.2
  malignant positional 386.2
  Ménière's (*see also* Disease, Ménière's)
    386.00
  menopausal 627.2
  otogenic 386.19
  paralytic 078.81
  paroxysmal positional, benign 386.11
  Pedersen's (epidemic) 386.12
  peripheral 386.10
    specified type NEC 386.19
  positional
    benign paroxysmal 386.11
    malignant 386.2
Verumontanitis (chronic) — *see also* Urethritis
  597.89
Vesania — *see also* Psychosis 298.9
Vesical — *see* condition
Vesicle
  cutaneous 709.8
  seminal — *see* condition

Vesicle — *continued*
  skin 709.8
Vesicocolic — *see* condition
Vesicoperineal — *see* condition
Vesicorectal — *see* condition
Vesicourethrorectal — *see* condition
Vesicovaginal — *see* condition
Vesicular — *see* condition
Vesiculitis (seminal) 608.0
  amebic 006.8
  gonorrheal (acute) 098.14
    chronic or duration of 2 months or over
      098.34
  trichomonal 131.09
  tuberculous (*see also* Tuberculosis)
    016.5 ☑ *[608.81]*
Vestibulitis (ear) — *see also* Labyrinthitis
  386.30
  nose (external) 478.19
  vulvar 625.71
Vestibulopathy, acute peripheral (recurrent)
  386.12
Vestige, vestigial — *see also* Persistence
  branchial 744.41
  structures in vitreous 743.51
Vibriosis NEC 027.9
Vidal's disease (lichen simplex chronicus)
  698.3
Video display tube syndrome 723.8
Vienna-type encephalitis 049.8
Villaret's syndrome 352.6
Villous — *see* condition
VIN I (vulvar intraepithelial neoplasia I) 624.01
VIN II (vulvar intraepithelial neoplasia II) 624.02
VIN III (vulvar intraepithelial neoplasia III)
  233.32
Vincent's
  angina 101
  bronchitis 101
  disease 101
  gingivitis 101
  infection (any site) 101
  laryngitis 101
  stomatitis 101
  tonsillitis 101
Vinson-Plummer syndrome (sideropenic
  dysphagia) 280.8
Viosterol deficiency — *see also* Deficiency,
  calciferol 268.9
Virchow's disease 733.99
Viremia 790.8
Virilism (adrenal) (female) NEC 255.2
  with
    3-beta-hydroxysteroid dehydrogenase
      defect 255.2
    11-hydroxylase defect 255.2
    21-hydroxylase defect 255.2
    adrenal
      hyperplasia 255.2
      insufficiency (congenital) 255.2
    cortical hyperfunction 255.2
Virilization (female) (suprarenal) — *see also*
  Virilism 255.2
  isosexual 256.4
Virulent bubo 099.0
Virus, viral — *see also* condition
  infection NEC (*see also* Infection, viral)
    079.99
  septicemia 079.99
  yaba monkey tumor 059.22
VISA (vancomycin intermediate staphylococcus
  aureus) V09.8 ☑
Viscera, visceral — *see* condition
Visceroptosis 569.89
Visible peristalsis 787.4
Vision, visual
  binocular, suppression 368.31
  blurred, blurring 368.8
    hysterical 300.11
  defect, defective (*see also* Impaired, vision)
    369.9
  disorientation (syndrome) 368.16
  disturbance NEC (*see also* Disturbance, vi-
    sion) 368.9
    hysterical 300.11
  examination V72.0

☑ **Additional Digit Required** — Refer to the Tabular List for Digit Selection   ▽ **Subterms under main terms may continue to next column or page**

294 — Volume 2   ▶◀ Revised Text   ● New Line   ▲ Revised Code   2013 ICD-9-CM

Vision, visual — *continued*
  field, limitation 368.40
  fusion, with defective steropsis 368.33
  hallucinations 368.16
  halos 368.16
  loss 369.9
    both eyes (*see also* Blindness, both eyes) 369.3
    complete (*see also* Blindness, both eyes) 369.00
    one eye 369.8
    sudden 368.16
    low (both eyes) 369.20
      one eye (other eye normal) (*see also* Impaired, vision) 369.70
      blindness, other eye 369.10
    perception, simultaneous without fusion 368.32
  tunnel 368.45
Vitality, lack or want of 780.79
  newborn 779.89
Vitamin deficiency NEC — *see also* Deficiency, vitamin 269.2
Vitelline duct, persistent 751.0
Vitiligo 709.01
  due to pinta (carate) 103.2
  eyelid 374.53
  vulva 624.8
Vitium cordis — *see* Disease, heart
Vitreous — *see also* condition
  touch syndrome 997.99
VLCAD (long chain/very long chain acyl CoA dehydrogenase deficiency, LCAD) 277.85
Vocal cord — *see* condition
Vocational rehabilitation V57.22
Vogt's (Cecile) disease or syndrome 333.7 ☑
Vogt-Koyanagi syndrome 364.24
Vogt-Spielmeyer disease (amaurotic familial idiocy) 330.1
Voice
  change (*see also* Dysphonia) 784.49
  loss (*see also* Aphonia) 784.41
Volhard-Fahr disease (malignant nephrosclerosis) 403.00
Volhynian fever 083.1
Volkmann's ischemic contracture or paralysis (complicating trauma) 958.6
Voluntary starvation 307.1
Volvulus (bowel) (colon) (intestine) 560.2
  with
    hernia (*see also* Hernia, by site, with obstruction)
      gangrenous — *see* Hernia, by site, with gangrene
    perforation 560.2
  congenital 751.5
  duodenum 537.3
  fallopian tube 620.5
  oviduct 620.5
  stomach (due to absence of gastrocolic ligament) 537.89
Vomiting 787.03
  with nausea 787.01
  allergic 535.4 ☑
  asphyxia 933.1
  bilious (cause unknown) 787.04
    following gastrointestinal surgery 564.3
    newborn 779.32
  blood (*see also* Hematemesis) 578.0
  causing asphyxia, choking, or suffocation (*see also* Asphyxia, food) 933.1
  cyclical 536.2
    associated with migraine 346.2 ☑
    psychogenic 306.4
  epidemic 078.82
  fecal matter 569.87
  following gastrointestinal surgery 564.3
  functional 536.8
    psychogenic 306.4
  habit 536.2
  hysterical 300.11
  nervous 306.4
  neurotic 306.4
  newborn 779.33
    bilious 779.32
  of or complicating pregnancy 643.9 ☑

Vomiting — *continued*
  of or complicating pregnancy — *continued*
    due to
      organic disease 643.8 ☑
      specific cause NEC 643.8 ☑
    early — *see* Hyperemesis, gravidarum
    late (after 22 completed weeks of gestation) 643.2 ☑
  pernicious or persistent 536.2
    complicating pregnancy — *see* Hyperemesis, gravidarum
  psychogenic 306.4
  physiological 787.03
    bilious 787.04
  psychic 306.4
  psychogenic 307.54
  stercoral 569.89
  uncontrollable 536.2
    psychogenic 306.4
  uremic — *see* Uremia
  winter 078.82
von Bechterew (-Strumpell) disease or syndrome (ankylosing spondylitis) 720.0
von Bezold's abscess 383.01
von Economo's disease (encephalitis lethargica) 049.8
von Eulenburg's disease (congenital paramyotonia) 359.29
von Gierke's disease (glycogenosis I) 271.0
von Gies' joint 095.8
von Graefe's disease or syndrome 378.72
von Hippel (-Lindau) disease or syndrome (retinocerebral angiomatosis) 759.6
von Jaksch's anemia or disease (pseudoleukemia infantum) 285.8
von Recklinghausen-Applebaum disease (hemochromatosis) — *see also* Hemochromatosis 275.03
von Recklinghausen's
  disease (nerves) (skin) (M9540/1) 237.71
    bones (osteitis fibrosa cystica) 252.01
  tumor (M9540/1) 237.71
von Schroetter's syndrome (intermittent venous claudication) 453.89
von Willebrand (-Jürgens) (-Minot) disease or syndrome (angiohemophilia) 286.4
von Zambusch's disease (lichen sclerosus et atrophicus) 701.0
Voorhoeve's disease or dyschondroplasia 756.4
Vossius' ring 921.3
  late effect 366.21
Voyeurism 302.82
VRE (vancomycin resistant enterococcus) V09.8 ☑
Vrolik's disease (osteogenesis imperfecta) 756.51
VRSA (vancomycin resistant staphylococcus aureus) V09.8 ☑
Vulva — *see* condition
Vulvismus 625.1
Vulvitis (acute) (allergic) (chronic) (gangrenous) (hypertrophic) (intertriginous) 616.10
  with
    abortion — *see* Abortion, by type, with sepsis
    ectopic pregnancy (*see also* categories 633.0–633.9) 639.0
    molar pregnancy (*see also* categories 630–632) 639.0
  adhesive, congenital 752.49
  blennorrhagic (acute) 098.0
    chronic or duration of 2 months or over 098.2
  chlamydial 099.53
  complicating pregnancy or puerperium 646.6 ☑
  due to Ducrey's bacillus 099.0
  following
    abortion 639.0
    ectopic or molar pregnancy 639.0
  gonococcal (acute) 098.0

Vulvitis — *continued*
  gonococcal — *continued*
    chronic or duration of 2 months or over 098.2
  herpetic 054.11
  leukoplakic 624.09
  monilial 112.1
  puerperal, postpartum, childbirth 646.6 ☑
  syphilitic (early) 091.0
    late 095.8
  trichomonal 131.01
Vulvodynia 625.70
  specified NEC 625.79
Vulvorectal — *see* condition
Vulvovaginitis — *see also* Vulvitis 616.10
  amebic 006.8
  chlamydial 099.53
  gonococcal (acute) 098.0
    chronic or duration of 2 months or over 098.2
  herpetic 054.11
  monilial 112.1
  trichomonal (Trichomonas vaginalis) 131.01

W

Waardenburg-Klein syndrome (ptosis-epicanthus) 270.2
Waardenburg's syndrome 756.89
  meaning ptosis-epicanthus 270.2
Wagner's disease (colloid milium) 709.3
Wagner (-Unverricht) syndrome (dermatomyositis) 710.3
Waiting list, person on V63.2
  undergoing social agency investigation V63.8
Wakefulness disorder — *see also* Hypersomnia 780.54
  nonorganic origin 307.43
Waldenström's
  disease (osteochondrosis, capital femoral) 732.1
  hepatitis (lupoid hepatitis) 571.49
  hypergammaglobulinemia 273.0
  macroglobulinemia 273.3
  purpura, hypergammaglobulinemic 273.0
  syndrome (macroglobulinemia) 273.3
Waldenström-Kjellberg syndrome (sideropenic dysphagia) 280.8
Walking
  difficulty 719.7
    psychogenic 307.9
  sleep 307.46
    hysterical 300.13
Wall, abdominal — *see* condition
Wallenberg's syndrome (posterior inferior cerebellar artery) — *see also* Disease, cerebrovascular, acute 436
Wallgren's
  disease (obstruction of splenic vein with collateral circulation) 459.89
  meningitis (*see also* Meningitis, aseptic) 047.9
Wandering
  acetabulum 736.39
  gallbladder 751.69
  in diseases classified elsewhere V40.31
  kidney, congenital 753.3
  organ or site, congenital NEC — *see* Malposition, congenital
  pacemaker (atrial) (heart) 427.89
  spleen 289.59
Wardrop's disease (with lymphangitis) 681.9
  finger 681.02
  toe 681.11
War neurosis 300.16
Wart (digitate) (filiform) (infectious) (viral) 078.10
  common 078.19
  external genital organs (venereal) 078.11
  fig 078.19
  flat 078.19
  genital 078.11
  Hassall-Henle's (of cornea) 371.41
  Henle's (of cornea) 371.41
  juvenile 078.19
  moist 078.10

Wart — *continued*
  Peruvian 088.0
  plantar 078.12
  prosector (*see also* Tuberculosis) 017.0 ☑
  seborrheic 702.19
    inflamed 702.11
  senile 702.0
  specified NEC 078.19
  syphilitic 091.3
  tuberculous (*see also* Tuberculosis) 017.0 ☑
  venereal (female) (male) 078.11
Warthin's tumor (salivary gland) (M8561/0) 210.2
Washerwoman's itch 692.4
Wassilieff's disease (leptospiral jaundice) 100.0
Wasting
  disease 799.4
    due to malnutrition 261
  extreme (due to malnutrition) 261
  muscular NEC 728.2
  palsy, paralysis 335.21
  pelvic muscle 618.83
Water
  clefts 366.12
  deprivation of 994.3
  in joint (*see also* Effusion, joint) 719.0 ☑
  intoxication 276.69
  itch 120.3
  lack of 994.3
  loading 276.69
  on
    brain — *see* Hydrocephalus
    chest 511.89
  poisoning 276.69
Waterbrash 787.1
Water-hammer pulse — *see also* Insufficiency, aortic 424.1
Waterhouse (-Friderichsen) disease or syndrome 036.3
Water-losing nephritis 588.89
Watermelon stomach 537.82
  with hemorrhage 537.83
  without hemorrhage 537.82
Wax in ear 380.4
Waxy
  degeneration, any site 277.39
  disease 277.39
  kidney 277.39 [583.81]
  liver (large) 277.39
  spleen 277.39
Weak, weakness (generalized) 780.79
  arches (acquired) 734
    congenital 754.61
  bladder sphincter 596.59
  congenital 779.89
  eye muscle — *see* Strabismus
  facial 781.94
  foot (double) — *see* Weak, arches
  heart, cardiac (*see also* Failure, heart) 428.9
    congenital 746.9
  mind 317
  muscle (generalized) 728.87
  myocardium (*see also* Failure, heart) 428.9
  newborn 779.89
  pelvic fundus
    pubocervical tissue 618.81
    rectovaginal tissue 618.82
  pulse 785.9
  senile 797
  urinary stream 788.62
  valvular — *see* Endocarditis
Wear, worn, tooth, teeth (approximal) (hard tissues) (interproximal) (occlusal) — *see also* Attrition, teeth 521.10
Weather, weathered
  effects of
    cold NEC 991.9
      specified effect NEC 991.8
    hot (*see also* Heat) 992.9
  skin 692.74
Weber-Christian disease or syndrome (nodular nonsuppurative panniculitis) 729.30
Weber-Cockayne syndrome (epidermolysis bullosa) 757.39

☑ **Additional Digit Required** — Refer to the Tabular List for Digit Selection   ▽ **Subterms under main terms may continue to next column or page**

2013 ICD-9-CM   ▶◀ **Revised Text**   ● **New Line**   ▲ **Revised Code**   **Volume 2 — 295**

Weber-Dimitri syndrome — Wound, open

Index

Weber-Dimitri syndrome 759.6
Weber-Gubler syndrome 344.89
Weber-Leyden syndrome 344.89
Weber-Osler syndrome (familial hemorrhagic telangiectasia) 448.0
Weber's paralysis or syndrome 344.89
Web, webbed (congenital) — *see also* Anomaly, specified type NEC
 canthus 743.63
 digits (*see also* Syndactylism) 755.10
 duodenal 751.5
 esophagus 750.3
 fingers (*see also* Syndactylism, fingers) 755.11
 larynx (glottic) (subglottic) 748.2
 neck (pterygium colli) 744.5
 Paterson-Kelly (sideropenic dysphagia) 280.8
 popliteal syndrome 756.89
 toes (*see also* Syndactylism, toes) 755.13
Wedge-shaped or wedging vertebra — *see also* Osteoporosis 733.00
Wegener's granulomatosis or syndrome 446.4
Wegner's disease (syphilitic osteochondritis) 090.0
Weight
 gain (abnormal) (excessive) 783.1
 during pregnancy 646.1 ☑
 insufficient 646.8 ☑
 less than 1000 grams at birth 765.0 ☑
 loss (cause unknown) 783.21
Weightlessness 994.9
Weil's disease (leptospiral jaundice) 100.0
Weill-Marchesani syndrome (brachymorphism and ectopia lentis) 759.89
Weingarten's syndrome (tropical eosinophilia) 518.3
Weir Mitchell's disease (erythromelalgia) 443.82
Weiss-Baker syndrome (carotid sinus syncope) 337.01
Weissenbach-Thibierge syndrome (cutaneous systemic sclerosis) 710.1
Wen — *see also* Cyst, sebaceous 706.2
Wenckebach's phenomenon, heart block (second degree) 426.13
Werdnig-Hoffmann syndrome (muscular atrophy) 335.0
Werlhof-Wichmann syndrome — *see also* Purpura, thrombocytopenic 287.39
Werlhof's disease — *see also* Purpura, thrombocytopenic 287.39
Wermer's syndrome or disease (polyendocrine adenomatosis) 258.01
Werner's disease or syndrome (progeria adultorum) 259.8
Werner-His disease (trench fever) 083.1
Werner-Schultz disease (agranulocytosis) 288.09
Wernicke's encephalopathy, disease, or syndrome (superior hemorrhagic polioencephalitis) 265.1
Wernicke-Korsakoff syndrome or psychosis (nonalcoholic) 294.0
 alcoholic 291.1
Wernicke-Posadas disease — *see also* Coccidioidomycosis 114.9
Wesselsbron fever 066.3
West African fever 084.8
West Nile
 encephalitis 066.41
 encephalomyelitis 066.41
 fever 066.40
 with
 cranial nerve disorders 066.42
 encephalitis 066.41
 optic neuritis 066.42
 other complications 066.49
 other neurologic manifestations 066.42
 polyradiculitis 066.42
 virus 066.40
Westphal-Strümpell syndrome (hepatolenticular degeneration) 275.1

Wet
 brain (alcoholic) (*see also* Alcoholism) 303.9 ☑
 feet, tropical (syndrome) (maceration) 991.4
 lung (syndrome)
 adult 518.52
 newborn 770.6
Wharton's duct — *see* condition
Wheal 709.8
Wheelchair confinement status V46.3
Wheezing 786.07
Whiplash injury or syndrome 847.0
Whipple's disease or syndrome (intestinal lipodystrophy) 040.2
Whipworm 127.3
"Whistling face" syndrome (craniocarpotarsal dystrophy) 759.89
White — *see also* condition
 kidney
 large — *see* Nephrosis
 small 582.9
 leg, puerperal, postpartum, childbirth 671.4 ☑
 nonpuerperal 451.19
 mouth 112.0
 patches of mouth 528.6
 sponge nevus of oral mucosa 750.26
 spot lesions, teeth 521.01
White's disease (congenital) (keratosis follicularis) 757.39
Whitehead 706.2
Whitlow (with lymphangitis) 681.01
 herpetic 054.6
Whitmore's disease or fever (melioidosis) 025
Whooping cough 033.9
 with pneumonia 033.9 *[484.3]*
 due to
 Bordetella
 bronchoseptica 033.8
 with pneumonia 033.8 *[484.3]*
 parapertussis 033.1
 with pneumonia 033.1 *[484.3]*
 pertussis 033.0
 with pneumonia 033.0 *[484.3]*
 specified organism NEC 033.8
 with pneumonia 033.8 *[484.3]*
 vaccination, prophylactic (against) V03.6
Wichmann's asthma (laryngismus stridulus) 478.75
Widal (-Abrami) syndrome (acquired hemolytic jaundice) 283.9
Widening aorta — *see also* Ectasia, aortic 447.70
 with aneurysm 441.9
 ruptured 441.5
Wilkie's disease or syndrome 557.1
Wilkinson-Sneddon disease or syndrome (subcorneal pustular dermatosis) 694.1
Willan's lepra 696.1
Willan-Plumbe syndrome (psoriasis) 696.1
Willebrand (-Jürgens) syndrome or thrombopathy (angiohemophilia) 286.4
Willi-Prader syndrome (hypogenital dystrophy with diabetic tendency) 759.81
Willis' disease (diabetes mellitus) — *see also* Diabetes 250.0 ☑
 due to secondary diabetes 249.0 ☑
Wilms' tumor or neoplasm (nephroblastoma) (M8960/3) 189.0
Wilson's
 disease or syndrome (hepatolenticular degeneration) 275.1
 hepatolenticular degeneration 275.1
 lichen ruber 697.0
Wilson-Brocq disease (dermatitis exfoliativa) 695.89
Wilson-Mikity syndrome 770.7
Window — *see also* Imperfect, closure aorticopulmonary 745.0
Winged scapula 736.89
Winter — *see also* condition
 vomiting disease 078.82
Wise's disease 696.2
Wiskott-Aldrich syndrome (eczema-thrombocytopenia) 279.12

Withdrawal symptoms, syndrome
 alcohol 291.81
 delirium (acute) 291.0
 chronic 291.1
 newborn 760.71
 drug or narcotic 292.0
 newborn, infant of dependent mother 779.5
 steroid NEC
 correct substance properly administered 255.41
 overdose or wrong substance given or taken 962.0
Withdrawing reaction, child or adolescent 313.22
Witts' anemia (achlorhydric anemia) 280.9
Witzelsucht 301.9
Woakes' syndrome (ethmoiditis) 471.1
Wohlfart-Kugelberg-Welander disease 335.11
Woillez's disease (acute idiopathic pulmonary congestion) 518.52
Wolff-Parkinson-White syndrome (anomalous atrioventricular excitation) 426.7
Wolhynian fever 083.1
Wolman's disease (primary familial xanthomatosis) 272.7
Wood asthma 495.8
Woolly, wooly hair (congenital) (nevus) 757.4
Wool-sorters' disease 022.1
Word
 blindness (congenital) (developmental) 315.01
 secondary to organic lesion 784.61
 deafness (secondary to organic lesion) 784.69
 developmental 315.31
Worm(s) (colic) (fever) (infection) (infestation) — *see also* Infestation 128.9
 guinea 125.7
 in intestine NEC 127.9
Worm-eaten soles 102.3
Worn out — *see also* Exhaustion 780.79
 artificial heart valve 996.02
 cardiac defibrillator (with synchronous cardiac pacemaker) V53.32
 cardiac pacemaker lead or battery V53.31
 joint prosthesis (*see also* Complications, mechanical, device NEC, prosthetic NEC, joint) 996.46
"Worried well" V65.5
Wound, open (by cutting or piercing instrument) (by firearms) (cut) (dissection) (incised) (laceration) (penetration) (perforating) (puncture) (with initial hemorrhage, not internal) 879.8

Note — For fracture with open wound, see Fracture.

For laceration, traumatic rupture, tear or penetrating wound of internal organs, such as heart, lung, liver, kidney, pelvic organs, etc., whether or not accompanied by open wound or fracture in the same region, see Injury, internal.

For contused wound, see Contusion. For crush injury, see Crush. For abrasion, insect bite (nonvenomous), blister, or scratch, see Injury, superficial.

Complicated includes wounds with:

 delayed healing

 delayed treatment

 foreign body

 primary infection

For late effect of open wound, see Late, effect, wound, open, by site.

 abdomen, abdominal (external) (muscle) 879.2
 complicated 879.3
 wall (anterior) 879.2
 complicated 879.3
 lateral 879.4
 complicated 879.5
 alveolar (process) 873.62

Wound, open — *continued*
 alveolar — *continued*
 complicated 873.72
 ankle 891.0
 with tendon involvement 891.2
 complicated 891.1
 anterior chamber, eye (*see also* Wound, open, intraocular) 871.9
 anus 863.89
 arm 884.0
 with tendon involvement 884.2
 complicated 884.1
 forearm 881.00
 with tendon involvement 881.20
 complicated 881.10
 multiple sites — *see* Wound, open, multiple, upper limb
 upper 880.03
 with tendon involvement 880.23
 complicated 880.13
 multiple sites (with axillary or shoulder regions) 880.09
 with tendon involvement 880.29
 complicated 880.19
 artery — *see* Injury, blood vessel, by site
 auditory
 canal (external) (meatus) 872.02
 complicated 872.12
 ossicles (incus) (malleus) (stapes) 872.62
 complicated 872.72
 auricle, ear 872.01
 complicated 872.11
 axilla 880.02
 with tendon involvement 880.22
 complicated 880.12
 with tendon involvement 880.29
 involving other sites of upper arm 880.09
 complicated 880.19
 back 876.0
 complicated 876.1
 bladder — *see* Injury, internal, bladder
 blood vessel — *see* Injury, blood vessel, by site
 brain — *see* Injury, intracranial, with open intracranial wound
 breast 879.0
 complicated 879.1
 brow 873.42
 complicated 873.52
 buccal mucosa 873.61
 complicated 873.71
 buttock 877.0
 complicated 877.1
 calf 891.0
 with tendon involvement 891.2
 complicated 891.1
 canaliculus lacrimalis 870.8
 with laceration of eyelid 870.2
 canthus, eye 870.8
 laceration — *see* Laceration, eyelid
 cavernous sinus — *see* Injury, intracranial
 cerebellum — *see* Injury, intracranial
 cervical esophagus 874.4
 complicated 874.5
 cervix — *see* Injury, internal, cervix
 cheek(s) (external) 873.41
 complicated 873.51
 internal 873.61
 complicated 873.71
 chest (wall) (external) 875.0
 complicated 875.1
 chin 873.44
 complicated 873.54
 choroid 363.63
 ciliary body (eye) (*see also* Wound, open, intraocular) 871.9
 clitoris 878.8
 complicated 878.9
 cochlea 872.64
 complicated 872.74
 complicated 879.9
 conjunctiva — *see* Wound, open, intraocular
 cornea (nonpenetrating) (*see also* Wound, open, intraocular) 871.9
 costal region 875.0
 complicated 875.1

☑ **Additional Digit Required** — Refer to the Tabular List for Digit Selection

🐾 **Subterms under main terms may continue to next column or page**

Wound, open — *continued*
Descemet's membrane (*see also* Wound, open, intraocular) 871.9
digit(s)
  foot 893.0
    with tendon involvement 893.2
    complicated 893.1
  hand 883.0
    with tendon involvement 883.2
    complicated 883.1
drumhead, ear 872.61
  complicated 872.71
ear 872.8
  canal 872.02
    complicated 872.12
  complicated 872.9
  drum 872.61
    complicated 872.71
  external 872.00
    complicated 872.10
  multiple sites 872.69
    complicated 872.79
  ossicles (incus) (malleus) (stapes) 872.62
    complicated 872.72
  specified part NEC 872.69
    complicated 872.79
elbow 881.01
  with tendon involvement 881.21
  complicated 881.11
epididymis 878.2
  complicated 878.3
epigastric region 879.2
  complicated 879.3
epiglottis 874.01
  complicated 874.11
esophagus (cervical) 874.4
  complicated 874.5
  thoracic — *see* Injury, internal, esophagus
Eustachian tube 872.63
  complicated 872.73
extremity
  lower (multiple) NEC 894.0
    with tendon involvement 894.2
    complicated 894.1
  upper (multiple) NEC 884.0
    with tendon involvement 884.2
    complicated 884.1
eye(s) (globe) — *see* Wound, open, intraocular
eyeball NEC 871.9
  laceration (*see also* Laceration, eyeball) 871.4
  penetrating (*see also* Penetrating wound, eyeball) 871.7
eyebrow 873.42
  complicated 873.52
eyelid NEC 870.8
  laceration — *see* Laceration, eyelid
face 873.40
  complicated 873.50
  multiple sites 873.49
    complicated 873.59
  specified part NEC 873.49
    complicated 873.59
fallopian tube — *see* Injury, internal, fallopian tube
finger(s) (nail) (subungual) 883.0
  with tendon involvement 883.2
  complicated 883.1
flank 879.4
  complicated 879.5
foot (any part except toe(s) alone) 892.0
  with tendon involvement 892.2
  complicated 892.1
forearm 881.00
  with tendon involvement 881.20
  complicated 881.10
forehead 873.42
  complicated 873.52
genital organs (external) NEC 878.8
  complicated 878.9
  internal — *see* Injury, internal, by site
globe (eye) (*see also* Wound, open, eyeball) 871.9
groin 879.4

Wound, open — *continued*
groin — *continued*
  complicated 879.5
gum(s) 873.62
  complicated 873.72
hand (except finger(s) alone) 882.0
  with tendon involvement 882.2
  complicated 882.1
head NEC 873.8
  with intracranial injury — *see* Injury, intracranial
  due to or associated with skull fracture — *see* Fracture, skull
  complicated 873.9
  scalp — *see* Wound, open, scalp
heel 892.0
  with tendon involvement 892.2
  complicated 892.1
high-velocity (grease gun) — *see* Wound, open, complicated, by site
hip 890.0
  with tendon involvement 890.2
  complicated 890.1
hymen 878.6
  complicated 878.7
hypochondrium 879.4
  complicated 879.5
hypogastric region 879.2
  complicated 879.3
iliac (region) 879.4
  complicated 879.5
incidental to
  dislocation — *see* Dislocation, open, by site
  fracture — *see* Fracture, open, by site
  intracranial injury — *see* Injury, intracranial, with open intracranial wound
  nerve injury — *see* Injury, nerve, by site
inguinal region 879.4
  complicated 879.5
instep 892.0
  with tendon involvement 892.2
  complicated 892.1
interscapular region 876.0
  complicated 876.1
intracranial — *see* Injury, intracranial, with open intracranial wound
intraocular 871.9
  with
    partial loss (of intraocular tissue) 871.2
    prolapse or exposure (of intraocular tissue) 871.1
    without prolapse (of intraocular tissue) 871.0
  laceration (*see also* Laceration, eyeball) 871.4
  penetrating 871.7
    with foreign body (nonmagnetic) 871.6
    magnetic 871.5
iris (*see also* Wound, open, eyeball) 871.9
jaw (fracture not involved) 873.44
  with fracture — *see* Fracture, jaw
  complicated 873.54
knee 891.0
  with tendon involvement 891.2
  complicated 891.1
labium (majus) (minus) 878.4
  complicated 878.5
lacrimal apparatus, gland, or sac 870.8
  with laceration of eyelid 870.2
larynx 874.01
  with trachea 874.00
    complicated 874.10
  complicated 874.11
leg (multiple) 891.0
  with tendon involvement 891.2
  complicated 891.1
  lower 891.0
    with tendon involvement 891.2
    complicated 891.1
  thigh 890.0
    with tendon involvement 890.2
    complicated 890.1

Wound, open — *continued*
leg — *continued*
  upper 890.0
    with tendon involvement 890.2
    complicated 890.1
lens (eye) (alone) (*see also* Cataract, traumatic) 366.20
  with involvement of other eye structures — *see* Wound, open, eyeball
limb
  lower (multiple) NEC 894.0
    with tendon involvement 894.2
    complicated 894.1
  upper (multiple) NEC 884.0
    with tendon involvement 884.2
    complicated 884.1
lip 873.43
  complicated 873.53
loin 876.0
  complicated 876.1
lumbar region 876.0
  complicated 876.1
malar region 873.41
  complicated 873.51
mastoid region 873.49
  complicated 873.59
mediastinum — *see* Injury, internal, mediastinum
midthoracic region 875.0
  complicated 875.1
mouth 873.60
  complicated 873.70
  floor 873.64
    complicated 873.74
  multiple sites 873.69
    complicated 873.79
  specified site NEC 873.69
    complicated 873.79
multiple, unspecified site(s) 879.8

> *Note — Multiple open wounds of sites classifiable to the same four-digit category should be classified to that category unless they are in different limbs.*
>
> *Multiple open wounds of sites classifiable to different four-digit categories, or to different limbs, should be coded separately.*

  complicated 879.9
  lower limb(s) (one or both) (sites classifiable to more than one three-digit category in 890 to 893) 894.0
    with tendon involvement 894.2
    complicated 894.1
  upper limb(s) (one or both) (sites classifiable to more than one three-digit category in 880 to 883) 884.0
    with tendon involvement 884.2
    complicated 884.1
muscle — *see* Sprain, by site
nail
  finger(s) 883.0
    complicated 883.1
  thumb 883.0
    complicated 883.1
  toe(s) 893.0
    complicated 893.1
nape (neck) 874.8
  complicated 874.9
  specified part NEC 874.8
    complicated 874.9
nasal (*see also* Wound, open, nose)
  cavity 873.22
    complicated 873.32
  septum 873.21
    complicated 873.31
  sinuses 873.23
    complicated 873.33
nasopharynx 873.22
  complicated 873.32
neck 874.8
  complicated 874.9
  nape 874.8
    complicated 874.9
  specified part NEC 874.8

Wound, open — *continued*
neck — *continued*
  specified part — *continued*
    complicated 874.9
nerve — *see* Injury, nerve, by site
non-healing surgical 998.83
nose 873.20
  complicated 873.30
  multiple sites 873.29
    complicated 873.39
  septum 873.21
    complicated 873.31
  sinuses 873.23
    complicated 873.33
occipital region — *see* Wound, open, scalp
ocular NEC 871.9
  adnexa 870.9
    specified region NEC 870.8
  laceration (*see also* Laceration, ocular) 871.4
  muscle (extraocular) 870.3
    with foreign body 870.4
    eyelid 870.1
    intraocular — *see* Wound, open, eyeball
  penetrating (*see also* Penetrating wound, ocular) 871.7
orbit 870.8
  penetrating 870.3
    with foreign body 870.4
orbital region 870.9
ovary — *see* Injury, internal, pelvic organs
palate 873.65
  complicated 873.75
palm 882.0
  with tendon involvement 882.2
  complicated 882.1
parathyroid (gland) 874.2
  complicated 874.3
parietal region — *see* Wound, open, scalp
pelvic floor or region 879.6
  complicated 879.7
penis 878.0
  complicated 878.1
perineum 879.6
  complicated 879.7
periocular area 870.8
  laceration of skin 870.0
pharynx 874.4
  complicated 874.5
pinna 872.01
  complicated 872.11
popliteal space 891.0
  with tendon involvement 891.2
  complicated 891.1
prepuce 878.0
  complicated 878.1
pubic region 879.2
  complicated 879.3
pudenda 878.8
  complicated 878.9
rectovaginal septum 878.8
  complicated 878.9
sacral region 877.0
  complicated 877.1
sacroiliac region 877.0
  complicated 877.1
salivary (ducts) (glands) 873.69
  complicated 873.79
scalp 873.0
  complicated 873.1
scalpel, fetus or newborn 767.8
scapular region 880.01
  with tendon involvement 880.21
  complicated 880.11
  involving other sites of upper arm 880.09
    with tendon involvement 880.29
    complicated 880.19
sclera (*see also* Wound, open, intraocular) 871.9
scrotum 878.2
  complicated 878.3
seminal vesicle — *see* Injury, internal, pelvic organs
shin 891.0
  with tendon involvement 891.2

Wound, open — *continued*
shin — *continued*
complicated 891.1
shoulder 880.00
with tendon involvement 880.20
complicated 880.10
involving other sites of upper arm 880.09
with tendon involvement 880.29
complicated 880.19
skin NEC 879.8
complicated 879.9
skull (*see also* Injury, intracranial, with open intracranial wound)
with skull fracture — *see* Fracture, skull
spermatic cord (scrotal) 878.2
complicated 878.3
pelvic region — *see* Injury, internal, spermatic cord
spinal cord — *see* Injury, spinal
sternal region 875.0
complicated 875.1
subconjunctival — *see* Wound, open, in-traocular
subcutaneous NEC 879.8
complicated 879.9
submaxillary region 873.44
complicated 873.54
submental region 873.44
complicated 873.54
subungual
finger(s) (thumb) — *see* Wound, open, finger
toe(s) — *see* Wound, open, toe
supraclavicular region 874.8
complicated 874.9
supraorbital 873.42
complicated 873.52
surgical, non-healing 998.83
temple 873.49
complicated 873.59
temporal region 873.49
complicated 873.59
testis 878.2
complicated 878.3
thigh 890.0
with tendon involvement 890.2
complicated 890.1
thorax, thoracic (external) 875.0
complicated 875.1
throat 874.8
complicated 874.9
thumb (nail) (subungual) 883.0
with tendon involvement 883.2
complicated 883.1
thyroid (gland) 874.2
complicated 874.3
toe(s) (nail) (subungual) 893.0
with tendon involvement 893.2
complicated 893.1
tongue 873.64
complicated 873.74
tonsil — *see* Wound, open, neck
trachea (cervical region) 874.02
with larynx 874.00
complicated 874.10
complicated 874.12
intrathoracic — *see* Injury, internal, tra-chea
trunk (multiple) NEC 879.6
complicated 879.7
specified site NEC 879.6
complicated 879.7

Wound, open — *continued*
tunica vaginalis 878.2
complicated 878.3
tympanic membrane 872.61
complicated 872.71
tympanum 872.61
complicated 872.71
umbilical region 879.2
complicated 879.3
ureter — *see* Injury, internal, ureter
urethra — *see* Injury, internal, urethra
uterus — *see* Injury, internal, uterus
uvula 873.69
complicated 873.79
vagina 878.6
complicated 878.7
vas deferens — *see* Injury, internal, vas def-erens
vitreous (humor) 871.2
vulva 878.4
complicated 878.5
wrist 881.02
with tendon involvement 881.22
complicated 881.12
Wright's syndrome (hyperabduction) 447.8
pneumonia 390 *[517.1]*
Wringer injury — *see* Crush injury, by site
Wrinkling of skin 701.8
Wrist — *see also* condition
drop (acquired) 736.05
Wrong drug (given in error) NEC 977.9
specified drug or substance — *see* Table of Drugs and Chemicals
Wry neck — *see also* Torticollis
congenital 754.1
Wuchereria infestation 125.0
bancrofti 125.0
Brugia malayi 125.1
malayi 125.1
Wuchereriasis 125.0
Wuchereriosis 125.0
Wuchernde struma langhans (M8332/3) 193

X

Xanthelasma 272.2
eyelid 272.2 *[374.51]*
palpebrarum 272.2 *[374.51]*
Xanthelasmatosis (essential) 272.2
Xanthelasmoidea 757.33
Xanthine stones 277.2
Xanthinuria 277.2
Xanthofibroma (M8831/0) — *see* Neoplasm, connective tissue, benign
Xanthoma(s), xanthomatosis 272.2
with
hyperlipoproteinemia
type I 272.3
type III 272.2
type IV 272.1
type V 272.3
bone 272.7
craniohypophyseal 277.89
cutaneotendinous 272.7
diabeticorum 250.8 ☑ *[272.2]*
due to secondary diabetes 249.8 ☑ *[272.2]*
disseminatum 272.7
eruptive 272.2
eyelid 272.2 *[374.51]*
familial 272.7
hereditary 272.7

Xanthoma(s), xanthomatosis — *continued*
hypercholesterinemic 272.0
hypercholesterolemic 272.0
hyperlipemic 272.4
hyperlipidemic 272.4
infantile 272.7
joint 272.7
juvenile 272.7
multiple 272.7
multiplex 272.7
primary familial 272.7
tendon (sheath) 272.7
tuberosum 272.2
tuberous 272.2
tubo-eruptive 272.2
Xanthosis 709.09
surgical 998.81
Xenophobia 300.29
Xeroderma (congenital) 757.39
acquired 701.1
eyelid 373.33
eyelid 373.33
pigmentosum 757.33
vitamin A deficiency 264.8
Xerophthalmia 372.53
vitamin A deficiency 264.7
Xerosis
conjunctiva 372.53
with Bitôt's spot 372.53
vitamin A deficiency 264.1
vitamin A deficiency 264.0
cornea 371.40
with corneal ulceration 370.00
vitamin A deficiency 264.3
vitamin A deficiency 264.2
cutis 706.8
skin 706.8
Xerostomia 527.7
Xiphodynia 733.90
Xiphoidalgia 733.90
Xiphoiditis 733.99
Xiphopagus 759.4
XO syndrome 758.6
X-ray
effects, adverse, NEC 990
of chest
for suspected tuberculosis V71.2
routine V72.5
XXX syndrome 758.81
XXXXY syndrome 758.81
XXY syndrome 758.7
Xyloketosuria 271.8
Xylosuria 271.8
Xylulosuria 271.8
XYY syndrome 758.81

Y

Yaba monkey tumor virus 059.22
Yawning 786.09
psychogenic 306.1
Yaws 102.9
bone or joint lesions 102.6
butter 102.1
chancre 102.0
cutaneous, less than five years after infec-tion 102.2
early (cutaneous) (macular) (maculopapular) (micropapular) (papular) 102.2
frambeside 102.2
skin lesions NEC 102.2

Yaws — *continued*
eyelid 102.9 *[373.4]*
ganglion 102.6
gangosis, gangosa 102.5
gumma, gummata 102.4
bone 102.6
gummatous
frambeside 102.4
osteitis 102.6
periostitis 102.6
hydrarthrosis 102.6
hyperkeratosis (early) (late) (palmar) (plan-tar) 102.3
initial lesions 102.0
joint lesions 102.6
juxta-articular nodules 102.7
late nodular (ulcerated) 102.4
latent (without clinical manifestations) (with positive serology) 102.8
mother 102.0
mucosal 102.7
multiple papillomata 102.1
nodular, late (ulcerated) 102.4
osteitis 102.6
papilloma, papillomata (palmar) (plantar) 102.1
periostitis (hypertrophic) 102.6
ulcers 102.4
wet crab 102.1
Yeast infection — *see also* Candidiasis 112.9
Yellow
atrophy (liver) 570
chronic 571.8
resulting from administration of blood, plasma, serum, or other biological substance (within 8 months of administration) — *see* Hepatitis, viral
fever — *see* Fever, yellow
jack (*see also* Fever, yellow) 060.9
jaundice (*see also* Jaundice) 782.4
vernix syndrome 762.2
Yersinia septica 027.8

Z

Zagari's disease (xerostomia) 527.7
Zahorsky's disease (exanthema subitum) (*see also* Exanthem subitum) 058.10
syndrome (herpangina) 074.0
Zellweger syndrome 277.86
Zenker's diverticulum (esophagus) 530.6
Ziehen-Oppenheim disease 333.6
Zieve's syndrome (jaundice, hyperlipemia, and hemolytic anemia) 571.1
Zika fever 066.3
Zollinger-Ellison syndrome (gastric hyper-secretion with pancreatic islet cell tu-mor) 251.5
Zona — *see also* Herpes, zoster 053.9
Zoophilia (erotica) 302.1
Zoophobia 300.29
Zoster (herpes) — *see also* Herpes, zoster 053.9
Zuelzer (-Ogden) anemia or syndrome (nu-tritional megaloblastic anemia) 281.2
Zygodactyly — *see also* Syndactylism 755.10
Zygomycosis 117.7
Zymotic — *see* condition

☑ **Additional Digit Required — Refer to the Tabular List for Digit Selection** | 🐧 **Subterms under main terms may continue to next column or page**

298 — Volume 2 | ▶◀ Revised Text | ● New Line | ▲ Revised Code | 2013 ICD-9-CM

SECTION 2

Alphabetic Index to Poisoning and External Causes of Adverse Effects of Drugs and Other Chemical Substances

TABLE OF DRUGS AND CHEMICALS

This table contains a classification of drugs and other chemical substances to identify poisoning states and external causes of adverse effects.

Each of the listed substances in the table is assigned a code according to the poisoning classification (960-989). These codes are used when there is a statement of poisoning, overdose, wrong substance given or taken, or intoxication.

The table also contains a listing of external causes of adverse effects. An adverse effect is a pathologic manifestation due to ingestion or exposure to drugs or other chemical substances (e.g., dermatitis, hypersensitivity reaction, aspirin gastritis). The adverse effect is to be identified by the appropriate code found in Section 1, Index to Diseases and Injuries. An external cause code can then be used to identify the circumstances involved. The table headings pertaining to external causes are defined below:

Accidental poisoning (E850-E869) — accidental overdose of drug, wrong substance given or taken, drug taken inadvertently, accidents in the usage of drugs and biologicals in medical and surgical procedures, and to show external causes of poisonings classifiable to 980-989.

Therapeutic use (E930-E949) — a correct substance properly administered in therapeutic or prophylactic dosage as the external cause of adverse effects.

Suicide attempt (E950-E952) — instances in which self-inflicted injuries or poisonings are involved.

Assault (E961-E962) — injury or poisoning inflicted by another person with the intent to injure or kill.

Undetermined (E980-E982) — to be used when the intent of the poisoning or injury cannot be determined whether it was intentional or accidental.

The American Hospital Formulary Service list numbers are included in the table to help classify new drugs not identified in the table by name. The AHFS list numbers are keyed to the continually revised American Hospital Formulary Service (AHFS).* These listings are found in the table under the main term **Drug**.

Excluded from the table are radium and other radioactive substances. The classification of adverse effects and complications pertaining to these substances will be found in Section 1, Index to Diseases and Injuries, and Section 3, Index to External Causes of Injuries.

Although certain substances are indexed with one or more subentries, the majority are listed according to one use or state. It is recognized that many substances may be used in various ways, in medicine and in industry, and may cause adverse effects whatever the state of the agent (solid, liquid, or fumes arising from a liquid). In cases in which the reported data indicates a use or state not in the table, or which is clearly different from the one listed, an attempt should be made to classify the substance in the form which most nearly expresses the reported facts.

*American Hospital Formulary Service, 2 vol. (Washington, D.C.: American Society of Hospital Pharmacists, 1959-)

☑ Additional Digit Required — Refer to the Tabular List for Digit Selection   Subterms under main terms may continue to next column or page

2013 ICD-9-CM   ►◄ Revised Text   ● New Line   ▲ Revised Code   Volume 2 — 299

	Poisoning	Accident	Therapeutic Use	Suicide Attempt	Assault	Undetermined
External Cause (E-Code)						
1-propanol	980.3	E860.4	—	E950.9	E962.1	E980.9
2-propanol	980.2	E860.3	—	E950.9	E962.1	E980.9
2, 4-D (dichlorophenoxyacetic acid)	989.4	E863.5	—	E950.6	E962.1	E980.7
2, 4-toluene diisocyanate	983.0	E864.0	—	E950.7	E962.1	E980.6
2, 4, 5-T (trichlorophenoxyacetic acid)	989.2	E863.5	—	E950.6	E962.1	E980.7
14-hydroxydihydromorphinone	965.09	E850.2	E935.2	E950.0	E962.0	E980.0
ABOB	961.7	E857	E931.7	E950.4	E962.0	E980.4
Abrus (seed)	988.2	E865.3	—	E950.9	E962.1	E980.9
Absinthe	980.0	E860.1	—	E950.9	E962.1	E980.9
beverage	980.0	E860.0	—	E950.9	E962.1	E980.9
Acenocoumarin, acenocoumarol	964.2	E858.2	E934.2	E950.4	E962.0	E980.4
Acepromazine	969.1	E853.0	E939.1	E950.3	E962.0	E980.3
Acetal	982.8	E862.4	—	E950.9	E962.1	E980.9
Acetaldehyde (vapor)	987.8	E869.8	—	E952.8	E962.2	E982.8
liquid	989.89	E866.8	—	E950.9	E962.1	E980.9
Acetaminophen	965.4	E850.4	E935.4	E950.0	E962.0	E980.0
Acetaminosalol	965.1	E850.3	E935.3	E950.0	E962.0	E980.0
Acetanilid(e)	965.4	E850.4	E935.4	E950.0	E962.0	E980.0
Acetarsol, acetarsone	961.1	E857	E931.1	E950.4	E962.0	E980.4
Acetazolamide	974.2	E858.5	E944.2	E950.4	E962.0	E980.4
Acetic						
acid	983.1	E864.1	—	E950.7	E962.1	E980.6
with sodium acetate (ointment)	976.3	E858.7	E946.3	E950.4	E962.0	E980.4
irrigating solution	974.5	E858.5	E944.5	E950.4	E962.0	E980.4
lotion	976.2	E858.7	E946.2	E950.4	E962.0	E980.4
anhydride	983.1	E864.1	—	E950.7	E962.1	E980.6
ether (vapor)	982.8	E862.4	—	E950.9	E962.1	E980.9
Acetohexamide	962.3	E858.0	E932.3	E950.4	E962.0	E980.4
Acetomenaphthone	964.3	E858.2	E934.3	E950.4	E962.0	E980.4
Acetomorphine	965.01	E850.0	E935.0	E950.0	E962.0	E980.0
Acetone (oils) (vapor)	982.8	E862.4	—	E950.9	E962.1	E980.9
Acetophenazine						
(maleate)	969.1	E853.0	E939.1	E950.3	E962.0	E980.3
Acetophenetidin	965.4	E850.4	E935.4	E950.0	E962.0	E980.0
Acetophenone	982.0	E862.4	—	E950.9	E962.1	E980.9
Acetorphine	965.09	E850.2	E935.2	E950.0	E962.0	E980.0
Acetosulfone (sodium)	961.8	E857	E931.8	E950.4	E962.0	E980.4
Acetrizoate (sodium)	977.8	E858.8	E947.8	E950.4	E962.0	E980.4
Acetylcarbromal	967.3	E852.2	E937.3	E950.2	E962.0	E980.2
Acetylcholine (chloride)	971.0	E855.3	E941.0	E950.4	E962.0	E980.4
Acetylcysteine	975.5	E858.6	E945.5	E950.4	E962.0	E980.4
Acetyldigitoxin	972.1	E858.3	E942.1	E950.4	E962.0	E980.4
Acetyldihydrocodeine	965.09	E850.2	E935.2	E950.0	E962.0	E980.0
Acetyldihydrocodeinone	965.09	E850.2	E935.2	E950.0	E962.0	E980.0
Acetylene (gas) (industrial)	987.1	E868.1	—	E951.8	E962.2	E981.8
incomplete combustion of — see Carbon monoxide, fuel, utility						
tetrachloride (vapor)	982.3	E862.4	—	E950.9	E962.1	E980.9
Acetyliodosalicylic acid	965.1	E850.3	E935.3	E950.0	E962.0	E980.0
Acetylphenylhydrazine	965.8	E850.8	E935.8	E950.0	E962.0	E980.0
Acetylsalicylic acid	965.1	E850.3	E935.3	E950.0	E962.0	E980.0
Achromycin	960.4	E856	E930.4	E950.4	E962.0	E980.4
ophthalmic preparation	976.5	E858.7	E946.5	E950.4	E962.0	E980.4
topical NEC	976.0	E858.7	E946.0	E950.4	E962.0	E980.4
Acidifying agents	963.2	E858.1	E933.2	E950.4	E962.0	E980.4
Acids (corrosive) NEC	983.1	E864.1	—	E950.7	E962.1	E980.6
Aconite (wild)	988.2	E865.4	—	E950.9	E962.1	E980.9
Aconitine (liniment)	976.8	E858.7	E946.8	E950.4	E962.0	E980.4
Aconitum ferox	988.2	E865.4	—	E950.9	E962.1	E980.9
Acridine	983.0	E864.0	—	E950.7	E962.1	E980.6
vapor	987.8	E869.8	—	E952.8	E962.2	E982.8
Acriflavine	961.9	E857	E931.9	E950.4	E962.0	E980.4
Acrisorcin	976.0	E858.7	E946.0	E950.4	E962.0	E980.4
Acrolein (gas)	987.8	E869.8	—	E952.8	E962.2	E982.8
liquid	989.89	E866.8	—	E950.9	E962.1	E980.9
Actaea spicata	988.2	E865.4	—	E950.9	E962.1	E980.9
Acterol	961.5	E857	E931.5	E950.4	E962.0	E980.4
ACTH	962.4	E858.0	E932.4	E950.4	E962.0	E980.4
Acthar	962.4	E858.0	E932.4	E950.4	E962.0	E980.4
Actinomycin (C) (D)	960.7	E856	E930.7	E950.4	E962.0	E980.4
Adalin (acetyl)	967.3	E852.2	E937.3	E950.2	E962.0	E980.2
Adenosine (phosphate)	977.8	E858.8	E947.8	E950.4	E962.0	E980.4
ADH	962.5	E858.0	E932.5	E950.4	E962.0	E980.4
Adhesives	989.89	E866.6	—	E950.9	E962.1	E980.9
External Cause (E-Code)						
Adicillin	960.0	E856	E930.0	E950.4	E962.0	E980.4
Adiphenine	975.1	E855.6	E945.1	E950.4	E962.0	E980.4
Adjunct, pharmaceutical	977.4	E858.8	E947.4	E950.4	E962.0	E980.4
Adrenal (extract, cortex or medulla) (glucocorticoids) (hormones) (mineralocorticoids)	962.0	E858.0	E932.0	E950.4	E962.0	E980.4
ENT agent	976.6	E858.7	E946.6	E950.4	E962.0	E980.4
ophthalmic preparation	976.5	E858.7	E946.5	E950.4	E962.0	E980.4
topical NEC	976.0	E858.7	E946.0	E950.4	E962.0	E980.4
Adrenalin	971.2	E855.5	E941.2	E950.4	E962.0	E980.4
Adrenergic blocking agents	971.3	E855.6	E941.3	E950.4	E962.0	E980.4
Adrenergics	971.2	E855.5	E941.2	E950.4	E962.0	E980.4
Adrenochrome (derivatives)	972.8	E858.3	E942.8	E950.4	E962.0	E980.4
Adrenocorticotropic hormone	962.4	E858.0	E932.4	E950.4	E962.0	E980.4
Adrenocorticotropin	962.4	E858.0	E932.4	E950.4	E962.0	E980.4
Adriamycin	960.7	E856	E930.7	E950.4	E962.0	E980.4
Aerosol spray — see Sprays						
Aerosporin	960.8	E856	E930.8	E950.4	E962.0	E980.4
ENT agent	976.6	E858.7	E946.6	E950.4	E962.0	E980.4
ophthalmic preparation	976.5	E858.7	E946.5	E950.4	E962.0	E980.4
topical NEC	976.0	E858.7	E946.0	E950.9	E962.0	E980.4
Aethusa cynapium	988.2	E865.4	—	E950.9	E962.1	E980.9
Afghanistan black	969.6	E854.1	E939.6	E950.3	E962.0	E980.3
Aflatoxin	989.7	E865.9	—	E950.9	E962.1	E980.9
African boxwood	988.2	E865.4	—	E950.9	E962.1	E980.9
Agar (-agar)	973.3	E858.4	E943.3	E950.4	E962.0	E980.4
Agricultural agent NEC	989.89	E863.9	—	E950.6	E962.1	E980.7
Agrypnal	967.0	E851	E937.0	E950.1	E962.0	E980.1
Air contaminant(s), source or type not specified	987.9	E869.9	—	E952.9	E962.2	E982.9
specified type — see specific substance						
Akee	988.2	E865.4	—	E950.9	E962.1	E980.9
Akrinol	976.0	E858.7	E946.0	E950.4	E962.0	E980.4
Alantolactone	961.6	E857	E931.6	E950.4	E962.0	E980.4
Albamycin	960.8	E856	E930.8	E950.4	E962.0	E980.4
Albumin (normal human serum)	964.7	E858.2	E934.7	E950.4	E962.0	E980.4
Albuterol	975.7	E858.6	E945.7	E950.4	E962.0	E980.4
Alcohol	980.9	E860.9	—	E950.9	E962.1	E980.9
absolute	980.0	E860.1	—	E950.9	E962.1	E980.9
beverage	980.0	E860.0	E947.8	E950.9	E962.1	E980.9
amyl	980.3	E860.4	—	E950.9	E962.1	E980.9
antifreeze	980.1	E860.2	—	E950.9	E962.1	E980.9
butyl	980.3	E860.4	—	E950.9	E962.1	E980.9
dehydrated	980.0	E860.1	—	E950.9	E962.1	E980.9
beverage	980.0	E860.0	E947.8	E950.9	E962.1	E980.9
denatured	980.0	E860.1	—	E950.9	E962.1	E980.9
deterrents	977.3	E858.8	E947.3	E950.4	E962.0	E980.4
diagnostic (gastric function)	977.8	E858.8	E947.8	E950.4	E962.0	E980.4
ethyl	980.0	E860.1	—	E950.9	E962.1	E980.9
beverage	980.0	E860.0	E947.8	E950.9	E962.1	E980.9
grain	980.0	E860.1	—	E950.9	E962.1	E980.9
beverage	980.0	E860.0	E947.8	E950.9	E962.1	E980.9
industrial	980.9	E860.9	—	E950.9	E962.1	E980.9
isopropyl	980.2	E860.3	—	E950.9	E962.1	E980.9
methyl	980.1	E860.2	—	E950.9	E962.1	E980.9
preparation for consumption	980.0	E860.0	E947.8	E950.9	E962.1	E980.9
propyl	980.3	E860.4	—	E950.9	E962.1	E980.9
secondary	980.2	E860.3	—	E950.9	E962.1	E980.9
radiator	980.1	E860.2	—	E950.9	E962.1	E980.9
rubbing	980.2	E860.3	—	E950.9	E962.1	E980.9
specified type NEC	980.8	E860.8	—	E950.9	E962.1	E980.9
surgical	980.9	E860.9	—	E950.9	E962.1	E980.9
vapor (from any type of alcohol)	987.8	E869.8	—	E952.8	E962.2	E982.8
wood	980.1	E860.2	—	E950.9	E962.1	E980.9
Alcuronium chloride	975.2	E858.6	E945.2	E950.4	E962.0	E980.4
Aldactone	974.4	E858.5	E944.4	E950.4	E962.0	E980.4
Aldicarb	989.3	E863.2	—	E950.6	E962.1	E980.7
Aldomet	972.6	E858.3	E942.6	E950.4	E962.0	E980.4
Aldosterone	962.0	E858.0	E932.0	E950.4	E962.0	E980.4
Aldrin (dust)	989.2	E863.0	—	E950.6	E962.1	E980.7
Algeldrate	973.0	E858.4	E943.0	E950.4	E962.0	E980.4
Alidase	963.4	E858.1	E933.4	E950.4	E962.0	Chemical
Aliphatic thiocyanates	989.0	E866.8	—	E950.9	E962.1	E980.9

	External Cause (E-Code)					
	Poisoning	Accident	Therapeutic Use	Suicide Attempt	Assault	Undeter-mined
Alkaline antiseptic solution (aromatic)	976.6	E858.7	E946.6	E950.4	E962.0	E980.4
Alkalinizing agents (medicinal)	963.3	E858.1	E933.3	E950.4	E962.0	E980.4
Alkalis, caustic	983.2	E864.2	—	E950.7	E962.1	E980.6
Alkalizing agents (medicinal)	963.3	E858.1	E933.3	E950.4	E962.0	E980.4
Alka-seltzer	965.1	E850.3	E935.3	E950.0	E962.0	E980.0
Alkavervir	972.6	E858.3	E942.6	E950.4	E962.0	E980.4
Allegron	969.05	E854.0	E939.0	E950.3	E962.0	E980.3
Alleve — Naproxen						
Allobarbital, allobarbitone	967.0	E851	E937.0	E950.1	E962.0	E980.1
Allopurinol	974.7	E858.5	E944.7	E950.4	E962.0	E980.4
Allylestrenol	962.2	E858.0	E932.2	E950.4	E962.0	E980.4
Allylisopropylacetylurea	967.8	E852.8	E937.8	E950.2	E962.0	E980.2
Allylisopropylmalonylurea	967.0	E851	E937.0	E950.1	E962.0	E980.1
Allyltribromide	967.3	E852.2	E937.3	E950.2	E962.0	E980.2
Aloe, aloes, aloin	973.1	E858.4	E943.1	E950.4	E962.0	E980.4
Alosetron	973.8	E858.4	E943.8	E950.4	E962.0	E980.4
Aloxidone	966.0	E855.0	E936.0	E950.4	E962.0	E980.4
Aloxiprin	965.1	E850.3	E935.3	E950.0	E962.0	E980.0
Alpha-1 blockers	971.3	E855.6	E941.3	E950.4	E962.0	E980.4
Alpha amylase	963.4	E858.1	E933.4	E950.4	E962.0	E980.4
Alphaprodine (hydrochloride)	965.09	E850.2	E935.2	E950.0	E962.0	E980.0
Alpha tocopherol	963.5	E858.1	E933.5	E950.4	E962.0	E980.4
Alseroxylon	972.6	E858.3	E942.6	E950.4	E962.0	E980.4
Alum (ammonium) (potassium)	983.2	E864.2	—	E950.7	E962.1	E980.6
medicinal (astringent) NEC	976.2	E858.7	E946.2	E950.4	E962.0	E980.4
Aluminium, aluminum (gel) (hydroxide)	973.0	E858.4	E943.0	E950.4	E962.0	E980.4
acetate solution	976.2	E858.7	E946.2	E950.4	E962.0	E980.4
aspirin	965.1	E850.3	E935.3	E950.0	E962.0	E980.0
carbonate	973.0	E858.4	E943.0	E950.4	E962.0	E980.4
glycinate	973.0	E858.4	E943.0	E950.4	E962.0	E980.4
nicotinate	972.2	E858.3	E942.2	E950.4	E962.0	E980.4
ointment (surgical) (topical)	976.3	E858.7	E946.3	E950.4	E962.0	E980.4
phosphate	973.0	E858.4	E943.0	E950.4	E962.0	E980.4
subacetate	976.2	E858.7	E946.2	E950.4	E962.0	E980.4
topical NEC	976.3	E858.7	E946.3	E950.4	E962.0	E980.4
Alurate	967.0	E851	E937.0	E950.1	E962.0	E980.1
Alverine (citrate)	975.1	E858.6	E945.1	E950.4	E962.0	E980.4
Alvodine	965.09	E850.2	E935.2	E950.0	E962.0	E980.0
Amanita phalloides	988.1	E865.5	—	E950.9	E962.1	E980.9
Amantadine (hydrochloride)	966.4	E855.0	E936.4	E950.4	E962.0	E980.4
Ambazone	961.9	E857	E931.9	E950.4	E962.0	E980.4
Ambenonium	971.0	E855.3	E941.0	E950.4	E962.0	E980.4
Ambutonium bromide	971.1	E855.4	E941.1	E950.4	E962.0	E980.4
Ametazole	977.8	E858.8	E947.8	E950.4	E962.0	E980.4
Amethocaine (infiltration) (topical)	968.5	E855.2	E938.5	E950.4	E962.0	E980.4
nerve block (peripheral) (plexus)	968.6	E855.2	E938.6	E950.4	E962.0	E980.4
spinal	968.7	E855.2	E938.7	E950.4	E962.0	E980.4
Amethopterin	963.1	E858.1	E933.1	E950.4	E962.0	E980.4
Amfepramone	977.0	E858.8	E947.0	E950.4	E962.0	E980.4
Amidon	965.02	E850.1	E935.1	E950.0	E962.0	E980.0
Amidopyrine	965.5	E850.5	E935.5	E950.0	E962.0	E980.0
Aminacrine	976.0	E858.7	E946.0	E950.4	E962.0	E980.4
Aminitrozole	961.5	E857	E931.5	E950.4	E962.0	E980.4
Aminoacetic acid	974.5	E858.5	E944.5	E950.4	E962.0	E980.4
Amino acids	974.5	E858.5	E944.5	E950.4	E962.0	E980.4
Aminocaproic acid	964.4	E858.2	E934.4	E950.4	E962.0	E980.4
Aminoethylisothiourium	963.8	E858.1	E933.8	E950.4	E962.0	E980.4
Aminoglutethimide	966.3	E855.0	E936.3	E950.4	E962.0	E980.4
Aminometradine	974.3	E858.5	E944.3	E950.4	E962.0	E980.4
Aminopentamide	971.1	E855.4	E941.1	E950.4	E962.0	E980.4
Aminophenazone	965.5	E850.5	E935.5	E950.0	E962.0	E980.0
Aminophenol	983.0	E864.0	—	E950.7	E962.1	E980.6
Aminophenylpyridone	969.5	E853.8	E939.5	E950.3	E962.0	E980.3
Aminophylline	975.7	E858.6	E945.7	E950.4	E962.0	E980.4
Aminopterin	963.1	E858.1	E933.1	E950.4	E962.0	E980.4
Aminopyrine	965.5	E850.5	E935.5	E950.0	E962.0	E980.0
Aminosalicylic acid	961.8	E857	E931.8	E950.4	E962.0	E980.4
Amiphenazole	970.1	E854.3	E940.1	E950.4	E962.0	E980.4
Amiquinsin	972.6	E858.3	E942.6	E950.4	E962.0	E980.4
Amisometradine	974.3	E858.5	E944.3	E950.4	E962.0	E980.4
Amitriptyline	969.05	E854.0	E939.0	E950.3	E962.0	E980.3
Ammonia (fumes) (gas) (vapor)	987.8	E869.8	—	E952.8	E962.2	E982.8
liquid (household) NEC	983.2	E861.4	—	E950.7	E962.1	E980.6
spirit, aromatic	970.89	E854.3	E940.8	E950.4	E962.0	E980.4
Ammoniated mercury	976.0	E858.7	E946.0	E950.4	E962.0	E980.4
Ammonium						
carbonate	983.2	E864.2	—	E950.7	E962.1	E980.6
chloride (acidifying agent)	963.2	E858.1	E933.2	E950.4	E962.0	E980.4
expectorant	975.5	E858.6	E945.5	E950.4	E962.0	E980.4
compounds (household) NEC	983.2	E861.4	—	E950.7	E962.1	E980.6
fumes (any usage)	987.8	E869.8	—	E952.8	E962.2	E982.8
industrial	983.2	E864.2	—	E950.7	E962.1	E980.6
ichthyosulfonate	976.4	E858.7	E946.4	E950.4	E962.0	E980.4
mandelate	961.9	E857	E931.9	E950.4	E962.0	E980.4
Amobarbital	967.0	E851	E937.0	E950.1	E962.0	E980.1
Amodiaquin(e)	961.4	E857	E931.4	E950.4	E962.0	E980.4
Amopyroquin(e)	961.4	E857	E931.4	E950.4	E962.0	E980.4
Amphenidone	969.5	E853.8	E939.5	E950.3	E962.0	E980.3
Amphetamine	969.72	E854.2	E939.7	E950.3	E962.0	E980.3
Amphomycin	960.8	E856	E930.8	E950.4	E962.0	E980.4
Amphotericin B	960.1	E856	E930.1	E950.4	E962.0	E980.4
topical	976.0	E858.7	E946.0	E950.4	E962.0	E980.4
Ampicillin	960.0	E856	E930.0	E950.4	E962.0	E980.4
Amprotropine	971.1	E855.4	E941.1	E950.4	E962.0	E980.4
Amygdalin	977.8	E858.8	E947.8	E950.4	E962.0	E980.4
Amyl						
acetate (vapor)	982.8	E862.4	—	E950.9	E962.1	E980.9
alcohol	980.3	E860.4	—	E950.9	E962.1	E980.9
nitrite (medicinal)	972.4	E858.3	E942.4	E950.4	E962.0	E980.4
Amylase (alpha)	963.4	E858.1	E933.4	E950.4	E962.0	E980.4
Amylene hydrate	980.8	E860.8	—	E950.9	E962.1	E980.9
Amylobarbitone	967.0	E851	E937.0	E950.1	E962.0	E980.1
Amylocaine	968.9	E855.2	E938.9	E950.4	E962.0	E980.4
infiltration (subcutaneous)	968.5	E855.2	E938.5	E950.4	E962.0	E980.4
nerve block (peripheral) (plexus)	968.6	E855.2	E938.6	E950.4	E962.0	E980.4
spinal	968.7	E855.2	E938.7	E950.4	E962.0	E980.4
topical (surface)	968.5	E855.2	E938.5	E950.4	E962.0	E980.4
Amytal (sodium)	967.0	E851	E937.0	E950.1	E962.0	E980.1
Analeptics	970.0	E854.3	E940.0	E950.4	E962.0	E980.4
Analgesics	965.9	E850.9	E935.9	E950.0	E962.0	E980.0
aromatic NEC	965.4	E850.4	E935.4	E950.0	E962.0	E980.0
non-narcotic NEC	965.7	E850.7	E935.7	E950.0	E962.0	E980.0
specified NEC	965.8	E850.8	E935.8	E950.0	E962.0	E980.0
Anamirta cocculus	988.2	E865.3	—	E950.9	E962.1	E980.9
Ancillin	960.0	E856	E930.0	E950.4	E962.0	E980.4
Androgens (anabolic congeners)	962.1	E858.0	E932.1	E950.4	E962.0	E980.4
Androstalone	962.1	E858.0	E932.1	E950.4	E962.0	E980.4
Androsterone	962.1	E858.0	E932.1	E950.4	E962.0	E980.4
Anemone pulsatilla	988.2	E865.4	—	E950.9	E962.1	E980.9
Anesthesia, anesthetic (general) NEC	968.4	E855.1	E938.4	E950.4	E962.0	E980.4
block (nerve) (plexus)	968.6	E855.2	E938.6	E950.4	E962.0	E980.4
gaseous NEC	968.2	E855.1	E938.2	E950.4	E962.0	E980.4
halogenated hydrocarbon derivatives NEC	968.2	E855.1	E938.2	E950.4	E962.0	E980.4
infiltration (intradermal) (subcutaneous) (submucosal)	968.5	E855.2	E938.5	E950.4	E962.0	E980.4
intravenous	968.3	E855.1	E938.3	E950.4	E962.0	E980.4
local NEC	968.9	E855.2	E938.9	E950.4	E962.0	E980.4
nerve blocking (peripheral) (plexus)	968.6	E855.2	E938.6	E950.4	E962.0	E980.4
rectal NEC	968.3	E855.1	E938.3	E950.4	E962.0	E980.4
spinal	968.7	E855.2	E938.7	E950.4	E962.0	E980.4
surface	968.5	E855.2	E938.5	E950.4	E962.0	E980.4
topical	968.5	E855.2	E938.5	E950.4	E962.0	E980.4
Aneurine	963.5	E858.1	E933.5	E950.4	E962.0	E980.4
Anginine — see Glyceryl trinitrate						
Angio-Conray	977.8	E858.8	E947.8	E950.4	E962.0	E980.4
Angiotensin	971.2	E855.5	E941.2	E950.4	E962.0	E980.4
Anhydrohydroxyprogesterone	962.2	E858.0	E932.2	E950.4	E962.0	E980.4
Anhydron	974.3	E858.5	E944.3	E950.4	E962.0	E980.4
Anileridine	965.09	E850.2	E935.2	E950.0	E962.0	E980.0

▽ Subterms under main terms may continue to next column or page

Substance	Poisoning	Accident	Therapeutic Use	Suicide Attempt	Assault	Undetermined
Aniline (dye) (liquid)	983.0	E864.0	—	E950.7	E962.1	E980.6
analgesic	965.4	E850.4	E935.4	E950.0	E962.0	E980.0
derivatives, therapeutic NEC	965.4	E850.4	E935.4	E950.0	E962.0	E980.0
vapor	987.8	E869.8	—	E952.8	E962.2	E982.8
Aniscorpine	971.1	E855.4	E941.1	E950.4	E962.0	E980.4
Anisindione	964.2	E858.2	E934.2	E950.4	E962.0	E980.4
Anorexic agents	977.0	E858.8	E947.0	E950.4	E962.0	E980.4
Ant (bite) (sting)	—	E905.5	—	E950.9	E962.1	E980.9
Antabuse	977.3	E858.8	E947.3	E950.4	E962.0	E980.4
Antacids	973.0	E858.4	E943.0	E950.4	E962.0	E980.4
Antazoline	963.0	E858.1	E933.0	E950.4	E962.0	E980.4
Anthralin	976.4	E858.7	E946.4	E950.4	E962.0	E980.4
Anthramycin	960.7	E856	E930.7	E950.4	E962.0	E980.4
Antiadrenergics	971.3	E855.6	E941.3	E950.4	E962.0	E980.4
Antiallergic agents	963.0	E858.1	E933.0	E950.4	E962.0	E980.4
Antianemic agents NEC	964.1	E858.2	E934.1	E950.4	E962.0	E980.4
Antiaris toxicaria	988.2	E865.4	—	E950.9	E962.1	E980.9
Antiarteriosclerotic agents	972.2	E858.3	E942.2	E950.4	E962.0	E980.4
Antiasthmatics	975.7	E858.6	E945.7	E950.4	E962.0	E980.4
Antibiotics	960.9	E856	E930.9	E950.4	E962.0	E980.4
antifungal	960.1	E856	E930.1	E950.4	E962.0	E980.4
antimycobacterial	960.6	E856	E930.6	E950.4	E962.0	E980.4
antineoplastic	960.7	E856	E930.7	E950.4	E962.0	E980.4
cephalosporin (group)	960.5	E856	E930.5	E950.4	E962.0	E980.4
chloramphenicol (group)	960.2	E856	E930.2	E950.4	E962.0	E980.4
macrolides	960.3	E856	E930.3	E950.4	E962.0	E980.4
specified NEC	960.8	E856	E930.8	E950.4	E962.0	E980.4
tetracycline (group)	960.4	E856	E930.4	E950.4	E962.0	E980.4
Anticancer agents NEC	963.1	E858.1	E933.1	E950.4	E962.0	E980.4
antibiotics	960.7	E856	E930.7	E950.4	E962.0	E980.4
Anticholinergics	971.1	E855.4	E941.1	E950.4	E962.0	E980.4
Anticholinesterase (organophosphorus) (reversible)	971.0	E855.3	E941.0	E950.4	E962.0	E980.4
Anticoagulants	964.2	E858.2	E934.2	E950.4	E962.0	E980.4
antagonists	964.5	E858.2	E934.5	E950.4	E962.0	E980.4
Anti-common cold agents NEC	975.6	E858.6	E945.6	E950.4	E962.0	E980.4
Anticonvulsants NEC	966.3	E855.0	E936.3	E950.4	E962.0	E980.4
Antidepressants	969.00	E854.0	E939.0	E950.3	E962.0	E980.3
monoamine oxidase inhibitors (MAOI)	969.01	E854.0	E939.0	E950.3	E962.0	E980.3
specified type NEC	969.09	E854.0	E939.0	E950.3	E962.0	E980.3
SSNRI (selective serotonin and norepinephrine reuptake inhibitors)	969.02	E854.0	E939.0	E950.3	E962.0	E980.3
SSRI (selective serotonin reuptake inhibitors)	969.03	E854.0	E939.0	E950.3	E962.0	E980.3
tetracyclic	969.04	E854.0	E939.0	E950.3	E962.0	E980.3
tricyclic	969.05	E854.0	E939.0	E950.3	E962.0	E980.3
Antidiabetic agents	962.3	E858.0	E932.3	E950.4	E962.0	E980.4
Antidiarrheal agents	973.5	E858.4	E943.5	E950.4	E962.0	E980.4
Antidiuretic hormone	962.5	E858.0	E932.5	E950.4	E962.0	E980.4
Antidotes NEC	977.2	E858.8	E947.2	E950.4	E962.0	E980.4
Antiemetic agents	963.0	E858.1	E933.0	E950.4	E962.0	E980.4
Antiepilepsy agent NEC	966.3	E855.0	E936.3	E950.4	E962.0	E980.4
Antifertility pills	962.2	E858.0	E932.2	E950.4	E962.0	E980.4
Antiflatulents	973.8	E858.4	E943.8	E950.4	E962.0	E980.4
Antifreeze	989.89	E866.8	—	E950.9	E962.1	E980.9
alcohol	980.1	E860.2	—	E950.9	E962.1	E980.9
ethylene glycol	982.8	E862.4	—	E950.9	E962.1	E980.9
Antifungals (nonmedicinal) (sprays)	989.4	E863.6	—	E950.6	E962.1	E980.7
medicinal NEC	961.9	E857	E931.9	E950.4	E962.0	E980.4
antibiotic	960.1	E856	E930.1	E950.4	E962.0	E980.4
topical	976.0	E858.7	E946.0	E950.4	E962.0	E980.4
Antigastric secretion agents	973.0	E858.4	E943.0	E950.4	E962.0	E980.4
Antihelmintics	961.6	E857	E931.6	E950.4	E962.0	E980.4
Antihemophilic factor (human)	964.7	E858.2	E934.7	E950.4	E962.0	E980.4
Antihistamine	963.0	E858.1	E933.0	E950.4	E962.0	E980.4
Antihypertensive agents NEC	972.6	E858.3	E942.6	E950.4	E962.0	E980.4
Anti-infectives NEC	961.9	E857	E931.9	E950.4	E962.0	E980.4
antibiotics	960.9	E856	E930.9	E950.4	E962.0	E980.4
specified NEC	960.8	E856	E930.8	E950.4	E962.0	E980.4
antihelmintic	961.6	E857	E931.6	E950.4	E962.0	E980.4
antimalarial	961.4	E857	E931.4	E950.4	E962.0	E980.4
antimycobacterial NEC	961.8	E857	E931.8	E950.4	E962.0	E980.4

Substance	Poisoning	Accident	Therapeutic Use	Suicide Attempt	Assault	Undetermined
Anti-infectives — continued						
antimycobacterial — continued						
antibiotics	960.6	E856	E930.6	E950.4	E962.0	E980.4
antiprotozoal NEC	961.5	E857	E931.5	E950.4	E962.0	—
blood	961.4	E857	E931.4	E950.4	E962.0	E980.4
antiviral	961.7	E857	E931.7	E950.4	E962.0	E980.4
arsenical	961.1	E857	E931.1	E950.4	E962.0	E980.4
ENT agents	976.6	E858.7	E946.6	E950.4	E962.0	E980.4
heavy metals NEC	961.2	E857	E931.2	E950.4	E962.0	E980.4
local	976.0	E858.7	E946.0	E950.4	E962.0	E980.4
ophthalmic preparation	976.5	E858.7	E946.5	E950.4	E962.0	E980.4
topical NEC	976.0	E858.7	E946.0	E950.4	E962.0	E980.4
Anti-inflammatory agents (topical)	976.0	E858.7	E946.0	E950.4	E962.0	E980.4
Antiknock (tetraethyl lead)	984.1	E862.1	—	E950.9	—	E980.9
Antilipemics	972.2	E858.3	E942.2	E950.4	E962.0	E980.4
Antimalarials	961.4	E857	E931.4	E950.4	E962.0	E980.4
Antimony (compounds) (vapor) NEC	985.4	E866.2	—	E950.9	E962.1	E980.9
anti-infectives	961.2	E857	E931.2	E950.4	E962.0	E980.4
pesticides (vapor)	985.4	E863.4	—	E950.6	E962.2	E980.7
potassium tartrate	961.2	E857	E931.2	E950.4	E962.0	E980.4
tartrated	961.2	E857	E931.2	E950.4	E962.0	E980.4
Antimuscarinic agents	971.1	E855.4	E941.1	E950.4	E962.0	E980.4
Antimycobacterials NEC	961.8	E857	E931.8	E950.4	E962.0	E980.4
antibiotics	960.6	E856	E930.6	E950.4	E962.0	E980.4
Antineoplastic agents	963.1	E858.1	E933.1	E950.4	E962.0	E980.4
antibiotics	960.7	E856	E930.7	E950.4	E962.0	E980.4
Anti-Parkinsonism agents	966.4	E855.0	E936.4	E950.4	E962.0	E980.4
Antiphlogistics	965.69	E850.6	E935.6	E950.0	E962.0	E980.0
Antiprotozoals NEC	961.5	E857	E931.5	E950.4	E962.0	E980.4
blood	961.4	E857	E931.4	E950.4	E962.0	E980.4
Antipruritics (local)	976.1	E858.7	E946.1	E950.4	E962.0	E980.4
Antipsychotic agents NEC	969.3	E853.8	E939.3	E950.3	E962.0	E980.3
Antipyretics	965.9	E850.9	E935.9	E950.0	E962.0	E980.0
specified NEC	965.8	E850.8	E935.8	E950.0	E962.0	E980.0
Antipyrine	965.5	E850.5	E935.5	E950.0	E962.0	E980.0
Antirabies serum (equine)	979.9	E858.8	E949.9	E950.4	E962.0	E980.4
Antirheumatics	965.69	E850.6	E935.6	E950.0	E962.0	E980.0
Antiseborrheics	976.4	E858.7	E946.4	E950.4	E962.0	E980.4
Antiseptics (external) (medicinal)	976.0	E858.7	E946.0	E950.4	E962.0	E980.4
Antistine	963.0	E858.1	E933.0	E950.4	E962.0	E980.4
Antithyroid agents	962.8	E858.0	E932.8	E950.4	E962.0	E980.4
Antitoxin, any	979.9	E858.8	E949.9	E950.4	E962.0	E980.4
Antituberculars	961.8	E857	E931.8	E950.4	E962.0	E980.4
antibiotics	960.6	E856	E930.6	E950.4	E962.0	E980.4
Antitussives	975.4	E858.6	E945.4	E950.4	E962.0	E980.4
Antivaricose agents (sclerosing)	972.7	E858.3	E942.7	E950.4	E962.0	E980.4
Antivenin (crotaline) (spider-bite)	979.9	E858.8	E949.9	E950.4	E962.0	E980.4
Antivert	963.0	E858.1	E933.0	E950.4	E962.0	E980.4
Antivirals NEC	961.7	E857	E931.7	E950.4	E962.0	E980.4
Ant poisons — see Pesticides						
Antrol	989.4	E863.4	—	E950.6	E962.1	E980.7
fungicide	989.4	E863.6	—	E950.6	E962.1	E980.7
Apomorphine hydrochloride (emetic)	973.6	E858.4	E943.6	E950.4	E962.0	E980.4
Appetite depressants, central	977.0	E858.8	E947.0	E950.4	E962.0	E980.4
Apresoline	972.6	E858.3	E942.6	E950.4	E962.0	E980.4
Aprobarbital, aprobarbitone	967.0	E851	E937.0	E950.1	E962.0	E980.1
Apronalide	967.8	E852.8	E937.8	E950.2	E962.0	E980.2
Aqua fortis	983.1	E864.1	—	E950.7	E962.1	E980.6
Arachis oil (topical)	976.3	E858.7	E946.3	E950.4	E962.0	E980.4
cathartic	973.2	E858.4	E943.2	E950.4	E962.0	E980.4
Aralen	961.4	E857	E931.4	E950.4	E962.0	E980.4
Arginine salts	974.5	E858.5	E944.5	E950.4	E962.0	E980.4
Argyrol	976.0	E858.7	E946.0	E950.4	E962.0	E980.4
ENT agent	976.6	E858.7	E946.6	E950.4	E962.0	E980.4
ophthalmic preparation	976.5	E858.7	E946.5	E950.4	E962.0	E980.4
Aristocort	962.0	E858.0	E932.0	E950.4	E962.0	E980.4
ENT agent	976.6	E858.7	E946.6	E950.4	E962.0	E980.4
ophthalmic preparation	976.5	E858.7	E946.5	E950.4	E962.0	E980.4
topical NEC	976.0	E858.7	E946.0	E950.4	E962.0	E980.4

External Cause (E-Code)

Substance	Poisoning	Accident	Therapeutic Use	Suicide Attempt	Assault	Undetermined
Aromatics, corrosive	983.0	E864.0	—	E950.7	E962.1	E980.6
disinfectants	983.0	E861.4	—	E950.7	E962.1	E980.6
Arsenate of lead (insecticide)	985.1	E863.4	—	E950.8	E962.1	E980.8
herbicide	985.1	E863.5	—	E950.8	E962.1	E980.8
Arsenic, arsenicals (compounds) (dust) (fumes) (vapor) NEC	985.1	E866.3	—	E950.8	E962.1	E980.8
anti-infectives	961.1	E857	E931.1	E950.4	E962.0	E980.4
pesticide (dust) (fumes)	985.1	E863.4	—	E950.8	E962.1	E980.8
Arsine (gas)	985.1	E866.3	—	E950.8	E962.1	E980.8
Arsphenamine (silver)	961.1	E857	E931.1	E950.4	E962.0	E980.4
Arsthinol	961.1	E857	E931.1	E950.4	E962.0	E980.4
Artane	971.1	E855.4	E941.1	E950.4	E962.0	E980.4
Arthropod (venomous) NEC	989.5	E905.5	—	E950.9	E962.1	E980.9
Asbestos	989.81	E866.8	—	E950.9	E962.1	E980.9
Ascaridole	961.6	E857	E931.6	E950.4	E962.0	E980.4
Ascorbic acid	963.5	E858.1	E933.5	E950.4	E962.0	E980.4
Asiaticoside	976.0	E858.7	E946.0	E950.4	E962.0	E980.4
Aspidium (oleoresin)	961.6	E857	E931.6	E950.4	E962.0	E980.4
Aspirin	965.1	E850.3	E935.3	E950.0	E962.0	E980.0
Astringents (local)	976.2	E858.7	E946.2	E950.4	E962.0	E980.4
Atabrine	961.3	E857	E931.3	E950.4	E962.0	E980.4
Ataractics	969.5	E853.8	E939.5	E950.3	E962.0	E980.3
Atonia drug, intestinal	973.3	E858.4	E943.3	E950.4	E962.0	E980.4
Atophan	974.7	E858.5	E944.7	E950.4	E962.0	E980.4
Atropine	971.1	E855.4	E941.1	E950.4	E962.0	E980.4
Attapulgite	973.5	E858.4	E943.5	E950.4	E962.0	E980.4
Attenuvax	979.4	E858.8	E949.4	E950.4	E962.0	E980.4
Aureomycin	960.4	E856	E930.4	E950.4	E962.0	E980.4
ophthalmic preparation	976.5	E858.7	E946.5	E950.4	E962.0	E980.4
topical NEC	976.0	E858.7	E946.0	E950.4	E962.0	E980.4
Aurothioglucose	965.69	E850.6	E935.6	E950.0	E962.0	E980.0
Aurothioglycanide	965.69	E850.6	E935.6	E950.0	E962.0	E980.0
Aurothiomalate	965.69	E850.6	E935.6	E950.0	E962.0	E980.0
Automobile fuel	981	E862.1	—	E950.9	E962.1	E980.9
Autonomic nervous system agents NEC	971.9	E855.9	E941.9	E950.4	E962.0	E980.4
Avlosulfon	961.8	E857	E931.8	E950.4	E962.0	E980.4
Avomine	967.8	E852.8	E937.8	E950.2	E962.0	E980.2
Azacyclonol	969.5	E853.8	E939.5	E950.3	E962.0	E980.3
Azapetine	971.3	E855.6	E941.3	E950.4	E962.0	E980.4
Azaribine	963.1	E858.1	E933.1	E950.4	E962.0	E980.4
Azaserine	960.7	E856	E930.7	E950.4	E962.0	E980.4
Azathioprine	963.1	E858.1	E933.1	E950.4	E962.0	E980.4
Azosulfamide	961.0	E857	E931.0	E950.4	E962.0	E980.4
Azulfidine	961.0	E857	E931.0	E950.4	E962.0	E980.4
Azuresin	977.8	E858.8	E947.8	E950.4	E962.0	E980.4
Bacimycin	976.0	E858.7	E946.0	E950.4	E962.0	E980.4
ophthalmic preparation	976.5	E858.7	E946.5	E950.4	E962.0	E980.4
Bacitracin	960.8	E856	E930.8	E950.4	E962.0	E980.4
ENT agent	976.6	E858.7	E946.6	E950.4	E962.0	E980.4
ophthalmic preparation	976.5	E858.7	E946.5	E950.4	E962.0	E980.4
topical NEC	976.0	E858.7	E946.0	E950.4	E962.0	E980.4
Baking soda	963.3	E858.1	E933.3	E950.4	E962.0	E980.4
BAL	963.8	E858.1	E933.8	E950.4	E962.0	E980.4
Bamethan (sulfate)	972.5	E858.3	E942.5	E950.4	E962.0	E980.4
Bamipine	963.0	E858.1	E933.0	E950.4	E962.0	E980.4
Baneberry	988.2	E865.4	—	E950.9	E962.1	E980.9
Banewort	988.2	E865.4	—	E950.9	E962.1	E980.9
Barbenyl	967.0	E851	E937.0	E950.1	E962.0	E980.1
Barbital, barbitone	967.0	E851	E937.0	E950.1	E962.0	E980.1
Barbiturates, barbituric acid	967.0	E851	E937.0	E950.1	E962.0	E980.1
anesthetic (intravenous)	968.3	E855.1	E938.3	E950.4	E962.0	E980.4
Barium (carbonate) (chloride) (sulfate)	985.8	E866.4	—	E950.9	E962.1	E980.9
diagnostic agent	977.8	E858.8	E947.8	E950.4	E962.0	E980.4
pesticide	985.8	E863.4	—	E950.6	E962.1	E980.7
rodenticide	985.8	E863.7	—	E950.6	E962.1	E980.7
Barrier cream	976.3	E858.7	E946.3	E950.4	E962.0	E980.4
Battery acid or fluid	983.1	E864.1	—	E950.7	E962.1	E980.6
Bay rum	980.8	E860.8	—	E950.9	E962.1	E980.9
BCG vaccine	978.0	E858.8	E948.0	E950.4	E962.0	E980.4
Bearsfoot	988.2	E865.4	—	E950.9	E962.1	E980.9
Beclamide	966.3	E855.0	E936.3	E950.4	E962.0	E980.4
Bee (sting) (venom)	989.5	E905.3	—	E950.9	E962.1	E980.9
Belladonna (alkaloids)	971.1	E855.4	E941.1	E950.4	E962.0	E980.4
Bemegride	970.0	E854.3	E940.0	E950.4	E962.0	E980.4
Benactyzine	969.8	E855.8	E939.8	E950.3	E962.0	E980.3
Benadryl	963.0	E858.1	E933.0	E950.4	E962.0	E980.4
Bendrofluazide	974.3	E858.5	E944.3	E950.4	E962.0	E980.4
Bendroflumethiazide	974.3	E858.5	E944.3	E950.4	E962.0	E980.4
Benemid	974.7	E858.5	E944.7	E950.4	E962.0	E980.4
Benethamine penicillin G	960.0	E856	E930.0	E950.4	E962.0	E980.4
Benisone	976.0	E858.7	E946.0	E950.4	E962.0	E980.4
Benoquin	976.8	E858.7	E946.8	E950.4	E962.0	E980.4
Benoxinate	968.5	E855.2	E938.5	E950.4	E962.0	E980.4
Bentonite	976.3	E858.7	E946.3	E950.4	E962.0	E980.4
Benzalkonium (chloride)	976.0	E858.7	E946.0	E950.4	E962.0	E980.4
ophthalmic preparation	976.5	E858.7	E946.5	E950.4	E962.0	E980.4
Benzamidosalicylate (calcium)	961.8	E857	E931.8	E950.4	E962.0	E980.4
Benzathine penicillin	960.0	E856	E930.0	E950.4	E962.0	E980.4
Benzcarbimine	963.1	E858.1	E933.1	E950.4	E962.0	E980.4
Benzedrex	971.2	E855.5	E941.2	E950.4	E962.0	E980.4
Benzedrine (amphetamine)	969.72	E854.2	E939.7	E950.3	E962.0	E980.3
Benzene (acetyl) (dimethyl) (methyl) (solvent) (vapor)	982.0	E862.4	—	E950.9	E962.1	E980.9
hexachloride (gamma) (insecticide) (vapor)	989.2	E863.0	—	E950.6	E962.1	E980.7
Benzethonium	976.0	E858.7	E946.0	E950.4	E962.0	E980.4
Benzhexol (chloride)	966.4	E855.0	E936.4	E950.4	E962.0	E980.4
Benzilonium	971.1	E855.4	E941.1	E950.4	E962.0	E980.4
Benzin(e) — see Ligroin						
Benziodarone	972.4	E858.3	E942.4	E950.4	E962.0	E980.4
Benzocaine	968.5	E855.2	E938.5	E950.4	E962.0	E980.4
Benzodiapin	969.4	E853.2	E939.4	E950.3	E962.0	E980.3
Benzodiazepines (tranquilizers) NEC	969.4	E853.2	E939.4	E950.3	E962.0	E980.3
Benzoic acid (with salicylic acid) (anti-infective)	976.0	E858.7	E946.0	E950.4	E962.0	E980.4
Benzoin	976.3	E858.7	E946.3	E950.4	E962.0	E980.4
Benzol (vapor)	982.0	E862.4	—	E950.9	E962.1	E980.9
Benzomorphan	965.09	E850.2	E935.2	E950.0	E962.0	E980.0
Benzonatate	975.4	E858.6	E945.4	E950.4	E962.0	E980.4
Benzothiadiazides	974.3	E858.5	E944.3	E950.4	E962.0	E980.4
Benzoylpas	961.8	E857	E931.8	E950.4	E962.0	E980.4
Benzperidol	969.5	E853.8	E939.5	E950.3	E962.0	E980.3
Benzphetamine	977.0	E858.8	E947.0	E950.4	E962.0	E980.4
Benzpyrinium	971.0	E855.3	E941.0	E950.4	E962.0	E980.4
Benzquinamide	963.0	E858.1	E933.0	E950.4	E962.0	E980.4
Benzthiazide	974.3	E858.5	E944.3	E950.4	E962.0	E980.4
Benztropine	971.1	E855.4	E941.1	E950.4	E962.0	E980.4
Benzyl acetate	982.8	E862.4	—	E950.9	E962.1	E980.9
benzoate (anti-infective)	976.0	E858.7	E946.0	E950.4	E962.0	E980.4
morphine	965.09	E850.2	E935.2	E950.0	E962.0	E980.0
penicillin	960.0	E856	E930.0	E950.4	E962.0	E980.4
Bephenium hydroxynapthoate	961.6	E857	E931.6	E950.4	E962.0	E980.4
Bergamot oil	989.89	E866.8	—	E950.9	E962.1	E980.9
Berries, poisonous	988.2	E865.3	—	E950.9	E962.1	E980.9
Beryllium (compounds) (fumes)	985.3	E866.4	—	E950.9	E962.1	E980.9
Beta-carotene	976.3	E858.7	E946.3	E950.4	E962.0	E980.4
Beta-Chlor	967.1	E852.0	E937.1	E950.2	E962.0	E980.2
Betamethasone	962.0	E858.0	E932.0	E950.4	E962.0	E980.4
topical	976.0	E858.7	E946.0	E950.4	E962.0	E980.4
Betazole	977.8	E858.8	E947.8	E950.4	E962.0	E980.4
Bethanechol	971.0	E855.3	E941.0	E950.4	E962.0	E980.4
Bethanidine	972.6	E858.3	E942.6	E950.4	E962.0	E980.4
Betula oil	976.3	E858.7	E946.3	E950.4	E962.0	E980.4
Bhang	969.6	E854.1	E939.6	E950.3	E962.0	E980.3
Bialamicol	961.5	E857	E931.5	E950.4	E962.0	E980.4
Bichloride of mercury — see Mercury, chloride						
Bichromates (calcium) (crystals) (potassium) (sodium)	983.9	E864.3	—	E950.7	E962.1	E980.6
fumes	987.8	E869.8	—	E952.8	E962.2	E982.8
Biguanide derivatives, oral	962.3	E858.0	E932.3	E950.4	E962.0	E980.4
Biligrafin	977.8	E858.8	E947.8	E950.4	E962.0	E980.4
Bilopaque	977.8	E858.8	E947.8	E950.4	E962.0	E980.4
Bioflavonoids	972.8	E858.3	E942.8	E950.4	E962.0	E980.4
Biological substance NEC	979.9	E858.8	E949.9	E950.4	E962.0	E980.4
Biperiden	966.4	E855.0	E936.4	E950.4	E962.0	E980.4
Bisacodyl	973.1	E858.4	E943.1	E950.4	E962.0	E980.4
Bishydroxycoumarin	964.2	E858.2	E934.2	E950.4	E962.0	E980.4

	Poisoning	Accident	Therapeutic Use	Suicide Attempt	Assault	Undetermined
Bismarsen	961.1	E857	E931.1	E950.4	E962.0	E980.4
Bismuth (compounds)						
NEC	985.8	E866.4	—	E950.9	E962.1	E980.9
anti-infectives	961.2	E857	E931.2	E950.4	E962.0	E980.4
subcarbonate	973.5	E858.4	E943.5	E950.4	E962.0	E980.4
sulfarsphenamine	961.1	E857	E931.1	E950.4	E962.0	E980.4
Bisphosphonates						
intravenous	963.1	E858.1	E933.7	E950.4	E962.0	E980.4
oral	963.1	E858.1	E933.6	E950.4	E962.0	E980.4
Bithionol	961.6	E857	E931.6	E950.4	E962.0	E980.4
Bitter almond oil	989.0	E866.8	—	E950.9	E962.1	E980.9
Bittersweet	988.2	E865.4	—	E950.9	E962.1	E930.9
Black						
flag	989.4	E863.4	—	E950.6	E962.1	E980.7
henbane	988.2	E865.4	—	E950.9	E962.1	E980.9
leaf (40)	989.4	E863.4	—	E950.6	E962.1	E980.7
widow spider (bite)	989.5	E905.1	—	E950.9	E962.1	E980.9
antivenin	979.9	E858.8	E949.9	E950.4	E962.0	E980.4
Blast furnace gas (carbon monoxide from)	986	E868.8	—	E952.1	E962.2	E982.1
Bleach NEC	983.9	E864.3	—	E950.7	E962.1	E980.6
Bleaching solutions	983.9	E864.3	—	E950.7	E962.1	E980.6
Bleomycin (sulfate)	960.7	E856	E930.7	E950.4	E962.0	E980.4
Blockain	968.9	E855.2	E938.9	E950.4	E962.0	E980.4
infiltration (subcutaneous)	968.5	E855.2	E938.5	E950.4	E962.0	E980.4
nerve block (peripheral) (plexus)	968.6	E855.2	E938.6	E950.4	E962.0	E980.4
topical (surface)	968.5	E855.2	E938.5	E950.4	E962.0	E980.4
Blood (derivatives) (natural) (plasma) (whole)	964.7	E858.2	E934.7	E950.4	E962.0	E980.4
affecting agent	964.9	E858.2	E934.9	E950.4	E962.0	E980.4
specified NEC	964.8	E858.2	E934.8	E950.4	E962.0	E980.4
substitute (macromolecular)	964.8	E858.2	E934.8	E950.4	E962.0	E980.4
Blue velvet	965.09	E850.2	E935.2	E950.0	E962.0	E980.0
Bone meal	989.89	E866.5	—	E950.9	E962.1	E980.9
Bonine	963.0	E858.1	E933.0	E950.4	E962.0	E980.4
Boracic acid	976.0	E858.7	E946.0	E950.4	E962.0	E980.4
ENT agent	976.6	E858.7	E946.6	E950.4	E962.0	E980.4
ophthalmic preparation	976.5	E858.7	E946.5	E950.4	E962.0	E980.4
Borate (cleanser) (sodium)	989.6	E861.3	—	E950.9	E962.1	E980.9
Borax (cleanser)	989.6	E861.3	—	E950.9	E962.1	E980.9
Boric acid	976.0	E858.7	E946.0	E950.4	E962.0	E980.4
ENT agent	976.6	E858.7	E946.6	E950.4	E962.0	E980.4
ophthalmic preparation	976.5	E858.7	E946.5	E950.4	E962.0	E980.4
Boron hydride NEC	989.89	E866.8	—	E950.9	E962.1	E980.9
fumes or gas	987.8	E869.8	—	E952.8	E962.2	E982.8
Botox	975.3	E858.6	E945.3	E950.4	E962.0	E980.4
Brake fluid vapor	987.8	E869.8	—	E952.8	E962.2	E982.8
Brass (compounds) (fumes)	985.8	E866.4	—	E950.9	E962.1	E980.9
Brasso	981	E861.3	—	E950.9	E962.1	E980.9
Bretylium (tosylate)	972.6	E858.3	E942.6	E950.4	E962.0	E980.4
Brevital (sodium)	968.3	E855.1	E938.3	E950.4	E962.0	E980.4
British antilewisite	963.8	E858.1	E933.8	E950.4	E962.0	E980.4
Bromal (hydrate)	967.3	E852.2	E937.3	E950.2	E962.0	E980.2
Bromelains	963.4	E858.1	E933.4	E950.4	E962.0	E980.4
Bromides NEC	967.3	E852.2	E937.3	E950.2	E962.0	E980.2
Bromine (vapor)	987.8	E869.8	—	E952.8	E962.2	E982.8
compounds (medicinal)	967.3	E852.2	E937.3	E950.2	E962.0	E980.2
Bromisovalum	967.3	E852.2	E937.3	E950.2	E962.0	E980.2
Bromobenzyl cyanide	987.5	E869.3	—	E952.8	E962.2	E982.8
Bromodiphenhydramine	963.0	E858.1	E933.0	E950.4	E962.0	E980.4
Bromoform	967.3	E852.2	E937.3	E950.2	E962.0	E980.2
Bromophenol blue reagent	977.8	E858.8	E947.8	E950.4	E962.0	E980.4
Bromosalicylhydroxamic acid	961.8	E857	E931.8	E950.4	E962.0	E980.4
Bromo-seltzer	965.4	E850.4	E935.4	E950.0	E962.0	E980.0
Brompheniramine	963.0	E858.1	E933.0	E950.4	E962.0	E980.4
Bromural	967.3	E852.2	E937.3	E950.2	E962.0	E980.2
Brown spider (bite) (venom)	989.5	E905.1	—	E950.9	E962.1	E980.9
Brucia	988.2	E865.3	—	E950.9	E962.1	E980.9
Brucine	989.1	E863.7	—	E950.6	E962.1	E980.7
Brunswick green — *see* Copper						
Bruten — *see* Ibuprofen						
Bryonia (alba) (dioica)	988.2	E865.4	—	E950.9	E962.1	E980.9
Buclizine	969.5	E853.8	E939.5	E950.3	E962.0	E980.3
Bufferin	965.1	E850.3	E935.3	E950.0	E962.0	E980.0
Bufotenine	969.6	E854.1	E939.6	E950.3	E962.0	E980.3
Buphenine	971.2	E855.5	E941.2	E950.4	E962.0	E980.4
Bupivacaine	968.9	E855.2	E938.9	E950.4	E962.0	E980.4
infiltration (subcutaneous)	968.5	E855.2	E938.5	E950.4	E962.0	E980.4
nerve block (peripheral) (plexus)	968.6	E855.2	E938.6	E950.4	E962.0	E980.4
Busulfan	963.1	E858.1	E933.1	E950.4	E962.0	E980.4
Butabarbital (sodium)	967.0	E851	E937.0	E950.1	E962.0	E980.1
Butabarbitone	967.0	E851	E937.0	E950.1	E962.0	E980.1
Butabarpal	967.0	E851	E937.0	E950.1	E962.0	E980.1
Butacaine	968.5	E855.2	E938.5	E950.4	E962.0	E980.4
Butallylonal	967.0	E851	E937.0	E950.1	E962.0	E980.1
Butane (distributed in mobile container)	987.0	E868.0	—	E951.1	E962.2	E981.1
distributed through pipes	987.0	E867	—	E951.0	E962.2	E981.0
incomplete combustion of — see Carbon monoxide, butane						
Butanol	980.3	E860.4	—	E950.9	E962.1	E980.9
Butanone	982.8	E862.4	—	E950.9	E962.1	E980.9
Butaperazine	969.1	E853.0	E939.1	E950.3	E962.0	E980.3
Butazolidin	965.5	E850.5	E935.5	E950.0	E962.0	E980.0
Butethal	967.0	E851	E937.0	E950.1	E962.0	E980.1
Butethamate	971.1	E855.4	E941.1	E950.4	E962.0	E980.4
Buthalitone (sodium)	968.3	E855.1	E938.3	E950.4	E962.0	E980.4
Butisol (sodium)	967.0	E851	E937.0	E950.1	E962.0	E980.1
Butobarbital, butobarbitone	967.0	E851	E937.0	E950.1	E962.0	E980.1
Butriptyline	969.05	E854.0	E939.0	E950.3	E962.0	E980.3
Buttercups	988.2	E865.4	—	E950.9	E962.1	E980.9
Butter of antimony — *see* Antimony						
Butyl						
acetate (secondary)	982.8	E862.4	—	E950.9	E962.1	E980.9
alcohol	980.3	E860.4	—	E950.9	E962.1	E980.9
carbinol	980.8	E860.8	—	E950.9	E962.1	E980.9
carbitol	982.8	E862.4	—	E950.9	E962.1	E980.9
cellosolve	982.8	E862.4	—	E950.9	E962.1	E980.9
chloral (hydrate)	967.1	E852.0	E937.1	E950.2	E962.0	E980.2
formate	982.8	E862.4	—	E950.9	E962.1	E980.9
scopolammonium bromide	971.1	E855.4	E941.1	E950.4	E962.0	E980.4
Butyn	968.5	E855.2	E938.5	E950.4	E962.0	E980.4
Butyrophenone (-based tranquilizers)	969.2	E853.1	E939.2	E950.3	E962.0	E980.3
Cacodyl, cacodylic acid — *see* Arsenic						
Cactinomycin	960.7	E856	E930.7	E950.4	E962.0	E980.4
Cade oil	976.4	E858.7	E946.4	E950.4	E962.0	E980.4
Cadmium (chloride) (compounds) (dust) (fumes) (oxide)	985.5	E866.4	—	E950.9	E962.1	E980.9
sulfide (medicinal) NEC	976.4	E858.7	E946.4	E950.4	E962.0	E980.4
Caffeine	969.71	E854.2	E939.7	E950.3	E962.0	E980.3
Calabar bean	988.2	E865.4	—	E950.9	E962.1	E980.9
Caladium seguinium	988.2	E865.4	—	E950.9	E962.1	E980.9
Calamine (liniment) (lotion)	976.3	E858.7	E946.3	E950.4	E962.0	E980.4
Calciferol	963.5	E858.1	E933.5	E950.4	E962.0	E980.4
Calcium (salts) NEC	974.5	E858.5	E944.5	E950.4	E962.0	E980.4
acetylsalicylate	965.1	E850.3	E935.3	E950.0	E962.0	E980.0
benzamidosalicylate	961.8	E857	E931.8	E950.4	E962.0	E980.4
carbaspirin	965.1	E850.3	E935.3	E950.0	E962.0	E980.0
carbimide (citrated)	977.3	E858.8	E947.3	E950.4	E962.0	E980.4
carbonate (antacid)	973.0	E858.4	E943.0	E950.4	E962.0	E980.4
cyanide (citrated)	977.3	E858.8	E947.3	E950.4	E962.0	E980.4
dioctyl sulfosuccinate	973.2	E858.4	E943.2	E950.4	E962.0	E980.4
disodium edathamil	963.8	E858.1	E933.8	E950.4	E962.0	E980.4
disodium edetate	963.8	E858.1	E933.8	E950.4	E962.0	E980.4
EDTA	963.8	E858.1	E933.8	E950.4	E962.0	E980.4
hydrate, hydroxide	983.2	E864.2	—	E950.7	E962.1	E980.6
mandelate	961.9	E857	E931.9	E950.4	E962.0	E980.4
oxide	983.2	E864.2	—	E950.7	E962.1	E980.6
Calomel — *see* Mercury, chloride						
Caloric agents NEC	974.5	E858.5	E944.5	E950.4	E962.0	E980.4
Calusterone	963.1	E858.1	E933.1	E950.4	E962.0	E980.4
Camoquin	961.4	E857	E931.4	E950.4	E962.0	E980.4
Camphor (oil)	976.1	E858.7	E946.1	E950.4	E962.0	E980.4

	Poisoning	Accident	Therapeutic Use	Suicide Attempt	Assault	Undetermined
Candeptin	976.0	E858.7	E946.0	E950.4	E962.0	E980.4
Candicidin	976.0	E858.7	E946.0	E950.4	E962.0	E980.4
Cannabinols	969.6	E854.1	E939.6	E950.3	E962.0	E980.3
Cannabis (derivatives) (indica) (sativa)	969.6	E854.1	E939.6	E950.3	E962.0	E980.3
Canned heat	980.1	E860.2	—	E950.9	E962.1	E980.9
Cantharides, cantharidin, cantharis	976.8	E858.7	E946.8	E950.4	E962.0	E980.4
Capillary agents	972.8	E858.3	E942.8	E950.4	E962.0	E980.4
Capreomycin	960.6	E856	E930.6	E950.4	E962.0	E980.4
Captodiame, captodi-amine	969.5	E853.8	E939.5	E950.3	E962.0	E980.3
Caramiphen (hydrochloride)	971.1	E855.4	E941.1	E950.4	E962.0	E980.4
Carbachol	971.0	E855.3	E941.0	E950.4	E962.0	E980.4
Carbacrylamine resins	974.5	E858.5	E944.5	E950.4	E962.0	E980.4
Carbamate (sedative)	967.8	E852.8	E937.8	E950.2	E962.0	E980.2
herbicide	989.3	E863.5	—	E950.6	E962.1	E980.7
insecticide	989.3	E863.2	—	E950.6	E962.1	E980.7
Carbamazepine	966.3	E855.0	E936.3	E950.4	E962.0	E980.4
Carbamic esters	967.8	E852.8	E937.8	E950.2	E962.0	E980.2
Carbamide	974.4	E858.5	E944.4	E950.4	E962.0	E980.4
topical	976.8	E858.7	E946.8	E950.4	E962.0	E980.4
Carbamylcholine chloride	971.0	E855.3	E941.0	E950.4	E962.0	E980.4
Carbarsone	961.1	E857	E931.1	E950.4	E962.0	E980.4
Carbaryl	989.3	E863.2	—	E950.6	E962.1	E980.7
Carbaspirin	965.1	E850.3	E935.3	E950.0	E962.0	E980.0
Carbazochrome	972.8	E858.3	E942.8	E950.4	E962.0	E980.4
Carbenicillin	960.0	E856	E930.0	E950.4	E962.0	E980.4
Carbenoxolone	973.8	E858.4	E943.8	E950.4	E962.0	E980.4
Carbetapentane	975.4	E858.6	E945.4	E950.4	E962.0	E980.4
Carbimazole	962.8	E858.0	E932.8	E950.4	E962.0	E980.4
Carbinol	980.1	E860.2	—	E950.9	E962.1	E980.9
Carbinoxamine	963.0	E858.1	E933.0	E950.4	E962.0	E980.4
Carbitol	982.8	E862.4	—	E950.9	E962.1	E980.9
Carbocaine	968.9	E855.2	E938.9	E950.4	E962.0	E980.4
infiltration (subcutaneous)	968.5	E855.2	E938.5	E950.4	E962.0	E980.4
nerve block (peripheral) (plexus)	968.6	E855.2	E938.6	E950.4	E962.0	E980.4
topical (surface)	968.5	E855.2	E938.5	E950.4	E962.0	E980.4
Carbol-fuchsin solution	976.0	E858.7	E946.0	E950.4	E962.0	E980.4
Carbolic acid — *see also* Phenol)	983.0	E864.0	—	E950.7	E962.1	E980.6
Carbomycin	960.8	E856	E930.8	E950.4	E962.0	E980.4
Carbon						
bisulfide (liquid) (vapor)	982.2	E862.4	—	E950.9	E962.1	E980.9
dioxide (gas)	987.8	E869.8	—	E952.8	E962.2	E982.8
disulfide (liquid) (vapor)	982.2	E862.4	—	E950.9	E962.1	E980.9
monoxide (from incomplete combustion of) (in)						
NEC	986	E868.9	—	E952.1	E962.2	E982.1
blast furnace gas	986	E868.8	—	E952.1	E962.2	E982.1
butane (distributed in mobile container)	986	E868.0	—	E951.1	E962.2	E981.1
distributed through pipes	986	E867	—	E951.0	E962.2	E981.0
charcoal fumes	986	E868.3	—	E952.1	E962.2	E982.1
coal						
gas (piped)	986	E867	—	E951.0	E962.2	E981.0
solid (in domestic stoves, fireplaces)	986	E868.3	—	E952.1	E962.2	E982.1
coke (in domestic stoves, fireplaces)	986	E868.3	—	E952.1	E962.2	E982.1
exhaust gas (motor) not in transit	986	E868.2	—	E952.0	E962.2	E982.0
combustion engine, any not in watercraft	986	E868.2	—	E952.0	E962.2	E982.0
farm tractor, not in transit	986	E868.2	—	E952.0	E962.2	E982.0
gas engine	986	E868.2	—	E952.0	E962.2	E982.0
motor pump	986	E868.2	—	E952.0	E962.2	E982.0
motor vehicle, not in transit	986	E868.2	—	E952.0	E962.2	E982.0
fuel (in domestic use)	986	E868.3	—	E952.1	E962.2	E982.1
gas (piped)	986	E867	—	E951.0	E962.2	E981.0
in mobile container	986	E868.0	—	E951.1	E962.2	E981.1
utility	986	E868.1	—	E951.8	E962.2	E981.1
in mobile container	986	E868.0	—	E951.1	E962.2	E981.1
piped (natural)	986	E867	—	E951.0	E962.2	E981.0
illuminating gas	986	E868.1	—	E951.8	E962.2	E981.8

	Poisoning	Accident	Therapeutic Use	Suicide Attempt	Assault	Undetermined
Carbon — *continued*						
monoxide — *continued*						
industrial fuels or gases, any	986	E868.8	—	E952.1	E962.2	E982.1
kerosene (in domestic stoves, fireplaces)	986	E868.3	—	E952.1	E962.2	E982.1
kiln gas or vapor	986	E868.8	—	E952.1	E962.2	E982.1
motor exhaust gas, not in transit	986	E868.2	—	E952.0	E962.2	E982.0
piped gas (manufactured) (natural)	986	E867	—	E951.0	E962.2	E981.0
producer gas	986	E868.8	—	E951.1	E962.2	E981.1
propane (distributed in mobile container)	986	E868.0	—	E951.1	E962.2	E981.1
distributed through pipes	986	E867	—	E951.0	E962.2	E981.0
specified source NEC	986	E868.8	—	E952.1	E962.2	E982.1
stove gas	986	E868.1	—	E951.8	E962.2	E981.8
piped	986	E867	—	E951.0	E962.2	E981.0
utility gas	986	E868.1	—	E951.8	E962.2	E981.8
piped	986	E867	—	E951.0	E962.2	E981.0
water gas	986	E868.1	—	E951.8	E962.2	E981.8
wood (in domestic stoves, fireplaces)	986	E868.3	—	E952.1	E962.2	E982.1
tetrachloride (vapor) NEC	987.8	E869.8	—	E952.8	E962.2	E982.8
liquid (cleansing agent)						
NEC	982.1	E861.3	—	E950.9	E962.1	E980.9
solvent	982.1	E862.4	—	E950.9	E962.1	E980.9
Carbonic acid (gas)	987.8	E869.8	—	E952.8	E962.2	E982.8
anhydrase inhibitors	974.2	E858.5	E944.2	E950.4	E962.0	E980.4
Carbowax	976.3	E858.7	E946.3	E950.4	E962.0	E980.4
Carbrital	967.0	E851	E937.0	E950.1	E962.0	E980.1
Carbromal (derivatives)	967.3	E852.2	E937.3	E950.2	E962.0	E980.2
Cardiac						
depressants	972.0	E858.3	E942.0	E950.4	E962.0	E980.4
rhythm regulators	972.0	E858.3	E942.0	E950.4	E962.0	E980.4
Cardiografin	977.8	E858.8	E947.8	E950.4	E962.0	E980.4
Cardio-green	977.8	E858.8	E947.8	E950.4	E962.0	E980.4
Cardiotonic glycosides	972.1	E858.3	E942.1	E950.4	E962.0	E980.4
Cardiovascular agents						
NEC	972.9	E858.3	E942.9	E950.4	E962.0	E980.4
Cardrase	974.2	E858.5	E944.2	E950.4	E962.0	E980.4
Carfusin	976.0	E858.7	E946.0	E950.4	E962.0	E980.4
Carisoprodol	968.0	E855.3	E938.0	E950.4	E962.0	E980.4
Carmustine	963.1	E858.1	E933.1	E950.4	E962.0	E980.4
Carotene	963.5	E858.1	E933.5	E950.4	E962.0	E980.4
Carphenazine (maleate)	969.1	E853.0	E939.1	E950.3	E962.0	E980.3
Carter's Little Pills	973.1	E858.4	E943.1	E950.4	E962.0	E980.4
Cascara (sagrada)	973.1	E858.4	E943.1	E950.4	E962.0	E980.4
Cassava	988.2	E865.4	—	E950.9	E962.1	E980.9
Castellani's paint	976.0	E858.7	E946.0	E950.4	E962.0	E980.4
Castor						
bean	988.2	E865.3	—	E950.9	E962.1	E980.9
oil	973.1	E858.4	E943.1	E950.4	E962.0	E980.4
Caterpillar (sting)	989.5	E905.5	—	E950.9	E962.1	E980.9
Catha (edulis)	970.89	E854.3	E940.8	E950.4	E962.0	E980.4
Cathartics NEC	973.3	E858.4	E943.3	E950.4	E962.0	E980.4
contact	973.1	E858.4	E943.1	E950.4	E962.0	E980.4
emollient	973.2	E858.4	E943.2	E950.4	E962.0	E980.4
intestinal irritants	973.1	E858.4	E943.1	E950.4	E962.0	E980.4
saline	973.3	E858.4	E943.3	E950.4	E962.0	E980.4
Cathomycin	960.8	E856	E930.8	E950.4	E962.0	E980.4
Caustic(s)	983.9	E864.4	—	E950.7	E962.1	E980.6
alkali	983.2	E864.2	—	E950.7	E962.1	E980.6
hydroxide	983.2	E864.2	—	E950.7	E962.1	E980.6
potash	983.2	E864.2	—	E950.7	E962.1	E980.6
soda	983.2	E864.2	—	E950.7	E962.1	E980.6
specified NEC	983.9	E864.3	—	E950.7	E962.1	E980.6
Ceepryn	976.0	E858.7	E946.0	E950.4	E962.0	E980.4
ENT agent	976.6	E858.7	E946.6	E950.4	E962.0	E980.4
lozenges	976.6	E858.7	E946.6	E950.4	E962.0	E980.4
Celestone	962.0	E858.0	E932.0	E950.4	E962.0	E980.4
topical	976.0	E858.7	E946.0	E950.4	E962.0	E980.4
Cellosolve	982.8	E862.4	—	E950.9	E962.1	E980.9
Cell stimulants and proliferants	976.8	E858.7	E946.8	E950.4	E962.0	E980.4
Cellulose derivatives, cathartic	973.3	E858.4	E943.3	E950.4	E962.0	E980.4
nitrates (topical)	976.3	E858.7	E946.3	E950.4	E962.0	E980.4
Centipede (bite)	989.5	E905.4	—	E950.9	E962.1	E980.9
Central nervous system						
depressants	968.4	E855.1	E938.4	E950.4	E962.0	E980.4

	Poisoning	Accident	Therapeutic Use	Suicide Attempt	Assault	Undetermined
External Cause (E-Code)						
Central nervous system — *continued*						
depressants — *continued*						
anesthetic (general)						
NEC	968.4	E855.1	E938.4	E950.4	E962.0	E980.4
gases NEC	968.2	E855.1	E938.2	E950.4	E962.0	E980.4
intravenous	968.3	E855.1	E938.3	E950.4	E962.0	E980.4
barbiturates	967.0	E851	E937.0	E950.1	E962.0	E980.1
bromides	967.3	E852.2	E937.3	E950.2	E962.0	E980.2
cannabis sativa	969.6	E854.1	E939.6	E950.3	E962.0	E980.3
chloral hydrate	967.1	E852.0	E937.1	E950.2	E962.0	E980.2
hallucinogenics	969.6	E854.1	E939.6	E950.3	E962.0	E980.3
hypnotics	967.9	E852.9	E937.9	E950.2	E962.0	E980.2
specified NEC	967.8	E852.8	E937.8	E950.2	E962.0	E980.2
muscle relaxants	968.0	E855.1	E938.0	E950.4	E962.0	E980.4
paraldehyde	967.2	E852.1	E937.2	E950.2	E962.0	E980.2
sedatives	967.9	E852.9	E937.9	E950.2	E962.0	E980.2
mixed NEC	967.6	E852.5	E937.6	E950.2	E962.0	E980.2
specified NEC	967.8	E852.8	E937.8	E950.2	E962.0	E980.2
muscle-tone depressants	968.0	E855.1	E938.0	E950.4	E962.0	E980.4
stimulants	970.9	E854.3	E940.9	E950.4	E962.0	E980.4
amphetamines	969.72	E854.2	E939.7	E950.3	E962.0	E980.3
analeptics	970.0	E854.3	E940.0	E950.4	E962.0	E980.4
antidepressants	969.00	E854.0	E939.0	E950.3	E962.0	E980.3
opiate antagonists	970.1	E854.3	E940.0	E950.4	E962.0	E980.4
specified NEC	970.89	E854.3	E940.8	E950.4	E962.0	E980.4
Cephalexin	960.5	E856	E930.5	E950.4	E962.0	E980.4
Cephaloglycin	960.5	E856	E930.5	E950.4	E962.0	E980.4
Cephaloridine	960.5	E856	E930.5	E950.4	E962.0	E980.4
Cephalosporins NEC	960.5	E856	E930.5	E950.4	E962.0	E980.4
N (adicillin)	960.0	E856	E930.0	E950.4	E962.0	E980.4
Cephalothin (sodium)	960.5	E856	E930.5	E950.4	E962.0	E980.4
Cerbera (odallam)	988.2	E865.4	—	E950.9	E962.1	E980.9
Cerberin	972.1	E858.3	E942.1	E950.4	E962.0	E980.4
Cerebral stimulants	970.9	E854.3	E940.9	E950.4	E962.0	E980.4
psychotherapeutic	969.79	E854.2	E939.7	E950.3	E962.0	E980.3
specified NEC	970.89	E854.3	E940.8	E950.4	E962.0	E980.4
Cetalkonium (chloride)	976.0	E858.7	E946.0	E950.4	E962.0	E980.4
Cetoxime	963.0	E858.1	E933.0	E950.4	E962.0	E980.4
Cetrimide	976.2	E858.7	E946.2	E950.4	E962.0	E980.4
Cetylpyridinium	976.0	E858.7	E946.0	E950.4	E962.0	E980.4
ENT agent	976.6	E858.7	E946.6	E950.4	E962.0	E980.4
lozenges	976.6	E858.7	E946.6	E950.4	E962.0	E980.4
Cevadilla — *see* Sabadilla						
Cevitamic acid	963.5	E858.1	E933.5	E950.4	E962.0	E980.4
Chalk, precipitated	973.0	E858.4	E943.0	E950.4	E962.0	E980.4
Charcoal						
fumes (carbon monoxide)	986	E868.3	—	E952.1	E962.2	E982.1
industrial	986	E868.8	—	E952.1	E962.2	E982.1
medicinal (activated)	973.0	E858.4	E943.0	E950.4	E962.0	E980.4
Chelating agents NEC	977.2	E858.8	E947.2	E950.4	E962.0	E980.4
Chelidonium majus	988.2	E865.4	—	E950.9	E962.1	E980.9
Chemical substance	989.9	E866.9	—	E950.9	E962.1	E980.9
specified NEC	989.89	E866.8	—	E950.9	E962.1	E980.9
Chemotherapy, antineoplastic	963.1	E858.1	E933.1	E950.4	E962.0	E980.4
Chenopodium (oil)	961.6	E857	E931.6	E950.4	E962.0	E980.4
Cherry laurel	988.2	E865.4	—	E950.9	E962.1	E980.9
Chiniofon	961.3	E857	E931.3	E950.4	E962.0	E980.4
Chlophedianol	975.4	E858.6	E945.4	E950.4	E962.0	E980.4
Chloral (betaine) (formamide) (hydrate)	967.1	E852.0	E937.1	E950.2	E962.0	E980.2
Chloralamide	967.1	E852.0	E937.1	E950.2	E962.0	E980.2
Chlorambucil	963.1	E858.1	E933.1	E950.4	E962.0	E980.4
Chloramphenicol	960.2	E856	E930.2	E950.4	E962.0	E980.4
ENT agent	976.6	E858.7	E946.6	E950.4	E962.0	E980.4
ophthalmic preparation	976.5	E858.7	E946.5	E950.4	E962.0	E980.4
topical NEC	976.0	E858.7	E946.0	E950.4	E962.0	E980.4
Chlorate(s) (potassium) (sodium) NEC	983.9	E864.3	—	E950.7	E962.1	E980.6
herbicides	989.4	E863.5	—	E950.6	E962.1	E980.7
Chlorcyclizine	963.0	E858.1	E933.0	E950.4	E962.0	E980.4
Chlordan(e) (dust)	989.2	E863.0	—	E950.6	E962.1	E980.7
Chlordantoin	976.0	E858.7	E946.0	E950.4	E962.0	E980.4
Chlordiazepoxide	969.4	E853.2	E939.4	E950.3	E962.0	E980.3
Chloresium	976.8	E858.7	E946.8	E950.4	E962.0	E980.4
Chlorethiazol	967.1	E852.0	E937.1	E950.2	E962.0	E980.2
Chlorethyl — *see* Ethyl, chloride						
Chloretone	967.1	E852.0	E937.1	E950.2	E962.0	E980.2
Chlorex	982.3	E862.4	—	E950.9	E962.1	E980.9

	Poisoning	Accident	Therapeutic Use	Suicide Attempt	Assault	Undetermined
External Cause (E-Code)						
Chlorhexadol	967.1	E852.0	E937.1	E950.2	E962.0	E980.2
Chlorhexidine (hydrochloride)	976.0	E858.7	E946.0	E950.4	E962.0	E980.4
Chlorhydroxyquinolin	976.0	E858.7	E946.0	E950.4	E962.0	E980.4
Chloride of lime (bleach)	983.9	E864.3	—	E950.7	E962.1	E980.6
Chlorinated						
camphene	989.2	E863.0	—	E950.6	E962.1	E980.7
diphenyl	989.89	E866.8	—	E950.9	E962.1	E980.9
hydrocarbons NEC	989.2	E863.0	—	E950.6	E962.1	E980.7
solvent	982.3	E862.4	—	E950.9	E962.1	E980.9
lime (bleach)	983.9	E864.3	—	E950.7	E962.1	E980.6
naphthalene — *see* Naphthalene						
pesticides NEC	989.2	E863.0	—	E950.6	E962.1	E980.7
soda — *see* Sodium, hypochlorite						
Chlorine (fumes) (gas)	987.6	E869.8	—	E952.8	E962.2	E982.8
bleach	983.9	E864.3	—	E950.7	E962.1	E980.6
compounds NEC	983.9	E864.3	—	E950.7	E962.1	E980.6
disinfectant	983.9	E861.4	—	E950.7	E962.1	E980.6
releasing agents NEC	983.9	E864.3	—	E950.7	E962.1	E980.6
Chlorisondamine	972.3	E858.3	E942.3	E950.4	E962.0	E980.4
Chlormadinone	962.2	E858.0	E932.2	E950.4	E962.0	E980.4
Chlormerodrin	974.0	E858.5	E944.0	E950.4	E962.0	E980.4
Chlormethiazole	967.1	E852.0	E937.1	E950.2	E962.0	E980.2
Chlormethylenecycline	960.4	E856	E930.4	E950.4	E962.0	E980.4
Chlormezanone	969.5	E853.8	E939.5	E950.3	E962.0	E980.3
Chloroacetophenone	987.5	E869.3	—	E952.8	E962.2	E982.8
Chloroaniline	983.0	E864.0	—	E950.7	E962.1	E980.6
Chlorobenzene, chlorobenzol	982.0	E862.4	—	E950.9	E962.1	E980.9
Chlorobutanol	967.1	E852.0	E937.1	E950.2	E962.0	E980.2
Chlorodinitrobenzene	983.0	E864.0	—	E950.7	E962.1	E980.6
dust or vapor	987.8	E869.8	—	E952.8	E962.2	E982.8
Chloroethane — *see* Ethyl, chloride						
Chloroform (fumes) (vapor)	987.8	E869.8	—	E952.8	E962.2	E982.8
anesthetic (gas)	968.2	E855.1	E938.2	E950.4	E962.0	E980.4
liquid NEC	968.4	E855.1	E938.4	E950.4	E962.0	E980.4
solvent	982.3	E862.4	—	E950.9	E962.1	E980.9
Chloroguanide	961.4	E857	E931.4	E950.4	E962.0	E980.4
Chloromycetin	960.2	E856	E930.2	E950.4	E962.0	E980.4
ENT agent	976.6	E858.7	E946.6	E950.4	E962.0	E980.4
ophthalmic preparation	976.5	E858.7	E946.5	E950.4	E962.0	E980.4
otic solution	976.6	E858.7	E946.6	E950.4	E962.0	E980.4
topical NEC	976.0	E858.7	E946.0	E950.4	E962.0	E980.4
Chloronitrobenzene	983.0	E864.0	—	E950.7	E962.1	E980.6
dust or vapor	987.8	E869.8	—	E952.8	E962.2	E982.8
Chlorophenol	983.0	E864.0	—	E950.7	E962.1	E980.6
Chlorophenothane	989.2	E863.0	—	E950.6	E962.1	E980.7
Chlorophyll (derivatives)	976.8	E858.7	E946.8	E950.4	E962.0	E980.4
Chloropicrin (fumes)	987.8	E869.8	—	E952.8	E962.2	E982.8
fumigant	989.4	E863.8	—	E950.6	E962.1	E980.7
fungicide	989.4	E863.6	—	E950.6	E962.1	E980.7
pesticide (fumes)	989.4	E863.4	—	E950.6	E962.1	E980.7
Chloroprocaine	968.9	E855.2	E938.9	E950.4	E962.0	E980.4
infiltration (subcutaneous)	968.5	E855.2	E938.5	E950.4	E962.0	E980.4
nerve block (peripheral) (plexus)	968.6	E855.2	E938.6	E950.4	E962.0	E980.4
Chloroptic	976.5	E858.7	E946.5	E950.4	E962.0	E980.4
Chloropurine	963.1	E858.1	E933.1	E950.4	E962.0	E980.4
Chloroquine (hydrochloride) (phosphate)	961.4	E857	E931.4	E950.4	E962.0	E980.4
Chlorothen	963.0	E858.1	E933.0	E950.4	E962.0	E980.4
Chlorothiazide	974.3	E858.5	E944.3	E950.4	E962.0	E980.4
Chlorotrianisene	962.2	E858.0	E932.2	E950.4	E962.0	E980.4
Chlorovinyldichloroarsine	985.1	E866.3	—	E950.8	E962.1	E980.8
Chloroxylenol	976.0	E858.7	E946.0	E950.4	E962.0	E980.4
Chlorphenesin (carbamate)	968.0	E855.1	E938.0	E950.4	E962.0	E980.4
topical (antifungal)	976.0	E858.7	E946.0	E950.4	E962.0	E980.4
Chlorpheniramine	963.0	E858.1	E933.0	E950.4	E962.0	E980.4
Chlorphenoxamine	966.4	E855.0	E936.4	E950.4	E962.0	E980.4
Chlorphentermine	977.0	E858.8	E947.0	E950.4	E962.0	E980.4
Chlorproguanil	961.4	E857	E931.4	E950.4	E962.0	E980.4
Chlorpromazine	969.1	E853.0	E939.1	E950.3	E962.0	E980.3
Chlorpropamide	962.3	E858.0	E932.3	E950.4	E962.0	E980.4
Chlorprothixene	969.3	E853.8	E939.3	E950.3	E962.0	E980.3
Chlorquinaldol	976.0	E858.7	E946.0	E950.4	E962.0	E980.4

	Poisoning	Accident	Therapeutic Use	Suicide Attempt	Assault	Undetermined
External Cause (E-Code)						
Chlortetracycline	960.4	E856	E930.4	E950.4	E962.0	E980.4
Chlorthalidone	974.4	E858.5	E944.4	E950.4	E962.0	E980.4
Chlortrianisene	962.2	E858.0	E932.2	E950.4	E962.0	E980.4
Chlor-Trimeton	963.0	E858.1	E933.0	E950.4	E962.0	E980.4
Chlorzoxazone	968.0	E855.1	E938.0	E950.4	E962.0	E980.4
Choke damp	987.8	E869.8	—	E952.8	E962.2	E982.8
Cholebrine	977.8	E858.8	E947.8	E950.4	E962.0	E980.4
Cholera vaccine	978.2	E858.8	E948.2	E950.4	E962.0	E980.4
Cholesterol-lowering agents	972.2	E858.3	E942.2	E950.4	E962.0	E980.4
Cholestyramine (resin)	972.2	E858.3	E942.2	E950.4	E962.0	E980.4
Cholic acid	973.4	E858.4	E943.4	E950.4	E962.0	E980.4
Choline						
dihydrogen citrate	977.1	E858.8	E947.1	E950.4	E962.0	E980.4
salicylate	965.1	E850.3	E935.3	E950.0	E962.0	E980.0
theophyllinate	974.1	E858.5	E944.1	E950.4	E962.0	E980.4
Cholinergics	971.0	E855.3	E941.0	E950.4	E962.0	E980.4
Cholografin	977.8	E858.8	E947.8	E950.4	E962.0	E980.4
Chorionic gonadotropin	962.4	E858.0	E932.4	E950.4	E962.0	E980.4
Chromates	983.9	E864.3	—	E950.7	E962.1	E980.6
dust or mist	987.8	E869.8	—	E952.8	E962.2	E982.8
lead	984.0	E866.0	—	E950.9	E962.1	E980.9
paint	984.0	E861.5	—	E950.9	E962.1	E980.9
Chromic acid	983.9	E864.3	—	E950.7	E962.1	E980.6
dust or mist	987.8	E869.8	—	E952.8	E962.2	E982.8
Chromium	985.6	E866.4	—	E950.9	E962.1	E980.9
compounds — see Chromates						
Chromonar	972.4	E858.3	E942.4	E950.4	E962.0	E980.4
Chromyl chloride	983.9	E864.3	—	E950.7	E962.1	E980.6
Chrysarobin (ointment)	976.4	E858.7	E946.4	E950.4	E962.0	E980.4
Chrysazin	973.1	E858.4	E943.1	E950.4	E962.0	E980.4
Chymar	963.4	E858.1	E933.4	E950.4	E962.0	E980.4
ophthalmic preparation	976.5	E858.7	E946.5	E950.4	E962.0	E980.4
Chymotrypsin	963.4	E858.1	E933.4	E950.4	E962.0	E980.4
ophthalmic preparation	976.5	E858.7	E946.5	E950.4	E962.0	E980.4
Cicuta maculata or virosa	988.2	E865.4	—	E950.9	E962.1	E980.9
Cigarette lighter fluid	981	E862.1	—	E950.9	E962.1	E980.9
Cinchocaine (spinal)	968.7	E855.2	E938.7	E950.4	E962.0	E980.4
topical (surface)	968.5	E855.2	E938.5	E950.4	E962.0	E980.4
Cinchona	961.4	E857	E931.4	E950.4	E962.0	E980.4
Cinchonine alkaloids	961.4	E857	E931.4	E950.4	E962.0	E980.4
Cinchophen	974.7	E858.5	E944.7	E950.4	E962.0	E980.4
Cinnarizine	963.0	E858.1	E933.0	E950.4	E962.0	E980.4
Citanest	968.9	E855.2	E938.9	E950.4	E962.0	E980.4
infiltration (subcutaneous)	968.5	E855.2	E938.5	E950.4	E962.0	E980.4
nerve block (peripheral) (plexus)	968.6	E855.2	E938.6	E950.4	E962.0	E980.4
Citric acid	989.89	E866.8	—	E950.9	E962.1	E980.9
Citrovorum factor	964.1	E858.2	E934.1	E950.4	E962.0	E980.4
Claviceps purpurea	988.2	E865.4	—	E950.9	E962.1	E980.9
Cleaner, cleansing agent, type not specified	989.89	E861.9	—	E950.9	E962.1	E980.9
of paint or varnish	982.8	E862.9	—	E950.9	E962.1	E980.9
specified type NEC	989.89	E861.3	—	E950.9	E962.1	E980.9
Clematis vitalba	988.2	E865.4	—	E950.9	E962.1	E980.9
Clemizole	963.0	E858.1	E933.0	E950.4	E962.0	E980.4
penicillin	960.0	E856	E930.0	E950.4	E962.0	E980.4
Clidinium	971.1	E855.4	E941.1	E950.4	E962.0	E980.4
Clindamycin	960.8	E856	E930.8	E950.4	E962.0	E980.4
Cliradon	965.09	E850.2	E935.2	E950.0	E962.0	E980.0
Clocortolone	962.0	E858.0	E932.0	E950.4	E962.0	E980.4
Clofedanol	975.4	E858.6	E945.4	E950.4	E962.0	E980.4
Clofibrate	972.2	E858.3	E942.2	E950.4	E962.0	E980.4
Clomethiazole	967.1	E852.0	E937.1	E950.2	E962.0	E980.2
Clomiphene	977.8	E858.8	E947.8	E950.4	E962.0	E980.4
Clonazepam	969.4	E853.2	E939.4	E950.3	E962.0	E980.3
Clonidine	972.6	E858.3	E942.6	E950.4	E962.0	E980.4
Clopamide	974.3	E858.5	E944.3	E950.4	E962.0	E980.4
Clorazepate	969.4	E853.2	E939.4	E950.3	E962.0	E980.3
Clorexolone	974.4	E858.5	E944.4	E950.4	E962.0	E980.4
Clorox (bleach)	983.9	E864.3	—	E950.7	E962.1	E980.6
Clortermine	977.0	E858.8	E947.0	E950.4	E962.0	E980.4
Clotrimazole	976.0	E858.7	E946.0	E950.4	E962.0	E980.4
Cloxacillin	960.0	E856	E930.0	E950.4	E962.0	E980.4
Coagulants NEC	964.5	E858.2	E934.5	E950.4	E962.0	E980.4
Coal (carbon monoxide from) — see also Carbon, monoxide, coal						
oil — see Kerosene						

	Poisoning	Accident	Therapeutic Use	Suicide Attempt	Assault	Undetermined
External Cause (E-Code)						
Coal — see also Carbon, monoxide, coal — continued						
tar NEC	983.0	E864.0	—	E950.7	E962.1	E980.6
fumes	987.8	E869.8	—	E952.8	E962.2	E982.8
medicinal (ointment)	976.4	E858.7	E946.4	E950.4	E962.0	E980.4
analgesics NEC	965.5	E850.5	E935.5	E950.0	E962.0	E980.0
naphtha (solvent)	981	E862.0	—	E950.9	E962.1	E980.9
Cobalt (fumes) (industrial)	985.8	E866.4	—	E950.9	E962.1	E980.9
Cobra (venom)	989.5	E905.0	—	E950.9	E962.1	E980.9
Coca (leaf)	970.81	E854.3	E940.8	E950.4	E962.0	E980.4
Cocaine (hydrochloride) (salt)	970.81	E854.3	E940.8	E950.4	E962.0	E980.4
topical anesthetic	968.5	E855.2	E938.5	E950.4	E962.0	E980.4
Coccidioidin	977.8	E858.8	E947.8	E950.4	E962.0	E980.4
Cocculus indicus	988.2	E865.3	—	E950.9	E962.1	E980.9
Cochineal	989.89	E866.8	—	E950.9	E962.1	E980.9
medicinal products	977.4	E858.8	E947.4	E950.4	E962.0	E980.4
Codeine	965.09	E850.2	E935.2	E950.0	E962.0	E980.0
Coffee	989.89	E866.8	—	E950.9	E962.1	E980.9
Cogentin	971.1	E855.4	E941.1	E950.4	E962.0	E980.4
Coke fumes or gas (carbon monoxide)	986	E868.3	—	E952.1	E962.2	E982.1
industrial use	986	E868.8	—	E952.1	E962.2	E982.1
Colace	973.2	E858.4	E943.2	E950.4	E962.0	E980.4
Colchicine	974.7	E858.5	E944.7	E950.4	E962.0	E980.4
Colchicum	988.2	E865.3	—	E950.9	E962.1	E980.9
Cold cream	976.3	E858.7	E946.3	E950.4	E962.0	E980.4
Colestipol	972.2	E858.3	E942.2	E950.4	E962.0	E980.4
Colistimethate	960.8	E856	E930.8	E950.4	E962.0	E980.4
Colistin	960.8	E856	E930.8	E950.4	E962.0	E980.4
Collagen	977.8	E866.8	E947.8	E950.9	E962.1	E980.9
Collagenase	976.8	E858.7	E946.8	E950.4	E962.0	E980.4
Collodion (flexible)	976.3	E858.7	E946.3	E950.4	E962.0	E980.4
Colocynth	973.1	E858.4	E943.1	E950.4	E962.0	E980.4
Coloring matter — see Dye(s)						
Combustion gas — see Carbon, monoxide						
Compazine	969.1	E853.0	E939.1	E950.3	E962.0	E980.3
Compound						
42 (warfarin)	989.4	E863.7	—	E950.6	E962.1	E980.7
269 (endrin)	989.2	E863.0	—	E950.6	E962.1	E980.7
497 (dieldrin)	989.2	E863.0	—	E950.6	E962.1	E980.7
1080 (sodium fluoroacetate)	989.4	E863.7	—	E950.6	E962.1	E980.7
3422 (parathion)	989.3	E863.1	—	E950.6	E962.1	E980.7
3911 (phorate)	989.3	E863.1	—	E950.6	E962.1	E980.7
3956 (toxaphene)	989.2	E863.0	—	E950.6	E962.1	E980.7
4049 (malathion)	989.3	E863.1	—	E950.6	E962.1	E980.7
4124 (dicapthon)	989.4	E863.4	—	E950.6	E962.1	E980.7
E (cortisone)	962.0	E858.0	E932.0	E950.4	E962.0	E980.4
F (hydrocortisone)	962.0	E858.0	E932.0	E950.4	E962.0	E980.4
Congo red	977.8	E858.8	E947.8	E950.4	E962.0	E980.4
Coniine, conine	965.7	E850.7	E935.7	E950.0	E962.0	E980.0
Conium (maculatum)	988.2	E865.4	—	E950.9	E962.1	E980.9
Conjugated estrogens (equine)	962.2	E858.0	E932.2	E950.4	E962.0	E980.4
Contac	975.6	E858.6	E945.6	E950.4	E962.0	E980.4
Contact lens solution	976.5	E858.7	E946.5	E950.4	E962.0	E980.4
Contraceptives (oral)	962.2	E858.0	E932.2	E950.4	E962.0	E980.4
vaginal	976.8	E858.7	E946.8	E950.4	E962.0	E980.4
Contrast media (roentgenographic)	977.8	E858.8	E947.8	E950.4	E962.0	E980.4
Convallaria majalis	988.2	E865.4	—	E950.9	E962.1	E980.9
Copper (dust) (fumes) (salts) NEC	985.8	E866.4	—	E950.9	E962.1	E980.9
arsenate, arsenite	985.1	E866.3	—	E950.8	E962.1	E980.8
insecticide	985.1	E863.4	—	E950.8	E962.1	E980.8
emetic	973.6	E858.4	E943.6	E950.4	E962.0	E980.4
fungicide	985.8	E863.6	—	E950.6	E962.1	E980.7
insecticide	985.8	E863.4	—	E950.6	E962.1	E980.7
oleate	976.0	E858.7	E946.0	E950.4	E962.0	E980.4
sulfate	983.9	E864.3	—	E950.7	E962.1	E980.6
cupric	973.6	E858.4	E943.6	E950.4	E962.0	E980.4
cuprous	983.9	E864.3	—	E950.7	E962.1	E980.6
fungicide	983.9	E863.6	—	E950.7	E962.1	E980.6
Copperhead snake (bite) (venom)	989.5	E905.0	—	E950.9	E962.1	E980.9
Coral (sting)	989.5	E905.6	—	E950.9	E962.1	E980.9
snake (bite) (venom)	989.5	E905.0	—	E950.9	E962.1	E980.9
Cordran	976.0	E858.7	E946.0	E950.4	E962.0	E980.4
Corn cures	976.4	E858.7	E946.4	E950.4	E962.0	E980.4
Cornhusker's lotion	976.3	E858.7	E946.3	E950.4	E962.0	E980.4

	Poisoning	Accident	Therapeutic Use	Suicide Attempt	Assault	Undetermined
External Cause (E-Code)						
Corn starch	976.3	E858.7	E946.3	E950.4	E962.0	E980.4
Corrosive	983.9	E864.4	—	E950.7	E962.1	E980.6
acids NEC	983.1	E864.1	—	E950.7	E962.1	E980.6
aromatics	983.0	E864.0	—	E950.7	E962.1	E980.6
disinfectant	983.0	E861.4	—	E950.7	E962.1	E980.6
fumes NEC	987.9	E869.9	—	E952.9	E962.2	E982.9
specified NEC	983.9	E864.3	—	E950.7	E962.1	E980.6
sublimate — see Mercury, chloride						
Cortate	962.0	E858.0	E932.0	E950.4	E962.0	E980.4
Cort-Dome	962.0	E858.0	E932.0	E950.4	E962.0	E980.4
ENT agent	976.6	E858.7	E946.6	E950.4	E962.0	E980.4
ophthalmic preparation	976.5	E858.7	E946.5	E950.4	E962.0	E980.4
topical NEC	976.0	E858.7	E946.0	E950.4	E962.0	E980.4
Cortef	962.0	E858.0	E932.0	E950.4	E962.0	E980.4
ENT agent	976.6	E858.7	E946.6	E950.4	E962.0	E980.4
ophthalmic preparation	976.5	E858.7	E946.5	E950.4	E962.0	E980.4
topical NEC	976.0	E858.7	E946.0	E950.4	E962.0	E980.4
Corticosteroids (fluorinated)	962.0	E858.0	E932.0	E950.4	E962.0	E980.4
ENT agent	976.6	E858.7	E946.6	E950.4	E962.0	E980.4
ophthalmic preparation	976.5	E858.7	E946.5	E950.4	E962.0	E980.4
topical NEC	976.0	E858.7	E946.0	E950.4	E962.0	E980.4
Corticotropin	962.4	E858.0	E932.4	E950.4	E962.0	E980.4
Cortisol	962.0	E858.0	E932.0	E950.4	E962.0	E980.4
ENT agent	976.6	E858.7	E946.6	E950.4	E962.0	E980.4
ophthalmic preparation	976.5	E858.7	E946.5	E950.4	E962.0	E980.4
topical NEC	976.0	E858.7	E946.0	E950.4	E962.0	E980.4
Cortisone derivatives (acetate)	962.0	E858.0	E932.0	E950.4	E962.0	E980.4
ENT agent	976.6	E858.7	E946.6	E950.4	E962.0	E980.4
ophthalmic preparation	976.5	E858.7	E946.5	E950.4	E962.0	E980.4
topical NEC	976.0	E858.7	E946.0	E950.4	E962.0	E980.4
Cortogen	962.0	E858.0	E932.0	E950.4	E962.0	E980.4
ENT agent	976.6	E858.7	E946.6	E950.4	E962.0	E980.4
ophthalmic preparation	976.5	E858.7	E946.5	E950.4	E962.0	E980.4
Cortone	962.0	E858.0	E932.0	E950.4	E962.0	E980.4
ENT agent	976.6	E858.7	E946.6	E950.4	E962.0	E980.4
ophthalmic preparation	976.5	E858.7	E946.5	E950.4	E962.0	E980.4
Cortril	962.0	E858.0	E932.0	E950.4	E962.0	E980.4
ENT agent	976.6	E858.7	E946.6	E950.4	E962.0	E980.4
ophthalmic preparation	976.5	E858.7	E946.5	E950.4	E962.0	E980.4
topical NEC	976.0	E858.7	E946.0	E950.4	E962.0	E980.4
Cosmetics	989.89	E866.7	—	E950.9	E962.1	E980.9
Cosyntropin	977.8	E858.8	E947.8	E950.4	E962.0	E980.4
Cotarnine	964.5	E858.2	E934.5	E950.4	E962.0	E980.4
Cottonseed oil	976.3	E858.7	E946.3	E950.4	E962.0	E980.4
Cough mixtures (antitussives)	975.4	E858.6	E945.4	E950.4	E962.0	E980.4
containing opiates	965.09	E850.2	E935.2	E950.0	E962.0	E980.0
expectorants	975.5	E858.6	E945.5	E950.4	E962.0	E980.4
Coumadin	964.2	E858.2	E934.2	E950.4	E962.0	E980.4
rodenticide	989.4	E863.7	—	E950.6	E962.1	E980.7
Coumarin	964.2	E858.2	E934.2	E950.4	E962.0	E980.4
Coumetarol	964.2	E858.2	E934.2	E950.4	E962.0	E980.4
Cowbane	988.2	E865.4	—	E950.9	E962.1	E980.9
Cozyme	963.5	E858.1	E933.5	E950.4	E962.0	E980.4
Crack	970.81	E854.3	E940.8	E950.4	E962.0	E980.4
Creolin	983.0	E864.0	—	E950.7	E962.1	E980.6
disinfectant	983.0	E861.4	—	E950.7	E962.1	E980.6
Creosol (compound)	983.0	E864.0	—	E950.7	E962.1	E980.6
Creosote (beechwood) (coal tar)	983.0	E864.0	—	E950.7	E962.1	E980.6
medicinal (expectorant)	975.5	E858.6	E945.5	E950.4	E962.0	E980.4
syrup	975.5	E858.6	E945.5	E950.4	E962.0	E980.4
Cresol	983.0	E864.0	—	E950.7	E962.1	E980.6
disinfectant	983.0	E861.4	—	E950.7	E962.1	E980.6
Cresylic acid	983.0	E864.0	—	E950.7	E962.1	E980.6
Cropropamide	965.7	E850.7	E935.7	E950.0	E962.0	E980.0
with crotethamide	970.0	E854.3	E940.0	E950.4	E962.0	E980.4
Crotamiton	976.0	E858.7	E946.0	E950.4	E962.0	E980.4
Crotethamide	965.7	E850.7	E935.7	E950.0	E962.0	E980.0
with cropropamide	970.0	E854.3	E940.0	E950.4	E962.0	E980.4
Croton (oil)	973.1	E858.4	E943.1	E950.4	E962.0	E980.4
chloral	967.1	E852.0	E937.1	E950.2	E962.0	E980.2
Crude oil	981	E862.1	—	E950.9	E962.1	E980.9
Cryogenine	965.8	E850.8	E935.8	E950.0	E962.0	E980.0
Cryolite (pesticide)	989.4	E863.4	—	E950.6	E962.1	E980.7
Cryptenamine	972.6	E858.3	E942.6	E950.4	E962.0	E980.4
Crystal violet	976.0	E858.7	E946.0	E950.4	E962.0	E980.4
Cuckoopint	988.2	E865.4	—	E950.9	E962.1	E980.9
Cumetharol	964.2	E858.2	E934.2	E950.4	E962.0	E980.4

	Poisoning	Accident	Therapeutic Use	Suicide Attempt	Assault	Undetermined
External Cause (E-Code)						
Cupric sulfate	973.6	E858.4	E943.6	E950.4	E962.0	E980.4
Cuprous sulfate	983.9	E864.3	—	E950.7	E962.1	E980.6
Curare, curarine	975.2	E858.6	E945.2	E950.4	E962.0	E980.4
Cyanic acid — see Cyanide(s)						
Cyanide(s) (compounds) (hydrogen) (potassium) (sodium) NEC	989.0	E866.8	—	E950.9	E962.1	E980.9
dust or gas (inhalation) NEC	987.7	E869.8	—	E952.8	E962.2	E982.8
fumigant	989.0	E863.8	—	E950.6	E962.1	E980.7
mercuric — see Mercury						
pesticide (dust) (fumes)	989.0	E863.4	—	E950.6	E962.1	E980.7
Cyanocobalamin	964.1	E858.2	E934.1	E950.4	E962.0	E980.4
Cyanogen (chloride) (gas) NEC	987.8	E869.8	—	E952.8	E962.2	E982.8
Cyclaine	968.5	E855.2	E938.5	E950.4	E962.0	E980.4
Cyclamen europaeum	988.2	E865.4	—	E950.9	E962.1	E980.9
Cyclandelate	972.5	E858.3	E942.5	E950.4	E962.0	E980.4
Cyclazocine	965.09	E850.2	E935.2	E950.0	E962.0	E980.0
Cyclizine	963.0	E858.1	E933.0	E950.4	E962.0	E980.4
Cyclobarbital, cyclobarbitone	967.0	E851	E937.0	E950.1	E962.0	E980.1
Cycloguanil	961.4	E857	E931.4	E950.4	E962.0	E980.4
Cyclohexane	982.0	E862.4	—	E950.9	E962.1	E980.9
Cyclohexanol	980.8	E860.8	—	E950.9	E962.1	E980.9
Cyclohexanone	982.8	E862.4	—	E950.9	E962.1	E980.9
Cyclomethycaine	968.5	E855.2	E938.5	E950.4	E962.0	E980.4
Cyclopentamine	971.2	E855.5	E941.2	E950.4	E962.0	E980.4
Cyclopenthiazide	974.3	E858.5	E944.3	E950.4	E962.0	E980.4
Cyclopentolate	971.1	E855.4	E941.1	E950.4	E962.0	E980.4
Cyclophosphamide	963.1	E858.1	E933.1	E950.4	E962.0	E980.4
Cyclopropane	968.2	E855.1	E938.2	E950.4	E962.0	E980.4
Cycloserine	960.6	E856	E930.6	E950.4	E962.0	E980.4
Cyclothiazide	974.3	E858.5	E944.3	E950.4	E962.0	E980.4
Cycrimine	966.4	E855.0	E936.4	E950.4	E962.0	E980.4
Cymarin	972.1	E858.3	E942.1	E950.4	E962.0	E980.4
Cyproheptadine	963.0	E858.1	E933.0	E950.4	E962.0	E980.4
Cyprolidol	969.09	E854.0	E939.0	E950.3	E962.0	E980.3
Cytarabine	963.1	E858.1	E933.1	E950.4	E962.0	E980.4
Cytisus						
laburnum	988.2	E865.4	—	E950.9	E962.1	E980.9
scoparius	988.2	E865.4	—	E950.9	E962.1	E980.9
Cytomel	962.7	E858.0	E932.7	E950.4	E962.0	E980.4
Cytosine (antineoplastic)	963.1	E858.1	E933.1	E950.4	E962.0	E980.4
Cytoxan	963.1	E858.1	E933.1	E950.4	E962.0	E980.4
Dacarbazine	963.1	E858.1	E933.1	E950.4	E962.0	E980.4
Dactinomycin	960.7	E856	E930.7	E950.4	E962.0	E980.4
DADPS	961.8	E857	E931.8	E950.4	E962.0	E980.4
Dakin's solution (external)	976.0	E858.7	E946.0	E950.4	E962.0	E980.4
Dalmane	969.4	E853.2	E939.4	E950.3	E962.0	E980.3
DAM	977.2	E858.8	E947.2	E950.4	E962.0	E980.4
Danilone	964.2	E858.2	E934.2	E950.4	E962.0	E980.4
Danthron	973.1	E858.4	E943.1	E950.4	E962.0	E980.4
Dantrolene	975.2	E858.6	E945.2	E950.4	E962.0	E980.4
Daphne (gnidium) (mezereum)	988.2	E865.4	—	E950.9	E962.1	E980.9
berry	988.2	E865.3	—	E950.9	E962.1	E980.9
Dapsone	961.8	E857	E931.8	E950.4	E962.0	E980.4
Daraprim	961.4	E857	E931.4	E950.4	E962.0	E980.4
Darnel	988.2	E865.3	—	E950.9	E962.1	E980.9
Darvon	965.8	E850.8	E935.8	E950.0	E962.0	E980.0
Daunorubicin	960.7	E856	E930.7	E950.4	E962.0	E980.4
DBI	962.3	E858.0	E932.3	E950.4	E962.0	E980.4
D-Con (rodenticide)	989.4	E863.7	—	E950.6	E962.1	E980.7
DDS	961.8	E857	E931.8	E950.4	E962.0	E980.4
DDT	989.2	E863.0	—	E950.6	E962.1	E980.7
Deadly nightshade	988.2	E865.4	—	E950.9	E962.1	E980.9
berry	988.2	E865.3	—	E950.9	E962.1	E980.9
Deanol	969.79	E854.2	E939.7	E950.3	E962.0	E980.3
Debrisoquine	972.6	E858.3	E942.6	E950.4	E962.0	E980.4
Decaborane	989.89	E866.8	—	E950.9	E962.1	E980.9
fumes	987.8	E869.8	—	E952.8	E962.2	E982.8
Decadron	962.0	E858.0	E932.0	E950.4	E962.0	E980.4
ENT agent	976.6	E858.7	E946.6	E950.4	E962.0	E980.4
ophthalmic preparation	976.5	E858.7	E946.5	E950.4	E962.0	E980.4
topical NEC	976.0	E858.7	E946.0	E950.4	E962.0	E980.4
Decahydronaphthalene	982.0	E862.4	—	E950.9	E962.1	E980.9
Decalin	982.0	E862.4	—	E950.9	E962.1	E980.9
Decamethonium	975.2	E858.6	E945.2	E950.4	E962.0	E980.4
Decholin	973.4	E858.4	E943.4	E950.4	E962.0	E980.4
sodium (diagnostic)	977.8	E858.8	E947.8	E950.4	E962.0	E980.4

	Poisoning	Accident	Therapeutic Use	Suicide Attempt	Assault	Undetermined
External Cause (E-Code)						
Declomycin	960.4	E856	E930.4	E950.4	E962.0	E980.4
Deferoxamine	963.8	E858.1	E933.8	E950.4	E962.0	E980.4
Dehydrocholic acid	973.4	E858.4	E943.4	E950.4	E962.0	E980.4
Dekalin	982.0	E862.4	—	E950.9	E962.1	E980.9
Delalutin	962.2	E858.0	E932.2	E950.4	E962.0	E980.4
Delphinium	988.2	E865.3	—	E950.9	E962.1	E980.9
Deltasone	962.0	E858.0	E932.0	E950.4	E962.0	E980.4
Deltra	962.0	E858.0	E932.0	E950.4	E962.0	E980.4
Delvinal	967.0	E851	E937.0	E950.1	E962.0	E980.1
Demecarium (bromide)	971.0	E855.3	E941.0	E950.4	E962.0	E980.4
Demeclocycline	960.4	E856	E930.4	E950.4	E962.0	E980.4
Demecolcine	963.1	E858.1	E933.1	E950.4	E962.0	E980.4
Demelanizing agents	976.8	E858.7	E946.8	E950.4	E962.0	E980.4
Demerol	965.09	E850.2	E935.2	E950.0	E962.0	E980.0
Demethylchlortetracy-cline	960.4	E856	E930.4	E950.4	E962.0	E980.4
Demethyltetracycline	960.4	E856	E930.4	E950.4	E962.0	E980.4
Demeton	989.3	E863.1	—	E950.6	E962.1	E980.7
Demulcents	976.3	E858.7	E946.3	E950.4	E962.0	E980.4
Demulen	962.2	E858.0	E932.2	E950.4	E962.0	E980.4
Denatured alcohol	980.0	E860.1	—	E950.9	E962.1	E980.9
Dendrid	976.5	E858.7	E946.5	E950.4	E962.0	E980.4
Dental agents, topical	976.7	E858.7	E946.7	E950.4	E962.0	E980.4
Deodorant spray (feminine hygiene)	976.8	E858.7	E946.8	E950.4	E962.0	E980.4
Deoxyribonuclease	963.4	E858.1	E933.4	E950.4	E962.0	E980.4
Depressants						
appetite, central	977.0	E858.8	E947.0	E950.4	E962.0	E980.4
cardiac	972.0	E858.3	E942.0	E950.4	E962.0	E980.4
central nervous system (anes-thetic)	968.4	E855.1	E938.4	E950.4	E962.0	E980.4
psychotherapeutic	969.5	E853.9	E939.5	E950.3	E962.0	E980.3
Dequalinium	976.0	E858.7	E946.0	E950.4	E962.0	E980.4
Dermolate	976.2	E858.7	E946.2	E950.4	E962.0	E980.4
DES	962.2	E858.0	E932.2	E950.4	E962.0	E980.4
Desenex	976.0	E858.7	E946.0	E950.4	E962.0	E980.4
Deserpidine	972.6	E858.3	E942.6	E950.4	E962.0	E980.4
Desipramine	969.05	E854.0	E939.0	E950.3	E962.0	E980.3
Deslanoside	972.1	E858.3	E942.1	E950.4	E962.0	E980.4
Desocodeine	965.09	E850.2	E935.2	E950.0	E962.0	E980.0
Desomorphine	965.09	E850.2	E935.2	E950.0	E962.0	E980.0
Desonide	976.0	E858.7	E946.0	E950.4	E962.0	E980.4
Desoxycorticosterone derivatives	962.0	E858.0	E932.0	E950.4	E962.0	E980.4
Desoxyephedrine	969.72	E854.2	E939.7	E950.3	E962.0	E980.3
DET	969.6	E854.1	E939.6	E950.3	E962.0	E980.3
Detergents (ingested) (synthet-ic)	989.6	E861.0	—	E950.9	E962.1	E980.9
ENT agent	976.6	E858.7	E946.6	E950.4	E962.0	E980.4
external medication	976.2	E858.7	E946.2	E950.4	E962.0	E980.4
ophthalmic preparation	976.5	E858.7	E946.5	E950.4	E962.0	E980.4
topical NEC	976.0	E858.7	E946.0	E950.4	E962.0	E980.4
Deterrent, alcohol	977.3	E858.8	E947.3	E950.4	E962.0	E980.4
Detrothyronine	962.7	E858.0	E932.7	E950.4	E962.0	E980.4
Dettol (external medica-tion)	976.0	E858.7	E946.0	E950.4	E962.0	E980.4
Dexamethasone	962.0	E858.0	E932.0	E950.4	E962.0	E980.4
Dexamphetamine	969.72	E854.2	E939.7	E950.3	E962.0	E980.3
Dexedrine	969.72	E854.2	E939.7	E950.3	E962.0	E980.3
Dexpanthenol	963.5	E858.1	E933.5	E950.4	E962.0	E980.4
Dextran	964.8	E858.2	E934.8	E950.4	E962.0	E980.4
Dextriferron	964.0	E858.2	E934.0	E950.4	E962.0	E980.4
Dextroamphetamine	969.72	E854.2	E939.7	E950.3	E962.0	E980.3
Dextro calcium pantothen-ate	963.5	E858.1	E933.5	E950.4	E962.0	E980.4
Dextromethorphan	975.4	E858.6	E945.4	E950.4	E962.0	E980.4
Dextromoramide	965.09	E850.2	E935.2	E950.0	E962.0	E980.0
Dextro pantothenyl alco-hol	963.5	E858.1	E933.5	E950.4	E962.0	E980.4
topical	976.8	E858.7	E946.8	E950.4	E962.0	E980.4
Dextropropoxyphene (hy-drochloride)	965.8	E850.8	E935.8	E950.0	E962.0	E980.0
Dextrorphan	965.09	E850.2	E935.2	E950.0	E962.0	E980.0
Dextrose NEC	974.5	E858.5	E944.5	E950.4	E962.0	E980.4
Dextrothyroxin	962.7	E858.0	E932.7	E950.4	E962.0	E980.4
DFP	971.0	E855.3	E941.0	E950.4	E962.0	E980.4
DHE-45	972.9	E858.3	E942.9	E950.4	E962.0	E980.4
Diabinese	962.3	E858.0	E932.3	E950.4	E962.0	E980.4
Diacetyl monoxime	977.2	E858.8	E947.2	E950.4	E962.0	E980.4
Diacetylmorphine	965.01	E850.0	E935.0	E950.0	E962.0	E980.0
Diagnostic agents	977.8	E858.8	E947.8	E950.4	E962.0	E980.4
Dial (soap)	976.2	E858.7	E946.2	E950.4	E962.0	E980.4
Dial — *continued*						
sedative	967.0	E851	E937.0	E950.1	E962.0	E980.1
Diallylbarbituric acid	967.0	E851	E937.0	E950.1	E962.0	E980.1
Diaminodiphenylsulfone	961.8	E857	E931.8	E950.4	E962.0	E980.4
Diamorphine	965.01	E850.0	E935.0	E950.0	E962.0	E980.0
Diamox	974.2	E858.5	E944.2	E950.4	E962.0	E980.4
Diamthazole	976.0	E858.7	E946.0	E950.4	E962.0	E980.4
Diaphenylsulfone	961.8	E857	E931.8	E950.4	E962.0	E980.4
Diasone (sodium)	961.8	E857	E931.8	E950.4	E962.0	E980.4
Diazepam	969.4	E853.2	E939.4	E950.3	E962.0	E980.3
Diazinon	989.3	E863.1	—	E950.6	E962.1	E980.7
Diazomethane (gas)	987.8	E869.8	—	E952.8	E962.2	E982.8
Diazoxide	972.5	E858.3	E942.5	E950.4	E962.0	E980.4
Dibenamine	971.3	E855.6	E941.3	E950.4	E962.0	E980.4
Dibenzheptropine	963.0	E858.1	E933.0	E950.4	E962.0	E980.4
Dibenzyline	971.3	E855.6	E941.3	E950.4	E962.0	E980.4
Diborane (gas)	987.8	E869.8	—	E952.8	E962.2	E982.8
Dibromomannitol	963.1	E858.1	E933.1	E950.4	E962.0	E980.4
Dibucaine (spinal)	968.7	E855.2	E938.7	E950.4	E962.0	E980.4
topical (surface)	968.5	E855.2	E938.5	E950.4	E962.0	E980.4
Dibunate sodium	975.4	E858.6	E945.4	E950.4	E962.0	E980.4
Dibutoline	971.1	E855.4	E941.1	E950.4	E962.0	E980.4
Dicapthon	989.4	E863.4	—	E950.6	E962.1	E980.7
Dichloralphenazone	967.1	E852.0	E937.1	E950.2	E962.0	E980.2
Dichlorodifluo-romethane	987.4	E869.8	—	E952.8	E962.2	E982.8
Dichloroethane	982.3	E862.4	—	E950.9	E962.1	E980.9
Dichloroethylene	982.3	E862.4	—	E950.9	E962.1	E980.9
Dichloroethyl sulfide	987.8	E869.8	—	E952.8	E962.2	E982.8
Dichlorohydrin	982.3	E862.4	—	E950.9	E962.1	E980.9
Dichloromethane (solvent) (vapor)	982.3	E862.4	—	E950.9	E962.1	E980.9
Dichlorophen(e)	961.6	E857	E931.6	E950.4	E962.0	E980.4
Dichlorphenamide	974.2	E858.5	E944.2	E950.4	E962.0	E980.4
Dichlorvos	989.3	E863.1	—	E950.6	E962.1	E980.7
Diclofenac sodium	965.69	E850.6	E935.6	E950.0	E962.0	E980.0
Dicoumarin, dicumarol	964.2	E858.2	E934.2	E950.4	E962.0	E980.4
Dicyanogen (gas)	987.8	E869.8	—	E952.8	E962.2	E982.8
Dicyclomine	971.1	E855.4	E941.1	E950.4	E962.0	E980.4
Dieldrin (vapor)	989.2	E863.0	—	E950.6	E962.1	E980.7
Dienestrol	962.2	E858.0	E932.2	E950.4	E962.0	E980.4
Dietetics	977.0	E858.8	E947.0	E950.4	E962.0	E980.4
Diethazine	966.4	E855.0	E936.4	E950.4	E962.0	E980.4
Diethyl						
barbituric acid	967.0	E851	E937.0	E950.1	E962.0	E980.1
carbamazine	961.6	E857	E931.6	E950.4	E962.0	E980.4
carbinol	980.8	E860.8	—	E950.9	E962.1	E980.9
carbonate	982.8	E862.4	—	E950.9	E962.1	E980.9
dioxide	982.8	E862.4	—	E950.9	E962.1	E980.9
ether (vapor) — see Ether(s)						
glycol (monoacetate) (mo-noethyl ether)	982.8	E862.4	—	E950.9	E962.1	E980.9
propion	977.0	E858.8	E947.0	E950.4	E962.0	E980.4
stilbestrol	962.2	E858.0	E932.2	E950.4	E962.0	E980.4
Diethylene						
dioxide	982.8	E862.4	—	E950.9	E962.1	E980.9
glycol (monoacetate) (mo-noethyl ether)	982.8	E862.4	—	E950.9	E962.1	E980.9
Diethylsulfone-diethyl-methane	967.8	E852.8	E937.8	E950.2	E962.0	E980.2
Difencloxazine	965.09	E850.2	E935.2	E950.0	E962.0	E980.0
Diffusin	963.4	E858.1	E933.4	E950.4	E962.0	E980.4
Diflos	971.0	E855.3	E941.0	E950.4	E962.0	E980.4
Digestants	973.4	E858.4	E943.4	E950.4	E962.0	E980.4
Digitalin(e)	972.1	E858.3	E942.1	E950.4	E962.0	E980.4
Digitalis glycosides	972.1	E858.3	E942.1	E950.4	E962.0	E980.4
Digitoxin	972.1	E858.3	E942.1	E950.4	E962.0	E980.4
Digoxin	972.1	E858.3	E942.1	E950.4	E962.0	E980.4
Dihydrocodeine	965.09	E850.2	E935.2	E950.0	E962.0	E980.0
Dihydrocodeinone	965.09	E850.2	E935.2	E950.0	E962.0	E980.0
Dihydroergocristine	972.9	E858.3	E942.9	E950.4	E962.0	E980.4
Dihydroergotamine	972.9	E858.3	E942.9	E950.4	E962.0	E980.4
Dihydroergotoxine	972.9	E858.3	E942.9	E950.4	E962.0	E980.4
Dihydrohydroxy-codeinone	965.09	E850.2	E935.2	E950.0	E962.0	E980.0
Dihydrohydroxymorphi-none	965.09	E850.2	E935.2	E950.0	E962.0	E980.0
Dihydroisocodeine	965.09	E850.2	E935.2	E950.0	E962.0	E980.0
Dihydromorphine	965.09	E850.2	E935.2	E950.0	E962.0	E980.0
Dihydromorphinone	965.09	E850.2	E935.2	E950.0	E962.0	E980.0
Dihydrostreptomycin	960.6	E856	E930.6	E950.4	E962.0	E980.4
Dihydrotachysterol	962.6	E858.0	E932.6	E950.4	E962.0	E980.4

	Poisoning	Accident	Therapeutic Use	Suicide Attempt	Assault	Undetermined
Dihydroxyan-						
thraquinone	973.1	E858.4	E943.1	E950.4	E962.0	E980.4
Dihydroxycodeinone	965.09	E850.2	E935.2	E950.0	E962.0	E980.0
Diiodohydroxyquin	961.3	E857	E931.3	E950.4	E962.0	E980.4
topical	976.0	E858.7	E946.0	E950.4	E962.0	E980.4
Diiodohydroxyquinoline	961.3	E857	E931.3	E950.4	E962.0	E980.4
Dilantin	966.1	E855.0	E936.1	E950.4	E962.0	E980.4
Dilaudid	965.09	E850.2	E935.2	E950.0	E962.0	E980.0
Diloxanide	961.5	E857	E931.5	E950.4	E962.0	E980.4
Dimefline	970.0	E854.3	E940.0	E950.4	E962.0	E980.4
Dimenhydrinate	963.0	E858.1	E933.0	E950.4	E962.0	E980.4
Dimercaprol	963.8	E858.1	E933.8	E950.4	E962.0	E980.4
Dimercaptopropanol	963.8	E858.1	E933.8	E950.4	E962.0	E980.4
Dimetane	963.0	E858.1	E933.0	E950.4	E962.0	E980.4
Dimethicone	976.3	E858.7	E946.3	E950.4	E962.0	E980.4
Dimethindene	963.0	E858.1	E933.0	E950.4	E962.0	E980.4
Dimethisoquin	968.5	E855.2	E938.5	E950.4	E962.0	E980.4
Dimethisterone	962.2	E858.0	E932.2	E950.4	E962.0	E980.4
Dimethoxanate	975.4	E858.6	E945.4	E950.4	E962.0	E980.4
Dimethyl						
arsine, arsinic acid — see Arsenic						
carbinol	980.2	E860.3	—	E950.9	E962.1	E980.9
diguanide	962.3	E858.0	E932.3	E950.4	E962.0	E980.4
ketone	982.8	E862.4	—	E950.9	E962.1	E980.9
vapor	987.8	E869.8	—	E952.8	E962.2	E982.8
meperidine	965.09	E850.2	E935.2	E950.0	E962.0	E980.0
parathion	989.3	E863.1	—	E950.6	E962.1	E980.7
polysiloxane	973.8	E858.4	E943.8	E950.4	E962.0	E980.4
sulfate (fumes)	987.8	E869.8	—	E952.8	E962.2	E982.8
liquid	983.9	E864.3	—	E950.7	E962.1	E980.6
sulfoxide NEC	982.8	E862.4	—	E950.9	E962.1	E980.9
medicinal	976.4	E858.7	E946.4	E950.4	E962.0	E980.4
triptamine	969.6	E854.1	E939.6	E950.3	E962.0	E980.3
tubocurarine	975.2	E858.6	E945.2	E950.4	E962.0	E980.4
Dindevan	964.2	E858.2	E934.2	E950.4	E962.0	E980.4
Dinitrobenzene	983.0	E864.0	—	E950.7	E962.1	E980.6
vapor	987.8	E869.8	—	E952.8	E962.2	E982.8
Dinitro (-ortho-) cresol (herbicide) (spray)	989.4	E863.5	—	E950.6	E962.1	E980.7
insecticide	989.4	E863.4	—	E950.6	E962.1	E980.7
Dinitro-orthocresol (herbicide)	989.4	E863.5	—	E950.6	E962.1	E980.7
insecticide	989.4	E863.4	—	E950.6	E962.1	E980.7
Dinitrophenol (herbicide) (spray)	989.4	E863.5	—	E950.6	E962.1	E980.7
insecticide	989.4	E863.4	—	E950.6	E962.1	E980.7
Dinoprost	975.0	E858.6	E945.0	E950.4	E962.0	E980.4
Dioctyl sulfosuccinate (calcium) (sodium)	973.2	E858.4	E943.2	E950.4	E962.0	E980.4
Diodoquin	961.3	E857	E931.3	E950.4	E962.0	E980.4
Dione derivatives NEC	966.3	E855.0	E936.3	E950.4	E962.0	E980.4
Dionin	965.09	E850.2	E935.2	E950.0	E962.0	E980.0
Dioxane	982.8	E862.4	—	E950.9	E962.1	E980.9
Dioxin — see Herbicide						
Dioxyline	972.5	E858.3	E942.5	E950.4	E962.0	E980.4
Dipentene	982.8	E862.4	—	E950.9	E962.1	E980.9
Diphemanil	971.1	E855.4	E941.1	E950.4	E962.0	E980.4
Diphenadione	964.2	E858.2	E934.2	E950.4	E962.0	E980.4
Diphenhydramine	963.0	E858.1	E933.0	E950.4	E962.0	E980.4
Diphenidol	963.0	E858.1	E933.0	E950.4	E962.0	E980.4
Diphenoxylate	973.5	E858.4	E943.5	E950.4	E962.0	E980.4
Diphenylchloroarsine	985.1	E866.3	—	E950.8	E962.1	E980.8
Diphenylhydantoin (sodium)	966.1	E855.0	E936.1	E950.4	E962.0	E980.4
Diphenylpyraline	963.0	E858.1	E933.0	E950.4	E962.0	E980.4
Diphtheria						
antitoxin	979.9	E858.8	E949.9	E950.4	E962.0	E980.4
toxoid	978.5	E858.8	E948.5	E950.4	E962.0	E980.4
with tetanus toxoid	978.9	E858.8	E948.9	E950.4	E962.0	E980.4
with pertussis component	978.6	E858.8	E948.6	E950.4	E962.0	E980.4
vaccine	978.5	E858.8	E948.5	E950.4	E962.0	E980.4
Dipipanone	965.09	E850.2	E935.2	E950.0	E962.0	E980.0
Diplovax	979.5	E858.8	E949.5	E950.4	E962.0	E980.4
Diprophylline	975.1	E858.6	E945.1	E950.4	E962.0	E980.4
Dipyridamole	972.4	E858.3	E942.4	E950.4	E962.0	E980.4
Dipyrone	965.5	E850.5	E935.5	E950.0	E962.0	E980.0
Diquat	989.4	E863.5	—	E950.6	E962.1	E980.7
Disinfectant NEC	983.9	E861.4	—	E950.7	E962.1	E980.6
alkaline	983.2	E861.4	—	E950.7	E962.1	E980.6
aromatic	983.0	E861.4	—	E950.7	E962.1	E980.6

	Poisoning	Accident	Therapeutic Use	Suicide Attempt	Assault	Undetermined
Disipal	966.4	E855.0	E936.4	E950.4	E962.0	E980.4
Disodium edetate	963.8	E858.1	E933.8	E950.4	E962.0	E980.4
Disulfamide	974.4	E858.5	E944.4	E950.4	E962.0	E980.4
Disulfanilamide	961.0	E857	E931.0	E950.4	E962.0	E980.4
Disulfiram	977.3	E858.8	E947.3	E950.4	E962.0	E980.4
Dithiazanine	961.6	E857	E931.6	E950.4	E962.0	E980.4
Dithioglycerol	963.8	E858.1	E933.8	E950.4	E962.0	E980.4
Dithranol	976.4	E858.7	E946.4	E950.4	E962.0	E980.4
Diucardin	974.3	E858.5	E944.3	E950.4	E962.0	E980.4
Diupres	974.3	E858.5	E944.3	E950.4	E962.0	E980.4
Diuretics NEC	974.4	E858.5	E944.4	E950.4	E962.0	E980.4
carbonic acid anhydrase inhibitors	974.2	E858.5	E944.2	E950.4	E962.0	E980.4
mercurial	974.0	E858.5	E944.0	E950.4	E962.0	E980.4
osmotic	974.4	E858.5	E944.4	E950.4	E962.0	E980.4
purine derivatives	974.1	E858.5	E944.1	E950.4	E962.0	E980.4
saluretic	974.3	E858.5	E944.3	E950.4	E962.0	E980.4
Diuril	974.3	E858.5	E944.3	E950.4	E962.0	E980.4
Divinyl ether	968.2	E855.1	E938.2	E950.4	E962.0	E980.4
D-lysergic acid diethylamide	969.6	E854.1	E939.6	E950.3	E962.0	E980.3
DMCT	960.4	E856	E930.4	E950.4	E962.0	E980.4
DMSO	982.8	E862.4	—	E950.9	E962.1	E980.9
DMT	969.6	E854.1	E939.6	E950.3	E962.0	E980.3
DNOC	989.4	E863.5	—	E950.6	E962.1	E980.7
DOCA	962.0	E858.0	E932.0	E950.4	E962.0	E980.4
Dolophine	965.02	E850.1	E935.1	E950.0	E962.0	E980.0
Doloxene	965.8	E850.8	E935.8	E950.0	E962.0	E980.0
DOM	969.6	E854.1	E939.6	E950.3	E962.0	E980.3
Domestic gas — see Gas, utility						
Domiphen (bromide) (lozenges)	976.6	E858.7	E946.6	E950.4	E962.0	E980.4
Dopa (levo)	966.4	E855.0	E936.4	E950.4	E962.0	E980.4
Dopamine	971.2	E855.5	E941.2	E950.4	E962.0	E980.4
Doriden	967.5	E852.4	E937.5	E950.2	E962.0	E980.2
Dormiral	967.0	E851	E937.0	E950.1	E962.0	E980.1
Dormison	967.8	E852.8	E937.8	E950.2	E962.0	E980.2
Dornase	963.4	E858.1	E933.4	E950.4	E962.0	E980.4
Dorsacaine	968.5	E855.2	E938.5	E950.4	E962.0	E980.4
Dothiepin hydrochloride	969.05	E854.0	E939.0	E950.3	E962.0	E980.3
Doxapram	970.0	E854.3	E940.0	E950.4	E962.0	E980.4
Doxepin	969.05	E854.0	E939.0	E950.3	E962.0	E980.3
Doxorubicin	960.7	E856	E930.7	E950.4	E962.0	E980.4
Doxycycline	960.4	E856	E930.4	E950.4	E962.0	E980.4
Doxylamine	963.0	E858.1	E933.0	E950.4	E962.0	E980.4
Dramamine	963.0	E858.1	E933.0	E950.4	E962.0	E980.4
Drano (drain cleaner)	983.2	E864.2	—	E950.7	E962.1	E980.6
Dromoran	965.09	E850.2	E935.2	E950.0	E962.0	E980.0
Dromostanolone	962.1	E858.0	E932.1	E950.4	E962.0	E980.4
Droperidol	969.2	E853.1	E939.2	E950.3	E962.0	E980.3
Drotrecogin alfa	964.2	E858.2	E934.2	E950.4	E962.0	E980.4
Drug	977.9	E858.9	E947.9	E950.5	E962.0	E980.5
AHFS List						
4:00 antihistamine drugs	963.0	E858.1	E933.0	E950.4	E962.0	E980.4
8:04 amebacides	961.5	E857	E931.5	E950.4	E962.0	E980.4
arsenical anti-infectives	961.1	E857	E931.1	E950.4	E962.0	E980.4
quinoline derivatives	961.3	E857	E931.3	E950.4	E962.0	E980.4
8:08 anthelmintics	961.6	E857	E931.6	E950.4	E962.0	E980.4
quinoline derivatives	961.3	E857	E931.3	E950.4	E962.0	E980.4
8:12.04 antifungal antibiotics	960.1	E856	E930.1	E950.4	E962.0	E980.4
8:12.06 cephalosporins	960.5	E856	E930.5	E950.4	E962.0	E980.4
8:12.08 chloramphenicol	960.2	E856	E930.2	E950.4	E962.0	E980.4
8:12.12 erythromycins	960.3	E856	E930.3	E950.4	E962.0	E980.4
8:12.16 penicillins	960.0	E856	E930.0	E950.4	E962.0	E980.4
8:12.20 streptomycins	960.6	E856	E930.6	E950.4	E962.0	E980.4
8:12.24 tetracyclines	960.4	E856	E930.4	E950.4	E962.0	E980.4
8:12.28 other antibiotics	960.8	E856	E930.8	E950.4	E962.0	E980.4
antimycobacterial	960.6	E856	E930.6	E950.4	E962.0	E980.4
macrolides	960.3	E856	E930.3	E950.4	E962.0	E980.4
8:16 antituberculars	961.8	E857	E931.8	E950.4	E962.0	E980.4
antibiotics	960.6	E856	E930.6	E950.4	E962.0	E980.4
8:18 antivirals	961.7	E857	E931.7	E950.4	E962.0	E980.4
8:20 plasmodicides (antimalarials)	961.4	E857	E931.4	E950.4	E962.0	E980.4
8:24 sulfonamides	961.0	E857	E931.0	E950.4	E962.0	E980.4
8:26 sulfones	961.8	E857	E931.8	E950.4	E962.0	E980.4
8:28 treponemicides	961.2	E857	E931.2	E950.4	E962.0	E980.4
8:32 trichomonacides	961.5	E857	E931.5	E950.4	E962.0	E980.4
nitrofuran derivatives	961.9	E857	E931.9	E950.4	E962.0	E980.4
quinoline derivatives	961.3	E857	E931.3	E950.4	E962.0	E980.4

Nontherapeutic use substance

Subterms under main terms may continue to next column or page

Drug — continued	Poisoning	Accident	Therapeutic Use	Suicide Attempt	Assault	Undetermined
8:36 urinary germicides	961.9	E857	E931.9	E950.4	E962.0	E980.4
quinoline derivatives	961.3	E857	E931.3	E950.4	E962.0	E980.4
8:40 other anti-infectives	961.9	E857	E931.9	E950.4	E962.0	E980.4
10:00 antineoplastic agents	963.1	E858.1	E933.1	E950.4	E962.0	E980.4
antibiotics	960.7	E856	E930.7	E950.4	E962.0	E980.4
progestogens	962.2	E858.0	E932.2	E950.4	E962.0	E980.4
12:04 parasympathomimetic (cholinergic) agents	971.0	E855.3	E941.0	E950.4	E962.0	E980.4
12:08 parasympatholytic (cholinergic-blocking) agents	971.1	E855.4	E941.1	E950.4	E962.0	E980.4
12:12 Sympathomimetic (adrenergic) agents	971.2	E855.5	E941.2	E950.4	E962.0	E980.4
12:16 sympatholytic (adrenergic-blocking) agents	971.3	E855.6	E941.3	E950.4	E962.0	E980.4
12:20 skeletal muscle relaxants						
central nervous system muscle-tone depressants	968.0	E855.1	E938.0	E950.4	E962.0	E980.4
myoneural blocking agents	975.2	E858.6	E945.2	E950.4	E962.0	E980.4
16:00 blood derivatives	964.7	E858.2	E934.7	E950.4	E962.0	E980.4
20:04.04 iron preparations	964.0	E858.2	E934.0	E950.4	E962.0	E980.4
20:04.08 liver and stomach preparations	964.1	E858.2	E934.1	E950.4	E962.0	E980.4
20:04 antianemia drugs	964.1	E858.2	E934.1	E950.4	E962.0	E980.4
20:12.04 anticoagulants	964.2	E858.2	E934.2	E950.4	E962.0	E980.4
20:12.08 antiheparin agents	964.5	E858.2	E934.5	E950.4	E962.0	E980.4
20:12.12 coagulants	964.5	E858.2	E934.5	E950.4	E962.0	E980.4
20:12.16 hemostatics NEC	964.5	E858.2	E934.5	E950.4	E962.0	E980.4
capillary active drugs	972.8	E858.3	E942.8	E950.4	E962.0	E980.4
24:04 cardiac drugs	972.9	E858.3	E942.9	E950.4	E962.0	E980.4
cardiotonic agents	972.1	E858.3	E942.1	E950.4	E962.0	E980.4
rhythm regulators	972.0	E858.3	E942.0	E950.4	E962.0	E980.4
24:06 antilipemic agents	972.2	E858.3	E942.2	E950.4	E962.0	E980.4
thyroid derivatives	962.7	E858.0	E932.7	E950.4	E962.0	E980.4
24:08 hypotensive agents	972.6	E858.3	E942.6	E950.4	E962.0	E980.4
adrenergic blocking agents	971.3	E855.6	E941.3	E950.4	E962.0	E980.4
ganglion blocking agents	972.3	E858.3	E942.3	E950.4	E962.0	E980.4
vasodilators	972.5	E858.3	E942.5	E950.4	E962.0	E980.4
24:12 vasodilating agents NEC	972.5	E858.3	E942.5	E950.4	E962.0	E980.4
coronary	972.4	E858.3	E942.4	E950.4	E962.0	E980.4
nicotinic acid derivatives	972.2	E858.3	E942.2	E950.4	E962.0	E980.4
24:16 sclerosing agents	972.7	E858.3	E942.7	E950.4	E962.0	E980.4
28:04 general anesthetics	968.4	E855.1	E938.4	E950.4	E962.0	E980.4
gaseous anesthetics	968.2	E855.1	E938.2	E950.4	E962.0	E980.4
halothane	968.1	E855.1	E938.1	E950.4	E962.0	E980.4
intravenous anesthetics	968.3	E855.1	E938.3	E950.4	E962.0	E980.4
28:08 analgesics and antipyretics	965.9	E850.9	E935.9	E950.0	E962.0	E980.0
antirheumatics	965.69	E850.6	E935.6	E950.0	E962.0	E980.0
aromatic analgesics	965.4	E850.4	E935.4	E950.0	E962.0	E980.0
non-narcotic NEC	965.7	E850.7	E935.7	E950.0	E962.0	E980.0
opium alkaloids	965.00	E850.2	E935.2	E950.0	E962.0	E980.0
heroin	965.01	E850.0	E935.0	E950.0	E962.0	E980.0
methadone	965.02	E850.1	E935.1	E950.0	E962.0	E980.0
specified type NEC	965.09	E850.2	E935.2	E950.0	E962.0	E980.0
pyrazole derivatives	965.5	E850.5	E935.5	E950.0	E962.0	E980.0
salicylates	965.1	E850.3	E935.3	E950.0	E962.0	E980.0
specified NEC	965.8	E850.8	E935.8	E950.0	E962.0	E980.0
28:10 narcotic antagonists	970.1	E854.3	E940.1	E950.4	E962.0	E980.4
28:12 anticonvulsants	966.3	E855.0	E936.3	E950.4	E962.0	E980.4
barbiturates	967.0	E851	E937.0	E950.1	E962.0	E980.1
benzodiazepine-based tranquilizers	969.4	E853.2	E939.4	E950.3	E962.0	E980.3
bromides	967.3	E852.2	E937.3	E950.2	E962.0	E980.2
hydantoin derivatives	966.1	E855.0	E936.1	E950.4	E962.0	E980.4
oxazolidine (derivatives)	966.0	E855.0	E936.0	E950.4	E962.0	E980.4
succinimides	966.2	E855.0	E936.2	E950.4	E962.0	E980.4
28:16.04 antidepressants	969.00	E854.0	E939.0	E950.3	E962.0	E980.3
28:16.08 tranquilizers	969.5	E853.9	E939.5	E950.3	E962.0	E980.3
benzodiazepine-based	969.4	E853.2	E939.4	E950.3	E962.0	E980.3
butyrophenone-based	969.2	E853.1	E939.2	E950.3	E962.0	E980.3
major NEC	969.3	E853.8	E939.3	E950.3	E962.0	E980.3
phenothiazine-based	969.1	E853.0	E939.1	E950.3	E962.0	E980.3
28:16.12 other psychotherapeutic agents	969.8	E855.8	E939.8	E950.3	E962.0	E980.3
28:20 respiratory and cerebral stimulants	970.9	E854.3	E940.9	E950.4	E962.0	E980.4
analeptics	970.0	E854.3	E940.0	E950.4	E962.0	E980.4
anorexigenic agents	977.0	E858.8	E947.0	E950.4	E962.0	E980.4
psychostimulants	969.70	E854.2	E939.7	E950.3	E962.0	E980.3
specified NEC	970.89	E854.3	E940.8	E950.4	E962.0	E980.4
28:24 sedatives and hypnotics	967.9	E852.9	E937.9	E950.2	E962.0	E980.2
barbiturates	967.0	E851	E937.0	E950.1	E962.0	E980.1
benzodiazepine-based tranquilizers	969.4	E853.2	E939.4	E950.3	E962.0	E980.3
chloral hydrate (group)	967.1	E852.0	E937.1	E950.2	E962.0	E980.2
glutethamide group	967.5	E852.4	E937.5	E950.2	E962.0	E980.2
intravenous anesthetics	968.3	E855.1	E938.3	E950.4	E962.0	E980.4
methaqualone (compounds)	967.4	E852.3	E937.4	E950.2	E962.0	E980.2
paraldehyde	967.2	E852.1	E937.2	E950.2	E962.0	E980.2
phenothiazine-based tranquilizers	969.1	E853.0	E939.1	E950.3	E962.0	E980.3
specified NEC	967.8	E852.8	E937.8	E950.2	E962.0	E980.2
thiobarbiturates	968.3	E855.1	E938.3	E950.4	E962.0	E980.4
tranquilizer NEC	969.5	E853.9	E939.5	E950.3	E962.0	E980.3
36:04 to 36:88 diagnostic agents	977.8	E858.8	E947.8	E950.4	E962.0	E980.4
40:00 electrolyte, caloric, and water balance agents NEC	974.5	E858.5	E944.5	E950.4	E962.0	E980.4
40:04 acidifying agents	963.2	E858.1	E933.2	E950.4	E962.0	E980.4
40:08 alkalinizing agents	963.3	E858.1	E933.3	E950.4	E962.0	E980.4
40:10 ammonia detoxicants	974.5	E858.5	E944.5	E950.4	E962.0	E980.4
40:12 replacement solutions	974.5	E858.5	E944.5	E950.4	E962.0	E980.4
plasma expanders	964.8	E858.2	E934.8	E950.4	E962.0	E980.4
40:16 sodium-removing resins	974.5	E858.5	E944.5	E950.4	E962.0	E980.4
40:18 potassium-removing resins	974.5	E858.5	E944.5	E950.4	E962.0	E980.4
40:20 caloric agents	974.5	E858.5	E944.5	E950.4	E962.0	E980.4
40:24 salt and sugar substitutes	974.5	E858.5	E944.5	E950.4	E962.0	E980.4
40:28 diuretics NEC	974.4	E858.5	E944.4	E950.4	E962.0	E980.4
carbonic acid anhydrase inhibitors	974.2	E858.5	E944.2	E950.4	E962.0	E980.4
mercurials	974.0	E858.5	E944.0	E950.4	E962.0	E980.4
purine derivatives	974.1	E858.5	E944.1	E950.4	E962.0	E980.4
saluretics	974.3	E858.5	E944.3	E950.4	E962.0	E980.4
thiazides	974.3	E858.5	E944.3	E950.4	E962.0	E980.4
40:36 irrigating solutions	974.5	E858.5	E944.5	E950.4	E962.0	E980.4
40:40 uricosuric agents	974.7	E858.5	E944.7	E950.4	E962.0	E980.4
44:00 enzymes	963.4	E858.1	E933.4	E950.4	E962.0	E980.4
fibrinolysis-affecting agents	964.4	E858.2	E934.4	E950.4	E962.0	E980.4
gastric agents	973.4	E858.4	E943.4	E950.4	E962.0	E980.4
48:00 expectorants and cough preparations						
antihistamine agents	963.0	E858.1	E933.0	E950.4	E962.0	E980.4
antitussives	975.4	E858.6	E945.4	E950.4	E962.0	E980.4
codeine derivatives	965.09	E850.2	E935.2	E950.0	E962.0	E980.0
expectorants	975.5	E858.6	E945.5	E950.4	E962.0	E980.4
narcotic agents NEC	965.09	E850.2	E935.2	E950.0	E962.0	E980.0
52:04.04 antibiotics (EENT)						
ENT agent	976.6	E858.7	E946.6	E950.4	E962.0	E980.4
ophthalmic preparation	976.5	E858.7	E946.5	E950.4	E962.0	E980.4
52:04.06 antivirals (EENT)						
ENT agent	976.6	E858.7	E946.6	E950.4	E962.0	E980.4
ophthalmic preparation	976.5	E858.7	E946.5	E950.4	E962.0	E980.4
52:04.08 sulfonamides (EENT)						
ENT agent	976.6	E858.7	E946.6	E950.4	E962.0	E980.4
ophthalmic preparation	976.5	E858.7	E946.5	E950.4	E962.0	E980.4
52:04.12 miscellaneous anti-infectives (EENT)						
ENT agent	976.6	E858.7	E946.6	E950.4	E962.0	E980.4

Nontherapeutic use substance

⬇ Subterms under main terms may continue to next column or page

Drug — continued	Poisoning	Accident	Therapeutic Use	Suicide Attempt	Assault	Undeter-mined
52:04.12 miscellaneous anti-infectives — continued						
ophthalmic preparation	976.5	E858.7	E946.5	E950.4	E962.0	E980.4
52:04 anti-infectives (EENT)						
ENT agent	976.6	E858.7	E946.6	E950.4	E962.0	E980.4
ophthalmic preparation	976.5	E858.7	E946.5	E950.4	E962.0	E980.4
52:08 anti-inflammatory agents (EENT)						
ENT agent	976.6	E858.7	E946.6	E950.4	E962.0	E980.4
ophthalmic preparation	976.5	E858.7	E946.5	E950.4	E962.0	E980.4
52:10 carbonic anhydrase inhibitors	974.2	E858.5	E944.2	E950.4	E962.0	E980.4
52:12 contact lens solutions	976.5	E858.7	E946.5	E950.4	E962.0	E980.4
52:16 local anesthetics (EENT)	968.5	E855.2	E938.5	E950.4	E962.0	E980.4
52:20 miotics	971.0	E855.3	E941.0	E950.4	E962.0	E980.4
52:24 mydriatics						
adrenergics	971.2	E855.5	E941.2	E950.4	E962.0	E980.4
anticholinergics	971.1	E855.4	E941.1	E950.4	E962.0	E980.4
antimuscarinics	971.1	E855.4	E941.1	E950.4	E962.0	E980.4
parasympatholytics	971.1	E855.4	E941.1	E950.4	E962.0	E980.4
spasmolytics	971.1	E855.4	E941.1	E950.4	E962.0	E980.4
sympathomimetics	971.2	E855.5	E941.2	E950.4	E962.0	E980.4
52:28 mouth washes and gargles	976.6	E858.7	E946.6	E950.4	E962.0	E980.4
52:32 vasoconstrictors (EENT)	971.2	E855.5	E941.2	E950.4	E962.0	E980.4
52:36 unclassified agents (EENT)						
ENT agent	976.6	E858.7	E946.6	E950.4	E962.0	E980.4
ophthalmic preparation	976.5	E858.7	E946.5	E950.4	E962.0	E980.4
56:04 antacids and adsorbents	973.0	E858.4	E943.0	E950.4	E962.0	E980.4
56:08 antidiarrhea agents	973.5	E858.4	E943.5	E950.4	E962.0	E980.4
56:10 antiflatulents	973.8	E858.4	E943.8	E950.4	E962.0	E980.4
56:12 cathartics NEC	973.3	E858.4	E943.3	E950.4	E962.0	E980.4
emollients	973.2	E858.4	E943.2	E950.4	E962.0	E980.4
irritants	973.1	E858.4	E943.1	E950.4	E962.0	E980.4
56:16 digestants	973.4	E858.4	E943.4	E950.4	E962.0	E980.4
56:20 emetics and antiemetics						
antiemetics	963.0	E858.1	E933.0	E950.4	E962.0	E980.4
emetics	973.6	E858.4	E943.6	E950.4	E962.0	E980.4
56:24 lipotropic agents	977.1	E858.8	E947.1	E950.4	E962.0	E980.4
56:40 miscellaneous G.I. drugs	973.8	E858.4	E943.8	E950.4	E962.0	E980.4
60:00 gold compounds	965.69	E850.6	E935.6	E950.0	E962.0	E980.0
64:00 heavy metal antagonists	963.8	E858.1	E933.8	E950.4	E962.0	E980.4
68:04 adrenals	962.0	E858.0	E932.0	E950.4	E962.0	E980.4
68:08 androgens	962.1	E858.0	E932.1	E950.4	E962.0	E980.4
68:12 contraceptives, oral	962.2	E858.0	E932.2	E950.4	E962.0	E980.4
68:16 estrogens	962.2	E858.0	E932.2	E950.4	E962.0	E980.4
68:18 gonadotropins	962.4	E858.0	E932.4	E950.4	E962.0	E980.4
68:20.08 insulins	962.3	E858.0	E932.3	E950.4	E962.0	E980.4
68:20 insulins and antidiabetic agents	962.3	E858.0	E932.3	E950.4	E962.0	E980.4
68:24 parathyroid	962.6	E858.0	E932.6	E950.4	E962.0	E980.4
68:28 pituitary (posterior)	962.5	E858.0	E932.5	E950.4	E962.0	E980.4
anterior	962.4	E858.0	E932.4	E950.4	E962.0	E980.4
68:32 progestogens	962.2	E858.0	E932.2	E950.4	E962.0	E980.4
68:34 other corpus luteum hormones NEC	962.2	E858.0	E932.2	E950.4	E962.0	E980.4
68:36 thyroid and antithyroid						
antithyroid	962.8	E858.0	E932.8	E950.4	E962.0	E980.4
thyroid (derivatives)	962.7	E858.0	E932.7	E950.4	E962.0	E980.4
72:00 local anesthetics NEC	968.9	E855.2	E938.9	E950.4	E962.0	E980.4
infiltration (intradermal) (subcutaneous) (submucosal)	968.5	E855.2	E938.5	E950.4	E962.0	E980.4
nerve blocking (peripheral) (plexus) (regional)	968.6	E855.2	E938.6	E950.4	E962.0	E980.4
spinal	968.7	E855.2	E938.7	E950.4	E962.0	E980.4
topical (surface)	968.5	E855.2	E938.5	E950.4	E962.0	E980.4
76:00 oxytocics	975.0	E858.6	E945.0	E950.4	E962.0	E980.4
78:00 radioactive agents	990	—	—	—	—	—
80:04 serums NEC	979.9	E858.8	E949.9	E950.4	E962.0	E980.4

Drug — continued	Poisoning	Accident	Therapeutic Use	Suicide Attempt	Assault	Undeter-mined
80:04 serums — continued						
immune gamma globulin (human)	964.6	E858.2	E934.6	E950.4	E962.0	E980.4
80:08 toxoids NEC	978.8	E858.8	E948.8	E950.4	E962.0	E980.4
diphtheria	978.5	E858.8	E948.5	E950.4	E962.0	E980.4
and diphtheria	978.9	E858.8	E948.9	E950.4	E962.0	E980.4
with pertussis component	978.6	E858.8	E948.6	E950.4	E962.0	E980.4
and tetanus	978.9	E858.8	E948.9	E950.4	E962.0	E980.4
with pertussis component	978.6	E858.8	E948.6	E950.4	E962.0	E980.4
tetanus	978.4	E858.8	E948.4	E950.4	E962.0	E980.4
80:12 vaccines	979.9	E858.8	E949.9	E950.4	E962.0	E980.4
bacterial NEC	978.8	E858.8	E948.8	E950.4	E962.0	E980.4
with other bacterial components	978.9	E858.8	E948.9	E950.4	E962.0	E980.4
pertussis component	978.6	E858.8	E948.6	E950.4	E962.0	E980.4
viral and rickettsial components	979.7	E858.8	E949.7	E950.4	E962.0	E980.4
rickettsial NEC	979.6	E858.8	E949.6	E950.4	E962.0	E980.4
with bacterial component	979.7	E858.8	E949.7	E950.4	E962.0	E980.4
pertussis component	978.6	E858.8	E948.6	E950.4	E962.0	E980.4
viral component	979.7	E858.8	E949.7	E950.4	E962.0	E980.4
viral NEC	979.6	E858.8	E949.6	E950.4	E962.0	E980.4
with bacterial component	979.7	E858.8	E949.7	E950.4	E962.0	E980.4
pertussis component	978.6	E858.8	E948.6	E950.4	E962.0	E980.4
rickettsial component	979.7	E858.8	E949.7	E950.4	E962.0	E980.4
84:04.04 antibiotics (skin and mucous membrane)	976.0	E858.7	E946.0	E950.4	E962.0	E980.4
84:04.08 fungicides (skin and mucous membrane)	976.0	E858.7	E946.0	E950.4	E962.0	E980.4
84:04.12 scabicides and pediculicides (skin and mucous membrane)	976.0	E858.7	E946.0	E950.4	E962.0	E980.4
84:04.16 miscellaneous local anti-infectives (skin and mucous membrane)	976.0	E858.7	E946.0	E950.4	E962.0	E980.4
84:06 anti-inflammatory agents (skin and mucous membrane)	976.0	E858.7	E946.0	E950.4	E962.0	E980.4
84:08 antipruritics and local anesthetics						
antipruritics	976.1	E858.7	E946.1	E950.4	E962.0	E980.4
local anesthetics	968.5	E855.2	E938.5	E950.4	E962.0	E980.4
84:12 astringents	976.2	E858.7	E946.2	E950.4	E962.0	E980.4
84:16 cell stimulants and proliferants	976.8	E858.7	E946.8	E950.4	E962.0	E980.4
84:20 detergents	976.2	E858.7	E946.2	E950.4	E962.0	E980.4
84:24 emollients, demulcents, and protectants	976.3	E858.7	E946.3	E950.4	E962.0	E980.4
84:28 keratolytic agents	976.4	E858.7	E946.4	E950.4	E962.0	E980.4
84:32 keratoplastic agents	976.4	E858.7	E946.4	E950.4	E962.0	E980.4
84:36 miscellaneous agents (skin and mucous membrane)	976.8	E858.7	E946.8	E950.4	E962.0	E980.4
86:00 spasmolytic agents	975.1	E858.6	E945.1	E950.4	E962.0	E980.4
antiasthmatics	975.7	E858.6	E945.7	E950.4	E962.0	E980.4
papaverine	972.5	E858.3	E942.5	E950.4	E962.0	E980.4
theophylline	974.1	E858.5	E944.1	E950.4	E962.0	E980.4
88:04 vitamin A	963.5	E858.1	E933.5	E950.4	E962.0	E980.4
88:08 vitamin B complex	963.5	E858.1	E933.5	E950.4	E962.0	E980.4
hematopoietic vitamin	964.1	E858.2	E934.1	E950.4	E962.0	E980.4
nicotinic acid derivatives	972.2	E858.3	E942.2	E950.4	E962.0	E980.4
88:12 vitamin C	963.5	E858.1	E933.5	E950.4	E962.0	E980.4
88:16 vitamin D	963.5	E858.1	E933.5	E950.4	E962.0	E980.4
88:20 vitamin E	963.5	E858.1	E933.5	E950.4	E962.0	E980.4
88:24 vitamin K activity	964.3	E858.2	E934.3	E950.4	E962.0	E980.4
88:28 multivitamin preparations	963.5	E858.1	E933.5	E950.4	E962.0	E980.4

Drug	Poisoning	Accident	Therapeutic Use	Suicide Attempt	Assault	Undetermined
Drug — *continued*						
92:00 unclassified therapeutic agents	977.8	E858.8	E947.8	E950.4	E962.0	E980.4
specified NEC	977.8	E858.8	E947.8	E950.4	E962.0	E980.4
Duboisine	971.1	E855.4	E941.1	E950.4	E962.0	E980.4
Dulcolax	973.1	E858.4	E943.1	E950.4	E962.0	E980.4
Duponol (C) (EP)	976.2	E858.7	E946.2	E950.4	E962.0	E980.4
Durabolin	962.1	E858.0	E932.1	E950.4	E962.0	E980.4
Dyclone	968.5	E855.2	E938.5	E950.4	E962.0	E980.4
Dyclonine	968.5	E855.2	E938.5	E950.4	E962.0	E980.4
Dydrogesterone	962.2	E858.0	E932.2	E950.4	E962.0	E980.4
Dyes NEC	989.89	E866.8	—	E950.9	E962.1	E980.9
diagnostic agents	977.8	E858.8	E947.8	E950.4	E962.0	E980.4
pharmaceutical NEC	977.4	E858.8	E947.4	E950.4	E962.0	E980.4
Dyfols	971.0	E855.3	E941.0	E950.4	E962.0	E980.4
Dymelor	962.3	E858.0	E932.3	E950.4	E962.0	E980.4
Dynamite	989.89	E866.8	—	E950.9	E962.1	E980.9
fumes	987.8	E869.8	—	E952.8	E962.2	E982.8
Dyphylline	975.1	E858.6	E945.1	E950.4	E962.0	E980.4
Ear preparations	976.6	E858.7	E946.6	E950.4	E962.0	E980.4
Echothiopate, ecothiopate	971.0	E855.3	E941.0	E950.4	E962.0	E980.4
Ecstasy	969.72	E854.2	E939.7	E950.3	E962.0	E980.3
Ectylurea	967.8	E852.8	E937.8	E950.2	E962.0	E980.2
Edathamil disodium	963.8	E858.1	E933.8	E950.4	E962.0	E980.4
Edecrin	974.4	E858.5	E944.4	E950.4	E962.0	E980.4
Edetate, disodium (calcium)	963.8	E858.1	E933.8	E950.4	E962.0	E980.4
Edrophonium	971.0	E855.3	E941.0	E950.4	E962.0	E980.4
Elase	976.8	E858.7	E946.8	E950.4	E962.0	E980.4
Elaterium	973.1	E858.4	E943.1	E950.4	E962.0	E980.4
Elder	988.2	E865.4	—	E950.9	E962.1	E980.9
berry (unripe)	988.2	E865.3	—	E950.9	E962.1	E980.9
Electrolytes NEC	974.5	E858.5	E944.5	E950.4	E962.0	E980.4
Electrolytic agent NEC	974.5	E858.5	E944.5	E950.4	E962.0	E980.4
Embramine	963.0	E858.1	E933.0	E950.4	E962.0	E980.4
Emetics	973.6	E858.4	E943.6	E950.4	E962.0	E980.4
Emetine (hydrochloride)	961.5	E857	E931.5	E950.4	E962.0	E980.4
Emollients	976.3	E858.7	E946.3	E950.4	E962.0	E980.4
Emylcamate	969.5	E853.8	E939.5	E950.3	E962.0	E980.3
Encyprate	969.09	E854.0	E939.0	E950.3	E962.0	E980.3
Endocaine	968.5	E855.2	E938.5	E950.4	E962.0	E980.4
Endrin	989.2	E863.0	—	E950.6	E962.1	E980.7
Enflurane	968.2	E855.1	E938.2	E950.4	E962.0	E980.4
Enovid	962.2	E858.0	E932.2	E950.4	E962.0	E980.4
ENT preparations (anti-infectives)	976.6	E858.7	E946.6	E950.4	E962.0	E980.4
Enzodase	963.4	E858.1	E933.4	E950.4	E962.0	E980.4
Enzymes NEC	963.4	E858.1	E933.4	E950.4	E962.0	E980.4
Epanutin	966.1	E855.0	E936.1	E950.4	E962.0	E980.4
Ephedra (tincture)	971.2	E855.5	E941.2	E950.4	E962.0	E980.4
Ephedrine	971.2	E855.5	E941.2	E950.4	E962.0	E980.4
Epiestriol	962.2	E858.0	E932.2	E950.4	E962.0	E980.4
Epilim — see Sodium valproate						
Epinephrine	971.2	E855.5	E941.2	E950.4	E962.0	E980.4
Epsom salt	973.3	E858.4	E943.3	E950.4	E962.0	E980.4
Equanil	969.5	E853.8	E939.5	E950.3	E962.0	E980.3
Equisetum (diuretic)	974.4	E858.5	E944.4	E950.4	E962.0	E980.4
Ergometrine	975.0	E858.6	E945.0	E950.4	E962.0	E980.4
Ergonovine	975.0	E858.6	E945.0	E950.4	E962.0	E980.4
Ergot NEC	988.2	E865.4	—	E950.9	E962.1	E980.9
medicinal (alkaloids)	975.0	E858.6	E945.0	E950.4	E962.0	E980.4
Ergotamine (tartrate) (for migraine) NEC	972.9	E858.3	E942.9	E950.4	E962.0	E980.4
Ergotrate	975.0	E858.6	E945.0	E950.4	E962.0	E980.4
Erythrityl tetranitrate	972.4	E858.3	E942.4	E950.4	E962.0	E980.4
Erythrol tetranitrate	972.4	E858.3	E942.4	E950.4	E962.0	E980.4
Erythromycin	960.3	E856	E930.3	E950.4	E962.0	E980.4
ophthalmic preparation	976.5	E858.7	E946.5	E950.4	E962.0	E980.4
topical NEC	976.0	E858.7	E946.0	E950.4	E962.0	E980.4
Eserine	971.0	E855.3	E941.0	E950.4	E962.0	E980.4
Eskabarb	967.0	E851	E937.0	E950.1	E962.0	E980.1
Eskalith	969.8	E855.8	E939.8	E950.3	E962.0	E980.3
Estradiol (cypionate) (dipropionate) (valerate)	962.2	E858.0	E932.2	E950.4	E962.0	E980.4
Estriol	962.2	E858.0	E932.2	E950.4	E962.0	E980.4
Estrogens (with progestogens)	962.2	E858.0	E932.2	E950.4	E962.0	E980.4
Estrone	962.2	E858.0	E932.2	E950.4	E962.0	E980.4
Etafedrine	971.2	E855.5	E941.2	E950.4	E962.0	E980.4
Ethacrynate sodium	974.4	E858.5	E944.4	E950.4	E962.0	E980.4
Ethacrynic acid	974.4	E858.5	E944.4	E950.4	E962.0	E980.4
Ethambutol	961.8	E857	E931.8	E950.4	E962.0	E980.4
Ethamide	974.2	E858.5	E944.2	E950.4	E962.0	E980.4
Ethamivan	970.0	E854.3	E940.0	E950.4	E962.0	E980.4
Ethamsylate	964.5	E858.2	E934.5	E950.4	E962.0	E980.4
Ethanol	980.0	E860.1	—	E950.9	E962.1	E980.9
beverage	980.0	E860.0	—	E950.9	E962.1	E980.9
Ethchlorvynol	967.8	E852.8	E937.8	E950.2	E962.0	E980.2
Ethebenecid	974.7	E858.5	E944.7	E950.4	E962.0	E980.4
Ether(s) (diethyl) (ethyl) (vapor)	987.8	E869.8	—	E952.8	E962.2	E982.8
anesthetic	968.2	E855.1	E938.2	E950.4	E962.0	E980.4
petroleum — see Ligroin						
solvent	982.8	E862.4	—	E950.9	E962.1	E980.9
Ethidine chloride (vapor)	987.8	E869.8	—	E952.8	E962.2	E982.8
liquid (solvent)	982.3	E862.4	—	E950.9	E962.1	E980.9
Ethinamate	967.8	E852.8	E937.8	E950.2	E962.0	E980.2
Ethinylestradiol	962.2	E858.0	E932.2	E950.4	E962.0	E980.4
Ethionamide	961.8	E857	E931.8	E950.4	E962.0	E980.4
Ethisterone	962.2	E858.0	E932.2	E950.4	E962.0	E980.4
Ethobral	967.0	E851	E937.0	E950.1	E962.0	E980.1
Ethocaine (infiltration) (topical)	968.5	E855.2	E938.5	E950.4	E962.0	E980.4
nerve block (peripheral) (plexus)	968.6	E855.2	E938.6	E950.4	E962.0	E980.4
spinal	968.7	E855.2	E938.7	E950.4	E962.0	E980.4
Ethoheptazine (citrate)	965.7	E850.7	E935.7	E950.0	E962.0	E980.0
Ethopropazine	966.4	E855.0	E936.4	E950.4	E962.0	E980.4
Ethosuximide	966.2	E855.0	E936.2	E950.4	E962.0	E980.4
Ethotoin	966.1	E855.0	E936.1	E950.4	E962.0	E980.4
Ethoxazene	961.9	E857	E931.9	E950.4	E962.0	E980.4
Ethoxzolamide	974.2	E858.5	E944.2	E950.4	E962.0	E980.4
Ethyl						
acetate (vapor)	982.8	E862.4	—	E950.9	E962.1	E980.9
alcohol	980.0	E860.1	—	E950.9	E962.1	E980.9
beverage	980.0	E860.0	—	E950.9	E962.1	E980.9
aldehyde (vapor)	987.8	E869.8	—	E952.8	E962.2	E982.8
liquid	989.89	E866.8	—	E950.9	E962.1	E980.9
aminobenzoate	968.5	E855.2	E938.5	E950.4	E962.0	E980.4
biscoumacetate	964.2	E858.2	E934.2	E950.4	E962.0	E980.4
bromide (anesthetic)	968.2	E855.1	E938.2	E950.4	E962.0	E980.4
carbamate (antineoplastic)	963.1	E858.1	E933.1	E950.4	E962.0	E980.4
carbinol	980.3	E860.4	—	E950.9	E962.1	E980.9
chaulmoograte	961.8	E857	E931.8	E950.4	E962.0	E980.4
chloride (vapor)	987.8	E869.8	—	E952.8	E962.2	E982.8
anesthetic (local)	968.5	E855.2	E938.5	E950.4	E962.0	E980.4
inhaled	968.2	E855.1	E938.2	E950.4	E962.0	E980.4
solvent	982.3	E862.4	—	E950.9	E962.1	E980.9
estranol	962.1	E858.0	E932.1	E950.4	E962.0	E980.4
ether — see Ether(s)						
formate (solvent) NEC	982.8	E862.4	—	E950.9	E962.1	E980.9
iodoacetate	987.5	E869.3	—	E952.8	E962.2	E982.8
lactate (solvent) NEC	982.8	E862.4	—	E950.9	E962.1	E980.9
methylcarbinol	980.8	E860.8	—	E950.9	E962.1	E980.9
morphine	965.09	E850.2	E935.2	E950.0	E962.0	E980.0
Ethylene (gas)	987.1	E869.8	—	E952.8	E962.2	E982.8
anesthetic (general)	968.2	E855.1	E938.2	E950.4	E962.0	E980.4
chlorohydrin (vapor)	982.3	E862.4	—	E950.9	E962.1	E980.9
dichloride (vapor)	982.3	E862.4	—	E950.9	E962.1	E980.9
glycol(s) (any) (vapor)	982.8	E862.4	—	E950.9	E962.1	E980.9
Ethylidene						
chloride NEC	982.3	E862.4	—	E950.9	E962.1	E980.9
diethyl ether	982.8	E862.4	—	E950.9	E962.1	E980.9
Ethynodiol	962.2	E858.0	E932.2	E950.4	E962.0	E980.4
Etidocaine	968.9	E855.2	E938.9	E950.4	E962.0	E980.4
infiltration (subcutaneous)	968.5	E855.2	E938.5	E950.4	E962.0	E980.4
nerve (peripheral) (plexus)	968.6	E855.2	E938.6	E950.4	E962.0	E980.4
Etilfen	967.0	E851	E937.0	E950.1	E962.0	E980.1
Etomide	965.7	E850.7	E935.7	E950.0	E962.0	E980.0
Etorphine	965.09	E850.2	E935.2	E950.0	E962.0	E980.0
Etoval	967.0	E851	E937.0	E950.1	E962.0	E980.1
Etryptamine	969.01	E854.0	E939.0	E950.3	E962.0	E980.3
Eucaine	968.5	E855.2	E938.5	E950.4	E962.0	E980.4
Eucalyptus (oil) NEC	975.5	E858.6	E945.5	E950.4	E962.0	E980.4
Eucatropine	971.1	E855.4	E941.1	E950.4	E962.0	E980.4
Eucodal	965.09	E850.2	E935.2	E950.0	E962.0	E980.0
Euneryl	967.0	E851	E937.0	E950.1	E962.0	E980.1
Euphthalmine	971.1	E855.4	E941.1	E950.4	E962.0	E980.4
Eurax	976.0	E858.7	E946.0	E950.4	E962.0	E980.4

Nontherapeutic use substance

▽ Subterms under main terms may continue to next column or page

	Poisoning	Accident	Therapeutic Use	Suicide Attempt	Assault	Undetermined
Euresol	976.4	E858.7	E946.4	E950.4	E962.0	E980.4
Euthroid	962.7	E858.0	E932.7	E950.4	E962.0	E980.4
Evans blue	977.8	E858.8	E947.8	E950.4	E962.0	E980.4
Evipal	967.0	E851	E937.0	E950.1	E962.0	E980.1
sodium	968.3	E855.1	E938.3	E950.4	E962.0	E980.4
Evipan	967.0	E851	E937.0	E950.1	E962.0	E980.1
sodium	968.3	E855.1	E938.3	E950.4	E962.0	E980.4
Exalgin	965.4	E850.4	E935.4	E950.0	E962.0	E980.0
Excipients, pharmaceutical	977.4	E858.8	E947.4	E950.4	E962.0	E980.4
Exhaust gas — see Carbon, monoxide						
Ex-Lax (phenolphthalein)	973.1	E858.4	E943.1	E950.4	E962.0	E980.4
Expectorants	975.5	E858.6	E945.5	E950.4	E962.0	E980.4
External medications (skin) (mucous membrane)	976.9	E858.7	E946.9	E950.4	E962.0	E980.4
dental agent	976.7	E858.7	E946.7	E950.4	E962.0	E980.4
ENT agent	976.6	E858.7	E946.6	E950.4	E962.0	E980.4
ophthalmic preparation	976.5	E858.7	E946.5	E950.4	E962.0	E980.4
specified NEC	976.8	E858.7	E946.8	E950.4	E962.0	E980.4
Eye agents (anti-infective)	976.5	E858.7	E946.5	E950.4	E962.0	E980.4
Factor IX complex (human)	964.5	E858.2	E934.5	E950.4	E962.0	E980.4
Fecal softeners	973.2	E858.4	E943.2	E950.4	E962.0	E980.4
Fenbutrazate	977.0	E858.8	E947.0	E950.4	E962.0	E980.4
Fencamfamin	970.89	E854.3	E940.8	E950.4	E962.0	E980.4
Fenfluramine	977.0	E858.8	E947.0	E950.4	E962.0	E980.4
Fenoprofen	965.61	E850.6	E935.6	E950.0	E962.0	E980.0
Fentanyl	965.09	E850.2	E935.2	E950.0	E962.0	E980.0
Fentazin	969.1	E853.0	E939.1	E950.3	E962.0	E980.3
Fenticlor, fentichlor	976.0	E858.7	E946.0	E950.4	E962.0	E980.4
Fer de lance (bite) (venom)	989.5	E905.0	—	E950.9	E962.1	E980.9
Ferric — see Iron						
Ferrocholinate	964.0	E858.2	E934.0	E950.4	E962.0	E980.4
Ferrous fumerate, gluconate, lactate, salt NEC, sulfate (medicinal)	964.0	E858.2	E934.0	E950.4	E962.0	E980.4
Ferrum — see Iron						
Fertilizers NEC	989.89	E866.5	—	E950.9	E962.1	E980.4
with herbicide mixture	989.4	E863.5	—	E950.6	E962.1	E980.7
Fibrinogen (human)	964.7	E858.2	E934.7	E950.4	E962.0	E980.4
Fibrinolysin	964.4	E858.2	E934.4	E950.4	E962.0	E980.4
Fibrinolysis-affecting agents	964.4	E858.2	E934.4	E950.4	E962.0	E980.4
Filix mas	961.6	E857	E931.6	E950.4	E962.0	E980.4
Fiorinal	965.1	E850.3	E935.3	E950.0	E962.0	E980.0
Fire damp	987.1	E869.8	—	E952.8	E962.2	E982.8
Fish, nonbacterial or noxious	988.0	E865.2	—	E950.9	E962.1	E980.9
shell	988.0	E865.1	—	E950.9	E962.1	E980.9
Flagyl	961.5	E857	E931.5	E950.4	E962.0	E980.4
Flavoxate	975.1	E858.6	E945.1	E950.4	E962.0	E980.4
Flaxedil	975.2	E858.6	E945.2	E950.4	E962.0	E980.4
Flaxseed (medicinal)	976.3	E858.7	E946.3	E950.4	E962.0	E980.4
Flomax	971.3	E855.6	E941.3	E950.4	E962.0	E980.4
Florantyrone	973.4	E858.4	E943.4	E950.4	E962.0	E980.4
Floraquin	961.3	E857	E931.3	E950.4	E962.0	E980.4
Florinef	962.0	E858.0	E932.0	E950.4	E962.0	E980.4
ENT agent	976.6	E858.7	E946.6	E950.4	E962.0	E980.4
ophthalmic preparation	976.5	E858.7	E946.5	E950.4	E962.0	E980.4
topical NEC	976.0	E858.7	E946.0	E950.4	E962.0	E980.4
Flowers of sulfur	976.4	E858.7	E946.4	E950.4	E962.0	E980.4
Floxuridine	963.1	E858.1	E933.1	E950.4	E962.0	E980.4
Flucytosine	961.9	E857	E931.9	E950.4	E962.0	E980.4
Fludrocortisone	962.0	E858.0	E932.0	E950.4	E962.0	E980.4
ENT agent	976.6	E858.7	E946.6	E950.4	E962.0	E980.4
ophthalmic preparation	976.5	E858.7	E946.5	E950.4	E962.0	E980.4
topical NEC	976.0	E858.7	E946.0	E950.4	E962.0	E980.4
Flumethasone	976.0	E858.7	E946.0	E950.4	E962.0	E980.4
Flumethiazide	974.3	E858.5	E944.3	E950.4	E962.0	E980.4
Flumidin	961.7	E857	E931.7	E950.4	E962.0	E980.4
Flunitrazepam	969.4	E853.2	E939.4	E950.3	E962.0	E980.3
Fluocinolone	976.0	E858.7	E946.0	E950.4	E962.0	E980.4
Fluocortolone	962.0	E858.0	E932.0	E950.4	E962.0	E980.4
Fluohydrocortisone	962.0	E858.0	E932.0	E950.4	E962.0	E980.4
ENT agent	976.6	E858.7	E946.6	E950.4	E962.0	E980.4
ophthalmic preparation	976.5	E858.7	E946.5	E950.4	E962.0	E980.4
topical NEC	976.0	E858.7	E946.0	E950.4	E962.0	E980.4
Fluonid	976.0	E858.7	E946.0	E950.4	E962.0	E980.4
Fluopromazine	969.1	E853.0	E939.1	E950.3	E962.0	E980.3

	Poisoning	Accident	Therapeutic Use	Suicide Attempt	Assault	Undetermined
Fluoracetate	989.4	E863.7	—	E950.6	E962.1	E980.7
Fluorescein (sodium)	977.8	E858.8	E947.8	E950.4	E962.0	E980.4
Fluoride(s) (pesticides) (sodium) NEC	989.4	E863.4	—	E950.6	E962.1	E980.7
hydrogen — see Hydrofluoric acid						
medicinal	976.7	E858.7	E946.7	E950.4	E962.0	E980.4
not pesticide NEC	983.9	E864.4	—	E950.7	E962.1	E980.6
stannous	976.7	E858.7	E946.7	E950.4	E962.0	E980.4
Fluorinated corticosteroids	962.0	E858.0	E932.0	E950.4	E962.0	E980.4
Fluorine (compounds) (gas)	987.8	E869.8	—	E952.8	E962.2	E982.8
salt — see Fluoride(s)						
Fluoristan	976.7	E858.7	E946.7	E950.4	E962.0	E980.4
Fluoroacetate	989.4	E863.7	—	E950.6	E962.1	E980.7
Fluorodeoxyuridine	963.1	E858.1	E933.1	E950.4	E962.0	E980.4
Fluorometholone (topical) NEC	976.0	E858.7	E946.0	E950.4	E962.0	E980.4
ophthalmic preparation	976.5	E858.7	E946.5	E950.4	E962.0	E980.4
Fluorouracil	963.1	E858.1	E933.1	E950.4	E962.0	E980.4
Fluothane	968.1	E855.1	E938.1	E950.4	E962.0	E980.4
Fluoxetine hydrochloride	969.03	E854.0	E939.0	E950.3	E962.0	E980.3
Fluoxymesterone	962.1	E858.0	E932.1	E950.4	E962.0	E980.4
Fluphenazine	969.1	E853.0	E939.1	E950.3	E962.0	E980.3
Fluprednisolone	962.0	E858.0	E932.0	E950.4	E962.0	E980.4
Flurandrenolide	976.0	E858.7	E946.0	E950.4	E962.0	E980.4
Flurazepam (hydrochloride)	969.4	E853.2	E939.4	E950.3	E962.0	E980.3
Flurbiprofen	965.61	E850.6	E935.6	E950.0	E962.0	E980.0
Flurobate	976.0	E858.7	E946.0	E950.4	E962.0	E980.4
Flurothyl	969.8	E855.8	E939.8	E950.3	E962.0	E980.3
Fluroxene	968.2	E855.1	E938.2	E950.4	E962.0	E980.4
Folacin	964.1	E858.2	E934.1	E950.4	E962.0	E980.4
Folic acid	964.1	E858.2	E934.1	E950.4	E962.0	E980.4
Follicle stimulating hormone	962.4	E858.0	E932.4	E950.4	E962.0	E980.4
Food, foodstuffs, nonbacterial or noxious	988.9	E865.9	—	E950.9	E962.1	E980.9
berries, seeds	988.2	E865.3	—	E950.9	E962.1	E980.9
fish	988.0	E865.2	—	E950.9	E962.1	E980.9
mushrooms	988.1	E865.5	—	E950.9	E962.1	E980.9
plants	988.2	E865.9	—	E950.9	E962.1	E980.9
specified type NEC	988.2	E865.4	—	E950.9	E962.1	E980.9
shellfish	988.0	E865.1	—	E950.9	E962.1	E980.9
specified NEC	988.8	E865.8	—	E950.9	E962.1	E980.9
Fool's parsley	988.2	E865.4	—	E950.9	E962.1	E980.9
Formaldehyde (solution)	989.89	E861.4	—	E950.9	E962.1	E980.9
fungicide	989.4	E863.6	—	E950.6	E962.1	E980.7
gas or vapor	987.8	E869.8	—	E952.8	E962.2	E982.8
Formalin	989.89	E861.4	—	E950.9	E962.1	E980.9
fungicide	989.4	E863.6	—	E950.6	E962.1	E980.7
vapor	987.8	E869.8	—	E952.8	E962.2	E982.8
Formic acid	983.1	E864.1	—	E950.7	E962.1	E980.6
automobile	981	E862.1	—	E950.9	E962.1	E980.9
exhaust gas, not in transit	986	E868.2	—	E952.0	E962.2	E982.0
vapor NEC	987.1	E869.8	—	E952.8	E962.2	E982.8
gas (domestic use) (see also Carbon, monoxide, fuel)						
utility	987.1	E868.1	—	E951.8	E962.2	E981.8
incomplete combustion of — see Carbon, monoxide, fuel, utility						
in mobile container	987.0	E868.0	—	E951.1	E962.2	E981.1
piped (natural)	987.1	E867	—	E951.0	E962.2	E981.0
industrial, incomplete combustion	986	E868.3	—	E952.1	E962.2	E982.1
vapor	987.8	E869.8	—	E952.8	E962.2	E982.8
Fowler's solution	985.1	E866.3	—	E950.8	E962.1	E980.8
Foxglove	988.2	E865.4	—	E950.9	E962.1	E980.9
Fox green	977.8	E858.8	E947.8	E950.4	E962.0	E980.4
Framycetin	960.8	E856	E930.8	E950.4	E962.0	E980.4
Frangula (extract)	973.1	E858.4	E943.1	E950.4	E962.0	E980.4
Frei antigen	977.8	E858.8	E947.8	E950.4	E962.0	E980.4
Freons	987.4	E869.2	—	E952.8	E962.2	E982.8
Fructose	974.5	E858.5	E944.5	E950.4	E962.0	E980.4
Frusemide	974.4	E858.5	E944.4	E950.4	E962.0	E980.4
FSH	962.4	E858.0	E932.4	E950.4	E962.0	E980.4
Fuel						
Fugillin	960.8	E856	E930.8	E950.4	E962.0	E980.4

	External Cause (E-Code)					
	Poisoning	Accident	Therapeutic Use	Suicide Attempt	Assault	Undetermined
Fulminate of mercury	985.0	E866.1	—	E950.9	E962.1	E980.9
Fulvicin	960.1	E856	E930.1	E950.4	E962.0	E980.4
Fumadil	960.8	E856	E930.8	E950.4	E962.0	E980.4
Fumagillin	960.8	E856	E930.8	E950.4	E962.0	E980.4
Fumes (from)	987.9	E869.9	—	E952.9	E962.2	E982.9
carbon monoxide — see Carbon, monoxide						
charcoal (domestic use)	986	E868.3	—	E952.1	E962.2	E982.1
chloroform — see Chloroform						
coke (in domestic stoves, fireplaces)	986	E868.3	—	E952.1	E962.2	E982.1
corrosive NEC	987.8	E869.8	—	E952.8	E962.2	E982.8
ether — see Ether(s)						
freons	987.4	E869.2	—	E952.8	E962.2	E982.8
hydrocarbons	987.1	E869.8	—	E952.8	E962.2	E982.8
petroleum (liquefied)	987.0	E868.0	—	E951.1	E962.2	E981.1
distributed through pipes (pure or mixed with air)	987.0	E867	—	E951.0	E962.2	E981.0
lead — see Lead						
metals — see specified metal						
nitrogen dioxide	987.2	E869.0	—	E952.8	E962.2	E982.8
pesticides — see Pesticides						
petroleum (liquefied)	987.0	E868.0	—	E951.1	E962.2	E981.1
distributed through pipes (pure or mixed with air)	987.0	E867	—	E951.0	E962.2	E981.0
polyester	987.8	E869.8	—	E952.8	E962.2	E982.8
specified, source other (see also substance specified)	987.8	E869.8	—	E952.8	E962.2	E982.8
sulfur dioxide	987.3	E869.1	—	E952.8	E962.2	E982.8
Fumigants	989.4	E863.8	—	E950.6	E962.1	E980.7
Fungicides — see also Antifungals	989.4	E863.6	—	E950.6	E962.1	E980.7
Fungi, noxious, used as food	988.1	E865.5	—	E950.9	E962.1	E980.9
Fungizone	960.1	E856	E930.1	E950.4	E962.0	E980.4
topical	976.0	E858.7	E946.0	E950.4	E962.0	E980.4
Furacin	976.0	E858.7	E946.0	E950.4	E962.0	E980.4
Furadantin	961.9	E857	E931.9	E950.4	E962.0	E980.4
Furazolidone	961.9	E857	E931.9	E950.4	E962.0	E980.4
Furnace (coal burning) (domestic), gas from	986	E868.3	—	E952.1	E962.2	E982.1
industrial	986	E868.8	—	E952.1	E962.2	E982.1
Furniture polish	989.89	E861.2	—	E950.9	E962.1	E980.9
Furosemide	974.4	E858.5	E944.4	E950.4	E962.0	E980.4
Furoxone	961.9	E857	E931.9	E950.4	E962.0	E980.4
Fusel oil (amyl) (butyl) (propyl)	980.3	E860.4	—	E950.9	E962.1	E980.9
Fusidic acid	960.8	E856	E930.8	E950.4	E962.0	E980.4
Gallamine	975.2	E858.6	E945.2	E950.4	E962.0	E980.4
Gallotannic acid	976.2	E858.7	E946.2	E950.4	E962.0	E980.4
Gamboge	973.1	E858.4	E943.1	E950.4	E962.0	E980.4
Gamimune	964.6	E858.2	E934.6	E950.4	E962.0	E980.4
Gamma-benzene hexachloride (vapor)	989.2	E863.0	—	E950.6	E962.1	E980.7
Gamma globulin	964.6	E858.2	E934.6	E950.4	E962.0	E980.4
Gamma hydroxy butyrate (GHB)	968.4	E855.1	E938.4	E950.4	E962.0	E980.4
Gamulin	964.6	E858.2	E934.6	E950.4	E962.0	E980.4
Ganglionic blocking agents	972.3	E858.3	E942.3	E950.4	E962.0	E980.4
Ganja	969.6	E854.1	E939.6	E950.3	E962.0	E980.3
Garamycin	960.8	E856	E930.8	E950.4	E962.0	E980.4
ophthalmic preparation	976.5	E858.7	E946.5	E950.4	E962.0	E980.4
topical NEC	976.0	E858.7	E946.0	E950.4	E962.0	E980.4
Gardenal	967.0	E851	E937.0	E950.1	E962.0	E980.1
Gardepanyl	967.0	E851	E937.0	E950.1	E962.0	E980.1
Gas	987.9	E869.9	—	E952.9	E962.2	E982.9
acetylene	987.1	E868.1	—	E951.8	E962.2	E981.8
incomplete combustion of — see Carbon, monoxide, fuel, utility						
air contaminants, source or type not specified	987.9	E869.9	—	E952.9	E962.2	E982.9
anesthetic (general) NEC	968.2	E855.1	E938.2	E950.4	E962.0	E980.4
blast furnace	986	E868.8	—	E952.1	E962.2	E982.1
butane — see Butane						
carbon monoxide — see Carbon, monoxide						

	External Cause (E-Code)					
	Poisoning	Accident	Therapeutic Use	Suicide Attempt	Assault	Undetermined
Gas — continued						
chlorine	987.6	E869.8	—	E952.8	E962.2	E982.8
coal — see Carbon, monoxide, coal						
cyanide	987.7	E869.8	—	E952.8	E962.2	E982.8
dicyanogen	987.8	E869.8	—	E952.8	E962.2	E982.8
domestic — see Gas, utility						
exhaust — see Carbon, monoxide, exhaust gas						
from wood- or coal-burning stove or fireplace	986	E868.3	—	E952.1	E962.2	E982.1
fuel (domestic use) (see also Carbon, monoxide, fuel)						
industrial use	986	E868.8	—	E952.1	E962.2	E982.1
utility	987.1	E868.1	—	E951.8	E962.2	E981.8
incomplete combustion of — see Carbon, monoxide, fuel, utility						
in mobile container	987.0	E868.0	—	E951.1	E962.2	E981.1
piped (natural)	987.1	E867	—	E951.0	E962.2	E981.0
garage	986	E868.2	—	E952.0	E962.2	E982.0
hydrocarbon NEC	987.1	E869.8	—	E952.8	E962.2	E982.8
incomplete combustion of — see Carbon, monoxide, fuel, utility						
liquefied (mobile container)	987.0	E868.0	—	E951.1	E962.2	E981.1
piped	987.0	E867	—	E951.0	E962.2	E981.0
hydrocyanic acid	987.7	E869.8	—	E952.8	E962.2	E982.8
illuminating — see Gas, utility						
incomplete combustion, any — see Carbon, monoxide						
kiln	986	E868.8	—	E952.1	E962.2	E982.1
lacrimogenic	987.5	E869.3	—	E952.8	E962.2	E982.8
marsh	987.1	E869.8	—	E952.8	E962.2	E982.8
motor exhaust, not in transit	986	E868.8	—	E952.1	E962.2	E982.1
mustard — see Mustard, gas						
natural	987.1	E867	—	E951.0	E962.2	E981.0
nerve (war)	987.9	E869.9	—	E952.9	E962.2	E982.9
oils	981	E862.1	—	E950.9	E962.1	E980.9
petroleum (liquefied) (distributed in mobile containers)	987.0	E868.0	—	E951.1	E962.2	E981.1
piped (pure or mixed with air)	987.0	E867	—	E951.1	E962.2	E981.1
piped (manufactured) (natural) NEC	987.1	E867	—	E951.0	E962.2	E981.0
producer	986	E868.8	—	E952.1	E962.2	E982.1
propane — see Propane						
refrigerant (freon)	987.4	E869.2	—	E952.8	E962.2	E982.8
not freon	987.9	E869.9	—	E952.9	E962.2	E982.9
sewer	987.8	E869.8	—	E952.8	E962.2	E982.8
specified source NEC (see also substance specified)	987.8	E869.8	—	E952.8	E962.2	E982.8
stove — see Gas, utility						
tear	987.5	E869.3	—	E952.8	E962.2	E982.8
utility (for cooking, heating, or lighting) (piped) NEC	987.1	E868.1	—	E951.8	E962.2	E981.8
incomplete combustion of — see Carbon, monoxide, fuel, utility						
in mobile container	987.0	E868.0	—	E951.1	E962.2	E981.1
piped (natural)	987.1	E867	—	E951.0	E962.2	E981.0
water	987.1	E868.1	—	E951.8	E962.2	E981.8
incomplete combustion of — see Carbon, monoxide, fuel, utility						
Gaseous substance — see Gas						
Gasoline, gasolene	981	E862.1	—	E950.9	E962.1	E980.9
vapor	987.1	E869.8	—	E952.8	E962.2	E982.8
Gastric enzymes	973.4	E858.4	E943.4	E950.4	E962.0	E980.4
Gastrografin	977.8	E858.8	E947.8	E950.4	E962.0	E980.4
Gastrointestinal agents	973.9	E858.4	E943.9	E950.4	E962.0	E980.4
specified NEC	973.8	E858.4	E943.8	E950.4	E962.0	E980.4
Gaultheria procumbens	988.2	E865.4	—	E950.9	E962.1	E980.9
Gelatin (intravenous)	964.8	E858.2	E934.8	E950.4	E962.0	E980.4
absorbable (sponge)	964.5	E858.2	E934.5	E950.4	E962.0	E980.4
Gelfilm	976.8	E858.7	E946.8	E950.4	E962.0	E980.4
Gelfoam	964.5	E858.2	E934.5	E950.4	E962.0	E980.4

■ Nontherapeutic use substance

▼ Subterms under main terms may continue to next column or page

Substance	Poisoning	Accident	Therapeutic Use	Suicide Attempt	Assault	Undetermined
Gelsemine	970.89	E854.3	E940.8	E950.4	E962.0	E980.4
Gelsemium (semper-virens)	988.2	E865.4	—	E950.9	E962.1	E980.9
Gemonil	967.0	E851	E937.0	E950.1	E962.0	E980.1
Gentamicin	960.8	E856	E930.8	E950.4	E962.0	E980.4
ophthalmic preparation	976.5	E858.7	E946.5	E950.4	E962.0	E980.4
topical NEC	976.0	E858.7	E946.0	E950.4	E962.0	E980.4
Gentian violet	976.0	E858.7	E946.0	E950.4	E962.0	E980.4
Gexane	976.0	E858.7	E946.0	E950.4	E962.0	E980.4
Gila monster (venom)	989.5	E905.0	—	E950.9	E962.1	E980.9
Ginger, Jamaica	989.89	E866.8	—	E950.9	E962.1	E980.9
Gitalin	972.1	E858.3	E942.1	E950.4	E962.0	E980.4
Gitoxin	972.1	E858.3	E942.1	E950.4	E962.0	E980.4
Glandular extract (medicinal) NEC	977.9	E858.9	E947.9	E950.5	E962.0	E980.5
Glaucarubin	961.5	E857	E931.5	E950.4	E962.0	E980.4
Globin zinc insulin	962.3	E858.0	E932.3	E950.4	E962.0	E980.4
Glucagon	962.3	E858.0	E932.3	E950.4	E962.0	E980.4
Glucochloral	967.1	E852.0	E937.1	E950.2	E962.0	E980.2
Glucocorticoids	962.0	E858.0	E932.0	E950.4	E962.0	E980.4
Glucose	974.5	E858.5	E944.5	E950.4	E962.0	E980.4
oxidase reagent	977.8	E858.8	E947.8	E950.4	E962.0	E980.4
Glucosulfone sodium	961.8	E857	E931.8	E950.4	E962.0	E980.4
Glue(s)	989.89	E866.6	—	E950.9	E962.1	E980.9
Glutamic acid (hydrochloride)	973.4	E858.4	E943.4	E950.4	E962.0	E980.4
Glutaraldehyde	989.89	E861.4	—	E950.9	E962.1	E980.9
Glutathione	963.8	E858.1	E933.8	E950.4	E962.0	E980.4
Glutethimide (group)	967.5	E852.4	E937.5	E950.2	E962.0	E980.2
Glycerin (lotion)	976.3	E858.7	E946.3	E950.4	E962.0	E980.4
Glycerol (topical)	976.3	E858.7	E946.3	E950.4	E962.0	E980.4
Glyceryl						
guaiacolate	975.5	E858.6	E945.5	E950.4	E962.0	E980.4
triacetate (topical)	976.0	E858.7	E946.0	E950.4	E962.0	E980.4
trinitrate	972.4	E858.3	E942.4	E950.4	E962.0	E980.4
Glycine	974.5	E858.5	E944.5	E950.4	E962.0	E980.4
Glycobiarsol	961.1	E857	E931.1	E950.4	E962.0	E980.4
Glycols (ether)	982.8	E862.4	—	E950.9	E962.1	E980.9
Glycopyrrolate	971.1	E855.4	E941.1	E950.4	E962.0	E980.4
Glymidine	962.3	E858.0	E932.3	E950.4	E962.0	E980.4
Gold (compounds) (salts)	965.69	E850.6	E935.6	E950.0	E962.0	E980.0
Golden sulfide of antimony	985.4	E866.2	—	E950.9	E962.1	E980.9
Goldylocks	988.2	E865.4	—	E950.9	E962.1	E980.9
Gonadal tissue extract	962.9	E858.0	E932.9	E950.4	E962.0	E980.4
female	962.2	E858.0	E932.2	E950.4	E962.0	E980.4
male	962.1	E858.0	E932.1	E950.4	E962.0	E980.4
Gonadotropin	962.4	E858.0	E932.4	E950.4	E962.0	E980.4
Grain alcohol	980.0	E860.1	—	E950.9	E962.1	E980.9
beverage	980.0	E860.0	—	E950.9	E962.1	E980.9
Gramicidin	960.8	E856	E930.8	E950.4	E962.0	E980.4
Gratiola officinalis	988.2	E865.4	—	E950.9	E962.1	E980.9
Grease	989.89	E866.8	—	E950.9	E962.1	E980.9
Green hellebore	988.2	E865.4	—	E950.9	E962.1	E980.9
Green soap	976.2	E858.7	E946.2	E950.4	E962.0	E980.4
Grifulvin	960.1	E856	E930.1	E950.4	E962.0	E980.4
Griseofulvin	960.1	E856	E930.1	E950.4	E962.0	E980.4
Growth hormone	962.4	E858.0	E932.4	E950.4	E962.0	E980.4
Guaiacol	975.5	E858.6	E945.5	E950.4	E962.0	E980.4
Guaiac reagent	977.8	E858.8	E947.8	E950.4	E962.0	E980.4
Guaifenesin	975.5	E858.6	E945.5	E950.4	E962.0	E980.4
Guaiphenesin	975.5	E858.6	E945.5	E950.4	E962.0	E980.4
Guanatol	961.4	E857	E931.4	E950.4	E962.0	E980.4
Guanethidine	972.6	E858.3	E942.6	E950.4	E962.0	E980.4
Guano	989.89	E866.5	—	E950.9	E962.1	E980.9
Guanochlor	972.6	E858.3	E942.6	E950.4	E962.0	E980.4
Guanoctine	972.6	E858.3	E942.6	E950.4	E962.0	E980.4
Guanoxan	972.6	E858.3	E942.6	E950.4	E962.0	E980.4
Hair treatment agent NEC	976.4	E858.7	E946.4	E950.4	E962.0	E980.4
Halcinonide	976.0	E858.7	E946.0	E950.4	E962.0	E980.4
Halethazole	976.0	E858.7	E946.0	E950.4	E962.0	E980.4
Hallucinogens	969.6	E854.1	E939.6	E950.3	E962.0	E980.3
Haloperidol	969.2	E853.1	E939.2	E950.3	E962.0	E980.3
Haloprogin	976.0	E858.7	E946.0	E950.4	E962.0	E980.4
Halotex	976.0	E858.7	E946.0	E950.4	E962.0	E980.4
Halothane	968.1	E855.1	E938.1	E950.4	E962.0	E980.4
Halquinols	976.0	E858.7	E946.0	E950.4	E962.0	E980.4
Hand sanitizer	976.0	E858.7	E946.0	E950.4	E962.0	E980.4
Harmonyl	972.6	E858.3	E942.6	E950.4	E962.0	E980.4
Hartmann's solution	974.5	E858.5	E944.5	E950.4	E962.0	E980.4
Hashish	969.6	E854.1	E939.6	E950.3	E962.0	E980.3
Hawaiian wood rose seeds	969.6	E854.1	E939.6	E950.3	E962.0	E980.3
Headache cures, drugs, powders NEC	977.9	E858.9	E947.9	E950.5	E962.0	E980.9
Heavenly Blue (morning glory)	969.6	E854.1	E939.6	E950.3	E962.0	E980.3
Heavy metal antagonists	963.8	E858.1	E933.8	E950.4	E962.0	E980.4
anti-infectives	961.2	E857	E931.2	E950.4	E962.0	E980.4
Hedaquinium	976.0	E858.7	E946.0	E950.4	E962.0	E980.4
Hedge hyssop	988.2	E865.4	—	E950.9	E962.1	E980.9
Heet	976.8	E858.7	E946.8	E950.4	E962.0	E980.4
Helenin	961.6	E857	E931.6	E950.4	E962.0	E980.4
Hellebore (black) (green) (white)	988.2	E865.4	—	E950.9	E962.1	E980.9
Hemlock	988.2	E865.4	—	E950.9	E962.1	E980.9
Hemostatics	964.5	E858.2	E934.5	E950.4	E962.0	E980.4
capillary active drugs	972.8	E858.3	E942.8	E950.4	E962.0	E980.4
Henbane	988.2	E865.4	—	E950.9	E962.1	E980.9
Heparin (sodium)	964.2	E858.2	E934.2	E950.4	E962.0	E980.4
Heptabarbital, heptabarbitone	967.0	E851	E937.0	E950.1	E962.0	E980.1
Heptachlor	989.2	E863.0	—	E950.6	E962.1	E980.7
Heptalgin	965.09	E850.2	E935.2	E950.0	E962.0	E980.0
Herbicides	989.4	E863.5	—	E950.6	E962.1	E980.7
Heroin	965.01	E850.0	E935.0	E950.0	E962.0	E980.0
Herplex	976.5	E858.7	E946.5	E950.4	E962.0	E980.4
HES	964.8	E858.2	E934.8	E950.4	E962.0	E980.4
Hetastarch	964.8	E858.2	E934.8	E950.4	E962.0	E980.4
Hexachlorocyclohexane	989.2	E863.0	—	E950.6	E962.1	E980.7
Hexachlorophene	976.2	E858.7	E946.2	E950.4	E962.0	E980.4
Hexadimethrine (bromide)	964.5	E858.2	E934.5	E950.4	E962.0	E980.4
Hexafluorenium	975.2	E858.6	E945.2	E950.4	E962.0	E980.4
Hexa-germ	976.2	E858.7	E946.2	E950.4	E962.0	E980.4
Hexahydrophenol	980.8	E860.8	—	E950.9	E962.1	E980.9
Hexalin	980.8	E860.8	—	E950.9	E962.1	E980.9
Hexamethonium	972.3	E858.3	E942.3	E950.4	E962.0	E980.4
Hexamethyleneamine	961.9	E857	E931.9	E950.4	E962.0	E980.4
Hexamine	961.9	E857	E931.9	E950.4	E962.0	E980.4
Hexanone	982.8	E862.4	—	E950.9	E962.1	E980.9
Hexapropymate	967.8	E852.8	E937.8	E950.2	E962.0	E980.2
Hexestrol	962.2	E858.0	E932.2	E950.4	E962.0	E980.4
Hexethal (sodium)	967.0	E851	E937.0	E950.1	E962.0	E980.1
Hexetidine	976.0	E858.7	E946.0	E950.4	E962.0	E980.4
Hexobarbital, hexobarbitone	967.0	E851	E937.0	E950.1	E962.0	E980.1
sodium (anesthetic)	968.3	E855.1	E938.3	E950.4	E962.0	E980.4
soluble	968.3	E855.1	E938.3	E950.4	E962.0	E980.4
Hexocyclium	971.1	E855.4	E941.1	E950.4	E962.0	E980.4
Hexoestrol	962.2	E858.0	E932.2	E950.4	E962.0	E980.4
Hexone	982.8	E862.4	—	E950.9	E962.1	E980.9
Hexylcaine	968.5	E855.2	E938.5	E950.4	E962.0	E980.4
Hexylresorcinol	961.6	E857	E931.6	E950.4	E962.0	E980.4
Hinkle's pills	973.1	E858.4	E943.1	E950.4	E962.0	E980.4
Histalog	977.8	E858.8	E947.8	E950.4	E962.0	E980.4
Histamine (phosphate)	972.5	E858.3	E942.5	E950.4	E962.0	E980.4
Histoplasmin	977.8	E858.8	E947.8	E950.4	E962.0	E980.4
Holly berries	988.2	E865.3	—	E950.9	E962.1	E980.9
Homatropine	971.1	E855.4	E941.1	E950.4	E962.0	E980.4
Homo-tet	964.6	E858.2	E934.6	E950.4	E962.0	E980.4
Hormones (synthetic substitute) NEC	962.9	E858.0	E932.9	E950.4	E962.0	E980.4
adrenal cortical steroids	962.0	E858.0	E932.0	E950.4	E962.0	E980.4
antidiabetic agents	962.3	E858.0	E932.3	E950.4	E962.0	E980.4
follicle stimulating	962.4	E858.0	E932.4	E950.4	E962.0	E980.4
gonadotropic	962.4	E858.0	E932.4	E950.4	E962.0	E980.4
growth	962.4	E858.0	E932.4	E950.4	E962.0	E980.4
ovarian (substitutes)	962.2	E858.0	E932.2	E950.4	E962.0	E980.4
parathyroid (derivatives)	962.6	E858.0	E932.6	E950.4	E962.0	E980.4
pituitary (posterior)	962.5	E858.0	E932.5	E950.4	E962.0	E980.4
anterior	962.4	E858.0	E932.4	E950.4	E962.0	E980.4
thyroid (derivative)	962.7	E858.0	E932.7	E950.4	E962.0	E980.4
Hornet (sting)	989.5	E905.3	—	E950.9	E962.1	E980.9
Horticulture agent NEC	989.4	E863.9	—	E950.6	E962.1	E980.7
Hyaluronidase	963.4	E858.1	E933.4	E950.4	E962.0	E980.4
Hyazyme	963.4	E858.1	E933.4	E950.4	E962.0	E980.4
Hycodan	965.09	E850.2	E935.2	E950.0	E962.0	E980.0
Hydantoin derivatives	966.1	E855.0	E936.1	E950.4	E962.0	E980.4
Hydeltra	962.0	E858.0	E932.0	E950.4	E962.0	E980.4
Hydergine	971.3	E855.6	E941.3	E950.4	E962.0	E980.4
Hydrabamine penicillin	960.0	E856	E930.0	E950.4	E962.0	E980.4

Nontherapeutic use substance

316 — Volume 2 · ▶◄ Revised Text · ● New Line · ▲ Revised Code · Subterms under main terms may continue to next column or page · 2013 ICD-9-CM

	Poisoning	External Cause (E-Code)				
		Accident	Therapeutic Use	Suicide Attempt	Assault	Undetermined
Hydralazine, hydral- lazine	972.6	E858.3	E942.6	E950.4	E962.0	E980.4
Hydrargaphen	976.0	E858.7	E946.0	E950.4	E962.0	E980.4
Hydrazine	983.9	E864.3	—	E950.7	E962.1	E980.6
Hydriodic acid	975.5	E858.6	E945.5	E950.4	E962.0	E980.4
Hydrocarbon gas	987.1	E869.8	—	E952.8	E962.2	E982.8
incomplete combustion of — see Carbon, monoxide, fu- el, utility						
liquefied (mobile contain- er)	987.0	E868.0	—	E951.1	E962.2	E981.1
piped (natural)	987.0	E867	—	E951.0	E962.2	E981.0
Hydrochloric acid (liquid)	983.1	E864.1	—	E950.7	E962.1	E980.6
medicinal	973.4	E858.4	E943.4	E950.4	E962.0	E980.4
vapor	987.8	E869.8	—	E952.8	E962.2	E982.8
Hydrochlorothiazide	974.3	E858.5	E944.3	E950.4	E962.0	E980.4
Hydrocodone	965.09	E850.2	E935.2	E950.0	E962.0	E980.0
Hydrocortisone	962.0	E858.0	E932.0	E950.4	E962.0	E980.4
ENT agent	976.6	E858.7	E946.6	E950.4	E962.0	E980.4
ophthalmic preparation	976.5	E858.7	E946.5	E950.4	E962.0	E980.4
topical NEC	976.0	E858.7	E946.0	E950.4	E962.0	E980.4
Hydrocortone	962.0	E858.0	E932.0	E950.4	E962.0	E980.4
ENT agent	976.6	E858.7	E946.6	E950.4	E962.0	E980.4
ophthalmic preparation	976.5	E858.7	E946.5	E950.4	E962.0	E980.4
topical NEC	976.0	E858.7	E946.0	E950.4	E962.0	E980.4
Hydrocyanic acid — see Cyanide(s)						
Hydroflumethiazide	974.3	E858.5	E944.3	E950.4	E962.0	E980.4
Hydrofluoric acid (liquid)	983.1	E864.1	—	E950.7	E962.1	E980.6
vapor	987.8	E869.8	—	E952.8	E962.2	E982.8
Hydrogen	987.8	E869.8	—	E952.8	E962.2	E982.8
arsenide	985.1	E866.3	—	E950.8	E962.1	E980.8
arseniureted	985.1	E866.3	—	E950.8	E962.1	E980.8
cyanide (salts)	989.0	E866.8	—	E950.9	E962.1	E980.9
gas	987.1	E869.8	—	E952.8	E962.2	E982.8
fluoride (liquid)	983.1	E864.1	—	E950.7	E962.1	E980.6
vapor	987.8	E869.8	—	E952.8	E962.2	E982.8
peroxide (solution)	976.6	E858.7	E946.6	E950.4	E962.0	E980.4
phosphureted	987.8	E869.8	—	E952.8	E962.2	E982.8
sulfide (gas)	987.8	E869.8	—	E952.8	E962.2	E982.8
arseniureted	985.1	E866.3	—	E950.8	E962.1	E980.8
sulfureted	987.8	E869.8	—	E952.8	E962.2	E982.8
Hydromorphinol	965.09	E850.2	E935.2	E950.0	E962.0	E980.0
Hydromorphinone	965.09	E850.2	E935.2	E950.0	E962.0	E980.0
Hydromorphone	965.09	E850.2	E935.2	E950.0	E962.0	E980.0
Hydromox	974.3	E858.5	E944.3	E950.4	E962.0	E980.4
Hydrophilic lotion	976.3	E858.7	E946.3	E950.4	E962.0	E980.4
Hydroquinone	983.0	E864.0	—	E950.7	E962.1	E980.6
vapor	987.8	E869.8	—	E952.8	E962.2	E982.8
Hydrosulfuric acid (gas)	987.8	E869.8	—	E952.8	E962.2	E982.8
Hydrous wool fat (lotion)	976.3	E858.7	E946.3	E950.4	E962.0	E980.4
Hydroxide, caustic	983.2	E864.2	—	E950.7	E962.1	E980.6
Hydroxocobalamin	964.1	E858.2	E934.1	E950.4	E962.0	E980.4
Hydroxyamphetamine	971.2	E855.5	E941.2	E950.4	E962.0	E980.4
Hydroxychloroquine	961.4	E857	E931.4	E950.4	E962.0	E980.4
Hydroxydihy- drocodeinone	965.09	E850.2	E935.2	E950.0	E962.0	E980.0
Hydroxyethyl starch	964.8	E858.2	E934.8	E950.4	E962.0	E980.4
Hydroxyphenamate	969.5	E853.8	E939.5	E950.3	E962.0	E980.3
Hydroxyphenylbutazone	965.5	E850.5	E935.5	E950.0	E962.0	E980.0
Hydroxyprogesterone	962.2	E858.0	E932.2	E950.4	E962.0	E980.4
Hydroxyquinoline deriva- tives	961.3	E857	E931.3	E950.4	E962.0	E980.4
Hydroxystilbamidine	961.5	E857	E931.5	E950.4	E962.0	E980.4
Hydroxyurea	963.1	E858.1	E933.1	E950.4	E962.0	E980.4
Hydroxyzine	969.5	E853.8	E939.5	E950.3	E962.0	E980.3
Hyoscine (hydrobromide)	971.1	E855.4	E941.1	E950.4	E962.0	E980.4
Hyoscyamine	971.1	E855.4	E941.1	E950.4	E962.0	E980.4
Hyoscyamus (albus) (niger)	988.2	E865.4	—	E950.9	E962.1	E980.9
Hypaque	977.8	E858.8	E947.8	E950.4	E962.0	E980.4
Hypertussis	964.6	E858.2	E934.6	E950.4	E962.0	E980.4
Hypnotics NEC	967.9	E852.9	E937.9	E950.2	E962.0	E980.2
Hypochlorites — see Sodium, hypochlorite						
Hypotensive agents NEC	972.6	E858.3	E942.6	E950.4	E962.0	E980.4
Ibufenac	965.69	E850.6	E935.6	E950.0	E962.0	E980.0
Ibuprofen	965.61	E850.6	E935.6	E950.0	E962.0	E980.0
ICG	977.8	E858.8	E947.8	E950.4	E962.0	E980.4
Ichthammol	976.4	E858.7	E946.4	E950.4	E962.0	E980.4
Ichthyol	976.4	E858.7	E946.4	E950.4	E962.0	E980.4
Idoxuridine	976.5	E858.7	E946.5	E950.4	E962.0	E980.4

	Poisoning	External Cause (E-Code)				
		Accident	Therapeutic Use	Suicide Attempt	Assault	Undetermined
IDU	976.5	E858.7	E946.5	E950.4	E962.0	E980.4
Iletin	962.3	E858.0	E932.3	E950.4	E962.0	E980.4
Ilex	988.2	E865.4	—	E950.9	E962.1	E980.9
Illuminating gas — see Gas, utility						
Ilopan	963.5	E858.1	E933.5	E950.4	E962.0	E980.4
Ilotycin	960.3	E856	E930.3	E950.4	E962.0	E980.4
ophthalmic preparation	976.5	E858.7	E946.5	E950.4	E962.0	E980.4
topical NEC	976.0	E858.7	E946.0	E950.4	E962.0	E980.4
Imipramine	969.05	E854.0	E939.0	E950.3	E962.0	E980.3
Immu-G	964.6	E858.2	E934.6	E950.4	E962.0	E980.4
Immuglobin	964.6	E858.2	E934.6	E950.4	E962.0	E980.4
Immune serum globulin	964.6	E858.2	E934.6	E950.4	E962.0	E980.4
Immunosuppressive agents	963.1	E858.1	E933.1	E950.4	E962.0	E980.4
Immu-tetanus	964.6	E858.2	E934.6	E950.4	E962.0	E980.4
Indandione (derivatives)	964.2	E858.2	E934.2	E950.4	E962.0	E980.4
Inderal	972.0	E858.3	E942.0	E950.4	E962.0	E980.4
Indian						
hemp	969.6	E854.1	E939.6	E950.3	E962.0	E980.3
tobacco	988.2	E865.4	—	E950.9	E962.1	E980.9
Indigo carmine	977.8	E858.8	E947.8	E950.4	E962.0	E980.4
Indocin	965.69	E850.6	E935.6	E950.0	E962.0	E980.0
Indocyanine green	977.8	E858.8	E947.8	E950.4	E962.0	E980.4
Indomethacin	965.69	E850.6	E935.6	E950.0	E962.0	E980.0
Industrial						
alcohol	980.9	E860.9	—	E950.9	E962.1	E980.9
fumes	987.8	E869.8	—	E952.8	E962.2	E982.8
solvents (fumes) (vapors)	982.8	E862.9	—	E950.9	E962.1	E980.9
Influenza vaccine	979.6	E858.8	E949.6	E950.4	E962.0	E982.8
Ingested substances NEC	989.9	E866.9	—	E950.9	E962.1	E980.9
INH (isoniazid)	961.8	E857	E931.8	E950.4	E962.0	E980.4
Inhalation, gas (noxious) — see Gas						
Ink	989.89	E866.8	—	E950.9	E962.1	E980.9
Innovar	967.6	E852.5	E937.6	E950.2	E962.0	E980.2
Inositol niacinate	972.2	E858.3	E942.2	E950.4	E962.0	E980.4
Inproquone	963.1	E858.1	E933.1	E950.4	E962.0	E980.4
Insecticides — see also Pesti- cides	989.4	E863.4	—	E950.6	E962.1	E980.7
chlorinated	989.2	E863.0	—	E950.6	E962.1	E980.7
mixtures	989.4	E863.3	—	E950.6	E962.1	E980.7
organochlorine (com- pounds)	989.2	E863.0	—	E950.6	E962.1	E980.7
organophosphorus (com- pounds)	989.3	E863.1	—	E950.6	E962.1	E980.7
Insect (sting), venomous	989.5	E905.5	—	E950.9	E962.1	E980.9
Insular tissue extract	962.3	E858.0	E932.3	E950.4	E962.0	E980.4
Insulin (amorphous) (globin) (isophane) (Lente) (NPH) (protamine) (Semilente) (Ul- tralente) (zinc)	962.3	E858.0	E932.3	E950.4	E962.0	E980.4
Intranarcon	968.3	E855.1	E938.3	E950.4	E962.0	E980.4
Inulin	977.8	E858.8	E947.8	E950.4	E962.0	E980.4
Invert sugar	974.5	E858.5	E944.5	E950.4	E962.0	E980.4
Inza — see Naproxen						
Iodide NEC — see also Io- dine	976.0	E858.7	E946.0	E950.4	E962.0	E980.4
mercury (ointment)	976.0	E858.7	E946.0	E950.4	E962.0	E980.4
methylate	976.0	E858.7	E946.0	E950.4	E962.0	E980.4
potassium (expectorant) NEC	975.5	E858.6	E945.5	E950.4	E962.0	E980.4
Iodinated glycerol	975.5	E858.6	E945.5	E950.4	E962.0	E980.4
Iodine (antiseptic, external) (tincture) NEC	976.0	E858.7	E946.0	E950.4	E962.0	E980.4
diagnostic	977.8	E858.8	E947.8	E950.4	E962.0	E980.4
for thyroid conditions (antithy- roid)	962.8	E858.0	E932.8	E950.4	E962.0	E980.4
vapor	987.8	E869.8	—	E952.8	E962.2	E982.8
Iodized oil	977.8	E858.8	E947.8	E950.4	E962.0	E980.4
Iodobismitol	961.2	E857	E931.2	E950.4	E962.0	E980.4
Iodochlorhydroxyquin	961.3	E857	E931.3	E950.4	E962.0	E980.4
topical	976.0	E858.7	E946.0	E950.4	E962.0	E980.4
Iodoform	976.0	E858.7	E946.0	E950.4	E962.0	E980.4
Iodopanoic acid	977.8	E858.8	E947.8	E950.4	E962.0	E980.4
Iodophthalein	977.8	E858.8	E947.8	E950.4	E962.0	E980.4
Ion exchange resins	974.5	E858.5	E944.5	E950.4	E962.0	E980.4
Iopanoic acid	977.8	E858.8	E947.8	E950.4	E962.0	E980.4
Iophendylate	977.8	E858.8	E947.8	E950.4	E962.0	E980.4
Iothiouracil	962.8	E858.0	E932.8	E950.4	E962.0	E980.4
Ipecac	973.6	E858.4	E943.6	E950.4	E962.0	E980.4
Ipecacuanha	973.6	E858.4	E943.6	E950.4	E962.0	E980.4

Nontherapeutic use substance

⬡ Subterms under main terms may continue to next column or page

Hydralazine, hydrallazine — Ipecacuanha

	Poisoning	Accident	Therapeutic Use	Suicide Attempt	Assault	Undetermined
External Cause (E-Code)						
Ipodate	977.8	E858.8	E947.8	E950.4	E962.0	E980.4
Ipral	967.0	E851	E937.0	E950.1	E962.0	E980.1
Ipratropium	975.1	E858.6	E945.1	E950.4	E962.0	E980.4
Iproniazid	969.01	E854.0	E939.0	E950.3	E962.0	E980.3
Iron (compounds) (medicinal)						
(preparations)	964.0	E858.2	E934.0	E950.4	E962.0	E980.4
dextran	964.0	E858.2	E934.0	E950.4	E962.0	E980.4
nonmedicinal (dust) (fumes) NEC	985.8	E866.4	—	E950.9	E962.1	E980.9
Irritant drug	977.9	E858.9	E947.9	E950.5	E962.0	E980.5
Ismelin	972.6	E858.3	E942.6	E950.4	E962.0	E980.4
Isoamyl nitrite	972.4	E858.3	E942.4	E950.4	E962.0	E980.4
Isobutyl acetate	982.8	E862.4	—	E950.9	E962.1	E980.9
Isocarboxazid	969.01	E854.0	E939.0	E950.3	E962.0	E980.3
Isoephedrine	971.2	E855.5	E941.2	E950.4	E962.0	E980.4
Isoetharine	971.2	E855.5	E941.2	E950.4	E962.0	E980.4
Isofluorophate	971.0	E855.3	E941.0	E950.4	E962.0	E980.4
Isoniazid (INH)	961.8	E857	E931.8	E950.4	E962.0	E980.4
Isopentaquine	961.4	E857	E931.4	E950.4	E962.0	E980.4
Isophane insulin	962.3	E858.0	E932.3	E950.4	E962.0	E980.4
Isopregnenone	962.2	E858.0	E932.2	E950.4	E962.0	E980.4
Isoprenaline	971.2	E855.5	E941.2	E950.4	E962.0	E980.4
Isopropamide	971.1	E855.4	E941.1	E950.4	E962.0	E980.4
Isopropanol	980.2	E860.3	—	E950.9	E962.1	E980.9
topical (germicide)	976.0	E858.7	E946.0	E950.4	E962.0	E980.4
Isopropyl						
acetate	982.8	E862.4	—	E950.9	E962.1	E980.9
alcohol	980.2	E860.3	—	E950.9	E962.1	E980.9
topical (germicide)	976.0	E858.7	E946.0	E950.4	E962.0	E980.4
ether	982.8	E862.4	—	E950.9	E962.1	E980.9
Isoproterenol	971.2	E855.5	E941.2	E950.4	E962.0	E980.4
Isosorbide dinitrate	972.4	E858.3	E942.4	E950.4	E962.0	E980.4
Isothipendyl	963.0	E858.1	E933.0	E950.4	E962.0	E980.4
Isoxazolyl penicillin	960.0	E856	E930.0	E950.4	E962.0	E980.4
Isoxsuprine hydrochloride	972.5	E858.3	E942.5	E950.4	E962.0	E980.4
I-thyroxine sodium	962.7	E858.0	E932.7	E950.4	E962.0	E980.4
Jaborandi (pilocarpus) (extract)	971.0	E855.3	E941.0	E950.4	E962.0	E980.4
Jalap	973.1	E858.4	E943.1	E950.4	E962.0	E980.4
Jamaica						
dogwood (bark)	965.7	E850.7	E935.7	E950.0	E962.0	E980.0
ginger	989.89	E866.8	—	E950.9	E962.1	E980.9
Jatropha	988.2	E865.4	—	E950.9	E962.1	E980.9
curcas	988.2	E865.3	—	E950.9	E962.1	E980.9
Jectofer	964.0	E858.2	E934.0	E950.4	E962.0	E980.4
Jellyfish (sting)	989.5	E905.6	—	E950.9	E962.1	E980.9
Jequirity (bean)	988.2	E865.3	—	E950.9	E962.1	E980.9
Jimson weed	988.2	E865.4	—	E950.9	E962.1	E980.9
seeds	988.2	E865.3	—	E950.9	E962.1	E980.9
Juniper tar (oil) (ointment)	976.4	E858.7	E946.4	E950.4	E962.0	E980.4
Kallikrein	972.5	E858.3	E942.5	E950.4	E962.0	E980.4
Kanamycin	960.6	E856	E930.6	E950.4	E962.0	E980.4
Kantrex	960.6	E856	E930.6	E950.4	E962.0	E980.4
Kaolin	973.5	E858.4	E943.5	E950.4	E962.0	E980.4
Karaya (gum)	973.3	E858.4	E943.3	E950.4	E962.0	E980.4
Kemithal	968.3	E855.1	E938.3	E950.4	E962.0	E980.4
Kenacort	962.0	E858.0	E932.0	E950.4	E962.0	E980.4
Keratolytics	976.4	E858.7	E946.4	E950.4	E962.0	E980.4
Keratoplastics	976.4	E858.7	E946.4	E950.4	E962.0	E980.4
Kerosene, kerosine (fuel) (solvent) NEC	981	E862.1	—	E950.9	E962.1	E980.9
insecticide	981	E863.4	—	E950.6	E962.1	E980.7
vapor	987.1	E869.8	—	E952.8	E962.2	E982.8
Ketamine	968.3	E855.1	E938.3	E950.4	E962.0	E980.4
Ketobemidone	965.09	E850.2	E935.2	E950.0	E962.0	E980.0
Ketols	982.8	E862.4	—	E950.9	E962.1	E980.9
Ketone oils	982.8	E862.4	—	E950.9	E962.1	E980.9
Ketoprofen	965.61	E850.6	E935.6	E950.0	E962.0	E980.0
Kiln gas or vapor (carbon monoxide)	986	E868.8	—	E952.1	E962.2	E982.1
Konsyl	973.3	E858.4	E943.3	E950.4	E962.0	E980.4
Kosam seed	988.2	E865.3	—	E950.9	E962.1	E980.9
Krait (venom)	989.5	E905.0	—	E950.9	E962.1	E980.9
Kwell (insecticide)	989.2	E863.0	—	E950.6	E962.1	E980.7
anti-infective (topical)	976.0	E858.7	E946.0	E950.4	E962.0	E980.4
Laburnum (flowers) (seeds)	988.2	E865.3	—	E950.9	E962.1	E980.9
leaves	988.2	E865.4	—	E950.9	E962.1	E980.9
Lacquers	989.89	E861.6	—	E950.9	E962.1	E980.9
Lacrimogenic gas	987.5	E869.3	—	E952.8	E962.2	E982.8
Lactic acid	983.1	E864.1	—	E950.7	E962.1	E980.6
Lactobacillus acidophilus	973.5	E858.4	E943.5	E950.4	E962.0	E980.4
Lactoflavin	963.5	E858.1	E933.5	E950.4	E962.0	E980.4
Lactuca (virosa) (extract)	967.8	E852.8	E937.8	E950.2	E962.0	E980.2
Lactucarium	967.8	E852.8	E937.8	E950.2	E962.0	E980.2
Laevulose	974.5	E858.5	E944.5	E950.4	E962.0	E980.4
Lanatoside (C)	972.1	E858.3	E942.1	E950.4	E962.0	E980.4
Lanolin (lotion)	976.3	E858.7	E946.3	E950.4	E962.0	E980.4
Largactil	969.1	E853.0	E939.1	E950.3	E962.0	E980.3
Larkspur	988.2	E865.3	—	E950.9	E962.1	E980.9
Laroxyl	969.05	E854.0	E939.0	E950.3	E962.0	E980.3
Lasix	974.4	E858.5	E944.4	E950.4	E962.0	E980.4
Latex	989.82	E866.8	—	E950.9	E962.1	E980.9
Lathyrus (seed)	988.2	E865.3	—	E950.9	E962.1	E980.9
Laudanum	965.09	E850.2	E935.2	E950.0	E962.0	E980.0
Laudexium	975.2	E858.6	E945.2	E950.4	E962.0	E980.4
Laurel, black or cherry	988.2	E865.4	—	E950.9	E962.1	E980.9
Laurolinium	976.0	E858.7	E946.0	E950.4	E962.0	E980.4
Lauryl sulfoacetate	976.2	E858.7	E946.2	E950.4	E962.0	E980.4
Laxatives NEC	973.3	E858.4	E943.3	E950.4	E962.0	E980.4
emollient	973.2	E858.4	E943.2	E950.4	E962.0	E980.4
L-dopa	966.4	E855.0	E936.4	E950.4	E962.0	E980.4
Lead (dust) (fumes) (vapor)						
NEC	984.9	E866.0	—	E950.9	E962.1	E980.9
acetate (dust)	984.1	E866.0	—	E950.9	E962.1	E980.9
anti-infectives	961.2	E857	E931.2	E950.4	E962.0	E980.4
antiknock compound (tetraethyl)	984.1	E862.1	—	E950.9	E962.1	E980.9
arsenate, arsenite (dust) (insecticide) (vapor)	985.1	E863.4	—	E950.8	E962.1	E980.8
herbicide	985.1	E863.5	—	E950.8	E962.1	E980.8
carbonate	984.0	E866.0	—	E950.9	E962.1	E980.9
paint	984.0	E861.5	—	E950.9	E962.1	E980.9
chromate	984.0	E866.0	—	E950.9	E962.1	E980.9
paint	984.0	E861.5	—	E950.9	E962.1	E980.9
dioxide	984.0	E866.0	—	E950.9	E962.1	E980.9
inorganic (compound)	984.0	E866.0	—	E950.9	E962.1	E980.9
paint	984.0	E861.5	—	E950.9	E962.1	E980.9
iodide	984.0	E866.0	—	E950.9	E962.1	E980.9
pigment (paint)	984.0	E861.5	—	E950.9	E962.1	E980.9
monoxide (dust)	984.0	E866.0	—	E950.9	E962.1	E980.9
paint	984.0	E861.5	—	E950.9	E962.1	E980.9
organic	984.1	E866.0	—	E950.9	E962.1	E980.9
oxide	984.0	E866.0	—	E950.9	E962.1	E980.9
paint	984.0	E861.5	—	E950.9	E962.1	E980.9
paint	984.0	E861.5	—	E950.9	E962.1	E980.9
salts	984.0	E866.0	—	E950.9	E962.1	E980.9
specified compound NEC	984.8	E866.0	—	E950.9	E962.1	E980.9
tetra-ethyl	984.1	E862.1	—	E950.9	E962.1	E980.9
Lebanese red	969.6	E854.1	E939.6	E950.3	E962.0	E980.3
Lente Iletin (insulin)	962.3	E858.0	E932.3	E950.4	E962.0	E980.4
Leptazol	970.0	E854.3	E940.0	E950.4	E962.0	E980.4
Leritine	965.09	E850.2	E935.2	E950.0	E962.0	E980.0
Letter	962.7	E858.0	E932.7	E950.4	E962.0	E980.4
Lettuce opium	967.8	E852.8	E937.8	E950.2	E962.0	E980.2
Leucovorin (factor)	964.1	E858.2	E934.1	E950.4	E962.0	E980.4
Leukeran	963.1	E858.1	E933.1	E950.4	E962.0	E980.4
Levalbuterol	975.7	E858.6	E945.7	E950.4	E962.0	E980.4
Levallorphan	970.1	E854.3	E940.1	E950.4	E962.0	E980.4
Levanil	967.8	E852.8	E937.8	E950.2	E962.0	E980.2
Levarterenol	971.2	E855.5	E941.2	E950.4	E962.0	E980.4
Levodopa	966.4	E855.0	E936.4	E950.4	E962.0	E980.4
Levo-dromoran	965.09	E850.2	E935.2	E950.0	E962.0	E980.0
Levoid	962.7	E858.0	E932.7	E950.4	E962.0	E980.4
Levo-iso-methadone	965.02	E850.1	E935.1	E950.0	E962.0	E980.0
Levomepromazine	967.8	E852.8	E937.8	E950.2	E962.0	E980.2
Levoprome	967.8	E852.8	E937.8	E950.2	E962.0	E980.2
Levopropoxyphene	975.4	E858.6	E945.4	E950.4	E962.0	E980.4
Levorphan, levophanol	965.09	E850.2	E935.2	E950.0	E962.0	E980.0
Levothyroxine (sodium)	962.7	E858.0	E932.7	E950.4	E962.0	E980.4
Levsin	971.1	E855.4	E941.1	E950.4	E962.0	E980.4
Levulose	974.5	E858.5	E944.5	E950.4	E962.0	E980.4
Lewisite (gas)	985.1	E866.3	—	E950.8	E962.1	E980.8
Librium	969.4	E853.2	E939.4	E950.3	E962.0	E980.3
Lidex	976.0	E858.7	E946.0	E950.4	E962.0	E980.4
Lidocaine (infiltration) (topical)	968.5	E855.2	E938.5	E950.4	E962.0	E980.4
nerve block (peripheral) (plexus)	968.6	E855.2	E938.6	E950.4	E962.0	E980.4
spinal	968.7	E855.2	E938.7	E950.4	E962.0	E980.4
Lighter fluid	981	E862.1	—	E950.9	E962.1	E980.9

	Poisoning	Accident	Therapeutic Use	Suicide Attempt	Assault	Undetermined
			External Cause (E-Code)			

Left column table:

	Poisoning	Accident	Therapeutic Use	Suicide Attempt	Assault	Undetermined
Lignocaine (infiltration) (topical)	968.5	E855.2	E938.5	E950.4	E962.0	E980.4
nerve block (peripheral) (plexus)	968.6	E855.2	E938.6	E950.4	E962.0	E980.4
spinal	968.7	E855.2	E938.7	E950.4	E962.0	E980.4
Ligroin(e) (solvent)	981	E862.0	—	E950.9	E962.1	E980.9
vapor	987.1	E869.8	—	E952.8	E962.2	E982.8
Ligustrum vulgare	988.2	E865.3	—	E950.9	E962.1	E980.9
Lily of the valley	988.2	E865.4	—	E950.9	E962.1	E980.9
Lime (chloride)	983.2	E864.2	—	E950.7	E962.1	E980.6
solution, sulferated	976.4	E858.7	E946.4	E950.4	E962.0	E980.4
Limonene	982.8	E862.4	—	E950.9	E962.1	E980.9
Lincomycin	960.8	E856	E930.8	E950.4	E962.0	E980.4
Lindane (insecticide) (vapor)	989.2	E863.0	—	E950.6	E962.1	E980.7
anti-infective (topical)	976.0	E858.7	E946.0	E950.4	E962.0	E980.4
Liniments NEC	976.9	E858.7	E946.9	E950.4	E962.0	E980.4
Linoleic acid	972.2	E858.3	E942.2	E950.4	E962.0	E980.4
Liothyronine	962.7	E858.0	E932.7	E950.4	E962.0	E980.4
Liotrix	962.7	E858.0	E932.7	E950.4	E962.0	E980.4
Lipancreatin	973.4	E858.4	E943.4	E950.4	E962.0	E980.4
Lipo-Lutin	962.2	E858.0	E932.2	E950.4	E962.0	E980.4
Lipotropic agents	977.1	E858.8	E947.1	E950.4	E962.0	E980.4
Liquefied petroleum gases	987.0	E868.0	—	E951.1	E962.2	E981.1
piped (pure or mixed with air)	987.0	E867	—	E951.0	E962.2	E981.0
Liquid petrolatum	973.2	E858.4	E943.2	E950.4	E962.0	E980.4
substance	989.9	E866.9	—	E950.9	E962.1	E980.9
specified NEC	989.89	E866.8	—	E950.9	E962.1	E980.9
Lirugen	979.4	E858.8	E949.4	E950.4	E962.0	E980.4
Lithane	969.8	E855.8	E939.8	E950.3	E962.0	E980.3
Lithium	985.8	E866.4	—	E950.9	E962.1	E980.9
carbonate	969.8	E855.8	E939.8	E950.3	E962.0	E980.3
Lithonate	969.8	E855.8	E939.8	E950.3	E962.0	E980.3
Liver (extract) (injection) (preparations)	964.1	E858.2	E934.1	E950.4	E962.0	E980.4
Lizard (bite) (venom)	989.5	E905.0	—	E950.9	E962.1	E980.9
LMD	964.8	E858.2	E934.8	E950.4	E962.0	E980.4
Lobelia	988.2	E865.4	—	E950.9	E962.1	E980.9
Lobeline	970.0	E854.3	E940.0	E950.4	E962.0	E980.4
Locorten	976.0	E858.7	E946.0	E950.4	E962.0	E980.4
Lolium temulentum	988.2	E865.3	—	E950.9	E962.1	E980.9
Lomotil	973.5	E858.4	E943.5	E950.4	E962.0	E980.4
Lomustine	963.1	E858.1	E933.1	E950.4	E962.0	E980.4
Lophophora williamsii	969.6	E854.1	E939.6	E950.3	E962.0	E980.3
Lorazepam	969.4	E853.2	E939.4	E950.3	E962.0	E980.3
Lotions NEC	976.9	E858.7	E946.9	E950.4	E962.0	E980.4
Lotronex	973.8	E858.4	E943.8	E950.4	E962.0	E980.4
Lotusate	967.0	E851	E937.0	E950.1	E962.0	E980.1
Lowila	976.2	E858.7	E946.2	E950.4	E962.0	E980.4
Loxapine	969.3	E853.8	E939.3	E950.3	E962.0	E980.3
Lozenges (throat)	976.6	E858.7	E946.6	E950.4	E962.0	E980.4
LSD (25)	969.6	E854.1	E939.6	E950.3	E962.0	E980.3
L-Tryptophan — see amino acid						
Lubricating oil NEC	981	E862.2	—	E950.9	E962.1	E980.9
Lucanthone	961.6	E857	E931.6	E950.4	E962.0	E980.4
Luminal	967.0	E851	E937.0	E950.1	E962.0	E980.1
Lung irritant (gas) NEC	987.9	E869.9	—	E952.9	E962.2	E982.9
Lutocylol	962.2	E858.0	E932.2	E950.4	E962.0	E980.4
Lutromone	962.2	E858.0	E932.2	E950.4	E962.0	E980.4
Lututrin	975.0	E858.6	E945.0	E950.4	E962.0	E980.4
Lye (concentrated)	983.2	E864.2	—	E950.7	E962.1	E980.6
Lygranum (skin test)	977.8	E858.8	E947.8	E950.4	E962.0	E980.4
Lymecycline	960.4	E856	E930.4	E950.4	E962.0	E980.4
Lymphogranuloma venereum antigen	977.8	E858.8	E947.8	E950.4	E962.0	E980.4
Lynestrenol	962.2	E858.0	E932.2	E950.4	E962.0	E980.4
Lyovac Sodium Edecrin	974.4	E858.5	E944.4	E950.4	E962.0	E980.4
Lypressin	962.5	E858.0	E932.5	E950.4	E962.0	E980.4
Lysergic acid (amide) (diethylamide)	969.6	E854.1	E939.6	E950.3	E962.0	E980.3
Lysergide	969.6	E854.1	E939.6	E950.3	E962.0	E980.3
Lysine vasopressin	962.5	E858.0	E932.5	E950.4	E962.0	E980.4
Lysol	983.0	E864.0	—	E950.7	E962.1	E980.6
Lytta (vitatta)	976.8	E858.7	E946.8	E950.4	E962.0	E980.4
Mace	987.5	E869.3	—	E952.8	E962.2	E982.8
Macrolides (antibiotics)	960.3	E856	E930.3	E950.4	E962.0	E980.4
Mafenide	976.0	E858.7	E946.0	E950.4	E962.0	E980.4
Magaldrate	973.0	E858.4	E943.0	E950.4	E962.0	E980.4
Magic mushroom	969.6	E854.1	E939.6	E950.3	E962.0	E980.3

	Poisoning	Accident	Therapeutic Use	Suicide Attempt	Assault	Undetermined
Magnamycin	960.8	E856	E930.8	E950.4	E962.0	E980.4
Magnesia magma	973.0	E858.4	E943.0	E950.4	E962.0	E980.4
Magnesium (compounds) (fumes) NEC	985.8	E866.4	—	E950.9	E962.1	E980.9
antacid	973.0	E858.4	E943.0	E950.4	E962.0	E980.4
carbonate	973.0	E858.4	E943.0	E950.4	E962.0	E980.4
cathartic	973.3	E858.4	E943.3	E950.4	E962.0	E980.4
citrate	973.3	E858.4	E943.3	E950.4	E962.0	E980.4
hydroxide	973.0	E858.4	E943.0	E950.4	E962.0	E980.4
oxide	973.0	E858.4	E943.0	E950.4	E962.0	E980.4
sulfate (oral)	973.3	E858.4	E943.3	E950.4	E962.0	E980.4
intravenous	966.3	E855.0	E936.3	E950.4	E962.0	E980.4
trisilicate	973.0	E858.4	E943.0	E950.4	E962.0	E980.4
Malathion (insecticide)	989.3	E863.1	—	E950.6	E962.1	E980.7
Male fern (oleoresin)	961.6	E857	E931.6	E950.4	E962.0	E980.4
Mandelic acid	961.9	E857	E931.9	E950.4	E962.0	E980.4
Manganese compounds (fumes) NEC	985.2	E866.4	—	E950.9	E962.1	E980.9
Mannitol (diuretic) (medicinal) NEC	974.4	E858.5	E944.4	E950.4	E962.0	E980.4
hexanitrate	972.4	E858.3	E942.4	E950.4	E962.0	E980.4
mustard	963.1	E858.1	E933.1	E950.4	E962.0	E980.4
Mannomustine	963.1	E858.1	E933.1	E950.4	E962.0	E980.4
MAO inhibitors	969.01	E854.0	E939.0	E950.3	E962.0	E980.3
Mapharsen	961.1	E857	E931.1	E950.4	E962.0	E980.4
Marcaine	968.9	E855.2	E938.9	E950.4	E962.0	E980.4
infiltration (subcutaneous)	968.5	E855.2	E938.5	E950.4	E962.0	E980.4
nerve block (peripheral) (plexus)	968.6	E855.2	E938.6	E950.4	E962.0	E980.4
Marezine	963.0	E858.1	E933.0	E950.4	E962.0	E980.4
Marihuana, marijuana (derivatives)	969.6	E854.1	E939.6	E950.3	E962.0	E980.3
Marine animals or plants (sting)	989.5	E905.6	—	E950.9	E962.1	E980.9
Marplan	969.01	E854.0	E939.0	E950.3	E962.0	E980.3
Marsh gas	987.1	E869.8	—	E952.8	E962.2	E982.8
Marsilid	969.01	E854.0	E939.0	E950.3	E962.0	E980.3
Matulane	963.1	E858.1	E933.1	E950.4	E962.0	E980.4
Mazindol	977.0	E858.8	E947.0	E950.4	E962.0	E980.4
MDMA	969.72	E854.2	E939.7	E950.3	E962.0	E980.3
Meadow saffron	988.2	E865.3	—	E950.9	E962.1	E980.9
Measles vaccine	979.4	E858.8	E949.4	E950.4	E962.0	E980.4
Meat, noxious or nonbacterial	988.8	E865.0	—	E950.9	E962.1	E980.9
Mebanazine	969.01	E854.0	E939.0	E950.3	E962.0	E980.3
Mebaral	967.0	E851	E937.0	E950.1	E962.0	E980.1
Mebendazole	961.6	E857	E931.6	E950.4	E962.0	E980.4
Mebeverine	975.1	E858.6	E945.1	E950.4	E962.0	E980.4
Mebhydroline	963.0	E858.1	E933.0	E950.4	E962.0	E980.4
Mebrophenhydramine	963.0	E858.1	E933.0	E950.4	E962.0	E980.4
Mebutamate	969.5	E853.8	E939.5	E950.3	E962.0	E980.3
Mecamylamine (chloride)	972.3	E858.3	E942.3	E950.4	E962.0	E980.4
Mechlorethamine hydrochloride	963.1	E858.1	E933.1	E950.4	E962.0	E980.4
Meclizene (hydrochloride)	963.0	E858.1	E933.0	E950.4	E962.0	E980.4
Meclofenoxate	970.0	E854.3	E940.0	E950.4	E962.0	E980.4
Meclozine (hydrochloride)	963.0	E858.1	E933.0	E950.4	E962.0	E980.4
Medazepam	969.4	E853.2	E939.4	E950.3	E962.0	E980.3
Medicine, medicinal substance	977.9	E858.9	E947.9	E950.5	E962.0	E980.5
specified NEC	977.8	E858.8	E947.8	E950.4	E962.0	E980.4
Medinal	967.0	E851	E937.0	E950.1	E962.0	E980.1
Medomin	967.0	E851	E937.0	E950.1	E962.0	E980.1
Medroxyprogesterone	962.2	E858.0	E932.2	E950.4	E962.0	E980.4
Medrysone	976.5	E858.7	E946.5	E950.4	E962.0	E980.4
Mefenamic acid	965.7	E850.7	E935.7	E950.0	E962.0	E980.0
Megahallucinogen	969.6	E854.1	E939.6	E950.3	E962.0	E980.3
Megestrol	962.2	E858.0	E932.2	E950.4	E962.0	E980.4
Meglumine	977.8	E858.8	E947.8	E950.4	E962.0	E980.4
Meladinin	976.3	E858.7	E946.3	E950.4	E962.0	E980.4
Melanizing agents	976.3	E858.7	E946.3	E950.4	E962.0	E980.4
Melarsoprol	961.1	E857	E931.1	E950.4	E962.0	E980.4
Melia azedarach	988.2	E865.3	—	E950.9	E962.1	E980.9
Mellaril	969.1	E853.0	E939.1	E950.3	E962.0	E980.3
Meloxine	976.3	E858.7	E946.3	E950.4	E962.0	E980.4
Melphalan	963.1	E858.1	E933.1	E950.4	E962.0	E980.4
Menadiol sodium diphosphate	964.3	E858.2	E934.3	E950.4	E962.0	E980.4
Menadione (sodium bisulfite)	964.3	E858.2	E934.3	E950.4	E962.0	E980.4
Menaphthone	964.3	E858.2	E934.3	E950.4	E962.0	E980.4

	Poisoning	Accident	Therapeutic Use	Suicide Attempt	Assault	Undeter-mined
External Cause (E-Code)						
Meningococcal vaccine	978.8	E858.8	E948.8	E950.4	E962.0	E980.4
Menningovax-C	978.8	E858.8	E948.8	E950.4	E962.0	E980.4
Menotropins	962.4	E858.0	E932.4	E950.4	E962.0	E980.4
Menthol NEC	976.1	E858.7	E946.1	E950.4	E962.0	E980.4
Mepacrine	961.3	E857	E931.3	E950.4	E962.0	E980.4
Meparfynol	967.8	E852.8	E937.8	E950.2	E962.0	E980.2
Mepazine	969.1	E853.0	E939.1	E950.3	E962.0	E980.3
Mepenzolate	971.1	E855.4	E941.1	E950.4	E962.0	E980.4
Meperidine	965.09	E850.2	E935.2	E950.0	E962.0	E980.0
Mephenamin(e)	966.4	E855.0	E936.4	E950.4	E962.0	E980.4
Mephenesin (carbamate)	968.0	E855.1	E938.0	E950.4	E962.0	E980.4
Mephenoxalone	969.5	E853.8	E939.5	E950.3	E962.0	E980.3
Mephentermine	971.2	E855.5	E941.2	E950.4	E962.0	E980.4
Mephenytoin	966.1	E855.0	E936.1	E950.4	E962.0	E980.4
Mephobarbital	967.0	E851	E937.0	E950.1	E962.0	E980.1
Mepiperphenidol	971.1	E855.4	E941.1	E950.4	E962.0	E980.4
Mepivacaine	968.9	E855.2	E938.9	E950.4	E962.0	E980.4
infiltration (subcuta-neous)	968.5	E855.2	E938.5	E950.4	E962.0	E980.4
nerve block (peripheral) (plexus)	968.6	E855.2	E938.6	E950.4	E962.0	E980.4
topical (surface)	968.5	E855.2	E938.5	E950.4	E962.0	E980.4
Meprednisone	962.0	E858.0	E932.0	E950.4	E962.0	E980.4
Meprobam	969.5	E853.8	E939.5	E950.3	E962.0	E980.3
Meprobamate	969.5	E853.8	E939.5	E950.3	E962.0	E980.3
Mepyramine (maleate)	963.0	E858.1	E933.0	E950.4	E962.0	E980.4
Meralluride	974.0	E858.5	E944.0	E950.4	E962.0	E980.4
Merbaphen	974.0	E858.5	E944.0	E950.4	E962.0	E980.4
Merbromin	976.0	E858.7	E946.0	E950.4	E962.0	E980.4
Mercaptomerin	974.0	E858.5	E944.0	E950.4	E962.0	E980.4
Mercaptopurine	963.1	E858.1	E933.1	E950.4	E962.0	E980.4
Mercumatilin	974.0	E858.5	E944.0	E950.4	E962.0	E980.4
Mercuramide	974.0	E858.5	E944.0	E950.4	E962.0	E980.4
Mercuranin	976.0	E858.7	E946.0	E950.4	E962.0	E980.4
Mercurochrome	976.0	E858.7	E946.0	E950.4	E962.0	E980.4
Mercury, mercuric, mer-curous (compounds) (cyanide) (fumes) (nonmedic-inal) (vapor) NEC	985.0	E866.1	—	E950.9	E962.1	E980.9
ammoniated	976.0	E858.7	E946.0	E950.4	E962.0	E980.4
anti-infective	961.2	E857	E931.2	E950.4	E962.0	E980.4
topical	976.0	E858.7	E946.0	E950.4	E962.0	E980.4
chloride (antiseptic) NEC	976.0	E858.7	E946.0	E950.4	E962.0	E980.4
fungicide	985.0	E863.6	—	E950.6	E962.1	E980.7
diuretic compounds	974.0	E858.5	E944.0	E950.4	E962.0	E980.4
fungicide	985.0	E863.6	—	E950.6	E962.1	E980.7
organic (fungicide)	985.0	E863.6	—	E950.6	E962.1	E980.7
Merethoxylline	974.0	E858.5	E944.0	E950.4	E962.0	E980.4
Mersalyl	974.0	E858.5	E944.0	E950.4	E962.0	E980.4
Merthiolate (topical)	976.0	E858.7	E946.0	E950.4	E962.0	E980.4
ophthalmic preparation	976.5	E858.7	E946.5	E950.4	E962.0	E980.4
Meruvax	979.4	E858.8	E949.4	E950.4	E962.0	E980.4
Mescal buttons	969.6	E854.1	E939.6	E950.3	E962.0	E980.3
Mescaline (salts)	969.6	E854.1	E939.6	E950.3	E962.0	E980.3
Mesoridazine besylate	969.1	E853.0	E939.1	E950.3	E962.0	E980.3
Mestanolone	962.1	E858.0	E932.1	E950.4	E962.0	E980.4
Mestranol	962.2	E858.0	E932.2	E950.4	E962.0	E980.4
Metacresylacetate	976.0	E858.7	E946.0	E950.4	E962.0	E980.4
Metaldehyde (snail killer) NEC	989.4	E863.4	—	E950.6	E962.1	E980.7
Metals (heavy) (nonmedici-nal) NEC	985.9	E866.4	—	E950.9	E962.1	E980.9
dust, fumes, or vapor NEC	985.9	E866.4	—	E950.9	E962.1	E980.9
light NEC	985.9	E866.4	—	E950.9	E962.1	E980.9
dust, fumes, or vapor NEC	985.9	E866.4	—	E950.9	E962.1	E980.9
pesticides (dust) (vapor)	985.9	E863.4	—	E950.6	E962.1	E980.7
Metamucil	973.3	E858.4	E943.3	E950.4	E962.0	E980.4
Metaphen	976.0	E858.7	E946.0	E950.4	E962.0	E980.4
Metaproterenol	975.1	E858.6	E945.1	E950.4	E962.0	E980.4
Metaraminol	972.8	E858.3	E942.8	E950.4	E962.0	E980.4
Metaxalone	968.0	E855.1	E938.0	E950.4	E962.0	E980.4
Metformin	962.3	E858.0	E932.3	E950.4	E962.0	E980.4
Methacycline	960.4	E856	E930.4	E950.4	E962.0	E980.4
Methadone	965.02	E850.1	E935.1	E950.0	E962.0	E980.0
Methallenestril	962.2	E858.0	E932.2	E950.4	E962.0	E980.4
Methamphetamine	969.72	E854.2	E939.7	E950.3	E962.0	E980.3
Methandienone	962.1	E858.0	E932.1	E950.4	E962.0	E980.4
Methandriol	962.1	E858.0	E932.1	E950.4	E962.0	E980.4
Methandrostenolone	962.1	E858.0	E932.1	E950.4	E962.0	E980.4
Methane gas	987.1	E869.8	—	E952.8	E962.2	E982.8

	Poisoning	Accident	Therapeutic Use	Suicide Attempt	Assault	Undeter-mined
External Cause (E-Code)						
Methanol	980.1	E860.2	—	E950.9	E962.1	E980.9
vapor	987.8	E869.8	—	E952.8	E962.2	E982.8
Methantheline	971.1	E855.4	E941.1	E950.4	E962.0	E980.4
Methaphenilene	963.0	E858.1	E933.0	E950.4	E962.0	E980.4
Methapyrilene	963.0	E858.1	E933.0	E950.4	E962.0	E980.4
Methaqualone (com-pounds)	967.4	E852.3	E937.4	E950.2	E962.0	E980.2
Metharbital, methar-bitone	967.0	E851	E937.0	E950.1	E962.0	E980.1
Methazolamide	974.2	E858.5	E944.2	E950.4	E962.0	E980.4
Methdilazine	963.0	E858.1	E933.0	E950.4	E962.0	E980.4
Methedrine	969.72	E854.2	E939.7	E950.3	E962.0	E980.3
Methenamine (mande-late)	961.9	E857	E931.9	E950.4	E962.0	E980.4
Methenolone	962.1	E858.0	E932.1	E950.4	E962.0	E980.4
Methergine	975.0	E858.6	E945.0	E950.4	E962.0	E980.4
Methiacil	962.8	E858.0	E932.8	E950.4	E962.0	E980.4
Methicillin (sodium)	960.0	E856	E930.0	E950.4	E962.0	E980.4
Methimazole	962.8	E858.0	E932.8	E950.4	E962.0	E980.4
Methionine	977.1	E858.8	E947.1	E950.4	E962.0	E980.4
Methisazone	961.7	E857	E931.7	E950.4	E962.0	E980.4
Methitural	967.0	E851	E937.0	E950.1	E962.0	E980.1
Methixene	971.1	E855.4	E941.1	E950.4	E962.0	E980.4
Methobarbital, methobarbi-tone	967.0	E851	E937.0	E950.1	E962.0	E980.1
Methocarbamol	968.0	E855.1	E938.0	E950.4	E962.0	E980.4
Methohexital, methohexi-tone (sodium)	968.3	E855.1	E938.3	E950.4	E962.0	E980.4
Methoin	966.1	E855.0	E936.1	E950.4	E962.0	E980.4
Methopholine	965.7	E850.7	E935.7	E950.0	E962.0	E980.0
Methorate	975.4	E858.6	E945.4	E950.4	E962.0	E980.4
Methoserpidine	972.6	E858.3	E942.6	E950.4	E962.0	E980.4
Methotrexate	963.1	E858.1	E933.1	E950.4	E962.0	E980.4
Methotrimeprazine	967.8	E852.8	E937.8	E950.2	E962.0	E980.2
Methoxa-Dome	976.3	E858.7	E946.3	E950.4	E962.0	E980.4
Methoxamine	971.2	E855.5	E941.2	E950.4	E962.0	E980.4
Methoxsalen	976.3	E858.7	E946.3	E950.4	E962.0	E980.4
Methoxybenzyl peni-cillin	960.0	E856	E930.0	E950.4	E962.0	E980.4
Methoxychlor	989.2	E863.0	—	E950.6	E962.1	E980.7
Methoxyflurane	968.2	E855.1	E938.2	E950.4	E962.0	E980.4
Methoxyphenamine	971.2	E855.5	E941.2	E950.4	E962.0	E980.4
Methoxypromazine	969.1	E853.0	E939.1	E950.3	E962.0	E980.3
Methoxypsoralen	976.3	E858.7	E946.3	E950.4	E962.0	E980.4
Methscopolamine (bro-mide)	971.1	E855.4	E941.1	E950.4	E962.0	E980.4
Methsuximide	966.2	E855.0	E936.2	E950.4	E962.0	E980.4
Methyclothiazide	974.3	E858.5	E944.3	E950.4	E962.0	E980.4
Methyl						
acetate	982.8	E862.4	—	E950.9	E962.1	E980.9
acetone	982.8	E862.4	—	E950.9	E962.1	E980.9
alcohol	980.1	E860.2	—	E950.9	E962.1	E980.9
amphetamine	969.72	E854.2	E939.7	E950.3	E962.0	E980.3
androstanolone	962.1	E858.0	E932.1	E950.4	E962.0	E980.4
atropine	971.1	E855.4	E941.1	E950.4	E962.0	E980.4
benzene	982.0	E862.4	—	E950.9	E962.1	E980.9
bromide (gas)	987.8	E869.8	—	E952.8	E962.2	E982.8
fumigant	987.8	E863.8	—	E950.6	E962.2	E980.7
butanol	980.8	E860.8	—	E950.9	E962.1	E980.9
carbinol	980.1	E860.2	—	E950.9	E962.1	E980.9
cellosolve	982.8	E862.4	—	E950.9	E962.1	E980.9
cellulose	973.3	E858.4	E943.3	E950.4	E962.0	E980.4
chloride (gas)	987.8	E869.8	—	E952.8	E962.2	E982.8
cyclohexane	982.8	E862.4	—	E950.9	E962.1	E980.9
cyclohexanone	982.8	E862.4	—	E950.9	E962.1	E980.9
dihydromorphinone	965.09	E850.2	E935.2	E950.0	E962.0	E980.0
ergometrine	975.0	E858.6	E945.0	E950.4	E962.0	E980.4
ergonovine	975.0	E858.6	E945.0	E950.4	E962.0	E980.4
ethyl ketone	982.8	E862.4	—	E950.9	E962.1	E980.9
hydrazine	983.9	E864.3	—	E950.7	E962.1	E980.6
isobutyl ketone	982.8	E862.4	—	E950.9	E962.1	E980.9
morphine NEC	965.09	E850.2	E935.2	E950.0	E962.0	E980.0
parafynol	967.8	E852.8	E937.8	E950.2	E962.0	E980.2
parathion	989.3	E863.1	—	E950.6	E962.1	E980.7
pentynol NEC	967.8	E852.8	E937.8	E950.2	E962.0	E980.2
peridol	969.2	E853.1	E939.2	E950.3	E962.0	E980.3
phenidate	969.73	E854.2	E939.7	E950.3	E962.0	E980.3
prednisolone	962.0	E858.0	E932.0	E950.4	E962.0	E980.4
ENT agent	976.6	E858.7	E946.6	E950.4	E962.0	E980.4
ophthalmic preparation	976.5	E858.7	E946.5	E950.4	E962.0	E980.4
topical NEC	976.0	E858.7	E946.0	E950.4	E962.0	E980.4
propylcarbinol	980.8	E860.8	—	E950.9	E962.1	E980.9

Subterms under main terms may continue to next column or page

►◄ Revised Text ● New Line ▲ Revised Code

Meningococcal vaccine — Methyl

Index

	Poisoning	Accident	Therapeutic Use	Suicide Attempt	Assault	Undeter-mined
Methyl — *continued*						
rosaniline NEC	976.0	E858.7	E946.0	E950.4	E962.0	E980.4
salicylate NEC	976.3	E858.7	E946.3	E950.4	E962.0	E980.4
sulfate (fumes)	987.8	E869.8	—	E952.8	E962.2	E982.8
liquid	983.9	E864.3	—	E950.7	E962.1	E980.6
sulfonal	967.8	E852.8	E937.8	E950.2	E962.0	E980.2
testosterone	962.1	E858.0	E932.1	E950.4	E962.0	E980.4
thiouracil	962.8	E858.0	E932.8	E950.4	E962.0	E980.4
Methylated spirit	980.0	E860.1	—	E950.9	E962.1	E980.9
Methyldopa	972.6	E858.3	E942.6	E950.4	E962.0	E980.4
Methylene						
blue	961.9	E857	E931.9	E950.4	E962.0	E980.4
chloride or dichloride (solvent) NEC	982.3	E862.4	—	E950.9	E962.1	E980.9
Methylhexabital	967.0	E851	E937.0	E950.1	E962.0	E980.1
Methylparaben (oph-thalmic)	976.5	E858.7	E946.5	E950.4	E962.0	E980.4
Methyprylon	967.5	E852.4	E937.5	E950.2	E962.0	E980.2
Methysergide	971.3	E855.6	E941.3	E950.4	E962.0	E980.4
Metoclopramide	963.0	E858.1	E933.0	E950.4	E962.0	E980.4
Metofoline	965.7	E850.7	E935.7	E950.0	E962.0	E980.0
Metopon	965.09	E850.2	E935.2	E950.0	E962.0	E980.0
Metronidazole	961.5	E857	E931.5	E950.4	E962.0	E980.4
Metycaine	968.9	E855.2	E938.9	E950.4	E962.0	E980.4
infiltration (subcuta-neous)	968.5	E855.2	E938.5	E950.4	E962.0	E980.4
nerve block (peripheral) (plexus)	968.6	E855.2	E938.6	E950.4	E962.0	E980.4
topical (surface)	968.5	E855.2	E938.5	E950.4	E962.0	E980.4
Metyrapone	977.8	E858.8	E947.8	E950.4	E962.0	E980.4
Mevinphos	989.3	E863.1	—	E950.6	E962.1	E980.7
Mezereon (berries)	988.2	E865.3	—	E950.9	E962.1	E980.9
Micatin	976.0	E858.7	E946.0	E950.4	E962.0	E980.4
Miconazole	976.0	E858.7	E946.0	E950.4	E962.0	E980.4
Midol	965.1	E850.3	E935.3	E950.0	E962.0	E980.0
Mifepristone	962.9	E858.0	E932.9	E950.4	E962.0	E980.4
Milk of magnesia	973.0	E858.4	E943.0	E950.4	E962.0	E980.4
Millipede (tropical) (ven-omous)	989.5	E905.4	—	E950.9	E962.1	E980.9
Miltown	969.5	E853.8	E939.5	E950.3	E962.0	E980.3
Mineral						
oil (medicinal)	973.2	E858.4	E943.2	E950.4	E962.0	E980.4
nonmedicinal	981	E862.1	—	E950.9	E962.1	E980.9
topical	976.3	E858.7	E946.3	E950.4	E962.0	E980.4
salts NEC	974.6	E858.5	E944.6	E950.4	E962.0	E980.4
spirits	981	E862.0	—	E950.9	E962.1	E980.9
Minocycline	960.4	E856	E930.4	E950.4	E962.0	E980.4
Mithramycin (antineoplas-tic)	960.7	E856	E930.7	E950.4	E962.0	E980.4
Mitobronitol	963.1	E858.1	E933.1	E950.4	E962.0	E980.4
Mitomycin (antineoplas-tic)	960.7	E856	E930.7	E950.4	E962.0	E980.4
Mitotane	963.1	E858.1	E933.1	E950.4	E962.0	E980.4
Moderil	972.6	E858.3	E942.6	E950.4	E962.0	E980.4
Mogadon — *see* Nitrazepam						
Molindone	969.3	E853.8	E939.3	E950.3	E962.0	E980.3
Monistat	976.0	E858.7	E946.0	E950.4	E962.0	E980.4
Monkshood	988.2	E865.4	—	E950.9	E962.1	E980.9
Monoamine oxidase in-hibitors	969.01	E854.0	E939.0	E950.3	E962.0	E980.3
Monochlorobenzene	982.0	E862.4	—	E950.9	E962.1	E980.9
Monosodium glutamate	989.89	E866.8	—	E950.9	E962.1	E980.9
Monoxide, carbon — *see* Car-bon, monoxide						
Moperone	969.2	E853.1	E939.2	E950.3	E962.0	E980.3
Morning glory seeds	969.6	E854.1	E939.6	E950.3	E962.0	E980.3
Moroxydine (hydrochlo-ride)	961.7	E857	E931.7	E950.4	E962.0	E980.4
Morphazinamide	961.8	E857	E931.8	E950.4	E962.0	E980.4
Morphinans	965.09	E850.2	E935.2	E950.0	E962.0	E980.0
Morphine NEC	965.09	E850.2	E935.2	E950.0	E962.0	E980.0
antagonists	970.1	E854.3	E940.1	E950.4	E962.0	E980.4
Morpholinylethylmor-phine	965.09	E850.2	E935.2	E950.0	E962.0	E980.0
Morrhuate sodium	972.7	E858.3	E942.7	E950.4	E962.0	E980.4
Moth balls — *see also* Pesti-cides	989.4	E863.4	—	E950.6	E962.1	E980.7
naphthalene	983.0	E863.4	—	E950.7	E962.1	E980.6
Motor exhaust gas — *see* Carbon, monoxide, exhaust gas						
Mouth wash	976.6	E858.7	E946.6	E950.4	E962.0	E980.4
Mucolytic agent	975.5	E858.6	E945.5	E950.4	E962.0	E980.4
Mucomyst	975.5	E858.6	E945.5	E950.4	E962.0	E980.4
Mucous membrane agents						
(external)	976.9	E858.7	E946.9	E950.4	E962.0	E980.4
specified NEC	976.8	E858.7	E946.8	E950.4	E962.0	E980.4
Mumps						
immune globulin (hu-man)	964.6	E858.2	E934.6	E950.4	E962.0	E980.4
skin test antigen	977.8	E858.8	E947.8	E950.4	E962.0	E980.4
vaccine	979.6	E858.8	E949.6	E950.4	E962.0	E980.4
Mumpsvax	979.6	E858.8	E949.6	E950.4	E962.0	E980.4
Muriatic acid — *see* Hydrochlo-ric acid						
Muscarine	971.0	E855.3	E941.0	E950.4	E962.0	E980.4
Muscle affecting agents						
NEC	975.3	E858.6	E945.3	E950.4	E962.0	E980.4
oxytocic	975.0	E858.6	E945.0	E950.4	E962.0	E980.4
relaxants	975.3	E858.6	E945.3	E950.4	E962.0	E980.4
central nervous system	968.0	E855.1	E938.0	E950.4	E962.0	E980.4
skeletal	975.2	E858.6	E945.2	E950.4	E962.0	E980.4
smooth	975.1	E858.6	E945.1	E950.4	E962.0	E980.4
Mushrooms, noxious	988.1	E865.5	—	E950.9	E962.1	E980.9
Mussel, noxious	988.0	E865.1	—	E950.9	E962.1	E980.9
Mustard (emetic)	973.6	E858.4	E943.6	E950.4	E962.0	E980.4
gas	987.8	E869.8	—	E952.8	E962.2	E982.8
nitrogen	963.1	E858.1	E933.1	E950.4	E962.0	E980.4
Mustine	963.1	E858.1	E933.1	E950.4	E962.0	E980.4
M-vac	979.4	E858.8	E949.4	E950.4	E962.0	E980.4
Mycifradin	960.8	E856	E930.8	E950.4	E962.0	E980.4
topical	976.0	E858.7	E946.0	E950.4	E962.0	E980.4
Mycitracin	960.8	E856	E930.8	E950.4	E962.0	E980.4
ophthalmic preparation	976.5	E858.7	E946.5	E950.4	E962.0	E980.4
Mycostatin	960.1	E856	E930.1	E950.4	E962.0	E980.4
topical	976.0	E858.7	E946.0	E950.4	E962.0	E980.4
Mydriacyl	971.1	E855.4	E941.1	E950.4	E962.0	E980.4
Myelobromal	963.1	E858.1	E933.1	E950.4	E962.0	E980.4
Myleran	963.1	E858.1	E933.1	E950.4	E962.0	E980.4
Myochrysin(e)	965.69	E850.6	E935.6	E950.0	E962.0	E980.0
Myoneural blocking agents	975.2	E858.6	E945.2	E950.4	E962.0	E980.4
Myristica fragrans	988.2	E865.3	—	E950.9	E962.1	E980.9
Myristicin	988.2	E865.3	—	E950.9	E962.1	E980.9
Mysoline	966.3	E855.0	E936.3	E950.4	E962.0	E980.4
Nafcillin (sodium)	960.0	E856	E930.0	E950.4	E962.0	E980.4
Nail polish remover	982.8	E862.4	—	E950.9	E962.1	E908.9
Nalidixic acid	961.9	E857	E931.9	E950.4	E962.0	E980.4
Nalorphine	970.1	E854.3	E940.1	E950.4	E962.0	E980.4
Naloxone	970.1	E854.3	E940.1	E950.4	E962.0	E980.4
Nandrolone (decanoate) (phenproprioate)	962.1	E858.0	E932.1	E950.4	E962.0	E980.4
Naphazoline	971.2	E855.5	E941.2	E950.4	E962.0	E980.4
Naphtha (painter's) (petroleum)	981	E862.0	—	E950.9	E962.1	E980.9
solvent	981	E862.0	—	E950.9	E962.1	E980.9
vapor	987.1	E869.8	—	E952.8	E962.2	E982.8
Naphthalene (chlorinat-ed)	983.0	E864.0	—	E950.7	E962.1	E980.6
insecticide or moth repel-lent	983.0	E863.4	—	E950.7	E962.1	E980.6
vapor	987.8	E869.8	—	E952.8	E962.2	E982.8
Naphthol	983.0	E864.0	—	E950.7	E962.1	E980.6
Naphthylamine	983.0	E864.0	—	E950.7	E962.1	E980.6
Naprosyn — *see* Naproxen						
Naproxen	965.61	E850.6	E935.6	E950.0	E962.0	E980.0
Narcotic (drug)	967.9	E852.9	E937.9	E950.2	E962.0	E980.2
analgesic NEC	965.8	E850.8	E935.8	E950.0	E962.0	E980.0
antagonist	970.1	E854.3	E940.1	E950.4	E962.0	E980.4
specified NEC	967.8	E852.8	E937.8	E950.2	E962.0	E980.2
Narcotine	975.4	E858.6	E945.4	E950.4	E962.0	E980.4
Nardil	969.01	E854.0	E939.0	E950.3	E962.0	E980.3
Natrium cyanide — *see* Cyanide(s)						
Natural						
blood (product)	964.7	E858.2	E934.7	E950.4	E962.0	E980.4
gas (piped)	987.1	E867	—	E951.0	E962.2	E981.0
incomplete combustion	986	E867	—	E951.0	E962.2	E981.0
Nealbarbital, nealbarbi-tone	967.0	E851	E937.0	E950.1	E962.0	E980.1
Nectadon	975.4	E858.6	E945.4	E950.4	E962.0	E980.4
Nematocyst (sting)	989.5	E905.6	—	E950.9	E962.1	E980.9
Nembutal	967.0	E851	E937.0	E950.1	E962.0	E980.1
Neoarsphenamine	961.1	E857	E931.1	E950.4	E962.0	E980.4

	Poisoning	Accident	Therapeutic Use	Suicide Attempt	Assault	Undetermined
External Cause (E-Code)						
Neocinchophen	974.7	E858.5	E944.7	E950.4	E962.0	E980.4
Neomycin	960.8	E856	E930.8	E950.4	E962.0	E980.4
ENT agent	976.6	E858.7	E946.6	E950.4	E962.0	E980.4
ophthalmic preparation	976.5	E858.7	E946.5	E950.4	E962.0	E980.4
topical NEC	976.0	E858.7	E946.0	E950.4	E962.0	E980.4
Neonal	967.0	E851	E937.0	E950.1	E962.0	E980.1
Neoprontosil	961.0	E857	E931.0	E950.4	E962.0	E980.4
Neosalvarsan	961.1	E857	E931.1	E950.4	E962.0	E980.4
Neosilversalvarsan	961.1	E857	E931.1	E950.4	E962.0	E980.4
Neosporin	960.8	E856	E930.8	E950.4	E962.0	E980.4
ENT agent	976.6	E858.7	E946.6	E950.4	E962.0	E980.4
opthalmic preparation	976.5	E858.7	E946.5	E950.4	E962.0	E980.4
topical NEC	976.0	E858.7	E946.0	E950.4	E962.0	E980.4
Neostigmine	971.0	E855.3	E941.0	E950.4	E962.0	E980.4
Neraval	967.0	E851	E937.0	E950.1	E962.0	E980.1
Neravan	967.0	E851	E937.0	E950.1	E962.0	E980.1
Nerium oleander	988.2	E865.4	—	E950.9	E962.1	E980.9
Nerve gases (war)	987.9	E869.9	—	E952.9	E962.2	E982.9
Nesacaine	968.9	E855.2	E938.9	E950.4	E962.0	E980.4
infiltration (subcutaneous)	968.5	E855.2	E938.5	E950.4	E962.0	E980.4
nerve block (peripheral) (plexus)	968.6	E855.2	E938.6	E950.4	E962.0	E980.4
Neurobarb	967.0	E851	E937.0	E950.1	E962.0	E980.1
Neuroleptics NEC	969.3	E853.8	E939.3	E950.3	E962.0	E980.3
Neuroprotective agent	977.8	E858.8	E947.8	E950.4	E962.0	E980.4
Neutral spirits	980.0	E860.1	—	E950.9	E962.1	E980.9
beverage	980.0	E860.0	—	E950.9	E962.1	E980.9
Niacin, niacinamide	972.2	E858.3	E942.2	E950.4	E962.0	E980.4
Nialamide	969.01	E854.0	E939.0	E950.3	E962.0	E980.3
Nickle (carbonyl) (compounds) (fumes) (tetracarbonyl) (vapor)	985.8	E866.4	—	E950.9	E962.1	E980.9
Niclosamide	961.6	E857	E931.6	E950.4	E962.0	E980.4
Nicomorphine	965.09	E850.2	E935.2	E950.0	E962.0	E980.0
Nicotinamide	972.2	E858.3	E942.2	E950.4	E962.0	E980.4
Nicotine (insecticide) (spray) (sulfate) NEC	989.4	E863.4	—	E950.6	E962.1	E980.7
not insecticide	989.89	E866.8	—	E950.9	E962.1	E980.9
Nicotinic acid (derivatives)	972.2	E858.3	E942.2	E950.4	E962.0	E980.4
Nicotinyl alcohol	972.2	E858.3	E942.2	E950.4	E962.0	E980.4
Nicoumalone	964.2	E858.2	E934.2	E950.4	E962.0	E980.4
Nifenazone	965.5	E850.5	E935.5	E950.0	E962.0	E980.0
Nifuraldezone	961.9	E857	E931.9	E950.4	E962.0	E980.4
Nightshade (deadly)	988.2	E865.4	—	E950.9	E962.1	E980.9
Nikethamide	970.0	E854.3	E940.0	E950.4	E962.0	E980.4
Nilstat	960.1	E856	E930.1	E950.4	E962.0	E980.4
topical	976.0	E858.7	E946.0	E950.4	E962.0	E980.4
Nimodipine	977.8	E858.8	E947.8	E950.4	E962.0	E980.4
Niridazole	961.6	E857	E931.6	E950.4	E962.0	E980.4
Nisentil	965.09	E850.2	E935.2	E950.0	E962.0	E980.0
Nitrates	972.4	E858.3	E942.4	E950.4	E962.0	E980.4
Nitrazepam	969.4	E853.2	E939.4	E950.3	E962.0	E980.3
Nitric						
acid (liquid)	983.1	E864.1	—	E950.7	E962.1	E980.6
vapor	987.8	E869.8	—	E952.8	E962.2	E982.8
oxide (gas)	987.2	E869.0	—	E952.8	E962.2	E982.8
Nitrite, amyl (medicinal) (vapor)	972.4	E858.3	E942.4	E950.4	E962.0	E980.4
Nitroaniline	983.0	E864.0	—	E950.7	E962.1	E980.6
vapor	987.8	E869.8	—	E952.8	E962.2	E982.8
Nitrobenzene, nitrobenzol	983.0	E864.0	—	E950.7	E962.1	E980.6
vapor	987.8	E869.8	—	E952.8	E962.2	E982.8
Nitrocellulose	976.3	E858.7	E946.3	E950.4	E962.0	E980.4
Nitrofuran derivatives	961.9	E857	E931.9	E950.4	E962.0	E980.4
Nitrofurantoin	961.9	E857	E931.9	E950.4	E962.0	E980.4
Nitrofurazone	976.0	E858.7	E946.0	E950.4	E962.0	E980.4
Nitrogen (dioxide) (gas) (oxide)	987.2	E869.0	—	E952.8	E962.2	E982.8
mustard (antineoplastic)	963.1	E858.1	E933.1	E950.4	E962.0	E980.4
nonmedicinal	989.89	E866.8	—	E950.9	E962.1	E980.9
fumes	987.8	E869.8	—	E952.8	E962.2	E982.8
Nitroglycerin, nitroglycerol (medicinal)	972.4	E858.3	E942.4	E950.4	E962.0	E980.4
Nitrohydrochloric acid	983.1	E864.1	—	E950.7	E962.1	E980.6
Nitromersol	976.0	E858.7	E946.0	E950.4	E962.0	E980.4
Nitronaphthalene	983.0	E864.0	—	E950.7	E962.1	E980.6
Nitrophenol	983.0	E864.0	—	E950.7	E962.2	E980.6
Nitrothiazol	961.6	E857	E931.6	E950.4	E962.0	E980.4
Nitrotoluene, nitrotoluol	983.0	E864.0	—	E950.7	E962.1	E980.6

	Poisoning	Accident	Therapeutic Use	Suicide Attempt	Assault	Undetermined
External Cause (E-Code)						
Nitrotoluene, nitrotoluol — continued						
vapor	987.8	E869.8	—	E952.8	E962.2	E982.8
Nitrous	968.2	E855.1	E938.2	E950.4	E962.0	E980.4
acid (liquid)	983.1	E864.1	—	E950.7	E962.1	E980.6
fumes	987.2	E869.0	—	E952.8	E962.2	E982.8
oxide (anesthetic) NEC	968.2	E855.1	E938.2	E950.4	E962.0	E980.4
Nitrozone	976.0	E858.7	E946.0	E950.4	E962.0	E980.4
Noctec	967.1	E852.0	E937.1	E950.2	E962.0	E980.2
Noludar	967.5	E852.4	E937.5	E950.2	E962.0	E980.2
Noptil	967.0	E851	E937.0	E950.1	E962.0	E980.1
Noradrenalin	971.2	E855.5	E941.2	E950.4	E962.0	E980.4
Noramidopyrine	965.5	E850.5	E935.5	E950.0	E962.0	E980.0
Norepinephrine	971.2	E855.5	E941.2	E950.4	E962.0	E980.4
Norethandrolone	962.1	E858.0	E932.1	E950.4	E962.0	E980.4
Norethindrone	962.2	E858.0	E932.2	E950.4	E962.0	E980.4
Norethisterone	962.2	E858.0	E932.2	E950.4	E962.0	E980.4
Norethynodrel	962.2	E858.0	E932.2	E950.4	E962.0	E980.4
Norlestrin	962.2	E858.0	E932.2	E950.4	E962.0	E980.4
Norlutin	962.2	E858.0	E932.2	E950.4	E962.0	E980.4
Normison — see Benzodiazepines						
Normorphine	965.09	E850.2	E935.2	E950.0	E962.0	E980.0
Nortriptyline	969.05	E854.0	E939.0	E950.3	E962.0	E980.3
Noscapine	975.4	E858.6	E945.4	E950.4	E962.0	E980.4
Nose preparations	976.6	E858.7	E946.6	E950.4	E962.0	E980.4
Novobiocin	960.8	E856	E930.8	E950.4	E962.0	E980.4
Novocain (infiltration) (topical)	968.5	E855.2	E938.5	E950.4	E962.0	E980.4
nerve block (peripheral) (plexus)	968.6	E855.2	E938.6	E950.4	E962.0	E980.4
spinal	968.7	E855.2	E938.7	E950.4	E962.0	E980.4
Noxythiolin	961.9	E857	E931.9	E950.4	E962.0	E980.4
NPH Iletin (insulin)	962.3	E858.0	E932.3	E950.4	E962.0	E980.4
Numorphan	965.09	E850.2	E935.2	E950.0	E962.0	E980.0
Nunol	967.0	E851	E937.0	E950.1	E962.0	E980.1
Nupercaine (spinal anesthetic)	968.7	E855.2	E938.7	E950.4	E962.0	E980.4
topical (surface)	968.5	E855.2	E938.5	E950.4	E962.0	E980.4
Nutmeg oil (liniment)	976.3	E858.7	E946.3	E950.4	E962.0	E980.4
Nux vomica	989.1	E863.7	—	E950.6	E962.1	E980.7
Nydrazid	961.8	E857	E931.8	E950.4	E962.0	E980.4
Nylidrin	971.2	E855.5	E941.2	E950.4	E962.0	E980.4
Nystatin	960.1	E856	E930.1	E950.4	E962.0	E980.4
topical	976.0	E858.7	E946.0	E950.4	E962.0	E980.4
Nytol	963.0	E858.1	E933.0	E950.4	E962.0	E980.4
Oblivion	967.8	E852.8	E937.8	E950.2	E962.0	E980.2
Octyl nitrite	972.4	E858.3	E942.4	E950.4	E962.0	E980.4
Oestradiol (cypionate) (dipropionate) (valerate)	962.2	E858.0	E932.2	E950.4	E962.0	E980.4
Oestriol	962.2	E858.0	E932.2	E950.4	E962.0	E980.4
Oestrone	962.2	E858.0	E932.2	E950.4	E962.0	E980.4
Oil (of) NEC	989.89	E866.8	—	E950.9	E962.1	E980.9
bitter almond	989.0	E866.8	—	E950.9	E962.1	E980.9
camphor	976.1	E858.7	E946.1	E950.4	E962.0	E980.4
colors	989.89	E861.6	—	E950.9	E962.1	E980.9
fumes	987.8	E869.8	—	E952.8	E962.2	E982.8
lubricating	981	E862.2	—	E950.9	E962.1	E980.9
specified source, other — see substance specified						
vitriol (liquid)	983.1	E864.1	—	E950.7	E962.1	E980.6
fumes	987.8	E869.8	—	E952.8	E962.2	E982.8
wintergreen (bitter) NEC	976.3	E858.7	E946.3	E950.4	E962.0	E980.4
Ointments NEC	976.9	E858.7	E946.9	E950.4	E962.0	E980.4
Oleander	988.2	E865.4	—	E950.9	E962.1	E980.9
Oleandomycin	960.3	E856	E930.3	E950.4	E962.0	E980.4
Oleovitamin A	963.5	E858.1	E933.5	E950.4	E962.0	E980.4
Oleum ricini	973.1	E858.4	E943.1	E950.4	E962.0	E980.4
Olive oil (medicinal) NEC	973.2	E858.4	E943.2	E950.4	E962.0	E980.4
OMPA	989.3	E863.1	—	E950.6	E962.1	E980.7
Oncovin	963.1	E858.1	E933.1	E950.4	E962.0	E980.4
Ophthaine	968.5	E855.2	E938.5	E950.4	E962.0	E980.4
Ophthetic	968.5	E855.2	E938.5	E950.4	E962.0	E980.4
Opiates, opioids, opium NEC	965.00	E850.2	E935.2	E950.0	E962.0	E980.0
antagonists	970.1	E854.3	E940.1	E950.4	E962.0	E980.4
Oracon	962.2	E858.0	E932.2	E950.4	E962.0	E980.4
Oragrafin	977.8	E858.8	E947.8	E950.4	E962.0	E980.4
Oral contraceptives	962.2	E858.0	E932.2	E950.4	E962.0	E980.4
Orciprenaline	975.1	E858.6	E945.1	E950.4	E962.0	E980.4
Organidin	975.5	E858.6	E945.5	E950.4	E962.0	E980.4
Organophosphates	989.3	E863.1	—	E950.6	E962.1	E980.7

Nontherapeutic use substance

Subterms under main terms may continue to next column or page

	Poisoning	Accident	Therapeutic Use	Suicide Attempt	Assault	Undeter-mined
Orimune	979.5	E858.8	E949.5	E950.4	E962.0	E980.4
Orinase	962.3	E858.0	E932.3	E950.4	E962.0	E980.4
Orphenadrine	966.4	E855.0	E936.4	E950.4	E962.0	E980.4
Ortal (sodium)	967.0	E851	E937.0	E950.1	E962.0	E980.1
Orthoboric acid	976.0	E858.7	E946.0	E950.4	E962.0	E980.4
ENT agent	976.6	E858.7	E946.6	E950.4	E962.0	E980.4
ophthalmic preparation	976.5	E858.7	E946.5	E950.4	E962.0	E980.4
Orthocaine	968.5	E855.2	E938.5	E950.4	E962.0	E980.4
Ortho-Novum	962.2	E858.0	E932.2	E950.4	E962.0	E980.4
Orthotolidine (reagent)	977.8	E858.8	E947.8	E950.4	E962.0	E980.4
Osmic acid (liquid)	983.1	E864.1	—	E950.7	E962.1	E980.6
fumes	987.8	E869.8	—	E952.8	E962.2	E982.8
Osmotic diuretics	974.4	E858.5	E944.4	E950.4	E962.0	E980.4
Ouabain	972.1	E858.3	E942.1	E950.4	E962.0	E980.4
Ovarian hormones (synthetic substitutes)	962.2	E858.0	E932.2	E950.4	E962.0	E980.4
Ovral	962.2	E858.0	E932.2	E950.4	E962.0	E980.4
Ovulation suppressants	962.2	E858.0	E932.2	E950.4	E962.0	E980.4
Ovulen	962.2	E858.0	E932.2	E950.4	E962.0	E980.4
Oxacillin (sodium)	960.0	E856	E930.0	E950.4	E962.0	E980.4
Oxalic acid	983.1	E864.1	—	E950.7	E962.1	E980.6
Oxanamide	969.5	E853.8	E939.5	E950.3	E962.0	E980.3
Oxandrolone	962.1	E858.0	E932.1	E950.4	E962.0	E980.4
Oxaprozin	965.61	E850.6	E935.6	E950.0	E962.0	E980.0
Oxazepam	969.4	E853.2	E939.4	E950.3	E962.0	E980.3
Oxazolidine derivatives	966.0	E855.0	E936.0	E950.4	E962.0	E980.4
Ox bile extract	973.4	E858.4	E943.4	E950.4	E962.0	E980.4
Oxedrine	971.2	E855.5	E941.2	E950.4	E962.0	E980.4
Oxeladin	975.4	E858.6	E945.4	E950.4	E962.0	E980.4
Oxethazaine NEC	968.5	E855.2	E938.5	E950.4	E962.0	E980.4
Oxidizing agents NEC	983.9	E864.3	—	E950.7	E962.1	E980.6
Oxolinic acid	961.3	E857	E931.3	E950.4	E962.0	E980.4
Oxophenarsine	961.1	E857	E931.1	E950.4	E962.0	E980.4
Oxsoralen	976.3	E858.7	E946.3	E950.4	E962.0	E980.4
Oxtriphylline	975.7	E858.6	E945.7	E950.4	E962.0	E980.4
Oxybuprocaine	968.5	E855.2	E938.5	E950.4	E962.0	E980.4
Oxybutynin	975.1	E858.6	E945.1	E950.4	E962.0	E980.4
Oxycodone	965.09	E850.2	E935.2	E950.0	E962.0	E980.0
Oxygen	987.8	E869.8	—	E952.8	E962.2	E982.8
Oxylone	976.0	E858.7	E946.0	E950.4	E962.0	E980.4
ophthalmic preparation	976.5	E858.7	E946.5	E950.4	E962.0	E980.4
Oxymesterone	962.1	E858.0	E932.1	E950.4	E962.0	E980.4
Oxymetazoline	971.2	E855.5	E941.2	E950.4	E962.0	E980.4
Oxymetholone	962.1	E858.0	E932.1	E950.4	E962.0	E980.4
Oxymorphone	965.09	E850.2	E935.2	E950.0	E962.0	E980.0
Oxypertine	969.09	E854.0	E939.0	E950.3	E962.0	E980.3
Oxyphenbutazone	965.5	E850.5	E935.5	E950.0	E962.0	E980.0
Oxyphencyclimine	971.1	E855.4	E941.1	E950.4	E962.0	E980.4
Oxyphenisatin	973.1	E858.4	E943.1	E950.4	E962.0	E980.4
Oxyphenonium	971.1	E855.4	E941.1	E950.4	E962.0	E980.4
Oxyquinoline	961.3	E857	E931.3	E950.4	E962.0	E980.4
Oxytetracycline	960.4	E856	E930.4	E950.4	E962.0	E980.4
Oxytocics	975.0	E858.6	E945.0	E950.4	E962.0	E980.4
Oxytocin	975.0	E858.6	E945.0	E950.4	E962.0	E980.4
Ozone	987.8	E869.8	—	E952.8	E962.2	E982.8
PABA	976.3	E858.7	E946.3	E950.4	E962.0	E980.4
Packed red cells	964.7	E858.2	E934.7	E950.4	E962.0	E980.4
Paint NEC	989.89	E861.6	—	E950.9	E962.1	E980.9
cleaner	982.8	E862.9	—	E950.9	E962.1	E980.9
fumes NEC	987.8	E869.8	—	E952.8	E962.1	E982.8
lead (fumes)	984.0	E861.5	—	E950.9	E962.1	E980.9
solvent NEC	982.8	E862.9	—	E950.9	E962.1	E980.9
stripper	982.8	E862.9	—	E950.9	E962.1	E980.9
Palfium	965.09	E850.2	E935.2	E950.0	E962.0	E980.0
Palivizumab	979.9	E858.8	E949.6	E950.4	E962.0	E980.4
Paludrine	961.4	E857	E931.4	E950.4	E962.0	E980.4
PAM	977.2	E855.8	E947.2	E950.4	E962.0	E980.4
Pamaquine (naphthoate)	961.4	E857	E931.4	E950.4	E962.0	E980.4
Pamprin	965.1	E850.3	E935.3	E950.0	E962.0	E980.0
Panadol	965.4	E850.4	E935.4	E950.0	E962.0	E980.0
Pancreatic dornase (mucolytic)	963.4	E858.1	E933.4	E950.4	E962.0	E980.4
Pancreatin	973.4	E858.4	E943.4	E950.4	E962.0	E980.4
Pancrelipase	973.4	E858.4	E943.4	E950.4	E962.0	E980.4
Pangamic acid	963.5	E858.1	E933.5	E950.4	E962.0	E980.4
Panthenol	963.5	E858.1	E933.5	E950.4	E962.0	E980.4
topical	976.8	E858.7	E946.8	E950.4	E962.0	E980.4
Pantopaque	977.8	E858.8	E947.8	E950.4	E962.0	E980.4
Pantopon	965.00	E850.2	E935.2	E950.0	E962.0	E980.0
Pantothenic acid	963.5	E858.1	E933.5	E950.4	E962.0	E980.4
Panwarfin	964.2	E858.2	E934.2	E950.4	E962.0	E980.4
Papain	973.4	E858.4	E943.4	E950.4	E962.0	E980.4
Papaverine	972.5	E858.3	E942.5	E950.4	E962.0	E980.4
Para-aminobenzoic acid	976.3	E858.7	E946.3	E950.4	E962.0	E980.4
Para-aminophenol derivatives	965.4	E850.4	E935.4	E950.0	E962.0	E980.0
Para-aminosalicylic acid (derivatives)	961.8	E857	E931.8	E950.4	E962.0	E980.4
Paracetaldehyde (medicinal)	967.2	E852.1	E937.2	E950.2	E962.0	E980.2
Paracetamol	965.4	E850.4	E935.4	E950.0	E962.0	E980.0
Paracodin	965.09	E850.2	E935.2	E950.0	E962.0	E980.0
Paradione	966.0	E855.0	E936.0	E950.4	E962.0	E980.4
Paraffin(s) (wax)	981	E862.3	—	E950.9	E962.1	E980.9
liquid (medicinal)	973.2	E858.4	E943.2	E950.4	E962.0	E980.4
nonmedicinal (oil)	981	E962.1	—	E950.9	—	E980.9
Paraldehyde (medicinal)	967.2	E852.1	E937.2	E950.2	E962.0	E980.2
Paramethadione	966.0	E855.0	E936.0	E950.4	E962.0	E980.4
Paramethasone	962.0	E858.0	E932.0	E950.4	E962.0	E980.4
Paraquat	989.4	E863.5	—	E950.6	E962.1	E980.7
Parasympatholytics	971.1	E855.4	E941.1	E950.4	E962.0	E980.4
Parasympathomimetics	971.0	E855.3	E941.0	E950.4	E962.0	E980.4
Parathion	989.3	E863.1	—	E950.6	E962.1	E980.7
Parathormone	962.6	E858.0	E932.6	E950.4	E962.0	E980.4
Parathyroid (derivatives)	962.6	E858.0	E932.6	E950.4	E962.0	E980.4
Paratyphoid vaccine	978.1	E858.8	E948.1	E950.4	E962.0	E980.4
Paredrine	971.2	E855.5	E941.2	E950.4	E962.0	E980.4
Paregoric	965.00	E850.2	E935.2	E950.0	E962.0	E980.0
Pargyline	972.3	E858.3	E942.3	E950.4	E962.0	E980.4
Paris green	985.1	E866.3	—	E950.8	E962.1	E980.8
insecticide	985.1	E863.4	—	E950.8	E962.1	E980.8
Parnate	969.01	E854.0	E939.0	E950.3	E962.0	E980.3
Paromomycin	960.8	E856	E930.8	E950.4	E962.0	E980.4
Paroxypropione	963.1	E858.1	E933.1	E950.4	E962.0	E980.4
Parzone	965.09	E850.2	E935.2	E950.0	E962.0	E980.0
PAS	961.8	E857	E931.8	E950.4	E962.0	E980.4
PCBs	981	E862.3	—	E950.9	E962.1	E980.9
PCP (pentachlorophenol)	989.4	E863.6	—	E950.6	E962.1	E980.7
herbicide	989.4	E863.5	—	E950.6	E962.1	E980.7
insecticide	989.4	E863.4	—	E950.6	E962.1	E980.7
phencyclidine	968.3	E855.1	E938.3	E950.4	E962.0	E980.4
Peach kernel oil (emulsion)	973.2	E858.4	E943.2	E950.4	E962.0	E980.4
Peanut oil (emulsion) NEC	973.2	E858.4	E943.2	E950.4	E962.0	E980.4
topical	976.3	E858.7	E946.3	E950.4	E962.0	E980.4
Pearly Gates (morning glory seeds)	969.6	E854.1	E939.6	E950.3	E962.0	E980.3
Pecazine	969.1	E853.0	E939.1	E950.3	E962.0	E980.3
Pecilocin	960.1	E856	E930.1	E950.4	E962.0	E980.4
Pectin (with kaolin) NEC	973.5	E858.4	E943.5	E950.4	E962.0	E980.4
Pelletierine tannate	961.6	E857	E931.6	E950.4	E962.0	E980.4
Pemoline	969.79	E854.2	E939.7	E950.3	E962.0	E980.3
Pempidine	972.3	E858.3	E942.3	E950.4	E962.0	E980.4
Penamecillin	960.0	E856	E930.0	E950.4	E962.0	E980.4
Penethamate hydriodide	960.0	E856	E930.0	E950.4	E962.0	E980.4
Penicillamine	963.8	E858.1	E933.8	E950.4	E962.0	E980.4
Penicillin (any type)	960.0	E856	E930.0	E950.4	E962.0	E980.4
Penicillinase	963.4	E858.1	E933.4	E950.4	E962.0	E980.4
Pentachlorophenol (fungicide)	989.4	E863.6	—	E950.6	E962.1	E980.7
herbicide	989.4	E863.5	—	E950.6	E962.1	E980.7
insecticide	989.4	E863.4	—	E950.6	E962.1	E980.7
Pentaerythritol	972.4	E858.3	E942.4	E950.4	E962.0	E980.4
chloral	967.1	E852.0	E937.1	E950.2	E962.0	E980.2
tetranitrate NEC	972.4	E858.3	E942.4	E950.4	E962.0	E980.4
Pentagastrin	977.8	E858.8	E947.8	E950.4	E962.0	E980.4
Pentalin	982.3	E862.4	—	E950.9	E962.1	E980.9
Pentamethonium (bromide)	972.3	E858.3	E942.3	E950.4	E962.0	E980.4
Pentamidine	961.5	E857	E931.5	E950.4	E962.0	E980.4
Pentanol	980.8	E860.8	—	E950.9	E962.1	E980.9
Pentaquine	961.4	E857	E931.4	E950.4	E962.0	E980.4
Pentazocine	965.8	E850.8	E935.8	E950.0	E962.0	E980.0
Penthienate	971.1	E855.4	E941.1	E950.4	E962.0	E980.4
Pentobarbital, pentobarbitone (sodium)	967.0	E851	E937.0	E950.1	E962.0	E980.1
Pentolinium (tartrate)	972.3	E858.3	E942.3	E950.4	E962.0	E980.4
Pentothal	968.3	E855.1	E938.3	E950.4	E962.0	E980.4
Pentylenetetrazol	970.0	E854.3	E940.0	E950.4	E962.0	E980.4
Pentylsalicylamide	961.8	E857	E931.8	E950.4	E962.0	E980.4
Pepsin	973.4	E858.4	E943.4	E950.4	E962.0	E980.4
Peptavlon	977.8	E858.8	E947.8	E950.4	E962.0	E980.4
Percaine (spinal)	968.7	E855.2	E938.7	E950.4	E962.0	E980.4

Substance	Poisoning	Accident	Therapeutic Use	Suicide Attempt	Assault	Undetermined
Percaine — *continued*						
topical (surface)	968.5	E855.2	E938.5	E950.4	E962.0	E980.4
Perchloroethylene (vapor)	982.3	E862.4	—	E950.9	E962.1	E980.9
medicinal	961.6	E857	E931.6	E950.4	E962.0	E980.4
Percodan	965.09	E850.2	E935.2	E950.0	E962.0	E980.0
Percogesic	965.09	E850.2	E935.2	E950.0	E962.0	E980.0
Percorten	962.0	E858.0	E932.0	E950.4	E962.0	E980.4
Pergonal	962.4	E858.0	E932.4	E950.4	E962.0	E980.4
Perhexiline	972.4	E858.3	E942.4	E950.4	E962.0	E980.4
Periactin	963.0	E858.1	E933.0	E950.4	E962.0	E980.4
Periclor	967.1	E852.0	E937.1	E950.2	E962.0	E980.2
Pericyazine	969.1	E853.0	E939.1	E950.3	E962.0	E980.3
Peritrate	972.4	E858.3	E942.4	E950.4	E962.0	E980.4
Permanganates NEC	983.9	E864.3	—	E950.7	E962.1	E980.6
potassium (topical)	976.0	E858.7	E946.0	E950.4	E962.0	E980.4
Pernocton	967.0	E851	E937.0	E950.1	E962.0	E980.1
Pernoston	967.0	E851	E937.0	E950.1	E962.0	E980.1
Peronin(e)	965.09	E850.2	E935.2	E950.0	E962.0	E980.0
Perphenazine	969.1	E853.0	E939.1	E950.3	E962.0	E980.3
Pertofrane	969.05	E854.0	E939.0	E950.3	E962.0	E980.3
Pertussis						
immune serum (human)	964.6	E858.2	E934.6	E950.4	E962.0	E980.4
vaccine (with diphtheria toxoid) (with tetanus toxoid)	978.6	E858.8	E948.6	E950.4	E962.0	E980.4
Peruvian balsam	976.8	E858.7	E946.8	E950.4	E962.0	E980.4
Pesticides (dust) (fumes) (vapor)	989.4	E863.4	—	E950.6	E962.1	E980.7
arsenic	985.1	E863.4	—	E950.8	E962.1	E980.8
chlorinated	989.2	E863.0	—	E950.6	E962.1	E980.7
cyanide	989.0	E863.4	—	E950.6	E962.1	E980.7
kerosene	981	E863.4	—	E950.6	E962.1	E980.7
mixture (of compounds)	989.4	E863.3	—	E950.6	E962.1	E980.7
naphthalene	983.0	E863.4	—	E950.7	E962.1	E980.6
organochlorine (compounds)	989.2	E863.0	—	E950.6	E962.1	E980.7
petroleum (distillate) (products) NEC	981	E863.4	—	E950.6	E962.1	E980.7
specified ingredient NEC	989.4	E863.4	—	E950.6	E962.1	E980.7
strychnine	989.1	E863.4	—	E950.6	E962.1	E980.7
thallium	985.8	E863.7	—	E950.6	E962.1	E980.7
Pethidine (hydrochloride)	965.09	E850.2	E935.2	E950.0	E962.0	E980.0
Petrichloral	967.1	E852.0	E937.1	E950.2	E962.0	E980.2
Petrol	981	E862.1	—	E950.9	E962.1	E980.9
vapor	987.1	E869.8	—	E952.8	E962.2	E982.8
Petrolatum (jelly) (ointment)	976.3	E858.7	E946.3	E950.4	E962.0	E980.4
hydrophilic	976.3	E858.7	E946.3	E950.4	E962.0	E980.4
liquid	973.2	E858.4	E943.2	E950.4	E962.0	E980.4
topical	976.3	E858.7	E946.3	E950.4	E962.0	E980.4
nonmedicinal	981	E862.1	—	E950.9	E962.1	E980.9
Petroleum (cleaners) (fuels) (products) NEC	981	E862.1	—	E950.9	E962.1	E980.9
benzin(e) — see Ligroin						
ether — see Ligroin						
jelly — see Petrolatum						
naphtha — see Ligroin						
pesticide	981	E863.4	—	E950.6	E962.1	E980.7
solids	981	E862.3	—	E950.9	E962.1	E980.9
solvents	981	E862.0	—	E950.9	E962.1	E980.9
vapor	987.1	E869.8	—	E952.8	E962.2	E982.8
Peyote	969.6	E854.1	E939.6	E950.3	E962.0	E980.3
Phanodorm, phanodorn	967.0	E851	E937.0	E950.1	E962.0	E980.1
Phanquinone, phanquone	961.5	E857	E931.5	E950.4	E962.0	E980.4
Pharmaceutical excipient or adjunct	977.4	E858.8	E947.4	E950.4	E962.0	E980.4
Phenacemide	966.3	E855.0	E936.3	E950.4	E962.0	E980.4
Phenacetin	965.4	E850.4	E935.4	E950.0	E962.0	E980.0
Phenadoxone	965.09	E850.2	E935.2	E950.0	E962.0	E980.0
Phenaglycodol	969.5	E853.8	E939.5	E950.3	E962.0	E980.3
Phenantoin	966.1	E855.0	E936.1	E950.4	E962.0	E980.4
Phenaphthazine reagent	977.8	E858.8	E947.8	E950.4	E962.0	E980.4
Phenazocine	965.09	E850.2	E935.2	E950.0	E962.0	E980.0
Phenazone	965.5	E850.5	E935.5	E950.0	E962.0	E980.0
Phenazopyridine	976.1	E858.7	E946.1	E950.4	E962.0	E980.4
Phenbenicillin	960.0	E856	E930.0	E950.4	E962.0	E980.4
Phenbutrazate	977.0	E858.8	E947.0	E950.4	E962.0	E980.4
Phencyclidine	968.3	E855.1	E938.3	E950.4	E962.0	E980.4
Phendimetrazine	977.0	E858.8	E947.0	E950.4	E962.0	E980.4
Phenelzine	969.01	E854.0	E939.0	E950.3	E962.0	E980.3
Phenergan	967.8	E852.8	E937.8	E950.2	E962.0	E980.2
Phenethicillin (potassium)	960.0	E856	E930.0	E950.4	E962.0	E980.4
Phenetsal	965.1	E850.3	E935.3	E950.0	E962.0	E980.0
Pheneturide	966.3	E855.0	E936.3	E950.4	E962.0	E980.4
Phenformin	962.3	E858.0	E932.3	E950.4	E962.0	E980.4
Phenglutarimide	971.1	E855.4	E941.1	E950.4	E962.0	E980.4
Phenicarbazide	965.8	E850.8	E935.8	E950.0	E962.0	E980.0
Phenindamine (tartrate)	963.0	E858.1	E933.0	E950.4	E962.0	E980.4
Phenindione	964.2	E858.2	E934.2	E950.4	E962.0	E980.4
Pheniprazine	969.01	E854.0	E939.0	E950.3	E962.0	E980.3
Pheniramine (maleate)	963.0	E858.1	E933.0	E950.4	E962.0	E980.4
Phenmetrazine	977.0	E858.8	E947.0	E950.4	E962.0	E980.4
Phenobal	967.0	E851	E937.0	E950.1	E962.0	E980.1
Phenobarbital	967.0	E851	E937.0	E950.1	E962.0	E980.1
Phenobarbitone	967.0	E851	E937.0	E950.1	E962.0	E980.1
Phenoctide	976.0	E858.7	E946.0	E950.4	E962.0	E980.4
Phenol (derivatives) NEC	983.0	E864.0	—	E950.7	E962.1	E980.6
disinfectant	983.0	E864.0	—	E950.7	E962.1	E980.6
pesticide	989.4	E863.4	—	E950.6	E962.1	E980.7
red	977.8	E858.8	E947.8	E950.4	E962.0	E980.4
Phenolphthalein	973.1	E858.4	E943.1	E950.4	E962.0	E980.4
Phenolsulfonphthalein	977.8	E858.8	E947.8	E950.4	E962.0	E980.4
Phenomorphan	965.09	E850.2	E935.2	E950.0	E962.0	E980.0
Phenonyl	967.0	E851	E937.0	E950.1	E962.0	E980.1
Phenoperidine	965.09	E850.2	E935.2	E950.0	E962.0	E980.0
Phenoquin	974.7	E858.5	E944.7	E950.4	E962.0	E980.4
Phenothiazines (tranquilizers) NEC	969.1	E853.0	E939.1	E950.3	E962.0	E980.3
insecticide	989.3	E863.4	—	E950.6	E962.1	E980.7
Phenoxybenzamine	971.3	E855.6	E941.3	E950.4	E962.0	E980.4
Phenoxymethyl penicillin	960.0	E856	E930.0	E950.4	E962.0	E980.4
Phenprocoumon	964.2	E858.2	E934.2	E950.4	E962.0	E980.4
Phensuximide	966.2	E855.0	E936.2	E950.4	E962.0	E980.4
Phentermine	977.0	E858.8	E947.0	E950.4	E962.0	E980.4
Phentolamine	971.3	E855.6	E941.3	E950.4	E962.0	E980.4
Phenyl						
butazone	965.5	E850.5	E935.5	E950.0	E962.0	E980.0
enediamine	983.0	E864.0	—	E950.7	E962.1	E980.6
hydrazine	983.0	E864.0	—	E950.7	E962.1	E980.6
antineoplastic	963.1	E858.1	E933.1	E950.4	E962.0	E980.4
mercuric compounds — see Mercury						
salicylate	976.3	E858.7	E946.3	E950.4	E962.0	E980.4
Phenylephrine	971.2	E855.5	E941.2	E950.4	E962.0	E980.4
Phenylethylbiguanide	962.3	E858.0	E932.3	E950.4	E962.0	E980.4
Phenylpropanolamine	971.2	E855.5	E941.2	E950.4	E962.0	E980.4
Phenylsulfthion	989.3	E863.1	—	E950.6	E962.1	E980.7
Phenyramidol, phenyramidon	965.7	E850.7	E935.7	E950.0	E962.0	E980.0
Phenytoin	966.1	E855.0	E936.1	E950.4	E962.0	E980.4
pHisoHex	976.2	E858.7	E946.2	E950.4	E962.0	E980.4
Pholcodine	965.09	E850.2	E935.2	E950.0	E962.0	E980.0
Phorate	989.3	E863.1	—	E950.6	E962.1	E980.7
Phosdrin	989.3	E863.1	—	E950.6	E962.1	E980.7
Phosgene (gas)	987.8	E869.8	—	E952.8	E962.2	E982.8
Phosphate (tricresyl)	989.89	E866.8	—	E950.9	E962.1	E980.9
organic	989.3	E863.1	—	E950.6	E962.1	E980.7
solvent	982.8	E862.4	—	E950.9	E926.1	E980.9
Phosphine	987.8	E869.8	—	E952.8	E962.2	E982.8
fumigant	987.8	E863.8	—	E950.6	E962.2	E980.7
Phospholine	971.0	E855.3	E941.0	E950.4	E962.0	E980.4
Phosphoric acid	983.1	E864.1	—	E950.7	E962.1	E980.6
Phosphorus (compounds) NEC	983.9	E864.3	—	E950.7	E962.1	E980.6
rodenticide	983.9	E863.7	—	E950.7	E962.1	E980.6
Phthalimidoglutarimide	967.8	E852.8	E937.8	E950.2	E962.0	E980.2
Phthalylsulfathiazole	961.0	E857	E931.0	E950.4	E962.0	E980.4
Phylloquinone	964.3	E858.2	E934.3	E950.4	E962.0	E980.4
Physeptone	965.02	E850.1	E935.1	E950.0	E962.0	E980.0
Physostigma venenosum	988.2	E865.4	—	E950.9	E962.1	E980.9
Physostigmine	971.0	E855.3	E941.0	E950.4	E962.0	E980.4
Phytolacca decandra	988.2	E865.4	—	E950.9	E962.1	E980.9
Phytomenadione	964.3	E858.2	E934.3	E950.4	E962.0	E980.4
Phytonadione	964.3	E858.2	E934.3	E950.4	E962.0	E980.4
Picric (acid)	983.0	E864.0	—	E950.7	E962.1	E980.6
Picrotoxin	970.0	E854.3	E940.0	E950.4	E962.0	E980.4
Pilocarpine	971.0	E855.3	E941.0	E950.4	E962.0	E980.4
Pilocarpus (jaborandi) extract	971.0	E855.3	E941.0	E950.4	E962.0	E980.4

Nontherapeutic use substance

▶◀ Revised Text   ● New Line   ▲ Revised Code

▽ Subterms under main terms may continue to next column or page

	Poisoning	Accident	Therapeutic Use	Suicide Attempt	Assault	Undeter-mined
Pimaricin	960.1	E856	E930.1	E950.4	E962.0	E980.4
Piminodine	965.09	E850.2	E935.2	E950.0	E962.0	E980.0
Pine oil, pinesol (disinfectant)	983.9	E861.4	—	E950.7	E962.1	E980.6
Pinkroot	961.6	E857	E931.6	E950.4	E962.0	E980.4
Pipadone	965.09	E850.2	E935.2	E950.0	E962.0	E980.0
Pipamazine	963.0	E858.1	E933.0	E950.4	E962.0	E980.4
Pipazethate	975.4	E858.6	E945.4	E950.4	E962.0	E980.4
Pipenzolate	971.1	E855.4	E941.1	E950.4	E962.0	E980.4
Piperacetazine	969.1	E853.0	E939.1	E950.3	E962.0	E980.3
Piperazine NEC	961.6	E857	E931.6	E950.4	E962.0	E980.4
estrone sulfate	962.2	E858.0	E932.2	E950.4	E962.0	E980.4
Piper cubeba	988.2	E865.4	—	E950.9	E962.1	E980.9
Piperidione	975.4	E858.6	E945.4	E950.4	E962.0	E980.4
Piperidolate	971.1	E855.4	E941.1	E950.4	E962.0	E980.4
Piperocaine	968.9	E855.2	E938.9	E950.4	E962.0	E980.4
infiltration (subcutaneous)	968.5	E855.2	E938.5	E950.4	E962.0	E980.4
nerve block (peripheral) (plexus)	968.6	E855.2	E938.6	E950.4	E962.0	E980.4
topical (surface)	968.5	E855.2	E938.5	E950.4	E962.0	E980.4
Pipobroman	963.1	E858.1	E933.1	E950.4	E962.0	E980.4
Pipradrol	970.89	E854.3	E940.8	E950.4	E962.0	E980.4
Piscidia (bark) (erythrina)	965.7	E850.7	E935.7	E950.0	E962.0	E980.0
Pitch	983.0	E864.0	—	E950.7	E962.1	E980.6
Pitkin's solution	968.7	E855.2	E938.7	E950.4	E962.0	E980.4
Pitocin	975.0	E858.6	E945.0	E950.4	E962.0	E980.4
Pitressin (tannate)	962.5	E858.0	E932.5	E950.4	E962.0	E980.4
Pituitary extracts (posterior)	962.5	E858.0	E932.5	E950.4	E962.0	E980.4
anterior	962.4	E858.0	E932.4	E950.4	E962.0	E980.4
Pituitrin	962.5	E858.0	E932.5	E950.4	E962.0	E980.4
Placental extract	962.9	E858.0	E932.9	E950.4	E962.0	E980.4
Placidyl	967.8	E852.8	E937.8	E950.2	E962.0	E980.2
Plague vaccine	978.3	E858.8	E948.3	E950.4	E962.0	E980.4
Plant foods or fertilizers NEC	989.89	E866.5	—	E950.9	E962.1	E980.9
mixed with herbicides	989.4	E863.5	—	E950.6	E962.1	E980.7
Plants, noxious, used as food	988.2	E865.9	—	E950.9	E962.1	E980.9
berries and seeds	988.2	E865.3	—	E950.9	E962.1	E980.9
specified type NEC	988.2	E865.4	—	E950.9	E962.1	E980.9
Plasma (blood)	964.7	E858.2	E934.7	E950.4	E962.0	E980.4
expanders	964.8	E858.2	E934.8	E950.4	E962.0	E980.4
Plasmanate	964.7	E858.2	E934.7	E950.4	E962.0	E980.4
Plegicil	969.1	E853.0	E939.1	E950.3	E962.0	E980.3
Podophyllin	976.4	E858.7	E946.4	E950.4	E962.0	E980.4
Podophyllum resin	976.4	E858.7	E946.4	E950.4	E962.0	E980.4
Poison NEC	989.9	E866.9	—	E950.9	E962.1	E980.9
Poisonous berries	988.2	E865.3	—	E950.9	E962.1	E980.9
Pokeweed (any part)	988.2	E865.4	—	E950.9	E962.1	E980.9
Poldine	971.1	E855.4	E941.1	E950.4	E962.0	E980.4
Poliomyelitis vaccine	979.5	E858.8	E949.5	E950.4	E962.0	E980.4
Poliovirus vaccine	979.5	E858.8	E949.5	E950.4	E962.0	E980.4
Polish (car) (floor) (furniture) (metal) (silver)	989.89	E861.2	—	E950.9	E962.1	E980.9
abrasive	989.89	E861.3	—	E950.9	E962.1	E980.9
porcelain	989.89	E861.3	—	E950.9	E962.1	E980.9
Poloxalkol	973.2	E858.4	E943.2	E950.4	E962.0	E980.4
Polyaminostyrene resins	974.5	E858.5	E944.5	E950.4	E962.0	E980.4
Polychlorinated biphenyl — see PCBs						
Polycycline	960.4	E856	E930.4	E950.4	E962.0	E980.4
Polyester resin hardener	982.8	E862.4	—	E950.9	E962.1	E980.9
fumes	987.8	E869.8	—	E952.8	E962.2	E982.8
Polyestradiol (phosphate)	962.2	E858.0	E932.2	E950.4	E962.0	E980.4
Polyethanolamine alkyl sulfate	976.2	E858.7	E946.2	E950.4	E962.0	E980.4
Polyethylene glycol	976.3	E858.7	E946.3	E950.4	E962.0	E980.4
Polyferose	964.0	E858.2	E934.0	E950.4	E962.0	E980.4
Polymyxin B	960.8	E856	E930.8	E950.4	E962.0	E980.4
ENT agent	976.6	E858.7	E946.6	E950.4	E962.0	E980.4
ophthalmic preparation	976.5	E858.7	E946.5	E950.4	E962.0	E980.4
topical NEC	976.0	E858.7	E946.0	E950.4	E962.0	E980.4
Polynoxylin(e)	976.0	E858.7	E946.0	E950.4	E962.0	E980.4
Polyoxymethyleneurea	976.0	E858.7	E946.0	E950.4	E962.0	E980.4
Polytetrafluoroethylene (inhaled)	987.8	E869.8	—	E952.8	E962.2	E982.8
Polythiazide	974.3	E858.5	E944.3	E950.4	E962.0	E980.4
Polyvinylpyrrolidone	964.8	E858.2	E934.8	E950.4	E962.0	E980.4

	Poisoning	Accident	Therapeutic Use	Suicide Attempt	Assault	Undeter-mined
Pontocaine (hydrochloride) (infiltration) (topical)	968.5	E855.2	E938.5	E950.4	E962.0	E980.4
nerve block (peripheral) (plexus)	968.6	E855.2	E938.6	E950.4	E962.0	E980.4
spinal	968.7	E855.2	E938.7	E950.4	E962.0	E980.4
Pot	969.6	E854.1	E939.6	E950.3	E962.0	E980.3
Potash (caustic)	983.2	E864.2	—	E950.7	E962.1	E980.6
Potassic saline injection (lactated)	974.5	E858.5	E944.5	E950.4	E962.0	E980.4
Potassium (salts) NEC	974.5	E858.5	E944.5	E950.4	E962.0	E980.4
aminosalicylate	961.8	E857	E931.8	E950.4	E962.0	E980.4
arsenite (solution)	985.1	E866.3	—	E950.8	E962.1	E980.8
bichromate	983.9	E864.3	—	E950.7	E962.1	E980.6
bisulfate	983.9	E864.3	—	E950.7	E962.1	E980.6
bromide (medicinal) NEC	967.3	E852.2	E937.3	E950.2	E962.0	E980.2
carbonate	983.2	E864.2	—	E950.7	E962.1	E980.6
chlorate NEC	983.9	E864.3	—	E950.7	E962.1	E980.6
cyanide — see Cyanide						
hydroxide	983.2	E864.2	—	E950.7	E962.1	E980.6
iodide (expectorant) NEC	975.5	E858.6	E945.5	E950.4	E962.0	E980.4
nitrate	989.89	E866.8	—	E950.9	E962.1	E980.9
oxalate	983.9	E864.3	—	E950.7	E962.1	E980.6
perchlorate NEC	977.8	E858.8	E947.8	E950.4	E962.0	E980.4
antithyroid	962.8	E858.0	E932.8	E950.4	E962.0	E980.4
permanganate	976.0	E858.7	E946.0	E950.4	E962.0	E980.4
nonmedicinal	983.9	E864.3	—	E950.7	E962.1	E980.6
Povidone-iodine (anti-infective) NEC	976.0	E858.7	E946.0	E950.4	E962.0	E980.4
Practolol	972.0	E858.3	E942.0	E950.4	E962.0	E980.4
Pralidoxime (chloride)	977.2	E858.8	E947.2	E950.4	E962.0	E980.4
Pramoxine	968.5	E855.2	E938.5	E950.4	E962.0	E980.4
Prazosin	972.6	E858.3	E942.6	E950.4	E962.0	E980.4
Prednisolone	962.0	E858.0	E932.0	E950.4	E962.0	E980.4
ENT agent	976.6	E858.7	E946.6	E950.4	E962.0	E980.4
ophthalmic preparation	976.5	E858.7	E946.5	E950.4	E962.0	E980.4
topical NEC	976.0	E858.7	E946.0	E950.4	E962.0	E980.4
Prednisone	962.0	E858.0	E932.0	E950.4	E962.0	E980.4
Pregnanediol	962.2	E858.0	E932.2	E950.4	E962.0	E980.4
Pregneninolone	962.2	E858.0	E932.2	E950.4	E962.0	E980.4
Preludin	977.0	E858.8	E947.0	E950.4	E962.0	E980.4
Premarin	962.2	E858.0	E932.2	E950.4	E962.0	E980.4
Prenylamine	972.4	E858.3	E942.4	E950.4	E962.0	E980.4
Preparation H	976.8	E858.7	E946.8	E950.4	E962.0	E980.4
Preservatives	989.89	E866.8	—	E950.9	E962.1	E980.9
Pride of China	988.2	E865.3	—	E950.9	E962.1	E980.9
Prilocaine	968.9	E855.2	E938.9	E950.4	E962.0	E980.4
infiltration (subcutaneous)	968.5	E855.2	E938.5	E950.4	E962.0	E980.4
nerve block (peripheral) (plexus)	968.6	E855.2	E938.6	E950.4	E962.0	E980.4
Primaquine	961.4	E857	E931.4	E950.4	E962.0	E980.4
Primidone	966.3	E855.0	E936.3	E950.4	E962.0	E980.4
Primula (veris)	988.2	E865.4	—	E950.9	E962.1	E980.9
Prinadol	965.09	E850.2	E935.2	E950.0	E962.0	E980.0
Priscol, Priscoline	971.3	E855.6	E941.3	E950.4	E962.0	E980.4
Privet	988.2	E865.4	—	E950.9	E962.1	E980.9
Privine	971.2	E855.5	E941.2	E950.4	E962.0	E980.4
Pro-Banthine	971.1	E855.4	E941.1	E950.4	E962.0	E980.4
Probarbital	967.0	E851	E937.0	E950.1	E962.0	E980.1
Probenecid	974.7	E858.5	E944.7	E950.4	E962.0	E980.4
Procainamide (hydrochloride)	972.0	E858.3	E942.0	E950.4	E962.0	E980.4
Procaine (hydrochloride) (infiltration) (topical)	968.5	E855.2	E938.5	E950.4	E962.0	E980.4
nerve block (peripheral) (plexus)	968.6	E855.2	E938.6	E950.4	E962.0	E980.4
penicillin G	960.0	E856	E930.0	E950.4	E962.0	E980.4
spinal	968.7	E855.2	E938.7	E950.4	E962.0	E980.4
Procalmidol	969.5	E853.8	E939.5	E950.3	E962.0	E980.3
Procarbazine	963.1	E858.1	E933.1	E950.4	E962.0	E980.4
Prochlorperazine	969.1	E853.0	E939.1	E950.3	E962.0	E980.3
Procyclidine	966.4	E855.0	E936.4	E950.4	E962.0	E980.4
Producer gas	986	E868.8	—	E952.1	E962.2	E982.1
Profenamine	966.4	E855.0	E936.4	E950.4	E962.0	E980.4
Profenil	975.1	E858.6	E945.1	E950.4	E962.0	E980.4
Progesterones	962.2	E858.0	E932.2	E950.4	E962.0	E980.4
Progestin	962.2	E858.0	E932.2	E950.4	E962.0	E980.4
Progestogens (with estrogens)	962.2	E858.0	E932.2	E950.4	E962.0	E980.4
Progestone	962.2	E858.0	E932.2	E950.4	E962.0	E980.4
Proguanil	961.4	E857	E931.4	E950.4	E962.0	E980.4
Prolactin	962.4	E858.0	E932.4	E950.4	E962.0	E980.4

	Poisoning	Accident	Therapeutic Use	Suicide Attempt	Assault	Undetermined
Proloid	962.7	E858.0	E932.7	E950.4	E962.0	E980.4
Proluton	962.2	E858.0	E932.2	E950.4	E962.0	E980.4
Promacetin	961.8	E857	E931.8	E950.4	E962.0	E980.4
Promazine	969.1	E853.0	E939.1	E950.3	E962.0	E980.3
Promedol	965.09	E850.2	E935.2	E950.0	E962.0	E980.0
Promethazine	967.8	E852.8	E937.8	E950.2	E962.0	E980.2
Promin	961.8	E857	E931.8	E950.4	E962.0	E980.4
Pronestyl (hydrochloride)	972.0	E858.3	E942.0	E950.4	E962.0	E980.4
Pronetalol, pronethalol	972.0	E858.3	E942.0	E950.4	E962.0	E980.4
Prontosil	961.0	E857	E931.0	E950.4	E962.0	E980.4
Propamidine isethionate	961.5	E857	E931.5	E950.4	E962.0	E980.4
Propanal (medicinal)	967.8	E852.8	E937.8	E950.2	E962.0	E980.2
Propane (gas) (distributed in mobile container)	987.0	E868.0	—	E951.1	E962.2	E981.1
distributed through pipes	987.0	E867	—	E951.0	E962.2	E981.0
incomplete combustion of — see Carbon monoxide, Propane						
Propanidid	968.3	E855.1	E938.3	E950.4	E962.0	E980.4
Propanol	980.3	E860.4	—	E950.9	E962.1	E980.9
Propantheline	971.1	E855.4	E941.1	E950.4	E962.0	E980.4
Proparacaine	968.5	E855.2	E938.5	E950.4	E962.0	E980.4
Propatyl nitrate	972.4	E858.3	E942.4	E950.4	E962.0	E980.4
Propicillin	960.0	E856	E930.0	E950.4	E962.0	E980.4
Propiolactone (vapor)	987.8	E869.8	—	E952.8	E962.2	E982.8
Propiomazine	967.8	E852.8	E937.8	E950.2	E962.0	E980.2
Propionaldehyde (medicinal)	967.8	E852.8	E937.8	E950.2	E962.0	E980.2
Propionate compound	976.0	E858.7	E946.0	E950.4	E962.0	E980.4
Propion gel	976.0	E858.7	E946.0	E950.4	E962.0	E980.4
Propitocaine	968.9	E855.2	E938.9	E950.4	E962.0	E980.4
infiltration (subcutaneous)	968.5	E855.2	E938.5	E950.4	E962.0	E980.4
nerve block (peripheral) (plexus)	968.6	E855.2	E938.6	E950.4	E962.0	E980.4
Propoxur	989.3	E863.2	—	E950.6	E962.1	E980.7
Propoxycaine	968.9	E855.2	E938.9	E950.4	E962.0	E980.4
infiltration (subcutaneous)	968.5	E855.2	E938.5	E950.4	E962.0	E980.4
nerve block (peripheral) (plexus)	968.6	E855.2	E938.6	E950.4	E962.0	E980.4
topical (surface)	968.5	E855.2	E938.5	E950.4	E962.0	E980.4
Propoxyphene (hydrochloride)	965.8	E850.8	E935.8	E950.0	E962.0	E980.0
Propranolol	972.0	E858.3	E942.0	E950.4	E962.0	E980.4
Propyl						
alcohol	980.3	E860.4	—	E950.9	E962.1	E980.9
carbinol	980.3	E860.4	—	E950.9	E962.1	E980.9
hexadrine	971.2	E855.5	E941.2	E950.4	E962.0	E980.4
iodone	977.8	E858.8	E947.8	E950.4	E962.0	E980.4
thiouracil	962.8	E858.0	E932.8	E950.4	E962.0	E980.4
Propylene	987.1	E869.8	—	E952.8	E962.2	E982.8
Propylparaben (ophthalmic)	976.5	E858.7	E946.5	E950.4	E962.0	E980.4
Proscillaridin	972.1	E858.3	E942.1	E950.4	E962.0	E980.4
Prostaglandins	975.0	E858.6	E945.0	E950.4	E962.0	E980.4
Prostigmin	971.0	E855.3	E941.0	E950.4	E962.0	E980.4
Protamine (sulfate)	964.5	E858.2	E934.5	E950.4	E962.0	E980.4
zinc insulin	962.3	E858.0	E932.3	E950.4	E962.0	E980.4
Protectants (topical)	976.3	E858.7	E946.3	E950.4	E962.0	E980.4
Protein hydrolysate	974.5	E858.5	E944.5	E950.4	E962.0	E980.4
Prothiaden — see Dothiepin hydrochloride						
Prothionamide	961.8	E857	E931.8	E950.4	E962.0	E980.4
Prothipendyl	969.5	E853.8	E939.5	E950.3	E962.0	E980.3
Protokylol	971.2	E855.5	E941.2	E950.4	E962.0	E980.4
Protopam	977.2	E858.8	E947.2	E950.4	E962.0	E980.4
Protoveratrine(s) (A) (B)	972.6	E858.3	E942.6	E950.4	E962.0	E980.4
Protriptyline	969.05	E854.0	E939.0	E950.3	E962.0	E980.3
Provera	962.2	E858.0	E932.2	E950.4	E962.0	E980.4
Provitamin A	963.5	E858.1	E933.5	E950.4	E962.0	E980.4
Proxymetacaine	968.5	E855.2	E938.5	E950.4	E962.0	E980.4
Proxyphylline	975.1	E858.6	E945.1	E950.4	E962.0	E980.4
Prozac — see Fluoxetine hydrochloride						
Prunus						
laurocerasus	988.2	E865.4	—	E950.9	E962.1	E980.9
virginiana	988.2	E865.4	—	E950.9	E962.1	E980.9
Prussic acid	989.0	E866.8	—	E950.9	E962.1	E980.9
vapor	987.7	E869.8	—	E952.8	E962.2	E982.8
Pseudoephedrine	971.2	E855.5	E941.2	E950.4	E962.0	E980.4

	Poisoning	Accident	Therapeutic Use	Suicide Attempt	Assault	Undetermined
Psilocin	969.6	E854.1	E939.6	E950.3	E962.0	E980.3
Psilocybin	969.6	E854.1	E939.6	E950.3	E962.0	E980.3
PSP	977.8	E858.8	E947.8	E950.4	E962.0	E980.4
Psychedelic agents	969.6	E854.1	E939.6	E950.3	E962.0	E980.3
Psychodysleptics	969.6	E854.1	E939.6	E950.3	E962.0	E980.3
Psychostimulants	969.70	E854.2	E939.7	E950.3	E962.0	E980.3
Psychotherapeutic agents	969.9	E855.9	E939.9	E950.3	E962.0	E980.3
antidepressants	969.00	E854.0	E939.0	E950.3	E962.0	E980.3
specified NEC	969.8	E855.8	E939.8	E950.3	E962.0	E980.3
tranquilizers NEC	969.5	E853.9	E939.5	E950.3	E962.0	E980.3
Psychotomimetic agents	969.6	E854.1	E939.6	E950.3	E962.0	E980.3
Psychotropic agents	969.9	E854.8	E939.9	E950.3	E962.0	E980.3
specified NEC	969.8	E854.8	E939.8	E950.3	E962.0	E980.3
Psyllium	973.3	E858.4	E943.3	E950.4	E962.0	E980.4
Pteroylglutamic acid	964.1	E858.2	E934.1	E950.4	E962.0	E980.4
Pteroyltriglutamate	963.1	E858.1	E933.1	E950.4	E962.0	E980.4
PTFE	987.8	E869.8	—	E952.8	E962.2	E982.8
Pulsatilla	988.2	E865.4	—	E950.9	E962.1	E980.9
Purex (bleach)	983.9	E864.3	—	E950.7	E962.1	E980.6
Purine diuretics	974.1	E858.5	E944.1	E950.4	E962.0	E980.4
Purinethol	963.1	E858.1	E933.1	E950.4	E962.0	E980.4
PVP	964.8	E858.2	E934.8	E950.4	E962.0	E980.4
Pyrabital	965.7	E850.7	E935.7	E950.0	E962.0	E980.0
Pyramidon	965.5	E850.5	E935.5	E950.0	E962.0	E980.0
Pyrantel (pamoate)	961.6	E857	E931.6	E950.4	E962.0	E980.4
Pyrathiazine	963.0	E858.1	E933.0	E950.4	E962.0	E980.4
Pyrazinamide	961.8	E857	E931.8	E950.4	E962.0	E980.4
Pyrazinoic acid (amide)	961.8	E857	E931.8	E950.4	E962.0	E980.4
Pyrazole (derivatives)	965.5	E850.5	E935.5	E950.0	E962.0	E980.0
Pyrazolone (analgesics)	965.5	E850.5	E935.5	E950.0	E962.0	E980.0
Pyrethrins, pyrethrum	989.4	E863.4	—	E950.6	E962.1	E980.7
Pyribenzamine	963.0	E858.1	E933.0	E950.4	E962.0	E980.4
Pyridine (liquid) (vapor)	982.0	E862.4	—	E950.9	E962.1	E980.9
aldoxime chloride	977.2	E858.8	E947.2	E950.4	E962.0	E980.4
Pyridium	976.1	E858.7	E946.1	E950.4	E962.0	E980.4
Pyridostigmine	971.0	E855.3	E941.0	E950.4	E962.0	E980.4
Pyridoxine	963.5	E858.1	E933.5	E950.4	E962.0	E980.4
Pyrilamine	963.0	E858.1	E933.0	E950.4	E962.0	E980.4
Pyrimethamine	961.4	E857	E931.4	E950.4	E962.0	E980.4
Pyrogallic acid	983.0	E864.0	—	E950.7	E962.1	E980.6
Pyroxylin	976.3	E858.7	E946.3	E950.4	E962.0	E980.4
Pyrrobutamine	963.0	E858.1	E933.0	E950.4	E962.0	E980.4
Pyrrocitine	968.5	E855.2	E938.5	E950.4	E962.0	E980.4
Pyrvinium (pamoate)	961.6	E857	E931.6	E950.4	E962.0	E980.4
PZI	962.3	E858.0	E932.3	E950.4	E962.0	E980.4
Quaalude	967.4	E852.3	E937.4	E950.2	E962.0	E980.2
Quaternary ammonium derivatives	971.1	E855.4	E941.1	E950.4	E962.0	E980.4
Quicklime	983.2	E864.2	—	E950.7	E962.1	E980.6
Quinacrine	961.3	E857	E931.3	E950.4	E962.0	E980.4
Quinaglute	972.0	E858.3	E942.0	E950.4	E962.0	E980.4
Quinalbarbitone	967.0	E851	E937.0	E950.1	E962.0	E980.1
Quinestradiol	962.2	E858.0	E932.2	E950.4	E962.0	E980.4
Quinethazone	974.3	E858.5	E944.3	E950.4	E962.0	E980.4
Quinidine (gluconate) (polygalacturonate) (salts) (sulfate)	972.0	E858.3	E942.0	E950.4	E962.0	E980.4
Quinine	961.4	E857	E931.4	E950.4	E962.0	E980.4
Quiniobine	961.3	E857	E931.3	E950.4	E962.0	E980.4
Quinolines	961.3	E857	E931.3	E950.4	E962.0	E980.4
Quotane	968.5	E855.2	E938.5	E950.4	E962.0	E980.4
Rabies						
immune globulin (human)	964.6	E858.2	E934.6	E950.4	E962.0	E980.4
vaccine	979.1	E858.8	E949.1	E950.4	E962.0	E980.4
Racemoramide	965.09	E850.2	E935.2	E950.0	E962.0	E980.0
Racemorphan	965.09	E850.2	E935.2	E950.0	E962.0	E980.0
Radiator alcohol	980.1	E860.2	—	E950.9	E962.1	E980.9
Radio-opaque (drugs) (materials)	977.8	E858.8	E947.8	E950.4	E962.0	E980.4
Ranunculus	988.2	E865.4	—	E950.9	E962.1	E980.9
Rat poison	989.4	E863.7	—	E950.6	E962.1	E980.7
Rattlesnake (venom)	989.5	E905.0	—	E950.9	E962.1	E980.9
Raudixin	972.6	E858.3	E942.6	E950.4	E962.0	E980.4
Rautensin	972.6	E858.3	E942.6	E950.4	E962.0	E980.4
Rautina	972.6	E858.3	E942.6	E950.4	E962.0	E980.4
Rautotal	972.6	E858.3	E942.6	E950.4	E962.0	E980.4
Rauwiloid	972.6	E858.3	E942.6	E950.4	E962.0	E980.4
Rauwoldin	972.6	E858.3	E942.6	E950.4	E962.0	E980.4
Rauwolfia (alkaloids)	972.6	E858.3	E942.6	E950.4	E962.0	E980.4
Realgar	985.1	E866.3	—	E950.8	E962.1	E980.8

	Poisoning	Accident	Therapeutic Use	Suicide Attempt	Assault	Undetermined
Red cells, packed	964.7	E858.2	E934.7	E950.4	E962.0	E980.4
Reducing agents, industrial NEC	983.9	E864.3	—	E950.7	E962.1	E980.6
Refrigerant gas (freon)	987.4	E869.2	—	E952.8	E962.2	E982.8
central nervous system	968.0	E855.1	E938.0	E950.4	E962.0	E980.4
not freon	987.9	E869.9	—	E952.9	E962.2	E982.9
Regroton	974.4	E858.5	E944.4	E950.4	E962.0	E980.4
Rela	968.0	E855.1	E938.0	E950.4	E962.0	E980.4
Relaxants, skeletal muscle (autonomic)	975.2	E858.6	E945.2	E950.4	E962.0	E980.4
Renese	974.3	E858.5	E944.3	E950.4	E962.0	E980.4
Renografin	977.8	E858.8	E947.8	E950.4	E962.0	E980.4
Replacement solutions	974.5	E858.5	E944.5	E950.4	E962.0	E980.4
Rescinnamine	972.6	E858.3	E942.6	E950.4	E962.0	E980.4
Reserpine	972.6	E858.3	E942.6	E950.4	E962.0	E980.4
Resorcin, resorcinol	976.4	E858.7	E946.4	E950.4	E962.0	E980.4
Respaire	975.5	E858.6	E945.5	E950.4	E962.0	E980.4
Respiratory agents NEC	975.8	E858.6	E945.8	E950.4	E962.0	E980.4
Retinoic acid	976.8	E858.7	E946.8	E950.4	E962.0	E980.4
Retinol	963.5	E858.1	E933.5	E950.4	E962.0	E980.4
Rh (D) immune globulin (human)	964.6	E858.2	E934.6	E950.4	E962.0	E980.4
Rhodine	965.1	E850.3	E935.3	E950.0	E962.0	E980.0
RhoGAM	964.6	E858.2	E934.6	E950.4	E962.0	E980.4
Riboflavin	963.5	E858.1	E933.5	E950.4	E962.0	E980.4
Ricin	989.89	E866.8	—	E950.9	E962.1	E980.9
Ricinus communis	988.2	E865.3	—	E950.9	E962.1	E980.9
Rickettsial vaccine NEC	979.6	E858.8	E949.6	E950.4	E962.0	E980.4
with viral and bacterial vaccine	979.7	E858.8	E949.7	E950.4	E962.0	E980.4
Rifampin	960.6	E856	E930.6	E950.4	E962.0	E980.4
Rimifon	961.8	E857	E931.8	E950.4	E962.0	E980.4
Ringer's injection (lactated)	974.5	E858.5	E944.5	E950.4	E962.0	E980.4
Ristocetin	960.8	E856	E930.8	E950.4	E962.0	E980.4
Ritalin	969.73	E854.2	E939.7	E950.3	E962.0	E980.3
Roach killers — see Pesticides						
Rocky Mountain spotted fever vaccine	979.6	E858.8	E949.6	E950.4	E962.0	E980.4
Rodenticides	989.4	E863.7	—	E950.6	E962.1	E980.7
Rohypnol	969.4	E853.2	E939.4	E950.3	E962.0	E980.3
Rolaids	973.0	E858.4	E943.0	E950.4	E962.0	E980.4
Rolitetracycline	960.4	E856	E930.4	E950.4	E962.0	E980.4
Romilar	975.4	E858.6	E945.4	E950.4	E962.0	E980.4
Rose water ointment	976.3	E858.7	E946.3	E950.4	E962.0	E980.4
Rosuvastatin calcium	972.1	E858.3	E942.2	E950.4	E962.0	E980.4
Rotenone	989.4	E863.7	—	E950.6	E962.1	E980.7
Rotoxamine	963.0	E858.1	E933.0	E950.4	E962.0	E980.4
Rough-on-rats	989.4	E863.7	—	E950.6	E962.1	E980.7
RU486	962.9	E858.0	E932.9	E950.4	E962.0	E980.4
Rubbing alcohol	980.2	E860.3	—	E950.9	E962.1	E980.9
Rubella virus vaccine	979.4	E858.8	E949.4	E950.4	E962.0	E980.4
Rubelogen	979.4	E858.8	E949.4	E950.4	E962.0	E980.4
Rubeovax	979.4	E858.8	E949.4	E950.4	E962.0	E980.4
Rubidomycin	960.7	E856	E930.7	E950.4	E962.0	E980.4
Rue	988.2	E865.4	—	E950.9	E962.1	E980.9
Ruta	988.2	E865.4	—	E950.9	E962.1	E980.9
Sabadilla (medicinal)	976.0	E858.7	E946.0	E950.4	E962.0	E980.4
pesticide	989.4	E863.4	—	E950.6	E962.1	E980.7
Sabin oral vaccine	979.5	E858.8	E949.5	E950.4	E962.0	E980.4
Saccharated iron oxide	964.0	E858.2	E934.0	E950.4	E962.0	E980.4
Saccharin	974.5	E858.5	E944.5	E950.4	E962.0	E980.4
Safflower oil	972.2	E858.3	E942.2	E950.4	E962.0	E980.4
Salbutamol sulfate	975.7	E858.6	E945.7	E950.4	E962.0	E980.4
Salicylamide	965.1	E850.3	E935.3	E950.0	E962.0	E980.0
Salicylate(s)	965.1	E850.3	E935.3	E950.0	E962.0	E980.0
methyl	976.3	E858.7	E946.3	E950.4	E962.0	E980.4
theobromine calcium	974.1	E858.5	E944.1	E950.4	E962.0	E980.4
Salicylazosulfapyridine	961.0	E857	E931.0	E950.4	E962.0	E980.4
Salicylhydroxamic acid	976.0	E858.7	E946.0	E950.4	E962.0	E980.4
Salicylic acid (keratolytic) NEC	976.4	E858.7	E946.4	E950.4	E962.0	E980.4
congeners	965.1	E850.3	E935.3	E950.0	E962.0	E980.0
salts	965.1	E850.3	E935.3	E950.0	E962.0	E980.0
Saliniazid	961.8	E857	E931.8	E950.4	E962.0	E980.4
Salol	976.3	E858.7	E946.3	E950.4	E962.0	E980.4
Salt (substitute) NEC	974.5	E858.5	E944.5	E950.4	E962.0	E980.4
Saluretics	974.3	E858.5	E944.3	E950.4	E962.0	E980.4
Saluron	974.3	E858.5	E944.3	E950.4	E962.0	E980.4
Salvarsan 606 (neosilver) (silver)	961.1	E857	E931.1	E950.4	E962.0	E980.4
Sambucus canadensis	988.2	E865.4	—	E950.9	E962.1	E980.9

	Poisoning	Accident	Therapeutic Use	Suicide Attempt	Assault	Undetermined
Sambucus canadensis — continued						
berry	988.2	E865.3	—	E950.9	E962.1	E980.9
Sandril	972.6	E858.3	E942.6	E950.4	E962.0	E980.4
Sanguinaria canadensis	988.2	E865.4	—	E950.9	E962.1	E980.9
Saniflush (cleaner)	983.9	E861.3	—	E950.7	E962.1	E980.6
Santonin	961.6	E857	E931.6	E950.4	E962.0	E980.4
Santyl	976.8	E858.7	E946.8	E950.4	E962.0	E980.4
Sarkomycin	960.7	E856	E930.7	E950.4	E962.0	E980.4
Saroten	969.05	E854.0	E939.0	E950.3	E962.0	E980.3
Saturnine — see Lead						
Savin (oil)	976.4	E858.7	E946.4	E950.4	E962.0	E980.4
Scammony	973.1	E858.4	E943.1	E950.4	E962.0	E980.4
Scarlet red	976.8	E858.7	E946.8	E950.4	E962.0	E980.4
Scheele's green	985.1	E866.3	—	E950.8	E962.1	E980.8
insecticide	985.1	E863.4	—	E950.8	E962.1	E980.8
Schradan	989.3	E863.1	—	E950.6	E962.1	E980.7
Schweinfurt(h) green	985.1	E866.3	—	E950.8	E962.1	E980.8
insecticide	985.1	E863.4	—	E950.8	E962.1	E980.8
Scilla — see Squill						
Sclerosing agents	972.7	E858.3	E942.7	E950.4	E962.0	E980.4
Scopolamine	971.1	E855.4	E941.1	E950.4	E962.0	E980.4
Scouring powder	989.89	E861.3	—	E950.9	E962.1	E980.9
Sea						
anemone (sting)	989.5	E905.6	—	E950.9	E962.1	E980.9
cucumber (sting)	989.5	E905.6	—	E950.9	E962.1	E980.9
snake (bite) (venom)	989.5	E905.0	—	E950.9	E962.1	E980.9
urchin spine (puncture)	989.5	E905.6	—	E950.9	E962.1	E980.9
Secbutabarbital	967.0	E851	E937.0	E950.1	E962.0	E980.1
Secbutabarbitone	967.0	E851	E937.0	E950.1	E962.0	E980.1
Secobarbital	967.0	E851	E937.0	E950.1	E962.0	E980.1
Seconal	967.0	E851	E937.0	E950.1	E962.0	E980.1
Secretin	977.8	E858.8	E947.8	E950.4	E962.0	E980.4
Sedatives, nonbarbiturate	967.9	E852.9	E937.9	E950.2	E962.0	E980.2
specified NEC	967.8	E852.8	E937.8	E950.2	E962.0	E980.2
Sedormid	967.8	E852.8	E937.8	E950.2	E962.0	E980.2
Seed (plant)	988.2	E865.3	—	E950.9	E962.1	E980.9
disinfectant or dressing	989.89	E866.5	—	E950.9	E962.1	E980.9
Selective serotonin and norepinephrine reuptake inhibitors (SSNRI)	969.02	E854.0	E939.0	E950.3	E962.0	E980.3
Selective serotonin reuptake inhibitors (SSRI)	969.03	E854.0	E939.0	E950.3	E962.0	E980.3
Selenium (fumes) NEC	985.8	E866.4	—	E950.9	E962.1	E980.9
disulfide or sulfide	976.4	E858.7	E946.4	E950.4	E962.0	E980.4
Selsun	976.4	E858.7	E946.4	E950.4	E962.0	E980.4
Senna	973.1	E858.4	E943.1	E950.4	E962.0	E980.4
Septisol	976.2	E858.7	E946.2	E950.4	E962.0	E980.4
Serax	969.4	E853.2	E939.4	E950.3	E962.0	E980.3
Serenesil	967.8	E852.8	E937.8	E950.2	E962.0	E980.2
Serenium (hydrochloride)	961.9	E857	E931.9	E950.4	E962.0	E980.4
Serepax — see Oxazepam						
Sernyl	968.3	E855.1	E938.3	E950.4	E962.0	E980.4
Serotonin	977.8	E858.8	E947.8	E950.4	E962.0	E980.4
Serpasil	972.6	E858.3	E942.6	E950.4	E962.0	E980.4
Sewer gas	987.8	E869.8	—	E952.8	E962.2	E982.8
Shampoo	989.6	E861.0	—	E950.9	E962.1	E980.9
Shellfish, nonbacterial or noxious	988.0	E865.1	—	E950.9	E962.1	E980.9
Silicones NEC	989.83	E866.8	E947.8	E950.9	E962.1	E980.9
Silvadene	976.0	E858.7	E946.0	E950.4	E962.0	E980.4
Silver (compound) (medicinal) NEC	976.0	E858.7	E946.0	E950.4	E962.0	E980.4
anti-infectives	976.0	E858.7	E946.0	E950.4	E962.0	E980.4
arsphenamine	961.1	E857	E931.1	E950.4	E962.0	E980.4
nitrate	976.0	E858.7	E946.0	E950.4	E962.0	E980.4
ophthalmic preparation	976.5	E858.7	E946.5	E950.4	E962.0	E980.4
toughened (keratolytic)	976.4	E858.7	E946.4	E950.4	E962.0	E980.4
nonmedicinal (dust)	985.8	E866.4	—	E950.9	E962.1	E980.9
protein (mild) (strong)	976.0	E858.7	E946.0	E950.4	E962.0	E980.4
salvarsan	961.1	E857	E931.1	E950.4	E962.0	E980.4
Simethicone	973.8	E858.4	E943.8	E950.4	E962.0	E980.4
Sinequan	969.05	E854.0	E939.0	E950.3	E962.0	E980.3
Singoserp	972.6	E858.3	E942.6	E950.4	E962.0	E980.4
Sintrom	964.2	E858.2	E934.2	E950.4	E962.0	E980.4
Sitosterols	972.2	E858.3	E942.2	E950.4	E962.0	E980.4
Skeletal muscle relaxants	975.2	E858.6	E945.2	E950.4	E962.0	E980.4
Skin						
agents (external)	976.9	E858.7	E946.9	E950.4	E962.0	E980.4
specified NEC	976.8	E858.7	E946.8	E950.4	E962.0	E980.4

Subterms under main terms may continue to next column or page

	Poisoning	Accident	Therapeutic Use	Suicide Attempt	Assault	Undetermined
Skin — *continued*						
test antigen	977.8	E858.8	E947.8	E950.4	E962.0	E980.4
Sleep-eze	963.0	E858.1	E933.0	E950.4	E962.0	E980.4
Sleeping draught (drug) (pill)						
(tablet)	967.9	E852.9	E937.9	E950.2	E962.0	E980.2
Smallpox vaccine	979.0	E858.8	E949.0	E950.4	E962.0	E980.4
Smelter fumes NEC	985.9	E866.4	—	E950.9	E962.1	E980.9
Smog	987.3	E869.1	—	E952.8	E962.2	E982.8
Smoke NEC	987.9	E869.9	—	E952.9	E962.2	E982.9
Smooth muscle relaxant	975.1	E858.6	E945.1	E950.4	E962.0	E980.4
Snail killer	989.4	E863.4	—	E950.6	E962.1	E980.7
Snake (bite) (venom)	989.5	E905.0	—	E950.9	E962.1	E980.9
Snuff	989.89	E866.8	—	E950.9	E962.1	E980.9
Soap (powder) (product)	989.6	E861.1	—	E950.9	E962.1	E980.9
bicarb	963.3	E858.1	E933.3	E950.4	E962.0	E980.4
chlorinated — see Sodium,						
hypochlorite						
medicinal, soft	976.2	E858.7	E946.2	E950.4	E962.0	E980.4
Soda (caustic)	983.2	E864.2	—	E950.7	E962.1	E980.6
Sodium						
acetosulfone	961.8	E857	E931.8	E950.4	E962.0	E980.4
acetrizoate	977.8	E858.8	E947.8	E950.4	E962.0	E980.4
amytal	967.0	E851	E937.0	E950.1	E962.0	E980.1
arsenate — see Arsenic						
bicarbonate	963.3	E858.1	E933.3	E950.4	E962.0	E980.4
bichromate	983.9	E864.3	—	E950.7	E962.1	E980.6
biphosphate	963.2	E858.1	E933.2	E950.4	E962.0	E980.4
bisulfate	983.9	E864.3	—	E950.7	E962.1	E980.6
borate (cleanser)	989.6	E861.3	—	E950.9	E962.1	E980.9
bromide NEC	967.3	E852.2	E937.3	E950.2	E962.0	E980.2
cacodylate (nonmedicinal)						
NEC	978.8	E858.8	E948.8	E950.4	E962.0	E980.4
anti-infective	961.1	E857	E931.1	E950.4	E962.0	E980.4
herbicide	989.4	E863.5	—	E950.6	E962.1	E980.7
calcium edetate	963.8	E858.1	E933.8	E950.4	E962.0	E980.4
carbonate NEC	983.2	E864.2	—	E950.7	E962.1	E980.6
chlorate NEC	983.9	E864.3	—	E950.7	E962.1	E980.6
herbicide	983.9	E863.5	—	E950.7	E962.1	E980.6
chloride NEC	974.5	E858.5	E944.5	E950.4	E962.0	E980.4
chromate	983.9	E864.3	—	E950.7	E962.1	E980.6
citrate	963.3	E858.1	E933.3	E950.4	E962.0	E980.4
cyanide — see Cyanide(s)						
cyclamate	974.5	E858.5	E944.5	E950.4	E962.0	E980.4
diatrizoate	977.8	E858.8	E947.8	E950.4	E962.0	E980.4
dibunate	975.4	E858.6	E945.4	E950.4	E962.0	E980.4
dioctyl sulfosuccinate	973.2	E858.4	E943.2	E950.4	E962.0	E980.4
edetate	963.8	E858.1	E933.8	E950.4	E962.0	E980.4
ethacrynate	974.4	E858.5	E944.4	E950.4	E962.0	E980.4
fluoracetate (dust) (rodenti-						
cide)	989.4	E863.7	—	E950.6	E962.1	E980.7
fluoride — see Fluoride(s)						
free salt	974.5	E858.5	E944.5	E950.4	E962.0	E980.4
glucosulfone	961.8	E857	E931.8	E950.4	E962.0	E980.4
hydroxide	983.2	E864.2	—	E950.7	E962.1	E980.6
hypochlorite (bleach)						
NEC	983.9	E864.3	—	E950.7	E962.1	E980.6
disinfectant	983.9	E861.4	—	E950.7	E962.1	E980.6
medicinal (anti-infective)						
(external)	976.0	E858.7	E946.0	E950.4	E962.0	E980.4
vapor	987.8	E869.8	—	E952.8	E962.2	E982.8
hyposulfite	976.0	E858.7	E946.0	E950.4	E962.0	E980.4
indigotindisulfonate	977.8	E858.8	E947.8	E950.4	E962.0	E980.4
iodide	977.8	E858.8	E947.8	E950.4	E962.0	E980.4
iothalamate	977.8	E858.8	E947.8	E950.4	E962.0	E980.4
iron edetate	964.0	E858.2	E934.0	E950.4	E962.0	E980.4
lactate	963.3	E858.1	E933.3	E950.4	E962.0	E980.4
lauryl sulfate	976.2	E858.7	E946.2	E950.4	E962.0	E980.4
L-triiodothyronine	962.7	E858.0	E932.7	E950.4	E962.0	E980.4
metrizoate	977.8	E858.8	E947.8	E950.4	E962.0	E980.4
monofluoracetate (dust) (ro-						
denticide)	989.4	E863.7	—	E950.6	E962.1	E980.7
morrhuate	972.7	E858.3	E942.7	E950.4	E962.0	E980.4
nafcillin	960.0	E856	E930.0	E950.4	E962.0	E980.4
nitrate (oxidizing agent)	983.9	E864.3	—	E950.7	E962.1	E980.6
nitrite (medicinal)	972.4	E858.3	E942.4	E950.4	E962.0	E980.4
nitroferricyanide	972.6	E858.3	E942.6	E950.4	E962.0	E980.4
nitroprusside	972.6	E858.3	E942.6	E950.4	E962.0	E980.4
para-aminohippurate	977.8	E858.8	E947.8	E950.4	E962.0	E980.4
perborate (nonmedicinal)						
NEC	989.89	E866.8	—	E950.9	E962.1	E980.9
medicinal	976.6	E858.7	E946.6	E950.4	E962.0	E980.4
soap	989.6	E861.1	—	E950.9	E962.1	E980.9

	Poisoning	Accident	Therapeutic Use	Suicide Attempt	Assault	Undetermined
Sodium — *continued*						
percarbonate — see Sodium,						
perborate						
phosphate	973.3	E858.4	E943.3	E950.4	E962.0	E980.4
polystyrene sulfonate	974.5	E858.5	E944.5	E950.4	E962.0	E980.4
propionate	976.0	E858.7	E946.0	E950.4	E962.0	E980.4
psylliate	972.7	E858.3	E942.7	E950.4	E962.0	E980.4
removing resins	974.5	E858.5	E944.5	E950.4	E962.0	E980.4
salicylate	965.1	E850.3	E935.3	E950.0	E962.0	E980.0
sulfate	973.3	E858.4	E943.3	E950.4	E962.0	E980.4
sulfoxone	961.8	E857	E931.8	E950.4	E962.0	E980.4
tetradecyl sulfate	972.7	E858.3	E942.7	E950.4	E962.0	E980.4
thiopental	968.3	E855.1	E938.3	E950.4	E962.0	E980.4
thiosalicylate	965.1	E850.3	E935.3	E950.0	E962.0	E980.0
thiosulfate	976.0	E858.7	E946.0	E950.4	E962.0	E980.4
tolbutamide	977.8	E858.8	E947.8	E950.4	E962.0	E980.4
tyropanoate	977.8	E858.8	E947.8	E950.4	E962.0	E980.4
valproate	966.3	E855.0	E936.3	E950.4	E962.0	E980.4
Solanine	977.8	E858.8	E947.8	E950.4	E962.0	E980.4
Solanum dulcamara	988.2	E865.4	—	E950.9	E962.1	E980.9
Solapsone	961.8	E857	E931.8	E950.4	E962.0	E980.4
Solasulfone	961.8	E857	E931.8	E950.4	E962.0	E980.4
Soldering fluid	983.1	E864.1	—	E950.7	E962.1	E980.6
Solid substance	989.9	E866.9	—	E950.9	E962.1	E980.9
specified NEC	989.9	E866.8	—	E950.9	E962.1	E980.9
Solvents, industrial	982.8	E862.9	—	E950.9	E962.1	E980.9
naphtha	981	E862.0	—	E950.9	E962.1	E980.9
petroleum	981	E862.0	—	E950.9	E962.1	E980.9
specified NEC	982.8	E862.4	—	E950.9	E962.1	E980.9
Soma	968.0	E855.1	E938.0	E950.4	E962.0	E980.4
Somatotropin	962.4	E858.0	E932.4	E950.4	E962.0	E980.4
Sominex	963.0	E858.1	E933.0	E950.4	E962.0	E980.4
Somnos	967.1	E852.0	E937.1	E950.2	E962.0	E980.2
Somonal	967.0	E851	E937.0	E950.1	E962.0	E980.1
Soneryl	967.0	E851	E937.0	E950.1	E962.0	E980.1
Soothing syrup	977.9	E858.9	E947.9	E950.5	E962.0	E980.5
Sopor	967.4	E852.3	E937.4	E950.2	E962.0	E980.2
Soporific drug	967.9	E852.9	E937.9	E950.2	E962.0	E980.2
specified type NEC	967.8	E852.8	E937.8	E950.2	E962.0	E980.2
Sorbitol NEC	977.4	E858.8	E947.4	E950.4	E962.0	E980.4
Sotradecol	972.7	E858.3	E942.7	E950.4	E962.0	E980.4
Spacoline	975.1	E858.6	E945.1	E950.4	E962.0	E980.4
Spanish fly	976.8	E858.7	E946.8	E950.4	E962.0	E980.4
Sparine	969.1	E853.0	E939.1	E950.3	E962.0	E980.3
Sparteine	975.0	E858.6	E945.0	E950.4	E962.0	E980.4
Spasmolytics	975.1	E858.6	E945.1	E950.4	E962.0	E980.4
anticholinergics	971.1	E855.4	E941.1	E950.4	E962.0	E980.4
Spectinomycin	960.8	E856	E930.8	E950.4	E962.0	E980.4
Speed	969.72	E854.2	E939.7	E950.3	E962.0	E980.3
Spermicides	976.8	E858.7	E946.8	E950.4	E962.0	E980.4
Spider (bite) (venom)	989.5	E905.1	—	E950.9	E962.1	E980.9
antivenin	979.9	E858.8	E949.9	E950.4	E962.0	E980.4
Spigelia (root)	961.6	E857	E931.6	E950.4	E962.0	E980.4
Spiperone	969.2	E853.1	E939.2	E950.3	E962.0	E980.3
Spiramycin	960.3	E856	E930.3	E950.4	E962.0	E980.4
Spirilene	969.5	E853.8	E939.5	E950.3	E962.0	E980.3
Spirit(s) (neutral) NEC	980.0	E860.1	—	E950.9	E962.1	E980.9
beverage	980.0	E860.0	—	E950.9	E962.1	E980.9
industrial	980.9	E860.9	—	E950.9	E962.1	E980.9
mineral	981	E862.0	—	E950.9	E962.1	E980.9
of salt — see Hydrochloric						
acid						
surgical	980.9	E860.9	—	E950.9	E962.1	E980.9
Spironolactone	974.4	E858.5	E944.4	E950.4	E962.0	E980.4
Sponge, absorbable						
(gelatin)	964.5	E858.2	E934.5	E950.4	E962.0	E980.4
Sporostacin	976.0	E858.7	E946.0	E950.4	E962.0	E980.4
Sprays (aerosol)	989.89	E866.8	—	E950.9	E962.1	E980.9
cosmetic	989.89	E866.7	—	E950.9	E962.1	E980.9
medicinal NEC	977.9	E858.9	E947.9	E950.5	E962.0	E980.5
pesticides — see Pesticides						
specified content — see sub-						
stance specified						
Spurge flax	988.2	E865.4	—	E950.9	E962.1	E980.9
Spurges	988.2	E865.4	—	E950.9	E962.1	E980.9
Squill (expectorant) NEC	975.5	E858.6	E945.5	E950.4	E962.0	E980.4
rat poison	989.4	E863.7	—	E950.6	E962.1	E980.7
Squirting cucumber (cathar-						
tic)	973.1	E858.4	E943.1	E950.4	E962.0	E980.4
SSNRI (selective serotonin and						
norepinephrine reuptake in-						
hibitors)	969.02	E854.0	E939.0	E950.3	E962.0	E980.3

Substance	Poisoning	Accident	Therapeutic Use	Suicide Attempt	Assault	Undetermined
SSRI (selective serotonin reuptake inhibitors)	969.03	E854.0	E939.0	E950.3	E962.0	E980.3
Stains	989.89	E866.8	—	E950.9	E962.1	E980.9
Stannous — see also Tin						
fluoride	976.7	E858.7	E946.7	E950.4	E962.0	E980.4
Stanolone	962.1	E858.0	E932.1	E950.4	E962.0	E980.4
Stanozolol	962.1	E858.0	E932.1	E950.4	E962.0	E980.4
Staphisagria or stavesacre (pediculicide)	976.0	E858.7	E946.0	E950.4	E962.0	E980.4
Stelazine	969.1	E853.0	E939.1	E950.3	E962.0	E980.3
Stemetil	969.1	E853.0	E939.1	E950.3	E962.0	E980.3
Sterculia (cathartic) (gum)	973.3	E858.4	E943.3	E950.4	E962.0	E980.4
Sternutator gas	987.8	E869.8	—	E952.8	E962.2	E982.8
Steroids NEC	962.0	E858.0	E932.0	E950.4	E962.0	E980.4
ENT agent	976.6	E858.7	E946.6	E950.4	E962.0	E980.4
ophthalmic preparation	976.5	E858.7	E946.5	E950.4	E962.0	E980.4
topical NEC	976.0	E858.7	E946.0	E950.4	E962.0	E980.4
Stibine	985.8	E866.4	—	E950.9	E962.1	E980.9
Stibophen	961.2	E857	E931.2	E950.4	E962.0	E980.4
Stilbamide, stilbamidine	961.5	E857	E931.5	E950.4	E962.0	E980.4
Stilbestrol	962.2	E858.0	E932.2	E950.4	E962.0	E980.4
Stimulants (central nervous system)	970.9	E854.3	E940.9	E950.4		E980.4
analeptics	970.0	E854.3	E940.0	E950.4	E962.0	E980.4
opiate antagonist	970.1	E854.3	E940.1	E950.4	E962.0	E980.4
psychotherapeutic NEC	969.09	E854.0	E939.0	E950.3	E962.0	E980.3
specified NEC	970.89	E854.3	E940.8	E950.4	E962.0	E980.4
Storage batteries (acid) (cells)	983.1	E864.1	—	E950.7	E962.1	E980.6
Stovaine	968.9	E855.2	E938.9	E950.4	E962.0	E980.4
infiltration (subcutaneous)	968.5	E855.2	E938.5	E950.4	E962.0	E980.4
nerve block (peripheral) (plexus)	968.6	E855.2	E938.6	E950.4	E962.0	E980.4
spinal	968.7	E855.2	E938.7	E950.4	E962.0	E980.4
topical (surface)	968.5	E855.2	E938.5	E950.4	E962.0	E980.4
Stovarsal	961.1	E857	E931.1	E950.4	E962.0	E980.4
Stove gas — see Gas, utility						
Stoxil	976.5	E858.7	E946.5	E950.4	E962.0	E980.4
STP	969.6	E854.1	E939.6	E950.3	E962.0	E980.3
Stramonium (medicinal) NEC	971.1	E855.4	E941.1	E950.4	E962.0	E980.4
natural state	988.2	E865.4	—	E950.9	E962.1	E980.9
Streptodornase	964.4	E858.2	E934.4	E950.4	E962.0	E980.4
Streptoduocin	960.6	E856	E930.6	E950.4	E962.0	E980.4
Streptokinase	964.4	E858.2	E934.4	E950.4	E962.0	E980.4
Streptomycin	960.6	E856	E930.6	E950.4	E962.0	E980.4
Streptozocin	960.7	E856	E930.7	E950.4	E962.0	E980.4
Stripper (paint) (solvent)	982.8	E862.9	—	E950.9	E962.1	E980.9
Strobane	989.2	E863.0	—	E950.6	E962.1	E980.7
Strophanthin	972.1	E858.3	E942.1	E950.4	E962.0	E980.4
Strophanthus hispidus or kombe	988.2	E865.4	—	E950.9	E962.1	E980.9
Strychnine (rodenticide) (salts)	989.1	E863.7	—	E950.6	E962.1	E980.7
medicinal NEC	970.89	E854.3	E940.8	E950.4	E962.0	E980.4
Strychnos (ignatii) — see Strychnine						
Styramate	968.0	E855.1	E938.0	E950.4	E962.0	E980.4
Styrene	983.0	E864.0	—	E950.7	E962.1	E980.6
Succinimide (anticonvulsant)	966.2	E855.0	E936.2	E950.4	E962.0	E980.4
mercuric — see Mercury						
Succinylcholine	975.2	E858.6	E945.2	E950.4	E962.0	E980.4
Succinylsulfathiazole	961.0	E857	E931.0	E950.4	E962.0	E980.4
Sucrose	974.5	E858.5	E944.5	E950.4	E962.0	E980.4
Sulfacetamide	961.0	E857	E931.0	E950.4	E962.0	E980.4
ophthalmic preparation	976.5	E858.7	E946.5	E950.4	E962.0	E980.4
Sulfachlorpyridazine	961.0	E857	E931.0	E950.4	E962.0	E980.4
Sulfacytine	961.0	E857	E931.0	E950.4	E962.0	E980.4
Sulfadiazine	961.0	E857	E931.0	E950.4	E962.0	E980.4
silver (topical)	976.0	E858.7	E946.0	E950.4	E962.0	E980.4
Sulfadimethoxine	961.0	E857	E931.0	E950.4	E962.0	E980.4
Sulfadimidine	961.0	E857	E931.0	E950.4	E962.0	E980.4
Sulfaethidole	961.0	E857	E931.0	E950.4	E962.0	E980.4
Sulfafurazole	961.0	E857	E931.0	E950.4	E962.0	E980.4
Sulfaguanidine	961.0	E857	E931.0	E950.4	E962.0	E980.4
Sulfamerazine	961.0	E857	E931.0	E950.4	E962.0	E980.4
Sulfameter	961.0	E857	E931.0	E950.4	E962.0	E980.4
Sulfamethizole	961.0	E857	E931.0	E950.4	E962.0	E980.4
Sulfamethoxazole	961.0	E857	E931.0	E950.4	E962.0	E980.4
Sulfamethoxydiazine	961.0	E857	E931.0	E950.4	E962.0	E980.4
Sulfamethoxypyridazine	961.0	E857	E931.0	E950.4	E962.0	E980.4
Sulfamethylthiazole	961.0	E857	E931.0	E950.4	E962.0	E980.4
Sulfamylon	976.0	E858.7	E946.0	E950.4	E962.0	E980.4
Sulfan blue (diagnostic dye)	977.8	E858.8	E947.8	E950.4	E962.0	E980.4
Sulfanilamide	961.0	E857	E931.0	E950.4	E962.0	E980.4
Sulfanilylguanidine	961.0	E857	E931.0	E950.4	E962.0	E980.4
Sulfaphenazole	961.0	E857	E931.0	E950.4	E962.0	E980.4
Sulfaphenylthiazole	961.0	E857	E931.0	E950.4	E962.0	E980.4
Sulfaproxyline	961.0	E857	E931.0	E950.4	E962.0	E980.4
Sulfapyridine	961.0	E857	E931.0	E950.4	E962.0	E980.4
Sulfapyrimidine	961.0	E857	E931.0	E950.4	E962.0	E980.4
Sulfarsphenamine	961.1	E857	E931.1	E950.4	E962.0	E980.4
Sulfasalazine	961.0	E857	E931.0	E950.4	E962.0	E980.4
Sulfasomizole	961.0	E857	E931.0	E950.4	E962.0	E980.4
Sulfasuxidine	961.0	E857	E931.0	E950.4	E962.0	E980.4
Sulfinpyrazone	974.7	E858.5	E944.7	E950.4	E962.0	E980.4
Sulfisoxazole	961.0	E857	E931.0	E950.4	E962.0	E980.4
ophthalmic preparation	976.5	E858.7	E946.5	E950.4	E962.0	E980.4
Sulfomyxin	960.8	E856	E930.8	E950.4	E962.0	E980.4
Sulfonal	967.8	E852.8	E937.8	E950.2	E962.0	E980.2
Sulfonamides (mixtures)	961.0	E857	E931.0	E950.4	E962.0	E980.4
Sulfones	961.8	E857	E931.8	E950.4	E962.0	E980.4
Sulfonethylmethane	967.8	E852.8	E937.8	E950.2	E962.0	E980.2
Sulfonmethane	967.8	E852.8	E937.8	E950.2	E962.0	E980.2
Sulfonphthal, sulfonphthol	977.8	E858.8	E947.8	E950.4	E962.0	E980.4
Sulfonylurea derivatives, oral	962.3	E858.0	E932.3	E950.4	E962.0	E980.4
Sulfoxone	961.8	E857	E931.8	E950.4	E962.0	E980.4
Sulfur, sulfureted, sulfuric, sulfurous, sulfuryl (compounds) NEC	989.89	E866.8	—	E950.9	E962.1	E980.9
acid	983.1	E864.1	—	E950.7	E962.1	E980.6
dioxide	987.3	E869.1	—	E952.8	E962.2	E982.8
ether — see Ether(s)						
hydrogen	987.8	E869.8	—	E952.8	E962.2	E982.8
medicinal (keratolytic) (ointment) NEC	976.4	E858.7	E946.4	E950.4	E962.0	E980.4
pesticide (vapor)	989.4	E863.4	—	E950.6	E962.1	E980.7
vapor NEC	987.8	E869.8	—	E952.8	E962.2	E982.8
Sulkowitch's reagent	977.8	E858.8	E947.8	E950.4	E962.0	E980.4
Sulphadione	961.8	E857	E931.8	E950.4	E962.0	E980.4
Sulph — see also Sulf-						
Sulthiame, sultiame	966.3	E855.0	E936.3	E950.4	E962.0	E980.4
Superinone	975.5	E858.6	E945.5	E950.4	E962.0	E980.4
Suramin	961.5	E857	E931.5	E950.4	E962.0	E980.4
Surfacaine	968.5	E855.2	E938.5	E950.4	E962.0	E980.4
Surital	968.3	E855.1	E938.3	E950.4	E962.0	E980.4
Sutilains	976.8	E858.7	E946.8	E950.4	E962.0	E980.4
Suxamethonium (bromide) (chloride) (iodide)	975.2	E858.6	E945.2	E950.4	E962.0	E980.4
Suxethonium (bromide)	975.2	E858.6	E945.2	E950.4	E962.0	E980.4
Sweet oil (birch)	976.3	E858.7	E946.3	E950.4	E962.0	E980.4
Sym-dichloroethyl ether	982.3	E862.4	—	E950.9	E962.1	E980.9
Sympatholytics	971.3	E855.6	E941.3	E950.4	E962.0	E980.4
Sympathomimetics	971.2	E855.5	E941.2	E950.4	E962.0	E980.4
Synagis	979.6	E858.8	E949.6	E950.4	E962.0	E980.4
Synalar	976.0	E858.7	E946.0	E950.4	E962.0	E980.4
Synthroid	962.7	E858.0	E932.7	E950.4	E962.0	E980.4
Syntocinon	975.0	E858.6	E945.0	E950.4	E962.0	—
Syrosingopine	972.6	E858.3	E942.6	E950.4	E962.0	E980.4
Systemic agents (primarily)	963.9	E858.1	E933.9	E950.4	E962.0	E980.4
specified NEC	963.8	E858.1	E933.8	E950.4	E962.0	E980.4
Tablets — see also specified substance	977.9	E858.9	E947.9	E950.5	E962.0	E980.5
Tace	962.2	E858.0	E932.2	E950.4	E962.0	E980.4
Tacrine	971.0	E855.3	E941.0	E950.4	E962.0	E980.4
Talbutal	967.0	E851	E937.0	E950.1	E962.0	E980.1
Talc	976.3	E858.7	E946.3	E950.4	E962.0	E980.4
Talcum	976.3	E858.7	E946.3	E950.4	E962.0	E980.4
Tamsulosin	971.3	E855.6	E941.3	E950.4	E962.0	E980.4
Tandearil, tanderil	965.5	E850.5	E935.5	E950.0	E962.0	E980.0
Tannic acid	983.1	E864.1	—	E950.7	E962.1	E980.6
medicinal (astringent)	976.2	E858.7	E946.2	E950.4	E962.0	E980.4
Tannin — see Tannic acid						
Tansy	988.2	E865.4	—	E950.9	E962.1	E980.9
TAO	960.3	E856	E930.3	E950.4	E962.0	E980.4
Tapazole	962.8	E858.0	E932.8	E950.4	E962.0	E980.4
Tar NEC	983.0	E864.0	—	E950.7	E962.1	E980.6
camphor — see Naphthalene						

	Poisoning	Accident	Therapeutic Use	Suicide Attempt	Assault	Undetermined
Tar — *continued*						
fumes	987.8	E869.8	—	E952.8	E962.2	E982.8
Taractan	969.3	E853.8	E939.3	E950.3	E962.0	E980.3
Tarantula (venomous)	989.5	E905.1	—	E950.9	E962.1	E980.9
Tartar emetic (anti-infective)	961.2	E857	E931.2	E950.4	E962.0	E980.4
Tartaric acid	983.1	E864.1	—	E950.7	E962.1	E980.6
Tartrated antimony (anti-infective)	961.2	E857	E931.2	E950.4	E962.0	E980.4
TCA — *see* Trichloroacetic acid						
TDI	983.0	E864.0	—	E950.7	E962.1	E980.6
vapor	987.8	E869.8	—	E952.8	E962.2	E982.8
Tear gas	987.5	E869.3	—	E952.8	E962.2	E982.8
Teclothiazide	974.3	E858.5	E944.3	E950.4	E962.0	E980.4
Tegretol	966.3	E855.0	E936.3	E950.4	E962.0	E980.4
Telepaque	977.8	E858.8	E947.8	E950.4	E962.0	E980.4
Tellurium	985.8	E866.4	—	E950.9	E962.1	E980.9
fumes	985.8	E866.4	—	E950.9	E962.1	E980.9
TEM	963.1	E858.1	E933.1	E950.4	E962.0	E980.4
Temazepan — *see* Benzodiazepines						
TEPA	963.1	E858.1	E933.1	E950.4	E962.0	E980.4
TEPP	989.3	E863.1	—	E950.6	E962.1	E980.7
Terbutaline	971.2	E855.5	E941.2	E950.4	E962.0	E980.4
Teroxalene	961.6	E857	E931.6	E950.4	E962.0	E980.4
Terpin hydrate	975.5	E858.6	E945.5	E950.4	E962.0	E980.4
Terramycin	960.4	E856	E930.4	E950.4	E962.0	E980.4
Tessalon	975.4	E858.6	E945.4	E950.4	E962.0	E980.4
Testosterone	962.1	E858.0	E932.1	E950.4	E962.0	E980.4
Tetanus (vaccine)	978.4	E858.8	E948.4	E950.4	E962.0	E980.4
antitoxin	979.9	E858.8	E949.9	E950.4	E962.0	E980.4
immune globulin (human)	964.6	E858.2	E934.6	E950.4	E962.0	E980.4
toxoid	978.4	E858.8	E948.4	E950.4	E962.0	E980.4
with diphtheria toxoid	978.9	E858.8	E948.9	E950.4	E962.0	E980.4
with pertussis	978.6	E858.8	E948.6	E950.4	E962.0	E980.4
Tetrabenazine	969.5	E853.8	E939.5	E950.3	E962.0	E980.3
Tetracaine (infiltration) (topical)	968.5	E855.2	E938.5	E950.4	E962.0	E980.4
nerve block (peripheral) (plexus)	968.6	E855.2	E938.6	E950.4	E962.0	E980.4
spinal	968.7	E855.2	E938.7	E950.4	E962.0	E980.4
Tetrachlorethylene — *see* Tetrachloroethylene						
Tetrachlormethiazide	974.3	E858.5	E944.3	E950.4	E962.0	E980.4
Tetrachloroethane (liquid) (vapor)	982.3	E862.4	—	E950.9	E962.1	E980.9
paint or varnish	982.3	E861.6	—	E950.9	E962.1	E980.9
Tetrachloroethylene (liquid) (vapor)	982.3	E862.4	—	E950.9	E962.1	E980.9
medicinal	961.6	E857	E931.6	E950.4	E962.0	E980.4
Tetrachloromethane — *see* Carbon, tetrachloride						
Tetracycline	960.4	E856	E930.4	E950.4	E962.0	E980.4
ophthalmic preparation	976.5	E858.7	E946.5	E950.4	E962.0	E980.4
topical NEC	976.0	E858.7	E946.0	E950.4	E962.0	E980.4
Tetraethylammonium chloride	972.3	E858.3	E942.3	E950.4	E962.0	E980.4
Tetraethyl lead (antiknock compound)	984.1	E862.1	—	E950.9	E962.1	E980.9
Tetraethyl pyrophosphate	989.3	E863.1	—	E950.6	E962.1	E980.7
Tetraethylthiuram disulfide	977.3	E858.8	E947.3	E950.4	E962.0	E980.4
Tetrahydroaminoacridine	971.0	E855.3	E941.0	E950.4	E962.0	E980.4
Tetrahydrocannabinol	969.6	E854.1	E939.6	E950.3	E962.0	E980.3
Tetrahydronaphthalene	982.0	E862.4	—	E950.9	E962.1	E980.9
Tetrahydrozoline	971.2	E855.5	E941.2	E950.4	E962.0	E980.4
Tetralin	982.0	E862.4	—	E950.9	E962.1	E980.9
Tetramethylthiuram (disulfide) NEC	989.4	E863.6	—	E950.6	E962.1	E980.7
medicinal	976.2	E858.7	E946.2	E950.4	E962.0	E980.4
Tetronal	967.8	E852.8	E937.8	E950.2	E962.0	E980.2
Tetryl	983.0	E864.0	—	E950.7	E962.1	E980.6
Thalidomide	967.8	E852.8	E937.8	E950.2	E962.0	E980.2
Thallium (compounds) (dust) NEC	985.8	E866.4	—	E950.9	E962.1	E980.9
pesticide (rodenticide)	985.8	E863.7	—	E950.6	E962.1	E980.7
THC	969.6	E854.1	E939.6	E950.3	E962.0	E980.3
Thebacon	965.09	E850.2	E935.2	E950.0	E962.0	E980.0
Thebaine	965.09	E850.2	E935.2	E950.0	E962.0	E980.0

	Poisoning	Accident	Therapeutic Use	Suicide Attempt	Assault	Undetermined
Theobromine (calcium salicylate)	974.1	E858.5	E944.1	E950.4	E962.0	E980.4
Theophylline (diuretic)	974.1	E858.5	E944.1	E950.4	E962.0	E980.4
ethylenediamine	975.7	E858.6	E945.7	E950.4	E962.0	E980.4
Thiabendazole	961.6	E857	E931.6	E950.4	E962.0	E980.4
Thialbarbital, thialbarbitone	968.3	E855.1	E938.3	E950.4	E962.0	E980.4
Thiamine	963.5	E858.1	E933.5	E950.4	E962.0	E980.4
Thiamylal (sodium)	968.3	E855.1	E938.3	E950.4	E962.0	E980.4
Thiazesim	969.09	E854.0	E939.0	E950.3	E962.0	E980.3
Thiazides (diuretics)	974.3	E858.5	E944.3	E950.4	E962.0	E980.4
Thiethylperazine	963.0	E858.1	E933.0	E950.4	E962.0	E980.4
Thimerosal (topical)	976.0	E858.7	E946.0	E950.4	E962.0	E980.4
ophthalmic preparation	976.5	E858.7	E946.5	E950.4	E962.0	E980.4
Thioacetazone	961.8	E857	E931.8	E950.4	E962.0	E980.4
Thiobarbiturates	968.3	E855.1	E938.3	E950.4	E962.0	E980.4
Thiobismol	961.2	E857	E931.2	E950.4	E962.0	E980.4
Thiocarbamide	962.8	E858.0	E932.8	E950.4	E962.0	E980.4
Thiocarbarsone	961.1	E857	E931.1	E950.4	E962.0	E980.4
Thiocarlide	961.8	E857	E931.8	E950.4	E962.0	E980.4
Thioguanine	963.1	E858.1	E933.1	E950.4	E962.0	E980.4
Thiomercaptomerin	974.0	E858.5	E944.0	E950.4	E962.0	E980.4
Thiomerin	974.0	E858.5	E944.0	E950.4	E962.0	E980.4
Thiopental, thiopentone (sodium)	968.3	E855.1	E938.3	E950.4	E962.0	E980.4
Thiopropazate	969.1	E853.0	E939.1	E950.3	E962.0	E980.3
Thioproperazine	969.1	E853.0	E939.1	E950.3	E962.0	E980.3
Thioridazine	969.1	E853.0	E939.1	E950.3	E962.0	E980.3
Thio-TEPA, thiotepa	963.1	E858.1	E933.1	E950.4	E962.0	E980.4
Thiothixene	969.3	E853.8	E939.3	E950.3	E962.0	E980.3
Thiouracil	962.8	E858.0	E932.8	E950.4	E962.0	E980.4
Thiourea	962.8	E858.0	E932.8	E950.4	E962.0	E980.4
Thiphenamil	971.1	E855.4	E941.1	E950.4	E962.0	E980.4
Thiram NEC	989.4	E863.6	—	E950.6	E962.1	E980.7
medicinal	976.2	E858.7	E946.2	E950.4	E962.0	E980.4
Thonzylamine	963.0	E858.1	E933.0	E950.4	E962.0	E980.4
Thorazine	969.1	E853.0	E939.1	E950.3	E962.0	E980.3
Thornapple	988.2	E865.4	—	E950.9	E962.1	E980.9
Throat preparation (lozenges) NEC	976.6	E858.7	E946.6	E950.4	E962.0	E980.4
Thrombin	964.5	E858.2	E934.5	E950.4	E962.0	E980.4
Thrombolysin	964.4	E858.2	E934.4	E950.4	E962.0	E980.4
Thymol	983.0	E864.0	—	E950.7	E962.1	E980.6
Thymus extract	962.9	E858.0	E932.9	E950.4	E962.0	E980.4
Thyroglobulin	962.7	E858.0	E932.7	E950.4	E962.0	E980.4
Thyroid (derivatives) (extract)	962.7	E858.0	E932.7	E950.4	E962.0	E980.4
Thyrolar	962.7	E858.0	E932.7	E950.4	E962.0	E980.4
Thyrothrophin, thyrotropin	977.8	E858.8	E947.8	E950.4	E962.0	E980.4
Thyroxin(e)	962.7	E858.0	E932.7	E950.4	E962.0	E980.4
Tigan	963.0	E858.1	E933.0	E950.4	E962.0	E980.4
Tigloidine	968.0	E855.1	E938.0	E950.4	E962.0	E980.4
Tin (chloride) (dust) (oxide) NEC	985.8	E866.4	—	E950.9	E962.1	E980.9
anti-infectives	961.2	E857	E931.2	E950.4	E962.0	E980.4
Tinactin	976.0	E858.7	E946.0	E950.4	E962.0	E980.4
Tincture, iodine — *see* Iodine						
Tindal	969.1	E853.0	E939.1	E950.3	E962.0	E980.3
Titanium (compounds) (vapor)	985.8	E866.4	—	E950.9	E962.1	E980.9
ointment	976.3	E858.7	E946.3	E950.4	E962.0	E980.4
Titroid	962.7	E858.0	E932.7	E950.4	E962.0	E980.4
TMTD — *see* Tetramethylthiuram disulfide						
TNT	989.89	E866.8	—	E950.9	E962.1	E980.9
fumes	987.8	E869.8	—	E952.8	E962.2	E982.8
Toadstool	988.1	E865.5	—	E950.9	E962.1	E980.9
Tobacco NEC	989.84	E866.8	—	E950.9	E962.1	E980.9
Indian	988.2	E865.4	—	E950.9	E962.1	E980.9
smoke, second-hand	987.8	E869.4	—	—	—	—
Tocopherol	963.5	E858.1	E933.5	E950.4	E962.0	E980.4
Tocosamine	975.0	E858.6	E945.0	E950.4	E962.0	E980.4
Tofranil	969.05	E854.0	E939.0	E950.3	E962.0	E980.3
Toilet deodorizer	989.89	E866.8	—	E950.9	E962.1	E980.9
Tolazamide	962.3	E858.0	E932.3	E950.4	E962.0	E980.4
Tolazoline	971.3	E855.6	E941.3	E950.4	E962.0	E980.4
Tolbutamide	962.3	E858.0	E932.3	E950.4	E962.0	E980.4
sodium	977.8	E858.8	E947.8	E950.4	E962.0	E980.4
Tolmetin	965.69	E850.6	E935.6	E950.0	E962.0	E980.0
Tolnaftate	976.0	E858.7	E946.0	E950.4	E962.0	E980.4
Tolpropamine	976.1	E858.7	E946.1	E950.4	E962.0	E980.4

Substance	Poisoning	Accident	Therapeutic Use	Suicide Attempt	Assault	Undetermined
Tolserol	968.0	E855.1	E938.0	E950.4	E962.0	E980.4
Toluene (liquid) (vapor)	982.0	E862.4	—	E950.9	E962.1	E980.9
diisocyanate	983.0	E864.0	—	E950.7	E962.1	E980.6
Toluidine	983.0	E864.0	—	E950.7	E962.1	E980.6
vapor	987.8	E869.8	—	E952.8	E962.2	E982.8
Toluol (liquid) (vapor)	982.0	E862.4	—	E950.9	E962.1	E980.9
Tolylene-2, 4-diiso- cyanate	983.0	E864.0	—	E950.7	E962.1	E980.6
Tonics, cardiac	972.1	E858.3	E942.1	E950.4	E962.0	E980.4
Toxaphene (dust) (spray)	989.2	E863.0	—	E950.6	E962.1	E980.7
Toxoids NEC	978.8	E858.8	E948.8	E950.4	E962.0	E980.4
Tractor fuel NEC	981	E862.1	—	E950.9	E962.1	E980.9
Tragacanth	973.3	E858.4	E943.3	E950.4	E962.0	E980.4
Tramazoline	971.2	E855.5	E941.2	E950.4	E962.0	E980.4
Tranquilizers	969.5	E853.9	E939.5	E950.3	E962.0	E980.3
benzodiazepine-based	969.4	E853.2	E939.4	E950.3	E962.0	E980.3
butyrophenone-based	969.2	E853.1	E939.2	E950.3	E962.0	E980.3
major NEC	969.3	E853.8	E939.3	E950.3	E962.0	E980.3
phenothiazine-based	969.1	E853.0	E939.1	E950.3	E962.0	E980.3
specified NEC	969.5	E853.8	E939.5	E950.3	E962.0	E980.3
Trantoin	961.9	E857	E931.9	E950.4	E962.0	E980.4
Tranxene	969.4	E853.2	E939.4	E950.3	E962.0	E980.3
Tranylcypromine (sul- fate)	969.01	E854.0	E939.0	E950.3	E962.0	E980.3
Trasentine	975.1	E858.6	E945.1	E950.4	E962.0	E980.4
Travert	974.5	E858.5	E944.5	E950.4	E962.0	E980.4
Trecator	961.8	E857	E931.8	E950.4	E962.0	E980.4
Tretinoin	976.8	E858.7	E946.8	E950.4	E962.0	E980.4
Triacetin	976.0	E858.7	E946.0	E950.4	E962.0	E980.4
Triacetyloleandomycin	960.3	E856	E930.3	E950.4	E962.0	E980.4
Triamcinolone	962.0	E858.0	E932.0	E950.4	E962.0	E980.4
ENT agent	976.6	E858.7	E946.6	E950.4	E962.0	E980.4
medicinal (keratolytic)	976.4	E858.7	E946.4	E950.4	E962.0	E980.4
ophthalmic preparation	976.5	E858.7	E946.5	E950.4	E962.0	E980.4
topical NEC	976.0	E858.7	E946.0	E950.4	E962.0	E980.4
Triamterene	974.4	E858.5	E944.4	E950.4	E962.0	E980.4
Triaziquone	963.1	E858.1	E933.1	E950.4	E962.0	E980.4
Tribromacetaldehyde	967.3	E852.2	E937.3	E950.2	E962.0	E980.2
Tribromoethanol	968.2	E855.1	E938.2	E950.4	E962.0	E980.4
Tribromomethane	967.3	E852.2	E937.3	E950.2	E962.0	E980.2
Trichlorethane	982.3	E862.4	—	E950.9	E962.1	E980.9
Trichlormethiazide	974.3	E858.5	E944.3	E950.4	E962.0	E980.4
Trichloroacetic acid	983.1	E864.1	—	E950.7	E962.1	E980.6
Trichloroethane	967.1	E852.0	E937.1	E950.2	E962.0	E980.2
Trichloroethylene (liquid) (va- por)	982.3	E862.4	—	E950.9	E962.1	E980.9
anesthetic (gas)	968.2	E855.1	E938.2	E950.4	E962.0	E980.4
Trichloroethyl phos- phate	967.1	E852.0	E937.1	E950.2	E962.0	E980.2
Trichlorofluoromethane NEC	987.4	E869.2	—	E952.8	E962.2	E982.8
Trichlorotriethylamine	963.1	E858.1	E933.1	E950.4	E962.0	E980.4
Trichomonacides NEC	961.5	E857	E931.5	E950.4	E962.0	E980.4
Trichomycin	960.1	E856	E930.1	E950.4	E962.0	E980.4
Triclofos	967.1	E852.0	E937.1	E950.2	E962.0	E980.2
Tricresyl phosphate	989.89	E866.8	—	E950.9	E962.1	E980.9
solvent	982.8	E862.4	—	E950.9	E962.1	E980.9
Tricyclamol	966.4	E855.0	E936.4	E950.4	E962.0	E980.4
Tridesilon	976.0	E858.7	E946.0	E950.4	E962.0	E980.4
Tridihexethyl	971.1	E855.4	E941.1	E950.4	E962.0	E980.4
Tridione	966.0	E855.0	E936.0	E950.4	E962.0	E980.4
Triethanolamine NEC	983.2	E864.2	—	E950.7	E962.1	E980.6
detergent	983.2	E861.0	—	E950.7	E962.1	E980.6
trinitrate	972.4	E858.3	E942.4	E950.4	E962.0	E980.4
Triethanomelamine	963.1	E858.1	E933.1	E950.4	E962.0	E980.4
Triethylene melamine	963.1	E858.1	E933.1	E950.4	E962.0	E980.4
Triethylenephospho- ramide	963.1	E858.1	E933.1	E950.4	E962.0	E980.4
Triethylenethiophospho- ramide	963.1	E858.1	E933.1	E950.4	E962.0	E980.4
Trifluoperazine	969.1	E853.0	E939.1	E950.3	E962.0	E980.3
Trifluperidol	969.2	E853.1	E939.2	E950.3	E962.0	E980.3
Triflupromazine	969.1	E853.0	E939.1	E950.3	E962.0	E980.3
Trihexyphenidyl	971.1	E855.4	E941.1	E950.4	E962.0	E980.4
Triiodothyronine	962.7	E858.0	E932.7	E950.4	E962.0	E980.4
Trilene	968.2	E855.1	E938.2	E950.4	E962.0	E980.4
Trimeprazine	963.0	E858.1	E933.0	E950.4	E962.0	E980.4
Trimetazidine	972.4	E858.3	E942.4	E950.4	E962.0	E980.4
Trimethadione	966.0	E855.0	E936.0	E950.4	E962.0	E980.4
Trimethaphan	972.3	E858.3	E942.3	E950.4	E962.0	E980.4
Trimethidinium	972.3	E858.3	E942.3	E950.4	E962.0	E980.4
Trimethobenzamide	963.0	E858.1	E933.0	E950.4	E962.0	E980.4

Substance	Poisoning	Accident	Therapeutic Use	Suicide Attempt	Assault	Undetermined
Trimethylcarbinol	980.8	E860.8	—	E950.9	E962.1	E980.9
Trimethylpsoralen	976.3	E858.7	E946.3	E950.4	E962.0	E980.4
Trimeton	963.0	E858.1	E933.0	E950.4	E962.0	E980.4
Trimipramine	969.05	E854.0	E939.0	E950.3	E962.0	E980.3
Trimustine	963.1	E858.1	E933.1	E950.4	E962.0	E980.4
Trinitrin	972.4	E858.3	E942.4	E950.4	E962.0	E980.4
Trinitrophenol	983.0	E864.0	—	E950.7	E962.1	E980.6
Trinitrotoluene	989.89	E866.8	—	E950.9	E962.1	E980.9
fumes	987.8	E869.8	—	E952.8	E962.2	E982.8
Trional	967.8	E852.8	E937.8	E950.2	E962.0	E980.2
Trioxide of arsenic — see Ar- senic						
Trioxsalen	976.3	E858.7	E946.3	E950.4	E962.0	E980.4
Tripelennamine	963.0	E858.1	E933.0	E950.4	E962.0	E980.4
Triperidol	969.2	E853.1	E939.2	E950.3	E962.0	E980.3
Triprolidine	963.0	E858.1	E933.0	E950.4	E962.0	E980.4
Trisoralen	976.3	E858.7	E946.3	E950.4	E962.0	E980.4
Troleandomycin	960.3	E856	E930.3	E950.4	E962.0	E980.4
Trolnitrate (phosphate)	972.4	E858.3	E942.4	E950.4	E962.0	E980.4
Trometamol	963.3	E858.1	E933.3	E950.4	E962.0	E980.4
Tromethamine	963.3	E858.1	E933.3	E950.4	E962.0	E980.4
Tronothane	968.5	E855.2	E938.5	E950.4	E962.0	E980.4
Tropicamide	971.1	E855.4	E941.1	E950.4	E962.0	E980.4
Troxidone	966.0	E855.0	E936.0	E950.4	E962.0	E980.4
Tryparsamide	961.1	E857	E931.1	E950.4	E962.0	E980.4
Trypsin	963.4	E858.1	E933.4	E950.4	E962.0	E980.4
Tryptizol	969.05	E854.0	E939.0	E950.3	E962.0	E980.3
Tuaminoheptane	971.2	E855.5	E941.2	E950.4	E962.0	E980.4
Tuberculin (old)	977.8	E858.8	E947.8	E950.4	E962.0	E980.4
Tubocurare	975.2	E858.6	E945.2	E950.4	E962.0	E980.4
Tubocurarine	975.2	E858.6	E945.2	E950.4	E962.0	E980.4
Turkish green	969.6	E854.1	E939.6	E950.3	E962.0	E980.3
Turpentine (spirits of) (liquid) (vapor)	982.8	E862.4	—	E950.9	E962.1	E980.9
Tybamate	969.5	E853.8	E939.5	E950.3	E962.0	E980.3
Tyloxapol	975.5	E858.6	E945.5	E950.4	E962.0	E980.4
Tymazoline	971.2	E855.5	E941.2	E950.4	E962.0	E980.4
Typhoid vaccine	978.1	E858.8	E948.1	E950.4	E962.0	E980.4
Typhus vaccine	979.2	E858.8	E949.2	E950.4	E962.0	E980.4
Tyrothricin	976.0	E858.7	E946.0	E950.4	E962.0	E980.4
ENT agent	976.6	E858.7	E946.6	E950.4	E962.0	E980.4
ophthalmic preparation	976.5	E858.7	E946.5	E950.4	E962.0	E980.4
Undecenoic acid	976.0	E858.7	E946.0	E950.4	E962.0	E980.4
Undecylenic acid	976.0	E858.7	E946.0	E950.4	E962.0	E980.4
Unna's boot	976.3	E858.7	E946.3	E950.4	E962.0	E980.4
Uracil mustard	963.1	E858.1	E933.1	E950.4	E962.0	E980.4
Uramustine	963.1	E858.1	E933.1	E950.4	E962.0	E980.4
Urari	975.2	E858.6	E945.2	E950.4	E962.0	E980.4
Urea	974.4	E858.5	E944.4	E950.4	E962.0	E980.4
topical	976.8	E858.7	E946.8	E950.4	E962.0	E980.4
Urethan(e) (antineoplas- tic)	963.1	E858.1	E933.1	E950.4	E962.0	E980.4
Urginea (maritima) (scilla) — see Squill						
Uric acid metabolism agents NEC	974.7	E858.5	E944.7	E950.4	E962.0	E980.4
Urokinase	964.4	E858.2	E934.4	E950.4	E962.0	E980.4
Urokon	977.8	E858.8	E947.8	E950.4	E962.0	E980.4
Urotropin	961.9	E857	E931.9	E950.4	E962.0	E980.4
Urtica	988.2	E865.4	—	E950.9	E962.1	E980.9
Utility gas — see Gas, utility						
Vaccine NEC	979.9	E858.8	E949.9	E950.4	E962.0	E980.4
bacterial NEC	978.8	E858.8	E948.8	E950.4	E962.0	E980.4
with						
other bacterial compo- nent	978.9	E858.8	E948.9	E950.4	E962.0	E980.4
pertussis component	978.6	E858.8	E948.6	E950.4	E962.0	E980.4
viral-rickettsial compo- nent	979.7	E858.8	E949.7	E950.4	E962.0	E980.4
mixed NEC	978.9	E858.8	E948.9	E950.4	E962.0	E980.4
BCG	978.0	E858.8	E948.0	E950.4	E962.0	E980.4
cholera	978.2	E858.8	E948.2	E950.4	E962.0	E980.4
diphtheria	978.5	E858.8	E948.5	E950.4	E962.0	E980.4
influenza	979.6	E858.8	E949.6	E950.4	E962.0	E980.4
measles	979.4	E858.8	E949.4	E950.4	E962.0	E980.4
meningococcal	978.8	E858.8	E948.8	E950.4	E962.0	E980.4
mumps	979.6	E858.8	E949.6	E950.4	E962.0	E980.4
paratyphoid	978.1	E858.8	E948.1	E950.4	E962.0	E980.4
pertussis (with diphtheria toxoid) (with tetanus tox- oid)	978.6	E858.8	E948.6	E950.4	E962.0	E980.4
plague	978.3	E858.8	E948.3	E950.4	E962.0	E980.4

Nontherapeutic use substance

Subterms under main terms may continue to next column or page

► ◄ Revised Text   ● New Line   ▲ Revised Code

Vaccine NEC — Zinc

		External Cause (E-Code)				
	Poisoning	Accident	Therapeutic Use	Suicide Attempt	Assault	Undeter-mined
Vaccine — *continued*						
poliomyelitis	979.5	E858.8	E949.5	E950.4	E962.0	E980.4
poliovirus	979.5	E858.8	E949.5	E950.4	E962.0	E980.4
rabies	979.1	E858.8	E949.1	E950.4	E962.0	E980.4
respiratory syncytial virus	979.6	E858.8	E949.6	E950.4	E962.0	E980.4
rickettsial NEC	979.6	E858.8	E949.6	E950.4	E962.0	E980.4
with						
bacterial component	979.7	E858.8	E949.7	E950.4	E962.0	E980.4
pertussis component	978.6	E858.8	E948.6	E950.4	E962.0	E980.4
viral component	979.7	E858.8	E949.7	E950.4	E962.0	E980.4
Rocky mountain spotted fever	979.6	E858.8	E949.6	E950.4	E962.0	E980.4
rotavirus	979.6	E858.8	E949.6	E950.4	E962.0	E980.4
rubella virus	979.4	E858.8	E949.4	E950.4	E962.0	E980.4
sabin oral	979.5	E858.8	E949.5	E950.4	E962.0	E980.4
smallpox	979.0	E858.8	E949.0	E950.4	E962.0	E980.4
tetanus	978.4	E858.8	E948.4	E950.4	E962.0	E980.4
typhoid	978.1	E858.8	E948.1	E950.4	E962.0	E980.4
typhus	979.2	E858.8	E949.2	E950.4	E962.0	E980.4
viral NEC	979.6	E858.8	E949.6	E950.4	E962.0	E980.4
with						
bacterial component	979.7	E858.8	E949.7	E950.4	E962.0	E980.4
pertussis component	978.6	E858.8	E948.6	E950.4	E962.0	E980.4
rickettsial component	979.7	E858.8	E949.7	E950.4	E962.0	E980.4
yellow fever	979.3	E858.8	E949.3	E950.4	E962.0	E980.4
Vaccinia immune globulin (human)	964.6	E858.2	E934.6	E950.4	E962.0	E980.4
Vaginal contraceptives	976.8	E858.7	E946.8	E950.4	E962.0	E980.4
Valethamate	971.1	E855.4	E941.1	E950.4	E962.0	E980.4
Valisone	976.0	E858.7	E946.0	E950.4	E962.0	E980.4
Valium	969.4	E853.2	E939.4	E950.3	E962.0	E980.3
Valmid	967.8	E852.8	E937.8	E950.2	E962.0	E980.2
Vanadium	985.8	E866.4	—	E950.9	E962.1	E980.9
Vancomycin	960.8	E856	E930.8	E950.4	E962.0	E980.4
Vapor — *see also* Gas	987.9	E869.9	—	E952.9	E962.2	E982.9
kiln (carbon monoxide)	986	E868.8	—	E952.1	E962.2	E982.1
lead — see Lead						
specified source NEC (see also specific substance)	987.8	E869.8	—	E952.8	E962.2	E982.8
Varidase	964.4	E858.2	E934.4	E950.4	E962.0	E980.4
Varnish	989.89	E861.6	—	E950.9	E962.1	E980.9
cleaner	982.8	E862.9	—	E950.9	E962.1	E980.9
Vaseline	976.3	E858.7	E946.3	E950.4	E962.0	E980.4
Vasodilan	972.5	E858.3	E942.5	E950.4	E962.0	E980.4
Vasodilators NEC	972.5	E858.3	E942.5	E950.4	E962.0	E980.4
coronary	972.4	E858.3	E942.4	E950.4	E962.0	E980.4
Vasopressin	962.5	E858.0	E932.5	E950.4	E962.0	E980.4
Vasopressor drugs	962.5	E858.0	E932.5	E950.4	E962.0	E980.4
Venom, venomous (bite) (sting)	989.5	E905.9	—	E950.9	E962.1	E980.9
arthropod NEC	989.5	E905.5	—	E950.9	E962.1	E980.9
bee	989.5	E905.3	—	E950.9	E962.1	E980.9
centipede	989.5	E905.4	—	E950.9	E962.1	E980.9
hornet	989.5	E905.3	—	E950.9	E962.1	E980.9
lizard	989.5	E905.0	—	E950.9	E962.1	E980.9
marine animals or plants	989.5	E905.6	—	E950.9	E962.1	E980.9
millipede (tropical)	989.5	E905.4	—	E950.9	E962.1	E980.9
plant NEC	989.5	E905.7	—	E950.9	E962.1	E980.9
marine	989.5	E905.6	—	E950.9	E962.1	E980.9
scorpion	989.5	E905.2	—	E950.9	E962.1	E980.9
snake	989.5	E905.0	—	E950.9	E962.1	E980.9
specified NEC	989.5	E905.8	—	E950.9	E962.1	E980.9
spider	989.5	E905.1	—	E950.9	E962.1	E980.9
wasp	989.5	E905.3	—	E950.9	E962.1	E980.9
Ventolin — *see* Salbutamol sulfate						
Veramon	967.0	E851	E937.0	E950.1	E962.0	E980.1
Veratrum						
album	988.2	E865.4	—	E950.9	E962.1	E980.9
alkaloids	972.6	E858.3	E942.6	E950.4	E962.0	E980.4
viride	988.2	E865.4	—	E950.9	E962.1	E980.9
Verdigris — *see also* Copper	985.8	E866.4	—	E950.9	E962.1	E980.9
Veronal	967.0	E851	E937.0	E950.1	E962.0	E980.1
Veroxil	961.6	E857	E931.6	E950.4	E962.0	E980.4
Versidyne	965.7	E850.7	E935.7	E950.0	E962.0	E980.0
Viagra	972.5	E858.3	E942.5	E950.4	E962.0	E980.4
Vienna						
green	985.1	E866.3	—	E950.8	E962.1	E980.8
insecticide	985.1	E863.4	—	E950.6	E962.1	E980.7
red	989.89	E866.8	—	E950.9	E962.1	E980.9
pharmaceutical dye	977.4	E858.8	E947.4	E950.4	E962.0	E980.4

		External Cause (E-Code)				
	Poisoning	Accident	Therapeutic Use	Suicide Attempt	Assault	Undeter-mined
Vinbarbital, vinbarbitone	967.0	E851	E937.0	E950.1	E962.0	E980.1
Vinblastine	963.1	E858.1	E933.1	E950.4	E962.0	E980.4
Vincristine	963.1	E858.1	E933.1	E950.4	E962.0	E980.4
Vinesthene, vinethene	968.2	E855.1	E938.2	E950.4	E962.0	E980.4
Vinyl						
bital	967.0	E851	E937.0	E950.1	E962.0	E980.1
ether	968.2	E855.1	E938.2	E950.4	E962.0	E980.4
Vioform	961.3	E857	E931.3	E950.4	E962.0	E980.4
topical	976.0	E858.7	E946.0	E950.4	E962.0	E980.4
Viomycin	960.6	E856	E930.6	E950.4	E962.0	E980.4
Viosterol	963.5	E858.1	E933.5	E950.4	E962.0	E980.4
Viper (venom)	989.5	E905.0	—	E950.9	E962.1	E980.9
Viprynium (embonate)	961.6	E857	E931.6	E950.4	E962.0	E980.4
Virugon	961.7	E857	E931.7	E950.4	E962.0	E980.4
Visine	976.5	E858.7	E946.5	E950.4	E962.0	E980.4
Vitamins NEC	963.5	E858.1	E933.5	E950.4	E962.0	E980.4
B_{12}	964.1	E858.2	E934.1	E950.4	E962.0	E980.4
hematopoietic	964.1	E858.2	E934.1	E950.4	E962.0	E980.4
K	964.3	E858.2	E934.3	E950.4	E962.0	E980.4
Vleminckx's solution	976.4	E858.7	E946.4	E950.4	E962.0	E980.4
Voltaren — *see* Diclofenac sodium						
Warfarin (potassium) (sodium)	964.2	E858.2	E934.2	E950.4	E962.0	E980.4
rodenticide	989.4	E863.7	—	E950.6	E962.1	E980.7
Wasp (sting)	989.5	E905.3	—	E950.9	E962.1	E980.9
Water						
balance agents NEC	974.5	E858.5	E944.5	E950.4	E962.0	E980.4
gas	987.1	E868.1	—	E951.8	E962.2	E981.8
incomplete combustion of — see Carbon, monoxide, fuel, utility						
hemlock	988.2	E865.4	—	E950.9	E962.1	E980.9
moccasin (venom)	989.5	E905.0	—	E950.9	E962.1	E980.9
Wax (paraffin) (petroleum)	981	E862.3	—	E950.9	E962.1	E980.9
automobile	989.89	E861.2	—	E950.9	E962.1	E980.9
floor	981	E862.0	—	E950.9	E962.1	E980.9
Weed killers NEC	989.4	E863.5	—	E950.6	E962.1	E980.7
Welldorm	967.1	E852.0	E937.1	E950.2	E962.0	E980.2
White						
arsenic — see Arsenic						
hellebore	988.2	E865.4	—	E950.9	E962.1	E980.9
lotion (keratolytic)	976.4	E858.7	E946.4	E950.4	E962.0	E980.4
spirit	981	E862.0	—	E950.9	E962.1	E980.9
Whitewashes	989.89	E861.6	—	E950.9	E962.1	E980.9
Whole blood	964.7	E858.2	E934.7	E950.4	E962.0	E980.4
Wild						
black cherry	988.2	E865.4	—	E950.9	E962.1	E980.9
poisonous plants NEC	988.2	E865.4	—	E950.9	E962.1	E980.9
Window cleaning fluid	989.89	E861.3	—	E950.9	E962.1	E980.9
Wintergreen (oil)	976.3	E858.7	E946.3	E950.4	E962.0	E980.4
Witch hazel	976.2	E858.7	E946.2	E950.4	E962.0	E980.4
Wood						
alcohol	980.1	E860.2	—	E950.9	E962.1	E980.9
spirit	980.1	E860.2	—	E950.9	E962.1	E980.9
Woorali	975.2	E858.6	E945.2	E950.4	E962.0	E980.4
Wormseed, American	961.6	E857	E931.6	E950.4	E962.0	E980.4
Xanthine diuretics	974.1	E858.5	E944.1	E950.4	E962.0	E980.4
Xanthocillin	960.0	E856	E930.0	E950.4	E962.0	E980.4
Xanthotoxin	976.3	E858.7	E946.3	E950.4	E962.0	E980.4
Xigris	964.2	E858.2	E934.2	E950.4	E962.0	E980.4
Xylene (liquid) (vapor)	982.0	E862.4	—	E950.9	E962.1	E980.9
Xylocaine (infiltration) (topical)	968.5	E855.2	E938.5	E950.4	E962.0	E980.4
nerve block (peripheral) (plexus)	968.6	E855.2	E938.6	E950.4	E962.0	E980.4
spinal	968.7	E855.2	E938.7	E950.4	E962.0	E980.4
Xylol (liquid) (vapor)	982.0	E862.4	—	E950.9	E962.1	E980.9
Xylometazoline	971.2	E855.5	E941.2	E950.4	E962.0	E980.4
Yellow						
fever vaccine	979.3	E858.8	E949.3	E950.4	E962.0	E980.4
jasmine	988.2	E865.4	—	E950.9	E962.1	E980.9
Yew	988.2	E865.4	—	E950.9	E962.1	E980.9
Zactane	965.7	E850.7	E935.7	E950.0	E962.0	E980.0
Zaroxolyn	974.3	E858.5	E944.3	E950.4	E962.0	E980.4
Zephiran (topical)	976.0	E858.7	E946.0	E950.4	E962.0	E980.4
ophthalmic preparation	976.5	E858.7	E946.5	E950.4	E962.0	E980.4
Zerone	980.1	E860.2	—	E950.9	E962.1	E980.9
Zinc (compounds) (fumes) (salts) (vapor) NEC	985.8	E866.4	—	E950.9	E962.1	E980.9
anti-infectives	976.0	E858.7	E946.0	E950.4	E962.0	E980.4

Nontherapeutic use substance

		External Cause (E-Code)				
	Poisoning	Accident	Therapeutic Use	Suicide Attempt	Assault	Undetermined
Zinc — *continued*						
antivaricose	972.7	E858.3	E942.7	E950.4	E962.0	E980.4
bacitracin	976.0	E858.7	E946.0	E950.4	E962.0	E980.4
chloride	976.2	E858.7	E946.2	E950.4	E962.0	E980.4
gelatin	976.3	E858.7	E946.3	E950.4	E962.0	E980.4
oxide	976.3	E858.7	E946.3	E950.4	E962.0	E980.4
peroxide	976.0	E858.7	E946.0	E950.4	E962.0	E980.4
pesticides	985.8	E863.4	—	E950.6	E962.1	E980.7
phosphide (rodenticide)	985.8	E863.7	—	E950.6	E962.1	E980.7
stearate	976.3	E858.7	E946.3	E950.4	E962.0	E980.4
sulfate (antivaricose)	972.7	E858.3	E942.7	E950.4	E962.0	E980.4
ENT agent	976.6	E858.7	E946.6	E950.4	E962.0	E980.4
ophthalmic solution	976.5	E858.7	E946.5	E950.4	E962.0	E980.4
topical NEC	976.0	E858.7	E946.0	E950.4	E962.0	E980.4
undecylenate	976.0	E858.7	E946.0	E950.4	E962.0	E980.4
Zovant	964.2	E858.2	E934.2	E950.4	E962.0	E980.4
Zoxazolamine	968.0	E855.1	E938.0	E950.4	E962.0	E980.4
Zygadenus (venenosus)	988.2	E865.4	—	E950.9	E962.1	E980.9
Zyprexa	969.3	E853.8	E939.3	E950.3	E962.0	E980.3

SECTION 3

Alphabetic Index to External Causes of Injury and Poisoning (E Code)

This section contains the index to the codes which classify environmental events, circumstances, and other conditions as the cause of injury and other adverse effects. Where a code from the section Supplementary Classification of External Causes of Injury and Poisoning (E800-E999) is applicable, it is intended that the E code shall be used in addition to a code from the main body of the classification, Chapters 1 to 17.

The alphabetic index to the E codes is organized by main terms which describe the accident, circumstance, event, or specific agent which caused the injury or other adverse effect.

Note — Transport accidents (E800-E848) include accidents involving:

- *aircraft and spacecraft (E840-E845)*
- *watercraft (E830-E838)*
- *motor vehicle (E810-E825)*
- *railway (E800-E807)*
- *other road vehicles (E826-E829)*

For definitions and examples related to transport accidents — see Volume 1 code categories E800-E848.

The fourth-digit subdivisions for use with categories E800-E848 to identify the injured person are found at the end of this section.

For identifying the place in which an accident or poisoning occurred (circumstances classifiable to categories E850-E869 and E880-E928) — see the listing in this section under "Accident, occurring."

See the Table of Drugs and Chemicals (Section 2 of this volume) for identifying the specific agent involved in drug overdose or a wrong substance given or taken in error, and for intoxication or poisoning by a drug or other chemical substance.

The specific adverse effect, reaction, or localized toxic effect to a correct drug or substance properly administered in therapeutic or prophylactic dosage should be classified according to the nature of the adverse effect (e.g., allergy, dermatitis, tachycardia) listed in Section 1 of this volume.

A

Abandonment
- causing exposure to weather conditions — *see* Exposure
- child, with intent to injure or kill E968.4
- helpless person, infant, newborn E904.0
  - with intent to injure or kill E968.4

Abortion, criminal, injury to child E968.8

Abuse (alleged) (suspected)
- adult
  - by
    - child E967.4
    - ex-partner E967.3
    - ex-spouse E967.3
    - father E967.0
    - grandchild E967.7
    - grandparent E967.6
    - mother E967.2
    - non-related caregiver E967.8
    - other relative E967.7
    - other specified person E967.1
    - partner E967.3
    - sibling E967.5
    - spouse E967.3
    - stepfather E967.0
    - stepmother E967.2
    - unspecified person E967.9
- child
  - by
    - boyfriend of parent or guardian E967.0
    - child E967.4
    - father E967.0
    - female partner of parent or guardian E967.2
    - girlfriend of parent or guardian E967.2
    - grandchild E967.7
    - grandparent E967.6
    - male partner of parent or guardian E967.0
    - mother E967.2
    - non-related caregiver E967.8
    - other relative E967.7
    - other specified person(s) E967.1
    - sibling E967.5
    - stepfather E967.0
    - stepmother E967.2
    - unspecified person E967.9

Accident (to) E928.9
- aircraft (in transit) (powered) E841 ☑
  - at landing, take-off E840 ☑
  - due to, caused by cataclysm — *see* categories E908 ☑, E909 ☑
  - late effect of E929.1
  - unpowered (*see also* Collision, aircraft, unpowered) E842 ☑
  - while alighting, boarding E843 ☑
- amphibious vehicle
  - on
    - land — *see* Accident, motor vehicle
    - water — *see* Accident, watercraft
- animal-drawn vehicle NEC E827 ☑
- animal, ridden NEC E828 ☑
- balloon (*see also* Collision, aircraft, unpowered) E842 ☑
- caused by, due to
  - abrasive wheel (metalworking) E919.3
  - animal NEC E906.9
    - being ridden (in sport or transport) E828 ☑
  - avalanche NEC E909.2
  - band saw E919.4
  - bench saw E919.4
  - bore, earth-drilling or mining (land) (seabed) E919.1
  - bulldozer E919.7
  - cataclysmic
    - earth surface movement or eruption E909.9
    - storm E908.9
  - chain
    - hoist E919.2
      - agricultural operations E919.0
      - mining operations E919.1

Accident (to) — *continued*
- caused by, due to — *continued*
  - chain — *continued*
    - saw E920.1
  - circular saw E919.4
  - cold (excessive) (*see also* Cold, exposure to) E901.9
  - combine E919.0
  - conflagration — *see* Conflagration
  - corrosive liquid, substance NEC E924.1
  - cotton gin E919.8
  - crane E919.2
    - agricultural operations E919.0
    - mining operations E919.1
  - cutting or piercing instrument (*see also* Cut) E920.9
  - dairy equipment E919.8
  - derrick E919.2
    - agricultural operations E919.0
    - mining operations E919.1
  - drill E920.1
    - earth (land) (seabed) E919.1
    - hand (powered) E920.1
      - not powered E920.4
    - metalworking E919.3
    - woodworking E919.4
  - earth(-)
    - drilling machine E919.1
    - moving machine E919.7
    - scraping machine E919.7
  - electric
    - current (*see also* Electric shock) E925.9
    - motor (*see also* Accident, machine, by type of machine)
      - current (of) — *see* Electric shock
  - elevator (building) (grain) E919.2
    - agricultural operations E919.0
    - mining operations E919.1
  - environmental factors NEC E928.9
  - excavating machine E919.7
  - explosive material (*see also* Explosion) E923.9
  - farm machine E919.0
  - firearm missile — *see* Shooting
  - fire, flames (*see also* Fire)
    - conflagration — *see* Conflagration
  - forging (metalworking) machine E919.3
  - forklift (truck) E919.2
    - agricultural operations E919.0
    - mining operations E919.1
  - gas turbine E919.5
  - harvester E919.0
  - hay derrick, mower, or rake E919.0
  - heat (excessive) (*see also* Heat) E900.9
  - hoist (*see also* Accident, caused by, due to, lift) E919.2
    - chain — *see* Accident, caused by, due to, chain
    - shaft E919.1
  - hot
    - liquid E924.0
      - caustic or corrosive E924.1
    - object (not producing fire or flames) E924.8
    - substance E924.9
      - caustic or corrosive E924.1
      - liquid (metal) NEC E924.0
      - specified type NEC E924.8
  - human bite E928.3
  - ignition — *see* Ignition
  - internal combustion engine E919.5
  - landslide NEC E909.2
  - lathe (metalworking) E919.3
    - turnings E920.8
    - woodworking E919.4
  - lift, lifting (appliances) E919.2
    - agricultural operations E919.0
    - mining operations E919.1
    - shaft E919.1
  - lightning NEC E907
  - machine, machinery (*see also* Accident, machine)
    - drilling, metal E919.3
    - manufacturing, for manufacture of beverages E919.8

Accident (to) — *continued*
- caused by, due to — *continued*
  - machine, machinery (*see also* Accident, machine) — *continued*
    - manufacturing, for manufacture of — *continued*
      - clothing E919.8
      - foodstuffs E919.8
      - paper E919.8
      - textiles E919.8
    - milling, metal E919.3
    - moulding E919.4
    - power press, metal E919.3
    - printing E919.8
    - rolling mill, metal E919.3
    - sawing, metal E919.3
    - specified type NEC E919.8
    - spinning E919.8
    - weaving E919.8
  - natural factor NEC E928.9
  - overhead plane E919.4
  - plane E920.4
    - overhead E919.4
  - powered
    - hand tool NEC E920.1
    - saw E919.4
      - hand E920.1
  - printing machine E919.8
  - pulley (block) E919.2
    - agricultural operations E919.0
    - mining operations E919.1
    - transmission E919.6
  - radial saw E919.4
  - radiation — *see* Radiation
  - reaper E919.0
  - road scraper E919.7
    - when in transport under its own power — *see* categories E810-E825 ☑
  - roller coaster E919.8
  - sander E919.4
  - saw E920.4
    - band E919.4
    - bench E919.4
    - chain E920.1
    - circular E919.4
    - hand E920.4
      - powered E920.1
    - powered, except hand E919.4
    - radial E919.4
  - sawing machine, metal E919.3
  - shaft
    - hoist E919.1
    - lift E919.1
    - transmission E919.6
  - shears E920.4
    - hand E920.4
      - powered E920.1
    - mechanical E919.3
  - shovel E920.4
    - steam E919.7
  - spinning machine E919.8
  - steam (*see also* Burning, steam)
    - engine E919.5
    - shovel E919.7
  - thresher E919.0
  - thunderbolt NEC E907
  - tractor E919.0
    - when in transport under its own power — *see* categories E810-E825 ☑
  - transmission belt, cable, chain, gear, pinion, pulley, shaft E919.6
  - turbine (gas) (water driven) E919.5
  - under-cutter E919.1
  - weaving machine E919.8
  - winch E919.2
    - agricultural operations E919.0
    - mining operations E919.1
- diving E883.0
  - with insufficient air supply E913.2
- glider (hang) (*see also* Collision, aircraft, unpowered) E842 ☑
- hovercraft
  - on
    - land — *see* Accident, motor vehicle

Accident (to) — *continued*
- hovercraft — *continued*
  - on — *continued*
    - water — *see* Accident, watercraft
- ice yacht (*see also* Accident, vehicle NEC) E848
- in
  - medical, surgical procedure
    - as, or due to misadventure — *see* Misadventure
    - causing an abnormal reaction or later complication without mention of misadventure — *see* Reaction, abnormal
- kite carrying a person (*see also* Collision, involving aircraft, unpowered) E842 ☑
- land yacht (*see also* Accident, vehicle NEC) E848
- late effect of — *see* Late effect
- launching pad E845 ☑
- machine, machinery (*see also* Accident, caused by, due to, by specific type of machine) E919.9
  - agricultural including animal-powered E919.0
  - earth-drilling E919.1
  - earth moving or scraping E919.7
  - excavating E919.7
  - involving transport under own power on highway or transport vehicle — *see* categories E810-E825 ☑, E840-E845 ☑
  - lifting (appliances) E919.2
  - metalworking E919.3
  - mining E919.1
  - prime movers, except electric motors E919.5
    - electric motors — *see* Accident, machine, by specific type of machine
  - recreational E919.8
  - specified type NEC E919.8
  - transmission E919.6
  - watercraft (deck) (engine room) (galley) (laundry) (loading) E836 ☑
  - woodworking or forming E919.4
- motor vehicle (on public highway) (traffic) E819 ☑
  - due to cataclysm — *see* categories E908 ☑, E909 ☑
  - involving
    - collision (*see also* Collision, motor vehicle) E812 ☑
    - nontraffic, not on public highway — *see* categories E820-E825 ☑
    - not involving collision — *see* categories E816-E819 ☑
- nonmotor vehicle NEC E829 ☑
  - nonroad — *see* Accident, vehicle NEC
  - road, except pedal cycle, animal-drawn vehicle, or animal being ridden E829 ☑
- nonroad vehicle NEC — *see* Accident, vehicle NEC
- not elsewhere classifiable involving
  - cable car (not on rails) E847
    - on rails E829 ☑
  - coal car in mine E846
  - hand truck — *see* Accident, vehicle NEC
  - logging car E846
  - sled(ge), meaning snow or ice vehicle E848
  - tram, mine or quarry E846
  - truck
    - mine or quarry E846
    - self-propelled, industrial E846
    - station baggage E846
  - tub, mine or quarry E846
  - vehicle NEC E848
    - snow and ice E848
    - used only on industrial premises E846
  - wheelbarrow E848
- occurring (at) (in)
  - apartment E849.0
  - baseball field, diamond E849.4

☑ **Additional Digit Required** — Refer to the Tabular List for Digit Selection

▽ **Subterms under main terms may continue to next column or page**

336 — Volume 2

►◄ Revised Text

● New Line

▲ Revised Code

2013 ICD-9-CM

Accident (to) — *continued*
  occurring — *continued*
    construction site, any E849.3
    dock E849.8
      yard E849.3
    dormitory E849.7
    factory (building) (premises) E849.3
    farm E849.1
      buildings E849.1
      house E849.0
    football field E849.4
    forest E849.8
    garage (place of work) E849.3
      private (home) E849.0
    gravel pit E849.2
    gymnasium E849.4
    highway E849.5
    home (private) (residential) E849.0
      institutional E849.7
    hospital E849.7
    hotel E849.6
    house (private) (residential) E849.0
      movie E849.6
      public E849.6
    institution, residential E849.7
    jail E849.7
    mine E849.2
    motel E849.6
    movie house E849.6
    office (building) E849.6
    orphanage E849.7
    park (public) E849.4
      mobile home E849.8
      trailer E849.8
    parking lot or place E849.8
    place
      industrial NEC E849.3
      parking E849.8
      public E849.8
        specified place NEC E849.5
      recreational NEC E849.4
      sport NEC E849.4
    playground (park) (school) E849.4
    prison E849.6
    public building NEC E849.6
    quarry E849.2
    railway
      line NEC E849.8
      yard E849.3
    residence
      home (private) E849.0
    resort (beach) (lake) (mountain)
      (seashore) (vacation) E849.4
    restaurant E849.6
    sand pit E849.2
    school (building) (private) (public) (state)
      E849.6
      reform E849.7
      riding E849.4
    seashore E849.8
      resort E849.4
    shop (place of work) E849.3
      commercial E849.6
    skating rink E849.4
    sports palace E849.4
    stadium E849.4
    store E849.6
    street E849.5
    swimming pool (public) E849.4
      private home or garden E849.0
    tennis court, public E849.4
    theatre, theater E849.6
    trailer court E849.8
    tunnel E849.8
      under construction E849.2
    warehouse E849.3
    yard
      dock E849.3
      industrial E849.3
      private (home) E849.0
      railway E849.3
  off-road type motor vehicle (not on public
    highway) NEC E821 ☑
    on public highway — *see* categories
      E810-E819 ☑
  pedal cycle E826 ☑

Accident (to) — *continued*
  railway E807 ☑
    due to cataclysm — *see* categories
      E908 ☑, E909 ☑
    involving
      avalanche E909.2
      burning by engine, locomotive, train
        (*see also* Explosion, railway
        engine) E803 ☑
      collision (*see also* Collision, railway)
        E800 ☑
      derailment (*see also* Derailment, rail-
        way) E802 ☑
      explosion (*see also* Explosion, railway
        engine) E803 ☑
      fall (*see also* Fall, from, railway rolling
        stock) E804 ☑
      fire (*see also* Explosion, railway en-
        gine) E803 ☑
      hitting by, being struck by
        object falling in, on, from, rolling
          stock, train, vehicle
          E806 ☑
        rolling stock, train, vehicle
          E805 ☑
      overturning, railway rolling stock,
        train, vehicle (*see also* Derail-
        ment, railway) E802 ☑
      running off rails, railway (*see also*
        Derailment, railway) E802 ☑
      specified circumstances NEC E806 ☑
      train or vehicle hit by
        avalanche E909.2
        falling object (earth, rock, tree)
          E806 ☑
          due to cataclysm — *see* cate-
            gories
            E908 ☑, E909 ☑
        landslide E909.2
  roller skate E885.1
  scooter (nonmotorized) E885.0
  skateboard E885.2
  ski(ing) E885.3
    jump E884.9
    lift or tow (with chair or gondola) E847
  snowboard E885.4
  snow vehicle, motor driven (not on public
    highway) E820 ☑
    on public highway — *see* categories
      E810-E819 ☑
  spacecraft E845 ☑
  specified cause NEC E928.8
  street car E829 ☑
  traffic NEC E819 ☑
  vehicle NEC (with pedestrian) E848
    battery powered
      airport passenger vehicle E846
      truck (baggage) (mail) E846
    powered commercial or industrial (with
      other vehicle or object within
      commercial or industrial premis-
      es) E846
  watercraft E838 ☑
    with
      drowning or submersion resulting
        from
        accident other than to watercraft
          E832 ☑
        accident to watercraft E830 ☑
      injury, except drowning or submer-
        sion, resulting from
        accident other than to watercraft
        — *see* categories
          E833-E838 ☑
        accident to watercraft E831 ☑
    due to, caused by cataclysm — *see* cate-
      gories E908 ☑, E909 ☑
    machinery E836 ☑

Acid throwing E961
Acosta syndrome E902.0
Activity (involving) E030
  aerobic and step exercise (class) E009.2
  alpine skiing E003.2
  animal care NEC E019.9
  arts and handcrafts NEC E012.9

Activity — *continued*
  athletics NEC E008.9
    played
      as a team or group NEC E007.9
      individually NEC E006.9
  baking E015.2
  ballet E005.0
  barbells E010.2
  baseball E007.3
  BASE (Building, Antenna, Span, Earth)
    jumping E004.2
  basketball E007.6
  bathing (personal) E013.0
  beach volleyball E007.7
  bike riding E006.4
  boogie boarding E002.7
  bowling E006.3
  boxing E008.0
  brass instrument playing E018.3
  building and construction E016.2
  bungee jumping E004.3
  calisthenics E009.1
  canoeing (in calm and turbulent water)
    E002.5
  capture the flag E007.8
  cardiorespiratory exercise NEC E009.9
  caregiving (providing) NEC E014.9
    bathing E014.0
    lifting E014.1
  cellular
    communication device E011.1
    telephone E011.1
  challenge course E009.4
  cheerleading E005.4
  circuit training E009.3
  cleaning
    floor E013.4
  climbing NEC E004.9
    mountain E004.0
    rock E004.0
    wall climbing E004.0
  combatives E008.4
  computer
    keyboarding E011.0
    technology NEC E011.9
  confidence course E009.4
  construction (building) E016.2
  cooking and baking E015.2
  cooking and grilling NEC E015.9
  cool down exercises E009.1
  cricket E007.9
  crocheting E012.0
  cross country skiing E003.3
  dancing (all types) E005.0
  digging
    dirt E016.0
  dirt digging E016.0
  dishwashing E015.0
  diving (platform) (springboard) E002.1
    underwater E002.4
  dodge ball E007.8
  downhill skiing E003.2
  drum playing E018.1
  dumbbells E010.2
  electronic
    devices NEC E011.9
      hand held interactive E011.1
    game playing (using) (with)
      interactive device E011.1
      keyboard or other stationary device
        E011.0
  elliptical machine E009.0
  exercise(s)
    machines (primarily for)
      cardiorespiratory conditioning
        E009.0
      muscle strengthening E010.0
    muscle strengthening (non-machine)
      NEC E010.9
  external motion NEC E017.9
    roller coaster E017.0
  field hockey E007.4
  figure skating (pairs) (singles) E003.0
  flag football E007.1
  floor mopping and cleaning E013.4
  food preparation and clean up E015.0

Activity — *continued*
  football (American) NOS E007.0
    flag E007.1
    tackle E007.0
    touch E007.1
  four square E007.8
  free weights E010.2
  frisbee (ultimate) E008.3
  furniture
    building E012.2
    finishing E012.2
    repair E012.2
  game playing (electronic)
    using
      interactive device E011.1
      keyboard or other stationary device
        E011.0
  gardening E016.1
  golf E006.2
  grass drills E009.5
  grilling and smoking food E015.1
  grooming and shearing an animal E019.2
  guerilla drills E009.5
  gymnastics (rhythmic) E005.2
  handball E008.2
  handcrafts NEC E012.9
  hand held interactive electronic device
    E011.1
  hang gliding E004.4
  hiking (on level or elevated terrain) E001.0
  hockey (ice) E003.1
    field E007.4
  horseback riding E006.1
  household maintenance NEC E013.9
  ice NEC E003.9
    dancing E003.0
    hockey E003.1
    skating E003.0
  inline roller skating E006.0
  ironing E013.3
  judo E008.4
  jumping (off) NEC E004.9
    BASE (Building, Antenna, Span, Earth)
      E004.2
    bungee E004.3
    jacks E009.1
    rope E006.5
  jumping jacks E009.1
  jumping rope E006.5
  karate E008.4
  kayaking (in calm and turbulent water)
    E002.5
  keyboarding (computer) E011.0
  kickball E007.8
  knitting E012.0
  lacrosse E007.4
  land maintenance NEC E016.9
  landscaping E016.1
  laundry E013.1
  machines (exercise) primarily for cardiores-
    piratory conditioning E009.0
  maintenance
    building E016.9
    household NEC E013.9
    land E016.9
    property E016.9
  marching (on level or elevated terrain)
    E001.0
  martial arts E008.4
  microwave oven E015.2
  milking an animal E019.1
  mopping (floor) E013.4
  mountain climbing E004.0
  muscle strengthening
    exercises (non-machine) NEC E010.9
    machines E010.0
  musical keyboard (electronic) playing E018.0
  nordic skiing E003.3
  obstacle course E009.4
  oven (microwave) E015.2
  packing up and unpacking in moving to a
    new residence E013.5
  parasailing E002.9
  percussion instrument playing NEC E018.1
  personal
    bathing and showering E013.0

☑ **Additional Digit Required** — Refer to the Tabular List for Digit Selection   ▽ **Subterms under main terms may continue to next column or page**

☑ **Additional Digit Required** — Refer to the Tabular List for Digit Selection ⏢ **Subterms under main terms may continue to next column or page**

338 — Volume 2 ▶◀ **Revised Text** ● **New Line** ▲ **Revised Code** 2013 ICD-9-CM

Collision (accidental)

Note — In the case of collisions between different types of vehicles, persons and objects, priority in classification is in the following order:

    Aircraft

    Watercraft

    Motor vehicle

    Railway vehicle

    Pedal cycle

    Animal-drawn vehicle

    Animal being ridden

    Streetcar or other nonmotor road vehicle

    Other vehicle

    Pedestrian or person using pedestrian conveyance

    Object (except where falling from or set in motion by vehicle etc. listed above)

In the listing below, the combinations are listed only under the vehicle etc. having priority. For definitions, see Supplementary Classification of External Causes of Injury and Poisoning (E800-E999).

aircraft (with object or vehicle) (fixed) (movable) (moving) E841 ☑
  with
    person (while landing, taking off) (without accident to aircraft) E844 ☑
    powered (in transit) (with unpowered aircraft) E841 ☑
      while landing, taking off E840 ☑
    unpowered E842 ☑
      while landing, taking off E840 ☑
animal being ridden (in sport or transport) E828 ☑
  and
    animal (being ridden) (herded) (unattended) E828 ☑
    nonmotor road vehicle, except pedal cycle or animal-drawn vehicle E828 ☑
    object (fallen) (fixed) (movable) (moving) not falling from or set in motion by vehicle of higher priority E828 ☑
    pedestrian (conveyance or vehicle) E828 ☑
animal-drawn vehicle E827 ☑
  and
    animal (being ridden) (herded) (unattended) E827 ☑
    nonmotor road vehicle, except pedal cycle E827 ☑
    object (fallen) (fixed) (movable) (moving) not falling from or set in motion by vehicle of higher priority E827 ☑
    pedestrian (conveyance or vehicle) E827 ☑
    streetcar E827 ☑
motor vehicle (on public highway) (traffic accident) E812 ☑
  after leaving, running off, public highway (without antecedent collision) (without re-entry) E816 ☑
  with antecedent collision on public highway — see categories E810-E815 ☑
    with re-entrance collision with another motor vehicle E811 ☑
  and
    abutment (bridge) (overpass) E815 ☑
    animal (herded) (unattended) E815 ☑

Collision — continued
motor vehicle — continued
  and — continued
    animal — continued
      carrying person, property E813 ☑
    animal-drawn vehicle E813 ☑
    another motor vehicle (abandoned) (disabled) (parked) (stalled) (stopped) E812 ☑
      with, involving re-entrance (on same roadway) (across median strip) E811 ☑
    any object, person, or vehicle off the public highway resulting from a noncollision motor vehicle nontraffic accident E816 ☑
    avalanche, fallen or not moving E815 ☑
      falling E909.2
    boundary fence E815 ☑
    culvert E815 ☑
    fallen
      stone E815 ☑
      tree E815 ☑
    guard post or guard rail E815 ☑
    inter-highway divider E815 ☑
    landslide, fallen or not moving E815 ☑
      moving E909 ☑
    machinery (road) E815 ☑
    nonmotor road vehicle NEC E813 ☑
    object (any object, person, or vehicle off the public highway resulting from a noncollision motor vehicle nontraffic accident) E815 ☑
      off, normally not on, public highway resulting from a noncollision motor vehicle traffic accident E816 ☑
    pedal cycle E813 ☑
    pedestrian (conveyance) E814 ☑
    person (using pedestrian conveyance) E814 ☑
    post or pole (lamp) (light) (signal) (telephone) (utility) E815 ☑
    railway rolling stock, train, vehicle E810 ☑
    safety island E815 ☑
    street car E813 ☑
    traffic signal, sign, or marker (temporary) E815 ☑
    tree E815 ☑
    tricycle E813 ☑
    wall of cut made for road E815 ☑
    due to cataclysm — see categories E908 ☑, E909 ☑
  not on public highway, nontraffic accident E822 ☑
  and
    animal (carrying person, property) (herded) (unattended) E822 ☑
    animal-drawn vehicle E822 ☑
    another motor vehicle (moving), except off-road motor vehicle E822 ☑
      stationary E823 ☑
    avalanche, fallen, not moving E823 ☑
      moving E909.2
    landslide, fallen, not moving E823 ☑
      moving E909.2
    nonmotor vehicle (moving) E822 ☑
      stationary E823 ☑
    object (fallen) (normally) (fixed) (movable but not in motion) (stationary) E823 ☑
      moving, except when falling from, set in motion by, aircraft or cataclysm E822 ☑
    pedal cycle (moving) E822 ☑

Collision — continued
motor vehicle — continued
  not on public highway, nontraffic accident — continued
  and — continued
    pedal cycle — continued
      stationary E823 ☑
    pedestrian (conveyance) E822 ☑
    person (using pedestrian conveyance) E822 ☑
    railway rolling stock, train, vehicle (moving) E822 ☑
      stationary E823 ☑
    road vehicle (any) (moving) E822 ☑
      stationary E823 ☑
    tricycle (moving) E822 ☑
      stationary E823 ☑
  off-road type motor vehicle (not on public highway) E821 ☑
  and
    animal (being ridden) (-drawn vehicle) E821 ☑
    another off-road motor vehicle, except snow vehicle E821 ☑
    other motor vehicle, not on public highway E821 ☑
    other object or vehicle NEC, fixed or movable, not set in motion by aircraft, motor vehicle on highway, or snow vehicle, motor driven E821 ☑
    pedal cycle E821 ☑
    pedestrian (conveyance) E821 ☑
    railway train E821 ☑
  on public highway — see Collision, motor vehicle
pedal cycle E826 ☑
  and
    animal (carrying person, property) (herded) (unherded) E826 ☑
    animal-drawn vehicle E826 ☑
    another pedal cycle E826 ☑
    nonmotor road vehicle E826 ☑
    object (fallen) (fixed) (movable) (moving) not falling from or set in motion by aircraft, motor vehicle, or railway train NEC E826 ☑
    pedestrian (conveyance) E826 ☑
    person (using pedestrian conveyance) E826 ☑
    street car E826 ☑
pedestrian(s) (conveyance) E917.9
  with fall E886.9
    in sports E886.0
  and
    crowd, human stampede E917.1
      with subsequent fall E917.6
    furniture E917.3
      with subsequent fall E917.7
    machinery — see Accident, machine
    object (fallen) (moving) not falling from NEC, fixed or set in motion by any vehicle classifiable to E800-E848 ☑, E917.9
      with subsequent fall E917.6
      caused by a crowd E917.1
        with subsequent fall E917.6
      furniture E917.3
        with subsequent fall E917.7
    in
      running water E917.2
        with drowning or submersion — see Submersion
      sports E917.0
        with subsequent fall E917.5
      stationary E917.4
        with subsequent fall E917.8
    vehicle, nonmotor, nonroad E848
  in
    running water E917.2

Collision — continued
pedestrian(s) — continued
  in — continued
    running water — continued
      with drowning or submersion — see Submersion
    sports E917.0
      with fall E886.0
  person(s) (using pedestrian conveyance) (see also Collision, pedestrian) E917.9
  railway (rolling stock) (train) (vehicle) (with (subsequent) derailment, explosion, fall or fire) E800 ☑
    with antecedent derailment E802 ☑
  and
    animal (carrying person) (herded) (unattended) E801 ☑
    another railway train or vehicle E800 ☑
    buffers E801 ☑
    fallen tree on railway E801 ☑
    farm machinery, nonmotor (in transport) (stationary) E801 ☑
    gates E801 ☑
    nonmotor vehicle E801 ☑
    object (fallen) (fixed) (movable) (moving) not falling from, set in motion by, aircraft or motor vehicle NEC E801 ☑
    pedal cycle E801 ☑
    pedestrian (conveyance) E805 ☑
    person (using pedestrian conveyance) E805 ☑
    platform E801 ☑
    rock on railway E801 ☑
    street car E801 ☑
  snow vehicle, motor-driven (not on public highway) E820 ☑
  and
    animal (being ridden) (-drawn vehicle) E820 ☑
    another off-road motor vehicle E820 ☑
    other motor vehicle, not on public highway E820 ☑
    other object or vehicle NEC, fixed or movable, not set in motion by aircraft or motor vehicle on highway E820 ☑
    pedal cycle E820 ☑
    pedestrian (conveyance) E820 ☑
    railway train E820 ☑
  on public highway — see Collision, motor vehicle
street car(s) E829 ☑
  and
    animal, herded, not being ridden, unattended E829 ☑
    nonmotor road vehicle NEC E829 ☑
    object (fallen) (fixed) (movable) (moving) not falling from or set in motion by aircraft, animal-drawn vehicle, animal being ridden, motor vehicle, pedal cycle, or railway train E829 ☑
    pedestrian (conveyance) E829 ☑
    person (using pedestrian conveyance) E829 ☑
vehicle
  animal-drawn — see Collision, animal-drawn vehicle
  motor — see Collision, motor vehicle
  nonmotor
    nonroad E848
    and
      another nonmotor, nonroad vehicle E848

☑ Additional Digit Required — Refer to the Tabular List for Digit Selection   ▽ Subterms under main terms may continue to next column or page

Collision — *continued*
  vehicle — *continued*
    nonmotor — *continued*
      nonroad — *continued*
        and — *continued*
          object (fallen) (fixed) (movable) (moving) not falling from or set in motion by aircraft, animal-drawn vehicle, animal being ridden, motor vehicle, nonmotor road vehicle, pedal cycle, railway train, or streetcar E848
        road, except animal being ridden, animal-drawn vehicle, or pedal cycle E829 ☑
        and
          animal, herded, not being ridden, unattended E829 ☑
          another nonmotor road vehicle, except animal being ridden, animal-drawn vehicle, or pedal cycle E829 ☑
          object (fallen) (fixed) (movable) (moving) not falling from or set in motion by, aircraft, animal-drawn vehicle, animal being ridden, motor vehicle, pedal cycle, or railway train E829 ☑
          pedestrian (conveyance) E829 ☑
          person (using pedestrian conveyance) E829 ☑
          vehicle, nonmotor, nonroad E829 ☑
  watercraft E838 ☑
    and
      person swimming or water skiing E838 ☑
    causing
      drowning, submersion E830 ☑
      injury except drowning, submersion E831 ☑
Combustion, spontaneous — *see* Ignition
Complication of medical or surgical procedure or treatment
  as an abnormal reaction — *see* Reaction, abnormal
  delayed, without mention of misadventure — *see* Reaction, abnormal
  due to misadventure — *see* Misadventure
Compression
  divers' squeeze E902.2
  trachea by
    food E911
    foreign body, except food E912
Conflagration
  building or structure, except private dwelling (barn) (church) (convalescent or residential home) (factory) (farm outbuilding) (hospital) (hotel) (institution) (educational) (domitory) (residential) (school) (shop) (store) (theater) E891.9
    with or causing (injury due to)
      accident or injury NEC E891.9
        specified circumstance NEC E891.8
      burns, burning E891.3
      carbon monoxide E891.2
      fumes E891.2
        polyvinylchloride (PVC) or similar material E891.1
      smoke E891.2
      causing explosion E891.0
    in terrorism E979.3
  not in building or structure E892

Conflagration — *continued*
  private dwelling (apartment) (boarding house) (camping place) (caravan) (farmhouse) (home (private)) (house) (lodging house) (private garage) (rooming house) (tenement) E890.9
    with or causing (injury due to)
      accident or injury NEC E890.9
        specified circumstance NEC E890.8
      burns, burning E890.3
      carbon monoxide E890.2
      fumes E890.2
        polyvinylchloride (PVC) or similar material E890.1
      smoke E890.2
      causing explosion E890.0
Constriction, external
  caused by
    hair E928.4
    other object E928.5
Contact with
  dry ice E901.1
  liquid air, hydrogen, nitrogen E901.1
Cramp(s)
  Heat — *see* Heat
  swimmers (*see also* category E910) E910.2
    not in recreation or sport E910.3
Cranking (car) (truck) (bus) (engine), injury by E917.9
Crash
  aircraft (in transit) (powered) E841 ☑
    at landing, take-off E840 ☑
    in
      terrorism E979.1
      war operations E994.9
    on runway NEC E840 ☑
    stated as
      homicidal E968.8
      suicidal E958.6
      undetermined whether accidental or intentional E988.6
    unpowered E842 ☑
  glider E842 ☑
  motor vehicle (*see also* Accident, motor vehicle)
    homicidal E968.5
    suicidal E958.5
    undetermined whether accidental or intentional E988.5
Crushed (accidentally) E928.9
  between
    boat(s), ship(s), watercraft (and dock or pier) (without accident to watercraft) E838 ☑
      after accident to, or collision, watercraft E831 ☑
    objects (moving) (stationary and moving) E918
  by
    avalanche NEC E909.2
    boat, ship, watercraft after accident to, collision, watercraft E831 ☑
    cave-in E916
      with asphyxiation or suffocation (*see also* Suffocation, due to, cave-in) E913.3
    crowd, human stampede E917.1
    falling
      aircraft (*see also* Accident, aircraft) E841 ☑
      in
        terrorism E979.1
        war operations E994.8
      earth, material E916
        with asphyxiation or suffocation (*see also* Suffocation, due to, cave-in) E913.3
      object E916
        on ship, watercraft E838 ☑
        while loading, unloading watercraft E838 ☑
    firearm E928.7
    landslide NEC E909.2
    lifeboat after abandoning ship E831 ☑
    machinery — *see* Accident, machine

Crushed — *continued*
  by — *continued*
    railway rolling stock, train, vehicle (part of) E805 ☑
    slide trigger mechanism, scope or other part of gun E928.7
    street car E829 ☑
    vehicle NEC — *see* Accident, vehicle NEC
  in
    machinery — *see* Accident, machine
    object E918
    transport accident — *see* categories E800-E848 ☑
  late effect of NEC E929.9
Cut, cutting (any part of body) (accidental) E920.9
  by
    arrow E920.8
    axe E920.4
    bayonet (*see also* Bayonet wound) E920.3
      in war operations E995.2
    blender E920.2
    broken glass E920.8
      following fall E888.0
    can opener E920.4
      powered E920.2
    chisel E920.4
    circular saw E919.4
    cutting or piercing instrument (*see also* category) E920 ☑
      following fall E888.0
      late effect of E929.8
    dagger E920.3
    dart E920.8
    drill — *see* Accident, caused by drill
    edge of stiff paper E920.8
    electric
      beater E920.2
      fan E920.2
      knife E920.2
      mixer E920.2
    firearm component E928.7
    fork E920.4
    garden fork E920.4
    hand saw or tool (not powered) E920.4
      powered E920.1
    hedge clipper E920.4
      powered E920.1
    hoe E920.4
    ice pick E920.4
    knife E920.3
      electric E920.2
      in war operations E995.2
    lathe turnings E920.8
    lawn mower E920.4
      powered E920.0
      riding E919.8
    machine — *see* Accident, machine
    meat
      grinder E919.8
      slicer E919.8
    nails E920.8
    needle E920.4
      hypodermic E920.5
    object, edged, pointed, sharp — *see* category E920 ☑
      following fall E888.0
    paper cutter E920.4
    piercing instrument (*see also* category) E920 ☑
      late effect of E929.8
    pitchfork E920.4
    powered
      can opener E920.2
      garden cultivator E920.1
        riding E919.8
      hand saw E920.1
      hand tool NEC E920.1
      hedge clipper E920.1
      household appliance or implement E920.2
      lawn mower (hand) E920.0
        riding E919.8
      rivet gun E920.1
      staple gun E920.1

Cut, cutting — *continued*
  by — *continued*
    rake E920.4
    saw
      circular E919.4
      hand E920.4
    scissors E920.4
    screwdriver E920.4
    sewing machine (electric) (powered) E920.2
      not powered E920.4
    shears E920.4
    shovel E920.4
    slide trigger mechanism, scope or other part of gun E928.7
    spade E920.4
    splinters E920.8
    sword E920.3
      in war operations E995.2
    tin can lid E920.8
    wood slivers E920.8
  homicide (attempt) E966
  inflicted by other person
    stated as
      intentional, homicidal E966
      undetermined whether accidental or intentional E986
  late effect of NEC E929.8
  legal
    execution E978
    intervention E974
  self-inflicted (unspecified whether accidental or intentional) E986
    stated as intentional, purposeful E956
  stated as undetermined whether accidental or intentional E986
  suicidal (attempt) E956
  terrorism E979.8
  war operations E995.2
Cyclone E908.1

D

Death due to injury occurring one year or more previous — *see* Late effect
Decapitation (accidental circumstances) NEC E928.9
  homicidal E966
  legal execution (by guillotine) E978
Deprivation — *see also* Privation
  homicidal intent E968.4
Derailment (accidental)
  railway (rolling stock) (train) (vehicle) (with subsequent collision) E802 ☑
    with
      collision (antecedent) (*see also* Collision, railway) E800 ☑
      explosion (subsequent) (without antecedent collision) E802 ☑
        antecedent collision E803 ☑
      fall (without collision (antecedent)) E802 ☑
      fire (without collision (antecedent)) E802 ☑
  street car E829 ☑
Descent
  parachute (voluntary) (without accident to aircraft) E844 ☑
    due to accident to aircraft — *see* categories E840-E842 ☑
Desertion
  child, with intent to injure or kill E968.4
  helpless person, infant, newborn E904.0
    with intent to injure or kill E968.4
Destitution — *see* Privation
Dirty bomb (*see also* War operations, injury due to, nuclear weapons) E996.9
Disability, late effect or sequela of injury — *see* Late effect
Disease
  Andes E902.0
  aviators' E902.1
  caisson E902.2
  range E902.0
Divers' disease, palsy, paralysis, squeeze E902.0

☑ Additional Digit Required — Refer to the Tabular List for Digit Selection   ▽ Subterms under main terms may continue to next column or page

2013 ICD-9-CM   ►◄ Revised Text   ● New Line   ▲ Revised Code   Volume 2 — 341

Dog bite E906.0
Dragged by
  cable car (not on rails) E847
    on rails E829 ☑
  motor vehicle (on highway) E814 ☑
    not on highway, nontraffic accident
      E825 ☑
  street car E829 ☑
Drinking poison (accidental) — *see* Table of
  Drugs and Chemicals
Drowning — *see* Submersion
Dust in eye E914

E

Earth falling (on) (with asphyxia or suffocation
  (by pressure)) — *see also* Suffocation,
  due to, cave-in E913.3
  as, or due to, a cataclysm (involving any
    transport vehicle) — *see* categories
    E908 ☑, E909 ☑
  not due to cataclysmic action E913.3
    motor vehicle (in motion) (on public
      highway) E813 ☑
      not on public highway E825 ☑
    nonmotor road vehicle NEC E829 ☑
    pedal cycle E826 ☑
    railway rolling stock, train, vehicle
      E806 ☑
    street car E829 ☑
    struck or crushed by E916
      with asphyxiation or suffocation
        E913.3
      with injury other than asphyxia, suf-
        focation E916
Earthquake (any injury) E909.0
Effect(s) (adverse) of
  air pressure E902.9
    at high altitude E902.9
      in aircraft E902.1
      residence or prolonged visit (causing
        conditions classifiable to
        E902.0) E902.0
    due to
      diving E902.2
      specified cause NEC E902.8
    in aircraft E902.1
  cold, excessive (exposure to) (*see also* Cold,
    exposure to) E901.9
  heat (excessive) (*see also* Heat) E900.9
  hot
    place — *see* Heat
    weather E900.0
  insulation — *see* Heat
  late — *see* Late effect of
  motion E903
  nuclear explosion or weapon
    in
      terrorism E979.5
      war operations (*see also* War opera-
        tions, injury due to, nuclear
        weapons) E996.9
  radiation — *see* Radiation
  terrorism, secondary E979.9
  travel E903
Electric shock, electrocution (accidental)
  (from exposed wire, faulty appliance,
  high voltage cable, live rail, open socket)
  (by) (in) E925.9
  appliance or wiring
    domestic E925.0
    factory E925.2
    farm (building) E925.8
      house E925.0
    home E925.0
    industrial (conductor) (control appara-
      tus) (transformer) E925.2
    outdoors E925.8
    public building E925.8
    residential institution E925.8
    school E925.8
    specified place NEC E925.8
  caused by other person
    stated as
      intentional, homicidal E968.8

Electric shock, electrocution — *continued*
  caused by other person — *continued*
    stated as — *continued*
      undetermined whether accidental or
        intentional E988.4
  electric power generating plant, distribution
    station E925.1
  electroshock gun (taser) (stun gun) E925.8
    caused by other person E968.8
    legal intervention E975
    stated as accidental E925.8
    stated as intentional E968.8
    due to legal intervention E975
    stated as intentional self-harm (suicidal
      attempt) E958.4
    stated as undetermined whether acciden-
      tal or intentional E988.4
    suicide (attempt) E958.4
  homicidal (attempt) E968.8
  legal execution E978
  lightning E907
  machinery E925.9
    domestic E925.0
    factory E925.2
    farm E925.8
    home E925.0
  misadventure in medical or surgical proce-
    dure
    in electroshock therapy E873.4
  self-inflicted (undetermined whether acci-
    dental or intentional) E988.4
    stated as intentional E958.4
    stated as undetermined whether accidental
      or intentional E988.4
  suicidal (attempt) E958.4
  transmission line E925.1
Electrocution — *see* Electric shock
Embolism
  air (traumatic) NEC — *see* Air, embolism
Encephalitis
  lead or saturnine E866.0
    from pesticide NEC E863.4
Entanglement
  in
    bedclothes, causing suffocation E913.0
    wheel of pedal cycle E826 ☑
Entry of foreign body, material, any — *see*
  Foreign body
Execution, legal (any method) E978
Exertion, excessive physical, from pro-
  longed activity E927.2
Exhaustion
  cold — *see* Cold, exposure to
  due to excessive exertion E927.2
  heat — *see* Heat
Explosion (accidental) (in) (of) (on) E923.9
  acetylene E923.2
  aerosol can E921.8
  aircraft (in transit) (powered) E841 ☑
    at landing, take-off E840 ☑
    in
      terrorism E979.1
      war operations
        from
          enemy fire or explosive(s)
            (device placed on air-
            craft) E994.0
          own onboard explosives
            E994.1
    unpowered E842 ☑
  air tank (compressed) (in machinery) E921.1
  anesthetic gas in operating theatre E923.2
  automobile tire NEC E921.8
    causing transport accident — *see* cate-
      gories E810-E825 ☑
  blasting (cap) (materials) E923.1
  boiler (machinery), not on transport vehicle
    E921.0
    steamship — *see* Explosion, watercraft
  bomb E923.8
    in
      terrorism E979.2
      war operations E993.8
        after cessation of hostilities
          E998.1

Explosion — *continued*
  bomb — *continued*
    in — *continued*
      war operations — *continued*
        atom, hydrogen or nuclear (*see*
          also War operations, injury
          due to, nuclear weapons)
          E996.9
        injury by fragments from E991.9
          antipersonnel bomb E991.3
  butane E923.2
  caused by
    other person
      stated as
        intentional, homicidal — *see* As-
          sault, explosive
        undetermined whether acciden-
          tal or homicidal E985.5
  coal gas E923.2
  detonator E923.1
  dynamite E923.1
  explosive (material) NEC E923.9
    gas(es) E923.2
    missile E923.8
      in
        terrorism E979.2
        war operations E993.1
          injury by fragments from
            E991.9
            antipersonnel bomb
              E991.3
    used in blasting operations E923.1
  fire-damp E923.2
  fireworks E923.0
  gas E923.2
    cylinder (in machinery) E921.1
    pressure tank (in machinery) E921.1
  gasoline (fumes) (tank) not in moving motor
    vehicle E923.2
  grain store (military) (munitions) E923.8
  grenade E923.8
    in
      terrorism E979.2
      war operations E993.8
        injury by fragments from E991.4
  homicide (attempt) — *see* Assault, explosive
  hot water heater, tank (in machinery) E921.0
  in mine (of explosive gases) NEC E923.2
  late effect of NEC E929.8
  machinery (*see also* Accident, machine)
    pressure vessel — *see* Explosion, pres-
      sure vessel
  methane E923.2
  missile E923.8
    in
      terrorism E979.2
      war operations E993.1
        injury by fragments from E991.4
  motor vehicle (part of)
    in motion (on public highway) E818 ☑
      not on public highway E825 ☑
  munitions (dump) (factory) E923.8
    in
      terrorism E979.2
      war operations E993.9
  of mine E923.8
    in
      terrorism
        at sea or in harbor E979.0
        land E979.2
        marine E979.0
      war operations
        after cessation of hostilities
          E998.0
        at sea or in harbor E992.2
        land E993.8
          after cessation of hostilities
            E998.0
          injury by fragments from
            E991.4
        marine E992.2
  own weapons
    in
      terrorism (*see also* Suicide) E979.2
      war operations E993.7
        injury by fragments from E991.9

Explosion — *continued*
  own weapons — *continued*
    in — *continued*
      war operations — *continued*
        injury by fragments from — *con-*
          tinued
          antipersonnel bomb E991.3
  pressure
    cooker E921.8
    gas tank (in machinery) E921.1
    vessel (in machinery) E921.9
      on transport vehicle — *see* cate-
        gories E800-E848 ☑
      specified type NEC E921.8
  propane E923.2
  railway engine, locomotive, train (boiler)
    (with subsequent collision, derail-
    ment, fall) E803 ☑
    with
      collision (antecedent) (*see also* Colli-
        sion, railway) E800 ☑
      derailment (antecedent) E802 ☑
      fire (without antecedent collision or
        derailment) E803 ☑
  secondary fire resulting from — *see* Fire
  self-inflicted (unspecified whether acciden-
    tal or intentional) E985.5
    stated as intentional, purposeful E955.5
  shell (artillery) E923.8
    in
      terrorism E979.2
      war operations E993.2
        injury by fragments from E991.4
  stated as undetermined whether caused
    accidentally or purposely inflicted
    E985.5
  steam or water lines (in machinery) E921.0
  suicide (attempted) E955.5
  terrorism — *see* Terrorism, explosion
  torpedo E923.8
    in
      terrorism E979.0
      war operations E992.0
  transport accident — *see* categories
    E800-E848 ☑
  war operations — *see* War operations, ex-
    plosion
  watercraft (boiler) E837 ☑
    causing drowning, submersion (after
      jumping from watercraft) E830 ☑
Exposure (weather) (conditions) (rain) (wind)
  E904.3
  with homicidal intent E968.4
  environmental
    to
      algae bloom E928.6
      blue-green algae bloom E928.6
      brown tide E928.6
      cyanobacteria bloom E928.6
      Florida red tide E928.6
      harmful alage
        and toxins E928.6
        bloom E928.6
      pfiesteria piscicida E928.6
      red tide E928.6
  excessive E904.3
    cold (*see also* Cold, exposure to) E901.9
      self-inflicted — *see* Cold, exposure
        to, self-inflicted
    heat (*see also* Heat) E900.9
  helpless person, infant, newborn due to
    abandonment or neglect E904.0
  noise E928.1
  prolonged in deep-freeze unit or refrigerator
    E901.1
  radiation — *see* Radiation
  resulting from transport accident — *see*
    categories E800-E848 ☑
  smoke from, due to
    fire — *see* Fire
    tobacco, second-hand E869.4
  vibration E928.2
External cause status E000.9
  child assisting in compensated work of
    other family member E000.8

☑ **Additional Digit Required** — Refer to the Tabular List for Digit Selection   🖝 **Subterms under main terms may continue to next column or page**

342 — Volume 2   ▶◀ Revised Text   ● New Line   ▲ Revised Code   2013 ICD-9-CM

External cause status — *continued*
  civilian
    done for
      financial or other compensation
        E000.0
      pay or income E000.0
    family member assisting in compensated
      work of other family member E000.8
    for income E000.0
    hobby or leisure E000.8
    military E000.1
      off duty E000.8
    off duty military E000.8
    recreation E000.8
    specified NEC E000.8
    sport not for income E000.8
    student E000.8
    volunteer E000.2

F

Fallen on by
  animal (horse) (not being ridden) E906.8
    being ridden (in sport or transport)
      E828 ☑
Fall, falling (accidental) E888.9
  building E916
    burning E891.8
      private E890.8
  down
    escalator E880.0
    ladder E881.0
      in boat, ship, watercraft E833 ☑
    staircase E880.9
    stairs, steps — *see* Fall, from, stairs
  earth (with asphyxia or suffocation (by
    pressure)) (*see also* Earth, falling)
    E913.3
  from, off
    aircraft (at landing, take-off) (in-transit)
      (while alighting, boarding)
      E843 ☑
      resulting from accident to aircraft —
        see categories E840-E842 ☑
    animal (in sport or transport) E828 ☑
    animal-drawn vehicle E827 ☑
    balcony E882
    bed E884.4
    bicycle E826 ☑
    boat, ship, watercraft (into water)
      E832 ☑
      after accident to, collision, fire on
        E830 ☑
        and subsequently struck by (part
          of) boat E831 ☑
      and subsequently struck by (part of)
        while alighting, boat E831 ☑
      burning, crushed, sinking E830 ☑
        and subsequently struck by (part
          of) boat E831 ☑
    bridge E882
    building E882
      burning (uncontrolled fire) E891.8
        in terrorism E979.3
      private E890.8
    bunk in boat, ship, watercraft E834 ☑
      due to accident to watercraft
        E831 ☑
    cable car (not on rails) E847
      on rails E829 ☑
    car — *see* Fall from motor vehicle
    chair E884.2
    cliff E884.1
    commode E884.6
    curb (sidewalk) E880.1
    elevation aboard ship E834 ☑
      due to accident to ship E831 ☑
    embankment E884.9
    escalator E880.0
    fire escape E882
    flagpole E882
    furniture NEC E884.5
    gangplank (into water) (*see also* Fall,
      from, boat) E832 ☑
      to deck, dock E834 ☑
    hammock on ship E834 ☑

Fall, falling — *continued*
  from, off — *continued*
    hammock on ship — *continued*
      due to accident to watercraft
        E831 ☑
    haystack E884.9
    heelies E885.1
    high place NEC E884.9
      stated as undetermined whether ac-
        cidental or intentional — *see*
        Jumping, from, high place
    horse (in sport or transport) E828 ☑
    in-line skates E885.1
    ladder E881.0
      in boat, ship, watercraft E833 ☑
        due to accident to watercraft
          E831 ☑
    machinery (*see also* Accident, machine)
      not in operation E884.9
    motorized
      mobility scooter E884.3
      wheelchair E884.3
    motor vehicle (in motion) (on public
      highway) E818 ☑
      not on public highway E825 ☑
        stationary, except while alighting,
          boarding, entering, leav-
          ing E884.9
        while alighting, boarding, enter-
          ing, leaving E824 ☑
      stationary, except while alighting,
        boarding, entering, leaving
        E884.9
      while alighting, boarding, entering,
        leaving, except off-road type
        motor vehicle E817 ☑
        off-road type — *see* Fall, from,
          off-road type motor vehi-
          cle
    nonmotor road vehicle (while alighting,
      boarding) NEC E829 ☑
      stationary, except while alighting,
        boarding, entering, leaving
        E884.9
    off road type motor vehicle (not on
      public highway) NEC E821 ☑
      on public highway E818 ☑
        while alighting, boarding, enter-
          ing, leaving E817 ☑
    snow vehicle — *see* Fall from snow
      vehicle, motor-driven
  one
    deck to another on ship E834 ☑
      due to accident to ship E831 ☑
    level to another NEC E884.9
      boat, ship, or watercraft E834 ☑
        due to accident to watercraft
          E831 ☑
    pedal cycle E826 ☑
    playground equipment E884.0
    railway rolling stock, train, vehicle (while
      alighting, boarding) E804 ☑
      with
        collision (*see also* Collision, rail-
          way) E800 ☑
        derailment (*see also* Derailment,
          railway) E802 ☑
        explosion (*see also* Explosion,
          railway engine) E803 ☑
    rigging (aboard ship) E834 ☑
      due to accident to watercraft
        E831 ☑
    roller skates E885.1
    scaffolding E881.1
    scooter (nonmotorized) E885.0
      motorized mobility E884.3
    sidewalk (curb) E880.1
      moving E885.9
    skateboard E885.2
    skis E885.3
    snowboard E885.4
    snow vehicle, motor-driven (not on
      public highway) E820 ☑
      on public highway E818 ☑

Fall, falling — *continued*
  from, off — *continued*
    snow vehicle, motor-driven — *contin-
      ued*
      on public highway — *continued*
        while alighting, boarding, enter-
          ing, leaving E817 ☑
    stairs, steps E880.9
      boat, ship, watercraft E833 ☑
        due to accident to watercraft
          E831 ☑
      motor bus, motor vehicle — *see* Fall,
        from, motor vehicle, while
        alighting, boarding
      street car E829 ☑
    stationary vehicle NEC E884.9
    stepladder E881.0
    street car (while boarding, alighting)
      E829 ☑
      stationary, except while boarding or
        alighting E884.9
    structure NEC E882
      burning (uncontrolled fire) E891.8
        in terrorism E979.3
    table E884.9
    toilet E884.6
    tower E882
    tree E884.9
    turret E882
    vehicle NEC (*see also* Accident, vehicle
      NEC)
      stationary E884.9
    viaduct E882
    wall E882
    wheelchair (electric) (motorized) E884.3
    wheelies E885.1
    window E882
  in, on
    aircraft (at landing, take-off) (in-transit)
      E843 ☑
      resulting from accident to aircraft —
        see categories E840-E842 ☑
    boat, ship, watercraft E835 ☑
      due to accident to watercraft
        E831 ☑
      one level to another NEC E834 ☑
      on ladder, stairs E833 ☑
    cutting or piercing instrument or ma-
      chine E888.0
    deck (of boat, ship, watercraft) E835 ☑
      due to accident to watercraft
        E831 ☑
    escalator E880.0
    gangplank E835 ☑
    glass, broken E888.0
    knife E888.0
    ladder E881.0
      in boat, ship, watercraft E833 ☑
        due to accident to watercraft
          E831 ☑
    object
      edged, pointed or sharp E888.0
      other E888.1
    pitchfork E888.0
    railway rolling stock, train, vehicle (while
      alighting, boarding) E804 ☑
      with
        collision (*see also* Collision, rail-
          way) E800 ☑
        derailment (*see also* Derailment,
          railway) E802 ☑
        explosion (see also Explosion,
          railway engine) E803 ☑
    scaffolding E881.1
    scissors E888.0
    staircase, stairs, steps (*see also* Fall, from,
      stairs) E880.9
    street car E829 ☑
    water transport (*see also* Fall, in, boat)
      E835 ☑
  into
    cavity E883.9
    dock E883.9
      from boat, ship, watercraft (*see also*
        Fall, from, boat) E832 ☑

Fall, falling — *continued*
  into — *continued*
    hold (of ship) E834 ☑
      due to accident to watercraft
        E831 ☑
    hole E883.9
    manhole E883.2
    moving part of machinery — *see* Acci-
      dent, machine
    opening in surface NEC E883.9
    pit E883.9
    quarry E883.9
    shaft E883.9
    storm drain E883.2
    tank E883.9
    water (with drowning or submersion)
      E910.9
    well E883.1
  late effect of NEC E929.3
  object (*see also* Hit by, object, falling) E916
  other E888.8
  over
    animal E885.9
    cliff E884.1
    embankment E884.9
    small object E885.9
  overboard (*see also* Fall, from, boat) E832 ☑
  resulting in striking against object E888.1
    sharp E888.0
  rock E916
  same level NEC E888.9
    aircraft (any kind) E843 ☑
      resulting from accident to aircraft —
        see categories E840-E842 ☑
    boat, ship, watercraft E835 ☑
      due to accident to, collision, water-
        craft E831 ☑
    from
      collision, pushing, shoving, by or
        with other person(s) E886.9
        as, or caused by, a crowd E917.6
        in sports E886.0
      in-line skates E885.1
      roller skates E885.1
      scooter (nonmotorized) E885.0
      skateboard E885.2
      slipping stumbling, tripping E885 ☑
      snowboard E885.4
  snowslide E916
    as avalanche E909.2
  stone E916
  through
    hatch (on ship) E834 ☑
      due to accident to watercraft
        E831 ☑
    roof E882
    window E882
  timber E916
  while alighting from, boarding, entering,
    leaving
    aircraft (any kind) E843 ☑
    motor bus, motor vehicle — *see* Fall,
      from, motor vehicle, while
      alighting, boarding
    nonmotor road vehicle NEC E829 ☑
    railway train E804 ☑
    street car E829 ☑
Fell or jumped from high place, so stated —
  see Jumping, from, high place
Felo-de-se — *see also* Suicide E958.9
Fever
  heat — *see* Heat
  thermic — *see* Heat
Fight (hand) (fist) (foot) — *see also* Assault,
  fight E960.0
Fire (accidental) (caused by great heat from
  appliance (electrical), hot object or hot
  substance) (secondary, resulting from
  explosion) E899
  conflagration — *see* Conflagration
  controlled, normal (in brazier, fireplace,
    furnace, or stove) (charcoal) (coal)
    (coke) (electric) (gas) (wood)
    bonfire E897
    brazier, not in building or structure E897

☑ **Additional Digit Required** — Refer to the Tabular List for Digit Selection   ⬝ **Subterms under main terms may continue to next column or page**

2013 ICD-9-CM   ▶◀ **Revised Text**   ● **New Line**   ▲ **Revised Code**   **Volume 2 — 343**

Fire, hot object or hot substance — *continued*
  controlled, normal — *continued*
    in building or structure, except private
      dwelling (barn) (church) (conva-
      lescent or residential home) (fac-
      tory) (farm outbuilding) (hospital)
      (hotel) (institution (educational)
      (dormitory) (residential) (private
      garage) (school) (shop) (store)
      (theatre) E896
    in private dwelling (apartment) (board-
      ing house) (camping place) (cara-
      van) (farmhouse) (home (private))
      (house) (lodging house) (rooming
      house) (tenement) E895
    not in building or structure E897
    trash E897
  forest (uncontrolled) E892
  grass (uncontrolled) E892
  hay (uncontrolled) E892
  homicide (attempt) E968.0
    late effect of E969
  in, of, on, starting in E892
    aircraft (in transit) (powered) E841 ☑
      at landing, take-off E840 ☑
      stationary E892
      unpowered (balloon) (glider)
        E842 ☑
    balloon E842 ☑
    boat, ship, watercraft — *see* categories
      E830 ☑, E831 ☑, E837 ☑
    building or structure, except private
      dwelling (barn) (church) (conva-
      lescent or residential home) (fac-
      tory) (farm outbuilding) (hospital)
      (hotel) (institution (educational)
      (dormitory) (residential)) (school)
      (shop) (store) (theatre) (*see also*
      Conflagration, building or struc-
      ture, except private dwelling)
      E891.9
    forest (uncontrolled) E892
    glider E842 ☑
    grass (uncontrolled) E892
    hay (uncontrolled) E892
    lumber (uncontrolled) E892
    machinery — *see* Accident, machine
    mine (uncontrolled) E892
    motor vehicle (in motion) (on public
      highway) E818 ☑
      not on public highway E825 ☑
      stationary E892
    prairie (uncontrolled) E892
    private dwelling (apartment) (boarding
      house) (camping place) (caravan)
      (farmhouse) (home (private))
      (house) (lodging house) (private
      garage) (rooming house) (tene-
      ment) (*see also* Conflagration,
      private dwelling) E890.9
    railway rolling stock, train, vehicle (*see
      also* Explosion, railway engine)
      E803 ☑
      stationary E892
    room NEC E898.1
    street car (in motion) E829 ☑
      stationary E892
    terrorism (by fire-producing device)
      E979.3
      fittings or furniture (burning build-
      ing) (uncontrolled fire) E979.3
      from nuclear explosion E979.5
    transport vehicle, stationary NEC E892
    tunnel (uncontrolled) E892
    war operations (by fire-producing device
      or conventional weapon) E990.9
      from nuclear explosion (*see also* War
      operations, injury due to, nu-
      clear weapons) E996.2
      incendiary bomb E990.0
      petrol bomb E990.0
  late effect of NEC E929.4
  lumber (uncontrolled) E892
  mine (uncontrolled) E892
  prairie (uncontrolled) E892

Fire, hot object or hot substance — *continued*
  self-inflicted (unspecified whether acciden-
    tal or intentional) E988.1
    stated as intentional, purposeful E958.1
  specified NEC E898.1
    with
      conflagration — *see* Conflagration
      ignition (of)
        clothing — *see* Ignition, clothes
        highly inflammable material
          (benzine) (fat) (gasoline)
          (kerosene) (paraffin)
          (petrol) E894
  started by other person
    stated as
      with intent to injure or kill E968.0
      undetermined whether or not with
        intent to injure or kill E988.1
  suicide (attempted) E958.1
    late effect of E959
  tunnel (uncontrolled) E892
Fireball effects from nuclear explosion
  in
    terrorism E979.5
    war operations (*see also* War operations,
      injury due to, nuclear weapons)
      E996.2
Fireworks (explosion) E923.0
Flash burns from explosion — *see also* Explosion E923.9
Flood (any injury) (resulting from storm) E908.2
  caused by collapse of dam or manmade
    structure E909.3
Forced landing (aircraft) E840 ☑
Foreign body, object or material (entrance
  into) (accidental)
  air passage (causing injury) E915
    with asphyxia, obstruction, suffocation
      E912
      food or vomitus E911
    nose (with asphyxia, obstruction, suffo-
      cation) E912
      causing injury without asphyxia, ob-
        struction, suffocation E915
  alimentary canal (causing injury) (with ob-
    struction) E915
    with asphyxia, obstruction respiratory
      passage, suffocation E912
      food E911
    mouth E915
      with asphyxia, obstruction, suffoca-
        tion E912
        food E911
    pharynx E915
      with asphyxia, obstruction, suffoca-
        tion E912
        food E911
  aspiration (with asphyxia, obstruction respi-
    ratory passage, suffocation) E912
    causing injury without asphyxia, obstruc-
      tion respiratory passage, suffoca-
      tion E915
    food (regurgitated) (vomited) E911
      causing injury without asphyxia, ob-
        struction respiratory passage,
        suffocation E915
    mucus (not of newborn) E912
    phlegm E912
  bladder (causing injury or obstruction) E915
  bronchus, bronchi — *see* Foreign body, air
    passages
  conjunctival sac E914
  digestive system — *see* Foreign body, ali-
    mentary canal
  ear (causing injury or obstruction) E915
  esophagus (causing injury or obstruction)
    (*see also* Foreign body, alimentary
    canal) E915
  eye (any part) E914
  eyelid E914
  hairball (stomach) (with obstruction) E915
  ingestion — *see* Foreign body, alimentary
    canal
  inhalation — *see* Foreign body, aspiration

Foreign body, object or material — *continued*
  intestine (causing injury or obstruction)
    E915
  iris E914
  lacrimal apparatus E914
  larynx — *see* Foreign body, air passage
  late effect of NEC E929.8
  lung — *see* Foreign body, air passage
  mouth — *see* Foreign body, alimentary
    canal, mouth
  nasal passage — *see* Foreign body, air pas-
    sage, nose
  nose — *see* Foreign body, air passage, nose
  ocular muscle E914
  operation wound (left in) — *see* Misadven-
    ture, foreign object
  orbit E914
  pharynx — *see* Foreign body, alimentary
    canal, pharynx
  rectum (causing injury or obstruction) E915
  stomach (hairball) (causing injury or obstruc-
    tion) E915
  tear ducts or glands E914
  trachea — *see* Foreign body, air passage
  urethra (causing injury or obstruction) E915
  vagina (causing injury or obstruction) E915
Found dead, injured
  from exposure (to) — *see* Exposure
  on
    public highway E819 ☑
    railway right of way E807 ☑
Fracture (circumstances unknown or unspecified) E887
  due to specified external means — *see*
    manner of accident
  late effect of NEC E929.3
  occurring in water transport NEC E835 ☑
Freezing — *see* Cold, exposure to
Frostbite E901.0
  due to manmade conditions E901.1
Frozen — *see* Cold, exposure to

G

Garrotting, homicidal (attempted) E963
Gored E906.8
Gunshot wound — *see also* Shooting E922.9

H

Hailstones, injury by E904.3
Hairball (stomach) (with obstruction) E915
Hanged himself — *see also* Hanging, self-inflicted E983.0
Hang gliding E842 ☑
Hanging (accidental) E913.8
  caused by other person
    in accidental circumstances E913.8
    stated as
      intentional, homicidal E963
      undetermined whether accidental or
        intentional E983.0
  homicide (attempt) E963
  in bed or cradle E913.0
  legal execution E978
  self-inflicted (unspecified whether acciden-
    tal or intentional) E983.0
    in accidental circumstances E913.8
    stated as intentional, purposeful E953.0
  stated as undetermined whether accidental
    or intentional E983.0
  suicidal (attempt) E953.0
Heat (apoplexy) (collapse) (cramps) (effects of)
  (excessive) (exhaustion) (fever) (prostration) (stroke) E900.9
  due to
    manmade conditions (as listed in E900.1,
      except boat, ship, watercraft)
      E900.1
    weather (conditions) E900.0
  from
    electric heating appartus causing burn-
      ing E924.8
    nuclear explosion
      in
        terrorism E979.5

Heat — *continued*
  from — *continued*
    nuclear explosion — *continued*
      in — *continued*
        war operations (*see also* War oper-
          ations, injury due to, nucle-
          ar weapons) E996.2
    generated in, boiler, engine, evaporator, fire
      room of boat, ship, watercraft
      E838 ☑
    inappropriate in local application or packing
      in medical or surgical procedure
      E873.5
  late effect of NEC E989
Hemorrhage
  delayed following medical or surgical
    treatment without mention of misad-
    venture — *see* Reaction, abnormal
  during medical or surgical treatment as
    misadventure — *see* Misadventure,
    cut
High
  altitude, effects E902.9
  level of radioactivity, effects — *see* Radia-
    tion
  pressure effects (*see also* Effects of, air pres-
    sure)
    from rapid descent in water (causing
      caisson or divers' disease, palsy,
      or paralysis) E902.2
  temperature, effects — *see* Heat
Hit, hitting (accidental) by
  aircraft (propeller) (without accident to air-
    craft) E844 ☑
    unpowered E842 ☑
  avalanche E909.2
  being thrown against object in or part of
    motor vehicle (in motion) (on public
      highway) E818 ☑
      not on public highway E825 ☑
    nonmotor road vehicle NEC E829 ☑
    street car E829 ☑
  boat, ship, watercraft
    after fall from watercraft E838 ☑
    damaged, involved in accident
      E831 ☑
    while swimming, water skiing E838 ☑
  bullet (*see also* Shooting) E922.9
    from air gun E922.4
    in
      terrorism E979.4
      war operations E991.2
        rubber E991.0
  flare, Verey pistol (*see also* Shooting) E922.8
  hailstones E904.3
  landslide E909.2
  law-enforcing agent (on duty) E975
    with blunt object (baton) (night stick)
      (stave) (truncheon) E973
  machine — *see* Accident, machine
  missile
    firearm (*see also* Shooting) E922.9
    in
      terrorism — *see* Terrorism, missile
      war operations — *see* War opera-
        tions, missile
  motor vehicle (on public highway) (traffic
    accident) E814 ☑
    not on public highway, nontraffic acci-
      dent E822 ☑
  nonmotor road vehicle NEC E829 ☑
  object
    falling E916
      from, in, on
        aircraft E844 ☑
          due to accident to aircraft —
            see categories
            E840-E842 ☑
          unpowered E842 ☑
        boat, ship, watercraft E838 ☑
          due to accident to watercraft
            E831 ☑
        building E916
          burning (uncontrolled fire)
            E891.8
            in terrorism E979.3

☑ Additional Digit Required — Refer to the Tabular List for Digit Selection   ▽ Subterms under main terms may continue to next column or page

344 — Volume 2   ▶◀ Revised Text   ● New Line   ▲ Revised Code   2013 ICD-9-CM

Hit, hitting by — *continued*
object — *continued*
falling — *continued*
from, in, on — *continued*
building — *continued*
burning — *continued*
private E890.8
cataclysmic
earth surface movement or
eruption E909.9
storm E908.9
cave-in E916
with asphyxiation or suffocation (*see also* Suffoca-
tion, due to, cave-in)
E913.3
earthquake E909.0
motor vehicle (in motion) (on
public highway) E818 ☑
not on public highway
E825 ☑
stationary E916
nonmotor road vehicle NEC
E829 ☑
pedal cycle E826 ☑
railway rolling stock, train, vehicle
E806 ☑
street car E829 ☑
structure, burning NEC E891.8
vehicle, stationary E916
moving NEC — *see* Striking against, object
projected NEC — *see* Striking against,
object
set in motion by
compressed air or gas, spring, striking, throwing — *see* Striking
against, object
explosion — *see* Explosion
thrown into, on, or towards
motor vehicle (in motion) (on public
highway) E818 ☑
not on public highway E825 ☑
nonmotor road vehicle NEC E829 ☑
pedal cycle E826 ☑
street car E829 ☑
off-road type motor vehicle (not on public
highway) E821 ☑
on public highway E814 ☑
other person(s) E917.9
with blunt or thrown object E917.9
in sports E917.0
with subsequent fall E917.5
intentionally, homicidal E968.2
as, or caused by, a crowd E917.1
with subsequent fall E917.6
in sports E917.0
pedal cycle E826 ☑
police (on duty) E975
with blunt object (baton) (nightstick)
(stave) (truncheon) E973
railway, rolling stock, train, vehicle (part of)
E805 ☑
shot — *see* Shooting
snow vehicle, motor-driven (not on
highway) E820 ☑
on public highway E814 ☑
street car E829 ☑
vehicle NEC — *see* Accident, vehicle NEC
Homicide, homicidal (attempt) (justifiable) —
see also Assault E968.9
Hot
liquid, object, substance, accident caused
by (*see also* Accident, caused by, hot,
by type of substance)
late effect of E929.8
place, effects — *see* Heat
weather, effects E900.0
Humidity, causing problem E904.3
Hunger E904.1
resulting from
abandonment or neglect E904.0
transport accident — *see* categories
E800-E848 ☑
Hurricane (any injury) E908.0

Hypobarism, hypobaropathy — *see* Effects
of, air pressure
Hypothermia — *see* Cold, exposure to

I

Ictus
caloris — *see* Heat
solaris E900.0
Ignition (accidental)
anesthetic gas in operating theatre E923.2
bedclothes
with
conflagration — *see* Conflagration
ignition (of)
clothing — *see* Ignition, clothes
highly inflammable material
(benzine) (fat) (gasoline)
(kerosene) (paraffin)
(petrol) E894
benzine E894
clothes, clothing (from controlled fire) (in
building) E893.9
with conflagration — *see* Conflagration
from
bonfire E893.2
highly inflammable material E894
sources or material as listed in E893.8
trash fire E893.2
uncontrolled fire — *see* Conflagration
in
private dwelling E893.0
specified building or structure, except private dwelling E893.1
not in building or structure E893.2
explosive material — *see* Explosion
fat E894
gasoline E894
kerosene E894
material
explosive — *see* Explosion
highly inflammable E894
with conflagration — *see* Conflagration
with explosion E923.2
nightdress — *see* Ignition, clothes
paraffin E894
petrol E894
Immersion — *see* Submersion
Implantation of quills of porcupine E906.8
Inanition (from) E904.9
hunger — *see* Lack of, food
resulting from homicidal intent E968.4
thirst — *see* Lack of, water
Inattention after, at birth E904.0
homicidal, infanticidal intent E968.4
Infanticide — *see also* Assault
Ingestion
foreign body (causing injury) (with obstruction) — *see* Foreign body, alimentary
canal
poisonous substance NEC — *see* Table of
Drugs and Chemicals
Inhalation
excessively cold substance, manmade
E901.1
foreign body — *see* Foreign body, aspiration
liquid air, hydrogen, nitrogen E901.1
mucus, not of newborn (with asphyxia, obstruction respiratory passage, suffocation) E912
phlegm (with asphyxia, obstruction respiratory passage, suffocation) E912
poisonous gas — *see* Table of Drugs and
Chemicals
smoke from, due to
fire — *see* Fire
tobacco, second-hand E869.4
vomitus (with asphyxia, obstruction respiratory passage, suffocation) E911
Injury, injured (accidental(ly)) NEC E928.9
by, caused by, from
air rifle (BB gun) E922.4
animal (not being ridden) NEC E906.9
being ridden (in sport or transport)
E828 ☑

Injury, injured — *continued*
by, caused by, from — *continued*
assault (*see also* Assault) E968.9
avalanche E909.2
bayonet (*see also* Bayonet wound)
E920.3
being thrown against some part of, or
object in
motor vehicle (in motion) (on public
highway) E818 ☑
not on public highway E825 ☑
nonmotor road vehicle NEC E829 ☑
off-road motor vehicle NEC E821 ☑
railway train E806 ☑
snow vehicle, motor-driven E820 ☑
street car E829 ☑
bending
due to
repetitive movement E927.3
sudden strenuous movement
E927.0
bite, human E928.3
broken glass E920.8
bullet — *see* Shooting
cave-in (*see also* Suffocation, due to,
cave-in) E913.3
without asphyxiation or suffocation
E916
earth surface movement or eruption
E909.9
storm E908.9
cloudburst E908.8
component of firearm or air gun E928.7
cutting or piercing instrument (*see also*
Cut) E920.9
cyclone E908.1
earthquake E909.0
earth surface movement or eruption
E909.9
electric current (*see also* Electric shock)
E925.9
explosion (*see also* Explosion) E923.9
of gun part E928.7
fire — *see* Fire
flare, Verey pistol E922.8
flood E908.2
foreign body — *see* Foreign body
gun recoil E928.7
hailstones E904.3
hurricane E908.0
landslide E909.2
law-enforcing agent, police, in course of
legal intervention — *see* Legal
intervention
lightning E907
live rail or live wire — *see* Electric shock
machinery (*see also* Accident, machine)
aircraft, without accident to aircraft
E844 ☑
boat, ship, watercraft (deck) (engine
room) (galley) (laundry)
(loading) E836 ☑
mechanism of firearm or air gun E928.7
missile
explosive E923.8
firearm — *see* Shooting
in
terrorism — *see* Terrorism, missile
war operations — *see* War operations, missile
moving part of motor vehicle (in motion)
(on public highway) E818 ☑
not on public highway, nontraffic
accident E825 ☑
while alighting, boarding, entering,
leaving — *see* Fall, from, motor vehicle, while alighting,
boarding
nail E920.8
needle (sewing) E920.4
hypodermic E920.5
noise E928.1

Injury, injured — *continued*
by, caused by, from — *continued*
object
fallen on
motor vehicle (in motion) (on
public highway) E818 ☑
not on public highway
E825 ☑
falling — *see* Hit by, object, falling
paintball gun E922.5
radiation — *see* Radiation
railway rolling stock, train, vehicle (part
of) E805 ☑
door or window E806 ☑
recoil of firearm E928.7
rotating propeller, aircraft E844 ☑
rough landing of off-road type motor
vehicle (after leaving ground or
rough terrain) E821 ☑
snow vehicle E820 ☑
saber (*see also* Wound, saber) E920.3
shot — *see* Shooting
sound waves E928.1
splinter or sliver, wood E920.8
straining
due to
repetitive movement E927.3
sudden strenuous movement
E927.0
street car (door) E829 ☑
suicide (attempt) E958.9
sword E920.3
terrorism — *see* Terrorism
third rail — *see* Electric shock
thunderbolt E907
tidal wave E909.4
caused by storm E908.0
tornado E908.1
torrential rain E908.2
twisting
due to
repetitive movement E927.3
sudden strenuous movement
E927.0
vehicle NEC — *see* Accident, vehicle NEC
vibration E928.2
volcanic eruption E909.1
weapon burst, in war operations E993.9
weightlessness (in spacecraft, real or
simulated) E928.0
wood splinter or sliver E920.8
due to
civil insurrection — *see* War operations
occurring after cessation of hostilities
E998.9
terrorism — *see* Terrorism
war operations — *see* War operations
occurring after cessation of hostilities
E998.9
weapon of mass destruction [WMD]
E997.3
homicidal (*see also* Assault) E968.9
inflicted (by)
in course of arrest (attempted), suppression of disturbance, maintenance
of order, by law enforcing agents
— *see* Legal intervention
law-enforcing agent (on duty) — *see*
Legal intervention
other person
stated as
accidental E928.9
homicidal, intentional — *see* Assault
undetermined whether accidental or intentional — *see*
Injury, stated as undetermined
police (on duty) — *see* Legal intervention
in, on
civil insurrection — *see* War operations
fight E960.0
parachute descent (voluntary) (without
accident to aircraft) E844 ☑

☑ Additional Digit Required — Refer to the Tabular List for Digit Selection   ▼ Subterms under main terms may continue to next column or page

Hit, hitting — Injury, injured

2013 ICD-9-CM   ►◄ Revised Text   ● New Line   ▲ Revised Code   Volume 2 — 345

Injury, injured — *continued*
  in, on — *continued*
    parachute descent — *continued*
      with accident to aircraft — *see* categories E840-E842 ☑
    public highway E819 ☑
    railway right of way E807 ☑
    terrorism — *see* Terrorism
    war operations — *see* War operations
  late effect of E929.9
  purposely (inflicted) by other person(s) — *see* Assault
  self-inflicted (unspecified whether accidental or intentional) E988.9
    stated as
      accidental E928.9
      intentionally, purposely E958.9
  specified cause NEC E928.8
  stated as
    hanging E983.0
    knife E986
    late effect of E989
    puncture (any part of body) E986
    shooting — *see* Shooting, stated as undetermined whether accidental or intentional
    specified means NEC E988.8
    stab (any part of body) E986
    strangulation — *see* Suffocation, stated as undetermined whether accidental or intentional
    submersion E984
    suffocation — *see* Suffocation, stated as undetermined whether accidental or intentional
  undetermined whether accidentally or purposely inflicted (by) E988.9
    cut (any part of body) E986
    cutting or piercing instrument (classifiable to E920) E986
    drowning E984
    explosive(s) (missile) E985.5
    falling from high place E987.9
      manmade structure, except residential E987.1
      natural site E987.2
      residential premises E987.0
  to child due to criminal abortion E968.8
Insufficient nourishment — *see also* Lack of, food
  homicidal intent E968.4
Insulation, effects — *see* Heat
Interruption of respiration by
  food lodged in esophagus E911
  foreign body, except food, in esophagus E912
Intervention, legal — *see* Legal intervention
Intoxication, drug or poison — *see* Table of Drugs and Chemicals
Irradiation — *see* Radiation

J

Jammed (accidentally)
  between objects (moving) (stationary and moving) E918
  in object E918
Jumped or fell from high place, so stated — *see* Jumping, from, high place, stated as in undetermined circumstances
Jumping
  before train, vehicle or other moving object (unspecified whether accidental or intentional) E988.0
    stated as
      intentional, purposeful E958.0
      suicidal (attempt) E958.0
  from
    aircraft
      by parachute (voluntarily) (without accident to aircraft) E844
      due to accident to aircraft — *see* categories E840-E842 ☑
    boat, ship, watercraft (into water)
      after accident to, fire on, watercraft E830 ☑

Jumping — *continued*
  from — *continued*
    boat, ship, watercraft — *continued*
      after accident to, fire on, watercraft — *continued*
        and subsequently struck by (part of) boat E831 ☑
      burning, crushed, sinking E830 ☑
        and subsequently struck by (part of) boat E831 ☑
      voluntarily, without accident (to boat) with injury other than drowning or submersion E883.0
    building (*see also* Jumping, from, high place)
      burning (uncontrolled fire) E891.8
        in terrorism E979.3
        private E890.8
    cable car (not on rails) E847
      on rails E829 ☑
    high place
      in accidental circumstances or in sport — *see* categories E880-E884 ☑
      stated as
        with intent to injure self E957.9
          man-made structures NEC E957.1
          natural sites E957.2
          residential premises E957.0
        in undetermined circumstances E987.9
          man-made structures NEC E987.1
          natural sites E987.2
          residential premises E987.0
        suicidal (attempt) E957.9
          man-made structures NEC E957.1
          natural sites E957.1
          residential premises E957.0
    motor vehicle (in motion) (on public highway) — *see* Fall, from, motor vehicle
    nonmotor road vehicle NEC E829 ☑
    street car E829 ☑
    structure (*see also* Jumping, from, high place)
      burning NEC (uncontrolled fire) E891.8
        in terrorism E979.3
  into water
    with injury other than drowning or submersion E883.0
    drowning or submersion — *see* Submersion
  from, off, watercraft — *see* Jumping, from, boat
Justifiable homicide — *see* Assault

K

Kicked by
  animal E906.8
  person(s) (accidentally) E917.9
    with intent to injure or kill E960.0
    as, or caused by a crowd E917.1
      with subsequent fall E917.6
    in fight E960.0
    in sports E917.0
      with subsequent fall E917.5
Kicking against
  object (moving) E917.9
    in sports E917.0
      with subsequent fall E917.5
    stationary E917.4
      with subsequent fall E917.8
  person — *see* Striking against, person
Killed, killing (accidentally) NEC — *see also* Injury E928.9
  in
    action — *see* War operations
    brawl, fight (hand) (fists) (foot) E960.0
      by weapon (*see also* Assault)
        cutting, piercing E966
        firearm — *see* Shooting, homicide

Killed, killing — *see also* Injury — *continued*
  self
    stated as
      accident E928.9
      suicide — *see* Suicide
      unspecified whether accidental or suicidal E988.9
Knocked down (accidentally) (by) NEC E928.9
  animal (not being ridden) E906.8
    being ridden (in sport or transport) E828 ☑
  blast from explosion (*see also* Explosion) E923.9
  crowd, human stampede E917.6
  late effect of — *see* Late effect
  person (accidentally) E917.9
    in brawl, fight E960.0
    in sports E917.5
  transport vehicle — *see* vehicle involved under Hit by
  while boxing E917.5

L

Laceration NEC E928.9
Lack of
  air (refrigerator or closed place), suffocation by E913.2
  care (helpless person) (infant) (newborn) E904.0
    homicidal intent E968.4
  food except as result of transport accident E904.1
    helpless person, infant, newborn due to abandonment or neglect E904.0
  water except as result of transport accident E904.2
    helpless person, infant, newborn due to abandonment or neglect E904.0
Landslide E909.2
  falling on, hitting
    motor vehicle (any) (in motion) (on or off public highway) E909.2
    railway rolling stock, train, vehicle E909.2
Late effect of
  accident NEC (accident classifiable to E928.9) E929.9
    specified NEC (accident classifiable to E9I0–E928.8) E929.8
  assault E969
  fall, accidental (accident classifiable to E880–E888) E929.3
  fire, accident caused by (accident classifiable to E890–E899) E929.4
  homicide, attempt (any means) E969
  injury due to terrorism E999.1
  injury undetermined whether accidentally or purposely inflicted (injury classifiable to E980–E988) E989
  legal intervention (injury classifiable to E970–E976) E977
  medical or surgical procedure, test or therapy
    as, or resulting in, or from
      abnormal or delayed reaction or complication — *see* Reaction, abnormal
      misadventure — *see* Misadventure
  motor vehicle accident (accident classifiable to E810–E825) E929.0
  natural or environmental factor, accident due to (accident classifiable to E900–E909) E929.5
  poisoning, accidental (accident classifiable to E850–E858, E860–E869) E929.2
  suicide, attempt (any means) E959
  transport accident NEC (accident classifiable to E800–E807, E826–E838, E840–E848) E929.1
  war operations, injury due to (injury classifiable to E990–E998) E999.0
Launching pad accident E845 ☑
Legal
  execution, any method E978
  intervention (by) (injury from) E976
    baton E973

Legal — *continued*
  intervention — *continued*
    bayonet E974
    blow E975
    blunt object (baton) (nightstick) (stave) (truncheon) E973
    cutting or piercing instrument E974
    dynamite E971
    execution, any method E973
    explosive(s) (shell) E971
    firearm(s) E970
    gas (asphyxiation) (poisoning) (tear) E972
    grenade E971
    late effect of E977
    machine gun E970
    manhandling E975
    mortar bomb E971
    nightstick E973
    revolver E970
    rifle E970
    specified means NEC E975
    stabbing E974
    stave E973
    truncheon E973
Lifting, injury
  due to
    repetitive movement E927.3
    sudden strenuous movement E927.0
Lightning (shock) (stroke) (struck by) E907
Liquid (noncorrosive) in eye E914
  corrosive E924.1
Loss of control
  motor vehicle (on public highway) (without antecedent collision) E816 ☑
    with
      antecedent collision on public highway — *see* Collision, motor vehicle
      involving any object, person or vehicle not on public highway E816 ☑
    not on public highway, nontraffic accident E825 ☑
      with antecedent collision — *see* Collision, motor vehicle, not on public highway
    on public highway — *see* Collision, motor vehicle
  off-road type motor vehicle (not on public highway) E821 ☑
    on public highway — *see* Loss of control, motor vehicle
  snow vehicle, motor-driven (not on public highway) E820 ☑
    on public highway — *see* Loss of control, motor vehicle
Lost at sea E832 ☑
  with accident to watercraft E830 ☑
  in war operations E995.8
Low
  pressure, effects — *see* Effects of, air pressure
  temperature, effects — *see* Cold, exposure to
Lying before train, vehicle or other moving object (unspecified whether accidental or intentional) E988.0
  stated as intentional, purposeful, suicidal (attempt) E958.0
Lynching — *see also* Assault E968.9

M

Malfunction, atomic power plant in water transport E838 ☑
Mangled (accidentally) NEC E928.9
Manhandling (in brawl, fight) E960.0
  legal intervention E975
Manslaughter (nonaccidental) — *see* Assault
Marble in nose E912
Mauled by animal E906.8
Medical procedure, complication of
  delayed or as an abnormal reaction without mention of misadventure — *see* Reaction, abnormal

Medical procedure, complication of — *continued*
  due to or as a result of misadventure — *see* Misadventure
Melting of fittings and furniture in burning
  in terrorism E979.3
Minamata disease E865.2
Misadventure(s) to patient(s) during surgical or medical care E876.9
  contaminated blood, fluid, drug or biological substance (presence of agents and toxins as listed in E875) E875.9
    administered (by) NEC E875.9
      infusion E875.0
      injection E875.1
      specified means NEC E875.2
      transfusion E875.0
      vaccination E875.1
  cut, cutting, puncture, perforation or hemorrhage (accidental) (inadvertent) (inappropriate) (during) E870.9
    aspiration of fluid or tissue (by puncture or catheterization, except heart) E870.5
    biopsy E870.8
      needle (aspirating) E870.5
    blood sampling E870.5
    catheterization E870.5
      heart E870.6
    dialysis (kidney) E870.2
    endoscopic examination E870.4
    enema E870.7
    infusion E870.1
    injection E870.3
    lumbar puncture E870.5
    needle biopsy E870.5
    paracentesis, abdominal E870.5
    perfusion E870.2
    specified procedure NEC E870.8
    surgical operation E870.0
    thoracentesis E870.5
    transfusion E870.1
    vaccination E870.3
  excessive amount of blood or other fluid during transfusion or infusion E873.0
  failure
    in dosage E873.9
      electroshock therapy E873.4
      inappropriate temperature (too hot or too cold) in local application and packing E873.5
      infusion
        excessive amount of fluid E873.0
        incorrect dilution of fluid E873.1
      insulin-shock therapy E873.4
      nonadministration of necessary drug or medicinal E873.6
      overdose (*see also* Overdose)
        radiation, in therapy E873.2
      radiation
        inadvertent exposure of patient (receiving radiation for test or therapy) E873.3
        not receiving radiation for test or therapy — *see* Radiation
        overdose E873.2
      specified procedure NEC E873.8
      transfusion
        excessive amount of blood E873.0
    mechanical, of instrument or apparatus (during procedure) E874.9
      aspiration of fluid or tissue (by puncture or catheterization, except of heart) E874.4
      biopsy E874.8
        needle (aspirating) E874.4
      blood sampling E874.4
      catheterization E874.4
        heart E874.5
      dialysis (kidney) E874.2
      endoscopic examination E874.3
      enema E874.8
      infusion E874.1
      injection E874.8
      lumbar puncture E874.4

Misadventure(s) to patient(s) during surgical or medical care — *continued*
  failure — *continued*
    mechanical, of instrument or apparatus — *continued*
      needle biopsy E874.4
      paracentesis, abdominal E874.4
      perfusion E874.2
      specified procedure NEC E874.8
      surgical operation E874.0
      thoracentesis E874.4
      transfusion E874.1
      vaccination E874.8
    sterile precautions (during procedure) E872.9
      aspiration of fluid or tissue (by puncture or catheterization, except heart) E872.5
      biopsy E872.8
        needle (aspirating) E872.5
      blood sampling E872.5
      catheterization E872.5
        heart E872.6
      dialysis (kidney) E872.2
      endoscopic examination E872.4
      enema E872.8
      infusion E872.1
      injection E872.3
      lumbar puncture E872.5
      needle biopsy E872.5
      paracentesis, abdominal E872.5
      perfusion E872.2
      removal of catheter or packing E872.8
      specified procedure NEC E872.8
      surgical operation E872.0
      thoracentesis E872.5
      transfusion E872.1
      vaccination E872.3
    suture or ligature during surgical procedure E876.2
    to introduce or to remove tube or instrument E876.4
    foreign object left in body — *see* Misadventure, foreign object
  foreign object left in body (during procedure) E871.9
    aspiration of fluid or tissue (by puncture or catheterization, except heart) E871.5
    biopsy E871.8
      needle (aspirating) E871.5
    blood sampling E871.5
    catheterization E871.5
      heart E871.6
    dialysis (kidney) E871.2
    endoscopic examination E871.4
    enema E871.8
    infusion E871.1
    injection E871.3
    lumbar puncture E871.5
    needle biopsy E871.5
    paracentesis, abdominal E871.5
    perfusion E871.2
    removal of catheter or packing E871.7
    specified procedure NEC E871.8
    surgical operation E871.0
    thoracentesis E871.5
    transfusion E871.1
    vaccination E871.3
  hemorrhage — *see* Misadventure, cut
  inadvertent exposure of patient to radiation (being received for test or therapy) E873.3
  inappropriate
    temperature (too hot or too cold) in local application or packing E873.5
  infusion (*see also* Misadventure, by specific type, infusion)
    excessive amount of fluid E873.0
    incorrect dilution of fluid E873.1
    wrong fluid E876.1
  mismatched blood in transfusion E876.0
  nonadministration of necessary drug or medicinal E873.6
  overdose (*see also* Overdose)

Misadventure(s) to patient(s) during surgical or medical care — *continued*
  overdose (*see also* Overdose) — *continued*
    radiation, in therapy E873.2
  perforation — *see* Misadventure, cut
  performance of correct operation (procedure) on wrong
    body part E876.7
    side E876.7
    site E876.7
  performance of operation (procedure)
    intended for another patient E876.6
    on patient not scheduled for surgery E876.6
    on wrong patient E876.6
  performance of wrong operation on correct patient E876.5
  puncture — *see* Misadventure, cut
  specified type NEC E876.8
    failure
      suture or ligature during surgical operation E876.2
      to introduce or to remove tube or instrument E876.4
      foreign object left in body E871.9
    infusion of wrong fluid E876.1
    performance of inappropriate operation E876.5
    transfusion of mismatched blood E876.0
    wrong
      fluid in infusion E876.1
      placement of endotracheal tube during anesthetic procedure E876.3
  transfusion (*see also* Misadventure, by specific type, transfusion)
    excessive amount of blood E873.0
    mismatched blood E876.0
  wrong
    device implanted into correct surgical site E876.5
    drug given in error — *see* Table of Drugs and Chemicals
    fluid in infusion E876.1
    placement of endotracheal tube during anesthetic procedure E876.3
    procedure (operation) performed on the correct patient E876.5
Motion (effects) E903
  sickness E903
Mountain sickness E902.0
Mucus aspiration or inhalation, not of newborn (with asphyxia, obstruction respiratory passage, suffocation) E912
Mudslide of cataclysmic nature E909.2
Murder (attempt) — *see also* Assault E968.9

N

Nail, injury by E920.8
Needlestick (sewing needle) E920.4
  hypodermic E920.5
Neglect — *see also* Privation
  criminal E968.4
  homicidal intent E968.4
Noise (causing injury) (pollution) E928.1
Nuclear weapon — *see also* War operations, injury due to, nuclear weapons E996.9

O

Object
  falling
    from, in, on, hitting
      aircraft E844 ☑
        due to accident to aircraft — *see* categories E840-E842 ☑
      machinery (*see also* Accident, machine)
        not in operation E916
      motor vehicle (in motion) (on public highway) E818 ☑
        not on public highway E825 ☑
        stationary E916
      nonmotor road vehicle NEC E829 ☑

Object — *continued*
  falling — *continued*
    from, in, on, hitting — *continued*
      motor vehicle — *continued*
        pedal cycle E826 ☑
        person E916
        railway rolling stock, train, vehicle E806 ☑
        street car E829 ☑
        watercraft E838 ☑
          due to accident to watercraft E831 ☑
    set in motion by
      accidental explosion of pressure vessel — *see* category E921 ☑
      firearm — *see* category E922 ☑
      machine(ry) — *see* Accident, machine
      transport vehicle — *see* categories E800-E848 ☑
    thrown from, in, on, towards
      aircraft E844 ☑
      cable car (not on rails) E847
        on rails E829 ☑
      motor vehicle (in motion) (on public highway) E818 ☑
        not on public highway E825 ☑
      nonmotor road vehicle NEC E829 ☑
      pedal cycle E826 ☑
      street car E829 ☑
      vehicle NEC — *see* Accident, vehicle NEC
Obstruction
  air passages, larynx, respiratory passages
    by
      external means NEC — *see* Suffocation
      food, any type (regurgitated) (vomited) E911
      material or object, except food E912
      mucus E912
      phlegm E912
      vomitus E911
  digestive tract, except mouth or pharynx
    by
      food, any type E915
      foreign body (any) E915
  esophagus
    without asphyxia or obstruction of respiratory passage E915
    food E911
    foreign body, except food E912
  mouth or pharynx
    by
      food, any type E911
      material or object, except food E912
  respiration — *see* Obstruction, air passages
Oil in eye E914
Overdose
  anesthetic (drug) — *see* Table of Drugs and Chemicals
  drug — *see* Table of Drugs and Chemicals
Overexertion E927.9
  from
    lifting
      repetitive movement E927.3
      sudden strenuous movement E927.0
    maintaining prolonged positions E927.1
      holding E927.1
      sitting E927.1
      standing E927.1
    prolonged static position E927.1
    pulling
      repetitive movement E927.3
      sudden strenuous movement E927.0
    pushing
      repetitive movement E927.3
      sudden strenuous movement E927.0
    specified NEC E927.8
    sudden strenuous movement E927.0
Overexposure (accidental) (to)
  cold (*see also* Cold, exposure to) E901.9
    due to manmade conditions E901.1
  heat (*see also* Heat) E900.9
  radiation — *see* Radiation
  radioactivity — *see* Radiation
  sun, except sunburn E900.0
  weather — *see* Exposure

☑ **Additional Digit Required** — Refer to the Tabular List for Digit Selection   ⍟ **Subterms under main terms may continue to next column or page**

Overexposure — *continued*
wind — *see* Exposure
Overheated — *see also* Heat E900.9
Overlaid E913.0
Overturning (accidental)
animal-drawn vehicle E827 ☑
boat, ship, watercraft
causing
drowning, submersion E830 ☑
injury except drowning, submersion E831 ☑
machinery — *see* Accident, machine
motor vehicle (*see also* Loss of control, motor vehicle) E816 ☑
with antecedent collision on public highway — *see* Collision, motor vehicle
not on public highway, nontraffic accident E825 ☑
with antecedent collision — *see* Collision, motor vehicle, not on public highway
nonmotor road vehicle NEC E829 ☑
off-road type motor vehicle — *see* Loss of control, off-road type motor vehicle
pedal cycle E826 ☑
railway rolling stock, train, vehicle (*see also* Derailment, railway) E802 ☑
street car E829 ☑
vehicle NEC — *see* Accident, vehicle NEC

P

Palsy, divers' E902.2
Parachuting (voluntary) (without accident to aircraft) E844 ☑
due to accident to aircraft — *see* categories E840-E842 ☑
Paralysis
divers' E902.2
lead or saturnine E866.0
from pesticide NEC E863.4
Pecked by bird E906.8
Performance of correct operation (procedure) **on wrong**
body part E876.7
side E876.7
site E876.7
Performance of operation (procedure)
intended for another patient E876.6
on patient not scheduled for surgery E876.6
on wrong patient E876.6
Performance of wrong operation on correct patient E876.5
Phlegm aspiration or inhalation (with asphyxia, obstruction respiratory passage, suffocation) E912
Piercing — *see also* Cut E920.9
by slide trigger mechanism, scope or other part of gun E928.7
Pinched
between objects (moving) (stationary and moving) E918
by slide trigger mechanism, scope or other part of gun E928.7
in object E918
Pinned under
machine(ry) — *see* Accident, machine
Place of occurrence of accident — *see* Accident (to), occurring (at) (in)
Plumbism E866.0
from insecticide NEC E863.4
Poisoning (accidental) (by) — *see also* Table of Drugs and Chemicals
carbon monoxide
generated by
aircraft in transit E844 ☑
motor vehicle
in motion (on public highway) E818 ☑
not on public highway E825 ☑
watercraft (in transit) (not in transit) E838 ☑

Poisoning — *see also* Table of Drugs and Chemicals — *continued*
caused by injection of poisons or toxins into or through skin by plant thorns, spines, or other mechanism E905.7
marine or sea plants E905.6
fumes or smoke due to
conflagration — *see* Conflagration
explosion or fire — *see* Fire
ignition — *see* Ignition
gas
in legal intervention E972
legal execution, by E978
on watercraft E838 ☑
used as anesthetic — *see* Table of Drugs and Chemicals
in
terrorism (chemical weapons) E979.7
war operations E997.2
execution E978
intervention
by gas E972
late effect of — *see* Late effect
legal
Pressure, external, causing asphyxia, suffocation — *see also* Suffocation E913.9
Privation E904.9
food (*see also* Lack of, food) E904.1
helpless person, infant, newborn due to abandonment or neglect E904.0
late effect of NEC E929.5
resulting from transport accident — *see* categories E800-E848 ☑
water (*see also* Lack of, water) E904.2
Projected objects, striking against or struck by — *see* Striking against, object
Prolonged stay in
high altitude (causing conditions as listed in E902.0) E902.0
weightless environment E928.0
Prostration
heat — *see* Heat
Pulling, injury
due to
repetitive movement E927.3
sudden strenuous movement E927.0
Puncture, puncturing — *see also* Cut E920.9
by
plant thorns or spines E920.8
toxic reaction E905.7
marine or sea plants E905.6
sea-urchin spine E905.6
Pushing (injury in) (overexertion)
by other person(s) (accidental) E917.9
with fall E886.9
in sports E886.0
as, or caused by, a crowd, human stampede E917.1
with subsequent fall E917.6
before moving vehicle or object
stated as
intentional, homicidal E968.5
undetermined whether accidental or intentional E988.8
from
high place
in accidental circum-stances — *see* categories E880-E884 ☑
stated as
intentional, homicidal E968.1
undetermined whether accidental or intentional E987.9
man-made structure, except residential E987.1
natural site E987.2
residential E987.0
motor vehicle (*see also* Fall, from, motor vehicle) E818 ☑
stated as
intentional, homicidal E968.5
undetermined whether accidental or intentional E988.8

Pushing — *continued*
by other person(s) — *continued*
in sports E917.0
with fall E886.0
due to
repetitive movement E927.3
sudden strenuous movement E927.0

R

Radiation (exposure to) E926.9
abnormal reaction to medical test or therapy E879.2
arc lamps E926.2
atomic power plant (malfunction) NEC E926.9
in water transport E838 ☑
electromagnetic, ionizing E926.3
gamma rays E926.3
in
terrorism (from or following nuclear explosion) (direct) (secondary) E979.5
laser E979.8
war operations (*see also* War operations, injury due to, nuclear weapons) E996.3
laser(s) E997.0
water transport E838 ☑
inadvertent exposure of patient (receiving test or therapy) E873.3
infrared (heaters and lamps) E926.1
excessive heat E900.1
ionized, ionizing (particles, artificially accelerated) E926.8
electromagnetic E926.3
isotopes, radioactive — *see* Radiation, radioactive isotopes
laser(s) E926.4
in
terrorism E979.8
war operations E997.0
misadventure in medical care — *see* Misadventure, failure, in dosage, radiation
late effect of NEC E929.8
excessive heat from — *see* Heat
light sources (visible) (ultraviolet) E926.2
misadventure in medical or surgical procedure — *see* Misadventure, failure, in dosage, radiation
overdose (in medical or surgical procedure) E873.2
radar E926.0
radioactive isotopes E926.5
atomic power plant malfunction E926.5
in water transport E838 ☑
misadventure in medical or surgical treatment — *see* Misadventure, failure, in dosage, radiation
radiobiologicals — *see* Radiation, radioactive isotopes
radiofrequency E926.0
radiopharmaceuticals — *see* Radiation, radioactive isotopes
radium NEC E926.9
sun E926.2
excessive heat from E900.0
tanning bed E926.2
welding arc or torch E926.2
excessive heat from E900.1
x-rays (hard) (soft) E926.3
misadventure in medical or surgical treatment — *see* Misadventure, failure, in dosage, radiation
Rape E960.1
Reaction, abnormal to or following (medical or surgical procedure) E879.9
amputation (of limbs) E878.5
anastomosis (arteriovenous) (blood vessel) (gastrojejunal) (skin) (tendon) (natural, artificial material, tissue) E878.2
external stoma, creation of E878.3
aspiration (of fluid) E879.4
tissue E879.8
biopsy E879.8

Reaction, abnormal to or following — *continued*
blood
sampling E879.7
transfusion
procedure E879.8
bypass — *see* Reaction, abnormal, anastomosis
catheterization
cardiac E879.0
urinary E879.6
colostomy E878.3
cystostomy E878.3
dialysis (kidney) E879.1
drugs or biologicals — *see* Table of Drugs and Chemicals
duodenostomy E878.3
electroshock therapy E879.3
formation of external stoma E878.3
gastrostomy E878.3
graft — *see* Reaction, abnormal, anastomosis
hypothermia E879.8
implant, implantation (of)
artificial
internal device (cardiac pacemaker) (electrodes in brain) (heart valve prosthesis) (orthopedic) E878.1
material or tissue (for anastomosis or bypass) E878.2
with creation of external stoma E878.3
natural tissues (for anastomosis or bypass) E878.2
with creation of external stoma E878.3
as transplantation — *see* Reaction, abnormal, transplant
infusion
procedure E879.8
injection
procedure E879.8
specific type of procedure E879.9
insertion of gastric or duodenal sound E879.5
insulin-shock therapy E879.3
lumbar puncture E879.4
perfusion E879.1
procedures other than surgical operation (*see also* Reaction, abnormal, by specified procedure NEC E879.8
radiological procedure or therapy E879.2
removal of organ (partial) (total) NEC E878.6
with
anastomosis, bypass or graft E878.2
formation of external stoma E878.3
implant of artificial internal device E878.1
transplant(ation)
partial organ E878.4
whole organ E878.0
sampling
blood E879.7
fluid NEC E879.4
tissue E879.8
shock therapy E879.3
surgical operation (*see also* Reaction, abnormal, by specified type of operation) E878.9
restorative NEC E878.4
with
anastomosis, bypass or graft E878.2
fomation of external stoma E878.3
implant(ation) — *see* Reaction, abnormal, implant
transplant(ation) — *see* Reaction, abnormal, transplant
specified operation NEC E878.8
thoracentesis E879.4
transfusion
procedure E879.8
transplant, transplantation (heart) (kidney) (liver) E878.0

Reaction, abnormal to or following — *continued*
　transplant, transplantation — *continued*
　　partial organ E878.4
　　ureterostomy E878.3
　　vaccination E879.8
Reduction in
　atmospheric pressure (*see also* Effects of, air pressure)
　　while surfacing from
　　　deep water diving causing caisson or divers' disease, palsy or paralysis E902.2
　　　underground E902.8
Repetitive movements NEC E927.8
Residual (effect) — *see* Late effect
Rock falling on or hitting (accidentally)
　motor vehicle (in motion) (on public highway) E818 ☑
　　not on public highway E825 ☑
　nonmotor road vehicle NEC E829 ☑
　pedal cycle E826 ☑
　person E916
　railway rolling stock, train, vehicle E806 ☑
Running off, away
　animal (being ridden) (in sport or transport) E828 ☑
　　not being ridden E906.8
　animal-drawn vehicle E827 ☑
　rails, railway (*see also* Derailment) E802 ☑
　roadway
　　motor vehicle (without antecedent collision) E816 ☑
　　　with
　　　　antecedent collision — *see* Collision motor vehicle
　　　　subsequent collision
　　　　　involving any object, person or vehicle not on public highway E816 ☑
　　　　　on public highway E811 ☑
　　　nontraffic accident E825 ☑
　　　　with antecedent collision — *see* Collision, motor vehicle, not on public highway
　　nonmotor road vehicle NEC E829 ☑
　　pedal cycle E826 ☑
Run over (accidentally) (by)
　animal (not being ridden) E906.8
　　being ridden (in sport or transport) E828 ☑
　animal-drawn vehicle E827 ☑
　machinery — *see* Accident, machine
　motor vehicle (on public highway) — *see* Hit by, motor vehicle
　nonmotor road vehicle NEC E829 ☑
　railway train E805 ☑
　street car E829 ☑
　vehicle NEC E848

S

Saturnism E866.0
　from insecticide NEC E863.4
Scald, scalding (accidental) (by) (from) (in) E924.0
　acid — *see* Scald, caustic
　boiling tap water E924.2
　caustic or corrosive liquid, substance E924.1
　　swallowed — *see* Table of Drugs and Chemicals
　homicide (attempt) — *see* Assault, burning
　inflicted by other person
　　stated as
　　　intentional or homicidal E968.3
　　　undetermined whether accidental or intentional E988.2
　late effect of NEC E929.8
　liquid (boiling) (hot) E924.0
　local application of externally applied substance in medical or surgical care E873.5
　molten metal E924.0
　self-inflicted (unspecified whether accidental or intentional) E988.2
　　stated as intentional, purposeful E958.2

Scald, scalding — *continued*
　stated as undetermined whether accidental or intentional E988.2
　steam E924.0
　tap water (boiling) E924.2
　transport accident — *see* categories E800-E848 ☑
　vapor E924.0
Scratch, cat E906.8
Sea
　sickness E903
Self-mutilation — *see* Suicide
Sequelae (of)
　in
　　terrorism E999.1
　　war operations E999.0
Shock
　anaphylactic (*see also* Table of Drugs and Chemicals) E947.9
　　due to
　　　bite (venomous) — *see* Bite, venomous NEC
　　　sting — *see* Sting
　electric (*see also* Electric shock) E925.9
　　from electric appliance or current (*see also* Electric shock) E925.9
Shooting, shot (accidental(ly)) E922.9
　air gun E922.4
　BB gun E922.4
　hand gun (pistol) (revolver) E922.0
　himself (*see also* Shooting, self-inflicted) E985.4
　　hand gun (pistol) (revolver) E985.0
　　military firearm, except hand gun E985.3
　　　hand gun (pistol) (revolver) E985.0
　　rifle (hunting) E985.2
　　　military E985.3
　　shotgun (automatic) E985.1
　　specified firearm NEC E985.4
　　Verey pistol E985.4
　homicide (attempt) E965.4
　　air gun E968.6
　　BB gun E968.6
　　hand gun (pistol) (revolver) E965.0
　　military firearm, except hand gun E965.3
　　　hand gun (pistol) (revolver) E965.0
　　paintball gun E965.4
　　rifle (hunting) E965.2
　　　military E965.3
　　shotgun (automatic) E965.1
　　specified firearm NEC E965.4
　　Verey pistol E965.4
　in
　　terrorism — *see* Terrorism, shooting
　　war operations — *see* War operations, shooting
　inflicted by other person
　　in accidental circumstances E922.9
　　　hand gun (pistol) (revolver) E922.0
　　　military firearm, except hand gun E922.3
　　　　hand gun (pistol) (revolver) E922.0
　　　rifle (hunting) E922.2
　　　　military E922.3
　　　shotgun (automatic) E922.1
　　　specified firearm NEC E922.8
　　　Verey pistol E922.8
　　stated as
　　　intentional, homicidal E965.4
　　　　hand gun (pistol) (revolver) E965.0
　　　　military firearm, except hand gun E965.3
　　　　　hand gun (pistol) (revolver) E965.0
　　　　paintball gun E965.4
　　　　rifle (hunting) E965.2
　　　　　military E965.3
　　　　shotgun (automatic) E965.1
　　　　specified firearm E965.4
　　　　Verey pistol E965.4
　　　undetermined whether accidental or intentional E985.4
　　　　air gun E985.6
　　　　BB gun E985.6

Shooting, shot — *continued*
　inflicted by other person — *continued*
　　stated as — *continued*
　　　undetermined whether accidental or intentional — *continued*
　　　　hand gun (pistol) (revolver) E985.0
　　　　military firearm, except hand gun E985.3
　　　　　hand gun (pistol) (revolver) E985.0
　　　　paintball gun E985.7
　　　　rifle (hunting) E985.2
　　　　shotgun (automatic) E985.1
　　　　specified firearm NEC E985.4
　　　　Verey pistol E985.4
　legal
　　execution E978
　　intervention E970
　military firearm, except hand gun E922.3
　　hand gun (pistol) (revolver) E922.0
　paintball gun E922.5
　rifle (hunting) E922.2
　　military E922.3
　self-inflicted (unspecified whether accidental or intentional) E985.4
　　air gun E985.6
　　BB gun E985.6
　　hand gun (pistol) (revolver) E985.0
　　military firearm, except hand gun E985.3
　　　hand gun (pistol) (revolver) E985.0
　　paintball gun E985.7
　　rifle (hunting) E985.2
　　　military E985.3
　　shotgun (automatic) E985.1
　　specified firearm NEC E985.4
　　stated as
　　　accidental E922.9
　　　　hand gun (pistol) (revolver) E922.0
　　　　military firearm, except hand gun E922.3
　　　　　hand gun (pistol) (revolver) E922.0
　　　　paintball gun E922.5
　　　　rifle (hunting) E922.2
　　　　　military E922.3
　　　　shotgun (automatic) E922.1
　　　　specified firearm NEC E922.8
　　　　Verey pistol E922.8
　　　intentional, purposeful E955.4
　　　　hand gun (pistol) (revolver) E955.0
　　　　military firearm, except hand gun E955.3
　　　　　hand gun (pistol) (revolver) E955.0
　　　　paintball gun E955.7
　　　　rifle (hunting) E955.2
　　　　　military E955.3
　　　　shotgun (automatic) E955.1
　　　　specified firearm NEC E955.4
　　　　Verey pistol E955.4
　　shotgun (automatic) E922.1
　　specified firearm NEC E922.8
　　stated as undetermined whether accidental or intentional E985.4
　　　hand gun (pistol) (revolver) E985.0
　　　military firearm, except hand gun E985.3
　　　　hand gun (pistol) (revolver) E985.0
　　　paintball gun E985.7
　　　rifle (hunting) E985.2
　　　　military E985.3
　　　shotgun (automatic) E985.1
　　　specified firearm NEC E985.4
　　　Verey pistol E985.4
　　suicidal (attempt) E955.4
　　　air gun E955.6
　　　BB gun E955.6
　　　hand gun (pistol) (revolver) E955.0
　　　military firearm, except hand gun E955.3
　　　　hand gun (pistol) (revolver) E955.0
　　　paintball gun E955.7
　　　rifle (hunting) E955.2
　　　　military E955.3
　　　shotgun (automatic) E955.1

Shooting, shot — *continued*
　suicidal — *continued*
　　specified firearm NEC E955.4
　　Verey pistol E955.4
　　Verey pistol E922.8
Shoving (accidentally) by other person — *see also* Pushing by other person E917.9
Sickness
　air E903
　alpine E902.0
　car E903
　motion E903
　mountain E902.0
　sea E903
　travel E903
Sinking (accidental)
　boat, ship, watercraft (causing drowning, submersion) E830 ☑
　　causing injury except drowning, submersion E831 ☑
Siriasis E900.0
Skydiving E844 ☑
Slashed wrists — *see also* Cut, self-inflicted E986
Slipping (accidental)
　on
　　deck (of boat, ship, watercraft) (icy) (oily) (wet) E835 ☑
　　ice E885.9
　　ladder of ship E833 ☑
　　　due to accident to watercraft E831 ☑
　　mud E885.9
　　oil E885.9
　　snow E885.9
　　stairs of ship E833 ☑
　　　due to accident to watercraft E831 ☑
　　surface
　　　slippery E885 ☑
　　　wet E885 ☑
Sliver, wood, injury by E920.8
Smothering, smothered — *see also* Suffocation E913.9
Smouldering building or structure in terrorism E979.3
Sodomy (assault) E960.1
Solid substance in eye (any part) or adnexa E914
Sound waves (causing injury) E928.1
Splinter, injury by E920.8
Stab, stabbing E966
　accidental — *see* Cut
Starvation E904.1
　helpless person, infant, newborn — *see* Lack of food
　homicidal intent E968.4
　late effect of NEC E929.5
　resulting from accident connected with transport — *see* categories E800-E848 ☑
Stepped on
　by
　　animal (not being ridden) E906.8
　　　being ridden (in sport or transport) E828 ☑
　　crowd E917.1
　　person E917.9
　　　in sports E917.0
　in sports E917.0
Stepping on
　object (moving) E917.9
　　in sports E917.0
　　　with subsequent fall E917.5
　　stationary E917.4
　　　with subsequent fall E917.8
　person E917.9
　　as, or caused by a crowd E917.1
　　　with subsequent fall E917.6
　　in sports E917.0
Sting E905.9
　ant E905.5
　bee E905.3
　caterpillar E905.5
　coral E905.6
　hornet E905.3

☑ **Additional Digit Required** — Refer to the Tabular List for Digit Selection　　　　　🔻 **Subterms under main terms may continue to next column or page**

2013 ICD-9-CM　　▶◀ **Revised Text**　　● **New Line**　　▲ **Revised Code**　　**Volume 2 — 349**

Sting — *continued*
- insect NEC E905.5
- jellyfish E905.6
- marine animal or plant E905.6
- nematocysts E905.6
- scorpion E905.2
- sea anemone E905.6
- sea cucumber E905.6
- wasp E905.3
- yellow jacket E905.3

Storm E908.9
- specified type NEC E908.8

Straining, injury
- due to
  - repetitive movement E927.3
  - sudden strenuous movement E927.0

Strangling — *see* Suffocation

Strangulation — *see* Suffocation

Strenuous movements (in recreational or other activities) NEC E927.8

Striking against
- bottom (when jumping or diving into water) E883.0
- object (moving) E917.9
  - caused by crowd E917.1
    - with subsequent fall E917.6
  - furniture E917.3
    - with subsequent fall E917.7
  - in
    - running water E917.2
      - with drowning or submersion — *see* Submersion
    - sports E917.0
      - with subsequent fall E917.5
    - stationary E917.4
      - with subsequent fall E917.8
- person(s) E917.9
  - with fall E886.9
    - in sports E886.0
  - as, or caused by, a crowd E917.1
    - with subsequent fall E917.6
    - in sports E917.0
      - with fall E886.0

Stroke
- heat — *see* Heat
- lightning E907

Struck by — *see also* Hit by
- bullet
  - in
    - terrorism E979.4
    - war operations E991.2
      - rubber E991.0
- lightning E907
- missile
  - in terrorism — *see* Terrorism, missile
- object
  - falling
    - from, in, on
      - building
        - burning (uncontrolled fire)
          - in terrorism E979.3
- thunderbolt E907

Stumbling over animal, carpet, curb, rug or (small) object (with fall) E885.9
- without fall — *see* Striking against, object

Submersion (accidental) E910.8
- boat, ship, watercraft (causing drowning, submersion) E830 ☑
  - causing injury except drowning, submersion E831 ☑
- by other person
  - in accidental circumstances — *see* category E910 ☑
  - intentional, homicidal E964
  - stated as undetermined whether accidental or intentional E984
- due to
  - accident
    - machinery — *see* Accident, machine
    - to boat, ship, watercraft E830 ☑
    - transport — *see* categories E800-E848 ☑
  - avalanche E909.2
  - cataclysmic
    - earth surface movement or eruption E909.9

Submersion (accidental) — *continued*
- due to — *continued*
  - cataclysmic — *continued*
    - storm E908.9
  - cloudburst E908.8
  - cyclone E908.1
  - fall
    - from
      - boat, ship, watercraft (not involved in accident) E832 ☑
        - burning, crushed E830 ☑
        - involved in accident, collision E830 ☑
      - gangplank (into water) E832 ☑
    - overboard NEC E832 ☑
  - flood E908.2
  - hurricane E908.0
  - jumping into water E910.8
    - from boat, ship, watercraft
      - burning, crushed, sinking E830 ☑
      - involved in accident, collision E830 ☑
      - not involved in accident, for swim E910.2
    - in recreational activity (without diving equipment) E910.2
      - with or using diving equipment E910.1
    - to rescue another person E910.3
- homicide (attempt) E964
- in
  - bathtub E910.4
  - specified activity, not sport, transport or recreational E910.3
  - sport or recreational activity (without diving equipment) E910.2
    - with or using diving equipment E910.1
    - water skiing E910.0
  - swimming pool NEC E910.8
  - terrorism E979.8
  - war operations E995.4
    - intentional E995.3
  - water transport E832 ☑
    - due to accident to boat, ship, watercraft E830 ☑
- landslide E909.2
- overturning boat, ship, watercraft E909.2
- sinking boat, ship, watercraft E909.2
- submersion boat, ship, watercraft E909.2
- tidal wave E909.4
  - caused by storm E908.0
- torrential rain E908.2
- late effect of NEC E929.8
- quenching tank E910.8
- self-inflicted (unspecified whether accidental or intentional) E984
  - in accidental circumstances — *see* category E910 ☑
  - stated as intentional, purposeful E954
- stated as undetermined whether accidental or intentional E984
- suicidal (attempted) E954
- while
  - attempting rescue of another person E910.3
  - engaged in
    - marine salvage E910.3
    - underwater construction or repairs E910.3
  - fishing, not from boat E910.2
  - hunting, not from boat E910.2
  - ice skating E910.2
  - pearl diving E910.3
  - placing fishing nets E910.3
  - playing in water E910.2
  - scuba diving E910.1
    - nonrecreational E910.3
  - skin diving E910.1
  - snorkel diving E910.2
  - spear fishing underwater E910.1
  - surfboarding E910.2
  - swimming (swimming pool) E910.2
  - wading (in water) E910.2
  - water skiing E910.0

Sucked
- into
  - jet (aircraft) E844 ☑

Suffocation (accidental) (by external means) (by pressure) (mechanical) E913.9
- caused by other person
  - in accidental circumstances — *see* category E913 ☑
  - stated as
    - intentional, homicidal E963
    - undetermined whether accidental or intentional E983.9
      - by, in
        - hanging E983.0
        - plastic bag E983.1
        - specified means NEC E983.8
- due to, by
  - avalanche E909.2
  - bedclothes E913.0
  - bib E913.0
  - blanket E913.0
  - cave-in E913.3
    - caused by cataclysmic earth surface movement or eruption E909.9
  - conflagration — *see* Conflagration
  - explosion — *see* Explosion
  - falling earth, other substance E913.3
  - fire — *see* Fire
  - food, any type (ingestion) (inhalation) (regurgitated) (vomited) E911
  - foreign body, except food (ingestion) (inhalation) E912
  - ignition — *see* Ignition
  - landslide E909.2
  - machine(ry) — *see* Accident, machine
  - material, object except food entering by nose or mouth, ingested, inhaled E912
  - mucus (aspiration) (inhalation), not of newborn E912
  - phlegm (aspiration) (inhalation) E912
  - pillow E913.0
  - plastic bag — *see* Suffocation, in, plastic bag
  - sheet (plastic) E913.0
  - specified means NEC E913.8
  - vomitus (aspiration) (inhalation) E911
- homicidal (attempt) E963
  - in war operations E995.3
- in
  - airtight enclosed place E913.2
  - baby carriage E913.0
  - bed E913.0
  - closed place E913.2
  - cot, cradle E913.0
  - perambulator E913.0
  - plastic bag (in accidental circumstances) E913.1
    - homicidal, purposely inflicted by other person E963
    - self-inflicted (unspecified whether accidental or intentional) E983.1
      - in accidental circumstances E913.1
      - intentional, suicidal E953.1
      - stated as undetermined whether accidentally or purposely inflicted E983.1
    - suicidal, purposely self-inflicted E953.1
  - refrigerator E913.2
  - war operations E995.3
- self-inflicted (*see also* Suffocation, stated as undetermined whether accidental or intentional) E953.9
  - in accidental circumstances — *see* category E913 ☑
  - stated as intentional, purposeful — *see* Suicide, suffocation
- stated as undetermined whether accidental or intentional E983.9
  - by, in
    - hanging E983.0
    - plastic bag E983.1
    - specified means NEC E983.8

Suffocation — *continued*
- suicidal — *see* Suicide, suffocation

Suicide, suicidal (attempted) (by) E958.9
- burning, burns E958.1
- caustic substance E958.7
  - poisoning E950.7
  - swallowed E950.7
- cold, extreme E958.3
- cut (any part of body) E956
- cutting or piercing instrument (classifiable to E920) E956
- drowning E954
- electrocution E958.4
- explosive(s) (classifiable to E923) E955.5
- fire E958.1
- firearm (classifiable to E922) — *see* Shooting, suicidal
- hanging E953.0
- jumping
  - before moving object, train, vehicle E958.0
  - from high place — *see* Jumping, from, high place, stated as, suicidal
- knife E956
- late effect of E959
- motor vehicle, crashing of E958.5
- poisoning — *see* Table of Drugs and Chemicals
- puncture (any part of body) E956
- scald E958.2
- shooting — *see* Shooting, suicidal
- specified means NEC E958.8
- stab (any part of body) E956
- strangulation — *see* Suicide, suffocation
- submersion E954
- suffocation E953.9
  - by, in
    - hanging E953.0
    - plastic bag E953.1
    - specified means NEC E953.8
- wound NEC E958.9

Sunburn E926.2

Sunstroke E900.0

Supersonic waves (causing injury) E928.1

Surgical procedure, complication of
- delayed or as an abnormal reaction without mention of misadventure — *see* Reaction, abnormal
- due to or as a result of misadventure — *see* Misadventure

Swallowed, swallowing
- foreign body — *see* Foreign body, alimentary canal
- poison — *see* Table of Drugs and Chemicals
- substance
  - caustic — *see* Table of Drugs and Chemicals
  - corrosive — *see* Table of Drugs and Chemicals
  - poisonous — *see* Table of Drugs and Chemicals

Swimmers cramp — *see also* category E910 E910.2
- not in recreation or sport E910.3

Syndrome, battered
- baby or child — *see* Abuse, child
- wife — *see* Assault

T

Tackle in sport E886.0

Terrorism (injury) (by) (in) E979.8
- air blast E979.2
- aircraft burned, destroyed, exploded, shot down E979.1
  - used as a weapon E979.1
- anthrax E979.6
- asphyxia from
  - chemical (weapons) E979.7
  - fire, conflagration (caused by fire-producing device) E979.3
  - from nuclear explosion E979.5
  - gas or fumes E979.7
- bayonet E979.8
- biological agents E979.6
- blast (air) (effects) E979.2
  - from nuclear explosion E979.5

☑ Additional Digit Required — Refer to the Tabular List for Digit Selection ▼ Subterms under main terms may continue to next column or page

Terrorism — *continued*
  blast — *continued*
    underwater E979.0
  bomb (antipersonnel) (mortar) (explosion) (fragments) E979.2
  bullet(s) (from carbine, machine gun, pistol, rifle, shotgun) E979.4
  burn from
    chemical E979.7
    fire, conflagration (caused by fire-producing device) E979.3
      from nuclear explosion E979.5
    gas E979.7
  burning aircraft E979.1
  chemical E979.7
  cholera E979.6
  conflagration E979.3
  crushed by falling aircraft E979.1
  depth-charge E979.0
  destruction of aircraft E979.1
  disability, as sequelae one year or more after injury E999.1
  drowning E979.8
  effect
    of nuclear weapon (direct) (secondary) E979.5
    secondary NEC E979.9
    sequelae E999.1
  explosion (artillery shell) (breech-block) (cannon block) E979.2
    aircraft E979.1
    bomb (antipersonnel) (mortar) E979.2
      nuclear (atom) (hydrogen) E979.5
    depth-charge E979.0
    grenade E979.2
    injury by fragments from E979.2
    land-mine E979.2
    marine weapon E979.0
    mine (land) E979.2
      at sea or in harbor E979.0
      marine E979.0
    missile (explosive) NEC E979.2
    munitions (dump) (factory) E979.2
    nuclear (weapon) E979.5
      other direct and secondary effects of E979.5
    sea-based artillery shell E979.0
    torpedo E979.0
  exposure to ionizing radiation from nuclear explosion E979.5
  falling aircraft E979.1
  firearms E979.4
  fireball effects from nuclear explosion E979.5
  fire or fire-producing device E979.3
  fragments from artillery shell, bomb NEC, grenade, guided missile, land-mine, rocket, shell, shrapnel E979.2
  gas or fumes E979.7
  grenade (explosion) (fragments) E979.2
  guided missile (explosion) (fragments) E979.2
    nuclear E979.5
  heat from nuclear explosion E979.5
  hot substances E979.3
  hydrogen cyanide E979.7
  land-mine (explosion) (fragments) E979.2
  laser(s) E979.8
  late effect of E999.1
  lewisite E979.7
  lung irritant (chemical) (fumes) (gas) E979.7
  marine mine E979.0
  mine E979.2
    at sea E979.0
    in harbor E979.0
    land (explosion) (fragments) E979.2
    marine E979.0
  missile (explosion) (fragments) (guided) E979.2
    marine E979.0
    nuclear weapons E979.5
  mortar bomb (explosion) (fragments) E979.2
  mustard gas E979.7
  nerve gas E979.7
  nuclear weapons E979.5
  pellets (shotgun) E979.4

Terrorism — *continued*
  petrol bomb E979.3
  phosgene E979.7
  piercing object E979.8
  poisoning (chemical) (fumes) (gas) E979.7
  radiation, ionizing from nuclear explosion E979.5
  rocket (explosion) (fragments) E979.2
  saber, sabre E979.8
  sarin E979.7
  screening smoke E979.7
  sequelae effect (of) E999.1
  shell (aircraft) (artillery) (cannon) (land-based) (explosion) (fragments) E979.2
    sea-based E979.0
  shooting E979.4
    bullet(s) E979.4
    pellet(s) (rifle) (shotgun) E979.4
  shrapnel E979.2
  smallpox E979.7
  stabbing object(s) E979.8
  submersion E979.8
  torpedo E979.0
  underwater blast E979.0
  vesicant (chemical) (fumes) (gas) E979.7
  weapon burst E979.2
Thermic fever E900.9
Thermoplegia E900.9
Thirst — *see also* Lack of water
  resulting from accident connected with transport — *see* categories E800-E848 ☑
Thrown (accidently)
  against object in or part of vehicle
    by motion of vehicle
      aircraft E844 ☑
      boat, ship, watercraft E838 ☑
      motor vehicle (on public highway) E818 ☑
        not on public highway E825 ☑
      off-road type (not on public highway) E821 ☑
        on public highway E818 ☑
      snow vehicle E820 ☑
        on public highway E818 ☑
      nonmotor road vehicle NEC E829 ☑
      railway rolling stock, train, vehicle E806 ☑
      street car E829 ☑
    from
      animal (being ridden) (in sport or transport) E828 ☑
      high place, homicide (attempt) E968.1
      machinery — *see* Accident, machine
      vehicle NEC — *see* Accident, vehicle NEC
      off — *see* Thrown, from
    overboard (by motion of boat, ship, watercraft) E832 ☑
      by accident to boat, ship, watercraft E830 ☑
Thunderbolt NEC E907
Tidal wave (any injury) E909.4
  caused by storm E908.0
Took
  overdose of drug — *see* Table of Drugs and Chemicals
  poison — *see* Table of Drugs and Chemicals
Tornado (any injury) E908.1
Torrential rain (any injury) E908.2
Traffic accident NEC E819 ☑
Trampled by animal E906.8
  being ridden (in sport or transport) E828 ☑
Trapped (accidently)
  between
    objects (moving) (stationary and moving) E918
  by
    door of
      elevator E918
      motor vehicle (on public highway) (while alighting, boarding) — *see* Fall, from, motor vehicle, while alighting
      railway train (underground) E806 ☑

Trapped — *continued*
  by — *continued*
    door of — *continued*
      street car E829 ☑
      subway train E806 ☑
    in object E918
Trauma
  cumulative
    from
      repetitive
        impact E927.4
        motion or movements E927.3
    sudden from strenuous movement E927.0
Travel (effects) E903
  sickness E903
Tree
  falling on or hitting E916
    motor vehicle (in motion) (on public highway) E818 ☑
      not on public highway E825 ☑
    nonmotor road vehicle NEC E829 ☑
    pedal cycle E826 ☑
    person E916
    railway rolling stock, train, vehicle E806 ☑
    street car E829 ☑
Trench foot E901.0
Tripping over animal, carpet, curb, rug, or small object (with fall) E885 ☑
  without fall — *see* Striking against, object
Tsunami E909.4
Twisting, injury
  due to
    repetitive movement E927.3
    sudden strenuous movement E927.0

V

Violence, nonaccidental — *see also* Assault E968.9
Volcanic eruption (any injury) E909.1
Vomitus in air passages (with asphyxia, obstruction or suffocation) E911

W

War operations (during hostilities) (injury) (by) (in) E995.9
  after cessation of hostilities, injury due to E998.9
  air blast E993.9
  aircraft burned, destroyed, exploded, shot down E994 ☑
  asphyxia from
    chemical E997.2
    fire, conflagration (caused by fire producing device or conventional weapon) E990.9
      from nuclear explosion (*see also* War operations, injury due to, nuclear weapons) E996.8
    incendiary bomb E990.0
    petrol bomb E990.0
    fumes E997.2
    gas E997.2
  baton (nightstick) E995.1
  battle wound NEC E995.8
  bayonet E995.2
  biological warfare agents E997.1
  blast (air) (effects) E993.9
    from nuclear explosion — *see* War operations, injury due to, nuclear weapons
    underwater E992.9
  bomb (mortar) (explosion) E993.2
    after cessation of hostilities E998.1
    fragments, injury by E991.4
      antipersonnel E991.3
  bullet(s) (from carbine, machine gun, pistol, rifle, shotgun) E991.2
    rubber E991.0
  burn from
    chemical E997.2
    fire, conflagration (caused by fire-producing device or conventional weapon) E990.9

War operations — *continued*
  burn from — *continued*
    fire, conflagration — *continued*
      from
        conventional weapon E990.3
        flamethrower E990.1
        incendiary bomb E990.0
        incendiary bullet E990.2
        nuclear explosion E996.2
      petrol bomb E990.0
    gas E997.2
  burning aircraft E994.3
  chemical E997.2
  chlorine E997.2
  conventional warfare, specified form NEC E995.8
  crushing by falling aircraft E994.8
  depth charge E992.1
  destruction of aircraft E994.9
  detonation of own munitions (ammunition) (artillery) (mortars), unintentional E993.6
  disability as sequela one year or more after injury E999.0
  discharge of own munitions launch device (autocannons) (automatic grenade launchers) (missile launchers) (small arms), unintentional E993.7
  drowning E995.4
  effect nuclear weapon (*see also* War operations, injury due to, nuclear weapons) E996.9
  explosion (breech block) (cannon shell) E993.9
    after cessation of hostilities
      bomb placed in war E998.1
      mine placed in war E998.0
    aircraft E994.1
      due to
        enemy fire or explosives E994.0
        own onboard explosives E994.1
    artillery shell E993.2
    bomb (mortar) E993.2
      aerial E993.0
      atom (*see also* War operations, injury due to, nuclear weapons) E996.9
      hydrogen (*see also* War operations, injury due to, nuclear weapons) E996.9
      injury by fragments from E991.4
        antipersonnel E991.3
      nuclear (*see also* War operations, injury due to, nuclear weapons) E996.9
    depth charge E992.1
    injury by fragments from E991.4
      antipersonnel E991.3
    marine weapon NEC E992.8
    mine
      at sea or in harbor E992.2
      land E993.8
        injury by fragments from E991.4
      marine E992.2
    missile, guided E993.1
    mortar E993.2
    munitions (accidental) (being used in war) (dump) (factory) E993.9
    own E993.7
      ammunition (artillery) (mortars) E993.6
      launch device (autocannons) (automatic grenade launchers) (missile launchers) (small arms) E993.7
    nuclear (weapon) (*see also* War operations, injury due to, nuclear weapons) E996.9
    own weapons (accidental) E993.7
      injury by fragments from E991.9
        antipersonnel E991.3
    sea-based artillery shell E992.3
    specified NEC E993.8
    torpedo E992.0

☑ **Additional Digit Required — Refer to the Tabular List for Digit Selection**

☝ **Subterms under main terms may continue to next column or page**

2013 ICD-9-CM

▶◀ Revised Text   ● New Line   ▲ Revised Code

Volume 2 — 351

Terrorism — War operations

War operations — *continued*
  exposure to ionizing radiation from nuclear explosion (*see also* War operations, injury due to, nuclear weapons) E996.3
  falling aircraft E994.8
  fireball effects from nuclear explosion E996.2
  fire or fire-producing device E990.9
    flamethrower E990.1
    incendiary bomb E990.0
    incendiary bullet E990.2
    indirectly caused from conventional weapon E990.3
    petrol bomb E990.0
  fragments from
    antipersonnel bomb E991.3
    artillery shell E991.4
    bomb NEC E991.4
    grenade E991.4
    guided missile E991.4
    land mine E991.4
    rocket E991.4
    shell E991.4
    shrapnel E991.9
  fumes E997.2
  gas E997.2
  grenade (explosion) E993.8
    fragments, injury by E991.4
  guided missile (explosion) E993.1
    fragments, injury by E991.4
    nuclear (*see also* War operations, injury due to, nuclear weapons) E996.9
  heat from nuclear explosion E996.2
  injury due to
    aerial bomb E993.0
    air blast E993.9
    aircraft shot down E994.0
    artillery shell E993.2
    blast E993.9
      wave E993.9
      wind E993.9
    bomb E993.8
    but occurring after cessation of hostilities
      explosion of bombs E998.1
      explosion of mines E998.0
      specified NEC E998.8
    conventional warfare E995.9
      specified form NEC E995.8
    depth charge E992.1
    destruction of aircraft E994.9
      due to
        air to air missile E994.0
        collision with other aircraft E994.2
        enemy fire or explosives E994.0
        on board explosion (explosives) E994.1
        on board fire E994.3
        rocket propelled grenade [RPG] E994.0
        small arms fire E994.0
        surface to air missile E994.0
      specified NEC E994.8
    dirty bomb (*see also* War operations, injury due to, nuclear weapons) E996.9
    drowning E995.4
    explosion (direct pressure) (indirect pressure) (due to) E993.9
      depth charge E992.1

War operations — *continued*
  injury due to — *continued*
    explosion — *continued*
      improvised explosive device [IED]
        person borne E993.3
        roadside E993.5
        specified NEC E993.5
        transport vehicle (air) (land) (water) borne E993.4
        vehicle (air) (land) (water) borne E993.4
      marine mines (in harbor) (at sea) E992.2
      marine weapons E992.9
        specified NEC E992.8
      sea based artillery shell E992.3
      specified NEC E993.8
      torpedo E992.0
      unintentional (of own)
        autocannons E993.7
        automatic grenade launchers E993.7
        launch device discharge E993.7
        missile launchers E993.7
        munitions detonation (ammunition) (artillery) (mortars) E993.6
        small arms E993.7
  fragments (from) E991.9
    artillery E991.8
    artillery shells E991.4
    autocannons E991.8
    automatic grenade launchers [AGL] E991.8
    bombs E991.4
      antipersonnel E991.3
    detonation of unexploded ordnance [UXO] E991.4
    grenade E991.4
    guided missile E991.4
    improvised explosive device [IED]
      person borne E991.5
      roadside E991.7
      specified NEC E991.7
      transport vehicle (air) (land) (water) borne E991.6
      vehicle (air) (land) (water) borne E991.6
    land mine E991.4
    missile launchers E991.8
    mortars E991.8
    munitions (artillery shells) (bombs) (grenades) (rockets) (shells) E991.4
    rockets E991.4
    shells E991.4
    small arms E991.8
    specified NEC E991.9
    weapons (artillery) (autocannons) (mortars) (small arms) E991.8
  grenade E993.8
  guided missile E993.1
  hand to hand combat, unarmed E995.0
  improvised explosive device [IED]
    person borne E993.3
    roadside E993.5
    specified NEC E993.5
    transport vehicle (air) (land) (water) borne E993.4
    vehicle (air) (land) (water) borne E993.4
  inability to surface or obtain air E995.4

War operations — *continued*
  injury due to — *continued*
    land mine E993.8
    marine mines (in harbor) (at sea) E992.2
    marine weapons E992.9
      specified NEC E992.8
    mortar E993.2
    nuclear weapons E996.9
      beta burns E996.3
      blast debris E996.1
      blast pressure E996.0
      burns due to thermal radiation E996.2
      direct blast effect E996.0
      fallout exposure E996.3
      fireball effect E996.2
      flash burns E996.2
      heat effect E996.2
      indirect blast effect E996.1
      nuclear radiation effects E996.3
      radiation exposure (acute) E996.3
      radiation sickness E996.3
      secondary effects E996.3
      specified effects NEC E996.8
      thermal radiation effect E996.2
    piercing object E995.2
    restriction of airway, intentional E995.3
    sea based artillery shell E992.3
    shrapnel E991.9
    stave E995.1
    strangulation E995.3
    strike by blunt object (baton) (nightstick) (stave) E995.1
    submersion (accidental) (unintentional) E995.4
      intentional E995.3
    suffocation E995.3
      accidental E995.4
    torpedo E992.0
    underwater blast E992.9
    weapon of mass destruction [WMD] E997.3
  knife E995.2
  lacrimator (gas) (chemical) E997.2
  land mine (explosion) E993.8
    after cessation of hostilities E998.0
    fragments, injury by E991.4
  laser(s) E997.0
  late effect of E999.0
  lewisite E997.2
  lung irritant (chemical) (fumes) (gas) E997.2
  marine mine E992.2
  mine
    after cessation of hostilities E998.0
    at sea E992.2
    in harbor E992.2
    land (explosion) E993.8
      fragments, injury by E991.4
    marine E992.2
  missile (guided) (explosion) E993.1
    fragments, injury by E991.4
    marine E992.8
    nuclear (*see also* War operations, injury due to, nuclear weapons) E996.9
  mortar bomb (explosion) E993.2
    fragments, injury by E991.4
  mustard gas E997.2
  nerve gas E997.2
  phosgene E997.2
  piercing object E995.2
  poisoning (chemical) (fumes) (gas) E997.2

War operations — *continued*
  radiation, ionizing from nuclear explosion (*see also* War operations, injury due to, nuclear weapons) E996.3
  rocket (explosion) E993.8
    fragments, injury by E991.4
  saber, sabre E995.2
  screening smoke E997.8
  shell (aircraft) (artillery) (cannon) (land based) (explosion) E993.2
    fragments, injury by E991.4
    sea-based E992.3
  shooting E991.2
    after cessation of hostilities E998.8
    bullet(s) E991.2
      rubber E991.0
    pellet(s) (rifle) E991.1
    shrapnel E991.9
    submersion E995 ☑
    torpedo E992 ☑
  stave E995.2
  strike by blunt object (baton) (nightstick) (stave) E995.1
  submersion E995.4
    intentional E995.3
  sword E995.2
  torpedo E992.0
  unconventional warfare, except by nuclear weapon E997.9
    biological (warfare) E997.1
    gas, fumes, chemicals E997.2
    laser(s) E997.0
    specified type NEC E997.8
  underwater blast E992.9
  vesicant (chemical) (fumes) (gas) E997.2
  weapon burst E993.9
Washed
  away by flood — *see* Flood
  away by tidal wave — *see* Tidal wave
  off road by storm (transport vehicle) E908.9
  overboard E832 ☑
Weapon of mass destruction [WMD] E997.3
Weather exposure — *see also* Exposure
  cold E901.0
  hot E900.0
Weightlessness (causing injury) (effects of) (in spacecraft, real or simulated) E928.0
Wound (accidental) NEC — *see also* Injury E928.9
  battle (*see also* War operations) E995.9
  bayonet E920.3
    in
      legal intervention E974
      war operations E995.2
  gunshot — *see* Shooting
  incised — *see* Cut
  saber, sabre E920.3
    in war operations E995.2
Wrong
  body part, performance of correct operation (procedure) on E876.7
  device implanted into correct surgical site E876.5
  patient, performance of operation (procedure) on E876.6
  procedure (operation) performed on correct patient E876.5
  side, performance of correct operation (procedure) on E876.7
  site, performance of correct operation (procedure) on E876.7

☑ **Additional Digit Required** — Refer to the Tabular List for Digit Selection   ▽ **Subterms under main terms may continue to next column or page**

352 — Volume 2   ▶◀ **Revised Text**   ● **New Line**   ▲ **Revised Code**   **2013 ICD-9-CM**

Railway Accidents (E800-E807)

The following fourth-digit subdivisions are for use with categories E800-E807 to identify the injured person:

.0 **Railway employee**
Any person who by virtue of his employment in connection with a railway, whether by the railway company or not, is at increased risk of involvement in a railway accident, such as:
catering staff on train
postal staff on train
driver
railway fireman
guard
shunter
porter
sleeping car attendant

.1 **Passenger on railway**
Any authorized person traveling on a train, except a railway employee
EXCLUDES *intending passenger waiting at station (.8)*
unauthorized rider on railway vehicle (.8)

.2 **Pedestrian** See definition (r), E-Codes-2

.3 **Pedal cyclist** See definition (p), E-Codes-2

.8 **Other specified person** Intending passenger waiting at station
Unauthorized rider on railway vehicle

.9 **Unspecified person**

Motor Vehicle Traffic and Nontraffic Accidents (E810-E825)

The following fourth-digit subdivisions are for use with categories E810-E819 and E820-E825 to identify the injured person:

.0 **Driver of motor vehicle other than motorcycle** See definition (1), E-Codes-2

.1 **Passenger in motor vehicle other than motorcycle** See definition (1), E-Codes-2

.2 **Motorcyclist** See definition (1), E-Codes-2

.3 **Passenger on motorcycle** See definition (1), E-Codes-2

.4 **Occupant of streetcar**

.5 **Rider of animal; occupant of animal-drawn vehicle**

.6 **Pedal cyclist** See definition (p), E-Codes-2

.7 **Pedestrian** See definition (r), E-Codes-2

.8 **Other specified person**
Occupant of vehicle other than above
Person in railway train involved in accident
Unauthorized rider of motor vehicle

.9 **Unspecified person**

Other Road Vehicle Accidents (E826-E829)

(animal-drawn vehicle, streetcar, pedal cycle, and other nonmotor road vehicle accidents)

The following fourth-digit subdivisions are for use with categories E826-E829 to identify the injured person:

.0 **Pedestrian** See definition (r), E-Codes-2

.1 **Pedal cyclist** (does not apply to codes E827, E828, E829) See definition (p), E-Codes-2

.2 **Rider of animal** (does not apply to code E829)

.3 **Occupant of animal-drawn vehicle** (does not apply to codes E828, E829)

.4 **Occupant of streetcar**

.8 **Other specified person**

.9 **Unspecified person**

Water Transport Accidents (E830-E838)

The following fourth-digit subdivisions are for use with categories E830-E838 to identify the injured person:

.0 **Occupant of small boat, unpowered**

.1 **Occupant of small boat, powered** See definition (t), E-Codes-2
EXCLUDES *water skier (.4)*

.2 **Occupant of other watercraft — crew**
Persons:
engaged in operation of watercraft
providing passenger services [cabin attendants, ship's physician, catering personnel]
working on ship during voyage in other capacity [musician in band, operators of shops and beauty parlors]

.3 **Occupant of other watercraft — other than crew**
Passenger
Occupant of lifeboat, other than crew, after abandoning ship

.4 **Water skier**

.5 **Swimmer**

.6 **Dockers, stevedores**
Longshoreman employed on the dock in loading and unloading ships

.8 **Other specified person**
Immigration and custom officials on board ship
Persons:
accompanying passenger or member of crew visiting boat
Pilot (guiding ship into port)

.9 **Unspecified person**

Air and Space Transport Accidents (E840-E845)

The following fourth-digit subdivisions are for use with categories E840-E845 to identify the injured person:

.0 **Occupant of spacecraft**
Crew
Passenger (civilian)
(military) } in military aircraft [air force] [army] [national guard] [navy]
Troops

.1 **Occupant of military aircraft, any**
EXCLUDES *occupants of aircraft operated under jurisdiction of police departments (.5) parachutist (.7)*

.2 **Crew of commercial aircraft (powered) in surface to surface transport**

.3 **Other occupant of commercial aircraft (powered) in surface to surface transport**
Flight personnel:
not part of crew
on familiarization flight
Passenger on aircraft

.4 **Occupant of commercial aircraft (powered) in surface to air transport**
Occupant [crew] [passenger] of aircraft (powered) engaged in activities, such as:
air drops of emergency supplies
air drops of parachutists, except from military craft
crop dusting
lowering of construction material [bridge or telephone pole]
sky writing

.5 **Occupant of other powered aircraft**
Occupant [crew] [passenger] of aircraft (powered) engaged in activities, such as:
aerial spraying (crops)(fire retardants)
aerobatic flying
aircraft racing
rescue operation
storm surveillance
traffic suveillance
Occupant of private plane NOS

.6 **Occupant of unpowered aircraft, except parachutist**
Occupant of aircraft classifiable to E842

.7 **Parachutist (military)(other)**
Person making voluntary descent
EXCLUDES *person making descent after accident to aircraft (.1-.6)*

.8 **Ground crew, airline employee**
Persons employed at airfields (civil)(military) or launching pads, not occupants of aircraft

.9 **Other person**

☑ **Additional Digit Required — Refer to the Tabular List for Digit Selection**   ▽ **Subterms under main terms may continue to next column or page**

2013 ICD-9-CM   ▶◀ Revised Text   ● New Line   ▲ Revised Code   Volume 2 — 353

1. Infectious and Parasitic Diseases (001-139)

> **NOTE** Categories for "late effects" of infectious and parasitic diseases are to be found at 137-139.

> **INCLUDES** diseases generally recognized as communicable or transmissible as well as a few diseases of unknown but possibly infectious origin

> **EXCLUDES** *acute respiratory infections (460-466)*
> *carrier or suspected carrier of infectious organism (V02.0-V02.9)*
> *certain localized infections*
> *influenza (487.0-487.8, 488.01-488.19)*

Intestinal Infectious Diseases (001-009)

> **EXCLUDES** *helminthiases (120.0-129)*

✓4th 001 Cholera
DEF: An acute infectious enteritis caused by a potent enterotoxin produced by *Vibrio cholerae*; changes the permeability of the mucosa of the intestines and leads to diarrhea and dehydration.

001.0 Due to Vibrio cholerae

001.1 Due to Vibrio cholerae el tor

001.9 Cholera, unspecified

✓4th 002 Typhoid and paratyphoid fevers
DEF: Typhoid fever: an acute generalized illness caused by *Salmonella typhi*; clinical features are fever, headache, abdominal pain, cough, toxemia, leukopenia, abnormal pulse, rose spots on the skin, bacteremia, hyperplasia of intestinal lymph nodes, mesenteric lymphadenopathy, and Peyer's patches in the intestines.
DEF: Paratyphoid fever: a prolonged febrile illness, caused by salmonella serotypes other than *S. typhi*, especially *S. enteritidis* serotypes paratyphi A and B and *S. choleraesuis*.

002.0 Typhoid fever
Typhoid (fever) (infection) [any site]

002.1 Paratyphoid fever A

002.2 Paratyphoid fever B

002.3 Paratyphoid fever C

002.9 Paratyphoid fever, unspecified

✓4th 003 Other salmonella infections
> **INCLUDES** infection or food poisoning by Salmonella [any serotype]

DEF: Infections caused by a genus of gram-negative, anaerobic bacteria of the family *Enterobacteriaceae*; major symptoms are enteric fevers, acute gastroenteritis and septicemia.

003.0 Salmonella gastroenteritis
Salmonellosis

003.1 Salmonella septicemia

✓5th 003.2 Localized salmonella infections

    003.20 Localized salmonella infection, unspecified

    003.21 Salmonella meningitis

    003.22 Salmonella pneumonia

    003.23 Salmonella arthritis

    003.24 Salmonella osteomyelitis

    003.29 Other

003.8 Other specified salmonella infections

003.9 Salmonella infection, unspecified

✓4th 004 Shigellosis
> **INCLUDES** bacillary dysentery

DEF: Acute infectious dysentery caused by the genus *Shigella*, of the family *Enterobacteriaceae*; affecting the colon causing blood-stained stools, tenesmus, abdominal cramps and fever.

004.0 Shigella dysenteriae
Infection by group A Shigella (Schmitz) (Shiga)

004.1 Shigella flexneri
Infection by group B Shigella

004.2 Shigella boydii
Infection by group C Shigella

004.3 Shigella sonnei
Infection by group D Shigella

004.8 Other specified Shigella infections

004.9 Shigellosis, unspecified

✓4th 005 Other food poisoning (bacterial)
> **EXCLUDES** *salmonella infections (003.0-003.9)*
> *toxic effect of:*
>   *food contaminants (989.7)*
>   *noxious foodstuffs (988.0-988.9)*

DEF: Enteritis caused by ingesting contaminated foods and characterized by diarrhea, abdominal pain, vomiting; symptoms may be mild or life threatening.

005.0 Staphylococcal food poisoning
Staphylococcal toxemia specified as due to food

005.1 Botulism food poisoning
Botulism NOS
Food poisoning due to Clostridium botulinum
> **EXCLUDES** *infant botulism (040.41)*
> *wound botulism (040.42)*

005.2 Food poisoning due to Clostridium perfringens [C. welchii]
Enteritis necroticans

005.3 Food poisoning due to other Clostridia

005.4 Food poisoning due to Vibrio parahaemolyticus

✓5th 005.8 Other bacterial food poisoning
> **EXCLUDES** *salmonella food poisoning (003.0-003.9)*

    005.81 Food poisoning due to Vibrio vulnificus

    005.89 Other bacterial food poisoning
    Food poisoning due to Bacillus cereus

005.9 Food poisoning, unspecified

✓4th 006 Amebiasis
> **INCLUDES** infection due to Entamoeba histolytica

> **EXCLUDES** *amebiasis due to organisms other than Entamoeba histolytica (007.8)*

DEF: Infection of the large intestine caused by *Entamoeba histolytica*; usually asymptomatic but symptoms may range from mild diarrhea to profound life-threatening dysentery. Extraintestinal complications include hepatic abscess, which may rupture, causing life-threatening infections.

006.0 Acute amebic dysentery without mention of abscess
Acute amebiasis
DEF: Sudden, severe *Entamoeba histolytica* infection causing bloody stools.

006.1 Chronic intestinal amebiasis without mention of abscess
Chronic:
    amebiasis
    amebic dysentery

006.2 Amebic nondysenteric colitis
DEF: *Entamoeba histolytica* infection with inflamed colon but no dysentery.

006.3 Amebic liver abscess
Hepatic amebiasis

006.4 Amebic lung abscess
Amebic abscess of lung (and liver)

006.5 Amebic brain abscess
Amebic abscess of brain (and liver) (and lung)

006.6 Amebic skin ulceration
Cutaneous amebiasis

006.8 Amebic infection of other sites
Amebic: Ameboma
    appendicitis
    balanitis
> **EXCLUDES** *specific infections by free-living amebae (136.21-136.29)*

006.9 Amebiasis, unspecified
Amebiasis NOS

Infectious and Parasitic Diseases

007–009.0

√4th **007 Other protozoal intestinal diseases**
> INCLUDES protozoal:
>> colitis
>> diarrhea
>> dysentery

007.0 Balantidiasis
> Infection by Balantidium coli

007.1 Giardiasis
> Infection by Giardia lamblia
> Lambliasis

007.2 Coccidiosis
> Infection by Isospora belli and Isospora hominis
> Isosporiasis

007.3 Intestinal trichomoniasis
> DEF: Colitis, diarrhea, or dysentery caused by the protozoa Trichomonas.

007.4 Cryptosporidiosis
> DEF: An intestinal infection by protozoan parasites causing intractable diarrhea in patients with AIDS and other immunosuppressed individuals.
> AHA: 4Q, '97, 30

007.5 Cyclosporiasis
> DEF: An infection of the small intestine by the protozoal organism, Cyclospora cayetenanesis, spread to humans through ingestion of contaminated water or food. Symptoms include watery diarrhea, loss of appetite, increased gas, stomach cramps, nausea, vomiting, muscle aches, low grade fever, and fatigue.
> AHA: 4Q, '00, 38

007.8 Other specified protozoal intestinal diseases
> Amebiasis due to organisms other than Entamoeba histolytica

007.9 Unspecified protozoal intestinal disease
> Flagellate diarrhea
> Protozoal dysentery NOS

√4th **008 Intestinal infections due to other organisms**
> INCLUDES any condition classifiable to 009.0-009.3 with mention of the responsible organisms
> EXCLUDES food poisoning by these organisms (005.0-005.9)

√5th **008.0 Escherichia coli [E. coli]**
> AHA: 4Q, '92, 17

008.00 E. coli, unspecified
> E. coli enteritis NOS

008.01 Enteropathogenic E. coli
> DEF: E. coli causing inflammation of intestines.

008.02 Enterotoxigenic E. coli
> DEF: A toxic reaction to E. coli of the intestinal mucosa, causing voluminous watery secretions.

008.03 Enteroinvasive E. coli
> DEF: E. coli infection penetrating intestinal mucosa.

008.04 Enterohemorrhagic E. coli
> DEF: E. coli infection penetrating the intestinal mucosa, producing microscopic ulceration and bleeding.
> AHA: ▶4Q, '11, 83◄

008.09 Other intestinal E. coli infections

008.1 Arizona group of paracolon bacilli

008.2 Aerobacter aerogenes
> Enterobacter aeogenes

008.3 Proteus (mirabilis) (morganii)

√5th **008.4 Other specified bacteria**
> AHA: 4Q, '92, 18

008.41 Staphylococcus
> Staphylococcal enterocolitis

008.42 Pseudomonas
> AHA: 2Q, '89, 10

008.43 Campylobacter

008.44 Yersinia enterocolitica

008.45 Clostridium difficile
> Pseudomembranous colitis
> DEF: An overgrowth of a species of bacterium that is a part of the normal colon flora in human infants and sometimes in adults; produces a toxin that causes pseudomembranous enterocolitis.; typically is seen in patients undergoing antibiotic therapy.
> A04.7 Enterocolitis due to clostridium difficile   I-10

008.46 Other anaerobes
> Anaerobic enteritis NOS
> Bacteroides (fragilis)
> Gram-negative anaerobes

008.47 Other gram-negative bacteria
> Gram-negative enteritis NOS
> EXCLUDES gram-negative anaerobes (008.46)

008.49 Other
> AHA: 2Q, '89, 10; 1Q, '88, 6

008.5 Bacterial enteritis, unspecified

√5th **008.6 Enteritis due to specified virus**
> AHA: 4Q, '92, 18

008.61 Rotavirus

008.62 Adenovirus

008.63 Norwalk virus
> Norovirus
> Norwalk-like agent

008.64 Other small round viruses [SRVs]
> Small round virus NOS

008.65 Calicivirus
> DEF: Enteritis due to a subgroup of Picornaviruses.

008.66 Astrovirus

008.67 Enterovirus NEC
> Coxsackie virus
> Echovirus
> EXCLUDES poliovirus (045.0-045.9)

008.69 Other viral enteritis
> Torovirus
> AHA: 1Q, '03, 10

008.8 Other organism, not elsewhere classified
> Viral:
>> enteritis NOS
>> gastroenteritis
> EXCLUDES influenza with involvement of gastrointestinal tract (487.8, 488.09, 488.19)
> A08.4 Viral intestinal infection unspecified   I-10

√4th **009 Ill-defined intestinal infections**
> EXCLUDES diarrheal disease or intestinal infection due to specified organism (001.0-008.8)
>> diarrhea following gastrointestinal surgery (564.4)
>> intestinal malabsorption (579.0-579.9)
>> ischemic enteritis (557.0-557.9)
>> other noninfectious gastroenteritis and colitis (558.1-558.9)
>> regional enteritis (555.0-555.9)
>> ulcerative colitis (556)

009.0 Infectious colitis, enteritis, and gastroenteritis
> Colitis
> Enteritis } septic
> Gastroenteritis
> Dysentery:
>> NOS
>> catarrhal
>> hemorrhagic
> DEF: Colitis: An inflammation of mucous membranes of the colon.
> DEF: Enteritis: An inflammation of mucous membranes of the small intestine.
> DEF: Gastroenteritis: An inflammation of mucous membranes of stomach and intestines.
> AHA: 3Q, '99, 4
> A09 Infectious gastroenteritis and colitis unspec   I-10

N Newborn Age: 0   P Pediatric Age: 0-17   M Maternity Age: 12-55   A Adult Age: 15-124

009.1 Colitis, enteritis, and gastroenteritis of presumed infectious origin

> **EXCLUDES** colitis NOS (558.9)
> enteritis NOS (558.9)
> gastroenteritis NOS (558.9)
> **AHA:** 3Q, '99, 6

009.2 Infectious diarrhea
Diarrhea:
    dysenteric
    epidemic
Infectious diarrheal disease NOS

009.3 Diarrhea of presumed infectious origin

> **EXCLUDES** diarrhea NOS (787.91)
> **AHA:** N-D, '87, 7

Tuberculosis (010-018)

INCLUDES infection by Mycobacterium tuberculosis (human) (bovine)

EXCLUDES congenital tuberculosis (771.2)
late effects of tuberculosis (137.0-137.4)

The following fifth digit subclassification is for use with categories 010-018:

  0 **unspecified**
  1 **bacteriological or histological examination not done**
  2 **bacteriological or histological examination unknown (at present)**
  3 **tubercle bacilli found (in sputum) by microscopy**
  4 **tubercle bacilli not found (in sputum) by microscopy, but found by bacterial culture**
  5 **tubercle bacilli not found by bacteriological examination, but tuberculosis confirmed histologically**
  6 **tubercle bacilli not found by bacteriological or histological examination but tuberculosis confirmed by other methods [inoculation of animals]**

DEF: An infection by Mycobacterium tuberculosis causing the formation of small, rounded nodules, called tubercles, that can disseminate throughout the body via lymph and blood vessels. Localized tuberculosis is most often seen in the lungs.

010 Primary tuberculous infection
DEF: Tuberculosis of the lungs occurring when the patient is first infected.

§ **010.0 Primary tuberculous infection**
[0-6] **EXCLUDES** nonspecific reaction to test for tuberculosis without active tuberculosis (795.51-795.52)
positive PPD (795.51)
positive tuberculin skin test without active tuberculosis (795.51)
DEF: Hilar or paratracheal lymph node enlargement in pulmonary tuberculosis.

§ **010.1 Tuberculous pleurisy in primary progressive**
[0-6] **tuberculosis**
DEF: Inflammation and exudation in the lining of the tubercular lung.

§ **010.8 Other primary progressive tuberculosis**
[0-6] **EXCLUDES** tuberculous erythema nodosum (017.1)

§ **010.9 Primary tuberculous infection, unspecified**
[0-6]

011 Pulmonary tuberculosis
Use additional code to identify any associated silicosis (502)

§ **011.0 Tuberculosis of lung, infiltrative**
[0-6]

§ **011.1 Tuberculosis of lung, nodular**
[0-6]

§ **011.2 Tuberculosis of lung with cavitation**
[0-6]

§ **011.3 Tuberculosis of bronchus**
[0-6] **EXCLUDES** isolated bronchial tuberculosis (012.2)

§ **011.4 Tuberculous fibrosis of lung**
[0-6]

§ **011.5 Tuberculous bronchiectasis**
[0-6]

§ **011.6 Tuberculous pneumonia [any form]**
[0-6] **DEF:** Inflammatory pulmonary reaction to tuberculous cells.

§ **011.7 Tuberculous pneumothorax**
[0-6] **DEF:** Spontaneous rupture of damaged tuberculous pulmonary tissue.

§ **011.8 Other specified pulmonary tuberculosis**
[0-6]

§ **011.9 Pulmonary tuberculosis, unspecified**
[0-6] Respiratory tuberculosis NOS
Tuberculosis of lung NOS

012 Other respiratory tuberculosis
EXCLUDES respiratory tuberculosis, unspecified (011.9)

§ **012.0 Tuberculous pleurisy**
[0-6] Tuberculosis of pleura
Tuberculous empyema
Tuberculous hydrothorax
EXCLUDES pleurisy with effusion without mention of cause (511.9)
tuberculous pleurisy in primary progressive tuberculosis (010.1)
DEF: Inflammation and exudation in the lining of the tubercular lung.

§ **012.1 Tuberculosis of intrathoracic lymph nodes**
[0-6] Tuberculosis of lymph nodes:
    hilar
    mediastinal
    tracheobronchial
Tuberculous tracheobronchial adenopathy
EXCLUDES that specified as primary (010.0-010.9)

§ **012.2 Isolated tracheal or bronchial tuberculosis**
[0-6]

§ **012.3 Tuberculous laryngitis**
[0-6] Tuberculosis of glottis

§ **012.8 Other specified respiratory tuberculosis**
[0-6] Tuberculosis of:
    mediastinum
    nasopharynx
    nose (septum)
    sinus [any nasal]

013 Tuberculosis of meninges and central nervous system

§ **013.0 Tuberculous meningitis**
[0-6] Tuberculosis of meninges (cerebral) (spinal)
Tuberculous:
    leptomeningitis
    meningoencephalitis
EXCLUDES tuberculoma of meninges (013.1)

§ **013.1 Tuberculoma of meninges**
[0-6]

§ **013.2 Tuberculoma of brain**
[0-6] Tuberculosis of brain (current disease)

§ **013.3 Tuberculous abscess of brain**
[0-6]

§ **013.4 Tuberculoma of spinal cord**
[0-6]

§ **013.5 Tuberculous abscess of spinal cord**
[0-6]

§ **013.6 Tuberculous encephalitis or myelitis**
[0-6]

§ **013.8 Other specified tuberculosis of central nervous system**
[0-6]

§ **013.9 Unspecified tuberculosis of central nervous system**
[0-6] Tuberculosis of central nervous system NOS

014 Tuberculosis of intestines, peritoneum, and mesenteric glands

§ **014.0 Tuberculous peritonitis**
[0-6] Tuberculous ascites
DEF: Tuberculous inflammation of the membrane lining the abdomen.

---

§ Requires fifth digit. Valid digits are in [brackets] under each code. See beginning of section 010-018 for codes and definitions.

Infectious and Parasitic Diseases

014.8–018

§ ✓5ᵗʰ **014.8 Other**
[0-6]   Tuberculosis (of):
      anus
      intestine (large) (small)
      mesenteric glands
      rectum
      retroperitoneal (lymph nodes)
    Tuberculous enteritis

✓4ᵗʰ **015   Tuberculosis of bones and joints**
    Use additional code to identify manifestation, as:
    tuberculous:
      arthropathy (711.4)
      necrosis of bone (730.8)
      osteitis (730.8)
      osteomyelitis (730.8)
      synovitis (727.01)
      tenosynovitis (727.01)

§ ✓5ᵗʰ **015.0 Vertebral column**
[0-6]   Pott's disease
      Use additional code to identify manifestation, as:
       curvature of spine [Pott's] (737.4)
       kyphosis (737.4)
       spondylitis (720.81)

§ ✓5ᵗʰ **015.1 Hip**
[0-6]

§ ✓5ᵗʰ **015.2 Knee**
[0-6]

§ ✓5ᵗʰ **015.5 Limb bones**
[0-6]   Tuberculous dactylitis

§ ✓5ᵗʰ **015.6 Mastoid**
[0-6]   Tuberculous mastoiditis

§ ✓5ᵗʰ **015.7 Other specified bone**
[0-6]

§ ✓5ᵗʰ **015.8 Other specified joint**
[0-6]

§ ✓5ᵗʰ **015.9 Tuberculosis of unspecified bones and joints**
[0-6]

✓4ᵗʰ **016   Tuberculosis of genitourinary system**

§ ✓5ᵗʰ **016.0 Kidney**
[0-6]   Renal tuberculosis
      Use additional code to identify manifestation, as:
      tuberculous:
       nephropathy (583.81)
       pyelitis (590.81)
       pyelonephritis (590.81)

§ ✓5ᵗʰ **016.1 Bladder**
[0-6]

§ ✓5ᵗʰ **016.2 Ureter**
[0-6]

§ ✓5ᵗʰ **016.3 Other urinary organs**
[0-6]

§ ✓5ᵗʰ **016.4 Epididymis**   ♂
[0-6]

§ ✓5ᵗʰ **016.5 Other male genital organs**   ♂
[0-6]   Use additional code to identify manifestation, as:
      tuberculosis of:
       prostate (601.4)
       seminal vesicle (608.81)
       testis (608.81)

§ ✓5ᵗʰ **016.6 Tuberculous oophoritis and salpingitis**   ♀
[0-6]

§ ✓5ᵗʰ **016.7 Other female genital organs**   ♀
[0-6]   Tuberculous:
      cervicitis
      endometritis

§ ✓5ᵗʰ **016.9 Genitourinary tuberculosis, unspecified**
[0-6]

✓4ᵗʰ **017   Tuberculosis of other organs**

§ ✓5ᵗʰ **017.0 Skin and subcutaneous cellular tissue**
[0-6]   Lupus: Tuberculosis:
      exedens   colliquativa
      vulgaris   cutis
    Scrofuloderma   lichenoides
                      papulonecrotica
                      verrucosa cutis

      EXCLUDES *lupus erythematosus (695.4)*
              disseminated (710.0)
        lupus NOS (710.0)
        nonspecific reaction to test for tuberculosis without
              active tuberculosis (795.51-795.52)
        positive PPD (795.51)
        positive tuberculin skin test without active
              tuberculosis (795.51)

§ ✓5ᵗʰ **017.1 Erythema nodosum with hypersensitivity**
[0-6] **reaction in tuberculosis**
    Bazin's disease
    Erythema:
      induratum
      nodosum, tuberculous
    Tuberculosis indurativa

      EXCLUDES *erythema nodosum NOS (695.2)*

      DEF: Tender, inflammatory, bilateral nodules appearing on the shins and thought to be an allergic reaction to tuberculotoxin.

§ ✓5ᵗʰ **017.2 Peripheral lymph nodes**
[0-6]   Scrofula
    Scrofulous abscess
    Tuberculous adenitis

      EXCLUDES *tuberculosis of lymph nodes:*
            bronchial and mediastinal (012.1)
            mesenteric and retroperitoneal (014.8)
            tuberculous tracheobronchial adenopathy (012.1)

      DEF: Scrofula: Old name for tuberculous cervical lymphadenitis.

§ ✓5ᵗʰ **017.3 Eye**
[0-6]   Use additional code to identify manifestation, as:
      tuberculous:
       chorioretinitis, disseminated (363.13)
       episcleritis (379.09)
       interstitial keratitis (370.59)
       iridocyclitis, chronic (364.11)
       keratoconjunctivitis (phlyctenular) (370.31)

§ ✓5ᵗʰ **017.4 Ear**
[0-6]   Tuberculosis of ear
    Tuberculous otitis media

      EXCLUDES *tuberculous mastoiditis (015.6)*

§ ✓5ᵗʰ **017.5 Thyroid gland**
[0-6]

§ ✓5ᵗʰ **017.6 Adrenal glands**
[0-6]   Addison's disease, tuberculous

§ ✓5ᵗʰ **017.7 Spleen**
[0-6]

§ ✓5ᵗʰ **017.8 Esophagus**
[0-6]

§ ✓5ᵗʰ **017.9 Other specified organs**
[0-6]   Use additional code to identify manifestation, as:
      tuberculosis of:
       endocardium [any valve] (424.91)
       myocardium (422.0)
       pericardium (420.0)

✓4ᵗʰ **018   Miliary tuberculosis**
      INCLUDES tuberculosis:
           disseminated
           generalized
           miliary, whether of a single specified site, multiple sites,
              or unspecified site
           polyserositis

      DEF: A form of tuberculosis caused by caseous material carried through the bloodstream planting seedlike tubercles in various body organs.

---

§   Requires fifth digit. Valid digits are in [brackets] under each code. See beginning of section 010-018 for codes and definitions.

Ⓝ Newborn Age: 0   Ⓟ Pediatric Age: 0-17   Ⓜ Maternity Age: 12-55   Ⓐ Adult Age: 15-124

§ ✓5ᵗʰ **018.0 Acute miliary tuberculosis**
[0-6]

§ ✓5ᵗʰ **018.8 Other specified miliary tuberculosis**
[0-6]

§ ✓5ᵗʰ **018.9 Miliary tuberculosis, unspecified**
[0-6]

Zoonotic Bacterial Diseases (020-027)

✓4ᵗʰ **020 Plague**
> INCLUDES infection by Yersinia [Pasteurella] pestis

020.0 Bubonic
> DEF: Most common acute and severe form of plague characterized by lymphadenopathy (buboes), chills, fever and headache.

020.1 Cellulocutaneous
> DEF: Plague characterized by inflammation and necrosis of skin.

020.2 Septicemic
> DEF: Plague characterized by massive infection in the bloodstream.

020.3 Primary pneumonic
> DEF: Plague characterized by massive pulmonary infection.

020.4 Secondary pneumonic
> DEF: Lung infection as a secondary complication of plague.

020.5 Pneumonic, unspecified

020.8 Other specified types of plague
> Abortive plague
> Ambulatory plague
> Pestis minor

020.9 Plague, unspecified

✓4ᵗʰ **021 Tularemia**
> INCLUDES deerfly fever
> infection by Francisella [Pasteurella] tularensis
> rabbit fever

> DEF: A febrile disease transmitted by the bites of deer flies, fleas and ticks, by inhalations of aerosolized *F. tularensis* or by ingestion of contaminated food or water; patients quickly develop fever, chills, weakness, headache, backache and malaise.

021.0 Ulceroglandular tularemia
> DEF: Lesions occur at the site *Francisella tularensis* organism enters body, usually the fingers or hands.

021.1 Enteric tularemia
> Tularemia:
> cryptogenic
> intestinal
> typhoidal

021.2 Pulmonary tularemia
> Bronchopneumonic tularemia

021.3 Oculoglandular tularemia
> DEF: Painful conjunctival infection by *Francisella tularensis* organism with possible corneal, preauricular lymph, or lacrimal involvement.

021.8 Other specified tularemia
> Tularemia:
> generalized or disseminated
> glandular

021.9 Unspecified tularemia

✓4ᵗʰ **022 Anthrax**
> DEF: An bacterial disease usually transmitted by contact with infected animals or their discharges; primary routes of inoculation are cutaneous, gastrointestinal and by inhalation.
> AHA: 4Q '02, 70

022.0 Cutaneous anthrax
> Malignant pustule

022.1 Pulmonary anthrax
> Respiratory anthrax
> Wool-sorters' disease

022.2 Gastrointestinal anthrax

022.3 Anthrax septicemia

022.8 Other specified manifestations of anthrax

022.9 Anthrax, unspecified

✓4ᵗʰ **023 Brucellosis**
> INCLUDES fever:
> Malta
> Mediterranean
> undulant

> DEF: An infectious disease caused by gram-negative, aerobic coccobacilli organisms transmitted to humans through contact with infected tissue or dairy products; fever, sweating, weakness and aching are symptoms.

023.0 Brucella melitensis
> DEF: Infection from direct or indirect contact with infected sheep or goats.

023.1 Brucella abortus
> DEF: Infection from direct or indirect contact with infected cattle.

023.2 Brucella suis
> DEF: Infection from direct or indirect contact with infected swine.

023.3 Brucella canis
> DEF: Infection from direct or indirect contact with infected dogs.

023.8 Other brucellosis
> Infection by more than one organism

023.9 Brucellosis, unspecified

024 Glanders
> Infection by:
> Actinobacillus mallei
> Malleomyces mallei
> Pseudomonas mallei
> Farcy
> Malleus
> DEF: Equine infection causing mucosal inflammation and skin ulcers in humans.

025 Melioidosis
> Infection by:
> Malleomyces pseudomallei
> Pseudomonas pseudomallei
> Whitmore's bacillus
> Pseudoglanders
> DEF: Rare infection caused by *Pseudomonas pseudomallei;* clinical symptoms range from localized infection to fatal septicemia.

✓4ᵗʰ **026 Rat-bite fever**

026.0 Spirillary fever
> Rat-bite fever due to Spirillum minor [S. minus]
> Sodoku

026.1 Streptobacillary fever
> Epidemic arthritic erythema
> Haverhill fever
> Rat-bite fever due to Streptobacillus moniliformis

026.9 Unspecified rat-bite fever

✓4ᵗʰ **027 Other zoonotic bacterial diseases**

027.0 Listeriosis
> Infection } by Listeria monocytogenes
> Septicemia }
> Use additional code to identify manifestation, as meningitis (320.7)
> EXCLUDES *congenital listeriosis (771.2)*

027.1 Erysipelothrix infection
> Erysipeloid (of Rosenbach)
> Infection } by Erysipelothrix insidiosa
> Septicemia } [E. rhusiopathiae]
> DEF: Usually associated with handling of fish, meat, or poultry; symptoms range from localized inflammation to septicemia.

027.2 Pasteurellosis
> Pasteurella pseudotuberculosis infection
> Mesenteric adenitis }
> Septic infection (cat bite) } by Pasteurella multocida
> (dog bite) } [P. septica]
> EXCLUDES infection by:
> *Francisella [Pasteurella] tularensis (021.0-021.9)*
> *Yersinia [Pasteurella] pestis (020.0-020.9)*
> DEF: Swelling, abscesses, or septicemia from *Pasteurella multocida,* commonly transmitted to humans by a dog or cat scratch.

027.8 Other specified zoonotic bacterial diseases

---

§ Requires fifth digit. Valid digits are in [brackets] under each code. See beginning of section 010-018 for codes and definitions.

✓4ᵗʰ / ✓5ᵗʰ Additional Digit Required   Unspecified Code   Other Specified Code   Manifestation Code   ▶◀ Revised Text   ● New Code   ▲ Revised Code Title

2013 ICD-9-CM   **Volume 1 – 5**

027.9　Unspecified zoonotic bacterial disease

Other Bacterial Diseases (030-041)

EXCLUDES *bacterial venereal diseases (098.0-099.9)*
bartonellosis (088.0)

✓4ᵗʰ **030　Leprosy**
INCLUDES Hansen's disease
infection by Mycobacterium leprae

030.0　Lepromatous [type L]
Lepromatous leprosy (macular) (diffuse) (infiltrated) (nodular) (neuritic)
DEF: Infectious, disseminated leprosy bacilli with lesions and deformities.

030.1　Tuberculoid [type T]
Tuberculoid leprosy (macular) (maculoanesthetic) (major) (minor) (neuritic)
DEF: Relatively benign, self-limiting leprosy with neuralgia and scales.

030.2　Indeterminate [group I]
Indeterminate [uncharacteristic] leprosy (macular) (neuritic)
DEF: Uncharacteristic leprosy, frequently an early manifestation.

030.3　Borderline [group B]
Borderline or dimorphous leprosy (infiltrated) (neuritic)
DEF: Transitional form of leprosy, neither lepromatous nor tuberculoid.

030.8　Other specified leprosy

030.9　Leprosy, unspecified

✓4ᵗʰ **031　Diseases due to other mycobacteria**

031.0　Pulmonary
Battey disease
Infection by Mycobacterium:
avium
intracellulare [Battey bacillus]
kansasii

031.1　Cutaneous
Buruli ulcer
Infection by Mycobacterium:
marinum [M. balnei]
ulcerans

031.2　Disseminated
Disseminated mycobacterium avium-intracellulare complex (DMAC)
Mycobacterium avium-intracellulare complex (MAC) bacteremia
DEF: Disseminated mycobacterium avium-intracellulare complex (DMAC): A serious systemic form of MAC commonly observed in patients in the late course of AIDS.
DEF: Mycobacterium avium-intracellulare complex (MAC) bacterium: Human pulmonary disease, lymphadenitis in children and systemic disease in immunocompromised individuals caused by a slow growing, gram-positive, aerobic organism.
AHA: 4Q, '97, 31

031.8　Other specified mycobacterial diseases

031.9　Unspecified diseases due to mycobacteria
Atypical mycobacterium infection NOS

✓4ᵗʰ **032　Diphtheria**
INCLUDES infection by Corynebacterium diphtheriae

032.0　Faucial diphtheria
Membranous angina, diphtheritic
DEF: Diphtheria of the throat.

032.1　Nasopharyngeal diphtheria

032.2　Anterior nasal diphtheria

032.3　Laryngeal diphtheria
Laryngotracheitis, diphtheritic

✓5ᵗʰ **032.8　Other specified diphtheria**

032.81　Conjunctival diphtheria
Pseudomembranous diphtheritic conjunctivitis

032.82　Diphtheritic myocarditis

032.83　Diphtheritic peritonitis

032.84　Diphtheritic cystitis

032.85　Cutaneous diphtheria

032.89　Other

032.9　Diphtheria, unspecified

✓4ᵗʰ **033　Whooping cough**
INCLUDES pertussis
Use additional code to identify any associated pneumonia (484.3)
DEF: An acute, highly contagious respiratory tract infection caused by *Bordetella pertussis* and *B. bronchiseptica*; characteristic paroxysmal cough.

033.0　Bordetella pertussis [B. pertussis]

033.1　Bordetella parapertussis [B. parapertussis]

033.8　Whooping cough due to other specified organism
Bordetella bronchiseptica [B. bronchiseptica]

033.9　Whooping cough, unspecified organism

✓4ᵗʰ **034　Streptococcal sore throat and scarlet fever**

034.0　Streptococcal sore throat

Septic:	Streptococcal:
angina	laryngitis
sore throat	pharyngitis
Streptococcal:	tonsillitis
angina	

J02.0 Streptococcal pharyngitis　　　　I-10

034.1　Scarlet fever
Scarlatina
EXCLUDES *parascarlatina (057.8)*
DEF: Streptococcal infection and fever with red rash spreading from trunk.

035　Erysipelas
EXCLUDES *postpartum or puerperal erysipelas (670.8)*
DEF: An acute superficial cellulitis involving the dermal lymphatics; it is often caused by group A streptococci.

✓4ᵗʰ **036　Meningococcal infection**

036.0　Meningococcal meningitis
Cerebrospinal fever (meningococcal)
Meningitis:
cerebrospinal
epidemic

036.1　Meningococcal encephalitis

036.2　Meningococcemia
Meningococcal septicemia

036.3　Waterhouse-Friderichsen syndrome, meningococcal
Meningococcal hemorrhagic adrenalitis
Meningococcic adrenal syndrome
Waterhouse-Friderichsen syndrome NOS

✓5ᵗʰ **036.4　Meningococcal carditis**

036.40　Meningococcal carditis, unspecified

036.41　Meningococcal pericarditis
DEF: Meningococcal infection of the outer membrane of the heart.

036.42　Meningococcal endocarditis
DEF: Meningococcal infection of the membranes lining the cavities of the heart.

036.43　Meningococcal myocarditis
DEF: Meningococcal infection of the muscle of the heart.

✓5ᵗʰ **036.8　Other specified meningococcal infections**

036.81　Meningococcal optic neuritis

036.82　Meningococcal arthropathy

036.89　Other

036.9　Meningococcal infection, unspecified
Meningococcal infection NOS

Ⓝ Newborn Age: 0　　　Ⓟ Pediatric Age: 0-17　　　Ⓜ Maternity Age: 12-55　　　Ⓐ Adult Age: 15-124

037 Tetanus

> **EXCLUDES** tetanus:
> complicating:
> abortion (634-638 with .0, 639.0)
> ectopic or molar pregnancy (639.0)
> neonatorum (771.3)
> puerperal (670.8)

DEF: An acute, often fatal, infectious disease caused by the anaerobic, spore-forming bacillus *Clostridium tetani;* the bacillus enters the body through a contaminated wound, burns, surgical wounds, or cutaneous ulcers. Symptoms: lockjaw, spasms, seizures, and paralysis.

✓4th 038 Septicemia

Use additional code for systemic inflammatory response syndrome (SIRS) (995.91-995.92)

> **EXCLUDES** bacteremia (790.7)
> during labor (659.3)
> following ectopic or molar pregnancy (639.0)
> following infusion, injection, transfusion, or vaccination (999.3)
> postpartum, puerperal (670)
> septicemia (sepsis) of newborn (771.81)
> that complicating abortion (634-638 with .0, 639.0)

DEF: A systemic disease associated with the presence and persistence of pathogenic microorganisms or their toxins in the blood.
AHA: ▶1Q, '12, 19;◀ 2Q, '10, 4; 2Q, '04, 16; 4Q, '88, 10; 3Q, '88, 12
TIP: When septicemia is due to a complication of care, sequence the complication code first (e.g., due to device or injury).

038.0 Streptococcal septicemia
AHA: 4Q, '03, 79; 2Q, '96, 5

✓5th 038.1 Staphylococcal septicemia
AHA: 4Q, '97, 32

038.10 Staphylococcal septicemia, unspecified

038.11 Methicillin susceptible Staphylococcus aureus septicemia
MSSA septicemia
Staphylococcus aureus septicemia NOS
AHA: 4Q, '08, 69-70; 1Q, '05, 7; 2Q, '00, 5; 4Q, '98, 42
A41.0 Sepsis due to Staphylococcus aureus   I-10

038.12 Methicillin resistant Staphylococcus aureus septicemia
AHA: 4Q, '11,153; 3Q, '11, 15; 4Q, '08, 69-73

038.19 Other staphylococcal septicemia
AHA: 2Q, '00, 5
A41.1 Sepsis due to other spec Staphylococcus   I-10

038.2 Pneumococcal septicemia [Streptococcus pneumoniae septicemia]
AHA: 2Q, '96, 5; 1Q, '91, 13

038.3 Septicemia due to anaerobes
Septicemia due to bacteroides
> **EXCLUDES** gas gangrene (040.0)
> that due to anaerobic streptococci (038.0)

DEF: Infection of blood by microorganisms that thrive without oxygen.

✓5th 038.4 Septicemia due to other gram-negative organisms
DEF: Infection of blood by microorganisms categorized as gram-negative by Gram's method of staining for identification of bacteria.

038.40 Gram-negative organism, unspecified
Gram-negative septicemia NOS

038.41 Hemophilus influenzae [H. influenzae]

038.42 Escherichia coli [E. coli]
AHA: 4Q, '03, 73
A41.51 Sepsis due to Escherichia coli [E coli]   I-10

038.43 Pseudomonas

038.44 Serratia

038.49 Other
A41.59 Other Gram-negative sepsis   I-10

038.8 Other specified septicemias
> **EXCLUDES** septicemia (due to):
> anthrax (022.3)
> gonococcal (098.89)
> herpetic (054.5)
> meningococcal (036.2)
> septicemic plague (020.2)

038.9 Unspecified septicemia
Septicemia NOS
> **EXCLUDES** bacteremia NOS (790.7)

AHA: 4Q, '07, 97; 2Q, '05, 18-19; 2Q, '04, 16; 4Q, '03, 79; 2Q, '00, 3; 3Q, '99, 5, 9; 1Q, '98, 5; 3Q, '96, 16; 2Q, '96, 6
TIP: Ensure that documentation includes clinical evidence of systemic infection; do not code if documentation indicates "urosepsis" only.
A41.9 Sepsis unspecified   I-10

✓4th 039 Actinomycotic infections
> **INCLUDES** actinomycotic mycetoma
> infection by Actinomycetales, such as species of Actinomyces, Actinomadura, Nocardia, Streptomyces
> maduromycosis (actinomycotic)
> schizomycetoma (actinomycotic)

DEF: Inflammatory lesions and abscesses at site of infection by *Actinomyces israelii.*

039.0 Cutaneous
Erythrasma
Trichomycosis axillaris

039.1 Pulmonary
Thoracic actinomycosis

039.2 Abdominal

039.3 Cervicofacial

039.4 Madura foot
> **EXCLUDES** madura foot due to mycotic infection (117.4)

039.8 Of other specified sites

039.9 Of unspecified site
Actinomycosis NOS
Maduromycosis NOS
Nocardiosis NOS

✓4th 040 Other bacterial diseases
> **EXCLUDES** bacteremia NOS (790.7)
> bacterial infection NOS (041.9)

040.0 Gas gangrene
Gas bacillus infection or gangrene
Infection by Clostridium:
  histolyticum
  oedematiens
  perfringens [welchii]
  septicum
  sordellii
Malignant edema
Myonecrosis, clostridial
Myositis, clostridial
AHA: 1Q, '95, 11

040.1 Rhinoscleroma
DEF: Growths on the nose and nasopharynx caused by *Klebsiella rhinoscleromatis.*

040.2 Whipple's disease
Intestinal lipodystrophy

040.3 Necrobacillosis
DEF: Infection with *Fusobacterium necrophorum* causing abscess or necrosis.
AHA: 4Q, '07, 85

Infectious and Parasitic Diseases

040.4–041.9

√5ᵗʰ **040.4 Other specified botulism**
Non-foodborne intoxication due to toxins of Clostridium
botulinum [C. botulinum]
> **EXCLUDES** botulism NOS (005.1)
> food poisoning due to toxins of Clostridium
> botulinum (005.1)

040.41 Infant botulism   P
> **DEF:** Colonization of Clostridium botulinum spores in the
> large intestine; release of neurotoxins results in
> constipation; may progress to neuromuscular paralysis;
> affects infants of less than six months.
> **AHA:** 4Q, '07, 60

040.42 Wound botulism
Non-foodborne botulism NOS
> Use additional code to identify complicated open
> wound
> **AHA:** 4Q, '07, 60

√5ᵗʰ **040.8 Other specified bacterial diseases**

040.81 Tropical pyomyositis

040.82 Toxic shock syndrome
> Use additional code to identify the organism
> **DEF:** Syndrome caused by staphylococcal exotoxin that may
> rapidly progress to severe and intractable shock; symptoms
> include sunburn-like rash with peeling of skin on palms
> and soles, sudden onset high fever, vomiting, diarrhea,
> myalgia, and hypotension.
> **AHA:** 4Q, '02, 44

040.89 Other
> **AHA:** N-D, '86, 7

√4ᵗʰ **041 Bacterial infection in conditions classified elsewhere and of
unspecified site**
> **NOTE** This category is provided to be used as an additional code to
> identify the bacterial agent in diseases classified elsewhere.
> This category will also be used to classify bacterial infections of
> unspecified nature or site.
> **EXCLUDES** septicemia (038.0-038.9)
> **AHA:** 2Q, '01, 12; J-A, '84, 19

√5ᵗʰ **041.0 Streptococcus**

041.00 Streptococcus, unspecified

041.01 Group A
> **AHA:** 1Q, '02, 3

041.02 Group B
> **B95.1** Streptococcus group B cause of dz class   I-10
> elsewhere

041.03 Group C

041.04 Group D [Enterococcus]
> **B95.2** Enterococcus as the cause of dz class elsewhere   I-10

041.05 Group G

041.09 Other Streptococcus
> **B95.4** Oth streptococcus cause of dz class elsewhere   I-10

√5ᵗʰ **041.1 Staphylococcus**

041.10 Staphylococcus, unspecified
> **AHA:** 2Q, '06, 15

041.11 Methicillin susceptible Staphylococcus aureus
MSSA
Staphylococcus aureus NOS
> **AHA:** 4Q, '08, 69-70; 2Q, '06, 16; 4Q, '03, 104, 106; 2Q, '01, 11;
> 4Q, '98, 42, 54; 4Q, '97, 32
> **B95.6** Staphylococcus aureus cause dz class   I-10
> elsewhere

041.12 Methicillin resistant Staphylococcus aureus
Methicillin-resistant staphylococcus aureus (MRSA)
> **AHA:** 4Q, '09, 98; 4Q, '08, 69-70, 73
> **TIP:** Do not assign if combination code (with localized
> infection) available, or if only colonization or carrier status
> documented.

041.19 Other Staphylococcus
> **AHA:** 2Q, '11, 7; 2Q, '08, 3
> **B95.7** Other staphylococcus cause of dz class elsewhere   I-10

041.2 Pneumococcus

041.3 Klebsiella pneumoniae
> **AHA:** 4Q, '08, 149

√5ᵗʰ **041.4 Escherichia coli [E. coli]**
> **AHA:** ▶4Q, '11, 81-83◀

**041.41 Shiga toxin-producing Escherichia coli [E. coli]
(STEC) O157**
> E. coli O157:H- (nonmotile) with confirmation of
> Shiga toxin
> E. coli O157 with confirmation of Shiga toxin when
> H antigen is unknown, or is not H7
> O157:H7 Escherichia coli [E.coli] with or without
> confirmation of Shiga toxin-production
> Shiga toxin-producing Escherichia coli [E.coli]
> O157:H7 with or without confirmation of Shiga
> toxin-production
> STEC O157:H7 with or without confirmation of Shiga
> toxin-production
> **AHA:** ▶4Q, '11, 83◀

**041.42 Other specified Shiga toxin-producing
Escherichia coli [E. coli] (STEC)**
> Non-O157 Shiga toxin-producing Escherichia coli
> [E.coli]
> Non-O157 Shiga toxin-producing Escherichia coli
> [E.coli] with known O group

**041.43 Shiga toxin-producing Escherichia coli [E. coli]
(STEC), unspecified**
> Shiga toxin-producing Escherichia coli [E. coli] with
> unspecified O group
> STEC NOS

041.49 Other and unspecified Escherichia coli [E. coli]
> Escherichia coli [E. coli] NOS
> Non-Shiga toxin-producing E. Coli
> **AHA:** ▶4Q, '11, 155◀
> **B96.2** Escherichia coli cause of dz class elsewhere   I-10

041.5 Hemophilus influenzae [H. influenzae]

041.6 Proteus (mirabilis) (morganii)

041.7 Pseudomonas
> **AHA:** 1Q, '10, 9; 4Q, '02, 45
> **B96.5** Pseudomonas as the cause of dz class elsewhere   I-10

√5ᵗʰ **041.8 Other specified bacterial infections**

041.81 Mycoplasma
Eaton's agent
Pleuropneumonia-like organisms [PPLO]

041.82 Bacteroides fragilis
> **DEF:** Anaerobic gram-negative bacilli of the gastrointestinal
> tract; frequently implicated in intra-abdominal infection;
> commonly resistant to antibiotics.

041.83 Clostridium perfringens

041.84 Other anaerobes
Gram-negative anaerobes
> **EXCLUDES** Helicobacter pylori (041.86)

041.85 Other gram-negative organisms
Aerobacter aerogenes
Gram-negative bacteria NOS
Mima polymorpha
Serratia
> **EXCLUDES** gram-negative anaerobes (041.84)
> **AHA:** 1Q, '95, 18

041.86 Helicobacter pylori [H. pylori]
> **AHA:** 4Q, '95, 60
> **B96.81** Helicobacter pylori cause of dz class elsewhere   I-10

041.89 Other specified bacteria
> **AHA:** 2Q, '06, 7; 2Q, '03, 7
> **A49.8** Other bacterial infections of unspec site   I-10

041.9 Bacterial infection, unspecified
> **AHA:** 2Q, '91, 9

N Newborn Age: 0   P Pediatric Age: 0-17   M Maternity Age: 12-55   A Adult Age: 15-124

Human Immunodeficiency Virus (HIV) Infection (042)

042 Human immunodeficiency virus [HIV] disease
Acquired immune deficiency syndrome
Acquired immunodeficiency syndrome
AIDS
AIDS-like syndrome
AIDS-related complex
ARC
HIV infection, symptomatic
Use additional code(s) to identify all manifestations of HIV
Use additional code to identify HIV-2 infection (079.53)

EXCLUDES asymptomatic HIV infection status (V08)
exposure to HIV virus (V01.79)
nonspecific serologic evidence of HIV (795.71)

AHA: 3Q, '10, 13; 4Q, '07, 63; 3Q, '06, 15; 1Q, '05, 7; 2Q, '04, 11; 1Q, '04, 5; 1Q, '03, 15; 1Q, '99, 14; 4Q, '97, 30, 31; 1Q, '93, 21; 2Q, '92, 11; 3Q, '90, 17; J-A, '87, 8
TIP: Code only confirmed cases of HIV infection/illness; may be coded from provider's diagnostic statement.
B20 Human immunodeficiency virus [HIV] disease

Poliomyelitis and Other Non-Arthropod-Borne Viral Diseases and Prion Diseases of Central Nervous System (045-049)

045 Acute poliomyelitis

EXCLUDES late effects of acute poliomyelitis (138)

The following fifth-digit subclassification is for use with category 045:
0 poliovirus, unspecified type
1 poliovirus type I
2 poliovirus type II
3 poliovirus type III

§ **045.0 Acute paralytic poliomyelitis specified as bulbar**
[0-3] Infantile paralysis (acute) } specified as
Poliomyelitis (acute) (anterior) } bulbar
Polioencephalitis (acute) (bulbar)
Polioencephalomyelitis (acute) (anterior) (bulbar)
DEF: Acute paralytic infection occurring where the brain merges with the spinal cord; affecting breathing, swallowing, and heart rate.

§ **045.1 Acute poliomyelitis with other paralysis**
[0-3] Paralysis:
acute atrophic, spinal
infantile, paralytic
Poliomyelitis (acute) } with paralysis except
anterior } bulbar
epidemic
DEF: Paralytic infection affecting peripheral or spinal nerves.

§ **045.2 Acute nonparalytic poliomyelitis**
[0-3] Poliomyelitis (acute)
anterior } specified as nonparalytic
epidemic
DEF: Nonparalytic infection causing pain, stiffness, and paresthesias.

§ **045.9 Acute poliomyelitis, unspecified**
[0-3] Infantile paralysis
Poliomyelitis (acute) } unspecified whether
anterior } paralytic or
epidemic } nonparalytic

046 Slow virus infections and prion diseases of central nervous system

046.0 Kuru
DEF: A chronic, progressive, fatal nervous system disorder; clinical symptoms include cerebellar ataxia, trembling, spasticity and progressive dementia.

046.1 Jakob-Creutzfeldt disease
Use additional code to identify dementia:
with behavioral disturbance (294.11)
without behavioral disturbance (294.10)

046.11 Variant Creutzfeldt-Jakob disease
vCJD
AHA: 4Q, '08, 73-75

046.19 Other and unspecified Creutzfeldt-Jacob disease
CJD
Familial Creutzfeldt-Jakob disease
Iatrogenic Creutzfeldt-Jakob disease
Jakob-Creutzfeldt disease, unspecified
Sporadic Creutzfeldt-Jakob disease
Subacute spongiform encephalopathy
EXCLUDES variant Creutzfeldt-Jakob disease (vCJD) (046.11)
DEF: Communicable, progressive spongiform encephalopathy thought to be caused by an infectious particle known as a "prion" (proteinaceous infection particle); a progressive, fatal disease manifested principally by mental deterioration.
AHA: 4Q, '08, 73-75

046.2 Subacute sclerosing panencephalitis
Dawson's inclusion body encephalitis
Van Bogaert's sclerosing leukoencephalitis
DEF: Progressive viral infection causing cerebral dysfunction, blindness, dementia, and death (SSPE).

046.3 Progressive multifocal leukoencephalopathy
Multifocal leukoencephalopathy NOS
DEF: Infection affecting cerebral cortex in patients with weakened immune systems.

046.7 Other specified prion diseases of central nervous system
EXCLUDES Creutzfeldt-Jakob disease (046.11-046.19)
Jakob-Creutzfeldt disease (046.11-046.19)
kuru (046.0)
variant Creutzfeldt-Jakob disease (vCJD) (046.11)

046.71 Gerstmann-Sträussler-Scheinker syndrome
GSS syndrome
AHA: 4Q, '08, 73-75

046.72 Fatal familial insomnia
FFI
AHA: 4Q, '08, 73-75

046.79 Other and unspecified prion disease of central nervous system

046.8 Other specified slow virus infection of central nervous system

046.9 Unspecified slow virus infection of central nervous system

047 Meningitis due to enterovirus
INCLUDES meningitis:
abacterial
aseptic
viral
EXCLUDES meningitis due to:
adenovirus (049.1)
arthropod-borne virus (060.0-066.9)
leptospira (100.81)
virus of:
herpes simplex (054.72)
herpes zoster (053.0)
lymphocytic choriomeningitis (049.0)
mumps (072.1)
poliomyelitis (045.0-045.9)
any other infection specifically classified elsewhere
AHA: J-F, '87, 6

047.0 Coxsackie virus

047.1 ECHO virus
Meningo-eruptive syndrome

047.8 Other specified viral meningitis

047.9 Unspecified viral meningitis
Viral meningitis NOS
A87.9 Viral meningitis unspecified

048 Other enterovirus diseases of central nervous system
Boston exanthem

---

§ Requires fifth digit. Valid digits are in [brackets] under each code. See category 045 for codes and definitions.

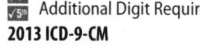 Additional Digit Required | Unspecified Code | Other Specified Code | Manifestation Code | ►◄ Revised Text | ● New Code | ▲ Revised Code Title

Infectious and Parasitic Diseases

049–054.2

☑4ᵗʰ **049 Other non-arthropod-borne viral diseases of central nervous system**

EXCLUDES *late effects of viral encephalitis (139.0)*

049.0 Lymphocytic choriomeningitis
Lymphocytic:
   meningitis (serous) (benign)
   meningoencephalitis (serous) (benign)

049.1 Meningitis due to adenovirus
DEF: Inflammation of lining of brain caused by Arenaviruses and usually occurring in adults in fall and winter months.

049.8 Other specified non-arthropod-borne viral diseases of central nervous system
Encephalitis: Encephalitis:
  acute: lethargica
    inclusion body   Rio Bravo
    necrotizing   von Economo's disease
    epidemic
EXCLUDES *human herpesvirus 6 encephalitis (058.21)*
other human herpesvirus encephalitis (058.29)

049.9 Unspecified non-arthropod-borne viral diseases of central nervous system
Viral encephalitis NOS

Viral Diseases Generally Accompanied by Exanthem (050-059)

EXCLUDES *arthropod-borne viral diseases (060.0-066.9)*
Boston exanthem (048)

☑4ᵗʰ **050 Smallpox**

050.0 Variola major
Hemorrhagic (pustular) smallpox
Malignant smallpox
Purpura variolosa
DEF: Form of smallpox known for its high mortality; exists only in laboratories.

050.1 Alastrim
Variola minor
DEF: Mild form of smallpox known for its low mortality rate.

050.2 Modified smallpox
Varioloid
DEF: Mild form occurring in patients with history of infection or vaccination.

050.9 Smallpox, unspecified

☑4ᵗʰ **051 Cowpox and paravaccinia**

☑5ᵗʰ **051.0 Cowpox and vaccinia not from vaccination**

051.01 Cowpox
DEF: A disease contracted by milking infected cows; vesicles usually appear on the fingers, hands and adjacent areas and usually disappear without scarring; other symptoms: local edema, lymphangitis, and regional lymphadenitis with or without fever.
AHA: 4Q, '08, 76-77

051.02 Vaccinia not from vaccination
EXCLUDES *vaccinia (generalized) (from vaccination) (999.0)*
AHA: 4Q, '08, 76-77

051.1 Pseudocowpox
Milkers' node
DEF: Hand lesions and mild fever in dairy workers caused by exposure to paravaccinia.

051.2 Contagious pustular dermatitis
Ecthyma contagiosum
Orf
DEF: Skin eruptions caused by exposure to poxvirus-infected sheep or goats.

051.9 Paravaccinia, unspecified

☑4ᵗʰ **052 Chickenpox**
DEF: Contagious infection by *Varicella-zoster* virus causing rash with pustules and fever.

052.0 Postvaricella encephalitis
Postchickenpox encephalitis

052.1 Varicella (hemorrhagic) pneumonitis

052.2 Postvaricella myelitis
Postchickenpox myelitis
AHA: 4Q, '06, 58-63

052.7 With other specified complications
AHA: 1Q, '02, 3

052.8 With unspecified complication

052.9 Varicella without mention of complication
Chickenpox NOS   Varicella NOS

☑4ᵗʰ **053 Herpes zoster**
INCLUDES shingles
                  zona
DEF: Self-limiting infection by *Varicella-zoster* virus causing unilateral eruptions and neuralgia along affected nerves.

053.0 With meningitis
DEF: *Varicella-zoster* virus infection causing inflammation of the lining of the brain and/or spinal cord.

☑5ᵗʰ **053.1 With other nervous system complications**

053.10 With unspecified nervous system complication

053.11 Geniculate herpes zoster
Herpetic geniculate ganglionitis
DEF: Unilateral eruptions and neuralgia along the facial nerve geniculum affecting face and outer and middle ear.

053.12 Postherpetic trigeminal neuralgia
DEF: Severe oral or nasal pain following a herpes zoster infection.

053.13 Postherpetic polyneuropathy
DEF: Multiple areas of pain following a herpes zoster infection.

053.14 Herpes zoster myelitis
AHA: 4Q, '06, 58-63

053.19 Other

☑5ᵗʰ **053.2 With ophthalmic complications**

053.20 Herpes zoster dermatitis of eyelid
Herpes zoster ophthalmicus

053.21 Herpes zoster keratoconjunctivitis

053.22 Herpes zoster iridocyclitis

053.29 Other

☑5ᵗʰ **053.7 With other specified complications**

053.71 Otitis externa due to herpes zoster

053.79 Other

053.8 With unspecified complication

053.9 Herpes zoster without mention of complication
Herpes zoster NOS
B02.9 Zoster without complications   I-10

☑4ᵗʰ **054 Herpes simplex**
EXCLUDES *congenital herpes simplex (771.2)*

054.0 Eczema herpeticum
Kaposi's varicelliform eruption
DEF: Herpes simplex virus invading site of preexisting skin inflammation.

☑5ᵗʰ **054.1 Genital herpes**
AHA: J-F, '87, 15, 16

054.10 Genital herpes, unspecified
Herpes progenitalis
AHA: 2Q, '10, 10
A60.00 Herpesviral infection urogenital system unspec   I-10

054.11 Herpetic vulvovaginitis   ♀

054.12 Herpetic ulceration of vulva   ♀

054.13 Herpetic infection of penis   ♂

054.19 Other

054.2 Herpetic gingivostomatitis

N Newborn Age: 0   P Pediatric Age: 0-17   M Maternity Age: 12-55   A Adult Age: 15-124

054.3 Herpetic meningoencephalitis
Herpes encephalitis   Simian B disease
EXCLUDES *human herpesvirus 6 encephalitis (058.21)*
other human herpesvirus encephalitis (058.29)
DEF: Inflammation of the brain and its lining, caused by infection of herpes simplex 1 in adults and simplex 2 in newborns.

√5ᵗʰ 054.4 With ophthalmic complications

054.40 With unspecified ophthalmic complication

054.41 Herpes simplex dermatitis of eyelid

054.42 Dendritic keratitis

054.43 Herpes simplex disciform keratitis

054.44 Herpes simplex iridocyclitis

054.49 Other

054.5 Herpetic septicemia
AHA: 2Q, '00, 5

054.6 Herpetic whitlow
Herpetic felon
DEF: A primary infection of the terminal segment of a finger by herpes simplex; intense itching and pain start the disease, vesicles form, and tissue ultimately is destroyed.

√5ᵗʰ 054.7 With other specified complications

054.71 Visceral herpes simplex

054.72 Herpes simplex meningitis

054.73 Herpes simplex otitis externa

054.74 Herpes simplex myelitis
AHA: 4Q, '06, 58-63

054.79 Other

054.8 With unspecified complication

054.9 Herpes simplex without mention of complication
B00.9 Herpesviral infection unspecified   I-10

√4ᵗʰ 055 Measles
INCLUDES morbilli
rubeola

055.0 Postmeasles encephalitis

055.1 Postmeasles pneumonia

055.2 Postmeasles otitis media

√5ᵗʰ 055.7 With other specified complications

055.71 Measles keratoconjunctivitis
Measles keratitis

055.79 Other

055.8 With unspecified complication

055.9 Measles without mention of complication

√4ᵗʰ 056 Rubella
INCLUDES German measles
EXCLUDES *congenital rubella (771.0)*
DEF: Acute but usually benign togavirus infection causing fever, sore throat, and rash; associated with complications to fetus as a result of maternal infection.

√5ᵗʰ 056.0 With neurological complications

056.00 With unspecified neurological complication

056.01 Encephalomyelitis due to rubella
Encephalitis
Meningoencephalitis   } due to rubella

056.09 Other

√5ᵗʰ 056.7 With other specified complications

056.71 Arthritis due to rubella

056.79 Other

056.8 With unspecified complications

056.9 Rubella without mention of complication

√4ᵗʰ 057 Other viral exanthemata
DEF: Skin eruptions or rashes and fever caused by viruses, including poxviruses.

057.0 Erythema infectiosum [fifth disease]
DEF: A moderately contagious, benign, epidemic disease, usually seen in children, of probable viral etiology; a red macular rash appears on face and may spread to the limbs and trunk.

057.8 Other specified viral exanthemata
Dukes (-Filatow) disease
Fourth disease
Parascarlatina
Pseudoscarlatina
EXCLUDES *exanthema subitum [sixth disease] (058.10-058.12)*
roseola infantum (058.10-058.12)

057.9 Viral exanthem, unspecified

√4ᵗʰ 058 Other human herpesvirus
EXCLUDES *congenital herpes (771.2)*
cytomegalovirus (078.5)
Epstein-Barr virus (075)
herpes NOS (054.0-054.9)
herpes simplex (054.0-054.9)
herpes zoster (053.0-053.9)
human herpesvirus NOS (054.0-054.9)
human herpesvirus 1 (054.0-054.9)
human herpesvirus 2 (054.0-054.9)
human herpesvirus 3 (052.0-053.9)
human herpesvirus 4 (075)
human herpesvirus 5 (078.5)
varicella (052.0-052.9)
varicella-zoster virus (052.0-053.9)
AHA: 4Q, '07, 61

√5ᵗʰ 058.1 Roseola infantum
Exanthema subitum [sixth disease]

058.10 Roseola infantum, unspecified   P
Exanthema subitum [sixth disease], unspecified
AHA: 4Q, '07, 63

058.11 Roseola infantum due to human herpesvirus 6   P
Exanthema subitum [sixth disease] due to human herpesvirus 6

058.12 Roseola infantum due to human herpesvirus 7   P
Exanthema subitum [sixth disease] due to human herpesvirus 7

√5ᵗʰ 058.2 Other human herpesvirus encephalitis
EXCLUDES *herpes encephalitis NOS (054.3)*
herpes simplex encephalitis (054.3)
human herpesvirus encephalitis NOS (054.3)
simian B herpesvirus encephalitis (054.3)

058.21 Human herpesvirus 6 encephalitis

058.29 Other human herpesvirus encephalitis
Human herpesvirus 7 encephalitis

√5ᵗʰ 058.8 Other human herpesvirus infections

058.81 Human herpesvirus 6 infection

058.82 Human herpesvirus 7 infection

058.89 Other human herpesvirus infection
Human herpesvirus 8 infection
Kaposi's sarcoma-associated herpesvirus infection
AHA: 4Q, '07, 63

√4ᵗʰ 059 Other poxvirus infections
EXCLUDES *contagious pustular dermatitis (051.2)*
cowpox (051.01)
ecthyma contagiosum (051.2)
milker's nodule (051.1)
orf (051.2)
paravaccinia NOS (051.9)
pseudocowpox (051.1)
smallpox (050.0-050.9)
vaccinia (generalized) (from vaccination) (999.0)
vaccinia not from vaccination (051.02)
AHA: 4Q, '08, 76-78

√5ᵗʰ 059.0 Other orthopoxvirus infections

059.00 Orthopoxvirus infection, unspecified

Infectious and Parasitic Diseases

059.01–066.40

059.01 **Monkeypox**

059.09 **Other orthopoxvirus infection**

√5ᵗʰ 059.1 **Other parapoxvirus infections**

059.10 **Parapoxvirus infection, unspecified**

059.11 **Bovine stomatitis**

059.12 **Sealpox**

059.19 **Other parapoxvirus infections**

√5ᵗʰ 059.2 **Yatapoxvirus infections**

059.20 **Yatapoxvirus infection, unspecified**

059.21 **Tanapox**

059.22 **Yaba monkey tumor virus**

059.8 **Other poxvirus infections**

059.9 **Poxvirus infections, unspecified**

Arthropod-borne Viral Diseases (060-066)

Use additional code to identify any associated meningitis (321.2)

EXCLUDES *late effects of viral encephalitis (139.0)*

√4ᵗʰ 060 **Yellow fever**

DEF: Fever and jaundice from infection by mosquito-borne virus of genus *Flavivirus.*

060.0 **Sylvatic**

Yellow fever:　　　Yellow fever:
　jungle　　　　　　sylvan

DEF: Yellow fever transmitted from animal to man, via mosquito.

060.1 **Urban**

DEF: Yellow fever transmitted from man to man, via mosquito.

060.9 **Yellow fever, unspecified**

061 **Dengue**

Breakbone fever

EXCLUDES *hemorrhagic fever caused by dengue virus (065.4)*

DEF: Acute, self-limiting infection by mosquito-borne virus characterized by fever and generalized aches.

√4ᵗʰ 062 **Mosquito-borne viral encephalitis**

062.0 **Japanese encephalitis**

Japanese B encephalitis

DEF: Flavivirus causing inflammation of the brain, with a wide range of clinical manifestations.

062.1 **Western equine encephalitis**

DEF: Alphavirus WEE infection causing inflammation of the brain, found in areas west of the Mississippi; transmitted horse to mosquito to man.

062.2 **Eastern equine encephalitis**

EXCLUDES *Venezuelan equine encephalitis (066.2)*

DEF: Alphavirus EEE causing inflammation of the brain and spinal cord, found from Canada to South America and Mexico; transmitted horse to mosquito to man.

062.3 **St. Louis encephalitis**

DEF: Epidemic form caused by Flavivirus and transmitted by mosquito, and characterized by fever, difficulty in speech, and headache.

062.4 **Australian encephalitis**

Australian arboencephalitis
Australian X disease
Murray Valley encephalitis

DEF: Flavivirus causing inflammation of the brain, occurring in Australia and New Guinea.

062.5 **California virus encephalitis**

Encephalitis:　　　Tahyna fever
　California
　La Crosse

DEF: Bunyamwere virus causing inflammation of the brain.

062.8 **Other specified mosquito-borne viral encephalitis**

Encephalitis by Ilheus virus

EXCLUDES *West Nile virus (066.40-066.49)*

062.9 **Mosquito-borne viral encephalitis, unspecified**

√4ᵗʰ 063 **Tick-borne viral encephalitis**

INCLUDES diphasic meningoencephalitis

063.0 **Russian spring-summer [taiga] encephalitis**

063.1 **Louping ill**

DEF: Inflammation of brain caused by virus transmitted sheep to tick to man; incidence usually limited to British Isles.

063.2 **Central European encephalitis**

DEF: Inflammation of brain caused by virus transmitted by tick; limited to central Europe and presenting with two distinct phases.

063.8 **Other specified tick-borne viral encephalitis**

Langat encephalitis　Powassan encephalitis

063.9 **Tick-borne viral encephalitis, unspecified**

064 **Viral encephalitis transmitted by other and unspecified arthropods**

Arthropod-borne viral encephalitis, vector unknown
Negishi virus encephalitis

EXCLUDES *viral encephalitis NOS (049.9)*

√4ᵗʰ 065 **Arthropod-borne hemorrhagic fever**

065.0 **Crimean hemorrhagic fever [CHF Congo virus]**

Central Asian hemorrhagic fever

065.1 **Omsk hemorrhagic fever**

065.2 **Kyasanur Forest disease**

065.3 **Other tick-borne hemorrhagic fever**

065.4 **Mosquito-borne hemorrhagic fever**

Chikungunya hemorrhagic fever
Dengue hemorrhagic fever

EXCLUDES *Chikungunya fever (066.3)*
　　　　　dengue (061)
　　　　　yellow fever (060.0-060.9)

065.8 **Other specified arthropod-borne hemorrhagic fever**

Mite-borne hemorrhagic fever

065.9 **Arthropod-borne hemorrhagic fever, unspecified**

Arbovirus hemorrhagic fever NOS

√4ᵗʰ 066 **Other arthropod-borne viral diseases**

066.0 **Phlebotomus fever**

Changuinola fever　　Sandfly fever

DEF: Sandfly-borne viral infection occurring in Asia, Mideast and South America.

066.1 **Tick-borne fever**

Nairobi sheep disease　　Tick fever:
Tick fever:　　　　　　　　Kemerovo
　American mountain　　　Quaranfil
　Colorado

066.2 **Venezuelan equine fever**

Venezuelan equine encephalitis

DEF: Alphavirus VEE infection causing inflammation of the brain, usually limited to South America, Mexico, and Florida; transmitted horse to mosquito to man.

066.3 **Other mosquito-borne fever**

Fever (viral):　　　　　Fever (viral):
　Bunyamwera　　　　　　Oropouche
　Bwamba　　　　　　　　Pixuna
　Chikungunya　　　　　　Rift valley
　Guama　　　　　　　　　Ross river
　Mayaro　　　　　　　　Wesselsbron
　Mucambo　　　　　　　Zika
　O'Nyong-Nyong

EXCLUDES *dengue (061)*
　　　　　yellow fever (060.0-060.9)

√5ᵗʰ 066.4 **West Nile fever**

AHA: 4Q, '02, 44

DEF: Mosquito-borne fever causing fatal inflammation of the brain, the lining of the brain, or of the lining of the brain and spinal cord.

066.40 **West Nile fever, unspecified**

West Nile fever NOS
West Nile fever without complications
West Nile virus NOS

066.41 West Nile fever with encephalitis
    West Nile encephalitis
    West Nile encephalomyelitis
    AHA: 4Q, '04, 51

066.42 West Nile fever with other neurologic manifestation
    Use additional code to specify the neurologic manifestation
    AHA: 4Q, '04, 51

066.49 West Nile fever with other complications
    Use additional code to specify the other conditions

066.8 Other specified arthropod-borne viral diseases
    Chandipura fever
    Piry fever

066.9 Arthropod-borne viral disease, unspecified
    Arbovirus infection NOS

Other Diseases Due to Viruses and Chlamydiae (070-079)

☑4ᵗʰ 070 Viral hepatitis
    INCLUDES viral hepatitis (acute) (chronic)
    EXCLUDES cytomegalic inclusion virus hepatitis (078.5)

    The following fifth-digit subclassification is for use with categories 070.2 and 070.3:
      0 acute or unspecified, without mention of hepatitis delta
      1 acute or unspecified, with hepatitis delta
      2 chronic, without mention of hepatitis delta
      3 chronic, with hepatitis delta

    DEF: Hepatitis A: HAV infection is self-limiting with flulike symptoms; transmission, fecal-oral.
    DEF: Hepatitis B: HBV infection can be chronic and systemic; transmission, bodily fluids.
    DEF: Hepatitis C: HCV infection can be chronic and systemic; transmission, blood transfusion and unidentified agents.
    DEF: Hepatitis D (delta): HDV occurs only in the presence of hepatitis B virus.
    DEF: Hepatitis E: HEV is epidemic form; transmission and nature under investigation.
    AHA: 2Q, '07, 5

070.0 Viral hepatitis A with hepatic coma

070.1 Viral hepatitis A without mention of hepatic coma
    Infectious hepatitis

§ ☑5ᵗʰ 070.2 Viral hepatitis B with hepatic coma
  [0-3] **AHA:** 4Q, '91, 28; **For code 070.20:** 2Q, '07, 6

§ ☑5ᵗʰ 070.3 Viral hepatitis B without mention of hepatic coma
  [0-3] Serum hepatitis
      AHA: 1Q, '93, 28; 4Q, '91, 28
      B16.9 Acute hep B w/o delta-agent & w/o hepatic coma   I-10

☑5ᵗʰ 070.4 Other specified viral hepatitis with hepatic coma
    AHA: 4Q, '91, 28

    070.41 Acute hepatitis C with hepatic coma

    070.42 Hepatitis delta without mention of active hepatitis B disease with hepatic coma
        Hepatitis delta with hepatitis B carrier state

    070.43 Hepatitis E with hepatic coma

    070.44 Chronic hepatitis C with hepatic coma
        AHA: 2Q, '07, 5

    070.49 Other specified viral hepatitis with hepatic coma

☑5ᵗʰ 070.5 Other specified viral hepatitis without mention of hepatic coma
    AHA: 4Q, '91, 28

    070.51 Acute hepatitis C without mention of hepatic coma

    070.52 Hepatitis delta without mention of active hepatititis B disease or hepatic coma

    070.53 Hepatitis E without mention of hepatic coma

    070.54 Chronic hepatitis C without mention of hepatic coma
        AHA: 1Q, '11, 23; 4Q, '08, 120; 3Q, '07, 7; 2Q, '06, 13
        B18.2 Chronic viral hepatitis C   I-10

070.59 Other specified viral hepatitis without mention of hepatic coma

070.6 Unspecified viral hepatitis with hepatic coma
    EXCLUDES unspecified viral hepatitis C with hepatic coma (070.71)

☑5ᵗʰ 070.7 Unspecified viral hepatitis C

    070.70 Unspecified viral hepatitis C without hepatic coma
        Unspecified viral hepatitis C NOS
        AHA: 4Q, '04, 52
        B19.20 Unspecified viral hepatitis C w/o hepatic coma   I-10

    070.71 Unspecified viral hepatitis C with hepatic coma
        AHA: 4Q, '04, 52

070.9 Unspecified viral hepatitis without mention of hepatic coma
    Viral hepatitis NOS
    EXCLUDES unspecified viral hepatitis C without hepatic coma (070.70)

071 Rabies
    Hydrophobia
    Lyssa
    DEF: Acute infectious disease of the CNS caused by a rhabdovirus; usually spread by bites by infected animals; progresses from fever, restlessness, and extreme excitability, to hydrophobia, seizures, confusion and death.

☑4ᵗʰ 072 Mumps
    DEF: Acute infectious disease caused by paramyxovirus; usually seen in children less than 15 years of age; salivary glands are typically enlarged, involves other organs, such as testes, pancreas and meninges.

    072.0 Mumps orchitis   ♂

    072.1 Mumps meningitis

    072.2 Mumps encephalitis
        Mumps meningoencephalitis

    072.3 Mumps pancreatitis

    ☑5ᵗʰ 072.7 Mumps with other specified complications

        072.71 Mumps hepatitis

        072.72 Mumps polyneuropathy

        072.79 Other

    072.8 Mumps with unspecified complication

    072.9 Mumps without mention of complication
        Epidemic parotitis
        Infectious parotitis

☑4ᵗʰ 073 Ornithosis
    INCLUDES parrot fever
        psittacosis
    DEF: Chlamydia psittaci infection often transmitted from birds to humans.

    073.0 With pneumonia
        Lobular pneumonitis due to ornithosis

    073.7 With other specified complications

    073.8 With unspecified complication

    073.9 Ornithosis, unspecified

☑4ᵗʰ 074 Specific diseases due to Coxsackie virus
    EXCLUDES Coxsackie virus:
        infection NOS (079.2)
        meningitis (047.0)

    074.0 Herpangina
        Vesicular pharyngitis
        DEF: Acute infectious coxsackie virus infection causing throat lesions, fever, and vomiting; generally affects children in summer.

    074.1 Epidemic pleurodynia
        Bornholm disease
        Devil's grip
        Epidemic:
          myalgia
          myositis
        DEF: Paroxysmal pain in chest, accompanied by fever and usually limited to children and young adults; caused by coxsackie virus.

---

§   Requires fifth digit. Valid digits are in [brackets] under each code. See category 070 for codes and definitions.

| ☑4ᵗʰ ☑5ᵗʰ Additional Digit Required | Unspecified Code | Other Specified Code | Manifestation Code | ►◄ Revised Text | ● New Code | ▲ Revised Code Title |

Infectious and Parasitic Diseases

074.2–078.81

√5ᵗʰ **074.2 Coxsackie carditis**

    074.20 Coxsackie carditis, unspecified

    074.21 Coxsackie pericarditis
        DEF: Coxsackie infection of the outer lining of the heart.

    074.22 Coxsackie endocarditis
        DEF: Coxsackie infection within the heart's cavities.

    074.23 Coxsackie myocarditis
        Aseptic myocarditis of newborn
        DEF: Coxsackie infection of the muscle of the heart.

074.3 Hand, foot, and mouth disease
    Vesicular stomatitis and exanthem
    DEF: Mild coxsackie infection causing lesions on hands, feet and oral mucosa, most commonly seen in preschool children.

074.8 Other specified diseases due to Coxsackie virus
    Acute lymphonodular pharyngitis

075 Infectious mononucleosis
    Glandular fever
    Monocytic angina
    Pfeiffer's disease
    DEF: Acute infection by Epstein-Barr virus causing fever, sore throat, enlarged lymph glands and spleen, and fatigue; usually seen in teens and young adults.
    AHA: 3Q, '01, 13; M-A, '87, 8

√4ᵗʰ **076 Trachoma**
    EXCLUDES late effect of trachoma (139.1)
    DEF: A chronic infectious disease of the cornea and conjunctiva caused by a strain of the bacteria *Chlamydia trachomatis*; the infection can cause photophobia, pain, excessive tearing and sometimes blindness.

    076.0 Initial stage
        Trachoma dubium

    076.1 Active stage
        Granular conjunctivitis (trachomatous)
        Trachomatous:
          follicular conjunctivitis
          pannus

    076.9 Trachoma, unspecified
        Trachoma NOS

√4ᵗʰ **077 Other diseases of conjunctiva due to viruses and Chlamydiae**
    EXCLUDES ophthalmic complications of viral diseases classified elsewhere

    077.0 Inclusion conjunctivitis
        Paratrachoma   Swimming pool conjunctivitis
        EXCLUDES inclusion blennorrhea (neonatal) (771.6)
        DEF: Pus in conjunctiva caused by *Chlamydiae trachomatis*.

    077.1 Epidemic keratoconjunctivitis
        Shipyard eye
        DEF: Highly contagious corneal or conjunctival infection caused by adenovirus type 8; symptoms include inflammation and corneal infiltrates.

    077.2 Pharyngoconjunctival fever
        Viral pharyngoconjunctivitis

    077.3 Other adenoviral conjunctivitis
        Acute adenoviral follicular conjunctivitis

    077.4 Epidemic hemorrhagic conjunctivitis
        Apollo:
          conjunctivitis
          disease
        Conjunctivitis due to enterovirus type 70
        Hemorrhagic conjunctivitis (acute) (epidemic)

    077.8 Other viral conjunctivitis
        Newcastle conjunctivitis

√5ᵗʰ **077.9 Unspecified diseases of conjunctiva due to viruses and Chlamydiae**

    077.98 Due to Chlamydiae

    077.99 Due to viruses
        Viral conjunctivitis NOS
        B30.9 Viral conjunctivitis, unspecified   I-10

√4ᵗʰ **078 Other diseases due to viruses and Chlamydiae**
    EXCLUDES viral infection NOS (079.0-079.9)
             viremia NOS (790.8)

078.0 Molluscum contagiosum
    DEF: Benign poxvirus infection causing small bumps on the skin or conjunctiva; transmitted by close contact.

√5ᵗʰ **078.1 Viral warts**
    Viral warts due to human papilloma virus
    DEF: A keratotic papilloma of the epidermis caused by the human papilloma virus; the superficial vegetative lesions last for varying durations and eventually regress spontaneously.
    AHA: 2Q, '97, 9; 4Q, '93, 22

    078.10 Viral warts, unspecified
        Verruca:
          NOS
          Vulgaris
        Warts (infectious)

    078.11 Condyloma acuminatum
        Condyloma NOS
        Genital warts NOS
        DEF: Clusters of mucosa or epidermal lesions on external genitalia; viral infection is sexually transmitted.

    078.12 Plantar wart
        Verruca plantaris
        AHA: 4Q, '08, 78-79

    078.19 Other specified viral warts
        Common wart
        Flat wart
        Verruca plana

078.2 Sweating fever
    Miliary fever
    Sweating disease
    DEF: A viral infection characterized by profuse sweating; various papular, vesicular and other eruptions cause the blockage of sweat glands.

078.3 Cat-scratch disease
    Benign lymphoreticulosis (of inoculation)
    Cat-scratch fever

078.4 Foot and mouth disease
    Aphthous fever
    Epizootic:
      aphthae
      stomatitis
    DEF: Ulcers on oral mucosa, legs, and feet after exposure to infected animal.

078.5 Cytomegaloviral disease
    Cytomegalic inclusion disease
    Salivary gland virus disease
    Use additional code to identify manifestation, as:
      cytomegalic inclusion virus:
        hepatitis (573.1)
        pneumonia (484.1)
      EXCLUDES congenital cytomegalovirus infection (771.1)
    DEF: A herpesvirus associated with serious disease morbidity including fever, leukopenia, pneumonia, retinitis, hepatitis and organ transplant; often leads to hepatomegaly, splenomegaly and thrombocytopenia; a common post-transplant complication.
    AHA: ▶3Q, '11, 5;◀ 1Q, '03, 10; 3Q, '98, 4; 2Q, '93, 11; 1Q, '89, 9

078.6 Hemorrhagic nephrosonephritis
    Hemorrhagic fever:
      epidemic
      Korean
      Russian
      with renal syndrome
    DEF: Viral infection causing kidney dysfunction and bleeding disorders.

078.7 Arenaviral hemorrhagic fever
    Hemorrhagic fever: Hemorrhagic fever:
      Argentine   Junin virus
      Bolivian   Machupo virus

√5ᵗʰ **078.8 Other specified diseases due to viruses and Chlamydiae**
    EXCLUDES epidemic diarrhea (009.2)
             lymphogranuloma venereum (099.1)

    078.81 Epidemic vertigo

N Newborn Age: 0   P Pediatric Age: 0-17   M Maternity Age: 12-55   A Adult Age: 15-124

078.82 Epidemic vomiting syndrome
Winter vomiting disease

078.88 Other specified diseases due to Chlamydiae
AHA: 4Q, '96, 22

078.89 Other specified diseases due to viruses
Epidemic cervical myalgia
Marburg disease

√4th **079 Viral and chlamydial infection in conditions classified elsewhere and of unspecified site**
NOTE This category is provided to be used as an additional code to identify the viral agent in diseases classifiable elsewhere. This category will also be used to classify virus infection of unspecified nature or site.

079.0 Adenovirus

079.1 ECHO virus
DEF: An "orphan" enteric RNA virus, certain serotypes of which are associated with human disease, especially aseptic meningitis.

079.2 Coxsackie virus
DEF: A heterogenous group of viruses associated with aseptic meningitis, myocarditis, pericarditis, and acute onset juvenile diabetes.

079.3 Rhinovirus
DEF: Rhinoviruses affect primarily the upper respiratory tract. Over 100 distinct types infect humans.

079.4 Human papillomavirus
DEF: Viral infection caused by the genus *Papillomavirus* causing cutaneous and genital warts, including verruca vulgaris and condyloma acuminatum; certain types are associated with cervical dysplasia, cancer and other genital malignancies.
AHA: 2Q, '97, 9; 4Q, '93, 22
TIP: Do not assign for viral warts; see instead subcategory 078.1.

√5th **079.5 Retrovirus**
EXCLUDES human immunodeficiency virus, type 1 [HIV-1] (042)
human T-cell lymphotrophic virus, type III [HTLV-III] (042)
lymphadenopathy-associated virus [LAV] (042)
DEF: A large group of RNA viruses that carry reverse transcriptase and include the leukoviruses and lentiviruses.
AHA: 4Q, '93, 22, 23

079.50 Retrovirus, unspecified

079.51 Human T-cell lymphotrophic virus, type I [HTLV-I]

079.52 Human T-cell lymphotrophic virus, type II [HTLV-II]

079.53 Human immunodeficiency virus, type 2 [HIV-2]

079.59 Other specified retrovirus

079.6 Respiratory syncytial virus [RSV]
DEF: The major respiratory pathogen of young children, causing severe bronchitis and bronchopneumonia, and minor infection in adults.
AHA: 4Q, '96, 27, 28

√5th **079.8 Other specified viral and chlamydial infections**
AHA: 1Q, '88, 12

079.81 Hantavirus
DEF: An infection caused by the Muerto Canyon virus whose primary rodent reservoir is the deer mouse Peromyscus maniculatus; commonly characterized by fever, myalgias, headache, cough.
AHA: 4Q, '95, 60

079.82 SARS-associated coronavirus
DEF: A life-threatening respiratory disease, severe acute respiratory syndrome (SARS); etiology coronavirus; presenting symptoms may range from mild to severe forms of flu-like conditions; fever, chills, cough, headache, myalgia; diagnosis of SARS is based upon clinical, laboratory, and epidemiological criteria.
AHA: 4Q, '03, 46

079.83 Parvovirus B19
Human parvovirus   Parvovirus NOS
EXCLUDES erythema infectiosum [fifth disease] (057.0)
DEF: The only known parvovirus to cause disease in humans; manifestation is erythema infectiosum; also associated with polyarthropathy, chronic anemia, red cell aplasia, and fetal hydrops.
AHA: 4Q, '07, 64

079.88 Other specified chlamydial infection

079.89 Other specified viral infection

√5th **079.9 Unspecified viral and chlamydial infections**
EXCLUDES viremia NOS (790.8)

079.98 Unspecified chlamydial infection
Chlamydial infections NOS

079.99 Unspecified viral infection
Viral infections NOS
B97.89 Other viral agents cause of dz class elsewhere   I-10

Rickettsioses and Other Arthropod-borne Diseases (080-088)
EXCLUDES arthropod-borne viral diseases (060.0-066.9)

080 Louse-borne [epidemic] typhus
Typhus (fever):
    classical
    epidemic
    exanthematic NOS
    louse-borne
DEF: *Rickettsia prowazekii;* causes severe headache, rash, high fever.

√4th **081 Other typhus**

081.0 Murine [endemic] typhus
Typhus (fever):
    endemic
    flea-borne
DEF: Milder typhus caused by *Rickettsia typhi (mooseri);* transmitted by rat flea.

081.1 Brill's disease
Brill-Zinsser disease
Recrudescent typhus (fever)

081.2 Scrub typhus
Japanese river fever
Kedani fever
Mite-borne typhus
Tsutsugamushi
DEF: Typhus caused by *Rickettsia tsutsugamushi* transmitted by chigger.

081.9 Typhus, unspecified
Typhus (fever) NOS

√4th **082 Tick-borne rickettsioses**

082.0 Spotted fevers
Rocky mountain spotted fever
Sao Paulo fever

082.1 Boutonneuse fever
African tick typhus
India tick typhus
Kenya tick typhus
Marseilles fever
Mediterranean tick fever

082.2 North Asian tick fever
Siberian tick typhus

082.3 Queensland tick typhus

√5th **082.4 Ehrlichiosis**
AHA: 3Q, '06, 11; 4Q, '00, 38

082.40 Ehrlichiosis, unspecified

082.41 Ehrlichiosis chaffeensis [E. chaffeensis]
DEF: A febrile illness caused by bacterial infection, also called human monocytic ehrlichiosis (HME). Causal organism is *Ehrlichia chaffeensis,* transmitted by the Lone Star tick. Symptoms include fever, chills, myalgia, nausea, vomiting, diarrhea, confusion, and severe headache occurring one week after a tick bite. Clinical findings are lymphadenopathy, rash, thrombocytopenia, leukopenia, and abnormal liver function tests.

082.49 Other ehrlichiosis

082.8 Other specified tick-borne rickettsioses
Lone star fever
AHA: 4Q, '99, 19

082.9 Tick-borne rickettsiosis, unspecified
Tick-borne typhus NOS

Infectious and Parasitic Diseases

083–088.0

☑4ᵗʰ **083 Other rickettsioses**

083.0 Q fever
DEF: Infection of *Coxiella burnettii* usually acquired through airborne organisms.

083.1 Trench fever
Quintan fever
Wolhynian fever

083.2 Rickettsialpox
Vesicular rickettsiosis
DEF: Infection of *Rickettsia akari* usually acquired through a mite bite.

083.8 Other specified rickettsioses

083.9 Rickettsiosis, unspecified

☑4ᵗʰ **084 Malaria**
NOTE Subcategories 084.0-084.6 exclude the listed conditions with mention of pernicious complications (084.8-084.9).
EXCLUDES *congenital malaria (771.2)*
DEF: Mosquito-borne disease causing high fever and prostration and cataloged by species of *Plasmodium: P. falciparum, P. malariae, P. ovale, and P. vivax.*

084.0 Falciparum malaria [malignant tertian]
Malaria (fever):
by Plasmodium falciparum
subtertian

084.1 Vivax malaria [benign tertian]
Malaria (fever) by Plasmodium vivax

084.2 Quartan malaria
Malaria (fever) by Plasmodium malariae
Malariae malaria

084.3 Ovale malaria
Malaria (fever) by Plasmodium ovale

084.4 Other malaria
Monkey malaria

084.5 Mixed malaria
Malaria (fever) by more than one parasite

084.6 Malaria, unspecified
Malaria (fever) NOS

084.7 Induced malaria
Therapeutically induced malaria
EXCLUDES *accidental infection from syringe, blood transfusion, etc. (084.0-084.6, above, according to parasite species)*
transmission from mother to child during delivery (771.2)

084.8 Blackwater fever
Hemoglobinuric:
fever (bilious)
malaria
Malarial hemoglobinuria
DEF: Severe hemic and renal complication of *Plasmodium falciparum* infection.

084.9 Other pernicious complications of malaria
Algid malaria
Cerebral malaria
Use additional code to identify complication, as:
malarial:
hepatitis (573.2)
nephrosis (581.81)

☑4ᵗʰ **085 Leishmaniasis**

085.0 Visceral [kala-azar]
Dumdum fever
Infection by Leishmania:
donovani
infantum
Leishmaniasis:
dermal, post-kala-azar
Mediterranean
visceral (Indian)

085.1 Cutaneous, urban
Aleppo boil
Baghdad boil
Delhi boil
Infection by Leishmania tropica (minor)
Leishmaniasis, cutaneous:
dry form
late
recurrent
ulcerating
Oriental sore

085.2 Cutaneous, Asian desert
Infection by Leishmania tropica major
Leishmaniasis, cutaneous:
acute necrotizing
rural
wet form
zoonotic form

085.3 Cutaneous, Ethiopian
Infection by Leishmania ethiopica
Leishmaniasis, cutaneous:
diffuse
lepromatous

085.4 Cutaneous, American
Chiclero ulcer
Infection by Leishmania mexicana
Leishmaniasis tegumentaria diffusa

085.5 Mucocutaneous (American)
Espundia
Infection by Leishmania braziliensis
Uta

085.9 Leishmaniasis, unspecified

☑4ᵗʰ **086 Trypanosomiasis**
Use additional code to identify manifestations, as:
trypanosomiasis:
encephalitis (323.2)
meningitis (321.3)

086.0 Chagas' disease with heart involvement
American trypanosomiasis ⎫
Infection by Trypanosoma cruzi ⎬ with heart involvement
Any condition classifiable to 086.2 with heart involvement

086.1 Chagas' disease with other organ involvement
American trypanosomiasis ⎫ with involvement of organ
Infection by Trypanosoma cruzi ⎭ other than heart
Any condition classifiable to 086.2 with involvement of organ other than heart

086.2 Chagas' disease without mention of organ involvement
American trypanosomiasis
Infection by Trypanosoma cruzi

086.3 Gambian trypanosomiasis
Gambian sleeping sickness
Infection by Trypanosoma gambiense

086.4 Rhodesian trypanosomiasis
Infection by Trypanosoma rhodesiense
Rhodesian sleeping sickness

086.5 African trypanosomiasis, unspecified
Sleeping sickness NOS

086.9 Trypanosomiasis, unspecified

☑4ᵗʰ **087 Relapsing fever**
INCLUDES recurrent fever
DEF: Infection of *Borrelia;* symptoms are episodic and include fever and arthralgia.

087.0 Louse-borne

087.1 Tick-borne

087.9 Relapsing fever, unspecified

☑4ᵗʰ **088 Other arthropod-borne diseases**

088.0 Bartonellosis
Carrión's disease   Verruga peruana
Oroya fever

N Newborn Age: 0   P Pediatric Age: 0-17   M Maternity Age: 12-55   A Adult Age: 15-124

√5ᵗʰ **088.8 Other specified arthropod-borne diseases**

   088.81 Lyme disease
      Erythema chronicum migrans
      DEF: A recurrent multisystem disorder caused by the spirochete *Borrelia burgdorferi* with the carrier being the tick; begins with lesions of erythema chronicum migrans; followed by arthritis of the large joints, myalgia, malaise, and neurological and cardiac manifestations.
      AHA: 4Q, '91, 15; 3Q, '90, 14; 2Q, '89, 10
      TIP: Do not assign if patient has been cured of Lyme disease but has residual chronic condition; refer instead to late-effect code 139.8.

   088.82 Babesiosis
      Babesiasis
      DEF: A tick-borne disease caused by infection of *Babesia*, characterized by fever, malaise, listlessness, severe anemia and hemoglobinuria.
      AHA: 4Q, '93, 23

   088.89 Other

  088.9 Arthropod-borne disease, unspecified

Syphilis and Other Venereal Diseases (090-099)

     EXCLUDES nonvenereal endemic syphilis (104.0)
              urogenital trichomoniasis (131.0)

√4ᵗʰ **090 Congenital syphilis**
   DEF: Infection by spirochete*Treponema pallidum* acquired in utero from the infected mother.

  090.0 Early congenital syphilis, symptomatic
     Congenital syphilitic: Congenital syphilitic:
      choroiditis   splenomegaly
      coryza (chronic)   Syphilitic (congenital):
      hepatomegaly   epiphysitis
      mucous patches   osteochondritis
      periostitis   pemphigus
     Any congenital syphilitic condition specified as early or manifest less than two years after birth

  090.1 Early congenital syphilis, latent
     Congenital syphilis without clinical manifestations, with positive serological reaction and negative spinal fluid test, less than two years after birth

  090.2 Early congenital syphilis, unspecified
     Congenital syphilis NOS, less than two years after birth

  090.3 Syphilitic interstitial keratitis
     Syphilitic keratitis:
      parenchymatous
      punctata profunda
     EXCLUDES interstitial keratitis NOS (370.50)

√5ᵗʰ **090.4 Juvenile neurosyphilis**
     Use additional code to identify any associated mental disorder
     DEF: *Treponema pallidum* infection involving the nervous system.

   090.40 Juvenile neurosyphilis, unspecified
      Congenital neurosyphilis
      Dementia paralytica juvenilis
      Juvenile:
        general paresis
        tabes
        taboparesis

   090.41 Congenital syphilitic encephalitis
      DEF: Congenital *Treponema pallidum* infection involving the brain.

   090.42 Congenital syphilitic meningitis
      DEF: Congenital *Treponema pallidum* infection involving the lining of the brain and/or spinal cord.

   090.49 Other

  090.5 Other late congenital syphilis, symptomatic
     Gumma due to congenital syphilis
     Hutchinson's teeth
     Syphilitic saddle nose
     Any congenital syphilitic condition specified as late or manifest two years or more after birth

  090.6 Late congenital syphilis, latent
     Congenital syphilis without clinical manifestations, with positive serological reaction and negative spinal fluid test, two years or more after birth

  090.7 Late congenital syphilis, unspecified
     Congenital syphilis NOS, two years or more after birth

  090.9 Congenital syphilis, unspecified

√4ᵗʰ **091 Early syphilis, symptomatic**
     EXCLUDES early cardiovascular syphilis (093.0-093.9)
              early neurosyphilis (094.0-094.9)

  091.0 Genital syphilis (primary)
     Genital chancre
     DEF: Genital lesion at the site of initial infection by *Treponema pallidum*.

  091.1 Primary anal syphilis
     DEF: Anal lesion at the site of initial infection by *Treponema pallidum*.

  091.2 Other primary syphilis
     Primary syphilis of: Primary syphilis of:
      breast   lip
      fingers   tonsils
     DEF: Lesion at the site of initial infection by *Treponema pallidum*.

  091.3 Secondary syphilis of skin or mucous membranes
     Condyloma latum   Secondary syphilis of:
     Secondary syphilis of: skin
      anus   tonsils
      mouth   vulva
      pharynx
     DEF: Transitory or chronic lesions following initial syphilis infection.

  091.4 Adenopathy due to secondary syphilis
     Syphilitic adenopathy (secondary)
     Syphilitic lymphadenitis (secondary)

√5ᵗʰ **091.5 Uveitis due to secondary syphilis**

   091.50 Syphilitic uveitis, unspecified

   091.51 Syphilitic chorioretinitis (secondary)
      DEF: Inflammation of choroid and retina as a secondary infection.

   091.52 Syphilitic iridocyclitis (secondary)
      DEF: Inflammation of iris and ciliary body as a secondary infection.

√5ᵗʰ **091.6 Secondary syphilis of viscera and bone**

   091.61 Secondary syphilitic periostitis
      DEF: Inflammation of outer layers of bone as a secondary infection.

   091.62 Secondary syphilitic hepatitis
      Secondary syphilis of liver

   091.69 Other viscera

  091.7 Secondary syphilis, relapse
     Secondary syphilis, relapse (treated) (untreated)
     DEF: Return of symptoms of syphilis following asymptomatic period.

√5ᵗʰ **091.8 Other forms of secondary syphilis**

   091.81 Acute syphilitic meningitis (secondary)
      DEF: Sudden, severe inflammation of the lining of the brain and/or spinal cord as a secondary infection.

   091.82 Syphilitic alopecia
      DEF: Hair loss following initial syphilis infection.

   091.89 Other

  091.9 Unspecified secondary syphilis

√4ᵗʰ **092 Early syphilis, latent**
     INCLUDES syphilis (acquired) without clinical manifestations, with positive serological reaction and negative spinal fluid test, less than two years after infection

  092.0 Early syphilis, latent, serological relapse after treatment

  092.9 Early syphilis, latent, unspecified

√4ᵗʰ **093 Cardiovascular syphilis**

  093.0 Aneurysm of aorta, specified as syphilitic
     Dilatation of aorta, specified as syphilitic

Infectious and Parasitic Diseases

093.1–098.2

093.1 Syphilitic aortitis
DEF: Inflammation of the aorta — the main artery leading from the heart.

☑5ᵗʰ **093.2 Syphilitic endocarditis**
DEF: Inflammation of the tissues lining the cavities of the heart.

093.20 Valve, unspecified
Syphilitic ostial coronary disease

093.21 Mitral valve

093.22 Aortic valve
Syphilitic aortic incompetence or stenosis

093.23 Tricuspid valve

093.24 Pulmonary valve

☑5ᵗʰ **093.8 Other specified cardiovascular syphilis**

093.81 Syphilitic pericarditis
DEF: Inflammation of the outer lining of the heart.

093.82 Syphilitic myocarditis
DEF: Inflammation of the muscle of the heart.

093.89 Other

093.9 Cardiovascular syphilis, unspecified

☑4ᵗʰ **094 Neurosyphilis**
Use additional code to identify any associated mental disorder

094.0 Tabes dorsalis
Locomotor ataxia (progressive)
Posterior spinal sclerosis (syphilitic)
Tabetic neurosyphilis
Use additional code to identify manifestation, as:
neurogenic arthropathy [Charcot's joint disease] (713.5)
DEF: Progressive degeneration of nerves associated with long-term syphilis; causing pain, wasting away, incontinence, and ataxia.

094.1 General paresis
Dementia paralytica
General paralysis (of the insane) (progressive)
Paretic neurosyphilis
Taboparesis
DEF: Degeneration of brain associated with long-term syphilis, causing loss of brain function, progressive dementia, and paralysis.

094.2 Syphilitic meningitis
Meningovascular syphilis
EXCLUDES *acute syphilitic meningitis (secondary) (091.81)*
DEF: Inflammation of the lining of the brain and/or spinal cord.

094.3 Asymptomatic neurosyphilis

☑5ᵗʰ **094.8 Other specified neurosyphilis**

094.81 Syphilitic encephalitis

094.82 Syphilitic Parkinsonism
DEF: Decreased motor function, tremors, and muscular rigidity.

094.83 Syphilitic disseminated retinochoroiditis
DEF: Inflammation of retina and choroid due to neurosyphilis.

094.84 Syphilitic optic atrophy
DEF: Degeneration of the eye and its nerves due to neurosyphilis.

094.85 Syphilitic retrobulbar neuritis
DEF: Inflammation of the posterior optic nerve due to neurosyphilis.

094.86 Syphilitic acoustic neuritis
DEF: Inflammation of acoustic nerve due to neurosyphilis.

094.87 Syphilitic ruptured cerebral aneurysm

094.89 Other

094.9 Neurosyphilis, unspecified
Gumma (syphilitic)
Syphilis (early) (late) } of central nervous system
Syphiloma } NOS

095 Other forms of late syphilis, with symptoms
INCLUDES gumma (syphilitic)
syphilis, late, tertiary, or unspecified stage

095.0 Syphilitic episcleritis

095.1 Syphilis of lung

095.2 Syphilitic peritonitis

095.3 Syphilis of liver

095.4 Syphilis of kidney

095.5 Syphilis of bone

095.6 Syphilis of muscle
Syphilitic myositis

095.7 Syphilis of synovium, tendon, and bursa
Syphilitic:
bursitis
synovitis

095.8 Other specified forms of late symptomatic syphilis
EXCLUDES *cardiovascular syphilis (093.0-093.9)*
neurosyphilis (094.0-094.9)

095.9 Late symptomatic syphilis, unspecified

096 Late syphilis, latent
Syphilis (acquired) without clinical manifestations, with positive serological reaction and negative spinal fluid test, two years or more after infection

☑4ᵗʰ **097 Other and unspecified syphilis**

097.0 Late syphilis, unspecified

097.1 Latent syphilis, unspecified
Positive serological reaction for syphilis

097.9 Syphilis, unspecified
Syphilis (acquired) NOS
EXCLUDES *syphilis NOS causing death under two years of age (090.9)*

☑4ᵗʰ **098 Gonococcal infections**
DEF: *Neisseria gonorrhoeae* infection generally acquired in utero or in sexual congress.

098.0 Acute, of lower genitourinary tract
Gonococcal:
Bartholinitis (acute)
urethritis (acute)
vulvovaginitis (acute)
Gonorrhea (acute):
NOS
genitourinary (tract) NOS

☑5ᵗʰ **098.1 Acute, of upper genitourinary tract**

098.10 Gonococcal infection (acute) of upper genitourinary tract, site unspecified

098.11 Gonococcal cystitis (acute) upper
Gonorrhea (acute) of bladder

098.12 Gonococcal prostatitis (acute) ♂

098.13 Gonococcal epididymo-orchitis (acute) ♂
Gonococcal orchitis (acute)
DEF: Acute inflammation of the testes.

098.14 Gonococcal seminal vesiculitis (acute) ♂
Gonorrhea (acute) of seminal vesicle

098.15 Gonococcal cervicitis (acute) ♀
Gonorrhea (acute) of cervix

098.16 Gonococcal endometritis (acute) ♀
Gonorrhea (acute) of uterus

098.17 Gonococcal salpingitis, specified as acute ♀
DEF: Acute inflammation of the fallopian tubes.

098.19 Other

098.2 Chronic, of lower genitourinary tract
Gonococcal:
Bartholinitis
urethritis } specified as chronic or with
vulvovaginitis } duration of two months
Gonorrhea: } or more
NOS
genitourinary (tract)
Any condition classifiable to 098.0 specified as chronic or with duration of two months or more

---

N Newborn Age: 0   P Pediatric Age: 0-17   M Maternity Age: 12-55   A Adult Age: 15-124

Infectious and Parasitic Diseases

✓5ᵗʰ **098.3 Chronic, of upper genitourinary tract**
> INCLUDES any condition classifiable to 098.1 stated as chronic or with a duration of two months or more

098.30 Chronic gonococcal infection of upper genitourinary tract, site unspecified

098.31 Gonococcal cystitis, chronic
Gonorrhea of bladder, chronic
Any condition classifiable to 098.11, specified as chronic

098.32 Gonococcal prostatitis, chronic ♂
Any condition classifiable to 098.12, specified as chronic

098.33 Gonococcal epididymo-orchitis, chronic ♂
Chronic gonococcal orchitis
Any condition classifiable to 098.13, specified as chronic
DEF: Chronic inflammation of the testes.

098.34 Gonococcal seminal vesiculitis, chronic ♂
Gonorrhea of seminal vesicle, chronic
Any condition classifiable to 098.14, specified as chronic

098.35 Gonococcal cervicitis, chronic ♀
Gonorrhea of cervix, chronic
Any condition classifiable to 098.15, specified as chronic

098.36 Gonococcal endometritis, chronic ♀
Any condition classifiable to 098.16, specified as chronic
DEF: Chronic inflammation of the uterus.

098.37 Gonococcal salpingitis (chronic) ♀
DEF: Chronic inflammation of the fallopian tubes.

098.39 Other

✓5ᵗʰ **098.4 Gonococcal infection of eye**

098.40 Gonococcal conjunctivitis (neonatorum)
Gonococcal ophthalmia (neonatorum)
DEF: Infection of conjunctiva present at birth.

098.41 Gonococcal iridocyclitis
DEF: Inflammation and infection of iris and ciliary body.

098.42 Gonococcal endophthalmia
DEF: Inflammation and infection of contents of eyeball.

098.43 Gonococcal keratitis
DEF: Inflammation and infection of the cornea.

098.49 Other

✓5ᵗʰ **098.5 Gonococcal infection of joint**

098.50 Gonococcal arthritis
Gonococcal infection of joint NOS

098.51 Gonococcal synovitis and tenosynovitis

098.52 Gonococcal bursitis
DEF: Inflammation of the sac-like cavities in a joint.

098.53 Gonococcal spondylitis

098.59 Other
Gonococcal rheumatism

098.6 Gonococcal infection of pharynx

098.7 Gonococcal infection of anus and rectum
Gonococcal proctitis

✓5ᵗʰ **098.8 Gonococcal infection of other specified sites**

098.81 Gonococcal keratosis (blennorrhagica)
DEF: Pustular skin lesions caused by Neisseria gonorrhoeae.

098.82 Gonococcal meningitis
DEF: Inflammation of lining of brain and/or spinal cord.

098.83 Gonococcal pericarditis
DEF: Inflammation of the outer lining of the heart.

098.84 Gonococcal endocarditis
DEF: Inflammation of tissues lining the cavities of heart.

098.85 Other gonococcal heart disease

098.86 Gonococcal peritonitis
DEF: Inflammation of the membrane lining the abdomen.

098.89 Other
Gonococcemia

✓4ᵗʰ **099 Other venereal diseases**

099.0 Chancroid
Bubo (inguinal):
  chancroidal
  due to Hemophilus ducreyi
Chancre:
  Ducrey's
  simple
  soft
Ulcus molle (cutis)(skin)
DEF: A sexually transmitted disease caused by Haemophilus ducreyi; identified by a painful primary ulcer at the site of inoculation (usually external genitalia) with related lymphadenitis.

099.1 Lymphogranuloma venereum
Climatic or tropical bubo
(Durand-) Nicolas-Favre disease
Esthiomene
Lymphogranuloma inguinale
DEF: Sexually transmitted infection of Chlamydia trachomatis causing skin lesions.

099.2 Granuloma inguinale
Donovanosis
Granuloma pudendi (ulcerating)
Granuloma venereum
Pudendal ulcer
DEF: Chronic, sexually transmitted infection of Calymmatobacterium granulomatis causing progressive, anogenital skin ulcers.

099.3 Reiter's disease
Reactive arthritis
Reiter's syndrome
Use additional code for associated:
  arthropathy (711.1)
  conjunctivitis (372.33)
DEF: A symptom complex of unknown etiology consisting of urethritis, conjunctivitis, arthritis and myocutaneous lesions; occurs most commonly in young men and patients with HIV. Also a form of reactive arthritis.

✓5ᵗʰ **099.4 Other nongonococcal urethritis [NGU]**

099.40 Unspecified
Nonspecific urethritis

099.41 Chlamydia trachomatis

099.49 Other specified organism

✓5ᵗʰ **099.5 Other venereal diseases due to Chlamydia trachomatis**
> EXCLUDES Chlamydia trachomatis infection of conjunctiva (076.0-076.9, 077.0, 077.9)
> Lymphogranuloma venereum (099.1)

DEF: Venereal diseases caused by Chlamydia trachomatis at other sites besides the urethra (e.g., pharynx, anus and rectum, conjunctiva and peritoneum).

099.50 Unspecified site

099.51 Pharynx

099.52 Anus and rectum

099.53 Lower genitourinary sites
Use additional code to specify site of infection, such as:
  bladder (595.4)
  cervix (616.0)
  vagina and vulva (616.11)
> EXCLUDES urethra (099.41)

099.54 Other genitourinary sites
Use additional code to specify site of infection, such as:
  pelvic inflammatory disease NOS (614.9)
  testis and epididymis (604.91)

099.55 Unspecified genitourinary site

099.56 Peritoneum
Perihepatitis

099.59 Other specified site

Infectious and Parasitic Diseases

099.8–110.2

099.8 Other specified venereal diseases

099.9 Venereal disease, unspecified

Other Spirochetal Diseases (100-104)

✓4ᵗʰ 100 Leptospirosis

DEF: A blood infection of any spirochete of the genus Leptospire; transmitted to humans by exposure to contaminated animal tissues or water. Patients present with flulike symptoms, characteristic muscle aches involving the thighs and low back.

100.0 Leptospirosis icterohemorrhagica
Leptospiral or spirochetal jaundice (hemorrhagic)
Weil's disease

✓5ᵗʰ 100.8 Other specified leptospiral infections

100.81 Leptospiral meningitis (aseptic)

100.89 Other
Fever:
Fort Bragg
pretibial
swamp
Infection by Leptospira:
australis
bataviae
pyrogenes

100.9 Leptospirosis, unspecified

101 Vincent's angina
Acute necrotizing ulcerative:
gingivitis
stomatitis
Fusospirochetal pharyngitis
Spirochetal stomatitis
Trench mouth
Vincent's:
gingivitis
infection [any site]
DEF: Painful ulceration with edema and hypermic patches of the oropharyngeal and throat membranes; it is caused by spreading of acute ulcerative gingivitis.

✓4ᵗʰ 102 Yaws

INCLUDES frambesia
pian
DEF: An infectious, endemic, tropical disease caused by *Treponema pertenue*; usually affects persons 15 years old or younger; a primary cutaneous lesion develops, then a granulomatous skin eruption, and occasionally lesions that destroy skin and bone.

102.0 Initial lesions
Chancre of yaws
Frambesia, initial or primary
Initial frambesial ulcer
Mother yaw

102.1 Multiple papillomata and wet crab yaws
Butter yaws
Frambesioma
Pianoma
Plantar or palmar papilloma of yaws

102.2 Other early skin lesions
Cutaneous yaws, less than five years after infection
Early yaws (cutaneous) (macular) (papular) (maculopapular) (micropapular)
Frambeside of early yaws

102.3 Hyperkeratosis
Ghoul hand
Hyperkeratosis, palmar or plantar (early) (late) due to yaws
Worm-eaten soles
DEF: Overgrowth of skin of palm or bottoms of feet, due to yaws.

102.4 Gummata and ulcers
Gummatous frambeside
Nodular late yaws (ulcerated)
DEF: Rubbery lesions and areas of dead skin caused by yaws.

102.5 Gangosa
Rhinopharyngitis mutilans
DEF: Massive, mutilating lesions of the nose and oral cavity caused by yaws.

102.6 Bone and joint lesions
Goundou
Gumma, bone } of yaws (late)
Gummatous osteitis or periostitis

Hydrarthrosis
Osteitis } of yaws (early) (late)
Periostitis (hypertrophic)

102.7 Other manifestations
Juxta-articular nodules of yaws
Mucosal yaws

102.8 Latent yaws
Yaws without clinical manifestations, with positive serology

102.9 Yaws, unspecified

✓4ᵗʰ 103 Pinta

DEF: A chronic form of treponematosis, endemic in areas of tropical America; it is identified by the presence of red, violet, blue, coffee-colored or white spots on the skin.

103.0 Primary lesions
Chancre (primary)
Papule (primary) } of pinta [carate]
Pintid

103.1 Intermediate lesions
Erythematous plaques
Hyperchronic lesions } of pinta [carate]
Hyperkeratosis

103.2 Late lesions
Cardiovascular lesions
Skin lesions:
achromic
cicatricial } of pinta [carate]
dyschromic
Vitiligo

103.3 Mixed lesions
Achromic and hyperchromic skin lesions of pinta [carate]

103.9 Pinta, unspecified

✓4ᵗʰ 104 Other spirochetal infection

104.0 Nonvenereal endemic syphilis
Bejel
Njovera
DEF: *Treponema pallidum, T. pertenue, or T. caroteum* infection transmitted non-sexually, causing lesions on mucosa and skin.

104.8 Other specified spirochetal infections
EXCLUDES relapsing fever (087.0-087.9)
syphilis (090.0-097.9)

104.9 Spirochetal infection, unspecified

Mycoses (110-118)

Use additional code to identify manifestation as:
arthropathy (711.6)
meningitis (321.0-321.1)
otitis externa (380.15)
EXCLUDES infection by Actinomycetales, such as species of Actinomyces, Actinomadura, Nocardia, Streptomyces (039.0-039.9)

✓4ᵗʰ 110 Dermatophytosis

INCLUDES infection by species of Epidermophyton, Microsporum, and Trichophyton
tinea, any type except those in 111
DEF: Superficial infection of the skin caused by a parasitic fungus.

110.0 Of scalp and beard
Kerion
Sycosis, mycotic
Trichophytic tinea [black dot tinea], scalp

110.1 Of nail
Dermatophytic onychia
Onychomycosis
Tinea unguium
B35.1 Tinea unguium   I-10

110.2 Of hand
Tinea manuum

N Newborn Age: 0   P Pediatric Age: 0-17   M Maternity Age: 12-55   A Adult Age: 15-124

110.3 **Of groin and perianal area**
Dhobie itch
Eczema marginatum
Tinea cruris

110.4 **Of foot**
Athlete's foot
Tinea pedis

110.5 **Of the body**
Herpes circinatus
Tinea imbricata [Tokelau]

110.6 **Deep seated dermatophytosis**
Granuloma trichophyticum
Majocchi's granuloma

110.8 **Of other specified sites**

110.9 **Of unspecified site**
Favus NOS
Microsporic tinea NOS
Ringworm NOS

√4ᵗʰ 111 **Dermatomycosis, other and unspecified**

111.0 **Pityriasis versicolor**
Infection by Malassezia [Pityrosporum] furfur
Tinea flava
Tinea versicolor

111.1 **Tinea nigra**
Infection by Cladosporium species
Keratomycosis nigricans
Microsporosis nigra
Pityriasis nigra
Tinea palmaris nigra

111.2 **Tinea blanca**
Infection by Trichosporon (beigelii) cutaneum
White piedra

111.3 **Black piedra**
Infection by Piedraia hortai

111.8 **Other specified dermatomycoses**

111.9 **Dermatomycosis, unspecified**

√4ᵗʰ 112 **Candidiasis**
[INCLUDES] infection by Candida species
moniliasis
[EXCLUDES] *neonatal monilial infection (771.7)*
DEF: Fungal infection caused by *Candida*; usually seen in mucous membranes or skin.

112.0 **Of mouth**
Thrush (oral)
B37.0 Candidal stomatitis I-10

112.1 **Of vulva and vagina** ♀
Candidal vulvovaginitis
Monilial vulvovaginitis
B37.3 Candidiasis of vulva and vagina I-10

112.2 **Of other urogenital sites**
Candidal balanitis
AHA: 4Q, '03, 105; 4Q, '96, 33

112.3 **Of skin and nails**
Candidal intertrigo
Candidal onychia
Candidal perionyxis [paronychia]
B37.2 Candidiasis of skin and nail I-10

112.4 **Of lung**
Candidal pneumonia
AHA: 2Q, '98, 7

112.5 **Disseminated**
Systemic candidiasis
AHA: 2Q, '00, 5; 2Q, '89, 10

√5ᵗʰ 112.8 **Of other specified sites**

112.81 **Candidal endocarditis**

112.82 **Candidal otitis externa**
Otomycosis in moniliasis

112.83 **Candidal meningitis**

112.84 **Candidal esophagitis**
AHA: 4Q, '92, 19
B37.81 Candidal esophagitis I-10

112.85 **Candidal enteritis**
AHA: 4Q, '92, 19

112.89 **Other**
AHA: 1Q, '92, 17; 3Q, '91, 20

112.9 **Of unspecified site**

√4ᵗʰ 114 **Coccidioidomycosis**
[INCLUDES] infection by Coccidioides (immitis)
Posada-Wernicke disease
DEF: A fungal disease caused by inhalation of dust particles containing arthrospores of *Coccidiodes immitis;* a self-limited respiratory infection; the primary form is known as San Joaquin fever, desert fever or valley fever.
AHA: 4Q, '93, 23

114.0 **Primary coccidioidomycosis (pulmonary)**
Acute pulmonary coccidioidomycosis
Coccidioidomycotic pneumonitis
Desert rheumatism
Pulmonary coccidioidomycosis
San Joaquin Valley fever
DEF: Acute, self-limiting *Coccidioides immitis* infection of the lung.
B38.0 Acute pulmonary coccidioidomycosis I-10

114.1 **Primary extrapulmonary coccidioidomycosis**
Chancriform syndrome
Primary cutaneous coccidioidomycosis
DEF: Acute, self-limiting *Coccidioides immitis* infection in nonpulmonary site.

114.2 **Coccidioidal meningitis**
DEF: *Coccidioides immitis* infection of the lining of the brain and/or spinal cord.

114.3 **Other forms of progressive coccidioidomycosis**
Coccidioidal granuloma
Disseminated coccidioidomycosis

114.4 **Chronic pulmonary coccidioidomycosis**

114.5 **Pulmonary coccidioidomycosis, unspecified**

114.9 **Coccidioidomycosis, unspecified**

√4ᵗʰ 115 **Histoplasmosis**
The following fifth-digit subclassification is for use with category 115:
0 **without mention of manifestation**
1 **meningitis**
2 **retinitis**
3 **pericarditis**
4 **endocarditis**
5 **pneumonia**
9 **other**

§ √5ᵗʰ 115.0 **Infection by Histoplasma capsulatum**
[0-5, 9] American histoplasmosis
Darling's disease
Reticuloendothelial cytomycosis
Small form histoplasmosis
DEF: Infection resulting from inhalation of fungal spores, causing acute pneumonia, an influenza-like illness, or a disseminated disease of the reticuloendothelial system. In immunocompromised patients it can reactivate, affecting lungs, meninges, heart, peritoneum and adrenals.

§ √5ᵗʰ 115.1 **Infection by Histoplasma duboisii**
[0-5, 9] African histoplasmosis
Large form histoplasmosis

§ √5ᵗʰ 115.9 **Histoplasmosis, unspecified**
[0-5, 9] Histoplasmosis NOS

√4ᵗʰ 116 **Blastomycotic infection**

116.0 **Blastomycosis**
Blastomycotic dermatitis
Chicago disease
Cutaneous blastomycosis
Disseminated blastomycosis
Gilchrist's disease
Infection by Blastomyces [Ajellomyces] dermatitidis
North American blastomycosis
Primary pulmonary blastomycosis

---

§ Requires fifth digit. Valid digits are in [brackets] under each code. See category 115 for codes and definitions.

√4ᵗʰ / √5ᵗʰ Additional Digit Required   Unspecified Code   Other Specified Code   Manifestation Code   ▶◀ Revised Text   ● New Code   ▲ Revised Code Title

Infectious and Parasitic Diseases

116.1 Paracoccidioidomycosis
Brazilian blastomycosis
Infection by Paracoccidioides [Blastomyces] brasiliensis
Lutz-Splendore-Almeida disease
Mucocutaneous-lymphangitic paracoccidioidomycosis
Pulmonary paracoccidioidomycosis
South American blastomycosis
Visceral paracoccidioidomycosis

116.2 Lobomycosis
Infections by Loboa [Blastomyces] loboi
Keloidal blastomycosis
Lobo's disease

✓4ᵗʰ **117 Other mycoses**

117.0 Rhinosporidiosis
Infection by Rhinosporidium seeberi

117.1 Sporotrichosis
Cutaneous sporotrichosis
Disseminated sporotrichosis
Infection by Sporothrix [Sporotrichum] schenckii
Lymphocutaneous sporotrichosis
Pulmonary sporotrichosis
Sporotrichosis of the bones

117.2 Chromoblastomycosis
Chromomycosis
Infection by Cladosporidium carrionii, Fonsecaea compactum, Fonsecaea pedrosoi, Phialophora verrucosa

117.3 Aspergillosis
Infection by Aspergillus species, mainly A. fumigatus, A. flavus group, A. terreus group
AHA: 4Q, '97, 40

117.4 Mycotic mycetomas
Infection by various genera and species of Ascomycetes and Deuteromycetes, such as Acremonium [Cephalosporium] falciforme, Neotestudina rosatii, Madurella grisea, Madurella mycetomii, Pyrenochaeta romeroi, Zopfia [Leptosphaeria] senegalensis
Madura foot, mycotic
Maduromycosis, mycotic
EXCLUDES actinomycotic mycetomas (039.0-039.9)

117.5 Cryptococcosis
Busse-Buschke's disease
European cryptococcosis
Infection by Cryptococcus neoformans
Pulmonary cryptococcosis
Systemic cryptococcosis
Torula

117.6 Allescheriosis [Petriellidosis]
Infections by Allescheria [Petriellidium] boydii [Monosporium apiospermum]
EXCLUDES mycotic mycetoma (117.4)

117.7 Zygomycosis [Phycomycosis or Mucormycosis]
Infection by species of Absidia, Basidiobolus, Conidiobolus, Cunninghamella, Entomophthora, Mucor, Rhizopus, Saksenaea

117.8 Infection by dematiacious fungi, [Phaeyphomycosis]
Infection by dematiacious fungi, such as Cladosporium trichoides [bantianum], Dreschlera hawaiiensis, Phialophora gougerotii, Phialophora jeanselmi

117.9 Other and unspecified mycoses

118 Opportunistic mycoses
Infection of skin, subcutaneous tissues, and/or organs by a wide variety of fungi generally considered to be pathogenic to compromised hosts only (e.g., infection by species of Alternaria, Dreschlera, Fusarium)
Use additional code to identify manifestation, such as:
keratitis (370.8)

Helminthiases (120-129)

✓4ᵗʰ **120 Schistosomiasis [bilharziasis]**
DEF: Infection caused by *Schistosoma*, a genus of flukes or trematode parasites.

120.0 Schistosoma haematobium
Vesical schistosomiasis NOS

120.1 Schistosoma mansoni
Intestinal schistosomiasis NOS

120.2 Schistosoma japonicum
Asiatic schistosomiasis NOS
Katayama disease or fever

120.3 Cutaneous
Cercarial dermatitis
Infection by cercariae of Schistosoma
Schistosome dermatitis
Swimmers' itch

120.8 Other specified schistosomiasis
Infection by Schistosoma:
bovis
intercalatum
mattheii
spindale
Schistosomiasis chestermani

120.9 Schistosomiasis, unspecified
Blood flukes NOS
Hemic distomiasis

✓4ᵗʰ **121 Other trematode infections**

121.0 Opisthorchiasis
Infection by:
cat liver fluke
Opisthorchis (felineus) (tenuicollis) (viverrini)

121.1 Clonorchiasis
Biliary cirrhosis due to clonorchiasis
Chinese liver fluke disease
Hepatic distomiasis due to Clonorchis sinensis
Oriental liver fluke disease

121.2 Paragonimiasis
Infection by Paragonimus
Lung fluke disease (oriental)
Pulmonary distomiasis

121.3 Fascioliasis
Infection by Fasciola:
gigantica
hepatica
Liver flukes NOS
Sheep liver fluke infection

121.4 Fasciolopsiasis
Infection by Fasciolopsis (buski)
Intestinal distomiasis

121.5 Metagonimiasis
Infection by Metagonimus yokogawai

121.6 Heterophyiasis
Infection by:
Heterophyes heterophyes
Stellantchasmus falcatus

121.8 Other specified trematode infections
Infection by:
Dicrocoelium dendriticum
Echinostoma ilocanum
Gastrodiscoides hominis

121.9 Trematode infection, unspecified
Distomiasis NOS
Fluke disease NOS

✓4ᵗʰ **122 Echinococcosis**
INCLUDES echinococciasis
hydatid disease
hydatidosis
DEF: Infection caused by larval forms of tapeworms of the genus *Echinococcus*.

122.0 Echinococcus granulosus infection of liver

122.1 Echinococcus granulosus infection of lung

122.2 Echinococcus granulosus infection of thyroid

122.3 Echinococcus granulosus infection, other

122.4 Echinococcus granulosus infection, unspecified

122.5 Echinococcus multilocularis infection of liver

122.6 Echinococcus multilocularis infection, other

122.7 Echinococcus multilocularis infection, unspecified

122.8 Echinococcosis, unspecified, of liver

122.9 Echinococcosis, other and unspecified

√4th **123 Other cestode infection**

123.0 Taenia solium infection, intestinal form
   Pork tapeworm (adult) (infection)

123.1 Cysticercosis
   Cysticerciasis
   Infection by Cysticercus cellulosae [larval form of Taenia solium]
   AHA: 2Q, '97, 8

123.2 Taenia saginata infection
   Beef tapeworm (infection)
   Infection by Taeniarhynchus saginatus

123.3 Taeniasis, unspecified

123.4 Diphyllobothriasis, intestinal
   Diphyllobothrium (adult) (latum) (pacificum) infection
   Fish tapeworm (infection)

123.5 Sparganosis [larval diphyllobothriasis]
   Infection by:
      Diphyllobothrium larvae
      Sparganum (mansoni) (proliferum)
      Spirometra larvae

123.6 Hymenolepiasis
   Dwarf tapeworm (infection)
   Hymenolepis (diminuta) (nana) infection
   Rat tapeworm (infection)

123.8 Other specified cestode infection
   Diplogonoporus (grandis) ⎫
   Dipylidium (caninum) ⎬ infection
   Dog tapeworm (infection) ⎭

123.9 Cestode infection, unspecified
   Tapeworm (infection) NOS

124 Trichinosis
   Trichinella spiralis infection
   Trichinellosis
   Trichiniasis
   DEF: Infection by *Trichinella spiralis*, the smallest of the parasitic nematodes.

√4th **125 Filarial infection and dracontiasis**

125.0 Bancroftian filariasis
   Chyluria ⎫
   Elephantiasis ⎪
   Infection ⎬ due to Wuchereria bancrofti
   Lymphadenitis ⎪
   Lymphangitis ⎭
   Wuchereriasis

125.1 Malayan filariasis
   Brugia filariasis ⎫
   Chyluria ⎪
   Elephantiasis ⎪
   Infection ⎬ due to Brugia [Wuchereria] malayi
   Lymphadenitis ⎪
   Lymphangitis ⎭

125.2 Loiasis
   Eyeworm disease of Africa
   Loa loa infection

125.3 Onchocerciasis
   Onchocerca volvulus infection
   Onchocercosis

125.4 Dipetalonemiasis
   Infection by:
      Acanthocheilonema perstans
      Dipetalonema perstans

125.5 Mansonella ozzardi infection
   Filariasis ozzardi

125.6 Other specified filariasis
   Dirofilaria infection
   Infection by:
      Acanthocheilonema streptocerca
      Dipetalonema streptocerca

125.7 Dracontiasis
   Guinea-worm infection
   Infection by Dracunculus medinensis

125.9 Unspecified filariasis

√4th **126 Ancylostomiasis and necatoriasis**
   [INCLUDES] cutaneous larva migrans due to Ancylostoma
      hookworm (disease) (infection)
      uncinariasis

126.0 Ancylostoma duodenale

126.1 Necator americanus

126.2 Ancylostoma braziliense

126.3 Ancylostoma ceylanicum

126.8 Other specified Ancylostoma

126.9 Ancylostomiasis and necatoriasis, unspecified
   Creeping eruption NOS
   Cutaneous larva migrans NOS

√4th **127 Other intestinal helminthiases**

127.0 Ascariasis
   Ascaridiasis
   Infection by Ascaris lumbricoides
   Roundworm infection

127.1 Anisakiasis
   Infection by Anisakis larva

127.2 Strongyloidiasis
   Infection by Strongyloides stercoralis
   [EXCLUDES] *trichostrongyliasis (127.6)*

127.3 Trichuriasis
   Infection by Trichuris trichiuria
   Trichocephaliasis
   Whipworm (disease) (infection)

127.4 Enterobiasis
   Infection by Enterobius vermicularis
   Oxyuriasis
   Oxyuris vermicularis infection
   Pinworm (disease) (infection)
   Threadworm infection

127.5 Capillariasis
   Infection by Capillaria philippinensis
   [EXCLUDES] *infection by Capillaria hepatica (128.8)*

127.6 Trichostrongyliasis
   Infection by Trichostrongylus species

127.7 Other specified intestinal helminthiasis
   Infection by:
      Oesophagostomum apiostomum and related species
      Ternidens diminutus
      other specified intestinal helminth
   Physalopteriasis

127.8 Mixed intestinal helminthiasis
   Infection by intestinal helminths classified to more than one
      of the categories 120.0-127.7
   Mixed helminthiasis NOS

127.9 Intestinal helminthiasis, unspecified

√4th **128 Other and unspecified helminthiases**

128.0 Toxocariasis
   Larva migrans visceralis
   Toxocara (canis) (cati) infection
   Visceral larva migrans syndrome

128.1 Gnathostomiasis
   Infection by Gnathostoma spinigerum and related species

√4th√5th Additional Digit Required   Unspecified Code   Other Specified Code   Manifestation Code   ►◄ Revised Text   ● New Code   ▲ Revised Code Title

2013 ICD-9-CM   **Volume 1 – 23**

Infectious and Parasitic Diseases

128.8–136.5

128.8 Other specified helminthiasis
Infection by:
Angiostrongylus cantonensis
Capillaria hepatica
other specified helminth

128.9 Helminth infection, unspecified
Helminthiasis NOS
Worms NOS

129 Intestinal parasitism, unspecified

Other Infectious and Parasitic Diseases (130–136)

✓4ᵗʰ 130 Toxoplasmosis
INCLUDES   infection by toxoplasma gondii
toxoplasmosis (acquired)
EXCLUDES   *congenital toxoplasmosis (771.2)*

130.0 Meningoencephalitis due to toxoplasmosis
Encephalitis due to acquired toxoplasmosis

130.1 Conjunctivitis due to toxoplasmosis

130.2 Chorioretinitis due to toxoplasmosis
Focal retinochoroiditis due to acquired toxoplasmosis

130.3 Myocarditis due to toxoplasmosis

130.4 Pneumonitis due to toxoplasmosis

130.5 Hepatitis due to toxoplasmosis

130.7 Toxoplasmosis of other specified sites

130.8 Multisystemic disseminated toxoplasmosis
Toxoplasmosis of multiple sites

130.9 Toxoplasmosis, unspecified

✓4ᵗʰ 131 Trichomoniasis
INCLUDES   infection due to Trichomonas (vaginalis)

✓5ᵗʰ 131.0 Urogenital trichomoniasis

131.00 Urogenital trichomoniasis, unspecified
Fluor (vaginalis)   } trichomonal or due to
Leukorrhea (vaginalis)   } Trichomonas
                 (vaginalis)
DEF: *Trichomonas vaginalis* infection of reproductive and urinary organs, transmitted through coitus.

131.01 Trichomonal vulvovaginitis   ♀
Vaginitis, trichomonal or due to Trichomonas (vaginalis)
DEF: *Trichomonas vaginalis* infection of vulva and vagina; often asymptomatic, transmitted through coitus.

131.02 Trichomonal urethritis
DEF: *Trichomonas vaginalis* infection of the urethra.

131.03 Trichomonal prostatitis   ♂
DEF: *Trichomonas vaginalis* infection of the prostate.

131.09 Other

131.8 Other specified sites
EXCLUDES   *intestinal (007.3)*

131.9 Trichomoniasis, unspecified

✓4ᵗʰ 132 Pediculosis and phthirus infestation

132.0 Pediculus capitis [head louse]

132.1 Pediculus corporis [body louse]

132.2 Phthirus pubis [pubic louse]
Pediculus pubis

132.3 Mixed infestation
Infestation classifiable to more than one of the categories 132.0-132.2

132.9 Pediculosis, unspecified

✓4ᵗʰ 133 Acariasis

133.0 Scabies
Infestation by Sarcoptes scabiei
Norwegian scabies
Sarcoptic itch

133.8 Other acariasis
Chiggers
Infestation by:
Demodex folliculorum
Trombicula

133.9 Acariasis, unspecified
Infestation by mites NOS

✓4ᵗʰ 134 Other infestation

134.0 Myiasis
Infestation by:
Dermatobia (hominis)
fly larvae
Gasterophilus (intestinalis)
maggots
Oestrus ovis

134.1 Other arthropod infestation
Infestation by: Jigger disease
chigoe   Scarabiasis
sand flea   Tungiasis
Tunga penetrans

134.2 Hirudiniasis
Hirudiniasis (external) (internal)
Leeches (aquatic) (land)

134.8 Other specified infestations

134.9 Infestation, unspecified
Infestation (skin) NOS   Skin parasites NOS

135 Sarcoidosis
Besnier-Boeck-Schaumann disease
Lupoid (miliary) of Boeck
Lupus pernio (Besnier)
Lymphogranulomatosis, benign (Schaumann's)
Sarcoid (any site):
NOS
Boeck
Darier-Roussy
Uveoparotid fever
DEF: A chronic, granulomatous reticulosis (abnormal increase in cells), affecting any organ or tissue; acute form has high rate of remission; chronic form is progressive.
D86.9 Sarcoidosis unspecified   I-10

✓4ᵗʰ 136 Other and unspecified infectious and parasitic diseases

136.0 Ainhum
Dactylolysis spontanea
DEF: A disease affecting the toes, especially the fifth digit, and the fingers, mostly seen in black adult males; characterized by a linear constriction around the affected digit leading to spontaneous amputation of the distal part of the digit.

136.1 Behçet's syndrome
DEF: A chronic inflammatory disorder of unknown etiology involving the small blood vessels; characterized by recurrent aphthous ulceration of the oral and pharyngeal mucous membranes and the genitalia, skin lesions, severe uveitis, retinal vascularitis and optic atrophy.

✓5ᵗʰ 136.2 Specific infections by free-living amebae
AHA: 4Q, '08, 79-81

136.21 Specific infection due to acanthamoeba
Use additional code to identify manifestation, such as:
keratitis (370.8)
AHA: 4Q, '08, 81

136.29 Other specific infections by free-living amebae
Meningoencephalitis due to Naegleria

136.3 Pneumocystosis
Pneumonia due to Pneumocystis carinii
Pneumonia due to Pneumocystis jiroveci
AHA: 1Q, '05, 7; 1Q, '03, 15; N-D, '87, 5-6
DEF: *Pneumocystis carinii* fungus causing pneumonia in immunocompromised patients; a leading cause of death among AIDS patients.

136.4 Psorospermiasis

136.5 Sarcosporidiosis
Infection by Sarcocystis lindemanni
DEF: *Sarcocystis* infection causing muscle cysts of intestinal inflammation.

N Newborn Age: 0   P Pediatric Age: 0-17   M Maternity Age: 12-55   A Adult Age: 15-124

136.8 Other specified infectious and parasitic diseases
Candiru infestation

136.9 Unspecified infectious and parasitic diseases
Infectious disease NOS
Parasitic disease NOS
AHA: 2Q, '91, 8

Late Effects of Infectious and Parasitic Diseases (137-139)

✓4ᵗʰ 137 Late effects of tuberculosis

NOTE This category is to be used to indicate conditions classifiable to 010-018 as the cause of late effects, which are themselves classified elsewhere. The "late effects" include those specified as such, as sequelae, or as due to old or inactive tuberculosis, without evidence of active disease.

137.0 Late effects of respiratory or unspecified tuberculosis

137.1 Late effects of central nervous system tuberculosis

137.2 Late effects of genitourinary tuberculosis

137.3 Late effects of tuberculosis of bones and joints

137.4 Late effects of tuberculosis of other specified organs

138 Late effects of acute poliomyelitis

NOTE This category is to be used to indicate conditions classifiable to 045 as the cause of late effects, which are themselves classified elsewhere. The "late effects" include conditions specified as such, or as sequelae, or as due to old or inactive poliomyelitis, without evidence of active disease.

B91 Sequelae of poliomyelitis   I-10

✓4ᵗʰ 139 Late effects of other infectious and parasitic diseases

NOTE This category is to be used to indicate conditions classifiable to categories 001-009, 020-041, 046-136 as the cause of late effects, which are themselves classified elsewhere. The "late effects" include conditions specified as such; they also include sequela of diseases classifiable to the above categories if there is evidence that the disease itself is no longer present.

139.0 Late effects of viral encephalitis
Late effects of conditions classifiable to 049.8-049.9, 062-064

139.1 Late effects of trachoma
Late effects of conditions classifiable to 076

139.8 Late effects of other and unspecified infectious and parasitic diseases
AHA: 2Q, '06, 17; 4Q, '91, 15; 3Q, '90, 14; M-A, '87, 8

✓4ᵗʰ
✓5ᵗʰ Additional Digit Required   Unspecified Code   Other Specified Code   Manifestation Code   ►◄ Revised Text   ● New Code   ▲ Revised Code Title
2013 ICD-9-CM   **Volume 1 – 25**

2. Neoplasms (140-239)

NOTES

1. Content

This chapter contains the following broad groups:

140-195	Malignant neoplasms, stated or presumed to be primary, of specified sites, except of lymphatic and hematopoietic tissue
196-198	Malignant neoplasms, stated or presumed to be secondary, of specified sites
199	Malignant neoplasms, without specification of site
200-208	Malignant neoplasms, stated or presumed to be primary, of lymphatic and hematopoietic tissue
209	Neuroendocrine tumors
210-229	Benign neoplasms
230-234	Carcinoma in situ
235-238	Neoplasms of uncertain behavior [see Note, above category 235]
239	Neoplasms of unspecified nature

2. Functional activity

All neoplasms are classified in this chapter, whether or not functionally active. An additional code from Chapter 3 may be used to identify such functional activity associated with any neoplasm, e.g.:

catecholamine-producing malignant pheochromocytoma of adrenal:

code 194.0, additional code 255.6

basophil adenoma of pituitary with Cushing's syndrome:

code 227.3, additional code 255.0

3. Morphology [Histology]

For those wishing to identify the histological type of neoplasms, a comprehensive coded nomenclature, which comprises the morphology rubrics of the ICD-Oncology, is given in Appendix A.

4. Malignant neoplasms overlapping site boundaries

Categories 140-195 are for the classification of primary malignant neoplasms according to their point of origin. A malignant neoplasm that overlaps two or more subcategories within a three-digit rubric and whose point of origin cannot be determined should be classified to the subcategory .8 "Other."

For example, "carcinoma involving tip and ventral surface of tongue" should be assigned to 141.8. On the other hand, "carcinoma of tip of tongue, extending to involve the ventral surface" should be coded to 141.2, as the point of origin, the tip, is known. Three subcategories (149.8, 159.8, 165.8) have been provided for malignant neoplasms that overlap the boundaries of three-digit rubrics within certain systems.

Overlapping malignant neoplasms that cannot be classified as indicated above should be assigned to the appropriate subdivision of category 195 (Malignant neoplasm of other and ill-defined sites).

> **DEF:** An abnormal growth; morphology determines behavior, i.e., whether it will remain intact (benign) or spread to adjacent tissue (malignant). The term mass is not synonymous with neoplasm, as it is often used to describe cysts and thickenings such as those occurring with hematoma or infection.
> **AHA:** 2Q, '90, 7

Malignant Neoplasm of Lip, Oral Cavity, and Pharynx (140-149)

EXCLUDES carcinoma in situ (230.0)

√4ᵗʰ **140 Malignant neoplasm of lip**

EXCLUDES malignant melanoma of skin of lip (172.0)
malignant neoplasm of skin of lip (173.00-173.09)

140.0 Upper lip, vermilion border
Upper lip:
NOS
external
lipstick area

140.1 Lower lip, vermilion border
Lower lip:
NOS
external
lipstick area

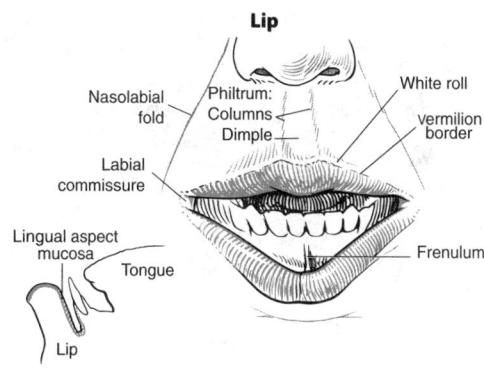

Lip

Nasolabial fold
Philtrum:
Columns
Dimple
White roll
vermilion border
Labial commissure
Lingual aspect mucosa
Tongue
Frenulum
Lip

140.3 Upper lip, inner aspect
Upper lip:
buccal aspect
frenulum
mucosa
oral aspect

140.4 Lower lip, inner aspect
Lower lip:
buccal aspect
frenulum
mucosa
oral aspect

140.5 Lip, unspecified, inner aspect
Lip, not specified whether upper or lower:
buccal aspect
frenulum
mucosa
oral aspect

140.6 Commissure of lip
Labial commissure

140.8 Other sites of lip
Malignant neoplasm of contiguous or overlapping sites of lip whose point of origin cannot be determined

140.9 Lip, unspecified, vermilion border
Lip, not specified as upper or lower:
NOS
external
lipstick area

√4ᵗʰ **141 Malignant neoplasm of tongue**

141.0 Base of tongue
Dorsal surface of base of tongue
Fixed part of tongue NOS
AHA: 4Q, '06, 90

141.1 Dorsal surface of tongue
Anterior two-thirds of tongue, dorsal surface
Dorsal tongue NOS
Midline of tongue
EXCLUDES dorsal surface of base of tongue (141.0)

141.2 Tip and lateral border of tongue

141.3 Ventral surface of tongue
Anterior two-thirds of tongue, ventral surface
Frenulum linguae

141.4 Anterior two-thirds of tongue, part unspecified
Mobile part of tongue NOS

141.5 Junctional zone
Border of tongue at junction of fixed and mobile parts at insertion of anterior tonsillar pillar

√4ᵗʰ √5ᵗʰ Additional Digit Required   Unspecified Code   Other Specified Code   Manifestation Code   ►◄ Revised Text   ● New Code   ▲ Revised Code Title

2013 ICD-9-CM   **Volume 1 – 27**

Tongue

Main Salivary Glands

Mouth

Oropharynx

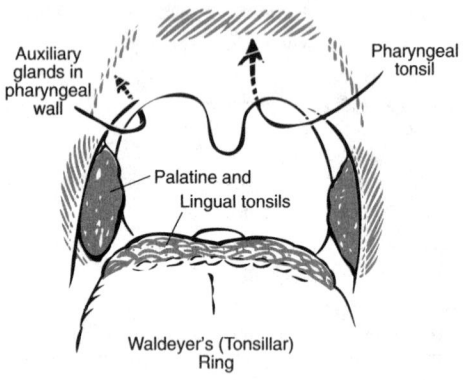

141.6 Lingual tonsil

141.8 Other sites of tongue
Malignant neoplasm of contiguous or overlapping sites of tongue whose point of origin cannot be determined

141.9 Tongue, unspecified
Tongue NOS

√4ᵗʰ 142 Malignant neoplasm of major salivary glands
INCLUDES salivary ducts
EXCLUDES malignant neoplasm of minor salivary glands:
NOS (145.9)
buccal mucosa (145.0)
soft palate (145.3)
tongue (141.0-141.9)
tonsil, palatine (146.0)

142.0 Parotid gland

142.1 Submandibular gland
Submaxillary gland

142.2 Sublingual gland

142.8 Other major salivary glands
Malignant neoplasm of contiguous or overlapping sites of salivary glands and ducts whose point of origin cannot be determined

142.9 Salivary gland, unspecified
Salivary gland (major) NOS

√4ᵗʰ 143 Malignant neoplasm of gum
INCLUDES alveolar (ridge) mucosa
gingiva (alveolar) (marginal)
interdental papillae
EXCLUDES malignant odontogenic neoplasms (170.0-170.1)

143.0 Upper gum

143.1 Lower gum

143.8 Other sites of gum
Malignant neoplasm of contiguous or overlapping sites of gum whose point of origin cannot be determined

143.9 Gum, unspecified

√4ᵗʰ 144 Malignant neoplasm of floor of mouth

144.0 Anterior portion
Anterior to the premolar-canine junction

144.1 Lateral portion

144.8 Other sites of floor of mouth
Malignant neoplasm of contiguous or overlapping sites of floor of mouth whose point of origin cannot be determined

144.9 Floor of mouth, part unspecified

√4ᵗʰ 145 Malignant neoplasm of other and unspecified parts of mouth
EXCLUDES mucosa of lips (140.0-140.9)

145.0 Cheek mucosa
Buccal mucosa
Cheek, inner aspect

145.1 Vestibule of mouth
Buccal sulcus (upper) (lower)
Labial sulcus (upper) (lower)

145.2 Hard palate

145.3 Soft palate
EXCLUDES nasopharyngeal [posterior] [superior] surface of soft palate (147.3)

145.4 Uvula

145.5 Palate, unspecified
Junction of hard and soft palate
Roof of mouth

145.6 Retromolar area

145.8 Other specified parts of mouth
Malignant neoplasm of contiguous or overlapping sites of mouth whose point of origin cannot be determined

145.9 Mouth, unspecified
Buccal cavity NOS
Minor salivary gland, unspecified site
Oral cavity NOS

Nasopharynx

Hypopharynx

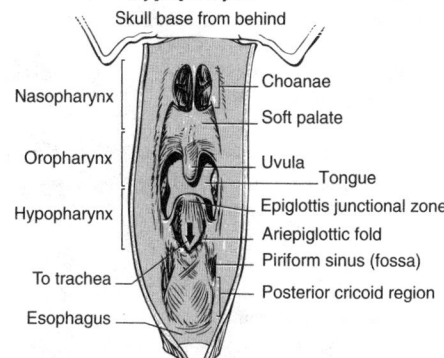

☑4ᵗʰ **146 Malignant neoplasm of oropharynx**

  146.0 Tonsil
Tonsil:
  NOS
  faucial
  palatine
EXCLUDES *lingual tonsil (141.6)*
pharyngeal tonsil (147.1)
AHA: S-O, '87, 8

  146.1 Tonsillar fossa

  146.2 Tonsillar pillars (anterior) (posterior)
Faucial pillar
Glossopalatine fold
Palatoglossal arch
Palatopharyngeal arch

  146.3 Vallecula
Anterior and medial surface of the pharyngoepiglottic fold

  146.4 Anterior aspect of epiglottis
Epiglottis, free border [margin]
Glossoepiglottic fold(s)
EXCLUDES *epiglottis:*
NOS (161.1)
suprahyoid portion (161.1)

  146.5 Junctional region
Junction of the free margin of the epiglottis, the aryepiglottic fold, and the pharyngoepiglottic fold

  146.6 Lateral wall of oropharynx

  146.7 Posterior wall of oropharynx

  146.8 Other specified sites of oropharynx
Branchial cleft
Malignant neoplasm of contiguous or overlapping sites of oropharynx whose point of origin cannot be determined

  146.9 Oropharynx, unspecified
AHA: 2Q, '02, 6

☑4ᵗʰ **147 Malignant neoplasm of nasopharynx**

  147.0 Superior wall
Roof of nasopharynx

  147.1 Posterior wall
Adenoid
Pharyngeal tonsil

  147.2 Lateral wall
Fossa of Rosenmüller
Opening of auditory tube
Pharyngeal recess

  147.3 Anterior wall
Floor of nasopharynx
Nasopharyngeal [posterior] [superior] surface of soft palate
Posterior margin of nasal septum and choanae

  147.8 Other specified sites of nasopharynx
Malignant neoplasm of contiguous or overlapping sites of nasopharynx whose point of origin cannot be determined

  147.9 Nasopharynx, unspecified
Nasopharyngeal wall NOS

☑4ᵗʰ **148 Malignant neoplasm of hypopharynx**

  148.0 Postcricoid region

  148.1 Pyriform sinus
Pyriform fossa

  148.2 Aryepiglottic fold, hypopharyngeal aspect
Aryepiglottic fold or interarytenoid fold:
  NOS
  marginal zone
EXCLUDES *aryepiglottic fold or interarytenoid fold, laryngeal aspect (161.1)*

  148.3 Posterior hypopharyngeal wall

  148.8 Other specified sites of hypopharynx
Malignant neoplasm of contiguous or overlapping sites of hypopharynx whose point of origin cannot be determined

  148.9 Hypopharynx, unspecified
Hypopharyngeal wall NOS
Hypopharynx NOS

☑4ᵗʰ **149 Malignant neoplasm of other and ill-defined sites within the lip, oral cavity, and pharynx**

  149.0 Pharynx, unspecified

  149.1 Waldeyer's ring

  149.8 Other
Malignant neoplasms of lip, oral cavity, and pharynx whose point of origin cannot be assigned to any one of the categories 140-148
EXCLUDES *"book leaf" neoplasm [ventral surface of tongue and floor of mouth] (145.8)*

  149.9 Ill-defined

Malignant Neoplasm of Digestive Organs and Peritoneum (150-159)

EXCLUDES *carcinoma in situ (230.1-230.9)*

☑4ᵗʰ **150 Malignant neoplasm of esophagus**

  150.0 Cervical esophagus

  150.1 Thoracic esophagus

  150.2 Abdominal esophagus
EXCLUDES *adenocarcinoma (151.0)*
cardio-esophageal junction (151.0)

  150.3 Upper third of esophagus
Proximal third of esophagus

  150.4 Middle third of esophagus

  150.5 Lower third of esophagus
Distal third of esophagus
EXCLUDES *adenocarcinoma (151.0)*
cardio-esophageal junction (151.0)

  150.8 Other specified part
Malignant neoplasm of contiguous or overlapping sites of esophagus whose point of origin cannot be determined

  150.9 Esophagus, unspecified

✓4ᵗʰ **151 Malignant neoplasm of stomach**

    EXCLUDES *benign carcinoid tumor of stomach (209.63)*
                    malignant carcinoid tumor of stomach (209.23)

151.0 Cardia
    Cardiac orifice
    Cardio-esophageal junction
    EXCLUDES *squamous cell carcinoma (150.2, 150.5)*

151.1 Pylorus
    Prepylorus
    Pyloric canal

151.2 Pyloric antrum
    Antrum of stomach NOS

151.3 Fundus of stomach

151.4 Body of stomach

151.5 Lesser curvature, unspecified
    Lesser curvature, not classifiable to 151.1-151.4

151.6 Greater curvature, unspecified
    Greater curvature, not classifiable to 151.0-151.4

151.8 Other specified sites of stomach
    Anterior wall, not classifiable to 151.0-151.4
    Posterior wall, not classifiable to 151.0-151.4
    Malignant neoplasm of contiguous or overlapping sites of
         stomach whose point of origin cannot be determined

151.9 Stomach, unspecified
    Carcinoma ventriculi
    Gastric cancer
    AHA: 2Q, '01, 17

✓4ᵗʰ **152 Malignant neoplasm of small intestine, including duodenum**

    EXCLUDES *benign carcinoid tumor of small intestine and duodenum*
                    (209.40-209.43)
                   malignant carcinoid tumor of small intestine and duodenum
                    (209.00-209.03)

152.0 Duodenum

152.1 Jejunum

152.2 Ileum
    EXCLUDES *ileocecal valve (153.4)*

152.3 Meckel's diverticulum

152.8 Other specified sites of small intestine
    Duodenojejunal junction
    Malignant neoplasm of contiguous or overlapping sites of
         small intestine whose point of origin cannot be
         determined

152.9 Small intestine, unspecified

✓4ᵗʰ **153 Malignant neoplasm of colon**

    EXCLUDES *benign carcinoid tumor of colon (209.50-209.56)*
                    malignant carcinoid tumor of colon (209.10-209.16)

153.0 Hepatic flexure

153.1 Transverse colon

153.2 Descending colon
    Left colon

153.3 Sigmoid colon
    Sigmoid (flexure)
    EXCLUDES *rectosigmoid junction (154.0)*

153.4 Cecum
    Ileocecal valve
    C18.0 Malignant neoplasm of cecum   I-10

153.5 Appendix

153.6 Ascending colon
    Right colon
    C18.2 Malignant neoplasm of ascending colon   I-10

153.7 Splenic flexure

153.8 Other specified sites of large intestine
    Malignant neoplasm of contiguous or overlapping sites of
         colon whose point of origin cannot be determined
    EXCLUDES *ileocecal valve (153.4)*
                    rectosigmoid junction (154.0)

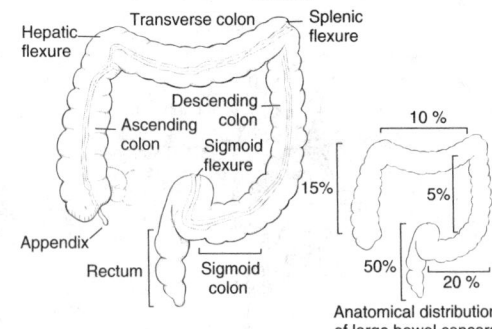

Colon

Anatomical distribution of large bowel cancers

153.9 Colon, unspecified
    Large intestine NOS
    AHA: 2Q, '10, 12
    C18.9 Malignant neoplasm of colon unspecified   I-10

✓4ᵗʰ **154 Malignant neoplasm of rectum, rectosigmoid junction, and anus**

    EXCLUDES *benign carcinoid tumor of rectum (209.57)*
                    malignant carcinoid tumor of rectum (209.17)

154.0 Rectosigmoid junction
    Colon with rectum
    Rectosigmoid (colon)

154.1 Rectum
    Rectal ampulla
    C20 Malignant neoplasm of rectum   I-10

154.2 Anal canal
    Anal sphincter
    EXCLUDES *malignant melanoma of skin of anus (172.5)*
                    malignant neoplasm of skin of anus (173.50-173.59)
    AHA: 1Q, '01, 8

154.3 Anus, unspecified
    EXCLUDES *malignant melanoma of:*
                    anus:
                       margin (172.5)
                       skin (172.5)
                    perianal skin (172.5)
                    malignant neoplasm of:
                    anus:
                       margin (173.50-173.59)
                       skin (173.50-173.59)
                    perianal skin (173.50-173.59)

154.8 Other
    Anorectum
    Cloacogenic zone
    Malignant neoplasm of contiguous or overlapping sites of
         rectum, rectosigmoid junction, and anus whose point of
         origin cannot be determined

✓4ᵗʰ **155 Malignant neoplasm of liver and intrahepatic bile ducts**

155.0 Liver, primary
    Carcinoma:
         hepatocellular
         liver cell
         liver, specified as primary
    Hepatoblastoma
    AHA: 4Q, '08, 82
    C22.0 Liver cell carcinoma   I-10

155.1 Intrahepatic bile ducts
    Canaliculi biliferi
    Interlobular:
         bile ducts
         biliary canals
    Intrahepatic:
         biliary passages
         canaliculi
         gall duct
    EXCLUDES *hepatic duct (156.1)*

155.2 Liver, not specified as primary or secondary

    N Newborn Age: 0   **P** Pediatric Age: 0-17   **M** Maternity Age: 12-55   **A** Adult Age: 15-124

Retroperitoneum and Peritoneum

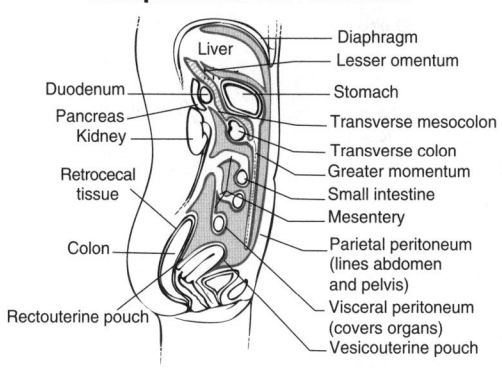

Liver
Diaphragm
Lesser omentum
Duodenum
Pancreas
Kidney
Stomach
Transverse mesocolon
Transverse colon
Greater momentum
Retrocecal tissue
Small intestine
Mesentery
Colon
Parietal peritoneum (lines abdomen and pelvis)
Rectouterine pouch
Visceral peritoneum (covers organs)
Vesicouterine pouch

√4ᵗʰ **156　Malignant neoplasm of gallbladder and extrahepatic bile ducts**

156.0　Gallbladder

156.1　Extrahepatic bile ducts
Biliary duct or passage NOS
Common bile duct
Cystic duct
Hepatic duct
Sphincter of Oddi

156.2　Ampulla of Vater
DEF: Malignant neoplasm in the area of dilation at the juncture of the common bile and pancreatic ducts near the opening into the lumen of the duodenum.

156.8　Other specified sites of gallbladder and extrahepatic bile ducts
Malignant neoplasm of contiguous or overlapping sites of gallbladder and extrahepatic bile ducts whose point of origin cannot be determined

156.9　Biliary tract, part unspecified
Malignant neoplasm involving both intrahepatic and extrahepatic bile ducts

√4ᵗʰ **157　Malignant neoplasm of pancreas**
AHA: 4Q, '07, 72

157.0　Head of pancreas
AHA: 2Q, '05, 9; 4Q, '00, 40

157.1　Body of pancreas

157.2　Tail of pancreas

157.3　Pancreatic duct
Duct of:
Santorini
Wirsung

157.4　Islets of Langerhans
Islets of Langerhans, any part of pancreas
Use additional code to identify any functional activity
DEF: Malignant neoplasm within the structures of the pancreas that produce insulin, somatostatin and glucagon.

157.8　Other specified sites of pancreas
Ectopic pancreatic tissue
Malignant neoplasm of contiguous or overlapping sites of pancreas whose point of origin cannot be determined

157.9　Pancreas, part unspecified
AHA: 4Q, '89, 11
C25.9　Malignant neoplasm of pancreas unspecified　　I-10

√4ᵗʰ **158　Malignant neoplasm of retroperitoneum and peritoneum**

158.0　Retroperitoneum
Periadrenal tissue　　Perirenal tissue
Perinephric tissue　　Retrocecal tissue

158.8　Specified parts of peritoneum
Cul-de-sac (of Douglas)
Malignant neoplasm of contiguous or overlapping sites of retroperitoneum and peritoneum whose point of origin cannot be determined
Mesentery
Mesocolon
Omentum
Peritoneum:
parietal
pelvic
Rectouterine pouch

158.9　Peritoneum, unspecified

√4ᵗʰ **159　Malignant neoplasm of other and ill-defined sites within the digestive organs and peritoneum**

159.0　Intestinal tract, part unspecified
Intestine NOS

159.1　Spleen, not elsewhere classified
Angiosarcoma ⎫ of spleen
Fibrosarcoma ⎭
EXCLUDES　*Hodgkin's disease (201.0-201.9)*
lymphosarcoma (200.1)
reticulosarcoma (200.0)

159.8　Other sites of digestive system and intra-abdominal organs
Malignant neoplasm of digestive organs and peritoneum whose point of origin cannot be assigned to any one of the categories 150-158
EXCLUDES　*anus and rectum (154.8)*
cardio-esophageal junction (151.0)
colon and rectum (154.0)

159.9　Ill-defined
Alimentary canal or tract NOS
Gastrointestinal tract NOS
EXCLUDES　*abdominal NOS (195.2)*
intra-abdominal NOS (195.2)

Neoplasm of Respiratory and Intrathoracic Organs (160-165)

EXCLUDES　*carcinoma in situ (231.0-231.9)*

√4ᵗʰ **160　Malignant neoplasm of nasal cavities, middle ear, and accessory sinuses**

160.0　Nasal cavities
Cartilage of nose　　Septum of nose
Conchae, nasal　　Vestibule of nose
Internal nose
EXCLUDES　*malignant melanoma of skin of nose (172.3)*
malignant neoplasm of skin of nose (173.30-173.39)
nasal bone (170.0)
nose NOS (195.0)
olfactory bulb (192.0)
posterior margin of septum and choanae (147.3)
turbinates (170.0)

160.1　Auditory tube, middle ear, and mastoid air cells
Antrum tympanicum
Eustachian tube
Tympanic cavity
EXCLUDES　*bone of ear (meatus) (170.0)*
cartilage of ear (171.0)
malignant melanoma of:
auditory canal (external) (172.2, 173.2)
ear (external) (skin) (172.2)
malignant neoplasm of:
auditory canal (external) (173.20-173.29)
ear (external) (skin) (173.20-173.29)

160.2　Maxillary sinus
Antrum (Highmore) (maxillary)

160.3　Ethmoidal sinus

160.4　Frontal sinus

160.5　Sphenoidal sinus

160.8　Other
Malignant neoplasm of contiguous or overlapping sites of nasal cavities, middle ear, and accessory sinuses whose point of origin cannot be determined

160.9 Accessory sinus, unspecified

✓4ᵗʰ **161 Malignant neoplasm of larynx**

161.0 Glottis
Intrinsic larynx
Laryngeal commissure (anterior) (posterior)
True vocal cord
Vocal cord NOS

161.1 Supraglottis
Aryepiglottic fold or interarytenoid fold, laryngeal aspect
Epiglottis (suprahyoid portion) NOS
Extrinsic larynx
False vocal cords
Posterior (laryngeal) surface of epiglottis
Ventricular bands

> **EXCLUDES** *anterior aspect of epiglottis (146.4)*
> *aryepiglottic fold or interarytenoid fold:*
> *NOS (148.2)*
> *hypopharyngeal aspect (148.2)*
> *marginal zone (148.2)*

161.2 Subglottis

161.3 Laryngeal cartilages
Cartilage: Cartilage:
arytenoid   cuneiform
cricoid   thyroid

161.8 Other specified sites of larynx
Malignant neoplasm of contiguous or overlapping sites of larynx whose point of origin cannot be determined
AHA: 3Q, '07, 7

161.9 Larynx, unspecified

✓4ᵗʰ **162 Malignant neoplasm of trachea, bronchus, and lung**
> **EXCLUDES** *benign carcinoid tumor of bronchus (209.61)*
> *malignant carcinoid tumor of bronchus (209.21)*

162.0 Trachea
Cartilage
Mucosa   } of trachea

162.2 Main bronchus
Carina   Hilus of lung

162.3 Upper lobe, bronchus or lung
AHA: 1Q, '04, 4
C34.10 Malig neoplasm upper lobe unspec bronchus/lung   I-10

162.4 Middle lobe, bronchus or lung

162.5 Lower lobe, bronchus or lung
AHA: 3Q, '10, 3

162.8 Other parts of bronchus or lung
Malignant neoplasm of contiguous or overlapping sites of bronchus or lung whose point of origin cannot be determined
AHA: 3Q, '06, 7

162.9 Bronchus and lung, unspecified
AHA: 2Q, '10, 14; 3Q, '06, 14-15; 2Q, '97, 3; 4Q, '96, 48
C34.90 Malig neoplasm unsp part of unspec bronchus/lung   I-10

✓4ᵗʰ **163 Malignant neoplasm of pleura**

163.0 Parietal pleura

163.1 Visceral pleura

163.8 Other specified sites of pleura
Malignant neoplasm of contiguous or overlapping sites of pleura whose point of origin cannot be determined

163.9 Pleura, unspecified

✓4ᵗʰ **164 Malignant neoplasm of thymus, heart, and mediastinum**

164.0 Thymus
> **EXCLUDES** *benign carcinoid tumor of the thymus (209.62)*
> *malignant carcinoid tumor of the thymus (209.22)*

Skull

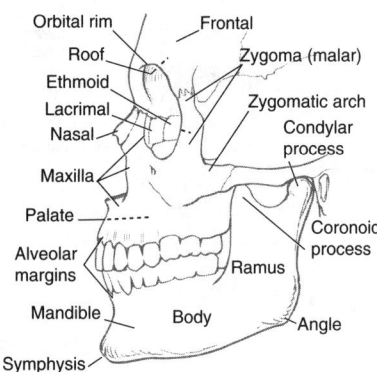

164.1 Heart
Endocardium   Myocardium
Epicardium   Pericardium
> **EXCLUDES** *great vessels (171.4)*

164.2 Anterior mediastinum

164.3 Posterior mediastinum

164.8 Other
Malignant neoplasm of contiguous or overlapping sites of thymus, heart, and mediastinum whose point of origin cannot be determined

164.9 Mediastinum, part unspecified

✓4ᵗʰ **165 Malignant neoplasm of other and ill-defined sites within the respiratory system and intrathoracic organs**

165.0 Upper respiratory tract, part unspecified

165.8 Other
Malignant neoplasm of respiratory and intrathoracic organs whose point of origin cannot be assigned to any one of the categories 160-164

165.9 Ill-defined sites within the respiratory system
Respiratory tract NOS
> **EXCLUDES** *intrathoracic NOS (195.1)*
> *thoracic NOS (195.1)*

Malignant Neoplasm of Bone, Connective Tissue, Skin, and Breast (170-176)

> **EXCLUDES** *carcinoma in situ:*
> *breast (233.0)*
> *skin (232.0-232.9)*

✓4ᵗʰ **170 Malignant neoplasm of bone and articular cartilage**
> **INCLUDES** cartilage (articular) (joint)
> periosteum
> **EXCLUDES** *bone marrow NOS (202.9)*
> *cartilage:*
> *ear (171.0)*
> *eyelid (171.0)*
> *larynx (161.3)*
> *nose (160.0)*
> *synovia (171.0-171.9)*

AHA: 4Q, '06, 103
TIP: Do not assign for bone metastasis; see instead code 198.5.

170.0 Bones of skull and face, except mandible
Bone: Bone:
ethmoid   sphenoid
frontal   temporal
malar   zygomatic
nasal   Maxilla (superior)
occipital   Turbinate
orbital   Upper jaw bone
parietal   Vomer
> **EXCLUDES** *carcinoma, any type except intraosseous or*
> *odontogenic:*
> *maxilla, maxillary (sinus) (160.2)*
> *upper jaw bone (143.0)*
> *jaw bone (lower) (170.1)*

170.1 Mandible
Inferior maxilla
Jaw bone NOS
Lower jaw bone
> EXCLUDES *carcinoma, any type except intraosseous or odontogenic:*
>   *jaw bone NOS (143.9)*
>   *lower (143.1)*
>   *upper jaw bone (170.0)*

170.2 Vertebral column, excluding sacrum and coccyx
Spinal column
Spine
Vertebra
> EXCLUDES *sacrum and coccyx (170.6)*

170.3 Ribs, sternum, and clavicle
Costal cartilage
Costovertebral joint
Xiphoid process

170.4 Scapula and long bones of upper limb
Acromion
Bones NOS of upper limb
Humerus
Radius
Ulna
AHA: 2Q, '99, 9

170.5 Short bones of upper limb

Carpal	Scaphoid (of hand)
Cuneiform, wrist	Semilunar or lunate
Metacarpal	Trapezium
Navicular, of hand	Trapezoid
Phalanges of hand	Unciform
Pisiform	

170.6 Pelvic bones, sacrum, and coccyx
Coccygeal vertebra
Ilium
Ischium
Pubic bone
Sacral vertebra

170.7 Long bones of lower limb
Bones NOS of lower limb
Femur
Fibula
Tibia

170.8 Short bones of lower limb

Astragalus [talus]	Navicular (of ankle)
Calcaneus	Patella
Cuboid	Phalanges of foot
Cuneiform, ankle	Tarsal
Metatarsal	

170.9 Bone and articular cartilage, site unspecified

√4ᵗʰ **171 Malignant neoplasm of connective and other soft tissue**
> INCLUDES blood vessel
>   bursa
>   fascia
>   fat
>   ligament, except uterine
>   muscle
>   peripheral, sympathetic, and parasympathetic nerves and ganglia
>   synovia
>   tendon (sheath)
> EXCLUDES *cartilage (of):*
>   *articular (170.0-170.9)*
>   *larynx (161.3)*
>   *nose (160.0)*
>   *connective tissue:*
>   *breast (174.0-175.9)*
>   *internal organs — code to malignant neoplasm of the site*
>   *[e.g., leiomyosarcoma of stomach, 151.9]*
>   *heart (164.1)*
>   *uterine ligament (183.4)*

171.0 Head, face, and neck
Cartilage of:
  ear
  eyelid
AHA: 2Q, '99, 6

171.2 Upper limb, including shoulder
Arm
Finger
Forearm
Hand

171.3 Lower limb, including hip
Foot
Leg
Popliteal space
Thigh
Toe

171.4 Thorax
Axilla
Diaphragm
Great vessels
> EXCLUDES *heart (164.1)*
>   *mediastinum (164.2-164.9)*
>   *thymus (164.0)*

171.5 Abdomen
Abdominal wall
Hypochondrium
> EXCLUDES *peritoneum (158.8)*
>   *retroperitoneum (158.0)*

171.6 Pelvis
Buttock
Groin
Inguinal region
Perineum
> EXCLUDES *pelvic peritoneum (158.8)*
>   *retroperitoneum (158.0)*
>   *uterine ligament, any (183.3-183.5)*

171.7 Trunk, unspecified
Back NOS
Flank NOS

171.8 Other specified sites of connective and other soft tissue
Malignant neoplasm of contiguous or overlapping sites of connective tissue whose point of origin cannot be determined

171.9 Connective and other soft tissue, site unspecified

√4ᵗʰ **172 Malignant melanoma of skin**
> INCLUDES melanocarcinoma
>   melanoma (skin) NOS
>   melanoma in situ of skin
> EXCLUDES *skin of genital organs (184.0-184.9, 187.1-187.9)*
>   *sites other than skin — code to malignant neoplasm of the site*

DEF: Malignant neoplasm of melanocytes; most common in skin, may involve oral cavity, esophagus, anal canal, vagina, leptomeninges, or conjunctiva.

172.0 Lip
> EXCLUDES *vermilion border of lip (140.0-140.1, 140.9)*

172.1 Eyelid, including canthus

172.2 Ear and external auditory canal
Auricle (ear)
Auricular canal, external
External [acoustic] meatus
Pinna

172.3 Other and unspecified parts of face
Cheek (external)
Chin
Eyebrow
Forehead
Nose, external
Temple

172.4 Scalp and neck

172.5 Trunk, except scrotum

Axilla	Perianal skin
Breast	Perineum
Buttock	Umbilicus
Groin	

> EXCLUDES *anal canal (154.2)*
>   *anus NOS (154.3)*
>   *scrotum (187.7)*

√4ᵗʰ / √5ᵗʰ   Additional Digit Required   Unspecified Code   Other Specified Code   Manifestation Code   ►◄ Revised Text   ● New Code   ▲ Revised Code Title

172.6 Upper limb, including shoulder

Arm	Forearm
Finger	Hand

172.7 Lower limb, including hip

Ankle	Leg
Foot	Popliteal area
Heel	Thigh
Knee	Toe

172.8 Other specified sites of skin

Malignant melanoma of contiguous or overlapping sites of skin whose point of origin cannot be determined

172.9 Melanoma of skin, site unspecified

√4th **173 Other and unspecified malignant neoplasm of skin**

INCLUDES malignant neoplasm of:
sebaceous glands
sudoriferous, sudoriparous glands
sweat glands

EXCLUDES *Kaposi's sarcoma (176.0-176.9)*
malignant melanoma of skin (172.0-172.9)
Merkel cell carcinoma of skin (209.31-209.36)
skin of genital organs (184.0-184.9, 187.1-187.9)

AHA: ▶4Q, '11, 83-87;◀ 1Q, '00, 18; 2Q, '96, 12

TIP: Do not assign for malignant neoplasm of skin documented as melanoma; see instead category 172.

√5th **173.0 Other and unspecified malignant neoplasm of skin of lip**

EXCLUDES *vermilion border of lip (140.0-140.1, 140.9)*

173.00 Unspecified malignant neoplasm of skin of lip

173.01 Basal cell carcinoma of skin of lip

173.02 Squamous cell carcinoma of skin of lip

173.09 Other specified malignant neoplasm of skin of lip

√5th **173.1 Other and unspecified malignant neoplasm of skin of eyelid, including canthus**

EXCLUDES *cartilage of eyelid (171.0)*

173.10 Unspecified malignant neoplasm of eyelid, including canthus

173.11 Basal cell carcinoma of eyelid, including canthus

173.12 Squamous cell carcinoma of eyelid, including canthus

173.19 Other specified malignant neoplasm of eyelid, including canthus

√5th **173.2 Other and unspecified malignant neoplasm of skin of ear and external auditory canal**

Auricle (ear)
Auricular canal, external
External meatus
Pinna

EXCLUDES *cartilage of ear (171.0)*

173.20 Unspecified malignant neoplasm of skin of ear and external auditory canal

173.21 Basal cell carcinoma of skin of ear and external auditory canal

173.22 Squamous cell carcinoma of skin of ear and external auditory canal

173.29 Other specified malignant neoplasm of skin of ear and external auditory canal

√5th **173.3 Other and unspecified malignant neoplasm of skin of other and unspecified parts of face**

Cheek, external	Forehead
Chin	Nose, external
Eyebrow	Temple

AHA: 1Q, '00, 3

173.30 Unspecified malignant neoplasm of skin of other and unspecified parts of face

173.31 Basal cell carcinoma of skin of other and unspecified parts of face

173.32 Squamous cell carcinoma of skin of other and unspecified parts of face

173.39 Other specified malignant neoplasm of skin of other and unspecified parts of face

√5th **173.4 Other and unspecified malignant neoplasm of scalp and skin of neck**

173.40 Unspecified malignant neoplasm of scalp and skin of neck

173.41 Basal cell carcinoma of scalp and skin of neck

173.42 Squamous cell carcinoma of scalp and skin of neck

173.49 Other specified malignant neoplasm of scalp and skin of neck

√5th **173.5 Other and unspecified malignant neoplasm of skin of trunk, except scrotum**

Axillary fold	Skin of:
Perianal skin	buttock
Skin of:	chest wall
abdominal wall	groin
anus	perineum
back	umbilicus
breast	

EXCLUDES *anal canal (154.2)*
anus NOS (154.3)
skin of scrotum (187.7)

AHA: 1Q, '01, 8

173.50 Unspecified malignant neoplasm of skin of trunk, except scrotum

173.51 Basal cell carcinoma of skin of trunk, except scrotum

173.52 Squamous cell carcinoma of skin of trunk, except scrotum

173.59 Other specified malignant neoplasm of skin of trunk, except scrotum

√5th **173.6 Other and unspecified malignant neoplasm of skin of upper limb, including shoulder**

Arm	Forearm
Finger	Hand

173.60 Unspecified malignant neoplasm of skin of upper limb, including shoulder

173.61 Basal cell carcinoma of skin of upper limb, including shoulder

173.62 Squamous cell carcinoma of skin of upper limb, including shoulder

173.69 Other specified malignant neoplasm of skin of upper limb, including shoulder

√5th **173.7 Other and unspecified malignant neoplasm of skin of lower limb, including hip**

Ankle	Leg
Foot	Popliteal area
Heel	Thigh
Knee	Toe

173.70 Unspecified malignant neoplasm of skin of lower limb, including hip

173.71 Basal cell carcinoma of skin of lower limb, including hip

173.72 Squamous cell carcinoma of skin of lower limb, including hip

173.79 Other specified malignant neoplasm of skin of lower limb, including hip

√5th **173.8 Other and unspecified malignant neoplasm of other specified sites of skin**

Malignant neoplasm of contiguous or overlapping sites of skin whose point of origin cannot be determined

173.80 Unspecified malignant neoplasm of other specified sites of skin

173.81 Basal cell carcinoma of other specified sites of skin

173.82 Squamous cell carcinoma of other specified sites of skin

173.89 Other specified malignant neoplasm of other specified sites of skin

√5th **173.9 Other and unspecified malignant neoplasm of skin, site unspecified**

173.90 Unspecified malignant neoplasm of skin, site unspecified

Malignant neoplasm of skin NOS

173.91 Basal cell carcinoma of skin, site unspecified

173.92 Squamous cell carcinoma of skin, site unspecified

N   Newborn Age: 0   P   Pediatric Age: 0-17   M   Maternity Age: 12-55   A   Adult Age: 15-124

173.99 Other specified malignant neoplasm of skin, site unspecified

√4ᵗʰ **174 Malignant neoplasm of female breast**

Use additional code to identify estrogen receptor status (V86.0, V86.1)

INCLUDES breast (female)
connective tissue
soft parts
Paget's disease of:
breast
nipple

EXCLUDES malignant melanoma of skin of breast (172.5)
malignant neoplasm of skin of breast (173.50-173.59)

AHA: 3Q, '97, 8; 4Q, '89, 11

TIP: For bilateral breast malignancy, do not assign two codes unless documentation indicates separate sites (i.e., different fourth digits).

174.0 Nipple and areola   ♀

174.1 Central portion   ♀

174.2 Upper-inner quadrant   ♀

174.3 Lower-inner quadrant   ♀

174.4 Upper-outer quadrant   ♀

AHA: 4Q, '08, 155; 1Q, '04, 3; 3Q, '97, 8

174.5 Lower-outer quadrant   ♀

174.6 Axillary tail   ♀

174.8 Other specified sites of female breast   ♀
Ectopic sites
Inner breast
Lower breast
Midline of breast
Outer breast
Upper breast
Malignant neoplasm of contiguous or overlapping sites of breast whose point of origin cannot be determined

174.9 Breast (female), unspecified   ♀
AHA: 3Q, '09, 3; 3Q, '05, 11; 2Q, '94, 10; 4Q, '89, 11
C50.911 Malig neoplasm of uns site of rt female breast   I-10

√4ᵗʰ **175 Malignant neoplasm of male breast**

Use additional code to identify estrogen receptor status (V86.0, V86.1)

EXCLUDES malignant melanoma of skin of breast (172.5)
malignant neoplasm of skin of breast (173.50-173.59)

175.0 Nipple and areola   ♂

175.9 Other and unspecified sites of male breast   ♂
Ectopic breast tissue, male

√4ᵗʰ **176 Kaposi's sarcoma**
AHA: 4Q, '91, 24

176.0 Skin
AHA: 4Q, '07, 63; 4Q. '94, 29; 4Q, '91, 24

176.1 Soft tissue
Blood vessel   Ligament
Connective tissue   Lymphatic(s) NEC
Fascia   Muscle
EXCLUDES lymph glands and nodes (176.5)

Female Breast

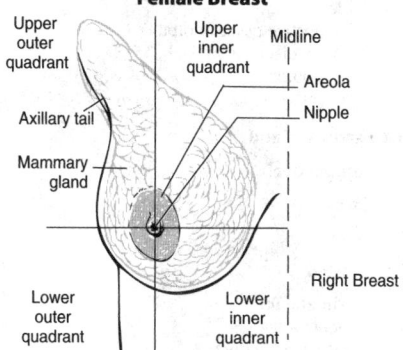

Upper outer quadrant
Upper inner quadrant
Midline
Areola
Nipple
Axillary tail
Mammary gland
Right Breast
Lower outer quadrant
Lower inner quadrant

176.2 Palate

176.3 Gastrointestinal sites

176.4 Lung

176.5 Lymph nodes

176.8 Other specified sites
Oral cavity NEC

176.9 Unspecified
Viscera NOS

Malignant Neoplasm of Genitourinary Organs (179-189)

EXCLUDES carcinoma in situ (233.1-233.9)

179 Malignant neoplasm of uterus, part unspecified   ♀

√4ᵗʰ **180 Malignant neoplasm of cervix uteri**
INCLUDES invasive malignancy [carcinoma]
EXCLUDES carcinoma in situ (233.1)

180.0 Endocervix   ♀
Cervical canal NOS
Endocervical canal
Endocervical gland

180.1 Exocervix   ♀

180.8 Other specified sites of cervix   ♀
Cervical stump
Squamocolumnar junction of cervix
Malignant neoplasm of contiguous or overlapping sites of cervix uteri whose point of origin cannot be determined

180.9 Cervix uteri, unspecified   ♀

181 Malignant neoplasm of placenta   ♀
Choriocarcinoma NOS
Chorioepithelioma NOS
EXCLUDES chorioadenoma (destruens) (236.1)
hydatidiform mole (630)
malignant (236.1)
invasive mole (236.1)
male choriocarcinoma NOS (186.0-186.9)

√4ᵗʰ **182 Malignant neoplasm of body of uterus**
EXCLUDES carcinoma in situ (233.2)

182.0 Corpus uteri, except isthmus   ♀
Cornu   Fundus
Endometrium   Myometrium
AHA: 3Q, '09, 5
C54.9 Malignant neoplasm of corpus uteri unspecified   I-10

182.1 Isthmus   ♀
Lower uterine segment

182.8 Other specified sites of body of uterus   ♀
Malignant neoplasm of contiguous or overlapping sites of body of uterus whose point of origin cannot be determined
EXCLUDES uterus NOS (179)

√4ᵗʰ **183 Malignant neoplasm of ovary and other uterine adnexa**
EXCLUDES Douglas' cul-de-sac (158.8)

183.0 Ovary   ♀
Use additional code to identify any functional activity
AHA: 4Q, '07, 96
C56.9 Malignant neoplasm of unspec ovary   I-10

183.2 Fallopian tube   ♀
Oviduct
Uterine tube

183.3 Broad ligament   ♀
Mesovarium
Parovarian region

183.4 Parametrium   ♀
Uterine ligament NOS
Uterosacral ligament

183.5 Round ligament   ♀
AHA: 3Q, '99, 5

√4ᵗʰ √5ᵗʰ Additional Digit Required   Unspecified Code   Other Specified Code   Manifestation Code   ►◄ Revised Text   ● New Code   ▲ Revised Code Title

2013 ICD-9-CM   Volume 1 – 35

Neoplasms

183.8 Other specified sites of uterine adnexa ♀
  Tubo-ovarian
  Utero-ovarian
  Malignant neoplasm of contiguous or overlapping sites of ovary and other uterine adnexa whose point of origin cannot be determined

183.9 Uterine adnexa, unspecified ♀

☑4ᵗʰ **184 Malignant neoplasm of other and unspecified female genital organs**
  EXCLUDES *carcinoma in situ (233.30-233.39)*

184.0 Vagina ♀
  Gartner's duct
  Vaginal vault

184.1 Labia majora ♀
  Greater vestibular [Bartholin's] gland

184.2 Labia minora ♀

184.3 Clitoris ♀

184.4 Vulva, unspecified ♀
  External female genitalia NOS
  Pudendum

184.8 Other specified sites of female genital ♀
  Malignant neoplasm of contiguous or overlapping sites of female genital organs whose point of origin cannot be determined

184.9 Female genital organ, site unspecified ♀
  Female genitourinary tract NOS

185 Malignant neoplasm of prostate ♂
  EXCLUDES *seminal vesicles (187.8)*
  AHA: 2Q, '10, 3; 3Q, '03, 13; 3Q, '99, 5; 3Q, '92, 7
  TIP: Assign as a secondary diagnosis if patient treated for BPH and incidental finding of carcinoma of the prostate is made.
  C61 Malignant neoplasm of prostate   I-10

☑4ᵗʰ **186 Malignant neoplasm of testis**
  Use additional code to identify any functional activity

186.0 Undescended testis ♂
  Ectopic testis
  Retained testis

186.9 Other and unspecified testis ♂
  Testis:
   NOS
   descended
   scrotal

☑4ᵗʰ **187 Malignant neoplasm of penis and other male genital organs**

187.1 Prepuce ♂
  Foreskin

187.2 Glans penis ♂

187.3 Body of penis ♂
  Corpus cavernosum

187.4 Penis, part unspecified ♂
  Skin of penis NOS

187.5 Epididymis ♂

187.6 Spermatic cord ♂
  Vas deferens

187.7 Scrotum ♂
  Skin of scrotum

187.8 Other specified sites of male genital organs ♂
  Seminal vesicle
  Tunica vaginalis
  Malignant neoplasm of contiguous or overlapping sites of penis and other male genital organs whose point of origin cannot be determined

187.9 Male genital organ, site unspecified ♂
  Male genital organ or tract NOS

☑4ᵗʰ **188 Malignant neoplasm of bladder**
  EXCLUDES *carcinoma in situ (233.7)*

188.0 Trigone of urinary bladder

188.1 Dome of urinary bladder

188.2 Lateral wall of urinary bladder

188.3 Anterior wall of urinary bladder

188.4 Posterior wall of urinary bladder

188.5 Bladder neck
  Internal urethral orifice

188.6 Ureteric orifice

188.7 Urachus

188.8 Other specified sites of bladder
  Malignant neoplasm of contiguous or overlapping sites of bladder whose point of origin cannot be determined

188.9 Bladder, part unspecified
  Bladder wall NOS
  AHA: 1Q, '00, 5
  C67.9 Malignant neoplasm of bladder unspecified   I-10

☑4ᵗʰ **189 Malignant neoplasm of kidney and other and unspecified urinary organs**
  EXCLUDES *benign carcinoid tumor of kidney (209.64)*
   malignant carcinoid tumor of kidney (209.24)

189.0 Kidney, except pelvis
  Kidney NOS
  Kidney parenchyma
  AHA: 2Q, '05, 4; 2Q, '04, 4
  C64.9 Malig neoplasm unspec kidney no renal pelvis   I-10

189.1 Renal pelvis
  Renal calyces
  Ureteropelvic junction

189.2 Ureter
  EXCLUDES *ureteric orifice of bladder (188.6)*

189.3 Urethra
  EXCLUDES *urethral orifice of bladder (188.5)*

189.4 Paraurethral glands

189.8 Other specified sites of urinary organs
  Malignant neoplasm of contiguous or overlapping sites of kidney and other urinary organs whose point of origin cannot be determined

189.9 Urinary organ, site unspecified
  Urinary system NOS

Malignant Neoplasm of Other and Unspecified Sites (190-199)
  EXCLUDES *carcinoma in situ (234.0-234.9)*

☑4ᵗʰ **190 Malignant neoplasm of eye**
  EXCLUDES *carcinoma in situ (234.0)*
   dark area on retina and choroid (239.81)
    cartilage (171.0)
   malignant melanoma of eyelid (skin) (172.1)
   malignant neoplasm of eyelid (skin) (173.10-173.19)
   optic nerve (192.0)
   orbital bone (170.0)
   retinal freckle (239.81)

190.0 Eyeball, except conjunctiva, cornea, retina, and choroid
  Ciliary body   Sclera
  Crystalline lens   Uveal tract
  Iris

190.1 Orbit
  Connective tissue of orbit
  Extraocular muscle
  Retrobulbar
  EXCLUDES *bone of orbit (170.0)*

190.2 Lacrimal gland

190.3 Conjunctiva

190.4 Cornea

190.5 Retina

190.6 Choroid

190.7 Lacrimal duct
  Lacrimal sac
  Nasolacrimal duct

Brain and Meninges

Midsagittal Section (between hemispheres) — Fourth ventricle, Cerebrum, Corpus callosum, Thalamus, Hypothalamus, Hypophysis, Pons, Medulla oblongata, Cerebellum

190.8 Other specified sites of eye

Malignant neoplasm of contiguous or overlapping sites of eye whose point of origin cannot be determined

190.9 Eye, part unspecified

✓4ᵗʰ 191 Malignant neoplasm of brain

EXCLUDES cranial nerves (192.0)
retrobulbar area (190.1)

AHA: 4Q, '07, 104

191.0 Cerebrum, except lobes and ventricles
Basal ganglia   Globus pallidus
Cerebral cortex   Hypothalamus
Corpus striatum   Thalamus

191.1 Frontal lobe
AHA: 4Q, '05, 118

191.2 Temporal lobe
Hippocampus
Uncus
AHA: 3Q, '09, 8; 4Q, '06, 123

191.3 Parietal lobe

191.4 Occipital lobe

191.5 Ventricles
Choroid plexus
Floor of ventricle

191.6 Cerebellum NOS
Cerebellopontine angle

191.7 Brain stem
Cerebral peduncle
Medulla oblongata
Midbrain
Pons

191.8 Other parts of brain
Corpus callosum
Tapetum
Malignant neoplasm of contiguous or overlapping sites of brain whose point of origin cannot be determined

191.9 Brain, unspecified
Cranial fossa NOS
AHA: 4Q, '09, 143

✓4ᵗʰ 192 Malignant neoplasm of other and unspecified parts of nervous system

EXCLUDES peripheral, sympathetic, and parasympathetic nerves and ganglia (171.0-171.9)

192.0 Cranial nerves
Olfactory bulb

192.1 Cerebral meninges
Dura (mater)   Meninges NOS
Falx (cerebelli) (cerebri)   Tentorium

192.2 Spinal cord
Cauda equina

192.3 Spinal meninges

192.8 Other specified sites of nervous system
Malignant neoplasm of contiguous or overlapping sites of other parts of nervous system whose point of origin cannot be determined

192.9 Nervous system, part unspecified
Nervous system (central) NOS
EXCLUDES meninges NOS (192.1)

193 Malignant neoplasm of thyroid gland
Thyroglossal duct
Use additional code to identify any functional activity
C73 Malignant neoplasm of thyroid gland   I-10

✓4ᵗʰ 194 Malignant neoplasm of other endocrine glands and related structures

EXCLUDES islets of Langerhans (157.4)
neuroendocrine tumors (209.00-209.69)
ovary (183.0)
testis (186.0-186.9)
thymus (164.0)

194.0 Adrenal gland
Adrenal cortex   Suprarenal gland
Adrenal medulla

194.1 Parathyroid gland

194.3 Pituitary gland and craniopharyngeal duct
Craniobuccal pouch   Rathke's pouch
Hypophysis   Sella turcica
AHA: J-A, '85, 9

194.4 Pineal gland

194.5 Carotid body

194.6 Aortic body and other paraganglia
Coccygeal body
Glomus jugulare
Para-aortic body

194.8 Other
Pluriglandular involvement NOS
NOTE If the sites of multiple involvements are known, they should be coded separately.

194.9 Endocrine gland, site unspecified

✓4ᵗʰ 195 Malignant neoplasm of other and ill-defined sites

INCLUDES malignant neoplasms of contiguous sites, not elsewhere classified, whose point of origin cannot be determined

EXCLUDES malignant neoplasm:
lymphatic and hematopoietic tissue (200.0-208.9)
secondary sites (196.0-198.8)
unspecified site (199.0-199.1)

195.0 Head, face, and neck
Cheek NOS   Nose NOS
Jaw NOS   Supraclavicular region NOS
AHA: 4Q, '03, 107

195.1 Thorax
Axilla
Chest (wall) NOS
Intrathoracic NOS

195.2 Abdomen
Intra-abdominal NOS
AHA: 2Q, '97, 3

195.3 Pelvis
Groin
Inguinal region NOS
Presacral region
Sacrococcygeal region
Sites overlapping systems within pelvis, as:
rectovaginal (septum)
rectovesical (septum)

195.4 Upper limb

195.5 Lower limb

195.8 Other specified sites
Back NOS
Flank NOS
Trunk NOS

✓4ᵗʰ
✓5ᵗʰ   Additional Digit Required   Unspecified Code   Other Specified Code   Manifestation Code   ►◄ Revised Text   ● New Code   ▲ Revised Code Title

2013 ICD-9-CM   **Volume 1 – 37**

Lymph Nodes

Head, neck, and face
Left subclavian vein
Intrathoracic
Intraabdominal
Cisterna chyli
Nodes generally accompany large blood vessels
Inguinal and lower limb

Thoracic duct empties into the left subclavian vein
Axillary and upper limb
Thoracic duct (transmits lymph through diaphragm using one-way valves)
Intrapelvic

✓4ᵗʰ **196 Secondary and unspecified malignant neoplasm of lymph nodes**

> **EXCLUDES** *any malignant neoplasm of lymph nodes, specified as primary (200.0-202.9)*
> *Hodgkin's disease (201.0-201.9)*
> *lymphosarcoma (200.1)*
> *other forms of lymphoma (202.0-202.9)*
> *reticulosarcoma (200.0)*
> *secondary neuroendocrine tumor of (distant) lymph nodes (209.71)*

AHA: 2Q, '92, 3; M-J, '85, 3

196.0 Lymph nodes of head, face, and neck

Cervical   Scalene
Cervicofacial   Supraclavicular

AHA: 3Q, '07, 7

C77.0 Sec & uns malig neo lymph nodes head face & neck   I-10

196.1 Intrathoracic lymph nodes

Bronchopulmonary   Mediastinal
Intercostal   Tracheobronchial

AHA: 3Q, '06, 7

196.2 Intra-abdominal lymph nodes

Intestinal   Retroperitoneal
Mesenteric

AHA: 4Q, '03, 111

C77.2 Sec & uns malig neoplasm intra-abd lymph nodes   I-10

196.3 Lymph nodes of axilla and upper limb

Brachial   Infraclavicular
Epitrochlear   Pectoral

196.5 Lymph nodes of inguinal region and lower limb

Femoral   Popliteal
Groin   Tibial

196.6 Intrapelvic lymph nodes

Hypogastric   Obturator
Iliac   Parametrial

196.8 Lymph nodes of multiple sites

196.9 Site unspecified

Lymph nodes NOS

✓4ᵗʰ **197 Secondary malignant neoplasm of respiratory and digestive systems**

> **EXCLUDES** *lymph node metastasis (196.0-196.9)*
> *secondary neuroendocrine tumor of liver (209.72)*
> *secondary neuroendocrine tumor of respiratory organs (209.79)*

AHA: M-J, '85, 3

197.0 Lung

Bronchus

AHA: 3Q, '10, 3; 1Q, '06, 4; 2Q, '99, 9

C78.00 Secondary malignant neoplasm of unspec lung   I-10

197.1 Mediastinum

AHA: 3Q, '06, 7

197.2 Pleura

AHA: 1Q, '08, 16; 3Q, '07, 3; 4Q, '03, 110; 4Q, '89, 11

TIP: Do not assign for malignant pleural effusion; see instead code 511.81.

C78.2 Secondary malignant neoplasm of pleura   I-10

197.3 Other respiratory organs

Trachea

197.4 Small intestine, including duodenum

197.5 Large intestine and rectum

197.6 Retroperitoneum and peritoneum

AHA: 3Q, '10, 3;2Q, '04, 4; 4Q, '89, 11

C78.6 Sec malignant neoplasm of retroperiton & periton   I-10

197.7 Liver, specified as secondary

AHA: 3Q, '10, 3; 1Q, '06, 4; 2Q, '05, 9

C78.7 Secondary malignant neoplasm of liver   I-10

197.8 Other digestive organs and spleen

AHA: 2Q, '97, 3; 2Q, '92, 3

✓4ᵗʰ **198 Secondary malignant neoplasm of other specified sites**

> **EXCLUDES** *lymph node metastasis (196.0-196.9)*
> *secondary neuroendocrine tumor of other specified sites (209.79)*

AHA: M-J, '85, 3

198.0 Kidney

198.1 Other urinary organs

198.2 Skin

Skin of breast

198.3 Brain and spinal cord

AHA: 3Q, '07, 4; 3Q, '99, 7

C79.31 Secondary malignant neoplasm of brain   I-10

198.4 Other parts of nervous system

Meninges (cerebral) (spinal)

AHA: J-F, '87, 7

198.5 Bone and bone marrow

AHA: 1Q, '07, 6; 4Q, '03, 110; 3Q, '99, 5; 2Q, '92, 3; 1Q, '91, 16; 4Q, '89, 10

C79.51 Secondary malignant neoplasm of bone   I-10

198.6 Ovary   ♀

198.7 Adrenal gland

Suprarenal gland

C79.70 Sec malignant neoplasm of unspec adrenal gland   I-10

✓5ᵗʰ **198.8 Other specified sites**

198.81 Breast

> **EXCLUDES** *skin of breast (198.2)*

198.82 Genital organs

198.89 Other

> **EXCLUDES** *retroperitoneal lymph nodes (196.2)*

AHA: 2Q, '05, 4; 2Q, '97, 4

TIP: Assign for intra-abdominal metastasis when no further specificity of site is documented.

C79.89 Secondary malignant neoplasm of other spec sites   I-10

✓4ᵗʰ **199 Malignant neoplasm without specification of site**

> **EXCLUDES** *malignant carcinoid tumor of unknown primary site (209.20)*
> *malignant (poorly differentiated) neuroendocrine carcinoma, any site (209.30)*
> *malignant (poorly differentiated) neuroendocrine tumor, any site (209.30)*
> *neuroendocrine carcinoma (high grade), any site (209.30)*

199.0 Disseminated

Carcinomatosis
Generalized:
  cancer   } unspecified site (primary)
  malignancy   (secondary)
Multiple cancer

AHA: 4Q, '89, 10

199.1 Other

Cancer   } unspecified site (primary)
Carcinoma   (secondary)
Malignancy

AHA: 3Q, '06, 14-15; 1Q, '06, 4

TIP: Assign if patient is assessed for a metastatic tumor but primary site is unknown.

C80.1 Malignant neoplasm unspecified   I-10

N Newborn Age: 0   P Pediatric Age: 0-17   M Maternity Age: 12-55   A Adult Age: 15-124

199.2 Malignant neoplasm associated with transplanted organ
Code first complication of transplanted organ (996.80-996.89)
Use additional code for specific malignancy
AHA: 4Q, '08, 82-83
TIP: Assign first the appropriate code from subcategory 996.8, Complications of transplanted organ; use additional code for the specific malignancy.

Malignant Neoplasm of Lymphatic and Hematopoietic Tissue (200-208)

EXCLUDES autoimmune lymphoproliferative syndrome (279.41)
secondary and unspecified neoplasm of lymph nodes (196.0-196.9)
secondary neoplasm of:
bone marrow (198.5)
spleen (197.8)

The following fifth-digit subclassification is for use with categories 200-202:
  0 unspecified site, extranodal and solid organ sites
  1 lymph nodes of head, face, and neck
  2 intrathoracic lymph nodes
  3 intra-abdominal lymph nodes
  4 lymph nodes of axilla and upper limb
  5 lymph nodes of inguinal region and lower limb
  6 intrapelvic lymph nodes
  7 spleen
  8 lymph nodes of multiple sites

√4th **200 Lymphosarcoma and reticulosarcoma and other specified malignant tumors of lymphatic tissue**
AHA: 4Q, '07, 65; 2Q, '92, 3; N-D, '86, 5

§ √5th **200.0 Reticulosarcoma**
[0-8] Lymphoma (malignant):   Reticulum cell sarcoma:
histiocytic (diffuse):   NOS
nodular   pleomorphic cell type
pleomorphic cell type
reticulum cell type
DEF: Malignant lymphoma of primarily histolytic cells; commonly originates in reticuloendothelium of lymph nodes.
AHA: For Code 200.03: 3Q, '01, 12; For Code 200.04: 3Q, '09, 4

§ √5th **200.1 Lymphosarcoma**
[0-8] Lymphoblastoma (diffuse)
Lymphoma (malignant):
lymphoblastic (diffuse)
lymphocytic (cell type) (diffuse)
lymphosarcoma type
Lymphosarcoma:
NOS
diffuse NOS
lymphoblastic (diffuse)
lymphocytic (diffuse)
prolymphocytic
EXCLUDES lymphosarcoma:
follicular or nodular (202.0)
mixed cell type (200.8)
lymphosarcoma cell leukemia (207.8)
DEF: Malignant lymphoma created from anaplastic lymphoid cells resembling lymphocytes or lymphoblasts.

§ √5th **200.2 Burkitt's tumor or lymphoma**
[0-8] Malignant lymphoma, Burkitt's type
DEF: Large osteolytic lesion most common in jaw or as abdominal mass; usually found in central Africa but reported elsewhere.

§ √5th **200.3 Marginal zone lymphoma**
[0-8] Extranodal marginal zone B-cell lymphoma
Mucosa associated lymphoid tissue [MALT]
Nodal marginal zone B-cell lymphoma
Splenic marginal zone B-cell lymphoma
AHA: 4Q, '07, 65

§ √5th **200.4 Mantle cell lymphoma**
[0-8] AHA: 4Q, '07, 65

§ √5th **200.5 Primary central nervous system lymphoma**
[0-8] AHA: 4Q, '07, 66

§ √5th **200.6 Anaplastic large cell lymphoma**
[0-8] AHA: 4Q, '07, 66

§ √5th **200.7 Large cell lymphoma**
[0-8] AHA: 4Q, '07, 66

§ √5th **200.8 Other named variants**
[0-8] Lymphoma (malignant):
lymphoplasmacytoid type
mixed lymphocytic-histiocytic (diffuse)
Lymphosarcoma, mixed cell type (diffuse)
Reticulolymphosarcoma (diffuse)

√4th **201 Hodgkin's disease**
DEF: Painless, progressive enlargement of lymph nodes, spleen and general lymph tissue; symptoms include anorexia, lassitude, weight loss, fever, pruritis, night sweats, anemia.
AHA: 2Q, '92, 3; N-D, '86, 5

§ √5th **201.0 Hodgkin's paragranuloma**
[0-8]

§ √5th **201.1 Hodgkin's granuloma**
[0-8] AHA: 2Q, '99, 7

§ √5th **201.2 Hodgkin's sarcoma**
[0-8]

§ √5th **201.4 Lymphocytic-histiocytic predominance**
[0-8]

§ √5th **201.5 Nodular sclerosis**
[0-8] Hodgkin's disease, nodular sclerosis:
NOS
cellular phase

§ √5th **201.6 Mixed cellularity**
[0-8]

§ √5th **201.7 Lymphocytic depletion**
[0-8] Hodgkin's disease, lymphocytic depletion:
NOS
diffuse fibrosis
reticular type

§ √5th **201.9 Hodgkin's disease, unspecified**
[0-8] Hodgkin's: Malignant:
disease NOS   lymphogranuloma
lymphoma NOS   lymphogranulomatosis

√4th **202 Other malignant neoplasms of lymphoid and histiocytic tissue**
AHA: 2Q, '92, 3; N-D, '86, 5

§ √5th **202.0 Nodular lymphoma**
[0-8] Brill-Symmers disease
Lymphoma:
follicular (giant) (large cell)
lymphocytic, nodular
Lymphosarcoma:
follicular (giant)
nodular
DEF: Lymphomatous cells clustered into nodules within the lymph node; usually occurs in older adults and may involve all nodes and possibly extranodal sites.
AHA: For code 202.04: 3Q, '09, 4

§ √5th **202.1 Mycosis fungoides**
[0-8] EXCLUDES peripheral T-cell lymphoma (202.7)
DEF: Type of cutaneous T-cell lymphoma; may evolve into generalized lymphoma; formerly thought to be of fungoid origin.
AHA: 2Q, '92, 4

§ √5th **202.2 Sézary's disease**
[0-8] DEF: Type of cutaneous T-cell lymphoma with erythroderma, intense pruritus, peripheral lymphadenopathy, abnormal hyperchromatic mononuclear cells in skin, lymph nodes and peripheral blood.
AHA: 2Q, '99, 7

§ √5th **202.3 Malignant histiocytosis**
[0-8] Histiocytic medullary reticulosis
Malignant:
reticuloendotheliosis
reticulosis

§ √5th **202.4 Leukemic reticuloendotheliosis**
[0-8] Hairy-cell leukemia
DEF: Chronic leukemia with large, mononuclear cells with "hairy" appearance in marrow, spleen, liver, blood.

§   Requires fifth digit. Valid digits are in [brackets] under each code. See appropriate category for codes and definitions.

√4th √5th Additional Digit Required   Unspecified Code   Other Specified Code   Manifestation Code   ▶◀ Revised Text   ● New Code   ▲ Revised Code Title

§ √5ᵗʰ **202.5 Letterer-Siwe disease**
[0-8]   Acute:
        differentiated progressive histiocytosis
        histiocytosis X (progressive)
        infantile reticuloendotheliosis
        reticulosis of infancy
     EXCLUDES *adult pulmonary Langerhans cell histiocytosis (516.5)*
          Hand-Schüller-Christian disease (277.89)
          histiocytosis (acute) (chronic) (277.89)
          histiocytosis X (chronic) (277.89)
     DEF: A recessive reticuloendotheliosis of early childhood, with a hemorrhagic tendency, eczema-like skin eruption, hepatosplenomegaly, lymph node enlargement, and progressive anemia; often a fatal disease with no established cause.

§ √5ᵗʰ **202.6 Malignant mast cell tumors**
[0-8]   Malignant: Mast cell sarcoma
        mastocytoma   Systemic tissue mast
        mastocytosis   cell disease
     EXCLUDES *mast cell leukemia (207.8)*

§ √5ᵗʰ **202.7 Peripheral T-cell lymphoma**
[0-8]   **AHA:** 4Q, '07, 66

§ √5ᵗʰ **202.8 Other lymphomas**
[0-8]   Lymphoma (malignant):
        NOS
        diffuse
     EXCLUDES *benign lymphoma (229.0)*
     AHA: 4Q, '06, 135; 2Q, '06, 20-21; 2Q, '92, 4; **For code 202.80:** 4Q, '08, 83; 1Q, '08, 16; 3Q, '07, 3
     C85.80 Oth spec types non-Hodgkins lymphoma unspec site   I-10

§ √5ᵗʰ **202.9 Other and unspecified malignant neoplasms of**
[0-8] **lymphoid and histiocytic tissue**
     Follicular dendritic cell sarcoma
     Interdigitating dendritic cell sarcoma
     Langerhans cell sarcoma
     Malignant neoplasm of bone marrow NOS

√4ᵗʰ **203 Multiple myeloma and immunoproliferative neoplasms**
     AHA: 4Q, '08, 83-84; 4Q, '91, 26

     The following fifth-digit subclassification is for use with category 203:
       0 without mention of having achieved remission
          Failed remission
       1 in remission
       2 in relapse

§ √5ᵗʰ **203.0 Multiple myeloma**
[0-2]   Kahler's disease   Myelomatosis
     EXCLUDES *solitary myeloma (238.6)*
     AHA: 1Q, '96, 16; 4Q, '89, 10; **For code 203.00:** 2Q, '10, 6; 2Q, '07, 8
     For code 203.01: 4Q, '08, 91
     C90.00 Multiple myeloma not in remission   I-10

§ √5ᵗʰ **203.1 Plasma cell leukemia**
[0-2]   Plasmacytic leukemia
     AHA: 4Q, '91, 26; S-0, '86, 12

§ √5ᵗʰ **203.8 Other immunoproliferative neoplasms**
[0-2]   **AHA:** 4Q, '90, 26; S-0, '86, 12

√4ᵗʰ **204 Lymphoid leukemia**
     INCLUDES leukemia:
          lymphatic
          lymphoblastic
          lymphocytic
          lymphogenous
     AHA: 4Q, '08, 83-84; 3Q, '93, 4

     The following fifth-digit subclassification is for use with category 204:
       0 without mention of having achieved remission
          Failed remission
       1 in remission
       2 in relapse

§ √5ᵗʰ **204.0 Acute**
[0-2]   **EXCLUDES** *acute exacerbation of chronic lymphoid leukemia (204.1)*
     AHA: 3Q, '99, 6; **For code 204.00:** 2Q, '11, 4;
     For code 204.02: ▶1Q, '12, 13◀

§ √5ᵗʰ **204.1 Chronic**
[0-2]   **C91.10** Chronic lymphocytic leukemia not in remission   I-10

§ √5ᵗʰ **204.2 Subacute**
[0-2]

§ √5ᵗʰ **204.8 Other lymphoid leukemia**
[0-2]   Aleukemic leukemia: Aleukemic leukemia:
        lymphatic   lymphoid
        lymphocytic
     AHA: 3Q, '09, 4
     TIP: Assign for T-cell large granular lymphocytic leukemia.

§ √5ᵗʰ **204.9 Unspecified lymphoid leukemia**
[0-2]

√4ᵗʰ **205 Myeloid leukemia**
     INCLUDES leukemia:
          granulocytic
          myeloblastic
          myelocytic
          myelogenous
          myelomonocytic
          myelosclerotic
          myelosis
     AHA: 4Q, '08, 83-84; 3Q, '93, 3; 4Q, '91, 26; 4Q, '90, 3; M-J, '85, 18

     The following fifth-digit subclassification is for use with category 205:
       0 without mention of having achieved remission
          Failed remission
       1 in remission
       2 in relapse

§ √5ᵗʰ **205.0 Acute**
[0-2]   Acute promyelocytic leukemia
     EXCLUDES *acute exacerbation of chronic myeloid leukemia (205.1)*
     AHA: 2Q, '06, 20-2; **For code 205.00:** 4Q, '09, 79
     C92.00 Acute myeloid leukemia not in remission   I-10

§ √5ᵗʰ **205.1 Chronic**
[0-2]   Eosinophilic leukemia
     Neutrophilic leukemia
     AHA: 1Q, '00, 6; J-A, '85, 13 ; **For code 205.10:** 4Q, '08, 142

§ √5ᵗʰ **205.2 Subacute**
[0-2]

§ √5ᵗʰ **205.3 Myeloid sarcoma**
[0-2]   Chloroma
     Granulocytic sarcoma

§ √5ᵗʰ **205.8 Other myeloid leukemia**
[0-2]   Aleukemic leukemia: Aleukemic leukemia:
        granulocytic   myeloid
        myelogenous   Aleukemic myelosis

§ √5ᵗʰ **205.9 Unspecified myeloid leukemia**
[0-2]

√4ᵗʰ **206 Monocytic leukemia**
     INCLUDES leukemia:
          histiocytic
          monoblastic
          monocytoid
     AHA: 4Q, '08, 83-84

     The following fifth-digit subclassification is for use with category 206:
       0 without mention of having achieved remission
          Failed remission
       1 in remission
       2 in relapse

§ √5ᵗʰ **206.0 Acute**
[0-2]   **EXCLUDES** *acute exacerbation of chronic monocytic leukemia (206.1)*

§ √5ᵗʰ **206.1 Chronic**
[0-2]

§ √5ᵗʰ **206.2 Subacute**
[0-2]

§ √5ᵗʰ **206.8 Other monocytic leukemia**
[0-2]   Aleukemic:
        monocytic leukemia
        monocytoid leukemia

---

§   Requires fifth digit. Valid digits are in [brackets] under each code. See appropriate category for codes and definitions.

N Newborn Age: 0   P Pediatric Age: 0-17   M Maternity Age: 12-55   A Adult Age: 15-124

§ ✓5ᵗʰ **206.9 Unspecified monocytic leukemia**
[0-2]

✓4ᵗʰ **207 Other specified leukemia**
> EXCLUDES leukemic reticuloendotheliosis (202.4)
> plasma cell leukemia (203.1)
>
> AHA: 4Q, '08, 83-85
>
> The following fifth-digit subclassification is for use with category 207:
> **0 without mention of having achieved remission**
> Failed remission
> **1 in remission**
> **2 in relapse**

§ ✓5ᵗʰ **207.0 Acute erythremia and erythroleukemia**
[0-2]   Acute erythremic myelosis
Di Guglielmo's disease
Erythremic myelosis
> DEF: Erythremia: polycythemia vera.
> DEF: Erythroleukemia: a malignant blood dyscrasia (a myeloproliferative disorder).

§ ✓5ᵗʰ **207.1 Chronic erythremia**
[0-2]   Heilmeyer-Schöner disease

§ ✓5ᵗʰ **207.2 Megakaryocytic leukemia**
[0-2]   Megakaryocytic myelosis
Thrombocytic leukemia

§ ✓5ᵗʰ **207.8 Other specified leukemia**
[0-2]   Lymphosarcoma cell leukemia

✓4ᵗʰ **208 Leukemia of unspecified cell type**
> AHA: 4Q, '08, 83-85
>
> The following fifth-digit subclassification is for use with category 208:
> **0 without mention of having achieved remission**
> Failed remission
> **1 in remission**
> **2 in relapse**

§ ✓5ᵗʰ **208.0 Acute**
[0-2]   Acute leukemia NOS   Stem cell leukemia
Blast cell leukemia
> EXCLUDES acute exacerbation of chronic unspecified leukemia (208.1)

§ ✓5ᵗʰ **208.1 Chronic**
[0-2]   Chronic leukemia NOS

§ ✓5ᵗʰ **208.2 Subacute**
[0-2]   Subacute leukemia NOS

§ ✓5ᵗʰ **208.8 Other leukemia of unspecified cell type**
[0-2]

§ ✓5ᵗʰ **208.9 Unspecified leukemia**
[0-2]   Leukemia NOS
> AHA: For code 208.90: ▶4Q, '11, 148◀

Neuroendocrine Tumors (209)

✓4ᵗʰ **209 Neuroendocrine tumors**
Code first any associated multiple endocrine neoplasia syndrome (258.01-258.03)
Use additional code to identify associated endocrine syndrome, such as:
carcinoid syndrome (259.2)
> EXCLUDES benign pancreatic islet cell tumors (211.7)
> malignant pancreatic islet cell tumors (157.4)
>
> AHA: 4Q, '09, 150; 4Q, '08, 85-89

✓5ᵗʰ **209.0 Malignant carcinoid tumors of the small intestine**

209.00 Malignant carcinoid tumor of the small intestine, unspecified portion

209.01 Malignant carcinoid tumor of the duodenum

209.02 Malignant carcinoid tumor of the jejunum

209.03 Malignant carcinoid tumor of the ileum

✓5ᵗʰ **209.1 Malignant carcinoid tumors of the appendix, large intestine, and rectum**

209.10 Malignant carcinoid tumor of the large intestine, unspecified portion
Malignant carcinoid tumor of the colon NOS

209.11 Malignant carcinoid tumor of the appendix

209.12 Malignant carcinoid tumor of the cecum

209.13 Malignant carcinoid tumor of the ascending colon

209.14 Malignant carcinoid tumor of the transverse colon

209.15 Malignant carcinoid tumor of the descending colon

209.16 Malignant carcinoid tumor of the sigmoid colon

209.17 Malignant carcinoid tumor of the rectum

✓5ᵗʰ **209.2 Malignant carcinoid tumors of other and unspecified sites**

209.20 Malignant carcinoid tumor of unknown primary site

209.21 Malignant carcinoid tumor of the bronchus and lung

209.22 Malignant carcinoid tumor of the thymus

209.23 Malignant carcinoid tumor of the stomach
> AHA: 4Q, '08, 89

209.24 Malignant carcinoid tumor of the kidney

209.25 Malignant carcinoid tumor of the foregut NOS

209.26 Malignant carcinoid tumor of the midgut NOS

209.27 Malignant carcinoid tumor of the hindgut NOS

209.29 Malignant carcinoid tumors of other sites

✓5ᵗʰ **209.3 Malignant poorly differentiated neuroendocrine tumors**
> AHA: 4Q, '09, 73-74

209.30 Malignant poorly differentiated neuroendocrine carcinoma, any site
High grade neuroendocrine carcinoma, any site
Malignant poorly differentiated neuroendocrine tumor NOS
> EXCLUDES Merkel cell carcinoma (209.31-209.36)

209.31 Merkel cell carcinoma of the face
Merkel cell carcinoma of the ear
Merkel cell carcinoma of the eyelid, including canthus
Merkel cell carcinoma of the lip

209.32 Merkel cell carcinoma of the scalp and neck

209.33 Merkel cell carcinoma of the upper limb

209.34 Merkel cell carcinoma of the lower limb

209.35 Merkel cell carcinoma of the trunk

209.36 Merkel cell carcinoma of other sites
Merkel cell carcinoma of the buttock
Merkel cell carcinoma of the genitals
Merkel cell carcinoma NOS
> AHA: 4Q, '09, 74

✓5ᵗʰ **209.4 Benign carcinoid tumors of the small intestine**

209.40 Benign carcinoid tumor of the small intestine, unspecified portion

209.41 Benign carcinoid tumor of the duodenum

209.42 Benign carcinoid tumor of the jejunum

209.43 Benign carcinoid tumor of the ileum

✓5ᵗʰ **209.5 Benign carcinoid tumors of the appendix, large intestine, and rectum**

209.50 Benign carcinoid tumor of the large intestine, unspecified portion
Benign carcinoid tumor of the colon NOS

209.51 Benign carcinoid tumor of the appendix

209.52 Benign carcinoid tumor of the cecum

209.53 Benign carcinoid tumor of the ascending colon

209.54 Benign carcinoid tumor of the transverse colon

209.55 Benign carcinoid tumor of the descending colon

209.56 Benign carcinoid tumor of the sigmoid colon

209.57 Benign carcinoid tumor of the rectum

---

§ Requires fifth digit. Valid digits are in [brackets] under each code. See appropriate category for codes and definitions.

✓4ᵗʰ/✓5ᵗʰ Additional Digit Required   Unspecified Code   Other Specified Code   Manifestation Code   ▶◀ Revised Text   ● New Code   ▲ Revised Code Title

✓5ᵗʰ **209.6 Benign carcinoid tumors of other and unspecified sites**

    209.60 Benign carcinoid tumor of unknown primary site
        Carcinoid tumor NOS
        Neuroendocrine tumor NOS

    209.61 Benign carcinoid tumor of the bronchus and lung
        AHA: 4Q, '09, 151

    209.62 Benign carcinoid tumor of the thymus

    209.63 Benign carcinoid tumor of the stomach

    209.64 Benign carcinoid tumor of the kidney

    209.65 Benign carcinoid tumor of the foregut NOS

    209.66 Benign carcinoid tumor of the midgut NOS

    209.67 Benign carcinoid tumor of the hindgut NOS

    209.69 Benign carcinoid tumors of other sites

✓5ᵗʰ **209.7 Secondary neuroendocrine tumors**
    Secondary carcinoid tumors
    AHA: 4Q, '09, 74

    209.70 Secondary neuroendocrine tumor, unspecified site

    209.71 Secondary neuroendocrine tumor of distant lymph nodes

    209.72 Secondary neuroendocrine tumor of liver

    209.73 Secondary neuroendocrine tumor of bone

    209.74 Secondary neuroendocrine tumor of peritoneum
        Mesentery metastasis of neuroendocrine tumor
        AHA: ▶4Q, '11, 181;◀ 4Q, '09, 150

    209.75 Secondary Merkel cell carcinoma
        Merkel cell carcinoma nodal presentation
        Merkel cell carcinoma visceral metastatic presentation
        Secondary Merkel cell carcinoma, any site

    209.79 Secondary neuroendocrine tumor of other sites

Benign Neoplasms (210-229)

✓4ᵗʰ **210 Benign neoplasm of lip, oral cavity, and pharynx**
    EXCLUDES *cyst (of):*
        jaw (526.0-526.2, 526.89)
        oral soft tissue (528.4)
        radicular (522.8)

    210.0 Lip
        Frenulum labii
        Lip (inner aspect) (mucosa) (vermilion border)
        EXCLUDES *labial commissure (210.4)*
                skin of lip (216.0)

    210.1 Tongue
        Lingual tonsil

    210.2 Major salivary glands
        Gland:
          parotid
          sublingual
          submandibular
        EXCLUDES *benign neoplasms of minor salivary glands:*
           NOS (210.4)
           buccal mucosa (210.4)
           lips (210.0)
           palate (hard) (soft) (210.4)
           tongue (210.1)
           tonsil, palatine (210.5)

    210.3 Floor of mouth

    210.4 Other and unspecified parts of mouth
        Gingiva   Oral mucosa
        Gum (upper) (lower)   Palate (hard) (soft)
        Labial commissure   Uvula
        Oral cavity NOS
        EXCLUDES *benign odontogenic neoplasms of bone*
           (213.0-213.1)
           developmental odontogenic cysts (526.0)
           mucosa of lips (210.0)
           nasopharyngeal [posterior] [superior] surface of soft palate (210.7)

    210.5 Tonsil
        Tonsil (faucial) (palatine)
        EXCLUDES *lingual tonsil (210.1)*
           pharyngeal tonsil (210.7)
           tonsillar:
             fossa (210.6)
             pillars (210.6)

    210.6 Other parts of oropharynx
        Branchial cleft or vestiges
        Epiglottis, anterior aspect
        Fauces NOS
        Mesopharynx NOS
        Tonsillar:
          fossa
          pillars
        Vallecula
        EXCLUDES *epiglottis:*
           NOS (212.1)
           suprahyoid portion (212.1)

    210.7 Nasopharynx
        Adenoid tissue
        Lymphadenoid tissue
        Pharyngeal tonsil
        Posterior nasal septum

    210.8 Hypopharynx
        Arytenoid fold   Postcricoid region
        Laryngopharynx   Pyriform fossa

    210.9 Pharynx, unspecified
        Throat NOS

✓4ᵗʰ **211 Benign neoplasm of other parts of digestive system**
    EXCLUDES *benign stromal tumors of digestive system (215.5)*

    211.0 Esophagus

    211.1 Stomach
        Body
        Cardia   } of stomach
        Fundus
        Cardiac orifice
        Pylorus
        EXCLUDES *benign carcinoid tumors of the stomach (209.63)*
        D13.1 Benign neoplasm of stomach   I-10

    211.2 Duodenum, jejunum, and ileum
        Small intestine NOS
        EXCLUDES *ampulla of Vater (211.5)*
           benign carcinoid tumors of the small intestine (209.40-209.43)
           ileocecal valve (211.3)

    211.3 Colon
        Appendix   Ileocecal valve
        Cecum   Large intestine NOS
        EXCLUDES *benign carcinoid tumors of the large intestine (209.50-209.56)*
           rectosigmoid junction (211.4)
        AHA: 2Q, '11, 9; 3Q, '05, 17; 2Q, '05, 16; 4Q, '01, 56
        D12.6 Benign neoplasm of colon unspecified   I-10

    211.4 Rectum and anal canal
        Anal canal or sphincter   Rectosigmoid junction
        Anus NOS
        EXCLUDES *anus:*
           margin (216.5)
           skin (216.5)
           benign carcinoid tumors of the rectum (209.57)
           perianal skin (216.5)
        AHA: 2Q, '11, 9

    211.5 Liver and biliary passages
        Ampulla of Vater   Gallbladder
        Common bile duct   Hepatic duct
        Cystic duct   Sphincter of Oddi

    211.6 Pancreas, except islets of Langerhans

    211.7 Islets of Langerhans
        Islet cell tumor
        Use additional code to identify any functional activity

---

N Newborn Age: 0   P Pediatric Age: 0-17   M Maternity Age: 12-55   A Adult Age: 15-124

211.8 Retroperitoneum and peritoneum
Mesentery
Mesocolon
Omentum
Retroperitoneal tissue

211.9 Other and unspecified site
Alimentary tract NOS
Digestive system NOS
Gastrointestinal tract NOS
Intestinal tract NOS
Intestine NOS
Spleen, not elsewhere classified

✓4ᵗʰ 212 Benign neoplasm of respiratory and intrathoracic organs

212.0 Nasal cavities, middle ear, and accessory sinuses
Cartilage of nose
Eustachian tube
Nares
Septum of nose
Sinus:
  ethmoidal
  frontal
  maxillary
  sphenoidal
EXCLUDES auditory canal (external) (216.2)
          bone of:
            ear (213.0)
            nose [turbinates] (213.0)
          cartilage of ear (215.0)
          ear (external) (skin) (216.2)
          nose NOS (229.8)
            skin (216.3)
          olfactory bulb (225.1)
          polyp of:
            accessory sinus (471.8)
            ear (385.30-385.35)
            nasal cavity (471.0)
          posterior margin of septum and choanae (210.7)

212.1 Larynx
Cartilage: Epiglottis (suprahyoid portion) NOS
  arytenoid   Glottis
  cricoid   Vocal cords (false)(true)
  cuneiform
  thyroid
EXCLUDES epiglottis, anterior aspect (210.6)
          polyp of vocal cord or larynx (478.4)

212.2 Trachea

212.3 Bronchus and lung
Carina
Hilus of lung
EXCLUDES benign carcinoid tumors of bronchus and lung
          (209.61)

212.4 Pleura

212.5 Mediastinum

212.6 Thymus
EXCLUDES benign carcinoid tumors of thymus (209.62)

212.7 Heart
EXCLUDES great vessels (215.4)

212.8 Other specified sites

212.9 Site unspecified
Respiratory organ NOS
Upper respiratory tract NOS
EXCLUDES intrathoracic NOS (229.8)
          thoracic NOS (229.8)

✓4ᵗʰ 213 Benign neoplasm of bone and articular cartilage
INCLUDES cartilage (articular) (joint)
          periosteum
EXCLUDES cartilage of:
            ear (215.0)
            eyelid (215.0))
            larynx (212.1)
            nose (212.0)
          exostosis NOS (726.91)
          synovia (215.0-215.9)

213.0 Bones of skull and face
EXCLUDES lower jaw bone (213.1)

213.1 Lower jaw bone

213.2 Vertebral column, excluding sacrum and coccyx

213.3 Ribs, sternum, and clavicle

213.4 Scapula and long bones of upper limb

213.5 Short bones of upper limb

213.6 Pelvic bones, sacrum, and coccyx

213.7 Long bones of lower limb

213.8 Short bones of lower limb

213.9 Bone and articular cartilage, site unspecified

✓4ᵗʰ 214 Lipoma
INCLUDES angiolipoma
          fibrolipoma
          hibernoma
          lipoma (fetal) (infiltrating) (intramuscular)
          myelolipoma
          myxolipoma
DEF: Benign tumor frequently composed of mature fat cells; may
occasionally be composed of fetal fat cells.

214.0 Skin and subcutaneous tissue of face

214.1 Other skin and subcutaneous tissue

214.2 Intrathoracic organs

214.3 Intra-abdominal organs

214.4 Spermatic cord   ♂

214.8 Other specified sites
AHA: 3Q, '94, 7

214.9 Lipoma, unspecified site

✓4ᵗʰ 215 Other benign neoplasm of connective and other soft tissue
INCLUDES blood vessel
          bursa
          fascia
          ligament
          muscle
          peripheral, sympathetic, and parasympathetic nerves and
            ganglia
          synovia
          tendon (sheath)
EXCLUDES cartilage:
            articular (213.0-213.9)
            larynx (212.1)
            nose (212.0)
          connective tissue of:
            breast (217)
            internal organ, except lipoma and hemangioma — code
              to benign neoplasm of the site
          lipoma (214.0-214.9)

215.0 Head, face, and neck

215.2 Upper limb, including shoulder

215.3 Lower limb, including hip

215.4 Thorax
EXCLUDES heart (212.7)
          mediastinum (212.5)
          thymus (212.6)

215.5 Abdomen
Abdominal wall
Benign stromal tumors of abdomen
Hypochondrium

215.6 Pelvis
  Buttock
  Groin
  Inguinal region
  Perineum
  EXCLUDES *uterine:*
    leiomyoma (218.0-218.9)
    ligament, any (221.0)

215.7 Trunk, unspecified
  Back NOS
  Flank NOS

215.8 Other specified sites

215.9 Site unspecified

√4ᵗʰ 216 Benign neoplasm of skin
  INCLUDES blue nevus
    dermatofibroma
    hydrocystoma
    pigmented nevus
    syringoadenoma
    syringoma
  EXCLUDES *skin of genital organs (221.0-222.9)*
  AHA: 1Q, '00, 21

216.0 Skin of lip
  EXCLUDES *vermilion border of lip (210.0)*

216.1 Eyelid, including canthus
  EXCLUDES *cartilage of eyelid (215.0)*

216.2 Ear and external auditory canal
  Auricle (ear)
  Auricular canal, external
  External meatus
  Pinna
  EXCLUDES *cartilage of ear (215.0)*

216.3 Skin of other and unspecified parts of face
  Cheek, external
  Eyebrow
  Nose, external
  Temple

216.4 Scalp and skin of neck
  AHA: 3Q, '91, 12

216.5 Skin of trunk, except scrotum
  Axillary fold   Skin of:
  Perianal skin   buttock
  Skin of: chest wall
    abdominal wall   groin
    anus   perineum
    back   Umbilicus
    breast
  EXCLUDES *anal canal (211.4)*
    anus NOS (211.4)
    skin of scrotum (222.4)

216.6 Skin of upper limb, including shoulder

216.7 Skin of lower limb, including hip

216.8 Other specified sites of skin

216.9 Skin, site unspecified

217 Benign neoplasm of breast
  Breast (male) (female):
    connective tissue
    glandular tissue
    soft parts
  EXCLUDES *adenofibrosis (610.2)*
    benign cyst of breast (610.0)
    fibrocystic disease (610.1)
    skin of breast (216.5)
  AHA: 1Q, '00, 4

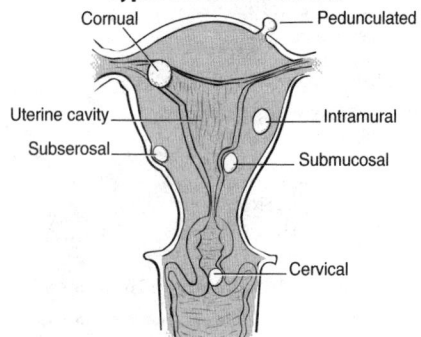

Types of Uterine Fibroids

√4ᵗʰ 218 Uterine leiomyoma
  INCLUDES fibroid (bleeding) (uterine)
    uterine:
      fibromyoma
      myoma
  DEF: Benign tumor primarily derived from uterine smooth muscle tissue; may contain fibrous, fatty, or epithelial tissue; also called uterine fibroid or myoma.

218.0 Submucous leiomyoma of uterus ♀

218.1 Intramural leiomyoma of uterus ♀
  Interstitial leiomyoma of uterus
  D25.1 Intramural leiomyoma of uterus **I-10**

218.2 Subserous leiomyoma of uterus ♀

218.9 Leiomyoma of uterus, unspecified ♀
  AHA: 1Q, '03, 4
  D25.9 Leiomyoma of uterus unspecified **I-10**

√4ᵗʰ 219 Other benign neoplasm of uterus

219.0 Cervix uteri ♀

219.1 Corpus uteri ♀
  Endometrium
  Fundus
  Myometrium

219.8 Other specified parts of uterus ♀

219.9 Uterus, part unspecified ♀

220 Benign neoplasm of ovary ♀
  Use additional code to identify any functional activity (256.0-256.1)
  EXCLUDES *cyst:*
    corpus albicans (620.2)
    corpus luteum (620.1)
    endometrial (617.1)
    follicular (atretic) (620.0)
    graafian follicle (620.0)
    ovarian NOS (620.2)
    retention (620.2)
  D27.9 Benign neoplasm of unspec ovary **I-10**

√4ᵗʰ 221 Benign neoplasm of other female genital organs
  INCLUDES adenomatous polyp
    benign teratoma
  EXCLUDES *cyst:*
    epoophoron (752.11)
    fimbrial (752.11)
    Gartner's duct (752.11)
    parovarian (752.11)

221.0 Fallopian tube and uterine ligaments ♀
  Oviduct
  Parametruim
  Uterine ligament (broad) (round) (uterosacral)
  Uterine tube

221.1 Vagina ♀

221.2 Vulva ♀
  Clitoris
  External female genitalia NOS
  Greater vestibular [Bartholin's] gland
  Labia (majora) (minora)
  Pudendum
  EXCLUDES *Bartholin's (duct) (gland) cyst (616.2)*

Neoplasms

221.8 **Other specified sites of female genital organs** ♀

221.9 **Female genital organ, site unspecified** ♀
Female genitourinary tract NOS

√4ᵗʰ **222** **Benign neoplasm of male genital organs**

222.0 **Testis** ♂
Use additional code to identify any functional activity

222.1 **Penis** ♂
Corpus cavernosum
Glans penis
Prepuce

222.2 **Prostate** ♂
EXCLUDES adenomatous hyperplasia of prostate
(600.20-600.21)
prostatic:
adenoma (600.20-600.21)
enlargement (600.00-600.01)
hypertrophy (600.00-600.01)

222.3 **Epididymis** ♂

222.4 **Scrotum** ♂
Skin of scrotum

222.8 **Other specified sites of male genital organs** ♂
Seminal vesicle
Spermatic cord

222.9 **Male genital organ, site unspecified** ♂
Male genitourinary tract NOS

√4ᵗʰ **223** **Benign neoplasm of kidney and other urinary organs**

223.0 **Kidney, except pelvis**
Kidney NOS
EXCLUDES benign carcinoid tumors of kidney (209.64)
renal:
calyces (223.1)
pelvis (223.1)

223.1 **Renal pelvis**

223.2 **Ureter**
EXCLUDES ureteric orifice of bladder (223.3)

223.3 **Bladder**

√5ᵗʰ **223.8** **Other specified sites of urinary organs**

223.81 **Urethra**
EXCLUDES urethral orifice of bladder (223.3)

223.89 **Other**
Paraurethral glands

223.9 **Urinary organ, site unspecified**
Urinary system NOS

√4ᵗʰ **224** **Benign neoplasm of eye**
EXCLUDES cartilage of eyelid (215.0)
eyelid (skin) (216.1)
optic nerve (225.1)
orbital bone (213.0)

224.0 **Eyeball, except conjunctiva, cornea, retina, and choroid**
Ciliary body
Iris
Sclera
Uveal tract

224.1 **Orbit**
EXCLUDES bone of orbit (213.0)

224.2 **Lacrimal gland**

224.3 **Conjunctiva**

224.4 **Cornea**

224.5 **Retina**
EXCLUDES hemangioma of retina (228.03)

224.6 **Choroid**

224.7 **Lacrimal duct**
Lacrimal sac
Nasolacrimal duct

224.8 **Other specified parts of eye**

Eyeball

Posterior segment
Vitreous
Optic nerve
Optic disc
Choroid
Sclera
Retina
Pars plana
Conjunctiva
Sclera
Lens
Cornea
Iris
Anterior chamber

224.9 **Eye, part unspecified**

√4ᵗʰ **225** **Benign neoplasm of brain and other parts of nervous system**
EXCLUDES hemangioma (228.02)
neurofibromatosis (237.70-237.79)
peripheral, sympathetic, and parasympathetic nerves and
ganglia (215.0-215.9)
retrobulbar (224.1)

225.0 **Brain**

225.1 **Cranial nerves**
Acoustic neuroma
AHA: 4Q, '04, 113

225.2 **Cerebral meninges**
Meninges NOS
Meningioma (cerebral)
D32.0 Benign neoplasm of cerebral meninges   I-10

225.3 **Spinal cord**
Cauda equina

225.4 **Spinal meninges**
Spinal meningioma

225.8 **Other specified sites of nervous system**

225.9 **Nervous system, part unspecified**
Nervous system (central) NOS
EXCLUDES meninges NOS (225.2)

226 **Benign neoplasm of thyroid glands**
Use additional code to identify any functional activity

√4ᵗʰ **227** **Benign neoplasm of other endocrine glands and related structures**
Use additional code to identify any functional activity
EXCLUDES ovary (220)
pancreas (211.6)
testis (222.0)

227.0 **Adrenal gland**
Suprarenal gland

227.1 **Parathyroid gland**

227.3 **Pituitary gland and craniopharyngeal duct (pouch)**
Craniobuccal pouch
Hypophysis
Rathke's pouch
Sella turcica

227.4 **Pineal gland**
Pineal body

227.5 **Carotid body**

227.6 **Aortic body and other paraganglia**
Coccygeal body
Glomus jugulare
Para-aortic body
AHA: N-D, '84, 17

227.8 **Other**

227.9 **Endocrine gland, site unspecified**

221.8-227.9

Neoplasms

228–232.3

☑4ᵗʰ **228 Hemangioma and lymphangioma, any site**
> INCLUDES angioma (benign) (cavernous) (congenital) NOS
> cavernous nevus
> glomus tumor
> hemangioma (benign) (congenital)
>
> EXCLUDES *benign neoplasm of spleen, except hemangioma and*
> *lymphangioma (211.9)*
> *glomus jugulare (227.6)*
> *nevus:*
> *NOS (216.0-216.9)*
> *blue or pigmented (216.0-216.9)*
> *vascular (757.32)*
>
> AHA: 1Q, '00, 21

☑5ᵗʰ **228.0 Hemangioma, any site**
> AHA: J-F, '85, 19
> DEF: A common benign tumor usually occurring in infancy;
> composed of newly formed blood vessels due to malformation of
> angioblastic tissue.

  228.00 Of unspecified site

  228.01 Of skin and subcutaneous tissue
  > AHA: 3Q, '10, 16

  228.02 Of intracranial structures

  228.03 Of retina

  228.04 Of intra-abdominal structures
  > Peritoneum
  > Retroperitoneal tissue

  228.09 Of other sites
  > Systemic angiomatosis
  > AHA: 3Q, '91, 20

228.1 Lymphangioma, any site
> Congenital lymphangioma
> Lymphatic nevus

☑4ᵗʰ **229 Benign neoplasm of other and unspecified sites**

229.0 Lymph nodes
> EXCLUDES *lymphangioma (228.1)*

229.8 Other specified sites
> Intrathoracic NOS
> Thoracic NOS

229.9 Site unspecified

Carcinoma In Situ (230-234)

> INCLUDES Bowen's disease
> erythroplasia
> Queyrat's erythroplasia
>
> EXCLUDES *leukoplakia — see Alphabetic Index*
> DEF: A neoplastic type; with tumor cells confined to epithelium of origin;
> without further invasion.

☑4ᵗʰ **230 Carcinoma in situ of digestive organs**

230.0 Lip, oral cavity, and pharynx
> Gingiva
> Hypopharynx
> Mouth [any part]
> Nasopharynx
> Oropharynx
> Salivary gland or duct
> Tongue
>
> EXCLUDES *aryepiglottic fold or interarytenoid fold, laryngeal*
> *aspect (231.0)*
> *epiglottis:*
> *NOS (231.0)*
> *suprahyoid portion (231.0)*
> *skin of lip (232.0)*

230.1 Esophagus

230.2 Stomach
> Body ⎫
> Cardia ⎬ of stomach
> Fundus ⎭
> Cardiac orifice
> Pylorus

230.3 Colon
> Appendix
> Cecum
> Ileocecal valve
> Large intestine NOS
>
> EXCLUDES *rectosigmoid junction (230.4)*

230.4 Rectum
> Rectosigmoid junction

230.5 Anal canal
> Anal sphincter

230.6 Anus, unspecified
> EXCLUDES *anus:*
> *margin (232.5)*
> *skin (232.5)*
> *perianal skin (232.5)*

230.7 Other and unspecified parts of intestine
> Duodenum
> Ileum
> Jejunum
> Small intestine NOS
>
> EXCLUDES *ampulla of Vater (230.8)*

230.8 Liver and biliary system
> Ampulla of Vater
> Common bile duct
> Cystic duct
> Gallbladder
> Hepatic duct
> Sphincter of Oddi

230.9 Other and unspecified digestive organs
> Digestive organ NOS
> Gastrointestinal tract NOS
> Pancreas
> Spleen

☑4ᵗʰ **231 Carcinoma in situ of respiratory system**

231.0 Larynx
> Cartilage:
> arytenoid
> cricoid
> cuneiform
> thyroid
> Epiglottis:
> NOS
> posterior surface
> suprahyoid portion
> Vocal cords (false)(true)
>
> EXCLUDES *aryepiglottic fold or interarytenoid fold:*
> *NOS (230.0)*
> *hypopharyngeal aspect (230.0)*
> *marginal zone (230.0)*

231.1 Trachea

231.2 Bronchus and lung
> Carina
> Hilus of lung

231.8 Other specified parts of respiratory system
> Accessory sinuses
> Middle ear
> Nasal cavities
> Pleura
>
> EXCLUDES *ear (external) (skin) (232.2)*
> *nose NOS (234.8)*
> *skin (232.3)*

231.9 Respiratory system, part unspecified
> Respiratory organ NOS

☑4ᵗʰ **232 Carcinoma in situ of skin**
> INCLUDES pigment cells
> EXCLUDES *melanoma in situ of skin (172.0-172.9)*

232.0 Skin of lip
> EXCLUDES *vermilion border of lip (230.0)*

232.1 Eyelid, including canthus

232.2 Ear and external auditory canal

232.3 Skin of other and unspecified parts of face

232.4 Scalp and skin of neck

232.5 Skin of trunk, except scrotum

Anus, margin	Skin of:
Axillary fold	breast
Perianal skin	buttock
Skin of:	chest wall
abdominal wall	groin
anus	perineum
back	Umbilicus

> **EXCLUDES** anal canal (230.5)
> anus NOS (230.6)
> skin of genital organs (233.30-233.39, 233.5-233.6)

232.6 Skin of upper limb, including shoulder

232.7 Skin of lower limb, including hip

232.8 Other specified sites of skin

232.9 Skin, site unspecified

√4ᵗʰ 233 Carcinoma in situ of breast and genitourinary system

> **TIP:** For patients with carcinoma in situ found incidentally when admitted for treatment of another condition, sequence the 233 code as a secondary condition.

233.0 Breast

> **EXCLUDES** Paget's disease (174.0-174.9)
> skin of breast (232.5)

> **TIP:** Assign for tumors specified as intraductal carcinoma.

233.1 Cervix uteri   ♀

Adenocarcinoma in situ of cervix
Cervical intraepithelial glandular neoplasia, grade III
Cervical intraepithelial neoplasia III [CIN III]
Severe dysplasia of cervix

> **EXCLUDES** cervical intraepithelial neoplasia II [CIN II] (622.12)
> cytologic evidence of malignancy without histologic confirmation (795.06)
> high grade squamous intraepithelial lesion (HGSIL) (795.04)
> moderate dysplasia of cervix (622.12)

> **AHA:** 3Q, '92, 7; 3Q, '92, 8; 1Q, '91, 11

233.2 Other and unspecified parts of uterus   ♀

√5ᵗʰ 233.3 Other and unspecified female genital organs

> **AHA:** 4Q, '07, 67

233.30 Unspecified female genital organ   ♀

233.31 Vagina   ♀

Severe dysplasia of vagina
Vaginal intraepithelial neoplasia III [VAIN III]

233.32 Vulva   ♀

Severe dysplasia of vulva
Vulvar intraepithelial neoplasia III [VIN III]

233.39 Other female genital organ   ♀

233.4 Prostate   ♂

233.5 Penis   ♂

233.6 Other and unspecified male genital organs   ♂

233.7 Bladder

233.9 Other and unspecified urinary organs

√4ᵗʰ 234 Carcinoma in situ of other and unspecified sites

234.0 Eye

> **EXCLUDES** cartilage of eyelid (234.8)
> eyelid (skin) (232.1)
> optic nerve (234.8)
> orbital bone (234.8)

234.8 Other specified sites
Endocrine gland [any]

234.9 Site unspecified
Carcinoma in situ NOS

Neoplasms of Uncertain Behavior (235-238)

> **NOTE** Categories 235–238 classify by site certain histomorphologically well-defined neoplasms, the subsequent behavior of which cannot be predicted from the present appearance.

> **TIP:** Typically assigned for cases in which the tumor is in transition and may be undergoing malignant transformation, but continued study is required for accurate classification.

√4ᵗʰ 235 Neoplasm of uncertain behavior of digestive and respiratory systems

> **EXCLUDES** stromal tumors of uncertain behavior of digestive system (238.1)

235.0 Major salivary glands
Gland:
  parotid
  sublingual
  submandibular

> **EXCLUDES** minor salivary glands (235.1)

235.1 Lip, oral cavity, and pharynx
Gingiva
Hypopharynx
Minor salivary glands
Mouth
Nasopharynx
Oropharynx
Tongue

> **EXCLUDES** aryepiglottic fold or interarytenoid fold, laryngeal aspect (235.6)
> epiglottis:
>   NOS (235.6)
>   suprahyoid portion (235.6)
> skin of lip (238.2)

235.2 Stomach, intestines, and rectum

235.3 Liver and biliary passages
Ampulla of Vater
Bile ducts [any]
Gallbladder
Liver

235.4 Retroperitoneum and peritoneum

235.5 Other and unspecified digestive organs
Anal:
  canal
  sphincter
Anus NOS
Esophagus
Pancreas
Spleen

> **EXCLUDES** anus:
>   margin (238.2)
>   skin (238.2)
> perianal skin (238.2)

235.6 Larynx

> **EXCLUDES** aryepiglottic fold or interarytenoid fold:
> NOS (235.1)
> hypopharyngeal aspect (235.1)
> marginal zone (235.1)

235.7 Trachea, bronchus, and lung

235.8 Pleura, thymus, and mediastinum

235.9 Other and unspecified respiratory organs
Accessory sinuses
Middle ear
Nasal cavities
Respiratory organ NOS

> **EXCLUDES** ear (external) (skin) (238.2)
> nose (238.8)
> skin (238.2)

√4ᵗʰ 236 Neoplasm of uncertain behavior of genitourinary organs

236.0 Uterus   ♀

236.1 Placenta   ♀
Chorioadenoma (destruens)
Invasive mole
Malignant hydatid mole
Malignant hydatidiform mole

√4ᵗʰ √5ᵗʰ Additional Digit Required   Unspecified Code   Other Specified Code   Manifestation Code   ►◄ Revised Text   ● New Code   ▲ Revised Code Title

2013 ICD-9-CM   **Volume 1 – 47**

Neoplasms

236.2 Ovary ♀
> Use additional code to identify any functional activity

236.3 Other and unspecified female genital organs ♀

236.4 Testis ♂
> Use additional code to identify any functional activity

236.5 Prostate ♂

236.6 Other and unspecified male genital organs ♂

236.7 Bladder

√5ᵗʰ **236.9 Other and unspecified urinary organs**

> **236.90 Urinary organ, unspecified**

> **236.91 Kidney and ureter**

> **236.99 Other**

√4ᵗʰ **237 Neoplasm of uncertain behavior of endocrine glands and nervous system**

> **237.0 Pituitary gland and craniopharyngeal duct**
>> Use additional code to identify any functional activity

> **237.1 Pineal gland**

> **237.2 Adrenal gland**
>> Suprarenal gland
>> Use additional code to identify any functional activity

> **237.3 Paraganglia**
>> Aortic body   Coccygeal body
>> Carotid body   Glomus jugulare
>> **AHA:** N-D, '84, 17

> **237.4 Other and unspecified endocrine glands**
>> Parathyroid gland
>> Thyroid gland

> **237.5 Brain and spinal cord**

> **237.6 Meninges**
>> Meninges:
>>> NOS
>>> cerebral
>>> spinal

√5ᵗʰ **237.7 Neurofibromatosis**
>> **DEF:** An inherited condition with developmental changes in the nervous system, muscles, bones and skin; multiple soft tumors (neurofibromas) distributed over the entire body.

> **237.70 Neurofibromatosis, unspecified**

> **237.71 Neurofibromatosis, type 1 [von Recklinghausen's disease]**
>> **AHA:** 4Q, '10, 76

> **237.72 Neurofibromatosis, type 2 [acoustic neurofibromatosis]**
>> **DEF:** Inherited condition with cutaneous lesions, benign tumors of peripheral nerves and bilateral 8th nerve masses.
>> **AHA:** 4Q, '10, 76

> **237.73 Schwannomatosis**
>> **DEF:** A genetic mutation (SMARCB1/INI1) causing multiple benign tumors along nerve pathways; characterized by the exception of 8th cranial nerve involvement.
>> **AHA:** 4Q, '10, 76-77

> **237.79 Other neurofibromatosis**
>> **AHA:** 4Q, '10, 76-77

> **237.9 Other and unspecified parts of nervous system**
>> Cranial nerves
>> *EXCLUDES* peripheral, sympathetic, and parasympathetic nerves and ganglia (238.1)

√4ᵗʰ **238 Neoplasm of uncertain behavior of other and unspecified sites and tissues**

> **238.0 Bone and articular cartilage**
>> *EXCLUDES* cartilage:
>>> ear (238.1)
>>> eyelid (238.1)
>>> larynx (235.6)
>>> nose (235.9)
>>> synovia (238.1)
>> **AHA:** 4Q, '04, 128

238.1 Connective and other soft tissue
> Peripheral, sympathetic, and parasympathetic nerves and ganglia
> Stromal tumors of digestive system
> *EXCLUDES* cartilage (of):
>> articular (238.0)
>> larynx (235.6)
>> nose (235.9)
>> connective tissue of breast (238.3)

238.2 Skin
> *EXCLUDES* anus NOS (235.5)
>> skin of genital organs (236.3, 236.6)
>> vermilion border of lip (235.1)
> **TIP:** Assign when documentation indicates keratoacanthoma only.

238.3 Breast
> *EXCLUDES* skin of breast (238.2)

238.4 Polycythemia vera
> **DEF:** Abnormal proliferation of all bone marrow elements, increased red cell mass and total blood volume; unknown etiology, frequently associated with splenomegaly, leukocytosis, and thrombocythemia.
> **D45** Polycythemia vera   I-10

238.5 Histiocytic and mast cells
> Mast cell tumor NOS
> Mastocytoma NOS

238.6 Plasma cells
> Plasmacytoma NOS
> Solitary myeloma

√5ᵗʰ **238.7 Other lymphatic and hematopoietic tissues**
> *EXCLUDES* acute myelogenous leukemia (205.0)
>> chronic myelomonocytic leukemia (205.1)
>> myelosclerosis NOS (289.89)
>> myelosis:
>>> NOS (205.9)
>>> megakaryocytic (207.2)
> **AHA:** 3Q, '01, 13; 1Q, '97, 5; 2Q, '89, 8

> **238.71 Essential thrombocythemia**
>> Essential hemorrhagic thrombocythemia
>> Essential thrombocytosis
>> Idiopathic (hemorrhagic) thrombocythemia
>> Primary thrombocytosis
>> **AHA:** 4Q, '06, 63-66
>> **D47.3** Essential (hemorrhagic) thrombocythemia   I-10

> **238.72 Low grade myelodysplastic syndrome lesions**
>> Refractory anemia (RA)
>> Refractory anemia with excess blasts-1 (RAEB-1)
>> Refractory anemia with ringed sideroblasts (RARS)
>> Refractory cytopenia with multilineage dysplasia (RCMD)
>> Refractory cytopenia with multilineage dysplasia and ringed sideroblasts (RCMD-RS)
>> **DEF:** Refractory anemia (RA): Form of bone marrow disorder (myelodysplastic syndrome) that interferes with red blood cell production in the bone marrow; unresponsive to hematinics; characteristic normal or hypercellular marrow with abnormal erythrocyte development and reticulocytopenia.
>> **AHA:** 4Q, '06, 63-66

> **238.73 High grade myelodysplastic syndrome lesions**
>> Refractory anemia with excess blasts-2 (RAEB-2)
>> **AHA:** 4Q, '06, 63-66

> **238.74 Myelodysplastic syndrome with 5q deletion**
>> 5q minus syndrome NOS
>> *EXCLUDES* constitutional 5q deletion (758.39)
>>> high grade myelodysplastic syndrome with 5q deletion (238.73)
>> **AHA:** 4Q, '06, 63-66

> **238.75 Myelodysplastic syndrome, unspecified**
>> **AHA:** 4Q, '06, 63-66
>> **D46.9** Myelodysplastic syndrome unspecified   I-10

N Newborn Age: 0   P Pediatric Age: 0-17   M Maternity Age: 12-55   A Adult Age: 15-124

238.76 Myelofibrosis with myeloid metaplasia
   Agnogenic myeloid metaplasia
   Idiopathic myelofibrosis (chronic)
   Myelosclerosis with myeloid metaplasia
   Primary myelofibrosis
   EXCLUDES *myelofibrosis NOS (289.83)*
              myelophthisic anemia (284.2)
              myelophthisis (284.2)
              secondary myelofibrosis (289.83)
   AHA: 4Q, '06, 63-66

238.77 Post-transplant lymphoproliferative disorder [PTLD]
   Code first complications of transplant (996.80-996.89)
   DEF: Excessive proliferation of B-cell lymphocytes following
   Epstein-Barr virus infection in organ transplant patients;
   may progress to non-Hodgkins lymphoma.
   AHA: 4Q, '08, 90-91

238.79 Other lymphatic and hematopoietic tissues
   Lymphoproliferative disease (chronic) NOS
   Megakaryocytic myelosclerosis
   Myeloproliferative disease (chronic) NOS
   Panmyelosis (acute)
   AHA: 4Q, '06, 63-66

238.8 Other specified sites
   Eye   Heart
   EXCLUDES *eyelid (skin) (238.2)*
              cartilage (238.1)

238.9 Site unspecified

Neoplasms of Unspecified Nature (239)

✓4ᵗʰ 239 Neoplasms of unspecified nature
   NOTE Category 239 classifies by site neoplasms of unspecified
   morphology and behavior. The term "mass," unless otherwise
   stated, is not to be regarded as a neoplastic growth.
   INCLUDES "growth" NOS
             neoplasm NOS
             new growth NOS
             tumor NOS
   TIP: Do not assign for inpatient cases; more information should be available.

239.0 Digestive system
   EXCLUDES *anus:*
              margin (239.2)
              skin (239.2)
              perianal skin (239.2)

239.1 Respiratory system

239.2 Bone, soft tissue, and skin
   EXCLUDES *anal canal (239.0)*
              anus NOS (239.0)
              bone marrow (202.9)
              cartilage:
                larynx (239.1)
                nose (239.1)
              connective tissue of breast (239.3)
              skin of genital organs (239.5)
              vermilion border of lip (239.0)

239.3 Breast
   EXCLUDES *skin of breast (239.2)*

239.4 Bladder

239.5 Other genitourinary organs

239.6 Brain
   EXCLUDES *cerebral meninges (239.7)*
              cranial nerves (239.7)

239.7 Endocrine glands and other parts of nervous system
   EXCLUDES *peripheral, sympathetic, and parasympathetic*
              nerves and ganglia (239.2)

✓5ᵗʰ 239.8 Other specified sites
   EXCLUDES *eyelid (skin) (239.2)*
              cartilage (239.2)
              great vessels (239.2)
              optic nerve (239.7)
   AHA: 4Q, '09, 75

   239.81 Retina and choroid
      Dark area on retina
      Retinal freckle
      TIP: Assign for documentation of retinal "freckles" or spots
      that may be indicative of malignant melanoma. Histologic
      confirmation is not required.

   239.89 Other specified sites

239.9 Site unspecified

3. Endocrine, Nutritional and Metabolic Diseases, and Immunity Disorders (240-279)

EXCLUDES *endocrine and metabolic disturbances specific to the fetus and newborn (775.0-775.9)*

NOTE All neoplasms, whether functionally active or not, are classified in Chapter 2. Codes in Chapter 3 (i.e., 242.8, 246.0, 251-253, 255-259) may be used to identify such functional activity associated with any neoplasm, or by ectopic endocrine tissue.

Disorders of Thyroid Gland (240-246)

✓4ʰ 240 Simple and unspecified goiter

    DEF: An enlarged thyroid gland often caused by an inadequate dietary intake of iodine.

    240.0 Goiter, specified as simple

        Any condition classifiable to 240.9, specified as simple

    240.9 Goiter, unspecified

        Enlargement of thyroid
        Goiter or struma:
          NOS
          diffuse colloid
          endemic
          hyperplastic
          nontoxic (diffuse)
          parenchymatous
          sporadic

        EXCLUDES *congenital (dyshormonogenic) goiter (246.1)*

✓4ʰ 241 Nontoxic nodular goiter

    EXCLUDES *adenoma of thyroid (226)*
                     cystadenoma of thyroid (226)

    241.0 Nontoxic uninodular goiter

        Thyroid nodule
        Uninodular goiter (nontoxic)

        DEF: Enlarged thyroid, commonly due to decreased thyroid production, with single nodule; no clinical hypothyroidism.

        E04.1 Nontoxic single thyroid nodule   I-10

    241.1 Nontoxic multinodular goiter

        Multinodular goiter (nontoxic)

        DEF: Enlarged thyroid, commonly due to decreased thyroid production with multiple nodules; no clinical hypothyroidism.

    241.9 Unspecified nontoxic nodular goiter

        Adenomatous goiter
        Nodular goiter (nontoxic) NOS
        Struma nodosa (simplex)

✓4ʰ 242 Thyrotoxicosis with or without goiter

    EXCLUDES *neonatal thyrotoxicosis (775.3)*

    DEF: A condition caused by excess quantities of thyroid hormones being introduced into the tissues

    The following fifth-digit subclassification is for use with categories 242:
      0 without mention of thyrotoxic crisis or storm
      1 with mention of thyrotoxic crisis or storm

§ ✓5ʰ 242.0 Toxic diffuse goiter
    [0-1]

        Basedow's disease
        Exophthalmic or toxic goiter NOS
        Graves' disease
        Primary thyroid hyperplasia

        DEF: Diffuse thyroid enlargement accompanied by hyperthyroidism, bulging eyes, and dermopathy.

§ ✓5ʰ 242.1 Toxic uninodular goiter
    [0-1]

        Thyroid nodule ⎫
        Uninodular goiter ⎬ toxic or with hyperthyroidism

        DEF: Symptomatic hyperthyroidism with a single nodule on the enlarged thyroid gland. Abrupt onset of symptoms; including extreme nervousness, insomnia, weight loss, tremors, and psychosis or coma.

§ ✓5ʰ 242.2 Toxic multinodular goiter
    [0-1]

        Secondary thyroid hyperplasia

        DEF: Symptomatic hyperthyroidism with multiple nodules on the enlarged thyroid gland. Abrupt onset of symptoms; including extreme nervousness, insomnia, weight loss, tremors, and psychosis or coma.

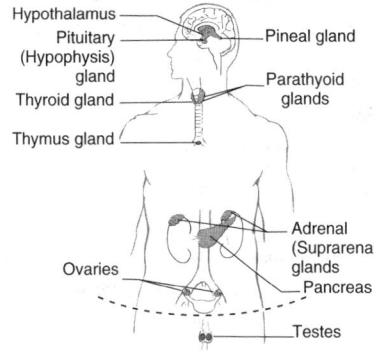

The Endocrine System

§ ✓5ʰ 242.3 Toxic nodular goiter, unspecified
    [0-1]

        Adenomatous goiter ⎫
        Nodular goiter ⎬ toxic or with hyperthyroidism
        Struma nodosa ⎭

        Any condition classifiable to 241.9 specified as toxic or with hyperthyroidism

§ ✓5ʰ 242.4 Thyrotoxicosis from ectopic thyroid nodule
    [0-1]

§ ✓5ʰ 242.8 Thyrotoxicosis of other specified origin
    [0-1]

        Overproduction of thyroid-stimulating hormone [TSH]
        Thyrotoxicosis:
          factitia from ingestion of excessive thyroid material

        Use additional E code to identify cause, if drug-induced

§ ✓5ʰ 242.9 Thyrotoxicosis without mention of goiter or other
    [0-1] **cause**

        Hyperthyroidism NOS
        Thyrotoxicosis NOS
        E05.90 Thyrotoxicosis uns w/o thyrotoxic crisis or storm   I-10

243 Congenital hypothyroidism

    Congenital thyroid insufficiency
    Cretinism (athyrotic) (endemic)

    Use additional code to identify associated intellectual disabilities

    EXCLUDES *congenital (dyshormonogenic) goiter (246.1)*

    DEF: Underproduction of thyroid hormone present from birth.

✓4ʰ 244 Acquired hypothyroidism

    INCLUDES athyroidism (acquired)
                  hypothyroidism (acquired)
                  myxedema (adult) (juvenile)
                  thyroid (gland) insufficiency (acquired)

    244.0 Postsurgical hypothyroidism

        DEF: Underproduction of thyroid hormone due to surgical removal of all or part of the thyroid gland.

        E89.0 Postprocedural hypothyroidism   I-10

    244.1 Other postablative hypothyroidism

        Hypothyroidism following therapy, such as irradiation

    244.2 Iodine hypothyroidism

        Hypothyroidism resulting from administration or ingestion of iodide

        EXCLUDES *hypothyroidism resulting from administration of radioactive iodine (244.1)*

        Use additional E code to identify drug

    244.3 Other iatrogenic hypothyroidism

        Hypothyroidism resulting from:
          P-aminosalicylic acid [PAS]
          Phenylbutazone
          Resorcinol
        Iatrogenic hypothyroidism NOS

        Use additional E code to identify drug

    244.8 Other specified acquired hypothyroidism

        Secondary hypothyroidism NEC

        AHA: J-A, '85, 9

---

§ Requires fifth digit. Valid digits are in [brackets] under each code. See category 242 for codes and definitions.

✓4ʰ / ✓5ʰ Additional Digit Required   Unspecified Code   Other Specified Code   Manifestation Code   ►◄ Revised Text   ● New Code   ▲ Revised Code Title

2013 ICD-9-CM   **Volume 1 – 51**

244.9 Unspecified hypothyroidism

Hypothyroidism⎫
Myxedema   ⎬ primary or NOS
            ⎭

AHA: 3Q, '99, 19; 4Q, '96, 29

E03.9 Hypothyroidism unspecified   I-10

245 Thyroiditis

245.0 Acute thyroiditis

Abscess of thyroid
Thyroiditis:
nonsuppurative, acute
pyogenic
suppurative

Use additional code to identify organism

DEF: Inflamed thyroid caused by infection, with abscess and liquid puris.

245.1 Subacute thyroiditis

Thyroiditis: Thyroiditis:
de Quervain's   granulomatous
giant cell   viral

DEF: Inflammation of the thyroid, characterized by fever and painful enlargement of the thyroid gland, with granulomas in the gland.

245.2 Chronic lymphocytic thyroiditis

Hashimoto's disease   Thyroiditis:
Struma lymphomatosa   autoimmune
                       lymphocytic (chronic)

DEF: Autoimmune disease of thyroid; lymphocytes infiltrate the gland and thyroid antibodies are produced; women more often affected.

245.3 Chronic fibrous thyroiditis

Struma fibrosa
Thyroiditis:
invasive (fibrous)
ligneous
Riedel's

DEF: Persistent fibrosing inflammation of thyroid with adhesions to nearby structures; rare condition

245.4 Iatrogenic thyroiditis

Use additional code to identify cause

DEF: Thyroiditis resulting from treatment or intervention by physician or in a patient intervention setting.

245.8 Other and unspecified chronic thyroiditis

Chronic thyroiditis: Chronicthyroiditis:
NOS   nonspecific

245.9 Thyroiditis, unspecified

Thyroiditis NOS

246 Other disorders of thyroid

246.0 Disorders of thyrocalcitonin secretion

Hypersecretion of calcitonin or thyrocalcitonin

246.1 Dyshormonogenic goiter

Congenital (dyshormonogenic) goiter
Goiter due to enzyme defect in synthesis of thyroid hormone
Goitrous cretinism (sporadic)

246.2 Cyst of thyroid

EXCLUDES cystadenoma of thyroid (226)

246.3 Hemorrhage and infarction of thyroid

246.8 Other specified disorders of thyroid

Abnormality of thyroid-binding globulin
Atrophy of thyroid
Hyper-TBG-nemia
Hypo-TBG-nemia

AHA: 2Q, '06, 5

246.9 Unspecified disorder of thyroid

E07.9 Disorder of thyroid unspecified   I-10

Diseases of Other Endocrine Glands (249-259)

249 Secondary diabetes mellitus

INCLUDES diabetes mellitus (due to) (in) (secondary) (with):
drug-induced or chemical induced infection

Use additional code to identify any associated insulin use (V58.67)

EXCLUDES gestational diabetes (648.8)
hyperglycemia NOS (790.29)
neonatal diabetes mellitus (775.1)
nonclinical diabetes (790.29)
Type I diabetes — see category 250
Type II diabetes — see category 250

The following fifth-digit subclassification is for use with category 249:
0 not stated as uncontrolled, or unspecified
1 uncontrolled

AHA: 4Q, '08, 91-95

TIP: If the secondary DM is due to pancreatectomy, code first 251.3 Postsurgical hypoinsulinemia; also assign a code from category 249 and any manifestations, and code V88.1x Acquired absence of pancreas.

§ 249.0 Secondary diabetes mellitus without mention
[0-1] of complication

Secondary diabetes mellitus without mention of complication or manifestation classifiable to 249.1-249.9
Secondary diabetes mellitus NOS

E09.9 Drug/chemical induced diabetes mellitus w/o comp   I-10

§ 249.1 Secondary diabetes mellitus with ketoacidosis
[0-1]

Secondary diabetes mellitus with diabetic acidosis without mention of coma
Secondary diabetes mellitus with diabetic ketosis without mention of coma

§ 249.2 Secondary diabetes mellitus with hyperosmolarity
[0-1]

Secondary diabetes mellitus with hyperosmolar (nonketotic) coma

§ 249.3 Secondary diabetes mellitus with other coma
[0-1]

Secondary diabetes mellitus with diabetic coma (with ketoacidosis)
Secondary diabetes mellitus with diabetic hypoglycemic coma
Secondary diabetes mellitus with insulin coma NOS

EXCLUDES secondary diabetes mellitus with hyperosmolar coma (249.2)

§ 249.4 Secondary diabetes mellitus with renal manifestations
[0-1]

Use additional code to identify manifestation, as:
chronic kidney disease (585.1-585.9)
diabetic nephropathy NOS (583.81)
diabetic nephrosis (581.81)
intercapillary glomerulosclerosis (581.81)
Kimmelstiel-Wilson syndrome (581.81)

§ 249.5 Secondary diabetes mellitus with ophthalmic
[0-1] manifestations

Use additional code to identify manifestation, as:
diabetic blindness (369.00-369.9)
diabetic cataract (366.41)
diabetic glaucoma (365.44)
diabetic macular edema (362.07)
diabetic retinal edema (362.07)
diabetic retinopathy (362.01-362.07)

§ 249.6 Secondary diabetes mellitus with neurological
[0-1] manifestations

Use additional code to identify manifestation, as:
diabetic amyotrophy (353.5)
diabetic gastroparalysis (536.3)
diabetic gastroparesis (536.3)
diabetic mononeuropathy (354.0-355.9)
diabetic neurogenic arthropathy (713.5)
diabetic peripheral autonomic neuropathy (337.1)
diabetic polyneuropathy (357.2)

AHA: For code 249.60: 4Q, '08, 94

§ 249.7 Secondary diabetes mellitus with peripheral
[0-1] circulatory disorders

Use additional code to identify manifestation, as:
diabetic gangrene (785.4)
diabetic peripheral angiopathy (443.81)

---

§ Requires fifth digit. Valid digits are in [brackets] under each code. See category 249 for codes and definitions.

N Newborn Age: 0   P Pediatric Age: 0-17   M Maternity Age: 12-55   A Adult Age: 15-124

Endocrine, Nutritional and Metabolic Diseases, and Immunity   249.8–251.0

§ ✓5ᵗʰ **249.8 Secondary diabetes mellitus with other specified**
[0-1] **manifestations**

     Secondary diabetic hypoglycemia in diabetes mellitus
     Secondary hypoglycemic shock in diabetes mellitus

     Use additional code to identify manifestation, as:
       any associated ulceration (707.10-707.19, 707.8, 707.9)
       diabetic bone changes (731.8)

§ ✓5ᵗʰ **249.9 Secondary diabetes mellitus with unspecified**
[0-1] **complication**

✓4ᵗʰ **250 Diabetes mellitus**

     EXCLUDES *gestational diabetes (648.8)*
             hyperglycemia NOS (790.29)
             neonatal diabetes mellitus (775.1)
             nonclinical diabetes (790.29)
             secondary diabetes (249.0-249.9)

     The following fifth-digit subclassification is for use with category 250:
     0 type II or unspecified type, not state as uncontrolled
       Fifth-digit 0 is for use for type II patients, even if the patient
         requires insulin
       Use additional code, if applicable, for associated long-term
         (current) insulin use V58.67
     1 type I [juvenile type], not stated as uncontrolled
     2 type II or unspecified type, uncontrolled
       Fifth-digit 2 is for use for type II patients, even if the patient
         requires insulin
       Use additional code, if applicable, for associated long-term
         (current) insulin use V58.67
     3 type I [juvenile type], uncontrolled

DEF: Diabetes mellitus: Inability to metabolize carbohydrates, proteins, and fats due to insufficient secretion of insulin. Symptoms may be unremarkable, with long-term complications, involving kidneys, nerves, blood vessels, and eyes.
DEF: Uncontrolled diabetes: A nonspecific term indicating that the current treatment regimen does not keep the blood sugar level of a patient within acceptable levels.
AHA: 1Q, '11, 9; 4Q, '04, 56; 2Q, '04, 17; 2Q, '02, 13; 2Q,'01, 16; 2Q,'98, 15; 4Q, '97, 32; 2Q, '97, 14; 3Q, '96, 5; 4Q, '93, 19; 2Q, '92, 5; 3Q, '91, 3; 2Q, '90, 22; N-D, '85, 11
TIP: Use of insulin does not ensure type I DM; if patient is on routine insulin, assign also V58.67 Long-term (current) use of insulin.

§ ✓5ᵗʰ **250.0 Diabetes mellitus without mention of complication**
[0-3]   Diabetes mellitus without mention of complication or
            manifestation classifiable to 250.1-250.9
     Diabetes (mellitus) NOS
     AHA: 1Q, '06, 14; 4Q, '97, 32; 3Q, '91, 3, 12; N-D, '85, 11; **For code 250.00:** 4Q, '09, 77; 1Q, '05, 15; 4Q, '04, 55; 4Q, '03, 105, 108; 2Q, '03, 16; 1Q, '02, 7, 11; **For code 250.01:** 4Q, '04, 55; 4Q, '03, 110; 2Q, '03, 6; **For code 250.02:** 1Q, '03, 5
     E11.9 Type 2 diabetes mellitus w/o comp   I-10

§ ✓5ᵗʰ **250.1 Diabetes with ketoacidosis**
[0-3]   Diabetic:
       acidosis   } without mention of coma
       ketosis
     DEF: Diabetic hyperglycemic crisis causing ketone presence in body fluids.
     AHA: 3Q, '91, 6; **For code 250.11:** 4Q, '03, 82; **For code 250.13:** 2Q, '06, 19-20
     E10.10 Type 1 diabetes mellitus w/ketoacidosis w/o coma   I-10

§ ✓5ᵗʰ **250.2 Diabetes with hyperosmolarity**
[0-3]   Hyperosmolar (nonketotic) coma
     AHA: 4Q, '93, 19; 3Q, '91, 7

§ ✓5ᵗʰ **250.3 Diabetes with other coma**
[0-3]   Diabetic coma (with ketoacidosis)
     Diabetic hypoglycemic coma
     Insulin coma NOS
     EXCLUDES *diabetes with hyperosmolar coma (250.2)*
     DEF: Coma (not hyperosmolar) caused by hyperglycemia or hypoglycemia as complication of diabetes.
     AHA: 3Q, '91, 7, 12

§ ✓5ᵗʰ **250.4 Diabetes with renal manifestations**
[0-3]   Use additional code to identify manifestation, as:
     chronic kidney disease (585.1-585.9)
     diabetic:
       nephropathy NOS (583.81)
       nephrosis (581.81)
     intercapillary glomerulosclerosis (581.81)
     Kimmelstiel-Wilson syndrome (581.81)
     AHA: 3Q, '91, 8, 12; S-O, '87, 9; S-O, '84, 3; **For code 250.40:** 1Q, '03, 20
     E11.22 Type 2 diabetes mellitus w/diabetic CKD   I-10

§ ✓5ᵗʰ **250.5 Diabetes with ophthalmic manifestations**
[0-3]   Use additional code to identify manifestation, as:
     diabetic:
       blindness (369.00-369.9)
       cataract (366.41)
       glaucoma (365.44)
       macular edema (362.07)
       retinal edema (362.07)
       retinopathy (362.01-362.07)
     AHA: 4Q, '05, 65; 3Q, '91, 8; S-O, '85, 11; **For code 250.50:** 4Q, '05, 67
     E10.36 Type 1 diabetes mellitus with diabetic cataract   I-10

§ ✓5ᵗʰ **250.6 Diabetes with neurological manifestations**
[0-3]   Use additional code to identify manifestation, as:
     diabetic:
       amyotrophy (353.5)
       gastroparalysis (536.3)
       gastroparesis (536.3)
       mononeuropathy (354.0-355.9)
       neurogenic arthropathy (713.5)
       peripheral autonomic neuropathy (337.1)
       polyneuropathy (357.2)
     AHA: 4Q, '09, 151; 2Q, '09, 13, 15; 3Q, '08, 5; 2Q, '93, 6; 2Q, '92, 15; 3Q, '91, 9; N-D, '84, 9; **For code 250.60:** 4Q, '03, 105; **For code 250.61:** 2Q, '04, 7
     E11.40 Type 2 diabetes mellitus w/diab neuropathy   I-10

§ ✓5ᵗʰ **250.7 Diabetes with peripheral circulatory disorders**
[0-3]   Use additional code to identify manifestation, as:
     diabetic:
       gangrene (785.4)
       peripheral angiopathy (443.81)
     DEF: Blood vessel damage or disease, usually in the feet, legs, or hands, as a complication of diabetes.
     AHA: 1Q, '96, 10; 3Q, '94, 5; 2Q, '94, 17; 3Q, '91, 10, 12; 3Q, '90, 15; **For code 250.70:** 1Q, '04, 14
     E10.51 Type 1 DM w/diab periph angiopathy w/o gangrene   I-10

§ ✓5ᵗʰ **250.8 Diabetes with other specified manifestations**
[0-3]   Diabetic hypoglycemia NOS
     Hypoglycemic shock NOS

     Use additional code to identify manifestation, as:
       any associated ulceration (707.10-707.19, 707.8, 707.9)
       diabetic bone changes (731.8)
     AHA: 4Q, '00, 44; 4Q, '97, 43; 2Q, '97, 16; 4Q, '93, 20; 3Q, '91, 10; **For code 250.80:** 1Q, '04, 14
     TIP: Assign for diabetic osteomyelitis, along with code 731.8 and the appropriate code from category 730.
     E11.618 Type 2 DM with other diabetic arthropathy   I-10

§ ✓5ᵗʰ **250.9 Diabetes with unspecified complication**
[0-3]   **AHA:** 2Q, '92, 15; 3Q, '91, 7, 12
     TIP: Do not assign with any other code in category 250.
     E10.8 Type 1 diabetes mellitus with unspecified comp   I-10

✓4ᵗʰ **251 Other disorders of pancreatic internal secretion**

     251.0 Hypoglycemic coma
     Iatrogenic hyperinsulinism
     Non-diabetic insulin coma

     Use additional E code to identify cause, if drug-induced
     EXCLUDES *hypoglycemic coma in diabetes mellitus (249.3, 250.3)*
     DEF: Coma induced by low blood sugar in non-diabetic patient.
     AHA: M-A, '85, 8

---

§   Requires fifth digit. Valid digits are in [brackets] under each code. See appropriate category for codes and definitions.

✓4ᵗʰ ✓5ᵗʰ Additional Digit Required	Unspecified Code	Other Specified Code	Manifestation Code	►◄ Revised Text	● New Code	▲ Revised Code Title

Endocrine, Nutritional and Metabolic Diseases, and Immunity

251.1–253.4

251.1 Other specified hypoglycemia

Hyperinsulinism: Hyperplasia of pancreatic
  NOS   islet beta cells NOS
  ectopic
  functional

Use additional E code to identify cause, if drug-induced

EXCLUDES *hypoglycemia:*
in diabetes mellitus (249.8, 250.8)
in infant of diabetic mother (775.0)
hypoglycemic coma (251.0)
neonatal hypoglycemia (775.6)

DEF: Excessive production of insulin by the pancreas; associated with obesity and insulin-producing tumors.
AHA: 1Q, '03, 10

251.2 Hypoglycemia, unspecified

Hypoglycemia: Hypoglycemia:
  NOS   spontaneous
  reactive

EXCLUDES *hypoglycemia:*
with coma (251.0)
in diabetes mellitus (249.8, 250.8)
leucine-induced (270.3)

AHA: M-A, '85, 8
E16.2 Hypoglycemia unspecified   I-10

251.3 Postsurgical hypoinsulinemia

Hypoinsulinemia following complete or partial pancreatectomy
Postpancreatectomy hyperglycemia

Use additional code to identify (any associated):
  acquired absence of pancreas (V88.11-V88.12)
  insulin use (V58.67)
  secondary diabetes mellitus (249.00-249.91)

EXCLUDES *transient hyperglycemia post procedure (790.29)*
transient hypoglycemia post procedure (251.2)

AHA: 3Q, '91, 6

251.4 Abnormality of secretion of glucagon

Hyperplasia of pancreatic islet alpha cells with glucagon excess

DEF: Production malfunction of a pancreatic hormone secreted by cells of the islets of Langerhans.

251.5 Abnormality of secretion of gastrin

Hyperplasia of pancreatic alpha cells with gastrin excess
Zollinger-Ellison syndrome

251.8 Other specified disorders of pancreatic internal secretion

AHA: 2Q, '98, 15; 3Q, '91, 6
E16.8 Oth spec d/o of pancreatic internal secretion   I-10

251.9 Unspecified disorder of pancreatic internal secretion

Islet cell hyperplasia NOS

✓4ᵗʰ 252 Disorders of parathyroid gland

EXCLUDES *hungry bone syndrome (275.5)*

✓5ᵗʰ 252.0 Hyperparathyroidism

EXCLUDES *ectopic hyperparathyroidism (259.3)*

DEF: Abnormally high secretion of parathyroid hormones causing bone deterioration, reduced renal function, kidney stones.

252.00 Hyperparathyroidism, unspecified

E21.3 Hyperparathyroidism unspecified   I-10

Dorsal View of Parathyroid Glands

Pharynx

Thyroid gland

Parathyroid glands

Trachea

Esophagus

Parathyroid glands
↓
Parathyroid hormone (PTH)
↓
Calcium in bones ⟶ Calcium in blood

252.01 Primary hyperparathyroidism

Hyperplasia of parathyroid

DEF: Parathyroid dysfunction commonly caused by hyperplasia of two or more glands; characteristic hypercalcemia and increased parathyroid hormone levels.

252.02 Secondary hyperparathyroidism, non-renal

EXCLUDES *secondary hyperparathyroidism (of renal origin) (588.81)*

DEF: Underlying disease of nonrenal origin decreases blood levels of calcium causing the parathyroid to release increased levels of parathyroid hormone; parathyroid hormone levels return to normal once underlying condition is treated and blood calcium levels are normal.
AHA: 4Q, '04, 57-59

252.08 Other hyperparathyroidism

Tertiary hyperparathyroidism

DEF: Tertiary hyperparathyroidism: chronic secondary hyperparathyroidism with adenomatous parathyroid causing irreversible abnormal production of parathyroid hormone (PTH); PTH remains high after the serum calcium levels are brought under control.

252.1 Hypoparathyroidism

Parathyroiditis (autoimmune)
Tetany:
  parathyroid
  parathyroprival

EXCLUDES *pseudohypoparathyroidism (275.4)*
pseudopseudohypoparathyroidism (275.4)
tetany NOS (781.7)
transitory neonatal hypoparathyroidism (775.4)

DEF: Abnormally low secretion of parathyroid hormones which causes decreased calcium and increased phosphorus in the blood, resulting in muscle cramps, tetany, urinary frequency and cataracts.

252.8 Other specified disorders of parathyroid gland

Cyst   } of parathyroid
Hemorrhage

252.9 Unspecified disorder of parathyroid gland

✓4ᵗʰ 253 Disorders of the pituitary gland and its hypothalamic control

INCLUDES the listed conditions whether the disorder is in the pituitary or the hypothalamus

EXCLUDES *Cushing's syndrome (255.0)*

253.0 Acromegaly and gigantism

Overproduction of growth hormone

DEF: Acromegaly: chronic, middle age condition; caused by hypersecretion of the pituitary growth hormone; enlarged parts of skeleton, especially the nose, ears, jaws, fingers and toes.
DEF: Gigantism: pituitary gigantism caused by excess growth of short flat bones; men may grow 78 to 80 inches tall.

253.1 Other and unspecified anterior pituitary hyperfunction

Forbes-Albright syndrome

EXCLUDES *overproduction of:*
ACTH (255.3)
thyroid-stimulating hormone [TSH] (242.8)

DEF: Spontaneous galactorrhea-amenorrhea syndrome unrelated to pregnancy; usually related to presence of pituitary tumor.
AHA: J-A, '85, 9

253.2 Panhypopituitarism

Cachexia, pituitary   Sheehan's syndrome
Necrosis of pituitary (postpartum)   Simmonds' disease
Pituitary insufficiency NOS

EXCLUDES *iatrogenic hypopituitarism (253.7)*

DEF: Damage to or absence of pituitary gland leading to impaired sexual function, weight loss, fatigue, bradycardia, hypotension, pallor, depression, and impaired growth in children; called Simmonds' disease if cachexia is prominent.

253.3 Pituitary dwarfism

Isolated deficiency of (human) growth hormone [HGH]
Lorain-Levi dwarfism

DEF: Dwarfism with infantile physical characteristics due to abnormally low secretion of growth hormone and gonadotropin deficiency.

253.4 Other anterior pituitary disorders

Isolated or partial deficiency of an anterior pituitary hormone, other than growth hormone
Prolactin deficiency

AHA: J-A, '85, 9

N Newborn Age: 0   P Pediatric Age: 0-17   M Maternity Age: 12-55   A Adult Age: 15-124

253.5 Diabetes insipidus
Vasopressin deficiency
EXCLUDES *nephrogenic diabetes insipidus (588.1)*
DEF: Metabolic disorder causing insufficient antidiuretic hormone release; symptoms include frequent urination, thirst, ravenous hunger, loss of weight, fatigue.

253.6 Other disorders of neurohypophysis
Syndrome of inappropriate secretion of antidiuretic hormone [ADH]
EXCLUDES *ectopic antidiuretic hormone secretion (259.3)*
E22.2 Synd inappropriate secrectn antidiuretic hormone   I-10

253.7 Iatrogenic pituitary disorders
Hypopituitarism:
hormone-induced
hypophysectomy-induced
postablative
radiotherapy-induced
Use additional E code to identify cause
DEF: Pituitary dysfunction that results from drug therapy, radiation therapy, or surgery, causing mild to severe symptoms.

253.8 Other disorders of the pituitary and other syndromes of diencephalohypophyseal origin
Abscess of pituitary   Cyst of Rathke's pouch
Adiposogenital dystrophy   Fröhlich's syndrome
EXCLUDES *craniopharyngioma (237.0)*

253.9 Unspecified
Dyspituitarism

✓4ᵗʰ 254 Diseases of thymus gland
EXCLUDES *aplasia or dysplasia with immunodeficiency (279.2)*
hypoplasia with immunodeficiency (279.2)
myasthenia gravis (358.00-358.01)

254.0 Persistent hyperplasia of thymus
Hypertrophy of thymus
DEF: Continued abnormal growth of the twin lymphoid lobes that produce T lymphocytes.

254.1 Abscess of thymus

254.8 Other specified diseases of thymus gland
Astrophy ⎫
Cyst   ⎬ of thymus
EXCLUDES *thymoma (212.6)*

254.9 Unspecified disease of thymus gland

✓4ᵗʰ 255 Disorders of adrenal glands
INCLUDES the listed conditions whether the basic disorder is in the adrenals or is pituitary-induced

255.0 Cushing's syndrome
Adrenal hyperplasia due to excess ACTH
Cushing's syndrome:
NOS
iatrogenic
idiopathic
pituitary-dependent
Ectopic ACTH syndrome
Iatrogenic syndrome of excess cortisol
Overproduction of cortisol
Use additional E code to identify cause, if drug-induced
EXCLUDES *congenital adrenal hyperplasia (255.2)*
DEF: Due to adrenal cortisol oversecretion or glucocorticoid medications; may cause excess fatty tissue of the face, neck and body; osteoporosis and curvature of spine, hypertension, diabetes mellitus, female genitourinary problems, male impotence, degeneration of muscle tissues, weakness.

✓5ᵗʰ 255.1 Hyperaldosteronism
DEF: Oversecretion of aldosterone causing fluid retention, hypertension.
AHA: 4Q, '03, 48

255.10 Hyperaldosteronism, unspecified
Aldosteronism NOS
Primary aldosteronism, unspecified
EXCLUDES *Conn's syndrome (255.12)*

255.11 Glucocorticoid-remediable aldosteronism
Familial aldosteronism type I
EXCLUDES *Conn's syndrome (255.12)*
DEF: Rare autosomal dominant familial form of primary aldosteronism in which the secretion of aldosterone is under the influence of adrenocortiotrophic hormone (ACTH) rather than the renin-angiotensin mechanism; moderate hypersecretion of aldosterone and suppressed plasma renin activity rapidly reversed by administration of glucosteroids; symptoms include hypertension and mild hypokalemia.

255.12 Conn's syndrome
DEF: A type of primary aldosteronism caused by an adenoma of the glomerulosa cells in the adrenal cortex; presence of hypertension.

255.13 Bartter's syndrome
DEF: A cluster of symptoms caused by a defect in the ability of the kidney to reabsorb potassium; signs include alkalosis (hypokalemic alkalosis), increased aldosterone, increased plasma renin, and normal blood pressure; symptoms include muscle cramping, weakness, constipation, frequency of urination, and failure to grow; also known as urinary potassium wasting or juxtaglomerular cell hyperplasia.

255.14 Other secondary aldosteronism
AHA: 3Q, '06, 24

255.2 Adrenogenital disorders
Achard-Thiers syndrome
Adrenogenital syndromes, virilizing or feminizing, whether acquired or associated with congenital adrenal hyperplasia consequent on inborn enzyme defects in hormone synthesis
Congenital adrenal hyperplasia
Female adrenal pseudohermaphroditism
Male:
macrogenitosomia praecox
sexual precocity with adrenal hyperplasia
Virilization (female) (suprarenal)
EXCLUDES *adrenal hyperplasia due to excess ACTH (255.0)*
isosexual virilization (256.4)

255.3 Other corticoadrenal overactivity
Acquired benign adrenal androgenic overactivity
Overproduction of ACTH

✓5ᵗʰ 255.4 Corticoadrenal insufficiency
EXCLUDES *tuberculous Addison's disease (017.6)*
DEF: Underproduction of adrenal hormones causing low blood pressure.
AHA: 4Q, '07, 68; 3Q, '06, 24

255.41 Glucocorticoid deficiency
Addisonian crisis
Addison's disease NOS
Adrenal atrophy (autoimmune)
Adrenal calcification
Adrenal crisis
Adrenal hemorrhage
Adrenal infarction
Adrenal insufficiency NOS
Combined glucocorticoid and mineralocorticoid deficiency
Corticoadrenal insufficiency NOS
DEF: Decreased function of the adrenal cortex resulting in insufficient production of glucocorticoid, the hormone regulating carbohydrate, fat, and protein metabolism; manifestations: hyponatremia, hyperpigmentation, orthostatic hypotension, anemia, loss of appetite, and malaise.
AHA: 4Q, '07, 68, 69
E27.1 Primary adrenocortical insufficiency   I-10

255.42 Mineralocorticoid deficiency
Hypoaldosteronism
EXCLUDES *combined glucocorticoid and mineralocorticoid deficiency (255.41)*
DEF: Decreased function of the adrenal cortex resulting in insufficient production of mineralocorticoid, which regulates electrolyte and water balance; manifestations: hyponatremia, hyperkalemia, and mild acidosis.

Endocrine, Nutritional and Metabolic Diseases, and Immunity

255.5–259.8

255.5 Other adrenal hypofunction
Adrenal medullary insufficiency

EXCLUDES *Waterhouse-Friderichsen syndrome (meningococcal) (036.3)*

255.6 Medulloadrenal hyperfunction
Catecholamine secretion by pheochromocytoma

255.8 Other specified disorders of adrenal glands
Abnormality of cortisol-binding globulin

255.9 Unspecified disorder of adrenal glands

√4th 256 Ovarian dysfunction
AHA: 4Q, '00, 51

256.0 Hyperestrogenism ♀
DEF: Excess secretion of estrogen by the ovaries; characterized by ovaries containing multiple follicular cysts filled with serous fluid.

256.1 Other ovarian hyperfunction ♀
Hypersecretion of ovarian androgens
AHA: 3Q, '95, 15

256.2 Postablative ovarian failure ♀
Ovarian failure:
  iatrogenic
  postirradiation
  postsurgical

Use additional code for states associated with artificial menopause (627.4)

EXCLUDES *acquired absence of ovary (V45.77)*
asymptomatic age-related (natural) postmenopausal status (V49.81)

DEF: Failed ovarian function after medical or surgical intervention.
AHA: 2Q, '02, 12

√5th 256.3 Other ovarian failure
Use additional code for states associated with natural menopause (627.2)

EXCLUDES *asymptomatic age-related (natural) postmenopausal status (V49.81)*

AHA: 4Q, '01, 41

256.31 Premature menopause Ⓐ♀
DEF: Permanent cessation of ovarian function before the age of 40 occuring naturally of unknown cause.

256.39 Other ovarian failure ♀
Delayed menarche
Ovarian hypofunction
Primary ovarian failure NOS

256.4 Polycystic ovaries ♀
Isosexual virilization
Stein-Leventhal syndrome
DEF: Multiple serous filled cysts of ovary; symptoms of infertility, hirsutism, oligomenorrhea or amenorrhea.
E28.2 Polycystic ovarian syndrome Ⓘ-10

256.8 Other ovarian dysfunction ♀

256.9 Unspecified ovarian dysfunction ♀

√4th 257 Testicular dysfunction

257.0 Testicular hyperfunction ♂
Hypersecretion of testicular hormones

257.1 Postablative testicular hypofunction ♂
Testicular hypofunction:
  iatrogenic
  postirradiation
  postsurgical

257.2 Other testicular hypofunction
Defective biosynthesis of testicular androgen
Eunuchoidism:
  NOS
  hypogonadotropic
Failure:
  Leydig's cell, adult
  seminiferous tubule, adult
Testicular hypogonadism
EXCLUDES *azoospermia (606.0)*

257.8 Other testicular dysfunction
EXCLUDES *androgen insensitivity syndromes (259.50-259.52)*

257.9 Unspecified testicular dysfunction ♂

√4th 258 Polyglandular dysfunction and related disorders

√5th 258.0 Polyglandular activity in multiple endocrine adenomatosis
Multiple endocrine neoplasia [MEN] syndromes

Use additional codes to identify any malignancies and other conditions associated with the syndromes
AHA: 4Q, '09, 150; 4Q, '07, 70

258.01 Multiple endocrine neoplasia [MEN] type I
Wermer's syndrome
DEF: Wermer's syndrome: A rare hereditary condition characterized by the presence of adenomas or hyperplasia in more than one endocrine gland causing premature aging.
AHA: 4Q, '08, 86, 89; 4Q, '07, 70, 72

258.02 Multiple endocrine neoplasia [MEN] type IIA
Sipple's syndrome
DEF: Sipple's syndrome: A hereditary disorder caused by a defect in the RET gene causing overactivity of the thyroid, adrenal, and parathyroid glands, resulting in adrenal pheochromocytoma and thyroid medullary carcinoma.

258.03 Multiple endocrine neoplasia [MEN] type IIB

258.1 Other combinations of endocrine dysfunction
Lloyd's syndrome
Schmidt's syndrome

258.8 Other specified polyglandular dysfunction

258.9 Polyglandular dysfunction, unspecified

√4th 259 Other endocrine disorders

259.0 Delay in sexual development and puberty, not elsewhere classified
Delayed puberty

259.1 Precocious sexual development and puberty, not elsewhere classified Ⓟ
Sexual precocity: Sexual precocity:
  NOS   cryptogenic
  constitutional   idiopathic

259.2 Carcinoid syndrome
Hormone secretion by carcinoid tumors
DEF: Presence of carcinoid tumors that spread to liver; characterized by cyanotic flushing of skin, diarrhea, bronchospasm, acquired tricuspid and pulmonary stenosis, sudden drops in blood pressure, edema, ascites.
AHA: 4Q, '08, 85-86, 89

259.3 Ectopic hormone secretion, not elsewhere classified
Ectopic:
  antidiuretic hormone secretion [ADH]
  hyperparathyroidism
EXCLUDES *ectopic ACTH syndrome (255.0)*
AHA: N-D, '85, 4

259.4 Dwarfism, not elsewhere classified
Dwarfism: Dwarfism:
  NOS   constitutional
EXCLUDES *dwarfism:*
achondroplastic (756.4)
intrauterine (759.7)
nutritional (263.2)
pituitary (253.3)
renal (588.0)
progeria (259.8)

√5th 259.5 Androgen insensitivity syndrome
DEF: X chromosome abnormality that prohibits the body from recognizing androgen; XY genotype with ambiguous genitalia.
AHA: 4Q, '08, 95-96; 4Q, '05, 53

259.50 Androgen insensitivity, unspecified

259.51 Androgen insensitivity syndrome
Complete androgen insensitivity
de Quervain's syndrome
Goldberg-Maxwell Syndrome

259.52 Partial androgen insensitivity
Partial androgen insensitivity syndrome
Reifenstein syndrome

259.8 Other specified endocrine disorders
Pineal gland dysfunction   Werner's syndrome
Progeria

Ⓝ Newborn Age: 0   Ⓟ Pediatric Age: 0-17   Ⓜ Maternity Age: 12-55   Ⓐ Adult Age: 15-124

259.9 Unspecified endocrine disorder
Disturbance:
   endocrine NOS
   hormone NOS
   Infantilism NOS

Nutritional Deficiencies (260-269)

EXCLUDES *deficiency anemias (280.0-281.9)*

TIP: Assign first a code for the underlying condition (e.g., anorexia nervosa) if specified.

260 Kwashiorkor
Nutritional edema with dyspigmentation of skin and hair

DEF: Syndrome, particulary of children; excessive carbohydrate with inadequate protein intake, inhibited growth potential, anomalies in skin and hair pigmentation, edema and liver disease.

AHA: 3Q, '09, 6

TIP: Do not assign when documentation indicates "mild or moderate protein malnutrition" only. Kwashiorkor is a rare severe protein deficiency.

E40 Kwashiorkor   `I-10`

261 Nutritional marasmus
Nutritional atrophy   Severe malnutrition NOS
Severe calorie deficiency

DEF: Protein-calorie malabsorption or malnutrition in children; characterized by tissue wasting, dehydration, and subcutaneous fat depletion; may occur with infectious disease; also called infantile atrophy.

AHA: 4Q, '07, 97; 3Q, '06, 14; 2Q, '06, 12

E41 Nutritional marasmus   `I-10`

262 Other severe, protein-calorie malnutrition
Nutritional edema without mention of dyspigmentation of skin and hair

AHA: 4Q, '92, 24; J-A, '85, 12

✓4ᵗʰ 263 Other and unspecified protein-calorie malnutrition
AHA: 4Q, '92, 24

   263.0 Malnutrition of moderate degree
     DEF: Malnutrition characterized by biochemical changes in electrolytes, lipids, blood plasma.
     AHA: 3Q, '09, 6; J-A, '85, 1

   263.1 Malnutrition of mild degree
     AHA: J-A, '85, 1

   263.2 Arrested development following protein-calorie malnutrition
     Nutritional dwarfism
     Physical retardation due to malnutrition

   263.8 Other protein-calorie malnutrition

   263.9 Unspecified protein-calorie malnutrition
     Dystrophy due to malnutrition
     Malnutrition (calorie) NOS
     EXCLUDES *nutritional deficiency NOS (269.9)*
     AHA: 4Q, '03, 109; N-D, '84, 19
     E46 Unspecified protein-calorie malnutrition   `I-10`

✓4ᵗʰ 264 Vitamin A deficiency

   264.0 With conjunctival xerosis
     DEF: Vitamin A deficiency with conjunctival dryness.

   264.1 With conjunctival xerosis and Bitot's spot
     Bitot's spot in the young child
     DEF: Vitamin A deficiency with conjunctival dryness, superficial spots of keratinized epithelium.

   264.2 With corneal xerosis
     DEF: Vitamin A deficiency with corneal dryness.

   264.3 With corneal ulceration and xerosis
     DEF: Vitamin A deficiency with corneal dryness, epithelial ulceration.

   264.4 With keratomalacia
     DEF: Vitamin A deficiency creating corneal dryness; progresses to corneal insensitivity, softness, necrosis; usually bilateral.

   264.5 With night blindness
     DEF: Vitamin A deficiency causing vision failure in dim light.

   264.6 With xerophthalmic scars of cornea
     DEF: Vitamin A deficiency with corneal scars from dryness.

   264.7 Other ocular manifestations of vitamin A deficiency
     Xerophthalmia due to vitamin A deficiency

   264.8 Other manifestations of vitamin A deficiency
     Follicular keratosis   } due to vitamin A deficiency
     Xeroderma

   264.9 Unspecified vitamin A deficiency
     Hypovitaminosis A NOS

✓4ᵗʰ 265 Thiamine and niacin deficiency states

   265.0 Beriberi
     DEF: Inadequate vitamin B_1 (thiamine) intake, affects heart and peripheral nerves; individual may become edematous and develop cardiac disease due to the excess fluid; affects alcoholics and people with a diet of excessive polished rice.

   265.1 Other and unspecified manifestations of thiamine deficiency
     Other vitamin B_1 deficiency states

   265.2 Pellagra
     Deficiency:
       niacin (-tryptophan)
       nicotinamide
       nicotinic acid
       vitamin PP
     Pellagra (alcoholic)
     DEF: Niacin deficiency causing dermatitis, inflammation of mucous membranes, diarrhea, and psychic disturbances.

✓4ᵗʰ 266 Deficiency of B-complex components

   266.0 Ariboflavinosis
     Riboflavin [vitamin B_2] deficiency
     DEF: Vitamin B_2 (riboflavin) deficiency marked by swollen lips and tongue fissures, corneal vascularization, scaling lesions, and anemia.
     AHA: S-O, '86, 10

   266.1 Vitamin B_6 deficiency
     Deficiency:
       pyridoxal
       pyridoxamine
       pyridoxine
     Vitamin B_6 deficiency syndrome
     EXCLUDES *vitamin B_6-responsive sideroblastic anemia (285.0)*
     DEF: Vitamin B_6 deficiency causing skin, lip, and tongue disturbances, peripheral neuropathy; and convulsions in infants.

   266.2 Other B-complex deficiencies
     Deficiency:
       cyanocobalamin
       folic acid
       vitamin B_{12}
     EXCLUDES *combined system disease with anemia (281.0-281.1)*
          deficiency anemias (281.0-281.9)
          subacute degeneration of spinal cord with anemia (281.0-281.1)
     E53.8 Deficiency of other specified B group vitamins   `I-10`

   266.9 Unspecified vitamin B deficiency

267 Ascorbic acid deficiency
Deficiency of vitamin C
Scurvy
EXCLUDES *scorbutic anemia (281.8)*
DEF: Vitamin C deficiency causing swollen gums, myalgia, weight loss, and weakness.

✓4ᵗʰ 268 Vitamin D deficiency
EXCLUDES *vitamin D-resistant:*
        osteomalacia (275.3)
        rickets (275.3)

   268.0 Rickets, active
     EXCLUDES *celiac rickets (579.0)*
          renal rickets (588.0)
     DEF: Inadequate vitamin D intake, usually in pediatrics, that affects bones most involved with muscular action; may cause nodules on ends and sides of bones; delayed closure of fontanels in infants; symptoms may include muscle soreness, and profuse sweating.

   268.1 Rickets, late effect
     Any condition specified as due to rickets and stated to be a late effect or sequela of rickets
     Code first the nature of late effect
     DEF: Distorted or demineralized bones as a result of vitamin D deficiency.

✓4ᵗʰ **✓5ᵗʰ** Additional Digit Required   Unspecified Code   Other Specified Code   Manifestation Code   ►◄ Revised Text   ● New Code   ▲ Revised Code Title

268.2 Osteomalacia, unspecified
DEF: Softening of bones due to decrease in calcium; marked by pain, tenderness, muscular weakness, anorexia, and weight loss.

268.9 Unspecified vitamin D deficiency
Avitaminosis D

✔4ᵗʰ 269 Other nutritional deficiencies

269.0 Deficiency of vitamin K
EXCLUDES deficiency of coagulation factor due to vitamin K deficiency (286.7)
vitamin K deficiency of newborn (776.0)

269.1 Deficiency of other vitamins
Deficiency:
  vitamin E
  vitamin P

269.2 Unspecified vitamin deficiency
Multiple vitamin deficiency NOS

269.3 Mineral deficiency, not elsewhere classified
Deficiency:
  calcium, dietary
  iodine
EXCLUDES deficiency:
  calcium NOS (275.4)
  potassium (276.8)
  sodium (276.1)

269.8 Other nutritional deficiency
EXCLUDES adult failure to thrive (783.7)
failure to thrive in childhood (783.41)
feeding problems (783.3)
newborn (779.31-779.34)

269.9 Unspecified nutritional deficiency

Other Metabolic and Immunity Disorders (270-279)
Use additional code to identify any associated intellectual disabilities

✔4ᵗʰ 270 Disorders of amino-acid transport and metabolism
EXCLUDES abnormal findings without manifest disease (790.0-796.9)
disorders of purine and pyrimidine metabolism (277.1-277.2)
gout (274.00-274.9)

270.0 Disturbances of amino-acid transport
Cystinosis
Cystinuria
Fanconi (-de Toni) (-Debré) syndrome
Glycinuria (renal)
Hartnup disease

270.1 Phenylketonuria [PKU]
Hyperphenylalaninemia
DEF: Inherited metabolic condition causing excess phenylpyruvic and other acids in urine; results in mental retardation, neurological manifestations, including spasticity and tremors, light pigmentation, eczema, and mousy odor.

270.2 Other disturbances of aromatic amino-acid metabolism
Albinism
Alkaptonuria
Alkaptonuric ochronosis
Disturbances of metabolism of tyrosine and tryptophan
Homogentisic acid defects
Hydroxykynureninuria
Hypertyrosinemia
Indicanuria
Kynureninase defects
Oasthouse urine disease
Ochronosis
Tyrosinosis
Tyrosinuria
Waardenburg syndrome
EXCLUDES vitamin B₆-deficiency syndrome (266.1)
AHA: 3Q, '99, 20

270.3 Disturbances of branched-chain amino-acid metabolism
Disturbances of metabolism of leucine, isoleucine, and valine
Hypervalinemia
Intermittent branched-chain ketonuria
Leucine-induced hypoglycemia
Leucinosis
Maple syrup urine disease
AHA: 3Q, '00, 8

270.4 Disturbances of sulphur-bearing amino-acid metabolism
Cystathioninemia
Cystathioninuria
Disturbances of metabolism of methionine, homocystine, and cystathionine
Homocystinuria
Hypermethioninemia
Methioninemia
AHA: 2Q, '07, 7;1Q, '04, 6

270.5 Disturbances of histidine metabolism
Carnosinemia
Histidinemia
Hyperhistidinemia
Imidazole aminoaciduria

270.6 Disorders of urea cycle metabolism
Argininosuccinic aciduria
Citrullinemia
Disorders of metabolism of ornithine, citrulline, argininosuccinic acid, arginine, and ammonia
Hyperammonemia
Hyperomithinemia

270.7 Other disturbances of straight-chain amino-acid metabolism
Glucoglycinuria
Glycinemia (with methyl-malonic acidemia)
Hyperglycinemia
Hyperlysinemia
Other disturbances of metabolism of glycine, threonine, serine, glutamine, and lysine
Pipecolic acidemia
Saccharopinuria
AHA: 3Q, '00, 8

270.8 Other specified disorders of amino-acid metabolism
Alaninemia	Iminoacidopathy
Ethanolaminuria	Prolinemia
Glycoprolinuria	Prolinuria
Hydroxyprolinemia	Sarcosinemia
Hyperprolinemia	

270.9 Unspecified disorder of amino-acid metabolism

✔4ᵗʰ 271 Disorders of carbohydrate transport and metabolism
EXCLUDES abnormality of secretion of glucagon (251.4)
diabetes mellitus (249.0-249.9, 250.0-250.9)
hypoglycemia NOS (251.2)
mucopolysaccharidosis (277.5)

271.0 Glycogenosis
Amylopectinosis
Glucose-6-phosphatase deficiency
Glycogen storage disease
McArdle's disease
Pompe's disease
von Gierke's disease
DEF: Excess glycogen storage; rare inherited trait affects liver, kidneys; causes various symptoms depending on type, though often weakness and muscle cramps.
AHA: 1Q, '98, 5

271.1 Galactosemia
Galactose-1-phosphate uridyl transferase deficiency
Galactosuria
DEF: Any of three genetic disorders due to defective galactose metabolism; symptoms include failure to thrive in infancy, jaundice, liver and spleen damage, cataracts, and mental retardation.

271.2 Hereditary fructose intolerance
Essential benign fructosuria
Fructosemia
DEF: Chromosome recessive disorder of carbohydrate metabolism; in infants, occurs after dietary sugar introduced; characterized by enlarged spleen, yellowish cast to skin, and progressive inability to thrive.

271.3 Intestinal disaccharidase deficiencies and disaccharide malabsorption
Intolerance or malabsorption (congenital) (of):
  glucose-galactose
  lactose
  sucrose-isomaltose
E73.9 Lactose intolerance unspecified [I-10]

| Ⓝ Newborn Age: 0 | Ⓟ Pediatric Age: 0-17 | Ⓜ Maternity Age: 12-55 | Ⓐ Adult Age: 15-124 |

271.4 Renal glycosuria

Renal diabetes

DEF: Persistent abnormal levels of glucose in urine, with normal blood glucose levels; caused by failure of the renal tubules to reabsorb glucose.

271.8 Other specified disorders of carbohydrate transport and metabolism

Essential benign pentosuria	Mannosidosis
Fucosidosis	Oxalosis
Glycolic aciduria	Xylosuria
Hyperoxaluria (primary)	Xylulosuria

271.9 Unspecified disorder of carbohydrate transport and metabolism

✓4ᵗʰ 272 Disorders of lipoid metabolism

    EXCLUDES *localized cerebral lipidoses (330.1)*

272.0 Pure hypercholesterolemia

Familial hypercholesterolemia
Fredrickson Type IIa hyperlipoproteinemia
Hyperbetalipoproteinemia
Hyperlipidemia, Group A
Low-density-lipoid-type [LDL] hyperlipoproteinemia

AHA: 4Q, '05, 71

E78.0 Pure hypercholesterolemia   **I-10**

272.1 Pure hyperglyceridemia

Endogenous hyperglyceridemia
Fredrickson Type IV hyperlipoproteinemia
Hyperlipidemia, Group B
Hyperprebetalipoproteinemia
Hypertriglyceridemia, essential
Very-low-density-lipoid-type [VLDL] hyperlipoproteinemia

272.2 Mixed hyperlipidemia

Broad- or floating-betalipoproteinemia
Combined hyperlipidemia
Elevated cholesterol with elevated triglycerides NEC
Fredrickson Type IIb or III hyperlipoproteinemia
Hypercholesterolemia with endogenous hyperglyceridemia
Hyperbetalipoproteinemia with prebetalipoproteinemia
Tubo-eruptive xanthoma
Xanthoma tuberosum

DEF: Elevated levels of lipoprotein, a complex of fats and proteins, in blood due to inherited metabolic disorder.

272.3 Hyperchylomicronemia

Bürger-Grütz syndrome
Fredrickson type I or V hyperlipoproteinemia
Hyperlipidemia, Group D
Mixed hyperglyceridemia

272.4 Other and unspecified hyperlipidemia

Alpha-lipoproteinemia	Hyperlipoproteinemia NOS
Hyperlipidemia NOS	

DEF: Hyperlipoproteinemia: elevated levels of transient chylomicrons in the blood which are a form of lipoproteins that transport dietary cholesterol and triglycerides from the small intestine to the blood.

AHA: 1Q, '05, 17

E78.4 Other hyperlipidemia   **I-10**

272.5 Lipoprotein deficiencies

Abetalipoproteinemia
Bassen-Kornzweig syndrome
High-density lipoid deficiency
Hypoalphalipoproteinemia
Hypobetalipoproteinemia (familial)

DEF: Abnormally low levels of lipoprotein, a complex of fats and protein, in the blood.

272.6 Lipodystrophy

Barraquer-Simons disease   Progressive lipodystrophy

Use additional E code to identify cause, if iatrogenic

    EXCLUDES *intestinal lipodystrophy (040.2)*

DEF: Disturbance of fat metabolism resulting in loss of fatty tissue in some areas of the body.

Lipid Metabolism

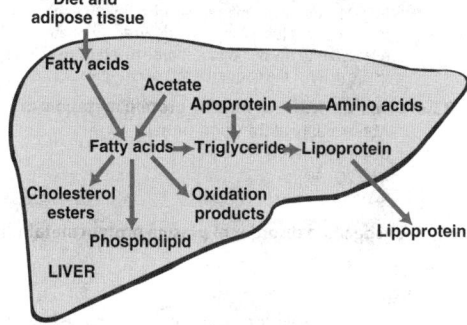

272.7 Lipidoses

Chemically-induced lipidosis
Disease:
    Anderson's
    Fabry's
    Gaucher's
    I cell [mucolipidosis I]
    lipoid storage NOS
    Niemann-Pick
    pseudo-Hurler's or mucolipdosis III
    triglyceride storage, Type I or II
    Wolman's or triglyceride storage, Type III
Mucolipidosis II
Primary familial xanthomatosis

    EXCLUDES *cerebral lipidoses (330.1)*
                Tay-Sachs disease (330.1)

DEF: Lysosomal storage diseases marked by an abnormal amount of lipids in reticuloendothelial cells.

272.8 Other disorders of lipoid metabolism

Hoffa's disease or liposynovitis prepatellaris
Launois-Bensaude's lipomatosis
Lipoid dermatoarthritis

272.9 Unspecified disorder of lipoid metabolism

✓4ᵗʰ 273 Disorders of plasma protein metabolism

    EXCLUDES *agammaglobulinemia and hypogammaglobulinemia*
                    (279.0-279.2)
            coagulation defects (286.0-286.9)
            hereditary hemolytic anemias (282.0-282.9)

273.0 Polyclonal hypergammaglobulinemia

Hypergammaglobulinemic purpura:
    benign primary
    Waldenström's

DEF: Elevated blood levels of gamma globulins, frequently found in patients with chronic infectious diseases.

273.1 Monoclonal paraproteinemia

Benign monoclonal hypergammaglobulinemia [BMH]
Monoclonal gammopathy:
    NOS
    associated with lymphoplasmacytic dyscrasias
    benign
Paraproteinemia:
    benign (familial)
    secondary to malignant or inflammatory disease

273.2 Other paraproteinemias

Cryoglobulinemic:
    purpura
    vasculitis
Mixed cryoglobulinemia

AHA: 2Q, '08, 17

273.3 Macroglobulinemia

Macroglobulinemia (idiopathic) (primary)
Waldenström's macroglobulinemia

DEF: Elevated blood levels of macroglobulins (plasma globulins of high weight); characterized by malignant neoplasms of bone marrow, spleen, liver, or lymph nodes; symptoms include weakness, fatigue, bleeding disorders, and vision problems.

✓4ᵗʰ ✓5ᵗʰ Additional Digit Required   Unspecified Code   Other Specified Code   Manifestation Code   ▶◀ Revised Text   ● New Code   ▲ Revised Code Title

2013 ICD-9-CM   **Volume 1 – 59**

Endocrine, Nutritional and Metabolic Diseases, and Immunity

273.4–276.1

273.4 Alpha-1-antitrypsin deficiency
AAT deficiency

DEF: Disorder of plasma protein metabolism that results in a deficiency of Alpha-1-antitrypsin, an acute-phase reactive protein, released into the blood in response to infection or injury to protect tissue against the harmful effect of enzymes.

273.8 Other disorders of plasma protein metabolism
Abnormality of transport protein
Bisalbuminemia

AHA: 2Q, '98, 11

E88.09 Oth disorders of plasma-protein metablolis NEC   I-10

273.9 Unspecified disorder of plasma protein metabolism

✓4ᵗʰ 274 Gout

EXCLUDES lead gout (984.0-984.9)

DEF: Purine and pyrimidine metabolic disorders; manifested by hyperuricemia and recurrent acute inflammatory arthritis; monosodium urate or monohydrate crystals may be deposited in and around the joints, leading to joint destruction, and severe crippling.

AHA: 2Q, '95, 4

✓5ᵗʰ 274.0 Gouty arthropathy
AHA: 4Q, '09, 76-77

274.00 Gouty arthropathy, unspecified
M10.00 Idiopathic gout unspecified site   I-10

274.01 Acute gouty arthropathy
Acute gout
Gout attack
Gout flare
Podagra

274.02 Chronic gouty arthropathy without mention of tophus (tophi)
Chronic gout

274.03 Chronic gouty arthropathy with tophus (tophi)
Chronic tophaceous gout
Gout with tophi NOS
AHA: 4Q, '09, 77

✓5ᵗʰ 274.1 Gouty nephropathy

274.10 Gouty nephropathy, unspecified
AHA: N-D, '85, 15

274.11 Uric acid nephrolithiasis
DEF: Sodium urate stones in the kidney.

274.19 Other

✓5ᵗʰ 274.8 Gout with other specified manifestations

274.81 Gouty tophi of ear
DEF: Chalky sodium urate deposit in the ear due to gout; produces chronic inflammation of external ear.

274.82 Gouty tophi of other sites
Gouty tophi of heart
EXCLUDES gout with tophi NOS (274.03)
gouty arthropathy with tophi (274.03)

274.89 Other
Use additional code to identify manifestations, as:
gouty:
iritis (364.11)
neuritis (357.4)

274.9 Gout, unspecified
M10.9 Gout unspecified   I-10

✓4ᵗʰ 275 Disorders of mineral metabolism
EXCLUDES abnormal findings without manifest disease (790.0-796.9)

✓5ᵗʰ 275.0 Disorders of iron metabolism
EXCLUDES anemia:
iron deficiency (280.0-280.9)
sideroblastic (285.0)
AHA: 4Q, '10, 77-78; 2Q, '97, 11

275.01 Hereditary hemochromatosis
Bronzed diabetes
Pigmentary cirrhosis (of liver)
Primary (hereditary) hemochromatosis
E83.110 Hereditary hemochromatosis   I-10

275.02 Hemochromatosis due to repeated red blood cell transfusions
Iron overload due to repeated red blood cell transfusions
Transfusion (red blood cell) associated hemochromatosis
AHA: 4Q, '10, 77-78
E83.111 Hemochromatosis due to repeated red blood   I-10
cell transfusions

275.03 Other hemochromatosis
Hemochromatosis NOS
E83.118 Other hemochromatosis   I-10

275.09 Other disorders of iron metabolism
E83.10 Disorder of iron-metabolism unspecified   I-10

275.1 Disorders of copper metabolism
Hepatolenticular degeneration
Wilson's disease

275.2 Disorders of magnesium metabolism
HypermagnesemiaHypomagnesemia
AHA: 1Q, '10, 14; 3Q, '09, 21
E83.40 Disorders of magnesium metabolism unspec   I-10

275.3 Disorders of phosphorus metabolism
Familial hypophosphatemia
Hypophosphatasia
Vitamin D-resistant:
osteomalacia
rickets

✓5ᵗʰ 275.4 Disorders of calcium metabolism
EXCLUDES hungry bone syndrome (275.5)
parathyroid disorders (252.00-252.9)
vitamin D deficiency (268.0-268.9)
AHA: 4Q, '97, 33

275.40 Unspecified disorder of calcium metabolism

275.41 Hypocalcemia
DEF: Abnormally decreased blood calcium level; symptoms include hyperactive deep tendon reflexes, muscle, abdominal cramps, and carpopedal spasm.
AHA: 3Q, '07, 5
E83.51 Hypocalcemia   I-10

275.42 Hypercalcemia
DEF: Abnormally increased blood calcium level; symptoms include muscle weakness, fatigue, nausea, depression, and constipation.
AHA: 4Q, '03, 110

275.49 Other disorders of calcium metabolism
Nephrocalcinosis
Pseudohypoparathyroidism
Pseudopseudohypoparathyroidism
DEF: Nephrocalcinosis: calcium phosphate deposits in the tubules of the kidney with resultant renal insufficiency.
DEF: Pseudohypoparathyroidism: inherited hypoparathyroidismdisorder; caused by inadequate response to parathyroid hormone, not hormonal deficiency; includes muscle cramps, tetany, urinary frequency, blurred vision due to cataracts, and dry scaly skin.
DEF: Pseudopseudohypoparathyroidism: clinical manifestations of hypoparathyroidism without affecting blood calcium levels.

275.5 Hungry bone syndrome
DEF: Marked and prolonged hypocalcemia; usually involves an extended history of elevated levels of parathyroid hormone, related bone demineralization causing the bone to sequester calcium.
AHA: 4Q, 08, 96-97

275.8 Other specified disorders of mineral metabolism

275.9 Unspecified disorder of mineral metabolism

✓4ᵗʰ 276 Disorders of fluid, electrolyte, and acid-base balance
EXCLUDES diabetes insipidus (253.5)
familial periodic paralysis (359.3)

276.0 Hyperosmolality and/or hypernatremia
Sodium [Na] excess
Sodium [Na] overload

276.1 Hyposmolality and/or hyponatremia
Sodium [Na] deficiency
E87.1 Hypo-osmolality and hyponatremia   I-10

N Newborn Age: 0   P Pediatric Age: 0-17   M Maternity Age: 12-55   A Adult Age: 15-124

276.2 Acidosis

Acidosis: Acidosis:
NOS metabolic
lactic respiratory

EXCLUDES *diabetic acidosis (249.1, 250.1)*

DEF: Disorder involves decrease of pH (hydrogen ion) concentration in blood and cellular tissues; caused by increase in acid and decrease in bicarbonate.

AHA: J-F, '87, 15

E87.2 Acidosis I-10

276.3 Alkalosis

Alkalosis: Alkalosis:
NOS respiratory
metabolic

DEF: Increased blood alkalinity (base) without relative loss of base in body fluids; caused by increased arterial plasma bicarbonate concentration or loss of carbon dioxide due to hyperventilation.

276.4 Mixed acid-base balance disorder

Hypercapnia with mixed acid-base disorder

√5ᵗʰ 276.5 Volume depletion

EXCLUDES *hypovolemic shock:*
postoperative (998.09)
traumatic (958.4)

AHA: 4Q, '05, 54; 2Q, '05, 9; 1Q, '03, 5, 22; 3Q, '02, 21; 4Q, '97, 30; 2Q, '88, 9

276.50 Volume depletion, unspecified

DEF: Depletion of total body water (dehydration) and/or contraction of total intravascular plasma (hypovolemia).

E86.9 Volume depletion unspecified I-10

276.51 Dehydration

DEF: Depletion of total body water; blood volume may be normal while fluid is pulled from other tissues.

AHA: 1Q, '08, 10

E86.0 Dehydration I-10

276.52 Hypovolemia

Depletion of volume of plasma

DEF: Depletion of volume plasma; depletion of total blood volume.

√5ᵗʰ 276.6 Fluid overload

EXCLUDES *ascites (789.51-789.59)*
localized edema (782.3)

AHA: 4Q, '10, 79; 3Q, '07, 9; 4Q, '06, 136

276.61 Transfusion associated circulatory overload

Fluid overload due to transfusion (blood) (blood components)

TACO

AHA: 4Q, '10, 79-80

E87.71 Transfusion associated circulatory overload I-10

276.69 Other fluid overload

Fluid retention

E87.79 Other fluid overload I-10

276.7 Hyperpotassemia

Hyperkalemia Potassium [K]:
Potassium [K]: intoxication
excess overload

DEF: Elevated blood levels of potassium; symptoms include abnormal EKG readings, weakness; related to defective renal excretion.

AHA: 2Q, '11, 6; 1Q, '05, 9; 2Q,'01, 12

E87.5 Hyperkalemia I-10

276.8 Hypopotassemia

Hypokalemia Potassium [K] deficiency

DEF: Decreased blood levels of potassium; symptoms include neuromuscular disorders.

E87.6 Hypokalemia I-10

276.9 Electrolyte and fluid disorders not elsewhere classified

Electrolyte imbalance Hypochloremia
Hyperchloremia

EXCLUDES *electrolyte imbalance:*
associated with hyperemesis gravidarum (643.1)
complicating labor and delivery (669.0)
following abortion and ectopic or molar pregnancy (634-638 with .4, 639.4)

AHA: J-F, '87, 15

E87.8 Oth disorders of electrolyte & fluid balance NEC I-10

√4ᵗʰ 277 Other and unspecified disorders of metabolism

√5ᵗʰ 277.0 Cystic fibrosis

Fibrocystic disease of the pancreas
Mucoviscidosis

DEF: Genetic disorder of infants, children, and young adults marked by exocrine gland dysfunction; characterized by chronic pulmonary disease with excess mucus production, pancreatic deficiency, and high levels of electrolytes in the sweat.

AHA: 4Q, '90, 16; 3Q, '90, 18

TIP: Sequencing of CF is determined by circumstances of admission. If a patient is admitted for CF, sequence the CF first. If admitted for a complication of CF (e.g., pneumothorax, acute bronchitis, or acute cor pulmonale), sequence the complication first.

277.00 Without mention of meconium ileus

Cystic fibrosis NOS

AHA: 2Q, '03, 12

E84.9 Cystic fibrosis unspecified I-10

277.01 With meconium ileus N

Meconium:
ileus (of newborn)
obstruction of intestine in mucoviscidosis

277.02 With pulmonary manifestations

Cystic fibrosis with pulmonary exacerbation

Use additional code to identify any infectious organism present, such as:
pseudomonas (041.7)

277.03 With gastrointestinal manifestations

EXCLUDES *with meconium ileus (277.01)*

AHA: 4Q, '02, 45

277.09 With other manifestations

277.1 Disorders of porphyrin metabolism

Hematoporphyria Porphyrinuria
Hematoporphyrinuria Protocoproporphyria
Hereditary coproporphyria Protoporphyria
Porphyria Pyrroloporphyria

277.2 Other disorders of purine and pyrimidine metabolism

Hypoxanthine-guanine-phosphoribosyltransferase deficiency [HG-PRT deficiency]
Lesch-Nyhan syndrome
Xanthinuria

EXCLUDES *gout (274.00-274.9)*
orotic aciduric anemia (281.4)

√5ᵗʰ 277.3 Amyloidosis

DEF: Conditions of diverse etiologies characterized by the accumulation of insoluble fibrillar proteins (amyloid) in various organs and tissues of the body, compromising vital functions.

AHA: 1Q, '96, 16

277.30 Amyloidosis, unspecified

Amyloidosis NOS

AHA: 4Q, '06, 66

277.31 Familial Mediterranean fever

Benign paroxysmal peritonitis
Hereditary amyloid nephropathy
Periodic familial polyserositis
Recurrent polyserositis

DEF: Early-life onset of recurrent attacks characterized by high fevers with pain and inflammation of chest and abdominal cavities, skin and joints, also rash or vasculitis. Etiology unknown, possibly genetic, but may be precipitated by stress, trauma or exertion.

AHA: 4Q, '06, 66

277.39 Other amyloidosis

Hereditary cardiac amyloidosis
Inherited systemic amyloidosis
Neuropathic (Portuguese) (Swiss) amyloidosis
Secondary amyloidosis

AHA: 1Q, '09, 9; 2Q, '08, 8; 4Q, '06, 66

√4ᵗʰ √5ᵗʰ Additional Digit Required Unspecified Code Other Specified Code Manifestation Code ▶◀ Revised Text ● New Code ▲ Revised Code Title

2013 ICD-9-CM **Volume 1 – 61**

Endocrine, Nutritional and Metabolic Diseases, and Immunity

277.4–278.2

277.4 Disorders of bilirubin excretion
Hyperbilirubinemia:
  congenital
  constitutional
Syndrome:
  Crigler-Najjar
  Dubin-Johnson
  Gilbert's
  Rotor's
EXCLUDES *hyperbilirubinemias specific to the perinatal period (774.0-774.7)*

277.5 Mucopolysaccharidosis
Gargoylism
Hunter's syndrome
Hurler's syndrome
Lipochondrodystrophy
Maroteaux-Lamy syndrome
Morquio-Brailsford disease
Osteochondrodystrophy
Sanfilippo's syndrome
Scheie's syndrome
DEF: Metabolic disorders evidenced by excretion of various mucopolysaccharides in urine and infiltration of these substances into connective tissue, with resulting defects of bone, cartilage and connective tissue.

277.6 Other deficiencies of circulating enzymes
Hereditary angioedema
AHA: 2Q, '10, 12

277.7 Dysmetabolic syndrome X
Use additional code for associated manifestation, such as:
  cardiovascular disease (414.00-414.07)
  obesity (278.00-278.03)
DEF: A specific group of metabolic disorders that are related to the state of insulin resistance (decreased cellular response to insulin) without elevated blood sugars; often related to elevated cholesterol and triglycerides, obesity, cardiovascular disease, and high blood pressure.
AHA: 4Q, '01, 42

✓5ᵗʰ 277.8 Other specified disorders of metabolism
AHA: 4Q, '03, 50; 2Q, '01, 18; S-O, '87, 9

277.81 Primary carnitine deficiency

277.82 Carnitine deficiency due to inborn errors of metabolism

277.83 Iatrogenic carnitine deficiency
Carnitine deficiency due to:
  hemodialysis
  valproic acid therapy

277.84 Other secondary carnitine deficiency

277.85 Disorders of fatty acid oxidation
Carnitine palmitoyltransferase deficiencies (CPT1, CPT2)
Glutaric aciduria type II (type IIA, IIB, IIC)
Long chain 3-hydroxyacyl CoA dehydrogenase deficiency (LCHAD)
Long chain/very long chain acyl CoA dehydrogenase deficiency (LCAD, VLCAD)
Medium chain acyl CoA dehydrogenase deficiency (MCAD)
Short chain acyl CoA dehydrogenase deficiency (SCAD)
EXCLUDES *primary carnitine deficiency (277.81)*

277.86 Peroxisomal disorders
Adrenomyeloneuropathy
Neonatal adrenoleukodystrophy
Rhizomelic chrondrodysplasia punctata
X-linked adrenoleukodystrophy
Zellweger syndrome
EXCLUDES *infantile Refsum disease (356.3)*

277.87 Disorders of mitochondrial metabolism
Kearns-Sayre syndrome
Mitochondrial Encephalopathy, Lactic Acidosis and Stroke-like episodes (MELAS syndrome)
Mitochondrial Neurogastrointestinal Encephalopathy syndrome (MNGIE)
Myoclonus with Epilepsy and with Ragged Red Fibers (MERRF syndrome)
Neuropathy, Ataxia and Retinitis Pigmentosa (NARP syndrome)
Use additional code for associated conditions
EXCLUDES *disorders of pyruvate metabolism (271.8)*
  Leber's optic atrophy (377.16)
  Leigh's subacute necrotizing encephalopathy (330.8)
  Reye's syndrome (331.81)
AHA: 4Q, '04, 62

277.88 Tumor lysis syndrome
Spontaneous tumor lysis syndrome
Tumor lysis syndrome following antineoplastic drug therapy
Use additional E code to identify cause, if drug-induced
DEF: A potentially fatal metabolic complication of tumor necrosis caused by either spontaneous or treatment-related accumulation of byproducts from dying cancer cells; symptoms include hyperkalemia, hyperphosphatemia, hypocalcemia, hyperuricemia, and hyperuricosuria.
AHA: 4Q, '09, 78-79

277.89 Other specified disorders of metabolism
Hand-Schüller-Christian disease
Histiocytosis (acute) (chronic)
Histiocytosis X (chronic)
EXCLUDES *histiocytosis:*
  acute differentiated progressive (202.5)
  adultpulmonaryLan
    gerhans cell (516.5)
  X, acute (progressive) (202.5)

277.9 Unspecified disorder of metabolism
Enzymopathy NOS

✓4ᵗʰ 278 Overweight, obesity and other hyperalimentation
EXCLUDES *hyperalimentation NOS (783.6)*
  poisoning by vitamins NOS (963.5)
  polyphagia (783.6)

✓5ᵗʰ 278.0 Overweight and obesity
Use additional code to identify Body Mass Index (BMI), if known (V85.0-V85.54)
EXCLUDES *adiposogenital dystrophy (253.8)*
  obesity of endocrine origin NOS (259.9)
AHA: ►3Q, '11, 4;◄ 4Q, '05, 97

278.00 Obesity, unspecified
Obesity NOS
DEF: BMI (body mass index) between 30.0 and 39.9.
AHA: 4Q, '01, 42; 1Q, '99, 5, 6

278.01 Morbid obesity
Severe obesity
DEF: BMI (body mass index) 40 or greater.
AHA: 4Q, '10, 81; 2Q, '09, 11; 2Q, '06, 5-6; 3Q, '03, 6-8
E66.01 Morbid (severe) obesity due to excess calories `I-10`

278.02 Overweight
DEF: BMI (body mass index) between 25 and 29.9.
AHA: 4Q, '05, 55
E66.3 Overweight `I-10`

278.03 Obesity hypoventilation syndrome
Pickwickian syndrome
DEF: Hypoventilation, somnolence and erythrocytosis due to excessive weight against the chest wall.
AHA: 4Q, '10, 80-81
E66.2 Morbid obesity w/alveolar hyperventilation `I-10`

278.1 Localized adiposity
Fat pad
AHA: 2Q, '06, 10

278.2 Hypervitaminosis A

N Newborn Age: 0   P Pediatric Age: 0-17   M Maternity Age: 12-55   A Adult Age: 15-124

278.3 Hypercarotinemia

DEF: Elevated blood carotene level due to ingesting excess carotenoids or the inability to convert carotenoids to vitamin A.

278.4 Hypervitaminosis D

DEF: Weakness, fatigue, loss of weight, and other symptoms resulting from ingesting excessive amounts of vitamin D.

278.8 Other hyperalimentation

AHA: 2Q, '09, 11

√4ᵗʰ **279 Disorders involving the immune mechanism**

Use additional code for associated manifestations

√5ᵗʰ **279.0 Deficiency of humoral immunity**

DEF: Inadequate immune response to bacterial infections with potential reinfection by viruses due to lack of circulating immunoglobulins (acquired antibodies).

279.00 Hypogammaglobulinemia, unspecified

Agammaglobulinemia NOS

279.01 Selective IgA immunodeficiency

279.02 Selective IgM immunodeficiency

279.03 Other selective immunoglobulin deficiencies

Selective deficiency of IgG

279.04 Congenital hypogammaglobulinemia

Agammaglobulinemia:
Bruton's type
X-linked

279.05 Immunodeficiency with increased IgM

Immunodeficiency with hyper-IgM:
autosomal recessive
X-linked

279.06 Common variable immunodeficiency

Dysgammaglobulinemia (acquired) (congenital) (primary)
Hypogammaglobulinemia:
acquired primary
congenital non-sex-linked
sporadic

279.09 Other

Transient hypogammaglobulinemia of infancy

√5ᵗʰ **279.1 Deficiency of cell-mediated immunity**

279.10 Immunodeficiency with predominant T-cell defect, unspecified

AHA: S-O, '87, 10

279.11 DiGeorge's syndrome

Pharyngeal pouch syndrome
Thymic hypoplasia

DEF: Congenital hypoplasia or aplasia of the thymus, parathyroid glands; related heart defects, anomalies of the great vessels, esophageal atresia, and abnormalities of facial structures.

279.12 Wiskott-Aldrich syndrome

DEF: A disease characterized by chronic conditions, such as eczema, suppurative otitis media and anemia; results from an X-linked recessive gene and is classified as an immune deficiency syndrome.

279.13 Nezelof's syndrome

Cellular immunodeficiency with abnormal immunoglobulin deficiency

DEF: Immune system disorder characterized by a pathological deficiency in cellular immunity and humoral antibodies resulting in inability to fight infectious diseases.

279.19 Other

EXCLUDES ataxia-telangiectasia (334.8)

279.2 Combined immunity deficiency

Agammaglobulinemia:
autosomal recessive
Swiss-type
x-linked recessive
Severe combined immunodeficiency [SCID]
Thymic:
alymphoplasia
aplasia or dysplasia with immunodeficiency

EXCLUDES thymic hypoplasia (279.11)

DEF: Agammaglobulinemia: No immunoglobulins in the blood.
DEF: Thymic alymphoplasia: Severe combined immunodeficiency; result of failed lymphoid tissue development.

AHA: ▶4Q, '11, 148◀

279.3 Unspecified immunity deficiency

√5ᵗʰ **279.4 Autoimmune disease, not elsewhere classified**

EXCLUDES transplant failure or rejection (996.80-996.89)

AHA: 4Q, '09, 80; 3Q, 08, 5

279.41 Autoimmune lymphoproliferative syndrome

ALPS

DEF: Rare genetic alteration of the *Fas* protein; impairs normal cellular apoptosis (normal cell death), causing abnormal accumulation of lymphocytes in the lymph glands, liver, and spleen; symptoms include neutropenia, anemia, and thrombocytopenia.

279.49 Autoimmune disease, not elsewhere classified

Autoimmune disease NOS

AHA: 2Q, '11, 15

√5ᵗʰ **279.5 Graft-versus-host disease**

Code first underlying cause, such as:
complication of blood transfusion (999.89)
complication of transplanted organ (996.80-996.89)

Use additional code to identify associated manifestations, such as:
desquamative dermatitis (695.89)
diarrhea (787.91)
elevated bilirubin (782.4)
hair loss (704.09)

DEF: A complication of transplantation, most commonly bone marrow; may involve skin, GI tract, liver and cause increased susceptibility to infection; results when donor cells responsible for immune response attack the cells of the transplant recipient.

AHA: 4Q, 08, 97-99, 154

279.50 Graft-versus-host disease, unspecified

AHA: 4Q, 08, 99

279.51 Acute graft-versus-host disease

AHA: ▶4Q, '11, 148;◀4Q, 08, 99

279.52 Chronic graft-versus-host disease

279.53 Acute on chronic graft-versus-host disease

279.8 Other specified disorders involving the immune mechanism

Single complement [C_1-C_9] deficiency or dysfunction

279.9 Unspecified disorder of immune mechanism

AHA: 3Q, '92, 13

√4ᵗʰ / √5ᵗʰ Additional Digit Required   Unspecified Code   Other Specified Code   Manifestation Code   ▶◀ Revised Text   ● New Code   ▲ Revised Code Title

4. Diseases of the Blood and Blood-Forming Organs (280-289)

EXCLUDES *anemia complicating pregnancy or the puerperium (648.2)*

✓4ᵗʰ 280 Iron deficiency anemias

INCLUDES anemia:
　　asiderotic
　　hypochromic-microcytic
　　sideropenic

EXCLUDES *familial microcytic anemia (282.49)*

280.0 Secondary to blood loss (chronic)
Normocytic anemia due to blood loss

EXCLUDES *acute posthemorrhagic anemia (285.1)*

AHA: 4Q, '93, 34

280.1 Secondary to inadequate dietary iron intake

280.8 Other specified iron deficiency anemias
Paterson-Kelly syndrome
Plummer-Vinson syndrome
Sideropenic dysphagia

280.9 Iron deficiency anemia, unspecified
Anemia:　　　　　Anemia:
　achlorhydric　　　idiopathic hypochromic
　chlorotic　　　　iron [Fe] deficiency NOS

✓4ᵗʰ 281 Other deficiency anemias

281.0 Pernicious anemia
Anemia:
　Addison's
　Biermer's
　congenital pernicious
Congenital intrinsic factor [Castle's] deficiency

EXCLUDES *combined system disease without mention of anemia (266.2)*
subacute degeneration of spinal cord without mention of anemia (266.2)

DEF: Chronic progressive anemia due to Vitamin B12 malabsorption; caused by lack of a secretion of intrinsic factor, which is produced by the gastric mucosa of the stomach.

AHA: N-D, '84, 1; S-O, '84, 16

281.1 Other vitamin B$_{12}$ deficiency anemia
Anemia:
　vegan's
　vitamin B$_{12}$ deficiency (dietary)
　due to selective vitamin B$_{12}$ malabsorption with proteinuria
Syndrome:
　Imerslund's
　Imerslund-Gräsbeck

EXCLUDES *combined system disease without mention of anemia (266.2)*
subacute degeneration of spinal cord without mention of anemia (266.2)

281.2 Folate-deficiency anemia
Congenital folate malabsorption
Folate or folic acid deficiency anemia:
　NOS
　dietary
　drug-induced
Goat's milk anemia
Nutritional megaloblastic anemia (of infancy)

Use additional E code to identify drug

DEF: Macrocytic anemia resembles pernicious anemia but without absence of hydrochloric acid secretions; responsive to folic acid therapy.

281.3 Other specified megaloblastic anemias not elsewhere classified
Combined B$_{12}$ and folate-deficiency anemia
Refractory megaloblastic anemia

DEF: Megaloblasts predominant in bone marrow with few normoblasts; rare familial type associated with proteinuria and genitourinary tract anomalies.

281.4 Protein-deficiency anemia
Amino-acid-deficiency anemia

281.8 Anemia associated with other specified nutritional deficiency
Scorbutic anemia

281.9 Unspecified deficiency anemia
Anemia:　　　　　Anemia:
　dimorphic　　　　nutritional NOS
　macrocytic　　　　simple chronic
　megaloblastic NOS

✓4ᵗʰ 282 Hereditary hemolytic anemias
DEF: Escalated rate of erythrocyte destruction; similar to all anemias, occurs when imbalance exists between blood loss and blood production.

282.0 Hereditary spherocytosis
Acholuric (familial) jaundice
Congenital hemolytic anemia (spherocytic)
Congenital spherocytosis
Minkowski-Chauffard syndrome
Spherocytosis (familial)

EXCLUDES *hemolytic anemia of newborn (773.0-773.5)*

DEF: Hereditary, chronic illness marked by abnormal red blood cell membrane; symptoms include enlarged spleen, jaundice; and anemia in severe cases.

282.1 Hereditary elliptocytosis
Elliptocytosis (congenital)
Ovalocytosis (congenital) (hereditary)

DEF: Genetic hemolytic anemia characterized by malformed, elliptical erythrocytes; there is increased destruction of red cells with resulting anemia.

282.2 Anemias due to disorders of glutathione metabolism
Anemia:
　6-phosphogluconic dehydrogenase deficiency
　enzyme deficiency, drug-induced
　erythrocytic glutathione deficiency
　glucose-6-phosphate dehydrogenase [G-6-PD] deficiency
　glutathione-reductase deficiency
　hemolytic nonspherocytic (hereditary), type I
Disorder of pentose phosphate pathway
Favism

282.3 Other hemolytic anemias due to enzyme deficiency
Anemia:
　hemolytic nonspherocytic (hereditary), type II
　hexokinase deficiency
　pyruvate kinase [PK] deficiency
　triosephosphate isomerase deficiency

✓5ᵗʰ 282.4 Thalassemias
EXCLUDES *sickle-cell:*
disease (282.60-282.69)
trait (282.5)

DEF: Inherited hemolytic disorders characterized by decreased production of at least one polypeptide globin chain results in defective hemoglobin synthesis; symptoms include severe anemia, expanded marrow spaces, transfusional and absorptive iron overload, impaired growth rate, thickened cranial bones, and pathologic fractures.

AHA: 4Q, '03, 51

282.40 Thalassemia, unspecified
Thalassemia NOS

AHA: ▶4Q, '11, 87-91◀

282.41 Sickle-cell thalassemia without crisis
Microdrepanocytosis
Sickle-cell thalassemia NOS
Thalassemia Hb-S disease without crisis

282.42 Sickle-cell thalassemia with crisis
Sickle-cell thalassemia with vaso-occlusive pain
Thalassemia Hb-S disease with crisis

Use additional code for type of crisis, such as:
　acute chest syndrome (517.3)
　splenic sequestration (289.52)

Diseases of the Blood and Blood-Forming Organs

282.43–282.69

282.43 Alpha thalassemia
Alpha thalassemia major
Hemoglobin H Constant Spring
Hemoglobin H disease
Hydrops fetalis due to alpha thalassemia
Severe alpha thalassemia
Triple gene defect alpha thalassemia

> **EXCLUDES** *alpha thalassemia trait or minor (282.46)*
> *hydrops fetalis due to isoimmunization (773.3)*
> *hydrops fetalis not due to immune hemolysis (778.0)*

DEF: ▶HBA1 and HBA2 genetic variant of chromosome 16 prevalent among Western African and South Asian descent; associated with a wide spectrum of anemic presentation, includes hemoglobin H disease subtypes.◀

AHA: ▶4Q, '11, 87-91◀

282.44 Beta thalassemia
Beta thalassemia major
Cooley's anemia
Homozygous beta thalassemia
Severe beta thalassemia
Thalassemia intermedia
Thalassemia major

> **EXCLUDES** *beta thalassemia minor (282.46)*
> *beta thalassemia trait (282.46)*
> *delta-beta thalassemia (282.45)*
> *hemoglobin E-beta thalassemia (282.47)*
> *sickle-cell beta thalassemia (282.41, 282.42)*

DEF: ▶Diversity of mutations of HBB gene on chromosome 11 prevalent among Mediterranean and certain South Asian descent with significant cellular damage, can result in toxicity and increased disease severity (e.g., severe beta thalassemia, thalassemia major).◀

AHA: ▶4Q, '11, 87-91◀

282.45 Delta-beta thalassemia
Homozygous delta-beta thalassemia

> **EXCLUDES** *delta-beta thalassemia trait (282.46)*

AHA: ▶4Q, '11, 87-91◀

282.46 Thalassemia minor
Alpha thalassemia minor
Alpha thalassemia trait
Alpha thalassemia silent carrier
Beta thalassemia minor
Beta thalassemia trait
Delta-beta thalassemia trait
Thalassemia trait NOS

> **EXCLUDES** *alpha thalassemia (282.43)*
> *beta thalassemia (282.44)*
> *delta-beta thalassemia (282.45)*
> *hemoglobin E-beta thalassemia (282.47)*
> *sickle-cell trait (282.5)*

DEF: ▶Solitary abnormal gene that identifies a carrier of the disease, yet with an absence of symptoms or a clinically mild anemic presentation.◀

AHA: ▶4Q, '11, 87-91◀

282.47 Hemoglobin E-beta thalassemia

> **EXCLUDES** *beta thalassemia (282.44)*
> *beta thalassemia minor (282.46)*
> *beta thalassemia trait (282.46)*
> *delta-beta thalassemia (282.45)*
> *delta-beta thalassemia trait (282.46)*
> *hemoglobin E disease (282.7)*
> *other hemoglobinopathies (282.7)*
> *sickle-cell beta thalassemia (282.41, 282.42)*

DEF: ▶Clinically similar phenotype to B thalassemia major prevalent among Southeast Asian and certain Indian descent; results in severe transfusion-dependent anemia when present with certain B mutations.◀

AHA: ▶4Q, '11, 87-91◀

282.49 Other thalassemia
Dominant thalassemia
Hemoglobin C thalassemia
Hereditary leptocytosis
Mediterranean anemia (with other hemoglobinopathy)
Mixed thalassemia
Thalassemia with other hemoglobinopathy

> **EXCLUDES** *hemoglobin C disease (282.7)*
> *hemoglobin E disease (282.7)*
> *other hemoglobinopathies (282.7)*
> *sickle-cell anemias (282.60-282.69)*
> *sickle-cell beta thalassemia (282.41-282.42)*

282.5 Sickle-cell trait
Hb-AS genotype   Heterozygous:
Hemoglobin S [Hb-S] trait   hemoglobin S
                                     Hb-S

> **EXCLUDES** *that with other hemoglobinopathy (282.60-282.69)*
> *that with thalassemia (282.41-282.42)*

DEF: Heterozygous genetic makeup characterized by one gene for normal hemoglobin and one for sickle-cell hemoglobin; clinical disease rarely present.

TIP: Do not assign along with another code for sickle-cell disease or thalassemia.

✓5ᵗʰ 282.6 Sickle-cell disease
Sickle-cell anemia

> **EXCLUDES** *sickle-cell thalassemia (282.41-282.42)*
> *sickle-cell trait (282.5)*

DEF: Inherited blood disorder; sickle-shaped red blood cells are hard and pointed, clogging blood flow; anemia characterized by periodic episodes of pain, acute abdominal discomfort, skin ulcerations of the legs, increased infections.

282.60 Sickle-cell disease, unspecified
Sickle-cell anemia NOS

AHA: 2Q, '97, 11

282.61 Hb-SS disease without crisis

282.62 Hb-SS disease with crisis
Hb-SS disease with vaso-occlusive pain
Sickle-cell crisis NOS

Use additional code for type of crisis, such as:
     acute chest syndrome (517.3)
     splenic sequestration (289.52)

AHA: 4Q, '10, 78; 4Q, '03, 56; 2Q, '98, 8; 2Q, '91, 15

282.63 Sickle-cell/Hb-C disease without crisis
Hb-S/Hb-C disease without crisis

282.64 Sickle-cell/Hb-C disease with crisis
Hb-S/Hb-C disease with crisis
Sickle-cell/Hb-C disease with vaso-occlusive pain

Use additional code for type of crisis, such as:
     acute chest syndrome (517.3)
     splenic sequestration (289.52)

AHA: 4Q, '03, 51

282.68 Other sickle-cell disease without crisis
Hb-S/Hb-D
Hb-S/Hb-E   } diseases without
Sickle-cell/Hb-D   crisis
Sickle-cell/Hb-E

AHA: 4Q, '03, 51

282.69 Other sickle-cell disease with crisis
Hb-S/Hb-D
Hb-S/Hb-E   } diseases with crisis
Sickle-cell/Hb-D
Sickle-cell/Hb-E

Other sickle-cell disease with vaso-occlusive pain

Use additional code for type of crisis, such as:
     acute chest syndrome (517.3)
     splenic sequestration (289.52)

Ⓝ Newborn Age: 0   Ⓟ Pediatric Age: 0-17   Ⓜ Maternity Age: 12-55   Ⓐ Adult Age: 15-124

282.7 Other hemoglobinopathies
Abnormal hemoglobin NOS
Congenital Heinz-body anemia
Disease:
    hemoglobin C [Hb-C]
    hemoglobin D [Hb-D]
    hemoglobin E [Hb-E]
    hemoglobin Zurich [Hb-Zurich]
Hemoglobinopathy NOS
Hereditary persistence of fetal hemoglobin [HPFH]
Unstable hemoglobin hemolytic disease

> **EXCLUDES** *familial polycythemia (289.6)*
> *hemoglobin E-beta thalassemia (282.47)*
> *hemoglobin M [Hb-M] disease (289.7)*
> *high-oxygen-affinity hemoglobin (289.0)*
> *other hemoglobinopathies with thalassemia (282.49)*

DEF: Any disorder of hemoglobin due to alteration of molecular structure; may include overt anemia.

282.8 Other specified hereditary hemolytic anemias
Stomatocytosis

282.9 Hereditary hemolytic anemia, unspecified
Hereditary hemolytic anemia NOS

√4ᵗʰ 283 Acquired hemolytic anemias
DEF: Non-hereditary anemia characterized by premature destruction of red blood cells; caused by infectious organisms, poisons, and physical agents.
AHA: N-D, '84, 1

283.0 Autoimmune hemolytic anemias
Autoimmune hemolytic disease (cold type) (warm type)
Chronic cold hemagglutinin disease
Cold agglutinin disease or hemoglobinuria
Hemolytic anemia:
    cold type (secondary) (symptomatic)
    drug-induced
    warm type (secondary) (symptomatic)
Use additional E code to identify cause, if drug-induced

> **EXCLUDES** *Evans' syndrome (287.32)*
> *hemolytic disease of newborn (773.0-773.5)*

AHA: 3Q, '08, 5

√5ᵗʰ 283.1 Non-autoimmune hemolytic anemias
Use additional E code to identify cause
DEF: Hemolytic anemia and thrombocytopenia with acute renal failure; relatively rare condition; 50 percent of patients require renal dialysis.
AHA: 4Q, '93, 25

283.10 Non-autoimmune hemolytic anemia, unspecified

283.11 Hemolytic-uremic syndrome
Use additional code to identify associated:
    E. coli infection (041.41-041.49)
    Pneumococcal pnemonia (481)
    Shigella dysenteriae (004.0)

283.19 Other non-autoimmune hemolytic anemias
Hemolytic anemia:
    mechanical
    microangiopathic
    toxic

283.2 Hemoglobinuria due to hemolysis from external causes
Acute intravascular hemolysis
Hemoglobinuria:
    from exertion
    march
    paroxysmal (cold) (nocturnal)
    due to other hemolysis
Marchiafava-Micheli syndrome
Use additional E code to identify cause

283.9 Acquired hemolytic anemia, unspecified
Acquired hemolytic anemia NOS
Chronic idiopathic hemolytic anemia

√4ᵗʰ 284 Aplastic anemia and other bone marrow failure syndromes
DEF: Bone marrow failure to produce the normal amount of blood components; generally non-responsive to usual therapy.
AHA: 1Q, '91, 14; N-D, '84, 1; S-0, '84, 16

√5ᵗʰ 284.0 Constitutional aplastic anemia
AHA: 1Q, '91, 14

284.01 Constitutional red blood cell aplasia
Aplasia, (pure) red cell:
    congenital
    of infants
    primary
Blackfan-Diamond syndrome
Familial hypoplastic anemia
AHA: 4Q, '06, 67-69

284.09 Other constitutional aplastic anemia
Fanconi's anemia
Pancytopenia with malformations
AHA: 4Q, '06, 67-69

√5ᵗʰ 284.1 Pancytopenia

> **EXCLUDES** *pancytopenia (due to) (with):*
> *aplastic anemia NOS (284.9)*
> *bone marrow infiltration (284.2)*
> *constitutional red blood cell aplasia (284.01)*
> *hairy cell leukemia (202.4)*
> *human immunodeficiency virus disease (042)*
> *leukoerythroblastic anemia (284.2)*
> *malformations (284.09)*
> *myelodysplastic syndromes (238.72-238.75)*
> *myeloproliferative disease (238.79)*
> *other constitutional aplastic anemia (284.09)*

AHA: ▶4Q, '11, 91-92;◀4Q, '06, 67-69

284.11 Antineoplastic chemotherapy induced pancytopenia

> **EXCLUDES** *aplastic anemia due to antineoplastic chemotherapy (284.89)*

AHA: ▶4Q, '11, 92◀

284.12 Other drug-induced pancytopenia
> **EXCLUDES** *aplastic anemia due to drugs (284.89)*

284.19 Other pancytopenia

284.2 Myelophthisis
Leukoerythroblastic anemia
Myelophthisic anemia

Code first the underlying disorder, such as:
    malignant neoplasm of breast (174.0-174.9, 175.0-175.9)
    tuberculosis (015.0-015.9)

> **EXCLUDES** *idiopathic myelofibrosis (238.76)*
> *myelofibrosis NOS (289.83)*
> *myelofibrosis with myeloid metaplasia (238.76)*
> *primary myelofibrosis (238.76)*
> *secondary myelofibrosis (289.83)*

DEF: A secondary disease process involving replacement of normal hematopoeitic tissue in the bone marrow with abnormal tissue, such as fibrous tissue or tumors. Occurs with advanced-stage neoplasms, granulomatous diseases such as miliary tuberculosis, and other inflammatory diseases.
AHA: 4Q, '06, 67-69

√5ᵗʰ 284.8 Other specified aplastic anemias
AHA: 4Q, '07, 72; 3Q, '05, 11; 1Q, '97, 5; 1Q, '92, 15; 1Q, '91, 14

284.81 Red cell aplasia (acquired) (adult) (with thymoma)
Red cell aplasia NOS

284.89 Other specified aplastic anemias
Aplastic anemia (due to):
    chronic systemic disease
    drugs
    infection
    radiation
    toxic (paralytic)
Use additional E code to identify cause
AHA: 1Q, '11, 6; 1Q, '09, 20; 2Q, '08, 6

284.9 Aplastic anemia, unspecified
Anemia:
    aplastic (idiopathic) NOS   Anemia:
    aregenerative   nonregenerative
    hypoplastic NOS   Medullary hypoplasia

> **EXCLUDES** *refractory anemia (238.72)*

Diseases of the Blood and Blood-Forming Organs

285–286.3

✓4th **285　Other and unspecified anemias**
　AHA: 1Q, '91, 14; N-D, '84, 1

285.0　Sideroblastic anemia
　Anemia:
　　hypochromic with iron loading
　　sideroachrestic
　　sideroblastic:
　　　acquired
　　　congenital
　　　hereditary
　　　primary
　　　secondary (drug-induced) (due to disease)
　　　sex-linked hypochromic
　　　vitamin B6-responsive
　Pyridoxine-responsive (hypochromic) anemia

　Use additional E code to identify cause, if drug induced

　EXCLUDES　refractory sideroblastic anemia (238.72)

　DEF: Characterized by a disruption of final heme synthesis; results in
　iron overload of reticuloendothelial tissues.

285.1　Acute posthemorrhagic anemia
　Anemia due to acute blood loss

　EXCLUDES　anemia due to chronic blood loss (280.0)
　　　　　　blood loss anemia NOS (280.0)

　AHA: ▶4Q, '11, 146;◀ 1Q. '07, 19; 2Q, '92, 15

✓4th **285.2　Anemia of chronic disease**
　Anemia in (due to) (with) chronic illness
　AHA: 4Q, '00, 39

285.21　Anemia in chronic kidney disease
　Anemia in end stage renal disease
　Erythropoietin-resistant anemia (EPO resistant
　anemia)

　TIP: Assign also a code for the chronic kidney disease
　(585.X).

285.22　Anemia in neoplastic disease

　EXCLUDES　anemia due to antineoplastic chemotherapy
　　　　　　(285.3)
　　　　　　aplastic anemia due to antineoplastic
　　　　　　chemotherapy (284.89)

　AHA: 4Q, '09, 81

　TIP: Assign also a code for the neoplasm causing the
　anemia. Do not assign if anemia is caused by
　chemotherapy drugs, which is instead reported with 285.3.
　D63.0 Anemia in neoplastic disease　　　　　I-10

285.29　Anemia of other chronic disease
　Anemia in other chronic illness

285.3　Antineoplastic chemotherapy induced anemia
　Anemia due to antineoplastic chemotherapy

　EXCLUDES　anemia due to drug NEC — code to type of anemia
　　　　　　anemia in neoplastic disease (285.22)
　　　　　　aplastic anemia due to antineoplastic chemotherapy
　　　　　　(284.89)

　DEF: Reversible adverse effect of chemotherapy, causing inhibition
　of bone marrow production; decrease in red blood cell production
　prevents adequate oxygenation of the tissues and organs causing
　fatigue, SOB, and exacerbation of other medical conditions.

　AHA: 4Q, '09, 80-82

285.8　Other specified anemias
　Anemia:
　　dyserythropoietic (congenital)
　　dyshematopoietic (congenital)
　　von Jaksch's
　Infantile pseudoleukemia
　AHA: 1Q, '91, 16

285.9　Anemia, unspecified
　Anemia:　　　　　　　　　Anemia:
　　NOS　　　　　　　　　　　profound
　　essential　　　　　　　　progressive
　　normocytic, not due　　　secondary
　　　to blood loss　　　　　Oligocythemia

　EXCLUDES　anemia (due to):
　　　　　　blood loss:
　　　　　　　acute (285.1)
　　　　　　　chronic or unspecified (280.0)
　　　　　　iron deficiency (280.0-280.9)

　AHA: 1Q, '11, 16; 1Q, '09, 17, 20; 1Q. '07, 19; 1Q, '02, 14; 2Q, '92, 16;
　M-A, '85, 13; N-D, '84, 1

　TIP: Assign for "postoperative anemia" if there is no mention of blood
　loss.

✓4th **286　Coagulation defects**
　AHA: 2Q, '06, 17

286.0　Congenital factor VIII disorder
　Antihemophilic globulin [AHG] deficiency
　Factor VIII (functional) deficiency
　Hemophilia:
　　NOS
　　A
　　classical
　　familial
　　hereditary
　Subhemophilia

　EXCLUDES　factor VIII deficiency with vascular defect (286.4)

　DEF: Hereditary, sex-linked, results in missing antihemophilic
　globulin (AHG) (factor VIII); causes abnormal coagulation
　characterized by increased bleeding, large bruises of skin, bleeding
　in mouth, nose, gastrointestinal tract; hemorrhages into joints,
　resulting in swelling and impaired function.

286.1　Congenital factor IX disorder
　Christmas disease
　Deficiency:
　　factor IX (functional)
　　plasma thromboplastin component [PTC]
　Hemophilia B

　DEF: Deficiency of plasma thromboplastin component (PTC) (factor
　IX) and plasma thromboplastin antecedent (PTA); PTC deficiency
　clinically indistinguishable from classical hemophilia.

286.2　Congenital factor XI deficiency
　Hemophilia C
　Plasma thromboplastin antecedent [PTA] deficiency
　Rosenthal's disease

286.3　Congenital deficiency of other clotting factors
　Congenital afibrinogenemia
　Deficiency:
　　AC globulin factor:
　　　I [fibrinogen]
　　　II [prothrombin]
　　　V [labile]
　　　VII [stable]
　　　X [Stuart-Prower]
　　　XII [Hageman]
　　　XIII [fibrin stabilizing]
　　Laki-Lorand factor
　　proaccelerin
　Disease:
　　Owren's
　　Stuart-Prower
　Dysfibrinogenemia (congenital)
　Dysprothrombinemia (constitutional)
　Hypoproconvertinemia
　Hypoprothrombinemia (hereditary)
　Parahemophilia

286.4 von Willebrand's disease
Angiohemophilia (A) (B)
Constitutional thrombopathy
Factor VIII deficiency with vascular defect
Pseudohemophilia type B
Vascular hemophilia
von Willebrand's (-Jürgens') disease
EXCLUDES factor VIII deficiency:
NOS (286.0)
with functional defect (286.0)
hereditary capillary fragility (287.8)
DEF: Abnormal blood coagulation caused by deficient blood Factor VII; congenital; symptoms include excess or prolonged bleeding.

√5ᵗʰ **286.5 Hemorrhagic disorder due to intrinsic circulating anticoagulants, antibodies, or inhibitors**
AHA: 4Q, '11, 93-95; 3Q, '04, 7; No.5, '93, 16; 3Q, '92, 15; 3Q, '90, 14
TIP: Do not assign a code from subcategory 286.5 for Coumadin/warfarin toxicity, poisoning or adverse effect. Follow coding guidelines for poisoning and adverse reactions.

286.52 Acquired hemophilia
Autoimmune hemophilia
Autoimmune inhibitors to clotting factors
Secondary hemophilia

286.53 Antiphospholipid antibody with hemorrhagic disorder
Lupus anticoagulant [LAC] with hemorrhagic disorder
Systemic lupus erythematosus [SLE] inhibitor with hemorrhagic disorder
EXCLUDES anti-phospholipid antibody, finding without diagnosis (795.79)
anti-phospholipid antibody syndrome (289.81)
anti-phospholipid antibody with hypercoagulable state (289.81)
lupus anticoagulant [LAC] finding without diagnosis (795.79)
lupus anticoagulant [LAC] with hypercoagulable state (289.81)
systemic lupus erythematosus [SLE] inhibitor finding without diagnosis (795.79)
systemic lupus erythematosus [SLE] inhibitor with hypercoagulable state (289.81)
TIP: ▶When a resulting associated hypercoagulable state is present, assign code 289.81.◀

286.59 Other hemorrhagic disorder due to intrinsic circulating anticoagulants, antibodies, or inhibitors
Antithrombinemia
Antithromboplastinemia
Antithromboplastinogenemia
Increase in:
anti-II (prothrombin)
anti-VIIIa
anti-IXa
anti-XIa

286.6 Defibrination syndrome
Afibrinogenemia, acquired
Consumption coagulopathy
Diffuse or disseminated intravascular coagulation [DIC syndrome]
Fibrinolytic hemorrhage, acquired
Hemorrhagic fibrinogenolysis
Pathologic fibrinolysis
Purpura:
fibrinolytic
fulminans
EXCLUDES that complicating:
abortion (634-638 with .1, 639.1)
pregnancy or the puerperium (641.3, 666.3)
disseminated intravascular coagulation in newborn (776.2)
DEF: Characterized by destruction of circulating fibrinogen; often precipitated by other conditions, such as injury, causing release of thromboplastic particles in blood stream.
AHA: 4Q, '93, 29

286.7 Acquired coagulation factor deficiency
Deficiency of coagulation factor due to:
liver disease
vitamin K deficiency
Hypoprothrombinemia, acquired
Use additional E code to identify cause, if drug induced
EXCLUDES vitamin K deficiency of newborn (776.0)
AHA: 4Q, '93, 29

286.9 Other and unspecified coagulation defects
Defective coagulation NOS   Disorder:
Deficiency, coagulation factor   coagulation
NOS   hemostasis
Delay, coagulation
EXCLUDES abnormal coagulation profile (790.92)
hemorrhagic disease of newborn (776.0)
that complicating:
abortion (634-638 with .1, 639.1)
pregnancy or the puerperium (641.3, 666.3)
AHA: 4Q, '99, 22; 4Q, '93, 29

√4ᵗʰ **287 Purpura and other hemorrhagic conditions**
EXCLUDES hemorrhagic thrombocythemia (238.79)
purpura fulminans (286.6)
AHA: 1Q, '91, 14

287.0 Allergic purpura
Peliosis rheumatica   Purpura:
Purpura: rheumatica
anaphylactoid   Schönlein-Henoch
autoimmune   vascular
Henoch's   Vasculitis, allergic
nonthrombocytopenic:
hemorrhagic
idiopathic
EXCLUDES hemorrhagic purpura (287.39)
purpura annularis telangiectodes (709.1)
DEF: Any hemorrhagic condition, thrombocytic or nonthrombocytopenic in origin, caused by a presumed allergic reaction.

287.1 Qualitative platelet defects
Thrombasthenia (hemorrhagic) (hereditary)
Thrombocytasthenia
Thrombocytopathy (dystrophic)
Thrombopathy (Bernard-Soulier)
EXCLUDES von Willebrand's disease (286.4)

287.2 Other nonthrombocytopenic purpuras
Purpura: Purpura:
NOS   simplex
senile

√5ᵗʰ **287.3 Primary thrombocytopenia**
EXCLUDES thrombotic thrombocytopenic purpura (446.6)
transient thrombocytopenia of newborn (776.1)
DEF: Decrease in number of blood platelets in circulating blood and purpural skin hemorrhages.
AHA: 4Q, '05, 56

287.30 Primary thrombocytopenia, unspecified
Megakaryocytic hypoplasia

287.31 Immune thrombocytopenic purpura
Idiopathic thrombocytopenic purpura
Tidal platelet dysgenesis
DEF: Tidal platelet dysgenesis: Platelet counts fluctuate from normal to very low within periods of 20 to 40 days and may involve autoimmune platelet destruction.
AHA: 4Q, '05, 57

287.32 Evans' syndrome
DEF: Combination of immunohemolytic anemia and autoimmune hemolytic anemia, sometimes with neutropenia.

287.33 Congenital and hereditary thrombocytopenic purpura
Congenital and hereditary thrombocytopenia
Thrombocytopenia with absent radii (TAR) syndrome
EXCLUDES *Wiskott-Aldrich syndrome (279.12)*
DEF: Thrombocytopenia with absent radii (TAR) syndrome: autosomal recessive syndrome characterized by thrombocytopenia and bilateral radial aplasia; manifestations include skeletal, gastrointestinal, hematologic, and cardiac system abnormalities.

287.39 Other primary thrombocytopenia

✓5ᵗʰ **287.4 Secondary thrombocytopenia**
Use additional E code to identify cause
EXCLUDES *heparin-induced thrombocytopenia (HIT) (289.84)*
transient thrombocytopenia of newborn (776.1)
AHA: 4Q, '10, 81-82; M-A, '85, 14

287.41 Posttransfusion purpura
Posttransfusion purpura from whole blood (fresh) or blood products
PTP
DEF: A potentially fatal transfusion complication characterized by sudden onset of severe thrombocytopenia, fever, chills, and cutaneous hemorrhaging.

287.49 Other secondary thrombocytopenia
Thrombocytopenia (due to):
dilutional
drugs
extracorporeal circulation of blood
massive blood transfusion
platelet alloimmunization
secondary NOS
DEF: Reduced number of platelets in circulating blood as consequence of an underlying disease or condition.

287.5 Thrombocytopenia, unspecified

287.8 Other specified hemorrhagic conditions
Capillary fragility (hereditary)
Vascular pseudohemophilia

287.9 Unspecified hemorrhagic conditions
Hemorrhagic diathesis (familial)

✓4ᵗʰ **288 Diseases of white blood cells**
EXCLUDES *leukemia (204.0-208.9)*
AHA: 4Q, '06, 69; 1Q, '91, 14

✓5ᵗʰ **288.0 Neutropenia**
Decreased absolute neutrophil count [ANC]
Use additional code for any associated:
fever (780.61)
mucositis (478.11, 528.00-528.09, 538, 616.81)
EXCLUDES *neutropenic splenomegaly (289.53)*
transitory neonatal neutropenia (776.7)
DEF: Sudden, severe condition characterized by reduced number of white blood cells; results in sores in the throat, stomach or skin; symptoms include chills, fever.
AHA: 4Q, '06, 69-73; 3Q, '05, 11; 3Q, '99, 6; 2Q, '99, 9; 3Q, '96, 16; 2Q, '96, 6

288.00 Neutropenia, unspecified
AHA: 4Q, '06, 69-73

288.01 Congenital neutropenia
Congenital agranulocytosis
Infantile genetic agranulocytosis
Kostmann's syndrome
AHA: 4Q, '06, 69-73

288.02 Cyclic neutropenia
Cyclic hematopoiesis Periodic neutropenia
AHA: 4Q, '06, 69-73

288.03 Drug induced neutropenia
Use additional E code to identify drug
AHA: 4Q, '06, 69-73
TIP: Assign for neutropenic fever due to chemotherapy drugs, along with codes for the fever, adverse effect, and the underlying malignancy.

288.04 Neutropenia due to infection
AHA: 4Q, '06, 69-73

288.09 Other neutropenia
Agranulocytosis
Neutropenia:
immune
toxic
AHA: 4Q, '06, 69-73

288.1 Functional disorders of polymorphonuclear neutrophils
Chronic (childhood) granulomatous disease
Congenital dysphagocytosis
Job's syndrome
Lipochrome histiocytosis (familial)
Progressive septic granulomatosis

288.2 Genetic anomalies of leukocytes
Anomaly (granulation) (granulocyte) or syndrome:
Alder's (-Reilly)
Chédiak-Steinbrinck (-Higashi)
Jordan's
May-Hegglin
Pelger-Huet
Hereditary:
hypersegmentation
hyposegmentation
leukomelanopathy

288.3 Eosinophilia
Eosinophilia: Eosinophilia:
allergic   secondary
hereditary   Eosinophilic leukocytosis
idiopathic
EXCLUDES *Löffler's syndrome (518.3)*
pulmonary eosinophilia (518.3)
DEF: Elevated number of eosinophils in the blood; characteristic of allergic states and various parasitic infections.
AHA: 3Q, '00, 11

288.4 Hemophagocytic syndromes
Familial hemophagocytic lymphohistiocytosis
Familial hemophagocytic reticulosis
Hemophagocytic syndrome, infection-associated
Histiocytic syndromes
Macrophage activation syndrome
AHA: 4Q, '06, 69-73

✓5ᵗʰ **288.5 Decreased white blood cell count**
EXCLUDES *neutropenia (288.01-288.09)*

288.50 Leukocytopenia, unspecified
Decreased leukocytes, unspecified
Decreased white blood cell count, unspecified
Leukopenia NOS
AHA: 4Q, '06, 69-73

288.51 Lymphocytopenia
Decreased lymphocytes
AHA: 4Q, '06, 69-73

288.59 Other decreased white blood cell count
Basophilic leukopenia
Eosinophilic leukopenia
Monocytopenia
Plasmacytopenia
AHA: 4Q, '06, 69-73

✓5ᵗʰ **288.6 Elevated white blood cell count**
EXCLUDES *eosinophilia (288.3)*

288.60 Leukocytosis, unspecified
Elevated leukocytes, unspecified
Elevated white blood cell count, unspecified
AHA: 4Q, '06, 69-73

288.61 Lymphocytosis (symptomatic)
Elevated lymphocytes
AHA: 4Q, '06, 69-73

288.62 Leukemoid reaction
Basophilic leukemoid reaction
Lymphocytic leukemoid reaction
Monocytic leukemoid reaction
Myelocytic leukemoid reaction
Neutrophilic leukemoid reaction
AHA: 4Q, '06, 69-73

Ⓝ Newborn Age: 0   Ⓟ Pediatric Age: 0-17   Ⓜ Maternity Age: 12-55   Ⓐ Adult Age: 15-124

288.63 Monocytosis (symptomatic)
  EXCLUDES *infectious mononucleosis (075)*
  AHA: 4Q, '06, 69-73

288.64 Plasmacytosis
  AHA: 4Q, '06, 69-73

288.65 Basophilia
  AHA: 4Q, '06, 69-73

288.66 Bandemia
  Bandemia without diagnosis of specific infection
  EXCLUDES *confirmed infection — code to infection*
    leukemia (204.00-208.9)
  DEF: Increase in early neutrophil cells, called band cells; may indicate infection.
  AHA: 4Q, '07, 73
  TIP: Do not assign based on lab values alone; physician must substantiate bandemia without evidence of corresponding infection.

288.69 Other elevated white blood cell count
  AHA: 4Q, '06, 69-73

288.8 Other specified disease of white blood cells
  EXCLUDES *decreased white blood cell counts (288.50-288.59)*
    elevated white blood cell counts (288.60-288.69)
    immunity disorders (279.0-279.9)
  AHA: M-A, '87, 12

288.9 Unspecified disease of white blood cells

✓4ᵗʰ 289 Other diseases of blood and blood-forming organs

289.0 Polycythemia, secondary
  High-oxygen-affinity hemoglobin
  Polycythemia:
    acquired
    benign
    due to:
      fall in plasma volume
      high altitude
    emotional
    erythropoietin
    hypoxemic
    nephrogenous
    relative
    spurious
    stress
  EXCLUDES *polycythemia:*
    neonatal (776.4)
    primary (238.4)
    vera (238.4)
  DEF: Elevated number of red blood cells in circulating blood as result of reduced oxygen supply to the tissues.
  D75.1 Secondary polycythemia   I-10

289.1 Chronic lymphadenitis
  Chronic:
    adenitis   ⎫ any lymph node, except
    lymphadenitis ⎰   mesenteric
  EXCLUDES *acute lymphadenitis (683)*
    mesenteric (289.2)
    enlarged glands NOS (785.6)
  DEF: Persistent inflammation of lymph node tissue; origin of infection is usually elsewhere.
  I88.1 Chronic lymphadenitis except mesenteric   I-10

289.2 Nonspecific mesenteric lymphadenitis
  Mesenteric lymphadenitis (acute) (chronic)
  DEF: Inflammation of the lymph nodes in peritoneal fold that encases abdominal organs; disease resembles acute appendicitis; unknown etiology.
  I88.0 Nonspecific mesenteric lymphadenitis   I-10

289.3 Lymphadenitis, unspecified, except mesenteric
  AHA: 2Q, '92, 8
  I88.9 Nonspecific lymphadenitis unspecified   I-10

289.4 Hypersplenism
  "Big spleen" syndrome
  Dyssplenism
  Hypersplenia
  EXCLUDES *primary splenic neutropenia (289.53)*
  DEF: An overactive spleen causing a deficiency of the peripheral blood components, an increase in bone marrow cells and sometimes a notable increase in the size of the spleen.
  D73.1 Hypersplenism   I-10

✓5ᵗʰ 289.5 Other diseases of spleen

289.50 Disease of spleen, unspecified
  D73.9 Disease of spleen unspecified   I-10

289.51 Chronic congestive splenomegaly
  D73.2 Chronic congestive splenomegaly   I-10

289.52 Splenic sequestration
  Code first sickle-cell disease in crisis (282.42, 282.62, 282.64, 282.69)
  DEF: Blood is entrapped in the spleen due to vessel occlusion; most often associated with sickle-cell disease; spleen becomes enlarged and there is a sharp drop in hemoglobin.
  AHA: 4Q, '03, 51

289.53 Neutropenic splenomegaly
  AHA: 4Q, '06, 73
  D73.81 Neutropenic splenomegaly   I-10

289.59 Other
  Lien migrans   Splenic:
  Perisplenitis   fibrosis
  Splenic: infarction
    abscess   rupture, nontraumatic
    atrophy   Splenitis
    cyst   Wandering spleen
  EXCLUDES *bilharzial splenic fibrosis (120.0-120.9)*
    hepatolienal fibrosis (571.5)
    splenomegaly NOS (789.2)
  D73.89 Other diseases of spleen   I-10

289.6 Familial polycythemia
  Familial:
    benign polycythemia
    erythrocytosis
  DEF: Elevated number of red blood cells.

289.7 Methemoglobinemia
  Congenital NADH [DPNH]-methemoglobin- reductase deficiency
  Hemoglobin M [Hb-M] disease
  Methemoglobinemia:
    NOS
    acquired (with sulfhemoglobinemia)
    hereditary
    toxic
  Stokvis' disease
  Sulfhemoglobinemia
  Use additional E code to identify cause
  DEF: Presence of blood methemoglobin, a chemically altered form of hemoglobin; causes cyanosis, headache, ataxia, dyspnea, tachycardia, nausea, stupor, and coma.
  D74.0 Congenital methemoglobinemia   I-10

✓4ᵗʰ / ✓5ᵗʰ Additional Digit Required   Unspecified Code   Other Specified Code   Manifestation Code   ►◄ Revised Text   ● New Code   ▲ Revised Code Title

Diseases of the Blood and Blood-Forming Organs

289.8–289.9

√5ᵗʰ **289.8 Other specified diseases of blood and blood-forming organs**
> **DEF:** Hypercoagulable states: a group of inherited or acquired abnormalities of specific proteins and anticoagulant factors; also called thromboembolic states or thrombotic disorders, result in abnormal development of blood clots.
> **AHA:** 4Q, '03, 56; 1Q, '02, 16; 2Q, '89, 8; M-A, '87, 12

289.81 Primary hypercoagulable state
Activated protein C resistance
Antiphospholipid antibody syndrome
Antithrombin III deficiency
Factor V Leiden mutation
Lupus anticoagulant with hypercoagulable state
Protein C deficiency
Protein S deficiency
Prothrombin gene mutation
Systemic lupus erythematosus [SLE] inhibitor with hypercoagulable state

> **EXCLUDES** *anti-phospholipid antibody, finding without diagnosis (795.79)*
> *anti-phospholipid antibody with hemorrhagic disorder (286.53)*
> *lupus anticoagulant [LAC] finding without diagnosis (795.79)*
> *lupus anticoagulant [LAC] with hemorrhagic disorder (286.53)*
> *secondary activated protein C resistance (289.82)*
> *secondary antiphospholipid antibody syndrome (289.82)*
> *secondary lupus anticoagulant with hypercoagulable state (289.82)*
> *secondary systemic lupus erythematosus [SLE] inhibitor with hypercoagulable state (289.82)*
> *systemic lupus erythematosus [SLE] inhibitor finding without diagnosis (795.79)*
> *systemic lupus erythematosus [SLE] inhibitor with hypercoagulable state (286.53)*

> **DEF:** Activated protein C resistance: decreased effectiveness of protein C to degrade factor V, necessary to inhibit clotting cascade; also called Factor V Leiden mutation.
> **DEF:** Antithrombin III deficiency: deficiency in plasma antithrombin III one of six naturally occurring antithrombins that limit coagulation.
> **DEF:** Factor V Leiden mutation: also called activated protein C resistance.
> **DEF:** Lupus anticoagulant: autoimmune deficiency in a circulating anticoagulant that inhibits the conversion of prothrombin into thrombin; also called anti-phospholipid syndrome.
> **DEF:** Protein C deficiency: deficiency of activated protein C which functions to bring the blood-clotting process into balance; same outcome as factor V Leiden mutation.
> **DEF:** Protein S deficiency: similar to protein C deficiency; protein S is a vitamin K dependent cofactor in the activation of protein C.
> **DEF:** Prothrombin gene mutation: increased levels of prothrombin, or factor II, a plasma protein that is converted to thrombin, which acts upon fibrinogen to form the fibrin.
> **AHA:** ▶4Q, '11, 93◀
> **D68.59** Other primary thrombophilia   I-10

289.82 Secondary hypercoagulable state
> **EXCLUDES** *heparin-induced thrombocytopenia (HIT) (289.84)*
> **D68.69** Other thrombophilia   I-10

289.83 Myelofibrosis
Myelofibrosis NOS   Secondary myelofibrosis
Code first the underlying disorder, such as:
> malignant neoplasm of breast (174.0-174.9, 175.0-175.9)

Use additional code for associated therapy-related myelodysplastic syndrome, if applicable (238.72, 238.73)
Use additional external cause code if due to antineoplastic chemotherapy (E933.1)

> **EXCLUDES** *idiopathic myelofibrosis (238.76)*
> *leukoerythroblastic anemia (284.2)*
> *myelofibrosis with myeloid metaplasia (238.76)*
> *myelophthisic anemia (284.2)*
> *myelophthisis (284.2)*
> *primary myelofibrosis (238.76)*

> **DEF:** A progressive bone marrow disease characterized by the replacement of bone marrow with the overgrowth of neoplastic stem cells and fibrotic tissue, also progressive anemia and enlarged spleen.
> **AHA:** 4Q, '06, 73
> **D75.81** Myelofibrosis   I-10

289.84 Heparin-induced thrombocytopenia [HIT]
> **DEF:** Immune-mediated reaction to heparin therapy causing an abrupt fall in platelet count and serious complications such as pulmonary embolism, stroke, AMI or DVT.
> **AHA:** 4Q, '08, 100-101

289.89 Other specified diseases of blood and blood-forming organs
Hypergammaglobulinemia
Pseudocholinesterase deficiency
D75.89 Oth specified dz of blood & blood-forming organs   I-10

289.9 Unspecified diseases of blood and blood-forming organs
Blood dyscrasia NOS   Erythroid hyperplasia
AHA: M-A, '85, 14
D75.9 Disease of blood and blood-forming organs unspecified   I-10

N Newborn Age: 0   P Pediatric Age: 0-17   M Maternity Age: 12-55   A Adult Age: 15-124

5. Mental, Behavioral and Neurodevelopmental Disorders (290-319)

Psychoses (290-299)

EXCLUDES *intellectual disabilities (317-319)*

Organic Psychotic Conditions (290-294)

INCLUDES psychotic organic brain syndrome
EXCLUDES *nonpsychotic syndromes of organic etiology (310.0-310.9)*
psychoses classifiable to 295-298 and without impairment of orientation, comprehension, calculation, learning capacity, and judgment, but associated with physical disease, injury, or condition affecting the brain [eg., following childbirth] (295.0-298.8)

√4ᵗʰ **290 Dementias**
Code first the associated neurological condition
EXCLUDES *dementia due to alcohol (291.0-291.2)*
dementia due to drugs (292.82)
dementia not classified as senile, presenile, or arteriosclerotic (294.10-294.11)
psychoses classifiable to 295-298 occurring in the senium without dementia or delirium (295.0-298.8)
senility with mental changes of nonpsychotic severity (310.1)
transient organic psychotic conditions (293.0-293.9)

290.0 Senile dementia, uncomplicated Ⓐ
Senile dementia:
NOS
simple type
EXCLUDES *mild memory disturbances, not amounting to dementia, associated with senile brain disease (310.89)*
senile dementia with:
delirium or confusion (290.3)
delusional [paranoid] features (290.20)
depressive features (290.21)
AHA: 4Q, '99, 4
F03 Unspecified dementia I-10

√5ᵗʰ **290.1 Presenile dementia**
Brain syndrome with presenile brain disease
EXCLUDES *arteriosclerotic dementia (290.40-290.43)*
dementia associated with other cerebral conditions (294.10-294.11)
AHA: N-D, '84, 20

290.10 Presenile dementia, uncomplicated Ⓐ
Presenile dementia:
NOS
simple type

290.11 Presenile dementia with delirium Ⓐ
Presenile dementia with acute confusional state
AHA: 1Q, '88, 3

290.12 Presenile dementia with delusional features Ⓐ
Presenile dementia, paranoid type

290.13 Presenile dementia with depressive features Ⓐ
Presenile dementia, depressed type

√5ᵗʰ **290.2 Senile dementia with delusional or depressive features**
EXCLUDES *senile dementia:*
NOS (290.0)
with delirium and/or confusion (290.3)

290.20 Senile dementia with delusional features Ⓐ
Senile dementia, paranoid type
Senile psychosis NOS

290.21 Senile dementia with depressive features Ⓐ

290.3 Senile dementia with delirium Ⓐ
Senile dementia with acute confusional state
EXCLUDES *senile:*
dementia NOS (290.0)
psychosis NOS (290.20)
AHA: 3Q, '09, 11

√5ᵗʰ **290.4 Vascular dementia**
Multi-infarct dementia or psychosis
Use additional code to identify cerebral atherosclerosis (437.0)
EXCLUDES *suspected cases with no clear evidence of arteriosclerosis (290.9)*
AHA: 1Q, '88, 3

290.40 Vascular dementia, uncomplicated Ⓐ
Arteriosclerotic dementia:
NOS
simple type
F01.50 Vascular dementia without behavioral disturbance I-10

290.41 Vascular dementia with delirium Ⓐ
Arteriosclerotic dementia with acute confusional state

290.42 Vascular dementia with delusions Ⓐ
Arteriosclerotic dementia, paranoid type

290.43 Vascular dementia with depressed mood Ⓐ
Arteriosclerotic dementia, depressed type

290.8 Other specified senile psychotic conditions
Presbyophrenic psychosis

290.9 Unspecified senile psychotic condition Ⓐ

√4ᵗʰ **291 Alcohol induced mental disorders**
EXCLUDES *alcoholism without psychosis (303.0-303.9)*
AHA: 1Q, '88, 3; S-O, '86, 3

291.0 Alcohol withdrawal delirium
Alcoholic delirium
Delirium tremens
EXCLUDES *alcohol withdrawal (291.81)*
AHA: 2Q, '91, 11
F10.921 Alcohol use unsp w/intox delirium I-10

291.1 Alcohol induced persisting amnestic disorder
Alcoholic polyneuritic psychosis
Korsakoff's psychosis, alcoholic
Wernicke-Korsakoff syndrome (alcoholic)
DEF: Prominent and lasting reduced memory span, disordered time appreciation and confabulation, occurring in alcoholics, as sequel to acute alcoholic psychosis.
AHA: 1Q, '88, 3

291.2 Alcohol induced persisting dementia
Alcoholic dementia NOS
Alcoholism associated with dementia NOS
Chronic alcoholic brain syndrome
F10.27 Alcohol depend alcohol-induced persist dementia I-10

291.3 Alcohol induced psychotic disorder with hallucinations
Alcoholic:
hallucinosis (acute)
psychosis with hallucinosis
EXCLUDES *alcohol withdrawal with delirium (291.0)*
schizophrenia (295.0-295.9) and paranoid states (297.0-297.9) taking the form of chronic hallucinosis with clear consciousness in an alcoholic
DEF: Psychosis lasting less than six months with slight or no clouding of consciousness in which auditory hallucinations predominate.
AHA: 2Q, '91, 11

291.4 Idiosyncratic alcohol intoxication
Pathologic:
alcohol intoxication
drunkenness
EXCLUDES *acute alcohol intoxication (305.0)*
in alcoholism (303.0)
simple drunkenness (305.0)
DEF: Unique behavioral patterns, like belligerence, after intake of relatively small amounts of alcohol; behavior not due to excess consumption.

291.5 Alcohol induced psychotic disorder with delusions
Alcoholic:
  paranoia
  psychosis, paranoid type
> EXCLUDES   *nonalcoholic paranoid states (297.0-297.9)*
> *schizophrenia, paranoid type (295.3)*

√5ᵗʰ **291.8 Other specified alcohol induced mental disorders**
AHA: 3Q, '94, 13; J-A, '85, 10

291.81 Alcohol withdrawal
Alcohol:
  abstinence syndrome or symptoms
  withdrawal syndrome or symptoms
> EXCLUDES   *alcohol withdrawal:*
> *delirium (291.0)*
> *hallucinosis (291.3)*
> *delirium tremens (291.0)*

AHA: 4Q, '96, 28; 2Q, '91, 11
F10.239 Alcohol dependence with withdrawal unspecified   I-10

291.82 Alcohol induced sleep disorders
Alcohol induced circadian rhythm sleep disorders
Alcohol induced hypersomnia
Alcohol induced insomnia
Alcohol induced parasomnia

291.89 Other
Alcohol induced anxiety disorder
Alcohol induced mood disorder
Alcohol induced sexual dysfunction

291.9 Unspecified alcohol induced mental disorders
Alcoholic:
  mania NOS
  psychosis NOS
Alcoholism (chronic) with psychosis
Alcohol related disorder NOS

√4ᵗʰ **292 Drug induced mental disorders**
> INCLUDES   organic brain syndrome associated with consumption of drugs

Use additional code for any associated drug dependence (304.0-304.9)
Use additional E code to identify drug
AHA: 3Q, '04, 8; 2Q, '91, 11; S-O, '86, 3

292.0 Drug withdrawal
Drug:
  abstinence syndrome or symptoms
  withdrawal syndrome or symptoms
AHA: 1Q, '97, 12; 1Q, '88, 3
TIP: Assign only for patients who suffer mental or behavioral disturbances due to drug withdrawal, regardless of the circumstances.
F19.939 Oth psychoactive sbstnc use uns w/withdraw uns   I-10

√5ᵗʰ **292.1 Drug induced psychotic disorders**

292.11 Drug induced psychotic disorder with delusions
Paranoid state induced by drugs

292.12 Drug induced psychotic disorder with hallucinations
Hallucinatory state induced by drugs
> EXCLUDES   *states following LSD or other hallucinogens, lasting only a few days or less ["bad trips"] (305.3)*

292.2 Pathological drug intoxication
Drug reaction:
  NOS   ⎫ resulting in brief psychotic
  idiosyncratic   ⎬   states
  pathologic   ⎭
> EXCLUDES   *expected brief psychotic reactions to hallucinogens ["bad trips"] (305.3)*
> *physiological side-effects of drugs (e.g., dystonias)*

√5ᵗʰ **292.8 Other specified drug induced mental disorders**

292.81 Drug induced delirium
AHA: 1Q, '88, 3
F19.921 Oth psychoactv sbstnc use uns intoxcat delirium   I-10

292.82 Drug induced persisting dementia

292.83 Drug induced persisting amnestic disorder

292.84 Drug induced mood disorder
Depressive state induced by drugs

292.85 Drug induced sleep disorders
Drug induced circadian rhythm sleep disorder
Drug induced hypersomnia
Drug induced insomnia
Drug induced parasomnia

292.89 Other
Drug induced anxiety disorder
Drug induced organic personality syndrome
Drug induced sexual dysfunction
Drug intoxication

292.9 Unspecified drug induced mental disorder
Drug related disorder NOS
Organic psychosis NOS due to or associated with drugs

√4ᵗʰ **293 Transient mental disorders due to conditions classified elsewhere**
> INCLUDES   transient organic mental disorders not associated with alcohol or drugs

Code first the associated physical or neurological condition
> EXCLUDES   *confusional state or delirium superimposed on senile dementia (290.3)*
> *dementia due to:*
> *alcohol (291.0-291.9)*
> *arteriosclerosis (290.40-290.43)*
> *drugs (292.82)*
> *senility (290.0)*

293.0 Delirium due to conditions classified elsewhere
Acute:
  confusional state
  infective psychosis
  organic reaction
  posttraumatic organic psychosis
  psycho-organic syndrome
Acute psychosis associated with endocrine, metabolic, or cerebrovascular disorder
Epileptic:
  confusional state
  twilight state
AHA: 1Q, '88, 3
F05 Delirium due to known physiological condition   I-10

293.1 Subacute delirium
Subacute:
  confusional state
  infective psychosis
  organic reaction
  posttraumatic organic psychosis
  psycho-organic syndrome
  psychosis associated with endocrine or metabolic disorder

√5ᵗʰ **293.8 Other specified transient mental disorders due to conditions classified elsewhere**

293.81 Psychotic disorder with delusions in conditions classified elsewhere
Transient organic psychotic condition, paranoid type
AHA: 1Q, '11, 12

293.82 Psychotic disorder with hallucinations in conditions classified elsewhere
Transient organic psychotic condition, hallucinatory type

293.83 Mood disorder in conditions classified elsewhere
Transient organic psychotic condition, depressive type

293.84 Anxiety disorder in conditions classified elsewhere
AHA: 4Q, '96, 29

293.89 Other
Catatonic disorder in conditions classified elsewhere

N Newborn Age: 0   P Pediatric Age: 0-17   M Maternity Age: 12-55   A Adult Age: 15-124

293.9 Unspecified transient mental disorder in conditions classified elsewhere
Organic psychosis:
   infective NOS
   posttraumatic NOS
   transient NOS
Psycho-organic syndrome

√4ʰ **294 Persistent mental disorders due to conditions classified elsewhere**
INCLUDES organic psychotic brain syndromes (chronic), not elsewhere classified
AHA: M-A, '85, 12

294.0 Amnestic disorder in conditions classified elsewhere
Korsakoff's psychosis or syndrome (nonalcoholic)
Code first underlying condition
EXCLUDES *alcoholic:*
   amnestic syndrome (291.1)
   Korsakoff's psychosis (291.1)

√5ʰ **294.1 Dementia in conditions classified elsewhere**
Dementia of the Alzheimer's type
Code first any underlying physical condition, as:
   Alzheimer's disease (331.0)
   cerebral lipidoses (330.1)
   dementia with Lewy bodies (331.82)
   dementia with Parkinsonism (331.82)
   epilepsy (345.0-345.9)
   frontal dementia (331.19)
   frontotemporal dementia (331.19)
   general paresis [syphilis] (094.1)
   hepatolenticular degeneration (275.1)
   Huntington's chorea (333.4)
   Jakob-Creutzfeldt disease (046.11-046.19)
   multiple sclerosis (340)
   Parkinson's disease (332.0)
   Pick's disease of the brain (331.11)
   polyarteritis nodosa (446.0)
   syphilis (094.1)
EXCLUDES *dementia:*
   arteriosclerotic (290.40-290.43)
   presenile (290.10-290.13)
   senile (290.0)
   epileptic psychosis NOS (294.8)
AHA: 4Q, '00, 40; 1Q, '99, 14; N-D, '85, 5

294.10 *Dementia in conditions classified elsewhere without behavioral disturbance*
Dementia in conditions classified elsewhere NOS
F02.80 Dementia in oth dz class elsw w/o behavrl distur I-10

294.11 *Dementia in conditions classified elsewhere with behavioral disturbance*
Aggressive behavior   Violent behavior
Combative behavior
Use additional code, where applicable, to identify:
   wandering in conditions classified elsewhere (V40.31)
AHA: 4Q, '00, 41
TIP: Review entire medical record for documentation of behavioral disturbance (aggressive, combative, violent behavior, wandering off); requires physician substantiation.

√5ʰ **294.2 Dementia, unspecified**
EXCLUDES *mild memory disturbances, not amounting to dementia (310.89)*
AHA: ▶4Q, '11, 95-96◀

294.20 Dementia, unspecified, without behavioral disturbance
Dementia NOS

294.21 Dementia, unspecified, with behavioral disturbance
Aggressive behavior
Combative behavior
Violent behavior
Use additional code, where applicable, to identify:
   wandering in conditions classified elsewhere (V40.31)
AHA: ▶4Q, '11, 95◀

294.8 Other persistent mental disorders due to conditions classified elsewhere
Amnestic disorder NOS
Epileptic psychosis NOS
Mixed paranoid and affective organic psychotic states
Use additional code for associated epilepsy (345.0-345.9)
EXCLUDES *mild memory disturbances, not amounting to dementia (310.89)*
AHA: 3Q, '09, 11; 3Q, '03, 14; 1Q, '88, 5
F06.8 Oth spec mental disord d/t known physiol cond I-10

294.9 Unspecified persistent mental disorders due to conditions classified elsewhere
Cognitive disorder NOS
Organic psychosis (chronic)
AHA: 2Q, '07, 4

Other Psychoses (295-299)

Use additional code to identify any associated physical disease, injury, or condition affecting the brain with psychoses classifiable to 295-298

√4ʰ **295 Schizophrenic disorders**
INCLUDES schizophrenia of the types described in 295.0-295.9 occurring in children
EXCLUDES *childhood type schizophrenia (299.9)*
   infantile autism (299.0)

The following fifth-digit subclassification is for use with category 295:
0 unspecified
1 subchronic
2 chronic
3 subchronic with acute exacerbation
4 chronic with acute exacerbation
5 in remission

DEF: Group of disorders with disturbances in thought (delusions, hallucinations), mood (blunted, flattened, inappropriate affect), sense of self; also bizarre, purposeless behavior, repetitive activity, or inactivity.

§ √5ʰ **295.0 Simple type**
[0-5]   Schizophrenia simplex
EXCLUDES *latent schizophrenia (295.5)*

§ √5ʰ **295.1 Disorganized type**
[0-5]   Hebephrenia   Hebephrenic type schizophrenia
DEF: Inappropriate behavior; results in extreme incoherence and disorganization of time, place and sense of social appropriateness; withdrawal from routine social interaction may occur.

§ √5ʰ **295.2 Catatonic type**
[0-5]   Catatonic (schizophrenia):   Schizophrenic:
   agitation   catalepsy
   excitation   catatonia
   excited type   flexibilitas cerea
   stupor
   withdrawn type
Schizophrenic:
DEF: Extreme changes in motor activity; one extreme is decreased response or reaction to the environment and the other is spontaneous activity.

§ √5ʰ **295.3 Paranoid type**
[0-5]   Paraphrenic schizophrenia
EXCLUDES *involutional paranoid state (297.2)*
   paranoia (297.1)
   paraphrenia (297.2)
DEF: Preoccupied with delusional suspicions and auditory hallucinations related to single theme; usually hostile, grandiose, overly religious, occasionally hypochondriacal.
F20.0 Paranoid schizophrenia I-10

§ √5ʰ **295.4 Schizophreniform disorder**
[0-5]   Oneirophrenia
Schizophreniform:
   attack
   psychosis, confusional type
EXCLUDES *acute forms of schizophrenia of:*
   catatonic type (295.2)
   hebephrenic type (295.1)
   paranoid type (295.3)
   simple type (295.0)
   undifferentiated type (295.8)

§ Requires fifth digit. Valid digits are in [brackets] under each code. See category 295 for codes and definitions.

√4ʰ Additional Digit Required   Unspecified Code   Other Specified Code   Manifestation Code   ▶◀ Revised Text   ● New Code   ▲ Revised Code Title
√5ʰ
2013 ICD-9-CM   February 2012 • Volume 1 – 75

§ ✓5ᵗʰ **295.5 Latent schizophrenia**
[0-5]   Latent schizophrenic reaction
Schizophrenia:
    borderline
    incipient
    prepsychotic
    prodromal
    pseudoneurotic
    pseudopsychopathic
    EXCLUDES *schizoid personality (301.20-301.22)*
    AHA: For code 295.50: 1Q, '06, 10

§ ✓5ᵗʰ **295.6 Residual type**
[0-5]   Chronic undifferentiated schizophrenia
Restzustand (schizophrenic)
Schizophrenic residual state
    AHA: For code 295.62: 4Q, '06, 78

§ ✓5ᵗʰ **295.7 Schizoaffective disorder**
[0-5]   Cyclic schizophrenia
Mixed schizophrenic and affective psychosis
Schizo-affective psychosis
Schizophreniform psychosis, affective type
    F25.9 Schizoaffective disorder unspecified   I-10

§ ✓5ᵗʰ **295.8 Other specified types of schizophrenia**
[0-5]   Acute (undifferentiated) schizophrenia
Atypical schizophrenia
Cenesthopathic schizophrenia
    EXCLUDES *infantile autism (299.0)*

§ ✓5ᵗʰ **295.9 Unspecified schizophrenia**
[0-5]   Schizophrenia:
    NOS
    mixed NOS
    undifferentiated NOS
    undifferentiated type
Schizophrenic reaction NOS
Schizophreniform psychosis NOS
    AHA: 3Q, '95, 6
    F20.9 Schizophrenia unspecified   I-10

✓4ᵗʰ **296 Episodic mood disorders**
    INCLUDES episodic affective disorders
    EXCLUDES *neurotic depression (300.4)*
       reactive depressive psychosis (298.0)
       reactive excitation (298.1)

The following fifth-digit subclassification is for use with categories 296.0-296.6:

0 unspecified
1 mild
2 moderate
3 severe, without mention of psychotic behavior
4 severe, specified as with psychotic behavior
5 in partial or unspecified remission
6 in full remission

    AHA: M-A, '85, 14

§ ✓5ᵗʰ **296.0 Bipolar I disorder, single manic episode**
[0-6]   Hypomania (mild) NOS
Hypomanic psychosis
Mania (monopolar) NOS   single episode or
Manic-depressive psychosis or reaction: unspecified
    hypomanic
    manic
    EXCLUDES *circular type, if there was a previous attack of depression (296.4)*
    DEF: Mood disorder identified by hyperactivity; may show extreme agitation or exaggerated excitability; speech and thought processes may be accelerated.

§ ✓5ᵗʰ **296.1 Manic disorder, recurrent episode**
[0-6]   Any condition classifiable to 296.0, stated to be recurrent
    EXCLUDES *circular type, if there was a previous attack of depression (296.4)*

§ ✓5ᵗʰ **296.2 Major depressive disorder, single episode**
[0-6]   Depressive psychosis
Endogenous depression
Involutional melancholia
Manic-depressive psychosis or   single episode or
    reaction, depressed type   unspecified
Monopolar depression
Psychotic depression
    EXCLUDES *circular type, if previous attack was of manic type (296.5)*
       depression NOS (311)
       reactive depression (neurotic) (300.4)
       psychotic (298.0)
    DEF: Mood disorder that produces depression; may exhibit as sadness, low self-esteem, or guilt feelings; other manifestations may be withdrawal from friends and family; interrupted sleep.
    AHA: For code 296.20: 3Q, '09, 18
    F32.9 Major depressive disorder single episode uns   I-10

§ ✓5ᵗʰ **296.3 Major depressive disorder, recurrent episode**
[0-6]   Any condition classifiable to 296.2, stated to be recurrent
    EXCLUDES *circular type, if previous attack was of manic type (296.5)*
       depression NOS (311)
       reactive depression (neurotic) (300.4)
       psychotic (298.0)
    F33.2 Maj dprsv disord recur sev w/o psychot features   I-10

§ ✓5ᵗʰ **296.4 Bipolar I disorder, most recent episode (or current) manic**
[0-6]   Bipolar disorder, now manic
Manic-depressive psychosis, circular type but currently manic
    EXCLUDES *brief compensatory or rebound mood swings (296.99)*
    F31.2 Bipolar d/o currnt epis mnic sev w/psychotc features   I-10

§ ✓5ᵗʰ **296.5 Bipolar I disorder, most recent episode (or current) depressed**
[0-6]
    Bipolar disorder, now depressed
Manic-depressive psychosis, circular type but currently depressed
    EXCLUDES *brief compensatory or rebound mood swings (296.99)*
    F31.30 Bipol disord currnt epis dprsd mild/mod sev uns   I-10

§ ✓5ᵗʰ **296.6 Bipolar I disorder, most recent episode (or current) mixed**
[0-6]   Manic-depressive psychosis, circular type, mixed

296.7 Bipolar I disorder, most recent episode (or current) unspecified
    Atypical bipolar affective disorder NOS
Manic-depressive psychosis, circular type, current condition not specified as either manic or depressive
    DEF: Manic-depressive disorder referred to as bipolar because of the mood range from manic to depressive.

✓5ᵗʰ **296.8 Other and unspecified bipolar disorders**

296.80 Bipolar disorder, unspecified
    Bipolar disorder NOS
Manic-depressive:
    reaction NOS
    syndrome NOS
    F31.9 Bipolar disorder unspecified   I-10

296.81 Atypical manic disorder

296.82 Atypical depressive disorder

296.89 Other
    Bipolar II disorder
Manic-depressive psychosis, mixed type
    F31.81 Bipolar II disorder   I-10

✓5ᵗʰ **296.9 Other and unspecified episodic mood disorder**
    EXCLUDES *psychogenic affective psychoses (298.0-298.8)*

296.90 Unspecified episodic mood disorder
    Affective psychosis NOS
Melancholia NOS
Mood disorder NOS
    AHA: M-A, '85, 14
    F39 Unspecified mood [affective] disorder   I-10

---

§   Requires fifth digit. Valid digits are in [brackets] under each code. See appropriate category for codes and definitions

    N Newborn Age: 0   P Pediatric Age: 0-17   M Maternity Age: 12-55   A Adult Age: 15-124

296.99 Other specified episodic mood disorder
Mood swings:
brief compensatory
rebound

√4ᵗʰ **297 Delusional disorders**
INCLUDES paranoid disorders
EXCLUDES *acute paranoid reaction (298.3)*
alcoholic jealousy or paranoid state (291.5)
paranoid schizophrenia (295.3)

297.0 Paranoid state, simple

297.1 Delusional disorder
Chronic paranoid psychosis
Sander's disease
Systematized delusions
EXCLUDES *paranoid personality disorder (301.0)*
F22 Delusional disorders   I-10

297.2 Paraphrenia
Involutional paranoid state
Late paraphrenia
Paraphrenia (involutional)
DEF: Paranoid schizophrenic disorder that persists over a prolonged period but does not distort personality despite persistent delusions.

297.3 Shared psychotic disorder
Folie à deux
Induced psychosis or paranoid disorder
DEF: Mental disorder two people share; first person with the delusional disorder convinces second person because of a close relationship and shared experiences to accept the delusions.

297.8 Other specified paranoid states
Paranoia querulans
Sensitiver Beziehungswahn
EXCLUDES *acute paranoid reaction or state (298.3)*
senile paranoid state (290.20)

297.9 Unspecified paranoid state
Paranoid:
disorder NOS
psychosis NOS
reaction NOS
state NOS
AHA: J-A, '85, 9

√4ᵗʰ **298 Other nonorganic psychoses**
INCLUDES psychotic conditions due to or provoked by:
emotional stress
environmental factors as major part of etiology

298.0 Depressive type psychosis
Psychogenic depressive psychosis
Psychotic reactive depression
Reactive depressive psychosis
EXCLUDES *manic-depressive psychosis, depressed type (296.2-296.3)*
neurotic depression (300.4)
reactive depression NOS (300.4)

298.1 Excitative type psychosis
Acute hysterical psychosis
Psychogenic excitation
Reactive excitation
EXCLUDES *manic-depressive psychosis, manic type (296.0-296.1)*
DEF: Affective disorder similar to manic-depressive psychosis, in the manic phase, seemingly brought on by stress.

298.2 Reactive confusion
Psychogenic confusion
Psychogenic twilight state
EXCLUDES *acute confusional state (293.0)*
DEF: Confusion, disorientation, cloudiness in consciousness; brought on by severe emotional upheaval.

298.3 Acute paranoid reaction
Acute psychogenic paranoid psychosis
Bouffée délirante
EXCLUDES *paranoid states (298.0-297.9)*

298.4 Psychogenic paranoid psychosis
Protracted reactive paranoid psychosis

298.8 Other and unspecified reactive psychosis
Brief psychotic disorder
Brief reactive psychosis NOS
Hysterical psychosis
Psychogenic psychosis NOS
Psychogenic stupor
EXCLUDES *acute hysterical psychosis (298.1)*

298.9 Unspecified psychosis
Atypical psychosis
Psychosis NOS
Psychotic disorder NOS
AHA: 3Q, '06, 22
F28 Oth psych d/o not d/t sbstnc/knwn physiolog cond   I-10

√4ᵗʰ **299 Pervasive developmental disorders**
EXCLUDES *adult type psychoses occurring in childhood, as:*
affective disorders (296.0-296.9)
manic-depressive disorders (296.0-296.9)
schizophrenia (295.0-295.9)

The following fifth-digit subclassification is for use with category 299:
0 current or active state
1 residual state

§ √5ᵗʰ **299.0 Autistic disorder**
[0-1] Childhood autism
Infantile psychosis
Kanner's syndrome
EXCLUDES *disintegrative psychosis (299.1)*
Heller's syndrome (299.1)
schizophrenic syndrome of childhood (299.9)
DEF: Severe mental disorder of children, results in impaired social behavior; abnormal development of communicative skills, appears to be unaware of the need for emotional support and little emotional response to family members.

§ √5ᵗʰ **299.1 Childhood disintegrative disorder**
[0-1] Heller's syndrome
Use additional code to identify any associated neurological disorder
EXCLUDES *infantile autism (299.0)*
schizophrenic syndrome of childhood (299.9)
DEF: Mental disease of children identified by impaired development of reciprocal social skills, verbal and nonverbal communication skills, imaginative play.

§ √5ᵗʰ **299.8 Other specified pervasive developmental disorders**
[0-1] Asperger's disorder
Atypical childhood psychosis
Borderline psychosis of childhood
EXCLUDES *simple stereotypes without psychotic disturbance (307.3)*

§ √5ᵗʰ **299.9 Unspecified pervasive developmental disorder**
[0-1] Child psychosis NOS
Pervasive developmental disorder NOS
Schizophrenia, childhood type NOS
Schizophrenic syndrome of childhood NOS
EXCLUDES *schizophrenia of adult type occurring in childhood (295.0-295.9)*

---

§ Requires fifth digit. Valid digits are in [brackets] under each code. See category 299 for codes and definitions.

√4ᵗʰ/√5ᵗʰ Additional Digit Required   Unspecified Code   Other Specified Code   Manifestation Code   ►◄ Revised Text   ● New Code   ▲ Revised Code Title

Mental, Behavioral and Neurodevelopmental Disorders

300–300.4

Neurotic Disorders, Personality Disorders, and Other Nonpsychotic Mental Disorders (300-316)

☑4ᵗʰ **300 Anxiety, dissociative and somatoform disorders**

☑5ᵗʰ **300.0 Anxiety states**

> **EXCLUDES** *anxiety in:*
> *acute stress reaction (308.0)*
> *transient adjustment reaction (309.24)*
> *neurasthenia (300.5)*
> *psychophysiological disorders (306.0-306.9)*
> *separation anxiety (309.21)*
>
> **DEF:** Mental disorder characterized by anxiety and avoidance behavior not particularly related to any specific situation or stimulus; symptoms include emotional instability, apprehension, fatigue.

300.00 Anxiety state, unspecified
Anxiety:
  neurosis
  reaction
  state (neurotic)
Atypical anxiety disorder
AHA: ▶3Q, '11, 6;◀2Q, '11, 5; 1Q, '02, 6
TIP: For chest pain due to anxiety, assign chest pain code first, because chest pain is not integral to the diagnosis of anxiety.
F41.9 Anxiety disorder unspecified   I-10

300.01 Panic disorder without agoraphobia
Panic:
  attack
  state
> **EXCLUDES** *panic disorder with agoraphobia (300.21)*
>
> **DEF:** Neurotic disorder characterized by recurrent panic or anxiety, apprehension, fear or terror; symptoms include shortness of breath, palpitations, dizziness, shakiness; fear of dying may persist.
F41.0 Panic d/o [epis paroxysmal anxiety] w/o   I-10
agoraphobia

300.02 Generalized anxiety disorder

300.09 Other

☑5ᵗʰ **300.1 Dissociative, conversion and factitious disorders**
> **EXCLUDES** *adjustment reaction (309.0-309.9)*
> *anorexia nervosa (307.1)*
> *gross stress reaction (308.0-308.9)*
> *hysterical personality (301.50-301.59)*
> *psychophysiologic disorders (306.0-306.9)*

300.10 Hysteria, unspecified

300.11 Conversion disorder
Astasia-abasia, hysterical
Conversion hysteria or reaction
Hysterical:
  blindness
  deafness
  paralysis
> **DEF:** Mental disorder that impairs physical functions with no physiological basis; sensory motor symptoms include seizures, paralysis, temporary blindness; increase in stress or avoidance of unpleasant responsibilities may precipitate onset of symptoms.
AHA: 2Q, '11, 5; N-D, '85, 15

300.12 Dissociative amnesia
Hysterical amnesia

300.13 Dissociative fugue
Hysterical fugue
> **DEF:** Dissociative hysteria; identified by loss of memory, flight from familiar surroundings; conscious activity is not associated with perception of surroundings, no later memory of episode.

300.14 Dissociative identity disorder

300.15 Dissociative disorder or reaction, unspecified
> **DEF:** Hysterical neurotic episode; sudden but temporary changes in perceived identity, memory, consciousness, segregated memory patterns exist separate from dominant personality.

300.16 Factitious disorder with predominantly psychological signs and symptoms
Compensation neurosis
Ganser's syndrome, hysterical
> **DEF:** A disorder characterized by the purposeful assumption of mental illness symptoms; which are acted out more often when another person is present.

300.19 Other and unspecified factitious illness
Factitious disorder (with combined psychological and physical signs and symptoms) (with predominantly physical signs and symptoms) NOS
> **EXCLUDES** *multiple operations or hospital addiction syndrome (301.51)*

☑5ᵗʰ **300.2 Phobic disorders**
> **EXCLUDES** *anxiety state not associated with a specific situation or object (300.00-300.09)*
> *obsessional phobias (300.3)*

300.20 Phobia, unspecified
Anxiety-hysteria NOS
Phobia NOS

300.21 Agoraphobia with panic disorder
Fear of:
  open spaces ⎫
  streets   ⎬ with panic attacks
  travel   ⎭
Panic disorder with agoraphobia
> **EXCLUDES** *agoraphobia without panic disorder (300.22)*
> *panic disorder without agoraphobia (300.01)*

300.22 Agoraphobia without mention of panic attacks
Any condition classifiable to 300.21 without mention of panic attacks

300.23 Social phobia
Fear of:
  eating in public
  public speaking
  washing in public

300.29 Other isolated or specific phobias
Acrophobia   Claustrophobia
Animal phobias   Fear of crowds

300.3 Obsessive-compulsive disorders
Anancastic neurosis
Compulsive neurosis
Obsessional phobia [any]
> **EXCLUDES** *obsessive-compulsive symptoms occurring in:*
> *endogenous depression (296.2-296.3)*
> *organic states (eg., encephalitis)*
> *schizophrenia (295.0-295.9)*

300.4 Dysthymic disorder
Anxiety depression
Depression with anxiety
Depressive reaction
Neurotic depressive state
Reactive depression
> **EXCLUDES** *adjustment reaction with depressive symptoms (309.0-309.1)*
> *depression NOS (311)*
> *manic-depressive psychosis, depressed type (296.2-296.3)*
> *reactive depressive psychosis (298.0)*
>
> **DEF:** Depression without psychosis; less severe depression related to personal change or unexpected circumstances; also referred to as "reactional depression."
AHA: ▶3Q, '11, 6◀
F34.1 Dysthymic disorder   I-10

300.5 Neurasthenia
Fatigue neurosis
Nervous debility
Psychogenic:
asthenia
general fatigue
Use additional code to identify any associated physical disorder

EXCLUDES anxiety state (300.00-300.09)
neurotic depression (300.4)
psychophysiological disorders (306.0-306.9)
specific nonpsychotic mental disorders following organic brain damage (310.0-310.9)

DEF: Physical and mental symptoms caused primarily by what is known as mental exhaustion; symptoms include chronic weakness, fatigue.

300.6 Depersonalization disorder
Derealization (neurotic)
Neurotic state with depersonalization episode

EXCLUDES depersonalization associated with:
anxiety (300.00-300.09)
depression (300.4)
manic-depressive disorder or psychosis (296.0-296.9)
schizophrenia (295.0-295.9)

DEF: Dissociative disorder characterized by feelings of strangeness about self or body image; symptoms include dizziness, anxiety, fear of insanity, loss of reality of surroundings.

300.7 Hypochondriasis
Body dysmorphic disorder

EXCLUDES hypochondriasis in:
hysteria (300.10-300.19)
manic-depressive psychosis, depressed type (296.2-296.3)
neurasthenia (300.5)
obsessional disorder (300.3)
schizophrenia (295.0-295.9)

300.8 Somatoform disorders

300.81 Somatization disorder
Briquet's disorder
Severe somatoform disorder

300.82 Undifferentiated somatoform disorder
Atypical somatoform disorder
Somatoform disorder NOS
DEF: Disorders in which patients have symptoms that suggest an organic disease but no evidence of physical disorder after repeated testing.
AHA: 4Q, '96, 29

300.89 Other somatoform disorders
Occupational neurosis, including writers' cramp
Psychasthenia
Psychasthenic neurosis

300.9 Unspecified nonpsychotic mental disorder
Psychoneurosis NOS

301 Personality disorders
INCLUDES character neurosis
Use additional code to identify any associated neurosis or psychosis, or physical condition

EXCLUDES nonpsychotic personality disorder associated with organic brain syndromes (310.0-310.9)

301.0 Paranoid personality disorder
Fanatic personality
Paranoid personality (disorder)
Paranoid traits

EXCLUDES acute paranoid reaction (298.3)
alcoholic paranoia (291.5)
paranoid schizophrenia (295.3)
paranoid states (297.0-297.9)

AHA: J-A, '85, 9

301.1 Affective personality disorder
EXCLUDES affective psychotic disorders (296.0-296.9)
neurasthenia (300.5)
neurotic depression (300.4)

301.10 Affective personality disorder, unspecified

301.11 Chronic hypomanic personality disorder
Chronic hypomanic disorder
Hypomanic personality

301.12 Chronic depressive personality disorder
Chronic depressive disorder
Depressive character or personality

301.13 Cyclothymic disorder
Cycloid personality
Cyclothymia
Cyclothymic personality

301.2 Schizoid personality disorder
EXCLUDES schizophrenia (295.0-295.9)

301.20 Schizoid personality disorder, unspecified

301.21 Introverted personality

301.22 Schizotypal personality disorder

301.3 Explosive personality disorder
Aggressive:
personality
reaction
Aggressiveness
Emotional instability (excessive)
Pathological emotionality
Quarrelsomeness

EXCLUDES dyssocial personality (301.7)
hysterical neurosis (300.10-300.19)

301.4 Obsessive-compulsive personality disorder
Anancastic personality
Obsessional personality

EXCLUDES obsessive-compulsive disorder (300.3)
phobic state (300.20-300.29)

301.5 Histrionic personality disorder
EXCLUDES hysterical neurosis (300.10-300.19)
DEF: Extreme emotional behavior, often theatrical; often concerned about own appeal; may demand attention, exhibit seductive behavior.

301.50 Histrionic personality disorder, unspecified
Hysterical personality NOS

301.51 Chronic factitious illness with physical symptoms
Hospital addiction syndrome
Multiple operations syndrome
Munchausen syndrome

301.59 Other histrionic personality disorder
Personality:
emotionally unstable
labile
psychoinfantile

301.6 Dependent personality disorder
Asthenic personality
Inadequate personality
Passive personality

EXCLUDES neurasthenia (300.5)
passive-aggressive personality (301.84)

DEF: Overwhelming feeling of helplessness; fears of abandonment may persist; difficulty in making personal decisions without confirmation by others; low self-esteem due to irrational sensitivity to criticism.

301.7 Antisocial personality disorder
Amoral personality
Asocial personality
Dyssocial personality
Personality disorder with predominantly sociopathic or asocial manifestation

EXCLUDES disturbance of conduct without specifiable personality disorder (312.0-312.9)
explosive personality (301.3)

DEF: Continuous antisocial behavior that violates rights of others; social traits include extreme aggression, total disregard for traditional social rules.

AHA: S-0, '84, 16

✓5ᵗʰ 301.8 Other personality disorders

301.81 Narcissistic personality disorder
DEF: Grandiose fantasy or behavior, lack of social empathy, hypersensitive to the lack of others' judgment, exploits others; need for continual admiration.

301.82 Avoidant personality disorder
DEF: Personality disorder marked by feelings of social inferiority; sensitivity to criticism, emotionally restrained due to fear of rejection.

301.83 Borderline personality disorder
DEF: Personality disorder characterized by unstable moods, self-image, and interpersonal relationships; uncontrolled anger, impulsive and self-destructive acts, fears of abandonment, feelings of emptiness and boredom, recurrent suicide threats or self-mutilation.
F60.3 Borderline personality disorder   **I-10**

301.84 Passive-aggressive personality
DEF: Pattern of procrastination and refusal to meet standards; introduce own obstacles to success and exploit failure.

301.89 Other
Personality: Personality:
eccentric   masochistic
"haltlose" type   psychoneurotic
immature
EXCLUDES psychoinfantile personality (301.59)

301.9 Unspecified personality disorder
Pathological personality NOS
Personality disorder NOS
Psychopathic:
constitutional state
personality (disorder)

✓4ᵗʰ 302 Sexual and gender identity disorders
EXCLUDES sexual disorder manifest in:
organic brain syndrome (290.0-294.9, 310.0-310.9)
psychosis (295.0-298.9)

302.0 Ego-dystonic sexual orientation
Ego-dystonic lesbianism
Sexual orientation conflict disorder
EXCLUDES homosexual pedophilia (302.2)

302.1 Zoophilia
Bestiality
DEF: A sociodeviant disorder marked by engaging in sexual intercourse with animals.

302.2 Pedophilia
DEF: A sociodeviant condition of adults characterized by sexual activity with children.

302.3 Transvestic fetishism
EXCLUDES trans-sexualism (302.5)
DEF: The desire to dress in clothing of opposite sex.

302.4 Exhibitionism
DEF: Sexual deviant behavior; exposure of genitals to strangers; behavior prompted by intense sexual urges and fantasies.

✓5ᵗʰ 302.5 Trans-sexualism
Sex reassignment surgery status
EXCLUDES transvestism (302.3)
DEF: Gender identity disturbance; overwhelming desire to change anatomic sex, due to belief that individual is a member of the opposite sex.

302.50 With unspecified sexual history

302.51 With asexual history

302.52 With homosexual history

302.53 With heterosexual history

302.6 Gender identity disorder in children
Feminism in boys
Gender identity disorder NOS
EXCLUDES gender identity disorder in adult (302.85)
trans-sexualism (302.50-302.53)
transvestism (302.3)

✓5ᵗʰ 302.7 Psychosexual dysfunction
EXCLUDES impotence of organic origin (607.84)
normal transient symptoms from ruptured hymen
transient or occasional failures of erection due to fatigue, anxiety, alcohol, or drugs

302.70 Psychosexual dysfunction, unspecified
Sexual dysfunction NOS

302.71 Hypoactive sexual desire disorder
EXCLUDES decreased sexual desire NOS (799.81)

302.72 With inhibited sexual excitement
Female sexual arousal disorder
Frigidity
Impotence
Male erectile disorder

302.73 Female orgasmic disorder   ♀

302.74 Male orgasmic disorder   ♂

302.75 Premature ejaculation   ♂

302.76 Dyspareunia, psychogenic   ♀
DEF: Difficult or painful sex due to psychosomatic state.

302.79 With other specified psychosexual dysfunctions
Sexual aversion disorder

✓5ᵗʰ 302.8 Other specified psychosexual disorders

302.81 Fetishism
DEF: Psychosexual disorder noted for intense sexual urges and arousal precipitated by fantasies; use of inanimate objects, such as clothing, to stimulate sexual arousal, orgasm.

302.82 Voyeurism
DEF: Psychosexual disorder characterized by uncontrollable impulse to observe others, without their knowledge, who are nude or engaged in sexual activity.

302.83 Sexual masochism
DEF: Psychosexual disorder noted for need to achieve sexual gratification through humiliating or hurtful acts inflicted on self.

302.84 Sexual sadism
DEF: Psychosexual disorder noted for need to achieve sexual gratification through humiliating or hurtful acts inflicted on someone else.

302.85 Gender identity disorder in adolescents or adults
Use additional code to identify sex reassignment surgery status (302.5)
EXCLUDES gender identity disorder NOS (302.6)
gender identity disorder in children (302.6)

302.89 Other
Frotteurism
Nymphomania
Satyriasis

302.9 Unspecified psychosexual disorder
Paraphilia NOS
Pathologic sexuality NOS
Sexual deviation NOS
Sexual disorder NOS

☑4ᵗʰ **303 Alcohol dependence syndrome**

Use additional code to identify any associated condition, as:
    alcoholic psychoses (291.0-291.9)
    drug dependence (304.0-304.9)
    physical complications of alcohol, such as:
      cerebral degeneration (331.7)
      cirrhosis of liver (571.2)
      epilepsy (345.0-345.9)
      gastritis (535.3)
      hepatitis (571.1)
      liver damage NOS (571.3)

EXCLUDES *drunkenness NOS (305.0)*

The following fifth-digit subclassification is for use with category 303:

  0 unspecified
  1 continuous
  2 episodic
  3 in remission

AHA: 1Q, '10, 20-21; 3Q, '95, 6; 2Q, '91, 9; 4Q, '88, 8; S-O, '86, 3
TIP: The patient has become physically addicted to alcohol and often experiences withdrawal symptoms when not drinking. Do not assign both 303.0X and 303.9X on the same encounter.

§ ☑5ᵗʰ **303.0 Acute alcoholic intoxication**
[0-3]   Acute drunkenness in alcoholism

§ ☑5ᵗʰ **303.9 Other and unspecified alcohol dependence**
[0-3]   Chronic alcoholism
       Dipsomania
       AHA: 2Q, '02, 4; 2Q, '89, 9; **For code 303.90:** 2Q, '07, 6
       F10.20 Alcohol dependence uncomplicated   I-10
       F10.21 Alcohol dependence in remission   I-10

☑4ᵗʰ **304 Drug dependence**

EXCLUDES *nondependent abuse of drugs (305.1-305.9)*

The following fifth-digit subclassification is for use with category 304:

  0 unspecified
  1 continuous
  2 episodic
  3 in remission

AHA: 1Q, '10, 20-21; 2Q, '91, 10; 4Q, '88, 8; S-O, '86, 3

§ ☑5ᵗʰ **304.0 Opioid type dependence**
[0-3]   Heroin
       Meperidine
       Methadone
       Morphine
       Opium
       Opium alkaloids and their derivatives
       Synthetics with morphine-like effects
       AHA: 2Q, '06, 7; **For code 304.00:** 1Q, '11, 15; 2Q, '10, 13

§ ☑5ᵗʰ **304.1 Sedative, hypnotic or anxiolytic dependence**
[0-3]   Barbiturates
       Nonbarbiturate sedatives and tranquilizers with a similar
          effect:
          chlordiazepoxide
          diazepam
          glutethimide
          meprobamate
          methaqualone

§ ☑5ᵗʰ **304.2 Cocaine dependence**
[0-3]   Coca leaves and derivatives
       F14.20 Cocaine dependence uncomplicated   I-10

§ ☑5ᵗʰ **304.3 Cannabis dependence**
[0-3]   Hashish
       Hemp
       Marihuana

§ ☑5ᵗʰ **304.4 Amphetamine and other psychostimulant dependence**
[0-3]   Methylphenidate
       Phenmetrazine

§ ☑5ᵗʰ **304.5 Hallucinogen dependence**
[0-3]   Dimethyltryptamine [DMT]
       Lysergic acid diethylamide [LSD] and derivatives
       Mescaline
       Psilocybin

§ ☑5ᵗʰ **304.6 Other specified drug dependence**
[0-3]   Absinthe addiction
       Glue sniffing
       Inhalant dependence
       Phencyclidine dependence
       EXCLUDES *tobacco dependence (305.1)*

§ ☑5ᵗʰ **304.7 Combinations of opioid type drug with any other**
[0-3]   **AHA:** M-A, '86, 12

§ ☑5ᵗʰ **304.8 Combinations of drug dependence excluding**
[0-3]   **opioid type drug**
       AHA: M-A, '86, 12

§ ☑5ᵗʰ **304.9 Unspecified drug dependence**
[0-3]   Drug addiction NOS
       Drug dependence NOS
       AHA: For code 304.90: 4Q, '03, 103

☑4ᵗʰ **305 Nondependent abuse of drugs**

NOTE Includes cases where a person, for whom no other diagnosis is possible, has come under medical care because of the maladaptive effect of a drug on which he is not dependent and that he has taken on his own initiative to the detriment of his health or social functioning.

EXCLUDES *alcohol dependence syndrome (303.0-303.9)*
       drug dependence (304.0-304.9)
       drug withdrawal syndrome (292.0)
       poisoning by drugs or medicinal substances (960.0-979.9)

The following fifth-digit subclassification is for use with codes 305.0, 305.2-305.9:

  0 unspecified
  1 continuous
  2 episodic
  3 in remission

AHA: 1Q, '10, 20-21; 2Q, '91, 10; 4Q, '88, 8; S-O, '86, 3

§ ☑5ᵗʰ **305.0 Alcohol abuse**
[0-3]   Drunkenness NOS
       Excessive drinking of alcohol NOS
       "Hangover" (alcohol)
       Inebriety NOS
       EXCLUDES *acute alcohol intoxication in alcoholism (303.0)*
          alcoholic psychoses (291.0-291.9)
       AHA: 3Q, '96, 16; **For code 305.00:** 4Q, '09, 112
       F10.10 Alcohol abuse uncomplicated   I-10

    305.1 Tobacco use disorder
       Tobacco dependence
       EXCLUDES *history of tobacco use (V15.82)*
          smoking complicating pregnancy (649.0)
          tobacco use disorder complicating pregnancy (649.0)
       AHA: 1Q, '09, 16; 2Q, '96, 10; N-D, '84, 12
       F17.210 Nicotine dependence cigarettes uncomplicated   I-10

§ ☑5ᵗʰ **305.2 Cannabis abuse**
[0-3]   **F12.10** Cannabis abuse uncomplicated   I-10

§ ☑5ᵗʰ **305.3 Hallucinogen abuse**
[0-3]   Acute intoxication from hallucinogens ["bad trips"]
       LSD reaction

§ ☑5ᵗʰ **305.4 Sedative, hypnotic or anxiolytic abuse**
[0-3]

§ ☑5ᵗʰ **305.5 Opioid abuse**
[0-3]

§ ☑5ᵗʰ **305.6 Cocaine abuse**
[0-3]   **AHA:** 1Q, '93, 25; **For code 305.60:** 1Q, '05, 6
       F14.10 Cocaine abuse uncomplicated   I-10

§ ☑5ᵗʰ **305.7 Amphetamine or related acting sympathomimetic**
[0-3]   **abuse**
       AHA: For code 305.70: 2Q, '03, 10-11

§ ☑5ᵗʰ **305.8 Antidepressant type abuse**
[0-3]

---

§ Requires fifth digit. Valid digits are in [brackets] under each code. See appropriate category for codes and definitions.

☑4ᵗʰ
☑5ᵗʰ Additional Digit Required   Unspecified Code   Other Specified Code   Manifestation Code   ►◄ Revised Text   ● New Code   ▲ Revised Code Title

§ ✓5ᵗʰ **305.9 Other, mixed, or unspecified drug abuse**
[0-3]   Caffeine intoxication
Inhalant abuse
"Laxative habit"
Misuse of drugs NOS
Nonprescribed use of drugs or patent medicinals
Phencyclidine abuse
AHA: 3Q, '99, 20

✓4ᵗʰ **306 Physiological malfunction arising from mental factors**
INCLUDES psychogenic:
physical symptoms ⎫
physiological ⎬ not involving tissue
manifestations ⎭ damage
EXCLUDES hysteria (300.11-300.19)
physical symptoms secondary to a psychiatric disorder classified elsewhere
psychic factors associated with physical conditions involving tissue damage classified elsewhere (316)
specific nonpsychotic mental disorders following organic brain damage (310.0-310.9)
DEF: Functional disturbances or interruptions due to mental or psychological causes; no tissue damage sustained in these conditions.

306.0 Musculoskeletal
Psychogenic paralysis   Psychogenic torticollis
EXCLUDES Gilles de la Tourette's syndrome (307.23)
paralysis as hysterical or conversion reaction (300.11)
tics (307.20-307.22)

306.1 Respiratory
Psychogenic: Psychogenic:
air hunger   hyperventilation
cough   yawning
hiccough
EXCLUDES psychogenic asthma (316 and 493.9)

306.2 Cardiovascular
Cardiac neurosis
Cardiovascular neurosis
Neurocirculatory asthenia
Psychogenic cardiovascular disorder
EXCLUDES psychogenic paroxysmal tachycardia (316 and 427.2)
DEF: Neurocirculatory asthenia: functional nervous and circulatory irregularities with palpitations, dyspnea, fatigue, rapid pulse, precordial pain, fear of effort, discomfort during exercise, anxiety; also called DaCosta's syndrome, Effort syndrome, Irritable or Soldier's Heart.
AHA: J-A, '85, 14

306.3 Skin
Psychogenic pruritus
EXCLUDES psychogenic:
alopecia (316 and 704.00)
dermatitis (316 and 692.9)
eczema (316 and 691.8 or 692.9)
urticaria (316 and 708.0-708.9)

306.4 Gastrointestinal
Aerophagy
Cyclical vomiting, psychogenic
Diarrhea, psychogenic
Nervous gastritis
Psychogenic dyspepsia
EXCLUDES cyclical vomiting NOS (536.2)
associated with migraine (346.2)
globus hystericus (300.11)
mucous colitis (316 and 564.9)
psychogenic:
cardiospasm (316 and 530.0)
duodenal ulcer (316 and 532.0-532.9)
gastric ulcer (316 and 531.0-531.9)
peptic ulcer NOS (316 and 533.0-533.9)
vomiting NOS (307.54)
DEF: Aerophagy: excess swallowing of air, usually unconscious; related to anxiety; results in distended abdomen or belching, often interpreted by the patient as a physical disorder.
AHA: 2Q, '89, 11

✓5ᵗʰ **306.5 Genitourinary**
EXCLUDES enuresis, psychogenic (307.6)
frigidity (302.72)
impotence (302.72)
psychogenic dyspareunia (302.76)

306.50 Psychogenic genitourinary malfunction, unspecified

306.51 Psychogenic vaginismus   ♀
Functional vaginismus
DEF: Psychogenic response resulting in painful contractions of vaginal canal muscles; can be severe enough to prevent sexual intercourse.

306.52 Psychogenic dysmenorrhea   ♀

306.53 Psychogenic dysuria

306.59 Other
AHA: M-A, '87, 11

306.6 Endocrine

306.7 Organs of special sense
EXCLUDES hysterical blindness or deafness (300.11)
psychophysical visual disturbances (368.16)

306.8 Other specified psychophysiological malfunction
Bruxism
Teeth grinding

306.9 Unspecified psychophysiological malfunction
Psychophysiologic disorder NOS
Psychosomatic disorder NOS

✓4ᵗʰ **307 Special symptoms or syndromes, not elsewhere classified**
NOTE This category is intended for use if the psychopathology is manifested by a single specific symptom or group of symptoms which is not part of an organic illness or other mental disorder classifiable elsewhere.
EXCLUDES those due to mental disorders classified elsewhere
those of organic origin

307.0 Adult onset fluency disorder
EXCLUDES childhood onset fluency disorder (315.35)x
dysphasia (784.59)
fluency disorder due to late effect of cerebrovascular accident (438.14)
fluency disorder in conditions classified elsewhere (784.52)
lisping or lalling (307.9)
retarded development of speech (315.31-315.39)
AHA: 4Q, '10, 83

307.1 Anorexia nervosa
EXCLUDES eating disturbance NOS (307.50)
feeding problem (783.3)
of nonorganic origin (307.59)
loss of appetite (783.0)
of nonorganic origin (307.59)
AHA: 2Q, '06, 12; 4Q, '89, 11
TIP: Assign an additional code for any associated malnutrition.

✓5ᵗʰ **307.2 Tics**
EXCLUDES nail-biting or thumb-sucking (307.9)
stereotypes occurring in isolation (307.3)
tics of organic origin (333.3)
DEF: Involuntary muscle response usually confined to the face, shoulders.

307.20 Tic disorder, unspecified
Tic disorder NOS

307.21 Transient tic disorder

307.22 Chronic motor or vocal tic disorder

307.23 Tourette's disorder
Motor-verbal tic disorder
DEF: Syndrome of facial and vocal tics in childhood; progresses to spontaneous or involuntary jerking, obscene utterances, other uncontrollable actions considered inappropriate.

---

§ Requires fifth digit. Valid digits are in [brackets] under each code. See category 305 for codes and definitions.

Ⓝ Newborn Age: 0   Ⓟ Pediatric Age: 0-17   Ⓜ Maternity Age: 12-55   Ⓐ Adult Age: 15-124

307.3 Stereotypic movement disorder
Body-rocking
Head banging
Spasmus nutans
Stereotypes NOS
EXCLUDES tics (307.20-307.23)
of organic origin (333.3)

√5ᵗʰ 307.4 Specific disorders of sleep of nonorganic origin
EXCLUDES narcolepsy (347.00-347.11)
organic hypersomnia (327.10-327.19)
organic insomnia (327.00-327.09)
those of unspecified cause (780.50-780.59)

307.40 Nonorganic sleep disorder, unspecified

307.41 Transient disorder of initiating or maintaining sleep
Adjustment insomnia
Hyposomnia ⎫ associated with intermittent
Insomnia ⎬ emotional reactions
Sleeplessness ⎭ or conflicts

307.42 Persistent disorder of initiating or maintaining sleep
Hyposomnia, insomnia, or sleeplessness associated with:
anxiety
conditioned arousal
depression (major) (minor)
psychosis
Idiopathic insomnia
Paradoxical insomnia
Primary insomnia
Psychophysiological insomnia

307.43 Transient disorder of initiating or maintaining wakefulness
Hypersomnia associated with acute or intermittent emotional reactions or conflicts

307.44 Persistent disorder of initiating or maintaining wakefulness
Hypersomnia associated with depression (major) (minor)
Insufficient sleep syndrome
Primary hypersomnia
EXCLUDES sleep deprivation (V69.4)

307.45 Circadian rhythm sleep disorder of nonorganic origin

307.46 Sleep arousal disorder
Night terror disorder
Night terrors
Sleep terror disorder
Sleepwalking
Somnambulism
DEF: Sleepwalking marked by extreme terror, panic, screaming, confusion; no recall of event upon arousal; term may refer to simply the act of sleepwalking.

307.47 Other dysfunctions of sleep stages or arousal from sleep
Nightmare disorder
Nightmares:
NOS
REM-sleep type
Sleep drunkenness

307.48 Repetitive intrusions of sleep
Repetitive intrusion of sleep with:
atypical polysomnographic features
environmental disturbances
repeated REM-sleep interruptions

307.49 Other
"Short-sleeper"
Subjective insomnia complaint

√5ᵗʰ 307.5 Other and unspecified disorders of eating
EXCLUDES anorexia:
nervosa (307.1)
of unspecified cause (783.0)
overeating, of unspecified cause (783.6)
vomiting:
NOS (787.03)
cyclical (536.2)
associated with migraine (346.2)
psychogenic (306.4)

307.50 Eating disorder, unspecified
Eating disorder NOS

307.51 Bulimia nervosa
Overeating of nonorganic origin
DEF: Mental disorder commonly characterized by binge eating followed by self-induced vomiting; perceptions of being fat; and fear the inability to stop eating voluntarily.

307.52 Pica
Perverted appetite of nonorganic origin
DEF: Compulsive eating disorder characterized by craving for substances other than food, such as paint chips or dirt.

307.53 Rumination disorder
Regurgitation, of nonorganic origin, of food with reswallowing
EXCLUDES obsessional rumination (300.3)

307.54 Psychogenic vomiting

307.59 Other
Feeding disorder of infancy or early childhood of nonorganic origin
Infantile feeding disturbances ⎫ of nonorganic
Loss of appetite ⎬ origin

307.6 Enuresis
Enuresis (primary) (secondary) of nonorganic origin
EXCLUDES enuresis of unspecified cause (788.3)
DEF: Involuntary urination past age of normal control; also called bedwetting; no trace to biological problem; focus on psychological issues.

307.7 Encopresis
Encopresis (continuous) (discontinuous) of nonorganic origin
EXCLUDES encopresis of unspecified cause (787.60-787.63)
DEF: Inability to control bowel movements; cause traced to psychological, not biological, problems.

√5ᵗʰ 307.8 Pain disorders related to psychological factors

307.80 Psychogenic pain, site unspecified

307.81 Tension headache
EXCLUDES headache:
NOS (784.0)
migraine (346.0-346.9)
syndromes (339.00-339.89)
tension type (339.10-339.12)
AHA: 4Q, '08, 103; N-D, '85, 16

307.89 Other
Code first to type or site of pain
EXCLUDES pain disorder exclusively attributed to psychological factors (307.80)
psychogenic pain (307.80)

307.9 Other and unspecified special symptoms or syndromes, not elsewhere classified
Communication disorder NOS
Hair plucking
Lalling
Lisping
Masturbation
Nail-biting
Thumb-sucking

✓4ᵗʰ **308   Acute reaction to stress**

> INCLUDES   combat and operational stress reaction
>
> EXCLUDES   *adjustment reaction or disorder (309.0-309.9)*
> *chronic stress reaction (309.1-309.9)*

308.0   Predominant disturbance of emotions

Anxiety
Emotional crisis   } as acute reaction to exceptional
Panic state   [gross] stress

308.1   Predominant disturbance of consciousness

Fugues as acute reaction to exceptional [gross] stress

308.2   Predominant psychomotor disturbance

Agitation states } as acute reaction to exceptional
Stupor   [gross] stress

308.3   Other acute reactions to stress

Acute situational disturbance
Acute stress disorder

> EXCLUDES   *prolonged posttraumatic emotional disturbance (309.81)*

308.4   Mixed disorders as reaction to stress

308.9   Unspecified acute reaction to stress

✓4ᵗʰ **309   Adjustment reaction**

> INCLUDES   adjustment disorders
> reaction (adjustment) to chronic stress
>
> EXCLUDES   *acute reaction to major stress (308.0-308.9)*
> *neurotic disorders (300.0-300.9)*

309.0   Adjustment disorder with depressed mood

Grief reaction

> EXCLUDES   *affective psychoses (296.0-296.9)*
> *neurotic depression (300.4)*
> *prolonged depressive reaction (309.1)*
> *psychogenic depressive psychosis (298.0)*
>
> F43.21 Adjustment disorder with depressed mood   I-10

309.1   Prolonged depressive reaction

> EXCLUDES   *affective psychoses (296.0-296.9)*
> *brief depressive reaction (309.0)*
> *neurotic depression (300.4)*
> *psychogenic depressive psychosis (298.0)*

✓5ᵗʰ **309.2   With predominant disturbance of other emotions**

309.21   Separation anxiety disorder

> **DEF:** Abnormal apprehension by a child when physically separated from support environment; byproduct of abnormal symbiotic child-parent relationship.

309.22   Emancipation disorder of adolescence and early adult life

> **DEF:** Adjustment reaction of late adolescence; conflict over independence from parental supervision; symptoms include difficulty in making decisions, increased reliance on parental advice, deliberate adoption of values in opposition of parents.

309.23   Specific academic or work inhibition

309.24   Adjustment disorder with anxiety

309.28   Adjustment disorder with mixed anxiety and depressed mood

Adjustment reaction with anxiety and depression

> F43.23 Adjustment d/o w/mixed anxiety & depressed   I-10
> mood

309.29   Other

Culture shock

309.3   Adjustment disorder with disturbance of conduct

Conduct disturbance } as adjustment reaction
Destructiveness

> EXCLUDES   *destructiveness in child (312.9)*
> *disturbance of conduct NOS (312.9)*
> *dyssocial behavior without manifest psychiatric disorder (V71.01-V71.02)*
> *personality disorder with predominantly sociopathic or asocial manifestations (301.7)*

309.4   Adjustment disorder with mixed disturbance of emotions and conduct

✓5ᵗʰ **309.8   Other specified adjustment reactions**

309.81   Posttraumatic stress disorder

Chronic posttraumatic stress disorder
Concentration camp syndrome
Posttraumatic stress disorder NOS
Post-traumatic stress disorder (PTSD)

> EXCLUDES   *acute stress disorder (308.3)*
> *posttraumatic brain syndrome:*
> *nonpsychotic (310.2)*
> *psychotic (293.0-293.9)*
>
> **DEF:** Preoccupation with traumatic events beyond normal experience; i.e., rape, personal assault, etc,; also recurring flashbacks of trauma; symptoms include difficulty remembering, sleeping, or concentrating, and guilt feelings for surviving.
> **AHA:** 2Q, '11, 5

309.82   Adjustment reaction with physical symptoms

309.83   Adjustment reaction with withdrawal

Elective mutism as adjustment reaction
Hospitalism (in children) NOS

309.89   Other

309.9   Unspecified adjustment reaction

Adaptation reaction NOS
Adjustment reaction NOS

✓4ᵗʰ **310   Specific nonpsychotic mental disorders due to brain damage**

> EXCLUDES   *neuroses, personality disorders, or other nonpsychotic conditions occurring in a form similar to that seen with functional disorders but in association with a physical condition (300.0-300.9, 301.0-301.9)*

310.0   Frontal lobe syndrome

Lobotomy syndrome
Postleucotomy syndrome [state]

> EXCLUDES   *postcontusion syndrome (310.2)*

310.1   Personality change due to conditions classified elsewhere

Cognitive or personality change of other type, of nonpsychotic severity
Organic psychosyndrome of nonpsychotic severity
Presbyophrenia NOS
Senility with mental changes of nonpsychotic severity

> EXCLUDES   *mild cognitive impairment (331.83)*
> *postconcussion syndrome (310.2)*
> *signs and symptoms involving emotional state (799.21-799.29)*
>
> **DEF:** Personality disorder caused by organic factors, such as brain lesions, head trauma, or cerebrovascular accident (CVA).
> **AHA:** 2Q, '05, 6

310.2   Postconcussion syndrome

Postcontusion syndrome or encephalopathy
Posttraumatic brain syndrome, nonpsychotic
Status postcommotio cerebri

Use additional code to identify associated post-traumatic headache, if applicable (339.20-339.22)

> EXCLUDES   *any organic psychotic conditions following head injury (293.0-294.0)*
> *frontal lobe syndrome (310.0)*
> *postencephalitic syndrome (310.89)*
>
> **DEF:** Nonpsychotic disorder due to brain trauma, causes symptoms unrelated to any disease process; symptoms include amnesia, serial headaches, rapid heartbeat, fatigue, disrupted sleep patterns, inability to concentrate.
> **AHA:** 4Q, '90, 24
> **TIP:** For treatment within 24 to 48 hours of the concussion, clarify with physician whether the concussion is still in the acute phase; if so, assign instead a code from 850.x subcategory.

✓5ᵗʰ **310.8   Other specified nonpsychotic mental disorders following organic brain damage**

> **AHA:** ▶4Q, '11, 96-97◀

310.81   Pseudobulbar affect

Involuntary emotional expression disorder

Code first underlying cause, if known, such as:
amyotrophic lateral sclerosis (335.20)
late effect of cerebrovascular accident (438.89)
late effect of traumatic brain injury (907.0)
mutiple sclerosis (340)

> **AHA:** ▶4Q, '11, 97◀

N   Newborn Age: 0   P   Pediatric Age: 0-17   M   Maternity Age: 12-55   A   Adult Age: 15-124

310.89 Other specified nonpsychotic mental disorders following organic brain damage
Mild memory disturbance
Other focal (partial) organic psychosyndromes
Postencephalitic syndrome
EXCLUDES *memory loss of unknown cause (780.93)*

310.9 Unspecified nonpsychotic mental disorder following organic brain damage
AHA: 4Q, '03, 103

311 Depressive disorder, not elsewhere classified
Depressive disorder NOS
Depressive state NOS
Depression NOS
EXCLUDES *acute reaction to major stress with depressive symptoms (308.0)*
affective personality disorder (301.10-301.13)
affective psychoses (296.0-296.9)
brief depressive reaction (309.0)
depressive states associated with stressful events (309.0-309.1)
disturbance of emotions specific to childhood and adolescence, with misery and unhappiness (313.1)
mixed adjustment reaction with depressive symptoms (309.4)
neurotic depression (300.4)
prolonged depressive adjustment reaction (309.1)
psychogenic depressive psychosis (298.0)
AHA: ▶3Q, '11, 6;◀ 4Q, '03, 75

✓4ᵗʰ 312 Disturbance of conduct, not elsewhere classified
EXCLUDES *adjustment reaction with disturbance of conduct (309.3)*
drug dependence (304.0-304.9)
dyssocial behavior without manifest psychiatric disorder (V71.01-V71.02)
personality disorder with predominantly sociopathic or asocial manifestations (301.7)
sexual deviations (302.0-302.9)

The following fifth-digit subclassification is for use with categories 312.0-312.2
   0 unspecified
   1 mild
   2 moderate
   3 severe

§ ✓5ᵗʰ **312.0 Undersocialized conduct disorder, aggressive type**
[0-3]   Aggressive outburst
   Anger reaction
   Unsocialized aggressive disorder
   DEF: Mental condition identified by behaviors disrespectful of others' rights and of age-appropriate social norms or rules; symptoms include bullying, vandalism, verbal and physical abusiveness, lying, stealing, defiance.

§ ✓5ᵗʰ **312.1 Undersocialized conduct disorder, unaggressive type**
[0-3]   Childhood truancy, unsocialized
   Solitary stealing
   Tantrums

§ ✓5ᵗʰ **312.2 Socialized conduct disorder**
[0-3]   Childhood truancy, socialized
   Group delinquency
   EXCLUDES *gang activity without manifest psychiatric disorder (V71.01)*

✓5ᵗʰ **312.3 Disorders of impulse control, not elsewhere classified**

   312.30 Impulse control disorder, unspecified

   312.31 Pathological gambling

   312.32 Kleptomania

   312.33 Pyromania

   312.34 Intermittent explosive disorder

   312.35 Isolated explosive disorder

   312.39 Other
      Trichotillomania

312.4 Mixed disturbance of conduct and emotions
Neurotic delinquency
EXCLUDES *compulsive conduct disorder (312.3)*

✓5ᵗʰ **312.8 Other specified disturbances of conduct, not elsewhere classified**

   312.81 Conduct disorder, childhood onset type

   312.82 Conduct disorder, adolescent onset type

   312.89 Other conduct disorder
      Conduct disorder of unspecified onset

312.9 Unspecified disturbance of conduct
Delinquency (juvenile)
Disruptive behavior disorder NOS
AHA: 2Q, '11, 5

✓4ᵗʰ **313 Disturbance of emotions specific to childhood and adolescence**
EXCLUDES *adjustment reaction (309.0-309.9)*
emotional disorder of neurotic type (300.0-300.9)
masturbation, nail-biting, thumbsucking, and other isolated symptoms (307.0-307.9)

313.0 Overanxious disorder
Anxiety and fearfulness } of childhood and
Overanxious disorder } adolescence
EXCLUDES *abnormal separation anxiety (309.21)*
anxiety states (300.00-300.09)
hospitalism in children (309.83)
phobic state (300.20-300.29)

313.1 Misery and unhappiness disorder
EXCLUDES *depressive neurosis (300.4)*

✓5ᵗʰ **313.2 Sensitivity, shyness, and social withdrawal disorder**
EXCLUDES *infantile autism (299.0)*
schizoid personality (301.20-301.22)
schizophrenia (295.0-295.9)

   313.21 Shyness disorder of childhood
      Sensitivity reaction of childhood or adolescence

   313.22 Introverted disorder of childhood
      Social withdrawal } of childhood and
      Withdrawal reaction } adolescence

   313.23 Selective mutism
      EXCLUDES *elective mutism as adjustment reaction (309.83)*

313.3 Relationship problems
Sibling jealousy
EXCLUDES *relationship problems associated with aggression, destruction, or other forms of conduct disturbance (312.0-312.9)*

✓5ᵗʰ **313.8 Other or mixed emotional disturbances of childhood or adolescence**

   313.81 Oppositional defiant disorder
      DEF: Mental disorder of children noted for pervasive opposition, defiance of authority.

   313.82 Identity disorder
      Identity problem
      DEF: Distress of adolescents caused by inability to form acceptable self-identity; uncertainty about career choice, sexual orientation, moral values.

   313.83 Academic underachievement disorder

   313.89 Other   P
      Reactive attachment disorder of infancy or early childhood

313.9 Unspecified emotional disturbance of childhood or adolescence   P
Mental disorder of infancy, childhood or adolescence NOS

---

§   Requires fifth digit. Valid digits are in [brackets] under each code. See category 312 for codes and definitions.

| ✓4ᵗʰ ✓5ᵗʰ Additional Digit Required | Unspecified Code | Other Specified Code | Manifestation Code | ▶◀ Revised Text | ● New Code | ▲ Revised Code Title |

Mental, Behavioral and Neurodevelopmental Disorders

314–319

✓4ᵗʰ **314 Hyperkinetic syndrome of childhood**
    EXCLUDES *hyperkinesis as symptom of underlying disorder — code the underlying disorder*

✓5ᵗʰ **314.0 Attention deficit disorder**
    Adult
    Child
    DEF: A behavioral disorder usually diagnosed at an early age; characterized by the inability to focus attention for a normal period of time.
    TIP: These codes may be assigned for patients of any age.

    314.00 Without mention of hyperactivity
        Predominantly inattentive type
        AHA: 1Q, '97, 8

    314.01 With hyperactivity
        Combined type
        Overactivity NOS
        Predominantly hyperactive/impulsive type
        Simple disturbance of attention with overactivity
        AHA: 2Q, '11, 5; 1Q, '97, 8
        F90.1 ADHD predominantly hyperactive type   I-10

314.1 Hyperkinesis with developmental delay
    Developmental disorder of hyperkinesis
    Use additional code to identify any associated neurological disorder

314.2 Hyperkinetic conduct disorder
    Hyperkinetic conduct disorder without developmental delay
    EXCLUDES *hyperkinesis with significant delays in specific skills (314.1)*

314.8 Other specified manifestations of hyperkinetic syndrome

314.9 Unspecified hyperkinetic syndrome
    Hyperkinetic reaction of childhood or adolescence NOS
    Hyperkinetic syndrome NOS

✓4ᵗʰ **315 Specific delays in development**
    EXCLUDES *that due to a neurological disorder (320.0-389.9)*

✓5ᵗʰ **315.0 Specific reading disorder**

    315.00 Reading disorder, unspecified

    315.01 Alexia
        DEF: Lack of ability to understand written language; manifestation of aphasia.

    315.02 Developmental dyslexia
        DEF: Serious impairment of reading skills unexplained in relation to general intelligence and teaching processes.

    315.09 Other
        Specific spelling difficulty

315.1 Mathematics disorder
    Dyscalculia

315.2 Other specific learning difficulties
    Disorder of written expression
    EXCLUDES *specific arithmetical disorder (315.1)*
                specific reading disorder (315.00-315.09)

✓5ᵗʰ **315.3 Developmental speech or language disorder**

    315.31 Expressive language disorder
        Developmental aphasia
        Word deafness
        EXCLUDES *acquired aphasia (784.3)*
                 elective mutism (309.83, 313.0, 313.23)

    315.32 Mixed receptive-expressive language disorder
        Central auditory processing disorder
        EXCLUDES *acquired auditory processing disorder (388.45)*

    315.34 Speech and language developmental delay due to hearing loss
        AHA: 4Q, '07, 80, 81

315.35 Childhood onset fluency disorder
    Cluttering NOS
    Stuttering NOS
    EXCLUDES *adult onset fluency disorder (307.0)*
              fluency disorder due to late effect of cerebrovascular accident (438.14)
              fluency disorder in conditions classified elsewhere (784.52)
    AHA: 4Q, '10, 83-84
    F80.81 Child onset fluency disorder   I-10

315.39 Other
    Developmental articulation disorder
    Dyslalia
    Phonological disorder
    EXCLUDES *lisping and lalling (307.9)*
    AHA: 3Q, '07, 7

315.4 Developmental coordination disorder
    Clumsiness syndrome
    Dyspraxia syndrome
    Specific motor development disorder

315.5 Mixed development disorder
    AHA: 2Q, '02, 11

315.8 Other specified delays in development
    F88 Other disorders of psychological development   I-10

315.9 Unspecified delay in development
    Developmental disorder NOS
    Learning disorder NOS

316 Psychic factors associated with diseases classified elsewhere
    Psychologic factors in physical conditions classified elsewhere
    Use additional code to identify the associated physical condition, as:
    psychogenic:
        asthma (493.9)
        dermatitis (692.9)
        duodenal ulcer (532.0-532.9)
        eczema (691.8, 692.9)
        gastric ulcer (531.0-531.9)
        mucous colitis (564.9)
        paroxysmal tachycardia (427.2)
        ulcerative colitis (556)
        urticaria (708.0-708.9)
    psychosocial dwarfism (259.4)
    EXCLUDES *physical symptoms and physiological malfunctions, not involving tissue damage, of mental origin (306.0-306.9)*

INTELLECTUAL DISABILITIES (317-319)

Use additional code(s) to identify any associated psychiatric or physical condition(s)
AHA: ▶4Q, '11, 98◀

317 Mild intellectual disabilities
    High-grade defect
    IQ 50-70
    Mild mental subnormality
    F70 Mild intellectual disabilities   I-10

✓4ᵗʰ **318 Other specified intellectual disabilities**
    AHA: ▶4Q, '11, 98◀

    318.0 Moderate intellectual disabilities
        IQ 35-49
        Moderate mental subnormality

    318.1 Severe intellectual disabilities
        IQ 20-34
        Severe mental subnormality

    318.2 Profound intellectual disabilities
        IQ under 20
        Profound mental subnormality

319 Unspecified intellectual disabilities
    Mental deficiency NOS
    Mental subnormality NOS
    AHA: ▶4Q, '11, 98◀
    F79 Unspecified intellectual disabilities   I-10

N Newborn Age: 0   P Pediatric Age: 0-17   M Maternity Age: 12-55   A Adult Age: 15-124

6. Diseases of the Nervous System and Sense Organs (320-389)

Inflammatory Diseases of the Central Nervous System (320-326)

✓4ᵗʰ 320 Bacterial meningitis

INCLUDES arachnoiditis
leptomeningitis
meningitis   } bacterial
meningoencephalitis
meningomyelitis
pachymeningitis

DEF: Bacterial infection causing inflammation of the lining of the brain and/or spinal cord.
AHA: J-F, '87, 6

320.0 Hemophilus meningitis
Meningitis due to Hemophilus influenzae [H. influenzae]

320.1 Pneumococcal meningitis

320.2 Streptococcal meningitis

320.3 Staphylococcal meningitis

320.7 Meningitis in other bacterial diseases classified elsewhere
Code first underlying disease, as:
actinomycosis (039.8)
listeriosis (027.0)
typhoid fever (002.0)
whooping cough (033.0-033.9)

EXCLUDES *meningitis (in):*
epidemic (036.0)
gonococcal (098.82)
meningococcal (036.0)
salmonellosis (003.21)
syphilis:
NOS (094.2)
congenital (090.42)
meningovascular (094.2)
secondary (091.81)
tuberculous (013.0)

✓5ᵗʰ 320.8 Meningitis due to other specified bacteria

320.81 Anaerobic meningitis
Bacteroides (fragilis)   Gram-negative anaerobes

320.82 Meningitis due to gram-negative bacteria, not elsewhere classified
Aerobacter aerogenes   Klebsiella
pneumoniae   Proteus morganii
Escherichia coli [E. coli]   Pseudomonas
Friedländer bacillus

EXCLUDES *gram-negative anaerobes (320.81)*
AHA: ▶4Q, '11, 155◀

320.89 Meningitis due to other specified bacteria
Bacillus pyocyaneus

320.9 Meningitis due to unspecified bacterium
Meningitis: Meningitis:
bacterial NOS   pyogenic NOS
purulent NOS   suppurative NOS

✓4ᵗʰ 321 Meningitis due to other organisms

INCLUDES arachnoiditis
leptomeningitis   } due to organisms other
meningitis   than bacterial
pachymeningitis

DEF: Infection causing inflammation of the lining of the brain and/or spinal cord, due to organisms other than bacteria.
AHA: J-F, '87, 6

321.0 Cryptococcal meningitis
Code first underlying disease (117.5)

321.1 Meningitis in other fungal diseases
Code first underlying disease (110.0-118)

EXCLUDES *meningitis in:*
candidiasis (112.83)
coccidioidomycosis (114.2)
histoplasmosis (115.01, 115.11, 115.91)

321.2 Meningitis due to viruses not elsewhere classified
Code first underlying disease, as:
meningitis due to arbovirus (060.0-066.9)

EXCLUDES *meningitis (due to):*
abacterial (047.0-047.9)
adenovirus (049.1)
aseptic NOS (047.9)
Coxsackie (virus)(047.0)
ECHO virus (047.1)
enterovirus (047.0-047.9)
herpes simplex virus (054.72)
herpes zoster virus (053.0)
lymphocytic choriomeningitis virus (049.0)
mumps (072.1)
viral NOS (047.9)
meningo-eruptive syndrome (047.1)

AHA: 4Q, '04, 51

321.3 Meningitis due to trypanosomiasis
Code first underlying disease (086.0-086.9)

321.4 Meningitis in sarcoidosis
Code first underlying disease (135)

321.8 Meningitis due to other nonbacterial organisms classified elsewhere
Code first underlying disease

EXCLUDES *leptospiral meningitis (100.81)*

✓4ᵗʰ 322 Meningitis of unspecified cause

INCLUDES arachnoiditis
leptomeningitis   } with no organism
meningitis   specified as cause
pachymeningitis

DEF: Infection causing inflammation of the lining of the brain and/or spinal cord, due to unspecified cause.
AHA: J-F, '87, 6

322.0 Nonpyogenic meningitis
Meningitis with clear cerebrospinal fluid

322.1 Eosinophilic meningitis

322.2 Chronic meningitis

322.9 Meningitis, unspecified

✓4ᵗʰ 323 Encephalitis, myelitis, and encephalomyelitis

INCLUDES acute disseminated encephalomyelitis
meningoencephalitis, except bacterial
meningomyelitis, except bacterial
myelitis:
ascending
transverse

EXCLUDES *acute transverse myelitis NOS (341.20)*
acute transverse myelitis in conditions classified elsewhere (341.21)
bacterial:
meningoencephalitis (320.0-320.9)
meningomyelitis (320.0-320.9)
idiopathic transverse myelitis (341.22)

DEF: Encephalitis: inflammation of brain tissues.
DEF: Myelitis: inflammation of the spinal cord.
DEF: Encephalomyelitis: inflammation of brain and spinal cord.

✓5ᵗʰ 323.0 Encephalitis, myelitis, and encephalomyelitis in viral diseases classified elsewhere
Code first underlying disease, as:
cat-scratch disease (078.3)
human immunodeficiency virus [HIV] disease (042)
infectious mononucleosis (075)
ornithosis (073.7)

Diseases of the Nervous System and Sense Organs

323.01–324.9

323.01 **Encephalitis and encephalomyelitis in viral diseases classified elsewhere**

> EXCLUDES   encephalitis (in):
> arthropod-borne viral (062.0-064)
> herpes simplex (054.3)
> mumps (072.2)
> other viral diseases of central nervous
>   system (049.8-049.9)
> poliomyelitis (045.0-045.9)
> rubella (056.01)
> slow virus infections of central nervous
>   system (046.0-046.9)
> viral NOS (049.9)
> West Nile (066.41)
>
> **AHA:** 3Q, '10, 13; 4Q, '06, 58-63

323.02 **Myelitis in viral diseases classified elsewhere**

> EXCLUDES   myelitis (in):
> herpes simplex (054.74)
> herpes zoster (053.14)
> poliomyelitis (045.0-045.9)
> rubella (056.01)
> other viral diseases of central nervous
>   system (049.8-049.9)
>
> **AHA:** 4Q, '06, 58-63

323.1 **Encephalitis, myelitis, and encephalomyelitis in rickettsial diseases classified elsewhere**

> Code first underlying disease (080-083.9)
> **DEF:** Inflammation of the brain caused by rickettsial disease carried by louse, tick, or mite.

323.2 **Encephalitis, myelitis, and encephalomyelitis in protozoal diseases classified elsewhere**

> Code first underlying disease, as:
>   malaria (084.0-084.9)
>   trypanosomiasis (086.0-086.9)
> **DEF:** Inflammation of the brain caused by protozoal disease carried by mosquitoes and flies.

√5ᵗʰ **323.4** **Other encephalitis, myelitis, and encephalomyelitis due to other infections classified elsewhere**

> Code first underlying disease

323.41 **Other encephalitis and encephalomyelitis due to other infections classified elsewhere**

> EXCLUDES   encephalitis (in):
> meningococcal (036.1)
> syphilis:
>   NOS (094.81)
>   congenital (090.41)
> toxoplasmosis (130.0)
> tuberculosis (013.6)
> meningoencephalitis due to free-living
>   ameba [Naegleria] (136.29)
>
> **AHA:** 4Q, '06, 58-63

323.42 **Other myelitis due to other infections classified elsewhere**

> EXCLUDES   myelitis (in):
> syphilis (094.89)
> tuberculosis (013.6)
>
> **AHA:** 4Q, '06, 58-63

√5ᵗʰ **323.5** **Encephalitis, myelitis, and encephalomyelitis following immunization procedures**

> Use additional E code to identify vaccine

323.51 **Encephalitis and encephalomyelitis following immunization procedures**

> Encephalitis postimmunization or postvaccinal
> Encephalomyelitis postimmunization or postvaccinal
> **AHA:** 4Q, '06, 58-63

323.52 **Myelitis following immunization procedures**

> Myelitis postimmunization or postvaccinal
> **AHA:** 4Q, '06, 58-63

√5ᵗʰ **323.6** **Postinfectious encephalitis, myelitis, and encephalomyelitis**

> Code first underlying disease
> **DEF:** Infection, inflammation of brain several weeks following the outbreak of a systemic infection.

323.61 **Infectious acute disseminated encephalomyelitis [ADEM]**

> Acute necrotizing hemorrhagic encephalopathy
> EXCLUDES   noninfectious acute disseminated
>   encephalomyelitis (ADEM) (323.81)
>
> **AHA:** 4Q, '06, 58-63

323.62 **Other postinfectious encephalitis and encephalomyelitis**

> EXCLUDES   encephalitis:
> postchickenpox (052.0)
> postmeasles (055.0)
>
> **AHA:** 4Q, '06, 58-63

323.63 **Postinfectious myelitis**

> EXCLUDES   postchickenpox myelitis (052.2)
> herpes simplex myelitis (054.74)
> herpes zoster myelitis (053.14)
>
> **AHA:** 4Q, '06, 58-63

√5ᵗʰ **323.7** **Toxic encephalitis, myelitis, and encephalomyelitis**

> Code first underlying cause, as:
>   carbon tetrachloride (982.1)
>   hydroxyquinoline derivatives (961.3)
>   lead (984.0-984.9)
>   mercury (985.0)
>   thallium (985.8)
> **AHA:** 2Q, '97, 8

323.71 **Toxic encephalitis and encephalomyelitis**

> **AHA:** 4Q, '06, 58-63

323.72 **Toxic myelitis**

> **AHA:** 4Q, '06, 58-63

√5ᵗʰ **323.8** **Other causes of encephalitis, myelitis, and encephalomyelitis**

323.81 **Other causes of encephalitis and encephalomyelitis**

> Noninfectious acute disseminated encephalomyelitis (ADEM)
> **AHA:** 1Q, '11, 12; 3Q, '10, 15; 4Q, '06, 58-63

323.82 **Other causes of myelitis**

> Transverse myelitis NOS
> **AHA:** 4Q, '06, 58-63

323.9 **Unspecified cause of encephalitis, myelitis, and encephalomyelitis**

√4ᵗʰ **324** **Intracranial and intraspinal abscess**

324.0 **Intracranial abscess**

> Abscess (embolic):
>   cerebellar
>   cerebral
> Abscess (embolic) of brain [any part]:
>   epidural
>   extradural
>   otogenic
>   subdural
> EXCLUDES   tuberculous (013.3)

324.1 **Intraspinal abscess**

> Abscess (embolic) of spinal cord [any part]:
>   epidural
>   extradural
>   subdural
> EXCLUDES   tuberculous (013.5)

324.9 **Of unspecified site**

> Extradural or subdural abscess NOS

N Newborn Age: 0   P Pediatric Age: 0-17   M Maternity Age: 12-55   A Adult Age: 15-124

325 Phlebitis and thrombophlebitis of intracranial venous sinuses

Embolism	of cavernous, lateral or other
Endophlebitis	intracranial or
Phlebitis, septic or suppurative	unspecified
Thrombophlebitis	intracranial venous
Thrombosis	sinus

> **EXCLUDES** that specified as:
>   complicating pregnancy, childbirth, or the puerperium
>   (671.5)
>   of nonpyogenic origin (437.6)

DEF: Inflammation and formation of blood clot in a vein within the brain or its lining.

326 Late effects of intracranial abscess or pyogenic infection

> **NOTE** This category is to be used to indicate conditions whose primary classification is to 320-325 [excluding 320.7, 321.0-321.8, 323.01-323.42, 323.6-323.7] as the cause of late effects, themselves classifiable elsewhere. The "late effects" include conditions specified as such, or as sequelae, which may occur at any time after the resolution of the causal condition.

Use additional code to identify condition, as:
    hydrocephalus (331.4)
    paralysis (342.0-342.9, 344.0-344.9)

Organic sleep disorders (327)

TIP: If the sleep disorder is not documented with the etiology related to an organic disease process, see instead subcategory 307.4.

√4ᵗʰ **327 Organic sleep disorders**

AHA: 4Q, '05, 59-64

√5ᵗʰ **327.0 Organic disorders of initiating and maintaining sleep [Organic insomnia]**

> **EXCLUDES** insomnia NOS (780.52)
>   insomnia not due to a substance or known
>   physiological condition (307.41-307.42)
>   insomnia with sleep apnea NOS (780.51)

327.00 Organic insomnia, unspecified

327.01 Insomnia due to medical condition classified elsewhere

> Code first underlying condition
> **EXCLUDES** insomnia due to mental disorder (327.02)

327.02 Insomnia due to mental disorder

> Code first mental disorder
> **EXCLUDES** alcohol induced insomnia (291.82)
>   drug induced insomnia (292.85)

327.09 Other organic insomnia

√5ᵗʰ **327.1 Organic disorder of excessive somnolence [Organic hypersomnia]**

> **EXCLUDES** hypersomnia NOS (780.54)
>   hypersomnia not due to a substance or known
>   physiological condition (307.43-307.44)
>   hypersomnia with sleep apnea NOS (780.53)

327.10 Organic hypersomnia, unspecified

327.11 Idiopathic hypersomnia with long sleep time

327.12 Idiopathic hypersomnia without long sleep time

327.13 Recurrent hypersomnia
    Kleine-Levin syndrome
    Menstrual related hypersomnia

327.14 Hypersomnia due to medical condition classified elsewhere

> Code first underlying condition
> **EXCLUDES** hypersomnia due to mental disorder (327.15)

327.15 Hypersomnia due to mental disorder

> Code first mental disorder
> **EXCLUDES** alcohol induced hypersomnia (291.82)
>   drug induced hypersomnia (292.85)

327.19 Other organic hypersomnia

√5ᵗʰ **327.2 Organic sleep apnea**

> **EXCLUDES** Cheyne-Stokes breathing (786.04)
>   hypersomnia with sleep apnea NOS (780.53)
>   insomnia with sleep apnea NOS (780.51)
>   sleep apnea in newborn (770.81-770.82)
>   sleep apnea NOS (780.57)

327.20 Organic sleep apnea, unspecified

327.21 Primary central sleep apnea

327.22 High altitude periodic breathing

327.23 Obstructive sleep apnea (adult) (pediatric)
    G47.33 Obstructive sleep apnea (adult) (pediatric)   I-10

327.24 Idiopathic sleep related nonobstructive alveolar hypoventilation
    Sleep related hypoxia

327.25 Congenital central alveolar hypoventilation syndrome

327.26 Sleep related hypoventilation/ hypoxemia in conditions classifiable elsewhere

> Code first underlying condition

327.27 Central sleep apnea in conditions classified elsewhere

> Code first underlying condition

327.29 Other organic sleep apnea

√4ᵗʰ **327.3 Circadian rhythm sleep disorder**
    Organic disorder of sleep wake cycle
    Organic disorder of sleep wake schedule

> **EXCLUDES** alcohol induced circadian rhythm sleep disorder
>   (291.82)
>   circadian rhythm sleep disorder of nonorganic origin
>   (307.45)
>   disruption of 24 hour sleep wake cycle NOS (780.55)
>   drug induced circadian rhythm sleep disorder
>   (292.85)

327.30 Circadian rhythm sleep disorder, unspecified

327.31 Circadian rhythm sleep disorder, delayed sleep phase type

327.32 Circadian rhythm sleep disorder, advanced sleep phase type

327.33 Circadian rhythm sleep disorder, irregular sleep-wake type

327.34 Circadian rhythm sleep disorder, free-running type

327.35 Circadian rhythm sleep disorder, jet lag type

327.36 Circadian rhythm sleep disorder, shift work type

327.37 Circadian rhythm sleep disorder in conditions classified elsewhere

> Code first underlying condition

327.39 Other circadian rhythm sleep disorder

√5ᵗʰ **327.4 Organic parasomnia**

> **EXCLUDES** alcohol induced parasomnia (291.82)
>   drug induced parasomnia (292.85)
>   parasomnia not due to a known physiological
>   condition (307.47)

327.40 Organic parasomnia, unspecified

327.41 Confusional arousals

327.42 REM sleep behavior disorder

327.43 Recurrent isolated sleep paralysis

327.44 Parasomnia in conditions classified elsewhere
> Code first underlying condition

327.49 Other organic parasomnia

√5ᵗʰ **327.5 Organic sleep related movement disorders**

> **EXCLUDES** restless legs syndrome (333.94)
>   sleep related movement disorder NOS (780.58)

327.51 Periodic limb movement disorder
    Periodic limb movement sleep disorder

327.52 Sleep related leg cramps

Diseases of the Nervous System and Sense Organs

327.53–331.82

    327.53 Sleep related bruxism

    327.59 Other organic sleep related movement disorders

  327.8 Other organic sleep disorders
      AHA: 2Q, '07, 6

Hereditary and Degenerative Diseases of the Central Nervous System (330-337)

> **EXCLUDES**   hepatolenticular degeneration (275.1)
> multiple sclerosis (340)
> other demyelinating diseases of central nervous system (341.0-341.9)

√4ᵗʰ **330 Cerebral degenerations usually manifest in childhood**

    Use additional code to identify associated intellectual disabilities

  330.0 Leukodystrophy

Krabbe's disease	Leukodystrophy:
Leukodystrophy:	sudanophilic
NOS	Pelizaeus-Merzbacher disease
globoid cell	Sulfatide lipidosis
metachromatic	

      DEF: Hereditary disease of arylsulfatase or cerebroside sulfatase; characterized by a diffuse loss of myelin in CNS; infantile form causes blindness, motor disturbances, rigidity, mental deterioration and, occasionally, convulsions.

  330.1 Cerebral lipidoses

Amaurotic (familial) idiocy	Disease:
Disease:	Spielmeyer-Vogt
Batten	Tay-Sachs
Jansky-Bielschowsky	Gangliosidosis
Kufs'	

      DEF: Genetic disorder causing abnormal lipid accumulation in the reticuloendothelial cells of the brain.

  330.2 Cerebral degeneration in generalized lipidoses

    Code first underlying disease, as:
      Fabry's disease (272.7)
      Gaucher's disease (272.7)
      Niemann-Pick disease (272.7)
      sphingolipidosis (272.7)

  330.3 Cerebral degeneration of childhood in other diseases classified elsewhere

    Code first underlying disease, as:
      Hunter's disease (277.5)
      mucopolysaccharidosis (277.5)

  330.8 Other specified cerebral degenerations in childhood
      Alpers' disease or gray-matter degeneration
      Infantile necrotizing encephalomyelopathy
      Leigh's disease
      Subacute necrotizing encephalopathy or encephalomyelopathy
      AHA: N-D, '85, 5

  330.9 Unspecified cerebral degeneration in childhood

√4ᵗʰ **331 Other cerebral degenerations**

    Use additional code, where applicable, to identify dementia:
    with behavioral disturbance (294.11)
    without behavioral disturbance (294.10)

  331.0 Alzheimer's disease
      DEF: Diffuse atrophy of cerebral cortex; causing a progressive decline in intellectual and physical functions, including memory loss, personality changes and profound dementia.
      AHA: 4Q, '00, 41; 4Q, '99, 7; N-D, '84, 20
      G30.9 Alzheimer's disease unspecified   I-10

√5ᵗʰ **331.1 Frontotemporal dementia**
      DEF: Rare, progressive degenerative brain disease, similar to Alzheimer's; cortical atrophy affects the frontal and temporal lobes.
      AHA: 4Q, '03, 57

    331.11 Pick's disease
        DEF: A progressive frontotemporal dementia with asymmetrical atrophy of the frontal and temporal regions of the cerebral cortex, abnormal rounded brain cells called Pick cells with the presence of abnormal staining of protein (called tau); symptoms include prominent apathy, behavioral changes such as disinhibition and restlessness, echolalia, impairment of language, memory, and intellect, increased carelessness, poor personal hygiene, and decreased attention span.

    331.19 Other frontotemporal dementia
        Frontal dementia

  331.2 Senile degeneration of brain
      EXCLUDES   senility NOS (797)

  331.3 Communicating hydrocephalus
      Secondary normal pressure hydrocephalus
      EXCLUDES   congenital hydrocephalus (742.3)
            idiopathic normal pressure hydrocephalus (331.5)
            normal pressure hydrocephalus (331.5)
            spina bifida with hydrocephalus (741.0)
      DEF: Subarachnoid hemorrhage and meningitis causing excess buildup of cerebrospinal fluid in cavities due to nonabsorption of fluid back through fluid pathways.
      AHA: S-O, '85, 12

  331.4 Obstructive hydrocephalus
      Acquired hydrocephalus NOS
      EXCLUDES   congenital hydrocephalus (742.3)
            idiopathic normal pressure hydrocephalus (331.5)
            normal pressure hydrocephalus (331.5)
            spina bifida with hydrocephalus (741.0)
      DEF: Obstruction of cerebrospinal fluid passage from brain into spinal canal.
      AHA: 4Q, '03, 106; 1Q, '99, 9
      G91.1 Obstructive hydrocephalus   I-10

  331.5 Idiopathic normal pressure hydrocephalus [INPH]
      Normal pressure hydrocephalus NOS
      EXCLUDES   congenital hydrocephalus (742.3)
            secondary normal pressure hydrocephalus (331.3)
            spina bifida with hydrocephalus (741.0)
      DEF: Abnormal increase of cerebrospinal fluid in the brain's ventricles; results in dementia, progressive mental impairment, gait disturbance, and impaired bladder control.
      AHA: 4Q, '07, 74

  331.6 Corticobasal degeneration
      AHA: ▶4Q, '11, 98◀

  331.7 Cerebral degeneration in diseases classified elsewhere
    Code first underlying disease, as:
      alcoholism (303.0-303.9)
      beriberi (265.0)
      cerebrovascular disease (430-438)
      congenital hydrocephalus (741.0, 742.3)
      myxedema (244.0-244.9)
      neoplastic disease (140.0-239.9)
      vitamin B12 deficiency (266.2)
      EXCLUDES   cerebral degeneration in:
            Jakob-Creutzfeldt disease (046.11-046.19)
            progressive multifocal leukoencephalopathy (046.3)
            subacute spongiform encephalopathy (046.1)

√5ᵗʰ **331.8 Other cerebral degeneration**

    331.81 Reye's syndrome   P
        DEF: Rare childhood illness, often developed after a viral upper respiratory infection; characterized by vomiting, elevated serum transaminase, changes in liver and other viscera; brain swelling, disturbances of consciousness and seizures; can be fatal.

    331.82 Dementia with Lewy bodies

Dementia with Parkinsonism	Lewy body disease
Lewy body dementia	

        DEF: A cerebral dementia with neurophysiologic changes, increased hippocampal volume, hypoperfusion in the occipital lobes, and beta amyloid deposits with neurofibrillarity tangles, atrophy of cortex and brainstem, hallmark neuropsychologic characteristics are fluctuating cognition with pronounced variation in attention and alertness; recurrent hallucinations; and parkinsonism.
        AHA: 4Q, '03, 57
        G31.83 Dementia with Lewy bodies   I-10

N Newborn Age: 0   P Pediatric Age: 0-17   M Maternity Age: 12-55   A Adult Age: 15-124

331.83 Mild cognitive impairment, so stated
> EXCLUDES altered mental status (780.97)
> cerebral degeneration (331.0-331.9)
> change in mental status (780.97)
> cognitive deficits following (late effects of)
>   cerebral hemorrhage or infarction
>   (438.0)
> cognitive impairment due to intracranial or
>   head injury (850-854, 959.01)
> cognitive impairment due to late effect of
>   intracranial injury (907.0)
> cognitive impairment due to skull fracture
>   (800-801, 803-804)
> dementia (290.0-290.43, 294.20-294.21)
> mild memory disturbance (310.89)
> neurologic neglect syndrome (781.8)
> personality change, nonpsychotic (310.1)

AHA: 4Q, '06, 75

331.89 Other
Cerebral ataxia

331.9 Cerebral degeneration, unspecified

332 Parkinson's disease
> EXCLUDES dementia with Parkinsonism (331.82)

332.0 Paralysis agitans
Parkinsonism or Parkinson's disease:
  NOS
  idiopathic
  primary
DEF: Form of progessive parkinsonism, characterized by masklike
facial expressions, in ability to stand or walk smoothly, muscle
weakness, and involuntary trembling movement.
AHA: M-A, '87, 7
G20 Parkinson's disease   I-10

332.1 Secondary Parkinsonism
Neuroleptic-induced Parkinsonism
Parkinsonism due to drugs
Use additional E code to identify drug, if drug-induced
> EXCLUDES Parkinsonism (in):
>   Huntington's disease (333.4)
>   progressive supranuclear palsy (333.0)
>   Shy-Drager syndrome (333.0)
>   syphilitic (094.82)

333 Other extrapyramidal disease and abnormal movement disorders
> INCLUDES other forms of extrapyramidal, basal ganglia, or
>   striatopallidal disease
> EXCLUDES abnormal movements of head NOS (781.0)
>   sleep related movement disorders (327.51-327.59)

333.0 Other degenerative diseases of the basal ganglia
Atrophy or degeneration:
  olivopontocerebellar [Déjérine-Thomas syndrome]
  pigmentary pallidal [Hallervorden-Spatz disease]
  striatonigral
Parkinsonian syndrome associated with:
  idiopathic orthostatic hypotension
  symptomatic orthostatic hypotension
Progressive supranuclear ophthalmoplegia
Shy-Drager syndrome
AHA: 3Q, '96, 8

333.1 Essential and other specified forms of tremor
Benign essential tremor
Familial tremor
Medication-induced postural tremor
Use additional E code to identify drug, if drug-induced
> EXCLUDES tremor NOS (781.0)

333.2 Myoclonus
Familial essential myoclonus   Palatal myoclonus
> EXCLUDES progressive myoclonic epilepsy (345.1)
>   Unverricht-Lundborg disease (345.1)
Use additional E code to identify drug, if drug-induced
DEF: Spontaneous movements or contractions of muscles.
AHA: 3Q, '97, 4; M-A, '87, 12

333.3 Tics of organic origin
Use additional E code to identify drug, if drug-induced
> EXCLUDES Gilles de la Tourette's syndrome (307.23)
>   habit spasm (307.22)
>   tic NOS (307.20)

333.4 Huntington's chorea
DEF: Genetic disease characterized by chronic progressive mental
deterioration; dementia and death within 15 years of onset.

333.5 Other choreas
Hemiballism(us)   Paroxysmal choreo-athetosis
Use additional E code to identify drug, if drug-induced
> EXCLUDES Sydenham's or rheumatic chorea (392.0-392.9)

333.6 Genetic torsion dystonia
Dystonia:
  deformans progressiva
  musculorum deformans
(Schwalbe-) Ziehen-Oppenheim disease
DEF: Sustained muscular contractions, causing twisting and
repetitive movements that result in abnormal postures of trunk and
limbs; etiology unknown.

333.7 Acquired torsion dystonia

333.71 Athetoid cerebral palsy
Double athetosis (syndrome)   Vogt's disease
> EXCLUDES infantile cerebral palsy (343.0-343.9)
AHA: 4Q, '06, 76-78

333.72 Acute dystonia due to drugs
Acute dystonic reaction due to drugs
Neuroleptic induced acute dystonia
Use additional E code to identify drug
> EXCLUDES blepharospasm due to drugs (333.85)
>   orofacial dyskinesia due to drugs (333.85)
>   secondary Parkinsonism (332.1)
>   subacute dyskinesia due to drugs (333.85)
>   tardive dyskinesia (333.85)
AHA: 4Q, '06, 76-78

333.79 Other acquired torsion dystonia
AHA: 4Q, '06, 76-78

333.8 Fragments of torsion dystonia
Use additional E code to identify drug, if drug-induced

333.81 Blepharospasm
> EXCLUDES blepharospasm due to drugs (333.85)
DEF: Uncontrolled winking or blinking due to orbicularis
oculi muscle spasm.

333.82 Orofacial dyskinesia
> EXCLUDES orofacial dyskinesia due to drugs (333.85)
DEF: Uncontrolled movement of mouth or facial muscles.

333.83 Spasmodic torticollis
> EXCLUDES torticollis:
>   NOS (723.5)
>   hysterical (300.11)
>   psychogenic (306.0)
DEF: Uncontrolled movement of head due to spasms of
neck muscle.

333.84 Organic writers' cramp
> EXCLUDES pychogenic (300.89)

333.85 Subacute dyskinesia due to drugs
Blepharospasm due to drugs
Orofacial dyskinesia due to drugs
Tardive dyskinesia
Use additional E code to identify drug
> EXCLUDES acute dystonia due to drugs (333.72)
>   acute dystonic reaction due to drugs (333.72)
>   secondary Parkinsonism (332.1)
AHA: 4Q, '06, 76-78

333.89 Other

Diseases of the Nervous System and Sense Organs

333.9–337.01

☑5ᵗʰ **333.9 Other and unspecified extrapyramidal diseases and abnormal movement disorders**

333.90 Unspecified extrapyramidal disease and abnormal movement disorder
Medication-induced movement disorders NOS
Use additional E code to identify drug, if drug-induced

333.91 Stiff-man syndrome

333.92 Neuroleptic malignant syndrome
Use additional E code to identify drug
EXCLUDES *neuroleptic induced Parkinsonism (332.1)*
AHA: 4Q, '94, 37

333.93 Benign shuddering attacks
AHA: 4Q, '94, 37

333.94 Restless legs syndrome [RLS]
DEF: Neurological disorder of unknown etiology with an irresistible urge to move the legs, which may temporarily relieve the symptoms, is accompanied by motor restlessness and sensations of pain, burning, prickling, or tingling.
AHA: 4Q, '06, 79
TIP: Assign an additional code if the underlying cause of the RLS is specified (e.g., iron deficiency anemia).
G25.81 Restless legs syndrome   I-10

333.99 Other
Neuroleptic-induced acute akathisia
Use additional E code to identify drug, if drug-induced
AHA: 4Q, '04, 95; 2Q, '04, 12; 4Q, '94, 37

☑4ᵗʰ **334 Spinocerebellar disease**
EXCLUDES *olivopontocerebellar degeneration (333.0)*
peroneal muscular atrophy (356.1)

334.0 Friedreich's ataxia
DEF: Genetic recessive disease of children; sclerosis of dorsal, lateral spinal cord columns; characterized by ataxia, speech impairment, swaying and irregular movements, with muscle paralysis, especially of lower limbs.

334.1 Hereditary spastic paraplegia

334.2 Primary cerebellar degeneration
Cerebellar ataxia:
   Marie's
   Sanger-Brown
Dyssynergia cerebellaris myoclonica
Primary cerebellar degeneration:
   NOS
   hereditary
   sporadic
AHA: M-A, '87, 9

334.3 Other cerebellar ataxia
Cerebellar ataxia NOS
Use additional E code to identify drug, if drug-induced

334.4 Cerebellar ataxia in diseases classified elsewhere
Code first underlying disease, as:
   alcoholism (303.0-303.9)
   myxedema (244.0-244.9)
   neoplastic disease (140.0-239.9)

334.8 Other spinocerebellar diseases
Ataxia-telangiectasia [Louis-Bar syndrome]
Corticostriatal-spinal degeneration

334.9 Spinocerebellar disease, unspecified

☑4ᵗʰ **335 Anterior horn cell disease**

335.0 Werdnig-Hoffmann disease
Infantile spinal muscular atrophy
Progressive muscular atrophy of infancy
DEF: Spinal muscle atrophy manifested in prenatal period or shortly after birth; symptoms include hypotonia, atrophy of skeletal muscle; death occurs in infancy.

☑5ᵗʰ **335.1 Spinal muscular atrophy**

335.10 Spinal muscular atrophy, unspecified

335.11 Kugelberg-Welander disease
Spinal muscular atrophy:
   familial
   juvenile
DEF: Hereditary; juvenile muscle atrophy; appears during first two decades of life; due to lesions of anterior horns of spinal cord; includes wasting, diminution of lower body muscles and twitching.

335.19 Other
Adult spinal muscular atrophy

☑5ᵗʰ **335.2 Motor neuron disease**

335.20 Amyotrophic lateral sclerosis   A
Motor neuron disease (bulbar) (mixed type)
AHA: 4Q, '95, 81

335.21 Progressive muscular atrophy
Duchenne-Aran muscular atrophy
Progressive muscular atrophy (pure)

335.22 Progressive bulbar palsy

335.23 Pseudobulbar palsy

335.24 Primary lateral sclerosis

335.29 Other

335.8 Other anterior horn cell diseases

335.9 Anterior horn cell disease, unspecified

☑4ᵗʰ **336 Other diseases of spinal cord**

336.0 Syringomyelia and syringobulbia
AHA: 1Q, '89, 10

336.1 Vascular myelopathies
Acute infarction of spinal cord (embolic) (nonembolic)
Arterial thrombosis of spinal cord
Edema of spinal cord
Hematomyelia
Subacute necrotic myelopathy

336.2 Subacute combined degeneration of spinal cord in diseases classified elsewhere
Code first underlying disease, as:
   pernicious anemia (281.0)
   other vitamin B12 deficiency anemia (281.1)
   vitamin B12 deficiency (266.2)

336.3 Myelopathy in other diseases classified elsewhere
Code first underlying disease, as:
   myelopathy in neoplastic disease (140.0-239.9)
EXCLUDES *myelopathy in:*
   intervertebral disc disorder (722.70-722.73)
   spondylosis (721.1, 721.41-721.42, 721.91)
AHA: 3Q, '99, 5

336.8 Other myelopathy
Myelopathy:
   drug-induced
   radiation-induced
Use additonal E code to identify cause

336.9 Unspecified disease of spinal cord
Cord compression NOS
Myelopathy NOS
EXCLUDES *myelitis (323.02, 323.1, 323.2, 323.42, 323.52, 323.63, 323.72, 323.82, 323.9)*
   spinal (canal) stenosis (723.0, 724.00-724.09)

☑4ᵗʰ **337 Disorders of the autonomic nervous system**
INCLUDES disorders of peripheral autonomic, sympathetic, parasympathetic, or vegetative system
EXCLUDES *familial dysautonomia [Riley-Day syndrome] (742.8)*

☑5ᵗʰ **337.0 Idiopathic peripheral autonomic neuropathy**

337.00 Idiopathic peripheral autonomic neuropathy, unspecified

337.01 Carotid sinus syndrome
Carotid sinus syncope
DEF: Vagal activation caused by pressure on the carotid sinus baroreceptors; sympathetic nerve impulses may cause sinus arrest or AV block.
AHA: 4Q, '08, 101-102

N Newborn Age: 0   P Pediatric Age: 0-17   M Maternity Age: 12-55   A Adult Age: 15-124

337.09 Other idiopathic peripheral autonomic neuropathy
Cervical sympathetic dystrophy or paralysis

337.1 Peripheral autonomic neuropathy in disorders classified elsewhere
Code first underlying disease, as:
amyloidosis (277.30-277.39)
diabetes (249.6, 250.6)
AHA: 2Q, '09, 13; 2Q, '93, 6; 3Q, '91, 9; N-D, '84, 9

✓5ᵗʰ **337.2 Reflex sympathetic dystrophy**
DEF: Disturbance of the sympathetic nervous system evidenced by sweating, pain, pallor and edema following injury to nerves or blood vessels.
AHA: 4Q, '93, 24

337.20 Reflex sympathetic dystrophy, unspecified
Complex regional pain syndrome type I, unspecified

337.21 Reflex sympathetic dystrophy of the upper limb
Complex regional pain syndrome type I of the upper limb

337.22 Reflex sympathetic dystrophy of the lower limb
Complex regional pain syndrome type I of the lower limb

337.29 Reflex sympathetic dystrophy of other specified site
Complex regional pain syndrome type I of other specified site

337.3 Autonomic dysreflexia
Use additional code to identify the cause, such as:
fecal impaction (560.32)
pressure ulcer (707.00-707.09)
urinary tract infection (599.0)
DEF: Noxious stimuli evokes paroxysmal hypertension, bradycardia, excess sweating, headache, pilomotor responses, facial flushing, and nasal congestion due to uncontrolled parasympathetic nerve response; occurs in patients with spinal cord injury above sympathetic outflow tract (T₆).
AHA: 4Q, '98, 37

337.9 Unspecified disorder of autonomic nervous system

Pain (338)

✓4ᵗʰ **338 Pain, not elsewhere classified**
Use additional code to identify:
pain associated with psychological factors (307.89)
EXCLUDES generalized pain (780.96)
headache syndromes (339.00-339.89)
localized pain, unspecified type — code to pain by site
migraines (346.0-346.9)
pain disorder exclusively attributed to psychological factors (307.80)
vulvar vestibulitis (625.71)
vulvodynia (625.70-625.79)
AHA: 2Q, '07, 12
TIP: Do not assign a 338 code if the pain is not specified as acute or chronic, unless post-thoracotomy, postoperative, neoplasm related or central pain syndrome.

338.0 Central pain syndrome
Déjérine-Roussy syndrome
Myelopathic pain syndrome
Thalamic pain syndrome (hyperesthetic)
AHA: 4Q, '06, 79-81

✓5ᵗʰ **338.1 Acute pain**

338.11 Acute pain due to trauma
AHA: 1Q, '07, 7; 4Q, '06, 79-81

338.12 Acute post-thoracotomy pain
Post-thoracotomy pain NOS
AHA: 4Q, '06, 79-81

338.18 Other acute postoperative pain
Postoperative pain NOS
AHA: 2Q, '07, 11; 4Q, '06, 79-81
G89.18 Other acute postprocedural pain   I-10

338.19 Other acute pain
EXCLUDES neoplasm related acute pain (338.3)
AHA: 2Q, '07, 11; 4Q, '06, 79-81

✓5ᵗʰ **338.2 Chronic pain**
EXCLUDES causalgia (355.9)
lower limb (355.71)
upper limb (354.4)
chronic pain syndrome (338.4)
myofascial pain syndrome (729.1)
neoplasm related chronic pain (338.3)
reflex sympathetic dystrophy (337.20-337.29)

338.21 Chronic pain due to trauma
AHA: 4Q, '06, 79-81

338.22 Chronic post-thoracotomy pain
AHA: 4Q, '06, 79-81

338.28 Other chronic postoperative pain
AHA: 4Q, '06, 79-81
G89.28 Other chronic postprocedural pain   I-10

338.29 Other chronic pain
AHA: 4Q, '06, 79-81

338.3 Neoplasm related pain (acute) (chronic)
Cancer associated pain
Pain due to malignancy (primary) (secondary)
Tumor associated pain
AHA: 2Q, '07, 11; 4Q, '06, 79-81
G89.3 Neoplasm related pain (acute) (chronic)   I-10

338.4 Chronic pain syndrome
Chronic pain associated with significant psychosocial dysfunction
AHA: 2Q, '07, 11; 4Q, '06, 79-81
G89.4 Chronic pain syndrome   I-10

Other Headache Syndromes (339)

✓4ᵗʰ **339 Other headache syndromes**
EXCLUDES headache:
NOS (784.0)
due to lumbar puncture (349.0)
migraine (346.0-346.9)
AHA: 4Q, '08, 102-105

✓5ᵗʰ **339.0 Cluster headaches and other trigeminal autonomic cephalgias**
TACS

339.00 Cluster headache syndrome, unspecified
Ciliary neuralgia
Cluster headache NOS
Histamine cephalgia
Lower half migraine
Migrainous neuralgia

339.01 Episodic cluster headache

339.02 Chronic cluster headache

339.03 Episodic paroxysmal hemicrania
Paroxysmal hemicrania NOS

339.04 Chronic paroxysmal hemicrania

339.05 Short lasting unilateral neuralgiform headache with conjunctival injection and tearing
SUNCT

339.09 Other trigeminal autonomic cephalgias

✓5ᵗʰ **339.1 Tension type headache**
EXCLUDES tension headache NOS (307.81)
tension headache related to psychological factors (307.81)
AHA: 4Q, '08, 103

339.10 Tension type headache, unspecified

339.11 Episodic tension type headache

339.12 Chronic tension type headache

✓5ᵗʰ **339.2 Post-traumatic headache**
TIP: Do not assign during the acute phase of the trauma (e.g., head injury). When assigning 339.2X, report also a late effect code (e.g., 907.0 for intracranial injury).

339.20 Post-traumatic headache, unspecified
AHA: 4Q, '08, 108

339.21 Acute post-traumatic headache

✓4ᵗʰ ✓5ᵗʰ Additional Digit Required   Unspecified Code   Other Specified Code   Manifestation Code   ▶◀ Revised Text   ● New Code   ▲ Revised Code Title

2013 ICD-9-CM   **Volume 1 – 93**

339.22 Chronic post-traumatic headache

339.3 Drug induced headache, not elsewhere classified
Medication overuse headache
Rebound headache

√5ᵗʰ **339.4 Complicated headache syndromes**

339.41 Hemicrania continua

339.42 New daily persistent headache
NDPH

339.43 Primary thunderclap headache

339.44 Other complicated headache syndrome

√5ᵗʰ **339.8 Other specified headache syndromes**

339.81 Hypnic headache

339.82 Headache associated with sexual activity
Orgasmic headache
Preorgasmic headache

339.83 Primary cough headache

339.84 Primary exertional headache

339.85 Primary stabbing headache

339.89 Other specified headache syndromes

Other Disorders of the Central Nervous System (340-349)

340 Multiple sclerosis
Disseminated or multiple sclerosis:
NOS
brain stem
cord
generalized
G35 Multiple sclerosis   I-10

√4ᵗʰ **341 Other demyelinating diseases of central nervous system**

341.0 Neuromyelitis optica

341.1 Schilder's disease
Baló's concentric sclerosis
Encephalitis periaxialis:
concentrica [Baló's]
diffusa [Schilder's]
DEF: Chronic leukoencephalopathy of children and adolescents; symptoms include blindness, deafness, bilateral spasticity and progressive mental deterioration.

√5ᵗʰ **341.2 Acute (transverse) myelitis**
EXCLUDES acute (transverse) myelitis (in) (due to):
following immunization procedures (323.52)
infection classified elsewhere (323.42)
postinfectious (323.63)
protozoal diseases classified elsewhere (323.2)
rickettsial diseases classified elsewhere (323.1)
toxic (323.72)
viral diseases classified elsewhere (323.02)
transverse myelitis NOS (323.82)

341.20 Acute (transverse) myelitis NOS
AHA: 4Q, '06, 58-63

341.21 Acute (transverse) myelitis in conditions classified elsewhere
Code first underlying condition
AHA: 4Q, '06, 58-63

341.22 Idiopathic transverse myelitis
AHA: 4Q, '06, 58-63

341.8 Other demyelinating diseases of central nervous system
Central demyelination of corpus callosum
Central pontine myelinosis
Marchiafava (-Bignami) disease
AHA: N-D, '87, 6

341.9 Demyelinating disease of central nervous system, unspecified

√4ᵗʰ **342 Hemiplegia and hemiparesis**
NOTE This category is to be used when hemiplegia (complete) (incomplete) is reported without further specification, or is stated to be old or long-standing but of unspecified cause. The category is also for use in multiple coding to identify these types of hemiplegia resulting from any cause.
EXCLUDES congenital (343.1)
hemiplegia due to late effect of cerebrovascular accident (438.20-438.22)
infantile NOS (343.4)

The following fifth-digits are for use with codes 342.0-342.9:
0 affecting unspecified side
1 affecting dominant side
2 affecting nondominant side

AHA: 4Q, '94, 38

§ √5ᵗʰ **342.0 Flaccid hemiplegia**
[0-2]

§ √5ᵗʰ **342.1 Spastic hemiplegia**
[0-2]

§ √5ᵗʰ **342.8 Other specified hemiplegia**
[0-2]

§ √5ᵗʰ **342.9 Hemiplegia, unspecified**
[0-2]   AHA: 3Q, '06, 5; 4Q, '98, 87
G81.90 Hemiplegia unspecified affect unspecified side   I-10

√4ᵗʰ **343 Infantile cerebral palsy**
INCLUDES cerebral:
palsy NOS
spastic infantile paralysis
congenital spastic paralysis (cerebral)
Little's disease
paralysis (spastic) due to birth injury:
intracranial
spinal
EXCLUDES athetoid cerebral palsy (333.71)
hereditary cerebral paralysis, such as:
hereditary spastic paraplegia (334.1)
Vogt's disease (333.71)
spastic paralysis specified as noncongenital or noninfantile (344.0-344.9)

343.0 Diplegic
Congenital diplegia
Congenital paraplegia
DEF: Paralysis affecting both sides of the body simultaneously.

343.1 Hemiplegic
Congenital hemiplegia
EXCLUDES infantile hemiplegia NOS (343.4)

343.2 Quadriplegic
Tetraplegic

343.3 Monoplegic

343.4 Infantile hemiplegia
Infantile hemiplegia (postnatal) NOS

343.8 Other specified infantile cerebral palsy

343.9 Infantile cerebral palsy, unspecified
Cerebral palsy NOS
AHA: 4Q, '05, 89
G80.9 Cerebral palsy unspecified   I-10

√4ᵗʰ **344 Other paralytic syndromes**
NOTE This category is to be used when the listed conditions are reported without further specification or are stated to be old or long-standing but of unspecified cause. The category is also for use in multiple coding to identify these conditions resulting from any cause.
INCLUDES paralysis (complete) (incomplete), except as classifiable to 342 and 343
EXCLUDES congenital or infantile cerebral palsy (343.0-343.9)
hemiplegia (342.0-342.9)
congenital or infantile (343.1, 343.4)

√5ᵗʰ **344.0 Quadriplegia and quadriparesis**
TIP: Assign also a code from subcategory 438.5 if late effect of CVA.

---

§ Requires fifth digit. Valid digits are in [brackets] under each code. See category 342 for codes and definitions.

N Newborn Age: 0   P Pediatric Age: 0-17   M Maternity Age: 12-55   A Adult Age: 15-124

344.00 Quadriplegia unspecified
　　AHA: 4Q, '03, 103; 4Q, '98, 38
　　G82.50 Quadriplegia unspecified　　I-10

344.01 C$_1$-C$_4$ complete

344.02 C$_1$-C$_4$ incomplete

344.03 C$_5$-C$_7$ complete

344.04 C$_5$-C$_7$ incomplete

344.09 Other
　　AHA: 1Q, '01, 12; 4Q, '98, 39

344.1 Paraplegia
　　Paralysis of both lower limbs　　Paraplegia (lower)
　　AHA: 4Q, '03, 110; M-A, '87, 10
　　G82.20 Paraplegia unspecified　　I-10

344.2 Diplegia of upper limbs
　　Diplegia (upper)　　Paralysis of both upper limbs

√5th **344.3 Monoplegia of lower limb**
　　Paralysis of lower limb
　　EXCLUDES monoplegia of lower limb due to late effect of
　　　　cerebrovascular accident (438.40-438.42)

344.30 Affecting unspecified side

344.31 Affecting dominant side

344.32 Affecting nondominant side

√5th **344.4 Monoplegia of upper limb**
　　Paralysis of upper limb
　　EXCLUDES monoplegia of upper limb due to late effect of
　　　　cerebrovascular accident (438.30-438.32)

344.40 Affecting unspecified side

344.41 Affecting dominant side

344.42 Affecting nondominant side

344.5 Unspecified monoplegia

√5th **344.6 Cauda equina syndrome**
　　DEF: Dull pain and paresthesias in sacrum, perineum and bladder
　　due to compression of spinal nerve roots; pain radiates down
　　buttocks, back of thigh, calf of leg and into foot with prickling,
　　burning sensations.

344.60 Without mention of neurogenic bladder

344.61 With neurogenic bladder
　　Acontractile bladder
　　Autonomic hyperreflexia of bladder
　　Cord bladder
　　Detrusor hyperreflexia
　　AHA: M-J, '87, 12; M-A, '87, 10

√5th **344.8 Other specified paralytic syndromes**

344.81 Locked-in state
　　DEF: State of consciousness where patients are paralyzed
　　and unable to respond to environmental stimuli; patients
　　have eye movements, and stimuli can enter the brain but
　　patients unable to respond.
　　AHA: 4Q, '93, 24

344.89 Other specified paralytic syndrome
　　AHA: 2Q, '99, 4

344.9 Paralysis, unspecified

√4th **345 Epilepsy and recurrent seizures**

The following fifth-digit subclassification is for use with categories
345.0, .1, .4-.9:
　0 without mention of intractable epilepsy
　1 with intractable epilepsy
　　pharmacoresistant (pharmacologically resistant)
　　poorly controlled
　　refractory (medically)
　　treatment resistant

EXCLUDES hippocampal sclerosis (348.81)
　　mesial temporal sclerosis (348.81)
　　temporal sclerosis (348.81)

DEF: Brain disorder characterized by electrical-like disturbances; may include
occasional impairment or loss of consciousness, abnormal motor
phenomena and psychic or sensory disturbances.
AHA: 4Q, '09, 82; 1Q, '93, 24; 2Q, '92, 8; 4Q, '92, 23

§ √5th **345.0 Generalized nonconvulsive epilepsy**
　[0-1]　Absences:　　　Pykno-epilepsy
　　atonic　　　　Seizures:
　　typical　　　　akinetic
　Minor epilepsy　　atonic
　Petit mal
　AHA: For code 345.00: 1Q, '04, 18

§ √5th **345.1 Generalized convulsive epilepsy**
　[0-1]　Epileptic seizures:　Grand mal
　　clonic　　　　Major epilepsy
　　myoclonic　　Progressive myoclonic epilepsy
　　tonic　　　　Unverricht-Lundborg disease
　　tonic-clonic

　　EXCLUDES convulsions:
　　　　NOS (780.39)
　　　　infantile (780.39)
　　　　newborn (779.0)
　　　　infantile spasms (345.6)

　DEF: Convulsive seizures with tension of limbs (tonic) or rhythmic
　contractions (clonic).
　AHA: 3Q, '97, 4

345.2 Petit mal status
　Epileptic absence status
　DEF: Minor myoclonic spasms and sudden momentary loss of
　consciousness in epilepsy.

345.3 Grand mal status
　Status epilepticus NOS
　EXCLUDES epilepsia partialis continua (345.7)
　　status:
　　　psychomotor (345.7)
　　　temporal lobe (345.7)
　DEF: Sudden loss of consciousness followed by generalized
　convulsions in epilepsy.
　AHA: 3Q, '05, 12
　G40.301 Gen idiopath epilep&epi syn not intractabl w/se　　I-10

§ √5th **345.4 Localization-related (focal) (partial) epilepsy and**
　[0-1]　**epileptic syndromes with complex partial seizures**
　　Epilepsy:
　　　limbic system
　　　partial:
　　　　secondarily generalized
　　　　with impairment of consciousness
　　　　with memory and ideational disturbances
　　　psychomotor
　　　psychosensory
　　　temporal lobe
　　Epileptic automatism
　　AHA: For code 345.41 4Q, '09, 83

§ √5th **345.5 Localization-related (focal) (partial) epilepsy and**
　[0-1]　**epileptic syndromes with simple partial seizures**
　　Epilepsy:　　　　Epilepsy:
　　　Bravais-Jacksonian NOS　somatomotor
　　　focal (motor) NOS　　somatosensory
　　　Jacksonian NOS　　visceral
　　　motor partial　　　visual
　　　partial NOS:
　　　　without impairment of consciousness
　　　sensory-induced

---

§　Requires fifth digit. Valid digits are in [brackets] under each code. See category 345 for codes and definitions.

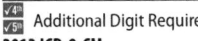

Diseases of the Nervous System and Sense Organs

345.6–348.4

§ ✓5ᵗʰ **345.6 Infantile spasms**
[0-1]   Hypsarrhythmia   Lightning spasms
           Salaam attacks
           EXCLUDES *salaam tic (781.0)*
           AHA: N-D, '84, 12

§ ✓5ᵗʰ **345.7 Epilepsia partialis continua**
[0-1]   Kojevnikov's epilepsy
           DEF: Continuous muscle contractions and relaxation; result of abnormal neural discharge.

§ ✓5ᵗʰ **345.8 Other forms of epilepsy and recurrent seizures**
[0-1]   Epilepsy:
           cursive [running]
           gelastic

§ ✓5ᵗʰ **345.9 Epilepsy, unspecified**
[0-1]   Epileptic convulsions, fits, or seizures NOS
           Seizure disorder NOS
           EXCLUDES *convulsion (convulsive) disorder (780.39)*
                   convulsive seizure or fit NOS (780.39)
                   recurrent convulsions (780.39)
           AHA: 1Q, '08, 17; N-D, '87, 12; For code 345.90: 2Q, '09, 10
           G40.909 Epilepsy uns not intractbl w/o status epilepticus   I-10

✓4ᵗʰ **346 Migraine**
           EXCLUDES *headache:*
                   NOS (784.0)
                   syndromes (339.00-339.89)
           AHA: 4Q, '08, 103, 105-107

The following fifth-digit subclassification is for use with category 346:
0 without mention of intractable migraine without mention of status migrainosus
     without mention of refractory migraine without mention of status migrainosus
1 with intractable migraine, so stated, without mention of status migrainosus
     with refractory migraine, so stated, without mention of status migrainosus
2 without mention of intractable migraine with status migrainosus
     without mention of refractory migraine with status migrainosus
3 with intractable migraine, so stated, with status migrainosus
     with refractory migraine, so stated, with status migrainosus

           DEF: Benign vascular headache of extreme pain; commonly associated with irritability, nausea, vomiting and often photophobia; premonitory visual hallucination of a crescent in the visual field (scotoma).

§ ✓5ᵗʰ **346.0 Migraine with aura**
[0-3]   Basilar migraine
           Classic migraine
           Migraine preceded or accompanied by transient focal neurological phenomena
           Migraine triggered seizures
           Migraine with acute-onset aura
           Migraine with aura without headache (migraine equivalents)
           Migraine with prolonged aura
           Migraine with typical aura
           Retinal migraine
           EXCLUDES *persistent migraine aura (346.5, 346.6)*

§ ✓5ᵗʰ **346.1 Migraine without aura**
[0-3]   Common migraine

§ ✓5ᵗʰ **346.2 Variants of migraine, not elsewhere classified**
[0-3]   Abdominal migraine
           Cyclical vomiting associated with migraine
           Ophthalmoplegic migraine
           Periodic headache syndromes in child or adolescent
           EXCLUDES *cyclical vomiting NOS (536.2)*
                   psychogenic cyclical vomiting (306.4)

§ ✓5ᵗʰ **346.3 Hemiplegic migraine**
[0-3]   Familial migraine   Sporadic migraine

§ ✓5ᵗʰ **346.4 Menstrual migraine**   ♀
[0-3]   Menstrual headache   Premenstrual migraine
           Menstrually related migraine   Pure menstrual migraine
           Premenstrual headache

§ ✓5ᵗʰ **346.5 Persistent migraine aura without cerebral infarction**
[0-3]   Persistent migraine aura NOS

§ ✓5ᵗʰ **346.6 Persistent migraine aura with cerebral infarction**
[0-3]   **AHA:** For code 346.60: 4Q, '08, 108
           TIP: Assign also a code for the specific type of cerebral infarction.

§ ✓5ᵗʰ **346.7 Chronic migraine without aura**
[0-3]   Transformed migraine without aura

§ ✓5ᵗʰ **346.8 Other forms of migraine**
[0-3]

§ ✓5ᵗʰ **346.9 Migraine, unspecified**
[0-3]   **AHA:** N-D, '85, 16
           G43.909 Migraine unspecified not intract w/o stat migran   I-10

✓4ᵗʰ **347 Cataplexy and narcolepsy**
           DEF: Cataplexy: Sudden onset of muscle weakness with loss of tone and strength; caused by aggressive or spontaneous emotions.
           DEF: Narcolepsy: Brief, recurrent, uncontrollable episodes of sound sleep.

✓5ᵗʰ **347.0 Narcolepsy**

           347.00 Without cataplexy
                Narcolepsy NOS

           347.01 With cataplexy

✓5ᵗʰ **347.1 Narcolepsy in conditions classified elsewhere**
           Code first underlying condition

           347.10 Without cataplexy

           347.11 With cataplexy

✓4ᵗʰ **348 Other conditions of brain**

           348.0 Cerebral cysts
                Arachnoid cyst   Porencephaly, acquired
                Porencephalic cyst   Pseudoporencephaly
                EXCLUDES *porencephaly (congenital) (742.4)*

           348.1 Anoxic brain damage
                Use additional E code to identify cause
                EXCLUDES *that occurring in:*
                         abortion (634-638 with .7, 639.8)
                         ectopic or molar pregnancy (639.8)
                         labor or delivery (668.2, 669.4)
                         that of newborn (767.0, 768.0-768.9, 772.1-772.2)
                DEF: Brain injury due to lack of oxygen, other than birth trauma.
                G93.1 Anoxic brain damage not elsewhere classified   I-10

           348.2 Benign intracranial hypertension
                Pseudotumor cerebri
                EXCLUDES *hypertensive encephalopathy (437.2)*
                DEF: Elevated pressure in brain due to fluid retention in brain cavities.

✓5ᵗʰ **348.3 Encephalopathy, not elsewhere classified**
                AHA: 4Q, '03, 58; 3Q, '97, 4

           348.30 Encephalopathy, unspecified
                G93.40 Encephalopathy unspecified   I-10

           348.31 Metabolic encephalopathy
                Septic encephalopathy
                EXCLUDES *toxic metabolic encephalopathy (349.82)*
                TIP: Physician documentation of "acute confusional state" denotes delirium inherent to the encephalopathy. Do not report an additional code for the delirium.

           348.39 Other encephalopathy
                EXCLUDES *encephalopathy:*
                       alcoholic (291.2)
                       hepatic (572.2)
                       hypertensive (437.2)
                       toxic (349.82)

           348.4 Compression of brain
                Compression   } brain (stem)
                Herniation   }
                Posterior fossa compression syndrome
                DEF: Elevated pressure in brain due to blood clot, tumor, fracture, abscess, other condition.
                AHA: ▶3Q, '11, 11;◀ 4Q, '94, 37
                TIP: Assign for Arnold-Chiari syndrome, Type I. For Type II, III, or IV, refer to categories 741 and 742.

---

§   Requires fifth digit. Valid digits are in [brackets] under each code. See appropriate category for codes and definitions.

     Ⓝ Newborn Age: 0   Ⓟ Pediatric Age: 0-17   Ⓜ Maternity Age: 12-55   Ⓐ Adult Age: 15-124

348.5 Cerebral edema

DEF: Elevated pressure in the brain due to fluid retention in brain tissues.
AHA: ▶4Q, '11, 99;◀ 1Q, '10, 8; 3Q, '09, 8
G93.6 Cerebral edema   I-10

✓5ᵗʰ 348.8 Other conditions of brain

AHA: S-O, '87, 9

348.81 Temporal sclerosis

Hippocampal sclerosis   Mesial temporal sclerosis
DEF: Abnormal hardening or scarring of frontal lobe tissues due to injury, tumor, congenital anomaly, or hypoxia, resulting in loss of functional neurons; commonly associated with temporal lobe epilepsy.
AHA: 4Q, '09, 83

348.82 Brain death

AHA: ▶4Q, '11, 99-100◀

348.89 Other conditions of brain

Cerebral: Cerebral:
  calcification   fungus
EXCLUDES brain death (348.82)

348.9 Unspecified condition of brain

✓4ᵗʰ 349 Other and unspecified disorders of the nervous system

AHA: 4Q, '08, 109

349.0 Reaction to spinal or lumbar puncture

Headache following lumbar puncture
AHA: 2Q, '99, 9; 3Q, '90, 18
G97.1 Other reaction to spinal and lumbar puncture   I-10

349.1 Nervous system complications from surgically implanted device

EXCLUDES immediate postoperative complications (997.00-997.09)
mechanical complications of nervous system device (996.2)

349.2 Disorders of meninges, not elsewhere classified

Adhesions, meningeal (cerebral) (spinal)
Cyst, spinal meninges
Meningocele, acquired
Pseudomeningocele, acquired
AHA: 1Q, '06, 15; 2Q, '98, 18; 3Q, '94, 4

✓5ᵗʰ 349.3 Dural tear

349.31 Accidental puncture or laceration of dura during a procedure

Incidental (inadvertent) durotomy
AHA: 4Q, '08, 109-110
TIP: Do not assign code 998.2 Accidental puncture or laceration during a procedure, for an incidental dural tear.

349.39 Other dural tear

✓5ᵗʰ 349.8 Other specified disorders of nervous system

349.81 Cerebrospinal fluid rhinorrhea

EXCLUDES cerebrospinal fluid otorrhea (388.61)
DEF: Cerebrospinal fluid discharging from the nose; caused by fracture of frontal bone with tearing of dura mater and arachnoid.

349.82 Toxic encephalopathy

Toxic metabolic encephalopathy
Use additional E code to identify cause
DEF: Brain tissue degeneration due to toxic substance.
AHA: 4Q, '93, 29
G92 Toxic encephalopathy   I-10

349.89 Other

349.9 Unspecified disorders of nervous system

Disorder of nervous system (central) NOS

Cranial Nerves

Olfactory bulb (I)
Optic nerve (II)
Oculomotor nerve (III)
Trochlear nerve (IV)
Trigeminal nerve (V)
Abducens nerve (VI)
Facial nerve (VII)
Vestibulocochlear nerve (VIII)
Glossopharyngeal nerve (IX)
Vagus nerve (X)
Accessory nerve (XI)
Hypoglossal nerve (XII)
Pons

Trigeminal and Facial Nerve Branches

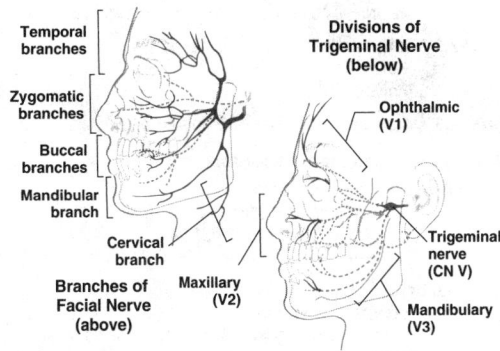

Temporal branches
Zygomatic branches
Buccal branches
Mandibular branch
Cervical branch
Branches of Facial Nerve (above)
Divisions of Trigeminal Nerve (below)
Ophthalmic (V1)
Maxillary (V2)
Trigeminal nerve (CN V)
Mandibulary (V3)

Disorders of the Peripheral Nervous System (350-359)

EXCLUDES diseases of:
acoustic [8th] nerve (388.5)
oculomotor [3rd, 4th, 6th] nerves (378.0-378.9)
optic [2nd] nerve (377.0-377.9)
peripheral autonomic nerves (337.0-337.9)
neuralgia
neuritis   } NOS or "rheumatic" (729.2)
radiculitis
peripheral neuritis in pregnancy (646.4)

✓4ᵗʰ 350 Trigeminal nerve disorders

INCLUDES disorders of 5th cranial nerve

350.1 Trigeminal neuralgia

Tic douloureux   Trigeminal neuralgia NOS
Trifacial neuralgia
EXCLUDES postherpetic (053.12)
G50.0 Trigeminal neuralgia   I-10

350.2 Atypical face pain

350.8 Other specified trigeminal nerve disorders

350.9 Trigeminal nerve disorder, unspecified

✓4ᵗʰ 351 Facial nerve disorders

INCLUDES disorders of 7th cranial nerve
EXCLUDES that in newborn (767.5)

351.0 Bell's palsy

Facial palsy
DEF: Unilateral paralysis of face due to lesion on facial nerve; produces facial distortion.
G51.0 Bell's palsy   I-10

351.1 Geniculate ganglionitis

Geniculate ganglionitis NOS
EXCLUDES herpetic (053.11)
DEF: Inflammation of tissue at bend in facial nerve.

351.8 Other facial nerve disorders

Facial myokymia
Melkersson's syndrome
AHA: 3Q, '02, 13

351.9 Facial nerve disorder, unspecified

Diseases of the Nervous System and Sense Organs

348.5–351.9

√4ᵗʰ **352 Disorders of other cranial nerves**

352.0 Disorders of olfactory [lst] nerve

352.1 Glossopharyngeal neuralgia
 DEF: Pain between throat and ear along petrosal and jugular ganglia.
 AHA: 2Q, '02, 8

352.2 Other disorders of glossopharyngeal [9th] nerve

352.3 Disorders of pneumogastric [10th] nerve
 Disorders of vagal nerve
 EXCLUDES paralysis of vocal cords or larynx (478.30-478.34)
 DEF: Nerve disorder affecting ear, tongue, pharynx, larynx,
 esophagus, viscera and thorax.

352.4 Disorders of accessory [11th] nerve
 DEF: Nerve disorder affecting palate, pharynx, larynx, thoracic
 viscera, sternocleidomastoid and trapezius muscles.

352.5 Disorders of hypoglossal [12th] nerve
 DEF: Nerve disorder affecting tongue muscles.

352.6 Multiple cranial nerve palsies
 Collet-Sicard syndrome
 Polyneuritis cranialis

352.9 Unspecified disorder of cranial nerves

√4ᵗʰ **353 Nerve root and plexus disorders**
 EXCLUDES conditions due to:
  intervertebral disc disorders (722.0-722.9)
  spondylosis (720.0-721.9)
  vertebrogenic disorders (723.0-724.9)

353.0 Brachial plexus lesions
 Cervical rib syndrome   Scalenus anticus syndrome
 Costoclavicular syndrome   Thoracic outlet syndrome
 EXCLUDES brachial neuritis or radiculitis NOS (723.4)
  that in newborn (767.6)
 DEF: Acquired disorder in tissue along nerves in shoulder; causes
 corresponding motor and sensory dysfunction.
 AHA: 3Q, '06, 12

353.1 Lumbosacral plexus lesions
 DEF: Acquired disorder in tissue along nerves in lower back; causes
 corresponding motor and sensory dysfunction.

353.2 Cervical root lesions, not elsewhere classified

353.3 Thoracic root lesions, not elsewhere classified

353.4 Lumbosacral root lesions, not elsewhere classified

353.5 Neuralgic amyotrophy
 Parsonage-Aldren-Turner syndrome
 Code first any associated underlying disease, such as:
  diabetes mellitus (249.6, 250.6)

353.6 Phantom limb (syndrome)
 DEF: Abnormal tingling or a burning sensation, transient aches, and
 intermittent or continuous pain perceived as originating in the
 absent limb.

353.8 Other nerve root and plexus disorders

353.9 Unspecified nerve root and plexus disorder

√4ᵗʰ **354 Mononeuritis of upper limb and mononeuritis multiplex**
 DEF: Inflammation of a single nerve; known as mononeuritis multiplex when
 several nerves in unrelated body areas are affected.

354.0 Carpal tunnel syndrome
 Median nerve entrapment
 Partial thenar atrophy
 DEF: Compression of median nerve by tendons; causes pain, tingling,
 numbness and burning sensation in hand.
 G56.00 Carpal tunnel syndrome unspec upper limb   I-10

354.1 Other lesion of median nerve
 Median nerve neuritis

354.2 Lesion of ulnar nerve
 Cubital tunnel syndrome   Tardy ulnar nerve palsy

354.3 Lesion of radial nerve
 Acute radial nerve palsy
 AHA: N-D, '87, 6

354.4 Causalgia of upper limb
 Complex regional pain syndrome type II of the upper limb
 EXCLUDES causalgia:
  NOS (355.9)
  lower limb (355.71)
  complex regional pain syndrome type II of the lower
  limb (355.71)
 DEF: Peripheral nerve damage, upper limb; usually due to injury;
 causes burning sensation and trophic skin changes.

354.5 Mononeuritis multiplex
 Combinations of single conditions classifiable to 354 or 355

354.8 Other mononeuritis of upper limb

354.9 Mononeuritis of upper limb, unspecified

√4ᵗʰ **355 Mononeuritis of lower limb**

355.0 Lesion of sciatic nerve
 EXCLUDES sciatica NOS (724.3)
 DEF: Acquired disorder of sciatic nerve; causes motor and sensory
 dysfunction in back, buttock and leg.
 AHA: 2Q, '89, 12

355.1 Meralgia paresthetica
 Lateral cutaneous femoral nerve of thigh compression or
  syndrome
 DEF: Inguinal ligament entraps lateral femoral cutaneous nerve;
 causes tingling, pain and numbness along outer thigh.

355.2 Other lesion of femoral nerve

355.3 Lesion of lateral popliteal nerve
 Lesion of common peroneal nerve

355.4 Lesion of medial popliteal nerve

Peripheral Nervous System

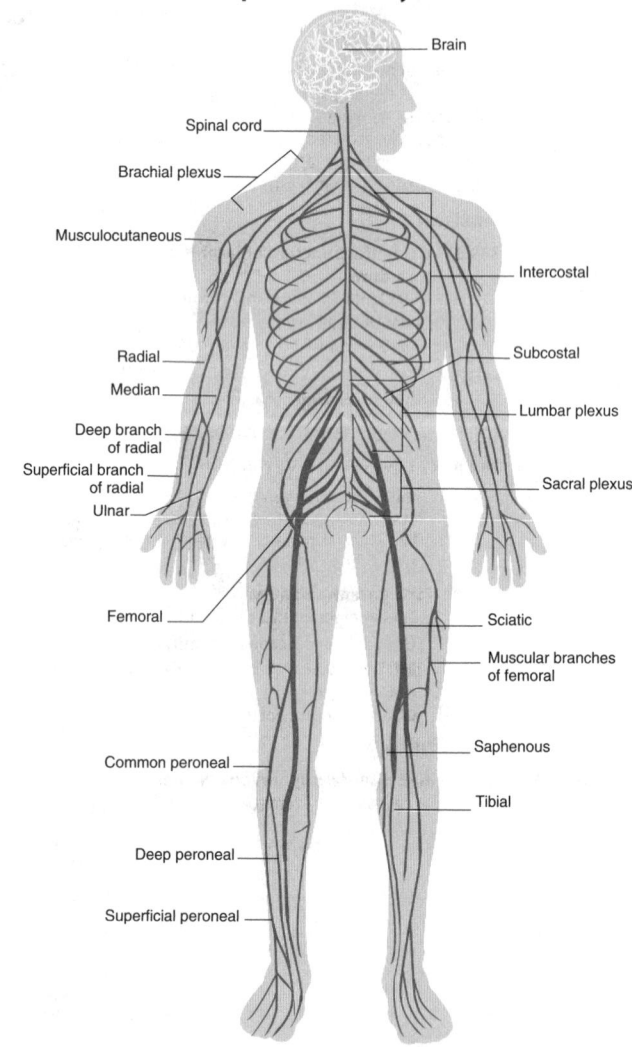

N Newborn Age: 0   P Pediatric Age: 0-17   M Maternity Age: 12-55   A Adult Age: 15-124

355.5 Tarsal tunnel syndrome
DEF: Compressed, entrapped posterior tibial nerve; causes tingling, pain and numbness in sole of foot.

355.6 Lesion of plantar nerve
Morton's metatarsalgia, neuralgia, or neuroma

√5ᵗʰ **355.7 Other mononeuritis of lower limb**

355.71 Causalgia of lower limb
EXCLUDES causalgia:
NOS (355.9)
upper limb (354.4)
complex regional pain syndrome type II of upper limb (354.4)
DEF: Dysfunction of lower limb peripheral nerve, usually due to injury; causes burning pain and trophic skin changes.

355.79 Other mononeuritis of lower limb

355.8 Mononeuritis of lower limb, unspecified

355.9 Mononeuritis of unspecified site
Causalgia NOS   Complex regional pain syndrome NOS
EXCLUDES causalgia:
lower limb (355.71)
upper limb (354.4)
complex regional pain syndrome:
lower limb (355.71)
upper limb (354.4)
G58.9 Mononeuropathy unspecified   I-10

√4ᵗʰ **356 Hereditary and idiopathic peripheral neuropathy**

356.0 Hereditary peripheral neuropathy
Déjérine-Sottas disease

356.1 Peroneal muscular atrophy
Charcôt-Marie-Tooth disease
Neuropathic muscular atrophy
DEF: Genetic disorder, in muscles innervated by peroneal nerves; symptoms include muscle wasting in lower limbs and locomotor difficulties.

356.2 Hereditary sensory neuropathy
DEF: Inherited disorder in dorsal root ganglia, optic nerve, and cerebellum, causing sensory losses, shooting pains, and foot ulcers.

356.3 Refsum's disease
Heredopathia atactica polyneuritiformis
DEF: Genetic disorder of lipid metabolism; causes persistent, painful inflammation of nerves and retinitis pigmentosa.

356.4 Idiopathic progressive polyneuropathy

356.8 Other specified idiopathic peripheral neuropathy
Supranuclear paralysis

356.9 Unspecified
G60.9 Hereditary & idiopathic neuropathy unspecified   I-10

√4ᵗʰ **357 Inflammatory and toxic neuropathy**

357.0 Acute infective polyneuritis
Guillain-Barré syndrome   Postinfectious polyneuritis
DEF: Guillain-Barré syndrome: acute demyelinating polyneuropathy preceded by viral illness (i.e., herpes, cytomegalovirus [CMV], Epstein-Barr virus [EBV]) or a bacterial illness; areflexic motor paralysis with mild sensory disturbance and acellular rise in spinal fluid protein.
AHA: 2Q, '98, 12

357.1 Polyneuropathy in collagen vascular disease
Code first underlying disease, as:
disseminated lupus erythematosus (710.0)
polyarteritis nodosa (446.0)
rheumatoid arthritis (714.0)

357.2 Polyneuropathy in diabetes
Code first underlying disease (249.6, 250.6)
AHA: 4Q, '09, 151; 2Q, '09, 13, 15; 3Q, '08, 5; 4Q, '03, 105; 2Q, '92, 15; 3Q, '91, 9

357.3 Polyneuropathy in malignant disease
Code first underlying disease (140.0-208.9)

357.4 Polyneuropathy in other diseases classified elsewhere
Code first underlying disease, as:
amyloidosis (277.30-277.39)
beriberi (265.0)
chronic uremia (585.9)
deficiency of B vitamins (266.0-266.9)
diphtheria (032.0-032.9)
hypoglycemia (251.2)
pellagra (265.2)
porphyria (277.1)
sarcoidosis (135)
uremia NOS (586)
EXCLUDES polyneuropathy in:
herpes zoster (053.13)
mumps (072.72)
AHA: 2Q, '08, 8; 2Q, '98, 15
G63 Polyneuropathy in dz classified elsewhere   I-10

357.5 Alcoholic polyneuropathy

357.6 Polyneuropathy due to drugs
Use additional E code to identify drug

357.7 Polyneuropathy due to other toxic agents
Use additional E code to identify toxic agent

√5ᵗʰ **357.8 Other**
AHA: 4Q, '02, 47; 2Q, '98, 12

357.81 Chronic inflammatory demyelinating polyneuritis
DEF: Inflammation of peripheral nerves resulting in destruction of myelin sheath; associated with diabetes mellitus, dysproteinemia, renal failure and malnutrition; symptoms include tingling, numbness, burning pain, diminished tendon reflexes, weakness of lower extremities.

357.82 Critical illness polyneuropathy
Acute motor neuropathy
DEF: An acute axonal neuropathy, both sensory and motor, that is associated with Systemic Inflammatory Response Syndrome (SIRS).
AHA: 4Q, '03, 111

357.89 Other inflammatory and toxic neuropathy

357.9 Unspecified

√4ᵗʰ **358 Myoneural disorders**

√5ᵗʰ **358.0 Myasthenia gravis**
DEF: Autoimmune disorder of acetylcholine at neuromuscular junction; causing fatigue of voluntary muscles.
AHA: 4Q, '03, 59

358.00 Myasthenia gravis without (acute) exacerbation
Myasthenia gravis NOS
G70.00 Myasthenia gravis w/o (acute) exacerbation   I-10

358.01 Myasthenia gravis with (acute) exacerbation
Myasthenia gravis in crisis
AHA: 4Q, '07, 109; 1Q, '05, 4; 4Q, '04, 139

358.1 Myasthenic syndromes in diseases classified elsewhere
Code first underlying disease, as:
botulism (005.1, 040.41-040.42)
hypothyroidism (244.0-244.9)
malignant neoplasm (140.0-208.9)
pernicious anemia (281.0)
thyrotoxicosis (242.0-242.9)

358.2 Toxic myoneural disorders
Use additional E code to identify toxic agent

√5ᵗʰ **358.3 Lambert-Eaton syndrome**
Eaton-Lambert syndrome
AHA: ▶4Q, '11, 100-101◀

358.30 Lambert-Eaton syndrome, unspecified
Lambert-Eaton syndrome NOS
AHA: ▶4Q, '11, 101◀

358.31 Lambert-Eaton syndrome in neoplastic disease
Code first the underlying neoplastic disease

358.39 Lambert-Eaton syndrome in other diseases classified elsewhere
Code first the underlying condition

358.8 Other specified myoneural disorders

358.9 Myoneural disorders, unspecified
AHA: 2Q, '02, 16

Diseases of the Nervous System and Sense Organs

359–360.03

✓4ᵗʰ **359 Muscular dystrophies and other myopathies**
    EXCLUDES *idiopathic polymyositis (710.4)*

359.0 Congenital hereditary muscular dystrophy
    Benign congenital myopathy   Myotubular myopathy
    Central core disease   Nemaline body disease
    Centronuclear myopathy
    EXCLUDES *arthrogryposis multiplex congenita (754.89)*
    DEF: Genetic disorder; causing progressive or nonprogressive muscle weakness.

359.1 Hereditary progressive muscular dystrophy
    Muscular dystrophy: Muscular dystrophy:
      NOS   Gower's
      distal   Landouzy-Déjérine
      Duchenne   limb-girdle
      Erb's   ocular
      fascioscapulohumeral   oculopharyngeal
    DEF: Genetic degenerative, muscle disease; causes progressive weakness, wasting of muscle with no nerve involvement.

✓5ᵗʰ **359.2 Myotonic disorders**
    EXCLUDES *periodic paralysis (359.3)*
    DEF: Impaired movement due to spasmatic, rigid muscles.
    AHA: 4Q, '07, 75

    359.21 Myotonic muscular dystrophy
      Dystrophia myotonica
      Myotonia atrophica
      Myotonic dystrophy
      Proximal myotonic myopathy [PROMM]
      Steinert's disease

    359.22 Myotonia congenita
      Acetazolamide responsive myotonia congenita
      Dominant form [Thomsen's disease]
      Myotonia levior
      Recessive form [Becker's disease]

    359.23 Myotonic chondrodystrophy
      Congenital myotonic chondrodystrophy
      Schwartz-Jampel disease

    359.24 Drug induced myotonia
      Use additional E code to identify drug

    359.29 Other specified myotonic disorder
      Myotonia fluctuans
      Myotonia permanens
      Paramyotonia congenita (of von Eulenburg)

359.3 Periodic paralysis
    Familial periodic paralysis
    Hypokalemic familial periodic paralysis
    Hyperkalemic periodic paralysis
    Hypokalemic periodic paralysis
    Potassium sensitive periodic paralysis
    EXCLUDES *paramyotonia congenita (of von Eulenburg) (359.29)*
    DEF: Genetic disorder; characterized by rapidly progressive flaccid paralysis; attacks often occur after exercise or exposure to cold or dietary changes.

359.4 Toxic myopathy
    Use additional E code to identify toxic agent
    DEF: Muscle disorder caused by toxic agent.
    AHA: 1Q, '88, 5

359.5 *Myopathy in endocrine diseases classified elsewhere*
    Code first underlying disease, as:
      Addison's disease (255.41)
      Cushing's syndrome (255.0)
      hypopituitarism (253.2)
      myxedema (244.0-244.9)
      thyrotoxicosis (242.0-242.9)
    DEF: Muscle disorder secondary to dysfunction in hormone secretion.

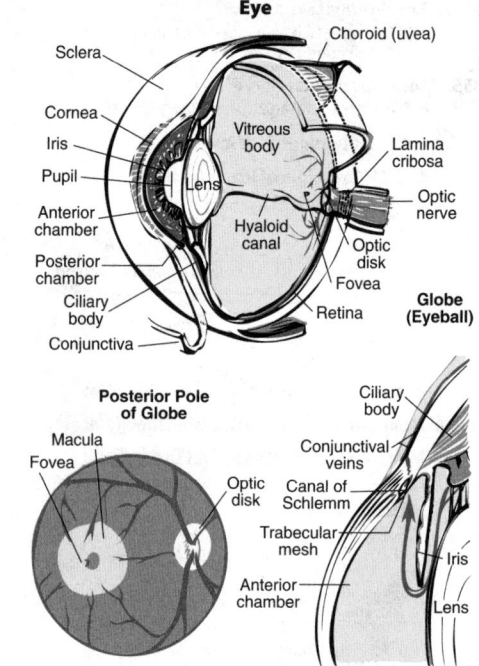

Eye

(Eye diagram labels: Sclera, Cornea, Iris, Pupil, Anterior chamber, Posterior chamber, Ciliary body, Conjunctiva, Choroid (uvea), Vitreous body, Lens, Hyaloid canal, Lamina cribosa, Optic nerve, Optic disk, Fovea, Retina, Globe (Eyeball))

Posterior Pole of Globe

(Labels: Macula, Fovea, Optic disk)

Flow of Aqueous Humor

(Labels: Ciliary body, Conjunctival veins, Canal of Schlemm, Trabecular mesh, Iris, Lens, Anterior chamber)

359.6 *Symptomatic inflammatory myopathy in diseases classified elsewhere*
    Code first underlying disease, as:
      amyloidosis (277.30-277.39)
      disseminated lupus erythematosus (710.0)
      malignant neoplasm (140.0-208.9)
      polyarteritis nodosa (446.0)
      rheumatoid arthritis (714.0)
      sarcoidosis (135)
      scleroderma (710.1)
      Sjögren's disease (710.2)

✓5ᵗʰ **359.7 Inflammatory and immune myopathies, NEC**
    359.71 Inclusion body myositis
      IBM
      DEF: Progressive, debilitating inflammatory muscle disease characterized by dysphagia, chronic muscle swelling, weakness, and atrophy (wasting); impairs fine motor functions.
      AHA: 4Q, '09, 84

    359.79 Other inflammatory and immune myopathies, NEC
      Inflammatory myopathy NOS

✓5ᵗʰ **359.8 Other myopathies**
    AHA: 4Q, '02, 47; 3Q, '90, 17

    359.81 Critical illness myopathy
      Acute necrotizing myopathy
      Acute quadriplegic myopathy
      Intensive care (ICU) myopathy
      Myopathy of critical illness

    359.89 Other myopathies

    359.9 Myopathy, unspecified

Disorders of the Eye and Adnexa (360-379)

Use additional external cause code, if applicable, to identify the cause of the eye condition

✓4ᵗʰ **360 Disorders of the globe**
    INCLUDES disorders affecting multiple structures of eye

✓5ᵗʰ **360.0 Purulent endophthalmitis**
    EXCLUDES *bleb associated endophthalmitis (379.63)*

    360.00 Purulent endophthalmitis, unspecified

    360.01 Acute endophthalmitis

    360.02 Panophthalmitis

    360.03 Chronic endophthalmitis

Adnexa

Upper eyelid
Orbicularis oculi muscle
Orbital septum
Tarsal plate (cartilage)
Conjunctival fornix
Lower eyelid
Tarsal plate
Orbital septum
Orbital floor
Orbital roof
Levator palpebri muscle
Müller's muscle
Globe (eyeball)
Optic nerve
Retrobulbar space
Fascia bulbi (Tenon's capsule)
Extraocular muscle

360.04 Vitreous abscess

360.1 Other endophthalmitis
> EXCLUDES *bleb associated endophthalmitis (379.63)*

360.11 Sympathetic uveitis
> DEF: Inflammation of vascular layer of uninjured eye; follows injury to other eye.

360.12 Panuveitis
> DEF: Inflammation of entire vascular layer of eye, including choroid, iris and ciliary body.

360.13 Parasitic endophthalmitis NOS
> DEF: Parasitic infection causing inflammation of the entire eye.

360.14 Ophthalmia nodosa
> DEF: Conjunctival inflammation caused by embedded hairs.

360.19 Other
> Phacoanaphylactic endophthalmitis

360.2 Degenerative disorders of globe
> AHA: 3Q, '91, 3

360.20 Degenerative disorder of globe, unspecified

360.21 Progressive high (degenerative) myopia
> Malignant myopia
> DEF: Severe, progressive nearsightedness in adults, complicated by serious disease of the choroid; leads to retinal detachment and blindness.

360.23 Siderosis
> DEF: Iron pigment deposits within tissue of eyeball; caused by high iron content of blood.

360.24 Other metallosis
> Chalcosis
> DEF: Metal deposits, other than iron, within eyeball tissues.

360.29 Other
> EXCLUDES *xerophthalmia (264.7)*

360.3 Hypotony of eye

360.30 Hypotony, unspecified
> DEF: Low osmotic pressure causing lack of tone, tension and strength.

360.31 Primary hypotony

360.32 Ocular fistula causing hypotony
> DEF: Low intraocular pressure due to leak through abnormal passage.

360.33 Hypotony associated with other ocular disorders

360.34 Flat anterior chamber
> DEF: Low pressure behind cornea, causing compression.

360.4 Degenerated conditions of globe

360.40 Degenerated globe or eye, unspecified

360.41 Blind hypotensive eye
> Atrophy of globe   Phthisis bulbi
> DEF: Vision loss due to extremely low intraocular pressure.

360.42 Blind hypertensive eye
> Absolute glaucoma
> DEF: Vision loss due to painful, high intraocular pressure.

360.43 Hemophthalmos, except current injury
> EXCLUDES *traumatic (871.0-871.9, 921.0-921.9)*
> DEF: Pool of blood within eyeball, not from current injury.

360.44 Leucocoria
> DEF: Whitish mass or reflex in the pupil behind lens; also called cat's eye reflex; often indicative of retinoblastoma.

360.5 Retained (old) intraocular foreign body, magnetic
> Use additional code to identify foreign body (V90.11)
> EXCLUDES *current penetrating injury with magnetic foreign body (871.5)*
> *retained (old) foreign body of orbit (376.6)*

360.50 Foreign body, magnetic, intraocular, unspecified

360.51 Foreign body, magnetic, in anterior chamber

360.52 Foreign body, magnetic, in iris or ciliary body

360.53 Foreign body, magnetic, in lens

360.54 Foreign body, magnetic, in vitreous

360.55 Foreign body, magnetic, in posterior wall

360.59 Foreign body, magnetic, in other or multiple sites

360.6 Retained (old) intraocular foreign body, nonmagnetic
> Retained (old) foreign body:
>   NOS
>   nonmagnetic
> Use additional code to identify foreign body (V90.01-V90.10, V90.12, V90.2-V90.9)
> EXCLUDES *current penetrating injury with (nonmagnetic) foreign body (871.6)*
> *retained (old) foreign body in orbit (376.6)*

360.60 Foreign body, intraocular, unspecified

360.61 Foreign body in anterior chamber

360.62 Foreign body in iris or ciliary body

360.63 Foreign body in lens

360.64 Foreign body in vitreous

360.65 Foreign body in posterior wall

360.69 Foreign body in other or multiple sites

360.8 Other disorders of globe

360.81 Luxation of globe
> DEF: Displacement of eyeball.

360.89 Other

360.9 Unspecified disorder of globe

361 Retinal detachments and defects
> DEF: Disorders of light-sensitive layer at back of eye, which separates from blood supply, disrupting vision.

361.0 Retinal detachment with retinal defect
> Rhegmatogenous retinal detachment
> EXCLUDES *detachment of retinal pigment epithelium (362.42-362.43)*
> *retinal detachment (serous) (without defect) (361.2)*

361.00 Retinal detachment with retinal defect, unspecified

361.01 Recent detachment, partial, with single defect

361.02 Recent detachment, partial, with multiple defects

361.03 Recent detachment, partial, with giant tear

361.04 Recent detachment, partial, with retinal dialysis
> Dialysis (juvenile) of retina (with detachment)

361.05 Recent detachment, total or subtotal

361.06 Old detachment, partial
> Delimited old retinal detachment

361.07 Old detachment, total or subtotal

Diseases of the Nervous System and Sense Organs

361.1–362.33

√5ᵗʰ **361.1 Retinoschisis and retinal cysts**

> EXCLUDES *juvenile retinoschisis (362.73)*
> *microcystoid degeneration of retina (362.62)*
> *parasitic cyst of retina (360.13)*

361.10 Retinoschisis, unspecified
> DEF: Separation of retina due to degenerative process of aging; should not be confused with acute retinal detachment.

361.11 Flat retinoschisis
> DEF: Slow, progressive split of retinal sensory layers.

361.12 Bullous retinoschisis
> DEF: Fluid retention between split retinal sensory layers.

361.13 Primary retinal cysts

361.14 Secondary retinal cysts

361.19 Other
> Pseudocyst of retina

361.2 Serous retinal detachment
> Retinal detachment without retinal defect
> EXCLUDES *central serous retinopathy (362.41)*
> *retinal pigment epithelium detachment (362.42-362.43)*

√5ᵗʰ **361.3 Retinal defects without detachment**

> EXCLUDES *chorioretinal scars after surgery for detachment (363.30-363.35)*
> *peripheral retinal degeneration without defect (362.60-362.66)*

361.30 Retinal defect, unspecified
> Retinal break(s) NOS

361.31 Round hole of retina without detachment

361.32 Horseshoe tear of retina without detachment
> Operculum of retina without mention of detachment

361.33 Multiple defects of retina without detachment

√5ᵗʰ **361.8 Other forms of retinal detachment**

361.81 Traction detachment of retina
> Traction detachment with vitreoretinal organization

361.89 Other
> AHA: 3Q, '99, 12

361.9 Unspecified retinal detachment
> AHA: N-D, '87, 10

√4ᵗʰ **362 Other retinal disorders**

> EXCLUDES *chorioretinal scars (363.30-363.35)*
> *chorioretinitis (363.0-363.2)*

√5ᵗʰ **362.0 Diabetic retinopathy**

> *Code first diabetes (249.5, 250.5)*
> DEF: Retinal changes in diabetes of long duration; causes hemorrhages, microaneurysms, waxy deposits and proliferative noninflammatory degenerative disease of retina.
> AHA: 4Q, '05, 65; 3Q, '91, 8

362.01 *Background diabetic retinopathy*
> Diabetic retinal microaneurysms
> Diabetic retinopathy NOS

362.02 *Proliferative diabetic retinopathy*
> DEF: Occurrence of the ischemic effects of vessel blockages result in neovascularization; new blood vessels begin to form to compensate for restricted blood flow; multiple areas of the retina and inner vitreous may be affected.
> AHA: 3Q, '96, 5

362.03 *Nonproliferative diabetic retinopathy NOS*

362.04 *Mild nonproliferative diabetic retinopathy*
> DEF: Early stages of degenerative condition of the retina due to diabetes; microaneurysm formation; small balloon-like swelling of the retinal vessels.

362.05 *Moderate nonproliferative diabetic retinopathy*
> DEF: Stage of degenerative condition of the retina due to diabetes with pronounced microaneurysms; vessel blockages can occur.

362.06 *Severe nonproliferative diabetic retinopathy*
> DEF: Stage of degenerative condition of the retina due to diabetes in which vascular breakdown in the retina results in multiple vascular blockages, or "beadings," with intraretinal hemorrhages.
> AHA: 4Q, '05, 67

362.07 *Diabetic macular edema*
> NOTE Code 362.07 must be used with a code for diabetic retinopathy (362.01-362.06)
> Diabetic retinal edema
> DEF: Leakage from retinal blood vessels causes swelling of the macula and impaired vision; exudates or plaques may develop in the posterior pole of the retina due to the breakdown of retinal vasculature.

√5ᵗʰ **362.1 Other background retinopathy and retinal vascular changes**

362.10 Background retinopathy, unspecified
> AHA: 1Q, '06, 12

362.11 Hypertensive retinopathy
> DEF: Retinal irregularities caused by systemic hypertension.
> AHA: 3Q, '90, 3

362.12 Exudative retinopathy
> Coats' syndrome
> AHA: 3Q, '99, 12

362.13 Changes in vascular appearance
> Vascular sheathing of retina
> Use additional code for any associated atherosclerosis (440.8)

362.14 Retinal microaneurysms NOS
> DEF: Microscopic dilation of retinal vessels in nondiabetic.

362.15 Retinal telangiectasia
> DEF: Dilation of blood vessels of the retina.

362.16 Retinal neovascularization NOS
> Neovascularization: Neovascularization:
> choroidal   subretinal
> DEF: New and abnormal vascular growth in the retina.

362.17 Other intraretinal microvascular abnormalities
> Retinal sclerosis
> Retinal varices

362.18 Retinal vasculitis
> Eales' disease   Retinal:
> Retinal: perivasculitis
> arteritis   phlebitis
> endarteritis
> DEF: Inflammation of retinal blood vessels.

√5ᵗʰ **362.2 Other proliferative retinopathy**
> AHA: 4Q, '08, 110-111

362.20 Retinopathy of prematurity, unspecified
> Retinopathy of prematurity NOS

362.21 Retrolental fibroplasia
> Cicatricial retinopathy of prematurity
> DEF: Fibrous tissue in vitreous, from retina to lens, causing blindness; associated with premature infants requiring high amounts of oxygen.

362.22 Retinopathy of prematurity, stage 0

362.23 Retinopathy of prematurity, stage 1

362.24 Retinopathy of prematurity, stage 2

362.25 Retinopathy of prematurity, stage 3

362.26 Retinopathy of prematurity, stage 4

362.27 Retinopathy of prematurity, stage 5

362.29 Other nondiabetic proliferative retinopathy
> AHA: 3Q, '96, 5

√5ᵗʰ **362.3 Retinal vascular occlusion**
> DEF: Obstructed blood flow to and from retina.

362.30 Retinal vascular occlusion, unspecified

362.31 Central retinal artery occlusion

362.32 Arterial branch occlusion

362.33 Partial arterial occlusion
> Hollenhorst plaque   Retinal microembolism

362.34 Transient arterial occlusion
Amaurosis fugax
AHA: 1Q, '00, 16

362.35 Central retinal vein occlusion
AHA: 2Q, '93, 6

362.36 Venous tributary (branch) occlusion

362.37 Venous engorgement
Occlusion:
incipient
partial } of retinal vein

√5th **362.4 Separation of retinal layers**
EXCLUDES   retinal detachment (serous) (361.2)
rhegmatogenous (361.00-361.07)

362.40 Retinal layer separation, unspecified

362.41 Central serous retinopathy
DEF: Serous-filled blister causing detachment of retina from pigment epithelium.

362.42 Serous detachment of retinal pigment epithelium
Exudative detachment of retinal pigment epithelium
DEF: Blister of fatty fluid causing detachment of retina from pigment epithelium.

362.43 Hemorrhagic detachment of retinal pigment epithelium
DEF: Blood-filled blister causing detachment of retina from pigment epithelium.

√5th **362.5 Degeneration of macula and posterior pole**
EXCLUDES   degeneration of optic disc (377.21-377.24)
hereditary retinal degeneration [dystrophy] (362.70-362.77)

362.50 Macular degeneration (senile), unspecified

362.51 Nonexudative senile macular degeneration
Senile macular degeneration:
atrophic
dry

362.52 Exudative senile macular degeneration
Kuhnt-Junius degeneration
Senile macular degeneration:
disciform
wet
DEF: Leakage in macular blood vessels with loss of visual acuity.

362.53 Cystoid macular degeneration
Cystoid macular edema
DEF: Retinal swelling and cyst formation in macula.

362.54 Macular cyst, hole, or pseudohole
AHA: ▶4Q, '11, 106◀

362.55 Toxic maculopathy
Use additional E code to identify drug, if drug induced

362.56 Macular puckering
Preretinal fibrosis

362.57 Drusen (degenerative)
DEF: White, hyaline deposits on Bruch's membrane (lamina basalis choroideae).

√5th **362.6 Peripheral retinal degenerations**
EXCLUDES   hereditary retinal degeneration [dystrophy] (362.70-362.77)
retinal degeneration with retinal defect (361.00-361.07)

362.60 Peripheral retinal degeneration, unspecified

362.61 Paving stone degeneration
DEF: Degeneration of peripheral retina; causes thinning through which choroid is visible.

362.62 Microcystoid degeneration
Blessig's cysts   Iwanoff's cysts

362.63 Lattice degeneration
Palisade degeneration of retina
DEF: Degeneration of retina; often bilateral, usually benign; characterized by lines intersecting at irregular intervals in peripheral retina; retinal thinning and retinal holes may occur.

362.64 Senile reticular degeneration
DEF: Net-like appearance of retina; sign of degeneration.

362.65 Secondary pigmentary degeneration
Pseudoretinitis pigmentosa

362.66 Secondary vitreoretinal degenerations

√5th **362.7 Hereditary retinal dystrophies**
DEF: Genetically induced progressive changes in retina.

362.70 Hereditary retinal dystrophy, unspecified

362.71 Retinal dystrophy in systemic or cerebroretinal lipidoses
Code first underlying disease, as:
cerebroretinal lipidoses (330.1)
systemic lipidoses (272.7)

362.72 Retinal dystrophy in other systemic disorders and syndromes
Code first underlying disease, as:
Bassen-Kornzweig syndrome (272.5)
Refsum's disease (356.3)

362.73 Vitreoretinal dystrophies
Juvenile retinoschisis

362.74 Pigmentary retinal dystrophy
Retinal dystrophy, albipunctate
Retinitis pigmentosa

362.75 Other dystrophies primarily involving the sensory retina
Progressive cone(-rod) dystrophy
Stargardt's disease

362.76 Dystrophies primarily involving the retinal pigment epithelium
Fundus flavimaculatus   Vitelliform dystrophy

362.77 Dystrophies primarily involving Bruch's membrane
Dystrophy:
hyaline
pseudoinflammatory foveal
Hereditary drusen

√5th **362.8 Other retinal disorders**
EXCLUDES   chorioretinal inflammations (363.0-363.2)
chorioretinal scars (363.30-363.35)

362.81 Retinal hemorrhage
Hemorrhage: Hemorrhage:
preretinal   subretinal
retinal (deep) (superficial)
AHA: 4Q, '96, 43

362.82 Retinal exudates and deposits

362.83 Retinal edema
Retinal:
cotton wool spots
edema (localized) (macular) (peripheral)
DEF: Retinal swelling due to fluid accumulation.

362.84 Retinal ischemia
DEF: Reduced retinal blood supply.

362.85 Retinal nerve fiber bundle defects

362.89 Other retinal disorders

362.9 Unspecified retinal disorder

√4th **363 Chorioretinal inflammations, scars, and other disorders of choroid**

√5th **363.0 Focal chorioretinitis and focal retinochoroiditis**
EXCLUDES   focal chorioretinitis or retinochoroiditis in:
histoplasmosis (115.02, 115.12, 115.92)
toxoplasmosis (130.2)
congenital infection (771.2)

363.00 Focal chorioretinitis, unspecified
Focal:
choroiditis or chorioretinitis NOS
retinitis or retinochoroiditis NOS

363.01 Focal choroiditis and chorioretinitis, juxtapapillary

363.03 Focal choroiditis and chorioretinitis of other posterior pole

√4th √5th Additional Digit Required   Unspecified Code   Other Specified Code   Manifestation Code   ▶◀ Revised Text   ● New Code   ▲ Revised Code Title

2013 ICD-9-CM   **February 2012 • Volume 1 – 103**

Diseases of the Nervous System and Sense Organs

363.04–364.10

363.04 Focal choroiditis and chorioretinitis, peripheral

363.05 Focal retinitis and retinochoroiditis, juxtapapillary
Neuroretinitis

363.06 Focal retinitis and retinochoroiditis, macular or paramacular

363.07 Focal retinitis and retinochoroiditis of other posterior pole

363.08 Focal retinitis and retinochoroiditis, peripheral

✓5ᵗʰ **363.1 Disseminated chorioretinitis and disseminated retinochoroiditis**
> **EXCLUDES** *disseminated choroiditis or chorioretinitis in secondary syphilis (091.51)*
> *neurosyphilitic disseminated retinitis or retinochoroiditis (094.83)*
> *retinal (peri)vasculitis (362.18)*

363.10 Disseminated chorioretinitis, unspecified
Disseminated:
choroiditis or chorioretinitis NOS
retinitis or retinochoroiditis NOS

363.11 Disseminated choroiditis and, chorioretinitis posterior pole

363.12 Disseminated choroiditis and chorioretinitis, peripheral

363.13 Disseminated choroiditis and chorioretinitis, generalized
Code first any underlying disease, as:
tuberculosis (017.3)

363.14 Disseminated retinitis and retinochoroiditis, metastatic

363.15 Disseminated retinitis and retinochoroiditis, pigment epitheliopathy
Acute posterior multifocal placoid pigment epitheliopathy
DEF: Widespread inflammation of retina and choroid; characterized by pigmented epithelium involvement.

✓5ᵗʰ **363.2 Other and unspecified forms of chorioretinitis and retinochoroiditis**
> **EXCLUDES** *panophthalmitis (360.02)*
> *sympathetic uveitis (360.11)*
> *uveitis NOS (364.3)*

363.20 Chorioretinitis, unspecified
Choroiditis NOS   Uveitis, posterior NOS
Retinitis NOS

363.21 Pars planitis
Posterior cyclitis
DEF: Inflammation of peripheral retina and ciliary body; characterized by bands of white cells.

363.22 Harada's disease
DEF: Retinal detachment and bilateral widespread exudative choroiditis; symptoms include headache, vomiting, increased lymphocytes in cerebrospinal fluid; with temporary or permanent deafness.

✓5ᵗʰ **363.3 Chorioretinal scars**
Scar (postinflammatory) (postsurgical) (posttraumatic):
choroid
retina

363.30 Chorioretinal scar, unspecified

363.31 Solar retinopathy
DEF: Retinal scarring caused by solar radiation.

363.32 Other macular scars

363.33 Other scars of posterior pole

363.34 Peripheral scars

363.35 Disseminated scars

✓5ᵗʰ **363.4 Choroidal degenerations**

363.40 Choroidal degeneration, unspecified
Choroidal sclerosis NOS

363.41 Senile atrophy of choroid
DEF: Wasting away of choroid; due to aging.

363.42 Diffuse secondary atrophy of choroid
DEF: Wasting away of choroid in systemic disease.

363.43 Angioid streaks of choroid
DEF: Degeneration of choroid; characterized by dark brown streaks radiating from optic disc; occurs with pseudoxanthoma, elasticum or Paget's disease.

✓5ᵗʰ **363.5 Hereditary choroidal dystrophies**
Hereditary choroidal atrophy:
partial [choriocapillaris]
total [all vessels]

363.50 Hereditary choroidal dystrophy or atrophy, unspecified

363.51 Circumpapillary dystrophy of choroid, partial

363.52 Circumpapillary dystrophy of choroid, total
Helicoid dystrophy of choroid

363.53 Central dystrophy of choroid, partial
Dystrophy, choroidal: Dystrophy, choroidal:
central areolar   circinate

363.54 Central choroidal atrophy, total
Dystrophy, choroidal: Dystrophy, choroidal:
central gyrate   serpiginous

363.55 Choroideremia
DEF: Hereditary choroid degeneration, occurs in first decade; characterized by constricted visual field and ultimately blindness in males; less debilitating in females.

363.56 Other diffuse or generalized dystrophy, partial
Diffuse choroidal sclerosis

363.57 Other diffuse or generalized dystrophy, total
Generalized gyrate atrophy, choroid

✓5ᵗʰ **363.6 Choroidal hemorrhage and rupture**

363.61 Choroidal hemorrhage, unspecified

363.62 Expulsive choroidal hemorrhage

363.63 Choroidal rupture

✓5ᵗʰ **363.7 Choroidal detachment**

363.70 Choroidal detachment, unspecified

363.71 Serous choroidal detachment
DEF: Detachment of choroid from sclera; due to blister of serous fluid.

363.72 Hemorrhagic choroidal detachment
DEF: Detachment of choroid from sclera; due to blood-filled blister.

363.8 Other disorders of choroid

363.9 Unspecified disorder of choroid

✓4ᵗʰ **364 Disorders of iris and ciliary body**

✓5ᵗʰ **364.0 Acute and subacute iridocyclitis**
Anterior uveitis
Cylitis   } acute, subacute
Iridocyclitis
Iritis
> **EXCLUDES** *gonococcal (098.41)*
> *herpes simplex (054.44)*
> *herpes zoster (053.22)*

364.00 Acute and subacute iridocyclitis, unspecified

364.01 Primary iridocyclitis

364.02 Recurrent iridocyclitis

364.03 Secondary iridocyclitis, infectious

364.04 Secondary iridocyclitis, noninfectious
Aqueous: Aqueous:
cells   flare
fibrin

364.05 Hypopyon
DEF: Accumulation of white blood cells between cornea and lens.

✓5ᵗʰ **364.1 Chronic iridocyclitis**
> **EXCLUDES** *posterior cyclitis (363.21)*

364.10 Chronic iridocyclitis, unspecified

364.11 Chronic iridocyclitis in diseases classified elsewhere

> Code first underlying disease, as:
> sarcoidosis (135)
> tuberculosis (017.3)
>
> EXCLUDES syphilitic iridocyclitis (091.52)
>
> **DEF:** Persistent inflammation of iris and ciliary body; due to underlying disease or condition.

364.2 Certain types of iridocyclitis

> EXCLUDES posterior cyclitis (363.21)
> sympathetic uveitis (360.11)

364.21 Fuchs' heterochromic cyclitis

> **DEF:** Chronic cyclitis characterized by differences in the color of the two irises; the lighter iris appears in the inflamed eye.

364.22 Glaucomatocyclitic crises

> **DEF:** An uncommon inflammatory unilateral eye condition, characteristic recurrent episodes of high intraocular pressure accompanied by mild inflammation.

364.23 Lens-induced iridocyclitis

> **DEF:** Inflammation of iris; due to immune reaction to proteins in lens following trauma or other lens abnormality.

364.24 Vogt-Koyanagi syndrome

> **DEF:** Uveomeningitis with exudative iridocyclitis and choroiditis; causes depigmentation of hair and skin, detached retina; tinnitus and loss of hearing.

364.3 Unspecified iridocyclitis

> Uveitis NOS

364.4 Vascular disorders of iris and ciliary body

364.41 Hyphema

> Hemorrhage of iris or ciliary body
> **DEF:** Hemorrhage in anterior chamber; also called hyphemia or "blood shot" eyes.

364.42 Rubeosis iridis

> Neovascularization of iris or ciliary body
> **DEF:** Blood vessel and connective tissue formation on surface of iris; symptomatic of diabetic retinopathy, central retinal vein occlusion and retinal detachment.

364.5 Degenerations of iris and ciliary body

364.51 Essential or progressive iris atrophy

364.52 Iridoschisis

> **DEF:** Splitting of the iris into two layers.

364.53 Pigmentary iris degeneration

> Acquired heterochromia
> Pigment dispersion syndrome } of iris
> Translucency

364.54 Degeneration of pupillary margin

> Atrophy of sphincter
> Ectropion of pigment epithelium } of iris

364.55 Miotic cysts of pupillary margin

> **DEF:** Serous-filled sacs in pupillary margin of iris.

364.56 Degenerative changes of chamber angle

364.57 Degenerative changes of ciliary body

364.59 Other iris atrophy

> Iris atrophy (generalized) (sector shaped)

364.6 Cysts of iris, ciliary body, and anterior chamber

> EXCLUDES miotic pupillary cyst (364.55)
> parasitic cyst (360.13)

364.60 Idiopathic cysts

> **DEF:** Fluid-filled sacs in iris or ciliary body; unknown etiology.

364.61 Implantation cysts

> Epithelial down-growth, anterior chamber
> Implantation cysts (surgical) (traumatic)

364.62 Exudative cysts of iris or anterior chamber

364.63 Primary cyst of pars plana

> **DEF:** Fluid-filled sacs of outermost ciliary ring.

364.64 Exudative cyst of pars plana

> **DEF:** Protein, fatty-filled sacs of outermost ciliary ring; due to fluid leak from blood vessels.

364.7 Adhesions and disruptions of iris and ciliary body

> EXCLUDES flat anterior chamber (360.34)

364.70 Adhesions of iris, unspecified

> Synechiae (iris) NOS

364.71 Posterior synechiae

> **DEF:** Adhesion binding iris to lens.

364.72 Anterior synechiae

> **DEF:** Adhesion binding the iris to cornea.

364.73 Goniosynechiae

> Peripheral anterior synechiae
> **DEF:** Adhesion binding the iris to cornea at the angle of the anterior chamber.

364.74 Pupillary membranes

> Iris bombé   Pupillary:
> Pupillary: seclusion
> occlusion
> **DEF:** Membrane traversing the pupil and blocking vision.

364.75 Pupillary abnormalities

> Deformed pupil   Rupture of sphincter, pupil
> Ectopic pupil

364.76 Iridodialysis

> **DEF:** Separation of the iris from the ciliary body base; due to trauma or surgical accident.

364.77 Recession of chamber angle

> **DEF:** Receding of anterior chamber angle of the eye; restricts vision.

364.8 Other disorders of iris and ciliary body

> AHA: 2Q, '07, 9

364.81 Floppy iris syndrome

> Intraoperative floppy iris syndrome [IFIS]
>
> Use additional E code to identify cause, such as:
> sympatholytics [antiadrenergics] causing adverse effect in therapeutic use (E941.3)
>
> **DEF:** Condition complicating cataract surgery for patients who have received alpha blocker treatment for urinary retention problems; iris dilator muscle fails to dilate, and the iris may billow or flap.
> AHA: 4Q, '07, 77, 79

364.82 Plateau iris syndrome

> **DEF:** A postoperative chronic angle-closure glaucoma characterized by closing of the anterior chamber angle secondary to a large or anteriorly positioned ciliary body that impairs the normal flow of aqueous fluid.
> AHA: 4Q, '08, 112

364.89 Other disorders of iris and ciliary body

> Prolapse of iris NOS
> EXCLUDES prolapse of iris in recent wound (871.1)

364.9 Unspecified disorder of iris and ciliary body

365 Glaucoma

> EXCLUDES blind hypertensive eye [absolute glaucoma] (360.42)
> congenital glaucoma (743.20-743.22)
> **DEF:** Rise in intraocular pressure restricting blood flow; multiple causes.

365.0 Borderline glaucoma [glaucoma suspect]

> AHA: 1Q, '90, 8

365.00 Preglaucoma, unspecified

365.01 Open angle with borderline findings, low risk

> Open angle, low risk
> **DEF:** Minor block of aqueous outflow from eye
> AHA: ►4Q, '11, 102◄

365.02 Anatomical narrow angle

> Primary angle closure suspect

365.03 Steroid responders

365.04 Ocular hypertension

> **DEF:** High fluid pressure within eye; no clear cause.

365.05 Open angle with borderline findings, high risk

> Open angle, high risk
> AHA: ►4Q, '11, 102-103◄

365.06 Primary angle closure without glaucoma damage

> AHA: ►4Q, '11, 102-103◄

√4ᵗʰ / √5ᵗʰ Additional Digit Required   Unspecified Code   Other Specified Code   Manifestation Code   ►◄ Revised Text   ● New Code   ▲ Revised Code Title

2013 ICD-9-CM   **February 2012 • Volume 1 – 105**

Plateau Iris Syndrome

Normal Aqueous Flow

Angle Closure Glaucoma

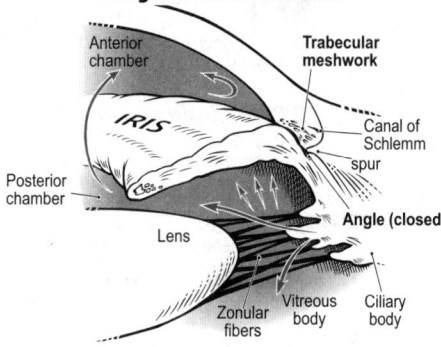

☑5ᵗʰ **365.1　Open-angle glaucoma**

　365.10　Open-angle glaucoma, unspecified
　　　Wide-angle glaucoma NOS
　　　Use additional code to identify glaucoma stage
　　　(365.70-365.74)

　365.11　Primary open angle glaucoma
　　　Chronic simple glaucoma
　　　Use additional code to identify glaucoma stage
　　　(365.70-365.74)
　　　DEF: High intraocular pressure, despite free flow of aqueous.

　365.12　Low tension glaucoma
　　　Use additional code to identify glaucoma stage
　　　(365.70-365.74)

　365.13　Pigmentary glaucoma
　　　Use additional code to identify glaucoma stage
　　　(365.70-365.74)
　　　DEF: High intraocular pressure; due to iris pigment granules blocking aqueous flow.

　365.14　Glaucoma of childhood
　　　Infantile or juvenile glaucoma

　365.15　Residual stage of open angle glaucoma

☑5ᵗʰ **365.2　Primary angle-closure glaucoma**
　　　DEF: Glaucoma caused by a shift in the position of the iris of the eye that blocks the surface of the trabecular meshwork causing impairment of the normal flow of aqueous fluid.

　365.20　Primary angle-closure glaucoma, unspecified
　　　Use additional code to identify glaucoma stage
　　　(365.70-365.74)

　365.21　Intermittent angle-closure glaucoma
　　　Angle-closure glaucoma:
　　　　interval
　　　　subacute
　　　DEF: Recurring attacks of high intraocular pressure; due to blocked aqueous flow.

　365.22　Acute angle-closure glaucoma
　　　Acute angle-closure glaucoma attack
　　　Acute angle-closure glaucoma crisis
　　　DEF: Sudden, severe rise in intraocular pressure due to blockage in aqueous drainage.

　365.23　Chronic angle-closure glaucoma
　　　Chronic primary angle closure glaucoma
　　　Use additional code to identify glaucoma stage
　　　(365.70-365.74)
　　　AHA: 2Q, '98, 16

　365.24　Residual stage of angle-closure glaucoma

☑5ᵗʰ **365.3　Corticosteroid-induced glaucoma**
　　　DEF: Elevated intraocular pressure; due to long-term corticosteroid therapy.

　365.31　Glaucomatous stage
　　　Use additional code to identify glaucoma stage
　　　(365.70-365.74)

　365.32　Residual stage

☑5ᵗʰ **365.4　Glaucoma associated with congenital anomalies, dystrophies, and systemic syndromes**

　365.41　Glaucoma associated with chamber angle anomalies

　365.42　Glaucoma associated with anomalies of iris

　365.43　Glaucoma associated with other anterior segment anomalies

　365.44　Glaucoma associated with systemic syndromes
　　　Code first associated disease, as
　　　　neurofibromatosis (237.70-237.79)
　　　　Sturge-Weber (-Dimitri) syndrome (759.6)

☑5ᵗʰ **365.5　Glaucoma associated with disorders of the lens**

　365.51　Phacolytic glaucoma
　　　DEF: Elevated intraocular pressure; due to lens protein blocking aqueous flow.

　365.52　Pseudoexfoliation glaucoma
　　　Use additional code to identify glaucoma stage
　　　(365.70-365.74)
　　　DEF: Glaucoma characterized by small grayish particles deposited on the lens.

　365.59　Glaucoma associated with other lens disorders

☑5ᵗʰ **365.6　Glaucoma associated with other ocular disorders**

　365.60　Glaucoma associated with unspecified ocular disorder

　365.61　Glaucoma associated with pupillary block
　　　DEF: Acute, open-angle glaucoma caused by mature cataract; aqueous flow is blocked by lens material and macrophages.

　365.62　Glaucoma associated with ocular inflammations
　　　Use additional code to identify glaucoma stage
　　　(365.70-365.74)

　365.63　Glaucoma associated with vascular disorders
　　　Use additional code to identify glaucoma stage
　　　(365.70-365.74)

　365.64　Glaucoma associated with tumors or cysts

　365.65　Glaucoma associated with ocular trauma
　　　Use additional code to identify glaucoma stage
　　　(365.70-365.74)

Ⓝ Newborn Age: 0　　　　Ⓟ Pediatric Age: 0-17　　　　Ⓜ Maternity Age: 12-55　　　　Ⓐ Adult Age: 15-124

√5ᵗʰ **365.7 Glaucoma stage**
Code first associated type of glaucoma (365.10-365.13, 365.20, 365.23, 365.31, 365.52, 365.62-365.63, 365.65)
AHA: 4Q, '11, 102-105
TIP: ▶If a patient has bilateral glaucoma with different stages or the stage evolves during the encounter from one stage to another, assign one code for the highest stage documented.◀

365.70 Glaucoma stage, unspecified
Glaucoma stage NOS

365.71 Mild stage glaucoma
Early stage glaucoma

365.72 Moderate stage glaucoma

365.73 Severe stage glaucoma
Advanced stage glaucoma   End-stage glaucoma

365.74 Indeterminate stage glaucoma

√5ᵗʰ **365.8 Other specified forms of glaucoma**

365.81 Hypersecretion glaucoma

365.82 Glaucoma with increased episcleral venous pressure

365.83 Aqueous misdirection
Malignant glaucoma
DEF: A form of secondary angle-closure glaucoma that occurs when aqueous humor flows into the posterior chamber of the eye (vitreous) rather than through the normal recycling channels.
AHA: 4Q, '02, 48

365.89 Other specified glaucoma
AHA: 2Q, '98, 16

365.9 Unspecified glaucoma
AHA: 3Q, '03, 14; 2Q, '01, 16
H40.9 Unspecified glaucoma   I-10

√4ᵗʰ **366 Cataract**
EXCLUDES congenital cataract (743.30-743.34)
DEF: A variety of conditions that create a cloudy, or calcified lens that obstructs vision.

√5ᵗʰ **366.0 Infantile, juvenile, and presenile cataract**

366.00 Nonsenile cataract, unspecified

366.01 Anterior subcapsular polar cataract
DEF: Defect within the front, center lens surface.

366.02 Posterior subcapsular polar cataract
DEF: Defect within the rear, center lens surface.

366.03 Cortical, lamellar, or zonular cataract
DEF: Opacities radiating from center to edge of lens; appear as thin, concentric layers of lens.

366.04 Nuclear cataract

366.09 Other and combined forms of nonsenile cataract

√5ᵗʰ **366.1 Senile cataract**
AHA: 3Q, '91, 9; S-0, '85, 10

366.10 Senile cataract, unspecified   ▲
AHA: 1Q, '03, 5

366.11 Pseudoexfoliation of lens capsule   ▲

366.12 Incipient cataract   ▲
Cataract: Cataract:
  coronary   punctate
  immature NOS   Water clefts
DEF: Minor disorders of lens not affecting vision; due to aging.

366.13 Anterior subcapsular polar senile cataract ▲

366.14 Posterior subcapsular polar senile cataract ▲

366.15 Cortical senile cataract   ▲

366.16 Nuclear sclerosis   ▲
Cataracta brunescens   Nuclear cataract
AHA: 4Q, '07, 79

366.17 Total or mature cataract   ▲

366.18 Hypermature cataract   ▲
Morgagni cataract

366.19 Other and combined forms of senile cataract ▲

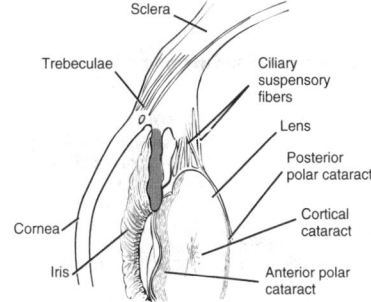

Cataract

(labels: Sclera, Trebeculae, Ciliary suspensory fibers, Lens, Posterior polar cataract, Cornea, Cortical cataract, Iris, Anterior polar cataract)

√5ᵗʰ **366.2 Traumatic cataract**

366.20 Traumatic cataract, unspecified

366.21 Localized traumatic opacities
Vossius' ring

366.22 Total traumatic cataract

366.23 Partially resolved traumatic cataract

√5ᵗʰ **366.3 Cataract secondary to ocular disorders**

366.30 Cataracta complicata, unspecified

366.31 Glaucomatous flecks (subcapsular)
Code first underlying glaucoma (365.0-365.9)

366.32 Cataract in inflammatory disorders
Code first underlying condition, as:
  chronic choroiditis (363.0-363.2)

366.33 Cataract with neovascularization
Code first underlying condition, as:
  chronic iridocyclitis (364.10)

366.34 Cataract in degenerative disorders
Sunflower cataract
Code first underlying condition, as:
  chalcosis (360.24)
  degenerative myopia (360.21)
  pigmentary retinal dystrophy (362.74)

√5ᵗʰ **366.4 Cataract associated with other disorders**

366.41 Diabetic cataract
Code first diabetes (249.5, 250.5)
AHA: 3Q, '91, 9; S-O, '85, 11

366.42 Tetanic cataract
Code first underlying disease, as:
  calcinosis (275.4)
  hypoparathyroidism (252.1)

366.43 Myotonic cataract
Code first underlying disorder (359.21, 359.23)

366.44 Cataract associated with other syndromes
Code first underlying condition, as:
  craniofacial dysostosis (756.0)
  galactosemia (271.1)

366.45 Toxic cataract
Drug-induced cataract
Use additional E code to identify drug or other toxic substance

366.46 Cataract associated with radiation and other physical influences
Use additional E code to identify cause

√5ᵗʰ **366.5 After-cataract**

366.50 After-cataract, unspecified
Secondary cataract NOS

366.51 Soemmering's ring
DEF: A donut-shaped lens remnant and a capsule behind the pupil as a result of cataract surgery or trauma.

366.52 Other after-cataract, not obscuring vision

366.53 After-cataract, obscuring vision

366.8 Other cataract
Calcification of lens

√4ᵗʰ
√5ᵗʰ Additional Digit Required   Unspecified Code   Other Specified Code   Manifestation Code   ▶◀ Revised Text   ● New Code   ▲ Revised Code Title

Diseases of the Nervous System and Sense Organs

366.9–368.53

366.9 Unspecified cataract
AHA: 4Q, '09, 131
H26.9 Unspecified cataract   I-10

☑4ᵗʰ **367 Disorders of refraction and accommodation**

367.0 Hypermetropia
Far-sightedness   Hyperopia
DEF: Refraction error, called also hyperopia, focal point is posterior to retina; abnormally short anteroposterior diameter or subnormal refractive power; causes farsightedness.

367.1 Myopia
Near-sightedness
DEF: Refraction error, focal point is anterior to retina; causes near-sightedness.

☑5ᵗʰ **367.2 Astigmatism**

367.20 Astigmatism, unspecified

367.21 Regular astigmatism

367.22 Irregular astigmatism

☑5ᵗʰ **367.3 Anisometropia and aniseikonia**

367.31 Anisometropia
DEF: Eyes with refractive powers that differ by at least one diopter.

367.32 Aniseikonia
DEF: Eyes with unequal retinal imaging; usually due to refractive error.

367.4 Presbyopia
DEF: Loss of crystalline lens elasticity; causes errors of accommodation; due to aging.

☑5ᵗʰ **367.5 Disorders of accommodation**

367.51 Paresis of accommodation
Cycloplegia
DEF: Partial paralysis of ciliary muscle, causing focus problems.

367.52 Total or complete internal ophthalmoplegia
DEF: Total paralysis of ciliary muscle; large pupil incapable of focus.

367.53 Spasm of accommodation
DEF: Abnormal contraction of ciliary muscle; causes focus problems.

☑5ᵗʰ **367.8 Other disorders of refraction and accommodation**

367.81 Transient refractive change

367.89 Other
Drug-induced ⎫ disorders of refraction and
Toxic   ⎭ accommodation

367.9 Unspecified disorder of refraction and accommodation

☑4ᵗʰ **368 Visual disturbances**
EXCLUDES electrophysiological disturbances (794.11-794.14)

☑5ᵗʰ **368.0 Amblyopia ex anopsia**
DEF: Vision impaired due to disuse; esotropia often cause.

368.00 Amblyopia, unspecified

368.01 Strabismic amblyopia
Suppression amblyopia

368.02 Deprivation amblyopia
DEF: Decreased vision associated with suppressed retinal image of one eye.

368.03 Refractive amblyopia

☑5ᵗʰ **368.1 Subjective visual disturbances**

368.10 Subjective visual disturbance, unspecified

368.11 Sudden visual loss

368.12 Transient visual loss
Concentric fading   Scintillating scotoma

368.13 Visual discomfort
Asthenopia   Photophobia
Eye strain

368.14 Visual distortions of shape and size
Macropsia   Micropsia
Metamorphopsia

368.15 Other visual distortions and entoptic phenomena
Photopsia   Refractive:
Refractive: polyopia
diplopia   Visual halos

368.16 Psychophysical visual disturbances
Prosopagnosia   Visual:
Visual: hallucinations
agnosia   object agnosia
disorientation syndrome

368.2 Diplopia
Double vision
H53.2 Diplopia   I-10

☑5ᵗʰ **368.3 Other disorders of binocular vision**

368.30 Binocular vision disorder, unspecified

368.31 Suppression of binocular vision

368.32 Simultaneous visual perception without fusion

368.33 Fusion with defective stereopsis
DEF: Faulty depth perception though normal ability to focus.

368.34 Abnormal retinal correspondence

☑5ᵗʰ **368.4 Visual field defects**

368.40 Visual field defect, unspecified

368.41 Scotoma involving central area
Scotoma: Scotoma:
central   paracentral
centrocecal
DEF: Vision loss (blind spot) in central five degrees of visual field.

368.42 Scotoma of blind spot area
Enlarged: Paracecal scotoma
angioscotoma
blind spot

368.43 Sector or arcuate defects
Scotoma: Scotoma:
arcuate   Seidel
Bjerrum
DEF: Arc-shaped blind spot caused by retinal nerve damage.

368.44 Other localized visual field defect
Scotoma: Visual field defect:
NOS   nasal step
ring   peripheral

368.45 Generalized contraction or constriction

368.46 Homonymous bilateral field defects
Hemianopsia (altitudinal) (homonymous)
Quadrant anopia
DEF: Disorders found in the corresponding vertical halves of the visual fields of both eyes.

368.47 Heteronymous bilateral field defects
Hemianopsia: Hemianopsia:
binasal   bitemporal
DEF: Disorders in the opposite halves of the visual fields of both eyes.

☑5ᵗʰ **368.5 Color vision deficiencies**
Color blindness

368.51 Protan defect
Protanomaly   Protanopia
DEF: Mild difficulty distinguishing green and red hues with shortened spectrum; sex-linked affecting one percent of males.

368.52 Deutan defect
Deuteranomaly   Deuteranopia
DEF: Male-only disorder; difficulty in distinguishing green and red, no shortened spectrum.

368.53 Tritan defect
Tritanomaly   Tritanopia
DEF: Difficulty in distinguishing blue and yellow; occurs often due to drugs, retinal detachment and central nervous system diseases.

368.54 Achromatopsia
Monochromatism (cone) (rod)
DEF: Complete color blindness; caused by disease, injury to retina, optic nerve or pathway.

368.55 Acquired color vision deficiencies

368.59 Other color vision deficiencies

√5ᵗʰ **368.6 Night blindness**
Nyctalopia
DEF: Nyctalopia: disorder of vision in dim light or night blindness.

368.60 Night blindness, unspecified

368.61 Congenital night blindness
Hereditary night blindness   Oguchi's disease

368.62 Acquired night blindness
EXCLUDES that due to vitamin A deficiency (264.5)

368.63 Abnormal dark adaptation curve
Abnormal threshold
Delayed adaptation } of cones or rods

368.69 Other night blindness

368.8 Other specified visual disturbances
Blurred vision NOS
AHA: 4Q, '02, 56

368.9 Unspecified visual disturbance
AHA: 3Q, '06, 22; 1Q, '04, 15

√4ᵗʰ **369 Blindness and low vision**
NOTE Visual impairment refers to a functional limitation of the eye (e.g., limited visual acuity or visual field). It should be distinguished from visual disability, indicating a limitation of the abilities of the individual (e.g., limited reading skills, vocational skills), and from visual handicap, indicating a limitation of personal and socioeconomic independence (e.g., limited mobility, limited employability).

The levels of impairment defined in the table on the next page are based on the recommendations of the WHO Study Group on Prevention of Blindness (Geneva, November 6-10, 1972; WHO Technical Report Series 518), and of the International Council of Ophthalmology (1976).

Note that definitions of blindness vary in different settings.

For international reporting WHO defines blindness as profound impairment. This definition can be applied to blindness of one eye (369.1, 369.6) and to blindness of the individual (369.0).

For determination of benefits in the U.S.A., the definition of legal blindness as severe impairment is often used. This definition applies to blindness of the individual only.

EXCLUDES correctable impaired vision due to refractive errors (367.0-367.9)

√5ᵗʰ **369.0 Profound impairment, both eyes**

369.00 Impairment level not further specified
Blindness:
NOS according to WHO definition
both eyes

369.01 Better eye: total impairment; lesser eye: total impairment

369.02 Better eye: near-total impairment; lesser eye: not further specified

369.03 Better eye: near-total impairment; lesser eye: total impairment

369.04 Better eye: near-total impairment; lesser eye: near-total impairment

369.05 Better eye: profound impairment; lesser eye: not further specified

369.06 Better eye: profound impairment; lesser eye: total impairment

369.07 Better eye: profound impairment; lesser eye: near-total impairment

369.08 Better eye: profound impairment; lesser eye: profound impairment

√4ᵗʰ **369.1 Moderate or severe impairment, better eye, profound impairment lesser eye**

369.10 Impairment level not further specified
Blindness, one eye, low vision other eye

369.11 Better eye: severe impairment; lesser eye: blind, not further specified

369.12 Better eye: severe impairment; lesser eye: total impairment

369.13 Better eye: severe impairment; lesser eye: near-total impairment

369.14 Better eye: severe impairment; lesser eye: profound impairment

369.15 Better eye: moderate impairment; lesser eye: blind, not further specified

369.16 Better eye: moderate impairment; lesser eye: total impairment

369.17 Better eye: moderate impairment; lesser eye: near-total impairment

369.18 Better eye: moderate impairment; lesser eye: profound impairment

√5ᵗʰ **369.2 Moderate or severe impairment, both eyes**

369.20 Impairment level not further specified
Low vision, both eyes NOS

369.21 Better eye: severe impairment; lesser eye: not further specified

369.22 Better eye: severe impairment; lesser eye: severe impairment

369.23 Better eye: moderate impairment; lesser eye: not further specified

369.24 Better eye: moderate impairment; lesser eye: severe impairment

369.25 Better eye: moderate impairment; lesser eye: moderate impairment

369.3 Unqualified visual loss, both eyes
EXCLUDES blindness NOS:
legal [U.S.A. definition] (369.4)
WHO definition (369.00)

369.4 Legal blindness, as defined in U.S.A.
Blindness NOS according to U.S.A. definition
EXCLUDES legal blindness with specification of impairment level (369.01-369.08, 369.11-369.14, 369.21-369.22)
H54.8 Legal blindness as defined in USA   **I-10**

√5ᵗʰ **369.6 Profound impairment, one eye**

369.60 Impairment level not further specified
Blindness, one eye

369.61 One eye: total impairment; other eye: not specified

369.62 One eye: total impairment; other eye: near normal vision

369.63 One eye: total impairment; other eye: normal vision

369.64 One eye: near-total impairment; other eye: not specified

369.65 One eye: near-total impairment; other eye: near-normal vision

369.66 One eye: near-total impairment; other eye: normal vision

369.67 One eye: profound impairment; other eye: not specified

369.68 One eye: profound impairment; other eye: near-normal vision

369.69 One eye: profound impairment; other eye: normal vision

√5ᵗʰ **369.7 Moderate or severe impairment, one eye**

369.70 Impairment level not further specified
Low vision, one eye

Classification		LEVELS OF VISUAL IMPAIRMENT	Additional descriptors which may be encountered
"legal"	WHO	Visual acuity and/or visual field limitation (whichever is worse)	
(NEAR-) NORMAL VISION		RANGE OF NORMAL VISION 20/10 20/13 20/16 20/20 20/25 2.0 1.6 1.25 1.0 0.8	
		NEAR-NORMAL VISION 20/30 20/40 20/50 20/60 0.7 0.6 0.5 0.4 0.3	
LOW VISION		MODERATE VISUAL IMPAIRMENT 20/70 20/80 20/100 20/125 20/160 0.25 0.20 0.16 0.12	Moderate low vision
		SEVERE VISUAL IMPAIRMENT 20/200 20/250 20/320 20/400 0.10 0.08 0.06 0.05 Visual field: 20 degrees or less	Severe low vision, "Legal" blindness
LEGAL BLINDNESS (U.S.A.) both eyes	BLINDNESS (WHO) one or both eyes	PROFOUND VISUAL IMPAIRMENT 20/500 20/630 20/800 20/1000 0.04 0.03 0.025 0.02 Count fingers at: less than 3m (10 ft.) Visual field: 10 degrees or less	Profound low vision, Moderate blindness
		NEAR-TOTAL VISUAL IMPAIRMENT Visual acuity: less than 0.02 (20/1000) Count fingers at: 1m (3 ft.) or less Hand movements: 5m (15 ft.) or less Light projection, light perception Visual field: 5 degrees or less	Severe blindness Near-total blindness
		TOTAL VISUAL IMPAIRMENT No light perception (NLP)	Total blindness

Visual acuity refers to best achievable acuity with correction.

Non-listed Snellen fractions may be classified by converting to the nearest decimal equivalent, e.g. 10/200 = 0.05, 6/30 = 0.20.

CF (count fingers) without designation of distance, may be classified to profound impairment.

HM (hand motion) without designation of distance, may be classified to near-total impairment.

Visual field measurements refer to the largest field diameter for a 1/100 white test object.

369.71 One eye: severe impairment; other eye: not specified

369.72 One eye: severe impairment; other eye: near-normal vision

369.73 One eye: severe impairment; other eye: normal vision

369.74 One eye: moderate impairment; other eye: not specified

369.75 One eye: moderate impairment; other eye: near-normal vision

369.76 One eye: moderate impairment; other eye: normal vision

369.8 Unqualified visual loss, one eye

369.9 Unspecified visual loss
AHA: 4Q, '02, 114; 3Q, '02, 20

√4ᵗʰ 370 Keratitis

√5ᵗʰ 370.0 Corneal ulcer
EXCLUDES that due to vitamin A deficiency (264.3)

370.00 Corneal ulcer, unspecified

370.01 Marginal corneal ulcer

370.02 Ring corneal ulcer

370.03 Central corneal ulcer

370.04 Hypopyon ulcer
Serpiginous ulcer
DEF: Corneal ulcer with an accumulation of pus in the eye's anterior chamber.

370.05 Mycotic corneal ulcer
DEF: Fungal infection causing corneal tissue loss.

370.06 Perforated corneal ulcer
DEF: Tissue loss through all layers of cornea.

370.07 Mooren's ulcer
DEF: Tissue loss, with chronic inflammation, at junction of cornea and sclera; seen in elderly.

√5ᵗʰ 370.2 Superficial keratitis without conjunctivitis
EXCLUDES dendritic [herpes simplex] keratitis (054.42)

370.20 Superficial keratitis, unspecified

370.21 Punctate keratitis
Thygeson's superficial punctate keratitis
DEF: Formation of cellular and fibrinous deposits (keratic precipitates) on posterior surface; deposits develop after injury or iridocyclitis.

370.22 Macular keratitis
Keratitis: Keratitis:
areolar   stellate
nummular   striate

370.23 Filamentary keratitis
DEF: Keratitis characterized by twisted filaments of mucoid material on the cornea's surface.

370.24 Photokeratitis
Snow blindness   Welders' keratitis
DEF: Painful, inflamed cornea; due to extended exposure to ultraviolet light.
AHA: 3Q, '96, 6

√5ᵗʰ 370.3 Certain types of keratoconjunctivitis

370.31 Phlyctenular keratoconjunctivitis
Phlyctenulosis
Use additional code for any associated tuberculosis (017.3)
DEF: Miniature blister on conjunctiva or cornea; associated with tuberculosis and malnutrition disorders.

370.32 Limbar and corneal involvement in vernal conjunctivitis
Use additional code for vernal conjunctivitis (372.13)
DEF: Corneal itching and inflammation in conjunctivitis; often limited to lining of eyelids.

370.33 Keratoconjunctivitis sicca, not specified as Sjögren's
EXCLUDES Sjögren's syndrome (710.2)
DEF: Inflammation of conjunctiva and cornea; characterized by "horny" looking tissue and excess blood in these areas; decreased flow of lacrimal (tear) is a contributing factor.

370.34 Exposure keratoconjunctivitis
DEF: Incomplete closure of eyelid causing dry, inflamed eye.

370.35 Neurotrophic keratoconjunctivitis

√5ᵗʰ 370.4 Other and unspecified keratoconjunctivitis

370.40 Keratoconjunctivitis, unspecified
Superficial keratitis with conjunctivitis NOS

370.44 Keratitis or keratoconjunctivitis in exanthema
Code first underlying condition (050.0-052.9)
EXCLUDES herpes simplex (054.43)
herpes zoster (053.21)
measles (055.71)

370.49 Other
EXCLUDES epidemic keratoconjunctivitis (077.1)

√5ᵗʰ 370.5 Interstitial and deep keratitis

370.50 Interstitial keratitis, unspecified

370.52 Diffuse interstitial keratitis
Cogan's syndrome
DEF: Inflammation of cornea; with deposits in middle corneal layers; may obscure vision.

370.54 Sclerosing keratitis
DEF: Chronic corneal inflammation leading to opaque scarring.

370.55 Corneal abscess
DEF: Pocket of pus and inflammation on the cornea.

370.59 Other
EXCLUDES disciform herpes simplex keratitis (054.43)
syphilitic keratitis (090.3)

√5ᵗʰ 370.6 Corneal neovascularization

370.60 Corneal neovascularization, unspecified

N Newborn Age: 0   P Pediatric Age: 0-17   M Maternity Age: 12-55   A Adult Age: 15-124

370.61 Localized vascularization of cornea
    DEF: Limited infiltration of cornea by new blood vessels.

370.62 Pannus (corneal)
    DEF: Buildup of superficial vascularization and granulated tissue under epithelium of cornea.
    AHA: 3Q, '02, 20

370.63 Deep vascularization of cornea
    DEF: Deep infiltration of cornea by new blood vessels.

370.64 Ghost vessels (corneal)

370.8 Other forms of keratitis
    Code first underlying condition, such as:
    Acanthamoeba (136.21)
    Fusarium (118)
    AHA: 4Q, '08, 80-81; 3Q, '94, 5

370.9 Unspecified keratitis

371 Corneal opacity and other disorders of cornea

  371.0 Corneal scars and opacities
    EXCLUDES *that due to vitamin A deficiency (264.6)*

    371.00 Corneal opacity, unspecified
      Corneal scar NOS

    371.01 Minor opacity of cornea
      Corneal nebula

    371.02 Peripheral opacity of cornea
      Corneal macula not interfering with central vision

    371.03 Central opacity of cornea
      Corneal:
        leucoma
        macula   } interfering with central vision

    371.04 Adherent leucoma
      DEF: Dense, opaque corneal growth adhering to the iris; also spelled as leukoma.

    371.05 *Phthisical cornea*
      Code first underlying tuberculosis (017.3)

  371.1 Corneal pigmentations and deposits

    371.10 Corneal deposit, unspecified

    371.11 Anterior pigmentations
      Stähli's lines

    371.12 Stromal pigmentations
      Hematocornea

    371.13 Posterior pigmentations
      Krukenberg spindle

    371.14 Kayser-Fleischer ring
      DEF: Copper deposits forming ring at outer edge of cornea; seen in Wilson's disease and other liver disorders.

    371.15 Other deposits associated with metabolic disorders

    371.16 Argentous deposits
      DEF: Silver deposits in cornea.

  371.2 Corneal edema

    371.20 Corneal edema, unspecified

    371.21 Idiopathic corneal edema
      DEF: Corneal swelling and fluid retention of unknown cause.

    371.22 Secondary corneal edema
      DEF: Corneal swelling and fluid retention caused by an underlying disease, injury, or condition.

    371.23 Bullous keratopathy
      DEF: Corneal degeneration; characterized by recurring, rupturing epithelial "blisters;" ruptured blebs expose corneal nerves; occurs in glaucoma, iridocyclitis and Fuchs' epithelial dystrophy.

    371.24 Corneal edema due to wearing of contact lenses

  371.3 Changes of corneal membranes

    371.30 Corneal membrane change, unspecified

    371.31 Folds and rupture of Bowman's membrane

    371.32 Folds in Descemet's membrane

    371.33 Rupture in Descemet's membrane

  371.4 Corneal degenerations

    371.40 Corneal degeneration, unspecified

    371.41 Senile corneal changes
      Arcus senilis   Hassall-Henle bodies

    371.42 Recurrent erosion of cornea
      EXCLUDES *Mooren's ulcer (370.07)*

    371.43 Band-shaped keratopathy
      DEF: Horizontal bands of superficial corneal calcium deposits.

    371.44 Other calcerous degenerations of cornea

    371.45 Keratomalacia NOS
      EXCLUDES *that due to vitamin A deficiency (264.4)*
      DEF: Destruction of the cornea by keratinization of the epithelium with ulceration and perforation of the cornea; seen in cases of vitamin A deficiency.

    371.46 Nodular degeneration of cornea
      Salzmann's nodular dystrophy

    371.48 Peripheral degenerations of cornea
      Marginal degeneration of cornea [Terrien's]

    371.49 Other
      Discrete colliquative keratopathy

  371.5 Hereditary corneal dystrophies
    DEF: Genetic disorder; leads to opacities, edema or lesions of cornea.

    371.50 Corneal dystrophy, unspecified

    371.51 Juvenile epithelial corneal dystrophy

    371.52 Other anterior corneal dystrophies
      Corneal dystrophy: Corneal dystrophy:
        microscopic cystic   ring-like

    371.53 Granular corneal dystrophy

    371.54 Lattice corneal dystrophy

    371.55 Macular corneal dystrophy

    371.56 Other stromal corneal dystrophies
      Crystalline corneal dystrophy

    371.57 Endothelial corneal dystrophy
      Combined corneal dystrophy
      Cornea guttata
      Fuchs' endothelial dystrophy

    371.58 Other posterior corneal dystrophies
      Polymorphous corneal dystrophy

  371.6 Keratoconus
    DEF: Bilateral bulging protrusion of anterior cornea; often due to noninflammatory thinning.

    371.60 Keratoconus, unspecified

    371.61 Keratoconus, stable condition

    371.62 Keratoconus, acute hydrops

  371.7 Other corneal deformities

    371.70 Corneal deformity, unspecified

    371.71 Corneal ectasia
      DEF: Bulging protrusion of thinned, scarred cornea.

    371.72 Descemetocele
      DEF: Protrusion of Descemet's membrane into cornea.

    371.73 Corneal staphyloma
      DEF: Protrusion of cornea into adjacent tissue.

  371.8 Other corneal disorders

    371.81 Corneal anesthesia and hypoesthesia
      DEF: Decreased or absent sensitivity of cornea.

    371.82 Corneal disorder due to contact lens
      EXCLUDES *corneal edema due to contact lens (371.24)*
      DEF: Contact lens wear causing cornea disorder, excluding swelling.

    371.89 Other
      AHA: 3Q, '99, 12

  371.9 Unspecified corneal disorder

Additional Digit Required   Unspecified Code   Other Specified Code   Manifestation Code   ►◄ Revised Text   ● New Code   ▲ Revised Code Title

√4ᵗʰ **372 Disorders of conjunctiva**
> **EXCLUDES** *keratoconjunctivitis (370.3-370.4)*

√5ᵗʰ **372.0 Acute conjunctivitis**

372.00 Acute conjunctivitis, unspecified

372.01 Serous conjunctivitis, except viral
> **EXCLUDES** *viral conjunctivitis NOS (077.9)*
> **AHA:** 3Q, '08, 6

372.02 Acute follicular conjunctivitis
Conjunctival folliculosis NOS
> **EXCLUDES** *conjunctivitis:*
> > *adenoviral (acute follicular) (077.3)*
> > *epidemic hemorrhagic (077.4)*
> > *inclusion (077.0)*
> > *Newcastle (077.8)*
> > *epidemic keratoconjunctivitis (077.1)*
> > *pharyngoconjunctival fever (077.2)*
> **DEF:** Severe conjunctival inflammation with dense infiltrations of lymphoid tissues of inner eyelids; may be traced to a viral or chlamydial etiology.

372.03 Other mucopurulent conjunctivitis
Catarrhal conjunctivitis
> **EXCLUDES** *blennorrhea neonatorum (gonococcal) (098.40)*
> > *neonatal conjunctivitis(771.6)*
> > *ophthalmia neonatorum NOS (771.6)*

372.04 Pseudomembranous conjunctivitis
Membranous conjunctivitis
> **EXCLUDES** *diphtheritic conjunctivitis (032.81)*
> **DEF:** Severe inflammation of conjunctiva; false membrane develops on inner surface of eyelid; membrane can be removed without harming epithelium, due to bacterial infections, toxic and allergic factors, and viral infections.

372.05 Acute atopic conjunctivitis
> **DEF:** Sudden, severe conjunctivitis due to allergens.

372.06 Acute chemical conjunctivitis
Acute toxic conjunctivitis
Use additional E code to identify the chemical or toxic agent
> **EXCLUDES** *burn of eye and adnexa (940.0-940.9)*
> > *chemical corrosion injury of eye (940.2-940.3)*
> **AHA:** 4Q, '09, 85

√5ᵗʰ **372.1 Chronic conjunctivitis**

372.10 Chronic conjunctivitis, unspecified

372.11 Simple chronic conjunctivitis

372.12 Chronic follicular conjunctivitis
> **DEF:** Persistent conjunctival inflammation with dense, localized infiltrations of lymphoid tissues of inner eyelids.

372.13 Vernal conjunctivitis
> **AHA:** 3Q, '96, 8

372.14 Other chronic allergic conjunctivitis
> **AHA:** 3Q, '96, 8

372.15 *Parasitic conjunctivitis*
Code first underlying disease, as:
> filariasis (125.0-125.9)
> mucocutaneous leishmaniasis (085.5)

√5ᵗʰ **372.2 Blepharoconjunctivitis**

372.20 Blepharoconjunctivitis, unspecified

372.21 Angular blepharoconjunctivitis
> **DEF:** Inflammation at junction of upper and lower eyelids; may block lacrimal secretions.

372.22 Contact blepharoconjunctivitis

√5ᵗʰ **372.3 Other and unspecified conjunctivitis**

372.30 Conjunctivitis, unspecified
> H10.9 Unspecified conjunctivitis   ⟨I-10⟩

372.31 *Rosacea conjunctivitis*
Code first underlying rosacea dermatitis (695.3)

372.33 *Conjunctivitis in mucocutaneous disease*
Code first underlying disease, as:
> erythema multiforme (695.10-695.19)
> Reiter's disease (099.3)
> **EXCLUDES** *ocular pemphigoid (694.61)*

372.34 Pingueculitis
> **EXCLUDES** *pinguecula (372.51)*
> **AHA:** 4Q, '08, 112-113

372.39 Other
> **AHA:** 2Q, '07, 9

√5ᵗʰ **372.4 Pterygium**
> **EXCLUDES** *pseudopterygium (372.52)*
> **DEF:** Wedge-shaped, conjunctival thickening that advances from the inner corner of the eye toward the cornea.

372.40 Pterygium, unspecified

372.41 Peripheral pterygium, stationary

372.42 Peripheral pterygium, progressive

372.43 Central pterygium

372.44 Double pterygium

372.45 Recurrent pterygium

√5ᵗʰ **372.5 Conjunctival degenerations and deposits**

372.50 Conjunctival degeneration, unspecified

372.51 Pinguecula
> **EXCLUDES** *pingueculitis (372.34)*
> **DEF:** Proliferative spot on the bulbar conjunctiva located near the sclerocorneal junction, usually on the nasal side; it is seen in elderly people.

372.52 Pseudopterygium
> **DEF:** Conjunctival scar joined to the cornea; it looks like a pterygium but is not attached to the tissue.

372.53 Conjunctival xerosis
> **EXCLUDES** *conjunctival xerosis due to vitamin A deficiency (264.0, 264.1, 264.7)*
> **DEF:** Dry conjunctiva due to vitamin A deficiency; related to Bitot's spots; may develop into xerophthalmia and keratomalacia.

372.54 Conjunctival concretions
> **DEF:** Calculus or deposit on conjunctiva.

372.55 Conjunctival pigmentations
Conjunctival argyrosis
> **DEF:** Color deposits in conjunctiva.

372.56 Conjunctival deposits

√5ᵗʰ **372.6 Conjunctival scars**

372.61 Granuloma of conjunctiva

372.62 Localized adhesions and strands of conjunctiva
> **DEF:** Abnormal fibrous connections in conjunctiva.

372.63 Symblepharon
Extensive adhesions of conjunctiva
> **DEF:** Adhesion of the eyelids to the eyeball.

372.64 Scarring of conjunctiva
Contraction of eye socket (after enucleation)

√5ᵗʰ **372.7 Conjunctival vascular disorders and cysts**

372.71 Hyperemia of conjunctiva
> **DEF:** Conjunctival blood vessel congestion causing eye redness.

372.72 Conjunctival hemorrhage
Hyposphagma   Subconjunctival hemorrhage

372.73 Conjunctival edema
Chemosis of conjunctiva   Subconjunctival edema
> **DEF:** Fluid retention and swelling in conjunctival tissue.

372.74 Vascular abnormalities of conjunctiva
Aneurysm(ata) of conjunctiva

372.75 Conjunctival cysts
> **DEF:** Abnormal sacs of fluid in conjunctiva.

Ⓝ Newborn Age: 0   Ⓟ Pediatric Age: 0-17   Ⓜ Maternity Age: 12-55   Ⓐ Adult Age: 15-124

✓5ᵗʰ **372.8 Other disorders of conjunctiva**

372.81 Conjunctivochalasis
DEF: Bilateral condition of redundant conjunctival tissue between globe and lower eyelid margin; may cover lower punctum, interfering with normal tearing.
AHA: 4Q, '00, 41

372.89 Other disorders of conjunctiva

372.9 Unspecified disorder of conjunctiva

✓4ᵗʰ **373 Inflammation of eyelids**

✓5ᵗʰ **373.0 Blepharitis**
EXCLUDES *blepharoconjunctivitis (372.20-372.22)*

373.00 Blepharitis, unspecified

373.01 Ulcerative blepharitis

373.02 Squamous blepharitis

✓5ᵗʰ **373.1 Hordeolum and other deep inflammation of eyelid**
DEF: Purulent, localized, staphylococcal infection in sebaceous glands of eyelids.

373.11 Hordeolum externum
Hordeolum NOS   Stye
DEF: Infection of the oil glands in the eyelash follicles.

373.12 Hordeolum internum
Infection of meibomian gland
DEF: Infection of the oil gland of the eyelid margin.

373.13 Abscess of eyelid
Furuncle of eyelid
DEF: Inflamed pocket of pus on the eyelid.

373.2 Chalazion
Meibomian (gland) cyst
EXCLUDES *infected meibomian gland (373.12)*
DEF: Chronic inflammation of the meibomian gland, causing an eyelid mass.

✓5ᵗʰ **373.3 Noninfectious dermatoses of eyelid**

373.31 Eczematous dermatitis of eyelid

373.32 Contact and allergic dermatitis of eyelid

373.33 Xeroderma of eyelid

373.34 Discoid lupus erythematosus of eyelid

373.4 Infective dermatitis of eyelid of types resulting in deformity
Code first underlying disease, as:
leprosy (030.0-030.9)
lupus vulgaris (tuberculous) (017.0)
yaws (102.0-102.9)

373.5 Other infective dermatitis of eyelid
Code first underlying disease, as:
actinomycosis (039.3)
impetigo (684)
mycotic dermatitis (110.0-111.9)
vaccinia (051.0)
postvaccination (999.0)
EXCLUDES *herpes:*
simplex (054.41)
zoster (053.20)

373.6 Parasitic infestation of eyelid
Code first underlying disease, as:
leishmaniasis (085.0-085.9)
loiasis (125.2)
onchocerciasis (125.3)
pediculosis (132.0)

373.8 Other inflammations of eyelids

373.9 Unspecified inflammation of eyelid

✓4ᵗʰ **374 Other disorders of eyelids**

✓5ᵗʰ **374.0 Entropion and trichiasis of eyelid**
DEF: Entropion: turning inward of eyelid edge toward eyeball.
DEF: Trichiasis: ingrowing eyelashes marked by irritation with possible distortion of sight.

374.00 Entropion, unspecified

374.01 Senile entropion ▲

Entropion and Ectropion

Ectropion

Normal eyelashes   Entropion

374.02 Mechanical entropion

374.03 Spastic entropion

374.04 Cicatricial entropion

374.05 Trichiasis without entropion

✓5ᵗʰ **374.1 Ectropion**
DEF: Turning outward (eversion) of eyelid edge; exposes palpebral conjunctiva; dryness irritation result.

374.10 Ectropion, unspecified

374.11 Senile ectropion ▲

374.12 Mechanical ectropion

374.13 Spastic ectropion

374.14 Cicatricial ectropion

✓5ᵗʰ **374.2 Lagophthalmos**
DEF: Incomplete closure of eyes; causes dry eye and other complications.

374.20 Lagophthalmos, unspecified

374.21 Paralytic lagophthalmos

374.22 Mechanical lagophthalmos

374.23 Cicatricial lagophthalmos

✓5ᵗʰ **374.3 Ptosis of eyelid**

374.30 Ptosis of eyelid, unspecified
AHA: 2Q, '96, 11

374.31 Paralytic ptosis
DEF: Drooping of upper eyelid due to nerve disorder.

374.32 Myogenic ptosis
DEF: Drooping of upper eyelid due to muscle disorder.

374.33 Mechanical ptosis
DEF: Outside force causes drooping of upper eyelid.

374.34 Blepharochalasis
Pseudoptosis
DEF: Loss of elasticity, thickened or indurated skin of eyelids associated with recurrent episodes of idiopathic edema causing intracellular tissue atrophy.

✓5ᵗʰ **374.4 Other disorders affecting eyelid function**
EXCLUDES *blepharoclonus (333.81)*
blepharospasm (333.81)
facial nerve palsy (351.0)
third nerve palsy or paralysis (378.51-378.52)
tic (psychogenic) (307.20-307.23)
organic (333.3)

374.41 Lid retraction or lag

374.43 Abnormal innervation syndrome
Jaw-blinking   Paradoxical facial movements

374.44 Sensory disorders

374.45 Other sensorimotor disorders
Deficient blink reflex

374.46 Blepharophimosis
Ankyloblepharon
DEF: Narrowing of palpebral fissure horizontally; caused by laterally displaced inner canthi; either acquired or congenital.

✓5ᵗʰ **374.5 Degenerative disorders of eyelid and periocular area**

374.50 Degenerative disorder of eyelid, unspecified

Diseases of the Nervous System and Sense Organs

372.8–374.50

374.51 Xanthelasma
Xanthoma (planum) (tuberosum) of eyelid
Code first underlying condition (272.0-272.9)
DEF: Fatty tumors of the eyelid linked to high fat content of blood.

374.52 Hyperpigmentation of eyelid
Chloasma   Dyspigmentation
DEF: Excess pigment of eyelid.

374.53 Hypopigmentation of eyelid
Vitiligo of eyelid
DEF: Lack of color pigment of the eyelid.

374.54 Hypertrichosis of eyelid
DEF: Excessive eyelash growth.

374.55 Hypotrichosis of eyelid
Madarosis of eyelid
DEF: Less than normal, or absent, eyelashes.

374.56 Other degenerative disorders of skin affecting eyelid

√5ᵗʰ **374.8 Other disorders of eyelid**

374.81 Hemorrhage of eyelid
EXCLUDES *black eye (921.0)*

374.82 Edema of eyelid
Hyperemia of eyelid
DEF: Swelling and fluid retention in eyelid.
AHA: 4Q, '08, 131

374.83 Elephantiasis of eyelid
DEF: Filarial disease causing dermatitis and enlargement of eyelid.

374.84 Cysts of eyelids
Sebaceous cyst of eyelid

374.85 Vascular anomalies of eyelid

374.86 Retained foreign body of eyelid
Use additional code to identify foreign body (V90.01-V90.9)

374.87 Dermatochalasis
DEF: Acquired form of connective tissue disorder associated with decreased elastic tissue and abnormal elastin formation resulting in loss of elasticity of the skin of the eyelid, generally associated with aging.

374.89 Other disorders of eyelid

374.9 Unspecified disorder of eyelid

√4ᵗʰ **375 Disorders of lacrimal system**

√5ᵗʰ **375.0 Dacryoadenitis**

375.00 Dacryoadenitis, unspecified

375.01 Acute dacryoadenitis
DEF: Severe, sudden inflammation of the lacrimal gland.

375.02 Chronic dacryoadenitis
DEF: Persistent inflammation of the lacrimal gland.

375.03 Chronic enlargement of lacrimal gland

√5ᵗʰ **375.1 Other disorders of lacrimal gland**

375.11 Dacryops
DEF: Overproduction and constant flow of tears; may cause distended lacrimal duct.

375.12 Other lacrimal cysts and cystic degeneration

375.13 Primary lacrimal atrophy

375.14 Secondary lacrimal atrophy
DEF: Wasting away of the lacrimal gland due to another disease.

375.15 Tear film insufficiency, unspecified
Dry eye syndrome
AHA: 3Q, '96, 6
DEF: Eye dryness and irritation from insufficient tear production.

375.16 Dislocation of lacrimal gland

√5ᵗʰ **375.2 Epiphora**
DEF: Abnormal development of tears due to stricture of lacrimal passages.

375.20 Epiphora, unspecified as to cause

375.21 Epiphora due to excess lacrimation
DEF: Tear overflow due to overproduction.

375.22 Epiphora due to insufficient drainage
DEF: Tear overflow due to blocked drainage.

√5ᵗʰ **375.3 Acute and unspecified inflammation of lacrimal passages**
EXCLUDES *neonatal dacryocystitis (771.6)*

375.30 Dacryocystitis, unspecified

375.31 Acute canaliculitis, lacrimal

375.32 Acute dacryocystitis
Acute peridacryocystitis

375.33 Phlegmonous dacryocystitis
DEF: Infection of the tear sac with pockets of pus.

√5ᵗʰ **375.4 Chronic inflammation of lacrimal passages**

375.41 Chronic canaliculitis

375.42 Chronic dacryocystitis

375.43 Lacrimal mucocele

√5ᵗʰ **375.5 Stenosis and insufficiency of lacrimal passages**

375.51 Eversion of lacrimal punctum
DEF: Abnormal turning outward of the tear duct.

375.52 Stenosis of lacrimal punctum
DEF: Abnormal narrowing of the tear duct.

375.53 Stenosis of lacrimal canaliculi

375.54 Stenosis of lacrimal sac
DEF: Abnormal narrowing of the tear sac.

375.55 Obstruction of nasolacrimal duct, neonatal
EXCLUDES *congenital anomaly of nasola- crimal duct (743.65)*
DEF: Acquired, abnormal obstruction of tear drainage system from the eye to the nose; in an infant.

375.56 Stenosis of nasolacrimal duct, acquired

375.57 Dacryolith
DEF: Concretion or stone anywhere in lacrimal system.

√5ᵗʰ **375.6 Other changes of lacrimal passages**

375.61 Lacrimal fistula
DEF: Abnormal communication from the lacrimal system.

375.69 Other

√5ᵗʰ **375.8 Other disorders of lacrimal system**

375.81 Granuloma of lacrimal passages
DEF: Abnormal nodules within lacrimal system.

375.89 Other

375.9 Unspecified disorder of lacrimal system

√4ᵗʰ **376 Disorders of the orbit**

√5ᵗʰ **376.0 Acute inflammation of orbit**

376.00 Acute inflammation of orbit, unspecified

376.01 Orbital cellulitis
Abscess of orbit
DEF: Infection of tissue between the orbital bone and eyeball.

376.02 Orbital periostitis
DEF: Inflammation of connective tissue covering the orbital bone.

376.03 Orbital osteomyelitis
DEF: Inflammation of the orbital bone.

376.04 Tenonitis

√5ᵗʰ **376.1 Chronic inflammatory disorders of orbit**

376.10 Chronic inflammation of orbit, unspecified

376.11 Orbital granuloma
Pseudotumor (inflammatory) of orbit
DEF: Abnormal nodule between orbital bone and eyeball.

Lacrimal System

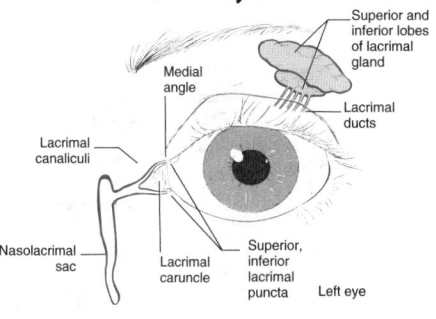

376.12 Orbital myositis
DEF: Painful inflammation of the muscles of the eye.

376.13 Parasitic infestation of orbit
Code first underlying disease, as:
hydatid infestation of orbit (122.3, 122.6, 122.9)
myiasis of orbit (134.0)

√5th **376.2 Endocrine exophthalmos**
Code first underlying thyroid disorder (242.0-242.9)

376.21 Thyrotoxic exophthalmos
DEF: Painful inflammation of eye muscles.

376.22 Exophthalmic ophthalmoplegia
DEF: Inability to rotate eye as a result of bulging eyes.

√5th **376.3 Other exophthalmic conditions**

376.30 Exophthalmos, unspecified
DEF: Abnormal protrusion of eyeball.

376.31 Constant exophthalmos
DEF: Continuous, abnormal protrusion or bulging of eyeball.

376.32 Orbital hemorrhage
DEF: Bleeding behind the eyeball, causing it to bulge forward.

376.33 Orbital edema or congestion
DEF: Fluid retention behind eyeball, causing forward bulge.

376.34 Intermittent exophthalmos

376.35 Pulsating exophthalmos
DEF: Bulge or protrusion; associated with a carotid-cavernous fistula.

376.36 Lateral displacement of globe
DEF: Abnormal displacement of the eyeball away from nose, toward temple.

√5th **376.4 Deformity of orbit**

376.40 Deformity of orbit, unspecified

376.41 Hypertelorism of orbit
DEF: Abnormal increase in interorbital distance; associated with congenital facial deformities; may be accompanied by mental deficiency.

376.42 Exostosis of orbit
DEF: Abnormal bony growth of orbit.

376.43 Local deformities due to bone disease
DEF: Acquired abnormalities of orbit; due to bone disease.

376.44 Orbital deformities associated with craniofacial deformities

376.45 Atrophy of orbit
DEF: Wasting away of bone tissue of orbit.

376.46 Enlargement of orbit

376.47 Deformity due to trauma or surgery

√5th **376.5 Enophthalmos**
DEF: Recession of eyeball deep into eye socket.

376.50 Enophthalmos, unspecified as to cause

376.51 Enophthalmos due to atrophy of orbital tissue

376.52 Enophthalmos due to trauma or surgery

376.6 Retained (old) foreign body following penetrating wound of orbit
Retrobulbar foreign body
Use additional code to identify foreign body (V90.01-V90.9)

√5th **376.8 Other orbital disorders**

376.81 Orbital cysts
Encephalocele of orbit
AHA: 3Q, '99, 13

376.82 Myopathy of extraocular muscles
DEF: Disease in the muscles that control eyeball movement.

376.89 Other

376.9 Unspecified disorder of orbit

√4th **377 Disorders of optic nerve and visual pathways**

√5th **377.0 Papilledema**

377.00 Papilledema, unspecified

377.01 Papilledema associated with increased intracranial pressure

377.02 Papilledema associated with decreased ocular pressure

377.03 Papilledema associated with retinal disorder

377.04 Foster-Kennedy syndrome
DEF: Retrobulbar optic neuritis, central scotoma and optic atrophy; caused by tumors in frontal lobe of brain that press downward.

√5th **377.1 Optic atrophy**

377.10 Optic atrophy, unspecified

377.11 Primary optic atrophy
EXCLUDES neurosyphilitic optic atrophy (094.84)

377.12 Postinflammatory optic atrophy
DEF: Adverse effect of inflammation causing wasting away of eye.

377.13 Optic atrophy associated with retinal dystrophies
DEF: Progressive changes in retinal tissue due to metabolic disorder causing wasting away of eye.

377.14 Glaucomatous atrophy [cupping] of optic disc

377.15 Partial optic atrophy
Temporal pallor of optic disc

377.16 Hereditary optic atrophy
Optic atrophy: Optic atrophy:
dominant hereditary   Leber's

√5th **377.2 Other disorders of optic disc**

377.21 Drusen of optic disc

377.22 Crater-like holes of optic disc

377.23 Coloboma of optic disc
DEF: Ocular malformation caused by the failure of fetal fissure of optic stalk to close.

377.24 Pseudopapilledema

√5th **377.3 Optic neuritis**
EXCLUDES meningococcal optic neuritis (036.81)

377.30 Optic neuritis, unspecified

377.31 Optic papillitis
DEF: Swelling and inflammation of the optic disc.

377.32 Retrobulbar neuritis (acute)
EXCLUDES syphilitic retrobulbar neuritis (094.85)
DEF: Inflammation of optic nerve immediately behind the eyeball.

377.33 Nutritional optic neuropathy
DEF: Malnutrition causing optic nerve disorder.

377.34 Toxic optic neuropathy
Toxic amblyopia
DEF: Toxic substance causing optic nerve disorder.

377.39 Other
EXCLUDES ischemic optic neuropathy (377.41)

√4th Additional Digit Required   Unspecified Code   Other Specified Code   Manifestation Code   ►◄ Revised Text   ● New Code   ▲ Revised Code Title
√5th

Diseases of the Nervous System and Sense Organs

377.4–378.54

√5ᵗʰ **377.4 Other disorders of optic nerve**

    377.41 Ischemic optic neuropathy
        DEF: Decreased blood flow affecting optic nerve.

    377.42 Hemorrhage in optic nerve sheaths
        DEF: Bleeding in meningeal lining of optic nerve.

    377.43 Optic nerve hypoplasia
        AHA: 4Q, '06, 81

    377.49 Other
        Compression of optic nerve

√5ᵗʰ **377.5 Disorders of optic chiasm**

    377.51 Associated with pituitary neoplasms and disorders
        DEF: Abnormal pituitary growth causing disruption in nerve chain from retina to brain.

    377.52 Associated with other neoplasms
        DEF: Abnormal growth, other than pituitary, causing disruption in nerve chain from retina to brain.

    377.53 Associated with vascular disorders
        DEF: Vascular disorder causing disruption in nerve chain from retina to brain.

    377.54 Associated with inflammatory disorders
        DEF: Inflammatory disease causing disruption in nerve chain from retina to brain.

√5ᵗʰ **377.6 Disorders of other visual pathways**

    377.61 Associated with neoplasms

    377.62 Associated with vascular disorders

    377.63 Associated with inflammatory disorders

√5ᵗʰ **377.7 Disorders of visual cortex**
    EXCLUDES visual:
        agnosia (368.16)
        hallucinations (368.16)
        halos (368.15)

    377.71 Associated with neoplasms

    377.72 Associated with vascular disorders

    377.73 Associated with inflammatory

    377.75 Cortical blindness
        DEF: Blindness due to brain disorder, rather than eye disorder.

    377.9 Unspecified disorder of optic nerve and visual pathways

√4ᵗʰ **378 Strabismus and other disorders of binocular eye movements**
    EXCLUDES nystagmus and other irregular eye movements (379.50-379.59)
    DEF: Misalignment of the eyes due to imbalance in extraocular muscles.

√5ᵗʰ **378.0 Esotropia**
    Convergent concomitant strabismus
    EXCLUDES intermittent esotropia (378.20-378.22)
    DEF: Visual axis deviation created by one eye fixing upon an image and the other eye deviating inward.

    378.00 Esotropia, unspecified

    378.01 Monocular esotropia

    378.02 Monocular esotropia with A pattern

    378.03 Monocular esotropia with V pattern

    378.04 Monocular esotropia with other noncomitancies
        Monocular esotropia with X or Y pattern

    378.05 Alternating esotropia

    378.06 Alternating esotropia with A pattern

    378.07 Alternating esotropia with V pattern

    378.08 Alternating esotropia with other noncomitancies
        Alternating esotropia with X or Y pattern

√5ᵗʰ **378.1 Exotropia**
    Divergent concomitant strabismus
    EXCLUDES intermittent exotropia (378.20, 378.23-378.24)
    DEF: Visual axis deviation created by one eye fixing upon an image and the other eye deviating outward.

    378.10 Exotropia, unspecified

Eye Musculature

Superior rectus
Superior oblique
Lateral rectus
Medial rectus
Inferior oblique
Inferior rectus
Muscles and actions (right eye)

R.   L.
Monocular (one eye only) esotropia (inward)

Monocular exotropia (outward)

Monocular hypertropia (upward)

    378.11 Monocular exotropia

    378.12 Monocular exotropia with A pattern

    378.13 Monocular exotropia with V pattern

    378.14 Monocular exotropia with other noncomitancies
        Monocular exotropia with X or Y pattern

    378.15 Alternating exotropia

    378.16 Alternating exotropia with A pattern

    378.17 Alternating exotropia with V pattern

    378.18 Alternating exotropia with other noncomitancies
        Alternating exotropia with X or Y pattern

√5ᵗʰ **378.2 Intermittent heterotropia**
    EXCLUDES vertical heterotropia (intermittent) (378.31)
    DEF: Deviation of eyes seen only at intervals; it is also called strabismus.

    378.20 Intermittent heterotropia, unspecified
        Intermittent: Intermittent:
        esotropia NOS   exotropia NOS

    378.21 Intermittent esotropia, monocular

    378.22 Intermittent esotropia, alternating

    378.23 Intermittent exotropia, monocular

    378.24 Intermittent exotropia, alternating

√5ᵗʰ **378.3 Other and unspecified heterotropia**

    378.30 Heterotropia, unspecified

    378.31 Hypertropia
        Vertical heterotropia (constant) (intermittent)

    378.32 Hypotropia

    378.33 Cyclotropia

    378.34 Monofixation syndrome
        Microtropia

    378.35 Accommodative component in esotropia

√5ᵗʰ **378.4 Heterophoria**
    DEF: Deviation occurring only when the other eye is covered.

    378.40 Heterophoria, unspecified

    378.41 Esophoria

    378.42 Exophoria

    378.43 Vertical heterophoria

    378.44 Cyclophoria

    378.45 Alternating hyperphoria

√6ᵗʰ **378.5 Paralytic strabismus**
    DEF: Deviation of the eye due to nerve paralysis affecting muscle.

    378.50 Paralytic strabismus, unspecified

    378.51 Third or oculomotor nerve palsy, partial
        AHA: 3Q, '91, 9

    378.52 Third or oculomotor nerve palsy, total
        AHA: 2Q, '89, 12

    378.53 Fourth or trochlear nerve palsy
        AHA: 2Q, '01, 21

    378.54 Sixth or abducens nerve palsy
        AHA: 2Q, '89, 12

N Newborn Age: 0   **P** Pediatric Age: 0-17   **M** Maternity Age: 12-55   **A** Adult Age: 15-124

378.55 External ophthalmoplegia

378.56 Total ophthalmoplegia

√5ʰ **378.6 Mechanical strabismus**
DEF: Deviation of the eye due to an outside force upon the extraocular muscles.

378.60 Mechanical strabismus, unspecified

378.61 Brown's (tendon) sheath syndrome
DEF: Congenital or acquired shortening of the anterior sheath of superior oblique muscle; eye is unable to move upward and inward; usually unilateral.

378.62 Mechanical strabismus from other musculofascial disorders

378.63 Limited duction associated with other conditions

√5ʰ **378.7 Other specified strabismus**

378.71 Duane's syndrome
DEF: Congenital, affects one eye; due to abnormal fibrous bands attached to rectus muscle; inability to abduct affected eye with retraction of globe.

378.72 Progressive external ophthalmoplegia
DEF: Paralysis progressing from one eye muscle to another.

378.73 Strabismus in other neuromuscular disorders

√5ʰ **378.8 Other disorders of binocular eye movements**
EXCLUDES nystagmus (379.50-379.56)

378.81 Palsy of conjugate gaze
DEF: Paralysis progressing from one eye muscle to another.

378.82 Spasm of conjugate gaze
DEF: Muscle contractions impairing parallel movement of eye.

378.83 Convergence insufficiency or palsy

378.84 Convergence excess or spasm

378.85 Anomalies of divergence

378.86 Internuclear ophthalmoplegia
DEF: Eye movement anomaly due to brainstem lesion.

378.87 Other dissociated deviation of eye movements
Skew deviation

378.9 Unspecified disorder of eye movements
Ophthalmoplegia NOS   Strabismus NOS
AHA: 2Q, '01, 21

√4ʰ **379 Other disorders of eye**

√5ʰ **379.0 Scleritis and episcleritis**
EXCLUDES syphilitic episcleritis (095.0)

379.00 Scleritis, unspecified
Episcleritis NOS

379.01 Episcleritis periodica fugax
DEF: Hyperemia (engorgement) of the sclera and overlying conjunctiva characterized by a sudden onset and short duration.

379.02 Nodular episcleritis
DEF: Inflammation of the outermost layer of the sclera, with formation of nodules.

379.03 Anterior scleritis

379.04 Scleromalacia perforans
DEF: Scleral thinning, softening and degeneration; seen with rheumatoid arthritis.

379.05 Scleritis with corneal involvement
Scleroperikeratitis

379.06 Brawny scleritis
DEF: Severe scleral inflammation with thickening corneal margins.

379.07 Posterior scleritis
Sclerotenonitis

379.09 Other
Scleral abscess

√5ʰ **379.1 Other disorders of sclera**
EXCLUDES blue sclera (743.47)

379.11 Scleral ectasia
Scleral staphyloma NOS
DEF: Protrusion of the contents of the eyeball where the sclera has thinned.

379.12 Staphyloma posticum
DEF: Ring-shaped protrusion or bulging of sclera and uveal tissue at posterior pole of eye.

379.13 Equatorial staphyloma
DEF: Ring-shaped protrusion or bulging of sclera and uveal tissue midway between front and back of eye.

379.14 Anterior staphyloma, localized

379.15 Ring staphyloma

379.16 Other degenerative disorders of sclera

379.19 Other

√5ʰ **379.2 Disorders of vitreous body**
DEF: Disorder of clear gel that fills space between retina and lens.

379.21 Vitreous degeneration
Vitreous: Vitreous:
cavitation   liquefaction
detachment

379.22 Crystalline deposits in vitreous
Asteroid hyalitis   Synchysis scintillans

379.23 Vitreous hemorrhage
AHA: 3Q, '91, 15

379.24 Other vitreous opacities
Vitreous floaters

379.25 Vitreous membranes and strands

379.26 Vitreous prolapse
DEF: Slipping of vitreous from normal position.

379.27 Vitreomacular adhesion   Ⓐ
Vitreomacular traction
EXCLUDES traction detachment with vitreoretinal organization (361.81)
AHA: ▶4Q, '11, 105-106◀

379.29 Other disorders of vitreous
EXCLUDES vitreous abscess (360.04)
AHA: 1Q, '99, 11

√5ʰ **379.3 Aphakia and other disorders of lens**
EXCLUDES after-cataract (366.50-366.53)

379.31 Aphakia
EXCLUDES cataract extraction status (V45.61)
DEF: Absence of eye's crystalline lens.

379.32 Subluxation of lens

379.33 Anterior dislocation of lens
DEF: Lens displaced toward iris.

379.34 Posterior dislocation of lens
DEF: Lens displaced backward toward vitreous.

379.39 Other disorders of lens

√5ʰ **379.4 Anomalies of pupillary function**

379.40 Abnormal pupillary function, unspecified

379.41 Anisocoria
DEF: Unequal pupil diameter.

379.42 Miosis (persistent), not due to miotics
DEF: Abnormal contraction of pupil less than 2 mil.

379.43 Mydriasis (persistent), not due to mydriatics
DEF: Morbid dilation of pupil.

379.45 Argyll Robertson pupil, atypical
Argyll Robertson phenomenon or pupil, nonsyphilitic
EXCLUDES Argyll Robertson pupil (syphilitic) (094.89)
DEF: Failure of pupil to respond to light; affects both eyes; may be caused by diseases such as syphilis of the central nervous system or miosis.

379.46 Tonic pupillary reaction
Adie's pupil or syndrome

379.49 Other
Hippus   Pupillary paralysis

✓5ᵗʰ 379.5 Nystagmus and other irregular eye movements

379.50 Nystagmus, unspecified
DEF: Involuntary, rapid, rhythmic movement of eyeball; vertical, horizontal, rotatory or mixed; cause may be congenital, acquired, physiological, neurological, myopathic, or due to ocular diseases.
AHA: 4Q, '02, 68; 2Q, '01, 21

379.51 Congenital nystagmus

379.52 Latent nystagmus

379.53 Visual deprivation nystagmus

379.54 Nystagmus associated with disorders of the vestibular system

379.55 Dissociated nystagmus

379.56 Other forms of nystagmus

379.57 Deficiencies of saccadic eye movements
Abnormal optokinetic response
DEF: Saccadic eye movements; small, rapid, involuntary movements by both eyes simultaneously, due to changing point of fixation on visualized object.

379.58 Deficiencies of smooth pursuit movements

379.59 Other irregularities of eye movements
Opsoclonus

✓5ᵗʰ 379.6 Inflammation (infection) of postprocedural bleb
Postprocedural blebitis

379.60 Inflammation (infection) of postprocedural bleb, unspecified
AHA: 4Q, '06, 82

379.61 Inflammation (infection) of postprocedural bleb, stage 1
AHA: 4Q, '06, 82

379.62 Inflammation (infection) of postprocedural bleb, stage 2
AHA: 4Q, '06, 82

379.63 Inflammation (infection) of postprocedural bleb, stage 3
Bleb associated endophthalmitis
AHA: 4Q, '06, 82

379.8 Other specified disorders of eye and adnexa

✓5ᵗʰ 379.9 Unspecified disorder of eye and adnexa

379.90 Disorder of eye, unspecified

379.91 Pain in or around eye

379.92 Swelling or mass of eye

379.93 Redness or discharge of eye

379.99 Other ill-defined disorders of eye
EXCLUDES blurred vision NOS (368.8)

Diseases of the Ear and Mastoid Process (380-389)

Use additional external cause code, if applicable, to identify the cause of the ear condition

✓4ᵗʰ 380 Disorders of external ear

✓5ᵗʰ 380.0 Perichondritis and chondritis of pinna
Chondritis of auricle   Perichondritis of auricle

380.00 Perichondritis of pinna, unspecified

380.01 Acute perichondritis of pinna

380.02 Chronic perichondritis of pinna

380.03 Chondritis of pinna
DEF: Infection that has progressed into the cartilage; presents as indurated and edematous skin over the pinna; vascular compromise occurs with tissue necrosis and deformity.
AHA: 4Q, '04, 76

Ear and Mastoid Process

Helix • Antihelix • Concha • Mastoid process • External auditory meatus • Tragus • Antitragus

✓5ᵗʰ 380.1 Infective otitis externa

380.10 Infective otitis externa, unspecified
Otitis externa (acute):   Otitis externa (acute):
  NOS   hemorrhagica
  circumscribed   infective NOS
  diffuse

380.11 Acute infection of pinna
EXCLUDES furuncular otitis externa (680.0)

380.12 Acute swimmers' ear
Beach ear   Tank ear
DEF: Otitis externa due to swimming.

380.13 Other acute infections of external ear
Code first underlying disease, as:
  erysipelas (035)
  impetigo (684)
  seborrheic dermatitis (690.10-690.18)
EXCLUDES herpes simplex (054.73)
         herpes zoster (053.71)

380.14 Malignant otitis externa
DEF: Severe necrotic otitis externa; due to bacteria.

380.15 Chronic mycotic otitis externa
Code first underlying disease, as:
  aspergillosis (117.3)
  otomycosis NOS (111.9)
EXCLUDES candidal otitis externa (112.82)

380.16 Other chronic infective otitis externa
Chronic infective otitis externa NOS

✓5ᵗʰ 380.2 Other otitis externa

380.21 Cholesteatoma of external ear
Keratosis obturans of external ear (canal)
EXCLUDES cholesteatoma NOS (385.30-385.35)
         postmastoidectomy (383.32)
DEF: Cystlike mass filled with debris, including cholesterol; rare, congenital condition.

380.22 Other acute otitis externa
Acute otitis externa: Acute otitis externa:
  actinic   eczematoid
  chemical   reactive
  contact

380.23 Other chronic otitis externa
Chronic otitis externa NOS

✓5ᵗʰ 380.3 Noninfectious disorders of pinna

380.30 Disorder of pinna, unspecified

380.31 Hematoma of auricle or pinna

380.32 Acquired deformities of auricle or pinna
EXCLUDES cauliflower ear (738.7)
AHA: 3Q, '03, 12

380.39 Other
EXCLUDES gouty tophi of ear (274.81)

380.4 Impacted cerumen
Wax in ear

✓5ᵗʰ 380.5 Acquired stenosis of external ear canal
Collapse of external ear canal

380.50 Acquired stenosis of external ear canal, unspecified as to cause

---

N Newborn Age: 0   P Pediatric Age: 0-17   M Maternity Age: 12-55   A Adult Age: 15-124

380.51 Secondary to trauma
DEF: Narrowing of the external ear canal; due to trauma.

380.52 Secondary to surgery
DEF: Postsurgical narrowing of the external ear canal.

380.53 Secondary to inflammation
DEF: Narrowing of the external ear canal; due to chronic inflammation.

√5ᵗʰ **380.8 Other disorders of external ear**

380.81 Exostosis of external ear canal

380.89 Other

380.9 Unspecified disorder of external ear

√4ᵗʰ **381 Nonsuppurative otitis media and Eustachian tube disorders**

√5ᵗʰ **381.0 Acute nonsuppurative otitis media**
Acute tubotympanic catarrh
Otitis media, acute or subacute:
catarrhal
exudative
transudative
with effusion
EXCLUDES otitic barotrauma (993.0)

381.00 Acute nonsuppurative otitis media, unspecified

381.01 Acute serous otitis media
Acute or subacute secretory otitis media
DEF: Sudden, severe infection of the middle ear.

381.02 Acute mucoid otitis media
Acute or subacute seromucinous otitis media
Blue drum syndrome
DEF: Sudden, severe infection of the middle ear, with mucous.

381.03 Acute sanguinous otitis media
DEF: Sudden, severe infection of the middle ear, with blood.

381.04 Acute allergic serous otitis media

381.05 Acute allergic mucoid otitis media

381.06 Acute allergic sanguinous otitis media

√5ᵗʰ **381.1 Chronic serous otitis media**
Chronic tubotympanic catarrh

381.10 Chronic serous otitis media, simple or unspecified
DEF: Persistent infection of the middle ear, without pus.

381.19 Other
Serosanguinous chronic otitis media

√5ᵗʰ **381.2 Chronic mucoid otitis media**
Glue ear
EXCLUDES adhesive middle ear disease (385.10-385.19)
DEF: Chronic condition; characterized by viscous fluid in middle ear; due to obstructed Eustachian tube.

381.20 Chronic mucoid otitis media, simple or unspecified

381.29 Other
Mucosanguinous chronic otitis media

381.3 Other and unspecified chronic nonsuppurative otitis media
Otitis media, chronic: Otitis media, chronic:
allergic   seromucinous
exudative   transudative
secretory   with effusion

381.4 Nonsuppurative otitis media, not specified as acute or chronic
Otitis media: Otitis media:
allergic   secretory
catarrhal   seromucinous
exudative   serous
mucoid   transudative
             with effusion

√6ᵗʰ **381.5 Eustachian salpingitis**

381.50 Eustachian salpingitis, unspecified

381.51 Acute Eustachian salpingitis
DEF: Sudden, severe inflammation of the Eustachian tube.

381.52 Chronic Eustachian salpingitis
DEF: Persistent inflammation of the Eustachian tube.

√5ᵗʰ **381.6 Obstruction of Eustachian tube**
Stenosis
Stricture   } of Eustachian tube

381.60 Obstruction of Eustachian tube, unspecified

381.61 Osseous obstruction of Eustachian tube
Obstruction of Eustachian tube from cholesteatoma, polyp, or other osseous lesion

381.62 Intrinsic cartilaginous obstruction of Eustachian tube
DEF: Blockage of Eustachian tube; due to cartilage overgrowth.

381.63 Extrinsic cartilaginous obstruction of Eustachian tube
Compression of Eustachian tube

381.7 Patulous Eustachian tube
DEF: Distended, oversized Eustachian tube.

√5ᵗʰ **381.8 Other disorders of Eustachian tube**

381.81 Dysfunction of Eustachian tube

381.89 Other

381.9 Unspecified Eustachian tube disorder

√4ᵗʰ **382 Suppurative and unspecified otitis media**

√5ᵗʰ **382.0 Acute suppurative otitis media**
Otitis media, acute: Otitis media, acute
necrotizing NOS   purulent

382.00 Acute suppurative otitis media without spontaneous rupture of ear drum
DEF: Sudden, severe inflammation of middle ear, with pus.

382.01 Acute suppurative otitis media with spontaneous rupture of ear drum
DEF: Sudden, severe inflammation of middle ear, with pressure tearing ear drum tissue.

382.02 *Acute suppurative otitis media in diseases classified elsewhere*
Code first underlying disease, as:
influenza (487.8, 488.09, 488.19)
scarlet fever (034.1)
EXCLUDES postmeasles otitis (055.2)

382.1 Chronic tubotympanic suppurative otitis media
Benign chronic suppurative
    ottis media   } (with anterior perforation
Chronic tubotympanic disease   } of ear drum)
DEF: Inflammation of tympanic cavity and auditory tube; with pus formation.

382.2 Chronic atticoantral suppurative otitis media
Chronic atticoantral disease   } (with posterior or superior
Persistent mucosal disease   } marginal perforation
                         of ear drum)
DEF: Inflammation of upper tympanic membrane and mastoid antrum with pus formation.

382.3 Unspecified chronic suppurative otitis media
Chronic purulent otitis media
EXCLUDES tuberculous otitis media (017.4)

382.4 Unspecified suppurative otitis media
Purulent otitis media NOS

382.9 Unspecified otitis media
Otitis media: Otitis media:
NOS   chronic NOS
acute NOS
AHA: N-D, '84, 16
H66.93 Otitis media unspecified bilateral   I-10

√4ᵗʰ **383 Mastoiditis and related conditions**

√5ᵗʰ **383.0 Acute mastoiditis**
Abscess of mastoid   Empyema of mastoid

383.00 Acute mastoiditis without complications
DEF: Sudden, severe inflammation of mastoid air cells.

√4ᵗʰ
√5ᵗʰ Additional Digit Required   Unspecified Code   Other Specified Code   Manifestation Code   ►◄ Revised Text   ● New Code   ▲ Revised Code Title
2013 ICD-9-CM   **Volume 1 – 119**

Diseases of the Nervous System and Sense Organs

383.01–385.24

383.01 Subperiosteal abscess of mastoid
DEF: Pocket of pus within the mastoid bone.

383.02 Acute mastoiditis with other complications
Gradenigo's syndrome

383.1 Chronic mastoiditis
Caries of mastoid   Fistula of mastoid
EXCLUDES tuberculous mastoiditis (015.6)
DEF: Persistent inflammation of the mastoid air cells.

√5ᵗʰ **383.2 Petrositis**
Coalescing osteitis
Inflammation   } of petrous bone
Osteomyelitis

383.20 Petrositis, unspecified

383.21 Acute petrositis
DEF: Sudden, severe inflammation of dense bone behind the ear.

383.22 Chronic petrositis
DEF: Persistent inflammation of dense bone behind the ear.

383.3 Complications following mastoidectomy

383.30 Postmastoidectomy complication, unspecified

383.31 Mucosal cyst of postmastoidectomy cavity
DEF: Mucous-lined cyst cavity following removal of mastoid bone.

383.32 Recurrent cholesteatoma of postmastoidectomy cavity
DEF: Cystlike mass of cell debris in cavity following removal of mastoid bone.

383.33 Granulations of postmastoidectomy cavity
Chronic inflammation of postmastoidectomy cavity
DEF: Granular tissue in cavity following removal of mastoid bone.

√5ᵗʰ **383.8 Other disorders of mastoid**

383.81 Postauricular fistula
DEF: Abnormal passage behind mastoid cavity.

383.89 Other

383.9 Unspecified mastoiditis

√4ᵗʰ **384 Other disorders of tympanic membrane**

√5ᵗʰ **384.0 Acute myringitis without mention of otitis media**

384.00 Acute myringitis, unspecified
Acute tympanitis NOS
DEF: Sudden, severe inflammation of ear drum.

384.01 Bullous myringitis
Myringitis bullosa hemorrhagica
DEF: Type of viral otitis media characterized by the appearance of serous or hemorrhagic blebs on the tympanic membrane.

384.09 Other

384.1 Chronic myringitis without mention of otitis media
Chronic tympanitis
DEF: Persistent inflammation of ear drum; with no evidence of middle ear infection.

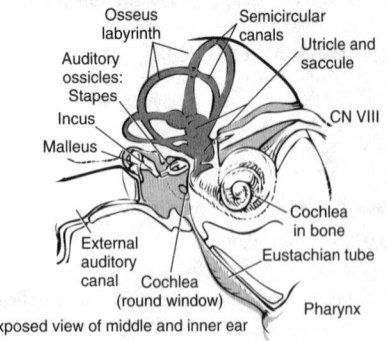

Middle and Inner Ear

Osseus labyrinth
Semicircular canals
Auditory ossicles:
Stapes
Incus
Malleus
Utricle and saccule
CN VIII
Cochlea in bone
External auditory canal
Cochlea (round window)
Eustachian tube
Pharynx

Exposed view of middle and inner ear

√5ᵗʰ **384.2 Perforation of tympanic membrane**
Perforation of ear drum: Perforation of ear drum:
NOS   postinflammatory
persistent posttraumatic
EXCLUDES otitis media with perforation of tympanic membrane (382.00-382.9)
traumatic perforation [current injury] (872.61)

384.20 Perforation of tympanic membrane, unspecified

384.21 Central perforation of tympanic membrane

384.22 Attic perforation of tympanic membrane
Pars flaccida

384.23 Other marginal perforation of tympanic membrane

384.24 Multiple perforations of tympanic membrane

384.25 Total perforation of tympanic membrane

√5ᵗʰ **384.8 Other specified disorders of tympanic membrane**

384.81 Atrophic flaccid tympanic membrane
Healed perforation of ear drum

384.82 Atrophic nonflaccid tympanic membrane

384.9 Unspecified disorder of tympanic membrane

√4ᵗʰ **385 Other disorders of middle ear and mastoid**
EXCLUDES mastoiditis (383.0-383.9)

√5ᵗʰ **385.0 Tympanosclerosis**

385.00 Tympanosclerosis, unspecified as to involvement

385.01 Tympanosclerosis involving tympanic membrane only
DEF: Tough, fibrous tissue impeding functions of ear drum.

385.02 Tympanosclerosis involving tympanic membrane and ear ossicles
DEF: Tough, fibrous tissue impeding functions of middle ear bones (stapes, malleus, incus).

385.03 Tympanosclerosis involving tympanic membrane, ear ossicles, and middle ear
DEF: Tough, fibrous tissue impeding functions of ear drum, middle ear bones and middle ear canal.

385.09 Tympanosclerosis involving other combination of structures

√5ᵗʰ **385.1 Adhesive middle ear disease**
Adhesive otitis   Otitis media:
Otitis media: fibrotic
chronic adhesive
EXCLUDES glue ear (381.20-381.29)
DEF: Adhesions of middle ear structures.

385.10 Adhesive middle ear disease, unspecified as to involvement

385.11 Adhesions of drum head to incus

385.12 Adhesions of drum head to stapes

385.13 Adhesions of drum head to promontorium

385.19 Other adhesions and combinations

√5ᵗʰ **385.2 Other acquired abnormality of ear ossicles**

385.21 Impaired mobility of malleus
Ankylosis of malleus

385.22 Impaired mobility of other ear ossicles
Ankylosis of ear ossicles, except malleus

385.23 Discontinuity or dislocation of ear ossicles
DEF: Disruption in auditory chain; created by malleus, incus and stapes.

385.24 Partial loss or necrosis of ear ossicles
DEF: Tissue loss in malleus, incus and stapes.

Cholesteatoma

Middle ear chamber

Cholesteatoma sac   Ear drum

√5ᵗʰ **385.3 Cholesteatoma of middle ear and mastoid**

Cholesterosis
Epidermosis
Keratosis
Polyp
} of (middle) ear

EXCLUDES cholesteatoma:
external ear canal (380.21)
recurrent of postmastoidectomy cavity (383.32)

DEF: Cystlike mass of middle ear and mastoid antrum filled with debris, including cholesterol.

385.30 Cholesteatoma, unspecified

385.31 Cholesteatoma of attic

385.32 Cholesteatoma of middle ear

385.33 Cholesteatoma of middle ear and mastoid
DEF: Cystlike mass of cell debris in middle ear and mastoid air cells behind ear.
AHA: 3Q, '00, 10

385.35 Diffuse cholesteatosis

√5ᵗʰ **385.8 Other disorders of middle ear and mastoid**

385.82 Cholesterin granuloma
DEF: Granuloma formed of fibrotic tissue; contains cholesterol crystals surrounded by foreign-body cells; found in the middle ear and mastoid area.

385.83 Retained foreign body of middle ear
Use additional code to identify foreign body (V90.01-V90.9)
AHA: 3Q, '94, 7; N-D, '87, 9

385.89 Other

385.9 Unspecified disorder of middle ear and mastoid

√4ᵗʰ **386 Vertiginous syndromes and other disorders of vestibular system**

EXCLUDES vertigo NOS (780.4)
AHA: M-A, '85, 12

√5ᵗʰ **386.0 Ménière's disease**
Endolymphatic hydrops   Ménière's syndrome or vertigo
Lermoyez's syndrome
DEF: Distended membranous labyrinth of middle ear from endolymphatic hydrops; causes ischemia, failure of nerve function; hearing and balance dysfunction; symptoms include fluctuating deafness, ringing in ears and dizziness.

386.00 Ménière's disease, unspecified
Ménière's disease (active)
H81.03 Ménière's disease bilateral   I-10

386.01 Active Ménière's disease, cochleovestibular

386.02 Active Ménière's disease, cochlear

386.03 Active Ménière's disease, vestibular

386.04 Inactive Ménière's disease
Ménière's disease in remission

√5ᵗʰ **386.1 Other and unspecified peripheral vertigo**
EXCLUDES epidemic vertigo (078.81)

386.10 Peripheral vertigo, unspecified

386.11 Benign paroxysmal positional vertigo
Benign paroxysmal positional nystagmus

386.12 Vestibular neuronitis
Acute (and recurrent) peripheral vestibulopathy
DEF: Transient benign vertigo, unknown cause; characterized by response to caloric stimulation on one side, nystagmus with rhythmic movement of eyes; normal auditory function present.

386.19 Other
Aural vertigo   Otogenic vertigo

386.2 Vertigo of central origin
Central positional nystagmus   Malignant positional vertigo

√5ᵗʰ **386.3 Labyrinthitis**

386.30 Labyrinthitis, unspecified

386.31 Serous labyrinthitis
Diffuse labyrinthitis
DEF: Inflammation of labyrinth; with fluid buildup.

386.32 Circumscribed labyrinthitis
Focal labyrinthitis

386.33 Suppurative labyrinthitis
Purulent labyrinthitis
DEF: Inflammation of labyrinth; with pus.

386.34 Toxic labyrinthitis
DEF: Inflammation of labyrinth; due to toxic reaction.

386.35 Viral labyrinthitis

√5ᵗʰ **386.4 Labyrinthine fistula**

386.40 Labyrinthine fistula, unspecified

386.41 Round window fistula

386.42 Oval window fistula

386.43 Semicircular canal fistula

386.48 Labyrinthine fistula of combined sites

√5ᵗʰ **386.5 Labyrinthine dysfunction**

386.50 Labyrinthine dysfunction, unspecified

386.51 Hyperactive labyrinth, unilateral
DEF: Abnormal increased sensitivity of labyrinth to stimuli such as sound, pressure or gravitational change, affecting one ear.

386.52 Hyperactive labyrinth, bilateral
DEF: Abnormal increased sensitivity of labyrinth to stimuli such as sound, pressure or gravitational change, affecting both ears.

386.53 Hypoactive labyrinth, unilateral
DEF: Abnormal decreased sensitivity of labyrinth to stimuli such as sound, pressure or gravitational change, affecting one ear.

386.54 Hypoactive labyrinth, bilateral
DEF: Abnormal decreased sensitivity of labyrinth to stimuli such as sound, pressure or gravitational change, affecting both ears.

386.55 Loss of labyrinthine reactivity, unilateral
DEF: Decreased function of the labyrinth sensors, affecting one ear

386.56 Loss of labyrinthine reactivity, bilateral
DEF: Decreased function of the labyrinth sensors, affecting both ears

386.58 Other forms and combinations

386.8 Other disorders of labyrinth
AHA: 1Q, '11, 6

386.9 Unspecified vertiginous syndromes and labyrinthine disorders

√4ᵗʰ **387 Otosclerosis**
INCLUDES otospongiosis
DEF: Synonym for otospongiosis, spongy bone formation in the labyrinth bones of the ear; it causes progressive hearing impairment.

387.0 Otosclerosis involving oval window, nonobliterative
DEF: Tough, fibrous tissue impeding functions of oval window.

387.1 Otosclerosis involving oval window, obliterative
DEF: Tough, fibrous tissue blocking oval window.

Diseases of the Nervous System and Sense Organs

387.2–389.9

387.2 Cochlear otosclerosis
Otosclerosis involving: Otosclerosis involving:
otic capsule   round window
DEF: Tough, fibrous tissue impeding functions of cochlea.

387.8 Other otosclerosis

387.9 Otosclerosis, unspecified

√4th **388 Other disorders of ear**

√5th **388.0 Degenerative and vascular disorders of ear**

     388.00 Degenerative and vascular disorders, unspecified

     388.01 Presbyacusis
DEF: Progressive, bilateral perceptive hearing loss caused by advancing age; it is also known as presbycusis.

     388.02 Transient ischemic deafness
DEF: Restricted blood flow to auditory organs causing temporary hearing loss.

√5th **388.1 Noise effects on inner ear**

     388.10 Noise effects on inner ear, unspecified

     388.11 Acoustic trauma (explosive) to ear
Otitic blast injury

     388.12 Noise-induced hearing loss

388.2 Sudden hearing loss, unspecified

√5th **388.3 Tinnitus**
DEF: Abnormal noises in ear; may be heard by others beside the affected individual; noises include ringing, clicking, roaring and buzzing.

     388.30 Tinnitus, unspecified

     388.31 Subjective tinnitus

     388.32 Objective tinnitus

√5th **388.4 Other abnormal auditory perception**

     388.40 Abnormal auditory perception, unspecified

     388.41 Diplacusis
DEF: Perception of a single auditory sound as two sounds at two different levels of intensity.

     388.42 Hyperacusis
DEF: Exceptionally acute sense of hearing caused by such conditions as Bell's palsy; this term may also refer to painful sensitivity to sounds.

     388.43 Impairment of auditory discrimination
DEF: Impaired ability to distinguish tone of sound.

     388.44 Recruitment
DEF: Perception of abnormally increased loudness caused by a slight increase in sound intensity; it is a term used in audiology.

     388.45 Acquired auditory processing disorder
Auditory processing disorder NOS
EXCLUDES *central auditory processing disorder (315.32)*
DEF: Difficulty in recognizing and interpreting sounds; a failure of the brain to process auditory information; due to neurological problems due to injury, infection, and degenerative conditions.
AHA: 4Q, '07, 79

388.5 Disorders of acoustic nerve
Acoustic neuritis
Degeneration   } of acoustic or eighth nerve
Disorder
EXCLUDES *acoustic neuroma (225.1)*
syphilitic acoustic neuritis (094.86)
AHA: M-A, '87, 8

√5th **388.6 Otorrhea**

     388.60 Otorrhea, unspecified
Discharging ear NOS

     388.61 Cerebrospinal fluid otorrhea
EXCLUDES *cerebrospinal fluid rhinorrhea (349.81)*
DEF: Spinal fluid leakage from ear.

     388.69 Other
Otorrhagia

√5th **388.7 Otalgia**

     388.70 Otalgia, unspecified
Earache NOS

     388.71 Otogenic pain

     388.72 Referred pain

388.8 Other disorders of ear

388.9 Unspecified disorder of ear

√4th **389 Hearing loss**

√5th **389.0 Conductive hearing loss**
Conductive deafness
EXCLUDES *mixed conductive and sensorineural hearing loss (389.20-389.22)*
DEF: Dysfunction in sound-conducting structures of external or middle ear causing hearing loss.
AHA: 4Q, '07, 80; 4Q, '89, 5

     389.00 Conductive hearing loss, unspecified

     389.01 Conductive hearing loss, external ear

     389.02 Conductive hearing loss, tympanic membrane

     389.03 Conductive hearing loss, middle ear

     389.04 Conductive hearing loss, inner ear

     389.05 Conductive hearing loss, unilateral

     389.06 Conductive hearing loss, bilateral
AHA: 4Q, '07, 81

     389.08 Conductive hearing loss of combined types

√5th **389.1 Sensorineural hearing loss**
Perceptive hearing loss or deafness
EXCLUDES *abnormal auditory perception (388.40-388.44)*
mixed conductive and sensorineural hearing loss (389.20-389.22)
psychogenic deafness (306.7)
DEF: Nerve conduction causing hearing loss.
AHA: 4Q, '07, 80; 4Q, '89, 5

     389.10 Sensorineural hearing loss, unspecified
AHA: 1Q, '93, 29

     389.11 Sensory hearing loss, bilateral

     389.12 Neural hearing loss, bilateral

     389.13 Neural hearing loss, unilateral

     389.14 Central hearing loss

     389.15 Sensorineural hearing loss, unilateral
AHA: 4Q, '06, 84

     389.16 Sensorineural hearing loss, asymmetrical
AHA: 4Q, '06, 84

     389.17 Sensory hearing loss, unilateral

     389.18 Sensorineural hearing loss, bilateral
AHA: 4Q, '06, 84

√5th **389.2 Mixed conductive and sensorineural hearing loss**
Deafness or hearing loss of type classifiable to 389.00-389.08 with type classifiable to 389.10-389.18
AHA: 4Q, '07, 80

     389.20 Mixed hearing loss, unspecified

     389.21 Mixed hearing loss, unilateral

     389.22 Mixed hearing loss, bilateral

389.7 Deaf, non-speaking, not elsewhere classifiable

389.8 Other specified forms of hearing loss

389.9 Unspecified hearing loss
Deafness NOS
AHA: 1Q, '04, 15
H91.93 Unspecified hearing loss bilateral   I-10

N Newborn Age: 0   P Pediatric Age: 0-17   M Maternity Age: 12-55   A Adult Age: 15-124

7. Diseases of the Circulatory System (390-459)

Acute Rheumatic Fever (390-392)

DEF: Febrile disease occurs mainly in children or young adults following throat infection by group A streptococci; symptoms include fever, joint pain, lesions of heart, blood vessels and joint connective tissue, abdominal pain, skin changes, and chorea.

390 Rheumatic fever without mention of heart involvement
Arthritis, rheumatic, acute or subacute
Rheumatic fever (active) (acute)
Rheumatism, articular, acute or subacute
EXCLUDES *that with heart involvement (391.0-391.9)*

✔4ᵗʰ 391 Rheumatic fever with heart involvement
EXCLUDES *chronic heart diseases of rheumatic origin (393-398.99) unless rheumatic fever is also present or there is evidence of recrudescence or activity of the rheumatic process*

391.0 Acute rheumatic pericarditis
Rheumatic:
    fever (active) (acute) with pericarditis
    pericarditis (acute)
Any condition classifiable to 390 with pericarditis
EXCLUDES *that not specified as rheumatic (420.0-420.9)*
DEF: Sudden, severe inflammation of heart lining due to rheumatic fever.

391.1 Acute rheumatic endocarditis
Rheumatic:
    endocarditis, acute
    fever (active) (acute) with endocarditis or valvulitis
    valvulitis acute
Any condition classifiable to 390 with endocarditis or valvulitis
DEF: Sudden, severe inflammation of heart cavities due to rheumatic fever.

391.2 Acute rheumatic myocarditis
Rheumatic fever (active) (acute) with myocarditis
Any condition classifiable to 390 with myocarditis
DEF: Sudden, severe inflammation of heart muscles due to rheumatic fever.

391.8 Other acute rheumatic heart disease
Rheumatic:
    fever (active) (acute) with other or multiple types of heart involvement
    pancarditis, acute
Any condition classifiable to 390 with other or multiple types of heart involvement

391.9 Acute rheumatic heart disease, unspecified
Rheumatic:
    carditis, acute
    fever (active) (acute) with unspecified type of heart involvement
    heart disease, active or acute
Any condition classifiable to 390 with unspecified type of heart involvement

Sections of Heart Muscle

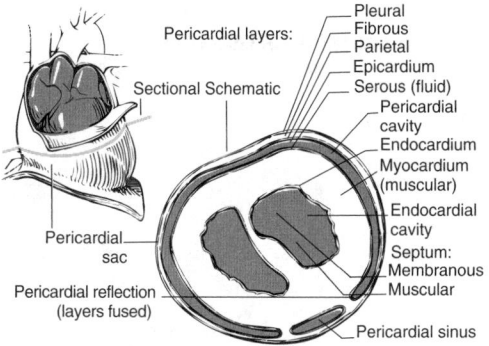

Pericardial layers:
  Pleural
  Fibrous
  Parietal
  Epicardium
  Serous (fluid)
Sectional Schematic
  Pericardial cavity
  Endocardium
  Myocardium (muscular)
  Endocardial cavity
Pericardial sac
  Septum:
    Membranous
    Muscular
Pericardial reflection (layers fused)
Pericardial sinus

✔4ᵗʰ 392 Rheumatic chorea
INCLUDES Sydenham's chorea
EXCLUDES *chorea:*
    NOS (333.5)
    Huntington's (333.4)
DEF: Childhood disease linked with rheumatic fever and streptococcal infections; symptoms include spasmodic, involuntary movements of limbs or facial muscles, psychic symptoms, and irritability.

392.0 With heart involvement
Rheumatic chorea with heart involvement of any type classifiable to 391

392.9 Without mention of heart involvement

Chronic Rheumatic Heart Disease (393-398)

393 Chronic rheumatic pericarditis
Adherent pericardium, rheumatic
Chronic rheumatic:
    mediastinopericarditis
    myopericarditis
EXCLUDES *pericarditis NOS or not specified as rheumatic (423.0-423.9)*
DEF: Persistent inflammation of heart lining due to rheumatic heart disease.

✔4ᵗʰ 394 Diseases of mitral valve
EXCLUDES *that with aortic valve involvement (396.0-396.9)*

394.0 Mitral stenosis
Mitral (valve):
    obstruction (rheumatic)
    stenosis NOS
DEF: Narrowing, of mitral valve between left atrium and left ventricle; due to rheumatic heart disease.
TIP: Assign when documentation indicates mitral valve stenosis or obstruction with no further specification of cause.

394.1 Rheumatic mitral insufficiency
Rheumatic mitral:
    incompetence
    regurgitation
EXCLUDES *that not specified as rheumatic (424.0)*
DEF: Malfunction of mitral valve between left atrium and left ventricle; due to rheumatic heart disease.
AHA: 2Q, '05, 14

394.2 Mitral stenosis with insufficiency
Mitral stenosis with incompetence or regurgitation
DEF: A narrowing or stricture of the mitral valve situated between the left atrium and left ventricle; valve does not completely close, is insufficient (inadequate) in preventing regurgitation into the atrium; also called incompetence.
AHA: 1Q, '07, 11

394.9 Other and unspecified mitral valve diseases
Mitral (valve):
    disease (chronic)
    failure

✔4ᵗʰ 395 Diseases of aortic valve
EXCLUDES *that not specified as rheumatic (424.1)*
    that with mitral valve involvement (396.0-396.9)

395.0 Rheumatic aortic stenosis
Rheumatic aortic (valve) obstruction
DEF: Narrowing of the aortic valve; results in backflow into ventricle; due to rheumatic heart disease.
AHA: 4Q, '88, 8

395.1 Rheumatic aortic insufficiency
Rheumatic aortic:
    incompetence
    regurgitation
DEF: Malfunction of the aortic valve; results in backflow into left ventricle; due to rheumatic heart disease.

395.2 Rheumatic aortic stenosis with insufficiency
Rheumatic aortic stenosis with incompetence or regurgitation
DEF: Malfunction and narrowing, of the aortic valve; results in backflow into left ventricle; due to rheumatic heart disease.

395.9 Other and unspecified rheumatic aortic diseases
Rheumatic aortic (valve) disease

✔4ᵗʰ ✔5ᵗʰ Additional Digit Required   Unspecified Code   Other Specified Code   Manifestation Code   ►◄ Revised Text   ● New Code   ▲ Revised Code Title

2013 ICD-9-CM   **Volume 1 – 123**

✓4ᵗʰ **396 Diseases of mitral and aortic valves**

INCLUDES involvement of both mitral and aortic valves, whether specified as rheumatic or not

AHA: N-D, '87, 8

396.0 Mitral valve stenosis and aortic valve stenosis
Atypical aortic (valve) stenosis
Mitral and aortic (valve) obstruction (rheumatic)

396.1 Mitral valve stenosis and aortic valve insufficiency

396.2 Mitral valve insufficiency and aortic valve stenosis
AHA: 2Q, '09, 17; 1Q, '09, 18; 2Q, '00, 16

396.3 Mitral valve insufficiency and aortic valve insufficiency
Mitral and aortic (valve):
  incompetence
  regurgitation
108.0 Rheumatic d/o of both mitral & aortic valves   I-10

396.8 Multiple involvement of mitral and aortic valves
Stenosis and insufficiency of mitral or aortic valve with stenosis or insufficiency, or both, of the other valve

396.9 Mitral and aortic valve diseases, unspecified

✓4ᵗʰ **397 Diseases of other endocardial structures**

397.0 Diseases of tricuspid valve
Tricuspid (valve) (rheumatic):
  disease
  insufficiency
  obstruction
  regurgitation
  stenosis
DEF: Malfunction of the valve between right atrium and right ventricle; due to rheumatic heart disease.
AHA: 3Q, '06, 7; 2Q, '00, 16
107.2 Rheumatic tricuspid stenosis and insufficiency   I-10

397.1 Rheumatic diseases of pulmonary valve
EXCLUDES that not specified as rheumatic (424.3)

397.9 Rheumatic diseases of endocardium, valve unspecified
Rheumatic:
  endocarditis (chronic)
  valvulitis (chronic)
EXCLUDES that not specified as rheumatic (424.90-424.99)

✓4ᵗʰ **398 Other rheumatic heart disease**

398.0 Rheumatic myocarditis
Rheumatic degeneration of myocardium
EXCLUDES myocarditis not specified as rheumatic (429.0)
DEF: Chronic inflammation of heart muscle; due to rheumatic heart disease.

✓5ᵗʰ **398.9 Other and unspecified rheumatic heart diseases**

398.90 Rheumatic heart disease, unspecified
Rheumatic:
  carditis
  heart disease NOS
EXCLUDES carditis not specified as rheumatic (429.89)
heart disease NOS not specified as rheumatic (429.9)

398.91 Rheumatic heart failure (congestive)
Rheumatic left ventricular failure
DEF: Decreased cardiac output, edema and hypertension; due to rheumatic heart disease.
AHA: 2Q, '05, 14; 1Q, '95, 6; 3Q, '88, 3
109.81 Rheumatic heart failure   I-10

398.99 Other

Hypertensive Disease (401-405)

EXCLUDES that complicating pregnancy, childbirth, or the puerperium (642.0-642.9)
that involving coronary vessels (410.00-414.9)
AHA: 3Q, '90, 3; 2Q, '89, 12; S-O, '87, 9; J-A, '84, 11

✓4ᵗʰ **401 Essential hypertension**

INCLUDES high blood pressure
hyperpiesia
hyperpiesis
hypertension (arterial) (essential) (primary) (systemic)
hypertensive vascular:
  degeneration
  disease

EXCLUDES elevated blood pressure without diagnosis of hypertension (796.2)
pulmonary hypertension (416.0-416.9)
that involving vessels of:
  brain (430-438)
  eye (362.11)

DEF: Hypertension that occurs without apparent organic cause; idiopathic.
AHA: 2Q, '92, 5

401.0 Malignant
DEF: Severe high arterial blood pressure; results in necrosis in kidney, retina, etc.; hemorrhages occur and death commonly due to uremia or rupture of cerebral vessel.
AHA: M-J, '85, 19

401.1 Benign
DEF: Mildly elevated arterial blood pressure.

401.9 Unspecified
AHA: ►1Q, '12, 14;◄ 4Q, '10,124,125, 135; 4Q, '09, 77, 129; 1Q, '09, 18; 2Q, '08, 16; 4Q, '05, 71; 3Q, '05, 8; 4Q, '04, 78; 4Q, '03, 105, 108, 111; 3Q, '03, 14; 2Q, '03, 16; 4Q, '97, 37
110 Essential (primary) hypertension   I-10

✓4ᵗʰ **402 Hypertensive heart disease**

INCLUDES hypertensive:
  cardiomegaly
  cardiopathy
  cardiovascular disease
  heart (disease) (failure)
any condition classifiable to 429.0-429.3, 429.8, 429.9 due to hypertension

Use additional code to specify type of heart failure (428.0-428.43), if known

AHA: 4Q, '02, 49; 2Q, '93, 9; N-D, '84, 18
TIP: Assign when a cardiac condition is stated (due to hypertension) or implied (hypertensive).

✓5ᵗʰ **402.0 Malignant**

402.00 Without heart failure

402.01 With heart failure
AHA: 4Q, '08, 180

✓5ᵗʰ **402.1 Benign**

402.10 Without heart failure

402.11 With heart failure

✓5ᵗʰ **402.9 Unspecified**

402.90 Without heart failure
111.9 Hypertensive heart disease without heart failure   I-10

402.91 With heart failure
AHA: 4Q, '02, 52; 1Q, '93, 19; 2Q, '89, 12

N Newborn Age: 0   P Pediatric Age: 0-17   M Maternity Age: 12-55   A Adult Age: 15-124

√4ᵗʰ **403 Hypertensive chronic kidney disease**

INCLUDES arteriolar nephritis
arteriosclerosis of:
   kidney
   renal arterioles
arteriosclerotic nephritis (chronic) (interstitial)
hypertensive:
   nephropathy
   renal failure
   uremia (chronic)
nephrosclerosis
renal sclerosis with hypertension

any condition classifiable to 585 and 587 with any condition classifiable to 401

EXCLUDES acute kidney failure (584.5-584.9)
renal disease stated as not due to hypertension
renovascular hypertension (405.0-405.9 with fifth-digit 1)

The following fifth-digit subclassification is for use with category 403:
0 with chronic kidney disease stage I through stage IV, or unspecified
   Use additional code to identify the stage of chronic kidney disease (585.1-585.4, 585.9)
1 with chronic kidney disease stage V or end stage renal disease
   Use additional code to identify the stage of chronic kidney disease (585.5, 585.6)

AHA: 4Q, '06, 84-86; 4Q, '05, 68; 4Q, '92, 22; 2Q, '92, 5
TIP: Assign whenever a patient has both chronic kidney disease and hypertension (presumed cause-and-effect relationship).

§ √5ᵗʰ **403.0 Malignant**
[0-1]

§ √5ᵗʰ **403.1 Benign**
[0-1]   AHA: For code 403.11: 3Q, '10, 12

§ √5ᵗʰ **403.9 Unspecified**
[0-1]   AHA: For code 403.90: 4Q, '10, 137; 1Q, '08, 10 ;2Q, '07, 3; 4Q, '06, 86; For code 403.91: 4Q, '10, 137; 1Q ,'08, 7; 4Q, '05, 69; 1Q, '04, 14; 1Q, '03, 20; 2Q, '01, 11; 3Q, '91, 8
   I12.9 HTN CKD w/stage I thru IV CKD/UNS CKD   I-10

√4ᵗʰ **404 Hypertensive heart and chronic kidney disease**

INCLUDES disease:
   cardiorenal
   cardiovascular renal

any condition classifiable to 402 with any condition classifiable to 403

Use additional code to specify type of heart failure (428.0-428.43), if known

The following fifth-digit subclassification is for use with category 404:
0 without heart failure and with chronic kidney disease stage I through stage IV, or unspecified
   Use additional code to identify the stage of chronic kidney disease (585.1-585.4, 585.9)
1 with heart failure and with chronic kidney disease stage I through stage IV, or unspecified
   Use additional code to identify the stage of chronic kidney disease (585.1-585.4, 585.9)
2 without heart failure and with chronic kidney disease stage V or end stage renal disease
   Use additional code to identify the stage of chronic kidney disease (585.5, 585.6)
3 with heart failure and chronic kidney disease stage V or end stage renal disease
   Use additional code to identify the stage of chronic kidney disease (585.5, 585.6)

AHA: 4Q, '06, 84-86; 4Q, '05, 68; 4Q, '02, 49; 3Q, '90, 3; J-A, '84, 14

§ √5ᵗʰ **404.0 Malignant**
[0-3]

§ √5ᵗʰ **404.1 Benign**
[0-3]

§ √5ᵗʰ **404.9 Unspecified**
[0-3]   I13.0 HTN heart & CKD HF & stage I thru IV CKD/UNS CKD   I-10

√4ᵗʰ **405 Secondary hypertension**

DEF: High arterial blood pressure due to or with a variety of primary diseases, such as renal disorders, CNS disorders, endocrine, and vascular diseases.
AHA: 3Q, '90, 3; S-O, '87, 9, 11; J-A, '84, 14

√5ᵗʰ **405.0 Malignant**

  405.01 Renovascular

  405.09 Other

√5ᵗʰ **405.1 Benign**

  405.11 Renovascular

  405.19 Other

√5ᵗʰ **405.9 Unspecified**

  405.91 Renovascular

  405.99 Other
     AHA: 3Q, '00, 4

Ischemic Heart Disease (410-414)

INCLUDES that with mention of hypertension

Use additional code to identify presence of hypertension (401.0-405.9)
AHA: 3Q, '91, 10; J-A, '84, 5

√4ᵗʰ **410 Acute myocardial infarction**

INCLUDES cardiac infarction
coronary (artery):
   embolism
   occlusion
   rupture
   thrombosis
infarction of heart, myocardium, or ventricle
rupture of heart, myocardium, or ventricle
ST elevation (STEMI) and non-ST elevation (NSTEMI) myocardial infarction

any condition classifiable to 414.1-414.9 specified as acute or with a stated duration of 8 weeks or less

The following fifth-digit subclassification is for use with category 410:
0 episode of care unspecified
   Use when the source document does not contain sufficient information for the assigment of fifth-digit 1 or 2.
1 initial episode of care
   Use fifth-digit 1 to designate the first episode of care (regardless of facility site) for a newly diagnosed myocardial infarction. The fifth-digit 1 is assigned regardless of the number of times a patient may be transferred during the initial episode of care.
2 subsequent episode of care
   Use fifth-digit 2 to designate an episode of care following the initial episode when the patient is admitted for further observation, evaluation or treatment for a myocardial infarction that has received initial treatment, but is still less than 8 weeks old.

DEF: A sudden insufficiency of blood supply to an area of the heart muscle; usually due to a coronary artery occlusion.
AHA: ▶1Q, '12, 7;◀ 2Q, '06, 9; 4Q, '05, 69; 3Q, '01, 21; 3Q, '98, 15; 4Q, '97, 37; 3Q, '95, 9; 4Q, 92, 24; 1Q, '92, 10; 3Q, '91, 18; 1Q, '91, 14; 3Q, '89, 3
TIP: Assign an acute MI code with a fifth digit of "1," initial episode of care, for all care provided before the AMI has resolved, regardless of type or number of transfers between facilities.

§ √5ᵗʰ **410.0 Of anterolateral wall**
[0-2]   ST elevation myocardial infarction (STEMI) of anterolateral wall
     AHA: For code 410.01: 4Q, '09, 129; 4Q, '08, 72

§ √5ᵗʰ **410.1 Of other anterior wall**
[0-2]   Infarction:
     anterior (wall) NOS   } (with contiguous portion of
     anteroapical   intraventricular
     anteroseptal   septum)
   ST elevation myocardial infarction (STEMI) of other anterior wall
     AHA: For code 410.11: 3Q, '03, 10

§ √5ᵗʰ **410.2 Of inferolateral wall**
[0-2]   ST elevation myocardial infarction (STEMI) of inferolateral wall

---

§   Requires fifth digit. Valid digits are in [brackets] under each code. See appropriate category for codes and definitions.

√4ᵗʰ √5ᵗʰ Additional Digit Required   Unspecified Code   Other Specified Code   Manifestation Code   ▶◀ Revised Text   ● New Code   ▲ Revised Code Title

Acute Myocardial Infarction

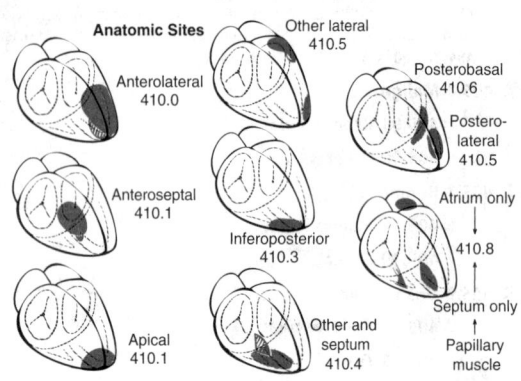

Anatomic Sites

Anterolateral 410.0

Other lateral 410.5

Posterobasal 410.6

Postero-lateral 410.5

Anteroseptal 410.1

Inferoposterior 410.3

Atrium only 410.8

Apical 410.1

Other and septum 410.4

Septum only

Papillary muscle

§ ✓5ᵗʰ **410.3 Of inferoposterior wall**
[0-2]   ST elevation myocardial infarction (STEMI) of inferoposterior wall

§ ✓5ᵗʰ **410.4 Of other inferior wall**
[0-2]   Infarction:
     diaphragmatic wall NOS ⎫ (with contiguous portion of
     inferior (wall) NOS   ⎭   intraventricular septum)
     ST elevation myocardial infarction (STEMI) of other inferior wall
     AHA: 1Q, '00, 7, 26; 4Q, '99, 9; 3Q, '97, 10; **For code 410.41:** 3Q, '09, 10; 2Q, '01, 8, 9
     I21.19 STEMI invlv oth coronary artery of inferior wall   I-10

§ ✓5ᵗʰ **410.5 Of other lateral wall**
[0-2]   Infarction:
     apical-lateral
     basal-lateral
     high lateral
     posterolateral
     ST elevation myocardial infarction (STEMI) of other lateral wall
     AHA: For code 410.51: 3Q, '09, 9

§ ✓5ᵗʰ **410.6 True posterior wall infarction**
[0-2]   Infarction:
     posterobasal
     strictly posterior
     ST elevation myocardial infarction (STEMI) of true posterior wall

§ ✓5ᵗʰ **410.7 Subendocardial infarction**
[0-2]   Non-ST elevation myocardial infarction (NSTEMI)
     Nontransmural infarction
     AHA: 1Q, '00, 7; **For code 410.71:** 2Q, '10, 8-9; 4Q, '05, 71; 2Q, '05, 19
     I21.4 Non-ST elevation (NSTEMI) myocardial infarction   I-10

§ ✓5ᵗʰ **410.8 Of other specified sites**
[0-2]   Infarction of:
     atrium
     papillary muscle
     septum alone
     ST elevation myocardial infarction (STEMI) of other specified sites

§ ✓5ᵗʰ **410.9 Unspecified site**
[0-2]   Acute myocardial infarction NOS
     Coronary occlusion NOS
     Myocardial infarction NOS
     AHA: 1Q, '96, 17; 1Q, '92, 9; **For code 410.91:** 2Q, '05, 18; 3Q, '02, 5
     I21.3 ST elevation myocardial infarction of uns site   I-10

✓4ᵗʰ **411 Other acute and subacute forms of ischemic heart disease**
     AHA: 4Q, '94, 55; 3Q, '91, 24

411.0 Postmyocardial infarction syndrome
     Dressler's syndrome
     DEF: Complication developing several days/weeks after myocardial infarction; symptoms include fever, leukocytosis, chest pain, pericarditis, pleurisy, and pneumonitis; tendency to recur.

411.1 Intermediate coronary syndrome
     Impending infarction   Preinfarction syndrome
     Preinfarction angina   Unstable angina
     EXCLUDES *angina (pectoris) (413.9)*
                decubitus (413.0)
     DEF: A condition representing an intermediate stage between angina of effort and acute myocardial infarction. It is often documented by the physician as "unstable angina."
     AHA: 3Q, '07, 9; 4Q, '05, 105; 2Q, '04, 3; 1Q, '03, 12; 3Q, '01, 15; 2Q, '01, 7, 9; 4Q, '98, 86; 2Q, '96, 10; 3Q, '91, 24; 1Q, '91, 14; 3Q, '90, 6; 4Q, '89, 10
     TIP: Do not assign code 411.1 on the same episode of care as an acute myocardial infarction (category 410). Assign 411.1 for accelerated angina.
     I20.0 Unstable angina   I-10

✓5ᵗʰ **411.8 Other**
     AHA: 3Q, '91, 18; 3Q, '89, 4

411.81 Acute coronary occlusion without myocardial infarction
     Acute coronary (artery):
       embolism   ⎫
       obstruction   ⎬ without or not resulting
       occlusion   ⎪ in myocardial
       thrombosis   ⎭ infarction
     EXCLUDES *obstruction without infarction due to atherosclerosis (414.00-414.07)*
                occlusion without infarction due to atherosclerosis (414.00-414.07)
     DEF: Interrupted blood flow to a portion of the heart; without tissue death.
     AHA: 3Q, '91, 24; 1Q, '91, 14

411.89 Other
     Coronary insufficiency (acute)
     Subendocardial ischemia
     AHA: 3Q, '01, 14; 1Q, '92, 9

412 Old myocardial infarction
     Healed myocardial infarction
     Past myocardial infarction diagnosed on ECG [EKG] or other special investigation, but currently presenting no symptoms
     AHA: 2Q, '03, 10; 2Q, '01, 9; 3Q, '98, 15; 2Q, '91, 22; 3Q, '90, 7
     TIP: Assign for any acute myocardial infarction stated to be older than 8 weeks.
     I25.2 Old myocardial infarction   I-10

✓4ᵗʰ **413 Angina pectoris**
     DEF: Severe constricting pain in the chest, often radiating from the precordium to the left shoulder and down the arm, due to ischemia of the heart muscle; usually caused by coronary disease; pain is often precipitated by effort or excitement.

413.0 Angina decubitus
     Nocturnal angina
     DEF: Angina occurring only in the recumbent position.

413.1 Prinzmetal angina
     Variant angina pectoris
     DEF: Angina occurring when patient is recumbent; associated with ST-segment elevations.
     AHA: 3Q, '06, 23

413.9 Other and unspecified angina pectoris
     Angina: Anginal syndrome
       NOS   Status anginosus
       cardiac   Stenocardia
       equivalent   Syncope anginosa
       of effort
     Use additional code(s) for symptoms associated with angina equivalent
     EXCLUDES *preinfarction angina (411.1)*
     AHA: 2Q, '08, 16; 3Q, '02, 4; 3Q, '91, 16; 3Q, '90, 6
     TIP: For patients with both angina and coronary artery disease, sequence the CAD (subcategory 414.0) code first.
     I20.9 Angina pectoris unspecified   I-10

---

§   Requires fifth digit. Valid digits are in [brackets] under each code. See category 410 for codes and definitions.

N Newborn Age: 0   P Pediatric Age: 0-17   M Maternity Age: 12-55   A Adult Age: 15-124

✓4ᵗʰ **414 Other forms of chronic ischemic heart disease**

> **EXCLUDES** *arteriosclerotic cardiovascular disease [ASCVD] (429.2)*
> *cardiovascular:*
> *arteriosclerosis or sclerosis (429.2)*
> *degeneration or disease (429.2)*

✓5ᵗʰ **414.0 Coronary atherosclerosis**

Arteriosclerotic heart disease [ASHD]
Atherosclerotic heart disease
Coronary (artery):
  arteriosclerosis

Coronary (artery):
  arteritis or endarteritis
  atheroma
  sclerosis
  stricture

Use additional code, if applicable, to identify chronic total occlusion of coronary artery (414.2)

> **EXCLUDES** *embolism of graft (996.72)*
> *occlusion NOS of graft (996.72)*
> *thrombus of graft (996.72)*

DEF: A chronic condition marked by thickening and loss of elasticity of the coronary artery; caused by deposits of plaque containing cholesterol, lipoid material and lipophages.
AHA: 2Q, '97, 13; 2Q, '95, 17; 4Q, '94, 49; 2Q, '94, 13; 1Q, '94, 6; 3Q, '90, 7

414.00 Of unspecified type of vessel, native or graft Ⓐ
  AHA: 1Q, '04, 24; 2Q, '03, 16; 3Q, '01, 15; 4Q, '99, 4; 3Q, '97, 15; 4Q, '96, 31

414.01 Of native coronary artery Ⓐ
  DEF: Plaque deposits in natural heart vessels.
  AHA: 3Q, '09, 9, 10; 3Q, '08, 10; 2Q, '08, 16; 3Q, '06, 25; 4Q, '05, 71; 2Q, '04, 3; 4Q, '03, 108; 3Q, '03, 9, 14; 3Q, '02, 4-9; 3Q, '01, 15; 2Q, '01, 8, 9; 3Q, '97, 15; 2Q, '96, 10; 4Q, '96, 31
  TIP: Assign for documentation of CAD NOS in a patient with no history of coronary artery bypass procedure.
  I25.10 ASHD of native cor artery w/o angina pectoris Ⅰ-10

414.02 Of autologous vein bypass graft Ⓐ
  AHA: 2Q, '10, 8-9
  DEF: Plaque deposit in grafted vein originating within patient.

414.03 Of nonautologous biological bypass graft Ⓐ
  DEF: Plaque deposits in grafted vessel originating outside patient.

414.04 Of artery bypass graft Ⓐ
  Internal mammary artery
  DEF: Plaque deposits in grafted artery originating within patient.
  AHA: 4Q, '96, 31

414.05 Of unspecified type of bypass graft Ⓐ
  Bypass graft NOS
  AHA: 3Q, '97, 15; 4Q, '96, 31

414.06 Of native coronary artery of transplanted heart
  AHA: 4Q, '03, 60; 4Q, '02, 53

414.07 Of bypass graft (artery) (vein) of transplanted heart Ⓐ

✓5ᵗʰ **414.1 Aneurysm and dissection of heart**
  AHA: 4Q, '02, 54

414.10 Aneurysm of heart (wall)
  Aneurysm (arteriovenous):
    mural
    ventricular

Arteries of the Heart

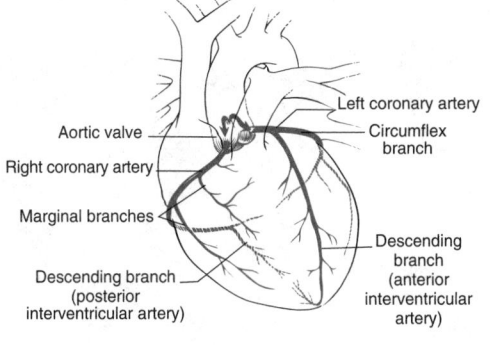

Aortic valve
Right coronary artery
Marginal branches
Descending branch (posterior interventricular artery)
Left coronary artery
Circumflex branch
Descending branch (anterior interventricular artery)

414.11 Aneurysm of coronary vessels
  Aneurysm (arteriovenous) of coronary vessels
  DEF: Dilatation of all three-vessel wall layers forming a sac filled with blood.
  AHA: 2Q, '10, 8-9; 3Q, '03, 10; 1Q, '99, 17

414.12 Dissection of coronary artery
  DEF: A tear in the intimal arterial wall of a coronary artery resulting in the sudden intrusion of blood within the layers of the wall.
  AHA: 1Q, '11, 3-4

414.19 Other aneurysm of heart
  Arteriovenous fistula, acquired, of heart

414.2 Chronic total occlusion of coronary artery
  Complete occlusion of coronary artery
  Total occlusion of coronary artery
  Code first coronary atherosclerosis (414.00-414.07)

> **EXCLUDES** *acute coronary occlusion with myo- cardial infarction (410.00-410.92)*
> *acute coronary occlusion without myocardial infarction (411.81)*

  DEF: Complete blockage of coronary artery due to plaque accumulation over an extended period of time; results in substantial reduction of blood flow.
  AHA: 4Q, '07, 82

414.3 Coronary atherosclerosis due to lipid rich plaque Ⓐ
  Code first coronary atherosclerosis (414.00-414.07)
  AHA: 4Q, '08, 113

414.4 Coronary atherosclerosis due to calcified coronary lesion Ⓐ
  Coronary atherosclerosis due to severely calcified coronary lesion
  Code first coronary atherosclerosis (414.00-414.07)
  AHA: ▶4Q, '11, 107◀

414.8 Other specified forms of chronic ischemic heart disease
  Chronic coronary insufficiency
  Ischemia, myocardial (chronic)
  Any condition classifiable to 410 specified as chronic, or presenting with symptoms after 8 weeks from date of infarction

> **EXCLUDES** *coronary insufficiency (acute) (411.89)*

  AHA: 3Q, '01, 15; 1Q, '92, 10; 3Q, '90, 7, 15; 2Q, '90, 19
  I25.89 Other forms of chronic ischemic heart disease Ⅰ-10

414.9 Chronic ischemic heart disease, unspecified
  Ischemic heart disease NOS

Diseases of Pulmonary Circulation (415-417)

✓4ᵗʰ **415 Acute pulmonary heart disease**

415.0 Acute cor pulmonale

> **EXCLUDES** *cor pulmonale NOS (416.9)*

  DEF: A heart-lung disease marked by dilation and failure of the right side of heart; due to pulmonary embolism; ventilatory function is impaired and pulmonary hypertension results.

✓5ᵗʰ **415.1 Pulmonary embolism and infarction**

Pulmonary (artery) (vein):
  apoplexy
  embolism

Pulmonary (artery) (vein):
  infarction (hemorrhagic)
  thrombosis

> **EXCLUDES** *chronic pulmonary embolism (416.2)*
> *personal history of pulmonary embolism (V12.55)*
> *that complicating:*
> *abortion (634-638 with .6, 639.6)*
> *ectopic or molar pregnancy (639.6)*
> *pregnancy, childbirth, or the puerperium (673.0-673.8)*

  DEF: Embolism: Closure of the pulmonary artery or branch; due to thrombosis (blood clot).
  DEF: Infarction: Necrosis of lung tissue; due to obstructed arterial blood supply, most often by pulmonary embolism.
  AHA: 4Q, '90, 25

415.11 Iatrogenic pulmonary embolism and infarction
  Use additional code for associated septic pulmonary embolism, if applicable, 415.12
  AHA: 4Q, '95, 58
  TIP: Do not report code 997.39 Other respiratory complications, with code 415.11.

415.12 Septic pulmonary embolism
Septic embolism NOS
Code first underlying infection, such as:
septicemia (038.0-038.9)
EXCLUDES septic arterial embolism (449)
AHA: 4Q, '07, 84-86

415.13 Saddle embolus of pulmonary artery
AHA: 4Q, '11, 107-108

415.19 Other
AHA: 3Q, '10, 10; 4Q, '09, 86
126.99 Other pulmonary embolism w/o acute   I-10
cor pulmonale

√4ᵗʰ **416 Chronic pulmonary heart disease**

416.0 Primary pulmonary hypertension
Idiopathic pulmonary arteriosclerosis
Pulmonary hypertension (essential) (idiopathic) (primary)
EXCLUDES pulmonary hypertension NOS (416.8)
secondary pulmonary hypertension (416.8)
DEF: A rare increase in pulmonary circulation, often resulting in right
ventricular failure or fatal syncope.
127.0 Primary pulmonary hypertension   I-10

416.1 Kyphoscoliotic heart disease
DEF: High blood pressure within the lungs as a result of curvature of
the spine.

416.2 Chronic pulmonary embolism
Use additional code, if applicable, for associated long-term
(current) use of anticoagulants (V58.61)
EXCLUDES personal history of pulmonary embolism (V12.55)
DEF: A long-standing condition commonly associated with
pulmonary hypertension in which small blood clots travel to the
lungs repeatedly over many weeks, months, or years, requiring
continuation of established anticoagulant or thrombolytic therapy.
AHA: 4Q, '09, 85-86

416.8 Other chronic pulmonary heart diseases
Pulmonary hypertension NOS
Pulmonary hypertension, secondary
AHA: ▶1Q, '12, 17;◀ 1Q, '11, 10; 3Q, '10, 12; 2Q, '10, 10
127.89 Other specified pulmonary heart diseases   I-10

416.9 Chronic pulmonary heart disease, unspecified
Chronic cardiopulmonary disease
Cor pulmonale (chronic) NOS

√4ᵗʰ **417 Other diseases of pulmonary circulation**

417.0 Arteriovenous fistula of pulmonary vessels
EXCLUDES congenital arteriovenous fistula (747.32)
DEF: Abnormal communication between blood vessels within lung.

417.1 Aneurysm of pulmonary artery
EXCLUDES congenital aneurysm (747.39)
congenital arteriovenous aneurysm (747.32)

417.8 Other specified diseases of pulmonary circulation
Pulmonary:
arteritis
endarteritis
Rupture } of pulmonary vessel
Stricture

417.9 Unspecified disease of pulmonary circulation

Anatomy

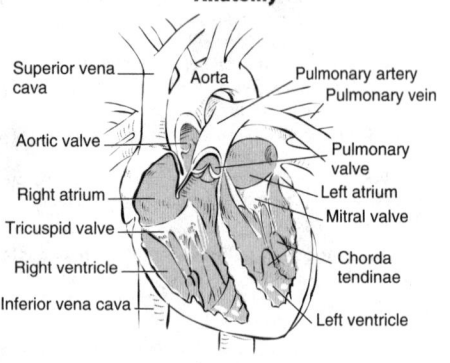

Superior vena cava
Aorta
Pulmonary artery
Pulmonary vein
Aortic valve
Pulmonary valve
Right atrium
Left atrium
Tricuspid valve
Mitral valve
Right ventricle
Chorda tendinae
Inferior vena cava
Left ventricle

Blood Flow

Other Forms of Heart Disease (420-429)

√4ᵗʰ **420 Acute pericarditis**
INCLUDES acute:
mediastinopericarditis
myopericarditis
pericardial effusion
pleuropericarditis
pneumopericarditis
EXCLUDES acute rheumatic pericarditis (391.0)
postmyocardial infarction syndrome [Dressler's] (411.0)
DEF: Inflammation of the pericardium (heart sac); pericardial friction rub
results from this inflammation and is heard as a scratchy or leathery sound.

420.0 Acute pericarditis in diseases classified elsewhere
Code first underlying disease, as:
actinomycosis (039.8)
amebiasis (006.8)
chronic uremia (585.9)
nocardiosis (039.8)
tuberculosis (017.9)
uremia NOS (586)
EXCLUDES pericarditis (acute) (in):
Coxsackie (virus) (074.21)
gonococcal (098.83)
histoplasmosis (115.0-115.9 with
fifth-digit 3)
meningococcal infection (036.41)
syphilitic (093.81)

√5ᵗʰ **420.9 Other and unspecified acute pericarditis**

420.90 Acute pericarditis, unspecified
Pericarditis (acute):   Periocarditis (acute):
NOS   sicca
infective NOS
AHA: 2Q, '89, 12

420.91 Acute idiopathic pericarditis
Pericarditis, acute: Periocarditis (acute):
benign   viral
nonspecific

420.99 Other
Pericarditis (acute):   Pericarditis (acute):
pneumococcal   suppurative
purulent   Pneumopyopericardium
staphylococcal   Pyopericardium
streptococcal
EXCLUDES pericarditis in diseases classified elsewhere
(420.0)

√4ᵗʰ **421** **Acute and subacute endocarditis**

DEF: Bacterial inflammation of the endocardium (intracardiac area); major symptoms include fever, fatigue, heart murmurs, splenomegaly, embolic episodes and areas of infarction.

421.0 **Acute and subacute bacterial endocarditis**
Endocarditis (acute)(chronic) (subacute):
bacterial
infective NOS
lenta
malignant
purulent
septic
ulcerative
vegetative
Infective aneurysm
Subacute bacterial endocarditis [SBE]

Use additional code to identify infectious organism [e.g., Streptococcus 041.0, Staphylococcus 041.1]

AHA: 4Q, '08, 73; 1Q, '99, 12; 1Q, '91, 15

I33.0 Acute and subacute infective endocarditis `I-10`

421.1 *Acute and subacute infective endocarditis in diseases classified elsewhere*

Code first underlying disease, as:
blastomycosis (116.0)
Q fever (083.0)
typhoid (fever) (002.0)

EXCLUDES *endocarditis (in):*
Coxsackie (virus) (074.22)
gonococcal (098.84)
histoplasmosis (115.0-115.9 with fifth-digit 4)
meningococcal infection (036.42)
monilial (112.81)

421.9 **Acute endocarditis, unspecified**
Endocarditis
Myoendocarditis } acute or subacute
Periendocarditis

EXCLUDES *acute rheumatic endocarditis (391.1)*

√4ᵗʰ **422** **Acute myocarditis**

EXCLUDES *acute rheumatic myocarditis (391.2)*

DEF: Acute inflammation of the muscular walls of the heart (myocardium).

422.0 *Acute myocarditis in diseases classified elsewhere*

Code first underlying disease, as:
myocarditis (acute):
influenzal (487.8, 488.09, 488.19)
tuberculous (017.9)

EXCLUDES *myocarditis (acute) (due to):*
aseptic, of newborn (074.23)
Coxsackie (virus) (074.23)
diphtheritic (032.82)
meningococcal infection (036.43)
syphilitic (093.82)
toxoplasmosis (130.3)

√5ᵗʰ **422.9** **Other and unspecified acute myocarditis**

422.90 **Acute myocarditis, unspecified**
Acute or subacute (interstitial) myocarditis

422.91 **Idiopathic myocarditis**
Myocarditis (acute or subacute):
Fiedler's
giant cell
isolated (diffuse) (granulomatous)
nonspecific granulomatous

422.92 **Septic myocarditis**
Myocarditis, acute or subacute:
pneumococcal
staphylococcal

Use additional code to identify infectious organism [e.g., Staphylococcus 041.1]

EXCLUDES *myocarditis, acute or subacute:*
in bacterial diseases classified elsewhere (422.0)
streptococcal (391.2)

Cardiac Tamponade

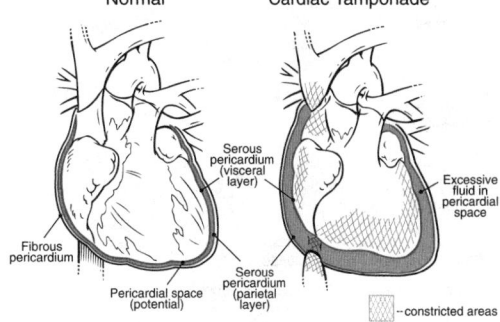

Normal   Cardiac Tamponade

422.93 **Toxic myocarditis**
DEF: Inflammation of the heart muscle due to an adverse reaction to certain drugs or chemicals reaching the heart through the bloodstream.

422.99 **Other**

√4ᵗʰ **423** **Other diseases of pericardium**
EXCLUDES *that specified as rheumatic (393)*

423.0 **Hemopericardium**
DEF: Blood in the pericardial sac (pericardium).

423.1 **Adhesive pericarditis**
Adherent pericardium   Pericarditis:
Fibrosis of pericardium   adhesive
Milk spots   obliterative
                                              Soldiers' patches
DEF: Two layers of serous pericardium adhere to each other by fibrous adhesions.

423.2 **Constrictive pericarditis**
Concato's disease
Pick's disease of heart (and liver)
DEF: Inflammation identified by a rigid, thickened and sometimes calcified pericardium; ventricles of the heart not adequately filled; congestive heart failure may result.

423.3 **Cardiac tamponade**
Code first the underlying cause
DEF: Life-threatening condition in which fluid or blood accumulates between the muscle of the heart (myocardium) and the outer sac (pericardium), resulting in compression of the heart, which decreases cardiac output.
AHA: 4Q, '07, 86, 87

423.8 **Other specified diseases of pericardium**
Calcification } of pericardium
Fistula
AHA: 2Q, '89, 12

423.9 **Unspecified disease of pericardium**
AHA: 1Q, '07, 11

√4ᵗʰ **424** **Other diseases of endocardium**
EXCLUDES *bacterial endocarditis (421.0-421.9)*
rheumatic endocarditis (391.1, 394.0-397.9)
syphilitic endocarditis (093.20-093.24)

424.0 **Mitral valve disorders**
Mitral (valve):
incompetence   } NOS of specified cause,
insufficiency   except rheumatic
regurgitation

EXCLUDES *mitral (valve):*
disease (394.9)
failure (394.9)
stenosis (394.0)
the listed conditions:
specified as rheumatic (394.1)
unspecified as to cause but with mention of:
diseases of aortic valve (396.0-396.9)
mitral stenosis or obstruction (394.2)
AHA: 3Q, '06, 7; 2Q, '00, 16; 3Q, '98, 11; N-D, '87, 8; N-D, '84, 8

I34.8 Other nonrheumatic mitral valve disorders `I-10`

√4ᵗʰ
√5ᵗʰ Additional Digit Required   Unspecified Code   Other Specified Code   Manifestation Code   ▶◀ Revised Text   ● New Code   ▲ Revised Code Title

2013 ICD-9-CM **Volume 1 – 129**

421–424.0

Diseases of the Circulatory System

424.1–426.10

Heart Valve Disorders

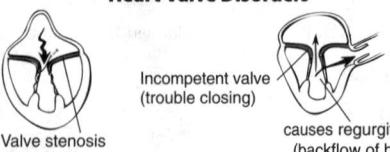

Valve stenosis
(trouble opening)

Incompetent valve
(trouble closing)

causes regurgitation
(backflow of blood)

Insufficient valve
(unable to close completely)

Shortened, fused
chorda tendinae

Ventricular hypertrophy

Normal Heart Valve Function

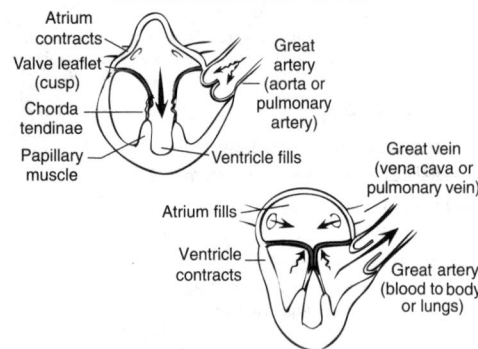

Atrium contracts

Valve leaflet (cusp)

Chorda tendinae

Papillary muscle

Great artery (aorta or pulmonary artery)

Ventricle fills

Great vein (vena cava or pulmonary vein)

Atrium fills

Ventricle contracts

Great artery (blood to body or lungs)

424.1 Aortic valve disorders

Aortic (valve):
  incompetence
  insufficiency   }   NOS of specified cause,
  regurgitation   except rheumatic
  stenosis

EXCLUDES *hypertrophic subaortic stenosis (425.11)*
that specified as rheumatic (395.0-395.9)
that of unspecified cause but with mention of diseases of mitral valve (396.0-396.9)

AHA: ▶4Q, '11, 152;◄ 4Q, '08, 179; 4Q, '88, 8; N-D, '87, 8

424.2 Tricuspid valve disorders, specified as nonrheumatic

Tricuspid valve:
  incompetence
  insufficiency   }   of specified cause, except
  regurgitation   rheumatic
  stenosis

EXCLUDES *rheumatic or of unspecified cause (397.0)*

424.3 Pulmonary valve disorders

Pulmonic: Pulmonic:
  incompetence NOS   regurgitation NOS
  insufficiency NOS   stenosis NOS

EXCLUDES *that specified as rheumatic (397.1)*

√5ᵗʰ 424.9 Endocarditis, valve unspecified

424.90 Endocarditis, valve unspecified, unspecified cause

Endocarditis (chronic):
  NOS
  nonbacterial thrombotic
Valvular:
  incompetence
  insufficiency   }   of unspecified valve,
  regurgitation   unspecified cause
  stenosis
Valvulitis (chronic)

I38 Endocarditis valve unspecified   [1-10]

424.91 *Endocarditis in diseases classified elsewhere*

Code first underlying disease as:
  atypical verrucous endocarditis [Libman-Sacks] (710.0)
  disseminated lupus erythematosus (710.0)
  tuberculosis (017.9)

EXCLUDES *syphilitic (093.20-093.24)*

424.99 Other

Any condition classifiable to 424.90 with specified cause, except rheumatic

EXCLUDES *endocardial fibroelastosis (425.3)*
that specified as rheumatic (397.9)

√4ᵗʰ 425 Cardiomyopathy

INCLUDES myocardiopathy

AHA: J-A, '85, 15

425.0 Endomyocardial fibrosis

√5ᵗʰ 425.1 Hypertrophic cardiomyopathy

EXCLUDES *ventricular hypertrophy (429.3)*

AHA: ▶4Q, '11, 109-110◄

425.11 Hypertrophic obstructive cardiomyopathy

Hypertrophic subaortic stenosis (idiopathic)

DEF: Cardiomyopathy marked by left ventricle hypertrophy, enlarged septum; results in obstructed blood flow.

425.18 Other hypertrophic cardiomyopathy

Nonobstructive hypertrophic cardiomyopathy

425.2 Obscure cardiomyopathy of Africa

Becker's disease
Idiopathic mural endomyocardial disease

425.3 Endocardial fibroelastosis

Elastomyofibrosis

DEF: A condition marked by left ventricle hypertrophy and conversion of the endocardium into a thick fibroelastic coat; capacity of the ventricle may be reduced, but is often increased.

425.4 Other primary cardiomyopathies

Cardiomyopathy: Cardiomyopathy:
  NOS   idiopathic
  congestive   obstructive
  constrictive   restrictive
  familial   Cardiovascular collagenosis

AHA: ▶4Q, '11, 109-110;◄ 4Q, '09, 141; 1Q, '07, 20; 2Q, '05, 14; 1Q, '00, 22; 4Q, '97, 55; 2Q, '90, 19

TIP: For congestive cardiomyopathy, assign first a code for the CHF (category 428) if the treatment is directed toward the CHF.

I42.8 Other cardiomyopathies   [1-10]

425.5 Alcoholic cardiomyopathy

DEF: Heart disease as result of excess alcohol consumption.

AHA: S-O, '85, 15

425.7 *Nutritional and metabolic cardiomyopathy*

Code first underlying disease, as:
  amyloidosis (277.30-277.39)
  beriberi (265.0)
  cardiac glycogenosis (271.0)
  mucopolysaccharidosis (277.5)
  thyrotoxicosis (242.0-242.9)

EXCLUDES *gouty tophi of heart (274.82)*

425.8 *Cardiomyopathy in other diseases classified elsewhere*

Code first underlying disease, as:
  Friedreich's ataxia (334.0)
  myotonia atrophica (359.21)
  progressive muscular dystrophy (359.1)
  sarcoidosis (135)

EXCLUDES *cardiomyopathy in Chagas' disease (086.0)*

AHA: 2Q, '93, 9

I43 Cardiomyopathy in diseases classified elsewhere   [1-10]

425.9 Secondary cardiomyopathy, unspecified

√4ᵗʰ 426 Conduction disorders

DEF: Disruption or disturbance in the electrical impulses that regulate heartbeats.

426.0 Atrioventricular block, complete

Third degree atrioventricular block

AHA: 2Q, '06, 14

TIP: Assign if documentation indicates intermittent complete heart block.

√5ᵗʰ 426.1 Atrioventricular block, other and unspecified

AHA: 2Q, '06, 14

TIP: Assign separate codes for each type of AV block documented.

426.10 Atrioventricular block, unspecified

Atrioventricular [AV] block (incomplete) (partial)

[N] Newborn Age: 0   [P] Pediatric Age: 0-17   [M] Maternity Age: 12-55   [A] Adult Age: 15-124

Nerve Conduction of the Heart

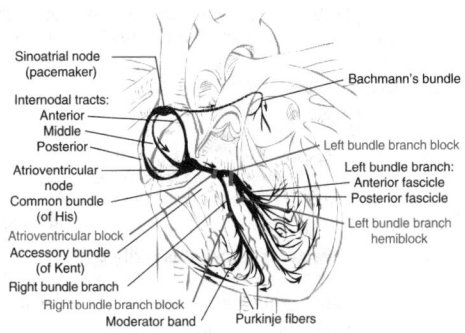

Normal and Long QT Electrocardiogram

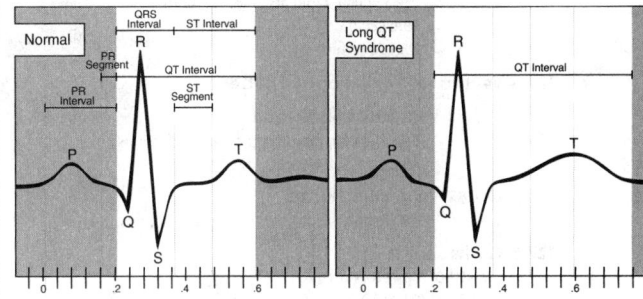

426.11 First degree atrioventricular block
Incomplete atrioventricular block, first degree
Prolonged P-R interval NOS
AHA: 2Q, '06, 14
I44.0 Atrioventricular block first degree   I-10

426.12 Mobitz (type) II atrioventricular block
Incomplete atrioventricular block:
Mobitz (type) II
second degree, Mobitz (type) II
DEF: Impaired conduction of excitatory impulse from
cardiac atrium to ventricle through AV node.
AHA: 2Q, '06, 14

426.13 Other second degree atrioventricular block
Incomplete atrioventricular block:
Mobitz (type) I [Wenckebach's]
second degree:
NOS
Mobitz (type) I
with 2:1 atrioventricular response [block]
Wenckebach's phenomenon
DEF: Wenckebach's phenomenon: impulses generated at
constant rate to sinus node, P-R interval lengthens; results
in cycle of ventricular inadequacy and shortened P-R
interval; second-degree A-V block commonly called
"Mobitz type 1."

426.2 Left bundle branch hemiblock
Block: Block:
left anterior fascicular   left posterior fascicular

426.3 Other left bundle branch block
Left bundle branch block:
NOS
anterior fascicular with posterior fascicular
complete
main stem
I44.7 Left bundle-branch block unspecified   I-10

426.4 Right bundle branch block
AHA: 3Q, '00, 3
I45.10 Unspecified right bundle-branch block   I-10

√5ᵗʰ **426.5 Bundle branch block, other and unspecified**

426.50 Bundle branch block, unspecified

**426.51 Right bundle branch block and left posterior
fascicular block**

**426.52 Right bundle branch block and left anterior
fascicular block**

426.53 Other bilateral bundle branch block
Bifascicular block NOS
Bilateral bundle branch block NOS
Right bundle branch with left bundle branch block
(incomplete) (main stem)

426.54 Trifascicular block

426.6 Other heart block
Intraventricular block:
NOS
diffuse
myofibrillar
Sinoatrial block
Sinoauricular block

426.7 Anomalous atrioventricular excitation
Atrioventricular conduction:
accelerated
accessory
pre-excitation
Ventricular pre-excitation
Wolff-Parkinson-White syndrome
DEF: Wolff-Parkinson-White: normal conduction pathway is
bypassed; results in short P-R interval on EKG; tendency to
supraventricular tachycardia.

√5ᵗʰ **426.8 Other specified conduction disorders**

426.81 Lown-Ganong-Levine syndrome
Syndrome of short P-R interval, normal QRS
complexes, and supraventricular tachycardias

426.82 Long QT syndrome
DEF: Condition characterized by recurrent syncope,
malignant arrhythmias, and sudden death; characteristic
prolonged Q-T interval on electrocardiogram.
AHA: 4Q, '05, 72

426.89 Other
Dissociation:
atrioventricular [AV]
interference
isorhythmic
Nonparoxysmal AV nodal tachycardia

426.9 Conduction disorder, unspecified
Heart block NOS
Stokes-Adams syndrome

√4ᵗʰ **427 Cardiac dysrhythmias**
EXCLUDES that complicating:
abortion (634-638 with .7, 639.8)
ectopic or molar pregnancy (639.8)
labor or delivery (668.1, 669.4)
DEF: Disruption or disturbance in the rhythm of heartbeats.
AHA: J-A, '85, 15

427.0 Paroxysmal supraventricular tachycardia
Paroxysmal tachycardia: Paroxysmal tachycardia:
atrial [PAT]   junctional
atrioventricular [AV]   nodal
DEF: Rapid atrial rhythm.

427.1 Paroxysmal ventricular tachycardia
Ventricular tachycardia (paroxysmal)
DEF: Rapid ventricular rhythm.
AHA: 2Q, '09, 14; 1Q, '08, 14; 2Q, '06, 15-16; 3Q, '95, 9; M-A, '86, 11
TIP: If a ventricular tachycardia is documented as sustained or
nonsustained but is induced during an EP study, assign 427.1.
I47.2 Ventricular tachycardia   I-10

427.2 Paroxysmal tachycardia, unspecified
Bouveret-Hoffmann syndrome
Paroxysmal tachycardia:
NOS
essential

√5ᵗʰ **427.3 Atrial fibrillation and flutter**
TIP: Assign V58.61 Long-term (current) use of anticoagulants, as a
secondary diagnosis if the patient is maintained on Coumadin.

427.31 Atrial fibrillation
DEF: Irregular, rapid atrial contractions.
AHA: ▶1Q, '12, 7;◀ 4Q, '08, 135; 3Q, '05, 8; 4Q, '04, 78, 121;
3Q, '04, 7; 4Q, '03, 95, 105; 1Q, '03, 8; 2Q, '99, 17; 3Q, '95, 8
I48.0 Atrial fibrillation   I-10

Diseases of the Circulatory System

427.32 Atrial flutter
DEF: Regular, rapid atrial contractions.
AHA: 4Q, '03, 94
I48.1 Atrial flutter   I-10

√5ᵗʰ **427.4 Ventricular fibrillation and flutter**

427.41 Ventricular fibrillation
DEF: Irregular, rapid ventricular contractions.
AHA: 2Q, '09, 14-15; 3Q, '02, 5

427.42 Ventricular flutter
DEF: Regular, rapid, ventricular contractions.

427.5 Cardiac arrest
Cardiorespiratory arrest
AHA: 3Q,'02, 5; 2Q, '00, 12; 3Q, '95, 8; 2Q, '88, 8
I46.9 Cardiac arrest cause unspecified   I-10

√5ᵗʰ **427.6 Premature beats**

427.60 Premature beats, unspecified
Ectopic beats
Extrasystoles
Extrasystolic arrhythmia
Premature contractions or systoles NOS

427.61 Supraventricular premature beats
Atrial premature beats, contractions, or systoles

427.69 Other
Ventricular premature beats, contractions, or systoles
AHA: 4Q, '93, 42

√5ᵗʰ **427.8 Other specified cardiac dysrhythmias**

427.81 Sinoatrial node dysfunction
Sinus bradycardia: Syndrome:
   persistent   sick sinus
   severe   tachycardia-bradycardia
EXCLUDES sinus bradycardia NOS (427.89)
DEF: Complex cardiac arrhythmia; appears as severe sinus
bradycardia, sinus bradycardia with tachycardia, or sinus
bradycardia with atrioventricular block.
AHA: 4Q, '11, 168; 3Q, '10, 9; 3Q, '00, 8
I49.5 Sick sinus syndrome   I-10

427.89 Other
Rhythm disorder:
   coronary sinus
   ectopic
   nodal
Wandering (atrial) pacemaker
EXCLUDES carotid sinus syncope (337.0)
     neonatal bradycardia (779.81)
     neonatal tachycardia (779.82)
     reflex bradycardia (337.0)
     tachycardia NOS (785.0)
I49.8 Other specified cardiac arrhythmias   I-10

427.9 Cardiac dysrhythmia, unspecified
Arrhythmia (cardiac) NOS
AHA: 2Q, '89, 10

Echocardiography of Heart Failure

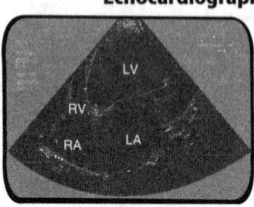

Four-chamber echocardiograms,
two-dimensional views.
LV: Left ventricle
RV: Right ventricle
RA: Right atrium
LA: Left atrium

Systolic dysfunction
with dilated LV

Diastolic dysfunction
with LV hypertrophy

√4ᵗʰ **428 Heart failure**
Code, if applicable, heart failure due to hypertension first
(402.0-402.9, with fifth-digit 1 or 404.0-404.9 with fifth-digit 1
or 3)
EXCLUDES following cardiac surgery (429.4)
     rheumatic (398.91)
     that complicating:
       abortion (634-638 with .7, 639.8)
       ectopic or molar pregnancy (639.8)
       labor or delivery (668.1, 669.4)
AHA: 4Q, '02, 49; 3Q, '98, 5; 2Q, '90, 16; 2Q, '90, 19; 2Q, '89, 10; 3Q, '88, 3

428.0 Congestive heart failure, unspecified
Congestive heart disease
Right heart failure (secondary to left heart failure)
EXCLUDES fluid overload NOS (276.69)
DEF: Mechanical inadequacy; caused by inability of heart to pump
and circulate blood; results in fluid collection in lungs, hypertension,
congestion and edema of tissue.
AHA: 4Q, '09, 141; 1Q, '09, 8, 18; 4Q, '08, 72, 180, 182; 3Q, '08, 12; 3Q,
'07, 9; 1Q, 07, 20; 3Q, '06, 7; 4Q, '05, 120; 3Q, '05, 8; 1Q, '05, 5, 9; 1Q,
'05, 5, 9; 4Q, '04, 140; 3Q, '04, 7;4Q, '03, 109; 1Q, '03, 9; 4Q, '02, 52; 2Q,
'01, 13; 4Q, '00, 48; 2Q, '00, 16; 1Q, '00, 22; 4Q, '99, 4; 1Q, '99, 11; 4Q,
'97, 55; 3Q, '97, 10; 3Q, '96, 9; 3Q, '91, 18; 3Q, '91, 19; 2Q, '89, 12
TIP: Assign additional code(s) from subcategory 428.2, 428.3, or
428.4 to specify the type of heart failure.
I50.9 Heart failure unspecified   I-10

428.1 Left heart failure
Acute edema of lung   } with heart disease NOS or
Acute pulmonary edema }   heart failure
Cardiac asthma
Left ventricular failure
DEF: Mechanical inadequacy of left ventricle; causing fluid in lungs.

√5ᵗʰ **428.2 Systolic heart failure**
EXCLUDES combined systolic and diastolic heart failure
     (428.40-428.43)
DEF: Heart failure due to a defect in expulsion of blood caused by an
abnormality in systolic function, or ventricular contractile
dysfunction.

428.20 Unspecified
I50.20 Unspecified systolic congestive heart failure   I-10

428.21 Acute
I50.21 Acute systolic congestive heart failure   I-10

428.22 Chronic
AHA: 4Q, '05, 120

428.23 Acute on chronic
AHA: 1Q, '09, 8, 18;1Q, '03, 9

√5ᵗʰ **428.3 Diastolic heart failure**
EXCLUDES combined systolic and diastolic heart failure
     (428.40-428.43)
DEF: Heart failure due to resistance to ventricular filling caused by an
abnormality in the diastolic function.
AHA: ▶1Q, '12, 7◀

428.30 Unspecified
AHA: 4Q, '02, 52
I50.30 Unspecified diastolic congestive heart failure   I-10

428.31 Acute

428.32 Chronic
AHA: 3Q, '08, 12
I50.32 Chronic diastolic congestive heart failure   I-10

428.33 Acute on chronic
AHA: 4Q, '09, 141; 3Q, '08, 12; 1Q, '07, 20
I50.33 Acute on chronic diastolic heart failure   I-10

√5ᵗʰ **428.4 Combined systolic and diastolic heart failure**

428.40 Unspecified

428.41 Acute
AHA: 4Q, '04, 140

428.42 Chronic

428.43 Acute on chronic
AHA: 3Q, '06, 7; 4Q, '02, 52

428.9 Heart failure, unspecified
Cardiac failure NOS   Myocardial failure NOS
Heart failure NOS   Weak heart
AHA: 2Q, '89, 10; N-D, '85, 14

☑4th 429 Ill-defined descriptions and complications of heart disease

429.0 Myocarditis, unspecified
Myocarditis
NOS
chronic (interstitial)   (with mention of
fibroid   arteriosclerosis)
senile

Use additional code to identify presence of arteriosclerosis
EXCLUDES acute or subacute (422.0-422.9)
rheumatic (398.0)
acute (391.2)
that due to hypertension (402.0-402.9)

429.1 Myocardial degeneration
Degeneration of heart or
myocardium:
fatty
mural   (with mention of
muscular   arteriosclerosis)
Myocardial:
degeneration
disease

Use additional code to identify presence of arteriosclerosis
EXCLUDES that due to hypertension (402.0-402.9)

429.2 Cardiovascular disease, unspecified
Arteriosclerotic cardiovascular disease [ASCVD]
Cardiovascular arteriosclerosis
Cardiovascular:
degeneration
disease   (with mention of
sclerosis   arteriosclerosis)

Use additional code to identify presence of arteriosclerosis
EXCLUDES that due to hypertension (402.0-402.9)

429.3 Cardiomegaly
Cardiac: Ventricular dilatation
dilatation
hypertrophy
EXCLUDES that due to hypertension (402.0-402.9)
I51.7 Cardiomegaly [I-10]

429.4 Functional disturbances following cardiac surgery
Cardiac insufficiency ⎱ following cardiac surgery or
Heart failure ⎰ due to prosthesis
Postcardiotomy syndrome
Postvalvulotomy syndrome
EXCLUDES cardiac failure in the immediate postoperative period
(997.1)
AHA: 2Q, '02, 12; N-D, '85, 6

429.5 Rupture of chordae tendineae
DEF: Torn tissue, between heart valves and papillary muscles.

429.6 Rupture of papillary muscle
DEF: Torn muscle, between chordae tendineae and heart wall.

☑5th 429.7 Certain sequelae of myocardial infarction, not elsewhere classified
Use additional code to identify the associated myocardial infarction:
with onset of 8 weeks or less (410.00-410.92)
with onset of more than 8 weeks (414.8)
EXCLUDES congenital defects of heart (745, 746)
coronary aneurysm (414.11)
disorders of papillary muscle (429.6, 429.81)
postmyocardial infarction syndrome (411.0)
rupture of chordae tendineae (429.5)
AHA: 3Q, '89, 5

429.71 Acquired cardiac septal defect Ⓐ
EXCLUDES acute septal infarction (410.00-410.92)
DEF: Abnormal communication, between opposite heart chambers; due to defect of septum; not present at birth.

429.79 Other Ⓐ
Mural thrombus (atrial) (ventricular), acquired, following myocardial infarction
AHA: 1Q, '92, 10

☑5th 429.8 Other ill-defined heart diseases

429.81 Other disorders of papillary muscle
Papillary muscle: Papillary muscle:
atrophy   incompetence
degeneration   incoordination
dysfunction   scarring

429.82 Hyperkinetic heart disease
DEF: Condition of unknown origin in young adults; marked by increased cardiac output at rest, increased rate of ventricular ejection; may lead to heart failure.

429.83 Takotsubo syndrome
Broken heart syndrome
Reversible left ventricular dysfunction following sudden emotional stress
Stress induced cardiomyopathy
Transient left ventricular apical ballooning syndrome
AHA: 4Q, '06, 87

429.89 Other
Carditis
EXCLUDES that due to hypertension (402.0-402.9)
AHA: 2Q, '06, 18; 3Q, '05, 14; 1Q, '92, 10

429.9 Heart disease, unspecified
Heart disease (organic) NOS   Morbus cordis NOS
EXCLUDES that due to hypertension (402.0-402.9)
AHA: 1Q, '09, 7; 1Q, '93, 19
I51.9 Heart disease unspecified [I-10]

Cerebrovascular Disease (430-438)

INCLUDES with mention of hypertension (conditions classifiable to 401-405)

Use additional code to identify presence of hypertension
EXCLUDES any condition classifiable to 430-434, 436, 437 occurring during pregnancy, childbirth, or the puerperium, or specified as puerperal (674.0)
iatrogenic cerebrovascular infarction or hemorrhage (997.02)
AHA: 1Q, '93, 27; 3Q, '91, 10; 3Q, '90, 3; 2Q, '89, 8; M-A, '85, 6

430 Subarachnoid hemorrhage
Meningeal hemorrhage   Ruptured:
Ruptured: (congenital) cerebral aneurysm NOS
berry aneurysm
EXCLUDES berry aneurysm, nonruptured (437.3)
syphilitic ruptured cerebral aneurysm (094.87)
AHA: 4Q, '04, 77
DEF: Bleeding in space between brain and lining.

431 Intracerebral hemorrhage
Hemorrhage (of):   Hemorrhage (of):
basilar   internal capsule
bulbar   intrapontine
cerebellar   pontine
cerebral   subcortical
cerebromeningeal   ventricular
corticalRupture of blood vessel in brain
DEF: Bleeding within the brain.
AHA: ▶1Q, '12, 14;◀ 3Q, '10, 5-6; 1Q, '10, 8; 3Q, '07, 4; 4Q, '04, 77
I61.9 Nontraumatic intracerebral hemorrhage unspec [I-10]

Berry Aneurysms

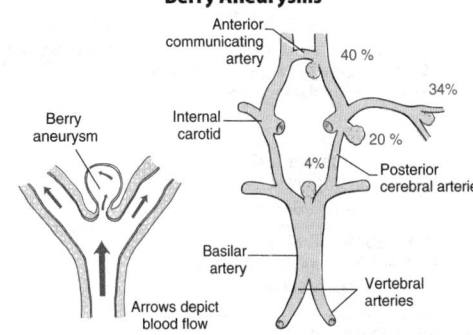

☑4th/☑5th Additional Digit Required   Unspecified Code   Other Specified Code   Manifestation Code   ▶◄ Revised Text   ● New Code   ▲ Revised Code Title

Diseases of the Circulatory System

432–437.4

Cerebrovascular Arteries

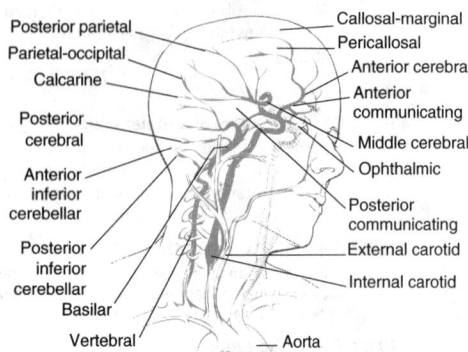

✓4ᵗʰ **432 Other and unspecified intracranial hemorrhage**
AHA: 4Q, '04, 7

432.0 Nontraumatic extradural hemorrhage
Nontraumatic epidural hemorrhage
DEF: Bleeding, nontraumatic, between skull and brain lining.

432.1 Subdural hemorrhage
Subdural hematoma, nontraumatic
DEF: Bleeding, between outermost and other layers of brain lining.

432.9 Unspecified intracranial hemorrhage
Intracranial hemorrhage NOS

✓4ᵗʰ **433 Occlusion and stenosis of precerebral arteries**

INCLUDES   embolism
       narrowing   ⎱ of basilar, carotid, and vertebral
       obstruction   ⎰   arteries
       thrombosis

Use additional code, if applicable, to identify status post administration of tPA (rtPA) in a different facility within the last 24 hours prior to admission to current facility (V45.88)

EXCLUDES   *insufficiency NOS of precerebral arteries (435.0-435.9)*

The following fifth-digit subclassification is for use with category 433:
   0 without mention of cerebral infarction
   1 with cerebral infarction

DEF: Blockage, stricture, arteries branching into brain.
AHA: 2Q, '95, 14; 3Q, '90, 16

§ ✓5ᵗʰ **433.0 Basilar artery**
[0-1]

§ ✓5ᵗʰ **433.1 Carotid artery**
[0-1]   AHA: 1Q, '00, 16; For code 433.10: 1Q, '06, 17; 1Q, '02, 7, 10
      165.29 Occlusion and stenosis of unspec carotid artery   I-10
      163.239 Cerbral infarct d/t usp occ/stenosis of uns carotid art   I-10
      163.449 Cerbral infarct d/t embo of uns cerebellar art   I-10

§ ✓5ᵗʰ **433.2 Vertebral artery**
[0-1]

§ ✓5ᵗʰ **433.3 Multiple and bilateral**
[0-1]   AHA: 2Q, '02, 19

§ ✓5ᵗʰ **433.8 Other specified precerebral artery**
[0-1]

§ ✓5ᵗʰ **433.9 Unspecified precerebral artery**
[0-1]   Precerebral artery NOS

✓4ᵗʰ **434 Occlusion of cerebral arteries**
Use additional code, if applicable, to identify status post administration of tPA (rtPA) in a different facility within the last 24 hours prior to admission to current facility (V45.88)

The following fifth-digit subclassification is for use with category 434:
   0 without mention of cerebral infarction
   1 with cerebral infarction

AHA: 2Q, '95, 14

§ ✓5ᵗʰ **434.0 Cerebral thrombosis**
[0-1]   Thrombosis of cerebral arteries
      AHA: For code 434.01: 4Q, '04, 77

§ ✓5ᵗʰ **434.1 Cerebral embolism**
[0-1]   AHA: For code 434.11: 4Q, '04, 77; 3Q, '97, 11
      163.449 Cerbral infarct d/t embo of uns cerebellar art   I-10

§ ✓5ᵗʰ **434.9 Cerebral artery occlusion, unspecified**
[0-1]   AHA: For code 434.91: 3Q, '10, 5-6; 4Q, '08, 108; 3Q, '07, 9; 1Q, '07, 23; 4Q, '04, 77-78; 4Q, '98, 87

✓4ᵗʰ **435 Transient cerebral ischemia**

INCLUDES   cerebrovascular insufficiency (acute) with transient focal neurological signs and symptoms
      insufficiency of basilar, carotid, and vertebral arteries
      spasm of cerebral arteries

EXCLUDES   *acute cerebrovascular insufficiency NOS (437.1)*
      that due to any condition classifiable to 433 (433.0-433.9)
DEF: Temporary restriction of blood flow to arteries branching into brain.

435.0 Basilar artery syndrome

435.1 Vertebral artery syndrome

435.2 Subclavian steal syndrome
DEF: Cerebrovascular insufficiency, due to occluded subclavian artery; symptoms include pain in mastoid and posterior head regions, flaccid paralysis of arm and diminished or absent radial pulse on affected side.

435.3 Vertebrobasilar artery syndrome
DEF: Transient ischemic attack; due to brainstem dysfunction; symptoms include confusion, vertigo, binocular blindness, diplopia, unilateral or bilateral weakness and paresthesis of extremities.
AHA: 4Q, '95, 60

435.8 Other specified transient cerebral ischemias

435.9 Unspecified transient cerebral ischemia
Impending cerebrovascular accident
Intermittent cerebral ischemia
Transient ischemic attack [TIA]
AHA: N-D, '85, 12
G45.9 Transient cerebral ischemic attack unspecified   I-10

436 Acute, but ill-defined, cerebrovascular disease
Apoplexy, apoplectic: Apoplexy, apoplectic:
   NOS   seizure
   attack   Cerebral seizure
   cerebral

EXCLUDES   *any condition classifiable to categories 430-435*
      cerebrovascular accident (434.91)
      CVA (ischemic) (434.91)
        embolic (434.11)
        hemorrhagic (430, 431, 432.0-432.9)
        thrombotic (434.01)
      postoperative cerebrovascular accident (997.02)
      stroke (ischemic) (434.91)
        embolic (434.11)
        hemorrhagic (430, 431, 432.0-432.9)
        thrombotic (434.01)
AHA: 4Q, '04, 77; 4Q, '99, 3
TIP: Do not assign when documentation indicates "CVA, stroke, or cerebral infarction." See instead default code 434.91.

✓4ᵗʰ **437 Other and ill-defined cerebrovascular disease**

437.0 Cerebral atherosclerosis   A
Atheroma of cerebral arteries
Cerebral arteriosclerosis
AHA: 3Q, '10, 15
167.2 Cerebral atherosclerosis   I-10

437.1 Other generalized ischemic cerebrovascular disease
Acute cerebrovascular insufficiency NOS
Cerebral ischemia (chronic)
AHA: 1Q, '09, 8

437.2 Hypertensive encephalopathy
DEF: Cerebral manifestations (such as visual disturbances and headache) due to high blood pressure.
AHA: J-A, '84, 14

437.3 Cerebral aneurysm, nonruptured
Internal carotid artery, intracranial portion
Internal carotid artery NOS
EXCLUDES   *congenital cerebral aneurysm, nonruptured (747.81)*
      internal carotid artery, extracranial portion (442.81)
AHA: 2Q, '09, 12

437.4 Cerebral arteritis
DEF: Inflammation of a cerebral artery or arteries.
AHA: 4Q, '99, 21

---

§   Requires fifth digit. Valid digits are in [brackets] under each code. See appropriate category for codes and definitions.

   N Newborn Age: 0   P Pediatric Age: 0-17   M Maternity Age: 12-55   A Adult Age: 15-124

437.5 Moyamoya disease
> **DEF:** Cerebrovascular ischemia; vessels occlude and rupture causing tiny hemorrhages at base of brain; predominantly affects Japanese.

437.6 Nonpyogenic thrombosis of intracranial venous sinus
> **EXCLUDES** pyogenic (325)

437.7 Transient global amnesia
> **DEF:** Episode of short-term memory loss, not often recurrent; pathogenesis unknown; with no signs or symptoms of neurological disorder.
> **AHA:** 4Q, '92, 20

437.8 Other

437.9 Unspecified
> Cerebrovascular disease or lesion NOS
> **AHA:** 1Q, '09, 9

√4ᵗʰ 438 Late effects of cerebrovascular disease
> **NOTE** This category is to be used to indicate conditions in 430-437 as the cause of late effects. The "late effects" include conditions specified as such, as sequelae, which may occur at any time after the onset of the causal condition.
>
> **EXCLUDES** personal history of:
>   cerebral infarction without residual deficits (V12.54)
>   PRIND [Prolonged reversible ischemic neurologic deficit] (V12.54)
>   RIND [Reversible ischemic neurological deficit] (V12.54)
>   transient ischemic attack [TIA] (V12.54)
> **AHA:** 3Q, '06, 3-4, 6; 4Q, '99, 4, 6, 7; 4Q, '98, 39, 88; 4Q, '97, 35, 37; 4Q, '92, 21;N-D,'86, 12; M-A, '86, 7
> **TIP:** Assign instead code V12.54 TIA and cerebral infarction without residual effects, if no residual deficits are present.

438.0 Cognitive deficits

√5ᵗʰ 438.1 Speech and language deficits

     438.10 Speech and language deficit, unspecified

     438.11 Aphasia
> **DEF:** Impairment or absence of the ability to communicate by speech, writing or signs or to comprehend the spoken or written language due to disease or injury to the brain.
> **AHA:** 4Q, '03, 105; 4Q, '97, 36

     438.12 Dysphasia
> **DEF:** Impaired speech; marked by inability to sequence language.
> **AHA:** 4Q, '99, 3, 9

     438.13 Dysarthria
> **DEF:** Speech disorder caused by paralysis, spasticity, or other nerve damage resulting in difficulty expressing words or sounds; characterized by slurring, interrupted rhythm of speech, or distorted vowel sounds.
> **AHA:** 4Q, '09, 87-88
> **TIP:** If dysarthria or other speech disturbances are not due to underlying cerebrovascular disease, see subcategory 784.5 codes.

     438.14 Fluency disorder
> Stuttering due to late effect of cerebrovascular accident
> **DEF:** Interruption in the flow of speech that significantly interferes with communication; characterized by primary sound and syllable repetitions, articulatory fixations, and abnormal prolongation of speech sounds.
> **AHA:** 4Q, '10, 83; 4Q, '09, 87-88

     438.19 Other speech and language deficits

√5ᵗʰ 438.2 Hemiplegia/hemiparesis
> **DEF:** Paralysis of one side of the body.
> **AHA:** 1Q, '10, 5

     438.20 Hemiplegia affecting unspecified side
> **AHA:** 4Q, '07, 94; 4Q, '03, 105; 4Q, '99, 3, 9
> **I69.959** Hemipl & hemiparesis flw uns CVD affect uns side   `I-10`

     438.21 Hemiplegia affecting dominant side

     438.22 Hemiplegia affecting nondominant side
> **AHA:** 4Q, '03, 105; 1Q, '02, 16

√5ᵗʰ 438.3 Monoplegia of upper limb
> **DEF:** Paralysis of one limb or one muscle group.

     438.30 Monoplegia of upper limb affecting unspecified side

     438.31 Monoplegia of upper limb affecting dominant side

     438.32 Monoplegia of upper limb affecting nondominant side

√5ᵗʰ 438.4 Monoplegia of lower limb

     438.40 Monoplegia of lower limb affecting unspecified side

     438.41 Monoplegia of lower limb affecting dominant side

     438.42 Monoplegia of lower limb affecting nondominant side

√5ᵗʰ 438.5 Other paralytic syndrome
> Use additional code to identify type of paralytic syndrome, such as:
>   locked-in state (344.81)
>   quadriplegia (344.00-344.09)
> **EXCLUDES** late effects of cerebrovascular accident with:
>   hemiplegia/hemiparesis (438.20-438.22)
>   monoplegia of lower limb (438.40-438.42)
>   monoplegia of upper limb (438.30-438.32)

     438.50 Other paralytic syndrome affecting unspecified side

     438.51 Other paralytic syndrome affecting dominant side

     438.52 Other paralytic syndrome affecting nondominant side

     438.53 Other paralytic syndrome, bilateral
> **AHA:** 4Q, '98, 39

438.6 Alterations of sensations
> Use additional code to identify the altered sensation

438.7 Disturbances of vision
> Use additional code to identify the visual disturbance
> **AHA:** 4Q, '02, 56

√5ᵗʰ 438.8 Other late effects of cerebrovascular disease

     438.81 Apraxia
> **DEF:** Inability to activate learned movements; no known sensory or motor impairment.

     438.82 Dysphagia
> Use additional code to identify the type of dysphagia, if known (787.20-787.29)
> **DEF:** Inability or difficulty in swallowing.
> **AHA:** 4Q, '07, 94
> **I69.991** Dysphagia following uns cerebrovascular dis   `I-10`

     438.83 Facial weakness
> Facial droop

     438.84 Ataxia
> **AHA:** 4Q, '02, 56

     438.85 Vertigo

     438.89 Other late effects of cerebrovascular disease
> Use additional code to identify the late effect
> **AHA:** 2Q, '09, 10; 1Q, '05, 13; 4Q, '98, 39
> **TIP:** Assign 438.89 and 728.87 Muscle weakness, for residual weakness secondary to late effect of CVA.
> **I69.998** Other sequelae flw uns cerebrovascular disease   `I-10`

438.9 Unspecified late effects of cerebrovascular disease

Diseases of the Circulatory System

440–440.22

Map of Major Arteries

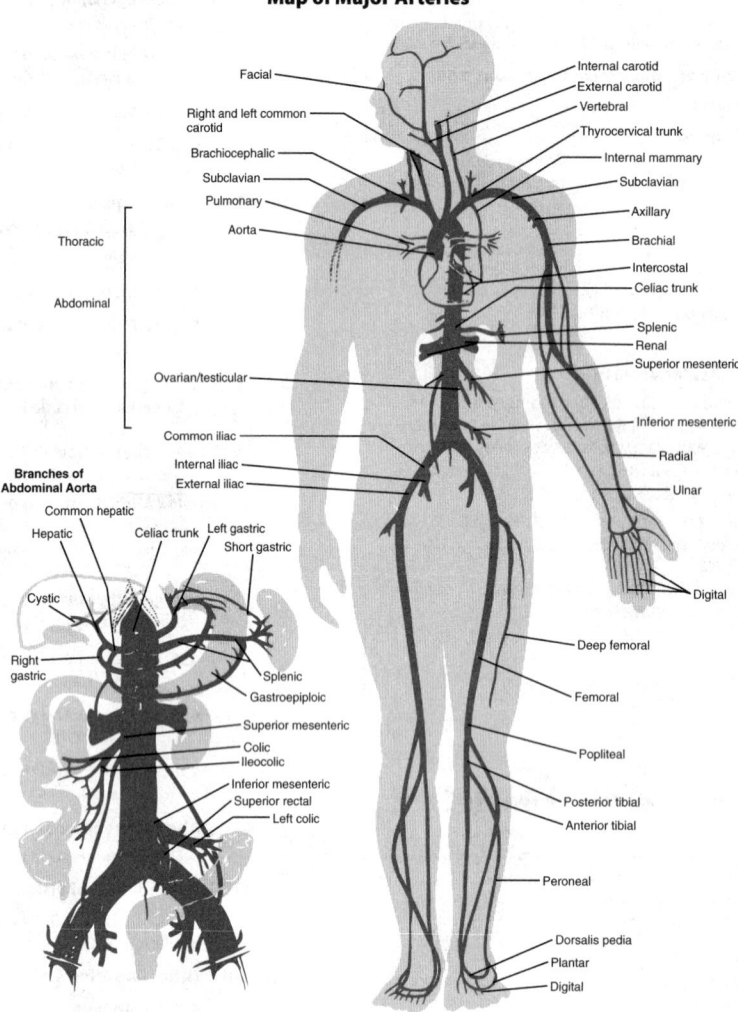

Branches of Abdominal Aorta

Diseases of Arteries, Arterioles, and Capillaries (440-449)

✓4ᵗʰ 440 Atherosclerosis

> INCLUDES arteriolosclerosis
> arteriosclerosis (obliterans) (senile)
> arteriosclerotic vascular disease
> atheroma
> degeneration:
>> arterial
>> arteriovascular
>> vascular
> endarteritis deformans or obliterans
> senile:
>> arteritis
>> endarteritis

> EXCLUDES atheroembolism (445.01-445.89)
> atherosclerosis of bypass graft of the extremities (440.30-440.32)

> DEF: Stricture and reduced elasticity of artery; due to plaque deposits.

440.0 Of aorta   A

> AHA: 2Q, '93, 7; 2Q, '93, 8; 4Q, '88, 8

440.1 Of renal artery   A

> EXCLUDES atherosclerosis of renal arterioles (403.00-403.91)

✓5ᵗʰ 440.2 Of native arteries of the extremities

> Use additional code, if applicable, to identify chronic total occlusion of artery of the extremities (440.4)

> EXCLUDES atherosclerosis of bypass graft of the extremities (440.30-440.32)

> AHA: 4Q, '94, 49; 4Q, '93, 27; 4Q, '92, 25; 3Q, '90, 15; M-A, '87, 6
> TIP: Codes are listed in order of increasing severity; all patients who have gangrene (regardless of whether ulceration, rest pain, and/or intermittent claudication are present) are coded to 440.24. Patients without gangrene, but with ulceration (regardless of whether they also suffer from rest pain or intermittent claudication) are coded to 440.23.

440.20 Atherosclerosis of the extremities, unspecified   A

> I70.209 Uns atherosclero natv art of extrem uns extrem   I-10

440.21 Atherosclerosis of the extremities with intermittent claudication   A

> DEF: Atherosclerosis; marked by pain, tension and weakness after walking; no symptoms while at rest.
> I70.219 Atherosclerosis native arteries ext interm claud uns ext   I-10

440.22 Atherosclerosis of the extremities with rest pain   A

> INCLUDES any condition classifiable to 440.21
> DEF: Atherosclerosis, marked by pain, tension and weakness while at rest.

N Newborn Age: 0   P Pediatric Age: 0-17   M Maternity Age: 12-55   A Adult Age: 15-124

440.23 Atherosclerosis of the extremities with ulceration   [A]

INCLUDES   any condition classifiable to 440.21 and 440.22

Use additional code for any associated ulceration (707.10-707.19, 707.8, 707.9)

AHA: 4Q, '00, 44

I70.249 Atherosclero natv art lt leg ulceration uns site   [I-10]

440.24 Atherosclerosis of the extremities with gangrene

INCLUDES   any condition classifiable to 440.21, 440.22, and 440.23 with ischemic gangrene 785.4

Use additional code for any associated ulceration (707.10-707.19, 707.8, 707.9)

EXCLUDES   gas gangrene (040.0)

AHA: 4Q, '03, 109; 3Q, '03, 14; 4Q, '95, 54; 1Q, '95, 11

440.29 Other   [A]

√5th **440.3 Of bypass graft of extremities**

EXCLUDES   atherosclerosis of native arteries of the extremities (440.21-440.24)

embolism [occlusion NOS] [thrombus] of graft (996.74)

AHA: 4Q, '94, 49

440.30 Of unspecified graft   [A]

440.31 Of autologous vein bypass graft   [A]

440.32 Of nonautologous biological bypass graft   [A]

440.4 Chronic total occlusion of artery of the extremities

Complete occlusion of artery of the extremities

Total occlusion of artery of the extremities

Code first atherosclerosis of arteries of the extremities (440.20-440.29, 440.30-440.32)

EXCLUDES   acute occlusion of artery of extremity (444.21-444.22)

AHA: 4Q, '07, 82

440.8 Of other specified arteries   [A]

EXCLUDES   basilar (433.0)
carotid (433.1)
cerebral (437.0)
coronary (414.00-414.07)
mesenteric (557.1)
precerebral (433.0-433.9)
pulmonary (416.0)
vertebral (433.2)

AHA: 3Q, '09, 9

TIP: Assign for arteriosclerosis of the iliac artery.

440.9 Generalized and unspecified atherosclerosis   [A]

Arteriosclerotic vascular disease NOS

EXCLUDES   arteriosclerotic cardiovascular disease [ASCVD] (429.2)

I70.91 Generalized atherosclerosis   [I-10]

√4th **441 Aortic aneurysm and dissection**

EXCLUDES   aortic ectasia (447.70-447.73)
syphilitic aortic aneurysm (093.0)
traumatic aortic aneurysm (901.0, 902.0)

√5th **441.0 Dissection of aorta**

DEF: Dissection or splitting of wall of the aorta; due to blood entering through intimal tear or interstitial hemorrhage.

AHA: 4Q, '89, 10

441.00 Unspecified site

441.01 Thoracic

AHA: 1Q, '09, 16; 4Q, '07, 87

441.02 Abdominal

441.03 Thoracoabdominal

441.1 Thoracic aneurysm, ruptured

441.2 Thoracic aneurysm without mention of rupture

AHA: 3Q, '92, 10

I71.2 Thoracic aortic aneurysm without rupture   [I-10]

441.3 Abdominal aneurysm, ruptured

I71.3 Abdominal aortic aneurysm, ruptured   [I-10]

Thoracic and Abdominal Aortic Aneurysm

Thoracic aneurysm — Aorta

Abdominal aneurysm

441.4 Abdominal aneurysm without mention of rupture

AHA: 4Q, '00, 64; 1Q, '99, 15, 16, 17; 3Q, '92, 10

I71.4 Abdominal aortic aneurysm without rupture   [I-10]

441.5 Aortic aneurysm of unspecified site, ruptured

Rupture of aorta NOS

441.6 Thoracoabdominal aneurysm, ruptured

441.7 Thoracoabdominal aneurysm, without mention of rupture

AHA: 2Q, '06, 16

441.9 Aortic aneurysm of unspecified site without mention of rupture

Aneurysm
Dilatation } of aorta
Hyaline necrosis

AHA: 4Q, '10, 84

√4th **442 Other aneurysm**

INCLUDES   aneurysm (ruptured) (cirsoid) (false) (varicose)
aneurysmal varix

EXCLUDES   arteriovenous aneurysm or fistula:
acquired (447.0)
congenital (747.60-747.69)
traumatic (900.0-904.9)

DEF: Dissection or splitting of arterial wall; due to blood entering through intimal tear or interstitial hemorrhage.

442.0 Of artery of upper extremity

442.1 Of renal artery

442.2 Of iliac artery

AHA: 1Q, '99, 16, 17

442.3 Of artery of lower extremity

Aneurysm: Aneurysm:
femoral artery   popliteal artery

AHA: 2Q, '08, 13; 3Q, '02, 24-26; 1Q, '99, 16

√5th **442.8 Of other specified artery**

442.81 Artery of neck

Aneurysm of carotid artery (common) (external) (internal, extracranial portion)

EXCLUDES   internal carotid artery, intra-cranial portion (437.3)

442.82 Subclavian artery

442.83 Splenic artery

442.84 Other visceral artery

Aneurysm:
celiac
gastroduodenal
gastroepiploic
hepatic } artery
pancreaticoduodenal
superior mesenteric

√4th
√5th   Additional Digit Required   Unspecified Code   Other Specified Code   Manifestation Code   ►◄ Revised Text   ● New Code   ▲ Revised Code Title

2013 ICD-9-CM   **Volume 1 – 137**

442.89 Other

Aneurysm:

mediastinal artery

spinal artery

EXCLUDES *cerebral (nonruptured) (437.3)*

congenital (747.81)

ruptured (430)

coronary (414.11)

heart (414.10)

pulmonary (417.1)

442.9 Of unspecified site

√4ᵗʰ **443 Other peripheral vascular disease**

443.0 Raynaud's syndrome

Raynaud's:

disease

phenomenon (secondary)

Use additional code to identify gangrene (785.4)

DEF: Constriction of the arteries, due to cold or stress; bilateral ischemic attacks of fingers, toes, nose or ears; symptoms include pallor, paresthesia and pain.

I73.00 Raynaud's syndrome without gangrene   I-10

443.1 Thromboangiitis obliterans [Buerger's disease]

Presenile gangrene

DEF: Inflammatory disease of extremity blood vessels, mainly the lower; occurs primarily in young men and leads to tissue ischemia and gangrene.

√5ᵗʰ **443.2 Other arterial dissection**

EXCLUDES *dissection of aorta (441.00-441.03)*

dissection of coronary arteries (414.12)

AHA: 4Q, '02, 54

443.21 Dissection of carotid artery

443.22 Dissection of iliac artery

443.23 Dissection of renal artery

443.24 Dissection of vertebral artery

443.29 Dissection of other artery

√5ᵗʰ **443.8 Other specified peripheral vascular diseases**

443.81 Peripheral angiopathy in diseases classified elsewhere

Code first underlying disease, as:

diabetes mellitus (249.7, 250.7)

AHA: 1Q, '04, 14; 3Q, '91, 10

I79.8 Oth d/o art arterioles & cap in dz clas elsw   I-10

443.82 Erythromelalgia

DEF: Rare syndrome of paroxysmal vasodilation; maldistribution of blood flow causes redness, pain, increased skin temperature, and burning sensations in various parts of the body.

AHA: 4Q, '05, 73

443.89 Other

Acrocyanosis   Erythrocyanosis

Acroparesthesia:

simple [Schultze's type]

vasomotor [Nothnagel's type]

EXCLUDES *chilblains (991.5)*

frostbite (991.0-991.3)

immersion foot (991.4)

AHA: 4Q, '07, 124

I73.89 Other specified peripheral vascular dz   I-10

443.9 Peripheral vascular disease, unspecified

Intermittent claudication NOS

Peripheral:

angiopathy NOS

vascular disease NOS

Spasm of artery

EXCLUDES *atherosclerosis of the arteries of the extremities (440.20-440.22)*

spasm of cerebral artery (435.0-435.9)

AHA: 4Q, '92, 25; 3Q, '91, 10

I73.9 Peripheral vascular disease unspecified   I-10

Arterial Diseases and Disorders

Lipids

Calcium deposits

Atherosclerosis narrowing lumen   Thrombus (clot) forming in lumen

Organization of thrombus and recanalization

Intimal proliferation

Aneurysm bypasses lumen or...

Embolus (from elsewhere) occluding lumen

...bulges from arterial wall

Arteriovenous fistula

√4ᵗʰ **444 Arterial embolism and thrombosis**

INCLUDES infarction:

embolic

thrombotic

occlusion

EXCLUDES *atheroembolism (445.01-445.89)*

that complicating:

abortion (634-638 with .6, 639.6)

ectopic or molar pregnancy (639.6)

pregnancy, childbirth, or the pueperium (673.0-673.8)

septic arterial embolism (449)

AHA: 2Q, '92, 11; 4Q, '90, 27

√5ᵗʰ **444.0 Of abdominal aorta**

AHA: ▶4Q, '11, 107-109;◀ 2Q, '93, 7; 4Q, '90, 27

444.01 Saddle embolus of abdominal aorta

AHA: ▶4Q, '11, 108◀

444.09 Other arterial embolism and thrombosis of abdominal aorta

Aortic bifurcation syndrome   Leriche's syndrome

Aortoiliac obstruction

444.1 Of thoracic aorta

Embolism or thrombosis of aorta (thoracic)

√5ᵗʰ **444.2 Of arteries of the extremities**

AHA: M-A, '87, 6

444.21 Upper extremity

444.22 Lower extremity

Arterial embolism or thrombosis:

femoral

peripheral NOS

popliteal

EXCLUDES *iliofemoral (444.81)*

AHA: 2Q, '11, 8; 4Q, '07, 85; 3Q, '03, 10; 1Q, '03, 17; 3Q, '90, 16

I74.3 Embo & thromb of arteries of the low extremities   I-10

√5ᵗʰ **444.8 Of other specified artery**

444.81 Iliac artery

AHA: 1Q, '03, 16

444.89 Other

EXCLUDES *basilar (433.0)*

carotid (433.1)

cerebral (434.0-434.9)

coronary (410.00-410.92)

mesenteric (557.0)

ophthalmic (362.30-362.34)

precerebral (433.0-433.9)

pulmonary (415.11-415.19)

renal (593.81)

retinal (362.30-362.34)

vertebral (433.2)

444.9 Of unspecified artery

√4ᵗʰ **445 Atheroembolism**

INCLUDES atherothrombotic microembolism

cholesterol embolism

AHA: 4Q, '02, 57

√5ᵗʰ **445.0 Of extremities**

445.01 Upper extremity

445.02 Lower extremity

☑5ᵗʰ **445.8 Of other sites**

445.81 Kidney
Use additional code for any associated acute kidney failure or chronic kidney disease (584, 585)

445.89 Other site

☑4ᵗʰ **446 Polyarteritis nodosa and allied conditions**

446.0 Polyarteritis nodosa
Disseminated necrotizing periarteritis
Panarteritis (nodosa)
Periarteritis (nodosa)
Necrotizing angiitis
DEF: Inflammation of small and mid-size arteries; symptoms related to involved arteries in kidneys, muscles, gastrointestinal tract and heart; results in tissue death.

446.1 Acute febrile mucocutaneous lymph node syndrome [MCLS]
Kawasaki disease
DEF: Acute febrile disease of children; marked by erythema of conjunctiva and mucous membranes of upper respiratory tract, skin eruptions and edema.

☑5ᵗʰ **446.2 Hypersensitivity angiitis**
EXCLUDES *antiglomerular basement membrane disease without pulmonary hemorrhage (583.89)*

446.20 Hypersensitivity angiitis, unspecified

446.21 Goodpasture's syndrome
Antiglomerular basement membrane antibody-mediated nephritis with pulmonary hemorrhage
Use additional code to identify renal disease (583.81)
DEF: Glomerulonephritis associated with hematuria, progresses rapidly; results in death from renal failure.

446.29 Other specified hypersensitivity angiitis
AHA: 1Q, '95, 3

446.3 Lethal midline granuloma
Malignant granuloma of face
DEF: Granulomatous lesion; in nose or paranasal sinuses; often fatal; occurs chiefly in males.
AHA: 3Q, '00, 11

446.4 Wegener's granulomatosis
Necrotizing respiratory granulomatosis
Wegener's syndrome
DEF: A disease occurring mainly in men; marked by necrotizing granulomas and ulceration of the upper respiratory tract; cause is a vasculitis affecting small vessels due to an immune disorder.
AHA: 3Q, '00, 11

446.5 Giant cell arteritis
Bagratuni's syndrome
Cranial arteritis
Horton's disease
Temporal arteritis
DEF: Inflammation of arteries; due to giant cells affecting carotid artery branches, resulting in occlusion; symptoms include fever, headache and neurological problems.
M31.6 Other giant cell arteritis   I-10

446.6 Thrombotic microangiopathy
Moschcowitz's syndrome
Thrombotic thrombocytopenic purpura
DEF: Blockage of small blood vessels; due to hyaline deposits; symptoms include purpura, CNS disorders; results in protracted disease or rapid death.

446.7 Takayasu's disease
Aortic arch arteritis
Pulseless disease
DEF: Progressive obliterative arteritis of brachiocephalic trunk, left subclavian, and left common carotid arteries above aortic arch; results in ischemia in brain, heart and arm.

☑4ᵗʰ **447 Other disorders of arteries and arterioles**

447.0 Arteriovenous fistula, acquired
Arteriovenous aneurysm, acquired
EXCLUDES *cerebrovascular (437.3)*
coronary (414.19)
pulmonary (417.0)
surgically created arteriovenous shunt or fistula:
complication (996.1, 996.61-996.62)
status or presence (V45.11)
traumatic (900.0-904.9)
DEF: Communication between an artery and vein caused by error in healing.

447.1 Stricture of artery
AHA: 2Q, '93, 8; M-A, '87, 6
I77.1 Stricture of artery   I-10

447.2 Rupture of artery
Erosion
Fistula, except arteriovenous ⎫ of artery
Ulcer ⎭
EXCLUDES *traumatic rupture of artery (900.0-904.9)*

447.3 Hyperplasia of renal artery
Fibromuscular hyperplasia of renal artery
DEF: Overgrowth of cells in muscular lining of renal artery.

447.4 Celiac artery compression syndrome
Celiac axis syndrome
Marable's syndrome

447.5 Necrosis of artery

447.6 Arteritis, unspecified
Aortitis NOS
Endarteritis NOS
EXCLUDES *arteritis, endarteritis:*
aortic arch (446.7)
cerebral (437.4)
coronary (414.00-414.07)
deformans (440.0-440.9)
obliterans (440.0-440.9)
pulmonary (417.8)
senile (440.0-440.9)
polyarteritis NOS (446.0)
syphilitic aortitis (093.1)
AHA: 1Q, '95, 3

☑5ᵗʰ **447.7 Aortic ectasia**
Ectasis aorta
EXCLUDES *aortic aneurysm and dissection (441.00-441.9)*
DEF: A diffuse, irregular dilation of the aorta less than 3 cm in diameter; increases the patient's risk of developing an aortic aneurysm.
AHA: 4Q, '10, 84-85

447.70 Aortic ectasia, unspecified site

447.71 Thoracic aortic ectasia

447.72 Abdominal aortic ectasia

447.73 Thoracoabdominal aortic ectasia

447.8 Other specified disorders of arteries and arterioles
Fibromuscular hyperplasia of arteries, except renal

447.9 Unspecified disorders of arteries and arterioles

☑4ᵗʰ **448 Disease of capillaries**

448.0 Hereditary hemorrhagic telangiectasia
Rendu-Osler-Weber disease
DEF: Genetic disease with onset after puberty; results in multiple telangiectases, dilated venules on skin and mucous membranes; recurrent bleeding may occur.

448.1 Nevus, non-neoplastic
Nevus:
araneus
senile
Nevus:
spider
stellar
EXCLUDES *neoplastic (216.0-216.9)*
port wine (757.32)
strawberry (757.32)
DEF: Enlarged or malformed blood vessels of skin; results in reddish swelling, skin patch, or birthmark.

448.9 Other and unspecified capillary diseases
Capillary:
hemorrhage
hyperpermeability
Capillary:
thrombosis
EXCLUDES *capillary fragility (hereditary) (287.8)*

449 Septic arterial embolism
Code first underlying infection, such as:
infective endocarditis (421.0)
lung abscess (513.0)
Use additional code to identify the site of the embolism (433.0-433.9, 444.01-444.9)
EXCLUDES *septic pulmonary embolism (415.12)*
AHA: 4Q, '07, 84-85

Diseases of Veins and Lymphatics, and Other Diseases of Circulatory System (451-459)

√4ᵗʰ **451 Phlebitis and thrombophlebitis**

INCLUDES endophlebitis
inflammation, vein
periphlebitis
suppurative phlebitis

Use additional E code to identify drug, if drug-induced

EXCLUDES *that complicating:*
abortion (634-638 with .7, 639.8)
ectopic or molar pregnancy (639.8)
pregnancy, childbirth, or the puerperium (671.0-671.9)
that due to or following:
implant or catheter device (996.61-996.62)
infusion, perfusion, or transfusion (999.2)

DEF: Inflammation of a vein (phlebitis) with formation of a thrombus (thrombophlebitis).

AHA: 1Q, '11, 19; 1Q, '92, 16

TIP: Assign an additional code from category 453 for thrombosis; if both conditions are present, assign codes from both categories 451 and 453.

451.0 Of superficial vessels of lower extremities
Saphenous vein (greater) (lesser)
AHA: 3Q, '91, 16

√5ᵗʰ **451.1 Of deep vessels of lower extremities**
AHA: 3Q, '91, 16

451.11 Femoral vein (deep) (superficial)

451.19 Other
Femoropopliteal vein   Tibial vein
Popliteal vein

451.2 Of lower extremities, unspecified
AHA: 4Q, '04, 80

√5ᵗʰ **451.8 Of other sites**
EXCLUDES *intracranial venous sinus (325)*
nonpyogenic (437.6)
portal (vein) (572.1)

451.81 Iliac vein

451.82 Of superficial veins of upper extremities
Antecubital vein   Cephalic vein
Basilic vein

451.83 Of deep veins of upper extremities
Brachial vein   Ulnar vein
Radial vein

451.84 Of upper extremities, unspecified

451.89 Other
Axillary vein
Jugular vein
Subclavian vein
Thrombophlebitis of breast (Mondor's disease)

451.9 Of unspecified site

452 Portal vein thrombosis
Portal (vein) obstruction
EXCLUDES *hepatic vein thrombosis (453.0)*
phlebitis of portal vein (572.1)
DEF: Formation of a blood clot in main vein of liver.

√4ᵗʰ **453 Other venous embolism and thrombosis**
EXCLUDES *that complicating:*
abortion (634-638 with .7, 639.8)
ectopic or molar pregnancy (639.8)
pregnancy, childbirth, or the puerperium (671.0-671.9)
AHA: 1Q, '11, 19-21; 1Q, '92, 16

453.0 Budd-Chiari syndrome
Hepatic vein thrombosis
DEF: Thrombosis or other obstruction of hepatic vein; symptoms include enlarged liver, extensive collateral vessels, intractable ascites and severe portal hypertension.

453.1 Thrombophlebitis migrans
DEF: Slow, advancing thrombophlebitis; appearing first in one vein then another.

453.2 Of inferior vena cava

453.3 Of renal vein

√5ᵗʰ **453.4 Acute venous embolism and thrombosis of deep vessels of lower extremity**
AHA: 4Q, '09, 88-92; 3Q, '08,16

453.40 Acute venous embolism and thrombosis of unspecified deep vessels of lower extremity
Deep vein thrombosis NOS
DVT NOS
AHA: ▶1Q, '12, 18◀
TIP: ▶Assign as the default code for "deep vein thrombosis," whether documented as acute or subacute.◀
I82.409 Ac embo & thrombo of uns deep veins of unsp [I-10] lower ext

453.41 Acute venous embolism and thrombosis of deep vessels of proximal lower extremity
Femoral   Thigh
Iliac   Upper leg NOS
Popliteal
AHA: 4Q, '04, 79

453.42 Acute venous embolism and thrombosis of deep vessels of distal lower extremity
Calf   Peroneal
Lower leg NOS   Tibial

√5ᵗʰ **453.5 Chronic venous embolism and thrombosis of deep vessels of lower extremity**
Use additional code, if applicable, for associated long-term (current) use of anticoagulants (V58.61)
EXCLUDES *personal history of venous thrombosis and embolism (V12.51)*
AHA: 4Q, '09, 88-92

453.50 Chronic venous embolism and thrombosis of unspecified deep vessels of lower

453.51 Chronic venous embolism and thrombosis of deep vessels of proximal lower extremity
Femoral   Thigh
Iliac   Upper leg NOS
Popliteal

453.52 Chronic venous embolism and thrombosis of deep vessels of distal lower extremity
Calf   Peroneal
Lower leg NOS   Tibial

453.6 Venous embolism and thrombosis of superficial vessels of lower extremity
Saphenous vein (greater) (lesser)
Use additional code, if applicable, for associated long-term (current) use of anticoagulants (V58.61)
AHA: 4Q, '09, 88-92

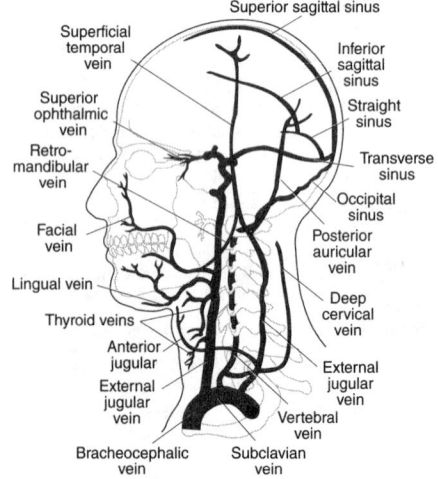

Veins of Head and Neck

Superior sagittal sinus
Superficial temporal vein
Inferior sagittal sinus
Superior ophthalmic vein
Straight sinus
Retro-mandibular vein
Transverse sinus
Facial vein
Occipital sinus
Posterior auricular vein
Lingual vein
Deep cervical vein
Thyroid veins
Anterior jugular
External jugular vein
External jugular vein
Vertebral vein
Bracheocephalic vein
Subclavian vein

Map of Major Veins

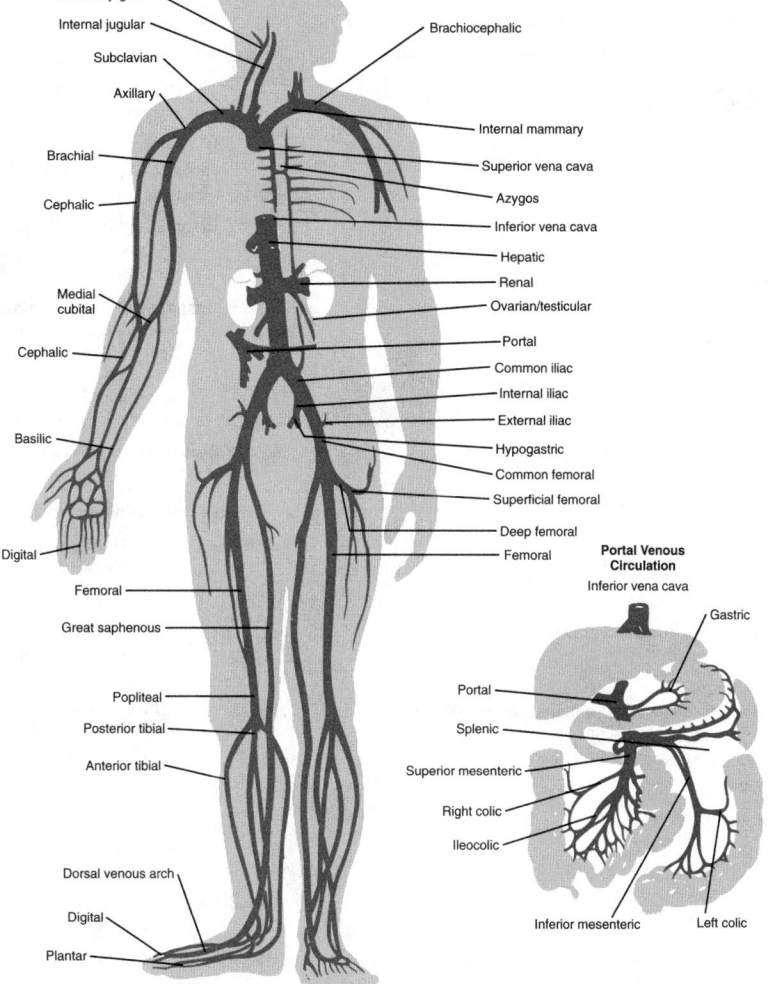

√5ᵗʰ **453.7 Chronic venous embolism and thrombosis of other specified vessels**

> Use additional code, if applicable, for associated long-term (current) use of anticoagulants (V58.61)
>
> **EXCLUDES** *personal history of venous thrombosis and embolism (V12.51)*
>
> **AHA:** 4Q, '09, 88-92

453.71 Chronic venous embolism and thrombosis of superficial veins of upper extremity
> Antecubital vein   Cephalic vein
> Basilic vein

453.72 Chronic venous embolism and thrombosis of deep veins of upper extremity
> Brachial vein   Ulnar vein
> Radial vein

453.73 Chronic venous embolism and thrombosis of upper extremity, unspecified

453.74 Chronic venous embolism and thrombosis of axillary veins

453.75 Chronic venous embolism and thrombosis of subclavian veins

453.76 Chronic venous embolism and thrombosis of internal jugular veins

453.77 Chronic venous embolism and thrombosis of other thoracic veins
> Brachiocephalic (innominate)
> Superior vena cava

453.79 Chronic venous embolism and thrombosis of other specified veins

√5ᵗʰ **453.8 Acute venous embolism and thrombosis of other specified veins**

> **EXCLUDES** *cerebral (434.0-434.9)*
> *coronary (410.00-410.92)*
> *intracranial venous sinus (325)*
> *nonpyogenic (437.6)*
> *mesenteric (557.0)*
> *portal (452)*
> *precerebral (433.0-433.9)*
> *pulmonary (415.19)*
>
> **AHA:** 4Q, '09, 88-92; 3Q, '91, 16; M-A, '87, 6

453.81 Acute venous embolism and thrombosis of superficial veins of upper extremity
> Antecubital vein
> Basilic vein
> Cephalic vein

453.82 Acute venous embolism and thrombosis of deep veins of upper extremity
> Brachial vein   Ulnar vein
> Radial vein

453.83 Acute venous embolism and thrombosis of upper extremity, unspecified

453.84 Acute venous embolism and thrombosis of axillary veins

453.85 Acute venous embolism and thrombosis of subclavian veins

453.86 Acute venous embolism and thrombosis of internal jugular veins

---

√4ᵗʰ / √5ᵗʰ Additional Digit Required   Unspecified Code   Other Specified Code   Manifestation Code   ►◄ Revised Text   ● New Code   ▲ Revised Code Title

453.87 Acute venous embolism and thrombosis of other thoracic veins
Brachiocephalic (innominate)
Superior vena cava

453.89 Acute venous embolism and thrombosis of other specified veins
I82.890 Ac embolism and thrombosis of other spec veins · I-10

453.9 Of unspecified site
Embolism of vein
Thrombosis (vein)
AHA: ▶1Q, '12, 18◀

✓4ᵗʰ **454 Varicose veins of lower extremities**
EXCLUDES *that complicating pregnancy, childbirth, or the puerperium (671.0)*
DEF: Dilated leg veins; due to incompetent vein valves that allow reversed blood flow and cause tissue erosion or weakness of wall; may be painful.
AHA: 2Q, '91, 20

454.0 With ulcer · A
Varicose ulcer (lower extremity, any part)
Varicose veins with ulcer of lower extremity [any part] or of unspecified site
Any condition classifiable to 454.9 with ulcer or specified as ulcerated
AHA: 4Q, '99, 18

454.1 With inflammation · A
Stasis dermatitis
Varicose veins with inflammation of lower extremity [any part] or of unspecified site
Any condition classifiable to 454.9 with inflammation or specified as inflamed

454.2 With ulcer and inflammation · A
Varicose veins with ulcer and inflammation of lower extremity [any part] or of unspecified site
Any condition classifiable to 454.9 with ulcer and inflammation

454.8 With other complications
Edema   Swelling
Pain
AHA: 4Q, '02, 58

454.9 Asymptomatic varicose veins · A
Phlebectasia ⎫
Varicose veins ⎬ of lower extremity [any part]
Varix ⎭   or of unspecified site
Varicose veins NOS
AHA: 4Q, '02, 58
TIP: Do not assign if patient seen for surgical treatment of varicose veins; query physician for specific symptom (inflammation, pain, edema, swelling).

✓4ᵗʰ **455 Hemorrhoids**
INCLUDES hemorrhoids (anus) (rectum)
piles
varicose veins, anus or rectum
EXCLUDES *that complicating pregnancy, childbirth, or the puerperium (671.8)*
DEF: Varicose condition of external hemorrhoidal veins causing painful swellings at the anus.

455.0 Internal hemorrhoids without mention of complication
AHA: 3Q, '05, 17
I84.21 Internal hemorrhoids without complication · I-10

455.1 Internal thrombosed hemorrhoids

455.2 Internal hemorrhoids with other complication
Internal hemorrhoids: Internal hemorrhoids:
bleeding   strangulated
prolapsed   ulcerated
AHA: 3Q, '05, 17; 1Q, '03, 8
I84.111 Internal bleeding hemorrhoids · I-10

455.3 External hemorrhoids without mention of complication
AHA: 1Q, '07, 13; 3Q, '05, 17
I84.22 External hemorrhoids without complicaton · I-10

455.4 External thrombosed hemorrhoids

455.5 External hemorrhoids with other complication
External hemorrhoids: External hemorrhoids:
bleeding   strangulated
prolapsed   ulcerated
AHA: 3Q, '05, 17; 1Q, '03, 8

455.6 Unspecified hemorrhoids without mention of complication
Hemorrhoids NOS

455.7 Unspecified thrombosed hemorrhoids
Thrombosed hemorrhoids, unspecified whether internal or external

455.8 Unspecified hemorrhoids with other complication
Hemorrhoids, unspecified whether internal or external:
bleeding
prolapsed
strangulated
ulcerated

455.9 Residual hemorrhoidal skin tags
Skin tags, anus or rectum

✓4ᵗʰ **456 Varicose veins of other sites**

456.0 Esophageal varices with bleeding
DEF: Distended, tortuous, veins of lower esophagus, usually due to portal hypertension.

456.1 Esophageal varices without mention of bleeding

✓5ᵗʰ **456.2 Esophageal varices in diseases classified elsewhere**
Code first underlying cause, as:
cirrhosis of liver (571.0-571.9)
portal hypertension (572.3)

456.20 With bleeding
AHA: N-D, '85, 14
I85.11 Secondary esophageal varices with bleeding · I-10

456.21 Without mention of bleeding
AHA: 3Q, '05, 15; 2Q, '02, 4

456.3 Sublingual varices
DEF: Distended, tortuous veins beneath tongue.

456.4 Scrotal varices · ♂
Varicocele

456.5 Pelvic varices
Varices of broad ligament

456.6 Vulval varices · ♀
Varices of perineum
EXCLUDES *that complicating pregnancy, childbirth, or the puerperium (671.1)*

456.8 Varices of other sites
Varicose veins of nasal septum (with ulcer)
EXCLUDES *placental varices (656.7)*
retinal varices (362.17)
varicose ulcer of unspecified site (454.0)
varicose veins of unspecified site (454.9)
AHA: 2Q, '02, 4

✓4ᵗʰ **457 Noninfectious disorders of lymphatic channels**

457.0 Postmastectomy lymphedema syndrome · A
Elephantiasis ⎫
Obliteration of lymphatic ⎬ due to mastectomy
vessel ⎭
DEF: Reduced lymphatic circulation following mastectomy; symptoms include swelling of the arm on the operative side.
AHA: 2Q, '02, 12

457.1 Other lymphedema

Elephantiasis (nonfilarial) NOS
Lymphangiectasis
Lymphedema:
   acquired (chronic)
   praecox
Lymphedema:
   secondary
Obliteration, lymphatic
   vessel

EXCLUDES *elephantiasis (nonfilarial):*
       congenital (757.0)
       eyelid (374.83)
       vulva (624.8)

DEF: Fluid retention due to reduced lymphatic circulation; due to other than mastectomy.
AHA: 3Q, '04, 5
I89.0 Lymphedema not elsewhere classified `I-10`

457.2 Lymphangitis

Lymphangitis:
   NOS
   chronic
Lymphangitis:
   subacute

EXCLUDES *acute lymphangitis (682.0-682.9)*

457.8 Other noninfectious disorders of lymphatic channels

Chylocele (nonfilarial)
Chylous:
   ascites
   cyst
Lymph node or vessel:
   fistula
   infarction
   rupture

EXCLUDES *chylocele:*
       filarial (125.0-125.9)
       tunica vaginalis (nonfilarial) (608.84)

AHA: 1Q, '04, 5; 3Q, '03, 17

457.9 Unspecified noninfectious disorder of lymphatic channels

√4ᵗʰ 458 Hypotension

INCLUDES hypopiesis

EXCLUDES *cardiovascular collapse (785.50)*
       maternal hypotension syndrome (669.2)
       shock (785.50-785.59)
       Shy-Drager syndrome (333.0)

458.0 Orthostatic hypotension

Hypotension:
   orthostatic (chronic)
Hypotension:
   postural
DEF: Low blood pressure; occurs when standing.
AHA: 3Q, '00, 8; 3Q, '91, 9
I95.1 Orthostatic hypotension `I-10`

458.1 Chronic hypotension

Permanent idiopathic hypotension
DEF: Persistent low blood pressure.

√5ᵗʰ 458.2 Iatrogenic hypotension

DEF: Abnormally low blood pressure; due to medical treatment.
AHA: 4Q, '03, 60; 3Q, '02, 12; 4Q, '95, 57

458.21 Hypotension of hemodialysis
Intra-dialytic hypotension
AHA: 4Q, '03, 61

458.29 Other iatrogenic hypotension
Postoperative hypotension
I95.81 Postprocedural hypotension `I-10`

458.8 Other specified hypotension
AHA: 4Q, '97, 37

458.9 Hypotension, unspecified
Hypotension (arterial) NOS
I95.9 Hypotension unspecified `I-10`

√4ᵗʰ 459 Other disorders of circulatory system

459.0 Hemorrhage, unspecified

Rupture of blood vessel NOS
Spontaneous hemorrhage NEC

EXCLUDES *hemorrhage:*
       gastrointestinal NOS (578.9)
       in newborn NOS (772.9)
       secondary or recurrent following trauma (958.2)
          traumatic rupture of blood vessel (900.0-904.9)
       nontraumatic hematoma of soft tissue (729.92)

AHA: 4Q, '90, 26
R58 Hemorrhage not elsewhere classified `I-10`

√5ᵗʰ 459.1 Postphlebitic syndrome

Chronic venous hypertension due to deep vein thrombosis

EXCLUDES *chronic venous hypertension without deep vein thrombosis (459.30-459.39)*

DEF: Various conditions following deep vein thrombosis; including edema, pain, stasis dermatitis, cellulitis, varicose veins and ulceration of the lower leg.
AHA: 4Q, '02, 58; 2Q, '91, 20

459.10 Postphlebitic syndrome without complications
Asymptomatic postphlebitic syndrome
Postphlebitic syndrome NOS

459.11 Postphlebitic syndrome with ulcer

459.12 Postphlebitic syndrome with inflammation

459.13 Postphlebitic syndrome with ulcer and inflammation

459.19 Postphlebitic syndrome with other complication

459.2 Compression of vein
Stricture of vein
Vena cava syndrome (inferior) (superior)

√5ᵗʰ 459.3 Chronic venous hypertension (idiopathic)

Stasis edema

EXCLUDES *chronic venous hypertension due to deep vein thrombosis (459.10-459.9)*
       varicose veins (454.0-454.9)

AHA: 4Q, '02, 59

459.30 Chronic venous hypertension without complications
Asymptomatic chronic venous hypertension
Chronic venous hypertension NOS

459.31 Chronic venous hypertension with ulcer
AHA: 4Q, '02, 43

459.32 Chronic venous hypertension with inflammation

459.33 Chronic venous hypertension with ulcer and inflammation

459.39 Chronic venous hypertension with other complication

√5ᵗʰ 459.8 Other specified disorders of circulatory system

459.81 Venous (peripheral) insufficiency, unspecified
Chronic venous insufficiency NOS

Use additional code for any associated ulceration (707.10-707.19, 707.8, 707.9)

DEF: Insufficient drainage, venous blood, any part of body, results in edema or dermatosis.
AHA: 3Q, '04, 5; 2Q, '91, 20; M-A, '87, 6
TIP: Assign for stasis dermatitis without varicose veins or past DVT.
I87.2 Venous insufficiency (chronic) (peripheral) `I-10`

459.89 Other
Collateral circulation (venous), any site
Phlebosclerosis
Venofibrosis

459.9 Unspecified circulatory system disorder

√4ᵗʰ
√5ᵗʰ Additional Digit Required   Unspecified Code   Other Specified Code   Manifestation Code   ►◄ Revised Text   ● New Code   ▲ Revised Code Title
2013 ICD-9-CM   **Volume 1 – 143**

8. Diseases of the Respiratory System (460-519)

Use additional code to identify infectious organism

Acute Respiratory Infections (460-466)

EXCLUDES *pneumonia and influenza (480.0-488.19)*

460 Acute nasopharyngitis [common cold]

Coryza (acute)   Rhinitis:
Nasal catarrh, acute   acute
Nasopharyngitis: infective
  NOS
  acute
  infective NOS

EXCLUDES *nasopharyngitis, chronic (472.2)*
pharyngitis:
* acute or unspecified (462)*
* chronic (472.1)*
rhinitis:
* allergic (477.0-477.9)*
* chronic or unspecified (472.0)*
sore throat:
* acute or unspecified (462)*
* chronic (472.1)*

DEF: Acute inflammation of mucous membranes; extends from nares to pharynx.
AHA: 1Q, '88, 12

✓4ᵗʰ 461 Acute sinusitis

INCLUDES abscess ⎫
empyema ⎪
infection ⎬ acute, of sinus
inflammation ⎪   (accessory) (nasal)
suppuration ⎭

EXCLUDES *chronic or unspecified sinusitis (473.0-473.9)*

461.0 Maxillary
Acute antritis

461.1 Frontal

461.2 Ethmoidal

461.3 Sphenoidal

461.8 Other acute sinusitis
Acute pansinusitis

461.9 Acute sinusitis, unspecified
Acute sinusitis NOS
J01.90 Acute sinusitis unspecified   I-10

462 Acute pharyngitis
Acute sore throat NOS
Pharyngitis (acute):
  NOS
  gangrenous
  infective
  phlegmonous
  pneumococcal
  staphylococcal
  suppurative
  ulcerative
Sore throat (viral) NOS
Viral pharyngitis

EXCLUDES *abscess:*
*   peritonsillar [quinsy] (475)*
*   pharyngeal NOS (478.29)*
*   retropharyngeal (478.24)*
* chronic pharyngitis (472.1)*
* infectious mononucleosis (075)*
* that specified as (due to):*
*   Coxsackie (virus) (074.0)*
*   gonococcus (098.6)*
*   herpes simplex (054.79)*
*   influenza (487.1, 488.02, 488.12)*
*   septic (034.0)*
*   streptococcal (034.0)*

AHA: 4Q, '99, 26; S-O, '85, 8
J02.9 Acute pharyngitis unspecified   I-10

Respiratory System

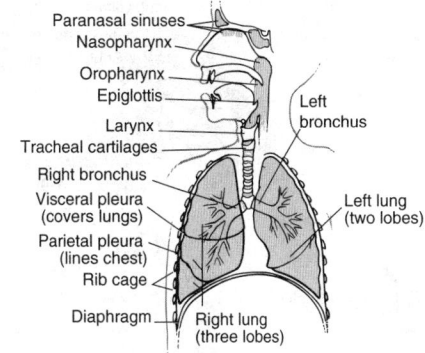

463 Acute tonsillitis

Tonsillitis (acute):   Tonsillitis (acute):
  NOS   septic
  follicular   staphylococcal
  gangrenous   suppurative
  infective   ulcerative
  pneumococcal   viral

EXCLUDES *chronic tonsillitis (474.0)*
hypertrophy of tonsils (474.1)
peritonsillar abscess [quinsy] (475)
sore throat:
* acute or NOS (462)*
* septic (034.0)*
streptococcal tonsillitis (034.0)

AHA: N-D, '84, 16

✓4ᵗʰ 464 Acute laryngitis and tracheitis

EXCLUDES *that associated with influenza (487.1, 488.02, 488.12)*
that due to Streptococcus (034.0)

✓5ᵗʰ 464.0 Acute laryngitis
Laryngitis (acute):
  NOS
  edematous
  Hemophilus influenzae [H. influenzae]
  pneumococcal
  septic
  suppurative
  ulcerative

EXCLUDES *chronic laryngitis (476.0-476.1)*
influenzal laryngitis (487.1, 488.02, 488.12)

AHA: 4Q, '01, 42

464.00 Without mention of obstruction

464.01 With obstruction

✓5ᵗʰ 464.1 Acute tracheitis
Tracheitis (acute):
  NOS
  catarrhal
  viral

EXCLUDES *chronic tracheitis (491.8)*

464.10 Without mention of obstruction

464.11 With obstruction

✓5ᵗʰ 464.2 Acute laryngotracheitis
Laryngotracheitis (acute)
Tracheitis (acute) with laryngitis (acute)

EXCLUDES *chronic laryngotracheitis (476.1)*

464.20 Without mention of obstruction

464.21 With obstruction

✓5ᵗʰ 464.3 Acute epiglottitis
Viral epiglottitis

EXCLUDES *epiglottitis, chronic (476.1)*

464.30 Without mention of obstruction

464.31 With obstruction

Upper Respiratory System

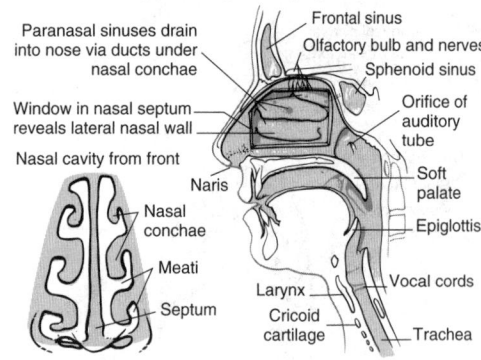

Paranasal sinuses drain into nose via ducts under nasal conchae

Window in nasal septum reveals lateral nasal wall

Nasal cavity from front

Frontal sinus
Olfactory bulb and nerves
Sphenoid sinus
Orifice of auditory tube
Soft palate
Epiglottis
Vocal cords
Trachea

Naris
Nasal conchae
Meati
Septum
Larynx
Cricoid cartilage

464.4 Croup
Croup syndrome
DEF: Acute laryngeal obstruction due to allergy, foreign body or infection; symptoms include barking cough, hoarseness and harsh, persistent high-pitched respiratory sound.
J05.0 Acute obstructive laryngitis [croup]   I-10

✓5ᵗʰ 464.5 Supraglottitis, unspecified
DEF: A rapidly advancing generalized upper respiratory infection of the lingual tonsillar area, epiglottic folds, false vocal cords, and the epiglottis.
AHA: 4Q, '01, 42

464.50 Without mention of obstruction
AHA: 4Q, '01, 43

464.51 With obstruction

✓4ᵗʰ 465 Acute upper respiratory infections of multiple or unspecified sites
EXCLUDES upper respiratory infection due to:
influenza (487.1, 488.02, 488.12)
Streptococcus (034.0)

465.0 Acute laryngopharyngitis
DEF: Acute infection of the vocal cords and pharynx.

465.8 Other multiple sites
Multiple URI
AHA: 4Q, '07, 85

465.9 Unspecified site
Acute URI NOS
Upper respiratory infection (acute)
J06.9 Acute upper respiratory infection unspecified   I-10

✓4ᵗʰ 466 Acute bronchitis and bronchiolitis
INCLUDES that with:
bronchospasm
obstruction

466.0 Acute bronchitis
Bronchitis, acute or subacute:
fibrinous
membranous
pneumococcal
purulent
septic
viral
with tracheitis
Croupous bronchitis
Tracheobronchitis, acute
EXCLUDES acute bronchitis with chronic obstructive pulmonary disease (491.22)
DEF: Acute inflammation of main branches of bronchial tree due to infectious or irritant agents; symptoms include cough with a varied production of sputum, fever, substernal soreness, and lung rales.
AHA: 4Q, '04, 137; 1Q, '04, 3; 4Q, '02, 46; 4Q, '96, 28; 4Q, '91, 24; 1Q, '88, 12
TIP: If documented with COPD, assign only 491.22 Obstructive chronic bronchitis with acute bronchitis.
J20.9 Acute bronchitis unspecified   I-10

✓5ᵗʰ 466.1 Acute bronchiolitis
Bronchiolitis (acute) Capillary pneumonia
EXCLUDES respiratory bronchiolitis interstitial lung disease (516.34)
DEF: Acute inflammation of the smallest branches of bronchial tree due to infectious or irritant agents; symptoms include cough, tachycardia, labored breathing, and lung crackles.

466.11 Acute bronchiolitis due to respiratory syncytial virus (RSV)
AHA: 1Q, '05, 10; 4Q, '96, 27
J21.0 Acute bronchiolitis d/t resp syncytial virus   I-10

466.19 Acute bronchiolitis due to other infectious organisms
Use additional code to identify organism
J21.8 Acute bronchiolitis d/t oth specified organisms   I-10

Other Diseases of the Upper Respiratory Tract (470-478)

470 Deviated nasal septum
Deflected septum (nasal) (acquired)
EXCLUDES congenital (754.0)

✓4ᵗʰ 471 Nasal polyps
EXCLUDES adenomatous polyps (212.0)

471.0 Polyp of nasal cavity
Polyp: Polyp:
choanal   nasopharyngeal

471.1 Polypoid sinus degeneration
Woakes' syndrome or ethmoiditis

471.8 Other polyp of sinus
Polyp of sinus: Polyp of sinus:
accessory   maxillary
ethmoidal   sphenoidal

471.9 Unspecified nasal polyp
Nasal polyp NOS

✓4ᵗʰ 472 Chronic pharyngitis and nasopharyngitis

472.0 Chronic rhinitis
Ozena   Rhinitis:
Rhinitis: hypertrophic
NOS   obstructive
atrophic   purulent
granulomatous   ulcerative
EXCLUDES allergic rhinitis (477.0-477.9)
DEF: Persistent inflammation of mucous membranes of nose.

472.1 Chronic pharyngitis
Chronic sore throat   Pharyngitis:
Pharyngitis: granular (chronic)
atrophic   hypertrophic

472.2 Chronic nasopharyngitis
EXCLUDES acute or unspecified nasopharyngitis (460)
DEF: Persistent inflammation of mucous membranes extending from nares to pharynx.

✓4ᵗʰ 473 Chronic sinusitis
INCLUDES abscess
empyema
infection } (chronic) of sinus (accessory) (nasal)
suppuration
EXCLUDES acute sinusitis (461.0-461.9)

473.0 Maxillary
Antritis (chronic)
J32.0 Chronic maxillary sinusitis   I-10

473.1 Frontal

473.2 Ethmoidal
EXCLUDES Woakes' ethmoiditis (471.1)

473.3 Sphenoidal

473.8 Other chronic sinusitis
Pansinusitis (chronic)

473.9 Unspecified sinusitis (chronic)
Sinusitis (chronic) NOS
J32.9 Chronic sinusitis unspecified   I-10

Paranasal Sinuses

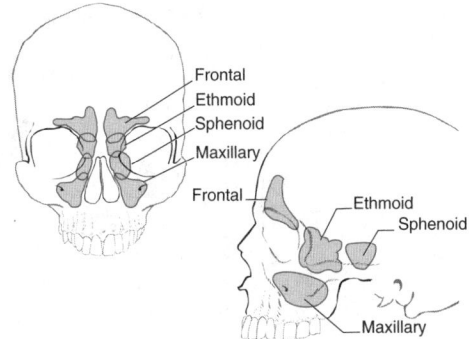

Frontal
Ethmoid
Sphenoid
Maxillary
Frontal
Ethmoid
Sphenoid
Maxillary

474 Chronic disease of tonsils and adenoids

474.0 Chronic tonsillitis and adenoiditis
EXCLUDES *acute or unspecified tonsillitis (463)*
AHA: 4Q, '97, 38

474.00 Chronic tonsillitis

474.01 Chronic adenoiditis

474.02 Chronic tonsillitis and adenoiditis

474.1 Hypertrophy of tonsils and adenoids
Enlargement
Hyperplasia } of tonsils or adenoids
Hypertrophy

EXCLUDES *that with:*
adenoiditis (474.01)
adenoiditis and tonsillitis (474.02)
tonsillitis (474.00)

474.10 Tonsils with adenoids
AHA: 2Q, '05, 16

474.11 Tonsils alone

474.12 Adenoids alone

474.2 Adenoid vegetations
DEF: Fungus-like growth of lymph tissue between the nares and
pharynx.

474.8 Other chronic disease of tonsils and adenoids
Amygdalolith
Calculus, tonsil
Cicatrix of tonsil (and adenoid)
Tonsillar tag
Ulcer, tonsil

474.9 Unspecified chronic disease of tonsils and adenoids
Disease (chronic) of tonsils (and adenoids)

475 Peritonsillar abscess
Abscess of tonsil
Peritonsillar cellulitis
Quinsy
EXCLUDES *tonsillitis:*
acute or NOS (463)
chronic (474.0)
J36 Peritonsillar abscess   I-10

476 Chronic laryngitis and laryngotracheitis

476.0 Chronic laryngitis
Laryngitis: Laryngitis:
  catarrhal   sicca
  hypertrophic

476.1 Chronic laryngotracheitis
Laryngitis, chronic, with tracheitis (chronic)
Tracheitis, chronic, with laryngitis
EXCLUDES *chronic tracheitis (491.8)*
laryngitis and tracheitis, acute or unspecified
(464.00-464.51)

477 Allergic rhinitis
INCLUDES allergic rhinitis (nonseasonal) (seasonal)
hay fever
spasmodic rhinorrhea
EXCLUDES *allergic rhinitis with asthma (bronchial) (493.0)*
DEF: True immunoglobulin E (IgE)-mediated allergic reaction of nasal
mucosa; seasonal (typical hay fever) or perennial (year-round allergens: dust,
food, dander).

477.0 Due to pollen
Pollinosis

477.1 Due to food
AHA: 4Q, '00, 42

477.2 Due to animal (cat) (dog) hair and dander

477.8 Due to other allergen

477.9 Cause unspecified
AHA: 2Q, '97, 9
J30.9 Allergic rhinitis unspecified   I-10

478 Other diseases of upper respiratory tract

478.0 Hypertrophy of nasal turbinates
DEF: Overgrowth, enlargement of shell-shaped bones in nasal cavity.

478.1 Other diseases of nasal cavity and sinuses
EXCLUDES *varicose ulcer of nasal septum (456.8)*

478.11 Nasal mucositis (ulcerative)
Use additional E code to identify adverse effects of
therapy, such as:
antineoplastic and immunosuppressive drugs
(E930.7, E933.1)
radiation therapy (E879.2)
AHA: 4Q, '06, 88-90

478.19 Other diseases of nasal cavity and sinuses
Abscess
Necrosis } of nose (septum)
Ulcer
Cyst or mucocele of sinus (nasal)
Rhinolith
AHA: 4Q, '06, 88-90
J34.1 Cyst and mucocele of nose and nasal sinus   I-10

478.2 Other diseases of pharynx, not elsewhere classified

478.20 Unspecified disease of pharynx

478.21 Cellulitis of pharynx or nasopharynx

478.22 Parapharyngeal abscess

478.24 Retropharyngeal abscess
DEF: Purulent infection, behind pharynx and front of
precerebral fascia.

478.25 Edema of pharynx or nasopharynx

478.26 Cyst of pharynx or nasopharynx

478.29 Other
Abscess of pharynx or nasopharynx
EXCLUDES *ulcerative pharyngitis (462)*

478.3 Paralysis of vocal cords or larynx
DEF: Loss of motor ability of vocal cords or larynx; due to nerve or
muscle damage.

478.30 Paralysis, unspecified
Laryngoplegia   Paralysis of glottis

478.31 Unilateral, partial

478.32 Unilateral, complete

478.33 Bilateral, partial

478.34 Bilateral, complete

478.4 Polyp of vocal cord or larynx
EXCLUDES *adenomatous polyps (212.1)*

Diseases of the Respiratory System

478.5–482.84

478.5 Other diseases of vocal cords

Abscess
Cellulitis
Granuloma } of vocal cords
Leukoplakia

Chorditis (fibrinous) (nodosa) (tuberosa)
Singers' nodes

478.6 Edema of larynx

Edema (of):   Edema (of):
glottis   supraglottic
subglottic

✓5ᵗʰ 478.7 Other diseases of larynx, not elsewhere classified

478.70 Unspecified disease of larynx

478.71 Cellulitis and perichondritis of larynx
DEF: Inflammation of deep soft tissues or lining of bone of the larynx.

478.74 Stenosis of larynx

478.75 Laryngeal spasm
Laryngismus (stridulus)
DEF: Involuntary muscle contraction of the larynx.

478.79 Other
Abscess
Necrosis
Obstruction } of larynx
Pachyderma
Ulcer
EXCLUDES ulcerative laryngitis (464.00-464.01)
AHA:3Q, '91, 20

478.8 Upper respiratory tract hypersensitivity reaction, site unspecified
EXCLUDES hypersensitivity reaction of lower respiratory tract, as:
extrinsic allergic alveolitis (495.0-495.9)
pneumoconiosis (500-505)

478.9 Other and unspecified diseases of upper respiratory tract
Abscess } of trachea
Cicatrix

Pneumonia and Influenza (480-488)
EXCLUDES pneumonia:
allergic or eosinophilic (518.3)
aspiration:
NOS (507.0)
newborn (770.18)
solids and liquids (507.0-507.8)
congenital (770.0)
lipoid (507.1)
passive (514)
rheumatic (390)
ventilator-associated (997.31)

✓4ᵗʰ 480 Viral pneumonia

480.0 Pneumonia due to adenovirus

480.1 Pneumonia due to respiratory syncytial virus
AHA: 4Q, '10, 98; 4Q, '96, 28; 1Q, '88, 12

480.2 Pneumonia due to parainfluenza virus

480.3 Pneumonia due to SARS-associated coronavirus
DEF: A severe adult respiratory syndrome caused by the coronavirus, specified as inflammation of the lungs with consolidation.
AHA: 4Q, '03, 46-47

480.8 Pneumonia due to other virus not elsewhere classified
EXCLUDES congenital rubella pneumonitis (771.0)
pneumonia complicating viral diseases classified elsewhere (484.1-484.8)

480.9 Viral pneumonia, unspecified
AHA: 3Q, '98, 5

481 Pneumococcal pneumonia [Streptococcus pneumoniae pneumonia]
Lobar pneumonia, organism unspecified
AHA: 2Q, '98, 7; 4Q, '92, 19; 1Q, '92, 18; 1Q, '91, 13; 1Q, '88, 13; M-A, '85, 6

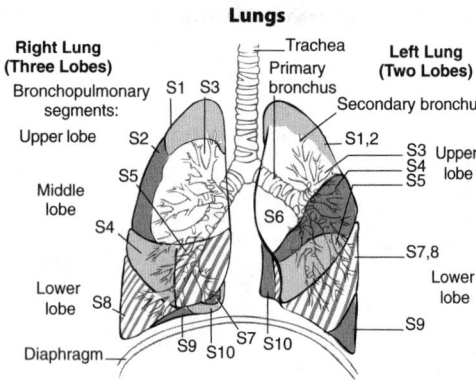

Lungs

Right Lung (Three Lobes)   Trachea   Left Lung (Two Lobes)
Bronchopulmonary segments: Primary bronchus
Upper lobe   S1 S3   Secondary bronchus
S2   S1,2
Middle lobe   S5   S3 Upper
S4   S6   S4 lobe
S5
Lower lobe   S8   S7,8
   Lower lobe
S9
Diaphragm   S9 S10   S7 S10

✓4ᵗʰ 482 Other bacterial pneumonia
AHA: 4Q, '93, 39

482.0 Pneumonia due to Klebsiella pneumoniae

482.1 Pneumonia due to Pseudomonas

482.2 Pneumonia due to Hemophilus influenzae [H. influenzae]
AHA: 2Q, '05, 19

✓5ᵗʰ 482.3 Pneumonia due to Streptococcus
EXCLUDES Streptococcus pneumoniae (481)
AHA: 1Q, '88, 13

482.30 Streptococcus, unspecified

482.31 Group A

482.32 Group B

482.39 Other Streptococcus

✓5ᵗʰ 482.4 Pneumonia due to Staphylococcus
AHA: 3Q, '91, 16

482.40 Pneumonia due to Staphylococcus, unspecified

482.41 Methicillin susceptible pneumonia due to Staphylococcus aureus
MSSA pneumonia
Pneumonia due to Staphylococcus aureus NOS
J15.21 Pneumonia due to staphylococcus aureus   I-10

482.42 Methicillin resistant pneumonia due to Staphylococcus aureus
AHA: 4Q, '08, 69, 71, 72

482.49 Other Staphylococcus pneumonia

✓5ᵗʰ 482.8 Pneumonia due to other specified bacteria
EXCLUDES pneumonia, complicating infectious disease classified elsewhere (484.1-484.8)
AHA: 3Q, '88, 11

482.81 Anaerobes
Bacteroides (melaninogenicus)
Gram-negative anaerobes

482.82 Escherichia coli [E. coli]

482.83 Other gram-negative bacteria
Gram-negative pneumonia NOS
Proteus
Serratia marcescens
EXCLUDES gram-negative anaerobes (482.81)
Legionnaires' disease (482.84)
AHA: 2Q, '98, 5; 3Q, '94, 9
TIP: Do not assign based solely on laboratory findings of gram-negative bacteria on gram-stain. Physician substantiation is required.
J15.6 Pneumonia d/t oth aerobic Gram-negative bacteria   I-10

482.84 Legionnaires' disease
DEF: Severe and often fatal infection by Legionella pneumophilia; symptoms include high fever, gastrointestinal pain, headache, myalgia, dry cough, and pneumonia; usually transmitted airborne via air conditioning systems.
AHA: 4Q, '97, 38

Diseases of the Respiratory System

482.89–488.09

482.89 Other specified bacteria
AHA: 2Q, '97, 6
TIP: Do not assign based on documentation of "mixed bacterial pneumonia" or "gram-positive pneumonia." See instead 482.9.

482.9 Bacterial pneumonia unspecified
AHA: 2Q, '98, 6; 2Q, '97, 6; 1Q, '94, 17
J15.9 Unspecified bacterial pneumonia   I-10

483 Pneumonia due to other specified organism
AHA: N-D, '87, 5
TIP: Do not assign if pneumonia due to candidiasis; see code 112.4.

483.0 Mycoplasma pneumoniae
Eaton's agent   Pleuropneumonia-like organism [PPLO]

483.1 Chlamydia
AHA: 4Q, '96, 31

483.8 Other specified organism

484 Pneumonia in infectious diseases classified elsewhere

484.1 Pneumonia in cytomegalic inclusion disease
Code first underlying disease (078.5)

484.3 Pneumonia in whooping cough
Code first underlying disease (033.0-033.9)

484.5 Pneumonia in anthrax
Code first underlying disease (022.1)

484.6 Pneumonia in aspergillosis
Code first underlying disease (117.3)
AHA: 4Q, '97, 40

484.7 Pneumonia in other systemic mycoses
Code first underlying disease
EXCLUDES pneumonia in:
    candidiasis (112.4)
    coccidioidomycosis (114.0)
    histoplasmosis (115.0-115.9 with fifth-digit 5)

484.8 Pneumonia in other infectious diseases classified elsewhere
Code first underlying disease, as:
    Q fever (083.0)
    typhoid fever (002.0)
EXCLUDES pneumonia in:
    actinomycosis (039.1)
    measles (055.1)
    nocardiosis (039.1)
    ornithosis (073.0)
    Pneumocystis carinii (136.3)
    salmonellosis (003.22)
    toxoplasmosis (130.4)
    tuberculosis (011.6)
    tularemia (021.2)
    varicella (052.1)

485 Bronchopneumonia, organism unspecified
Bronchopneumonia: Pneumonia:
    hemorrhagic   lobular
    terminal   segmental
Pleurobronchopneumonia
EXCLUDES bronchiolitis (acute) (466.11-466.19)
    chronic (491.8)
    lipoid pneumonia (507.1)

486 Pneumonia, organism unspecified
EXCLUDES hypostatic or passive pneumonia (514)
    inhalation or aspiration pneumonia due to foreign materials (507.0-507.8)
    pneumonitis due to fumes and vapors (506.0)
AHA: 4Q, '10, 135; 1Q, '10, 3, 12; 3Q, '09, 16; 4Q, '08, 142; 4Q, '99, 6; 3Q, '99, 9; 3Q, '98, 7; 2Q, '98, 4, 5; 1Q, '98, 8; 3Q, '97, 9; 3Q, '94, 10; 3Q, '88, 11
TIP: Never assume a causal organism based on laboratory or radiology findings alone.
J18.9 Pneumonia unspecified organism   I-10

487 Influenza
Influenza caused by unspecified influenza virus
EXCLUDES Hemophilus influenzae [H. influenzae]:
    infection NOS (041.5)
    influenza due to identified avian influenza virus (488.01-488.09)
    influenza due to 2009 H1N1 [swine] influenza virus (488.11-488.19)
    influenza due to identified (novel) 2009 H1N1 influenza virus (488.11-488.19)
    laryngitis (464.00-464.01)
    meningitis (320.0)

487.0 With pneumonia
Influenza with pneumonia, any form   Influenzal:
Influenzal: pneumonia
    bronchopneumonia
Use additional code to identify the type of pneumonia (480.0-480.9, 481, 482.0-482.9, 483.0-483.8, 485)
AHA: 1Q, '06, 18; 2Q, '05, 18
TIP: Selection of the principal diagnosis will be dependent on the circumstances of admission

487.1 With other respiratory manifestations
Influenza NEC   Influenzal:
Influenza NOS   pharyngitis
Influenzal: respiratory infection (upper) (acute)
    laryngitis
AHA: ▶4Q, '11, 114;◀ 1Q, '10, 4; 1Q, '06, 18; 2Q, '05, 18; 4Q, '99, 26
J10.1 Influenza d/t oth influenza virus w/resp manifst   I-10

487.8 With other manifestations
Encephalopathy due to influenza
Influenza with involvement of gastrointestinal tract
EXCLUDES "intestinal flu" [viral gastroenteritis] (008.8)

488 Influenza due to certain identified influenza viruses
EXCLUDES influenza caused by unspecified or seasonal influenza viruses (487.0-487.8)
AHA: 4Q, '09, 92-93
TIP: Do not assign a code from this category unless the specified influenza virus is confirmed.

488.0 Influenza due to identified avian influenza virus
Avian influenza
Bird flu
Influenza A/H5N1
DEF: Infection caused by contact with bird influenza viruses; results in flu-like symptoms that may progress to other severe and life-threatening complications.
AHA: 4Q, '10, 85-87; 4Q, '07, 87

488.01 Influenza due to identified avian influenza virus with pneumonia
Avian influenzal:
    bronchopneumonia
    pneumonia
Influenza due to identified avian influenza virus with pneumonia, any form
Use additional code to identify the type of pneumonia (480.0- 480.9, 481, 482.0-482.9, 483.0-483.8, 485)
J09.019 Influenza d/t ident avian influenza virus w/ unspec pneumonia   I-10

488.02 Influenza due to identified avian influenza virus with other respiratory manifestations
Avian influenzal: Identified avian influenza NOS
    laryngitis
    pharyngitis
    respiratory infection (acute) (upper)
J09.02 Influenza due to identified avian influenza virus with other respiratory manifestations   I-10

488.09 Influenza due to identified avian influenza virus with other manifestations
Avian influenza with involvement of gastrointestinal tract
Encephalopathy due to identified avian influenza
EXCLUDES "intestinal flu" [viral gastroenteritis] (008.8)

Bronchioli and Alveoli

✓5ᵗʰ 488.1 Influenza due to identified 2009 H1N1 influenza virus

2009 H1N1 swine influenza virus   Novel H1N1 influenza
(Novel) 2009 influenza H1N1   Novel influenza A/H1N1

> **EXCLUDES**   bird influenza virus infection (488.01-488.09)
>   influenza A/H5N1 (488.01-488.09)
>   other human infection with influenza virus of animal
>   origin (488.81-488.89)
>   swine influenza virus infection (488.81-488.89)

> **AHA:** ▶4Q, '11, 110-112, 114;◀4Q, '10, 85-87; 1Q, '10, 3-4

488.11 Influenza due to identified 2009 H1N1 influenza virus with pneumonia

Influenza due to identified (novel) 2009 H1N1 with
pneumonia, any form
(Novel) 2009 H1N1 influenzal:
   bronchopneumonia
   pneumonia
Use additional code to identify the type of
   pneumonia (480.0- 480.9, 481, 482.0-482.9,
   483.0-483.8, 485)

J09.119 Influenza d/t ident novel H1N1 influenza virus   [I-10]
w/ unspec pneumonia

488.12 Influenza due to identified 2009 H1N1 influenza virus with other respiratory manifestations

(Novel) 2009 H1N1 influenza NOS
(Novel) 2009 H1N1 influenzal:
   laryngitis
   pharyngitis
   respiratory infection (acute) (upper)

J09.12 Influenza due to identified novel H1N1   [I-10]
influenza virus with other respiratory manifestations

488.19 Influenza due to identified 2009 H1N1 influenza virus with other manifestations

Encephalopathy due to identified (novel) 2009 H1N1
   influenza
(Novel) 2009 H1N1 influenza with involvement of
   gastrointestinal tract

> **EXCLUDES**   "intestinal flu" [viral gastroenteritis] (008.8)

✓5ᵗʰ 488.8 Influenza due to novel influenza A

Influenza due to animal origin influenza virus
Infection with influenza viruses occurring in pigs or other
   animals
Other novel influenza A viruses not previously found in
   humans

> **EXCLUDES**   bird influenza virus infection (488.01-488.09)
>   influenza A/H5N1 (488.01-488.09)
>   influenza due to identified 2009 H1N1 influenza virus
>   (488.11- 488.19)

> **AHA:** ▶4Q, '11, 110-114◀

488.81 Influenza due to identified novel influenza A virus with pneumonia

Influenza due to animal origin influenza virus with
   pneumonia, any form
Novel influenza A:
   bronchopneumonia
   pneumonia
Use additional code to identify the type of
   pneumonia (480.0-480.9, 481, 482.0-482.9,
   483.0-483.8, 485)

488.82 Influenza due to identified novel influenza A virus with other respiratory manifestations

Influenza due to animal origin influenza A virus with
   other respiratory manifestations
Novel influenza A:
   laryngitis
   pharyngitis
   respiratory infection (acute) (upper)

488.89 Influenza due to identified novel influenza A virus with other manifestations

Encephalopathy due to novel influenza A
Influenza due to animal origin influenza virus with
   encephalopathy
Influenza due to animal origin influenza virus with
   involvement of gastrointestinal tract
Novel influenza A with involvement of
   gastrointestinal tract

> **EXCLUDES**   "intestinal flu" [viral gastroenteritis] (008.8)

Chronic Obstructive Pulmonary Disease and Allied Conditions (490-496)

AHA: 3Q, '88, 5

TIP: Due to the overlapping nature of conditions that make up COPD, it's
essential that the coder review all instructional notes carefully.

490 Bronchitis, not specified as acute or chronic

Bronchitis NOS: Tracheobronchitis NOS
   catarrhal
   with tracheitis NOS

> **EXCLUDES**   bronchitis:
>   allergic NOS (493.9)
>   asthmatic NOS (493.9)
>   due to fumes and vapors (506.0)

J40 Bronchitis not specified as acute or chronic   [I-10]

✓4ᵗʰ 491 Chronic bronchitis

> **EXCLUDES**   chronic obstructive asthma (493.2)

491.0 Simple chronic bronchitis

Catarrhal bronchitis, chronic   Smokers' cough

J41.0 Simple chronic bronchitis   [I-10]

491.1 Mucopurulent chronic bronchitis

Bronchitis (chronic) (recurrent):
   fetid
   mucopurulent
   purulent

DEF: Chronic bronchial infection characterized by both mucus and
pus secretions in the bronchial tree; recurs after asymptomatic
periods; signs are coughing, expectoration and secondary changes
in the lung.

AHA: 3Q, '88, 12

✓5ᵗʰ 491.2 Obstructive chronic bronchitis

Bronchitis: Bronchitis with:
   emphysematous   chronic airway obstruction
   obstructive (chronic)   emphysema
   (diffuse)

> **EXCLUDES**   asthmatic bronchitis (acute) NOS (493.9)
>   chronic obstructive asthma (493.2)

AHA: 3Q, '97, 9; 4Q, '91, 25; 2Q, '91, 21

491.20 Without exacerbation

Emphysema with chronic bronchitis

AHA: 3Q, '97, 9

J44.9 Chronic obst pulmonary disease, unspecified   [I-10]

Interrelationship Between Chronic Airway Obstruction, Chronic Bronchitis, and Emphysema

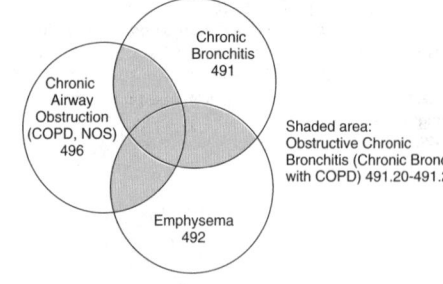

491.21 With (acute) exacerbation
  Acute exacerbation of chronic obstructive pulmonary disease [COPD]
  Decompensated chronic obstructive pulmonary disease [COPD]
  Decompensated chronic obstructive pulmonary disease [COPD] with exacerbation
  EXCLUDES *chronic obstructive asthma with acute exacerbation (493.22)*
  AHA: 1Q, '10, 12; 1Q, '04, 3; 3Q, '02, 18, 19; 4Q, '01, 43; 2Q, '96, 10
  J44.1 Chronic obst pulmonary disease with exacerbation [I-10]

491.22 With acute bronchitis
  AHA: 3Q, '06, 20; 4Q, '04, 82
  J44.0 Chronic obst pulmonary disease w/exacerbation [I-10]

491.8 Other chronic bronchitis
  Chronic: Chronic:
    tracheitis   tracheobronchitis

491.9 Unspecified chronic bronchitis
  J42 Unspecified chronic bronchitis [I-10]

√4ᵗʰ 492 Emphysema
  AHA: 2Q, '91, 21

492.0 Emphysematous bleb
  Giant bullous emphysema
  Ruptured emphysematous bleb
  Tension pneumatocele
  Vanishing lung
  DEF: Formation of vesicle or bulla in emphysematous lung, more than one millimeter; contains serum or blood.
  AHA: 2Q, '93, 3

492.8 Other emphysema
  Emphysema (lung or pulmonary):
    NOS
    centriacinar
    centrilobular
    obstructive
    panacinar
    panlobular
    unilateral
    vesicular
  MacLeod's syndrome
  Swyer-James syndrome
  Unilateral hyperlucent lung
  EXCLUDES *emphysema:*
    with chronic bronchitis (491.20-491.22)
    compensatory (518.2)
    due to fumes and vapors (506.4)
    interstitial (518.1)
      newborn (770.2)
    mediastinal (518.1)
    surgical (subcutaneous) (998.81)
    traumatic (958.7)
  AHA: 4Q, '08, 175; 1Q, '05, 4; 4Q, '93, 41; J-A, '84, 17
  J43.9 Emphysema unspecified [I-10]

√4ᵗʰ 493 Asthma
  EXCLUDES *wheezing NOS (786.07)*

  The following fifth-digit subclassification is for use with codes 493.0-493.2, 493.9:
    0 unspecified
    1 with status asthmaticus
    2 with (acute) exacerbation

  DEF: Status asthmaticus: severe, intractable episode of asthma unresponsive to normal therapeutic measures.
  AHA: 4Q, '04, 137; 4Q, '03, 62; 4Q, '01, 43; 4Q, '00, 42; 1Q, '91, 13; 3Q, '88, 9; J-A, '85, 8; N-D, '84, 17
  TIP: If documentation indicates both exacerbation and status asthmaticus, assign only the code for status asthmaticus.

§ √5ᵗʰ 493.0 Extrinsic asthma
  [0-2] Asthma:
    allergic with stated cause
    atopic
    childhood
    hay
    platinum
  Hay fever with asthma
  EXCLUDES *asthma:*
    allergic NOS (493.9)
    detergent (507.8)
    miners' (500)
    wood (495.8)
  DEF: Transient stricture of airway diameters of bronchi; due to environmental factor; also called allergic (bronchial) asthma.
  J45.20 Mild intermittent asthma uncomplicated [I-10]

§ √5ᵗʰ 493.1 Intrinsic asthma
  [0-2] Late-onset asthma
  DEF: Transient stricture of airway diameters of bronchi; due to pathophysiological disturbances.
  AHA: 3Q, '88, 9; M-A, '85, 7

§ √5ᵗʰ 493.2 Chronic obstructive asthma
  [0-2] Asthma with chronic obstructive pulmonary disease [COPD]
  Chronic asthmatic bronchitis
  EXCLUDES *acute bronchitis (466.0)*
    chronic obstructive bronchitis (491.20-491.22)
  DEF: Persistent narrowing of airway diameters in the bronchial tree, restricting airflow and causing constant labored breathing.
  AHA: 2Q, '91, 21; 2Q, '90, 20; **For code 493.20:** 4Q, '03, 108; **For code 493.22:** 1Q, '09, 17; 3Q, '06, 20

√5ᵗʰ 493.8 Other forms of asthma
  AHA: 4Q, '03, 62

  493.81 Exercise induced bronchospasm

  493.82 Cough variant asthma

§ √5ᵗʰ 493.9 Asthma, unspecified
  [0-2] Asthma (bronchial) (allergic NOS)
  Bronchitis:
    allergic
    asthmatic
  AHA: 4Q, '97, 40, **For code 493.90:** 4Q, '04, 137; 4Q, '03, 108; 4Q, '99, 25; 1Q, '97, 7; **For code 493.91:** 1Q, '05, 5; **For code 493.92:** 1Q, '03, 9
  J45.909 Unspecified asthma uncomplicated [I-10]
  J45.901 Unspecified asthma with acute exacerbation [I-10]

√4ᵗʰ 494 Bronchiectasis
  Bronchiectasis (fusiform) (postinfectious) (recurrent)
  Bronchiolectasis
  EXCLUDES *congenital (748.61)*
    tuberculous bronchiectasis (current disease) (011.5)
  DEF: Dilation of bronchi; due to infection or chronic conditions; causes decreased lung capacity and recurrent infections of lungs.
  AHA: 4Q, '00, 42

494.0 Bronchiectasis without acute exacerbation
  J47.9 Bronchiectasis uncomplicated [I-10]

494.1 Bronchiectasis with acute exacerbation

---

§ Requires fifth digit. Valid digits are in [brackets] under each code. See category 493 for codes and definitions.

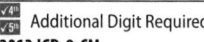

Diseases of the Respiratory System

495–507.0

☑4ᵗʰ **495 Extrinsic allergic alveolitis**

> **INCLUDES** allergic alveolitis and pneumonitis due to inhaled organic dust particles of fungal, thermophilic actinomycete, or other origin

> **DEF:** Pneumonitis due to particles inhaled into lung, often at workplace; symptoms include cough, chills, fever, increased heart and respiratory rates; develops within hours of exposure.

495.0 Farmers' lung

495.1 Bagassosis

495.2 Bird-fanciers' lung
> Budgerigar-fanciers' disease or lung
> Pigeon-fanciers' disease or lung

495.3 Suberosis
> Cork-handlers' disease or lung

495.4 Malt workers' lung
> Alveolitis due to Aspergillus clavatus

495.5 Mushroom workers' lung

495.6 Maple bark-strippers' lung
> Alveolitis due to Cryptostroma corticale

495.7 "Ventilation" pneumonitis
> Allergic alveolitis due to fungal, thermophilic actinomycete, and other organisms growing in ventilation [air conditioning] systems

495.8 Other specified allergic alveolitis and pneumonitis

Cheese-washers' lung	Grain-handlers' disease or lung
Coffee workers' lung	Pituitary snuff-takers' disease
Fish-meal workers' lung	Sequoiosis or red-cedar asthma
Furriers' lung	Wood asthma

495.9 Unspecified allergic alveolitis and pneumonitis
> Alveolitis, allergic (extrinsic)   Hypersensitivity pneumonitis

496 Chronic airway obstruction, not elsewhere classified

> **NOTE** This code is not to be used with any code from categories 491-493

> Chronic:
> nonspecific lung disease
> obstructive lung disease
> obstructive pulmonary disease [COPD] NOS

> **EXCLUDES** chronic obstructive lung disease [COPD] specified (as) (with):
> allergic alveolitis (495.0-495.9)
> asthma (493.20-493.22)
> bronchiectasis (494.0-494.1)
> bronchitis (491.20-491.22)
> with emphysema (491.20-491.22)
> decompensated (491.21)
> emphysema (492.0-492.8)

> **AHA:** 1Q, '10, 5, 18; 1Q, '09, 16; 3Q, '07, 10; 4Q, '03, 109; 2Q, '00, 15; 2Q, '92, 16; 2Q, '91, 21; 3Q, '88, 56

> **TIP:** COPD is a nonspecific term that encompasses many different respiratory conditions; review medical record and query physician for more specific documentation of emphysema, bronchitis, asthma, etc.

> **J44.9** Chronic obstructive pulmonary disease unspec   I-10

Pneumoconioses and Other Lung Diseases Due to External Agents (500-508)

> **DEF:** Permanent deposits of particulate matter, within lungs; due to occupational or environmental exposure; results in chronic induration and fibrosis. (See specific listings in 500-508 code range).

500 Coal workers' pneumoconiosis   A

Anthracosilicosis	Coal workers' lung
Anthracosis	Miner's asthma
Black lung disease	

501 Asbestosis   A

502 Pneumoconiosis due to other silica or silicates
> Pneumoconiosis due to talc
> Silicotic fibrosis (massive) of lung
> Silicosis (simple) (complicated)

503 Pneumoconiosis due to other inorganic dust

Aluminosis (of lung)	Graphite fibrosis (of lung)
Baritosis	Siderosis
Bauxite fibrosis (of lung)	Stannosis
Berylliosis	

504 Pneumonopathy due to inhalation of other dust

Byssinosis	Flax-dressers' disease
Cannabinosis	

> **EXCLUDES** allergic alveolitis (495.0-495.9)
> asbestosis (501)
> bagassosis (495.1)
> farmers' lung (495.0)

505 Pneumoconiosis, unspecified

☑4ᵗʰ **506 Respiratory conditions due to chemical fumes and vapors**

> Use additional code to identify associated respiratory conditions, such as:
> acute respiratory failure (518.81)

506.0 Bronchitis and pneumonitis due to fumes and vapors
> Chemical bronchitis (acute)
> **AHA:** 3Q. '10, 19; 3Q, '08, 7

506.1 Acute pulmonary edema due to fumes and vapors
> Chemical pulmonary edema (acute)
> **EXCLUDES** acute pulmonary edema NOS (518.4)
> chronic or unspecified pulmonary edema (514)
> **AHA:** 3Q, '88, 4

506.2 Upper respiratory inflammation due to fumes and vapors
> **AHA:** 3Q, '05, 10

506.3 Other acute and subacute respiratory conditions due to fumes and vapors
> **AHA:** 3Q, '10, 19

506.4 Chronic respiratory conditions due to fumes and vapors

> Emphysema (diffuse) (chronic) ⎫
> Obliterative bronchiolitis   ⎬ due to inhalation
> (chronic) (subacute)   ⎬ of chemical
> Pulmonary fibrosis (chronic) ⎭ fumes and vapors

506.9 Unspecified respiratory conditions due to fumes and vapors
> Silo-fillers' disease

☑4ᵗʰ **507 Pneumonitis due to solids and liquids**

> **EXCLUDES** fetal aspiration pneumonitis (770.18)
> postprocedural pneumonitis (997.32)
> **AHA:** 3Q, '91, 16

507.0 Due to inhalation of food or vomitus
> Aspiration pneumonia (due to):
> NOS
> food (regurgitated)
> gastric secretions
> milk
> saliva
> vomitus
> **AHA:** 4Q, '11, 150; 1Q, '11, 16; 1Q, '08, 18; 1Q, '89,10
> **TIP:** ▶If postprocedural or postoperative aspiration pneumonia is specified, assign instead 997.32.◀
> **J69.0** Pneumonitis due to inhalation of food and vomit   I-10

N Newborn Age: 0   P Pediatric Age: 0-17   M Maternity Age: 12-55   A Adult Age: 15-124

507.1 Due to inhalation of oils and essences
Lipoid pneumonia (exogenous)
EXCLUDES *endogenous lipoid pneumonia (516.8)*

507.8 Due to other solids and liquids
Detergent asthma

✓4ᵗʰ **508 Respiratory conditions due to other and unspecified external agents**
Use additional code to identify associated respiratory conditions, such as:
acute respiratory failure (518.81)

508.0 Acute pulmonary manifestations due to radiation
Radiation pneumonitis
AHA: 2Q, '88, 4

508.1 Chronic and other pulmonary manifestations due to radiation
Fibrosis of lung following radiation

508.2 Respiratory conditions due to smoke inhalation
Smoke inhalation NOS
EXCLUDES *smoke inhalation due to chemical fumes and vapors (506.9)*
AHA: ▶4Q, '11, 114-115◀
TIP: ▶Assign for smoke inhalation, along with the appropriate E code describing the source of the smoke and fumes.◀

508.8 Respiratory conditions due to other specified external agents

508.9 Respiratory conditions due to unspecified external agent

Other Diseases of Respiratory System (510-519)

✓4ᵗʰ **510 Empyema**
Use additional code to identify infectious organism (041.0-041.9)
EXCLUDES *abscess of lung (513.0)*
DEF: Purulent infection within pleural space.

510.0 With fistula
Fistula:	Fistula:
bronchocutaneous	mediastinal
bronchopleural	pleural
hepatopleural	thoracic

Any condition classifiable to 510.9 with fistula
DEF: Purulent infection of respiratory cavity, with communication from cavity to another structure.

510.9 Without mention of fistula
Abscess:	Pleurisy:
pleura	purulent
thorax	septic
Empyema (chest) (lung)	seropurulent
(pleura)	suppurative
Fibrinopurulent pleurisy	Pyopneumothorax
	Pyothorax

AHA: 4Q, '07, 113; 3Q, '94, 6
J86.9 Pyothorax without fistula   I-10

✓4ᵗʰ **511 Pleurisy**
EXCLUDES *pleurisy with mention of tuberculosis, current disease (012.0)*
DEF: Inflammation of serous membrane of lungs and lining of thoracic cavity; causes exudation in cavity or membrane surface.

511.0 Without mention of effusion or current tuberculosis
Adhesion, lung or pleura	Pleurisy:
Calcification of pleura	NOS
Pleurisy (acute) (sterile):	pneumococcal
diaphragmatic	staphylococcal
fibrinous	streptococcal
interlobar	Thickening of pleura

AHA: 3Q, '94, 5

511.1 With effusion, with mention of a bacterial cause other than tuberculosis
Pleurisy with effusion (exudative) (serous):
pneumococcal
staphylococcal
streptococcal
other specified nontuberculous bacterial cause

►Lower Respiratory System◄

✓5ᵗʰ **511.8 Other specified forms of effusion, except tuberculous**
EXCLUDES *traumatic (860.2-860.5, 862.29, 862.39)*
AHA: 4Q, '08, 113-114; 1Q, '97, 10

511.81 Malignant pleural effusion
Code first malignant neoplasm, if known
J91.0 Malignant pleural effusion   I-10

511.89 Other specified forms of effusion, except tuberculous
Encysted pleurisy	Hydropneumothorax
Hemopneumothorax	Hydrothorax
Hemothorax	

511.9 Unspecified pleural effusion
Pleural effusion NOS	Pleurisy:
Pleurisy:	serous
exudative	with effusion NOS
serofibrinous	

AHA: 2Q, '03, 7; 3Q, '91, 19; 4Q, '89, 11
TIP: Do not assign when the pleural effusion is a symptom of CHF and no therapeutic treatment (e.g., thoracentesis) is directed towards the pleural effusion.
J90 Pleural effusion not elsewhere classified   I-10

✓4ᵗʰ **512 Pneumothorax and air leak**
DEF: Collapsed lung; due to gas or air in pleural space.
AHA: ▶4Q, '11, 115-116◀

512.0 Spontaneous tension pneumothorax
DEF: Leaking air from lung into lining causing collapse.
AHA: 3Q, '94, 5

512.1 Iatrogenic pneumothorax
Postoperative pneumothorax
DEF: Air trapped in the lining of the lung following surgery.
AHA: 1Q, '11, 14; 4Q, '94, 40
TIP: Pneumothorax is a known risk associated with most thoracic surgery; do not assign based on radiology findings alone, without physician substantiation.
J95.81 Postprocedural pneumothorax   I-10

512.2 Postoperative air leak
AHA: ▶4Q, '11, 115-117◀

✓5ᵗʰ **512.8 Other pneumothorax and air leak**
Pneumothorax:	Pneumothorax:
NOS	chronic
acute	

EXCLUDES *pneumothorax:*
congenital (770.2)
traumatic (860.0-860.1, 860.4-860.5)
tuberculous, current disease (011.7)
AHA: ▶4Q, '11, 115-117◀ 2Q, '93, 3
J93.9 Pneumothorax unspecified   I-10

512.81 Primary spontaneous pneumothorax

Diseases of the Respiratory System

512.82 Secondary spontaneous pneumothorax
Code first underlying condition, such as:
cancer metastatic to lung (197.0)
catamenial pneumothorax due to endometriosis (617.8)
cystic fibrosis (277.02)
eosinophilic pneumonia (518.3)
lymphangioleiomyomatosis (516.4)
Marfan syndrome (759.82)
pneumocystis carinii pneumonia (136.3)
primary lung cancer (162.3-162.9)
spontaneous rupture of the esophagus (530.4)

512.83 Chronic pneumothorax

512.84 Other air leak
Persistent air leak

512.89 Other pneumothorax
Acute pneumothorax
Spontaneous pneumothorax NOS
Pneumothorax NOS
J93.9 Pneumothorax unspecified   I-10

√4ᵗʰ **513 Abscess of lung and mediastinum**

513.0 Abscess of lung
Abscess (multiple) of lung
Gangrenous or necrotic pneumonia
Pulmonary gangrene or necrosis
AHA: 4Q, '07, 85; 2Q, '98, 7

513.1 Abscess of mediastinum

514 Pulmonary congestion and hypostasis
Hypostatic: Pulmonary edema:
  bronchopneumonia   NOS
  pneumonia   chronic
Passive pneumonia
Pulmonary congestion (chronic) (passive)
EXCLUDES *acute pulmonary edema:*
NOS (518.4)
with mention of heart disease or failure (428.1)
hypostatic pneumonia due to or specified as a specific type of pneumonia— code to the type of pneumonia (480.0-480.9, 481, 482.0-482.9, 483.0-483.8, 487.0, 488.01, 488.11)
DEF: Excessive retention of interstitial fluid in the lungs and pulmonary vessels; due to poor circulation.
AHA: 2Q, '98, 6; 3Q, '88, 5
J81.1 Chronic pulmonary edema   I-10

515 Postinflammatory pulmonary fibrosis
Cirrhosis of lung
Fibrosis of lung (atrophic)
    (confluent) (massive) } chronic or unspecified
    (perialveolar) (peribronchial)
Induration of lung
DEF: Fibrosis and scarring of the lungs due to inflammatory reaction.
J84.1 Other interstitial pulmonary diseases w/fibrosis   I-10

√4ᵗʰ **516 Other alveolar and parietoalveolar pneumonopathy**

516.0 Pulmonary alveolar proteinosis
DEF: Reduced ventilation; due to proteinaceous deposits on alveoli; symptoms include dyspnea, cough, chest pain, weakness, weight loss, and hemoptysis.

516.1 Idiopathic pulmonary hemosiderosis
Code first underlying disease (275.01-275.09)
Essential brown induration of lung
EXCLUDES *acute idiopathic pulmonary hemorrhage in infants [AIPHI] (786.31)*
DEF: Fibrosis of alveolar walls; marked by abnormal amounts hemosiderin in lungs; primarily affects children; symptoms include anemia, fluid in lungs, and blood in sputum; etiology unknown.

516.2 Pulmonary alveolar microlithiasis
DEF: Small calculi in pulmonary alveoli resembling sand-like particles on x-ray.

√5ᵗʰ **516.3 Idiopathic interstitial pneumonia**
AHA: ▶4Q, '11, 117-119◀

516.30 Idiopathic interstitial pneumonia, not otherwise specified
Idiopathic fibrosing alveolitis

516.31 Idiopathic pulmonary fibrosis
Cryptogenic fibrosing alveolitis
DEF: ▶Chronic disease of unknown causation characterized by scarring and thickening of the lungs affecting males over 50◀

516.32 Idiopathic non-specific interstitial pneumonitis
EXCLUDES *non-specific interstitial pneumonia NOS, or due to known underlying cause (516.8)*

516.33 Acute interstitial pneumonitis
Hamman Rich syndrome
EXCLUDES *pneumocystis pneumonia (136.3)*

516.34 Respiratory bronchiolitis interstitial lung disease

516.35 Idiopathic lymphoid interstitial pneumonia
Idiopathic lymphocytic interstitial pneumonitis
EXCLUDES *lymphoid interstitial pneumonia NOS, or due to known underlying cause (516.8)*
pneumocystis pneumonia (136.3)

516.36 Cryptogenic organizing pneumonia
EXCLUDES *organizing pneumonia NOS, or due to known underlying cause (516.8)*

516.37 Desquamative interstitial pneumonia

516.4 Lymphangioleiomyomatosis   ♀
Lymphangiomyomatosis
AHA: ▶4Q, '11, 119◀

516.5 Adult pulmonary Langerhans cell histiocytosis   A
Adult PLCH
AHA: ▶4Q, '11, 119◀

√5ᵗʰ **516.6 Interstitial lung diseases of childhood**
AHA: ▶4Q, '11, 120-123◀

516.61 Neuroendocrine cell hyperplasia of infancy

516.62 Pulmonary interstitial glycogenosis

516.63 Surfactant mutations of the lung
DEF: ▶Genetic disorders resulting in insufficient secretion of a complex mixture of phospholipids and proteins that reduce surface tension in the alveoli following the onset of breathing to facilitate lung expansion in the newborn; leading indication for pediatric lung transplantation. ◀

516.64 Alveolar capillary dysplasia with vein misalignment

516.69 Other interstitial lung diseases of childhood

516.8 Other specified alveolar and parietoalveolar pneumonopathies
Endogenous lipoid pneumonia
Interstitial pneumonia
Lymphoid interstitial pneumonia due to known underlying cause
Lymphoid interstitial pneumonia NOS
Non-specific interstitial pneumonia due to known underlying cause
Non-specific interstitial pneumonia NOS
Organizing pneumonia due to known underlying cause
Organizing pneumonia NOS
Code first, if applicable, underlying cause of pneumonopathy, if known
Use additional E code, if applicable, for drug-induced or toxic pneumonopathy
EXCLUDES *cryptogenic organizing pneumonia (516.36)*
idiopathic lymphoid interstitial pneumonia (516.35)
idiopathic non-specific interstitial pneumonitis (516.32)
lipoid pneumonia, exogenous or unspecified (507.1)
AHA: 1Q, '11, 16; 1Q, '10, 6; 2Q, '06, 20; 1Q, '92, 12

516.9 Unspecified alveolar and parietoalveolar pneumonopathy

√4ᵗʰ **517 Lung involvement in conditions classified elsewhere**
EXCLUDES *rheumatoid lung (714.81)*

517.1 Rheumatic pneumonia
Code first underlying disease (390)

517.2 Lung involvement in systemic sclerosis
Code first underlying disease (710.1)

517.3 Acute chest syndrome
Code first sickle-cell disease in crisis (282.42, 282.62, 282.64, 282.69)
AHA: 4Q, '03, 51, 56

512.82–517.3 (side tab)

517.8 **Lung involvement in other diseases classified elsewhere**

Code first underlying disease, as:
 amyloidosis (277.30-277.39)
 polymyositis (710.4)
 sarcoidosis (135)
 Sjögren's disease (710.2)
 systemic lupus erythematosus (710.0)
 EXCLUDES *syphilis (095.1)*
 AHA: 2Q, '03, 7

518 Other diseases of lung

518.0 Pulmonary collapse
 Atelectasis   Middle lobe syndrome
 Collapse of lung
 EXCLUDES *atelectasis:*
 congenital (partial) (770.5)
 primary (770.4)
 tuberculous, current disease (011.8)
 AHA: 4Q, '90, 25
 J98.11 Atelectasis   I-10

518.1 Interstitial emphysema
 Mediastinal emphysema
 EXCLUDES *surgical (subcutaneous) emphysema (998.81)*
 that in fetus or newborn (770.2)
 traumatic emphysema (958.7)
 DEF: Escaped air from the alveoli trapped in the interstices of the lung; trauma or cough may cause the disease.

518.2 Compensatory emphysema
 DEF: Distention of all or part of the lung caused by disease processes or surgical intervention that decreased volume in another part of the lung; overcompensation reaction to the loss of capacity in another part of the lung.

518.3 Pulmonary eosinophilia
 Eosinophilic asthma   Pneumonia:
 Löffler's syndrome   eosinophilic
 Pneumonia: Tropical eosinophilia
  allergic
 EXCLUDES *pulmonary infiltrate NOS (793.19)*
 DEF: Infiltration, into pulmonary parenchyma of eosinophils; results in cough, fever, and dyspnea.
 AHA: ►4Q, '11, 139◄

518.4 Acute edema of lung, unspecified
 Acute pulmonary edema NOS
 Pulmonary edema, postoperative
 EXCLUDES *pulmonary edema:*
 acute, with mention of heart disease or failure (428.1)
 chronic or unspecified (514)
 due to external agents (506.0-508.9)
 DEF: Severe, sudden fluid retention within lung tissues.
 TIP: Do not assign separately if associated with CHF or heart disease; it is incorporated into those codes.

518.5 Pulmonary insufficiency following trauma and surgery
 EXCLUDES *adult respiratory distress syndrome associated with other conditions (518.82)*
 pneumonia:
 aspiration (507.0)
 hypostatic (514)
 respiratory failure in other conditions (518.81, 518.83-518.84)
 AHA: ►4Q, '11, 123-125;◄ 3Q. '10, 19; 4Q, '04, 139; 3Q, '88, 3; 3Q, '88, 7; S-O, '87, 1

518.51 Acute respiratory failure following trauma and surgery
 Respiratory failure, not otherwise specified, following trauma and surgery
 EXCLUDES *acute respiratory failure in other conditions (518.81)*
 J95.82 Postprocedural respiratory failure   I-10

518.52 Other pulmonary insufficiency, not elsewhere classified, following trauma and surgery
 Adult respiratory distress syndrome
 Pulmonary insufficiency following surgery
 Pulmonary insufficiency following trauma
 Shock lung related to trauma and surgery
 EXCLUDES *adult respiratory distress syndrome associated with other conditions (518.82)*
 aspiration pneumonia (507.0)
 hypostatic pneumonia (514)
 shock lung, not related to trauma or surgery (518.82)

518.53 Acute and chronic respiratory failure following trauma and surgery
 EXCLUDES *acute and chronic respiratory failure in other conditions (518.84)*

518.6 Allergic bronchopulmonary aspergillosis
 DEF: Noninvasive hypersensitive reaction; due to allergic reaction to *Aspergillus fumigatus* (mold).
 AHA: 4Q, '97, 39

518.7 Transfusion related acute lung injury [TRALI]
 DEF: A relatively rare, but serious pulmonary complication of blood transfusion, with acute respiratory distress, noncardiogenic pulmonary edema, cyanosis, hypoxemia, hypotension, fever and chills.
 AHA: 4Q, '06, 91

518.8 Other diseases of lung

518.81 Acute respiratory failure
 Respiratory failure NOS
 EXCLUDES *acute and chronic respiratory failure (518.84)*
 acute respiratory distress (518.82)
 acute respiratory failure following trauma and surgery (518.51)
 chronic respiratory failure (518.83)
 respiratory arrest (799.1)
 respiratory failure, newborn (770.84)
 AHA: 4Q, '10, 80; 1Q, '10, 18-19; 3Q, '09, 14; 2Q, '09, 11; 1Q, '08, 18; 3Q, '07, 6; 2Q, '06, 25; 4Q, '05, 96; 2Q, '05, 19; 1Q, '05, 3-8; 1Q, '05, 3-8; 4Q, '04, 139; 1Q, '03, 15; 4Q, '98, 41; 3Q, '91, 14; 2Q, '91, 3; 4Q, '90, 25; 2Q, '90, 20; 3Q, '88, 7; 3Q, '88, 10; S-O, '87, 1
 TIP: If both respiratory failure and another acute condition are equally responsible for admission, either may be sequenced as principal diagnosis in the absence of chapter-specific guidelines to the contrary.
 J96.01 Acute respiratory failure with hypoxia   I-10

518.82 Other pulmonary insufficiency, not elsewhere classified
 Acute respiratory distress
 Acute respiratory insufficiency
 Adult respiratory distress syndrome NEC
 EXCLUDES *acute interstitial pneumonitis (516.33)*
 adult respiratory distress syndrome associated with trauma or surgery (518.52)
 pulmonary insufficiency following trauma or surgery (518.52)
 respiratory distress:
 NOS (786.09)
 newborn (770.89)
 syndrome, newborn (769)
 AHA: 4Q, '03, 105; 2Q, '91, 21; 3Q, '88, 7
 J80 Acute respiratory distress syndrome   I-10

518.83 Chronic respiratory failure
 AHA: 4Q, '05, 96; 4Q, '03, 103, 111
 J96.10 Chronic respiratory failure, unsp w/   I-10
 hypox or hypercap

518.84 Acute and chronic respiratory failure
 Acute on chronic respiratory failure
 EXCLUDES *acute and chronic respiratory failure following trauma or surgery (518.53)*
 AHA: 2Q, '11, 7
 J96.20 Ac & chr resp failure unsp w/hypox or hypercap   I-10

Diseases of the Respiratory System

518.89 Other diseases of lung, not elsewhere classified
Broncholithiasis   Lung disease NOS
Calcification of lung   Pulmolithiasis
DEF: Broncholithiasis: calculi in lumen of transbronchial tree.
DEF: Pulmolithiasis: calculi in lung.
AHA: 3Q, '90, 18; 4Q, '88, 6
TIP: ▶Do not assign for solitary lung nodule; see instead code 793.11.◀
J98.4 Other disorders of lung   `I-10`

√4th **519 Other diseases of respiratory system**

√5th **519.0 Tracheostomy complications**

519.00 Tracheostomy complication, unspecified

519.01 Infection of tracheostomy
Use additional code to identify type of infection, such as:
   abscess or cellulitis of neck (682.1)
   septicemia (038.0-038.9)
Use additional code to identify organism (041.00-041.9)
AHA: 4Q, '98, 41

519.02 Mechanical complication of tracheostomy
Tracheal stenosis due to tracheostomy

519.09 Other tracheostomy complications
Hemorrhage due to tracheostomy
Tracheoesophageal fistula due to tracheostomy

√5th **519.1 Other diseases of trachea and bronchus, not elsewhere classified**
AHA: 3Q, '02, 18; 3Q, '88, 6

519.11 Acute bronchospasm
Bronchospasm NOS
EXCLUDES acute bronchitis with bronchospasm (466.0)
     asthma (493.00-493.92)
     exercise induced bronchospasm (493.81)
AHA: 4Q, '06, 92

519.19 Other diseases of trachea and bronchus
Calcification ⎫
Stenosis   ⎬ of bronchus or trachea
Ulcer   ⎭
AHA: 4Q, '06, 92

519.2 Mediastinitis
DEF: Inflammation of tissue between organs behind sternum.

519.3 Other diseases of mediastinum, not elsewhere classified
Fibrosis ⎫
Hernia   ⎬ of mediastinum
Retraction ⎭

519.4 Disorders of diaphragm
Diaphragmitis   Relaxation of diaphragm
Paralysis of diaphragm
EXCLUDES congenital defect of diaphragm (756.6)
     diaphragmatic hernia (551-553 with .3)
     congenital (756.6)

519.8 Other diseases of respiratory system, not elsewhere classified
AHA: 4Q, '89, 12

519.9 Unspecified disease of respiratory system
Respiratory disease (chronic) NOS

N Newborn Age: 0   P Pediatric Age: 0-17   M Maternity Age: 12-55   A Adult Age: 15-124

9. Diseases of the Digestive System (520-579)

Diseases of Oral Cavity, Salivary Glands, and Jaws (520-529)

√4ᵗʰ 520 Disorders of tooth development and eruption

520.0 Anodontia
Absence of teeth (complete) (congenital) (partial)
Hypodontia
Oligodontia
EXCLUDES acquired absence of teeth (525.10-525.19)

520.1 Supernumerary teeth
Distomolar
Fourth molar
Mesiodens
Paramolar
Supplemental teeth
EXCLUDES supernumerary roots (520.2)

520.2 Abnormalities of size and form
Concrescence
Fusion } of teeth
Gemination

Dens evaginatus
Dens in dente
Dens invaginatus
Enamel pearls
Macrodontia
Microdontia
Peg-shaped [conical] teeth
Supernumerary roots
Taurodontism
Tuberculum paramolare
EXCLUDES that due to congenital syphilis (090.5)
tuberculum Carabelli, which is regarded as a normal variation

520.3 Mottled teeth
Mottling of enamel
Dental fluorosis
Nonfluoride enamel opacities

Digestive System

The Oral Cavity

Teeth

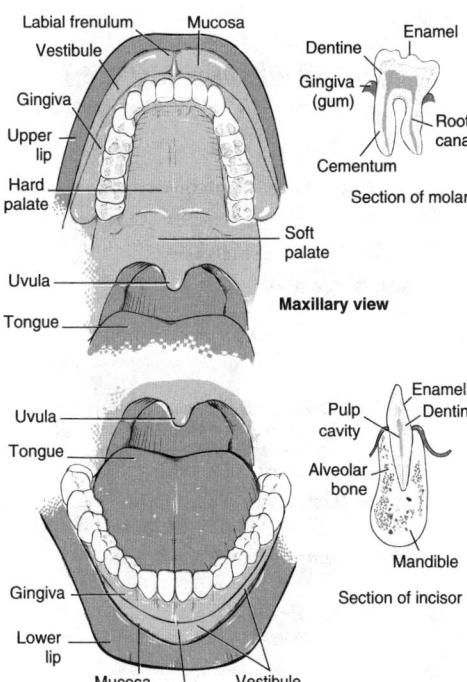

Maxillary view

Mandibulary view

520.4 Disturbances of tooth formation
Aplasia and hypoplasia of cementum
Dilaceration of tooth
Enamel hypoplasia (neonatal) (postnatal) (prenatal)
Horner's teeth
Hypocalcification of teeth
Regional odontodysplasia
Turner's tooth
EXCLUDES Hutchinson's teeth and mulberry molars in congenital syphilis (090.5)
mottled teeth (520.3)

520.5 Hereditary disturbances in tooth structure, not elsewhere classified
Amelogensis
Dentinogenesis } imperfecta
Odontogenesis

Dentinal dysplasia
Shell teeth

520.6 Disturbances in tooth eruption
Teeth:
  embedded
  impacted
  natal
  neonatal
  prenatal
  primary [deciduous]:
    persistent
    shedding, premature
Tooth eruption:
  late
  obstructed
  premature
EXCLUDES exfoliation of teeth (attributable to disease of surrounding tissues) (525.0-525.19)
AHA: 1Q, '06, 18; 2Q, '05, 15

520.7 Teething syndrome

520.8 Other specified disorders of tooth development and eruption
Color changes during tooth formation
Pre-eruptive color changes
EXCLUDES posteruptive color changes (521.7)

520.9 Unspecified disorder of tooth development and eruption

Diseases of the Digestive System *(left margin)*

521–522.8 *(left margin)*

√4th **521 Diseases of hard tissues of teeth**

√5th **521.0 Dental caries**
> AHA: 4Q, '01, 44

521.00 Dental caries, unspecified

521.01 Dental caries limited to enamel
> Initial caries
> White spot lesion

521.02 Dental caries extending into dentine

521.03 Dental caries extending into pulp

521.04 Arrested dental caries

521.05 Odontoclasia
> Infantile melanodontia
> Melanodontoclasia
> EXCLUDES *internal and external resorption of teeth (521.40-521.49)*
> DEF: A pathological dental condition described as stained areas, loss of tooth substance, and hypoplasia linked to nutritional deficiencies during tooth development and to cariogenic oral conditions.

521.06 Dental caries pit and fissure
> Primary dental caries, pit and fissure origin

521.07 Dental caries of smooth surface
> Primary dental caries, smooth surface origin

521.08 Dental caries of root surface
> Primary dental caries, root surface

521.09 Other dental caries
> AHA: 3Q, '02, 14

√5th **521.1 Excessive attrition (approximal wear) (occlusal wear)**

521.10 Excessive attrition, unspecified

521.11 Excessive attrition, limited to enamel

521.12 Excessive attrition, extending into dentine

521.13 Excessive attrition, extending into pulp

521.14 Excessive attrition, localized

521.15 Excessive attrition, generalized

√5th **521.2 Abrasion**
> Abrasion:
>   dentifrice
>   habitual
>   occupational } of teeth
>   ritual
>   traditional
> Wedge defect NOS

521.20 Abrasion, unspecified

521.21 Abrasion, limited to enamel

521.22 Abrasion, extending into dentine

521.23 Abrasion, extending into pulp

521.24 Abrasion, localized

521.25 Abrasion, generalized

√5th **521.3 Erosion**
> Erosion of teeth:
>   NOS
>   due to:
>   medicine
>   persistent vomiting
>   idiopathic
>   occupational

521.30 Erosion, unspecified

521.31 Erosion, limited to enamel

521.32 Erosion, extending into dentine

521.33 Erosion, extending into pulp

521.34 Erosion, localized

521.35 Erosion, generalized

√5th **521.4 Pathological resorption**
> DEF: Loss of dentin and cementum due to disease process.

521.40 Pathological resorption, unspecified

521.41 Pathological resorption, internal

521.42 Pathological resorption, external

521.49 Other pathological resorption
> Internal granuloma of pulp

521.5 Hypercementosis
> Cementation hyperplasia
> DEF: Excess deposits of cementum, on tooth root.

521.6 Ankylosis of teeth
> DEF: Adhesion of tooth to surrounding bone.

521.7 Intrinsic posteruptive color changes
> Staining [discoloration] of teeth:
>   NOS
>   due to:
>   drugs
>   metals
>   pulpal bleeding
> EXCLUDES *accretions [deposits] on teeth (523.6)*
> *extrinsic color changes (523.6)*
> *pre-eruptive color changes (520.8)*

√5th **521.8 Other specified diseases of hard tissues of teeth**

521.81 Cracked tooth
> EXCLUDES *asymptomatic craze lines in enamel — omit code*
> *broken tooth due to trauma (873.63, 873.73)*
> *fractured tooth due to trauma (873.63, 873.73)*

521.89 Other specified diseases of hard tissues of teeth
> Irradiated enamel
> Sensitive dentin

521.9 Unspecified disease of hard tissues of teeth

√4th **522 Diseases of pulp and periapical tissues**

522.0 Pulpitis
> Pulpal: Pulpitis:
>   abscess   acute
>   polyp   chronic (hyperplastic) (ulcerative)
>   suppurative

522.1 Necrosis of the pulp
> Pulp gangrene
> DEF: Death of pulp tissue.

522.2 Pulp degeneration
> Denticles   Pulp stones
> Pulp calcifications

522.3 Abnormal hard tissue formation in pulp
> Secondary or irregular dentin

522.4 Acute apical periodontitis of pulpal origin
> DEF: Severe inflammation of periodontal ligament due to pulpal inflammation or necrosis.

522.5 Periapical abscess without sinus
> Abscess:
>   dental
>   dentoalveolar
> EXCLUDES *periapical abscess with sinus (522.7)*

522.6 Chronic apical periodontitis
> Apical or periapical granuloma
> Apical periodontitis NOS

522.7 Periapical abscess with sinus
> Fistula:
>   alveolar process
>   dental

522.8 Radicular cyst
> Cyst:
>   apical (periodontal)
>   periapical
>   radiculodental
>   residual radicular
> DEF: Cyst in tissue around tooth apex due to chronic infection of granuloma around root.

N Newborn Age: 0   P Pediatric Age: 0-17   M Maternity Age: 12-55   A Adult Age: 15-124

522.9 Other and unspecified diseases of pulp and periapical tissues

✓4ᵗʰ 523 Gingival and periodontal diseases

✓5ᵗʰ 523.0 Acute gingivitis
> **EXCLUDES** acute necrotizing ulcerative gingivitis (101)
> herpetic gingivostomatitis (054.2)

523.00 Acute gingivitis, plaque induced
Acute gingivitis NOS

523.01 Acute gingivitis, non-plaque induced

✓5ᵗʰ 523.1 Chronic gingivitis
Gingivitis (chronic):
desquamative
hyperplastic
simple marginal
ulcerative
> **EXCLUDES** herpetic gingivostomatitis (054.2)

523.10 Chronic gingivitis, plaque induced
Chronic gingivitis NOS
Gingivitis NOS

523.11 Chronic gingivitis, non-plaque induced

✓5ᵗʰ 523.2 Gingival recession
Gingival recession (postinfective) (postoperative)

523.20 Gingival recession, unspecified

523.21 Gingival recession, minimal

523.22 Gingival recession, moderate

523.23 Gingival recession, severe

523.24 Gingival recession, localized

523.25 Gingival recession, generalized

✓5ᵗʰ 523.3 Aggressive and acute periodontitis
Acute:
pericementitis
pericoronitis
> **EXCLUDES** acute apical periodontitis (522.4)
> periapical abscess (522.5, 522.7)
DEF: Severe inflammation of tissues supporting teeth.

523.30 Aggressive periodontitis, unspecified

523.31 Aggressive periodontitis, localized
Periodontal abscess

523.32 Aggressive periodontitis, generalized

523.33 Acute periodontitis

✓5ᵗʰ 523.4 Chronic periodontitis
Chronic pericoronitis
Pericementitis (chronic)
Periodontitis:
NOS
complex
simplex
> **EXCLUDES** chronic apical periodontitis (522.6)

523.40 Chronic periodontitis, unspecified

523.41 Chronic periodontitis, localized

523.42 Chronic periodontitis, generalized

523.5 Periodontosis

523.6 Accretions on teeth
Dental calculus:
subgingival
supragingival
Deposits on teeth:
betel
materia alba
soft
tartar
tobacco
Extrinsic discoloration of teeth
> **EXCLUDES** intrinsic discoloration of teeth (521.7)
DEF: Foreign material on tooth surface, usually plaque or calculus.

523.8 Other specified periodontal diseases
Giant cell:
epulis
peripheral granuloma
Gingival:
cysts
enlargement NOS
fibromatosis
Gingival polyp
Periodontal lesions due to traumatic occlusion
Peripheral giant cell granuloma
> **EXCLUDES** leukoplakia of gingiva (528.6)

523.9 Unspecified gingival and periodontal disease
AHA: 3Q ,'02, 14

✓4ᵗʰ 524 Dentofacial anomalies, including malocclusion

✓5ᵗʰ 524.0 Major anomalies of jaw size
> **EXCLUDES** hemifacial atrophy or hypertrophy (754.0)
> unilateral condylar hyperplasia or hypoplasia of mandible (526.89)

524.00 Unspecified anomaly
DEF: Unspecified deformity of jaw size.

524.01 Maxillary hyperplasia
DEF: Overgrowth or over development of upper jaw bone.

524.02 Mandibular hyperplasia
DEF: Overgrowth or over development of lower jaw bone.

524.03 Maxillary hypoplasia
DEF: Incomplete or underdeveloped upper jaw bone.

524.04 Mandibular hypoplasia
DEF: Incomplete or underdeveloped lower jaw bone.

524.05 Macrogenia
DEF: Enlarged jaw, especially chin; affects bone, soft tissue, or both.

524.06 Microgenia
DEF: Underdeveloped mandible, characterized by an extremely small chin.

524.07 Excessive tuberosity of jaw
Entire maxillary tuberosity

524.09 Other specified anomaly

✓5ᵗʰ 524.1 Anomalies of relationship of jaw to cranial base

524.10 Unspecified anomaly
Prognathism
Retrognathism
DEF: Prognathism: protrusion of lower jaw.
DEF: Retrognathism: jaw is located posteriorly to a normally positioned jaw; backward position of mandible.

524.11 Maxillary asymmetry
DEF: Absence of symmetry of maxilla.

524.12 Other jaw asymmetry

524.19 Other specified anomaly

Angle's Classification of Malocclusion

Normal occlusion   Class I Malocclusion

Class II Malocclusion   Class III Malocclusion

Diseases of the Digestive System

524.2–525.19

√5ᵗʰ **524.2 Anomalies of dental arch relationship**
Anomaly of dental arch
EXCLUDES *hemifacial atrophy or hypertrophy (754.0)*
soft tissue impingement (524.81-524.82)
unilateral condylar hyperplasia or hypoplasia of
mandible (526.89)

524.20 Unspecified anomaly of dental arch relationship

524.21 Malocclusion, Angle's class I
Neutro-occlusion

524.22 Malocclusion, Angle's class II
Disto-occlusion Division I
Disto-occlusion Division II

524.23 Malocclusion, Angle's class III
Mesio-occlusion

524.24 Open anterior occlusal relationship
Anterior open bite

524.25 Open posterior occlusal relationship
Posterior open bite

524.26 Excessive horizontal overlap
Excessive horizontal overjet

524.27 Reverse articulation
Anterior articulation
Crossbite
Posterior articulation

524.28 Anomalies of interarch distance
Excessive interarch distance
Inadequate interarch distance

524.29 Other anomalies of dental arch relationship
Other anomalies of dental arch

√5ᵗʰ **524.3 Anomalies of tooth position of fully erupted teeth**
EXCLUDES *impacted or embedded teeth with abnormal position*
of such teeth or adjacent teeth (520.6)

524.30 Unspecified anomaly of tooth position
Diastema of teeth NOS
Displacement of teeth NOS
Transposition of teeth NOS

524.31 Crowding of teeth

524.32 Excessive spacing of teeth

524.33 Horizontal displacement of teeth
Tipped teeth
Tipping of teeth

524.34 Vertical displacement of teeth
Extruded tooth
Infraeruption of teeth
Intruded tooth
Supraeruption of teeth

524.35 Rotation of tooth/teeth

524.36 Insufficient interocclusal distance of teeth (ridge)
Lack of adequate intermaxillary vertical dimension

524.37 Excessive interocclusal distance of teeth
Excessive intermaxillary vertical dimension
Loss of occlusal vertical dimension

524.39 Other anomalies of tooth position

524.4 Malocclusion, unspecified
DEF: Malposition of top and bottom teeth; interferes with chewing.

√5ᵗʰ **524.5 Dentofacial functional abnormalities**

524.50 Dentofacial functional abnormality, unspecified

524.51 Abnormal jaw closure

524.52 Limited mandibular range of motion

524.53 Deviation in opening and closing of the mandible

524.54 Insufficient anterior guidance
Insufficient anterior occlusal guidance

524.55 Centric occlusion maximum intercuspation discrepancy
Centric occlusion of teeth discrepancy

524.56 Non-working side interference
Balancing side interference

524.57 Lack of posterior occlusal support

524.59 Other dentofacial functional abnormalities
Abnormal swallowing'   Sleep postures
Mouth breathing   Tongue, lip, or finger habits

√5ᵗʰ **524.6 Temporomandibular joint disorders**
EXCLUDES *current temporomandibular joint:*
dislocation (830.0-830.1)
strain (848.1)

524.60 Temporomandibular joint disorders, unspecified
Temporomandibular joint-pain-dysfunction syndrome [TMJ]

524.61 Adhesions and ankylosis (bony or fibrous)
DEF: Stiffening or union of temporomandibular joint due to bony or fibrous union across joint.

524.62 Arthralgia of temporomandibular joint
DEF: Pain in temporomandibular joint; not inflammatory in nature.

524.63 Articular disc disorder (reducing or non-reducing)

524.64 Temporomandibular joint sounds on opening and/or closing the jaw

524.69 Other specified temporomandibular joint disorders

√5ᵗʰ **524.7 Dental alveolar anomalies**

524.70 Unspecified alveolar anomaly

524.71 Alveolar maxillary hyperplasia
DEF: Excessive tissue formation in the dental alveoli of upper jaw.

524.72 Alveolar mandibular hyperplasia
DEF: Excessive tissue formation in the dental alveoli of lower jaw.

524.73 Alveolar maxillary hypoplasia
DEF: Incomplete or underdeveloped alveolar tissue of upper jaw.

524.74 Alveolar mandibular hypoplasia
DEF: Incomplete or underdeveloped alveolar tissue of lower jaw.

524.75 Vertical displacement of alveolus and teeth
Extrusion of alveolus and teeth

524.76 Occlusal plane deviation

524.79 Other specified alveolar anomaly

√5ᵗʰ **524.8 Other specified dentofacial anomalies**

524.81 Anterior soft tissue impingement

524.82 Posterior soft tissue impingement

524.89 Other specified dentofacial anomalies

524.9 Unspecified dentofacial anomalies

√4ᵗʰ **525 Other diseases and conditions of the teeth and supporting structures**

525.0 Exfoliation of teeth due to systemic causes
DEF: Deterioration of teeth and surrounding structures due to systemic disease.

√5ᵗʰ **525.1 Loss of teeth due to trauma, extraction, or periodontal disease**
Code first class of edentulism (525.40-525.44, 525.50-525.54)
AHA: 4Q, '05, 74; 4Q, '01, 44

525.10 *Acquired absence of teeth, unspecified*
Tooth extraction status, NOS

525.11 *Loss of teeth due to trauma*

525.12 *Loss of teeth due to periodontal disease*

525.13 *Loss of teeth due to caries*

525.19 *Other loss of teeth*

Diseases of the Digestive System

525.2–526.3

✓5ᵗʰ **525.2 Atrophy of edentulous alveolar ridge**

  525.20 Unspecified atrophy of edentulous alveolar ridge
    Atrophy of the mandible NOS
    Atrophy of the maxilla NOS

  525.21 Minimal atrophy of the mandible

  525.22 Moderate atrophy of the mandible

  525.23 Severe atrophy of the mandible

  525.24 Minimal atrophy of the maxilla

  525.25 Moderate atrophy of the maxilla

  525.26 Severe atrophy of the maxilla

525.3 Retained dental root

✓5ᵗʰ **525.4 Complete edentulism**
  Use additional code to identify cause of edentulism (525.10-525.19)
  AHA: 4Q, '05, 74

  525.40 Complete edentulism, unspecified
    Edentulism NOS

  525.41 Complete edentulism, class I

  525.42 Complete edentulism, class II

  525.43 Complete edentulism, class III

  525.44 Complete edentulism, class IV

✓5ᵗʰ **525.5 Partial edentulism**
  Use additional code to identify cause of edentulism (525.10-525.19)
  AHA: 4Q, '05, 74

  525.50 Partial edentulism, unspecified

  525.51 Partial edentulism, class I

  525.52 Partial edentulism, class II

  525.53 Partial edentulism, class III

  525.54 Partial edentulism, class IV

✓5ᵗʰ **525.6 Unsatisfactory restoration of tooth**
  Defective bridge, crown, fillings
  Defective dental restoration
  EXCLUDES *dental restoration status (V45.84)*
    unsatisfactory endodontic treatment (526.61-526.69)

  525.60 Unspecified unsatisfactory restoration of tooth
    Unspecified defective dental restoration

  525.61 Open restoration margins
    Dental restoration failure of marginal integrity
    Open margin on tooth restoration

  525.62 Unrepairable overhanging of dental restorative materials
    Overhanging of tooth restoration

  525.63 Fractured dental restorative material without loss of material
    EXCLUDES *cracked tooth (521.81)*
      fractured tooth (873.63, 873.73)

  525.64 Fractured dental restorative material with loss of material
    EXCLUDES *cracked tooth (521.81)*
      fractured tooth (873.63, 873.73)

  525.65 Contour of existing restoration of tooth biologically incompatible with oral health
    Dental restoration failure of periodontal anatomical integrity
    Unacceptable contours of existing restoration
    Unacceptable morphology of existing restoration

  525.66 Allergy to existing dental restorative material
    Use additional code to identify the specific type of allergy

  525.67 Poor aesthetics of existing restoration
    Dental restoration aesthetically inadequate or displeasing

  525.69 Other unsatisfactory restoration of existing tooth

✓5ᵗʰ **525.7 Endosseous dental implant failure**

  525.71 Osseointegration failure of dental implant
    Failure of dental implant due to infection
    Failure of dental implant due to unintentional loading
    Failure of dental implant osseointegration due to premature loading
    Failure of dental implant to osseointegrate prior to intentional prosthetic loading
    Hemorrhagic complications of dental implant placement
    Iatrogenic osseointegration failure of dental implant
    Osseointegration failure of dental implant due to complications of systemic disease
    Osseointegration failure of dental implant due to poor bone quality
    Pre-integration failure of dental implant NOS
    Pre-osseointegration failure of dental implant

  525.72 Post-osseointegration biological failure of dental implant
    Failure of dental implant due to lack of attached gingiva
    Failure of dental implant due to occlusal trauma (caused by poor prosthetic design)
    Failure of dental implant due to parafunctional habits
    Failure of dental implant due to periodontal infection (peri-implantitis)
    Failure of dental implant due to poor oral hygiene
    Failure of dental implant to osseointegrate following intentional prosthetic loading
    Iatrogenic post-osseointegration failure of dental implant
    Post-osseointegration failure of dental implant due to complications of systemic disease

  525.73 Post-osseointegration mechanic failure of dental implant
    Failure of dental prosthesis causing loss of dental implant
    Fracture of dental implant
    Mechanical failure of dental implant NOS
    EXCLUDES *cracked tooth (521.81)*
      fractured dental restorative material with loss of material (525.64)
      fractured dental restorative material without loss of material (525.63)
      fractured tooth (873.63, 873.73)

  525.79 Other endosseous dental implant failure
    Dental implant failure NOS

525.8 Other specified disorders of the teeth and supporting structures
  Enlargement of alveolar ridge NOS
  Irregular alveolar process

525.9 Unspecified disorder of the teeth and supporting structures

✓4ᵗʰ **526 Diseases of the jaws**

526.0 Developmental odontogenic cysts
  Cyst: Cyst:
    dentigerous   lateral periodontal
    eruption   primordial
    follicular   Keratocyst
    lateral developmental
  EXCLUDES *radicular cyst (522.8)*

526.1 Fissural cysts of jaw
  Cyst: Cyst:
    globulomaxillary   median palatal
    incisor canal   nasopalatine
    median anterior maxillary   palatine of papilla
  EXCLUDES *cysts of oral soft tissues (528.4)*

526.2 Other cysts of jaws
  Cyst of jaw: Cyst of jaw:
    NOS   hemorrhagic
    aneurysmal   traumatic

526.3 Central giant cell (reparative) granuloma
  EXCLUDES *peripheral giant cell granuloma (523.8)*

Diseases of the Digestive System

526.4 Inflammatory conditions

Abscess
Osteitis
Osteomyelitis (neonatal)
Periostitis
} of jaw (acute) (chronic) (suppurative)

Sequestrum of jaw bone

EXCLUDES *alveolar osteitis (526.5)*
osteonecrosis of jaw (733.45)

526.5 Alveolitis of jaw

Alveolar osteitis   Dry socket

DEF: Inflammation of alveoli or tooth socket.

✓5ᵗʰ 526.6 Periradicular pathology associated with previous endodontic treatment

526.61 Perforation of root canal space

526.62 Endodontic overfill

526.63 Endodontic underfill

526.69 Other periradicular pathology associated with previous endodontic treatment

✓5ᵗʰ 526.8 Other specified diseases of the jaws

526.81 Exostosis of jaw

Torus mandibularis   Torus palatinus

DEF: Spur or bony outgrowth on the jaw.

526.89 Other

Cherubism
Fibrous dysplasia
Latent bone cyst
Osteoradionecrosis
} of jaw(s)

Unilateral condylar hyperplasia or hypoplasia of mandible

526.9 Unspecified disease of the jaws

AHA: 4Q, '10, 93-94

✓4ᵗʰ 527 Diseases of the salivary glands

527.0 Atrophy

DEF: Wasting away, necrosis of salivary gland tissue.

527.1 Hypertrophy

DEF: Overgrowth or overdeveloped salivary gland tissue.

527.2 Sialoadenitis

Parotitis: Sialoangitis
     NOS   Sialodochitis
     allergic
     toxic

EXCLUDES *epidemic or infectious parotitis (072.0-072.9)*
uveoparotid fever (135)

DEF: Inflammation of salivary gland.

527.3 Abscess

527.4 Fistula

EXCLUDES *congenital fistula of salivary gland (750.24)*

527.5 Sialolithiasis

Calculus
Stone
} of salivary gland or duct

Sialodocholithiasis

527.6 Mucocele

Mucous:
     extravasation cyst of salivary gland
     retention cyst of salivary gland
Ranula

DEF: Dilated salivary gland cavity filled with mucous.

527.7 Disturbance of salivary secretion

Hyposecretion   Sialorrhea
Ptyalism   Xerostomia

527.8 Other specified diseases of the salivary glands

Benign lymphoepithelial lesion of salivary gland
Sialectasia
Sialosis
Stenosis
Stricture
} of salivary duct

527.9 Unspecified disease of the salivary glands

✓4ᵗʰ 528 Diseases of the oral soft tissues, excluding lesions specific for gingiva and tongue

✓5ᵗʰ 528.0 Stomatitis and mucositis (ulcerative)

EXCLUDES *cellulitis and abscess of mouth (528.3)*
diphtheritic stomatitis (032.0)
epizootic stomatitis (078.4)
gingivitis (523.0-523.1)
oral thrush (112.0)
Stevens-Johnson syndrome (695.13)
stomatitis:
     acute necrotizing ulcerative (101)
     aphthous (528.2)
     gangrenous (528.1)
     herpetic (054.2)
     Vincent's (101)

DEF: Stomatitis: Inflammation of oral mucosa; labial and buccal mucosa, tongue, palate, floor of the mouth, and gingivae.

AHA: 2Q, '99, 9

TIP: Do not assign if documented as fungal oral thrush, or as due to candidiasis. See instead 112.0.

528.00 Stomatitis and mucositis, unspecified

Mucositis NOS
Ulcerative mucositis NOS
Ulcerative stomatitis NOS
Vesicular stomatitis NOS

AHA: 4Q, '06, 88-90

528.01 Mucositis (ulcerative) due to antineoplastic therapy

Use additional E code to identify adverse effects of therapy, such as:
     antineoplastic and immunosuppressive drugs (E930.7, E933.1)
     radiation therapy (E879.2)

AHA: 4Q, '06, 88-90

528.02 Mucositis (ulcerative) due to other drugs

Use additional E code to identify drug

AHA: 4Q, '06, 88-90

528.09 Other stomatitis and mucositis (ulcerative)

AHA: 4Q, '06, 88-90

528.1 Cancrum oris

Gangrenous stomatitis
Noma

DEF: A severely gangrenous lesion of mouth due to fusospirochetal infection; destroys buccal, labial and facial tissues; can be fatal; found primarily in debilitated and malnourished children.

528.2 Oral aphthae

Aphthous stomatitis
Canker sore
Periadenitis mucosa necrotica recurrens
Recurrent aphthous ulcer
Stomatitis herpetiformis

EXCLUDES *herpetic stomatitis (054.2)*

DEF: Small oval or round ulcers of the mouth marked by a grayish exudate and a red halo effect.

528.3 Cellulitis and abscess

Cellulitis of mouth (floor)
Ludwig's angina
Oral fistula

EXCLUDES *abscess of tongue (529.0)*
cellulitis or abscess of lip (528.5)
fistula (of):
     dental (522.7)
     lip (528.5)
gingivitis (523.00-523.11)

528.4 Cysts

Dermoid cyst
Epidermoid cyst
Epstein's pearl
Lymphoepithelial cyst
Nasoalveolar cyst
Nasolabial cyst
} of mouth

EXCLUDES *cyst:*
     gingiva (523.8)
     tongue (529.8)

528.5 Diseases of lips

Abscess ⎫
Cellulitis ⎬ of lips
Fistula ⎪
Hypertrophy ⎭

Cheilitis:
  NOS
  angular
Cheilodynia
Cheilosis

EXCLUDES *actinic cheilitis (692.79)*
congenital fistula of lip (750.25)
leukoplakia of lips (528.6)

AHA: S-O, '86, 10

528.6 Leukoplakia of oral mucosa, including tongue

Leukokeratosis of oral mucosa
Leukoplakia of:
  gingiva
  lips
  tongue

EXCLUDES *carcinoma in situ (230.0, 232.0)*
leukokeratosis nicotina palati (528.79)

DEF: Thickened white patches of epithelium on mucous membranes of mouth.

√5ᵗʰ **528.7 Other disturbances of oral epithelium, including tongue**

EXCLUDES *carcinoma in situ (230.0, 232.0)*
leukokeratosis NOS (702.8)

528.71 Minimal keratinized residual ridge mucosa
Minimal keratinization of alveolar ridge mucosa

528.72 Excessive keratinized residual ridge mucosa
Excessive keratinization of alveolar ridge mucosa

528.79 Other disturbances of oral epithelium, including tongue
Erythroplakia of mouth or tongue
Focal epithelial hyperplasia of mouth or tongue
Leukoedema of mouth or tongue
Leukokeratosis nicotina palate
Other oral epithelium disturbances

528.8 Oral submucosal fibrosis, including of tongue

528.9 Other and unspecified diseases of the oral soft tissues
Cheek and lip biting
Denture sore mouth
Denture stomatitis
Melanoplakia
Papillary hyperplasia of palate

Eosinophilic granuloma ⎫
Irritative hyperplasisa ⎬ of oral mucosa
Pyogenic granuloma ⎪
Ulcer (traumatic) ⎭

√4ᵗʰ **529 Diseases and other conditions of the tongue**

529.0 Glossitis

Abscess ⎫ of tongue
Ulceration (traumatic) ⎭

EXCLUDES *glossitis:*
benign migratory (529.1)
Hunter's (529.4)
median rhomboid (529.2)
Moeller's (529.4)

529.1 Geographic tongue
Benign migratory glossitis
Glossitis areata exfoliativa

DEF: Chronic glossitis; marked by filiform papillae atrophy and inflammation; no known etiology.

529.2 Median rhomboid glossitis

DEF: A noninflammatory, congenital disease characterized by rhomboid-like lesions at the middle third of the tongue's dorsal surface.

529.3 Hypertrophy of tongue papillae
Black hairy tongue
Coated tongue
Hypertrophy of foliate papillae
Lingua villosa nigra

529.4 Atrophy of tongue papillae
Bald tongue
Glazed tongue
Glossitis:
  Hunter's
  Moeller's
Glossodynia exfoliativa
Smooth atrophic tongue

529.5 Plicated tongue

Fissured ⎫
Furrowed ⎬ tongue
Scrotal ⎭

EXCLUDES *fissure of tongue, congenital (750.13)*

DEF: Cracks, fissures or furrows, on dorsal surface of tongue.

529.6 Glossodynia
Glossopyrosis
Painful tongue

EXCLUDES *glossodynia exfoliativa (529.4)*

529.8 Other specified conditions of the tongue

Atrophy ⎫
Crenated ⎬ (of) tongue
Enlargement ⎪
Hypertrophy ⎭

Glossocele
Glossoptosis

EXCLUDES *erythroplasia of tongue (528.79)*
leukoplakia of tongue (528.6)
macroglossia (congenital) (750.15)
microglossia (congenital) (750.16)
oral submucosal fibrosis (528.8)

529.9 Unspecified condition of the tongue

Diseases of Esophagus, Stomach, and Duodenum (530-539)

√4ᵗʰ **530 Diseases of esophagus**

EXCLUDES *esophageal varices (456.0-456.2)*

530.0 Achalasia and cardiospasm
Achalasia (of cardia)
Aperistalsis of esophagus
Megaesophagus

EXCLUDES *congenital cardiospasm (750.7)*

DEF: Failure of smooth muscle fibers to relax at gastrointestinal junctures, such as esophagogastric sphincter when swallowing.

√5ᵗʰ **530.1 Esophagitis**

Esophagitis: Esphagitis:
  chemical   postoperative
  peptic   regurgitant

Use additional E code to identify cause, if induced by chemical

EXCLUDES *tuberculous esophagitis (017.8)*

AHA: 4Q, '93, 27; 1Q, '92, 17; 3Q, '91, 20

TIP: Do not assign if esophagitis due to candidiasis; see instead code 112.84.

530.10 Esophagitis, unspecified
Esophagitis NOS

AHA: 3Q, '05, 17

Esophagus

Pharyngeal constrictors
Front view
Epiglottis
Cricoid cartilage
C6
Trachea
Pharyngoesophageal sphincter
Side view
Gastroesophageal sphincter
Diaphragm
Stomach

√4ᵗʰ √5ᵗʰ Additional Digit Required   Unspecified Code   Other Specified Code   Manifestation Code   ►◄ Revised Text   ● New Code   ▲ Revised Code Title

2013 ICD-9-CM   **Volume 1 – 163**

Diseases of the Digestive System

530.11–531.4

530.11 Reflux esophagitis
DEF: Inflammation of lower esophagus; due to regurgitated gastric acid.
AHA: 4Q, '95, 82
K21.0 Gastro-esophageal reflux disease w/esophagitis ⟨I-10⟩

530.12 Acute esophagitis
DEF: An acute inflammation of the mucous lining or submucosal coat of the esophagus.
AHA: 4Q, '01, 45

530.13 Eosinophilic esophagitis
AHA: 4Q, '08, 115-116

530.19 Other esophagitis
Abscess of esophagus
AHA: 3Q, '01, 10
K20.8 Other esophagitis ⟨I-10⟩

✓5th 530.2 Ulcer of esophagus
Ulcer of esophagus:
  fungal
  peptic
Ulcer of esophagus due to ingestion of:
  aspirin
  chemicals
  medicines
Use additional E code to identify cause, if induced by chemical or drug
AHA: 4Q, '03, 63

530.20 Ulcer of esophagus without bleeding
Ulcer of esophagus NOS

530.21 Ulcer of esophagus with bleeding
EXCLUDES bleeding esophageal varices (456.0, 456.20)

530.3 Stricture and stenosis of esophagus
Compression of esophagus
Obstruction of esophagus
EXCLUDES congenital stricture of esophagus (750.3)
AHA: ▶1Q, '12, 15;◀ 2Q, '01, 4; 2Q, '97, 3; 1Q, '88, 13
TIP: If esophageal obstruction is due to impacted foreign body, such as meat or other substance, assign instead code 935.1.
K22.2 Esophageal obstruction ⟨I-10⟩

530.4 Perforation of esophagus
Rupture of esophagus
EXCLUDES traumatic perforation of esophagus (862.22, 862.32, 874.4-874.5)

530.5 Dyskinesia of esophagus
Corkscrew esophagus
Curling esophagus
Esophagospasm
Spasm of esophagus
EXCLUDES cardiospasm (530.0)
DEF: Difficulty performing voluntary esophageal movements.
AHA: 1Q, '88, 13; N-D, '84, 19

530.6 Diverticulum of esophagus, acquired
Diverticulum, acquired:
  epiphrenic
  pharyngoesophageal
  pulsion
  subdiaphragmatic
  traction
  Zenker's (hypopharyngeal)
Esophageal pouch, acquired
Esophagocele, acquired
EXCLUDES congenital diverticulum of esophagus (750.4)
AHA: J-F, '85, 3

530.7 Gastroesophageal laceration-hemorrhage syndrome
Mallory-Weiss syndrome
DEF: Laceration of distal esophagus and proximal stomach due to vomiting, hiccups or other sustained activity.

✓5th 530.8 Other specified disorders of esophagus

530.81 Esophageal reflux
Gastroesophageal reflux
EXCLUDES reflux esophagitis (530.11)
DEF: Regurgitation of the gastric contents into esophagus and possibly pharynx.
AHA: 4Q, '10, 97; 2Q, '01, 4; 1Q, '95, 7; 4Q, '92, 27
K21.9 Gastro-esophageal reflux dz w/o esophagitis ⟨I-10⟩

530.82 Esophageal hemorrhage
EXCLUDES hemorrhage due to esophageal varices (456.0-456.2)
AHA: 1Q, '05, 17

530.83 Esophageal leukoplakia

530.84 Tracheoesophageal fistula
EXCLUDES congenital tracheoesophageal fistula (750.3)

530.85 Barrett's esophagus
DEF: A metaplastic disorder in which specialized columnar epithelial cells replace the normal squamous epithelial cells; secondary to chronic gastroesophageal reflux damage to the mucosa; increases risk of developing adenocarcinoma.
AHA: 4Q, '03, 63
K22.70 Barrett's esophagus w/o dysphagia ⟨I-10⟩

530.86 Infection of esophagostomy
Use additional code to specify infection

530.87 Mechanical complication of esophagostomy
Malfunction of esophagostomy

530.89 Other
EXCLUDES Paterson-Kelly syndrome (280.8)

530.9 Unspecified disorder of esophagus

✓4th 531 Gastric ulcer
INCLUDES ulcer (peptic):
  prepyloric
  pylorus
  stomach
Use additional E code to identify drug, if drug-induced
EXCLUDES peptic ulcer NOS (533.0-533.9)

The following fifth-digit subclassification is for use with category 531:
  0 without mention of obstruction
  1 with obstruction

DEF: Destruction of tissue in lumen of stomach due to action of gastric acid and pepsin on gastric mucosa decreasing resistance to ulcers.
AHA: 1Q, '91, 15; 4Q, '90, 27

§ ✓5th **531.0 Acute with hemorrhage**
[0-1]   **AHA:** N-D, '84, 15

§ ✓5th **531.1 Acute with perforation**
[0-1]

§ ✓5th **531.2 Acute with hemorrhage and perforation**
[0-1]

§ ✓5th **531.3 Acute without mention of hemorrhage or perforation**
[0-1]

§ ✓5th **531.4 Chronic or unspecified with hemorrhage**
[0-1]   **AHA:** 4Q, '90, 22
K25.4 Chronic/unspec gastric ulcer w/hemorrhage ⟨I-10⟩

Stomach

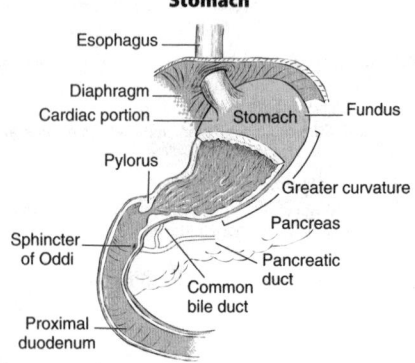

§ Requires fifth digit. Valid digits are in [brackets] under each code. See category 531 for codes and definitions.

⟨N⟩ Newborn Age: 0   ⟨P⟩ Pediatric Age: 0-17   ⟨M⟩ Maternity Age: 12-55   ⟨A⟩ Adult Age: 15-124

164 – Volume 1 • October 2012   **2013 ICD-9-CM**

§ ✓5ᵗʰ **531.5 Chronic or unspecified with perforation**
[0-1]

§ ✓5ᵗʰ **531.6 Chronic or unspecified with hemorrhage and**
[0-1] **perforation**

§ ✓5ᵗʰ **531.7 Chronic without mention of hemorrhage or**
[0-1] **perforation**

§ ✓5ᵗʰ **531.9 Unspecified as acute or chronic, without mention**
[0-1] **of hemorrhage or perforation**
     K25.9 Gastric ulcer uns acute/chronic w/o hem/perf   I-10

✓4ᵗʰ **532 Duodenal ulcer**
    INCLUDES   erosion (acute) of duodenum
                ulcer (peptic):
                   duodenum
                   postpyloric
    Use additional E code to identify drug, if drug-induced
    EXCLUDES   *peptic ulcer NOS (533.0-533.9)*

    The following fifth-digit subclassification is for use with category 532:
     0 without mention of obstruction
     1 with obstruction

    DEF: Ulcers in duodenum due to action of gastric acid and pepsin on mucosa decreasing resistance to ulcers.
    AHA: 4Q, '90, 27; 1Q, '91, 15

§ ✓5ᵗʰ **532.0 Acute with hemorrhage**
[0-1]   **AHA:** 4Q, '90, 22

§ ✓5ᵗʰ **532.1 Acute with perforation**
[0-1]

§ ✓5ᵗʰ **532.2 Acute with hemorrhage and perforation**
[0-1]

§ ✓5ᵗʰ **532.3 Acute without mention of hemorrhage or perforation**
[0-1]

§ ✓5ᵗʰ **532.4 Chronic or unspecified with hemorrhage**
[0-1]   K26.4 Chronic/unspecified duodenal ulcer w/hemorrhage   I-10

§ ✓5ᵗʰ **532.5 Chronic or unspecified with perforation**
[0-1]

§ ✓5ᵗʰ **532.6 Chronic or unspecified with hemorrhage and**
[0-1] **perforation**

§ ✓5ᵗʰ **532.7 Chronic without mention of hemorrhage or**
[0-1] **perforation**

§ ✓5ᵗʰ **532.9 Unspecified as acute or chronic, without mention**
[0-1] **of hemorrhage or perfortaion**
     K26.9 Duodenal ulcer uns acute/chronic w/o hem/perf   I-10

✓4ᵗʰ **533 Peptic ulcer, site unspecified**
    INCLUDES   gastroduodenal ulcer NOS
                peptic ulcer NOS
                stress ulcer NOS
    Use additional E code to identify drug, if drug-induced
    EXCLUDES   *peptic ulcer:*
            duodenal (532.0-532.9)
            gastric (531.0-531.9)

    The following fifth-digit subclassification is for use with category 533:
     0 without mention of obstruction
     1 with obstruction

    DEF: Ulcer of mucous membrane of esophagus, stomach or duodenum due to gastric acid secretion.
    AHA: 1Q, '91, 15; 4Q, '90, 27

§ ✓5ᵗʰ **533.0 Acute with hemorrhage**
[0-1]

§ ✓5ᵗʰ **533.1 Acute with perforation**
[0-1]

§ ✓5ᵗʰ **533.2 Acute with hemorrhage and perforation**
[0-1]

§ ✓5ᵗʰ **533.3 Acute without mention of hemorrhage and**
[0-1] **perforation**

§ ✓5ᵗʰ **533.4 Chronic or unspecified with hemorrhage**
[0-1]

§ ✓5ᵗʰ **533.5 Chronic or unspecified with perforation**
[0-1]

§ ✓5ᵗʰ **533.6 Chronic or unspecified with hemorrhage and**
[0-1] **perforation**

§ ✓5ᵗʰ **533.7 Chronic without mention of hemorrhage or**
[0-1] **perforation**
     AHA: 2Q, '89, 16

§ ✓5ᵗʰ **533.9 Unspecified as acute or chronic, without**
[0-1] **mention of hemorrhage or perforation**

✓4ᵗʰ **534 Gastrojejunal ulcer**
    INCLUDES   ulcer (peptic) or erosion:
              anastomotic
              gastrocolic
              gastrointestinal
              gastrojejunal
              jejunal
              marginal
              stomal
    EXCLUDES   *primary ulcer of small intestine (569.82)*

    The following fifth-digit subclassification is for use with category 534:
     0 without mention of obstruction
     1 with obstruction

    AHA: 1Q, '91, 15; 4Q, '90, 27

§ ✓5ᵗʰ **534.0 Acute with hemorrhage**
[0-1]

§ ✓5ᵗʰ **534.1 Acute with perforation**
[0-1]

§ ✓5ᵗʰ **534.2 Acute with hemorrhage and perforation**
[0-1]

§ ✓5ᵗʰ **534.3 Acute without mention of hemorrhage or perforation**
[0-1]

§ ✓5ᵗʰ **534.4 Chronic or unspecified with hemorrhage**
[0-1]

§ ✓5ᵗʰ **534.5 Chronic or unspecified with perforation**
[0-1]

§ ✓5ᵗʰ **534.6 Chronic or unspecified with hemorrhage and perforation**
[0-1]

§ ✓5ᵗʰ **534.7 Chronic without mention of hemorrhage or perforation**
[0-1]

§ ✓5ᵗʰ **534.9 Unspecified as acute or chronic, without mention**
[0-1] **of hemorrhage or perforation**

✓4ᵗʰ **535 Gastritis and duodenitis**
    The following fifth-digit subclassification is for use with category 535:
     0 without mention of hemorrhage
     1 with hemorrhage

    AHA: 2Q, '92, 9; 4Q, '91, 25

§ ✓5ᵗʰ **535.0 Acute gastritis**
[0-1]   **AHA:** 2Q, '92, 8; N-D, '86, 9

§ ✓5ᵗʰ **535.1 Atrophic gastritis**
[0-1]   Gastritis:
          atrophic-hyperplastic
          chronic (atrophic)
      DEF: Inflammation of stomach, with mucous membrane atrophy and peptic gland destruction.
      AHA: 1Q, '94, 18
      K29.50 Unspecified chronic gastritis without bleeding   I-10

§ ✓5ᵗʰ **535.2 Gastric mucosal hypertrophy**
[0-1]   Hypertrophic gastritis

§ ✓5ᵗʰ **535.3 Alcoholic gastritis**
[0-1]

§ ✓5ᵗʰ **535.4 Other specified gastritis**
[0-1]   Gastritis: Gastritis:
        allergic   superficial
        bile induced   toxic
        irritant
      EXCLUDES   *eosinophilic gastritis (535.7)*
      AHA: 4Q, '90, 27

---

§   Requires fifth digit. Valid digits are in [brackets] under each code. See appropriate category for codes and definitions.

✓4ᵗʰ ✓5ᵗʰ Additional Digit Required   Unspecified Code   Other Specified Code   Manifestation Code   ▶◀ Revised Text   ● New Code   ▲ Revised Code Title

Diseases of the Digestive System

535.5–537.9

§ ✓5ᵗʰ **535.5 Unspecified gastritis and gastroduodenitis**
[0-1]   AHA: For code 535.50: 3Q, '05, 17; 4Q, '99, 25

§ ✓5ᵗʰ **535.6 Duodenitis**
[0-1]   DEF: Inflammation of intestine, between pylorus and jejunum.
AHA: For code 535.60: 3Q, '05, 17
K29.80 Duodenitis without bleeding   I-10

§ ✓5ᵗʰ **535.7 Eosinophilic gastritis**
[0-1]   AHA: 4Q, '08, 115-116

✓4ᵗʰ **536 Disorders of function of stomach**
     EXCLUDES *functional disorders of stomach specified as psychogenic (306.4)*

536.0 Achlorhydria
     DEF: Absence of gastric acid due to gastric mucosa atrophy; unresponsive to histamines; also known as gastric anacidity.

536.1 Acute dilatation of stomach
     Acute distention of stomach

536.2 Persistent vomiting
     Cyclical vomiting
     Habit vomiting
     Persistent vomiting [not of pregnancy]
     Uncontrollable vomiting
     EXCLUDES *bilious emesis (vomiting) (787.04)*
       excessive vomiting in pregnancy (643.0-643.9)
       vomiting NOS (787.03)
        cyclical, associated with migraine (346.2)
       vomiting of fecal matter (569.87)

536.3 Gastroparesis
     Gastroparalysis
     Code first underlying disease, if known, such as:
       diabetes mellitus (249.6, 250.6)
     DEF: Slight degree of paralysis within muscular coat of stomach.
     AHA: 4Q, '08, 94; 2Q, '04, 7; 2Q, '01, 4; 4Q, '94, 42

✓5ᵗʰ **536.4 Gastrostomy complications**
     AHA: 4Q, '98, 42
     TIP: Do not assign code 997.4 Digestive system complications, for any gastrostomy complications.

     536.40 Gastrostomy complication, unspecified

     536.41 Infection of gastrostomy
       Use additional code to identify organism (041.00-041.9)
       Use additional code to specify type of infection, such as:
         abscess or cellulitis of abdomen (682.2)
         septicemia (038.0-038.9)
       AHA: 4Q, '98, 42

     536.42 Mechanical complication of gastrostomy

     536.49 Other gastrostomy complications
       AHA: 4Q, '98, 42

536.8 Dyspepsia and other specified disorders of function of stomach
     Achylia gastrica   Hypochlorhydria
     Hourglass contraction of stomach   Indigestion
     Hyperacidity   Tachygastria
     Hyperchlorhydria
     EXCLUDES *achlorhydria (536.0)*
       heartburn (787.1)
     AHA: 2Q, '93, 6; 2Q, '89, 16; N-D, '84, 9
     K30 Functional dyspepsia   I-10

536.9 Unspecified functional disorder of stomach
     Functional gastrointestinal:
       disorder
       disturbance
       irritation

✓4ᵗʰ **537 Other disorders of stomach and duodenum**

537.0 Acquired hypertrophic pyloric stenosis
     Constriction ⎫
     Obstruction ⎬ of pylorus, acquired or adult
     Stricture ⎭
     EXCLUDES *congenital or infantile pyloric stenosis (750.5)*
     AHA: 2Q, '01, 4; J-F, '85, 14

Duodenum

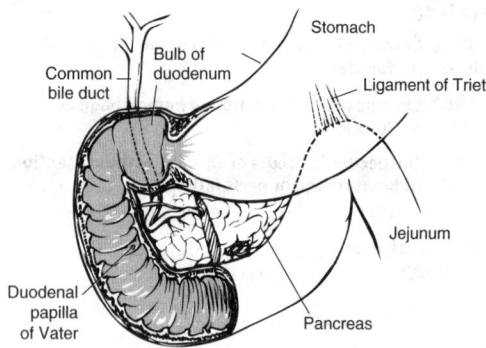

537.1 Gastric diverticulum
     EXCLUDES *congenital diverticulum of stomach (750.7)*
     DEF: Herniated sac or pouch within stomach or duodenum.
     AHA: J-F, '85, 4

537.2 Chronic duodenal ileus
     DEF: Persistent obstruction between pylorus and jejunum.

537.3 Other obstruction of duodenum
     Cicatrix ⎫
     Stenosis ⎬ of duodenum
     Stricture ⎪
     Volvulus ⎭
     EXCLUDES *congenital obstruction of duodenum (751.1)*

537.4 Fistula of stomach or duodenum
     Gastrocolic fistula
     Gastrojejunocolic fistula
     AHA: ▶1Q, '12, 10◄
     TIP: ▶Assign when a previous G-tube site has failed to spontaneously close and requires further treatment.◄

537.5 Gastroptosis
     DEF: Downward displacement of stomach.

537.6 Hourglass stricture or stenosis of stomach
     Cascade stomach
     EXCLUDES *congenital hourglass stomach (750.7)*
       hourglass contraction of stomach (536.8)

✓5ᵗʰ **537.8 Other specified disorders of stomach and duodenum**
     AHA: 4Q, '91, 25

     537.81 Pylorospasm
       EXCLUDES *congenital pylorospasm (750.5)*
       DEF: Spasm of the pyloric sphincter.

     537.82 Angiodysplasia of stomach and duodenum (without mention of hemorrhage)
       AHA: 2Q, '07, 7; 3Q, '96, 10; 4Q, '90, 4

     537.83 Angiodysplasia of stomach and duodenum with hemorrhage
       DEF: Bleeding of stomach and duodenum due to vascular abnormalities.
       AHA: 2Q, '07, 7

     537.84 Dieulafoy lesion (hemorrhagic) of stomach and duodenum
       DEF: An abnormally large and convoluted submucosal artery protruding through a defect in the mucosa in the stomach or intestines that can erode the epithelium causing hemorrhaging.
       AHA: 4Q, '02, 60

     537.89 Other
       Gastric or duodenal:
         prolapse
         rupture
       Intestinal metaplasia of gastric mucosa
       Passive congestion of stomach
       EXCLUDES *diverticula of duodenum (562.00-562.01)*
         gastrointestinal hemorrhage (578.0-578.9)
       AHA: 1Q, '11, 10-11; 3Q, '05, 15; N-D, '84, 7
       TIP: Assign for congestive portal gastropathy or portal hypertensive gastropathy.

537.9 Unspecified disorder of stomach and duodenum

N   Newborn Age: 0   P   Pediatric Age: 0-17   M   Maternity Age: 12-55   A   Adult Age: 15-124

538 Gastrointestinal mucositis (ulcerative)

Use additional E code to identify adverse effects of therapy, such as:
antineoplastic and immunosuppressive drugs (E930.7, E933.1)
radiation therapy (E879.2)

EXCLUDES *mucositis (ulcerative) of mouth and oral soft tissue (528.00-528.09)*

AHA: 4Q, '06, 88-90

√4ᵗʰ 539 Complications of bariatric procedures

TIP: ▶ If associated dumping syndrome is documented, assign also code 564.2.◀

√5ᵗʰ 539.0 Complications of gastric band procedure

AHA: 4Q, '11, 125-127

539.01 Infection due to gastric band procedure

Use additional code to specify type of infection,
such as:
abscess or cellulitis of abdomen (682.2)
septicemia (038.0-038.9)
Use additional code to identify organism
(041.00-041.9)

AHA: 4Q, '11, 127

539.09 Other complications of gastric band procedure

Use additional code(s) to further specify the
complication

√5ᵗʰ 539.8 Complications of other bariatric procedure

EXCLUDES *complications of gastric band procedure
(539.01-539.09)*

AHA: 4Q, '11, 125-127

539.81 Infection due to other bariatric procedure

Use additional code to specify type of infection,
such as:
abscess or cellulitis of abdomen (682.2)
septicemia (038.0-038.9)
Use additional code to identify organism
(041.00-041.9)

539.89 Other complications of other bariatric procedure

Use additional code(s) to further specify the
complication

Appendicitis (540-543)

√4ᵗʰ 540 Acute appendicitis

DEF: Inflammation of vermiform appendix due to fecal obstruction,
neoplasm or foreign body of appendiceal lumen; causes infection, edema
and infarction of appendiceal wall; may result in mural necrosis, and
perforation.

AHA: N-D, '84, 19

540.0 With generalized peritonitis

Appendicitis ⎱ perforation ⎰ ⎱ fulminating
(acute) ⎰ peritonitis (generalized) ⎱ gangrenous
with: ⎰ rupture ⎰ obstructive

Cecitis (acute) with perforation, peritonitis (generalized),
rupture
Rupture of appendix

EXCLUDES *acute appendicitis with peritoneal abscess (540.1)*

K35.2 Acute appendicitis w/generalized peritonitis   I-10

540.1 With peritoneal abscess

Abscess of appendix   With generalized peritonitis

AHA: N-D, '84, 19

Appendix

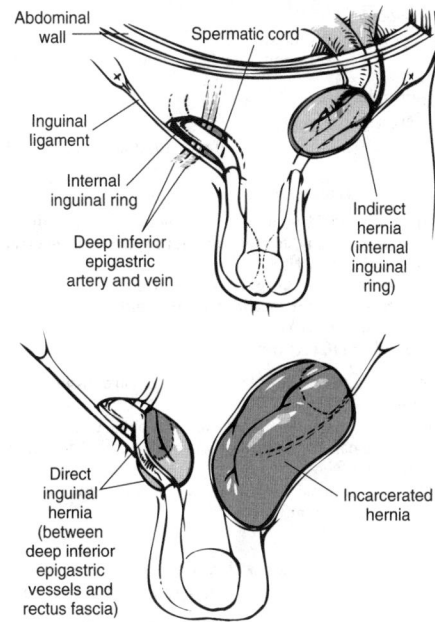

Appendicular artery
Mesoappendix
Cecum
Vermiform appendix

Inguinal Hernias

Abdominal wall
Spermatic cord
Inguinal ligament
Internal inguinal ring
Deep inferior epigastric artery and vein
Indirect hernia (internal inguinal ring)
Direct inguinal hernia (between deep inferior epigastric vessels and rectus fascia)
Incarcerated hernia

540.9 Without mention of peritonitis

Acute appendicitis without mention of perforation,
peritonitis, or rupture:
fulminating
gangrenous
inflamed
obstructive

Acute cecitis without mention of perforation, peritonitis, or
rupture

AHA: 1Q, '01, 15; 4Q, '97, 52

K35.80 Unspecified acute appendicitis   I-10

541 Appendicitis, unqualified

AHA: 2Q, '90, 26

TIP: Do not assign for normal appendix found at appendectomy. Assign
instead symptom code (e.g., abdominal pain).

542 Other appendicitis

Appendicitis: Appendicitis:
chronic   relapsing
recurrent   subacute

EXCLUDES *hyperplasia (lymphoid) of appendix (543.0)*

AHA: 1Q, '01, 15

√4ᵗʰ 543 Other diseases of appendix

543.0 Hyperplasia of appendix (lymphoid)

DEF: Proliferation of cells in appendix tissue.

543.9 Other and unspecified diseases of appendix

Appendicular or appendiceal:
colic
concretion
fistula

Diverticulum ⎱
Fecalith ⎱
Intussusception ⎰ of appendix
Mucocele ⎰
Stercolith ⎰

√4ᵗʰ Additional Digit Required   **√5ᵗʰ**   Unspecified Code   Other Specified Code   Manifestation Code   ▶◀ Revised Text   ● New Code   ▲ Revised Code Title

2013 ICD-9-CM   **October 2012 · Volume 1 – 167**

Diseases of the Digestive System

550–552.9

Hernia of Abdominal Cavity (550-553)

INCLUDES hernia:
    acquired
    congenital, except diaphragmatic or hiatal

√4ᵗʰ **550 Inguinal hernia**

INCLUDES bubonocele
    inguinal hernia (direct) (double) (indirect) (oblique)
      (sliding)
    scrotal hernia

The following fifth-digit subclassification is for use with category 550:
  0 unilateral or unspecified (not specified as recurrent)
    Unilateral NOS
  1 unilateral or unspecified, recurrent
  2 bilateral (not specified as recurrent)
    Bilateral NOS
  3 bilateral, recurrent

DEF: Hernia protrusion of an abdominal organ or tissue through inguinal canal.
DEF: Indirect inguinal hernia: (external or oblique) leaves abdomen through deep inguinal ring, passes through inguinal canal lateral to the inferior epigastric artery.
DEF: Direct inguinal hernia: (internal) emerges between inferior epigastric artery and rectus muscle edge.
AHA: N-D, '85, 12

§ √5ᵗʰ **550.0 Inguinal hernia, with gangrene**
[0-3]   Inguinal hernia with gangrene (and obstruction)

§ √5ᵗʰ **550.1 Inguinal hernia, with obstruction, without mention**
[0-3]   **of gangrene**
    Inguinal hernia with mention of incarceration, irreducibility, or strangulation

§ √5ᵗʰ **550.9 Inguinal hernia, without mention of obstruction**
[0-3]   **or gangrene**
    Inguinal hernia NOS
    AHA: For code 550.91: 3Q, '03, 10; 1Q, '03, 4
    K40.90 Uni ingin hernia w/o obst/gangrene not spec recur I-10

√4ᵗʰ **551 Other hernia of abdominal cavity, with gangrene**

INCLUDES that with gangrene (and obstruction)

√5ᵗʰ **551.0 Femoral hernia with gangrene**

    551.00 Unilateral or unspecified (not specified as recurrent)
      Femoral hernia NOS with gangrene

    551.01 Unilateral or unspecified, recurrent

    551.02 Bilateral (not specified as recurrent)

    551.03 Bilateral, recurrent

  551.1 Umbilical hernia with gangrene
    Parumbilical hernia specified as gangrenous

√5ᵗʰ **551.2 Ventral hernia with gangrene**

    551.20 Ventral, unspecified, with gangrene

    551.21 Incisional, with gangrene
      Hernia:
        postoperative } specified as
        recurrent, ventral }   gangrenous

    551.29 Other
      Epigastric hernia specified as gangrenous

Hernias of Abdominal Cavity

Hiatal hernia
Diaphragm
Epigastric hernia
Incisional hernia
Umbilical hernia
Inguinal hernia

Femoral Hernia

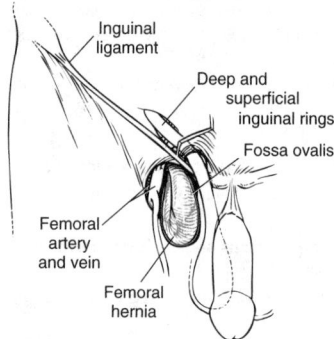

Inguinal ligament
Deep and superficial inguinal rings
Fossa ovalis
Femoral artery and vein
Femoral hernia

551.3 Diaphragmatic hernia with gangrene
    Hernia:
      hiatal (esophageal) (sliding) }
      paraesophageal } specified as
      Thoracic stomach }   gangrenous
    EXCLUDES *congenital diaphragmatic hernia (756.6)*

551.8 Hernia of other specified sites, with gangrene
    Any condition classifiable to 553.8 if specified as gangrenous

551.9 Hernia of unspecified site, with gangrene
    Any condition classifiable to 553.9 if specified as gangrenous

√4ᵗʰ **552 Other hernia of abdominal cavity, with obstruction, but without mention of gangrene**
    EXCLUDES *that with mention of gangrene (551.0-551.9)*

√5ᵗʰ **552.0 Femoral hernia with obstruction**
    Femoral hernia specified as incarcerated, irreducible, strangulated, or causing obstruction

    552.00 Unilateral or unspecified (not specified as recurrent)

    552.01 Unilateral or unspecified, recurrent

    552.02 Bilateral (not specified as recurrent)

    552.03 Bilateral, recurrent

  552.1 Umbilical hernia with obstruction
    Parumbilical hernia specified as incarcerated, irreducible, strangulated, or causing obstruction

√5ᵗʰ **552.2 Ventral hernia with obstruction**
    Ventral hernia specified as incarcerated, irreducible, strangulated, or causing obstruction

    552.20 Ventral, unspecified, with obstruction
      AHA: 2Q, '11, 18

    552.21 Incisional, with obstruction
      Hernia:
        postoperative } specified as incarcerated,
        recurrent, }   irreducible, strangulated,
        ventral }   or causing obstruction
      AHA: ▶1Q, '12, 8;◀ 3Q, '03, 11

    552.29 Other
      Epigastric hernia specified as incarcerated, irreducible, strangulated, or causing obstruction

  552.3 Diaphragmatic hernia with obstruction
    Hernia:
      hiatal (esophageal) } specified as caracerated,
        (sliding) }   irreducible,
      paraesophageal }   strangulated, or
      Thoracic stomach }   causing obstruction
    EXCLUDES *congenital diaphragmatic hernia (756.6)*

552.8 Hernia of other specified sites, with obstruction
    Any condition classifiable to 553.8 if specified as incarcerated, irreducible, strangulated, or causing obstruction
    AHA: 1Q, '04, 10

552.9 Hernia of unspecified site, with obstruction
    Any condition classifiable to 553.9 if specified as incarcerated, irreducible, strangulated, or causing obstruction

---

§ Requires fifth digit. Valid digits are in [brackets] under each code. See category 550 for codes and definitions.

  N Newborn Age: 0   P Pediatric Age: 0-17   M Maternity Age: 12-55   A Adult Age: 15-124

Diaphragmatic Hernias

- Esophagus
- Stomach
- Gastroesophageal junction (remains in place)
- Diaphragm
- Gastroesophageal junction (slides up and down)
- **Paraesophageal Hiatal Hernia**
- **Sliding Hiatal Hernia**

√4ᵗʰ **553　Other hernia of abdominal cavity without mention of obstruction or gangrene**

EXCLUDES the listed conditions with mention of:
　gangrene (and obstruction) (551.0-551.9)
　obstruction (552.0-552.9)

√5ᵗʰ **553.0　Femoral hernia**

553.00　Unilateral or unspecified (not specified as recurrent)
　Femoral hernia NOS

553.01　Unilateral or unspecified, recurrent

553.02　Bilateral (not specified as recurrent)

553.03　Bilateral, recurrent

553.1　Umbilical hernia
　Parumbilical hernia
　K42.9 Umbilical hernia without obstruction/gangrene　I-10

√5ᵗʰ **553.2　Ventral hernia**

553.20　Ventral, unspecified
　AHA: 2Q, '06, 10; 3Q, '03, 6

553.21　Incisional
　Hernia:
　　postoperative
　　recurrent, ventral
　AHA: 3Q, '03, 6
　K43.91 Incisional hernia w/o obstruction or gangrene　I-10

553.29　Other
　Hernia:
　　epigastric
　　spigelian

553.3　Diaphragmatic hernia
　Hernia:
　　hiatal (esophageal) (sliding)
　　paraesophageal
　Thoracic stomach
　EXCLUDES congenital:
　　　diaphragmatic hernia (756.6)
　　　hiatal hernia (750.6)
　　　esophagocele (530.6)
　AHA: 2Q, '01, 6; 1Q, '00, 6
　K44.9 Diaphragmatic hernia w/o obstruction/gangrene　I-10

553.8　Hernia of other specified sites
　Hernia:
　　ischiatic
　　ischiorectal
　　lumbar
　　obturator
　　pudendal
　　retroperitoneal
　　sciatic
　Other abdominal hernia of specified site
　EXCLUDES vaginal enterocele (618.6)

553.9　Hernia of unspecified site

Enterocele	Hernia:
Epiplocele	intestinal
Hernia:	intra-abdominal
NOS	Rupture (nontraumatic)
interstitial	Sarcoepiplocele

Noninfectious Enteritis and Colitis (555-558)

√4ᵗʰ **555　Regional enteritis**

INCLUDES　Crohn's disease
　　　　　Granulomatous enteritis

EXCLUDES ulcerative colitis (556)

DEF: Inflammation of intestine; classified to site.

TIP: Assign separate code for fistula, if present. Sequence 555 code as first-listed/principal diagnosis (if underlying cause of fistula).

555.0　Small intestine

Ileitis:	Regional enteritis or Crohn's disease of:
regional	duodenum
segmental	ileum
terminal	jejunum

555.1　Large intestine
　Colitis:
　　granulmatous
　　regional
　　transmural
　Regional enteritis or Crohn's disease of:
　　colon
　　large bowel
　　rectum
　AHA: 3Q, '99, 8

555.2　Small intestine with large intestine
　Regional ileocolitis
　AHA: 1Q, '03, 18

555.9　Unspecified site
　Crohn's disease NOS
　Regional enteritis NOS
　AHA: 1Q, '09, 5; 2Q, '05, 11; 3Q, '99, 8; 4Q, '97, 42; 2Q, '97, 3
　K50.90 Crohns disease unspecified w/o complications　I-10

√4ᵗʰ **556　Ulcerative colitis**

DEF: Chronic inflammation of mucosal lining of intestinal tract; may be single area or entire colon.

AHA: 3Q, '99, 8

556.0　Ulcerative (chronic) enterocolitis

556.1　Ulcerative (chronic) ileocolitis

556.2　Ulcerative (chronic) proctitis

556.3　Ulcerative (chronic) proctosigmoiditis

556.4　Pseudopolyposis of colon

556.5　Left-sided ulcerative (chronic) colitis

556.6　Universal ulcerative (chronic) colitis
　Pancolitis

556.8　Other ulcerative colitis

556.9　Ulcerative colitis, unspecified
　Ulcerative enteritis NOS
　AHA: 1Q, '03, 10
　K51.90 Ulcerative colitis unspecified w/o complications　I-10

Large Intestine

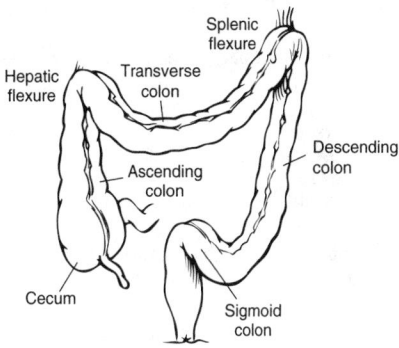

- Splenic flexure
- Hepatic flexure
- Transverse colon
- Descending colon
- Ascending colon
- Cecum
- Sigmoid colon

√4ᵗʰ √5ᵗʰ　Additional Digit Required　　Unspecified Code　　Other Specified Code　　Manifestation Code　　▶◀ Revised Text　　● New Code　　▲ Revised Code Title

2013 ICD-9-CM　　　**Volume 1 – 169**

Diseases of the Digestive System

557–560.39

√4ᵗʰ **557   Vascular insufficiency of intestine**

> **EXCLUDES** *necrotizing enterocolitis of the newborn (777.50-777.53)*
> **DEF:** Inadequacy of intestinal vessels.

557.0   Acute vascular insufficiency of intestine

> Acute:
>   hemorrhagic enterocolitis
>   ischemic colitis, enteritis, or enterocolitis
>   massive necrosis of intestine
> Bowel infarction
> Embolism of mesenteric artery
> Fulminant enterocolitis
> Hemorrhagic necrosis of intestine
> Infarction of appendices epiploicae
> Intestinal gangrene
> Intestinal infarction (acute) (agnogenic) (hemorrhagic)
>   (nonocclusive)
> Mesenteric infarction (embolic) (thrombotic)
> Necrosis of intestine
> Terminal hemorrhagic enteropathy
> Thrombosis of mesenteric artery
> **AHA:** 3Q, '11, 11; 2Q, '08, 15; 4Q, '01, 53
> **TIP:** Do not assign an additional code for GI bleeding; it is inherent in 557.0.
> **K55.0** Acute vascular disorders of intestine   I-10

557.1   Chronic vascular insufficiency of intestine

> Angina, abdominal
> Chronic ischemic colitis, enteritis, or enterocolitis
> Ischemic stricture of intestine
> Mesenteric:
>   angina
>   artery syndrome (superior)
>   vascular insufficiency
> **AHA:** 3Q, '96, 9; 4Q, '90, 4; N-D, '86, 11; N-D, '84, 7

557.9   Unspecified vascular insufficiency of intestine

> Alimentary pain due to vascular insufficiency
> Ischemic colitis, enteritis, or enterocolitis NOS
> **K55.9** Vascular disorder of intestine unspecified   I-10

√4ᵗʰ **558   Other and unspecified noninfectious gastroenteritis and colitis**

> **EXCLUDES** *infectious:*
>   *colitis, enteritis, or gastroenteritis (009.0-009.1)*
>   *diarrhea (009.2-009.3)*

558.1   Gastroenteritis and colitis due to radiation

> Radiation enterocolitis

558.2   Toxic gastroenteritis and colitis

> Use additional E code to identify cause

558.3   Allergic gastroenteritis and colitis

> Use additional code to identify type of food allergy
>   (V15.01-V15.05)
> **DEF:** True immunoglobulin E (IgE)-mediated allergic reaction of the lining of the stomach, intestines, or colon to food proteins; causes nausea, vomiting, diarrhea, and abdominal cramping.
> **AHA:** 4Q, '08, 116; 1Q, '03, 12; 4Q, '00, 42

√5ᵗʰ **558.4   Eosinophilic gastroenteritis and colitis**

> **AHA:** 4Q, '08, 116

558.41   Eosinophilic gastroenteritis

> Eosinophilic enteritis
> **AHA:** 4Q, '08, 116

558.42   Eosinophilic colitis

> **AHA:** 4Q, '08, 115-116

558.9   Other and unspecified noninfectious gastroenteritis and colitis

> Colitis ⎫
> Enteritis ⎪
> Gastroenteritis ⎬ NOS, dietetic, or
> Ileitis ⎪   noninfectious
> Jejunitis ⎪
> Sigmoiditis ⎭
> **AHA:** 3Q, '11, 11; 2Q, '08, 10; 1Q, '08, 10; 3Q, '99, 4, 6; N-D, '87, 7
> **K52.9** Noninfective gastroenteritis & colitis unspec   I-10

Other Diseases of Intestines and Peritoneum (560-569)

√4ᵗʰ **560   Intestinal obstruction without mention of hernia**

> **EXCLUDES** *duodenum (537.2-537.3)*
>   *inguinal hernia with obstruction (550.1)*
>   *intestinal obstruction complicating hernia (552.0-552.9)*
>   *mesenteric:*
>   *embolism (557.0)*
>   *infarction (557.0)*
>   *thrombosis (557.0)*
>   *neonatal intestinal obstruction (277.01, 777.1-777.2, 777.4)*
> **TIP:** If intestinal obstruction is due to abdominal carcinomatosis or Crohn's disease, sequence that condition first.

560.0   Intussusception

> Intussusception (colon) (intestine) (rectum)
> Invagination of intestine or colon
> **EXCLUDES** *intussusception of appendix (543.9)*
> **DEF:** Prolapse of a bowel section into adjacent section; occurs primarily in children; symptoms include paroxysmal pain, vomiting, presence of blood, and mucous passage from rectum.
> **AHA:** 4Q, '98, 82

560.1   Paralytic ileus

> Adynamic ileus
> Ileus (of intestine) (of bowel) (of colon)
> Paralysis of intestine or colon
> **EXCLUDES** *gallstone ileus (560.31)*
> **DEF:** Obstruction of ileus due to inhibited bowel motility.
> **AHA:** ▶1Q, '12, 6;◀ J-F, '87, 13
> **K56.0** Paralytic ileus   I-10

560.2   Volvulus

> Knotting ⎫
> Strangulation ⎪
> Torsion ⎬ if intestine, bowel, or colon
> Twist ⎭
> **DEF:** Entanglement of bowel; causes obstruction; may compromise bowel circulation.

√5ᵗʰ **560.3   Impaction of intestine**

560.30   Impaction of intestine, unspecified

> Impaction of colon

560.31   Gallstone ileus

> Obstruction of intestine by gallstone

560.32   Fecal impaction

> **EXCLUDES** *constipation (564.00-564.09)*
>   *incomplete defecation (787.61)*
> **AHA:** 4Q, '10, 87-89
> **K56.41** Fecal impaction   I-10

560.39   Other

> Concretion of intestine
> Enterolith
> **AHA:** 4Q, '98, 38
> **K56.49** Other impaction of intestine   I-10

Volvulus and Diverticulitis

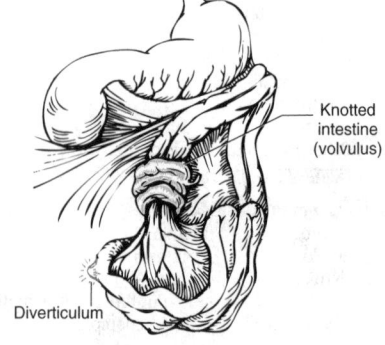

Knotted intestine (volvulus)

Diverticulum

√5ᵗʰ **560.8 Other specified intestinal obstruction**

560.81 Intestinal or peritoneal adhesions with obstruction (postoperative) (postinfection)

> **EXCLUDES** *adhesions without obstruction (568.0)*
>
> **DEF:** Obstruction of peritoneum or intestine due to abnormal union of tissues.
>
> **AHA:** 1Q, '10, 11; 4Q, '95, 55; 3Q, '95, 6; N-D, '87, 9
>
> **TIP:** Do not assign additional code from subcategory 997.4 Digestive system complications.
>
> **K56.5** Intestinal adhes [bands] w/obst (postproc) (postinfec)   I-10

560.89 Other

> Acute pseudo-obstruction of intestine
> Mural thickening causing obstruction
>
> **EXCLUDES** *ischemic stricture of intestine (557.1)*
>
> **AHA:** 2Q, '97, 3; 1Q, '88, 6

560.9 Unspecified intestinal obstruction

> Enterostenosis
> Obstruction
> Occlusion   } of intestine or colon
> Stenosis
> Stricture
>
> **EXCLUDES** *congenital stricture or stenosis of intestine (751.1-751.2)*
>
> **K56.60** Unspecified intestinal obstruction   I-10

√4ᵗʰ **562 Diverticula of intestine**

> Use additional code to identify any associated:
> peritonitis (567.0-567.9)
>
> **EXCLUDES** *congenital diverticulum of colon (751.5)*
> *diverticulum of appendix (543.9)*
> *Meckel's diverticulum (751.0)*
>
> **AHA:** 4Q, '91, 25; J-F, '85, 1

√5ᵗʰ **562.0 Small intestine**

562.00 Diverticulosis of small intestine (without mention of hemorrhage)

> Diverticulosis:
> duodenum
> ileum   } without mention of diverticulitis
> jejunum
>
> **DEF:** Saclike herniations of mucous lining of small intestine.

562.01 Diverticulitis of small intestine (without mention of hemorrhage)

> Diverticulitis (with diverticulosis):
> duodenum
> ileum
> jejunum
> small intestine
>
> **DEF:** Inflamed saclike herniations of mucous lining of small intestine.

562.02 Diverticulosis of small intestine with hemorrhage

562.03 Diverticulitis of small intestine with hemorrhage

√5ᵗʰ **562.1 Colon**

562.10 Diverticulosis of colon (without mention of hemorrhage)

> Diverticulosis:
> NOS
> intestine (large)   } without metion of diverticulitis
> Diverticular disease (colon)
>
> **DEF:** Saclike herniations of mucous lining of large intestine.
>
> **AHA:** 3Q, '05, 17; 3Q, '02, 15; 4Q, '90, 21; J-F, '85, 5
>
> **K57.30** Divrticulos lg intest uns w/o perf/absc w/o bldg   I-10

562.11 Diverticulitis of colon (without mention of hemorrhage)

> Diverticulitis (with diverticulosis):
> NOS
> colon
> intestine (large)
>
> **DEF:** Inflamed saclike herniations of mucosal lining of large intestine.
>
> **AHA:** 1Q, '96, 14; J-F, '85, 5
>
> **K57.32** Divrticulit lg intest uns w/o perf/absc w/o bldg   I-10

562.12 Diverticulosis of colon with hemorrhage

562.13 Diverticulitis of colon with hemorrhage

√4ᵗʰ **564 Functional digestive disorders, not elsewhere classified**

> **EXCLUDES** *functional disorders of stomach (536.0-536.9)*
> *those specified as psychogenic (306.4)*

√5ᵗʰ **564.0 Constipation**

> **EXCLUDES** *fecal impaction (560.32)*
> *incomplete defecation (787.61)*
>
> **AHA:** 4Q, '01, 45

564.00 Constipation, unspecified

> **K59.00** Constipation unspecified   I-10

564.01 Slow transit constipation

> **DEF:** Delay in the transit of fecal material through the colon secondary to smooth muscle dysfunction or decreased peristaltic contractions along the colon: also called colonic inertia or delayed transit.

564.02 Outlet dysfunction constipation

> **DEF:** Failure to relax the paradoxical contractions of the striated pelvic floor muscles during the attempted defecation.

564.09 Other constipation

564.1 Irritable bowel syndrome

> Irritable colon
> Spastic colon
>
> **DEF:** Functional gastrointestinal disorder (FGID); symptoms include diarrhea, constipation, abdominal pain, gas, distended abdomen, nausea, vomiting, emotional distress, and depression.
>
> **AHA:** 1Q, '88, 6
>
> **K58.9** Irritable bowel syndrome without diarrhea   I-10

564.2 Postgastric surgery syndromes

> Dumping syndrome
> Jejunal syndrome
> Postgastrectomy syndrome
> Postvagotomy syndrome
>
> **EXCLUDES** *malnutrition following gastrointestinal surgery (579.3)*
> *postgastrojejunostomy ulcer (534.0-534.9)*
>
> **AHA:** 1Q, '95, 11

564.3 Vomiting following gastrointestinal surgery

> Vomiting (bilious) following gastrointestinal surgery

564.4 Other postoperative functional disorders

> Diarrhea following gastrointestinal surgery
>
> **EXCLUDES** *colostomy and enterostomy complications (569.60-569.69)*

564.5 Functional diarrhea

> **EXCLUDES** *diarrhea:*
> *NOS (787.91)*
> *psychogenic (306.4)*
>
> **DEF:** Diarrhea with no detectable organic cause.

564.6 Anal spasm

> Proctalgia fugax

564.7 Megacolon, other than Hirschsprung's

> Dilatation of colon
>
> **EXCLUDES** *megacolon:*
> *congenital [Hirschsprung's] (751.3)*
> *toxic (556)*
>
> **DEF:** Enlarged colon; congenital or acquired; can occur acutely or become chronic.

√5ᵗʰ **564.8 Other specified functional disorders of intestine**

> **EXCLUDES** *malabsorption (579.0-579.9)*
>
> **AHA:** 1Q, '88, 6

564.81 Neurogenic bowel

> **DEF:** Disorder of bowel due to spinal cord lesion above conus medullaris; symptoms include precipitous micturition, nocturia, headache, sweating, nasal obstruction and spastic contractions.
>
> **AHA:** 1Q, '01, 12; 4Q, '98, 45

564.89 Other functional disorders of intestine

> Atony of colon
>
> **DEF:** Absence of normal bowel tone or strength.

564.9 Unspecified functional disorder of intestine

√4ᵗʰ √5ᵗʰ Additional Digit Required   Unspecified Code   Other Specified Code   Manifestation Code   ▶◀ Revised Text   ● New Code   ▲ Revised Code Title

2013 ICD-9-CM   **Volume 1 – 171**

Diseases of the Digestive System

565–567.9

Anal Fistula and Abscess

Psoas Muscle Abscess

☑4ᵗʰ 565 Anal fissure and fistula

565.0 Anal fissure

EXCLUDES anal sphincter tear (healed) (non-traumatic) (old)
(569.43)
traumatic (863.89, 863.99)

DEF: Ulceration of cleft at anal mucosa; causes pain, itching, bleeding, infection, and sphincter spasm; may occur with hemorrhoids.

565.1 Anal fistula

Fistula:
anorectal
rectal
rectum to skin

EXCLUDES fistula of rectum to internal organs — see Alphabetic Index
ischiorectal fistula (566)
rectovaginal fistula (619.1)

DEF: Abnormal opening on cutaneous surface near anus; may lack connection with rectum.

AHA: 1Q, '07, 13

566 Abscess of anal and rectal regions

Abscess: Cellulitis:
ischiorectal   anal
perianal   perirectal
perirectal   rectal
              Ischiorectal fistula

☑4ᵗʰ 567 Peritonitis and retroperitoneal infections

EXCLUDES peritonitis:
benign paroxysmal (277.31)
pelvic, female (614.5, 614.7)
periodic familial (277.31)
puerperal (670.8)
with or following:
abortion (634-638 with .0, 639.0)
appendicitis (540.0-540.1)
ectopic or molar pregnancy (639.0)

DEF: Inflammation of the peritoneal cavity.

567.0 Peritonitis in infectious diseases classified elsewhere

Code first underlying disease

EXCLUDES peritonitis:
gonococcal (098.86)
syphilitic (095.2)
tuberculous (014.0)

567.1 Pneumococcal peritonitis

☑5ᵗʰ 567.2 Other suppurative peritonitis

AHA: 4Q, '05, 74; 2Q, '01, 11, 12; 3Q, '99, 9; 2Q, '98, 19

567.21 Peritonitis (acute) generalized

Pelvic peritonitis, male

TIP: For pelvic peritonitis in a female patient, refer to code 614.5.

567.22 Peritoneal abscess

Abscess (of):
abdominopelvic
mesenteric
omentum
peritoneum
retrocecal
subdiaphragmatic
subhepatic
subphrenic

K65.1 Peritoneal abscess   I-10

567.23 Spontaneous bacterial peritonitis

EXCLUDES bacterial peritonitis NOS (567.29)

567.29 Other suppurative peritonitis

Subphrenic peritonitis

AHA: 2Q, '10, 4

☑5ᵗʰ 567.3 Retroperitoneal infections

AHA: 4Q, '05, 74

567.31 Psoas muscle abscess

DEF: Infection that extends into or around the psoas muscle that connects the lumbar vertebrae to the femur.

567.38 Other retroperitoneal abscess

AHA: 4Q, '05, 77

567.39 Other retroperitoneal infections

☑5ᵗʰ 567.8 Other specified peritonitis

AHA: 4Q, '05, 74

567.81 Choleperitonitis

Peritonitis due to bile

DEF: Inflammation or infection due to presence of bile in the peritoneum resulting from rupture of the bile passages or gallbladder.

567.82 Sclerosing mesenteritis

Fat necrosis of peritoneum
(Idiopathic) sclerosing mesenteric fibrosis
Mesenteric lipodystrophy
Mesenteric panniculitis
Retractile mesenteritis

DEF: Inflammatory processes involving the mesenteric fat; progresses to fibrosis and necrosis of tissue.

AHA: 4Q, '05, 77

567.89 Other specified peritonitis

Chronic proliferative peritonitis
Mesenteric saponification
Peritonitis due to urine

567.9 Unspecified peritonitis

Peritonitis NOS
Peritonitis of unspecified cause

AHA: 1Q, '04, 10

√4ᵗʰ **568 Other disorders of peritoneum**

568.0 Peritoneal adhesions (postoperative) (postinfection)
Adhesions (of):
abdominal (wall)
diaphragm
intestine
male pelvis
mesenteric
omentum
stomach
Adhesive bands

EXCLUDES *adhesions:*
pelvic, female (614.6)
with obstruction:
duodenum (537.3)
intestine (560.81)

DEF: Abnormal union of tissues in peritoneum.
AHA: ▶1Q, '12, 8;◄ 2Q, '11, 18; 3Q, '03, 7, 11; 4Q, '95, 55; 3Q, '95, 7;
S-O, '85, 11
TIP: Do not assign additional code from subcategory 997.4 Digestive
system complications.
K66.0 Peritoneal adhesns (postprocedural) (postinfection) I-10

√5ᵗʰ **568.8 Other specified disorders of peritoneum**

568.81 Hemoperitoneum (nontraumatic)

568.82 Peritoneal effusion (chronic)
EXCLUDES *ascites NOS (789.51-789.59)*
DEF: Persistent leakage of fluid within peritoneal cavity.

568.89 Other
Peritoneal:
cyst
granuloma

568.9 Unspecified disorder of peritoneum

√4ᵗʰ **569 Other disorders of intestine**

569.0 Anal and rectal polyp
Anal and rectal polyp NOS
EXCLUDES *adenomatous anal and rectal polyp (211.4)*

569.1 Rectal prolapse
Procidentia: Prolapse:
anus (sphincter)   anal canal
rectum (sphincter)   rectal mucosa
Proctoptosis
EXCLUDES *prolapsed hemorrhoids (455.2, 455.5)*

569.2 Stenosis of rectum and anus
Stricture of anus (sphincter)

569.3 Hemorrhage of rectum and anus
EXCLUDES *gastrointestinal bleeding NOS (578.9)*
melena (578.1)
AHA: 3Q, '05, 17
K62.5 Hemorrhage of anus and rectum I-10

√5ᵗʰ **569.4 Other specified disorders of rectum and anus**

569.41 Ulcer of anus and rectum
Solitary ulcer ⎫ of anus (sphincter) or
Stercoral ulcer ⎭ rectum (sphincter)

569.42 Anal or rectal pain
AHA: 1Q, '03, 8; 1Q, '96, 13

Rectum and Anus

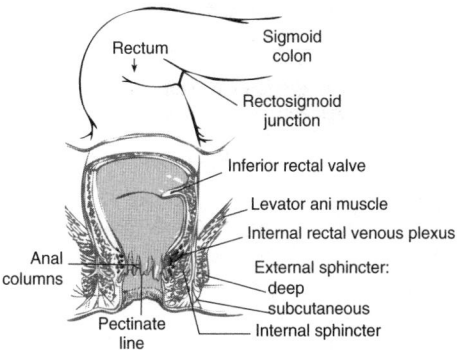

Rectum
Sigmoid colon
Rectosigmoid junction
Inferior rectal valve
Levator ani muscle
Internal rectal venous plexus
Anal columns
External sphincter:
deep
subcutaneous
Internal sphincter
Pectinate line

569.43 Anal sphincter tear (healed) (old)
Tear of anus, nontraumatic
Use additional code for any associated fecal
incontinence (787.60-787.63)
EXCLUDES *anal fissure (565.0)*
anal sphincter tear (healed) (old)
complicating delivery (654.8)
AHA: 4Q, '07, 88

569.44 Dysplasia of anus
Anal intraepithelial neoplasia I and II (AIN I and II)
(histologically confirmed)
Dysplasia of anus NOS
Mild and moderate dysplasia of anus (histologically
confirmed)
EXCLUDES *abnormal results from anal cytologic*
examination without histologic
confirmation (796.70-796.79)
anal intraepithelial neoplasia III (230.5,
230.6)
carcinoma in situ of anus (230.5, 230.6)
HGSIL of anus (796.74)
severe dysplasia of anus (230.5, 230.6)
AHA: 4Q, '08, 117

569.49 Other
Granuloma ⎫
Rupture   ⎭ of rectum (sphincter)
Hypertrophy of anal papillae
Proctitis NOS
Use additional code for any associated fecal
incontinence (787.60-787.63)
EXCLUDES *fistula of rectum to:*
internal organs — see Alphabetic Index
skin (565.1)
hemorrhoids (455.0-455.9)

569.5 Abscess of intestine
EXCLUDES *appendiceal abscess (540.1)*
K63.0 Abscess of intestine I-10

√5ᵗʰ **569.6 Colostomy and enterostomy complications**
DEF: Complication in a surgically created opening, from intestine to
surface skin.
AHA: 4Q, '95, 58
TIP: Do not assign additional code from subcategory 997.4 Digestive
system complications.

**569.60 Colostomy and enterostomy
complication, unspecified**

569.61 Infection of colostomy or enterostomy
Use additional code to identify organism
(041.00-041.9)
Use additional code to specify type of infection, such
as:
abscess or cellulitis of abdomen (682.2)
septicemia (038.0-038.9)

**569.62 Mechanical complication of colostomy and
enterostomy**
Malfunction of colostomy and enterostomy
AHA: 2Q, '05, 11 ; 1Q, '03, 10; 4Q, '98, 44

569.69 Other complication
Fistula   Prolapse
Hernia
AHA: 3Q, '98, 16

√5ᵗʰ **569.7 Complications of intestinal pouch**
TIP: Do not assign code from subcategory 997.4 Digestive system
complications in addition to a code from this subcategory.

569.71 Pouchitis
Inflammation of internal ileoanal pouch
DEF: Inflammatory complication of an existing surgically
created ileoanal pouch, resulting in multiple GI complaints,
including diarrhea, abdominal pain, rectal bleeding, fecal
urgency, or incontinence.
AHA: 4Q, '09, 94

569.79 Other complications of intestinal pouch

Diseases of the Digestive System

569.8–572.0

√5ᵗʰ **569.8 Other specified disorders of intestine**
AHA: 4Q, '91, 25

569.81 Fistula of intestine, excluding rectum and anus

Fistula:	Fistula:
abdominal wall	enteroenteric
enterocolic	ileorectal

EXCLUDES   *fistula of intestine to internal organs — see Alphabetic Index*
persistent postoperative fistula (998.6)
AHA: 3Q, '99, 8

569.82 Ulceration of intestine
Primary ulcer of intestine
Ulceration of colon
EXCLUDES   *that with perforation (569.83)*

569.83 Perforation of intestine

569.84 Angiodysplasia of intestine (without mention of hemorrhage)
DEF: Small vascular abnormalities of the intestinal tract without bleeding problems.
AHA: 3Q, '96, 10; 4Q, '90, 4; 4Q, '90, 21
TIP: Assign code 569.84 or 569.85 for documentation of either intestinal arteriovenous (AV) malformation or angiodysplasia.

569.85 Angiodysplasia of intestine with hemorrhage
DEF: Small vascular abnormalities of the intestinal tract with bleeding problems.
AHA: 3Q, '96, 9

569.86 Dieulafoy lesion (hemorrhagic) of intestine
AHA: 4Q, '02, 60-61

569.87 Vomiting of fecal matter
DEF: Spasmodic expulsion of partially digested substance with similar odor to fecal matter; often suggestive of bowel obstruction or other underlying causal pathology.
AHA: 4Q, '09, 105

569.89 Other
Enteroptosis
Granuloma ⎫
Prolapse ⎬ of intestine
  ⎭
Pericolitis
Perisigmoiditis
Visceroptosis
EXCLUDES   *gangrene of intestine, mesentery, or omentum (557.0)*
hemorrhage of intestine NOS (578.9)
obstruction of intestine (560.0-560.9)
AHA: 3Q, '96, 9

569.9 Unspecified disorder of intestine

Other Diseases of Digestive System (570-579)

570 Acute and subacute necrosis of liver
Acute hepatic failure
Acute or subacute hepatitis, not specified as infective
Necrosis of liver (acute) (diffuse) (massive) (subacute)
Parenchymatous degeneration of liver
Yellow atrophy (liver) (acute) (subacute)
EXCLUDES   *icterus gravis of newborn (773.0-773.2)*
serum hepatitis (070.2-070.3)
that with:
abortion (634-638 with .7, 639.8)
ectopic or molar pregnancy (639.8)
pregnancy, childbirth, or the puerperium (646.7)
viral hepatitis (070.0-070.9)
AHA: 2Q, '05, 9; 1Q, '00, 22
K72.00 Acute and subacute hepatic failure without coma   I-10

√4ᵗʰ **571 Chronic liver disease and cirrhosis**

571.0 Alcoholic fatty liver   A

571.1 Acute alcoholic hepatitis   A
Acute alcoholic liver disease
AHA: 2Q, '02, 4

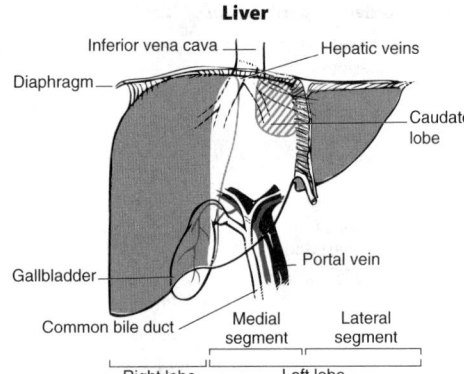

Liver

Inferior vena cava — Hepatic veins
Diaphragm
Caudate lobe
Gallbladder
Portal vein
Common bile duct
Medial segment — Lateral segment
Right lobe — Left lobe

571.2 Alcoholic cirrhosis of liver   A
Florid cirrhosis
Laennec's cirrhosis (alcoholic)
DEF: Fibrosis and dysfunction of liver due to alcoholic liver disease.
AHA: 1Q, '11, 23; 3Q, '07, 7; 2Q, '07, 6; 2Q, '02, 4; 1Q, '02, 3; N-D, '85, 14
TIP: For a patient admitted for bleeding esophageal varices due to alcoholic liver cirrhosis, sequence the liver cirrhosis first.
K70.30 Alcoholic cirrhosis of liver without ascites   I-10

571.3 Alcoholic liver damage, unspecified   A

√5ᵗʰ **571.4 Chronic hepatitis**
EXCLUDES   *viral hepatitis (acute) (chronic) (070.0-070.9)*

571.40 Chronic hepatitis, unspecified

571.41 Chronic persistent hepatitis

571.42 Autoimmune hepatitis
AHA: 4Q, '08, 120

571.49 Other
Chronic hepatitis:
active
aggressive
Recurrent hepatitis
AHA: 3Q, '99, 19; N-D, '85, 14

571.5 Cirrhosis of liver without mention of alcohol
Cirrhosis of liver:
NOS
cryptogenic
macronodular
micronodular
posthepatitic
postnecrotic
Healed yellow atrophy (liver)
Portal cirrhosis
Code first, if applicable, viral hepatitis (acute) (chronic) (070.0-070.9)
DEF: Fibrosis and dysfunction of liver; not alcohol related.
AHA: 1Q, '11, 23; 3Q, '07, 7; 2Q, '07, 5
TIP: For a patient admitted for bleeding esophageal varices due to liver cirrhosis, sequence the liver cirrhosis first.

571.6 Biliary cirrhosis
Chronic nonsuppurative destructive cholangitis
Cirrhosis:
cholangitic
cholestatic

571.8 Other chronic nonalcoholic liver disease
Chronic yellow atrophy (liver)
Fatty liver, without mention of alcohol
AHA: 2Q, '96, 12

571.9 Unspecified chronic liver disease without mention of alcohol

√4ᵗʰ **572 Liver abscess and sequelae of chronic liver disease**

572.0 Abscess of liver
EXCLUDES   *amebic liver abscess (006.3)*

572.1 Portal pyemia
Phlebitis of portal vein   Pylephlebitis
Portal thrombophlebitis   Pylethrombophlebitis
DEF: Inflammation of portal vein or branches; may be due to intestinal disease; symptoms include fever, chills, jaundice, sweating, and abscess in various body parts.

572.2 Hepatic encephalopathy
Hepatic coma
Hepatocerebral intoxication
Portal-systemic encephalopathy
EXCLUDES *hepatic coma associated with viral hepatitis — see category 070*
AHA: 2Q, '07, 5; 2Q, '05, 9; 1Q, '02, 3; 3Q, '95, 14
TIP: Do not assign if hepatic coma is documented with viral hepatitis; see category 070 with fourth digit indicating hepatic coma.
K72.91 Hepatic failure unspecified with coma   I-10

572.3 Portal hypertension
Use additional code for any associated complications, such as:
portal hypertensive gastropathy (537.89)
DEF: Abnormally high blood pressure in the portal vein.
AHA: 3Q, '05, 15
K76.6 Portal hypertension   I-10

572.4 Hepatorenal syndrome
EXCLUDES *that following delivery (674.8)*
DEF: Hepatic and renal failure characterized by cirrhosis with ascites or obstructive jaundice, oliguria, and low sodium concentration.
AHA: 3Q, '93, 15

572.8 Other sequelae of chronic liver disease
EXCLUDES *hepatopulmonary syndrome (573.5)*

573 Other disorders of liver
EXCLUDES *amyloid or lardaceous degeneration of liver (277.39)*
congenital cystic disease of liver (751.62)
glycogen infiltration of liver (271.0)
hepatomegaly NOS (789.1)
portal vein obstruction (452)

573.0 Chronic passive congestion of liver
DEF: Blood accumulation in liver tissue.

573.1 Hepatitis in viral diseases classified elsewhere
Code first underlying disease as:
Coxsackie virus disease (074.8)
cytomegalic inclusion virus disease (078.5)
infectious mononucleosis (075)
EXCLUDES *hepatitis (in):*
mumps (072.71)
viral (070.0-070.9)
yellow fever (060.0-060.9)

573.2 Hepatitis in other infectious diseases classified elsewhere
Code first underlying disease, as:
malaria (084.9)
EXCLUDES *hepatitis in:*
late syphilis (095.3)
secondary syphilis (091.62)
toxoplasmosis (130.5)

▶Hepatic portal veins◀

Gallbladder and Bile Ducts

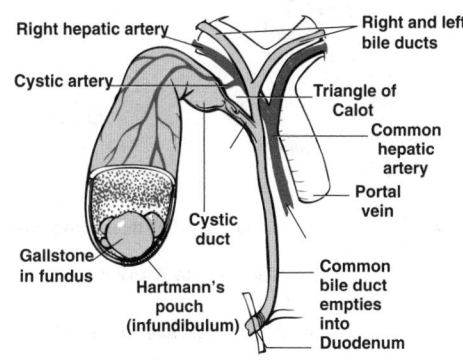

573.3 Hepatitis, unspecified
Toxic (noninfectious) hepatitis
Use additional E code to identify cause
AHA: 3Q, '98, 3, 4; 4Q, '90, 26
K75.9 Inflammatory liver disease unspecified   I-10

573.4 Hepatic infarction

573.5 Hepatopulmonary syndrome
Code first underlying liver disease, such as:
alcoholic cirrhosis of liver (571.2)
cirrhosis of liver without mention of alcohol (571.5)
AHA: ▶4Q, '11, 127-128◀

573.8 Other specified disorders of liver
Hepatoptosis

573.9 Unspecified disorder of liver

574 Cholelithiasis
The following fifth-digit subclassification is for use with category 574:
   0 without mention of obstruction
   1 with obstruction
EXCLUDES *retained cholelithiasis following cholecystectomy (997.41)*

§ 574.0 Calculus of gallbladder with acute cholecystitis
[0-1]
Biliary calculus
Calculus of cystic duct } with acute cholecystitis
Cholelithiasis
Any condition classifiable to 574.2 with acute cholecystitis
AHA: 4Q, '96, 32
K80.00 Calculus of GB w/acute cholecystitis w/o obst   I-10

§ 574.1 Calculus of gallbladder with other cholecystitis
[0-1]
Biliary calculus
Calculus of cystic duct } with cholecystitis
Cholelithiasis
Cholecystitis with cholelithiasis NOS
Any condition classifiable to 574.2 with cholecystitis (chronic)
AHA: 3Q, '99, 9; 4Q, '96, 32, 69; 2Q, '96, 13; **For code 574.10:** 1Q, '03, 5
K80.10 Calculus of GB w/chronic cholecystitis w/o obst   I-10

§ 574.2 Calculus of gallbladder without mention of cholecystitis
[0-1]
Biliary:
calculus NOS
colic NOS
Calculus of cystic duct
Cholelithiasis NOS
Colic (recurrent) of gallbladder
Gallstone (impacted)
AHA: For code 574.20: 1Q, '88, 14
K80.20 Calculus of GB w/o cholecystitis w/o obst   I-10

§ 574.3 Calculus of bile duct with acute cholecystitis
[0-1]
Calculus of bile duct (any) } with acute cholecystitis
Choledocholithiasis
Any condition classifiable to 574.5 with acute cholecystitis

§ 574.4 Calculus of bile duct with other cholecystitis
[0-1]
Calculus of bile duct
(any) } with cholecystitis (chronic)
Choledocholithiasis
Any condition classifiable to 574.5 with cholecystitis (chronic)

§ Requires fifth digit. Valid digits are in [brackets] under each code. See category 574 for codes and definitions.

Diseases of the Digestive System

574.5–576.9

§ ✔5ᵗʰ **574.5 Calculus of bile duct without mention of cholecystitis**
[0-1]   Calculus of:
         bile duct [any]
         common duct
         hepatic duct
     Choledocholithiasis
     Hepatic:
         colic (recurrent)
         lithiasis
     AHA: 3Q, '94, 11

§ ✔5ᵗʰ **574.6 Calculus of gallbladder and bile duct with acute**
[0-1]   **cholecystitis**
     Any condition classifiable to 574.0 and 574.3
     AHA: 4Q, '96, 32

§ ✔5ᵗʰ **574.7 Calculus of gallbladder and bile duct with**
[0-1]   **other cholecytitis**
     Any condition classifiable to 574.1 and 574.4
     AHA: 4Q, '96, 32

§ ✔5ᵗʰ **574.8 Calculus of gallbladder and bile duct with acute**
[0-1]   **and chronic cholcystitis**
     Any condition classifiable to 574.6 and 574.7
     AHA: 4Q, '96, 32

§ ✔5ᵗʰ **574.9 Calculus of gallbladder and bile duct without cholecystitis**
[0-1]   Any condition classifiable to 574.2 and 574.5
     AHA: 4Q, '96, 32

✔4ᵗʰ **575 Other disorders of gallbladder**

575.0 Acute cholecystitis
     Abscess of gallbladder ⎫
     Angiocholecystitis   ⎪
     Cholecystitis: ⎪
         emphysematous (acute) ⎬ without mention of
         gangrenous   ⎪   calculus
         suppurative   ⎪
     Empyema of gallbladder ⎪
     Gangrene of gallbladder ⎭

     EXCLUDES *that with:*
         acute and chronic cholecystitis (575.12)
         choledocholithiasis (574.3)
         choledocholithiasis and cholelithiasis (574.6)
         cholelithiasis (574.0)
     AHA: 3Q, '91, 17
     TIP: Do not assign a separate cholecystitis code from category 575 with a code from category 574.
     K81.0 Acute cholecystitis   I-10

✔5ᵗʰ **575.1 Other cholecystitis**
     Cholecystitis: ⎫
         NOS   ⎬ without mention of calculus
         chronic   ⎭

     EXCLUDES *that with:*
         choledocholithiasis (574.4)
         choledocholithiasis and cholelithiasis (574.8)
         cholelithiasis (574.1)
     AHA: 4Q, '96, 32

     575.10 Cholecystitis, unspecified
         Cholecystitis NOS

     575.11 Chronic cholecystitis
         K81.1 Chronic cholecystitis   I-10

     575.12 Acute and chronic cholecystitis
         AHA: 4Q, '97, 52; 4Q, '96, 32

575.2 Obstruction of gallbladder
     Occlusion   ⎫
     Stenosis   ⎬ of cystic duct or gallbladder without
     Stricture   ⎭   mention of calculus

     EXCLUDES *that with calculus (574.0-574.2 with*
         fifth-digit 1)

575.3 Hydrops of gallbladder
     Mucocele of gallbladder
     DEF: Serous fluid accumulation in bladder.
     AHA: 2Q, '89, 13

575.4 Perforation of gallbladder
     Rupture of cystic duct or gallbladder

575.5 Fistula of gallbladder
     Fistula:
         cholecystoduodenal
         cholecystoenteric

575.6 Cholesterolosis of gallbladder
     Strawberry gallbladder
     DEF: Cholesterol deposits in gallbladder tissue.
     AHA: 4Q, '90, 17

575.8 Other specified disorders of gallbladder
     Adhesions   ⎫
     Atrophy   ⎪
     Cyst   ⎬ of cystic duct or gallbladder
     Hypertrophy   ⎪
     Nonfunctioning ⎪
     Ulcer   ⎭

     Biliary dyskinesia
     EXCLUDES *Hartmann's pouch of intestine (V44.3)*
         nonvisualization of gallbladder (793.3)
     AHA: 4Q, '90, 26; 2Q, '89, 13

575.9 Unspecified disorder of gallbladder

✔4ᵗʰ **576 Other disorders of biliary tract**
     EXCLUDES *that involving the:*
         cystic duct (575.0-575.9)
         gallbladder (575.0-575.9)

576.0 Postcholecystectomy syndrome
     DEF: Jaundice or abdominal pain following cholecystectomy.
     AHA: 1Q, '88, 10
     TIP: Do not assign additional code from subcategory 997.4 Digestive system complications.

576.1 Cholangitis
     Cholangitis: Cholangitis:
         NOS   recurrent
         acute   sclerosing
         ascending   secondary
         chronic   stenosing
         primary   suppurative
     AHA: 2Q, '99, 13
     K83.0 Cholangitis   I-10

576.2 Obstruction of bile duct
     Occlusion   ⎫
     Stenosis   ⎬ of bile duct, except cystic duct, without
     Stricture   ⎭   mention of calculus

     EXCLUDES *congenital (751.61)*
         that with calculus (574.3-574.5 with
         fifth-digit 1)
     AHA: 3Q, '03, 17-18; 1Q, '01, 8; 2Q, '99, 13
     K83.1 Obstruction of bile duct   I-10

576.3 Perforation of bile duct
     Rupture of bile duct, except cystic duct

576.4 Fistula of bile duct
     Choledochoduodenal fistula

576.5 Spasm of sphincter of Oddi

576.8 Other specified disorders of biliary tract
     Adhesions   ⎫
     Atrophy   ⎪
     Cyst   ⎬ of bile duct (any)
     Hypertrophy   ⎪
     Nonfunctioning ⎪
     Ulcer   ⎭

     EXCLUDES *congenital choledochal cyst (751.69)*
     AHA: 3Q, '03, 17; 2Q, '99, 14

576.9 Unspecified disorder of biliary tract

---

§   Requires fifth digit. Valid digits are in [brackets] under each code. See category 574 for codes and definitions.

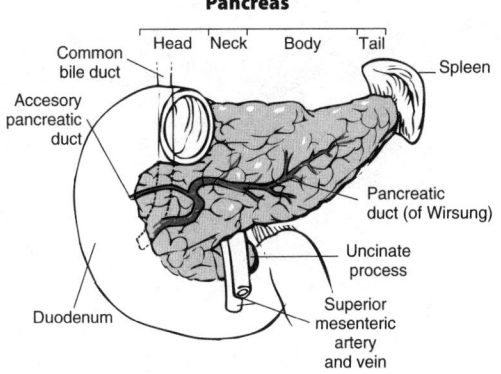

Pancreas

✓4ᵗʰ 577 Diseases of pancreas

577.0 Acute pancreatitis
Abscess of pancreas
Necrosis of pancreas:
  acute
  infective
Pancreatitis:
  NOS
  acute (recurrent)
  apoplectic
  hemorrhagic
  subacute
  suppurative
> **EXCLUDES** *mumps pancreatitis (072.3)*

AHA: 3Q, '99, 9; 2Q, '98, 19; 2Q, '96, 13; 2Q, '89, 9
K85.0 Idiopathic acute pancreatitis   `I-10`

577.1 Chronic pancreatitis
Chronic pancreatitis:
  NOS
  infectious
  interstitial
Pancreatitis:
  painless
  recurrent
  relapsing
AHA: 1Q, '01, 8; 2Q, '96, 13; 3Q, '94, 11
K86.1 Other chronic pancreatitis   `I-10`

577.2 Cyst and pseudocyst of pancreas
K86.2 Cyst of pancreas   `I-10`

577.8 Other specified diseases of pancreas
Atrophy ⎫
Calculus ⎬ of pancreas
Cirrhosis ⎪
Fibrosis ⎭
Pancreatic:
  infantilism
  necrosis:
    NOS
    aseptic
    fat
Pancreatolithiasis
> **EXCLUDES** *fibrocystic disease of pancreas (277.00-277.09)*
> *islet cell tumor of pancreas (211.7)*
> *pancreatic steatorrhea (579.4)*

AHA: 1Q, '01, 8

577.9 Unspecified disease of pancreas

✓4ᵗʰ 578 Gastrointestinal hemorrhage
> **EXCLUDES** *that with mention of:*
> *angiodysplasia of stomach and duodenum (537.83)*
> *angiodysplasia of intestine (569.85)*
> *diverticulitis, intestine:*
> *large (562.13)*
> *small (562.03)*
> *diverticulosis, intestine:*
> *large (562.12)*
> *small (562.02)*
> *gastritis and duodenitis (535.0-535.6)*
> *ulcer:*
> *duodenal, gastric, gastrojejuunal or peptic*
> *(531.00-534.91)*

AHA: 2Q, '92, 9; 4Q, '90, 20

578.0 Hematemesis
Vomiting of blood
AHA: 2Q, '02, 4

578.1 Blood in stool
Melena
> **EXCLUDES** *melena of the newborn (772.4, 777.3)*
> *occult blood (792.1)*

AHA: 2Q, '06, 17; 2Q, '92, 8
K91.2 Melena   `I-10`

578.9 Hemorrhage of gastrointestinal tract, unspecified
Gastric hemorrhage
Intestinal hemorrhage
AHA: 4Q, '06, 91; 3Q, '05, 17; N-D, '86, 9
TIP: Assign 578.9 if the physician does not establish a causal link between GI bleeding and any possible causes found on endoscopy.
K92.2 Gastrointestinal hemorrhage unspecified   `I-10`

✓4ᵗʰ 579 Intestinal malabsorption

579.0 Celiac disease
Celiac: Gee (-Herter) disease
  crisis   Gluten enteropathy
  infantilism   Idiopathic steatorrhea
  rickets   Nontropical sprue
DEF: Malabsorption syndrome due to gluten consumption; symptoms include fetid, bulky, frothy, oily stools, distended abdomen, gas, asthenia, electrolyte depletion and vitamin B, D and K deficiency.

579.1 Tropical sprue
Sprue:
  NOS
  tropical
Tropical steatorrhea
DEF: Diarrhea, occurs in tropics; may be due to enteric infection and malnutrition.

579.2 Blind loop syndrome
Postoperative blind loop syndrome
DEF: Obstruction or impaired passage in small intestine due to alterations, from strictures or surgery; causes stasis, abnormal bacterial flora, diarrhea, weight loss, multiple vitamin deficiency, and megaloblastic anemia.
TIP: Do not assign additional code from subcategory 997.4 Digestive system complications.

579.3 Other and unspecified postsurgical nonabsorption
Hypoglycemia ⎫ following gastrointestinal
Malnutrition ⎬ surgery
AHA: 4Q, '03, 104

579.4 Pancreatic steatorrhea
DEF: Excess fat in feces due to absence of pancreatic secretions in intestine.

579.8 Other specified intestinal malabsorption
Enteropathy:
  exudative
  protein-losing
Steatorrhea (chronic)
AHA: 1Q, '88, 6

579.9 Unspecified intestinal malabsorption
Malabsorption syndrome NOS
AHA: 2Q, '11, 15; 4Q, '04, 59

10. Diseases of the Genitourinary System (580-629)

Nephritis, Nephrotic Syndrome, and Nephrosis (580-589)

> **EXCLUDES** *hypertensive chronic kidney disease (403.00-403.91, 404.00-404.93)*

☑4ᵗʰ 580 Acute glomerulonephritis

INCLUDES acute nephritis

DEF: Acute, severe inflammation in tuft of capillaries that filter the kidneys.

580.0 With lesion of proliferative glomerulonephritis
Acute (diffuse) proliferative glomerulonephritis
Acute poststreptococcal glomerulonephritis

580.4 With lesion of rapidly progressive glomerulonephritis
Acute nephritis with lesion of necrotizing glomerulitis

DEF: Acute glomerulonephritis; progresses to ESRD with diffuse epithelial proliferation.

☑5ᵗʰ 580.8 With other specified pathological lesion in kidney

580.81 *Acute glomerulonephritis in diseases classified elsewhere*

Code first underlying disease, as:
infectious hepatitis (070.0-070.9)
mumps (072.79)
subacute bacterial endocarditis (421.0)
typhoid fever (002.0)

580.89 Other
Glomerulonephritis, acute, with lesion of:
exudative nephritis
interstitial (diffuse) (focal) nephritis

580.9 Acute glomerulonephritis with unspecified pathological lesion in kidney
Glomerulonephritis
NOS
hemorrhagic } specified as acute
Nephritis
Nephropathy

☑4ᵗʰ 581 Nephrotic syndrome

DEF: Disease process marked by symptoms such as extensive edema, notable proteinuria, hypoalbuminemia, and susceptibility to intercurrent infections.

581.0 With lesion of proliferative glomerulonephritis

581.1 With lesion of membranous glomerulonephritis
Epimembranous nephritis
Idiopathic membranous glomerular disease
Nephrotic syndrome with lesion of:
focal glomerulosclerosis
sclerosing membranous glomerulonephritis
segmental hyalinosis

581.2 With lesion of membranoproliferative glomerulonephritis
Nephrotic syndrome with lesion (of):
endothelial
hypocomplementemic persistent
lobular
mesangiocapillary } glomerulonephritis
mixed membranous and
    proliferative

DEF: Glomerulonephritis combined with clinical features of nephrotic syndrome; characterized by uneven thickening of glomerular capillary walls and mesangial cell increase; slowly progresses to ESRD.

581.3 With lesion of minimal change glomerulonephritis
Foot process disease
Lipoid nephrosis
Minimal change:
glomerular disease
glomerulitis
nephrotic syndrome

AHA: 1Q, '07, 23

Kidney

(anatomical diagram labels:) Renal cortex, Fibrous capsule, Nephron, Medulla (pyramid), Renal column, Renal sinus, Pelvis, Renal hilum, Major calyx, Minor calyx, Ureter

☑5ᵗʰ 581.8 With other specified pathological lesion in kidney

581.81 *Nephrotic syndrome in diseases classified elsewhere*

Code first underlying disease, as:
amyloidosis (277.30-277.39)
diabetes mellitus (249.4, 250.4)
tes mellitus (250.4)
malaria (084.9)
polyarteritis (446.0)
systemic lupus erythematosus (710.0)

> **EXCLUDES** *nephrosis in epidemic hemorrhagic fever (078.6)*

AHA: 3Q, '91, 8, 12; S-O, '85, 3

581.89 Other
Glomerulonephritis with edema and lesion of:
exudative nephritis
interstitial (diffuse) (focal) nephritis

581.9 Nephrotic syndrome with unspecified pathological lesion in kidney
Glomerulonephritis with edema NOS
Nephritis:
nephrotic NOS
with edema NOS
Nephrosis NOS
Renal disease with edema NOS

☑4ᵗʰ 582 Chronic glomerulonephritis

INCLUDES chronic nephritis

DEF: Slow progressive type of nephritis characterized by inflammation of the capillary loops in the glomeruli of the kidney, which leads to renal failure.

582.0 With lesion of proliferative glomerulonephritis
Chronic (diffuse) proliferative glomerulonephritis

582.1 With lesion of membranous glomerulonephritis
Chronic glomerulonephritis:
membranous
sclerosing
Focal glomerulosclerosis
Segmental hyalinosis

AHA: S-O, '84, 16

Nephron

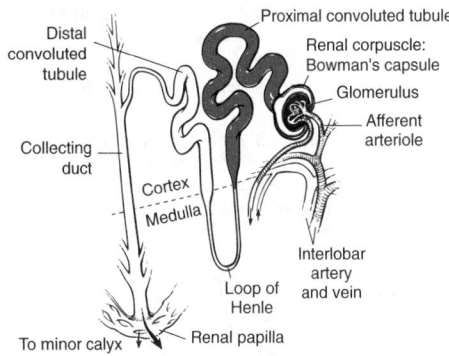

(anatomical diagram labels:) Distal convoluted tubule, Proximal convoluted tubule, Renal corpuscle: Bowman's capsule, Glomerulus, Afferent arteriole, Collecting duct, Cortex, Medulla, Interlobar artery and vein, Loop of Henle, To minor calyx, Renal papilla

☑4ᵗʰ / ☑5ᵗʰ Additional Digit Required   Unspecified Code   Other Specified Code   Manifestation Code   ►◄ Revised Text   ● New Code   ▲ Revised Code Title

2013 ICD-9-CM   **Volume 1 – 179**

582.2 With lesion of membranoproliferative glomerulonephritis
Chronic glomerulonephritis:
   endothelial
   hypocomplementemic persistent
   lobular
   membranoproliferative
   mesangiocapillary
   mixed membranous and proliferative
DEF: Chronic glomerulonephritis with mesangial cell proliferation.

582.4 With lesion of rapidly progressive glomerulonephritis
Chronic nephritis with lesion of necrotizing glomerulitis
DEF: Chronic glomerulonephritis rapidly progresses to ESRD; marked by diffuse epithelial proliferation.

√5ᵗʰ 582.8 With other specified pathological lesion in kidney

  582.81 Chronic glomerulonephritis in diseases classified elsewhere
    Code first underlying disease, as:
      amyloidosis (277.30-277.39)
      systemic lupus erythematosus (710.0)

  582.89 Other
    Chronic glomerulonephritis with lesion of:
      exudative nephritis
      interstitial (diffuse) (focal) nephritis

582.9 Chronic glomerulonephritis with unspecified pathological lesion in kidney
Glomerulonephritis:
  NOS
  hemorrhagic } specified as chronic
Nephritis
Nephropathy
AHA: 2Q, '01, 12

√4ᵗʰ 583 Nephritis and nephropathy, not specified as acute or chronic
INCLUDES "renal disease" so stated, not specified as acute or chronic but with stated pathology or cause

583.0 With lesion of proliferative glomerulonephritis
Proliferative:
  glomerulonephritis (diffuse) NOS
  nephritis NOS
  nephropathy NOS

583.1 With lesion of membranous glomerulonephritis
Membranous:
  glomerulonephritis NOS
  nephritis NOS
Membranous nephropathy NOS
DEF: Kidney inflammation or dysfunction with deposits on glomerular capillary basement membranes.
N05.2 Uns nephritic syndr w/ diffuse membranous gln   I-10

583.2 With lesion of membranoproliferative glomerulonephritis
Membranoproliferative:
  glomerulonephritis NOS
  nephritis NOS
  nephropathy NOS
Nephritis NOS, with lesion of:
  hypocomplementemic persistent
  lobular
  mesangiocapillary } glomerulonephritis
  mixed membranous and proliferative
DEF: Kidney inflammation or dysfunction with mesangial cell proliferation.

583.4 With lesion of rapidly progressive glomerulonephritis
Necrotizing or rapidly progressive:
  glomerulitis NOS
  glomerulonephritis NOS
  nephritis NOS
  nephropathy NOS
Nephritis, unspecified, with lesion of necrotizing glomerulitis
DEF: Kidney inflammation or dysfunction; rapidly progresses to ESRD marked by diffuse epithelial proliferation.

583.6 With lesion of renal cortical necrosis
Nephritis, NOS
Nephropathy NOS } with (renal) cortical necrosis
Renal cortical necrosis NOS

583.7 With lesion of renal medullary necrosis
Nephritis, NOS
Nephropathy NOS } with (renal) medullary [papillary] necrosis

√5ᵗʰ 583.8 With other specified pathological lesion in kidney

  583.81 Nephritis and nephropathy, not specified as acute or chronic, in diseases classified elsewhere
    Code first underlying disease, as:
      amyloidosis (277.30-277.39)
      diabetes mellitus (249.4, 250.4)
      gonococcal infection (098.19)
      Goodpasture's syndrome (446.21)
      systemic lupus erythematosus (710.0)
      tuberculosis (016.0)
    EXCLUDES gouty nephropathy (274.10)
      syphilitic nephritis (095.4)
    AHA: 2Q, '03, 7; 3Q, '91, 8; S-O, '85, 3

  583.89 Other
    Glomerulitis
    Glomerulonephritis
    Nephritis } with lesions of:
    Nephropathy   exudative nephritis
    Renal disease   interstitial nephritis

583.9 With unspecified pathological lesion in kidney
Glomerulitis
Glomerulonephritis } NOS
Nephritis
Nephropathy
EXCLUDES nephropathy complicating pregnancy, labor, or the puerperium (642.0-642.9, 646.2)
renal disease NOS with no stated cause (593.9)

√4ᵗʰ 584 Acute kidney failure
INCLUDES acute renal failure
EXCLUDES following labor and delivery (669.3)
posttraumatic (958.5)
that complicating:
  abortion (634-638 with .3, 639.3)
  ectopic or molar pregnancy (639.3)
DEF: State resulting from increasing urea and related substances from the blood (azotemia), often with urine output of less than 500 ml per day.
AHA: 2Q, '11, 15; 3Q, '10, 15; 1Q, '93, 18; 2Q, '92, 5; 4Q, '92, 22
TIP: Report acute renal failure separately when documented in addition to or in association with hypertensive renal disease..

584.5 Acute kidney failure with lesion of tubular necrosis
Lower nephron nephrosis
Renal failure with (acute) tubular necrosis
Tubular necrosis:
  NOS
  acute
DEF: Acute decline in kidney efficiency with destruction of tubules.
N17.0 Acute renal failure with tubular necrosis   I-10

584.6 Acute kidney failure with lesion of renal cortical necrosis
DEF: Acute decline in kidney efficiency with destruction of renal tissues that filter blood.

584.7 Acute kidney failure with lesion of renal medullary [papillary] necrosis
Necrotizing renal papillitis
DEF: Acute decline in kidney efficiency with destruction of renal tissues that collect urine.

584.8 Acute kidney failure with other specified pathological lesion in kidney
AHA: ▶3Q, '11, 16-17;◀ N-D, '85, 1

584.9 Acute kidney failure, unspecified
Acute kidney injury (nontraumatic)
EXCLUDES traumatic kidney injury (866.00-866.13)
AHA: ▶3Q, '11, 16-17;◀ 4Q, '09, 98; 4Q, '08, 192; 4Q, '07, 97; 2Q, '05, 18; 2Q, '03, 7; 1Q, '03, 22; 3Q, '02, 21, 28; 2Q, '01, 14; 1Q, '00, 22; 3Q, '96, 9; 4Q, '88, 1
N17.9 Acute renal failure unspecified   I-10

√4ᵗʰ **585 Chronic kidney disease [CKD]**
Chronic uremia

Code first hypertensive chronic kidney disease, if applicable,
(403.00-403.91, 404.00-404.93)

Use additional code to identify kidney transplant status, if applicable
(V42.0)

Use additional code to identify manifestation as:
uremic:
neuropathy (357.4)
pericarditis (420.0)

AHA: 4Q, '06, 84-86; 4Q, '05, 68, 77; 1Q, '04, 5; 4Q, '03, 61, 111; 2Q, '03, 7; 2Q, '01, 12, 13; 1Q, '01, 3; 4Q, '98, 55; 3Q, '98, 6, 7; 2Q, '98, 20; 3Q, '96, 9; 1Q, '93, 18; 3Q, '91, 8; 4Q, '89, 1; N-D, '85, 15; S-O, '84, 3

585.1 Chronic kidney disease, Stage I
DEF: Some kidney damage; normal or slightly increased GFR (> 90).

585.2 Chronic kidney disease, Stage II (mild)
DEF: Kidney damage with mild decrease in GFR (60–89).

585.3 Chronic kidney disease, Stage III (moderate)
AHA: 4Q, '05, 69
DEF: Kidney damage with moderate decrease in GFR (30–59).
N18.3 Chronic kidney disease stage 3 (moderate) | I-10

585.4 Chronic kidney disease, Stage IV (severe)
DEF: Kidney damage with severe decrease in GFR (15–29).
N18.4 Chronic kidney disease stage 4 (severe) | I-10

585.5 Chronic kidney disease, Stage V
EXCLUDES chronic kidney disease, stage V requiring chronic dialysis (585.6)
DEF: Kidney failure with GFR value of less than 15.
AHA: 4Q, '10, 137

585.6 End stage renal disease
Chronic kidney disease requiring chronic dialysis
DEF: Federal government indicator of a stage V CKD patient undergoing treatment by dialysis or transplantation.
AHA: ▶3Q, '11,15;◀ 2Q, '11, 6; 3Q, '10, 12, 15; 4Q, '08, 193; 1Q, '08, 7; 4Q, '07, 86; 3Q, '07, 5, 9; 4Q, '06, 136; 4Q, '05, 79
N18.6 End stage renal disease | I-10

585.9 Chronic kidney disease, unspecified
Chronic renal disease   Chronic renal insufficiency
Chronic renal failure NOS
AHA: 1Q, '08, 10; 2Q, '07, 3; 4Q, '06, 86; 4Q, '05, 79
N18.9 Chronic kidney disease unspecified | I-10

586 Renal failure, unspecified
Uremia NOS
EXCLUDES following labor and delivery (669.3)
posttraumatic renal failure (958.5)
that complicating:
abortion (634-638 with .3, 639.3)
ectopic or molar pregnancy (639.3)
uremia:
extrarenal (788.9)
prerenal (788.9)
DEF: Renal failure: kidney functions cease; malfunction may be due to inability to excrete metabolized substances or retain level of electrolytes.
DEF: Uremia: excess urea, creatinine and other nitrogenous products of protein and amino acid metabolism in blood due to reduced excretory function in bilateral kidney disease; also called azotemia.
AHA: 3Q, '98, 6; 1Q, '93, 18; 1Q, '88, 3
N19 Unspecified renal failure | I-10

Genitourinary System

Inferior vena cava — Aorta
Right kidney — Left kidney
Anterior division of internal iliac artery — Ureter
Superior and Inferior vesicular arteries — Ovarian or testicular artery and vein
Ureteral orifice — Urinary bladder
Urethra — Urogenital diaphragm

587 Renal sclerosis, unspecified
Atrophy of kidney
Contracted kidney
Renal:
cirrhosis
fibrosis
AHA: 4Q, '10, 137

√4ᵗʰ **588 Disorders resulting from impaired renal function**

588.0 Renal osteodystrophy
Azotemic osteodystrophy
Phosphate-losing tubular disorders
Renal:
dwarfism
infantilism
rickets
DEF: Condition resulting from chronic renal failure results in osteomalacia, osteoporosis or osteosclerosis; an abnormal level of phosphorus in the blood and impaired stimulation of the parathyroid.

588.1 Nephrogenic diabetes insipidus
EXCLUDES diabetes insipidus NOS (253.5)
DEF: Type of diabetes due to renal tubules inability to reabsorb water; not responsive to vasopressin; may develop into chronic renal insufficiency.

√5ᵗʰ **588.8 Other specified disorders resulting from impaired renal function**
EXCLUDES secondary hypertension (405.0-405.9)

588.81 Secondary hyperparathyroidism (of renal origin)
Secondary hyperparathyroidism NOS
DEF: Parathyroid dysfunction caused by chronic renal failure; phosphate clearance is impaired, phosphate is released from bone, vitamin D is not produced, intestinal calcium absorption is low, and blood levels of calcium are lowered causing excessive production of parathyroid hormone.
AHA: 4Q, '04, 58-59
N25.81 Secondary hyperparathyroidism of renal origin | I-10

588.89 Other specified disorders resulting from impaired renal function
Hypokalemic nephropathy

588.9 Unspecified disorder resulting from impaired renal function

√4ᵗʰ **589 Small kidney of unknown cause**

589.0 Unilateral small kidney

589.1 Bilateral small kidneys

589.9 Small kidney, unspecified

Other Diseases of Urinary System (590-599)

√4ᵗʰ **590 Infections of kidney**
Use additional code to identify organism, such as Escherichia coli [E. coli] (041.41-041.49)

√5ᵗʰ **590.0 Chronic pyelonephritis**
Chronic pyelitis
Chronic pyonephrosis
Code if applicable, any casual condition first

590.00 Without lesion of renal medullary necrosis

590.01 With lesion of renal medullary necrosis

√5ᵗʰ **590.1 Acute pyelonephritis**
Acute pyelitis
Acute pyonephrosis

590.10 Without lesion of renal medullary necrosis

590.11 With lesion of renal medullary necrosis

590.2 Renal and perinephric abscess
Abscess:
kidney
nephritic
perirenal
Carbuncle of kidney

√4ᵗʰ Additional Digit Required   Unspecified Code   Other Specified Code   Manifestation Code   ▶◀ Revised Text   ● New Code   ▲ Revised Code Title
√5ᵗʰ

Diseases of the Genitourinary System

590.3–594.9

590.3 Pyeloureteritis cystica
Infection of renal pelvis and ureter
Ureteritis cystica
DEF: Inflammation and formation of submucosal cysts in the kidney, pelvis, and ureter.

√5ᵗʰ **590.8 Other pyelonephritis or pyonephrosis, not specified as acute or chronic**

590.80 Pyelonephritis, unspecified
Pyelitis NOS
Pyelonephritis NOS
AHA: 1Q, '98, 10; 4Q, '97, 40
N11.9 Chronic tubulo-interstitial nephritis uns   I-10

590.81 Pyelitis or pyelonephritis in diseases classified elsewhere
Code first underlying disease, as:
tuberculosis (016.0)

590.9 Infection of kidney, unspecified
EXCLUDES urinary tract infection NOS (599.0)

591 Hydronephrosis
Hydrocalycosis
Hydronephrosis
Hydroureteronephrosis
EXCLUDES congenital hydronephrosis (753.29)
hydroureter (593.5)
DEF: Distention of kidney and pelvis, with urine build-up due to ureteral obstruction; pyonephrosis may result.
AHA: 2Q, '98, 9
TIP: Hydronephrosis is not inherent in urinary obstructions and should be coded separately.
N13.30 Unspecified hydronephrosis   I-10

√4ᵗʰ **592 Calculus of kidney and ureter**
EXCLUDES nephrocalcinosis (275.4)

592.0 Calculus of kidney
Nephrolithiasis NOS
Renal calculus or stone
Staghorn calculus
Stone in kidney
EXCLUDES uric acid nephrolithiasis (274.11)
AHA: 1Q, '00, 4
N20.0 Calculus of kidney   I-10

592.1 Calculus of ureter
Ureteric stone
Ureterolithiasis
AHA: 2Q, '98, 9; 1Q, '98, 10; 1Q, '91, 11
N20.1 Calculus of ureter   I-10

592.9 Urinary calculus, unspecified
AHA: 1Q, '98, 10; 4Q, '97, 40

√4ᵗʰ **593 Other disorders of kidney and ureter**

593.0 Nephroptosis
Floating kidney
Mobile kidney

593.1 Hypertrophy of kidney

593.2 Cyst of kidney, acquired
Cyst (multiple) (solitary) of kidney, not congenital
Peripelvic (lymphatic) cyst
EXCLUDES calyceal or pyelogenic cyst of kidney (591)
congenital cyst of kidney (753.1)
polycystic (disease of) kidney (753.1)
DEF: Abnormal, fluid-filled sac in the kidney, not present at birth.
AHA: 4Q, '90, 3
N28.1 Cyst of kidney acquired   I-10

593.3 Stricture or kinking of ureter
Angulation } of ureter (post-operative)
Constriction
Stricture of pelviureteric junction
DEF: Stricture or knot in tube connecting kidney to bladder.
AHA: 2Q, '98, 9

593.4 Other ureteric obstruction
Idiopathic retroperitoneal fibrosis
Occlusion NOS of ureter
EXCLUDES that due to calculus (592.1)
AHA: 1Q, '10, 9; 2Q, '97, 4

593.5 Hydroureter
EXCLUDES congenital hydroureter (753.22)
hydroureteronephrosis (591)

593.6 Postural proteinuria
Benign postural proteinuria
Orthostatic proteinuria
EXCLUDES proteinuria NOS (791.0)
DEF: Excessive amounts of serum protein in the urine caused by the body position, e.g., orthostatic and lordotic.

√5ᵗʰ **593.7 Vesicoureteral reflux**
DEF: Backflow of urine, from bladder into ureter due to obstructed bladder neck.
AHA: 4Q, '94, 42

593.70 Unspecified or without reflux nephropathy

593.71 With reflux nephropathy, unilateral

593.72 With reflux nephropathy, bilateral

593.73 With reflux nephropathy NOS

√5ᵗʰ **593.8 Other specified disorders of kidney and ureter**

593.81 Vascular disorders of kidney
Renal (artery):
embolism
hemorrhage
thrombosis
Renal infarction

593.82 Ureteral fistula
Intestinoureteral fistula
EXCLUDES fistula between ureter and female genital tract (619.0)
DEF: Abnormal communication, between tube connecting kidney to bladder and another structure.

593.89 Other
Adhesions, kidney or ureter
Periureteritis
Polyp of ureter
Pyelectasia
Ureterocele
EXCLUDES tuberculosis of ureter (016.2)
ureteritis cystica (590.3)

593.9 Unspecified disorder of kidney and ureter
Acute renal disease
Acute renal insufficiency
Renal disease NOS
Salt-losing nephritis or syndrome
EXCLUDES chronic renal insufficiency (585.9)
cystic kidney disease (753.1)
nephropathy, so stated (583.0-583.9)
renal disease:
arising in pregnancy or the puerperium
(642.1-642.2, 642.4-642.7, 646.2)
not specified as acute or chronic, but with stated
pathology or cause (583.0-583.9)
AHA: 4Q, '05, 79; 1Q, '93, 17
N28.9 Disorder of kidney and ureter unspecified   I-10

√4ᵗʰ **594 Calculus of lower urinary tract**

594.0 Calculus in diverticulum of bladder
DEF: Stone or mineral deposit in abnormal sac on the bladder wall.

594.1 Other calculus in bladder
Urinary bladder stone
EXCLUDES staghorn calculus (592.0)
DEF: Stone or mineral deposit in bladder.

594.2 Calculus in urethra
DEF: Stone or mineral deposit in tube that empties urine from bladder.

594.8 Other lower urinary tract calculus
AHA: J-F, '85, 16

594.9 Calculus of lower urinary tract, unspecified
EXCLUDES calculus of urinary tract NOS (592.9)

Bladder

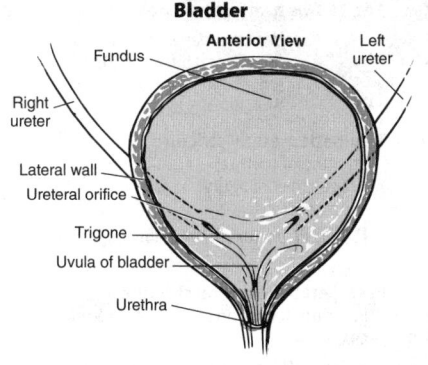

Anterior View

Fundus

Right ureter

Left ureter

Lateral wall

Ureteral orifice

Trigone

Uvula of bladder

Urethra

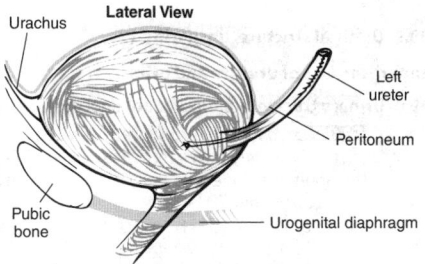

Lateral View

Urachus

Left ureter

Peritoneum

Pubic bone

Urogenital diaphragm

✓4th 595 Cystitis

> **EXCLUDES** *prostatocystitis (601.3)*
>
> Use additional code to identify organism, such as Escherichia coli [E. coli] (041.41-041.49)

595.0 Acute cystitis

> **EXCLUDES** *trigonitis (595.3)*
> **DEF:** Acute inflammation of bladder.
> **AHA:** 2Q, '99, 15
> N30.00 Acute cystitis without hematuria   I-10

595.1 Chronic interstitial cystitis

> Hunner's ulcer
> Panmural fibrosis of bladder
> Submucous cystitis
> **DEF:** Inflamed lesion affecting bladder wall; symptoms include urinary frequency, pain on bladder filling, nocturia, and distended bladder.

595.2 Other chronic cystitis

> Chronic cystitis NOS
> Subacute cystitis
> **EXCLUDES** *trigonitis (595.3)*
> **DEF:** Persistent inflammation of bladder.

595.3 Trigonitis

> Follicular cystitis
> Trigonitis (acute) (chronic)
> Urethrotrigonitis
> **DEF:** Inflammation of the triangular area of the bladder called the trigonum vesicae.

595.4 Cystitis in diseases classified elsewhere

> *Code first underlying disease, as:*
> actinomycosis (039.8)
> amebiasis (006.8)
> bilharziasis (120.0-120.9)
> Echinococcus infestation (122.3, 122.6)
> **EXCLUDES** *cystitis:*
> *diphtheritic (032.84)*
> *gonococcal (098.11, 098.31)*
> *monilial (112.2)*
> *trichomonal (131.09)*
> *tuberculous (016.1)*

✓5th 595.8 Other specified types of cystitis

595.81 Cystitis cystica

> **DEF:** Inflammation of the bladder characterized by formation of multiple cysts.

595.82 Irradiation cystitis

> Use additional E code to identify cause
> **DEF:** Inflammation of the bladder due to effects of radiation.

595.89 Other

> Abscess of bladder:
> Cystitis:
> bullous
> emphysematous
> glandularis

595.9 Cystitis, unspecified

✓4th 596 Other disorders of bladder

> Use additional code to identify urinary incontinence (625.6, 788.30-788.39)
> **AHA:** M-A, '87, 10

596.0 Bladder neck obstruction

> Contracture (acquired) ⎫ of bladder neck or
> Obstruction (acquired) ⎬ vesicourethral
> Stenosis (acquired) ⎭ orifice
>
> **EXCLUDES** *congenital (753.6)*
> **DEF:** Bladder outlet and vesicourethral obstruction; occurs as a consequence of benign prostatic hypertrophy or prostatic cancer; may also occur in either sex due to strictures, following radiation, cystoscopy, catheterization, injury, infection, blood clots, bladder cancer, impaction or disease compressing bladder neck.
> **AHA:** 3Q, '02, 28; 2Q, '01, 14; N-D, '86, 10
> N32.0 Bladder-neck obstruction   I-10

596.1 Intestinovesical fistula

> Fistula:
> enterovesical
> vesicocolic
> vesicoenteric
> vesicorectal
> **DEF:** Abnormal communication, between intestine and bladder.

596.2 Vesical fistula, not elsewhere classified

> Fistula:
> bladder NOS
> urethrovesical
> vesicocutaneous
> vesicoperineal
> **EXCLUDES** *fistula between bladder and female genital tract (619.0)*
> **DEF:** Abnormal communication between bladder and another structure.

596.3 Diverticulum of bladder

> Diverticulitis ⎫ of bladder
> Diverticulum (acquired) (false) ⎬
> **EXCLUDES** *that with calculus in diverticulum of bladder (594.0)*
> **DEF:** Abnormal pouch in bladder wall.

596.4 Atony of bladder

> High compliance bladder
> Hypotonicity ⎫ of bladder
> Inertia ⎭
> **EXCLUDES** *neurogenic bladder (596.54)*
> **DEF:** Distended, bladder with loss of expulsive force; linked to CNS disease.

✓5th 596.5 Other functional disorders of bladder

> **EXCLUDES** *cauda equina syndrome with neurogenic bladder (344.61)*

596.51 Hypertonicity of bladder

> Hyperactivity
> Overactive bladder
> **DEF:** Abnormal tension of muscular wall of bladder; may appear after surgery of voluntary nerve.
> N32.81 Overactive bladder   I-10

596.52 Low bladder compliance

> **DEF:** Low bladder capacity; causes increased pressure and frequent urination.

596.53 Paralysis of bladder

> **DEF:** Impaired bladder motor function due to nerve or muscle damage.

596.54 Neurogenic bladder NOS

> **DEF:** Unspecified dysfunctional bladder due to lesion of central, peripheral nervous system; may result in incontinence, residual urine retention, urinary infection, stones and renal failure.
> **AHA:** 1Q, '01, 12
> N31.9 Neuromuscular dysfunction of   I-10
> bladder unspecified

✓4th ✓5th   Additional Digit Required   Unspecified Code   Other Specified Code   Manifestation Code   ►◄ Revised Text   ● New Code   ▲ Revised Code Title

2013 ICD-9-CM   **Volume 1 – 183**

596.55 Detrusor sphincter dyssynergia
> **DEF:** Instability of the urinary bladder sphincter muscle associated with urinary incontinence.

596.59 Other functional disorder of bladder
> Detrusor instability
> **DEF:** Detrusor instability: instability of bladder; marked by uninhibited contractions often leading to incontinence.

596.6 Rupture of bladder, nontraumatic

596.7 Hemorrhage into bladder wall
> Hyperemia of bladder
> **EXCLUDES** acute hemorrhagic cystitis (595.0)

√5ᵗʰ **596.8 Other specified disorders of bladder**
> **EXCLUDES** cystocele, female (618.01-618.02, 618.09, 618.2-618.4)
> hernia or prolapse of bladder, female (618.01-618.02, 618.09, 618.2-618.4)
> **AHA:** 4Q, '11, 128-129; J-F, '85, 8

596.81 Infection of cystostomy
> Use additional code to specify type of infection, such as:
> abscess or cellulitis of abdomen (682.2)
> septicemia (038.0-038.9)
> Use additional code to identify organism (041.00-041.9)
> **AHA:** 4Q, '11, 129

596.82 Mechanical complication of cystostomy
> Malfunction of cystostomy

596.83 Other complication of cystostomy
> Fistula
> Hernia
> Prolapse

596.89 Other specified disorders of bladder
> Bladder hemorrhage
> Bladder hypertrophy
> Calcified bladder
> Contracted bladder

596.9 Unspecified disorder of bladder
> **AHA:** J-F, '85, 8

√4ᵗʰ **597 Urethritis, not sexually transmitted, and urethral syndrome**
> **EXCLUDES** nonspecific urethritis, so stated (099.4)

597.0 Urethral abscess
> Abscess:　　　　　　Abscess of:
> periurethral　　　　Cowper's gland
> urethral (gland)　　Littré's gland
> Abscess of:　　　　Periurethral cellulitis
> bulbourethral gland
> **EXCLUDES** urethral caruncle (599.3)
> **DEF:** Pocket of pus in tube that empties urine from the bladder.

√5ᵗʰ **597.8 Other urethritis**

597.80 Urethritis, unspecified

597.81 Urethral syndrome NOS

597.89 Other
> Adenitis, Skene's glands
> Cowperitis
> Meatitis, urethral
> Ulcer, urethra (meatus)
> Verumontanitis
> **EXCLUDES** trichomonal (131.02)

√4ᵗʰ **598 Urethral stricture**
> Use additional code to identify urinary incontinence (625.6, 788.30-788.39)
> **INCLUDES** pinhole meatus
> stricture of urinary meatus
> **EXCLUDES** congenital stricture of urethra and urinary meatus (753.6)
> **DEF:** Narrowing of tube that empties urine from bladder.

√5ᵗʰ **598.0 Urethral stricture due to infection**

598.00 Due to unspecified infection

598.01 Due to infective diseases classified elsewhere
> Code first underlying disease, as:
> gonococcal infection (098.2)
> schistosomiasis (120.0-120.9)
> syphilis (095.8)

598.1 Traumatic urethral stricture
> Stricture of urethra:
> late effect of injury
> postobstetric
> **EXCLUDES** postoperative following surgery on genitourinary tract (598.2)

598.2 Postoperative urethral stricture
> Postcatheterization stricture of urethra
> **AHA:** 3Q, '97, 6

598.8 Other specified causes of urethral stricture
> **AHA:** N-D, '84, 9

598.9 Urethral stricture, unspecified

√4ᵗʰ **599 Other disorders of urethra and urinary tract**

599.0 Urinary tract infection, site not specified
> **EXCLUDES** candidiasis of urinary tract (112.2)
> urinary tract infection of newborn (771.82)
> Use additional code to identify organism, such as Escherichia coli [E. coli] (041.41-041.49)
> **AHA:** ▶1Q, '12, 11;◀4Q, '11, 129; 1Q, '10, 9; 3Q, '09, 10-11; 3Q, '05, 12; 2Q, '04, 13; 4Q, '03, 79; 4Q, '99, 6; 2Q, '99, 15;1Q, '98, 5; 2Q, '96, 7; 4Q, '96, 33; 2Q, '95, 7; 1Q, '92, 13
> N39.0 Urinary tract infection site not specified　　I-10

599.1 Urethral fistula
> Fistula:　　　　　　　　Urinary fistula NOS
> urethroperineal
> urethrorectal
> **EXCLUDES** fistula:
> urethroscrotal (608.89)
> urethrovaginal (619.0)
> urethrovesicovaginal (619.0)
> **AHA:** 2Q, '11, 13; 3Q, '97, 6

599.2 Urethral diverticulum
> **DEF:** Abnormal pouch in urethral wall.

599.3 Urethral caruncle
> Polyp of urethra

599.4 Urethral false passage
> **DEF:** Abnormal opening in urethra due to surgery; trauma or disease.

599.5 Prolapsed urethral mucosa
> Prolapse of urethra　　　Urethrocele
> **EXCLUDES** urethrocele, female (618.03, 618.09, 618.2-618.4)

√5ᵗʰ **599.6 Urinary obstruction**
> Use additional code to identify urinary incontinence (625.6, 788.30-788.39)
> **EXCLUDES** obstructive nephropathy NOS (593.89)
> **AHA:** 4Q, '05, 80

599.60 Urinary obstruction, unspecified
> Obstructive uropathy NOS
> Urinary (tract) obstruction NOS
> N13.9 Obstructive and reflux uropathy unspec　　I-10

599.69 Urinary obstruction, not elsewhere classified
> Code, if applicable, any causal condition first, such as:
> hyperplasia of prostate (600.0-600.9 with fifth-digit 1)
> **AHA:** 4Q, '06, 93

√5ᵗʰ **599.7 Hematuria**
> Hematuria (benign) (essential)
> **EXCLUDES** hemoglobinuria (791.2)
> **AHA:** 4Q, '08, 121; 1Q, '00, 5; 3Q, '95, 8

599.70 Hematuria, unspecified
> R31.9 Hematuria unspecified　　I-10

599.71 Gross hematuria
> **AHA:** 2Q, '10, 3; 2Q, '10, 3

599.72 Microscopic hematuria

N Newborn Age: 0　　　　P Pediatric Age: 0-17　　　　M Maternity Age: 12-55　　　　A Adult Age: 15-124

✓5ᵗʰ 599.8 Other specified disorders of urethra and urinary tract
Use additional code to identify urinary incontinence (625.6, 788.30-788.39), if present

> **EXCLUDES** symptoms and other conditions classifiable to 788.0-788.2, 788.4-788.9, 791.0-791.9

599.81 Urethral hypermobility
     DEF: Hyperactive urethra.

599.82 Intrinsic (urethral) sphincter deficiency [ISD]
     DEF: Malfunctioning urethral sphincter.
     AHA: 2Q, '96, 15

599.83 Urethral instability
     DEF: Inconsistent functioning of urethra.

599.84 Other specified disorders of urethra
Rupture of urethra (nontraumatic)
Urethral:
     cyst
     granuloma
     DEF: Rupture of urethra due to herniation or breaking down of tissue; not due to trauma.
     DEF: Urethral cyst: abnormal sac in urethra; usually fluid filled.
     DEF: Granuloma: inflammatory cells forming small nodules in urethra.
     AHA: 1Q, '09, 15

599.89 Other specified disorders of urinary tract

599.9 Unspecified disorder of urethra and urinary tract

Diseases of Male Genital Organs (600-608)

✓4ᵗʰ 600 Hyperplasia of prostate
     INCLUDES enlarged prostate
     DEF: Fibrostromal proliferation in periurethral glands, causes blood in urine; etiology unknown.
     AHA: 3Q, '05, 20; 4Q, '00, 43; 3Q, '94, 12; 3Q, '92, 7; N-D, '86, 10

✓5ᵗʰ 600.0 Hypertrophy (benign) of prostate
Benign prostatic hypertrophy   Soft enlarged prostate
Enlargement of prostate
Smooth enlarged prostate
     AHA: 4Q, '06, 93-95; 3Q, '05, 20; 4Q, '03, 63; 1Q, '03, 6; 3Q, '02, 28; 2Q, '01, 14

600.00 Hypertrophy (benign) of prostate without urinary obstruction and other lower urinary tract symptoms [LUTS]   Ⓐ ♂
Hypertrophy (benign) of prostate NOS
     N40.0 Enlarged prostate without LUTS   [I-10]

600.01 Hypertrophy (benign) of prostate with urinary obstruction and other lower urinary tract symptoms [LUTS]   Ⓐ ♂
Hypertrophy (benign) of prostate with urinary retention
Use additional code to identify symptoms:
     incomplete bladder emptying (788.21)
     nocturia (788.43)
     straining on urination (788.65)
     urinary frequency (788.41)
     urinary hesitancy (788.64)
     urinary incontinence (788.30-788.39)
     urinary obstruction (599.69)
     urinary retention (788.20)
     urinary urgency (788.63)
     weak urinary stream (788.62)
     AHA: 4Q, '06, 93-95; 4Q, '03, 64

✓5ᵗʰ 600.1 Nodular prostate
Hard, firm prostate
Multinodular prostate
     EXCLUDES malignant neoplasm of prostate (185)
     DEF: Hard, firm nodule in prostate.
     AHA: 4Q, '03, 63

600.10 Nodular prostate without urinary obstruction   Ⓐ ♂
Nodular prostate NOS

600.11 Nodular prostate with urinary obstruction   Ⓐ ♂
Nodular prostate with urinary retention

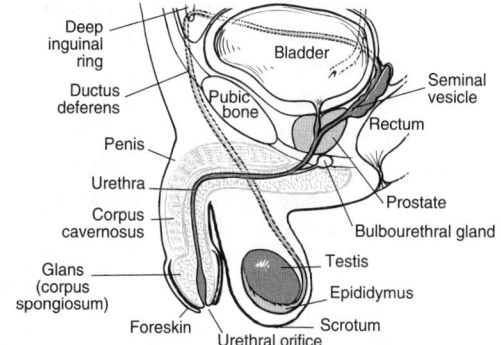

Male Pelvic Organs

Deep inguinal ring — Bladder — Seminal vesicle — Ductus deferens — Pubic bone — Rectum — Penis — Prostate — Urethra — Bulbourethral gland — Corpus cavernosus — Testis — Glans (corpus spongiosum) — Epididymus — Foreskin — Scrotum — Urethral orifice

✓5ᵗʰ 600.2 Benign localized hyperplasia of prostate
Adenofibromatous hypertrophy of prostate
Adenoma of prostate
Fibroadenoma of prostate
Fibroma of prostate
Myoma of prostate
Polyp of prostate
     EXCLUDES benign neoplasms of prostate (222.2)
         hypertrophy of prostate (600.00-600.01)
         malignant neoplasm of prostate (185)
     DEF: Benign localized hyperplasia clearly defined epithelial tumor.
     AHA: 4Q, '06, 93-95; 4Q, '03, 63

600.20 Benign localized hyperplasia of prostate without urinary obstruction and other lower urinary tract symptoms [LUTS]   Ⓐ ♂
Benign localized hyperplasia of prostate NOS

600.21 Benign localized hyperplasia of prostate with urinary obstruction and other lower urinary tract symptoms [LUTS]   Ⓐ ♂
Benign localized hyperplasia of prostate with urinary retention
Use additional code to identify symptoms:
     incomplete bladder emptying (788.21)
     nocturia (788.43)
     straining on urination (788.65)
     urinary frequency (788.41)
     urinary hesitancy (788.64)
     urinary incontinence (788.30-788.39)
     urinary obstruction (599.69)
     urinary retention (788.20)
     urinary urgency (788.63)
     weak urinary stream (788.62)

600.3 Cyst of prostate   Ⓐ ♂
     DEF: Sacs of fluid, which differentiate this from either nodular or adenomatous tumors.

✓5ᵗʰ 600.9 Hyperplasia of prostate, unspecified
Median bar
Prostatic obstruction NOS
     AHA: 4Q, '06, 93-95; 4Q, '03, 63

600.90 Hyperplasia of prostate, unspecified, without urinary obstruction and other lower urinary tract symptoms [LUTS]   Ⓐ ♂
Hyperplasia of prostate NOS

600.91 Hyperplasia of prostate, unspecified with urinary obstruction and other lower urinary tract symptoms [LUTS]   Ⓐ ♂
Hyperplasia of prostate, unspecified, with urinary retention
Use additional code to identify symptoms:
     incomplete bladder emptying (788.21)
     nocturia (788.43)
     straining on urination (788.65)
     urinary frequency (788.41)
     urinary hesitancy (788.64)
     urinary incontinence (788.30-788.39)
     urinary obstruction (599.69)
     urinary retention (788.20)
     urinary urgency (788.63)
     weak urinary stream (788.62)

✓4ᵗʰ / ✓5ᵗʰ Additional Digit Required   Unspecified Code   Other Specified Code   Manifestation Code   ►◄ Revised Text   ● New Code   ▲ Revised Code Title

2013 ICD-9-CM   **Volume 1 – 185**

Diseases of the Genitourinary System

601–606.9

√4ᵗʰ **601 Inflammatory diseases of prostate**

Use additional code to identify organism, such as Staphylococcus (041.1), or Streptococcus (041.0)

601.0 Acute prostatitis   A ♂

601.1 Chronic prostatitis   A ♂

601.2 Abscess of prostate   A ♂

601.3 Prostatocystitis   A ♂

601.4 Prostatitis in diseases classified elsewhere   A ♂

Code first underlying disease, as:
actinomycosis (039.8)
blastomycosis (116.0)
syphilis (095.8)
tuberculosis (016.5)

EXCLUDES *prostatitis:*
gonococcal (098.12, 098.32)
monilial (112.2)
trichomonal (131.03)

601.8 Other specified inflammatory diseases of prostate   A ♂

Prostatitis:
cavitary
diverticular
granulomatous

601.9 Prostatitis, unspecified   A ♂

Prostatitis NOS

√4ᵗʰ **602 Other disorders of prostate**

602.0 Calculus of prostate   A ♂

Prostatic stone

DEF: Stone or mineral deposit in prostate.

602.1 Congestion or hemorrhage of prostate   A ♂

DEF: Bleeding or fluid collection in prostate.

602.2 Atrophy of prostate   A ♂

602.3 Dysplasia of prostate   ♂

Prostatic intraepithelial neoplasia I (PIN I)
Prostatic intraepithelial neoplasia II (PIN II)

EXCLUDES *prostatic intraepithelial neoplasia III (PIN III) (233.4)*

DEF: Abnormality of shape and size of the intraepithelial tissues of the prostate; premalignant condition characterized by stalks and absence of a basilar cell layer; synonyms are intraductal dysplasia, large acinar atypical hyperplasia, atypical primary hyperplasia, hyperplasia with malignant changes, marked atypia, or duct-acinar dysplasia.

AHA: 4Q, '01, 46

602.8 Other specified disorders of prostate   A ♂

Fistula
Infarction } of prostate
Stricture
Periprostatic adhesions

602.9 Unspecified disorder of prostate   A ♂

√4ᵗʰ **603 Hydrocele**

INCLUDES hydrocele of spermatic cord, testis or tunica vaginalis

EXCLUDES *congenital (778.6)*

DEF: Circumscribed collection of fluid in tunica vaginalis, spermatic cord or testis.

603.0 Encysted hydrocele   ♂

603.1 Infected hydrocele   ♂

Use additional code to identify organism

603.8 Other specified types of hydrocele   ♂

603.9 Hydrocele, unspecified   ♂

Common Inguinal Canal Anomalies

√4ᵗʰ **604 Orchitis and epididymitis**

Use additional code to identify organism, such as:
Escherichia coli [E. coli] (041.41-041.49)
Staphylococcus (041.10-041.19)
Streptococcus (041.00-041.09)

604.0 Orchitis, epididymitis, and epididymo-orchitis, with abscess   ♂

Abscess of epididymis or testis

√5ᵗʰ **604.9 Other orchitis, epididymitis, and epididymo-orchitis, without mention of abscess**

604.90 Orchitis and epididymitis, unspecified   ♂

604.91 Orchitis and epididymitis in diseases classified elsewhere   ♂

Code first underlying disease, as:
diphtheria (032.89)
filariasis (125.0-125.9)
syphilis (095.8)

EXCLUDES *orchitis:*
gonococcal (098.13, 098.33)
mumps (072.0)
tuberculous (016.5)
tuberculous epididymitis (016.4)

604.99 Other   ♂

605 Redundant prepuce and phimosis   ♂

Adherent prepuce
Paraphimosis
Phimosis (congenital)
Tight foreskin

DEF: Constriction of preputial orifice causing inability of the prepuce to be drawn back over the glans; it may be congenital or caused by infection.

AHA: 3Q, '08, 9

√4ᵗʰ **606 Infertility, male**

AHA: 2Q, '96, 9

606.0 Azoospermia   A ♂

Absolute infertility
Infertility due to:
germinal (cell) aplasia
spermatogenic arrest (complete)

DEF: Absence of spermatozoa in the semen or inability to produce spermatozoa.

606.1 Oligospermia   A ♂

Infertility due to:
germinal cell desquamation
hypospermatogenesis
incomplete spermatogenic arrest

DEF: Insufficient number of sperm in semen.

606.8 Infertility due to extratesticular causes   A ♂

Infertility due to:
drug therapy
infection
obstruction of efferent ducts
radiation
systemic disease

606.9 Male infertility, unspecified   A ♂

N Newborn Age: 0   P Pediatric Age: 0-17   M Maternity Age: 12-55   A Adult Age: 15-124

√4ᵗʰ 607 Disorders of penis

EXCLUDES phimosis (605)

607.0 Leukoplakia of penis   ♂
Kraurosis of penis

EXCLUDES carcinoma in situ of penis (233.5)
erythroplasia of Queyrat (233.5)

DEF: White, thickened patches on glans penis.

607.1 Balanoposthitis   ♂
Balanitis

Use additional code to identify organism

DEF: Inflammation of glans penis and prepuce.

607.2 Other inflammatory disorders of penis   ♂
Abscess
Boil   of corpus cavernosum or
Carbuncle   penis
Cellulitis
Cavernitis (penis)

Use additional code to identify organism

EXCLUDES herpetic infection (054.13)

607.3 Priapism   ♂
Painful erection

DEF: Prolonged penile erection without sexual stimulation.

√5ᵗʰ 607.8 Other specified disorders of penis

607.81 Balanitis xerotica obliterans   ♂
Induratio penis plastica

DEF: Inflammation of the glans penis, caused by stricture of the opening of the prepuce.

607.82 Vascular disorders of penis   ♂
Embolism
Hematoma   of corpus
  (nontraumatic)   cavernosum
Hemorrhage   or penis
Thrombosis

607.83 Edema of penis   ♂

DEF: Fluid retention within penile tissues.

607.84 Impotence of organic origin   A ♂

EXCLUDES nonorganic (302.72)

DEF: Physiological cause interfering with erection.

AHA: 3Q, '91, 11

TIP: If impotence is a result of previous radical prostatectomy, report code 997.99 first.

607.85 Peyronie's disease   ♂

DEF: A severe curvature of the erect penis due to fibrosis of the cavernous sheaths.

AHA: 4Q, '03, 64

607.89 Other   ♂
Atrophy
Fibrosis   of corpus cavernosum or
Hypertrophy   penis
Ulcer (chronic)

607.9 Unspecified disorder of penis   ♂

√4ᵗʰ 608 Other disorders of male genital organs

608.0 Seminal vesiculitis   ♂
Abscess   of seminal vesicle
Cellulitis

Vesiculitis (seminal)

Use additional code to identify organism

EXCLUDES gonococcal infection (098.14, 098.34)

DEF: Inflammation of seminal vesicle.

608.1 Spermatocele   ♂

DEF: Cystic enlargement of the epididymis or the testis; the cysts contain spermatozoa.

√5ᵗʰ 608.2 Torsion of testis

DEF: Twisted or rotated testis; may compromise blood flow.

608.20 Torsion of testis, unspecified   ♂

AHA: 4Q, '06, 95

Torsion of the Testis

608.21 Extravaginal torsion of spermatic cord   ♂

DEF: Torsion of the spermatic cord just below the tunica vaginalis attachments.

AHA: 4Q, '06, 95

608.22 Intravaginal torsion of spermatic cord   ♂
Torsion of spermatic cord NOS

DEF: Torsion within the tunica vaginalis also called the "bell-clapper" anomaly. It usually occurs in older children.

AHA: 4Q, '06, 95

608.23 Torsion of appendix testis   ♂

DEF: Torsion of small solid projection of tissue on the upper outer surface of the testis (hydatid of Morgagni); a remnant of the embryologic Müllerian duct.

AHA: 4Q, '06, 95

608.24 Torsion of appendix epididymis   ♂

DEF: Torsion of small stalked appendage of the head of the epididymis (pedunculated hydatid); a detached embryologic efferent duct.

AHA: 4Q, '06, 95

608.3 Atrophy of testis   ♂

608.4 Other inflammatory disorders of male genital organs   ♂
Abscess
Boil   of scrotum, spermatic cord, testis
Carbuncle   [except abscess], tunica
Cellulitis   vaginalis, or vas deferens
Vasitis

Use additional code to identify organism

EXCLUDES abscess of testis (604.0)

√5ᵗʰ 608.8 Other specified disorders of male genital organs

608.81 Disorders of male genital organs in diseases classified elsewhere   ♂

Code first underlying disease, as:
filariasis (125.0-125.9)
tuberculosis (016.5)

608.82 Hematospermia   ♂

DEF: Presence of blood in the ejaculate; relatively common, affecting men of any age after puberty; cause is often the result of a viral or bacterial infection and inflammation.

AHA: 4Q, '01, 46

608.83 Vascular disorders   ♂
Hematoma (non-   of seminal vessel, spermatic
  traumatic)   cord, testis, scrotum,
Hemorrhage   tunica vaginalis, or vas
Thrombosis   deferens
Hematocele NOS, male

AHA: 4Q, '03, 110

TIP: Assign for Fournier's gangrene, which is a result of an infection in the genital area.

608.84 Chylocele of tunica vaginalis   ♂

DEF: Chylous effusion into tunica vaginalis; due to infusion of lymphatic fluids.

608.85 Stricture   ♂
Stricture of:
spermatic cord
tunica vaginalis
vas deferens

608.86 Edema   ♂

Diseases of the Genitourinary System

608.87–612.1

608.87 Retrograde ejaculation   ♂
> **DEF:** Condition where the semen travels to the bladder rather than out through the urethra due to damaged nerves causing the bladder neck to remain open during ejaculation.
> **AHA:** 4Q, '01, 46

608.89 Other   ♂
> Atrophy   ⎤ of seminal vessel, spermatic
> Fibrosis   ⎬ cord, testis, scrotum,
> Hypertrophy   ⎬ tunica vaginalis, or vas
> Ulcer   ⎦ deferens
> **EXCLUDES** *atrophy of testis (608.3)*

608.9 Unspecified disorder of male genital organs   ♂

Disorders of Breast (610-612)

☑4ᵗʰ **610 Benign mammary dysplasias**

610.0 Solitary cyst of breast
> Cyst (solitary) of breast

610.1 Diffuse cystic mastopathy   A
> Chronic cystic mastitis
> Cystic breast
> Fibrocystic disease of
>   breast
> **DEF:** Extensive formation of nodular cysts in breast tissue; symptoms include tenderness, change in size and hyperplasia of ductal epithelium.
> **AHA:** 2Q, '06, 10
> **TIP:** Assign in addition to screening mammography V code; is a normal variant, commonly found in normal breasts and not a pathological condition.

610.2 Fibroadenosis of breast
> Fibroadenosis of breast:
>   NOS
>   chronic
>   cystic
>   diffuse
>   periodic
>   segmental
> **DEF:** Non-neoplastic nodular condition of breast.

610.3 Fibrosclerosis of breast
> **DEF:** Fibrous tissue in breast.

610.4 Mammary duct ectasia
> Comedomastitis
> Duct ectasia
> Mastitis:
>   periductal
>   plasma cell
> **DEF:** Atrophy of duct epithelium; causes distended collecting ducts of mammary gland, drying up of breast secretion, intraductal inflammation and periductal and interstitial chronic inflammatory reaction.

610.8 Other specified benign mammary dysplasias
> Mazoplasia
> Sebaceous cyst of breast
> **AHA:** 2Q, '09, 9

610.9 Benign mammary dysplasia, unspecified

☑4ᵗʰ **611 Other disorders of breast**
> **EXCLUDES** *that associated with lactation or the puerperium (675.0-676.9)*

611.0 Inflammatory disease of breast
> Abscess (acute) (chronic) (nonpuerperal) of:
>   areola
>   breast
> Mammillary fistula
> Mastitis (acute) (subacute) (nonpuerperal):
>   NOS
>   infective
>   retromammary
>   submammary
> **EXCLUDES** *carbuncle of breast (680.2)*
> *chronic cystic mastitis (610.1)*
> *neonatal infective mastitis (771.5)*
> *thrombophlebitis of breast [Mondor's disease] (451.89)*

611.1 Hypertrophy of breast
> Gynecomastia
> Hypertrophy of breast:
>   NOS
>   massive pubertal
> **EXCLUDES** *breast engorgement in newborn (778.7)*
> *disproportion of reconstructed breast (612.1)*

611.2 Fissure of nipple

611.3 Fat necrosis of breast
> Fat necrosis (segmental) of breast
> Code first breast necrosis due to breast graft (996.79)
> **DEF:** Splitting of neutral fats in adipose tissue cells as a result of trauma; a firm circumscribed mass is then formed in the breast.

611.4 Atrophy of breast

611.5 Galactocele
> **DEF:** Milk-filled cyst in breast due to blocked duct.

611.6 Galactorrhea not associated with childbirth
> **DEF:** Flow of milk not associated with childbirth or pregnancy.

☑5ᵗʰ **611.7 Signs and symptoms in breast**

611.71 Mastodynia
> Pain in breast

611.72 Lump or mass in breast
> **AHA:** 4Q, '09, 106; 2Q, '03, 4-5
> **TIP:** Do not assign if the underlying cause of the breast lump or mass is determined and documented during the episode of care.

611.79 Other
> Induration of breast
> Inversion of nipple
> Nipple discharge
> Retraction of nipple

☑5ᵗʰ **611.8 Other specified disorders of breast**
> **AHA:** 4Q, '08, 121-122

611.81 Ptosis of breast   A
> **EXCLUDES** *ptosis of native breast in relation to reconstructed breast (612.1)*

611.82 Hypoplasia of breast   A
> Micromastia
> **EXCLUDES** *congenital absence of breast (757.6)*
> *hypoplasia of native breast in relation to reconstructed breast (612.1)*

611.83 Capsular contracture of breast implant   A
> **TIP:** Do not assign additional code from category 996 Complications peculiar to certain specified procedures.

611.89 Other specified disorders of breast
> Hematoma (nontraumatic) of breast
> Infarction of breast
> Occlusion of breast duct
> Subinvolution of breast (postlactational) (postpartum)

611.9 Unspecified breast disorder

☑4ᵗʰ **612 Deformity and disproportion of reconstructed breast**
> **AHA:** 4Q, '08, 123

612.0 Deformity of reconstructed breast   A
> Contour irregularity in reconstructed breast
> Excess tissue in reconstructed breast
> Misshapen reconstructed breast

612.1 Disproportion of reconstructed breast   A
> Breast asymmetry between native breast and reconstructed breast
> Disproportion between native breast and reconstructed breast

---

N   Newborn Age: 0   P   Pediatric Age: 0-17   M   Maternity Age: 12-55   A   Adult Age: 15-124

Inflammatory Disease of Female Pelvic Organs (614-616)

Use additional code to identify organism, such as Staphylococcus (041.1), or Streptococcus (041.0)

EXCLUDES *that associated with pregnancy, abortion, childbirth, or the puerperium (630-676.9)*

✓4ᵗʰ 614 Inflammatory disease of ovary, fallopian tube, pelvic cellular tissue, and peritoneum

EXCLUDES *endometritis (615.0-615.9)*
major infection following delivery (670.0-670.8)
that complicating:
abortion (634-638 with .0, 639.0)
ectopic or molar pregnancy (639.0)
pregnancy or labor (646.6)

614.0 Acute salpingitis and oophoritis   ♀
Any condition classifiable to 614.2, specified as acute or subacute

DEF: Acute inflammation of ovary and fallopian tube.

614.1 Chronic salpingitis and oophoritis   ♀
Hydrosalpinx
Salpingitis:
   follicularis
   isthmica nodosa
Any condition classifiable to 614.2, specified as chronic

DEF: Persistent inflammation of ovary and fallopian tube.

614.2 Salpingitis and oophoritis not specified as acute, subacute, or chronic   ♀
Abscess (of):
   fallopian tube
   ovary
   tubo-ovarian
Oophoritis
Perioophoritis
Perisalpingitis
Pyosalpinx
Salpingitis
Salpingo-oophoritis
Tubo-ovarian inflammatory disease

EXCLUDES *gonococcal infection (chronic) (098.37)*
acute (098.17)
tuberculous (016.6)

AHA: 2Q, '91, 5

614.3 Acute parametritis and pelvic cellulitis   ♀
Acute inflammatory pelvic disease
Any condition classifiable to 614.4, specified as acute

DEF: Parametritis: inflammation of the parametrium; pelvic cellulitis is a synonym for parametritis.

614.4 Chronic or unspecified parametritis and pelvic cellulitis   ♀
Abscess (of):
   broad ligament ⎫
   parametrium   ⎬ chronic or NOS
   pelvis, femal |
   pouch of Douglas ⎭
Chronic inflammatory pelvic disease
Pelvic cellulitis, female

EXCLUDES *tuberculous (016.7)*

614.5 Acute or unspecified pelvic peritonitis, female   ♀
AHA: 4Q, '05, 74
TIP: For pelvic peritonitis in a male patient, refer to code 567.21.

614.6 Pelvic peritoneal adhesions, female (postoperative) (postinfection)   ♀
Adhesions:
   peritubal
   tubo-ovarian
Use additional code to identify any associated infertility (628.2)

DEF: Fibrous scarring abnormally joining structures within abdomen.
AHA: 2Q, '11, 19; 3Q, '03, 6; 1Q, '03, 4; 3Q, '95, 7; 3Q, '94, 12
N73.6 Female pelvic peritoneal adhesions (postinfective)   I-10

614.7 Other chronic pelvic peritonitis, female   ♀
EXCLUDES *tuberculous (016.7)*

614.8 Other specified inflammatory disease of female pelvic organs and tissues   ♀

614.9 Unspecified inflammatory disease of female pelvic organs and tissues   ♀
Pelvic infection or inflammation, female NOS
Pelvic inflammatory disease [PID]

✓4ᵗʰ 615 Inflammatory diseases of uterus, except cervix
EXCLUDES *following delivery (670.0-670.8)*
hyperplastic endometritis (621.30-621.35)
that complicating:
abortion (634-638 with .0, 639.0)
ectopic or molar pregnancy (639.0)
pregnancy or labor (646.6)

615.0 Acute   ♀
Any condition classifiable to 615.9, specified as acute or subacute

615.1 Chronic   ♀
Any condition classifiable to 615.9, specified as chronic

615.9 Unspecified inflammatory disease of uterus   ♀
Endometritis   Myometritis
Endomyometritis   Perimetritis
Intrauterine infection   Pyometra
Metritis   Uterine abscess
N71.9 Inflammatory disease of uterus unspecified   I-10

✓4ᵗʰ 616 Inflammatory disease of cervix, vagina, and vulva
EXCLUDES *that complicating:*
abortion (634-638 with .0, 639.0)
ectopic or molar pregnancy (639.0)
pregnancy, childbirth, or the puerperium (646.6)

616.0 Cervicitis and endocervicitis   ♀
Cervicitis   ⎫ with or without mention of
Endocervicitis ⎬   erosion or ectropion
Nabothian (gland) cyst or follicle

EXCLUDES *erosion or ectropion without mention of cervicitis (622.0)*
N72 Inflammatory disease of cervix uteri   I-10

✓5ᵗʰ 616.1 Vaginitis and vulvovaginitis
EXCLUDES *vulvar vestibulitis (625.71)*
DEF: Inflammation or infection of vagina or external female genitalia.

616.10 Vaginitis and vulvovaginitis, unspecified   ♀
Vaginitis:
   NOS
   postirradiation
Vulvitis NOS
Vulvovaginitis NOS

Use additional code to identify organism, such as:
   Escherichia coli [E. coli] (041.41-041.49)
   Staphylococcus (041.10-041.19)
   Streptococcus (041.00-041.09)

EXCLUDES *noninfective leukorrhea (623.5)*
postmenopausal or senile vaginitis (627.3)

616.11 Vaginitis and vulvovaginitis in diseases classified elsewhere   ♀
Code first underlying disease, as:
   pinworm vaginitis (127.4)

EXCLUDES *herpetic vulvovaginitis (054.11)*
monilial vulvovaginitis (112.1)
trichomonal vaginitis or vulvovaginitis (131.01)

616.2 Cyst of Bartholin's gland   ♀
Bartholin's duct cyst
DEF: Fluid-filled sac within gland of vaginal orifice.

616.3 Abscess of Bartholin's gland   ♀
Vulvovaginal gland abscess

616.4 Other abscess of vulva   ♀
Abscess   ⎫
Carbuncle   ⎬ of vulva
Furuncle   ⎭

Diseases of the Genitourinary System

616.5–618.09

√5th **616.5 Ulceration of vulva**

616.50 Ulceration of vulva, unspecified ♀
Ulcer NOS of vulva

616.51 Ulceration of vulva in diseases classified elsewhere ♀
Code first underlying disease, as:
Behçet's syndrome (136.1)
tuberculosis (016.7)
EXCLUDES *vulvar ulcer (in):*
gonococcal (098.0)
herpes simplex (054.12)
syphilitic (091.0)

√5th **616.8 Other specified inflammatory diseases of cervix, vagina, and vulva**
EXCLUDES *noninflammatory disorders of:*
cervix (622.0-622.9)
vagina (623.0-623.9)
vulva (624.0-624.9)

616.81 Mucositis (ulcerative) of cervix, vagina, and vulva ♀
Use additional E code to identify adverse effects of therapy, such as:
antineoplastic and immunosuppressive drugs (E930.7, E933.1)
radiation therapy (E879.2)
AHA: 4Q, '06, 88-90

616.89 Other inflammatory disease of cervix, vagina and vulva ♀
Caruncle, vagina or labium
Ulcer, vagina
AHA: 4Q, '06, 88-90

616.9 Unspecified inflammatory disease of cervix, vagina, and vulva ♀

Other Disorders of Female Genital Tract (617-629)

√4th **617 Endometriosis**

617.0 Endometriosis of uterus ♀
Adenomyosis
Endometriosis:
cervix
internal
myometrium
EXCLUDES *stromal endometriosis (236.0)*
DEF: Aberrant uterine mucosal tissue; creating products of menses and inflamed uterine tissues.
AHA: 3Q, '92, 7
N80.0 Endometriosis of uterus   [I-10]

617.1 Endometriosis of ovary ♀
Chocolate cyst of ovary
Endometrial cystoma of ovary
DEF: Aberrant uterine tissue; creating products of menses and inflamed ovarian tissues.
N80.1 Endometriosis of ovary   [I-10]

617.2 Endometriosis of fallopian tube ♀
DEF: Aberrant uterine tissue; creating products of menses and inflamed tissues of fallopian tubes.

617.3 Endometriosis of pelvic peritoneum ♀
Endometriosis:
broad ligament
cul-de-sac (Douglas')
parametrium
round ligament
DEF: Aberrant uterine tissue; creating products of menses and inflamed peritoneum tissues.

617.4 Endometriosis of rectovaginal septum and vagina ♀
DEF: Aberrant uterine tissue; creating products of menses and inflamed tissues in and behind vagina.

617.5 Endometriosis of intestine ♀
Endometriosis: Endometriosis:
appendix   rectum
colon
DEF: Aberrant uterine tissue; creating products of menses and inflamed intestinal tissues.

Female Genitourinary System

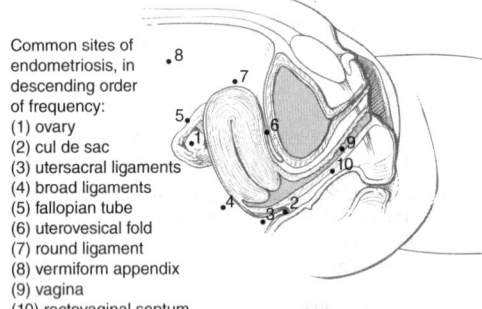

Uterine (fallopian) tube — Ovary — Rectouterine pouch (of Douglas) — Uterus (fundus) — Cervix — Bladder — Rectum — Pubic bone — Clitoris — Urogenital diaphragm — Urethral orifice (meatus) — Labia minora — Labia majora — Anus — Vaginal canal

Common Sites of Endometriosis

Common sites of endometriosis, in descending order of frequency:
(1) ovary
(2) cul de sac
(3) utersacral ligaments
(4) broad ligaments
(5) fallopian tube
(6) uterovesical fold
(7) round ligament
(8) vermiform appendix
(9) vagina
(10) rectovaginal septum

617.6 Endometriosis in scar of skin ♀

617.8 Endometriosis of other specified sites ♀
Endometriosis: Endometriosis:
bladder   umbilicus
lung   vulva

617.9 Endometriosis, site unspecified ♀

√4th **618 Genital prolapse**
Use additional code to identify urinary incontinence (625.6, 788.31, 788.33-788.39)
EXCLUDES *that complicating pregnancy, labor, or delivery (654.4)*

√5th **618.0 Prolapse of vaginal walls without mention of uterine prolapse**
EXCLUDES *that with uterine prolapse (618.2-618.4)*
enterocele (618.6)
vaginal vault prolapse following hysterectomy (618.5)

618.00 Unspecified prolapse of vaginal walls ♀
Vaginal prolapse NOS

618.01 Cystocele, midline ♀
Cystocele NOS
DEF: Defect in the pubocervical fascia, the supportive layer of the bladder, causing bladder drop and herniated into the vagina along the midline.
N81.11 Cystocele midline   [I-10]

618.02 Cystocele, lateral ♀
Paravaginal
DEF: Loss of support of the lateral attachment of the vagina at the arcus tendinous results in bladder drop; bladder herniates into the vagina laterally.

618.03 Urethrocele ♀

618.04 Rectocele ♀
Proctocele
Use additional code for any associated fecal incontinence (787.60-787.63)
N81.6 Rectocele   [I-10]

618.05 Perineocele ♀

618.09 Other prolapse of vaginal walls without mention of uterine prolapse ♀
Cystourethrocele

[N] Newborn Age: 0   [P] Pediatric Age: 0-17   [M] Maternity Age: 12-55   [A] Adult Age: 15-124

Diseases of the Genitourinary System

618.1–620.3

Vaginal Midline Cystocele

Vaginal Lateral Cystocele

Types of Vaginal Hernias

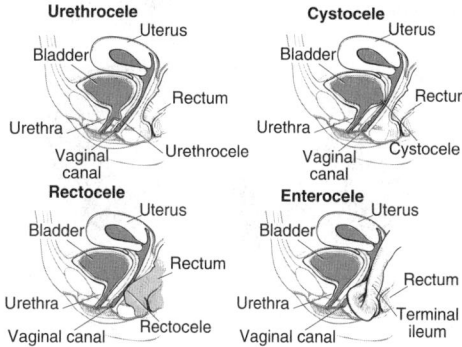

618.1 Uterine prolapse without mention of vaginal wall prolapse ♀

Descensus uteri

Uterine prolapse:
NOS
complete

Uterine prolapse:
first degree
second degree
third degree

EXCLUDES *that with mention of cystocele, urethrocele, or rectocele (618.2-618.4)*

618.2 Uterovaginal prolapse, incomplete ♀

DEF: Downward displacement of uterus downward into vagina.

N81.2 Incomplete uterovaginal prolapse   `I-10`

618.3 Uterovaginal prolapse, complete ♀

DEF: Downward displacement of uterus exposed within external genitalia.

618.4 Uterovaginal prolapse, unspecified ♀

N81.4 Uterovaginal prolapse unspecified   `I-10`

618.5 Prolapse of vaginal vault after hysterectomy ♀

N99.3 Prolapse of vaginal vault after hysterectomy   `I-10`

618.6 Vaginal enterocele, congenital or acquired ♀

Pelvic enterocele, congenital or acquired

DEF: Vaginal vault hernia formed by the loop of the small intestine protruding into the rectal vaginal pouch; can also accompany uterine prolapse or follow hysterectomy.

N81.5 Vaginal enterocele   `I-10`

618.7 Old laceration of muscles of pelvic floor ♀

√5ᵗʰ **618.8 Other specified genital prolapse**

618.81 Incompetence or weakening of pubocervical tissue ♀

618.82 Incompetence or weakening of rectovaginal tissue ♀

618.83 Pelvic muscle wasting ♀

Disuse atrophy of pelvic muscles and anal sphincter

618.84 Cervical stump prolapse ♀

AHA: 4Q, '06, 97

618.89 Other specified genital prolapse ♀

618.9 Unspecified genital prolapse ♀

√4ᵗʰ **619 Fistula involving female genital tract**

EXCLUDES *vesicorectal and intestinovesical fistula (596.1)*

619.0 Urinary-genital tract fistula, female ♀

Fistula:
cervicovesical
ureterovaginal
urethrovaginal
urethrovesicovaginal

Fistula:
uteroureteric
uterovesical
vesicocervicovaginal
vesicovaginal

619.1 Digestive-genital tract fistula, female ♀

Fistula:
intestinouterine
intestinovaginal
rectovaginal

Fistula:
rectovulval
sigmoidovaginal
uterorectal

619.2 Genital tract-skin fistula, female ♀

Fistula:
uterus to abdominal wall
vaginoperineal

619.8 Other specified fistulas involving female genital tract ♀

Fistula:
cervix
cul-de-sac (Douglas')
uterus
vagina

DEF: Abnormal communication between female reproductive tract and skin.

619.9 Unspecified fistula involving female genital tract ♀

√4ᵗʰ **620 Noninflammatory disorders of ovary, fallopian tube, and broad ligament**

EXCLUDES *hydrosalpinx (614.1)*

620.0 Follicular cyst of ovary ♀

Cyst of graafian follicle

DEF: Fluid-filled, encapsulated cyst due to occluded follicle duct that secretes hormones into ovaries.

N83.0 Follicular cyst of ovary   `I-10`

620.1 Corpus luteum cyst or hematoma ♀

Corpus luteum hemorrhage or rupture
Lutein cyst

DEF: Fluid-filled cyst due to serous developing from corpus luteum or clotted blood.

N83.1 Corpus luteum cyst   `I-10`

620.2 Other and unspecified ovarian cyst ♀

Cyst:
NOS
corpus albicans
retention NOS } of ovary
serous
theca-lutein

Simple cystoma of ovary

EXCLUDES *cystadenoma (benign) (serous) (220)*
developmental cysts (752.0)
neoplastic cysts (220)
polycystic ovaries (256.4)
Stein-Leventhal syndrome (256.4)

N83.20 Unspecified ovarian cysts   `I-10`

620.3 Acquired atrophy of ovary and fallopian tube ♀

Senile involution of ovary

√4ᵗʰ √5ᵗʰ Additional Digit Required   Unspecified Code   Other Specified Code   Manifestation Code   ▶◀ Revised Text   ● New Code   ▲ Revised Code Title

2013 ICD-9-CM   **Volume 1 – 191**

Diseases of the Genitourinary System

620.4–622.11

Uterus and Ovaries

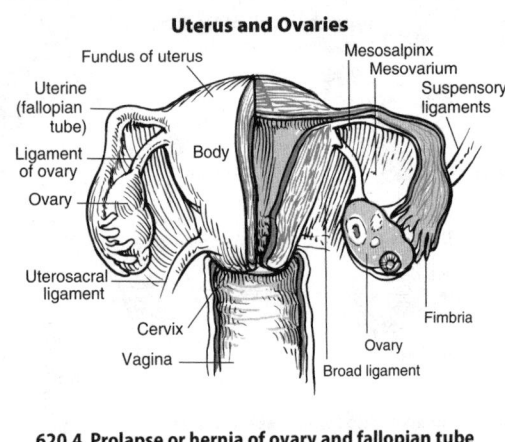

Fundus of uterus

Uterine
(fallopian
tube)

Ligament
of ovary

Ovary

Uterosacral
ligament

Cervix

Vagina

Body

Mesosalpinx
Mesovarium
Suspensory
ligaments

Fimbria

Ovary

Broad ligament

620.4 Prolapse or hernia of ovary and fallopian tube ♀
    Displacement of ovary and fallopian tube
    Salpingocele

620.5 Torsion of ovary, ovarian pedicle, or fallopian tube ♀
    Torsion:
      accessory tube
      hydatid of Morgagni

620.6 Broad ligament laceration syndrome ♀
    Masters-Allen syndrome

620.7 Hematoma of broad ligament ♀
    Hematocele, broad ligament
    DEF: Blood within peritoneal fold that supports uterus.

**620.8 Other noninflammatory disorders of ovary,
fallopian tube, and broad ligament** ♀
    Cyst   } of broad ligament or
    Polyp   }   fallopian tube

    Infarction }
    Rupture   } of ovary or fallopian tube
    Hematosalpinx
    EXCLUDES *hematosalpinx in ectopic pregnancy (639.2)*
            peritubal adhesions (614.6)
            *torsion of ovary, ovarian pedicle, or fallopian tube
              (620.5)*

**620.9 Unspecified noninflammatory disorder of
ovary, fallopian tube, and broad ligament** ♀

√4ᵗʰ **621 Disorders of uterus, not elsewhere classified**

621.0 Polyp of corpus uteri ♀
    Polyp:
      endometrium
      uterus NOS
    EXCLUDES *cervical polyp NOS (622.7)*
    N84.0 Polyp of corpus uteri   I-10

621.1 Chronic subinvolution of uterus ♀
    EXCLUDES *puerperal (674.8)*
    DEF: Abnormal size of uterus after delivery; the uterus does not
    return to its normal size after the birth of a child.
    AHA: 1Q, '91, 11

621.2 Hypertrophy of uterus ♀
    Bulky or enlarged uterus
    EXCLUDES *puerperal (674.8)*

√5ᵗʰ **621.3 Endometrial hyperplasia**
    DEF: Abnormal cystic overgrowth of endometrial tissue.

    621.30 Endometrial hyperplasia, unspecified ♀
        Endometrial hyperplasia NOS
        Hyperplasia (adenomatous) (cystic) (glandular) of
            endometrium
        Hyperplastic endometritis

    621.31 Simple endometrial hyperplasia without atypia ♀
        EXCLUDES *benign endometrial hyperplasia (621.34)*

    **621.32 Complex endometrial hyperplasia
without atypia** ♀
        EXCLUDES *benign endometrial hyperplasia (621.34)*

    621.33 Endometrial hyperplasia with atypia ♀
        EXCLUDES *endometrial intraepithelial neoplasia [EIN]*
             (621.35)

    621.34 Benign endometrial hyperplasia ♀
        DEF: Excessive cell growth of the endometrium due to
        primary hormonal changes (menopause) that result in
        secondary effects to the endometrial stroma and
        associated structures.
        AHA: 4Q, '09, 95-96

    621.35 Endometrial intraepithelial neoplasia [EIN] ♀
        EXCLUDES *malignant neoplasm of endometrium with*
             endometrial intraepithelial neoplasia
             [EIN] (182.0)
        DEF: Abnormal premalignant neoplastic changes of the
        endometrial glands prone to malignant transformation.
        AHA: 4Q, '09, 95-96
        TIP: Do not confuse (EIN) with unrelated serous
        intraepithelial carcinoma (serous EIC), which is an early
        phase of (Type II) papillary serous adenocarcinoma of the
        endometrium.

621.4 Hematometra ♀
    Hemometra
    EXCLUDES *that in congenital anomaly (752.2-752.39)*
    DEF: Accumulated blood in uterus.

621.5 Intrauterine synechiae ♀
    Adhesions of uterus   Band(s) of uterus

621.6 Malposition of uterus ♀
    Anteversion
    Retroflexion } of uterus
    Retroversion
    EXCLUDES *malposition complicating pregnancy, labor, or*
            delivery (654.3-654.4)
            prolapse of uterus (618.1-618.4)

621.7 Chronic inversion of uterus ♀
    EXCLUDES *current obstetrical trauma (665.2)*
            prolapse of uterus (618.1-618.4)

**621.8 Other specified disorders of uterus, not
elsewhere classified** ♀
    Atrophy, acquired
    Cyst
    Fibrosis NOS   } of uterus
    Old laceration (postpartum)
    Ulcer
    EXCLUDES *bilharzial fibrosis (120.0-120.9)*
            endometriosis (617.0)
            fistulas (619.0-619.8)
            inflammatory diseases (615.0-615.9)

621.9 Unspecified disorder of uterus ♀

√4ᵗʰ **622 Noninflammatory disorders of cervix**
    EXCLUDES *abnormality of cervix complicating pregnancy, labor, or*
            delivery (654.5-654.6)
            fistula (619.0-619.8)

622.0 Erosion and ectropion of cervix ♀
    Eversion   } of cervix
    Ulcer   }
    EXCLUDES *that in chronic cervicitis (616.0)*
    DEF: Ulceration or turning outward of uterine cervix.

√5ᵗʰ **622.1 Dysplasia of cervix (uteri)**
    EXCLUDES *abnormal results from cervical cytologic examination*
            without histologic confirmation
            (795.00-795.09)
            carcinoma in situ of cervix (233.1)
            cervical intraepithelial neoplasia III [CIN III] (233.1)
            HGSIL of cervix (795.04)
    DEF: Abnormal cell structures in portal between uterus and vagina.
    AHA: 1Q, '91, 11

    622.10 Dysplasia of cervix, unspecified ♀
        Anaplasia of cervix Cervical dysplasia NOS
        Cervical atypism

    622.11 Mild dysplasia of cervix ♀
        Cervical intraepithelial neoplasia I [CIN I]

N Newborn Age: 0   P Pediatric Age: 0-17   M Maternity Age: 12-55   A Adult Age: 15-124

622.12 Moderate dysplasia of cervix ♀
Cervical intraepithelial neoplasia II [CIN II]
EXCLUDES   *carcinoma in situ of cervix (233.1)*
     cervical intraepithelial neoplasia III [CIN III]
       (233.1)
     severe dysplasia (233.1)

622.2 Leukoplakia of cervix (uteri) ♀
EXCLUDES   *carcinoma in situ of cervix (233.1)*
DEF: Thickened, white patches on portal between uterus and vagina.

622.3 Old laceration of cervix ♀
Adhesions
Band(s)   } of cervix
Cicatrix (postpartum)
EXCLUDES   *current obstetrical trauma (665.3)*
DEF: Scarring or other evidence of old wound on cervix.

622.4 Stricture and stenosis of cervix ♀
Atresia (acquired)
Contracture   } of cervix
Occlusion
Pinpoint os uteri
EXCLUDES   *congenital (752.49)*
     that complicating labor (654.6)

622.5 Incompetence of cervix ♀
EXCLUDES   *complicating pregnancy (654.5)*
     that affecting fetus or newborn (761.0)
DEF: Inadequate functioning of cervix; marked by abnormal
widening during pregnancy; causing miscarriage.

622.6 Hypertrophic elongation of cervix ♀
DEF: Overgrowth of cervix tissues extending down into vagina.

622.7 Mucous polyp of cervix ♀
Polyp NOS of cervix
EXCLUDES   *adenomatous polyp of cervix (219.0)*

622.8 Other specified noninflammatory disorders of cervix ♀
Atrophy (senile)
Cyst   } of cervix
Fibrosis
Hemorrhage
EXCLUDES   *endometriosis (617.0)*
     fistula (619.0-619.8)
     inflammatory diseases (616.0)

622.9 Unspecified noninflammatory disorder of cervix ♀

√4ᵗʰ **623 Noninflammatory disorders of vagina**
√5ᵗʰ
EXCLUDES   *abnormality of vagina complicating pregnancy, labor, or*
     delivery (654.7)
     congenital absence of vagina (752.49)
     congenital diaphragm or bands (752.49)
     fistulas involving vagina (619.0-619.8)

623.0 Dysplasia of vagina ♀
Mild and moderate dysplasia of vagina
Vaginal intraepithelial neoplasia I and II [VAIN I and II]
EXCLUDES   *abnormal results from vaginal cytological*
     examination without histologic confirmation
     (795.10-795.19)
     carcinoma in situ of vagina (233.31)
     HGSIL of vagina (795.14)
     severe dysplasia of vagina (233.31)
     vaginal intraepithelial neoplasia III [VAIN III] (233.31)

623.1 Leukoplakia of vagina ♀
DEF: Thickened white patches on vaginal canal.

623.2 Stricture or atresia of vagina ♀
Adhesions (postoperative) (postradiation) of vagina
Occlusion of vagina
Stenosis, vagina
Use additional E code to identify any external cause
EXCLUDES   *congenital atresia or stricture (752.49)*

623.3 Tight hymenal ring ♀
Rigid hymen
Tight hymenal ring   } acquired or congenital
Tight introitus
EXCLUDES   *imperforate hymen (752.42)*

623.4 Old vaginal laceration ♀
EXCLUDES   *old laceration involving muscles of pelvic floor (618.7)*
DEF: Scarring or other evidence of old wound on vagina.

623.5 Leukorrhea, not specified as infective ♀
Leukorrhea NOS of vagina
Vaginal discharge NOS
EXCLUDES   *trichomonal (131.00)*
DEF: Viscid whitish discharge from vagina.

623.6 Vaginal hematoma ♀
EXCLUDES   *current obstetrical trauma (665.7)*

623.7 Polyp of vagina ♀

623.8 Other specified noninflammatory disorders of vagina ♀
Cyst   } of vagina
Hemorrhage

623.9 Unspecified noninflammatory disorder of vagina ♀

√4ᵗʰ **624 Noninflammatory disorders of vulva and perineum**
EXCLUDES   *abnormality of vulva and perineum complicating pregnancy,*
     labor, or delivery (654.8)
     condyloma acuminatum (078.11)
     fistulas involving:
       perineum — see Alphabetic Index
       vulva (619.0-619.8)
     vulval varices (456.6)
     vulvar involvement in skin conditions (690-709.9)

√5ᵗʰ **624.0 Dystrophy of vulva**
EXCLUDES   *carcinoma in situ of vulva (233.32)*
     severe dysplasia of vulva (233.32)
     vulvar intraepithelial neoplasia III [VIN III] (233.32)
AHA: 4Q, '07, 90

624.01 Vulvar intraepithelial neoplasia I [VIN I] ♀
Mild dysplasia of vulva

624.02 Vulvar intraepithelial neoplasia II [VIN II] ♀
Moderate dysplasia of vulva
AHA: 4Q, '07, 91

624.09 Other dystrophy of vulva ♀
Kraurosis of vulva
Leukoplakia of vulva

624.1 Atrophy of vulva ♀

624.2 Hypertrophy of clitoris ♀
EXCLUDES   *that in endocrine disorders (255.2, 256.1)*

624.3 Hypertrophy of labia ♀
Hypertrophy of vulva NOS
DEF: Overgrowth of fleshy folds on either side of vagina.

624.4 Old laceration or scarring of vulva ♀
DEF: Scarring or other evidence of old wound on external female
genitalia.

624.5 Hematoma of vulva ♀
EXCLUDES   *that complicating delivery (664.5)*
DEF: Blood in tissue of external genitalia.

624.6 Polyp of labia and vulva ♀

624.8 Other specified noninflammatory disorders of vulva and perineum ♀
Cyst
Edema   } of vulva
Stricture
AHA: 1Q, '03, 13; 1Q, '95, 8

624.9 Unspecified noninflammatory disorder of vulva and perineum ♀

√4ᵗʰ **625 Pain and other symptoms associated with female genital organs**

625.0 Dyspareunia ♀
EXCLUDES   *psychogenic dyspareunia (302.76)*
DEF: Difficult or painful sexual intercourse.

625.1 Vaginismus ♀
Colpospasm
Vulvismus
EXCLUDES   *psychogenic vaginismus (306.51)*
DEF: Vaginal spasms; due to involuntary contraction of musculature;
prevents intercourse.

√4ᵗʰ
√5ᵗʰ Additional Digit Required   Unspecified Code   Other Specified Code   Manifestation Code   ►◄ Revised Text   ● New Code   ▲ Revised Code Title
2013 ICD-9-CM   **Volume 1 – 193**

Diseases of the Genitourinary System

625.2–628.3

625.2 Mittelschmerz ♀
Intermenstrual pain
Ovulation pain
DEF: Pain occurring between menstrual periods.

625.3 Dysmenorrhea ♀
Painful menstruation
EXCLUDES psychogenic dysmenorrhea (306.52)
AHA: 2Q, '94, 12
N94.6 Dysmenorrhea unspecified   I-10

625.4 Premenstrual tension syndromes ♀
Menstrual molimen
Premenstrual dysphoric disorder
Premenstrual syndrome
Premenstrual tension NOS
EXCLUDES menstrual migraine (346.4)
AHA: 4Q, '03, 116

625.5 Pelvic congestion syndrome ♀
Congestion-fibrosis syndrome
Taylor's syndrome
DEF: Excessive accumulation of blood in vessels of pelvis; may occur
after orgasm; causes abnormal menstruation, lower back pain and
vaginal discharge.

625.6 Stress incontinence, female ♀
EXCLUDES mixed incontinence (788.33)
stress incontinence, male (788.32)
DEF: Involuntary leakage of urine due to insufficient sphincter
control; occurs upon sneezing, laughing, coughing, sudden
movement or lifting.
N39.3 Stress incontinence(female) (male)   I-10

√5ᵗʰ **625.7 Vulvodynia**
DEF: Vulvar pain without an identifiable cause that persists for three
months or longer.
AHA: 4Q, '08, 124

625.70 Vulvodynia, unspecified ♀
Vulvodynia NOS

625.71 Vulvar vestibulitis ♀

625.79 Other vulvodynia ♀

**625.8 Other specified symptoms associated with
female genital organs** ♀
AHA: N-D, '85, 16

**625.9 Unspecified symptom associated with female
genital organs** ♀
AHA: 4Q, '06, 110
R10.2 Pelvic and perineal pain   I-10

√4ᵗʰ **626 Disorders of menstruation and other abnormal bleeding from
female genital tract**
EXCLUDES menopausal and premenopausal bleeding (627.0)
pain and other symptoms associated with menstrual cycle
(625.2-625.4)
postmenopausal bleeding (627.1)
precocious puberty (259.1)

626.0 Absence of menstruation ♀
Amenorrhea (primary) (secondary)

626.1 Scanty or infrequent menstruation ♀
Hypomenorrhea   Oligomenorrhea

626.2 Excessive or frequent menstruation ♀
Heavy periods   Menorrhagia
Menometrorrhagia   Plymenorrhea
EXCLUDES premenopausal (627.0)
that in puberty (626.3)
AHA: ▶4Q, '11, 146◀
N92.0 Excess & frequent menstruation w/regular cycle   I-10

626.3 Puberty bleeding ♀
Excessive bleeding associated with onset of menstrual
periods
Pubertal menorrhagia

626.4 Irregular menstrual cycle ♀
Irregular: Irregular:
bleeding NOS   periods
menstruation

626.5 Ovulation bleeding ♀
Regular intermenstrual bleeding

626.6 Metrorrhagia ♀
Bleeding unrelated to menstrual cycle
Irregular intermenstrual bleeding

626.7 Postcoital bleeding ♀
DEF: Bleeding from vagina after sexual intercourse.

626.8 Other ♀
Dysfunctional or functional uterine hemorrhage NOS
Menstruation:
retained
suppression of
N92.5 Other specified irregular menstruation   I-10

626.9 Unspecified ♀

√4ᵗʰ **627 Menopausal and postmenopausal disorders**
EXCLUDES asymptomatic age-related (natural) postmenopausal status
(V49.81)

627.0 Premenopausal menorrhagia ♀
Excessive bleeding associated with onset of menopause
Menorrhagia:
climacteric
menopausal
preclimacteric

627.1 Postmenopausal bleeding ♀
N95.0 Postmenopausal bleeding   I-10

627.2 Symptomatic menopausal or female climacteric states ♀
Symptoms, such as flushing, sleeplessness, headache, lack
of concentration, associated with the menopause

627.3 Postmenopausal atrophic vaginitis ♀
Senile (atrophic) vaginitis

**627.4 Symptomatic states associated with artificial
menopause** ♀
Postartificial menopause syndromes
Any condition classifiable to 627.1, 627.2, or 627.3 which
follows induced menopause
DEF: Conditions arising after hysterectomy.

**627.8 Other specified menopausal and postmenopausal
disorders** ♀
EXCLUDES premature menopause NOS (256.31)

**627.9 Unspecified menopausal and postmenopausal
disorder** ♀

√4ᵗʰ **628 Infertility, female**
INCLUDES primary and secondary sterility
DEF: Infertility: inability to conceive for at least one year with regular
intercourse.
DEF: Primary infertility: occurring in patients who have never conceived.
DEF: Secondary infertility: occurring in patients who have previously
conceived.
AHA: 2Q, '96, 9; 1Q, '95, 7

628.0 Associated with anovulation ♀
Anovulatory cycle
Use additional code for any associated Stein-Leventhal
syndrome (256.4)

628.1 Of pituitary-hypothalamic origin ♀
Code first underlying cause, as:
adiposogenital dystrophy (253.8)
anterior pituitary disorder (253.0-253.4)

628.2 Of tubal origin ♀
Infertility associated with congenital anomaly of tube
Tubal:
block
occlusion
stenosis
Use additional code for any associated peritubal adhesions
(614.6)

628.3 Of uterine origin ♀
Infertility associated with congenital anomaly of uterus
Nonimplantation
Use additional code for any associated tuberculous
endometritis (016.7)

N Newborn Age: 0   P Pediatric Age: 0-17   M Maternity Age: 12-55   A Adult Age: 15-124

628.4 Of cervical or vaginal origin ♀
Infertility associated with:
anomaly of cervical mucus
congenital structural anomaly
dysmucorrhea

628.8 Of other specified origin ♀

628.9 Of unspecified origin ♀

√4ᵗʰ **629 Other disorders of female genital organs**

629.0 Hematocele, female, not elsewhere classified ♀
EXCLUDES hematocele or hematoma:
broad ligament (620.7)
fallopian tube (620.8)
that associated with ectopic pregnancy (633.00-633.91)
uterus (621.4)
vagina (623.6)
vulva (624.5)

629.1 Hydrocele, canal of Nuck ♀
Cyst of canal of Nuck (acquired)
EXCLUDES *congenital (752.41)*

√5ᵗʰ **629.2 Female genital mutilation status**
Female circumcision status
Female genital cutting
AHA: 4Q, '04, 88

629.20 Female genital mutilation status, unspecified ♀
Female genital cutting status, unspecified
Female genital mutilation status NOS

629.21 Female genital mutilation Type I status ♀
Clitorectomy status
Female genital cutting Type I status
DEF: Female genital mutilation involving clitorectomy, with part or all of the clitoris removed.

629.22 Female genital mutilation Type II status ♀
Clitorectomy with excision of labia minora status
Female genital cutting Type II status
DEF: Female genital mutilation involving clitoris and the labia minora amputation.
AHA: 4Q, '04, 90

629.23 Female genital mutilation Type III status ♀
Female genital cutting Type III status
Infibulation status
DEF: Female genital mutilation involving removal, most or all of the labia minora excised, labia majora incised which is then made into a hood of skin over the urethral and vaginal opening.
AHA: 4Q, '04, 90

629.29 Other female genital mutilation status ♀
Female genital cutting Type IV status
Female genital mutilation Type IV status
Other female genital cutting status
AHA: 4Q, '06, 97

√5ᵗʰ **629.3 Complication of implanted vaginal mesh and other prosthetic materials**
AHA: ▶4Q, '11, 130-131◀

629.31 Erosion of implanted vaginal mesh and other prosthetic materials to surrounding organ or tissue ♀
Erosion of implanted vaginal mesh and other prosthetic materials into pelvic floor muscles

629.32 Exposure of implanted vaginal mesh and other prosthetic materials into vagina ♀
Exposure of vaginal mesh and other prosthetic materials through vaginal wall

√5ᵗʰ **629.8 Other specified disorders of female genital organs**

629.81 Recurrent pregnancy loss without current pregnancy ♀
EXCLUDES *recurrent pregnancy loss with current pregnancy (646.3)*
AHA: 4Q, '06, 98

629.89 Other specified disorders of female genital organs ♀
AHA: 4Q, '06, 98

629.9 Unspecified disorder of female genital organs ♀

√4ᵗʰ
√5ᵗʰ Additional Digit Required   Unspecified Code   Other Specified Code   Manifestation Code   ▶◀ Revised Text   ● New Code   ▲ Revised Code Title
2013 ICD-9-CM   **February 2012 • Volume 1 – 195**

11. Complications of Pregnancy, Childbirth, and the Puerperium (630-679)

Ectopic and Molar Pregnancy (630-633)

Use additional code from category 639 to identify any complications

630 Hydatidiform mole   Ⓜ♀
Trophoblastic disease NOS
Vesicular mole

> **EXCLUDES** *chorioadenoma (destruens) (236.1)*
> *chorionepithelioma (181)*
> *malignant hydatidiform mole (236.1)*

DEF: Abnormal product of pregnancy; marked by mass of cysts resembling bunch of grapes due to chorionic villi proliferation, and dissolution; must be surgically removed.

✓4ᵗʰ 631 Other abnormal product of conception
AHA: ▶4Q, '11, 131-132◀

631.0 Inappropriate change in quantitative human chorionic Ⓜ♀ gonadotropin (hCG) in early pregnancy
Biochemical pregnancy
Chemical pregnancy
Inappropriate level of quantitative human chorionic gonadotropin (hCG) for gestational age in early pregnancy

> **EXCLUDES** *blighted ovum (631.8)*
> *molar pregnancy (631.8)*

631.8 Other abnormal products of conception   Ⓜ♀
Blighted ovum

632 Missed abortion   Ⓜ♀
Early fetal death before completion of 22 weeks' gestation with retention of dead fetus
Retained products of conception, not following spontaneous or induced abortion or delivery

> **EXCLUDES** *failed induced abortion (638.0-638.9)*
> *fetal death (intrauterine) (late) (656.4)*
> *missed delivery (656.4)*
> *that with hydatidiform mole (630)*
> *that with other abnormal products of conception (631.8)*

AHA: 1Q, '01, 5

002.1 Missed abortion   [1-10]

✓4ᵗʰ 633 Ectopic pregnancy
INCLUDES ruptured ectopic pregnancy
DEF: Fertilized egg develops outside uterus.
AHA: 4Q, '02, 61

✓5ᵗʰ 633.0 Abdominal pregnancy
Intraperitoneal pregnancy

633.00 Abdominal pregnancy without intrauterine pregnancy   Ⓜ♀

633.01 Abdominal pregnancy with intrauterine pregnancy   Ⓜ♀

✓5ᵗʰ 633.1 Tubal pregnancy
Fallopian pregnancy
Rupture of (fallopian) tube due to pregnancy
Tubal abortion
AHA: 2Q, '90, 27

633.10 Tubal pregnancy without intrauterine pregnancy   Ⓜ♀
000.1 Tubal pregnancy   [1-10]

633.11 Tubal pregnancy with intrauterine pregnancy   Ⓜ♀

✓5ᵗʰ 633.2 Ovarian pregnancy

633.20 Ovarian pregnancy without intrauterine pregnancy   Ⓜ♀

633.21 Ovarian pregnancy with intrauterine pregnancy   Ⓜ♀

✓5ᵗʰ 633.8 Other ectopic pregnancy
Pregnancy:
cervical
combined
cornual
intraligamentous
mesometric
mural

633.80 Other ectopic pregnancy without intrauterine pregnancy   Ⓜ♀

633.81 Other ectopic pregnancy with intrauterine pregnancy   Ⓜ♀

✓5ᵗʰ 633.9 Unspecified ectopic pregnancy

633.90 Unspecified ectopic pregnancy without intrauterine pregnancy   Ⓜ♀

633.91 Unspecified ectopic pregnancy with intrauterine pregnancy   Ⓜ♀

Other Pregnancy with Abortive Outcome (634-639)

The following fourth-digit subdivisions are for use with categories 634-638:

.0 Complicated by genital tract and pelvic infection
Endometritis
Salpingo-oophoritis
Sepsis NOS
Septicemia NOS
Any condition classifiable to 639.0 with condition classifiable to 634-638
> **EXCLUDES** *urinary tract infection (634-638 with .7)*

.1 Complicated by delayed or excessive hemorrhage
Afibrinogenemia
Defibrination syndrome
Intravascular hemolysis
Any condition classifiable to 639.1 with condition classifiable to 634-638

.2 Complicated by damage to pelvic organs and tissues
Laceration, perforation, or tear of:
bladder
uterus
Any condition classifiable to 639.2 with condition classifiable to 634-638

.3 Complicated by renal failure
Oliguria
Uremia
Any condition classifiable to 639.3, with condition classifiable to 634-638

.4 Complicated by metabolic disorder
Electrolyte imbalance with conditions classfiable to 634-638

.5 Complicated by shock
Circulatory collapse
Shock (postoperative) (septic)
Any condition classifiable to 639.5 with condition classifiable to 634-638

.6 Complicated by embolism
Embolism:
NOS
amniotic fluid
pulmonary
Any condition classifiable to 639.6, with condition classifiable to 634-638

.7 With other specified complications
Cardiac arrest or failure
Urinary tract infection
Any condition classiable to 639.8 with condition classifiable to 634-638

.8 With unspecified complication
.9 Without mention of complication

§ ✓4ᵗʰ 634 Spontaneous abortion
Requires fifth-digit to identify stage:
  0 unspecified
  1 incomplete
  2 complete

INCLUDES miscarriage
  spontaneous abortion

DEF: Spontaneous premature expulsion of the products of conception from the uterus.
AHA: ▶4Q, '11, 181;◀ 2Q, '91, 16

§§ ✓5ᵗʰ 634.0 Complicated by genital tract and pelvic infection   Ⓜ♀
[0-2]

§§ ✓5ᵗʰ 634.1 Complicated by delayed or excessive hemorrhage   Ⓜ♀
[0-2]   AHA: For Code 634.11: 1Q, '03, 6

---

§ See beginning of section 634-639 for fourth-digit definitions.
§§ Requires fifth digit. Valid digits are in [brackets] under each code. See appropriate category for codes and definitions.

✓4ᵗʰ ✓5ᵗʰ Additional Digit Required   Unspecified Code   Other Specified Code   Manifestation Code   ▶◀ Revised Text   ● New Code   ▲ Revised Code Title

Complications of Pregnancy, Childbirth, and the Puerperium

634.2–638

Ectopic Pregnancy Sites

§§ ✓5ᵗʰ **634.2 Complicated by damage to pelvic organs or tissues** [0-2] Ⓜ♀

§§ ✓5ᵗʰ **634.3 Complicated by renal failure** [0-2] Ⓜ♀

§§ ✓5ᵗʰ **634.4 Complicated by metabolic disorder** [0-2] Ⓜ♀

§§ ✓5ᵗʰ **634.5 Complicated by shock** [0-2] Ⓜ♀

§§ ✓5ᵗʰ **634.6 Complicated by embolism** [0-2] Ⓜ♀

§§ ✓5ᵗʰ **634.7 With other specified complications** [0-2] Ⓜ♀

§§ ✓5ᵗʰ **634.8 With unspecified complication** [0-2] Ⓜ♀

§§ ✓5ᵗʰ **634.9 Without mention of complication** [0-2] Ⓜ♀

§ ✓4ᵗʰ **635 Legally induced abortion**

Requires fifth-digit to identify stage:
0 unspecified
1 incomplete
2 complete

INCLUDES abortion or termination of pregnancy:
elective
legal
therapeutic

EXCLUDES *menstrual extraction or regulation (V25.3)*

DEF: Intentional expulsion of products of conception from uterus performed by medical professionals inside boundaries of law.

AHA: ▶4Q, '11, 181;◀ 2Q, '94, 14

§§ ✓5ᵗʰ **635.0 Complicated by genital tract and pelvic infection** [0-2] Ⓜ♀

§§ ✓5ᵗʰ **635.1 Complicated by delayed or excessive hemorrhage** [0-2] Ⓜ♀

§§ ✓5ᵗʰ **635.2 Complicated by damage to pelvic organs or tissues** [0-2] Ⓜ♀

§§ ✓5ᵗʰ **635.3 Complicated by renal failure** [0-2] Ⓜ♀

§§ ✓5ᵗʰ **635.4 Complicated by metabolic disorder** [0-2] Ⓜ♀

§§ ✓5ᵗʰ **635.5 Complicated by shock** [0-2] Ⓜ♀

§§ ✓5ᵗʰ **635.6 Complicated by embolism** [0-2] Ⓜ♀

§§ ✓5ᵗʰ **635.7 With other specified complications** [0-2] Ⓜ♀

§§ ✓5ᵗʰ **635.8 With unspecified complication** [0-2] Ⓜ♀

§§ ✓5ᵗʰ **635.9 Without mention of complication** [0-2] Ⓜ♀   AHA: For code 635.92: 2Q, '10, 6-7; 2Q, '94, 14

§ ✓4ᵗʰ **636 Illegally induced abortion**

Requires fifth-digit to identify stage:
0 unspecified
1 incomplete
2 complete

INCLUDES abortion:
criminal
illegal
self-induced

DEF: Intentional expulsion of products of conception from uterus; outside boundaries of law.

AHA: ▶4Q, '11, 181◀

§§ ✓5ᵗʰ **636.0 Complicated by genital tract and pelvic infection** [0-2] Ⓜ♀

§§ ✓5ᵗʰ **636.1 Complicated by delayed or excessive hemorrhage** [0-2] Ⓜ♀

§§ ✓5ᵗʰ **636.2 Complicated by damage to pelvic organs or tissues** [0-2] Ⓜ♀

§§ ✓5ᵗʰ **636.3 Complicated by renal failure** [0-2] Ⓜ♀

§§ ✓5ᵗʰ **636.4 Complicated by metabolic disorder** [0-2] Ⓜ♀

§§ ✓5ᵗʰ **636.5 Complicated by shock** [0-2] Ⓜ♀

§§ ✓5ᵗʰ **636.6 Complicated by embolism** [0-2] Ⓜ♀

§§ ✓5ᵗʰ **636.7 With other specified complications** [0-2] Ⓜ♀

§§ ✓5ᵗʰ **636.8 With unspecified complication** [0-2] Ⓜ♀

§§ ✓5ᵗʰ **636.9 Without mention of complication** [0-2] Ⓜ♀

§ ✓4ᵗʰ **637 Unspecified abortion**

Requires fifth-digit to identify stage:
0 unspecified
1 incomplete
2 complete

INCLUDES abortion NOS
retained products of conception following abortion, not classifiable elsewhere

AHA: ▶4Q, '11, 181◀

§§ ✓5ᵗʰ **637.0 Complicated by genital tract and pelvic infection** [0-2] Ⓜ♀

§§ ✓5ᵗʰ **637.1 Complicated by delayed or excessive hemorrhage** [0-2] Ⓜ♀

§§ ✓5ᵗʰ **637.2 Complicated by damage to pelvic organs or tissues** [0-2] Ⓜ♀

§§ ✓5ᵗʰ **637.3 Complicated by renal failure** [0-2] Ⓜ♀

§§ ✓5ᵗʰ **637.4 Complicated by metabolic disorder** [0-2] Ⓜ♀

§§ ✓5ᵗʰ **637.5 Complicated by shock** [0-2] Ⓜ♀

§§ ✓5ᵗʰ **637.6 Complicated by embolism** [0-2] Ⓜ♀

§§ ✓5ᵗʰ **637.7 With other specified complications** [0-2] Ⓜ♀

§§ ✓5ᵗʰ **637.8 With unspecified complication** [0-2] Ⓜ♀

§§ ✓5ᵗʰ **637.9 Without mention of complication** [0-2] Ⓜ♀

§ ✓4ᵗʰ **638 Failed attempted abortion**

INCLUDES failure of attempted induction of (legal) abortion

EXCLUDES *incomplete abortion (634.0-637.9)*

DEF: Continued pregnancy despite an attempted legal abortion.

---

§ See beginning of section 634-639 for fourth-digit definitions.
§§ Requires fifth digit. Valid digits are in [brackets] under each code. See appropriate category for codes and definitions.

Ⓝ Newborn Age: 0   Ⓟ Pediatric Age: 0-17   Ⓜ Maternity Age: 12-55   Ⓐ Adult Age: 15-124

638.0 Complicated by genital tract and pelvic infection Ⓜ♀

638.1 Complicated by delayed or excessive hemorrhage Ⓜ♀

638.2 Complicated by damage to pelvic organs or tissues Ⓜ♀

638.3 Complicated by renal failure Ⓜ♀

638.4 Complicated by metabolic disorder Ⓜ♀

638.5 Complicated by shock Ⓜ♀

638.6 Complicated by embolism Ⓜ♀

638.7 With other specified complications Ⓜ♀

638.8 With unspecified complication Ⓜ♀

638.9 Without mention of complication Ⓜ♀

✓4ᵗʰ **639 Complications following abortion and ectopic and molar pregnancies**

> **NOTE** This category is provided for use when it is required to classify separately the complications classifiable to the fourth-digit level in categories 634-638; for example:
>
> a) when the complication itself was responsible for an episode of medical care, the abortion, ectopic or molar pregnancy itself having been dealt with at a previous episode
>
> b) when these conditions are immediate complications of ectopic or molar pregnancies classifiable to 630-633 where they cannot be identified at fourth-digit level.

639.0 Genital tract and pelvic infection Ⓜ♀

Endometritis
Parametritis
Pelvic peritonitis
Salpingitis
Salpingo-oophoritis
Sepsis NOS
Septicemia NOS
} following conditions classifiable to 630-638

> **EXCLUDES** urinary tract infection (639.8)

639.1 Delayed or excessive hemorrhage Ⓜ♀

Afibrinogenemia
Defibrination syndrome
Intravascular
} following conditions classfiable to 630-638

639.2 Damage to pelvic organs and tissues Ⓜ♀

Laceration, perforation, or tear of:
bladder
bowel
broad ligament
cervix
periurethral tissue
uterus
vagina
} following conditions classifiable to 630-638

639.3 Kidney failure Ⓜ♀

Oliguria
Renal (kidney):
failure (acute)
shutdown
tubular necrosis
Uremia
} following conditions classifiable to 630-638

639.4 Metabolic disorders Ⓜ♀

Electrolyte imbalance following conditions classifiable to 630-638

639.5 Shock Ⓜ♀

Circulatory collapse
Shock (postoperative)
(septic)
} following conditions classifiable to 630-638

639.6 Embolism Ⓜ♀

Embolism:
NOS
air
amniotic fluid
blood-clot
fat
pulmonary
pyemic
septic
soap
} following conditions classifiable to 630-638

639.8 Other specified complications following abortion or ectopic and molar pregnancy Ⓜ♀

Acute yellow atrophy
or necrosis of
liver
Cardiac arrest or failure
Cerebral anoxia
Urinary tract infection
} following conditons classifiable to 630-638

639.9 Unspecified complication following abortion or ectopic and molar pregnancy Ⓜ♀

Complication(s) not further specified following conditions classifiable to 630-638

Complications Mainly Related to Pregnancy (640-649)

> **INCLUDES** the listed conditions even if they arose or were present during labor, delivery, or the puerperium
>
> AHA: 2Q, '90, 11

The following fifth-digit subclassification is for use with categories 640-649 to denote the current episode of care. Valid fifth-digits are in [brackets] under each code.

0 unspecified as to episode of care or not applicable
1 delivered, with or without mention of antepartum condition
Antepartum condition with delivery
Delivery NOS (with mention of antepartum complication during current episode of care)
Intrapartum obstetric condition (with mention of antepartum complication during current episode of care)
Pregnancy, delivered (with mention of antepartum complication during current episode of care)
2 delivered, with mention of postpartum complication
Delivery with mention of puerperal complication during current episode of care
3 antepartum condition or complication
Antepartum obstetric condtion, not delivered during the current episode of care
4 postpartum condition of complication
Postpartum or puerperal obstetric condition or complication following delivery that occurred:
during previous episode of care
outside hospital, with subsequent admission for observation or care

✓4ᵗʰ **640 Hemorrhage in early pregnancy**

> **INCLUDES** hemorrhage before completion of 22 weeks' gestation

§ ✓5ᵗʰ **640.0 Threatened abortion** Ⓜ♀
[0,1,3] **DEF:** Bloody discharge during pregnancy; cervix may be dilated and pregnancy is threatened, but the pregnancy is not terminated.

§ ✓5ᵗʰ **640.8 Other specified hemorrhage in early pregnancy** Ⓜ♀
[0,1,3]

§ ✓5ᵗʰ **640.9 Unspecified hemorrhage in early pregnancy** Ⓜ♀
[0,1,3]

✓4ᵗʰ **641 Antepartum hemorrhage, abruptio placentae, and placenta previa**

§ ✓5ᵗʰ **641.0 Placenta previa without hemorrhage** Ⓜ♀
[0,1,3]
Low impantation of placenta
Placenta previa noted:
during pregnancy
before labor (and delivered by caesarean delivery)
} without hemorrhage

DEF: Placenta implanted in lower segment of uterus; commonly causes hemorrhage in the last trimester of pregnancy.

Placenta Previa

Low (marginal) implantation   Partial placenta previa   Total placenta previa

---

§ Requires fifth digit. Valid digits are in [brackets] under each code. See beginning of section 640-649 for codes and definitions.

✓4ᵗʰ / ✓5ᵗʰ Additional Digit Required   Unspecified Code   Other Specified Code   Manifestation Code   ▶◀ Revised Text   ● New Code   ▲ Revised Code Title

2013 ICD-9-CM   **Volume 1 – 199**

Complications of Pregnancy, Childbirth, and the Puerperium

641.1–643.2

Abruptio Placentae

Partial separation (concealed bleeding)   Partial separation (apparent hemorrhage)   Complete separation (concealed hemorrhage)

§ √5ᵗʰ **641.1 Hemorrhage from placenta previa**   Ⓜ♀
[0,1,3]

Low-lying placenta
Placenta previa
  incomplete
  marginal   NOS or with hemorrhage (intrapartum)
  partial
  total

> **EXCLUDES** *hemorrhage from vasa previa (663.5)*

§ √5ᵗʰ **641.2 Premature separation of placenta**   Ⓜ♀
[0,1,3]

Ablatio placentae
Abruptio placentae
Accidental antepartum hemorrhage
Couvelaire uterus
Detachment of placenta (premature)
Premature separation of normally implanted placenta
DEF: Abruptio placentae: premature detachment of the placenta, characterized by shock, oliguria and decreased fibrinogen.
045.90 Premature sep of placenta unspec, uns trimester   I-10

§ √5ᵗʰ **641.3 Antepartum hemorrhage associated**   Ⓜ♀
[0,1,3] **with coagulation defects**

Antepartum or intrapartum hemorrhage associated with:
  afibrinogenemia
  hyperfibrinolysis
  hypofibrinogenemia
> **EXCLUDES** *coagulation defects not associated with antepartum hemorrhage (649.3)*
DEF: Uterine hemorrhage prior to delivery.

§ √5ᵗʰ **641.8 Other antepartum hemorrhage**   Ⓜ♀
[0,1,3]

Antepartum or intrapartum hemorrhage associated with:
  trauma
  uterine leiomyoma

§ √5ᵗʰ **641.9 Unspecified antepartum hemorrhage**   Ⓜ♀
[0,1,3]

Hemorrhage:
  antepartum NOS
  intrapartum NOS
  of pregnancy NOS

√4ᵗʰ **642 Hypertension complicating pregnancy, childbirth, and the puerperium**

§ √5ᵗʰ **642.0 Benign essential hypertension complicating**   Ⓜ♀
[0-4] **pregnancy, childbirth, and the puerperium**

Hypertension
  benign essential
  chronic NOS   specified as complicating, or as reason for obstetric care during pregnancy, childbirth, or the puerperium
  essential
  pre-existing NOS

010.02 Pre-exist essential hypertension comp childbirth   I-10

§ √5ᵗʰ **642.1 Hypertension secondary to renal disease,**   Ⓜ♀
[0-4] **complicating pregnancy, childbirth, and the puerperium**

Hypertension secondary to renal disease, specified as complicating, or as a reason for obstetric care during pregnancy, childbirth, or the puerperium

§ √5ᵗʰ **642.2 Other pre-existing hypertension complicating**   Ⓜ♀
[0-4] **pregnancy, childbirth, and the puerperium**

Hypertensive
  chronic kidney disease
  heart and chronic
    kidney disease   specified as complicating, or as a reason for obstetric care during pregnancy, childbirth, or the puerperium
  heart disease
Malignant hypertension

§ √5ᵗʰ **642.3 Transient hypertension of pregnancy**   Ⓜ♀
[0-4]

Gestational hypertension
Transient hypertension, so described, in pregnancy, childbirth, or the puerperium
AHA: 3Q, '90, 4
013.9 Gestatnl pg-inducd HTN w/o sig protnuria uns tri   I-10

§ √5ᵗʰ **642.4 Mild or unspecified pre-eclampsia**   Ⓜ♀
[0-4]

Hypertension in pregnancy, childbirth, or the puerperium, not specified as pre-existing, with either albuminuria or edema, or both; mild or unspecified
Pre-eclampsia:
  NOS
  mild
Toxemia (pre-eclamptic):
  NOS
  mild
> **EXCLUDES** *albuminuria in pregnancy, without mention of hypertension (646.2)*
> *edema in pregnancy, without mention of hypertension (646.1)*
AHA: For code 642.41: 4Q, '09, 153
014.00 Mild to moderate pre-eclampsia unspec trimester   I-10

§ √5ᵗʰ **642.5 Severe pre-eclampsia**   Ⓜ♀
[0-4]

Hypertension in pregnancy, childbirth, or the puerperium, not specified as pre-existing, with either albuminuria or edema, or both; specified as severe
Pre-eclampsia, severe
Toxemia (pre-eclamptic), severe
AHA: N-D, '85, 3

§ √5ᵗʰ **642.6 Eclampsia**   Ⓜ♀
[0-4]

Toxemia:
  eclamptic
  with convulsions

§ √5ᵗʰ **642.7 Pre-eclampsia or eclampsia superimposed**   Ⓜ♀
[0-4] **on pre-existing hypertension**

Conditions classifiable to 642.4-642.6, with conditions classifiable to 642.0-642.2

§ √5ᵗʰ **642.9 Unspecified hypertension complicating**   Ⓜ♀
[0-4] **pregnancy, childbirth, or the puerperium**

Hypertension NOS, without mention of albuminuria or edema, complicating pregnancy, childbirth, or the puerperium
AHA: For code 642.94: 1Q, '09, 17

√4ᵗʰ **643 Excessive vomiting in pregnancy**

> **INCLUDES** hyperemesis
> vomiting:
>   persistent   arising during pregnancy
>   vicious
> hyperemesis gravidarum

§ √5ᵗʰ **643.0 Mild hyperemesis gravidarum**   Ⓜ♀
[0,1,3]

Hyperemesis gravidarum, mild or unspecified, starting before the end of the 22nd week of gestation
DEF: Detrimental vomiting and nausea.

§ √5ᵗʰ **643.1 Hyperemesis gravidarum with metabolic**   Ⓜ♀
[0,1,3] **disturbance**

Hyperemesis gravidarum, starting before the end of the 22nd week of gestation, with metabolic disturbance, such as:
  carbohydrate depletion
  dehydration
  electrolyte imbalance

§ √5ᵗʰ **643.2 Late vomiting of pregnancy**   Ⓜ♀
[0,1,3]

Excessive vomiting starting after 22 completed weeks of gestation

---

§   Requires fifth digit. Valid digits are in [brackets] under each code. See beginning of section 640-649 for codes and definitions.

Ⓝ Newborn Age: 0   Ⓟ Pediatric Age: 0-17   Ⓜ Maternity Age: 12-55   Ⓐ Adult Age: 15-124

200 – Volume 1   **2013 ICD-9-CM**

§ ✓5ᵗʰ **643.8 Other vomiting complicating pregnancy** Ⓜ♀
[0,1,3]   Vomiting due to organic disease or other cause, specified as complicating pregnancy, or as a reason for obstetric care during pregnancy
       Use additional code to specify cause

§ ✓5ᵗʰ **643.9 Unspecified vomiting of pregnancy** Ⓜ♀
[0,1,3]   Vomiting as a reason for care during pregnancy, length of gestation unspecified

✓4ᵗʰ **644 Early or threatened labor**

§ ✓5ᵗʰ **644.0 Threatened premature labor** Ⓜ♀
[0,3]   Premature labor after 22 weeks, but before 37 completed weeks of gestation without delivery
       EXCLUDES *that occurring before 22 completed weeks of gestation (640.0)*
       060.00 Preterm labor without delivery unspec trimester   I-10

§ ✓5ᵗʰ **644.1 Other threatened labor** Ⓜ♀
[0,3]   False labor:
       NOS
       after 37 completed weeks of gestation ⎫ without delivery
       Threatened labor NOS ⎭

§ ✓5ᵗʰ **644.2 Early onset of delivery** Ⓜ♀
[0,1]   Onset (spontaneous) of delivery ⎫ before 37 completed
       Premature labor with onset of ⎬ weeks of
       delivery ⎭ gestation
       AHA: 2Q, '91, 16; For code 644.21: ▶3Q, '11, 3◀
       TIP: Assign if an attempted termination of pregnancy results in a liveborn fetus.
       060.14x0 Pt labor 3rd tri w/pt del 3rd tri not applic/uns   I-10

✓4ᵗʰ **645 Late pregnancy**
     AHA: 4Q, '00, 43; 4Q, '91, 26

§ ✓5ᵗʰ **645.1 Post term pregnancy** Ⓜ♀
[0,1,3]   Pregnancy over 40 completed weeks to 42 completed weeks gestation
       048.0 Post-term pregnancy   I-10

§ ✓5ᵗʰ **645.2 Prolonged pregnancy** Ⓜ♀
[0,1,3]   Pregnancy which has advanced beyond 42 completed weeks gestation

✓4ᵗʰ **646 Other complications of pregnancy, not elsewhere classified**
     Use additional code(s) to further specify complication
     AHA: 4Q, '95, 59

§ ✓5ᵗʰ **646.0 Papyraceous fetus** Ⓜ♀
[0,1,3]   DEF: Fetus that dies in the second trimester of pregnancy and is retained in the uterus, with subsequent atrophy and mummification; commonly occurs in twin pregnancy, nonviable fetus becomes compressed by growth of living twin.

§ ✓5ᵗʰ **646.1 Edema or excessive weight gain in** Ⓜ♀
[0-4]   **pregnancy, without mention of hypertension**
       Gestational edema
       Maternal obesity syndrome
       EXCLUDES *that with mention of hypertension (642.0-642.9)*

§ ✓5ᵗʰ **646.2 Unspecified renal disease in pregnancy,** Ⓜ♀
[0-4]   **without mention of hypertension**
       Albuminuria ⎫ in pregnancy or the
       Nephropathy NOS ⎪ puerperium, without
       Renal disease NOS ⎬ mention of
       Uremia ⎭ hypertension
       Gestational proteinuria
       EXCLUDES *that with mention of hypertension (642.0-642.9)*

§ ✓5ᵗʰ **646.3 Recurrent pregnancy loss** Ⓜ♀
[0,1,3]   **EXCLUDES** *with current abortion (634.0-634.9)*
                without current pregnancy (629.81)
       DEF: Three or more consecutive spontaneous abortions.

§ ✓5ᵗʰ **646.4 Peripheral neuritis in pregnancy** Ⓜ♀
[0-4]

§ ✓5ᵗʰ **646.5 Asymptomatic bacteriuria in pregnancy** Ⓜ♀
[0-4]

§ ✓5ᵗʰ **646.6 Infections of genitourinary tract in pregnancy** Ⓜ♀
[0-4]   Conditions classifiable to 590, 595, 597, 599.0, 616 complicating pregnancy, childbirth, or the puerperium
       Conditions classifiable to 614.0-614.5, 614.7-614.9, 615 complicating pregnancy or labor
       EXCLUDES *major puerperal infection (670.0-670.8)*
       AHA: For code 646.63: 4Q, '04, 90
       023.90 Unspec GU tract infection in pregnancy uns tri   I-10

§ ✓5ᵗʰ **646.7 Liver and biliary tract disorders in pregnancy** Ⓜ♀
[0,1,3]   Acute yellow atrophy of liver ⎫
       (obstetric) (true) ⎬ of pregnancy
       Icterus gravis ⎪
       Necrosis of liver ⎭
       EXCLUDES *hepatorenal syndrome following delivery (674.8)*
                viral hepatitis (647.6)

§ ✓5ᵗʰ **646.8 Other specified complications of pregnancy** Ⓜ♀
[0-4]   Fatigue during pregnancy
       Herpes gestationis
       Insufficient weight gain of pregnancy
       AHA: 3Q, '98, 16; J-F, '85, 15

§ ✓5ᵗʰ **646.9 Unspecified complication of pregnancy** Ⓜ♀
[0,1,3]

✓4ᵗʰ **647 Infectious and parasitic conditions in the mother classifiable elsewhere, but complicating pregnancy, childbirth, or the puerperium**
     INCLUDES the listed conditions when complicating the pregnant state, aggravated by the pregnancy, or when a main reason for obstetric care
     Use additional code(s) to further specify complication
     EXCLUDES *those conditions in the mother known or suspected to have affected the fetus (655.0-655.9)*

§ ✓5ᵗʰ **647.0 Syphilis** Ⓜ♀
[0-4]   Conditions classifiable to 090-097

§ ✓5ᵗʰ **647.1 Gonorrhea** Ⓜ♀
[0-4]   Conditions classifiable to 098

§ ✓5ᵗʰ **647.2 Other venereal diseases** Ⓜ♀
[0-4]   Conditions classifiable to 099

§ ✓5ᵗʰ **647.3 Tuberculosis** Ⓜ♀
[0-4]   Conditions classifiable to 010-018

§ ✓5ᵗʰ **647.4 Malaria** Ⓜ♀
[0-4]   Conditions classifiable to 084

§ ✓5ᵗʰ **647.5 Rubella** Ⓜ♀
[0-4]   Conditions classifiable to 056

§ ✓5ᵗʰ **647.6 Other viral diseases** Ⓜ♀
[0-4]   Conditions classifiable to 042, 050-055, 057-079, 795.05, 795.15, 796.75
       AHA: J-F, '85, 15; For code 647.61: 2Q, '10, 10
       TIP: Assign when pregnant patient has any HIV-related condition or is stated to have an asymptomatic HIV infection.
       098.52 Other viral diseases complicating childbirth   I-10

§ ✓5ᵗʰ **647.8 Other specified infectious and parasitic** Ⓜ♀
[0-4]   **diseases**

§ ✓5ᵗʰ **647.9 Unspecified infection or infestation** Ⓜ♀
[0-4]

✓4ᵗʰ **648 Other current conditions in the mother classifiable elsewhere, but complicating pregnancy, childbirth, or the puerperium**
     INCLUDES the listed conditions when complicating the pregnant state, aggravated by the pregnancy, or when a main reason for obstetric care
     Use additional code(s) to identify the condition
     EXCLUDES *those conditions in the mother known or suspected to have affected the fetus (655.0-655.9)*

§ ✓5ᵗʰ **648.0 Diabetes mellitus** Ⓜ♀
[0-4]   Conditions classifiable to 249, 250
       EXCLUDES *gestational diabetes (648.8)*
       AHA: 3Q, '91, 5, 11
       024.32 Uns pre-existing diabetes mellitus in childbirth   I-10

---

§   Requires fifth digit. Valid digits are in [brackets] under each code. See beginning of section 640-649 for codes and definitions.

✓4ᵗʰ
✓5ᵗʰ Additional Digit Required   Unspecified Code   Other Specified Code   Manifestation Code   ▶◀ Revised Text   ● New Code   ▲ Revised Code Title

Complications of Pregnancy, Childbirth, and the Puerperium

648.1–650

§ ✓5ᵗʰ **648.1 Thyroid dysfunction** Ⓜ♀
[0-4] Conditions classifiable to 240-246

§ ✓5ᵗʰ **648.2 Anemia** Ⓜ♀
[0-4] Conditions classifiable to 280-285
AHA: For Code 648.22: 1Q, '02, 14; For code 648.24: 1Q, '09, 17
TIP: Assign with fifth digit 2 for postpartum anemia.
099.013 Anemia complicating pregnancy third trimester ｜-10

§ ✓5ᵗʰ **648.3 Drug dependence** Ⓜ♀
[0-4] Conditions classifiable to 304
AHA: 2Q, '98, 13; 4Q, '88, 8

§ ✓5ᵗʰ **648.4 Mental disorders** Ⓜ♀
[0-4] Conditions classifiable to 290-303, 305.0, 305.2-305.9,
306-316, 317-319
AHA: 2Q, '98, 13; 4Q, '95, 63
099.314 Alcohol use complicating childbirth ｜-10

§ ✓5ᵗʰ **648.5 Congenital cardiovascular disorders** Ⓜ♀
[0-4] Conditions classifiable to 745-747

§ ✓5ᵗʰ **648.6 Other cardiovascular diseases** Ⓜ♀
[0-4] Conditions classifiable to 390-398, 410-429
EXCLUDES cerebrovascular disorders in the puerperium (674.0)
peripartum cardiomyopathy (674.5)
venous complications (671.0-671.9)
AHA: 3Q, '98, 11

§ ✓5ᵗʰ **648.7 Bone and joint disorders of back, pelvis, and** Ⓜ♀
[0-4] **lower limbs**
Conditions classifiable to 720-724, and those classifiable to
711-719 or 725-738, specified as affecting the lower
limbs

§ ✓5ᵗʰ **648.8 Abnormal glucose tolerance** Ⓜ♀
[0-4] Conditions classifiable to 790.21-790.29
Gestational diabetes
Use additional code, if applicable, for associated long-term
(current) insulin use (V58.67)
DEF: Glucose intolerance arising in pregnancy, resolving at end of
pregnancy.
AHA: 3Q, '91, 5; For code 648.83: 4Q, '04, 56
TIP: Do not assign if patient was diabetic before becoming pregnant;
should never be assigned in combination with code 648.0X.
024.429 Gestational diab mellitus childbirth uns cntrl ｜-10

§ ✓5ᵗʰ **648.9 Other current conditions classifiable elsewhere** Ⓜ♀
[0-4] Conditions classifiable to 440-459, 795.01-795.04, 795.06,
795.10-795.14, 795.16, 796.70-796.74, 796.76
Nutritional deficiencies [conditions classifiable to 260-269]
AHA: 3Q, '06, 14; 4Q, '04, 88; N-D, '87, 10; For code 648.91: 1Q, '02, 14;
For code 648.93: 4Q, '04, 90; For code 648.94: 1Q, '09, 17
TIP: Assign for group B streptococcus carrier patients, along with
code V02.51 Carrier or suspected carrier of infectious diseases.

✓4ᵗʰ **649 Other conditions or status of the mother complicating**
pregnancy, childbirth, or the puerperium
AHA: 4Q, '06, 99

§ ✓5ᵗʰ **649.0 Tobacco use disorder complicating pregnancy,** Ⓜ♀
[0-4] **childbirth, or the puerperium**
Smoking complicating pregnancy, childbirth, or the
puerperium
AHA: 4Q, '06, 99
099.334 Smoking tobacco complicating childbirth ｜-10

§ ✓5ᵗʰ **649.1 Obesity complicating pregnancy, childbirth,** Ⓜ♀
[0-4] **or the puerperium**
Use additional code to identify the obesity (278.00- 278.03)
AHA: 4Q, '06, 99
099.214 Obesity complicating childbirth ｜-10

§ ✓5ᵗʰ **649.2 Bariatric surgery status complicating** Ⓜ♀
[0-4] **pregnancy, childbirth, or the puerperium**
Gastric banding status complicating pregnancy, childbirth, or
the puerperium
Gastric bypass status for obesity complicating pregnancy,
childbirth, or the puerperium
Obesity surgery status complicating pregnancy, childbirth, or
the puerperium
AHA: 4Q, '06, 99, 118

§ ✓5ᵗʰ **649.3 Coagulation defects complicating pregnancy,** Ⓜ♀
[0-4] **childbirth, or the puerperium**
Conditions classifiable to 286, 287, 289
Use additional code to identify the specific coagulation defect
(286.0-286.9, 287.0-287.9, 289.0-289.9)
EXCLUDES coagulation defects causing antepartum
hemorrhage (641.3)
postpartum coagulation defects (666.3)
AHA: 4Q, '06, 99

§ ✓5ᵗʰ **649.4 Epilepsy complicating pregnancy, childbirth,** Ⓜ♀
[0-4] **or the puerperium**
Conditions classifiable to 345
Use additional code to identify the specific type of epilepsy
(345.00-345.91)
EXCLUDES eclampsia (642.6)
AHA: 4Q, '06, 99

§ ✓5ᵗʰ **649.5 Spotting complicating pregnancy** Ⓜ♀
[0,1,3] **EXCLUDES** antepartum hemorrhage (641.0-641.9)
hemorrhage in early pregnancy (640.0-640.9)
AHA: 4Q, '06, 99

§ ✓5ᵗʰ **649.6 Uterine size date discrepancy** Ⓜ♀
[0-4] **EXCLUDES** suspected problem with fetal growth not found
(V89.04)
AHA: 4Q, '06, 99

§ ✓5ᵗʰ **649.7 Cervical shortening** Ⓜ♀
[0,1,3] **EXCLUDES** suspected cervical shortening not found (V89.05)
DEF: A cervix that has shortened to < 25 mm in length by the 16th
week of pregnancy; warning sign for impending premature delivery;
treated by cervical cerclage placement or progesterone.
AHA: 4Q, '08, 124-125; For code 649.73: 4Q, '08, 125

§ ✓5ᵗʰ **649.8 Onset (spontaneous) of labor after 37 completed** Ⓜ♀
[1,2] **weeks of gestation but before 39 completed weeks**
gestation, with delivery by (planned) cesarean section
Delivery by (planned) cesarean section occurring after 37
completed weeks of gestation but before 39 completed
weeks gestation due to (spontaneous) onset of labor
Use additional code to specify reason for planned cesarean
section such as:
cephalopelvic disproportion (normally formed fetus)
(653.4)
previous cesarean delivery (654.2)
AHA: ▶4Q, '11, 132-133; For code 649.81: 4Q, '11, 133◀

Normal Delivery, and Other Indications for Care in Pregnancy, Labor, and Delivery (650-659)

The following fifth-digit subclassification is for use with categories 651-659 to
denote the current episode of care. Valid fifth-digits are in [brackets] under each
code.
0 unspecified as to episode of care or not applicable
1 delivered, with or without mention of antepartum condition
2 delivered, with mention of postpartum complication
3 antepartum condition or complication
4 postpartum condition or complication

650 Normal delivery Ⓜ♀
NOTE Delivery requiring minimal or no assistance, with or without
episiotomy, without fetal manipulation [e.g., rotation version]
or instrumentation [forceps] of spontaneous, cephalic, vaginal,
full-term, single, live-born infant. This code is for use as a single
diagnosis code and is not to be used with any other code in the
range 630-676.
Use additional code to indicate outcome of delivery (V27.0)
EXCLUDES breech delivery (assisted) (spontaneous) NOS (652.2)
delivery by vacuum extractor, forceps, cesarean section, or
breech extraction, without specified complication
(669.5-669.7)
AHA: 2Q, '02, 10; 3Q, '01, 12; 3Q, '00, 5; 4Q, '95, 28, 59
TIP: Code 650 is to be assigned only for the episode of care during which the
patient delivers and may be assigned if the patient is admitted for induction
of labor.
080 Encounter for full-term uncomplicated delivery ｜-10

§ Requires fifth digit. Valid digits are in [brackets] under each code. See beginning of section 640-649 for codes and definitions.

Ⓝ Newborn Age: 0   Ⓟ Pediatric Age: 0-17   Ⓜ Maternity Age: 12-55   Ⓐ Adult Age: 15-124

Malposition and Malpresentation

Breech

Mother's pelvis

Face (mentum)

Shoulder (arm prolapse)

Compound (extremity together with head)

Oblique

Cephalopelvic Disproportion

Pubic symphysis

Ischial tuberosity

Contraction of pelvic outlet (from below)

Cephalopelvic disproportion due to: Contraction of pelvic inlet, or large fetus, or hydrocephalus

Pubic symphysis

Pelvic inlet from above

✓4ᵗʰ **651 Multiple gestation**
Use additional code to specify placenta status (V91.00-V91.99)

§ ✓5ᵗʰ **651.0 Twin pregnancy**   Ⓜ♀
[0,1,3]   **EXCLUDES** *fetal conjoined twins (678.1)*
AHA: 3Q, '06, 16
030.009 Twin preg unspec numb of placenta & unspec numb amniotic sacs unspec tri   I-10

§ ✓5ᵗʰ **651.1 Triplet pregnancy**   Ⓜ♀
[0,1,3]

§ ✓5ᵗʰ **651.2 Quadruplet pregnancy**   Ⓜ♀
[0,1,3]

§ ✓5ᵗʰ **651.3 Twin pregnancy with fetal loss and retention of one**   Ⓜ♀
[0,1,3] **fetus**
Vanishing twin syndrome (651.33)

§ ✓5ᵗʰ **651.4 Triplet pregnancy with fetal loss and retention of one**   Ⓜ♀
[0,1,3] **or more fetus(es)**

§ ✓5ᵗʰ **651.5 Quadruplet pregnancy with fetal loss and retention**   Ⓜ♀
[0,1,3] **of one or more fetus(es)**

§ ✓5ᵗʰ **651.6 Other multiple pregnancy with fetal loss and**   Ⓜ♀
[0,1,3] **retention of one or more fetus(es)**

§ ✓5ᵗʰ **651.7 Multiple gestation following (elective)**   Ⓜ♀
[0,1,3] **fetal reduction**
Fetal reduction of multiple fetuses reduced to single fetus
AHA: 3Q, '06, 18; **For code 651.71:** 4Q, '05, 81

§ ✓5ᵗʰ **651.8 Other specified multiple gestation**   Ⓜ♀
[0,1,3]

§ ✓5ᵗʰ **651.9 Unspecified multiple gestation**   Ⓜ♀
[0,1,3]

✓4ᵗʰ **652 Malposition and malpresentation of fetus**
Code first any associated obstructed labor (660.0)

§ ✓5ᵗʰ **652.0 Unstable lie**   Ⓜ♀
[0,1,3]   **DEF:** Changing fetal position.

§ ✓5ᵗʰ **652.1 Breech or other malpresentation successfully**   Ⓜ♀
[0,1,3] **converted to cephalic presentation**
Cephalic version NOS

§ ✓5ᵗʰ **652.2 Breech presentation without mention of version**   Ⓜ♀
[0,1,3] Breech delivery (assisted) (spontaneous) NOS
Buttocks presentation
Complete breech
Frank breech
EXCLUDES *footling presentation (652.8)*
incomplete breech (652.8)
DEF: Fetal presentation of buttocks or feet at birth canal.
032.1xx0 Maternal care breech presentation not applic/uns   I-10

§ ✓5ᵗʰ **652.3 Transverse or oblique presentation**   Ⓜ♀
[0,1,3] Oblique lie   Transverse lie
EXCLUDES *transverse arrest of fetal head (660.3)*
DEF: Delivery of fetus, shoulder first.

§ ✓5ᵗʰ **652.4 Face or brow presentation**   Ⓜ♀
[0,1,3] Mentum presentation

§ ✓5ᵗʰ **652.5 High head at term**   Ⓜ♀
[0,1,3] Failure of head to enter pelvic brim
032.4xx0 Maternal care high head at term not applic/uns   I-10

§ ✓5ᵗʰ **652.6 Multiple gestation with malpresentation**   Ⓜ♀
[0,1,3] **of one fetus or more**

§ ✓5ᵗʰ **652.7 Prolapsed arm**   Ⓜ♀
[0,1,3]

§ ✓5ᵗʰ **652.8 Other specified malposition or malpresentation**   Ⓜ♀
[0,1,3] Compound presentation

§ ✓5ᵗʰ **652.9 Unspecified malposition or malpresentation**   Ⓜ♀
[0,1,3]

✓4ᵗʰ **653 Disproportion**
Code first any associated obstructed labor (660.1)

§ ✓5ᵗʰ **653.0 Major abnormality of bony pelvis, not**   Ⓜ♀
[0,1,3] **further specified**
Pelvic deformity NOS

§ ✓5ᵗʰ **653.1 Generally contracted pelvis**   Ⓜ♀
[0,1,3] Contracted pelvis NOS

§ ✓5ᵗʰ **653.2 Inlet contraction of pelvis**   Ⓜ♀
[0,1,3] Inlet contraction (pelvis)

§ ✓5ᵗʰ **653.3 Outlet contraction of pelvis**   Ⓜ♀
[0,1,3] Outlet contraction (pelvis)

§ ✓5ᵗʰ **653.4 Fetopelvic disproportion**   Ⓜ♀
[0,1,3] Cephalopelvic disproportion NOS
Disproportion of mixed maternal and fetal origin, with
normally formed fetus
033.4xx0 Mtrn care dispropor mtrn & fetal orig not applic   I-10

§ ✓5ᵗʰ **653.5 Unusually large fetus causing disproportion**   Ⓜ♀
[0,1,3] Disproportion of fetal origin with normally formed fetus
Fetal disproportion NOS
EXCLUDES *that when the reason for medical care was concern*
for the fetus (656.6)

§ ✓5ᵗʰ **653.6 Hydrocephalic fetus causing disproportion**   Ⓜ♀
[0,1,3] **EXCLUDES** *that when the reason for medical care was concern*
for the fetus (655.0)

§ ✓5ᵗʰ **653.7 Other fetal abnormality causing disproportion**   Ⓜ♀
[0,1,3] Fetal:
ascites
hydrops
myelomeningocele
sacral teratoma
tumor
EXCLUDES *conjoined twins causing disproportion (678.1)*

§ ✓5ᵗʰ **653.8 Disproportion of other origin**   Ⓜ♀
[0,1,3] **EXCLUDES** *shoulder (girdle) dystocia (660.4)*

§ ✓5ᵗʰ **653.9 Unspecified disproportion**   Ⓜ♀
[0,1,3]

---

§   Requires fifth digit. Valid digits are in [brackets] under each code. See beginning of section 640-649 for codes and definitions.

| ✓4ᵗʰ ✓5ᵗʰ Additional Digit Required | Unspecified Code | Other Specified Code | Manifestation Code | ▶◀ Revised Text | ● New Code | ▲ Revised Code Title |

Complications of Pregnancy, Childbirth, and the Puerperium

654–656.5

✓4ᵗʰ 654   Abnormality of organs and soft tissues of pelvis
> **INCLUDES** the listed conditions during pregnancy, childbirth, or the puerperium
> Code first any associated obstructed labor (660.2)
> **EXCLUDES** *trauma to perineum and vulva complicating current delivery (664.0-664.9)*

§ ✓5ᵗʰ **654.0 Congenital abnormalities of uterus**   M ♀
[0-4]   Double uterus
     Uterus bicornis

§ ✓5ᵗʰ **654.1 Tumors of body of uterus**   M ♀
[0-4]   Uterine fibroids

§ ✓5ᵗʰ **654.2 Previous cesarean delivery**   M ♀
[0,1,3]   Uterine scar from previous cesarean delivery
     AHA: 1Q, '92, 8; For code 654.21: ▶4Q, '11, 133◀
     034.21 Maternal care for scar from prev cesarean del   I-10

§ ✓5ᵗʰ **654.3 Retroverted and incarcerated gravid uterus**   M ♀
[0-4]   **DEF:** Retroverted: tilted back uterus; no change in angle of longitudinal axis.
     DEF: Incarcerated: immobile, fixed uterus.

§ ✓5ᵗʰ **654.4 Other abnormalities in shape or position of**   M ♀
[0-4]   **gravid uterus and of neighboring structures**
     Cystocele
     Pelvic floor repair
     Pendulous abdomen
     Prolapse of gravid uterus
     Rectocele
     Rigid pelvic floor

§ ✓5ᵗʰ **654.5 Cervical incompetence**   M ♀
[0-4]   Presence of Shirodkar suture with or without mention of cervical incompetence
     DEF: Abnormal cervix; tendency to dilate in second trimester; causes premature fetal expulsion.
     DEF: Shirodkar suture: purse-string suture used to artificially close incompetent cervix.

§ ✓5ᵗʰ **654.6 Other congenital or acquired abnormality of cervix**   M ♀
[0-4]   Cicatricial cervix
     Polyp of cervix
     Previous surgery to cervix
     Rigid cervix (uteri)
     Stenosis or stricture of cervix
     Tumor of cervix

§ ✓5ᵗʰ **654.7 Congenital or acquired abnormality of vagina**   M ♀
[0-4]   Previous surgery to vagina
     Septate vagina
     Stenosis of vagina (acquired) (congenital)
     Stricture of vagina
     Tumor of vagina

§ ✓5ᵗʰ **654.8 Congenital or acquired abnormality of vulva**   M ♀
[0-4]   Anal sphincter tear (healed) (old) complicating delivery
     Fibrosis of perineum
     Persistent hymen
     Previous surgery to perineum or vulva
     Rigid perineum
     Tumor of vulva
     EXCLUDES *anal sphincter tear (healed) (old) not associated with delivery (569.43)*
     varicose veins of vulva (671.1)
     AHA: 1Q, '03, 14

§ ✓5ᵗʰ **654.9 Other and unspecified**   M ♀
[0-4]   Uterine scar NEC

✓4ᵗʰ 655   Known or suspected fetal abnormality affecting management of mother
> **INCLUDES** the listed conditions in the fetus as a reason for observation or obstetrical care of the mother, or for termination of pregnancy
> **AHA:** 3Q, '90, 4
> **TIP:** Only assign when the fetal condition affects the management of the mother. Assign on mother's chart when in utero procedures are performed on the fetus.

§ ✓5ᵗʰ **655.0 Central nervous system malformation in fetus**   M ♀
[0,1,3]   Fetal or suspected fetal:
     anencephaly
     hydrocephalus
     spina bifida (with myelomeningocele)

§ ✓5ᵗʰ **655.1 Chromosomal abnormality in fetus**   M ♀
[0,1,3]

§ ✓5ᵗʰ **655.2 Hereditary disease in family possibly**   M ♀
[0,1,3] **affecting fetus**

§ ✓5ᵗʰ **655.3 Suspected damage to fetus from viral disease**   M ♀
[0,1,3] **in the mother**
     Suspected damage to fetus from maternal rubella

§ ✓5ᵗʰ **655.4 Suspected damage to fetus from other disease in**   M ♀
[0,1,3] **the mother**
     Suspected damage to fetus from maternal:
     alcohol addiction
     listeriosis
     toxoplasmosis

§ ✓5ᵗʰ **655.5 Suspected damage to fetus from drugs**   M ♀
[0,1,3]

§ ✓5ᵗʰ **655.6 Suspected damage to fetus from radiation**   M ♀
[0,1,3]

§ ✓5ᵗʰ **655.7 Decreased fetal movements**   M ♀
[0,1,3]   **AHA:** 4Q, '97, 41

§ ✓5ᵗʰ **655.8 Other known or suspected fetal abnormality, not**   M ♀
[0,1,3] **elsewhere classified**
     Suspected damage to fetus from:
     environmental toxins
     intrauterine contraceptive device
     AHA: 3Q, '06, 16, 18

§ ✓5ᵗʰ **655.9 Unspecified**   M ♀
[0,1,3]   **AHA:** For code 655.93: 2Q, '10, 6-7

✓4ᵗʰ 656   Other known or suspected fetal and placental problems affecting management of mother
> **EXCLUDES** *fetal hematologic conditions (678.0)*
> *suspected placental problems not found (V89.02)*

§ ✓5ᵗʰ **656.0 Fetal-maternal hemorrhage**   M ♀
[0,1,3]   Leakage (microscopic) of fetal blood into maternal circulation

§ ✓5ᵗʰ **656.1 Rhesus isoimmunization**   M ♀
[0,1,3]   Anti-D [Rh] antibodies
     Rh incompatibility
     DEF: Antibodies developing against Rh factor; mother with Rh negative develops antibodies against Rh positive fetus.
     036.0190 Mtrn care anti-D Rh antibods uns tri not applic   I-10

§ ✓5ᵗʰ **656.2 Isoimmunization from other and unspecified**   M ♀
[0,1,3] **blood-group incompatibility**
     ABO isoimmunization
     AHA: 4Q, '06, 135

§ ✓5ᵗʰ **656.3 Fetal distress**   M ♀
[0,1,3]   Fetal metabolic acidemia
     EXCLUDES *abnormal fetal acid-base balance (656.8)*
     abnormality in fetal heart rate or rhythm (659.7)
     fetal bradycardia (659.7)
     fetal tachycardia (659.7)
     meconium in liquor (656.8)
     DEF: Life-threatening disorder; fetal anoxia, hemolytic disease and other miscellaneous diseases cause fetal distress.
     AHA: N-D, '86, 4

§ ✓5ᵗʰ **656.4 Intrauterine death**   M ♀
[0,1,3]   Fetal death:
     NOS
     after completion of 22 weeks' gestation
     late
     Missed delivery
     EXCLUDES *missed abortion (632)*

§ ✓5ᵗʰ **656.5 Poor fetal growth**   M ♀
[0,1,3]   "Light-for-dates"
     "Placental insufficiency"
     "Small-for-dates"
     036.5190 Mtrn care known/spct placental insuff uns tri   I-10

---

§   Requires fifth digit. Valid digits are in [brackets] under each code. See beginning of section 640-649 for codes and definitions.

N Newborn Age: 0   P Pediatric Age: 0-17   M Maternity Age: 12-55   A Adult Age: 15-124

§ ✓5ᵗʰ **656.6 Excessive fetal growth**   Ⓜ♀
    [0,1,3]
        "Large-for-dates"
        036.60x0 Mtrn care excess fetl grwth uns tri not applic   I-10

§ ✓5ᵗʰ **656.7 Other placental conditions**   Ⓜ♀
    [0,1,3]
        Abnormal placenta
        Placental infarct
        EXCLUDES *placental polyp (674.4)*
                    placentitis (658.4)

§ ✓5ᵗʰ **656.8 Other specified fetal and placental problems**   Ⓜ♀
    [0,1,3]
        Abnormal acid-base balance
        Intrauterine acidosis
        Lithopedian
        Meconium in liquor
        Subchorionic hematoma
        DEF: Lithopedion: Calcified fetus; not expelled by mother.
        036.20x0 Mtrn care hydrops fetalis uns tri not applic/uns   I-10

§ ✓5ᵗʰ **656.9 Unspecified fetal and placental problem**   Ⓜ♀
    [0,1,3]

✓4ᵗʰ **657 Polyhydramnios**   Ⓜ♀
    [0,1,3]

§ ✓5ᵗʰ   Use 0 as fourth-digit for this category
        Hydramnios
        EXCLUDES *suspected polyhydramnios not found (V89.01)*
        DEF: Excess amniotic fluid.
        AHA: 3Q, '06, 16; 4Q, '91, 26
        040.9xx0 Polyhydraminos uns trimester not applicable/uns   I-10

✓4ᵗʰ **658 Other problems associated with amniotic cavity and membranes**
        EXCLUDES *amniotic fluid embolism (673.1)*
                    suspected problems with amniotic cavity and membranes
                          not found (V89.01)

§ ✓5ᵗʰ **658.0 Oligohydramnios**   Ⓜ♀
    [0,1,3]
        Oligohydramnios without mention of rupture of membranes
        DEF: Deficient amount of amniotic fluid.
        AHA: 3Q, '06, 16
        041.00x0 Oligohydraminos uns trimester not applicable/uns   I-10

§ ✓5ᵗʰ **658.1 Premature rupture of membranes**   Ⓜ♀
    [0,1,3]
        Rupture of amniotic sac less than 24 hours prior
            to the onset of labor
        AHA: For code 658.13: 1Q, '01, 5; 4Q, '98, 77
        042.00 Prmat rom ool w/in 24 hrs of rup uns wks gestatn   I-10

§ ✓5ᵗʰ **658.2 Delayed delivery after spontaneous or unspecified rupture of membranes**   Ⓜ♀
    [0,1,3]
        Prolonged rupture of membranes NOS
        Rupture of amniotic sac 24 hours or more prior to the
            onset of labor

§ ✓5ᵗʰ **658.3 Delayed delivery after artificial rupture of membranes**   Ⓜ♀
    [0,1,3]

§ ✓5ᵗʰ **658.4 Infection of amniotic cavity**   Ⓜ♀
    [0,1,3]
        Amnionitis
        Chorioamnionitis
        Membranitis
        Placentitis
        041.1090 Inf amniotic sac & memb uns, uns tri not applic/uns   I-10

§ ✓5ᵗʰ **658.8 Other**   Ⓜ♀
    [0,1,3]
        Amnion nodosum
        Amniotic cyst

§ ✓5ᵗʰ **658.9 Unspecified**   Ⓜ♀
    [0,1,3]

✓4ᵗʰ **659 Other indications for care or intervention related to labor and delivery, not elsewhere classified**

§ ✓5ᵗʰ **659.0 Failed mechanical induction**   Ⓜ♀
    [0,1,3]
        Failure of induction of labor by surgical or other
            instrumental methods

§ ✓5ᵗʰ **659.1 Failed medical or unspecified induction**   Ⓜ♀
    [0,1,3]
        Failed induction NOS
        Failure of induction of labor by medical methods,
            such as oxytocic drugs
        061.9 Failed induction of labor unspecified   I-10

§ ✓5ᵗʰ **659.2 Maternal pyrexia during labor, unspecified**   Ⓜ♀
    [0,1,3]   **DEF:** Fever during labor.
        075.2 Pyrexia during labor not elsewhere classified   I-10

§ ✓5ᵗʰ **659.3 Generalized infection during labor**   Ⓜ♀
    [0,1,3]
        Septicemia during labor

§ ✓5ᵗʰ **659.4 Grand multiparity**   Ⓜ♀
    [0,1,3]   **EXCLUDES** *supervision only, in pregnancy (V23.3)*
                    without current pregnancy (V61.5)
        DEF: Having borne six or more children previously.

§ ✓5ᵗʰ **659.5 Elderly primigravida**   Ⓜ♀
    [0,1,3]
        First pregnancy in a woman who will be 35 years of age or
            older at expected date of delivery
        EXCLUDES *supervision only, in pregnancy (V23.81)*
        AHA: 3Q, '01, 12
        009.519 Supervisn of elderly primigravida uns trimester   I-10

§ ✓5ᵗʰ **659.6 Elderly multigravida**   Ⓜ♀
    [0,1,3]
        Second or more pregnancy in a woman who will be 35 years
            of age or older at expected date of delivery
        EXCLUDES *elderly primigravida 659.5*
                    supervision only, in pregnancy (V23.82)
        AHA: 3Q, '01, 12
        009.529 Supervisn of elderly multigravida uns trimester   I-10

§ ✓5ᵗʰ **659.7 Abnormality in fetal heart rate or rhythm**   Ⓜ♀
    [0,1,3]
        Depressed fetal heart tones
        Fetal:
            bradycardia
            tachycardia
        Fetal heart rate decelerations
        Non-reassuring fetal heart rate or rhythm
        AHA: 4Q, '98, 48
        076 Abn in fetal heart rate & rhythm comp L&D   I-10

§ ✓5ᵗʰ **659.8 Other specified indications for care or intervention related to labor and delivery**   Ⓜ♀
    [0,1,3]
        Pregnancy in a female less than 16 years
            old at expected date of delivery
        Very young maternal age
        AHA: 3Q, '01, 12

§ ✓5ᵗʰ **659.9 Unspecified indication for care or intervention related to labor and delivery**   Ⓜ♀
    [0,1,3]

Complications Occurring Mainly in the Course of Labor and Delivery (660-669)

The following fifth-digit subclassification is for use with categories 660-669 to denote the current episode of care. Valid fifth-digits are in [brackets] under each code.
    0   unspecified as to episode of care or not applicable
    1   delivered, with or without mention of antepartum condition
    2   delivered, with mention of postpartum complication
    3   antepartum condition or complication
    4   postpartum condition or complication

✓4ᵗʰ **660 Obstructed labor**
    AHA: 3Q, '95, 10

§ ✓5ᵗʰ **660.0 Obstruction caused by malposition of fetus at onset of labor**   Ⓜ♀
    [0,1,3]
        Any condition classifiable to 652, causing obstruction during
            labor
        Use additional code from 652.0-652.9 to identify condition

§ ✓5ᵗʰ **660.1 Obstruction by bony pelvis**   Ⓜ♀
    [0,1,3]
        Any condition classifiable to 653, causing obstruction during
            labor
        Use additional code from 653.0-653.9 to identify condition

§ ✓5ᵗʰ **660.2 Obstruction by abnormal pelvic soft tissues**   Ⓜ♀
    [0,1,3]
        Prolapse of anterior lip of cervix
        Any condition classifiable to 654, causing obstruction during
            labor
        Use additional code from 654.0-654.9 to identify condition

§ ✓5ᵗʰ **660.3 Deep transverse arrest and persistent occipitoposterior position**   Ⓜ♀
    [0,1,3]
        064.0xx0 Obst labor incpl rotat of fetal head not applic   I-10

---

§   Requires fifth digit. Valid digits are in [brackets] under each code. See beginning of section 640-649 for codes and definitions.

✓4ᵗʰ/✓5ᵗʰ Additional Digit Required   Unspecified Code   Other Specified Code   Manifestation Code   ▶◀ Revised Text   ● New Code   ▲ Revised Code Title

§ ✓5ᵗʰ **660.4 Shoulder (girdle) dystocia**   Ⓜ♀
[0,1,3]   Impacted shoulders
DEF: Obstructed labor due to impacted fetal shoulders.
O66.0 Obstructed labor due to shoulder dystocia   I-10

§ ✓5ᵗʰ **660.5 Locked twins**   Ⓜ♀
[0,1,3]

§ ✓5ᵗʰ **660.6 Failed trial of labor, unspecified**   Ⓜ♀
[0,1,3]   Failed trial of labor, without mention of condition or suspected condition

§ ✓5ᵗʰ **660.7 Failed forceps or vacuum extractor,**   Ⓜ♀
[0,1,3] **unspecified**
   Application of ventouse or forceps, without mention of condition

§ ✓5ᵗʰ **660.8 Other causes of obstructed labor**   Ⓜ♀
[0,1,3]   Use additional code to identify condition
AHA: 4Q, '04, 88

§ ✓5ᵗʰ **660.9 Unspecified obstructed labor**   Ⓜ♀
[0,1,3]   Dystocia:
    NOS
    fetal NOS
    maternal NOS

✓4ᵗʰ **661 Abnormality of forces of labor**

§ ✓5ᵗʰ **661.0 Primary uterine inertia**   Ⓜ♀
[0,1,3]   Failure of cervical dilation
   Hypotonic uterine dysfunction, primary
   Prolonged latent phase of labor
DEF: Lack of efficient contractions during labor causing prolonged labor.
O62.0 Primary inadequate contractions   I-10

§ ✓5ᵗʰ **661.1 Secondary uterine inertia**   Ⓜ♀
[0,1,3]   Arrested active phase of labor
   Hypotonic uterine dysfunction, secondary
O62.1 Secondary uterine inertia   I-10

§ ✓5ᵗʰ **661.2 Other and unspecified uterine inertia**   Ⓜ♀
[0,1,3]   Atony of uterus without hemorrhage
   Desultory labor
   Irregular labor
   Poor contractions
   Slow slope active phase of labor
EXCLUDES *atony of uterus with hemorrhage (666.1)*
postpartum atony of uterus without hemorrhage (669.8)

§ ✓5ᵗʰ **661.3 Precipitate labor**   Ⓜ♀
[0,1,3]   **DEF:** Rapid labor and delivery.

§ ✓5ᵗʰ **661.4 Hypertonic, incoordinate, or prolonged**   Ⓜ♀
[0,1,3] **uterine contractions**
   Cervical spasm
   Contraction ring (dystocia)
   Dyscoordinate labor
   Hourglass contraction of uterus
   Hypertonic uterine dysfunction
   Incoordinate uterine action
   Retraction ring (Bandl's) (pathological)
   Tetanic contractions
   Uterine dystocia NOS
   Uterine spasm

§ ✓5ᵗʰ **661.9 Unspecified abnormality of labor**   Ⓜ♀
[0,1,3]

✓4ᵗʰ **662 Long labor**

§ ✓5ᵗʰ **662.0 Prolonged first stage**   Ⓜ♀
[0,1,3]

§ ✓5ᵗʰ **662.1 Prolonged labor, unspecified**   Ⓜ♀
[0,1,3]

§ ✓5ᵗʰ **662.2 Prolonged second stage**   Ⓜ♀
[0,1,3]

§ ✓5ᵗʰ **662.3 Delayed delivery of second twin, triplet, etc.**   Ⓜ♀
[0,1,3]

✓4ᵗʰ **663 Umbilical cord complications**

§ ✓5ᵗʰ **663.0 Prolapse of cord**   Ⓜ♀
[0,1,3]   Presentation of cord
DEF: Abnormal presentation of fetus; marked by protruding umbilical cord during labor; can cause fetal death.

§ ✓5ᵗʰ **663.1 Cord around neck, with compression**   Ⓜ♀
[0,1,3]   Cord tightly around neck
O69.1xx0 L&D comp by cord arnd neck with comprs not applic/uns   I-10

§ ✓5ᵗʰ **663.2 Other and unspecified cord entanglement,**   Ⓜ♀
[0,1,3] **with compression**
   Entanglement of cords of twins in mono-amniotic sac
   Knot in cord (with compression)

§ ✓5ᵗʰ **663.3 Other and unspecified cord entanglement,**   Ⓜ♀
[0,1,3] **without mention of compression**
AHA: For code 663.31: 2Q, '03, 9
O69.82x0 L&D comp by oth cord entanglement w/o comprs unsp. fetus   I-10

§ ✓5ᵗʰ **663.4 Short cord**   Ⓜ♀
[0,1,3]

§ ✓5ᵗʰ **663.5 Vasa previa**   Ⓜ♀
[0,1,3]   **DEF:** Abnormal presentation of fetus marked by blood vessels of umbilical cord in front of fetal head.

§ ✓5ᵗʰ **663.6 Vascular lesions of cord**   Ⓜ♀
[0,1,3]   Bruising of cord
   Hematoma of cord
   Thrombosis of vessels of cord

§ ✓5ᵗʰ **663.8 Other umbilical cord complications**   Ⓜ♀
[0,1,3]   Velamentous insertion of umbilical cord

§ ✓5ᵗʰ **663.9 Unspecified umbilical cord complication**   Ⓜ♀
[0,1,3]

✓4ᵗʰ **664 Trauma to perineum and vulva during delivery**
INCLUDES damage from instruments
that from extension of episiotomy
AHA: 1Q, '92, 11; N-D, '84, 10

§ ✓5ᵗʰ **664.0 First-degree perineal laceration**   Ⓜ♀
[0,1,4]   Perineal laceration, rupture, or tear involving:
    fourchette
    hymen
    labia
    skin
    vagina
    vulva
O70.0 First degree perineal laceration during delivery   I-10

§ ✓5ᵗʰ **664.1 Second-degree perineal laceration**   Ⓜ♀
[0,1,4]   Perineal laceration, rupture, or tear (following episiotomy) involving:
    pelvic floor
    perineal muscles
    vaginal muscles
EXCLUDES *that involving anal sphincter (664.2)*
AHA: For code 664.11: 4Q, '08, 192
O70.1 Second degree perineal laceration dur delivery   I-10

§ ✓5ᵗʰ **664.2 Third-degree perineal laceration**   Ⓜ♀
[0,1,4]   Perineal laceration, rupture, or tear (following episiotomy) involving:
    anal sphincter
    rectovaginal septum
    sphincter NOS
EXCLUDES *anal sphincter tear during delivery not associated with third-degree perineal laceration (664.6)*
that with anal or rectal mucosal laceration (664.3)
O70.2 Third degree perineal laceration during delivery   I-10

§ ✓5ᵗʰ **664.3 Fourth-degree perineal laceration**   Ⓜ♀
[0,1,4]   Perineal laceration, rupture, or tear as classifiable to 664.2 and involving also:
    anal mucosa
    rectal mucosa

§ ✓5ᵗʰ **664.4 Unspecified perineal laceration**   Ⓜ♀
[0,1,4]   Central laceration
AHA: 1Q, '92, 8

Ⓝ Newborn Age: 0   Ⓟ Pediatric Age: 0-17   Ⓜ Maternity Age: 12-55   Ⓐ Adult Age: 15-124

Perineal Lacerations

First degree
Second degree
Anus
Third degree
Fourth degree

§ ✓5ᵗʰ **664.5 Vulval and perineal hematoma** Ⓜ♀
[0,1,4] AHA: N-D, '84, 10

§ ✓5ᵗʰ **664.6 Anal sphincter tear complicating delivery,** Ⓜ♀
[0,1,4] **not associated with third-degree perineal laceration**
EXCLUDES third-degree perineal laceration (664.2)
AHA: For code 664.61: 4Q, '07, 88, 90

§ ✓5ᵗʰ **664.8 Other specified trauma to perineum and vulva** Ⓜ♀
[0,1,4] Periurethral trauma
AHA: For code 664.81: 4Q, '07, 125
TIP: Assign when documentation indicates periurethral laceration only.

§ ✓5ᵗʰ **664.9 Unspecified trauma to perineum and vulva** Ⓜ♀
[0,1,4]

✓4ᵗʰ **665 Other obstetrical trauma**
INCLUDES damage from instruments

§ ✓5ᵗʰ **665.0 Rupture of uterus before onset of labor** Ⓜ♀
[0,1,3]

§ ✓5ᵗʰ **665.1 Rupture of uterus during labor** Ⓜ♀
[0,1] Rupture of uterus NOS

§ ✓5ᵗʰ **665.2 Inversion of uterus** Ⓜ♀
[0,2,4]

§ ✓5ᵗʰ **665.3 Laceration of cervix** Ⓜ♀
[0,1,4]

§ ✓5ᵗʰ **665.4 High vaginal laceration** Ⓜ♀
[0,1,4] Laceration of vaginal wall or sulcus without mention of perineal laceration
071.4 Obstetric high vaginal laceration alone I-10

§ ✓5ᵗʰ **665.5 Other injury to pelvic organs** Ⓜ♀
[0,1,4] **EXCLUDES** periurethral trauma (664.8)
Injury to:
bladder
urethra
AHA: M-A, '87, 10
071.5 Other obstetric injury to pelvic organs I-10

§ ✓5ᵗʰ **665.6 Damage to pelvic joints and ligaments** Ⓜ♀
[0,1,4] Avulsion of inner symphyseal cartilage
Damage to coccyx
Separation of symphysis (pubis)
AHA: N-D, '84, 12

§ ✓5ᵗʰ **665.7 Pelvic hematoma** Ⓜ♀
[0,1,2,4] Hematoma of vagina

§ ✓5ᵗʰ **665.8 Other specified obstetrical trauma** Ⓜ♀
[0-4]

§ ✓5ᵗʰ **665.9 Unspecified obstetrical trauma** Ⓜ♀
[0-4]

✓4ᵗʰ **666 Postpartum hemorrhage**
AHA: 1Q, '88, 14

§ ✓5ᵗʰ **666.0 Third-stage hemorrhage** Ⓜ♀
[0,2,4] Hemorrhage associated with retained, trapped, or adherent placenta
Retained placenta NOS

§ ✓5ᵗʰ **666.1 Other immediate postpartum hemorrhage** Ⓜ♀
[0,2,4] Atony of uterus with hemorrhage
Hemorrhage within the first 24 hours following delivery of placenta
Postpartum atony of uterus with hemorrhage
Postpartum hemorrhage (atonic) NOS
EXCLUDES atony of uterus without hemorrhage (661.2)
postpartum atony of uterus without hemorrhage (669.8)
072.1 Other immediate postpartum hemorrhage I-10

§ ✓5ᵗʰ **666.2 Delayed and secondary postpartum hemorrhage** Ⓜ♀
[0,2,4] Hemorrhage:
after the first 24 hours following delivery
associated with retained portions of placenta or membranes
Postpartum hemorrhage specified as delayed or secondary
Retained products of conception NOS, following delivery

§ ✓5ᵗʰ **666.3 Postpartum coagulation defects** Ⓜ♀
[0,2,4] Postpartum:
afibrinogenemia
fibrinolysis

✓4ᵗʰ **667 Retained placenta or membranes, without hemorrhage**
NOTE Requires fith digit; valid digits are in [brackets] under each code. See beginning of section 660-669 for definitions.
DEF: Postpartum condition resulting from failure to expel placental membrane tissues due to failed contractions of uterine wall.
AHA: 1Q, '88, 14
TIP: A retained placenta is one that has not separated or been expelled within one hour after completion of the second stage of labor (birth of the fetus).

§ ✓5ᵗʰ **667.0 Retained placenta without hemorrhage** Ⓜ♀
[0,2,4] Placenta accreta
Retained placenta: } without hemorrhage
NOS
total
073.0 Retained placenta without hemorrhage I-10

§ ✓5ᵗʰ **667.1 Retained portions of placenta or** Ⓜ♀
[0,2,4] **membranes, without hemorrhage**
Retained products of conception following delivery, without hemorrhage

✓4ᵗʰ **668 Complications of the administration of anesthetic or other sedation in labor and delivery**
INCLUDES complications arising from the administration of a general or local anesthetic, analgesic, or other sedation in labor and delivery
EXCLUDES reaction to spinal or lumbar puncture (349.0)
spinal headache (349.0)
Use additional code(s) to further specify complication

§ ✓5ᵗʰ **668.0 Pulmonary complications** Ⓜ♀
[0-4] Inhalation (aspiration) of stomach contents or secretions } following anesthesia or other sedation in
Mendelson's syndrome labor or delivery
Pressure collapse of lung

§ ✓5ᵗʰ **668.1 Cardiac complications** Ⓜ♀
[0-4] Cardiac arrest or failure following anesthesia or other sedation in labor and delivery

§ ✓5ᵗʰ **668.2 Central nervous system complications** Ⓜ♀
[0-4] Cerebral anoxia following anesthesia or other sedation in labor and delivery

§ ✓5ᵗʰ **668.8 Other complications of anesthesia or** Ⓜ♀
[0-4] **other sedation in labor and delivery**
AHA: 2Q, '99, 9

§ ✓5ᵗʰ **668.9 Unspecified complication of anesthesia** Ⓜ♀
[0-4] **and other sedation**

✓4ᵗʰ **669 Other complications of labor and delivery, not elsewhere classified**

§ ✓5ᵗʰ **669.0 Maternal distress** Ⓜ♀
[0-4] Metabolic disturbance in labor and delivery

§ Requires fifth digit. Valid digits are in [brackets] under each code. See beginning of section 640-649 for codes and definitions.

✓4ᵗʰ/✓5ᵗʰ Additional Digit Required | Unspecified Code | Other Specified Code | Manifestation Code | ▶◀ Revised Text | ● New Code | ▲ Revised Code Title
2013 ICD-9-CM | **Volume 1 – 207**

Complications of Pregnancy, Childbirth, and the Puerperium

669.1–673.2

§ ✓5ᵗʰ **669.1 Shock during or following labor and delivery** Ⓜ♀
[0-4]   Obstetric shock

§ ✓5ᵗʰ **669.2 Maternal hypotension syndrome** Ⓜ♀
[0-4]   **DEF:** Low arterial blood pressure in mother during labor and delivery.

§ ✓5ᵗʰ **669.3 Acute kidney failure following labor and delivery** Ⓜ♀
[0,2,4]

§ ✓5ᵗʰ **669.4 Other complications of obstetrical surgery** Ⓜ♀
[0-4] **and procedures**
   Cardiac:
     arrest   } following cesarean or other obstetrical
     failure   surgery or procedure, including
     Cerebral anoxia   delivery NOS
   EXCLUDES complications of obstetrical surgical wounds (674.1-674.3)

§ ✓5ᵗʰ **669.5 Forceps or vacuum extractor delivery** Ⓜ♀
[0,1] **without mention of indication**
   Delivery by ventouse, without mention of indication

§ ✓5ᵗʰ **669.6 Breech extraction, without mention of** Ⓜ♀
[0,1] **indication**
   EXCLUDES breech delivery NOS (652.2)

§ ✓5ᵗʰ **669.7 Cesarean delivery, without mention of indication** Ⓜ♀
[0,1]   **AHA: For code 669.71:** 1Q, '01, 11
   O82 Encounter for cesarean delivery w/o indication   I-10

§ ✓5ᵗʰ **669.8 Other complications of labor and delivery** Ⓜ♀
[0-4]   **AHA:** 4Q, '06, 135

§ ✓5ᵗʰ **669.9 Unspecified complication of labor and delivery** Ⓜ♀
[0-4]

Complications of the Puerperium (670-677)

NOTE Categories 671 and 673-676 include the listed conditions even if they occur during pregnancy or childbirth.

The following fifth-digit subclassification is for use with categories 670-676 to denote the current episode of care. Valid fifth-digits are in [brackets] under each code.
0   unspecified as to episode of care or not applicable
1   delivered, with or without mention of antepartum condition
2   delivered, with mention of postpartum complication
3   antepartum condition or complication
4   postpartum condition or complication

✓4ᵗʰ **670 Major puerperal infection**
   EXCLUDES infection following abortion (639.0)
     minor genital tract infection following delivery (646.6)
     puerperal pyrexia NOS (672)
     puerperal fever NOS (672)
     puerperal pyrexia of unknown origin (672)
     urinary tract infection following delivery (646.6)
   DEF: Infection and inflammation following childbirth.
   AHA: 4Q, '91, 26; 2Q, '91, 7

§ ✓5ᵗʰ **670.0 Major puerperal infection, unspecified** Ⓜ♀
[0,2,4]   **AHA: For code 670.02:** 3Q, '07, 8

§ ✓5ᵗʰ **670.1 Puerperal endometritis** Ⓜ♀
[0,2,4]

§ ✓5ᵗʰ **670.2 Puerperal sepsis** Ⓜ♀
[0,2,4]   Puerperal pyemia
   Use additional code to identify severe sepsis (995.92) and any associated acute organ dysfunction, if applicable
   AHA: For code 670.24: 4Q, '09, 98
   TIP: Do not assign a code from category 038 or 995.91 Sepsis, along with a code from this subcategory. If applicable, assign additional codes to indicate severe sepsis (995.92), and any associated acute organ dysfunction.

§ ✓5ᵗʰ **670.3 Puerperal septic thrombophlebitis** Ⓜ♀
[0,2,4]

§ ✓5ᵗʰ **670.8 Other major puerperal infection** Ⓜ♀
[0,2,4]   Puerperal: Puerperal:
     pelvic cellulitis   salpingitis
     peritonitis

✓4ᵗʰ **671 Venous complications in pregnancy and the puerperium**
   EXCLUDES personal history of venous complications prior to pregnancy, such as:
     thrombophlebitis (V12.52)
     thrombosis and embolism (V12.51)

§ ✓5ᵗʰ **671.0 Varicose veins of legs** Ⓜ♀
[0-4]   Varicose veins NOS
   DEF: Distended, tortuous veins on legs associated with pregnancy.

§ ✓5ᵗʰ **671.1 Varicose veins of vulva and perineum** Ⓜ♀
[0-4]   **DEF:** Distended, tortuous veins on external female genitalia associated with pregnancy.

§ ✓5ᵗʰ **671.2 Superficial thrombophlebitis** Ⓜ♀
[0-4]   Phlebitis NOS
   Thrombophlebitis (superficial)
   Thrombosis NOS
   Use additional code to identify the superficial thrombophlebitis (453.6, 453.71, 453.81)

§ ✓5ᵗʰ **671.3 Deep phlebothrombosis, antepartum** Ⓜ♀
[0,1,3]   Deep vein thrombosis antepartum
   Use additional code to identify the deep vein thrombosis (453.40-453.42, 453.50-453.52, 453.72-453.79, 453.82-453.89)
   Use additional code for long term (current) use of anticoagulants, if applicable (V58.61)

§ ✓5ᵗʰ **671.4 Deep phlebothrombosis, postpartum** Ⓜ♀
[0,2,4]   Deep-vein thrombosis, postpartum
   Pelvic thrombophlebitis, postpartum
   Phlegmasia alba dolens (puerperal)
   Use additional code to identify the deep vein thrombosis (453.40-453.42, 453.50-453.52, 453.72-453.79, 453.82-453.89)
   Use additional code for long term (current) use of anticoagulants, if applicable (V58.61)

§ ✓5ᵗʰ **671.5 Other phlebitis and thrombosis** Ⓜ♀
[0-4]   Cerebral venous thrombosis
   Thrombosis of intracranial venous sinus

§ ✓5ᵗʰ **671.8 Other venous complications** Ⓜ♀
[0-4]   Hemorrhoids

§ ✓5ᵗʰ **671.9 Unspecified venous complication** Ⓜ♀
[0-4]

✓4ᵗʰ **672 Pyrexia of unknown origin during the puerperium** Ⓜ♀
[0,2,4]
§ ✓5ᵗʰ Use 0 as fourth-digit for this category
   Postpartum fever NOS
   Puerperal fever NOS
   Puerperal pyrexia NOS
   DEF: Fever of unknown origin experienced by the mother after childbirth.
   AHA: 4Q, '91, 26
   O86.4 Pyrexia of unknown origin following delivery   I-10

✓4ᵗʰ **673 Obstetrical pulmonary embolism**
   INCLUDES pulmonary emboli in pregnancy, childbirth, or the puerperium, or specified as puerperal
   EXCLUDES embolism following abortion (639.6)

§ ✓5ᵗʰ **673.0 Obstetrical air embolism** Ⓜ♀
[0-4]   **DEF:** Sudden blocking of pulmonary artery with air or nitrogen bubbles during puerperium.

§ ✓5ᵗʰ **673.1 Amniotic fluid embolism** Ⓜ♀
[0-4]   **DEF:** Sudden onset of pulmonary artery blockage from amniotic fluid entering the mother's circulation near the end of pregnancy due to strong uterine contractions.

§ ✓5ᵗʰ **673.2 Obstetrical blood-clot embolism** Ⓜ♀
[0-4]   Puerperal pulmonary embolism NOS
   AHA: For code 673.24: 1Q, '05, 6
   DEF: Blood clot blocking artery in the lung; associated with pregnancy.
   TIP: If a pregnant or postpartum patient develops a pulmonary embolism that progresses to acute respiratory failure, the code for the pregnancy/delivery complication (673.2X) should be sequenced first.

§ Requires fifth digit. Valid digits are in [brackets] under each code. See beginning of section 640-649 for codes and definitions.

Ⓝ Newborn Age: 0   Ⓟ Pediatric Age: 0-17   Ⓜ Maternity Age: 12-55   Ⓐ Adult Age: 15-124

§ ✓5ᵗʰ **673.3 Obstetrical pyemic and septic embolism**   Ⓜ♀
[0-4]

§ ✓5ᵗʰ **673.8 Other pulmonary embolism**   Ⓜ♀
[0-4]   Fat embolism

✓4ᵗʰ **674 Other and unspecified complications of the puerperium, not elsewhere classified**

§ ✓5ᵗʰ **674.0 Cerebrovascular disorders in the puerperium**   Ⓜ♀
[0-4]   Any condition classifiable to 430-434, 436-437 occurring during pregnancy, childbirth, or the puerperium, or specified as puerperal
     EXCLUDES *intracranial venous sinus thrombosis (671.5)*

§ ✓5ᵗʰ **674.1 Disruption of cesarean wound**   Ⓜ♀
[0,2,4]   Dehiscence or disruption of uterine wound
     EXCLUDES *uterine rupture before onset of labor (665.0)*
                 uterine rupture during labor (665.1)

§ ✓5ᵗʰ **674.2 Disruption of perineal wound**   Ⓜ♀
[0,2,4]   Breakdown of perineum
     Disruption of wound of:
       episiotomy
       perineal laceration
     Secondary perineal tear
     AHA: For code 674.24: 1Q, '97, 9

§ ✓5ᵗʰ **674.3 Other complications of obstetrical surgical**   Ⓜ♀
[0,2,4] **wounds**
     Hematoma ⎫
     Hemorrhage ⎬ of cesarean section or
     Infection ⎭   perineal wound
     EXCLUDES *damage from instruments in delivery (664.0-665.9)*
     AHA: For code 674.32: 2Q, '91, 7; For code 674.34: 4Q, '09, 98

§ ✓5ᵗʰ **674.4 Placental polyp**   Ⓜ♀
[0,2,4]

§ ✓5ᵗʰ **674.5 Peripartum cardiomyopathy**   Ⓜ♀
[0-4]   Postpartum cardiomyopathy
     DEF: Any structural or functional abnormality of the ventricular myocardium, non-inflammatory disease of obscure or unknown etiology with onset during the postpartum period.
     AHA: 4Q, '03, 65

§ ✓5ᵗʰ **674.8 Other**   Ⓜ♀
[0,2,4]   Hepatorenal syndrome, following delivery
     Postpartum:
       subinvolution of uterus
       uterine hypertrophy
     AHA: 3Q, '98, 16

§ ✓5ᵗʰ **674.9 Unspecified**   Ⓜ♀
[0,2,4]   Sudden death of unknown cause during the puerperium

✓4ᵗʰ **675 Infections of the breast and nipple associated with childbirth**
     INCLUDES the listed conditions during pregnancy, childbirth, or the puerperium

§ ✓5ᵗʰ **675.0 Infections of nipple**   Ⓜ♀
[0-4]   Abscess of nipple

§ ✓5ᵗʰ **675.1 Abscess of breast**   Ⓜ♀
[0-4]   Abscess: Abscess:
       mammary   purulent
       subareolar   retromammary
       submammary   submammary

§ ✓5ᵗʰ **675.2 Nonpurulent mastitis**   Ⓜ♀
[0-4]   Lymphangitis of breast
     Mastitis:
       NOS
       interstitial
       parenchymatous

§ ✓5ᵗʰ **675.8 Other specified infections of the breast and**   Ⓜ♀
[0-4] **nipple**

§ ✓5ᵗʰ **675.9 Unspecified infection of the breast and nipple**   Ⓜ♀
[0-4]

Lactation Process: Ejection Reflex Arc

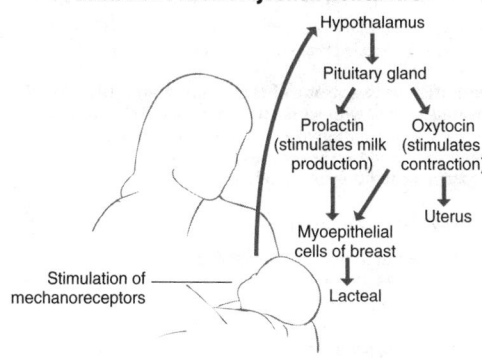

✓4ᵗʰ **676 Other disorders of the breast associated with childbirth and disorders of lactation**
     INCLUDES the listed conditions during pregnancy, the puerperium, or lactation

§ ✓5ᵗʰ **676.0 Retracted nipple**   Ⓜ♀
[0-4]

§ ✓5ᵗʰ **676.1 Cracked nipple**   Ⓜ♀
[0-4]   Fissure of nipple

§ ✓5ᵗʰ **676.2 Engorgement of breasts**   Ⓜ♀
[0-4]   **DEF:** Abnormal accumulation of milk in ducts of breast.

§ ✓5ᵗʰ **676.3 Other and unspecified disorder of breast**   Ⓜ♀
[0-4]

§ ✓5ᵗʰ **676.4 Failure of lactation**   Ⓜ♀
[0-4]   Agalactia
     DEF: Abrupt ceasing of milk secretion by breast.

§ ✓5ᵗʰ **676.5 Suppressed lactation**   Ⓜ♀
[0-4]

§ ✓5ᵗʰ **676.6 Galactorrhea**   Ⓜ♀
[0-4]   **EXCLUDES** *galactorrhea not associated with childbirth (611.6)*
     DEF: Excessive or persistent milk secretion by breast; may be in absence of nursing.

§ ✓5ᵗʰ **676.8 Other disorders of lactation**   Ⓜ♀
[0-4]   Galactocele
     DEF: Galactocele: Obstructed mammary gland, creating retention cyst, results in milk-filled cysts enlarging mammary gland.

§ ✓5ᵗʰ **676.9 Unspecified disorder of lactation**   Ⓜ♀
[0-4]

677 Late effect of complication of pregnancy, childbirth, and the puerperium   ♀
     NOTE This category is to be used to indicate conditions in 632-648.9 and 651-676.9 as the cause of the late effect, themselves classifiable elsewhere. The "late effects" include conditions specified as such, or as sequelae, which may occur at any time after puerperium.
     Code first any sequelae
     AHA: 1Q, '97, 9; 4Q, '94, 42
     TIP: Sequence as a secondary diagnosis, after the code for the late effect complication. May be assigned at any time after the initial postpartum period (six weeks following delivery).

---

§   Requires fifth digit. Valid digits are in [brackets] under each code. See beginning of section 640-649 for codes and definitions.

✓4ᵗʰ
✓5ᵗʰ   Additional Digit Required   Unspecified Code   Other Specified Code   Manifestation Code   ▶◀ Revised Text   ● New Code   ▲ Revised Code Title

Other Maternal and Fetal Complications (678-679)

The following fifth-digit subclassification is for use with categories 678-679 to denote the current episode of care. Valid fifth-digits are in [brackets] under each code.

   0 **unspecified as to episode of care or not applicable**
   1 **delivered, with or without mention of antepartum condition**
   2 **delivered, with mention of postpartum complication**
   3 **antepartum condition or complication**
   4 **postpartum condition or complication**

✓4ᵗʰ **678**   **Other fetal conditions**

§ ✓5ᵗʰ **678.0** **Fetal hematologic conditions**   Ⓜ♀
   [0,1,3]   Fetal anemia
              Fetal thrombocytopenia
              Fetal twin to twin transfusion

          EXCLUDES *fetal and neonatal hemorrhage (772.0-772.9)*
                   fetal hematologic disorders affecting newborn (776.0-776.9)
                   fetal-maternal hemorrhage (656.00-656.03)
                   isoimmunization incompatibility (656.10-656.13, 656.20-656.23)

          AHA: 4Q, '08, 125-127

§ ✓5ᵗʰ **678.1** **Fetal conjoined twins**   Ⓜ♀
   [0,1,3]   **AHA:** 4Q, '08, 125-127

✓4ᵗʰ **679**   **Complications of in utero procedures**
      AHA: 4Q, '08, 127-128, 158

§ ✓5ᵗʰ **679.0** **Maternal complications from in utero procedure**   Ⓜ♀
   [0-4]   **EXCLUDES** *maternal history of in utero procedure during previous pregnancy (V23.86)*

§ ✓5ᵗʰ **679.1** **Fetal complications from in utero procedure**   Ⓜ♀
   [0-4]   Fetal complications from amniocentesis

          EXCLUDES *newborn affected by in utero procedure (760.61-760.64)*

          TIP: Assign only on the mother's record. Although there is a fetal complication, it affects the mother's pregnancy.

---

§   Requires fifth digit. Valid digits are in [brackets] under each code. See beginning of section 640-649 for codes and definitions.

Ⓝ Newborn Age: 0   Ⓟ Pediatric Age: 0-17   Ⓜ Maternity Age: 12-55   Ⓐ Adult Age: 15-124

12. Diseases of the Skin and Subcutaneous Tissue (680-709)

Infections of Skin and Subcutaneous Tissue (680-686)

EXCLUDES *certain infections of skin classified under "Infectious and Parasitic Diseases," such as:*
erysipelas (035)
erysipeloid of Rosenbach (027.1)
herpes:
    simplex (054.0-054.9)
    zoster (053.0-053.9)
molluscum contagiosum (078.0)
viral warts (078.10-078.19)

✓4th 680 Carbuncle and furuncle

INCLUDES boil
furunculosis

DEF: Carbuncle: necrotic boils in skin and subcutaneous tissue of neck or back mainly due to staphylococcal infection.
DEF: Furuncle: circumscribed inflammation of corium and subcutaneous tissue due to staphylococcal infection.

680.0 Face
Ear [any part]
Face [any part, except eye]
Nose (septum)
Temple (region)
EXCLUDES *eyelid (373.13)*
lacrimal apparatus (375.31)
orbit (376.01)

680.1 Neck

680.2 Trunk
Abdominal wall
Back [any part, except buttocks]
Breast
Chest wall
Flank
Groin
Pectoral region
Perineum
Umbilicus
EXCLUDES *buttocks (680.5)*
external genital organs:
female (616.4)
male (607.2, 608.4)

680.3 Upper arm and forearm
Arm [any part, except hand]
Axilla
Shoulder

680.4 Hand
Finger [any]
Thumb
Wrist

680.5 Buttock
Anus
Gluteal region

680.6 Leg, except foot
Ankle
Hip
Knee
Thigh

680.7 Foot
Heel
Toe

680.8 Other specified sites
Head [any part, except face]
Scalp
EXCLUDES *external genital organs:*
female (616.4)
male (607.2, 608.4)

680.9 Unspecified site
Boil NOS
Carbuncle NOS
Furuncle NOS

Skin and Subcutaneous Layer

✓4th 681 Cellulitis and abscess of finger and toe

INCLUDES that with lymphangitis

Use additional code to identify organism, such as Staphylococcus (041.1)

DEF: Acute suppurative inflammation and edema in subcutaneous tissue or muscle of finger or toe.
AHA: 2Q, '91, 5; J-F, '87, 12
TIP: Coding of cellulitis due to superficial injury, burn, or frostbite requires two codes, one for the injury and one for the cellulitis. Sequencing depends on the circumstances of the admission.

✓5th 681.0 Finger

681.00 Cellulitis and abscess, unspecified
L03.019 Cellulitis of unspecified finger I-10

681.01 Felon
Pulp abscess
Whitlow
EXCLUDES *herpetic whitlow (054.6)*
DEF: Painful abscess of fingertips caused by infection in the closed space of terminal phalanx.

681.02 Onychia and paronychia of finger
Panaritium
Perionychia } of finger
DEF: Onychia: inflammation of nail matrix; causes nail loss.
DEF: Paronychia: inflammation of tissue folds around nail.

✓5th 681.1 Toe

681.10 Cellulitis and abscess, unspecified
AHA: 1Q, '05, 14
L03.039 Cellulitis of unspecified toe I-10

681.11 Onychia and paronychia of toe
Panaritium
Perionychia } of toe

681.9 Cellulitis and abscess of unspecified digit
Infection of nail NOS

✓4th 682 Other cellulitis and abscess

INCLUDES abscess (acute)
cellulitis (diffuse) } (with lymphangitis) except
lymphangitis, acute   of finger or toe

Use additional code to identify organism, such as Staphylococcus (041.1)

EXCLUDES *lymphangitis (chronic) (subacute) (457.2)*
DEF: Cellulitis: Acute suppurative inflammation of deep subcutaneous tissue and sometimes muscle due to infection of wound, burn or other lesion.
AHA: 2Q, '91, 5; J-F, '87, 12; S-O, '85, 10
TIP: Coding of cellulitis due to superficial injury, burn, or frostbite requires two codes, one for the injury and one for the cellulitis. Sequencing depends on the circumstances of the admission.

682.0 Face
Cheek, external   Nose, external
Chin   Submandibular
Forehead   Temple (region)
EXCLUDES *ear [any part] (380.10-380.16)*
eyelid (373.13)
lacrimal apparatus (375.31)
lip (528.5)
mouth (528.3)
nose (internal) (478.1)
orbit (376.01)
L03.211 Cellulitis of face I-10

682.1 Neck
L03.221 Cellulitis of neck   `I-10`

682.2 Trunk
Abdominal wall
Back [any part, except buttock]
Chest wall
Flank
Groin
Pectoral region
Perineum
Umbilicus, except newborn

EXCLUDES   anal and rectal regions (566)
       breast:
         NOS (611.0)
         puerperal (675.1)
       external genital organs:
         female (616.3-616.4)
         male (604.0, 607.2, 608.4)
       umbilicus, newborn (771.4)

AHA: 4Q, '98, 42

L03.319 Cellulitis of trunk unspecified   `I-10`

682.3 Upper arm and forearm
Arm [any part, except hand]
Axilla
Shoulder

EXCLUDES   hand (682.4)

AHA: 2Q, '03, 7

L03.113 Cellulitis of right upper limb   `I-10`

682.4 Hand, except fingers and thumb
Wrist

EXCLUDES   finger and thumb (681.00-681.02)

682.5 Buttock
Gluteal region

EXCLUDES   anal and rectal regions (566)

L03.317 Cellulitis of buttock   `I-10`

682.6 Leg, except foot
Ankle
Hip
Knee
Thigh

AHA: 1Q, '09, 10; 3Q, '04, 5; 4Q, '03, 108

L03.115 Cellulitis of right lower limb   `I-10`

682.7 Foot, except toes
Heel

EXCLUDES   toe (681.10-681.11)

682.8 Other specified sites
Head [except face]
Scalp

EXCLUDES   face (682.0)

682.9 Unspecified site
Abscess NOS
Cellulitis NOS
Lymphangitis, acute NOS

EXCLUDES   lymphangitis NOS (457.2)

683 Acute lymphadenitis
Abscess (acute)   } lymph gland or node,
Adenitis, acute   }   except
Lymphadenitis, acute   }   mesenteric

Use additional code to identify organism, such as Staphylococcus (041.1)

EXCLUDES   enlarged glands NOS (785.6)
       lymphadenitis:
         chronic or subacute, except mesenteric (289.1)
         mesenteric (acute) (chronic) (subacute) (289.2)
         unspecified (289.3)

DEF: Acute inflammation of lymph nodes due to primary infection located elsewhere in the body.

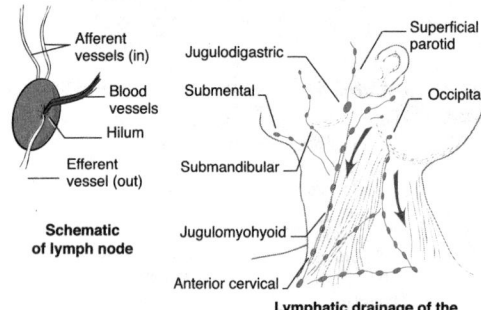

Lymphatic System of Head and Neck

Afferent vessels (in)
Blood vessels
Hilum
Efferent vessel (out)
Jugulodigastric
Submental
Submandibular
Jugulomyohyoid
Anterior cervical
Superficial parotid
Occipital

Schematic of lymph node

Lymphatic drainage of the head, neck, and face

684 Impetigo
Impetiginization of other dermatoses
Impetigo (contagiosa) [any site] [any organism]:
   bullous
   circinate
   neonatorum
   simplex
Pemphigus neonatorum

EXCLUDES   impetigo herpetiformis (694.3)

DEF: Infectious skin disease commonly occurring in children; caused by group A streptococci or *Staphylococcus aureus;* skin lesions usually appear on the face and consist of subcorneal vesicles and bullae that burst and form yellow crusts.

✓4ᵗʰ 685 Pilonidal cyst
INCLUDES   fistula   } coccygeal or pilonidal
            sinus   }

DEF: Hair-containing cyst or sinus in the tissues of the sacrococcygeal area; often drains through opening at the postanal dimple.

685.0 With abscess

685.1 Without mention of abscess
AHA: ▶3Q, '11, 9◀

✓4ᵗʰ 686 Other local infections of skin and subcutaneous tissue
Use additional code to identify any infectious organism (041.0-041.8)

✓5ᵗʰ 686.0 Pyoderma
Dermatitis: Dermatitis:
   purulent   suppurative
   septic

DEF: Nonspecific purulent skin disease related most to furuncles, pustules, or possibly carbuncles.

686.00 Pyoderma, unspecified

686.01 Pyoderma gangrenosum
DEF: Persistent debilitating skin disease characterized by irregular, boggy, blue-red ulcerations, with central healing and undermined edges.

AHA: 4Q, '97, 42

686.09 Other pyoderma

686.1 Pyogenic granuloma
Granuloma: Granuloma:
   septic   telangiectaticum
   suppurative

EXCLUDES   pyogenic granuloma of oral mucosa (528.9)

DEF: Solitary polypoid capillary hemangioma often associated with local irritation, trauma, and superimposed inflammation; located on the skin and gingival or oral mucosa.

Stages of Pilonidal Disease

Normal follicle
Stretched follicle
Infected follicle
Acute abscess
Chronic abscess
Epithelial tube

686.8 Other specified local infections of skin and subcutaneous tissue
Bacterid (pustular)
Dermatitis vegetans
Ecthyma
Perlèche
EXCLUDES *dermatitis infectiosa eczematoides (690.8)*
panniculitis (729.30-729.39)

686.9 Unspecified local infection of skin and subcutaneous tissue
Fistula of skin NOS
Skin infection NOS
EXCLUDES *fistula to skin from internal organs — see Alphabetic Index*

Other Inflammatory Conditions of Skin and Subcutaneous Tissue (690-698)

EXCLUDES *panniculitis (729.30-729.39)*

√4ᵗʰ 690 Erythematosquamous dermatosis
EXCLUDES *eczematous dermatitis of eyelid (373.31)*
parakeratosis variegata (696.2)
psoriasis (696.0-696.1)
seborrheic keratosis (702.11-702.19)

√5ᵗʰ 690.1 Seborrheic dermatitis
AHA: 4Q, '95, 58

690.10 Seborrheic dermatitis, unspecified
Seborrheic dermatitis NOS
L21.9 Seborrheic dermatitis unspecified   I-10

690.11 Seborrhea capitis   P
Cradle cap

690.12 Seborrheic infantile dermatitis   P

690.18 Other seborrheic dermatitis

690.8 Other erythematosquamous dermatosis

√4ᵗʰ 691 Atopic dermatitis and related conditions
DEF: Atopic dermatitis: chronic, pruritic, inflammatory skin disorder found on the face and antecubital and popliteal fossae; often accompanied by allergic rhinitis, hay fever, asthma, and extreme itching; also called allergic dermatitis, or disseminated neurodermatitis.

691.0 Diaper or napkin rash
Ammonia dermatitis
Diaper or napkin:
dermatitis
erythema
rash
Psoriasiform napkin eruption

691.8 Other atopic dermatitis and related conditions
Atopic dermatitis
Besnier's prurigo
Eczema:
atopic
flexural
intrinsic (allergic)
Neurodermatitis:
atopic
diffuse (of Brocq)

√4ᵗʰ 692 Contact dermatitis and other eczema
INCLUDES dermatitis:
NOS
contact
occupational
venenata
eczema (acute) (chronic):
NOS
allergic
erythematous
occupational
EXCLUDES *allergy NOS (995.3)*
contact dermatitis of eyelids (373.32)
dermatitis due to substances taken internally (693.0-693.9)
eczema of external ear (380.22)
perioral dermatitis (695.3)
urticarial reactions (708.0-708.9, 995.1)
DEF: Contact dermatitis: acute or chronic dermatitis caused by initial irritant effect of a substance, or by prior sensitization to a substance coming once again in contact with skin.

692.0 Due to detergents

692.1 Due to oils and greases

692.2 Due to solvents
Dermatitis due to solvents of:
chlorocompound
cyclohexane
ester
glycol } group
hydrocarbon
ketone

692.3 Due to drugs and medicines in contact with skin
Dermatitis (allergic) (contact) due to:
arnica
fungicides
iodine
keratolytics
mercurials
neomycin
pediculocides
phenols
scabicides
any drug applied to skin
Dermatitis medicamentosa due to drug applied to skin
Use additional E code to identify drug
EXCLUDES *allergy NOS due to drugs (995.27)*
dermatitis due to ingested drugs (693.0)
dermatitis medicamentosa NOS (693.0)

692.4 Due to other chemical products
Dermatitis due to:
acids
adhesive plaster
alkalis
caustics
dichromate
insecticide
nylon
plastic
rubber
AHA: 3Q, '08, 6-7; 2Q, '89, 16

692.5 Due to food in contact with skin
Dermatitis, contact, due to:
cereals
fish
flour
fruit
meat
milk
EXCLUDES *dermatitis due to:*
dyes (692.89)
ingested foods (693.1)
preservatives (692.89)

Diseases of the Skin and Subcutaneous Tissue

692.6–693.9

692.6 Due to plants [except food]
Dermatitis due to:
lacquer tree [Rhus verniciflua]
poison:
ivy [Rhus toxicodendron]
oak [Rhus diversiloba]
sumac [Rhus venenata]
vine [Rhus radicans]
primrose [Primula]
ragweed [Senecio jacobae]
other plants in contact with the skin
EXCLUDES *allergy NOS due to pollen (477.0)*
nettle rash (708.8)

✓5ᵗʰ 692.7 Due to solar radiation
EXCLUDES *sunburn due to other ultraviolet radiation exposure (692.82)*

692.70 Unspecified dermatitis due to sun

692.71 Sunburn
First degree sunburn
Sunburn NOS
AHA: 4Q, '01, 47
TIP: Do not assign if sunburn is due to tanning bed use; see instead code 692.82.

692.72 Acute dermatitis due to solar radiation
Acute solar skin damage NOS
Berlogue dermatitis
Photoallergic response
Phototoxic response
Polymorphus light eruption
Use additional E code to identify drug, if drug induced
EXCLUDES *sunburn (692.71, 692.76-692.77)*
DEF: Berloque dermatitis: Phytophotodermatitis due to sun exposure after use of a product containing bergamot oil; causes red patches, that turn brown.
DEF: Photoallergic response: Dermatitis due to hypersensitivity to the sun; causes papulovesicular, eczematous or exudative eruptions.
DEF: Phototoxic response: Chemically induced sensitivity to sun causes burn-like reaction, occasionally vesiculation and subsequent hyperpigmentation.
DEF: Polymorphous light eruption: Inflammatory skin eruptions due to sunlight exposure; eruptions differ in size and shape.
DEF: Acute solar skin damage (NOS): Rapid, unspecified injury to skin from sun.

692.73 Actinic reticuloid and actinic granuloma
DEF: Actinic reticuloid: Dermatosis aggravated by light, causes chronic eczema-like eruption on exposed skin which extends to other unexposed surfaces; occurs in the elderly.
DEF: Actinic granuloma: Inflammatory response of skin to sun causing small nodule of microphages.

692.74 Other chronic dermatitis due to solar radiation
Chronic solar skin damage NOS
Solar elastosis
EXCLUDES *actinic [solar] keratosis (702.0)*
DEF: Solar elastosis: Premature aging of skin of light-skinned people; causes inelasticity, thinning or thickening, wrinkling, dryness, scaling and hyperpigmentation.
DEF: Chronic solar skin damage (NOS): Chronic skin impairment due to exposure to the sun, not otherwise specified.

692.75 Disseminated superficial actinic porokeratosis [DSAP]
DEF: Autosomal dominant skin condition occurring in skin that has been overexposed to the sun; characterized by superficial annular, keratotic, brownish-red spots or thickenings with depressed centers and sharp, ridged borders, may evolve into squamous cell carcinoma.
AHA: 4Q, '00, 43

692.76 Sunburn of second degree
AHA: 4Q, '01, 47
TIP: Do not assign if sunburn is due to tanning bed use; see instead code 692.82.

692.77 Sunburn of third degree
AHA: 4Q, '01, 47
TIP: Do not assign if sunburn is due to tanning bed use; see instead code 692.82.

692.79 Other dermatitis due to solar radiation
Hydroa aestivale
Photodermatitis
Photosensitiveness } (due to sun)
Solar skin damage NOS

✓5ᵗʰ 692.8 Due to other specified agents

692.81 Dermatitis due to cosmetics

692.82 Dermatitis due to other radiation
Infrared rays
Light, except from sun
Radiation NOS
Tanning bed
Ultraviolet rays, except from sun
X-rays
EXCLUDES *solar radiation (692.70-692.79)*
AHA: 4Q, '01, 47; 3Q, '00, 5

692.83 Dermatitis due to metals
Jewelry

692.84 Due to animal (cat) (dog) dander
Due to animal (cat) (dog) hair

692.89 Other
Dermatitis due to:
cold weather
dyes
hot weather
preservatives
EXCLUDES *allergy (NOS) (rhinitis) due to animal hair or dander (477.2)*
allergy to dust (477.8)
sunburn (692.71, 692.76-692.77)

692.9 Unspecified cause
Dermatitis:
NOS
contact NOS
venenata NOS
Eczema NOS
L23.9 Allergic contact dermatitis unspecified cause   ʰ¹⁰

✓4ᵗʰ 693 Dermatitis due to substances taken internally
EXCLUDES *adverse effect NOS of drugs and medicines (995.20)*
allergy NOS (995.3)
contact dermatitis (692.0-692.9)
urticarial reactions (708.0-708.9, 995.1)
DEF: Inflammation of skin due to ingested substance.

693.0 Due to drugs and medicines
Dermatitis medicamentosa NOS
Use additional E code to identify drug
EXCLUDES *that due to drugs in contact with skin (692.3)*
AHA: 2Q, '07, 8
TIP: Assign for palmar plantar erythrodysesthesia (PPE) or hand-foot syndrome due to chemotherapy drugs.
L27.0 Gen skin eruption d/t Rx & med taken internally   ʰ¹⁰

693.1 Due to food

693.8 Due to other specified substances taken internally

693.9 Due to unspecified substance taken internally
EXCLUDES *dermatitis NOS (692.9)*

☑4ᵗʰ **694**   **Bullous dermatoses**

694.0   **Dermatitis herpetiformis**
Dermatosis herpetiformis
Duhring's disease
Hydroa herpetiformis
> **EXCLUDES**   *herpes gestationis (646.8)*
> *dermatitis herpetiformis:*
> *juvenile (694.2)*
> *senile (694.5)*

DEF: Chronic, multisystem disease manifested most in the cutaneous system; seen as an extremely pruritic eruption of various lesions that frequently heal leaving hyperpigmentation or hypopigmentation and occasionally scarring; usually associated with an asymptomatic gluten-sensitive enteropathy, and immunogenic factors.

694.1   **Subcorneal pustular dermatosis**
Sneddon-Wilkinson disease or syndrome
DEF: Chronic relapses of sterile pustular blebs beneath the horny skin layer of the trunk and skin folds; resembles dermatitis herpetiformis.

694.2   **Juvenile dermatitis herpetiformis**
Juvenile pemphigoid

694.3   **Impetigo herpetiformis**
DEF: Rare dermatosis associated with pregnancy; marked by itching pustules in third trimester, hypocalcemia, tetany, fever and lethargy; may result in maternal or fetal death.

694.4   **Pemphigus**
Pemphigus:
NOS
erythematosus
foliaceus
malignant
vegetans
vulgaris
> **EXCLUDES**   *pemphigus neonatorum (684)*

DEF: Chronic, relapsing, sometimes fatal skin diseases; causes vesicles, bullae; autoantibodies against intracellular connections cause acantholysis.

694.5   **Pemphigoid**
Benign pemphigus NOS
Bullous pemphigoid
Herpes circinatus bullosus
Senile dermatitis herpetiformis

☑5ᵗʰ **694.6**   **Benign mucous membrane pemphigoid**
Cicatricial pemphigoid
Mucosynechial atrophic bullous dermatitis

    694.60   **Without mention of ocular involvement**

    694.61   **With ocular involvement**
Ocular pemphigus
DEF: Mild self-limiting, subepidermal blistering of mucosa including the conjunctiva, seen predominantly in the elderly, produces adhesions and scarring.

694.8   **Other specified bullous dermatoses**
> **EXCLUDES**   *herpes gestationis (646.8)*

694.9   **Unspecified bullous dermatoses**

☑4ᵗʰ **695**   **Erythematous conditions**

695.0   **Toxic erythema**
Erythema venenatum

☑5ᵗʰ **695.1**   **Erythema multiforme**
Use additional code to identify associated manifestations, such as:
arthropathy associated with dermatological disorders (713.3)
conjunctival edema (372.73)
conjunctivitis (372.04, 372.33)
corneal scars and opacities (371.00-371.05)
corneal ulcer (370.00-370.07)
edema of eyelid (374.82)
inflammation of eyelid (373.8)
keratoconjunctivitis sicca (370.33)
mechanical lagophthalmos (374.22)
mucositis (478.11, 528.00, 538, 616.81)
stomatitis (528.00)
symblepharon (372.63)

Use additional E code to identify drug, if drug-induced

Use additional code to identify percentage of skin exfoliation (695.50-695.59)
> **EXCLUDES**   *(Staphylococcal) scalded skin syndrome (695.81)*

DEF: Symptom complex with varied skin eruption pattern of macular, bullous, papular, nodose, or vesicular lesions on the neck, face, and legs; gastritis and rheumatic pains; secondary to number of factors, including infections, ingestants, physical agents, malignancy and pregnancy.
AHA: 4Q, '08, 128-130

    695.10   **Erythema multiforme, unspecified**
Erythema iris
Herpes iris

    695.11   **Erythema multiforme minor**

    695.12   **Erythema multiforme major**

    695.13   **Stevens-Johnson syndrome**

    695.14   **Stevens-Johnson syndrome-toxic epidermal necrolysis overlap syndrome**
SJS-TEN overlap syndrome
AHA: 4Q, '08, 131

    695.15   **Toxic epidermal necrolysis**
Lyell's syndrome

    695.19   **Other erythema multiforme**

695.2   **Erythema nodosum**
> **EXCLUDES**   *tuberculous erythema nodosum (017.1)*

DEF: Panniculitis (an inflammatory reaction of the subcutaneous fat) of women, usually seen as a hypersensitivity reaction to infections, drugs, sarcoidosis, and specific enteropathies; the acute stage associated with fever, malaise, and arthralgia; the lesions are pink to blue in color as tender nodules and are found on the front of the legs below the knees.

695.3   **Rosacea**
Acne:
erythematosa
rosacea
Perioral dermatitis
Rhinophyma
DEF: Chronic skin disease, usually of the face, characterized by persistent erythema and telangiectasis with acute episodes of edema, engorgement papules, and pustules.

695.4   **Lupus erythematosus**
Lupus:
erythematodes (discoid)
erythematosus (discoid), not disseminated
> **EXCLUDES**   *lupus (vulgaris) NOS (017.0)*
> *systemic [disseminated] lupus erythematosus (710.0)*

DEF: Group of connective tissue disorders occurring as various cutaneous diseases of unknown origin; it primarily affects women between the ages of 20 and 40.

☑4ᵗʰ / ☑5ᵗʰ Additional Digit Required   Unspecified Code   Other Specified Code   Manifestation Code   ►◄ Revised Text   ● New Code   ▲ Revised Code Title

2013 ICD-9-CM   **Volume 1 – 215**

√5ᵗʰ **695.5 Exfoliation due to erythematous conditions according to extent of body surface involved**

Code first erythematous condition causing exfoliation, such as:
     Ritter's disease (695.81)
     (Staphylococcal) scalded skin syndrome (695.81)
     Stevens-Johnson syndrome (695.13)
     Stevens-Johnson syndrome-toxic epidermal necrolysis overlap syndrome (695.14)
     toxic epidermal necrolysis (695.15)

AHA: 4Q, '08, 128-131

695.50 Exfoliation due to erythematous condition involving less than 10 percent of body surface

Exfoliation due to erythematous condition NOS

695.51 Exfoliation due to erythematous condition involving 10-19 percent of body surface

695.52 Exfoliation due to erythematous condition involving 20-29 percent of body surface

695.53 Exfoliation due to erythematous condition involving 30-39 percent of body surface

AHA: 4Q, '08, 131

695.54 Exfoliation due to erythematous condition involving 40-49 percent of body surface

695.55 Exfoliation due to erythematous condition involving 50-59 percent of body surface

695.56 Exfoliation due to erythematous condition involving 60-69 percent of body surface

695.57 Exfoliation due to erythematous condition involving 70-79 percent of body surface

695.58 Exfoliation due to erythematous condition involving 80-89 percent of body surface

695.59 Exfoliation due to erythematous condition involving 90 percent or more of body surface

√5ᵗʰ **695.8 Other specified erythematous conditions**

695.81 Ritter's disease

Dermatitis exfoliativa neonatorum
(Staphylococcal) Scalded skin syndrome
Use additional code to identify percentage of skin exfoliation (695.50-695.59)

DEF: Infectious skin disease of young children marked by eruptions ranging from a localized bullous to widespread of easily ruptured fine vesicles and bullae; results in exfoliation of large planes of skin and leaves raw areas.

695.89 Other

Erythema intertrigo
Intertrigo
Pityriasis rubra (Hebra)

EXCLUDES mycotic intertrigo (111.0-111.9)

AHA: S-O, '86, 10

695.9 Unspecified erythematous condition

Erythema NOS
Erythroderma (secondary)

√4ᵗʰ **696 Psoriasis and similar disorders**

696.0 Psoriatic arthropathy

DEF: Psoriasis associated with inflammatory arthritis; often involves interphalangeal joints.

696.1 Other psoriasis

Acrodermatitis continua
Dermatitis repens
Psoriasis:
     NOS
     any type, except arthropathic

EXCLUDES psoriatic arthropathy (696.0)

L40.9 Psoriasis unspecified   I-10

696.2 Parapsoriasis

Parakeratosis variegata
Parapsoriasis lichenoides chronica
Pityriasis lichenoides et varioliformis

DEF: Erythrodermas similar to lichen, planus and psoriasis; symptoms include redness and itching; resistant to treatment.

696.3 Pityriasis rosea

Pityriasis circinata (et maculata)

DEF: Common, self-limited rash of unknown etiology marked by a solitary erythematous, salmon or fawn-colored herald plaque on the trunk, arms or thighs; followed by development of papular or macular lesions that tend to peel and form a scaly collarette.

696.4 Pityriasis rubra pilaris

Devergie's disease
Lichen ruber acuminatus

EXCLUDES pityriasis rubra (Hebra) (695.89)

DEF: Inflammatory disease of hair follicles; marked by firm, red lesions topped by horny plugs; may form patches; occurs on fingers elbows, knees.

696.5 Other and unspecified pityriasis

Pityriasis:
     NOS
     alba
     streptogenes

EXCLUDES pityriasis:
     simplex (690.18)
     versicolor (111.0)

696.8 Other

√4ᵗʰ **697 Lichen**

EXCLUDES lichen:
     obtusus corneus (698.3)
     pilaris (congenital) (757.39)
     ruber acuminatus (696.4)
     sclerosus et atrophicus (701.0)
     scrofulosus (017.0)
     simplex chronicus (698.3)
     spinulosus (congenital) (757.39)
     urticatus (698.2)

697.0 Lichen planus

Lichen: Lichen:
     planopilaris   ruber planus

DEF: Inflammatory, pruritic skin disease; marked by angular, flat-top, violet-colored papules; may be acute and widespread or chronic and localized.

697.1 Lichen nitidus

Pinkus' disease

DEF: Chronic, inflammatory, asymptomatic skin disorder, characterized by numerous glistening, flat-topped, discrete, skin-colored micropapules most often on penis, lower abdomen, inner thighs, wrists, forearms, breasts and buttocks.

697.8 Other lichen, not elsewhere classified

Lichen:
     ruber moniliforme
     striata

697.9 Lichen, unspecified

√4ᵗʰ **698 Pruritus and related conditions**

EXCLUDES pruritus specified as psychogenic (306.3)

DEF: Pruritus: Intense, persistent itching due to irritation of sensory nerve endings from organic or psychogenic causes.

698.0 Pruritus ani

Perianal itch

698.1 Pruritus of genital organs

698.2 Prurigo

Lichen urticatus
Prurigo:
     NOS
     Hebra's
     mitis
     simplex
Urticaria papulosa (Hebra)

EXCLUDES prurigo nodularis (698.3)

698.3 Lichenification and lichen simplex chronicus
Hyde's disease
Neurodermatitis (circumscripta) (local)
Prurigo nodularis

> EXCLUDES *neurodermatitis, diffuse (of Brocq) (691.8)*

> **DEF:** Lichenification: thickening of skin due to prolonged rubbing or scratching.

> **DEF:** Lichen simplex chronicus: eczematous dermatitis, of face, neck, extremities, scrotum, vulva, and perianal region due to repeated itching, rubbing and scratching; spontaneous or evolves with other dermatoses.

698.4 Dermatitis factitia [artefacta]
Dermatitis ficta
Neurotic excoriation

> Use additional code to identify any associated mental disorder

> **DEF:** Various types of self-inflicted skin lesions characterized in appearance as an erythema to a gangrene.

698.8 Other specified pruritic conditions
Pruritus:
  hiemalis
  senilis
Winter itch

698.9 Unspecified pruritic disorder
Itch NOS
Pruritus NOS

> L29.9 Pruritus unspecified   [I-10]

Other Diseases of Skin and Subcutaneous Tissue (700-709)

> EXCLUDES *conditions confined to eyelids (373.0-374.9)*
> *congenital conditions of skin, hair, and nails (757.0-757.9)*

700 Corns and callosities
Callus
Clavus

> **DEF:** Corns: Conical or horny thickening of skin on toes, due to friction, pressure from shoes and hosiery; pain and inflammation may develop.
> **DEF:** Callosities: Localized overgrowth (hyperplasia) of the horny epidermal layer due to pressure or friction.

√4ᵗʰ 701 Other hypertrophic and atrophic conditions of skin

> EXCLUDES *dermatomyositis (710.3)*
> *hereditary edema of legs (757.0)*
> *scleroderma (generalized) (710.1)*

701.0 Circumscribed scleroderma
Addison's keloid
Dermatosclerosis, localized
Lichen sclerosus et atrophicus
Morphea
Scleroderma, circumscribed or localized

> **DEF:** Thickened, hardened, skin and subcutaneous tissue; may involve musculoskeletal system.

701.1 Keratoderma, acquired
Acquired:
  ichthyosis
  keratoderma palmaris et plantaris
Elastosis perforans serpiginosa
Hyperkeratosis:
  NOS
  follicularis in cutem penetrans
  palmoplantaris climacterica
Keratoderma:
  climactericum
  tylodes, progressive
Keratosis (blennorrhagica)

> EXCLUDES *Darier's disease [keratosis follicularis] (congenital) (757.39)*
> *keratosis:*
> *arsenical (692.4)*
> *gonococcal (098.81)*

> AHA: 4Q, '94, 48

701.2 Acquired acanthosis nigricans
Keratosis nigricans

> **DEF:** Diffuse velvety hyperplasia of the spinous skin layer of the axilla and other body folds marked by gray, brown, or black pigmentation; in adult form often associated with malignant acanthosis nigricans in a benign, nevoid form relatively generalized.

701.3 Striae atrophicae
Atrophic spots of skin
Atrophoderma maculatum
Atrophy blanche (of Milian)
Degenerative colloid atrophy
Senile degenerative atrophy
Striae distensae

> **DEF:** Bands of atrophic, depressed, wrinkled skin associated with stretching of skin from pregnancy, obesity, or rapid growth during puberty.

701.4 Keloid scar
Cheloid
Hypertrophic scar
Keloid

> **DEF:** Overgrowth of scar tissue due to excess amounts of collagen during connective tissue repair; occurs mainly on upper trunk, face.

701.5 Other abnormal granulation tissue
Excessive granulation

701.8 Other specified hypertrophic and atrophic conditions of skin
Acrodermatitis atrophicans chronica
Atrophia cutis senilis
Atrophoderma neuriticum
Confluent and reticulate papillomatosis
Cutis laxa senilis
Elastosis senilis
Folliculitis ulerythematosa reticulata
Gougerot-Carteaud syndrome or disease

> AHA: 1Q, '08, 7

> **TIP:** Assign for nephrogenic fibrosing dermopathy (NFD) or nephrogenic systemic dermopathy (NSD), a systemic condition occurring only in patients with kidney disease.

701.9 Unspecified hypertrophic and atrophic conditions of skin
Atrophoderma
Skin tag

√4ᵗʰ 702 Other dermatoses

> EXCLUDES *carcinoma in situ (232.0-232.9)*

702.0 Actinic keratosis

> **DEF:** Wart-like growth, red or skin-colored; may form a cutaneous horn.

> AHA: 1Q, '92, 18

√5ᵗʰ 702.1 Seborrheic keratosis

> **DEF:** Common, benign, lightly pigmented, warty growth composed of basaloid cells.

702.11 Inflamed seborrheic keratosis

> AHA: 4Q, '94, 48

702.19 Other seborrheic keratosis
Seborrheic keratosis NOS

702.8 Other specified dermatoses

√4ᵗʰ 703 Diseases of nail

> EXCLUDES *congenital anomalies (757.5)*
> *onychia and paronychia (681.02, 681.11)*

703.0 Ingrowing nail
Ingrowing nail with infection
Unguis incarnatus

> EXCLUDES *infection, nail NOS (681.9)*

703.8 Other specified diseases of nail
Dystrophia unguium
Hypertrophy of nail
Koilonychia
Leukonychia (punctata) (striata)
Onychauxis
Onychogryposis
Onycholysis

703.9 Unspecified disease of nail

√4ᵗʰ
√5ᵗʰ Additional Digit Required   Unspecified Code   Other Specified Code   Manifestation Code   ►◄ Revised Text   ● New Code   ▲ Revised Code Title

2013 ICD-9-CM   **Volume 1 – 217**

Diseases of the Skin and Subcutaneous Tissue

704–706.1

√4ᵗʰ **704 Diseases of hair and hair follicles**
> **EXCLUDES** congenital anomalies (757.4)

√5ᵗʰ **704.0 Alopecia**
> **EXCLUDES** madarosis (374.55)
> syphilitic alopecia (091.82)
> **DEF:** Lack of hair, especially on scalp; often called baldness; may be partial or total; occurs at any age.

    704.00 Alopecia, unspecified
> Baldness   Loss of hair

    704.01 Alopecia areata
> Ophiasis
> **DEF:** Alopecia areata: usually reversible, inflammatory, patchy hair loss found in beard or scalp.
> **DEF:** Ophiasis: alopecia areata of children; marked by band around temporal and occipital scalp margins.

    704.02 Telogen effluvium
> **DEF:** Shedding of hair from premature telogen development in follicles due to stress, including shock, childbirth, surgery, drugs or weight loss.

    704.09 Other
> Folliculitis decalvans
> Hypotrichosis:
>   NOS
>   postinfectional NOS
> Pseudopelade

704.1 Hirsutism
> Hypertrichosis: Polytrichia
>   NOS
>   lanuginosa, acquired
> **EXCLUDES** hypertrichosis of eyelid (374.54)
> **DEF:** Excess hair growth; often in unexpected places and amounts.

704.2 Abnormalities of the hair
> Atrophic hair
> Clastothrix
> Fragilitas crinium
> Trichiasis:
>   NOS
>   cicatrical
> Trichorrhexis (nodosa)
> **EXCLUDES** trichiasis of eyelid (374.05)

704.3 Variations in hair color
> Canities (premature)
> Grayness, hair (premature)
> Heterochromia of hair
> Poliosis:
>   NOS
>   circumscripta, acquired

√5ᵗʰ **704.4 Pilar and trichilemmal cysts**
> **AHA:** ▶4Q, '11, 134-135◀

    704.41 Pilar cyst

    704.42 Trichilemmal cyst
> Trichilemmal proliferating cyst
> **AHA:** ▶4Q, '11, 135◀

704.8 Other specified diseases of hair and hair follicles
> Folliculitis:
>   NOS
>   abscedens et suffodiens
>   pustular
> Perifolliculitis:
>   NOS
>   capitis abscedens et suffodiens
>   scalp
> Sycosis:
>   NOS
>   barbae [not parasitic]
>   lupoid
>   vulgaris
> **AHA:** 1Q, '11, 8

704.9 Unspecified disease of hair and hair follicles

√4ᵗʰ **705 Disorders of sweat glands**

705.0 Anhidrosis
> Hypohidrosis   Oligohidrosis
> **DEF:** Lack or deficiency of ability to sweat.

705.1 Prickly heat
> Heat rash
> Miliaria rubra (tropicalis)
> Sudamina

√5ᵗʰ **705.2 Focal hyperhidrosis**
> **EXCLUDES** generalized (secondary) hyperhidrosis (780.8)

    705.21 Primary focal hyperhidrosis
> Focal hyperhidrosis NOS
> Hyperhidrosis NOS
> Hyperhidrosis of:
>   axilla
>   face
>   palms
>   soles
> **DEF:** A rare disorder of the sweat glands resulting in excessive production of sweat; occurs in the absence of any underlying condition, almost always focal, confined to one or more specific areas of the body.
> **AHA:** 4Q, '04, 91

    705.22 Secondary focal hyperhidrosis
> Frey's syndrome
> **DEF:** Secondary focal hyperhidrosis: a symptom of an underlying disease process resulting in excessive sweating beyond what the body requires to maintain thermal control, confined to one or more specific areas of the body.
> **DEF:** Frey's syndrome: an auriculotemporal syndrome due to lesion on the parotid gland; characteristic redness and excessive sweating on the cheek in connection with eating.
> **AHA:** 4Q, '04, 91

√5ᵗʰ **705.8 Other specified disorders of sweat glands**

    705.81 Dyshidrosis
> Cheiropompholyx
> Pompholyx
> **DEF:** Vesicular eruption, on hands, feet causing itching and burning.

    705.82 Fox-Fordyce disease
> **DEF:** Chronic, usually pruritic disease evidenced by small follicular papular eruptions, especially in the axillary and pubic areas; develops from the closure and rupture of the affected apocrine glands' intraepidermal portion of the ducts.

    705.83 Hidradenitis
> Hidradenitis suppurativa
> **DEF:** Inflamed sweat glands.

    705.89 Other
> Bromhidrosis
> Chromhidrosis
> Granulosis rubra nasi
> Urhidrosis
> **EXCLUDES** generalized hyperhidrosis (780.8)
>   hidrocystoma (216.0-216.9)
> **DEF:** Bromhidrosis: foul-smelling axillary sweat due to decomposed bacteria.
> **DEF:** Chromhidrosis: secretion of colored sweat.
> **DEF:** Granulosis rubra nasi: idiopathic condition of children; causes redness, sweating around nose, face and chin; tends to end by puberty.
> **DEF:** Urhidrosis: urinous substance, such as uric acid, in sweat; occurs in uremia.

705.9 Unspecified disorder of sweat glands
> Disorder of sweat glands NOS

√4ᵗʰ **706 Diseases of sebaceous glands**

706.0 Acne varioliformis
> Acne:
>   frontalis
>   necrotica
> **DEF:** Rare form of acne characterized by persistent brown papulo-pustules usually on the brow and temporoparietal part of the scalp.

706.1 Other acne
> Acne: Acne:
>   NOS   vulgaris
>   conglobata   Blackhead
>   cystic   Comedo
>   pustular
> **EXCLUDES** acne rosacea (695.3)

Ⓝ Newborn Age: 0   Ⓟ Pediatric Age: 0-17   Ⓜ Maternity Age: 12-55   Ⓐ Adult Age: 15-124

706.2 Sebaceous cyst
Atheroma, skin
Keratin cyst
Wen

EXCLUDES pilar cyst (704.41)
trichilemmal (proliferating) cyst (704.42)

DEF: Benign epidermal cyst, contains sebum and keratin; presents as firm, circumscribed nodule.

706.3 Seborrhea

EXCLUDES seborrhea:
capitis (690.11)
sicca (690.18)
seborrheic
dermatitis (690.10)
keratosis (702.11-702.19)

DEF: Seborrheic dermatitis marked by excessive secretion of sebum; the sebum forms an oily coating, crusts, or scales on the skin; it is also called hypersteatosis.

706.8 Other specified diseases of sebaceous glands
Asteatosis (cutis)
Xerosis cutis

706.9 Unspecified disease of sebaceous glands

√4th **707 Chronic ulcer of skin**

INCLUDES non-infected sinus of skin
non-healing ulcer

EXCLUDES varicose ulcer (454.0, 454.2)

AHA: 4Q, '04, 92

√5th **707.0 Pressure ulcer**
Bed sore
Decubitus ulcer
Plaster ulcer

Use additional code to identify pressure ulcer stage (707.20-707.25)

AHA: 4Q, '08, 132-133; 1Q, '04, 14; 4Q, '03, 110; 4Q, '99, 20; 1Q, '96, 15; 3Q, '90, 15; N-D, '87, 9

707.00 Unspecified site

707.01 Elbow

707.02 Upper back
Shoulder blades

707.03 Lower back
Coccyx
Sacrum
AHA: 3Q, '08, 17; 1Q, '05, 16
L89.159 Pressure ulcer of sacral region uns stage   I-10

707.04 Hip
L89.209 Pressure ulcer of unspecified hip uns stage   I-10

707.05 Buttock
L89.309 Pressure ulcer of unspecified buttock uns stage   I-10

707.06 Ankle

707.07 Heel
AHA: 4Q, '09, 150; 1Q, '05, 16
L89.609 Pressure ulcer of unspecified heel uns stage   I-10

707.09 Other site
Head
L89.899 Pressure ulcer of other site unspecified stage   I-10

Four Stages of Pressure Ulcers

First Stage
Persistent focal erythema

Second Stage
Partial thickness skin loss involving epidermis, dermis, or both

Third Stage
Full thickness skin loss extending through subcutaneous tissue

Fourth Stage
Necrosis of soft tissue extending to muscle and bone

Cutaneous Lesions

Surface Lesions
Fissure   Polyp growth   Ulcer

Solid Lesions
Flat macule   Slightly elevated wheal   Solid papule

Sac Lesions
Cyst   Clear fluid vesicle   Pustule

√5th **707.1 Ulcer of lower limbs, except pressure ulcer**
Ulcer, chronic:
neurogenic } of lower limb
trophic

Code, if applicable, any causal condition first:
atherosclerosis of the extremities with ulceration (440.23)
chronic venous hypertension with ulcer (459.31)
chronic venous hypertension with ulcer and inflammation (459.33)
diabetes mellitus (249.80-249.81, 250.80-250.83)
postphlebitic syndrome with ulcer (459.11)
postphlebitic syndrome with ulcer and inflammation (459.13)

AHA: 4Q, '00, 44; 4Q, '99, 15

707.10 Ulcer of lower limb, unspecified
AHA: 3Q, '04, 5; 4Q, '02, 43
L97.901 Non-prss chr ulcr uns part uns lw leg brkdwn skn   I-10

707.11 Ulcer of thigh

707.12 Ulcer of calf
L97.229 Non-press chronic ulcer left calf w/uns severity   I-10

707.13 Ulcer of ankle
L97.309 Non-press chronic ulcer uns ankle uns severity   I-10

707.14 Ulcer of heel and midfoot
Plantar surface of midfoot
L97.409 Non-press chr ulcer uns heel & midft uns sevrity   I-10

707.15 Ulcer of other part of foot
Toes
L97.509 Non-press chr ulcer oth part uns ft uns severity   I-10

707.19 Ulcer of other part of lower limb
L97.819 Non-press chr ulcer oth part rt low leg uns sevr   I-10

√5th **707.2 Pressure ulcer stages**
Code first site of pressure ulcer (707.00-707.09)
AHA: 4Q, '08, 132-134
TIP: If a pressure ulcer progresses during an admission from one stage to another, assign only the code for the higher stage.

707.20 Pressure ulcer, unspecified stage
Healing pressure ulcer NOS
Healing pressure ulcer, unspecified stage

707.21 Pressure ulcer stage I
Healing pressure ulcer, stage I
Pressure pre-ulcer skin changes limited to persistent focal erythema

707.22 Pressure ulcer stage II
Healing pressure ulcer, stage II
Pressure ulcer with abrasion, blister, partial thickness skin loss involving epidermis and/or dermis

707.23 Pressure ulcer stage III
Healing pressure ulcer, stage III
Pressure ulcer with full thickness skin loss involving damage or necrosis of subcutaneous tissue
AHA: 4Q, '09, 150

√4th √5th Additional Digit Required   Unspecified Code   Other Specified Code   Manifestation Code   ►◄ Revised Text   ● New Code   ▲ Revised Code Title

2013 ICD-9-CM   **Volume 1 – 219**

707.24 Pressure ulcer stage IV
Healing pressure ulcer, stage IV
Pressure ulcer with necrosis of soft tissues through to underlying muscle, tendon, or bone

707.25 Pressure ulcer, unstageable
TIP: Assign only if ulcer is covered by eschar, has been treated with skin or other graft, or is documented as a deep tissue injury but not documented as due to trauma.

707.8 Chronic ulcer of other specified sites
Ulcer, chronic:
neurogenic | of other specified sites
trophic
L98.499 Non-press chr ulcer skin oth sites uns severity   I-10

707.9 Chronic ulcer of unspecified site
Chronic ulcer NOS   Tropical ulcer NOS
Trophic ulcer NOS   Ulcer of skin NOS

√4ᵗʰ **708 Urticaria**
EXCLUDES edema:
angioneurotic (995.1)
Quincke's (995.1)
hereditary angioedema (277.6)
urticaria:
giant (995.1)
papulosa (Hebra) (698.2)
pigmentosa (juvenile) (congenital) (757.33)
DEF: Skin disorder marked by raised edematous patches of skin or mucous membrane with intense itching; also called hives.

708.0 Allergic urticaria

708.1 Idiopathic urticaria

708.2 Urticaria due to cold and heat
Thermal urticaria

708.3 Dermatographic urticaria
Dermatographia
Factitial urticaria

708.4 Vibratory urticaria

708.5 Cholinergic urticaria

708.8 Other specified urticaria
Nettle rash
Urticaria:
chronic
recurrent periodic

708.9 Urticaria, unspecified
Hives NOS

√4ᵗʰ **709 Other disorders of skin and subcutaneous tissue**

√5ᵗʰ **709.0 Dyschromia**
EXCLUDES albinism (270.2)
pigmented nevus (216.0-216.9)
that of eyelid (374.52-374.53)
DEF: Pigment disorder of skin or hair.

709.00 Dyschromia, unspecified

709.01 Vitiligo
DEF: Persistent, progressive development of nonpigmented white patches on otherwise normal skin.

709.09 Other

709.1 Vascular disorders of skin
Angioma serpiginosum
Purpura (primary)annularis telangiectodes

709.2 Scar conditions and fibrosis of skin
Adherent scar (skin)
Cicatrix
Disfigurement (due to scar)
Fibrosis, skin NOS
Scar NOS
EXCLUDES keloid scar (701.4)
AHA: N-D, '84, 19

709.3 Degenerative skin disorders
Calcinosis: Degeneration, skin
circumscripta   Deposits, skin
cutis   Senile dermatosis NOS
Colloid milium   Subcutaneous calcification

709.4 Foreign body granuloma of skin and subcutaneous tissue
Use additional code to identify foreign body (V90.01-V90.9)
EXCLUDES residual foreign body without granuloma of skin and subcutaneous tissue (729.6)
that of muscle (728.82)

709.8 Other specified disorders of skin
Epithelial hyperplasia
Menstrual dermatosis
Vesicular eruption
DEF: Epithelial hyperplasia: increased number of epithelial cells.
DEF: Vesicular eruption: liquid-filled structures appearing through skin.
AHA: 4Q, '08, 99; N-D, '87, 6
L98.8 Other spec disorders skin & subcutaneous tissue   I-10

709.9 Unspecified disorder of skin and subcutaneous tissue
Dermatosis NOS

13. Diseases of the Musculoskeletal System and Connective Tissue (710-739)

Use additional external cause code, if applicable, to identify the cause of the musculoskeletal condition

The following fifth-digit subclassification is for use with categories 711-712, 715-716, 718-719, and 730:

0 site unspecified
1 shoulder region
    Acromioclavicular joint(s)
    Clavicle
    Glenohumeral joint(s)
    Scapula
    Sternoclavicular joint(s)
2 upper arm
    Elbow joint
    Humerus
3 forearm
    Radius
    Ulna
    Wrist joint
4 hand
    Carpus
    Metacarpus
    Phalanges [fingers]
5 pelvic region and thigh
    Buttock
    Femur
    Hip (joint)
6 lower leg
    Fibula
    Knee joint
    Patella
    Tibia
7 ankle and foot
    Ankle joint
    Digits [toes]
    Metatarsus
    Phalanges, foot
    Tarsus
    Other joints in foot
8 other specified sites
    Head
    Neck
    Ribs
    Skull
    Trunk
    Vertebral column
9 multiple sites

Arthropathies and Related Disorders (710-719)

> **EXCLUDES** *disorders of spine (720.0-724.9)*

✓4ᵗʰ 710 Diffuse diseases of connective tissue

> **INCLUDES** all collagen diseases whose effects are not mainly confined to a single system
>
> **EXCLUDES** *those affecting mainly the cardiovascular system, i.e., polyarteritis nodosa and allied conditions (446.0-446.7)*

710.0 Systemic lupus erythematosus
Disseminated lupus erythematosus
Libman-Sacks disease

Use additional code to identify manifestation, as:
    endocarditis (424.91)
    nephritis (583.81)
        chronic (582.81)
    nephrotic syndrome (581.81)

> **EXCLUDES** *lupus erythematosus (discoid) NOS (695.4)*

DEF: A chronic multisystemic inflammatory disease affecting connective tissue; marked by anemia, leukopenia, muscle and joint pains, fever, rash of a butterfly pattern around cheeks and forehead area; of unknown etiology.
AHA: 2Q, '03, 7-8; 2Q, '97, 8
M32.9 Systemic lupus erythematosus unspecified `I-10`

710.1 Systemic sclerosis
Acrosclerosis
CRST syndrome
Progressive systemic sclerosis
Scleroderma

Use additional code to identify manifestation, as:
    lung involvement (517.2)
    myopathy (359.6)

> **EXCLUDES** *circumscribed scleroderma (701.0)*

DEF: Systemic disease, involving excess fibrotic collagen build-up; symptoms include thickened skin, fibrotic degenerative changes in various organs, and vascular abnormalities; condition occurs more often in females.
AHA: 1Q, '88, 6

710.2 Sicca syndrome
Keratoconjunctivitis sicca
Sjögren's disease

DEF: Autoimmune disease; associated with keratoconjunctivitis, laryngopharyngitis, rhinitis, dry mouth, enlarged parotid gland, and chronic polyarthritis.

710.3 Dermatomyositis
Poikilodermatomyositis
Polymyositis with skin involvement

DEF: Polymyositis characterized by flat-top purple papules on knuckles; upper eyelid rash, edema of eyelids and orbit area, red rash on forehead, neck, shoulders, trunk and arms; symptoms include fever, weight loss, aching muscles; visceral cancer.

710.4 Polymyositis

DEF: Chronic, progressive, inflammatory skeletal muscle disease; causes weakness of limb girdles, neck, pharynx; may precede or follow scleroderma, Sjogren's disease, systemic lupus erythematosus, arthritis, or malignancy.

710.5 Eosinophilia myalgia syndrome
Toxic oil syndrome

Use additional E code to identify drug, if drug induced

DEF: Eosinophilia myalgia syndrome (EMS): inflammatory, multisystem fibrosis; associated with ingesting elementary L-tryptophan; symptoms include myalgia, weak limbs and bulbar muscles, distal sensory loss, areflexia, arthralgia, cough, fever, fatigue, skin rashes, myopathy, and eosinophil counts greater than 1000/microliter.
DEF: Toxic oil syndrome: syndrome similar to EMS due to ingesting contaminated cooking oil.
AHA: 4Q, '92, 21

710.8 Other specified diffuse diseases of connective tissue
Multifocal fibrosclerosis (idiopathic) NEC
Systemic fibrosclerosing syndrome
AHA: M-A, '87, 12

710.9 Unspecified diffuse connective tissue disease
Collagen disease NOS

✓4ᵗʰ 711 Arthropathy associated with infections

> **INCLUDES** arthritis
> arthropathy
> polyarthritis   associated with conditions
> polyarthropathy   classifiable below
>
> **EXCLUDES** *rheumatic fever (390)*

The following fifth-digit subclassification is for use with category 711; valid digits are in [brackets] under each code. See list at beginning of chapter for definitions.

0 site unspecified
1 shoulder region
2 upper arm
3 forearm
4 hand
5 pelvic region and thigh
6 lower leg
7 ankle and foot
8 other specified sites
9 multiple sites

AHA: 1Q, '92, 17

§ ✓5ᵗʰ 711.0 Pyogenic arthritis
[0-9] Arthritis or polyarthritis (due to):
    coliform [Escherichia coli]
    Hemophilus influenzae [H. influenzae]
    pneumococcal
    Pseudomonas
    staphylococcal
    streptococcal
Pyarthrosis

Use additional code to identify infectious organism (041.0-041.8)

DEF: Infectious arthritis caused by various bacteria; marked by inflamed synovial membranes, and purulent effusion in joints.
AHA: 1Q, '92, 16; 1Q, '91, 15
M00.869 Arthritis due to other bacteria unspecified knee `I-10`

§ ✓5ᵗʰ 711.1 Arthropathy associated with Reiter's disease and
[0-9] nonspecific urethritis

Code first underlying disease as:
    nonspecific urethritis (099.4)
    Reiter's disease (099.3)

DEF: Reiter's disease: joint disease marked by diarrhea, urethritis, conjunctivitis, keratosis and arthritis; of unknown etiology; affects young males.
DEF: Urethritis: inflamed urethra.

---

§ Requires fifth digit. Valid digits are in [brackets] under each code. See beginning of section 710-739 for codes and defintions.

Diseases of the Musculoskeletal System and Connective Tissue

711.2–713.3

Joint Structures

Muscle — Periosteum (covers bone) — Cortical bone — Medullary bone — Fascia over Muscle — Sesamoid bone — Bursa (with synovial fluid) — Tendon (muscle to bone) — Muscle insertion into bone (crosses one or more joints) — Retinaculum — Tendon sheath around Tendon — Synovium lines — Joint capsule around — Synovial cavity (with fluid) — Articular cartilage — Ligament (bone to bone) — Bursa — Bone covered with periosteum

§ ✓5th **711.2 Arthropathy in Behçet's syndrome**
[0-9]   *Code first underlying disease (136.1)*
     DEF: Behçet's syndrome: Chronic inflammatory disorder, of unknown etiology; affects small blood vessels; causes ulcers of oral and pharyngeal mucous membranes and genitalia, skin lesions, retinal vasculitis, optic atrophy and severe uveitis.

§ ✓5th **711.3 Postdysenteric arthropathy**
[0-9]   *Code first underlying disease as:*
     dysentery (009.0)
     enteritis, infectious (008.0-009.3)
     paratyphoid fever (002.1-002.9)
     typhoid fever (002.0)
     EXCLUDES *salmonella arthritis (003.23)*

§ ✓5th **711.4 Arthropathy associated with other bacterial diseases**
[0-9]   *Code first underlying disease as:*
     diseases classifiable to 010-040, 090-099, except as in 711.1, 711.3, and 713.5
     leprosy (030.0-030.9)
     tuberculosis (015.0-015.9)
     EXCLUDES *gonococcal arthritis (098.50)*
              meningococcal arthritis (036.82)

§ ✓5th **711.5 Arthropathy associated with other viral diseases**
[0-9]   *Code first underlying disease as:*
     diseases classifiable to 045-049, 050-079, 480, 487
     O'nyong nyong (066.3)
     EXCLUDES *that due to rubella (056.71)*

§ ✓5th **711.6 Arthropathy associated with mycoses**
[0-9]   *Code first underlying disease (110.0-118)*

§ ✓5th **711.7 Arthropathy associated with helminthiasis**
[0-9]   *Code first underlying disease as:*
     filariasis (125.0-125.9)

§ ✓5th **711.8 Arthropathy associated with other infectious and parasitic diseases**
[0-9]   *Code first underlying disease as:*
     diseases classifiable to 080-088, 100-104, 130-136
     EXCLUDES *arthropathy associated with sarcoidosis (713.7)*
     AHA: 4Q, '91, 15; 3Q, '90, 14

§ ✓5th **711.9 Unspecified infective arthritis**
[0-9]   Infective arthritis or polyarthritis (acute) (chronic) (subacute) NOS

✓4th **712 Crystal arthropathies**
   INCLUDES crystal-induced arthritis and synovitis
   EXCLUDES *gouty arthropathy (274.00-274.03)*
   DEF: Joint disease due to urate crystal deposit in joints or synovial membranes.

   The following fifth-digit subclassification is for use with category 712; valid digits are in [brackets] under each code. See list at beginning of chapter for definitions.
     0 site unspecified
     1 shoulder region
     2 upper arm
     3 forearm
     4 hand
     5 pelvic region and thigh
     6 lower leg
     7 ankle and foot
     8 other specified sites
     9 multiple sites

§ ✓5th **712.1 Chondrocalcinosis due to dicalcium phosphate crystals**
[0-9]   Chondrocalcinosis due to dicalcium phosphate crystals (with other crystals)
     Code first underlying disease (275.4)

§ ✓5th **712.2 Chondrocalcinosis due to pyrophosphate crystals**
[0-9]   *Code first underlying disease (275.4)*

§ ✓5th **712.3 Chondrocalcinosis, unspecified**
[0-9]   *Code first underlying disease (275.4)*

§ ✓5th **712.8 Other specified crystal arthropathies**
[0-9]

§ ✓5th **712.9 Unspecified crystal arthropathy**
[0-9]

✓4th **713 Arthropathy associated with other disorders classified elsewhere**
   INCLUDES arthritis / arthropathy / polyarthritis / polyarthropathy — associated with conditions classifiable below

713.0 Arthropathy associated with other endocrine and metabolic disorders
   Code first underlying disease as:
     acromegaly (253.0)
     hemochromatosis (275.01-275.09)
     hyperparathyroidism (252.00-252.08)
     hypogammaglobulinemia (279.00-279.09)
     hypothyroidism (243-244.9)
     lipoid metabolism disorder (272.0-272.9)
     ochronosis (270.2)
     EXCLUDES *arthropathy associated with:*
         amyloidosis (713.7)
         crystal deposition disorders, except gout (712.1-712.9)
         diabetic neuropathy (713.5)
         gout (274.00-274.03)

713.1 Arthropathy associated with gastrointestinal conditions other than infections
   Code first underlying disease as:
     regional enteritis (555.0-555.9)
     ulcerative colitis (556)

713.2 Arthropathy associated with hematological disorders
   Code first underlying disease as:
     hemoglobinopathy (282.4-282.7)
     hemophilia (286.0-286.2)
     leukemia (204.0-208.9)
     malignant reticulosis (202.3)
     multiple myelomatosis (203.0)
     EXCLUDES *arthropathy associated with Henoch-Schönlein purpura (713.6)*

713.3 Arthropathy associated with dermatological disorders
   Code first underlying disease as:
     erythema multiforme (695.10-695.19)
     erythema nodosum (695.2)
     EXCLUDES *psoriatic arthropathy (696.0)*

---

§ Requires fifth digit. Valid digits are in [brackets] under each code. See beginning of section 710-739 for codes and definitions.

713.4 Arthropathy associated with respiratory disorders

Code first underlying disease as:
diseases classifiable to 490-519

EXCLUDES arthropathy associated with respiratory infections (711.0, 711.4-711.8)

713.5 Arthropathy associated with neurological disorders

Charcôt's arthropathy ⎫ associated with diseases
Neuropathic arthritis ⎬ classifiable elsewhere

Code first underlying disease as:
neuropathic joint disease [Charcôt's joints]:
NOS (094.0)
diabetic (249.6, 250.6)
syringomyelic (336.0)
tabetic [syphilitic] (094.0)

713.6 Arthropathy associated with hypersensitivity reaction

Code first underlying disease as:
Henoch (-Schönlein) purpura (287.0)
serum sickness (999.51-999.59)

EXCLUDES allergic arthritis NOS (716.2)

713.7 Other general diseases with articular involvement

Code first underlying disease as:
amyloidosis (277.30-277.39)
familial Mediterranean fever (277.31)
sarcoidosis (135)

AHA: 2Q, '97, 12

713.8 Arthropathy associated with other condition classifiable elsewhere

Code first underlying disease as:
conditions classifiable elsewhere except as in 711.1-711.8, 712, and 713.0-713.7

✓4ᵗʰ **714 Rheumatoid arthritis and other inflammatory polyarthropathies**

EXCLUDES rheumatic fever (390)
rheumatoid arthritis of spine NOS (720.0)

AHA: 2Q, '95, 3

714.0 Rheumatoid arthritis

Arthritis or polyarthritis:
atrophic
rheumatic (chronic)

Use additional code to identify manifestation, as:
myopathy (359.6)
polyneuropathy (357.1)

EXCLUDES juvenile rheumatoid arthritis NOS (714.30)

DEF: Chronic systemic disease principally of joints, manifested by inflammatory changes in articular structures and synovial membranes, atrophy, and loss in bone density.

AHA: 2Q, '06, 20; 1Q, '90, 5

M06.9 Rheumatoid arthritis unspecified   I-10

714.1 Felty's syndrome

Rheumatoid arthritis with splenoadenomegaly and leukopenia

DEF: Syndrome marked by rheumatoid arthritis, splenomegaly, leukopenia, pigmented spots on lower extremity skin, anemia, and thrombocytopenia.

714.2 Other rheumatoid arthritis with visceral or systemic involvement

Rheumatoid carditis

✓5ᵗʰ **714.3 Juvenile chronic polyarthritis**

DEF: Rheumatoid arthritis of more than one joint; lasts longer than six weeks in age 17 or younger; symptoms include fever, erythematous rash, weight loss, lymphadenopathy, hepatosplenomegaly and pericarditis.

714.30 Polyarticular juvenile rheumatoid arthritis, chronic or unspecified

Juvenile rheumatoid arthritis NOS
Still's disease

714.31 Polyarticular juvenile rheumatoid arthritis, acute

714.32 Pauciarticular juvenile rheumatoid arthritis

714.33 Monoarticular juvenile rheumatoid arthritis

714.4 Chronic postrheumatic arthropathy

Chronic rheumatoid nodular fibrositis
Jaccoud's syndrome

DEF: Persistent joint disorder; follows previous rheumatic infection.

✓5ᵗʰ **714.8 Other specified inflammatory polyarthropathies**

714.81 Rheumatoid lung

Caplan's syndrome
Diffuse interstitial rheumatoid disease of lung
Fibrosing alveolitis, rheumatoid

DEF: Lung disorders associated with rheumatoid arthritis.

714.89 Other

714.9 Unspecified inflammatory polyarthropathy

Inflammatory polyarthropathy or polyarthritis NOS

EXCLUDES polyarthropathy NOS (716.5)

✓4ᵗʰ **715 Osteoarthrosis and allied disorders**

NOTE Localized, in the subcategories below, includes bilateral involvement of the same site.

INCLUDES arthritis or polyarthritis:
degenerative
hypertrophic
degenerative joint disease
osteoarthritis

EXCLUDES Marie-Strümpell spondylitis (720.0)
osteoarthrosis [osteoarthritis] of spine (721.0-721.9)

The following fifth-digit subclassification is for use with category 715; valid digits are in [brackets] under each code. See list at beginning of chapter for definitions.

0 site unspecified
1 shoulder region
2 upper arm
3 forearm
4 hand
5 pelvic region and thigh
6 lower leg
7 ankle and foot
8 other specified sites
9 multiple sites

§ ✓5ᵗʰ **715.0 Osteoarthrosis, generalized**
[0,4,9]   Degenerative joint disease, involving multiple joints
Primary generalized hypertrophic osteoarthrosis

DEF: Chronic noninflammatory arthritis; marked by degenerated articular cartilage and enlarged bone; symptoms include pain and stiffness with activity.

§ ✓5ᵗʰ **715.1 Osteoarthrosis, localized, primary**
[0-8]   Localized osteoarthropathy, idiopathic
M17.0 Bilateral primary osteoarthritis of knee   I-10

§ ✓5ᵗʰ **715.2 Osteoarthrosis, localized, secondary**
[0-8]   Coxae malum senilis

§ ✓5ᵗʰ **715.3 Osteoarthrosis, localized, not specified whether**
[0-8]   **primary or secondary**
Otto's pelvis

AHA: For code 715.35: 3Q, '04, 12; 2Q, '04, 15; **For code 715.36:** 4Q, '03, 118; 2Q, '95, 5

M16.9 Osteoarthritis of hip unspecified   I-10

§ ✓5ᵗʰ **715.8 Osteoarthrosis involving, or with mention of**
[0,9]   **more than one site, but not specified as generalized**

§ ✓5ᵗʰ **715.9 Osteoarthrosis, unspecified whether**
[0-8]   **generalized or localized**

AHA: For code 715.90: 2Q, '97, 12

M19.90 Unspecified osteoarthritis unspecified site   I-10
M17.9 Osteoarthritis of knee unspecified   I-10

---

§ Requires fifth digit. Valid digits are in [brackets] under each code. See beginning of section 710-739 for codes and defintions.

✓4ᵗʰ/✓5ᵗʰ Additional Digit Required   Unspecified Code   Other Specified Code   Manifestation Code   ▶◀ Revised Text   ● New Code   ▲ Revised Code Title

2013 ICD-9-CM   **Volume 1 – 223**

☑4ᵗʰ **716 Other and unspecified arthropathies**

> EXCLUDES cricoarytenoid arthropathy (478.79)

> The following fifth-digit subclassification is for use with category 716; valid digits are in [brackets] under each code. See list at beginning of chapter for definitions.
> 0 site unspecified
> 1 shoulder region
> 2 upper arm
> 3 forearm
> 4 hand
> 5 pelvic region and thigh
> 6 lower leg
> 7 ankle and foot
> 8 other specified sites
> 9 multiple sites

> AHA: 2Q, '95, 3

§ ☑5ᵗʰ **716.0 Kaschin-Beck disease**
[0-9]   Endemic polyarthritis
> DEF: Chronic degenerative disease of spine and peripheral joints; occurs in eastern Siberian, northern Chinese, and Korean youth; may be a mycotoxicosis caused by eating cereals infected with fungus.

§ ☑5ᵗʰ **716.1 Traumatic arthropathy**
[0-9]   AHA: For Code 716.11: 1Q, '02, 9; For code 716.15: 2Q, '09, 11

§ ☑5ᵗʰ **716.2 Allergic arthritis**
[0-9]   EXCLUDES arthritis associated with Henoch-Schönlein purpura or serum sickness (713.6)

§ ☑5ᵗʰ **716.3 Climacteric arthritis**   ♀
[0-9]   Menopausal arthritis
> DEF: Ovarian hormone deficiency; causes pain in small joints, shoulders, elbows or knees; affects females at menopause; also called arthropathia ovaripriva.

§ ☑5ᵗʰ **716.4 Transient arthropathy**
[0-9]   EXCLUDES palindromic rheumatism (719.3)

§ ☑5ᵗʰ **716.5 Unspecified polyarthropathy or polyarthritis**
[0-9]

§ ☑5ᵗʰ **716.6 Unspecified monoarthritis**
[0-8]   Coxitis

§ ☑5ᵗʰ **716.8 Other specified arthropathy**
[0-9]

§ ☑5ᵗʰ **716.9 Arthropathy, unspecified**
[0-9]   Arthritis
         Arthropathy } (acute) (chronic) (subacute)
         Articular rheumatism (chronic)
         Inflammation of joint NOS
         M12.9 Arthropathy unspecified   I-10

☑4ᵗʰ **717 Internal derangement of knee**
> INCLUDES   degeneration
>   rupture, old   } of articular cartilage or
>   tear, old   meniscus of knee

> EXCLUDES acute derangement of knee (836.0-836.6)
>   ankylosis (718.5)
>   contracture (718.4)
>   current injury (836.0-836.6)
>   deformity (736.4-736.6)
>   recurrent dislocation (718.3)

717.0 Old bucket handle tear of medial meniscus
Old bucket handle tear of unspecified cartilage

717.1 Derangement of anterior horn of medial meniscus

717.2 Derangement of posterior horn of medial meniscus

717.3 Other and unspecified derangement of medial meniscus
Degeneration of internal semilunar cartilage

Disruption and Tears of Meniscus

Bucket-handle   Flap-type   Peripheral / Radial

Horizontal cleavage   Vertical   Congenital discoid meniscus

Internal Derangements of Knee

Disruptions of Cruciate Ligament
Anterior
Posterior

Chondromalacia of Patella
"Kissing" lesion of femur

☑5ᵗʰ **717.4 Derangement of lateral meniscus**

717.40 Derangement of lateral meniscus, unspecified

717.41 Bucket handle tear of lateral meniscus

717.42 Derangement of anterior horn of lateral meniscus

717.43 Derangement of posterior horn of lateral meniscus

717.49 Other

717.5 Derangement of meniscus, not elsewhere classified
Congenital discoid meniscus
Cyst of semilunar cartilage
Derangement of semilunar cartilage NOS

717.6 Loose body in knee
Joint mice, knee
Rice bodies, knee (joint)
> DEF: The presence in the joint synovial area of a small, frequently calcified, loose body created from synovial membrane, organized fibrin fragments of articular cartilage or arthritis osteophytes.

717.7 Chondromalacia of patella
Chondromalacia patellae
Degeneration [softening] of articular cartilage of patella
> DEF: Softened patella cartilage.
> AHA: M-A, '85, 14; N-D, '84, 9

☑5ᵗʰ **717.8 Other internal derangement of knee**

717.81 Old disruption of lateral collateral ligament

717.82 Old disruption of medial collateral ligament

717.83 Old disruption of anterior cruciate ligament

717.84 Old disruption of posterior cruciate ligament

717.85 Old disruption of other ligaments of knee
Capsular ligament of knee

717.89 Other
Old disruption of ligaments NOS

717.9 Unspecified internal derangement of knee
Derangement NOS of knee

---

§ Requires fifth digit. Valid digits are in [brackets] under each code. See beginning of section 710-739 for codes and defintions.

✓4ᵗʰ **718 Other derangement of joint**

> *EXCLUDES*   current injury (830.0-848.9)
> jaw (524.60-524.69)

The following fifth-digit subclassification is for use with category 718; valid digits are in [brackets] under each code. See list at beginning of chapter for definitions.
- **0 site unspecified**
- **1 shoulder region**
- **2 upper arm**
- **3 forearm**
- **4 hand**
- **5 pelvic region and thigh**
- **6 lower leg**
- **7 ankle and foot**
- **8 other specified sites**
- **9 multiple sites**

§ ✓5ᵗʰ **718.0 Articular cartilage disorder**
[0-5,7-9] Meniscus:
     disorder
     rupture, old
     tear, old
Old rupture of ligament(s) of joint NOS
> *EXCLUDES*   articular cartilage disorder:
>   in ochronosis (270.2)
>   knee (717.0-717.9)
>   chondrocalcinosis (275.4)
>   metastatic calcification (275.4)

§ ✓5ᵗʰ **718.1 Loose body in joint**
[0-5,7-9] Joint mice
> *EXCLUDES*   knee (717.6)

DEF: Calcified loose bodies in synovial fluid; due to arthritic osteophytes.
AHA: For code 718.17: 2Q, '01, 15

§ ✓5ᵗʰ **718.2 Pathological dislocation**
[0-9] Dislocation or displacement of joint, not recurrent and not current injury
Spontaneous dislocation (joint)

§ ✓5ᵗʰ **718.3 Recurrent dislocation of joint**
[0-9] **AHA:** N-D, '87, 7

§ ✓5ᵗʰ **718.4 Contracture of joint**
[0-9] **AHA:** 4Q, '98, 40
TIP: Assign an additional code from category 438 if the contracture is a result of a CVA.

§ ✓5ᵗʰ **718.5 Ankylosis of joint**
[0-9] Ankylosis of joint (fibrous) (osseous)
> *EXCLUDES*   spine (724.9)
> stiffness of joint without mention of ankylosis (719.5)

DEF: Immobility and solidification of joint; due to disease, injury or surgical procedure.

§ ✓5ᵗʰ **718.6 Unspecified intrapelvic protrusion of acetabulum**
[5] Protrusio acetabuli, unspecified
DEF: Sinking of the floor of acetabulum, causing femoral head to protrude, limits hip movement; of unknown etiology.

§ ✓5ᵗʰ **718.7 Developmental dislocation of joint**
[0-9] *EXCLUDES*   congenital dislocation of joint (754.0-755.8)
    traumatic dislocation of joint (830-839)
AHA: 4Q, '01, 48

Joint Derangements and Disorders

Loose body in joint

Dislocation of joint

Joint contracture   Ankylosis of joint   Synovial effusion (fluid)   Hemarthrosis (blood)

§ ✓5ᵗʰ **718.8 Other joint derangement, not elsewhere classified**
[0-9] Flail joint (paralytic)   Instability of joint
> *EXCLUDES*   deformities classifiable to 736 (736.0-736.9)

AHA: For code 718.81: 2Q, '00, 14
TIP: Assign 718.81 for multidirectional shoulder instability.

§ ✓5ᵗʰ **718.9 Unspecified derangement of joint**
[0-5,7-9] *EXCLUDES*   knee (717.9)

✓4ᵗʰ **719 Other and unspecified disorders of joint**
> *EXCLUDES*   jaw (524.60-524.69)

The following fifth-digit subclassification is for use with codes 719.0-719.6, 719.8-719.9; valid digits are in [brackets] under each code. See list at beginning of chapter for definitions.
- **0 site unspecified**
- **1 shoulder region**
- **2 upper arm**
- **3 forearm**
- **4 hand**
- **5 pelvic region and thigh**
- **6 lower leg**
- **7 ankle and foot**
- **8 other specified sites**
- **9 multiple sites**

§ ✓5ᵗʰ **719.0 Effusion of joint**
[0-9] Hydrarthrosis
Swelling of joint, with or without pain
> *EXCLUDES*   intermittent hydrarthrosis (719.3)

M25.469 Effusion unspecified knee   I-10

§ ✓5ᵗʰ **719.1 Hemarthrosis**
[0-9] *EXCLUDES*   current injury (840.0-848.9)

§ ✓5ᵗʰ **719.2 Villonodular synovitis**
[0-9] **DEF:** Overgrowth of synovial tissue, especially at knee joint; due to macrophage infiltration of giant cells in synovial villi and fibrous nodules.

§ ✓5ᵗʰ **719.3 Palindromic rheumatism**
[0-9] Hench-Rosenberg syndrome
Intermittent hydrarthrosis
DEF: Recurrent episodes of afebrile arthritis and periarthritis marked by their complete disappearance after a few days or hours; causes swelling, redness, and disability usually affecting only one joint; no known cause.

§ ✓5ᵗʰ **719.4 Pain in joint**
[0-9] Arthralgia
AHA: For code 719.46: 1Q, '01, 3
TIP: Assign 719.46 for patellofemoral syndrome, a chronic knee pain common among athletes.
M25.519 Pain in unspecified shoulder   I-10
M25.552 Pain in left hip   I-10

§ ✓5ᵗʰ **719.5 Stiffness of joint, not elsewhere classified**
[0-9]

§ ✓5ᵗʰ **719.6 Other symptoms referable to joint**
[0-9] Joint crepitus
Snapping hip
AHA: 1Q, '94, 15; **For code 719.66:** 2Q, '07, 6
TIP: Assign 719.66 for patellar clunk syndrome, which is a fibrous reaction caused by chronic pressure on the patella, S/P knee replacement surgery.

719.7 Difficulty in walking
> *EXCLUDES*   abnormality of gait (781.2)

AHA: 2Q, '04, 15; 4Q, '03, 66
R26.2 Difficulty in walking not elsewhere classified   I-10

§ ✓5ᵗʰ **719.8 Other specified disorders of joint**
[0-9] Calcification of joint
Fistula of joint
> *EXCLUDES*   temporomandibular joint-pain-dysfunction syndrome [Costen's syndrome] (524.60)

§ ✓5ᵗʰ **719.9 Unspecified disorder of joint**
[0-9]

---

§   Requires fifth digit. Valid digits are in [brackets] under each code. See beginning of section 710-739 for codes and defintions.

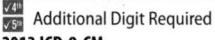

✓4ᵗʰ/✓5ᵗʰ Additional Digit Required   Unspecified Code   Other Specified Code   Manifestation Code   ▶◀ Revised Text   ● New Code   ▲ Revised Code Title

Dorsopathies (720-724)

EXCLUDES curvature of spine (737.0-737.9)
osteochondrosis of spine (juvenile) (732.0)
adult (732.8)

√4ᵗʰ 720 Ankylosing spondylitis and other inflammatory spondylopathies

720.0 Ankylosing spondylitis
Rheumatoid arthritis of spine NOS
Spondylitis:
  Marie-Strümpell
  rheumatoid
DEF: Rheumatoid arthritis of spine and sacroiliac joints; fusion and deformity in spine follows; affects mainly males; cause unknown.

720.1 Spinal enthesopathy
Disorder of peripheral ligamentous or muscular attachments of spine
Romanus lesion
DEF: Tendinous or muscular vertebral bone attachment abnormality.

720.2 Sacroiliitis, not elsewhere classified
Inflammation of sacroiliac joint NOS
DEF: Pain due to inflammation in joint, at juncture of sacrum and hip.

√5ᵗʰ 720.8 Other inflammatory spondylopathies

720.81 Inflammatory spondylopathies in diseases classified elsewhere
Code first underlying disease as:
  tuberculosis (015.0)

720.89 Other

720.9 Unspecified inflammatory spondylopathy
Spondylitis NOS

√4ᵗʰ 721 Spondylosis and allied disorders
DEF: Degenerative changes in spinal joint.
AHA: 2Q, '89, 14

721.0 Cervical spondylosis without myelopathy
Cervical or cervicodorsal:
  arthritis
  osteoarthritis
  spondylarthritis

721.1 Cervical spondylosis with myelopathy
Anterior spinal artery compression syndrome
Spondylogenic compression of cervical spinal cord
Vertebral artery compression syndrome
M47.12 Other spondylosis w/myelopathy cervical region   I-10

721.2 Thoracic spondylosis without myelopathy
Thoracic:
  arthritis
  osteoarthritis
  spondylarthritis

721.3 Lumbosacral spondylosis without myelopathy
Lumbar or lumbosacral:
  arthritis
  osteoarthritis
  spondylarthritis
AHA: 4Q, '02, 107
M47.817 Spondylosis w/o myelopath/radiculopath lumboscrl   I-10

√5ᵗʰ 721.4 Thoracic or lumbar spondylosis with myelopathy

721.41 Thoracic region
Spondylogenic compression of thoracic spinal cord

721.42 Lumbar region

721.5 Kissing spine
Baastrup's syndrome
DEF: Compression of spinous processes of adjacent vertebrae; due to mutual contact.

721.6 Ankylosing vertebral hyperostosis

721.7 Traumatic spondylopathy
Kümmell's disease or spondylitis

721.8 Other allied disorders of spine

√5ᵗʰ 721.9 Spondylosis of unspecified site

721.90 Without mention of myelopathy
Spinal:
  arthritis (deformans) (degenerative) (hypertrophic)
  osteoarthritis NOS
Spondylarthrosis NOS

721.91 With myelopathy
Spondylogenic compression of spinal cord NOS

√4ᵗʰ 722 Intervertebral disc disorders
AHA: 1Q, '88, 10

722.0 Displacement of cervical intervertebral disc without myelopathy
Neuritis (brachial) or radiculitis due to displacement or rupture of cervical intervertebral disc
Any condition classifiable to 722.2 of the cervical or cervicothoracic intervertebral disc
M50.20 Other cerv disc displacement uns cerv region   I-10

√5ᵗʰ 722.1 Displacement of thoracic or lumbar intervertebral disc without myelopathy

722.10 Lumbar intervertebral disc without myelopathy
Lumbago or sciatica due to displacement of intervertebral disc
Neuritis or radiculitis due to displacement or rupture of lumbar intervertebral disc
Any condition classifiable to 722.2 of the lumbar or lumbosacral intervertebral disc
AHA: 4Q, '08, 184; 1Q, '07, 9; 3Q, '03, 12; 1Q, '03, 7; 4Q, '02, 107
M51.26 Oth intervertebral disc displcmnt lumbar region   I-10

722.11 Thoracic intervertebral disc without myelopathy
Any condition classifiable to 722.2 of thoracic intervertebral disc

722.2 Displacement of intervertebral disc, site unspecified, without myelopathy
Discogenic syndrome NOS
Herniation of nucleus pulposus NOS
Intervertebral disc NOS:
  extrusion
  prolapse
  protrusion
  rupture
Neuritis or radiculitis due to displacement or rupture of intervertebral disc

√5ᵗʰ 722.3 Schmorl's nodes
DEF: Irregular bone defect in the margin of the vertebral body; causes herniation into end plate of vertebral body.

722.30 Unspecified region

722.31 Thoracic region

722.32 Lumbar region

722.39 Other

Normal Anatomy of Vertebral Disc

Lamina
Ligamentum flavum
Disk annulus
Nucleus pulposus
Normal Top View

Spinal canal
Spinal cord in dural sac
Intervertebral disk
Annulus
Nucleus pulposus
Vertebral body
Spinal nerve
Lamina
Normal Side View

N Newborn Age: 0   P Pediatric Age: 0-17   M Maternity Age: 12-55   A Adult Age: 15-124

Derangement of Vertebral Disc

Stenosis in Cervical Region

722.4 Degeneration of cervical intervertebral disc
Degeneration of cervicothoracic intervertebral disc
M50.30 Other cerv disc degeneration uns cerv region [I-10]

√5ᵗʰ **722.5 Degeneration of thoracic or lumbar intervertebral disc**

722.51 Thoracic or thoracolumbar intervertebral disc
AHA: 2Q, '11, 8

722.52 Lumbar or lumbosacral intervertebral disc
AHA: 2Q, '06, 18; 4Q, '04, 133
M51.37 Oth intervertebral disc degen lumbosacral region [I-10]

722.6 Degeneration of intervertebral disc, site unspecified
Degenerative disc disease NOS
Narrowing of intervertebral disc or space NOS

√5ᵗʰ **722.7 Intervertebral disc disorder with myelopathy**

722.70 Unspecified region

722.71 Cervical region

722.72 Thoracic region

722.73 Lumbar region

√5ᵗʰ **722.8 Postlaminectomy syndrome**
DEF: Spinal disorder due to spinal laminectomy surgery.
AHA: J-F, '87, 7
TIP: Assign if documentation indicates that pain is due to scar tissue formation following disc surgery.

722.80 Unspecified region

722.81 Cervical region

722.82 Thoracic region

722.83 Lumbar region
AHA: 2Q, '97, 15
M96.1 Postlaminectomy syndrome NEC [I-10]

√5ᵗʰ **722.9 Other and unspecified disc disorder**
Calcification of intervertebral cartilage or disc
Discitis

722.90 Unspecified region
AHA: N-D, '84, 19

722.91 Cervical region

722.92 Thoracic region

722.93 Lumbar region
M51.86 Other intervertebral disc disorder lumbar region [I-10]

√4ᵗʰ **723 Other disorders of cervical region**
EXCLUDES conditions due to:
intervertebral disc disorders (722.0-722.9)
spondylosis (721.0-721.9)
AHA: 3Q, '94, 14; 2Q, '89, 14

723.0 Spinal stenosis in cervical region
AHA: 4Q, '03, 101
M48.02 Spinal stenosis cervical region [I-10]

723.1 Cervicalgia
Pain in neck
DEF: Pain in cervical spine or neck region.
M54.2 Cervicalgia [I-10]

723.2 Cervicocranial syndrome
Barré-Liéou syndrome
Posterior cervical sympathetic syndrome
DEF: Neurologic disorder of upper cervical spine and nerve roots.

723.3 Cervicobrachial syndrome (diffuse)
DEF: Complex of symptoms due to scalenus anterior muscle compressing the brachial plexus; pain radiates from shoulder to arm or back of neck.
AHA: N-D, '85, 12

723.4 Brachial neuritis or radiculitis NOS
Cervical radiculitis　　Radicular syndrome of upper limbs

723.5 Torticollis, unspecified
Contracture of neck
EXCLUDES congenital (754.1)
due to birth injury (767.8)
hysterical (300.11)
ocular torticollis (781.93)
psychogenic (306.0)
spasmodic (333.83)
traumatic, current (847.0)
DEF: Abnormally positioned neck relative to head due to cervical muscle or fascia contractions; also called wryneck.
AHA: 2Q, '01, 21; 1Q, '95, 7

723.6 Panniculitis specified as affecting neck
DEF: Inflammation of the panniculus adiposus (subcutaneous fat) in the neck.

723.7 Ossification of posterior longitudinal ligament in cervical region

723.8 Other syndromes affecting cervical region
Cervical syndrome NEC　　Occipital neuralgia
Klippel's disease
AHA: 1Q, '00, 7

723.9 Unspecified musculoskeletal disorders and symptoms referable to neck
Cervical (region) disorder NOS

√4ᵗʰ **724 Other and unspecified disorders of back**
EXCLUDES collapsed vertebra (code to cause, e.g., osteoporosis, 733.00-733.09)
conditions due to:
intervertebral disc disorders (722.0-722.9)
spondylosis (721.0-721.9)
AHA: 2Q, '89, 14

√5ᵗʰ **724.0 Spinal stenosis, other than cervical**

724.00 Spinal stenosis, unspecified region
M48.00 Spinal stenosis site unspecified [I-10]

724.01 Thoracic region

724.02 Lumbar region, without neurogenic claudication
Lumbar region NOS
AHA: 4Q, '08, 109; 4Q, '07, 120; 1Q, '07, 10, 20; 4Q, '99, 13
M48.06 Spinal stenosis lumbar region [I-10]

724.03 Lumbar region, with neurogenic claudication
DEF: Spinal canal narrowing with nerve root compression causing muscle pain, fatigue, and weakness during extension of the lumbar spine; pain is relieved by sitting or bending.
AHA: 2Q, '11, 10; 4Q, '10, 89

724.09 Other

724.1 Pain in thoracic spine

724.2 Lumbago
Low back pain
Low back syndrome
Lumbalgia
AHA: 2Q, '07, 11; N-D, '85, 12
M54.5 Low back pain   I-10

724.3 Sciatica
Neuralgia or neuritis of sciatic nerve
EXCLUDES specified lesion of sciatic nerve (355.0)
AHA: 2Q, '89, 12
M54.30 Sciatica unspecified side   I-10

724.4 Thoracic or lumbosacral neuritis or radiculitis, unspecified
Radicular syndrome of lower limbs
AHA: 2Q, '99, 3
M51.14 Intervertebral disc d/o w/radiculopathy thoracic   I-10

724.5 Backache, unspecified
Vertebrogenic (pain) syndrome NOS
M54.9 Dorsalgia unspecified   I-10

724.6 Disorders of sacrum
Ankylosis
Instability } lumbosacral or sacroiliac (joint)

√5ᵗʰ **724.7 Disorders of coccyx**

724.70 Unspecified disorder of coccyx

724.71 Hypermobility of coccyx

724.79 Other
Coccygodynia

724.8 Other symptoms referable to back
Ossification of posterior longitudinal ligament NOS
Panniculitis specified as sacral or affecting back

724.9 Other unspecified back disorders
Ankylosis of spine NOS
Compression of spinal nerve root NEC
Spinal disorder NOS
EXCLUDES sacroiliitis (720.2)

Rheumatism, Excluding the Back (725-729)

INCLUDES disorders of muscles and tendons and their attachments, and of other soft tissues

725 Polymyalgia rheumatica
DEF: Joint and muscle pain, pelvis, and shoulder girdle stiffness, high sedimentation rate and temporal arteritis; occurs in elderly.
M35.3 Polymyalgia rheumatica   I-10

√4ᵗʰ **726 Peripheral enthesopathies and allied syndromes**
NOTE Enthesopathies are disorders of peripheral ligamentous or muscular attachments.
EXCLUDES spinal enthesopathy (720.1)

726.0 Adhesive capsulitis of shoulder

√5ᵗʰ **726.1 Rotator cuff syndrome of shoulder and allied disorders**

726.10 Disorders of bursae and tendons in shoulder region, unspecified
Rotator cuff syndrome NOS
Supraspinatus syndrome NOS
AHA: 2Q, '01, 11
M75.11 Rotator cuff syndrome right shoulder   I-10

726.11 Calcifying tendinitis of shoulder

726.12 Bicipital tenosynovitis

726.13 Partial tear of rotator cuff
EXCLUDES complete rupture of rotator cuff, nontraumatic (727.61)
AHA: ▶4Q, '11, 135-136◄

726.19 Other specified disorders
EXCLUDES complete rupture of rotator cuff, nontraumatic (727.61)

726.2 Other affections of shoulder region, not elsewhere classified
Periarthritis of shoulder
Scapulohumeral fibrositis

√5ᵗʰ **726.3 Enthesopathy of elbow region**

726.30 Enthesopathy of elbow, unspecified

726.31 Medial epicondylitis

726.32 Lateral epicondylitis
Epicondylitis NOS
Golfers' elbow
Tennis elbow

726.33 Olecranon bursitis
Bursitis of elbow

726.39 Other

726.4 Enthesopathy of wrist and carpus
Bursitis of hand or wrist
Periarthritis of wrist

726.5 Enthesopathy of hip region
Bursitis of hip
Gluteal tendinitis
Iliac crest spur
Psoas tendinitis
Trochanteric tendinitis

√5ᵗʰ **726.6 Enthesopathy of knee**

726.60 Enthesopathy of knee, unspecified
Bursitis of knee NOS

726.61 Pes anserinus tendinitis or bursitis
DEF: Inflamed tendons of sartorius, gracilis and semitendinosus muscles of medial aspect of knee.

726.62 Tibial collateral ligament bursitis
Pellegrini-Stieda syndrome

726.63 Fibular collateral ligament bursitis

726.64 Patellar tendinitis

726.65 Prepatellar bursitis
AHA: 2Q, '06, 15

726.69 Other
Bursitis:
infrapatellar
subpatellar

√5ᵗʰ **726.7 Enthesopathy of ankle and tarsus**

726.70 Enthesopathy of ankle and tarsus, unspecified
Metatarsalgia NOS
EXCLUDES Morton's metatarsalgia (355.6)

726.71 Achilles bursitis or tendinitis

726.72 Tibialis tendinitis
Tibialis (anterior) (posterior) tendinitis

726.73 Calcaneal spur
DEF: Overgrowth of calcaneus bone; causes pain on walking; due to chronic avulsion injury of plantar fascia from calcaneus.

726.79 Other
Peroneal tendinitis

726.8 Other peripheral enthesopathies

√5ᵗʰ **726.9 Unspecified enthesopathy**

726.90 Enthesopathy of unspecified site
Capsulitis NOS
Periarthritis NOS
Tendinitis NOS

726.91 Exostosis of unspecified site
Bone spur NOS
AHA: 2Q, '01, 15

√4ᵗʰ **727 Other disorders of synovium, tendon, and bursa**

√5ᵗʰ **727.0 Synovitis and tenosynovitis**

727.00 Synovitis and tenosynovitis, unspecified
Synovitis NOS
Tenosynovitis NOS
M65.9 Synovitis and tenosynovitis unspecified   I-10

727.01 **Synovitis and tenosynovitis in diseases classified elsewhere**

     Code first underlying disease as:
       tuberculosis (015.0-015.9)
     EXCLUDES *crystal-induced (275.4)*
         gonococcal (098.51)
         gout (274.00-274.03)
         syphilitic (095.7)

727.02 Giant cell tumor of tendon sheath

727.03 Trigger finger (acquired)
     DEF: Stenosing tenosynovitis or nodule in flexor tendon; cessation of flexion or extension movement in finger, followed by snapping into place.

727.04 Radial styloid tenosynovitis
     de Quervain's disease

727.05 Other tenosynovitis of hand and wrist

727.06 Tenosynovitis of foot and ankle

727.09 Other

727.1 Bunion
     DEF: Enlarged first metatarsal head due to inflamed bursa; results in laterally displaced great toe.

727.2 Specific bursitides often of occupational origin
     Beat: Chronic crepitant synovitis of wrist
       elbow   Miners':
       hand   elbow
       knee   knee

727.3 Other bursitis
     Bursitis NOS
     EXCLUDES *bursitis:*
         gonococcal (098.52)
         subacromial (726.19)
         subcoracoid (726.19)
         subdeltoid (726.19)
         syphilitic (095.7)
         "frozen shoulder" (726.0)

√5ᵗʰ **727.4 Ganglion and cyst of synovium, tendon, and bursa**

     727.40 Synovial cyst, unspecified
       EXCLUDES *that of popliteal space (727.51)*
       AHA: 2Q, '97, 6

     727.41 Ganglion of joint

     727.42 Ganglion of tendon sheath

Bunion

Normal metatarsophalangeal joint

Exostosis

Ganglia

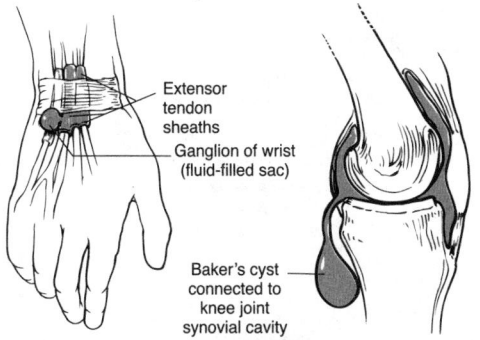

Extensor tendon sheaths

Ganglion of wrist (fluid-filled sac)

Baker's cyst connected to knee joint synovial cavity

727.43 Ganglion, unspecified

727.49 Other
     Cyst of bursa

√5ᵗʰ **727.5 Rupture of synovium**

     727.50 Rupture of synovium, unspecified

     727.51 Synovial cyst of popliteal space
       Baker's cyst (knee)

     727.59 Other

√5ᵗʰ **727.6 Rupture of tendon, nontraumatic**

     727.60 Nontraumatic rupture of unspecified tendon

     727.61 Complete rupture of rotator cuff
       EXCLUDES *partial tear of rotator cuff (726.13)*
       AHA: ▶4Q, '11, 136◀

     727.62 Tendons of biceps (long head)

     727.63 Extensor tendons of hand and wrist

     727.64 Flexor tendons of hand and wrist

     727.65 Quadriceps tendon

     727.66 Patellar tendon

     727.67 Achilles tendon

     727.68 Other tendons of foot and ankle

     727.69 Other

√5ᵗʰ **727.8 Other disorders of synovium, tendon, and bursa**

     727.81 Contracture of tendon (sheath)
       Short Achilles tendon (acquired)

     727.82 Calcium deposits in tendon and bursa
       Calcification of tendon NOS
       Calcific tendinitis NOS
       EXCLUDES *peripheral ligamentous or muscular attachments (726.0-726.9)*

     727.83 Plica syndrome
       Plica knee
       DEF: A fold in the synovial tissue formed before birth, creating a septum between two pockets of synovial tissue; most common are the medial patellar plica and the suprapatellar plica. Plica syndrome, or plica knee, refers to symptomatic plica.
       AHA: 4Q, '00, 44

     727.89 Other
       Abscess of bursa or tendon
       EXCLUDES *xanthomatosis localized to tendons (272.7)*
       AHA: 2Q, '89, 15

     727.9 Unspecified disorder of synovium, tendon, and bursa

√4ᵗʰ **728 Disorders of muscle, ligament, and fascia**
     EXCLUDES *enthesopathies (726.0-726.9)*
         muscular dystrophies (359.0-359.1)
         myoneural disorders (358.00-358.9)
         myopathies (359.2-359.9)
         nontraumatic hematoma of muscle (729.92)
         old disruption of ligaments of knee (717.81-717.89)

     728.0 Infective myositis
       Myositis:
         purulent
         suppurative
       EXCLUDES *myositis:*
           epidemic (074.1)
           interstitial (728.81)
           syphilitic (095.6)
           tropical (040.81)
       DEF: Inflamed connective septal tissue of muscle.

√5ᵗʰ **728.1 Muscular calcification and ossification**

     728.10 Calcification and ossification, unspecified
       Massive calcification (paraplegic)

     728.11 Progressive myositis ossificans
       DEF: Progressive myositic disease; marked by bony tissue formed by voluntary muscle; occurs among very young.

√4ᵗʰ √5ᵗʰ   Additional Digit Required   Unspecified Code   Other Specified Code   Manifestation Code   ▶◀ Revised Text   ● New Code   ▲ Revised Code Title

2013 ICD-9-CM   **February 2012 · Volume 1 – 229**

Diseases of the Musculoskeletal System and Connective Tissue

728.12–729.6

728.12 Traumatic myositis ossificans
Myositis ossificans (circumscripta)

728.13 Postoperative heterotopic calcification
DEF: Abnormal formation of calcium deposits in muscular tissue after surgery, marked by a corresponding loss of muscle tone and tension.

728.19 Other
Polymyositis ossificans

728.2 Muscular wasting and disuse atrophy, not elsewhere classified
Amyotrophia NOS
Myofibrosis
EXCLUDES neuralgic amyotrophy (353.5)
pelvic muscle wasting and disuse atrophy (618.83)
progressive muscular atrophy (335.0-335.9)

728.3 Other specific muscle disorders
Arthrogryposis
Immobility syndrome (paraplegic)
EXCLUDES arthrogryposis multiplex congenita (754.89)
stiff-man syndrome (333.91)

728.4 Laxity of ligament

728.5 Hypermobility syndrome

728.6 Contracture of palmar fascia   [A]
Dupuytren's contracture
DEF: Dupuytren's contracture: flexion deformity of finger, due to shortened, thickened fibrosing of palmar fascia; cause unknown; associated with long-standing epilepsy.

√5ᵗʰ **728.7 Other fibromatoses**

728.71 Plantar fascial fibromatosis
Contracture of plantar fascia
Plantar fasciitis (traumatic)
DEF: Plantar fascia fibromatosis; causes nodular swelling and pain; not associated with contractures.

728.79 Other
Garrod's or knuckle pads
Nodular fasciitis
Pseudosarcomatous fibromatosis (proliferative) (subcutaneous)
DEF: Knuckle pads: Pea-size nodules on dorsal surface of interphalangeal joints; new growth of fibrous tissue with thickened dermis and epidermis.

√5ᵗʰ **728.8 Other disorders of muscle, ligament, and fascia**

728.81 Interstitial myositis
DEF: Inflammation of septal connective parts of muscle tissue.

728.82 Foreign body granuloma of muscle
Talc granuloma of muscle
Use additional code to identify foreign body (V90.01-V90.9)

728.83 Rupture of muscle, nontraumatic

728.84 Diastasis of muscle
Diastasis recti (abdomen)
EXCLUDES diastasis recti complicating pregnancy, labor, and delivery (665.8)
DEF: Muscle separation, such as recti abdominis after repeated pregnancies.

728.85 Spasm of muscle
M62.838 Other muscle spasm   [I-10]

728.86 Necrotizing fasciitis
Use additional code to identify:
gangrene (785.4), if applicable
infectious organism (041.00-041.89)
DEF: Fulminating infection begins with extensive cellulitis, spreads to superficial and deep fascia; causes thrombosis of subcutaneous vessels, and gangrene of underlying tissue.
AHA: 4Q, '95, 54

728.87 Muscle weakness (generalized)
EXCLUDES generalized weakness (780.79)
AHA: 1Q, '05, 13; 4Q, '03, 66
TIP: Assign an additional code from category 438 if the weakness is a result of a CVA.

728.88 Rhabdomyolysis
DEF: A disintegration or destruction of muscle; an acute disease characterized by the excretion of myoglobin into the urine.
AHA: 4Q, '03, 66

728.89 Other
Eosinophilic fasciitis
Use additional E code to identify drug, if drug induced
DEF: Eosinophilic fasciitis: inflammation of fascia of extremities associated with eosinophilia, edema, and swelling; occurs alone or as part of myalgia syndrome.
AHA: 3Q, '06, 13; 3Q, '02, 28; 2Q, '01, 14, 15

728.9 Unspecified disorder of muscle, ligament, and fascia

√4ᵗʰ **729 Other disorders of soft tissues**
EXCLUDES acroparesthesia (443.89)
carpal tunnel syndrome (354.0)
disorders of the back (720.0-724.9)
entrapment syndromes (354.0-355.9)
palindromic rheumatism (719.3)
periarthritis (726.0-726.9)
psychogenic rheumatism (306.0)

729.0 Rheumatism, unspecified and fibrositis
DEF: General term describes diseases of muscle, tendon, nerve, joint, or bone; symptoms include pain and stiffness.

729.1 Myalgia and myositis, unspecified
Fibromyositis NOS
DEF: Myalgia: muscle pain.
DEF: Myositis: inflamed voluntary muscle.
DEF: Fibromyositis: inflamed fibromuscular tissue.
M79.1 Myalgia   [I-10]

729.2 Neuralgia, neuritis, and radiculitis, unspecified
EXCLUDES brachial radiculitis (723.4)
cervical radiculitis (723.4)
lumbosacral radiculitis (724.4)
mononeuritis (354.0-355.9)
radiculitis due to intervertebral disc involvement (722.0-722.2, 722.7)
sciatica (724.3)
DEF: Neuralgia: paroxysmal pain along nerve; symptoms include brief pain and tenderness at point nerve exits.
DEF: Neuritis: inflamed nerve, symptoms include paresthesia, paralysis and loss of reflexes at nerve site.
DEF: Radiculitis: inflamed nerve root.

√5ᵗʰ **729.3 Panniculitis, unspecified**
DEF: Inflammatory reaction of subcutaneous fat; causes nodules; often develops in abdominal region.

729.30 Panniculitis, unspecified site
Weber-Christian disease
DEF: Febrile, nodular, nonsuppurative, relapsing inflammation of subcutaneous fat.

729.31 Hypertrophy of fat pad, knee
Hypertrophy of infrapatellar fat pad

729.39 Other site
EXCLUDES panniculitis specified as (affecting):
back (724.8)
neck (723.6)
sacral (724.8)
AHA: 2Q, '11, 3

729.4 Fasciitis, unspecified
EXCLUDES necrotizing fasciitis (728.86)
nodular fasciitis (728.79)
AHA: 2Q, '94, 13

729.5 Pain in limb
AHA: 2Q, '07, 11
M79.609 Pain in unspecified limb   [I-10]

729.6 Residual foreign body in soft tissue
Use additional code to identify foreign body (V90.01-V90.9)
EXCLUDES foreign body granuloma:
muscle (728.82)
skin and subcutaneous tissue (709.4)

[N]   Newborn Age: 0   [P]   Pediatric Age: 0-17   [M]   Maternity Age: 12-55   [A]   Adult Age: 15-124

✓5ᵗʰ 729.7 Nontraumatic compartment syndrome

Code first, if applicable, postprocedural complication (998.89)

EXCLUDES   *compartment syndrome NOS (958.90)*
traumatic compartment syndrome (958.90-958.99)

DEF: Compression of nerves and blood vessels within an enclosed space, leading to impaired blood flow and muscle and nerve damage.

729.71 Nontraumatic compartment syndrome of upper extremity

Nontraumatic compartment syndrome of shoulder, arm, forearm, wrist, hand, and fingers

AHA: 4Q, '06, 100-102

729.72 Nontraumatic compartment syndrome of lower extremity

Nontraumatic compartment syndrome of hip, buttock, thigh, leg, foot, and toes

AHA: 4Q, '06, 100-102

729.73 Nontraumatic compartment syndrome of abdomen

AHA: 4Q, '06, 100-102

729.79 Nontraumatic compartment syndrome of other sites

AHA: 4Q, '06, 100-102

✓5ᵗʰ 729.8 Other musculoskeletal symptoms referable to limbs

TIP: Assign for pseudothrombophlebitis, which involves painful swelling of the lower extremity and mimics deep vein thrombosis (DVT).

729.81 Swelling of limb

AHA: 4Q, '88, 6

TIP: Assign for hyperalgesic pseudothrombophlebitis, which involves painful swelling of the lower extremity and mimics deep vein thrombosis (DVT).

729.82 Cramp

729.89 Other

EXCLUDES   *abnormality of gait (781.2)*
tetany (781.7)
transient paralysis of limb (781.4)

AHA: 4Q, '88, 12

R29.898 Oth symptoms & signs involv musculo sys   [I-10]

✓5ᵗʰ 729.9 Other and unspecified disorders of soft tissue

AHA: 4Q, '08, 134-136

729.90 Disorders of soft tissue, unspecified

729.91 Post-traumatic seroma

EXCLUDES   *seroma complicating a procedure (998.13)*

729.92 Nontraumatic hematoma of soft tissue

Nontraumatic hematoma of muscle

AHA: 4Q, '08, 135

TIP: Assign an additional E code for a drug adverse effect if caused by Coumadin or other anticoagulants.

729.99 Other disorders of soft tissue

Polyalgia

Osteopathies, Chondropathies, and Acquired Musculoskeletal Deformities (730-739)

✓4ᵗʰ 730 Osteomyelitis, periostitis, and other infections involving bone

EXCLUDES   *jaw (526.4-526.5)*
petrous bone (383.2)

Use additional code to identify organism, such as Staphylococcus (041.1)

The following fifth-digit subclassification is for use with category 730; valid digits are in [brackets] under each code. See list at beginning of chapter for definitions.

  0 site unspecified
  1 shoulder region
  2 upper arm
  3 forearm
  4 hand
  5 pelvic region and thigh
  6 lower leg
  7 ankle and foot
  8 other specified sites
  9 multiple sites

DEF: Osteomyelitis: bacterial inflammation of bone tissue and marrow.
DEF: Periostitis: inflammation of specialized connective tissue; causes swelling of bone and aching pain.
AHA: 4Q, '97, 43

§ ✓5ᵗʰ **730.0 Acute osteomyelitis**
[0-9] Abscess of any bone except accessory sinus, jaw, or mastoid
  Acute or subacute osteomyelitis, with or without mention of periostitis

  Use additional code to identify major osseous defect, if applicable (731.3)

  AHA: 4Q, '06, 103; **For code 730.06:** 1Q, '02, 4; **For code 730.07:** 1Q, '04, 14

§ ✓5ᵗʰ **730.1 Chronic osteomyelitis**
[0-9] Brodie's abscess
  Chronic or old osteomyelitis, with or without mention of periostitis
  Sclerosing osteomyelitis of Garré
  Sequestrum of bone

  Use additional code to identify major osseous defect, if applicable (731.3)

  EXCLUDES   *aseptic necrosis of bone (733.40-733.49)*

  AHA: 4Q, '06, 103; **For code 730.17:** ▶3Q, '11, 15; ◀3Q, '00, 4

§ ✓5ᵗʰ **730.2 Unspecified osteomyelitis**
[0-9] Osteitis or osteomyelitis NOS, with or without mention of periostitis

  Use additional code to identify major osseous defect, if applicable (731.3)

  AHA: 4Q, '06, 103

  M86.9 Osteomyelitis unspecified   [I-10]

§ ✓5ᵗʰ **730.3 Periostitis without mention of osteomyelitis**
[0-9] Abscess of periosteum ⎫ without mention of
  Periostosis   ⎭ osteomyelitis

  EXCLUDES   *that in secondary syphilis (091.61)*

§ ✓5ᵗʰ **730.7 Osteopathy resulting from poliomyelitis**
[0-9] *Code first underlying disease (045.0-045.9)*

§ ✓5ᵗʰ **730.8 Other infections involving bone in diseases classified elsewhere**
[0-9] *Code first underlying disease as:*
    tuberculosis (015.0-015.9)
    typhoid fever (002.0)

  EXCLUDES   *syphilis of bone NOS (095.5)*

  AHA: 2Q, '97, 16; 3Q, '91, 10

§ ✓5ᵗʰ **730.9 Unspecified infection of bone**
[0-9]

---

§ Requires fifth digit. Valid digits are in [brackets] under each code. See beginning of section 710-739 for codes and defintions.

| ✓4ᵗʰ ✓5ᵗʰ Additional Digit Required | Unspecified Code | Other Specified Code | Manifestation Code | ▶◀ Revised Text | ● New Code | ▲ Revised Code Title |

Diseases of the Musculoskeletal System and Connective Tissue

731–733.03

✓4ᵗʰ 731 Osteitis deformans and osteopathies associated with other disorders classified elsewhere

DEF: Osteitis deformans: Bone disease marked by episodes of increased bone loss, excessive repair attempts; causes weakened, deformed bones with increased mass, bowed long bones, deformed flat bones, pain and pathological fractures; may be fatal if associated with congestive heart failure, giant cell tumors or bone sarcoma; also called Paget's disease.

731.0 Osteitis deformans without mention of bone tumor
Paget's disease of bone

731.1 Osteitis deformans in diseases classified elsewhere

Code first underlying disease as:
    malignant neoplasm of bone (170.0-170.9)

731.2 Hypertrophic pulmonary osteoarthropathy
Bamberger-Marie disease
DEF: Clubbing of fingers and toes; related to enlarged ends of long bones, due to chronic lung and heart disease.

731.3 Major osseous defects
Code first underlying disease, if known, such as:
    aseptic necrosis (733.40-733.49)
    malignant neoplasm of bone (170.0-170.9)
    osteomyelitis (730.00-730.29)
    osteoporosis (733.00-733.09)
    peri-prosthetic osteolysis (996.45)
AHA: 4Q, '06, 103

731.8 Other bone involvement in diseases classified elsewhere

Code first underlying disease as:
    diabetes mellitus (249.8, 250.8)

Use additional code to specify bone condition, such as:
    acute osteomyelitis (730.00-730.09)
AHA: 2Q, '10, 6; 1Q, '04, 14; 4Q, '97, 43; 2Q, '97, 16
TIP: For diabetic osteomyelitis, assign a total of three codes: 250.8X, 731.8, and a code from category 730.
M90.89 Osteopathy dz classified elsewhere multiple site   `I-10`

✓4ᵗʰ 732 Osteochondropathies
DEF: Conditions related to both bone and cartilage, or conditions in which cartilage is converted to bone (enchondral ossification).

732.0 Juvenile osteochondrosis of spine
Juvenile osteochondrosis (of):
    marginal or vertebral epiphysis (of Scheuermann)
    spine NOS
Vertebral epiphysitis
    EXCLUDES adolescent postural kyphosis (737.0)

732.1 Juvenile osteochondrosis of hip and pelvis
Coxa plana
Ischiopubic synchondrosis (of van Neck)
Osteochondrosis (juvenile) of:
    acetabulum
    head of femur (of Legg-Calvé-Perthes)
    iliac crest (of Buchanan)
    symphysis pubis (of Pierson)
Pseudocoxalgia

732.2 Nontraumatic slipped upper femoral epiphysis
Slipped upper femoral epiphysis NOS

732.3 Juvenile osteochondrosis of upper extremity
Osteochondrosis (juvenile) of:
    capitulum of humerus (of Panner)
    carpal lunate (of Kienbock)
    hand NOS
    head of humerus (of Haas)
    heads of metacarpals (of Mauclaire)
    lower ulna (of Burns)
    radial head (of Brailsford)
    upper extremity NOS

732.4 Juvenile osteochondrosis of lower extremity, excluding foot
Osteochondrosis (juvenile) of:
    lower extremity NOS
    primary patellar center (of Köhler)
    proximal tibia (of Blount)
    secondary patellar center (of Sinding-Larsen)
    tibial tubercle (of Osgood-Schlatter)
Tibia vara

Slipped Femoral Epiphysis

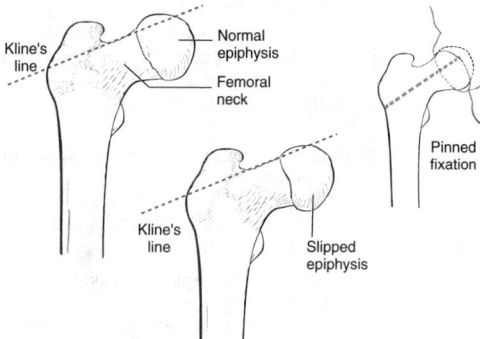

Kline's line — Normal epiphysis
Femoral neck
Pinned fixation
Kline's line — Slipped epiphysis

732.5 Juvenile osteochondrosis of foot
Calcaneal apophysitis
Epiphysitis, os calcis
Osteochondrosis (juvenile) of:
    astragalus (of Diaz)
    calcaneum (of Sever)
    foot NOS
    metatarsal
        second (of Freiberg)
        fifth (of Iselin)
    os tibiale externum (of Haglund)
    tarsal navicular (of Köhler)

732.6 Other juvenile osteochondrosis
Apophysitis
Epiphysitis   } specified as juvenile, of other
Osteochondritis   } site, or site NOS
Osteochondrosis

732.7 Osteochondritis dissecans

732.8 Other specified forms of osteochondropathy
Adult osteochondrosis of spine

732.9 Unspecified osteochondropathy
Apophysitis   } NOS
Epiphysitis   } not specified as adult or juvenile, of
Osteochondritis } unspecified site
Osteochondrosis

✓4ᵗʰ 733 Other disorders of bone and cartilage
EXCLUDES bone spur (726.91)
    cartilage of, or loose body in, joint (717.0-717.9, 718.0-718.9)
    giant cell granuloma of jaw (526.3)
    osteitis fibrosa cystica generalisata (252.01)
    osteomalacia (268.2)
    polyostotic fibrous dysplasia of bone (756.54)
    prognathism, retrognathism (524.1)
    xanthomatosis localized to bone (272.7)

✓5ᵗʰ 733.0 Osteoporosis
Use additional code to identify major osseous defect, if applicable (731.3)
Use additional code to identify personal history of pathologic (healed) fracture (V13.51)
DEF: Bone mass reduction that ultimately results in fractures after minimal trauma; dorsal kyphosis or loss of height often occur.
AHA: 4Q, '06, 103

733.00 Osteoporosis, unspecified
Wedging of vertebra NOS
AHA: 4Q, '07, 92;1Q, '07, 22; 3Q, '01, 19; 2Q, '98, 12
M81.8 Other osteoporosis w/o current pathological fx   `I-10`

733.01 Senile osteoporosis
Postmenopausal osteoporosis
AHA: 1Q, '07, 5, 6
M81.0 Age-related osteoporosis without current pathological fracture   `I-10`

733.02 Idiopathic osteoporosis

733.03 Disuse osteoporosis

733.09 Other
Drug-induced osteoporosis
Use additional E code to identify drug
AHA: 4Q, '03, 108
M81.6 Localized osteoporosis [Lequesne]   [I-10]

√5ᵗʰ 733.1 Pathologic fracture
Chronic fracture
Spontaneous fracture
EXCLUDES *stress fracture (733.93-733.95)*
traumatic fracture (800-829)
DEF: Fracture due to bone structure weakening by pathological
processes (e.g., osteoporosis, neoplasms and osteomalacia).
AHA: 4Q, '08, 158; 1Q, '07, 3-4; 4Q, '93, 25; N-D, '86, 10;
N-D, '85, 16
TIP: Assign only for newly diagnosed fractures; refer to V code
aftercare categories if patient is receiving routine care during
healing or recovery phase.

733.10 Pathologic fracture, unspecified site

733.11 Pathologic fracture of humerus
AHA: 2Q, '10, 6

733.12 Pathologic fracture of distal radius and ulna
Wrist NOS

733.13 Pathologic fracture of vertebrae
Collapse of vertebra NOS
AHA: 3Q, '08, 4; 1Q, '07, 5, 6, 22; 3Q, '99, 5
TIP: Assign for a chronic vertebral pathological fracture for
which the patient is receiving medication.
M48.53xA Collapsed vertebra NEC cervicothorac   [I-10]
initial enc

733.14 Pathologic fracture of neck of femur
Femur NOS
Hip NOS
AHA: 1Q, '01, 1; 1Q, '96, 16

**733.15 Pathologic fracture of other specified part of
femur**
AHA: 2Q, '98, 12
M84.453A Pathological fracture, unspec femur,   [I-10]
initial encounter for fx

733.16 Pathologic fracture of tibia or fibula
Ankle NOS

733.19 Pathologic fracture of other specified site

√5ᵗʰ 733.2 Cyst of bone

733.20 Cyst of bone (localized), unspecified

733.21 Solitary bone cyst
Unicameral bone cyst

733.22 Aneurysmal bone cyst
DEF: Solitary bone lesion, bulges into periosteum; marked
by calcified rim.

733.29 Other
Fibrous dysplasia (monostotic)
EXCLUDES *cyst of jaw (526.0-526.2, 526.89)*
osteitis fibrosa cystica (252.01)
polyostotic fibrousdyplasia of bone (756.54)

733.3 Hyperostosis of skull
Hyperostosis interna frontalis
Leontiasis ossium
DEF: Abnormal bone growth on inner aspect of cranial bones.

√5ᵗʰ 733.4 Aseptic necrosis of bone
Use additional code to identify major osseous defect, if
applicable (731.3)
EXCLUDES *osteochondropathies (732.0-732.9)*
DEF: Infarction of bone tissue due to a noninfectious etiology, such as
a fracture, ischemic disorder or administration of
immunosuppressive drugs; leads to degenerative joint disease or
nonunion of fractures.
AHA: 4Q, '06, 103

733.40 Aseptic necrosis of bone, site unspecified

733.41 Head of humerus

733.42 Head and neck of femur
Femur NOS
EXCLUDES *Legg-Calvé-Perthes disease (732.1)*
M87.256 Osteonecrosis due to previous   [I-10]
trauma uns femur

733.43 Medial femoral condyle

733.44 Talus

733.45 Jaw
Use additional E code to identify drug, if
drug-induced
EXCLUDES *osteoradionecrosis of jaw (526.89)*
AHA: 4Q, '07, 91

733.49 Other

733.5 Osteitis condensans
Piriform sclerosis of ilium
DEF: Idiopathic condition marked by low back pain; associated with
oval or triangular sclerotic, opaque bone next to sacroiliac joints in
the ileum.

733.6 Tietze's disease
Costochondral junction syndrome
Costochondritis
DEF: Painful, idiopathic, nonsuppurative, swollen costal cartilage
sometimes confused with cardiac symptoms because the anterior
chest pain resembles that of coronary artery disease.
M94.0 Chondrocostal junction syndrome (Tietze dz)   [I-10]

733.7 Algoneurodystrophy
Disuse atrophy of bone
Sudeck's atrophy
DEF: Painful, idiopathic complex reflex sympathetic dystrophy, a
chronic progressive disease characterized by severe pain, swelling,
and changes in the skin.

√5ᵗʰ 733.8 Malunion and nonunion of fracture
AHA: 2Q, '94, 5

733.81 Malunion of fracture

733.82 Nonunion of fracture
Pseudoarthrosis (bone)

√5ᵗʰ 733.9 Other unspecified disorders of bone and cartilage
AHA: 4Q, '08, 136-137

733.90 Disorder of bone and cartilage unspecified
M89.9 Disorder of bone, unspecified   [I-10]

733.91 Arrest of bone development or growth
Epiphyseal arrest

733.92 Chondromalacia
Chondromalacia:
NOS
localized, except patella
systemic
tibial plateau
EXCLUDES *chondromalacia of patella (717.7)*
DEF: Articular cartilage softening.

733.93 Stress fracture of tibia or fibula
Stress reaction of tibia or fibula
Use additional external cause code(s) to identify the
cause of the stress fracture
AHA: 4Q, '08, 158; 4Q, '01, 48

733.94 Stress fracture of the metatarsals
Stress reaction of metatarsals
Use additional external cause code(s) to identify the
cause of the stress fracture
AHA: 4Q, '08, 158; 4Q, '01, 48

733.95 Stress fracture of other bone
Stress reaction of other bone
Use additional external cause code(s) to identify the
cause of the stress fracture
EXCLUDES *stress fracture of:*
femoral neck (733.96)
fibula (733.93)
metatarsals (733.94)
pelvis (733.98)
shaft of femur (733.97)
tibia (733.93)
AHA: 4Q, '08, 158; 4Q, '01, 48

733.96 Stress fracture of femoral neck
Stress reaction of femoral neck

Use additional external cause code(s) to identify the cause of the stress fracture

AHA: 4Q, '08, 158

733.97 Stress fracture of shaft of femur
Stress reaction of shaft of femur

Use additional external cause code(s) to identify the cause of the stress fracture

AHA: 4Q, '08, 158

733.98 Stress fracture of pelvis
Stress reaction of pelvis

Use additional external cause code(s) to identify the cause of the stress fracture

AHA: 4Q, '08, 158

733.99 Other
Diaphysitis
Hypertrophy of bone
Relapsing polychondritis

AHA: 1Q, '11, 6; J-F, '87, 14

734 Flat foot
Pes planus (acquired)
Talipes planus (acquired)

EXCLUDES   congenital (754.61)
rigid flat foot (754.61)
spastic (everted) flat foot (754.61)

√4ᵗʰ 735 Acquired deformities of toe
EXCLUDES   congenital (754.60-754.69, 755.65-755.66)

735.0 Hallux valgus (acquired)
DEF: Angled displacement of the great toe, causing it to ride over or under other toes.

735.1 Hallux varus (acquired)
DEF: Angled displacement of the great toe toward the body midline, away from the other toes.

735.2 Hallux rigidus
DEF: Limited flexion movement at metatarsophalangeal joint of great toe; due to degenerative joint disease.

735.3 Hallux malleus
DEF: Extended proximal phalanx, flexed distal phalanges of great toe; foot resembles claw or hammer.

735.4 Other hammer toe (acquired)

735.5 Claw toe (acquired)
DEF: Hyperextended proximal phalanges, flexed middle and distal phalanges.

735.8 Other acquired deformities of toe
AHA: 4Q, '07, 123
TIP: Assign for hallux limitus, a deformity of the first metatarsophalangeal joint, which restricts the range of motion and can lead to stiffness and pain in the joint.

735.9 Unspecified acquired deformity of toe

√4ᵗʰ 736 Other acquired deformities of limbs
EXCLUDES   congenital (754.3-755.9)

√5ᵗʰ 736.0 Acquired deformities of forearm, excluding fingers

736.00 Unspecified deformity
Deformity of elbow, forearm, hand, or wrist (acquired) NOS

736.01 Cubitus valgus (acquired)
DEF: Deviation of the elbow away from the body midline upon extension; it occurs when the palm is turning outward.

736.02 Cubitus varus (acquired)
DEF: Elbow joint displacement angled laterally; when the forearm is extended, it is deviated toward the midline of the body; also called "gun stock" deformity.

736.03 Valgus deformity of wrist (acquired)
DEF: Abnormal angulation away from the body midline.

736.04 Varus deformity of wrist (acquired)
DEF: Abnormal angulation toward the body midline.

Acquired Deformities of Toe

Hallux valgus

Hallux varus

Hallux malleus
(hammer of big toe)

Hammertoe

Acquired Deformities of Forearm

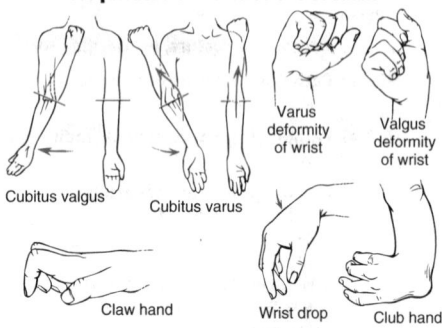

Varus deformity of wrist

Valgus deformity of wrist

Cubitus valgus

Cubitus varus

Claw hand

Wrist drop

Club hand

736.05 Wrist drop (acquired)
DEF: Inability to extend the hand at the wrist due to extensor muscle paralysis.

736.06 Claw hand (acquired)
DEF: Flexion and atrophy of the hand and fingers; found in ulnar nerve lesions, syringomyelia, and leprosy.

736.07 Club hand, acquired
DEF: Twisting of the hand out of shape or position; caused by the congenital absence of the ulna or radius.

736.09 Other

736.1 Mallet finger
DEF: Permanently flexed distal phalanx.

√5ᵗʰ 736.2 Other acquired deformities of finger

736.20 Unspecified deformity
Deformity of finger (acquired) NOS

736.21 Boutonniere deformity
DEF: A deformity of the finger caused by flexion of the proximal interphalangeal joint and hyperextension of the distal joint; also called buttonhole deformity.

736.22 Swan-neck deformity
DEF: Flexed distal and hyperextended proximal interphalangeal joint.

736.29 Other
EXCLUDES   trigger finger (727.03)
AHA: 2Q, '05, 7; 2Q, '89, 13

√5ᵗʰ 736.3 Acquired deformities of hip

736.30 Unspecified deformity
Deformity of hip (acquired) NOS

736.31 Coxa valga (acquired)
DEF: Increase of at least 140 degrees in the angle formed by the axis of the head and the neck of the femur, and the axis of its shaft.

736.32 Coxa vara (acquired)
DEF: The bending downward of the neck of the femur, causing difficulty in movement; a right angle or less may be formed by the axis of the head and neck of the femur, and the axis of its shaft.

736.39 Other
AHA: 2Q, '08, 4; 2Q, '91, 18
TIP: Assign as principal diagnosis for follow-up visit for patient with hip methylmethacrylate cement spacer, following removal of infected joint prosthesis.

Deformities of Lower Limb

Kyphosis and Lordosis

✓5ᵗʰ **736.4 Genu valgum or varum (acquired)**

    736.41 Genu valgum (acquired)
        DEF: Abnormally close together and an abnormally large space between the ankles; also called "knock-knees."

    736.42 Genu varum (acquired)
        DEF: Abnormally separated knees and the inward bowing of the legs; it is also called "bowlegs."

736.5 Genu recurvatum (acquired)
    DEF: Hyperextended knees; also called "backknee."

736.6 Other acquired deformities of knee
    Deformity of knee (acquired) NOS

✓5ᵗʰ **736.7 Other acquired deformities of ankle and foot**
    EXCLUDES deformities of toe (acquired) (735.0-735.9)
                 pes planus (acquired) (734)

    736.70 Unspecified deformity of ankle and foot, acquired

    736.71 Acquired equinovarus deformity
        Clubfoot, acquired
        EXCLUDES clubfoot not specified as acquired (754.5-754.7)

    736.72 Equinus deformity of foot, acquired
        DEF: A plantar flexion deformity that forces people to walk on their toes.

    736.73 Cavus deformity of foot
        EXCLUDES that with claw foot (736.74)
        DEF: Abnormally high longitudinal arch of the foot.

    736.74 Claw foot, acquired
        DEF: High foot arch with hyperextended toes at metatarsophalangeal joint and flexed toes at distal joints; also called "main en griffe."

    736.75 Cavovarus deformity of foot, acquired
        DEF: Inward turning of the heel from the midline of the leg and an abnormally high longitudinal arch.

    736.76 Other calcaneus deformity

    736.79 Other
        Acquired:
           pes
           talipes   } not elsewhere classified

✓5ᵗʰ **736.8 Acquired deformities of other parts of limbs**

    736.81 Unequal leg length (acquired)

    736.89 Other
        Deformity (acquired):
           arm or leg, not elsewhere classified
           shoulder
        AHA: 2Q, '08, 5
        TIP: Assign as principal diagnosis for follow-up visit for patient with humeral methylmethacrylate cement spacer, following removal of infected joint prosthesis.

736.9 Acquired deformity of limb, site unspecified

✓4ᵗʰ **737 Curvature of spine**
    EXCLUDES congenital (754.2)

    737.0 Adolescent postural kyphosis
        EXCLUDES osteochondrosis of spine (juvenile) (732.0)
                 adult (732.8)

✓5ᵗʰ   **737.1 Kyphosis (acquired)**

    737.10 Kyphosis (acquired) (postural)
        M40.05 Postural kyphosis thoracolumbar region   [I-10]

    737.11 Kyphosis due to radiation

    737.12 Kyphosis, postlaminectomy
        AHA: J-F, '87, 7
        M96.3 Postlaminectomy kyphosis   [I-10]

    737.19 Other
        EXCLUDES that associated with conditions classifiable elsewhere (737.41)
        AHA: 1Q, '07, 20

✓5ᵗʰ   **737.2 Lordosis (acquired)**
    DEF: Swayback appearance created by an abnormally increased spinal curvature; it is also referred to as "hollow back" or "saddle back."

    737.20 Lordosis (acquired) (postural)

    737.21 Lordosis, postlaminectomy

    737.22 Other postsurgical lordosis

    737.29 Other
        EXCLUDES that associated with conditions classifiable elsewhere (737.42)

✓5ᵗʰ   **737.3 Kyphoscoliosis and scoliosis**
    DEF: Kyphoscoliosis: backward and lateral curvature of the spinal column; it is found in vertebral osteochondrosis.
    DEF: Scoliosis: an abnormal deviation of the spine to the left or right of the midline.

    737.30 Scoliosis [and kyphoscoliosis], idiopathic
        AHA: 3Q, '03, 19
        M41.115 Juvenile idiopathic scoliosis thoracolumbar region   [I-10]

    737.31 Resolving infantile idiopathic scoliosis

    737.32 Progressive infantile idiopathic scoliosis
        AHA: 3Q, '02, 12

Scoliosis and Kyphoscoliosis

Scoliosis   Kyphoscoliosis

✓4ᵗʰ / ✓5ᵗʰ Additional Digit Required   Unspecified Code   Other Specified Code   Manifestation Code   ▶◀ Revised Text   ● New Code   ▲ Revised Code Title

2013 ICD-9-CM   **Volume 1 – 235**

Diseases of the Musculoskeletal System and Connective Tissue

737.33–739.9

737.33 Scoliosis due to radiation

737.34 Thoracogenic scoliosis

737.39 Other

> **EXCLUDES** *that associated with conditions classifiable elsewhere (737.43)*
> *that in kyphoscoliotic heart disease (416.1)*
>
> **AHA:** 2Q, '02, 16

√5ᵗʰ **737.4 Curvature of spine associated with other conditions**

> *Code first associated condition as:*
> Charcôt-Marie-Tooth disease (356.1)
> mucopolysaccharidosis (277.5)
> neurofibromatosis (237.70-237.79)
> osteitis deformans (731.0)
> osteitis fibrosa cystica (252.01)
> osteoporosis (733.00-733.09)
> poliomyelitis (138)
> tuberculosis [Pott's curvature] (015.0)

737.40 Curvature of spine, unspecified

737.41 Kyphosis

737.42 Lordosis

737.43 Scoliosis

737.8 Other curvatures of spine

737.9 Unspecified curvature of spine

> Curvature of spine (acquired) (idiopathic) NOS
> Hunchback, acquired
> **EXCLUDES** *deformity of spine NOS (738.5)*

√4ᵗʰ **738 Other acquired deformity**

> **EXCLUDES** *congenital (754.0-756.9, 758.0-759.9)*
> *dentofacial anomalies (524.0-524.9)*

738.0 Acquired deformity of nose

> Deformity of nose (acquired)
> Overdevelopment of nasal bones
> **EXCLUDES** *deflected or deviated nasal septum (470)*

√5ᵗʰ **738.1 Other acquired deformity of head**

738.10 Unspecified deformity

738.11 Zygomatic hyperplasia

> **DEF:** Abnormal enlargement of the zygoma (processus zygomaticus temporalis).

738.12 Zygomatic hypoplasia

> **DEF:** Underdevelopment of the zygoma (processus zygomaticus temporalis).

738.19 Other specified deformity

> **AHA:** 1Q, '06, 8; 2Q, '03, 13

738.2 Acquired deformity of neck

738.3 Acquired deformity of chest and rib

> Deformity:
> chest (acquired)
> rib (acquired)
> Pectus:
> carinatum, acquired
> excavatum, acquired

738.4 Acquired spondylolisthesis

> Degenerative spondylolisthesis
> Spondylolysis, acquired
> **EXCLUDES** *congenital (756.12)*
> **DEF:** Vertebra displaced forward over another; due to bilateral defect in vertebral arch, eroded articular surface of posterior facets and elongated pedicle between fifth lumbar vertebra and sacrum.
> **AHA:** 4Q, '07, 120; 1Q, '07, 10
> **M43.10** Spondylolisthesis site unspecified `I-10`

738.5 Other acquired deformity of back or spine

> Deformity of spine NOS
> **EXCLUDES** *curvature of spine (737.0-737.9)*
> **AHA:** 1Q, '08, 11
> **TIP:** Assign for post procedural flat back syndrome, which may be the result of a previous spinal fusion surgery. Do not assign a surgical complication code.

738.6 Acquired deformity of pelvis

> Pelvic obliquity
> **EXCLUDES** *intrapelvic protrusion of acetabulum (718.6)*
> *that in relation to labor and delivery (653.0-653.4, 653.8-653.9)*
> **DEF:** Pelvic obliquity: slanting or inclination of the pelvis at an angle between 55 and 60 degrees between the plane of the pelvis and the horizontal plane.

738.7 Cauliflower ear

> **DEF:** Abnormal external ear; due to injury, subsequent perichondritis.

738.8 Acquired deformity of other specified site

> Deformity of clavicle
> **AHA:** 2Q, '01, 15

738.9 Acquired deformity of unspecified site

√4ᵗʰ **739 Nonallopathic lesions, not elsewhere classified**

> **INCLUDES** segmental dysfunction
> somatic dysfunction
> **DEF:** Disability, loss of function or abnormality of a body part that is neither classifiable to a particular system nor brought about therapeutically to counteract another disease.

739.0 Head region

> Occipitocervical region

739.1 Cervical region

> Cervicothoracic region

739.2 Thoracic region

> Thoracolumbar region

739.3 Lumbar region

> Lumbosacral region

739.4 Sacral region

> Sacrococcygeal region
> Sacroiliac region

739.5 Pelvic region

> Hip region
> Pubic region

739.6 Lower extremities

739.7 Upper extremities

> Acromioclavicular region
> Sternoclavicular region

739.8 Rib cage

> Costochondral region
> Costovertebral region
> Sternochondral region

739.9 Abdomen and other

> **AHA:** 2Q, '89, 14

N Newborn Age: 0   P Pediatric Age: 0-17   M Maternity Age: 12-55   A Adult Age: 15-124

14. Congenital Anomalies (740-759)

TIP: Codes from chapter 14 may be assigned throughout the life of the patient, whenever the congenital anomaly is diagnosed.

√4ᵗʰ 740　Anencephalus and similar anomalies

740.0　Anencephalus
　　Acrania
　　Amyelencephalus
　　Hemicephaly
　　Hemianencephaly
　　DEF: Fetus without cerebrum, cerebellum and flat bones of skull.

740.1　Craniorachischisis
　　DEF: Congenital slit in cranium and vertebral column.

740.2　Iniencephaly
　　DEF: Spinal cord passes through enlarged occipital bone (foramen magnum); absent vertebral bone layer and spinal processes; resulting in both reduction in number and proper fusion of the vertebrae.

√4ᵗʰ 741　Spina bifida

　　EXCLUDES spina bifida occulta (756.17)

　　The following fifth-digit subclassification is for use with category 741:
　　　　0　unspecified region
　　　　1　cervical region
　　　　2　dorsal [thoracic] region
　　　　3　lumbar region

　　DEF: Lack of closure of spinal cord's bony encasement; marked by cord protrusion into lumbosacral area; evident by elevated alpha-fetoprotein of amniotic fluid.
　　AHA: 3Q, '94, 7
　　TIP: For Arnold-Chiari syndrome, Type I, refer to code 348.4.

§ √5ᵗʰ 741.0　With hydrocephalus
　　[0-3]　Arnold-Chiari syndrome, type II
　　　　Chiari malformation, type II
　　　　Any condition classifiable to 741.9 with any condition classifiable to 742.3
　　　　AHA: 4Q, '97, 51; 4Q, '94, 37; S-O, '87, 10
　　　　Q05.4 Unspecified spina bifida with hydrocephalus　　I-10

§ √5ᵗʰ 741.9　Without mention of hydrocephalus
　　[0-3]　Hydromeningocele (spinal)
　　　　Hydromyelocele
　　　　Meningocele (spinal)
　　　　Meningomyelocele
　　　　Myelocele
　　　　Myelocystocele
　　　　Rachischisis
　　　　Spina bifida (aperta)
　　　　Syringomyelocele
　　　　Q05.8 Sacral spina bifida without hydrocephalus　　I-10

√4ᵗʰ 742　Other congenital anomalies of nervous system
　　EXCLUDES congenital central alveolar hypoventilation syndrome (327.25)

742.0　Encephalocele
　　Encephalocystocele
　　Encephalomyelocele
　　Hydroencephalocele
　　Hydromeningocele, cranial
　　Meningocele, cerebral
　　Meningoencephalocele
　　DEF: Brain tissue protrudes through skull defect.
　　AHA: 4Q, '94, 37

742.1　Microcephalus
　　Hydromicrocephaly
　　Micrencephaly
　　DEF: Extremely small head or brain.

Spina Bifida

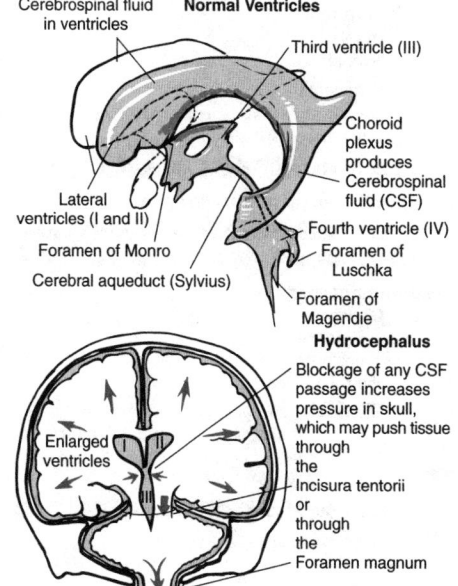

742.2　Reduction deformities of brain
　　Absence
　　Agenesis ⎫
　　Aplasia　⎬ of part of brain
　　Hypoplasia ⎭

　　Agyria
　　Arhinencephaly
　　Holoprosencephaly
　　Microgyria
　　AHA: 3Q, '03, 15; 4Q, '94, 37
　　TIP: Assign for septo-optic dysplasia.

742.3　Congenital hydrocephalus
　　Aqueduct of Sylvius:
　　　　anomaly
　　　　obstruction, congenital
　　　　stenosis
　　Atresia of foramina of Magendie and Luschka
　　Hydrocephalus in newborn
　　EXCLUDES hydrocephalus:
　　　　acquired (331.3-331.4)
　　　　due to congenital toxoplasmosis (771.2)
　　　　with any condition classifiable to 741.9 (741.0)
　　DEF: Fluid accumulation within the skull; involves subarachnoid (external) or ventricular (internal) brain spaces.
　　AHA: 4Q, '05, 83
　　Q03.9 Congenital hydrocephalus unspecified　　I-10

742.4　Other specified anomalies of brain
　　Congenital cerebral cyst　　　Multiple anomalies of brain NOS
　　Macroencephaly　　　　　　　Porencephaly
　　Macrogyria　　　　　　　　　　Ulegyria
　　Megalencephaly
　　AHA: 1Q, '99, 9; 3Q, '92, 12

Normal Ventricles and Hydrocephalus

§ Requires fifth digit. Valid digits are in [brackets] under each code. See category 741 for codes and definitions.

√4ᵗʰ Additional Digit Required　　Unspecified Code　　Other Specified Code　　Manifestation Code　　▶◀ Revised Text　　● New Code　　▲ Revised Code Title
√5ᵗʰ

2013 ICD-9-CM　　　**Volume 1 – 237**

Congenital Anomalies

742.5–743.59

√5ᵗʰ **742.5 Other specified anomalies of spinal cord**

    742.51 Diastematomyelia
        DEF: Congenital anomaly often associated with spina bifida; the spinal cord is separated into halves by a bony tissue resembling a "spike" (a spicule), each half surrounded by a dural sac.

    742.53 Hydromyelia
        Hydrorhachis
        DEF: Dilated central spinal cord canal; characterized by increased fluid accumulation.

    742.59 Other
        Amyelia
        Atelomyelia
        Congenital anomaly of spinal meninges
        Defective development of cauda equina
        Hypoplasia of spinal cord
        Myelatelia
        Myelodysplasia
        AHA: 2Q, '91, 14; 1Q, '89, 10
        TIP: Assign for tethered spinal cord syndrome, regardless of when it is diagnosed.

742.8 Other specified anomalies of nervous system
    Agenesis of nerve
    Displacement of brachial plexus
    Familial dysautonomia
    Jaw-winking syndrome
    Marcus-Gunn syndrome
    Riley-Day syndrome
      EXCLUDES neurofibromatosis (237.70-237.79)

742.9 Unspecified anomaly of brain, spinal cord, and nervous system
    Anomaly
    Congenital: brain
      disease   of: nervous system
      lesion   spinal cord
    Deformity

√4ᵗʰ **743 Congenital anomalies of eye**

√5ᵗʰ **743.0 Anophthalmos**
    DEF: Complete absence of the eyes or the presence of vestigial eyes.

    743.00 Clinical anophthalmos, unspecified
        Agenesis
        Cogenital absence   of eye
        Anophthalmos NOS

    743.03 Cystic eyeball, congenital

    743.06 Cryptophthalmos
        DEF: Skin is continuous over eyeball, results in apparent absence of eyelids.

√5ᵗʰ **743.1 Microphthalmos**
    Dysplasia
    Hypoplasia   of eye
    Rudimentary eye
    DEF: Abnormally small eyeballs, may be opacities of cornea and lens; scarring of choroid and retina.

    743.10 Microphthalmos, unspecified

    743.11 Simple microphthalmos

    743.12 Microphthalmos associated with other anomalies of eye and adnexa

√5ᵗʰ **743.2 Buphthalmos**
    Glaucoma:
      congenital
      newborn
    Hydrophthalmos
      EXCLUDES glaucoma of childhood (365.14)
                   traumatic glaucoma due to birth injury (767.8)
    DEF: Distended, enlarged fibrous coats of eye; due to intraocular pressure of congenital glaucoma.

    743.20 Buphthalmos, unspecified

    743.21 Simple buphthalmos

    743.22 Buphthalmos associated with other ocular anomalies
        Keratoglobus, cogenital
                      associated with buphthalmos
        Megalocornea

√5ᵗʰ **743.3 Congenital cataract and lens anomalies**
      EXCLUDES infantile cataract (366.00-366.09)
    DEF: Opaque eye lens.

    743.30 Congenital cataract, unspecified

    743.31 Capsular and subcapsular cataract

    743.32 Cortical and zonular cataract

    743.33 Nuclear cataract

    743.34 Total and subtotal cataract, congenital

    743.35 Congenital aphakia
        Congenital absence of lens

    743.36 Anomalies of lens shape
        Microphakia
        Spherophakia

    743.37 Congenital ectopic lens

    743.39 Other

√5ᵗʰ **743.4 Coloboma and other anomalies of anterior segment**
    DEF: Coloboma: ocular tissue defect associated with defect of ocular fetal intraocular fissure; may cause small pit on optic disk, major defects of iris, ciliary body, choroid, and retina.

    743.41 Anomalies of corneal size and shape
        Microcornea
        EXCLUDES that associated with buphthalmos (743.22)

    743.42 Corneal opacities, interfering with vision, congenital

    743.43 Other corneal opacities, congenital

    743.44 Specified anomalies of anterior chamber, chamber angle, and related structures
        Anomaly:
          Axenfeld's
          Peters'
          Rieger's

    743.45 Aniridia
        DEF: Incompletely formed or absent iris; affects both eyes; dominant trait; also called congenital absence of iris.
        AHA: 2Q, '10, 4-5; 3Q, '02, 20

    743.46 Other specified anomalies of iris and ciliary body
        Anisocoria, congenital
        Atresia of pupil
        Coloboma of iris
        Corectopia

    743.47 Specified anomalies of sclera

    743.48 Multiple and combined anomalies of anterior segment

    743.49 Other

√5ᵗʰ **743.5 Congenital anomalies of posterior segment**

    743.51 Vitreous anomalies
        Congenital vitreous opacity

    743.52 Fundus coloboma
        DEF: Absent retinal and choroidal tissue; occurs in lower fundus; a bright white ectatic zone of exposed sclera extends into and changes the optic disk.

    743.53 Chorioretinal degeneration, congenital

    743.54 Congenital folds and cysts of posterior segment

    743.55 Congenital macular changes

    743.56 Other retinal changes, congenital
        AHA: 3Q, '99, 12

    743.57 Specified anomalies of optic disc
        Coloboma of optic disc (congenital)

    743.58 Vascular anomalies
        Congenital retinal aneurysm

    743.59 Other

☑5ᵗʰ **743.6 Congenital anomalies of eyelids, lacrimal system, and orbit**

743.61 Congenital ptosis
DEF: Drooping of eyelid.

743.62 Congenital deformities of eyelids
Ablepharon
Absence of eyelid
Accessory eyelid
Congenital:
  ectropion
  entropion
AHA: 1Q, '00, 22
TIP: Assign for epiblepharon, in which a redundant horizontal skin fold under the eyelid causes an abnormal vertical orientation of the eyelashes; may result in the eyelashes touching the eyeball.

743.63 Other specified congenital anomalies of eyelid
Absence, agenesis, of cilia

743.64 Specified congenital anomalies of lacrimal gland

743.65 Specified congenital anomalies of lacrimal passages
Absence, agenesis of:
  lacrimal apparatus
  punctum lacrimale
Accessory lacrimal canal

743.66 Specified congenital anomalies of orbit

743.69 Other
Accessory eye muscles

743.8 Other specified anomalies of eye
EXCLUDES congenital nystagmus (379.51)
ocular albinism (270.2)
optic nerve hypoplasia (377.43)
retinitis pigmentosa (362.74)

743.9 Unspecified anomaly of eye
Congenital:
  anomaly NOS ⎱ of eye (any part)
  deformity NOS ⎰

☑4ᵗʰ **744 Congenital anomalies of ear, face, and neck**
EXCLUDES anomaly of:
cervical spine (754.2, 756.10-756.19)
larynx (748.2-748.3)
nose (748.0-748.1)
parathyroid gland (759.2)
thyroid gland (759.2)
cleft lip (749.10-749.25)

☑5ᵗʰ **744.0 Anomalies of ear causing impairment of hearing**
EXCLUDES congenital deafness without mention of cause (389.0-389.9)

744.00 Unspecified anomaly of ear with impairment of hearing

744.01 Absence of external ear
Absence of:
  auditory canal (external)
  auricle (ear) (with stenosis or atresia of auditory canal)

744.02 Other anomalies of external ear with impairment of hearing
Atresia or stricture of auditory canal (external)

744.03 Anomaly of middle ear, except ossicles
Atresia or stricture of osseous meatus (ear)

744.04 Anomalies of ear ossicles
Fusion of ear ossicles

744.05 Anomalies of inner ear
Congenital anomaly of:
  membranous labyrinth
  organ of Corti

744.09 Other
Absence of ear, congenital

744.1 Accessory auricle
Accessory tragus   Supernumerary:
Polyotia   ear
Preauricular appendage   lobule
DEF: Redundant tissue or structures of ear.

☑5ᵗʰ **744.2 Other specified anomalies of ear**
EXCLUDES that with impairment of hearing (744.00-744.09)

744.21 Absence of ear lobe, congenital

744.22 Macrotia
DEF: Abnormally large pinna of ear.

744.23 Microtia
DEF: Hypoplasia of pinna; associated with absent or closed auditory canal.

744.24 Specified anomalies of Eustachian tube
Absence of Eustachian tube

744.29 Other
Bat ear
Darwin's tubercle
Pointed ear
Prominence of auricle
Ridge ear
EXCLUDES preauricular sinus (744.46)

744.3 Unspecified anomaly of ear
Congenital:
  anomaly NOS ⎱ of ear, not elsewhere
  deformity NOS ⎰   classified

☑5ᵗʰ **744.4 Branchial cleft cyst or fistula; preauricular sinus**

744.41 Branchial cleft sinus or fistula
Branchial:
  sinus (external) (internal)
  vestige
DEF: Cyst due to failed closure of embryonic branchial cleft.

744.42 Branchial cleft cyst

744.43 Cervical auricle

744.46 Preauricular sinus or fistula

744.47 Preauricular cyst

744.49 Other
Fistula (of):
  auricle, congenital
  cervicoaural

744.5 Webbing of neck
Pterygium colli
DEF: Thick, triangular skinfold, stretches from lateral side of neck across shoulder; associated with Turner's and Noonan's syndromes.

☑5ᵗʰ **744.8 Other specified anomalies of face and neck**

744.81 Macrocheilia
Hypertrophy of lip, congenital
DEF: Abnormally large lips.

744.82 Microcheilia
DEF: Abnormally small lips.

744.83 Macrostomia
DEF: Bilateral or unilateral anomaly of mouth due to malformed maxillary and mandibular processes; results in mouth extending toward ear.

744.84 Microstomia
DEF: Abnormally small mouth.

744.89 Other
EXCLUDES congenital fistula of lip (750.25)
musculoskeletal anomalies (754.0-754.1, 756.0)

744.9 Unspecified anomalies of face and neck
Congenital:
  anomaly NOS ⎱ of face [any part] or neck [any
  deformity NOS ⎰   part]

Congenital Anomalies

745–746.7

☑4ᵗʰ 745 Bulbus cordis anomalies and anomalies of cardiac septal closure

745.0 Common truncus

Absent septum ⎫ between aorta and
Communication (abnormal) ⎬ pulmonary artery

Aortic septal defect
Common aortopulmonary trunk
Persistent truncus arteriosus

☑5ᵗʰ 745.1 Transposition of great vessels

745.10 Complete transposition of great vessels

Transposition of great vessels:
NOS
classical

745.11 Double outlet right ventricle

Dextratransposition of aorta
Incomplete transposition of great vessels
Origin of both great vessels from right ventricle
Taussig-Bing syndrome or defect

745.12 Corrected transposition of great vessels

745.19 Other

745.2 Tetralogy of Fallot

Fallot's pentalogy
Ventricular septal defect with pulmonary stenosis or atresia,
dextraposition of aorta, and hypertrophy of right
ventricle

EXCLUDES *Fallot's triad (746.09)*

DEF: Obstructed cardiac outflow causes pulmonary stenosis,
interventricular septal defect and right ventricular hypertrophy.

745.3 Common ventricle

Cor triloculare biatriatum
Single ventricle

745.4 Ventricular septal defect

Eisenmenger's defect or complex
Gerbo dedefect
Interventricular septal defect
Left ventricular-right atrial communication
Roger's disease

EXCLUDES *common atrioventricular canal type (745.69)*
single ventricle (745.3)

Q21.0 Ventricular septal defect   I-10

745.5 Ostium secundum type atrial septal defect

Defect: Patent or persistent:
   atrium secundum   foramen ovale
   fossa ovalis   ostium secundum
Lutembacher's syndrome

DEF: Opening in atrial septum due to failure of the septum
secundum and the endocardial cushions to fuse; there is a rim of
septum surrounding the defect.

AHA: 3Q, '09, 17; 3Q, '09, 17

Q21.1 Atrial septal defect   I-10

☑5ᵗʰ 745.6 Endocardial cushion defects

DEF: Atrial and/or ventricular septal defects causing abnormal fusion
of cushions in atrioventricular canal.

745.60 Endocardial cushion defect, unspecified type

DEF: Septal defect due to imperfect fusion of endocardial
cushions.

Heart Defects

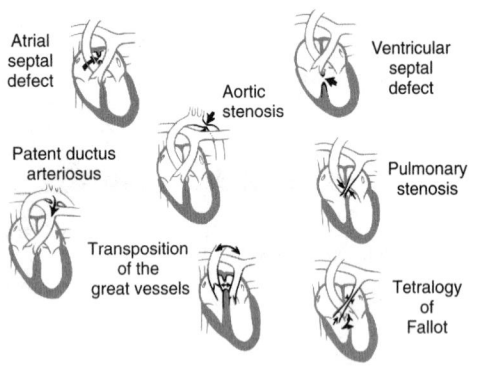

Atrial septal defect
Ventricular septal defect
Aortic stenosis
Patent ductus arteriosus
Pulmonary stenosis
Transposition of the great vessels
Tetralogy of Fallot

745.61 Ostium primum defect

Persistent ostium primum

DEF: Opening in low, posterior septum primum; causes cleft
in basal portion of atrial septum; associated with cleft
mitral valve.

745.69 Other

Absence of atrial septum
Atrioventricular canal type ventricular septal defect
Common atrioventricular canal
Common atrium

745.7 Cor biloculare

Absence of atrial and ventricular septa

DEF: Atrial and ventricular septal defect; marked by heart with two
cardiac chambers (one atrium, one ventricle), and one
atrioventricular valve.

745.8 Other

745.9 Unspecified defect of septal closure

Septal defect NOS

☑4ᵗʰ 746 Other congenital anomalies of heart

EXCLUDES *endocardial fibroelastosis (425.3)*

☑5ᵗʰ 746.0 Anomalies of pulmonary valve

EXCLUDES *infundibular or subvalvular pulmonic stenosis*
(746.83)
tetralogy of Fallot (745.2)

746.00 Pulmonary valve anomaly, unspecified

746.01 Atresia, congenital

Congenital absence of pulmonary valve

746.02 Stenosis, congenital

DEF: Stenosis of opening between pulmonary artery and
right ventricle; causes obstructed blood outflow from right
ventricle.

746.09 Other

Congenital insufficiency of pulmonary valve
Fallot's triad or trilogy

746.1 Tricuspid atresia and stenosis, congenital

Absence of tricuspid valve

746.2 Ebstein's anomaly

DEF: Malformation of the tricuspid valve characterized by septal and
posterior leaflets attaching to the wall of the right ventricle; causing
the right ventricle to fuse with the atrium into a large right atrium
and a small ventricle; causes heart failure and abnormal cardiac
rhythm.

746.3 Congenital stenosis of aortic valve

Congenital aortic stenosis

EXCLUDES *congenital:*
subaortic stenosis (746.81)
supravalvular aortic stenosis (747.22)

DEF: Stenosis of orifice of aortic valve; obstructs blood outflow from
left ventricle.

AHA: 4Q, '88, 8

746.4 Congenital insufficiency of aortic valve

Bicuspid aortic valve
Congenital aortic insufficiency

DEF: Impaired functioning of aortic valve due to incomplete closure;
causes backflow (regurgitation) of blood from aorta to left ventricle.

Q23.1 Congenital insufficiency of aortic valve   I-10

746.5 Congenital mitral stenosis

Fused commissure ⎫
Parachute deformity ⎬ of mitral valve
Supernumerary cusps ⎭

DEF: Stenosis of left atrioventricular orifice.

AHA: 3Q, '07, 3

746.6 Congenital mitral insufficiency

DEF: Impaired functioning of mitral valve due to incomplete closure;
causes backflow of blood from left ventricle to left atrium.

746.7 Hypoplastic left heart syndrome

Atresia, or marked hypoplasia, of aortic orifice or valve, with
hypoplasia of ascending aorta and defective
development of left ventricle (with mitral valve atresia)

Ⓝ Newborn Age: 0   Ⓟ Pediatric Age: 0-17   Ⓜ Maternity Age: 12-55   Ⓐ Adult Age: 15-124

√5ᵗʰ **746.8 Other specified anomalies of heart**

746.81 Subaortic stenosis
>**DEF:** Stenosis, of left ventricular outflow tract due to fibrous tissue ring or septal hypertrophy below aortic valve.
>**AHA:** 3Q, '07, 3

746.82 Cor triatriatum
>**DEF:** Transverse septum divides left atrium due to failed resorption of embryonic common pulmonary vein; results in three atrial chambers.

746.83 Infundibular pulmonic stenosis
>Subvalvular pulmonic stenosis
>**DEF:** Stenosis of right ventricle outflow tract within infundibulum due to fibrous diaphragm below valve or long, narrow fibromuscular channel.

746.84 Obstructive anomalies of heart, not elsewhere classified
>Shone's syndrome
>Uhl's disease
>Use additional code for associated anomalies, such as:
>coarctation of aorta (747.10)
>congenital mitral stenosis (746.5)
>subaortic stenosis (746.81)

746.85 Coronary artery anomaly
>Anomalous origin or communication of coronary artery
>Arteriovenous malformation of coronary artery
>Coronary artery:
>absence
>arising from aorta or pulmonary trunk
>single
>**AHA:** N-D, '85, 3

746.86 Congenital heart block
>Complete or incomplete atrioventricular [AV] block
>**DEF:** Impaired conduction of electrical impulses; due to maldeveloped junctional tissue.

746.87 Malposition of heart and cardiac apex
>Abdominal heart
>Dextrocardia
>Ectopia cordis
>Levocardia (isolated)
>Mesocardia
>**EXCLUDES** dextrocardia with complete transposition of viscera (759.3)

746.89 Other
>Atresia ⎱
>Hypoplasia ⎰ of cardiac vein
>Congenital:
>cardiomegaly
>diverticulum, left ventricle
>pericardial defect
>**AHA:** 3Q, '00, 3; 1Q, '99, 11; J-F, '85, 3
>**TIP:** Assign for Brugada syndrome. Additional codes may be required.
>**Q24.8** Oth specified congenital malformations of heart I-10

746.9 Unspecified anomaly of heart
>Congenital:
>anomaly of heart NOS
>heart disease NOS

√4ᵗʰ **747 Other congenital anomalies of circulatory system**

747.0 Patent ductus arteriosus
>Patent ductus Botalli
>Persistent ductus arteriosus
>**DEF:** Open lumen in ductus arteriosus causes arterial blood recirculation in lungs; inhibits blood supply to aorta; symptoms such as shortness of breath more noticeable upon activity.
>**AHA:** 3Q, '09, 17
>**Q25.0** Patent ductus arteriosus I-10

√5ᵗʰ **747.1 Coarctation of aorta**
>**DEF:** Localized deformity of aortic media seen as a severe constriction of the vessel lumen; major symptom is high blood pressure in the arms and low pressure in the legs; may result in a CVA, rupture of the aorta, bacterial endocarditis or congestive heart failure.

747.10 Coarctation of aorta (preductal) (postductal)
>Hypoplasia of aortic arch
>**AHA:** 3Q, '07, 3; 1Q, '99, 11; 4Q, '88, 8

747.11 Interruption of aortic arch

√5ᵗʰ **747.2 Other anomalies of aorta**

747.20 Anomaly of aorta, unspecified

747.21 Anomalies of aortic arch
>Anomalous origin, right subclavian artery
>Dextraposition of aorta
>Double aortic arch
>Kommerell's diverticulum
>Overriding aorta
>Persistent:
>convolutions, aortic arch
>right aortic arch
>Vascular ring
>**EXCLUDES** hypoplasia of aortic arch (747.10)
>**AHA:** 1Q, '03, 15

747.22 Atresia and stenosis of aorta
>Absence ⎱
>Aplasia ⎱
>Hypoplasia ⎰ of aorta
>Stricture ⎰
>Supra (valvular)-aortic stenosis
>**EXCLUDES** congenital aortic (valvular) stenosis or stricture, so stated (746.3)
>hypoplasia of aorta in hypoplastic left heart syndrome (746.7)

747.29 Other
>Aneurysm of sinus of Valsalva
>Congenital:
>aneurysm ⎱
>dilation ⎰ of aorta

√5ᵗʰ **747.3 Anomalies of pulmonary artery**
>**AHA:** ▶4Q, '11, 137-138◀

747.31 Pulmonary artery coarctation and atresia
>Agenesis of pulmonary artery
>Atresia of pulmonary artery
>Coarctation of pulmonary artery
>Hypoplasia of pulmonary artery
>Stenosis of pulmonary artery

747.32 Pulmonary arteriovenous malformation
>Pulmonary arteriovenous aneurysm
>**EXCLUDES** acquired pulmonary arteriovenous fistula (417.0)
>**AHA:** ▶4Q, '11, 138◀

747.39 Other anomalies of pulmonary artery and pulmonary circulation
>Anomaly of pulmonary artery

√5ᵗʰ **747.4 Anomalies of great veins**

747.40 Anomaly of great veins, unspecified
>Anomaly NOS of:
>pulmonary veins
>vena cava

747.41 Total anomalous pulmonary venous connection
>Total anomalous pulmonary venous return [TAPVR]:
>subdiaphragmatic
>supradiaphragmatic

747.42 Partial anomalous pulmonary venous connection
>Partial anomalous pulmonary venous return

747.49 Other anomalies of great veins
>Absence ⎱
>Congenital ⎱ of vena cava (inferior)
>stenosis ⎰ (superior)
>Persistent:
>left posterior cardinal vein
>left superior vena cava
>Scimitar syndrome
>Transposition of pulmonary veins NOS

747.5 Absence or hypoplasia of umbilical artery
>Single umbilical artery

√4ᵗʰ/√5ᵗʰ Additional Digit Required   Unspecified Code   Other Specified Code   Manifestation Code   ▶◀ Revised Text   ● New Code   ▲ Revised Code Title

2013 ICD-9-CM   **February 2012 • Volume 1 – 241**

Congenital Anomalies

747.6–748.4

√5ᵗʰ **747.6 Other anomalies of peripheral vascular system**

Absence
Anomaly } of artery or vein, NEC
Atresia

Arteriovenous aneurysm (peripheral)
Arteriovenous malformation of the peripheral vascular system
Congenital:
  aneurysm (peripheral)
  phlebectasia
  stricture, artery
  varix
Multiple renal arteries

EXCLUDES *anomalies of:*
    cerebral vessels (747.81)
    pulmonary artery (747.39)
    congenital retinal aneurysm (743.58)
    hemangioma (228.00-228.09)
    lymphangioma (228.1)

747.60 Anomaly of the peripheral vascular system, unspecified site

747.61 Gastrointestinal vessel anomaly
  AHA: 3Q, '96, 10
  TIP: Do not assign for gastric or intestinal AV malformation or angiodysplasia not stated to be congenital. See instead code 537.82, 537.83, 569.84, or 569.85.

747.62 Renal vessel anomaly

747.63 Upper limb vessel anomaly

747.64 Lower limb vessel anomaly

747.69 Anomalies of other specified sites of peripheral vascular system

√5ᵗʰ **747.8 Other specified anomalies of circulatory system**

747.81 Anomalies of cerebrovascular system
  Arteriovenous malformation of brain
  Cerebral arteriovenous aneurysm, congenital
  Congenital anomalies of cerebral vessels
  EXCLUDES *ruptured cerebral (arteriovenous) aneurysm (430)*
  Q28.3 Other malformations of cerebral vessels   I-10

747.82 Spinal vessel anomaly
  Arteriovenous malformation of spinal vessel
  AHA: 3Q, '95, 5

747.83 Persistent fetal circulation   N
  Persistent pulmonary hypertension
  Primary pulmonary hypertension of newborn
  DEF: A return to fetal circulation due to constriction of pulmonary arterioles and opening of the ductus arteriosus and foramen ovale, right-to-left shunting, oxygenation of the blood does not occur, and the lungs remain constricted after birth; is seen in term or post-term infants; causes include asphyxiation, meconium aspiration syndrome, acidosis, sepsis, and developmental immaturity.
  AHA: 4Q, '02, 62

Persistent Fetal Circulation

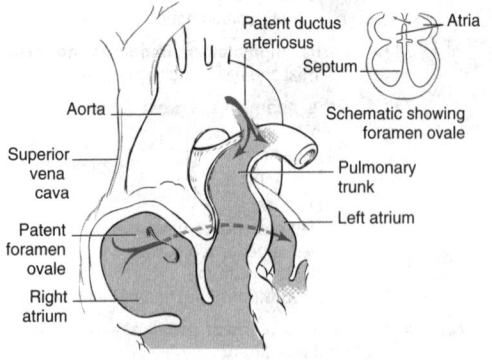

Patent ductus arteriosus
Atria
Septum
Schematic showing foramen ovale
Aorta
Pulmonary trunk
Superior vena cava
Left atrium
Patent foramen ovale
Right atrium

747.89 Other
Aneurysm, congenital, specified site not elsewhere classified
  EXCLUDES *congenital aneurysm:*
    coronary (746.85)
    peripheral (747.6)
    pulmonary (747.39)
    arteriovenous (747.32)
    retinal (743.58)
  AHA: 4Q, '02, 63

747.9 Unspecified anomaly of circulatory system

√4ᵗʰ **748 Congenital anomalies of respiratory system**
  EXCLUDES *congenital central alveolar hypoventilation syndrome (327.25)*
    congenital defect of diaphragm (756.6)

748.0 Choanal atresia
Atresia
Congenital stenosis } of nares (anterior) (posterior)
  DEF: Occluded posterior nares (choana), bony or membranous due to failure of embryonic bucconasal membrane to rupture.

748.1 Other anomalies of nose
Absent nose
Accessory nose
Cleft nose
Congenital:
  deformity of nose
  notching of tip of nose
  perforation of wall of nasal sinus
Deformity of wall of nasal sinus
  EXCLUDES *congenital deviation of nasal septum (754.0)*

748.2 Web of larynx
Web of larynx:
  NOS
  glottic
  subglottic
  DEF: Malformed larynx; marked by thin, translucent, or thick, fibrotic spread between vocal folds; affects speech.

748.3 Other anomalies of larynx, trachea, and bronchus
Absence or agenesis of:
  bronchus
  larynx
  trachea
Anomaly (of):
  cricoid cartilage
  epiglottis
  thyroid cartilage
  tracheal cartilage
Atresia (of):
  epiglottis
  glottis
  larynx
  trachea
Cleft thyroid, cartilage, congenital
Congenital:
  dilation, trachea
  stenosis:
    larynx
    trachea
  tracheocele
Diverticulum:
  bronchus
  trachea
Fissure of epiglottis
Laryngocele
Posterior cleft of cricoid cartilage (congenital)
Rudimentary tracheal bronchus
Stridor, laryngeal, congenital
  AHA: 1Q, '99, 14
  Q32.4 Other congenital malformations of bronchus   I-10

748.4 Congenital cystic lung
Disease, lung:
  cystic, congenital
  polycystic, congenital
Honeycomb lung, congenital
  EXCLUDES *acquired or unspecified cystic lung (518.89)*
  DEF: Enlarged air spaces of lung parenchyma.

N Newborn Age: 0   P Pediatric Age: 0-17   M Maternity Age: 12-55   A Adult Age: 15-124

748.5 Agenesis, hypoplasia, and dysplasia of lung
Absence of lung (fissures) (lobe) (lobe)
Aplasia of lung
Hypoplasia of lung
Sequestration of lung

√5ᵗʰ **748.6 Other anomalies of lung**

748.60 Anomaly of lung, unspecified

748.61 Congenital bronchiectasis

748.69 Other
Accessory lung (lobe)
Azygos lobe (fissure), lung

748.8 Other specified anomalies of respiratory system
Abnormal communication between pericardial and pleural
sacs
Anomaly, pleural folds
Atresia of nasopharynx
Congenital cyst of mediastinum

748.9 Unspecified anomaly of respiratory system
Anomaly of respiratory system NOS

√4ᵗʰ **749 Cleft palate and cleft lip**

√5ᵗʰ **749.0 Cleft palate**

749.00 Cleft palate, unspecified

749.01 Unilateral, complete

749.02 Unilateral, incomplete
Cleft uvula

749.03 Bilateral, complete

749.04 Bilateral, incomplete

√5ᵗʰ **749.1 Cleft lip**
Cheiloschisis
Congenital fissure of lip
Harelip
Labium leporinum

749.10 Cleft lip, unspecified

749.11 Unilateral, complete

749.12 Unilateral, incomplete

749.13 Bilateral, complete

749.14 Bilateral, incomplete

√5ᵗʰ **749.2 Cleft palate with cleft lip**
Cheilopalatoschisis

749.20 Cleft palate with cleft lip, unspecified

749.21 Unilateral, complete

749.22 Unilateral, incomplete

Cleft Lip and Palate

Unilateral cleft lip

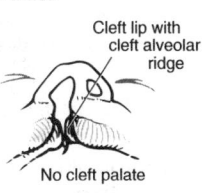
Cleft lip with
cleft alveolar
ridge

No cleft palate

No cleft palate

Unilateral cleft lip
and cleft palate

Alveolar ridge

Cleft palate

Prolabium

Bilateral
cleft lip and
cleft palate

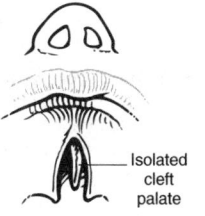
Isolated
cleft
palate

749.23 Bilateral, complete
AHA: 1Q, '96, 14

749.24 Bilateral, incomplete

749.25 Other combinations

√4ᵗʰ **750 Other congenital anomalies of upper alimentary tract**
EXCLUDES dentofacial anomalies (524.0-524.9)

750.0 Tongue tie
Ankyloglossia
DEF: Restricted tongue movement due to lingual frenum extending
toward tip of tongue. Tongue may be fused to mouth floor affecting
speech.

√5ᵗʰ **750.1 Other anomalies of tongue**

750.10 Anomaly of tongue, unspecified

750.11 Aglossia
DEF: Absence of tongue.

750.12 Congenital adhesions of tongue

750.13 Fissure of tongue
Bifid tongue
Double tongue

750.15 Macroglossia
Congenital hypertrophy of tongue

750.16 Microglossia
Hypoplasia of tongue

750.19 Other

√5ᵗʰ **750.2 Other specified anomalies of mouth and pharynx**

750.21 Absence of salivary gland

750.22 Accessory salivary gland

750.23 Atresia, salivary duct
Imperforate salivary duct

750.24 Congenital fistula of salivary gland

750.25 Congenital fistula of lip
Congenital (mucus) lip pits

750.26 Other specified anomalies of mouth
Absence of uvula

750.27 Diverticulum of pharynx
Pharyngeal pouch

750.29 Other specified anomalies of pharynx
Imperforate pharynx

750.3 Tracheoesophageal fistula, esophageal atresia and stenosis
Absent esophagus
Atresia of esophagus
Congenital:
esophageal ring
stenosis of esophagus
stricture of esophagus
Congenital fistula:
esophagobronchial
esophagotracheal
Imperforate esophagus
Webbed esophagus
AHA: ▶1Q, '12, 15◀

750.4 Other specified anomalies of esophagus
Dilatation, congenital
Displacement, congenital
Diverticulum ⎫
Duplication ⎬ (of) esophagus
Giant ⎭

Esophageal pouch
EXCLUDES congenital hiatus hernia (750.6)
AHA: J-F, '85, 3

√4ᵗʰ/√5ᵗʰ Additional Digit Required   Unspecified Code   Other Specified Code   Manifestation Code   ▶◀ Revised Text   ● New Code   ▲ Revised Code Title

2013 ICD-9-CM   **October 2012 • Volume 1 – 243**

748.5–750.4

Congenital Anomalies

750.5–751.8

750.5 Congenital hypertrophic pyloric stenosis

Congenital or infantile:

constriction
hypertrophy
spasm   } of pylorus
stenosis
stricture

DEF: Obstructed pylorus due to overgrowth of pyloric muscle.
Q40.0 Congenital hypertrophic pyloric stenosis   [I-10]

750.6 Congenital hiatus hernia

Displacement of cardia through esophageal hiatus

EXCLUDES   *congenital diaphragmatic hernia (756.6)*

750.7 Other specified anomalies of stomach

Congenital:
cardiospasm
hourglass stomach
Displacement of stomach
Diverticulum of stomach, congenital
Duplication of stomach
Megalogastria
Microgastria
Transposition of stomach

750.8 Other specified anomalies of upper alimentary tract

750.9 Unspecified anomaly of upper alimentary tract

Congenital:
anomaly NOS   } of upper alimentary tract [any
deformity NOS }   part, except tongue]

[√4th] 751 Other congenital anomalies of digestive system

751.0 Meckel's diverticulum

Meckel's diverticulum (displaced) (hypertrophic)
Persistent:
omphalomesenteric duct
vitelline duct

DEF: Malformed sacs or appendages of ileum of small intestine; can
cause strangulation, volvulus and intussusception.
AHA: 1Q, '04, 10
TIP: Assign for mesodiverticular band, a fibrous band connecting the
tip of the diverticulum to the mesentery; can cause small bowel
herniation and obstruction.

751.1 Atresia and stenosis of small intestine   [P]

Atresia of:
duodenum
ileum
intestine NOS
Congenital:
absence
obstruction   } of small intestine or intestine
stenosis   NOS
stricture

Imperforate jejunum

751.2 Atresia and stenosis of large intestine rectum, and anal canal   [P]

Absence:
anus (congenital)
appendix, congenital
large intestine, congenital
rectum
Atresia of:
anus
colon
rectum
Congenital or infantile:
obstruction of large intestine
occlusion of anus
stricture of anus
Imperforate:
anus
rectum
Stricture of rectum, congenital
AHA: 2Q, '11, 13; 2Q, '98, 16

751.3 Hirschsprung's disease and other congenital functional disorders of colon

Aganglionosis   Congenital megacolon
Congenital dilation of colon   Macrocolon

DEF: Hirschsprung's disease: enlarged or dilated colon (megacolon),
with absence of ganglion cells in the narrowed wall distally; causes
inability to defecate.

751.4 Anomalies of intestinal fixation

Congenital adhesions: Rotation of cecum or colon:
   omental, anomalous   failure of
   peritoneal   incomplete
Jackson's membrane   insufficient
Malrotation of colon   Universal mesentery

751.5 Other anomalies of intestine

Congenital diverticulum, colon   Megaloappendix
Dolichocolon   Megaloduodenum
Duplication of: Microcolon
   anus   Persistent cloaca
   appendix   Transposition of:
   cecum   appendix
   intestine   colon
Ectopic anus   intestine

AHA: 2Q, '10, 12; 3Q, '02, 11; 3Q, '01, 8
Q43.9 Congenital malformation of intestine unspecified   [I-10]

[√5th] 751.6 Anomalies of gallbladder, bile ducts, and liver

751.60 Unspecified anomaly of gallbladder, bile ducts, and liver

751.61 Biliary atresia   [P]

Congenital:
absence
hypoplasia } of bile duct
obstruction } (common) of
stricture   } passage

AHA: S-O, '87, 8

751.62 Congenital cystic disease of liver

Congenital polycystic disease of liver
Fibrocystic disease of liver

751.69 Other anomalies of gallbladder, bile ducts, and liver

Absence of:
gallbladder, congenital
liver (lobe)
Accessory:
hepatic ducts
liver
Congenital:
choledochal cyst
hepatomegaly
Duplication of:
biliary duct
cystic duct
gallbladder
liver
Floating:
gallbladder
liver
Intrahepatic gallbladder
AHA: S-O, '87, 8

751.7 Anomalies of pancreas

Absence
Accessory
Agenesis   } (of) pancreas
Annular
Hypoplasia

Ectopic pancreatic tissue
Pancreatic heterotopia

EXCLUDES   *diabetes mellitus (249.0-249.9, 250.0-250.9)*
           fibrocystic disease of pancreas
              (277.00-277.09)
           neonatal diabetes mellitus (775.1)

751.8 Other specified anomalies of digestive system

Absence (complete) (partial) of alimentary tract NOS
Duplication   } of digestive organs NOS
Malposition, congenital }

EXCLUDES   *congenital diaphragmatic hernia (756.6)*
           congenital hiatus hernia (750.6)

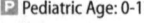

[N] Newborn Age: 0   [P] Pediatric Age: 0-17   [M] Maternity Age: 12-55   [A] Adult Age: 15-124

751.9 Unspecified anomaly of digestive system
Congenital:
anomaly NOS
deformity NOS } of digestive system NOS

√4th **752 Congenital anomalies of genital organs**
EXCLUDES syndromes associated with anomalies in the number and form of chromosomes (758.0-758.9)

752.0 Anomalies of ovaries ♀
Absence, congenital
Accessory
Ectopic
Streak } (of) ovary

√5th **752.1 Anomalies of fallopian tubes and broad ligaments**

752.10 Unspecified anomaly of fallopian tubes and broad ligaments ♀

752.11 Embryonic cyst of fallopian tubes and broad ligaments ♀
Cyst: Cyst:
epoophoron   parovarian
fimbrial
AHA: S-O, '85, 13

752.19 Other ♀
Absence
Accessory
Atresia } (of) fallopian tube or broad ligament

752.2 Doubling of uterus ♀
Didelphic uterus
Doubling of uterus [any degree] (associated with doubling of cervix and vagina)

√5th **752.3 Other anomalies of uterus**
AHA: 4Q, '10, 90-91; 3Q, '06, 18

752.31 Agenesis of uterus ♀
Congenital absence of uterus
Q51.0 Congenital absence of uterus I-10

752.32 Hypoplasia of uterus ♀
Q51.811 Hypoplasia of uterus I-10

752.33 Unicornuate uterus ♀
Unicornuate uterus with or without a separate uterine horn
Uterus with only one functioning horn
Q51.4 Unicornuate uterus I-10

752.34 Bicornuate uterus ♀
Bicornuate uterus, complete or partial
Q51.3 Bicornuate uterus I-10

752.35 Septate uterus ♀
Septate uterus, complete or partial

752.36 Arcuate uterus ♀
Q51.810 Arcuate uterus I-10

752.39 Other anomalies of uterus ♀
Aplasia of uterus NOS
Müllerian anomaly of the uterus, NEC
EXCLUDES anomaly of uterus due to exposure to diethylstilbestrol [DES] in utero (760.76)
didelphic uterus (752.2)
doubling of uterus (752.2)
DEF: Müllerian anomalies: The failure or disruption of female embryonic Müllerian ducts to transform into the upper vagina, cervix uterus, and oviducts, resulting in anomalous organ development.

√5th **752.4 Anomalies of cervix, vagina, and external female genitalia**

752.40 Unspecified anomaly of cervix, vagina, and external female genitalia ♀

752.41 Embryonic cyst of cervix, vagina, and external female genitalia ♀
Cyst of:
canal of Nuck, congenital
Gartner's duct
vagina, embryonal
vulva, congenital
DEF: Embryonic fluid-filled cysts of cervix, vagina or external female genitalia.

Hypospadias and Epispadias

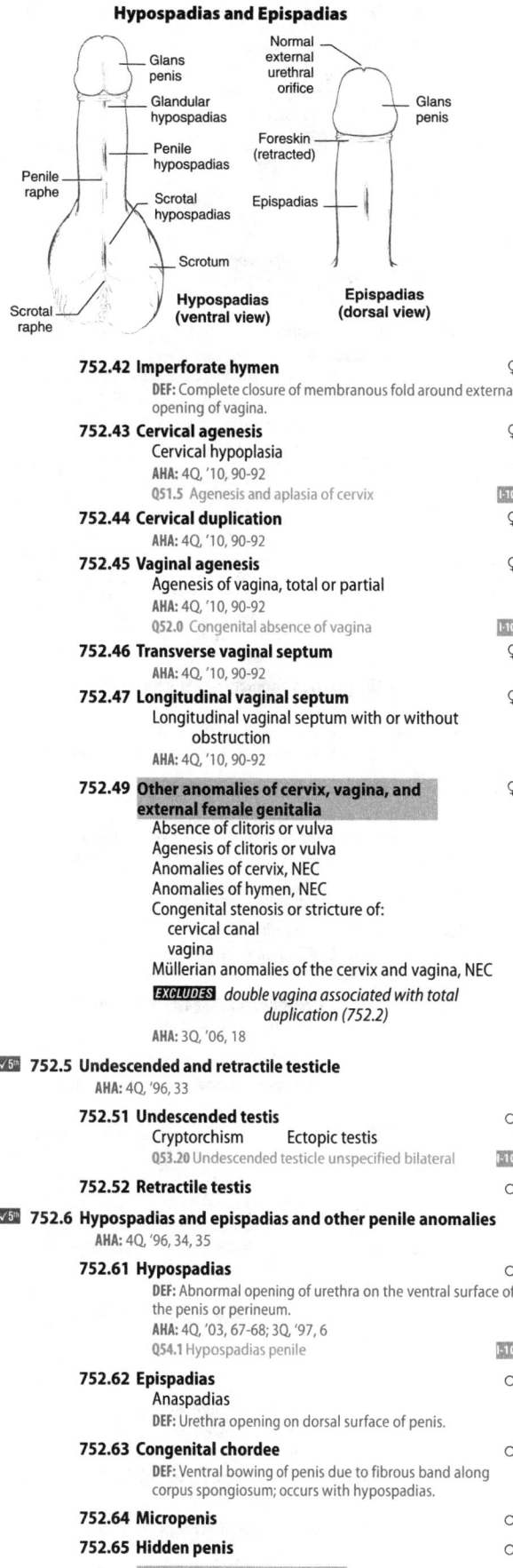

Hypospadias (ventral view)   Epispadias (dorsal view)

752.42 Imperforate hymen ♀
DEF: Complete closure of membranous fold around external opening of vagina.

752.43 Cervical agenesis ♀
Cervical hypoplasia
AHA: 4Q, '10, 90-92
Q51.5 Agenesis and aplasia of cervix I-10

752.44 Cervical duplication ♀
AHA: 4Q, '10, 90-92

752.45 Vaginal agenesis ♀
Agenesis of vagina, total or partial
AHA: 4Q, '10, 90-92
Q52.0 Congenital absence of vagina I-10

752.46 Transverse vaginal septum ♀
AHA: 4Q, '10, 90-92

752.47 Longitudinal vaginal septum ♀
Longitudinal vaginal septum with or without obstruction
AHA: 4Q, '10, 90-92

752.49 Other anomalies of cervix, vagina, and external female genitalia ♀
Absence of clitoris or vulva
Agenesis of clitoris or vulva
Anomalies of cervix, NEC
Anomalies of hymen, NEC
Congenital stenosis or stricture of:
cervical canal
vagina
Müllerian anomalies of the cervix and vagina, NEC
EXCLUDES double vagina associated with total duplication (752.2)
AHA: 3Q, '06, 18

√5th **752.5 Undescended and retractile testicle**
AHA: 4Q, '96, 33

752.51 Undescended testis ♂
Cryptorchism   Ectopic testis
Q53.20 Undescended testicle unspecified bilateral I-10

752.52 Retractile testis ♂

√5th **752.6 Hypospadias and epispadias and other penile anomalies**
AHA: 4Q, '96, 34, 35

752.61 Hypospadias ♂
DEF: Abnormal opening of urethra on the ventral surface of the penis or perineum.
AHA: 4Q, '03, 67-68; 3Q, '97, 6
Q54.1 Hypospadias penile I-10

752.62 Epispadias ♂
Anaspadias
DEF: Urethra opening on dorsal surface of penis.

752.63 Congenital chordee ♂
DEF: Ventral bowing of penis due to fibrous band along corpus spongiosum; occurs with hypospadias.

752.64 Micropenis ♂

752.65 Hidden penis ♂

752.69 Other penile anomalies ♂

Congenital Anomalies

752.7 Indeterminate sex and pseudohermaphroditism
Gynandrism
Hermaphroditism
Ovotestis
Pseudohermaphroditism (male) (female)
Pure gonadal dysgenesis
>EXCLUDES androgen insensitivity (259.50-259.52)
>pseudohermaphroditism:
> female, with adrenocortical disorder (255.2)
> male, with gonadal disorder (257.8)
> with specified chromosomal anomaly
>   (758.0-758.9)
>testicular feminization syndrome (259.50-259.52)
DEF: Pseudohermaphroditism: presence of gonads of one sex and external genitalia of other sex.

√5ᵗʰ 752.8 Other specified anomalies of genital organs
>EXCLUDES congenital hydrocele (778.6)
>penile anomalies (752.61-752.69)
>phimosis or paraphimosis (605)

752.81 Scrotal transposition ♂
AHA: 4Q, '03, 67-68

752.89 Other specified anomalies of genital organs
Absence of: Atresia of:
  prostate   ejaculatory duct
  spermatic cord   vas deferens
  vas deferens   Fusion of testes
Anorchism   Hypoplasia of testis
Aplasia (congenital) of: Monorchism
  prostate   Polyorchism
  round ligament
  testicle

752.9 Unspecified anomaly of genital organs
Congenital:
  anomaly NOS } of genital organ, not
  deformity NOS }   elsewhere classified

√4ᵗʰ 753 Congenital anomalies of urinary system

753.0 Renal agenesis and dysgenesis
Atrophy of kidney: Congenital absence of kidney(s)
  congenital   Hypoplasia of kidney(s)
  infantile
Q60.2 Renal agenesis unspecified   I-10

√5ᵗʰ 753.1 Cystic kidney disease
>EXCLUDES acquired cyst of kidney (593.2)
AHA: 4Q, '90, 3

753.10 Cystic kidney disease, unspecified
Q61.9 Cystic kidney disease unspecified   I-10

753.11 Congenital single renal cyst

753.12 Polycystic kidney, unspecified type
Q61.3 Polycystic kidney unspecified   I-10

753.13 Polycystic kidney, autosomal dominant
DEF: Slow progressive disease characterized by bilateral cysts causing increased kidney size and impaired function.

753.14 Polycystic kidney, autosomal recessive
DEF: Rare disease characterized by multiple cysts involving kidneys and liver, producing renal and hepatic failure in childhood or adolescence.

753.15 Renal dysplasia

753.16 Medullary cystic kidney
Nephronopthisis
DEF: Diffuse kidney disease results in uremia onset prior to age 20.

753.17 Medullary sponge kidney
DEF: Dilated collecting tubules; usually asymptomatic but calcinosis in tubules may cause renal insufficiency.

753.19 Other specified cystic kidney disease
Multicystic kidney

√5ᵗʰ 753.2 Obstructive defects of renal pelvis and ureter
AHA: 4Q, '96, 35

753.20 Unspecified obstructive defect of renal pelvis and ureter

753.21 Congenital obstruction of ureteropelvic junction
DEF: Stricture at junction of ureter and renal pelvis.

753.22 Congenital obstruction of ureterovesical junction
Adynamic ureter
Congenital hydroureter
DEF: Stricture at junction of ureter and bladder.

753.23 Congenital ureterocele

753.29 Other
Q62.39 Other obstructive defects renal pelvis & ureter   I-10

753.3 Other specified anomalies of kidney
Accessory kidney   Fusion of kidneys
Congenital: Giant kidney
  calculus of kidney   Horseshoe kidney
  displaced kidney   Hyperplasia of kidney
Discoid kidney   Lobulation of kidney
Double kidney with   Malrotation of kidney
  double pelvis   Trifid kidney (pelvis)
Ectopic kidney
AHA: 1Q, '07, 23
TIP: Assign for Finnish-type congenital nephrosis, along with code 581.3 Nephrotic syndrome.
Q63.8 Oth specified congenital malformations of kidney   I-10

753.4 Other specified anomalies of ureter
Absent ureter
Accessory ureter
Deviation of ureter
Displaced ureteric orifice
Double ureter
Ectopic ureter
Implantation, anomalous of ureter

753.5 Exstrophy of urinary bladder
Ectopia vesicae
Extroversion of bladder
DEF: Absence of lower abdominal and anterior bladder walls with posterior bladder wall protrusion.

753.6 Atresia and stenosis of urethra and bladder neck
Congenital obstruction:
  bladder neck
  urethra
Congenital stricture of:
  urethra (valvular)
  urinary meatus
  vesicourethral orifice
Imperforate urinary meatus
Impervious urethra
Urethral valve formation

753.7 Anomalies of urachus
Cyst
Fistula } (of) urachussinus
Patent }
Persistent umbilical sinus

753.8 Other specified anomalies of bladder and urethra
Absence, congenital of:
  bladder
  urethra
Accessory:
  bladder
  urethra
Congenital:
  diverticulum of bladder
  hernia of bladder
  prolapse of:
    bladder (mucosa)
    urethra
  urethrorectal fistula
Double:
  urethra
  urinary meatus

753.9 Unspecified anomaly of urinary system
Congenital:
  anomaly NOS } of urinary system [any part,
  deformity NOS }   except urachus]
AHA: 2Q, '11, 6

✓4ᵗʰ **754 Certain congenital musculoskeletal deformities**

INCLUDES nonteratogenic deformities which are considered to be due to intrauterine malposition and pressure

754.0 Of skull, face, and jaw
Asymmetry of face
Compression facies
Depressions in skull
Deviation of nasal septum, congenital
Dolichocephaly
Plagiocephaly
Potter's facies
Squashed or bent nose, congenital
EXCLUDES dentofacial anomalies (524.0-524.9)
syphilitic saddle nose (090.5)

754.1 Of sternocleidomastoid muscle
Congenital sternomastoid torticollis
Congenital wryneck
Contracture of sternocleidomastoid (muscle)
Sternomastoid tumor

754.2 Of spine
Congenital postural:
lordosis
scoliosis

✓5ᵗʰ **754.3 Congenital dislocation of hip**

754.30 Congenital dislocation of hip, unilateral
Congenital dislocation of hip NOS

754.31 Congenital dislocation of hip, bilateral

754.32 Congenital subluxation of hip, unilateral
Congenital flexion deformity, hip or thigh
Predislocation status of hip at birth
Preluxation of hip, congenital

754.33 Congenital subluxation of hip, bilateral

754.35 Congenital dislocation of one hip with subluxation of other hip

✓5ᵗʰ **754.4 Congenital genu recurvatum and bowing of long bones of leg**

754.40 Genu recurvatum
DEF: Backward curving of knee joint.

754.41 Congenital dislocation of knee (with genu recurvatum)

754.42 Congenital bowing of femur

754.43 Congenital bowing of tibia and fibula

754.44 Congenital bowing of unspecified long bones of leg

✓5ᵗʰ **754.5 Varus deformities of feet**
EXCLUDES acquired (736.71, 736.75, 736.79)

754.50 Talipes varus
Congenital varus deformity of foot, unspecified
Pes varus
DEF: Inverted foot marked by outer sole resting on ground.

754.51 Talipes equinovarus
Equinovarus (congenital)
DEF: Elevated, outward rotation of heel; also called clubfoot.

754.52 Metatarsus primus varus
DEF: Malformed first metatarsal bone, with bone angled toward body.

754.53 Metatarsus varus

754.59 Other
Talipes calcaneovarus

✓5ᵗʰ **754.6 Valgus deformities of feet**
EXCLUDES valgus deformity of foot (acquired) (736.79)

754.60 Talipes valgus
Congenital valgus deformity of foot, unspecified

754.61 Congenital pes planus
Congenital rocker bottom flat foot
Flat foot, congenital
EXCLUDES pes planus (acquired) (734)

754.62 Talipes calcaneovalgus

754.69 Other
Talipes:
equinovalgus
planovalgus

✓5ᵗʰ **754.7 Other deformities of feet**
EXCLUDES acquired (736.70-736.79)

754.70 Talipes, unspecified
Congenital deformity of foot NOS

754.71 Talipes cavus
Cavus foot (congenital)

754.79 Other
Asymmetric talipes
Talipes:
calcaneus
equinus

✓5ᵗʰ **754.8 Other specified nonteratogenic anomalies**

754.81 Pectus excavatum
Congenital funnel chest

754.82 Pectus carinatum
Congenital pigeon chest [breast]

754.89 Other
Club hand (congenital)
Congenital:
deformity of chest wall
dislocation of elbow
Generalized flexion contractures of lower limb joints, congenital
Spade-like hand (congenital)

✓4ᵗʰ **755 Other congenital anomalies of limbs**
EXCLUDES those deformities classifiable to 754.0-754.8

✓5ᵗʰ **755.0 Polydactyly**

755.00 Polydactyly, unspecified digits
Supernumerary digits

755.01 Of fingers
Accessory fingers

755.02 Of toes
Accessory toes

✓5ᵗʰ **755.1 Syndactyly**
Symphalangy
Webbing of digits

755.10 Of multiple and unspecified sites

755.11 Of fingers without fusion of bone

755.12 Of fingers with fusion of bone

755.13 Of toes without fusion of bone

755.14 Of toes with fusion of bone

✓5ᵗʰ **755.2 Reduction deformities of upper limb**

755.20 Unspecified reduction deformity of upper limb
Ectromelia NOS ⎫
Hemimelia NOS ⎬ of upper limb
Shortening of arm, congenital

755.21 Transverse deficiency of upper limb
Amelia of upper limb
Congenital absence of:
fingers, all (complete or partial)
forearm, including hand and fingers
upper limb, complete
Congenital amputation of upper limb
Transverse hemimelia of upper limb

755.22 Longitudinal deficiency of upper limb, not elsewhere classified
Phocomelia NOS of upper limb
Rudimentary arm

755.23 Longitudinal deficiency, combined, involving humerus, radius, and ulna (complete or incomplete)
Congenital absence of arm and forearm (complete or incomplete) with or without metacarpal deficiency and/or phalangeal deficiency, incomplete
Phocomelia, complete, of upper limb

755.24 Longitudinal deficiency, humeral, complete or partial (with or without distal deficiencies, incomplete)
Congenital absence of humerus (with or without absence of some [but not all] distal elements)
Proximal phocomelia of upper limb

755.25 Longitudinal deficiency, radioulnar, complete or partial (with or without distal deficiencies, incomplete)
Congenital absence of radius and ulna (with or without absence of some [but not all] distal elements)
Distal phocomelia of upper limb

755.26 Longitudinal deficiency, radial, complete or partial (with or without distal deficiencies, incomplete)
Agenesis of radius
Congenital absence of radius (with or without absence of some [but not all] distal elements)

755.27 Longitudinal deficiency, ulnar, complete or partial (with or without distal deficiencies, incomplete)
Agenesis of ulna
Congenital absence of ulna (with or without absence of some [but not all] distal elements)

755.28 Longitudinal deficiency, carpals or metacarpals, complete or partial (with or without incomplete phalangeal deficiency)

755.29 Longitudinal deficiency, phalanges, complete or partial
Absence of finger, congenital
Aphalangia of upper limb, terminal, complete or partial
EXCLUDES terminal deficiency of all five digits (755.21)
transverse deficiency of phalanges (755.21)

√5ᵗʰ **755.3 Reduction deformities of lower limb**

755.30 Unspecified reduction deformity of lower limb
Ectromelia NOS ⎫
Hemimelia NOS ⎬ of lower limb
Shortening of leg, congenital

755.31 Transverse deficiency of lower limb
Amelia of lower limb
Congenital absence of:
  foot
  leg, including foot and toes
  lower limb, complete
  toes, all, complete
Transverse hemimelia of lower limb

755.32 Longitudinal deficiency of lower limb, not elsewhere classified
Phocomelia NOS of lower limb

755.33 Longitudinal deficiency, combined, involving femur, tibia, and fibula (complete or incomplete)
Congenital absence of thigh and (lower) leg (complete or incomplete) with or without metacarpal deficiency and/or phalangeal deficiency, incomplete
Phocomelia, complete, of lower limb

755.34 Longitudinal deficiency, femoral, complete or partial (with or without distal deficiencies, incomplete)
Congenital absence of femur (with or without absence of some [but not all] distal elements)
Proximal phocomelia of lower limb

755.35 Longitudinal deficiency, tibiofibular, complete or partial (with or without distal deficiencies, incomplete)
Congenital absence of tibia and fibula (with or without absence of some [but not all] distal elements)
Distal phocomelia of lower limb

755.36 Longitudinal deficiency, tibia, complete or partial (with or without distal deficiencies, incomplete)
Agenesis of tibia
Congenital absence of tibia (with or without absence of some [but not all] distal elements)

755.37 Longitudinal deficiency, fibular, complete or partial (with or without distal deficiencies, incomplete)
Agenesis of fibula
Congenital absence of fibula (with or without absence of some [but not all] distal elements)

755.38 Longitudinal deficiency, tarsals or metatarsals, complete or partial (with or without incomplete phalangeal deficiency)

755.39 Longitudinal deficiency, phalanges, complete or partial
Absence of toe, congenital
Aphalangia of lower limb, terminal, complete or partial
EXCLUDES terminal deficiency of all five digits (755.31)
transverse deficiency of phalanges (755.31)

755.4 Reduction deformities, unspecified limb
Absence, congenital (complete or partial) of limb NOS
Amelia ⎫
Ectromelia ⎬ of unspecified limb
Hemimelia ⎪
Phocomelia ⎭

√5ᵗʰ **755.5 Other anomalies of upper limb, including shoulder girdle**

755.50 Unspecified anomaly of upper limb

755.51 Congenital deformity of clavicle

755.52 Congenital elevation of scapula
Sprengel's deformity

755.53 Radioulnar synostosis
DEF: Osseous adhesion of radius and ulna.

755.54 Madelung's deformity
DEF: Distal ulnar overgrowth or radial shortening; also called carpus curvus.

755.55 Acrocephalosyndactyly
Apert's syndrome
DEF: Premature cranial suture fusion (craniostenosis); marked by cone-shaped or pointed (acrocephaly) head and webbing of the fingers (syndactyly); similar to craniofacial dysostosis.

755.56 Accessory carpal bones

755.57 Macrodactylia (fingers)
DEF: Abnormally large fingers, toes.

755.58 Cleft hand, congenital
Lobster-claw hand
DEF: Extended separation between fingers into metacarpus; also may refer to large fingers and absent middle fingers of hand.

755.59 Other
Cleidocranial dysostosis
Cubitus:
  valgus, congenital
  varus, congenital
EXCLUDES club hand (congenital) (754.89)
congenital dislocation of elbow (754.89)

√5ᵗʰ **755.6 Other anomalies of lower limb, including pelvic girdle**

755.60 Unspecified anomaly of lower limb

755.61 Coxa valga, congenital
DEF: Abnormally wide angle between the neck and shaft of the femur.

755.62 Coxa vara, congenital
DEF: Diminished angle between neck and shaft of femur.

755.63 Other congenital deformity of hip (joint)
Congenital anteversion of femur (neck)
EXCLUDES congenital dislocation of hip (754.30-754.35)
AHA: 1Q, '94, 15; S-O, '84, 15
Q65.9 Congenital deformity of hip unspecified   I-10

755.64 Congenital deformity of knee (joint)
Congenital:
  absence of patella
  genu valgum [knock-knee]
  genu varum [bowleg]
Rudimentary patella

755.65 Macrodactylia of toes
> DEF: Abnormally large toes.

755.66 Other anomalies of toes
> Congenital:
>> hallux valgus
>> hallux varus
>> hammer toe

755.67 Anomalies of foot, not elsewhere classified
> Astragaloscaphoid synostosis
> Calcaneonavicular bar
> Coalition of calcaneus
> Talonavicular synostosis
> Tarsal coalitions

755.69 Other
> Congenital:
>> angulation of tibia
>> deformity (of):
>>> ankle (joint)
>>> sacroiliac (joint)
>> fusion of sacroiliac joint

755.8 Other specified anomalies of unspecified limb

755.9 Unspecified anomaly of unspecified limb
> Congenital:
>> anomaly NOS
>> deformity NOS } of unspecified limb

> EXCLUDES reduction deformity of unspecified limb (755.4)

√4th **756 Other congenital musculoskeletal anomalies**
> EXCLUDES congenital myotonic chondrodystrophy (359.23)
>> those deformities classifiable to 754.0-754.8

756.0 Anomalies of skull and face bones
> Absence of skull bones
> Acrocephaly
> Congenital deformity of forehead
> Craniosynostosis
> Crouzon's disease
> Hypertelorism
> Imperfect fusion of skull
> Oxycephaly
> Platybasia
> Premature closure of cranial sutures
> Tower skull
> Trigonocephaly

> EXCLUDES acrocephalosyndactyly [Apert's syndrome] (755.55)
>> dentofacial anomalies (524.0-524.9)
>> skull defects associated with brain anomalies, such
>>> as:
>>>> anencephalus (740.0)
>>>> encephalocele (742.0)
>>>> hydrocephalus (742.3)
>>>> microcephalus (742.1)

> AHA: 3Q, '98, 9; 3Q, '96, 15
> TIP: Assign for Nager syndrome (preaxial acrofacial dysostosis), along with codes for any additional features that are not captured in the code.
> Q75.8 Other spec cong malformations skull & face bones   I-10

√5th **756.1 Anomalies of spine**

756.10 Anomaly of spine, unspecified

756.11 Spondylolysis, lumbosacral region
> Prespondylolisthesis (lumbosacral)
> DEF: Bilateral or unilateral defect through the pars interarticularis of a vertebra causes spondylolisthesis.

756.12 Spondylolisthesis
> DEF: Downward slipping of lumbar vertebra over next vertebra; usually related to pelvic deformity.
> Q76.2 Congenital spondylolisthesis   I-10

756.13 Absence of vertebra, congenital

756.14 Hemivertebra
> DEF: Incomplete development of one side of a vertebra.

756.15 Fusion of spine [vertebra], congenital

756.16 Klippel-Feil syndrome
> DEF: Short, wide neck; limits range of motion due to abnormal number of cervical vertebra or fused hemivertebrae.

756.17 Spina bifida occulta
> EXCLUDES spina bifida (aperta) (741.0-741.9)
> DEF: Spina bifida marked by a bony spinal canal defect without a protrusion of the cord or meninges; it is diagnosed by radiography and has no symptoms.

756.19 Other
> Platyspondylia
> Supernumerary vertebra

756.2 Cervical rib
> Supernumerary rib in the cervical region
> DEF: Costa cervicalis: extra rib attached to cervical vertebra.

756.3 Other anomalies of ribs and sternum
> Congenital absence of:
>> rib
>> sternum
> Congenital:
>> fissure of sternum
>> fusion of ribs
> Sternum bifidum
> EXCLUDES nonteratogenic deformity of chest wall
>> (754.81-754.89)

756.4 Chondrodystrophy
> Achondroplasia   Enchondromatosis
> Chondrodystrophia (fetalis)   Ollier's disease
> Dyschondroplasia
> EXCLUDES congenital myotonic chondrodystrophy (359.23)
>> lipochondrodystrophy [Hurler's syndrome] (277.5)
>> Morquio's disease (277.5)

> DEF: Abnormal development of cartilage.
> AHA: 2Q, '02, 16; S-O, '87, 10
> TIP: Assign for Jeune's syndrome, and also for cartilage-hair syndrome (cartilage-hair hypoplasia).

√5th **756.5 Osteodystrophies**

756.50 Osteodystrophy, unspecified

756.51 Osteogenesis imperfecta
> Fragilitas ossium
> Osteopsathyrosis
> DEF: A collagen disorder commonly characterized by brittle, osteoporotic, easily fractured bones, hypermobility of joints, blue sclerae, and a tendency to hemorrhage.

756.52 Osteopetrosis
> DEF: Abnormally dense bone, optic atrophy, hepatosplenomegaly, deafness; sclerosing depletes bone marrow and nerve foramina of skull; often fatal.

756.53 Osteopoikilosis
> DEF: Multiple sclerotic foci on ends of long bones, stippling in round, flat bones; identified by x-ray.

756.54 Polyostotic fibrous dysplasia of bone
> DEF: Fibrous tissue displaces bone results in segmented ragged-edge café-au-lait spots; occurs in girls of early puberty.

756.55 Chondroectodermal dysplasia
> Ellis-van Creveld syndrome
> DEF: Inadequate enchondral bone formation; impaired development of hair and teeth, polydactyly, and cardiac septum defects.

756.56 Multiple epiphyseal dysplasia

756.59 Other
> Albright (-McCune)-Sternberg syndrome

√4th
√5th Additional Digit Required   Unspecified Code   Other Specified Code   Manifestation Code   ►◄ Revised Text   ● New Code   ▲ Revised Code Title

2013 ICD-9-CM   **Volume 1 – 249**

Congenital Anomalies

756.6–757.8

Omphalocele

peritoneum
amniotic membrane
Herniated organs
Umbilicus
Omphalocele
amniotic membrane
skin
distal
proximal
DEFECT

756.6 Anomalies of diaphragm
Absence of diaphragm
Congenital hernia:
  diaphragmatic
  foramen of Morgagni
Eventration of diaphragm
EXCLUDES congenital hiatus hernia (750.6)

√5ᵗʰ **756.7 Anomalies of abdominal wall**

756.70 Anomaly of abdominal wall, unspecified

756.71 Prune belly syndrome
Eagle-Barrett syndrome
Prolapse of bladder mucosa
DEF: Prune belly syndrome: absence of lower rectus abdominis muscle and lower and medial oblique muscles; results in dilated bladder and ureters, dysplastic kidneys and hydronephrosis; common in male infants with undescended testicles.
AHA: 4Q, '97, 44

756.72 Omphalocele
Exomphalos
DEF: Exomphalos: umbilical hernia prominent navel.
DEF: Omphalocele: hernia of umbilicus due to impaired abdominal wall; results in membrane-covered intestine protruding through peritoneum and amnion.
AHA: 4Q, '09, 98-99

756.73 Gastroschisis
DEF: Fissure of abdominal wall, results in protruding small or large intestine.
AHA: 4Q, '09, 98-99

756.79 Other congenital anomalies of abdominal wall
EXCLUDES umbilical hernia (551-553 with .1)

√5ᵗʰ **756.8 Other specified anomalies of muscle, tendon, fascia, and connective tissue**

756.81 Absence of muscle and tendon
Absence of muscle (pectoral)
AHA: 1Q, '10, 13

756.82 Accessory muscle

756.83 Ehlers-Danlos syndrome
DEF: Danlos syndrome: connective tissue disorder causes hyperextended skin and joints; results in fragile blood vessels with bleeding, poor wound healing and subcutaneous pseudotumors.

Gastroschisis

Herniated small bowel (gastroschisis)
Rectus abdominus m.
Umbilicus
skin
distal
proximal
DEFECT

756.89 Other
Amyotrophia congenita
Congenital shortening of tendon
AHA: 3Q, '99, 16
TIP: Assign for Stickler's syndrome, a hereditary progressive arthro-ophthalmopathy, along with codes for the specific manifestations.

756.9 Other and unspecified anomalies of musculoskeletal system
Congenital:
  anomaly NOS ⎱ of musculoskeletal system, not
  deformity NOS ⎰ elsewhere classified

√4ᵗʰ **757 Congenital anomalies of the integument**
INCLUDES anomalies of skin, subcutaneous tissue, hair, nails, and breast
EXCLUDES hemangioma (228.00-228.09)
  pigmented nevus (216.0-216.9)

757.0 Hereditary edema of legs
Congenital lymphedema
Hereditary trophedema
Milroy's disease

757.1 Ichthyosis congenita
Congenital ichthyosis
Harlequin fetus
Ichthyosiform erythroderma
DEF: Overproduction of skin cells causes scaling of skin; may result in stillborn fetus or death soon after birth.

757.2 Dermatoglyphic anomalies
Abnormal palmar creases
DEF: Abnormal skin-line patterns of fingers, palms, toes and soles; initial finding of possible chromosomal abnormalities.

√5ᵗʰ **757.3 Other specified anomalies of skin**

757.31 Congenital ectodermal dysplasia
DEF: Tissues and structures originate in embryonic ectoderm; includes anhidrotic and hidrotic ectodermal dysplasia and EEC syndrome.

757.32 Vascular hamartomas
Birthmarks   Strawberry nevus
Port-wine stain
DEF: Benign tumor of blood vessels; due to malformed angioblastic tissues.
Q82.5 Congenital non-neoplastic nevus   I-10

757.33 Congenital pigmentary anomalies of skin
Congenital poikiloderma
Urticaria pigmentosa
Xeroderma pigmentosum
EXCLUDES albinism (270.2)
Q82.2 Mastocytosis   I-10

757.39 Other
Accessory skin tags, congenital
Congenital scar
Epidermolysis bullosa
Keratoderma (congenital)
EXCLUDES pilonidal cyst (685.0-685.1)
Q82.8 Other specified congenital malformations of skin   I-10

757.4 Specified anomalies of hair
Congenital: Congenital:
  alopecia   hypertrichosis
  atrichosis   monilethrix
  beaded hair   Persistent lanugo

757.5 Specified anomalies of nails
Anonychia   Congenital:
Congenital: leukonychia
  clubnail   onychauxis
  koilonychia   pachyonychia

757.6 Specified congenital anomalies of breast
Accessory ⎫
Congenital absent ⎬ breast or nipple
Supernumerary ⎭
EXCLUDES absence of pectoral muscle (756.81)
  hypoplasia of breast (611.82)
  micromastia (611.82)

757.8 Other specified anomalies of the integument

757.9 Unspecified anomaly of the integument
Congenital:
anomaly NOS
deformity NOS } of integument

√4ᵗʰ **758 Chromosomal anomalies**
INCLUDES syndromes associated with anomalies in the number and form of chromosomes
Use additional codes for conditions associated with the chromosomal anomalies

758.0 Down syndrome
Mongolism
Translocation Down syndrome
Trisomy:
21 or 22
G
Q90.9 Down syndrome unspecified I-10

758.1 Patau's syndrome
Trisomy:
13
D_1
DEF: Trisomy of 13th chromosome; characteristic failure to thrive, severe mental impairment, seizures, abnormal eyes, low-set ears and sloped forehead.

758.2 Edwards' syndrome
Trisomy:
18
E_3
DEF: Trisomy of 18th chromosome; characteristic mental and physical impairments; mainly affects females.

√5ᵗʰ **758.3 Autosomal deletion syndromes**

758.31 Cri-du-chat syndrome
Deletion 5p
DEF: Hereditary congenital syndrome caused by a microdeletion of short arm of chromosome 5; characterized by catlike cry in newborn, microencephaly, severe mental deficiency, and hypertelorism.

758.32 Velo-cardio-facial syndrome
Deletion 22q11.2
DEF: Microdeletion syndrome affecting multiple organs; characteristic cleft palate, heart defects, elongated face with almond-shaped eyes, wide nose, small ears, weak immune systems, weak musculature, hypothyroidism, short stature, and scoliosis; deletion at q11.2 on the long arm of the chromosome 22.

758.33 Other microdeletions
Miller-Dieker syndrome
Smith-Magenis syndrome
DEF: Miller-Dieker syndrome: deletion from the short arm of chromosome 17; characteristic mental retardation, speech and motor development delays, neurological complications, and multiple abnormalities affecting the kidneys, heart, gastrointestinal tract; death in infancy or early childhood.
DEF: Smith-Magenis syndrome: deletion in a certain area of chromosome 17 that results in craniofacial changes, speech delay, hoarse voice, hearing loss and behavioral problems, such as self-destructive head banging, wrist biting, and tearing at nails.

758.39 Other autosomal deletions

758.4 Balanced autosomal translocation in normal individual

758.5 Other conditions due to autosomal anomalies
Accessory autosomes NEC

758.6 Gonadal dysgenesis
Ovarian dysgenesis   XO syndrome
Turner's syndrome
EXCLUDES pure gonadal dysgenesis (752.7)

758.7 Klinefelter's syndrome   ♂
XXY syndrome
DEF: Impaired embryonic development of seminiferous tubes; results in small testes, azoospermia, infertility and enlarged mammary glands.

√5ᵗʰ **758.8 Other conditions due to chromosome anomalies**

758.81 Other conditions due to sex chromosome anomalies

758.89 Other
Q99.8 Other specified chromosome abnormalities I-10

758.9 Conditions due to anomaly of unspecified chromosome

√4ᵗʰ **759 Other and unspecified congenital anomalies**

759.0 Anomalies of spleen
Aberrant
Absent } spleen
Accessory
Congenital splenomegaly
Ectopic spleen
Lobulation of spleen

759.1 Anomalies of adrenal gland
Aberrant
Absent } adrenal gland
Accessory
EXCLUDES adrenogenital disorders (255.2)
congenital disorders of steroid metabolism (255.2)

759.2 Anomalies of other endocrine glands
Absent parathyroid gland
Accessory thyroid gland
Persistent thyroglossal or thyrolingual duct
Thyroglossal (duct) cyst
EXCLUDES congenital:
goiter (246.1)
hypothyroidism (243)

759.3 Situs inversus
Situs inversus or transversus:
abdominalis
thoracis
Transposition of viscera:
abdominal
thoracic
EXCLUDES dextrocardia without mention of complete transposition (746.87)
DEF: Laterally transposed thoracic and abdominal viscera.

759.4 Conjoined twins
Craniopagus   Thoracopagus
Dicephalus   Xiphopagus
Pygopagus

759.5 Tuberous sclerosis
Bourneville's disease
Epiloia
DEF: Hamartomas of brain, retina and viscera, impaired mental ability, seizures and adenoma sebaceum.

759.6 Other hamartoses, not elsewhere classified
Syndrome:
Peutz-Jeghers
Sturge-Weber (-Dimitri)
von Hippel-Lindau
EXCLUDES neurofibromatosis (237.70-237.79)
DEF: Peutz-Jeghers: hereditary syndrome characterized by hamartomas of small intestine.
DEF: Sturge-Weber: congenital syndrome characterized by unilateral port-wine stain over trigeminal nerve, underlying meninges and cerebral cortex.
DEF: von Hipple-Lindau: hereditary syndrome of congenital angiomatosis of the retina and cerebellum.
AHA: 3Q, '92, 12

759.7 Multiple congenital anomalies, so described
Congenital:
anomaly, multiple NOS
deformity, multiple NOS

√5ᵗʰ **759.8 Other specified anomalies**
AHA: S-O, '87, 9; S-O, '85, 11

759.81 Prader-Willi syndrome

759.82 Marfan syndrome
AHA: 3Q, '93, 11

759.83 Fragile X syndrome
AHA: 4Q, '94, 41

759.89 Other

Congenital malformation syndromes affecting multiple systems, not elsewhere classified

Laurence-Moon-Biedl syndrome

AHA: 3Q, '08, 3; 3Q, '06, 21; 2Q, '05, 17; 2Q, '04, 12; 1Q, '01, 3; 3Q, '99, 17, 18; 3Q, '98, 8

TIP: Assign for the following syndromes: cardiofaciocutaneous (CFC), Borjeson-Forssman-Lehmann syndrome (BFLS), Alagille syndrome, startle disease, Alport's syndrome, branchio-oto-renal (BOR) syndrome, Costello syndrome, Williams syndrome, Antley-Bixler syndrome, and multiple pterygium syndrome. Assign additional codes for any documented manifestations.

759.9 Congenital anomaly, unspecified

15. Certain Conditions Originating in the Perinatal Period (760-779)

INCLUDES conditions which have their origin in the perinatal period, before birth through the first 28 days after birth, even though death or morbidity occurs later

Use additional code(s) to further specify condition

Maternal Causes of Perinatal Morbidity and Mortality (760-763)

AHA: 2Q, '89, 14; 3Q, '90, 5

TIP: A newborn condition is clinically significant when it has implications for the newborn's *future* health care. This is an exception to the UHDDS guidelines.

√4ᵗʰ 760 Fetus or newborn affected by maternal conditions which may be unrelated to present pregnancy

INCLUDES the listed maternal conditions only when specified as a cause of mortality or morbidity of the fetus or newborn

EXCLUDES maternal endocrine and metabolic disorders affecting fetus or newborn (775.0-775.9)

AHA: 1Q, '94, 8; 2Q, '92, 12; N-D, '84, 11

TIP: Do not assign unless the mother's condition has actually affected the fetus or newborn.

760.0 Maternal hypertensive disorders
Fetus or newborn affected by maternal conditions classifiable to 642

760.1 Maternal renal and urinary tract diseases
Fetus or newborn affected by maternal conditions classifiable to 580-599

760.2 Maternal infections
Fetus or newborn affected by maternal infectious disease classifiable to 001-136 and 487, but fetus or newborn not manifesting that disease

EXCLUDES congenital infectious diseases (771.0-771.8)
maternal genital tract and other localized infections (760.8)

760.3 Other chronic maternal circulatory and respiratory diseases
Fetus or newborn affected by chronic maternal conditions classifiable to 390-459, 490-519, 745-748

760.4 Maternal nutritional disorders
Fetus or newborn affected by:
maternal disorders classifiable to 260-269
maternal malnutrition NOS

EXCLUDES fetal malnutrition (764.10-764.29)

760.5 Maternal injury
Fetus or newborn affected by maternal conditions classifiable to 800-995

√5ᵗʰ 760.6 Surgical operation on mother and fetus

EXCLUDES cesarean section for present delivery (763.4)
damage to placenta from amniocentesis, cesarean section, or surgical induction (762.1)

AHA: 4Q, '08, 137-138

TIP: These codes include existing conditions present at the time of birth that are related to procedures performed before the time of delivery.

760.61 Newborn affected by amniocentesis
EXCLUDES fetal complications from amniocentesis (679.1)

760.62 Newborn affected by other in utero procedure
EXCLUDES fetal complications of in utero procedure (679.1)

760.63 Newborn affected by other surgical operations on mother during pregnancy
EXCLUDES newborn affected by previous surgical procedure on mother not associated with pregnancy (760.64)

760.64 Newborn affected by previous surgical procedure on mother not associated with pregnancy

√5ᵗʰ 760.7 Noxious influences affecting fetus or newborn via placenta or breast milk
Fetus or newborn affected by noxious substance transmitted via placenta or breast milk

EXCLUDES anesthetic and analgesic drugs administered during labor and delivery (763.5)
drug withdrawal syndrome in newborn (779.5)

AHA: 3Q, '91, 21

760.70 Unspecified noxious substance
Fetus or newborn affected by:
Drug NEC

760.71 Alcohol
Fetal alcohol syndrome

760.72 Narcotics

760.73 Hallucinogenic agents

760.74 Anti-infectives
Antibiotics   Antifungals

760.75 Cocaine
AHA: 3Q, '94, 6; 2Q, '92, 12; 4Q, '91, 26
TIP: If documentation indicates drug withdrawal in the newborn, also assign code 779.5 Drug withdrawal syndrome in newborn.

760.76 Diethylstilbestrol [DES]
AHA: 4Q, '94, 45

760.77 Anticonvulsants   N
Carbamazepine   Phenytoin
Phenobarbital   Valproic acid
AHA: 4Q, '05, 82

760.78 Antimetabolic agents   N
Methotrexate
Retinoic acid
Statins
AHA: 4Q, '05, 82-83

760.79 Other
Fetus or newborn affected by:
immune sera   } transmitted via
medicinal agents NEC }   placenta
toxic substance NEC }   or breast
AHA: 1Q, '10, 14; 3Q, '09, 21
P04.8 Newborn (suspected) affected by oth   I-10
maternl noxious subst

760.8 Other specified maternal conditions affecting fetus or newborn
Maternal genital tract and other localized infection affecting fetus or newborn, but fetus or newborn not manifesting that disease

EXCLUDES maternal urinary tract infection affecting fetus or newborn (760.1)

760.9 Unspecified maternal condition affecting fetus or newborn

√4ᵗʰ 761 Fetus or newborn affected by maternal complications of pregnancy
INCLUDES the listed maternal conditions only when specified as a cause of mortality or morbidity of the fetus or newborn

761.0 Incompetent cervix
DEF: Inadequate functioning of uterine cervix.

761.1 Premature rupture of membranes

761.2 Oligohydramnios
EXCLUDES that due to premature rupture of membranes (761.1)
DEF: Deficient amniotic fluid.

761.3 Polyhydramnios
Hydramnios (acute) (chronic)
DEF: Excess amniotic fluid.

761.4 Ectopic pregnancy
Pregnancy:
abdominal
intraperitoneal
tubal

761.5 Multiple pregnancy
Triplet (pregnancy)   Twin (pregnancy)

√4ᵗʰ / √5ᵗʰ Additional Digit Required   Unspecified Code   Other Specified Code   Manifestation Code   ►◄ Revised Text   ● New Code   ▲ Revised Code Title

Certain Conditions Originating in the Perinatal Period

761.6–763.9

761.6 Maternal death

761.7 Malpresentation before labor

Breech presentation
External version
Oblique lie } before labor
Transverse lie
Unstable lie

761.8 Other specified maternal complications of pregnancy affecting fetus or newborn

Spontaneous abortion, fetus

761.9 Unspecified maternal complication of pregnancy affecting fetus or newborn

√4ᵗʰ **762 Fetus or newborn affected by complications of placenta, cord, and membranes**

INCLUDES the listed maternal conditions only when specified as a cause of mortality or morbidity in the fetus or newborn

AHA: 1Q, '94, 8

762.0 Placenta previa   N

DEF: Placenta developed in lower segment of uterus; causes hemorrhaging in last trimester.

762.1 Other forms of placental separation and hemorrhage   N

Abruptio placentae
Antepartum hemorrhage
Damage to placenta from amniocentesis, cesarean section, or surgical induction
Maternal blood loss
Premature separation of placenta
Rupture of marginal sinus

762.2 Other and unspecified morphological and functional abnormalities of placenta   N

Placental:
dysfunction
infarction
insufficiency

762.3 Placental transfusion syndromes   N

Placental and cord abnormality resulting in twin-to-twin or other transplacental transfusion

Use additional code to indicate resultant condition in newborn:
fetal blood loss (772.0)
polycythemia neonatorum (776.4)

762.4 Prolapsed cord   N

Cord presentation

762.5 Other compression of umbilical cord   N

Cord around neck
Entanglement of cord
Knot in cord
Torsion of cord

AHA: 2Q, '03, 9

TIP: Assign only if the cord compression or entanglement was documented as having affected the fetus/newborn.

P02.5 Newborn (suspected) affected by oth compression umb cord   I-10

762.6 Other and unspecified conditions of umbilical cord   N

Short cord
Thrombosis
Varices } of umbilical cord
Velamentous insertion

Vasa previa

EXCLUDES infection of umbilical cord (771.4)
single umbilical artery (747.5)

P02.69 Newborn (suspected) affected by oth cond umbil cord   I-10

762.7 Chorioamnionitis   N

Amnionitis   Placentitis
Membranitis

DEF: Inflamed fetal membrane.

762.8 Other specified abnormalities of chorion and amnion   N

762.9 Unspecified abnormality of chorion and amnion   N

√4ᵗʰ **763 Fetus or newborn affected by other complications of labor and delivery**

INCLUDES the listed conditions only when specified as a cause of mortality or morbidity in the fetus or newborn

EXCLUDES newborn affected by surgical procedures on mother (760.61-760.64)

AHA: 1Q, '94, 8

763.0 Breech delivery and extraction   N

763.1 Other malpresentation, malposition, and disproportion during labor and delivery   N

Fetus or newborn affected by:
abnormality of bony pelvis
contracted pelvis
persistent occipitoposterior position
shoulder presentation
transverse lie
Fetus or newborn affected by conditions classifiable to 652, 653, and 660

763.2 Forceps delivery   N

Fetus or newborn affected by forceps extraction

763.3 Delivery by vacuum extractor   N

763.4 Cesarean delivery   N

EXCLUDES placental separation or hemorrhage from cesarean section (762.1)

763.5 Maternal anesthesia and analgesia   N

Reactions and intoxications from maternal opiates and tranquilizers during labor and delivery

EXCLUDES drug withdrawal syndrome in newborn (779.5)

763.6 Precipitate delivery   N

Rapid second stage

763.7 Abnormal uterine contractions   N

Fetus or newborn affected by:
contraction ring
hypertonic labor
hypotonic uterine dysfunction
uterine inertia or dysfunction
Fetus or newborn affected by conditions classifiable to 661, except 661.3

√5ᵗʰ **763.8 Other specified complications of labor and delivery affecting fetus or newborn**

AHA: 4Q, '98, 46

763.81 Abnormality in fetal heart rate or rhythm before the onset of labor   N

763.82 Abnormality in fetal heart rate or rhythm during labor   N

AHA: 4Q, '98, 46

763.83 Abnormality in fetal heart rate or rhythm, unspecified as to time of onset   N

763.84 Meconium passage during delivery   N

EXCLUDES meconium aspiration (770.11, 770.12)
meconium staining (779.84)

DEF: Fetal intestinal activity that increases in response to a distressed state during delivery; anal sphincter relaxes, and meconium is passed into the amniotic fluid.

AHA: 4Q, '05, 83

TIP: If the meconium was documented as aspirated or had any effect on the newborn, see codes 770.11 and 770.12.

763.89 Other specified complications of labor and delivery affecting fetus or newborn   N

Fetus or newborn affected by:
abnormality of maternal soft tissues
destructive operation on live fetus to facilitate delivery
induction of labor (medical)
other procedures used in labor and delivery
Fetus or newborn affected by other conditions classifiable to 650-669

763.9 Unspecified complication of labor and delivery affecting fetus or newborn   N

N Newborn Age: 0   P Pediatric Age: 0-17   M Maternity Age: 12-55   A Adult Age: 15-124

Other Conditions Originating in the Perinatal Period (764-779)

The following fifth-digit subclassification is for use with category 764 and codes 765.0-765.1 to denote birthweight:
0 **unspecified [weight]**
1 **less than 500 grams**
2 **500-749 grams**
3 **750-999 grams**
4 **1,000-1,249 grams**
5 **1,250-1,499 grams**
6 **1,500-1,749 grams**
7 **1,750-1,999 grams**
8 **2,000-2,499 grams**
9 **2,500 grams and over**

√4ᵗʰ **764 Slow fetal growth and fetal malnutrition**
      AHA: 1Q, '09, 13; 3Q, '04, 4; 4Q, '02, 63; 1Q,'94, 8; 2Q, '91, 19; 2Q, '89, 15

§ √5ᵗʰ **764.0 "Light-for-dates" without mention of fetal malnutrition** N
      [0-9]   Infants underweight for gestational age
               "Small-for-dates"
               P05.00 Newborn light for gest age unsp weight   I-10

§ √5ᵗʰ **764.1 "Light-for-dates" with signs of fetal malnutrition** N
      [0-9]   Infants "light-for-dates" classifiable to 764.0, who in addition
               show signs of fetal malnutrition, such as dry peeling
               skin and loss of subcutaneous tissue

§ √5ᵗʰ **764.2 Fetal malnutrition without mention of "light-for-dates"** N
      [0-9]   Infants, not underweight for gestational age, showing signs of
               fetal malnutrition, such as dry peeling skin and loss of
               subcutaneous tissue
               Intrauterine malnutrition

§ √5ᵗʰ **764.9 Fetal growth retardation, unspecified** N
      [0-9]   Intrauterine growth retardation
               AHA: For code 764.97: 1Q, '97, 6

√4ᵗʰ **765 Disorders relating to short gestation and low birthweight**
      INCLUDES the listed conditions, without further specification, as
                   causes of mortality, morbidity, or additional care, in
                   fetus or newborn
      AHA: 1Q, '97, 6; 1Q, '94, 8; 2Q, '91, 19; 2Q, '89, 15

§ √5ᵗʰ **765.0 Extreme immaturity** N
      [0-9]   **NOTE** Usually implies a birthweight of less than 1000 grams.
               Use additional code for weeks of gestation (765.20-765.29)
               AHA: 1Q, '09, 13; 3Q, '04, 4; 4Q, '02, 63; For code 765.03: 4Q, '01, 51

§ √5ᵗʰ **765.1 Other preterm infants** N
      [0-9]   **NOTE** Usually implies a birthweight of 1000-2499 grams.
               Prematurity NOS
               Prematurity or small size, not classifiable to 765.0 or as
               "light-for-dates" in 764
               Use additional code for weeks of gestation (765.20-765.29)
               AHA: 1Q, '09, 13; 3Q, '04, 4; 4Q, '02, 63; For code 765.10: 1Q, '09, 15; 1Q,
               '94, 14; For code 765.17: 4Q, '08, 139; 1Q, '97, 6;
               For code 765.18: 4Q, '02, 64
               P07.10 Other low birth weight newborn uns weight   I-10

√5ᵗʰ **765.2 Weeks of gestation**
      AHA: 3Q, '04, 4; 4Q, '02, 63
      TIP: Assign as an additional code with category 764 and codes from
      765.0 and 765.1, as documented by the provider.

      765.20 Unspecified weeks of gestation N

      765.21 Less than 24 completed weeks of gestation N

      765.22 24 completed weeks of gestation N

      765.23 25-26 completed weeks of gestation N
               AHA: 1Q, '09, 14

      765.24 27-28 completed weeks of gestation N

      765.25 29-30 completed weeks of gestation N
               P07.31 Other preterm newborn 28-31 complete weeks   I-10

      765.26 31-32 completed weeks of gestation N
               AHA: 1Q, '09, 14; 4Q, '08, 139

      765.27 33-34 completed weeks of gestation N
               AHA: 4Q, '10, 97

      765.28 35-36 completed weeks of gestation N
               AHA: 4Q, '02, 64
               P07.32 Other preterm newborn 32-36 complete weeks   I-10

      765.29 37 or more completed weeks of gestation N

√4ᵗʰ **766 Disorders relating to long gestation and high birthweight**
      INCLUDES the listed conditions, without further specification, as
                   causes of mortality, morbidity, or additional care, in
                   fetus or newborn

      766.0 Exceptionally large baby N
             NOTE Usually implies a birthweight of 4500 grams or more.

      766.1 Other "heavy-for-dates" infants N
             Other fetus or infant "heavy-" or "large-for-dates" regardless
             of period of gestation
             P08.1 Other heavy for gestational age newborn   I-10

√5ᵗʰ **766.2 Late infant, not "heavy-for-dates"**
      AHA: 2Q, '06, 12; 4Q, '03, 69
      TIP: May be assigned based on gestational age alone, without
      documentation of any related specific condition or disorder.

      766.21 Post-term infant N
               Infant with gestation period over 40 completed
               weeks to 42 completed weeks
               AHA: 1Q, '09, 12;
               P08.21 Post-term newborn   I-10

      766.22 Prolonged gestation of infant N
               Infant with gestation period over 42 completed
               weeks
               Postmaturity NOS
               AHA: 1Q, '09, 12

√4ᵗʰ **767 Birth trauma**

      767.0 Subdural and cerebral hemorrhage N
             Subdural and cerebral hemorrhage, whether described as due
             to birth trauma or to intrapartum anoxia or hypoxia
             Subdural hematoma (localized)
             Tentorial tear
             Use additional code to identify cause
             EXCLUDES intraventricular hemorrhage (772.10-772.14)
                          subarachnoid hemorrhage (772.2)

√5ᵗʰ **767.1 Injuries to scalp**
      AHA: 4Q, '03, 69

      767.11 Epicranial subaponeurotic hemorrhage N
               (massive)
               Subgaleal hemorrhage
               DEF: A hemorrhage that occurs within the space between
               the galea aponeurotica, or epicranial aponeurosis, a thin
               tendinous structure that is attached to the skull laterally,
               and the periosteum of the skull.

      767.19 Other injuries to scalp N
               Caput succedaneum
               Cephalhematoma
               Chignon (from vacuum extraction)
               P12.89 Other birth injuries to scalp   I-10

      767.2 Fracture of clavicle N

      767.3 Other injuries to skeleton N
             Fracture of: Fracture of:
             long bones   skull
             EXCLUDES congenital dislocation of hip (754.30-754.35)
                          fracture of spine, congenital (767.4)

      767.4 Injury to spine and spinal cord N
             Dislocation ⎤
             Fracture   ⎥ of spine or spinal cord due to
             Laceration   ⎥ birth trauma
             Rupture   ⎦

      767.5 Facial nerve injury N
             Facial palsy

      767.6 Injury to brachial plexus N
             Palsy or paralysis: Palsy or paralysis:
             brachial   Klumpke (-Déjérine)
             Erb (-Duchenne)

      767.7 Other cranial and peripheral nerve injuries N
             Phrenic nerve paralysis

───

§ Requires fifth digit. Valid digits are in [brackets] under each code. See beginning of section 764-779 for codes and definitions.

√4ᵗʰ
√5ᵗʰ Additional Digit Required   Unspecified Code   Other Specified Code   Manifestation Code   ▶◀ Revised Text   ● New Code   ▲ Revised Code Title

Epicranial Aponeurosis

767.8 Other specified birth trauma   N

Eye damage	Rupture of:
Hematoma of:	liver
liver (subcapsular)	spleen
testes	Scalpel wound
vulva	Traumatic glaucoma

EXCLUDES   *hemorrhage classifiable to 772.0-772.9*

767.9 Birth trauma, unspecified   N
Birth injury NOS

√4th 768 Intrauterine hypoxia and birth asphyxia

NOTE Use only when associated with newborn morbidity classifiable elsewhere

EXCLUDES   *acidemia NOS of newborn (775.81)*
acidosis NOS of newborn (775.81)
cerebral ischemia NOS (779.2)
hypoxia NOS of newborn (770.88)
mixed metabolic and respiratory acidosis of newborn (775.81)
respiratory arrest of newborn (770.87)

DEF: Oxygen intake insufficiency due to interrupted placental circulation or premature separation of placenta.
AHA: 4Q, '92, 20

768.0 Fetal death from asphyxia or anoxia before onset of labor or at unspecified time   N

768.1 Fetal death from asphyxia or anoxia during labor   N

768.2 Fetal distress before onset of labor, in liveborn infant   N
Fetal metabolic acidemia before onset of labor, in liveborn infant

768.3 Fetal distress first noted during labor and delivery, in liveborn infant   N
Fetal metabolic acidemia first noted during labor and delivery, in liveborn infant

768.4 Fetal distress, unspecified as to time of onset, in liveborn infant   N
Fetal metabolic acidemia unspecified as to time of onset, in liveborn infant
AHA: N-D, '86, 10

768.5 Severe birth asphyxia   N
Birth asphyxia with neurologic involvement
EXCLUDES   *hypoxic-ischemic encephalopathy [HIE] (768.70-768.73)*
AHA: N-D, '86, 3

768.6 Mild or moderate birth asphyxia   N
Other specified birth asphyxia (without mention of neurologic involvement)
EXCLUDES   *hypoxic-ischemic encephalopathy [HIE] (768.70-768.73)*
AHA: N-D, '86, 3

√5th 768.7 Hypoxic-ischemic encephalopathy [HIE]
AHA: 4Q, '09, 99-101; 4Q, '06, 104

768.70 Hypoxic-ischemic encephalopathy, unspecified   N

768.71 Mild hypoxic-ischemic encephalopathy   N

768.72 Moderate hypoxic-ischemic encephalopathy   N
AHA: 4Q, '09, 101

768.73 Severe hypoxic-ischemic encephalopathy   N

768.9 Unspecified birth asphyxia in liveborn infant   N
Anoxia
Asphyxia } NOS, in liveborn infant

769 Respiratory distress syndrome   N
Cardiorespiratory distress syndrome of newborn
Hyaline membrane disease (pulmonary)
Idiopathic respiratory distress syndrome [IRDS or RDS] of newborn
Pulmonary hypoperfusion syndrome
EXCLUDES   *transient tachypnea of newborn (770.6)*
DEF: Severe chest contractions upon air intake and expiratory grunting; infant appears blue due to oxygen deficiency and has rapid respiratory rate; formerly called hyaline membrane disease.
AHA: 1Q, '89, 10; N-D, '86, 6
TIP: Do not assign if documentation specifies Type II respiratory distress syndrome, which usually resolves within six to 24 hours after birth; see instead 770.6.
P22.0 Respiratory distress syndrome of newborn   I-10

√4th 770 Other respiratory conditions of fetus and newborn

770.0 Congenital pneumonia   N
Infective pneumonia acquired prenatally
EXCLUDES   *pneumonia from infection acquired after birth (480.0-486)*
AHA: 1Q, '05, 10

√5th 770.1 Fetal and newborn aspiration
EXCLUDES   *aspiration of postnatal stomach contents (770.85, 770.86)*
meconium passage during delivery (763.84)
meconium staining (779.84)
AHA: 4Q, '05, 83

770.10 Fetal and newborn aspiration, unspecified   N

770.11 Meconium aspiration without respiratory symptoms   N
Meconium aspiration NOS

770.12 Meconium aspiration with respiratory symptoms   N
Meconium aspiration pneumonia
Meconium aspiration pneumonitis
Meconium aspiration syndrome NOS
Use additional code to identify any secondary pulmonary hypertension (416.8), if applicable
DEF: Meconium aspiration syndrome: aspiration of fetal intestinal material during or prior to delivery, usually a complication of placental insufficiency, causing pneumonitis and bronchial obstruction (inflammatory reaction of lungs).

770.13 Aspiration of clear amniotic fluid without respiratory symptoms   N
Aspiration of clear amniotic fluid NOS

770.14 Aspiration of clear amniotic fluid with respiratory symptoms   N
Aspiration of clear amniotic fluid with pneumonia
Aspiration of clear amniotic fluid with pneumonitis
Use additional code to identify any secondary pulmonary hypertension (416.8), if applicable

770.15 Aspiration of blood without respiratory symptoms   N
Aspiration of blood NOS

770.16 Aspiration of blood with respiratory symptoms   N
Aspiration of blood with pneumonia
Aspiration of blood with pneumonitis
Use additional code to identify any secondary pulmonary hypertension (416.8), if applicable

770.17 Other fetal and newborn aspiration without respiratory symptoms   N

770.18 Other fetal and newborn aspiration with respiratory symptoms   N
Other aspiration pneumonia
Other aspiration pneumonitis
Use additional code to identify any secondary pulmonary hypertension (416.8), if applicable

---

N Newborn Age: 0   P Pediatric Age: 0-17   M Maternity Age: 12-55   A Adult Age: 15-124

770.2 Interstitial emphysema and related conditions `N`
> Pneumomediastinum
> Pneumopericardium } originating in the perinatal
> Pneumothorax } period

P25.0 Interstitial emphysema origin perinatal period `I-10`

770.3 Pulmonary hemorrhage `N`
> Hemorrhage:
> alveolar (lung)
> intra-alveolar (lung) } originating in the
> massive pulmonary } perinatal period

770.4 Primary atelectasis `N`
> Pulmonary immaturity NOS

DEF: Alveoli fail to expand causing insufficient air intake by newborn.

770.5 Other and unspecified atelectasis `N`
> Atelectasis:
> NOS
> partial } originating in the perinatal
> secondary } period
> Pulmonary collapse

770.6 Transitory tachypnea of newborn `N`
> Idiopathic tachypnea of newborn
> Wet lung syndrome

EXCLUDES respiratory distress syndrome (769)

DEF: Quick, shallow breathing of newborn; short-term problem.
AHA: 4Q, '95, 4; 1Q, '94, 12; 3Q, '93, 7; 1Q, '89, 10; N-D, '86, 6
P22.1 Transient tachypnea of newborn `I-10`

770.7 Chronic respiratory disease arising in the perinatal period
> Bronchopulmonary dysplasia
> Interstitial pulmonary fibrosis of prematurity
> Wilson-Mikity syndrome

AHA: 1Q, '11, 16; 2Q, '91, 19; N-D, '86, 11
P27.8 Other chronic resp dz origin perinatal period `I-10`

√5ᵗʰ 770.8 Other respiratory problems after birth

EXCLUDES mixed metabolic and respiratory acidosis of newborn (775.81)

AHA: 4Q, '02, 65; 2Q, '98, 10; 2Q, '96, 10

770.81 Primary apnea of newborn `N`
> Apneic spells of newborn NOS
> Essential apnea of newborn
> Sleep apnea of newborn

DEF: Cessation of breathing when a neonate makes no respiratory effort for 15 seconds, resulting in cyanosis and bradycardia.
P28.3 Primary sleep apnea of newborn `I-10`

770.82 Other apnea of newborn `N`
> Obstructive apnea of newborn

770.83 Cyanotic attacks of newborn `N`

770.84 Respiratory failure of newborn `N`
EXCLUDES respiratory distress syndrome (769)
AHA: 4Q, '08, 99

770.85 Aspiration of postnatal stomach contents without respiratory symptoms `N`
> Aspiration of postnatal stomach contents NOS
AHA: 4Q, '05, 83

770.86 Aspiration of postnatal stomach contents with respiratory symptoms `N`
> Aspiration of postnatal stomach contents with pneumonia
> Aspiration of postnatal stomach contents with pneumonitis
> Use additional code to identify any secondary pulmonary hypertension (416.8), if applicable
AHA: 4Q, '05, 83

770.87 Respiratory arrest of newborn `N`
AHA: 4Q, '06, 104-106

770.88 Hypoxemia of newborn `N`
> Hypoxia NOS of newborn
AHA: 4Q, '06, 104-106

770.89 Other respiratory problems after birth `N`
AHA: 3Q, '09, 20
P28.89 Oth specified respiratory conditions of newborn `I-10`

770.9 Unspecified respiratory condition of fetus and newborn `N`

√4ᵗʰ 771 Infections specific to the perinatal period
INCLUDES infections acquired before or during birth or via the umbilicus or during the first 28 days after birth

EXCLUDES congenital pneumonia (770.0)
> congenital syphilis (090.0-090.9)
> infant botulism (040.41)
> maternal infectious disease as a cause of mortality or morbidity in fetus or newborn, but fetus or newborn not manifesting the disease (760.2)
> ophthalmia neonatorum due to gonococcus (098.40)
> other infections not specifically classified to this category

AHA: N-D, '85, 4

771.0 Congenital rubella `N`
> Congenital rubella pneumonitis

771.1 Congenital cytomegalovirus infection `N`
> Congenital cytomegalic inclusion disease

771.2 Other congenital infections `N`
> Congenital: Congenital:
> herpes simplex   toxoplasmosis
> listeriosis   tuberculosis
> malaria

771.3 Tetanus neonatorum `N`
> Tetanus omphalitis

EXCLUDES hypocalcemic tetany (775.4)

DEF: Severe infection of central nervous system; due to exotoxin of tetanus bacillus from navel infection prompted by nonsterile technique during umbilical ligation.

771.4 Omphalitis of the newborn `N`
> Infection:
> navel cord
> umbilical stump

EXCLUDES tetanus omphalitis (771.3)

DEF: Inflamed umbilicus.
AHA: 4Q, '09, 102

771.5 Neonatal infective mastitis `N`
EXCLUDES noninfective neonatal mastitis (778.7)

771.6 Neonatal conjunctivitis and dacryocystitis `N`
> Ophthalmia neonatorum NOS
EXCLUDES ophthalmia neonatorum due to gonococcus (098.40)

771.7 Neonatal Candida infection `N`
> Neonatal moniliasis
> Thrush in newborn

√5ᵗʰ 771.8 Other infection specific to the perinatal period
> Use additional code to identify organism or specific infection
AHA: 4Q, '02, 66

771.81 Septicemia [sepsis] of newborn `N`
> Use additional codes to identify severe sepsis (995.92) and any associated acute organ dysfunction, if applicable
AHA: 4Q, '08, 99
TIP: Assign instead of 038 or 995.91.
P36.9 Bacterial sepsis newborn unspecified `I-10`

771.82 Urinary tract infection of newborn `N`

771.83 Bacteremia of newborn `N`

771.89 Other infections specific to the perinatal period `N`
> Intra-amniotic infection of fetus NOS
> Infection of newborn NOS

☑4ᵗʰ 772   Fetal and neonatal hemorrhage

> **EXCLUDES** *fetal hematologic conditions complicating pregnancy (678.0)*
> *hematological disorders of fetus and newborn (776.0-776.9)*

772.0   Fetal blood loss affecting newborn   N
> Fetal blood loss from:
>   cut end of co-twin's cord
>   placenta
>   ruptured cord
>   vasa previa
> Fetal exsanguination
> Fetal hemorrhage into:
>   co-twin
>   mother's circulation

☑5ᵗʰ 772.1   Intraventricular hemorrhage
> Intraventricular hemorrhage from any perinatal cause
> **AHA:** 4Q, '01, 49; 3Q, '92, 8; 4Q, '88, 8

> **772.10   Unspecified grade**   N

> **772.11   Grade I**   N
> > Bleeding into germinal matrix

> **772.12   Grade II**   N
> > Bleeding into ventricle

> **772.13   Grade III**   N
> > Bleeding with enlargement of ventricle
> > **AHA:** 4Q, '01, 51

> **772.14   Grade IV**   N
> > Bleeding into cerebral cortex

772.2   Subarachnoid hemorrhage   N
> Subarachnoid hemorrhage from any perinatal cause
> **EXCLUDES** *subdural and cerebral hemorrhage (767.0)*

772.3   Umbilical hemorrhage after birth   N
> Slipped umbilical ligature

772.4   Gastrointestinal hemorrhage   N
> **EXCLUDES** *swallowed maternal blood (777.3)*

772.5   Adrenal hemorrhage   N

772.6   Cutaneous hemorrhage   N
> Bruising
> Ecchymoses   } in fetus or newborn
> Petechiae
> Superficial hematoma
> **P54.5** Neonatal cutaneous hemorrhage   I-10

772.8   Other specified hemorrhage of fetus or newborn   N
> **EXCLUDES** *hemorrhagic disease of newborn (776.0)*
> *pulmonary hemorrhage (770.3)*

772.9   Unspecified hemorrhage of newborn   N

☑4ᵗʰ 773   Hemolytic disease of fetus or newborn, due to isoimmunization
> **DEF:** Hemolytic anemia of fetus or newborn due to maternal antibody formation against fetal erythrocytes; infant blood contains nonmaternal antigen.
> **TIP:** Do not assign unless the physician substantiates confirmation by a positive Coomb's (direct antibody or direct antiglobulin) test.

773.0   Hemolytic disease due to Rh isoimmunization   N
> Anemia   } due to RH:
> Erythroblastosis (fetalis)   antibodies
> Hemolytic disease (fetus)   isoimmunization
>   (newborn)   maternal/fetal
> Jaundice   incompatibility
>
> Rh hemolytic disease
> Rh isoimmunization

773.1   Hemolytic disease due to ABO isoimmunization   N
> ABO hemolytic disease
> ABO isoimmunization
> Anemia   } due to ABO:
> Erythroblastosis (fetalis)   antibodies
> Hemolytic disease (fetus)   isoimmunization
>   (newborn)   maternal/fetal
> Jaundice   incompatibility
> **DEF:** Incompatible Rh fetal-maternal blood grouping; prematurely destroys red blood cells; detected by Coombs test.
> **AHA:** 3Q, '92, 8
> **P55.1** ABO isoimmunization of newborn   I-10

773.2   Hemolytic disease due to other and unspecified isoimmunization   N
> Eythroblastosis (fetalis) (neonatorum) NOS
> Hemolytic disease (fetus) (newborn) NOS
> Jaundice or anemia due to other and unspecified blood-group
>   incompatibility
> **AHA:** 1Q, '94, 13
> **P55.9** Hemolytic disease of newborn unspecified   I-10

773.3   Hydrops fetalis due to isoimmunization   N
> Use additional code to identify type of isoimmunization
>   (773.0-773.2)
> **DEF:** Massive edema of entire body and severe anemia; may result in fetal death or stillbirth.

773.4   Kernicterus due to isoimmunization   N
> Use additional code to identify type of isoimmunization
>   (773.0-773.2)
> **DEF:** Complication of erythroblastosis fetalis associated with severe neural symptoms, high blood bilirubin levels and nerve cell destruction; results in bilirubin-pigmented gray matter of central nervous system.

773.5   Late anemia due to isoimmunization   N

☑4ᵗʰ 774   Other perinatal jaundice

774.0   *Perinatal jaundice from hereditary hemolytic anemias*   N
> *Code first underlying disease (282.0-282.9)*

774.1   Perinatal jaundice from other excessive hemolysis   N
> Fetal or neonatal jaundice from:
>   bruising
>   drugs or toxins transmitted from mother
>   infection
>   polycythemia
>   swallowed maternal blood
> Use additional code to identify cause
> **EXCLUDES** *jaundice due to isoimmunization (773.0-773.2)*

774.2   Neonatal jaundice associated with preterm delivery   N
> Hyperbilirubinemia of prematurity
> Jaundice due to delayed conjugation associated with preterm
>   delivery
> **AHA:** 3Q, '91, 21
> **P59.0** Neonatal jaundice associated w/preterm delivery   I-10

☑5ᵗʰ 774.3   Neonatal jaundice due to delayed conjugation from other causes

> **774.30   Neonatal jaundice due to delayed conjugation, cause unspecified**   N
> > **DEF:** Jaundice of newborn with abnormal bilirubin metabolism; causes excess accumulated unconjugated bilirubin in blood.

> **774.31   *Neonatal jaundice due to delayed conjugation in diseases classified elsewhere***   N
> > *Code first underlying diseases as:*
> >   congenital hypothyroidism (243)
> >   Crigler-Najjar syndrome (277.4)
> >   Gilbert's syndrome (277.4)

> **774.39   Other**   N
> > Jaundice due to delayed conjugation from causes,
> >   such as:
> >   breast milk inhibitors
> >   delayed development of conjugating system

774.4   Perinatal jaundice due to hepatocellular damage   N
> Fetal or neonatal hepatitis
> Giant cell hepatitis
> Inspissated bile syndrome

774.5   *Perinatal jaundice from other causes*   N
> *Code first underlying cause as:*
>   congenital obstruction of bile duct (751.61)
>   galactosemia (271.1)
>   mucoviscidosis (277.00-277.09)

774.6   Unspecified fetal and neonatal jaundice   N
> Icterus neonatorum
> Neonatal hyperbilirubinemia (transient)
> Physiologic jaundice NOS in newborn
> **EXCLUDES** *that in preterm infants (774.2)*
> **AHA:** 1Q, '94, 13; 2Q, '89, 15
> **P59.9** Neonatal jaundice unspecified   I-10

N   Newborn Age: 0   P   Pediatric Age: 0-17   M   Maternity Age: 12-55   A   Adult Age: 15-124

774.7 Kernicterus not due to isoimmunization [N]
Bilirubin encephalopathy
Kernicterus of newborn NOS
EXCLUDES *kernicterus due to isoimmunization (773.4)*

√4ᵗʰ **775 Endocrine and metabolic disturbances specific to the fetus and newborn**
INCLUDES transitory endocrine and metabolic disturbances caused by the infant's response to maternal endocrine and metabolic factors, its removal from them, or its adjustment to extrauterine existence

775.0 Syndrome of "infant of a diabetic mother" [N]
Maternal diabetes mellitus affecting fetus or newborn (with hypoglycemia)
AHA: 1Q, '04, 7-8; 3Q, '91, 5
TIP: Do not assign if the infant has no manifestations or symptoms of the syndrome; refer instead to code V18.0 Family history, diabetes mellitus.
P70.1 Syndrome of infant of diabetic mother [I-10]

775.1 Neonatal diabetes mellitus [N]
Diabetes mellitus syndrome in newborn infant
AHA: 3Q, '91, 6

775.2 Neonatal myasthenia gravis [N]

775.3 Neonatal thyrotoxicosis [N]
Neonatal hyperthyroidism (transient)

775.4 Hypocalcemia and hypomagnesemia of newborn [N]
Cow's milk hypocalcemia
Hypocalcemic tetany, neonatal
Neonatal hypoparathyroidism
Phosphate-loading hypocalcemia

775.5 Other transitory neonatal electrolyte disturbances [N]
Dehydration, neonatal
AHA: 1Q, '10, 14; 3Q, '09, 21; 1Q, '05, 9
TIP: If the patient has neonatal hyperkalemia, assign also code 276.7 Hyperpotassemia.
P74.1 Dehydration of newborn [I-10]

775.6 Neonatal hypoglycemia [N]
EXCLUDES *infant of mother with diabetes mellitus (775.0)*
AHA: 1Q '94, 8
P70.4 Other neonatal hypoglycemia [I-10]

775.7 Late metabolic acidosis of newborn [N]

√5ᵗʰ **775.8 Other neonatal endocrine and metabolic disturbances**

775.81 Other acidosis of newborn [N]
Acidemia NOS of newborn
Acidosis of newborn NOS
Mixed metabolic and respiratory acidosis of newborn
AHA: 4Q, '06, 104-106

775.89 Other neonatal endocrine and metabolic disturbances [N]
Amino-acid metabolic disorders described as transitory
AHA: 4Q, '06, 104-106

775.9 Unspecified endocrine and metabolic disturbances specific to the fetus and newborn [N]

√4ᵗʰ **776 Hematological disorders of newborn**
INCLUDES disorders specific to the newborn though possibly originating in utero
EXCLUDES *fetal hematologic conditions (678.0)*

776.0 Hemorrhagic disease of newborn [N]
Hemorrhagic diathesis of newborn
Vitamin K deficiency of newborn
EXCLUDES *fetal or neonatal hemorrhage (772.0-772.9)*

776.1 Transient neonatal thrombocytopenia [N]
Neonatal thrombocytopenia due to:
exchange transfusion
idiopathic maternal thrombocytopenia
isoimmunization
DEF: Temporary decrease in blood platelets of newborn.
P61.0 Transient neonatal thrombocytopenia [I-10]

776.2 Disseminated intravascular coagulation in newborn [N]
DEF: Disseminated intravascular coagulation of newborn: clotting disorder due to excess thromboplastic agents in blood as a result of disease or trauma; causes blood clotting within vessels and reduces available elements necessary for blood coagulation.

776.3 Other transient neonatal disorders of coagulation [N]
Transient coagulation defect, newborn

776.4 Polycythemia neonatorum [N]
Plethora of newborn
Polycythemia due to:
donor twin transfusion
maternal-fetal transfusion
DEF: Abnormal increase of total red blood cells of newborn.

776.5 Congenital anemia [N]
Anemia following fetal blood loss
EXCLUDES *anemia due to isoimmunization (773.0-773.2, 773.5)*
hereditary hemolytic anemias (282.0-282.9)

776.6 Anemia of prematurity [N]
P61.2 Anemia of prematurity [I-10]

776.7 Transient neonatal neutropenia [N]
Isoimmune neutropenia   Maternal transfer neutropenia
EXCLUDES *congenital neutropenia (nontransient) (288.01)*
DEF: Decreased neutrophilic leukocytes in blood of newborn.

776.8 Other specified transient hematological disorders [N]

776.9 Unspecified hematological disorder specific to newborn [N]

√4ᵗʰ **777 Perinatal disorders of digestive system**
INCLUDES disorders specific to the fetus and newborn
EXCLUDES *intestinal obstruction classifiable to 560.0-560.9*

777.1 Meconium obstruction [N]
Congenital fecaliths
Delayed passage of meconium
Meconium ileus NOS
Meconium plug syndrome
EXCLUDES *meconium ileus in cystic fibrosis (277.01)*
DEF: Meconium blocked digestive tract of newborn.

777.2 Intestinal obstruction due to inspissated milk [N]

777.3 Hematemesis and melena due to swallowed maternal blood [N]
Swallowed blood syndrome in newborn
EXCLUDES *that not due to swallowed maternal blood (772.4)*

777.4 Transitory ileus of newborn [N]
EXCLUDES *Hirschsprung's disease (751.3)*

√5ᵗʰ **777.5 Necrotizing enterocolitis in newborn**
DEF: Serious intestinal infection and inflammation in preterm infants; severity is measured by stages and may progress to life-threatening perforation or peritonitis; resection surgical treatment may be necessary.
AHA: 4Q, '08, 138-140

777.50 Necrotizing enterocolitis in newborn, unspecified [N]
Necrotizing enterocolitis in newborn, NOS

777.51 Stage I necrotizing enterocolitis in newborn [N]
Necrotizing enterocolitis without pneumatosis, without perforation
DEF: Broad-spectrum symptoms with non-specific signs including feeding intolerance, sepsis, gastroenteritis, ileus, metabolic abnormalities.

777.52 Stage II necrotizing enterocolitis in newborn [N]
Necrotizing enterocolitis with pneumatosis, without perforation
DEF: Radiographic confirmation of necrotizing enterocolitis showing intestinal dilatation, fixed loops of bowels, pneumatosis intestinalis, metabolic acidosis, and thrombocytopenia.

777.53 Stage III necrotizing enterocolitis in newborn [N]
Necrotizing enterocolitis with perforation
Necrotizing enterocolitis with pneumatosis and perforation
DEF: Advanced stage in which infant demonstrates signs of bowel perforation, septic shock, metabolic acidosis, ascites, disseminated intravascular coagulopathy, neutropenia.
AHA: 4Q, '08, 139

Certain Conditions Originating in the Perinatal Period

777.6–779.9

777.6 Perinatal intestinal perforation   N
  Meconium peritonitis

777.8 Other specified perinatal disorders of digestive system   N
  AHA: 4Q, '10, 97

777.9 Unspecified perinatal disorder of digestive system   N

√4ᵗʰ **778 Conditions involving the integument and temperature regulation of fetus and newborn**

778.0 Hydrops fetalis not due to isoimmunization   N
  Idiopathic hydrops
  EXCLUDES *hydrops fetalis due to isoimmunization (773.3)*
  DEF: Edema of entire body, unrelated to immune response.

778.1 Sclerema neonatorum   N
  Subcutaneous fat necrosis
  DEF: Diffuse, rapidly progressing white, waxy, nonpitting hardening of tissue, usually of legs and feet, life-threatening; found in preterm or debilitated infants; unknown etiology.

778.2 Cold injury syndrome of newborn   N

778.3 Other hypothermia of newborn   N

778.4 Other disturbances of temperature regulation of newborn   N
  Dehydration fever in newborn
  Environmentally-induced pyrexia
  Hyperthermia in newborn
  Transitory fever of newborn
  P81.9 Disturbance of temp regulation newborn uns   I-10

778.5 Other and unspecified edema of newborn   N
  Edema neonatorum

778.6 Congenital hydrocele   N
  Congenital hydrocele of tunica vaginalis
  P83.5 Congenital hydrocele   I-10

778.7 Breast engorgement in newborn   N
  Noninfective mastitis of newborn
  EXCLUDES *infective mastitis of newborn (771.5)*

778.8 Other specified conditions involving the integument of fetus and newborn   N
  Urticaria neonatorum
  EXCLUDES *impetigo neonatorum (684)*
  pemphigus neonatorum (684)
  P83.8 Oth spec conditions integument specific to newborn   I-10

778.9 Unspecified condition involving the integument and temperature regulation of fetus and newborn   N

√4ᵗʰ **779 Other and ill-defined conditions originating in the perinatal period**

779.0 Convulsions in newborn   N
  Fits ⎫
  Seizures ⎬ in newborn
  AHA: N-D, '84, 11
  TIP: Clarify with the physician that convulsions are not actually infantile spasms; if so, refer to subcategory 345.6.

779.1 Other and unspecified cerebral irritability in newborn   N

779.2 Cerebral depression, coma, and other abnormal cerebral signs   N
  Cerebral ischemia NOS of newborn
  CNS dysfunction in newborn NOS
  EXCLUDES *cerebral ischemia due to birth trauma (767.0)*
  intrauterine cerebral ischemia (768.2-768.9)
  intraventricular hemorrhage (772.10-772.14)

√5ᵗʰ **779.3 Disorder of stomach function and feeding problems in newborn**
  AHA: 2Q, '89, 15

779.31 Feeding problems in newborn   N
  Slow feeding in newborn
  EXCLUDES *feeding problem in child over 28 days old (783.3)*
  AHA: 4Q, '09, 102
  P92.9 Feeding problem of newborn unspecified   I-10

779.32 Bilious vomiting in newborn   N
  EXCLUDES *bilious vomiting in child over 28 days old (787.04)*

779.33 Other vomiting in newborn   N
  Regurgitation of food in newborn
  EXCLUDES *vomiting in child over 28 days old (536.2, 787.01-787.04)*

779.34 Failure to thrive in newborn   N
  EXCLUDES *failure to thrive in child over 28 days old (783.41)*

779.4 Drug reactions and intoxications specific to newborn   N
  Gray syndrome from chloramphenicol administration in newborn
  EXCLUDES *fetal alcohol syndrome (760.71)*
  reactions and intoxications from maternal opiates and tranquilizers (763.5)

779.5 Drug withdrawal syndrome in newborn   N
  Drug withdrawal syndrome in infant of dependent mother
  EXCLUDES *fetal alcohol syndrome (760.71)*
  AHA: 3Q, '94, 6
  TIP: If the infant is asymptomatic but has a positive drug screen (e.g., for cocaine), assign instead 760.75.

779.6 Termination of pregnancy (fetus)   N
  Fetal death due to:
   induced abortion
   termination of pregnancy
  EXCLUDES *spontaneous abortion (fetus) (761.8)*

779.7 Periventricular leukomalacia
  DEF: Necrosis of white matter adjacent to lateral ventricles with the formation of cysts; cause of PVL has not been firmly established, but thought to be related to inadequate blood flow in certain areas of the brain.
  AHA: 4Q, '01, 50, 51

√5ᵗʰ **779.8 Other specified conditions originating in the perinatal period**
  AHA: 4Q, '02, 67; 1Q, '94, 15

779.81 Neonatal bradycardia   N
  EXCLUDES *abnormality in fetal heart rate or rhythm complicating labor and delivery (763.81-763.83)*
  bradycardia due to birth asphyxia (768.5-768.9)
  P29.12 Neonatal bradycardia   I-10

779.82 Neonatal tachycardia   N
  EXCLUDES *abnormality in fetal heart rate or rhythm complicating labor and delivery (763.81-763.83)*

779.83 Delayed separation of umbilical cord   N
  AHA: 4Q, '03, 71

779.84 Meconium staining   N
  EXCLUDES *meconium aspiration (770.11, 770.12)*
  meconium passage during delivery (763.84)
  AHA: 4Q, '05, 83, 88
  P96.83 Meconium staining   I-10

779.85 Cardiac arrest of newborn   N
  AHA: 4Q, '06, 104-106

779.89 Other specified conditions originating in the perinatal period   N
  Use additional code to specify condition
  AHA: ▶3Q, '11, 3-4;◀ 2Q, '11, 13; 1Q, '06, 18; 2Q, '05, 15; 1Q, '05, 9
  P96.89 Oth spec conditions originating perinatal period   I-10

779.9 Unspecified condition originating in the perinatal period   N
  Congenital debility NOS
  Stillbirth NEC

N Newborn Age: 0   P Pediatric Age: 0-17   M Maternity Age: 12-55   A Adult Age: 15-124

16. Symptoms, Signs, and Ill-Defined Conditions (780-799)

This section includes symptoms, signs, abnormal results of laboratory or other investigative procedures, and ill-defined conditions regarding which no diagnosis classifiable elsewhere is recorded.

Signs and symptoms that point rather definitely to a given diagnosis are assigned to some category in the preceding part of the classification. In general, categories 780-796 include the more ill-defined conditions and symptoms that point with perhaps equal suspicion to two or more diseases or to two or more systems of the body, and without the necessary study of the case to make a final diagnosis. Practically all categories in this group could be designated as "not otherwise specified," or as "unknown etiology," or as "transient." The Alphabetic Index should be consulted to determine which symptoms and signs are to be allocated here and which to more specific sections of the classification; the residual subcategories numbered .9 are provided for other relevant symptoms which cannot be allocated elsewhere in the classification.

The conditions and signs or symptoms included in categories 780-796 consist of: (a) cases for which no more specific diagnosis can be made even after all facts bearing on the case have been investigated; (b) signs or symptoms existing at the time of initial encounter that proved to be transient and whose causes could not be determined; (c) provisional diagnoses in a patient who failed to return for further investigation or care; (d) cases referred elsewhere for investigation or treatment before the diagnosis was made; (e) cases in which a more precise diagnosis was not available for any other reason; (f) certain symptoms which represent important problems in medical care and which it might be desired to classify in addition to a known cause.

AHA: 3Q, '11, 12

Symptoms (780-789)

AHA: 1Q, '91, 12; 2Q, '90, 3; 2Q, '90, 5; 2Q, '90, 15; M-A, '85, 3

√4ᵗʰ **780 General symptoms**

√5ᵗʰ **780.0 Alteration of consciousness**

EXCLUDES alteration of consciousness due to:
intracranial injuries (850.0-854.19)
skull fractures (800.00-801.99, 803.00-804.99)
coma:
diabetic (249.2-249.3, 250.2-250.3)
hepatic (572.2)
originating in the perinatal period (779.2)

AHA: 4Q, '92, 20

780.01 Coma
DEF: State of unconsciousness from which the patient cannot be awakened.
AHA: ▶1Q, '12, 14;◀ 3Q, '96, 16
TIP: ▶Although found in the symptoms and signs chapter, coma is not inherent in other conditions and should be reported whenever appropriately documented.◀

780.02 Transient alteration of awareness
DEF: Temporary, recurring spells of reduced consciousness.

780.03 Persistent vegetative state
DEF: Persistent wakefulness without consciousness due to nonfunctioning cerebral cortex.

780.09 Other
Drowsiness
Semicoma
Somnolence
Stupor
Unconsciousness
R40.1 Stupor   I-10

780.1 Hallucinations
Hallucinations:
NOS
auditory
gustatory
olfactory
tactile

EXCLUDES those associated with mental disorders, as functional psychoses (295.0-298.9)
organic brain syndromes (290.0-294.9, 310.0-310.9)
visual hallucinations (368.16)

DEF: Perception of external stimulus in absence of stimulus; inability to distinguish between real and imagined.

780.2 Syncope and collapse
Blackout
Fainting
(Near) (Pre) syncope
Vasovagal attack

EXCLUDES carotid sinus syncope (337.0)
heat syncope (992.1)
neurocirculatory asthenia (306.2)
orthostatic hypotension (458.0)
shock NOS (785.50)

DEF: Sudden unconsciousness due to reduced blood flow to brain.
AHA: 1Q, '02, 6; 3Q, '00, 12; 4Q, '95, 42; 3Q, '95, 14; N-D, '85, 12
R55 Syncope and collapse   I-10

√5ᵗʰ **780.3 Convulsions**

EXCLUDES convulsions:
epileptic (345.10-345.91)
in newborn (779.0)

DEF: Sudden, involuntary contractions of the muscles.
AHA: 2Q, '97, 8; 1Q, '97, 12; 3Q, '94, 9; 1Q, '93, 24; 4Q, '92, 23; N-D, '87, 12

780.31 Febrile convulsions (simple), unspecified
Febrile seizure NOS
AHA: 4Q, '97, 45

780.32 Complex febrile convulsions
Febrile seizure:
atypical
complex
complicated
EXCLUDES status epilepticus (345.3)
AHA: 4Q, '06, 106

780.33 Post traumatic seizures
EXCLUDES post traumatic epilepsy (345.00-345.91)
AHA: 4Q, '10, 92-93

780.39 Other convulsions
Convulsive disorder NOS
Fit NOS
Recurrent convulsions NOS
Seizure NOS
AHA: 2Q, '11, 5; 1Q, '08, 17; 3Q, '06, 22; 4Q, '04, 51; 1Q, '03, 7; 2Q, '99, 17; 4Q, '98, 39
R56.9 Unspecified convulsions   I-10

780.4 Dizziness and giddiness
Light-headedness
Vertigo NOS
EXCLUDES Ménière's disease and other specified vertiginous syndromes (386.0-386.9)
DEF: Whirling sensations in head with feeling of falling.
AHA: 2Q, '03, 11; 3Q, '00, 12; 2Q, '97, 9; 2Q, '91, 17
R42 Dizziness and giddiness   I-10

√5ᵗʰ **780.5 Sleep disturbances**

EXCLUDES circadian rhythm sleep disorders (327.30-327.39)
organic hypersomnia (327.10-327.19)
organic insomnia (327.00-327.09)
organic sleep apnea (327.20-327.29)
organic sleep related movement disorders (327.51-327.59)
parasomnias (327.40-327.49)
that of nonorganic origin (307.40-307.49)
AHA: 4Q, '05, 59

780.50 Sleep disturbance, unspecified

780.51 Insomnia with sleep apnea, unspecified
DEF: Transient cessation of breathing disturbing sleep.

780.52 Insomnia, unspecified
DEF: Inability to maintain adequate sleep cycle.
G47.00 Insomnia unspecified   I-10

780.53 Hypersomnia with sleep apnea, unspecified
DEF: Autonomic response inhibited during sleep; causes insufficient oxygen intake, acidosis and pulmonary hypertension.
AHA: 1Q, '93, 28; N-D, '85, 4

780.54 Hypersomnia, unspecified
DEF: Prolonged sleep cycle.

780.55 Disruptions of 24 hour sleep wake cycle, unspecified

√4ᵗʰ/√5ᵗʰ Additional Digit Required   Unspecified Code   Other Specified Code   Manifestation Code   ▶◀ Revised Text   ● New Code   ▲ Revised Code Title

Symptoms, Signs, and Ill-Defined Conditions

780.56–780.93

780.56 Dysfunctions associated with sleep stages or arousal from sleep

780.57 Unspecified sleep apnea
AHA: 1Q, '01, 6 ; 1Q, '97, 5; 1Q, '93, 28
G47.30 Sleep apnea unspecified   I-10

780.58 Sleep related movement disorder, unspecified
EXCLUDES *restless legs syndrome (333.94)*
AHA: 4Q, '04, 95

780.59 Other

√5ᵗʰ **780.6 Fever and other physiologic disturbances of temperature regulation**
EXCLUDES *effects of reduced environmental temperature (991.0-991.9)*
effects of heat and light (992.0-992.9)
fever, chills or hypothermia associated with confirmed infection — code to infection
AHA: 4Q, '08,140-142; 3Q, '05, 16; 3Q, '00,13; 4Q, '99, 26; 2Q, '91, 8

780.60 Fever, unspecified
Chills with fever
Fever NOS
Fever of unknown origin (FUO)
Hyperpyrexia NOS
Pyrexia NOS
Pyrexia of unknown origin
EXCLUDES *chills without fever (780.64)*
neonatal fever (778.4)
pyrexia of unknown origin (during):
in newborn (778.4)
labor (659.2)
the puerperium (672)
R50.9 Fever unspecified   I-10

780.61 Fever presenting with conditions classified elsewhere
Code first underlying condition when associated fever is present, such as with:
leukemia (conditions classifiable to 204-208)
neutropenia (288.00-288.09)
sickle-cell disease (282.60-282.69)
AHA: 4Q, '08, 142

780.62 Postprocedural fever
EXCLUDES *posttransfusion fever (780.66)*
postvaccination fever (780.63)
TIP: Do not assign a code from category 998 for post-procedural fever.

780.63 Postvaccination fever
Postimmunization fever

780.64 Chills (without fever)
Chills NOS
EXCLUDES *chills with fever (780.60)*

780.65 Hypothermia not associated with low environmental temperature
EXCLUDES *hypothermia:*
associated with low environmental temperature (991.6)
due to anesthesia (995.89)
of newborn (778.2, 778.3)

780.66 Febrile nonhemolytic transfusion reaction
FNHTR
Posttransfusion fever
AHA: 4Q, '10, 99-100

√5ᵗʰ **780.7 Malaise and fatigue**
EXCLUDES *debility, unspecified (799.3)*
fatigue (during):
combat (308.0-308.9)
heat (992.6)
pregnancy (646.8)
neurasthenia (300.5)
senile asthenia (797)
AHA: 4Q, '88, 12; M-A, '87, 8

780.71 Chronic fatigue syndrome
DEF: Persistent fatigue, symptoms include weak muscles, sore throat, lymphadenitis, headache, depression and mild fever; no known cause; also called chronic mononucleosis, benign myalgic encephalomyelitis, Iceland disease and neurosthenia.
AHA: 4Q, '98, 48

780.72 Functional quadriplegia
Complete immobility due to severe physical disability or frailty
EXCLUDES *hysterical paralysis (300.11)*
immobility syndrome (728.3)
neurologic quadriplegia (344.00-344.09)
quadriplegia NOS (344.00)
DEF: Inability to move due to another condition such as dementia, severe contractures, or arthritis, not a physiologic one; no mental ability to move independently; typically found in severely demented patients.
AHA: 4Q, '08, 143
TIP: The functional quadriplegic patient typically has severe dementia and the quadriplegia will be due to a nonneurologic condition.

780.79 Other malaise and fatigue
Asthenia NOS   Postviral (asthenic) syndrome
Lethargy   Tiredness
DEF: Asthenia: Any weakness, lack of strength or loss of energy, especially neuromuscular.
DEF: Lethargy: Listlessness, drowsiness, stupor and apathy.
DEF: Malaise: Vague feeling of debility or lack of good health.
DEF: Postviral (asthenic) syndrome: Listlessness, drowsiness, stupor and apathy; follows acute viral infection.
DEF: Tiredness: General exhaustion or fatigue.
AHA: 4Q, '04, 78; 1Q, '00, 6; 4Q, '99, 26
R53.83 Other fatigue   I-10

780.8 Generalized hyperhidrosis
Diaphoresis   Secondary hyperhidrosis
Excessive sweating
EXCLUDES *focal (localized) (primary) (secondary) hyperhidrosis (705.21-705.22)*
Frey's syndrome (705.22)
DEF: Excessive sweating, appears as droplets on skin; general or localized.

√5ᵗʰ **780.9 Other general symptoms**
EXCLUDES *hypothermia:*
NOS (accidental) (991.6)
due to anesthesia (995.89)
of newborn (778.2-778.3)
memory disturbance as part of a pattern of mental disorder
AHA: 4Q, '02, 67; 4Q, '99, 10; 3Q, '93, 11; N-D, '85, 12

780.91 Fussy infant (baby)   P

780.92 Excessive crying of infant (baby)   N
EXCLUDES *excessive crying of child, adolescent or adult (780.95)*

780.93 Memory loss
Amnesia (retrograde)
Memory loss NOS
EXCLUDES *memory loss due to:*
intracranial injuries (850.0-854.19)
skull fractures (800.00-801.99, 803.00-804.99)
mild memory disturbance due to organic brain damage (310.89)
transient global amnesia (437.7)
AHA: 4Q, '03, 71

N Newborn Age: 0   P Pediatric Age: 0-17   M Maternity Age: 12-55   A Adult Age: 15-124

780.94 Early satiety
DEF: The premature feeling of being full; mechanism of satiety is multifactorial.
AHA: 4Q, '03, 72

780.95 Excessive crying of child, adolescent, or adult
EXCLUDES excessive crying of infant (baby) (780.92)
AHA: 4Q, '05, 89

780.96 Generalized pain
Pain NOS
AHA: 4Q, '06, 79-81
TIP: For pain syndromes, refer to category 338; if site is specified, refer to index.

780.97 Altered mental status
Change in mental status
EXCLUDES altered level of consciousness (780.01-780.09)
altered mental status due to known condition — code to condition
delirium NOS (780.09)
AHA: 4Q, '06, 107
R41.82 Altered mental status unspecified I-10

780.99 Other general symptoms
AHA: 4Q, '03, 103

√4ᵗʰ **781 Symptoms involving nervous and musculoskeletal systems**
EXCLUDES depression NOS (311)
disorders specifically relating to:
back (724.0-724.9)
hearing (388.0-389.9)
joint (718.0-719.9)
limb (729.0-729.9)
neck (723.0-723.9)
vision (368.0-369.9)
pain in limb (729.5)

781.0 Abnormal involuntary movements
Abnormal head movements   Spasms NOS
Fasciculation   Tremor NOS
EXCLUDES abnormal reflex (796.1)
chorea NOS (333.5)
infantile spasms (345.60-345.61)
spastic paralysis (342.1, 343.0-344.9)
specified movement disorders classifiable to 333 (333.0-333.9)
that of nonorganic origin (307.2-307.3)
R25.9 Unspecified abnormal involuntary movements I-10

781.1 Disturbances of sensation of smell and taste
Anosmia   Parosmia
Parageusia
DEF: Anosmia: loss of sense of smell due to organic factors, including loss of olfactory nerve conductivity, cerebral disease, nasal fossae formation and peripheral olfactory nerve diseases; can also be psychological disorder.
DEF: Parageusia: distorted sense of taste, or bad taste in mouth.
DEF: Parosmia: distorted sense of smell.

781.2 Abnormality of gait
Gait: Gait:
ataxic   spastic
paralytic   staggering
EXCLUDES ataxia:
NOS (781.3)
locomotor (progressive) (094.0)
difficulty in walking (719.7)
DEF: Abnormal, asymmetric gait.
AHA: 1Q, '11, 9; 2Q, '05, 6; 2Q, '04, 15
TIP: If the patient's gait abnormality is due to a joint problem, refer to code 719.7 Difficulty in walking.
R26.9 Unspecified abnormalities of gait and mobility I-10

781.3 Lack of coordination
Ataxia NOS
Muscular incoordination
EXCLUDES ataxic gait (781.2)
cerebellar ataxia (334.0-334.9)
difficulty in walking (719.7)
vertigo NOS (780.4)
AHA: 4Q, '04, 51; 3Q, '97, 12

781.4 Transient paralysis of limb
Monoplegia, transient NOS
EXCLUDES paralysis (342.0-344.9)

781.5 Clubbing of fingers
DEF: Enlarged soft tissue of distal fingers.

781.6 Meningismus
Dupré's syndrome
Meningism
DEF: Condition with signs and symptoms that resemble meningeal irritation; it is associated with febrile illness and dehydration with no evidence of infection.
AHA: 3Q, '00,13; J-F, '87, 7

781.7 Tetany
Carpopedal spasm
EXCLUDES tetanus neonatorum (771.3)
tetany:
hysterical (300.11)
newborn (hypocalcemic) (775.4)
parathyroid (252.1)
psychogenic (306.0)
DEF: Nerve and muscle hyperexcitability; symptoms include muscle spasms, twitching, cramps, laryngospasm with inspiratory stridor, hyperreflexia and choreiform movements.

781.8 Neurologic neglect syndrome
Asomatognosia   Left-sided neglect
Hemi-akinesia   Sensory extinction
Hemi-inattention   Sensory neglect
Hemispatial neglect   Visuospatial neglect
EXCLUDES visuospatial deficit (799.53)
AHA: 4Q, '94, 37
TIP: If documented as sequelae of a CVA, assign also a code from category 438.

√5ᵗʰ **781.9 Other symptoms involving nervous and musculoskeletal systems**
AHA: 4Q, '00, 45

781.91 Loss of height
EXCLUDES osteoporosis (733.00-733.09)

781.92 Abnormal posture

781.93 Ocular torticollis
DEF: Abnormal head posture as a result of a contracted state of cervical muscles to correct a visual disturbance; either double vision or a visual field defect.
AHA: 4Q, '02, 68

781.94 Facial weakness
Facial droop
EXCLUDES facial weakness due to late effect of cerebrovascular accident (438.83)
AHA: 4Q, '03, 72
TIP: Do not assign if facial droop or weakness is due to Bell's palsy; see instead code 351.0.
R29.810 Facial weakness I-10

781.99 Other symptoms involving nervous and musculoskeletal systems

√4ᵗʰ **782 Symptoms involving skin and other integumentary tissue**
EXCLUDES symptoms relating to breast (611.71-611.79)

782.0 Disturbance of skin sensation
Anesthesia of skin   Hypoesthesia
Burning or prickling   Numbness
sensation   Paresthesia
Hyperesthesia   Tingling
R20.9 Unspecified disturbances of skin sensation I-10

782.1 Rash and other nonspecific skin eruption
Exanthem
EXCLUDES vesicular eruption (709.8)
AHA: 4Q, '08, 99

782.2 Localized superficial swelling, mass, or lump
Subcutaneous nodules
EXCLUDES localized adiposity (278.1)

Symptoms, Signs, and Ill-Defined Conditions

780.94–782.2

782.3 Edema
Anasarca   Localized edema NOS
Dropsy

EXCLUDES ascites (789.51-789.59)
edema of:
newborn NOS (778.5)
pregnancy (642.0-642.9, 646.1)
fluid retention (276.69)
hydrops fetalis (773.3, 778.0)
hydrothorax (511.81-511.89)
nutritional edema (260, 262)

DEF: Edema: excess fluid in intercellular body tissue.
DEF: Anasarca: massive edema in all body tissues.
DEF: Dropsy: serous fluid accumulated in body cavity or cellular tissue.
DEF: Localized edema: edema in specific body areas.
AHA: 2Q, '00, 18
R60.9 Edema unspecified   I-10

782.4 Jaundice, unspecified, not of newborn
Cholemia NOS
Icterus NOS

EXCLUDES jaundice in newborn (774.0-774.7)
due to isoimmunization (773.0-773.2, 773.4)

DEF: Bilirubin deposits of skin, causing yellow cast.
R17 Unspecified jaundice   I-10

782.5 Cyanosis
EXCLUDES newborn (770.83)
DEF: Deficient oxygen of blood; causes blue cast to skin.

√5ʰ **782.6 Pallor and flushing**

782.61 Pallor

782.62 Flushing
Excessive blushing

782.7 Spontaneous ecchymoses
Petechiae
EXCLUDES ecchymosis in fetus or newborn (772.6)
purpura (287.0-287.9)
DEF: Hemorrhagic spots of skin; resemble freckles.

782.8 Changes in skin texture
Induration } of skin
Thickening

782.9 Other symptoms involving skin and integumentary tissues

√4ʰ **783 Symptoms concerning nutrition, metabolism, and development**

783.0 Anorexia
Loss of appetite
EXCLUDES anorexia nervosa (307.1)
loss of appetite of nonorganic origin (307.59)
R63.0 Anorexia   I-10

783.1 Abnormal weight gain
EXCLUDES excessive weight gain in pregnancy (646.1)
obesity (278.00)
morbid (278.01)

√5ʰ **783.2 Abnormal loss of weight and underweight**
Use additional code to identify Body Mass Index (BMI), if known (V85.0-V85.54)
AHA: 4Q, '00, 45

783.21 Loss of weight
AHA: 4Q, '05, 96
R63.4 Abnormal weight loss   I-10

783.22 Underweight
AHA: 4Q, '05, 96

783.3 Feeding difficulties and mismanagement
Feeding problem (elderly) (infant)
EXCLUDES feeding disturbance or problems:
in newborn (779.31-779.34)
of nonorganic origin (307.50-307.59
AHA: 3Q, '97, 12

√5ʰ **783.4 Lack of expected normal physiological development in childhood**
EXCLUDES delay in sexual development and puberty (259.0)
gonadal dysgenesis (758.6)
pituitary dwarfism (253.3)
slow fetal growth and fetal malnutrition (764.00-764.99)
specific delays in mental development (315.0-315.9)
AHA: 4Q, '00, 45; 3Q, '97, 4

783.40 Lack of normal physiological development, unspecified
Inadequate development
Lack of development

783.41 Failure to thrive   P
Failure to gain weight
EXCLUDES failure to thrive in newborn (779.34)
DEF: Organic failure to thrive: acute or chronic illness that interferes with nutritional intake, absorption, metabolism excretion and energy requirements. Nonorganic FTT is symptom of neglect or abuse.
AHA: 1Q, '03, 12

783.42 Delayed milestones   P
Late talker
Late walker

783.43 Short stature
Growth failure   Lack of growth
Growth retardation   Physical retardation
DEF: Constitutional short stature: stature inconsistent with chronological age. Genetic short stature is when skeletal maturation matches chronological age.

783.5 Polydipsia
Excessive thirst

783.6 Polyphagia
Excessive eating
Hyperalimentation NOS
EXCLUDES disorders of eating of nonorganic origin (307.50-307.59)

783.7 Adult failure to thrive   A
R62.7 Adult failure to thrive   I-10

783.9 Other symptoms concerning nutrition, metabolism, and development
Hypometabolism
EXCLUDES abnormal basal metabolic rate (794.7)
dehydration (276.51)
other disorders of fluid, electrolyte, and acid-base balance (276.0-276.9)
AHA: 2Q, '04, 3

√4ʰ **784 Symptoms involving head and neck**
EXCLUDES encephalopathy NOS (348.30)
specific symptoms involving neck classifiable to 723 (723.0-723.9)

784.0 Headache
Facial pain
Pain in head NOS
EXCLUDES atypical face pain (350.2)
migraine (346.0-346.9)
tension headache (307.81)
AHA: 3Q, '06, 22; 2Q, '06, 17; 3Q, '00, 13; 1Q, '90, 4; 3Q, '92, 14
TIP: Do not assign if headache syndrome has been diagnosed, refer to category 339.
R51 Headache   I-10

784.1 Throat pain
EXCLUDES dysphagia (787.20-787.29)
neck pain (723.1)
sore throat (462)
chronic (472.1)

784.2 Swelling, mass, or lump in head and neck
Space-occupying lesion, intracranial NOS
AHA: 1Q, '03, 8

N Newborn Age: 0   P Pediatric Age: 0-17   M Maternity Age: 12-55   A Adult Age: 15-124

784.3 Aphasia
> **EXCLUDES** *aphasia due to late effects of cerebrovascular disease (438.11)*
> *developmental aphasia (315.31)*
>
> **DEF:** Inability to communicate through speech, written word, or sign language.
> **AHA:** 3Q, '10, 5; 4Q, '04, 78; 4Q, '98, 87; 3Q, '97, 12
> **R47.01** Aphasia   I-10

√5ᵗʰ 784.4 Voice and resonance disorders
> **AHA:** 4Q, '09, 102-103

> **784.40 Voice and resonance disorder, unspecified**

> **784.41 Aphonia**
> Loss of voice

> **784.42 Dysphonia**
> Hoarseness

> **784.43 Hypernasality**

> **784.44 Hyponasality**

> **784.49 Other voice and resonance disorders**
> Change in voice

√5ᵗʰ 784.5 Other speech disturbance
> **EXCLUDES** *speech disorder due to late effect of cerebrovascular accident (438.10-438.19)*
> *stuttering (315.35)*
> **AHA:** 4Q, '09, 87-88

> **784.51 Dysarthria**
> > **EXCLUDES** *dysarthria due to late effect of cerebrovascular accident (438.13)*

> **784.52 Fluency disorder in conditions classified elsewhere**
> Stuttering in conditions classified elsewhere
> *Code first underlying disease or condition, such as:*
> Parkinson's disease (332.0)
> > **EXCLUDES** *adult onset fluency disorder (307.0)*
> > *childhood onset fluency disorder (315.35)*
> > *fluency disorder due to late effect of cerebrovascular accident (438.14)*
> **AHA:** 4Q, '10, 83-84

> **784.59 Other speech disturbance**
> Dysphasia
> Slurred speech
> Speech disturbance NOS
> **R47.89** Other speech disturbances   I-10

√5ᵗʰ 784.6 Other symbolic dysfunction
> **EXCLUDES** *developmental learning delays (315.0-315.9)*

> **784.60 Symbolic dysfunction, unspecified**

> **784.61 Alexia and dyslexia**
> Alexia (with agraphia)
> **DEF:** Alexia: Inability to understand written word due to central brain lesion.
> **DEF:** Dyslexia: Ability to recognize letters but inability to read, spell, and write words; genetic.

> **784.69 Other**
> Acalculia   Agraphia NOS
> Agnosia   Apraxia

784.7 Epistaxis
> Hemorrhage from nose
> Nosebleed
> **AHA:** 3Q, '04, 7
> **R04.0** Epistaxis   I-10

784.8 Hemorrhage from throat
> **EXCLUDES** *hemoptysis (786.30-786.39)*

√5ᵗʰ 784.9 Other symptoms involving head and neck

> **784.91 Postnasal drip**
> **AHA:** 4Q, '06, 108

> **784.92 Jaw pain**
> Mandibular pain
> Maxilla pain
> > **EXCLUDES** *temporomandibular joint arthralgia (524.62)*
> **AHA:** 4Q, '10, 93-94
> **R68.84** Jaw pain

784.99 Other symptoms involving head and neck
> Choking sensation
> Feeling of foreign body in throat
> Halitosis
> Mouth breathing
> Sneezing
> > **EXCLUDES** *foreign body in throat (933.0)*
> **AHA:** 4Q, '06, 108

√4ᵗʰ 785 Symptoms involving cardiovascular system
> **EXCLUDES** *heart failure NOS (428.9)*

> **785.0 Tachycardia, unspecified**
> Rapid heart beat
> > **EXCLUDES** *neonatal tachycardia (779.82)*
> > *paroxysmal tachycardia (427.0-427.2)*
> **DEF:** Excessively rapid heart rate.
> **AHA:** 2Q, '03, 11
> **R00.0** Tachycardia unspecified   I-10

> **785.1 Palpitations**
> Awareness of heart beat
> > **EXCLUDES** *specified dysrhythmias (427.0-427.9)*
> **R00.2** Palpitations   I-10

> **785.2 Undiagnosed cardiac murmurs**
> Heart murmurs NOS
> **AHA:** 4Q, '92, 16
> **R01.1** Cardiac murmur unspecified   I-10

> **785.3 Other abnormal heart sounds**
> Cardiac dullness, increased or decreased
> Friction fremitus, cardiac
> Precordial friction

> **785.4 Gangrene**
> Gangrene: Gangrenous cellulitis
>   NOS   Phagedena
>   spreading cutaneous
> *Code first any associated underlying condition*
> > **EXCLUDES** *gangrene of certain sites — see Alphabetic Index*
> > *gangrene with atherosclerosis of the extremities (440.24)*
> > *gas gangrene (040.0)*
> **DEF:** Gangrene: necrosis of skin tissue due to bacterial infection, diabetes, embolus and vascular supply loss.
> **DEF:** Gangrenous cellulitis: group A streptococcal infection; begins with severe cellulitis, spreads to superficial and deep fascia; produces gangrene of underlying tissues.
> **AHA:** 1Q, '04, 14; 3Q, '91, 12; 3Q, '90, 15; M-A, '86, 12
> **I96** Gangrene not elsewhere classified   I-10

√5ᵗʰ 785.5 Shock without mention of trauma

> **785.50 Shock, unspecified**
> Failure of peripheral circulation
> **DEF:** Peripheral circulatory failure due to heart insufficiencies.
> **AHA:** 2Q, '96, 10

> **785.51 Cardiogenic shock**
> **DEF:** Shock syndrome: associated with myocardial infarction, cardiac tamponade and massive pulmonary embolism; symptoms include mental confusion, reduced blood pressure, tachycardia, pallor and cold, clammy skin.
> **AHA:** 4Q, '08, 182; 3Q, '05, 14
> **R57.0** Cardiogenic shock   I-10

> **785.52 Septic shock**
> Shock:
>   endotoxic
>   gram-negative
> *Code first underlying infection*
> Use additional code, if applicable, to identify systemic inflammatory response syndrome due to infectious process with organ dysfunction (995.92)
> **AHA:** 2Q, '10, 4; 4Q, '08, 99; 4Q, '06, 113; 2Q, '05, 18-19; 4Q, '03, 73, 79
> **TIP:** The diagnosis of septic shock indicates the presence of severe sepsis; code 785.52 should not be assigned without first assigning code 995.92.

Symptoms, Signs, and Ill-Defined Conditions

785.59–786.9

785.59 Other
Shock:
hypovolemic
EXCLUDES *shock (due to):*
anesthetic (995.4)
anaphylactic (995.0)
due to serum (999.41-999.49)
electric (994.8)
following abortion (639.5)
lightning (994.0)
obstetrical (669.1)
postoperative (998.00-998.09)
traumatic (958.4)
AHA: 2Q, '00, 3

785.6 Enlargement of lymph nodes
Lymphadenopathy
"Swollen glands"
EXCLUDES *lymphadenitis (chronic) (289.1-289.3)*
acute (683)
R59.9 Enlarged lymph nodes unspecified   I-10

785.9 Other symptoms involving cardiovascular system
Bruit (arterial)
Weak pulse

786 Symptoms involving respiratory system and other chest symptoms

786.0 Dyspnea and respiratory abnormalities

786.00 Respiratory abnormality, unspecified

786.01 Hyperventilation
EXCLUDES *hyperventilation, psychogenic (306.1)*
DEF: Rapid breathing causes carbon dioxide loss from blood.

786.02 Orthopnea
DEF: Difficulty breathing except in upright position.

786.03 Apnea
EXCLUDES *apnea of newborn (770.81, 770.82)*
sleep apnea (780.51, 780.53, 780.57)
DEF: Cessation of breathing.
AHA: 4Q, '98, 50

786.04 Cheyne-Stokes respiration
DEF: Rhythmic increase of depth and frequency of breathing with apnea; occurs in frontal lobe and diencephalic dysfunction.
AHA: 4Q, '98, 50

786.05 Shortness of breath
DEF: Inability to take in sufficient oxygen.
AHA: 4Q, '99, 25; 1Q, '99, 6; 4Q, '98, 50
R06.02 Shortness of breath   I-10

786.06 Tachypnea
EXCLUDES *transitory tachypnea of newborn (770.6)*
DEF: Abnormal rapid respiratory rate; called hyperventilation.
AHA: 1Q, '11, 16-17; 4Q, '98, 50

786.07 Wheezing
EXCLUDES *asthma (493.00-493.92)*
DEF: Stenosis of respiratory passageway; causes whistling sound; due to asthma, coryza, croup, emphysema, hay fever, edema, and pleural effusion.
AHA: 4Q, '98, 50

786.09 Other
Respiratory:
distress
insufficiency
EXCLUDES *respiratory distress:*
following trauma and surgery (518.52)
newborn (770.89)
syndrome (newborn) (769)
adult (518.52)
respiratory failure (518.81, 518.83-518.84)
newborn (770.84)
AHA: 4Q, '05, 90; 2Q, '98, 10; 1Q, '97, 7; 1Q, '90, 9
R06.00 Dyspnea, unspecified   I-10

786.1 Stridor
EXCLUDES *congenital laryngeal stridor (748.3)*
DEF: Obstructed airway causes harsh sound.

786.2 Cough
EXCLUDES *cough:*
psychogenic (306.1)
smokers' (491.0)
with hemorrhage (786.39)
AHA: 4Q, '99, 26
R05 Cough   I-10

786.3 Hemoptysis
DEF: Coughing up blood or blood-stained sputum.
AHA: ▶3Q, '11, 12;◄ 4Q, '10, 94-95; 2Q, '06, 17; 4Q, '90, 26

786.30 Hemoptysis, unspecified
Pulmonary hemorrhage NOS
R04.2 Hemoptysis   I-10

786.31 Acute idiopathic pulmonary hemorrhage in infants [AIPHI]   P
Acute idiopathic pulmonary hemorrhage in infant over 28 days old
EXCLUDES *pulmonary hemorrhage of newborn under 28 days old (770.3)*
von Willebrand's disease (286.4)
DEF: An abrupt onset of bleeding or blood in the airway with acute respiratory distress or failure in a patient with no prior history of an identifiable causal condition.
R04.81 Acute idiopathic pulmonary hemorrhage in infants

786.39 Other hemoptysis
Cough with hemorrhage
R04.89 Hemorrhage from othr site in resp passages   I-10

786.4 Abnormal sputum
Abnormal:
amount
color   } (of) sputum
odor
Excessive

786.5 Chest pain

786.50 Chest pain, unspecified
AHA: 1Q, '07, 19; 2Q, '06, 7; 1Q, '03, 6; 1Q, '02, 4; 4Q, '99, 25
R07.9 Chest pain unspecified   I-10

786.51 Precordial pain
DEF: Chest pain over heart and lower thorax.

786.52 Painful respiration
Pain:
anterior chest wall
pleuritic
Pleurodynia
EXCLUDES *epidemic pleurodynia (074.1)*
AHA: N-D, '84, 17
R07.1 Chest pain on breathing   I-10

786.59 Other
Discomfort
Pressure   } in chest
Tightness
EXCLUDES *pain in breast (611.71)*
AHA: 1Q, '02, 6
TIP: Assign for chest pain due to anxiety, along with an additional code for anxiety. Chest pain is not integral to the diagnosis of anxiety.
R07.89 Other chest pain   I-10

786.6 Swelling, mass, or lump in chest
EXCLUDES *lump in breast (611.72)*
R22.2 Localized swelling, mass, lump, trunk   I-10

786.7 Abnormal chest sounds
Abnormal percussion, chest   Rales
Friction sounds, chest   Tympany, chest
EXCLUDES *wheezing (786.07)*

786.8 Hiccough
EXCLUDES *psychogenic hiccough (306.1)*

786.9 Other symptoms involving respiratory system and chest
Breath-holding spell

√4ʰ **787 Symptoms involving digestive system**
     EXCLUDES *constipation (564.00-564.09)*
              pylorospasm (537.81)
              congenital (750.5)

√5ʰ **787.0 Nausea and vomiting**
      Emesis
      EXCLUDES *hematemesis NOS (578.0)*
            vomiting:
               bilious, following gastrointestinal surgery (564.3)
               cyclical (536.2)
                  associated with migraine (346.2)
                  psychogenic (306.4)
               excessive, in pregnancy (643.0-643.9)
               fecal matter (569.87)
               habit (536.2)
               of newborn (779.32, 779.33)
               persistent (536.2)
               psychogenic NOS (307.54)
      AHA: M-A, '85, 11

     787.01 Nausea with vomiting
          AHA: 1Q, '03, 5
          R11.2 Nausea with vomiting, unspecified   I-10

     787.02 Nausea alone
          AHA: 3Q, '00, 12; 2Q, '97, 9
          R11.0 Nausea alone   I-10

     787.03 Vomiting alone

     787.04 Bilious emesis
          Bilious vomiting
          EXCLUDES *bilious emesis (vomiting) in newborn*
                   (779.32)
          AHA: 4Q, '09, 103-104

787.1 Heartburn
      Pyrosis   Waterbrash
      EXCLUDES *dyspepsia or indigestion (536.8)*
      AHA: 2Q, '01, 6

√5ʰ **787.2 Dysphagia**
      Code first, if applicable, dysphagia due to late effect of
        cerebrovascular accident (438.82)
      AHA: 4Q, '07, 92-94; 3Q, '07, 7; 4Q, '03, 103, 109; 2Q, '01, 4

     787.20 Dysphagia, unspecified
          Difficulty in swallowing NOS

     787.21 Dysphagia, oral phase

     787.22 Dysphagia, oropharyngeal phase
          AHA: 4Q, '07, 94

     787.23 Dysphagia, pharyngeal phase

     787.24 Dysphagia, pharyngoesophageal phase

     787.29 Other dysphagia
          Cervical dysphagia
          Neurogenic dysphagia
          R13.19 Other dysphagia   I-10

787.3 Flatulence, eructation, and gas pain
      Abdominal distention (gaseous)
      Bloating
      Tympanites (abdominal) (intestinal)
      EXCLUDES *aerophagy (306.4)*
      DEF: Flatulence: excess air or gas in intestine or stomach.
      DEF: Eructation: belching, expelling gas through mouth.
      DEF: Gas pain: gaseous pressure affecting gastrointestinal system.

787.4 Visible peristalsis
      Hyperperistalsis
      DEF: Increase in involuntary movements of intestines.

787.5 Abnormal bowel sounds
      Absent bowel sounds
      Hyperactive bowel sounds

√5ʰ **787.6 Incontinence of feces**
      Encopresis NOS
      Incontinence of sphincter ani
      EXCLUDES *that of nonorganic origin (307.7)*
      AHA: 4Q, '10, 87-89; 1Q, '97, 9

     787.60 Full incontinence of feces
          Fecal incontinence NOS
          R15.9 Full incontinence of feces   I-10

     787.61 Incomplete defecation
          EXCLUDES *constipation (564.00-564.09)*
                  fecal impaction (560.32)

     787.62 Fecal smearing
          Fecal soiling

     787.63 Fecal urgency
          R15.2 Fecal urgency

787.7 Abnormal feces
      Bulky stools
      EXCLUDES *abnormal stool content (792.1)*
             melena:
               NOS (578.1)
               newborn (772.4, 777.3)

√5ʰ **787.9 Other symptoms involving digestive system**
      EXCLUDES *gastrointestinal hemorrhage (578.0-578.9)*
            intestinal obstruction (560.0-560.9)
            specific functional digestive disorders:
               esophagus (530.0-530.9)
               stomach and duodenum (536.0-536.9)
               those not elsewhere classified (564.00-564.9)

     787.91 Diarrhea
          Diarrhea NOS
          AHA: 2Q, '10, 12; 4Q, '08, 99; 4Q, '95, 54
          R19.7 Diarrhea unspecified   I-10

     787.99 Other
          Change in bowel habits
          Tenesmus (rectal)
          DEF: Tenesmus: Painful, ineffective straining at the rectum
          with limited passage of fecal matter.

√4ʰ **788 Symptoms involving urinary system**
      EXCLUDES *hematuria (599.70-599.72)*
            nonspecific findings on examination of the urine
               (791.0-791.9)
            small kidney of unknown cause (589.0-589.9)
            uremia NOS (586)
            urinary obstruction (599.60, 599.69)

788.0 Renal colic
      Colic (recurrent) of:
        kidney
        ureter
      DEF: Kidney pain.
      AHA: 3Q, '04, 8
      TIP: Do not assign if renal colic is due to calculus; see category 592.

788.1 Dysuria
      Painful urination
      Strangury

Phases of Swallowing

Oral phase

Oropharyngeal phase

Pharyngeal phase   Pharyngeoesophageal phase

√4ʰ √5ʰ Additional Digit Required   Unspecified Code   Other Specified Code   Manifestation Code   ►◄ Revised Text   ● New Code   ▲ Revised Code Title

2013 ICD-9-CM   **Volume 1 – 267**

√5ᵗʰ **788.2 Retention of urine**

Code, if applicable, any causal condition first, such as:
hyperplasia of prostate (600.0-600.9 with fifth-digit 1)
DEF: Accumulation of urine in the bladder due to inability to void.

788.20 Retention of urine, unspecified

AHA: 4Q, '06, 93, 95; 2Q, '04, 18; 3Q, '03, 12-13; 1Q, '03, 6; 3Q, '96, 10

R33.9 Retention of urine unspecified   I-10

788.21 Incomplete bladder emptying

AHA: 4Q, '06, 93

788.29 Other specified retention of urine

√5ᵗʰ **788.3 Urinary incontinence**

Code, if applicable, any causal condition first, such as:
congenital ureterocele (753.23)
genital prolapse (618.00-618.9)
hyperplasia of prostate (600.0-600.9 with fifth-digit 1)
EXCLUDES *functional urinary incontinence (788.91)*
that of nonorganic origin (307.6)
urinary incontinence associated with cognitive
impairment (788.91)
AHA: 4Q, '06, 93; 4Q, '92, 22

788.30 Urinary incontinence, unspecified

Enuresis NOS
AHA: 1Q, '09, 15

R32 Unspecified urinary incontinence   I-10

788.31 Urge incontinence

DEF: Inability to control urination, upon urge to urinate.
AHA: 1Q, '00, 19

788.32 Stress incontinence, male   ♂

EXCLUDES *stress incontinence, female (625.6)*
DEF: Inability to control urination associated with weak sphincter in males.

788.33 Mixed incontinence, (male) (female)

Urge and stress
DEF: Urge, stress incontinence: involuntary discharge of urine due to anatomic displacement.

788.34 Incontinence without sensory awareness

DEF: Involuntary discharge of urine without sensory warning.

788.35 Post-void dribbling

DEF: Involuntary discharge of residual urine after voiding.

788.36 Nocturnal enuresis

DEF: Involuntary discharge of urine during the night.

788.37 Continuous leakage

DEF: Continuous, involuntary urine seepage.

788.38 Overflow incontinence

DEF: Leakage caused by pressure of retained urine in the bladder after the bladder has fully contracted due to weakened bladder muscles or an obstruction of the urethra.

788.39 Other urinary incontinence

√5ᵗʰ **788.4 Frequency of urination and polyuria**

Code, if applicable, any causal condition first, such as:
hyperplasia of prostate (600.0-600.9 with fifth-digit 1)

788.41 Urinary frequency

Frequency of micturition
AHA: 4Q, '06, 93

788.42 Polyuria

DEF: Excessive urination.

788.43 Nocturia

DEF: Urination affecting sleep patterns.
AHA: 4Q, '06, 93

788.5 Oliguria and anuria

Deficient secretion of urine
Suppression of urinary secretion
EXCLUDES *that complicating:*
abortion (634-638 with .3, 639.3)
ectopic or molar pregnancy (639.3)
pregnancy, childbirth, or the puerperium
(642.0-642.9, 646.2)
DEF: Oliguria: diminished urinary secretion related to fluid intake.
DEF: Anuria: lack of urinary secretion due to renal failure or obstructed urinary tract.

√5ᵗʰ **788.6 Other abnormality of urination**

Code, if applicable, any causal condition first, such as:
hyperplasia of prostate (600.0-600.9 with fifth-digit 1)

788.61 Splitting of urinary stream

Intermittent urinary stream

788.62 Slowing of urinary stream

Weak stream
AHA: 4Q, '06, 93

788.63 Urgency of urination

EXCLUDES *urge incontinence (788.31, 788.33)*
DEF: Feeling of intense need to urinate; abrupt sensation of imminent urination.
AHA: 4Q, '06, 93; 4Q, '03, 74

788.64 Urinary hesitancy

AHA: 4Q, '06, 93, 109

788.65 Straining on urination

AHA: 4Q, '06, 93, 109

788.69 Other

788.7 Urethral discharge

Penile discharge
Urethrorrhea

788.8 Extravasation of urine

DEF: Leaking or infiltration of urine into tissues.

√5ᵗʰ **788.9 Other symptoms involving urinary system**

AHA: 1Q, '05, 12; 4Q, '88, 1

788.91 Functional urinary incontinence

Urinary incontinence due to cognitive impairment, or severe physical disability or immobility
EXCLUDES *urinary incontinence due to physiologic condition (788.30-788.39)*
AHA: 4Q, '08, 144-145

788.99 Other symptoms involving urinary system

Extrarenal uremia
Vesical:
pain
tenesmus

√4ᵗʰ **789 Other symptoms involving abdomen and pelvis**

EXCLUDES *symptoms referable to genital organs:*
female (625.0-625.9)
male (607.0-608.9)
psychogenic (302.70-302.79)

The following fifth-digit subclassification is to be used for codes 789.0, 789.3, 789.4, 789.6:
0 unspecified site
1 right upper quadrant
2 left upper quadrant
3 right lower quadrant
4 left lower quadrant
5 periumbilic
6 epigastric
7 generalized
9 other specified site
Multiple sites

§ √5ᵗʰ **789.0 Abdominal pain**

[0-7, 9]   Cramps, abdominal
AHA: 1Q, '95, 3; **For code 789.06:** 1Q, '02, 5

R10.9 Unspecified abdominal pain   I-10
R10.31 Right lower quadrant pain   I-10
R10.13 Epigastric pain   I-10
R10.84 Generalized abdominal pain   I-10

---

§   Requires fifth digit. Valid digits are in [brackets] under each code. See category 789 for codes and definitions.

789.1 Hepatomegaly
Enlargement of liver

789.2 Splenomegaly
Enlargement of spleen

§ √5ᵗʰ **789.3 Abdominal or pelvic swelling, mass, or lump**
[0-7, 9] Diffuse or generalized swelling or mass:
abdominal NOS
umbilical
EXCLUDES abdominal distention (gaseous) (787.3)
ascites (789.51-789.59)

§ √5ᵗʰ **789.4 Abdominal rigidity**
[0-7, 9]

√5ᵗʰ **789.5 Ascites**
Fluid in peritoneal cavity
DEF: Serous fluid effusion and accumulation in abdominal cavity.
AHA: 4Q, '07, 95; 2Q, '05, 8; 4Q, '89, 11

789.51 Malignant ascites
Code first malignancy, such as:
malignant neoplasm of ovary (183.0)
secondary malignant neoplasm of retroperitoneum
and peritoneum (197.6)
AHA: 4Q, '07, 96
R18.0 Malignant ascites   [I-10]

789.59 Other ascites
AHA: 4Q, '08, 99
R18.8 Other ascites   [I-10]

§ √5ᵗʰ **789.6 Abdominal tenderness**
[0-7, 9] Rebound tenderness

789.7 Colic   [P]
Colic NOS   Infantile colic
EXCLUDES colic in adult and child over 12 months old (789.0)
renal colic (788.0)
DEF: Inconsolable crying in an otherwise well-fed and healthy infant
for more than three hours a day, three days a week, for more than
three weeks.
AHA: 4Q, '09, 104-105

789.9 Other symtoms involving abdomen and pelvis
Umbilical:
bleeding
discharge

Nonspecific Abnormal Findings (790-796)
AHA: 3Q, '11, 4; 2Q, '90, 16

√4ᵗʰ **790 Nonspecific findings on examination of blood**
EXCLUDES abnormality of:
platelets (287.0-287.9)
thrombocytes (287.0-287.9)
white blood cells (288.00-288.9)

√5ᵗʰ **790.0 Abnormality of red blood cells**
EXCLUDES anemia:
congenital (776.5)
newborn, due to isoimmunization (773.0-773.2,
773.5)
of premature infant (776.6)
other specified types (280.0-285.9)
hemoglobin disorders (282.5-282.7)
polycythemia:
familial (289.6)
neonatorum (776.4)
secondary (289.0)
vera (238.4)
AHA: 4Q, '00, 46

790.01 Precipitous drop in hematocrit
Drop in hematocritDrop in hemoglobin
TIP: Typically reported as a reason for encounter at a dialysis
center.

790.09 Other abnormality of red blood cells
Abnormal red cell morphology NOS
Abnormal red cell volume NOS
Anisocytosis
Poikilocytosis

790.1 Elevated sedimentation rate

√5ᵗʰ **790.2 Abnormal glucose**
EXCLUDES diabetes mellitus (249.00-249.91, 250.00-250.93)
dysmetabolic syndrome X (277.7)
gestational diabetes (648.8)
glycosuria (791.5)
hypoglycemia (251.2)
that complicating pregnancy, childbirth, or
puerperium (648.8)
AHA: 1Q, '11, 9; 4Q, '03, 74; 3Q, '91, 5
TIP: These codes are typically assigned on encounters before a
patient is diagnosed with diabetes mellitus.

790.21 Impaired fasting glucose
Elevated fasting glucose

790.22 Impaired glucose tolerance test (oral)
Elevated glucose tolerance test

790.29 Other abnormal glucose
Abnormal glucose NOS
Abnormal non-fasting glucose
Hyperglycemia NOS
Pre-diabetes NOS
AHA: ▶1Q, '12, 17;◀3Q, '09, 5; 2Q, '05, 21
TIP: Assign for any stress hyperglycemia for which no causal
condition is determined including postoperative
hyperglycemia that is not specifically documented as a
complication of the procedure.
R73.09 Other abnormal glucose   [I-10]

790.3 Excessive blood level of alcohol
Elevated blood-alcohol
AHA: S-O, '86, 3

**790.4 Nonspecific elevation of levels of transaminase or lactic
acid dehydrogenase [LDH]**
R74.0 Nonspecific elevation levels transaminase & LDH   [I-10]

790.5 Other nonspecific abnormal serum enzyme levels
Abnormal serum level of:
acid phosphatase
alkaline phosphatase
amylase
lipase
EXCLUDES deficiency of circulating enzymes (277.6)
R74.8 Abnormal levels of other serum enzymes   [I-10]

790.6 Other abnormal blood chemistry
Abnormal blood level of:
cobalt
copper
iron
lead
lithium
magnesium
mineral
zinc
EXCLUDES abnormality of electrolyte or acid-base balance
(276.0-276.9)
hypoglycemia NOS (251.2)
lead poisoning (984.0-984.9)
specific finding indicating abnormality of:
amino-acid transport and metabolism
(270.0-270.9)
carbohydrate transport and metabolism
(271.0-271.9)
lipid metabolism (272.0-272.9)
uremia NOS (586)
AHA: 4Q, '88, 1
TIP: If only azotemia is documented (indexed to 790.6), clarify with
physician; if due to uremia or renal failure, code to those conditions
instead.
R78.89 Finding oth spec substances not norm found blood   [I-10]

---

§ Requires fifth digit. Valid digits are in [brackets] under each code. See category 789 for codes and definitions.

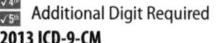

√4ᵗʰ / √5ᵗʰ Additional Digit Required   Unspecified Code   Other Specified Code   Manifestation Code   ▶◀ Revised Text   ● New Code   ▲ Revised Code Title

Symptoms, Signs, and Ill-Defined Conditions

790.7 Bacteremia

> EXCLUDES *bacteremia of newborn (771.83)*
> *septicemia (038)*

Use additional code to identify organism (041)

DEF: Laboratory finding of bacteria in the blood in the absence of two or more signs of sepsis; transient in nature, progresses to septicemia with severe infectious process.

AHA: 2Q, '11, 7; 2Q, '03, 7; 4Q, '93, 29; 3Q, '88, 12

TIP: If clinical signs or symptoms indicating systemic disease exist, query physician for the presence of sepsis; code to category 038 if documented.

790.8 Viremia, unspecified

DEF: Presence of a virus in the blood stream.

AHA: 4Q, '88, 10

√5th 790.9 Other nonspecific findings on examination of blood

AHA: 4Q, '93, 29

790.91 Abnormal arterial blood gases

790.92 Abnormal coagulation profile

Abnormal or prolonged:
  bleeding time
  coagulation time
  partial thromboplastin time [PTT]
  prothrombin time [PT]

> EXCLUDES *coagulation (hemorrhagic) disorders (286.0-286.9)*

R79.1 Abnormal coagulaton profile   I-10

790.93 Elevated prostate specific antigen, [PSA]   A♂

790.94 Euthyroid sick syndrome

DEF: Transient alteration of thyroid hormone metabolism due to nonthyroid illness or stress.

AHA: 4Q, '97, 45

790.95 Elevated C-reactive protein [CRP]

DEF: Inflammation in an arterial wall results in elevated C-reactive protein (CRP) in the blood; CRP is a recognized risk factor in cardiovascular disease.

790.99 Other

AHA: 3Q, '11, 4; 2Q, '03, 14

√4th 791 Nonspecific findings on examination of urine

> EXCLUDES *hematuria NOS (599.70-599.72)*
> *specific findings indicating abnormality of:*
> *amino-acid transport and metabolism (270.0-270.9)*
> *carbohydrate transport and metabolism (271.0-271.9)*

791.0 Proteinuria

Albuminuria
Bence-Jones proteinuria

> EXCLUDES *postural proteinuria (593.6)*
> *that arising during pregnancy or the puerperium (642.0-642.9, 646.2)*

DEF: Excess protein in urine.

AHA: 3Q, '91, 8

791.1 Chyluria

> EXCLUDES *filarial (125.0-125.9)*

DEF: Excess chyle in urine.

791.2 Hemoglobinuria

DEF: Free hemoglobin in blood due to rapid hemolysis of red blood cells.

791.3 Myoglobinuria

DEF: Myoglobin (oxygen-transporting pigment) in urine.

791.4 Biliuria

DEF: Bile pigments in urine.

791.5 Glycosuria

> EXCLUDES *renal glycosuria (271.4)*

DEF: Sugar in urine.

791.6 Acetonuria

Ketonuria

DEF: Excess acetone in urine.

791.7 Other cells and casts in urine

791.9 Other nonspecific findings on examination of urine

Crystalluria
Elevated urine levels of:
  17-ketosteroids
  catecholamines
  indolacetic acid
  vanillylmandelic acid [VMA]
Melanuria

AHA: 1Q, '05, 12

√4th 792 Nonspecific abnormal findings in other body substances

> EXCLUDES *that in chromosomal analysis (795.2)*

792.0 Cerebrospinal fluid

792.1 Stool contents

Abnormal stool color	Occult stool
Fat in stool	Pus in stool
Mucus in stool	

> EXCLUDES *blood in stool [melena] (578.1)*
> *newborn (772.4, 777.3)*

AHA: 2Q, '92, 9

792.2 Semen   ♂

Abnormal spermatozoa

> EXCLUDES *azoospermia (606.0)*
> *oligospermia (606.1)*

792.3 Amniotic fluid   M♀

DEF: Nonspecific abnormal findings in amniotic fluid.

AHA: N-D, '86, 4

792.4 Saliva

> EXCLUDES *that in chromosomal analysis (795.2)*

792.5 Cloudy (hemodialysis) (peritoneal) dialysis effluent

AHA: 4Q, '00, 46

792.9 Other nonspecific abnormal findings in body substances

Peritoneal fluid
Pleural fluid
Synovial fluid
Vaginal fluids

√4th 793 Nonspecific (abnormal) findings on radiological and other examination of body structure

> INCLUDES nonspecific abnormal findings of:
> thermography
> ultrasound examination [echogram]
> x-ray examination

> EXCLUDES *abnormal results of function studies and radioisotope scans (794.0-794.9)*

793.0 Skull and head

> EXCLUDES *nonspecific abnormal echoencephalogram (794.01)*

AHA: 3Q, '06, 22

√5th 793.1 Lung field

AHA: 4Q, '11, 138-139

793.11 Solitary pulmonary nodule

Coin lesion lung
Solitary pulmonary nodule, subsegmental branch of the bronchial tree

793.19 Other nonspecific abnormal finding of lung field

Pulmonary infiltrate NOS
Shadow, lung
AHA: 4Q, '11, 139

793.2 Other intrathoracic organ

Abnormal:
  echocardiogram
  heart shadow
  ultrasound cardiogram
Mediastinal shift
AHA: ▶1Q, '12, 17◀

793.3 Biliary tract

Nonvisualization of gallbladder

793.4 Gastrointestinal tract

793.5 Genitourinary organs

Filling defect:
  bladder
  kidney
  ureter

N Newborn Age: 0   P Pediatric Age: 0-17   M Maternity Age: 12-55   A Adult Age: 15-124

Symptoms, Signs, and Ill-Defined Conditions

793.6 **Abdominal area, including retroperitoneum**

793.7 **Musculoskeletal system**

√5ᵗʰ 793.8 **Breast**
> AHA: 4Q, '01, 51

793.80 **Abnormal mammogram, unspecified**

793.81 **Mammographic microcalcification**
> EXCLUDES mammographic calcification (793.89)
>   mammographic calculus (793.89)
> DEF: Calcium and cellular debris deposits in the breast that cannot be felt but can be detected on a mammogram; can be a sign of cancer, benign conditions, or changes in the breast tissue as a result of inflammation, injury, or obstructed duct.

793.82 **Inconclusive mammogram**
> Dense breasts NOS
> Inconclusive mammogram NEC
> Inconclusive mammography due to dense breasts
> Inconclusive mammography NEC
> AHA: 4Q, '09, 105-106

793.89 **Other (abnormal) findings on radiological examination of breast**
> Mammographic calcification
> Mammographic calculus

√5ᵗʰ 793.9 **Other**
> EXCLUDES abnormal finding by radioisotope localization of placenta (794.9)
> TIP: Sequence a code for the sign or symptom that was the reason for the imaging or radiological test first.

793.91 **Image test inconclusive due to excess body fat**
> Use additional code to identify Body Mass Index (BMI), if known (V85.0-V85.54)
> AHA: 4Q, '06, 109

793.99 **Other nonspecific (abnormal) findings on radiological and other examinations of body structure**
> Abnormal:
>   placental finding by x-ray or ultrasound method
>   radiological findings in skin and subcutaneous tissue
> AHA: 4Q, '06, 109

√4ᵗʰ 794 **Nonspecific abnormal results of function studies**
> INCLUDES radioisotope:
>   scans
>   uptake studies
>   scintiphotography

√5ᵗʰ 794.0 **Brain and central nervous system**

794.00 **Abnormal function study, unspecified**

794.01 **Abnormal echoencephalogram**

794.02 **Abnormal electroencephalogram [EEG]**

794.09 **Other**
> Abnormal brain scan

√5ᵗʰ 794.1 **Peripheral nervous system and special senses**

794.10 **Abnormal response to nerve stimulation, unspecified**

794.11 **Abnormal retinal function studies**
> Abnormal electroretinogram [ERG]

794.12 **Abnormal electro-oculogram [EOG]**

794.13 **Abnormal visually evoked potential**

794.14 **Abnormal oculomotor studies**

794.15 **Abnormal auditory function studies**
> AHA: 1Q, '04, 15-16
> TIP: If the reason for the encounter was for a hearing examination, sequence a code from subcategory V72.1 first. When nonspecific hearing loss is documented, assign 389.9 instead of 794.15.

794.16 **Abnormal vestibular function studies**

794.17 **Abnormal electromyogram [EMG]**
> EXCLUDES that of eye (794.14)

794.19 **Other**

794.2 **Pulmonary**
> Abnormal lung scan
> Reduced:
>   ventilatory capacity
>   vital capacity

√5ᵗʰ 794.3 **Cardiovascular**

794.30 **Abnormal function study, unspecified**

794.31 **Abnormal electrocardiogram [ECG] [EKG]**
> EXCLUDES long QT syndrome (426.82)
> R94.31 Abnormal electrocardiogram [ECG] [EKG]   I-10

794.39 **Other**
> Abnormal:
>   ballistocardiogram
>   phonocardiogram
>   vectorcardiogram
> R94.39 Abnormal result oth cardiovasculr function study   I-10

794.4 **Kidney**
> Abnormal renal function test

794.5 **Thyroid**
> Abnormal thyroid:
>   scan
>   uptake

794.6 **Other endocrine function study**

794.7 **Basal metabolism**
> Abnormal basal metabolic rate [BMR]

794.8 **Liver**
> Abnormal liver scan
> R94.5 Abnormal results of liver function studies   I-10

794.9 **Other**
> Bladder   Placenta
> Pancreas   Spleen

√4ᵗʰ 795 **Other and nonspecific abnormal cytological, histological, immunological and DNA test findings**
> EXCLUDES abnormal cytologic smear of anus and anal HPV (796.70-796.79)
> nonspecific abnormalities of red blood cells (790.01-790.09)

√5ᵗʰ 795.0 **Abnormal Papanicolaou smear of cervix and cervical HPV**
> Abnormal thin preparation smear of cervix
> Abnormal cervical cytology
> EXCLUDES abnormal cytologic smear of vagina and vaginal HPV (795.10-795.19)
> carcinoma in situ of cervix (233.1)
> cervical intraepithelial neoplasia I (CIN I) (622.11)
> cervical intraepithelial neoplasia II (CIN II) (622.12)
> cervical intraepithelial neoplasia III (CIN III) (233.1)
> dysplasia (histologically confirmed) of cervix (uteri) NOS (622.10)
> mild cervical dysplasia (histologically confirmed) (622.11)
> moderate cervical dysplasia (histologically confirmed) (622.12)
> severe cervical dysplasia (histologically confirmed) (233.1)
> AHA: 4Q, '08, 145-146; 4Q, '02, 69

795.00 **Abnormal glandular Papanicolaou smear of cervix**   ♀
> Atypical endocervical cells NOS
> Atypical endometrial cells NOS
> Atypical cervical glandular cells NOS

795.01 **Papanicolaou smear of cervix with atypical squamous cells of undetermined significance [ASC-US]**   ♀
> AHA: 2Q, '06, 4

795.02 **Papanicolaou smear of cervix with atypical squamous cells cannot exclude high grade squamous intraepithelial lesion [ASC-H]**   ♀

795.03 **Papanicolaou smear of cervix with low grade squamous intraepithelial lesion [LGSIL]**   ♀

795.04 **Papanicolaou smear of cervix with high grade squamous intraepithelial lesion [HGSIL]**   ♀

√4ᵗʰ √5ᵗʰ Additional Digit Required   Unspecified Code   Other Specified Code   Manifestation Code   ▶◀ Revised Text   ● New Code   ▲ Revised Code Title

2013 ICD-9-CM   Volume 1 – 271

793.6–795.04

795.05 Cervical high risk human papillomavirus [HPV] DNA test positive ♀

795.06 Papanicolaou smear of cervix with cytologic evidence of malignancy ♀
  AHA: 4Q, '06, 110

795.07 Satisfactory cervical smear but lacking transformation zone ♀

795.08 Unsatisfactory cervical cytology smear ♀
  Inadequate cervical cytology sample
  AHA: 2Q, '06, 4

795.09 Other abnormal Papanicolaou smear of cervix and cervical HPV ♀
  Cervical low risk human papillomavirus (HPV) DNA test positive
  Use additional code for associated human papillomavirus (079.4)
  EXCLUDES *encounter for Papanicolaou cervical smear to confirm findings of recent normal smear following initial abnormal smear (V72.32)*

√5ᵗʰ **795.1 Abnormal Papanicolaou smear of vagina and vaginal HPV**
  Abnormal thin preparation smear of vagina NOS
  Abnormal vaginal cytology NOS
  Use additional code to identify acquired absence of uterus and cervix, if applicable (V88.01-V88.03)
  EXCLUDES *abnormal cytologic smear of cervix and cervical HPV (795.00-795.09)*
    carcinoma in situ of vagina (233.31)
    carcinoma in situ of vulva (233.32)
    dysplasia (histologically confirmed) of vagina NOS (623.0, 233.31)
    dysplasia (histologically confirmed) of vulva NOS (624.01, 624.02, 233.32)
    mild vaginal dysplasia (histologically confirmed) (623.0)
    mild vulvar dysplasia (histologically confirmed) (624.01)
    moderate vaginal dysplasia (histologically confirmed) (623.0)
    moderate vulvar dysplasia (histologically confirmed) (624.02)
    severe vaginal dysplasia (histologically confirmed) (233.31)
    severe vulvar dysplasia (histologically confirmed) (233.32)
    vaginal intraepithelial neoplasia I (VAIN I) (623.0)
    vaginal intraepithelial neoplasia II (VAIN II) (623.0)
    vaginal intraepithelial neoplasia III (VAIN III) (233.31)
    vulvar intraepithelial neoplasia I (VIN I) (624.01)
    vulvar intraepithelial neoplasia II (VIN II) (624.02)
    vulvar intraepithelial neoplasia III (VIN III) (233.32)
  AHA: 4Q, '08, 145-148

795.10 Abnormal glandular Papanicolaou smear of vagina ♀
  Atypical vaginal glandular cells NOS

795.11 Papanicolaou smear of vagina with atypical squamous cells of undetermined significance [ASC-US] ♀

795.12 Papanicolaou smear of vagina with atypical squamous cells cannot exclude high grade squamous intraepithelial lesion [ASC-H] ♀

795.13 Papanicolaou smear of vagina with low grade squamous intraepithelial lesion [LGSIL] ♀

795.14 Papanicolaou smear of vagina with high grade squamous intraepithelial lesion [HGSIL] ♀

795.15 Vaginal high risk human papillomavirus [HPV] DNA test positive ♀
  EXCLUDES *condyloma acuminatum (078.11)*
    genital warts (078.11)

795.16 Papanicolaou smear of vagina with cytologic evidence of malignancy ♀

795.18 Unsatisfactory vaginal cytology smear ♀
  Inadequate vaginal cytology sample

795.19 Other abnormal Papanicolaou smear of vagina and vaginal HPV ♀
  Vaginal low risk human papillomavirus (HPV) DNA test positive
  Use additional code for associated human papillomavirus (079.4)

795.2 Nonspecific abnormal findings on chromosomal analysis
  Abnormal karyotype

√5ᵗʰ **795.3 Nonspecific positive culture findings**
  Positive culture findings in:
    nose   sputum
    throat   wound
  EXCLUDES *that of:*
    blood (790.7-790.8)
    urine (791.9)

795.31 Nonspecific positive findings for anthrax
  Positive findings by nasal swab
  AHA: 4Q, '02, 70
  TIP: If the patient has been exposed only to anthrax, assign instead V01.81. If a patient has not been exposed but fears anthrax and tests negative, assign instead V71.82.

795.39 Other nonspecific positive culture findings
  EXCLUDES *colonization status (V02.0-V02.9)*

795.4 Other nonspecific abnormal histological findings

√5ᵗʰ **795.5 Nonspecific reaction to test for tuberculosis**
  AHA: 4Q, '11, 140-141

795.51 Nonspecific reaction to tuberculin skin test without active tuberculosis
  Abnormal result of Mantoux test
  PPD positive
  Tuberculin (skin test) positive
  Tuberculin (skin test) reactor
  EXCLUDES *nonspecific reaction to cell mediated immunity measurement of gamma interferon antigen response without active tuberculosis (795.52)*
  AHA: 4Q, '11, 182
  TIP: ►Assign when documentation indicates "latent tuberculosis."◄

795.52 Nonspecific reaction to cell mediated immunity measurement of gamma interferon antigen response without active tuberculosis
  Nonspecific reaction to QuantiFERON-TB test (QFT) without active tuberculosis
  EXCLUDES *nonspecific reaction to tuberculin skin test without active tuberculosis (795.51)*
    positive tuberculin skin test (795.51)

795.6 False positive serological test for syphilis
  False positive Wassermann reaction

√5ᵗʰ **795.7 Other nonspecific immunological findings**
  EXCLUDES *abnormal tumor markers (795.81-795.89)*
    elevated prostate specific antigen [PSA] (790.93)
    elevated tumor associated antigens (795.81-795.89)
    isoimmunization, in pregnancy (656.1-656.2)
    affecting fetus or newborn (773.0-773.2)
  AHA: 2Q, '93, 6

795.71 Nonspecific serologic evidence of human immunodeficiency virus [HIV]
  Inclusive human immunodeficiency [HIV] test (adult) (infant)
  NOTE This code is **only** to be used when a test finding is reported as nonspecific. Asymptomatic positive findings are coded to V08. If any HIV infection symptom or condition is present, see code 042. Negative findings are not coded.
  EXCLUDES *acquired immunodeficiency syndrome [AIDS] (042)*
    asymptomatic human immunodeficiency virus, [HIV] infection status (V08)
    HIV infection, symptomatic (042)
    human immunodeficiency virus [HIV] disease (042)
    positive (status) NOS (V08)
  AHA: 2Q, '04, 11; 1Q, '93, 21; 1Q, '93, 22; 2Q, '92, 11; J-A, '87, 24

Ⓝ Newborn Age: 0   Ⓟ Pediatric Age: 0-17   Ⓜ Maternity Age: 12-55   Ⓐ Adult Age: 15-124

795.79 Other and unspecified nonspecific immunological findings
Raised antibody titer
Raised level of immunoglobulins
AHA: ▶4Q, '11, 93◀

√5th **795.8 Abnormal tumor markers**
Elevated tumor associated antigens [TAA]
Elevated tumor specific antigens [TSA]
EXCLUDES *elevated prostate specific antigen [PSA] (790.93)*

795.81 Elevated carcinoembryonic antigen [CEA]
AHA: 4Q, '06, 111

795.82 Elevated cancer antigen 125 [CA 125] ♀
AHA: 4Q, '06, 111

795.89 Other abnormal tumor markers
AHA: 4Q, '06, 111

√4th **796 Other nonspecific abnormal findings**

796.0 Nonspecific abnormal toxicological findings
Abnormal levels of heavy metals or drugs in blood, urine, or other tissue
Use additional code for retained foreign body, if applicable, (V90.01-V90.9)
EXCLUDES *excessive blood level of alcohol (790.3)*
AHA: 1Q, '97, 16

796.1 Abnormal reflex

796.2 Elevated blood pressure reading without diagnosis of hypertension
NOTE This category is to be used to record an episode of elevated blood pressure in a patient in whom no formal diagnosis of hypertension has been made, or as an incidental finding.
AHA: 2Q, '03, 11; 3Q, '90, 4; J-A, '84, 12
TIP: Assign an additional E code for poisoning or adverse effect of a drug if the documentation indicates it's the underlying cause of the elevated blood pressure.
R03.0 Elevated blood-pressure reading without dx HTN   I-10

796.3 Nonspecific low blood pressure reading

796.4 Other abnormal clinical findings
AHA: 1Q, '97, 16

796.5 Abnormal finding on antenatal screening ♀ M
AHA: 4Q, '97, 46

796.6 Abnormal findings on neonatal screening N
EXCLUDES *nonspecific serologic evidence of human immunodeficiency virus [HIV] (795.71)*
AHA: 4Q, '04, 99

√5th **796.7 Abnormal cytologic smear of anus and anal HPV**
EXCLUDES *abnormal cytologic smear of cervix and cervical HPV (795.00-795.09)*
abnormal cytologic smear of vagina and vaginal HPV (795.10-795.19)
anal intraepithelial neoplasia I (AIN I) (569.44)
anal intraepithelial neoplasia II (AIN II) (569.44)
anal intraepithelial neoplasia III (AIN III) (230.5, 230.6)
carcinoma in situ of anus (230.5, 230.6)
dysplasia (histologically confirmed) of anus NOS (569.44)
mild anal dysplasia (histologically confirmed) (569.44)
moderate anal dysplasia (histologically confirmed) (569.44)
severe anal dysplasia (histologically confirmed) (230.5, 230.6)
AHA: 4Q, '08, 117-119

796.70 Abnormal glandular Papanicolaou smear of anus
Atypical anal glandular cells NOS

796.71 Papanicolaou smear of anus with atypical squamous cells of undetermined significance [ASC-US]

796.72 Papanicolaou smear of anus with atypical squamous cells cannot exclude high grade squamous intraepithelial lesion [ASC-H]

796.73 Papanicolaou smear of anus with low grade squamous intraepithelial lesion [LGSIL]

796.74 Papanicolaou smear of anus with high grade squamous intraepithelial lesion [HGSIL]

796.75 Anal high risk human papillomavirus [HPV] DNA test positive

796.76 Papanicolaou smear of anus with cytologic evidence of malignancy

796.77 Satisfactory anal smear but lacking transformation zone

796.78 Unsatisfactory anal cytology smear
Inadequate anal cytology sample

796.79 Other abnormal Papanicolaou smear of anus and anal HPV
Anal low risk human papillomavirus (HPV) DNA test positive
Use additional code for associated human papillomavirus (079.4)

796.9 Other

Ill-Defined and Unknown Causes of Morbidity and Mortality (797-799)

797 Senility without mention of psychosis
Frailty   Senile asthenia
Old age   Senile:
Senescence   debility
                   exhaustion
EXCLUDES *senile psychoses (290.0-290.9)*

√4th **798 Sudden death, cause unknown**

798.0 Sudden infant death syndrome P
Cot death
Crib death
Sudden death of nonspecific cause in infancy
DEF: Death of infant under age one due to nonspecific cause.

798.1 Instantaneous death

798.2 Death occurring in less than 24 hours from onset of symptoms, not otherwise explained
Death known not to be violent or instantaneous, for which no cause could be discovered
Died without sign of disease

798.9 Unattended death
Death in circumstances where the body of the deceased was found and no cause could be discovered
Found dead

√4th **799 Other ill-defined and unknown causes of morbidity and mortality**

√5th **799.0 Asphyxia and hypoxemia**
EXCLUDES *asphyxia and hypoxemia (due to):*
carbon monoxide (986)
hypercapnia (786.09)
inhalation of food or foreign body (932-934.9)
newborn (768.0-768.9)
traumatic (994.7)

799.01 Asphyxia
DEF: Lack of oxygen in inspired air, causing a deficiency of oxygen in tissues (hypoxia) and elevated levels of arterial carbon dioxide (hypercapnia).
AHA: 4Q, '05, 90

799.02 Hypoxemia
DEF: Deficient oxygenation of the blood.
AHA: 3Q, '09, 20; 2Q, '06, 24, 25; 4Q, '05, 90
TIP: Hypoxia is not inherent in COPD (496) and may be assigned in addition, if applicable.
R09.02 Hypoxemia   I-10

799.1 Respiratory arrest
Cardiorespiratory failure
EXCLUDES cardiac arrest (427.5)
failure of peripheral circulation (785.50)
respiratory distress:
NOS (786.09)
acute (518.82)
following trauma and surgery (518.52)
newborn (770.89)
syndrome (newborn) (769)
adult (following trauma and surgery) (518.52)
other (518.82)
respiratory failure (518.81, 518.83-518.84)
newborn (770.84)
respiratory insufficiency (786.09)
acute (518.82)

√5ᵗʰ **799.2 Signs and symptoms involving emotional state**
EXCLUDES anxiety (293.84, 300.00-300.09)
depression (311)
AHA: 4Q, '09,107
TIP: If associated with underlying history of traumatic brain injury (TBI), assign in addition to a code for the late effect of TBI (e.g., 905.0 or 907.0).

799.21 Nervousness
Nervous
AHA: 4Q, '09,108

799.22 Irritability
Irritable
AHA: 4Q, '09,108

799.23 Impulsiveness
Impulsive
EXCLUDES impulsive neurosis (300.3)

799.24 Emotional lability

799.25 Demoralization and apathy
Apathetic

799.29 Other signs and symptoms involving emotional state

799.3 Debility, unspecified
EXCLUDES asthenia (780.79)
nervous debility (300.5)
neurasthenia (300.5)
senile asthenia (797)

799.4 Cachexia
Wasting disease
Code first underlying condition, if known
DEF: General ill health and poor nutrition.
AHA: 3Q, '06, 14, 15; 3Q, '90, 17
TIP: Assign an additional code for any associated malnutrition, if documented.
R64 Cachexia   I-10

√5ᵗʰ **799.5 Signs and symptoms involving cognition**
EXCLUDES amnesia (780.93)
amnestic syndrome (294.0)
attention deficit disorder (314.00-314.01)
late effects of cerebrovascular disease (438.0)
memory loss (780.93)
mild cognitive impairment, so stated (331.83)
specific problems in developmental delay (315.00-315.9)
transient global amnesia (437.7)
visuospatial neglect (781.8)
AHA: 4Q, '10, 95-96

799.51 Attention or concentration deficit

799.52 Cognitive communication deficit

799.53 Visuospatial deficit

799.54 Psychomotor deficit
AHA: 4Q, '10, 95-97

799.55 Frontal lobe and executive function deficit

799.59 Other signs and symptoms involving cognition

√5ᵗʰ **799.8 Other ill-defined conditions**

799.81 Decreased libido   A
Decreased sexual desire
EXCLUDES psychosexual dysfunction with inhibited sexual desire (302.71)
AHA: 4Q, '03, 75

799.82 Apparent life threatening event in infant   P
ALTE
Apparent life threatening event in newborn and infant
Code first confirmed diagnosis, if known
Use additional code(s) for associated signs and symptoms if no confirmed diagnosis established, or if signs and symptoms are not associated routinely with confirmed diagnosis, or provide additional information for cause of ALTE
AHA: 4Q, '10, 97-98; 4Q, '09, 109

799.89 Other ill-defined conditions

799.9 Other unknown and unspecified cause
Undiagnosed disease, not specified as to site or system involved
Unknown cause of morbidity or mortality
AHA: 1Q, '98,.4; 1Q, '90, 20

N Newborn Age: 0   P Pediatric Age: 0-17   M Maternity Age: 12-55   A Adult Age: 15-124

17. Injury and Poisoning (800-999)

Use additional code for retained foreign body, if applicable, (V90.01-V90.9)

Use E code(s) to identify the cause and intent of the injury or poisoning (E800-E999)

NOTE

1. The principle of multiple coding of injuries should be followed wherever possible. Combination categories for multiple injuries are provided for use when there is insufficient detail as to the nature of the individual conditions, or for primary tabulation purposes when it is more convenient to record a single code; otherwise, the component injuries should be coded separately.

   Where multiple sites of injury are specified in the titles, the word "with" indicates involvement of both sites, and the word "and" indicates involvement of either or both sites. The word "finger" includes thumb.

2. Categories for "late effect" of injuries are to be found at 905-909.

FRACTURES (800-829)

EXCLUDES   malunion (733.81)
     nonunion (733.82)
     pathological or spontaneous fracture (733.10-733.19)
     stress fractures (733.93-733.95)

NOTE The terms "condyle," "coronoid process," "ramus," and "symphysis" indicate the portion of the bone fractured, not the name of the bone involved.

The descriptions "closed" and "open" used in the fourth-digit subdivisions include the following terms:

closed (with or without delayed healing):
comminuted	impacted
depressed	linear
elevated	simple
fissured	slipped epiphysis
fracture NOS	spiral
greenstick	

open (with or without delayed healing):
compound	puncture
infected	with foreign body
missile	

NOTE A fracture not indicated as closed or open should be classified as closed.

AHA: 4Q, '08, 158; 1Q, '07, 3-4; 4Q, '90, 26; 3Q, '90, 5; 3Q, '90, 13; 2Q, '90, 7; 2Q, '89, 15, S-O, '85, 3

TIP: Assign the acute fracture codes only while the patient is receiving active treatment for the fracture, such as during surgical care, an ED encounter, or evaluation and treatment by a new physician. Otherwise, refer to aftercare category V54.

Fracture of Skull (800-804)

INCLUDES   traumatic brain injury due to fracture of skull

The following fifth-digit subclassification is for use with the appropriate codes in category 800, 801, 803, and 804:
0 unspecified state of consciousness
1 with no loss of consciousness
2 with brief [less than one hour] loss of consciousness
3 with moderate [1-24 hours] loss of consciousness
4 with prolonged [more than 24 hours] loss of consciousness and return to pre-existing conscious level
5 with prolonged [more than 24 hours] loss of consciousness, without return to pre-existing conscious level
    Use fifth-digit 5 to designate when a patient is unconscious and dies before regaining consciousness, regardless of the duration of the loss of consciousness
6 with loss of consciousness of unspecified duration
9 with concussion, unspecified

√4ᵗʰ **800**   **Fracture of vault of skull**
    INCLUDES   frontal bone
                 parietal bone
    DEF: Fracture of bone that forms skull dome and protects brain.
    AHA: 4Q,'96, 36

§ √5ᵗʰ **800.0 Closed without mention of intracranial injury**
    [0-6, 9]

§ √5ᵗʰ **800.1 Closed with cerebral laceration and contusion**
    [0-6, 9]

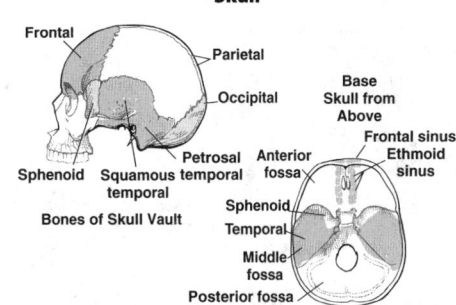

Skull

§ √5ᵗʰ **800.2 Closed with subarachnoid, subdural, and extradural**
    [0-6, 9]**hemorrhage**

§ √5ᵗʰ **800.3 Closed with other and unspecified intracranial**
    [0-6, 9]**hemorrhage**

§ √5ᵗʰ **800.4 Closed with intracranial injury of other and**
    [0-6, 9]**unspecified nature**

§ √5ᵗʰ **800.5 Open without mention of intracranial injury**
    [0-6, 9]

§ √5ᵗʰ **800.6 Open with cerebral laceration and contusion**
    [0-6, 9]

§ √5ᵗʰ **800.7 Open with subarachnoid, subdural, and**
    [0-6, 9]**extradural hemorrhage**

§ √5ᵗʰ **800.8 Open with other and unspecified intracranial**
    [0-6, 9]**hemorrhage**

§ √5ᵗʰ **800.9 Open with intracranial injury of other and**
    [0-6, 9]**unspecified nature**

√4ᵗʰ **801**   **Fracture of base of skull**
    INCLUDES   fossa:
               anterior
               middle
               posterior
              occiput bone
              orbital roof
              sinus:
               ethmoid
               frontal
              sphenoid bone
              temporal bone
    DEF: Fracture of bone that forms skull floor.
    AHA: 4Q, '96, 36

§ √5ᵗʰ **801.0 Closed without mention of intracranial injury**
    [0-6, 9]

§ √5ᵗʰ **801.1 Closed with cerebral laceration and contusion**
    [0-6, 9]   **AHA: For code 801.15:** 4Q, '96, 36

§ √5ᵗʰ **801.2 Closed with subarachnoid, subdural, and**
    [0-6, 9]**extradural hemorrhage**

§ √5ᵗʰ **801.3 Closed with other and unspecified intracranial**
    [0-6, 9]**hemorrhage**

§ √5ᵗʰ **801.4 Closed with intracranial injury of other and**
    [0-6, 9]**unspecified nature**

§ √5ᵗʰ **801.5 Open without mention of intracranial injury**
    [0-6, 9]

§ √5ᵗʰ **801.6 Open with cerebral laceration and contusion**
    [0-6, 9]

§ √5ᵗʰ **801.7 Open with subarachnoid, subdural, and**
    [0-6, 9]**extradural hemorrhage**

§ √5ᵗʰ **801.8 Open with other and unspecified intracranial**
    [0-6, 9]**hemorrhage**

§ √5ᵗʰ **801.9 Open with intracranial injury of other and**
    [0-6, 9]**unspecified nature**

§   Requires fifth digit. Valid digits are in [brackets] under each code. See beginning of section 800-804 for codes and definitions.

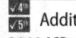 Additional Digit Required   Unspecified Code   Other Specified Code   Manifestation Code   ▶◀ Revised Text   ● New Code   ▲ Revised Code Title

Injury and Poisoning

802–804.9

Fractures

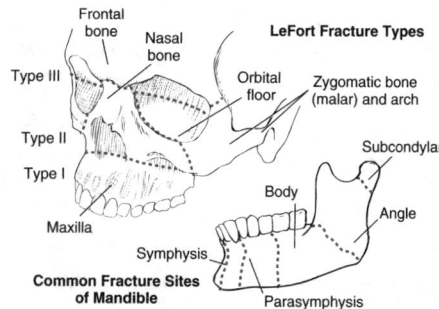

Avulsion   Fracture-dislocation   Impacted

Open (skin broken)

Oblique

Closed spiral

Epiphyseal

March

Linear (fissured)

Greenstick

Depressed

Comminuted

Facial Fracture

Frontal bone   Nasal bone

Type III

Type II

Type I

Maxilla

LeFort Fracture Types

Orbital floor   Zygomatic bone (malar) and arch

Subcondylar

Body

Angle

Symphysis

Parasymphysis

Common Fracture Sites of Mandible

☑4ᵗʰ **802 Fracture of face bones**
  AHA: 4Q, '96, 36

802.0 Nasal bones, closed
  S02.2xxA Fracture nasal bones initial encounter closed fx   I-10

802.1 Nasal bones, open

☑5ᵗʰ **802.2 Mandible, closed**
  Inferior maxilla   Lower jaw (bone)

  802.20 Unspecified site

  802.21 Condylar process

  802.22 Subcondylar

  802.23 Coronoid process

  802.24 Ramus, unspecified

  802.25 Angle of jaw

  802.26 Symphysis of body

  802.27 Alveolar border of body

  802.28 Body, other and unspecified

  802.29 Multiple sites

☑5ᵗʰ **802.3 Mandible, open**

  802.30 Unspecified site

  802.31 Condylar process

  802.32 Subcondylar

  802.33 Coronoid process

  802.34 Ramus, unspecified

  802.35 Angle of jaw

  802.36 Symphysis of body

  802.37 Alveolar border of body

  802.38 Body, other and unspecified

  802.39 Multiple sites

802.4 Malar and maxillary bones, closed
  Superior maxilla   Zygoma
  Upper jaw (bone)   Zygomatic arch
  S02.400A Malar fx uns initial enc closed fx   I-10
  S02.401A Maxillary fx uns initial enc closed fx   I-10
  S02.402A Zygomatic fx uns initial enc closed fx   I-10

802.5 Malar and maxillary bones, open

802.6 Orbital floor (blow-out), closed
  S02.3xxA Fracture orbital floor initial encounter clos fx   I-10

802.7 Orbital floor (blow-out), open

802.8 Other facial bones, closed
  Alveolus
  Orbit:
    NOS
    part other than roof or floor
  Palate
  EXCLUDES orbital:
        floor (802.6)
        roof (801.0-801.9)
  S02.42xA Fx of alveolus of maxilla initial enc closed fx   I-10

802.9 Other facial bones, open

☑4ᵗʰ **803 Other and unqualified skull fractures**
  INCLUDES skull NOS
        skull multiple NOS
  AHA: 4Q, '96, 36

§ ☑5ᵗʰ **803.0 Closed without mention of intracranial injury**
  [0-6, 9]

§ ☑5ᵗʰ **803.1 Closed with cerebral laceration and contusion**
  [0-6, 9]

§ ☑5ᵗʰ **803.2 Closed with subarachnoid, subdural, and**
  [0-6, 9] **extradural hemorrhage**

§ ☑5ᵗʰ **803.3 Closed with other and unspecified intracranial**
  [0-6, 9] **hemorrhage**

§ ☑5ᵗʰ **803.4 Closed with intracranial injury of other and**
  [0-6, 9] **unspecified nature**

§ ☑5ᵗʰ **803.5 Open without mention of intracranial injury**
  [0-6, 9]

§ ☑5ᵗʰ **803.6 Open with cerebral laceration and contusion**
  [0-6, 9]

§ ☑5ᵗʰ **803.7 Open with subarachnoid, subdural, and**
  [0-6, 9] **extradural hemorrhage**

§ ☑5ᵗʰ **803.8 Open with other and unspecified intracranial**
  [0-6, 9] **hemorrhage**

§ ☑5ᵗʰ **803.9 Open with intracranial injury of other and**
  [0-6, 9] **unspecified nature**

☑4ᵗʰ **804 Multiple fractures involving skull or face with other bones**
  AHA: 4Q, '96, 36

§ ☑5ᵗʰ **804.0 Closed without mention of intracranial injury**
  [0-6, 9]

§ ☑5ᵗʰ **804.1 Closed with cerebral laceration and contusion**
  [0-6, 9]   AHA: For code 804.10: 1Q, '06, 6

§ ☑5ᵗʰ **804.2 Closed with subarachnoid, subdural, and**
  [0-6, 9] **extradural hemorrhage**

§ ☑5ᵗʰ **804.3 Closed with other and unspecified intracranial**
  [0-6, 9] **hemorrhage**

§ ☑5ᵗʰ **804.4 Closed with intracranial injury of other and**
  [0-6, 9] **unspecified nature**

§ ☑5ᵗʰ **804.5 Open without mention of intracranial injury**
  [0-6, 9]

§ ☑5ᵗʰ **804.6 Open with cerebral laceration and contusion**
  [0-6, 9]

§ ☑5ᵗʰ **804.7 Open with subarachnoid, subdural, and**
  [0-6, 9] **extradural hemorrage**

§ ☑5ᵗʰ **804.8 Open with other and unspecified intracranial**
  [0-6, 9] **hemorrhage**

§ ☑5ᵗʰ **804.9 Open with intracranial injury of other and**
  [0-6, 9] **unspecified nature**

§   Requires fifth digit. Valid digits are in [brackets] under each code. See beginning of section 800-804 for codes and definitions.

N Newborn Age: 0   P Pediatric Age: 0-17   M Maternity Age: 12-55   A Adult Age: 15-124

Fracture of Neck and Trunk (805-809)

✓4ᵗʰ **805 Fracture of vertebral column without mention of spinal cord injury**

    INCLUDES   neural arch
                  spine
                  spinous process
                  transverse process
                  vertebra

The following fifth-digit subclassification is for use with codes 805.0-805.1:

   0 cervical vertebra, unspecified level
   1 first cervical vertebra
   2 second cervical vertebra
   3 third cervical vertebra
   4 fourth cervical vertebra
   5 fifth cervical vertebra
   6 sixth cervical vertebra
   7 seventh cervical vertebra
   8 multiple cervical vertebrae

§ ✓5ᵗʰ **805.0 Cervical, closed**
[0-8]   Atlas
         Axis
         S12.101A Uns nondisplcd fx 2nd cerv vert initial enc closed fx   I-10

§ ✓5ᵗʰ **805.1 Cervical, open**
[0-8]

805.2 Dorsal [thoracic], closed
    S22.008A Oth fx uns thoracic vertebra initial enc clos fx   I-10

805.3 Dorsal [thoracic], open

805.4 Lumbar, closed
    AHA: 1Q, '07, 7; 4Q, '99, 12
    S32.008A Oth fx uns lumbar vertebra initial enc closed fx   I-10

805.5 Lumbar, open

805.6 Sacrum and coccyx, closed
    S32.19xA Other fx of sacrum initial encounter closed fx   I-10

805.7 Sacrum and coccyx, open

805.8 Unspecified, closed

805.9 Unspecified, open

Vertebral Column

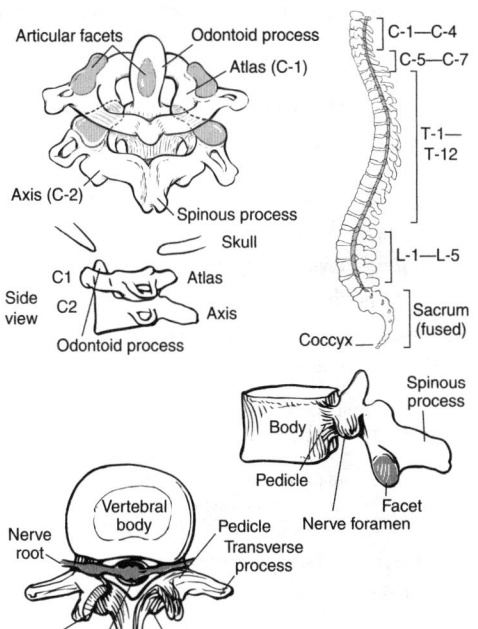

✓4ᵗʰ **806 Fracture of vertebral column with spinal cord injury**

    INCLUDES any condition classifiable to 805 with:
          complete or incomplete transverse lesion (of cord)
          hematomyelia
          injury to:
              cauda equina
              nerve
          paralysis
          paraplegia
          quadriplegia
          spinal concussion

✓5ᵗʰ **806.0 Cervical, closed**

    806.00 C_1-C_4 level with unspecified spinal cord injury
        Cervical region NOS with spinal cord injury NOS

    806.01 C_1-C_4 level with complete lesion of cord

    806.02 C_1-C_4 level with anterior cord syndrome

    806.03 C_1-C_4 level with central cord syndrome

    806.04 C_1-C_4 level with other specified spinal cord injury
        C_1-C_4 level with:
          incomplete spinal cord lesion NOS
          posterior cord syndrome

    806.05 C_5-C_7 level with unspecified spinal cord injury

    806.06 C_5-C_7 level with complete lesion of cord

    806.07 C_5-C_7 level with anterior cord syndrome

    806.08 C_5-C_7 level with central cord syndrome

    806.09 C_5-C_7 level with other specified spinal cord injury
        C_5-C_7 level with:
          incomplete spinal cord lesion NOS
          posterior cord syndrome

✓5ᵗʰ **806.1 Cervical, open**

    806.10 C_1-C_4 level with unspecified spinal cord injury

    806.11 C_1-C_4 level with complete lesion of cord

    806.12 C_1-C_4 level with anterior cord syndrome

    806.13 C_1-C_4 level with central cord syndrome

    806.14 C_1-C_4 level with other specified spinal cord injury
        C_1-C_4 level with:
          incomplete spinal cord lesion NOS
          posterior cord syndrome

    806.15 C_5-C_7 level with unspecified spinal cord injury

    806.16 C_5-C_7 level with complete lesion of cord

    806.17 C_5-C_7 level with anterior cord syndrome

    806.18 C_5-C_7 level with central cord syndrome

    806.19 C_5-C_7 level with other specified spinal cord injury
        C_5-C_7 level with:
          incomplete spinal cord lesion NOS
          posterior cord syndrome

✓5ᵗʰ **806.2 Dorsal [thoracic], closed**

    806.20 T_1-T_6 level with unspecified spinal cord injury
        Thoracic region NOS with spinal cord injury NOS

    806.21 T_1-T_6 level with complete lesion of cord

    806.22 T_1-T_6 level with anterior cord syndrome

    806.23 T_1-T_6 level with central cord syndrome

    806.24 T_1-T_6 level with other specified spinal cord injury
        T_1-T_6 level with:
          incomplete spinal cord lesion NOS
          posterior cord syndrome

    806.25 T_7-T_{12} level with unspecified spinal cord injury

    806.26 T_7-T_{12} level with complete lesion of cord

    806.27 T_7-T_{12} level with anterior cord syndrome

    806.28 T_7-T_{12} level with central cord syndrome

    806.29 T_7-T_{12} level with other specified spinal cord injury
        T_7-T_{12} level with:
          incomplete spinal cord lesion NOS
          posterior cord syndrome

---

§ Requires fifth digit. Valid digits are in [brackets] under each code. See category 805 for codes and definitions.

✓4ᵗʰ ✓5ᵗʰ Additional Digit Required   Unspecified Code   Other Specified Code   Manifestation Code   ►◄ Revised Text   ● New Code   ▲ Revised Code Title

Injury and Poisoning

806.3–809.1

✓5ᵗʰ **806.3 Dorsal [thoracic], open**

     806.30 T_1-T_6 level with unspecified spinal cord injury

     806.31 T_1-T_6 level with complete lesion of cord

     806.32 T_1-T_6 level with anterior cord syndrome

     806.33 T_1-T_6 level with central cord syndrome

     806.34 T_1-T_6 level with other specified spinal cord injury
        T_1-T_6 level with:
          incomplete spinal cord lesion NOS
          posterior cord syndrome

     806.35 T_7-T_{12} level with unspecified spinal cord injury

     806.36 T_7-T_{12} level with complete lesion of cord

     806.37 T_7-T_{12} level with anterior cord syndrome

     806.38 T_7-T_{12} level with central cord syndrome

     806.39 T_7-T_{12} level with other specified spinal cord injury
        T_7-T_{12} level with:
          incomplete spinal cord lesion NOS
          posterior cord syndrome

806.4 Lumbar, closed
     AHA: 4Q, '99, 11, 13

806.5 Lumbar, open

✓5ᵗʰ **806.6 Sacrum and coccyx, closed**

     806.60 With unspecified spinal cord injury

     806.61 With complete cauda equina lesion

     806.62 With other cauda equina injury

     806.69 With other spinal cord injury

✓5ᵗʰ **806.7 Sacrum and coccyx, open**

     806.70 With unspecified spinal cord injury

     806.71 With complete cauda equina lesion

     806.72 With other cauda equina injury

     806.79 With other spinal cord injury

806.8 Unspecified, closed

806.9 Unspecified, open

✓4ᵗʰ **807 Fracture of rib(s), sternum, larynx, and trachea**

     The following fifth-digit subclassification is for use with codes 807.0-807.1:
       0   rib(s) unspecifed
       1   one rib
       2   two ribs
       3   three ribs
       4   four ribs
       5   five ribs
       6   six ribs
       7   seven ribs
       8   eight or more ribs
       9   multiple ribs, unspecified

§ ✓5ᵗʰ **807.0 Rib(s), closed**
     [0-9]   S22.31xA Fracture one rib right side, initial encounter closed fx   I-10
           S22.43xG Mx fx ribs bilat subseqnt enc fx delayed healing   I-10

§ ✓5ᵗʰ **807.1 Rib(s), open**
     [0-9]

Ribs, Sternum, Larynx, and Trachea

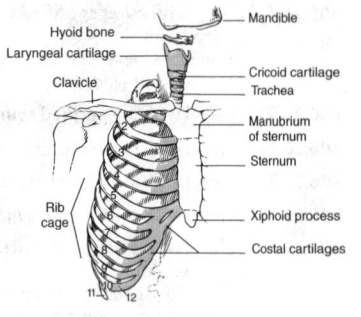

807.2 Sternum, closed
     DEF: Break in flat bone (breast bone) in anterior thorax.

807.3 Sternum, open
     DEF: Break, with open wound, in flat bone in mid anterior thorax.

807.4 Flail chest

807.5 Larynx and trachea, closed
     Hyoid bone
     Thyroid cartilage
     Trachea

807.6 Larynx and trachea, open

✓4ᵗʰ **808 Fracture of pelvis**

808.0 Acetabulum, closed

808.1 Acetabulum, open

808.2 Pubis, closed
     AHA: 1Q, '08, 9
     S32.509A Unspec fx unspec pubis initial encounter closed fx   I-10

808.3 Pubis, open

✓5ᵗʰ **808.4 Other specified part, closed**

     808.41 Ilium

     808.42 Ischium

     808.43 Multiple closed pelvic fractures with disruption of pelvic circle
        Multiple closed pelvic fractures with disruption of pelvic ring
        AHA: 1Q, '08, 9
        TIP: To assign, documentation must indicate multiple pelvic fractures with complete disruption of the pelvic circle.

     808.44 Multiple closed pelvic fractures without disruption of pelvic circle
        Multiple closed pelvic fractures without disruption of pelvic ring
        AHA: ▶4Q, '11, 141-142◀

     808.49 Other
        Innominate bone
        Pelvic rim

✓5ᵗʰ **808.5 Other specified part, open**

     808.51 Ilium

     808.52 Ischium

     808.53 Multiple open pelvic fractures with disruption of pelvic circle
        Multiple open pelvic fractures with disruption of pelvic ring

     808.54 Multiple open pelvic fractures without disruption of pelvic circle
        Multiple open pelvic fractures without disruption of pelvic ring
        AHA: ▶4Q, '11, 141-142◀

     808.59 Other

808.8 Unspecified, closed

808.9 Unspecified, open

✓4ᵗʰ **809 Ill-defined fractures of bones of trunk**
     INCLUDES   bones of trunk with other bones except those of skull and face
            multiple bones of trunk

     EXCLUDES   *multiple fractures of:*
            pelvic bones alone (808.0-808.9)
            ribs alone (807.0-807.1, 807.4)
            ribs or sternum with limb bones (819.0-819.1, 828.0-828.1)
            skull or face with other bones (804.0-804.9)

809.0 Fracture of bones of trunk, closed

809.1 Fracture of bones of trunk, open

---

§   Requires fifth digit. Valid digits are in [brackets] under each code. See category 807 for codes and definitions.

Pelvis and Pelvic Fractures

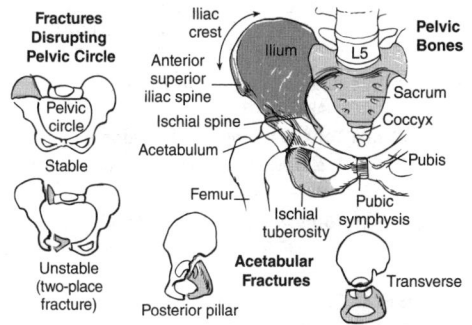

Right Clavicle and Scapula, Anterior View

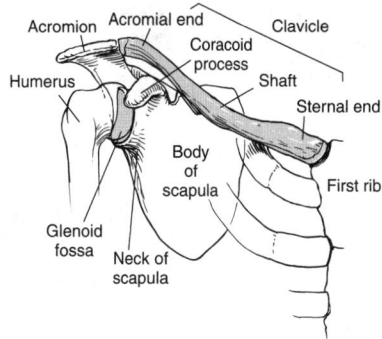

Fracture of Upper Limb (810-819)

√4ᵗʰ 810 Fracture of clavicle

> **INCLUDES** collar bone
> interligamentous part of clavicle

> The following fifth-digit subclassification is for use with category 810:
> **0 unspecified part**
>   Clavicle NOS
> **1 sternal end of clavicle**
> **2 shaft of clavicle**
> **3 acromial end of clavicle**

§ **√5ᵗʰ 810.0 Closed**
[0-3]

§ **√5ᵗʰ 810.1 Open**
[0-3]

√4ᵗʰ 811 Fracture of scapula

> **INCLUDES** shoulder blade

> The following fifth-digit subclassification is for use with category 811:
> **0 unspecified part**
> **1 acromial process**
>   Acromion (process)
> **2 coracoid process**
> **3 glenoid cavity and neck of scapula**
> **9 other**

§ **√5ᵗʰ 811.0 Closed**
[0-3, 9]

§ **√5ᵗʰ 811.1 Open**
[0-3, 9]

√4ᵗʰ 812 Fracture of humerus

√5ᵗʰ 812.0 Upper end, closed

> **812.00 Upper end, unspecified part**
>   Proximal end   Shoulder

> **812.01 Surgical neck**
>   Neck of humerus NOS
>   **S42.214A** Uns nondsplcd fx surg neck rt   **I-10**
>   humerus inital enc closed fx

> **812.02 Anatomical neck**

> **812.03 Greater tuberosity**

> **812.09 Other**
>   Head   Upper epiphysis
>   Lesser tuberosity
>   **S42.294A** Oth nondsplcd fx up end rt humerus   **I-10**
>   initial enc clos fx

√5ᵗʰ 812.1 Upper end, open

> **812.10 Upper end, unspecified part**

> **812.11 Surgical neck**

> **812.12 Anatomical neck**

> **812.13 Greater tuberosity**

> **812.19 Other**

Right Humerus, Anterior View

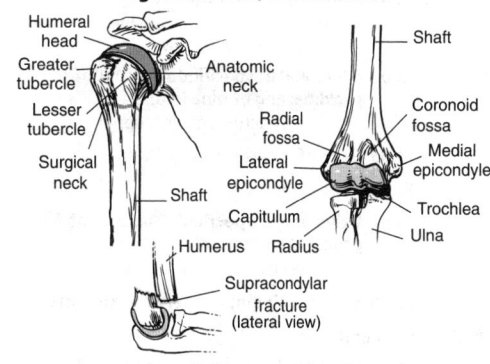

√5ᵗʰ 812.2 Shaft or unspecified part, closed

> **812.20 Unspecified part of humerus**
>   Humerus NOS   Upper arm NOS

> **812.21 Shaft of humerus**
>   **AHA:** 4Q, '05, 129; 3Q, '99, 14

√5ᵗʰ 812.3 Shaft or unspecified part, open

> **812.30 Unspecified part of humerus**

> **812.31 Shaft of humerus**

√5ᵗʰ 812.4 Lower end, closed
   Distal end of humerus   Elbow

> **812.40 Lower end, unspecified part**

> **812.41 Supracondylar fracture of humerus**

> **812.42 Lateral condyle**
>   External condyle

> **812.43 Medial condyle**
>   Internal epicondyle

> **812.44 Condyle(s), unspecified**
>   Articular process NOS   Lower epiphysis NOS

> **812.49 Other**
>   Multiple fractures of lower end   Trochlea

√5ᵗʰ 812.5 Lower end, open

> **812.50 Lower end, unspecified part**

> **812.51 Supracondylar fracture of humerus**

> **812.52 Lateral condyle**

> **812.53 Medial condyle**

> **812.54 Condyle(s), unspecified**

> **812.59 Other**

√4ᵗʰ 813 Fracture of radius and ulna

√5ᵗʰ 813.0 Upper end, closed
   Proximal end

> **813.00 Upper end of forearm, unspecified**

> **813.01 Olecranon process of ulna**

> **813.02 Coronoid process of ulna**

---

§   Requires fifth digit. Valid digits are in [brackets] under each code. See appropriate category for codes and definitions.

Right Radius and Ulna, Anterior View

813.03 Monteggia's fracture
DEF: Fracture near the head of the ulnar shaft, causing dislocation of the radial head.

813.04 Other and unspecified fractures of proximal end of ulna (alone)
Multiple fractures of ulna, upper end

813.05 Head of radius

813.06 Neck of radius

813.07 Other and unspecified fractures of proximal end of radius (alone)
Multiple fractures of radius, upper end

813.08 Radius with ulna, upper end [any part]

√5ᵗʰ **813.1 Upper end, open**

813.10 Upper end of forearm, unspecified

813.11 Olecranon process of ulna

813.12 Coronoid process of ulna

813.13 Monteggia's fracture

813.14 Other and unspecified fractures of proximal end of ulna (alone)

813.15 Head of radius

813.16 Neck of radius

813.17 Other and unspecified fractures of proximal end of radius (alone)

813.18 Radius with ulna, upper end [any part]

√5ᵗʰ **813.2 Shaft, closed**

813.20 Shaft, unspecified

813.21 Radius (alone)

813.22 Ulna (alone)

813.23 Radius with ulna
AHA: 4Q, '09, 120

√5ᵗʰ **813.3 Shaft, open**

813.30 Shaft, unspecified

813.31 Radius (alone)

813.32 Ulna (alone)

813.33 Radius with ulna

√5ᵗʰ **813.4 Lower end, closed**
Distal end

813.40 Lower end of forearm, unspecified

813.41 Colles' fracture
Smith's fracture
DEF: Break of lower end of radius; associated with backward movement of the radius lower section.

813.42 Other fractures of distal end of radius (alone)
Dupuytren's fracture, radius   Radius, lower end
DEF: Dupuytren's fracture: fracture and dislocation of the forearm; the fracture is of the radius above the wrist, and the dislocation is of the ulna at the lower end.
S52.501A Uns fx lower end rt radius initial enc closed fx   I-10

813.43 Distal end of ulna (alone)
Ulna:	Ulna:
head	lower epiphysis
lower end	styloid process

813.44 Radius with ulna, lower end
AHA: 1Q, '07, 7

813.45 Torus fracture of radius (alone)
EXCLUDES   torus fracture of radius and ulna (813.47)
AHA: 4Q, '02, 70

813.46 Torus fracture of ulna (alone)
EXCLUDES   torus fracture of radius and ulna (813.47)
AHA: 4Q, '09, 110

813.47 Torus fracture of radius and ulna
AHA: 4Q, '09, 110

√5ᵗʰ **813.5 Lower end, open**

813.50 Lower end of forearm, unspecified

813.51 Colles' fracture

813.52 Other fractures of distal end of radius (alone)

813.53 Distal end of ulna (alone)

813.54 Radius with ulna, lower end

√5ᵗʰ **813.8 Unspecified part, closed**

813.80 Forearm, unspecified

813.81 Radius (alone)
AHA: 2Q, '98, 19

813.82 Ulna (alone)

813.83 Radius with ulna

√5ᵗʰ **813.9 Unspecified part, open**

813.90 Forearm, unspecified

813.91 Radius (alone)

813.92 Ulna (alone)

813.93 Radius with ulna

√4ᵗʰ **814 Fracture of carpal bone(s)**
The following fifth-digit subclassification is for use with category 814:
- **0 carpal bone, unspecified**
  Wrist NOS
- **1 navicular [scaphoid] of wrist**
- **2 lunate [semilunar] bone of wrist**
- **3 triquetral [cuneiform] bone of wrist**
- **4 pisiform**
- **5 trapezium bone [larger multangular]**
- **6 trapezoid bone [smaller multangular]**
- **7 capitate bone [os magnum]**
- **8 hamate [unciform] bone**
- **9 other**

§ √5ᵗʰ **814.0 Closed**
[0-9]

§ √5ᵗʰ **814.1 Open**
[0-9]

Hand Fractures

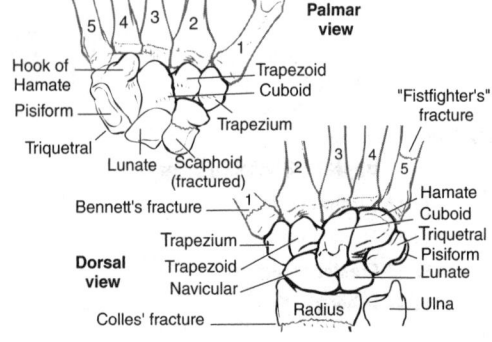

§ Requires fifth digit. Valid digits are in [brackets] under each code. See category 814 for codes and definitions.

N Newborn Age: 0   P Pediatric Age: 0-17   M Maternity Age: 12-55   A Adult Age: 15-124

280 – Volume 1   2013 ICD-9-CM

✓4ᵗʰ **815　Fracture of metacarpal bone(s)**
　　　[INCLUDES]　hand [except finger]
　　　　　　　　metacarpus

　　　The following fifth-digit subclassification is for use with category 815:
　　　　0　metacarpal bone(s), site unspecified
　　　　1　base of thumb [first] metacarpal
　　　　　　Bennett's fracture
　　　　2　base of other metacarpal bone(s)
　　　　3　shaft of metacarpal bone(s)
　　　　4　neck of metacarpal bone(s)
　　　　9　multiple sites of metacarpus

§ ✓5ᵗʰ **815.0　Closed**
　　　[0-4, 9]

§ ✓5ᵗʰ **815.1　Open**
　　　[0-4, 9]

✓4ᵗʰ **816　Fracture of one or more phalanges of hand**
　　　[INCLUDES]　finger(s)
　　　　　　　　thumb

　　　The following fifth-digit subclassification is for use with category 816:
　　　　0　phalanx or phalanges, unspecified
　　　　1　middle or proximal phalanx or phalanges
　　　　2　distal phalanx or phalanges
　　　　3　multiple sites

　　　TIP: If phalangeal fracture(s) are due to crushing injury, sequence that code (927.3) first.

§ ✓5ᵗʰ **816.0　Closed**
　　　[0-3]

§ ✓5ᵗʰ **816.1　Open**
　　　[0-3]　　**AHA: For code 816.12:** 4Q, '03, 77

✓4ᵗʰ **817　Multiple fractures of hand bones**
　　　[INCLUDES]　metacarpal bone(s) with phalanx or phalanges of same
　　　　　　　　hand

　　　817.0　Closed

　　　817.1　Open

✓4ᵗʰ **818　Ill-defined fractures of upper limb**
　　　[INCLUDES]　arm NOS
　　　　　　　　multiple bones of same upper limb
　　　[EXCLUDES]　*multiple fractures of:*
　　　　　　　　metacarpal bone(s) with phalanx or phalanges
　　　　　　　　(817.0-817.1)
　　　　　　　　phalanges of hand alone (816.0-816.1)
　　　　　　　　radius with ulna (813.0-813.9)

　　　818.0　Closed

　　　818.1　Open

✓4ᵗʰ **819　Multiple fractures involving both upper limbs, and upper limb with rib(s) and sternum**
　　　[INCLUDES]　arm(s) with rib(s) or sternum
　　　　　　　　both arms [any bones]

　　　819.0　Closed

　　　819.1　Open

Fracture of Lower Limb (820-829)

✓4ᵗʰ **820　Fracture of neck of femur**

　✓5ᵗʰ **820.0　Transcervical fracture, closed**

　　　820.00　Intracapsular section, unspecified

　　　820.01　Epiphysis (separation) (upper)
　　　　　　Transepiphyseal

　　　820.02　Midcervical section
　　　　　　Transcervical NOS
　　　　　　AHA: 3Q, '03, 12

　　　820.03　Base of neck
　　　　　　Cervicotrochanteric section

　　　820.09　Other
　　　　　　Head of femur　　　Subcapital
　　　　　　S72.064A Nondsplcd art fx head rt femur　　[I-10]
　　　　　　initial enc closed fx

　✓5ᵗʰ **820.1　Transcervical fracture, open**

　　　820.10　Intracapsular section, unspecified

　　　820.11　Epiphysis (separation) (upper)

　　　820.12　Midcervical section

　　　820.13　Base of neck

　　　820.19　Other

　✓5ᵗʰ **820.2　Pertrochanteric fracture, closed**

　　　820.20　Trochanteric section, unspecified
　　　　　　Trochanter:
　　　　　　NOS
　　　　　　greater
　　　　　　lesser

　　　820.21　Intertrochanteric section

　　　820.22　Subtrochanteric section
　　　　　　S72.25xA Nondsplcd subtrochant fx lt femur　　[I-10]
　　　　　　inital enc closed fx

　✓5ᵗʰ **820.3　Pertrochanteric fracture, open**

　　　820.30　Trochanteric section, unspecified

　　　820.31　Intertrochanteric section

　　　820.32　Subtrochanteric section

　　　820.8　Unspecified part of neck of femur, closed
　　　　　Hip NOS　　　　　Neck of femur NOS
　　　　　S72.002A Fx uns part neck left femur initial enc clos fx　　[I-10]

　　　820.9　Unspecified part of neck of femur, open

✓4ᵗʰ **821　Fracture of other and unspecified parts of femur**

　✓5ᵗʰ **821.0　Shaft or unspecified part, closed**

　　　821.00　Unspecified part of femur
　　　　　　Thigh　　　　Upper leg
　　　　　　[EXCLUDES]　*hip NOS (820.8)*

　　　821.01　Shaft
　　　　　　AHA: 1Q, '07, 4; 1Q, '99, 5
　　　　　　S72.331A Displaced obl fx shaft rt femur initial　　[I-10]
　　　　　　enc clos fx

　✓5ᵗʰ **821.1　Shaft or unspecified part, open**

　　　821.10　Unspecified part of femur

　　　821.11　Shaft

　✓5ᵗʰ **821.2　Lower end, closed**
　　　　Distal end

　　　821.20　Lower end, unspecified part

　　　821.21　Condyle, femoral

　　　821.22　Epiphysis, lower (separation)

　　　821.23　Supracondylar fracture of femur

　　　821.29　Other
　　　　　　Multiple fractures of lower end

　✓5ᵗʰ **821.3　Lower end, open**

　　　821.30　Lower end, unspecified part

　　　821.31　Condyle, femoral

　　　821.32　Epiphysis, lower (separation)

　　　821.33　Supracondylar fracture of femur

　　　821.39　Other

✓4ᵗʰ **822　Fracture of patella**

　　　822.0　Closed
　　　　　　S82.001A Uns fx right patella initial encounter closed fx　　[I-10]

　　　822.1　Open

---

§　Requires fifth digit. Valid digits are in [brackets] under each code. See appropriate category for codes and definitions.

✓4ᵗʰ ✓5ᵗʰ Additional Digit Required　　Unspecified Code　　Other Specified Code　　Manifestation Code　　▶◀ Revised Text　　● New Code　　▲ Revised Code Title

2013 ICD-9-CM　　　　　　　　　　　　　　　　　　　　　　　　　　　　　　　　**Volume 1 – 281**

Injury and Poisoning

823–825.29

Right Femur, Anterior View

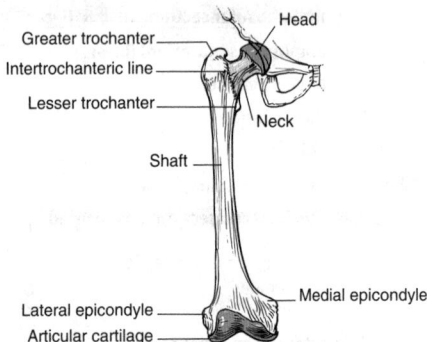

Head
Greater trochanter
Intertrochanteric line
Lesser trochanter
Neck
Shaft
Lateral epicondyle
Medial epicondyle
Articular cartilage

Right Tibia and Fibula, Anterior View

Patella
Tibial plateau
Tibial tubercle
Shaft of fibula
Tibia
Pott's fracture
Lateral (fibular) malleolus
Medial (tibial) malleolus

Torus Fracture

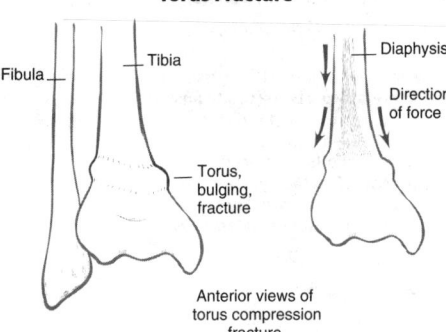

Fibula
Tibia
Diaphysis
Direction of force
Torus, bulging, fracture

Anterior views of
torus compression
fracture

✓4ᵗʰ **823 Fracture of tibia and fibula**

> **EXCLUDES** Dupuytren's fracture (824.4-824.5)
> ankle (824.4-824.5)
> radius (813.42, 813.52)
> Pott's fracture (824.4-824.5)
> that involving ankle (824.0-824.9)

The following fifth-digit subclassification is for use with category 823:

0   tibia alone
1   fibula alone
2   fibula with tibia

§ ✓5ᵗʰ **823.0 Upper end, closed**
[0-2]   Head
Proximal end
Tibia:
condyles
tuberosity
S82.121A Displcd fx lat condyle rt tibia initial enc clos fx   I-10

§ ✓5ᵗʰ **823.1 Upper end, open**
[0-2]

§ ✓5ᵗʰ **823.2 Shaft, closed**
[0-2]

§ ✓5ᵗʰ **823.3 Shaft, open**
[0-2]

§ ✓5ᵗʰ **823.4 Torus fracture**
[0-2]   **DEF:** A bone deformity in children, occurring commonly in the tibia and fibula, in which the bone bends and buckles but does not fracture.
AHA: 4Q, '02, 70

§ ✓5ᵗʰ **823.8 Unspecified part, closed**
[0-2]   Lower leg NOS
AHA: For code 823.82: 1Q, '97, 8

§ ✓5ᵗʰ **823.9 Unspecified part, open**
[0-2]

✓4ᵗʰ **824 Fracture of ankle**

> **TIP:** If ankle fracture also includes syndesmotic injury, assign also code 845.03 Sprains and strains of tibiofibular (ligament), distal.

824.0 Medial malleolus, closed
Tibia involving:
ankle
malleolus
AHA: 1Q, '04, 9

824.1 Medial malleolus, open

824.2 Lateral malleolus, closed
Fibula involving:
ankle
malleolus
AHA: 2Q, '02, 3

824.3 Lateral malleolus, open

824.4 Bimalleolar, closed
Dupuytren's fracture, fibula   Pott's fracture
DEF: Bimalleolar, closed: Breaking of both nodules (malleoli) on either side of ankle joint, without an open wound.
DEF: Dupuytren's fracture (Pott's fracture): The breaking of the farthest end of the lower leg bone (fibula), with injury to the farthest end joint of the other lower leg bone (tibia).
S82.841A Displcd bimalleolar fx rt lw leg initial enc clos fx   I-10

824.5 Bimalleolar, open

824.6 Trimalleolar, closed
Lateral and medial malleolus with anterior or posterior lip of tibia
S82.855G Nondsplcd trimalleolr fx lt lw leg subsq clo delay healing   I-10

824.7 Trimalleolar, open

824.8 Unspecified, closed
Ankle NOS
AHA: 3Q, '00, 12
S89.302A Uns physeal fx low end lt fibula initial enc clo fx   I-10

824.9 Unspecified, open

✓4ᵗʰ **825 Fracture of one or more tarsal and metatarsal bones**

825.0 Fracture of calcaneus, closed
Heel bone   Os calcis

825.1 Fracture of calcaneus, open

✓5ᵗʰ **825.2 Fracture of other tarsal and metatarsal bones, closed**

825.20 Unspecified bone(s) of foot [except toes]
Instep

825.21 Astragalus
Talus

825.22 Navicular [scaphoid], foot

825.23 Cuboid

825.24 Cuneiform, foot

825.25 Metatarsal bone(s)

825.29 Other
Tarsal with metatarsal bone(s) only
EXCLUDES calcaneus (825.0)

§   Requires fifth digit. Valid digits are in [brackets] under each code. See category 823 for codes and definitions.

N Newborn Age: 0   P Pediatric Age: 0-17   M Maternity Age: 12-55   A Adult Age: 15-124

282 – Volume 1   2013 ICD-9-CM

Right Foot, Dorsal

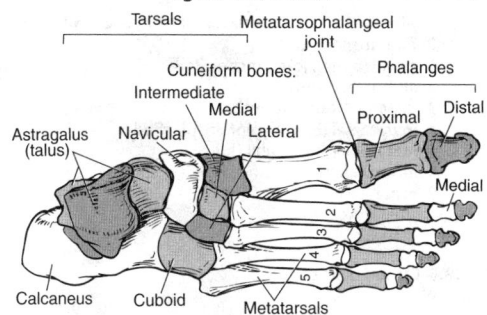

✓5ᵗʰ **825.3 Fracture of other tarsal and metatarsal bones, open**

825.30 Unspecified bone(s) of foot [except toes]

825.31 Astragalus

825.32 Navicular [scaphoid], foot

825.33 Cuboid

825.34 Cuneiform, foot

825.35 Metatarsal bone(s)

825.39 Other

✓4ᵗʰ **826 Fracture of one or more phalanges of foot**
     INCLUDES   toe(s)

826.0 Closed

826.1 Open

✓4ᵗʰ **827 Other, multiple, and ill-defined fractures of lower limb**
     INCLUDES   leg NOS
                multiple bones of same lower limb
     EXCLUDES   *multiple fractures of:*
                ankle bones alone (824.4-824.9)
                phalanges of foot alone (826.0-826.1)
                tarsal with metatarsal bones (825.29, 825.39)
                tibia with fibula (823.0-823.9 with fifth-digit 2)

827.0 Closed

827.1 Open

✓4ᵗʰ **828 Multiple fractures involving both lower limbs, lower with upper limb, and lower limb(s) with rib(s) and sternum**
     INCLUDES   arm(s) with leg(s) [any bones]
                both legs [any bones]
                leg(s) with rib(s) or sternum

828.0 Closed

828.1 Open

✓4ᵗʰ **829 Fracture of unspecified bones**

829.0 Unspecified bone, closed

829.1 Unspecified bone, open

Dislocation (830-839)

     INCLUDES   displacement
                subluxation
     EXCLUDES   *congenital dislocation (754.0-755.8)*
                pathological dislocation (718.2)
                recurrent dislocation (718.3)

     NOTE The descriptions "closed" and "open," used in the fourth-digit subdivisions, include the following terms:

closed:	open:
complete	compound
dislocation NOS	infected
partial	with foreign body
simple	
uncomplicated	

A dislocation not indicated as closed or open should be classified as closed.

AHA: 3Q, '90, 12

TIP: Do not assign if documentation indicates developmental dislocation; see instead subcategory 718.7.

✓4ᵗʰ **830 Dislocation of jaw**
     INCLUDES   jaw (cartilage) (meniscus)
                mandible
                maxilla (inferior)
                temporomandibular (joint)

830.0 Closed dislocation

830.1 Open dislocation

✓4ᵗʰ **831 Dislocation of shoulder**
     EXCLUDES   *sternoclavicular joint (839.61, 839.71)*
                sternum (839.61, 839.71)

The following fifth-digit subclassification is for use with category 831:
   0 shoulder, unspecified
      Humerus NOS
   1 anterior dislocation of humerus
   2 posterior dislocation of humerus
   3 inferior dislocation of humerus
   4 acromioclavicular (joint)
      Clavicle
   9 other
      Scapula

TIP: Do not assign if documentation indicates recurrent shoulder dislocation; see instead code 718.31.

§ ✓5ᵗʰ **831.0 Closed dislocation**
[0-4, 9]

§ ✓5ᵗʰ **831.1 Open dislocation**
[0-4, 9]

✓4ᵗʰ **832 Dislocation of elbow**
The following fifth-digit subclassification is for use with subcategories 832.0 and 832.1:
   0 elbow, unspecified
   1 anterior dislocation of elbow
   2 posterior dislocation of elbow
   3 medial dislocation of elbow
   4 lateral dislocation of elbow
   9 other

§ ✓5ᵗʰ **832.0 Closed dislocation**
[0-4, 9]

§ ✓5ᵗʰ **832.1 Open dislocation**
[0-4, 9]

832.2 Nursemaid's elbow
     Subluxation of radial head
     AHA: 4Q, '09, 110-111

✓4ᵗʰ **833 Dislocation of wrist**
The following fifth-digit subclassification is for use with category 833:
   0 wrist unspecified part
      Carpal (bone)
      Radius, distal end
   1 radioulnar (joint), distal
   2 radiocarpal (joint)
   3 midcarpal (joint)
   4 carpometacarpal (joint)
   5 metacarpal (bone), proximal end
   9 other
      Ulna, distal end

§ ✓5ᵗʰ **833.0 Closed dislocation**
[0-5, 9]

§ ✓5ᵗʰ **833.1 Open dislocation**
[0-5, 9]

✓4ᵗʰ **834 Dislocation of finger**
     INCLUDES   finger(s)
                phalanx of hand
                thumb

The following fifth-digit subclassification is for use with category 834:
   0 finger unspecified part
   1 metacarpophalangeal (joint)
      Metacarpal (bone), distal end
   2 interphalangeal (joint), hand

§ ✓5ᵗʰ **834.0 Closed dislocation**
[0-2]

§ ✓5ᵗʰ **834.1 Open dislocation**
[0-2]

§   Requires fifth digit. Valid digits are in [brackets] under each code. See appropriate category for codes and definitions.

✓4ᵗʰ ✓5ᵗʰ Additional Digit Required   Unspecified Code   Other Specified Code   Manifestation Code   ►◄ Revised Text   ● New Code   ▲ Revised Code Title

Injury and Poisoning

835–839.59

√4ᵗ **835 Dislocation of hip**

The following fifth-digit subclassification is for use with category 835:
 0 **dislocation of hip, unspecified**
 1 **posterior dislocation**
 2 **obturator dislocation**
 3 **other anterior dislocation**

§ √5ᵗ **835.0 Closed dislocation**
[0-3]

§ √5ᵗ **835.1 Open dislocation**
[0-3]

√4ᵗ **836 Dislocation of knee**

EXCLUDES dislocation of knee:
old or pathological (718.2)
recurrent (718.3)
internal derangement of knee joint (717.0-717.5,
717.8-717.9)
old tear of cartilage or meniscus of knee (717.0-717.5,
717.8-717.9)

836.0 Tear of medial cartilage or meniscus of knee, current
Bucket handle tear:
NOS } current injury
medial meniscus

836.1 Tear of lateral cartilage or meniscus of knee, current

836.2 Other tear of cartilage or meniscus of knee, current
Tear of:
cartilage
(semilunar) } current injury, not specified as
meniscus medial or lateral

836.3 Dislocation of patella, closed

836.4 Dislocation of patella, open

√5ᵗ **836.5 Other dislocation of knee, closed**

836.50 Dislocation of knee, unspecified

836.51 Anterior dislocation of tibia, proximal end
Posterior dislocation of femur, distal end, closed

836.52 Posterior dislocation of tibia, proximal end
Anterior dislocation of femur, distal end, closed

836.53 Medial dislocation of tibia, proximal end

836.54 Lateral dislocation of tibia, proximal end

836.59 Other

√5ᵗ **836.6 Other dislocation of knee, open**

836.60 Dislocation of knee, unspecified

836.61 Anterior dislocation of tibia, proximal end
Posterior dislocation of femur, distal end, open

836.62 Posterior dislocation of tibia, proximal end
Anterior dislocation of femur, distal end, open

836.63 Medial dislocation of tibia, proximal end

836.64 Lateral dislocation of tibia, proximal end

836.69 Other

√4ᵗ **837 Dislocation of ankle**

INCLUDES astragalus
fibula, distal end
navicular, foot
scaphoid, foot
tibia, distal end

837.0 Closed dislocation

837.1 Open dislocation

√4ᵗ **838 Dislocation of foot**

The following fifth-digit subclassification is for use with category 838:
 0 **foot unspecified**
 1 **tarsal (bone), joint unspecified**
 2 **midtarsal (joint)**
 3 **tarsometatarsal (joint)**
 4 **metatarsal (bone), joint unspecified**
 5 **metatarsophalangeal (joint)**
 6 **interphalangeal (joint), foot**
 9 **other**
 Phalanx of foot
 Toe(s)

§ √5ᵗ **838.0 Closed dislocation**
[0-6, 9]

§ √5ᵗ **838.1 Open dislocation**
[0-6, 9]

√4ᵗ **839 Other, multiple, and ill-defined dislocations**

√5ᵗ **839.0 Cervical vertebra, closed**
Cervical spine
Neck

839.00 Cervical vertebra, unspecified

839.01 First cervical vertebra

839.02 Second cervical vertebra

839.03 Third cervical vertebra

839.04 Fourth cervical vertebra

839.05 Fifth cervical vertebra

839.06 Sixth cervical vertebra

839.07 Seventh cervical vertebra

839.08 Multiple cervical vertebrae

√5ᵗ **839.1 Cervical vertebra, open**

839.10 Cervical vertebra, unspecified

839.11 First cervical vertebra

839.12 Second cervical vertebra

839.13 Third cervical vertebra

839.14 Fourth cervical vertebra

839.15 Fifth cervical vertebra

839.16 Sixth cervical vertebra

839.17 Seventh cervical vertebra

839.18 Multiple cervical vertebrae

√5ᵗ **839.2 Thoracic and lumbar vertebra, closed**

839.20 Lumbar vertebra

839.21 Thoracic vertebra
Dorsal [thoracic] vertebra

√5ᵗ **839.3 Thoracic and lumbar vertebra, open**

839.30 Lumbar vertebra

839.31 Thoracic vertebra

√5ᵗ **839.4 Other vertebra, closed**

839.40 Vertebra, unspecified site
Spine NOS

839.41 Coccyx

839.42 Sacrum
Sacroiliac (joint)

839.49 Other

√5ᵗ **839.5 Other vertebra, open**

839.50 Vertebra, unspecified site

839.51 Coccyx

839.52 Sacrum

839.59 Other

§ Requires fifth digit. Valid digits are in [brackets] under each code. See appropriate category for codes and definitions.

N Newborn Age: 0 P Pediatric Age: 0-17 M Maternity Age: 12-55 A Adult Age: 15-124

✓5ᵗʰ 839.6 Other location, closed

    839.61 Sternum
        Sternoclavicular joint

    839.69 Other
        Pelvis

✓5ᵗʰ 839.7 Other location, open

    839.71 Sternum

    839.79 Other

839.8 Multiple and ill-defined, closed
    Arm
    Back
    Hand
    Multiple locations, except fingers or toes alone
    Other ill-defined locations
    Unspecified location

839.9 Multiple and ill-defined, open

Sprains and Strains of Joints and Adjacent Muscles (840-848)

INCLUDES
avulsion
hemarthrosis
laceration   of:
rupture   joint capsule
sprain   ligament
strain   muscle
tear   tendon

EXCLUDES *laceration of tendon in open wounds (880-884 and 890-894 with .2)*

✓4ᵗʰ 840 Sprains and strains of shoulder and upper arm

    840.0 Acromioclavicular (joint) (ligament)

    840.1 Coracoclavicular (ligament)

    840.2 Coracohumeral (ligament)

    840.3 Infraspinatus (muscle) (tendon)

    840.4 Rotator cuff (capsule)
        EXCLUDES *complete rupture of rotator cuff, nontraumatic (727.61)*

    840.5 Subscapularis (muscle)

    840.6 Supraspinatus (muscle) (tendon)

    840.7 Superior glenoid labrum lesion
        SLAP lesion
        AHA: 4Q,'01, 52
        DEF: Detachment injury of the superior aspect of the glenoid labrum which is the ring of fibrocartilage attached to the rim of the glenoid cavity of the scapula.

    840.8 Other specified sites of shoulder and upper arm

    840.9 Unspecified site of shoulder and upper arm
        Arm NOS
        Shoulder NOS

✓4ᵗʰ 841 Sprains and strains of elbow and forearm

    841.0 Radial collateral ligament

    841.1 Ulnar collateral ligament

    841.2 Radiohumeral (joint)

    841.3 Ulnohumeral (joint)

    841.8 Other specified sites of elbow and forearm

    841.9 Unspecified site of elbow and forearm
        Elbow NOS

✓4ᵗʰ 842 Sprains and strains of wrist and hand

    ✓5ᵗʰ 842.0 Wrist

        842.00 Unspecified site

        842.01 Carpal (joint)

        842.02 Radiocarpal (joint) (ligament)

        842.09 Other
            Radioulnar joint, distal

    ✓5ᵗʰ 842.1 Hand

        842.10 Unspecified site

        842.11 Carpometacarpal (joint)

        842.12 Metacarpophalangeal (joint)

        842.13 Interphalangeal (joint)

        842.19 Other
            Midcarpal (joint)

✓4ᵗʰ 843 Sprains and strains of hip and thigh

    843.0 Iliofemoral (ligament)

    843.1 Ischiocapsular (ligament)

    843.8 Other specified sites of hip and thigh

    843.9 Unspecified site of hip and thigh
        Hip NOS   Thigh NOS

✓4ᵗʰ 844 Sprains and strains of knee and leg

    844.0 Lateral collateral ligament of knee

    844.1 Medial collateral ligament of knee

    844.2 Cruciate ligament of knee

    844.3 Tibiofibular (joint) (ligament), superior

    844.8 Other specified sites of knee and leg

    844.9 Unspecified site of knee and leg
        Knee NOS   Leg NOS

✓4ᵗʰ 845 Sprains and strains of ankle and foot

    ✓5ᵗʰ 845.0 Ankle

        845.00 Unspecified site
            AHA: 2Q, '02, 3

        845.01 Deltoid (ligament), ankle
            Internal collateral (ligament), ankle

        845.02 Calcaneofibular (ligament)

        845.03 Tibiofibular (ligament), distal
            AHA: 1Q, '04, 9

        845.09 Other
            Achilles tendon

    ✓5ᵗʰ 845.1 Foot

        845.10 Unspecified site

        845.11 Tarsometatarsal (joint) (ligament)

        845.12 Metatarsophalangeal (joint)

        845.13 Interphalangeal (joint), toe

        845.19 Other

✓4ᵗʰ 846 Sprains and strains of sacroiliac region

    846.0 Lumbosacral (joint) (ligament)

    846.1 Sacroiliac ligament

    846.2 Sacrospinatus (ligament)

    846.3 Sacrotuberous (ligament)

    846.8 Other specified sites of sacroiliac region

    846.9 Unspecified site of sacroiliac region

✓4ᵗʰ 847 Sprains and strains of other and unspecified parts of back
    EXCLUDES *lumbosacral (846.0)*

    847.0 Neck
        Anterior longitudinal (ligament), cervical
        Atlanto-axial (joints)
        Atlanto-occipital (joints)
        Whiplash injury
        EXCLUDES *neck injury NOS (959.0)*
                   thyroid region (848.2)
        S13.4xxA Sprain ligaments cervical spine initial encounter   I-10

    847.1 Thoracic

    847.2 Lumbar

    847.3 Sacrum
        Sacrococcygeal (ligament)

    847.4 Coccyx

    847.9 Unspecified site of back
        Back NOS

✓4ᵗʰ ✓5ᵗʰ Additional Digit Required   Unspecified Code   Other Specified Code   Manifestation Code   ►◄ Revised Text   ● New Code   ▲ Revised Code Title

Injury and Poisoning

848–852.5

✓4ᵗʰ **848 Other and ill-defined sprains and strains**

848.0 Septal cartilage of nose

848.1 Jaw
Temporomandibular (joint) (ligament)

848.2 Thyroid region
Cricoarytenoid (joint) (ligament)   Thyroid cartilage
Cricothyroid (joint) (ligament)

848.3 Ribs
Chondrocostal (joint) } without mention of injury
Costal cartilage   to sternum

✓5ᵗʰ **848.4 Sternum**

848.40 Unspecified site

848.41 Sternoclavicular (joint) (ligament)

848.42 Chondrosternal (joint)

848.49 Other
Xiphoid cartilage

848.5 Pelvis
Symphysis pubis
EXCLUDES *that in childbirth (665.6)*

848.8 Other specified sites of sprains and strains

848.9 Unspecified site of sprain and strain

Intracranial Injury, Excluding those with Skull Fracture (850-854)

INCLUDES traumatic brain injury without skull fracture

EXCLUDES *intracranial injury with skull fracture (800-801 and 803-804, except .0 and .5)*
open wound of head without intracranial injury (870.0-873.9)
skull fracture alone (800-801 and 803-804 with .0, .5)

NOTE The description "with open intracranial wound," used in the fourth-digit subdivisions, includes those specified as open or with mention of infection or foreign body.

The following fifth-digit subclassification is for use with categories 851-854:
0 unspecified state of consciousness
1 with no loss of consciousness
2 with brief [less than one hour] loss of consciousness
3 with moderate [1-24 hours] loss of consciousness
4 with prolonged [more than 24 hours] loss of consciousness and return to pre-existing conscious level
5 with prolonged [more than 24 hours] loss of consciousness without return to pre-existing conscious level
Use fifth-digit 5 to designate when a patient is unconscious and dies before regaining consciousness, regardless of the duration of the loss of consciousness
6 with loss of consciousness of unspecified duration
9 with concussion, unspecified

AHA: 1Q, '93, 22
TIP: If documentation specifies only "head injury," with no further specificity, and is self-limiting, assign instead code 959.01 Head injury, unspecified.

✓4ᵗʰ **850 Concussion**

INCLUDES commotio cerebri

EXCLUDES *concussion with:*
cerebral laceration or contusion (851.0-851.9)
cerebral hemorrhage (852-853)
head injury NOS (959.01)

AHA: 2Q, '96, 6; 4Q, '90, 24
TIP: When a patient is treated for symptoms within 24 to 48 hours of the concussion, clarify with the physician whether the concussion is still in the acute phase or is a postconcussion syndrome; if so, assign instead code 310.2.

850.0 With no loss of consciousness
Concussion with mental confusion or disorientation, without loss of consciousness

✓5ᵗʰ **850.1 With brief loss of consciousness**
Loss of consciousness for less than one hour
AHA: 4Q, '03, 76; 1Q, '99, 10; 2Q, '92, 5

850.11 With loss of consciousness of 30 minutes or less
S06.0x1A Concussion w/loc 30 min/less initial encounter **I-10**

850.12 With loss of consciousness from 31 to 59 minutes
AHA: 4Q, '10, 111

850.2 With moderate loss of consciousness
Loss of consciousness for 1-24 hours

850.3 With prolonged loss of consciousness and return to pre-existing conscious level
Loss of consciousness for more than 24 hours with complete recovery

850.4 With prolonged loss of consciousness, without return to pre-existing conscious level

850.5 With loss of consciousness of unspecified duration
S06.0x9A Concussion w/loc uns duration initial encounter **I-10**

850.9 Concussion, unspecified

✓4ᵗʰ **851 Cerebral laceration and contusion**
AHA: 4Q, '96, 36; 1Q, '93, 22; 4Q, '90, 24

§ ✓5ᵗʰ **851.0 Cortex (cerebral) contusion without mention of**
[0-6, 9] **open intracranial wound**
AHA: For code 851.00: 4Q, '10, 93

§ ✓5ᵗʰ **851.1 Cortex (cerebral) contusion with open**
[0-6, 9] **intracranial wound**
AHA: 1Q, '92, 9

§ ✓5ᵗʰ **851.2 Cortex (cerebral) laceration without mention of**
[0-6, 9] **open intracranial wound**
S06.5x0A Traumatic subdurl hemorrhage w/o loc initial enc **I-10**

§ ✓5ᵗʰ **851.3 Cortex (cerebral) laceration with open intracranial wound**
[0-6, 9]

§ ✓5ᵗʰ **851.4 Cerebellar or brain stem contusion without mention of**
[0-6, 9] **open intracranial wound**

§ ✓5ᵗʰ **851.5 Cerebellar or brain stem contusion with open**
[0-6, 9] **intracranial wound**

§ ✓5ᵗʰ **851.6 Cerebellar or brain stem laceration without**
[0-6, 9] **mention of open intracranial wound**

§ ✓5ᵗʰ **851.7 Cerebellar or brain stem laceration with open**
[0-6, 9] **intracranial wound**

§ ✓5ᵗʰ **851.8 Other and unspecified cerebral laceration and**
[0-6, 9] **contusion, without mention of open intracranial wound**
Brain (membrane) NOS
AHA: 4Q, '96, 37

§ ✓5ᵗʰ **851.9 Other and unspecified cerebral laceration and**
[0-6, 9] **contusion, with open intracranial wound**

✓4ᵗʰ **852 Subarachnoid, subdural, and extradural hemorrhage, following injury**
EXCLUDES *cerebral contusion or laceration (with hemorrhage) (851.0-851.9)*
DEF: Bleeding from lining of brain; due to injury.

§ ✓5ᵗʰ **852.0 Subarachnoid hemorrhage following injury**
[0-6, 9] **without mention of open intracranial wound**
Middle meningeal hemorrhage following injury

§ ✓5ᵗʰ **852.1 Subarachnoid hemorrhage following injury with**
[0-6, 9] **open intracranial wound**

§ ✓5ᵗʰ **852.2 Subdural hemorrhage following injury without**
[0-6, 9] **mention of open intracranial wound**
AHA: For code 852.25: ▶4Q, '11, 99;◄ 4Q, '96, 43; For codes 852.21-852.29: 4Q, '07, 107

§ ✓5ᵗʰ **852.3 Subdural hemorrhage following injury with**
[0-6, 9] **open intracranial wound**

§ ✓5ᵗʰ **852.4 Extradural hemorrhage following injury without**
[0-6, 9] **mention of open intracranial wound**
Epidural hematoma following injury

§ ✓5ᵗʰ **852.5 Extradural hemorrhage following injury with**
[0-6, 9] **open intracranial wound**

§ Requires fifth digit. Valid digits are in [brackets] under each code. See beginning of section 850-854 for codes and definitions.

N Newborn Age: 0   **P** Pediatric Age: 0-17   **M** Maternity Age: 12-55   **A** Adult Age: 15-124

Brain

✓4ᵗʰ 853 Other and unspecified intracranial hemorrhage following injury

§　✓5ᵗʰ **853.0 Without mention of open intracranial wound**
[0-6, 9]　Cerebral compression due to injury
　　　　　Intracranial hematoma following injury
　　　　　Traumatic cerebral hemorrhage
　　　　　AHA: 3Q, '90, 14

§　✓5ᵗʰ **853.1 With open intracranial wound**
[0-6, 9]

✓4ᵗʰ 854 Intracranial injury of other and unspecified nature

INCLUDES　injury:
　　　　　　brain NOS
　　　　　　cavernous sinus
　　　　　　intracranial
　　　　　　traumatic brain NOS

EXCLUDES　any condition classifiable to 850-853
　　　　　　head injury NOS (959.01)

AHA: 1Q, '99, 10; 2Q, '92, 6
TIP: Assign a code from category 854 for traumatic brain injury (TBI) with diffuse axonal injury (DAI), also known as a shear injury.

§　✓5ᵗʰ **854.0 Without mention of open intracranial wound**
[0-6, 9]　**AHA:** For code 854.00: 4Q, '09, 108; 2Q, '05, 6

§　✓5ᵗʰ **854.1 With open intracranial wound**
[0-6, 9]

Internal Injury of Thorax, Abdomen, and Pelvis (860-869)

INCLUDES　blast injuries
　　　　　　blunt trauma
　　　　　　bruise
　　　　　　concussion injuries (except cerebral)
　　　　　　crushing　　　　　　　　　　of internal
　　　　　　hematoma　　　　　　　　　organs
　　　　　　laceration
　　　　　　puncture
　　　　　　tear
　　　　　　traumatic rupture

EXCLUDES　concussion NOS (850.0-850.9)
　　　　　　flail chest (807.4)
　　　　　　foreign body entering through orifice (930.0-939.9)
　　　　　　injury to blood vessels (901.0-902.9)

NOTE The description "with open wound," used in the fourth-digit subdivisions, includes those with mention of infection or foreign body.

✓4ᵗʰ 860 Traumatic pneumothorax and hemothorax

DEF: Traumatic pneumothorax: air or gas leaking into pleural space of lung due to trauma.
DEF: Traumatic hemothorax: blood buildup in pleural space of lung due to trauma.
AHA: 2Q, '93, 4
TIP: If there's no mention of trauma associated with pneumothorax, see instead category 512.

860.0 Pneumothorax without mention of open wound into thorax
　　S27.0xxA Traumatic pneumothorax initial encounter　　I-10

860.1 Pneumothorax with open wound into thorax

860.2 Hemothorax without mention of open wound into thorax

860.3 Hemothorax with open wound into thorax

860.4 Pneumohemothorax without mention of open wound into thorax

860.5 Pneumohemothorax with open wound into thorax

✓4ᵗʰ 861 Injury to heart and lung

EXCLUDES　injury to blood vessels of thorax (901.0-901.9)

✓5ᵗʰ **861.0 Heart, without mention of open wound into thorax**
　　AHA: 1Q, '92, 9

　　861.00 Unspecified injury

　　861.01 Contusion
　　　　Cardiac contusion
　　　　Myocardial contusion
　　　　DEF: Bruising within the pericardium with no mention of open wound.

　　861.02 Laceration without penetration of heart chambers
　　　　DEF: Tearing injury of heart tissue, without penetration of chambers; no open wound.

　　861.03 Laceration with penetration of heart chambers

✓5ᵗʰ **861.1 Heart, with open wound into thorax**

　　861.10 Unspecified injury

　　861.11 Contusion

　　861.12 Laceration without penetration of heart chambers

　　861.13 Laceration with penetration of heart chambers

✓5ᵗʰ **861.2 Lung, without mention of open wound into thorax**

　　861.20 Unspecified injury

　　861.21 Contusion
　　　　DEF: Bruising of lung without mention of open wound.
　　　　S27.321A Contusion of lung unilateral initial encounter　　I-10

　　861.22 Laceration

✓5ᵗʰ **861.3 Lung, with open wound into thorax**

　　861.30 Unspecified injury

　　861.31 Contusion

　　861.32 Laceration

✓4ᵗʰ 862 Injury to other and unspecified intrathoracic organs

EXCLUDES　injury to blood vessels of thorax (901.0-901.9)

862.0 Diaphragm, without mention of open wound into cavity

862.1 Diaphragm, with open wound into cavity

✓5ᵗʰ **862.2 Other specified intrathoracic organs, without mention of open wound into cavity**

　　862.21 Bronchus

　　862.22 Esophagus

　　862.29 Other
　　　　Pleura
　　　　Thymus gland

✓5ᵗʰ **862.3 Other specified intrathoracic organs, with open wound into cavity**

　　862.31 Bronchus

　　862.32 Esophagus

　　862.39 Other

---

§　Requires fifth digit. Valid digits are in [brackets] under each code. See beginning of section 850-854 for codes and definitions.

✓4ᵗʰ
✓5ᵗʰ　Additional Digit Required　　Unspecified Code　　Other Specified Code　　Manifestation Code　　▶◀ Revised Text　　● New Code　　▲ Revised Code Title

Injury and Poisoning

862.8–867.7

862.8 Multiple and unspecified intrathoracic organs, without mention of open wound into cavity
> Crushed chest   Multiple intrathoracic organs

862.9 Multiple and unspecified intrathoracic organs, with open wound into cavity

✓4ᵗʰ **863 Injury to gastrointestinal tract**
> *EXCLUDES*   *anal sphincter laceration during delivery (664.2)*
> *bile duct (868.0-868.1 with fifth-digit 2)*
> *gallbladder (868.0-868.1 with fifth-digit 2)*

863.0 Stomach, without mention of open wound into cavity

863.1 Stomach, with open wound into cavity

✓5ᵗʰ **863.2 Small intestine, without mention of open wound into cavity**

     863.20 Small intestine, unspecified site

     863.21 Duodenum

     863.29 Other

✓5ᵗʰ **863.3 Small intestine, with open wound into cavity**

     863.30 Small intestine, unspecified site

     863.31 Duodenum

     863.39 Other

✓5ᵗʰ **863.4 Colon or rectum, without mention of open wound into cavity**

     863.40 Colon, unspecified site

     863.41 Ascending [right] colon

     863.42 Transverse colon

     863.43 Descending [left] colon

     863.44 Sigmoid colon

     863.45 Rectum

     863.46 Multiple sites in colon and rectum

     863.49 Other

✓5ᵗʰ **863.5 Colon or rectum, with open wound into cavity**

     863.50 Colon, unspecified site

     863.51 Ascending [right] colon

     863.52 Transverse colon

     863.53 Descending [left] colon

     863.54 Sigmoid colon

     863.55 Rectum

     863.56 Multiple sites in colon and rectum

     863.59 Other

✓5ᵗʰ **863.8 Other and unspecified gastrointestinal sites, without mention of open wound into cavity**

     863.80 Gastrointestinal tract, unspecified site

     863.81 Pancreas, head

     863.82 Pancreas, body

     863.83 Pancreas, tail

     863.84 Pancreas, multiple and unspecified sites

     863.85 Appendix

     863.89 Other
>   Intestine NOS

✓5ᵗʰ **863.9 Other and unspecified gastrointestinal sites, with open wound into cavity**

     863.90 Gastrointestinal tract, unspecified site

     863.91 Pancreas, head

     863.92 Pancreas, body

     863.93 Pancreas, tail

     863.94 Pancreas, multiple and unspecified sites

     863.95 Appendix

863.99 Other

✓4ᵗʰ **864 Injury to liver**
> The following fifth-digit subclassification is for use with category 864:
> **0 unspecified injury**
> **1 hematoma and contusion**
> **2 laceration, minor**
>   Laceration involving capsule only, or without significant involvement of hepatic parenchyma [i.e., less than 1 cm deep]
> **3 laceration, moderate**
>   Laceration involving parenchyma but without major disruption of parenchyma [i.e., less than 10 cm long and less than 3 cm deep]
> **4 laceration, major**
>   Laceration with significant disruption of hepatic parenchyma [i.e., 10 cm long and 3 cm deep]
>   Multiple moderate lacerations, with or without hematoma
>   Stellate lacerations of liver
> **5 laceration, unspecified**
> **9 other**

§ ✓5ᵗʰ **864.0 Without mention of open wound into cavity**
> [0-5, 9]

§ ✓5ᵗʰ **864.1 With open wound into cavity**
> [0-5, 9]

✓4ᵗʰ **865 Injury to spleen**
> The following fifth-digit subclassification is for use with category 865:
> **0 unspecified injury**
> **1 hematoma without rupture of capsule**
> **2 capsular tears, without major disruption of parenchyma**
> **3 laceration extending into parenchyma**
> **4 massive parenchymal disruption**
> **9 other**

§ ✓5ᵗʰ **865.0 Without mention of wound into cavity**
> [0-4, 9]

§ ✓5ᵗʰ **865.1 With open wound into cavity**
> [0-4, 9]

✓4ᵗʰ **866 Injury to kidney**
> *EXCLUDES*   *acute kidney injury (nontraumatic) (584.9)*
> The following fifth-digit subclassification is for use with category 866:
> **0 unspecified injury**
> **1 hematoma without rupture of capsule**
> **2 laceration**
> **3 complete disruption of kidney parenchyma**

> **AHA:** 4Q, '08, 192

§ ✓5ᵗʰ **866.0 Without mention of open wound into cavity**
> [0-3]

§ ✓5ᵗʰ **866.1 With open wound into cavity**
> [0-3]

✓4ᵗʰ **867 Injury to pelvic organs**
> *EXCLUDES*   *injury during delivery (664.0-665.9)*

867.0 Bladder and urethra, without mention of open wound into cavity
> **AHA:** N-D, '85, 15
> **TIP:** Assign for urethral injury due to patient's pulling out indwelling urinary catheter.
> S37.20xA Unspecified injury of bladder initial encounter   I-10

867.1 Bladder and urethra, with open wound into cavity

867.2 Ureter, without mention of open wound into cavity

867.3 Ureter, with open wound into cavity

867.4 Uterus, without mention of open wound into cavity   ♀

867.5 Uterus, with open wound into cavity   ♀

867.6 Other specified pelvic organs, without mention of open wound into cavity
> Fallopian tube   Seminal vesicle
> Ovary   Vas deferens
> Prostate

867.7 Other specified pelvic organs, with open wound into cavity

---

§   Requires fifth digit. Valid digits are in [brackets] under each code. See appropriate category for codes and definitions.

Ⓝ Newborn Age: 0   Ⓟ Pediatric Age: 0-17   Ⓜ Maternity Age: 12-55   Ⓐ Adult Age: 15-124

867.8 **Unspecified pelvic organ, without mention of open wound into cavity**

867.9 **Unspecified pelvic organ, with open wound into cavity**

√4th 868 **Injury to other intra-abdominal organs**

The following fifth-digit subclassification is for use with category 868:
   0 unspecified intra-abdominal organ
   1 adrenal gland
   2 bile duct and gallbladder
   3 peritoneum
   4 retroperitoneum
   9 other and multiple intra-abdominal organs

§ √5th 868.0 **Without mention of open wound into cavity**
[0-4, 9]

§ √5th 868.1 **With open wound into cavity**
[0-4, 9]

√4th 869 **Internal injury to unspecified or ill-defined organs**

INCLUDES   internal injury NOS
           multiple internal injury NOS

869.0 **Without mention of open wound into cavity**

869.1 **With open wound into cavity**
AHA: 2Q, '89, 15

Open Wound (870-897)

INCLUDES   animal bite
           avulsion
           cut
           laceration
           puncture wound
           traumatic amputation

EXCLUDES   burn (940.0-949.5)
           crushing (925-929.9)
           puncture of internal organs (860.0-869.1)
           superficial injury (910.0-919.9)
           that incidental to:
              dislocation (830.0-839.9)
              fracture (800.0-829.1)
              internal injury (860.0-869.1)
              intracranial injury (851.0-854.1)

NOTE The description "complicated" used in the fourth-digit subdivisions includes those with mention of delayed healing, delayed treatment, foreign body, or infection.
AHA: 4Q, '01, 52
TIP: Do not assign a code designated as "complicated" based only on physician documentation of complicated. For coding purposes, there must be indications of delayed healing, delayed treatment, infection, or foreign body.

Open Wound of Head, Neck, and Trunk (870-879)

√4th 870 **Open wound of ocular adnexa**

870.0 **Laceration of skin of eyelid and periocular area**

870.1 **Laceration of eyelid, full-thickness, not involving lacrimal passages**

870.2 **Laceration of eyelid involving lacrimal passages**

870.3 **Penetrating wound of orbit, without mention of foreign body**

870.4 **Penetrating wound of orbit with foreign body**
EXCLUDES   retained (old) foreign body in orbit (376.6)

870.8 **Other specified open wounds of ocular adnexa**

870.9 **Unspecified open wound of ocular adnexa**

√4th 871 **Open wound of eyeball**

EXCLUDES   2nd cranial nerve [optic] injury (950.0-950.9)
           3rd cranial nerve [oculomotor] injury (951.0)

871.0 **Ocular laceration without prolapse of intraocular tissue**
DEF: Tear in ocular tissue without displacing structures.
AHA: 3Q, '96, 7

871.1 **Ocular laceration with prolapse or exposure of intraocular tissue**

871.2 **Rupture of eye with partial loss of intraocular tissue**
DEF: Forcible tearing of eyeball, with tissue loss.

871.3 **Avulsion of eye**
Traumatic enucleation
DEF: Traumatic extraction of eyeball from socket.

871.4 **Unspecified laceration of eye**

871.5 **Penetration of eyeball with magnetic foreign body**
EXCLUDES   retained (old) magnetic foreign body in globe (360.50-360.59)

871.6 **Penetration of eyeball with (nonmagnetic) foreign body**
EXCLUDES   retained (old) (nonmagnetic) foreign body in globe (360.60-360.69)

871.7 **Unspecified ocular penetration**

871.9 **Unspecified open wound of eyeball**

√4th 872 **Open wound of ear**

√5th 872.0 **External ear, without mention of complication**

872.00 **External ear, unspecified site**

872.01 **Auricle, ear**
Pinna
DEF: Open wound of fleshy, outer ear.

872.02 **Auditory canal**
DEF: Open wound of passage from external ear to eardrum.

√5th 872.1 **External ear, complicated**

872.10 **External ear, unspecified site**

872.11 **Auricle, ear**

872.12 **Auditory canal**

√5th 872.6 **Other specified parts of ear, without mention of complication**

872.61 **Ear drum**
Drumhead   Tympanic membrane

872.62 **Ossicles**

872.63 **Eustachian tube**
DEF: Open wound of channel between nasopharynx and tympanic cavity.

872.64 **Cochlea**
DEF: Open wound of snail shell shaped tube of inner ear.

872.69 **Other and multiple sites**

√5th 872.7 **Other specified parts of ear, complicated**

872.71 **Ear drum**

872.72 **Ossicles**

872.73 **Eustachian tube**

872.74 **Cochlea**

872.79 **Other and multiple sites**

872.8 **Ear, part unspecified, without mention of complication**
Ear NOS

872.9 **Ear, part unspecified, complicated**

√4th 873 **Other open wound of head**

873.0 **Scalp, without mention of complication**
S01.01xA Laceration w/o foreign body scalp initial enc   I-10

873.1 **Scalp, complicated**

√5th 873.2 **Nose, without mention of complication**

873.20 **Nose, unspecified site**

873.21 **Nasal septum**
DEF: Open wound between nasal passages.

873.22 **Nasal cavity**
DEF: Open wound of nostrils.

873.23 **Nasal sinus**
DEF: Open wound of mucous-lined respiratory cavities.

873.29 **Multiple sites**

√5th 873.3 **Nose, complicated**

873.30 **Nose, unspecified site**

§ Requires fifth digit. Valid digits are in [brackets] under each code. See category 868 for codes and definitions.

√4th
√5th Additional Digit Required   Unspecified Code   Other Specified Code   Manifestation Code   ▶◀ Revised Text   ● New Code   ▲ Revised Code Title
2013 ICD-9-CM   **Volume 1 – 289**

Injury and Poisoning

873.31–879.5

873.31 **Nasal septum**

873.32 **Nasal cavity**

873.33 **Nasal sinus**

873.39 **Multiple sites**

√5ᵗʰ 873.4 **Face, without mention of complication**

    873.40 **Face, unspecified site**

    873.41 **Cheek**

    873.42 **Forehead**
        Eyebrow
        AHA: 4Q, '96, 43
        S01.81xA Laceration w/o FB other part head   I-10
        initial enc

    873.43 **Lip**

    873.44 **Jaw**

    873.49 **Other and multiple sites**

√5ᵗʰ 873.5 **Face, complicated**

    873.50 **Face, unspecified site**

    873.51 **Cheek**

    873.52 **Forehead**

    873.53 **Lip**

    873.54 **Jaw**

    873.59 **Other and multiple sites**

√5ᵗʰ 873.6 **Internal structures of mouth, without mention of complication**

    873.60 **Mouth, unspecified site**

    873.61 **Buccal mucosa**
        DEF: Open wound of inside of cheek.

    873.62 **Gum (alveolar process)**

    873.63 **Tooth (broken) (fractured) (due to trauma)**
        EXCLUDES cracked tooth (521.81)
        AHA: 1Q, '04, 17

    873.64 **Tongue and floor of mouth**

    873.65 **Palate**
        DEF: Open wound of roof of mouth.

    873.69 **Other and multiple sites**

√5ᵗʰ 873.7 **Internal structures of mouth, complicated**

    873.70 **Mouth, unspecified site**

    873.71 **Buccal mucosa**

    873.72 **Gum (alveolar process)**

    873.73 **Tooth (broken) (fractured) (due to trauma)**
        EXCLUDES cracked tooth (521.81)
        AHA: 1Q, '04, 17

    873.74 **Tongue and floor of mouth**

    873.75 **Palate**

    873.79 **Other and multiple sites**

873.8 **Other and unspecified open wound of head without mention of complication**
    Head NOS

873.9 **Other and unspecified complicated open wound of head**

√4ᵗʰ 874 **Open wound of neck**

√5ᵗʰ 874.0 **Larynx and trachea, without mention of complication**

    874.00 **Larynx with trachea**

    874.01 **Larynx**

    874.02 **Trachea**

√5ᵗʰ 874.1 **Larynx and trachea, complicated**

    874.10 **Larynx with trachea**

    874.11 **Larynx**

    874.12 **Trachea**

874.2 **Thyroid gland, without mention of complication**

874.3 **Thyroid gland, complicated**

874.4 **Pharynx, without mention of complication**
    Cervical esophagus

874.5 **Pharynx, complicated**

874.8 **Other and unspecified parts, without mention of complication**
    Nape of neck
    Supraclavicular region
    Throat NOS

874.9 **Other and unspecified parts, complicated**

√4ᵗʰ 875 **Open wound of chest (wall)**
    EXCLUDES open wound into thoracic cavity (860.0-862.9)
        traumatic pneumothorax and hemothorax (860.1, 860.3, 860.5)
    AHA: 3Q, '95, 17; 3Q, '93, 17

875.0 **Without mention of complication**

875.1 **Complicated**

√4ᵗʰ 876 **Open wound of back**
    INCLUDES loin
        lumbar region
    EXCLUDES open wound into thoracic cavity (860.0-862.9)
        traumatic pneumothorax and hemothorax (860.1, 860.3, 860.5)

876.0 **Without mention of complication**

876.1 **Complicated**

√4ᵗʰ 877 **Open wound of buttock**
    INCLUDES sacroiliac region

877.0 **Without mention of complication**

877.1 **Complicated**

√4ᵗʰ 878 **Open wound of genital organs (external), including traumatic amputation**
    EXCLUDES injury during delivery (664.0-665.9)
        internal genital organs (867.0-867.9)

878.0 **Penis, without mention of complication** ♂

878.1 **Penis, complicated** ♂

878.2 **Scrotum and testes, without mention of complication** ♂

878.3 **Scrotum and testes, complicated** ♂

878.4 **Vulva, without mention of complication** ♀
    Labium (majus) (minus)

878.5 **Vulva, complicated** ♀

878.6 **Vagina, without mention of complication** ♀

878.7 **Vagina, complicated** ♀

878.8 **Other and unspecified parts, without mention of complication**

878.9 **Other and unspecified parts, complicated**

√4ᵗʰ 879 **Open wound of other and unspecified sites, except limbs**

879.0 **Breast, without mention of complication**

879.1 **Breast, complicated**

879.2 **Abdominal wall, anterior, without mention of complication**
    Abdominal wall NOS   Pubic region
    Epigastric region   Umbilical region
    Hypogastric region
    AHA: 2Q, '91, 22; 3Q, '90, 5
    TIP: If the abdominal wall open wound results in aortic rupture, sequence code 902.0 first.

879.3 **Abdominal wall, anterior, complicated**

879.4 **Abdominal wall, lateral, without mention of complication**
    Flank   Iliac (region)
    Groin   Inguinal region
    Hypochondrium

879.5 **Abdominal wall, lateral, complicated**

879.6 Other and unspecified parts of trunk, without mention of complication
Pelvic region   Trunk NOS
Perineum

879.7 Other and unspecified parts of trunk, complicated

879.8 Open wound(s) (multiple) of unspecified site(s) without mention of complication
Multiple open wounds NOS   Open wound NOS

879.9 Open wound(s) (multiple) of unspecified site(s), complicated

Open Wound of Upper Limb (880-887)

AHA: N-D, '85, 5
TIP: For degloving injuries, assign code for open wound of the specified site, most often involving extremities.

√4ᵗʰ **880 Open wound of shoulder and upper arm**
The following fifth-digit subclassification is for use with category 880:
  0 shoulder region
  1 scapular region
  2 axillary region
  3 upper arm
  9 multiple sites

§ √5ᵗʰ **880.0 Without mention of complication**
[0-3, 9]

§ √5ᵗʰ **880.1 Complicated**
[0-3, 9]   **AHA:** For code 880.13: 2Q, '06, 7

§ √5ᵗʰ **880.2 With tendon involvement**
[0-3, 9]

√4ᵗʰ **881 Open wound of elbow, forearm, and wrist**
The following fifth-digit subclassification is for use with category 881:
  0 forearm
  1 elbow
  2 wrist

§ √5ᵗʰ **881.0 Without mention of complication**
[0-2]

§ √5ᵗʰ **881.1 Complicated**
[0-2]

§ √5ᵗʰ **881.2 With tendon involvement**
[0-2]

√4ᵗʰ **882 Open wound of hand except finger(s) alone**

882.0 Without mention of complication

882.1 Complicated
AHA: 4Q, '08, 152

882.2 With tendon involvement

√4ᵗʰ **883 Open wound of finger(s)**
INCLUDES fingernail
        thumb (nail)

883.0 Without mention of complication

883.1 Complicated

883.2 With tendon involvement

√4ᵗʰ **884 Multiple and unspecified open wound of upper limb**
INCLUDES arm NOS
        multiple sites of one upper limb
        upper limb NOS

884.0 Without mention of complication

884.1 Complicated

884.2 With tendon involvement

√4ᵗʰ **885 Traumatic amputation of thumb (complete) (partial)**
INCLUDES thumb(s) (with finger(s) of either hand)

885.0 Without mention of complication
AHA: 1Q, '03, 7

885.1 Complicated

√4ᵗʰ **886 Traumatic amputation of other finger(s) (complete) (partial)**
INCLUDES finger(s) of one or both hands, without mention of thumb(s)

886.0 Without mention of complication

886.1 Complicated

√4ᵗʰ **887 Traumatic amputation of arm and hand (complete) (partial)**

887.0 Unilateral, below elbow, without mention of complication

887.1 Unilateral, below elbow, complicated

887.2 Unilateral, at or above elbow, without mention of complication

887.3 Unilateral, at or above elbow, complicated

887.4 Unilateral, level not specified, without mention of complication

887.5 Unilateral, level not specified, complicated

887.6 Bilateral [any level], without mention of complication
One hand and other arm

887.7 Bilateral [any level], complicated

Open Wound of Lower Limb (890-897)

AHA: N-D, '85, 5

√4ᵗʰ **890 Open wound of hip and thigh**

890.0 Without mention of complication

890.1 Complicated

890.2 With tendon involvement

√4ᵗʰ **891 Open wound of knee, leg [except thigh], and ankle**
INCLUDES leg NOS
        multiple sites of leg, except thigh
EXCLUDES that of thigh (890.0-890.2)
        with multiple sites of lower limb (894.0-894.2)

891.0 Without mention of complication
S81.031A Puncture wound w/o FB rt knee initial   I-10
encounter

891.1 Complicated

891.2 With tendon involvement

√4ᵗʰ **892 Open wound of foot except toe(s) alone**
INCLUDES heel

892.0 Without mention of complication

892.1 Complicated

892.2 With tendon involvement

√4ᵗʰ **893 Open wound of toe(s)**
INCLUDES toenail

893.0 Without mention of complication

893.1 Complicated
AHA: 4Q, '08, 73

893.2 With tendon involvement

√4ᵗʰ **894 Multiple and unspecified open wound of lower limb**
INCLUDES lower limb NOS
        multiple sites of one lower limb, with thigh

894.0 Without mention of complication

894.1 Complicated

894.2 With tendon involvement

√4ᵗʰ **895 Traumatic amputation of toe(s) (complete) (partial)**
INCLUDES toe(s) of one or both feet

895.0 Without mention of complication

895.1 Complicated

√4ᵗʰ **896 Traumatic amputation of foot (complete) (partial)**

896.0 Unilateral, without mention of complication

896.1 Unilateral, complicated

---

§ Requires fifth digit. Valid digits are in [brackets] under each code. See appropriate category for codes and definitions.

√4ᵗʰ/√5ᵗʰ Additional Digit Required   Unspecified Code   Other Specified Code   Manifestation Code   ►◄ Revised Text   ● New Code   ▲ Revised Code Title

896.2 Bilateral, without mention of complication
> EXCLUDES one foot and other leg (897.6-897.7)

896.3 Bilateral, complicated

√4ᵗʰ **897 Traumatic amputation of leg(s) (complete) (partial)**

897.0 Unilateral, below knee, without mention of complication

897.1 Unilateral, below knee, complicated

897.2 Unilateral, at or above knee, without mention of complication

897.3 Unilateral, at or above knee, complicated

897.4 Unilateral, level not specified, without mention of complication

897.5 Unilateral, level not specified, complicated

897.6 Bilateral [any level], without mention of complication
> One foot and other leg

897.7 Bilateral [any level], complicated
> AHA: 3Q, '90, 5

Injury to Blood Vessels (900-904)

> INCLUDES arterial hematoma
> avulsion
> cut
> laceration   of blood vessel
> rupture   secondary to other
> traumatic aneurysm or fistula   injuries, e.g.;
> (arteriovenous)   fracture or open
>   wound

> EXCLUDES accidental puncture or laceration during medical procedure (998.2)
> intracranial hemorrhage following injury (851.0-854.1)
> AHA: 3Q, '90, 5

√4ᵗʰ **900 Injury to blood vessels of head and neck**

√5ᵗʰ **900.0 Carotid artery**

900.00 Carotid artery, unspecified

900.01 Common carotid artery

900.02 External carotid artery

900.03 Internal carotid artery

900.1 Internal jugular vein

√5ᵗʰ **900.8 Other specified blood vessels of head and neck**

900.81 External jugular vein
> Jugular vein NOS

900.82 Multiple blood vessels of head and neck

900.89 Other

900.9 Unspecified blood vessel of head and neck

√4ᵗʰ **901 Injury to blood vessels of thorax**
> EXCLUDES traumatic hemothorax (860.2-860.5)

901.0 Thoracic aorta

901.1 Innominate and subclavian arteries

901.2 Superior vena cava

901.3 Innominate and subclavian veins

√5ᵗʰ **901.4 Pulmonary blood vessels**

901.40 Pulmonary vessel(s), unspecified

901.41 Pulmonary artery

901.42 Pulmonary vein

√5ᵗʰ **901.8 Other specified blood vessels of thorax**

901.81 Intercostal artery or vein

901.82 Internal mammary artery or vein

901.83 Multiple blood vessels of thorax

901.89 Other
> Azygos vein   Hemiazygos vein

901.9 Unspecified blood vessel of thorax

√4ᵗʰ **902 Injury to blood vessels of abdomen and pelvis**

902.0 Abdominal aorta

√5ᵗʰ **902.1 Inferior vena cava**

902.10 Inferior vena cava, unspecified

902.11 Hepatic veins

902.19 Other

√5ᵗʰ **902.2 Celiac and mesenteric arteries**

902.20 Celiac and mesenteric arteries, unspecified

902.21 Gastric artery

902.22 Hepatic artery

902.23 Splenic artery

902.24 Other specified branches of celiac axis

902.25 Superior mesenteric artery (trunk)

902.26 Primary branches of superior mesenteric artery
> Ileocolic artery

902.27 Inferior mesenteric artery

902.29 Other

√5ᵗʰ **902.3 Portal and splenic veins**

902.31 Superior mesenteric vein and primary subdivisions
> Ileocolic vein

902.32 Inferior mesenteric vein

902.33 Portal vein

902.34 Splenic vein

902.39 Other
> Cystic vein   Gastric vein

√5ᵗʰ **902.4 Renal blood vessels**

902.40 Renal vessel(s), unspecified

902.41 Renal artery

902.42 Renal vein

902.49 Other
> Suprarenal arteries

√5ᵗʰ **902.5 Iliac blood vessels**

902.50 Iliac vessel(s), unspecified

902.51 Hypogastric artery

902.52 Hypogastric vein

902.53 Iliac artery

902.54 Iliac vein

902.55 Uterine artery ♀

902.56 Uterine vein ♀

902.59 Other

√5ᵗʰ **902.8 Other specified blood vessels of abdomen and pelvis**

902.81 Ovarian artery ♀

902.82 Ovarian vein ♀

902.87 Multiple blood vessels of abdomen and pelvis

902.89 Other

902.9 Unspecified blood vessel of abdomen and pelvis

√4ᵗʰ **903 Injury to blood vessels of upper extremity**

√5ᵗʰ **903.0 Axillary blood vessels**

903.00 Axillary vessel(s), unspecified

903.01 Axillary artery

903.02 Axillary vein

903.1 Brachial blood vessels

903.2 Radial blood vessels

903.3 Ulnar blood vessels

903.4 Palmar artery

903.5 Digital blood vessels

N Newborn Age: 0   P Pediatric Age: 0-17   M Maternity Age: 12-55   A Adult Age: 15-124

903.8 Other specified blood vessels of upper extremity
Multiple blood vessels of upper extremity

903.9 Unspecified blood vessel of upper extremity

√4ᵗʰ **904 Injury to blood vessels of lower extremity and unspecified sites**

904.0 **Common femoral artery**
Femoral artery above profunda origin

904.1 **Superficial femoral artery**

904.2 **Femoral veins**

904.3 **Saphenous veins**
Saphenous vein (greater) (lesser)

√5ᵗʰ 904.4 **Popliteal blood vessels**

904.40 **Popliteal vessel(s), unspecified**

904.41 **Popliteal artery**

904.42 **Popliteal vein**

√5ᵗʰ 904.5 **Tibial blood vessels**

904.50 **Tibial vessel(s), unspecified**

904.51 **Anterior tibial artery**

904.52 **Anterior tibial vein**

904.53 **Posterior tibial artery**

904.54 **Posterior tibial vein**

904.6 **Deep plantar blood vessels**

904.7 **Other specified blood vessels of lower extremity**
Multiple blood vessels of lower extremity

904.8 **Unspecified blood vessel of lower extremity**

904.9 **Unspecified site**
Injury to blood vessel NOS

Late Effects of Injuries, Poisonings, Toxic Effects, and Other External Causes (905-909)

NOTE These categories are to be used to indicate conditions classifiable to 800-999 as the cause of late effects, which are themselves classified elsewhere. The "late effects" include those specified as such, or as sequelae, which may occur at any time after the acute injury.

√4ᵗʰ **905 Late effects of musculoskeletal and connective tissue injuries**
AHA: 1Q, '95, 10; 2Q, '94, 3

905.0 **Late effect of fracture of skull and face bones**
Late effect of injury classifiable to 800-804
AHA: 3Q, '97, 12

905.1 **Late effect of fracture of spine and trunk without mention of spinal cord lesion**
Late effect of injury classifiable to 805, 807-809
AHA: 1Q, '07, 20

905.2 **Late effect of fracture of upper extremities**
Late effect of injury classifiable to 810-819

905.3 **Late effect of fracture of neck of femur**
Late effect of injury classifiable to 820

905.4 **Late effect of fracture of lower extremities**
Late effect of injury classifiable to 821-827
S79.001S Uns physeal fx upper end right femur sequela I-10

905.5 **Late effect of fracture of multiple and unspecified bones**
Late effect of injury classifiable to 828-829

905.6 **Late effect of dislocation**
Late effect of injury classifiable to 830-839

905.7 **Late effect of sprain and strain without mention of tendon injury**
Late effect of injury classifiable to 840-848, except tendon injury

905.8 **Late effect of tendon injury**
Late effect of tendon injury due to:
open wound [injury classifiable to 880-884 with .2, 890-894 with .2]
sprain and strain [injury classifiable to 840-848]
AHA: 2Q, '89, 13; 2Q, '89, 15

905.9 **Late effect of traumatic amputation**
Late effect of injury classifiable to 885-887, 895-897
EXCLUDES late amputation stump complication (997.60-997.69)

√4ᵗʰ **906 Late effects of injuries to skin and subcutaneous tissues**

906.0 **Late effect of open wound of head, neck, and trunk**
Late effect of injury classifiable to 870-879

906.1 **Late effect of open wound of extremities without mention of tendon injury**
Late effect of injury classifiable to 880-884, 890-894 except .2

906.2 **Late effect of superficial injury**
Late effect of injury classifiable to 910-919

906.3 **Late effect of contusion**
Late effect of injury classifiable to 920-924

906.4 **Late effect of crushing**
Late effect of injury classifiable to 925-929

906.5 **Late effect of burn of eye, face, head, and neck**
Late effect of injury classifiable to 940-941
AHA: 4Q, '04, 76

906.6 **Late effect of burn of wrist and hand**
Late effect of injury classifiable to 944
AHA: 4Q, '94, 22

906.7 **Late effect of burn of other extremities**
Late effect of injury classifiable to 943 or 945
AHA: 4Q, '94, 22

906.8 **Late effect of burns of other specified sites**
Late effect of injury classifiable to 942, 946-947
AHA: 4Q, '94, 22

906.9 **Late effect of burn of unspecified site**
Late effect of injury classifiable to 948-949
AHA: 4Q, '94, 22

√4ᵗʰ **907 Late effects of injuries to the nervous system**

907.0 **Late effect of intracranial injury without mention of skull fracture**
Late effect of injury classifiable to 850-854
AHA: ▶4Q, '11, 97;◀ 4Q, '10, 96; 4Q, '09, 108; 4Q, '08, 108; 4Q, '03, 103; 3Q, '90, 14
S06.2x1S Diffuse traumatic brain inj loc 30 min/less sequela I-10

907.1 **Late effect of injury to cranial nerve**
Late effect of injury classifiable to 950-951

907.2 **Late effect of spinal cord injury**
Late effect of injury classifiable to 806, 952
AHA: 4Q, '03, 103; 4Q, '98, 38
S34.114S Complete lesion L4 of lumbar spinal cord sequela I-10

907.3 **Late effect of injury to nerve root(s), spinal plexus(es), and other nerves of trunk**
Late effect of injury classifiable to 953-954
AHA: 2Q, '07, 11

907.4 **Late effect of injury to peripheral nerve of shoulder girdle and upper limb**
Late effect of injury classifiable to 955

907.5 **Late effect of injury to peripheral nerve of pelvic girdle and lower limb**
Late effect of injury classifiable to 956

907.9 **Late effect of injury to other and unspecified nerve**
Late effect of injury classifiable to 957

√4ᵗʰ **908 Late effects of other and unspecified injuries**

908.0 **Late effect of internal injury to chest**
Late effect of injury classifiable to 860-862

908.1 **Late effect of internal injury to intra-abdominal organs**
Late effect of injury classifiable to 863-866, 868

908.2 **Late effect of internal injury to other internal organs**
Late effect of injury classifiable to 867 or 869

908.3 **Late effect of injury to blood vessel of head, neck, and extremities**
Late effect of injury classifiable to 900, 903-904

908.4 **Late effect of injury to blood vessel of thorax, abdomen, and pelvis**
Late effect of injury classifiable to 901-902

903.8–908.4

√4ᵗʰ √5ᵗʰ Additional Digit Required | Unspecified Code | Other Specified Code | Manifestation Code | ▶◀ Revised Text | ● New Code | ▲ Revised Code Title

2013 ICD-9-CM | February 2012 • Volume 1 – 293

Injury and Poisoning

908.5–914.3

908.5 Late effect of foreign body in orifice
Late effect of injury classifiable to 930-939

908.6 Late effect of certain complications of trauma
Late effect of complications classifiable to 958

908.9 Late effect of unspecified injury
Late effect of injury classifiable to 959
AHA: 3Q, '00, 4

√4ᵗʰ **909 Late effects of other and unspecified external causes**

909.0 Late effect of poisoning due to drug, medicinal or biological substance
Late effect of conditions classifiable to 960-979
EXCLUDES late effect of adverse effect of drug, medicinal or biological substance (909.5)
AHA: 4Q, '03, 103

909.1 Late effect of toxic effects of nonmedical substances
Late effect of conditions classifiable to 980-989

909.2 Late effect of radiation
Late effect of conditions classifiable to 990

909.3 Late effect of complications of surgical and medical care
Late effect of conditions classifiable to 996-999
AHA: 1Q, '93, 29

909.4 Late effect of certain other external causes
Late effect of conditions classifiable to 991-994

909.5 Late effect of adverse effect of drug, medical or biological substance
EXCLUDES late effect of poisoning due to drug, medicinal or biological substance (909.0)
AHA: 4Q, '94, 48

909.9 Late effect of other and unspecified external causes

Superficial Injury (910-919)

EXCLUDES burn (blisters) (940.0-949.5)
contusion (920-924.9)
foreign body:
granuloma (728.82)
inadvertently left in operative wound (998.4)
residual in soft tissue (729.6)
insect bite, venomous (989.5)
open wound with incidental foreign body (870.0-897.7)
AHA: 2Q, '89, 15
TIP: Do not code separately when associated with more severe injuries of the same site.

√4ᵗʰ **910 Superficial injury of face, neck, and scalp except eye**
INCLUDES cheek
ear
gum
lip
nose
throat
EXCLUDES eye and adnexa (918.0-918.9)

910.0 Abrasion or friction burn without mention of infection
S00.01xA Abrasion of scalp initial encounter I-10

910.1 Abrasion or friction burn, infected

910.2 Blister without mention of infection

910.3 Blister, infected

910.4 Insect bite, nonvenomous, without mention of infection

910.5 Insect bite, nonvenomous, infected

910.6 Superficial foreign body (splinter) without major open wound and without mention of infection

910.7 Superficial foreign body (splinter) without major open wound, infected

910.8 Other and unspecified superficial injury of face, neck, and scalp without mention of infection

910.9 Other and unspecified superficial injury of face, neck, and scalp, infected

√4ᵗʰ **911 Superficial injury of trunk**
INCLUDES abdominal wall · interscapular region
anus · labium (majus) (minus)
back · penis
breast · perineum
buttock · scrotum
chest wall · testis
flank · vagina
groin · vulva
EXCLUDES hip (916.0-916.9)
scapular region (912.0-912.9)

911.0 Abrasion or friction burn without mention of infection
AHA: 3Q, '01, 10

911.1 Abrasion or friction burn, infected

911.2 Blister without mention of infection

911.3 Blister, infected

911.4 Insect bite, nonvenomous, without mention of infection

911.5 Insect bite, nonvenomous, infected

911.6 Superficial foreign body (splinter) without major open wound and without mention of infection

911.7 Superficial foreign body (splinter) without major open wound, infected

911.8 Other and unspecified superficial injury of trunk without mention of infection

911.9 Other and unspecified superficial injury of trunk, infected

√4ᵗʰ **912 Superficial injury of shoulder and upper arm**
INCLUDES axilla
scapular region

912.0 Abrasion or friction burn without mention of infection

912.1 Abrasion or friction burn, infected

912.2 Blister without mention of infection

912.3 Blister, infected

912.4 Insect bite, nonvenomous, without mention of infection

912.5 Insect bite, nonvenomous, infected

912.6 Superficial foreign body (splinter) without major open wound and without mention of infection

912.7 Superficial foreign body (splinter) without major open wound, infected

912.8 Other and unspecified superficial injury of shoulder and upper arm without mention of infection

912.9 Other and unspecified superficial injury of shoulder and upper arm infected

√4ᵗʰ **913 Superficial injury of elbow, forearm, and wrist**

913.0 Abrasion or friction burn without mention of infection

913.1 Abrasion or friction burn, infected

913.2 Blister without mention of infection

913.3 Blister, infected

913.4 Insect bite, nonvenomous, without mention of infection

913.5 Insect bite, nonvenomous, infected

913.6 Superficial foreign body (splinter) without major open wound and without mention of infection

913.7 Superficial foreign body (splinter) without major open wound, infected

913.8 Other and unspecified superficial injury of elbow, forearm, and wrist without mention of infection

913.9 Other and unspecified superficial injury of elbow, forearm, and wrist, infected

√4ᵗʰ **914 Superficial injury of hand(s) except finger(s) alone**

914.0 Abrasion or friction burn without mention of infection

914.1 Abrasion or friction burn, infected

914.2 Blister without mention of infection

914.3 Blister, infected

914.4   Insect bite, nonvenomous, without mention of infection

914.5   Insect bite, nonvenomous, infected

914.6   Superficial foreign body (splinter) without major open wound and without mention of infection

914.7   Superficial foreign body (splinter) without major open wound, infected

914.8   Other and unspecified superficial injury of hand without mention of infection

914.9   Other and unspecified superficial injury of hand, infected

✓4ᵗʰ **915   Superficial injury of finger(s)**

    INCLUDES   fingernail
                 thumb (nail)

915.0   Abrasion or friction burn without mention of infection

915.1   Abrasion or friction burn, infected

915.2   Blister without mention of infection

915.3   Blister, infected

915.4   Insect bite, nonvenomous, without mention of infection

915.5   Insect bite, nonvenomous, infected

915.6   Superficial foreign body (splinter) without major open wound and without mention of infection

915.7   Superficial foreign body (splinter) without major open wound, infected

915.8   Other and unspecified superficial injury of fingers without mention of infection

        AHA: 3Q, '01, 10

915.9   Other and unspecified superficial injury of fingers, infected

✓4ᵗʰ **916   Superficial injury of hip, thigh, leg, and ankle**

916.0   Abrasion or friction burn without mention of infection

        S80.812A Abrasion left lower leg initial encounter   I-10

916.1   Abrasion or friction burn, infected

916.2   Blister without mention of infection

916.3   Blister, infected

916.4   Insect bite, nonvenomous, without mention of infection

916.5   Insect bite, nonvenomous, infected

916.6   Superficial foreign body (splinter) without major open wound and without mention of infection

916.7   Superficial foreign body (splinter) without major open wound, infected

916.8   Other and unspecified superficial injury of hip, thigh, leg, and ankle without mention of infection

916.9   Other and unspecified superficial injury of hip, thigh, leg, and ankle, infected

✓4ᵗʰ **917   Superficial injury of foot and toe(s)**

    INCLUDES   heel
                 toenail

917.0   Abrasion or friction burn without mention of infection

917.1   Abrasion or friction burn, infected

917.2   Blister without mention of infection

917.3   Blister, infected

917.4   Insect bite, nonvenomous, without mention of infection

917.5   Insect bite, nonvenomous, infected

917.6   Superficial foreign body (splinter) without major open wound and without mention of infection

917.7   Superficial foreign body (splinter) without major open wound, infected

917.8   Other and unspecified superficial injury of foot and toes without mention of infection

        AHA: 1Q, '03, 13

917.9   Other and unspecified superficial injury of foot and toes infected

        AHA: 1Q, '03, 13

        TIP: Assign for hair strangulation of toe, with infection.

✓4ᵗʰ **918   Superficial injury of eye and adnexa**

    EXCLUDES   burn (940.0-940.9)
                 foreign body on external eye (930.0-930.9)

918.0   Eyelids and periocular area

        Abrasion
        Insect bite
        Superficial foreign body (splinter)

918.1   Cornea

        Corneal abrasion   Superficial laceration
        EXCLUDES   corneal injury due to contact lens (371.82)

918.2   Conjunctiva

918.9   Other and unspecified superficial injuries of eye

        Eye (ball) NOS

✓4ᵗʰ **919   Superficial injury of other, multiple, and unspecified sites**

    EXCLUDES   multiple sites classifiable to the same three-digit category (910.0-918.9)

919.0   Abrasion or friction burn without mention of infection

919.1   Abrasion or friction burn, infected

919.2   Blister without mention of infection

919.3   Blister, infected

919.4   Insect bite, nonvenomous, without mention of infection

919.5   Insect bite, nonvenomous, infected

919.6   Superficial foreign body (splinter) without major open wound and without mention of infection

919.7   Superficial foreign body (splinter) without major open wound, infected

919.8   Other and unspecified superficial injuries without mention of infection

919.9   Other and unspecified superficial injury, infected

Contusion with Intact Skin Surface (920-924)

    INCLUDES   bruise   } without fracture or open
                 hematoma }   wound

    EXCLUDES   concussion (850.0-850.9)
                 hemarthrosis (840.0-848.9)
                 internal organs (860.0-869.1)
                 that incidental to:
                     crushing injury (925-929.9)
                     dislocation (830.0-839.9)
                     fracture (800.0-829.1)
                     internal injury (860.0-869.1)
                     intracranial injury (850.0-854.1)
                     nerve injury (950.0-957.9)
                     open wound (870.0-897.7)

920   Contusion of face, scalp, and neck except eye(s)

        Cheek   Mandibular joint area
        Ear (auricle)   Nose
        Gum   Throat
        Lip
        S00.33xA Contusion of nose initial encounter   I-10

✓4ᵗʰ **921   Contusion of eye and adnexa**

921.0   Black eye, not otherwise specified

921.1   Contusion of eyelids and periocular area

921.2   Contusion of orbital tissues

921.3   Contusion of eyeball

        TIP: If iridodialysis (rupture of the root of the iris) is present and is due to the eyeball contusion, assign also code 364.76.

921.9   Unspecified contusion of eye

        Injury of eye NOS

✓4ᵗʰ **922   Contusion of trunk**

922.0   Breast

922.1   Chest wall

        S20.212A Contusion left front wall thorax initial enc   I-10

✓4ᵗʰ
✓5ᵗʰ Additional Digit Required   Unspecified Code   Other Specified Code   Manifestation Code   ▶◀ Revised Text   ● New Code   ▲ Revised Code Title

2013 ICD-9-CM   **Volume 1 – 295**

Injury and Poisoning

922.2–928.3

922.2 **Abdominal wall**
Flank   Groin

✓5ᵗʰ 922.3 **Back**
AHA: 4Q, '96, 39

922.31 **Back**
EXCLUDES *interscapular region (922.33)*
AHA: 3Q, '99, 14

922.32 **Buttock**

922.33 **Interscapular region**

922.4 **Genital organs**
Labium (majus) (minus)
Penis
Perineum
Scrotum
Testis
Vagina
Vulva

922.8 **Multiple sites of trunk**

922.9 **Unspecified part**
Trunk NOS

✓4ᵗʰ 923 **Contusion of upper limb**

✓5ᵗʰ 923.0 **Shoulder and upper arm**

923.00 **Shoulder region**

923.01 **Scapular region**

923.02 **Axillary region**

923.03 **Upper arm**

923.09 **Multiple sites**

✓5ᵗʰ 923.1 **Elbow and forearm**

923.10 **Forearm**

923.11 **Elbow**

✓5ᵗʰ 923.2 **Wrist and hand(s), except finger(s) alone**

923.20 **Hand(s)**

923.21 **Wrist**

923.3 **Finger**
Fingernail   Thumb (nail)

923.8 **Multiple sites of upper limb**

923.9 **Unspecified part of upper limb**
Arm NOS

✓4ᵗʰ 924 **Contusion of lower limb and of other and unspecified sites**

✓5ᵗʰ 924.0 **Hip and thigh**

924.00 **Thigh**
AHA: 1Q, '09, 10

924.01 **Hip**
S70.02xA Contusion of left hip initial encounter   I-10

✓5ᵗʰ 924.1 **Knee and lower leg**

924.10 **Lower leg**

924.11 **Knee**

✓5ᵗʰ 924.2 **Ankle and foot, excluding toe(s)**

924.20 **Foot**
Heel

924.21 **Ankle**

924.3 **Toe**
Toenail

924.4 **Multiple sites of lower limb**

924.5 **Unspecified part of lower limb**
Leg NOS

924.8 **Multiple sites, not elsewhere classified**
AHA: 1Q, '03, 7
S70.10xA Contusion of unspecified thigh initial encounter   I-10

924.9 **Unspecified site**

Crushing Injury (925-929)

Use additional code to identify any associated injuries, such as:
fractures (800-829)
internal injuries (860.0-869.1)
intracranial injuries (850.0-854.1)
AHA: 4Q, '03, 77; 2Q, '93, 7

✓4ᵗʰ 925 **Crushing injury of face, scalp, and neck**
Cheek   Pharynx
Ear   Throat
Larynx

925.1 **Crushing injury of face and scalp**
Cheek   Ear

925.2 **Crushing injury of neck**
Larynx
Pharynx
Throat

✓4ᵗʰ 926 **Crushing injury of trunk**

926.0 **External genitalia**
Labium (majus) (minus)
Penis
Scrotum
Testis
Vulva

✓5ᵗʰ 926.1 **Other specified sites**

926.11 **Back**

926.12 **Buttock**

926.19 **Other**
Breast

926.8 **Multiple sites of trunk**

926.9 **Unspecified site**
Trunk NOS

✓4ᵗʰ 927 **Crushing injury of upper limb**

✓5ᵗʰ 927.0 **Shoulder and upper arm**

927.00 **Shoulder region**

927.01 **Scapular region**

927.02 **Axillary region**

927.03 **Upper arm**

927.09 **Multiple sites**

✓5ᵗʰ 927.1 **Elbow and forearm**

927.10 **Forearm**

927.11 **Elbow**

✓5ᵗʰ 927.2 **Wrist and hand(s), except finger(s) alone**

927.20 **Hand(s)**

927.21 **Wrist**

927.3 **Finger(s)**
AHA: 4Q, '03, 77

927.8 **Multiple sites of upper limb**

927.9 **Unspecified site**
Arm NOS

✓4ᵗʰ 928 **Crushing injury of lower limb**

✓5ᵗʰ 928.0 **Hip and thigh**

928.00 **Thigh**

928.01 **Hip**

✓5ᵗʰ 928.1 **Knee and lower leg**

928.10 **Lower leg**

928.11 **Knee**

✓5ᵗʰ 928.2 **Ankle and foot, excluding toe(s) alone**

928.20 **Foot**
Heel

928.21 **Ankle**

928.3 **Toe(s)**

N Newborn Age: 0   P Pediatric Age: 0-17   M Maternity Age: 12-55   A Adult Age: 15-124

928.8 **Multiple sites of lower limb**

928.9 **Unspecified site**
Leg NOS

✓4ᵗʰ 929 **Crushing injury of multiple and unspecified sites**

929.0 **Multiple sites, not elsewhere classified**

929.9 **Unspecified site**

Effects Of Foreign Body Entering Through Orifice (930-939)

EXCLUDES foreign body:
granuloma (728.82)
inadvertently left in operative wound (998.4, 998.7)
in open wound (800-839, 851-897)
residual in soft tissues (729.6)
superficial without major open wound (910-919
with .6 or .7)

✓4ᵗʰ 930 **Foreign body on external eye**
EXCLUDES foreign body in penetrating wound of:
eyeball (871.5-871.6)
retained (old) (360.5-360.6)
ocular adnexa (870.4)
retained (old) (376.6)

930.0 **Corneal foreign body**

930.1 **Foreign body in conjunctival sac**

930.2 **Foreign body in lacrimal punctum**

930.8 **Other and combined sites**

930.9 **Unspecified site**
External eye NOS

931 **Foreign body in ear**
Auditory canal   Auricle

932 **Foreign body in nose**
Nasal sinus   Nostril

✓4ᵗʰ 933 **Foreign body in pharynx and larynx**

933.0 **Pharynx**
Nasopharynx   Throat NOS

933.1 **Larynx**
Asphyxia due to foreign body
Choking due to:
food (regurgitated)
phlegm
TIP: Assign for mucous plug causing asphyxia; otherwise, for
tracheobronchial, refer to code 519.19 Other diseases of trachea and
bronchus.

✓4ᵗʰ 934 **Foreign body in trachea, bronchus, and lung**

934.0 **Trachea**

934.1 **Main bronchus**
AHA: 3Q, '02, 18

934.8 **Other specified parts**
Bronchioles
Lung

934.9 **Respiratory tree, unspecified**
Inhalation of liquid or vomitus, lower respiratory tract NOS

✓4ᵗʰ 935 **Foreign body in mouth, esophagus, and stomach**

935.0 **Mouth**

935.1 **Esophagus**
AHA: 1Q, '88, 13
TIP: If esophageal obstruction is due to stenosis, caustic stricture
(e.g., lye ingestion), or tumor, assign instead code 530.3.

935.2 **Stomach**

936 **Foreign body in intestine and colon**

937 **Foreign body in anus and rectum**
Rectosigmoid (junction)

938 **Foreign body in digestive system, unspecified**
Alimentary tract NOS
Swallowed foreign body

✓4ᵗʰ 939 **Foreign body in genitourinary tract**

939.0 **Bladder and urethra**

939.1 **Uterus, any part**   ♀
EXCLUDES intrauterine contraceptive device:
complications from (996.32, 996.65)
presence of (V45.51)

939.2 **Vulva and vagina**   ♀

939.3 **Penis**   ♂

939.9 **Unspecified site**

Burns (940-949)

INCLUDES burns from:
electrical heating appliance
electricity
flame
hot object
lightning
radiation
chemical burns (external) (internal)
scalds
EXCLUDES friction burns (910-919 with .0, .1)
sunburn (692.71, 692.76-692.77)
AHA: 4Q, 94, 22; 2Q, '90, 7; 4Q, '88, 3; M-A, '86, 9
TIP: Nonhealing burns are coded as acute burns, as is necrosis of burned skin.
Assign code 958.3 for any documented infected burn site.

✓4ᵗʰ 940 **Burn confined to eye and adnexa**

940.0 **Chemical burn of eyelids and periocular area**

940.1 **Other burns of eyelids and periocular area**

940.2 **Alkaline chemical burn of cornea and conjunctival sac**

940.3 **Acid chemical burn of cornea and conjunctival sac**

940.4 **Other burn of cornea and conjunctival sac**

940.5 **Burn with resulting rupture and destruction of eyeball**

940.9 **Unspecified burn of eye and adnexa**

✓4ᵗʰ 941 **Burn of face, head, and neck**
EXCLUDES mouth (947.0)

The following fifth-digit subclassification is for use with category 941:
0 **face and head, unspecified site**
1 **ear [any part]**
2 **eye (with other parts of face, head, and neck)**
3 **lip(s)**
4 **chin**
5 **nose (septum)**
6 **scalp [any part]**
Temple (region)
7 **forehead and cheek**
8 **neck**
9 **multiple sites [except with eye] of face, head and neck**

AHA: 4Q, '94, 22; M-A, '86, 9

§ ✓5ᵗʰ 941.0 **Unspecified degree**
[0-9]

§ ✓5ᵗʰ 941.1 **Erythema [first degree]**
[0-9]   AHA: For code 941.11: 3Q, '10, 19; For code 941.19: 3Q, '05, 10

§ ✓5ᵗʰ 941.2 **Blisters, epidermal loss [second degree]**
[0-9]

§ ✓5ᵗʰ 941.3 **Full-thickness skin loss [third degree NOS]**
[0-9]

§ ✓5ᵗʰ 941.4 **Deep necrosis of underlying tissues [deep third**
[0-9]   **degree] without mention of loss of a body part**

§ ✓5ᵗʰ 941.5 **Deep necrosis of underlying tissues [deep third**
[0-9]   **degree] with loss of a body part**

---

§ Requires fifth digit. Valid digits are in [brackets] under each code. See category 941 for codes and definitions.

Injury and Poisoning

942–947.9

√4ᵗʰ **942 Burn of trunk**

> EXCLUDES *scapular region (943.0-943.5 with fifth-digit 6)*
>
> The following fifth-digit subclassificaiton is for use with category 942:
>
> 0 **trunk, unspecified site**
> 1 **breast**
> 2 **chest wall, excluding breast and nipple**
> 3 **abdominal wall**
> > Flank
> > Groin
> 4 **back [any part]**
> > Buttock
> > Interscapular region
> 5 **genitalia**
> > Labium (majus) (minus
> > Penis
> > Perineum
> > Scrotum
> > Testis
> > Vulva
> 9 **other and multiple sites of trunk**
>
> AHA: 4Q, '94, 22; M-A, '86, 9

§ √5ᵗʰ **942.0 Unspecified degree**
[0-5, 9]

§ √5ᵗʰ **942.1 Erythema [first degree]**
[0-5, 9]

§ √5ᵗʰ **942.2 Blisters, epidermal loss [second degree]**
[0-5, 9]

§ √5ᵗʰ **942.3 Full-thickness skin loss [third degree NOS]**
[0-5, 9]

§ √5ᵗʰ **942.4 Deep necrosis of underlying tissues [deep third**
[0-5, 9] **degree] without mention of loss of a body part**

§ √5ᵗʰ **942.5 Deep necrosis of underlying tissues [deep third**
[0-5, 9] **degree] with loss of a body part**

√4ᵗʰ **943 Burn of upper limb, except wrist and hand**

> The following fifth-digit subclassificaiton is for use with category 943:
>
> 0 **upper limb, unspecified site**
> 1 **forearm**
> 2 **elbow**
> 3 **upper arm**
> 4 **axilla**
> 5 **shoulder**
> 6 **scapular region**
> 9 **multiple sites of upper limb, except wrist and hand**
>
> AHA: 4Q, '94, 22; M-A, '86, 9

§ √5ᵗʰ **943.0 Unspecified degree**
[0-6, 9] AHA: For code 943.00: 3Q, '10, 19

§ √5ᵗʰ **943.1 Erythema [first degree]**
[0-6, 9]

§ √5ᵗʰ **943.2 Blisters, epidermal loss [second degree]**
[0-6, 9]

§ √5ᵗʰ **943.3 Full-thickness skin loss [third degree NOS]**
[0-6, 9]

§ √5ᵗʰ **943.4 Deep necrosis of underlying tissues [deep third**
[0-6, 9] **degree] without mention of loss of a body part**

§ √5ᵗʰ **943.5 Deep necrosis of underlying tissues [deep third**
[0-6, 9] **degree] with loss of a body part**

√4ᵗʰ **944 Burn of wrist(s) and hand(s)**

> The following fifth-digit subclassification is for use with category 944:
>
> 0 **hand, unspecified site**
> 1 **single digit [finger (nail)] other than thumb**
> 2 **thumb (nail)**
> 3 **two or more digits, not including thumb**
> 4 **two or more digits including thumb**
> 5 **palm**
> 6 **back of hand**
> 7 **wrist**
> 8 **multiple sites of wrist(s) and hand(s)**

§ √5ᵗʰ **944.0 Unspecified degree**
[0-8]

§ √5ᵗʰ **944.1 Erythema [first degree]**
[0-8]

§ √5ᵗʰ **944.2 Blisters, epidermal loss [second degree]**
[0-8]

§ √5ᵗʰ **944.3 Full-thickness skin loss [third degree NOS]**
[0-8]

§ √5ᵗʰ **944.4 Deep necrosis of underlying tissues [deep third**
[0-8] **degree] without mention of loss of a body part**

§ √5ᵗʰ **944.5 Deep necrosis of underlying tissues [deep third**
[0-8] **degree] with loss of a body part**

√4ᵗʰ **945 Burn of lower limb(s)**

> The following fifth-digit subclassification is for use with category 945:
>
> 0 **lower limb [leg], unspecified site**
> 1 **toe(s) (nail)**
> 2 **foot**
> 3 **ankle**
> 4 **lower leg**
> 5 **knee**
> 6 **thigh [any part]**
> 9 **multiple sites of lower limb(s)**
>
> AHA: 4Q, '94, 22; M-A, '86, 9

§ √5ᵗʰ **945.0 Unspecified degree**
[0-6, 9]

§ √5ᵗʰ **945.1 Erythema [first degree]**
[0-6, 9]

§ √5ᵗʰ **945.2 Blisters, epidermal loss [second degree]**
[0-6, 9]

§ √5ᵗʰ **945.3 Full-thickness skin loss [third degree NOS]**
[0-6, 9]

§ √5ᵗʰ **945.4 Deep necrosis of underlying tissues [deep third**
[0-6, 9] **degree] without mention of loss of a body part**

§ √5ᵗʰ **945.5 Deep necrosis of underlying tissues [deep third**
[0-6, 9] **degree] with loss of a body part**

√4ᵗʰ **946 Burns of multiple specified sites**

> INCLUDES burns of sites classifiable to more than one three-digit
> category in 940-945
>
> EXCLUDES *multiple burns NOS (949.0-949.5)*
> AHA: 4Q, '94, 22; M-A, '86, 9
> TIP: Only assign if the specific sites of the multiple burns are not specified.

946.0 Unspecified degree

946.1 Erythema [first degree]

946.2 Blisters, epidermal loss [second degree]

946.3 Full-thickness skin loss [third degree NOS]

946.4 Deep necrosis of underlying tissues [deep third degree]
without mention of loss of a body part

946.5 Deep necrosis of underlying tissues [deep third degree]
with loss of a body part

√4ᵗʰ **947 Burn of internal organs**

> INCLUDES burns from chemical agents (ingested)
> AHA: 4Q, '94, 22; M-A, '86, 9

947.0 Mouth and pharynx
> Gum   Tongue

947.1 Larynx, trachea, and lung

947.2 Esophagus

947.3 Gastrointestinal tract
> Colon   Small intestine
> Rectum   Stomach

947.4 Vagina and uterus   ♀

947.8 Other specified sites

947.9 Unspecified site

---

§ Requires fifth digit. Valid digits are in [brackets] under each code. See appropriate category for codes and definitions.

N Newborn Age: 0   P Pediatric Age: 0-17   M Maternity Age: 12-55   A Adult Age: 15-124

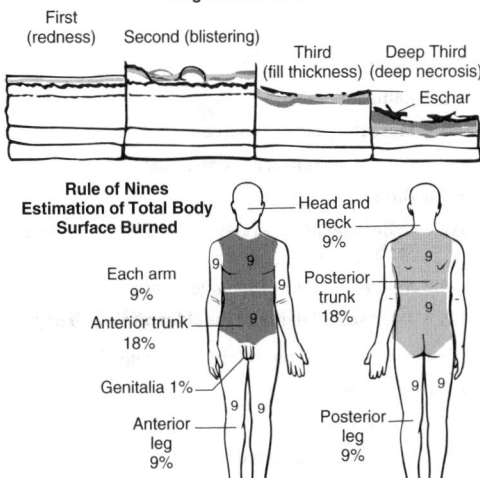

Burns
Degrees of Burns

First (redness)   Second (blistering)   Third (fill thickness)   Deep Third (deep necrosis)   Eschar

Rule of Nines
Estimation of Total Body Surface Burned

Head and neck 9%
Each arm 9%
Anterior trunk 18%
Posterior trunk 18%
Genitalia 1%
Anterior leg 9%
Posterior leg 9%

949.1 Erythema [first degree]

949.2 Blisters, epidermal loss [second degree]

949.3 Full-thickness skin loss [third degree NOS]

949.4 Deep necrosis of underlying tissues [deep third degree] without mention of loss of a body part

949.5 Deep necrosis of underlying tissues [deep third degree] with loss of a body part

Injury to Nerves and Spinal Cord (950-957)

> **INCLUDES**   division of nerve
> lesion in continuity
> traumatic neuroma   (with open wound)
> traumatic transient paralysis
>
> **EXCLUDES**   *accidental puncture or laceration during medical procedure (998.2)*

√4ᵗʰ **950 Injury to optic nerve and pathways**

    950.0 Optic nerve injury
       Second cranial nerve

    950.1 Injury to optic chiasm

    950.2 Injury to optic pathways

    950.3 Injury to visual cortex

    950.9 Unspecified
       Traumatic blindness NOS

√4ᵗʰ **951 Injury to other cranial nerve(s)**

    951.0 Injury to oculomotor nerve
       Third cranial nerve

    951.1 Injury to trochlear nerve
       Fourth cranial nerve

    951.2 Injury to trigeminal nerve
       Fifth cranial nerve

    951.3 Injury to abducens nerve
       Sixth cranial nerve

    951.4 Injury to facial nerve
       Seventh cranial nerve

    951.5 Injury to acoustic nerve
       Auditory nerve
       Eighth cranial nerve
       Traumatic deafness NOS

    951.6 Injury to accessory nerve
       Eleventh cranial nerve

    951.7 Injury to hypoglossal nerve
       Twelfth cranial nerve

    951.8 Injury to other specified cranial nerves
       Glossopharyngeal [9th cranial] nerve
       Olfactory [1st cranial] nerve
       Pneumogastric [10th cranial] nerve
       Traumatic anosmia NOS
       Vagus [10th cranial] nerve

    951.9 Injury to unspecified cranial nerve

√4ᵗʰ **952 Spinal cord injury without evidence of spinal bone injury**

    √5ᵗʰ **952.0 Cervical**

      952.00 C_1-C_4 level with unspecified spinal cord injury
         Spinal cord injury, cervical region NOS

      952.01 C_1-C_4 level with complete lesion of spinal cord

      952.02 C_1-C_4 level with anterior cord syndrome

      952.03 C_1-C_4 level with central cord syndrome

      952.04 C_1-C_4 level with other specified spinal cord injury
         Incomplete spinal cord lesion at C_1-C_4 level:
           NOS
           with posterior cord syndrome

      952.05 C_5-C_7 level with unspecified spinal cord injury

      952.06 C_5-C_7 level with complete lesion of spinal cord

      952.07 C_5-C_7 level with anterior cord syndrome

√4ᵗʰ **948 Burns classified according to extent of body surface involved**

     NOTE This category is to be used when the site of the burn is unspecified, or with categories 940-947 when the site is specified.

     EXCLUDES *sunburn (692.71, 692.76-692.77)*

     The following fifth-digit subclassification is for use with category 948 to indicate the percent of body surface with third degree burn; valid digits are in [brackets] under each code:
       0 less than 10 percent or unspecified
       1 10-19%
       2 20-29%
       3 30-39%
       4 40-49%
       5 50-59%
       6 60-69%
       7 70-79%
       8 80-89%
       9 90% or more of body surface

     AHA: 4Q, '94, 22; 4Q, '88, 3; M-A, '86, 9; N-D, '84, 13

§ √5ᵗʰ **948.0 Burn [any degree] involving less than 10**
[0]   **percent of body surface**
       T31.0 Burns involving less than 10% of body surface   I-10

§ √5ᵗʰ **948.1 10-19 percent of body surface**
[0-1]

§ √5ᵗʰ **948.2 20-29 percent of body surface**
[0-2]

§ √5ᵗʰ **948.3 30-39 percent of body surface**
[0-3]

§ √5ᵗʰ **948.4 40-49 percent of body surface**
[0-4]

§ √5ᵗʰ **948.5 50-59 percent of body surface**
[0-5]

§ √5ᵗʰ **948.6 60-69 percent of body surface**
[0-6]

§ √5ᵗʰ **948.7 70-79 percent of body surface**
[0-7]

§ √5ᵗʰ **948.8 80-89 percent of body surface**
[0-8]

§ √5ᵗʰ **948.9 90 percent or more of body surface**
[0-9]

√4ᵗʰ **949 Burn, unspecified**

     INCLUDES   burn NOS
         multiple burns NOS

     EXCLUDES *burn of unspecified site but with statement of the extent of body surface involved (948.0-948.9)*

     AHA: 4Q, '94, 22; M-A, '86, 9

    949.0 Unspecified degree

§   Requires fifth digit. Valid digits are in [brackets] under each code. See category 948 for codes and definitions.

√4ᵗʰ √5ᵗʰ Additional Digit Required   Unspecified Code   Other Specified Code   Manifestation Code   ▶◀ Revised Text   ● New Code   ▲ Revised Code Title

2013 ICD-9-CM   **Volume 1 – 299**

Spinal Nerve Roots

952.08 C₅-C₇ level with central cord syndrome

952.09 C₅-C₇ level with other specified spinal cord injury
Incomplete spinal cord lesion at C₅-C₇ level:
NOS
with posterior cord syndrome

√5ᵗʰ 952.1 **Dorsal [thoracic]**

952.10 T_1-T_6 level with unspecified spinal cord injury
Spinal cord injury, thoracic region NOS

952.11 T_1-T_6 level with complete lesion of spinal cord

952.12 T_1-T_6 level with anterior cord syndrome

952.13 T_1-T_6 level with central cord syndrome

952.14 T_1-T_6 level with other specified spinal cord injury
Incomplete spinal cord lesion at T_1-T_6 level:
NOS
with posterior cord syndrome

952.15 T_7-T_{12} level with unspecified spinal cord injury

952.16 T_7-T_{12} level with complete lesion of spinal cord

952.17 T_7-T_{12} level with anterior cord syndrome

952.18 T_7-T_{12} level with central cord syndrome

952.19 T_7-T_{12} level with other specified spinal cord injury
Incomplete spinal cord lesion at T_7-T_{12} level:
NOS
with posterior cord syndrome

952.2 **Lumbar**

952.3 **Sacral**

952.4 **Cauda equina**

952.8 **Multiple sites of spinal cord**

952.9 **Unspecified site of spinal cord**

√4ᵗʰ 953 **Injury to nerve roots and spinal plexus**

953.0 **Cervical root**

953.1 **Dorsal root**

953.2 **Lumbar root**

953.3 **Sacral root**

953.4 **Brachial plexus**

953.5 **Lumbosacral plexus**

953.8 **Multiple sites**

953.9 **Unspecified site**

√4ᵗʰ 954 **Injury to other nerve(s) of trunk, excluding shoulder and pelvic girdles**

954.0 **Cervical sympathetic**

954.1 **Other sympathetic**
Celiac ganglion or plexus
Inferior mesenteric plexus
Splanchnic nerve(s)
Stellate ganglion

954.8 **Other specified nerve(s) of trunk**

954.9 **Unspecified nerve of trunk**

√4ᵗʰ 955 **Injury to peripheral nerve(s) of shoulder girdle and upper limb**

955.0 **Axillary nerve**

955.1 **Median nerve**

955.2 **Ulnar nerve**

955.3 **Radial nerve**

955.4 **Musculocutaneous nerve**

955.5 **Cutaneous sensory nerve, upper limb**

955.6 **Digital nerve**

955.7 **Other specified nerve(s) of shoulder girdle and upper limb**

955.8 **Multiple nerves of shoulder girdle and upper limb**

955.9 **Unspecified nerve of shoulder girdle and upper limb**

√4ᵗʰ 956 **Injury to peripheral nerve(s) of pelvic girdle and lower limb**

956.0 **Sciatic nerve**

956.1 **Femoral nerve**

956.2 **Posterior tibial nerve**

956.3 **Peroneal nerve**

956.4 **Cutaneous sensory nerve, lower limb**

956.5 **Other specified nerve(s) of pelvic girdle and lower limb**

956.8 **Multiple nerves of pelvic girdle and lower limb**

956.9 **Unspecified nerve of pelvic girdle and lower limb**

√4ᵗʰ 957 **Injury to other and unspecified nerves**

957.0 **Superficial nerves of head and neck**

957.1 **Other specified nerve(s)**

957.8 **Multiple nerves in several parts**
Multiple nerve injury NOS

957.9 **Unspecified site**
Nerve injury NOS

Certain Traumatic Complications and Unspecified Injuries (958-959)

√4ᵗʰ 958 **Certain early complications of trauma**

EXCLUDES *adult respiratory distress syndrome (518.52)*
flail chest (807.4)
post-traumatic seroma (729.91)
shock lung related to trauma and surgery (518.52)
that occurring during or following medical procedures (996.0-999.9)

958.0 **Air embolism**
Pneumathemia

EXCLUDES *that complicating:*
abortion (634-638 with .6, 639.6)
ectopic or molar pregnancy (639.6)
pregnancy, childbirth, or the puerperium (673.0)

DEF: Arterial obstruction due to introduction of air bubbles into the veins following surgery or trauma.

958.1 **Fat embolism**

EXCLUDES *that complicating:*
abortion (634-638 with .6, 639.6)
pregnancy, childbirth, or the puerperium (673.8)

DEF: Arterial blockage due to the entrance of fat in circulatory system, after fracture of large bones or administration of corticosteroids.

958.2 **Secondary and recurrent hemorrhage**

958.3 **Posttraumatic wound infection, not elsewhere classified**

EXCLUDES *infected open wounds — code to complicated open wound of site*

AHA: 4Q, '01, 53; S-O, '85, 10

TIP: Do not assign if the infection is documented as due to cellulitis; see instead categories 681 and 682 and complicated wound codes.

958.4 Traumatic shock
Shock (immediate) (delayed) following injury
EXCLUDES shock:
anaphylactic (995.0)
due to serum (999.41-999.49)
anesthetic (995.4)
electric (994.8)
following abortion (639.5)
lightning (994.0)
nontraumatic NOS (785.50)
obstetric (669.1)
postoperative (998.00-998.09)
DEF: Shock, immediate or delayed following injury.

958.5 Traumatic anuria
Crush syndrome   Renal failure following crushing
EXCLUDES that due to a medical procedure (997.5)
DEF: Complete suppression of urinary secretion by kidneys due to trauma.

958.6 Volkmann's ischemic contracture
Posttraumatic muscle contracture
DEF: Muscle deterioration due to loss of blood supply from injury or tourniquet; causes muscle contraction and results in inability to extend the muscles fully.

958.7 Traumatic subcutaneous emphysema
EXCLUDES subcutaneous emphysema resulting from a procedure (998.81)

958.8 Other early complications of trauma
AHA: 2Q, '92, 13

√5ᵗʰ **958.9 Traumatic compartment syndrome**
EXCLUDES nontraumatic compartment syndrome (729.71-729.79)
DEF: Compression of nerves and blood vessels within an enclosed space due to previous trauma, which leads to impaired blood flow and muscle and nerve damage.
TIP: If the compartment syndrome is specified as chronic or exercise-induced, see instead subcategory 729.7.

958.90 Compartment syndrome, unspecified
AHA: 4Q, '06, 100-102

958.91 Traumatic compartment syndrome of upper extremity
Traumatic compartment syndrome of shoulder, arm, forearm, wrist, hand, and fingers
AHA: 4Q, '06, 100-102

958.92 Traumatic compartment syndrome of lower extremity
Traumatic compartment syndrome of hip, buttock, thigh, leg, foot, and toes
AHA: 4Q, '06, 100-102

958.93 Traumatic compartment syndrome of abdomen
AHA: 4Q, '06, 100-102

958.99 Traumatic compartment syndrome of other sites
AHA: 4Q, '06, 100-102

√4ᵗʰ **959 Injury, other and unspecified**
INCLUDES injury NOS
EXCLUDES injury NOS of:
blood vessels (900.0-904.9)
eye (921.0-921.9)
internal organs (860.0-869.1)
intracranial sites (854.0-854.1)
nerves (950.0-951.9, 953.0-957.9)
spinal cord (952.0-952.9)

√5ᵗʰ **959.0 Head, face and neck**

959.01 Head injury, unspecified
EXCLUDES concussion (850.1-850.9)
with head injury NOS (850.1-850.9)
head injury NOS with loss of consciousness (850.1-850.5)
specified head injuries (850.0-854.1)
AHA: 4Q, '08, 108; 4Q, '97, 46
S09.90xA Unspecified injury of head initial encounter [I-10]

959.09 Injury of face and neck
Cheek   Mouth
Ear   Nose
Eyebrow   Throat
Lip
AHA: 4Q, '97, 46

√5ᵗʰ **959.1 Trunk**
EXCLUDES scapular region (959.2)
AHA: 4Q, '03, 78; 1Q, '99, 10

959.11 Other injury of chest wall

959.12 Other injury of abdomen

959.13 Fracture of corpus cavernosum penis   ♂

959.14 Other injury of external genitals

959.19 Other injury of other sites of trunk
Injury of trunk NOS

959.2 Shoulder and upper arm
Axilla   Scapular region

959.3 Elbow, forearm, and wrist
AHA: 1Q, '97, 8

959.4 Hand, except finger

959.5 Finger
Fingernail   Thumb (nail)

959.6 Hip and thigh
Upper leg

959.7 Knee, leg, ankle, and foot

959.8 Other specified sites, including multiple
EXCLUDES multiple sites classifiable to the same four-digit category (959.0-959.7)

959.9 Unspecified site

Poisoning by Drugs, Medicinal and Biological Substances (960-979)

INCLUDES overdose of these substances
wrong substance given or taken in error
Use additional code to specify the effects of the poisoning
EXCLUDES adverse effects ["hypersensitivity," "reaction," etc.] of correct substance properly administered. Such cases are to be classified according to the nature of the adverse effect, such as:
adverse effect NOS (995.20)
allergic lymphadenitis (289.3)
aspirin gastritis (535.4)
blood disorders (280.0-289.9)
dermatitis:
contact (692.0-692.9)
due to ingestion (693.0-693.9)
nephropathy (583.9)
[The drug giving rise to the adverse effect may be identified by use of categories E930-E949.]
drug dependence (304.0-304.9)
drug reaction and poisoning affecting the newborn (760.0-779.9)
nondependent abuse of drugs (305.0-305.9)
pathological drug intoxication (292.2)
AHA: 2Q, '90, 11
TIP: Assign a poisoning code for interaction between prescribed drug and alcohol or prescribed drug and other nonprescribed drug or medicinal agent. Sequence poisoning code first, then code for manifestation of poisoning.
If respiratory failure is due to a poisoning, the poisoning code must be sequenced first.

√4ᵗʰ **960 Poisoning by antibiotics**
EXCLUDES antibiotics:
ear, nose, and throat (976.6)
eye (976.5)
local (976.0)

960.0 Penicillins
Ampicillin
Carbenicillin
Cloxacillin
Penicillin G

960.1 Antifungal antibiotics
Amphotericin B
Griseofulvin
Nystatin
Trichomycin
EXCLUDES *preparations intended for topical use (976.0-976.9)*

960.2 Chloramphenicol group
Chloramphenicol
Thiamphenicol

960.3 Erythromycin and other macrolides
Oleandomycin
Spiramycin

960.4 Tetracycline group
Doxycycline
Minocycline
Oxytetracycline

960.5 Cephalosporin group
Cephalexin
Cephaloglycin
Cephaloridine
Cephalothin

960.6 Antimycobacterial antibiotics
Cycloserine
Kanamycin
Rifampin
Streptomycin

960.7 Antineoplastic antibiotics
Actinomycin such as:
Bleomycin
Cactinomycin
Dactinomycin
Daunorubicin
Mitomycin

960.8 Other specified antibiotics

960.9 Unspecified antibiotic

√4ᵗʰ **961 Poisoning by other anti-infectives**
EXCLUDES *anti-infectives:*
ear, nose, and throat (976.6)
eye (976.5)
local (976.0)

961.0 Sulfonamides
Sulfadiazine
Sulfafurazole
Sulfamethoxazole

961.1 Arsenical anti-infectives

961.2 Heavy metal anti-infectives
Compounds of:
antimony
bismuth
lead
mercury
EXCLUDES *mercurial diuretics (974.0)*

961.3 Quinoline and hydroxyquinoline derivatives
Chiniofon
Diiodohydroxyquin
EXCLUDES *antimalarial drugs (961.4)*

961.4 Antimalarials and drugs acting on other blood protozoa
Chloroquine
Cycloguanil
Primaquine
Proguanil [chloroguanide]
Pyrimethamine
Quinine

961.5 Other antiprotozoal drugs
Emetine

961.6 Anthelmintics
Hexylresorcinol
Piperazine
Thiabendazole

961.7 Antiviral drugs
Methisazone
EXCLUDES *amantadine (966.4)*
cytarabine (963.1)
idoxuridine (976.5)

961.8 Other antimycobacterial drugs
Ethambutol
Ethionamide
Isoniazid
Para-aminosalicylic acid derivatives
Sulfones

961.9 Other and unspecified anti-infectives
Flucytosine
Nitrofuran derivatives

√4ᵗʰ **962 Poisoning by hormones and synthetic substitutes**
EXCLUDES *oxytocic hormones (975.0)*

962.0 Adrenal cortical steroids
Cortisone derivatives
Desoxycorticosterone derivatives
Fluorinated corticosteroids

962.1 Androgens and anabolic congeners
Methandriol
Nandrolone
Oxymetholone
Testosterone

962.2 Ovarian hormones and synthetic substitutes
Contraceptives, oral
Estrogens
Estrogens and progestogens, combined
Progestogens

962.3 Insulins and antidiabetic agents
Acetohexamide
Biguanide derivatives, oral
Chlorpropamide
Glucagon
Insulin
Phenformin
Sulfonylurea derivatives, oral
Tolbutamide
AHA: 4Q, '93, 19; M-A, '85, 8
TIP: Assign only if documentation indicates overdose of insulin; if due to diabetic adjusting dosage, assign instead 250.8X or 249.8X and E932.3 for adverse reaction to insulin, if applicable.

962.4 Anterior pituitary hormones
Corticotropin
Gonadotropin
Somatotropin [growth hormone]

962.5 Posterior pituitary hormones
Vasopressin
EXCLUDES *oxytocic hormones (975.0)*

962.6 Parathyroid and parathyroid derivatives

962.7 Thyroid and thyroid derivatives
Dextrothyroxin
Levothyroxine sodium
Liothyronine
Thyroglobulin

962.8 Antithyroid agents
Iodides
Thiouracil
Thiourea

962.9 Other and unspecified hormones and synthetic substitutes

√4ᵗʰ **963 Poisoning by primarily systemic agents**

963.0 Antiallergic and antiemetic drugs
Antihistamines
Chlorpheniramine
Diphenhydramine
Diphenylpyraline
Thonzylamine
Tripelennamine
EXCLUDES *phenothiazine-based tranquilizers (969.1)*

963.1 Antineoplastic and immunosuppressive drugs
  Azathioprine
  Busulfan
  Chlorambucil
  Cyclophosphamide
  Cytarabine
  Fluorouracil
  Mercaptopurine
  thio-TEPA
  EXCLUDES *antineoplastic antibiotics (960.7)*

963.2 Acidifying agents

963.3 Alkalizing agents

963.4 Enzymes, not elsewhere classified
  Penicillinase

963.5 Vitamins, not elsewhere classified
  Vitamin A
  Vitamin D
  EXCLUDES *nicotinic acid (972.2)*
            vitamin K (964.3)

963.8 Other specified systemic agents
  Heavy metal antagonists

963.9 Unspecified systemic agent

☑4ᵗʰ **964 Poisoning by agents primarily affecting blood constituents**

964.0 Iron and its compounds
  Ferric salts
  Ferrous sulfate and other ferrous salts

964.1 Liver preparations and other antianemic agents
  Folic acid

964.2 Anticoagulants
  Coumarin
  Heparin
  Phenindione
  Warfarin sodium
  AHA: 1Q, '94, 22
  TIP: If documentation indicates an adverse reaction to Coumadin,
  assign instead manifestation (e.g., hematuria or epistaxis), code
  790.92 if abnormal coagulation profile is documented, and E934.2.

964.3 Vitamin K [phytonadione]

964.4 Fibrinolysis-affecting drugs
  Aminocaproic acid
  Streptodornase
  Streptokinase
  Urokinase

964.5 Anticoagulant antagonists and other coagulants
  Hexadimethrine
  Protamine sulfate

964.6 Gamma globulin

964.7 Natural blood and blood products
  Blood plasma
  Human fibrinogen
  Packed red cells
  Whole blood
  EXCLUDES *transfusion reactions (999.41-999.8)*

964.8 Other specified agents affecting blood constituents
  Macromolecular blood substitutes
  Plasma expanders

964.9 Unspecified agent affecting blood constituents

☑4ᵗʰ **965 Poisoning by analgesics, antipyretics, and antirheumatics**
  EXCLUDES *drug dependence (304.0-304.9)*
            nondependent abuse (305.0-305.9)

☑5ᵗʰ **965.0 Opiates and related narcotics**

  965.00 Opium (alkaloids), unspecified
    AHA: 3Q, '07, 6

  965.01 Heroin
    Diacetylmorphine

  965.02 Methadone

  965.09 Other
    Codeine [methylmorphine]
    Meperidine [pethidine]
    Morphine
    AHA: 3Q, '07, 6
    T40.4x1A Poisoning oth synthetic narc accidnt initial enc 1-10

965.1 Salicylates
  Acetylsalicylic acid [aspirin]
  Salicylic acid salts
  AHA: N-D, '94, 15

965.4 Aromatic analgesics, not elsewhere classified
  Acetanilid
  Paracetamol [acetaminophen]
  Phenacetin [acetophenetidin]

965.5 Pyrazole derivatives
  Aminophenazone [aminopyrine]
  Phenylbutazone

☑5ᵗʰ **965.6 Antirheumatics [antiphlogistics]**
  EXCLUDES *salicylates (965.1)*
            steroids (962.0-962.9)
  AHA: 4Q, '98, 50

  965.61 Propionic acid derivatives
    Fenoprofen
    Flurbiprofen
    Ibuprofen
    Ketoprofen
    Naproxen
    Oxaprozin
    AHA: 4Q, '98, 50

  965.69 Other antirheumatics
    Gold salts
    Indomethacin

965.7 Other non-narcotic analgesics
  Pyrabital

965.8 Other specified analgesics and antipyretics
  Pentazocine

965.9 Unspecified analgesic and antipyretic

☑4ᵗʰ **966 Poisoning by anticonvulsants and anti-Parkinsonism drugs**

966.0 Oxazolidine derivatives
  Paramethadione
  Trimethadione

966.1 Hydantoin derivatives
  Phenytoin

966.2 Succinimides
  Ethosuximide
  Phensuximide

966.3 Other and unspecified anticonvulsants
  Primidone
  EXCLUDES *barbiturates (967.0)*
            sulfonamides (961.0)

966.4 Anti-Parkinsonism drugs
  Amantadine
  Ethopropazine [profenamine]
  Levodopa [L-dopa]

☑4ᵗʰ **967 Poisoning by sedatives and hypnotics**
  EXCLUDES *drug dependence (304.0-304.9)*
            nondependent abuse (305.0-305.9)

967.0 Barbiturates
  Amobarbital [amylobarbitone]
  Barbital [barbitone]
  Butabarbital [butabarbitone]
  Pentobarbital [pentobarbitone]
  Phenobarbital [phenobarbitone]
  Secobarbital [quinalbarbitone]
  EXCLUDES *thiobarbiturate anesthetics (968.3)*

967.1 Chloral hydrate group

967.2 Paraldehyde

967.3 Bromine compounds
  Bromide
  Carbromal (derivatives)

Injury and Poisoning

967.4–971.3

967.4 Methaqualone compounds

967.5 Glutethimide group

967.6 Mixed sedatives, not elsewhere classified

967.8 Other sedatives and hypnotics

967.9 Unspecified sedative or hypnotic
Sleeping:
drug
pill } NOS
tablet

√4ᵗʰ **968 Poisoning by other central nervous system depressants and anesthetics**
EXCLUDES *drug dependence (304.0-304.9)*
nondependent abuse (305.0-305.9)

968.0 Central nervous system muscle-tone depressants
Chlorphenesin (carbamate)
Mephenesin
Methocarbamol

968.1 Halothane

968.2 Other gaseous anesthetics
Ether
Halogenated hydrocarbon derivatives, except halothane
Nitrous oxide

968.3 Intravenous anesthetics
Ketamine
Methohexital [methohexitone]
Thiobarbiturates, such as thiopental sodium

968.4 Other and unspecified general anesthetics

968.5 Surface (topical) and infiltration anesthetics
Cocaine (topical)
Lidocaine (lignocaine)
Procaine
Tetracaine
EXCLUDES *poisoning by cocaine used as a central nervous system stimulant (970.81)*
AHA: 1Q, '93, 25

968.6 Peripheral nerve- and plexus-blocking anesthetics

968.7 Spinal anesthetics

968.9 Other and unspecified local anesthetics
T41.44xA Poisoning uns anesthetic undetermind initial enc   I-10

√4ᵗʰ **969 Poisoning by psychotropic agents**
EXCLUDES *drug dependence (304.0-304.9)*
nondependent abuse (305.0-305.9)

√5ᵗʰ **969.0 Antidepressants**
AHA: 4Q, '09, 111-112

969.00 Antidepressant, unspecified
AHA: 3Q, '07, 6; #5, '94, 9; 3Q, '91, 14; N-D, '84, 14

969.01 Monoamine oxidase inhibitors
MAOI

969.02 Selective serotonin and norepinephrine reuptake inhibitors
SSNRI antidepressants
TIP: Assign for serotonin syndrome due to poisoning, along with 333.99 and E854.0, for accidental poisoning.

969.03 Selective serotonin reuptake inhibitors
SSRI antidepressants
TIP: Assign for serotonin syndrome due to poisoning, along with 333.99 and E854.0, for accidental poisoning.

969.04 Tetracyclic antidepressants

969.05 Tricyclic antidepressants
AHA: 4Q, '09, 112

969.09 Other antidepressants

969.1 Phenothiazine-based tranquilizers
Chlorpromazine
Fluphenazine
Prochlorperazine
Promazine

969.2 Butyrophenone-based tranquilizers
Haloperidol
Spiperone
Trifluperidol

969.3 Other antipsychotics, neuroleptics, and major tranquilizers

969.4 Benzodiazepine-based tranquilizers
Chlordiazepoxide
Diazepam
Flurazepam
Lorazepam
Medazepam
Nitrazepam
AHA: 4Q, '09, 112
T42.4x1D Poisoning benzodiazepines accidental subseq enc   I-10

969.5 Other tranquilizers
Hydroxyzine
Meprobamate

969.6 Psychodysleptics [hallucinogens]
Cannabis (derivatives)
Lysergide [LSD]
Marihuana (derivatives)
Mescaline
Psilocin
Psilocybin

√5ᵗʰ **969.7 Psychostimulants**
EXCLUDES *central appetite depressants (977.0)*
AHA: 4Q, '09, 113-114

969.70 Psychostimulant, unspecified
AHA: 2Q, '03, 11

969.71 Caffeine

969.72 Amphetamines
Methamphetamines
TIP: Assign for overdose and poisoning by the club drug ecstasy.

969.73 Methylphenidate

969.79 Other psychostimulants

969.8 Other specified psychotropic agents

969.9 Unspecified psychotropic agent

√4ᵗʰ **970 Poisoning by central nervous system stimulants**

970.0 Analeptics
Lobeline
Nikethamide

970.1 Opiate antagonists
Levallorphan
Nalorphine
Naloxone

√5ᵗʰ **970.8 Other specified central nervous system stimulants**
AHA: 4Q, '10, 98-99; 1Q, '05, 6

970.81 Cocaine
Crack

970.89 Other central nervous system stimulants

970.9 Unspecified central nervous system stimulant

√4ᵗʰ **971 Poisoning by drugs primarily affecting the autonomic nervous system**

971.0 Parasympathomimetics [cholinergics]
Acetylcholine
Anticholinesterase:
organophosphorus
reversible
Pilocarpine

971.1 Parasympatholytics [anticholinergics and antimuscarinics] and spasmolytics
Atropine
Homatropine
Hyoscine [scopolamine]
Quaternary ammonium derivatives
EXCLUDES *papaverine (972.5)*

971.2 Sympathomimetics [adrenergics]
Epinephrine [adrenalin]
Levarterenol [noradrenalin]

971.3 Sympatholytics [antiadrenergics]
Phenoxybenzamine
Tolazoline hydrochloride

N Newborn Age: 0   P Pediatric Age: 0-17   M Maternity Age: 12-55   A Adult Age: 15-124

971.9 **Unspecified drug primarily affecting autonomic nervous system**

✓4th 972 **Poisoning by agents primarily affecting the cardiovascular system**

972.0 **Cardiac rhythm regulators**
Practolol
Procainamide
Propranolol
Quinidine
EXCLUDES lidocaine (968.5)

972.1 **Cardiotonic glycosides and drugs of similar action**
Digitalis glycosides
Digoxin
Strophanthins

972.2 **Antilipemic and antiarteriosclerotic drugs**
Clofibrate
Nicotinic acid derivatives

972.3 **Ganglion-blocking agents**
Pentamethonium bromide

972.4 **Coronary vasodilators**
Dipyridamole
Nitrates [nitroglycerin]
Nitrites

972.5 **Other vasodilators**
Cyclandelate
Diazoxide
Papaverine
EXCLUDES nicotinic acid (972.2)

972.6 **Other antihypertensive agents**
Clonidine
Guanethidine
Rauwolfia alkaloids
Reserpine

972.7 **Antivaricose drugs, including sclerosing agents**
Sodium morrhuate
Zinc salts

972.8 **Capillary-active drugs**
Adrenochrome derivatives
Metaraminol

972.9 **Other and unspecified agents primarily affecting the cardiovascular system**

✓4th 973 **Poisoning by agents primarily affecting the gastrointestinal system**

973.0 **Antacids and antigastric secretion drugs**
Aluminum hydroxide
Magnesium trisilicate
AHA: 1Q, '03, 19

973.1 **Irritant cathartics**
Bisacodyl
Castor oil
Phenolphthalein

973.2 **Emollient cathartics**
Dioctyl sulfosuccinates

973.3 **Other cathartics, including intestinal atonia drugs**
Magnesium sulfate

973.4 **Digestants**
Pancreatin
Papain
Pepsin

973.5 **Antidiarrheal drugs**
Kaolin
Pectin
EXCLUDES anti-infectives (960.0-961.9)

973.6 **Emetics**

973.8 **Other specified agents primarily affecting the gastrointestinal system**

973.9 **Unspecified agent primarily affecting the gastrointestinal system**

✓4th 974 **Poisoning by water, mineral, and uric acid metabolism drugs**

974.0 **Mercurial diuretics**
Chlormerodrin
Mercaptomerin
Mersalyl

974.1 **Purine derivative diuretics**
Theobromine
Theophylline
EXCLUDES aminophylline [theophylline ethylenediamine] (975.7)
caffeine (969.71)

974.2 **Carbonic acid anhydrase inhibitors**
Acetazolamide

974.3 **Saluretics**
Benzothiadiazides
Chlorothiazide group

974.4 **Other diuretics**
Ethacrynic acid
Furosemide

974.5 **Electrolytic, caloric, and water-balance agents**

974.6 **Other mineral salts, not elsewhere classified**

974.7 **Uric acid metabolism drugs**
Allopurinol
Colchicine
Probenecid

✓4th 975 **Poisoning by agents primarily acting on the smooth and skeletal muscles and respiratory system**

975.0 **Oxytocic agents**
Ergot alkaloids
Oxytocin
Prostaglandins

975.1 **Smooth muscle relaxants**
Adiphenine
Metaproterenol [orciprenaline]
EXCLUDES papaverine (972.5)

975.2 **Skeletal muscle relaxants**

975.3 **Other and unspecified drugs acting on muscles**

975.4 **Antitussives**
Dextromethorphan
Pipazethate

975.5 **Expectorants**
Acetylcysteine
Guaifenesin
Terpin hydrate

975.6 **Anti-common cold drugs**

975.7 **Antiasthmatics**
Aminophylline [theophylline ethylenediamine]

975.8 **Other and unspecified respiratory drugs**

✓4th 976 **Poisoning by agents primarily affecting skin and mucous membrane, ophthalmological, otorhinolaryngological, and dental drugs**

976.0 **Local anti-infectives and anti-inflammatory drugs**

976.1 **Antipruritics**

976.2 **Local astringents and local detergents**

976.3 **Emollients, demulcents, and protectants**

976.4 **Keratolytics, keratoplastics, other hair treatment drugs and preparations**

976.5 **Eye anti-infectives and other eye drugs**
Idoxuridine

976.6 **Anti-infectives and other drugs and preparations for ear, nose, and throat**

976.7 **Dental drugs topically applied**
EXCLUDES anti-infectives (976.0)
local anesthetics (968.5)

976.8 **Other agents primarily affecting skin and mucous membrane**
Spermicides [vaginal contraceptives]

976.9 Unspecified agent primarily affecting skin and mucous membrane

☑4ᵗʰ **977 Poisoning by other and unspecified drugs and medicinal substances**

977.0 Dietetics
Central appetite depressants

977.1 Lipotropic drugs

977.2 Antidotes and chelating agents, not elsewhere classified

977.3 Alcohol deterrents

977.4 Pharmaceutical excipients
Pharmaceutical adjuncts

977.8 Other specified drugs and medicinal substances
Contrast media used for diagnostic x-ray procedures
Diagnostic agents and kits

977.9 Unspecified drug or medicinal substance

☑4ᵗʰ **978 Poisoning by bacterial vaccines**

978.0 BCG

978.1 Typhoid and paratyphoid

978.2 Cholera

978.3 Plague

978.4 Tetanus

978.5 Diphtheria

978.6 Pertussis vaccine, including combinations with a pertussis component

978.8 Other and unspecified bacterial vaccines

978.9 Mixed bacterial vaccines, except combinations with a pertussis component

☑4ᵗʰ **979 Poisoning by other vaccines and biological substances**
EXCLUDES *gamma globulin (964.6)*

979.0 Smallpox vaccine

979.1 Rabies vaccine

979.2 Typhus vaccine

979.3 Yellow fever vaccine

979.4 Measles vaccine

979.5 Poliomyelitis vaccine

979.6 Other and unspecified viral and rickettsial vaccines
Mumps vaccine

979.7 Mixed viral-rickettsial and bacterial vaccines, except combinations with a pertussis component
EXCLUDES *combinations with a pertussis component (978.6)*

979.9 Other and unspecified vaccines and biological substances

Toxic Effects of Substances Chiefly Nonmedicinal as to Source (980-989)

Use additional code to identify:
personal history of retained foreign body fully removed (V15.53)
retained foreign body status, if applicable, (V90.01-V90.9)

Use additional code to specify the nature of the toxic effect

EXCLUDES *burns from chemical agents (ingested) (947.0-947.9)*
localized toxic effects indexed elsewhere (001.0-799.9)
respiratory conditions due to external agents (506.0-508.9)
respiratory conditions due to smoke inhalation NOS (508.2)
AHA: 3Q, '10, 19

☑4ᵗʰ **980 Toxic effect of alcohol**

980.0 Ethyl alcohol
Denatured alcohol   Grain alcohol
Ethanol

Use additional code to identify any associated:
acute alcohol intoxication (305.0)
in alcoholism (303.0)
drunkenness (simple) (305.0)
pathological (291.4)
AHA: 4Q, '09, 112; 3Q, '96, 16
T51.0x1A Toxic effect ethanol accidental initial encountr   I-10

980.1 Methyl alcohol
Methanol
Wood alcohol

980.2 Isopropyl alcohol
Dimethyl carbinol
Isopropanol
Rubbing alcohol

980.3 Fusel oil
Alcohol:
amyl
butyl
propyl

980.8 Other specified alcohols

980.9 Unspecified alcohol

981 Toxic effect of petroleum products
Benzine   Petroleum:
Gasoline   ether
Kerosene   naphtha
Paraffin wax   spirit

☑4ᵗʰ **982 Toxic effect of solvents other than petroleum-based**

982.0 Benzene and homologues

982.1 Carbon tetrachloride

982.2 Carbon disulfide
Carbon bisulfide

982.3 Other chlorinated hydrocarbon solvents
Tetrachloroethylene
Trichloroethylene
EXCLUDES *chlorinated hydrocarbon preparations other than solvents (989.2)*
AHA: 3Q, '08, 6-7

982.4 Nitroglycol

982.8 Other nonpetroleum-based solvents
Acetone

☑4ᵗʰ **983 Toxic effect of corrosive aromatics, acids, and caustic alkalis**

983.0 Corrosive aromatics
Carbolic acid or phenol
Cresol

983.1 Acids
Acid:
hydrochloric
nitric
sulfuric

983.2 Caustic alkalis
Lye
Potassium hydroxide
Sodium hydroxide

983.9 Caustic, unspecified

☑4ᵗʰ **984 Toxic effect of lead and its compounds (including fumes)**
INCLUDES that from all sources except medicinal substances

984.0 Inorganic lead compounds
Lead dioxide
Lead salts

984.1 Organic lead compounds
Lead acetate
Tetraethyl lead

984.8 Other lead compounds

984.9 Unspecified lead compound

☑4ᵗʰ **985 Toxic effect of other metals**
INCLUDES that from all sources except medicinal substances

985.0 Mercury and its compounds
Minamata disease

985.1 Arsenic and its compounds

985.2 Manganese and its compounds

985.3 Beryllium and its compounds

985.4 Antimony and its compounds

985.5 Cadmium and its compounds

985.6 Chromium

985.8 Other specified metals
   Brass fumes
   Copper salts
   Iron compounds
   Nickel compounds
   AHA: 1Q, '88, 5
   TIP: Assign for aluminum overloading or excessive concentration of aluminum in the body, along with E879.1 if due to renal dialysis and E879.8 if due to total parenteral nutrition.

985.9 Unspecified metal

986 Toxic effect of carbon monoxide
   Carbon monoxide from any source

√4ᵗʰ **987 Toxic effect of other gases, fumes, or vapors**

987.0 Liquefied petroleum gases
   Butane
   Propane

987.1 Other hydrocarbon gas

987.2 Nitrogen oxides
   Nitrogen dioxide
   Nitrous fumes

987.3 Sulfur dioxide

987.4 Freon
   Dichloromonofluoromethane

987.5 Lacrimogenic gas
   Bromobenzyl cyanide
   Chloroacetophenone
   Ethyliodoacetate

987.6 Chlorine gas

987.7 Hydrocyanic acid gas

987.8 Other specified gases, fumes, or vapors
   Phosgene
   Polyester fumes

987.9 Unspecified gas, fume, or vapor
   AHA: 4Q, '11, 114; 3Q, '05, 10
   TIP: ►Do not assign for conditions due to smoke inhalation; assign instead code 508.2.◄

988 Toxic effect of noxious substances eaten as food
   EXCLUDES allergic reaction to food, such as:
      gastroenteritis (558.3)
      rash (692.5, 693.1)
      food poisoning (bacterial) (005.0-005.9)
      toxic effects of food contaminants, such as:
         aflatoxin and other mycotoxin (989.7)
         mercury (985.0)

988.0 Fish and shellfish

988.1 Mushrooms

988.2 Berries and other plants

988.8 Other specified noxious substances eaten as food

988.9 Unspecified noxious substance eaten as food

√4ᵗʰ **989 Toxic effect of other substances, chiefly nonmedicinal as to source**

989.0 Hydrocyanic acid and cyanides
   Potassium cyanide
   Sodium cyanide
   EXCLUDES gas and fumes (987.7)

989.1 Strychnine and salts

989.2 Chlorinated hydrocarbons
   Aldrin
   Chlordane
   DDT
   Dieldrin
   EXCLUDES chlorinated hydrocarbon solvents (982.0-982.3)

989.3 Organophosphate and carbamate
   Carbaryl
   Dichlorvos
   Malathion
   Parathion
   Phorate
   Phosdrin

989.4 Other pesticides, not elsewhere classified
   Mixtures of insecticides

989.5 Venom
   Bites of venomous snakes, lizards, and spiders
   Tick paralysis

989.6 Soaps and detergents

989.7 Aflatoxin and other mycotoxin [food contaminants]

√5ᵗʰ **989.8 Other substances, chiefly nonmedicinal as to source**
   AHA: 4Q, '95, 60

   989.81 Asbestos
      EXCLUDES asbestosis (501)
                exposure to asbestos (V15.84)

   989.82 Latex

   989.83 Silicone
      EXCLUDES silicone used in medical devices, implants and grafts (996.00-996.79)

   989.84 Tobacco

   989.89 Other

989.9 Unspecified substance, chiefly nonmedicinal as to source

Other and Unspecified Effects of External Causes (990-995)

990 Effects of radiation, unspecified
   Complication of:
      phototherapy
      radiation therapy
   Radiation sickness
   [The type of radiation giving rise to the adverse effect may be identified by use of the E codes.]
   EXCLUDES specified adverse effects of radiation. Such conditions are to be classified according to the nature of the adverse effect, as:
      burns (940.0-949.5)
      dermatitis (692.7-692.8)
      leukemia (204.0-208.9)
      pneumonia (508.0)
      sunburn (692.71, 692.76-692.77)

√4ᵗʰ **991 Effects of reduced temperature**

991.0 Frostbite of face

991.1 Frostbite of hand

991.2 Frostbite of foot

991.3 Frostbite of other and unspecified sites

991.4 Immersion foot
   Trench foot
   DEF: Paresthesia, edema, blotchy cyanosis of foot, the skin is soft (macerated), pale and wrinkled, and the sole is swollen with surface ridging and following sustained immersion in water.

991.5 Chilblains
   Erythema pernio
   Perniosis
   DEF: Red, swollen, itchy skin; follows damp cold exposure; also associated with pruritus and a burning feeling in hands, feet, ears, and face in children, legs and toes in women, and hands and fingers in men.

991.6 Hypothermia
   Hypothermia (accidental)
   EXCLUDES hypothermia following anesthesia (995.89)
             hypothermia not associated with low environmental temperature (780.65)
   DEF: Reduced body temperature due to low environmental temperatures.

991.8 Other specified effects of reduced temperature

Injury and Poisoning

991.9–995.21

991.9 Unspecified effect of reduced temperature
Effects of freezing or excessive cold NOS

✓4ᵗʰ **992 Effects of heat and light**
    EXCLUDES *burns (940.0-949.5)*
       diseases of sweat glands due to heat (705.0-705.9)
       malignant hyperpyrexia following anesthesia (995.86)
       sunburn (692.71, 692.76-692.77)

992.0 Heat stroke and sunstroke
Heat apoplexy	Siriasis
Heat pyrexia	Thermoplegia
Ictus solaris	

Use additional code(s) to identify any associated complication of heat stroke, such as:
    alterations of consciousness (780.01-780.09)
    systemic inflammatory response syndrome (995.93-995.94)
DEF: Headache, vertigo, cramps and elevated body temperature due to high environmental temperatures.

992.1 Heat syncope
Heat collapse

992.2 Heat cramps

992.3 Heat exhaustion, anhydrotic
Heat prostration due to water depletion
    EXCLUDES *that associated with salt depletion (992.4)*

992.4 Heat exhaustion due to salt depletion
Heat prostration due to salt (and water) depletion

992.5 Heat exhaustion, unspecified
Heat prostration NOS

992.6 Heat fatigue, transient

992.7 Heat edema
DEF: Fluid retention due to high environmental temperatures.

992.8 Other specified heat effects

992.9 Unspecified

✓4ᵗʰ **993 Effects of air pressure**

993.0 Barotrauma, otitic
Aero-otitis media
Effects of high altitude on ears
DEF: Ringing ears, deafness, pain and vertigo due to air pressure changes.

993.1 Barotrauma, sinus
Aerosinusitis
Effects of high altitude on sinuses

993.2 Other and unspecified effects of high altitude
Alpine sickness	Hypobaropathy
Andes disease	Mountain sickness
Anoxia due to high altitude	

AHA: 3Q, '88, 4

993.3 Caisson disease
Bends
Compressed-air disease
Decompression sickness
Divers' palsy or paralysis
DEF: Rapid reduction in air pressure while breathing compressed air; symptoms include skin lesions, joint pains, respiratory and neurological problems.

993.4 Effects of air pressure caused by explosion

993.8 Other specified effects of air pressure

993.9 Unspecified effect of air pressure

✓4ᵗʰ **994 Effects of other external causes**
    EXCLUDES *certain adverse effects not elsewhere classified (995.0-995.8)*

994.0 Effects of lightning
Shock from lightning
Struck by lightning NOS
    EXCLUDES *burns (940.0-949.5)*

994.1 Drowning and nonfatal submersion
Bathing cramp
Immersion
AHA: 3Q, '09, 14; 3Q, '88, 4
TIP: When near-drowning results in acute respiratory edema, assign also code 518.5 Post-traumatic pulmonary insufficiency.

994.2 Effects of hunger
Deprivation of food
Starvation

994.3 Effects of thirst
Deprivation of water

994.4 Exhaustion due to exposure

994.5 Exhaustion due to excessive exertion
Exhaustion due to overexertion

994.6 Motion sickness
Air sickness	Travel sickness
Seasickness	

994.7 Asphyxiation and strangulation
Suffocation (by):	Suffocation (by):
bedclothes	plastic bag
cave-in	pressure
constriction	strangulation
mechanical	

    EXCLUDES *asphyxia from:*
       carbon monoxide (986)
       inhalation of food or foreign body (932-934.9)
       other gases, fumes, and vapors (987.0-987.9)

994.8 Electrocution and nonfatal effects of electric current
Shock from electric current
Shock from electroshock gun (taser)
    EXCLUDES *electric burns (940.0-949.5)*

994.9 Other effects of external causes
Effects of:
    abnormal gravitational [G] forces or states
    weightlessness

✓4ᵗʰ **995 Certain adverse effects not elsewhere classified**
    EXCLUDES *complications of surgical and medical care (996.0-999.9)*

995.0 Other anaphylactic reaction
Allergic shock
Anaphylactic reaction
Anaphylactic shock NOS or due to adverse effect of correct medicinal substance properly administered
Anaphylactoid reaction, NOS
Anaphylaxis

Use additional E code to identify external cause, such as:
    adverse effects of correct medicinal substance properly administered [E930-E949]
    EXCLUDES *anaphylactic reaction to serum (999.41-999.49)*
       anaphylactic shock or reaction due to adverse food reaction (995.60-995.69)
DEF: Immediate sensitivity response after exposure to specific antigen; results in life-threatening respiratory distress; usually followed by vascular collapse, shock, urticaria, angioedema and pruritus.
AHA: 4Q, '93, 30

995.1 Angioneurotic edema
Allergic angioedema
Giant urticaria
    EXCLUDES *urticaria:*
       due to serum (999.51-999.59)
       other specified (698.2, 708.0-708.9, 757.33)
DEF: Circulatory response of deep dermis, subcutaneous or submucosal tissues; causes localized edema and wheals.

✓5ᵗʰ **995.2 Other and unspecified adverse effect of drug, medicinal and biological substance**
    EXCLUDES *pathological drug intoxication (292.2)*
AHA: 2Q, '97, 12; 3Q, '95, 13; 3Q, '92, 16
TIP: Codes from this subcategory should not be assigned for inpatient cases; their use is limited to certain outpatient cases in which there is no documentation of specific symptoms associated with the adverse effect.

995.20 Unspecified adverse effect of unspecified drug, medicinal and biological substance
Unspecified adverse effect of unspecified medicinal substance properly administered
AHA: 4Q, '06, 112

995.21 Arthus phenomenon
Arthus reaction
AHA: 4Q, '06, 112

995.22 Unspecified adverse effect of anesthesia
AHA: 4Q, '06, 112

995.23 Unspecified adverse effect of insulin
AHA: 4Q, '06, 112

995.24 Failed moderate sedation during procedure
Failed conscious sedation during procedure
AHA: 4Q, '09, 114
TIP: If documentation indicates a personal history of failed moderate sedation, assign instead code V15.80 History of failed moderate sedation.

995.27 Other drug allergy
Allergic reaction NEC (due) to correct medical substance properly administered
Drug allergy NOS
Drug hypersensitivity NOS
Hypersensitivity (due) to correct medical substance properly administered
AHA: 4Q, '06, 112

995.29 Unspecified adverse effect of other drug, medicinal and biological substance
Unspecified adverse effect of medicinal substance NEC properly administered
AHA: 4Q, '06, 112

995.3 Allergy, unspecified
Allergic reaction NOS   Idiosyncrasy NOS
Hypersensitivity NOS
EXCLUDES *allergic reaction NOS to correct medicinal substance properly administered (995.27)*
allergy to existing dental restorative materials (525.66)
specific types of allergic reaction, such as:
allergic diarrhea (558.3)
dermatitis (691.0-693.9)
hayfever (477.0-477.9)

995.4 Shock due to anesthesia
Shock due to anesthesia in which the correct substance was properly administered
EXCLUDES *complications of anesthesia in labor or delivery (668.0-668.9)*
overdose or wrong substance given (968.0-969.9)
postoperative shock NOS (998.00)
specified adverse effects of anesthesia classified elsewhere, such as:
anoxic brain damage (348.1)
hepatitis (070.0-070.9), etc.
unspecified adverse effect of anesthesia (995.22)

√5ᵗʰ **995.5 Child maltreatment syndrome**
Use additional code(s), if applicable, to identify any associated injuries

Use additional E code to identify:
nature of abuse (E960-E968)
perpetrator (E967.0-E967.9)
AHA: 1Q, '98, 11
TIP: Although separate codes for any associated injuries should be assigned, codes from this subcategory may be assigned alone if there are no documented injuries or associated conditions.

995.50 Child abuse, unspecified P

995.51 Child emotional/psychological abuse P
AHA: 4Q, '96, 38, 40

995.52 Child neglect (nutritional) P
AHA: 4Q, '96, 38, 40

995.53 Child sexual abuse P
AHA: 4Q, '96, 39, 40

995.54 Child physical abuse P
Battered baby or child syndrome
EXCLUDES *shaken infant syndrome (995.55)*
AHA: 3Q, '99, 14; 4Q, '96, 39, 40

995.55 Shaken infant syndrome P
Use additional code(s) to identify any associated injuries
AHA: 4Q, '96, 40, 43

995.59 Other child abuse and neglect P
Multiple forms of abuse

√5ᵗʰ **995.6 Anaphylactic reaction due to food**
Anaphylactic reaction due to adverse food reaction
Anaphylactic shock or reaction due to nonpoisonous foods
Anaphylactoid reaction due to food
AHA: ▶4Q, '11, 142-145;◀ 4Q, '93, 30
TIP: Codes from this subcategory may be assigned not only for anaphylactic shock, but also for any documentation of anaphylactic reaction to food.

995.60 Anaphylactic reaction due to unspecified food

995.61 Anaphylactic reaction due to peanuts

995.62 Anaphylactic reaction due to crustaceans

995.63 Anaphylactic reaction due to fruits and vegetables

995.64 Anaphylactic reaction due to tree nuts and seeds
AHA: 1Q, '08, 12

995.65 Anaphylactic reaction due to fish

995.66 Anaphylactic reaction due to food additives

995.67 Anaphylactic reaction due to milk products

995.68 Anaphylactic reaction due to eggs

995.69 Anaphylactic reaction due to other specified food

995.7 Other adverse food reactions, not elsewhere classified
Use additional code to identify the type of reaction, such as:
hives (708.0)
wheezing (786.07)
EXCLUDES *anaphylactic reaction or shock due to adverse food reaction (995.60-995.69)*
asthma (493.0, 493.9)
dermatitis due to food (693.1)
in contact with skin (692.5)
gastroenteritis and colitis due to food (558.3)
rhinitis due to food (477.1)

√5ᵗʰ **995.8 Other specified adverse effects, not elsewhere classified**

995.80 Adult maltreatment, unspecified A
Abused person NOS
Use additional code to identify:
any associated injury
perpetrator (E967.0-E967.9)
AHA: 4Q, '96, 41, 43

995.81 Adult physical abuse A
Battered:
person syndrome NEC
man
spouse
woman
Use additional code to identify:
any association injury
nature of abuse (E960-E968)
perpetrator (E967.0-E967.9)
AHA: 4Q, '96, 42, 43

995.82 Adult emotional/psychological abuse A
Use additional E code to identify perpetrator (E967.0-E967.9)

995.83 Adult sexual abuse A
Use additional code(s) to identify:
any associated injury
perpetrator (E967.0-E967.9)

995.84 Adult neglect (nutritional) A
Use additional code(s) to identify:
intent of neglect (E904.0, E968.4)
perpetrator (E967.0-E967.9)

Continuum of Illness Due to Infection

Bacteremia ➡ Septicemia ➡ Sepsis

Severe Sepsis with Septic Shock ⬅ Severe Sepsis ⬅

MODS (Multiple Organ Dysfunction Syndrome) ➡ Death

995.85 Other adult abuse and neglect   [A]
Multiple forms of abuse and neglect

Use additional code(s) to identify
  any associated injury
  intent of neglect (E904.0, E968.4)
  nature of abuse (E960-E968)
  perpetrator (E967.0-E967.9)

995.86 Malignant hyperthermia
Malignant hyperpyrexia due to anesthesia
AHA: 4Q, '98, 51

995.89 Other
Hypothermia due to anesthesia
AHA: 2Q, '04, 18; 3Q, '03, 12

√5ᵗʰ 995.9 Systemic inflammatory response syndrome (SIRS)
DEF: Clinical response to infection or trauma that can trigger an acute inflammatory reaction and progresses to coagulation, impaired fibrinolysis, and organ failure; manifested by two or more of the following symptoms: fever, tachycardia, tachypnea, leukocytosis or leukopenia.
AHA: 4Q, '06, 113-116; 2Q, '04, 16; 4Q, '02, 71
TIP: Coding these conditions requires a minimum of two codes: the underlying cause (e.g., Infection or trauma) is sequenced first, followed by a code from subcategory 995.9.

995.90 Systemic inflammatory response syndrome, unspecified
SIRS NOS

995.91 Sepsis
Systemic inflammatory response syndrome due to infectious process without acute organ dysfunction

Code first underlying infection
EXCLUDES sepsis with acute organ dysfunction (995.92)
  sepsis with multiple organ dysfunction (995.92)
  severe sepsis (995.92)
AHA: ▶3Q, '11, 15;◀4Q, '08, 72; 4Q, '07, 86; 4Q, '06, 113-116; 2Q, '04, 16; 4Q, '03, 79

995.92 Severe sepsis
Sepsis with acute organ dysfunction
Sepsis with multiple organ dysfunction (MOD)
Systemic inflammatory response syndrome due to infectious process with acute organ dysfunction

Code first underlying infection
Use additional code to specify acute organ dysfunction, such as:
  acute kidney failure (584.5-584.9)
  acute respiratory failure (518.81)
  critical illness myopathy (359.81)
  critical illness polyneuropathy (357.82)
  disseminated intravascular coagulopathy [DIC] (286.6)
  encephalopathy (348.31)
  hepatic failure (570)
  septic shock (785.52)
AHA: ▶4Q, '11, 153;◀2Q, '10, 4; 4Q, '09, 98; 4Q, '08, 99; 4Q, '07, 97; 4Q, '06, 113-116; 2Q, '05, 18-19; 1Q, '05, 7; 1Q, '05, 7; 2Q, '04, 16; 4Q, '03, 73, 79
R65.21 Severe sepsis with septic shock   [I-10]

995.93 Systemic inflammatory response syndrome due to noninfectious process without acute organ dysfunction
Code first underlying conditions, such as:
  acute pancreatitis (577.0)
  trauma
EXCLUDES systemic inflammatory response syndrome due to noninfectious process with acute organ dysfunction (995.94)
AHA: 1Q, '11, 22; 1Q, '10, 10-11; 4Q, '06, 113-116

995.94 Systemic inflammatory response syndrome due to noninfectious process with acute organ dysfunction
Code first underlying conditions, such as:
  acute pancreatitis (577.0)
  heat stroke (992.0)
  trauma
Use additional code to specify acute organ dysfunction, such as:
  acute kidney failure (584.5-584.9)
  acute respiratory failure (518.81)
  critical illness myopathy (359.81)
  critical illness polyneuropathy (357.82)
  disseminated intravascular coagulopathy [DIC] syndrome (286.6)
  encephalopathy (348.31)
  hepatic failure (570)
EXCLUDES severe sepsis (995.92)
AHA: 1Q, '10, 10; 4Q, '06, 113-116; 4Q, '03, 79

Complications of Surgical and Medical Care, Not Elsewhere Classified (996-999)
EXCLUDES adverse effects of medicinal agents (001.0-799.9, 995.0-995.8)
  burns from local applications and irradiation (940.0-949.5)
  complications of:
    conditions for which the procedure was performed
    surgical procedures during abortion, labor, and delivery (630-676.9)
  poisoning and toxic effects of drugs and chemicals (960.0-989.9)
  postoperative conditions in which no complications are present, such as:
    artificial opening status (V44.0-V44.9)
    closure of external stoma (V55.0-V55.9)
    fitting of prosthetic device (V52.0-V52.9)
  specified complications classified elsewhere
    anesthetic shock (995.4)
    electrolyte imbalance (276.0-276.9)
    postlaminectomy syndrome (722.80-722.83)
    postmastectomy lymphedema syndrome (457.0)
    postoperative psychosis (293.0-293.9)
  any other condition classified elsewhere in the Alphabetic Index when described as due to a procedure

√4ᵗʰ 996 Complications peculiar to certain specified procedures
INCLUDES complications, not elsewhere classified, in the use of artificial substitutes [e.g., Dacron, metal, Silastic, Teflon] or natural sources [e.g., bone] involving:
  anastomosis (internal)
  graft (bypass) (patch)
  implant
  internal device:
    catheter
    electronic
    fixation
    prosthetic
  reimplant
  transplant
EXCLUDES accidental puncture or laceration during procedure (998.2)
  capsular contracture of breast implant (611.83)
  complications of internal anastomosis of:
    gastrointestinal tract (997.49)
    urinary tract (997.5)
  endosseous dental implant failures (525.71-525.79)
  intraoperative floppy iris syndrome [IFIS] (364.81)
  mechanical complication of respirator (V46.14)
  other specified complications classified elsewhere, such as:
    hemolytic anemia (283.1)
    functional cardiac disturbances (429.4)
    serum hepatitis (070.2-070.3)
AHA: 1Q, '94, 3

| N Newborn Age: 0 | P Pediatric Age: 0-17 | M Maternity Age: 12-55 | A Adult Age: 15-124 |

√5ᵗʰ **996.0 Mechanical complication of cardiac device, implant, and graft**

Breakdown (mechanical)	Obstruction, mechanical
Displacement	Perforation
Leakage	Protrusion

AHA: 2Q, '08, 9; 2Q, '93, 9

TIP: If the documentation indicates that the cardiac device (e.g., pacemaker, heart valve prosthesis) has reached its normally occurring end of life, do not assign a complication code; see instead subcategory V53.3.

996.00 Unspecified device, implant, and graft

996.01 Due to cardiac pacemaker (electrode)
> AHA: 2Q, '06, 15; 2Q, '99, 11
> T82.120A Displacement cardiac electrode initial encounter   I-10

996.02 Due to heart valve prosthesis

996.03 Due to coronary bypass graft
> EXCLUDES   atherosclerosis of graft (414.02, 414.03)
> embolism [occlusion NOS] [thrombus] of graft (996.72)
> AHA: 2Q, '95, 17; N-D, '86, 5

996.04 Due to automatic implantable cardiac defibrillator
> AHA: 2Q, '05, 3

996.09 Other
> AHA: 2Q, '93, 9

996.1 Mechanical complication of other vascular device, implant, and graft

Mechanical complications involving:
> aortic (bifurcation) graft (replacement)
> arteriovenous:
>> dialysis catheter
>> fistula   } surgically created
>> shunt
>
> balloon (counterpulsation) device, intra-aortic
> carotid artery bypass graft
> femoral-popliteal bypass graft
> umbrella device, vena cava

> EXCLUDES   atherosclerosis of biological graft (440.30-440.32)
> embolism [occlusion NOS] [thrombus] of (biological) (synthetic) graft (996.74)
> peritoneal dialysis catheter (996.56)

AHA: ►1Q, '12, 18;◄ 1Q, '11, 5; 1Q, '06, 10; 2Q, '05, 8; 1Q, '02, 13; 1Q, '95, 3

TIP: Assign for a nonmaturing AV fistula and also for postprocedural reduction in transjugular intrahepatic portosystemic shunt flow in a patient with a TIPS catheter.

T82.330A Leakage aortic bifurcation graft initial enc   I-10

996.2 Mechanical complication of nervous system device, implant, and graft

Mechanical complications involving:
> dorsal column stimulator
> electrodes implanted in brain [brain "pacemaker"]
> peripheral nerve graft
> ventricular (communicating) shunt

AHA: 2Q, '99, 4; S-O, '87, 10

√5ᵗʰ **996.3 Mechanical complication of genitourinary device, implant, and graft**
> AHA: 3Q, '01, 13; S-O, '85, 3

996.30 Unspecified device, implant, and graft

996.31 Due to urethral [indwelling] catheter

996.32 Due to intrauterine contraceptive device   ♀

996.39 Other
> Prosthetic reconstruction of vas deferens
> Repair (graft) of ureter without mention of resection
> EXCLUDES   complications due to:
>> external stoma of urinary tract (596.81-596.83)
>> internal anastomosis of urinary tract (997.5)

√5ᵗʰ **996.4 Mechanical complication of internal orthopedic device, implant, and graft**

Mechanical complications involving:
> external (fixation) device utilizing internal screw(s), pin(s) or other methods of fixation
> grafts of bone, cartilage, muscle, or tendon
> internal (fixation) device such as nail, plate, rod, etc.

Use additional code to identify prosthetic joint with mechanical complication (V43.60-V43.69)

> EXCLUDES   complications of external orthopedic device, such as: pressure ulcer due to cast (707.00-707.09)

AHA: 4Q, '05, 91; 2Q, '99, 10; 2Q, '98, 19; 2Q, '96, 11; 3Q, '95, 16; N-D, '85, 11

TIP: Since these codes may be used for any joint device complications, assign an additional code from subcategory V43.6 to specify the joint involved.

996.40 Unspecified mechanical complication of internal orthopedic device, implant, and graft

996.41 Mechanical loosening of prosthetic joint
> Aseptic loosening
> AHA: 4Q, '05, 112
> T84.031A Mech loosening int lt hip prosth jnt initial enc   I-10

996.42 Dislocation of prosthetic joint
> Instability of prosthetic joint
> Subluxation of prosthetic joint
> T84.020D Displacment internal right hip prosth subsqt enc   I-10

996.43 Broken prosthetic joint implant
> Breakage (fracture) of prosthetic joint

996.44 Peri-prosthetic fracture around prosthetic joint
> AHA: 4Q, '05, 93

996.45 Peri-prosthetic osteolysis
> Use additional code to identify major osseous defect, if applicable (731.3)
> AHA: 4Q, '06, 103

996.46 Articular bearing surface wear of prosthetic joint

996.47 Other mechanical complication of prosthetic joint implant
> Mechanical complication of prosthetic joint NOS
> Prosthetic joint implant failure NOS

996.49 Other mechanical complication of other internal orthopedic device, implant, and graft
> Breakage of internal fixation device in bone
> Dislocation of internal fixation device in bone
> EXCLUDES   mechanical complication of prosthetic joint implant (996.41-996.47)
> AHA: 1Q, '10, 7

√5ᵗʰ **996.5 Mechanical complication of other specified prosthetic device, implant, and graft**

Mechanical complications involving:
> nonabsorbable surgical material NOS
> other graft, implant, and internal device, not elsewhere classified
> prosthetic implant in:
>> bile duct
>> breast
>> chin
>> orbit of eye

AHA: 1Q, '98, 11

996.51 Due to corneal graft
> AHA: 2Q, '10, 4-5

996.52 Due to graft of other tissue, not elsewhere classified
> Skin graft failure or rejection
> EXCLUDES   failure of artificial skin graft (996.55)
> failure of decellularized allodermis (996.55)
> sloughing of temporary skin allografts or xenografts (pigskin) — omit code
> AHA: 1Q, '96, 10

996.53 Due to ocular lens prosthesis
> EXCLUDES   contact lenses — code to condition
> AHA: 1Q, '00, 9

√4ᵗʰ
√5ᵗʰ Additional Digit Required   Unspecified Code   Other Specified Code   Manifestation Code   ►◄ Revised Text   ● New Code   ▲ Revised Code Title

2013 ICD-9-CM   **October 2012 • Volume 1 – 311**

Injury and Poisoning

996.54–996.72

996.54 Due to breast prosthesis
Breast capsule (prosthesis)
Mammary implant
AHA: 2Q, '98, 14; 3Q, '92, 4
TIP: If documentation indicates capsular contracture of breast implant, see instead code 611.83.

996.55 Due to artificial skin graft and decellularized allodermis
Dislodgement
Displacement
Failure
Non-adherence
Poor incorporation
Shearing
AHA: 4Q, '98, 52

996.56 Due to peritoneal dialysis catheter
EXCLUDES *mechanical complication of arteriovenous dialysis catheter (996.1)*
AHA: 4Q, '98, 54

996.57 Due to insulin pump
AHA: 4Q, '03, 81-82

996.59 Due to other implant and internal device, not elsewhere classified
Nonabsorbable surgical material NOS
Prosthetic implant in:
  bile duct
  chin
  orbit of eye
AHA: 1Q, '11, 10-11; 2Q, '99, 13; 3Q, '94, 7
TIP: Assign for clogged biliary stent and also for nonfunctioning pressure equalization (PE) tubes.

√5ᵗʰ **996.6 Infection and inflammatory reaction due to internal prosthetic device, implant, and graft**
Infection (causing obstruction) } due to (presence of) any device,
Inflammation implant, and graft
classifiable to 996.0-996.5
Use additional code to identify specified infections
AHA: 2Q, '89, 16; J-F, '87, 14

996.60 Due to unspecified device, implant, and graft

996.61 Due to cardiac device, implant, and graft
Cardiac pacemaker or defibrillator:
  electrode(s), lead(s)
  pulse generator
  subcutaneous pocket
Coronary artery bypass graft
Heart valve prosthesis

996.62 Due to other vascular device, implant, and graft
Arterial graft
Arteriovenous fistula or shunt
Infusion pump
Vascular catheter (arterial) (dialysis) (peripheral venous)
EXCLUDES *infection due to:*
  central venous catheter (999.31-999.32)
  Hickman catheter (999.31-999.32)
  peripherally inserted central catheter [PICC] (999.31-999.32)
  portacath (port-a-cath) (999.31-999.32)
  triple lumen catheter (999.31-999.32)
  umbilical venous catheter (999.31-999.32)
AHA: 2Q, '10, 8; 4Q, '07, 86; 2Q, '04, 16; 1Q, '04, 5; 4Q, '03, 107, 111; 2Q, '03, 7; 2Q, '94, 13
T82.7xxA Inf & inflam react oth card vasc dev gft initial enc [I-10]

996.63 Due to nervous system device, implant, and graft
Electrodes implanted in brain
Peripheral nerve graft
Spinal canal catheter
Ventricular (communicating) shunt (catheter)

996.64 Due to indwelling urinary catheter
Use additional code to identify specified infections, such as:
  cystitis (595.0-595.9)
  sepsis (038.0-038.9)
EXCLUDES *complications due to:*
  external stoma of urinary tract (596.81-596.83)
AHA: ▶1Q, '12, 11;◄ 3Q, '09, 10-11; 3Q, '93, 6
TIP: Assign for documented infection due to the presence of an indwelling urinary catheter, whether Foley, suprapubic, or other type.
T83.51xD Inf & inflam react indwll urinary cath subsq enc [I-10]

996.65 Due to other genitourinary device implant, and graft
Intrauterine contraceptive device
AHA: 1Q, '00, 15

996.66 Due to internal joint prosthesis
Use additional code to identify infected prosthetic joint (V43.60-V43.69)
AHA: 2Q, '08, 3-5; 2Q, '07, 7; 4Q, '05, 91, 113; 2Q, '91, 18
TIP: Do not assign for the second admission of a staged procedure whereby the infected prosthesis has been previously removed and the patient now returns for placement of a new prosthesis; see instead codes from category 736.
T84.51xA Inf & inflam reaction int rt hip pros initial enc [I-10]

996.67 Due to other internal orthopedic device, implant, and graft
Bone growth stimulator (electrode)
Internal fixation device (pin) (rod) (screw)

996.68 Due to peritoneal dialysis catheter
Exit-site infection or inflammation
AHA: 4Q, '98, 54

996.69 Due to other internal prosthetic device, implant, and graft
Breast prosthesis
Ocular lens prosthesis
Prosthetic orbital implant
AHA: 1Q, '11, 10; 2Q, '08, 11; 4Q, '03, 108; 4Q, '98, 52

√5ᵗʰ **996.7 Other complications of internal (biological) (synthetic) prosthetic device, implant, and graft**
Complication NOS
Occlusion NOS
Embolism
Fibrosis } due to (presence of) any device,
Hemorrhage implant, and graft
Pain classifiable to 996.0-996.5
Stenosis
Thrombus
Use additional code to identify complication, such as:
  pain due to presence of device, implant or graft (338.18-338.19, 338.28-338.29)
  venous embolism and thrombosis (453.2-453.9)
EXCLUDES *disruption (dehiscence) of internal suture material (998.31)*
  transplant rejection (996.80-996.89)
AHA: 2Q, '07, 12; 4Q, '05, 94; 1Q, '89, 9; N-D, '86, 5

996.70 Due to unspecified device, implant, and graft

996.71 Due to heart valve prosthesis

996.72 Due to other cardiac device, implant, and graft
Cardiac pacemaker or defibrillator:
  electrode(s), lead(s)
  subcutaneous pocket
Coronary artery bypass (graft)
EXCLUDES *occlusion due to atherosclerosis (414.02-414.06)*
AHA: 2Q, '10, 8-9; 3Q, '08, 10; 3Q, '06, 8, 25; 3Q, '01, 20
TIP: Assign for in-stent stenosis of previously placed coronary artery stent.
T82.847A Pain cardiac prosth devc impl graft initial enc [I-10]

N Newborn Age: 0   P Pediatric Age: 0-17   M Maternity Age: 12-55   A Adult Age: 15-124

996.73 Due to renal dialysis device, implant, and graft
AHA: 2Q, '91, 18
T82.858A Stenosis vasc prosth devc impl graft initial enc `I-10`

996.74 Due to other vascular device, implant, and graft
EXCLUDES   *occlusion of biological graft due to atherosclerosis (440.30-440.32)*
AHA: ▶1Q, '12, 18;◀ 2Q, '11, 8;1Q, '03, 16, 17
TIP: ▶Assign for clotted peripherally inserted central catheter (PICC) line.◀

996.75 Due to nervous system device, implant, and graft

996.76 Due to genitourinary device, implant, and graft
EXCLUDES   *complications of implanted vaginal mesh (629.31-629.32)*
AHA: 1Q, '09, 15; 1Q, '00, 15
T83.83xA Hemorrhage GU prosth devc impl graft initial enc `I-10`

996.77 Due to internal joint prosthesis
Use additional code to identify prosthetic joint (V43.60-V43.69)
AHA: 4Q, '05, 91
T84.84xA Pain int ortho prosth devc impl gft initial enc `I-10`

996.78 Due to other internal orthopedic device, implant, and graft
AHA: 2Q, '03, 14

996.79 Due to other internal prosthetic device, implant, and graft
AHA: 2Q, '04, 7; 1Q,'01, 8; 3Q, '95, 14; 3Q, '92, 4

√5ᵗʰ **996.8 Complications of transplanted organ**
Transplant failure or rejection
Use additional code to identify nature of complication, such as:
cytomegalovirus (CMV) infection (078.5)
graft-versus-host disease (279.50-279.53)
malignancy associated with organ transplant (199.2)
post-transplant lymphoproliferative disorder (PTLD) (238.77)
AHA: 4Q, '08, 82-83; 3Q, '01, 12; 3Q, '93, 3, 4; 2Q, '93, 11; 1Q, '93, 24
TIP: Assign only if the complication affects the function of the transplanted organ. Assign also a code for the specific complication.

996.80 Transplanted organ, unspecified

996.81 Kidney
AHA: 2Q, '11, 6; 1Q, '10, 9; 4Q, '08, 83; 3Q, '03, 16; 3Q, '98, 6, 7; 3Q, '94, 8; 2Q, '94, 9; 1Q, '93, 24
TIP: Do not assign for chronic kidney disease (CKD) status following kidney transplant. The provider must indicate transplant failure, rejection, or other complication to support assignment of this code.
T86.11 Kidney transplant rejection `I-10`

996.82 Liver
AHA: 4Q, '08, 82, 99; 3Q, '03, 17; 3Q, '98, 3, 4

996.83 Heart
AHA: 3Q, '03, 16; 4Q, '02, 53; 3Q, '98, 5

996.84 Lung
AHA: 2Q, '03, 12; 3Q, '98, 5

996.85 Bone marrow
AHA: ▶1Q, '12, 13;◀ 4Q, '08, 91; 4Q, '90, 4
TIP: ▶Do not assign for recurrence or relapse of hematopoietic or lymphatic malignancy following bone marrow/stem cell transplant.◀

996.86 Pancreas

996.87 Intestine

996.88 Stem cell
Complications from stem cells from:
peripheral blood
umbilical cord
AHA: 4Q, '11, 147-148

996.89 Other specified transplanted organ
AHA: 1Q, '11, 8; 3Q, '94, 5

√5ᵗʰ **996.9 Complications of reattached extremity or body part**

996.90 Unspecified extremity

996.91 Forearm

996.92 Hand

996.93 Finger(s)

996.94 Upper extremity, other and unspecified

996.95 Foot and toe(s)

996.96 Lower extremity, other and unspecified

996.99 Other specified body part

√4ᵗʰ **997 Complications affecting specified body systems, not elsewhere classified**
Use additional code to identify complications
EXCLUDES   *the listed conditions when specified as:*
causing shock (998.00-998.09)
complications of:
anesthesia:
adverse effect (001.0-799.9, 995.0-995.8)
in labor or delivery (668.0-668.9)
poisoning (968.0-969.9)
implanted device or graft (996.0-996.9)
obstetrical procedures (669.0-669.4)
reattached extremity (996.90-996.96)
transplanted organ (996.80-996.89)
AHA: 1Q, '94, 4; 1Q, '93, 26

√5ᵗʰ **997.0 Nervous system complications**

997.00 Nervous system complication, unspecified

997.01 Central nervous system complication
Anoxic brain damage
Cerebral hypoxia
EXCLUDES   *cerebrovascular hemorrhage or infarction (997.02)*
AHA: 1Q, '07, 22; 1Q, '06, 15
TIP: Assign for hyperperfusion syndrome, a complication of carotid endarterectomy.

997.02 Iatrogenic cerebrovascular infarction or hemorrhage
Postoperative stroke
AHA: 3Q, '10, 5; 3Q, '06, 6; 2Q, '04, 8; 4Q, '95, 57
TIP: Assign an additional code to specify the type of postoperative stroke involved.
I97.810 Intraop cerebrovascular infarct during card surg `I-10`

997.09 Other nervous system complications
G97.0 Cerebrospinal fluid leak from spinal puncture `I-10`

997.1 Cardiac complications
Cardiac:
arrest
insufficiency
Cardiorespiratory failure
Heart failure
} during or resulting from a procedure
EXCLUDES   *the listed conditions as long-term effects of cardiac surgery or due to the presence of cardiac prosthetic device (429.4)*
AHA: 1Q, '11, 3-4; 4Q, '08, 179; 2Q, '02, 12
I97.711 Intraoperative cardiac arrest during oth surgery `I-10`

997.2 Peripheral vascular complications
Phlebitis or thrombophlebitis during or resulting from a procedure
EXCLUDES   *the listed conditions due to:*
implant or catheter device (996.62)
infusion, perfusion, or transfusion (999.2)
complications affecting blood vessels (997.71-997.79)
AHA: 1Q, '03, 6; 3Q, '02, 24-26
T81.72xA Complication of vein following a procedure NEC init. enc `I-10`

√4ᵗʰ √5ᵗʰ Additional Digit Required   Unspecified Code   Other Specified Code   Manifestation Code   ▶◀ Revised Text   ● New Code   ▲ Revised Code Title

Injury and Poisoning

997.3–997.99

✓5ᵗʰ 997.3 Respiratory complications

EXCLUDES   iatrogenic [postoperative] pneumothorax (512.1)
     iatrogenic pulmonary embolism (415.11)
     specified complications classified elsewhere, such as:
        adult respiratory distress syndrome (518.52)
        pulmonary edema, postoperative (518.4)
        respiratory insufficiency, acute, postoperative
          (518.52)
        shock lung related to trauma and surgery (518.52)
        tracheostomy complications (519.00-519.09)
        transfusion related acute lung injury [TRALI] (518.7)

AHA: 4Q, '11, 148-150; 1Q, '97, 10; 2Q, '93, 3; 2Q, '93, 9; 4Q, '90, 25

997.31 Ventilator associated pneumonia
Ventilator associated pneumonitis

Use additional code to identify organism

AHA: 4Q, '08, 148-149

TIP: Do not assign unless the provider has documented the relationship between the pneumonia and ventilation status.

997.32 Postprocedural aspiration pneumonia
Chemical pneumonitis resulting from a procedure
Mendelson's syndrome resulting from a procedure

EXCLUDES   aspiration pneumonia during labor and delivery (668.0)

DEF: Mendelson's syndrome: acid pneumonitis due to aspiration of gastric acids, may occur after anesthesia or sedation.

AHA: 4Q, '11, 150

TIP: ▶Do not also assign code 507.0; aspiration pneumonia is fully captured with this code.◀

997.39 Other respiratory complications

AHA: 1Q, '11, 16

J95.4 Chem pneumonitis d/t anesthesia [Mendelson syndrm]   I-10

✓5ᵗʰ 997.4 Digestive system complications

Complications of:
     intestinal (internal) anastomosis and bypass, not elsewhere classified, except that involving urinary tract

Hepatic failure
Hepatorenal syndrome   } specified as due to a procedure
Intestinal obstruction NOS

EXCLUDES   complications of gastric band procedure
        (539.01-539.09)
     complications of other bariatric procedure
        (539.81-539.89)
     gastrostomy complications (536.40-536.49)
     specified gastrointestinal complications classified
        elsewhere, such as:
        blind loop syndrome (579.2)
        colostomy and enterostomy complications
          (569.60-569.69)
        complications of intestinal pouch (569.71-569.79)
        gastrojejunal ulcer (534.0-534.9)
        infection of esophagostomy (530.86)
        infection of external stoma (569.61)
        mechanical complication of esophagostomy
          (530.87)
        pelvic peritoneal adhesions, female (614.6)
        peritoneal adhesions (568.0)
        peritoneal adhesions with obstruction (560.81)
        postcholecystectomy syndrome (576.0)
        postgastric surgery syndromes (564.2)
        pouchitis (569.71)
        vomiting following gastrointestinal surgery (564.3)

AHA: 4Q, '11, 125, 148-150; 2Q, '01, 4-6; 3Q, '99, 4; 2Q, '99, 14; 3Q, '97, 7; 1Q, '97, 11; 2Q, '95, 7; 1Q, '93, 26; 3Q, '92, 15; 2Q, '89, 15; 1Q, '88, 14

997.41 Retained cholelithiasis following cholecystectomy

997.49 Other digestive system complications

AHA: ▶1Q, '12, 6◀

TIP: ▶Assign for ileus following gastrointestinal surgery; physician documentation of the cause-and-effect relationship is not required.◀

K91.89 Oth postproc comp & disorder of digest syst   I-10

997.5 Urinary complications

Complications of:
     internal anastomosis and bypass of urinary tract, including that involving intestinal tract

Oliguria or anuria
Renal (kidney):   } specified as due to
   failure (acute)   procedure
   insufficiency (acute)
Tubular necrosis (acute)

EXCLUDES   complications of cystostomy (596.81-596.83)
     complications of external stoma of urinary tract
        (596.81-596.83)
     specified complications classified elsewhere, such as:
        postoperative stricture of:
          ureter (593.3)
          urethra (598.2)

AHA: ▶1Q, '12, 11;◀ 3Q, '03, 13; 3Q, '96, 10, 15; 4Q, '95, 73; 1Q, '92, 13; 2Q, '89, 16; M-A, '87, 10; S-O, '85, 3

TIP: ▶Assign for a urostomy-associated urinary tract infection with poor self-catheterization technique/hygiene.◀

N99.0 Postprocedural (acute) (chronic) renal failure   I-10

✓5ᵗʰ 997.6 Amputation stump complication

EXCLUDES   admission for treatment for a current traumatic amputation — code to complicated traumatic amputation
     phantom limb (syndrome) (353.6)

AHA: 4Q, '95, 82

997.60 Unspecified complication

997.61 Neuroma of amputation stump

DEF: Hyperplasia generated nerve cell mass following amputation.

997.62 Infection (chronic)

Use additional code to identify the organism

AHA: 1Q, '05, 15 4Q, '96, 46

TIP: If cellulitis is specified as a manifestation of the infection, assign an additional code from category 681 or 682.

T87.43 Infection amputation stump right lower extremity   I-10

997.69 Other

AHA: 1Q, '05, 15

✓5ᵗʰ 997.7 Vascular complications of other vessels

EXCLUDES   peripheral vascular complications (997.2)

997.71 Vascular complications of mesenteric artery

AHA: 4Q, '01, 53

TIP: For postoperative mesenteric artery embolism, assign also code 557.0 Acute vascular insufficiency of intestine.

997.72 Vascular complications of renal artery

997.79 Vascular complications of other vessels

✓5ᵗʰ 997.9 Complications affecting other specified body systems, not elsewhere classified

EXCLUDES   specified complications classified elsewhere, such as:
     broad ligament laceration syndrome (620.6)
     postartificial menopause syndrome (627.4)
     postoperative stricture of vagina (623.2)

997.91 Hypertension

EXCLUDES   essential hypertension (401.0-401.9)

AHA: 4Q, '95, 57

997.99 Other

Vitreous touch syndrome

DEF: Vitreous touch syndrome: vitreous protruding through pupil and attaches to corneal epithelium; causes aqueous fluid in vitreous body; marked by corneal edema, loss of lucidity; complication of cataract surgery.

AHA: 2Q, '94, 12; 1Q, '94, 17

N   Newborn Age: 0   P   Pediatric Age: 0-17   M   Maternity Age: 12-55   A   Adult Age: 15-124

Injury and Poisoning

✓4ᵗʰ **998 Other complications of procedures, not elsewhere classified**

     EXCLUDES *fluid overload due to transfusion (blood) (276.61)*
         TACO (276.61)
         transfusion associated circulatory overload (276.61)
     AHA: 1Q, '94, 4

✓5ᵗʰ **998.0 Postoperative shock**
     Shock during or resulting from a surgical procedure
     EXCLUDES *shock:*
         anaphylactic due to serum (999.41-999.49)
         anesthetic (995.4)
         electric (994.8)
         following abortion (639.5)
         obstetric (669.1)
         traumatic (958.4)
     AHA: 4Q, '11, 150-153

     998.00 Postoperative shock, unspecified
         Collapse, not otherwise specified, during or resulting
            from a surgical procedure
         Failure of peripheral circulation, postoperative

     998.01 Postoperative shock, cardiogenic
         AHA: 4Q, '11, 152

     998.02 Postoperative shock, septic
         Postoperative endotoxic shock
         Postoperative gram-negative shock

         Code first underlying infection

         Use additional code, to identify severe sepsis (995.92)
            and any associated acute organ dysfunction, if
            applicable
         AHA: 4Q, '11, 153

     998.09 Postoperative shock, other
         Postoperative hypovolemic shock

✓5ᵗʰ **998.1 Hemorrhage or hematoma or seroma complicating a procedure**
     EXCLUDES *hemorrhage, hematoma, or seroma:*
         complicating cesarean section or puerperal
            perineal wound (674.3)
         due to implanted device or graft (996.70-996.79)

     998.11 Hemorrhage complicating a procedure
         AHA: 1Q, '11, 13; 3Q '03, 13; 1Q, '03, 4; 4Q, '97, 52; 1Q, '97, 10
         I97.410 Intraop hemorrhage circ sys organ   `I-10`
         comp card cath

     998.12 Hematoma complicating a procedure
         AHA: 1Q, '11, 13; 3Q, '06, 12; 1Q, '03, 6; 3Q, '02, 24, 26

     998.13 Seroma complicating a procedure
         AHA: 4Q, '96, 46; 1Q, '93, 26; 2Q, '92, 15; S-O, '87, 8

     998.2 Accidental puncture or laceration during a procedure
         Accidental perforation by catheter or other instrument during
            a procedure on:
         blood vessel
         nerve
         organ
     EXCLUDES *iatrogenic [postoperative] pneumothorax (512.1)*
         puncture or laceration caused by implanted device
            intentionally left in operation wound
            (996.0-996.5)
         specified complications classified elsewhere, such as:
            broad ligament laceration syndrome (620.6)
            dural tear (349.31)
            incidental durotomy (349.31)
            trauma from instruments during delivery
            (664.0-665.9)
         AHA: 1Q, '10, 8, 11; 2Q, '07, 9; 1Q, '06, 15; 3Q, '02, 24, 26; 3Q, '94, 6; 3Q,
         '90, 17; 3Q, '90, 18
         I97.51 Accidentl punct lac circ sys organ dur circ proc   `I-10`

✓5ᵗʰ **998.3 Disruption of wound**
     Dehiscence ⎫
     Rupture   ⎬ of operation wound
     Disruption of any suture materials or other closure method
     EXCLUDES *disruption of:*
         cesarean wound (674.1)
         perineal wound, puerperal (674.2)
     AHA: 4Q, '08, 149-152; 4Q, '02, 73; 1Q, '93, 19

     998.30 Disruption of wound, unspecified
         Disruption of wound NOS

     998.31 Disruption of internal operation (surgical) wound
         Disruption or dehiscence of closure of:
            fascia, superficial or muscular
            internal organ
            muscle or muscle flap
            ribs or rib cage
            skull or craniotomy
            sternum or sternotomy
            tendon or ligament
          Deep disruption or dehiscence of operation wound
            NOS

         EXCLUDES *complications of internal anastomosis of:*
            gastrointestinal tract (997.49)
            urinary tract (997.5)
          AHA: 4Q, '10,131

     998.32 Disruption of external operation (surgical) wound
         Disruption of operation wound NOS
         Disruption or dehiscence of closure of:
            cornea
            mucosa
            skin
            subcutaneous tissue
         Full-thickness skin disruption or dehiscence
         Superficial disruption or dehiscence of operation
            wound
         AHA: 1Q, '06, 8; 1Q, '05, 11; 4Q, '03, 104, 106
         T81.31xA Disruption ext operation wound   `I-10`
         NEC initial enc

     998.33 Disruption of traumatic injury wound repair
         Disruption or dehiscence of closure of traumatic
            laceration (external) (internal)
         AHA: 4Q, '08, 151, 152

     998.4 Foreign body accidentally left during a procedure
     Adhesions   ⎫ due to foreign body accidentally left in
     Obstruction   ⎬ operative wound or body cavity
     Perforation   ⎭ during a procedure
     EXCLUDES *obstruction or perforation caused by implanted*
         device intentionally left in body (996.0-996.5)
     AHA: ▶1Q, '12, 12;◀1Q, '11, 5-6; 1Q, '09,18; 1Q, '89, 9
     TIP: ▶Report for an unintended retention of a foreign object
     following any type of procedure, in any type of setting..◀

✓5ᵗʰ **998.5 Postoperative infection**
     EXCLUDES *bleb associated endophthalmitis (379.63)*
         infection due to:
            implanted device (996.60-996.69)
            infusion, perfusion, or transfusion (999.31-999.39)
         postoperative obstetrical wound infection (674.3)

     998.51 Infected postoperative seroma
         Use additional code to identify organism
         AHA: 4Q, '96, 46

     998.59 Other postoperative infection
         Abscess:
            intra-abdominal ⎫
            stitch   ⎬ postoperative
            subphrenic   ⎪
            wound   ⎭
         Septicemia
         Use additional code to identify infection
         AHA: 4Q, '11, 153; 2Q, '06, 23; 4Q, '04, 76; 4Q, '03, 104,
         106-107; 3Q, '98, 3; 3Q, '95, 5; 2Q, '95, 7; 3Q, '94, 6; 1Q, '93,
         19; J-F, '87, 14
         TIP: Do not assign if the infection is related to an internal
         prosthetic device, implant, or graft; see instead
         subcategory 996.6.
         T81.4xxA Infection following procedure initl encounter   `I-10`

     998.6 Persistent postoperative fistula
         AHA: J-F, '87, 14
         T81.83xD Persistent postprocedural fistula subsequent enc   `I-10`

     998.7 Acute reaction to foreign substance accidentally left during a procedure
         Peritonitis:
            aseptic
            chemical

✓5ᵗʰ **998.8 Other specified complications of procedures, not elsewhere classified**
     AHA: 4Q, '94, 46; 1Q, '89, 9

✓4ᵗʰ / ✓5ᵗʰ Additional Digit Required   Unspecified Code   Other Specified Code   Manifestation Code   ▶◀ Revised Text   ● New Code   ▲ Revised Code Title

2013 ICD-9-CM   **October 2012 · Volume 1 – 315**

Injury and Poisoning

998.81–999.4

998.81 Emphysema (subcutaneous) (surgical) resulting from a procedure

998.82 Cataract fragments in eye following cataract surgery

998.83 Non-healing surgical wound
> AHA: 4Q, '96, 47

998.89 Other specified complications
> AHA: 2Q, '09, 11; 3Q, '06, 9; 3Q, '05, 16; 3Q, '99, 13; 2Q, '98, 16
> TIP: Assign for cases in which a procedure is performed on the wrong body site (e.g., right leg versus left leg), along with E876.5-E876.7.
> T81.89xA Other complications of procedures NEC, init enc   I-10

998.9 Unspecified complication of procedure, not elsewhere classified
> Postoperative complication NOS
> EXCLUDES   *complication NOS of obstetrical, surgery or procedure (669.4)*
> AHA: 4Q, '93, 37

✓4ᵗʰ **999 Complications of medical care, not elsewhere classified**
> INCLUDES   complications, not elsewhere classified, of:
>> dialysis (hemodialysis) (peritoneal) (renal)
>> extracorporeal circulation
>> hyperalimentation therapy
>> immunization
>> infusion
>> inhalation therapy
>> injection
>> inoculation
>> perfusion
>> transfusion
>> vaccination
>> ventilation therapy
>
> Use additional code, where applicable, to identify specific complication
>
> EXCLUDES   *specified complications classified elsewhere such as:*
>> *complications of implanted device (996.0-996.9)*
>> *contact dermatitis due to drugs (692.3)*
>> *dementia dialysis (294.8)*
>> *transient (293.9)*
>> *dialysis disequilibrium syndrome (276.0-276.9)*
>> *poisoning and toxic effects of drugs and chemicals (960.0-989.9)*
>> *postvaccinal encephalitis (323.51)*
>> *water and electrolyte imbalance (276.0-276.9)*

999.0 Generalized vaccinia
> EXCLUDES   *vaccinia not from vaccine (051.02)*
> DEF: Skin eruption, self-limiting; follows vaccination; due to transient viremia with virus localized in skin.

999.1 Air embolism
> Air embolism to any site following infusion, perfusion, or transfusion
> EXCLUDES   *embolism specified as:*
>> *complicating:*
>>> *abortion (634-638 with .6, 639.6)*
>>> *ectopic or molar pregnancy (639.6)*
>>> *pregnancy, childbirth, or the puerperium (673.0)*
>> *due to implanted device (996.7)*
>> *traumatic (958.0)*

999.2 Other vascular complications
> Phlebitis
> Thromboembolism } following infusion, perfusion,
> Thrombophlebitis   or transfusion
>
> EXCLUDES   *extravasation of vesicant drugs (999.81, 999.82)*
>> *the listed conditions when specified as:*
>>> *due to implanted device (996.61-996.62. 996.72-996.74)*
>>> *postoperative NOS (997.2, 997.71-997.79)*
> AHA: 2Q, '97, 5
> TIP: Do not assign for IV infiltration; if the infiltration is severe enough to cause other complications, a code for the specific complication should be assigned. For chemotherapy extravasation, see code 999.81.
> T80.1xxA Vasc comp follw inf transfusn tx inj initial enc   I-10

✓5ᵗʰ **999.3 Other infection**
> Infection
> Sepsis } following infusion, injection,
> Septicemia   transfusion, or vaccination
>
> Use additional code to identify the specified infection, such as:
>> septicemia (038.0-038.9)
> EXCLUDES   *the listed conditions when specified as:*
>> *due to implanted device (996.60-996.69)*
>> *postoperative NOS (998.51-998.59)*
> AHA: 4Q, '07, 96; 2Q, '01, 11, 12; 2Q, '97, 5; J-F, '87, 14

999.31 Other and unspecified infection due to central venous catheter
> Central line-associated infection
> Infection due to:
>> central venous catheter NOS
>> Hickman catheter
>> peripherally inserted central catheter (PICC)
>> triple lumen catheter
>> umbilical venous catheter
> EXCLUDES   *infection due to:*
>> *arterial catheter (996.62)*
>> *catheter NOS (996.69)*
>> *peripheral venous catheter (996.62)*
>> *urinary catheter (996.64)*
> AHA: 2Q, '11, 7; 4Q, '08, 72, 193; 4Q, '07, 97

999.32 Bloodstream infection due to central venous catheter
> Bloodstream infection due to:
>> Hickman catheter
>> peripherally inserted central catheter (PICC)
>> portacath (port-a-cath)
>> triple lumen catheter
>> umbilical venous catheter
> Catheter-related bloodstream infection (CRBSI) NOS
> Central line-associated bloodstream infection (CLABSI)
> AHA: 4Q, '11, 153-155

999.33 Local infection due to central venous catheter
> Exit or insertion site infection
> Local infection due to:
>> Hickman catheter
>> peripherally inserted central catheter (PICC)
>> portacath (port-a-cath)
>> triple lumen catheter
>> umbilical venous catheter
> Port or reservoir infection
> Tunnel infection
> AHA: 4Q, '11, 153-155

999.34 Acute infection following transfusion, infusion, or injection of blood and blood products
> AHA: 4Q, '11, 153-155
> TIP: ▶If the acute infection transmitted via transfusion, infusion, or injection is HIV, sequence code 042 first.◀

999.39 Infection following other infusion, injection, transfusion, or vaccination
> AHA: 4Q, '08, 99

✓5ᵗʰ **999.4 Anaphylactic reaction due to serum**
> Allergic shock
> Anaphylactic shock due to serum
> Anaphylactoid reaction due to serum
> Anaphylaxis
> EXCLUDES   *ABO incompatibility reaction due to transfusion of blood or blood products (999.60-999.69)*
>> *reaction:*
>>> *allergic NOS (995.0)*
>>> *anaphylactic:*
>>>> *NOS (995.0)*
>>>> *due to drugs and chemicals (995.0)*
>>> *other serum (999.51-999.59)*
>> *shock:*
>>> *allergic NOS (995.0)*
>>> *anaphylactic:*
>>>> *NOS (995.0)*
>>>> *due to drugs and chemicals (995.0)*
> DEF: Life-threatening hypersensitivity to foreign serum; causes respiratory distress, vascular collapse, and shock.
> AHA: 4Q, '11, 142-147

N Newborn Age: 0   P Pediatric Age: 0-17   M Maternity Age: 12-55   A Adult Age: 15-124

999.41 Anaphylactic reaction due to administration of blood and blood products
    AHA: 4Q, '11, 146

999.42 Anaphylactic reaction due to vaccination

999.49 Anaphylactic reaction due to other serum

√5ᵗʰ **999.5 Other serum reaction**
    Intoxication by serum
    Protein sickness
    Serum rash
    Serum sickness
    Urticaria due to serum
    EXCLUDES *serum hepatitis (070.2-070.3)*
    DEF: Serum sickness: Hypersensitivity to foreign serum; causes fever, hives, swelling, and lymphadenopathy.
    AHA: 4Q, '11, 142-146

999.51 Other serum reaction due to administration of blood and blood products

999.52 Other serum reaction due to vaccination

999.59 Other serum reaction

√5ᵗʰ **999.6 ABO incompatibility reaction due to transfusion of blood or blood products**
    EXCLUDES *minor blood group antigens reactions (Duffy) (E) (K(ell)) (Kidd) (Lewis) (M) (N) (P) (S) (999.75-999.79)*
    AHA: 4Q, '10, 99-102

999.60 ABO incompatibility reaction, unspecified
    ABO incompatible blood transfusion NOS
    Reaction to ABO incompatibility from transfusion NOS

999.61 ABO incompatibility with hemolytic transfusion reaction not specified as acute or delayed
    ABO incompatibility with hemolytic transfusion reaction at unspecified time after transfusion
    Hemolytic transfusion reaction (HTR) due to ABO incompatibility

999.62 ABO incompatibility with acute hemolytic transfusion reaction
    ABO incompatibility with hemolytic transfusion reaction less than 24 hours after transfusion
    Acute hemolytic transfusion reaction (AHTR) due to ABO incompatibility

999.63 ABO incompatibility with delayed hemolytic transfusion reaction
    ABO incompatibility with hemolytic transfusion reaction 24 hours or more after transfusion
    Delayed hemolytic transfusion reaction (DHTR) due to ABO incompatibility

999.69 Other ABO incompatibility reaction
    Delayed serologic transfusion reaction (DSTR) from ABO incompatibility
    Other ABO incompatible blood transfusion
    Other reaction to ABO incompatibility from transfusion

√5ᵗʰ **999.7 Rh and other non-ABO incompatibility reaction due to transfusion of blood or blood products**
    Elevation of Rh titer
    AHA: 4Q, '10, 99-100,102-105

999.70 Rh incompatibility reaction, unspecified
    Reaction due to Rh factor in transfusion NOS
    Rh incompatible blood transfusion NOS
    Unspecified reaction due to incompatibility related to Rh antigens (C) (c) (D) (E) (e)
    Unspecified reaction to Rh incompatibility

999.71 Rh incompatibility with hemolytic transfusion reaction not specified as acute or delayed
    Hemolytic transfusion reaction (HTR) due to Rh incompatibility
    HTR due to incompatibility related to Rh antigens (C) (c) (D) (E) (e), not specified as acute or delayed
    Rh incompatibility with hemolytic transfusion reaction at unspecified time after transfusion

999.72 Rh incompatibility with acute hemolytic transfusion reaction
    Acute hemolytic transfusion reaction (AHTR) due to Rh incompatibility
    AHTR due to incompatibility related to Rh antigens (C) (c) (D) (E) (e)
    Rh incompatibility with hemolytic transfusion reaction less than 24 hours after transfusion

999.73 Rh incompatibility with delayed hemolytic transfusion reaction
    Delayed hemolytic transfusion reaction (DHTR) due to Rh incompatibility
    DHTR due to incompatibility related to Rh antigens (C) (c) (D) (E) (e)
    Rh incompatibility with hemolytic transfusion reaction 24 hours or more after transfusion

999.74 Other Rh incompatibility reaction
    Delayed serologic transfusion reaction (DSTR) from Rh incompatibility
    Other reaction due to incompatibility related to Rh antigens (C) (c) (D) (E) (e)
    Other reaction to Rh incompatible blood transfusion

999.75 Non-ABO incompatibility reaction, unspecified
    Non-ABO incompatible blood transfusion NOS
    Reaction to non-ABO antigen incompatibility from transfusion NOS
    Unspecified reaction due to incompatibility related to minor antigens (Duffy) (Kell) (Kidd) (Lewis) (M) (N) (P) (S)

999.76 Non-ABO incompatibility with hemolytic transfusion reaction not specified as acute or delayed
    Hemolytic transfusion reaction (HTR) due to non-ABO incompatibility
    HTR from incompatibility related to minor antigens (Duffy) (Kell) (Kidd) (Lewis) (M) (N) (P) (S)
    Non-ABO incompatibility with hemolytic transfusion reaction at unspecified time after transfusion

999.77 Non-ABO incompatibility with acute hemolytic transfusion reaction
    Acute hemolytic transfusion reaction (AHTR) due to non-ABO incompatibility
    AHTR from incompatibility related to minor antigens (Duffy) (Kell) (Kidd) (Lewis) (M) (N) (P) (S)
    Non-ABO incompatibility with hemolytic transfusion reaction less than 24 hours after transfusion

999.78 Non-ABO incompatibility with delayed hemolytic transfusion reaction
    Delayed hemolytic transfusion reaction(DHTR) due to non-ABO incompatibility
    DHTR from incompatibility related to minor antigens (Duffy) (Kell) (Kidd) (Lewis) (M) (N) (P) (S)
    Non-ABO incompatibility with hemolytic transfusion reaction 24 hours or more after transfusion

999.79 Other non-ABO incompatibility reaction
    Delayed serologic transfusion reaction (DSTR) from non-ABO incompatibility
    Other non-ABO incompatible blood transfusion
    Other reaction due to incompatibility related to minor antigens (Duffy) (Kell) (Kidd) (Lewis) (M) (N) (P) (S)
    Other reaction to non-ABO incompatibility from transfusion

Injury and Poisoning

999.8–999.9

√5ᵗʰ **999.8 Other and unspecified infusion and transfusion reaction**

EXCLUDES   ABO incompatibility reactions (999.60-999.69)
     febrile nonhemolytic transfusion reaction (FNHTR)
        (780.66)
     hemochromatosis due to repeated red blood cell
        transfusions (275.02)
     non-ABO incompatibility reactions (999.70-999.79)
     postoperative shock (998.00-998.09)
     posttransfusion purpura (287.41)
     Rh incompatibility reactions (999.70-999.74)
     transfusion associated circulatory overload (TACO)
        (276.61)
     transfusion related acute lung injury [TRALI] (518.7)

AHA: 4Q, '08, 152-155; 3Q, '00, 9

999.80 Transfusion reaction, unspecified
Incompatible blood transfusion NOS
Reaction to blood group incompatibility in infusion or
     transfusion NOS
AHA: 4Q, '10, 99-100, 106-107

999.81 Extravasation of vesicant chemotherapy
Infiltration of vesicant chemotherapy
AHA: 4Q, '08, 155

999.82 Extravasation of other vesicant agent
Infiltration of other vesicant agent

**999.83 Hemolytic transfusion reaction,
incompatibility unspecified**
Hemolytic transfusion reaction (HTR) with antigen
     incompatibility unspecified, not specified as
     acute or delayed
HTR with incompatibility unspecified at unspecified
     time after transfusion
AHA: 4Q, '10, 99-100, 106-107

**999.84 Acute hemolytic transfusion reaction,
incompatibility unspecified**
Acute hemolytic transfusion reaction (AHTR) with
     antigen incompatibility unspecified
AHTR, incompatibility unspecified
AHA: 4Q, '10, 99-100, 106-107

**999.85 Delayed hemolytic transfusion reaction,
incompatibility unspecified**
Delayed hemolytic transfusion reaction (DHTR) with
     antigen incompatibility unspecified
DHTR, incompatibility unspecified
AHA: 4Q, '10, 99-100, 106-107

999.88 Other infusion reaction

999.89 Other transfusion reaction
Delayed serologic transfusion reaction (DSTR),
     incompatibility unspecified
Use additional code to identify graft-versus-host
     reaction (279.5)
AHA: 4Q, '08, 99, 154

**999.9 Other and unspecified complications of medical
care, not elsewhere classified**
Complications, not elsewhere classified, of:
     electroshock   ⎫
     inhalation   ⎬ therapy
     ultrasound   ⎪
     ventilation   ⎭
Unspecified misadventure of medical care

EXCLUDES   unspecified complication of:
     phototherapy (990)
     radiation therapy (999)
     ventilator associated pneumonia (997.31)

AHA: 3Q, '06, 25; 1Q, '03, 19; 2Q, '97, 5

Ⓝ Newborn Age: 0   Ⓟ Pediatric Age: 0-17   Ⓜ Maternity Age: 12-55   Ⓐ Adult Age: 15-124

Supplementary Classification of Factors Influencing Health Status and Contact with Health Services (V01-V91)

This classification is provided to deal with occasions when circumstances other than a disease or injury classifiable to categories 001-999 (the main part of ICD) are recorded as "diagnoses" or "problems." This can arise mainly in three ways:

a) When a person who is not currently sick encounters the health services for some specific purpose, such as to act as a donor of an organ or tissue, to receive prophylactic vaccination, or to discuss a problem which is in itself not a disease or injury. This will be a fairly rare occurrence among hospital inpatients, but will be relatively more common among hospital outpatients and patients of family practitioners, health clinics, etc.

b) When a person with a known disease or injury, whether it is current or resolving, encounters the health care system for a specific treatment of that disease or injury (e.g., dialysis for renal disease; chemotherapy for malignancy; cast change).

c) When some circumstance or problem is present which influences the person's health status but is not in itself a current illness or injury. Such factors may be elicited during population surveys, when the person may or may not be currently sick, or be recorded as an additional factor to be borne in mind when the person is receiving care for some current illness or injury classifiable to categories 001-999.

In the latter circumstances the V code should be used only as a supplementary code and should not be the one selected for use in primary, single cause tabulations. Examples of these circumstances are a personal history of certain diseases, or a person with an artificial heart valve in situ.

AHA: J-F, '87, 8

Persons with Potential Health Hazards Related to Communicable Diseases (V01-V06)

EXCLUDES family history of infectious and parasitic diseases (V18.8)
personal history of infectious and parasitic diseases (V12.0)

√4ᵗʰ **V01 Contact with or exposure to communicable diseases**
TIP: Do not assign if the patient shows signs or symptoms of the disease to which he or she was exposed.

V01.0 Cholera
Conditions classifiable to 001

V01.1 Tuberculosis
Conditions classifiable to 010-018

V01.2 Poliomyelitis
Conditions classifiable to 045

V01.3 Smallpox
Conditions classifiable to 050

V01.4 Rubella
Conditions classifiable to 056

V01.5 Rabies
Conditions classifiable to 071

V01.6 Venereal diseases
Conditions classifiable to 090-099
AHA: 4Q, '07, 125

√5ᵗʰ **V01.7 Other viral diseases**
Conditions classifiable to 042-078 and V08, except as above
AHA: 2Q, '92, 11

V01.71 Varicella

V01.79 Other viral diseases

√5ᵗʰ **V01.8 Other communicable diseases**
Conditions classifiable to 001-136, except as above
AHA: J-A, '87, 24

V01.81 Anthrax
AHA: 4Q, '02, 70, 78

V01.82 Exposure to SARS-associated coronavirus
AHA: 4Q, '03, 46-47

V01.83 Escherichia coli (E. coli)

V01.84 Meningococcus
Z20.811 Contact with and exposure to meningococcus I-10

V01.89 Other communicable diseases

V01.9 Unspecified communicable diseases

√4ᵗʰ **V02 Carrier or suspected carrier of infectious diseases**
INCLUDES colonization status
AHA: 3Q, '95, 18; 3Q, '94, 4

V02.0 Cholera

V02.1 Typhoid

V02.2 Amebiasis

V02.3 Other gastrointestinal pathogens

V02.4 Diphtheria

√5ᵗʰ **V02.5 Other specified bacterial diseases**

V02.51 Group B streptococcus
AHA: 3Q, '06, 14; 1Q, '02, 14; 4Q, '98, 56

V02.52 Other streptococcus

V02.53 Methicillin susceptible Staphylococcus aureus
MSSA colonization
AHA: 4Q, '08, 69, 71, 156

V02.54 Methicillin resistant Staphylococcus aureus
MRSA colonization
AHA: 4Q, '08, 69, 71, 72, 156

V02.59 Other specified bacterial diseases
Meningococcal
Staphylococcal

√5ᵗʰ **V02.6 Viral hepatitis**
Hepatitis Australian-antigen [HAA] [SH] carrier
Serum hepatitis carrier

V02.60 Viral hepatitis carrier, unspecfied
AHA: 4Q, '97, 47

V02.61 Hepatitis B carrier
AHA: 4Q, '97, 47
Z22.51 Carrier of viral hepatitis B I-10

V02.62 Hepatitis C carrier
AHA: 4Q, '97, 47

V02.69 Other viral hepatitis carrier
AHA: 4Q, '97, 47

V02.7 Gonorrhea

V02.8 Other venereal diseases

V02.9 Other specified infectious organism
AHA: 3Q, '95, 18; 1Q, '93, 22; J-A, '87, 24

√4ᵗʰ **V03 Need for prophylactic vaccination and inoculation against bacterial diseases**
EXCLUDES vaccination not carried out (V64.00-V64.09)
vaccines against combinations of diseases (V06.0-V06.9)

V03.0 Cholera alone

V03.1 Typhoid-paratyphoid alone [TAB]

V03.2 Tuberculosis [BCG]

V03.3 Plague

V03.4 Tularemia

V03.5 Diphtheria alone

V03.6 Pertussis alone

V03.7 Tetanus toxoid alone

√5ᵗʰ **V03.8 Other specified vaccinations against single bacterial diseases**

V03.81 Hemophilus influenza, type B [Hib]

V03.82 Streptococcus pneumoniae [pneumococcus]

V03.89 Other specified vaccination
AHA: 2Q, '00, 9
TIP: Assign for vaccination against Lyme disease.

V03.9 Unspecified single bacterial disease

√4ᵗʰ **V04 Need for prophylactic vaccination and inoculation against certain viral diseases**
EXCLUDES vaccines against combinations of diseases (V06.0-V06.9)

V04.0 Poliomyelitis

V04.1 Smallpox

√4ᵗʰ √5ᵗʰ Additional Digit Required   Unspecified Code   Other Specified Code   Manifestation Code   ▶◀ Revised Text   ● New Code   ▲ Revised Code Title

2013 ICD-9-CM   **Volume 1 – 319**

V Codes

V04.2–V08

V04.2 Measles alone

V04.3 Rubella alone

V04.4 Yellow fever

V04.5 Rabies

V04.6 Mumps alone

V04.7 Common cold

√5ᵗʰ **V04.8 Other viral diseases**
AHA: 4Q, '03, 83

     V04.81 Influenza

     V04.82 Respiratory syncytial virus (RSV)
         AHA: 1Q, '09, 14

     V04.89 Other viral diseases
         AHA: 2Q, '07, 9
         TIP: Assign for vaccination against human papilloma virus (HPV).

√4ᵗʰ **V05 Need for other prophylactic vaccination and inoculation against single diseases**
     EXCLUDES *vaccines against combinations of diseases (V06.0-V06.9)*

V05.0 Athropod-borne viral encephalitis

V05.1 Other arthropod-borne viral diseases

V05.2 Leshmaniasis

V05.3 Viral hepatitis

V05.4 Varicella
     Chickenpox

V05.8 Other specified disease
     AHA: 1Q, '01, 4; 3Q, '91, 20

V05.9 Unspecified single disease

√4ᵗʰ **V06 Need for prophylactic vaccination and inoculation against combinations of diseases**
     NOTE Use additional single vaccination codes from categories V03-V05 to identify any vaccinations not included in a combination code.

V06.0 Cholera with typhoid-paratyphoid [cholera+TAB]

V06.1 Diphtheia-tetanus-pertussis, combined [DTP] [DTaP]
     AHA: 4Q, '03, 83; 3Q, '98, 13

V06.2 Diphtheria-tetanus-pertussis with typhoid-paratyphoid [DTP+TAB]

V06.3 Diphtheria-tetanus-pertussis with poliomyelitis [DTP+polio]

V06.4 Measles-mumps-rubella [MMR]

V06.5 Tetanus-diphtheria [Td] [DT]
     AHA: 4Q, '03, 83

V06.6 Streptococcus pneumoniae [pneumococcus] and influenza

V06.8 Other combinations
     EXCLUDES *multiple single vaccination codes (V03.0-V05.9)*
     AHA: ▶1Q, '12, 11;◀ 1Q, '94, 19

V06.9 Unspecified combined vaccine

Persons with Need for Isolation, Other Potential Health Hazards and Prophylactic Measures (V07-V09)

√4ᵗʰ **V07 Need for isolation and other prophylactic or treatment measures**
     EXCLUDES *long-term (current) (prophylactic) use of certain specific drugs (V58.61-V58.69)*
         prophylactic organ removal (V50.41-V50.49)

V07.0 Isolation
     Admission to protect the individual from his surroundings or for isolation of individual after contact with infectious diseases

V07.1 Desensitization to allergens

V07.2 Prophylactic immunotherapy
     Administration of:
         antivenin
         immune sera [gamma globulin]
         RhoGAM
         tetanus antitoxin

√5ᵗʰ **V07.3 Other prophylactic chemotherapy**

     V07.31 Prophylactic fluoride administration

     V07.39 Other prophylactic chemotherapy
         EXCLUDES *maintenance chemotherapy following disease (V58.11)*

V07.4 Hormone replacement therapy (postmenopausal) ♀
     Z79.890 Hormone replacement therapy postmenopausal   I-10

√5ᵗʰ **V07.5 Use of agents affecting estrogen receptors and estrogen levels**
     Code first, if applicable:
         malignant neoplasm of breast (174.0-174.9, 175.0-175.9)
         malignant neoplasm of prostate (185)
     Use additional code, if applicable, to identify:
         estrogen receptor positive status (V86.0)
         family history of breast cancer (V16.3)
         genetic susceptibility to cancer (V84.01-V84.09)
         personal history of breast cancer (V10.3)
         personal history of prostate cancer (V10.46)
         postmenopausal status (V49.81)
     EXCLUDES *hormone replacement therapy (postmenopausal) (V07.4)*
     AHA: 4Q, '10, 108; 4Q, '08, 156

     V07.51 Use of selective estrogen receptor modulators [SERMs]
         Use of:
            raloxifene (Evista)
            tamoxifen (Nolvadex)
            toremifene (Fareston)
         Z79.810 Lng term sel estrogen receptor   I-10
         modulators SERMS

     V07.52 Use of aromatase inhibitors
         Use of:
            anastrozole (Arimidex)
            exemestane (Aromasin)
            letrozole (Femara)

     V07.59 Use of other agents affecting estrogen receptors and estrogen levels
         Use of:
            estrogen receptor downregulators
            fulvestrant (Faslodex)
            gonadotropin-releasing hormone (GnRH) agonist
            goserelin acetate (Zoladex)
            leuprolide acetate (leuprorelin) (Lupron)
            megestrol acetate (Megace)

V07.8 Other specified prophylactic or treatment measure
     AHA: 2Q, '10, 6, 14; 1Q, '92, 11
     TIP: Assign for patients having prophylactic breast removal because of a strong family history of breast cancer, along with code V16.3 Family history of breast cancer.

V07.9 Unspecified prophylactic or treatment measure

V08 Asymptomatic human immunodeficiency virus [HIV] infection status
     HIV positive NOS
     NOTE This code is only to be used when no HIV infection symptoms or conditions are present. If any HIV infection symptoms or conditions are present, see code 042.
     EXCLUDES *AIDS (042)*
         human immunodeficiency virus [HIV] disease (042)
         exposure to HIV (V01.79)
         nonspecific serologic evidence of HIV (795.71)
         symptomatic human immunodeficiency virus [HIV] infection (042)
     AHA: 2Q, '04, 11; 2Q, '99, 8; 3Q, '95, 18
     Z21 Asymptomatic HIV infection status   I-10

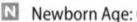

☑4ᵗʰ **V09 Infection with drug-resistant microorganisms**
> **NOTE** This category is intended for use as an additional code for infectious conditions classified elsewhere to indicate the presence of drug-resistance of the infectious organism.
> AHA: 3Q, '94, 4; 4Q, '93, 22

V09.0 Infection with microorganisms resistant to penicillins
> AHA: 2Q, '06, 16; 4Q, '03, 104, 106

V09.1 Infection with microorganisms resistant to cephalosporins and other B-lactam antibiotics

V09.2 Infection with microorganisms resistant to macrolides

V09.3 Infection with microorganisms resistant to tetracyclines

V09.4 Infection with microorganisms resistant to aminoglycosides

☑5ᵗʰ **V09.5 Infection with microorganisms resistant to quinolones and fluoroquinolones**

> **V09.50 Without mention of resistance to multiple quinolones and fluoroquinoles**

> **V09.51 With resistance to multiple quinolones and fluoroquinoles**

V09.6 Infection with microorganisms resistant to sulfonamides

☑5ᵗʰ **V09.7 Infection with microorganisms resistant to other specified antimycobacterial agents**
> **EXCLUDES** Amikacin (V09.4)
> Kanamycin (V09.4)
> Streptomycin [SM] (V09.4)

> **V09.70 Without mention of resistance to multiple antimycobacterial agents**

> **V09.71 With resistance to multiple antimycobacterial agents**

☑5ᵗʰ **V09.8 Infection with microorganisms resistant to other specified drugs**
> Vancomycin (glycopeptide) intermediate staphylococcus aureus (VISA/GISA)
> Vancomycin (glycopeptide) resistant enterococcus (VRE)
> Vancomycin (glycopeptide) resistant staphylococcus aureus (VRSA/GRSA)

> **V09.80 Without mention of resistance to multiple drugs**

> **V09.81 With resistance to multiple drugs**

☑5ᵗʰ **V09.9 Infection with drug-resistant microorganisms, unspecified**
> Drug resistance, NOS

> **V09.90 Without mention of multiple drug resistance**
> > **Z16** Infection with drug resistant microorganisms I-10

> **V09.91 With multiple drug resistance**
> > Multiple drug resistance NOS

Persons with Potential Health Hazards Related to Personal and Family History (V10-V19)

> **EXCLUDES** obstetric patients where the possibility that the fetus might be affected is the reason for observation or management during pregnancy (655.0-655.9)
> AHA: J-F, '87, 1

☑4ᵗʰ **V10 Personal history of malignant neoplasm**
> AHA: 4Q, '02, 80; 4Q, '98, 69; 1Q, '95, 4; 3Q, '92, 5; M-J, '85, 10; 2Q, '90, 9
> TIP: Assign the codes in this category only for a personal history of primary malignancy (not metastatic malignancies).

☑5ᵗʰ **V10.0 Gastrointestinal tract**
> History of conditions classifiable to 140-159
> **EXCLUDES** personal history of malignant carcinoid tumor (V10.91)
> personal history of malignant neuroendocrine tumor (V10.91)

> **V10.00 Gastrointestinal tract, unspecified**

> **V10.01 Tongue**

> **V10.02 Other and unspecified oral cavity and pharynx**

> **V10.03 Esophagus**

V10.04 Stomach

V10.05 Large intestine
> AHA: 3Q, '99, 7; 1Q, '95, 4
> **Z85.038** Personal hx othr malig neoplasm large intestine I-10

V10.06 Rectum, rectosigmoid junction, and anus

V10.07 Liver

V10.09 Other
> AHA: 4Q, '03, 111

☑5ᵗʰ **V10.1 Trachea, bronchus, and lung**
> History of conditions classifiable to 162
> **EXCLUDES** personal history of malignant carcinoid tumor (V10.91)
> personal history of malignant neuroendocrine tumor (V10.91)

> **V10.11 Bronchus and lung**

> **V10.12 Trachea**

☑5ᵗʰ **V10.2 Other respiratory and intrathoracic organs**
> History of conditions classifiable to 160, 161, 163-165

> **V10.20 Respiratory organ, unspecified**

> **V10.21 Larynx**
> > AHA: 4Q, '03, 108, 110

> **V10.22 Nasal cavities, middle ear, and accessory sinuses**

> **V10.29 Other**

V10.3 Breast
> History of conditions classifiable to 174 and 175
> AHA: ▶1Q, '12, 11;◀ 2Q, '11, 12; 3Q, '07, 4; 1Q, '07, 6; 2Q, '03, 5; 4Q, '01, 66; 4Q, '98, 65; 4Q, '97, 50; 1Q, '91, 16; 1Q, '90, 21
> TIP: ▶Do not assign for personal history of ductal carcinoma in situ (DCIS); assign code V13.89.◀
> **Z85.3** Personal history primary malig neoplasm breast I-10

☑5ᵗʰ **V10.4 Genital organs**
> History of conditions classifiable to 179-187

> **V10.40 Female genital organ, unspecfied** ♀

> **V10.41 Cervix uteri** ♀
> > AHA: 4Q, '07, 99

> **V10.42 Other parts of uterus** ♀

> **V10.43 Ovary** ♀

> **V10.44 Other female genital organs** ♀

> **V10.45 Male genital organ, unspecfied** ♂

> **V10.46 Prostate** ♂
> > AHA: 1Q, '09, 15

> **V10.47 Testis** ♂
> > **Z85.47** Personal history primary malig neoplasm testis I-10

> **V10.48 Epididymis** ♂

> **V10.49 Other male genital organs** ♂

☑5ᵗʰ **V10.5 Urinary organs**
> History of conditions classifiable to 188 and 189
> **EXCLUDES** personal history of malignant carcinoid tumor (V10.91)
> personal history of malignant neuroendocrine tumor (V10.91)

> **V10.50 Urinary organ, unspecified**

> **V10.51 Bladder**

> **V10.52 Kidney**
> > **EXCLUDES** renal pelvis (V10.53)
> > AHA: 2Q, '04, 4

> **V10.53 Renal pelvis**
> > AHA: 4Q, '01, 55

> **V10.59 Other**

☑5ᵗʰ **V10.6 Leukemia**
> Conditions classifiable to 204-208
> **EXCLUDES** leukemia in remission (204-208)
> AHA: 2Q, '92, 13; 4Q, '91, 26; 4Q, '90, 3

> **V10.60 Leukemia, unspecified**

V10.61 **Lymphoid leukemia**

V10.62 **Myeloid leukemia**

V10.63 **Monocytic leukemia**

V10.69 Other

✓5ᵗʰ V10.7 **Other lymphatic and hematopoietic neoplasms**
Conditions classifiable to 200-203
EXCLUDES *listed conditions in 200-203 in remission*
AHA: M-J, '85, 18

V10.71 **Lymphosarcoma and reticulosarcoma**

V10.72 **Hodgkin's disease**

V10.79 Other

✓5ᵗʰ V10.8 **Personal history of malignant neoplasm of other sites**
History of conditions classifiable to 170-173, 190-195
EXCLUDES *personal history of malignant carcinoid tumor (V10.91)*
personal history of malignant neuroendocrine tumor (V10.91)

V10.81 **Bone**
AHA: 2Q, '03, 13

V10.82 **Malignant melanoma of skin**

V10.83 Other malignant neoplasm of skin

V10.84 **Eye**

V10.85 **Brain**
AHA: 1Q, '01, 6

V10.86 Other parts of the nervous system
EXCLUDES *peripheral sympathetic, and parasympathetic nerves (V10.89)*

V10.87 **Thyroid**

V10.88 Other endocrine glands and related structures

V10.89 Other

✓5ᵗʰ V10.9 **Other and unspecified personal history of malignant neoplasm**
AHA: 4Q, '09, 115

V10.90 Personal history of unspecified malignant neoplasm
Personal history of malignant neoplasm NOS
EXCLUDES *personal history of malignant carcinoid tumor (V10.91)*
personal history of malignant neuroendocrine tumor (V10.91)
personal history of Merkel cell carcinoma (V10.91)

V10.91 **Personal history of malignant neuroendocrine tumor**
Personal history of malignant carcinoid tumor NOS
Personal history of malignant neuroendocrine tumor NOS
Personal history of Merkel cell carcinoma NOS
Code first any continuing functional activity, such as: carcinoid syndrome (259.2)

✓4ᵗʰ **V11 Personal history of mental disorder**

V11.0 **Schizophrenia**
EXCLUDES *that in remission (295.0-295.9 with fifth-digit 5)*

V11.1 **Affective disorders**
Personal history of manic-depressive psychosis
EXCLUDES *that in remission (296.0-296.6 with fifth-digit 5, 6)*

V11.2 **Neurosis**

V11.3 **Alcoholism**

V11.4 **Combat and operational stress reaction**   Ⓐ
AHA: 4Q, '10, 108

V11.8 Other mental disorders

V11.9 Unspecified mental disorder

✓4ᵗʰ **V12 Personal history of certain other diseases**
AHA: 3Q, '92, 11

✓5ᵗʰ V12.0 **Infectious and parasitic diseases**
EXCLUDES *personal history of infectious diseases specific to a body system*

V12.00 Unspecified infectious and parasitic disease

V12.01 **Tuberculosis**

V12.02 **Poliomyelitis**
Z86.12 Personal history of poliomyelitis   I-10

V12.03 **Malaria**

V12.04 **Methicillin resistant Staphylococcus aureus**
MRSA
AHA: 4Q, '08, 69, 71

V12.09 Other

V12.1 **Nutritional deficiency**

✓5ᵗʰ V12.2 **Endocrine, metabolic, and immunity disorders**
AHA: ▶4Q, '11, 156◀

V12.21 **Gestational diabetes**   ♀

V12.29 Other endocrine, metabolic, and immunity disorders

V12.3 **Diseases of blood and blood-forming organs**

✓5ᵗʰ V12.4 **Disorders of nervous system and sense organs**

V12.40 Unspecified disorder of nervous system and sense organs

V12.41 **Benign neoplasm of the brain**
AHA: 4Q, '97, 48
TIP: Benign neoplasms of the brain are tracked separately because, besides being potentially life-threatening, they often recur and can be difficult to treat.

V12.42 **Infections of the central nervous system**
Encephalitis   Meningitis
AHA: 4Q, '05, 95

V12.49 Other disorders of nervous system and sense organs
AHA: 4Q, '98, 59

✓5ᵗʰ V12.5 **Diseases of circulatory system**
EXCLUDES *history of anaphylactic shock (V13.81)*
old myocardial infarction (412)
postmyocardial infarction syndrome (411.0)
AHA: 4Q, '95, 61

V12.50 Unspecified circulatory disease

V12.51 **Venous thrombosis and embolism**
EXCLUDES *pulmonary embolism (V12.55)*
AHA: 1Q, '11, 20; 3Q, '06, 12; 4Q, '03, 108; 1Q, '02, 15

V12.52 **Thrombophlebitis**

V12.53 **Sudden cardiac arrest**
Sudden cardiac death successfully resuscitated
AHA: 4Q, '07, 98

V12.54 **Transient ischemic attack [TIA], and cerebral infarction without residual deficits**
Prolonged reversible ischemic neurological deficit [PRIND]
Reversible ischemic neurologic deficit [RIND]
Stroke NOS without residual deficits
EXCLUDES *history of traumatic brain injury (V15.52)*
late effects of cerebrovascular disease (438.0-438.9)
AHA: 4Q, '07, 98
TIP: Assign for old CVA for which the patient has no residual deficits; if deficits are present, see category 438.
Z86.73 Personal hx TIA & cerebral infarct w/o deficits   I-10

V12.55 **Pulmonary embolism**
AHA: ▶4Q, '11, 156◀

V12.59 Other
AHA: 2Q, '07, 3; 4Q, '99, 4; 4Q, '98, 88; 4Q, '97, 37

✓5ᵗʰ V12.6 **Diseases of respiratory system**
EXCLUDES *tuberculosis (V12.01)*

V12.60 Unspecified disease of respiratory system

V12.61 **Pneumonia (recurrent)**
   AHA: 4Q, '05, 95

V12.69 **Other diseases of respiratory system**

√5ᵗʰ V12.7 **Diseases of digestive system**
   AHA: 1Q, '95, 3; 2Q, '89, 16

V12.70 **Unspecified digestive disease**

V12.71 **Peptic ulcer disease**

V12.72 **Colonic polyps**
   AHA: 3Q, '02, 15
   Z86.010 Personal history of colonic polyps   I-10

V12.79 **Other**

√4ᵗʰ **V13   Personal history of other diseases**

√5ᵗʰ V13.0 **Disorders of urinary system**

V13.00 **Unspecified urinary disorder**

V13.01 **Urinary calculi**

V13.02 **Urinary (tract) infection**
   AHA: 4Q, '05, 95

V13.03 **Nephrotic syndrome**
   AHA: 4Q, '05, 95

V13.09 **Other**

V13.1 **Trophoblastic disease**   ♀
   EXCLUDES supervision during a current pregnancy (V23.1)

√5ᵗʰ V13.2 **Other genital system and obstetric disorders**
   EXCLUDES recurrent pregnancy loss (646.3)
      without current pregnancy (629.81)
      supervision during a current pregnancy of a woman
         with poor obstetric history (V23.0-V23.9)

V13.21 **Personal history of pre-term labor**   ♀
   EXCLUDES current pregnancy with history of pre-term
      labor (V23.41)
   AHA: 4Q, '02, 78

V13.22 **Personal history of cervical dysplasia**   ♀
   Personal history of conditions classifiable to
      622.10-622.12
   EXCLUDES personal history of malignant neoplasm of
      cervix uteri (V10.41)
   AHA: 4Q, '07, 98

V13.23 **Personal history of vaginal dysplasia**   ♀
   Personal history of conditions classifiable to 623.0
   EXCLUDES personal history of malignant neoplasm of
      vagina (V10.44)
   AHA: 4Q, '10, 108

V13.24 **Personal history of vulvar dysplasia**   ♀
   Personal history of conditions classifiable to
      624.01-624.02
   EXCLUDES personal history of malignant neoplasm of
      vulva (V10.44)
   AHA: 4Q, '10, 108

V13.29 **Other genital system and obstetric disorders**   ♀

V13.3 **Diseases of skin and subcutaneous tissue**

V13.4 **Arthritis**

√5ᵗʰ V13.5 **Other musculoskeletal disorders**
   AHA: 4Q, '08, 158
   TIP: Personal histories of pathological, stress, or traumatic fractures
   are separately classified because a patient with such a history is at
   much higher risk of refracture of the same site.

V13.51 **Pathologic fracture**
   Healed pathologic fracture
   EXCLUDES personal history of traumatic fracture
      (V15.51)

V13.52 **Stress fracture**
   Healed stress fracture
   EXCLUDES personal history of traumatic fracture
      (V15.51)

V13.59 **Other musculoskeletal disorders**

√5ᵗʰ V13.6 **Congenital (corrected) malformations**
   AHA: 4Q, '10, 108, 136; 4Q, '98, 63

V13.61 **Personal history of (corrected) hypospadias**   ♂

V13.62 **Personal history of other (corrected) congenital malformations of genitourinary system**

V13.63 **Personal history of (corrected) congenital malformations of nervous system**

V13.64 **Personal history of (corrected) congenital malformations of eye, ear, face and neck**
   Corrected cleft lip and palate

V13.65 **Personal history of (corrected) congenital malformations of heart and circulatory system**

V13.66 **Personal history of (corrected) congenital malformations of respiratory system**

V13.67 **Personal history of (corrected) congenital malformations of digestive system**

V13.68 **Personal history of (corrected) congenital malformations of integument, limbs, and musculoskeletal systems**

V13.69 **Personal history of other (corrected) congenital malformations**
   AHA: 4Q, '10, 108; 1Q, '04, 16

V13.7 **Perinatal problems**
   EXCLUDES low birth weight status (V21.30-V21.35)

√5ᵗʰ V13.8 **Other specified diseases**
   AHA: 4Q, '11, 156

V13.81 **Anaphylaxis**

V13.89 **Other specified diseases**
   AHA: ▶1Q, '12, 11◀

V13.9 **Unspecified disease**
   AHA: 4Q, '06, 117

√4ᵗʰ **V14   Personal history of allergy to medicinal agents**

V14.0 **Penicillin**
   Z88.0 Allergy status to penicillin   I-10

V14.1 **Other antibiotic agent**

V14.2 **Sulfonamides**

V14.3 **Other anti-infective agent**

V14.4 **Anesthetic agent**

V14.5 **Narcotic agent**

V14.6 **Analgesic agent**

V14.7 **Serum or vaccine**

V14.8 **Other specified medicinal agents**

V14.9 **Unspecified medicinal agent**

√4ᵗʰ **V15   Other personal history presenting hazards to health**
   EXCLUDES personal history of drug therapy (V87.41-V87.49)

√5ᵗʰ V15.0 **Allergy, other than to medicinal agents**
   EXCLUDES allergy to food substance used as base for medicinal
      agent (V14.0-V14.9)
   AHA: 4Q, '00, 42, 49
   TIP: A person who has had an allergic episode to a substance in the
   past should always be considered allergic to the substance.

V15.01 **Allergy to peanuts**
   Z91.010 Allergy to peanuts   I-10

V15.02 **Allergy to milk products**
   EXCLUDES lactose intolerance (271.3)
   AHA: 1Q, '03, 12

V15.03 **Allergy to eggs**

V15.04 **Allergy to seafood**
   Seafood (octopus) (squid) ink   Shellfish

V15.05 **Allergy to other foods**
   Food additives   Nuts other than peanuts

V15.06 **Allergy to insects and arachnids**
   Bugs   Spiders
   Insect bites and stings

V15.07 **Allergy to latex**
   Latex sensitivity

√4ᵗʰ √5ᵗʰ Additional Digit Required   Unspecified Code   Other Specified Code   Manifestation Code   ▶◀ Revised Text   ● New Code   ▲ Revised Code Title
2013 ICD-9-CM   **October 2012 · Volume 1 – 323**

V12.61–V15.07

V Codes

V15.08–V16.6

V15.08 Allergy to radiographic dye
Contrast media used for diagnostic x-ray procedures

V15.09 Other allergy, other than to medicinal agents

V15.1 Surgery to heart and great vessels
EXCLUDES replacement by transplant or other means (V42.1-V42.2, V43.2-V43.4)
AHA: 1Q, '04, 16

√5ᵗʰ **V15.2 Surgery to other organs**
EXCLUDES replacement by transplant or other means (V42.0-V43.8)
AHA: 4Q, '08, 158

V15.21 Personal history of undergoing in utero procedure during pregnancy ♀
AHA: 4Q, '08, 158

V15.22 Personal history of undergoing in utero procedure while a fetus
AHA: 4Q, '08, 158

V15.29 Surgery to other organs

V15.3 Irradiation
Previous exposure to therapeutic or other ionizing radiation
AHA: 2Q, '11, 12;

√5ᵗʰ **V15.4 Psychological trauma**
EXCLUDES history of condition classifiable to 290-316 (V11.0-V11.9)

V15.41 History of physical abuse
Rape
AHA: 3Q, '99, 15

V15.42 History of emotional abuse
Neglect
AHA: 3Q, '99, 15

V15.49 Other
AHA: 3Q, '99, 15

√5ᵗʰ **V15.5 Injury**
AHA: 4Q, '08, 158

V15.51 Traumatic fracture
Healed traumatic fracture
EXCLUDES personal history of pathologic and stress fracture (V13.51, V13.52)
TIP: Personal histories of pathological, stress, or traumatic fractures are separately classified because a patient with such a history is at much higher risk of refracture of the same site.

V15.52 History of traumatic brain injury
EXCLUDES personal history of cerebrovascular accident (cerebral infarction) without residual deficits (V12.54)
AHA: 4Q, '09, 115

V15.53 Personal history of retained foreign body fully removed
AHA: 4Q, '10, 108

V15.59 Other injury

V15.6 Poisoning

V15.7 Contraception
*EXCLUDES current contraceptive management (V25.0-V25.4)
presence of intrauterine contraceptive device as incidental finding (V45.5)*

√5ᵗʰ **V15.8 Other specified personal history presenting hazards to health**
*EXCLUDES contact with and (suspected) exposure to:
aromatic compounds and dyes (V87.11-V87.19)
arsenic and other metals (V87.01-V87.09)
molds (V87.31)*
AHA: 4Q, '95, 62

V15.80 History of failed moderate sedation
History of failed conscious sedation
AHA: 4Q, '09, 115

V15.81 Noncompliance with medical treatment
EXCLUDES noncompliance with renal dialysis (V45.12)
AHA: 3Q, '07, 9; 4Q, '06, 136; 2Q, '03, 7; 2Q, '01, 11, 12, 13; 2Q, '99, 17; 2Q, '97, 11; 1Q, '97, 12; 3Q, '96, 9

V15.82 History of tobacco use
EXCLUDES tobacco dependence (305.1)
AHA: 1Q, '09, 17
Z87.891 Personal history of nicotine dependence   I-10

V15.83 Underimmunization status
Delinquent immunization status
Lapsed immunization schedule status
AHA: 4Q, '09, 115

V15.84 Contact with and (suspected) exposure to asbestos
AHA: 4Q, '09, 116

V15.85 Contact with and (suspected) exposure to potentially hazardous body fluids
AHA: 4Q, '09, 116

V15.86 Contact with and (suspected) exposure to lead
AHA: 4Q, '09, 116

V15.87 History of extracorporeal membrane oxygenation [ECMO]
AHA: 4Q, '03, 84

V15.88 History of fall
At risk for falling
AHA: 4Q, '05, 95
Z91.81 History of falling   I-10

V15.89 Other
*EXCLUDES contact with and (suspected) exposure to other potentially hazardous:
chemicals (V87.2)
substances (V87.39)*
AHA: 3Q, '08, 7; 3Q, '07, 5; 1Q, '90, 21; N-D, '84, 12

V15.9 Unspecified personal history presenting hazards to health

√4ᵗʰ **V16 Family history of malignant neoplasm**

V16.0 Gastrointestinal tract
Family history of condition classifiable to 140-159
AHA: 1Q, '99, 4
TIP: Family history of colon cancer is a condition that meets the criteria of "high risk" for a screening colonoscopy.

V16.1 Trachea, bronchus, and lung
Family history of condition classifiable to 162

V16.2 Other respiratory and intrathoracic organs
Family history of condition classifiable to 160-161, 163-165

V16.3 Breast
Family history of condition classifiable to 174
AHA: 4Q, '04, 107; 2Q, '03, 4; 2Q, '00, 8; 1Q, '92, 11
Z80.3 Family history of malignant neoplasm of breast   I-10

√5ᵗʰ **V16.4 Genital organs**
Family history of condition classifiable to 179-187
AHA: 4Q, '97, 48

V16.40 Genital organ, unspecified

V16.41 Ovary
AHA: 3Q, '09, 5

V16.42 Prostate
Z80.42 Family history of malignant neoplasm of prostate   I-10

V16.43 Testis

V16.49 Other
AHA: 2Q, '06, 2

√5ᵗʰ **V16.5 Urinary organs**
Family history of condition classifiable to 188-189

V16.51 Kidney

V16.52 Bladder
AHA: 4Q, '07, 98

V16.59 Other

V16.6 Leukemia
Family history of condition classifiable to 204-208

V16.7 Other lymphatic and hematopoietic neoplasms
　　Family history of condition classifiable to 200-203

V16.8 Other specified malignant neoplasm
　　Family history of other condition classifiable to 140-199

V16.9 Unspecified malignant neoplasm

☑4ᵗʰ **V17 Family history of certain chronic disabling diseases**

V17.0 Psychiatric condition
　　EXCLUDES *family history of intellectual disabilities (V18.4)*

V17.1 Stroke (cerebrovascular)
　　Z82.3 Family history of stroke   I-10

V17.2 Other neurological diseases
　　Epilepsy
　　Huntington's chorea

V17.3 Ischemic heart disease

☑5ᵗʰ **V17.4 Other cardiovascular diseases**
　　AHA: 1Q, '04, 6

　　V17.41 Family history of sudden cardiac death [SCD]
　　　　EXCLUDES *family history of ischemic heart disease (V17.3)*
　　　　　　family history of myocardial infarction (V17.3)
　　　　AHA: 4Q, '07, 98

　　V17.49 Family history of other cardiovascular diseases
　　　　Family history of cardiovascular disease NOS

V17.5 Asthma

V17.6 Other chronic respiratory conditions

V17.7 Arthritis

☑5ᵗʰ **V17.8 Other musculoskeletal diseases**

　　V17.81 Osteoporosis
　　　　AHA: 4Q, '05, 95

　　V17.89 Other musculoskeletal diseases

☑4ᵗʰ **V18 Family history of certain other specific conditions**

V18.0 Diabetes mellitus
　　AHA: 1Q, '04, 8
　　TIP: Assign for a normal infant born to a diabetic mother who presents with no manifestations of the syndrome.

☑5ᵗʰ **V18.1 Other endocrine and metabolic diseases**

　　V18.11 Multiple endocrine neoplasia [MEN] syndrome
　　　　AHA: 4Q, '07, 98, 100

　　V18.19 Other endocrine and metabolic diseases

V18.2 Anemia

V18.3 Other blood disorders

V18.4 Intellectual disabilities

☑5ᵗʰ **V18.5 Digestive disorders**

　　V18.51 Colonic polyps
　　　　EXCLUDES *family history of malignant neoplasm of gastrointestinal tract (V16.0)*
　　　　AHA: 4Q, '06, 117
　　　　Z83.71 Family history of colonic polyps   I-10

　　V18.59 Other digestive disorders

☑5ᵗʰ **V18.6 Kidney diseases**

　　V18.61 Polycystic kidney

　　V18.69 Other kidney diseases

V18.7 Other genitourinary diseases

V18.8 Infectious and parasitic diseases

V18.9 Genetic disease carrier
　　AHA: 4Q, '05, 95

☑4ᵗʰ **V19 Family history of other conditions**

V19.0 Blindness or visual loss

☑5ᵗʰ **V19.1 Other eye disorders**
　　AHA: ▶4Q, '11, 156◄

　　V19.11 Glaucoma

　　V19.19 Other specified eye disorder

V19.2 Deafness or hearing loss

V19.3 Other ear disorders

V19.4 Skin conditions

V19.5 Congenital anomalies

V19.6 Allergic disorders

V19.7 Consanguinity

V19.8 Other condition

Persons Encountering Health Services in Circumstances Related to Reproduction and Development (V20-V29)

☑4ᵗʰ **V20 Health supervision of infant or child**

V20.0 Foundling   PDx P

V20.1 Other healthy infant or child receiving care   PDx P
　　Medical or nursing care supervision of healthy infant in cases of:
　　　maternal illness, physical or psychiatric
　　　socioeconomic adverse condition at home
　　　too many children at home preventing or interfering with normal care
　　AHA: 1Q, '00, 25; 3Q, '89, 14

V20.2 Routine infant or child health check   PDx P
　　Developmental testing of infant or child
　　Health check for child over 28 days old
　　Immunizations appropriate for age
　　Routine vision and hearing testing
　　Use additional code(s) to identify:
　　　special screening examination(s) performed (V73.0-V82.9)
　　EXCLUDES *health check for child under 29 days old (V20.31-V20.32)*
　　　　newborn health supervision (V20.31-V20.32)
　　　　special screening for developmental handicaps (V79.3)
　　AHA: 4Q, '09, 115; 1Q, '09, 15; 1Q, '04, 15

☑5ᵗʰ **V20.3 Newborn health supervision**
　　Health check for child under 29 days old
　　EXCLUDES *health check for child over 28 days old (V20.2)*
　　AHA: 4Q, '09, 117

　　V20.31 Health supervision for newborn under 8 days old   PDx N
　　　　Health check for newborn under 8 days old

　　V20.32 Health supervision for newborn 8 to 28 days old   PDx N
　　　　Health check for newborn 8 to 28 days old
　　　　Newborn weight check
　　　　AHA: 4Q, '09, 102, 117

☑4ᵗʰ **V21 Constitutional states in development**

V21.0 Period of rapid growth in childhood

V21.1 Puberty

V21.2 Other adolescence

☑5ᵗʰ **V21.3 Low birth weight status**
　　EXCLUDES *history of perinatal problems*
　　AHA: 4Q, '00, 51
　　TIP: There are no age restrictions on these V codes after the perinatal period; assign for patients without the initial condition who may continue to manifest the consequences of it.

　　V21.30 Low birth weight status, unspecified

　　V21.31 Low birth weight status, less than 500 grams

　　V21.32 Low birth weight status, 500-999 grams

　　V21.33 Low birth weight status, 1000-1499 grams

　　V21.34 Low birth weight status, 1500-1999 grams

　　V21.35 Low birth weight status, 2000-2500 grams

V21.8 Other specified constitutional states in development

V21.9 Unspecified constitutional state in development

☑4ᵗʰ/☑5ᵗʰ Additional Digit Required   Unspecified Code   Other Specified Code   Manifestation Code   ▶◄ Revised Text   ● New Code   ▲ Revised Code Title

2013 ICD-9-CM   **February 2012 • Volume 1 – 325**

☑4ᵗʰ **V22 Normal pregnancy**

EXCLUDES *pregnancy examination or test, pregnancy unconfirmed (V72.40)*

AHA: ▶1Q, '12, 10;◀ 4Q, '07, 125

TIP: Do not assign with any code from chapter 11, "Complications of Pregnancy, Childbirth, and the Puerperium."

V22.0 Supervision of normal first pregnancy PDx ♀

AHA: 3Q, '99, 16

Z34.00 Encounter suprvisn norm 1 pregnancy uns trimestr I-10

V22.1 Supervision of other normal pregnancy PDx ♀

AHA: 3Q, '99, 16

V22.2 Pregnant state, incidental ♀

Pregnant state NOS

☑4ᵗʰ **V23 Supervision of high-risk pregnancy**

AHA: ▶1Q, '12, 10;◀ 1Q, '90, 10

V23.0 Pregnancy with history of infertility M ♀

V23.1 Pregnancy with history of trophoblastic disease M ♀

Pregnancy with history of:

hydatidiform mole

vesicular mole

EXCLUDES *that without current pregnancy (V13.1)*

V23.2 Pregnancy with history of abortion M ♀

Pregnancy with history of conditions classifiable to 634-638

EXCLUDES *recurrent pregnancy loss:*

care during pregnancy (646.3)

that without current pregnancy (629.81)

V23.3 Grand multiparity M ♀

EXCLUDES *care in relation to labor and delivery (659.4)*

that without current pregnancy (V61.5)

☑5ᵗʰ **V23.4 Pregnancy with other poor obstetric history**

Pregnancy with history of other conditions classifiable to 630-676

V23.41 Pregnancy with history of labor pre-term M ♀

AHA: 4Q, '02, 79

V23.42 Pregnancy with history of ectopic pregnancy M ♀

AHA: 4Q, '11, 157

V23.49 Pregnancy with other poor obstetric history M ♀

V23.5 Pregnancy with other poor reproductive history M ♀

Pregnancy with history of stillbirth or neonatal death

V23.7 Insufficient prenatal care M ♀

History of little or no prenatal care

☑5ᵗʰ **V23.8 Other high-risk pregnancy**

AHA: 4Q, '08, 158; 4Q, '98, 56, 63

V23.81 Elderly primigravida M ♀

First pregnancy in a woman who will be 35 years of age or older at expected date of delivery

EXCLUDES *elderly primigravida complicating pregnancy (659.5)*

V23.82 Elderly multigravida M ♀

Second or more pregnancy in a woman who will be 35 years of age or older at expected date of delivery

EXCLUDES *elderly multigravida complicating pregnancy (659.6)*

AHA: 4Q, '11, 133

V23.83 Young primigravida M ♀

First pregnancy in a female less than 16 years old at expected date of delivery

EXCLUDES *young primigravida complicating pregnancy (659.8)*

V23.84 Young multigravida M ♀

Second or more pregnancy in a female less than 16 years old at expected date of delivery

EXCLUDES *young multigravida complicating pregnancy (659.8)*

V23.85 Pregnancy resulting from assisted reproductive technology M ♀

Pregnancy resulting from in vitro fertilization

AHA: 4Q, '08, 160

V23.86 Pregnancy with history of in utero procedure during previous pregnancy M ♀

EXCLUDES *management of pregnancy affected by in utero procedure during current pregnancy (679.0-679.1)*

AHA: 4Q, '08, 158, 160

V23.87 Pregnancy with inconclusive fetal viability M ♀

Encounter to determine fetal viability of pregnancy

AHA: 4Q, '11, 157

V23.89 Other high-risk pregnancy M ♀

AHA: 3Q, '06, 14

V23.9 Unspecified high-risk pregnancy M ♀

☑4ᵗʰ **V24 Postpartum care and examination**

V24.0 Immediately after delivery PDx M ♀

Care and observation in uncomplicated cases

AHA: 3Q, '06, 11

V24.1 Lactating mother PDx ♀

Supervision of lactation

V24.2 Routine postpartum follow-up PDx ♀

☑4ᵗʰ **V25 Encounter for contraceptive management**

AHA: 4Q, '92, 24

☑5ᵗʰ **V25.0 General counseling and advice**

V25.01 Prescription of oral contraceptives ♀

V25.02 Initiation of other contraceptive measures

Fitting of diaphragm

Prescription of foams, creams, or other agents

AHA: 3Q, '97, 7

V25.03 Encounter for emergency contraceptive counseling and prescription

Encounter for postcoital contraceptive counseling and prescription

AHA: 4Q, '03, 84

V25.04 Counseling and instruction in natural family planning to avoid pregnancy

AHA: 4Q, '07, 99

Z30.02 Counsel & instruct natural family plan avoid pg I-10

V25.09 Other

Family planning advice

☑5ᵗʰ **V25.1 Encounter for insertion or removal of intrauterine contraceptive device**

EXCLUDES *encounter for routine checking of intrauterine contraceptive device (V25.42)*

AHA: 4Q, '10, 109

V25.11 Encounter for insertion of intrauterine contraceptive device ♀

V25.12 Encounter for removal of intrauterine contraceptive device ♀

V25.13 Encounter for removal and reinsertion of intrauterine contraceptive device ♀

Encounter for replacement of intrauterine contraceptive device

V25.2 Sterilization

Admission for interruption of fallopian tubes or vas deferens

V25.3 Menstrual extraction ♀

Menstrual regulation

☑5ᵗʰ **V25.4 Surveillance of previously prescribed contraceptive methods**

Checking, reinsertion, or removal of contraceptive device

Repeat prescription for contraceptive method

Routine examination in connection with contraceptive maintenance

V25.40 Contraceptive surveillance, unspecified

V25.41 Contraceptive pill ♀

V Codes

V25.42 Intrauterine contraceptive device ♀
　Checking of intrauterine device
　　EXCLUDES insertion or removal of intrauterine
　　　contraceptive device (V25.11-V25.13)
　　　presence of intrauterine contraceptive device
　　　as incidental finding (V45.51)
　　AHA: 4Q, '10, 109-110

V25.43 Implantable subdermal contraceptive ♀

V25.49 Other contraceptive method
　　AHA: 3Q, '97, 7

V25.5 Insertion of implantable subdermal contraceptive ♀
　AHA: 3Q, '92, 9

V25.8 Other specified contraceptive management
　Postvasectomy sperm count
　　EXCLUDES sperm count following sterilization reversal (V26.22)
　　　sperm count for fertility testing (V26.21)
　　AHA: 3Q, '96, 9

V25.9 Unspecified contraceptive management

✓4th **V26 Procreative management**

V26.0 Tuboplasty or vasoplasty after previous sterilization
　AHA: 2Q, '95, 10
　TIP: Assign for encounters for tubal ligation or vasectomy reversal
　procedures.

V26.1 Artificial insemination ♀

✓5th **V26.2 Investigation and testing**
　　EXCLUDES postvasectomy sperm count (V25.8)
　AHA: 4Q, '00, 56

V26.21 Fertility testing
　Fallopian insufflation
　Sperm count for fertility testing
　　EXCLUDES genetic counseling and testing
　　　(V26.31-V26.39)

V26.22 Aftercare following sterilization reversal
　Fallopian insufflation following sterilization reversal
　Sperm count following sterilization reversal

V26.29 Other investigation and testing
　　AHA: 2Q, '96, 9; N-D, '85, 15

✓5th **V26.3 Genetic counseling and testing**
　　EXCLUDES fertility testing (V26.21)
　　　nonprocreative genetic screening (V82.71, V82.79)
　AHA: 4Q, '05, 96

V26.31 Testing of female for genetic disease ♀
　carrier status
　　AHA: 4Q, '06, 117

V26.32 Other genetic testing of female ♀
　Use additional code to identify recurrent pregnancy
　　loss (629.81, 646.3)
　AHA: 4Q, '06, 117
　Z31.438 Encounter oth genetic test female [I-10]
　procreative mngmnt

V26.33 Genetic counseling

V26.34 Testing of male for genetic disease ♂
　carrier status
　　AHA: 4Q, '06, 117

V26.35 Encounter for testing of male partner of female ♂
　with recurrent pregnancy loss
　　AHA: 4Q, '06, 117

V26.39 Other genetic testing of male ♂
　　AHA: 4Q, '06, 117

✓5th **V26.4 General counseling and advice**

V26.41 Procreative counseling and advice using natural
　family planning
　　AHA: 4Q, '07, 99

V26.42 Encounter for fertility preservation counseling
　Encounter for fertility preservation counseling prior
　　to cancer therapy
　Encounter for fertility preservation counseling
　　prior to surgical removal of gonads
　　AHA: 4Q, '09, 117

V26.49 Other procreative management,
　counseling and advice

✓5th **V26.5 Sterilization status**

V26.51 Tubal ligation status ♀
　　EXCLUDES infertility not due to previous tubal ligation
　　　(628.0-628.9)
　Z98.51 Tubal ligation status [I-10]

V26.52 Vasectomy status ♂

✓5th **V26.8 Other specified procreative management**

V26.81 Encounter for assisted reproductive [PDx] ♀
　fertility procedure cycle
　Patient undergoing in vitro fertilization cycle
　Use additional code to identify the type of infertility
　　EXCLUDES pre-cycle diagnosis and testing — code to
　　　reason for encounter
　　AHA: 4Q, '07, 99

V26.82 Encounter for fertility preservation procedure [PDx]
　Encounter for fertility preservation procedure prior to
　　cancer therapy
　Encounter for fertility preservation procedure prior to
　　surgical removal of gonads
　　AHA: 4Q, '09, 117

V26.89 Other specified procreative management

V26.9 Unspecified procreative management

✓4th **V27 Outcome of delivery**
　NOTE This category is intended for the coding of the outcome of
　　delivery on the mother's record.
　AHA: 2Q, '91, 16
　TIP: Assign on the maternal chart for every admission during which a deliv-
　ery occurs.

V27.0 Single liveborn [M] ♀
　AHA: ▶4Q, '11, 133;◀ 4Q, '08, 192; 4Q, '05, 81; 2Q, '03, 9; 2Q, '02, 10;
　　1Q, '01, 10; 3Q, '00, 5; 4Q, '98, 77; 4Q, '95, 59; 1Q, '92, 9
　Z37.0 Single live birth [I-10]

V27.1 Single stillborn [M] ♀

V27.2 Twins, both liveborn [M] ♀
　Z37.2 Twins both liveborn [I-10]

V27.3 Twins, one liveborn and one stillborn [M] ♀

V27.4 Twins, both stillborn [M] ♀

V27.5 Other multiple birth, all liveborn [M] ♀

V27.6 Other multiple birth, some liveborn [M] ♀

V27.7 Other multiple birth, all stillborn [M] ♀

V27.9 Unspecified outcome of delivery [M] ♀
　Single birth ⎱ outcome to infant unspecified
　Multiple birth ⎰

✓4th **V28 Encounter for antenatal screening of mother**
　　EXCLUDES abnormal findings on screening — code to findings
　　　routine prenatal care (V22.0-V23.9)
　　　suspected fetal conditions affecting management of
　　　　pregnancy (655.00-655.93, 656.00- 656.93,
　　　　657.00-657.03, 658.00, 658.93)
　　　suspected fetal conditions not found (V89.01-V89.09)
　AHA: 4Q, '06, 117; 1Q, '04, 11

V28.0 Screening for chromosomal anomalies by [M] ♀
　amniocentesis

V28.1 Screening for raised alpha-fetoprotein [M] ♀
　levels in amniotic fluid

V28.2 Other screening based on amniocentesis [M] ♀

V28.3 Encounter for routine screening for malformation ♀
　using ultrasonics
　Encounter for routine fetal ultrasound NOS
　　EXCLUDES encounter for fetal anatomic survey (V28.81)
　　　genetic counseling and testing (V26.31-V26.39)

V28.4 Screening for fetal growth retardation ♀
　using ultrasonics

V28.5 Screening for isoimmunization ♀

V25.42–V28.5

V Codes (side tab)

V28.6–V42.83 (side tab)

V28.6 Screening for Streptococcus B Ⓜ♀
AHA: 4Q, '97, 46

✓5ᵗʰ **V28.8 Other specified antenatal screening**
AHA: 4Q, '08, 159; 3Q, '99, 16

V28.81 Encounter for fetal anatomic survey Ⓜ♀

V28.82 Encounter for screening for risk of pre-term labor Ⓜ♀

V28.89 Other specified antenatal screening Ⓜ♀
Chorionic villus sampling
Genomic screening
Nuchal translucency testing
Proteomic screening

V28.9 Unspecified antenatal screening ♀

✓4ᵗʰ **V29 Observation and evaluation of newborns and infants for suspected condition not found**
NOTE This category is to be used for newborns, within the neonatal period, (the first 28 days of life) who are suspected of having an abnormal condition resulting from exposure from the mother or the birth process, but without signs or symptoms, and, which after examination and observation, is found not to exist.
EXCLUDES suspected fetal conditions not found (V89.01-V89.09)
AHA: 1Q, '00, 25; 4Q, '94, 47; 1Q, '94, 9; 4Q, '92, 21
TIP: Do not assign if the infant shows any signs or symptoms.

¹ **V29.0 Observation for suspected infectious condition** Ⓝ
AHA: 1Q, '01, 10

¹ **V29.1 Observation for suspected neurological condition** Ⓝ

¹ **V29.2 Observation for suspected respiratory condition** Ⓝ

¹ **V29.3 Observation for suspected genetic or metabolic condition** Ⓝ
AHA: 2Q, '05, 21; 4Q, '98, 59, 68

¹ **V29.8 Observation for other specified suspected condition** Ⓝ
AHA: 2Q, '03, 15

¹ **V29.9 Observation for unspecified suspected condition** Ⓝ
AHA: 1Q, '02, 6

Liveborn Infants According to Type of Birth (V30-V39)

NOTE These categories are intended for the coding of liveborn infants who are consuming health care [e.g., crib or bassinet occupancy].

The following fourth-digit subdivisions are for use with categories V30-V39:

✓5ᵗʰ 0 Born in hospital Ⓝ
1 Born before admission to hospital Ⓝ
2 Born outside hospital and not hospitalized
The following two fifth-digits are for use with the fourth-digit .0, Born in hospital:

0 delivered without mention of cesarean delivery
1 delivered by cesarean delivery

AHA: 1Q, '01, 10

§ ✓4ᵗʰ **V30 Single liveborn** PDx
AHA: 2Q, '03, 9; 4Q, '98, 46, 59; 1Q, '94, 9; For code V30.00: 1Q, '04, 8, 16; 4Q, '03, 68; For code V30.01: 4Q, '09, 101; 4Q, '05, 88; For code V30.10: 3Q, '06, 10
Z38.00 Single liveborn infant delivered vaginally I-10

§ ✓4ᵗʰ **V31 Twin, mate liveborn** PDx
AHA: 3Q, '92, 10
Z38.31 Twin liveborn infant delivered by cesarean I-10

§ ✓4ᵗʰ **V32 Twin, mate stillborn** PDx

§ ✓4ᵗʰ **V33 Twin, unspecified** PDx

§ ✓4ᵗʰ **V34 Other multiple, mates all liveborn** PDx

§ ✓4ᵗʰ **V35 Other multiple, mates all stillborn** PDx

§ ✓4ᵗʰ **V36 Other multiple, mates live and stillborn** PDx

§ ✓4ᵗʰ **V37 Other multiple, unspecified** PDx

§ ✓4ᵗʰ **V39 Unspecified** PDx

Persons with a Condition Influencing their Health Status (V40-V49)

NOTE These categories are intended for use when these conditions are recorded as "diagnoses" or "problems."
TIP: Includes patients with a carrier status or who have sequelae or residual of a past condition or disease, which may affect current or future treatment.

✓4ᵗʰ **V40 Mental and behavioral problems**

V40.0 Problems with learning

V40.1 Problems with communication [including speech]

V40.2 Other mental problems

✓5ᵗʰ **V40.3 Other behavioral problems**
AHA: 4Q, '11, 158

V40.31 Wandering in diseases classified elsewhere
Code first underlying disorder such as:
Alzheimer's disease (331.0)
autism or pervasive developmental disorder (299.0-299.9)
dementia, unspecified, with behavioral disturbance (294.21)
intellectual disabilities (317-319)

V40.39 Other specified behavioral problem

V40.9 Unspecified mental or behavioral problem

✓4ᵗʰ **V41 Problems with special senses and other special functions**

V41.0 Problems with sight

V41.1 Other eye problems

V41.2 Problems with hearing

V41.3 Other ear problems

V41.4 Problems with voice production

V41.5 Problems with smell and taste

V41.6 Problems with swallowing and mastication

V41.7 Problems with sexual function
EXCLUDES marital problems (V61.10)
psychosexual disorders (302.0-302.9)

V41.8 Other problems with special functions

V41.9 Unspecified problem with special functions

✓4ᵗʰ **V42 Organ or tissue replaced by transplant**
INCLUDES homologous or heterologous (animal) (human) transplant organ status
AHA: 3Q, '11, 5; 3Q, '98, 3, 4
TIP: Do not assign if the patient has a complication of the transplanted organ; the code from subcategory 996.8 provides the information.

V42.0 Kidney
AHA: 1Q, '08, 10; 1Q, '03, 10; 3Q, '01, 12
Z94.0 Kidney transplant status I-10

V42.1 Heart
AHA: 3Q, '03, 16; 3Q, '01, 13

V42.2 Heart valve

V42.3 Skin

V42.4 Bone

V42.5 Cornea

V42.6 Lung

V42.7 Liver
AHA: 3Q, '11, 5
Z94.4 Liver transplant status I-10

✓5ᵗʰ **V42.8 Other specified organ or tissue**
AHA: 4Q, '98, 64; 4Q, '97, 49

V42.81 Bone marrow
AHA: ▶1Q, '12, 13◀

V42.82 Peripheral stem cells

V42.83 Pancreas
AHA: 1Q, '03, 10; 2Q, '01, 16

---

¹ A code from the V30–V39 series may be sequenced before the V29 on the newborn medical record.
§ Require fourth and fifth digits. See beginning of section V30-V39 for codes and definitions.

 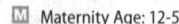

V42.84 Intestines
> AHA: 4Q, '00, 48, 50

V42.89 Other

V42.9 Unspecified organ or tissue

√4ᵗʰ **V43 Organ or tissue replaced by other means**

> INCLUDES   organ or tissue assisted by other means
> replacement of organ by:
>> artificial device
>> mechanical device
>> prosthesis

> EXCLUDES   cardiac pacemaker in situ (V45.01)
> fitting and adjustment of prosthetic device (V52.0-V52.9)
> renal dialysis status (V45.11)

V43.0 Eye globe

V43.1 Lens
> Pseudophakos
> AHA: 4Q, '98, 65

√5ᵗʰ **V43.2 Heart**
> Fully implantable artificial heart
> Heart assist device
> AHA: 4Q, '03, 85

    V43.21 Heart assist device

    V43.22 Fully implantable artificial heart

V43.3 Heart valve
> AHA: 3Q, '06, 7; 3Q, '02, 13, 14
> **TIP:** If the status post heart valve replacement information includes "porcine" or mention of other homologous or heterologous tissue, assign instead V42.2.
> Z95.2 Presence of prosthetic heart valve   I-10

V43.4 Blood vessel

V43.5 Bladder

√5ᵗʰ **V43.6 Joint**
> AHA: 4Q, '05, 91

    V43.60 Unspecified joint

    V43.61 Shoulder

    V43.62 Elbow

    V43.63 Wrist

    V43.64 Hip
> AHA: 1Q, '09, 6; 2Q, '08, 3-5; 3Q, '06, 4, 5; 4Q, '05, 93, 112; 2Q, '04, 15
> Z96.641 Presence of right artificial hip joint   I-10

    V43.65 Knee
> AHA: 3Q, '06, 5

    V43.66 Ankle

    V43.69 Other

V43.7 Limb

√5ᵗʰ **V43.8 Other organ or tissue**

    V43.81 Larynx
> AHA: 4Q, '95, 55

    V43.82 Breast
> AHA: 4Q, '95, 55
> Z98.82 Breast implant status   I-10

    V43.83 Artificial skin

    V43.89 Other

√4ᵗʰ **V44 Artificial opening status**

> EXCLUDES   artificial openings requiring attention or management (V55.0-V55.9)

> **TIP:** Do not assign if the patient has a complication of the artificial opening, such as infection or obstruction; assign only the complication code.

V44.0 Tracheostomy
> AHA: 4Q, '03, 103, 107, 111; 1Q, '01, 6

V44.1 Gastrostomy
> AHA: 4Q, '03, 103, 107-108, 110; 1Q, '01, 12; 3Q, '97, 12; 1Q, '93, 26

V44.2 Ileostomy

V44.3 Colostomy
> AHA: 4Q, '03, 110
> Z93.3 Colostomy status   I-10

V44.4 Other artificial opening of gastrointestinal tract

√5ᵗʰ **V44.5 Cystostomy**

    V44.50 Cystostomy, unspecified

    V44.51 Cutaneous-vesicostomy

    V44.52 Appendico-vesicostomy

    V44.59 Other cystostomy

V44.6 Other artificial opening of urinary tract
> Nephrostomy   Urethrostomy
> Ureterostomy

V44.7 Artificial vagina

V44.8 Other artificial opening status

V44.9 Unspecified artificial opening status

√4ᵗʰ **V45 Other postprocedural states**

> EXCLUDES   aftercare management (V51-V58.9)
> malfunction or other complication — code to condition

> AHA: 4Q, '03, 85

√5ᵗʰ **V45.0 Cardiac device in situ**

> EXCLUDES   artificial heart (V43.22)
> heart assist device (V43.21)

    V45.00 Unspecified cardiac device

    V45.01 Cardiac pacemaker
> EXCLUDES   cardiac defibrillator with synchronous cardiac pacemaker (V45.02)

    V45.02 Automatic implantable cardiac defibrillator
> With synchronous cardiac pacemaker
> Z95.810 Presence auto implantable cardiac defibrillator   I-10

    V45.09 Other specified cardiac device
> Carotid sinus pacemaker in situ

√5ᵗʰ **V45.1 Renal dialysis status**

> EXCLUDES   admission for dialysis treatment or session (V56.0)
> AHA: 4Q, '08, 157; 1Q, '08, 7; 4Q, '07, 86; 3Q, '07, 9; 4Q, '06, 136; 4Q, '05, 96; 2Q, '03, 7; 2Q, '01, 12, 13

    V45.11 Renal dialysis status
> Hemodialysis status
> Patient requiring intermittent renal dialysis
> Peritoneal dialysis status
> Presence of arterial-venous shunt (for dialysis)
> AHA: ▶3Q, '11, 15;◀ 4Q, '08, 157, 193
> Z99.2 Dependence on renal dialysis   I-10

    V45.12 Noncompliance with renal dialysis

    V45.2 Presence of cerebrospinal fluid drainage device
> Cerebral ventricle (communicating) shunt, valve, or device in situ
> EXCLUDES   malfunction (996.2)
> AHA: 4Q, '03, 106

    V45.3 Intestinal bypass or anastomosis status
> EXCLUDES   bariatric surgery status (V45.86)
> gastric bypass status (V45.86)
> obesity surgery status (V45.86)

    V45.4 Arthrodesis status
> AHA: N-D, '84, 18
> **TIP:** If there is a complication of the fusion graft site that requires refusion or revision, assign instead a code from subcategory 996.4.

√5ᵗʰ **V45.5 Presence of contraceptive device**

    V45.51 Intrauterine contraceptive device   ♀
> EXCLUDES   checking of device (V25.42)
> complication from device (996.32)
> insertion and removal of device (V25.11-V25.13)
> Z97.5 Presence of intrauterine contraceptive device   I-10

    V45.52 Subdermal contraceptive implant

    V45.59 Other

√4ᵗʰ √5ᵗʰ Additional Digit Required   Unspecified Code   Other Specified Code   Manifestation Code   ▶◀ Revised Text   ● New Code   ▲ Revised Code Title

2013 ICD-9-CM   **February 2012 · Volume 1 – 329**

V42.84-V45.59

√5ᵗʰ **V45.6 States following surgery of eye and adnexa**

Cataract extraction
Filtering bleb
Surgical eyelid adhesion
} state following eye surgery

EXCLUDES aphakia (379.31)
artificial eye globe (V43.0)
AHA: 4Q, '98, 65; 4Q, '97, 49

V45.61 Cataract extraction status
Use additional code for associated artificial lens status (V43.1)

V45.69 Other states following surgery of eye and adnexa
AHA: 2Q, '01, 16; 1Q, '98, 10; 4Q, '97, 19

√5ᵗʰ **V45.7 Acquired absence of organ**
AHA: 4Q, '98, 65; 4Q, '97, 50

V45.71 Acquired absence of breast and nipple
EXCLUDES congenital absence of breast and nipple (757.6)
AHA: 4Q, '08, 159; 4Q, '01, 66

V45.72 Acquired absence of intestine (large)(small)

V45.73 Acquired absence of kidney

V45.74 Other parts of urinary tract
Bladder
AHA: 4Q, '00, 51

V45.75 Stomach
AHA: 4Q, '00, 51

V45.76 Lung
AHA: 4Q, '00, 51

V45.77 Genital organs
EXCLUDES acquired absence of cervix and uterus (V88.01-V88.03)
female genital mutilation status (629.20-629.29)
AHA: 1Q, '03, 13, 14; 4Q, '00, 51

V45.78 Eye
AHA: 4Q, '00, 51

V45.79 Other acquired absence of organ
EXCLUDES acquired absence of pancreas (V88.11-V88.12)
AHA: 4Q, '00, 51

√5ᵗʰ **V45.8 Other postprocedural status**

V45.81 Aortocoronary bypass status
AHA: ▶4Q, '11, 153;◀ 4Q, '10, 131; 4Q, '03, 105; 3Q, '01, 15; 3Q, '97, 16

V45.82 Percutaneous transluminal coronary angioplasty status

V45.83 Breast implant removal status
AHA: 4Q, '95, 55

V45.84 Dental restoration status
Dental crowns status   Dental fillings status
AHA: 4Q, '01, 54

V45.85 Insulin pump status

V45.86 Bariatric surgery status
Gastric banding status
Gastric bypass status for obesity
Obesity surgery status
EXCLUDES bariatric surgery status complicating pregnancy, childbirth or the puerperium (649.2)
intestinal bypass or anastomosis status (V45.3)
AHA: 2Q, '09, 10; 4Q, '06, 118
Z98.84 Bariatric surgery status   I-10

V45.87 Transplanted organ removal status
Transplanted organ previously removed due to complication, failure, rejection or infection
EXCLUDES encounter for removal of transplanted organ — code to complication of transplanted organ (996.80-996.89)
AHA: 4Q, '08, 157

V45.88 Status post administration of tPA (rtPA) in a different facility within the last 24 hours prior to admission to current facility
Code first condition requiring tPA administration, such as:
acute cerebral infarction (433.0-433.9 with fifth-digit 1, 434.0-434.9 with fifth digit 1)
acute myocardial infarction (410.00-410.92)
AHA: 4Q, '08, 157
TIP: Assign only on receiving facility record; assign even if the patient is still receiving tPA at the time of transfer.

V45.89 Other
Presence of neuropacemaker or other electronic device
EXCLUDES artificial heart valve in situ (V43.3)
vascular prosthesis in situ (V43.4)
AHA: 1Q, '95, 11

√4ᵗʰ **V46 Other dependence on machines and devices**

V46.0 Aspirator

√5ᵗʰ **V46.1 Respirator [Ventilator]**
Iron lung
AHA: 4Q, '05, 96; 4Q, '03, 103; 1Q, '01, 12; J-F, '87, 7 3

V46.11 Dependence on respirator, status
AHA: 4Q, '04, 100
Z99.11 Dependence on respirator ventilator status   I-10

V46.12 Encounter for respirator dependence during power failure   PDx
AHA: 4Q, '04, 100

V46.13 Encounter for weaning from respirator [ventilator]   PDx

V46.14 Mechanical complication of respirator [ventilator]
Mechanical failure of respirator [ventilator]

V46.2 Supplemental oxygen
Long-term oxygen therapy
AHA: 4Q, '03, 108; 4Q, '02, 79

V46.3 Wheelchair dependence
Wheelchair confinement status
Code first cause of dependence, such as:
muscular dystrophy (359.1)
obesity (278.00-278.03)
AHA: 4Q, '08, 157

V46.8 Other enabling machines
Hyperbaric chamber
Possum [Patient-Operated-Selector-Mechanism]
EXCLUDES cardiac pacemaker (V45.0)
kidney dialysis machine (V45.11)

V46.9 Unspecified machine dependence
AHA: 4Q, '06, 117

√4ᵗʰ **V47 Other problems with internal organs**

V47.0 Deficiencies of internal organs

V47.1 Mechanical and motor problems with internal organs

V47.2 Other cardiorespiratory problems
Cardiovascular exercise intolerance with pain (with):
at rest
less than ordinary activity
ordinary activity

V47.3 Other digestive problems

V47.4 Other urinary problems

V47.5 Other genital problems

V47.9 Unspecified

√4ᵗʰ **V48 Problems with head, neck, and trunk**

V48.0 Deficiencies of head
EXCLUDES deficiencies of ears, eyelids, and nose (V48.8)

V48.1 Deficiencies of neck and trunk

V48.2 Mechanical and motor problems with head

V48.3 Mechanical and motor problems with neck and trunk

V48.4 Sensory problem with head

V48.5 **Sensory problem with neck and trunk**

V48.6 **Disfigurements of head**

V48.7 **Disfigurements of neck and trunk**

V48.8 Other problems with head, neck, and trunk

V48.9 Unspecified problem with head, neck, or trunk

✓4ᵗʰ **V49 Other conditions influencing health status**

V49.0 **Deficiencies of limbs**

V49.1 **Mechanical problems with limbs**

V49.2 **Motor problems with limbs**

V49.3 **Sensory problems with limbs**

V49.4 **Disfigurements of limbs**

V49.5 Other problems of limbs

✓5ᵗʰ V49.6 **Upper limb amputation status**
AHA: 4Q, '05, 94; 4Q, '98, 42; 4Q, '94, 39

    V49.60 **Unspecified level**
Z89.201 Acquired absence of right upper limb   I-10
uns level

    V49.61 **Thumb**

    V49.62 **Other finger(s)**
AHA: 2Q, '05, 7

    V49.63 **Hand**

    V49.64 **Wrist**
Disarticulation of wrist

    V49.65 **Below elbow**

    V49.66 **Above elbow**
Disarticulation of elbow

    V49.67 **Shoulder**
Disarticulation of shoulder

✓5ᵗʰ V49.7 **Lower limb amputation status**
AHA: 3Q, '06, 5; 4Q, '05, 94; 4Q, '98, 42; 4Q, '94, 39

    V49.70 **Unspecified level**

    V49.71 **Great toe**

    V49.72 **Other toe(s)**

    V49.73 **Foot**

    V49.74 **Ankle**
Disarticulation of ankle

    V49.75 **Below knee**
Z89.52 Acquired absence of left leg below knee   I-10

    V49.76 **Above knee**
Disarticulation of knee

    V49.77 **Hip**
Disarticulation of hip

✓5ᵗʰ V49.8 **Other specified conditions influencing health status**
AHA: 4Q, '00, 51

    V49.81 **Asymptomatic postmenopausal status**   A♀
(age-related) (natural)
EXCLUDES menopausal and premenopausal disorder
(627.0-627.9)
postsurgical menopause (256.2)
premature menopause (256.31)
symptomatic menopause (627.0-627.9)
AHA: 4Q, '09, 106; 4Q, '02, 79; 4Q, '00, 54

    V49.82 **Dental sealant status**
AHA: 4Q, '01, 54

    V49.83 **Awaiting organ transplant status**

    V49.84 **Bed confinement status**
AHA: 4Q, '05, 96

    V49.85 **Dual sensory impairment**
Blindness with deafness
Combined visual hearing impairment
Code first:
hearing impairment (389.00-389.9)
visual impairment (369.00-369.9)
AHA: 4Q, '07, 100

V49.86 **Do not resuscitate status**
AHA: ▶1Q, '12, 14;◀ 4Q, '10, 108
Z66 Do not resuscitate   I-10

V49.87 **Physical restraints status**
EXCLUDES restraint due to a procedure – omit code
AHA: 4Q, '10, 108-109

V49.89 Other specified conditions
influencing health status
AHA: 4Q, '05, 94

V49.9 Unspecified

Persons Encountering Health Services for Specific Procedures and Aftercare (V50-V59)

NOTE Categories V51-V59 are intended for use to indicate a reason
for care in patients who may have already been treated for
some disease or injury not now present, or who are receiving
care to consolidate the treatment, to deal with residual states,
or to prevent recurrence.

EXCLUDES follow-up examination for medical surveillance following
treatment (V67.0-V67.9)

✓4ᵗʰ **V50 Elective surgery for purposes other than remedying health
states**

V50.0 **Hair transplant**

V50.1 Other plastic surgery for unacceptable cosmetic
appearance
Breast augmentation or reduction
Face-lift
EXCLUDES encounter for breast reduction (611.1)
plastic surgery following healed injury or operation
(V51.0-V51.8)

V50.2 **Routine or ritual circumcision**   ♂
Circumcision in the absence of significant medical indication

V50.3 **Ear piercing**

✓5ᵗʰ V50.4 **Prophylactic organ removal**
EXCLUDES organ donations (V59.0-V59.9)
therapeutic organ removal — code to condition
AHA: 4Q, '94, 44
TIP: Assign an additional code, such as one from category V16 Family
history of malignant neoplasm, to indicate the reason for the
prophylactic organ removal.

    V50.41 **Breast**
AHA: 2Q, '11, 12; 4Q, '04, 107

    V50.42 **Ovary**   ♀
AHA: 3Q, '09, 5

    V50.49 Other
AHA: 3Q, '09, 5

V50.8 Other
Z40.8 Encounter for other prophylactic surgery   I-10

V50.9 Unspecified

✓4ᵗʰ **V51 Aftercare involving the use of plastic surgery**
Plastic surgery following healed injury or operation
EXCLUDES cosmetic plastic surgery (V50.2)
plastic surgery as treatment for current condition or injury —
code to condition or injury
repair of scarred tissue — code to scar
AHA: 4Q, '08, 159

V51.0 **Encounter for breast reconstruction**   PDx A
following mastectomy
EXCLUDES deformity and disproportion of reconstructed breast
(612.0-612.1)
AHA: 4Q, '08, 159-160

V51.8 Other aftercare involving the use of plastic surgery

✓4ᵗʰ **V52 Fitting and adjustment of prosthetic device and implant**
INCLUDES removal of device
EXCLUDES malfunction or complication of prosthetic device
(996.0-996.7)
status only, without need for care (V43.0-V43.8)
AHA: 4Q, '05, 94; 4Q, '95, 55 ; 1Q, '90, 7

V52.0 **Artificial arm (complete) (partial)**

✓4ᵗʰ Additional Digit Required   Unspecified Code   Other Specified Code   Manifestation Code   ▶◀ Revised Text   ● New Code   ▲ Revised Code Title
✓5ᵗʰ

2013 ICD-9-CM   October 2012 • Volume 1 – 331

V48.5–V52.0

V Codes

V52.1–V54.19

V52.1 Artificial leg (complete) (partial)

V52.2 Artificial eye

V52.3 Dental prosthetic device

V52.4 Breast prosthesis and implant ♀
Elective implant exchange (different material) (different size)
Removal of tissue expander without synchronous insertion of permanent implant

> EXCLUDES *admission for initial breast implant insertion for breast augmentation (V50.1)*
> *complications of breast implant (996.54, 996.69, 996.79)*
> *encounter for breast reconstruction following mastectomy (V51.0)*

AHA: 4Q, '95, 80, 81

V52.8 Other specified prosthetic device
AHA: 2Q, '02, 12, 16

V52.9 Unspecified prosthetic device

√4ᵗʰ V53 Fitting and adjustment of other device
> INCLUDES removal of device
> replacement of device
> EXCLUDES *status only, without need for care (V45.0-V45.8)*

√5ᵗʰ V53.0 Devices related to nervous system and special senses
AHA: 4Q, '98, 66; 4Q, '97, 51

V53.01 Fitting and adjustment of cerebral ventricular (communicating) shunt
AHA: 4Q, '97, 51

V53.02 Neuropacemaker (brain) (peripheral nerve) (spinal cord)

V53.09 Fitting and adjustment of other devices related to nervous system and special senses
Auditory substitution device
Visual substitution device
AHA: 2Q, '99, 4

V53.1 Spectacles and contact lenses

V53.2 Hearing aid

√5ᵗʰ V53.3 Cardiac device
Reprogramming
AHA: 3Q, '92, 3; 1Q, '90, 7; M-J, '87, 8 ; N-D, '84, 18
TIP: Assign for cardiac device replacement when the device has reached normal end-of-life parameters.

V53.31 Cardiac pacemaker
> EXCLUDES *automatic implantable cardiac defibrillator with synchronous cardiac pacemaker (V53.32)*
> *mechanical complication of cardiac pacemaker (996.01)*
AHA: 3Q, '10, 9; 1Q, '02, 3

V53.32 Automatic implantable cardiac defibrillator
With synchronous cardiac pacemaker
AHA: 3Q, '05, 8

V53.39 Other cardiac device
AHA: 4Q, '10, 124,125; 2Q, '08, 9; 1Q, '07, 20

V53.4 Orthodontic devices

√5ᵗʰ V53.5 Other gastrointestinal appliance and device
> EXCLUDES *colostomy (V55.3)*
> *ileostomy (V55.2)*
> *other artificial opening of digestive tract (V55.4)*
AHA: 4Q, '09, 116

V53.50 Fitting and adjustment of intestinal appliance and device

V53.51 Fitting and adjustment of gastric lap band

V53.59 Fitting and adjustment of other gastrointestinal appliance and device

V53.6 Urinary devices
Urinary catheter
> EXCLUDES *cystostomy (V55.5)*
> *nephrostomy (V55.6)*
> *ureterostomy (V55.6)*
> *urethrostomy (V55.6)*

V53.7 Orthopedic devices
Orthopedic: Orthopedic:
brace   corset
cast   shoes
> EXCLUDES *other orthopedic aftercare (V54)*

V53.8 Wheelchair

√5ᵗʰ V53.9 Other and unspecified device
AHA: 2Q, '03, 6

V53.90 Unspecified device

V53.91 Fitting and adjustment of insulin pump
Insulin pump titration

V53.99 Other device

AHA: 2Q, '09, 10

√4ᵗʰ V54 Other orthopedic aftercare
> EXCLUDES *fitting and adjustment of orthopedic devices (V53.7)*
> *malfunction of internal orthopedic device (996.40-996.49)*
> *other complication of nonmechanical nature (996.60-996.79)*
AHA: 4Q, '08, 158; 1Q, '07, 3-4; 3Q, '95, 3

√5ᵗʰ V54.0 Aftercare involving internal fixation device
> EXCLUDES *malfunction of internal orthopedic device (996.40-996.49)*
> *other complication of nonmechanical nature (996.60-996.79)*
> *removal of external fixation device (V54.89)*
AHA: 4Q, '03, 87

V54.01 Encounter for removal of internal fixation device

V54.02 Encounter for lengthening/adjustment of growth rod

V54.09 Other aftercare involving internal fixation device

√5ᵗʰ V54.1 Aftercare for healing traumatic fracture
> EXCLUDES *aftercare following joint replacement (V54.81)*
> *aftercare for amputation stump (V54.89)*
AHA: 4Q, '02, 80
TIP: Assign for follow-up and treatment during the healing phase of the fracture; an aftercare code should be used for all subsequent encounters after the initial encounter for care of a fracture.

V54.10 Aftercare for healing traumatic fracture of arm, unspecified

V54.11 Aftercare for healing traumatic fracture of upper arm

V54.12 Aftercare for healing traumatic fracture of lower arm
AHA: 1Q, '07, 7

V54.13 Aftercare for healing traumatic fracture of hip
AHA: 1Q, '09, 6; 4Q, '03, 103, 105; 2Q, '03, 16

V54.14 Aftercare for healing traumatic fracture of leg, unspecified

V54.15 Aftercare for healing traumatic fracture of upper leg
> EXCLUDES *aftercare for healing traumatic fracture of hip (V54.13)*
AHA: 3Q, '06, 6

V54.16 Aftercare for healing traumatic fracture of lower leg

V54.17 Aftercare for healing traumatic fracture of vertebrae

V54.19 Aftercare for healing traumatic fracture of other bone
AHA: 1Q, '05, 13; 4Q, '02, 80

☑5ᵗʰ **V54.2 Aftercare for healing pathologic fracture**

> EXCLUDES *aftercare following joint replacement (V54.81)*
> AHA: 4Q, '02, 80

V54.20 Aftercare for healing pathologic fracture of arm, unspecified

V54.21 Aftercare for healing pathologic fracture of upper arm

V54.22 Aftercare for healing pathologic fracture of lower arm

V54.23 Aftercare for healing pathologic fracture of hip

V54.24 Aftercare for healing pathologic fracture of leg, unspecified

V54.25 Aftercare for healing pathologic fracture of upper leg

> EXCLUDES *aftercare for healing pathologic fracture of hip (V54.23)*

V54.26 Aftercare for healing pathologic fracture of lower leg

V54.27 Aftercare for healing pathologic fracture of vertebrae
> AHA: 1Q, '07, 6; 4Q, '03, 108

V54.29 Aftercare for healing pathologic fracture of other bone
> AHA: 4Q, '02, 80

☑5ᵗʰ **V54.8 Other orthopedic aftercare**
> AHA: 3Q, '01, 19; 4Q, '99, 5

V54.81 Aftercare following joint replacement
> Use additional code to identify joint replacement site (V43.60-V43.69)
> AHA: 1Q, '11, 9; 1Q, '09, 6; 3Q, '06, 4; 2Q, '04, 15; 4Q, '02, 80

V54.82 Aftercare following explantation of joint prosthesis
> Aftercare following explantation of joint prosthesis, staged procedure
> Encounter for joint prosthesis insertion following prior explantation of joint prosthesis
> AHA: 4Q, '11, 156
> TIP: ▶Assign also a code from subcategory V88.2 to identify the specific joint.◀

V54.89 Other orthopedic aftercare
> Aftercare for healing fracture NOS

V54.9 Unspecified orthopedic aftercare

☑4ᵗʰ **V55 Attention to artificial openings**

> INCLUDES adjustment or repositioning of catheter
> closure
> passage of sounds or bougies
> reforming
> removal or replacement of catheter
> toilet or cleansing

> EXCLUDES *complications of external stoma (519.00-519.09, 569.60-569.69, 596.81-596.83, 997.49)*
> *status only, without need for care (V44.0-V44.9)*

V55.0 Tracheostomy

V55.1 Gastrostomy
> AHA: 4Q, '99, 9; 3Q, '97, 7, 8; 1Q, '96, 14; 3Q, '95, 13
> TIP: Assign for gastrostomy or PEG tube that has been dislodged or clogged, for which simple irrigation or replacement is performed.

V55.2 Ileostomy

V55.3 Colostomy
> AHA: 1Q, '09, 5; 2Q, '05, 4; 3Q, '97, 9
> Z43.3 Encounter for attention to colostomy `I-10`

V55.4 Other artificial opening of digestive tract
> AHA: 2Q, '05, 14; 1Q, '03, 10

V55.5 Cystostomy

V55.6 Other artificial opening of urinary tract
> Nephrostomy   Urethrostomy
> Ureterostomy

V55.7 Artificial vagina

V55.8 Other specified artificial opening

V55.9 Unspecified artificial opening

☑4ᵗʰ **V56 Encounter for dialysis and dialysis catheter care**

> Use additional code to identify the associated condition
> EXCLUDES *dialysis preparation — code to condition*
> AHA: 4Q, '98, 66; 1Q, '93, 29

V56.0 Extracorporeal dialysis `PDx`
> Dialysis (renal) NOS
> EXCLUDES *dialysis status (V45.11)*
> AHA: 4Q, '05, 79; 1Q, '04, 23; 4Q, '00, 40; 3Q, '98, 6; 2Q, '98, 20

V56.1 Fitting and adjustment of extracorporeal dialysis catheter
> Removal or replacement of catheter
> Toilet or cleansing
> Use additional code for any concurrent extracorporeal dialysis (V56.0)
> AHA: 2Q, '98, 20

V56.2 Fitting and adjustment of peritoneal dialysis catheter
> Use additional code for any concurrent peritoneal dialysis (V56.8)
> AHA: 4Q, '98, 55

☑5ᵗʰ **V56.3 Encounter for adequacy testing for dialysis**
> AHA: 4Q, '00, 55

V56.31 Encounter for adequacy testing for hemodialysis

V56.32 Encounter for adequacy testing for peritoneal dialysis
> Peritoneal equilibration test

V56.8 Other dialysis
> Peritoneal dialysis
> AHA: 4Q, '98, 55

☑4ᵗʰ **V57 Care involving use of rehabilitation procedures**

> Use additional code to identify underlying condition
> AHA: 3Q, '06, 3; 1Q, '02, 19; 3Q, '97, 12; 1Q, '90, 6; S-O, '86, 3
> TIP: Assign codes from this category for episodes of care related to rehabilitation.

V57.0 Breathing exercises `PDx`

V57.1 Other physical therapy `PDx`
> Therapeutic and remedial exercises, except breathing
> AHA: 3Q, '06, 4; 2Q, '04, 15; 4Q, '02, 56; 4Q, '99, 5

☑5ᵗʰ **V57.2 Occupational therapy and vocational rehabilitation**

V57.21 Encounter for occupational therapy `PDx`
> AHA: 4Q, '99, 7

V57.22 Encounter for vocational therapy `PDx`

V57.3 Speech-language therapy `PDx`
> AHA: 4Q, '97, 36

V57.4 Orthoptic training `PDx`

☑5ᵗʰ **V57.8 Other specified rehabilitation procedure**

V57.81 Orthotic training `PDx`
> Gait training in the use of artificial limbs

V57.89 Other `PDx`
> Multiple training or therapy
> AHA: 4Q, '07, 94; 3Q, '06, 6; 4Q, '03, 105-106, 108; 2Q, '03, 16; 1Q, '02, 16; 3Q, '01, 21; 3Q, '97, 11, 12; S-O, '86, 4

V57.9 Unspecified rehabilitation procedure `PDx`

☑4ᵗʰ **V58 Encounter for other and unspecified procedures and aftercare**

> EXCLUDES *convalescence and palliative care (V66)*
> TIP: If a patient is admitted for both radiation therapy and chemotherapy, either code V58.0 or V58.11 may be sequenced as the principal diagnosis.

V58.0 Radiotherapy `PDx`
> Encounter or admission for radiotherapy
> EXCLUDES *encounter for radioactive implant — code to condition*
> *radioactive iodine therapy — code to condition*
> AHA: 3Q, '92, 5; 2Q, '90, 7; J-F, '87, 13
> Z51.0 Encounter for antineoplastic radiation therapy `I-10`

V Codes

V58.1–V58.75

√5ᵗʰ **V58.1 Encounter for antineoplastic chemotherapy and immunotherapy**
Encounter or admission for chemotherapy
EXCLUDES *chemotherapy and immunotherapy for nonneoplastic conditions — code to condition*
AHA: 1Q, '04, 13; 2Q, '03, 16; 3Q, '93, 4; 2Q, '92, 6; 2Q, '91, 17; 2Q, '90, 7; S-O, '84, 5

V58.11 Encounter for antineoplastic chemotherapy PDx
AHA: ▶1Q, '12, 13;◀ 2Q, '11, 4; 4Q, '09, 79; 4Q, '08, 82, 155; 4Q, '07, 104; 2Q, '06, 20-21; 4Q, '05, 98
Z51.11 Encounter for antineoplastic chemotherapy I-10

V58.12 Encounter for antineoplastic immunotherapy PDx
AHA: 4Q, '05, 98

V58.2 Blood transfusion, without reported diagnosis

√5ᵗʰ **V58.3 Attention to dressings and sutures**
Change or removal of wound packing
EXCLUDES *attention to drains (V58.49)*
planned postoperative wound closure (V58.41)
AHA: 2Q, '05, 14

V58.30 Encounter for change or removal of nonsurgical wound dressing
Encounter for change or removal of wound dressing NOS
AHA: 4Q, '09, 150; 4Q, '06, 117

V58.31 Encounter for change or removal of surgical wound dressing
AHA: 4Q, '06, 117
Z48.01 Encounter change/removal surgical wound dressing I-10

V58.32 Encounter for removal of sutures
Encounter for removal of staples
AHA: 4Q, '06, 117
Z48.02 Encounter for removal of sutures I-10

√5ᵗʰ **V58.4 Other aftercare following surgery**
NOTE Codes from this subcategory should be used in conjunction with other aftercare codes to fully identify the reason for the aftercare encounter
EXCLUDES *aftercare following sterilization reversal surgery (V26.22)*
attention to artificial openings (V55.0-V55.9)
orthopedic aftercare (V54.0-V54.9)
AHA: 4Q, '99, 9; N-D, '87, 9

V58.41 Encounter for planned postoperative wound closure
EXCLUDES *disruption of operative wound (998.31-998.32)*
encounter for dressings and suture aftercare (V58.30-V58.32)
AHA: 4Q, '99, 15

V58.42 Aftercare following surgery for neoplasm
Conditions classifiable to 140-239
AHA: 4Q, '02, 80

V58.43 Aftercare following surgery for injury and trauma
Conditions classifiable to 800-999
EXCLUDES *aftercare for healing traumatic fracture (V54.10-V54.19)*
AHA: 4Q, '02, 80

V58.44 Aftercare following organ transplant
Use additional code to identify the organ transplanted (V42.0-V42.9)
AHA: 3Q, '11, 5; 4Q, '04, 101

V58.49 Other specified aftercare following surgery
Change or removal of drains
AHA: 1Q, '96, 8, 9

V58.5 Orthodontics
EXCLUDES *fitting and adjustment of orthodontic device (V53.4)*

√5ᵗʰ **V58.6 Long-term (current) drug use**
Long-term (current) prophylactic drug use
EXCLUDES *drug abuse and dependence complicating pregnancy (648.3-648.4)*
drug abuse (305.00-305.93)
drug dependence (304.00-304.93)
hormone replacement therapy (postmenopausal) (V07.4)
use of agents affecting estrogen receptors and estrogen levels (V07.51-V07.59)
AHA: 1Q, '11, 15; 4Q, '08, 159; 4Q, '03, 85; 4Q, '02, 84; 3Q, '02, 15; 4Q, '95, 61
TIP: Do not assign for patients on detoxification drugs or maintenance programs to prevent withdrawal symptoms related to drug dependence; assign instead drug dependence code(s).

V58.61 Long-term (current) use of anticoagulants
EXCLUDES *long-term (current) use of aspirin (V58.66)*
AHA: 4Q, '08, 135; 3Q, '06, 13; 3Q, '04, 7; 4Q, '03, 108; 3Q, '02, 13-16; 1Q, '02, 15, 16
Z79.01 Long term (current) use of anticoagulants I-10

V58.62 Long-term (current) use of antibiotics
AHA: 4Q, '98, 59

V58.63 Long-term (current) use of antiplatelets/ antithrombotics
EXCLUDES *long-term (current) use of aspirin (V58.66)*

V58.64 Long-term (current) use of non-steroidal anti-inflammatories (NSAID)
EXCLUDES *long-term (current) use of aspirin (V58.66)*

V58.65 Long-term (current) use of steroids
Z79.52 Long term (current) use of systemic steroids I-10

V58.66 Long-term (current) use of aspirin
AHA: 4Q, '04, 102

V58.67 Long-term (current) use of insulin
AHA: 4Q, '04, 55-56, 103
Z79.4 Long term (current) use of insulin I-10

V58.68 Long term (current) use of bisphosphonates
AHA: 4Q, '11, 157

V58.69 Long-term (current) use of other medications
Other high-risk medications
Long term current use of methadone for pain control
Long term current use of opiate analgesic
EXCLUDES *methadone maintenance NOS (304.00)*
methadone use NOS (304.00)
AHA: 2Q, '11, 7; 2Q, '10, 10, 13; 4Q, '09, 83; 3Q, '09, 3; 4Q, '08, 156; 2Q, '04, 10; 1Q, '04, 13; 1Q, '03, 11; 2Q, '00, 8; 3Q, '99, 13; 2Q, '99, 17; 1Q, '97, 12; 2Q, '96, 7

√5ᵗʰ **V58.7 Aftercare following surgery to specified body systems, not elsewhere classified**
NOTE Codes from this subcategory should be used in conjunction with other aftercare codes to fully identify the reason for the aftercare encounter
EXCLUDES *aftercare following organ transplant (V58.44)*
aftercare following surgery for neoplasm (V58.42)
AHA: 4Q, '03, 104; 4Q, '02, 80

V58.71 Aftercare following surgery of the sense organs, NEC
Conditions classifiable to 360-379, 380-389

V58.72 Aftercare following surgery of the nervous system, NEC
Conditions classifiable to 320-359
EXCLUDES *aftercare following surgery of the sense organs, NEC (V58.71)*

V58.73 Aftercare following surgery of the circulatory system, NEC
Conditions classifiable to 390-459
AHA: 2Q, '09, 12; 4Q, '03, 105

V58.74 Aftercare following surgery of the respiratory system, NEC
Conditions classifiable to 460-519

V58.75 Aftercare following surgery of the teeth, oral cavity and digestive system, NEC
Conditions classifiable to 520-579
AHA: 2Q, '05, 14

V58.76 Aftercare following surgery of the genitourinary system, NEC
  Conditions classifiable to 580-629
    EXCLUDES *aftercare following sterilization reversal (V26.22)*
  AHA: 1Q, '05, 11-12

V58.77 Aftercare following surgery of the skin and subcutaneous tissue, NEC
  Conditions classifiable to 680-709

V58.78 Aftercare following surgery of the musculoskeletal system, NEC
  Conditions classifiable to 710-739
    EXCLUDES *orthopedic aftercare (V54.01-V54.9)*

√5ᵗʰ **V58.8 Other specified procedures and aftercare**
  AHA: 4Q, '94, 45; 2Q, '94, 8

  V58.81 Fitting and adjustment of vascular catheter
    Removal or replacement of catheter
    Toilet or cleansing
      EXCLUDES *complication of renal dialysis (996.73)*
        complication of vascular catheter (996.74)
        dialysis preparation — code to condition
        encounter for dialysis (V56.0-V56.8)
        fitting and adjustment of dialysis catheter (V56.1)
    AHA: 2Q, '11, 4

  V58.82 Fitting and adjustment of nonvascular catheter, NEC
    Removal or replacement of catheter
    Toilet or cleansing
      EXCLUDES *fitting and adjustment of peritoneal dialysis catheter (V56.2)*
        fitting and adjustment of urinary catheter (V53.6)

  V58.83 Encounter for therapeutic drug monitoring
    Use additional code for any associated long- term (current) drug use (V58.61-V58.69)
      EXCLUDES *blood-drug testing for medico- legal reasons (V70.4)*
    DEF: Drug monitoring: Measurement of the level of a specific drug in the body or measurement of a specific function to assess effectiveness of a drug.
    AHA: 4Q, '08, 156; 2Q, '04, 10; 1Q, '04, 13;4Q, '03, 85; 4Q, '02, 84; 3Q, '02, 13-16

  V58.89 Other specified aftercare
    AHA: 4Q, '98, 59

V58.9 Unspecified aftercare

√4ᵗʰ **V59 Donors**
  EXCLUDES *examination of potential donor (V70.8)*
    self-donation of organ or tissue — code to condition
  AHA: 4Q, '95, 62; 1Q, '90, 10; N-D, '84,
  TIP: Assign only for living donations to other individuals, not for self-donation or for cadaveric donations.

√5ᵗʰ **V59.0 Blood**
  V59.01 Whole blood   PDx
  V59.02 Stem cells   PDx
  V59.09 Other   PDx
  V59.1 Skin   PDx
  V59.2 Bone   PDx
  V59.3 Bone marrow   PDx
  V59.4 Kidney   PDx
  V59.5 Cornea   PDx
  V59.6 Liver   PDx

√5ᵗʰ **V59.7 Egg (oocyte) (ovum)**
  AHA: 4Q, '05, 99

  V59.70 Egg (oocyte) (ovum) donor, unspecified   PDx ♀
  V59.71 Egg (oocyte) (ovum) donor, under age 35, anonymous recipient   PDx ♀
    Egg donor, under age 35 NOS

V59.72 Egg (oocyte) (ovum) donor, under age 35, designated recipient   PDx ♀

V59.73 Egg (oocyte) (ovum) donor, age 35 and over, anonymous recipient   PDx ♀
  Egg donor, age 35 and over NOS

V59.74 Egg (oocyte) (ovum) donor, age 35 and over, designated recipient   PDx ♀

V59.8 Other specified organ or tissue   PDx
  AHA: 3Q, '02, 20

V59.9 Unspecified organ or tissue   PDx

Persons Encountering Health Services in Other Circumstances (V60-V69)

√4ᵗʰ **V60 Housing, household, and economic circumstances**

  V60.0 Lack of housing
    Hobos   Transients
    Social migrants   Vagabonds
    Tramps

  V60.1 Inadequate housing
    Lack of heating
    Restriction of space
    Technical defects in home preventing adequate care

  V60.2 Inadequate material resources
    Economic problem   Poverty NOS

  V60.3 Person living alone

  V60.4 No other household member able to render care
    Person requiring care (has) (is):
      family member too handicapped, ill, or otherwise unsuited to render care
      partner temporarily away from home
      temporarily away from usual place of abode
      EXCLUDES *holiday relief care (V60.5)*

  V60.5 Holiday relief care
    Provision of health care facilities to a person normally cared for at home, to enable relatives to take a vacation

  V60.6 Person living in residential institution
    Boarding school resident

  √5ᵗʰ **V60.8 Other specified housing or economic circumstances**
    AHA: 4Q, '09, 118
    V60.81 Foster care (status)
    V60.89 Other specified housing or economic circumstances

  V60.9 Unspecified housing or economic circumstance

√4ᵗʰ **V61 Other family circumstances**
  INCLUDES when these circumstances or fear of them, affecting the person directly involved or others, are mentioned as the reason, justified or not, for seeking or receiving medical advice or care
  AHA: 1Q, '90, 9

  √5ᵗʰ **V61.0 Family disruption**
    AHA: 4Q, '08, 160

    V61.01 Family disruption due to family member on military deployment
      Individual or family affected by other family member being on deployment
        EXCLUDES *family disruption due to family member on non-military extended absence from home (V61.08)*

    V61.02 Family disruption due to return of family member from military deployment
      Individual or family affected by other family member having returned from deployment (current or past conflict)

    V61.03 Family disruption due to divorce or legal separation

    V61.04 Family disruption due to parent-child estrangement
        EXCLUDES *other family estrangement (V61.09)*

    V61.05 Family disruption due to child in welfare custody

√4ᵗʰ/√5ᵗʰ Additional Digit Required | Unspecified Code | Other Specified Code | Manifestation Code | ►◄ Revised Text | ● New Code | ▲ Revised Code Title

V Codes

V61.06 Family disruption due to child in foster care or in care of non-parental family member

V61.07 Family disruption due to death of family member
> EXCLUDES *bereavement (V62.82)*
> AHA: 4Q, '09, 117

V61.08 Family disruption due to other extended absence of family member
> EXCLUDES *family disruption due to family member on military deployment (V61.01)*
> AHA: 4Q, '09, 117

V61.09 Other family disruption
> Family estrangement NOS

√5ᵗʰ **V61.1 Counseling for marital and partner problems**
> EXCLUDES *problems related to:*
> *psychosexual disorders (302.0-302.9)*
> *sexual function (V41.7)*

V61.10 Counseling for marital and partner problems, unspecified
> Marital conflict
> Marital relationship problem
> Partner conflict
> Partner relationship problem

V61.11 Counseling for victim of spousal and partner abuse
> EXCLUDES *encounter for treatment of current injuries due to abuse (995.80-995.85)*

V61.12 Counseling for perpetrator of spousal and partner abuse

√5ᵗʰ **V61.2 Parent-child problems**

V61.20 Counseling for parent-child problem, unspecified
> Concern about behavior of child
> Parent-child conflict
> Parent-child relationship problem

V61.21 Counseling for victim of child abuse
> Child battering   Child neglect
> EXCLUDES *current injuries due to abuse (995.50-995.59)*

V61.22 Counseling for perpetrator of parental child abuse
> EXCLUDES *counseling for non-parental abuser (V62.83)*

V61.23 Counseling for parent-biological child problem
> Concern about behavior of biological child
> Parent-biological child conflict
> Parent-biological child relationship problem
> AHA: 4Q, '09, 117

V61.24 Counseling for parent-adopted child problem
> Concern about behavior of adopted child
> Parent-adopted child conflict
> Parent-adopted child relationship problem
> AHA: 4Q, '09, 117

V61.25 Counseling for parent (guardian)-foster child problem
> Concern about behavior of foster child
> Parent (guardian)-foster child conflict
> Parent (guardian)-foster child relationship problem
> AHA: 4Q, '09, 117

V61.29 Other parent-child problems
> AHA: 3Q, '99, 16

V61.3 Problems with aged parents or in-laws

√5ᵗʰ **V61.4 Health problems within family**

V61.41 Alcoholism in family

V61.42 Substance abuse in family
> AHA: 4Q, '09, 117

V61.49 Other
> Care of   ⎫ sick or handicapped person
> Presence of ⎬ in family or household

V61.5 Multiparity

V61.6 Illegitimacy or illegitimate pregnancy   Ⓜ ♀

V61.7 Other unwanted pregnancy   Ⓜ ♀

V61.8 Other specified family circumstances
> Problems with family members NEC
> Sibling relationship problem

V61.9 Unspecified family circumstance

√4ᵗʰ **V62 Other psychosocial circumstances**
> INCLUDES those circumstances or fear of them, affecting the person directly involved or others, mentioned as the reason, justified or not, for seeking or receiving medical advice or care
> EXCLUDES *previous psychological trauma (V15.41-V15.49)*

V62.0 Unemployment
> EXCLUDES *circumstances when main problem is economic inadequacy or poverty (V60.2)*

V62.1 Adverse effects of work environment

√5ᵗʰ **V62.2 Other occupational circumstances or maladjustment**
> AHA: 4Q, '08, 160

V62.21 Personal current military deployment status Ⓐ
> Individual (civilian or military) currently deployed in theater or in support of military war, peacekeeping and humanitarian operations

V62.22 Personal history of return from military deployment Ⓐ
> Individual (civilian or military) with past history of military war, peacekeeping and humanitarian deployment (current or past conflict)

V62.29 Other occupational circumstances or maladjustment Ⓐ
> Career choice problem
> Dissatisfaction with employment
> Occupational problem

V62.3 Educational circumstances
> Academic problem
> Dissatisfaction with school environment
> Educational handicap

V62.4 Social maladjustment
> Acculturation problem
> Cultural deprivation
> Political, religious, or sex discrimination
> Social:
> isolation
> persecution

V62.5 Legal circumstances
> Imprisonment   Litigation
> Legal investigation   Prosecution

V62.6 Refusal of treatment for reasons of religion or conscience

√5ᵗʰ **V62.8 Other psychological or physical stress, not elsewhere classified**

V62.81 Interpersonal problems, not elsewhere classified
> Relational problem NOS

V62.82 Bereavement, uncomplicated
> EXCLUDES *bereavement as adjustment reaction (309.0)*
> *family disruption due to death of family member (V61.07)*

V62.83 Counseling for perpetrator of physical/sexual abuse
> EXCLUDES *counseling for perpetrator of parental child abuse (V61.22)*
> *counseling for perpetrator of spousal and partner abuse (V61.12)*

V62.84 Suicidal ideation
> EXCLUDES *suicidal tendencies (300.9)*
> DEF: Thoughts of committing suicide; no actual attempt of suicide has been made.
> AHA: 4Q, '05, 96
> TIP: Assign for patients who have not attempted suicide, and who may not be considered a suicide risk, but who have indicated thoughts about suicide.
> R45.851 Suicidal ideations   I-10

V62.85 Homicidal ideation
> AHA: 4Q, '10, 110
> R45.850 Homicidal ideations

V62.89 Other
    Borderline intellectual functioning
    Life circumstance problems
    Phase of life problems
    Religious or spiritual problem

V62.9 Unspecified psychosocial circumstance

√4ᵗʰ **V63 Unavailability of other medical facilities for care**
    AHA: 1Q, '91, 21

V63.0 Residence remote from hospital or other health care facility

V63.1 Medical services in home not available
    EXCLUDES no other household member able to render care
        (V60.4)
    AHA: 4Q, '01, 67; 1Q, '01, 12

V63.2 Person awaiting admission to adequate facility elsewhere

V63.8 Other specified reasons for unavailability of medical facilities
    Person on waiting list undergoing social agency investigation

V63.9 Unspecified reason for unavailability of medical facilities

√4ᵗʰ **V64 Persons encountering health services for specific procedures, not carried out**

√5ᵗʰ **V64.0 Vaccination not carried out**
    AHA: 4Q, '05, 99

V64.00 Vaccination not carried out, unspecified reason

V64.01 Vaccination not carried out because of acute illness

V64.02 Vaccination not carried out because of chronic illness or condition

V64.03 Vaccination not carried out because of immune compromised state

V64.04 Vaccination not carried out because of allergy to vaccine or component
    Z28.04 Immunization not carried out pt allergy vaccine I-10

V64.05 Vaccination not carried out because of caregiver refusal
    Guardian refusal   Parent refusal
    EXCLUDES vaccination not carried out because of
        caregiver refusal for religious reasons
        (V64.07)
    AHA: 4Q, '09, 115; 1Q, '07, 12

V64.06 Vaccination not carried out because of patient refusal

V64.07 Vaccination not carried out for religious reasons

V64.08 Vaccination not carried out because patient had disease being vaccinated against

V64.09 Vaccination not carried out for other reason

V64.1 Surgical or other procedure not carried out because of contraindication
    TIP: Assign an additional code to indicate the contraindication (reason the surgery or other procedure was canceled).

V64.2 Surgical or other procedure not carried out because of patient's decision
    AHA: 2Q, '01, 8

V64.3 Procedure not carried out for other reasons

√5ᵗʰ **V64.4 Closed surgical procedure converted to open procedure**
    AHA: 4Q, '03, 87; 4Q, '98, 68; 4Q, '97, 52

V64.41 Laparoscopic surgical procedure converted to open procedure
    AHA: 1Q, '11, 14-15

V64.42 Thoracoscopic surgical procedure converted to open procedure

V64.43 Arthroscopic surgical procedure converted to open procedure

√4ᵗʰ **V65 Other persons seeking consultation**

V65.0 Healthy person accompanying sick person
    Boarder

√5ᵗʰ **V65.1 Person consulting on behalf of another person**
    Advice or treatment for nonattending third party
    EXCLUDES concern (normal) about sick person in family
        (V61.41-V61.49)
    AHA: 4Q, '03, 84

V65.11 Pediatric pre-birth visit for expectant parent(s)
    Pre-adoption visit for adoptive parent(s)

V65.19 Other person consulting on behalf of another person

V65.2 Person feigning illness
    Malingerer   Peregrinating patient
    AHA: 3Q, '99, 20
    TIP: Assign for patients engaged in what is documented as "drug-seeking behavior."

V65.3 Dietary surveillance and counseling
    Dietary surveillance and counseling (in):
        NOS
        colitis
        diabetes mellitus
        food allergies or intolerance
        gastritis
        hypercholesterolemia
        hypoglycemia
        obesity
    Use additional code to identify Body Mass Index (BMI), if known (V85.0-V85.54)
    AHA: 4Q, '05, 96

√5ᵗʰ **V65.4 Other counseling, not elsewhere classified**
    Health:
        advice
        education
        instruction
    EXCLUDES counseling (for):
        contraception (V25.40-V25.49)
        genetic (V26.31-V26.39)
        on behalf of third party (V65.11-V65.19)
        procreative management (V26.41-V26.49)

V65.40 Counseling NOS

V65.41 Exercise counseling

V65.42 Counseling on substance use and abuse
    Z71.6 Tobacco abuse counseling I-10

V65.43 Counseling on injury prevention

V65.44 Human immunodeficiency virus [HIV] counseling

V65.45 Counseling on other sexually transmitted diseases

V65.46 Encounter for insulin pump training
    Z46.81 Encounter for fitting & adjustment insulin pump I-10

V65.49 Other specified counseling
    AHA: 4Q, '08, 156; 2Q, '00, 8

V65.5 Person with feared complaint in whom no diagnosis was made
    Feared condition not demonstrated
    Problem was normal state
    "Worried well"

V65.8 Other reasons for seeking consultation
    EXCLUDES specified symptoms
    AHA: 3Q, '92, 4

V65.9 Unspecified reason for consultation

√4ᵗʰ **V66 Convalescence and palliative care**

V66.0 Following surgery PDx

V66.1 Following radiotherapy PDx

V66.2 Following chemotherapy PDx

V66.3 Following psychotherapy and other treatment for mental disorder PDx

V66.4 Following treatment of fracture PDx

V66.5 Following other treatment PDx

V66.6 Following combined treatment PDx

V66.7 Encounter for palliative care
End of life care
Hospice care
Terminal care
Code first underlying disease
AHA: ▶1Q, '12, 14;◀ 3Q, '10, 18; 3Q, '08, 13; 2Q, '05, 9; 4Q, '03, 107; 1Q, '98, 11; 4Q, '96, 47, 48
TIP: Assign as secondary diagnosis when treatment is focused on management of pain and symptoms in a patient with an incurable disease.
Z51.5 Encounter for palliative care   I-10

V66.9 Unspecified convalescence   PDx
AHA: 4Q, '99, 8

☑4ᵗʰ **V67 Follow-up examination**
INCLUDES surveillance only following completed treatment
EXCLUDES surveillance of contraception (V25.40-V25.49)
AHA: 4Q, '08, 157; 2Q, '03, 5; 4Q, '94, 98

☑5ᵗʰ **V67.0 Following surgery**
AHA: 4Q, '00, 56; 4Q, '98, 69; 4Q, '97, 50; 2Q, '95, 8;1Q, '95, 4; 3Q, '92, 11

V67.00 Following surgery, unspecified

V67.01 Follow-up vaginal pap smear   ♀
Vaginal pap-smear, status-post hysterectomy for malignant condition
Use additional code to identify:
acquired absence of uterus (V88.01-V88.03)
personal history of malignant neoplasm (V10.40-V10.44)
EXCLUDES vaginal pap smear status-post hysterectomy for non-malignant condition (V76.47)
AHA: 4Q, '08, 157

V67.09 Following other surgery
EXCLUDES sperm count following sterilization reversal (V26.22)
sperm count for fertility testing (V26.21)
AHA: 3Q, '08, 6; 3Q, '03, 16; 3Q, '02, 15

V67.1 Following radiotherapy

V67.2 Following chemotherapy
Cancer chemotherapy follow-up

V67.3 Following psychotherapy and other treatment for mental disorder

V67.4 Following treatment of healed fracture
EXCLUDES current (healing) fracture aftercare (V54.0-V54.9)
AHA: 1Q, '09, 6; 1Q, '90, 7

☑5ᵗʰ **V67.5 Following other treatment**

V67.51 Following completed treatment with high-risk medications, not elsewhere classified
EXCLUDES long-term (current) drug use (V58.61-V58.69)
AHA: 1Q, '99, 5, 6;4Q, '95, 61 ; 1Q, '90, 18

V67.59 Other

V67.6 Following combined treatment

V67.9 Unspecified follow-up examination

☑4ᵗʰ **V68 Encounters for administrative purposes**

☑5ᵗʰ **V68.0 Issue of medical certificates**
EXCLUDES encounter for general medical examination (V70.0-V70.9)

V68.01 Disability examination   PDx
Use additional code(s) to identify specific examination(s), screening and testing performed (V72.0-V82.9)
AHA: 4Q, '07, 101

V68.09 Other issue of medical certificates   PDx

V68.1 Issue of repeat prescriptions   PDx
Issue of repeat prescription for:
appliance
glasses
medications
EXCLUDES repeat prescription for contraceptives (V25.41-V25.49)

V68.2 Request for expert evidence   PDx

☑5ᵗʰ **V68.8 Other specified administrative purpose**

V68.81 Referral of patient without examination or treatment   PDx

V68.89 Other   PDx

V68.9 Unspecified administrative purpose   PDx

☑4ᵗʰ **V69 Problems related to lifestyle**
AHA: 4Q, '94, 48

V69.0 Lack of physical exercise

V69.1 Inappropriate diet and eating habits
EXCLUDES anorexia nervosa (307.1)
bulimia (783.6)
malnutrition and other nutritional deficiencies (260-269.9)
other and unspecified eating disorders (307.50-307.59)

V69.2 High-risk sexual behavior

V69.3 Gambling and betting
EXCLUDES pathological gambling (312.31)

V69.4 Lack of adequate sleep
Sleep deprivation
EXCLUDES insomnia (780.52)

V69.5 Behavioral insomnia of childhood   P
DEF: Behaviors on the part of the child or caregivers that cause negative compliance with a child's sleep schedule; results in lack of adequate sleep.
AHA: 4Q, '05, 99

V69.8 Other problems related to lifestyle
Self-damaging behavior

V69.9 Problem related to lifestyle, unspecified

Persons without Reported Diagnosis Encountered During Examination and Investigation of Individuals and Populations (V70-V82)

NOTE Nonspecific abnormal findings disclosed at the time of these examinations are classifiable to categories 790-796.

☑4ᵗʰ **V70 General medical examination**
Use additional code(s) to identify any special screening examination(s) performed (V73.0-V82.9)

V70.0 Routine general medical examination at a health care facility   PDx
Health checkup
EXCLUDES health checkup of infant or child over 28 days old (V20.2)
health supervision of newborn 8 to 28 days old (V20.32)
health supervision of newborn under 8 days old (V20.31)
pre-procedural general physical examination (V72.83)

V70.1 General psychiatric examination, requested by the authority   PDx

V70.2 General psychiatric examination, other and unspecified   PDx

---

N Newborn Age: 0   P Pediatric Age: 0-17   M Maternity Age: 12-55   A Adult Age: 15-124   PDx Primary Diagnosis

V70.3 Other medical examination for administrative purposes `PDx`

General medical examination for:
- admission to old age home
- adoption
- camp
- driving license
- immigration and naturalization
- insurance certification
- marriage
- prison
- school admission
- sports competition

EXCLUDES *attendance for issue of medical certificates (V68.0)*
pre-employment screening (V70.5)

AHA: 3Q, '08, 6; 1Q, '90, 6

Z02.6 Encounter for exam for insurance purposes `I-10`

V70.4 Examination for medicolegal reasons `PDx`

Blood-alcohol tests   Paternity testing
Blood-drug tests

EXCLUDES *examination and observation following:*
accidents (V71.3, V71.4)
assault (V71.6)
rape (V71.5)

V70.5 Health examination of defined subpopulations `PDx`

- Armed forces personnel
- Inhabitants of institutions
- Occupational healthexaminations
- Pre-employment screening
- Preschool children
- Prisoners
- Prostitutes
- Refugees
- School children
- Students

V70.6 Health examination in population surveys `PDx`

EXCLUDES *special screening (V73.0-V82.9)*

V70.7 Examination of participant in clinical trial

Examination of participant or control in clinical research

AHA: 2Q, '06, 5-6; 4Q, '01, 55

V70.8 Other specified general medical examinations `PDx`

Examination of potential donor of organ or tissue

V70.9 Unspecified general medical examination `PDx`

`√4ᵗʰ` **V71 Observation and evaluation for suspected conditions not found**

INCLUDES This category is to be used when persons without a diagnosis are suspected of having an abnormal condition, without signs or symptoms, which requires study, but after examination and observation, is found not to exist. This category is also for use for administrative and legal observation status.

EXCLUDES *suspected maternal and fetal conditions not found (V89.01-V89.09)*

AHA: 4Q, '94, 47; 2Q, '90, 5; M-A, '87, 1

TIP: Assign observation codes only as principal/first-listed diagnosis and only if there is no documentation of any signs or symptoms.

`√5ᵗʰ` **V71.0 Observation for suspected mental condition**

V71.01 Adult antisocial behavior `A` `PDx`
Dyssocial behavior or gang activity in adult without manifest psychiatric disorder

V71.02 Childhood or adolescent antisocial behavior `PDx`
Dyssocial behavior or gang activity in child or adolescent without manifest psychiatric disorder

V71.09 Other suspected mental condition `PDx`

V71.1 Observation for suspected malignant neoplasm `PDx`

V71.2 Observation for suspected tuberculosis `PDx`

V71.3 Observation following accident at work `PDx`

V71.4 Observation following other accident `PDx`
Examination of individual involved in motor vehicle traffic accident

AHA: 1Q, '06, 9

V71.5 Observation following alleged rape or seduction `PDx`
Examination of victim or culprit

V71.6 Observation following other inflicted injury `PDx`
Examination of victim or culprit

V71.7 Observation for suspected cardiovascular disease `PDx`
AHA: 1Q, '04, 6; 3Q, '90, 10; S-O, '87, 10

`√5ᵗʰ` **V71.8 Observation and evaluation for other specified suspected conditions**

EXCLUDES *contact with and (suspected) exposure to (potentially) hazardous substances (V15.84-V15.86, V87.0-V87.31)*

AHA: 4Q, '00, 54 ; 1Q, '90, 19

V71.81 Abuse and neglect `PDx`
EXCLUDES *adult abuse and neglect (995.80-995.85)*
child abuse and neglect (995.50-995.59)
AHA: 4Q, '00, 55

V71.82 Observation and evaluation for suspected exposure to anthrax `PDx`
AHA: 4Q, '02, 70, 85

V71.83 Observation and evaluation for suspected exposure to other biological agent `PDx`
AHA: 4Q, '03, 47

V71.89 Other specified suspected conditions `PDx`
AHA: 2Q, '11, 4; 3Q, '08, 7; 2Q, '03, 15

V71.9 Observation for unspecified suspected condition `PDx`
AHA: 1Q, '02, 6

`√4ᵗʰ` **V72 Special investigations and examinations**

INCLUDES routine examination of specific system

Use additional code(s) to identify any special screening examination(s) performed (V73.0-V82.9)

EXCLUDES *general medical examination (V70.0-V70.4)*
general screening examination of defined population groups (V70.5, V70.6, V70.7)
health supervision of newborn 8 to 28 days old (V20.32)
health supervision of newborn under 8 days old (V20.31)
routine examination of infant or child over 28 days old (V20.2)

V72.0 Examination of eyes and vision
AHA: 1Q, '04, 15

`√5ᵗʰ` **V72.1 Examination of ears and hearing**
AHA: 1Q, '04, 15

V72.11 Encounter for hearing examination following failed hearing screening
AHA: ►3Q, '11, 3;◄ 4Q, '06, 118
Z01.110 Encounter hearing exam follow failed hearing scr `I-10`

V72.12 Encounter for hearing conservation and treatment
AHA: 4Q, '07, 100

V72.19 Other examination of ears and hearing

V72.2 Dental examination

`√5ᵗʰ` **V72.3 Gynecological examination**
EXCLUDES *cervical Papanicolaou smear without general gynecological examination (V76.2)*
routine examination in contraceptive management (V25.40-V25.49)

V72.31 Routine gynecological examination ♀
General gynecological examination with or without Papanicolaou cervical smear
Pelvic examination (annual) (periodic)
Use additional code to identify:
human papillomavirus (HPV) screening (V73.81)
routine vaginal Papanicolaou smear (V76.47)
AHA: 2Q, '06, 2-3; 4Q, '05, 98

`√4ᵗʰ`
`√5ᵗʰ` Additional Digit Required   Unspecified Code   Other Specified Code   Manifestation Code   ►◄ Revised Text   ● New Code   ▲ Revised Code Title

2013 ICD-9-CM   **February 2012 • Volume 1 – 339**

V72.32 Encounter for Papanicolaou cervical smear to confirm findings of recent normal smear following initial abnormal smear ♀
　　AHA: 2Q, '06, 4

√5ᵗʰ **V72.4 Pregnancy examination or test**
　　AHA: 4Q, '05, 98

　　V72.40 Pregnancy examination or test, pregnancy unconfirmed ♀
　　　　Possible pregnancy, not (yet) confirmed

　　V72.41 Pregnancy examination or test, negative result ♀

　　V72.42 Pregnancy examination or test, positive result ♀ Ⓜ

V72.5 Radiological examination, not elsewhere classified
　　Routine chest x-ray
　　EXCLUDES radiologic examinations as part of pre-procedural testing (V72.81-V72.84)
　　AHA: 1Q, '90, 19

√5ᵗʰ **V72.6 Laboratory examination**
　　Encounters for blood and urine testing
　　AHA: 4Q, '09, 117-118; 2Q, '06, 4; 1Q, '90, 22

　　V72.60 Laboratory examination, unspecified

　　V72.61 Antibody response examination
　　　　Immunity status testing
　　　　EXCLUDES encounter for allergy testing (V72.7)

　　V72.62 Laboratory examination ordered as part of a routine general medical examination
　　　　Blood tests for routine general physical examination

　　V72.63 Pre-procedural laboratory examination
　　　　Blood tests prior to treatment or procedure
　　　　Pre-operative laboratory examination

　　V72.69 Other laboratory examination

V72.7 Diagnostic skin and sensitization tests
　　Allergy tests
　　Skin tests for hypersensitivity
　　EXCLUDES diagnostic skin tests for bacterial diseases (V74.0-V74.9)

√5ᵗʰ **V72.8 Other specified examinations**
　　EXCLUDES pre-procedural laboratory examinations (V72.63)

　　V72.81 Pre-operative cardiovascular examination
　　　　Pre-procedural cardiovascular examination
　　　　Z01.810 Encounter for preprocedural cardiovascular exam　I-10

　　V72.82 Pre-operative respiratory examination
　　　　Pre-procedural respiratory examination
　　　　AHA: 3Q, '96, 14

　　V72.83 Other specified pre-operative examination
　　　　Examination prior to chemotherapy
　　　　Other pre-procedural examination
　　　　Pre-procedural general physical examination
　　　　EXCLUDES routine general medical examination (V70.0)
　　　　AHA: 3Q, '96, 14

　　V72.84 Pre-operative examination, unspecified
　　　　Pre-procedural examination, unspecified

　　V72.85 Other specified examination
　　　　AHA: ▶1Q, '12, 10;◀ 4Q, '05, 96; 1Q, '04, 12

　　V72.86 Encounter for blood typing

V72.9 Unspecified examination
　　AHA: 4Q, '06, 117

√4ᵗʰ **V73 Special screening examination for viral and chlamydial diseases**
　　AHA: 1Q, '04, 11

　　V73.0 Poliomyelitis

　　V73.1 Smallpox

　　V73.2 Measles

　　V73.3 Rubella

　　V73.4 Yellow fever

V73.5 Other arthropod-borne viral diseases
　　Dengue fever
　　Hemorrhagic fever
　　Viral encephalitis:
　　　　mosquito-borne
　　　　tick-borne

V73.6 Trachoma

√5ᵗʰ **V73.8 Other specified viral and chlamydial diseases**

　　V73.81 Human papillomavirus [HPV]
　　　　AHA: 4Q, '07, 100

　　V73.88 Other specified chlamydial diseases
　　　　AHA: 4Q, '07, 124

　　V73.89 Other specified viral diseases

√5ᵗʰ **V73.9 Unspecified viral and chlamydial disease**

　　V73.98 Unspecified chlamydial disease

　　V73.99 Unspecified viral disease

√4ᵗʰ **V74 Special screening examination for bacterial and spirochetal diseases**
　　INCLUDES diagnostic skin tests for these diseases
　　AHA: 1Q, '04, 11

　　V74.0 Cholera

　　V74.1 Pulmonary tuberculosis

　　V74.2 Leprosy [Hansen's disease]

　　V74.3 Diphtheria

　　V74.4 Bacterial conjunctivitis

　　V74.5 Venereal disease
　　　　Screening for bacterial and spirochetal sexually transmitted diseases
　　　　Screening for sexually transmitted diseases NOS
　　　　EXCLUDES special screening for nonbacterial sexually transmitted diseases (V73.81-V73.89, V75.4, V75.8)
　　　　AHA: 4Q, '07, 124

　　V74.6 Yaws

　　V74.8 Other specified bacterial and spirochetal diseases
　　　　Brucellosis
　　　　Leptospirosis
　　　　Plague
　　　　Tetanus
　　　　Whooping cough

　　V74.9 Unspecified bacterial and spirochetal disease

√4ᵗʰ **V75 Special screening examination for other infectious diseases**
　　AHA: 1Q, '04, 11

　　V75.0 Rickettsial diseases

　　V75.1 Malaria

　　V75.2 Leishmaniasis

　　V75.3 Trypanosomiasis
　　　　Chagas' disease
　　　　Sleeping sickness

　　V75.4 Mycotic infections

　　V75.5 Schistosomiasis

　　V75.6 Filariasis

　　V75.7 Intestinal helminthiasis

　　V75.8 Other specified parasitic infections

　　V75.9 Unspecified infectious disease

√4ᵗʰ **V76 Special screening for malignant neoplasms**
　　AHA: 1Q, '04, 11
　　TIP: Whenever a screening examination is performed, the screening code is the first-listed code, regardless of the findings or any procedure that is performed as a result of the findings.

　　V76.0 Respiratory organs

√5ᵗʰ **V76.1 Breast**
　　AHA: 4Q, '98, 67

　　V76.10 Breast screening, unspecified

Ⓝ Newborn Age: 0　　　　Ⓟ Pediatric Age: 0-17　　　　Ⓜ Maternity Age: 12-55　　　　Ⓐ Adult Age: 15-124　　　　PDx Primary Diagnosis

V Codes

V76.11 Screening mammogram for high-risk patient ♀
    AHA: 2Q, '03, 4

V76.12 Other screening mammogram
    AHA: 4Q, '09, 106; 2Q, '06, 10; 2Q, '03, 3-4

V76.19 Other screening breast examination

V76.2 Cervix ♀
Routine cervical Papanicolaou smear
> EXCLUDES special screening for human papillomavirus (V73.81)
> that as part of a general gynecological examination
> (V72.31)

V76.3 Bladder

✓5ᵗʰ **V76.4 Other sites**

  V76.41 Rectum

  V76.42 Oral cavity

  V76.43 Skin

  V76.44 Prostate ♂
    Z12.5 Encounter screening malignant neoplasm `I-10`
    prostate

  V76.45 Testis ♂

  V76.46 Ovary ♀
    AHA: 4Q, '00, 52

  V76.47 Vagina ♀
  Vaginal pap smear status-post hysterectomy for
    non-malignant condition
  Use additional code to identify acquired absence of
    uterus (V88.01-V88.03)
>   EXCLUDES vaginal pap smear status-post hysterectomy
>   for malignant condition (V67.01)
    AHA: 4Q, '08, 157; 4Q, '00, 52

  V76.49 Other sites
    AHA: 1Q, '99, 4

✓5ᵗʰ **V76.5 Intestine**
  AHA: 4Q, '00, 52

  V76.50 Intestine, unspecified

  V76.51 Colon
  Screening colonoscopy NOS
>   EXCLUDES rectum (V76.41)
    AHA: 4Q, '01, 56
    Z12.11 Encounter screening malignant neoplasm `I-10`
    of colon

  V76.52 Small intestine

✓5ᵗʰ **V76.8 Other neoplasm**
  AHA: 4Q, '00, 52

  V76.81 Nervous system

  V76.89 Other neoplasm

V76.9 Unspecified

✓4ᵗʰ **V77 Special screening for endocrine, nutritional, metabolic, and immunity disorders**
  AHA: 1Q, '04, 11

V77.0 Thyroid disorders

V77.1 Diabetes mellitus

V77.2 Malnutrition

V77.3 Phenylketonuria [PKU]

V77.4 Galactosemia

V77.5 Gout

V77.6 Cystic fibrosis
Screening for mucoviscidosis

V77.7 Other inborn errors of metabolism

V77.8 Obesity

✓5ᵗʰ **V77.9 Other and unspecified endocrine, nutritional, metabolic, and immunity disorders**
  AHA: 4Q, '00, 53

  V77.91 Screening for lipoid disorders
  Screening for cholesterol level
  Screening for hypercholesterolemia
  Screening for hyperlipidemia

  V77.99 Other and unspecified endocrine nutritional metabolic and immunity disorders

✓4ᵗʰ **V78 Special screening for disorders of blood and blood-forming organs**
  AHA: 1Q, '04, 11

V78.0 Iron deficiency anemia

V78.1 Other and unspecified deficiency anemia

V78.2 Sickle cell disease or trait

V78.3 Other hemoglobinopathies

V78.8 Other disorders of blood and blood-forming organs

V78.9 Unspecified disorder of blood and blood-forming organs

✓4ᵗʰ **V79 Special screening for mental disorders and developmental handicaps**
  AHA: 1Q, '04, 11

V79.0 Depression

V79.1 Alcoholism

V79.2 Intellectual disabilities

V79.3 Developmental handicaps in early childhood

V79.8 Other specified mental disorders and developmental handicaps

V79.9 Unspecified mental disorder and developmental handicap

✓4ᵗʰ **V80 Special screening for neurological, eye, and ear diseases**
  AHA: 1Q, '04, 11

✓5ᵗʰ **V80.0 Neurological conditions**
  AHA: 4Q, '09, 116

  V80.01 Traumatic brain injury

  V80.09 Other neurological conditions

V80.1 Glaucoma

V80.2 Other eye conditions
Screening for:
  cataract
  congenital anomaly of eye
  senile macular lesions
> EXCLUDES general vision examination (V72.0)

V80.3 Ear diseases
> EXCLUDES general hearing examination (V72.11-V72.19)

✓4ᵗʰ **V81 Special screening for cardiovascular, respiratory, and genitourinary diseases**
  AHA: 1Q, '04, 11

V81.0 Ischemic heart disease

V81.1 Hypertension

V81.2 Other and unspecified cardiovascular conditions

V81.3 Chronic bronchitis and emphysema

V81.4 Other and unspecified respiratory conditions
> EXCLUDES screening for:
>   lung neoplasm (V76.0)
>   pulmonary tuberculosis (V74.1)

V81.5 Nephropathy
Screening for asymptomatic bacteriuria

V81.6 Other and unspecified genitourinary conditions

✓4ᵗʰ **V82 Special screening for other conditions**
  AHA: 1Q, '04, 11

V82.0 Skin conditions

V82.1 Rheumatoid arthritis

V82.2 Other rheumatic disorders

V76.11–V82.2

V82.3 **Congenital dislocation of hip**

V82.4 **Maternal postnatal screening for chromosomal anomalies** ♀

EXCLUDES *antenatal screening by amniocentesis (V28.0)*

V82.5 **Chemical poisoning and other contamination**
Screening for:
heavy metal poisoning
ingestion of radioactive substance
poisoning from contaminated water supply
radiation exposure

V82.6 **Multiphasic screening**

✓5ᵗʰ V82.7 **Genetic screening**

EXCLUDES *genetic testing for procreative management (V26.31-V26.39)*

V82.71 **Screening for genetic disease carrier status**
AHA: 4Q, '06, 118

V82.79 **Other genetic screening**
AHA: 4Q, '06, 118

✓5ᵗʰ V82.8 **Other specified conditions**
AHA: 4Q, '00, 53

V82.81 **Osteoporosis**
Use additional code to identify:
hormone replacement therapy (postmenopausal) status (V07.4)
postmenopausal (age-related) (natural) status (V49.81)
AHA: 4Q, '00, 54

V82.89 **Other specified conditions**

V82.9 **Unspecified condition**

Genetics (V83-V84)

✓4ᵗʰ **V83 Genetic carrier status**
AHA: 4Q, '02, 79; 4Q, '01, 54
TIP: The patient does not have the disease or carry a risk of developing it, but may genetically pass it to offspring who then may develop it.

✓5ᵗʰ V83.0 **Hemophilia A carrier**

V83.01 **Asymptomatic hemophilia A carrier**

V83.02 **Symptomatic hemophilia A carrier**

✓5ᵗʰ V83.8 **Other genetic carrier status**

V83.81 **Cystic fibrosis gene carrier**

V83.89 **Other genetic carrier status**

✓4ᵗʰ **V84 Genetic susceptibility to disease**
INCLUDES confirmed abnormal gene
EXCLUDES *chromosomal anomalies (758.0-758.9)*
Use additional code, if applicable, for any associated family history of the disease (V16-V19)
AHA: 4Q, '04, 106
TIP: The patient has a gene that increases the risk of developing a specific disease; assign only as a secondary condition.

✓5ᵗʰ V84.0 **Genetic susceptibility to malignant neoplasm**
Code first, if applicable, any current malignant neoplasms (140.0-195.8, 200.0-208.9, 230.0-234.9)
Use additional code, if applicable, for any personal history of malignant neoplasm (V10.0-V10.9)

V84.01 **Genetic susceptibility to malignant neoplasm of breast**
AHA: 2Q, '11, 12; 4Q, '04, 107
Z15.01 Genetic susceptibility malignant neoplasm breast I-10

V84.02 **Genetic susceptibility to malignant neoplasm of ovary** ♀

V84.03 **Genetic susceptibility to malignant neoplasm of prostate** ♂

V84.04 **Genetic susceptibility to malignant neoplasm of endometrium** ♀

V84.09 **Genetic susceptibility to other malignant neoplasm**

✓5ᵗʰ V84.8 **Genetic susceptibility to other disease**

V84.81 **Genetic susceptibility to multiple endocrine neoplasia [MEN]**
EXCLUDES *multiple endocrine neoplasia [MEN] syndromes (258.01-258.03)*
AHA: 4Q, '07, 100

V84.89 **Genetic susceptibility to other disease**

Body Mass Index (V85)

✓4ᵗʰ **V85 Body Mass Index [BMI]**
Kilograms per meters squared
NOTE BMI adult codes are for use for persons over 20 years old
AHA: ▶3Q, '11, 4-5;◀ 2Q, '10, 15; 4Q, '08, 191; 4Q, '05, 97
TIP: While BMI may be coded from dietician or other caregiver documentation, the diagnosis of being overweight or obese must be coded from physician documentation.

V85.0 **Body Mass Index less than 19, adult** A

V85.1 **Body Mass Index between 19-24, adult** A

✓5ᵗʰ V85.2 **Body Mass Index between 25-29, adult**

V85.21 **Body Mass Index 25.0-25.9, adult** A

V85.22 **Body Mass Index 26.0-26.9, adult** A

V85.23 **Body Mass Index 27.0-27.9, adult** A

V85.24 **Body Mass Index 28.0-28.9, adult** A

V85.25 **Body Mass Index 29.0-29.9, adult** A

✓5ᵗʰ V85.3 **Body Mass Index between 30-39, adult**

V85.30 **Body Mass Index 30.0-30.9, adult** A

V85.31 **Body Mass Index 31.0-31.9, adult** A

V85.32 **Body Mass Index 32.0-32.9, adult** A

V85.33 **Body Mass Index 33.0-33.9, adult** A

V85.34 **Body Mass Index 34.0-34.9, adult** A

V85.35 **Body Mass Index 35.0-35.9, adult** A

V85.36 **Body Mass Index 36.0-36.9, adult** A

V85.37 **Body Mass Index 37.0-37.9, adult** A

V85.38 **Body Mass Index 38.0-38.9, adult** A

V85.39 **Body Mass Index 39.0-39.9, adult** A

✓5ᵗʰ V85.4 **Body Mass Index 40 and over, adult**
AHA: 4Q, '10, 81, 109

V85.41 **Body Mass Index 40.0-44.9, adult** A
AHA: 4Q, '10, 109

V85.42 **Body Mass Index 45.0-49.9, adult** A

V85.43 **Body Mass Index 50.0-59.9, adult** A

V85.44 **Body Mass Index 60.0-69.9, adult** A

V85.45 **Body Mass Index 70 and over, adult** A

✓5ᵗʰ V85.5 **Body Mass Index, pediatric**
NOTE BMI pediatric codes are for use for persons age 2-20 years old. These percentiles are based on the growth charts published by the Centers for Disease Control and Prevention (CDC)
AHA: 4Q, '06, 118

V85.51 **Body Mass Index, pediatric, less than 5th percentile for age** P

V85.52 **Body Mass Index, pediatric, 5th percentile to less than 85th percentile for age** P

V85.53 **Body Mass Index, pediatric, 85th percentile to less than 95th percentile for age** P

V85.54 **Body Mass Index, pediatric, greater than or equal to 95th percentile for age** P
Z68.54 Body mass index (BMI) ≥ 95% for age I-10

V Codes

Estrogen Receptor Status (V86)

√4ᵗʰ **V86** **Estrogen receptor status**
Code first malignant neoplasm of breast (174.0-174.9, 175.0-175.9)
AHA: 4Q, '06, 118

V86.0 **Estrogen receptor positive status [ER+]**

V86.1 **Estrogen receptor negative status [ER-]**

Other Specified Personal Exposures and History Presenting Hazards to Health (V87)

√4ᵗʰ **V87** **Other specified personal exposures and history presenting hazards to health**

√5ᵗʰ **V87.0** **Contact with and (suspected) exposure to hazardous metals**
EXCLUDES *exposure to lead (V15.86)*
toxic effect of metals (984.0-985.9)
AHA: 4Q, '08, 158

V87.01 **Arsenic**

V87.02 **Contact with and (suspected) exposure to uranium**
EXCLUDES *retained depleted uranium fragments (V90.01)*
AHA: ▶4Q, '11, 156◄

V87.09 **Other hazardous metals**
Chromium compounds Nickel dust

√5ᵗʰ **V87.1** **Contact with and (suspected) exposure to hazardous aromatic compounds**
EXCLUDES *toxic effects of aromatic compounds (982.0, 983.0)*
AHA: 4Q, '08, 158

V87.11 **Aromatic amines**

V87.12 **Benzene**

V87.19 **Other hazardous aromatic compounds**
Aromatic dyes NOS
Polycyclic aromatic hydrocarbons

V87.2 **Contact with and (suspected) exposure to other potentially hazardous chemicals**
Dyes NOS
EXCLUDES *exposure to asbestos (V15.84)*
toxic effect of chemicals (980-989)
AHA: 4Q, '08, 158

√5ᵗʰ **V87.3** **Contact with and (suspected) exposure to other potentially hazardous substances**
EXCLUDES *contact with and (suspected) exposure to potentially hazardous body fluids (V15.85)*
personal history of retained foreign body fully removed (V15.53)
toxic effect of substances (980-989)

V87.31 **Exposure to mold**

V87.32 **Contact with and (suspected) exposure to algae bloom**
AHA: 4Q, '09, 116

V87.39 **Contact with and (suspected) exposure to other potentially hazardous substances**

√5ᵗʰ **V87.4** **Personal history of drug therapy**
EXCLUDES *long-term (current) drug use (V58.61-V58.69)*
AHA: 4Q, '09, 116; 4Q, '08, 159

V87.41 **Personal history of antineoplastic chemotherapy**
Z92.21 Personal hx antineoplastic chemotherapy I-10

V87.42 **Personal history of monoclonal drug therapy**

V87.43 **Personal history of estrogen therapy**

V87.44 **Personal history of inhaled steroid therapy**

V87.45 **Personal history of systemic steroid therapy**
Personal history of steroid therapy NOS

V87.46 **Personal history of immunosuppression therapy**
EXCLUDES *personal history of steroid therapy (V87.44, V87.45)*

V87.49 **Personal history of other drug therapy**

Acquired Absence of Other Organs and Tissue (V88)

√4ᵗʰ **V88** **Acquired absence of other organs and tissue**

√5ᵗʰ **V88.0** **Acquired absence of cervix and uterus**
AHA: 4Q, '08, 157

V88.01 **Acquired absence of both cervix and uterus** ♀
Acquired absence of uterus NOS
Status post total hysterectomy

V88.02 **Acquired absence of uterus with remaining cervical stump** ♀
Status post partial hysterectomy with remaining cervical stump

V88.03 **Acquired absence of cervix with remaining uterus** ♀

√5ᵗʰ **V88.1** **Acquired absence of pancreas**
Use additional code to identify any associated:
insulin use (V58.67)
secondary diabetes mellitus (249.00-249.91)
AHA: 4Q, '10, 109

V88.11 **Acquired total absence of pancreas**
Acquired absence of pancreas NOS

V88.12 **Acquired partial absence of pancreas**

√5ᵗʰ **V88.2** **Acquired absence of joint**
Acquired absence of joint following prior explantation of joint prosthesis
Joint prosthesis explantation status
AHA: ▶4Q, '11, 156-157◄

V88.21 **Acquired absence of hip joint**
Acquired absence of hip joint following explantation of joint prosthesis, with or without presence of antibiotic-impregnated cement spacer

V88.22 **Acquired absence of knee joint**
Acquired absence of knee joint following explantation of joint prosthesis, with or without presence of antibiotic-impregnated cement spacer

V88.29 **Acquired absence of other joint**
Acquired absence of other joint following explantation of joint prosthesis, with or without presence of antibiotic-impregnated cement spacer

Other Suspected Conditions Not Found (V89)

√4ᵗʰ **V89** **Other suspected conditions not found**

√5ᵗʰ **V89.0** **Suspected maternal and fetal conditions not found**
EXCLUDES *known or suspected fetal anomalies affecting management of mother, not ruled out (655.00, 655.93, 656.00-656.93, 657.00-657.03, 658.00-658.93)*
newborn and perinatal conditions — code to condition
AHA: 4Q, '08, 159
TIP: These investigations are performed while the fetus is in utero; the codes should be assigned only on the mother's medical record.

V89.01 **Suspected problem with amniotic cavity and membrane not found** M♀
Suspected oligohydramnios not found
Suspected polyhydramnios not found

V89.02 **Suspected placental problem not found** M♀

V89.03 **Suspected fetal anomaly not found** M♀

V89.04 **Suspected problem with fetal growth not found** M♀

V89.05 **Suspected cervical shortening not found** M♀

V89.09 **Other suspected maternal and fetal condition not found** M♀

Retained Foreign Body (V90)

√4ᵗʰ **V90 Retained foreign body**
Embedded fragment (status)
Embedded splinter (status)
Retained foreign body status

> **EXCLUDES** artificial joint prosthesis status (V43.60-V43.69)
> foreign body accidentally left during a procedure (998.4)
> foreign body entering through orifice (930.0-939.9)
> in situ cardiac devices (V45.00-V45.09)
> organ or tissue replaced by other means (V43.0-V43.89)
> organ or tissue replaced by transplant (V42.0-V42.9)
> personal history of retained foreign body removed (V15.53)
> superficial foreign body (splinter) (categories 910-917 and
> 919 with 4ᵗʰ character 6 or 7, 918.0)

> **AHA:** 4Q, '10, 109

√5ᵗʰ **V90.0 Retained radioactive fragment**
V90.01 Retained depleted uranium fragments
V90.09 Other retained radioactive fragments
Other retained depleted isotope fragments
Retained nontherapeutic radioactive fragments

√5ᵗʰ **V90.1 Retained metal fragments**
> **EXCLUDES** retained radioactive metal fragments
> (V90.01-V90.09)

V90.10 Retained metal fragments, unspecified
Retained metal fragment NOS
V90.11 Retained magnetic metal fragments
V90.12 Retained nonmagnetic metal fragments

V90.2 Retained plastic fragments
Acrylics fragments
Diethylhexylphthalates fragments
Isocyanate fragments

√5ᵗʰ **V90.3 Retained organic fragments**
V90.31 Retained animal quills or spines
V90.32 Retained tooth
V90.33 Retained wood fragments
V90.39 Other retained organic fragments

√5ᵗʰ **V90.8 Other specified retained foreign body**
V90.81 Retained glass fragments
V90.83 Retained stone or crystalline fragments
Retained concrete or cement fragments
V90.89 Other specified retained foreign body

V90.9 Retained foreign body, unspecified material

Multiple Gestation Placenta Status (V91)

√4ᵗʰ **V91 Multiple gestation placenta status**
Code first multiple gestation (651.0-651.9)
> **AHA:** 4Q, '10, 110

√5ᵗʰ **V91.0 Twin gestation placenta status**
V91.00 Twin gestation, unspecified number of Ⓜ♀
placenta, unspecified number of amniotic sacs
V91.01 Twin gestation, monochorionic/monoamniotic Ⓜ♀
(one placenta, one amniotic sac)
V91.02 Twin gestation, monochorionic/diamniotic Ⓜ♀
(one placenta, two amniotic sacs)
V91.03 Twin gestation, dichorionic/diamniotic (two Ⓜ♀
placentae, two amniotic sacs)
V91.09 Twin gestation, unable to determine number Ⓜ♀
of placenta and number of amniotic sacs

√5ᵗʰ **V91.1 Triplet gestation placenta status**
V91.10 Triplet gestation, unspecified number of Ⓜ♀
placenta and unspecified number of amniotic
sacs
V91.11 Triplet gestation, with two or more Ⓜ♀
monochorionic fetuses
V91.12 Triplet gestation, with two or more Ⓜ♀
monoamniotic fetuses
V91.19 Triplet gestation, unable to determine number Ⓜ♀
of placenta and number of amniotic sacs

√5ᵗʰ **V91.2 Quadruplet gestation placenta status**
V91.20 Quadruplet gestation, unspecified number Ⓜ♀
of placenta and unspecified number of
amniotic sacs
V91.21 Quadruplet gestation, with two or more Ⓜ♀
monochorionic fetuses
V91.22 Quadruplet gestation, with two or more Ⓜ♀
monoamniotic fetuses
V91.29 Quadruplet gestation, unable to determine Ⓜ♀
number of placenta and number of amniotic sacs

√5ᵗʰ **V91.9 Other specified multiple gestation placenta status**
Placenta status for multiple gestations greater than
quadruplets
V91.90 Other specified multiple gestation, Ⓜ♀
unspecified number of placenta and
unspecified number of amniotic sacs
V91.91 Other specified multiple gestation, with Ⓜ♀
two or more monochorionic fetuses
V91.92 Other specified multiple gestation, with two Ⓜ♀
or more monoamniotic fetuses
V91.99 Other specified multiple gestation, unable to Ⓜ♀
determine number of placenta and number of
amniotic sacs

Supplementary Classification of External Causes of Injury and Poisoning (E000-E999)

This section is provided to permit the classification of environmental events, circumstances, and conditions as the cause of injury, poisoning, and other adverse effects. Where a code from this section is applicable, it is intended that it shall be used in addition to a code from one of the main chapters of ICD-9-CM, indicating the nature of the condition. Certain other conditions which may be stated to be due to external causes are classified in Chapters 1 to 16 of ICD-9-CM. For these, the "E" code classification should be used as an additional code for more detailed analysis.

Machinery accidents [other than those connected with transport] are classifiable to category E919, in which the fourth digit allows a broad classification of the type of machinery involved.

Categories for "late effects" of accidents and other external causes are to be found at E929, E959, E969, E977, E989, and E999.

External Cause Status (E000)

NOTE A code from category E000 may be used in conjunction with the external cause code(s) assigned to a record to indicate the status of the person at the time the event occurred. A single code from category E000 should be assigned for an encounter.

√4ᵗʰ **E000 External cause status**

    E000.0 Civilian activity done for income or pay
        Civilian activity done for financial or other compensation
        EXCLUDES *military activity (E000.1)*

    E000.2 Volunteer activity
        EXCLUDES *activity of child or other family member assisting in compensated work of other family member (E000.8)*

    E000.1 Military activity
        EXCLUDES *activity of off-duty military personnel (E000.8)*

    E000.8 Other external cause status
        Activity of child or other family member assisting in compensated work of other family member
        Activity NEC
        Hobby not done for income
        Leisure activity
        Off-duty activity of military personnel
        Recreation or sport not for income or while a student
        Student activity
        EXCLUDES *civilian activity done for income or compensation (E000.0)*
                       military activity (E000.1)

    E000.9 Unspecified external cause status

Activity (E001-E030)

NOTE Categories E001 to E030 are provided for use to indicate the activity of the person seeking healthcare for an injury or health condition, such as a heart attack while shoveling snow, which resulted from, or was contributed to, by the activity. These codes are appropriate for use for both acute injuries, such as those from chapter 17, and conditions that are due to the long-term, cumulative affects of an activity, such as those from chapter 13. They are also appropriate for use with external cause codes for cause and intent if identifying the activity provides additional information on the event.

These codes should be used in conjunction with other external cause codes for external cause status (E000) and place of occurrence (E849).

This section contains the following broad activity categories:

E001   Activities involving walking and running
E002   Activities involving water and water craft
E003   Activities involving ice and snow
E004   Activities involving climbing, rappelling, and jumping off
E005   Activities involving dancing and other rhythmic movement
E006   Activities involving other sports and athletics played individually
E007   Activities involving other sports and athletics played as a team or group
E008   Activities involving other specified sports and athletics
E009   Activity involving other cardiorespiratory exercise
E010   Activity involving other muscle strengthening exercises
E011   Activities involving computer technology and electronic devices
E012   Activities involving arts and handcrafts
E013   Activities involving personal hygiene and household maintenance
E014   Activities involving person providing caregiving
E015   Activities involving food preparation, cooking and grilling
E016   Activities involving property and land maintenance, building and construction
E017   Activities involving roller coasters and other types of external motion
E018   Activities involving playing musical instrument
E019   Activities involving animal care
E029   Other activity
E030   Unspecified activity

√4ᵗʰ **E001 Activities involving walking and running**
        EXCLUDES *walking an animal (E019.0)*
                   walking or running on a treadmill (E009.0)

    E001.0 Walking, marching and hiking
        Walking, marching and hiking on level or elevated terrain
        EXCLUDES *mountain climbing (E004.0)*

    E001.1 Running

√4ᵗʰ **E002 Activities involving water and water craft**
        EXCLUDES *activities involving ice (E003.0-E003.9)*
                   boating and other watercraft transport accidents (E830-E838)

    E002.0 Swimming

    E002.1 Springboard and platform diving

    E002.2 Water polo

    E002.3 Water aerobics and water exercise

    E002.4 Underwater diving and snorkeling
        SCUBA diving

    E002.5 Rowing, canoeing, kayaking, rafting and tubing
        Canoeing, kayaking, rafting and tubing in calm and turbulent water

    E002.6 Water skiing and wake boarding

    E002.7 Surfing, windsurfing and boogie boarding

    E002.8 Water sliding

    E002.9 Other activity involving water and watercraft
        Activity involving water NOS
        Parasailing
        Water survival training and testing

√4ᵗʰ **E003 Activities involving ice and snow**
        EXCLUDES *shoveling ice and snow (E016.0)*

    E003.0 Ice skating
        Figure skating (singles) (pairs)
        Ice dancing
        EXCLUDES *ice hockey (E003.1)*

    E003.1 Ice hockey

    E003.2 Snow (alpine) (downhill) skiing, snow boarding, sledding, tobogganing and snow tubing
        EXCLUDES *cross country skiing (E003.3)*

    E003.3 Cross country skiing
        Nordic skiing

    E003.9 Other activity involving ice and snow
        Activity involving ice and snow NOS

√4ᵗʰ **E004 Activities involving climbing, rappelling, and jumping off**
        EXCLUDES *hiking on level or elevated terrain (E001.0)*
                   jumping rope (E006.5)
                   sky diving (E840-E844)
                   trampoline jumping (E005.3)

    E004.0 Mountain climbing, rock climbing and wall climbing

    E004.1 Rappelling

    E004.2 BASE jumping
        Building, Antenna, Span, Earth jumping

    E004.3 Bungee jumping

    E004.4 Hang gliding

    E004.9 Other activity involving climbing, rappelling and jumping off

---

√4ᵗʰ Fourth-digit Required   ►◄ Revised Text   ● New Code   ▲ Revised Code TitleDx

☑4ᵗʰ **E005 Activities involving dancing and other rhythmic movement**
     EXCLUDES *martial arts (E008.4)*

E005.0 Dancing

E005.1 Yoga

E005.2 Gymnastics
     Rhythmic gymnastics
     EXCLUDES *trampoline (E005.3)*

E005.3 Trampoline

E005.4 Cheerleading

E005.9 Other activity involving dancing and other rhythmic movements

☑4ᵗʰ **E006 Activities involving other sports and athletics played individually**
     EXCLUDES *dancing (E005.0)*
             gymnastic (E005.2)
             trampoline (E005.3)
             yoga (E005.1)

E006.0 Roller skating (inline) and skateboarding

E006.1 Horseback riding

E006.2 Golf

E006.3 Bowling

E006.4 Bike riding
     EXCLUDES *transport accident involving bike riding (E800-E829)*

E006.5 Jumping rope

E006.6 Non-running track and field events
     EXCLUDES *running (any form) (E001.1)*

E006.9 Other activity involving other sports and athletics played individually
     EXCLUDES *activities involving climbing, rappelling, and jumping (E004.0-E004.9)*
             activities involving ice and snow (E003.0-E003.9)
             activities involving walking and running (E001.0-E001.9)
             activities involving water and watercraft (E002.0-E002.9)

☑4ᵗʰ **E007 Activities involving other sports and athletics played as a team or group**
     EXCLUDES *ice hockey (E003.1)*
             water polo (E002.2)

E007.0 American tackle football
     Football NOS

E007.1 American flag or touch football

E007.2 Rugby

E007.3 Baseball
     Softball

E007.4 Lacrosse and field hockey

E007.5 Soccer

E007.6 Basketball

E007.7 Volleyball (beach) (court)

E007.8 Physical games generally associated with school recess, summer camp and children
     Capture the flag
     Dodge ball
     Four square
     Kickball

E007.9 Other activity involving other sports and athletics played as a team or group
     Cricket

☑4ᵗʰ **E008 Activities involving other specified sports and athletics**

E008.0 Boxing

E008.1 Wrestling

E008.2 Racquet and hand sports
     Handball
     Racquetball
     Squash
     Tennis

E008.3 Frisbee
     Ultimate frisbee

E008.4 Martial arts
     Combatives

E008.9 Other specified sports and athletics activity
     EXCLUDES *sports and athletics activities specified in categories E001-E007*

☑4ᵗʰ **E009 Activity involving other cardiorespiratory exercise**
     Activity involving physical training

E009.0 Exercise machines primarily for cardiorespiratory conditioning
     Elliptical and stepper machines
     Stationary bike
     Treadmill

E009.1 Calisthenics
     Jumping jacks
     Warm up and cool down

E009.2 Aerobic and step exercise

E009.3 Circuit training

E009.4 Obstacle course
     Challenge course
     Confidence course

E009.5 Grass drills
     Guerilla drills

E009.9 Other activity involving cardiorespiratory exercise
     EXCLUDES *activities involving cardiorespiratory exercise specified in categories E001-E008*

☑4ᵗʰ **E010 Activity involving other muscle strengthening exercises**

E010.0 Exercise machines primarily for muscle strengthening

E010.1 Push-ups, pull-ups, sit-ups

E010.2 Free weights
     Barbells
     Dumbbells

E010.3 Pilates

E010.9 Other activity involving other muscle strengthening exercises
     EXCLUDES *activities involving muscle strengthening specified in categories E001-E009*

☑4ᵗʰ **E011 Activities involving computer technology and electronic devices**
     EXCLUDES *electronic musical keyboard or instruments (E018.0)*

E011.0 Computer keyboarding
     Electronic game playing using keyboard or other stationary device

E011.1 Hand held interactive electronic device
     Cellular telephone and communication device
     Electronic game playing using interactive device
     EXCLUDES *electronic game playing using keyboard or other stationary device (E011.0)*

E011.9 Other activity involving computer technology and electronic devices

☑4ᵗʰ **E012 Activities involving arts and handcrafts**
     EXCLUDES *activities involving playing musical instrument (E018.0-E018.3)*

E012.0 Knitting and crocheting

E012.1 Sewing

E012.2 Furniture building and finishing
     Furniture repair

E012.9 Activity involving other arts and handcrafts

☑4ᵗʰ Fourth-digit Required   ►◄ Revised Text   ● New Code   ▲ Revised Code TitleDx

☑4ᵗʰ **E013 Activities involving personal hygiene and household maintenance**

> EXCLUDES *activities involving cooking and grilling (E015.0-E015.9)*
> *activities involving property and land maintenance, building and construction (E016.0-E016.9)*
> *activity involving persons providing caregiving (E014.0-E014.9)*
> *dishwashing (E015.0)*
> *food preparation (E015.0)*
> *gardening (E016.1)*

E013.0 Personal bathing and showering

E013.1 Laundry

E013.2 Vacuuming

E013.3 Ironing

E013.4 Floor mopping and cleaning

E013.5 Residential relocation
> Packing up and unpacking involved in moving to a new residence

E013.8 Other personal hygiene activity

E013.9 Other household maintenance

☑4ᵗʰ **E014 Activities involving person providing caregiving**

E014.0 Caregiving involving bathing

E014.1 Caregiving involving lifting

E014.9 Other activity involving person providing caregiving

☑4ᵗʰ **E015 Activities involving food preparation, cooking and grilling**

E015.0 Food preparation and clean up
> Dishwasing

E015.1 Grilling and smoking food

E015.2 Cooking and baking
> Use of stove, oven and microwave oven

E015.9 Other activity involving cooking and grilling

☑4ᵗʰ **E016 Activities involving property and land maintenance, building and construction**

E016.0 Digging, shoveling and raking
> Dirt digging
> Raking leaves
> Snow shoveling

E016.1 Gardening and landscaping
> Pruning, trimming shrubs, weeding

E016.2 Building and construction

E016.9 Other activity involving property and land maintenance, building and construction

☑4ᵗʰ **E017 Activities involving roller coasters and other types of external motion**

E017.0 Roller coaster riding

E017.9 Other activity involving external motion

☑4ᵗʰ **E018 Activities involving playing musical instrument**
> Activity involving playing electric musical instrument

E018.0 Piano playing
> Musical keyboard (electronic) playing

E018.1 Drum and other percussion instrument playing

E018.2 String instrument playing

E018.3 Wind and brass instrument playing

☑4ᵗʰ **E019 Activities involving animal care**

> EXCLUDES *horseback riding (E006.1)*

E019.0 Walking an animal

E019.1 Milking an animal

E019.2 Grooming and shearing an animal

E019.9 Other activity involving animal care

☑4ᵗʰ **E029 Other activity**

E029.0 Refereeing a sports activity

E029.1 Spectator at an event

E029.2 Rough housing and horseplay

E029.9 Other activity

E030 Unspecified activity

Transport Accidents (E800-E848)

Definitions and Examples Related to Transport Accidents

(a) A **transport accident** (E800-E848) is any accident involving a device designed primarily for, or being used at the time primarily for, conveying persons or goods from one place to another.

> INCLUDES accidents involving:
> aircraft and spacecraft (E840-E845)
> watercraft (E830-E838)
> motor vehicle (E810-E825)
> railway (E800-E807)
> other road vehicles (E826-E829)

In classifying accidents which involve more than one kind of transport, the above order of precedence of transport accidents should be used.

Accidents involving agricultural and construction machines, such as tractors, cranes, and bulldozers, are regarded as transport accidents only when these vehicles are under their own power on a highway [otherwise the vehicles are regarded as machinery]. Vehicles which can travel on land or water, such as hovercraft and other amphibious vehicles, are regarded as watercraft when on the water, as motor vehicles when on the highway, and as off-road motor vehicles when on land, but off the highway.

> EXCLUDES *accidents:*
> *in sports which involve the use of transport but where the transport vehicle itself was not involved in the accident*
> *involving vehicles which are part of industrial equipment used entirely on industrial premises*
> *occurring during transportation but unrelated to the hazards associated with the means of transportation [e.g., injuries received in a fight on board ship; transport vehicle involved in a cataclysm such as an earthquake]*
> *to persons engaged in the maintenance or repair of transport equipment or vehicle not in motion, unless injured by another vehicle in motion*

(b) A **railway accident** is a transport accident involving a railway train or other railway vehicle operated on rails, whether in motion or not.

> EXCLUDES *accidents:*
> *in repair shops*
> *in roundhouse or on turntable*
> *on railway premises but not involving a train or other railway vehicle*

(c) A **railway train** or **railway vehicle** is any device with or without cars coupled to it, desiged for traffic on a railway.

> INCLUDES interurban:
> electric car } (operated chiefly on its own
> street car   right-of-way, not open to other traffic)
> railway train, any power [diesel] [electric] [steam]:
> funicular
> monorail or two-rail
> subterranean or elevated
> other vehicle designed to run on a railway track
>> EXCLUDES *interurban electric cars [streetcars] specified to be operating on a right-of-way that forms part of the public street or highway [definition (h)]*

(d) A **railway** or **railroad** is a right-of-way designed for traffic on rails, which is used by carriages or wagons transporting passengers or freight, and by other rolling stock, and which is not open to other public vehicular traffic.

(e) A **motor vehicle accident** is a transport accident involving a motor vehicle. It is defined as a motor vehicle traffic accident or as a motor vehicle nontraffic accident according to whether the accident occurs on a public highway or elsewhere.

> EXCLUDES *injury or damage due to cataclysm*
> *injury or damage while a motor vehicle, not under its own power, is being loaded on, or unloaded from, another conveyance*

(f) A **motor vehicle traffic accident** is any motor vehicle accident occurring on a public highway [i.e., originating, terminating, or involving a vehicle partially on the highway]. A motor vehicle accident is assumed to have occurred on the highway unless another place is specified, except in the case of accidents involving only off-road motor vehicles which are classified as nontraffic accidents unless the contrary is stated.

☑4ᵗʰ Fourth-digit Required   ▶◀ Revised Text   ● New Code   ▲ Revised Code TitleDx

(g) A **motor vehicle nontraffic accident** is any motor vehicle accident which occurs entirely in any place other than a public highway.

(h) A **public highway [trafficway]** or **street** is the entire width between property lines [or other boundary lines] of every way or place, of which any part is open to the use of the public for purposes of vehicular traffic as a matter of right or custom. A **roadway** is that part of the public highway designed, improved, and ordinarily used, for vehicular travel.

INCLUDES approaches (public) to:
  docks
  public building
  station

EXCLUDES driveway (private)
  parking lot
  ramp
  roads in:
    airfield
    farm
    industrial premises
    mine
    private grounds
    quarry

(i) A **motor vehicle** is any mechanically or electrically powered device, not operated on rails, upon which any person or property may be transported or drawn upon a highway. Any object such as a trailer, coaster, sled, or wagon being towed by a motor vehicle is considered a part of the motor vehicle.

INCLUDES automobile [any type]
  bus
  construction machinery, farm and industrial machinery, steam roller, tractor, army tank, highway grader, or similar vehicle on wheels or treads, while in transport under own power
  fire engine (motorized)
  motorcycle
  motorized bicycle [moped] or scooter
  trolley bus not operating on rails
  truck
  van

EXCLUDES devices used solely to move persons or materials within the confines of a building and its premises, such as:
  building elevator
  coal car in mine
  electric baggage or mail truck used solely within a railroad station
  electric truck used solely within an industrial plant
  moving overhead crane

(j) A **motorcycle** is a two-wheeled motor vehicle having one or two riding saddles and sometimes having a third wheel for the support of a sidecar. The sidecar is considered part of the motorcycle.

INCLUDES motorized:
  bicycle [moped]
  scooter
  tricycle

(k) An **off-road motor vehicle** is a motor vehicle of special design, to enable it to negotiate rough or soft terrain or snow. Examples of special design are high construction, special wheels and tires, driven by treads, or support on a cushion of air.

INCLUDES all terrain vehicle [ATV]
  army tank
  hovercraft, on land or swamp
  snowmobile

(l) A **driver** of a motor vehicle is the occupant of the motor vehicle operating it or intending to operate it. A **motorcyclist** is the driver of a motorcycle. Other authorized occupants of a motor vehicle are **passengers**.

(m) An **other road vehicle** is any device, except a motor vehicle, in, on, or by which any person or property may be transported on a highway.

INCLUDES animal carrying a person or goods
  animal-drawn vehicles
  animal harnessed to conveyance
  bicycle [pedal cycle]
  streetcar
  tricycle (pedal)

EXCLUDES pedestrian conveyance [definition (q)]

(n) A **streetcar** is a device designed and used primarily for transporting persons within a municipality, running on rails, usually subject to normal traffic control signals, and operated principally on a right-of-way that forms part of the traffic way. A trailer being towed by a streetcar is considered a part of the streetcar.

INCLUDES interurban or intraurban electric or streetcar, when specified to be operating on a street or public highway
  tram (car)
  trolley (car)

(o) A **pedal cycle** is any road transport vehicle operated solely by pedals.

INCLUDES bicycle
  pedal cycle
  tricycle

EXCLUDES motorized bicycle [definition (j)]

(p) A **pedal cyclist** is any person riding on a pedal cycle or in a sidecar attached to such a vehicle.

(q) A **pedestrian conveyance** is any human powered device by which a pedestrian may move other than by walking or by which a walking person may move another pedestrian.

INCLUDES baby carriage
  coaster wagon
  heelies, wheelies
  ice skates
  motorized mobility scooter
  perambulator
  pushcart
  pushchair
  roller skates
  scooter
  skateboard
  skis
  sled
  wheelchair (electric)

(r) A **pedestrian** is any person involved in an accident who was not at the time of the accident riding in or on a motor vehicle, railroad train, streetcar, animal-drawn or other vehicle, or on a bicycle or animal.

INCLUDES person:
  changing tire of vehicle
  in or operating a pedestrian conveyance
  making adjustment to motor of vehicle
  on foot

(s) A **watercraft** is any device for transporting passengers or goods on the water.

(t) A **small boat** is any watercraft propelled by paddle, oars, or small motor, with a passenger capacity of less than ten.

INCLUDES boat NOS
  canoe
  coble
  dinghy
  punt
  raft
  rowboat
  rowing shell
  scull
  skiff
  small motorboat

EXCLUDES barge
  lifeboat (used after abandoning ship)
  raft (anchored) being used as a diving platform
  yacht

(u) An **aircraft** is any device for transporting passengers or goods in the air.

INCLUDES airplane [any type]
  balloon
  bomber
  dirigible
  glider (hang)
  military aircraft
  parachute

(v) A **commercial transport aircraft** is any device for collective passenger or freight transportation by air, whether run on commercial lines for profit or by government authorities, with the exception of military craft.

Railway Accidents (E800-E807)

NOTE For definitions of railway accident and related terms see definitions (a) to (d).

EXCLUDES accidents involving railway train and:
> aircraft (E840.0-E845.9)
> motor vehicle (E810.0-E825.9)
> watercraft (E830.0-E838.9)

The following fourth digit subdivisions are for use with categories E800-E807 to identify the injured person:

.0 Railway employee
> Any person who by virtue of his employment in connection with a railway, whether by the railway company or not, is at increased risk of involvement in a railway accident, such as:
> catering staff of train
> driver
> guard
> porter
> postal staff on train
> railway fireman
> shunter
> sleeping car attendant

.1 Passenger on railway
> Any authorized person traveling on a train, except a railway employee.
> **EXCLUDES** intending passenger waiting at station (.8)
> unauthorized rider on railway vehicle (.8)

.2 Pedestrian
> See definition (r)

.3 Pedal cyclist
> See definition (p)

.8 Other specified person
> Intending passenger or bystander waiting at station
> Unauthorized rider on railway vehicle

.9 Unspecified person

§ ☑4ᵗʰ **E800 Railway accident involving collision with rolling stock**

INCLUDES collision between railway trains or railway vehicles, any kind
collision NOS on railway
derailment with antecedent collision with rolling stock or NOS

§ ☑4ᵗʰ **E801 Railway accident involving collision with other object**

INCLUDES collision of railway train with:
> buffers
> fallen tree on railway
> gates
> platform
> rock on railway
> streetcar
> other nonmotor vehicle
> other object

EXCLUDES collision with:
> aircraft (E840.0-E842.9)
> motor vehicle (E810.0-E810.9, E820.0-E822.9)

§ ☑4ᵗʰ **E802 Railway accident involving derailment without antecedent collision**

§ ☑4ᵗʰ **E803 Railway accident involving explosion, fire, or burning**

EXCLUDES explosion or fire, with antecedent derailment (E802.0-E802.9)
explosion or fire, with mention of antecedent collision (E800.0-E801.9)

§ ☑4ᵗʰ **E804 Fall in, on, or from railway train**

INCLUDES fall while alighting from or boarding railway train

EXCLUDES fall related to collision, derailment, or explosion of railway train (E800.0-E803.9)

§ ☑4ᵗʰ **E805 Hit by rolling stock**

INCLUDES crushed
injured
killed   } by railway train or part
knocked down
run over

EXCLUDES pedestrian hit by object set in motion by railway train (E806.0-E806.9)

§ ☑4ᵗʰ **E806 Other specified railway accident**

INCLUDES hit by object falling in railway train
injured by door or window on railway train
nonmotor road vehicle or pedestrian hit by object set in motion by railway train
railway train hit by falling:
> earth NOS
> rock
> tree
> other object

EXCLUDES railway accident due to cataclysm (E908-E909)

§ ☑4ᵗʰ **E807 Railway accident of unspecified nature**

INCLUDES found dead   }
injured   } on railway right-of-way NOS
railway accident NOS

Motor Vehicle Traffic Accidents (E810-E819)

NOTE For definitions of motor vehicle traffic accident, and related terms, see definitions (e) to (k).

EXCLUDES accidents involving motor vehicle and aircraft (E840.0-E845.9)

The following fourth digit subdivisions are for use with categories E810-E819 to identify the injured person:

.0 Driver of motor vehicle other than motorcycle
> See definition (l)

.1 Passenger in motor vehicle other than motorcycle
> See definition (l)

.2 Motorcyclist
> See definition (l)

.3 Passenger on motorcycle
> See definition (l)

.4 Occupant of streetcar

.5 Rider of animal; occupant of animal-drawn vehicle

.6 Pedal cyclist
> See definition (p)

.7 Pedestrian
> See definition (r)

.8 Other specified person
> Occupant of vehicle other than above
> Person in railway train involved in accident
> Unauthorized rider of motor vehicle

.9 Unspecified person

§ ☑4ᵗʰ **E810 Motor vehicle traffic accident involving collision with train**

EXCLUDES motor vehicle collision with object set in motion by railway train (E815.0-E815.9)
railway train hit by object set in motion by motor vehicle (E818.0-E818.9)

§ ☑4ᵗʰ **E811 Motor vehicle traffic accident involving re-entrant collision with another motor vehicle**

INCLUDES collision between motor vehicle which accidentally leaves the roadway then re-enters the same roadway, or the opposite roadway on a divided highway, and another motor vehicle

EXCLUDES collision on the same roadway when none of the motor vehicles involved have left and re-entered the highway (E812.0-E812.9)

§ ☑4ᵗʰ **E812 Other motor vehicle traffic accident involving collision with motor vehicle**

INCLUDES collision with another motor vehicle parked, stopped, stalled, disabled, or abandoned on the highway
motor vehicle collision NOS

EXCLUDES collision with object set in motion by another motor vehicle (E815.0-E815.9)
re-entrant collision with another motor vehicle (E811.0-E811.9)

---

§ Requires fourth digit. See beginning of appropriate section for codes and definitions.

☑4ᵗʰ Fourth-digit Required   ►◄ Revised Text   ● New Code   ▲ Revised Code TitleDx

E Codes

E813–E819

§ ☑4ᵗʰ **E813 Motor vehicle traffic accident involving collision with other vehicle**

INCLUDES   collision between motor vehicle, any kind, and:
    other road (nonmotor transport) vehicle, such as:
      animal carrying a person
      animal-drawn vehicle
      pedal cycle
      streetcar

EXCLUDES   *collision with:*
    object set in motion by nonmotor road vehicle
      (E815.0-E815.9)
    pedestrian (E814.0-E814.9)
    nonmotor road vehicle hit by object set in motion by motor
      vehicle (E818.0-E818.9)

§ ☑4ᵗʰ **E814 Motor vehicle traffic accident involving collision with pedestrian**

INCLUDES   collision between motor vehicle, any kind, and:
    pedestrian
    pedestrian dragged, hit, or run over by motor vehicle, any kind

EXCLUDES   *pedestrian hit by object set in motion by motor vehicle (E818.0-E818.9)*

§ ☑4ᵗʰ **E815 Other motor vehicle traffic accident involving collision on the highway**

INCLUDES   collision (due to loss of control) (on highway) between motor vehicle, any kind, and:
    abutment (bridge) (overpass)
    animal (herded) (unattended)
    fallen stone, traffic sign, tree, utility pole
    guard rail or boundary fence
    interhighway divider
    landslide (not moving)
    object set in motion by railway train or road vehicle (motor) (nonmotor)
    object thrown in front of motor vehicle
    other object, fixed, movable, or moving
    safety island
    temporary traffic sign or marker
    wall of cut made for road

EXCLUDES   *collision with:*
    any object off the highway (resulting from loss of control) (E816.0-E816.9)
    any object which normally would have been off the highway and is not stated to have been on it (E816.0-E816.9)
    motor vehicle parked, stopped, stalled, disabled, or abandoned on highway (E812.0-E812.9)
    moving landslide (E909)
    motor vehicle hit by object:
      set in motion by railway train or road vehicle (motor) (nonmotor) (E818.0-E818.9)
      thrown into or on vehicle (E818.0-E818.9)

§ ☑4ᵗʰ **E816 Motor vehicle traffic accident due to loss of control, without collision on the highway**

INCLUDES   motor vehicle:
    failing to make curve
    going out of control (due to):   and:
      blowout   coliding with object off the highway
      burst tire   overturning
      driver falling asleep   stopping abruptly off the highway
      drive inattention
      excessive speed
      failure of mechanical part

EXCLUDES   *collision on highway following loss of control (E810.0-E815.9)*
    loss of control of motor vehicle following collision on the highway (E810.0-E815.9)

§ ☑4ᵗʰ **E817 Noncollision motor vehicle traffic accident while boarding or alighting**

INCLUDES   fall down stairs of motor bus
    fall from car in street
    injured by moving part of the vehicle
    trapped by door of motor bus
     } while boarding or alighting

§ ☑4ᵗʰ **E818 Other noncollision motor vehicle traffic accident**

INCLUDES   accidental poisoning from exhaust gas generated by
    breakage of any part of
    explosion of any part of
    fall, jump, or being accidentally pushed from
    fire starting in
    hit by object thrown into or on
    injured by being thrown against some part of, or object in
    injury from moving part of
    object falling in or on
    object thrown on
     } motor vehicle while in motion

    collision of railway train or road vehicle except motor vehicle, with object set in motion by motor vehicle
    motor vehicle hit by object set in motion by railway train or road vehicle (motor) (nonmotor)
    pedestrian, railway train, or road vehicle (motor) (nonmotor) hit by object set in motion by motor vehicle

EXCLUDES   *collision between motor vehicle and:*
    object set in motion by railway train or road vehicle (motor) (nonmotor) (E815.0-E815.9)
    object thrown towards the motor vehicle (E815.0-E815.9)
    person overcome by carbon monoxide generated by stationary motor vehicle off the roadway with motor running (E868.2)

§ ☑4ᵗʰ **E819 Motor vehicle traffic accident of unspecified nature**

INCLUDES   motor vehicle traffic accident NOS
    traffic accident NOS

Motor Vehicle Nontraffic Accidents (E820-E825)

NOTE   For definitions of motor vehicle nontraffic accident and related terms see definition (a) to (k).

INCLUDES   accidents involving motor vehicles being used in recreational or sporting activities off the highway
    collision and noncollision motor vehicle accidents occurring entirely off the highway

EXCLUDES   *accidents involving motor vehicle and:*
    aircraft (E840.0-E845.9)
    watercraft (E830.0-E838.9)
    accidents, not on the public highway, involving agricultural and construction machinery but not involving another motor vehicle (E919.0, E919.2, E919.7)

The following fourth digit subdivisions are for use with categories E820-E825 to identify the injured person:

.0 Driver of motor vehicle other than motorcycle
    See definition (l)
.1 Passenger in motor vehicle other than motorcycle
    See definition (l)
.2 Motorcyclist
    See definition (l)
.3 Passenger on motorcycle
    See definition (l)
.4 Occupant of streetcar
.5 Rider of animal; occupant of animal-drawn vehicle
.6 Pedal cyclist
    See definition (p)
.7 Pedestrian
    See definition (r)
.8 Other specified person
    Occupant of vehicle other than above
    Person in railway train involved in accident
    Unauthorized rider of motor vehicle
.9 Unspecified person

§   Requires fourth digit. See beginning of appropriate section for codes and definitions.

☑4ᵗʰ Fourth-digit Required   ▶◀ Revised Text   ● New Code   ▲ Revised Code TitleDx

6 – E Codes   2013 ICD-9-CM

§ ✓4ᵗʰ **E820 Nontraffic accident involving motor-driven snow vehicle**

INCLUDES
breakage of part of
fall from
hit by   }   motor-driven snow
overturning of   vehicle (not on
run over or dragged by   public highway)

collision of motor-driven snow vehicle with:
    animal (being ridden) (-drawn vehicle)
    another off-road motor vehicle
    other motor vehicle, not on public highway
    railway train
    other object, fixed or movable
injury caused by rough landing of motor-driven snow
    vehicle (after leaving ground on rough terrain)

EXCLUDES   *accident on the public highway involving motor driven*
                snow vehicle (E810.0-E819.9)

§ ✓4ᵗʰ **E821 Nontraffic accident involving other off-road motor vehicle**

INCLUDES
breakage of part of
fall from
hit by   off-road motorvehicle
overturning of   }   except snow
run over or dragged by   vehicle (not on
thrown against some part   public highway
    of or object in

collision with:
    animal (being ridden) (-drawn vehicle)
    another off-road motor vehicle, except snow vehicle
    other motor vehicle, not on public highway
    other object, fixed or movable

EXCLUDES   *accident on public highway involving off-road motor*
                vehicle (E810.0-E819.9)
                collision between motor driven snow vehicle and other
                off-road motor vehicle (E820.0-E820.9)
                hovercraft accident on water (E830.0-E838.9)

§ ✓4ᵗʰ **E822 Other motor vehicle nontraffic accident involving collision with moving object**

INCLUDES   collision, not on public highway, between motor vehicle,
                except off-road motor vehicle and:
    animal
    nonmotor vehicle
    other motor vehicle, except off-road motor vehicle
    pedestrian
    railway train
    other moving object

EXCLUDES   *collision with:*
                motor-driven snow vehicle (E820.0-E820.9)
                other off-road motor vehicle (E821.0-E821.9)

§ ✓4ᵗʰ **E823 Other motor vehicle nontraffic accident involving collision with stationary object**

INCLUDES   collision, not on public highway, between motor vehicle,
                except off-road motor vehicle, and any object,
                fixed or movable, but not in motion

§ ✓4ᵗʰ **E824 Other motor vehicle nontraffic accident while boarding and alighting**

INCLUDES
fall
injury from oving part   while boarding or alighting
    of motor   }   from motor vehicle,
    vehicle   except off-road motor
trapped by door of   vehicle, not on public
    motor vehhicle   highway

§ ✓4ᵗʰ **E825 Other motor vehicle nontraffic accident of other and unspecified nature**

INCLUDES   accidental poisoning from carbon
            monoxide generated by
breakage of any part of
explosion of any part of
fall, jump, or being accidentally   motor vehicle
    pushed from   while in
fire starting in   }   motion, not
hit by object thrown into, towards,   on public
    or on   highway
injured by being thrown against
    some part of, or object in
injury from moving part of
object falling in or on
motor vehicle nontraffic accident NOS

EXCLUDES   *fall from or in stationary motor vehicle (E884.9, E885.9)*
                overcome by carbon monoxide or exhaust gas generated by
                stationary motor vehicle off the roadway with motor
                running (E868.2)
                struck by falling object from or in stationary motor vehicle
                (E916)

Other Road Vehicle Accidents (E826-E829)

NOTE   Other road vehicle accidents are transport accidents involving road
       vehicles other than motor vehicles. For definitions of other road
       vehicle and related terms see definitions (m) to (o).

INCLUDES   accidents involving other road vehicles being used in recreational
            or sporting activities

EXCLUDES   *collision of other road vehicle [any] with:*
            aircraft (E840.0-E845.9)
            motor vehicle (E813.0-E813.9, E820.0-E822.9)
            railway train (E801.0-E801.9))

> The following fourth digit subdivisions are for use with categories E826-E829
> to identify the injured person:
> **.0 Pedestrian**
>   See definition (r)
> **.1 Pedal cyclist**
>   See definition (p)
> **.2 Rider of animal**
> **.3 Occupant of animal-drawn vehicle**
> **.4 Occupant of streetcar**
> **.8 Other specified person**
> **.9 Unspecified person**

§ ✓4ᵗʰ **E826 Pedal cycle accident**

[0-9]   INCLUDES   breakage of any part of pedal cycle
                collision between pedal cycle and:
                  animal (being ridden) (herded) (unattended)
                  another pedal cycle
                  any pedestrian
                  nonmotor road vehicle
                  other object, fixed, movable, or moving, not set in
                     motion by motor vehicle, railway train, or aircraft
                entanglement in wheel of pedal cycle
                fall from pedal cycle
                hit by object falling or thrown on the pedal cycle
                pedal cycle accident NOS
                pedal cycle overturned

§ ✓4ᵗʰ **E827 Animal-drawn vehicle accident**

[0,2,4,8,9]   INCLUDES   breakage of any part of vehicle
                collision between animal-drawn vehicle and:
                  animal (being ridden) (herded) (unattended)
                  nonmotor road vehicle, except pedal cycle
                  pedestrian, pedestrian conveyance, or pedestrian
                     vehicle
                  other object, fixed, movable, or moving, not set in
                     motion by motor vehicle, railway train, or aircraft
fall from
knocked down by
overturning of   }   animal drawn vehicle
running over by
thrown from

EXCLUDES   *collision of animal-drawn vehicle with pedal cycle*
                (E826.0-E826.9)

---

§   Requires fourth digit. See beginning of appropriate section for codes and definitions.

§ ✓4ᵗʰ **E828 Accident involving animal being ridden**

[0,2,4,8,9] INCLUDES collision between animal being ridden and:
- another animal
- nonmotor road vehicle, except pedal cycle, and animal-drawn vehicle
- pedestrian, pedestrian conveyance, or pedestrian vehicle
- other object, fixed, movable, or moving, not set in motion by motor vehicle, railway train, or aircraft

fall from	
knocked down by	animal being ridden
thrown from	
trampled by	

ridden animal stumbled and fell

EXCLUDES collision of animal being ridden with:
- animal-drawn vehicle (E827.0-E827.9)
- pedal cycle (E826.0-E826.9)

§ ✓4ᵗʰ **E829 Other road vehicle accidents**

[0,4,8,9] INCLUDES accident while boarding

or alighting from	
blow from object in	streetcar
breakage of any part of	nonmotor road vehicle
caught in door of	not classifiable to
derailment of	E826-E828
fall in, on, or from	
fire in	

collision between streetcar or nonmotor road vehicle, except as in E826-E828, and:
- animal (not being ridden)
- another nonmotor road vehicle not classifiable to E826-E828
- pedestrian
- other object, fixed, movable, or moving, not set in motion by motor vehicle, railway train, or aircraft

nonmotor road vehicle accident NOS
streetcar accident NOS

EXCLUDES collision with:
- animal being ridden (E828.0-E828.9)
- animal-drawn vehicle (E827.0-E827.9)
- pedal cycle (E826.0-E826.9)

Water Transport Accidents (E830-E838)

NOTE For definitions of water transport accident and related terms see definitions (a), (s), and (t).

INCLUDES watercraft accidents in the course of recreational activities

EXCLUDES accidents involving both aircraft, including objects set in motion by aircraft, and watercraft (E840.0-E845.9)

The following fourth digit subdivisions are for use with categories E830-E838 to identify the injured person:

.0 Occupant of small boat, unpowered
.1 Occupant of small boat, powered
  See definition (t)
  EXCLUDES water skier (.4)
.2 Occupant of other watercraft — crew
  Persons:
    engaged in operation of watercraft
    providing passenger services [cabin attendants, ship's physician, catering personnel]
    working on ship during voyage in other capacity [musician in band, operators of shops and beauty parlors
.3 Occupant of other watercraft — other than crew
  Passenger
  Occupant of lifeboat, other than crew, after abandoning ship
.4 Water skier
.5 Swimmer
.6 Dockers, stevedores
  Longshoreman employed on the dock in loading and unloading ships
.7 Occupant of military watercraft, any type
.8 Other specified person
  Immigration and custom officials on board ship
  Person:
    accompanying passenger or member of crew visiting boat
  Pilot (guiding ship into port)
.9 Unspecified person

§ ✓4ᵗʰ **E830 Accident to watercraft causing submersion**

INCLUDES submersion and drowning due to:
- boat overturning
- boat submerging
- falling or jumping from burning ship
- falling or jumping from crushed watercraft
- ship sinking
- other accident to watercraft

§ ✓4ᵗʰ **E831 Accident to watercraft causing other injury**

INCLUDES any injury, except submersion and drowning, as a result of an accident to watercraft
- burned while ship on fire
- crushed between ships in collision
- crushed by lifeboat after abandoning ship
- fall due to collision or other accident to watercraft
- hit by falling object due to accident to watercraft
- injured in watercraft accident involving collision
- struck by boat or part thereof after fall or jump from damaged boat

EXCLUDES burns from localized fire or explosion on board ship (E837.0-E837.9)

§ ✓4ᵗʰ **E832 Other accidental submersion or drowning in water transport accident**

INCLUDES submersion or drowning as a result of an accident other than accident to the watercraft, such as:
- fall:
  - from gangplank
  - from ship
  - overboard
- thrown overboard by motion of ship
- washed overboard

EXCLUDES submersion or drowning of swimmer or diver who voluntarily jumps from boat not involved in an accident (E910.0-E910.9)

§ ✓4ᵗʰ **E833 Fall on stairs or ladders in water transport**

EXCLUDES fall due to accident to watercraft (E831.0-E831.9)

§ ✓4ᵗʰ **E834 Other fall from one level to another in water transport**

EXCLUDES fall due to accident to watercraft (E831.0-E831.9)

§ ✓4ᵗʰ **E835 Other and unspecified fall in water transport**

EXCLUDES fall due to accident to watercraft (E831.0-E831.9)

§ ✓4ᵗʰ **E836 Machinery accident in water transport**

INCLUDES injuries in water transport caused by:

deck	
engine room	
galley	machinery
laundry	
loading	

§ ✓4ᵗʰ **E837 Explosion, fire, or burning in watercraft**

INCLUDES explosion of boiler on steamship
localized fire on ship

EXCLUDES burning ship (due to collision or explosion) resulting in:
- submersion or drowning (E830.0-E830.9)
- other injury (E831.0-E831.9)

§ ✓4ᵗʰ **E838 Other and unspecified water transport accident**

INCLUDES accidental poisoning by gases or fumes on ship
atomic power plant malfunction in watercraft
crushed between ship and stationary object [wharf]
crushed between ships without accident to watercraft
crushed by falling object on ship or while loading or unloading
hit by boat while water skiing
struck by boat or part thereof (after fall from boat)
watercraft accident NOS

---

§   Requires fourth digit. Valid digits are in [brackets] under each code. See beginning of appropriate section for codes and definitions.

Air and Space Transport Accidents (E840-E845)

NOTE For definition of aircraft and related terms see definitions (u) and (v).

The following fourth digit subdivisions are for use with categories E840-E845 to identify the injured person. Valid fourth digits are in [brackets] under codes E842-E845:

.0 Occupant of spacecraft
.1 Occupant of military aircraft, any
   Crew in military aircraft [air force] [army] [national guard] [navy]
   Passenger (civilian) (military) in military aircraft [air force] [army] [national guard] [navy]
   Troops in military aircraft [air force] [army] [national guard] [navy]
   EXCLUDES occupants of aircraft operated under jurisdiction of police departments (.5)
   parachutist (.7)
.2 Crew of commercial aircraft (powered) in surface to surface transport
.3 Other occupant of commercial aircraft (powered) in surface to surface transport
   Flight personnel:
      not part of crew
      on familiarization flight
   Passenger on aircraft (powered) NOS
.4 Occupant of commercial aircraft (powered) in surface to air transport
   Occupant [crew] [passenger] of aircraft (powered) engaged in activities, such as:
      aerial spraying (crops) (fire retardants)
      air drops of emergency supplies
      air drops of parachutists, except from military craft
      crop dusting
      lowering of construction material [bridge or telephone pole]
      sky writing
.5 Occupant of other powered aircraft
   Occupant [crew] [passenger] of aircraft (powered) engaged in activities, such as:
      aerobatic flying
      aircraft racing
      rescue operation
      storm surveillance
      traffic surveillance
   Occupant of private plane NOS
.6 Occupant of unpowered aircraft, except parachutist
   Occupant of aircraft classifiable to E842
.7 Parachutist (military) (other)
   Person making voluntary descent
   EXCLUDES person making descent after accident to aircraft (.1-.6)
.8 Ground crew, airline employee
   Persons employed at airfields (civil) (military) or launching pads, not occupants of aircraft
.9 Other person

§ ☑4ᵗʰ **E840 Accident to powered aircraft at takeoff or landing**
   INCLUDES collision of aircraft with any object, fixed, movable, or moving
      crash
      explosion on aircraft   while taking off or landing
      fire on aircraft
      forced landing

§ ☑4ᵗʰ **E841 Accident to powered aircraft, other and unspecified**
   INCLUDES aircraft accident NOS
      aircraft crash or wreck NOS
      any accident to powered aircraft while in transit or when not specified whether in transit, taking off, or landing
      collision of aircraft with another aircraft, bird, or any object, while in transit
      explosion on aircraft while in transit
      fire on aircraft while in transit

§ ☑4ᵗʰ **E842 Accident to unpowered aircraft**
   [6-9] **INCLUDES** any accident, except collision with powered aircraft, to:
      balloon
      glider
      hang glider
      kite carrying a person
      hit by object falling from unpowered aircraft

§ ☑4ᵗʰ **E843 Fall in, on, or from aircraft**
   [0-9] **INCLUDES** accident in boarding or alighting from aircraft, any kind
      fall in, on, or from aircraft [any kind], while in transit, taking off, or landing, except when as a result of an accident to aircraft

§ ☑4ᵗʰ **E844 Other specified air transport accidents**
   [0-9] **INCLUDES** hit by:
      aircraft
      object falling from aircraft
   injury by or from:
      machinery of aircraft
      rotating propeller   without accident to aircraft
      voluntary parachute descent
   poisoning by carbon monoxide from aircraft while in transit
   sucked into jet
   any accident involving other transport vehicle (motor) (nonmotor) due to being hit by object set in motion by aircraft (powered)
   EXCLUDES air sickness (E903)
      effects of:
         high altitude (E902.0-E902.1)
         pressure change (E902.0-E902.1)
      injury in parachute descent due to accident to aircraft (E840.0-E842-9)

§ ☑4ᵗʰ **E845 Accident involving spacecraft**
   [0,8,9] **INCLUDES** launching pad accident
      EXCLUDES effects of weightlessness in spacecraft (E928.0)

Vehicle Accidents Not Elsewhere Classifiable (E846-E848)

E846 Accidents involving powered vehicles used solely within the buildings and premises of industrial or commercial establishment
   Accident to, on, or involving:
      battery powered airport passenger vehicle
      battery powered trucks (baggage) (mail)
      coal car in mine
      logging car
      self propelled truck, industrial
      station baggage truck (powered)
      tram, truck, or tub (powered) in mine or quarry
   Collision with:
      pedestrian
      other vehicle or object within premises
   Explosion of
   Fall from   powered vehicle, industrial or
   Overturning of   commercial
   Struck by
   EXCLUDES accidental poisoning by exhaust gas from vehicle not elsewhere classifiable (E868.2)
      injury by crane, lift (fork), or elevator (E919.2)

E847 Accidents involving cable cars not running on rails
   Accident to, on, or involving:
      cable car, not on rails
      ski chair-lift
      ski-lift with gondola
      téléférique
   Breakage of cable
   Caught or dragged by
   Fall or jump from   cable car, not on rails
   Object thrown from or in

E848 Accidents involving other vehicles, not elsewhere classifiable
   Accident to, on, or involving:
      ice yacht
      land yacht
      nonmotor, nonroad vehicle NOS

---

§ Requires fourth digit. See beginning of appropriate section for codes and definitions.

Place of Occurrence (E849)

✓4ᵗʰ **E849　Place of Occurrence**

NOTE The following category is for use to denote the place where the injury or poisoning occurred.

E849.0　Home
　　Apartment
　　Boarding house
　　Farm house
　　Home premises
　　House (residential)
　　Noninstitutional place of residence
　　Private:
　　　driveway
　　　garage
　　　garden
　　　home
　　　walk
　　Swimming pool in private house or garden
　　Yard of home
　　EXCLUDES home under construction but not yet occupied
　　　　　　(E849.3)
　　　　　　institutional place of residence (E849.7)

E849.1　Farm
　　Farm:
　　　buildings
　　　land under cultivation
　　EXCLUDES farm house and home premises of farm (E849.0)

E849.2　Mine and quarry
　　Gravel pit
　　Sand pit
　　Tunnel under construction

E849.3　Industrial place and premises
　　Building under construction
　　Dockyard
　　Dry dock
　　Factory
　　　building
　　　premises
　　Garage (place of work)
　　Industrial yard
　　Loading platform (factory) (store)
　　Plant, industrial
　　Railway yard
　　Shop (place of work)
　　Warehouse
　　Workhouse

E849.4　Place for recreation and sport
　　Amusement park　　　Playground, including school
　　Baseball field　　　　　　playground
　　Basketball court　　　Public park
　　Beach resort　　　　　Racecourse
　　Cricket ground　　　　Resort NOS
　　Fives court　　　　　　Riding school
　　Football field　　　　Rifle range
　　Golf course　　　　　Seashore resort
　　Gymnasium　　　　　Skating rink
　　Hockey field　　　　　Sports palace
　　Holiday camp　　　　Stadium
　　Ice palace　　　　　　Swimming pool, public
　　Lake resort　　　　　Tennis court
　　Mountain resort　　　Vacation resort
　　EXCLUDES that in private house or garden (E849.0)

E849.5　Street and highway

E849.6　Public building
　　Building (including adjacent grounds) used by the general
　　　　public or by a particular group of the public, such as:
　　airport
　　bank
　　café
　　casino
　　church
　　cinema
　　clubhouse
　　courthouse
　　dance hall
　　garage building (for car storage)
　　hotel
　　market (grocery or other commodity)
　　movie house
　　music hall
　　nightclub
　　office
　　office building
　　opera house
　　post office
　　public hall
　　radio broadcasting station
　　restaurant
　　school (state) (public) (private)
　　shop, commercial
　　station (bus) (railway)
　　store
　　theater
　　EXCLUDES home garage (E849.0)
　　　　　　industrial building or workplace (E849.3)

E849.7　Residential institution
　　Children's home
　　Dormitory
　　Hospital
　　Jail
　　Old people's home
　　Orphanage
　　Prison
　　Reform school

E849.8　Other specified places
　　Beach NOS　　　　　　Pond or pool (natural)
　　Canal　　　　　　　　Prairie
　　Caravan site NOS　　Public place NOS
　　Derelict house　　　Railway line
　　Desert　　　　　　　Reservoir
　　Dock　　　　　　　　River
　　Forest　　　　　　　Sea
　　Harbor　　　　　　　Seashore NOS
　　Hill　　　　　　　　Stream
　　Lake NOS　　　　　　Swamp
　　Mountain　　　　　Trailer court
　　Parking lot　　　　Woods
　　Parking place

E849.9　Unspecified place

Accidental Poisoning by Drugs, Medicinal Substances, and Biologicals (E850-E858)

INCLUDES accidental overdose of drug, wrong drug given or taken in error, and drug taken inadvertently
accidents in the use of drugs and biologicals in medical and surgical procedures

EXCLUDES *administration with suicidal or homicidal intent or intent to harm, or in circumstances classifiable to E980-E989 (E950.0-E950.5, E962.0, E980.0-E980.5)*
correct drug properly administered in therapeutic or prophylactic dosage, as the cause of adverse effect (E930.0-E949.9)

NOTE See Alphabetic Index for more complete list of specific drugs to be classified under the fourth digit subdivisions. The American Hospital Formulary numbers can be used to classify new drugs listed by the American Hospital Formulary Service (AHFS). See Appendix C.

√4th E850 Accidental poisoning by analgesics, antipyretics, and antirheumatics

E850.0 Heroin
Diacetylmorphine

E850.1 Methadone

E850.2 Other opiates and related narcotics
Codeine [methylmorphine]
Meperidine [pethidine]
Morphine
Opium (alkaloids)

E850.3 Salicylates
Acetylsalicylic acid [aspirin]
Amino derivatives of salicylic acid
Salicylic acid salts

E850.4 Aromatic analgesics, not elsewhere classified
Acetanilid
Paracetamol [acetaminophen]
Phenacetin [acetophenetidin]

E850.5 Pyrazole derivatives
Aminophenazone [amidopyrine]
Phenylbutazone

E850.6 Antirheumatics [antiphlogistics]
Gold salts
Indomethacin
EXCLUDES *salicylates (E850.3)*
steroids (E858.0)

E850.7 Other non-narcotic analgesics
Pyrabital

E850.8 Other specified analgesics and antipyretics
Pentazocine

E850.9 Unspecified analgesic or antipyretic

E851 Accidental poisoning by barbiturates
Amobarbital [amylobarbitone]
Barbital [barbitone]
Butabarbital [butabarbitone]
Pentobarbital [pentobarbitone]
Phenobarbital [phenobarbitone]
Secobarbital [quinalbarbitone]
EXCLUDES *thiobarbiturates (E855.1)*

√4th E852 Accidental poisoning by other sedatives and hypnotics

E852.0 Chloral hydrate group

E852.1 Paraldehyde

E852.2 Bromine compounds
Bromides
Carbromal (derivatives)

E852.3 Methaqualone compounds

E852.4 Glutethimide group

E852.5 Mixed sedatives, not elsewhere classified

E852.8 Other specified sedatives and hypnotics

E852.9 Unspecified sedative or hypnotic
Sleeping:
drug
pill } NOS
tablet

√4th E853 Accidental poisoning by tranquilizers

E853.0 Phenothiazine-based tranquilizers
Chlorpromazine   Prochlorperazine
Fluphenazine   Promazine

E853.1 Butyrophenone-based tranquilizers
Haloperidol   Trifluperidol
Spiperone

E853.2 Benzodiazepine-based tranquilizers
Chlordiazepoxide   Lorazepam
Diazepam   Medazepam
Flurazepam   Nitrazepam

E853.8 Other specified tranquilizers
Hydroxyzine   Meprobamate

E853.9 Unspecified tranquilizer

√4th E854 Accidental poisoning by other psychotropic agents

E854.0 Antidepressants
Amitriptyline
Imipramine
Monoamine oxidase [MAO] inhibitors

E854.1 Psychodysleptics [hallucinogens]
Cannabis derivatives   Mescaline
Lysergide [LSD]   Psilocin
Marihuana (derivatives)   Psilocybin

E854.2 Psychostimulants
Amphetamine
Caffeine
EXCLUDES *central appetite depressants (E858.8)*

E854.3 Central nervous system stimulants
Analeptics
Opiate antagonists

E854.8 Other psychotropic agents

√4th E855 Accidental poisoning by other drugs acting on central and autonomic nervous system

E855.0 Anticonvulsant and anti-Parkinsonism drugs
Amantadine
Hydantoin derivatives
Levodopa [L-dopa]
Oxazolidine derivatives [paramethadione] [trimethadione]
Succinimides

E855.1 Other central nervous system depressants
Ether
Gaseous anesthetics
Halogenated hydrocarbon derivatives
Intravenous anesthetics
Thiobarbiturates, such as thiopental sodium

E855.2 Local anesthetics
Cocaine   Procaine
Lidocaine [lignocaine]   Tetracaine

E855.3 Parasympathomimetics [cholinergics]
Acetylcholine   Anticholinesterase:
Anticholinesterase: reversible
  organophosphorus   Pilocarpine

E855.4 Parasympatholytics [anticholinergics and antimuscarinics] and spasmolytics
Atropine   Hyoscine [scopolamine]
Homatropine   Quaternary ammonium derivatives

E855.5 Sympathomimetics [adrenergics]
Epinephrine [adrenalin]
Levarterenol [noradrenalin]

E855.6 Sympatholytics [antiadrenergics]
Phenoxybenzamine
Tolazoline hydrochloride

E855.8 Other specified drugs acting on central and autonomic nervous systems

E855.9 Unspecified drug acting on central and autonomic nervous systems

E856 Accidental poisoning by antibiotics

E857 Accidental poisoning by other anti-infectives

✔4ᵗʰ **E858 Accidental poisoning by other drugs**

E858.0 Hormones and synthetic substitutes

E858.1 Primarily systemic agents

E858.2 Agents primarily affecting blood constituents

E858.3 Agents primarily affecting cardiovascular system

E858.4 Agents primarily affecting gastrointestinal system

E858.5 Water, mineral, and uric acid metabolism drugs

E858.6 Agents primarily acting on the smooth and skeletal muscles and respiratory system

E858.7 Agents primarily affecting skin and mucous membrane, ophthalmological, otorhinolaryngological, and dental drugs

E858.8 Other specified drugs
Central appetite depressants

E858.9 Unspecified drug

Accidental Poisoning by Other Solid and Liquid Substances, Gases, and Vapors (E860–E869)

NOTE Categories in this section are intended primarily to indicate the external cause of poisoning states classifiable to 980-989. They may also be used to indicate external causes of localized effects classifiable to 001-799.

✔4ᵗʰ **E860 Accidental poisoning by alcohol, not elsewhere classified**

E860.0 Alcoholic beverages
Alcohol in preparations intended for consumption

E860.1 Other and unspecified ethyl alcohol and its products
Denatured alcohol   Grain alcohol NOS
Ethanol NOS   Methylated spirit

E860.2 Methyl alcohol
Methanol   Wood alcohol

E860.3 Isopropyl alcohol
Dimethyl carbinol   Rubbing alcohol subsitute
Isopropanol   Secondary propyl alcohol

E860.4 Fusel oil
Alcohol: Alcohol:
  amyl   propyl
  butyl

E860.8 Other specified alcohols

E860.9 Unspecified alcohol

✔4ᵗʰ **E861 Accidental poisoning by cleansing and polishing agents, disinfectants, paints, and varnishes**

E861.0 Synthetic detergents and shampoos

E861.1 Soap products

E861.2 Polishes

E861.3 Other cleansing and polishing agents
Scouring powders

E861.4 Disinfectants
Household and other disinfectants not ordinarily used on the person
EXCLUDES *carbolic acid or phenol (E864.0)*

E861.5 Lead paints

E861.6 Other paints and varnishes
Lacquers   Paints, other than lead
Oil colors   White washes

E861.9 Unspecified

✔4ᵗʰ **E862 Accidental poisoning by petroleum products, other solvents and their vapors, not elsewhere classified**

E862.0 Petroleum solvents
Petroleum: Petroleum:
  ether   naphtha
  benzine

E862.1 Petroleum fuels and cleaners
Antiknock additives to petroleum fuels
Gas oils
Gasoline or petrol
Kerosene
EXCLUDES *kerosene insecticides (E863.4)*

E862.2 Lubricating oils

E862.3 Petroleum solids
Paraffin wax

E862.4 Other specified solvents
Benzene

E862.9 Unspecified solvent

✔4ᵗʰ **E863 Accidental poisoning by agricultural and horticultural chemical and pharmaceutical preparations other than plant foods and fertilizers**
EXCLUDES *plant foods and fertilizers (E866.5)*

E863.0 Insecticides of organochlorine compounds
Benzene hexachloride   Dieldrin
Chlordane   Endrine
DDT   Toxaphene

E863.1 Insecticides of organophosphorus compounds
Demeton   Parathion
Diazinon   Phenylsulphthion
Dichlorvos   Phorate
Malathion   Phosdrin
Methyl parathion

E863.2 Carbamates
Aldicarb   Propoxur
Carbaryl

E863.3 Mixtures of insecticides

E863.4 Other and unspecified insecticides
Kerosene insecticides

E863.5 Herbicides
2, 4-Dichlorophenoxyacetic acid [2, 4-D]
2, 4, 5-Trichlorophenoxyacetic acid [2, 4, 5-T]
Chlorates
Diquat
Mixtures of plant foods and fertilizers with herbicides
Paraquat

E863.6 Fungicides
Organic mercurials (used in seed dressing)
Pentachlorophenols

E863.7 Rodenticides
Fluoroacetates   Warfarin
Squill and derivatives   Zinc phosphide
Thallium

E863.8 Fumigants
Cyanides   Phosphine
Methyl bromide

E863.9 Other and unspecified

✔4ᵗʰ **E864 Accidental poisoning by corrosives and caustics, not elsewhere classified**
EXCLUDES *those as components of disinfectants (E861.4)*

E864.0 Corrosive aromatics
Carbolic acid or phenol

E864.1 Acids
Acid:
  hydrochloric
  nitric
  sulfuric

E864.2 Caustic alkalis
Lye

E864.3 Other specified corrosives and caustics

E864.4 Unspecified corrosives and caustics

☑4ᵗʰ **E865 Accidental poisoning from poisonous foodstuffs and poisonous plants**

> **INCLUDES** any meat, fish, or shellfish
> plants, berries, and fungi eaten as, or in mistake for, food, or by a child

> **EXCLUDES** *anaphylactic shock due to adverse food reaction (995.60-995.69)*
> *food poisoning (bacterial) (005.0-005.9)*
> *poisoning and toxic reactions to venomous plants (E905.6-E905.7)*

E865.0 Meat

E865.1 Shellfish

E865.2 Other fish

E865.3 Berries and seeds

E865.4 Other specified plants

E865.5 Mushrooms and other fungi

E865.8 Other specified foods

E865.9 Unspecified foodstuff or poisonous plant

☑4ᵗʰ **E866 Accidental poisoning by other and unspecified solid and liquid substances**

> **EXCLUDES** *these substances as a component of:*
> *medicines (E850.0-E858.9)*
> *paints (E861.5-E861.6)*
> *pesticides (E863.0-E863.9)*
> *petroleum fuels (E862.1)*

E866.0 Lead and its compounds and fumes

E866.1 Mercury and its compounds and fumes

E866.2 Antimony and its compounds and fumes

E866.3 Arsenic and its compounds and fumes

E866.4 Other metals and their compounds and fumes
> Beryllium (compounds)
> Brass fumes
> Cadmium (compounds)
> Copper salts
> Iron (compounds)
> Manganese (compounds)
> Nickel (compounds)
> Thallium (compounds)

E866.5 Plant foods and fertilizers
> **EXCLUDES** *mixtures with herbicides (E863.5)*

E866.6 Glues and adhesives

E866.7 Cosmetics

E866.8 Other specified solid or liquid substances

E866.9 Unspecified solid or liquid substance

E867 Accidental poisoning by gas distributed by pipeline
> Carbon monoxide from incomplete combustion of piped gas
> Coal gas NOS
> Liquefied petroleum gas distributed through pipes (pure or mixed with air)
> Piped gas (natural) (manufactured)

☑4ᵗʰ **E868 Accidental poisoning by other utility gas and other carbon monoxide**

E868.0 Liquefied petroleum gas distributed in mobile containers
> Butane
> Liquefied hydrocarbon gas NOS
> Propane
> } or carbon monoxide from incomplete combustion of these gases

E868.1 Other and unspecified utility gas
> Acetylene
> Gas NOS used for lighting, heating, or cooking
> Water gas
> } or carbon monoxide from incomplete combustion of these gases

E868.2 Motor vehicle exhaust gas
> Exhaust gas from:
> any type of combustion engine not in watercraft
> farm tractor, not in transit
> gas engine
> motor pump
> motor vehicle, not in transit

> **EXCLUDES** *poisoning by carbon monoxide from:*
> *aircraft while in transit (E844.0-E844.9)*
> *motor vehicle while in transit (E818.0-E818.9)*
> *watercraft whether or not in transit (E838.0-E838.9)*

E868.3 Carbon monoxide from incomplete combustion of other domestic fuels
> Carbon monoxide from incomplete combustion of:
> coal
> coke
> kerosene
> wood
> } in domestic stove or fireplace

> **EXCLUDES** *carbon monoxide from smoke and fumes due to conflagration (E890.0-E893.9)*

E868.8 Carbon monoxide from other sources
> Carbon monoxide from:
> blast furnace gas
> incomplete combustion of fuels in industrial use
> kiln vapor

E868.9 Unspecified carbon monoxide

☑4ᵗʰ **E869 Accidental poisoning by other gases and vapors**

> **EXCLUDES** *effects of gases used as anesthetics (E855.1, E938.2)*
> *fumes from heavy metals (E866.0-E866.4)*
> *smoke and fumes due to conflagration or explosion (E890.0-E899)*

E869.0 Nitrogen oxides

E869.1 Sulfur dioxide

E869.2 Freon

E869.3 Lacrimogenic gas [tear gas]
> Bromobenzyl cyanide
> Chloroacetophenone
> Ethyliodoacetate

E869.4 Second-hand tobacco smoke

E869.8 Other specified gases and vapors
> Chlorine
> Hydrocyanic acid gas

E869.9 Unspecified gases and vapors

Misadventures to Patients During Surgical and Medical Care (E870-E876)

> **EXCLUDES** *accidental overdose of drug and wrong drug given in error (E850.0-E858.9)*
> *surgical and medical procedures as the cause of abnormal reaction by the patient, without mention of misadventure at the time of procedure (E878.0-E879.9)*

☑4ᵗʰ **E870 Accidental cut, puncture, perforation, or hemorrhage during medical care**

E870.0 Surgical operation

E870.1 Infusion or transfusion

E870.2 Kidney dialysis or other perfusion

E870.3 Injection or vaccination

E870.4 Endoscopic examination

E870.5 Aspiration of fluid or tissue, puncture, and catheterization
> Abdominal paracentesis
> Aspirating needle biopsy
> Blood sampling
> Lumbar puncture
> Thoracentesis
> **EXCLUDES** *heart catheterization (E870.6)*

E870.6 Heart catheterization

E870.7 Administration of enema

☑4ᵗʰ Fourth-digit Required   ▶◀ Revised Text   ● New Code   ▲ Revised Code TitleDx

E Codes

E870.8–E876.9

E870.8 **Other specified medical care**

E870.9 **Unspecified medical care**

☑4ᵗʰ **E871 Foreign object left in body during procedure**

E871.0 **Surgical operation**

E871.1 **Infusion or transfusion**

E871.2 **Kidney dialysis or other perfusion**

E871.3 **Injection or vaccination**

E871.4 **Endoscopic examination**

E871.5 **Aspiration of fluid or tissue, puncture, and catheterization**
Abdominal paracentesis
Aspiration needle biopsy
Blood sampling
Lumbar puncture
Thoracentesis
EXCLUDES *heart catheterization (E871.6)*

E871.6 **Heart catheterization**

E871.7 **Removal of catheter or packing**

E871.8 **Other specified procedures**

E871.9 **Unspecified procedure**

☑4ᵗʰ **E872 Failure of sterile precautions during procedure**

E872.0 **Surgical operation**

E872.1 **Infusion or transfusion**

E872.2 **Kidney dialysis and other perfusion**

E872.3 **Injection or vaccination**

E872.4 **Endoscopic examination**

E872.5 **Aspiration of fluid or tissue, puncture, and catheterization**
Abdominal paracentesis
Aspiration needle biopsy
Blood sampling
Lumbar puncture
Thoracentesis
EXCLUDES *heart catheterization (E872.6)*

E872.6 **Heart catheterization**

E872.8 **Other specified procedures**

E872.9 **Unspecified procedure**

☑4ᵗʰ **E873 Failure in dosage**
EXCLUDES *accidental overdose of drug, medicinal or biological substance (E850.0-E858.9)*

E873.0 **Excessive amount of blood or other fluid during transfusion or infusion**

E873.1 **Incorrect dilution of fluid during infusion**

E873.2 **Overdose of radiation in therapy**

E873.3 **Inadvertent exposure of patient to radiation during medical care**

E873.4 **Failure in dosage in electroshock or insulin-shock therapy**

E873.5 **Inappropriate [too hot or too cold] temperature in local application and packing**

E873.6 **Nonadministration of necessary drug or medicinal substance**

E873.8 **Other specified failure in dosage**

E873.9 **Unspecified failure in dosage**

☑4ᵗʰ **E874 Mechanical failure of instrument or apparatus during procedure**

E874.0 **Surgical operation**

E874.1 **Infusion and transfusion**
Air in system

E874.2 **Kidney dialysis and other perfusion**

E874.3 **Endoscopic examination**

E874.4 **Aspiration of fluid or tissue, puncture, and catheterization**
Abdominal paracentesis   Lumbar puncture
Aspiration needle biopsy   Thoracentesis
Blood sampling
EXCLUDES *heart catheterization (E874.5)*

E874.5 **Heart catheterization**

E874.8 **Other specified procedures**

E874.9 **Unspecified procedure**

☑4ᵗʰ **E875 Contaminated or infected blood, other fluid, drug, or biological substance**
INCLUDES presence of:
bacterial pyrogens
endotoxin-producing bacteria
serum hepatitis-producing agent

E875.0 **Contaminated substance transfused or infused**

E875.1 **Contaminated substance injected or used for vaccination**

E875.2 **Contaminated drug or biological substance administered by other means**

E875.8 **Other**

E875.9 **Unspecified**

☑4ᵗʰ **E876 Other and unspecified misadventures during medical care**

E876.0 **Mismatched blood in transfusion**

E876.1 **Wrong fluid in infusion**

E876.2 **Failure in suture and ligature during surgical operation**

E876.3 **Endotracheal tube wrongly placed during anesthetic procedure**

E876.4 **Failure to introduce or to remove other tube or instrument**
EXCLUDES *foreign object left in body during procedure (E871.0-E871.9)*

* E876.5 **Performance of wrong operation (procedure) on correct patient**
Wrong device implanted into correct surgical site
EXCLUDES *correct operation (procedure) performed on wrong body part (E876.7)*

* E876.6 **Performance of operation (procedure) on patient not scheduled for surgery**
Performance of operation (procedure) intended for another patient
Performance of operation (procedure) on wrong patient

* E876.7 **Performance of correct operation (procedure) on wrong side/body part**
Performance of correct operation (procedure) on wrong side
Performance of correct operation (procedure) on wrong site

E876.8 **Other specified misadventures during medical care**
Performance of inappropriate treatment NEC

E876.9 **Unspecified misadventure during medical care**

---

* Wrong surgery edit applies.

Surgical and Medical Procedures as the Cause of Abnormal Reaction of Patient or Later Complication, Without Mention of Misadventure at the Time of Procedure (E878-E879)

INCLUDES   procedures as the cause of abnormal reaction, such as:
- displacement or malfunction of prosthetic device
- hepatorenal failure, postoperative
- malfunction of external stoma
- postoperative intestinal obstruction
- rejection of transplanted organ

EXCLUDES   anesthetic management properly carried out as the cause of adverse effect (E937.0-E938.9)
infusion and transfusion, without mention of misadventure in the technique of procedure (E930.0-E949.9)

✓4ᵗʰ **E878 Surgical operation and other surgical procedures as the cause of abnormal reaction of patient, or of later complication, without mention of misadventure at the time of operation**

    E878.0 Surgical operation with transplant of whole organ
        Transplantation of:
          heart
          kidney
          liver

    E878.1 Surgical operation with implant of artificial internal device
        Cardiac pacemaker
        Electrodes implanted in brain
        Heart valve prosthesis
        Internal orthopedic device

    E878.2 Surgical operation with anastomosis, bypass, or graft, with natural or artificial tissues used as implant
        Anastomosis:
          arteriovenous
          gastrojejunal
        Graft of blood vessel, tendon, or skin
        EXCLUDES   external stoma (E878.3)

    E878.3 Surgical operation with formation of external stoma
        Colostomy   Gastrostomy
        Cystostomy   Ureterostomy
        Duodenostomy

    E878.4 Other restorative surgery

    E878.5 Amputation of limb(s)

    E878.6 Removal of other organ (partial) (total)

    E878.8 Other specified surgical operations and procedures

    E878.9 Unspecified surgical operations and procedures

✓4ᵗʰ **E879 Other procedures, without mention of misadventure at the time of procedure, as the cause of abnormal reaction of patient, or of later complication**

    E879.0 Cardiac catheterization

    E879.1 Kidney dialysis

    E879.2 Radiological procedure and radiotherapy
        EXCLUDES   radio-opaque dyes for diagnostic x-ray procedures (E947.8)

    E879.3 Shock therapy
        Electroshock therapy
        Insulin-shock therapy

    E879.4 Aspiration of fluid
        Lumbar puncture
        Thoracentesis

    E879.5 Insertion of gastric or duodenal sound

    E879.6 Urinary catheterization

    E879.7 Blood sampling

    E879.8 Other specified procedures
        Blood transfusion

    E879.9 Unspecified procedure

Accidental Falls (E880-E888)

EXCLUDES   falls (in or from):
    burning building (E890.8, E891.8)
    into fire (E890.0-E899)
    into water (with submersion or drowning) (E910.0-E910.9)
    machinery (in operation) (E919.0-E919.9)
    on edged, pointed, or sharp object (E920.0-E920.9)
    transport vehicle (E800.0-E845.9)
    vehicle not elsewhere classifiable (E846-E848)

✓4ᵗʰ **E880 Fall on or from stairs or steps**

    E880.0 Escalator

    E880.1 Fall on or from sidewalk curb
        EXCLUDES   fall from moving sidewalk (E885.9)

    E880.9 Other stairs or steps

✓4ᵗʰ **E881 Fall on or from ladders or scaffolding**

    E881.0 Fall from ladder

    E881.1 Fall from scaffolding

E882 Fall from or out of building or other structure
    Fall from: Fall from:
      balcony   turret
      bridge   viaduct
      building   wall
      flagpole   window
      tower   Fall through roof
    EXCLUDES   collapse of a building or structure (E916)
                   fall or jump from burning building (E890.8, E891.8)

✓4ᵗʰ **E883 Fall into hole or other opening in surface**
    INCLUDES   fall into: fall into:
          cavity   shaft
          dock   swimming pool
          hole   tank
          pit   well
          quarry
    EXCLUDES   fall into water NOS (E910.9)
                   that resulting in drowning or submersion without mention of injury (E910.0-E910.9)

    E883.0 Accident from diving or jumping into water [swimming pool]
        Strike or hit:
          against bottom when jumping or diving into water
          wall or board of swimming pool
          water surface
        EXCLUDES   diving with insufficient air supply (E913.2)
                   effects of air pressure from diving (E902.2)

    E883.1 Accidental fall into well

    E883.2 Accidental fall into storm drain or manhole

    E883.9 Fall into other hole or other opening in surface

✓4ᵗʰ **E884 Other fall from one level to another**

    E884.0 Fall from playground equipment
        EXCLUDES   recreational machinery (E919.8)

    E884.1 Fall from cliff

    E884.2 Fall from chair

    E884.3 Fall from wheelchair
        Fall from motorized mobility scooter
        Fall from motorized wheelchair

    E884.4 Fall from bed

    E884.5 Fall from other furniture

    E884.6 Fall from commode
        Toilet

    E884.9 Other fall from one level to another
        Fall from: Fall from:
          embankment   stationary vehicle
          haystack   tree

✓4ᵗʰ **E885 Fall on same level from slipping, tripping, or stumbling**

    E885.0 Fall from (nonmotorized) scooter
        EXCLUDES   fall from motorized mobility scooter (E884.3)

E Codes

E885.1–E893.2

E885.1 Fall from roller skates
Heelies
In-line skates
Wheelies

E885.2 Fall from skateboard

E885.3 Fall from skis

E885.4 Fall from snowboard

E885.9 Fall from other slipping, tripping, or stumbling
Fall on moving sidewalk

☑4ᵗʰ E886 Fall on same level from collision, pushing, or shoving, by or with other person
> **EXCLUDES** *crushed or pushed by a crowd or human stampede (E917.1, E917.6)*

E886.0 In sports
Tackles in sports
> **EXCLUDES** *kicked, stepped on, struck by object, in sports (E917.0, E917.5)*

E886.9 Other and unspecified
Fall from collision of pedestrian (conveyance) with another pedestrian (conveyance)

E887 Fracture, cause unspecified

☑4ᵗʰ E888 Other and unspecified fall
Accidental fall NOS
Fall on same level NOS

E888.0 Fall resulting in striking against sharp object
Use additional external cause code to identify object (E920)

E888.1 Fall resulting in striking against other object

E888.8 Other fall

E888.9 Unspecified fall
Fall NOS

Accidents Caused by Fire and Flames (E890-E899)
> **INCLUDES** asphyxia or poisoning due to conflagration or ignition
> burning by fire
> secondary fires resulting from explosion
> **EXCLUDES** *arson (E968.0)*
> *fire in or on:*
> *machinery (in operation) (E919.0-E919.9)*
> *transport vehicle other than stationary vehicle (E800.0-E845.9)*
> *vehicle not elsewhere classifiable (E846-E848)*

☑4ᵗʰ E890 Conflagration in private dwelling
> **INCLUDES** conflagration in:
> apartment
> boarding house
> camping place
> caravan
> farmhouse
> house
> lodging house
> mobile home
> private garage
> rooming house
> tenement
> conflagration originating from sources classifiable to E893-E898 in the above buildings

E890.0 Explosion caused by conflagration

E890.1 Fumes from combustion of polyvinylchloride [PVC] and similar material in conflagration

E890.2 Other smoke and fumes from conflagration
Carbon monoxide ⎫
Fumes NOS   ⎬ from conflagration in private building
Smoke NOS   ⎭

E890.3 Burning caused by conflagration

E890.8 Other accident resulting from conflagration
Collapse of   ⎫
Fall from   ⎬ burning private
Hit by object falling from   building
Jump from   ⎭

E890.9 Unspecified accident resulting from conflagration in private dwelling

☑4ᵗʰ E891 Conflagration in other and unspecified building or structure
Conflagration in:
barn
church
convalescent and other residential home
dormitory of educational institution
factory
farm outbuildings
hospital
hotel
school
store
theater
Conflagration originating from sources classifiable to E893-E898, in the above buildings

E891.0 Explosion caused by conflagration

E891.1 Fumes from combustion of polyvinylchloride [PVC] and similar material in conflagration

E891.2 Other smoke and fumes from conflagration
Carbon monoxide ⎫
Fumes NOS   ⎬ from conflagration in private building or structure
Smoke NOS   ⎭

E891.3 Burning caused by conflagration

E891.8 Other accident resulting from conflagration
Collapse of   ⎫
Fall from   ⎬ burning private building or structure
Hit by object falling from
Jump from   ⎭

E891.9 Unspecified accident resulting from conflagration of other and unspecified building or structure

E892 Conflagration not in building or structure
Fire (uncontrolled) (in) (of):
forest
grass
hay
lumber
mine
prairie
transport vehicle [any], except while in transit
tunnel

☑4ᵗʰ E893 Accident caused by ignition of clothing
> **EXCLUDES** *ignition of clothing:*
> *from highly inflammable material (E894)*
> *with conflagration (E890.0-E892)*

E893.0 From controlled fire in private dwelling
Ignition of clothing from:
normal fire (charcoal) (coal) ⎫
(electric) (gas) (wood) in: ⎬ in private dwelling (as listed in E890)
brazier
fireplace
furnace
stove   ⎭

E893.1 From controlled fire in other building or structure
Ignition of clothing from:
normal fire (charcoal) (coal) ⎫
(electric) (gas) (wood) in: ⎬ in other building or structure (as listed in E891)
brazier
fireplace
furnace
stove   ⎭

E893.2 From controlled fire not in building or structure
Ignition of clothing from:
bonfire (controlled)
brazier fire (controlled), not in building or structure
trash fire (controlled)
> **EXCLUDES** *conflagration not in building (E892)*
> *trash fire out of control (E892)*

☑4ᵗʰ Fourth-digit Required   ►◄ Revised Text   ● New Code   ▲ Revised Code TitleDx

E893.8 From other specified sources

Ignition of clothing from: Ignition of clothing from:
- blowlamp
- blowtorch
- burning bedspread
- candle
- cigar

- cigarette
- lighter
- matches
- pipe
- welding torch

E893.9 Unspecified source

Ignition of clothing (from controlled fire NOS) (in building NOS) NOS

E894 Ignition of highly inflammable material

Ignition of:
- benzine
- gasoline
- fat
- kerosene
- paraffin
- petrol

} (with ignition of clothing)

EXCLUDES ignition of highly inflammable material with:
conflagration (E890.0-E892)
explosion (E923.0-E923.9)

E895 Accident caused by controlled fire in private dwelling

Burning by (flame of) normal fire (charcoal) (coal) (electric) (gas) (wood) in:
- brazier
- fireplace
- furnace
- stove

} in private dwelling (as listed in E890)

EXCLUDES burning by hot objects not producing fire or flames (E924.0-E924.9)
ignition of clothing from these sources (E893.0)
poisoning by carbon monoxide from incomplete combustion of fuel (E867-E868.9)
that with conflagration (E890.0-E890.9)

E896 Accident caused by controlled fire in other and unspecified building or structure

Burning by (flame of) normal fire (charcoal) (coal)(electric)(gas)(wood) in:
- brazier
- fireplace
- furnace
- stove

} in other building or structure (as listed in E891)

EXCLUDES burning by hot objects not producing fire or flames (E924.0-E924.9)
ignition of clothing from these sources (E893.1)
poisoning by carbon monoxide from incomplete combustion of fuel (E867-E868.9)
that with conflagration (E891.0-E891.9)

E897 Accident caused by controlled fire not in building or structure

Burns from flame of:
- bonfire
- brazier fire, not in building or structure
- trash fire

} controlled

EXCLUDES ignition of clothing from these sources (E893.2)
trash fire out of control (E892)
that with conflagration (E892)

☑4ᵗʰ E898 Accident caused by other specified fire and flames

EXCLUDES conflagration (E890.0-E892)
that with ignition of:
clothing (E893.0-E893.9)
highly inflammable material (E894)

E898.0 Burning bedclothes

Bed set on fire NOS

E898.1 Other

Burning by: Burning by:
- blowlamp
- blowtorch
- candle
- cigar
- cigarette
- fire in room NOS

- lamp
- lighter
- matches
- pipe
- welding torch

E899 Accident caused by unspecified fire

Burning NOS

Accidents Due to Natural and Environmental Factors (E900-E909)

☑4ᵗʰ E900 Excessive heat

E900.0 Due to weather conditions

Excessive heat as the external cause of:
- ictus solaris
- siriasis
- sunstroke

E900.1 Of man-made origin

Heat (in):
- boiler room
- drying room
- factory
- furnace room
- generated in transport vehicle
- kitchen

E900.9 Of unspecified origin

☑4ᵗʰ E901 Excessive cold

E901.0 Due to weather conditions

Excessive cold as the cause of:
- chilblains NOS
- immersion foot

E901.1 Of man-made origin

Contact with or inhalation of:
- dry ice
- liquid air
- liquid hydrogen
- liquid nitrogen

Prolonged exposure in:
- deep freeze unit
- refrigerator

E901.8 Other specified origin

E901.9 Of unspecified origin

☑4ᵗʰ E902 High and low air pressure and changes in air pressure

E902.0 Residence or prolonged visit at high altitude

Residence or prolonged visit at high altitude as the cause of:
- Acosta syndrome
- Alpine sickness
- altitude sickness
- Andes disease
- anoxia, hypoxia
- barotitis, barodontalgia, barosinusitis, otitic barotrauma
- hypobarism, hypobaropathy
- mountain sickness
- range disease

E902.1 In aircraft

Sudden change in air pressure in aircraft during ascent or descent as the cause of:
- aeroneurosis
- aviators' disease

E902.2 Due to diving

High air pressure from rapid descent in water
Reduction in atmospheric pressure while surfacing from deep water diving

} as the cause of:
- caisson disease
- divers' disease
- divers' palsy or paralysis

E902.8 Due to other specified causes

Reduction in atmospheric pressure while surfacing from underground

E902.9 Unspecified cause

E903 Travel and motion

E Codes

E904–E909.3

☑4ᵗʰ **E904 Hunger, thirst, exposure, and neglect**

> **EXCLUDES** *any condition resulting from homicidal intent (E968.0-E968.9)*
> *hunger, thirst, and exposure resulting from accidents connected with transport (E800.0-E848)*

E904.0 Abandonment or neglect of infants and helpless persons

Exposure to weather conditions ⎫
Hunger or thirst ⎬ resulting from abandonment or neglect
Desertion of newborn
Inattention at or after birth
Lack of care (helpless person) (infant)

> **EXCLUDES** *criminal [purposeful] neglect (E968.4)*

E904.1 Lack of food

Lack of food as the cause of:
　inanition
　insufficient nourishment
　starvation

> **EXCLUDES** *hunger resulting from abandonment or neglect (E904.0)*

E904.2 Lack of water

Lack of water as the cause of:
　dehydration
　inanition

> **EXCLUDES** *dehydration due to acute fluid loss (276.51)*

E904.3 Exposure (to weather conditions), not elsewhere classifiable

Exposure NOS
Humidity
Struck by hailstones

> **EXCLUDES** *struck by lightning (E907)*

E904.9 Privation, unqualified

Destitution

☑4ᵗʰ **E905 Venomous animals and plants as the cause of poisoning and toxic reactions**

> **INCLUDES** chemical released by animal
> insects
> release of venom through fangs, hairs, spines, tentacles, and other venom apparatus

> **EXCLUDES** *eating of poisonous animals or plants (E865.0-E865.9)*

E905.0 Venomous snakes and lizards

Cobra	Mamba
Copperhead snake	Rattlesnake
Coral snake	Sea snake
Fer de lance	Snake (venomous)
Gila monster	Viper
Krait	Water moccasin

> **EXCLUDES** *bites of snakes and lizards known to be nonvenomous (E906.2)*

E905.1 Venomous spiders

Black widow spider
Brown spider
Tarantula (venomous)

E905.2 Scorpion

E905.3 Hornets, wasps, and bees

Yellow jacket

E905.4 Centipede and venomous millipede (tropical)

E905.5 Other venomous arthropods

Sting of:
　ant
　caterpillar

E905.6 Venomous marine animals and plants

Puncture by sea urchin spine
Sting of:
　coral
　jelly fish
　nematocysts
　sea anemone
　sea cucumber
　other marine animal or plant

> **EXCLUDES** *bites and other injuries caused by nonvenomous marine animal (E906.2-E906.8)*
> *bite of sea snake (venomous) (E905.0)*

E905.7 Poisoning and toxic reactions caused by other plants

Injection of poisons or toxins into or through skin by plant thorns, spines, or other mechanisms

> **EXCLUDES** *puncture wound NOS by plant thorns or spines (E920.8)*

E905.8 Other specified

E905.9 Unspecified

Sting NOS
Venomous bite NOS

☑4ᵗʰ **E906 Other injury caused by animals**

> **EXCLUDES** *poisoning and toxic reactions caused by venomous animals and insects (E905.0-E905.9)*
> *road vehicle accident involving animals (E827.0-E828.9)*
> *tripping or falling over an animal (E885.9)*

E906.0 Dog bite

E906.1 Rat bite

E906.2 Bite of nonvenomous snakes and lizards

E906.3 Bite of other animal except arthropod

Cats	Rodents, except rats
Moray eel	Shark

E906.4 Bite of nonvenomous arthropod

Insect bite NOS

E906.5 Bite by unspecified animal

Animal bite NOS

E906.8 Other specified injury caused by animal

Butted by animal
Fallen on by horse or other animal, not being ridden
Gored by animal
Implantation of quills of porcupine
Pecked by bird
Run over by animal, not being ridden
Stepped on by animal, not being ridden

> **EXCLUDES** *injury by animal being ridden (E828.0-E828.9)*

E906.9 Unspecified injury caused by animal

E907 Lightning

> **EXCLUDES** *injury from:*
> *fall of tree or other object caused by lightning (E916)*
> *fire caused by lightning (E890.0-E892)*

☑4ᵗʰ **E908 Cataclysmic storms, and floods resulting from storms**

> **EXCLUDES** *collapse of dam or man-made structure causing flood (E909.3)*

E908.0 Hurricane

Storm surge
"Tidal wave" caused by storm action
Typhoon

E908.1 Tornado

Cyclone
Twisters

E908.2 Floods

Torrential rainfall
Flash flood

> **EXCLUDES** *collapse of dam or man-made structure causing flood (E909.3)*

E908.3 Blizzard (snow)(ice)

E908.4 Dust storm

E908.8 Other cataclysmic storms

Cloudburst

E908.9 Unspecified cataclysmic storms, and floods resulting from storms

Storm NOS

☑4ᵗʰ **E909 Cataclysmic earth surface movements and eruptions**

E909.0 Earthquakes

E909.1 Volcanic eruptions

Burns from lava
Ash inhalation

E909.2 Avalanche, landslide, or mudslide

E909.3 Collapse of dam or man-made structure

☑4ᵗʰ Fourth-digit Required　　　　▶◀ Revised Text　　　　● New Code　　　　▲ Revised Code TitleDx

E909.4 Tidalwave caused by earthquake
Tidalwave NOS
Tsunami
EXCLUDES tidalwave caused by tropical storm (E908.0)

E909.8 Other cataclysmic earth surface movements and eruptions

E909.9 Unspecified cataclysmic earth surface movements and eruptions

Accidents Caused by Submersion, Suffocation, and Foreign Bodies (E910-E915)

☑4ᵗʰ E910 Accidental drowning and submersion
INCLUDES immersion
swimmers' cramp
EXCLUDES *diving accident (NOS) (resulting in injury except drowning) (E883.0)*
diving with insufficient air supply (E913.2)
drowning and submersion due to:
cataclysm (E908-E909)
machinery accident (E919.0-E919.9)
transport accident (E800.0-E845.9)
effect of high and low air pressure (E902.2)
injury from striking against objects while in running water (E917.2)

E910.0 While water-skiing
Fall from water skis with submersion or drowning
EXCLUDES *accident to water-skier involving a watercraft and resulting in submersion or other injury (E830.4, E831.4)*

E910.1 While engaged in other sport or recreational activity with diving equipment
Scuba diving NOS
Skin diving NOS
Underwater spear fishing NOS

E910.2 While engaged in other sport or recreational activity without diving equipment
Fishing or hunting, except from boat or with diving equipment
Ice skating
Playing in water
Surfboarding
Swimming NOS
Voluntarily jumping from boat, not involved in accident, for swim NOS
Wading in water
EXCLUDES *jumping into water to rescue another person (E910.3)*

E910.3 While swimming or diving for purposes other than recreation or sport
Marine salvage
Pearl diving
Placement of fishing nets
Rescue (attempt) of another person
Underwater construction or repairs
(with diving equipment)

E910.4 In bathtub

E910.8 Other accidental drowning or submersion
Drowning in:
quenching tank
swimming pool

E910.9 Unspecified accidental drowning or submersion
Accidental fall into water NOS
Drowning NOS

E911 Inhalation and ingestion of food causing obstruction of respiratory tract or suffocation
Aspiration and inhalation of food [any] (into respiratory tract) NOS
Asphyxia by
Choked on
Suffocation by
} food [including bone, seed in food, regurgitated food]
Compression of trachea
Interruption of respiration
Obstruction of respiration
} by food lodged in esophagus
Obstruction of pharynx by food (bolus)
EXCLUDES *injury, except asphyxia and obstruction of respiratory passage, caused by food (E915)*
obstruction of esophagus by food without mention of asphyxia or obstruction of respiratory passage (E915)

E912 Inhalation and ingestion of other object causing obstruction of respiratory tract or suffocation
Aspiration and inhalation of foreign body except food (into respiratory tract) NOS
Foreign object [bean] [marble] in nose
Obstruction of pharynx by foreign body
Compression
Interruption of respiration
Obstruction of respiration
} by foreign body in esophagus
EXCLUDES *injury, except asphyxia and obstruction of respiratory passage, caused by foreign body (E915)*
obstruction of esophagus by foreign body without mention of asphyxia or obstruction in respiratory passage (E915)

☑4ᵗʰ E913 Accidental mechanical suffocation
EXCLUDES *mechanical suffocation from or by:*
accidental inhalation or ingestion of:
food (E911)
foreign object (E912)
cataclysm (E908-E909)
explosion (E921.0-E921.9, E923.0-E923.9)
machinery accident (E919.0-E919.9)

E913.0 In bed or cradle
EXCLUDES *suffocation by plastic bag (E913.1)*

E913.1 By plastic bag

E913.2 Due to lack of air (in closed place)
Accidentally closed up in refrigerator or other airtight enclosed space
Diving with insufficient air supply
EXCLUDES *suffocation by plastic bag (E913.1)*

E913.3 By falling earth or other substance
Cave-in NOS
EXCLUDES *cave-in caused by cataclysmic earth surface movements and eruptions (E909)*
struck by cave-in without asphyxiation or suffocation (E916)

E913.8 Other specified means
Accidental hanging, except in bed or cradle

E913.9 Unspecified means
Asphyxia, mechanical NOS
Strangulation NOS
Suffocation NOS

E914 Foreign body accidentally entering eye and adnexa
EXCLUDES *corrosive liquid (E924.1)*

E915 Foreign body accidentally entering other orifice
EXCLUDES *aspiration and inhalation of foreign body, any, (into respiratory tract) NOS (E911-E912)*

Other Accidents (E916-E928)

E916   Struck accidentally by falling object
     Collapse of building, except on fire
     Falling:
         rock
         snowslide NOS
         stone
         tree
     Object falling from:
         machine, not in operation
         stationary vehicle
     Code first:
         collapse of building on fire (E890.0-E891.9)
         falling object in:
         cataclysm (E908-E909)
         machinery accidents (E919.0-E919.9)
         transport accidents (E800.0-E845.9)
         vehicle accidents not elsewhere classifiable (E846-E848)
         object set in motion by:
         explosion (E921.0-E921.9, E923.0-E923.9)
         firearm (E922.0-E922.9)
         projected object (E917.0-E917.9)

√4ᵗʰ E917   Striking against or struck accidentally by objects or persons
     INCLUDES   bumping into or
               against
         colliding with
         kicking against
         stepping on
         struck by

         object (moving) (projected)
            (stationary)
         pedestrian conveyance
         person

     EXCLUDES   *fall from:*
         collision with another person, except when caused by a
            crowd (E886.0-E886.9)
         stumbling over object (E885.9)
         fall resulting in striking against object (E888.0, E888.1)
         injury caused by:
         assault (E960.0-E960.1, E967.0-E967.9)
         cutting or piercing instrument (E920.0-E920.9)
         explosion (E921.0-E921.9, E923.0-E923.9)
         firearm (E922.0-E922.9)
         machinery (E919.0-E919.9)
         transport vehicle (E800.0-E845.9)
         vehicle not elsewhere classifiable (E846-E848)

E917.0   In sports without subsequent fall
     Kicked or stepped on during game (football) (rugby)
     Struck by hit or thrown ball
     Struck by hockey stick or puck

E917.1   Caused by a crowd, by collective fear or panic without subsequent fall
     Crushed
     Pushed   } by crowd or human
     Stepped on   stampede

E917.2   In running water without subsequent fall
     EXCLUDES   *drowning or submersion (E910.0-E910.9)*
             that in sports (E917.0, E917.5)

E917.3   Furniture without subsequent fall
     EXCLUDES   *fall from furniture (E884.2, E884.4-E884.5)*

E917.4   Other stationary object without subsequent fall
     Bath tub
     Fence
     Lamp-post

E917.5   Object in sports with subsequent fall
     Knocked down while boxing

E917.6   Caused by a crowd, by collective fear or panic with subsequent fall

E917.7   Furniture with subsequent fall
     EXCLUDES   *fall from furniture (E884.2, E884.4-E884.5)*

E917.8   Other stationary object with subsequent fall
     Bath tub
     Fence
     Lamp-post

E917.9   Other striking against with or without subsequent fall

E918   Caught accidentally in or between objects
     Caught, crushed, jammed, or pinched in or between moving or
         stationary objects, such as:
     escalator
     folding object
     hand tools, appliances, or implements
     sliding door and door frame
     under packing crate
     washing machine wringer
     EXCLUDES   *injury caused by:*
         cutting or piercing instrument (E920.0-E920.9)
         machinery (E919.0-E919.9)
         mechanism or component of firearm and air gun
            (E928.7)
         transport vehicle (E800.0-E845.9)
         vehicle not elsewhere classifiable (E846-E848)
         struck accidentally by:
         falling object (E916)
         object (moving) (projected) (E917.0-E917.9)

√4ᵗʰ E919   Accidents caused by machinery
     INCLUDES   burned by
         caught in (moving parts of)
         collapse of
         crushed by
         cut or pierced by
         drowning or submersion caused by
         explosion of, on, in
         fall from or into moving part of   } machinery
         fire starting in or on   (accident)
         mechanical suffocation caused by
         object falling from, on, in motion
            by
         overturning of
         pinned under
         run over by
         struck by
         thrown from

     caught between machinery and other object
     machinery accident NOS
     EXCLUDES   *accidents involving machinery, not in operation (E884.9,*
            E916-E918)
         injury caused by:
         electric current in connection with machinery
            (E925.0-E925.9)
         escalator (E880.0, E918)
         explosion of pressure vessel in connection with
            machinery (E921.0-E921.9)
         mechanism or component of firearm and air gun
            (E928.7)
         moving sidewalk (E885.9)
         powered hand tools, appliances, and implements
            (E916-E918, E920.0-E921.9, E923.0-E926.9)
         transport vehicle accidents involving machinery
            (E800.0-E848)
         poisoning by carbon monoxide generated by machine
            (E868.8)

E919.0   Agricultural machines

Animal-powered	Farm tractor
agricultural machine	Harvester
Combine	Hay mower or rake
Derrick, hay	Reaper
Farm machinery NOS	Thresher

     EXCLUDES   *that in transport under own power on the highway*
            (E810.0-E819.9)
         that being towed by another vehicle on the
            highway (E810.0-E819.9, E827.0-E827.9,
            E829.0-E829.9)
         that involved in accident classifiable to E820-E829
            (E820.0-E829.9)

E919.1   Mining and earth-drilling machinery
     Bore or drill (land) (seabed)
     Shaft hoist
     Shaft lift
     Under-cutter
     EXCLUDES   *coal car, tram, truck, and tub in mine (E846)*

E919.2 Lifting machines and appliances

Chain hoist	
Crane	
Derrick	
Elevator (building) (grain)	except in agricultural or mining operations
Forklift truck	
Lift	
Pulley block	
Winch	

EXCLUDES *that being towed by another vehicle on the highway (E810.0-E819.9, E827.0-E827.9, E829.0-829.9)*
that in transport under own power on the highway (E810.0-E819.9)
that involved in accident classifiable to E820-E829 (E820.0-E829.9)

E919.3 Metalworking machines

Abrasive wheel	Metal:
Forging machine	milling machine
Lathe	power press
Mechanical shears	rolling-mill
Metal:	sawing machine
drilling machine	

E919.4 Woodworking and forming machines

Band saw	Overhead plane
Bench saw	Powered saw
Circular saw	Radial saw
Molding machine	Sander

EXCLUDES *hand saw (E920.1)*

E919.5 Prime movers, except electrical motors

Gas turbine
Internal combustion engine
Steam engine
Water driven turbine

EXCLUDES *that being towed by other vehicle on the highway (E810.0-E819.9, E827.0-E827.9, E829.0-E829.9)*
that in transport under own power on the highway (E810.0-E819.9)

E919.6 Transmission machinery

Transmission:	Transmission:
belt	pinion
cable	pulley
chain	shaft
gear	

E919.7 Earth moving, scraping, and other excavating machines

Bulldozer	Steam shovel
Road scraper	

EXCLUDES *that being towed by other vehicle on the highway (E810.0-E819.9, E827.0-E827.9, E829.0-E829.9)*
that in transport under own power on the highway (E810.0-E819.9)

E919.8 Other specified machinery

Machines for manufacture of:
  clothing
  foodstuffs and beverages
  paper
Printing machine
Recreational machinery
Spinning, weaving, and textile machines

E919.9 Unspecified machinery

✔4ᵗʰ E920 Accidents caused by cutting and piercing instruments or objects

INCLUDES		
accidental injury (by) object	edged pointed sharp

EXCLUDES *injury caused by mechanism or component of firearm and air gun (E928.7)*

E920.0 Powered lawn mower

E920.1 Other powered hand tools

Any powered hand tool [compressed air] [electric] [explosive cartridge] [hydraulic power], such as:
  drill
  hand saw
  hedge clipper
  rivet gun
  snow blower
  staple gun

EXCLUDES *band saw (E919.4)*
bench saw (E919.4)

E920.2 Powered household appliances and implements

Blender	Electric:
Electric:	knife
beater or mixer	sewing machine
can opener	Garbage disposal appliance
fan	

E920.3 Knives, swords, and daggers

E920.4 Other hand tools and implements

Axe	Paper cutter
Can opener NOS	Pitchfork
Chisel	Rake
Fork	Scissors
Hand saw	Screwdriver
Hoe	Sewing machine, not powered
Ice pick	Shovel
Needle (sewing)	

E920.5 Hypodermic needle

Contaminated needle
Needle stick

E920.8 Other specified cutting and piercing instruments or objects

Arrow	Nail
Broken glass	Plant thorn
Dart	Splinter
Edge of stiff paper	Tin can lid
Lathe turnings	

EXCLUDES *animal spines or quills (E906.8)*
flying glass due to explosion (E921.0-E923.9)

E920.9 Unspecified cutting and piercing instrument or object

✔4ᵗʰ E921 Accident caused by explosion of pressure vessel

INCLUDES accidental explosion of pressure vessels, whether or not part of machinery

EXCLUDES *explosion of pressure vessel on transport vehicle (E800.0-E845.9)*

E921.0 Boilers

E921.1 Gas cylinders

Air tank	Pressure gas tank

E921.8 Other specified pressure vessels

Aerosol can	Tin can lid
Automobile tire	

E921.9 Unspecified pressure vessel

✔4ᵗʰ E922 Accident caused by firearm, and air gun missile

EXCLUDES *injury caused by mechanism or component of firearm and air gun (E928.7)*

E922.0 Handgun

Pistol	Revolver

EXCLUDES *Verey pistol (E922.8)*

E922.1 Shotgun (automatic)

E922.2 Hunting rifle

E922.3 Military firearms

Army rifle	Machine gun

E922.4 Air gun

BB gun	Pellet gun

E922.5 Paintball gun

E922.8 Other specified firearm missile

Verey pistol [flare]

E922.9 Unspecified firearm missile

Gunshot wound NOS
Shot NOS

E Codes

E923–E926.5

✓4ᵗʰ **E923 Accident caused by explosive material**

INCLUDES flash burns and other injuries resulting from explosion of explosive material
ignition of highly explosive material with explosion

EXCLUDES explosion:
in or on machinery (E919.0-E919.9)
on any transport vehicle, except stationary motor vehicle (E800.0-E848)
with conflagration (E890.0, E891.0,E892)
injury caused by mechanism or component of firearm and air gun (E928.7)
secondary fires resulting from explosion (E890.0-E899)

E923.0 Fireworks

E923.1 Blasting materials

Blasting cap   Dynamite
Detonator   Explosive [any] used in blasting operations

E923.2 Explosive gases

Acetylene   Fire damp
Butane   Gasoline fumes
Coal gas   Methane
Explosion in mine NOS   Propane

E923.8 Other explosive materials

Bomb   Torpedo
Explosive missile   Explosion in munitions:
Grenade   dump
Mine   factory
Shell

E923.9 Unspecified explosive material

Explosion NOS

✓4ᵗʰ **E924 Accident caused by hot substance or object, caustic or corrosive material, and steam**

EXCLUDES burning NOS (E899)
chemical burn resulting from swallowing a corrosive substance (E860.0-E864.4)
fire caused by these substances and objects (E890.0-E894)
radiation burns (E926.0-E926.9)
therapeutic misadventures (E870.0-E876.9)

E924.0 Hot liquids and vapors, including steam

Burning or scalding by:
boiling water
hot or boiling liquids not primarily caustic or corrosive
liquid metal
steam
other hot vapor

EXCLUDES hot (boiling) tap water (E924.2)

E924.1 Caustic and corrosive substances

Burning by:
acid [any kind]
ammonia
caustic oven cleaner or other substance
corrosive substance
lye
vitriol

E924.2 Hot (boiling) tap water

E924.8 Other

Burning by:
heat from electric heating appliance
hot object NOS
light bulb
steam pipe

E924.9 Unspecified

✓4ᵗʰ **E925 Accident caused by electric current**

INCLUDES electric current from exposed wire, faulty appliance, high voltage cable, live rail, or open electric socket as the cause of:
burn
cardiac fibrillation
convulsion
electric shock
electrocution
puncture wound
respiratory paralysis

EXCLUDES burn by heat from electrical appliance (E924.8)
lightning (E907)

E925.0 Domestic wiring and appliances

E925.1 Electric power generating plants, distribution stations, transmission lines

Broken power line

E925.2 Industrial wiring, appliances, and electrical machinery

Conductors
Control apparatus
Electrical equipment and machinery
Transformers

E925.8 Other electric current

Wiring and appliances in or on:
farm [not farmhouse]
outdoors
public building
residential institutions
schools

E925.9 Unspecified electric current

Burns or other injury from electric current NOS
Electric shock NOS
Electrocution NOS

✓4ᵗʰ **E926 Exposure to radiation**

EXCLUDES abnormal reaction to or complication of treatment without mention of misadventure (E879.2)
atomic power plant malfunction in water transport (E838.0-E838.9)
misadventure to patient in surgical and medical procedures (E873.2-E873.3)
use of radiation in war operations (E996-E997.9)

E926.0 Radiofrequency radiation

Overexposure to:	from:
microwave radiation	high-powered radio and
radar radiation	television transmitters
radiofrequency	industrial radiofrequency
radiofrequency	induction heaters
radiation [any]	radar installations

E926.1 Infrared heaters and lamps

Exposure to infrared radiation from heaters and lamps as the cause of:
blistering
burning
charring
inflammatory change

EXCLUDES physical contact with heater or lamp (E924.8)

E926.2 Visible and ultraviolet light sources

Arc lamps
Black light sources
Electrical welding arc
Oxygas welding torch
Sun rays
Tanning bed

EXCLUDES excessive heat from these sources (E900.1-E900.9)

E926.3 X-rays and other electromagnetic ionizing radiation

Gamma rays
X-rays (hard) (soft)

E926.4 Lasers

E926.5 Radioactive isotopes

Radiobiologicals
Radiopharmaceuticals

✓4ᵗʰ Fourth-digit Required   ►◄ Revised Text   ● New Code   ▲ Revised Code TitleDx

E926.8 Other specified radiation
    Artificially accelerated beams of ionized particles generated by:
        betatrons
        synchrotrons

E926.9 Unspecified radiation
    Radiation NOS

☑4ᵗʰ E927 Overexertion and strenuous and repetitive movements or loads
    Use additional code to identify activity (E001-E030)

E927.0 Overexertion from sudden strenuous movement
    Sudden trauma from strenuous movement

E927.1 Overexertion from prolonged static position
    Overexertion from maintaining prolonged positions, such as:
        holding
        sitting
        standing

E927.2 Excessive physical exertion from prolonged activity

E927.3 Cumulative trauma from repetitive motion
    Cumulative trauma from repetitive movements

E927.4 Cumulative trauma from repetitive impact

E927.8 Other overexertion and strenuous and repetitive movements or loads

E927.9 Unspecified overexertion and strenuous and repetitive movements or loads

☑4ᵗʰ E928 Other and unspecified environmental and accidental causes

E928.0 Prolonged stay in weightless environment
    Weightlessness in spacecraft (simulator)

E928.1 Exposure to noise
    Noise (pollution)
    Sound waves
    Supersonic waves

E928.2 Vibration

E928.3 Human bite

E928.4 External constriction caused by hair

E928.5 External constriction caused by other object

E928.6 Environmental exposure to harmful algae and toxins
    Algae bloom NOS   Florida red tide
    Blue-green algae bloom   Harmful algae bloom
    Brown tide   Pfiesteria piscicida
    Cyanobacteria bloom   Red tide

E928.7 Mechanism or component of firearm and air gun
    Injury due to:
        explosion of gun parts
        recoil
    Pierced, cut, crushed, or pinched by slide, trigger mechanism, scope, or other gun part
    Powder burn from firearm or air gun
    EXCLUDES accident caused by firearm and air gun missile (E922.0-E922.9)

E928.8 Other

E928.9 Unspecified accident
    Accident NOS ⎤
    Blow NOS   ⎥ stated as accidentally
    Casualty (not due to war) ⎥ inflicted
    Decapitation ⎦

    Knocked down ⎤
    Killed   ⎥ stated as accidentally
    Injury [any part of body, or ⎥ inflicted, but not
        unspecified] ⎥ otherwise
    Mangled   ⎥ specified
    Wound   ⎦
    EXCLUDES fracture, cause unspecified (E887)
        injuries undetermined whether accidentally or purposely inflicted (E980.0-E989)

Late Effects Of Accidental Injury (E929)

NOTE This category is to be used to indicate accidental injury as the cause of death or disability from late effects, which are themselves classifiable elsewhere. The "late effects" include conditions reported as such, or as sequelae which may occur at any time after the attempted suicide or self-inflicted injury.

☑4ᵗʰ E929 Late effects of accidental injury
    EXCLUDES late effects of:
        surgical and medical procedures (E870.0-E879.9)
        therapeutic use of drugs and medicines (E930.0-E949.9)

E929.0 Late effects of motor vehicle accident
    Late effects of accidents classifiable to E810-E825

E929.1 Late effects of other transport accident
    Late effects of accidents classifiable to E800-E807, E826-E838, E840-E848

E929.2 Late effects of accidental poisoning
    Late effects of accidents classifiable to E850-E858, E860-E869

E929.3 Late effects of accidental fall
    Late effects of accidents classifiable to E880-E888

E929.4 Late effects of accident caused by fire
    Late effects of accidents classifiable to E890-E899

E929.5 Late effects of accident due to natural and environmental factors
    Late effects of accidents classifiable to E900-E909

E929.8 Late effects of other accidents
    Late effects of accidents classifiable to E910-E928.8

E929.9 Late effects of unspecified accident
    Late effects of accidents classifiable to E928.9

Drugs, Medicinal And Biological Substances Causing Adverse Effects In Therapeutic Use (E930-E949)

INCLUDES correct drug properly administered in therapeutic or prophylactic dosage, as the cause of any adverse effect including allergic or hypersensitivity reactions

EXCLUDES *accidental overdose of drug and wrong drug given or taken in error (E850.0-E858.9)*
    accidents in the technique of administration of drug or biological substance, such as accidental puncture during injection, or contamination of drug (E870.0-E876.9)
    administration with suicidal or homicidal intent or intent to harm, or in circumstances classifiable to E950.0-E950.5, E962.0, E980.0-E980.5

NOTE See Alphabetic Index for more complete list of specific drugs to be classified under the fourth digit subdivisions. The American Hospital Formulary numbers can be used to classify new drugs listed by the American Hospital Formulary Service (AHFS). See Appendix C.

☑4ᵗʰ E930 Antibiotics
    EXCLUDES that used as eye, ear, nose, and throat [ENT], and local anti-infectives (E946.0-E946.9)

E930.0 Penicillins
    Natural   Semisynthetic, such as:
    Synthetic   cloxacillin
    Semisynthetic, such as: nafcillin
        ampicillin   oxacillin

E930.1 Antifungal antibiotics
    Amphotericin B   Hachimycin [trichomycin]
    Griseofulvin   Nystatin

E930.2 Chloramphenicol group
    Chloramphenicol   Thiamphenicol

E930.3 Erythromycin and other macrolides
    Oleandomycin   Spiramycin

E930.4 Tetracycline group
    Doxycycline   Oxytetracycline
    Minocycline

E930.5 Cephalosporin group
    Cephalexin   Cephaloridine
    Cephaloglycin   Cephalothin

E930.6 Antimycobacterial antibiotics
    Cycloserine   Rifampin
    Kanamycin   Streptomycin

E930.7 Antineoplastic antibiotics
Actinomycins, such as:
Bleomycin
Cactinomycin
Dactinomycin
Daunorubicin
Mitomycin
EXCLUDES other antineoplastic drugs (E933.1)

E930.8 Other specified antibiotics

E930.9 Unspecified antibiotic

✓4ᵗʰ **E931 Other anti-infectives**
EXCLUDES ENT, and local anti-infectives (E946.0-E946.9)

E931.0 Sulfonamides
Sulfadiazine
Sulfafurazole
Sulfamethoxazole

E931.1 Arsenical anti-infectives

E931.2 Heavy metal anti-infectives
Compounds of:
antimony
bismuth
lead
mercury
EXCLUDES mercurial diuretics (E944.0)

E931.3 Quinoline and hydroxyquinoline derivatives
Chiniofon
Diiodohydroxyquin
EXCLUDES antimalarial drugs (E931.4)

E931.4 Antimalarials and drugs acting on other blood protozoa
Chloroquine phosphate   Proguanil [chloroguanide]
Cycloguanil   Pyrimethamine
Primaquine   Quinine (sulphate)

E931.5 Other antiprotozoal drugs
Emetine

E931.6 Anthelmintics
Hexylresorcinol   Piperazine
Male fern oleoresin   Thiabendazole

E931.7 Antiviral drugs
Methisazone
EXCLUDES amantadine (E936.4)
cytarabine (E933.1)
idoxuridine (E946.5)

E931.8 Other antimycobacterial drugs
Ethambutol
Ethionamide
Isoniazid
Para-aminosalicylic acid derivatives
Sulfones

E931.9 Other and unspecified anti-infectives
Flucytosine
Nitrofuranderivatives

✓4ᵗʰ **E932 Hormones and synthetic substitutes**

E932.0 Adrenal cortical steroids
Cortisone derivatives
Desoxycorticosterone derivatives
Fluorinated corticosteroid

E932.1 Androgens and anabolic congeners
Nandrolone phenpropionate
Oxymetholone
Testosterone and preparations

E932.2 Ovarian hormones and synthetic substitutes
Contraceptives, oral
Estrogens
Estrogens and progestogens combined
Progestogens

E932.3 Insulins and antidiabetic agents
Acetohexamide
Biguanide derivatives, oral
Chlorpropamide
Glucagon
Insulin
Phenformin
Sulfonylurea derivatives, oral
Tolbutamide
EXCLUDES adverse effect of insulin administered for shock therapy (E879.3)

E932.4 Anterior pituitary hormones
Corticotropin
Gonadotropin
Somatotropin [growth hormone]

E932.5 Posterior pituitary hormones
Vasopressin
EXCLUDES oxytocic agents (E945.0)

E932.6 Parathyroid and parathyroid derivatives

E932.7 Thyroid and thyroid derivatives
Dextrothyroxine
Levothyroxine sodium
Liothyronine
Thyroglobulin

E932.8 Antithyroid agents
Iodides
Thiouracil
Thiourea

E932.9 Other and unspecified hormones and synthetic substitutes

✓4ᵗʰ **E933 Primarily systemic agents**

E933.0 Antiallergic and antiemetic drugs
Antihistamines   Diphenylpyraline
Chlorpheniramine   Thonzylamine
Diphenhydramine   Tripelennamine
EXCLUDES phenothiazine-based tranquilizers (E939.1)

E933.1 Antineoplastic and immunosuppressive drugs
Azathioprine
Busulfan
Chlorambucil
Cyclophosphamide
Cytarabine
Fluorouracil
Mechlorethamine hydrochloride
Mercaptopurine
Triethylenethiophosphoramide [thio-TEPA]
EXCLUDES antineoplastic antibiotics (E930.7)

E933.2 Acidifying agents

E933.3 Alkalizing agents

E933.4 Enzymes, not elsewhere classified
Penicillinase

E933.5 Vitamins, not elsewhere classified
Vitamin A
Vitamin D
EXCLUDES nicotinic acid (E942.2)
vitamin K (E934.3)

E933.6 Oral bisphosphonates

E933.7 Intravenous bisphosphonates

E933.8 Other systemic agents, not elsewhere classified
Heavy metal antagonists

E933.9 Unspecified systemic agent

✓4ᵗʰ **E934 Agents primarily affecting blood constituents**

E934.0 Iron and its compounds
Ferric salts
Ferrous sulphate and other ferrous salts

E934.1 Liver preparations and other antianemic agents
Folic acid

E934.2 Anticoagulants
    Coumarin
    Heparin
    Phenindione
    Prothrombin synthesis inhibitor
    Warfarin sodium

E934.3 Vitamin K [phytonadione]

E934.4 Fibrinolysis-affecting drugs
    Aminocaproic acid   Streptokinase
    Streptodornase   Urokinase

E934.5 Anticoagulant antagonists and other coagulants
    Hexadimethrine bromide
    Protamine sulfate

E934.6 Gamma globulin

E934.7 Natural blood and blood products
    Blood plasma
    Human fibrinogen
    Packed red cells
    Whole blood

E934.8 Other agents affecting blood constituents
    Macromolecular blood substitutes

E934.9 Unspecified agent affecting blood constituents

✓4ᵗʰ **E935 Analgesics, antipyretics, and antirheumatics**

E935.0 Heroin
    Diacetylmorphine

E935.1 Methadone

E935.2 Other opiates and related narcotics
    Codeine [methylmorphine]
    Meperidine [pethidine]
    Morphine
    Opium (alkaloids)

E935.3 Salicylates
    Acetylsalicylic acid [aspirin]
    Amino derivatives of salicylic acid
    Salicylic acid salts

E935.4 Aromatic analgesics, not elsewhere classified
    Acetanilid
    Paracetamol [acetaminophen]
    Phenacetin [acetophenetidin]

E935.5 Pyrazole derivatives
    Aminophenazone [aminopyrine]
    Phenylbutazone

E935.6 Antirheumatics [antiphlogistics]
    Gold salts
    Indomethacin
    EXCLUDES   salicylates (E935.3)
              steroids (E932.0)

E935.7 Other non-narcotic analgesics
    Pyrabital

E935.8 Other specified analgesics and antipyretics
    Pentazocine

E935.9 Unspecified analgesic and antipyretic

✓4ᵗʰ **E936 Anticonvulsants and anti-Parkinsonism drugs**

E936.0 Oxazolidine derivatives
    Paramethadione
    Trimethadione

E936.1 Hydantoin derivatives
    Phenytoin

E936.2 Succinimides
    Ethosuximide
    Phensuximide

E936.3 Other and unspecified anticonvulsants
    Beclamide
    Primidone

E936.4 Anti-Parkinsonism drugs
    Amantadine
    Ethopropazine [profenamine]
    Levodopa [L-dopa]

✓4ᵗʰ **E937 Sedatives and hypnotics**

E937.0 Barbiturates
    Amobarbital [amylobarbitone]
    Barbital [barbitone]
    Butabarbital [butabarbitone]
    Pentobarbital [pentobarbitone]
    Phenobarbital [phenobarbitone]
    Secobarbital [quinalbarbitone]
    EXCLUDES   thiobarbiturates (E938.3)

E937.1 Chloral hydrate group

E937.2 Paraldehyde

E937.3 Bromine compounds
    Bromide
    Carbromal (derivatives)

E937.4 Methaqualone compounds

E937.5 Glutethimide group

E937.6 Mixed sedatives, not elsewhere classified

E937.8 Other sedatives and hypnotics

E937.9 Unspecified
    Sleeping:
        drug
        pill   } NOS
        tablet

✓4ᵗʰ **E938 Other central nervous system depressants and anesthetics**

E938.0 Central nervous system muscle-tone depressants
    Chlorphenesin (carbamate)
    Mephenesin
    Methocarbamol

E938.1 Halothane

E938.2 Other gaseous anesthetics
    Ether
    Halogenated hydrocarbon derivatives, except halothane
    Nitrous oxide

E938.3 Intravenous anesthetics
    Ketamine
    Methohexital [methohexitone]
    Thiobarbiturates, such as thiopental sodium

E938.4 Other and unspecified general anesthetics

E938.5 Surface and infiltration anesthetics
    Cocaine
    Lidocaine [lignocaine]
    Procaine
    Tetracaine

E938.6 Peripheral nerve- and plexus-blocking anesthetics

E938.7 Spinal anesthetics

E938.9 Other and unspecified local anesthetics

✓4ᵗʰ **E939 Psychotropic agents**

E939.0 Antidepressants
    Amitriptyline
    Imipramine
    Monoamine oxidase [MAO] inhibitors

E939.1 Phenothiazine-based tranquilizers
    Chlorpromazine   Prochlorperazine
    Fluphenazine   Promazine
    Phenothiazine

E939.2 Butyrophenone-based tranquilizers
    Haloperidol
    Spiperone
    Trifluperidol

E939.3 Other antipsychotics, neuroleptics, and major tranquilizers

E939.4 Benzodiazepine-based tranquilizers
    Chlordiazepoxide   Lorazepam
    Diazepam   Medazepam
    Flurazepam   Nitrazepam

E939.5 Other tranquilizers
    Hydroxyzine
    Meprobamate

E934.2–E939.5

E939.6 Psychodysleptics [hallucinogens]
Cannabis (derivatives)   Mescaline
Lysergide [LSD]   Psilocin
Marihuana (derivatives)   Psilocybin

E939.7 Psychostimulants
Amphetamine
Caffeine
EXCLUDES central appetite depressants (E947.0)

E939.8 Other psychotropic agents

E939.9 Unspecified psychotropic agent

E940 Central nervous system stimulants

E940.0 Analeptics
Lobeline
Nikethamide

E940.1 Opiate antagonists
Levallorphan
Nalorphine
Naloxone

E940.8 Other specified central nervous system stimulants

E940.9 Unspecified central nervous system stimulant

E941 Drugs primarily affecting the autonomic nervous system

E941.0 Parasympathomimetics [cholinergics]
Acetylcholine
Anticholinesterase:
   organophosphorus
   reversible
Pilocarpine

E941.1 Parasympatholytics [anticholinergics and antimuscarinics] and spasmolytics
Atropine
Homatropine
Hyoscine [scopolamine]
Quaternary ammonium derivatives
EXCLUDES papaverine (E942.5)

E941.2 Sympathomimetics [adrenergics]
Epinephrine [adrenalin]
Levarterenol [noradrenalin]

E941.3 Sympatholytics [antiadrenergics]
Phenoxybenzamine
Tolazolinehydrochloride

E941.9 Unspecified drug primarily affecting the autonomic nervous system

E942 Agents primarily affecting the cardiovascular system

E942.0 Cardiac rhythm regulators
Practolol   Propranolol
Procainamide   Quinidine

E942.1 Cardiotonic glycosides and drugs of similar action
Digitalis glycosides   Strophanthins
Digoxin

E942.2 Antilipemic and antiarteriosclerotic drugs
Cholestyramine   Nicotinic acid derivatives
Clofibrate   Sitosterols
EXCLUDES dextrothyroxine (E932.7)

E942.3 Ganglion-blocking agents
Pentamethonium bromide

E942.4 Coronary vasodilators
Dipyridamole   Nitrites
Nitrates [nitroglycerin]   Prenylamine

E942.5 Other vasodilators
Cyclandelate   Hydralazine
Diazoxide   Papaverine

E942.6 Other antihypertensive agents
Clonidine   Rauwolfia alkaloids
Guanethidine   Reserpine

E942.7 Antivaricose drugs, including sclerosing agents
Monoethanolamine
Zinc salts

E942.8 Capillary-active drugs
Adrenochrome derivatives
Bioflavonoids
Metaraminol

E942.9 Other and unspecified agents primarily affecting the cardiovascular system

E943 Agents primarily affecting gastrointestinal system

E943.0 Antacids and antigastric secretion drugs
Aluminum hydroxide
Magnesium trisilicate

E943.1 Irritant cathartics
Bisacodyl
Castor oil
Phenolphthalein

E943.2 Emollient cathartics
Sodium dioctyl sulfosuccinate

E943.3 Other cathartics, including intestinal atonia drugs
Magnesium sulfate

E943.4 Digestants
Pancreatin
Papain
Pepsin

E943.5 Antidiarrheal drugs
Bismuth subcarbonate
Pectin
Kaolin
EXCLUDES anti-infectives (E930.0-E931.9)

E943.6 Emetics

E943.8 Other specified agents primarily affecting the gastrointestinal system

E943.9 Unspecified agent primarily affecting the gastrointestinal system

E944 Water, mineral, and uric acid metabolism drugs

E944.0 Mercurial diuretics
Chlormerodrin   Mercurophylline
Mercaptomerin   Mersalyl

E944.1 Purine derivative diuretics
Theobromine
Theophylline
EXCLUDES aminophylline [theophylline ethylenediamine] (E945.7)

E944.2 Carbonic acid anhydrase inhibitors
Acetazolamide

E944.3 Saluretics
Benzothiadiazides
Chlorothiazide group

E944.4 Other diuretics
Ethacrynic acid   Furosemide

E944.5 Electrolytic, caloric, and water-balance agents

E944.6 Other mineral salts, not elsewhere classified

E944.7 Uric acid metabolism drugs
Cinchophen and congeners
Colchicine
Phenoquin
Probenecid

E945 Agents primarily acting on the smooth and skeletal muscles and respiratory system

E945.0 Oxytocic agents
Ergot alkaloids
Prostaglandins

E945.1 Smooth muscle relaxants
Adiphenine
Metaproterenol [orciprenaline]
EXCLUDES papaverine (E942.5)

E945.2 Skeletal muscle relaxants
Alcuronium chloride
Suxamethonium chloride

E945.3 Other and unspecified drugs acting on muscles

E Codes

E945.4 **Antitussives**
   Dextromethorphan
   Pipazethate hydrochloride

E945.5 **Expectorants**
   Acetylcysteine
   Cocillana
   Guaifenesin [glyceryl guaiacolate]
   Ipecacuanha
   Terpin hydrate

E945.6 **Anti-common cold drugs**

E945.7 **Antiasthmatics**
   Aminophylline [theophylline ethylenediamine]

E945.8 **Other and unspecified respiratory drugs**

☑4ᵗʰ E946 **Agents primarily affecting skin and mucous membrane, ophthalmological, otorhinolaryngological, and dental drugs**

E946.0 **Local anti-infectives and anti-inflammatory drugs**

E946.1 **Antipruritics**

E946.2 **Local astringents and local detergents**

E946.3 **Emollients, demulcents, and protectants**

E946.4 **Keratolytics, kerstoplastics, other hair treatment drugs and preparations**

E946.5 **Eye anti-infectives and other eye drugs**
   Idoxuridine

E946.6 **Anti-infectives and other drugs and preparations for ear, nose, and throat**

E946.7 **Dental drugs topically applied**

E946.8 **Other agents primarily affecting skin and mucous membrane**
   Spermicides

E946.9 **Unspecified agent primarily affecting skin and mucous membrane**

☑4ᵗʰ E947 **Other and unspecified drugs and medicinal substances**

E947.0 **Dietetics**

E947.1 **Lipotropic drugs**

E947.2 **Antidotes and chelating agents, not elsewhere classified**

E947.3 **Alcohol deterrents**

E947.4 **Pharmaceutical excipients**

E947.8 **Other drugs and medicinal substances**
   Contrast media used for diagnostic x-ray procedures
   Diagnostic agents and kits

E947.9 **Unspecified drug or medicinal substance**

☑4ᵗʰ E948 **Bacterial vaccines**

E948.0 **BCG vaccine**

E948.1 **Typhoid and paratyphoid**

E948.2 **Cholera**

E948.3 **Plague**

E948.4 **Tetanus**

E948.5 **Diphtheria**

E948.6 **Pertussis vaccine, including combinations with a pertussis component**

E948.8 **Other and unspecified bacterial vaccines**

E948.9 **Mixed bacterial vaccines, except combinations with a pertussis component**

☑4ᵗʰ E949 **Other vaccines and biological substances**
   EXCLUDES *gamma globulin (E934.6)*

E949.0 **Smallpox vaccine**

E949.1 **Rabies vaccine**

E949.2 **Typhus vaccine**

E949.3 **Yellow fever vaccine**

E949.4 **Measles vaccine**

E949.5 **Poliomyelitis vaccine**

E949.6 **Other and unspecified viral and rickettsial vaccines**
   Mumps vaccine

E949.7 **Mixed viral-rickettsial and bacterial vaccines, except combinations with a pertussis component**
   EXCLUDES *combinations with a pertussis component (E948.6)*

E949.9 **Other and unspecified vaccines and biological substances**

Suicide and Self-inflicted Injury (E950-E959)

INCLUDES injuries in suicide and attempted suicide
self-inflicted injuries specified as intentional

☑4ᵗʰ E950 **Suicide and self-inflicted poisoning by solid or liquid substances**

E950.0 **Analgesics, antipyretics, and antirheumatics**

E950.1 **Barbiturates**

E950.2 **Other sedatives and hypnotics**

E950.3 **Tranquilizers and other psychotropic agents**

E950.4 **Other specified drugs and medicinal substances**

E950.5 **Unspecified drug or medicinal substance**

E950.6 **Agricultural and horticultural chemical and pharmaceutical preparations other than plant foods and fertilizers**

E950.7 **Corrosive and caustic substances**
   Suicide and self-inflicted poisoning by substances classifiable to E864

E950.8 **Arsenic and its compounds**

E950.9 **Other and unspecified solid and liquid substances**

☑4ᵗʰ E951 **Suicide and self-inflicted poisoning by gases in domestic use**

E951.0 **Gas distributed by pipeline**

E951.1 **Liquefied petroleum gas distributed in mobile containers**

E951.8 **Other utility gas**

☑4ᵗʰ E952 **Suicide and self-inflicted poisoning by other gases and vapors**

E952.0 **Motor vehicle exhaust gas**

E952.1 **Other carbon monoxide**

E952.8 **Other specified gases and vapors**

E952.9 **Unspecified gases and vapors**

☑4ᵗʰ E953 **Suicide and self-inflicted injury by hanging, strangulation, and suffocation**

E953.0 **Hanging**

E953.1 **Suffocation by plastic bag**

E953.8 **Other specified means**

E953.9 **Unspecified means**

E954 **Suicide and self-inflicted injury by submersion [drowning]**

☑4ᵗʰ E955 **Suicide and self-inflicted injury by firearms, air guns and explosives**

E955.0 **Handgun**

E955.1 **Shotgun**

E955.2 **Hunting rifle**

E955.3 **Military firearms**

E955.4 **Other and unspecified firearm**
   Gunshot NOS
   Shot NOS

E955.5 **Explosives**

E955.6 **Air gun**
   BB gun
   Pellet gun

E955.7 **Paintball gun**

E955.9 **Unspecified**

E956 **Suicide and self-inflicted injury by cutting and piercing instrument**

☑4ᵗʰ Fourth-digit Required   ►◄ Revised Text   ● New Code   ▲ Revised Code TitleDx

E Codes

E957–E968.8

☑4ᵗʰ **E957 Suicide and self-inflicted injuries by jumping from high place**

    E957.0 Residential premises

    E957.1 Other man-made structures

    E957.2 Natural sites

    E957.9 Unspecified

☑4ᵗʰ **E958 Suicide and self-inflicted injury by other and unspecified means**

    E958.0 Jumping or lying before moving object

    E958.1 Burns, fire

    E958.2 Scald

    E958.3 Extremes of cold

    E958.4 Electrocution

    E958.5 Crashing of motor vehicle

    E958.6 Crashing of aircraft

    E958.7 Caustic substances, except poisoning

        EXCLUDES *poisoning by caustic substance (E950.7)*

    E958.8 Other specified means

    E958.9 Unspecified means

E959 Late effects of self-inflicted injury

    NOTE This category is to be used to indicate circumstances classifiable to E950-E958 as the cause of death or disability from late effects, which are themselves classifiable elsewhere. The "late effects" include conditions reported as such, or as sequelae which may occur at any time after the attempted suicide or self-inflicted injury.

Homicide and Injury Purposely Inflicted by Other Persons (E960-E969)

    INCLUDES injuries inflicted by another person with intent to injure or kill, by any means

    EXCLUDES *injuries due to:*
        legal intervention (E970-E978)
        operations of war (E990-E999)
        terrorism (E979)

☑4ᵗʰ **E960 Fight, brawl, rape**

    E960.0 Unarmed fight or brawl
        Beatings NOS
        Brawl or fight with hands, fists, feet
        Injured or killed in fight NOS
        EXCLUDES *homicidal:*
          injury by weapons (E965.0-E966, E969)
          strangulation (E963)
          submersion (E964)

    E960.1 Rape

E961 Assault by corrosive or caustic substance, except poisoning
    Injury or death purposely caused by corrosive or caustic substance, such as:
    acid [any]
    corrosive substance
    vitriol
    EXCLUDES *burns from hot liquid (E968.3)*
        chemical burns from swallowing a corrosive substance (E962.0-E962.9)

☑4ᵗʰ **E962 Assault by poisoning**

    E962.0 Drugs and medicinal substances
        Homicidal poisoning by any drug or medicinal substance

    E962.1 Other solid and liquid substances

    E962.2 Other gases and vapors

    E962.9 Unspecified poisoning

E963 Assault by hanging and strangulation
    Homicidal (attempt):
        garrotting or ligature
        hanging
        strangulation
        suffocation

E964 Assault by submersion [drowning]

☑4ᵗʰ **E965 Assault by firearms and explosives**

    E965.0 Handgun
        Pistol
        Revolver

    E965.1 Shotgun

    E965.2 Hunting rifle

    E965.3 Military firearms

    E965.4 Other and unspecified firearm

    E965.5 Antipersonnel bomb

    E965.6 Gasoline bomb

    E965.7 Letter bomb

    E965.8 Other specified explosive
        Bomb NOS (placed in):
          car
          house
        Dynamite

    E965.9 Unspecified explosive

E966 Assault by cutting and piercing instrument
    Assassination (attempt), homicide (attempt) by any instrument classifiable under E920
    Homicidal:
      cut
      puncture } any part of the body
      stab
    Stabbed any part of the body

☑4ᵗʰ **E967 Perpetrator of child and adult abuse**
    NOTE Selection of the correct perpetrator code is based on the relationship between the perpetrator and the victim

    E967.0 By father, stepfather, or boyfriend
        Male partner of child's parent or guardian

    E967.1 By other specified person

    E967.2 By mother, stepmother, or girlfriend
        Female partner of child's parent or guardian

    E967.3 By spouse or partner
        Abuse of spouse or partner by ex-spouse or ex-partner

    E967.4 By child

    E967.5 By sibling

    E967.6 By grandparent

    E967.7 By other relative

    E967.8 By non-related caregiver

    E967.9 By unspecified person

☑4ᵗʰ **E968 Assault by other and unspecified means**

    E968.0 Fire
        Arson
        Homicidal burns NOS
        EXCLUDES *burns from hot liquid (E968.3)*

    E968.1 Pushing from a high place

    E968.2 Striking by blunt or thrown object

    E968.3 Hot liquid
        Homicidal burns by scalding

    E968.4 Criminal neglect
        Abandonment of child, infant, or other helpless person with intent to injure or kill

    E968.5 Transport vehicle
        Being struck by other vehicle or run down with intent to injure
        Pushed in front of, thrown from, or dragged by moving vehicle with intent to injure

    E968.6 Air gun
        BB gun
        Pellet gun

    E968.7 Human bite

    E968.8 Other specified means

☑4ᵗʰ Fourth-digit Required   ►◄ Revised Text   ● New Code   ▲ Revised Code TitleDx

E968.9 Unspecified means
  Assassination (attempt) NOS
  Homicidal (attempt):
    injury NOS
    wound NOS
  Manslaughter (nonaccidental)
  Murder (attempt) NOS
  Violence, non-accidental

E969 Late effects of injury purposely inflicted by other person
  NOTE This category is to be used to indicate circumstances classifiable to E960-E968 as the cause of death or disability from late effects, which are themselves classifiable elsewhere. The "late effects" include conditions reported as such, or as sequelae which may occur at any time after injury purposely inflicted by another person.

Legal Intervention (E970-E978)

  INCLUDES injuries inflicted by the police or other law-enforcing agents, including military on duty, in the course of arresting or attempting to arrest lawbreakers, suppressing disturbances, maintaining order, and other legal action
       legal execution
  EXCLUDES injuries caused by civil insurrections (E990.0-E999)

E970 Injury due to legal intervention by firearms
  Gunshot wound
  Injury by:
    machine gun
    revolver
    rifle pellet or rubber bullet
    shot NOS

E971 Injury due to legal intervention by explosives
  Injury by:
    dynamite
    explosive shell
    grenade
    mortar bomb

E972 Injury due to legal intervention by gas
  Asphyxiation by gas
  Injury by tear gas
  Poisoning by gas

E973 Injury due to legal intervention by blunt object
  Hit, struck by:
    baton (nightstick)
    blunt object
    stave

E974 Injury due to legal intervention by cutting and piercing instrument
  Cut
  Incised wound
  Injured by bayonet
  Stab wound

E975 Injury due to legal intervention by other specified means
  Blow
  Manhandling

E976 Injury due to legal intervention by unspecified means

E977 Late effects of injuries due to legal intervention
  NOTE This category is to be used to indicate circumstances classifiable to E970-E976 as the cause of death or disability from late effects, which are themselves classifiable elsewhere. The "late effects" include conditions reported as such, or as sequelae, which may occur at any time after the injury due to legal intervention.

E978 Legal execution
  All executions performed at the behest of the judiciary or ruling authority [whether permanent or temporary] as:
    asphyxiation by gas
    beheading, decapitation (by guillotine)
    capital punishment
    electrocution
    hanging
    poisoning
    shooting
    other specified means

Terrorism (E979)

☑4ᵗʰ **E979 Terrorism**
  Injuries resulting from the unlawful use of force or violence against persons or property to intimidate or coerce a Government, the civilian population, or any segment thereof, in furtherance of political or social objective

E979.0 Terrorism involving explosion of marine weapons
  Depth-charge
  Marine mine
  Mine NOS, at sea or in harbour
  Sea-based artillery shell
  Torpedo
  Underwater blast

E979.1 Terrorism involving destruction of aircraft
  Aircraft used as a weapon
  Aircraft:
    burned
    exploded
    shot down
  Crushed by falling aircraft

E979.2 Terrorism involving other explosions and fragments
  Antipersonnel bomb (fragments)
  Blast NOS
  Explosion (of):
    artillery shell
    breech-block
    cannon block
    mortar bomb
    munitions being used in terrorism
    NOS
  Fragments from:
    artillery shell
    bomb
    grenade
    guided missile
    land-mine
    rocket
    shell
    shrapnel
  Mine NOS

E979.3 Terrorism involving fires, conflagration and hot substances
  Burning building or structure:
    collapse of
    fall from
    hit by falling object in
    jump from
  Conflagration NOS
  Fire (causing):
    Asphyxia
    Burns
    NOS
    Other injury
  Melting of fittings and furniture in burning
  Petrol bomb
  Smouldering building or structure

E979.4 Terrorism involving firearms
  Bullet:
    carbine
    machine gun
    pistol
    rifle
    rubber (rifle)
  Pellets (shotgun)

E979.5 Terrorism involving nuclear weapons
  Blast effects
  Exposure to ionizing radiation from nuclear weapon
  Fireball effects
  Heat from nuclear weapon
  Other direct and secondary effects of nuclear weapons

E979.6 Terrorism involving biological weapons
  Anthrax
  Cholera
  Smallpox

☑4ᵗʰ Fourth-digit Required   ►◄ Revised Text   ● New Code   ▲ Revised Code TitleDx

E979.7 Terrorism involving chemical weapons
Gases, fumes, chemicals
Hydrogen cyanide
Phosgene
Sarin

E979.8 Terrorism involving other means
Drowning and submersion
Lasers
Piercing or stabbing instruments
Terrorism NOS

E979.9 Terrorism, secondary effects
NOTE This code is for use to identify conditions occurring subsequent to a terrorist attack not those that are due to the initial terrorist act
EXCLUDES late effect of terrorist attack (E999.1)

Injury Undetermined Whether Accidentally or Purposely Inflicted (E980-E989)

NOTE Categories E980-E989 are for use when it is unspecified or it cannot be determined whether the injuries are accidental (unintentional), suicide (attempted), or assault.

E980 Poisoning by solid or liquid substances, undetermined whether accidentally or purposely inflicted

E980.0 Analgesics, antipyretics, and antirheumatics

E980.1 Barbiturates

E980.2 Other sedatives and hypnotics

E980.3 Tranquilizers and other psychotropic agents

E980.4 Other specified drugs and medicinal substances

E980.5 Unspecified drug or medicinal substance

E980.6 Corrosive and caustic substances
Poisoning, undetermined whether accidental or purposeful, by substances classifiable to E864

E980.7 Agricultural and horticultural chemical and pharmaceutical preparations other than plant foods and fertilizers

E980.8 Arsenic and its compounds

E980.9 Other and unspecified solid and liquid substances

E981 Poisoning by gases in domestic use, undetermined whether accidentally or purposely inflicted

E981.0 Gas distributed by pipeline

E981.1 Liquefied petroleum gas distributed in mobile containers

E981.8 Other utility gas

E982 Poisoning by other gases, undetermined whether accidentally or purposely inflicted

E982.0 Motor vehicle exhaust gas

E982.1 Other carbon monoxide

E982.8 Other specified gases and vapors

E982.9 Unspecified gases and vapors

E983 Hanging, strangulation, or suffocation, undetermined whether accidentally or purposely inflicted

E983.0 Hanging

E983.1 Suffocation by plastic bag

E983.8 Other specified means

E983.9 Unspecified means

E984 Submersion [drowning], undetermined whether accidentally or purposely inflicted

E985 Injury by firearms, air guns and explosives, undetermined whether accidentally or purposely inflicted

E985.0 Handgun

E985.1 Shotgun

E985.2 Hunting rifle

E985.3 Military firearms

E985.4 Other and unspecified firearm

E985.5 Explosives

E985.6 Air gun
BB gun   Pellet gun

E985.7 Paintball gun

E986 Injury by cutting and piercing instruments, undetermined whether accidentally or purposely inflicted

E987 Falling from high place, undetermined whether accidentally or purposely inflicted

E987.0 Residential premises

E987.1 Other man-made structures

E987.2 Natural sites

E987.9 Unspecified site

E988 Injury by other and unspecified means, undetermined whether accidentally or purposely inflicted

E988.0 Jumping or lying before moving object

E988.1 Burns, fire

E988.2 Scald

E988.3 Extremes of cold

E988.4 Electrocution

E988.5 Crashing of motor vehicle

E988.6 Crashing of aircraft

E988.7 Caustic substances, except poisoning

E988.8 Other specified means

E988.9 Unspecified means

E989 Late effects of injury, undetermined whether accidentally or purposely inflicted
NOTE This category is to be used to indicate circumstances classifiable to E980-E988 as the cause of death or disability from late effects, which are themselves classifiable elsewhere. The "late effects" include conditions reported as such, or as sequelae, which may occur at any time after injury, undetermined whether accidentally or purposely inflicted.

Injury Resulting from Operations of War (E990-E999)

INCLUDES injuries to military personnel and civilians caused by war and civil insurrections and occurring during the time of war and insurrection, and peacekeeping missions

EXCLUDES accidents during training of military personnel manufacture of war material and transport, unless attributable to enemy action

E990 Injury due to war operations by fires and conflagrations
INCLUDES asphyxia, burns, or other injury originating from fire caused by a fire-producing device or indirectly by any conventional weapon

E990.0 From gasoline bomb
Incendiary bomb

E990.1 From flamethrower

E990.2 From incendiary bullet

E990.3 From fire caused indirectly from conventional weapon
EXCLUDES fire aboard military aircraft (E994.3)

E990.9 From other and unspecified source

E991 Injury due to war operations by bullets and fragments
EXCLUDES injury due to bullets and fragments due to war operations, but occurring after cessation of hostilities (E998.0)
injury due to explosion of artillery shells and mortars (E993.2)
injury due to explosion of improvised explosive device [IED] (E993.3-E993.5)
injury due to sea-based artillery shell (E992.3)

E991.0 Rubber bullets (rifle)

E991.1 Pellets (rifle)

E991.2 Other bullets
Bullet [any, except rubber bullets and pellets]:
carbine
machine gun
pistol
rifle
shotgun

E991.3 Antipersonnel bomb (fragments)

E991.4 Fragments from munitions
Fragments from:
artillery shell
bombs, except antipersonnel
detonation of unexploded ordnance [UXO]
grenade
guided missile
land mine
rockets
shell

E991.5 Fragments from person-borne improvised explosive device [IED]

E991.6 Fragments from vehicle-borne improvised explosive device [IED]
IED borne by land, air, or water transport vehicle

E991.7 Fragments from other improvised explosive device [IED]
Roadside IED

E991.8 Fragments from weapons
Fragments from:
artillery
autocannons
automatic grenade launchers
missile launchers
mortars
small arms

E991.9 Other and unspecified fragments
Shrapnel NOS

✓4ᵗʰ **E992 Injury due to war operations by explosion of marine weapons**

E992.0 Torpedo

E992.1 Depth charge

E992.2 Marine mines
Marine mines at sea or in harbor

E992.3 Sea-based artillery shell

E992.8 Other marine weapons

E992.9 Unspecified marine weapon
Underwater blast NOS

✓4ᵗʰ **E993 Injury due to war operations by other explosion**
Injuries due to direct or indirect pressure or air blast of an explosion occurring during war operations
EXCLUDES *injury due to fragments resulting from an explosion (E991.0-E991.9)*
injury due to detonation of unexploded ordnance but occurring after cessation of hostilities (E998.0-E998.9)
injury due to nuclear weapons (E996.0-E996.9)

E993.0 Aerial bomb

E993.1 Guided missile

E993.2 Mortar
Artillery shell

E993.3 Person-borne improvised explosive device [IED]

E993.4 Vehicle-borne improvised explosive device [IED]
IED borne by land, air, or water transport vehicle

E993.5 Other improvised explosive device [IED]
Roadside IED

E993.6 Unintentional detonation of own munitions
Unintentional detonation of own ammunition (artillery) (mortars)

E993.7 Unintentional discharge of own munitions launch device
Unintentional explosion of own:
autocannons
automatic grenade launchers
missile launchers
small arms

E993.8 Other specified explosion
Bomb
Grenade
Land mine

E993.9 Unspecified explosion
Air blast NOS
Blast NOS
Blast wave NOS
Blast wind NOS
Explosion NOS

✓4ᵗʰ **E994 Injury due to war operations by destruction of aircraft**

E994.0 Destruction of aircraft due to enemy fire or explosives
Air to air missile
Explosive device placed on aircraft
Rocket propelled grenade [RPG]
Small arms fire
Surface to air missile

E994.1 Unintentional destruction of aircraft due to own onboard explosives

E994.2 Destruction of aircraft due to collision with other aircraft

E994.3 Destruction of aircraft due to onboard fire

E994.8 Other destruction of aircraft

E994.9 Unspecified destruction of aircraft

✓4ᵗʰ **E995 Injury due to war operations by other and unspecified forms of conventional warfare**

E995.0 Unarmed hand-to-hand combat
EXCLUDES *intentional restriction of airway (E995.3)*

E995.1 Struck by blunt object
Baton (nightstick)
Stave

E995.2 Piercing object
Bayonet
Knife
Sword

E995.3 Intentional restriction of air and airway
Intentional submersion
Strangulation
Suffocation

E995.4 Unintentional drowning due to inability to surface or obtain air
Submersion

E995.8 Other forms of conventional warfare

E995.9 Unspecified form of conventional warfare

✓4ᵗʰ **E996 Injury due to war operations by nuclear weapons**
Dirty bomb NOS
EXCLUDES *late effects of injury due to nuclear weapons (E999.0, E999.1)*

E996.0 Direct blast effect of nuclear weapon
Injury to bodily organs due to blast pressure

E996.1 Indirect blast effect of nuclear weapon
Injury due to being thrown by blast
Injury due to being struck or crushed by blast debris

E996.2 Thermal radiation effect of nuclear weapon
Burns due to thermal radiation
Fireball effects
Flash burns
Heat effects

E996.3 Nuclear radiation effects
Acute radiation exposure
Beta burns
Fallout exposure
Radiation sickness
Secondary effects of nuclear weapons

E996.8 Other effects of nuclear weapons

E996.9 Unspecified effect of nuclear weapon

☑4ᵗʰ **E997   Injury due to war operations by other forms of unconventional warfare**

     E997.0   Lasers

     E997.1   Biological warfare

     E997.2   Gases, fumes, and chemicals

     E997.3   Weapon of mass destruction [WMD], unspecified

     E997.8   Other specified forms of unconventional warfare

     E997.9   Unspecified form of unconventional warfare

☑4ᵗʰ **E998   Injury due to war operations but occurring after cessation of hostilities**

     Injuries due to operations of war but occurring after cessation of hostilities by any means classifiable under E990-E997

     Injuries by explosion of bombs or mines placed in the course of operations of war, if the explosion occurred after cessation of hostilities

     E998.0   Explosion of mines

     E998.1   Explosion of bombs

     E998.8   Injury due to other war operations but occurring after cessation of hostilities

     E998.9   Injury due to unspecified war operations but occurring after cessation of hostilities

☑4ᵗʰ **E999   Late effect of injury due to war operations and terrorism**

     NOTE This category is to be used to indicate circumstances classifiable to E979, E990-E998 as the cause of death or disability from late effects, which are themselves classifiable elsewhere. The "late effects" include conditions reported as such, or as sequelae, which may occur at any time after the injury, resulting from operations of war or terrorism

     E999.0   Late effect of injury due to war operations

     E999.1   Late effect of injury due to terrorism

☑4ᵗʰ Fourth-digit Required   ▶◀ Revised Text   ● New Code   ▲ Revised Code TitleDx

Appendix A: Morphology of Neoplasms

The World Health Organization has published an adaptation of the International Classification of Diseases for oncology (ICD-O). It contains a coded nomenclature for the morphology of neoplasms, which is reproduced here for those who wish to use it in conjunction with Chapter 2 of the International Classification of Diseases, 9th Revision, Clinical Modification.

The morphology code numbers consist of five digits; the first four identify the histological type of the neoplasm and the fifth indicates its behavior. The one-digit behavior code is as follows:

/0 Benign
/1 Uncertain whether benign or malignant
    Borderline malignancy
/2 Carcinoma in situ
    Intraepithelial
    Noninfiltrating
    Noninvasive
/3 Malignant, primary site
/6 Malignant, metastatic site
    Secondary site
/9 Malignant, uncertain whether primary or metastatic site

In the nomenclature below, the morphology code numbers include the behavior code appropriate to the histological type of neoplasm, but this behavior code should be changed if other reported information makes this necessary. For example, "chordoma (M9370/3)" is assumed to be malignant; the term "benign chordoma" should be coded M9370/0. Similarly, "superficial spreading adenocarcinoma (M8143/3)" described as "noninvasive" should be coded M8143/2 and "melanoma (M8720/3)" described as "secondary" should be coded M8720/6.

The following table shows the correspondence between the morphology code and the different sections of Chapter 2:

Morphology Code Histology/Behavior		ICD-9-CM Chapter 2	
Any	0	210-229	Benign neoplasms
M8000-M8004	1	239	Neoplasms of unspecified nature
M8010+	1	235-238	Neoplasms of uncertain behavior
Any	2	230-234	Carcinoma in situ
Any	3	140-195 200-208	Malignant neoplasms, stated or presumed to be primary
Any	6	196-198	Malignant neoplasms, stated or presumed to be secondary

The ICD-O behavior digit /9 is inapplicable in an ICD context, since all malignant neoplasms are presumed to be primary (/3) or secondary (/6) according to other information on the medical record.the first-listed term of the full ICD-O morphology nomenclature appears against each code number in the list below. The ICD-9-CM Alphabetical Index (Volume 2), however, includes all the ICD-O synonyms as well as a number of other morphological names still likely to be encountered on medical records but omitted from ICD-O as outdated or otherwise undesirable.

A coding difficulty sometimes arises where a morphological diagnosis contains two qualifying adjectives that have different code numbers. An example is "transitional cell epidermoid carcinoma." "Transitional cell carcinoma NOS" is M8120/3 and "epidermoid carcinoma NOS" is M8070/3. In such circumstances, the higher number (M8120/3 in this example) should be used, as it is usually more specific.

Coded Nomenclature for Morphology of Neoplasms

M800	**Neoplasms NOS**
M8000/0	Neoplasm, benign
M8000/1	Neoplasm, uncertain whether benign or malignant
M8000/3	Neoplasm, malignant
M8000/6	Neoplasm, metastatic
M8000/9	Neoplasm, malignant, uncertain whether primary or metastatic
M8001/0	Tumor cells, benign
M8001/1	Tumor cells, uncertain whether benign or malignant
M8001/3	Tumor cells, malignant
M8002/3	Malignant tumor, small cell type
M8003/3	Malignant tumor, giant cell type
M8004/3	Malignant tumor, fusiform cell type

M801-M804	**Epithelial neoplasms NOS**
M8010/0	Epithelial tumor, benign
M8010/2	Carcinoma in situ NOS
M8010/3	Carcinoma NOS
M8010/6	Carcinoma, metastatic NOS
M8010/9	Carcinomatosis
M8011/0	Epithelioma, benign
M8011/3	Epithelioma, malignant
M8012/3	Large cell carcinoma NOS
M8020/3	Carcinoma, undifferentiated type NOS
M8021/3	Carcinoma, anaplastic type NOS
M8022/3	Pleomorphic carcinoma
M8030/3	Giant cell and spindle cell carcinoma
M8031/3	Giant cell carcinoma
M8032/3	Spindle cell carcinoma
M8033/3	Pseudosarcomatous carcinoma
M8034/3	Polygonal cell carcinoma
M8035/3	Spheroidal cell carcinoma
M8040/1	Tumorlet
M8041/3	Small cell carcinoma NOS
M8042/3	Oat cell carcinoma
M8043/3	Small cell carcinoma, fusiform cell type

M805-M808	**Papillary and squamous cell neoplasms**
M8050/0	Papilloma NOS (except Papilloma of urinary bladder M8120/1)
M8050/2	Papillary carcinoma in situ
M8050/3	Papillary carcinoma NOS
M8051/0	Verrucous papilloma
M8051/3	Verrucous carcinoma NOS
M8052/0	Squamous cell papilloma
M8052/3	Papillary squamous cell carcinoma
M8053/0	Inverted papilloma
M8060/0	Papillomatosis NOS
M8070/2	Squamous cell carcinoma in situ NOS
M8070/3	Squamous cell carcinoma NOS
M8070/6	Squamous cell carcinoma, metastatic NOS
M8071/3	Squamous cell carcinoma, keratinizing type NOS
M8072/3	Squamous cell carcinoma, large cell, nonkeratinizing type
M8073/3	Squamous cell carcinoma, small cell, nonkeratinizing type
M8074/3	Squamous cell carcinoma, spindle cell type
M8075/3	Adenoid squamous cell carcinoma
M8076/2	Squamous cell carcinoma in situ with questionable stromal invasion
M8076/3	Squamous cell carcinoma, microinvasive
M8080/2	Queyrat's erythroplasia
M8081/2	Bowen's disease
M8082/3	Lymphoepithelial carcinoma

M809-M811	**Basal cell neoplasms**
M8090/1	Basal cell tumor
M8090/3	Basal cell carcinoma NOS
M8091/3	Multicentric basal cell carcinoma
M8092/3	Basal cell carcinoma, morphea type
M8093/3	Basal cell carcinoma, fibroepithelial type
M8094/3	Basosquamous carcinoma
M8095/3	Metatypical carcinoma
M8096/0	Intraepidermal epithelioma of Jadassohn
M8100/0	Trichoepithelioma
M8101/0	Trichofolliculoma
M8102/0	Tricholemmoma
M8110/0	Pilomatrixoma

M812-M813	**Transitional cell papillomas and carcinomas**
M8120/0	Transitional cell papilloma NOS
M8120/1	Urothelial papilloma
M8120/2	Transitional cell carcinoma in situ
M8120/3	Transitional cell carcinoma NOS
M8121/0	Schneiderian papilloma
M8121/1	Transitional cell papilloma, inverted type
M8121/3	Schneiderian carcinoma
M8122/3	Transitional cell carcinoma, spindle cell type
M8123/3	Basaloid carcinoma
M8124/3	Cloacogenic carcinoma
M8130/3	Papillary transitional cell carcinoma

M814-M838	**Adenomas and adenocarcinomas**
M8140/0	Adenoma NOS
M8140/1	Bronchial adenoma NOS
M8140/2	Adenocarcinoma in situ
M8140/3	Adenocarcinoma NOS
M8140/6	Adenocarcinoma, metastatic NOS
M8141/3	Scirrhous adenocarcinoma
M8142/3	Linitis plastica
M8143/3	Superficial spreading adenocarcinoma
M8144/3	Adenocarcinoma, intestinal type
M8145/3	Carcinoma, diffuse type
M8146/0	Monomorphic adenoma
M8147/0	Basal cell adenoma
M8150/0	Islet cell adenoma
M8150/3	Islet cell carcinoma
M8151/0	Insulinoma NOS
M8151/3	Insulinoma, malignant
M8152/0	Glucagonoma NOS
M8152/3	Glucagonoma, malignant
M8153/1	Gastrinoma NOS
M8153/3	Gastrinoma, malignant
M8154/3	Mixed islet cell and exocrine adenocarcinoma
M8160/0	Bile duct adenoma
M8160/3	Cholangiocarcinoma

M8161/0	Bile duct cystadenoma
M8161/3	Bile duct cystadenocarcinoma
M8170/0	Liver cell adenoma
M8170/3	Hepatocellular carcinoma NOS
M8180/0	Hepatocholangioma, benign
M8180/3	Combined hepatocellular carcinoma and cholangiocarcinoma
M8190/0	Trabecular adenoma
M8190/3	Trabecular adenocarcinoma
M8191/0	Embryonal adenoma
M8200/0	Eccrine dermal cylindroma
M8200/3	Adenoid cystic carcinoma
M8201/3	Cribriform carcinoma
M8210/0	Adenomatous polyp NOS
M8210/3	Adenocarcinoma in adenomatous polyp
M8211/0	Tubular adenoma NOS
M8211/3	Tubular adenocarcinoma
M8220/0	Adenomatous polyposis coli
M8220/3	Adenocarcinoma in adenomatous polyposis coli
M8221/0	Multiple adenomatous polyps
M8230/3	Solid carcinoma NOS
M8231/3	Carcinoma simplex
M8240/1	Carcinoid tumor NOS
M8240/3	Carcinoid tumor, malignant
M8241/1	Carcinoid tumor, argentaffin NOS
M8241/3	Carcinoid tumor, argentaffin, malignant
M8242/1	Carcinoid tumor, nonargentaffin NOS
M8242/3	Carcinoid tumor, nonargentaffin, malignant
M8243/3	Mucocarcinoid tumor, malignant
M8244/3	Composite carcinoid
M8250/1	Pulmonary adenomatosis
M8250/3	Bronchiolo-alveolar adenocarcinoma
M8251/0	Alveolar adenoma
M8251/3	Alveolar adenocarcinoma
M8260/0	Papillary adenoma NOS
M8260/3	Papillary adenocarcinoma NOS
M8261/1	Villous adenoma NOS
M8261/3	Adenocarcinoma in villous adenoma
M8262/3	Villous adenocarcinoma
M8263/0	Tubulovillous adenoma
M8270/0	Chromophobe adenoma
M8270/3	Chromophobe carcinoma
M8280/0	Acidophil adenoma
M8280/3	Acidophil carcinoma
M8281/0	Mixed acidophil-basophil adenoma
M8281/3	Mixed acidophil-basophil carcinoma
M8290/0	Oxyphilic adenoma
M8290/3	Oxyphilic adenocarcinoma
M8300/0	Basophil adenoma
M8300/3	Basophil carcinoma
M8310/0	Clear cell adenoma
M8310/3	Clear cell adenocarcinoma NOS
M8311/1	Hypernephroid tumor
M8312/3	Renal cell carcinoma
M8313/0	Clear cell adenofibroma
M8320/3	Granular cell carcinoma
M8321/0	Chief cell adenoma
M8322/0	Water-clear cell adenoma
M8322/3	Water-clear cell adenocarcinoma
M8323/0	Mixed cell adenoma
M8323/3	Mixed cell adenocarcinoma
M8324/0	Lipoadenoma
M8330/0	Follicular adenoma
M8330/3	Follicular adenocarcinoma NOS
M8331/3	Follicular adenocarcinoma, well differentiated type
M8332/3	Follicular adenocarcinoma, trabecular type

M8333/0	Microfollicular adenoma
M8334/0	Macrofollicular adenoma
M8340/3	Papillary and follicular adenocarcinoma
M8350/3	Nonencapsulated sclerosing carcinoma
M8360/1	Multiple endocrine adenomas
M8361/1	Juxtaglomerular tumor
M8370/0	Adrenal cortical adenoma NOS
M8370/3	Adrenal cortical carcinoma
M8371/0	Adrenal cortical adenoma, compact cell type
M8372/0	Adrenal cortical adenoma, heavily pigmented variant
M8373/0	Adrenal cortical adenoma, clear cell type
M8374/0	Adrenal cortical adenoma, glomerulosa cell type
M8375/0	Adrenal cortical adenoma, mixed cell type
M8380/0	Endometrioid adenoma NOS
M8380/1	Endometrioid adenoma, borderline malignancy
M8380/3	Endometrioid carcinoma
M8381/0	Endometrioid adenofibroma NOS
M8381/1	Endometrioid adenofibroma, borderline malignancy
M8381/3	Endometrioid adenofibroma, malignant

M839-M842 Adnexal and skin appendage neoplasms

M8390/0	Skin appendage adenoma
M8390/3	Skin appendage carcinoma
M8400/0	Sweat gland adenoma
M8400/1	Sweat gland tumor NOS
M8400/3	Sweat gland adenocarcinoma
M8401/0	Apocrine adenoma
M8401/3	Apocrine adenocarcinoma
M8402/0	Eccrine acrospiroma
M8403/0	Eccrine spiradenoma
M8404/0	Hidrocystoma
M8405/0	Papillary hydradenoma
M8406/0	Papillary syringadenoma
M8407/0	Syringoma NOS
M8410/0	Sebaceous adenoma
M8410/3	Sebaceous adenocarcinoma
M8420/0	Ceruminous adenoma
M8420/3	Ceruminous adenocarcinoma

M843 Mucoepidermoid neoplasms

M8430/1	Mucoepidermoid tumor
M8430/3	Mucoepidermoid carcinoma

M844-M849 Cystic, mucinous, and serous neoplasms

M8440/0	Cystadenoma NOS
M8440/3	Cystadenocarcinoma NOS
M8441/0	Serous cystadenoma NOS
M8441/1	Serous cystadenoma, borderline malignancy
M8441/3	Serous cystadenocarcinoma NOS
M8450/0	Papillary cystadenoma NOS
M8450/1	Papillary cystadenoma, borderline malignancy
M8450/3	Papillary cystadenocarcinoma NOS
M8460/0	Papillary serous cystadenoma NOS
M8460/1	Papillary serous cystadenoma, borderline malignancy
M8460/3	Papillary serous cystadenocarcinoma
M8461/0	Serous surface papilloma NOS
M8461/1	Serous surface papilloma, borderline malignancy
M8461/3	Serous surface papillary carcinoma
M8470/0	Mucinous cystadenoma NOS
M8470/1	Mucinous cystadenoma, borderline malignancy

M8470/3	Mucinous cystadenocarcinoma NOS
M8471/0	Papillary mucinous cystadenoma NOS
M8471/1	Papillary mucinous cystadenoma, borderline malignancy
M8471/3	Papillary mucinous cystadenocarcinoma
M8480/0	Mucinous adenoma
M8480/3	Mucinous adenocarcinoma
M8480/6	Pseudomyxoma peritonei
M8481/3	Mucin-producing adenocarcinoma
M8490/3	Signet ring cell carcinoma
M8490/6	Metastatic signet ring cell carcinoma

M850-M854 Ductal, lobular, and medullary neoplasms

M8500/2	Intraductal carcinoma, noninfiltrating NOS
M8500/3	Infiltrating duct carcinoma
M8501/2	Comedocarcinoma, noninfiltrating
M8501/3	Comedocarcinoma NOS
M8502/3	Juvenile carcinoma of the breast
M8503/0	Intraductal papilloma
M8503/2	Noninfiltrating intraductal papillary adenocarcinoma
M8504/0	Intracystic papillary adenoma
M8504/2	Noninfiltrating intracystic carcinoma
M8505/0	Intraductal papillomatosis NOS
M8506/0	Subareolar duct papillomatosis
M8510/3	Medullary carcinoma NOS
M8511/3	Medullary carcinoma with amyloid stroma
M8512/3	Medullary carcinoma with lymphoid stroma
M8520/2	Lobular carcinoma in situ
M8520/3	Lobular carcinoma NOS
M8521/3	Infiltrating ductular carcinoma
M8530/3	Inflammatory carcinoma
M8540/3	Paget's disease, mammary
M8541/3	Paget's disease and infiltrating duct carcinoma of breast
M8542/3	Paget's disease, extramammary (except Paget's disease of bone)

M855 Acinar cell neoplasms

M8550/0	Acinar cell adenoma
M8550/1	Acinar cell tumor
M8550/3	Acinar cell carcinoma

M856-M858 Complex epithelial neoplasms

M8560/3	Adenosquamous carcinoma
M8561/0	Adenolymphoma
M8570/3	Adenocarcinoma with squamous metaplasia
M8571/3	Adenocarcinoma with cartilaginous and osseous metaplasia
M8572/3	Adenocarcinoma with spindle cell metaplasia
M8573/3	Adenocarcinoma with apocrine metaplasia
M8580/0	Thymoma, benign
M8580/3	Thymoma, malignant

M859-M867 Specialized gonadal neoplasms

M8590/1	Sex cord-stromal tumor
M8600/0	Thecoma NOS
M8600/3	Theca cell carcinoma
M8610/0	Luteoma NOS
M8620/1	Granulosa cell tumor NOS
M8620/3	Granulosa cell tumor, malignant
M8621/1	Granulosa cell-theca cell tumor
M8630/0	Androblastoma, benign
M8630/1	Androblastoma NOS
M8630/3	Androblastoma, malignant
M8631/0	Sertoli-Leydig cell tumor

Code	Description
M8632/1	Gynandroblastoma
M8640/0	Tubular androblastoma NOS
M8640/3	Sertoli cell carcinoma
M8641/0	Tubular androblastoma with lipid storage
M8650/0	Leydig cell tumor, benign
M8650/1	Leydig cell tumor NOS
M8650/3	Leydig cell tumor, malignant
M8660/0	Hilar cell tumor
M8670/0	Lipid cell tumor of ovary
M8671/0	Adrenal rest tumor

M868-M871 Paragangliomas and glomus tumors

Code	Description
M8680/1	Paraganglioma NOS
M8680/3	Paraganglioma, malignant
M8681/1	Sympathetic paraganglioma
M8682/1	Parasympathetic paraganglioma
M8690/1	Glomus jugulare tumor
M8691/1	Aortic body tumor
M8692/1	Carotid body tumor
M8693/1	Extra-adrenal paraganglioma NOS
M8693/3	Extra-adrenal paraganglioma, malignant
M8700/0	Pheochromocytoma NOS
M8700/3	Pheochromocytoma, malignant
M8710/3	Glomangiosarcoma
M8711/0	Glomus tumor
M8712/0	Glomangioma

M872-M879 Nevi and melanomas

Code	Description
M8720/0	Pigmented nevus NOS
M8720/3	Malignant melanoma NOS
M8721/3	Nodular melanoma
M8722/0	Balloon cell nevus
M8722/3	Balloon cell melanoma
M8723/0	Halo nevus
M8724/0	Fibrous papule of the nose
M8725/0	Neuronevus
M8726/0	Magnocellular nevus
M8730/0	Nonpigmented nevus
M8730/3	Amelanotic melanoma
M8740/0	Junctional nevus
M8740/3	Malignant melanoma in junctional nevus
M8741/2	Precancerous melanosis NOS
M8741/3	Malignant melanoma in precancerous melanosis
M8742/2	Hutchinson's melanotic freckle
M8742/3	Malignant melanoma in Hutchinson's melanotic freckle
M8743/3	Superficial spreading melanoma
M8750/0	Intradermal nevus
M8760/0	Compound nevus
M8761/1	Giant pigmented nevus
M8761/3	Malignant melanoma in giant pigmented nevus
M8770/0	Epithelioid and spindle cell nevus
M8771/3	Epithelioid cell melanoma
M8772/3	Spindle cell melanoma NOS
M8773/3	Spindle cell melanoma, type A
M8774/3	Spindle cell melanoma, type B
M8775/3	Mixed epithelioid and spindle cell melanoma
M8780/0	Blue nevus NOS
M8780/3	Blue nevus, malignant
M8790/0	Cellular blue nevus

M880 Soft tissue tumors and sarcomas NOS

Code	Description
M8800/0	Soft tissue tumor, benign
M8800/3	Sarcoma NOS
M8800/9	Sarcomatosis NOS
M8801/3	Spindle cell sarcoma
M8802/3	Giant cell sarcoma (except of bone M9250/3)
M8803/3	Small cell sarcoma
M8804/3	Epithelioid cell sarcoma

M881-M883 Fibromatous neoplasms

Code	Description
M8810/0	Fibroma NOS
M8810/3	Fibrosarcoma NOS
M8811/0	Fibromyxoma
M8811/3	Fibromyxosarcoma
M8812/0	Periosteal fibroma
M8812/3	Periosteal fibrosarcoma
M8813/0	Fascial fibroma
M8813/3	Fascial fibrosarcoma
M8814/3	Infantile fibrosarcoma
M8820/0	Elastofibroma
M8821/1	Aggressive fibromatosis
M8822/1	Abdominal fibromatosis
M8823/1	Desmoplastic fibroma
M8830/0	Fibrous histiocytoma NOS
M8830/1	Atypical fibrous histiocytoma
M8830/3	Fibrous histiocytoma, malignant
M8831/0	Fibroxanthoma NOS
M8831/1	Atypical fibroxanthoma
M8831/3	Fibroxanthoma, malignant
M8832/0	Dermatofibroma NOS
M8832/1	Dermatofibroma protuberans
M8832/3	Dermatofibrosarcoma NOS

M884 Myxomatous neoplasms

Code	Description
M8840/0	Myxoma NOS
M8840/3	Myxosarcoma

M885-M888 Lipomatous neoplasms

Code	Description
M8850/0	Lipoma NOS
M8850/3	Liposarcoma NOS
M8851/0	Fibrolipoma
M8851/3	Liposarcoma, well differentiated type
M8852/0	Fibromyxolipoma
M8852/3	Myxoid liposarcoma
M8853/3	Round cell liposarcoma
M8854/3	Pleomorphic liposarcoma
M8855/3	Mixed type liposarcoma
M8856/0	Intramuscular lipoma
M8857/0	Spindle cell lipoma
M8860/0	Angiomyolipoma
M8860/3	Angiomyoliposarcoma
M8861/0	Angiolipoma NOS
M8861/1	Angiolipoma, infiltrating
M8870/0	Myelolipoma
M8880/0	Hibernoma
M8881/0	Lipoblastomatosis

M889-M892 Myomatous neoplasms

Code	Description
M8890/0	Leiomyoma NOS
M8890/1	Intravascular leiomyomatosis
M8890/3	Leiomyosarcoma NOS
M8891/1	Epithelioid leiomyoma
M8891/3	Epithelioid leiomyosarcoma
M8892/1	Cellular leiomyoma
M8893/0	Bizarre leiomyoma
M8894/0	Angiomyoma
M8894/3	Angiomyosarcoma
M8895/0	Myoma
M8895/3	Myosarcoma
M8900/0	Rhabdomyoma NOS
M8900/3	Rhabdomyosarcoma NOS
M8901/3	Pleomorphic rhabdomyosarcoma
M8902/3	Mixed type rhabdomyosarcoma
M8903/0	Fetal rhabdomyoma
M8904/0	Adult rhabdomyoma
M8910/3	Embryonal rhabdomyosarcoma
M8920/3	Alveolar rhabdomyosarcoma

M893-M899 Complex mixed and stromal neoplasms

Code	Description
M8930/3	Endometrial stromal sarcoma
M8931/1	Endolymphatic stromal myosis
M8932/0	Adenomyoma
M8940/0	Pleomorphic adenoma
M8940/3	Mixed tumor, malignant NOS
M8950/3	Mullerian mixed tumor
M8951/3	Mesodermal mixed tumor
M8960/1	Mesoblastic nephroma
M8960/3	Nephroblastoma NOS
M8961/3	Epithelial nephroblastoma
M8962/3	Mesenchymal nephroblastoma
M8970/3	Hepatoblastoma
M8980/3	Carcinosarcoma NOS
M8981/3	Carcinosarcoma, embryonal type
M8982/0	Myoepithelioma
M8990/0	Mesenchymoma, benign
M8990/1	Mesenchymoma NOS
M8990/3	Mesenchymoma, malignant
M8991/3	Embryonal sarcoma

M900-M903 Fibroepithelial neoplasms

Code	Description
M9000/0	Brenner tumor NOS
M9000/1	Brenner tumor, borderline malignancy
M9000/3	Brenner tumor, malignant
M9010/0	Fibroadenoma NOS
M9011/0	Intracanalicular fibroadenoma NOS
M9012/0	Pericanalicular fibroadenoma
M9013/0	Adenofibroma NOS
M9014/0	Serous adenofibroma
M9015/0	Mucinous adenofibroma
M9020/0	Cellular intracanalicular fibroadenoma
M9020/1	Cystosarcoma phyllodes NOS
M9020/3	Cystosarcoma phyllodes, malignant
M9030/0	Juvenile fibroadenoma

M904 Synovial neoplasms

Code	Description
M9040/0	Synovioma, benign
M9040/3	Synovial sarcoma NOS
M9041/3	Synovial sarcoma, spindle cell type
M9042/3	Synovial sarcoma, epithelioid cell type
M9043/3	Synovial sarcoma, biphasic type
M9044/3	Clear cell sarcoma of tendons and aponeuroses

M905 Mesothelial neoplasms

Code	Description
M9050/0	Mesothelioma, benign
M9050/3	Mesothelioma, malignant
M9051/0	Fibrous mesothelioma, benign
M9051/3	Fibrous mesothelioma, malignant
M9052/0	Epithelioid mesothelioma, benign
M9052/3	Epithelioid mesothelioma, malignant
M9053/0	Mesothelioma, biphasic type, benign
M9053/3	Mesothelioma, biphasic type, malignant
M9054/0	Adenomatoid tumor NOS

M906-M909 Germ cell neoplasms

Code	Description
M9060/3	Dysgerminoma
M9061/3	Seminoma NOS
M9062/3	Seminoma, anaplastic type
M9063/3	Spermatocytic seminoma
M9064/3	Germinoma
M9070/3	Embryonal carcinoma NOS
M9071/3	Endodermal sinus tumor
M9072/3	Polyembryoma
M9073/1	Gonadoblastoma
M9080/0	Teratoma, benign
M9080/1	Teratoma NOS
M9080/3	Teratoma, malignant NOS
M9081/3	Teratocarcinoma

Appendix A: Morphology of Neoplasms

M9082/3	Malignant teratoma, undifferentiated type
M9083/3	Malignant teratoma, intermediate type
M9084/0	Dermoid cyst
M9084/3	Dermoid cyst with malignant transformation
M9090/0	Struma ovarii NOS
M9090/3	Struma ovarii, malignant
M9091/1	Strumal carcinoid

M910 Trophoblastic neoplasms

M9100/0	Hydatidiform mole NOS
M9100/1	Invasive hydatidiform mole
M9100/3	Choriocarcinoma
M9101/3	Choriocarcinoma combined with teratoma
M9102/3	Malignant teratoma, trophoblastic

M911 Mesonephromas

M9110/0	Mesonephroma, benign
M9110/1	Mesonephric tumor
M9110/3	Mesonephroma, malignant
M9111/1	Endosalpingioma

M912-M916 Blood vessel tumors

M9120/0	Hemangioma NOS
M9120/3	Hemangiosarcoma
M9121/0	Cavernous hemangioma
M9122/0	Venous hemangioma
M9123/0	Racemose hemangioma
M9124/3	Kupffer cell sarcoma
M9130/0	Hemangioendothelioma, benign
M9130/1	Hemangioendothelioma NOS
M9130/3	Hemangioendothelioma, malignant
M9131/0	Capillary hemangioma
M9132/0	Intramuscular hemangioma
M9140/3	Kaposi's sarcoma
M9141/0	Angiokeratoma
M9142/0	Verrucous keratotic hemangioma
M9150/0	Hemangiopericytoma, benign
M9150/1	Hemangiopericytoma NOS
M9150/3	Hemangiopericytoma, malignant
M9160/0	Angiofibroma NOS
M9161/1	Hemangioblastoma

M917 Lymphatic vessel tumors

M9170/0	Lymphangioma NOS
M9170/3	Lymphangiosarcoma
M9171/0	Capillary lymphangioma
M9172/0	Cavernous lymphangioma
M9173/0	Cystic lymphangioma
M9174/0	Lymphangiomyoma
M9174/1	Lymphangiomyomatosis
M9175/0	Hemolymphangioma

M918-M920 Osteomas and osteosarcomas

M9180/0	Osteoma NOS
M9180/3	Osteosarcoma NOS
M9181/3	Chondroblastic osteosarcoma
M9182/3	Fibroblastic osteosarcoma
M9183/3	Telangiectatic osteosarcoma
M9184/3	Osteosarcoma in Paget's disease of bone
M9190/3	Juxtacortical osteosarcoma
M9191/0	Osteoid osteoma NOS
M9200/0	Osteoblastoma

M921-M924 Chondromatous neoplasms

M9210/0	Osteochondroma
M9210/1	Osteochondromatosis NOS
M9220/0	Chondroma NOS
M9220/1	Chondromatosis NOS
M9220/3	Chondrosarcoma NOS
M9221/0	Juxtacortical chondroma
M9221/3	Juxtacortical chondrosarcoma
M9230/0	Chondroblastoma NOS
M9230/3	Chondroblastoma, malignant
M9240/3	Mesenchymal chondrosarcoma
M9241/0	Chondromyxoid fibroma

M925 Giant cell tumors

M9250/1	Giant cell tumor of bone NOS
M9250/3	Giant cell tumor of bone, malignant
M9251/1	Giant cell tumor of soft parts NOS
M9251/3	Malignant giant cell tumor of soft parts

M926 Miscellaneous bone tumors

M9260/3	Ewing's sarcoma
M9261/3	Adamantinoma of long bones
M9262/0	Ossifying fibroma

M927-M934 Odontogenic tumors

M9270/0	Odontogenic tumor, benign
M9270/1	Odontogenic tumor NOS
M9270/3	Odontogenic tumor, malignant
M9271/0	Dentinoma
M9272/0	Cementoma NOS
M9273/0	Cementoblastoma, benign
M9274/0	Cementifying fibroma
M9275/0	Gigantiform cementoma
M9280/0	Odontoma NOS
M9281/0	Compound odontoma
M9282/0	Complex odontoma
M9290/0	Ameloblastic fibro-odontoma
M9290/3	Ameloblastic odontosarcoma
M9300/0	Adenomatoid odontogenic tumor
M9301/0	Calcifying odontogenic cyst
M9310/0	Ameloblastoma NOS
M9310/3	Ameloblastoma, malignant
M9311/0	Odontoameloblastoma
M9312/0	Squamous odontogenic tumor
M9320/0	Odontogenic myxoma
M9321/0	Odontogenic fibroma NOS
M9330/0	Ameloblastic fibroma
M9330/3	Ameloblastic fibrosarcoma
M9340/0	Calcifying epithelial odontogenic tumor

M935-M937 Miscellaneous tumors

M9350/1	Craniopharyngioma
M9360/1	Pinealoma
M9361/1	Pineocytoma
M9362/3	Pineoblastoma
M9363/0	Melanotic neuroectodermal tumor
M9370/3	Chordoma

M938-M948 Gliomas

M9380/3	Glioma, malignant
M9381/3	Gliomatosis cerebri
M9382/3	Mixed glioma
M9383/1	Subependymal glioma
M9384/1	Subependymal giant cell astrocytoma
M9390/0	Choroid plexus papilloma NOS
M9390/3	Choroid plexus papilloma, malignant
M9391/3	Ependymoma NOS
M9392/3	Ependymoma, anaplastic type
M9393/1	Papillary ependymoma
M9394/1	Myxopapillary ependymoma
M9400/3	Astrocytoma NOS
M9401/3	Astrocytoma, anaplastic type
M9410/3	Protoplasmic astrocytoma
M9411/3	Gemistocytic astrocytoma
M9420/3	Fibrillary astrocytoma
M9421/3	Pilocytic astrocytoma
M9422/3	Spongioblastoma NOS
M9423/3	Spongioblastoma polare
M9430/3	Astroblastoma

M9440/3	Glioblastoma NOS
M9441/3	Giant cell glioblastoma
M9442/3	Glioblastoma with sarcomatous component
M9443/3	Primitive polar spongioblastoma
M9450/3	Oligodendroglioma NOS
M9451/3	Oligodendroglioma, anaplastic type
M9460/3	Oligodendroblastoma
M9470/3	Medulloblastoma NOS
M9471/3	Desmoplastic medulloblastoma
M9472/3	Medullomyoblastoma
M9480/3	Cerebellar sarcoma NOS
M9481/3	Monstrocellular sarcoma

M949-M952 Neuroepitheliomatous neoplasms

M9490/0	Ganglioneuroma
M9490/3	Ganglioneuroblastoma
M9491/0	Ganglioneuromatosis
M9500/3	Neuroblastoma NOS
M9501/3	Medulloepithelioma NOS
M9502/3	Teratoid medulloepithelioma
M9503/3	Neuroepithelioma NOS
M9504/3	Spongioneuroblastoma
M9505/1	Ganglioglioma
M9506/0	Neurocytoma
M9507/0	Pacinian tumor
M9510/3	Retinoblastoma NOS
M9511/3	Retinoblastoma, differentiated type
M9512/3	Retinoblastoma, undifferentiated type
M9520/3	Olfactory neurogenic tumor
M9521/3	Esthesioneurocytoma
M9522/3	Esthesioneuroblastoma
M9523/3	Esthesioneuroepithelioma

M953 Meningiomas

M9530/0	Meningioma NOS
M9530/1	Meningiomatosis NOS
M9530/3	Meningioma, malignant
M9531/0	Meningotheliomatous meningioma
M9532/0	Fibrous meningioma
M9533/0	Psammomatous meningioma
M9534/0	Angiomatous meningioma
M9535/0	Hemangioblastic meningioma
M9536/0	Hemangiopericytic meningioma
M9537/0	Transitional meningioma
M9538/1	Papillary meningioma
M9539/3	Meningeal sarcomatosis

M954-M957 Nerve sheath tumor

M9540/0	Neurofibroma NOS
M9540/1	Neurofibromatosis NOS
M9540/3	Neurofibrosarcoma
M9541/0	Melanotic neurofibroma
M9550/0	Plexiform neurofibroma
M9560/0	Neurilemmoma NOS
M9560/1	Neurinomatosis
M9560/3	Neurilemmoma, malignant
M9570/0	Neuroma NOS

M958 Granular cell tumors and alveolar soft part sarcoma

M9580/0	Granular cell tumor NOS
M9580/3	Granular cell tumor, malignant
M9581/3	Alveolar soft part sarcoma

M959-M963 Lymphomas, NOS or diffuse

M9590/0	Lymphomatous tumor, benign
M9590/3	Malignant lymphoma NOS
M9591/3	Malignant lymphoma, non Hodgkin's type
M9600/3	Malignant lymphoma, undifferentiated cell type NOS
M9601/3	Malignant lymphoma, stem cell type

M9602/3	Malignant lymphoma, convoluted cell type NOS
M9610/3	Lymphosarcoma NOS
M9611/3	Malignant lymphoma, lymphoplasmacytoid type
M9612/3	Malignant lymphoma, immunoblastic type
M9613/3	Malignant lymphoma, mixed lymphocytic-histiocytic NOS
M9614/3	Malignant lymphoma, centroblastic-centrocytic, diffuse
M9615/3	Malignant lymphoma, follicular center cell NOS
M9620/3	Malignant lymphoma, lymphocytic, well differentiated NOS
M9621/3	Malignant lymphoma, lymphocytic, intermediate differentiation NOS
M9622/3	Malignant lymphoma, centrocytic
M9623/3	Malignant lymphoma, follicular center cell, cleaved NOS
M9630/3	Malignant lymphoma, lymphocytic, poorly differentiated NOS
M9631/3	Prolymphocytic lymphosarcoma
M9632/3	Malignant lymphoma, centroblastic type NOS
M9633/3	Malignant lymphoma, follicular center cell, noncleaved NOS

M964   *Reticulosarcomas*

M9640/3	Reticulosarcoma NOS
M9641/3	Reticulosarcoma, pleomorphic cell type
M9642/3	Reticulosarcoma, nodular

M965-M966   *Hodgkin's disease*

M9650/3	Hodgkin's disease NOS
M9651/3	Hodgkin's disease, lymphocytic predominance
M9652/3	Hodgkin's disease, mixed cellularity
M9653/3	Hodgkin's disease, lymphocytic depletion NOS
M9654/3	Hodgkin's disease, lymphocytic depletion, diffuse fibrosis
M9655/3	Hodgkin's disease, lymphocytic depletion, reticular type
M9656/3	Hodgkin's disease, nodular sclerosis NOS
M9657/3	Hodgkin's disease, nodular sclerosis, cellular phase
M9660/3	Hodgkin's paragranuloma
M9661/3	Hodgkin's granuloma
M9662/3	Hodgkin's sarcoma

M969   **Lymphomas, nodular or follicular**

M9690/3	Malignant lymphoma, nodular NOS
M9691/3	Malignant lymphoma, mixed lymphocytic-histiocytic, nodular
M9692/3	Malignant lymphoma, centroblastic-centrocytic, follicular
M9693/3	Malignant lymphoma, lymphocytic, well differentiated, nodular
M9694/3	Malignant lymphoma, lymphocytic, intermediate differentiation, nodular
M9695/3	Malignant lymphoma, follicular center cell, cleaved, follicular
M9696/3	Malignant lymphoma, lymphocytic, poorly differentiated, nodular
M9697/3	Malignant lymphoma, centroblastic type, follicular
M9698/3	Malignant lymphoma, follicular center cell, noncleaved, follicular

M970   **Mycosis fungoides**

M9700/3	Mycosis fungoides
M9701/3	Sezary's disease

M971-M972   **Miscellaneous reticuloendothelial neoplasms**

M9710/3	Microglioma
M9720/3	Malignant histiocytosis
M9721/3	Histiocytic medullary reticulosis
M9722/3	Letterer-Siwe's disease

M973   **Plasma cell tumors**

M9730/3	Plasma cell myeloma
M9731/0	Plasma cell tumor, benign
M9731/1	Plasmacytoma NOS
M9731/3	Plasma cell tumor, malignant

M974   **Mast cell tumors**

M9740/1	Mastocytoma NOS
M9740/3	Mast cell sarcoma
M9741/3	Malignant mastocytosis

M975   **Burkitt's tumor**

M9750/3	Burkitt's tumor

M980-M994   **Leukemias NOS**

M9800/3	Leukemias NOS
M9800/3	Leukemia NOS
M9801/3	Acute leukemia NOS
M9802/3	Subacute leukemia NOS
M9803/3	Chronic leukemia NOS
M9804/3	Aleukemic leukemia NOS

M981   **Compound leukemias**

M9810/3	Compound leukemia

M982   **Lymphoid leukemias**

M9820/3	Lymphoid leukemia NOS
M9821/3	Acute lymphoid leukemia
M9822/3	Subacute lymphoid leukemia
M9823/3	Chronic lymphoid leukemia
M9824/3	Aleukemic lymphoid leukemia
M9825/3	Prolymphocytic leukemia

M983   **Plasma cell leukemias**

M9830/3	Plasma cell leukemia

M984   **Erythroleukemias**

M9840/3	Erythroleukemia
M9841/3	Acute erythremia
M9842/3	Chronic erythremia

M985   **Lymphosarcoma cell leukemias**

M9850/3	Lymphosarcoma cell leukemia

M986   **Myeloid leukemias**

M9860/3	Myeloid leukemia NOS
M9861/3	Acute myeloid leukemia
M9862/3	Subacute myeloid leukemia
M9863/3	Chronic myeloid leukemia
M9864/3	Aleukemic myeloid leukemia
M9865/3	Neutrophilic leukemia
M9866/3	Acute promyelocytic leukemia

M987   **Basophilic leukemias**

M9870/3	Basophilic leukemia

M988   **Eosinophilic leukemias**

M9880/3	Eosinophilic leukemia

M989   **Monocytic leukemias**

M9890/3	Monocytic leukemia NOS
M9891/3	Acute monocytic leukemia
M9892/3	Subacute monocytic leukemia
M9893/3	Chronic monocytic leukemia
M9894/3	Aleukemic monocytic leukemia

M990-M994   **Miscellaneous leukemias**

M9900/3	Mast cell leukemia
M9910/3	Megakaryocytic leukemia
M9920/3	Megakaryocytic myelosis
M9930/3	Myeloid sarcoma
M9940/3	Hairy cell leukemia

M995-M997   **Miscellaneous myeloproliferative and lymphoproliferative disorders**

M9950/1	Polycythemia vera
M9951/1	Acute panmyelosis
M9960/1	Chronic myeloproliferative disease
M9961/1	Myelosclerosis with myeloid metaplasia
M9962/1	Idiopathic thrombocythemia
M9970/1	Chronic lymphoproliferative disease

Appendix B: Glossary of Mental Disorders

was officially deleted October 1, 2004

Appendix C: Classification of Drugs by American Hospital Formulary Service List Number and Their ICD-9-CM Equivalents

The coding of adverse effects of drugs is keyed to the continually revised Hospital Formulary of the American Hospital Formulary Service (AHFS) published under the direction of the American Society of Hospital Pharmacists.

The following section gives the ICD-9-CM diagnosis code for each AHFS list.

AHFS* List	ICD-9-CM Dx Code
4:00 ANTIHISTAMINE DRUGS	963.0
8:00 ANTI-INFECTIVE AGENTS	
8:04 Amebacides	961.5
hydroxyquinoline derivatives	961.3
arsenical anti-infectives	961.1
quinoline derivatives	961.3
8:12.04 Antifungal Antibiotics	960.1
nonantibiotics	961.9
8:12.06 Cephalosporins	960.5
8:12.08 Chloramphenicol	960.2
8:12.12 The Erythromycins	960.3
8:12.16 The Penicillins	960.0
8:12.20 The Streptomycins	960.6
8:12.24 The Tetracyclines	960.4
8:12.28 Other Antibiotics	960.8
antimycobacterial antibiotics	960.6
macrolides	960.3
8:16 Antituberculars	961.8
antibiotics	960.6
8:18 Antivirals	961.7
8:20 Plasmodicides (antimalarials)	961.4
8:24 Sulfonamides	961.0
8:26 The Sulfones	961.8
8:28 Treponemicides	961.2
8:32 Trichomonacides	961.5
hydroxyquinoline derivatives	961.3
nitrofuran derivatives	961.9
8:36 Urinary Germicides	961.9
quinoline derivatives	961.3
8:40 Other Anti-Infectives	961.9
10:00 ANTINEOPLASTIC AGENTS	963.1
antibiotics	960.7
progestogens	962.2
12:00 AUTONOMIC DRUGS	
12:04 Parasympathomimetic (Cholinergic) Agents	971.0
12:08 Parasympatholytic (Cholinergic Blocking Agents	971.1
12:12 Sympathomimetic (Adrenergic) Agents	971.2
12:16 Sympatholytic (Adrenergic Blocking) Agents	971.3
12:20 Skeletal Muscle Relaxants	975.2
central nervous system	
muscle-tone depressants	968.0
16:00 BLOOD DERIVATIVES	964.7
20:00 BLOOD FORMATION AND COAGULATION	
20:04 Antianemia Drugs	964.1
20:04.04 Iron Preparations	964.0
20:04.08 Liver and Stomach Preparations	964.1
20:12.04 Anticoagulants	964.2
20:12.08 Antiheparin Agents	964.5
20:12.12 Coagulants	964.5
20.12.16 Hemostatics	964.5
capillary-active drugs	972.8
fibrinolysis-affecting agents	964.4
natural products	964.7
24:00 CARDIOVASCULAR DRUGS	
24:04 Cardiac Drugs	972.9
cardiotonic agents	972.1
rhythm regulators	972.0
24:06 Antilipemic Agents	972.2
thyroid derivatives	962.7

AHFS* List	ICD-9-CM Dx Code
24:08 Hypotensive Agents	972.6
adrenergic blocking agents	971.3
ganglion-blocking agents	972.3
vasodilators	972.5
24:12 Vasodilating Agents	972.5
coronary	972.4
nicotinic acid derivatives	972.2
24:16 Sclerosing Agents	972.7
28:00 CENTRAL NERVOUS SYSTEM DRUGS	
28:04 General Anesthetics	968.4
gaseous anesthetics	968.2
halothane	968.1
intravenous anesthetics	968.3
28:08 Analgesics and Antipyretics	965.9
antirheumatics	965.61-965.69
aromatic analgesics	965.4
non-narcotics NEC	965.7
opium alkaloids	965.00
heroin	965.01
methadone	965.02
specified type NEC	965.09
pyrazole derivatives	965.5
salicylates	965.1
specified type NEC	965.8
28:10 Narcotic Antagonists	970.1
28:12 Anticonvulsants	966.3
barbiturates	967.0
benzodiazepine-based tranquilizers	969.4
bromides	967.3
hydantoin derivatives	966.1
oxazolidine derivative	966.0
succinimides	966.2
28:16.04 Antidepressants	969.00-969.09
28:16.08 Tranquilizers	969.5
benzodiazepine-based	969.4
butyrophenone-based	969.2
major NEC	969.3
phenothiazine-based	969.1
28:16.12 Other Psychotherapeutic Agents	969.8
28:20 Respiratory and Cerebral Stimulants	970.9
analeptics	970.0
anorexigenic agents	977.0
psychostimulants	969.70-969.79
specified type NEC	970.8
28:24 Sedatives and Hypnotics	967.9
barbiturates	967.0
benzodiazepine-based tranquilizers	969.4
chloral hydrate group	967.1
glutethamide group	967.5
intravenous anesthetics	968.3
methaqualone	967.4
paraldehyde	967.2
phenothiazine-based tranquilizers	969.1
specified type NEC	967.8
thiobarbiturates	968.3
tranquilizer NEC	969.5
36:00 DIAGNOSTIC AGENTS	977.8
40:00 ELECTROLYTE, CALORIC, AND WATER BALANCE AGENTS NEC	974.5
40:04 Acidifying Agents	963.2
40:08 Alkalinizing Agents	963.3
40:10 Ammonia Detoxicants	974.5
40:12 Replacement Solutions NEC	974.5
plasma volume expanders	964.8
40:16 Sodium-Removing Resins	974.5
40:18 Potassium-Removing Resins	974.5
40:20 Caloric Agents	974.5
40:24 Salt and Sugar Substitutes	974.5
40:28 Diuretics NEC	974.4
carbonic acid anhydrase inhibitors	974.2
mercurials	974.0
purine derivatives	974.1
saluretics	974.3

AHFS* List		ICD-9-CM Dx Code		AHFS* List		ICD-9-CM Dx Code
40:36	Irrigating Solutions	974.5		68:34	Other Corpus Luteum Hormones	962.2
40:40	Uricosuric Agents	974.7		68:36	Thyroid and Antithyroid	
44:00	ENZYMES NEC	963.4			antithyroid	962.8
	fibrinolysis-affecting agents	964.4			thyroid	962.7
	gastric agents	973.4		72:00	LOCAL ANESTHETICS NEC	968.9
48:00	EXPECTORANTS AND COUGH PREPARATIONS				topical (surface) agents	968.5
	antihistamine agents	963.0			infiltrating agents (intradermal)	
	antitussives	975.4			(subcutaneous) (submucosal)	968.5
	codeine derivatives	965.09			nerve blocking agents (peripheral) (plexus) (regional)	968.6
	expectorants	975.5			spinal	968.7
	narcotic agents NEC	965.09		76:00	OXYTOCICS	975.0
52:00	EYE, EAR, NOSE, AND THROAT PREPARATIONS			78:00	RADIOACTIVE AGENTS	990
52:04	Anti-Infectives			80:00	SERUMS, TOXOIDS, AND VACCINES	
	ENT	976.6		80:04	Serums	979.9
	ophthalmic	976.5			immune globulin (gamma) (human)	964.6
52:04.04	Antibiotics			80:08	Toxoids NEC	978.8
	ENT	976.6			diphtheria	978.5
	ophthalmic	976.5			and tetanus	978.9
52:04.06	Antivirals				with pertussis component	978.6
	ENT	976.6			tetanus	978.4
	ophthalmic	976.5			and diphtheria	978.9
52:04.08	Sulfonamides				with pertussis component	978.6
	ENT	976.6		80:12	Vaccines NEC	979.9
	ophthalmic	976.5			bacterial NEC	978.8
52:04.12	Miscellaneous Anti-Infectives				with other bacterial component	978.9
	ENT	976.6			pertussis component	978.6
	ophthalmic	976.5			viral and rickettsial component	979.7
52:08	Anti-Inflammatory Agents				rickettsial NEC	979.6
	ENT	976.6			with bacterial component	979.7
	ophthalmic	976.5			pertussis component	978.6
52:10	Carbonic Anhydrase Inhibitors	974.2			viral component	979.7
52:12	Contact Lens Solutions	976.5			viral NEC	979.6
52:16	Local Anesthetics	968.5			with bacterial component	979.7
52:20	Miotics	971.0			pertussis component	978.6
52:24	Mydriatics				rickettsial component	979.7
	adrenergics	971.2		84:00	SKIN AND MUCOUS MEMBRANE PREPARATIONS	
	anticholinergics	971.1		84:04	Anti-Infectives	976.0
	antimuscarinics	971.1		84:04.04	Antibiotics	976.0
	parasympatholytics	971.1		84:04.08	Fungicides	976.0
	spasmolytics	971.1		84:04.12	Scabicides and Pediculicides	976.0
	sympathomimetics	971.2		84:04.16	Miscellaneous Local Anti-Infectives	976.0
52:28	Mouth Washes and Gargles	976.6		84:06	Anti-Inflammatory Agents	976.0
52:32	Vasoconstrictors	971.2		84:08	Antipruritics and Local Anesthetics	
52:36	Unclassified Agents				antipruritics	976.1
	ENT	976.6			local anesthetics	968.5
	ophthalmic	976.5		84:12	Astringents	976.2
56:00	GASTROINTESTINAL DRUGS			84:16	Cell Stimulants and Proliferants	976.8
56:04	Antacids and Absorbents	973.0		84:20	Detergents	976.2
56:08	Anti-Diarrhea Agents	973.5		84:24	Emollients, Demulcents, and Protectants	976.3
56:10	Antiflatulents	973.8		84:28	Keratolytic Agents	976.4
56:12	Cathartics NEC	973.3		84:32	Keratoplastic Agents	976.4
	emollients	973.2		84:36	Miscellaneous Agents	976.8
	irritants	973.1		86:00	SPASMOLYTIC AGENTS	975.1
56:16	Digestants	973.4			antiasthmatics	975.7
56:20	Emetics and Antiemetics				papaverine	972.5
	antiemetics	963.0			theophyllin	974.1
	emetics	973.6		88:00	VITAMINS	
56:24	Lipotropic Agents	977.1		88:04	Vitamin A	963.5
60:00	GOLD COMPOUNDS	965.69		88:08	Vitamin B Complex	963.5
64:00	HEAVY METAL ANTAGONISTS	963.8			hematopoietic vitamin	964.1
68:00	HORMONES AND SYNTHETIC SUBSTITUTES				nicotinic acid derivatives	972.2
68:04	Adrenals	962.0		88:12	Vitamin C	963.5
68:08	Androgens	962.1		88:16	Vitamin D	963.5
68:12	Contraceptives	962.2		88:20	Vitamin E	963.5
68:16	Estrogens	962.2		88:24	Vitamin K Activity	964.3
68:18	Gonadotropins	962.4		88:28	Multivitamin Preparations	963.5
68:20	Insulins and Antidiabetic Agents	962.3		92:00	UNCLASSIFIED THERAPEUTIC AGENTS	977.8
68:20.08	Insulins	962.3		* American Hospital Formulary Service		
68:24	Parathyroid	962.6				
68:28	Pituitary					
	anterior	962.4				
	posterior	962.5				
68:32	Progestogens	962.2				

Appendix D: Classification of Industrial Accidents According to Agency

Annex B to the Resolution concerning Statistics of Employment Injuries adopted by the Tenth International Conference of Labor Statisticians on 12 October 1962

1 Machines

11	Prime-Movers, except Electrical Motors
111	Steam engines
112	Internal combustion engines
119	Others
12	Transmission Machinery
121	Transmission shafts
122	Transmission belts, cables, pulleys, pinions, chains, gears
129	Others
13	Metalworking Machines
131	Power presses
132	Lathes
133	Milling machines
134	Abrasive wheels
135	Mechanical shears
136	Forging machines
137	Rolling-mills
139	Others
14	Wood and Assimilated Machines
141	Circular saws
142	Other saws
143	Molding machines
144	Overhand planes
149	Others
15	Agricultural Machines
151	Reapers (including combine reapers)
152	Threshers
159	Others
16	Mining Machinery
161	Under-cutters
169	Others
19	Other Machines Not Elsewhere Classified
191	Earth-moving machines, excavating and scraping machines, except means of transport
192	Spinning, weaving and other textile machines
193	Machines for the manufacture of food- stuffs and beverages
194	Machines for the manufacture of paper
195	Printing machines
199	Others

2 Means of Transport and Lifting Equipment

21	Lifting Machines and Appliances
211	Cranes
212	Lifts and elevators
213	Winches
214	Pulley blocks
219	Others
22	Means of Rail Transport
221	Inter-urban railways
222	Rail transport in mines, tunnels, quarries, industrial establishments, docks, etc.
229	Others
23	Other Wheeled Means of Transport, Excluding Rail Transport
231	Tractors
232	Lorries
233	Trucks
234	Motor vehicles, not elsewhere classified
235	Animal-drawn vehicles
236	Hand-drawn vehicles
239	Others
24	Means of Air Transport
25	Means of Water Transport
251	Motorized means of water transport
252	Non-motorized means of water transport
26	Other Means of Transport
261	Cable-cars
262	Mechanical conveyors, except cable-cars
269	Others

3 Other Equipment

31	Pressure Vessels
311	Boilers
312	Pressurized containers
313	Pressurized piping and accessories
314	Gas cylinders
315	Caissons, diving equipment
319	Others
32	Furnaces, Ovens, Kilns
321	Blast furnaces
322	Refining furnaces
323	Other furnaces
324	Kilns
325	Ovens
33	Refrigerating Plants
34	Electrical Installations, Including Electric Motors, but Excluding Electric Hand Tools
341	Rotating machines
342	Conductors
343	Transformers
344	Control apparatus
349	Others
35	Electric Hand Tools
36	Tools, Implements, and Appliances, Except Electric Hand Tools
361	Power-driven hand tools, except electrichand tools
362	Hand tools, not power-driven
369	Others
37	Ladders, Mobile Ramps
38	Scaffolding
39	Other Equipment, Not Elsewhere Classified

4 Materials, Substances and Radiations

41	Explosives
42	Dusts, Gases, Liquids and Chemicals, Excluding Explosives
421	Dusts
422	Gases, vapors, fumes
423	Liquids, not elsewhere classified
424	Chemicals, not elsewhere classified
43	Flying Fragments
44	Radiations
441	Ionizing radiations
449	Others
49	Other Materials and Substances Not Elsewhere Classified

5 Working Environment

51	Outdoor
511	Weather
512	Traffic and working surfaces
513	Water
519	Others
52	Indoor
521	Floors
522	Confined quarters
523	Stairs
524	Other traffic and working surfaces
525	Floor openings and wall openings
526	Environmental factors (lighting, ventilation, temperature, noise, etc.)
529	Others
53	Underground
531	Roofs and faces of mine roads and tunnels, etc.
532	Floors of mine roads and tunnels, etc.
533	Working-faces of mines, tunnels, etc.
534	Mine shafts
535	Fire
536	Water
539	Others

6 Other Agencies, Not Elsewhere Classified

61	Animals
611	Live animals
612	Animal products
69	Other Agencies, Not Elsewhere Classified

7 Agencies Not Classified for Lack of Sufficient Data

Appendix E: List of Three-digit Categories

1. Infectious and Parasitic Diseases

Intestinal infectious diseases (001-009)
001 Cholera
002 Typhoid and paratyphoid fevers
003 Other salmonella infections
004 Shigellosis
005 Other food poisoning (bacterial)
006 Amebiasis
007 Other protozoal intestinal diseases
008 Intestinal infections due to other organisms
009 Ill-defined intestinal infections

Tuberculosis (010-018)
010 Primary tuberculous infection
011 Pulmonary tuberculosis
012 Other respiratory tuberculosis
013 Tuberculosis of meninges and central nervous system
014 Tuberculosis of intestines, peritoneum, and mesenteric glands
015 Tuberculosis of bones and joints
016 Tuberculosis of genitourinary system
017 Tuberculosis of other organs
018 Miliary tuberculosis

Zoonotic bacterial diseases (020-027)
020 Plague
021 Tularemia
022 Anthrax
023 Brucellosis
024 Glanders
025 Melioidosis
026 Rat-bite fever
027 Other zoonotic bacterial diseases

Other bacterial diseases (030-041)
030 Leprosy
031 Diseases due to other mycobacteria
032 Diphtheria
033 Whooping cough
034 Streptococcal sore throat and scarlet fever
035 Erysipelas
036 Meningococcal infection
037 Tetanus
038 Septicemia
039 Actinomycotic infections
040 Other bacterial diseases
041 Bacterial infection in conditions classified elsewhere and of unspecified site

Human immunodeficiency virus (042)
042 Human immunodeficiency virus [HIV] disease

Poliomyelitis and other non-arthropod-borne viral diseases and prion diseases of central nervous system (045-049)
045 Acute poliomyelitis
046 Slow virus infections and prion diseases of central nervous system
047 Meningitis due to enterovirus
048 Other enterovirus diseases of central nervous system
049 Other non-arthropod-borne viral diseases of central nervous system

Viral diseases generally accompanied by exanthem (050-059)
050 Smallpox
051 Cowpox and paravaccinia
052 Chickenpox
053 Herpes zoster
054 Herpes simplex
055 Measles
056 Rubella
057 Other viral exanthemata
058 Other human herpesvirus
059 Other poxvirus infections

Arthropod-borne viral diseases (060-066)
060 Yellow fever
061 Dengue
062 Mosquito-borne viral encephalitis
063 Tick-borne viral encephalitis
064 Viral encephalitis transmitted by other and unspecified arthropods
065 Arthropod-borne hemorrhagic fever
066 Other arthropod-borne viral diseases

Other diseases due to viruses and Chlamydiae (070-079)
070 Viral hepatitis
071 Rabies
072 Mumps
073 Ornithosis
074 Specific diseases due to Coxsackie virus
075 Infectious mononucleosis
076 Trachoma
077 Other diseases of conjunctiva due to viruses and Chlamydiae
078 Other diseases due to viruses and Chlamydiae
079 Viral and chlamydial infection in conditions classified elsewhere and of unspecified site

Rickettsioses and other arthropod-borne diseases (080-088)
080 Louse-borne [epidemic] typhus
081 Other typhus
082 Tick-borne rickettsioses
083 Other rickettsioses
084 Malaria
085 Leishmaniasis
086 Trypanosomiasis
087 Relapsing fever
088 Other arthropod-borne diseases

Syphilis and other venereal diseases (090-099)
090 Congenital syphilis
091 Early syphilis, symptomatic
092 Early syphilis, latent
093 Cardiovascular syphilis
094 Neurosyphilis
095 Other forms of late syphilis, with symptoms
096 Late syphilis, latent
097 Other and unspecified syphilis
098 Gonococcal infections
099 Other venereal diseases

Other spirochetal diseases (100-104)
100 Leptospirosis
101 Vincent's angina
102 Yaws
103 Pinta
104 Other spirochetal infection

Mycoses (110-118)
110 Dermatophytosis
111 Dermatomycosis, other and unspecified
112 Candidiasis
114 Coccidioidomycosis
115 Histoplasmosis
116 Blastomycotic infection
117 Other mycoses
118 Opportunistic mycoses

Helminthiases (120-129)
120 Schistosomiasis [bilharziasis]
121 Other trematode infections
122 Echinococcosis
123 Other cestode infection
124 Trichinosis
125 Filarial infection and dracontiasis
126 Ancylostomiasis and necatoriasis
127 Other intestinal helminthiases
128 Other and unspecified helminthiases
129 Intestinal parasitism, unspecified

Other infectious and parasitic diseases (130-136)
130 Toxoplasmosis
131 Trichomoniasis
132 Pediculosis and phthirus infestation
133 Acariasis
134 Other infestation
135 Sarcoidosis
136 Other and unspecified infectious and parasitic diseases

Late effects of infectious and parasitic diseases (137-139)
137 Late effects of tuberculosis
138 Late effects of acute poliomyelitis
139 Late effects of other infectious and parasitic diseases

2. Neoplasms

Malignant neoplasm of lip, oral cavity, and pharynx (140-149)
140 Malignant neoplasm of lip
141 Malignant neoplasm of tongue
142 Malignant neoplasm of major salivary glands
143 Malignant neoplasm of gum
144 Malignant neoplasm of floor of mouth
145 Malignant neoplasm of other and unspecified parts of mouth
146 Malignant neoplasm of oropharynx
147 Malignant neoplasm of nasopharynx
148 Malignant neoplasm of hypopharynx
149 Malignant neoplasm of other and ill-defined sites within the lip, oral cavity, and pharynx

Malignant neoplasm of digestive organs and peritoneum (150-159)
150 Malignant neoplasm of esophagus
151 Malignant neoplasm of stomach
152 Malignant neoplasm of small intestine, including duodenum
153 Malignant neoplasm of colon
154 Malignant neoplasm of rectum, rectosigmoid junction, and anus
155 Malignant neoplasm of liver and intrahepatic bile ducts
156 Malignant neoplasm of gallbladder and extrahepatic bile ducts
157 Malignant neoplasm of pancreas
158 Malignant neoplasm of retroperitoneum and peritoneum
159 Malignant neoplasm of other and ill-defined sites within the digestive organs and peritoneum

Malignant neoplasm of respiratory and intrathoracic organs (160-165)
160 Malignant neoplasm of nasal cavities, middle ear, and accessory sinuses
161 Malignant neoplasm of larynx
162 Malignant neoplasm of trachea, bronchus, and lung
163 Malignant neoplasm of pleura
164 Malignant neoplasm of thymus, heart, and mediastinum
165 Malignant neoplasm of other and ill-defined sites within the respiratory system and intrathoracic organs

Malignant neoplasm of bone, connective tissue, skin, and breast (170-176)
170 Malignant neoplasm of bone and articular cartilage
171 Malignant neoplasm of connective and other soft tissue
172 Malignant melanoma of skin
173 Other and unspecified malignant neoplasm of skin
174 Malignant neoplasm of female breast
175 Malignant neoplasm of male breast
176 Kaposi's sarcoma

Malignant neoplasm of genitourinary organs (179-189)
179 Malignant neoplasm of uterus, part unspecified
180 Malignant neoplasm of cervix uteri
181 Malignant neoplasm of placenta
182 Malignant neoplasm of body of uterus
183 Malignant neoplasm of ovary and other uterine adnexa
184 Malignant neoplasm of other and unspecified female genital organs
185 Malignant neoplasm of prostate
186 Malignant neoplasm of testis
187 Malignant neoplasm of penis and other male genital organs
188 Malignant neoplasm of bladder
189 Malignant neoplasm of kidney and other unspecified urinary organs

Malignant neoplasm of other and unspecified sites (190-199)
190 Malignant neoplasm of eye
191 Malignant neoplasm of brain
192 Malignant neoplasm of other and unspecified parts of nervous system
193 Malignant neoplasm of thyroid gland
194 Malignant neoplasm of other endocrine glands and related structures
195 Malignant neoplasm of other and ill-defined sites
196 Secondary and unspecified malignant neoplasm of lymph nodes
197 Secondary malignant neoplasm of respiratory and digestive systems
198 Secondary malignant neoplasm of other specified sites
199 Malignant neoplasm without specification of site

Malignant neoplasm of lymphatic and hematopoietic tissue (200-208)
200 Lymphosarcoma and reticulosarcoma and other specified malignant tumors of lymphatic tissue
201 Hodgkin's disease
202 Other malignant neoplasm of lymphoid and histiocytic tissue
203 Multiple myeloma and immunoproliferative neoplasms
204 Lymphoid leukemia
205 Myeloid leukemia
206 Monocytic leukemia
207 Other specified leukemia
208 Leukemia of unspecified cell type

Neuroendocrine tumors (209)
209 Neuroendocrine tumors

Benign neoplasms (210-229)
210 Benign neoplasm of lip, oral cavity, and pharynx
211 Benign neoplasm of other parts of digestive system
212 Benign neoplasm of respiratory and intrathoracic organs
213 Benign neoplasm of bone and articular cartilage
214 Lipoma
215 Other benign neoplasm of connective and other soft tissue
216 Benign neoplasm of skin
217 Benign neoplasm of breast
218 Uterine leiomyoma
219 Other benign neoplasm of uterus
220 Benign neoplasm of ovary
221 Benign neoplasm of other female genital organs
222 Benign neoplasm of male genital organs
223 Benign neoplasm of kidney and other urinary organs
224 Benign neoplasm of eye
225 Benign neoplasm of brain and other parts of nervous system
226 Benign neoplasm of thyroid gland

227 Benign neoplasm of other endocrine glands and related structures
228 Hemangioma and lymphangioma, any site
229 Benign neoplasm of other and unspecified sites

Carcinoma in situ (230-234)
230 Carcinoma in situ of digestive organs
231 Carcinoma in situ of respiratory system
232 Carcinoma in situ of skin
233 Carcinoma in situ of breast and genitourinary system
234 Carcinoma in situ of other and unspecified sites

Neoplasms of uncertain behavior (235-238)
235 Neoplasm of uncertain behavior of digestive and respiratory systems
236 Neoplasm of uncertain behavior of genitourinary organs
237 Neoplasm of uncertain behavior of endocrine glands and nervous system
238 Neoplasm of uncertain behavior of other and unspecified sites and tissues

Neoplasms of unspecified nature (239)
239 Neoplasm of unspecified nature

3. Endocrine, Nutritional and Metabolic Diseases, and Immunity Disorders

Disorders of thyroid gland (240-246)
240 Simple and unspecified goiter
241 Nontoxic nodular goiter
242 Thyrotoxicosis with or without goiter
243 Congenital hypothyroidism
244 Acquired hypothyroidism
245 Thyroiditis
246 Other disorders of thyroid

Diseases of other endocrine glands (249-259)
249 Secondary diabetes mellitus
250 Diabetes mellitus
251 Other disorders of pancreatic internal secretion
252 Disorders of parathyroid gland
253 Disorders of the pituitary gland and its hypothalamic control
254 Diseases of thymus gland
255 Disorders of adrenal glands
256 Ovarian dysfunction
257 Testicular dysfunction
258 Polyglandular dysfunction and related disorders
259 Other endocrine disorders

Nutritional deficiencies (260-269)
260 Kwashiorkor
261 Nutritional marasmus
262 Other severe protein-calorie malnutrition
263 Other and unspecified protein-calorie malnutrition
264 Vitamin A deficiency
265 Thiamine and niacin deficiency states
266 Deficiency of B-complex components
267 Ascorbic acid deficiency
268 Vitamin D deficiency
269 Other nutritional deficiencies

Other metabolic disorders and immnity disorders (270-279)
270 Disorders of amino-acid transport and metabolism
271 Disorders of carbohydrate transport and metabolism
272 Disorders of lipoid metabolism
273 Disorders of plasma protein metabolism
274 Gout
275 Disorders of mineral metabolism
276 Disorders of fluid, electrolyte, and acid-base balance
277 Other and unspecified disorders of metabolism

278 Overweight, obesity and other hyperalimentation
279 Disorders involving the immune mechanism

4. Diseases of Blood and Blood-forming Organs (280-289)
280 Iron deficiency anemias
281 Other deficiency anemias
282 Hereditary hemolytic anemias
283 Acquired hemolytic anemias
284 Aplastic anemia and other bone marrow failure syndromes
285 Other and unspecified anemias
286 Coagulation defects
287 Purpura and other hemorrhagic conditions
288 Diseases of white blood cells
289 Other diseases of blood and blood-forming organs

5. Mental, Behavioral and Neurodevelopmental Disorders

Organic psychotic conditions (290-294)
290 Dementias
291 Alcoholic induced mental disorders
292 Drug induced mental disorders
293 Transient mental disorders due to conditions classified elsewhere
294 Persistent mental disorders due to conditions classified elsewhere

Other psychoses (295-299)
295 Schizophrenic disorders
296 Episodic mood disorders
297 Delusional disorders
298 Other nonorganic psychoses
299 Pervasive developmental disorders

Neurotic disorders, personality disorders, and other nonpsychotic mental disorders (300-316)
300 Anxiety, dissociative and somatoform disorders
301 Personality disorders
302 Sexual and gender identity disorders
303 Alcohol dependence syndrome
304 Drug dependence
305 Nondependent abuse of drugs
306 Physiological malfunction arising from mental factors
307 Special symptoms or syndromes, not elsewhere classified
308 Acute reaction to stress
309 Adjustment reaction
310 Specific nonpsychotic mental disorders due to brain damage
311 Depressive disorder, not elsewhere classified
312 Disturbance of conduct, not elsewhere classified
313 Disturbance of emotions specific to childhood and adolescence
314 Hyperkinetic syndrome of childhood
315 Specific delays in development
316 Psychic factors associated with diseases classified elsewhere

Intellectual Disabilities (317-319)
317 Mild intellectual disabilities
318 Other specified intellectual disabilities
319 Unspecified intellectual disabilities

6. Diseases of the Nervous System and Sense Organs

Inflammatory diseases of the central nervous system (320-326)
320 Bacterial meningitis
321 Meningitis due to other organisms
322 Meningitis of unspecified cause
323 Encephalitis, myelitis, and encephalomyelitis

324   Intracranial and intraspinal abscess
325   Phlebitis and thrombophlebitis of intracranial venous sinuses
326   Late effects of intracranial abscess or pyogenic infection

Organic Sleep Disorders (327)
327   Organic sleep disorders

Hereditary and degenerative diseases of the central nervous system (330-337)
330   Cerebral degenerations usually manifest in childhood
331   Other cerebral degenerations
332   Parkinson's disease
333   Other extrapyramidal diseases and abnormal movement disorders
334   Spinocerebellar disease
335   Anterior horn cell disease
336   Other diseases of spinal cord
337   Disorders of the autonomic nervous system

Pain (338)
338   Pain, not elsewhere classified

Other headache syndromes (339)
339   Other headache syndromes

Other disorders of the central nervous system (340-349)
340   Multiple sclerosis
341   Other demyelinating diseases of central nervous system
342   Hemiplegia and hemiparesis
343   Infantile cerebral palsy
344   Other paralytic syndromes
345   Epilepsy and recurrent seizures
346   Migraine
347   Cataplexy and narcolepsy
348   Other conditions of brain
349   Other and unspecified disorders of the nervous system

Disorders of the peripheral nervous system (350-359)
350   Trigeminal nerve disorders
351   Facial nerve disorders
352   Disorders of other cranial nerves
353   Nerve root and plexus disorders
354   Mononeuritis of upper limb and mononeuritis multiplex
355   Mononeuritis of lower limb
356   Hereditary and idiopathic peripheral neuropathy
357   Inflammatory and toxic neuropathy
358   Myoneural disorders
359   Muscular dystrophies and other myopathies

Disorders of the eye and adnexa (360-379)
360   Disorders of the globe
361   Retinal detachments and defects
362   Other retinal disorders
363   Chorioretinal inflammations and scars and other disorders of choroid
364   Disorders of iris and ciliary body
365   Glaucoma
366   Cataract
367   Disorders of refraction and accommodation
368   Visual disturbances
369   Blindness and low vision
370   Keratitis
371   Corneal opacity and other disorders of cornea
372   Disorders of conjunctiva
373   Inflammation of eyelids
374   Other disorders of eyelids
375   Disorders of lacrimal system
376   Disorders of the orbit
377   Disorders of optic nerve and visual pathways
378   Strabismus and other disorders of binocular eye movements
379   Other disorders of eye

Diseases of the ear and mastoid process (380-389)
380   Disorders of external ear
381   Nonsuppurative otitis media and Eustachian tube disorders
382   Suppurative and unspecified otitis media
383   Mastoiditis and related conditions
384   Other disorders of tympanic membrane
385   Other disorders of middle ear and mastoid
386   Vertiginous syndromes and other disorders of vestibular system
387   Otosclerosis
388   Other disorders of ear
389   Hearing loss

7. Diseases of the Circulatory System

Acute rheumatic fever (390-392)
390   Rheumatic fever without mention of heart involvement
391   Rheumatic fever with heart involvement
392   Rheumatic chorea

Chronic rheumatic heart disease (393-398)
393   Chronic rheumatic pericarditis
394   Diseases of mitral valve
395   Diseases of aortic valve
396   Diseases of mitral and aortic valves
397   Diseases of other endocardial structures
398   Other rheumatic heart disease

Hypertensive disease (401-405)
401   Essential hypertension
402   Hypertensive heart disease
403   Hypertensive chronic kidney disease
404   Hypertensive heart and chronic kidney disease
405   Secondary hypertension

Ischemic heart disease (410-414)
410   Acute myocardial infarction
411   Other acute and subacute forms of ischemic heart disease
412   Old myocardial infarction
413   Angina pectoris
414   Other forms of chronic ischemic heart disease

Diseases of pulmonary circulation (415-417)
415   Acute pulmonary heart disease
416   Chronic pulmonary heart disease
417   Other diseases of pulmonary circulation

Other forms of heart disease (420-429)
420   Acute pericarditis
421   Acute and subacute endocarditis
422   Acute myocarditis
423   Other diseases of pericardium
424   Other diseases of endocardium
425   Cardiomyopathy
426   Conduction disorders
427   Cardiac dysrhythmias
428   Heart failure
429   Ill-defined descriptions and complications of heart disease

Cerebrovascular disease (430-438)
430   Subarachnoid hemorrhage
431   Intracerebral hemorrhage
432   Other and unspecified intracranial hemorrhage
433   Occlusion and stenosis of precerebral arteries
434   Occlusion of cerebral arteries
435   Transient cerebral ischemia
436   Acute, but ill-defined, cerebrovascular disease
437   Other and ill-defined cerebrovascular disease
438   Late effects of cerebrovascular disease

Diseases of arteries, arterioles, and capillaries (440-449)
440   Atherosclerosis
441   Aortic aneurysm and dissection
442   Other aneurysm
443   Other peripheral vascular disease
444   Arterial embolism and thrombosis
445   Atheroembolism
446   Polyarteritis nodosa and allied conditions
447   Other disorders of arteries and arterioles
448   Diseases of capillaries
449   Septic arterial embolism

Diseases of veins and lymphatics, and other diseases of circulatory system (451-459)
451   Phlebitis and thrombophlebitis
452   Portal vein thrombosis
453   Other venous embolism and thrombosis
454   Varicose veins of lower extremities
455   Hemorrhoids
456   Varicose veins of other sites
457   Noninfectious disorders of lymphatic channels
458   Hypotension
459   Other disorders of circulatory system

8. Diseases of the Respiratory System

Acute respiratory infections (460-466)
460   Acute nasopharyngitis [common cold]
461   Acute sinusitis
462   Acute pharyngitis
463   Acute tonsillitis
464   Acute laryngitis and tracheitis
465   Acute upper respiratory infections of multiple or unspecified sites
466   Acute bronchitis and bronchiolitis

Other diseases of upper respiratory tract (470-478)
470   Deviated nasal septum
471   Nasal polyps
472   Chronic pharyngitis and nasopharyngitis
473   Chronic sinusitis
474   Chronic disease of tonsils and adenoids
475   Peritonsillar abscess
476   Chronic laryngitis and laryngotracheitis
477   Allergic rhinitis
478   Other diseases of upper respiratory tract

Pneumonia and influenza (480-488)
480   Viral pneumonia
481   Pneumococcal pneumonia [Streptococcus pneumoniae pneumonia]
482   Other bacterial pneumonia
483   Pneumonia due to other specified organism
484   Pneumonia in infectious diseases classified elsewhere
485   Bronchopneumonia, organism unspecified
486   Pneumonia, organism unspecified
487   Influenza
488   Influenza due to certain identified influenza viruses

Chronic obstructive pulmonary disease and allied conditions (490-496)
490   Bronchitis, not specified as acute or chronic
491   Chronic bronchitis
492   Emphysema
493   Asthma
494   Bronchiectasis
495   Extrinsic allergic alveolitis
496   Chronic airways obstruction, not elsewhere classified

Pneumoconioses and other lung diseases due to external agents (500-508)
500   Coal workers' pneumoconiosis
501   Asbestosis
502   Pneumoconiosis due to other silica or silicates
503   Pneumoconiosis due to other inorganic dust
504   Pneumopathy due to inhalation of other dust
505   Pneumoconiosis, unspecified
506   Respiratory conditions due to chemical fumes and vapors
507   Pneumonitis due to solids and liquids
508   Respiratory conditions due to other and unspecified external agents

Other diseases of respiratory system (510-519)
510 Empyema
511 Pleurisy
512 Pneumothorax and air leak
513 Abscess of lung and mediastinum
514 Pulmonary congestion and hypostasis
515 Postinflammatory pulmonary fibrosis
516 Other alveolar and parietoalveolar pneumopathy
517 Lung involvement in conditions classified elsewhere
518 Other diseases of lung
519 Other diseases of respiratory system

9. Diseases of the Digestive System

Diseases of oral cavity, salivary glands, and jaws (520-529)
520 Disorders of tooth development and eruption
521 Diseases of hard tissues of teeth
522 Diseases of pulp and periapical tissues
523 Gingival and periodontal diseases
524 Dentofacial anomalies, including malocclusion
525 Other diseases and conditions of the teeth and supporting structures
526 Diseases of the jaws
527 Diseases of the salivary glands
528 Diseases of the oral soft tissues, excluding lesions specific for gingiva and tongue
529 Diseases and other conditions of the tongue

Diseases of esophagus, stomach, and duodenum (530-539)
530 Diseases of esophagus
531 Gastric ulcer
532 Duodenal ulcer
533 Peptic ulcer, site unspecified
534 Gastrojejunal ulcer
535 Gastritis and duodenitis
536 Disorders of function of stomach
537 Other disorders of stomach and duodenum
538 Gastrointestinal mucositis (ulcerative)
539 Complications of bariatric procedures

Appendicitis (540-543)
540 Acute appendicitis
541 Appendicitis, unqualified
542 Other appendicitis
543 Other diseases of appendix

Hernia of abdominal cavity (550-553)
550 Inguinal hernia
551 Other hernia of abdominal cavity, with gangrene
552 Other hernia of abdominal cavity, with obstruction, but without mention of gangrene
553 Other hernia of abdominal cavity without mention of obstruction or gangrene

Noninfective enteritis and colitis (555-558)
555 Regional enteritis
556 Ulcerative colitis
557 Vascular insufficiency of intestine
558 Other noninfective gastroenteritis and colitis

Other diseases of intestines and peritoneum (560-569)
560 Intestinal obstruction without mention of hernia
562 Diverticula of intestine
564 Functional digestive disorders, not elsewhere classified
565 Anal fissure and fistula
566 Abscess of anal and rectal regions
567 Peritonitis and retroperitoneal infections
568 Other disorders of peritoneum
569 Other disorders of intestine

Other diseases of digestive system (570-579)
570 Acute and subacute necrosis of liver
571 Chronic liver disease and cirrhosis
572 Liver abscess and sequelae of chronic liver disease
573 Other disorders of liver
574 Cholelithiasis
575 Other disorders of gallbladder
576 Other disorders of biliary tract
577 Diseases of pancreas
578 Gastrointestinal hemorrhage
579 Intestinal Malabsorption

10. Diseases of the Genitourinary System

Nephritis, nephrotic syndrome, and nephrosis (580-589)
580 Acute gloerulonephritis
581 Nephrotic syndrome
582 Chronic glomerulonephritis
583 Nephritis and nephropathy, not specified as acute or chronic
584 Acute kidney failure
585 Chronic kidney disease (CKD)
586 Renal failure, unspecified
587 Renal sclerosis, unspecified
588 Disorders resulting from impaired renal function
589 Small kidney of unknown cause

Other diseases of urinary system (590-599)
590 Infections of kidney
591 Hydronephrosis
592 Calculus of kidney and ureter
593 Other disorders of kidney and ureter
594 Calculus of lower urinary tract
595 Cystitis
596 Other disorders of bladder
597 Urethritis, not sexually transmitted, and urethral syndrome
598 Urethral stricture
599 Other disorders of urethra and urinary tract

Diseases of male genital organs (600-608)
600 Hyperplasia of prostate
601 Inflammatory diseases of prostate
602 Other disorders of prostate
603 Hydrocele
604 Orchitis and epididymitis
605 Redundant prepuce and phimosis
606 Infertility, male
607 Disorders of penis
608 Other disorders of male genital organs

Disorders of breast (610-612)
610 Benign mammary dysplasias
611 Other disorders of breast
612 Deformity and disproportion of reconstructed breast

Inflammatory disease of female pelvic organs (614-616)
614 Inflammatory disease of ovary, fallopian tube, pelvic cellular tissue, and peritoneum
615 Inflammatory diseases of uterus, except cervix
616 Inflammatory disease of cervix, vagina, and vulva

Other disorders of female genital tract (617-629)
617 Endometriosis
618 Genital prolapse
619 Fistula involving female genital tract
620 Noninflammatory disorders of ovary, fallopian tube, and broad ligament
621 Disorders of uterus, not elsewhere classified
622 Noninflammatory disorders of cervix
623 Noninflammatory disorders of vagina
624 Noninflammatory disorders of vulva and perineum
625 Pain and other symptoms associated with female genital organs
626 Disorders of menstruation and other abnormal bleeding from female genital tract
627 Menopausal and postmenopausal disorders
628 Infertility, female
629 Other disorders of female genital organs

11. Complications of Pregnancy, Childbirth and the Puerperium

Ectopic and molar pregnancy (630-633)
630 Hydatidiform mole
631 Other abnormal product of conception
632 Missed abortion
633 Ectopic pregnancy

Other pregnancy with abortive outcome (634-639)
634 Spontaneous abortion
635 Legally induced abortion
636 Illegally induced abortion
637 Unspecified abortion
638 Failed attempted abortion
639 Complications following abortion and ectopic and molar pregnancies

Complications mainly related to pregnancy (640-649)
640 Hemorrhage in early pregnancy
641 Antepartum hemorrhage, abruptio placentae, and placenta previa
642 Hypertension complicating pregnancy, childbirth, and the puerperium
643 Excessive vomiting in pregnancy
644 Early or threatened labor
645 Late pregnancy
646 Other complications of pregnancy, not elsewhere classified
647 Infectious and parasitic conditions in the mother classifiable elsewhere, but complicating pregnancy, childbirth, and the puerperium
648 Other current conditions in the mother classifiable elsewhere, but complicating pregnancy, childbirth, and the puerperium
649 Other conditions or status of the mother complicating pregnancy, childbirth, or the puerperium

Normal delivery, and other indications for care in pregnancy, labor, and delivery (650-659)
650 Normal delivery
651 Multiple gestation
652 Malposition and malpresentation of fetus
653 Disproportion
654 Abnormality of organs and soft tissues of pelvis
655 Known or suspected fetal abnormality affecting management of mother
656 Other known or suspected fetal and placental problems affecting management of mother
657 Polyhydramnios
658 Other problems associated with amniotic cavity and membranes
659 Other indications for care or intervention related to labor and delivery, not elsewhere classified

Complications occurring mainly in the course of labor and delivery (660-669)
660 Obstructed labor
661 Abnormality of forces of labor
662 Long labor
663 Umbilical cord complications
664 Trauma to perineum and vulva during delivery
665 Other obstetrical trauma
666 Postpartum hemorrhage
667 Retained placenta or membranes, without hemorrhage
668 Complications of the administration of anesthetic or other sedation in labor and delivery
669 Other complications of labor and delivery, not elsewhere classified

Complications of the puerperium (670-677)
670 Major puerperal infection

671 Venous complications in pregnancy and the puerperium
672 Pyrexia of unknown origin during the puerperium
673 Obstetrical pulmonary embolism
674 Other and unspecified complications of the puerperium, not elsewhere classified
675 Infections of the breast and nipple associated with childbirth
676 Other disorders of the breast associated with childbirth, and disorders of lactation
677 Late effect of complication of pregnancy, childbirth, and the puerperium

Other maternal and fetal complications (678-679)
678 Other fetal conditions
679 Complications of in utero procedures

12. Diseases of the Skin and Subcutaneous Tissue

Infections of skin and subcutaneous tissue (680-686)
680 Carbuncle and furuncle
681 Cellulitis and abscess of finger and toe
682 Other cellulitis and abscess
683 Acute lymphadenitis
684 Impetigo
685 Pilonidal cyst
686 Other local infections of skin and subcutaneous tissue

Other inflammatory conditions of skin and subcutaneous tissue (690-698)
690 Erythematosquamous dermatosis
691 Atopic dermatitis and related conditions
692 Contact dermatitis and other eczema
693 Dermatitis due to substances taken internally
694 Bullous dermatoses
695 Erythematous conditions
696 Psoriasis and similar disorders
697 Lichen
698 Pruritus and related conditions

Other diseases of skin and subcutaneous tissue (700-709)
700 Corns and callosities
701 Other hypertrophic and atrophic conditions of skin
702 Other dermatoses
703 Diseases of nail
704 Diseases of hair and hair follicles
705 Disorders of sweat glands
706 Diseases of sebaceous glands
707 Chronic ulcer of skin
708 Urticaria
709 Other disorders of skin and subcutaneous tissue

13. Diseases of the Musculoskeletal System and Connective Tissue

Arthropathies and related disorders (710-719)
710 Diffuse diseases of connective tissue
711 Arthropathy associated with infections
712 Crystal arthropathies
713 Arthropathy associated with other disorders classified elsewhere
714 Rheumatoid arthritis and other inflammatory polyarthropathies
715 Osteoarthrosis and allied disorders
716 Other and unspecified arthropathies
717 Internal derangement of knee
718 Other derangement of joint
719 Other and unspecified disorder of joint

Dorsopathies (720-724)
720 Ankylosing spondylitis and other inflammatory spondylopathies
721 Spondylosis and allied disorders
722 Intervertebral disc disorders
723 Other disorders of cervical region
724 Other and unspecified disorders of back

Rheumatism, excluding the back (725-729)
725 Polymyalgia rheumatica
726 Peripheral enthesopathies and allied syndromes
727 Other disorders of synovium, tendon, and bursa
728 Disorders of muscle, ligament, and fascia
729 Other disorders of soft tissues

Osteopathies, chondropathies, and acquired musculoskeletal deformities (730-739)
730 Osteomyelitis, periostitis, and other infections involving bone
731 Osteitis deformans and osteopathies associated with other disorders classified elsewhere
732 Osteochondropathies
733 Other disorders of bone and cartilage
734 Flat foot
735 Acquired deformities of toe
736 Other acquired deformities of limbs
737 Curvature of spine
738 Other acquired deformity
739 Nonallopathic lesions, not elsewhere classified

14. Congenital Anomalies

740 Anencephalus and similar anomalies
741 Spina bifida
742 Other congenital anomalies of nervous system
743 Congenital anomalies of eye
744 Congenital anomalies of ear, face, and neck
745 Bulbus cordis anomalies and anomalies of cardiac septal closure
746 Other congenital anomalies of heart
747 Other congenital anomalies of circulatory system
748 Congenital anomalies of respiratory system
749 Cleft palate and cleft lip
750 Other congenital anomalies of upper alimentary tract
751 Other congenital anomalies of digestive system
752 Congenital anomalies of genital organs
753 Congenital anomalies of urinary system
754 Certain congenital musculoskeletal deformities
755 Other congenital anomalies of limbs
756 Other congenital musculoskeletal anomalies
757 Congenital anomalies of the integument
758 Chromosomal anomalies
759 Other and unspecified congenital anomalies

15. Certain Conditions Originating in the Perinatal Period

Maternal causes of perinatal morbidity and mortality (760-763)
760 Fetus or newborn affected by maternal conditions which may be unrelated to present pregnancy
761 Fetus or newborn affected by maternal complications of pregnancy
762 Fetus or newborn affected by complications of placenta, cord, and membranes
763 Fetus or newborn affected by other complications of labor and delivery

Other conditions originating in the perinatal period (764-779)
764 Slow fetal growth and fetal malnutrition
765 Disorders relating to short gestation and unspecified low birthweight
766 Disorders relating to long gestation and high birthweight
767 Birth trauma
768 Intrauterine hypoxia and birth asphyxia
769 Respiratory distress syndrome
770 Other respiratory conditions of fetus and newborn
771 Infections specific to the perinatal period
772 Fetal and neonatal hemorrhage
773 Hemolytic disease of fetus or newborn, due to isoimmunization
774 Other perinatal jaundice
775 Endocrine and metabolic disturbances specific to the fetus and newborn
776 Hematological disorders of newborn
777 Perinatal disorders of digestive system
778 Conditions involving the integument and temperature regulation of fetus and newborn
779 Other and ill-defined conditions originating in the perinatal period

16. Symptoms, Signs, and Ill-defined Conditions

Symptoms (780-789)
780 General symptoms
781 Symptoms involving nervous and musculoskeletal systems
782 Symptoms involving skin and other integumentary tissue
783 Symptoms concerning nutrition, metabolism, and development
784 Symptoms involving head and neck
785 Symptoms involving cardiovascular system
786 Symptoms involving respiratory system and other chest symptoms
787 Symptoms involving digestive system
788 Symptoms involving urinary system
789 Other symptoms involving abdomen and pelvis

Nonspecific abnormal findings (790-796)
790 Nonspecific findings on examination of blood
791 Nonspecific findings on examination of urine
792 Nonspecific abnormal findings in other body substances
793 Nonspecific (abnormal) findings on radiological and other examination of body structure
794 Nonspecific abnormal results of function studies
795 Other and nonspecific abnormal cystological, histological, immunological and DNA test findings
796 Other nonspecific abnormal findings

Ill-defined and unknown causes of morbidity and mortality (797-799)
797 Senility without mention of psychosis
798 Sudden death, cause unknown
799 Other ill-defined and unknown causes of morbidity and mortality

17. Injury and Poisoning

Fracture of skull (800-804)
800 Fracture of vault of skull
801 Fracture of base of skull
802 Fracture of face bones
803 Other and unqualified skull fractures
804 Multiple fractures involving skull or face with other bones

Fracture of spine and trunk (805-809)
805 Fracture of vertebral column without mention of spinal cord injury
806 Fracture of vertebral column with spinal cord injury
807 Fracture of rib(s), sternum, larynx, and trachea
808 Fracture of pelvis
809 Ill-defined fractures of bones of trunk

Fracture of upper limb (810-819)
810 Fracture of clavicle
811 Fracture of scapula
812 Fracture of humerus
813 Fracture of radius and ulna
814 Fracture of carpal bone(s)
815 Fracture of metacarpal bone(s)

Appendix E: List of Three-digit Categories

816 Fracture of one or more phalanges of hand
817 Multiple fractures of hand bones
818 Ill-defined fractures of upper limb
819 Multiple fractures involving both upper limbs, and upper limb with rib(s) and sternum

Fracture of lower limb (820-829)
820 Fracture of neck of femur
821 Fracture of other and unspecified parts of femur
822 Fracture of patella
823 Fracture of tibia and fibula
824 Fracture of ankle
825 Fracture of one or more tarsal and metatarsal bones
826 Fracture of one or more phalanges of foot
827 Other, multiple, and ill-defined fractures of lower limb
828 Multiple fractures involving both lower limbs, lower with upper limb, and lower limb(s) with rib(s) and sternum
829 Fracture of unspecified bones

Dislocation (830-839)
830 Dislocation of jaw
831 Dislocation of shoulder
832 Dislocation of elbow
833 Dislocation of wrist
834 Dislocation of finger
835 Dislocation of hip
836 Dislocation of knee
837 Dislocation of ankle
838 Dislocation of foot
839 Other, multiple, and ill-defined dislocations

Sprains and strains of joints and adjacent muscles (840-848)
840 Sprains and strains of shoulder and upper arm
841 Sprains and strains of elbow and forearm
842 Sprains and strains of wrist and hand
843 Sprains and strains of hip and thigh
844 Sprains and strains of knee and leg
845 Sprains and strains of ankle and foot
846 Sprains and strains of sacroiliac region
847 Sprains and strains of other and unspecified parts of back
848 Other and ill-defined sprains and strains

Intracranial injury, excluding those with skull fracture (850-854)
850 Concussion
851 Cerebral laceration and contusion
852 Subarachnoid, subdural, and extradural hemorrhage, following injury
853 Other and unspecified intracranial hemorrhage following injury
854 Intracranial injury of other and unspecified nature

Internal injury of thorax, abdomen, and pelvis (860-869)
860 Traumatic pneumothorax and hemothorax
861 Injury to heart and lung
862 Injury to other and unspecified intrathoracic organs
863 Injury to gastrointestinal tract
864 Injury to liver
865 Injury to spleen
866 Injury to kidney
867 Injury to pelvic organs
868 Injury to other intra-abdominal organs
869 Internal injury to unspecified or ill-defined organs

Open wound of head, neck, and trunk (870-879)
870 Open wound of ocular adnexa
871 Open wound of eyeball
872 Open wound of ear
873 Other open wound of head
874 Open wound of neck
875 Open wound of chest (wall)

876 Open wound of back
877 Open wound of buttock
878 Open wound of genital organs (external), including traumatic amputation
879 Open wound of other and unspecified sites, except limbs

Open wound of upper limb (880-887)
880 Open wound of shoulder and upper arm
881 Open wound of elbow, forearm, and wrist
882 Open wound of hand except finger(s) alone
883 Open wound of finger(s)
884 Multiple and unspecified open wound of upper limb
885 Traumatic amputation of thumb (complete) (partial)
886 Traumatic amputation of other finger(s) (complete) (partial)
887 Traumatic amputation of arm and hand (complete) (partial)

Open wound of lower limb (890-897)
890 Open wound of hip and thigh
891 Open wound of knee, leg [except thigh], and ankle
892 Open wound of foot except toe(s) alone
893 Open wound of toe(s)
894 Multiple and unspecified open wound of lower limb
895 Traumatic amputation of toe(s) (complete) (partial)
896 Traumatic amputation of foot (complete) (partial)
897 Traumatic amputation of leg(s) (complete) (partial)

Injury to blood vessels (900-904)
900 Injury to blood vessels of head and neck
901 Injury to blood vessels of thorax
902 Injury to blood vessels of abdomen and pelvis
903 Injury to blood vessels of upper extremity
904 Injury to blood vessels of lower extremity and unspecified sites

Late effects of injuries, poisonings, toxic effects, and other external causes (905-909)
905 Late effects of musculoskeletal and connective tissue injuries
906 Late effects of injuries to skin and subcutaneous tissues
907 Late effects of injuries to the nervous system
908 Late effects of other and unspecified injuries
909 Late effects of other and unspecified external causes

Superficial injury (910-919)
910 Superficial injury of face, neck, and scalp except eye
911 Superficial injury of trunk
912 Superficial injury of shoulder and upper arm
913 Superficial injury of elbow, forearm, and wrist
914 Superficial injury of hand(s) except finger(s) alone
915 Superficial injury of finger(s)
916 Superficial injury of hip, thigh, leg, and ankle
917 Superficial injury of foot and toe(s)
918 Superficial injury of eye and adnexa
919 Superficial injury of other, multiple, and unspecified sites

Contusion with intact skin surface (920-924)
920 Contusion of face, scalp, and neck except eye(s)
921 Contusion of eye and adnexa
922 Contusion of trunk
923 Contusion of upper limb
924 Contusion of lower limb and of other and unspecified sites

Crushing injury (925-929)
925 Crushing injury of face, scalp, and neck
926 Crushing injury of trunk

927 Crushing injury of upper limb
928 Crushing injury of lower limb
929 Crushing injury of multiple and unspecified sites

Effects of foreign body entering through orifice (930-939)
930 Foreign body on external eye
931 Foreign body in ear
932 Foreign body in nose
933 Foreign body in pharynx and larynx
934 Foreign body in trachea, bronchus, and lung
935 Foreign body in mouth, esophagus, and stomach
936 Foreign body in intestine and colon
937 Foreign body in anus and rectum
938 Foreign body in digestive system, unspecified
939 Foreign body in genitourinary tract

Burns (940-949)
940 Burn confined to eye and adnexa
941 Burn of face, head, and neck
942 Burn of trunk
943 Burn of upper limb, except wrist and hand
944 Burn of wrist(s) and hand(s)
945 Burn of lower limb(s)
946 Burns of multiple specified sites
947 Burn of internal organs
948 Burns classified according to extent of body surface involved
949 Burn, unspecified

Injury to nerves and spinal cord (950-957)
950 Injury to optic nerve and pathways
951 Injury to other cranial nerve(s)
952 Spinal cord injury without evidence of spinal bone injury
953 Injury to nerve roots and spinal plexus
954 Injury to other nerve(s) of trunk excluding shoulder and pelvic girdles
955 Injury to peripheral nerve(s) of shoulder girdle and upper limb
956 Injury to peripheral nerve(s) of pelvic girdle and lower limb
957 Injury to other and unspecified nerves

Certain traumatic complications and unspecified injuries (958-959)
958 Certain early complications of trauma
959 Injury, other and unspecified

Poisoning by drugs, medicinals and biological substances (960-979)
960 Poisoning by antibiotics
961 Poisoning by other anti-infectives
962 Poisoning by hormones and synthetic substitutes
963 Poisoning by primarily systemic agents
964 Poisoning by agents primarily affecting blood constituents
965 Poisoning by analgesics, antipyretics, and antirheumatics
966 Poisoning by anticonvulsants and anti-Parkinsonism drugs
967 Poisoning by sedatives and hypnotics
968 Poisoning by other central nervous system depressants and anesthetics
969 Poisoning by psychotropic agents
970 Poisoning by central nervous system stimulants
971 Poisoning by drugs primarily affecting the autonomic nervous system
972 Poisoning by agents primarily affecting the cardiovascular system
973 Poisoning by agents primarily affecting the gastrointestinal system
974 Poisoning by water, mineral, and uric acid metabolism drugs
975 Poisoning by agents primarily acting on the smooth and skeletal muscles and respiratory system

976   Poisoning by agents primarily affecting skin and mucous membrane, ophthalmological, otorhinolaryngological, and dental drugs

977   Poisoning by other and unspecified drugs and medicinals

978   Poisoning by bacterial vaccines

979   Poisoning by other vaccines and biological substances

Toxic effects of substances chiefly nonmedicinal as to source (980-989)

980   Toxic effect of alcohol

981   Toxic effect of petroleum products

982   Toxic effect of solvents other than petroleum-based

983   Toxic effect of corrosive aromatics, acids, and caustic alkalis

984   Toxic effect of lead and its compounds (including fumes)

985   Toxic effect of other metals

986   Toxic effect of carbon monoxide

987   Toxic effect of other gases, fumes, or vapors

988   Effect of noxious substances eaten as food

989   Toxic effect of other substances, chiefly nonmedicinal as to source

Other and unspecified effects of external causes (990-995)

990   Effects of radiation, unspecified

991   Effects of reduced temperature

992   Effects of heat and light

993   Effects of air pressure

994   Effects of other external causes

995   Certain adverse effects, not elsewhere classified

Complications of surgical and medical care, not elsewhere classified (996-999)

996   Complications peculiar to certain specified procedures

997   Complications affecting specified body systems, not elsewhere classified

998   Other complications of procedures, not elsewhere classified

999   Complications of medical care, not elsewhere classified

Supplementary Classification of Factors Influencing Health Status and Contact With Health Services

Persons with potential health hazards related to communicable diseases (V01-V06)

V01   Contact with or exposure to communicable diseases

V02   Carrier or suspected carrier of infectious diseases

V03   Need for prophylactic vaccination and inoculation against bacterial diseases

V04   Need for prophylactic vaccination and inoculation against certain viral diseases

V05   Need for other prophylactic vaccination and inoculation against single diseases

V06   Need for prophylactic vaccination and inoculation against combinations of diseases

Persons with need for isolation, other potential health hazards, and prophylactic measures (V07-V09)

V07   Need for isolation and other prophylactic or treatment measures

V08   Asymptomatic human immunodeficiency virus [HIV] infection status

V09   Infection with drug-resistant microorganisms

Persons with potential health hazards related to personal and family history (V10-V19)

V10   Personal history of malignant neoplasm

V11   Personal history of mental disorder

V12   Personal history of certain other diseases

V13   Personal history of other diseases

V14   Personal history of allergy to medicinal agents

V15   Other personal history presenting hazards to health

V16   Family history of malignant neoplasm

V17   Family history of certain chronic disabling diseases

V18   Family history of certain other specific conditions

V19   Family history of other conditions

Persons encountering health services in circumstances related to reproduction and development (V20-V29)

V20   Health supervision of infant or child

V21   Constitutional states in development

V22   Normal pregnancy

V23   Supervision of high-risk pregnancy

V24   Postpartum care and examination

V25   Encounter for contraceptive management

V26   Procreative management

V27   Outcome of delivery

V28   Encounter for antenatal screening of mother

V29   Observation and evaluation of newborns and infants for suspected condition not found

Liveborn infants according to type of birth (V30-V39)

V30   Single liveborn

V31   Twin, mate liveborn

V32   Twin, mate stillborn

V33   Twin, unspecified

V34   Other multiple, mates all liveborn

V35   Other multiple, mates all stillborn

V36   Other multiple, mates live and stillborn

V37   Other multiple, unspecified

V39   Unspecified

Persons with a condition influencing their health status (V40-V49)

V40   Mental and behavioral problems

V41   Problems with special senses and other special functions

V42   Organ or tissue replaced by transplant

V43   Organ or tissue replaced by other means

V44   Artificial opening status

V45   Other postprocedural states

V46   Other dependence on machines and devices

V47   Other problems with internal organs

V48   Problems with head, neck, and trunk

V49   Other conditions influencing health status

Persons encountering health services for specific procedures and aftercare (V50-V59)

V50   Elective surgery for purposes other than remedying health states

V51   Aftercare involving the use of plastic surgery

V52   Fitting and adjustment of prosthetic device and implant

V53   Fitting and adjustment of other device

V54   Other orthopedic aftercare

V55   Attention to artificial openings

V56   Encounter for dialysis and dialysis catheter care

V57   Care involving use of rehabilitation procedures

V58   Encounter for other and unspecified procedures and aftercare

V59   Donors

Persons encountering health services in other circumstances (V60-V69)

V60   Housing, household, and economic circumstances

V61   Other family circumstances

V62   Other psychosocial circumstances

V63   Unavailability of other medical facilities for care

V64   Persons encountering health services for specific procedures, not carried out

V65   Other persons seeking consultation

V66   Convalescence and palliative care

V67   Follow-up examination

V68   Encounters for administrative purposes

V69   Problems related to lifestyle

Persons without reported diagnosis encountered during examination and investigation of individuals and populations (V70-V82)

V70   General medical examination

V71   Observation and evaluation for suspected conditions not found

V72   Special investigations and examinations

V73   Special screening examination for viral and chlamydial diseases

V74   Special screening examination for bacterial and spirochetal diseases

V75   Special screening examination for other infectious diseases

V76   Special screening for malignant neoplasms

V77   Special screening for endocrine, nutritional, metabolic, and immunity disorders

V78   Special screening for disorders of blood and blood-forming organs

V79   Special screening for mental disorders and developmental handicaps

V80   Special screening for neurological, eye, and ear diseases

V81   Special screening for cardiovascular, respiratory, and genitourinary diseases

V82   Special screening for other conditions

Genetics (V83-V84)

V83   Genetic carrier status

V84   Genetic susceptibility to disease

Body mass index (V85)

V85   Body Mass Index [BMI]

Estrogen receptor status (V86)

V86   Estrogen receptor status

Other specified personal exposures and history presenting hazards to health (V87)

V87   Other specified personal exposures and history presenting hazards to health

Acquired absence of other organs and tissue (V88)

V88   Acquired absence of other organs and tissue

Other suspected conditions not found (V89)

V89   Other suspected conditions not found

Retained Foreign Body (V90)

V90   Retained foreign body

Multiple Gestation Placenta Status (V91)

V91   Multiple gestation placenta status

Supplementary Classification of External Causes of Injury and Poisoning

External Cause Status (E000)

E000   External cause status

Activity (E001-E030)

E001   Activities involving walking and running

E002   Activities involving water and water craft

E003   Activities involving ice and snow

E004   Activities involving climbing, rappelling, and jumping off

E005   Activities involving dancing and other rhythmic movement

E006   Activities involving other sports and athletics played individually

E007   Activities involving other sports and athletics played as a team or group

E008   Activities involving other specified sports and athletics

E009   Activity involving other cardiorespiratory exercise

E010   Activity involving other muscle strengthening exercises

E011　Activities involving computer technology and electronic devices
E012　Activities involving arts and handcrafts
E013　Activities involving personal hygiene and household maintenance
E014　Activities involving person providing caregiving
E015　Activities involving food preparation, cooking and grilling
E016　Activities involving property and land maintenance, building and construction
E017　Activities involving roller coasters and other types of external motion
E018　Activities involving playing musical instrument
E019　Activities involving animal care
E029　Other activity
E030　Unspecified activity

Transport Accidents (E800-E848)

Railway accidents (E800-E807)
E800　Railway accident involving collision with roling stock
E801　Railway accident involving collision with other object
E802　Railway accident involving derailment without antecedent collision
E803　Railway accident involving explosion, fire, or burning
E804　Fall in, on, or from railway train
E805　Hit by rolling stock
E806　Other specified railway accident
E807　Railway accident of unspecified nature

Motor vehicle traffic accidents (E810-E819)
E810　Motor vehicle traffic accident involving collision with train
E811　Motor vehicle traffic accident involving re-entrant collision with another motor vehicle
E812　Other motor vehicle traffic accident involving collision with another motor vehicle
E813　Motor vehicle traffic accident involving collision with other vehicle
E814　Motor vehicle traffic accident involving collision with pedestrian
E815　Other motor vehicle traffic accident involving collision on the highway
E816　Motor vehicle traffic accident due to loss of control, without collision on the highway
E817　Noncollision motor vehicle traffic accident while boarding or alighting
E818　Other noncollision motor vehicle traffic accident
E819　Motor vehicle traffic accident of unspecified nature

Motor vehicle nontraffic accidents (E820-E825)
E820　Nontraffic accident involving motor-driven snow vehicle
E821　Nontraffic accident involving other off-road motor vehicle
E822　Other motor vehicle nontraffic accident involving collision with moving object
E823　Other motor vehicle nontraffic accident involving collision with stationary object
E824　Other motor vehicle nontraffic accident while boarding and alighting
E825　Other motor vehicle nontraffic accident of other and unspecified nature

Other road vehicle accidents (E826-E829)
E826　Pedal cycle accident
E827　Animal-drawn vehicle accident
E828　Accident involving animal being ridden
E829　Other road vehicle accidents

Water transport accidents (E830-E838)
E830　Accident to watercraft causing submersion
E831　Accident to watercraft causing other injury
E832　Other accidental submersion or drowning in water transport accident
E833　Fall on stairs or ladders in water transport
E834　Other fall from one level to another in water transport
E835　Other and unspecified fall in water transport
E836　Machinery accident in water transport
E837　Explosion, fire, or burning in watercraft
E838　Other and unspecified water transport accident

Air and space transport accidents (E840-E845)
E840　Accident to powered aircraft at takeoff or landing
E841　Accident to powered aircraft, other and unspecified
E842　Accident to unpowered aircraft
E843　Fall in, on, or from aircraft
E844　Other specified air transport accidents
E845　Accident involving spacecraft

Vehicle accidents, not elsewhere classfiable (E846-E849)
E846　Accidents involving powered vehicles used solely within the buildings and premises of an industrial or commercial establishment
E847　Accidents involving cable cars not running on rails
E848　Accidents involving other vehicles, not elsewhere classifiable
E849　Place of occurrence

Accidental poisoning by drugs, medicinal substances, and biologicals (E850-E858)
E850　Accidental poisoning by analgesics, antipyretics, and antirheumatics
E851　Accidental poisoning by barbiturates
E852　Accidental poisoning by other sedatives and hypnotics
E853　Accidental poisoning by tranquilizers
E854　Accidental poisoning by other psychotropic agents
E855　Accidental poisoning by other drugs acting on central and autonomic nervous systems
E856　Accidental poisoning by antibiotics
E857　Accidental poisoning by anti-infectives
E858　Accidental poisoning by other drugs

Accidental poisoning by other solid and liquid substances, gases, and vapors (E860-E869)
E860　Accidental poisoning by alcohol, not elsewhere classified
E861　Accidental poisoning by cleansing and polishing agents, disinfectants, paints, and varnishes
E862　Accidental poisoning by petroleum products, other solvents and their vapors, not elsewhere classified
E863　Accidental poisoning by agricultural and horticultural chemical and pharmaceutical preparations other than plant foods and fertilizers
E864　Accidental poisoning by corrosives and caustics, not elsewhere classified
E865　Accidental poisoning from poisonous foodstuffs and poisonous plants
E866　Accidental poisoning by other and unspecified solid and liquid substances
E867　Accidental poisoning by gas distributed by pipeline
E868　Accidental poisoning by other utility gas and other carbon monoxide
E869　Accidental poisoning by other gases and vapors

Misadventures to patients during surgical and medical care (E870-E876)
E870　Accidental cut, puncture, perforation, or hemorrhage during medical care
E871　Foreign object left in body during procedure
E872　Failure of sterile precautions during procedure
E873　Failure in dosage
E874　Mechanical failure of instrument or apparatus during procedure
E875　Contaminated or infected blood, other fluid, drug, or biological substance
E876　Other and unspecified misadventures during medical care

Surgical and medical procedures as the cause of abnormal reaction of patient or later complication, without mention of misadventure at the time of procedure (E878-E879)
E878　Surgical operation and other surgical procedures as the cause of abnormal reaction of patient, or of later complication, without mention of misadventure at the time of operation
E879　Other procedures, without mention of misadventure at the time of procedure, as the cause of abnormal reaction of patient, or of later complication

Accidental falls (E880-E888)
E880　Fall on or from stairs or steps
E881　Fall on or from ladders or scaffolding
E882　Fall from or out of building or other structure
E883　Fall into hole or other opening in surface
E884　Other fall from one level to another
E885　Fall on same level from slipping, tripping, or stumbling
E886　Fall on same level from collision, pushing or shoving, by or with other person
E887　Fracture, cause unspecified
E888　Other and unspecified fall

Accidents caused by fire and flames (E890-E899)
E890　Conflagration in private dwelling
E891　Conflagration in other and unspecified building or structure
E892　Conflagration not in building or structure
E893　Accident caused by ignition of clothing
E894　Ignition of highly inflammable material
E895　Accident caused by controlled fire in private dwelling
E896　Accident caused by controlled fire in other and unspecified building or structure
E897　Accident caused by controlled fire not in building or structure
E898　Accident caused by other specified fire and flames
E899　Accident caused by unspecified fire

Accidents due to natural and environmental factors (E900-E909)
E900　Excessive heat
E901　Excessive cold
E902　High and low air pressure and changes in air pressure
E903　Travel and motion
E904　Hunger, thirst, exposure, and neglect
E905　Venomous animals and plants as the cause of poisoning and toxic reactions
E906　Other injury caused by animals
E907　Lightning
E908　Cataclysmic storms, and floods resulting from storms
E909　Cataclysmic earth surface movements and eruptions

Accidents caused by submersion, suffocation, and foreign bodies (E910-E915)
E910　Accidental drowning and submersion
E911　Inhalation and ingestion of food causing obstruction of respiratory tract or suffocation
E912　Inhalation and ingestion of other object causing obstruction of respiratory tract or suffocation
E913　Accidental mechanical suffocation
E914　Foreign body accidentally entering eye and adnexa
E915　Foreign body accidentally entering other orifice

Other accidents (E916-E928)
E916　Struck accidentally by falling object

E917 Striking against or struck accidentally by objects or persons
E918 Caught accidentally in or between objects
E919 Accidents caused by machinery
E920 Accidents caused by cutting and piercing instruments or objects
E921 Accident caused by explosion of pressure vessel
E922 Accident caused by firearm and air gun missile
E923 Accident caused by explosive material
E924 Accident caused by hot substance or object, caustic or corrosive material, and steam
E925 Accident caused by electric current
E926 Exposure to radiation
E927 Overexertion and strenuous and repetitive movements or loads
E928 Other and unspecified environmental and accidental causes

Late effects of accidental injury (E929)
E929 Late effects of accidental injury

Drugs, medicinal and biological substances causing adverse effects in therapeutic use (E930-E949)
E930 Antibiotics
E931 Other anti-infectives
E932 Hormones and synthetic substitutes
E933 Primarily systemic agents
E934 Agents primarily affecting blood constituents
E935 Analgesics, antipyretics, and antirheumatics
E936 Anticonvulsants and anti-Parkinsonism drugs
E937 Sedatives and hypnotics
E938 Other central nervous system depressants and anesthetics
E939 Psychotropic agents
E940 Central nervous system stimulants
E941 Drugs primarily affecting the autonomic nervous system
E942 Agents primarily affecting the cardiovascular system
E943 Agents primarily affecting gastrointestinal system
E944 Water, mineral, and uric acid metabolism drugs
E945 Agents primarily acting on the smooth and skeletal muscles and respiratory system
E946 Agents primarily affecting skin and mucous membrane, ophthalmological, otorhinolaryngological, and dental drugs
E947 Other and unspecified drugs and medicinal substances
E948 Bacterial vaccines
E949 Other vaccines and biological substances

Suicide and self-inflicted injury (E950-E959)
E950 Suicide and self-inflicted poisoning by solid or liquid substances
E951 Suicide and self-inflicted poisoning by gases in domestic use
E952 Suicide and self-inflicted poisoning by other gases and vapors
E953 Suicide and self-inflicted injury by hanging, strangulation, and suffocation
E954 Suicide and self-inflicted injury by submersion [drowning]
E955 Suicide and self-inflicted injury by firearms, air guns and explosives
E956 Suicide and self-inflicted injury by cutting and piercing instruments
E957 Suicide and self-inflicted injuries by jumping from high place
E958 Suicide and self-inflicted injury by other and unspecified means
E959 Late effects of self-inflicted injury

Homicide and injury purposely inflicted by other persons (E960-E969)
E960 Fight, brawl, and rape
E961 Assault by corrosive or caustic substance, except poisoning
E962 Assault by poisoning
E963 Assault by hanging and strangulation
E964 Assault by submersion [drowning]
E965 Assault by firearms and explosives
E966 Assault by cutting and piercing instrument
E967 Perpetrator of child and adult abuse
E968 Assault by other and unspecified means
E969 Late effects of injury purposely inflicted by other person

Legal intervention (E970-E978)
E970 Injury due to legal intervention by firearms
E971 Injury due to legal intervention by explosives
E972 Injury due to legal intervention by gas
E973 Injury due to legal intervention by blunt object
E974 Injury due to legal intervention by cutting and piercing instruments
E975 Injury due to legal intervention by other specified means
E976 Injury due to legal intervention by unspecified means
E977 Late effects of injuries due to legal intervention
E978 Legal execution

Terrorism (E979)
E979 Terrorism

Injury undetermined whether accidentally or purposely inflicted (E980-E989)
E980 Poisoning by solid or liquid substances, undetermined whether accidentally or purposely inflicted
E981 Poisoning by gases in domestic use, undetermined whether accidentally or purposely inflicted
E982 Poisoning by other gases, undetermined whether accidentally or purposely inflicted
E983 Hanging, strangulation, or suffocation, undetermined whether accidentally or purposely inflicted
E984 Submersion [drowning], undetermined whether accidentally or purposely inflicted
E985 Injury by firearms and explosives, undetermined whether accidentally or purposely inflicted
E986 Injury by cutting and piercing instruments, undetermined whether accidentally or purposely inflicted
E987 Falling from high place, undetermined whether accidentally or purposely inflicted
E988 Injury by other and unspecified means, undetermined whether accidentally or purposely inflicted
E989 Late effects of injury, undetermined whether accidentally or purposely inflicted

Injury resulting from operations of war (E990-E999)
E990 Injury due to war operations by fires and conflagrations
E991 Injury due to war operations by bullets and fragments
E992 Injury due to war operations by explosion of marine weapons
E993 Injury due to war operations by other explosion
E994 Injury due to war operations by destruction of aircraft
E995 Injury due to war operations by other and unspecified forms of conventional warfare
E996 Injury due to war operations by nuclear weapons
E997 Injury due to war operations by other forms of unconventional warfare
E998 Injury due to war operations but occurring after cessation of hostilities
E999 Late effects of injury due to war operations and terrorism

10 Steps to Correct Coding

Follow the 10 steps below to correctly code encounters for healthcare services.

Step 1: Identify the reason for the visit or encounter (i.e., a sign, symptom, diagnosis and/or condition).

The medical record documentation should accurately reflect the patient's condition, using terminology that includes specific diagnoses and symptoms, or clearly states the reasons for the encounter.

Choosing the main term that best describes the reason chiefly responsible for the service provided is the most important step in coding. If symptoms are present and documented, but a definitive diagnosis has not yet been determined, code the symptoms. **Do not code conditions that are referred to as "rule out," "suspected," "probable" or "questionable."** Diagnoses often are not established at the time of the initial encounter/visit. Two or more visits may be necessary to establish the diagnosis. Code only what is documented in the available records and only to the highest degree of certainty known at the time of the patient's visit.

Step 2: After selecting the reason for the encounter, always consult the Alphabetic Index, Volume 2, before verifying code selection in the Tabular section.

The most critical rule is to begin the code selection process in the *Alphabetic Index*. Never turn first to the Tabular List (Volume 1). The Index provides cross references, essential and non-essential modifiers, and inclusion terms not found in the Tabular List. To prevent coding errors, always use both the Alphabetic Index and the Tabular List when locating and assigning a code. Always verify the code found in the Alphabetic Index in the Tabular List. First, the Index does not include the important instructional notes found in the Tabular. Second, the advantage of a classification system is that like items are grouped together. A quick scan of the Tabular might provide coding options for the coder that would have been missed.

Step 3: Locate the main term entry.

The Alphabetic Index is a listing of conditions. Conditions may be expressed as nouns or eponyms, with critical use of adjectives. Some conditions have multiple entries under synonyms. Reasons for encounters may be located under general terms such as admission, encounter, and examination. Other general terms such as history of or status post are used to locate factors influencing health.

Step 4: Read and interpret any notes listed with the main term or the subterm.

Notes such as common fifth-digit references and cross references are identified by italicized type. Always check any cross-references to ensure that all alternative terms are researched.

Step 5: Review entries for modifiers.

Nonessential modifiers are the terms located within parentheses following the main term entry. These parenthetical terms are supplementary words or explanatory information that may either be present or absent in the diagnostic statement and do not affect code selection. The subterms listed under the main term are essential modifiers that do affect coding assignment. Each line of indent represents a more specific code entry.

Step 6: Interpret abbreviations, cross-references, fifth digits, and brackets.

The cross-references used are "see," "see category" and "see also" which indicate alternative term choices for code searches. The abbreviation NEC may follow main terms or subterms. NEC (not elsewhere classified) indicates that there is no specific code for the condition even though the medical documentation may be very specific. Is a fifth digit required? You MUST refer to the Tabular List to discover the correct code. Italicized brackets *[ ]* enclose a second code that must be used along with the code immediately preceding it, with the bracketed code sequenced as the secondary code. This is a mandatory multiple code situation. Both the underlying condition and the manifestation (code in the slanted bracket) must be reported.

Step 7: Choose a potential code and locate it in the Tabular List.

The coder must follow any Includes, Excludes notes, and other instructional notes, such as "Code first" and "Use additional code," listed in the Tabular for the chapter, category, subcategory, and subclassification level of code selection which direct the coder to use a different or additional code.

Any codes in the Tabular range, 001.0 through 999.9, may be used to identify the diagnostic reason for the encounter. The Tabular encompasses many codes describing disease and injury classifications (e.g., infectious and parasitic diseases, neoplasms, symptoms, signs and ill-defined conditions, etc.).

Codes that describe symptoms and signs, as opposed to definitive diagnoses, should be used for reporting purposes when an established diagnosis has not been made (confirmed) by the physician. Chapter 16 of the ICD-9-CM code book, "Symptoms, Signs, and Ill-Defined Conditions" (codes 780.01-799.9) contains many, but not all, codes for symptoms.

ICD-9-CM classifies encounters with health care providers for circumstances other than a disease or injury using codes in the Supplementary Classification of Factors Influencing Health Status and Contact with Health Services (V01.0-V91.99). There are many occasions when circumstances other than a disease or injury are recorded as chiefly responsible for the encounter.

Step 8: Determine whether the code is at the highest level of specificity.

A code is invalid if it has not been coded to the full number of digits (greatest level of specificity) required. A three-digit code is to be used only if the category is not further subdivided. Assign four-digit codes (subcategory codes) only if there are no five-digit codes for that category. Assign five-digit codes (fifth-digit subclassification codes) for those categories mandating the use of five digits.

Step 9: Assign the code.

Having reviewed all relevant information concerning the possible code choices, assign the code that most completely describes the condition.

Repeat steps one through nine for all additional documented conditions that meet the following criteria:

- Conditions that currently exist at the time of the visit.

- Conditions that require or affect patient care, treatment or management.

Step 10: Sequence codes correctly.

Sequencing is defined as the order in which the codes are listed on the claim. List first the ICD-9-CM code for the diagnosis, condition, problem or other reason for the encounter/visit, which is shown in the medical record to be chiefly responsible for the services provided. List additional codes that describe any coexisting conditions. Follow the official coding guidelines (See Section IV Diagnostic Coding and Reporting Guidelines for Outpatient Services) concerning proper sequencing of codes.

Coding Examples

Diagnosis: Anorexia
- Step 1: The reason for the encounter was the condition, anorexia.

- Step 2: Consult the Index to Diseases.

- Step 3: Locate the main term "Anorexia."

- Step 4: There are no italicized instructional notes to interpret.

- Step 5: Note that there are two possible subterms (essential modifiers), "hysterical" and "nervosa," neither of which is documented in this instance and therefore cannot be used in code selection. The code listed next to the main term is called the default code selection.

- Step 6: There are no abbreviations, cross-references, fifth-digit notations, or brackets.

- Step 7: Turn to code 783.0 in the Tabular List and read the instructional notes. In this case the "Excludes" note indicates that anorexia determined to be of non-organic origin should be coded to Chapter 5. The diagnostic statement does not indicate non-organic origin.

- Step 8: There is no further division of the category past the fourth digit subcategory. Therefore, the subcategory code level is the highest level of specificity.

- Step 9: The default code, 783.0 is the correct code selection.

- Step 10: Since anorexia is listed as the chief reason for the healthcare encounter, the first-listed or principal diagnosis is 783.0.

Diagnosis: Acute bronchitis
- Step 1: The reason for the encounter was the condition, acute bronchitis.

- Step 2. Consult the Index to Diseases.

- Step 3: Locate the main term "Bronchitis."

- Step 4: There are no italicized instructional notes to interpret.

- Step 5: Review entries for modifiers. Since "acute" is not listed as a nonessential modifier, read past the "with" modifier until you find the subterm "acute or subacute" with code 466.0.

- Step 6: There are no abbreviations, cross-references, fifth digit notations, or brackets.

- Step 7: Since there are no more appropriate subterms, turn to code 466.0 in the Tabular List. The Includes note under category 466 does refer to possible infective organism, and other alternative terms for acute bronchitis. Note that inclusion term list is not exhaustive, but is only a representative selection of diagnoses that are included in the subcategory. At the beginning of chapter 8, "Diseases of the Respiratory System," you will notice the "use additional code" note that tells you to assign a code to identify the infectious organism. This instructional note applies to the entire chapter.

- Step 8: There is no further division of the category past the fourth- digit subcategory. Therefore, the subcategory code level is the highest level of specificity.

- Step 9: Assign code 466.0.

- Step 10: Repeat steps 1-9 for any additional code assignments.

Diagnosis: Acute bronchitis due to staphylococcus

- Step 1: The reason for the encounter was the condition, acute bronchitis due to staphylococcus.

- Step 2: Follow the steps listed in the above example for the diagnosis of acute bronchitis. You will now start the search for code identifying the underlying infectious organism, which in this case is staphylococcus.

- Step 3. Consult the Index to Diseases.

- Step 4: Locate the main term Staphylococcus, staphylococcal.

- Step 5: The italicized instructional notes states see condition. Locate the main term "Infection, infected, infective".

- Step 6: Review entries for modifiers. Locate the subterm "staphylococcal NEC," where you will find code 041.10 referenced. The abbreviation NEC indicates that a review of the medical record may be necessary to determine if there is documentation concerning the specific type of staphylococcus.

- Step 7: Verify code 041.10 in the Tabular List. The code title is Staphylococcus, unspecified. If there is additional information identifying the organism as aureus or other, assign the appropriate code; 041.11–041.19. Otherwise, assign code 041.10, Staphylococcus, unspecified, as an additional code.

- Step 8: There is no further division of the category past the fifth-digit subclassification level. Therefore, the subclassification code level is the highest level of specificity. The final code assignment would be 041.10.

- Step 9: Assign code 041.10.

- Step 10: Sequence codes as directed by the instructional note for category 466. Code first 466.0 and assign code 041.10 as an additional condition.

Diagnosis: Traveler's diarrhea

- Step 1: The reason for the encounter was the condition, Traveler's diarrhea.

- Step 2: Consult the Index to Diseases.

- Step 3: Locate the main term "Diarrhea" in the Alphabetic Index.

- Step 4: There are no italicized instructional notes to interpret.

- Step 5: Review entries for modifiers. Note that the nonessential modifiers (in parentheses) after the main term do not include the term "Traveler's," which means that the coder should search the subterms for the term "Traveler's." The subterm "Traveler's" has a possible code selection, 009.2, and suggests the subterm "due to specified organism NEC 008.8." The diagnostic statement does not include the infectious agent; therefore, code 008.8 does not apply.

- Step 6: There are no abbreviations, cross-references, fifth-digit notations, or brackets.

- Step 7: Locate code 009.2 in the Tabular List and read all instructional notes under the main category and subcategories. The Includes notes does not list the term "Traveler's" under code 009.2. As instructed by the Alphabetic Index, you should code the condition to 009.2. The ICD-9-CM code book implies that "Traveler's diarrhea" is the same as infectious diarrhea when it is not attributed to any specified infectious agent.

- Step 8: There is no further division of the category past the fourth-digit subcategory level. Therefore, the subcategory code level is the highest level of specificity. The final code assignment would be 009.2.

- Step 9: Assign code 009.2.

- Step 10: Since infectious diarrhea is listed as the chief reason for the healthcare encounter, the first-listed or principal diagnosis is 009.2.

Diagnosis: Ingrown toenail, infected

- Step 1: The reason for the encounter was the condition, infected ingrown toenail.

- Step 2. Consult the Index to Diseases.

- Step 3: First you must decide what the searchable main term should be. Reminder: search for condition, not anatomical site. The Alphabetic Index helps you determine the main term. Refer to "toenail" in the Alphabetic Index; the closest match is "Toe," which includes the instruction "see condition." Locate the main term "Infection" in the Alphabetic Index. The subterm toe has a subterm "nail" which refers the coder to category 681, Cellulitis and abscess of finger and toe. This does not indicate the condition ingrown toenail. The main term, therefore, is "Ingrown." A review of the Alphabetic Index takes you to "Ingrowing."

- Step 4: There are no italicized instructional notes to interpret.

- Step 5: Review the subterms. The subterm "nail" appears and lists nonessential modifiers (in parentheses) as "finger," "toe" and "infected." These nonessential modifiers complete the diagnostic statement.

- Step 6: There are no abbreviations, cross-references, fifth-digit notations, or brackets.

- Step 7: Verify code 703.0 in the Tabular List Before assigning the code, review all instructional notes under category 703 and under code 703.0. The note, "Excludes: infection, nail NOS (681.9)," can be ignored because the diagnostic statement specifies the infection is due to the ingrowing nail.

- Step 8: Therefore, the subcategory code level is the highest level of specificity. The final code assignment would be 703.0.

- Step 9: The correct code choice is 703.0, Ingrowing nail with infection.

- Step 10: Since infectious infected ingrown toenail is listed as the chief reason for the healthcare encounter, the first-listed or principal diagnosis is 703.0.

Valid Three-digit ICD-9-CM Codes

Three-digit ICD-9-CM codes are used to identify a condition or disease only when a fourth or fifth digit is not available. The following are the only ICD-9-CM codes that are valid without further specificity.

024	Glanders
025	Melioidosis
035	Erysipelas
037	Tetanus
042	Human immunodeficiency virus (HIV) disease
048	Other enterovirus diseases of central nervous system
061	Dengue
064	Viral encephalitis transmitted by other and unspecified arthropods
071	Rabies
075	Infectious mononucleosis
080	Louse-borne [epidemic] typhus
096	Late syphilis, latent
101	Vincent's angina
118	Opportunistic mycoses
124	Trichinosis
129	Intestinal parasitism, unspecified
135	Sarcoidosis
138	Late effects of acute poliomyelitis
179	Malignant neoplasm of uterus, part unspecified
181	Malignant neoplasm of placenta
185	Malignant neoplasm of prostate
193	Malignant neoplasm of thyroid gland
217	Benign neoplasm of breast
220	Benign neoplasm of ovary
226	Benign neoplasm of thyroid glands
243	Congenital hypothyroidism
260	Kwashiorkor
261	Nutritional marasmus
262	Other severe, protein-calorie malnutrition
267	Ascorbic acid deficiency
311	Depressive disorder, not elsewhere classified

316	Psychic factors associated with diseases classified elsewhere
317	Mild intellectual disabilities
319	Unspecified intellectual disabilities
325	Phlebitis and thrombophlebitis of intracranial venous sinuses
326	Late effects of intracranial abscess or pyogenic infection
340	Multiple sclerosis
390	Rheumatic fever without mention of heart involvement
393	Chronic rheumatic pericarditis
412	Old myocardial infarction
430	Subarachnoid hemorrhage
431	Intracerebral hemorrhage
436	Acute, but ill-defined, cerebrovascular disease
449	Septic arterial embolism
452	Portal vein thrombosis
460	Acute nasopharyngitis [common cold]
462	Acute pharyngitis
463	Acute tonsillitis
470	Deviated nasal septum
475	Peritonsillar abscess
481	Pneumococcal pneumonia [Streptococcus pneumoniae pneumonia]
485	Bronchopneumonia, organism unspecified
486	Pneumonia, organism unspecified
490	Bronchitis, not specified as acute or chronic
496	Chronic airway obstruction, not elsewhere classified
500	Coal workers' pneumoconiosis
501	Asbestosis
502	Pneumoconiosis due to other silica or silicates
503	Pneumoconiosis due to other inorganic dust
504	Pneumonopathy due to inhalation of other dust

505	Pneumoconiosis, unspecified
514	Pulmonary congestion and hypostasis
515	Postinflammatory pulmonary fibrosis
538	Gastrointestinal mucositis (ulcerative)
541	Appendicitis, unqualified
542	Other appendicitis
566	Abscess of anal and rectal regions
570	Acute and subacute necrosis of liver
586	Renal failure, unspecified
587	Renal sclerosis, unspecified
591	Hydronephrosis
605	Redundant prepuce and phimosis
630	Hydatidiform mole
632	Missed abortion
650	Normal delivery
677	Late effect of complication of pregnancy, childbirth, and the puerperium
683	Acute lymphadenitis
684	Impetigo
700	Corns and callosities
725	Polymyalgia rheumatica
734	Flat foot
769	Respiratory distress syndrome
797	Senility without mention of psychosis
920	Contusion of face, scalp, and neck except eye(s)
931	Foreign body in ear
932	Foreign body in nose
936	Foreign body in intestine and colon
937	Foreign body in anus and rectum
938	Foreign body in digestive system, unspecified
981	Toxic effect of petroleum products
986	Toxic effect of carbon monoxide
990	Effects of radiation, unspecified
V08	Asymptomatic HIV infection status

Coding Tables

Abortion—Spontaneous/Legally Induced	Spontaneous Abortion (accidental) (early) (late) (miscarriage) (recurrent)				Legal Abortion (legal indication) (medical indication)(under medical supervision)			
	Incomplete (part of the products of conception are retained)	Complete (all of the products of conception are expelled)	Complication following abortion (separate episode of care)	Unspecified	Incomplete (part of the products of conception are retained)	Complete (all of the products of conception are expelled)	Unspecified	Complication following abortion (separate episode of care)
Without complication	634.91	634.92	634.90		635.91	635.92	635.90	
With complication of:								
Afibrinogenemia						635.12	635.10	639.1
Atrophy, acute yellow	634.71	634.72	634.70	639.8	635.71	635.72	635.70	639.8
Cardiac arrest	634.71	634.72	634.70	639.8	635.71	635.72	635.70	639.8
Cardiac failure	634.71	634.72	634.70	639.8	635.71	635.72	635.70	639.8
Cerebral anoxia	634.71	634.72	634.70	639.8	635.71	635.72	635.70	639.8
Circulatory collapse	634.51	634.52	634.50	639.5	635.51	635.52	635.50	639.5
Defibrination syndrome	634.11	634.12	634.10	639.1	635.11	635.12	635.10	639.1
Electrolyte imbalance	634.41	634.42	634.40	639.4	635.41	635.42	635.40	639.4
Embolism (any type)	634.61	634.62	634.60	639.6	635.61	635.62	635.60	639.6
Endometritis	634.01	634.02	634.00	639.0	635.01	635.02	635.00	639.0
Genital tract infection	634.01	634.02	634.00	639.0	635.01	635.02	635.00	639.0
Hemorrhage, delayed or excessive	634.11	634.12	634.10	639.1	635.11	635.12	635.10	639.1
Intravascular hemolysis	634.11	634.12	634.10	639.1	635.11	635.12	635.10	639.1
Kidney failure (acute)	634.31	634.32	634.30	639.3	635.31	635.32	635.30	639.3
Laceration of:								
pelvic organs	634.21	634.22	634.20	639.2	635.21	635.22	635.20	639.2
Metabolic disorder	634.41	634.42	634.40	639.4	635.41	635.42	635.40	639.4
Necrosis of liver	634.71	634.72	634.70	639.8	635.71	635.72	635.70	639.8
Oliguria	634.31	634.32	634.30	639.3	635.31	635.32	635.30	639.3
Other specified complication	634.71	634.72	634.70	639.8	635.71	635.72	635.70	639.8
Parametritis	634.01	634.02	634.00	639.0	635.01	635.02	635.00	639.0
Pelvic infection	634.01	634.02	634.00	639.0	635.01	635.02	635.00	639.0
Pelvic peritonitis	634.01	634.02	634.00	639.0	635.01	635.02	635.00	639.0
Perforation — see Abortion, by type, laceration								
Renal shutdown	634.31	634.32	634.30	639.3	635.31	635.32	635.30	639.3
Renal tubular necrosis	634.31	634.32	634.30	639.3	635.31	635.32	635.30	639.3
Salpingitis	634.01	634.02	634.00	639.0	635.01	635.02	635.00	639.0
Salpingo-oophoritis	634.01	634.02	634.00	639.0	635.01	635.02	635.00	639.0
Sepsis NOS	634.01	634.02	634.00	639.0	635.01	635.02	635.00	639.0
Septicemia NOS	634.01	634.02	634.00	639.0	635.01	635.02	635.00	639.0
Shock (postoperative)(septic)	634.51	634.52	634.50	639.5	635.51	635.52	635.50	639.5
Tear — see Abortion, by type, laceration								
Unspecified complications	634.81	634.82	634.80	639.9	635.81	635.82	635.80	639.9
Uremia	634.31	634.32	634.30	639.3	635.31	635.32	635.30	639.3
Urinary tract infection	634.71	634.72	634.70	639.8	635.71	635.72	635.70	639.8
UTI (urinary tract infection)	634.71	634.72	634.70	639.8	635.71	635.72	635.70	639.8

Abortion—Illegally Induced/Unspecified	Illegally Induced Abortion (criminal) (homicidal) (self-induced)				Unspecified Abortion — Retained products of conception following abortion, not classifiable elsewhere or not otherwise specified			
	Incomplete (part of the products of conception are retained)	Complete (all of the products of conception are expelled)	Unspecified	Complication following abortion (separate episode of care)	Incomplete (part of the products of conception are retained)	Complete (all of the products of conception are expelled)	Unspecified	Complication following abortion (separate episode of care)
Without complication	636.91	636.92	636.90		637.91	637.92	637.90	
With complication of:								
Afibrinogenemia	636.11	636.12	636.10	639.1	637.11	637.12	637.10	639.1
Atrophy, acute yellow	636.71	636.72	636.70	639.8	637.71	637.72	637.70	639.8
Cardiac arrest	636.71	636.72	636.70	639.8	637.71	637.72	637.70	639.8
Cardiac failure	636.71	636.72	636.70	639.8	637.71	637.72	637.70	639.8
Cerebral anoxia	636.71	636.72	636.70	639.8	637.71	637.72	637.70	639.8
Circulatory collapse	636.51	636.52	636.50	639.5	637.51	637.52	637.50	639.5
Defibrination syndrome	636.11	636.12	636.10	639.1	637.11	637.12	637.10	639.1
Electrolyte imbalance	636.41	636.42	636.40	639.4	637.41	637.42	637.40	639.4
Embolism (any type)	636.61	636.62	636.60	639.6	637.61	637.62	637.60	639.6
Endometritis	636.01	636.02	636.00	639.0	637.01	637.02	637.00	639.0

Coding Tables

Abortion

Abortion—Illegally Induced/Unspecified

With complication of: — continued	Illegally Induced Abortion (criminal) (homicidal) (self-induced)				Unspecified Abortion — Retained products of conception following abortion, not classifiable elsewhere or not otherwise specified			
	Incomplete (part of the products of conception are retained)	Complete (all of the products of conception are expelled)	Unspecified	Complication following abortion (separate episode of care)	Incomplete (part of the products of conception are retained)	Complete (all of the products of conception are expelled)	Unspecified	Complication following abortion (separate episode of care)
Genital tract infection	636.01	636.02	636.00	639.0	637.01	637.02	637.00	639.0
Hemorrhage, delayed or excessive	636.11	636.12	636.10	639.1	637.11	637.12	637.10	639.1
Intravascular hemolysis	636.11	636.12	636.10	639.1	637.11	637.12	637.10	639.1
Kidney failure (acute)	636.31	636.32	636.30	639.3	637.31	637.32	637.30	639.3
Laceration of:								
pelvic organs	636.21	636.22	636.20	639.2	637.21	637.22	637.20	639.2
Metabolic disorder	636.41	636.42	636.40	639.4	637.41	637.42	637.40	639.4
Necrosis of liver	636.71	636.72	636.70	639.8	637.71	637.72	637.70	639.8
Oliguria	636.31	636.32	636.30	639.3	637.31	637.32	637.30	639.3
Other specified complication	636.71	636.72	636.70	639.8	637.71	637.72	637.70	639.8
Parametritis	636.01	636.02	636.00	639.0	637.01	637.02	637.00	639.0
Pelvic infection	636.01	636.02	636.00	639.0	637.01	637.02	637.00	639.0
Pelvic peritonitis	636.01	636.02	636.00	639.0	637.01	637.02	637.00	639.0
Perforation — see Abortion, by type, laceration								
Renal shutdown	636.31	636.32	636.30	639.3	637.31	637.32	637.30	639.3
Renal tubular necrosis	636.31	636.32	636.30	639.3	637.31	637.32	637.30	639.3
Salpingitis	636.01	636.02	636.00	639.0	637.01	637.02	637.00	639.0
Salpingo-oophoritis	636.01	636.02	636.00	639.0	637.01	637.02	637.00	639.0
Sepsis NOS	636.01	636.02	636.00	639.0	637.01	637.02	637.00	639.0
Septicemia NOS	636.01	636.02	636.00	639.0	637.01	637.02	637.00	639.0
Shock (postoperative) (septic)	636.51	636.52	636.50	639.5	637.51	637.52	637.50	639.5
Specified complication NEC	636.71	636.72	636.70	639.8	637.71	637.72	637.70	639.8
Tear — see Abortion, by type, laceration								
Unspecified complications	636.81	636.82	636.80	639.9	637.81	637.82	637.80	639.9
Uremia	636.31	636.32	636.30	639.3	637.31	637.32	637.30	639.3
Urinary tract infection	636.71	636.72	636.70	639.8	637.71	637.72	637.70	639.8
UTI (urinary tract infection)	636.71	636.72	636.70	639.8	637.71	637.72	637.70	639.8

Abortion—Other Specified

	Failed Attempted Abortion / Hydatidiform Mole / Missed Abortion / Other Abnormal Product of Conception			
	Failed Attempted Abortion	Hydatidiform Mole	Missed Abortion (all products of conception retained)	Other abnormal product of conception (blighted ovum, chemical, fleshy mole, stone mole, carneous mole, mole NOS)
Without complication	638.9	630	632	
inappropriate level of hCG (chemical, false positive)				631.0
other abnormal products of conception				631.8
With complication of:				
Afibrinogenemia	638.1	639.1	639.1	639.1
Atrophy, acute yellow	638.7	639.8	639.8	639.8
Cardiac arrest	638.7	639.8	639.8	639.8
Cardiac failure	638.7	639.8	639.8	639.8
Cerebral anoxia	638.7	639.8	639.8	639.8
Circulatory collapse	638.5	639.5	639.5	639.5
Defibrination syndrome	638.1	639.1	639.1	639.1
Electrolyte imbalance	638.4	639.4	639.4	639.4
Embolism (any type)	638.6	639.6	639.6	639.6
Endometritis	638.0	639.0	639.0	639.0
Genital tract infection	638.0	639.0	639.0	639.0
Hemorrhage, delayed or excessive	638.1	639.1	639.1	639.1
Intravascular hemolysis	638.1	639.1	639.1	639.1
Kidney failure (acute)	638.3	639.3	639.3	639.3
Laceration of:				
pelvic organs	638.2	639.2	639.2	639.2
Metabolic disorder	638.4	639.4	639.4	639.4
Necrosis of liver	638.7	639.8	639.8	639.8
Oliguria	638.3	639.3	639.3	639.3

Abortion—Other Specified	Failed Attempted Abortion Hydatidiform Mole Missed Abortion Other Abnormal Product of Conception			
	Failed Attempted Abortion	Hydatidiform Mole	Missed Abortion (all products of conception retained)	Other abnormal product of conception (blighted ovum, chemical, fleshy mole, stone mole, carneous mole, mole NOS)
With complication of: — *continued*				
Other specified complications	638.7	639.8	639.8	639.8
Parametritis	638.0	639.0	639.0	639.0
Pelvic infection	638.0	639.0	639.0	639.0
Pelvic peritonitis	638.0	639.0	639.0	639.0
Perforation — *see* Abortion, by type, laceration				
Renal shutdown	638.3	639.3	639.3	639.3
Renal tubular necrosis	638.3	639.3	639.3	639.3
Salpingitis	638.0	639.0	639.0	639.0
Salpingo-oophoritis	638.0	639.0	639.0	639.0
Sepsis NOS	638.0	639.0	639.0	639.0
Septicemia NOS	638.0	639.0	639.0	639.0
Shock (postoperative) (septic)	638.5	639.5	639.5	639.5
Tear — *see* Abortion, by type, laceration				
Unspecified complications	638.8	639.9	639.9	639.9
Urinary tract infection	638.7	639.8	639.8	639.8
UTI (urinary tract infection)	638.7	639.8	639.8	639.8

Burn (acid) (cathode ray) (caustic) (chemical) (electric heating appliance) (electricity) (fire) (flame) (hot liquid or object) (irradiation) (lime) (radiation) (steam) (thermal) (x-ray)	Unspecified Degree	First Degree [erythema]	Second Degree [blisters, epidermal loss]	Third Degree NOS [full-thickness skin loss]	Deep Third Degree [without mention of loss of body part]	Deep Third Degree [with loss of a body part]
Abdomen, abdominal (wall) (muscle)	942.03	942.13	942.23	942.33	942.43	942.53
with trunk	942.09	942.19	942.29	942.39	942.49	942.59
Ankle	945.03	945.13	945.23	945.33	945.43	945.53
with lower limb	945.09	945.19	945.29	945.39	945.49	945.59
Anus	942.09	942.19	942.29	942.39	942.49	942.59
Arm(s)	943.00	943.10	943.20	943.30	943.40	943.50
lower	943.01	943.11	943.21	943.31	943.41	943.51
multiple sites, except hand(s) or wrist(s)	943.09	943.19	943.29	943.39	943.49	943.59
upper	943.03	943.13	943.23	943.33	943.43	943.53
Auditory canal (external)	941.01	941.11	941.21	941.31	941.41	941.51
with face or head	941.09	941.19	941.29	941.39	941.49	941.59
Auricle (ear)	941.01	941.11	941.21	941.31	941.41	941.51
with face or head	941.09	941.19	941.29	941.39	941.49	941.59
Axilla	943.04	943.14	943.24	943.34	943.44	943.54
with upper limb, except hand(s) or wrist(s)	943.09	943.19	943.29	943.39	943.49	943.59
Back	942.04	942.14	942.24	942.34	942.44	942.54
with trunk	942.09	942.19	942.29	942.39	942.49	942.59
Biceps						
brachii	943.03	943.13	943.23	943.33	943.43	943.53
femoris	945.06	945.16	945.26	945.36	945.46	945.56
Breast(s)	942.01	942.11	942.21	942.31	942.41	942.51
with trunk	942.09	942.19	942.29	942.39	942.49	942.59
Brow	941.07	941.17	941.27	941.37	941.47	941.57
Buttock(s)	942.04	942.14	942.24	942.34	942.44	942.54
Cheek (cutaneous)	941.07	941.17	941.27	941.37	941.47	941.57
with face or head	941.09	941.19	941.29	941.39	941.49	941.59
Chest wall (anterior)	942.02	942.12	942.22	942.32	942.42	942.52
with trunk	942.09	942.19	942.29	942.39	942.49	942.59
Chin	941.04	941.14	941.24	941.34	941.44	941.54
with face or head	941.09	941.19	941.29	941.39	941.49	941.59
Clitoris	942.05	942.15	942.25	942.35	942.45	942.55
Ear (drum) (external)	941.01	941.11	941.21	941.31	941.41	941.51
with face or head	941.09	941.19	941.29	941.39	941.49	941.59
Elbow	943.02	943.12	943.22	943.32	943.42	943.52
with hand(s) and wrist(s)	946.0	946.1	946.2	946.3	946.4	946.5
with upper limb, except hand(s) or wrist(s)	943.09	943.19	943.29	943.39	943.49	943.59
Entire body	946.0	946.1	946.2	946.3	946.4	946.5
Epididymis	942.05	942.15	942.25	942.35	942.45	942.55
Epigastric region	942.03	942.13	942.23	942.33	942.43	942.53

Burn

Coding Tables

Burn

Burn (acid) (cathode ray) (caustic) (chemical) (electric heating appliance) (electricity) (fire) (flame) (hot liquid or object) (irradiation) (lime) (radiation) (steam) (thermal) (x-ray)	Unspecified Degree	First Degree [erythema]	Second Degree [blisters, epidermal loss]	Third Degree NOS [full-thickness skin loss]	Deep Third Degree [without mention of loss of body part]	Deep Third Degree [with loss of a body part]
Extremity						
arm	943.00	943.10	943.20	943.30	943.40	943.50
lower	943.01	943.11	943.21	943.31	943.41	943.51
multiple sites	943.09	943.19	943.29	943.39	943.49	943.59
upper	943.03	943.13	943.23	943.33	943.43	943.53
leg	945.00	945.10	945.20	945.30	945.40	945.50
lower	945.04	945.14	945.24	945.34	945.44	945.54
multiple sites	945.09	945.19	945.29	945.39	945.49	945.59
upper	945.06	945.16	945.26	945.36	945.46	945.56
Eye(s), only — *see* Eye, eyeball, burn						
with						
face, head or neck	941.02	941.12	941.22	941.32	941.42	941.52
other sites	946.0	946.1	946.2	946.3	946.4	946.5
Face	941.00	941.10	941.20	941.30	941.40	941.50
multiple sites	941.09	941.19	941.29	941.39	941.49	941.59
with eye(s)	941.02	941.12	941.22	941.32	941.42	941.52
Finger (nail) (subungual)	944.01	944.11	944.21	944.31	944.41	944.41
with						
hand(s)	944.08	944.18	944.28	944.38	944.48	944.58
other sites	946.0	946.1	946.2	946.3	946.4	946.5
thumb	944.04	944.14	944.24	944.34	944.44	944.54
multiple digits	944.03	944.13	944.23	944.33	944.43	944.53
with thumb	944.04	944.14	944.24	944.34	944.44	944.54
Foot	945.02	945.12	945.22	945.32	945.42	945.52
with lower limb	945.09	945.19	945.29	945.39	945.49	945.59
Forearm(s)	943.01	943.11	943.21	943.31	943.41	943.51
with upper limb, except hand(s) or wrist(s)	943.09	943.19	943.29	943.39	943.49	943.59
Forehead	941.07	941.17	941.27	941.37	941.47	941.57
with face or head	941.09	941.19	941.29	941.39	941.49	941.59
Genitourinary organ(s)						
external	942.05	942.15	942.25	942.35	942.45	942.55
internal—*see* specific organ or site, burn						
Groin	942.03	942.13	942.23	942.33	942.43	942.53
Hand(s) (and wrist)	944.00	944.10	944.20	944.30	944.40	944.50
back (doral surface)	944.06	944.16	944.26	944.36	944.46	944.56
multiple sites	944.08	944.18	944.28	944.38	944.48	944.58
Head (and face)	941.00	941.10	941.20	941.30	941.40	941.50
multiple sites	941.09	941.19	941.29	941.39	941.49	941.59
Heel	945.02	945.12	945.22	945.32	945.42	945.52
Hip	942.09	942.19	942.29	942.39	942.49	942.59
Internal organ(s) — *see* specific organ or site, burn						
Knee	945.05	945.15	945.25	945.35	945.45	945.55
with lower limb	945.09	945.19	945.29	945.39	945.49	945.59
Labium (majus) (minus)	942.05	942.15	942.25	942.35	942.45	942.55
Leg	945.00	945.10	945.20	945.30	945.40	945.50
lower, unspecified site	945.04	945.14	945.24	945.34	945.44	945.54
multiple sites	945.09	945.19	945.29	945.39	945.49	945.59
upper (thigh) (any part)	945.06	945.16	945.26	945.36	945.46	945.56
Lip(s)	941.03	941.13	941.23	941.33	941.43	941.53
with face or head	941.09	941.19	941.29	941.39	941.49	941.59
Lumbar region	942.04	942.14	942.24	942.34	942.44	942.54
Malar region	941.07	941.17	941.27	941.37	941.47	941.57
Mastoid region	941.06	941.16	941.26	941.36	941.46	941.56
Membrane, tympanic	941.01	941.11	941.21	941.31	941.41	941.51
Multiple, specified sites, classifiable to more than one category in 940–945	946.0	946.1	946.2	946.3	946.4	946.5
Nasal (septum)	941.05	941.15	941.25	941.35	941.45	941.55
Neck	941.08	941.18	941.28	941.38	941.48	941.58
with face or head	941.09	941.19	941.29	941.39	941.49	941.59
Nose	941.05	941.15	941.25	941.35	941.45	941.55
with face or head	941.09	941.19	941.29	941.39	941.49	941.59
Palm(s)	944.05	944.15	944.25	944.35	944.45	944.55
with hand(s) or wrist(s)	944.08	944.18	944.28	944.38	944.48	944.58
Penis	942.05	942.15	942.25	942.35	942.45	942.55
Perineum	942.05	942.15	942.25	942.35	942.45	942.55
Pubic region	942.05	942.15	942.25	942.35	942.45	942.55

Burn (acid) (cathode ray) (caustic) (chemical) (electric heating appliance) (electricity) (fire) (flame) (hot liquid or object) (irradiation) (lime) (radiation) (steam) (thermal) (x-ray)	Unspecified Degree	First Degree [erythema]	Second Degree [blisters, epidermal loss]	Third Degree NOS [full-thickness skin loss]	Deep Third Degree [without mention of loss of body part]	Deep Third Degree [with loss of a body part]
Sacral region	942.04	942.14	942.24	942.34	942.44	942.54
Scalp	941.06	941.16	941.26	941.36	941.46	941.56
with face or head	941.09	941.19	941.29	941.39	941.49	941.59
Scapular region	943.06	943.16	943.26	943.36	943.46	943.56
with upper limb, except hand(s) or wrist(s)	943.09	943.19	943.29	943.39	943.49	943.59
Scrotum	942.05	942.15	942.25	942.35	942.45	942.55
Shoulder(s)	943.05	943.15	943.25	943.35	943.45	943.55
with						
hand(s) and wrist(s)	946.0	946.1	946.2	946.3	946.4	946.5
upper limb, except hand(s) or wrist(s)	943.09	943.19	943.29	943.39	943.49	943.59
Skin, unspecified site	949.0	949.1	949.2	949.3	949.4	949.5
Skull	941.00	941.10	941.20	941.30	941.40	941.50
Submental region	941.04	941.14	941.24	941.34	941.44	941.54
Supraclavicular fossa	941.08	941.18	941.28	941.38	941.48	941.58
Temple	941.06	941.16	941.26	941.36	941.46	941.56
Testicle	942.05	942.15	942.25	942.35	942.45	942.55
Thigh	945.06	945.16	945.26	945.36	945.46	945.56
with lower limb	945.09	945.19	945.29	945.39	945.49	945.59
Thumb(s) (nail)	944.02	944.12	944.22	944.32	944.42	944.52
with finger(s)	944.04	944.14	944.24	944.34	944.44	944.54
with hand(s) or wrist(s)	944.08	944.18	944.28	944.38	944.48	944.58
Toe (nail)	945.01	945.11	945.21	945.31	945.41	945.51
with lower limb	945.09	945.19	945.29	945.39	945.49	945.59
Trunk	942.00	942.10	942.20	942.30	942.40	942.50
multiple sites	942.09	942.19	942.29	942.39	942.49	942.59
specified site, NEC	942.09	942.19	942.29	942.39	942.49	942.59
Tunica vaginalis	942.05	942.15	942.25	942.35	942.45	942.55
Unspecified site	949.0	949.1	949.2	949.3	949.4	949.5
Vulva	942.05	942.15	942.25	942.35	942.45	942.55
Wrist(s)	944.07	944.17	944.27	944.37	944.47	944.57
with hand(s)	944.08	944.18	944.28	944.38	944.48	944.58

Complications due to (presence of)	Mechanical	Infection/inflammatory reaction	Other
Aortocoronary bypass graft	996.03	996.61	996.72
Arteriovenous			
fistula	996.1	996.62	996.74
shunt	996.1	996.62	996.74
Artificial heart	996.09	996.61	996.72
Artificial skin graft	996.55	996.69	996.79
Bariatric procedure			
gastric band		539.01	539.09
other		539.81	539.89
Bile duct	996.59	996.69	996.79
Blood vessel graft	996.1	996.62	996.74
Bone growth stimulator	996.40	996.67	996.78
Bone marrow transplant	996.85	996.85	996.85
Breast implant	996.54	996.69	996.79
Bypass graft			
aortocoronary	996.03	996.61	996.72
blood vessel	996.1	996.62	996.74
carotid artery	996.1	996.62	996.74
coronary artery	996.03	996.61	996.72
femoral-popliteal	996.1	996.62	996.74
Cardiac			
defibrillator	996.04	996.61	996.72
pulse generator	996.04	996.61	996.72
subcutaneous pocket	996.04	996.61	996.72
pacemaker		996.61	996.72
pulse generator	996.09	996.61	996.72
subcutaneous pocket	996.09	996.61	996.72
valve prosthesis	996.02	996.61	996.71
Carotid artery bypass graft	996.1	996.62	996.74
Catheter			
central venous	996.1	999.31	996.74
cystostomy	596.82	996.65	996.76

Coding Tables (sidebar)

Complications due to (sidebar)

Complications due to (presence of)	Mechanical	Infection/inflammatory reaction	Other
Catheter — continued			
dialysis (hemodialysis)	996.1	996.62	996.73
peritoneal	996.56	996.68	996.73
Hickman	996.1	999.31	996.74
PICC	996.1	999.31	996.74
spinal	996.2	996.63	996.75
urinary, indwelling	996.31	996.64	996.76
triple lumen	996.1	999.31	996.74
vascular (peripheral)	996.1	996.62	996.74
Chin implant	996.59	996.69	996.79
Contraceptive device (intrauterine)	996.32	996.65	996.76
Corneal graft	996.51	996.69	996.79
retroprosthetic membrane	996.51		
Coronary artery bypass graft	996.03	996.61	996.72
Cystostomy	596.82	596.81	596.83
Decellularized alodermis	996.55	996.69	996.79
Dialysis catheter (hemodialysis)	996.1	996.62	996.73
peritoneal	996.56	996.68	996.73
Dorsal column stimulator	996.2	996.63	996.75
Electrodes			
brain	996.2	996.63	996.75
heart	996.01	996.61	996.72
Esophagostomy	530.87	530.86	
External fixator device	996.40	996.67	996.78
Genitourinary device	996.39	996.65	996.76
unspecified	996.30	996.65	996.70
Graft			
artificial skin	996.52	996.69	996.79
blood vessel	996.1	996.62	996.74
bone	996.40	996.67	996.78
cartilage	996.40	996.67	996.78
carotid artery	996.1	996.62	996.74
corneal	996.51	996.69	996.79
retroprosthetic membrane	996.51		
coronary artery	996.03	996.61	996.72
femoral-popliteal	996.1	996.62	996.74
muscle	996.40	996.67	996.78
peripheral nerve	996.2	996.62	996.75
skin	996.52	996.69	996.79
tendon	996.40	996.67	996.78
ureter	996.39	996.65	996.76
Heart assist device	996.09	996.61	996.72
Heart transplant	996.83	996.83	996.83
Infusion pump	996.59	996.62	996.74
Insulin pump	996.57	996.69	996.57
Internal fixator device			
nail	996.40	996.67	996.78
plate	996.40	996.67	996.78
rod	996.40	996.67	996.78
screw	996.40	996.67	996.78
Intraaortic balloon	996.1	996.62	996.74
Joint prosthesis, internal			
Articular bearing surface wear	996.46	996.66	996.77
Aseptic loosening	996.41	996.66	996.77
Breakage (fracture) of prosthetic joint	996.43	996.66	996.77
Dislocation of prosthetic joint	996.42	996.66	996.77
Failure of prosthetic joint implant	996.47	996.66	996.77
Instability of prosthetic joint	996.42	996.66	996.77
Loosening of prosthetic joint	996.41	996.66	996.77
Peri-prosthetic fracture	996.44	996.66	996.77
Peri-prosthetic osteolysis	996.45	996.66	996.77
Subluxation of prosthetic joint	996.42	996.66	996.77
Liver transplant	996.82	996.82	996.82
Lung transplant	996.84	996.84	996.84
Mammary implant	996.54	996.69	996.79
Nervous system device	996.2	996.63	996.75
Nonabsorbable surgical material NOS	996.59	996.69	996.79
Other vascular device	996.1	996.62	996.74

Complications due to (presence of)	Mechanical	Infection/inflammatory reaction	Other
Pancreas transplant	996.86	996.86	996.86
Prosthetic implant			
bile duct	996.59	996.69	996.79
breast	996.54	996.69	996.79
chin	996.59	996.69	996.79
ocular lens	996.53	996.69	996.79
orbit of eye	996.59	996.69	996.79
vaginal mesh			
erosion			629.31
exposure			629.32
vas deferens	996.39	996.65	996.76
Shunt			
arteriovenous	996.1	996.62	996.74
ventricular	996.2	996.63	996.75
Transfusion			
anaphylactic reaction			999.41
febrile			780.66
hemochromatosis			275.02
hemolytic reaction			999.83
acute			999.84
delayed			999.85
incompatibility reaction			
ABO			999.60
with HTR			999.61
acute			999.62
delayed			999.63
non-specified			999.61
specified type NEC			999.69
non-ABO			
with HTR			999.76
acute			999.77
delayed			999.78
non-specified			999.75
specified type NEC			999.79
Rh			
with HTR			999.71
acute			999.72
delayed			999.73
non-specified			999.70
specified type NEC			999.74
overload			
circulatory (TACO)			276.61
fluid			276.61
iron			275.02
purpura			287.41
serum reaction			999.51
specified reaction NEC			999.89
Transplanted organ			
bone marrow	996.85	996.85	996.85
heart	996.83	996.83	996.83
liver	996.82	996.82	996.82
lung	996.84	996.84	996.84
other specified organ	996.89	996.89	996.89
pancreas	996.86	996.86	996.86
stem cell	996.88	996.88	996.88
unspecified organ	996.80	996.80	996.80
Umbrella device, vena cava	996.1	996.62	996.74
Unspecified cardiac device	996.00	996.60	996.72
Vascular catheter (peripheral)	996.1	996.62	996.74
Ventricular shunt	996.2	996.63	996.75

Diabetes (brittle) (congenital) (familial) (mellitus) (severe) (slight)	**TYPE I**		**TYPE II or unspecified type. The codes found in these columns are for use even if the patient requires insulin.**			**Additional Code Required**
	Controlled or not stated as uncontrolled	Uncontrolled	Controlled or not stated as uncontrolled	Uncontrolled	Other metabolic disorders or conditions	List these codes after the diabetes code
Without complication or manifestation	250.01	250.03	250.00	250.02		
With complication or manifestation						
coma (ketoacidosis)	250.31	250.33	250.30	250.32		
hyperosmolar (nonketotic)	250.21	250.23	250.20	250.22		
complication NOS	250.91	250.93	250.90	250.92		
specified NEC	250.81	250.83	250.80	250.82		
gangrene	250.71	250.73	250.70	250.72		785.4
hyperosmolarity	250.21	250.23	250.20	250.22		
ketosis, ketoacidosis	250.11	250.13	250.10	250.12		
osteomyelitis	250.81	250.83	250.80	250.82		731.8
specified manifestations NEC	250.81	250.83	250.80	250.82		
Abnormal glucose NOS						
NOS					790.29	
non-fasting					790.29	
fasting					790.21	
tolerance test					790.22	
Abnormal glucose tolerance test (GTT), **elevated glucose tolerance test**					790.22	
Acetonemia	250.11	250.13	250.10	250.12		
Acidosis	250.11	250.13	250.10	250.12		
Amyotrophy	250.61	250.63	250.60	250.62		353.1
Angiopathia, angiopathy (peripheral)	250.71	250.73	250.70	250.72		443.81
retinalis (juvenilis)	250.51	250.53	250.50	250.52		362.01
Arthritis, arthropathy	250.61	250.63	250.60	250.62		713.5
Charcôt's	250.61	250.63	250.60	250.62		713.5
neuropathic (Charcôt's)	250.61	250.63	250.60	250.62		713.5
Asymptomatic elevated (abnormal glucose)					790.29	
Ataxia, ataxy, ataxic, locomotor (progressive)	250.61	250.63	250.60	250.62		337.1
Autonomic neuropathy (peripheral)	250.61	250.63	250.60	250.62		337.1
Bone change	250.81	250.83	250.80	250.82		731.8
Bronze, bronzed					275.01	
Cataract diabetic	250.51	250.53	250.50	250.52		366.41
senile (non diabetic)	250.01	250.03	250.00	250.02		366.17
snowflake	250.51	250.53	250.50	250.52		366.41
Charcôt's joint (disease)	250.61	250.63	250.60	250.62		713.5
Chemical					790.29	
Coma (with ketoacidosis)	250.31	250.33	250.30	250.32		
hyperglycemic	250.31	250.33	250.30	250.32		
hyperosmolar (nonketotic)	250.21	250.23	250.20	250.22		
hypoglycemic	250.31	250.33	250.30	250.32		
nondiabetic					251.0	
insulin	250.31	250.33	250.30	250.32		
nondiabetic					251.0	
Kussmaul's	250.31	250.33	250.30	250.32		
prediabetic	250.21	250.23	250.20	250.22		
Complication NOS	250.91	250.93	250.90	250.92		
specified NEC	250.81	250.83	250.80	250.82		
Dermopathy	250.81	250.83	250.80	250.82		709.8
Dietary supervision					V65.3	
Ebstein's disease	250.41	250.43	250.40	250.42		581.81
Edema (macula) (retina)	250.51	250.53	250.50	250.52		362.01
Family History					V18.0	
Gangrene	250.71	250.73	250.70	250.72		785.4
Gastroparalysis/Gastroparesis	250.61	250.63	250.60	250.62		536.3
Gestational diabetes						
antepartum					648.83	
delivered w/o antepartum condition					648.81	
postpartum					648.84	
unspecified. episode. of care					648.80	
with antepartum condition					648.82	
with long term (current) insulin use						V58.67
Glaucoma	250.51	250.53	250.50	250.52		365.44
Glomeruiohyalinosis — diabetic syndrome	250.41	250.43	250.40	250.42		581.81

Diabetes (brittle) (congenital) (familial) (mellitus) (severe) (slight)	TYPE I		TYPE II or unspecified type. The codes found in these columns are for use even if the patient requires insulin.			Additional Code Required
	Controlled or not stated as uncontrolled	Uncontrolled	Controlled or not stated as uncontrolled	Uncontrolled	Other metabolic disorders or conditions	List these codes after the diabetes code
Glomerulonephritis, chronic	250.41	250.43	250.40	250.42		583.81
with nephrotic syndrome	250.41	250.43	250.40	250.42		581.81
Glomerulosclerosis (intercapillary)	250.41	250.43	250.40	250.42		581.81
Glucose Intolerance					790.22	
Glycogenosis, secondary	250.81	250.83	250.80	250.82		259.8
Hemochromatosis						
hereditary	275.01					
primary	275.01					
specified type	275.03					
transfusion associated (red cell)	275.02					
Hirschfeld's disease	250.01	250.01	250.00	250.02		
Hyperglycemia						
with coma	250.31	250.33	250.30	250.32		
diabetic	250.11	250.13	250.10	250.12		
neonatal (transient)					775.1	
nondiabetic					790.6	
postpancreatectomy					251.3	
Hyperosmolar coma	250.21	250.23	250.20	250.22		
Hyperosmolarity	250.21	250.23	250.20	250.22		
Hypertension nephrosis syndrome	250.41	250.43	250.40	250.42		581.81
Hypoglycemia (diabetic) without coma	250.81	250.83	250.80	250.82		
with coma	250.31	250.33	250.30	250.32		
neonatal, transient					775.0	
nondiabetic						
with coma					251.0	
without coma					251.1	
NOS (spontaneous)					251.2	
Hypoglycemic shock	250.81	250.83	250.80	250.82		
Hypoinsulinemia, postsurgical					251.3	
Impaired fasting glucose					790.21	
Impotence	250.61	250.63	250.60	250.62		607.84
Insipidus					253.5	
nephrogenic					588.1	
pituitary					253.5	
vasopressin-resistant					588.1	
Insulin, long term (current) use						V58.67
Insulin overdose	250.x1	250.x3	250.x0	250.x2	962.3	
Insulin underdose (code to diabetes only)						
Intercapillary glomerulosclerosis	250.41	250.43	250.40	250.42		581.81
Iridis rubeosis/Iritis	250.51	250.53	250.50	250.53		364.42
Ketosis, ketoacidosis	250.11	250.13	250.10	250.12		
Kidney disease, chronic	250.41	250.43	250.40	250.42		585.9
End Stage	250.41	250.43	250.40	250.42		585.6
Stage I	250.41	250.43	250.40	250.42		585.1
Stage II	250.41	250.43	250.40	250.42		585.2
Stage III	250.41	250.43	250.40	250.42		585.3
Stage IV	250.41	250.43	250.40	250.42		585.4
Stage V	250.41	250.43	250.40	250.42		585.5
Kimmelstiel (-Wilson) disease or syndrome	250.41	250.43	250.40	250.42		581.81
Kussmaul's coma	250.31	250.33	250.30	250.32		
Lancereaux's (diabetes mellitus with marked emaciation)	250.81	250.83	250.80	250.82		261
Latent (chemical)					790.29	
Lipoidosis	250.81	250.83	250.80	250.82		272.7
Macular edema	250.51	250.53	250.50	250.52		362.01
Microangiopathy (peripheral)	250.71	250.73	250.70	250.72		443.81
Mononeuropathy, mononeuritis, unspecified site	250.61	250.63	250.60	250.62		355.9
lower limb, unspecified	250.61	250.63	250.60	250.62		355.8
upper limb, unspecified	250.61	250.63	250.60	250.62		354.9
Myelopathy	250.61	250.63	250.60	250.62		336.3
Necrobiosis lipoidica	250.81	250.83	250.80	250.82		709.3
Neonatal, transient hyperglycemia					775.1	
hypoglycemia					775.0	
Nephritis, chronic	250.41	250.43	250.40	250.42		583.81
with nephrotic syndrome	250.41	250.43	250.40	250.42		581.81

Coding Tables

Diabetes (side tab)

Diabetes (brittle) (congenital) (familial) (mellitus) (severe) (slight)	TYPE I		TYPE II or unspecified type. The codes found in these columns are for use even if the patient requires insulin.			Additional Code Required
	Controlled or not stated as uncontrolled	Uncontrolled	Controlled or not stated as uncontrolled	Uncontrolled	Other metabolic disorders or conditions	List these codes after the diabetes code
Nephropathy	250.41	250.43	250.40	250.42		583.81
Nephrosis (Ebsteins) (syndrome)	250.41	250.43	250.40	250.42		581.81
Neuralgia	250.61	250.63	250.60	250.62		357.2
Neuritis	250.61	250.63	250.60	250.62		357.2
Neurogenic arthropathy	250.61	250.63	250.60	250.62		713.5
Neuropathic arthritis	250.61	250.63	250.60	250.62	713.5	
Neuropathy	250.61	250.63	250.60	250.62		357.2
autonomic (peripheral)	250.61	250.63	250.60	250.62		337.1
Neurophthisis	250.61	250.63	250.60	250.62		357.2
Nonclinical					790.29	
Ophthalmoplegia	250.51	250.53	250.50	250.52		378.86
Osteomyelitis	250.81	250.83	250.80	250.82		731.8
Peripheral angiopathy	250.71	250.73	250.70	250.72		443.81
Peripheral autonomic neuropathy	250.61	250.63	250.60	250.62		337.1
Peripheral vascular disease (occlusive)	250.71	250.73	250.70	250.72		443.81
Pre-diabetes NOS					790.29	
Phosphate					275.3	
Polyneuropathy, polyneuritis	250.61	250.63	250.60	250.62		357.2
Postpancreatectomy					251.3	
Postsurgical (hypoinsulinemia)					251.3	
Prediabetes					790.29	
Pseudotabes	250.61	250.63	250.60	250.62		337.1
Renal glycosuria (true)					271.4	
Retinal						
edema	250.51	250.53	250.50	250.52		362.07
hemorrhage	250.51	250.53	250.50	250.52		362.01
Retinitis	250.51	250.53	250.50	250.52		362.01
Retinopathy	250.51	250.53	250.50	250.52		362.01
background (simple)	250.51	250.53	250.50	250.52		362.01
nonproliferative, NOS	250.51	250.53	250.50	250.52		362.03
nonproliferative, mild	250.51	250.53	250.50	250.52		362.04
nonproliferative, moderate	250.51	250.53	250.50	250.52		362.05
nonproliferative, severe	250.51	250.53	250.50	250.52		362.06
proliferative	250.51	250.53	250.50	250.52		362.02
Rubeosis iridis	250.51	250.53	250.50	250.52		364.42
Secondary						
postsurgical					251.3	
steroid induced					251.8	E932.0
Skin						
dermopathy	250.81	250.83	250.80	250.82		709.8
necrobiosis lipoidica diabeticorum	250.81	250.83	250.80	250.82		709.3
Screening					V77.1	
Steroid induced						
correct substance properly administered					251.8	E932.0
overdose or wrong substance given or taken					962.0	
Stress					790.29	
Subclinical					790.29	
Subliminal					790.29	
Syndrome						
diabetes-dwarfism-obesity (juvenile)					258.1	
diabetes mellitus in newborn						
infant					775.1	
diabetes-nephrosis	250.41	250.43	250.40	250.42		581.81
diabetic amyotrophy	250.61	250.63	250.60	250.62		353.1
Hanot-Chauffard (-Troisier) (bronze diabetes)					275.01	
nephrotic	250.41	250.43	250.40	250.42		581.81
Oppenheim-Urbach (necrobiosis lipoidica diabeticorum)	250.81	250.83	250.80	250.82		709.3
Pierre Mauriac's (diabetes-dwarfism-obesity)					258.1	
renal glomerulohyalinosis-diabetic	250.41	250.43	250.40	250.42		581.81
Troisier-Hanot-Chauffard (bronze diabetes)					275.01	
Urbach-Oppenheim (necrobiosis lipoidica diabeticorum)	250.81	250.83	250.80	250.82		709.3

Diabetes (brittle) (congenital) (familial) (mellitus) (severe) (slight)	TYPE I		TYPE II or unspecified type. The codes found in these columns are for use even if the patient requires insulin.			Additional Code Required
	Controlled or not stated as uncontrolled	Uncontrolled	Controlled or not stated as uncontrolled	Uncontrolled	Other metabolic disorders or conditions	List these codes after the diabetes code
Ulcer (skin), **except pressure, unspecified site**	250.81	250.83	250.80	250.82		707.9
lower extremity, unspecified	250.81	250.83	250.80	250.82		707.19
lower extremity, ankle	250.81	250.83	250.80	250.82		707.13
lower extremity, calf	250.81	250.83	250.80	250.82		707.12
lower extremity, heel and midfoot	250.81	250.83	250.80	250.82		707.14
lower extremity, thigh	250.81	250.83	250.80	250.82		707.11
lower extremity, toes	250.81	250.83	250.80	250.82		707.15
specified site NEC	250.81	250.83	250.80	250.82		707.8
unspecified complication	250.91	250.93	250.90	250.92		
Willis' disease	250.01	250.03	250.00	250.02		
Xanthoma diabeticorum, xanthomatosis	250.81	250.83	250.80	250.82		272.2

Site of Hernia	Without Obstruction	With Obstruction	Gangrene (with or without obstruction)
Abdomen (wall)	553.20	552.20	551.20
recurrent	553.21	552.21	551.21
Abdominal, specified site NEC	553.8	552.8	551.8
Appendix	553.8	552.8	551.8
Bilateral — see Hernia, by site			
Bladder (sphincter)			
congenital (female) (male)	756.71		
female			
lateral	618.02		
midline	618.01		
male		596.89	
Brain (acquired) (stem)	348.4		
congenital	742.0		
Broad ligament	553.8		
Bubonocele — see Hernia, inguinal			
Cecocele — see also Hernia, by site	553.9	552.9	551.9
Cerebral (acquired)	348.4		
congenital (endaural)	742.0		
Ciliary body (acquired)	364.89		
traumatic	871.1		
Colic	553.9	552.9	551.9
Colon	553.9	552.9	551.9
Colostomy	569.69		
Cooper's	553.8	552.8	551.8
Crural — see Hernia, femoral			
Diaphragm(atic)	553.3	552.3	551.3
congenital (gross defect)	756.6		
traumatic	862.0		
with open wound	862.1		
Direct — see Hernia, inguinal			
Disc, intervertebral — see Displacement, intervertebral disc			
Diverticulum (intestine)	553.9	552.9	551.9
Double — see Hernia, inguinal			
Duodenojejunal	553.8	552.8	551.8
Encysted — see Hernia, inguinal			
En glissade — see Hernia, inguinal			
Enterocele – see also Hernia, by site	553.9	552.9	551.9
Enterostomy	569.69		
Epigastric	553.29	552.29	551.29
recurrent	553.21	552.21	551.21
Epigastrocele	553.29	552.29	551.29
recurrent	553.21	552.21	551.21
Epiplocele	553.9	552.9	551.9
Epiplosarcomphalocele	553.1	552.1	551.1
Esophageal (hiatal)	553.3	552.3	551.3
congenital	750.6		
Eventration (chest to colon)	553.3	552.3	551.3
congenital (gross defect)	756.6		
External — see Hernia, inguinal			

Site of Hernia	Without Obstruction	With Obstruction	Gangrene (with or without obstruction)
Fallopian tube	620.4		
Fascia	728.89		
Fat (pad)	729.30		
eye, eyelid	374.34		
knee		729.31	
orbit		374.34	
retro-orbital	374.34		
retropatellar	729.31		
specified site NEC	729.39		
Female			
complete	618.3		
cystocele			
lateral	618.02		
midline	618.01		
with prolapse	618.4		
incomplete	618.2		
fallopian tube	620.4		
ovary, oviduct	620.4		
rectovaginal	618.6		
uterus	621.8		
vaginal	618.6		
vesical			
congenital	756.71		
lateral	618.02		
midline	618.01		
Femoral (unilateral)	553.00	552.00	551.00
bilateral	553.02	552.02	551.02
recurrent	553.03	552.03	551.03
recurrent (unilateral)	553.01	552.01	551.01
Foramen			
Bochdale (acquired)	553.3	552.3	551.3
congenital	756.6		
magnum	348.4		
Morgagni (an) (acquired)	553.3	552.3	551.3
congenital	756.6		
Furnicular (umbilical)	553.1	552.1	551.1
spermatic cord—*see* Hernia, inguinal			
Gastric mucosa	537.89		
Gastrointestinal tract	553.9	552.9	551.9
Gluteal — *see* Hernia, femoral			
Gruber's	553.8	552.8	551.8
Hesselbach's	553.8	552.8	551.8
Hiatal (esophageal) (sliding)	553.3	552.3	551.3
Holthouse's — *see* Hernia, inguinal			
Incarcerated — *see* Hernia, by site, with obstruction			
Incisional	553.21	552.21	551.21
lumbar	553.8	552.8	551.8
Indirect — *see* Hernia, inguinal			
Infantile — *see* Hernia, inguinal			
Infrapatellar fat pad	729.31		
Inguinal (unilateral) (direct) (double) ((encysted) (external) (furnicular) (indirect) (infantile) (internal) (interstial) (oblique) (scrotal) (sliding)	550.90	550.10	550.00
bilateral	550.92	550.12	550.02
recurrent	550.93	550.13	550.03
recurrent (unilateral)	550.91	550.11	550.01
Internal	553.8	552.8	551.8
Interstitial	553.9	552.9	551.9
Intervertebral cartilage — *see* Displacement, intervertebral disc			
Intestine(al)	553.9	552.9	551.9
Intra-abdominal	553.9	552.9	551.9
Intraparietal	553.9	552.9	551.9
Iris (acquired)	364.89		
traumatic	871.1		
Irreducible — *see* Hernia, by site, with obstruction			
Ischiatic	553.8	552.8	551.8

Site of Hernia

Site of Hernia	Without Obstruction	With Obstruction	Gangrene (with or without obstruction)
Lens (acquired)	379.32		
traumatic	871.1		
Linea alba	553.29	552.29	551.29
recurrent	553.21	552.21	551.21
Linea semilunaris	553.29	552.29	551.29
Littre's	553.9	552.9	551.9
Lumbar	553.8	552.8	551.8
intervertebral disc	722.10		
Lung (acquired)	518.89		
congenital	748.69		
Male			
chylocele	608.84		
cystocele	596.89		
scrotal - *see* Hernia, inguinal			
spermatocele	608.1		
congenital	752.8		
testis	550.90	550.10	550.00
bilateral	550.92	550.12	550.02
recurrent	550.93	550.13	550.03
recurrent (unilateral)	550.91	550.11	550.01
vesical	596.89		
congenital	756.71		
Mediastinum	519.3		
Merocele — *see* Hernia, femoral			
Mesenteric (internal)	553.8	552.8	551.8
Mesocolon	553.8	552.8	551.8
Muscle (sheath)	728.89		
Nucleus polpous — *see* Displacement, intervertebral disc			
Oblique — *see* Hernia, inguinal			
Obstructive — *see* Hernia, by site with obstruction			
Orbturator	553.8	552.8	551.8
Omental	553.8	552.8	551.8
Omentocele	553.8	552.8	551.8
Orbital fat pad	374.34		
Ovary, oviduct	620.4		
Paracolostomy	569.69		
Paraduodenal	553.8	552.8	551.8
Paraesophageal	553.8	552.8	551.8
congenital	750.6		
Parahiatal	553.8	552.8	551.8
Paraumbilical	553.1	552.1	551.1
Parietal	553.9	552.9	551.9
Perineal	553.8	552.8	551.8
Peritoneal sac, lesser	553.8	552.8	551.8
Petit's	553.8	552.8	551.8
intervertebral disc	722.10		
Popliteal fat pad	729.31		
Postoperative	553.21	552.21	551.21
Prevesical	596.89		
Properitoneal	553.8	552.8	551.8
Pudendal	553.8	552.8	551.8
Rectovaginal	618.6		
Retroperitoneal	553.8	552.8	551.8
Richter's	553.9	552.9	551.9
Rieux's, Reix's	553.8	552.8	551.8
Saint's, triad — *see* Hernia, Diaphragm			
Sarcopiplocele	553.9	552.9	551.9
Sarcoepiplomphalocele	553.9	552.9	551.9
Sciatic	553.8	552.8	551.8
Scrotum, scrotal — *see* Hernia, inguinal			
Sliding			
hiatal	553.3	552.3	551.3
congenital	750.6		
inguinal — *see* Hernia, inguinal			
Spermatocele	608.1		
congenital	752.8		
Spigelian	553.29	552.29	551.29
Spinal — *see* Spina Bifida			

Coding Tables

Site of Hernia	Without Obstruction	With Obstruction	Gangrene (with or without obstruction)
Strangulated — *see* Hernia, by site, wth obstruction			
Supraumbilicus	553.29	552.29	551.29
recurrent	553.21	552.21	551.21
Tendon	727.9		
Testis (nontraumatic)	550.90	550.10	550.00
bilateral	550.92	550.12	550.02
recurrent	550.93	550.13	550.03
recurrent (unilateral)	550.91	550.11	550.01
Thoracic stomach	553.8	552.8	551.8
Treitz's	553.8	552.8	551.8
Triad, Saint's — *see* Hernia, diaphragm			
Umbilical, umbilicus	553.1	552.1	551.1
Unspecified site NEC	553.9	552.9	551.9
Ureter	593.89	593.4	
Uterus NOS	621.8		
pregnant — *see* herniation of uterus—pregnancy table			
Vaginal	618.6		
Velpeau's — *see* Hernia, femoral			
Ventral	553.20	552.20	551.20
incisional	553.21	552.21	551.21
recurrent	553.21	552.21	551.21
Vertebral cartilage — *see* Displacement, intervertebral disc			
Vesical			
congenital (female) (male)	756.71		
female			
lateral	618.02		
midline	618.01		
male		596.89	
Vitreous (acquired)	379.21		
traumatic	871.1		

Ectopic Pregnancy

Ectopic Pregnancy	Abdominal pregnancy (Intraperitoneal pregnancy)	Tubal pregnancy (Fallopian pregnancy, rupture of fallopian tube due to pregnancy, tubal abortion)	Ovarian pregnancy	Other ectopic pregnancy (Includes the following pregnancy(s): cervical, cornual mural mesometric intraligamentous)	Unspecified ectopic pregnancy
Without complication					
with intrauterine pregnancy	633.01	633.11	633.21	633.81	633.91
without intrauterine pregnancy	633.00	633.10	633.20	633.80	633.90
With complication of:					
Afibrinogenemia	639.1	639.1	639.1	639.1	639.1
Atrophy, acute yellow	639.8	639.8	639.8	639.8	639.8
Cardiac arrest	639.8	639.8	639.8	639.8	639.8
Cardiac failure	639.8	639.8	639.8	639.8	639.8
Cerebral anoxia	639.8	639.8	639.8	639.8	639.8
Circulatory collapse	639.5	639.5	639.5	639.5	639.5
Defibrination syndrome	639.1	639.1	639.1	639.1	639.1
Electrolyte imbalance	639.4	639.4	639.4	639.4	639.4
Embolism (any type)	639.6	639.6	639.6	639.6	639.6
Endometritis	639.0	639.0	639.0	639.0	639.0
Genital tract infection	639.0	639.0	639.0	639.0	639.0
Hemorrhage, delayed or excessive	639.1	639.1	639.1	639.1	639.1
Intravascular hemolysis	639.1	639.1	639.1	639.1	639.1
Kidney failure (acute)	639.3	639.3	639.3	639.3	639.3
Laceration of:					
pelvic organs	639.2	639.2	639.2	639.2	639.2
Metabolic disorder	639.4	639.4	639.4	639.4	639.4
Necrosis of liver	639.8	639.8	639.8	639.8	639.8
Oliguria	639.3	639.3	639.3	639.3	639.3
Other specified complication	639.8	639.8	639.8	639.8	639.8
Parametritis	639.0	639.0	639.0	639.0	639.0
Pelvic infection	639.0	639.0	639.0	639.0	639.0
Pelvic peritonitis	639.0	639.0	639.0	639.0	639.0
Renal shutdown	639.3	639.3	639.3	639.3	639.3
Renal tubular necrosis	639.3	639.3	639.3	639.3	639.3
Salpingitis	639.0	639.0	639.0	639.0	639.0
Salpingo-oophoritis	639.0	639.0	639.0	639.0	639.0

Coding Tables

Ectopic Pregnancy (side tab)

Ectopic Pregnancy

Ectopic Pregnancy	Abdominal pregnancy (Intraperitoneal pregnancy)	Tubal pregnancy (Fallopian pregnancy, rupture of fallopian tube due to pregnancy, tubal abortion)	Ovarian pregnancy	Other ectopic pregnancy (Includes the following pregnancy(s): cervical, cornual mural mesometric intraligamentous)	Unspecified ectopic pregnancy
With complication of: — *continued*					
Sepsis NOS	639.0	639.0	639.0	639.0	639.0
Septicemia NOS	639.0	639.0	639.0	639.0	639.0
Shock (postoperative)(septic)	639.5	639.5	639.5	639.5	639.5
Unspecified complications	639.9	639.9	639.9	639.9	639.9
Urinary tract infection (UTI)	639.8	639.8	639.8	639.8	639.8

Normal Pregnancy

Pregnancy/Delivery, current (Normal) (Single) (Uterine) (without Sickness)	Code	Special Notes
Assisted reproductive technology	V23.85	
Counseling (for)		
illegitimate	V61.6	
multiparity	V61.5	
unwanted pregnancy, NEC	V61.7	
Examination (pregnancy test)		
negative results	V72.41	
positive results	V72.42	
unconfirmed	V72.40	
Normal delivery	650	This code is always a primary diagnosis.
Normal pregnancy		
with other condition not affecting the pregnancy	V22.2	V22.2 should be used in place of any other pregnancy codes and listed second on the claim form. The condition, which does not affect the pregnancy, must be listed first.
first pregnancy	V22.0	Codes V22.0 and V22.1 should never be used in conjunction with any codes from cataegories 640-648 and 651-676.
second or other normal pregnancy	V22.1	Meaning 2nd, 3rd, 4th etc. pregnancy
Postpartum care and examination		
immediately after delivery	V24.0	Normal uncomplicated cases
lactating mother	V24.1	Supervision of lactating mother
routine postpartum follow-up	V24.2	Care within 6 weeks after delivery
Previous (not affecting current pregnancy)		These codes may be used in conjunction with chapter 11 codes. A thorough review of any pertinent excludes notes (found in the tabular list) is necessary to be certain that these V codes are being used properly.
abortion	V23.2	Excludes recurrent pregnancy loss (646.3x)
difficult delivery	V23.49	
ectopic pregnancy	V23.42	
forceps delivery	V23.49	
hemorrhage, antepartum or postpartum	V23.49	
hydatidiform mole	V23.1	
infertility	V23.0	
in utero procedure	V23.86	Current pregnancy with history of in utero procedure during a prior pregnancy. Report a history of in utero procedure in a nongravid uterus with code V15.21
malignancy NEC	V23.89	
neonatal death	V23.5	
nonobstetrical conditions	V23.89	
premature delivery	V23.41	
pre-term labor	V23.41	
specified NEC	V23.89	
stillbirth	V23.5	
trophoblastic disease	V23.1	
unspecified condition	V23.9	
vesicular mole	V23.1	
Screening, prenatal (for)		If the abnormal finding is known—code the screening and the findings as additional codes
by		
amniocentesis		
chromosomal anomalies	V28.0	
raised alpha-fetoprotein levels (amniotic fluid)	V28.1	
specified, NEC	V28.2	
fetal anatomic survey	V28.81	
ultrasound		
amniocentesis — *continued*		
fetal growth retardation	V28.4	
malformation	V28.3	

Coding Tables

Normal Pregnancy

Pregnancy/Delivery, current (Normal) (Single) (Uterine) (without Sickness)	Code	Special Notes
Screening, prenatal (for) — *continued*		
isoimmunization	V28.5	
other specified screening	V28.89	
Streptococcus B	V28.6	
unspecified, screening	V28.9	
Supervision (of) (for)		These codes may be used in conjunction with chapter 11 codes. A thorough review of any pertinent excludes notes (found in the tabular list) is necessary to be certain that these V codes are being used properly.
high-risk, NOS	V23.9	
insufficient prenatal care	V23.7	
specified problem NEC	V23.89	
inconclusive fetal viability	V23.87	
multigravida		Second or more pregnancy
elderly	V23.82	35 years of age or older at expected date of delivery
young	V23.84	Younger than 16 years of age at expected date of delivery
multiparity	V23.3	
normal NEC	V22.1	
first pregnancy	V22.0	
poor		
obstetric history	V23.49	
reproductive history	V23.5	
primigravida		First pregnancy
elderly	V23.81	35 years of age or older at expected date of delivery
young	V23.83	Younger than 16 years of age at expected date of delivery
unconfirmed	V72.40	
undelivered (no other diagnosis)	V22.2	
with false labor	644.1	
high risk	V23.9	
specified problems NEC	V23.89	
Suspected problem not found		
amniotic cavity and membrane	V89.01	
cervical shortening	V89.05	
fetal anomaly	V89.03	
fetal growth	V89.04	
placental	V89.02	

Antepartum Pregnancy

Condition or Complication; affecting management of mother	Antepartum condition or complication	Delivered, with or without mention of antepartum condition	Unspecified episode of care	Assign additional code to describe the...	Affecting fetus (coded on the newborn chart only)
Ablatio placentae	641.23	641.21	641.20		762.1
Abnormal, NEC	646.93	646.91	646.90		761.8
amnion	658.93	658.91	658.90		762.9
cervix	654.63	654.61	654.60		763.89
causing obstructed labor	660.23	660.21	660.20	cause	763.1
change in	631.0				
quantitative human chorionic gonadotropin (hCG) in early pregnancy					
chorion	658.93	658.91	658.90		762.9
cord (umbilical)	663.93	663.91	663.90		762.6
fetal chromosomes (suspected)	655.13	655.11	655.10		758.89
fetal					
heart rate	659.73	659.71	659.70		763.83
before onset of labor	659.73	659.71	659.70		763.81
during labor	659.73	659.71	659.70		763.82
heart rhythm	659.73	659.71	659.70		763.8
before onset of labor	659.73	659.71	659.70		763.81
during labor	659.73	659.71	659.70		763.82
fetus, fetal (suspected) NEC	655.93	655.91	655.90		779.9
acid-base balance	656.83	656.81	656.80		768.4
causing disproportion	653.73	653.71	653.70		763.1
causing obstructed labor	660.13	660.11	660.10	cause	763.1
specified NEC	655.83	655.81	655.80		779.8

Antepartum Pregnancy Condition or Complication; affecting management of mother	Antepartum condition or complication	Delivered, with or without mention of antepartum condition	Unspecified episode of care	Assign additional code to describe the…	Affecting fetus (coded on the newborn chart only)
Abnormal, NEC — *continued*					
findings, nonspecific (a code from 640-648 should be used first when the management of the mother is affected by the abnormal findings)	796.5				
glucose tolerance test	648.83	648.81	648.80	condition	775.0
labor (forces of) NEC	661.93	661.91	661.90	condition	763.7
pelvic organs or tissues NEC	654.93	654.91	654.90		763.89
causing obstructed labor	660.23	660.21	660.20	cause	763.1
pelvis (bony)	653.03	653.01	653.00		763.1
causing obstructed labor	660.13	660.11	660.10	cause	763.1
perineum or vulva	654.83	654.81	654.80		763.89
causing obstructed labor	660.23	660.21	660.20	cause	763.1
placenta, placental (vessel)	656.73	656.71	656.70		762.2
with hemorrhage	641.83	641.81	641.80		762.1
position					
cervix	654.43	654.41	654.40		763.89
causing obstructed labor	660.23	660.21	660.20	cause	763.1
fetus	652.93	652.91	652.90		763.1
causing obstructed labor	660.03	660.01	660.00	cause	763.1
placenta (low implantation) (previa)	641.03	641.01	641.00		762.0
with hemorrhage	641.13	641.11	641.10		762.1
uterus	654.43	654.41	654.40		763.89
causing obstructed labor	660.23	660.21	660.20	cause	763.1
product(s) of conception NEC	631.8				
quality of milk	676.83	676.81	676.80		
shape of uterus	654.43	654.41	654.40		763.89
causing obstructed labor	660.23	660.21	660.20	cause	763.1
size of fetus	653.53	653.51	653.50		763.1
causing obstructed labor	660.13	660.11	660.10	cause	763.1
umbilical cord NEC	663.83	663.81	663.80		762.6
uterus (congenital)	654.03	654.01	654.00		763.89
causing obstructed labor	660.23	660.21	660.20	cause	763.1
vagina	654.73	654.71	654.70		763.89
causing obstructed labor	660.23	660.21	660.20	cause	763.1
vulva (acquired) (congenital)	654.83	654.81	654.80		763.89
causing obstructed labor	660.23	660.21	660.20	cause	763.1
weight gain	646.13	646.11	646.10	condition	761.8
with					
hypertension (mild) (pre-eclamptic)	642.43	642.41	642.40		760.0
convulsions	642.63	642.61	642.60		760.0
pre-existing hypertension	642.73	642.71	642.70		760.0
severe hypertension	642.53	642.51	642.50		760.0
Aborter, recurrent	646.33	646.31	646.30	condition	761.8
Abruption of placenta	641.23	641.21	641.20		762.1
Abscess					
areola (acute) (chronic)	675.13	675.11	675.10		
Bartholin's gland	646.63	646.61	646.60	condition	760.8
bladder	646.63	646.61	646.60	condition	760.1
breast (acute) (chronic)	675.13	675.11	675.10		
kidney	646.63	646.61	646.60	condition	760.1
labium (majus) (minus)	646.63	646.61	646.60	condition	760.8
milk	675.13	675.11	675.10		
nipple	675.03	675.01	675.00		
subareolar	675.13	675.11	675.10		
urethra	646.63	646.61	646.60	condition	760.1
vulva	646.63	646.61	646.60	condition	760.8
Absorption (of) (through placenta)					
suspected damage to fetus					
chemical	655.53	655.51	655.50		760.70
drug	655.53	655.51	655.50		760.70
Acidosis (fetal) (intrauterine)	656.83	656.81	656.80		768.4
Addiction					
alcoholic	648.43	648.41	648.40	condition	760.71
suspected fetal damage	655.43	655.41	655.40		760.71

Coding Tables

Antepartum Pregnancy

Antepartum Pregnancy Condition or Complication; affecting management of mother	Antepartum condition or complication	Delivered, with or without mention of antepartum condition	Unspecified episode of care	Assign additional code to describe the…	Affecting fetus (coded on the newborn chart only)
Adhesion(s), adhesive					
amnion to fetus	658.83	658.81	658.80		762.8
uterus to abdominal wall	654.43	654.41	654.40		763.89
causing obstructed labor	660.23	660.21	660.20	cause	763.1
Advanced maternal age (multigravida)	659.63	659.61	659.60		761.8
primigravida	659.53	659.51	659.50		761.8
Aerocele	673.03	673.01	673.00		
AFP (screening for raised levels in amniotic fluid)	V28.1				
Agalactia	676.43	676.41	676.40		
Air embolism	673.03	673.01	673.00		
Age					
elderly (35 years of age or older at expected date of delivery)					
multigravida (second or more pregnancy)	659.63	659.61	659.60		
primigravida (first pregnancy)	659.53	659.51	659.50		
young (less than 16 years old at expected date of delivery)	659.83	659.81	659.80		
Albuminuria (gravidarum)	646.23	646.21	646.20	condition	760.1
with hypertension (and edema)					760.1
mild	642.43	642.41	642.40		760.0
severe	642.53	642.51	642.50		760.0
gestational	646.23	646.21	646.20	condition	760.1
pre-eclamptic (mild)	642.23	642.21	642.20		760.0
severe	642.53	642.51	642.50		760.0
Alcohol, alcoholic					
addiction (maternal)	648.43	648.41	648.40	condition	760.71
with suspected fetal damage	655.43	655.41	655.40		760.71
Alphafetoprotein (screening for raised levels in amniotic fluid)	V28.1				
Amnion (nodosum)	658.83	658.81	658.80		762.9
Amnionitis	658.43	658.41	658.40		762.7
Amniotic fluid embolism	673.13	673.11	673.10		
Amputation of cervix	654.63	654.61	654.60		763.89
causing obstructed labor	660.23	660.21	660.20	cause	763.1
Android pelvis					
with disproportion (fetopelvic)	653.33	653.31	653.30		763.1
causing obstructed labor	660.13	660.11	660.10	cause	763.1
Anemia	648.23	648.21	648.20	condition	760.8
aplastic	648.23	648.21	648.20	condition	760.8
iron (Fe) deficiency	648.23	648.21	648.20	condition	760.8
macrocytic	648.23	648.21	648.20	condition	760.8
megaloblastic	648.23	648.21	648.20	condition	760.8
pernicious	648.23	648.21	648.20	condition	760.8
postpartum	648.23	648.21	648.20	condition	
Anencephalus, anencephaly (fetal)	655.03	655.01	655.00		
Anesthesia, anesthetic					
complications NEC	668.83	668.81	668.80	condition	
cardiac	668.13	668.11	668.10	condition	763.5
central nervous system	668.23	668.21	668.20	condition	763.5
pulmonary	668.03	668.01	668.00	condition	763.5
death (from) during delivery	668.93	668.91	668.90	condition	761.6
Anomaly, anomalous (congenital)					
cardiovascular system	648.53	648.51	648.50	condition	
cervix	654.63	654.61	654.60		763.89
causing obstructed labor	660.23	660.21	660.20	cause	763.1
pelvis (bony)	653.03	653.01	653.00		763.1
causing obstructed labor	660.13	660.11	660.10	cause	763.1
uterus	654.03	654.01	654.00		763.89
causing obstructed labor	660.23	660.21	660.20	cause	763.1
Anoxia cerebral					
complicating delivery (cesarean) (instrumental)	669.43	669.41	669.40		
due to obstetric anesthesia or sedation	668.23	668.21	668.20	complication	
Anteversion					
uterus, uterine (cervix)	654.43	654.41	654.40		763.89
causing obstructed labor	660.23	660.21	660.20	cause	763.1

Antepartum Pregnancy Condition or Complication; affecting management of mother	Antepartum condition or complication	Delivered, with or without mention of antepartum condition	Unspecified episode of care	Assign additional code to describe the...	Affecting fetus (coded on the newborn chart only)
Anthropoid pelvis					
with disproportion (fetopelvic)	653.23	653.21	653.20		763.1
causing obstructed labor	660.13	660.11	660.10	cause	763.1
Antibodies (incompatibility)					
ABO	656.23	656.21	656.20		773.2
anti-C	656.13	656.11	656.10		773.0
anti-D, cord blood	656.13	656.11	656.10		773.0
anti-E	656.13	656.11	656.10		773.0
blood group (ABO)	656.23	656.21	656.20		773.1
Rh (blood group) (factor)	656.13	656.11	656.10		773.0
Apoplexia, apoplexy, apoplectic					
placenta	641.23	641.21	641.20		762.1
uteroplacental	641.23	641.21	641.20		762.1
Arrest, arrested					
active phase of labor	661.13	661.11	661.10		763.7
any plane in pelvis complicating delivery	660.13	660.11	660.10	cause	763.1
cardiac					
anesthesia, complicating	668.13	668.11	668.10		
delivery (cesarean) (instrumental)	669.43	669.41	669.40		
deep transverse	660.33	660.31	660.30	cause	763.1
development or growth of fetus	656.53	656.51	656.50		764.90
transverse (deep)	660.33	660.31	660.30	cause	763.1
Ascites					
fetal, causing fetopelvic disproportion	653.73	653.71	653.70		763.1
causing obstructed labor	660.13	660.11	660.10	cause	763.1
Aspiration					
acid-pulmonary (syndrome)	668.03	668.01	668.00	complication	
pneumonitis	668.03	668.01	668.00	complication	
Assimilation, pelvis					
with disproportion	653.23	653.21	653.20		763.1
causing obstructed labor	660.13	660.11	660.10	cause	763.1
Asymmetry					
pelvis with disproportion	653.03	653.01	653.00		763.1
causing obstructed labor	660.13	660.11	660.10	cause	763.1
Atonia, atony, atonic (intrapartum)					
w/o hemmorage	661.23	661.21	661.20		
Atresia, atretic					
cervix	654.63	654.61	654.60		763.89
causing obstructed labor	660.23	660.21	660.20	cause	763.1
Atrophy, atrophic					
breast	676.33	676.31	676.30		
liver (acute) (subacute) (yellow)	646.73	646.71	646.70	complication	
Avulsion (traumatic)					
symphyseal cartilage (inner)		665.61	665.60		
Bacilluria, asymptomatic	646.53	646.51	646.50	complication	
Bacteremia					
during labor	659.33	659.31	659.30		
during pregnancy	647.83	647.81	647.80	condition	
Bacteriuria, asymptomatic	646.53	646.51	646.50	complication	760.1
Band(s), amniotic	658.83	658.81	658.80		762.8
Bandl's ring (contraction)	661.43	661.41	661.40		763.7
Bariatric surgery	649.23	649.21	649.20		
Bicornis or Bicornuate uterus	654.03	654.01	654.00		763.89
causing obstructed labor	660.23	660.21	660.20	cause	763.1
Bleeding	641.93	641.91	641.90		
accidental	641.23	641.21	641.20		762.1
before 22 completed weeks gestation NEC	640.93	640.91	640.90		
cerebrovascular	674.03	674.01	674.00		
due to					
afibrinogenemia or other coagulation defect	641.33	641.31	641.30		
fibroids	641.83	641.81	641.80		762.1
marginal sinus (rupture)	641.23	641.21	641.20		762.1
premature separation, placenta	641.23	641.21	641.20		762.1
trauma	641.83	641.81	641.80		
early (before 22 completed weeks gestation)	640.93	640.91	640.90		
threatened abortion	640.03	640.01	640.00		

Coding Tables

Antepartum Pregnancy

Antepartum Pregnancy Condition or Complication; affecting management of mother	Antepartum condition or complication	Delivered, with or without mention of antepartum condition	Unspecified episode of care	Assign additional code to describe the…	Affecting fetus (coded on the newborn chart only)
Bleeding — *continued*					
unavoidable	641.13	641.11	641.10		
Bone disorders	648.73	648.71	648.70	condition	
Borderline pelvis	653.13	653.11	653.10		763.1
with obstruction during labor	660.13	660.11	660.10	cause	763.1
Braxton Hicks contractions	644.13		644.10		
Breech presentation (buttocks) (complete) (frank)	652.23	652.21	652.20		761.7
with successful version	652.13	652.11	652.10		763.1
before labor	652.23	652.21	652.20		761.7
during labor	652.23	652.21	652.20		763.0
Brow presentation					
complicating delivery	652.43	652.41	652.40		763.1
Bruise					
umbilical cord	663.63	663.61	663.60		762.6
Caked breast	676.23	676.21	676.20		
Cardiomyopathy	674.53	674.51	674.50		
Cardiovascular disease	648.63	648.61	648.60	condition	
congenital	648.53	648.51	648.50	condition	
Cellulitis, breast	675.13	675.11	675.10		
Cephalopelvic disproportion NOS	653.43	653.41	653.40		763.1
with obstruction during labor	660.13	660.11	660.10	cause	763.1
Cerebrovascular disorders	674.03	674.01	674.00	condition	
Cervical Shortening	649.73	649.71	649.70		
Cervicitis	646.63	646.61	646.60	condition	760.8
Cervix					
adhesions	654.63	654.61	654.60		
anaplasia	654.63	654.61	654.60		
atypism	654.63	654.61	654.60		
bands	654.63	654.61	654.60		
with obstruction during labor	660.23	660.21	660.20	cause	763.1
cervicitis	654.63	654.61	654.60		
cicatrix	654.63	654.61	654.60		
cyst		654.61	654.60		
dysplasia	654.63	654.61	654.60		
ectropion	654.63	654.61	654.60		
endocervicitis	654.63	654.61	654.60		
erosion	654.63	654.61	654.60		
hypertrophic elongation	654.63	654.61	654.60		
incompetence	654.53	654.51	654.50		761.0
leukoplakia	654.63	654.61	654.60		
Nabothian (gland) cyst or follicle	654.63	654.61	654.60		
polyp		654.61	654.60		
stricture and stenosis	654.63	654.61	654.60		
ulcer		654.61	654.60		
Cesarean delivery, section NEC		669.71	669.70		763.4
post mortem		669.71	669.70		761.6
previous	654.23	654.21	654.20		
causing obstructed labor	660.23	660.21	660.20	cause	763.1
Chiari-Frommel syndrome	676.63	676.61	676.60		
Chloasma (gravidarum)	646.83	646.81	646.80	condition	
Chorioamnionitis	658.43	658.41	658.40		762.7
Cicatrix					
cervix	654.63	654.61	654.60		
causing obstructed labor	660.23	660.21	660.20	cause	763.1
vagina	654.73	654.71	654.70		
causing obstructed labor	660.23	660.21	660.20	cause	763.1
Coagulation defects	649.33	649.31	649.30	286.0-286.9, 287.0-287.9, 289.0-289.9	
Collapse (during or after labor and delivery)					
circulatory (peripheral)	669.13	669.11	669.10		779.8
lung		668.01	668.00		
vascular (peripheral)	669.13	669.11	669.10		
Colporrhexis		665.41	665.40		
Complications NEC	646.93	646.91	646.90	condition	761.9
delivery	669.93	669.91	669.90		

Antepartum Pregnancy Condition or Complication; affecting management of mother	Antepartum condition or complication	Delivered, with or without mention of antepartum condition	Unspecified episode of care	Assign additional code to describe the…	Affecting fetus (coded on the newborn chart only)
Complications NEC — *continued*					
labor and delivery					
procedure (instrumental) (manual) (surgical)	669.43	669.41	669.40		
specified type NEC	669.83	669.81	669.80		
umbilical cord	663.93	663.91	663.90		762.6
specified type NEC	663.83	663.81	663.80		762.6
in utero procedure					
fetal	679.13	679.11	679.10		
maternal	679.03	679.01	679.00		
intrauterine contraceptive device (IUD)	655.83	655.81	655.80		
labor and delivery	669.93	669.91	669.90		
anesthesia (sedation)	668.93	668.91	668.90		763.5
cardiac	668.13	668.11	668.10		
central nervous system	668.23	668.21	668.20		
pulmonary	668.03	668.01	668.00		
specified type NEC	668.83	668.81	668.80		
specified condition NEC	669.83	669.81	669.80		
Compound presentation					
complicating delivery	652.83	652.81	652.80		763.1
causing obstructed labor	660.03	660.01	660.00	cause	763.1
Compression, umbilical cord					
complicating delivery	663.23	663.21	663.20		762.5
cord around neck	663.13	663.11	663.10		762.5
cord prolapsed	663.03	663.01	663.00		762.4
Conjoined twins	678.10	678.11	678.10		
causing disproportion (fetopelvic)	653.73	653.71	653.70		763.1
with obstruction during labor	660.13	661.00	660.10	cause	763.1
Constriction					
ring (uterus)	661.43	661.41	661.40		763.7
Contractions					
before 37 weeks	644.03		644.00		
Braxton Hicks	644.13		644.10		
Hicks'	644.13		644.10		
hourglass uterus	661.43	661.41	661.40		763.7
pelvis, complicating delivery	653.13	653.11	653.10		763.1
causing obstructed labor	660.13	660.11	660.10	cause	763.1
generally contracted	653.13	653.11	653.10		763.1
causing obstructed labor	660.13	660.11	660.10	cause	763.1
inlet	653.23	653.21	653.20		763.1
causing obstructed labor	660.13	660.11	660.10	cause	763.1
midpelvic	653.83	653.81	653.80		763.1
causing obstructed labor	660.13	660.11	660.10	cause	763.1
midplane	653.83	653.81	653.80		763.1
causing obstructed labor	660.13	660.11	660.10	cause	763.1
outlet	653.33	653.31	653.30		763.1
causing obstructed labor	660.13	660.11	660.10	cause	763.1
ring (Bandl's)	661.43	661.41	661.40		763.7
uterus					
abnormal	661.93	661.91	661.90		763.7
clonic, hourglass or tetanic	661.43	661.41	661.40		763.7
dyscoordinate	661.43	661.41	661.40		763.7
hourglass	661.43	661.41	661.40		763.7
incoordinate	661.43	661.41	661.40		763.7
inefficient or poor	661.23	661.21	661.20		763.7
irregular	661.23	661.21	661.20		763.7
tetanic	661.43	661.41	661.40		763.7
Convulsions (eclamptic) (uremic)	642.63	642.61	642.60		760.0
with pre-existing hypertension	642.73	642.71	642.70		760.0
Cord, complicating delivery					
around neck (tightly) (with compression)	663.13	663.11	663.10		762.5
without compression	663.33	663.31	663.30		762.6
prolapse, complicating delivery	663.03	663.01	663.00		762.4
Cornual — *see* Ectopic pregnancy					761.4
CPD	653.43	653.41	653.40		763.1
causing obstructed labor	653.43	653.41	653.40		763.1
Cracked nipple	676.13	676.11	676.10		

Coding Tables

Antepartum Pregnancy

Antepartum Pregnancy Condition or Complication; affecting management of mother	Antepartum condition or complication	Delivered, with or without mention of antepartum condition	Unspecified episode of care	Assign additional code to describe the...	Affecting fetus (coded on the newborn chart only)
Cretin, pelvis (with disproportion) (fetopelvic)	653.13	653.11	653.10		763.1
causing obstructed labor	660.13	660.11	660.10	cause	763.1
Cross birth (of fetus) **complicating delivery**	652.33	652.31	652.30		763.1
with successful version	652.13	652.11	652.10		763.1
causing obstructed labor	660.03	660.01	660.00	cause	763.1
Cyst					
amnion, amniotic	658.83	658.81	658.80		763.89
chorion	658.83	658.81	658.80		763.89
ovary	654.43	654.41	654.40		763.89
causing obstructed labor	660.23	660.21	660.20	cause	763.1
pelvic	654.43	654.41	654.40		763.89
causing obstructed labor	660.23	660.21	660.20	cause	763.1
Cystitis	646.63	646.61	646.60	condition	760.1
Cystocele	654.43	654.41	654.40		763.89
causing obstructed labor	660.23	660.21	660.20	cause	763.1
Damage					
coccyx, complicating delivery		665.61	665.60		763.89
pelvic (during delivery)					
joint or ligament		665.61	665.60		763.89
organ		665.51	665.50		
Dates vs uterine size discrepancy	646.83	646.81	646.80		
Dead, fetus					
retained in utero (after 22 completed weeks' gestation)	656.43	656.41	656.40		779.9
before 22 weeks — *see* Abortion, missed					
syndrome	641.33	641.31	641.30		779.9
Death					
fetal NEC	646.93	646.91	646.90	condition	779.9
early before 22 weeks gestation — *see* Abortion, missed					
near term	656.43	656.41	656.40		779.9
maternal, NEC	646.93	646.91	646.90	condition	761.6
during delivery	668.93	668.91	668.90		
sudden, during delivery	669.93	669.91	669.90		761.6
under anesthesia NEC	668.93	668.91	668.90		761.6
Deciduitis	646.63	646.61	646.60		760.8
Decreased fetal movements	655.73	655.71	655.70		
Defect, defective					
coagulation (factor)	641.33	641.31	641.30		762.1
causing hemorrhage of pregnancy or delivery	641.33	641.31	641.30		762.1
Deficiency, deficient					
coagulation (factor)	641.33	641.31	641.30		762.1
causing hemorrhage of pregnancy or delivery	641.33	641.31	641.30		762.1
Deformity					
fetal					
with fetopelvic disproportion	653.73	653.71	653.70		763.1
causing obstructed labor	660.13	660.11	660.10		763.1
known or suspected	655.93	655.91	655.90		763.89
pelvic, pelvis					
with disproportion (fetopelvic)	653.03	653.01	653.00		763.1
causing obstructed labor	660.13	660.11	660.10	cause	763.1
soft part, organs or tissues NEC	654.93	654.91	654.90	cause	763.89
causing obstructed labor	660.23	660.21	660.20	cause	763.1
Delay, delayed					
any plane in pelvis, complicating delivery	660.13	660.11	660.10	cause	763.1
birth or delivery NEC	662.13	662.11	662.10		763.89
second twin, triplet, or multiple mate	662.33	662.31	662.30		763.89
Dependence, maternal					
alcohol, with suspected fetal damage	655.43	655.41	655.40		779.5
drug	648.33	648.31	648.30	condition	779.5
suspected damage to fetus	655.53	655.51	655.50		779.5
Depression	648.43	648.41	648.40	condition	
Dermatitis, gestationis	646.83	646.81	646.80	condition	
Detachment					
cervix, annular		665.31	665.30		763.89

Antepartum Pregnancy Condition or Complication; affecting management of mother	Antepartum condition or complication	Delivered, with or without mention of antepartum condition	Unspecified episode of care	Assign additional code to describe the…	Affecting fetus (coded on the newborn chart only)
Development					
incomplete (fetus or newborn)	656.53	656.51	656.50		763.89
Diabetes					
condition present before pregnancy	648.03	648.01	648.00	condition	775.0
gestational (chemical) (latent)	648.83	648.81	648.80	condition	775.0
with long term (current) insulin use				V58.67	775.0
Diastasis, recti (abdomen) **complicating delivery**	665.83	665.81	665.80		763.89
Difficult delivery NEC	669.93	669.91	669.90		763.89
Dilatation					
bladder (sphincter)	654.43	654.41	654.40		763.89
causing obstructed labor	660.23	660.21	660.20	cause	763.1
cervix, complicating delivery	654.63	654.61	654.60		763.89
incomplete, poor, slow	661.03	661.01	661.00		763.7
Discrepancy-uterine size to dates	646.83	646.81	646.80		
Disease, diseased NEC	646.93	646.91	646.90	condition	
breast NEC	676.33	676.31	676.30		
cerebrovascular, NEC	674.03	674.01	674.00		
Frommel's	676.63	676.61	676.60		
heart					
placenta	656.73	656.71	656.70		762.2
renal NEC	646.23	646.21	646.20	condition	760.1
Valsuani's (progressive pernicious anemia, puerperal)	648.23	648.21	648.20	condition	
venereal NEC	647.23	647.21	647.20	condition	
virus NEC	647.63	647.61	647.60	condition	
with fetal damage	655.33	655.31	655.30		763.89
Disorders					
breast	676.33	676.31	676.30		
genital tract or organ	646.63	646.61	646.60	condition	760.8
lactation	676.93	676.91	676.90		
liver	646.73	646.71	646.70	condition	760.8
mental	648.43	648.41	648.40	condition	
metabolism NEC (in labor and delivery)	669.03	669.01	669.00		763.89
Displacement, uterus NEC	654.43	654.41	654.40		763.89
causing obstructed labor	660.23	660.21	660.20	cause	763.1
Disproportion	653.93	653.91	653.90		763.1
caused by					
conjoined twins	653.73	653.71	653.70		763.1
contraction, pelvis (general)	653.13	653.11	653.10		763.1
inlet	653.23	653.21	653.20		763.1
midpelvic	653.83	653.81	653.80		763.1
midplane	653.83	653.81	653.80		763.1
outlet	653.33	653.31	653.30		763.1
fetal NEC	653.53	653.51	653.50		763.1
ascites	653.73	653.71	653.70		763.1
hydrocephalus	653.63	653.61	653.60		763.1
hydrops	653.73	653.71	653.70		763.1
meningomyelocele	653.73	653.71	653.70		763.1
sacral teratoma	653.73	653.71	653.70		763.1
tumor	653.73	653.71	653.70		763.1
hydrocephalic fetus	653.63	653.61	653.60		763.1
pelvis, pelvic, abnormality (bony) NEC	653.03	653.01	653.00		763.1
unusually large fetus	653.53	653.51	653.50		763.1
causing obstructed labor	660.13	660.11	660.10	cause	763.1
cephalopelvic, normally formed fetus	653.43	653.41	653.40		763.1
fetopelvic, normally formed fetus	653.43	653.41	653.40		763.1
causing obstructed labor	660.13	660.11	660.10	cause	763.1
pelvis, pelvic (bony) NEC	653.13	653.11	653.10		763.1
causing obstructed labor	660.13	660.11	660.10	cause	763.1
specified type NEC	653.83	653.81	653.80		763.1
Distortion					
lumbar spine					
with disproportion (fetopelvic)	653.03	653.01	653.00		763.1
causing obstructed labor	660.13	660.11	660.10	cause	763.1
maternal	669.03	669.01	669.00		
Distress (fetal)	656.83	656.81	656.80		763.89

Antepartum Pregnancy Condition or Complication; affecting management of mother	Antepartum condition or complication	Delivered, with or without mention of antepartum condition	Unspecified episode of care	Assign additional code to describe the...	Affecting fetus (coded on the newborn chart only)
Double uterus	654.03	654.01	654.00		763.89
causing obstructed labor	660.23	660.21	660.20	cause	763.1
Dropsy, amnion	657.03	657.01	657.00		761.3
Drug dependence	648.33	648.31	648.30	condition	
Dyscrasia, blood					
with antepartum hemorrhage	641.33	641.31	641.30		762.1
Dysfunction					
thyroid	648.13	648.11	648.10	condition	
uterus, complicating delivery	661.93	661.91	661.90		763.7
hypertonic	661.43	661.41	661.40		763.7
hypotonic, primary	661.03	661.01	661.00		763.7
secondary	661.13	661.11	661.10		763.7
Dysplasia of cervix	654.63	654.61	654.60		763.89
causing obstructed labor	660.23	660.21	660.20	cause	763.1
Dystocia	660.93	660.91	660.90	cause	763.1
cervical	661.23	661.21	661.20		763.7
contraction ring	661.43	661.41	661.40		763.7
fetal	660.93	660.91	660.90	cause	763.1
abnormal size	653.53	653.51	653.50		763.1
causing obstructed labor	660.13	660.11	660.10	cause	763.1
deformity	653.73	653.71	653.70		763.1
causing obstructed labor	660.13	660.11	660.10	cause	763.1
maternal	660.93	660.91	660.90		763.1
positional	660.03	660.01	660.00	cause	763.1
shoulder (girdle)	660.43	660.41	660.40	cause	763.1
uterine NEC	661.43	661.41	661.40		763.7
Early onset of delivery (spontaneous)		644.21	644.20		
Preterm neonate birthweight					
Extreme immaturity (code also weeks of gestation, codes 765.20-765.29)					
unspecified (weight)					765.00
< 500 gms					765.11
500-749 gms					765.02
750-999 gms					765.03
1,000-1,249 gms					765.04
1,250-1,499 gms					765.05
1,500-1,749 gms					765.06
1,750-1,999 gms					765.07
2,000-2,499 gms					765.08
≥ 2,500 gms					765.09
Other preterm (code also weeks of gestation, codes 765.20-765.29)					
unspecified (weight)					765.10
< 500 gms					765.11
500-749 gms					765.12
750-999 gms					765.13
1,000-1,249 gms					765.14
1,250-1,499 gms					765.15
1,500-1,749 gms					765.16
1,750-1,999 gms					765.17
2,000-2,499 gms					765.18
≥ 2,500 gms					765.19
Preterm neonate weeks of gestation (code in addition to birthweight, subcategory codes 765.0 and 765.1)					
unspecified weeks of gestation					765.20
< 24 completed weeks of gestation					765.21
24 completed weeks of gestation					765.22
25-26 completed weeks of gestation					765.23
27-28 completed weeks of gestation					765.24
29-30 completed weeks of gestation					765.25
31-32 completed weeks of gestation					765.26
33-34 completed weeks of gestation					765.27
35-36 completed weeks of gestation					765.28
≥ 37 completed weeks of gestation					765.29

Antepartum Pregnancy Condition or Complication; affecting management of mother	Antepartum condition or complication	Delivered, with or without mention of antepartum condition	Unspecified episode of care	Assign additional code to describe the...	Affecting fetus (coded on the newborn chart only)
Eclampsia, eclamptic (coma) (convulsions) (delirium)	642.63	642.61	642.60		760.0
with pre-existing hypertension	642.73	642.71	642.70		760.0
Edema	646.13	646.11	646.10	condition	
with hypertension — *see* Pregnancy, toxemia					
Effect, adverse					
anesthetic (in labor and delivery) NEC	668.93	668.91	668.90		763.5
radiation (suspected damage to fetus)	655.63	655.61	655.60	condition	
Effusion, amniotic fluid	658.13	658.11	658.10		761.1
delayed delivery following	658.23	658.21	658.20		761.1
Electrolyte imbalance with hyperemesis gravidarum (before 22 completed weeks' gestation)	643.13	643.11	643.10		761.8
Embolism					
air (pulmonary)	673.03	673.01	673.00		
amniotic fluid	673.13	673.11	673.10		
blood clot	673.23	673.21	673.20		
brain	674.03	674.01	674.00		
cerebral	674.03	674.01	674.00		
fat (cerebral) (pulmonary) (systemic)	673.83	673.81	673.80		
intracranial (venous sinus) (nonpyogenic)	671.53	671.51	671.50		
pulmonary NEC	673.23	673.21	673.20		
pyemic	673.33	673.31	673.30		
septic	673.33	673.31	673.30		
Emesis (gravidarum) — *see* Pregnancy, vomiting					
Endometritis	646.63	646.61	646.60	condition	760.8
decidual	646.63	646.61	646.60	condition	760.8
Engorgement, breast	676.23	676.21	676.20		
Entanglement, umbilical cord(s)	663.33	663.31	663.30		762.5
with compression	663.23	663.21	663.20		762.5
around neck with compression	663.13	663.11	663.10		762.5
twins in monoamniotic sac	663.23	663.21	663.20		762.5
Epilepsy	649.43	649.41	649.40	345.00-345.91	
Excessive					
large (fetus)	656.63	656.61	656.60		766.0
with obstructed labor	660.13	660.11	660.10	cause	763.1
causing disproportion	653.53	653.51	653.50		763.1
causing obstructed labor	660.13	660.11	660.10	cause	763.1
milk secretion	676.63	676.61	676.60		
weight gain	646.13	646.11	646.10	condition	
Exhaustion (complicating delivery)	669.83	669.81	669.80		763.89
Extraction					
breech NEC		669.61	669.60		763.0
manual NEC	669.83	669.81	669.80		763.89
Face presentation	652.43	652.41	652.40		763.1
causing obstructed labor	660.03	660.01	660.00	cause	763.1
Failure, failed					
cervical dilation in labor	661.03	661.01	661.00		763.7
descent of head (at term)	652.53	652.51	652.50		763.1
in labor	660.03	660.01	660.00	cause	763.1
engagement of head NEC	652.53	652.51	652.50		763.1
in labor	660.03	660.01	660.00	cause	763.1
fetal head to enter pelvic brim	652.53	652.51	652.50		763.1
in labor	660.03	660.01	660.00	cause	763.1
forceps NEC	660.73	660.71	660.70	cause	763.1
heart, complicating					
delivery (cesarean) (instrumental)	669.43	669.41	669.40		
obstetric anesthesia or sedation	668.13	668.11	668.10		
induction (of labor)	659.13	659.11	659.10		763.89
by oxytocic drugs (Pitocin)	659.13	659.11	659.10		763.89
instrumental	659.03	659.01	659.00		763.89
mechanical	659.03	659.01	659.00		763.89
medical	659.13	659.11	659.10		763.89
surgical	659.03	659.01	659.00		763.89
lactation	676.43	676.41	676.40		
to progress	661.23	661.21	661.20		763.89
trial of labor NOS	660.63	660.61	660.60	cause	763.1

Coding Tables (left margin)

Antepartum Pregnancy (left margin)

Antepartum Pregnancy Condition or Complication; affecting management of mother	Antepartum condition or complication	Delivered, with or without mention of antepartum condition	Unspecified episode of care	Assign additional code to describe the...	Affecting fetus (coded on the newborn chart only)
Failure, failed — *continued*					
vacuum extraction delivery NOS	660.73	660.71	660.70	cause	763.1
ventouse NOS	660.73	660.71	660.70	cause	763.1
False labor (pains)	644.13		644.10		
False positive pregnancy	631.0				
Fatigue	646.83	646.81	646.80	condition	
Fatty metamorphosis of liver	646.73	646.71	646.70	condition	760.8
Female genital mutilation	649.93	648.91	648.90	629.20-629	
Fetal					
acidosis	656.33	656.31	656.30		763.89
anemia	678.03	678.01	678.00		
following blood loss (affecting newborn)					776.5
bradycardia	659.73	659.71	659.70		763.83
before onset of labor	659.73	659.71	659.70		763.81
during labor	659.73	659.71	659.70		763.82
complication from in utero procedure	679.13	679.11	679.10		
decreased movements	655.73	655.71	655.70		763.89
demise (near term)	656.43	656.41	656.40	cause	
early (before 22 weeks completed gestation)	632				761.8
deformity	653.73	653.71	653.70		763.1
causing obstructed labor	660.13	660.11	660.10	cause	763.1
distress	656.83	656.81	656.80		
heart rate, abnormal	659.73	659.71	659.70		763.83
before onset of labor	659.73	659.71	659.70		763.81
during labor	659.73	659.71	659.70		763.82
heart rhythm, abnormal	659.73	659.71	659.70		763.83
before onset of labor	659.73	659.71	659.70		763.81
during labor	659.73	659.71	659.70		763.82
hematologic conditions	678.03	678.01	678.00		
movements, decreased	655.73	655.71	655.70		
thrombocytopenia	678.03	678.01	678.00		
twin to twin transfusion	678.03	678.01	678.00		
Fetomaternal hemorrhage	656.03	656.01	656.00		772.0
Fibrinolysis	641.33	641.31	641.30		762.1
Fibroid tumor(s)	654.13	654.11	654.10		763.89
causing obstructed labor	660.23	660.21	660.20	cause	763.1
Fibromyoma (uterus)	654.13	654.11	654.10		763.89
causing obstructed labor	660.23	660.21	660.20	cause	763.1
Fibrosis, fibrotic					
amnion	658.83	658.81	658.80		
chorion	658.83	658.81	658.80		
perineum	654.83	654.81	654.80		763.8
causing obstructed labor	660.23	660.21	660.20	cause	763.1
Fissure, nipple	676.13	676.11	676.10		
Fistula					
breast	675.13	675.11	675.10		
mammary gland	675.13	675.11	675.10		
Flat, pelvis					
with disproportion (fetopelvic)	653.23	653.21	653.20		763.1
causing obstructed labor	660.13	660.11	660.10	cause	763.1
Footling presentation	652.83	652.81	652.80		
with successful version	652.13	652.11	652.10		
Forced birth or delivery NEC		669.81	669.80		763.89
Forceps delivery NEC		669.51	669.50		763.2
Fractured coccyx complicating delivery		665.61	665.60		
Frommel's disease	676.63	676.61	676.60		
Frommel-Chiari syndrome	676.63	676.61	676.60		
Funnel pelvis with disproportion (fetopelvic)	653.33	653.31	653.30		763.1
causing obstructed labor	660.13	660.11	660.10	cause	763.1
Fusion, hymeno-urethral					
causing obstructed labor	660.13	660.11	660.10	cause	763.1
Galactocele (breast)	676.83	676.81	676.80		
Galactorrhea	676.63	676.61	676.60		
Genital (female) **mutilation**	648.93	648.91	648.90	629.20-629.29	
Goiter	648.13	648.11	648.10	condition	
Gonococcal infection	647.13	647.11	647.10	condition	760.2

Antepartum Pregnancy Condition or Complication; affecting management of mother	Antepartum condition or complication	Delivered, with or without mention of antepartum condition	Unspecified episode of care	Assign additional code to describe the...	Affecting fetus (coded on the newborn chart only)
Gonorrhea	647.13	647.11	647.10	condition	760.2
Grand multiparity, affecting labor and delivery	659.43	659.41	659.40		
Growth fetal (poor)	656.53	656.51	656.50		764.90
Heart (fetal)					
abnormal					
rate	659.73	659.71	659.70		763.81
before onset of labor	659.73	659.71	659.70		763.81
during labor	659.73	659.71	659.70		763.82
rhythm	659.73	659.71	659.70		763.83
before onset of labor	659.73	659.71	659.70		763.81
during labor	659.73	659.71	659.70		763.82
HELLP (Hemolysis, Elevated Liver function and Low Platelets)	642.53	642.51	642.50		
Hematoma					
amnion	658.83	658.81	658.80		
broad ligament		665.71	665.70		
complicating delivery (perineum) (vulva)		664.51	664.50		
pelvic		665.71	665.70	665.71	
vagina		665.71	665.70		
pelvis, complicating delivery		665.71	665.70		
perineal wound complicating delivery		664.51	664.50		
umbilical cord	663.63	663.61	663.60		762.6
vagina		665.71	665.70		
vulva, complicating delivery		664.51	664.50		767.8
Hemolysis, intravascular	641.33	641.31	641.30		762.1
Hemolysis, elevated liver function, low platelets syndrome (HELLP)	642.53	642.51	642.50		
Hemorrhage					
accidental	641.23	641.21	641.20		762.1
before 22 completed weeks gestation NEC	640.93	640.91	640.90		
brain	674.03	674.01	674.00		
cerebrovascular	674.03	674.01	674.00		
complicating delivery	641.93	641.91	641.90		762.1
associated with					
afibrinogenemia	641.33	641.31	641.30		763.89
coagulation defect	641.33	641.31	641.30		763.89
hyperfibrinolysis	641.33	641.31	641.30		763.89
hypofibrinogenemia	641.33	641.31	641.30		763.89
concealed	641.93	641.91	641.90		762.1
due to					
afibrinogenemia or other coagulation defect	641.33	641.31	641.30	condition	763.89
fibroids	641.83	641.81	641.80		763.89
low-lying placenta	641.13	641.11	641.10		762.0
marginal sinus (rupture)	641.23	641.21	641.20		762.1
placenta previa	641.13	641.11	641.10		762.0
premature separation, placenta	641.23	641.21	641.20		762.1
trauma	641.83	641.81	641.80		763.89
umbilicus, umbilical cord	663.83	663.81	663.80		772.0
due to					
afibrinogenemia or other coagulation defect	641.33	641.31	641.30	condition	762.1
fibroids	641.83	641.81	641.80		762.1
low-lying placenta	641.13	641.11	641.10		762.1
marginal sinus					
(rupture)	641.23	641.21	641.20		762.1
placenta previa	641.13	641.11	641.10		762.0
premature separation, placenta	641.23	641.21	641.20		762.1
trauma	641.83	641.81	641.80		763.89
umbilicus, umbilical cord	663.83	663.81	663.80		772.0
early (before 22 completed weeks gestation)	640.93	640.91	640.90		762.1
fetomaternal	656.03	656.01	656.00		772.0
funis (complicating delivery)	663.83	663.81	663.80		772.0
intracranial	674.03	674.01	674.00		
marginal sinus	641.23	641.21	641.20		762.1
placenta NEC	641.93	641.91	641.90		762.1
from surgical or instrumental damage	641.83	641.81	641.80		762.1
previa	641.13	641.11	641.10		762.0

Antepartum Pregnancy Condition or Complication; affecting management of mother	Antepartum condition or complication	Delivered, with or without mention of antepartum condition	Unspecified episode of care	Assign additional code to describe the...	Affecting fetus (coded on the newborn chart only)
Hemorrhage — *continued*					
retroplacental	641.23	641.21	641.20		762.1
subarachnoid	674.03	674.01	674.00		
subdural	674.03	674.01	674.00		
threatened abortion	640.03	640.01	640.00		
umbilicus, umbilical cord (complicating delivery)	663.83	663.81	663.80		772.0
unavoidable	641.13	641.11	641.10		762.0
vasa previa	663.53	663.51	663.50		772.0
Hemorrhoids	671.83	671.81	671.80		
Hepatitis	646.73	646.71	646.70	condition	
viral	647.63	647.61	647.60	condition	
Herniation of uterus	654.43	654.41	654.40		
causing obstructed labor	660.23	660.21	660.20	cause	763.1
Herpes, herpetic	647.63	647.61	647.60	condition	
gestationis	646.83	646.81	646.80	condition	
High head at term	652.43	652.41	652.40		763.1
HIV	647.63	647.61	647.60	042	
asymptomatic	647.63	647.61	647.60	V08	
Hourglass uterus	661.43	661.41	661.40		763.7
Hydatidiform mole	630				
previous pregnancy, affecting management of current pregnancy	V23.1	V23.1	V23.1		
Hydramnios	657.03	657.01	657.00		761.3
Hydroa gestationis	646.83	646.81	646.80	condition	
Hydrocephalic fetus	655.03	655.01	655.00		763.1
causing disproportion	653.63	653.61	653.60		763.1
with obstructed labor	660.13	660.11	660.10	cause	763.1
Hydrops amnii	657.03	657.01	657.00		
Hydrorrhea	658.13	658.11	658.10		
Hyperemesis					
before 22 completed weeks of gestation	643.03	643.01	643.00		761.8
with					
carbohydrate depletion	643.13	643.11	643.10		761.8
dehydration	643.13	643.11	643.10		761.8
electrolyte imbalance	643.13	643.11	643.10		761.8
metabolic disturbance	643.13	643.11	643.10		761.8
mild	643.03	643.01	643.00		761.8
severe with metabolic disturbance	643.13	643.11	643.10		761.8
late (starting 23rd week of gestation)	643.23	643.21	643.20		761.8
Hypersecretion of milk	676.63	676.61	676.60		
Hypertension	642.93	642.91	642.90		760.0
with					
albuminuria (and edema) (mild)	642.43	642.41	642.40		760.0
severe	642.53	642.51	642.50		760.0
edema (mild)	642.43	642.41	642.40		760.0
severe	642.53	642.51	642.50		760.0
heart disease	642.23	642.21	642.20		760.0
and renal disease	642.23	642.21	642.20		760.0
pre-eclampsia or eclampsia	642.73	642.71	642.70		760.0
renal disease	642.23	642.21	642.20		760.0
and heart disease	642.23	642.21	642.20		760.0
benign	642.03	642.01	642.00		760.0
chronic	642.03	642.01	642.00		760.0
pre-existing	642.03	642.01	642.00		760.0
chronic	642.03	642.01	642.00		760.0
essential	642.03	642.01	642.00		760.0
with pre-eclampsia or eclampsia	642.73	642.71	642.70		760.0
gestational	642.33	642.31	642.30		
malignant	642.23	642.21	642.20		760.0
chronic	642.23	642.21	642.20		760.0
with pre-eclampsia or eclampsia	642.73	642.71	642.70		760.0
pre-existing	642.23	642.21	642.20		760.0
pre-existing	642.03	642.01	642.00		
secondary to renal disease	642.13	642.11	642.10		760.0
with pre-eclampsia or eclampsia	642.73	642.71	642.70		760.0
transient	642.33	642.31	642.30		

Antepartum Pregnancy Condition or Complication; affecting management of mother	Antepartum condition or complication	Delivered, with or without mention of antepartum condition	Unspecified episode of care	Assign additional code to describe the...	Affecting fetus (coded on the newborn chart only)
Hypertensive					
heart and renal disease	642.23	642.21	642.20		760.0
heart disease	642.23	642.21	642.20		760.0
renal disease	642.23	642.21	642.20		760.0
Hyperthyroidism	648.13	648.11	648.10	condition	
Hypertonicity	648.13	648.11	648.10	condition	763.7
Hypertrophy					
breast	676.33	676.31	676.30		
Hypotension (following labor and delivery)	669.23	669.21	669.20		
Hypothyroidism	648.13	648.11	648.10	condition	
Hysteralgia	646.83	646.81	646.80	condition	
Icterus gravis	646.73	646.71	646.70	condition	760.8
Illegitimate	V61.6	V61.6	V61.6		
Imbalance					
electrolyte with hyperemesis gravidarum (before 22 completed weeks' gestation)	643.13	643.11	643.10		
Immunization					
ABO	656.23	656.21	656.20		773.1
Rh factor	656.13	656.11	656.10		773.0
Immunodeficiency to Rh factor	656.13	656.11	656.10		773.0
Impacted shoulder	660.43	660.41	660.40	cause	763.1
Inadequate development of fetus	656.53	656.51	656.50		764.90
Incarceration, uterus	654.33	654.31	654.30		763.1
causing obstructed labor	660.23	660.21	660.20	cause	763.1
Incompatibility, blood groups (ABO)					
ABO	656.23	656.21	656.20		773.1
Blood (group) (Duffy) (E) (K(ell)) (Kidd) (Lewis) (M) (N) (P) (S) NEC	656.23	656.21	656.20		773.2
Rh(esus) (blood group) (factor)	656.13	656.11	656.10		773.0
Incompetent cervix (os)	654.53	654.51	654.50		761.0
causing obstructed labor	660.23	660.21	660.20	cause	763.1
Incoordinate uterus (action) (contractions)	661.43	661.41	661.40		763.7
In double uterus	654.03	654.01	654.00		
causing obstructed labor	660.23	660.21	660.20	cause	763.1
Induced					
failed by method of					
drugs	659.13	659.11	659.10		
mechanical	659.03	659.01	659.00		
successful — assign code to indicate the reason for the induction					763.89
Indurated breast	676.33	676.31	676.30		
Inertia, uterus NEC					
primary	661.03	661.01	661.00		763.7
secondary	661.13	661.11	661.10		763.7
Infantile					
genitalia, genitals	654.43	654.41	654.40		763.89
causing obstructed labor	660.23	660.21	660.20	cause	763.1
pelvis	653.13	653.11	653.10		763.1
causing obstructed labor	660.13	660.11	660.10	cause	763.1
Infarct, infarction					
amnion	658.83	658.81	658.80		
brain (stem)	674.03	674.01	674.00		
chorion	658.83	658.81	658.80		
lung — *see* Pregnancy, embolism					
placenta	656.73	656.71	656.70		762.2
Infection	647.93	647.91	647.90	condition	760.2
amniotic fluid	658.43	658.41	658.40	condition	762.7
bladder	646.63	646.61	646.60	condition	
breast (mammary gland)	675.23	675.21	675.20		
with nipple	675.93	675.91	675.90		
specified type NEC	675.83	675.81	675.80		
nonpurulent	675.23	675.21	675.20		
purulent	675.13	675.11	675.10		
chorionic plate	658.83	658.81	658.80		
genital organs	646.63	646.61	646.60	condition	760.8
minor or localized	646.63	646.61	646.60	condition	760.8

Coding Tables *(side tab)*

Antepartum Pregnancy *(side tab)*

Antepartum Pregnancy Condition or Complication; affecting management of mother	Antepartum condition or complication	Delivered, with or without mention of antepartum condition	Unspecified episode of care	Assign additional code to describe the...	Affecting fetus (coded on the newborn chart only)
Infection — *continued*					
intrauterine, complicating delivery	646.63	646.61	646.60	condition	
kidney	646.63	646.61	646.60	condition	760.1
nipple	675.03	675.01	675.00		
with breast	675.93	675.91	675.90		
specified type NEC	675.83	675.81	675.80		
perineal wound minor	646.63	646.61	646.60	condition	760.1
urinary (tract)	646.63	646.61	646.60	condition	760.1
asymptomatic	646.53	646.51	646.50	condition	760.1
UTI	646.63	646.61	646.60	condition	760.1
asymptomatic	646.53	646.51	646.50	condition	760.1
Infective and parasitic diseases NEC	647.83	647.81	647.80	complication	
Infestation	647.93	647.91	647.90	condition	760.8
Inflammation					
areola	675.03	675.01	675.00		
bladder	646.63	646.61	646.60	condition	760.8
breast (mammary gland)	675.23	675.21	675.20		
fetal membranes (acute)	658.43	658.41	658.40		762.7
genital organ	646.63	646.61	646.60	condition	760.8
urinary tract NEC	646.63	646.61	646.60	condition	760.8
Inhalation of stomach contents or secretions in labor and delivery	668.03	668.01	668.00		
Injury	648.93	648.91	648.90	condition	
birth canal NEC	665.93	665.91	665.90		763.89
coccyx, complicating delivery		665.61	665.60		
genital organs, obstetrical					
trauma NEC	665.93	665.91	665.90		763.89
instrumental, obstetrical NEC	665.93	665.91	665.90		763.89
bladder		665.51	665.50		763.89
cervix		665.31	665.30		763.89
high vaginal		665.41	665.40		763.89
perineal NEC		664.91	664.90		763.89
urethra		665.51	665.50		763.89
uterus		665.51	665.50		763.89
obstetrical NEC	665.93	665.91	665.90		763.89
floor		664.11	664.10		763.89
joint or ligament		665.61	665.60		763.89
organs		665.51	665.50		763.89
periurethral tissue, complicating delivery		665.51	665.50		763.89
symphysis pubis, complicating delivery		665.61	665.60		763.89
Insertion of umbilical cord, lateral or velamentous	663.53	663.51	663.50		762.6
Insufficient					
prenatal care	V23.7				
weight gain	646.83	646.81	646.80	condition	
Interstitial — *see* Ectopic pregnancy	633.8x				
Intoxication					
chemical via placenta or breast milk, suspected	655.53	655.51	655.50		760.70
drug					
obstetric anesthetic or sedation	668.93	668.91	668.90		763.5
via placenta or breast milk, suspected	655.53	655.51	655.50		760.70
septic					
during labor	659.33	659.31	659.30		
Intraligamentous — *see* Ectopic pregnancy	633.8x				
Intramural — *see* Ectopic pregnancy	633.8x				
Intraperitoneal — *see* Ectopic pregnancy	633.0x				
Intrauterine fetal death					
early (before 22 completed weeks of gestation)	632				
near term NEC	656.43	656.41	656.40		
In utero procedure					
fetal complication	679.13	679.11	679.10		
maternal complication	679.03	679.01	679.00		
Inversion					
nipple	676.33	676.31	676.30		
Ischemia, cerebral	674.03	674.01	674.00		
Isoimmunization (ABO)	656.23	656.21	656.20		
Rh(esus)	656.13	656.11	656.10		

Antepartum Pregnancy Condition or Complication; affecting management of mother	Antepartum condition or complication	Delivered, with or without mention of antepartum condition	Unspecified episode of care	Assign additional code to describe the...	Affecting fetus (coded on the newborn chart only)
Isthmian (with rupture) — *see* Ectopic Pregnancy	633.1x				
Joint disorders	648.73	648.71	648.70	condition	
Kidney					
disease or failure NEC	646.23	646.21	646.20	condition	
with secondary hypertension	642.13	642.11	642.10		
hypertensive	642.23	642.21	642.20		
Knot, umbilical cord (true)	663.23	663.21	663.20		762.5
Labor					
abnormal NEC	661.93	661.91	661.90		763.7
arrested active phase	661.13	661.11	661.10		763.7
desultory	661.23	661.21	661.20		763.7
dyscoordinate	661.43	661.41	661.40		763.7
early onset (22-36 weeks gestation)		644.21	644.20		763.7
failed					763.7
induction	659.13	659.11	659.10		763.89
mechanical	659.03	659.01	659.00		763.89
medical (drug)	659.13	659.11	659.10		763.89
surgical	659.03	659.01	659.00		763.89
trial (vaginal delivery)	660.63	660.61	660.60	cause	763.1
false	644.13		644.10		
hypertonic	661.43	661.41	661.40		763.7
hypotonic, primary	661.03	661.01	661.00		763.7
secondary	661.13	661.11	661.10		763.7
incoordinate	661.43	661.41	661.40		763.7
irregular	661.23	661.21	661.20		763.7
long	662.13	662.11	662.10		763.89
first stage	662.03	662.01	662.00		763.89
second stage	662.23	662.21	662.20		763.89
missed (at or near term)	656.43	656.41	656.40		
obstructed NEC	660.93	660.91	660.90	cause	763.1
specified cause NEC	660.83	660.81	660.80	cause	763.1
onset (spontaneous) after 37 completed weeks of gestation but before 39 completed weeks of gestation, with delivery by (planned) cesarean section		649.81			
pains, spurious	644.13		644.10		
precipitate	661.33	661.31	661.30		763.6
premature		644.21	644.20		
threatened	644.03		644.00		
prolonged or protracted	662.13	662.11	662.10		763.89
first stage	662.03	662.01	662.00		763.89
second stage	662.23	662.21	662.20		763.89
threatened NEC	644.13		644.10		
undelivered	644.13		644.10		
Laceration (obstetrical trauma)					
Anus, anal (sphincter)complicating delivery					
with third degree perineal laceration		664.21	664.20		763.89
w/mucosa		664.31	664.30		763.89
w/o third degree perineal laceration		664.61	664.60		763.89
old (healed)		654.81	654.80		763.89
bladder		665.51	665.50		
bowel		665.51	665.50		
broad ligament		665.61	665.60		
central, complicating delivery		664.41	664.40		
cervix (uteri)		665.31	665.30		
fourchette, complicating delivery		664.01	664.00		
labia, complicating delivery		664.01	664.00		
pelvic (complicating delivery)					
floor (muscles)		664.11	664.10		
organ NEC (obstetrical trauma)		665.51	665.50		763.89
perineum, complicating delivery		664.41	664.40		
first degree		664.01	664.00		
second degree		664.11	664.10		
third degree		664.21	664.20		
fourth degree		664.31	664.30		

Antepartum Pregnancy Condition or Complication; affecting management of mother	Antepartum condition or complication	Delivered, with or without mention of antepartum condition	Unspecified episode of care	Assign additional code to describe the…	Affecting fetus (coded on the newborn chart only)
Laceration (obstetrical trauma) — *continued*					
perineum, complicating delivery — *continued*					
involving					
anal sphincter		664.21	664.20		
fourchette		664.01	664.00		
hymen		664.01	664.00		
labia		664.01	664.00		
pelvic floor		664.11	664.10		
perineal muscles		664.11	664.10		
rectovaginal with septum		664.21	664.20		
with anal mucosa		664.31	664.30		
skin		664.01	664.00		
sphincter (anal)		664.21	664.20		
with anal mucosa		664.31	664.30		
vagina		664.01	664.00		
vaginal muscles		664.11	664.10		
vulva		664.01	664.00		
peritoneum (obstetrical trauma)		665.51	665.50		
periurethral tissue (obstetrical trauma)		665.51	665.50		
rectovaginal septum		665.41	665.40		
with perineum		664.21	664.20		
involving anal or rectal mucosa		664.31	664.30		
urethra (obstetrical trauma)		665.51	665.50		
uterus (obstetrical trauma NEC)		665.11	665.10		
vagina (complicating delivery)		665.41	665.40		
with perineal involvement		664.01	664.00		
first degree		664.01	664.00		
second degree		664.11	664.10		
third degree		664.21	664.20		
fourth degree		664.31	664.30		
high		664.41	664.40		
muscles		664.11	664.10		
sulcus		665.41	665.40		
wall		665.41	665.40		
vulva (complicating delivery)		664.01	664.00		
Lactation, lactating (breast)					
defective	676.43	676.41	676.40		
disorder	676.93	676.91	676.90		
specified type NEC	676.83	676.81	676.80		
examination and/or care of mother	V24.1	V24.1	V24.1		
excessive	676.63	676.61	676.60		
failed	676.43	676.41	676.40		
mastitis NEC	675.23	675.21	675.20		
suppressed	676.53	676.51	676.50		
Large					
fetus causing disproportion	653.53	653.51	653.50		763.1
with obstructed labor	660.13	660.11	660.10	cause	763.1
for-dates (fetus)	656.63	656.61	656.60		766.1
exceptionally (weight of 4500 grams or more)	656.63	656.61	656.60		766.0
childbirth complication(s)	677	677	677	condition	
Late effect(s) (of)					
complication(s) of					
childbirth	677	677	677	condition	
delivery	677	677	677	condition	
postpartum	677	677	677	condition	
pregnancy	677	677	677	condition	
puerperium	677	677	677	condition	
Lateroversion, uterus	654.43	654.41	654.40		763.89
causing obstructed labor	660.23	660.21	660.20	cause	763.1
Leakage					
amniotic fluid	658.13	658.11	658.10		761.1
with delayed delivery	658.23	658.21	658.20		761.1
blood (microscopic), fetal, into maternal circulation	656.03	656.01	656.00		
Lesion, vascular of umbilical cord	663.63	663.61	663.60		762.6
Light-for-dates	656.53	656.51	656.50		764.00
with signs of fetal malnutrition	656.53	656.51	656.50		764.10

Antepartum Pregnancy Condition or Complication; affecting management of mother	Antepartum condition or complication	Delivered, with or without mention of antepartum condition	Unspecified episode of care	Assign additional code to describe the…	Affecting fetus (coded on the newborn chart only)
Listeriosis, suspected fetal damage	655.43	655.41	655.40		771.2
Lithopedion	656.83	656.81	656.80		
Locked twins	660.53	660.51	660.50	cause	763.1
Lymphadenitis, breast	675.23	675.21	675.20		
breast	675.23	675.21	675.20		
Malaria	647.43	647.41	647.40	condition	
Male type pelvis with disproportion (fetopelvic)	653.23	653.21	653.20		763.1
causing obstructed labor	660.13	660.11	660.10	cause	763.1
Malformation					
pelvic organs or tissues	654.93	654.91	654.90		763.89
causing obstructed labor	660.23	660.21	660.20	cause	763.1
placenta	656.73	656.71	656.70		
umbilical cord (complicating delivery)	663.93	663.91	663.90		762.6
uterus (congenital)	654.03	654.01	654.00		
causing obstructed labor	660.23	660.21	660.20	cause	763.1
Malnutrition	648.93	648.91	648.90	condition	
Fetal malnutrition					
Without mention of "light-for dates"					
unspecified (weight)					764.20
< 500 gms					764.21
500-749 gms					764.22
750-999 gms					764.23
1,000-1,249 gms					764.24
1,250-1,499 gms					764.25
1,500-1,749 gms					764.26
1,750-1,999 gms					764.27
2,000-2,499 gms					764.28
≥ 2,500 gms					764.29
With mention of "light-for dates" unspecified (weight)					764.10
< 500 gms					764.11
500-749 gms					764.12
750-999 gms					764.13
1,000-1,249 gms					764.14
1,250-1,499 gms					764.15
1,500-1,749 gms					764.16
1,750-1,999 gms					764.17
2,000-2,499 gms					764.18
≥ 2,500 gms					764.19
Malposition					
fetal NEC	652.93	652.91	652.90		763.1
with successful version	652.13	652.11	652.10		763.1
before labor	652.93	652.91	652.90		763.1
in multiple gestation	652.63	652.61	652.60		763.1
with locking	660.53	660.51	660.50	cause	763.1
causing obstructed labor	660.03	660.01	660.00	cause	763.1
pelvic organs or tissues	654.43	654.41	654.40		763.89
causing obstructed labor	660.23	660.21	660.20	cause	763.1
specified type NEC	652.83	652.81	652.80		763.1
causing obstructed labor	660.03	660.01	660.00	cause	763.1
uterus or cervix	654.43	654.41	654.40		763.89
causing obstructed labor	660.23	660.21	660.20	cause	763.1
Malpresentation					
fetal	652.93	652.91	652.90		763.1
with successful version	652.13	652.11	652.10		763.1
in multiple gestation	652.63	652.61	652.60		763.1
specified type NEC	652.83	652.81	652.80		763.1
causing obstructed labor	660.03	660.01	660.00	cause	763.1
uterus or cervix	654.43	654.41	654.40		
causing obstructed labor	660.03	660.01	660.00	cause	763.1
Mammillitis, puerperal	675.23	675.21	675.20		
Mammitis, puerperal	675.23	675.21	675.20		
Marginal sinus hemorrhage or rupture	641.23	641.21	641.20		762.1
Mastitis					
lactational	675.23	675.21	675.20		

Coding Tables

Antepartum Pregnancy

Antepartum Pregnancy Condition or Complication; affecting management of mother	Antepartum condition or complication	Delivered, with or without mention of antepartum condition	Unspecified episode of care	Assign additional code to describe the...	Affecting fetus (coded on the newborn chart only)
Mastitis — *continued*					
puerperal, (interstitial) (nonpurulent) (parenchymatous)	675.23	675.21	675.20		
purulent	675.13	675.11	675.10		
stagnation	675.23	675.21	675.20		
puerperalis	675.23	675.21	675.20		
retromammary	675.13	675.11	675.10		
submammary	675.13	675.11	675.10		
Maternal obesity syndrome	646.13	646.11	646.10	condition	
Meconium in liquor (staining)	656.83	656.81	656.80		
Membranitis, fetal	658.43	658.41	658.40		762.7
Mendelson's syndrome	668.03	668.01	668.00		
Menstruation during pregnancy	640.83	640.81	640.80		
Mental disorders	648.43	648.41	648.40	condition	
Mentum presentation	652.43	652.41	652.40		763.1
causing obstructed labor	660.03	660.01	660.00	cause	763.1
Metaplasia squamous cell amnion	658.83	658.81	658.80		763.89
Milk					
excess secretion	676.63	676.61	676.60		
Milk leg (deep vessels)	671.33	671.31	671.30		
Missed					
delivery (at or near term)	656.43	656.41	656.40		763.89
labor (at or near term)	656.43	656.41	656.40		763.89
Morning sickness	643.03	643.01	643.00		
Multiparity (grand)	659.43	659.41	659.40		763.89
Myelomeningocele fetal, causing fetopelvic disproportion	653.73	653.71	653.70		763.1
causing obstructed labor	660.13	660.11	660.10	cause	763.1
Myoma uterus (cervix) (corpus)	654.13	654.11	654.10		763.89
causing obstructed labor	660.23	660.21	660.20	cause	763.1
Nägele's pelvis with disproportion (fetopelvic)	653.03	653.01	653.00		763.1
causing obstructed labor	660.13	660.11	660.10	cause	763.1
Necrosis					
genital organ or tract	646.63	646.61	646.60	condition	760.8
kidney, cortical (acute)	646.23	646.21	646.20	condition	760.1
tubular	646.23	646.21	646.20	condition	760.1
liver	646.73	646.71	646.70	condition	760.8
placenta	656.73	656.71	656.70		762.2
renal, cortical	646.23	646.21	646.20	condition	760.1
Nephritis, nephrosis	646.23	646.21	646.20	condition	760.1
with hypertension	642.13	642.11	642.10		760.0
Nephropathy NEC	646.23	646.21	646.20	condition	
Neuritis (peripheral)	646.43	646.41	646.40	condition	
Nonengagement of head NEC	652.53	652.51	652.50		763.1
in labor	660.03	660.01	660.00	cause	763.1
Noxious substances transmitted through placenta or breast milk, suspected, unspecified	655.53	655.51	655.50		760.70
Nuchal hitch (arm)	652.83	652.81	652.80		763.1
causing obstructed labor	660.03	660.01	660.00	cause	763.1
Nutritional deficiency	648.93	648.91	648.90	condition	
Obesity					
excessive weight gain during pregnancy	646.13	646.11	646.10	complication	
morbid	649.13	649.11	649.10	278.00, 278.01-278.03, V85.30-V85.45	
Oblique lie or presentation	652.33	652.31	652.30		763.1
with successful version	652.13	652.11	652.10		763.1
causing obstructed labor	660.03	660.01	660.00	cause	763.1
Obstetrical trauma NEC (complicating delivery)	665.93	665.91	665.90		763.89
Obstruction, obstructed, obstructive					
labor	660.93	660.91	660.90	cause	763.1
borderline pelvis	660.13	660.11	660.10	cause	763.1
by					
bony pelvis	660.13	660.11	660.10	cause	763.1
deep transverse arrest	660.33	660.31	660.30	cause	763.1
impacted shoulder	660.43	660.41	660.40	cause	763.1

Antepartum Pregnancy Condition or Complication; affecting management of mother	Antepartum condition or complication	Delivered, with or without mention of antepartum condition	Unspecified episode of care	Assign additional code to describe the…	Affecting fetus (coded on the newborn chart only)
Obstruction, obstructed, obstructive — *continued*					
locked twins	660.53	660.51	660.50	cause	763.1
malposition (fetus)	660.03	660.01	660.00	cause	763.1
head during labor	660.33	660.31	660.30	cause	763.1
persistent occipitoposterior position	660.33	660.31	660.30	cause	763.1
soft tissue, pelvic	660.23	660.21	660.20	cause	763.1
Occlusion, precerebral artery NEC	674.03	674.01	674.00	condition	
Oligohydramnios NEC	658.03	658.01	658.00		761.2
due to premature rupture of membranes	658.13	658.11	658.10		761.2
Oliguria	646.23	646.21	646.20	condition	
with hypertension — *see* Pregnancy, toxemia					
Oophoritis	646.63	646.61	646.60	condition	
Oversize fetus (weight of 4500 grams or more)	656.63	656.61	656.60		766.0
causing disproportion	653.53	653.51	653.50		763.1
with obstructed labor	660.13	660.11	660.10	cause	763.1
Pain(s)	646.83	646.81	646.80	condition	
false labor	644.13		644.10		
Papyraceous fetus	646.03	646.01	646.00	condition	779.8
Paralysis, bladder		665.51	665.50		
Patent cervix	654.53	654.51	654.50		761.0
causing obstructed labor	660.23	660.21	660.20	cause	763.1
Pendulous	654.43	654.41	654.40		763.89
causing obstructed labor	660.23	660.21	660.20	cause	763.1
complication of delivery		665.11	665.10		763.89
Perforation					
bladder		665.51	665.50		
bowel		665.51	665.50		
broad ligament		665.61	665.60		
cervix		665.31	665.30		
instrumental (complicating delivery)	665.93	665.91	665.90		
pelvic (floor)		664.11	664.10		
organ		665.51	665.50		763.89
urethral		665.51	665.50		763.89
uterus		665.51	665.50		763.89
Persistence					
hymen (tag)	654.83	654.81	654.80		
causing obstructed labor	660.23	660.21	660.20	cause	763.1
occiput (anterior or posterior)	660.33	660.31	660.30	cause	763.1
Phlebitis	671.93	671.91	671.90		760.3
deep	671.33	671.31	671.30	DVT code, anticoag use (V58.61)	760.3
intracranial	671.53	671.51	671.50		
lower extremities	671.23	671.21	671.20	453.6, 453.71, 453.81	760.3
specified site NEC	671.53	671.51	671.50		
superficial	671.23	671.21	671.20	453.6, 453.71, 453.81	760.3
Phlegmasia	671.33	671.31	671.30	DVT code, anticoag use (V58.61)	760.3
PID	646.63	646.61	646.60	condition	
Pithecoid pelvis (fetopelvic)	653.23	653.21	653.20		763.1
obstructed labor	660.13	660.11	660.10	cause	763.1
Placenta, placental					
abnormal	656.73	656.71	656.70		762.2
with hemorrhage	641.83	641.81	641.80		762.1
abruptio or ablatio	641.23	641.21	641.20		762.1
absorption (suspected) of					
chemical	655.53	655.51	655.50		760.79
drug (NEC)	655.53	655.51	655.50		760.79
accessory lobe	656.73	656.71	656.70		762.2
with hemorrhage	641.83	641.81	641.80		762.1
apoplexy	641.23	641.21	641.20		762.1
battledore	656.73	656.71	656.70		762.2
with hemorrhage	641.83	641.81	641.80		762.1
bilobate	656.73	656.71	656.70		762.2
with hemorrhage	641.83	641.81	641.80		762.1
bipartita	656.73	656.71	656.70		762.2
with hemorrhage	641.83	641.81	641.80		762.1

Antepartum Pregnancy Condition or Complication; affecting management of mother	Antepartum condition or complication	Delivered, with or without mention of antepartum condition	Unspecified episode of care	Assign additional code to describe the...	Affecting fetus (coded on the newborn chart only)
Placenta, placental — *continued*					
centralis	641.03	641.01	641.00		762.0
with hemorrhage	641.13	641.11	641.10		762.1
circumvallata	656.73	656.71	656.70		762.2
with hemorrhage	641.83	641.81	641.80		762.1
cyst (amniotic)	656.73	656.71	656.70		762.2
with hemorrhage	641.83	641.81	641.80		762.1
deficiency	656.53	656.51	656.50		762.2
degeneration	656.53	656.51	656.50		762.2
detachment	641.23	641.21	641.20		762.1
dimidiata	656.73	656.71	656.70		762.2
with hemorrhage	641.83	641.81	641.80		762.1
disease	656.73	656.71	656.70		762.2
with hemorrhage	641.83	641.81	641.80		762.1
duplex	656.73	656.71	656.70		762.2
with hemorrhage	641.83	641.81	641.80		762.1
dysfunction	656.53	656.51	656.50		762.2
fenestrata	656.73	656.71	656.70		762.2
with hemorrhage	641.83	641.81	641.80		762.1
fibrosis	656.73	656.71	656.70		762.2
with hemorrhage	641.83	641.81	641.80		762.1
hematoma	656.73	656.71	656.70		762.2
with hemorrhage	641.83	641.81	641.80		762.1
hemorrhage	641.23	641.21	641.20		762.1
hormone disturbance	656.73	656.71	656.70		762.2
with hemorrhage	641.83	641.81	641.80		762.1
hyperplasia	656.73	656.71	656.70		762.2
with hemorrhage	641.83	641.81	641.80		762.1
infarct	656.73	656.71	656.70		762.2
with hemorrhage	641.83	641.81	641.80		762.1
insertion, vicious	641.03	641.01	641.00		762.0
with hemorrhage	641.13	641.11	641.10		762.1
insufficiency	656.53	656.51	656.50		762.2
lateral	641.03	641.01	641.00		762.0
with hemorrhage	641.13	641.11	641.10		762.1
low implantation	641.03	641.01	641.00		762.0
with hemorrhage	641.13	641.11	641.10		762.1
low lying	641.03	641.01	641.00		762.0
with hemorrhage	641.13	641.11	641.10		762.1
malformation	656.73	656.71	656.70		762.2
with hemorrhage	641.83	641.81	641.80		762.1
malposition	641.03	641.01	641.00		762.2
with hemorrhage	641.13	641.11	641.10		762.1
marginalis, marginata	641.03	641.01	641.00		762.0
with hemorrhage	641.13	641.11	641.10		762.1
marginal sinus (hemorrhage)	641.23	641.21	641.20		762.1
membranacea	656.73	656.71	656.70		762.2
with hemorrhage	641.83	641.81	641.80		762.1
multiload	656.73	656.71	656.70		762.2
with hemorrhage	641.83	641.81	641.80		762.1
necrosis	656.73	656.71	656.70		762.2
with hemorrhage	641.83	641.81	641.80		762.1
previa	641.03	641.01	641.00		762.0
with hemorrhage	641.13	641.11	641.10		762.1
separation (premature) (undelivered)	641.23	641.21	641.20		762.1
septuplex	656.73	656.71	656.70		762.2
with hemorrhage	641.83	641.81	641.80		762.1
small	656.53	656.51	656.50		762.2
softening	656.73	656.71	656.70		762.2
with hemorrhage	641.83	641.81	641.80		762.1
spuria	656.73	656.71	656.70		762.2
with hemorrhage	641.83	641.81	641.80		762.1
succenturiata	656.73	656.71	656.70		762.2
with hemorrhage	641.83	641.81	641.80		762.1
syphilitic	647.03	647.01	647.00	condition	760.2
manifest syphilis in the infant or fetus	647.03	647.01	647.00	condition	090.0

Antepartum Pregnancy Condition or Complication; affecting management of mother	Antepartum condition or complication	Delivered, with or without mention of antepartum condition	Unspecified episode of care	Assign additional code to describe the…	Affecting fetus (coded on the newborn chart only)
Placenta, placental — *continued*					
transfusion syndromes (fetus)					762.3
transmission of chemical substance (suspected, affecting pregnancy)	655.53	655.51	655.50		760.70
trilobate	656.73	656.71	656.70		762.2
with hemorrhage	641.83	641.81	641.80		762.1
triplex	656.73	656.71	656.70		762.2
with hemorrhage	641.83	641.81	641.80		762.1
varicose vessel	656.73	656.71	656.70		762.2
with hemorrhage	641.83	641.81	641.80		762.1
vicious insertion	641.03	641.01	641.00		
with hemorrhage	641.13	641.11	641.10		762.0
Placentitis	658.43	658.41	658.40		762.7
Platypelloid pelvis (disproportion)	653.23	653.21	653.20		763.1
obstructed labor	660.13	660.11	660.10	cause	763.1
Pneumonitis					
aspiration	668.03	668.01	668.00	condition	770.18
postanesthetic	668.03	668.01	668.00	condition	
postoperative	668.03	668.01	668.00		
Polygalactia	676.63	676.61	676.60		
Polyhydramnios	657.03	657.01	657.00		761.3
Polyp					
cervix	654.63	654.61	654.60		763.89
obstructed labor	660.23	660.21	660.20	cause	763.1
uterus	654.13	654.11	654.10		763.89
obstructed labor	660.23	660.21	660.20	cause	763.1
Poor					
contractions labor	661.23	661.21	661.20		763.7
fetal growth, affecting management	656.53	656.51	656.50		
Fetal growth retardation					
unspecified (weight)					764.90
< 500 gms					764.91
500-749 gms					764.92
750-999 gms					764.93
1,000-1,249 gms					764.94
1,250-1,499 gms					764.95
1,500-1,749 gms					764.96
1,750-1,999 gms					764.97
2,000-2,499 gms					764.98
≥ 2,500 gms					764.99
obstetrical history	V23.4				
Position – *see* also Presentation, fetal	652.93	652.91	652.90		763.1
causing obstructed labor	660.03	660.01	660.00	cause	763.1
Post-term (over 40 to 42 completed weeks)	645.13	645.11	645.10		766.21
Prediabetes	648.83	648.81	648.80	condition	
Prolonged (over 42 completed weeks)	645.23	645.21	645.20		766.22
Pre-eclampsia (mild)	642.43	642.41	642.40		760.0
with convulsions	642.63	642.61	642.60		760.0
severe	642.53	642.51	642.50		760.0
superimposed on pre-existing hypertensive disease	642.73	642.71	642.70		760.0
Pre-existing condition (prior to pregnancy) **affecting current pregnancy**					
abnormal glucose tolerance	648.83	648.81	648.80	condition	
anemia	648.23	648.21	648.20	condition	
bone and joint (lower limb)	648.73	648.71	648.70	condition	
cardiovascular	648.63	648.61	648.60	condition	
congenital	648.53	648.51	648.50	condition	
cerebrovascular	674.03	674.01	674.00		
diabetic	648.03	648.01	648.00	condition	
drug dependence	648.33	648.31	648.30	condition	
genital organ or tract	646.63	646.61	646.60	condition	
gonorrheal	647.13	647.11	647.10	condition	
hypertensive	642.23	642.21	642.20		
renal	642.13	642.11	642.10		
infectious	647.93	647.91	647.90	condition	
specified type NEC	647.83	647.81	647.80	condition	

Antepartum Pregnancy

Condition or Complication; affecting management of mother	Antepartum condition or complication	Delivered, with or without mention of antepartum condition	Unspecified episode of care	Assign additional code to describe the…	Affecting fetus (coded on the newborn chart only)
Pre-existing condition (prior to pregnancy) **affecting current pregnancy** — *continued*					
liver	646.73	646.71	646.70	condition	
malarial	647.43	647.41	647.40	condition	
nutritional deficiency	648.93	648.91	648.90	condition	
parasitic NEC	647.83	647.81	647.80	condition	
renal	646.23	646.21	646.20	condition	
hypertensive	642.13	642.11	642.10		
rubella	647.53	647.51	647.50	condition	
specified condition NEC	648.93	648.91	648.90	condition	
syphilitic	647.03	647.01	647.00	condition	
thyroid	648.13	648.11	648.10	condition	
tuberculous	647.33	647.31	647.30	condition	
urinary	646.63	646.61	646.60	condition	
venereal	647.23	647.21	647.20	condition	
viral NEC	647.63	647.61	647.60	condition	
Premature					
labor		644.21	644.20		
threatened	644.03		644.00		
rupture of membranes or amnion	658.13	658.11	658.10		761.1
with delayed delivery	658.23	658.21	658.20		
Presentation, fetal					
abnormal	652.93	652.91	652.90		763.1
with successful version	652.13	652.11	652.10		761.7
causing obstructed labor	660.03	660.01	660.00	cause	763.1
in multiple gestation (one or more)	652.63	652.61	652.60		763.1
causing obstructed labor	660.03	660.01	660.00	cause	763.1
specified NEC	652.83	652.81	652.80		763.1
causing obstructed labor	660.03	660.01	660.00	cause	763.1
arm	652.73	652.71	652.70		763.1
causing obstructed labor	660.03	660.01	660.00	cause	763.1
breech	652.23	652.21	652.20		761.7
with successful version	652.13	652.11	652.10		761.7
causing obstructed labor	660.03	660.01	660.00	cause	763.0
brow	652.43	652.41	652.40		763.1
causing obstructed labor	660.03	660.01	660.00	cause	763.1
cord	663.03	663.01	663.00		762.5
extended head	652.43	652.41	652.40		763.1
causing obstructed labor	660.03	660.01	660.00	cause	763.1
face	652.43	652.41	652.40		763.1
causing obstructed labor	660.03	660.01	660.00	cause	763.1
to pubes	652.83	652.81	652.80		763.1
causing obstructed labor	660.33	660.31	660.30	cause	763.1
hand, leg, or foot NEC	652.83	652.81	652.80		763.1
causing obstructed labor	660.03	660.01	660.00	cause	763.1
mentum	652.43	652.41	652.40		763.1
causing obstructed labor	660.03	660.01	660.00	cause	763.1
multiple gestation (one fetus or more)	652.63	652.61	652.60		763.1
causing obstructed labor	660.03	660.01	660.00	cause	763.1
oblique	652.33	652.31	652.30		763.1
with successful version	652.13	652.11	652.10		763.1
causing obstructed labor	660.03	660.01	660.00	cause	763.1
shoulder	652.83	652.81	652.80		763.1
causing obstructed labor	660.03	660.01	660.00	cause	763.1
transverse	652.33	652.31	652.30		763.1
with successful version	652.13	652.11	652.10		763.1
causing obstructed labor	660.03	660.01	660.00	cause	763.1
umbilical cord	663.03	663.01	663.00		
unstable	652.03	652.01	652.00		763.1
causing obstructed labor	660.03	660.01	660.00	cause	763.1
Previous					
abortion	V23.2				
infertility	V23.0				
nonobstetric condition	V23.89				
poor obstetrical history	V23.49				
premature delivery	V23.41				

Antepartum Pregnancy Condition or Complication; affecting management of mother	Antepartum condition or complication	Delivered, with or without mention of antepartum condition	Unspecified episode of care	Assign additional code to describe the...	Affecting fetus (coded on the newborn chart only)
Previous — *continued*					
recurrent pregnancy loss	646.33	646.31	646.30		
trophoblastic disease	V23.1				
Primigravida, elderly	659.53	659.51	659.50		763.89
Primipara, old	659.53	659.51	659.50		763.89
Problem (with)					
fetus NOS	656.93	656.91	656.90		779.9
specified type NEC	656.83	656.81	656.80		779.8
placenta NOS	656.93	656.91	656.90		762.2
specified type NEC	656.83	656.81	656.80		762.2
Prolapse, prolapsed					
arm or hand, complicating delivery	652.73	652.71	652.70		763.1
causing obstructed labor	660.03	660.01	660.00	cause	763.1
cervix, anterior lip (obstructing labor)	660.23	660.21	660.20	cause	763.1
fetal extremity, complicating delivery	652.83	652.81	652.80		763.1
causing obstructed labor	660.03	660.01	660.00	cause	763.1
leg, complicating delivery	652.83	652.81	652.80		763.1
causing obstructed labor	660.03	660.01	660.00	cause	763.1
umbilical cord, complicating delivery	663.03	663.01	663.00		762.4
causing obstructed labor	660.23	660.21	660.20	cause	763.1
Prolonged					
labor	662.13	662.11	662.10		
first stage	662.03	662.01	662.00		763.89
second stage	662.23	662.21	662.20		763.89
pregnancy over 40 completed weeks to 42 completed weeks	645.13	645.11	645.10		766.21
pregnancy over 42 completed weeks	645.23	645.21	645.20		766.22
rupture of membranes (24 hours or more prior to onset of labor)	658.23	658.21	658.20		761.8
uterine contractions in labor	661.43	661.41	661.40		763.7
PROM	658.13	658.11	658.10		761.1
with delayed delivery	658.23	658.21	658.20		761.8
Prominence, ischial spine or sacral promontory					
with disproportion (fetopelvic)	653.33	653.31	653.30		763.1
causing obstructed labor	660.13	660.11	660.10	cause	763.1
Proteinuria (gestational)	646.23	646.21	646.20	condition	
with toxemia (mild) (pre-eclamptic)	642.43	642.41	642.40		760.0
convulsions	642.63	642.61	642.60		760.0
pre-existing hypertension	642.73	642.71	642.70		760.0
severe	642.53	642.51	642.50		760.0
Pruritus, pruritic	646.83	646.81	646.80	condition	
Psychosis or psychoneurosis	648.43	648.41	648.40	condition	
Ptyalism	646.83	646.81	646.80	condition	
Pyelitis	646.63	646.61	646.60	condition	760.1
Pyrexia (of unknown origin) (PUO), **during labor**	659.23	659.21	659.20		
Quadruplet NEC	651.23	651.21	651.20	V91.20-V91.29	761.5
with fetal loss and retention of one or more fetus(es)	651.53	651.51	651.50	V91.20-V91.29	
reduction, multiple gestation (elective)	651.73	651.71	651.70	V91.20-V91.29	
Quintuplet NEC	651.83	651.81	651.80	V91.90-V91.99	761.5
with fetal loss and retention of one or more fetus(es)	651.63	651.61	651.60	V91.90-V91.99	
reduction, multiple gestation (elective)	651.73	651.71	651.70	V91.90-V91.99	
Rachitic with disproportion (fetopelvic)	653.23	653.21	653.20		763.1
causing obstructed labor	660.13	660.11	660.10	cause	763.1
Rapid second stage (delivery)	661.33	661.31	661.30		763.6
Reaction obstetric anesthetic or analgesic NEC	668.93	668.91	668.90		763.5
Rectocele	654.43	654.41	654.40		763.1
causing obstructed labor	660.23	660.21	660.20	cause	763.1
Recurrent pregnancy loss	646.33	646.31	646.30		
Reduction, multiple gestation (elective)	651.73	651.71	651.70	placenta status	
Repair of pelvic floor, previous	654.43	654.41	654.40		763.89
causing obstructed labor	660.23	660.21	660.20	cause	763.1
Retardation fetal growth (intrauterine)	656.53	656.51	656.50		764.90
Retention, retained					
dead					
fetus (after 22 completed weeks gestation)	656.43	656.41	656.40		cause

Coding Tables

Antepartum Pregnancy

Antepartum Pregnancy Condition or Complication; affecting management of mother	Antepartum condition or complication	Delivered, with or without mention of antepartum condition	Unspecified episode of care	Assign additional code to describe the…	Affecting fetus (coded on the newborn chart only)
Retention, retained — *continued*					
early fetal death (before 22 completed weeks gestation)	632				
ovum		631.8			
Retinitis	646.83	646.81	646.80	condition	
Retraction					
nipple	676.03	676.01	676.00		
ring, uterus (Bandl's) (pathological)	661.43	661.41	661.40		763.7
Retroversion, uterus	654.33	654.31	654.30		763.89
causing obstructed labor	660.23	660.21	660.20	cause	763.1
Rh immunization, incompatibility, or sensitization	656.13	656.11	656.10		773.0
Rigid, rigidity					
cervix	654.63	654.61	654.60		763.89
causing obstructed labor	660.23	660.21	660.20	cause	763.1
pelvic floor	654.43	654.41	654.40		763.89
causing obstructed labor	660.23	660.21	660.20	cause	763.1
Ring(s), complicating delivery					
perineum or vulva	654.83	654.81	654.80		763.89
causing obstructed labor	660.23	660.21	660.20	cause	763.1
vagina	654.73	654.71	654.70		763.89
causing obstructed labor	660.23	660.21	660.20	cause	763.1
Bandl's	661.43	661.41	661.40		763.7
contraction	661.43	661.41	661.40		763.7
retraction, uterus, pathological	661.43	661.41	661.40		763.7
Robert's pelvis with disproportion (fetopelvic)	653.03	653.01	653.00		763.1
causing obstructed labor	660.13	660.11	660.10	cause	763.1
Rubella (German measles)	647.53	647.51	647.50	condition	760.2
with suspected fetal damage	655.33	655.31	655.30		771.0
Rupture					
abdominal viscera (obstetrical trauma)		665.51	665.50		
amnion (premature)	658.13	658.11	658.10		763.89
with delayed delivery	658.23	658.21	658.20		763.89
bladder (sphincter), obstetrical trauma		665.51	665.50		
cervix (uteri), obstetrical trauma		665.31	665.30		
marginal sinus (hemorrhage)	641.23	641.21	641.20		762.1
membranes (premature)	658.13	658.11	658.10		761.1
with delayed delivery	658.23	658.21	658.20		761.1
artificial with delayed delivery following	658.33	658.31	658.30		761.1
pelvic floor, complicating delivery		664.11	664.10		
perineum during delivery		664.41	664.40		
umbilical cord	663.83	663.81	663.80		772.0
urethra (obstetrical trauma)		665.51	665.50		
uterus					
before onset of labor	665.03	665.01	665.00		763.89
during labor		665.11	665.10		763.89
vulva, complicating delivery		664.01	664.00		
Sacculation, complicating delivery	654.43	654.41	654.40		763.1
causing obstructed labor	660.23	660.21	660.20	cause	763.1
Salivation (excessive)	646.83	646.81	646.80	condition	
Salpingitis	646.63	646.61	646.60	condition	760.8
Salpingo-oophoritis	646.63	646.61	646.60	condition	760.8
Scar, scarring					
cervix	654.63	654.61	654.60		763.89
causing obstructed labor	660.23	660.21	660.20	cause	763.1
uterus NEC	654.93	654.91	654.90		763.89
from previous cesarean delivery	654.23	654.21	654.20		763.89
causing obstructed labor	660.23	660.21	660.20	cause	763.1
Scoliotic pelvis with disproportion (fetopelvic)	653.03	653.01	653.00		763.1
causing obstructed labor	660.13	660.11	660.10	cause	763.1
Screening, prenatal (for)					
If the abnormal finding is known — code the findings					
by					
amniocentesis					
chromosomal anomalies	V28.0				

Antepartum Pregnancy Condition or Complication; affecting management of mother	Antepartum condition or complication	Delivered, with or without mention of antepartum condition	Unspecified episode of care	Assign additional code to describe the...	Affecting fetus (coded on the newborn chart only)
Screening, prenatal (for) — *continued*					
If the abnormal finding is known — code the findings — *continued*					
by — *continued*					
amniocentesis — *continued*					
raised alpha-fetoprotein levels (amniotic fluid)	V28.1				
specified, NEC	V28.2				
ultrasound					
fetal growth retardation	V28.4				
malformation	V28.3				
isoimmunization	V28.5				
other specified screening	V28.89				
Streptococcus B	V28.6				
unspecified, screening	V28.9				
Separation (obstetrical trauma)					
pubic bone		665.61	665.60		
symphysis pubis		665.61	665.60		
Sepsis, complicating labor	659.33	659.31	659.30		
Septicemia	647.83	647.81	647.80	condition	
Septum, vagina	654.73	654.71	654.70		763.89
causing obstructed labor	660.23	660.21	660.20	cause	763.1
Sextuplet NEC	651.83	651.81	651.80	V91.90-V91.99	761.5
with fetal loss and retention of one or more fetus(es)	651.63	651.61	651.60	V91.90-V91.99	
reduction, multiple gestation (elective)	651.73	651.71	651.70	V91.90-V91.99	
Shirodkar suture	654.53	654.51	654.50		
causing obstructed labor	660.23	660.21	660.20	cause	763.1
Shock					
complicating labor and delivery	669.13	669.11	669.10		
following labor and delivery	669.13	669.11	669.10		
Short, shortening, shortness	663.43	663.41	663.40		762.6
cervix	649.73	649.71	649.70	complication	
umbilical cord	663.43	663.41	663.40		762.6
Sinus, marginal, rupture or bleeding	641.23	641.21	641.20		762.1
Slow fetal growth	656.53	656.51	656.50		764.90
Small					
for-dates fetus	656.53	656.51	656.50		764.00
pelvis					
with disproportion (fetopelvic)	653.13	653.11	653.10		763.1
causing obstructed labor	660.13	660.11	660.10	cause	763.1
Spasms					
cervix, complicating delivery	661.43	661.41	661.40		763.7
uterus	646.83	646.81	646.80	condition	
complicating delivery	661.43	661.41	661.40		763.7
complicating labor	661.43	661.41	661.40		763.7
Specified condition NEC	646.83	646.81	646.80	condition	
Spina bifida (aperta)**, suspected fetal**	655.03	655.01	655.00		
Spondylolisthesis with disproportion (fetopelvic)	653.33	653.31	653.30		763.1
causing obstructed labor	660.13	660.11	660.10	cause	763.1
Spondylolysis with disproportion (fetopelvic)	653.33	653.31	653.30		763.1
causing obstructed labor	660.13	660.11	660.10	cause	763.1
Spondylosis with disproportion (fetopelvic)	653.33	653.31	653.30		763.1
causing obstructed labor	660.13	660.11	660.10	cause	763.1
Spotting					
antepartum hemorrhage	641.93	641.91	641.90		
spotting	649.53	649.51	649.50		
Spurious labor pains	644.13		644.10		
Stenosis (cicatricial)					
cervix, cervical (canal)	654.63	654.61	654.60		763.89
causing obstructed labor	660.23	660.21	660.20	cause	763.1
vagina	654.73	654.71	654.70		763.89
causing obstructed labor	660.23	660.21	660.20	cause	763.1
Stricture, cervix (canal)	654.63	654.61	654.60		763.89
causing obstructed labor	660.23	660.21	660.20	cause	763.1
Sudden death					
during childbirth	669.93	669.91	669.90		

Coding Tables

Antepartum Pregnancy

Antepartum Pregnancy Condition or Complication; affecting management of mother	Antepartum condition or complication	Delivered, with or without mention of antepartum condition	Unspecified episode of care	Assign additional code to describe the…	Affecting fetus (coded on the newborn chart only)
Supervision (of) (for)					
high-risk	V23.9				
insufficient prenatal care	V23.7				
specified problem NEC	V23.89				
multiparity	V23.3				
normal NEC	V22.1				
first pregnancy	V22.0				
poor					
obstetric history	V23.49				
reproductive history	V23.5				
Suppression of lactation	676.53	676.51	676.50		
Suppurative, breast, mammary gland	675.13	675.11	675.10		
Surgery, previous					
cervix	654.63	654.61	654.60		763.89
causing obstructed labor	660.23	660.21	660.20	cause	763.1
pelvic soft tissues NEC	654.93	654.91	654.90		763.89
causing obstructed labor	660.23	660.21	660.20	cause	763.1
perineum or vulva	654.83	654.81	654.80		
uterus NEC	654.93	654.91	654.90		763.89
causing obstructed labor	660.23	660.21	660.20	cause	763.1
from previous cesarean delivery	654.23	654.21	654.20		
causing obstructed labor	660.23	660.21	660.20	cause	763.1
vagina	654.73	654.71	654.70		
causing obstructed labor	660.23	660.21	660.20	cause	763.1
Suspended uterus	654.43	654.41	654.40		763.89
causing obstructed labor	660.23	660.21	660.20	cause	763.1
Suture, Shirodkar (with or without cervical incompetence)	654.53	654.51	654.50		
causing obstructed labor	660.23	660.21	660.20	cause	763.1
Syncope complicating delivery	669.23	669.21	669.20		
Syndrome					
acid pulmonary aspiration (Mendelson's)	668.03	668.01	668.00		
Chiari-Frommel	676.63	676.61	676.60		
dead fetus	641.33	641.31	641.30		
dystocia, dystrophia	654.93	654.91	654.90		
causing obstructed labor	660.23	660.21	660.20	cause	763.1
Frommel-Chiari	676.63	676.61	676.60		
H.E.L.L.P (Hemolysis, Elevated Liver function and Low Platelets)	642.53	642.51	642.50		
hypotension, maternal	669.23	669.21	669.20		
maternal hypotension	669.23	669.21	669.20		
Mendelson's (during labor) (obstetric)	668.03	668.01	668.00		
vanishing twin	651.33			V91.00-V91.09	
Syphilis	647.03	647.01	647.00	condition	760.2
Tear, torn					
Anus, anal (sphincter)complicating delivery					
with third degree perineal laceration		664.21	664.20		763.89
w/mucosa		664.31	664.30		763.89
w/o third degree perineal laceration		664.61	664.60		763.89
old (healed)		654.81	654.80		763.89
bladder, obstetrical trauma		665.51	665.50		763.89
bowel, obstetrical trauma		665.51	665.50		763.89
broad ligament, obstetrical trauma		665.51	665.50		763.89
cervix, obstetrical trauma		665.31	665.30		763.89
pelvic					
floor, complicating delivery		664.11	664.10		763.89
organ NEC, obstetrical trauma		665.51	665.50		763.89
perineum, obstetrical trauma		665.51	665.50		763.89
periurethral, obstetrical trauma		664.81	664.80		763.89
umbilical cord, complicating delivery	663.83	663.81	663.80		772.0
urethra, obstetrical trauma		665.51	665.50		
vulva, complicating delivery		664.01	664.00		763.89
Teratoma, fetal sacral, causing fetopelvic disproportion	653.73	653.71	653.70		763.1
causing obstructed labor	660.23	660.21	660.20	cause	763.1
Thelitis	675.03	675.01	675.00		

Antepartum Pregnancy Condition or Complication; affecting management of mother	Antepartum condition or complication	Delivered, with or without mention of antepartum condition	Unspecified episode of care	Assign additional code to describe the...	Affecting fetus (coded on the newborn chart only)
Threatened					
abortion or miscarriage	640.03	640.01	640.00		762.1
labor	644.13		644.10		761.8
before 22 completed weeks gestation	640.03	640.01	640.00		762.1
premature delivery		644.21	644.20		761.8
premature labor	644.03		644.00		761.8
Thrombophlebitis	671.23	671.21	671.20	453.6, 453.71, 453.81	760.3
cerebral (sinus) (vein), nonpyogenic	671.53	671.51	671.50		760.3
deep	671.33	671.31	671.30	DVT code, anticoag use (V58.61)	760.3
intracranial venous sinus, nonpyogenic	671.53	671.51	671.50		760.3
specified site NEC	671.53	671.51	671.50		760.3
superficial	671.23	671.21	671.20	453.6, 453.71, 453.81	760.3
Thrombosis	671.93	671.91	671.90		
brain (artery) (stem)	674.03	674.01	674.00		
intracranial, venous sinus (nonpyogenic origin)	671.53	671.51	671.50		
deep	671.33	671.31	671.30	DVT code, anticoag use (V58.61)	760.3
spinal cord	671.53	671.51	671.50		
superficial	671.23	671.21	671.20	453.6, 453.71, 453.81	
umbilical cord (vessels)	663.63	663.61	663.60		762.6
venous (superficial)	671.23	671.21	671.20	453.6, 453.71, 453.81	
Thyroid dysfunction	648.13	648.11	648.10	condition	
Thyroiditis	648.13	648.11	648.10	condition	
Thyrotoxicosis	648.13	648.11	648.10	condition	
Tipping pelvis with disproportion (fetopelvic)	653.03	653.01	653.00		763.1
causing obstructed labor	660.13	660.11	660.10	cause	763.1
Tobacco use disorder	649.03	649.01	649.00		
Torsion of uterus	654.43	654.41	654.40		
causing obstructed labor	660.23	660.21	660.20	cause	763.1
Toxemia (mild) (pre-eclamptic)	642.43	642.41	642.40		760.0
with					760.0
convulsions	642.63	642.61	642.60		760.0
pre-existing hypertension	642.73	642.71	642.70		760.0
Toxemia (mild) (pre-eclamptic)	642.43	642.41	642.40		760.0
eclamptic	642.63	642.61	642.60		760.0
with pre-existing hypertension	642.73	642.71	642.70		760.0
severe	642.53	642.51	642.50		760.0
Transmission of chemical substances through the placenta, suspected	655.53	655.51	655.50		760.70
Transverse					
arrest (deep), in labor	660.33	660.31	660.30	cause	763.1
lie or presentation	652.33	652.31	652.30		761.7
with successful version	652.13	652.11	652.10		763.1
causing obstructed labor	660.03	660.01	660.00	cause	763.1
Trauma	648.93	648.91	648.90	condition	
causing hemorrhage	641.83	641.81	641.80		760.5
during delivery NEC	665.93	665.91	665.90		760.5
obstetrical	665.93	665.91	665.90		760.5
previous pregnancy (major), affecting management of current pregnancy, childbirth or puerperium	V23.89	V23.89	V23.89		
Triplet NEC	651.13	651.11	651.10	V91.10-V91.19	761.5
with fetal loss and retention of one or more fetus(es)	651.43	651.41	651.40	V91.10-V91.19	761.5
reduction, multiple gestation (elective)	651.73	651.71	651.70	V91.10-V91.19	
Trophoblastic disease	630				
previous pregnancy, affecting management of current pregnancy	V23.1	V23.1	V23.1		
Tubal (with rupture)					761.4
w/ intrauterine pregnancy	633.11				
w/o intrauterine pregnancy	633.10				
Tuberculosis	647.33	647.31	647.30	condition	760.2
Tumor					
cervix	654.63	654.61	654.60		763.89
causing obstructed labor	660.23	660.21	660.20	cause	763.1
fetal, causing disproportion	653.73	653.71	653.70		763.1
causing obstructed labor	660.13	660.11	660.10	cause	763.1

Antepartum Pregnancy

Antepartum Pregnancy Condition or Complication; affecting management of mother	Antepartum condition or complication	Delivered, with or without mention of antepartum condition	Unspecified episode of care	Assign additional code to describe the...	Affecting fetus (coded on the newborn chart only)
Tumor — *continued*					
ovary	654.43	654.41	654.40		763.89
causing obstructed labor	660.23	660.21	660.20	cause	763.1
pelvic	654.93	654.91	654.90		763.89
causing obstructed labor	660.23	660.21	660.20	cause	763.1
pelvic organs or tissue NEC	654.43	654.41	654.40		763.89
causing obstructed labor	660.23	660.21	660.20	cause	763.1
uterus	654.13	654.11	654.10		763.89
causing obstructed labor	660.23	660.21	660.20	cause	763.1
vagina	654.73	654.71	654.70		763.89
causing obstructed labor	660.23	660.21	660.20	cause	763.1
vulva	654.83	654.81	654.80		763.89
causing obstructed labor	660.23	660.21	660.20	cause	763.1
Twin NEC	651.03	651.01	651.00	V91.00-V91.09	761.5
with fetal loss and retention of one or more fetus(es)	651.33	651.31	651.30	V91.00-V91.09	761.5
reduction, multiple gestation (elective)	651.73	651.71	651.70	V91.00-V91.09	
conjoined (siamese)	678.13	678.11	678.10		759.4
Unstable lie	652.03	652.01	652.00		761.7
causing obstructed labor	660.03	660.01	660.00	cause	763.1
Unwanted NEC	V61.7				
Uremia (renal disease or failure) **NEC**	646.23	646.21	646.20	condition	760.1
with secondary hypertension	642.13	642.11	642.10		760.0
hypertensive	642.23	642.21	642.20		760.0
Urethritis	646.63	646.61	646.60	condition	760.1
Uterine size date discrepancy	649.63	649.61	649.60		
UTI	646.63	646.61	646.60	condition	760.1
Vaginitis or vulvitis	646.63	646.61	646.60	condition	760.8
Valsuani's disease	648.23	648.21	648.20	condition	
Vanishing twin	651.33			V91.00-V91.09	
Varicose					
placental vessels	656.73	656.71	656.70		
veins (legs)	671.03	671.01	671.00		
perineum	671.13	671.11	671.10		
vulva	671.13	671.11	671.10		
Varicosity, labia or vulva	671.13	671.11	671.10		
Varix (lower extremity)	671.03	671.01	671.00		
perineum	671.13	671.11	671.10		
Vulva	671.13	671.11	671.10		
Vasa previa	663.53	663.51	663.50		762.6
hemorrhage	663.53	663.51	663.50		772.0
Venereal disease NEC	647.23	647.21	647.20	disease	
Venous, unspecified	671.93	671.91	671.90		
Ventouse delivery NEC		669.51	669.50		763.3
Version					
before labor	652.13	652.11	652.10		761.7
causing obstructed labor	660.03	660.01	660.00	cause	763.1
cephalic (correcting previous malposition)	652.13	652.11	652.10		763.1
causing obstructed labor	660.03	660.01	660.00	cause	763.1
Viral disease NEC	647.63	647.61	647.60	disease	
Vomiting	643.93	643.91	643.90		761.8
due to					
organic disease or other cause	643.83	643.81	643.80		761.8
specific cause NEC	643.83	643.81	643.80		761.8
early (mild) (before 22 completed weeks gestation)	643.03	643.01	643.00		761.8
with					761.8
carbohydrate depletion	643.13	643.11	643.10		761.8
dehydration	643.13	643.11	643.10		761.8
electrolyte imbalance	643.13	643.11	643.10		761.8
late (after 22 completed weeks gestation)	643.23	643.21	643.20		761.8
severe (with metabolic disturbance)	643.13	643.11	643.10		761.8
Vulvitis	646.63	646.61	646.60	condition	760.8
Weight gain	646.13	646.11	646.10	condition	
insufficient	646.83	646.81	646.80	condition	
Young maternal age	659.83	659.81	659.80		

Coding Tables

Postpartum Pregnancy

Postpartum Pregnancy Condition or Complication; affecting management of mother	Postpartum condition or complication	Delivered with mention of postpartum complication	Unspecified episode of care	Assign additional code to describe the…	Affecting newborn (coded on the newborn chart only)
Abnormal NEC					
cervix	654.64	654.62	654.60		763.89
glucose tolerance test	648.84	648.82	648.80	condition	775.0
pelvic organs or tissues NEC	654.94	654.92	654.90		763.89
perineum or vulva	654.84	654.82	654.80		763.89
position					
cervix	654.44	654.42	654.40		763.89
uterus	654.44	654.42	654.40		763.89
quality of milk	676.84	676.82	676.80		
shape of uterus	654.44	654.42	654.40		763.89
uterus (congenital)	654.04	654.02	654.00		763.89
vagina	654.74	654.72	654.70		763.89
vulva (acquired) (congenital)	654.84	654.82	654.80		763.89
weight gain	646.14	646.12	646.10	condition	761.8
with hypertension (mild) (pre-eclamptic)	642.44	642.42	642.40		760.0
with					
convulsions	642.64	642.62	642.60		760.0
pre-existing hypertension	642.74	642.72	642.70		760.0
with severe hypertension	642.54	642.52	642.50		760.0
Abscess					
areola (acute) (chronic)	675.14	675.12	675.10		
Bartholin's gland	646.64	646.62	646.60	condition	760.8
bladder	646.64	646.62	646.60	condition	760.1
breast (acute) (chronic)	675.14	675.12	675.10		
cervix (uteri)	670.84	670.82	670.80		
fallopian tube	670.84	670.82	670.80		
genital organ or tract NEC (postpartum)	670.84	670.82	670.80		
kidney	646.64	646.62	646.60	condition	760.1
labium (majus) (minus)	646.64	646.62	646.60	condition	760.8
mesosalpinx	670.84	670.82	670.80		
milk	675.14	675.12	675.10		
nabothian	646.64	646.62	646.60	condition	
nipple	675.04	675.02	675.00		
ovary	670.84	670.82	670.80		
oviduct	670.84	670.82	670.80		
para-uterine	670.84	670.82	670.80		
pelvic	670.84	670.82	670.80		
perimetric	670.84	670.82	670.80		
peritoneum, peritoneal (perforated) (ruptured) postpartum	670.84	670.82	670.80		
periuterine	670.84	670.82	670.80		
retro-uterine	670.84	670.82	670.80		
subareolar postpartum	675.14	675.12	675.10		
suprapelvic	670.84	670.82	670.80		
tubal (ruptured)	670.84	670.82	670.80		
tubo-ovarian	67084	670.82	670.80		
urethra	646.64	646.62	646.60	condition	760.1
urinary tract NEC	646.64	646.62	646.60	condition	
uterine, uterus	670.84	670.82	670.80		
vagina (wall)	646.64	646.62	646.60	condition	
vaginorectal	646.64	646.62	646.60	condition	
vulva	646.64	646.62	646.60	condition	760.8
vulvovaginal gland	646.64	646.62	646.60	condition	
Accreta placenta	667.04	667.02	667.00		
with hemorrhage	666.04	666.02	666.00		
Accident	674.94	674.92	674.90		
Addiction					
alcoholic	648.44	648.42	648.40	condition	760.71
Adherent placenta	667.04	667.02	667.00		
with hemorrhage	666.04	666.02	666.00		
Adhesion(s), adhesive					
cervicovaginal (postpartum)	674.84	674.82	674.80		
uterus to abdominal wall	654.44	654.42	654.40		763.89
Adnexitis	670.84	670.82	670.80		
Aerocele	673.04	673.02	673.00		

Coding Tables

Postpartum Pregnancy

Postpartum Pregnancy Condition or Complication; affecting management of mother	Postpartum condition or complication	Delivered with mention of postpartum complication	Unspecified episode of care	Assign additional code to describe the...	Affecting newborn (coded on the newborn chart only)
Afibrinogenemia (postpartum)	666.34	666.32	666.30		
AFP (screening for raised levels in amniotic fluid)	V28.1				
Agalactia	676.44	676.42	676.40		
Air embolism	673.04	673.02	673.00		
Albuminuria (gravidarum)	646.24	646.22	646.20	condition	760.1
with hypertension (and edema)					760.1
mild	642.44	642.42	642.40		760.0
severe	642.54	642.52	642.50		760.0
gestational	646.24	646.22	646.20	condition	760.1
pre-eclamptic (mild)	642.24	642.22	642.20		760.0
severe	642.54	642.52	642.50		760.0
Alcohol, alcoholic					
addiction (maternal)	648.44	648.42	648.40	condition	760.71
Alphafetoprotein (screening for raised levels in amniotic fluid)	V28.1				
Amniotic fluid embolism	673.14	673.12	673.10		
Amputation of cervix	654.64	654.62	654.60		763.8
Anemia	648.24	648.22	648.20	condition	760.8
aplastic	648.24	648.22	648.20	condition	760.8
iron (Fe) deficiency	648.24	648.22	648.20	condition	760.8
macrocytic	648.24	648.22	648.20	condition	760.8
megaloblastic	648.24	648.22	648.20	condition	760.8
pernicious	648.24	648.22	648.20	condition	760.8
postpartum	648.24	648.22	648.20	condition	
Anesthesia, anesthetic					
complications NEC	668.84	668.82	668.80	condition	763.5
cardiac	668.14	668.12	668.10	condition	763.5
central nervous system	668.24	668.22	668.20	condition	763.5
pulmonary	668.04	668.02	668.00	condition	763.5
death (from) during delivery	668.94	668.92	668.90	condition	761.6
Anomaly, anomalous (congenital)					
cardiovascular system	648.54	648.52	648.50	condition	
cervix	654.64	654.62	654.60		763.89
uterus	654.04	654.02	654.00		763.89
Anoxia cerebral					
complicating delivery (cesarean) (instrumental)	669.44	669.42	669.40		
due to obstetric anesthesia or sedation	668.24	668.22	668.20	complication	
Anteversion					
uterus, uterine (cervix)	654.44	654.42	654.40		763.89
Anuria, postpartum	669.34	669.32	669.30		
Apoplexy	674.04	674.02	674.00		
Arrest, arrested					
cardiac					
anesthesia, complicating delivery (cesarean)	668.14	668.12	668.10		
(instrumental)	669.44	669.42	669.40		
Aspiration					
acid-pulmonary (syndrome)	668.04	668.02	668.00	complication	
pneumonitis	668.04	668.02	668.00	complication	
Atonia, atony, atonic					
w/hemorrhage	666.14	666.12	666.10		
w/o hemorrhage	669.84	669.82	669.80		
Atresia, atretic					
cervix	654.64	654.62	654.60		763.89
Atrophy, atrophic					
breast, postpartum	676.34	676.32	676.30		
postpartum	674.84	674.82	674.80		
Avulsion (traumatic)					
symphyseal cartilage (inner)	665.64		665.60		
Bacilluria, asymptomatic	646.54	646.52	646.50	complication	760.1
Bacteremia	647.84	647.82	647.80	condition	
Bacteriuria, asymptomatic	646.54	646.52	646.50	complication	760.1
Bariatric surgery	649.24	649.22	649.20		
Bicornis or Bicornuate uterus	654.04	654.02	654.00		763.89
Bleeding					
atonic, following delivery	666.14	666.12	666.10		
cerebrovascular	674.04	674.02	674.00		

Postpartum Pregnancy Condition or Complication; affecting management of mother	Postpartum condition or complication	Delivered with mention of postpartum complication	Unspecified episode of care	Assign additional code to describe the...	Affecting newborn (coded on the newborn chart only)
Bleeding — *continued*					
due to					
subinvolution, postpartum	666.24	666.22	666.20		
Blood, dyscrasia (postpartum)	666.34	666.32	666.30		
Bone disorders	648.74	648.72	648.70	condition	
Breakdown, perineum	674.24	674.22	674.20		
Breastfeeding difficulties	676.84	676.82	676.80		
Caked breast (postpartum)	676.24	676.22	676.20		
Cardiomyopathy	674.54	674.52	674.50		
Cardiovascular disease	648.64	648.62	648.60	condition	
congenital	648.54	648.52	648.50	condition	
Cellulitis (postpartum)					
breast	675.14	675.12	675.10		
pelvis	670.84	670.82	670.80		
Cerebrovascular disorders	674.04	674.02	674.00	condition	
Cervical shortening		649.70			
Cervicitis	646.64	646.62	646.60	condition	760.8
Cervix					
adhesions	654.64	654.62	654.60		
anaplasia	654.64	654.62	654.60		
atypism	654.64	654.62	654.60		
bands	654.64	654.62	654.60		
cervicitis	654.64	654.62	654.60		
cicatrix	654.64	654.62	654.60		
cyst	654.64	654.62	654.60		
dysplasia	654.64	654.62	654.60		
ectropion	654.64	654.62	654.60		
endocervicitis	654.64	654.62	654.60		
erosion	654.64	654.62	654.60		
hypertrophic elongation	654.64	654.62	654.60		
incompetence	654.54	654.52	654.50		761.0
leukoplakia	654.64	654.62	654.60		
Nabothian (gland) cyst or follicle	654.64	654.62	654.60		
old laceration	654.64	654.62	654.60		
polyp	654.64	654.62	654.60		
stricture and stenosis	654.64	654.62	654.60		
ulcer	654.64	654.62	654.60		
Chiari-Frommel syndrome	676.64	676.62	676.60		
Childbed fever	670.24	670.22	670.20	Sepsis, 995.92, organ failure,	
Chloasma (gravidarum)	646.84	646.82	646.80	condition	
Cicatrix					
cervix	654.64	654.62	654.60		
vagina	654.74	654.72	654.70		
Circulating anticoagulants	666.34	666.32	666.30		
Coagulation defects	649.34	649.32	649.30	286.0-286.9	
Collapse (during or after labor and delivery)					
circulatory (peripheral)	669.14	669.12	669.10		779.8
lung	668.04	668.02	668.00		
vascular (peripheral)	669.14	669.12	669.10		
Colporrhexis	665.44		665.40		
Complications NEC					
cesarean section wound	674.34	674.32	674.30		
delivery	669.94	669.92	669.90		
procedure (instrumental) (manual) (surgical)	669.44	669.42	669.40		
specified type NEC	669.84	669.82	669.80		
fetal	679.13	679.11	679.10		
labor and delivery	669.94	669.92	669.90		
anesthesia (sedation)	668.94	668.92	668.90		763.5
cardiac	668.14	668.12	668.10		
central nervous system	668.24	668.22	668.20		
pulmonary	668.04	668.02	668.00		
specified type NEC	668.84	668.82	668.80		
specified condition NEC	669.84	669.82	669.80		
maternal	679.03	679.01	679.00		
perineal repair	674.34	674.32	674.30		

Coding Tables

Postpartum Pregnancy

Postpartum Pregnancy Condition or Complication; affecting management of mother	Postpartum condition or complication	Delivered with mention of postpartum complication	Unspecified episode of care	Assign additional code to describe the...	Affecting newborn (coded on the newborn chart only)
Complications NEC — *continued*					
perineal repair — *continued*					
disruption	674.24	674.22	674.20		
postpartum NEC	674.94	674.92	674.90		
surgical wound	674.34	674.32	674.30		
Convulsions (eclamptic) (uremic)	642.64	642.62	642.60		760.0
with pre-existing hypertension	642.74	642.72	642.70		760.0
Cracked nipple (postpartum)	676.14	676.12	676.10		
Cyst					
ovary	654.44	654.42	654.40		763.89
pelvic	654.44	654.42	654.40		763.89
Cystitis	646.64	646.62	646.60	condition	760.1
Cystocele	654.44	654.42	654.40		763.89
Damage					
coccyx, complicating delivery	665.64		665.60		763.89
pelvic (during delivery)					
joint or ligament	665.64		665.60		763.89
organ	665.54		665.50		763.89
Death, maternal, NEC					
during delivery	668.94	668.92	668.90		761.6
postpartum (cause not stated) (sudden)	674.94	674.92	674.90		
under anesthesia NEC	668.94	668.92	668.90		761.6
Deciduitis	646.64	646.62	646.60		760.8
postpartum	670.84	670.82	670.80		
Defect, defective coagulation (factor)					
postpartum	666.34	666.32	666.30		
Deficiency, deficient coagulation (factor)					
postpartum	666.34	666.32	666.30		
Deformity					
pelvic, pelvis					
soft part, organs or tissues NEC	654.94	654.92	654.90	cause	763.89
Dehiscence (postpartum)					
cesarean wound	674.14	674.12	674.10		
episiotomy	674.24	674.22	674.20		
perineal wound	674.24	674.22	674.20		
uterine wound	674.14	674.12	674.10		
Dependence, maternal					
drug	648.34	648.32	648.30	condition	779.5
Depression, postpartum	648.44	648.42	648.40	condition	
Dermatitis, gestationis	646.84	646.82	646.80	condition	
Detachment					
cervix, annular	665.34		665.30		763.89
Diabetes					
with long term (current) insulin use				V58.67	775.0
condition present before pregnancy	648.04	648.02	648.00	condition	775.0
gestational (chemical) (latent)	648.84	648.82	648.80	condition	775.0
Diastasis, recti (abdomen) **complicating delivery**	665.84	665.82	665.80		763.89
Difficult delivery NEC	669.94	669.92	669.90		763.89
Difficulty with breast feeding	676.84	676.82	676.80		
Dilatation					
bladder (sphincter)	654.44	654.42	654.40		763.89
Disease, NEC (postpartum)	674.94	674.92	674.90		
breast NEC	676.34	676.32	676.30		
cerebrovascular, NEC	674.04	674.02	674.00		
Frommel's	676.64	676.62	676.60		
heart	648.64	648.62	648.60	condition	760.8
postpartum	674.84	674.82	674.80		
renal NEC	646.24	646.22	646.20	condition	760.1
Valsuani's (progressive pernicious anemia, puerperal)	648.24	648.22	648.20	condition	
venereal NEC	647.24	647.22	647.20	condition	
virus NEC	647.64	647.62	647.60	condition	
Disorders					
breast, postpartum	676.34	676.32	676.30		
genital tract or organ	646.64	646.62	646.60	condition	760.8
lactation	676.94	676.92	676.90		
mental	648.44	648.42	648.40	condition	

Postpartum Pregnancy Condition or Complication; affecting management of mother	Postpartum condition or complication	Delivered with mention of postpartum complication	Unspecified episode of care	Assign additional code to describe the...	Affecting newborn (coded on the newborn chart only)
Disorders — *continued*					
metabolism NEC (in labor and delivery)	669.04	669.02	669.00		763.8
specified type NEC	676.84	676.82	676.80		
Displacement, uterus NEC	654.44	654.42	654.40		763.8
Disruption, wound					
cesarean operation	674.14	674.12	674.10		
episiotomy	674.24	674.22	674.20		
perineal (obstetric)	674.24	674.22	674.20		
uterine	674.14	674.12	674.10		
Distortion					
maternal	669.04	669.02	669.00		
Double uterus	654.04	654.02	654.00		763.89
Drug dependence	648.34	648.32	648.30	condition	
Dyscrasia, blood					
postpartum	666.34	666.32	666.30		
Dysfunction					
thyroid	648.14	648.12	648.10	condition	
Dysplasia of cervix	654.64	654.62	654.60		763.89
Eclampsia, eclamptic	642.64	642.62	642.60		760.0
with pre-existing hypertension	642.74	642.72	642.70		760.0
Edema	646.14	646.12	646.10	condition	
with hypertension — *see* Pregnancy, toxemia					
cervix (postpartum)	674.84	674.82	674.80		
Effect, adverse					
anesthetic (in labor and delivery) NEC	668.94	668.92	668.90		763.5
Embolism					
air (pulmonary)	673.04	673.02	673.00		
amniotic fluid	673.14	673.12	673.10		
blood clot	673.24	673.22	673.20		
brain (postpartum)	674.04	674.02	674.00		
cerebral (postpartum)	674.04	674.02	674.00		
fat (cerebral) (pulmonary) (systemic)	673.84	673.82	673.80		
heart	674.84	674.82	674.80		
intracranial (venous sinus) (nonpyogenic)	671.54	671.52	671.50		
pulmonary NEC	673.24	673.22	673.20		
pyemic	673.34	673.32	673.30		
septic	673.34	673.32	673.30		
specified NEC	674.84	674.82	674.80		
spinal cord	671.54	671.52	671.50		
Emesis (gravidarum) — *see* Pregnancy, vomiting					
Endometritis	670.14	670.12	670.10	condition	760.8
decidual	670.14	670.12	670.10	condition	760.8
postpartum	670.14	670.12	670.10		
puerperal	670.14	670.12	670.10		
Engorgement, breast (postpartum)	676.24	676.22	676.20		
Epilepsy	649.44	649.42	649.40	345.00-345.91	
Erysipelas (postpartum, childbirth)	670.84	670.82	670.80		
Eversion, uterus					
complicating delivery	665.24	665.22	665.20		763.89
postpartum	674.84	674.82	674.80		
Excessive					
milk secretion	676.64	676.62	676.60		
weight gain	646.14	646.12	646.10	condition	
Exhaustion (complicating delivery)	669.84	669.82	669.80		763.89
Extraction					
manual NEC	669.84	669.82	669.80		763.89
Extroversion, uterus (complicating delivery)	665.24	665.22	665.20		763.89
Failure, failed					
heart, complicating					
delivery (cesarean) (instrumental)	669.44	669.42	669.40		
obstetric anesthesia or sedation	668.14	668.12	668.10		
lactation	676.44	676.42	676.40		
renal following labor and delivery (acute)	669.34	669.32	669.30		
Fatigue	646.84	646.82	646.80	condition	
Febris puerperalis	672.04	672.02	672.00		
Female genital mutilation	648.94	648.92	648.90	629.20-629.29	

Coding Tables

Postpartum Pregnancy

Postpartum Pregnancy Condition or Complication; affecting management of mother	Postpartum condition or complication	Delivered with mention of postpartum complication	Unspecified episode of care	Assign additional code to describe the…	Affecting newborn (coded on the newborn chart only)
Fever	672.04	672.02	672.00		
childbed	670.24	670.22	670.20	Sepsis, 995.92, organ failure	
milk	672.04	672.02	672.00		
sepsis	670.24	670.22	670.20	Sepsis, 995.92, organ failure	
Fibrinolysis postpartum	666.34	666.32	666.30		
Fibroid tumor(s)	654.14	654.12	654.10		763.89
Fibromyoma (uterus)	654.14	654.12	654.10		763.89
Fibrosis, fibrotic					
perineum	654.84	654.82	654.80		763.89
Fissure, nipple (postpartum)	676.14	676.12	676.10		
Fistula (postpartum)					
breast, mammary gland	675.14	675.12	675.10		
nipple	675.04	675.02	675.00		
Forced birth or delivery NEC	669.84	669.82	669.80		763.89
Fractured coccyx complicating delivery	665.64		665.60		
Frommel's disease	676.64	676.62	676.60		
Frommel-Chiari syndrome	676.64	676.62	676.60		
Galactocele (breast), **postpartum**	676.84	676.82	676.80		
Galactorrhea	676.64	676.62	676.60		
Gangrene					
gas (bacillus) postpartum, childbirth	670.84	670.82	670.80		
Genital (female) **mutilation**	648.94	648.92	648.90	629.20-629.29	
Goiter	648.14	648.12	648.10	condition	
Gonococcal infection	647.14	647.12	647.10	condition	760.2
Gonorrhea	647.14	647.12	647.10	condition	760.2
HELLP	642.54	642.52	642.50		
Hematoma					
broad ligament	665.74	665.72	665.70		
cesarean section wound	674.34	674.32	674.30		
complicating delivery (perineum) (vulva)	664.54		664.50		
pelvic	665.74	665.72	665.70		
vagina	665.74	665.72	665.70		
episiotomy	674.34	674.32	674.30		
obstetrical surgical wound	674.34	674.32	674.30		
pelvis, complicating delivery	665.74	665.72	665.70		
perineal wound	674.34	674.32	674.30		
complicating delivery	664.54		664.50		
vagina	665.74	665.72	665.70		
vulva, complicating delivery	664.54		664.50		767.8
Hematosalpinx, infectional	670.84	670.82	670.80		
Hemiplegia, cerebral	674.04	674.02	674.00		
Hemolysis, liver dysfunction, low platelets syndrome	642.54	642.52	642.50		
Hemorrhage					
brain (postpartum, childbirth)	674.04	674.02	674.00		
bulbar	674.04	674.02	674.00		
cerebrovascular	674.04	674.02	674.00		
cesarean section wound	674.34	674.32	674.30		
retained					
placenta	666.04	666.02	666.00		
secundines	666.24	666.22	666.20		
delayed, postpartum	666.24	666.22	666.20		
due to					
episiotomy	674.34	674.32	674.30		
extradural	674.04	674.02	674.00		
internal capsule	674.04	674.02	674.00		
intracranial, postpartum, childbirth	674.04	674.02	674.00		
intrapontine	674.04	674.02	674.00		
obstetrical surgical wound	674.34	674.32	674.30		
perineal wound	674.34	674.32	674.30		
postpartum (atonic) (following delivery of placenta)	666.14	666.12	666.10		
pontine	674.04	674.02	674.00		
subarachnoid	674.04	674.02	674.00		
subcortical	674.04	674.02	674.00		

Postpartum Pregnancy Condition or Complication; affecting management of mother	Postpartum condition or complication	Delivered with mention of postpartum complication	Unspecified episode of care	Assign additional code to describe the…	Affecting newborn (coded on the newborn chart only)
Hemorrhage — *continued*					
subdural	674.04	674.02	674.00		
delayed or secondary (after 24 hours)	666.24	666.22	666.20		
retained placenta	666.04	666.02	666.00		
third stage	666.04	666.02	666.00		
subarachnoid, postpartum, childbirth	674.04	674.02	674.00		
subdural, postpartum, childbirth	674.04	674.02	674.00		
third stage	666.04	666.02	666.00		
uterine, delayed	666.24	666.22	666.20		
ventricular	674.04	674.02	674.00		
Hemorrhoids	671.84	671.82	671.80		
Hepatitis, viral	647.64	647.62	647.60	condition	
Hepatorenal syndrome	674.84	674.82	674.80		
Herniation of uterus	654.44	654.42	654.40		
Herpes, herpetic	647.64	647.62	647.60	condition	
gestationis	646.84	646.82	646.80	condition	
Hydroa gestationis	646.84	646.82	646.80	condition	
Hypersecretion of milk	676.64	676.62	676.60		
Hypertension	642.94	642.92	642.90		760.0
with					
albuminuria (and edema) (mild)	642.44	642.42	642.40		760.0
severe	642.54	642.52	642.50		760.0
edema (mild)	642.44	642.42	642.40		760.0
severe	642.54	642.52	642.50		760.0
heart disease	642.24	642.22	642.20		760.0
and renal disease	642.24	642.22	642.20		760.0
pre-eclampsia or eclampsia	642.74	642.72	642.70		760.0
renal disease	642.24	642.22	642.20		760.0
and heart disease	642.24	642.22	642.20		760.0
benign	642.04	642.02	642.00		760.0
chronic	642.04	642.02	642.00		760.0
pre-existing	642.04	642.02	642.00		760.0
chronic	642.04	642.02	642.00		760.0
essential	642.04	642.02	642.00		760.0
with pre-eclampsia or eclampsia	642.74	642.72	642.70		760.0
gestational	642.34	642.32	642.30		
malignant	642.24	642.22	642.20		760.0
chronic	642.24	642.22	642.20		760.0
with pre-eclampsia or eclampsia	642.74	642.72	642.70		760.0
pre-existing	642.24	642.22	642.20		760.0
pre-existing	642.04	642.02	642.00		
secondary to renal disease	642.14	642.12	642.10		760.0
with pre-eclampsia or eclampsia	642.74	642.72	642.70		760.0
transient	642.34	642.32	642.30		
Hypertensive					
heart and renal disease	642.24	642.22	642.20		760.0
heart disease	642.24	642.22	642.20		760.0
renal disease	642.24	642.22	642.20		760.0
Hyperthyroidism	648.14	648.12	648.10	condition	
Hypotonic uterus	666.14	666.12	666.10		
Hypertonicity	648.14	648.12	648.10	condition	763.7
Hypertrophy					
breast (postpartum)	676.34	676.32	676.30		
uterus (postpartum)	674.84	674.82	674.80		
Hypotension (following labor and delivery)	669.24	669.22	669.20		
Hypothyroidism	648.14	648.12	648.10	condition	
Hysteralgia	646.84	646.82	646.80	condition	
Incarceration, uterus	654.34	654.32	654.30		763.1
Incompetent cervix (os)	654.54	654.52	654.50		761.0
Increased anticoagulants (postpartum)	666.34	666.32	666.30		
In double uterus	654.04	654.02	654.00		763.89
Indurated breast (postpartum)	676.34	676.32	676.30		
Inertia of uterus	666.14	666.12	666.10		
Infantile					
genitalia, genitals	654.44	654.42	654.40		763.89

Coding Tables

Postpartum Pregnancy

Coding Tables

Postpartum Pregnancy

Postpartum Pregnancy Condition or Complication; affecting management of mother	Postpartum condition or complication	Delivered with mention of postpartum complication	Unspecified episode of care	Assign additional code to describe the...	Affecting newborn (coded on the newborn chart only)
Infarct, infarction					
brain (stem), postpartum, childbirth	674.04	674.02	674.00		
Infection	647.94	647.92	647.90	condition	760.2
Bartholin's gland	646.64	646.62	646.60	condition	
bladder	646.64	646.62	646.60	condition	
breast (mammary gland), postpartum	675.24	675.22	675.20		
with nipple	675.94	675.92	675.90		
specified type NEC	675.84	675.82	675.80		
nonpurulent	675.24	675.22	675.20		
purulent	675.14	675.12	675.10		
cervix (uteri)	646.64	646.62	646.60	condition	
cesarean section wound	674.34	674.32	674.30		
endocervix	646.64	646.62	646.60	condition	
episiotomy	674.34	674.32	674.30		
fallopian tube	670.84	670.82	670.80		
generalized	670.04	670.02	670.00		
genital organs	646.64	646.62	646.60	condition	760.8
postpartum, childbirth	670.04	670.02	670.00		760.8
major (unspec.)	670.04	670.02	670.00		760.8
minor or localized	646.64	646.62	646.60	condition	760.8
intrauterine, complicating delivery	646.64	646.62	646.60	condition	
kidney	646.64	646.62	646.60	condition	760.1
nipple	675.04	675.02	675.00		
with breast	675.94	675.92	675.90		
specified type NEC	675.84	675.82	675.80		
ovary	670.84	670.82	670.80		
pelvic	670.84	670.82	670.80		
perineal wound (obstetrical)	674.34	674.32	674.30		
postpartum (major) (unspec.)	670.04	670.02	670.00		
minor	646.64	646.62	646.60	condition	
other	670.84	670.82	670.80		
puerperal (major) (unspec.)	670.04	670.02	670.00		
renal	646.64	646.62	646.60	condition	
tubo-ovarian	670.84	670.82	670.80		
urinary (tract)	646.64	646.62	646.60	condition	760.1
asymptomatic	646.54	646.52	646.50	condition	760.1
UTI	646.64	646.62	646.60	condition	760.1
asymptomatic	646.54	646.52	646.50	condition	760.1
vagina	646.64	646.62	646.60	condition	
Infective and parasitic diseases NEC	647.84	647.82	647.80	complication	
Infestation	647.94	647.92	647.90	condition	760.8
Inflammation					
areola, postpartum	675.04	675.02	675.00		
Bartholin's gland	646.64	646.62	646.60	condition	
bladder	646.64	646.62	646.60	condition	760.8
breast (mammary gland), postpartum	675.24	675.22	675.20		
cervix (uteri)	646.64	646.62	646.60	condition	
fallopian tube	670.84	670.82	670.80		
genital organ	646.64	646.62	646.60	condition	760.8
urinary tract NEC	646.64	646.62	646.60	condition	760.8
Inhalation of stomach contents or secretions in labor and delivery	668.04	668.02	668.00		
Injury	648.94	648.92	648.90	condition	
birth canal NEC	665.94	665.92	665.90		763.89
coccyx, complicating delivery	665.64		665.60		
genital organs, obstetrical trauma NEC	665.94	665.92	665.90		763.89
instrumental, obstetrical NEC	665.94	665.92	665.90		763.89
bladder	665.54		665.50		763.89
cervix	665.34		665.30		763.89
high vaginal	665.44		665.40		763.89
perineal NEC	664.94		664.90		763.89
periurethral	664.84		664.80		763.89
urethra	665.54		665.50		763.89
uterus	665.54		665.50		763.89
obstetrical NEC	665.94	665.92	665.90		763.89

Postpartum Pregnancy Condition or Complication; affecting management of mother	Postpartum condition or complication	Delivered with mention of postpartum complication	Unspecified episode of care	Assign additional code to describe the…	Affecting newborn (coded on the newborn chart only)
Injury — *continued*	648.94	648.92	648.90	condition	
pelvic, complicating delivery					
floor	664.14		664.10		763.89
joint or ligament	665.64		665.60		763.89
organs	665.54		665.50		763.89
periurethral tissue, complicating delivery	664.84		664.80		763.89
symphysis pubis, complicating delivery	665.64		665.60		763.89
Insufficient					
prenatal care	V23.7				
weight gain	646.84	646.82	646.80	condition	
Newborn "light-for-dates" without mention of fetal malnutrition					
unspecified (weight)					764.00
< 500 gms					764.01
500-749 gms					764.02
750-999 gms					764.03
1,000-1,249 gms					764.04
1,250-1,499 gms					764.05
1,500-1,749 gms					764.06
1,750-1,999 gms					764.07
2,000-2,499 gms					764.08
≥ 2,500 gms					764.09
Intoxication					
drug					
obstetric anesthetic or sedation	668.94	668.92	668.90		763.5
septic, postpartum, childbirth	670.24	670.22	670.20	Sepsis, 995.92, organ failure	
Inversion					
nipple, postpartum	676.34	676.32	676.30		
uterus, complicating delivery	665.24	665.22	665.20		763.89
Ischemia, cerebral (postpartum, childbirth)	674.04	674.02	674.00		
Joint disorders	648.74	648.72	648.70	condition	
Labor		649.82			
onset (spontaneous) after 37 completed weeks of gestation but before 39 completed weeks of gestation, with delivery by (planned) cesarean section					
Laceration (obstetrical trauma)					
Anus, anal (sphincter)complicating delivery					
with third degree perineal laceration	664.24		664.20		
w/mucosa	664.34		664.30		
w/o third degree perineal laceration	664.64		664.60		
old (healed)	654.84		654.80		
bladder	665.54		665.50		
bowel	665.54		665.50		
broad ligament	665.64		665.60		
central	664.44		664.40		
cervix (uteri)	665.34		665.30		
fourchette	664.04		664.00		
labia	664.04		664.00		
pelvic					
floor (muscles)	664.14		664.10		
organ NEC	665.54		665.50		
perineum	664.44		664.40		
first degree	664.04		664.00		
second degree	664.14		664.10		
third degree	664.24		664.20		
fourth degree	664.34		664.30		
central	664.44		664.40		
involving					
anal sphincter	664.24		664.20		
fourchette	664.04		664.00		
hymen	664.04		664.00		
labia	664.04		664.00		
pelvic floor	664.14		664.10		
perineal muscles	664.14		664.10		

Postpartum Pregnancy Condition or Complication; affecting management of mother	Postpartum condition or complication	Delivered with mention of postpartum complication	Unspecified episode of care	Assign additional code to describe the…	Affecting newborn (coded on the newborn chart only)
Laceration — *continued*					
perineum — *continued*					
involving — *continued*					
rectovaginal with septum	664.24		664.20		
with anal mucosa	664.34		664.30		
skin	664.04		664.00		
sphincter (anal)	664.24		664.20		
with anal mucosa	664.34		664.30		
vagina	664.04		664.00		
vaginal muscles	664.14		664.10		
vulva	664.04		664.00		
secondary	674.24	674.22	674.20		
peritoneum (obstetrical trauma)	665.54		665.50		
periurethral tissue (obstetrical trauma)	664.84		664.80		
rectovaginal septum	665.44		665.40		
with perineum	664.24		664.20		
involving anal or rectal mucosa	664.34		664.30		
urethra (obstetrical trauma)	665.54		665.50		
vagina (complicating delivery)	665.44		665.40		
with perineal involvement	664.04		664.00		
first degree	664.04		664.00		
second degree	664.14		664.10		
third degree	664.24		664.20		
fourth degree	664.34		664.30		
high	664.44		664.40		
muscles	664.14		664.10		
sulcus	665.44		665.40		
wall	665.44		665.40		
vulva (complicating delivery)	664.04		664.00		
Lactation, lactating (breast) (postpartum)					
defective	676.44	676.42	676.40		
disorder	676.94	676.92	676.90		
specified type NEC	676.84	676.82	676.80		
examination and/or care of mother	V24.1	V24.1	V24.1		
excessive	676.64	676.62	676.60		
failed	676.44	676.42	676.40		
mastitis NEC	675.24	675.22	675.20		
suppressed	676.54	676.52	676.50		
Late effect(s) (of)					
childbirth complication(s)	677	677	677	condition	
complication(s) of					
childbirth	677	677	677	condition	
delivery	677	677	677	condition	
postpartum	677	677	677	condition	
pregnancy	677	677	677	condition	
puerperium	677	677	677	condition	
Lateroversion, uterus	654.44	654.42	654.40		763.89
Lymphadenitis, breast postpartum	675.24	675.22	675.20		
Lymphangitis (postpartum)	670.84	670.82	670.80		
breast	675.24	675.22	675.20		
Malaria	647.44	647.42	647.40	condition	
Malformation					
pelvic organs or tissues	654.94	654.92	654.90		763.89
uterus (congenital)	654.04	654.02	654.00		
Malnutrition	648.94	648.92	648.90	condition	
Malposition					
pelvic organs or tissues	654.44	654.42	654.40		763.89
uterus or cervix	654.44	654.42	654.40		763.89
Malpresentation					
uterus or cervix	654.44	654.42	654.40		
Mammillitis, puerperal, postpartum	675.24	675.22	675.20		
Mammitis, puerperal, postpartum	675.24	675.22	675.20		
Mastitis					
lactational	675.24	675.22	675.20		
puerperal, postpartum, (interstitial) (nonpurulent) (parenchymatous)	675.24	675.22	675.20		

Coding Tables (right margin)

Postpartum Pregnancy (right margin)

Postpartum Pregnancy Condition or Complication; affecting management of mother	Postpartum condition or complication	Delivered with mention of postpartum complication	Unspecified episode of care	Assign additional code to describe the…	Affecting newborn (coded on the newborn chart only)
Mastitis — *continued*					
puerperal, postpartum, (interstitial) (nonpurulent) (parenchymatous) — *continued*					
purulent	675.14	675.12	675.10		
stagnation	675.24	675.22	675.20		
puerperalis	675.24	675.22	675.20		
retromammary (puerperal, postpartum)	675.14	675.12	675.10		
submammary (puerperal, postpartum)	675.14	675.12	675.10		
Maternal obesity syndrome	646.14	646.12	646.10	condition	
Membrane, retained (complicating delivery) (with hemorrhage)	666.24	666.22	666.20		
without hemorrhage	667.14	667.12	667.10		
Mendelson's syndrome	668.04	668.02	668.00		
Mental disorders	648.44	648.42	648.40	condition	
Metritis (puerperal, postpartum, childbirth)	670.14	670.12	670.10		
Metroperitonitis	670.84	670.82	670.80		
Metrorrhagia	666.24	666.22	666.20		
Metrorrhagia, postpartum	666.24	666.22	666.20		
Metrosalpingitis	670.84	670.82	670.80		
Metrovaginitis	670.84	670.82	670.80		
Milk					
excess secretion	676.64	676.62	676.60		
fever	672.04	672.02	672.00		
retention	672.04	672.02	672.00		
Milk leg (deep vessels)	671.44	671.42	671.40		
Monoplegia, cerebral	674.04	674.02	674.00		
Myocardiopathy (postpartum)	674.84	674.82	674.80		
Myoma uterus (cervix) (corpus)	654.14	654.12	654.10		763.89
Myxedema (postpartum)	674.84	674.82	674.80		
Necrosis					
genital organ or tract	646.64	646.62	646.60	condition	760.8
kidney, cortical (acute)	646.24	646.22	646.20	condition	760.1
following labor and delivery	669.34	669.32	669.30		
liver, puerperal, postpartum	674.84	674.82	674.80		
ovary	670.84	670.82	670.80		
renal, cortical	646.24	646.22	646.20	condition	760.1
tubular	646.24	646.22	646.20	condition	760.1
following labor and delivery	669.34	669.32	669.30		
Nephritis, nephrosis	646.24	646.22	646.20	condition	760.1
with hypertension	642.14	642.12	642.10		760.0
Nephropathy NEC	646.24	646.22	646.20	condition	
Neuritis (peripheral)	646.44	646.42	646.40	condition	
puerperal, postpartum	646.44	646.42	646.40	condition	
Nutritional deficiency	648.94	648.92	648.90	condition	
Obesity					
excessive weight gain during pregnancy	646.14	646.12	646.10	complication	
morbid	649.14	649.12	649.10	278.00, 278.01, 278.03, V85.39-V85.45	
Obstetrical trauma NEC (complicating delivery)	665.94	665.92	665.90		763.89
Occlusion, precerebral artery NEC (puerperal, postpartum, childbirth)	674.04	674.02	674.00	condition	
Oliguria	646.24	646.22	646.20	condition	
with hypertension — *see* Pregnancy, toxemia					
following labor and delivery (postpartum)	669.34	669.32	669.30		
Oophoritis	646.64	646.62	646.60	condition	
Pain(s),	646.84	646.82	646.80	condition	
Paralysis, bladder	665.54		665.50		
Paralytic stroke	674.04	674.02	674.00		
Parametritis	670.84	670.82	670.80		
Paravaginitis	646.64	646.62	646.60	condition	
Patent cervix	654.54	654.52	654.50		761.0
Pelvic inflammatory disease	646.64	646.62	646.60	condition	
Pelviperitonitis	670.84	670.82	670.80		
Pendulous abdomen	654.44	654.42	654.40		763.89

Coding Tables (side margin)

Postpartum Pregnancy (side margin)

Postpartum Pregnancy Condition or Complication; affecting management of mother	Postpartum condition or complication	Delivered with mention of postpartum complication	Unspecified episode of care	Assign additional code to describe the...	Affecting newborn (coded on the newborn chart only)
Perforation					
bladder	665.54		665.50		
bowel	665.54		665.50		
broad ligament	665.64		665.60		
cervix	665.34		665.30		
instrumental (complicating delivery)	665.94	665.92	665.90		
pelvic (floor)	664.14		664.10		
organ	665.54		665.50		763.89
urethral	665.54		665.50		763.89
uterus	665.54		665.50		763.89
Perimetritis	670.14	670.12	670.10		
Perimetrosalpingitis	670.84	670.82	670.80		
Perinephritis	646.64	646.62	646.60	condition	
Perioophoritis	670.84	670.82	670.80		
Perisalpingitis	670.84	670.82	670.80		
Peritoneal infection	670.84	670.82	670.80		
Peritonitis	670.84	670.82	670.80		
Perivaginitis	670.84	670.82	670.80	condition	
Persistence					
hymen (tag)	654.84	654.82	654.80		
Phlebitis	671.94	671.92	671.90		760.3
deep, postpartum	671.44	671.42	671.40		
intracranial	671.54	671.52	671.50		
lower extremities	671.24	671.22	671.20	453.6, 453.71, 453.81	760.3
specified site NEC	671.54	671.52	671.50		
superficial	671.24	671.22	671.20	453.6, 453.71, 453.81	760.3
Phlegmasia alba dolens	671.44	671.42	671.40		
PID	646.64	646.62	646.60	condition	
Placenta, placental					
accreta	667.04	667.02	667.00		
with hemorrhage	666.04	666.02	666.00		
adherent	667.04	667.02	667.00		
with hemorrhage	666.04	666.02	666.00		
increta	667.04	667.02	667.00		
with hemorrhage	666.04	666.02	666.00		
percreta	667.04	667.02	667.00		
with hemorrhage	666.04	666.02	666.00		
polyp	674.44	674.42	674.40		
retention (without hemorrhage)	667.04	667.02	667.00		
fragments (delayed hemorrhage)	666.24	666.22	666.20		
without hemorrhage	667.14	667.12	667.10		
hemorrhage	666.04	666.02	666.00		
postpartum	666.24	666.22	666.20		
syphilitic	647.04	647.02	647.00	condition	760.2
manifest syphilis in the infant or fetus	647.04	647.02	647.00	condition	090.0
trapped	667.04	667.02	667.00		
with hemorrhage	666.04	666.02	666.00		
Pneumonitis					
aspiration	668.04	668.02	668.00	condition	770.18
postanesthetic	668.04	668.02	668.00	condition	
postoperative	668.04	668.02	668.00		
Polygalactia	676.64	676.62	676.60		
Polyp					
cervix	654.64	654.62	654.60		763.89
placenta	674.44	674.42	674.40		
uterus	654.14	654.12	654.10		763.89
Pyelocystitis	646.64	646.62	646.60	condition	
Pyelohydronephrosis	646.64	646.62	646.60	condition	
Pyelonephritis	646.64	646.62	646.60	condition	
Pyelonephrosis	646.64	646.62	646.60	condition	
Pyemia	670.24	670.22	670.20	Sepsis, 995.92, organ failure	
Pyocystitis	670.84	670.82	670.80	condition	
Pyohemia	670.04	670.02	670.00		
Pyometra	670.04	670.02	670.00		
Pyonephritis	670.84	670.82	670.80	condition	

Postpartum Pregnancy Condition or Complication; affecting management of mother	Postpartum condition or complication	Delivered with mention of postpartum complication	Unspecified episode of care	Assign additional code to describe the…	Affecting newborn (coded on the newborn chart only)
Pyonephrosis	670.84	670.82	670.80	condition	
Pyo-oophoritis	670.84	670.82	670.80		
Pyosalpingitis	670.84	670.82	670.80		
Pyosalpinx	670.84	670.82	670.80		
Prediabetes	648.84	648.82	648.80	condition	
Pre-eclampsia (mild)	642.44	642.42	642.40		760.0
with convulsions	642.64	642.62	642.60		760.0
severe	642.54	642.52	642.50		760.0
superimposed on pre-existing hypertensive disease	642.74	642.72	642.70		760.0
Pre-existing condition (prior to pregnancy) **affecting current pregnancy**					
abnormal glucose tolerance	648.84	648.82	648.80	condition	
anemia	648.24	648.22	648.20	condition	
bone and joint (lower limb)	648.74	648.72	648.70	condition	
cardiovascular	648.64	648.62	648.60	condition	
congenital	648.54	648.52	648.50	condition	
cerebrovascular	674.04	674.02	674.00		
diabetic	648.04	648.02	648.00	condition	
drug dependence	648.34	648.32	648.30	condition	
genital organ or tract	646.64	646.62	646.60	condition	
gonorrheal	647.14	647.12	647.10	condition	
hypertensive	642.24	642.22	642.20		
renal	642.14	642.12	642.10		
infectious	647.94	647.92	647.90	condition	
specified type NEC	647.84	647.82	647.80	condition	
malarial	647.44	647.42	647.40	condition	
nutritional deficiency	648.94	648.92	648.90	condition	
parasitic NEC	647.84	647.82	647.80	condition	
renal	646.24	646.22	646.20	condition	
hypertensive	642.14	642.12	642.10		
rubella	647.54	647.52	647.50	condition	
specified condition NEC	648.94	648.92	648.90	condition	
syphilitic	647.04	647.02	647.00	condition	
thyroid	648.14	648.12	648.10	condition	
tuberculous	647.34	647.32	647.30	condition	
urinary	646.64	646.62	646.60	condition	
venereal	647.24	647.22	647.20	condition	
viral NEC	647.64	647.62	647.60	condition	
Proteinuria (gestational)	646.24	646.22	646.20	condition	
with toxemia (mild) (pre-eclamptic)	642.44	642.42	642.40		760.0
with convulsion	642.64	642.62	642.60		760.0
with pre-existing hypertension	642.74	642.72	642.70		760.0
severe	642.54	642.52	642.50		760.0
Pruritus, pruritic	646.84	646.82	646.80	condition	
Psychosis or psychoneurosis	648.44	648.42	648.40	condition	
Ptyalism	646.84	646.82	646.80	condition	
Pyelitis	646.64	646.62	646.60	condition	760.1
Pyrexia (of unknown origin) (PUO)					
postpartum	672.04	672.02	672.00		
Reaction obstetric anesthetic or analgesic NEC	668.94	668.92	668.90		763.5
Rectocele	654.44	654.42	654.40		763.1
Renal					
disease or failure NEC	646.24	646.22	646.20	condition	
with secondary hypertension	642.14	642.12	642.10		
hypertensive	642.24	642.22	642.20		
shutdown following labor and delivery	669.34	669.32	669.30		
Repair of pelvic floor, previous	654.44	654.42	654.40		763.89
Retention, retained					
decidua (following delivery) (fragments)	667.14	667.12	667.10		
with hemorrhage	666.24	666.22	666.20		
membranes (following delivery)	667.14	667.12	667.10		
with hemorrhage	666.24	666.22	666.20		
milk (postpartum)	676.24	676.22	676.20		
placenta (total) (without hemorrhage)	667.04	667.02	667.00		
with hemorrhage	666.04	666.02	666.00		

Postpartum Pregnancy Condition or Complication; affecting management of mother	Postpartum condition or complication	Delivered with mention of postpartum complication	Unspecified episode of care	Assign additional code to describe the…	Affecting newborn (coded on the newborn chart only)
Retention, retained — *continued*					
portions or fragments	667.14	667.12	667.10		
with hemorrhage	666.24	666.22	666.20		
secundines (following delivery)	667.14	667.12	667.10		
with hemorrhage	666.24	666.22	666.20		
complicating puerperium (delayed hemorrhage)	666.24	666.22	666.20		
Retinitis	646.84	646.82	646.80	condition	
Retraction					
nipple (postpartum)	676.04	676.02	676.00		
Retroversion, uterus	654.34	654.32	654.30		763.89
Rigid, rigidity					
cervix	654.64	654.62	654.60		763.89
pelvic floor	654.44	654.42	654.40		763.89
perineum or vulva	654.84	654.82	654.80		763.89
vagina	654.74	654.72	654.70		763.89
Rubella (German measles)	647.54	647.52	647.50	condition	760.2
Rupture					
abdominal viscera	665.54		665.50		
bladder (sphincter)	665.54		665.50		
cervix (uteri	665.34		665.30		
pelvic floor	664.14		664.10		
perineum	664.44		664.40		
urethra	665.54		665.50		
vulva	664.04		664.00		
Sacculation	654.44	654.42	654.40		763.1
Salivation (excessive)	646.84	646.82	646.80	condition	
Salpingitis	646.64	646.62	646.60	condition	760.8
postpartum	670.84	670.82	670.80		
Salpingo-oophoritis	646.64	646.62	646.60	condition	760.8
postpartum	670.84	670.82	670.80		
Scar, scarring					
cervix	654.64	654.62	654.60		763.89
uterus NEC	654.94	654.92	654.90		763.89
Separation (obstetrical trauma)					
pubic bone	665.64		665.60		
symphysis pubis	665.64		665.60		
Sepsis					
postpartum	670.24	670.22	670.20	Sepsis, 995.92, organ failure	
puerperal	670.24	670.22	670.20	Sepsis, 995.92, organ failure	
Septicemia	647.84	647.82	647.80	condition	771.81
postpartum	670.24	670.22	670.20	Sepsis, 995.92, organ failure	
Septum, vagina	654.74	654.72	654.70		763.89
Shirodkar suture	654.54	654.52	654.50		
Shock					
complicating labor and delivery	669.14	669.12	669.10		
following labor and delivery	669.14	669.12	669.10		
Spasms					
uterus	646.84	646.82	646.80	condition	
Specified condition NEC	646.84	646.82	646.80	condition	
Stenosis (cicatricial)					
cervix, cervical (canal)	654.64	654.62	654.60		763.89
vagina	654.74	654.72	654.70		763.89
Stricture, cervix (canal)	654.64	654.62	654.60		763.89
Subinvolution of uterus (postpartum)	674.84	674.82	674.80		
Sudden death					
during childbirth	669.94	669.92	669.90		
postpartum	674.94	674.92	674.90		
Suppression of lactation	676.54	676.52	676.50		
Suppuration, suppurative of breast or mammary gland (postpartum)	675.14	675.12	675.10		
Surgery, previous					
cervix	654.64	654.62	654.60		763.89

Postpartum Pregnancy Condition or Complication; affecting management of mother	Postpartum condition or complication	Delivered with mention of postpartum complication	Unspecified episode of care	Assign additional code to describe the...	Affecting newborn (coded on the newborn chart only)
Surgery, previous — *continued*					
pelvic soft tissues NEC	654.94	654.92	654.90		763.89
perineum or vulva	654.84	654.82	654.80		
uterus NEC	654.94	654.92	654.90		763.89
vagina	654.74	654.72	654.70		
Suspended uterus	654.44	654.42	654.40		763.89
Suture, Shirodkar (with or without cervical incompetence)	654.54	654.52	654.50		
Syncope complicating delivery	669.24	669.22	669.20		
Syndrome					
acid pulmonary aspiration (Mendelson's)	668.04	668.02	668.00		
Chiari-Frommel	676.64	676.62	676.60		
dystocia, dystrophia	654.94	654.92	654.90		
Frommel-Chiari	676.64	676.62	676.60		
H.E.L.L.P (Hemolysis, Elevated Liver function and Low Platelets)	642.54	642.52	642.50		
hepatorenal following delivery	674.84	674.82	674.80		
hypotension, maternal	669.24	669.22	669.20		
maternal hypotension	669.24	669.22	669.20		
Mendelson's (during labor) (obstetric)	668.04	668.02	668.00		
Syphilis	647.04	647.02	647.00	condition	760.2
Tear, torn					
Anus, anal (sphincter)					
with third degree perineal laceration	664.24		664.20		
w/mucosa	664.34		664.30		
w/o third degree perineal laceration	664.64		664.60		
old (healed)	654.84		654.80		
bladder	665.54		665.50		763.89
bowel	665.54		665.50		763.89
broad ligament	665.54		665.50		763.89
cervix	665.34		665.30		763.89
pelvic					
floor	664.14		664.10		763.89
organ NEC	665.54		665.50		763.89
perineum	665.54		665.50		763.89
periurethral	664.84		664.80		763.89
urethra	665.54		665.50		
vulva	664.04		664.00		763.89
Tetanus, tetanic (puerperal, postpartum, childbirth)	670.84	670.82	670.80		
Thelitis (puerperal, postpartum)	675.04	675.02	675.00		
Thrombocytopenia (postpartum)	666.34	666.32	666.30		
Thrombophlebitis	671.24	671.22	671.20	453.6, 453.71, 453.81	760.3
cerebral (sinus) (vein), nonpyogenic	671.54	671.52	671.50		760.3
intracranial venous sinus, nonpyogenic	671.54	671.52	671.50		760.3
pelvic, postpartum	671.44	671.42	671.40		
septic (puerperal)	670.34	670.32	670..30		
specified site NEC	671.54	671.52	671.50		760.3
superficial	671.24	671.22	671.20	453.6, 453.71, 453.81	760.3
Thrombosis	671.94	671.92	671.90		
brain (artery) (stem)	674.04	674.02	674.00		
intracranial, venous sinus (nonpyogenic origin)	671.54	671.52	671.50		
pelvic	671.44	671.42	671.40		
postpartum	671.94	671.92	671.90		
brain (artery) (stem)	674.04	674.02	674.00		
venous	671.54	671.52	671.50		760.3
cardiac	674.84	674.82	674.80		
cerebral (artery)	674.04	674.02	674.00		
venous	671.54	671.52	671.50		760.3
deep (vein)	671.44	671.42	671.40		
intracranial sinus (nonpyogenic) (venous)	671.54	671.52	671.50		760.3
pulmonary (artery)	673.24	673.22	673.20		
specified site NEC	671.54	671.52	671.50		
superficial	671.24	671.22	671.20	453.6, 453.71, 453.81	
spinal cord	671.54	671.52	671.50		
superficial	671.24	671.22	671.20	453.6, 453.71, 453.81	

Postpartum Pregnancy Condition or Complication; affecting management of mother	Postpartum condition or complication	Delivered with mention of postpartum complication	Unspecified episode of care	Assign additional code to describe the…	Affecting newborn (coded on the newborn chart only)
Thrombosis — *continued*					
venous (superficial)	671.24	671.22	671.20	453.6, 453.71, 453.81	
Thyroid dysfunction	648.14	648.12	648.10	condition	
Thyroiditis	648.14	648.12	648.10	condition	
Thyrotoxicosis	648.14	648.12	648.10	condition	
Tobacco use disorder	649.04	649.02	649.00		
Torsion of uterus	654.44	654.42	654.40		
Toxemia (mild) (pre-eclamptic)	642.44	642.42	642.40		760.0
with					760.0
convulsions	642.64	642.62	642.60		760.0
pre-existing hypertension	642.74	642.72	642.70		760.0
eclamptic	642.64	642.62	642.60		760.0
with pre-existing hypertension	642.74	642.72	642.70		760.0
severe	642.54	642.52	642.50		760.0
Trapped placenta (without hemorrhage)	666.04	666.02	666.00		
with hemorrhage	667.04	667.02	667.00		
Trauma	648.94	648.92	648.90	condition	
during delivery NEC	665.94	665.92	665.90		760.5
obstetrical	665.94	665.92	665.90		760.5
previous pregnancy (major), affecting childbirth or postpartum management	V23.89	V23.89	V23.89		
Tuberculosis	647.34	647.32	647.30	condition	760.2
Tumor					
cervix	654.64	654.62	654.60		763.89
ovary	654.44	654.42	654.40		763.89
pelvic	654.94	654.92	654.90		763.89
pelvic organs or tissue NEC	654.44	654.42	654.40		763.89
uterus	654.14	654.12	654.10		763.89
vagina	654.74	654.72	654.70		763.89
vulva	654.84	654.82	654.80		763.89
Uremia (renal disease or failure) **NEC**	646.24	646.22	646.20	condition	760.1
with secondary hypertension	642.14	642.12	642.10		760.0
complicating labor and delivery	669.34	669.32	669.30		
hypertensive	642.24	642.22	642.20		760.0
Urethritis	646.64	646.62	646.60	condition	760.1
Urinary Tract Infection	646.64	646.62	646.60	condition	760.1
Uterine size date discrepancy	649.64	649.62	649.60		
UTI	646.64	646.62	646.60	condition	760.1
Vaginitis or vulvitis	646.64	646.62	646.60	condition	760.8
Valsuani's disease (progressive pernicious anemia, puerperal)	648.24	648.22	648.20	condition	
Varicose					
veins (legs)	671.04	671.02	671.00		
perineum	671.14	671.12	671.10		
vulva	671.14	671.12	671.10		
Varicosity, labia or vulva	671.14	671.12	671.10		
Varix (lower extremity)	671.04	671.02	671.00		
perineum	671.14	671.12	671.10		
vulva	671.14	671.12	671.10		
Venereal disease NEC	647.24	647.22	647.20	disease	
Viral disease NEC	647.64	647.62	647.60	disease	
Vulvitis	646.64	646.62	646.60	condition	760.8
Weight gain	646.14	646.12	646.10	condition	
insufficient	646.84	646.82	646.80	condition	
White leg, postpartum, childbirth	671.44	671.42	671.40		

Personal and Family History	Personal	Family	Notes
Abuse			
emotional	V15.42		Subcategory VI5.4 excludes history of conditions classifiable to 290-316 (see V11.0-V11.9)
neglect	V15.42		Subcategory VI5.4 excludes history of conditions classifiable to 290-316 (see V11.0-V11.9)
physical	V15.41		Subcategory VI5.4 excludes history of conditions classifiable to 290-316 (see V11.0-V11.9)

Personal and Family History	Personal	Family	Notes
Abuse — *continued*			
sexual	V15.41		Subcategory VI5.4 excludes history of conditions classifiable to 290-316 (see V11.0-V11.9)
Affective psychosis	V11.1	V17.0	V11.1 includes personal history of manic-depressive psychosis
			V17.0 excludes family history of mental retardation (see code V18.4)
Alcoholism	V11.3	V61.41	V17.0 excludes family history of mental retardation (see code V18.4)
Allergy to			
analgesic agent NEC	V14.6	V19.6	
anesthetic NEC	V14.4	V19.6	
antibiotic agent NEC	V14.1	V19.6	
anti-infective agent NEC	V14.3	V19.6	
arachnid bite	V15.06	V19.6	
diathesis	V15.09	V19.6	
drug allergy	V14.9	V19.6	
drug allergy, specified type NEC	V14.8	V19.6	
eggs	V15.03	V19.6	
food additives	V15.05	V19.6	
insect bite	V15.06	V19.6	
latex	V15.07	V19.6	
medicinal agents	V14.9	V19.6	
medicinal agents, specified type NEC	V14.8	V19.6	
milk products	V15.02	V19.6	
narcotic agent NEC	V14.5	V19.6	
nuts	V15.05	V19.6	
peanuts	V15.01	V19.6	
penicillin	V14.0	V19.6	
radiographic dye	V15.08	V19.6	
seafood	V15.04	V19.6	
serum	V14.7	V19.6	
specified food NEC	V15.05	V19.6	
specified nonmedicinal agents NEC	V15.09	V19.6	
spider bite	V15.06	V19.6	
sulfa	V14.2	V19.6	
sulfonamides	V14.2	V19.6	
therapeutic agent	V15.09	V19.6	
vaccine	V14.7	V19.6	
Anaphylactic shock	V15.09		
Anaphylaxis	V13.81	V19.6	
Anemia	V12.3	V18.2	For family history of other blood disorders, see code V18.3
Anomaly (corrected)			
circulatory system	V13.65	V19.5	
cleft lip, palate	V13.64	V19.5	V13.64 also includes malformations (corrected) of eye, ear, face and neck
digestive system	V13.67	V19.5	
genitourinary system	V13.62	V19.5	
musculoskeletal system	V13.68	V19.5	V13.68 includes malformations of integument and limbs
nervous system	V13.63	V19.5	
respiratory system	V13.66	V19.5	
Arrest, sudden cardiac	V12.53	V17.41	V12.5 excludes old myocardial infarction (412) and postmyocardial infarction syndrome (411.0)
			V12.53 includes successfully resuscitated sudden cardiac death
Arteriosclerosis (cardiovascular)	code to condition	V17.49	
Arthritis	V13.4	V17.7	
Asthma	code to condition	V17.5	
attack, transient ischemic (TIA)	V12.54	V17.1	V12.54 includes unspecified stroke without residual deficits
Benign neoplasm of brain	V12.41		
Blindness	code to condition	V19.0	
Blood disease	V12.3	V18.3	
Calculi, urinary	V13.01	V18.7	
Cardiovascular disease	V12.50	V17.49	
myocardial infarction	412	V17.3	
Carrier, genetic disease	V83.01-V83.89	V18.9	See category V84 for Genetic susceptibility to disease
Chemotherapy, antineoplastic	V87.41		V87.41 excludes long-term current drug use(see codes V58.61-V58.69)
Child abuse	V15.41		
Chronic respiratory condition NEC	V12.60	V17.6	
Cigarette smoking	V15.82		V15.82 excludes tobacco dependence (see code 305.1)
Circulatory system disease	V12.50	V17.3	V12.5 excludes old myocardial infarction (412) and postmyocardial infarction syndrome (411.0)
myocardial infarction	412	V17.3	

Coding Tables

Personal and Family History

Personal and Family History	Personal	Family	Notes
Colonic polyps	V12.72	V18.51	
Combat and operational stress reaction	V11.4		
Congenital (corrected) malformation	V13.69	V19.5	
circulatory system	V13.65	V19.5	
digestive system	V13.67	V19.5	
ear	V13.64	V19.5	
eye	V13.64	V19.5	
face	V13.64	V19.5	
genitourinary system	V13.62	V19.5	
heart	V13.65	V19.5	
hypospadias	V13.61	V19.5	
integument (skin)	V13.68	V19.5	
limbs	V13.68	V19.5	
lip (cleft)	V13.64	V19.5	
musculsoskeletal	V13.68	V19.59	
nervous system	V13.63	V19.5	
palate (cleft)	V13.64	V19.5	
respiratory system	V13.66	V19.5	
specified type	V13.69	V19.5	
Consanguinity		V19.7	
Contact (exposure) (suspected)			
asbestos	V15.84		
bodily fluids, potentially hazardous	V15.85		
lead	V15.86		
Contraception	V15.7		
Coronary artery disease	V12.50	V17.3	V12.5 excludes old myocardial infarction (412) and postmyocardial infarction syndrome (411.0)
Cystic fibrosis	V12.69	V18.19	
Deafness	code to condition	V19.2	
Death, sudden, successfully resuscitated	V12.53	V17.41	V12.5 excludes old myocardial infarction (412) and postmyocardial infarction syndrome (411.0)
Deficit			
prolonged reversible ischemic neurologic (PRIND)	V12.54	V17.1, V17.2	V12.54 includes unspecified stroke without residual deficits
reversible ischemic neurologic (RIND)	V12.54	V17.1, V17.2	V12.54 includes unspecified stroke without residual deficits
Diabetes mellitus	code to condition	V18.0	
gestational	V12.21	V18.0	
Diathesis, allergic	V15.09	V19.6	
Digestive system disease	V12.70	V18.59	
peptic ulcer	V12.71	V18.59	
polyps, colonic	V12.72	V18.51	For family history of malignant neoplasm of gastrointestinal tract see code V16.0
specified NEC	V12.79	V18.59	
Disease (of)	V13.9	V19.8	
blood	V12.3	V18.3	
blood-forming organs	V12.3	V18.3	
cardiovascular system	V12.50	V17.49	
cerebrovascular system	V12.59	V17.2	
circulatory system	V12.50	V17.1, V17.3	
circulatory, specified NEC	V12.59	V17.1	
coronary artery	V12.50	V17.3	V12.5 excludes old myocardial infarction (412) and postmyocardial infarction syndrome (411.0)
digestive system	V12.70	V18.59	
peptic ulcer	V12.71	V18.59	
polyps, colonic	V12.72	V18.51	For family history of malignant neoplasm of gastrointestinal tract see code V16.0
digestive, specified NEC	V12.79	V18.59	
ear NEC	V12.49	V19.3	
eye NEC	V12.49	V19.19	
glaucoma	code to condition	V19.11	
hypertensive	V12.59	V17.49	
infectious	V12.00	V18.8	
malaria	V12.03	V18.8	
methicillin resistant Staphylococcus aureus (MRSA) V12.04	V12.04	V18.8	
MRSA (methicillin resistant Staphylococcus aureus) V12.04	V12.04	V18.8	
poliomyelitis	V12.02	V18.8	

Personal and Family History	Personal	Family	Notes
Disease (of) — *continued*			
infectious — *continued*			
specified NEC	V12.09	V18.8	
tuberculosis	V12.01	V18.8	
ischemic heart	V12.59	V17.3	
parasitic	V12.00	V18.8	V18.8 Infectious and parasitic diseases
infectious/parasitic, specified NEC V12.09	V12.09	V18.8	V18.8 Infectious and parasitic diseases
respiratory system	V12.60	V17.6	AHA CC Q2 1992 History of COPD is coded to 496, Chronic airway obstruction, not elsewhere classified.
pneumonia	V12.61	V18.8	
respiratory, specified NEC	V12.69	V17.6	
skin	V13.3	V19.4	
other, specified site NEC	V13.89	V19.8	
subcutaneous tissue	V13.3	V19.8	
trophoblastic	V13.1	V19.8	
affecting management of pregnancy	V23.1		
vaginal dysplasia	V13.23		
vulvar dysplasia	V13.24		
Disorder (of)	V13.9		
endocrine	V12.29	V18.19	
diabetes mellitus	code to condition	V18.0	
gestational diabetes	V12.21		
multiple neoplasia [MEN] syndrome	V12.29	V18.11	
genital system	V13.29	V18.7	
vaginal dysplasia	V13.23		
vulvar dysplasia	V13.24		
hematological	V12.3	V18.3	
immunity	V12.29	V19.8	V12.29 Personal history of endocrine, metabolic, and immunity disorders
kidney	code to condition	V18.69	
polycystic	code to condition	V18.61	
mental	V11.9	V17.0	V17.0 excludes family history of mental retardation (see code V18.4)
	V11.1	V17.0	V11.1 includes a personal history of manic-depressive psychosis
affective type			V17.0 excludes family history of mental retardation (see code V18.4)
combat and operational stress reaction	V11.4		
	V11.1	V17.0	V11.1 includes a personal history of manic-depressive psychosis
manic-depressive			V17.0 excludes family history of mental retardation (see code V18.4)
neurosis	V11.2	V17.0	V17.0 excludes family history of mental retardation (see code V18.4)
schizophrenia	V11.0	V17.0	V17.0 excludes family history of mental retardation (see code V18.4)
mental, specified type NEC	V11.8	V17.0	
metabolic	V12.29	V18.19	
musculoskeletal NEC	V13.59	V17.89	
osteoporosis	code to condition	V17.81	
nervous system	V12.40	V17.2	
nervous, specified type NEC	V12.49	V17.2	
obstetric	V13.29		
affecting management of current pregnancy	V23.49		
pre-term labor	V23.41		
pre-term labor	V13.21		
psychiatric condition	V11.9	V17.0	
sense organs	V12.40	V19.0-V19.4	
sense organs, specified type NEC	V12.49	V19.0-V19.4	
other, specified site NEC	V13.89	V19.8	
urinary system	V13.00	V18.61, V18.69, V18.7	
calculi	V13.01	V18.69, V18.7	
infection	V13.02	V18.69, V18.7	
nephrotic syndrome	V13.03	V18.69	
urinary, specified NEC	V13.09	V18.61, V18.69, V18.7	
Drug therapy			See code 305.9 for patent, nonprescribed (see also Abuse, drugs, nondependent)
antineoplastic chemotherapy	V87.41		
estrogen therapy	V87.43		
immunosuppression therapy	V87.46		
monoclonal drug therapy	V87.42		
other drug therapy	V87.49		
steroid therapy NOS	V87.45		
inhaled	V87.44		

Personal and Family History	Personal	Family	Notes
Drug therapy — *continued*			
steroid therapy NOS — *continued*			
systemic	V87.45		
Dysplasia			
cervical	V13.22	V18.7	V13.22 includes conditions in subcategories 622.10-622.12
vaginal	V13.23		Personal history of conditions classifiable to 623.0
vulvar	V13.24		Personal history of conditions classifiable to 624.01-624.02
Effect NEC of external cause	V15.89	V19.8	
Embolism (pulmonary)	V12.55	V19.8	
Emotional abuse	V15.42		
Encephalitis	V12.42	V18.8	
Endocrine disorder	V12.29	V18.19	
multiple neoplasia [MEN] syndrome	V12.29	V18.11	
Epilepsy	code to condition	V17.2	
Extracorporeal membrane oxygenation (ECMO)	V15.87		
Failed conscious/moderate sedation	V15.80		
Falling	V15.88		Code V15.88 can be reported as either 1st-listed or secondary.
Foreign body, retained, fully removed	V15.53		
Fracture, healed			
pathologic	V13.51	V17.89	
stress	V13.52	V17.89	
traumatic	V15.51	V17.89	
Genetic disease carrier	V83.01-V83.89	V18.9	
Genital system disorder	V13.29	V18.7	
pre-term labor	V13.21		
Glaucoma	code to condition	V19.11	
Glomerulonephritis	code to condition	V18.69	
Gout	V12.29	V18.19	
Hay fever	V12.69	V17.6	
Health hazard	V15.9		
falling	V15.88		
specified cause NEC	V15.89		
Hearing loss	code to condition	V19.2	
Hematopoietic neoplasia	V10.79	V16.7	
Hepatitis, B or C	V12.09	V18.8	
Hodgkin's disease	V10.72	V16.7	
Huntington's chorea	code to condition	V17.2	
Hydrocephalus	code to condition	V19.5	
Hypertension	V12.59	V17.49	
Hypospadias (corrected)	V13.61	V19.5	
Immunity disorder	V12.29	V19.8	
Infarction, cerebral, without residual deficits	V12.54	V17.1	
Infarction, myocardial	412	V17.3	
Infection			
central nervous system	V12.42	V18.8	
urinary (tract)	V13.02	V18.7, V18.8	
Infectious disease	V12.00	V18.8	
malaria	V12.03	V18.8	
methicillin resistant Staphylococcus aureus (MRSA)	V12.04	V18.8	
MRSA (methicillin resistant Staphylococcus aureus)	V12.04	V18.8	
poliomyelitis	V12.02	V18.8	
specified NEC	V12.09	V18.8	
tuberculosis	V12.01	V18.8	
Injury NEC	V15.59		
fracture, healed			
pathologic	V13.51	V17.89	
stress	V13.52	V17.89	
traumatic	V15.51	V17.89	
traumatic brain	V15.52		
Insufficient prenatal care	V23.7		
In utero procedure			
during pregnancy	V15.21		
while a fetus	V15.22		
Irradiation	V15.3		
Ischemic heart disease	V12.59	V17.3	

Personal and Family History	Personal	Family	Notes
Kidney disease	code to condition	V18.69	
polycystic	code to condition	V18.61	
Leukemia	V10.60	V16.6	
lymphoid	V10.61	V16.6	
monocytic	V10.63	V16.6	
myeloid	V10.62	V16.6	
specified type NEC	V10.69	V16.6	
Little or no prenatal care	V23.7		
Low birth weight	V21.30		Also see Status, low birth weight
Lymphatic malignant neoplasia NEC	V10.79	V16.7	
Lymphosarcoma	V10.71	V16.7	V10.7 includes conditions in categories 200-203 except those in remission
			V16.7 includes family history of conditons in categories 200-203
Malaria	V12.03	V18.8	V12.0 excludes personal history of specific body system infectious diseases
Malformations (corrected)			
circulatory system	V13.65		
cleft lip, palate	V13.64		V13.64 also includes malformations (corrected) of eye, ear, face and neck
digestive system	V13.67		
genitourinary system	V13.62		
musculoskeletal system	V13.68		V13.68 includes malformations of integument and limbs
nervous system	V13.63		
respiratory system	V13.66		
Malignant neoplasm (of)	V10.90	V16.9	
accessory sinus	V10.22	V16.2	
adrenal	V10.88	V16.7	V10.8 includes history of conditions in categories 170-173, 190-195
			V16.7 includes family history of conditons in categories 200-203
anorectal	V10.06	V16.0	
anus	V10.06	V16.0	V16.0 includes family history of conditions in categories 140-159
appendix	V10.09	V16.0	
bile duct	V10.09		V10.0 includes history of conditions in categories 140-159
bladder	V10.51	V16.52	V16.5 incudes family history of condition in categories 160-161, 163-165
bone	V10.81	V16.8	V16.8 includes family history of conditons in categories 140-199
brain	V10.85	V16.8	
breast	V10.3	V16.3	
male	V10.3	V16.8	
bronchus	V10.11	V16.1	V10.1 includes history of conditions in category 162
carcinoid tumor	V10.91	V16.8	Code V10.91 secondary to any continuing functional activity (e.g., 259.2)
cecum	V10.05	V16.0	
cervix uteri	V10.41	V16.49	
colon	V10.05	V16.0	
connective tissue NEC	V10.89	V16.8	
corpus uteri	V10.42	V16.49	
digestive system	V10.00	V16.0	
digestive, specified part NEC	V10.09	V16.0	
duodenum	V10.09	V16.0	
endocrine gland NEC	V10.88	V16.8	
epididymis	V10.48	V16.49	
esophagus	V10.03	V16.0	
eye	V10.84	V16.8	
fallopian tube	V10.44	V16.49	
female genital organ	V10.40	V16.40	
female genital, specified site NEC	V10.44	V16.49	
gallbladder	V10.09	V16.0	
gastrointestinal tract	V10.00	V16.0	
genital organs	V10.40, V10.45	V16.40	
gum	V10.02	V16.0	
hematopoietic NEC	V10.79	V16.7	
hypopharynx	V10.02	V16.0	
ileum	V10.09	V16.0	
ilium	V10.81	V16.8	
intestine	V10.05, V10.06	V16.0	
intrathoracic organs NEC	V10.20	V16.2	
jejunum	V10.09	V16.0	
kidney	V10.52	V16.51	
large intestine	V10.05	V16.0	
larynx	V10.21	V16.2	
lip	V10.02	V16.0	
liver	V10.07	V16.0	
lung	V10.11	V16.1	V10.1 includes history of conditions in category 162

Personal and Family History	Personal	Family	Notes
Malignant neoplasm (of) — *continued*			
lymph glands or nodes NEC	V10.79	V16.7	
lymphatic NEC	V10.79	V16.7	
male genital organ	V10.45	V16.40	
male genital, specified site NEC	V10.49	V16.49	
mediastinum	V10.29	V16.2	
melanoma (of skin)	V10.82	V16.8	
Merkel cell carcinoma	V10.91	V16.8	Code V10.91 secondary to any continuing functional activity (e.g., 259.2)
middle ear	V10.22	V16.2	
mouth	V10.02	V16.0	
mouth, specified part NEC	V10.02	V16.0	
nasal cavities	V10.22	V16.2	
nasopharynx	V10.02	V16.2	
nervous system NEC	V10.86	V16.8	
neuroendocrine tumor	V10.91	V16.8	Code V10.91 secondary to any continuing functional activity (e.g., 259.2)
nose	V10.22	V16.2	
oropharynx	V10.02	V16.0	
ovary	V10.43	V16.41	
oviduct	V10.44	V16.41	
pancreas	V10.09	V16.0	
parathyroid	V10.88	V16.8	
penis	V10.49	V16.49	
pharynx	V10.02	V16.0	
pineal	V10.88	V16.8	
pituitary	V10.88	V16.8	
placenta	V10.44	V16.49	
pleura	V10.29	V16.2	
prostate	V10.46	V16.42	
rectosigmoid junction	V10.06	V16.0	
rectum	V10.06	V16.0	
renal pelvis	V10.53	V16.59	
respiratory organs NEC	V10.20	V16.2	
salivary gland	V10.02	V16.0	
skin	V10.83	V16.8	
melanoma	V10.82	V16.8	
small intestine NEC	V10.09	V16.0	
soft tissue NEC	V10.89	V16.8	
specified site NEC	V10.89	V16.8	
stomach	V10.04	V16.0	
testis	V10.47	V16.43	
thymus	V10.29	V16.2	
thyroid	V10.87	V16.8	
tongue	V10.01	V16.0	
trachea	V10.12	V16.1	V10.1 includes history of conditions in category 162
ureter	V10.59	V16.59	
urethra	V10.59	V16.59	
urinary organ	V10.50	V16.59	
uterine adnexa	V10.44	V16.49	
uterus	V10.42	V16.49	
vagina	V10.44	V16.49	
vulva	V10.44	V16.49	
Manic-depressive psychosis	V11.1	V17.0	V17.0 excludes family history of mental retardation (see code V18.4)
Meningitis	V12.42	V18.8	
Mental disorder	V11.9	V17.0	V17.0 excludes family history of mental retardation (see code V18.4)
affective type	V11.1	V17.0	V17.0 excludes family history of mental retardation (see code V18.4)
combat and operational stress reaction	V11.4		
manic-depressive	V11.1	V17.0	V17.0 excludes family history of mental retardation (see code V18.4)
neurosis	V11.2	V17.0	V17.0 excludes family history of mental retardation (see code V18.4)
schizophrenia	V11.0	V17.0	V17.0 excludes family history of mental retardation (see code V18.4)
specified type NEC	V11.8	V17.0	V17.0 excludes family history of mental retardation (see code V18.4)
Mental retardation	code to condition	V18.4	
Merkel cell carcinoma	V10.91	V16.8	Code V10.91 secondary to any continuing functional activity (e.g., 259.2)
Metabolic disorder	V12.29	V18.19	
Methicillin resistant Staphylococcus aureus (MRSA)	V12.04	V18.8	
Mongolism	code to condition	V19.5	
Monoclonal drug therapy	V87.42		

Personal and Family History	Personal	Family	Notes
MRSA (methicillin resistant Staphylococcus aureus)	V12.04	V18.8	
Multiple endocrine neoplasia [MEN] syndrome	V12.29	V18.11	
Musculoskeletal disorder NEC	V13.59	V17.89	
osteoporosis	code to condition	V17.81	
Myeloma	V10.79	V16.7	
Myocardial infarction	412	V17.3	
Neglect (emotional)	V15.42		
Nephritis	V13.03	V18.69	
Nephrosis	V13.09	V18.69	
Nephrotic syndrome	V13.03	V18.69	
Nervous system disorder	V12.40	V17.2	
Nervous, specified type NEC	V12.49	V17.2	
Neurosis	V11.2	V17.0	V17.0 excludes family history of mental retardation (see code V18.4)
Noncompliance with medical treatment	V15.81		
Nutritional deficiency	V12.1		
Obstetric disorder	V13.89		
affecting management of current pregnancy	V23.49		
history of pre-term labor	V13.21		
pregnancy with history of ectopic pregnancy	V23.42		
pregnancy with history of pre-term labor	V23.41		
pregnancy with inconclusive fetal viability	V23.87		
Osteoporosis	code to condition	V17.81	
Parasitic disease	V12.00	V18.8	
parasitic/infectious, specified NEC	V12.09	V18.8	
Perinatal problems	V13.7		
low birth weight	V12.30		For V21.30 low birth weight see also Status, low birth weight
Physical abuse	V15.41		
Poisoning	V15.6		
Poliomyelitis	V12.02	V18.8	
Polycystic kidney disease	code to condition	V18.61	
Polyps, colonic	V12.72	V18.51	
Poor obstetric	V13.29		
affecting management of current pregnancy	V23.49		
history of pre-term labor	V13.21		
pregnancy with history of ectopic pregnancy	V23.42		
pregnancy with history of pre-term labor	V23.41		
pregnancy with inconclusive fetal viability	V23.87		
Prolonged reversible ischemic neurologic deficit (PRIND)	V12.54	V17.1, V17.2	
Psychiatric disorder	V11.9	V17.0	V17.0 excludes family history of mental retardation (see code V18.4)
affective type	V11.1	V17.0	V17.0 excludes family history of mental retardation (see code V18.4)
manic-depressive	V11.1	V17.0	V17.0 excludes family history of mental retardation (see code V18.4)
neurosis	V11.2	V17.0	V17.0 excludes family history of mental retardation (see code V18.4)
schizophrenia	V11.0	V17.0	V17.0 excludes family history of mental retardation (see code V18.4)
psychiatric , specified type NEC	V11.8	V17.0	V17.0 excludes family history of mental retardation (see code V18.4)
Psychological trauma	V15.49		
emotional abuse	V15.42		
neglect	V15.42		
physical abuse	V15.41		
rape	V15.41		
stress, combat and operational	V11.4		
Psychoneurosis	V11.2	V17.0	V17.0 excludes family history of mental retardation (see code V18.4)
Radiation therapy	V15.3		
Rape	V15.41		
Respiratory system disease	V12.60	V17.5, V17.6	
pneumonia	V12.61	V18.8	
respiratory , specified NEC	V12.69	V17.5, V17.6	
Retardation, mental	code to condition	V18.4	
Reticulosarcoma	V10.71	V16.7	V16.7 includes family history of conditions in cateogries 200-203
Retinitis pigmentosa	V12.49	V19.19	
Return from military deployment	V62.22		
Reversible ischemic neurologic deficit (RIND)	V12.54	V17.1, V17.2	
Schizophrenia	V11.0	V17.0	V17.0 excludes family history of mental retardation (see code V18.4)
Skin disease	V13.3	V19.4	
Smoking (tobacco)	V15.82		V15.82 excludes tobacco dependence (see code 305.1)

Personal and Family History	Personal	Family	Notes
Stress, combat and operational	V11.4		
Status, low birth weight			
> 500 grams	V21.31		
500-999 grams	V21.32		
1000-1499 grams	V21.33		
1500-1999 grams	V21.34		
2000-2500	V21.35		
unspecified	V21.30		
Stroke without residual deficits	V12.54	V17.1	
Subcutaneous tissue disease	V13.3	V19.8	
Sudden			
cardiac arrest	V12.53	V17.41	V17.41 excludes family history of ischemic heart disease and myocardial infarction (see V17.3)
cardiac death (successfully resuscitated)	V12.53	V17.41	
Surgery to			
surgery, great vessels	V15.1		
surgery, heart	V15.1		
surgery, during pregnancy	V15.21		
surgery, while a fetus	V15.22		
surgery, organs NEC	V15.29		
Syndrome, nephrotic	V13.03	V18.69	
Therapy			
antineoplastic drug	V87.41		
drug NEC	V87.49		
estrogen	V87.43		
immunosuppression	V87.46		
monoclonal drug	V87.42		
steroid therapy NOS	V87.45		
inhaled	V87.44		
systemic	V87.45		
Thrombophlebitis	V12.52	V18.3	
Thrombosis	V12.51	V18.3	
Tobacco use	V15.82		V15.82 excludes tobacco dependence (see code 305.1)
Traumatic brain injury	V15.52		
Trophoblastic disease	V13.1	V19.8	
trophoblastic, affecting management of pregnancy	V23.1		
Tuberculosis	V12.01	V18.8	
Ulcer, peptic	V12.71	V18.59	
Underimmunization	V15.83		
Urinary system disorder	V13.00	V18.7	
calculi	V13.01	V18.7	
infection	V13.02	V18.7, V18.8	
nephrotic syndrome	V13.03	V18.69	
specified NEC	V13.09	V18.7	
Vaginal dysplasia	V13.23		
Visual loss	code to condition	V19.0	
Vulvar dysplasia	V13.24		

Y0-CDR-786

Word 6.0
for Windows

A Professional Approach

Author

Deborah A. Hinkle
Instructor, Microcomputing
Forsyth Technical
Community College

McGraw-Hill

New York, New York   Columbus, Ohio   Mission Hills, California   Peoria, Illinois

Screens were captured using SnapPRO! from Window Painters, Ltd., Minneapolis, MN.

This program has been prepared with the assistance of Gleason Group, Inc., Norwalk, CT.
  Project Manager: Pamela Ross
  Copy Editor: Chris Begley
  Proof Reader: Sandra Huggard
  Desktop Publisher: PDS Associates, Allenhurst, NJ
  Film: Pulsar Photographics, Ltd., New York, NY

Hinkle, Deborah A.
    Word 6.0 for Windows : a professional approach / Deborah A. Hinkle
        p.   cm.
    Includes index.
    ISBN 0-02-803085-0
    1. Microsoft Word for Windows. 2. Word processing. I. Title.
Z52.5.M523H566 1995
652.5'536--dc20   94-5260
                                                             CIP

Word 6.0 for Windows: A Professional Approach

Printed in the United States of America

Send all inquiries to:

Glencoe/McGraw-Hill
936 Eastwind Drive
Westerville, OH 43081
ISBN 0-02-803085-0

4 5 6 7 8 9 10 POH 00 99 98 97 96

Microsoft and MS-DOS are registered trademarks.

Microsoft Windows is a product of Microsoft Corporation.

PostScript is a registered trademark of Adobe Systems, Inc.

TrueType is a registered trademark of Apple Computer, Inc.

Table of Contents

Module 2:
Basic
Formatting

Module 3: Working with Text and Documents

Module 4:
Page
Formatting

Module 5:
Printing

Module 6:
Advanced Character Formatting

Module 8:
Styles,
Templates
and Macros

Module 9: Merging and Sorting

Module 10: Graphics

Module 11: File Management

Appendices

A Word to the Student

Word 6.0 for Windows: A Professional Approach has been written to help you master Microsoft Word for Windows. The text is designed to present the Word concept and then to present a step-by-step procedure that walks you through the actual use of that concept. This "explain and do" format provides you with a chance to practice each important Word feature before being introduced to the next one.

There are eleven modules in the text. Each module is divided into smaller lessons. Each lesson begins with a list of the lesson's objectives and includes detailed explanations of Word concepts and step-by-step procedures that lead you through these concepts. Key terms in the lesson are defined. A list of key terms also is compiled at the end of the lesson for review purposes. Keyboard shortcuts for Word also are listed at the end of each lesson. Special "Feature Boxes" provide you with tips and hints to increase your efficiency.

To reinforce your understanding, four exercises follow each lesson in the first ten modules. The exercises provide realistic practice by incorporating documents from a fictional business ("Duke City Gateway Travel Agency," located in Albuquerque, New Mexico). Exercises one and two provide a comprehensive review of the concepts introduced in the lesson. Exercise three often requires more extensive keying and the use of proofreader's marks. Exercise four is the most challenging. It is designed to give you an opportunity to practice word-processing features on your own, without step-by-step instructions.

A project concludes each of the first ten modules. This provides you with a very challenging assignment—to create realistic business documents independently. Procedures and explanations are limited to basic instructions. The project is a "test" of your knowledge of Word.

Module 1 is introductory. It is designed to give you such basic skills as entering text, editing text, and character formatting.

Module 2 introduces basic paragraph formatting, working with tabs, and using indents. *Module 3* explains how to cut and copy text in the same document or between multiple documents. The Find and Replace features also are presented in this module.

Module 4 focuses on page formatting, including the use of page and section breaks, page numbering, and headers and footers. *Module 5* emphasizes printing and special printing features.

Module 6 discusses advanced character formatting, including fonts, type size, and special characters. *Module 7* focuses on creating tables and columns.

Module 8 includes the advanced features of styles, macros, and templates. *Module 9* contains an important professional feature—mail merging.

Module 10 introduces the use of graphics and teaches how to create forms. *Module 11* discusses Word file management and focuses on the Find File feature.

As you read about and practice each concept, illustrations of the screens have been provided to help you follow the instructions. (Don't worry if your screen looks somewhat different from the screen illustration. These differences are the result of varying system and computer configurations.)

The *Appendices* help you become familiar with the correct business-document format for letters, memorandum, and envelopes. An Appendix is also provided as a brief tutorial for basic Windows skills. Additionally, a *Glossary* provides a definition of all the key terms encountered in the lessons. The Glossary also indicates the lesson in which the term was used first. The inside front and back covers of the text provide a description of the Word screen and a reference list of keyboard shortcuts. A Word keyboard template also is provided.

The student data disk contains all the files used in the lesson and the exercises. The files used in the projects are available from your instructor.

We would like to thank our reviewers for their valuable assistance: Kathleene Basil, Los Angeles Pierce College, Los Angeles, California; Susan Olson, Northwest Technical College, East Grand Forks, MN; and Kay Stephan, University of Akron/Wayne College, Orville, OH.

Deborah A. Hinkle

Professional Approach Series
Editorial Advisory Board

The following individuals have helped shape the editorial and pedagogical content of the texts in the Professional Approach Series.

Kathleene Basil
Los Angeles Pierce College
Los Angeles, CA

Vicky Charlston
Portland Community College
Portland, OR

Marie Cimineri
Bryant & Stratton Business Institute
Rochester, NY

Hannah Darling
Boston Education Corporation
Somerville, MA

Rosemarie DeCaprio
Katharine Gibbs School
Norwalk, CT

Anne Emmerson
Nassau Community College
Garden City, NY

Lynne Groves
South Central Technical College
North Mankato, MN

Bruce Hager
Ohio State University
Columbus, OH

Gary Howlett
Spokane Community College
Spokane, WA

Ron Kapper
College of DuPage
Glen Ellyn, IL

Barbara Lesko
Scottsdale Community College
Scottsdale, AZ

Dan Light
Northwest State Community College
Archbold, OH

Vivian Mejias
Valencia Community College
Orlando, FL

Carol Messer
Tulsa Junior College
Tulsa, OK

Susan Olson
Northwest Technical College
East Grand Forks, MN

Glen Parker
Lansing Community College
Lansing, MI

Scott Persky
McHenry County College
McHenry, IL

Tom Sanfilippo
Rio Salado Community College
Mesa, AZ

Kay Stephan
University of Akron-Wayne College
Orville, OH

Professional Approach Series

Desktop Publishing with PageMaker 5.0 (1995)
Deborah A. Hinkle
     Forsyth Technical Community College, Winston-Salem, NC

Desktop Publishing with PageMaker 4.0 (1993)
Deborah A. Hinkle
     Forsyth Technical Community College, Winston-Salem, NC

Excel 5.0 for Windows (1995)
Judith J. Lambrecht
     University of Minnesota, Minneapolis-St. Paul, MN
Nina M. Edgmand
     Salt Lake Community College, Salt Lake City, UT

Word 6.0 for Windows (1995)
Deborah A. Hinkle
     Forsyth Technical Community College, Winston-Salem, NC

Word 2.0 for Windows (1994)
Deborah A. Hinkle
     Forsyth Technical Community College, Winston-Salem, NC

WordPerfect 6.0 for MS-DOS (1995)
Deborah A. Hinkle
     Forsyth Technical Community College, Winston-Salem, NC

WordPerfect 6.0 for Windows (1995)
Deborah A. Hinkle
     Forsyth Technical Community College, Winston-Salem, NC

WordPerfect 5.2 for Windows (1994)
Deborah A. Hinkle
     Forsyth Technical Community College, Winston-Salem, NC

Basic Word For Windows Skills

A Guided Tour

Objectives

- Learn what you need to operate Word.

- Become familiar with the Word screen.

- Start Word, and create a new document.

- Name and save a document.

- Use Word Help.

- Print a document.

- Close a document and exit Word.

This module is an introduction to the basic features of Word for Windows. Word is a versatile, easy-to-use program. It is very different from typing on a typewriter, and it is more sophisticated than traditional word-processing programs. After learning the basics, you will quickly become a productive Word user.

Lesson 1 begins with an overview of what the Word screen looks like. Windows skills will help you navigate through the program. (Refer to Appendix E: "Basic Windows Skills", if necessary.) This lesson will teach the steps involved in creating a document, including keying, simple editing, naming, saving, and closing the document. It will also explain the use of Word Help. Different methods for performing tasks will be taught, using both the keyboard and the mouse. As you become more familiar with the program, you will use the method that you find most comfortable.

What You Need to Operate Word for Windows

The minimum software and hardware requirements needed to run Word are:

- A personal computer with an 80286 microprocessor (an 80386 or higher microprocessor is preferred)

- A hard-disk drive and a floppy-disk drive

- 4 MB of RAM (random-access memory)

- An EGA (enhanced graphics adapter) monitor

- Microsoft Windows version 3.1 or later

- A mouse or pointing device (while this is recommended to operate Word, it is required for the purpose of this course)

Starting Word

Before beginning Word, the program must be loaded into the computer's memory from Windows. First, open Windows, if you have not already done so.

To start Word:

Note: You can start Word automatically from the DOS prompt (c:\>) by keying **win winword**. This command opens both Windows and Word.

1. Open Windows by keying **win** at the DOS prompt (c:\>) and pressing **Enter**, or follow your instructor's directions to start Word.

Microsoft
Word

Word icon

2.   At the Program Manager window, double-click the Word icon.

Depending upon how Word was installed, the Word icon may appear as part of the Microsoft Office program group.

In a few seconds, the program is loaded, and the opening Word screen appears.

Tip of the Day

Each time you start Word, a tip is shown in the Word screen to help you become more familiar with the program. The tip appears in the Tip of the Day dialog box.

Figure 1-1
The Tip of the Day dialog box

Note: A Word tip will not appear if this option has been previously turned off by clearing the check box at the bottom of the Tip of the Day dialog box. To view Word tips, choose Tip of the Day from the Help menu. Word Help is discussed later in this lesson.

To close the Tip of the Day dialog box:

1.   Move the mouse pointer to the OK button in the dialog box.

Notice the arrow shape of the pointer when it is pointing to a button.

2.   Click the left mouse button.

Word closes the dialog box.

The Word Screen

The following is an illustration of the opening Word screen, or desktop. Parts of the Word screen, such as the Minimize and Maximize buttons, are the same as they are in Windows. See Figure 1-2 on page 5.

Some of the important parts of the Word screen are:

- Title bar
  The program name, "Microsoft Word," and the name of the document appear in the top center of the screen. The opening screen of Word is always a blank document called "Document1."

Title bar
Menu bar
Toolbars
Ruler

Text area

Vertical scroll bar

Horizontal scroll bar

Status bar

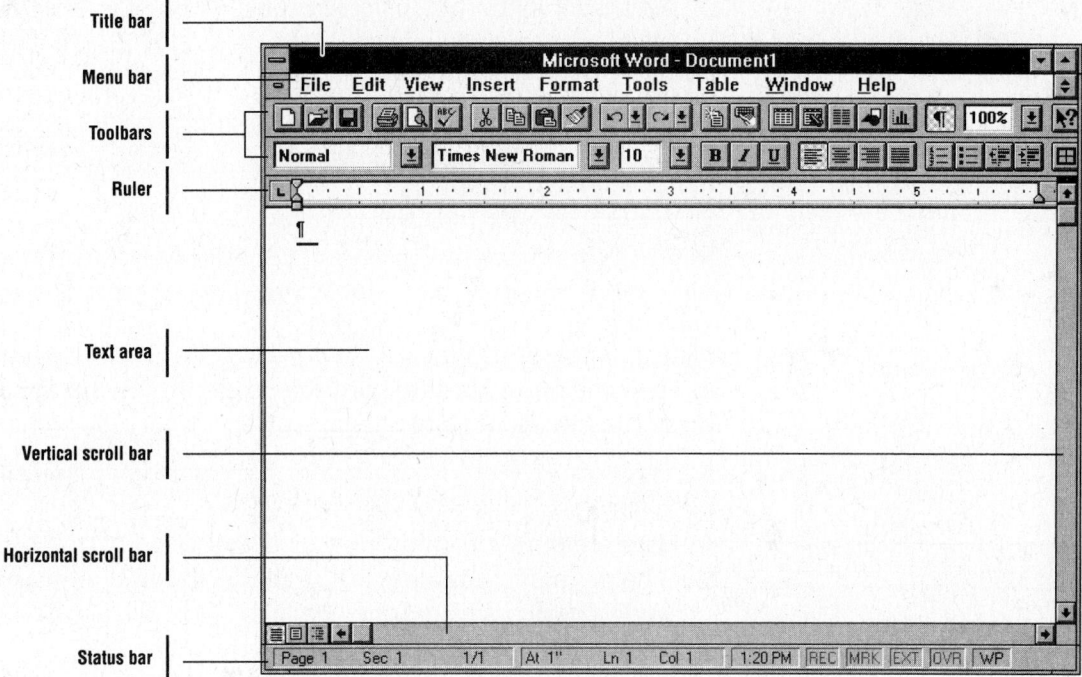

Figure 1-2
The Word screen

- Menu bar
  The Word menu bar displays the names of the menus from which you can select options to perform various tasks. The menus are File, Edit, View, Insert, Format, Table, Window, and Help. These menus can be accessed with the mouse or the keyboard.

- Toolbars
  A toolbar consists of a row of buttons that allows instant access to a wide range of commands, from formatting to file management. Each button is represented by an icon and is accessed with the mouse. The Word screen displays the Standard and Formatting toolbars just below the menu bar.

Figure 1-3
The Standard and Formatting toolbars

Identifying a button

To identify a button, use the mouse to point to it. Word will display the button name.

• Ruler
The ruler, which appears horizontally across the screen, is useful when working with indents, margins, and tabs.

Note: The toolbars and the ruler can be taken off the screen to make more room for your document. For example, to hide the ruler, open the View menu, and click Ruler to uncheck it. To hide toolbars, choose Toolbars from the View menu, and clear the check box of the toolbar you wish to hide, or click the check box of the toolbar you wish to display.

• Text area
The main, rectangular section of the screen that displays text and graphics is called the text area. This is where a document is viewed.

• Scroll bars
The scroll bars operate the same way in Word as they do in Windows. The scroll arrows and scroll boxes are used with the mouse to move right or left and up or down through a document. The horizontal scroll bar also contains buttons to change the view of a document (for example, from normal to outline view).

• Status bar
At the bottom of the screen, the status bar displays information about a document or about a task you are performing. It also displays the current time.

Creating a New Document

New button

When you open Word, a new document window called "Document1" opens automatically. This is the document's name until you name it and save it.

A new document can also be created by clicking the New button on the Standard toolbar or by opening the File menu and choosing New. Each time you create a new document, Word gives it the next new document name, such as "Document2".

Template
The framework upon which a document is created.

When you create a new document by choosing New from the File menu, Word displays the New document dialog box. This allows you to choose a *template* for the new document. All documents are based on templates, which determine the standard formats of documents. For example, you can choose a template to create a particular type of document, such as a memo or a letter.

File menu

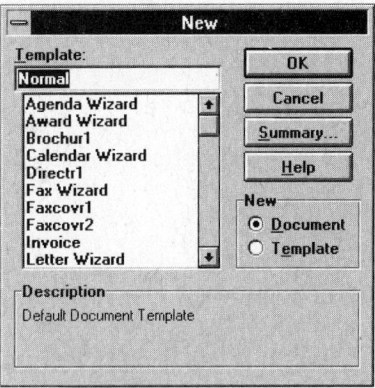

Figure 1-4
The New dialog box

Default settings
Settings predefined by
Word if the user does not
specify settings.

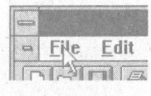

Menu bar

Insertion point
A vertical blinking bar on the
Word screen that indicates
where an action will begin.

End mark
A short horizontal bar on the
Word screen that indicates
the end of the document.

Paragraph mark
The symbol on the Word screen
inserted each time you press
Enter to indicate a new paragraph or start a new line.

New documents are automatically created using the NORMAL template, unless another template is chosen. The NORMAL template
contains Word's *default settings*. This means that a new document
is automatically set for standard 8½" × 11" paper, with 1.25-inch left
and right margins and 1-inch top and bottom margins. Future lessons will explain how to change the default settings to customize a
document.

To create a new document:

1. Move the mouse pointer to the menu bar, and click File to
    open the File menu.

2. Click New to choose that option.

    The New dialog box appears.

3. Click OK to confirm use of the NORMAL template.

    Word opens a new document.

Keying Text

The Word screen contains symbols that are integral to your keying
actions. The point where you begin keying text is the *insertion point*.
This is indicated by the vertical blinking bar in the upper left corner
of the text area. The *end mark*, a short horizontal line, moves as you
key text and indicates the end of the document. The mouse pointer
takes on different shapes depending on where it is moved. When you
point in the text area, the pointer is in the shape of an I-beam. When
you point to areas of the screen outside of the text area, the pointer
is in the shape of an arrow. The insertion point moves when you click
the mouse in different lines or paragraphs. The *paragraph mark* is a
character that marks the beginning of a new paragraph. The importance of this mark and the information it contains is discussed in
Lesson 2.

To create a document and observe these symbols:

1. Key the words **Duke City Gateway**

Note: If you press the
wrong key, use the **Backspace** key and start
again.

    After keying the text, notice that the insertion point and the
    paragraph mark move to the last letter keyed.

2. Continue keying:

    **is New Mexico's leading full-service travel agency, located
    on Montgomery Boulevard in Albuquerque.**

Wordwrap
The automatic placement
of text on the next line.

Notice how the text moved to the beginning of the next line
when it reached the end of the line. This is known as *wordwrap*,
and it marks an important difference between word processing
and typing. With a typewriter, you must press the Return key
at the end of each line. In Word, text moves to the next line
automatically. You only need to press **Enter** to start a new
paragraph or to insert a blank line.

Note: In addition to not pressing **Enter** at the end of each line,
you should not press the **Spacebar** to move the insertion point
through the text. Instead, use the Arrow keys or click the mouse
to the desired location in the text. The **Spacebar** is used to insert
a space in the text, indicated on the screen by a dot between
words.

---

3. Continue by keying the following sentence (insert only one
    space between sentences):

    **It is the southwestern franchise division of Gateway Travel,
    an international travel agency with 49 offices throughout
    the United States, Canada, and Europe.**

This is now a one-paragraph document. The end mark is now
located under the last line of this paragraph, and one space
appears between sentences (after the period). Throughout this
text, one space is used after a period to separate sentences.
This is in keeping with standard word-processing practices.
Extra spaces can cause problems when using various fonts and
paragraph alignments. Fonts are discussed in Lesson 16, and
paragraph alignment is discussed in Lesson 5. See Figure 1-5
on page 9.

Note: Paragraph marks can be either displayed or hidden on the
screen. If the paragraph mark, as it appears in Figure 1-5, does
not appear on the screen, click the Show/Hide ¶ button on the
Standard toolbar to make it appear.

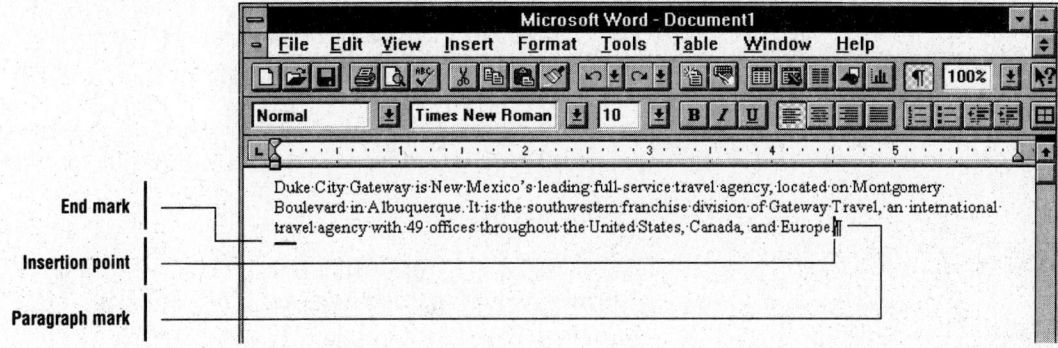

Figure 1-5
The Word screen

Editing Text

In Word, it is very easy to edit text. This lesson reviews the methods of deleting, revising, and inserting text using the following keys:

- **Delete** key
  Used to delete characters to the right of the insertion point.

- **Backspace** key
  Used to delete characters to the left of the insertion point.

- **Insert** key
  Used to toggle between insert mode and overtype mode. When you want to insert or add text, use insert mode. When you want to key over text, use overtype mode. Overtype mode is indicated on the right side of the status bar as "OVR". When "OVR" is dimmed, insert mode is on.

> **Note**: You can also switch between insert and overtype mode by double-clicking "OVR" on the status bar.

To insert text in the document:

1. Look at the status bar to make sure that "OVR"—the overtype-mode indicator—is not turned on. If it is, press the **Insert** key once. This will return you to regular insert mode.

2. Move the insertion point to the left of the "A" in "Albuquerque". (Use the mouse to move the I-beam into place, and then click the mouse.)

Position the I-beam and click.

3. Key **downtown**, and press the **Spacebar** once to leave a space between the two words.

   The text now reads "downtown Albuquerque".

To create two paragraphs:

1. Move the insertion point to the left of the word "It" at the beginning of the second sentence. (Be sure the insertion point is to the right of the space.)

2. Press **Enter** once to indicate the start of a new paragraph. Press **Enter** again to create a blank line between the two paragraphs.

To revise text using the **Backspace** key:

1. Move the insertion point to the right of the word "It" in the second paragraph.

2. Press the **Backspace** key twice to delete both characters.

3. Key **Duke City Gateway**

    The second paragraph now begins "Duke City Gateway is the southwestern franchise division".

To revise text using the **Delete** key:

1. Move the insertion point to the left of the number "49".

2. Press the **Delete** key twice.

3. Key **50**

The **Caps Lock** key on your keyboard can be used to key text in all uppercase letters.

To change the words "Duke City Gateway" to all uppercase letters using the **Caps Lock** key and the "OVR" mode:

1. Move the insertion point to the beginning of the document, to the left of "Duke". (Position the insertion point with the mouse and click.)

2. Double-click "OVR" on the status bar to switch to overtype mode.

    "OVR" changes from gray to black on the status bar.

Note: Most keyboards have a light indicator to show when Caps Lock is turned on.

3. Press the **Caps Lock** key.

4. Key **duke city gateway**, and then press the **Caps Lock** key to turn off the Caps Lock mode.

    "Duke City Gateway" is now in all uppercase letters. Repeat the process for "Duke City Gateway" in the second paragraph.

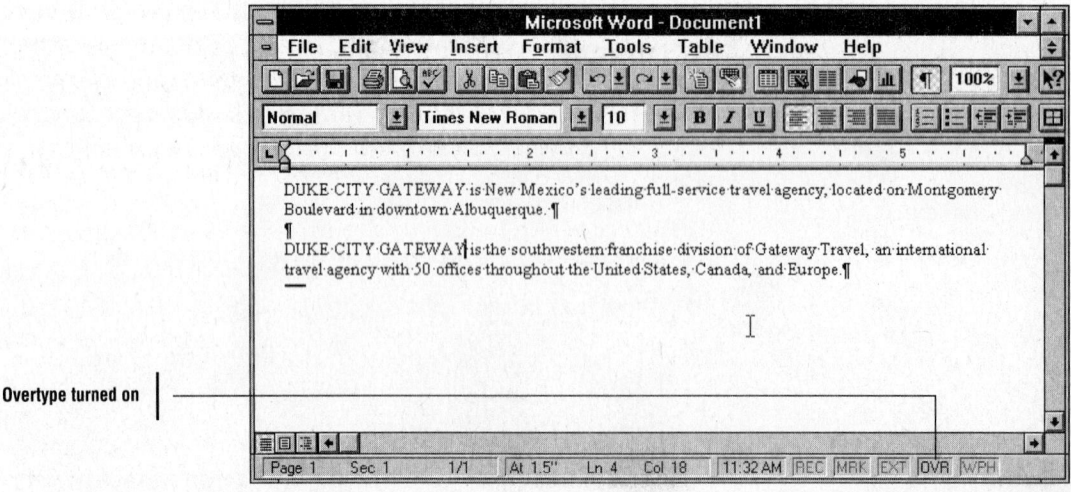

Overtype turned on

Figure 1-6
The edited document

Naming and Saving a Document

The document you are creating, called "Document1," is a temporary document that is stored in the computer's temporary memory. Until you name it and save it to disk, it can be lost to a power failure or to a computer-hardware problem. It is always a good idea to save your work frequently.

Note: If you are not used to working on a computer, it is easy to forget that documents must be saved. If you do forget, Word reminds you. When you try to exit the program, Word asks if you want to save the document(s) on which you were working.

The first step in saving a document for future use is to name it. When you name a document, you are giving it a *filename*. In Word, all documents are referred to and saved as *files*.

Filename
The unique name given to a document that is saved in Word.

File
A document that has been created and then saved under a unique filename.

Filenames can be one to eight characters long and are generally followed by a period and a one- to three-character extension. Filename extensions are used to distinguish different types of files. For example, document files have the extension .DOC, and document templates have the extension .DOT.

Throughout the lessons and exercises in this course, when you save a document, the document name will consist of three parts:

- *[Your three-letter identifier]*, which may be your initials or the identifier your instructor asks you to use, such as **RST**

- The number of the document, such as **4-1**

  RST4-1

- The extension that Word uses automatically for documents: **.DOC**

  RST4-1.DOC

File menu

Save button

A document can be saved by using either the Save command or the Save As command. Both commands are available from the File menu. The Save As command is used to name and save a document for the first time or to save an existing document under a new name. The Save command is used to resave an existing document as you key and edit.

You can also save a document by clicking the Save button on the Standard toolbar. When you are saving a document for the first time, the button will execute the Save As command. When you use the Save button for a document that has already been saved, it will execute the Save command and update the document with your most recent changes.

Before you save a new document, it is important to determine where you plan to save it. Word will save a document in the current drive and directory, which is the default drive and directory, unless you specify otherwise. If you do not want to save a document to the current drive and directory, which is most likely c:\winword, but wish to save it to a floppy disk, you need to change the default drive to either a: or b:, whichever is appropriate for your computer. Your instructor will advise you on the proper drive and directory.

To name and save the document created in this lesson:

1.   Click File to open the File menu.

2. Choose Save As.

    The Save As dialog box appears.

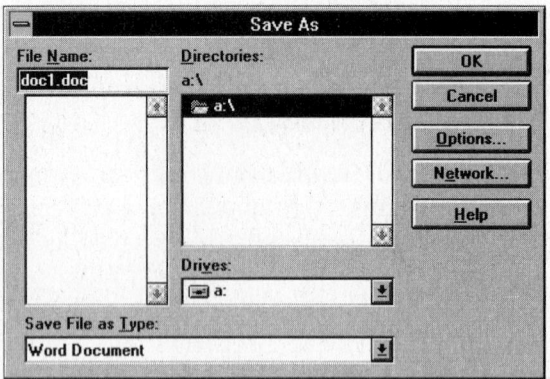

Figure 1-7
The Save As dialog box

3. In the File Name text box, use the **Delete** key to delete any
    existing text, and then key *[your three-letter identifier]***1-0**

    Use the **Right** or **Left Arrow** key or the **Backspace** key to
    correct any mistakes made while keying the name. It is not
    necessary to key the .DOC extension—Word automatically
    adds it to the filename unless you specify another extension.

4. Click OK if you are saving the document to the current drive
    and directory.

    When saving a document to a floppy disk, click the arrow in
    the Drives box. Make sure you have a formatted disk in the
    floppy-disk drive, and then click the appropriate drive. Word
    reads the disk in the floppy drive and is ready to copy the file
    to it. Click OK.

    The document is named *[your three-letter identifier]*1-0.doc and
    is saved for future use.

Using Word Help

Word Help provides complete on-line reference information to explain every feature of the program. While working in Word, use
Help to:

- Explain the procedures for a task you are performing

- Find a definition for a term you do not understand

- Learn about a Word command or area of the screen

- View an on-line demonstration of a procedure

The easiest way to access Word Help is to press the **F1** key. When you
press **F1**, Word displays the Word Help Contents window.

Word Help Contents

The opening Word Help Contents window gives an overview of what is in Help. You can click a topic in this window for more detailed information.

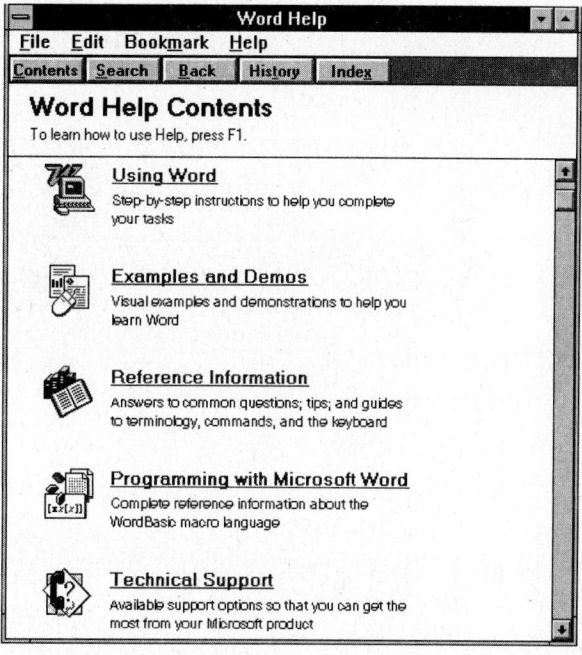

Figure 1-8
The Word Help Contents window

When using Help, you will notice that topics appear underlined. They also appear in color, if you have a color monitor. When you click on a word with a solid underline, you can move quickly around the Help system, going from one term to a cross-reference. These are called *jump terms*.

When you click on a word with a dotted underline, a definition of that term pops up in a box in the window.

To access Help and navigate Word Help Contents:

1. Press the **F1** key, or choose Contents from the Help menu.

    The Word Help Contents window appears.

2. Point to <u>Using Word</u> (the pointer will change to a hand symbol) and click.

    A new Help screen, Using Word, is displayed.

    Notice that clicking a solid-underline jump term opens a new Help screen.

3. At the new screen, click <u>Typing and Revising</u>.

    A new Help screen, Typing and Revising, is displayed.

Jump term
A Help topic that is linked to other Help topics or to more information, usually identified by an underline and a color.

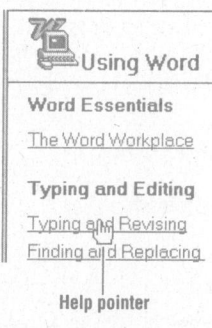

Help pointer as hand symbol

How To window

Double-click to close window

Help button

4. Click the topic <u>Inserting text into a document</u>.

    Help displays a How To window for this topic. A How To window provides step-by-step procedures. The window can be viewed while you work by clicking the On Top button. This places the window on top of your document window. You can then move or resize the How To window, as needed.

5. In the How To window, click the term "insertion point", which appears with a dotted underline.

    Notice that clicking a dotted-underline jump term displays a definition.

6. Click again to clear the definition.

7. Click the Close button in the How To window.

8. Close Word Help by double-clicking the Control-menu box in the upper-left corner of the window, or by choosing Exit from the window's File menu.

The Search Feature

When you know the topic you want to locate, use the Search feature to find it. To use the Search feature, double-click the Help button on the Standard toolbar, or choose Search For Help On from the Help menu. To search for a specific topic, key a word or phrase, or scroll through a list of topics.

To use the Search feature:

1. Double-click the Help button on the Standard toolbar.

    The Search dialog box appears.

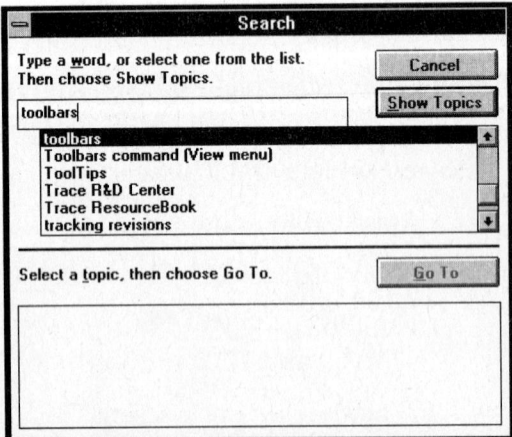

Figure 1-9
The Search dialog box

2. Key **toolbars** in the text box.

3. Click the Show Topics button.

   A list of related Help topics concerning the toolbars is found. You can choose from any of the topics by highlighting the line and pressing Go To or by double-clicking the topic.

4. Double-click the topic Parts of the Word Screen and Toolbars.

   Word displays the Help screen for this topic.

5. Close the Help screen by choosing Exit from the File menu.

Context-Sensitive Help

While working in Word, you may come to a command, a key, a dialog box, or even an area of the screen about which you have a question. Word Help is context-sensitive. This means that it provides help on an as-needed basis—while you are performing a procedure or before you begin a procedure.

This can be done in two ways. To get help on a menu item or a dialog box, display the item or dialog box and press the **F1** key, or click the Help button that appears in every dialog box. Word Help goes directly to that subject with an explanation.

To get help on a menu item:

1. Click File. With the File menu displayed, press the **Down Arrow** key to move the highlight to Save As.

2. Press the **F1** key.

   Help about the Save As command from the File menu is displayed.

3. Exit Help.

To get help on a command, a key, or a screen region, click the Help button or press **Shift+F1**. A question mark appears with the pointer. Press the key or command, or point to the area in question. Help goes directly to that topic.

To get help on a command:

1. Click the Help button.

   The pointer changes to a question mark.

2. Move the pointer to the New button on the Standard toolbar and click.

   A Help screen about creating a new document is displayed.

3. Exit Help.

Help pointer with question mark

Note: To change the Help pointer back to the regular I-beam, press the **Esc** key.

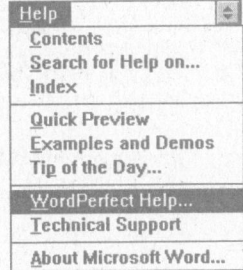

Help menu

WordPerfect Help

There is a special Word Help feature for those familiar with WordPerfect. It allows you to choose from a list of WordPerfect commands and teaches you how to carry out the commands in Word. You can also press a WordPerfect command key, such as a function key, and Help will show the Word equivalent. WordPerfect Help either shows in text how to carry out the command or demonstrates the command in a speed you can regulate. You can also ask for more detailed information about a given command, which opens the regular Help utility.

To access the WordPerfect Help feature:

1. Choose WordPerfect Help from the Help menu.

    The Help for WordPerfect Users dialog box appears.

2. Look at the command list on the left, and use the down arrow to scroll down and highlight the word "Save".

    A description of the Save command appears.

3. Click the Demo button.

    Word demonstrates the Save command by going through the save steps and then displays the Save As dialog box.

4. Click OK.

Demonstrations in Word

Word provides online demonstrations of procedures that are both informative and enjoyable to view. New Word users or users familiar with earlier versions of Word can choose Quick Preview from the Help menu and watch the "Getting Started" or "What's New" demo. Users switching from WordPerfect can choose the "Tips for WordPerfect Users" demo.

The Help menu also contains the Examples and Demos option. When you choose this option, Word Help displays a window listing all the procedures of which you can view demonstrations. For example, you can view a wide variety of demonstrations on such topics as Formatting Text, Working with Tables, and Mail Merge.

Take the time to learn how Word features work by viewing some of these demonstrations.

Printing a Document

Once you have created a document, it is easy to print it.

You can use the Print command by:

*   Choosing Print from the File menu

*   Pressing **Ctrl+P**

- Clicking the Print button on the Standard toolbar

When you choose Print from the File menu or press **Ctrl+P**, Word displays the Print dialog box from which you can choose different Print options.

When you choose the Print command from the Standard toolbar, Word sends the document directly to the printer, using the default settings.

To print the document:

1. Choose Print from the File menu.

    Word displays the Print dialog box containing the default print settings.

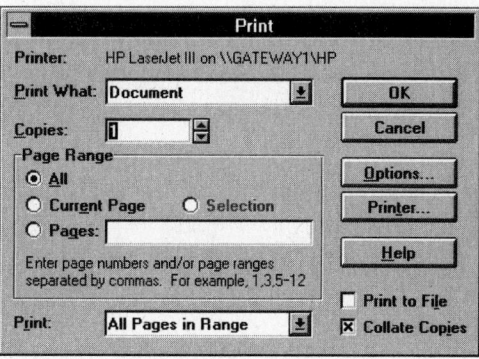

Figure 1-10
The Print dialog box

2. Click OK or press **Enter**.

    Word sends the document to the printer. Notice the changes in the status bar as the document is sent to the printer, and as the printer is actually printing.

Closing a Document and Exiting Word

When you are finished working on a document and have saved it, you can close it and open another, or you can exit the program. In Word, a document does not have to be closed to open another. In the Windows environment, you can open several documents, or files, and keep them open throughout the Word session.

You can close a document by:

- Choosing Close from the File menu

- Double-clicking the document Control-menu box in the upper left corner of the document window or clicking the box and choosing Close

- Pressing **Ctrl+F4** or **Ctrl+W**

Application Control-menu box

Document Control-menu box

Control-menu boxes

You can exit Word by:

- Choosing Exit from the File menu

- Double-clicking the application Control-menu box or clicking the box and choosing Close

- Pressing **Alt+F4**

To close the document and exit Word:

1. Double-click the document Control-menu box.

   Word closes the document.

2. Click the File menu and choose Exit.

   Word closes and the Windows opening screen appears.

Table 1-1: Keyboard Shortcuts for Introductory Word Skills	
Keyboard Shortcut	Action
F1	Open Help Contents
Shift+F1	Open context-sensitive Help
Ctrl+P	Access Print command
Ctrl+F4 or **Ctrl+W**	Close a document
Alt+F4	Exit Word

Key Terms

Default settings	Jump term
End mark	Paragraph mark
File	Template
Filename	Wordwrap
Insertion point	

Exercises

Exercise 1.1

1. Start Word:

   A. At the DOS prompt c:\>, key **win** to open Windows and press **Enter** (or follow your instructor's directions to open Windows).

   B. At the Windows Program Manager screen, double-click the Word icon.

2. Key the text in Figure 1-11.

Figure 1-11

Duke City Gateway has just celebrated its 25th anniversary in the travel
business. The agency has proudly served over 45,000 area residents and
visitors to New Mexico from all over the world. Duke City Gateway has been
at its current location for all of its 25 years.

3. Move the insertion point to the right of the word "residents"
    in the second sentence.

4. Make sure the overtype mode is not turned on.

5. After the word "residents", key:

    , business travelers,

6. Move the insertion point to the right of the space following
    the word "for" in the last sentence.

7. Use the **Delete** key to delete the text "all of its"and the space
    following "its".

8. Change the number "45,000" to "50,000" using overtype
    mode:

    A. Move the insertion point to the left of "45,000".

    B. Press the **Insert** key to switch to overtype mode.

    C. Key **50** over "45".

    D. Press **Insert** again to switch back to insert mode.

9. Save the document as *[your three-letter identifier]*1-1.doc:

    A. From the File menu, choose Save As.

    B. In the Save As dialog box, key the name of the document
        and click OK.

10. Print the document:

    A. Choose Print from the File menu.

    B. In the Print dialog box, click OK.

11. Before closing the document, look up the Close file menu
    command in Help:

    A. Double-click the Help button.

    B. In the Search dialog box, key **close**

    C. Click Show Topics, and then click Go To.

12. After reviewing the information, close Help by double-
    clicking the Control-menu box.

13.　Close the document and exit Word using the File menu:

    A.　Choose Close from the File menu.

    B.　Choose Exit from the File menu.

Exercise 1.2

1.　Start Word.

2.　Create a new document from the File menu:

    A.　Click File and then click New.

    B.　In the New dialog box, click OK to confirm use of the NORMAL template.

3.　Key the text in Figure 1-12.

Figure 1-12

As its slogan says, Duke City Gateway truly is the gateway to the Southwest, offering the greatest number of specialized tours to New Mexico, Arizona, and Colorado. The agency's tour planners and tour guides are considered experts in the history and culture of this area.

4.　Move the insertion point to the left of the "A" in "Arizona" in the first sentence.

5.　Press the **Insert** key to switch to overtype mode.

6.　Key **Colorado, and Arizona.**

7.　Switch back to insert mode, and move the insertion point to the left of the apostrophe in the word "agency's".

8.　Use the **Backspace** key to delete "The agency". Then key **Duke City Gateway**

9.　In the last sentence, key **remarkable** before the word "area".

10.　Save the document as *[your three-letter identifier]*1-2.doc.

11.　Print the document using the Print button on the Standard toolbar.

12.　Close the document and quit Word using the keyboard shortcuts (unless you will be doing the following exercises immediately):

    A.　Press **Ctrl+F4** to close the document.

    B.　Press **Alt+F4** to exit Word.

Exercise 1.3

1. Start Word, if necessary.

2. Create a new document using the File menu.

3. Key the text in Figure 1-13.

Figure 1-13

TO THE STAFF:

The lower airfares are good for travel between June 15 and September 15 only. Travelers must stay over one Saturday night to qualify. The reservation policy is first come, first served. Remember: Groups booked on these low fare flights will not necessarily be booked on the same carrier and will not necessarily arrive at the same time.

---

4. In the first, key **new** to the left of the word "lower". Add a comma after "new". Then delete the word "lower" and key **reduced** (make sure you are in insert mode).

5. Switch to overtype mode, and insert a hyphen between "low" and "fare" in the last sentence.

6. In the last sentence, delete the colon after "Remember". Switch to insert mode, key **that**, and make the "G" in "Groups" lowercase.

7. Insert a blank line after "TO THE STAFF".

8. Save the document as *[your three-letter identifier]*1-3.doc.

9. Print the document.

10. Close the document.

11. Exit Word (unless you will be doing the following exercises immediately).

Exercise 1.4: Challenge Yourself

First, practice navigating in Word Help by using context-sensitive Help to find out about the Save button on the Standard toolbar. Once in Help with the Save command window open, scroll to the end of the window, and jump to <u>Opening, Saving, and Protecting Documents</u>. Then, jump to the <u>Overview</u> topic, scroll to the information on saving, review the information, and close Help.

Next, create a new document and key the text in Figure 1-14, which appears at the end of this exercise. After keying the text, switch to overtype mode, and rekey the word "Reminder" in all capital letters using the **Caps Lock** key. In the first sentence, delete the word "one" and key **person**. After the word "office", key **be sure to**. Create a new paragraph out of each sentence. Before "Thank you!" insert another paragraph by keying: **And don't forget to turn on the alarm and lock the door.** Insert a blank line between each line of text.

Save the document as *[your three-letter identifier]*1-4.doc and print it. Close the document and exit Word.

Figure 1-14

Reminder:

Will the last one to leave the office:

Turn off all computers and monitors. Turn on the answering machine. Turn

on the FAX machine. Turn off the coffee machine. Turn off the lights.

Thank you!

Revising Text

Objectives

- Open an existing document.
- Merge and split paragraphs.
- Move within a document.
- Use the Undo, Redo, and Repeat commands.
- Select text.
- Delete and replace selected text.
- Learn more about saving documents.

Open button

Once you are familiar with the basics of Word, it is easy to revise text in a document. This lesson teaches how to move through a document quickly, make changes to a document, undo changes, and save a revised document using a number of different save options.

Opening an Existing Document

In this lesson, instead of creating a new document, you will open an existing document. As you learned, Word automatically opens to a new document window when the program is started. To open an existing document, you can use one of two methods:

- Choose Open from the File menu

- Click the Open button on the Standard toolbar

With either option, Word displays the Open dialog box.

Figure 2-1
The Open dialog box

Under File Name, you can key the name of the file you want to open in the text box, or you can choose a file in the current directory from the list box. You can change the directory, the drive, or the type of file, if needed, to locate a file.

Follow your instructor's directions as to the disk drive and directory of the files you will open in this lesson and in future lessons.

To open the file 2-0.doc:

1. From the menu bar, click File to open the File menu.

Notice the list of filenames at the bottom of the File menu. This list represents the last four files opened. When the file you are looking for is listed, it can be chosen from this list.

2. Choose Open.

    The Open dialog box appears.

Choosing a drive

3. Click the scroll arrow in the Drives drop-down list box to choose the appropriate drive for your computer, according to your instructor's directions. If you are using a floppy disk, make sure a disk is in the floppy drive.

4. Double-click the appropriate drive.

5. If your instructor has directed you to open a specific directory, choose the appropriate directory from the Directories box.

6. From the File Name list box, choose the file 2-0.doc.

7. Click OK. (You can also double-click the filename to open the file.)

    Word opens the file 2-0.doc.

Word, Sentence, Paragraph: Some Definitions

When document 2-0.doc appears on the screen, you will notice a variety of symbols in the text. These are *nonprinting characters*, which are displayed on the screen but will not appear in the printed document. They represent the definition and spacing of the words, lines, sentences, and paragraphs in the document.

Nonprinting character
A symbol for a tab, paragraph, or space that appears on the screen but not in the printed document.

A word includes the space character that follows it. A sentence includes the end-of-sentence punctuation and at least one space. A paragraph is any amount of text followed by a paragraph mark.

Note: If the nonprinting characters are not displayed on your screen, press the Show/Hide ¶ button on the Standard toolbar.

The Show/Hide ¶ button on the Standard toolbar can make all nonprinting characters disappear from the document window. However, while working in the document, it is often helpful to see these characters. It makes it easier, for example, to check that you have entered a space between sentences and after commas.

Show/Hide ¶ button

Wordwrap selects the best place to break text and start a new line from these spaces. However, there may be occasions where you want two words to appear together in a sentence and not be separated by wordwrap. For example, in keying a date such as July 4, you would not want wordwrap to break the date and place the "4" on the next line. You also would not want a name like "Mr. Smith" to be divided between two lines in a document. In these instances, you would insert a *nonbreaking space* between the two words by pressing **Ctrl+Shift+Spacebar** instead of just the **Spacebar**.

Nonbreaking space
A space between two words, defined by a special character, that prevents Word from breaking a line between the two words.

Table 2-1: Nonprinting Characters	
Character	Command
Tab (→)	**Tab** key
Space (·)	**Spacebar**
Nonbreaking space (∘)	**Ctrl+Shift+Spacebar**
Paragraph mark (¶)	**Enter** key
Line-break character (↵)	**Shift+Enter** keys

As explained in Lesson 1, you press the **Enter** key to start a new line and create a new paragraph. However, there may be instances where you want to create a line break within a paragraph. An example of this is an address, which may consist of three lines. To accommodate all three lines as one paragraph, press **Shift+Enter**, and the *line-break character* appears on the screen. Using this method of line breaking, all the characters will share the same formatting, which is contained in the paragraph symbol. Paragraph formatting is explained in further detail in Lesson 5: "Changing Margins and Formatting Paragraphs."

Line-break character
A symbol entered to start a new line within a paragraph.

To practice keying some of these nonprinting characters:

1. Move the insertion point to the end of the document, press **Enter**, and then begin a new paragraph by keying:

   Duke City Gateway Travel Agency has been a member in good standing of the IATA for 25

Note: In this textbook, a period appears after text to be keyed only if that period is also to be keyed.

2. Insert a nonbreaking space after "25" by pressing **Ctrl+Shift+Spacebar**. Then key **years.** (including the period)

   Notice the appearance of the nonbreaking-space character. Word now treats these two words as one inseparable unit.

3. Press **Enter** twice.

4. Key the following as one paragraph at the end of the document. Press **Shift+Enter** at the end of each line instead of **Enter**:

   Duke City Gateway
   15 Montgomery Boulevard
   Albuquerque, NM 87111

   Notice the appearance of the line-break characters.

5. Press the Show/Hide ¶ button once, and then press it once again to see how all the nonprinting characters in the document disappear and reappear in view.

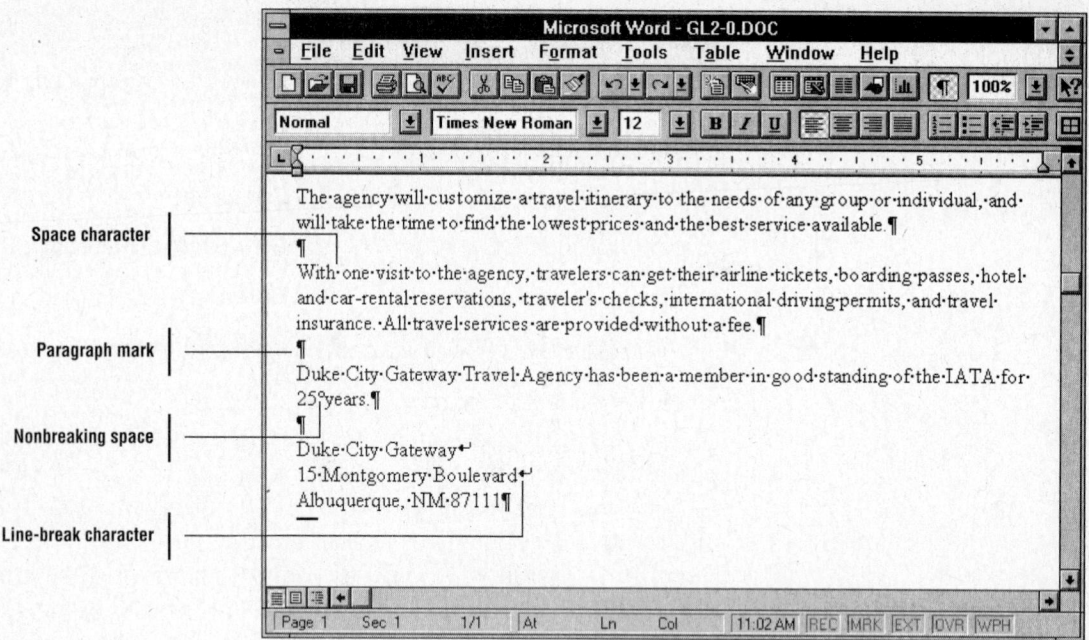

Figure 2-2
Nonprinting characters

Merging and Splitting Paragraphs

In the last lesson, you practiced creating new paragraphs. Now that you have a better understanding of the space character and the paragraph mark, you can practice revising a document by merging and splitting paragraphs.

To merge paragraphs:

1. Move the insertion point to the left of the paragraph mark at the end of the paragraph that begins "The agency will customize" (after the period following the word "available").

2. Press the **Delete** key twice to delete the two paragraph marks.

    The paragraphs are merged. Notice, however, that there is no space between the sentences at the point of the merge.

3. Press the **Spacebar** once.

To split the paragraph:

1. In the second sentence of your merged paragraph, place the insertion point to the left of the word "With" and to the right of the space character.

2. Press **Enter** twice.

Moving Within a Document

As explained in Lesson 1, when you key text, it is inserted at the insertion point. As you continue keying text, Word automatically scrolls through the document, keeping the section in which you are working visible.

You can move to different parts of the document using four methods:

- Using the mouse
- Pressing **Shift+F5** to return to a previous editing location
- Using the keyboard
- Using the scroll bars

Moving the Insertion Point Using the Mouse

To move the insertion point—the blinking vertical bar—position the I-beam with the mouse and click. This is the easiest way to move around the portion of the document displayed in the document window.

Returning to a Previous Editing Location

Word remembers the last three locations in the document where you edited or keyed text. The keyboard shortcut **Shift+F5** returns the insertion point to these locations. This is particularly helpful, for example, when opening a document you were working on yesterday. **Shift+F5** can be used to return to the exact point in the document where you were last working, before you saved and closed the document.

Moving the Insertion Point Using the Keyboard

Certain keys on the keyboard can move the insertion point. The Arrow keys, for example, can move the insertion point up or down one line, or one character to the left or to the right. Other keys and key combinations can move the insertion point to specified locations in the document quickly.

Table 2-2: Keys to Move the Insertion Point	
To Move	Press
One word to the left	**Ctrl+Left Arrow**
One word to the right	**Ctrl+Right Arrow**
Beginning of the line	**Home**
End of the line	**End**
One paragraph up	**Ctrl+Up Arrow**
One paragraph down	**Ctrl+Down Arrow**

Continued on next page

Table 2-2—Continued	
To Move	Press
Up one window	**PgUp**
Down one window	**PgDn**
Top of the window	**Ctrl+PgUp**
Bottom of the window	**Ctrl+PgDn**
Beginning of the document	**Ctrl+Home**
End of the document	**Ctrl+End**

To practice moving the insertion point in document 2-0.doc:

1. Make sure the insertion point is at the beginning of the document. Press the **End** key to move to the end of the line.

2. Press **Ctrl+End** to move to the end of the document.

3. Press **Ctrl+Up Arrow** several times, until you are at the top of the document.

Scrolling

You can use the vertical scroll bar at the right of the document window to move through a document. The position of the scroll box indicates the approximate location in the document, which is particularly helpful in long documents.

To view and move through a document that is wider than the document window, use the horizontal scroll bar at the bottom of the document window.

Note: Remember that scrolling through a document does not move the insertion point. It moves only the portion of the document you are currently viewing in the document window.

Table 2-3: Scrolling Through a Document	
To Move	Do This
Up one line	Click the up scroll arrow
Down one line	Click the down scroll arrow
Up one screen	Click the scroll bar above the scroll box
Down one screen	Click the scroll bar below the scroll box
To any relative position	Drag the scroll box up or down
To the right	Click the right scroll arrow
To the left	Click the left scroll arrow
Into the left margin	Hold down the **Shift** key and click the left scroll arrow

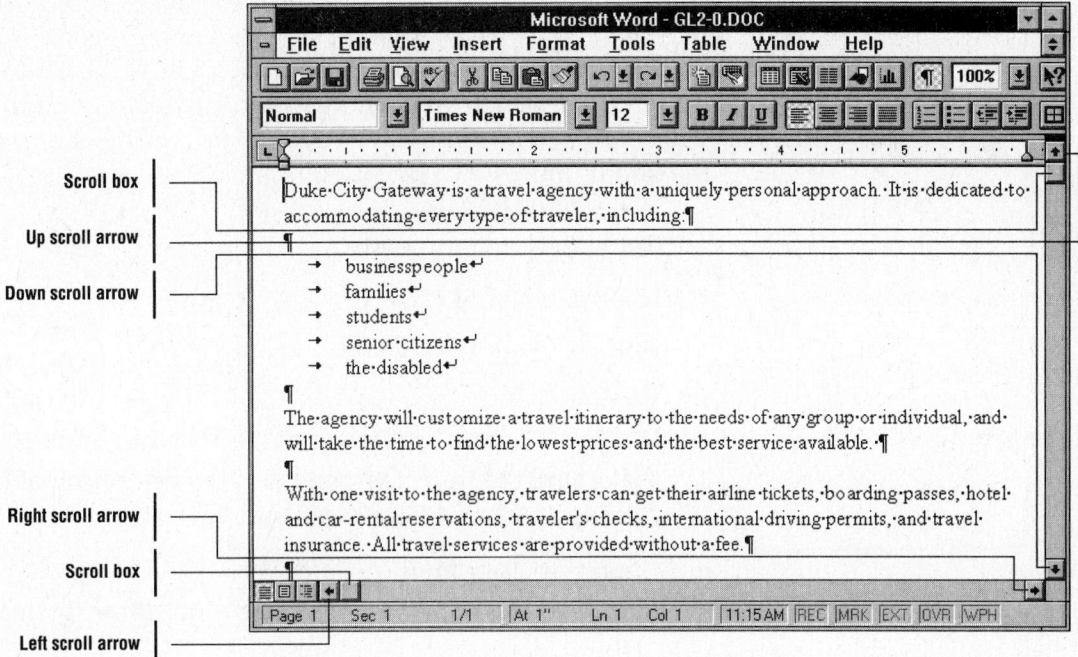

Figure 2-3
Using the scroll bars

To practice scrolling within the document:

1. Click below the vertical scroll box to move down one screen.

2. Drag the box back up to the top of the scroll bar.

3. Click the down scroll arrow on the scroll bar twice to move down two lines.

4. Press and hold the **Shift** key while clicking the left scroll arrow on the horizontal scroll bar once.

5. Click the right scroll arrow once to return to the correct horizontal position.

6. Press the up scroll arrow on the vertical scroll bar twice to bring the document back into full view.

   Notice that, throughout this scrolling movement, the insertion point remained in the same place, at the top of the document.

Undo, Redo, and Repeat Commands

Word remembers the changes you make in a document and allows you to undo, redo, or repeat the change easily.

Undo and Redo buttons

Undo and Redo Commands

If you accidentally delete some text, you can use the Undo command to reverse the action and restore the document to its original form. If you change your mind and decide to keep the deletion, you can use the Redo command to reverse the canceled action.

There are three ways to undo an action:

* Click the Undo button on the Standard toolbar
* Choose Undo from the Edit menu
* Press **Ctrl+Z**

There are three ways to redo an action:

* Click the Redo button on the Standard toolbar
* Choose Redo from the Edit menu
* Press **Ctrl+Y**

Word can undo the last several actions

You can also undo or redo the last several actions you took. To do this, click the arrow to the right of the Undo or Redo button, and then choose the actions you wish to reverse from the drop-down list. The actions on the drop-down list are listed in reverse order of their occurrences (so that the most recent action is at the top of the list, followed by the action that took place immediately before it, and so on).

To practice using the Undo and Redo commands:

1. Delete the first word in the document, "Duke", by first moving the insertion point to the right of the space after "Duke" and then pressing the **Backspace** key five times. (Remember that a word includes the space following it.)

2. Click the Undo button on the Standard toolbar.

   The word "Duke" is restored.

3. Move the insertion point to the left of the word "one" in the paragraph that begins "With one visit".

4. Key **just** and press the **Spacebar** once.

   The text now reads "With just one visit".

5. Open the Edit menu, and choose Undo Typing. (Notice the reminder of the keyboard command for the same action, **Ctrl+Z**.)

   The word "just" is deleted.

6. Click the Redo button.

   The word "just" is restored.

Note: If you have clicked the down arrow next to the Undo button, click "Typing" at the top of the Undo drop-down list, which represents the last action.

Edit	
<u>U</u>ndo Typing	Ctrl+Z
<u>R</u>epeat Typing	Ctrl+Y
Cu<u>t</u>	Ctrl+X
<u>C</u>opy	Ctrl+C
<u>P</u>aste	Ctrl+V
Paste <u>S</u>pecial...	
Clea<u>r</u>	Delete
Select A<u>ll</u>	Ctrl+A
<u>F</u>ind...	Ctrl+F
R<u>e</u>place...	Ctrl+H
<u>G</u>o To...	Ctrl+G
A<u>u</u>toText...	
<u>B</u>ookmark...	
Lin<u>k</u>s...	
Ob<u>j</u>ect	

Edit menu

The Repeat Command

Suppose you key text in a document that you want to repeat in other areas of the document. Instead of rekeying the same text, the Repeat command can duplicate the text. This feature is also helpful in repeating other commands and keystrokes, as explained in Lesson 3: "Character Formatting."

There are two ways to use the Repeat command:

- Press the **F4**, or **Ctrl+Y** key

- Choose Repeat from the Edit menu

To practice using the Repeat command:

1. In the paragraph that begins "The agency will", position the insertion point to the left of the word "agency".

2. Key **travel** and press the **Spacebar** once.

   The sentence now begins "The travel agency will".

3. Move the insertion point to the left of the word "agency" in the next paragraph.

4. Press the **F4** key.

   The word "travel" is repeated.

5. Save the document as *[your three-letter identifier]*2-0.doc.

Note: To undo, redo, or re-peat your last action, do so immediately before pressing any other keys.

Selecting Text

Selecting text is an important, basic technique that adds speed and ease to revising documents. Future lessons will teach how to move, copy, save, and even print a selected portion of a document. In this lesson, you will delete and replace selected text.

You have deleted text using the **Delete** and **Backspace** keys, one character at a time. In this lesson, you will select a word, a sentence, or a paragraph, and delete it with one keystroke.

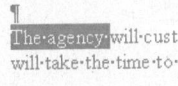

The·agency·will·cust will·take·the·time·to·

Selected text

You have replaced text by pressing the **Insert** key to change to overtype mode. This lesson explains how selecting the text you want to replace offers more flexibility.

There are many different methods for selecting text, using both the keyboard and the mouse. As you work more in Word, the method best suited to the task will become apparent.

Selection
The selected portion of a document (or the whole document), which appears highlighted on the screen.

When you select text, that area of the document is called the *selection*, and it appears highlighted on the screen. The selected text remains highlighted until you cancel the selection.

Selecting with the Mouse

You can choose from several methods of text selection using the mouse, depending on the size of the area to be selected.

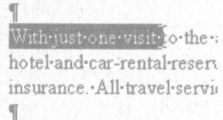

Dragging the I-beam

- Dragging

  The standard method of selection is to drag the mouse over text. This is done by positioning the mouse pointer at one end of the area you want to select, holding down the left mouse button, and dragging the I-beam to the end of the selection.

- **Shift**+click

  With this method of selection, you position the pointer and click at one end of the desired selection, such as the beginning of a sentence. Then you hold down the **Shift** key while clicking at the other end.

- Double-click a word

  To select a word, you position the pointer anywhere on the word and double-click the mouse.

Selection bar
An unmarked area at the left edge of a document window, used to select text with the mouse.

To select single or multiple lines, paragraphs, or the whole document, the *selection bar* is used. It is the unmarked area along the left side of the document window. When you move the mouse pointer to this area, it changes from an I-beam to an arrow that points toward the text. If the arrow is not pointing to the text but is pointing to the left (as it does, for example, in the toolbars), you are not in the selection bar area.

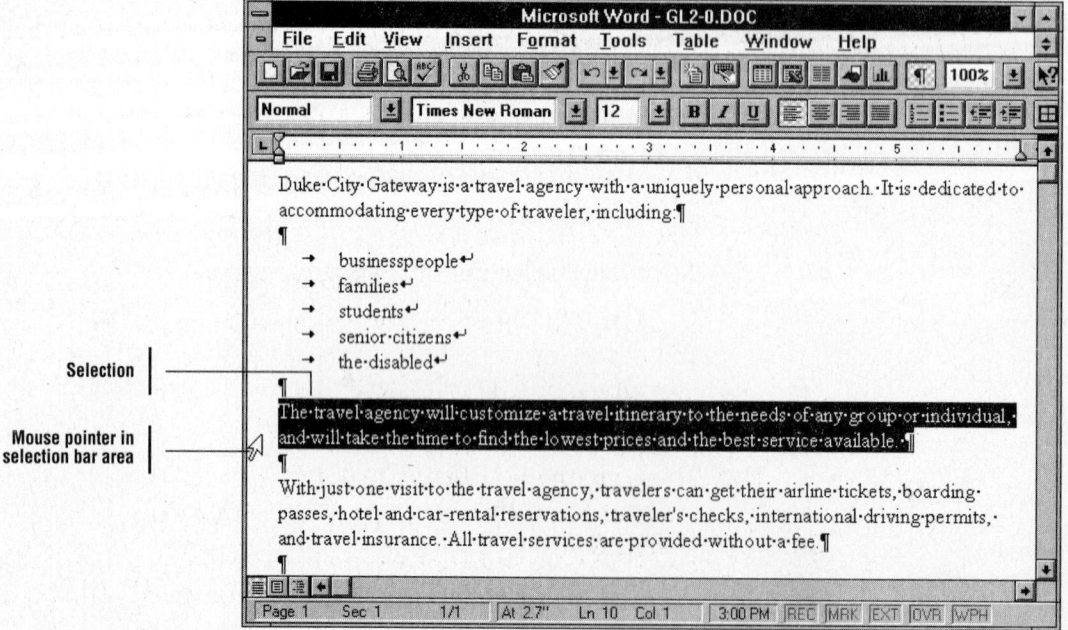

Figure 2-4
Using the selection bar to select text

Table 2-4: Mouse Selection	
To Select	Use the Mouse To
A series of characters	Click and drag, or click one end and then click the other end while holding down the **Shift** key.
A word	Double-click the word.
A sentence	Hold down the **Ctrl** key while clicking anywhere in the sentence.
A line of text	Point to the line in the selection bar and click. To select multiple lines, drag in the selection bar.
A paragraph	Point to the paragraph in the selection bar and double-click. To select multiple paragraphs, drag in the selection bar.
The entire document	Hold down the **Ctrl** key while clicking anywhere in the selection bar, or triple-click in the selection bar.

Once a selection is made, you can adjust the amount of text selected or cancel the selection.

To adjust a mouse selection:

- Hold down the **Shift** key, and click where you want the selection to end, either beyond the highlighted area to lengthen the selection or within the highlighted area to shorten the selection

- Hold down the **Shift** key, and press any Arrow key to lengthen or shorten the selection

To cancel a mouse selection:

- Click anywhere in the document

- Press an Arrow key

To practice selecting text using the mouse:

1. Select the first word by double-clicking it.

   Notice that the space following the word is also selected.

2. Cancel the selection by clicking anywhere in the document.

3. Position the insertion point at the beginning of the sentence that starts "With just one visit" and click.

4. Select the sentence by pressing the left mouse button and dragging to the end of the sentence. Release the mouse button.

   As you drag the mouse, notice that Word selects the sentence word by word, including the space after each word. When the

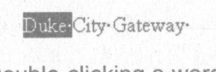

Double-clicking a word

whole sentence is selected, Word includes the space at the end of the sentence as part of the selection.

5. Adjust the selection to include the second sentence by holding down the **Shift** key and then moving the pointer to the end of the second sentence. Click.

6. Press any Arrow key to clear the selection. (If you use an Arrow key from the numeric keypad, make sure Num Lock is not on.)

7. Move the pointer in the selection bar area to the left of the same paragraph, and then double-click to select the paragraph.

    Notice that the first click selects the first line, and the second click selects the paragraph, including the paragraph mark.

8. Move the pointer anywhere in the selection bar, and then hold down the **Ctrl** key and click.

    The entire document is selected.

Selecting with the Keyboard

You can use a variety of keyboard commands to select text. Most of these selections use the **Shift** key.

Table 2-5: Keyboard Selection	
To Select	**Press**
One character to the right	**Shift+Right Arrow**
One character to the left	**Shift+Left Arrow**
To the end of a word	**Ctrl+Shift+Right Arrow**
To the beginning of a word	**Ctrl+Shift+Left Arrow**
To the end of a line	**Shift+End**
To the beginning of a line	**Shift+Home**
One line up	**Shift+Up Arrow**
One line down	**Shift+Down Arrow**
To the end of a paragraph	**Ctrl+Shift+Down Arrow**
To the beginning of a paragraph	**Ctrl+Shift+Up Arrow**
One screen down	**Shift+PgDn**
One screen up	**Shift+PgUp**
To the end of a document	**Ctrl+Shift+End**
To the beginning of a document	**Ctrl+Shift+Home**
An entire document	**Ctrl+5** (on keypad)

You can also use the function key **F8** for text selection and adjustment. The **F8** key turns on extend mode. Once in extend mode,

Shift+F8 reduces the size of a selection, and the **F8** key extends a selection.

*   **Shift+F8**

    To adjust an area of text that is too large, press **Shift+F8**. Each time you press this combination, Word reduces the selection first to a paragraph, then to a sentence, then to a word.

*   The **F8** key

    To extend an area of text, press the **F8** key to turn on extend mode. The status bar shows "EXT" turned on. Each time the key is pressed, Word extends the selection first by a sentence, then by a paragraph, then to the whole document.

To cancel a selection made with the **F8** key, press the **Esc** key to turn off extend mode, and then press an Arrow key to cancel the selection.

Deleting and Replacing a Selection

Once text is selected, you can delete it by pressing the **Delete** key. You can also replace it by keying over the selected text. Unlike using the overtype mode, when you key over selected text, the keyed text can be longer or shorter than the selection. Whatever length it is, Word will replace the selected text with the newly keyed text.

Note: While keying over selected text is an excellent editing feature, it is sometimes the cause of accidental deletions. Remember, when there is selected text in a document (or even in a dialog box), and you begin keying text, Word deletes all the selected text with your first keystroke. If you key text without realizing that a portion of the document is selected, use the Undo command to restore the text.

To practice deleting and replacing selected text:

1. Select the first paragraph.

2. Press the **Delete** key.

    The paragraph is deleted.

3. Click the Undo button.

    The paragraph is restored.

4. In the paragraph that begins "With just one visit", select the words "the travel agency".

5. Key **Duke City Gateway Travel**

    The selected text is replaced with the agency's name.

More Ways to Save a Document

In Lesson 1, you named and saved a new document. In this lesson, after revising an existing document, you will save it, close it, and rename it. Word's additional save options will also be reviewed.

Saving a Revised Document

Saving a revised document is as easy as saving a new one. You can either click the Save button on the Standard toolbar or choose Save from the File menu. This command will automatically save the document with all the changes made to it, replacing the old file with the revised file.

The Save As Command

You may wish to save the revised document under a new name and retain the original document without the revisions. This can be done using the Save As command. When you use this command, you are actually renaming the document with the revisions. The original document remains unchanged.

To use the Save As command:

1. Choose Save As from the File menu. (You can also press the **F12** key.)

    The Save As dialog box appears.

2. In the File Name text box, move the insertion point to the right of the "0" and before the period and key **r**

3. Click OK.

    The revised document is saved as *[your three-letter identifier]*2-0r.doc. Notice the change in the title bar on the screen. The original document file is automatically closed, and the revised document file with the new name remains open.

The document *[your three-letter identifier]*2-0.doc has been revised, and the revision has been saved as a new version of the document. The original document remains unchanged.

The Save All Command

Another command on the File menu is the Save All command. When several documents are open, this command can be used to save changes to all of them. Word prompts you through the process if this is the first time you are saving a particular document, or if you have made any "global" changes that affect other files. These changes include glossary or macro entries and command changes, which are discussed in future lessons.

Saving vs. Closing a Document

In the last lesson, you closed a document. Remember that closing is different from saving. When you are finished working on a document, you save it. Then you close it, so that it does not take up unnecessary memory, especially when working with several open documents. It is best to close all open documents before exiting Word.

Save Options

Like many of the features in Word, the Save feature can be customized by choosing from a list of options. These options allow you to control the way Word saves documents.

There are two ways to choose Save options:

- Choose Options from the Tools menu, and then click the Save tab

- Click the Options button in the Save As dialog box

Both methods open the Options dialog box for Save settings.

Save tab

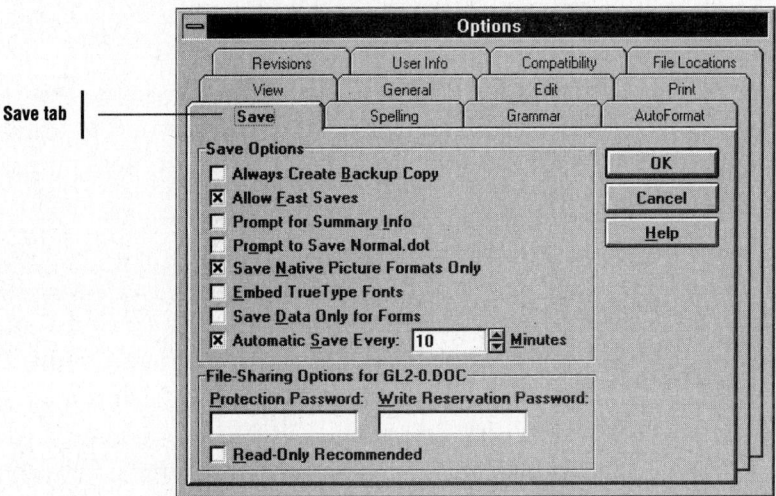

Figure 2-5
The Save tab in the Options dialog box

To view the Save options:

1. Choose Options from the Tools menu.

2. Click the Save tab.

The Options dialog box allows you to choose your own Save options. For example:

- Always Create Backup Copy
  This is a safety feature, in which Word creates a backup copy every time you save a document. Word gives the backup copy the filename extension .bak.

- Allow Fast Saves
  This option speeds up the saving process by saving just the revisions made to a document.

- Prompt for Summary Info
  This option reminds you to save a document with summary information, such as the title or author of the document. Summary information can be used to search for a specific document. Searching is discussed in Lesson 28: "Word File Management."

- Prompt to Save Normal.dot
  This option asks if you want to save any changes you may have made to the NORMAL.DOT template when you exit Word.

- Automatic Save
  With this option, Word saves documents at regular intervals that you specify.

- File-Sharing Options
  This option allows you to assign a password to a document to protect it from changes. You can only open a password-protected document with the password.

- Read-Only Recommended
  This option recommends to anyone who opens up a document that the document should be read-only, that is, no changes should be made to the document unless necessary.

Note: Word is flexible in that it allows you to change its default settings in a variety of option categories. However, any changes made in the Options dialog box apply from that point forward, until you change the setting back. If you are sharing a computer with other users, do not change any options unless you are advised to do so by your instructor.

Automatic Save

Automatic Save is an excellent safety feature. You can specify the interval, such as every five or ten minutes, at which Word saves a document.

In the event of a power outage or a system failure, you can retrieve the document from the autosave backup file.

However, even with the automatic save feature, a document should still be saved with the Save command before closing it and exiting Word. The Save command performs a complete save with all the most recent revisions to the document, from the time of the last automatic save.

Remember, if you forget to save a document before closing it, Word asks if you want to save the changes to the document. When you click "Yes," Word performs the save and closes the document.

To perform a final save of the revised document and exit Word:

1. Click the Save button.

2. Close the document and exit Word (unless you will be doing the following exercises immediately).

Table 2-6: Keyboard Shortcuts for Revising Text

Keyboard Shortcut	Action
Ctrl+Shift+Spacebar	Insert nonbreaking space
Shift+Enter	Insert line-break character
Shift+F5	Return to previous editing location
Ctrl+Z	Undo
Ctrl+Y	Redo or Repeat
F4	Repeat
Ctrl+F12	Open
Shift+F12	Save
F12	Save As

Keyboard Shortcut	To Move the Insertion Point
Ctrl+Left Arrow	One word to the left
Ctrl+Right Arrow	One word to the right
Home	Beginning of the line
End	End of the line
Ctrl+Up Arrow	One paragraph up
Ctrl+Down Arrow	One paragraph down
PgUp	Up one window
PgDn	Down one window
Ctrl+PgUp	To the top of the window
Ctrl+PgDn	To the bottom of the window
Ctrl+Home	Beginning of the document
Ctrl+End	End of the document

Keyboard Shortcut	To Select Text
Shift+Right Arrow	One character to the right
Shift+Left Arrow	One character to the left
Ctrl+Shift+Right Arrow	To the end of a word
Ctrl+Shift+Left Arrow	To the start of a word
Shift+End	To the end of a line
Shift+Home	To the start of a line
Shift+Up Arrow	One line up
Shift+Down Arrow	One line down

Continued on next page

Table 2-6—Continued	
Keyboard Shortcut	To Select Text
Ctrl+Shift+Down Arrow	To the end of a paragraph
Ctrl+Shift+Up Arrow	To the start of a paragraph
Shift+PgDn	One screen down
Shift+PgUp	One screen up
Ctrl+Shift+End	To the end of a document
Ctrl+Shift+Home	To the start of a document
Ctrl+5 (on keypad)	The entire document

Key Terms

Line-break character   Selection

Nonbreaking space   Selection bar

Nonprinting character

Exercises

Exercise 2.1

1. Start Word, if necessary.

2. Open the file 2-1.doc:

    A. Click the Open button on the Standard toolbar.

    B. Choose the drive appropriate for your computer.

    C. Look for the filename, and double-click it.

3. In the second sentence, select the words "the agency" by dragging with the mouse.

4. Key in their place **Duke City Gateway**

5. Move the insertion point to the left of the word "Customers" in the last sentence.

6. Use the Repeat command to change "Customers" to "Duke City Gateway customers":

    A. Click before the "C" of the word, and press the **F4** key.

    B. Enter a space after "Gateway", and change the "C" in "Customers" to lowercase.

7. Replace the first two words of the second sentence, "The videos" with "These travelogues":

    A. Select the words by dragging with the mouse.

    B. Key **These travelogues**

8. Press **Ctrl+End** to move to the end of the document.

9. Press **Enter** twice. Then key the following text, using a line break (**Shift+Enter**) for each new line:

Our most popular travelogues are:
The Grand Canyon
Aloha Hawaii
Paris, City of Light

10. Save the revised document as *[your three-letter identifier]*2-1.doc.

11. Print the document.

12. Close the document and exit Word (unless you will be doing the following exercises immediately).

Exercise 2.2

1. Start Word, if necessary.

2. Open the file 2-2.doc.

3. Select the entire document:

    A. Move the pointer into the selection bar.

    B. Hold down the **Ctrl** key and then click.

4. Delete the text by pressing the **Delete** key.

5. Restore the text by clicking the Undo button on the Standard toolbar.

6. Cancel the selection by clicking anywhere in the document.

7. In the next-to-last sentence, double-click the word "stunt" to select it, and then delete the word.

8. In the last sentence, insert a nonbreaking space between "must" and "see":

    A. Move the insertion point to the space between the two words, and delete the space.

    B. Hold down the **Ctrl+Shift** keys, and press the **Spacebar**.

9. Create a second paragraph with the sentence that begins "For children". Insert a blank line between the two paragraphs.

10. In the last paragraph, replace the word "this" with "the International Balloon Fiesta".

11. Save the document as *[your three-letter identifier]*2-2.doc.

12. Print the document.

13. Close the document and exit Word (unless you will be doing the following exercises immediately).

Exercise 2.3

1. Start Word, if necessary.

2. Open the file 2-3.doc.

3. Revise the document as shown in Figure 2-6.

Figure 2-6

Summer is a great time to visit Albuquerque. ~~In June, there's~~ the New
Mexico Arts & Crafts Fair, ~~featuring~~ *in June features* more than 150 artists and
craftspeople. *Visitors can* Enjoy free working exhibitions, live entertainment, and
wonderful ethnic food.

in Albuquerque
The July 4th fireworks are a special treat. Dozens of aerial displays and
fantastic ground displays are all part of the American Legion Fireworks
Spectacular at University Stadium.

In August, the Cowboy Classic Art Show comes to the New Mexico State
Fairgrounds. Also in August, the Inter-Tribal Ceremonial presents 50
tribes in a dazzling display of parades and dances at Red Rock State Park.

4. In the second sentence of the last paragraph, change the ending to "more than 200 New Mexican craftspeople and artists."

5. In the third sentence, replace "wonderful" with "a wide variety of".

6. In the second sentence of the second paragraph, revise the sentence, so that it begins "Dozens of fantastic aerial and ground displays".

7. Change the last paragraph, so that it is three lines of text as follows (use line breaks to start a new line):

   Coming in August:
   The Cowboy Classic Art Show at the State Fairgrounds
   The Inter-Tribal Ceremonial at Red Rock State Park

8. Save the document as *[your three-letter identifier]*2-3.doc.

9. Print the document.

10. Close the document and exit Word (unless you will be doing the following exercise immediately).

Exercise 2.4: Challenge Yourself

Open the file 2-4.doc. In the first paragraph, create a new paragraph at the sentence that begins "For shoppers". Insert a blank line before the new paragraph, and then merge the second paragraph with the third paragraph.

In the second paragraph, spell out "You'll" and "it's". Replace "the best of" with "superb". Add the following sentence to the end of the paragraph:

Choose from the colorful array of T-shirts, turquoise, Apache baskets, Navajo wool rugs, and much more.

In the last paragraph, change "278 years" to "280 years", and add a nonbreaking space between "280" and "years". Between the first and second sentences, insert the following text:

The church sits at the northern edge of Old Town Plaza and is the scene for events like the Blessing of the Animals in May and the Old Town Fiesta in June.

Save the document as *[your three-letter identifier]*2-4.doc and print it. Close the document and exit Word.

Character Formatting

The previous lessons have taught the fundamentals of using Word to create and revise documents. So far, though, you have keyed only standard text. This lesson is an introduction to creating text with different character attributes, such as bold, italic, and underline.

What Are Character Attributes and Formats?

A *character attribute* is an option that determines the appearance of the characters that make up a word or a block of text. Suppose you want to emphasize a word in a paragraph. You can do this by giving the word a different character attribute than the other text in the paragraph. For example, you can apply the bold attribute to the word.

This lesson shows how to apply the following character attributes to text:

- Bold
- Italic
- Underline
- All capitals

It also shows how to turn off these attributes to create normal text. Lesson 17: "Symbols, Special Characters, and Attributes" shows how to work with additional character attributes.

Table 3-1: Character-Attribute Options

Attribute	Example	Comments
Normal	This is a sample.	Normal text uses the standard character attributes.
Bold	**This is a sample.**	Bold text is darker and heavier than normal text.
Italic	*This is a sample.*	Italic text is slanted to the right and is somewhat lighter than normal text.
Single underline	<u>This is a sample</u>.	Single-underlined text is underscored with one continuous line.
All capitals	THIS IS A SAMPLE.	All-capitals text appears uppercase regardless of whether you use the **Shift** or **Caps Lock** key to key the text.

Character attributes are often combined. For example, text can be both bold and underlined. All the character attributes you apply to text make up the *character format* of that text.

Character format
The combined character attributes of text.

Table 3-2: Character Formats with Multiple Character Attributes	
Character Format	Example
Bold, italic, and all capitals	***THIS IS A SAMPLE.***
Single underlined and bold	**This is a sample.**
Single underlined and italic	*This is a sample*.
Bold and italic	***This is a sample.***

Word includes features that allow you to repeat a single character attribute or an entire character format of selected text without specifying the attributes individually. You can also copy an existing character format to another block of existing text.

Specifying Character Attributes

There are several ways to specify character attributes, using either the mouse or key combinations. You can specify character attributes for text before keying it or for existing text.

Using the Font Dialog Box

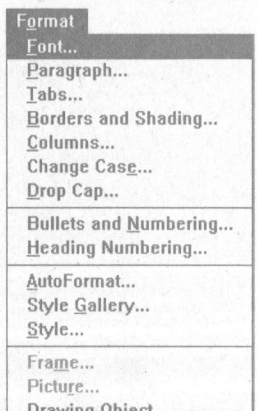

. Format menu

Font
A type design, such as Times New Roman or Courier.

Note: Fonts are discussed in more detail in Lesson 16: "Fonts and Type Sizes."

The Font dialog box can be used to turn on or off all optional character attributes. To display the Font dialog box, choose Font from the Format menu. *Font* refers to the design of type, such as Times New Roman or Courier. Character attributes, such as bold or italic, affect the font style.

The Font dialog box contains check boxes and list boxes that you can use to specify any character attribute. It also shows a preview of text with the specified attributes. See Figure 3-1 on page 47.

The Font Style list box allows you to choose italic, bold, bold italic, or regular (no character attribute). The Underline drop-down list box allows you to choose from several types of underline styles. The Effects group contains check boxes to choose additional character attributes, such as All Caps, which is discussed in this lesson. All other character attributes in this group are discussed in Lesson 17: "Symbols, Special Characters, and Attributes."

The Preview box in the Font dialog box shows how text looks with the character attributes that are turned on. The appearance of the text in the Preview box changes whenever you turn on or off an attribute option. This allows you to experiment with different character attributes before you click OK to specify a character format.

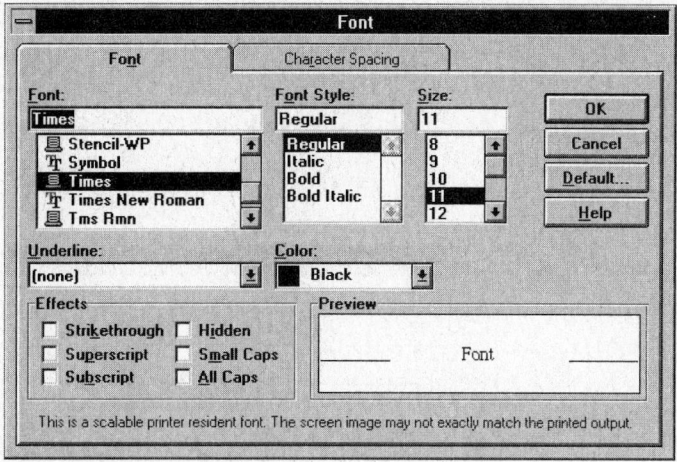

Figure 3-1
The Font dialog box

Note: When working with check boxes in a dialog box, click the check box to turn on an option. An X will appear in the check box. Click a check box to turn off an option and clear the check box.

To specify character attributes for new text using the Font dialog box:

1. Start Word, if necessary.

2. Open the file 3-0.doc.

3. Move the insertion point to the end of the first line. Remember, to go to the end of the line, press the **End** key.

4. Press **Enter** twice.

5. Choose Font from the Format menu.

   The Font dialog box appears.

6. Click the Font tab, if necessary.

7. Choose Bold from the Font Style list, and click the All Caps check box.

   The text in the Preview box appears in bold capital letters.

8. Click OK to close the Character dialog box.

9. Key **culture is alive in the desert!**

   The text appears in bold capital letters.

You can also change the character attributes of existing text using the Font dialog box.

To turn on or off character attributes for existing text:

1. In the paragraph that begins "July 1", select "Madame Butterfly".

2. Choose Font from the Format menu.

3. Choose the Bold and All Caps character attributes.

4. Click OK to close the dialog box.

The selected text appears in bold capital letters.

5. With the text still selected, open the Font dialog box again.

6. Click the All Caps check box to turn off this attribute.

7. Click OK to close the dialog box.

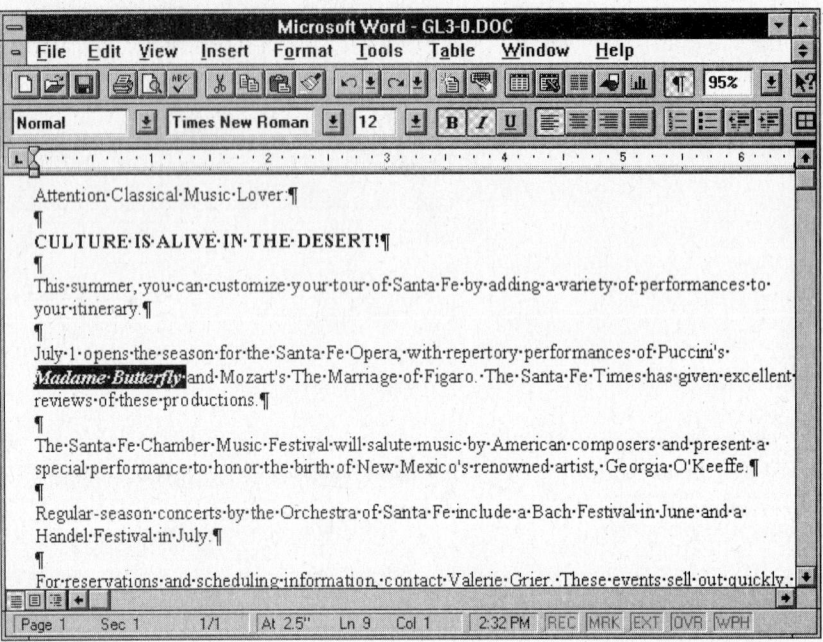

Figure 3-2
Applying character formatting

Using the Shortcut Menu

In addition to opening the Font dialog box using the menu bar, you can also open it using the shortcut menu. Shortcut menus access the most common Word commands and save the time it would take to search for the command on the regular menus.

To open a shortcut menu, click the right mouse button. To use the shortcut menu to access the Font dialog box, select the text you wish to format (or position the insertion point where you wish to key formatted text), click the right mouse button, and then choose Font from the shortcut menu. Once in the Font dialog box, choose the desired character attributes.

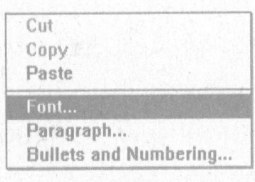

Shortcut menu

To open the Font dialog box using the shortcut menu:

1. With the text "Madame Butterfly" still selected, click the right mouse button.

   Word displays the shortcut menu.

2. Choose Font from the shortcut menu.

   Word opens the Font dialog box.

3. Choose the font style Bold Italic.

   The text in the Preview box appears in bold italic letters.

4. Click OK to close the dialog box.

Using the Formatting Toolbar

Character-attribute buttons on the Formatting toolbar

You can click buttons on the Formatting toolbar to switch on and off the bold, italic, and underline options. Clicking the buttons is generally faster than using the Font dialog box.

When you click a button on the Formatting toolbar to switch on an option, the button is highlighted. Click a highlighted button to turn off the option.

For example, to create italic text, click the Italic button. The text you key when the Italic button is highlighted appears in italics. To return to keying text that is not in italics, click the Italic button again to turn off the option.

If you select existing text with a character format that includes bold, italics, or continuous single underlining, the button for that optional attribute is highlighted. You can click the button to switch the bold, italic, or underline options on or off for selected text.

When you click the Underline button to specify underlining, the text appears with a continuous single underline.

To specify character attributes for new and existing text using the Formatting toolbar:

1. In the paragraph that begins "July 1", select "The Marriage of Figaro".

Italic and Underline buttons highlighted

2. Click the Italic and Underline buttons.

   The buttons appear highlighted. The selected text appears underlined and in italic letters.

3. Click the Underline button to turn the option off, and then click the Bold button.

   The selected text appears in bold italics.

4. Move the insertion point to the end of the paragraph, and press the **Spacebar** once.

5. Key **Its production of**, press the **Spacebar** once, and then click the Bold and Italic buttons.

   The buttons are highlighted.

6. Key **La Boheme**, and then click the Bold and Italic buttons to turn them off.

7. Press the **Spacebar** once, and key **won a rave review from Opera News magazine.**

Using Keyboard Shortcuts

In addition to the Font dialog box and the Formatting toolbar, there are keyboard shortcuts to switch on and off the bold, italic, and underline character-attribute options. The keyboard shortcut for the bold, italic, or underline options consists of the **Ctrl** key and the option's initial letter. For example, **Ctrl+B** is the keyboard shortcut for switching on and off the bold option. The keyboard shortcut for the all-capitals option is **Ctrl+Shift+A**. To remove character attributes from text, press **Ctrl+Spacebar**. Using keyboard shortcuts is faster than using the Font dialog box to specify character attributes.

To use keyboard shortcuts for new and existing text:

1. Move the insertion point to the end of the document, and then press **Enter** twice to start a new paragraph. (Remember, you can press **Ctrl+End** to go to the end of a document.)

2. Press **Ctrl+Shift+A** to turn on the all-capitals option, and then press **Ctrl+B** to turn on the bold option.

3. Key **jazz fans note:**

   The text appears in bold capital letters. Note that the Bold button on the Formatting toolbar is highlighted.

4. Press **Ctrl+Shift+A** to turn off the all-capitals option.

5. Press the **Spacebar**, and then key the following:

   The first annual Desert Bloom Jazz Festival, featuring some of the world's greatest musicians, will be held in Santa Fe next May 1-15.

   The text appears in bold capital and lowercase letters.

A Shortcut for Changing the Case of Characters

To change the case of characters quickly and easily, use the keyboard shortcut **Shift+F3**. This key combination acts as a three-way toggle that can change text to uppercase, lowercase, and mixed case (words with the first letter uppercase).

For example, to change all lowercase characters to uppercase characters, select the text, and then press **Shift+F3**. The text becomes all uppercase. Press **Shift+F3** again, and the text changes to words with the first letter uppercase and all other characters lowercase. Press **Shift+F3** again, and the text changes back to all lowercase.

Select	Keyboard Shortcut	Result
this text	Press **Shift+F3**	THIS TEXT
THIS TEXT	Press **Shift+F3**	This Text
This Text	Press **Shift+F3**	this text

To change the case of just a word, you can place the insertion point anywhere in the word (instead of selecting the word) and press **Shift+F3**.

6. Select the last sentence of the preceding paragraph.

7. Press **Ctrl+I** to turn on the italic option.

The selected text appears in italics.

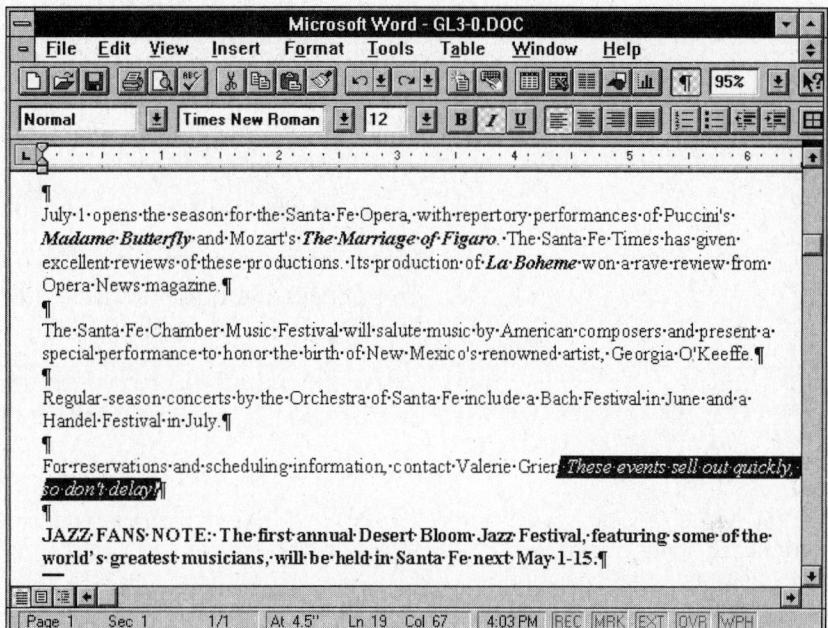

Figure 3-3
The document with additional character formatting

8. Select the first line of the document, and then press **Ctrl+Shift+A**.

The selected text appears in all-capital letters.

Repeating Character Attributes

If you have just applied a character attribute to selected text, you can repeat that attribute for other selected or new text. This can be done by either choosing the Repeat command from the Edit menu or using the keyboard shortcut **Ctrl+Y** or the **F4** key.

For example, if you have just used the Formatting toolbar or a keyboard shortcut to apply the bold attribute, Repeat Bold will appear on the Edit menu. You can choose this menu option to repeat the formatting for other text. This option remains on the Edit menu only until text is keyed, or until the Font dialog box is used to create another format. Therefore, if you want to repeat an attribute, you must do so immediately after you apply it.

Use the Repeat option to repeat only the last attribute you applied, not an entire format consisting of several attributes. For example, suppose you select text, press **Ctrl+B** to apply bold to the selected text, and then press **Ctrl+I** to apply italics to the text. The Repeat

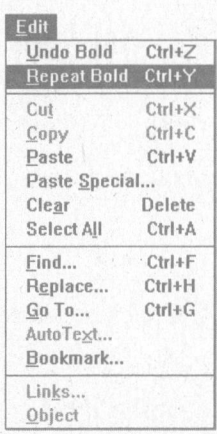

Edit menu with Repeat
Bold option

option would repeat only the italic attribute, not the entire bold italic format.

To practice repeating character attributes for new and existing text:

1. Select the paragraph that begins "This summer" (double-click in the left margin to select it), and then click the Bold button on the Formatting toolbar.

    The paragraph appears bold.

2. Select the text "Santa Fe Chamber Music Festival".

3. Choose Repeat Bold from the Edit menu.

    The selected text appears bold.

4. In the paragraph that begins "July 1", select "repertory", and then press **Ctrl+I** to apply italics to the selected word.

5. Move the insertion point to the next paragraph, before the word "special", and press the **F4** key.

    Notice that the Italic button is highlighted.

6. Make sure that Word is in insert mode, key **very**, and press the **Spacebar** once.

    The word appears in italics.

Repeating Character Formats

Suppose you use the Font dialog box to apply a character format to selected text, and you want to apply the same format to other new or existing text. Perhaps the format is a complicated one, calling for bold, italic, all-capital characters. You can choose Repeat Font Formatting from the Edit menu, or you can press the **F4** key or **Ctrl+Y** to repeat the format.

Repeat Font Formatting appears on the Edit menu after using the Font dialog box to specify a character attribute. This option remains on the Edit menu only until text is keyed, or until a keyboard shortcut or a Formatting toolbar button is used to apply an optional character attribute.

To repeat character formats for new and existing text:

1. Select the first line, click the right mouse button, and then choose Font from the shortcut menu.

    Word displays the Font dialog box.

2. Choose the Bold font style, and leave the All Caps check box checked. Click OK to close the dialog box.

3. Select the paragraph that begins "Regular-season", and choose Repeat Font Formatting from the Edit menu.

Note: Remember, Word is in insert mode unless "OVR" appears in black letters on the status bar. Use the **Insert** key or double-click "OVR" on the status bar to switch between insert and overtype mode.

Edit	
Undo Font Formatting	Ctrl+Z
Repeat Font Formatting	Ctrl+Y
Cut	Ctrl+X
Copy	Ctrl+C
Paste	Ctrl+V
Paste Special...	
Clear	Delete
Select All	Ctrl+A
Find...	Ctrl+F
Replace...	Ctrl+H
Go To...	Ctrl+G
AutoText...	
Bookmark...	
Links...	
Object	

Edit menu with Repeat Font Formatting option

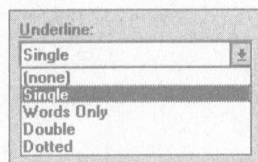

Underline options in the Font dialog box

Note: Punctuation marks, such as periods or exclamation marks, should not be underlined.

The paragraph appears in a bold, all-capitals format.

4. Select the second line, which begins "Culture is", and then choose Font from the shortcut menu.

5. Choose the Italic font style.

6. Click the down arrow on the Underline drop-down list box, and then choose Single from the drop-down list.

7. Click OK to close the dialog box.

    The selected line appears in all capitals and underlined italics.

8. Move the insertion point to the end of the document, and then press the **F4** key.

    Notice that the Italic and Underline buttons are highlighted.

9. Press the **Spacebar** once, and then key:

    We will send out performance schedules around the end of this year.

    The text appears in underlined italics.

10. Click the Underline button on the Formatting toolbar to turn off that attribute, and then key a period.

11. Select the space character at the beginning of the sentence (to the left of "_We_"), and click the Underline button to turn it off.

12. Select the exclamation point in the second line, and click the Underline button to remove the underline.

Copying Character Formats

You can copy a character format and apply it to selected text. This can be faster than assigning individual character-format options to the selected text, especially if the format uses several optional attributes.

Format Painter button

Paintbrush pointer

To copy a character format to selected text, use the Format Painter button on the Standard toolbar. For example, to copy the character formatting from sentence "A" to sentence "B", select sentence "A", and then click the Format Painter button. The mouse pointer changes to a paintbrush with an I-beam pointer. Use the paintbrush pointer to select sentence "B". Word will copy the character formatting.

You may wish to use the Format Painter button to copy character formatting to several selections in a document. To do this, select the text with the desired formatting, and double-click the Format Painter button. Then, each time you select text with the paintbrush pointer, the formatting is copied. To restore the pointer to the normal I-beam, press the **Esc** key, or click the Format Painter button.

To copy a character format using the Format Painter button:

1. In the paragraph that begins "July 1", select "The Santa Fe Times".

2. Click the Underline button on the Formatting toolbar to underline the publication name.

3. Click the Format Painter button on the Standard toolbar.

   The pointer changes to a paintbrush with an I-beam.

4. Use the paintbrush pointer to select "Opera News" in the next sentence.

   Word underlines the selected text.

5. Select the bold all-capitals word "REGULAR" two paragraphs down.

6. Double-click the Format Painter button, so it can be used repeatedly.

7. Select the first sentence in the last paragraph (through "May 1-15.").

   Word copies the formatting to the sentence.

8. Select the last sentence in the last paragraph.

   The entire paragraph is in bold and all-capital letters.

9. Press the **Esc** key to restore the I-beam pointer.

10. Save the document as *[your three-letter identifier]*3-0.doc.

11. Print the document.

12. Close the document and exit Word (unless you will be doing the following exercises immediately).

Note: When using Format Painter to copy formatting to a paragraph or line of text, you can move the paintbrush pointer to the selection bar. When the pointer changes to an arrow, you can select the text quickly. For example, you can double-click in the selection bar to select the paragraph, instead of dragging the paintbrush pointer through the entire paragraph.

Table 3-3: Keyboard Shortcuts for Character Attributes	
Keyboard Shortcut	Action
Ctrl+B	Turn on or off the bold option
Ctrl+I	Turn on or off the italic option
Ctrl+U	Turn on or off single, continuous underlining
Ctrl+Shift+A	Turn on or off the all-capitals option
Ctrl+Spacebar	Turn off the bold, italic, underline, or all-capitals option
Shift+F3	Change the case of characters
F4 or **Ctrl+Y**	Repeat a character attribute or a character format

Key Terms

Character attribute   Font

Character format

Exercises

Exercise 3.1

1. Start Word, if necessary.

2. Open the file 3-1.doc.

3. Select the first line, and apply the bold character attribute by using the Font dialog box:

    A. Choose Font from the Format menu.

    B. Choose the Bold font style, and then click OK to close the dialog box.

4. Move the insertion point to the end of the document, and press **Enter** twice to start a new paragraph.

5. Press **Ctrl+Shift+A** to turn on the all-capitals attribute, and then key:

    rates do not include tax or insurance charges.

6. Move the insertion point to the end of the second line, before the colon. Press the **Spacebar** and key **(except for**

7. Press the **Spacebar**, click the Italic button on the Formatting toolbar, and then key **holiday**

8. Press **Ctrl+I** to turn off the italic option, and then press the **Spacebar** and key **weekends)**

9. Double-click the word "holiday", and click the Underline button.

10. Copy the character format from the word "holiday" to the sentence that begins "We try our best":

    A. Select the word "holiday".

    B. Click the Format Painter button on the Standard toolbar.

    C. Use the paintbrush pointer to select the sentence that begins "We try our best".

11. Save the document as *[your three-letter identifier]*3-1.doc.

12. Print the document.

13. Close the document and exit Word (unless you will be doing the following exercises immediately).

Exercise 3.2

1. Start Word, if necessary.

2. Open the file 3-2.doc.

3. Select the first line, and then use the keyboard shortcuts **Ctrl+B** to apply the bold attribute and **Ctrl+Shift+A** to apply the all-capitals attribute.

4. Select "101 Reasons to Visit the Caribbean" in the next paragraph, and then use the Italic button to apply the italic attribute.

5. Position the insertion point in the next paragraph, before the word "interesting", and repeat the previously selected character formatting:

    A. From the Edit menu, choose Repeat Italic. (You can also press the **F4** key.)

    B. Check the status bar to be sure that Word is in insert mode, key **very**, and press the **Spacebar**.

6. Position the insertion point at the beginning of the last line.

7. Key **This book is**, and press the **Spacebar**.

8. Select the entire last line, and then use the shortcut menu to open the Font dialog box:

    A. Click the right mouse button.

    B. Choose Font from the shortcut menu.

9. Choose the bold italic and all-capitals attributes from the Font dialog box, and then click OK.

10. Use the Formatting toolbar to add the bold attribute to the book title in the second paragraph.

11. Save the document as *[your three-letter identifier]*3-2.doc.

12. Print the document.

13. Close the document and exit Word (unless you will be doing the following exercises immediately).

Exercise 3.3

1. Start Word, if necessary.

2. Open the file 3-3.doc.

3. Apply the all-capitals and underline attributes to the first line.

4.   Add the bold and all-capitals attributes to the word "Hotel" (above "Crown Beach Resort").

5.   Change the first hotel name, "Crown Beach Resort", to italic, all-capital letters.

6.   Use the Format Painter button to copy the all-capitals and italics character formatting to the next four hotel names. (Remember to double-click the Format Painter button for multiple copying and to press the **Esc** key when you are done copying.)

7.   Position the insertion point at the end of the document. Press **Enter** to start a new paragraph, and then key in bold italics:

     Payment must be made before ticketing.

8.   Turn the bold and italic attributes off, press the **Spacebar**, and then key:

     All major credit cards are accepted.

9.   Remove the underlining from the first paragraph, and apply the bold attribute.

10. Save the document as *[your three-letter identifier]*3-3.doc.

11. Print the document.

12. Close the document and exit Word (unless you will be doing the following exercise immediately).

Exercise 3.4: Challenge Yourself

Create a new document, and key the text in Figure 3-4, which appears at the end of this exercise. Include the corrections.

Apply the all-capitals attribute to "Tourist/Budget" in the first line. Then copy this formatting to the words "Moderate", "First Class", "Deluxe", and "Luxury". Beginning with "MODERATE", create four new paragraphs from each of the words with the copied formatting. Insert a blank line between each of the paragraphs.

At the beginning of the document, as a separate paragraph, key the following, using the bold and all-capitals attributes:

guide to hotel classification

Leave a blank line between this line and the next paragraph. In the second paragraph, apply the bold attribute to "the lowest possible prices". Repeat this formatting for the words "the world's finest" in the last paragraph. Select the entire document, and apply the italic attribute.

Save the document as *[your three-letter identifier]*3-4.doc and print it. Close the document and exit Word.

58

LESSON 3

Figure 3-4

In hotel classificatoin, Tourist/Budget is geared to those seeking the lowest possible prices. This type of property has limited ~~services~~ *amenities*, yet offers functional accommodations. Moderate means the hotel is suitable for cost conscious clients. The rooms are simple and comfortable. First Class hotels offer a selective variety of facilities ~~and services~~ *STET* that will please a majority of travellers. Deluxe hotels are outstanding properties with fine rooms, public areas, and services. They are the better hotels in the area and will satisfy most discriminating travellers. Luxury hotels are the exceptional hotels, offering the highest standard of service and facilities. *They are classified as the world's finest.*

Writing Tools

Objectives

- Correct spelling errors automatically.

- Use the spelling-check tool.

- Use the grammar-check tool.

- Choose grammar and spelling options.

- Use the thesaurus.

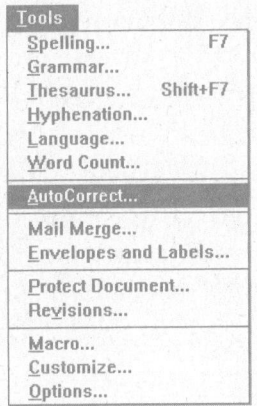

Tools menu

Word provides writing tools to help you correct spelling and grammar errors. Word also provides a thesaurus to help you improve your writing vocabulary.

Correcting Spelling Errors Automatically

The AutoCorrect feature in Word corrects commonly misspelled words automatically, as you key text. For example, if you key a sentence with the word "teh" for "the", Word will automatically change the spelling to "the".

To see how AutoCorrect works:

1. Start Word, if necessary.

2. Create a new document.

3. To make sure AutoCorrect is turned on, choose AutoCorrect from the Tools menu.

   Word displays the AutoCorrect dialog box.

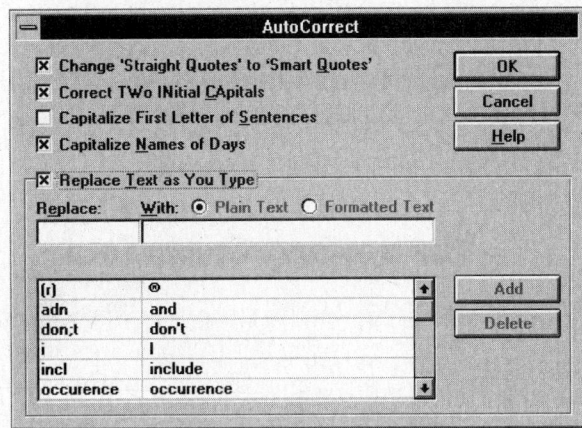

Figure 4-1
The AutoCorrect dialog box

4. Check the Replace Text as You Type check box, if necessary, and click OK to close the dialog box.

5. Key the following sentence with the spelling as shown:

   i am testing teh AutoCorrect feature.

   Word corrects "i" and "teh" automatically.

59

In addition to correcting commonly misspelled words, AutoCorrect can make additional types of automatic corrections. The following options may be chosen from the AutoCorrect dialog box:

- Change 'Straight Quotes' to 'Smart Quotes'

  This option automatically changes straight quotation marks to the type that open and close, which are used by typesetters.

- Correct TWo INitial Capitals

  This option corrects words typed accidentally with two initial capital letters, such as "WOrd" or "THis".

- Capitalize First Letter of Sentences

  This option corrects any word at the beginning of a sentence that is not keyed with a capital letter.

- Capitalize Names of Days

  This option corrects a day spelled without an initial capital letter. For example, "monday" will be corrected to "Monday" automatically.

If there are words that you commonly misspell that are not already on the AutoCorrect list (which is shown in the AutoCorrect dialog box), you can add them to the list. To do this, key the misspelled word in the Replace box, and key the corrected word in the With box.

Note: AutoCorrect corrects newly keyed text. An AutoCorrect option cannot be used to correct an existing document. To correct the spelling of an existing document, use the spelling-check tool.

The Spelling-Check Tool

Checking spelling is a word-processing procedure that should become a routine step in proofing documents. You can check spelling while working on or after completing a document. Word's spelling-check tool compares the spelling in a document with the spelling in the program's internal dictionary. If a word in the document does not match up with a word in the dictionary, Word brings it to your attention. The Spelling dialog box appears, from which you can choose an action to take. For example, you can:

- Choose from a list of words that may be offered for the correct spelling, and instruct Word to make the change

- Leave the word unchanged by instructing Word to ignore it

- Add the word to a custom dictionary that can be set up for special words (including names and abbreviations) not contained in Word's dictionary

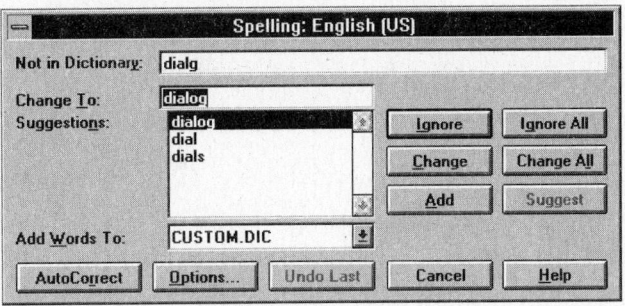

Figure 4-2
The Spelling dialog box

What Spelling Check Can and Cannot Do

Word's spelling-check tool can find many mistakes and provide useful suggestions, but it is important to understand what it can and cannot do.

Along with finding regular misspellings, spelling check can find:

- Repeated words, such as "the the" in a sentence

- Words that should have their first letter capitalized, such as "colorado"

- Words with unusual capitalization, such as "vAcation"

Spelling check has some limitations. It cannot find:

- A word that is correctly spelled but incorrectly keyed

  For example, you key "sue" when you meant to key "use".

- A word that is correctly spelled but incorrectly used

  For example, if you use the word "your" instead of "you're" in a sentence, a spelling check will not catch it. In this case, proofreading is essential.

- Special words, such as proper names, technical terms, acronyms, or abbreviations, that are not in Word's dictionary

  This means that every one of these unfamiliar words will be questioned during the spelling-check process. To minimize this, you can add the words to a custom dictionary, which is discussed later in this lesson.

Using Spelling Check

Spelling check can confirm the spelling of a single word, a group of words, or all the words in a document. There are three ways to issue the spelling-check command:

- Choose Spelling from the Tools menu

Spelling button

- Click the Spelling button on the Standard toolbar

- Press the **F7** key

To begin the process:

1. Close the open document without saving it.

2. Open the file 4-0.doc.

   When you issue the Spelling command, it starts spell-checking from where the insertion point is in the document. (It is now at the beginning.) If you select just a word or sentence to spell-check, Word will check just that selection.

To spell-check a word in the document:

1. Select the word "profesionals" at the end of the paragraph that begins "Their are field".

2. Click the Spelling button on the Standard toolbar, or press the **F7** key.

   Word displays the Spelling dialog box when it finds a word that is not in the spelling-check dictionary. A list of suggested words is shown. The first word on the list is usually the most probable spelling. This word is highlighted and displayed in the Change To box.

   Behind the dialog box, Word scrolls to the portion of the document containing the word and highlights the word. See Figure 4-3 on page 63.

From the Spelling dialog box, you can:

- Change the spelling

   To accept the correction Word suggests, click the Change button. To correct all occurrences of the word in the document, click the Change All button.

- Choose from suggested words

   To choose one of the suggested words, click it, and click the Change button or the Change All button (or double-click the word).

   When Word cannot suggest a correction, you can choose the Suggest button for possible word ideas that are close to the spelling of the word.

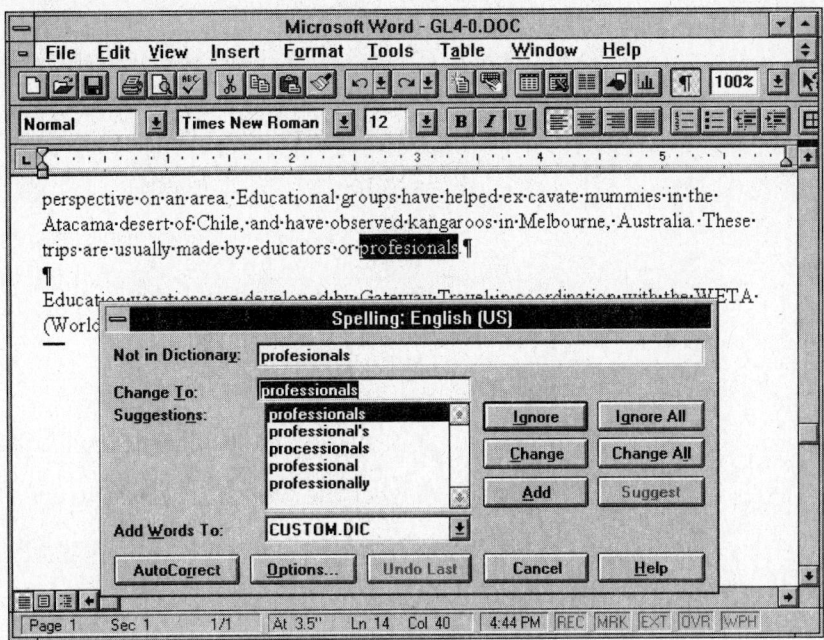

Figure 4-3
Spelling check finds a misspelled word

- Leave the word unchanged

  To leave the word unchanged and continue with the spelling check, click the Ignore button. To ignore all occurrences of the word in the document, click the Ignore All button.

- Delete a repeated word

  If Word finds a repeated word, click the Delete button to remove the repeated word. If your intention is to repeat the word, click the Ignore button, and continue with the spelling check.

- Add the word to a custom dictionary

  If Word does not recognize a word or term you use, you can add it to a custom dictionary. You can create several dictionaries for different types of words, such as one dictionary for technical terms and one for foreign words or names. Once added to a dictionary, these words are not questioned during a spelling check.

- Add a word to the AutoCorrect list

  To have Word correct a misspelling automatically in the future, click the AutoCorrect button. This adds the misspelled word and its correction to the AutoCorrect list. Use this option for words you frequently misspell.

- Interrupt spelling check to edit the document

  To interrupt the spelling check temporarily to make some changes in the document, click outside the dialog box in the document window or press **Ctrl+Tab**. This allows you to make changes or scroll through the now-active document window. To restart the spelling check, click the Start button in the Spelling dialog box.

- Undo the last correction

  After changing the spelling of word during a spelling check, you can click the Undo Last button to undo the correction. The Undo Last button will undo only the most recent change made.

- Cancel spelling check

  To end the spelling check at any time, click the Cancel or Close button, or press the **Esc** key.

To correct the word displayed in the Spelling dialog box:

1. Click Change to correct the spelling.

   Word changes the spelling in the document, and displays a dialog box to say it has completed checking the word selected. It asks if you want to continue checking from the beginning of the document.

2. Click No to return to the document.

To practice using spelling check and its various features by spell-checking a sentence:

1. Select the sentence that contains the word "professionals".

2. Press the **F7** key.

   Word does not show the Spelling dialog box, indicating that all words are spelled correctly. It displays a box that asks if you want to continue checking the rest of the document. Click No to return to the document.

To spell-check the entire document:

1. Move the insertion point to the beginning of the document. Click the Spelling button on the Standard toolbar.

   The Spelling dialog box shows a misspelled word, "formaal".

2. Click the Change box to correct the spelling.

   Word makes the correction and moves on to "11AM", with no suggested spellings.

3. Since the travel agency often uses this time format, click Ignore All. Spelling options for this usage are changed later in the lesson.

   Word finds a repeated word, "as as".

4. Click Delete.

Word removes the repeated word in the sentence, and then stops on "cavate". This is not a word, but the result of a wrongly placed space in the word "excavate".

5. Click in the text area outside the dialog box to interrupt the spelling check temporarily and activate the document window.

    Notice the change in the Spelling dialog box. The text can now be edited.

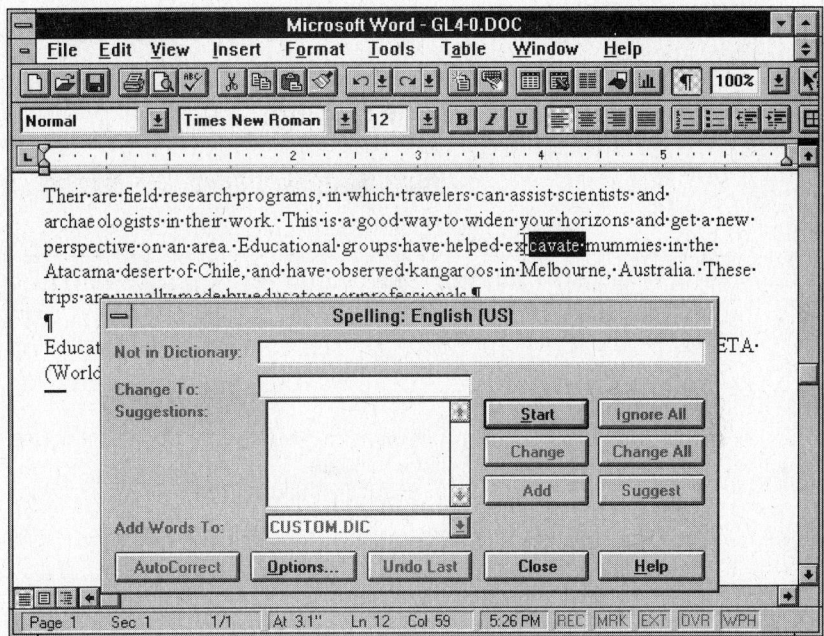

Figure 4-4

Activating the document window during a spelling check

6. Move the insertion point to the space between "ex" and "cavate". Delete the space.

7. Click Start in the dialog box to reactivate the spelling check for the remainder of the document.

    Word stops on "Atacama". This is a correctly spelled name that is not in Word's dictionary. A custom dictionary for this word is created later in the lesson.

8. Click Ignore.

    Word stops on "WETA". This is an acronym not in the Word dictionary. Spelling options for this word are changed later in the lesson.

9. Click Ignore.

    Word indicates that the spelling check is complete. Click OK to return to the document.

Choosing Spelling Options

You can control how Word checks spelling by choosing options for the Spelling command. Using the Options dialog box for spelling, you can instruct Word to ignore certain types of words and create custom dictionaries for special words. There are two ways to choose spelling options:

- Before you spell-check a document, choose Options from the Tools menu, and click the Spelling tab

- After you start the spelling check, click the Options button in the Spelling dialog box

Figure 4-5
Spelling options

Words to Ignore

There are two categories of words you can instruct Word to ignore during the spelling check:

- Words in uppercase

  This includes words in all-uppercase letters and any combination of uppercase letters and numbers, such as "TWA" or "RTE66".

- Words with numbers

  This includes any combination of characters that include numbers, such as "DC-10" or "12PM".

To choose spelling options:

1. Choose Options from the Tools menu, and click the Spelling tab.

   The Options dialog box for spelling is displayed.

2. Choose Words in UPPERCASE from the Ignore box.

   This makes Word ignore the acronym "WETA" in the document.

3. Choose Words with Numbers from the Ignore box.

   This makes Word ignore "11AM" and similar combinations in the document.

4. Click OK to return to the document.

Note: Remember, changes made in any Options dialog box remain in effect even after you quit Word. For this course, when options are changed for practice purposes, you will be directed to reset the original options before the lesson is completed.

Custom Dictionaries

Word uses a standard dictionary that may not contain the special words, names, or abbreviations you commonly use. By adding these words to a custom dictionary, Word will not question them during spelling checks.

Word has already created a custom dictionary called CUSTOM.DIC. You can add words to this dictionary throughout the spelling-check process. Additional custom dictionaries can be created for special categories of words, such as the names of clients and associates, foreign words, or technical terms. You can create as many custom dictionaries as needed.

Like a document filename, a custom-dictionary filename can be no more than eight letters. Unlike document filenames, which have the extension ".doc", dictionary filenames end with ".dic".

To create a custom dictionary:

1. Make sure the insertion point is at the beginning of the document, and press the **F7** key to start the spelling check.

   Notice how Word accepts all the changes made thus far and stops on "Atacama". At this point, you can either add the word to the existing custom dictionary called CUSTOM.DIC or create a new custom dictionary.

2. From the Spelling dialog box, click Options.

   The Options dialog box for spelling appears.

3. In the Custom Dictionaries option group, click New.

   The Create Custom Dictionary dialog box appears.

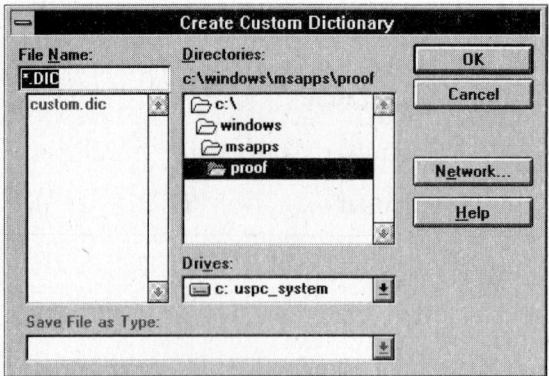

Figure 4-6
The Create Custom Dictionary dialog box

Note: You can also just
key the drive and the filename in the text box. For
example, key **a:world.dic**

4. Change to the appropriate drive to create the custom
    dictionary on your floppy disk and not on the hard drive.
    Then key **world.dic** in the File Name text box.

5. Click OK.

    Word creates a custom dictionary called WORLD.DIC and
    adds it to the list of dictionaries in the Options dialog box.

6. Click OK in the Options dialog box.

    Word returns to the Spelling dialog box.

7. Click the arrow in the Add Words To drop-down list box to
    reveal the new dictionary.

8. Choose the new dictionary and click Add.

    "Atacama" is added to the new dictionary, WORLD.DIC. Word
    completes the spelling check, skipping over the previously
    questioned items "11AM" and "WETA" because of the change
    in spelling options.

Note: You can always delete a word from a custom
dictionary by opening the
dictionary file. A dictionary
file is simply a text file. It is
a list of words, any of
which can be selected and
deleted.

9. Click OK to return to the document.

Selective Spell-Checking

Another way to control how Word spell-checks a document is by selecting portions of a document that you do not want spell-checked.
For example, suppose your document contains a table of technical
terms that you do not want to add to a custom dictionary. You also do
not want Word to flag each of these words during a spelling check of
the document.

You can eliminate this portion of the document from the spelling
check. To do this, select the text, and then choose Language from the
Format menu. In the Language dialog box, the Mark Selected Text As
list box is set for English (U.S.). This is the dictionary used during the
spell check. Scroll up the list box, and choose the first option (no
proofing). When you spell-check the document, Word will ignore the
selected text.

The Grammar-Check Tool

Grammar check is another valuable Word tool that can improve the quality of a document. The Grammar command checks sentences for:

• Grammatical errors

• Stylistic errors

• Readability

Grammar check suggests corrections, just like spelling check. From the Grammar dialog box, you can choose the correction and have Word change the sentence, or you can ignore the suggestion, find out more about the error, or make changes directly in the document.

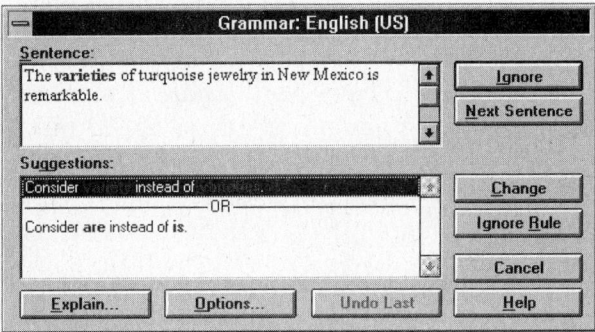

Figure 4-7
The Grammar dialog box

Grammar check also checks for spelling. If it finds a questionable word, the Spelling dialog box is temporarily displayed over the Grammar dialog box, so that the correction can be made.

Like spelling check, grammar check has an Options feature that allows you to customize the Grammar command by changing the particular rules observed during the checking process.

Using Grammar Check

You can use grammar check for a single sentence or for an entire document. To check the grammar of a document, choose Grammar from the Tools menu. Word checks all of the document beginning at the insertion point. To check a portion of the document, such as a sentence or paragraph, select that portion before choosing the Grammar command.

To start grammar check:

1.   Move the insertion point to the beginning of the document 4-0.doc.

Tools menu

2. Choose Grammar from the Tools menu.

Word displays the Grammar dialog box when it finds questionable usage. In the dialog box, it displays the sentence in the Sentence box with the questionable word(s) in bold and lists suggestions. Behind the dialog box, Word scrolls to and highlights the sentence in the document.

From the Grammar dialog box, you can:

- Change the sentence

  To accept the correction Word suggests, click the Change button or double-click the suggestion. Word then updates the document.

- Leave the sentence unchanged

  To leave the found word or phrase unchanged and continue with the grammar check, click the Ignore button. Word moves on to the rest of the sentence. To leave the entire sentence unchanged, click the Next Sentence button.

  To have Word ignore all similar occurrences of the grammatical error it has found, click the Ignore Rule button. For example, if Word questions the use of a passive verb, you can allow passive verb usage for the remainder of the grammar check by choosing Ignore Rule.

- Ask Word to explain the error

  For more information about the error, click the Explain button. Word displays a dialog box describing the rule of grammar or style in question.

- Interrupt the grammar check to edit the sentence

  When Word cannot suggest a correction, you can interrupt the grammar check temporarily to type a correction directly in the document. To do this, click outside the dialog box or press **Ctrl+Tab** to activate the document window. Once the change is make, restart Grammar check by clicking the Start button in the dialog box.

In the dialog box on the screen, Word is pointing out a grammatical error in the use of the word "are", which is in bold. (If you have a color monitor, the bold text is red.)

To change the word to "is" and continue checking grammar in the document:

1. Click the Change button.

   Word makes the change in the document and moves on to the next sentence. In the new sentence, the words "are held" are in bold. No suggestion is given, only the indication that this is the use of a passive verb.

2.   Click the Explain button for further information.

     A window describing usage of the passive voice appears.

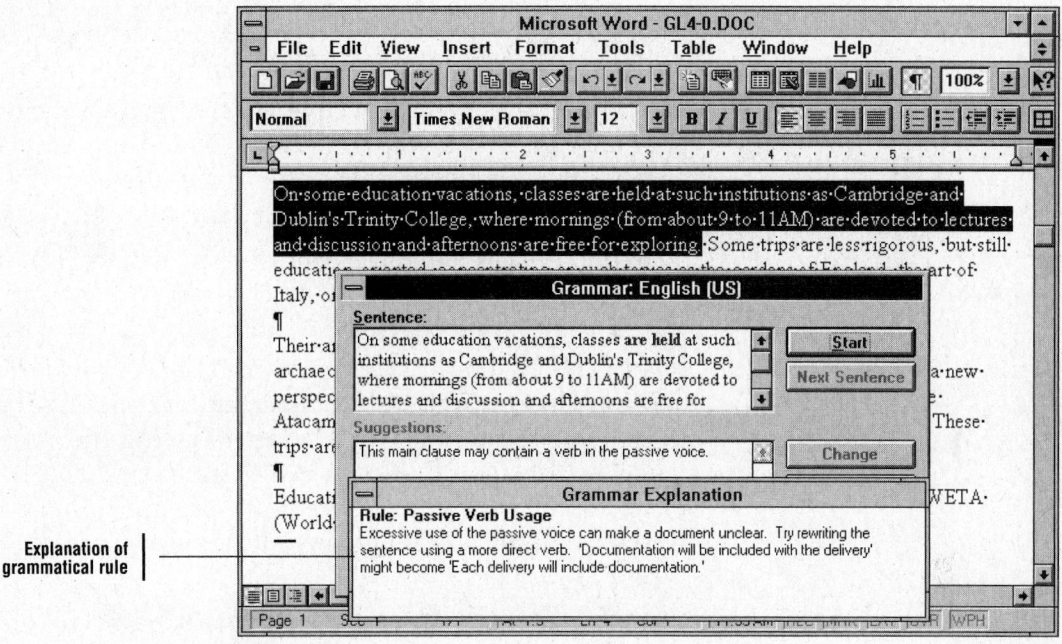

Explanation of
grammatical rule

Figure 4-8
Viewing an explanation in the Grammar dialog box

3.   After reading the explanation, close the Grammar Explanation
     window to return to the dialog box.

4.   Click the Ignore button.

     Within the same sentence, the words "are devoted" are now in
     bold, indicating another instance of a passive verb.

5.   Click the Ignore Rule button to allow use of the passive voice
     throughout the document.

     Word questions the use of the phrase "education-oriented".

6.   Click the Next Sentence button to skip over this entire sentence
     and continue with the grammar check.

     Word finds the incorrect usage of the word "Their".

7.   Click the Change button to change the word to "There".

8.   Continue with the grammar check to the end of the document.

     Word flags the words "perspective" and "desert", which are
     often misused. In this case, however, they are used correctly.

9.   Click Ignore for both words. When the grammar check is
     complete, click OK to return to the document.

Choosing Grammar Options

You can control the way Word checks a document by choosing the rules of style and grammar observed during the grammar check. For example, while checking a document, you may want Word to use the grammar and style rules that apply to business writing.

Rules of style are often subjective, based upon what you are writing about and for whom you are writing. Rules of grammar are more concrete. However, there may be instances that justify ignoring a grammatical rule. For example, grammar check questions every use of a passive verb. Yet, in some types of writing, you may prefer to say: "Tickets must be paid for in advance" rather than "You must pay for tickets in advance."

You can choose grammar options before starting grammar check by choosing Options from the Tools menu and clicking the Grammar tab. To choose grammar options after issuing the Grammar command, click the Options button in the Grammar dialog box. Remember, any options chosen are saved by Word and applied to all future documents until you change the settings again.

Figure 4-9
Grammar options

You can choose a particular rule group to apply to a document. A rule group is a set of grammar and style rules. Depending upon the nature of the document, there are three built-in options from which to choose:

- Strictly (all rules)
  Word applies every style and grammar rule.

- For Business Writing
  Word applies only the rules appropriate to business writing.

- For Casual Writing
  Word applies the fewest rules. This is for informal writing.

You can further specify the rules within these rule groups and create your own rule groups. To create your own rule group, choose Custom 1, Custom 2, or Custom 3 from the list box, and then click the Customize Settings button. In the Customize Grammar Settings dialog box, you can choose or remove the desired options.

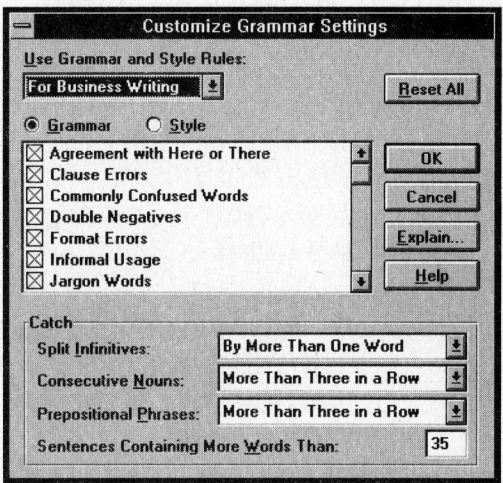

Figure 4-10
The Customize Grammar Settings dialog box

To choose grammar options:

1. Choose Options from the Tools menu, and click the Grammar tab.

    The Options dialog box for grammar is displayed.

2. Make sure the rule group For Business Writing is chosen.

3. Click the Customize Settings button.

    The Customize Grammar Settings dialog box appears.

4. Click the Grammar option button, if necessary, and scroll down the list box to clear the Jargon Words check box.

    This will make Word ignore expressions like "education-oriented" in the document.

5. Scroll down to Passive Verb Usage and clear the check box.

    This will make Word ignore all uses of the passive voice in the document.

6. Click OK to return to the Options dialog box.

7. Click OK to return to the document.

8. Choose Grammar from the Tools menu to begin the grammar check.

    Word ignores the previously questioned usages as a result of the grammar options chosen, but it still flags "perspective".

9. Click the Options button, and then click the Customize Settings button.

    Word displays the rule Possible Word Confusions, for which the grammar check continues to look.

10. Clear the Possible Word Confusions check box, and return to the Grammar dialog box.

11. When the grammar check is complete, click OK.

To reset the original grammar and spelling options:

1. Choose Options from the Tools menu.

2. In the Options dialog box, click the Grammar tab, if necessary, and then click the Customize Settings button.

3. Click the Reset All button to restore the default settings.

4. Click OK to return to the Options dialog box.

5. Click the Spelling tab.

6. Clear the check boxes for Words in UPPERCASE and Words with Numbers.

7. Click OK to return to the document.

Readability Statistics

Another grammar option you can choose from the Options dialog box is Show Readability Statistics. When chosen, Word displays a dialog box called Readability Statistics after completing the grammar check. This information helps to evaluate how easy a document is to understand.

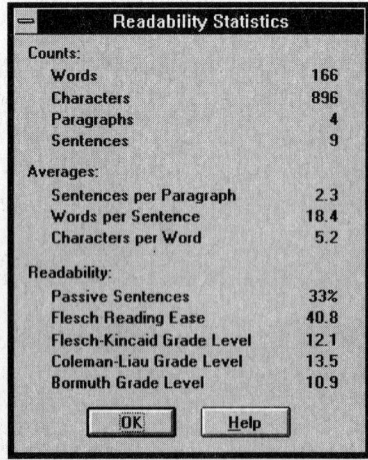

Figure 4-11
The Readability Statistics dialog box

The first category of statistics shows the word count, character count, and so on. The second category shows several averages, such as the average number of sentences per paragraph and words per sentence. The final category—Readability—measures the overall readability of a document based on standard indicators applied to writing samples.

Table 4-1: Readability Indicators	
Indicator	Description
Passive Sentences	Indicates the percentage of sentences that contain passive verbs. Writing experts generally advise against excessive use of passive verbs.
Flesch Reading Ease	A measurement of readability based on the average number of words per sentence and syllables per word, expressed from 0 to 100. For example, 60-70 is for standard text, 0-30 is for very difficult text, and 90-100 is for very easy text.
Flesch-Kincaid Grade Level	A measurement of readability based on the average number of words per sentence and syllables per word, expressed in reading grade level. For example, 7 indicates writing that can be understood by a person who has completed the 7th grade, 4 is very easy writing understood by a 4th grader, and 15 is very difficult writing understood by college-level readers.
Coleman-Liau Grade Level	Uses word length in characters and sentence length in words to determine a grade level.
Bormuth Grade Level	Another readability measurement that uses word length and sentence length to determine a grade level.

The Thesaurus Tool

The thesaurus is a tool that can add interest and variety to your writing. Use the thesaurus to look up a synonym (a word with a similar meaning) for a selected word. The thesaurus will offer several different meanings of the word, such as the word's noun and verb meanings, as well as a list of synonyms from which to choose. You can then replace the selected word with one of the suggested synonyms.

The thesaurus sometimes displays antonyms (words with the opposite meaning) and related words. You can look up synonyms for any of these words to get more word ideas.

Using the Thesaurus

The thesaurus is used for individual words in a document. To look up a word, select it, or place the insertion point in the word or to the right or left of the word.

Tools menu

The Thesaurus command can be issued two ways:

- Choose Thesaurus from the Tools menu

- Press **Shift+F7**

To use the thesaurus:

1. Select the word "range" in the first paragraph.

2. Choose Thesaurus from the Tools menu.

   The Thesaurus dialog box appears. It shows the possible meanings for "range" as a noun and a verb, along with a list of synonyms. The first synonym recommended is "extent".

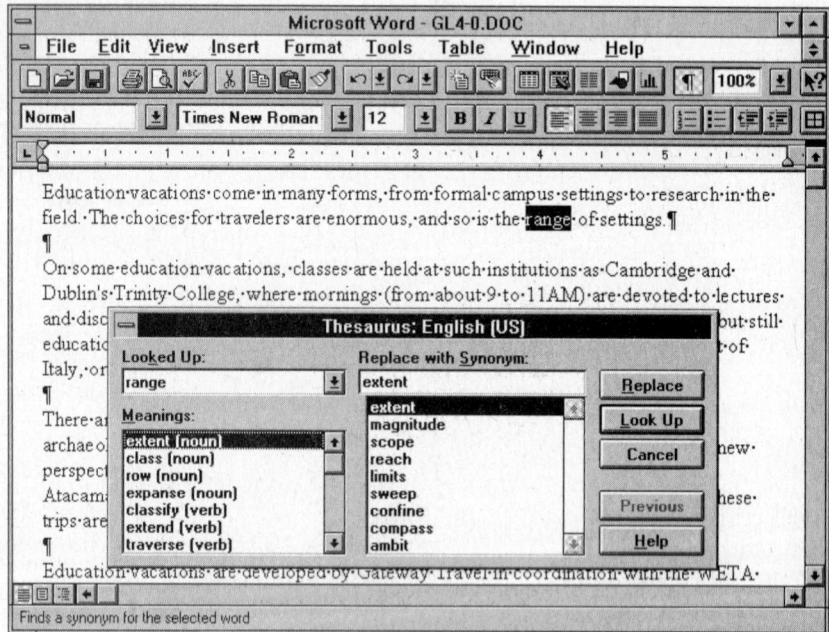

Figure 4-12
Using the thesaurus

3. Scroll down to review the Meanings list, and then scroll back up. Notice that antonyms are included in the list.

4. Click the word "expanse" in the Meanings list.

   A list of synonyms for this word appears in the Synonyms list.

5. Click the Look Up button.

   A list of more meanings and synonyms appears.

6. Double-click the word "amplitude" from either of the boxes where it is highlighted.

7. From the new list of synonyms, click the word "magnitude".

8. Click the Replace button.

Word replaces "range" with "magnitude" and returns to the document.

9. Save the document as *[your three-letter identifier]*4-0.doc.

10. Print the document.

11. Close the document and exit Word (unless you will be doing the following exercises immediately).

Table 4-2: Keyboard Shortcuts for Writing Tools	
Keyboard Shortcut	Action
F7	Spell-check a word
Ctrl+Tab	Activate document window during grammar or spelling check
Shift+F7	Start thesaurus

Exercises

Exercise 4.1

1. Start Word, if necessary.

2. Open the file 4-1.doc.

3. Click the Spelling button on the Standard toolbar.

4. In the Spelling dialog box, click the Change button to correct the spelling of "itinerary".

5. At the next misspelling, click the Change All button to correct all occurrences of "gratuities".

6. At the next misspelling, click the Change button to correct the spelling of "incidental".

7. Click the Delete button to remove the repeat of the word "to".

8. Interrupt the spelling check to remove the space in the word "availability":

    A. Click outside the dialog box in the text area to activate the document window.

    B. Click the word to remove the highlight. Then delete the space before "vailability".

    C. Click the Start button in the Spelling dialog box.

9. Save the document as *[your three-letter identifier]*4-1.doc.

10. Print the document.

11. Close the document and exit Word (unless you will be doing the following exercises immediately).

Exercise 4.2

1. Start Word, if necessary.

2. Open the file 4-2.doc.

3. Change the spelling options to ignore words with numbers:

   A. Choose Options from the Tools menu, and click the Spelling tab.

   B. In the Ignore box, click the Words with Numbers check box.

   C. Click OK.

4. Click the Spelling button on the Standard toolbar.

5. When Word finds the incorrect spellings of "experience" and "significance", change the spelling.

6. When Word questions "Tesuque", create a new custom dictionary for Southwest names called "SWEST":

   A. Click the Options button in the Spelling dialog box.

   B. In the Custom Dictionaries box, click the New button.

   C. In the Create Custom Dictionary dialog box, select the appropriate drive and key **swest.dic**

   D. Click OK.

   E. In the Options dialog box, click OK.

7. Add "Tesuque" to the new Southwest dictionary:

   A. Click the scroll arrow in the Add Word To drop-down list box.

   B. Choose the new dictionary, SWEST.DIC, so it is now the dictionary displayed.

   C. Click the Add button.

8. When the spelling check stops on the pueblo names "Pojoque", "Nambe", "Ildefonso", "Clara", "Puye", and "Picuris", add each name to the new Southwest dictionary:

9. Open the Options dialog box for spelling, and clear the Words with Numbers check box. Click OK to return to the document.

10. Save the document as *[your three-letter identifier]*4-2.doc.

11. Print the document.

12. Close the document and exit Word (unless you will be doing the following exercises immediately).

Exercise 4.3

1. Start Word, if necessary.

2. Open the file 4-3.doc.

3. After the paragraph that begins "The hotel has two", start a new paragraph by keying the text in Figure 4-13. Include the corrections.

Figure 4-13

The Red River has an *heated* indoor pool as well as a heated outdoor pool. It also has full health=club facilities, including 10 racquetball courts, 5 tennis courts, nautilus equipment, computerized treadmills, *a* steam room, and *a* sauna. Spa services, such as massage*s* and facials, can be scheduled. *as well as the services of a personal weight trainer.*

4. Grammar-check and spell-check from the beginning of the document.

5. At the first instance of a passive verb, customize the grammar rules to accept passive verb usage.

6. When Word stops on "Mariachi", add it to the world dictionary.

7. Ignore any run-on sentences that Word may find.

8. Reset the grammar options to restore the default settings.

9. Save the document as *[your three-letter identifier]*4-3.doc.

10. Print the document.

11. Close the document and exit Word (unless you will be doing the following exercise immediately).

Exercise 4.4: Challenge Yourself

Open the file 4-4.doc. Change grammar options to casual writing, and clear the options to show readability statistics and to spell-check the document. Then, use the grammar-check tool.

After completing the grammar check, use the thesaurus to look up the word "loveliest" in the first sentence of the paragraph that begins "On Day 1". Find the nearest definition by looking up "lovely" in the Alphabetic list, and then look up "charming" from the Synonyms list. Replace "loveliest" with the first selection in the Synonyms list box.

In the same sentence, key **most** after "Canada's". Apply the italic, single-underline attributes to the first sentence in the document, and then split the first paragraph after the first sentence. Change "Day 1" in the third paragraph to bold, all-capital letters, and copy this formatting for all the other day numbers.

Restore all the grammar options changed at the start of the exercise. Save the document as *[your three-letter identifier]*4-4.doc and print it. Close the document and exit Word.

An Information Sheet

Background

Duke City Gateway Travel prepares information sheets on Albuquerque, Santa Fe, and Taos to distribute to customers who call or stop by for information. Separate information sheets are prepared for restaurants, hotels, shops, events, and sightseeing excursions for each city.

Business Purpose

Create an information sheet about Albuquerque's popular restaurants.

Procedures

1. Start Word, if necessary.

2. Open the file p1-1.doc, and complete the information sheet. The paragraphs are single spaced, and there is a blank line after each heading.

3. Key **Northern** before the heading "New Mexican Cuisine".

4. Press **Enter** after "Jorge's", and key the following description:

   Jorge's is an upscale New Mexican restaurant serving seafood and chicken specialties in a formal atmosphere. Daily specialties are your best bet at this restaurant. Jeans and sneakers are not appropriate for dining at Jorge's. The meal prices range from moderate to expensive, but they are well worth it.

5. Press **Enter** after "Pete's Bar & Grill", and key the following description:

   Pete's Bar & Grill serves everyone's favorites, including hamburgers, hot dogs, club sandwiches, and an assortment of soups and salads. Even the picky eater is sure to find something delicious at Pete's Bar & Grill. The dress is casual, and the prices are inexpensive.

6. Press **Enter** after "St. Germain's", and key the following description:

> **St. Germain's is the place for a classic French meal, with fine, gourmet food and many old favorites. The atmosphere is surprisingly casual, and the prices are moderate.**

7. Scroll to the top of the page, and then merge the two paragraphs beneath the heading "Casa Jovita".

8. At the bottom of the page, move the insertion point after the first sentence in the description of Luna's, and insert a blank line.

9. Undo the last action using the Undo command.

10. At the bottom of the page, key a new paragraph:

> **Remember: When dining out in Albuquerque, it is customary to tip the restaurant servers 15% to 20%.**

11. Select "Remember:", and replace it with "Important:".

12. Spell-check the document. Create a custom dictionary on your floppy disk named Food for all references to food. Do not change any of the restaurant names or add the names to a custom dictionary.

13. Use the thesaurus to change the word "genuine" (in the paragraph describing Charley's Saloon) to the replacement that Word suggests. (If necessary, change the "a" preceding the new word to "an" in the sentence.)

14. At the top of the page, make the heading "Dining Out: Albuquerque" bold and all-capital letters.

15. Make the heading "Northern New Mexican Cuisine" bold.

16. Repeat this formatting for "American Cuisine" and "International Cuisine".

17. Underline the heading "Casa Jovita".

18. Use the Format Painter button to copy this formatting for "Jorge's", "Charley's Saloon", "Pete's Bar & Grill", "Luna's," and "St. Germain's".

19. Make the last sentence on the page bold and italicized.

20. Make any changes you feel will improve the appearance of the document.

21. Save the document as *[your three-letter identifier]*p1-1.doc and print it.

22. Close the document and exit Word.

Tips and Hints

- Use bold, underline, all-capitals, or italic character attributes for headings, but limit the use of these character attributes in your document.

- Always proof and spell-check your documents.

- Include proper names and business names in a custom dictionary. This will help speed up the spell-checking process.

- Use the Save As command to save different versions of a document. Remember to give each version a new name.

- Use Print Preview to see how your document looks before printing it.

Module 2

Basic Formatting

Changing Margins and Formatting Paragraphs

In Word, there are many ways to make a document more professional looking and more readable. One way is to vary the placement of text on a page by changing margins and formatting paragraphs. By doing so, you can significantly change the look of a document.

Documents and Sections

You can change the margins and formatting either for an entire document or for only a portion of a document. In Word, documents can be divided into *sections*, and each section can have its own separate formatting. Every document consists of at least one section. Separate sections in a document are defined by *section breaks*, which appear as double-dotted lines on the screen. This lesson explains the importance of sections in formatting portions of a document. Section breaks are also discussed in Lesson 11: "Controlling Page and Section Breaks".

Changing Margins

In a Word document, text is keyed and printed within the boundaries of the *margins*. The margins are the spaces at the top, bottom, left, and right between the edges of the text and the edges of the paper. Margins can be adjusted to change the appearance of a document. For example, widening left and right margins shortens the lines of text, which often improves readability. Reducing margins increases the amount of text on a page, which can change the length of a document. Margins may also be adjusted to allow extra space for binding.

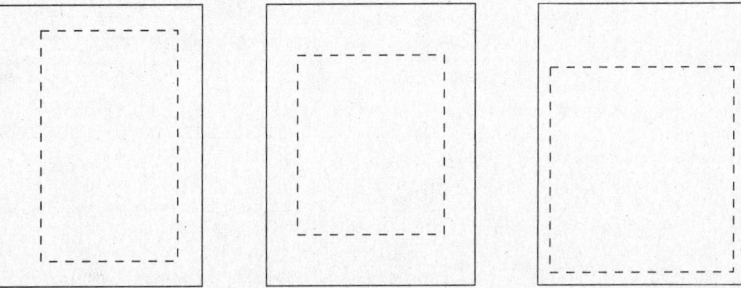

Figure 5-1
Variations in margin settings

Objectives

- Change margins.
- Format paragraphs.
- Align paragraphs.
- Adjust line spacing in and between paragraphs.
- Hyphenate paragraphs.
- Insert the date and time.

Section
A portion of a document that has its own formatting.

Section breaks
The double-dotted lines that appear on the screen to indicate the beginning and end of a section.

Margins
The distances between the text and the top, bottom, left, and right edges of the paper.

Default margin settings

Actual workspace using
default margins and
standard-size paper

Word has default settings for margins that are automatically set for
each new document you create. These settings are:

- Top margin   1 inch

- Bottom margin   1 inch

- Left margin   1.25 inches

- Right margin   1.25 inches

Using standard-size paper (8½" x 11") and Word's default margins
settings, the actual printing space for text is 6" x 9".

You can change the margins in a document by using the Page Setup
dialog box or by using the rulers in either page layout view or print
preview.

Changing Margins Using the Page Setup Dialog Box

To change margins using the Page Setup dialog box, choose Page
Setup from the File menu, and click the Margins tab. Then set the
figures in the text boxes to the desired measurements. You can key
in the new margin settings or use the arrow buttons to increase or
decrease the existing settings. In the Apply To box, indicate whether
you wish to change the whole document or a portion of the document. For example, you can change margins for:

- A whole document

- Selected text

- Selected sections

- From the insertion point forward

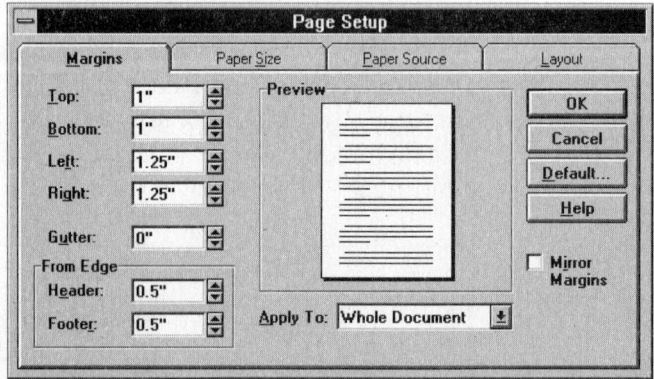

Figure 5-2
The Page Setup dialog box

To change the margins of a portion of a document, select the text,
and then choose Page Setup from the File menu. Click the Margins
tab. In the dialog box, set the margins, and then choose Selected Text
from the Apply To box. Word applies the change and automatically

inserts section breaks before and after the selection to indicate a new section. The new section starts on a new page.

Once a document has section breaks, change the margins of a section by selecting it or by placing the insertion point anywhere in the section before opening the Page Setup dialog box.

You can also apply a margin formatting change from the insertion point to the end of the document. When you do this, Word inserts a section break at the insertion point to create a new section, and applies the formatting change. The new section starts on a new page.

To set margins for an entire document using the Page Setup dialog box:

1. Start Word, if necessary.

2. Open the file 5-0.doc.

3. Choose Page Setup from the File menu.

4. Click the Margins tab, if necessary.

5. Edit the margin text boxes as follows (or click the arrow boxes to change the settings):

   Top   **1.5**

   Bottom   **1.5**

   Left   **2**

   Right   **2**

   Notice the changes in the Preview box. Notice also that the Apply To box reads Whole Document.

6. Click OK.

   The margins of the entire document are changed.

To set margins for selected text using the Page Setup dialog box:

1. Select the second and third paragraphs.

2. Choose Page Setup from the File menu.

3. Change the margins to the following settings:

   Top   2

   Bottom   2

   Left   1

   Right   1

   Notice that the Apply To box reads Selected Text.

4. Click OK.

   Word applies the margin changes to the selected text and creates a new section by inserting section breaks before and after the selected text.

File

New...   Ctrl+N
Open...   Ctrl+O
Close

Save   Ctrl+S
Save As...
Save All

Find File...
Summary Info...
Templates...

Page Setup...
Print Preview
Print...   Ctrl+P

Send...
Add Routing Slip...

1 4-1.DOC
2 4-2.DOC
3 4-3.DOC
4 4-4.DOC

Exit

File menu

Note: Use the **Tab** key to move from one margin text box to the next.

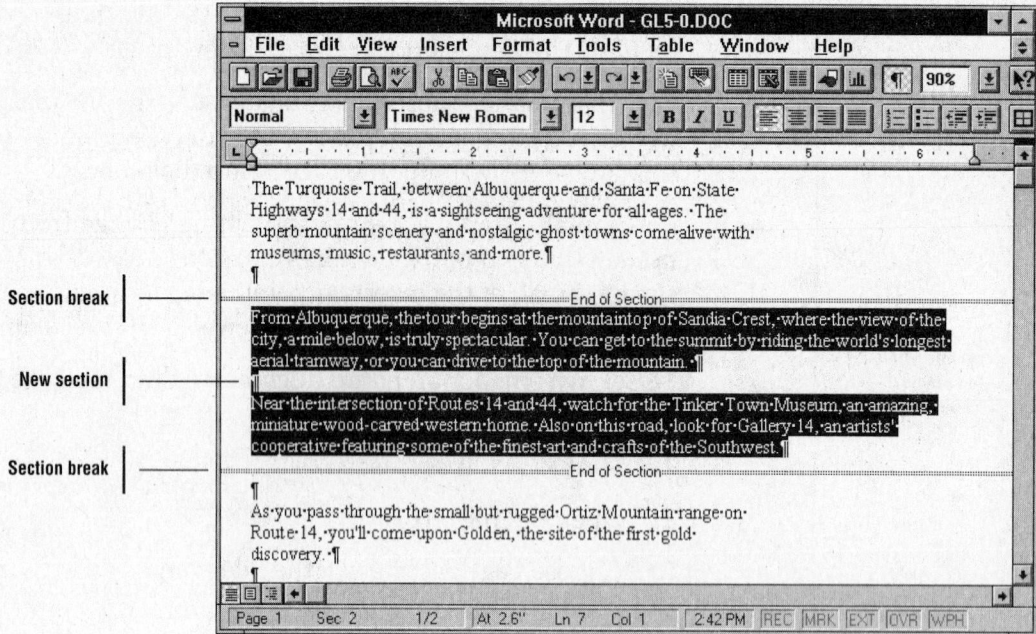

Figure 5-3
Changing margins of a selection creates section breaks.

5. Move the insertion point anywhere in the new section.

6. Choose Page Setup from the File menu.

7. Click the arrow in the Apply To drop-down list box.

    Notice that, by placing the insertion point in the section, Word can format the whole section. Word also offers This Point Forward as a formatting choice.

8. Click Cancel to close the dialog box.

9. Close the document without saving the changes.

Changing Margins in Page Layout View

Thus far, you have worked with documents in normal view. You can change the view to page layout view for the purpose of changing margins. Page layout view lets you see how a document will look when it is printed. It is useful when working with other print elements, such as headers and footers (which are discussed in Lesson 12).

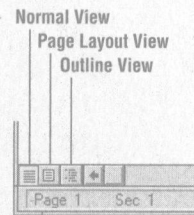

View buttons on the horizontal scroll bar

View buttons on the horizontal scroll bar let you switch between page layout and normal view. You can change views by choosing Page Layout or Normal from the View menu.

Once in page layout view, use the rulers to change the margins. The horizontal ruler on top of the screen controls the left and right margins, while the vertical ruler on the left of the screen controls the top and bottom margins. To change a margin, move the pointer over one of the margin boundaries on the ruler. When the pointer changes to a double-headed arrow, drag the margin boundary to the desired position. As you drag, a dotted line indicates the margin boundary. When you release the mouse button, Word adjusts the margin.

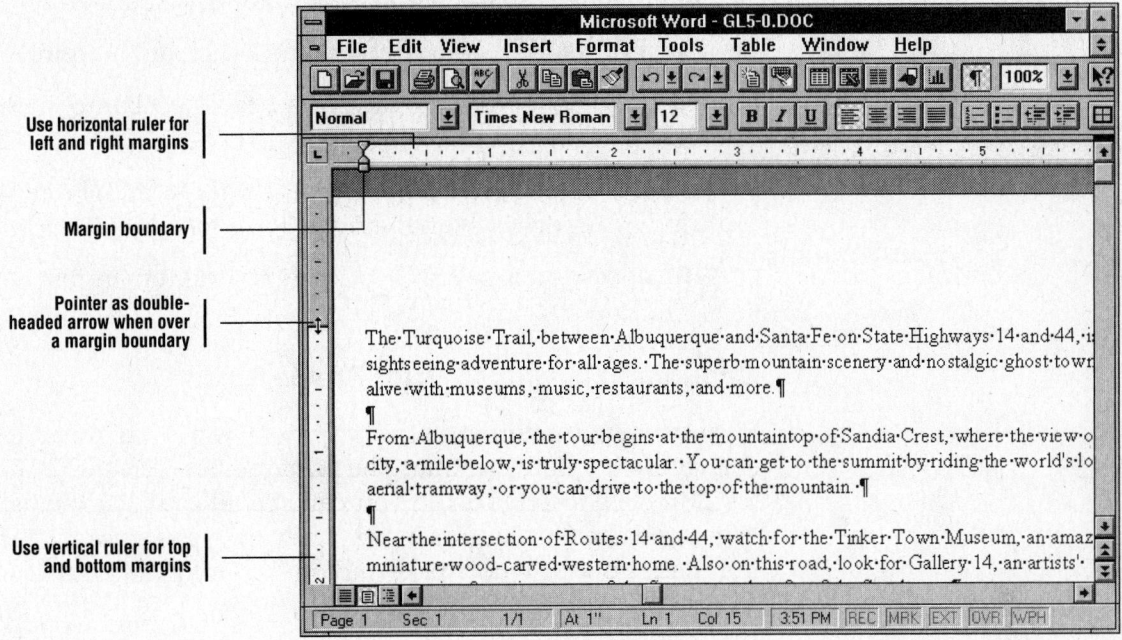

Figure 5-4
Changing margins in page layout view

Pointer over left margin boundary

Adjusting the left margin

If you hold down the **Alt** key as you drag a margin boundary, Word displays the measurements of the margin and the text area as you move the pointer.

To change margins using the rulers:

1. Open the file 5-0.doc.

2. Click the Page Layout View button on the horizontal scroll bar.

   The document changes to page layout view, and a vertical ruler appears.

3. Position the pointer over the left margin boundary on the left of the horizontal ruler.

   The pointer changes to a double-headed arrow.

4. Press and hold down the left mouse button.

   The margin boundary appears as a dotted vertical line.

5. Drag the margin boundary slightly to the right, and release the mouse button.

   Word adjusts the left margin.

6. Hold down the **Alt** key, and begin dragging the left margin boundary again.

The ruler shows margin and text-area measurements. The margin portion of the ruler is shaded.

7. Drag the margin boundary until it is 2 inches from the left, and then release the **Alt** key and the mouse button.

   Word shifts the text to adjust to the 2-inch left margin.

8. Click the right arrow on the horizontal scroll bar to view the right margin boundary.

9. Using the same procedure, drag the right margin boundary until it is 2 inches from the right.

   The document now has 2-inch left and right margins.

Changing Margins in Print Preview

Print preview is another useful way to view a document and make changes to it before printing. The print-preview screen shows entire pages in a reduced size, so you can see all four margins at once. When you change margins in print preview, you can see the effect of the change on the whole page and on the entire document.

Print Preview button

To switch to print preview, click the Print Preview button on the Standard toolbar, or choose Print Preview from the File menu. Changing margins in print preview is very similar to changing margins in page layout view. You use the vertical and horizontal rulers to drag the margins to the desired positions.

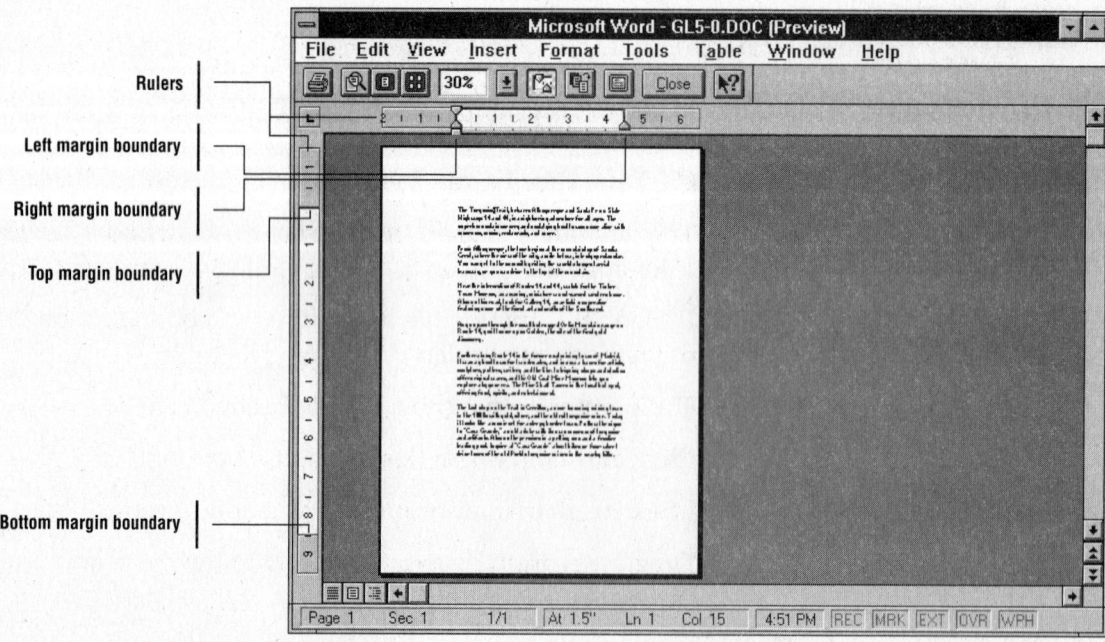

Figure 5-5
A page shown in print preview

To change margins in print preview:

1. Click the Print Preview button on the Standard toolbar.

   Word displays the document in print preview. The pointer in print preview is in the shape of a magnifying glass when it is over the document.

2. Click the View Ruler button to display the rulers, if necessary.

3. Move the pointer to the top margin boundary on the vertical ruler.

   The pointer changes to the double-headed arrow.

4. Hold down the **Alt** key as you drag the margin boundary down to 2 inches on the shaded portion of the ruler.

   Word adjusts the top margin to 2 inches.

5. Use the same procedure to change the bottom margin to 2 inches.

   The document now has 2-inch top, bottom, left, and right margins.

6. To return to normal view, click the Normal View button at the bottom left of the print-preview screen. This is a shortcut that closes print preview and returns the document to normal view.

Mirror Margins and Gutter Margins

When you are creating a bound document—one that is to be read like a book—Word provides two types of margins.

For documents with printing on both sides of the paper, choose the Mirror Margins option in the Page Setup dialog box. With this option, the margins on facing pages mirror each other, and the left and right margins change to inside and outside margins.

Sometimes, extra space is needed in the inside margin area for binding a document. This extra space is called a *gutter margin*, which can be inserted between the inside margins of two facing pages (or to the left of a single-sided page).

To set up facing pages and add a gutter margin:

1. Choose Page Setup from the File menu.

2. Click the Mirror Margins check box.

   Notice the change in the Preview box.

3. Set the gutter margin to .5 inches.

   The Preview box changes again to reflect the gutter margin.

4. Click OK to return to the document.

5. Close the document without saving the changes.

Outside margins

Inside margins

Mirror margins on facing pages

Gutter margin
Extra space added to a margin to allow for binding.

Outside margins

Inside margins

Gutter margin
Facing pages with gutter margin

Paragraph Formatting

Using Word's paragraph-formatting options, you can add interest to a document by varying the look of the paragraphs. Word provides several options for controlling the appearance of the paragraphs in a document. As with character formatting, paragraph formatting can be applied to paragraphs before you key them or to paragraphs that already exist. Paragraph-formatting options include changing paragraph alignment, adding line spacing in or between paragraphs, and adding hyphenation to paragraphs.

Paragraph Marks

Word stores the instructions for paragraph formatting in the paragraph mark. As discussed in Lesson 1, a paragraph mark is a nonprinting symbol that is inserted each time you press **Enter**. When you press **Enter**, Word copies the formatting instructions in the current paragraph mark and applies them to the new paragraph.

It is a good practice to display paragraph marks while working on a document. If the paragraph marks are not displayed, you may accidentally delete a paragraph mark and the formatting information it contains.

Remember, to display paragraph marks and other nonprinting characters, click the Show/Hide ¶ button on the Standard toolbar.

Note: If you accidentally delete a paragraph mark, immediately click the Undo button to restore the paragraph mark and the formatting.

Show/Hide ¶ button

Paragraph Alignment

In Word, you can change the alignment of paragraphs to specify how you want text to align. There are four different types of paragraph alignment:

- Left

    Each line of text is aligned with the left margin, leaving the right edge of each line uneven, or *ragged*. Left alignment is Word's default setting.

- Centered

    Each line of text is aligned between the left and right margins. Headings and titles in a document often have center alignment.

- Right

    Each line of text is aligned with the right margin, leaving the left edge ragged.

- Justified

    Each line of text is aligned with both the right and left margins. In *justified* text, the spacing between words is

Ragged
The uneven edge of text that is not aligned with a margin.

Justified
Text that is aligned with both the left and right margins by adjusting the spacing between words.

adjusted to create text with even left and right margins. Justified text has a neat appearance and is often used in professional publications.

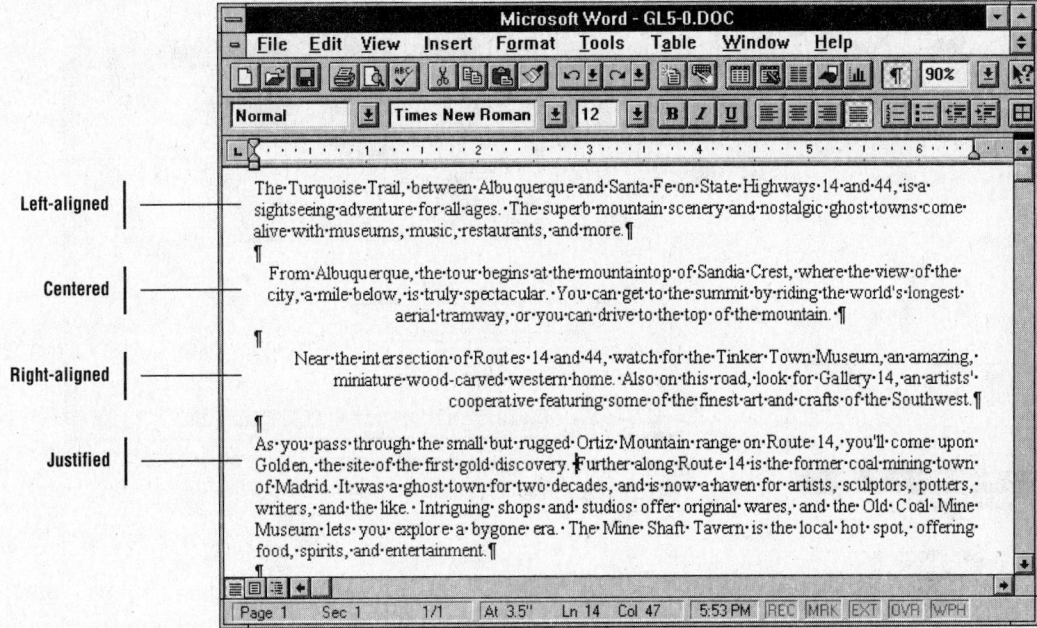

Figure 5-6
Paragraph-alignment options

There are three ways to change paragraph alignment:

* By choosing an alignment option from the Paragraph dialog box

* By using the alignment buttons on the Formatting toolbar

* By using keyboard commands:

  Ctrl+L   Left-align

  Ctrl+E   Center-align

  Ctrl+R   Right-align

  Ctrl+J   Justify

To change paragraph alignment using all three methods:

1. Open the file 5-0.doc.

2. Position the insertion point in the paragraph that begins "From Albuquerque".

Note: You do not have to select a paragraph to change its formatting. You only need to place the insertion point within the paragraph, before its paragraph mark. Paragraph formats affect the entire paragraph.

Format menu

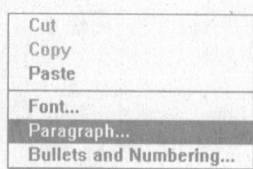

Shortcut menu

3. Choose Paragraph from the Format menu, or choose Paragraph from the shortcut menu. (Remember, to open the shortcut menu, click the right mouse button.)

The Paragraph dialog box appears.

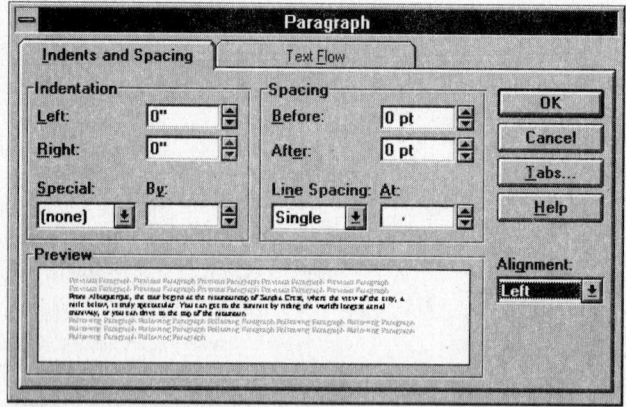

Figure 5-7
The Paragraph dialog box

4. In the bottom right of the dialog box, click the arrow to the right of the Alignment box to reveal the paragraph-alignment options.

5. Choose Right from the Alignment drop-down list.

6. Click OK to return to the document.

The paragraph is right-aligned.

7. Position the insertion point in the paragraph that begins "Near the intersection".

8. Click the Center button on the Formatting toolbar.

The paragraph is centered.

9. Combine the fourth and fifth paragraphs into one paragraph.

10. With the insertion point in the paragraph, press **Ctrl+J**.

The paragraph is justified.

11. Select the entire document.

12. Click the Align Left button on the Formatting toolbar.

The paragraphs are left-aligned again.

Alignment buttons on the Formatting toolbar

Line Spacing

Line space
The amount of vertical space used by characters in one line of text.

Word allows you to adjust the space between paragraphs and between the lines of text in paragraphs. This is another way to improve the look of a document or make it more readable. *Line space* is the amount of vertical space used by the characters in one line of text. It is based on the height of the characters, or it can be set to a specific value.

Changing Line Spacing in a Paragraph

Line-spacing options in the Paragraph dialog box

To change the spacing of lines in a paragraph, choose an option from the Line Spacing drop-down list box contained in the Paragraph dialog box. Line-spacing options are:

*   Single

    A single line space

*   1.5 Lines

    1½ line spaces

*   Double

    A double line space (one extra line space between each pair of lines)

*   At Least

    A minimum line-space measurement that you enter, and that Word can increase if necessary to accommodate larger fonts or graphics

*   Exactly

    A fixed line-space measurement that you enter, and that Word does not adjust

*   Multiple

    A line-space measurement that you enter, which increases or decreases the spacing by a percentage

Figure 5-8
Paragraph line-spacing options

In addition to using the Paragraph dialog box, you can use the following keyboard commands to change line spacing in a paragraph:

Single-space	**Ctrl+1**
Double-space	**Ctrl+2**
One-and-one-half space	**Ctrl+5**

To change line spacing in a paragraph:

1. Position the insertion point in the paragraph that begins "The Turquoise Trail".

2. Choose Paragraph from the Format menu.

3. Choose Double from the Line Spacing drop-down list box.

   Notice the change in the Preview box.

4. Click OK.

   The paragraph is double-spaced.

5. Move the insertion point to the paragraph that begins "Near the intersection".

6. Choose Paragraph from the shortcut menu.

7. Choose the Line Spacing option Multiple.

8. In the At box, key **1.20** and click OK.

   Word increases the line spacing by 20 percent.

Changing Line Spacing Between Paragraphs

You can add extra space between the paragraphs in a document by using the Paragraph dialog box. For example, you may want to separate a heading from a paragraph by inserting extra space after the heading. Instead of pressing **Enter** several times, use the Before and After spacing options in the Paragraph dialog box to set the exact amount of space you want.

Line spacing between paragraphs is set in points. If a document has 12-point text, as the current document does, then one line space is 12 points (12 pt). Likewise, two line spaces is 24 points (24 pt). Point sizes are discussed in more detail in Lesson 16: "Fonts and Type Sizes".

To adjust the spacing between paragraphs:

1. Move the insertion point to the beginning of the document, and press **Ctrl+1** to change the first paragraph (which begins "The Turquoise Trail") back to single spacing.

2. Key **The Turquoise Trail** and press **Enter**.

3. Select the paragraph you just keyed. (Remember, a paragraph is any amount of text followed by the paragraph mark.)

4. Open the Paragraph dialog box.

5. In the Spacing options group, change the Before text box to 12 pt (you can click the up arrow twice).

6. Set the After text box to 24 pt.

7. Click OK.

    The heading now has one line space before it and is separated from the text by two line spaces.

8. Click the Center button to center the heading, and then make the heading all capital letters.

Hyphenation

Hyphenating words, which can give text a less ragged appearance, is another way to improve the look of a document. In justified text, which does not have ragged edges, hyphenation reduces the amount of space Word has to insert between words on each line. Hyphens are used to join compound words and to split long words between lines. Hyphenation is especially useful in documents with narrow columns of text, such as newsletters.

In Word, there are three types of hyphens:

- Normal

- Nonbreaking

- Optional

Normal hyphens are used for words that should always be hyphenated, such as "twenty-three" or "mother-in-law".

Nonbreaking hyphen
A hyphen in a hyphenated word that prevents the word from dividing at a line break.

A *nonbreaking hyphen* is used when a hyphenated word should not be divided at a line break. For example, you could use a nonbreaking hyphen in a hyphenated proper name, such as "Minneapolis-St. Paul". Nonbreaking hyphens are similar in purpose to nonbreaking spaces, which are discussed in Lesson 2.

To insert normal and nonbreaking hyphens:

1. Scroll to the last paragraph, which begins "The last stop". In the sentence that begins "Follow the signs", position the insertion point to the immediate right of the word "old" and key:

    , 20-room,

    This is a normal hyphen.

2. After the word "adobe", key **bed**, and then key a nonbreaking hyphen by pressing **Ctrl+Shift+** the **Hyphen** (-) key.

3. Key **and-breakfast**, inserting another nonbreaking hyphen between the two words.

Optional hyphen
A hyphen that shows
where a word should be
divided if the word falls at
the end of a line.

Notice that the nonbreaking hyphens appear longer than the normal hyphen on the screen. However, nonbreaking hyphens are printed as normal hyphens.

An *optional hyphen* is used to indicate where a word should be divided if the word falls at the end of a line. If the word does not fall at the end of a line, the optional hyphen disappears from the screen and is not printed.

To insert an optional hyphen:

1. In the last sentence of the paragraph that begins "The last stop", position the insertion point between the "r" and "q" of "turquoise".

2. Press **Ctrl**+ the **Hyphen** (-) key.

    Word inserts an optional hyphen. Notice the difference between this hyphen and the others in the paragraph.

To control the ragged edges at the ends of paragraph lines, or to reduce the amount of space Word inserts in justified text, hyphenate a document. Choose Hyphenation from the Tools menu. The Hyphenation dialog box allows you to:

*   Automatically hyphenate the document as you key text

*   Hyphenate words written in all-capital letters

*   Set a Hyphenation Zone measurement to control the amount of raggedness in the right margin. The default setting is .25". A lower number reduces the raggedness, and a higher number reduces the amount of hyphenation.

*   Limit the number of consecutive hyphens in lines of text by a number you enter

*   Manually hyphenate a document. This allows you to confirm each hyphenation.

20-room¶

bed—and—breakfast¶

tur¬quoise¶

Normal, nonbreaking, and
optional hyphens

Figure 5-9
The Hyphenation dialog box

To hyphenate the document:

1. Move the insertion point to the beginning of the document.

2. Choose Hyphenation from the Tools menu.

The Hyphenation dialog box appears.

3. Click the Manual button.

   Word starts the hyphenation process and changes the document to page layout view. It asks for confirmation for the word "sightseeing" and indicates where it plans to place the hyphen. You can move the hyphenation point by clicking another point in the word.

4. Click Yes to accept the hyphenation and the hyphenation point.

   Word asks for confirmation for the word "cooperative".

5. Click Yes.

   A dialog box appears to tell you the hyphenation is complete.

6. Click OK to return to the document.

Hyphenation Guidelines

The Gregg Reference Manual contains several guidelines for the preferred practices of hyphenation. When hyphenating a document, do not:

- End more than two consecutive lines with hyphens

- Hyphenate the last word on a page

- Hyphenate at the end of the first line or at the end of the last full line in a paragraph

- Hyphenate a word to create a one-letter syllable (for example, a-ware)

- Hyphenate an abbreviation (such as "approx.") or a contraction (such as "shouldn't")

- Hyphenate within the prefix of a word (for example, use intro-duce instead of in-troduce)

- Hyphenate within the suffix of a word (for example, use (appli-cable instead of applica-ble)

For more information about hyphenation, see Section 9: "Word Division" in *The Gregg Reference Manual*.

Inserting the Date and Time

You can insert the current date or time in a document without keying it. With the Insert Date and Time command, Word inserts the date or time at the insertion point and uses the current date and time from the computer's clock. When you print the document, the date and time that appear indicate when the document was printed.

Date and Time Formats

Several formats for listing the date and time are available. To access the formats, choose Date and Time from the Insert menu. The Date and Time dialog box offers 13 different options from which to choose.

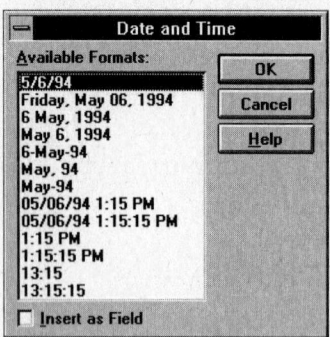

Figure 5-10
The Date and Time dialog box

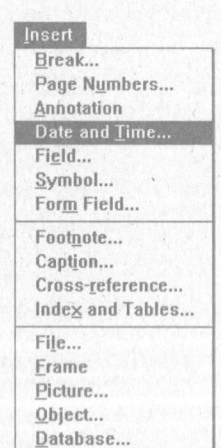

Insert menu

To insert the date and time:

1.   Move the insertion point to the left of the heading, and press **Enter** to insert a blank line.

2.   Move the insertion point up to the blank line.

3.   Choose Date and Time from the Insert menu.

4.   From the Date and Time dialog box, choose a format that includes both the date and the time. (For this document, choose the 8th choice.)

5.   Click OK.

The date and time appear at the top of the screen.

Fields

You can instruct Word to insert items into a document automatically through the use of *fields*. A field is a set of codes used for inserting the date, the time, page numbers, and other information in a document. The advantage of inserting items such as the date and time as a field is that Word updates the field each time you open or print the document. Fields, which are used extensively in Word, are discussed in future lessons.

Field
A set of hidden codes in a Word document that tell Word where to insert specific text or graphics.

Note: If you open a document with a date field, the onscreen date will show the date the document was last printed. When you print the document, the date field will update automatically to the current date. You can always update a field on the screen by clicking it and then pressing the **F9** key.

Fields can be displayed within a document in one of two ways: as field results or as field codes. A field result is the actual contents of the field, the way it appears on the printed document. For example, a date field looks the same as ordinary text, except when you click it, the text is shaded gray to indicate that it is a field. A field code is actually a group of characters representing a field.

Field characters
Brackets that show the beginning and end of a field.

Field type
The action the field is to perform in a document.

Field instructions
Instructions in a field that tell Word how to perform the action.

Field codes have three parts: field characters, field types, and field instructions. *Field characters* look like brackets. They show the beginning and end of a field. The *field type* indicates the action you want the field to perform in a document, such as insert the date and time. *Field instructions* tell Word how to perform the action.

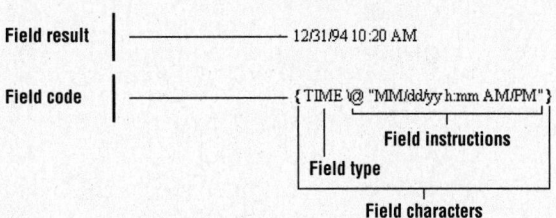

Figure 5-11
A field result and a field code

To insert the date and time as a field:

1. Delete the date and time you inserted, but keep the paragraph mark for spacing.

2. With the insertion at the paragraph mark, choose Date and Time from the Insert menu.

3. Choose the same date format you chose before, and check the Insert as Field check box. Click OK.

    Word inserts the date and time as a field.

4. Click within the field.

    Word shades the text to indicate that it is a field.

To view the date and time as a field code:

1. Choose Options from the Tools menu.

2. Click the View tab, if necessary.

3. In the Show options group, click the Field Codes check box and click OK.

    The date and time now appear as a field code.

Note: When you print a document with a field code, Word prints the field result, not the field code.

---

4. Save the document as *[your three-letter identifier]*5-0.doc.

5. Print the document.

6. Choose Options from the Tools menu again, and clear the Field Codes check box.

7. Close the document and exit Word (unless you will be doing the following exercises immediately).

**Table 5-1: Keyboard Shortcuts for Changing Margins
and Formatting Paragraphs**

Keyboard Shortcut	Action
Ctrl+L	Left-align
Ctrl+E	Center-align
Ctrl+R	Right-align
Ctrl+J	Justify
Ctrl+1	Single-space
Ctrl+2	Double-space
Ctrl+5	1½ space
Ctrl+Shift+Hyphen (-) key	Insert nonbreaking hyphen
Ctrl+Hyphen (-) key	Insert optional hyphen

Key Terms

Field	Margins
Field characters	Nonbreaking hyphen
Field instructions	Optional hyphen
Field type	Ragged
Gutter margin	Section
Justified	Section breaks
Line space	

Exercises

Exercise 5.1

1. Start Word, if necessary.

2. At the new document window, click the Centered Text button.

3. Key the following two lines of text in all-uppercase letters:

   **Family Vacations in the Southwest
   Transportation, Accommodations, Activities**

4. Press **Enter** twice, and then press **Ctrl+L** to left-align the insertion point.

5. Key the following lines of text as one paragraph (enter a line break after each of the first five lines, and press **Enter** after the telephone number):

For More Information:
Tom Carey
Duke City Gateway Travel Agency
15 Montgomery Boulevard
Albuquerque, New Mexico 87111
(505) 555-1234

6. Change the margins of the document:

   A. Choose Page Setup from the File menu.

   B. Set the top and bottom margins to 2 inches and the left and right margins to 3 inches.

   C. Click OK.

7. Change the line spacing of the paragraph that begins "For More Information":

   A. Place the insertion point within a line of the paragraph, and then choose Paragraph from the Format menu.

   B. From the Paragraph dialog box, change line spacing to 1.5 lines.

   C. Click OK.

8. Move the insertion point to the end of the document, and press **Enter** to insert 5 blank lines.

9. Insert the Date and Time as a field:

   A. Choose Date and Time from the Insert menu.

   B. Select the eighth available format.

   C. Click the Insert as Field check box, and then click OK.

   D. Click within the field to view its shading.

10. Right-align the date using the Align Right button on the Formatting toolbar.

11. Save the document as *[your three-letter identifier]*5-1.doc.

12. Print the document.

13. Close the document and exit Word (unless you will be doing the following exercises immediately).

Exercise 5.2

1. Start Word, if necessary.

2. Open the file 5-2.doc.

3. Change paragraph formatting to double spaced with one line after paragraphs:

   A. Select the entire document.

B.   Choose Paragraph from the Format menu or the shortcut
     menu.

C.   Change Line Spacing to Double.

D.   Set the After text box to 12 pt, and then click OK.

4.   Use print preview to change the top and bottom margins to
     2 inches:

     A.   Click the Print Preview button on the Standard toolbar.

     B.   Position the pointer over the top margin boundary on the
          vertical ruler.

     C.   Press the left mouse button, and hold down the **Alt** key.
          Then drag the margin boundary to 2 inches on the
          shaded portion of the ruler.

     D.   Use the same technique to change the bottom margin to
          2 inches.

     E.   Click Close.

5.   Use the ruler in page layout view to increase the left and right
     margins from 1.25 inches to 1.5 inches (thereby changing the
     text area from 6 inches to 5.5 inches):

     A.   Click the Page Layout View button on the horizontal
          scroll bar.

     B.   While holding down the **Alt** key, drag the left margin
          boundary until the text area is 5.75 inches on the ruler.

     C.   Drag the right margin boundary until the text area is
          5.5 inches on the ruler.

6.   Format the first paragraph of the document, which begins
     "Tour prices include", to have 2-inch left and right margins:

     A.   Switch to normal view by clicking the Normal View button.

     B.   Select the first paragraph.

     C.   Choose Page Setup from the File menu.

     D.   Change the left and right margins to 2 inches.

     E.   Make sure the Apply To box is set for Selected Text, and
          then click OK.

7.   Add a .5-inch gutter margin to the document:

     A.   Choose Page Setup from the File menu.

     B.   Set the Gutter text box to .5 inches.

     C.   Choose Whole Document from the Apply To box and
          click OK.

8. In the first sentence, after "hotel accommodations," use a nonbreaking hyphen and key **half-price city tours,**

9. Hyphenate the first section:

   A. Select the first section.

   B. Choose Hyphenation from the Tools menu.

   C. Click the Manual button in the dialog box.

   D. Confirm the suggestions. Click No when Word asks if you want to hyphenate the rest of the document. Then click OK to return to the document.

10. Save the document as *[your three-letter identifier]*5-2.doc.

11. Print the document.

12. Close the document and exit Word (unless you will be doing the following exercises immediately).

Exercise 5.3

1. Start Word, if necessary.

2. Open the file 5-3.doc.

3. After the paragraph that begins "I received some", begin a new paragraph. Key the text in Figure 5-12, including the corrections.

Figure 5-12

The new spa is called "The Ojo Caliente Hot Springs." It is 100 miles from Alburquerque International airport, and only one hour from Santa Fe. Ojo Caliente is a very quaint commuinty, surrounded by rugged desert *and* ~~and~~ mountains. There are 3 different springs on the grounds, and they offer several of the spa services you enjoy such as massage and aromatherapy. They have 25 lovely rooms in the main facility and 5 *separate* cottages. Their restaurant offers delicious, healthy meals, and there is also a gift shop *on the grounds* that showcases the work of local artists.

4. In the fourth sentence of the paragraph just keyed, add an optional hyphen between "aroma" and "therapy" of the word "aromatherapy".

5. Change the margins for the entire document to 1 inch left and right, 2 inches top, and 1 inch bottom.

6. Change the alignment to left-aligned text.

7. Change the line spacing to single-spaced.

8. Delete the date, and insert the date as a field code, using the same format.

9. Hyphenate the document automatically. Set the Hyphenation Zone to .5.

10. Grammar-check the document. Allow use of the passive voice.

11. Add your own reference initials and an enclosure notation at the bottom of the letter.

12. Save the document as *[your three-letter identifier]*5-3.doc.

13. Print the document.

14. Close the document and exit Word (unless you will be doing the following exercise immediately).

Exercise 5.4: Challenge Yourself

Open the file 5-4.doc. Format the first line in bold, capital letters, and center the line. Change the line spacing from the second line (which begins "Airfares") through "*All meals are included" to double spaced.

Select the rest of the document, from "Itinerary" to the end, and format it as a separate section with 1-inch left and right margins. Change the paragraph spacing of this section to 1 line (12 points) after paragraphs and the page setup to facing pages (using mirror margins) with a .5 inch gutter.

Change the formatting of "Itinerary" from bold italic to bold uppercase letters. Center the word, and then insert three blank lines after it. In this section, center and underline all the lines that begin with "Day", such as "Day 1: Arrive Albuquerque".

Spell-check the document, adding the names and words that Word questions to the Southwest dictionary created in Lesson 4. (If you did not create this custom dictionary, do so now, using your floppy disk and not the computer's hard disk.) Save the document as *[your three-letter identifier]*5-4.doc. Print the document, close it, and exit Word.

Tabs and Tabbed Columns

Objectives

- Set tabs.
- Set leaders.
- Clear tabs.
- Adjust tabs.
- Set up tabbed columns.

Tab
A set amount of space that is used to align text in a document.

Tab stop
The stopping point of a tab.

Tabs are a paragraph-formatting feature used to align text. With tabs, you can create documents according to a proper format, such as a business memo, and you can create lists of information and columns. As with other paragraph-formatting features, tabs are stored in the paragraph marks at the end of each paragraph. In Word, you can set, change, and clear tabs.

What Is a Tab?

A *tab* is a set amount of space between two words, characters, or numbers in a line of text, or between a word, character, or number and the left or right margin. To create a tab, press the **Tab** key. When you press the **Tab** key on a typewriter, the carrier moves a set amount of space to the right. When you press the **Tab** key in Word, the insertion point moves to the right. The distance the insertion point moves is determined by a *tab stop*. When you press the **Tab** key, Word inserts a tab character to represent the onscreen space between the insertion point and the tab stop.

Note: In Word, you cannot press the **Spacebar** to simulate a tab as you can with a typewriter. Characters and spaces do not necessarily occupy the same amount of space on a line. Tabs must be used to align text properly in a printed document.

To insert a tab in a document:

1. Start Word, if necessary.

2. In the new document screen, key **Word for Windows**, and press the **Tab** key.

   Word inserts a tab character and moves the insertion point to the right.

3. Key **Version 6.0**

Tab character

Like the paragraph mark, tabs are nonprinting characters that can be displayed or hidden from view. If you plan to include tabs in a document, it is a good idea to display them so you can see where they are on the screen. Remember, to display or hide nonprinting characters, click the Show/Hide ¶ button on the Standard toolbar.

Default and Custom Tabs

When you create a new document, default tab stops are set at .5-inch intervals from the left margin.

There are two ways to change default tab stops. You can instruct Word to change the distance between default tab stops from .5 inches to another increment, such as 2 inches, or you can create a *custom tab* by choosing any measurement other than a .5-inch default increment. When you set a custom tab, Word clears all default tabs to the left of the tab stop. For example, if you set a custom tab at 1.25 inches, the .5-inch default tab stops up to that point are cleared. Custom tab settings are indicated on the horizontal ruler by *tab markers*.

Note: It is important to set up your documents correctly and to not rely on default tabs. For example, if you have a line of text that you want to align at the 2-inch mark on the ruler, do not press the **Tab** key four times to reach the 2-inch default tab stop. This inserts extraneous tab characters that clutter the document. Instead, create a 2-inch custom tab, and then press the **Tab** key once. Only one tab character will appear in the document.

Custom tab
A tab that is set to replace default tab settings.

Tab marker
A symbol on the horizontal ruler that indicates a custom tab setting.

1.25" custom tab setting

Types of Tabs

You can insert four different types of tabs in Word documents. They are based on the alignment of text on the tab stop. The four types of tabs are:

- Left-aligned

  The left edge of the text lines up with the tab stop.

- Centered

  The text is centered at the tab stop.

- Right-aligned

  The right edge of the text lines up with the tab stop.

- Decimal

  The decimal point lines up with the tab stop. This is useful for creating columns of dollar amounts.

Setting Tabs

When you set tabs in a document, the tabs are stored in the paragraph mark at the end of the paragraph. Each time you press **Enter**, the tabs and their settings are copied to the next paragraph. You can set tabs either before you key text or for existing text.

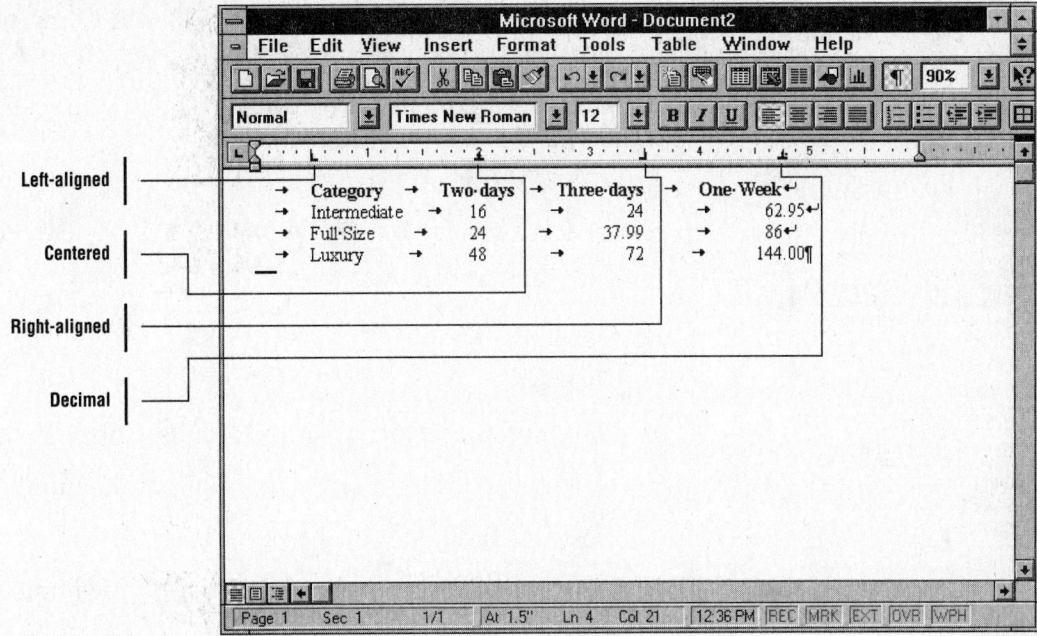

Figure 6-1
Types of tabs

There are two ways to set tabs:

• Use the Tabs dialog box.

• Click the Tab Alignment button on the horizontal ruler.

Setting Tabs Using the Tabs Dialog Box

The most precise method of setting tabs is using the Tabs dialog box.
To access the Tabs dialog box, choose Tabs from the Format menu.

Figure 6-2
The Tabs dialog box

The Tabs dialog box allows you to change the distance between
default tab stops or to set a new tab-stop position.

To set tabs with the Tabs dialog box:

1. Close the open document without saving it, and then open the file 6-0.doc.

2. After the memo heading, double-click in the selection bar (the left margin area) to select the paragraph from "1.Accommodations" to "car rental".

3. Choose Tabs from Format menu.

4. Key **.4** in the Tab Stop Position box.

   The alignment is already set to Left, by default.

5. Click OK.

   The ruler shows the tab marker at just under .5 inches.

6. Move the insertion point to the right of the number "1."

7. Press the **Tab** key.

8. Move the insertion point to the right of the number "2."

9. Press the **Tab** key.

10. Do the same for the numbers "3." and "4."

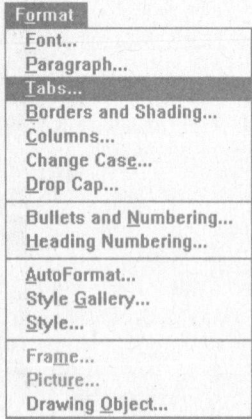

Format menu

Setting Tabs Using the Ruler

You can set tabs using the horizontal ruler. To do this, first click the Tab Alignment button at the left of the ruler until it reflects the tab alignment you want. Each time you click the button, it changes its display.

Table 6-1: Tab Alignment Buttons	
Type of Tab	Button Display
Left-aligned	⌊
Centered	⊥
Right-aligned	⌟
Decimal	⊥

When the Tab Alignment button displays the type of tab you want, click the ruler where you want to set the tab stop.

To set tabs with the ruler:

1. Move the insertion point to the left of "Avenue Inn".

2. Click the Tab Alignment button on the horizontal ruler until it shows right alignment, and then click the ruler at 1.5 inches.

   Word inserts a right-aligned tab marker at 1.5 inches and deletes the tab markers to the left of it.

Tab Alignment button on ruler showing right alignment

3. With the insertion point to the left of "Avenue Inn", press the **Tab** key.

   Word right-aligns "Avenue Inn" at the 1.5-inch tab stop.

4. Click the Tab Alignment button until it changes to decimal alignment, and then click the ruler at 3 inches, 4 inches, and 5 inches.

5. Move the insertion point to the right of "Avenue Inn".

6. Key the following figures, pressing the **Tab** key before each figure:

   99.50   216.00   278.00

7. Press **Shift+Enter** to start a new line.

8. Key the following, pressing the **Tab** key before the hotel name and before each figure:

   Hotel Westport   245.75   389.00   519.50

   Word right-aligns the hotel names and aligns the rate figures according to the decimal tab stops.

9. Move the insertion point to the line that begins "Per person rates".

Note: Remember, you can use the Center button on the Formatting toolbar to center text between the left and right margins.

10. Click the Tab Alignment button until it shows center alignment, and then click the ruler at 3 inches.

11. Press the **Tab** key to center the line at the tab stop.

Figure 6-3
The document with tabbed text

Setting Leaders

Leader
Patterns of dots or dashes
added to fill the tab
spaces in a document.

Dotted .... leader
Dashed ----------- leader
Solid _____ leader

Leader patterns

Note: You can place the insertion point anywhere in
the paragraph and then
choose the tab setting and
leader pattern from the Tabs
dialog box. Remember,
placing the insertion point in
a paragraph is all that is
necessary when applying
formatting to the paragraph,
including tab settings.

Word allows you to set *leaders* in a document. Leaders are patterns of dots or dashes that fill the tab spaces and lead the reader's eye from left to right. Leaders are often found in a table of contents, in which dotted lines fill the space between the headings on the left and the page numbers on the right. To add a tab-stop leader, use the Tabs dialog box.

There are three different leader patterns available in Word: dotted line, dashed line, and solid line.

To set a leader:

1. Move the insertion point to the right of "Avenue Inn".
2. Choose Tabs from the Format menu.
3. Choose 3" from the Tab Stop Position list box.
4. Click the second leader pattern (the dotted line).
5. Click Set, and then click OK.

   A dotted-line leader appears to the left of the tab setting and fills the tab space for both lines of the paragraph.

Clearing Tabs

Custom tabs can be cleared either all at once or individually. When custom tabs are cleared, Word restores the default tab stops to the left of the custom tab stop. Use the Tabs dialog box or the ruler to clear tabs.

To clear tabs in a line of text or a paragraph, simply place the insertion point anywhere in the line or paragraph. To clear tabs in more than one line of text (separate paragraphs), select the text.

To clear an individual tab using the Tabs dialog box:

1. Position the insertion point in the line of text that begins "Per person rates".
2. Choose Tabs from the Format menu.

   The 3-inch tab is highlighted in the Tab Stop Position box.
3. Click the Clear button, and then click OK.

   Word clears the 3-inch custom tab and restores the .5-inch default tabs.
4. Delete the tab character to the left of "Per person rates".

You can clear tabs with the ruler by positioning the pointer on the tab marker and dragging the tab marker off the ruler.

To clear a tab using the ruler:

1. Scroll down toward the end of the document to the line of tabbed text that begins "Luxury".

2. Place the insertion point in the line.

    Notice that the last figure, "24", is center-aligned, and all the other figures are right-aligned.

3. Position the pointer on the 5.5-inch centered tab marker.

4. Drag the tab marker down and off the ruler.

    The custom tab is cleared, and the .5 inch default tab setting is restored.

5. Change the Tab Alignment button to right alignment, and then click the ruler at 5.5 inches.

    The figure is right-aligned.

You can clear all the tabs in the document or in selected text using the Tabs dialog box.

To clear all the tabs in a few selected paragraphs using the Tabs dialog box:

1. Select the text from "Category" to "same location" (including the period and the paragraph mark).

2. Choose Tabs from the Format menu.

3. Click the Clear All button. (To clear an individual tab, you can key a specific tab stop in the Tab Stop Position box.) Click OK.

    Word clears all the custom tabs in the selected paragraphs and restores the default tab stops. Remember, to completely remove tabs from text, you must delete the tab characters.

4. Click the Undo button on the Standard toolbar to restore the tab settings.

Adjusting Tab Settings

Any tabs inserted in a document can be adjusted after they are set. You can adjust the position of the tab or change the type of tab using either the Tabs dialog box or the ruler.

To adjust tabs using the Tabs dialog box:

1. Position the insertion point in the paragraph that begins "Avenue Inn".

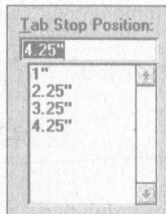

Tab settings in the Tabs
dialog box

Note: In this case, right
alignment and decimal
alignment will produce the
same results.

Note: When changing tab
settings with the ruler,
make sure to drag the tab
marker to the right or left
only. Do not drag the tab
marker up or down, which
may clear it from the ruler.
If you clear the tab
marker, insert another tab
marker and try again, or
click the Undo button from
the Standard toolbar.

2. Choose Tabs from the Format menu.

3. Click the Clear All button to clear the existing tabs.

4. In the Tab Stop Position box, key **1**, choose Center alignment,
    and then click the Set button.

5. In the Tab Stop Position box, key **2.25**, choose Right alignment,
    and then click the Set button.

6. In the Tab Stop Position box, key **3.25**, leave right alignment
    selected, and click the Set button.

7. In the Tab Stop Position box, key **4.25**, leave right alignment
    selected, and click the Set button.

    All four tab settings appear in the Tab Stop Position dialog box.

8. Click OK.

    Word applies the new tab settings.

To adjust tabs with the ruler:

1. With the insertion point in the same paragraph, click the tab-stop
    marker at 2.25 inches, and drag it to 2.5 inches on the ruler.

    The tab stop is changed from 2.25 inches to 2.5 inches.

2. Click the tab-stop marker at 3.25 inches, and drag it to 3.5
    inches on the ruler.

3. Click the tab-stop marker at 4.25 inches, and drag it to 4.5
    inches on the ruler.

    The tab stops are adjusted to the new settings.

Changing the Ruler's Unit of Measure

In Word, the ruler's unit of measure is normally shown in inches. If
inches do not provide sufficiently detailed measurements in a particular document, you can change the ruler to smaller increments,
such as centimeters, picas, or points. There are 2.54 centimeters to
1 inch, 6 picas to 1 inch, and 72 points to 1 inch.

To change the ruler's unit of measure, choose Options from the Tools
menu, and click the General tab. In the Options dialog box, choose
the desired setting from the Measurement Units drop-down list. The
measurement unit you choose will be reflected on the ruler when you
close the dialog box.

Figure 6-4

The ruler changed from inches to points

Tabbed Columns

Tabs can be used to create tabbed columns (side-by-side vertical lists of information) in documents. Information in a document that is presented in a column format, separate from the body text, is often easy to read.

You can use tabbed columns to set up a table, as illustrated in the document 6-0.doc. When setting up a table with tabbed columns, there are general rules that apply. These rules, based on *The Gregg Reference Manual*, are:

- The table should be centered horizontally within the margins.

- Columns within the table should be between six and ten spaces apart.

- The width of a table should not exceed the width of the document's body text.

- There should be at least one blank line separating the top and the bottom of the table and the body text of the document.

The standard procedure for centering tabbed columns horizontally is provided in *The Gregg Reference Manual* ("Centering Tables Horizontally"). This method, derived from typing, can be used in Word. However, there is a more efficient method that takes advantage of the highly visual and graphical qualities of Windows.

When using Word's Table feature, the recommended procedure for creating a horizontally centered table from tabbed columns is as follows:

- Create a guide line.

  From the columns you wish to set up, look for the item in each column with the most characters. This could be the column heading or the column text. Key the items as one line of text, inserting six space characters between each item. (You can, however, insert more spaces to make the table more readable.) Center the line, and position it directly below the ruler.

- Set the tabs.

  Clear all existing tabs from the ruler. To set a left-aligned tab, click the Tab Alignment button for left alignment, move the I-beam to the left of the first letter of the item, and click the corresponding point on the ruler. To set a right-aligned tab, click the Tab Alignment button for right alignment, move the I-beam to the right of the last letter of the item, and click the ruler above that point. To set a center tab, click the Tab Alignment button for center alignment, and then click the ruler above the middle of the item. To set a decimal tab, click the Tab Alignment button for decimal alignment, then click the

Note: To set up a sizable amount of text and numbers in columnar form, it is generally easier to use the Table feature, which is discussed in Lesson 18: "Working with Tables". The Table feature allows for more precisely centered columns.

ruler at a point that will allow for the alignment of the decimal point and the numbers to the right and left of it.

You can also move existing tabs into the correct position and adjust the tabs after the text is keyed.

• Create the columnar text.

Delete the text in the guide line, which was used for measuring purposes only. Do not delete the paragraph mark, which contains the tab information. Left-align the insertion point, and begin keying the text, using the **Tab** key for positioning.

Location	Lateness	Late Fee
Albuquerque	1 day	$1.00
Phoenix	2 days	$1.75

Figure 6-5

Example of a centered table

To insert the above table horizontally in document 6-0.doc using tabbed columns:

1. Press **Enter** twice after the line that ends "same location" at the end of the document. Delete all tabs.

2. Key **Charges for cars returned late:**, and press **Enter** twice.

3. Begin creating a guide line that contains the longest item in each column. Key the following items, and insert ten spaces between each item:

   Albuquerque   Lateness   Late Fee

Center button

4. Click the Center button on the Formatting toolbar to center the line.

5. Scroll down until the guide line is directly below the ruler.

6. Change the Tab Alignment button to center alignment, and then set three center-aligned tabs. Use the I-beam as a guide, and click the ruler in the center of each item.

Use the I-beam as a guide, and then click the ruler directly above.

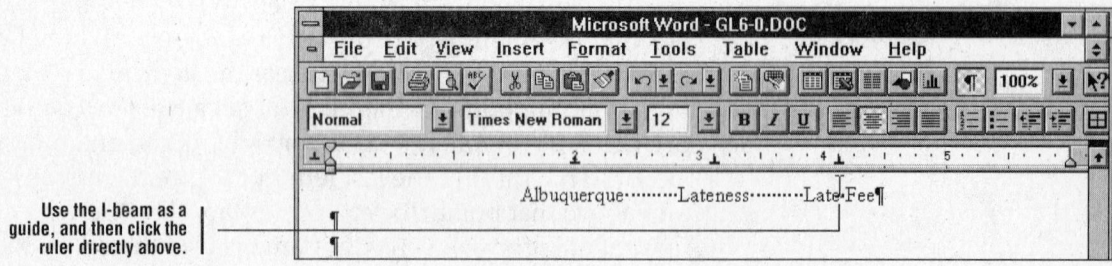

Figure 6-6

Guide line for centering tabbed columns

7. Delete the text in the guide line up to the paragraph mark.

8. Click the Align Left button to left-align the insertion point. Key the table text, pressing the **Tab** key before each item and single-spacing each line:

Location	**Lateness**	**Late Fee**
Albuquerque	**1 day**	**$1.00**
Phoenix	**2 days**	**$1.75**

9. Apply the underline attribute to each heading.

10. Key your reference initials at the bottom of the document.

11. Save the document as *[your three-letter identifier]*6-0.doc.

12. Print the document.

13. Close the document and exit Word (unless you will be doing the following exercises immediately).

Key Terms

Custom tab   Tab stop

Leader   Tab marker

Tab

Exercises

Exercise 6.1

1. Start Word, if necessary.

2. Create a new document.

3. In all-capital letters, key the heading **PARADISE ISLAND HOTELS - PEAK SEASON RATES**, and press **Enter** three times.

4. Switch to lowercase letters. Press the **Tab** key, and key **3 nights, double occupancy**

5. Press the **Tab** key again, and key **Single add-on per night**

6. Use the Tabs dialog box to set this line with 3- and 5-inch center tabs:

   A. With the insertion point in the line, choose Tabs from the Format menu.

   B. In the Stop Tab Position box, key **3**, choose Center alignment, and click the Set button.

C. In the Stop Tab Position box, key **5**, click the Set button, and then click OK.

7. Double space after this line, and then key the following text, pressing the **Tab** key before each dollar amount:

Crown Beach Resort	**$378**	**$36.75**
Turtle Bay Inn	**$432**	**$42**
Reef Villas	**$455**	**$43.75**
Ocean Resort	**$398**	**$38**

8. Change the tabs for the dollar amounts to decimal alignment, and add dotted leaders:

A. Select the text from "Crown Beach Resort" to "$38".

B. Choose Tabs from the Format menu.

C. With the 3-inch tab highlighted in the Stop Tab Position box, choose Decimal alignment and the dotted leader. Click the Set button.

D. Click the 5-inch tab, and then choose Decimal alignment and the dotted leader. Click the Set button, and then click OK.

9. Tab each of the hotel names .5 inches from the left margin:

A. Select the text from "Crown Beach Resort" to "$38".

B. Choose Tabs from the Format menu.

C. In the Stop Tab Position box, key **.5**, choose Left alignment, click the Set button, and then click OK.

D. Move the insertion point to the left of each hotel name, and press the **Tab** key.

10. Center the first line heading, and then underline the headings above the tabbed figures.

11. Change the top margin to 2 inches.

12. Save the document as *[your three-letter identifier]*6-1.doc.

13. Print the document.

14. Close the document and exit Word (unless you will be doing the following exercises immediately).

Exercise 6.2

1. Start Word, if necessary.

2. Open the file 6-2.doc.

3. Change the left and right margins to 1 inch and the top margin to 2 inches.

4. Center the first line, and add the bold attribute.

5. Format the remaining text in one right-aligned and two left-aligned columns:

   A. Place the insertion point within the text (which is all one paragraph).

   B. Clear all tabs by dragging the tab-stop markers off the ruler.

   C. Click the Tab Alignment button until it displays right alignment, and then click the ruler at .75 inches.

   D. Change the Tab Alignment button to left alignment, and then click the ruler at 1.25 inches and 4.25 inches.

6. Set up the flight information as tabbed columns:

   A. Press the **Tab** key to insert one tab character to the left of "Day", "Leaving", and "Flight". ("Day" will not move to the tab setting until you insert a tab before "Flight".)

   B. In the next line, insert a tab character to the left of "Mon", "Depart", and "Southwest".

   C. Do the same for the rest of the lines, inserting a tab character before the day, before the word "Depart", and before the airline name.

7. Underline the headings "Day", "Flight Times", and "Leaving On".

8. Save the document as *[your three-letter identifier]*6-2.doc.

9. Print the document.

10. Close the document and exit Word (unless you will be doing the following exercises immediately).

Exercise 6.3

1. Start Word, if necessary.

2. Create a new document with 2-inch top and bottom margins and 1-inch right and left margins.

3. Key the first line of Figure 6-7 (see next page) in bold, all-capital letters.

Figure 6-7

Travel Mode Comparisons

Washington, D.C. to Philadelphia, PA

Air		Rail	
Taxi to terminal	20 min.	Taxi to station	10 min.
In flight	55 min.	On Metroliner	102 min.
In terminal	30 min.	In station	10 min.
Taxi to destination	<u>30 min.</u>	Taxi to destination	<u>10 min.</u>
	135 min.		132 min.
	(2 hr. 15 min.)		(2 hr. 12 min.)

4. Press **Enter** twice, and then key the second line in bold. Center the first and second lines.

5. Triple space, and left-align the insertion point.

6. Set centered tabs at 1.5 inches and 5 inches.

7. Key the headings in the third line ("Air" and "Rail") in bold, underlined letters, aligning them at the centered tab stops.

8. Press **Enter** twice, turn off the bold and underline attributes (press **Ctrl+Spacebar**), and clear all prior custom tab settings.

9. Key the next four lines as single-spaced tabbed columns. Left-align the first column at .5 inches, right-align the second column at 2.5 inches, left-align the third column at 4 inches, and right-align the last column at 6 inches.

10. Underline "30 min." and "10 min." as shown.

11. For the last two lines, delete the .5-inch and 4-inch tabs, and then key the text using single spacing.

12. Change the line spacing for the last six lines of text to 1.5 lines.

13. Spell-check the document.

14. Save the document as *[your three-letter identifier]*6-3.doc.

15. Print the document.

16. Close the document and exit Word (unless you will be doing the following exercise immediately).

Exercise 6.4: Challenge Yourself

Create a new document with a 2-inch top margin and 1-inch left, right, and bottom margins. Key the heading **FAMILIARIZATION TRIP** in bold, all capitals, and center it. Press **Enter** three times, and then key the first paragraph in Figure 6-8, which appears at the end of this exercise (include the correction). Press **Enter** twice, and then key the next nine lines (from "Location:" through "Mountain Top Restaurant") as two single-spaced tabbed columns, with the first column right-aligned at 1.25 inches, and the second column left-aligned at 1.75 inches. Include the corrections. Press **Enter** twice, and then key the rest of the text in the figure. Press **Enter** twice, and then key in italics **RSVP** and **(303) 555-4587** as two single-spaced, centered lines.

From "Location:" to "Mountain Top Restaurant", change the line spacing to 1.5 lines. For the entire document, change the paragraph spacing to 6 points after each paragraph.

Use print preview to see how the document looks on the page. Then spell-check the document and save it as *[your three-letter identifier]*6-4.doc. Print the document, close it, and exit Word.

Figure 6-8 (bf)

The Rocky Mountain Hot Springs Ranch has invited Duke City ~~Gateway~~ travel counselors to visit their new facility in Gunnison, Colorado.

(bf)
Location: 15 Country Road, Gunnison, Colorado

(bf)
Date: August 8, 1995

Schedule:

9:30 a.m.   Welcome Breakfast

10:15-12:15   Tour of the exercise rooms, swimming areas, spa, tennis courts

12:30   Lunch by the lake patio

2:00-3:30   Tour of the guest rooms and cottages, ski area, hot springs, stables

3:30-6:00   Leisure time to ~~indulge in any of the services and~~ *enjoy the ranch's* facilities

7:00   Dinner at the Mountain Top Restaurant

Guests are invited to spend the night with us in their choice of rooms or cottages. A full country breakfast will be served in the morning. Return transportation to the airport will be provided.

Indents and Advanced Paragraph Formatting

Indent

The distance between the sides of a paragraph and the margins.

Along with line spacing, margins, and tabs, indents are another paragraph-formatting feature used to emphasize or separate paragraphs in a document. Word provides additional tools for this purpose, including borders, shading, and bulleted and numbered lists, all of which are discussed in this lesson.

Indents

An *indent* is the distance between the sides of a paragraph and the margins. While margin settings generally apply to an entire document or section, indent settings apply to individual paragraphs within a document or section. Indented paragraphs appear to have different margin settings from the rest of the document or section. For example, if a document has a 1-inch left margin, and you format one of the paragraphs with a .5-inch left indent, the paragraph prints 1.5 inches from the left edge of the page.

Indents may appear to be similar to tabs, but a tab affects only one line of text within a paragraph, while indents affect the whole paragraph. Indents are a paragraph-formatting feature stored in the paragraph mark at the end of a paragraph. When you press **Enter**, the indents are copied to the next paragraph.

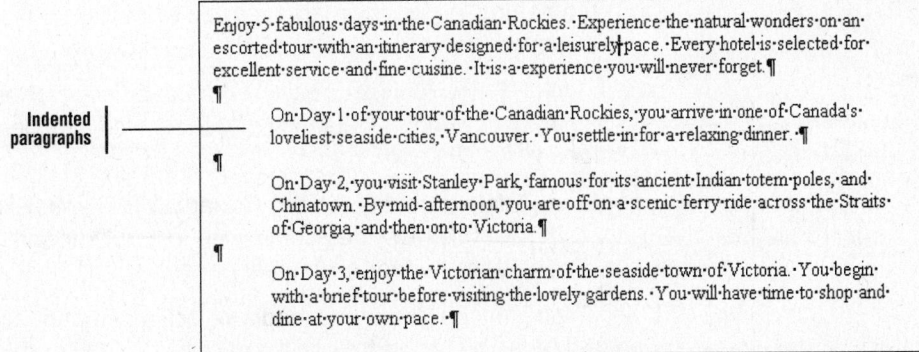

Indented paragraphs

Figure 7-1
Indented paragraphs

Types of Indents

Word provides a variety of indents to emphasize paragraphs in a document. Each type of indent relates to one or both margins. The five types of indents are:

- Left indent
- Right indent
- First-line indent
- Hanging indent
- Negative indent

A *left indent* increases a paragraph's distance from the left margin. A *right indent* increases a paragraph's distance from the right margin. A *first-line indent* affects only the first line of a paragraph, indenting it from the left margin. This is similar to pressing the **Tab** key at the beginning of a paragraph. A *hanging indent* is one in which the first line of a paragraph aligns on the left, and the rest of the paragraph is indented from the first line. This type of indent is often used to create numbered lists.

All of these are considered *positive indents*, in that they occur within the left and right margins of a document. A *negative indent* causes a paragraph to extend outside the left or right margin. This type of indent is often used to make titles stand out from body text.

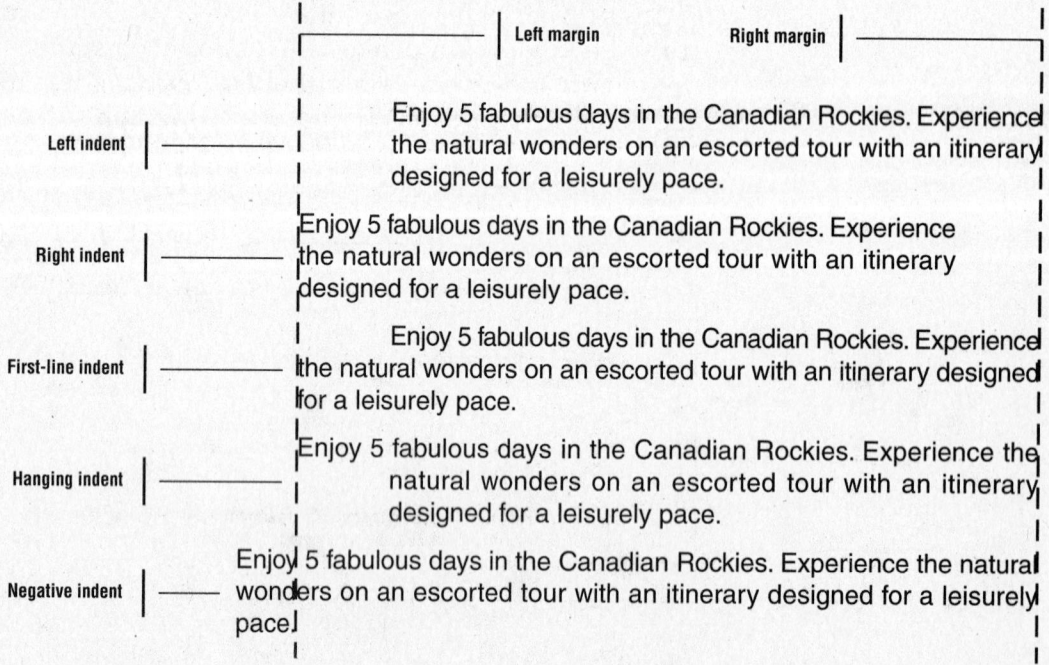

Figure 7-2
Types of indentation

Indenting Paragraphs

To set an indent, select the paragraph, or place the insertion point in the paragraph you want to indent. For text not yet keyed, place the insertion point where you want indenting to start. There are four methods for formatting paragraphs with indents:

- Using the Paragraph dialog box

- Using the ruler

- Using the Indent buttons on the Formatting toolbar

- Using the keyboard

Setting Indents with the Paragraph Dialog Box

The most precise way to set indents is to use the Paragraph dialog box. When you choose Paragraph from the Format menu or the shortcut menu, Word presents the left and right indentation options and a drop-down list box for first-line and hanging indents under the word "Special".

Indentation options

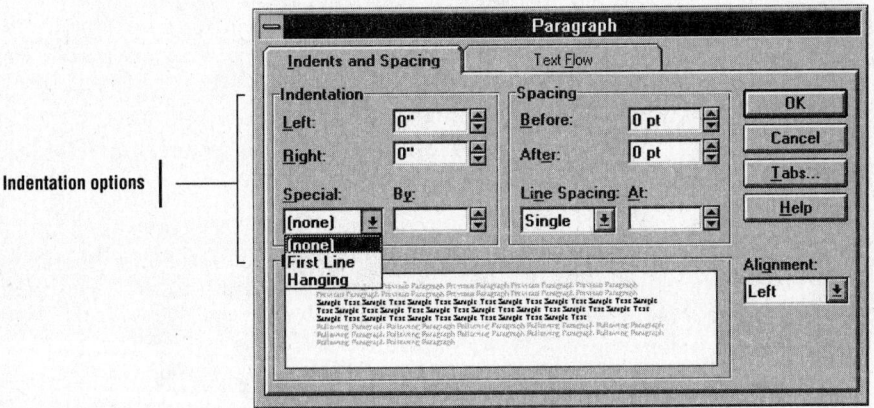

Figure 7-3
The Paragraph dialog box

Note: Remember, when selecting paragraphs to format, you do not have to select the entire paragraph. For example, to select two consecutive paragraphs, you can click in the last line of the first paragraph and drag into the first line of the second paragraph. Any formatting you then apply is applied to both paragraphs.

To set an indent using the Paragraph dialog box:

1. Start Word, if necessary.

2. Open the file 7-0.doc.

3. Select the two paragraphs under "Deadlines".

4. Choose Paragraph from the Format menu. Click the Indents and Spacing tab, if necessary.

5. Key **.5** in both the Left and Right text boxes (you can also click the arrow instead of keying).

   The text in the Preview box reflects the settings.

6. Click OK.

   Word indents the paragraphs .5 inches from both margins.

7. Place the insertion point anywhere in the opening paragraph (which begins "I would like to").

8. Click the right mouse button, and then choose Paragraph from the shortcut menu.

9. Choose First Line from the Special drop-down list box. Key **.25** in the By box and click OK.

   Word creates a first-line indent .25 inches from the left margin.

Setting Indents with the Ruler

You can set indents by dragging the *indent markers* on the horizontal ruler. There are three indent markers:

Indent markers
Markers that appear at the left and right margins on the ruler.

First-line indent marker

Left indent marker

Right indent marker

- First-line indent marker

  This marker appears at the top left of the ruler. When you drag it to the right, you create a first-line indent.

- Left indent marker

  This marker appears at the bottom left of the ruler and has a small box attached to it. You can drag the triangular portion of the left indent marker to set a left indent, or drag the small box to move both the left and first-line indent markers at once.

- Right indent marker

  This marker appears at the right margin on the ruler. Drag it to the left to create a right indent, which affects all lines of the paragraph.

Figure 7-4
Indent markers on the ruler

To set indents with the ruler:

1. Position the insertion point in the paragraph at the bottom of page 1, which begins "Write these deadlines".

2. Position the pointer on the right indent marker, and drag it to 5.5 inches on the ruler.

   The paragraph is indented from the right margin.

3. Position the pointer on the small box below the left indent marker. Drag it to the right 1 inch.

The left and first-line indent markers move together to indent the entire paragraph 1 inch from the left margin.

4. Select the paragraph that begins "July 1" and the four paragraphs below it, ending with the text "Give them the option".

5. Position the pointer on the left indent marker (just above the small box), and drag it to the right to .5 inches on the ruler.

   You have set a hanging indent. The first line of each paragraph remains at the left margin, and the rest of the paragraph aligns at the .5-inch indent.

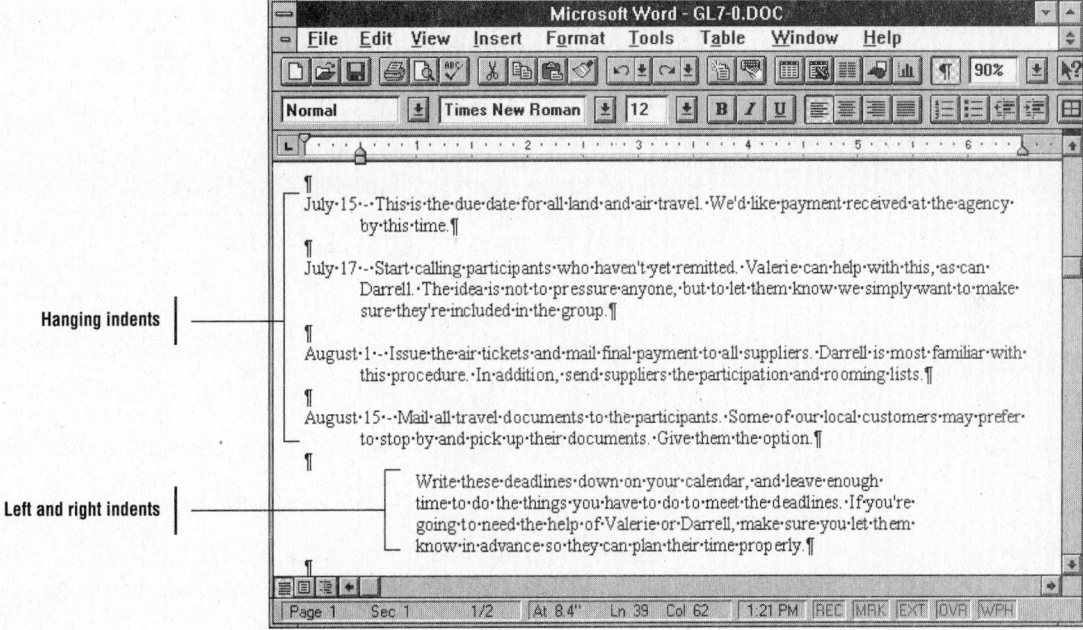

Figure 7-5
The document with indented paragraphs

Setting Indents with the Formatting Toolbar

Indent buttons on the
Formatting toolbar

Another way to set left indents is to use the Indent buttons on the Formatting toolbar. When you click the Increase Indent button, the selected paragraphs (or the paragraph containing the insertion point) move to the right, to the first tab stop. If default tabs are in use, the paragraph or paragraphs moves to the right .5 inches. If you click the Increase Indent button again, the paragraph moves to the next tab stop.

To decrease or undo the indent, click the Decrease Indent button. The paragraph moves to the left, one tab stop at a time.

To indent paragraphs using the indent buttons:

1. Select the text at the beginning of the document, from "MEMO TO:" to "Group Travel".

2. Click the Increase Indent button.

    The paragraphs move to the first tab stop (a 1-inch custom tab).

3. Click the Increase Indent button again.

    The paragraphs move to the 1.5-inch default tab stop.

4. Click the Decrease Indent button until the paragraphs align with the left margin (the 0 mark on the ruler).

Setting Indents with the Keyboard

The keyboard offers some shortcuts for setting indents. To use keyboard shortcuts, first select the paragraph to indent, or place the insertion point in the paragraph. Press **Ctrl+M** to set a left indent at the next tab stop, and press **Ctrl+Shift+M** to decrease the indent to the previous tab stop or to the left margin. To set a hanging indent, press **Ctrl+T**. Press it again to move the indent to the next tab stop, and press **Ctrl+Shift+T** to move the text back again.

To indent paragraphs using the keyboard:

1. Select the same text, from "MEMO TO:" to "Group Travel".

2. Press **Ctrl+M**.

    The paragraphs move to the first tab stop.

3. Press **Ctrl+M** again.

    The paragraphs move to the next tab stop.

4. Press **Ctrl+Shift+M** (or click the Decrease Indent button) to move the paragraphs back to the left margin.

Bulleted and Numbered Lists

Bulleted list
A hanging indent, in which lines of text are preceded by bullet characters.

Numbered list
A hanging indent, in which lines of text are preceded by sequential numbers or letters.

Numbering and Bullets buttons on the Formatting toolbar

Word provides two additional indenting options: *bulleted* and *numbered lists*. Both are types of hanging indents and are useful in organizing important details in a document.

In a bulleted list, each paragraph is preceded by a character known as a *bullet* (•). In a numbered list, each paragraph is preceded by a sequential number or letter.

To create a bulleted or numbered list, select the information to which you wish to add bullets or numbers. Then use the Bullets and Numbering command on the Format menu or the Bullets and Numbering buttons on the Formatting toolbar. Word adds bullets or numbers in sequence and automatically sets a .25-inch hanging indent.

You can also click the Bullets or Numbering button before you key text. Then the text you key is formatted with either bullets or numbers. When you finish keying the list, press **Enter**, and click the same button to turn off the formatting.

Bulleted Lists

The quickest way to create a bulleted list is to use the Bullets button on the Formatting toolbar. This method uses the standard bullet format (•). Other formats are available, such as a larger bullet character or a diamond-shaped character. To use another format, choose the Bullets and Numbering command from the Format menu. This opens the Bullets and Numbering dialog box, from which you can choose other formats and modify a bullet's shape, size, and color.

Figure 7-6
Bullet options in the Bullets and Numbering dialog box

To create a bulleted list:

1. On page 2 of document 7-0.doc, select the text from "Airline tickets" to "Flight bag".

2. Click the Bullets button on the Formatting toolbar.

   Word formats the list with the standard bullet and indents each paragraph line .25 inches.

3. With the list still selected, choose Bullets and Numbering from the Format menu.

4. Click the Bulleted tab, if necessary, and then choose one of the diamond-shaped bullets.

5. Click OK.

   Word reformats the list with diamond-shaped bullets.

Format menu

Numbered Lists

Create a numbered list the same way you create a bulleted list. The quickest method is to use the Numbering button on the Formatting toolbar. This method uses the standard numbering format, which is an Arabic numeral followed by a period (1.). To use another format, such as letters or Roman numerals, choose the Bullets and Numbering command from the Format menu. Click the Numbered tab, if necessary, and then choose a numbering formats.

Figure 7-7
Numbering options in the Bullets and Numbering dialog box

To create a numbered list:

1. Select the last three paragraphs in the document, from "Gateway Travel Agency" to "IATA".

2. Click the Numbering button.

    Word formats the list using the standard numbering style.

3. With the list still selected, choose Bullets and Numbering from the Format menu.

4. Click the Numbered tab, if necessary, choose the Roman numeral format, and click OK.

    Word reformats the list with Roman numerals.

Changing a Bulleted or Numbered List

Word's bulleting and numbering feature is very flexible. Once a list has been bulleted or numbered, you can change it in several ways. For example, you can:

*   Convert bullets to numbers or numbers to bullets in a list.

*   Add or remove items in a bulleted or numbered list. If you add or remove items in a numbered list, Word renumbers the list automatically. To add items to a bulleted or numbered list, press **Enter** after the last item to continue the formatting, and key the new text.

*   Interrupt a bulleted or numbered list to create several shorter lists. For example, a list numbered 1 through 10 can be interrupted by stopping the numbering midway. Word will then automatically start numbering the second half of the list at number 1.

*   Modify the bullet or list formatting. For example, you can add text such as "Number" before the numeral, change the symbol

used for bullets, or change the alignment and spacing of the bullets and numbers.

To convert bullets to numbers and rearrange items in a list:

1. Select the bulleted list in the document.

   You cannot select the bullets, just the text in the list.

2. Choose Bullets and Numbering from the Format menu.

3. Click the Numbered tab, and choose the first numbered format. Click OK.

   Word changes the bullets to numbers.

4. Select and delete the sixth item in the list, "Baggage tags."

   Word renumbers the list.

5. Place the insertion point at the end of the last item (after "supplier").

6. Press **Enter**, and key **Baggage tags**

   The formatting is carried to the new line.

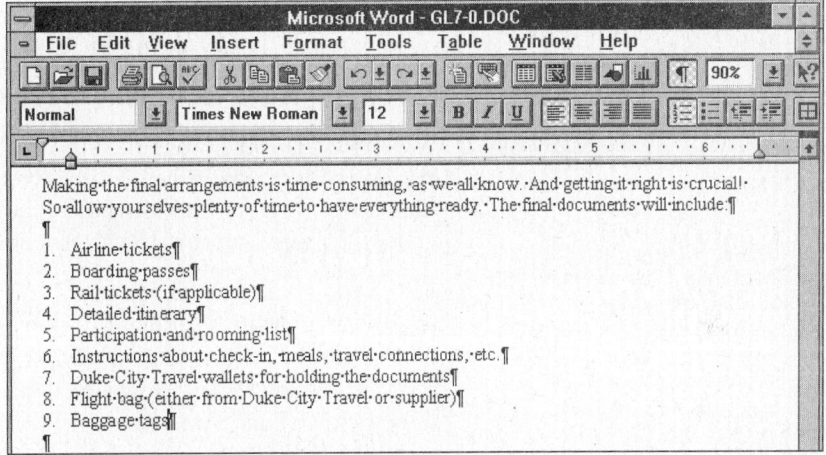

Figure 7-8
The numbered and rearranged list

The shortcut menu is used to interrupt a list. Place the insertion point where you want to break up the list, click the right mouse button, and then choose Stop Numbering from the shortcut menu.

To interrupt the numbered list:

1. Position the insertion point in the sixth item in the list.

2. Click the right mouse button, and choose Stop Numbering.

   Word interrupts the list by removing the numbering from the item and starting a new list under it.

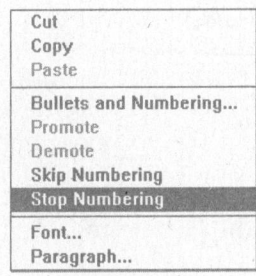

Shortcut menu

3. Click the Numbering button to restore the numbering for that line (you can also click the Undo button).

To modify list formatting, click the Modify button in the Bullets and Numbering dialog box. Then choose from a variety of options to change the appearance and spacing of the bullets or numbers.

Figure 7-9
The Modify Bulleted List dialog box

Choosing Special Bullets

Not only can you change the size, color, and spacing of a bullet, but you can also choose a new bullet shape. In the Modify Bulleted List dialog box, you can click the Bullets button. This button allows you to choose a special symbol to use as a bullet character.

When you click the Bullets button, Word displays the Symbol dialog box over the Modify Bulleted List dialog box. Depending upon the fonts installed with your printer, you can choose a symbol character, such as a heart (♥), an arrow (⇨), or a happy face (☺), for use in your documents. When you select a symbol, it appears as a bullet character in the Bullets and Numbering dialog box for future use.

Symbols are discussed further in Lesson 17: "Symbols, Special Characters, and Attributes".

Removing Bullets or Numbers

Once applied, bullets or numbers can easily be removed. To remove bullets or numbering from lists, select the text, and then choose one of three methods:

*   Click the Bullets or Numbering button on the Formatting toolbar to deselect it.

*   Choose Stop Numbering from the shortcut menu.

*   Click Remove in the Bullets and Numbering dialog box.

To remove numbers:

1. At the end of the document, select the list with the Roman numerals.

    Notice the Numbering button is selected on the Formatting toolbar.

2. Click the Numbering button to turn off the number formatting.

    Word removes the number formatting.

Introduction to Borders and Shading

Border

A line or box applied to paragraphs or sections in a document.

Note: Colors for borders and shading are not visible without a color monitor and cannot be printed without a color printer.

You can add visual interest to paragraphs in Word by adding a *border*, such as a line or a box. For example, you can add lines to separate sections within a document or place a box around a paragraph or a group of paragraphs. Another option is the application of shading to emphasize paragraphs. Shading can appear as a shade of gray, as a pattern, or as a color. Borders can appear in black or in color.

Figure 7-10

Variations in borders and shading

Borders and shading, once applied, become part of a paragraph's formatting. Like all paragraph formatting, the information about a paragraph's borders or shading is contained in the paragraph mark.

There are two ways to apply borders and shading to a paragraph:

*   Using the Borders button on the Formatting toolbar

*   Using the Borders and Shading command on the Format menu

Borders button

When you click the Borders button, Word opens the Borders toolbar, from which you can apply commonly used borders and shading to selected paragraphs. For more border and shading options, choose Borders and Shading from the Format menu.

Borders

The Borders toolbar allows you to apply borders such as top, bottom, or side rules to a paragraph, as well as box borders. You can choose from a variety of thicknesses for the lines, as well as dotted or dashed lines.

Figure 7-11
The Borders toolbar

If you choose Borders and Shading from the Format menu to open the Paragraph Borders and Shading dialog box, you can apply additional options, such as a shadow for a box border, or a border color. You can also change the spacing between borders and text.

To apply a border to a paragraph:

1. Place the insertion point in the paragraph on page 2 that begins "A booking should".

2. Click the Borders button on the Formatting toolbar.

    The Borders toolbar appears above the Standard toolbar.

3. Click the Outside Border button.

    Word adds a box border around the paragraph.

4. Move the insertion point to the paragraph below it that begins "Making the final".

5. Click the arrow to the right of the Line Style box on the Borders toolbar.

6. Choose the dotted-line border, and then click the Bottom Border button.

    A dotted-line border appears at the bottom of the paragraph.

Borders extend from the left margin to the right margin or, if indents are set, from the left indent to the right indent. To adjust the length of a paragraph border, you can change the indents in the Paragraph dialog box or use the indent marker on the ruler.

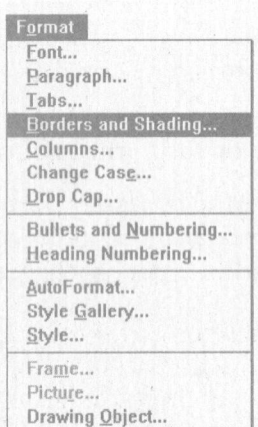

Format menu

To adjust a border:

1. Select the heading "Deadlines" on the first page, and remove the underlining.

2. Choose Borders and Shading from the Format menu.

    The Paragraph Borders and Shading dialog box appears.

3. In the Presets box, click Shadow.

4. Click the arrow to open the Color drop-down list, and then choose red. Click OK.

Figure 7-12
Border options in the Paragraph Borders and Shading dialog box

Right indent marker

Adjusting a border

Word applies a red box border with a shadow that extends from the left margin to the right margin.

5. Drag the right indent marker to the left, to .75 inches on the ruler.

    The box is adjusted to fit the heading.

To remove a border from a paragraph, select the paragraph, or place the insertion point in the paragraph. Click the No Border button on the Borders toolbar, if it is open, or click None in the Presets box in the Paragraph Borders and Shadow dialog box.

To remove a border:

1. Place the insertion point in the paragraph on page 2 with the dotted bottom-line border.

2. Click the No Border button on the Borders toolbar. You can also click the Bottom Border button to deselect it.

3. Place the insertion point in the paragraph with the box border (which begins "A booking should").

4. Choose Borders and Shading from the Format menu.

3. Click None in the Presets box, and then click OK.

    Word removes the border.

Shading

Shading can be used to offset a paragraph or column of text from the body text in the document. When you apply shading to a paragraph, the shading begins at the left margin and extends to the right margin. If a paragraph is left- and right-indented, the shading extends from the left indent to the right indent.

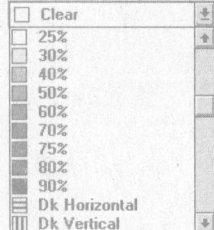

Background shading
options on the Borders
toolbar

Note: Shading may affect
the readability of text. It is
a good idea to use a
larger type size and bold
characters when you plan
to add shading to a para-
graph.

To apply background shading, select a paragraph, or place the insertion point in the paragraph. Then click an option from the Shading
box on the Borders toolbar. From the drop-down list, you can choose
a shade of gray from 5 to 90 percent, or a pattern, such as vertical
lines or a grid.

For more shading varieties, choose Borders and Shading from the
Format menu, and click the Shading tab. The dialog box allows you
to choose custom shading options, including both background and
foreground shading. You can preview these custom combinations in
the Preview box before choosing them.

To apply shading to a paragraph:

1. Select the text "<u>Deposits/Cancellations</u>" and the paragraph
   that follows it.

2. Click the arrow to the right of the Shading button on the
   Borders toolbar.

3. Choose a light-gray shading of 10%.

   The paragraph is lightly shaded.

4. Place the insertion point in the box around "Deadlines" on
   page 1.

5. Choose Borders and Shading from the Format menu, and click
   the Shading tab.

Figure 7-13
Shading options in the Paragraph Borders and Shading dialog box

6. In the dialog box, choose Yellow from the Foreground drop-
   down list. Choose 20% from the Shading box.

   The Preview box shows yellow dots against a white background,
   producing a light-yellow shading.

7. Click OK.

Word applies the light-yellow shading to the text within the border.

Removing shading is similar to removing a border. Use the None option in the Paragraph Borders and Shading dialog box. You may also use the Clear option in the Shading box on the Borders toolbar.

To remove shading from a paragraph:

1. Place the insertion point in the yellow-shaded text.

2. Choose Borders and Shading from the Format menu.

3. Choose Clear from the Shading list box.

    Notice that the Preview box is cleared of shading. Clear can also be chosen from the Shading box on the Borders toolbar.

4. Click the None option button.

    This clears all previous color selections and restores the original settings for the dialog box for this paragraph.

5. Click OK.

    Word removes the shading.

Shortcuts to Repeat, Copy, and Remove Paragraph Formats

Paragraph formatting can be quickly repeated, copied, or removed using many of the techniques taught in Lesson 3 for character formatting. For example, the **F4** key can be used to repeat paragraph formatting, and the Format Painter button can be used to copy paragraph formatting. Using these shortcuts to repeat and copy paragraph formatting is particularly helpful when several formats have been applied to a particular paragraph, such as indents, borders, and shading.

To repeat paragraph formatting:

1. Place the insertion point in the indented paragraph on page 1, which begins "Write these deadlines".

2. Choose Borders and Shading from the Format menu. Click the Borders tab, if necessary.

3. Apply a blue box border and click OK.

4. Move the insertion point to the paragraph below it that begins "All correspondence".

5. Press the **F4** key (or choose Repeat Border Outside from the Edit menu, or press **Ctrl+Y**).

    Word repeats the border formatting in the paragraph.

6. Click the Undo button.

Remember, the Repeat command is only used to repeat formatting that was just applied. In this example, the **F4** key repeated only the border, not the other paragraph formatting (the indents) applied to the paragraph earlier in the lesson. You can copy the paragraph formatting to copy all formats from one paragraph to another.

In addition, the Repeat command can repeat multiple formats chosen in a dialog box, such as the box border and the color. However, it can repeat only the last single format chosen using a toolbar button.

To copy paragraph formatting:

1. Select the indented paragraph that begins "Write these deadlines", including the paragraph mark. You can also just select the paragraph mark, which contains all the paragraph formatting.

Format Painter button

2. Click the Format Painter button on the Standard toolbar.

3. Move the painter pointer into the paragraph that begins "All correspondence" and click.

   Word copies all the formatting, including the indents, from one paragraph to the other.

To remove formatting from a paragraph:

1. Place the insertion point in the paragraph you just formatted (which begins "All correspondence").

2. Press **Ctrl+Q**.

   All the paragraph formatting is removed.

3. Click the Borders button to close the Borders toolbar.

4. Spell-check the document.

5. Add your reference initials to the end of the document.

6. Save the document as *[your three-letter identifier]*7-0.doc.

7. Print the document.

8. Close the document and exit Word (unless you will be doing the following exercises immediately).

Table 7-1: Keyboard Shortcuts for Paragraph Formatting

Keyboard Shortcut	Action
Ctrl+M	Indent from left margin
Ctrl+Shift+M	Decrease indent
Ctrl+T	Set hanging indent
Ctrl+Shift+T	Decrease hanging indent
Ctrl+Q	Remove paragraph formatting

Key Terms

Border	Indent marker
Bullet	Left indent
Bulleted list	Negative indent
First-line indent	Numbered list
Hanging indent	Positive indent
Indent	Right indent

Exercises

Exercise 7.1

1. Start Word, if necessary.

2. Open the file 7-1.doc.

3. Set a first-line indent:

   A. Select the entire document.

   B. Choose Paragraph from the Format menu.

   C. Choose First Line from the Special drop-down list box.

   D. Set the indent to .5", if necessary, and click OK.

4. Set a left and right indent for paragraphs 2-6:

   A. Select paragraphs 2-6 (from the start of the paragraph that begins "On Day 1" to the end of the paragraph that begins "Day 5").

   B. Click the Increase Indent button on the Formatting toolbar to create a left indent.

   C. Drag the right indent marker to 5.5 inches on the ruler.

5. Remove the paragraph formatting from the first paragraph:

   A. Place the insertion point in the paragraph that begins "Enjoy 5 fabulous".

   B. Press **Ctrl+Q**.

6. Add a border and shading to the first paragraph:

   A. With the insertion point in the paragraph, click the Borders button on the Formatting toolbar.

   B. Click the Outside Border button on the Borders toolbar.

   C. Choose the 10% shade of gray from the Shading box.

7. Center-align the text in the paragraph that begins "Enjoy 5 fabulous".

8. Click the Borders button to close the Borders toolbar.

9. Spell-check the document.

10. Save the document as *[your three-letter identifier]*7-1.doc.

11. Print the document.

12. Close the document and exit Word (unless you will be doing the following exercises immediately).

Exercise 7.2

1. Start Word, if necessary.

2. Open the file 7-2.doc.

3. Set a hanging indent and a right indent:

    A. Select the paragraphs with underlined headings on the first page, from "<u>Churches and religious organizations</u>" through "<u>Singles Clubs</u>".

    B. Drag the left indent marker to .25 inches on the ruler.

    C. Drag the right indent marker to 6 inches on the ruler.

4. Create a negative indent:

    A. Scroll to the paragraph that begins "First, identify". Place the insertion point to the right of the colon after "following", and press **Enter** twice.

    B. Key **Community Groups**

    C. With the insertion point in the "Community Groups" paragraph, choose Paragraph from the Format menu.

    D. Key **-.25** in the Left text box and click OK.

5. Create a bulleted list:

    A. Select the list at the bottom of the second page, from "Annual visits" to "theater weekend".

    B. Choose Bullets and Numbering from the Format menu.

    C. Click the Bulleted tab, if necessary.

    D. Choose the diamond bullet and click OK.

6. Copy the paragraph formatting from the paragraph that begins "<u>Singles Clubs</u>" at the bottom of page 1 to the paragraph that begins "<u>Businesses</u>" on the next page:

    A. Select the paragraph mark for the paragraph that begins "<u>Singles Clubs</u>".

    B. Click the Format Painter button on the Standard toolbar.

    C. Move the pointer into the paragraph that begins "<u>Businesses</u>", and click the left mouse button.

7. Set a left indent for the next paragraph, which begins "Group travel", using the keyboard shortcut:

   A. Place the insertion point in the paragraph.

   B. Press **Ctrl+M**.

8. Apply a double-underline border to the first paragraph:

   A. Place the insertion point in the paragraph.

   B. Click the Borders button.

   C. Choose the ¾ pt double-underline border from the Line Style box.

   D. Click the Bottom Border button.

   E. Close the Borders toolbar.

9. Spell-check the document.

10. Save the document as *[your three-letter identifier]*7-2.doc.

11. Print the document.

12. Close the document and exit Word (unless you will be doing the following exercises immediately).

Exercise 7.3

1. Start Word, if necessary.

2. Open the file 7-3.doc.

3. Set the left and right margins to 1.25 inches (the default settings).

4. Edit the second paragraph as shown in Figure 7-14.

Figure 7-14

the   (STET)   *we offer*

Our local area tours are ~~some of our most~~ popular special-interest tours.

The treasures of New Mexico make for excellent itineraries focusing on

architecture, arch*a*eology, Native American culture, and nature. *Some of the Southwest attractions are* ~~We have~~

~~arranged photography tours, museum sponsored tours, cycling tours, and~~

~~student tours~~

Monument Valley

The Taos Pueblos

Petroglyph State Park

The Grand Canyon

The

Rio Grande

The Cliff Palace Ruins

5. Using the Bullets and Numbering dialog box, format the three lists that begin "Monument Valley", "The Great Sphinx", and "Hawaii" with the standard bullet. (Remember, use the Repeat command.)

6. Format each of the paragraphs in the document, but not the lists, with a first-line indent of .5 inches.

7. Using the Paragraph dialog box, reformat the bulleted lists by creating a 2-inch indent from the left margin and 3-point spacing before paragraphs.

8. Make the last sentence in the document a separate paragraph. Place a box border around it using the thinnest double line, and delete the period.

9. Adjust the length of the border by removing the first-line indent and setting .75-inch left and right indents. Center-align the text within the box.

10. If the box moves to the second page, change the bottom margin to .75 inches.

11. Spell-check the document, adding foreign names to the world or Southwest dictionary, if necessary.

12. Save the document as *[your three-letter identifier]*7-3.doc.

13. Print the document.

14. Close the document and exit Word (unless you will be doing the following exercise immediately.)

Exercise 7.4: Challenge Yourself

Open the file 7-4.doc, and clear all paragraph formatting, including tabs, indents, shading, borders, and character attributes. Left-align the document.

Format the document as a standard business memo to Nina Chavez from Valerie Grier. The subject is Toronto bed-and-breakfast accommodations. Insert the date as a field, and add a 2¼-point bottom border below the memo heading (add it to the blank paragraph under "SUBJECT:").

Format the three paragraphs that begin "The Fountaines" to "Lowter House" as a numbered list, using the uppercase-letter format with periods. Add the following paragraph to the numbered list, keying it after the paragraph that begins "The St. Clair":

"The Brookside" is a charming Edwardian home in the University area of Toronto. It has a beautiful parlor room with a piano that is available to guests. A full breakfast is served on weekends and a continental breakfast on weekdays. They offer a large bedroom with a fireplace and antique furniture. The room has a private bath and is $50 per night.

Change the hanging indent of the numbered list to .5 inches. (Hint: Click the Modify button in the Bullets and Numbering dialog box, and then edit the Distance from Indent to Text box.) Change line spacing to 6 points after paragraphs.

Change the hyphens in the first paragraph to nonbreaking hyphens, and then spell-check and grammar-check the document. Allow the passive voice, and add names to the world dictionary, if necessary.

Save the document as *[your three-letter identifier]*7-4.doc and print it. Close the document and exit Word.

An Announcement and a Memo

Background

The Duke City Gateway Travel Agency is known worldwide for its unique special-interest tour packages. These special-interest tours range from local tours of New Mexican pueblos to exotic international archaeological tours. In honor of its 25th anniversary in business, Duke City Gateway Travel is offering its customers low rates on their special-interest tours.

Duke City Gateway Travel's manager, Susan Allen, will notify customers of the new tour rates with an announcement, and will notify Duke City Gateway Travel's agents with a memo.

Business Purpose

Create an announcement for Duke City Gateway Travel customers to inform them of the special tour prices. Then create a memo to inform Duke City Gateway Travel agents of the special tour prices.

Procedures

1. Start Word, if necessary.
2. Open the file p2-1.doc.
3. Center the heading "ATTENTION TRAVELERS", and make it bold.
4. Apply a double-line box border and a light-gray background shade to the heading.
5. Make the next line of text bold and centered.
6. Make the headings "Local-Interest Tour", "International Tour", "Naturalist Tour", and "Music Tour" italic.
7. Make the paragraph that begins "Take Advantage" bold.
8. Center and make bold the text from "For more information" through "(505) 555-1234". Then apply a double-line box border to the text.
9. Indent the text from "Local-Interest Tour" through "Radio City Music Hall" .5 inches from the left and from the right.

10. For the same text, set a 5-inch left-aligned tab with a dotted leader.

11. After "New Mexican Indian Pueblos", insert the tab leader by pressing the **Tab** key, and then key **$199**

12. After "Greece", insert the tab leader and key **$699**

13. After "Alaska", insert the tab leader and key **$850**

14. After "New York City", insert the tab leader and key **$249**

15. Use print preview to change the top margin to 1.5 inches.

16. Make any changes you feel will improve the appearance of the document.

17. Spell-check the document.

18. Save the document as [*your three-letter identifier*]p2-1.doc and print it.

19. Close the document, and then create a new file.

20. Using the standard form as shown in Appendix C, format a memo to the Duke City Gateway Travel agents from Susan Allen. The subject of the memo is the low rates on special-interest tours. Insert the date as a field.

21. After the memo headings, key the sentence:

    In celebration of our 25th anniversary in business, we will lower our prices on the following special-interest tours:

22. Press **Enter** twice, and key the following list:

    Local-Interest Tour: New Mexican Pueblos

    International Tour: Greece

    Naturalist Tour: Alaska

    Music Tour: New York City

23. Indent the list 1 inch from the left. Then format it as a bulleted list (using a standard bullet and the default bullet indent of .25 inches), and change the line spacing to 1.5 lines.

24. Press **Enter** twice after the bulleted list, clear the bullet formatting from the paragraph mark, and key **Tour**. Press the **Tab** key, and key **Former Price**. Then press the **Tab** key, and key **New Low Price**

25. Change the tabs for this line to two centered tabs, spacing the text evenly between the margins.

26. Press **Enter,** and create tabbed columns by keying the following information:

New Mexican Pueblos	$215.00	$199.00
Greece	$799.00	$699.00
Alaska	$999.00	$850.00
New York City	$299.00	$249.00

27. Change the line spacing of the tabbed columns (including the heading for each column) to double spacing.

28. Underline the entire line of text that contains "Tour", "Former Price", and "New Low Price".

29. Make any change you feel will improve the appearance of the document.

30. Spell-check the document.

31. Save the document as *[your three-letter identifier]*p2-2.doc and print it.

32. Close the document and exit Word.

Tips and Hints

- Use borders to emphasize the important information in your document.

- When shading text, it is best to use a light shade. If you use a shade that is darker than 5 percent, make the text bold.

- Create tabbed columns for lists of information to give your documents an organized appearance.

- Use the paragraph-alignment settings to distinguish one part of the document from another. For example, center the headings in your document to separate them from the body text.

- To give your memos a uniform appearance, single-space the paragraphs in the body of the memo, and leave one blank line between paragraphs.

Working with Text and Documents

Moving and Copying Text

One of the most useful features of word processing is the ability to move text from one part of a document to another and to copy text from one part of a document to another without having to rekey the entire document. In Word, there are several ways to move and copy text quickly. This lesson introduces the Cut, Copy, and Paste commands, drag-and-drop editing, and a special Windows feature—the Clipboard.

Moving Text

Moving text means cutting it from one location and pasting it to another. Text can be moved using a variety of methods:

- The Cut and Paste commands—available from the Edit menu, the shortcut menu, the Standard toolbar, and by using keyboard shortcuts. The Cut and Paste commands involve use of the Clipboard, and can be used to move text from one document to another.

Note: To undo the moving of text, click the Undo button, or choose Undo Move from the Edit menu immediately after the procedure.

- The drag-and-drop method, which involves use of the mouse

Using the Clipboard to Cut and Paste

A common way to move text is to use the Cut and Paste commands. The Cut command deletes selected text from a document, and the Paste command inserts the text into a new location. When the text is deleted from a document using the Cut command, it is placed on the Clipboard. The *Clipboard* is a temporary storage area. Text stored on the Clipboard can be moved to any location in a document and can be inserted as many times as you wish. Text remains on the Clipboard until another selection is cut (using the Cut command) or copied. The new selection replaces the text previously stored on the Clipboard.

Clipboard
A temporary storage area used to hold text that is cut or copied.

Selections generally stay on the Clipboard even after you quit Word. This allows you to paste the Clipboard material into another application. When you have moved or copied a large amount of text using the Clipboard, you may get a screen message asking if you want to save the Clipboard contents. Save the contents if you plan to use them, or click No to clear the Clipboard.

By using the Clipboard to cut and paste text, you eliminate the need to rekey many documents and sections within documents. There are three ways to access the Cut and Paste commands for moving text:

- Choose the Cut and Paste commands from the Edit menu or the shortcut menu.

- Click the Cut and Paste buttons on the Standard toolbar.

- Use the keyboard commands **Ctrl+X** to cut and **Ctrl+V** to paste.

The first step in moving text is to select it. Selecting text correctly is important and saves editing steps after cutting and pasting. Whenever text is selected, remember to include the punctuation, paragraph mark, or blank line adjacent to the word, sentence, or paragraph to be moved.

To move text using the Cut and Paste commands from the Edit menu:

1. Start Word, if necessary.

2. Open the file 8-0.doc.

3. On the subject line of the memo, select "New York".

4. Choose Cut from the Edit menu.

   The text is deleted from the document and stored on the Clipboard.

5. Position the insertion point to the left of "Night on the Town".

6. Choose Paste from the Edit menu.

   Word moves the text to the new location.

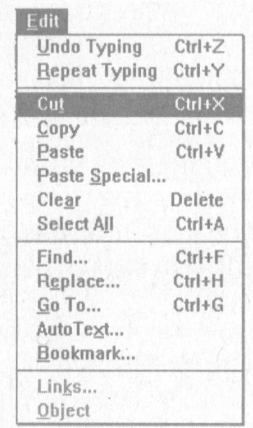

Edit menu

Note: You may have noticed in earlier lessons that when you select a word or words, such as "New York" in this procedure, Word selects the entire word and the space character after each word. This is the result of the editing option Automatic Word Selection. In this procedure, when you pasted the text, Word pasted it with the space character, eliminating the need to enter a space with the **Spacebar**.

After using the Cut command, the text "New York" remains on the Clipboard until new text is selected and cut.

Clipboard icon

Viewing the Clipboard

You can view the contents of the Clipboard in Windows. To do this, switch to Windows Program Manager and open the Main window. Double-click the Clipboard icon. The Clipboard Viewer window displays the text or graphics you last cut or copied using the Cut or Copy commands.

Cut, Copy, and Paste
buttons on the Standard
toolbar

Note: When using the Cut
and Paste commands to
move text, the Undo com-
mand will undo the inser-
tion of the text to the new
location, but it will not automatically restore the text
deleted from the old location. Remember, though,
that the text is stored on the
Clipboard. Use the Paste
command to insert the text
at its original location.

Drag-and-drop editing
A method of editing that
allows you to move or
copy text by dragging,
without cutting, copying,
or pasting.

You can also move text using the Cut and Paste buttons on the Standard toolbar and the cut and paste keyboard shortcuts.

Use these additional cut and paste methods to move text:

1. Select the text "New York" (and the space following it) again.

2. Click the Cut button on the Standard toolbar.

3. Move the insertion point to the left of "Weekends".

4. Click the Paste button.

5. Scroll down to the paragraph that begins "All the hotels".
   Select the paragraph, including the paragraph mark below it
   (selecting the second paragraph mark will delete and move the
   blank line).

6. Press **Ctrl+X** to cut the selection.

7. Move the insertion point to the left of "Please" in the last
   paragraph.

8. Press **Ctrl+V** to paste the selection.

Using Drag-and-Drop Editing to Move Text

Drag-and-drop editing allows you to move or copy text to a new location by dragging the selection. It involves no cutting, copying, or
pasting.

Dragging text to move it is useful when moving a short distance.

To use drag-and-drop editing to move text:

1. In the paragraph that begins "Rates are based", select the text
   "per night".

2. Point to the selection, and then hold down the left mouse
   button to display a small, dotted box and a dotted insertion
   point. Drag the dotted insertion point to the right of the word
   "more". Release the mouse button.

   The selection is inserted at the new location. See Figure 8-1 on
   page 154.

You may need to move text to another location that is too far to use
the drag-and-drop method. In that case, use Cut and Paste, or select
the text you want to move, hold down the **Ctrl** key, and click the right
mouse button at the new location. This method and the drag-and-
drop method do not involve the Clipboard. Therefore, they are useful when you do not want to replace what is currently on the
Clipboard.

To move text using the mouse and the **Ctrl** key:

1. Select the last paragraph, which begins "Please refer", and the
   paragraph mark below it.

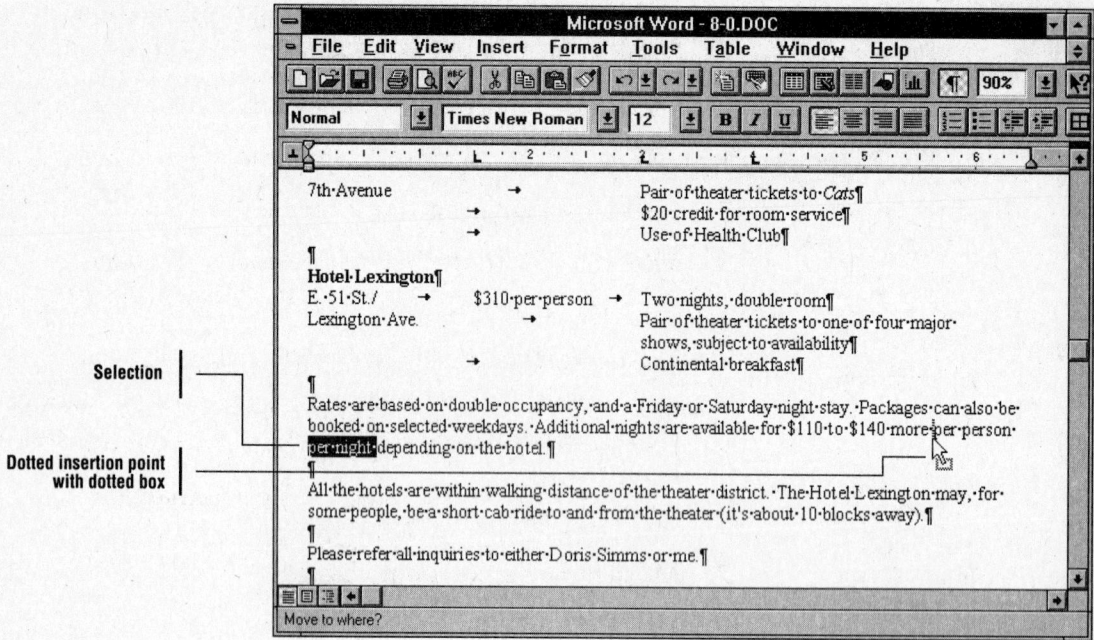

Selection

Dotted insertion point with dotted box

Figure 8-1
Dragging to move text

2. Scroll to the top of the document. Hold down the **Ctrl** key, and, in the selection bar, point to the paragraph beginning "There are three". Click the right mouse button.

    Word moves the paragraph to the new location.

Copying Text

Copying text means making a copy of the selected text and inserting it in another location, leaving the original unchanged. Text can be copied using a variety of methods:

Note: To undo the copying of text, click the Undo button, or choose Undo from the Edit menu immediately after the procedure.

*   The Copy and Paste commands—available from the Edit menu, the shortcut menu, the Standard toolbar, and by using keyboard shortcuts. Like the Cut and Paste commands, Copy and Paste involve use of the Clipboard and can be used to copy text from one document to another.

*   The drag-and-drop method, which involves use of the mouse

Using the Clipboard to Copy and Paste

Copy and Paste are similar to Cut and Paste. The difference is between Cut and Copy: the Cut command deletes a selection, while the Copy command duplicates a selection. Both commands store the selection on the Clipboard, so it can be pasted to a new location. Remember, a selection remains on the Clipboard until you use the Copy or Cut command again, which replaces the selection.

Using the Copy and Paste command saves time and rekeying when text needs to be repeated throughout a document or copied from one document to another (see Lesson 9: "Working with Multiple Document Windows").

There are three ways to access the Copy and Paste commands:

- Choose the Copy and Paste commands from the Edit menu or shortcut menu.

- Click the Copy and Paste buttons on the Standard toolbar.

- Use the keyboard commands **Ctrl+C** to copy and **Ctrl+V** to paste.

Whether you are copying a word, a sentence, or a paragraph, remember to select the appropriate punctuation or paragraph marks.

To copy text using the Copy and Paste commands:

1. Under "Peabody Hotel", select the line of text containing the headings, along with the paragraph mark.

2. Click the right mouse button, and choose Copy from the shortcut menu.

3. Place the insertion point to the left of "W. 47 St." under "Renaissance Hotel".

4. Choose Paste from the Edit menu.

    Word copies the text to the new location. The selected text remains on the Clipboard and can be copied again.

5. Move the insertion point to the left of "E. 51 St." below "Hotel Lexington".

6. Click the Paste button on the Standard toolbar.

    The text is repeated in the new location.

7. Under the package description of Hotel Lexington, select the text "subject to availability". Include the comma and the space character preceding it, but not the paragraph mark following it.

8. Press **Ctrl+C** to copy the selection.

9. Under the package description for the Renaissance Hotel, move the insertion point to the right of "Cats".

10. Press **Ctrl+V** to paste the selection. See Figure 8-2 on page 156.

Shortcut menu

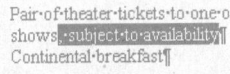

Selection

Using Drag-and-Drop Editing to Copy Text

You can use the drag-and-drop method to copy text by selecting the text, holding down the **Ctrl** key, and then dragging the selection. Another way to copy text is to select the text, hold down the **Ctrl** and **Shift** keys, and click the right mouse button at the new location. These methods do not involve the Clipboard, and they can be used when you want to preserve what is currently on the Clipboard.

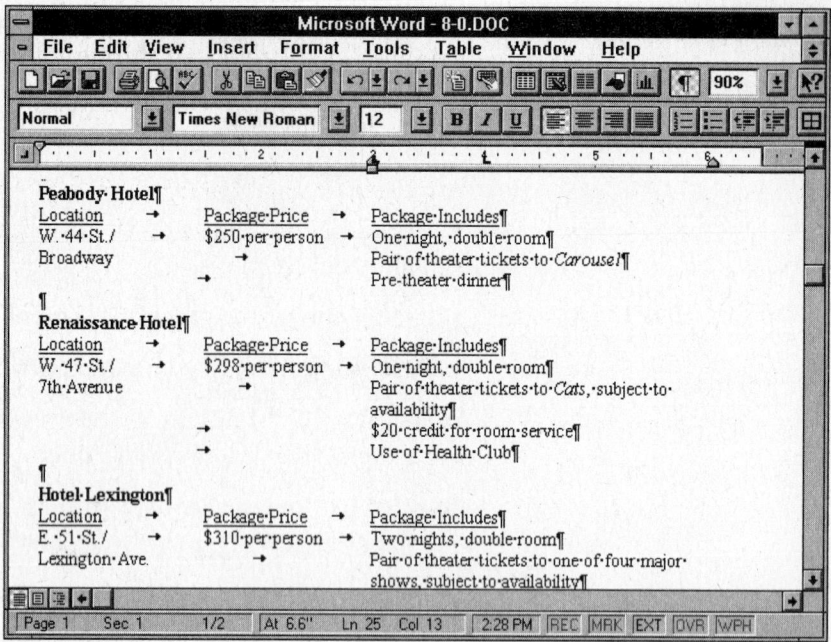

Figure 8-2
The document with copied text

To use the drag-and-drop method and the **Ctrl+Shift** method to copy text:

1. Select the text you have just copied, including the comma and the space character but not the paragraph mark.

2. Hold down the **Ctrl** key, point to the selection, and hold down the left mouse button.

3. Drag the dotted insertion point to the right of "Carousel" in the Peabody Hotel package description. Release the mouse button and the **Ctrl** key.

    Word copies the text to the new location.

4. Click the Undo button.

5. With the text still selected, hold down the **Ctrl** and **Shift** keys, move the insertion point to the right of "Carousel", and click the right mouse button.

    The selection is once again copied to the new location.

Smart Cut and Paste

Whenever you cut, paste, or copy text using either the Cut, Paste, and Copy commands or drag-and-drop editing, Word adjusts the spaces between words. For example, if you delete a word at the end of a sentence, Word will automatically delete the space before the word. If you insert a word in the middle of a sentence, Word will make sure there is one space before and one space after the word. This is called

Smart Cut and Paste. It is a special editing feature that is turned on when you start Word. To make sure it is turned on, choose Options from the Tools menu, click the Edit tab, and check the Smart Cut and Paste check box.

Figure 8-3
Editing options

In addition to Smart Cut and Paste, other default editing options in the Options dialog box are Typing Replaces Selection, which deletes selected text as soon as you key text; Drag-and-Drop Text Editing, which allows you to use the drag-and-drop method taught in this lesson; and Automatic Word Selection, which was described earlier.

To observe Smart Cut and Paste in action:

1. In the second paragraph after the memo heading, delete the word "either".

2. Select the text at the end of the sentence "or me", not including the space character before "or" or the period after "me".

3. Cut the text.

    Word closes up the space before the period.

4. With the insertion point before the period, insert the text again by pasting it from the Clipboard.

    Word inserts the text and inserts a space character before it.

Figure 8-4
Smart Cut and Paste adjusts word spacing

Moving and Copying Columns

In Word, you can move and copy columns to a new location in a document. The technique described in this lesson is for moving and copying tabbed columns.

To move or copy a column, first select the text. The technique for selecting a vertical block of text, such as a column, is to hold down the **Alt** key, place the insertion point at one corner, and drag to the opposite corner. After selecting the tabbed column, use one of the move or copy methods to position the selection.

To move a tabbed column:

1. At the end of document 8-0.doc, double space after the last paragraph. Clear all tabs, and then set .5- and 2.5-inch left-aligned tabs.

2. Beginning at the left margin, key the following text, pressing the **Tab** key after each number (for example, after "1.") and before the last item in each line (for example, before "How many people?"):

   For immediate telephone bookings:
   1. Ask for show preference   Theater?
   2. Ask for hotel preference   How many people?
   3. Ask for major credit card   Credit-card payment?

3. To move the column that begins "Theater?", select it along with the preceding tab characters. To do this, place the insertion point to the left of the tab character before "Theater?", hold down the **Alt** key, and drag down to the opposite corner ("payment?"). Extend the selection to the right to include all three paragraph marks. Release the **Alt** key and the mouse button. See Figure 8-5 on page 159.

4. Click the Cut button.

5. Move the insertion point to the right of the period in "1.", and click the Paste button.

   The tabbed column is moved to the new location.

6. To make the memo fit on one page, delete the paragraphs that begin "There are three" and "All the hotels". Delete the "Hotel Peabody" package, add your own reference initials to the memo, and change the top margin to 2 inches.

7. Spell-check the document.

8. Save the document as *[your three-letter identifier]*8-0.doc.

9. Print the document.

10. Close the document and exit Word (unless you will be doing the following exercises immediately).

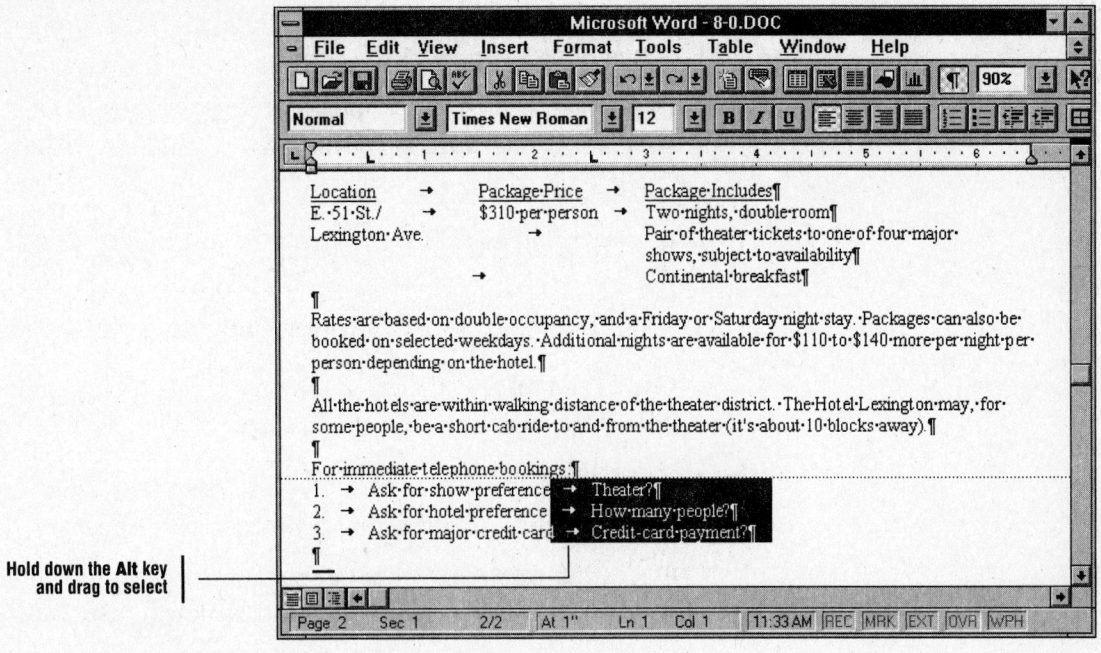

Hold down the Alt key and drag to select

Figure 8-5
Selecting a tabbed column to move it

Table 8-1: Keyboard Shortcuts for Moving and Copying Text	
Keyboard Shortcut	Action
Ctrl+X	Cut text
Ctrl+V	Paste text
Ctrl+C	Copy text

Key Terms

Clipboard   Drag-and-drop editing

Exercises

Exercise 8.1

1. Start Word, if necessary.

2. Open the file 8-1.doc.

3. In the first paragraph after the salutation, move the first sentence using the Cut and Paste commands from the Edit menu:

   A. Select the sentence beginning "I received" and the space character following it.

   B. Choose Cut from the Edit menu.

C.   Move the insertion point to the end of the paragraph, and choose Paste from the Edit menu.

4.   In the next paragraph, copy "Hot Springs" from the first sentence to the third sentence using keyboard shortcuts:

A.   Select "Hot Springs".

B.   Press **Ctrl+C** to copy the text.

C.   Move the insertion point to the right of "Caliente" on the next line, and then press **Ctrl+V**.

5.   Copy the name of the spa to the next-to-the-last paragraph before the closing using the buttons on the Standard toolbar:

A.   Select the text "Ojo Caliente Hot Springs".

B.   Click the Copy button on the Standard toolbar.

C.   In the paragraph that begins "Our manager", delete the word "there", and key **at**, and click the Paste button.

6.   In the paragraph that begins "The new spa", reverse the order of the fourth and fifth sentences using the drag-and-drop method:

A.   Select the fourth sentence, which begins "There are 3", and the space that follows it.

B.   Point to the sentence, hold down the left mouse button, and drag the dotted insertion point to the left of the sentence beginning "Their restaurant".

7.   In the last sentence of this paragraph, reverse the order of "artists" and "craftspeople" using the drag-and-drop method of moving text.

8.   Add your own reference initials to the document and an enclosure notation.

9.   Spell-check the document.

10.   Save the document as *[your three-letter identifier]*8-1.doc.

11.   Print the document.

12.   Close the document and exit Word (unless you will be doing the following exercises immediately).

Exercise 8.2

1.   Start Word, if necessary.

2.   Open the original file 7-2.doc, which was used in the last lesson.

3.   Move the first paragraph on page 2 to page 1 using the **Ctrl** key:

A. Scroll to the paragraph on page 2 that begins "<u>Businesses</u>", and select the paragraph, including the paragraph mark below it.

B. Hold down the **Ctrl** key, scroll to the top of the document, and position the insertion point to the left of "<u>Churches</u>".

C. Click the right mouse button.

4. At the end of the paragraph that begins "<u>Sports clubs</u>", key:

(Use local directory for listings.)

5. Copy the text you just keyed to the end of the next three paragraphs using the Copy button on the Standard toolbar:

A. Select the text, excluding the paragraph mark at the end of it.

B. Click the Copy button on the Standard toolbar.

C. Move the insertion point to the end of the next paragraph, then click the Paste button on the Standard toolbar.

D. With the text still on the Clipboard, repeat the previous step for the next two paragraphs.

6. Move the paragraphs that begin "<u>Recreation clubs</u>" and "<u>Singles clubs</u>" above the paragraph that begins "<u>Ethnic groups</u>" using keyboard shortcuts:

A. Select the two paragraphs, including the paragraph mark below the second paragraph.

B. Press **Ctrl+X**.

C. Scroll up, place the insertion point to the left of "<u>Ethnic groups</u>", and press **Ctrl+V**.

7. Move the text in the list at the end of the document to create two columns:

A. Select the list, clear any tabs, and set a 3.5-inch left-aligned tab.

B. Place a tab character at the end of each of the first four lines of the list.

C. Hold down the **Alt** key, and drag to select the last four lines of the list. Release the **Alt** key.

D. Choose Cut from the shortcut menu.

E. Move the insertion point to the right of the tab character following "Holy Land", and then choose Paste from the shortcut menu.

8. Remove any extra paragraph marks between paragraphs, and then spell-check the document.

9.   Save the document as *[your three-letter identifier]*8-2.doc.

10.   Print the document.

11.   Close the document and exit Word (unless you will be doing the following exercises immediately).

Exercise 8.3

1.   Start Word, if necessary.

2.   Open the file 5-0.doc.

3.   Edit the last paragraph, as shown in Figure 8-6. Include the corrections.

Figure 8-6

From Santa Fe, the tour begins at

The last stop on the Trail is Cerrillos, a once booming mining
town in the 1880s with gold, silver, and the oldest turquoise
mine. Today it looks like a movie set for a sleepy border town.
Follow the signs to "Casa Grande," an old *20 = room* adobe with its own
museum of *and* turquoise and artifacts. Also on the premises is a
petting zoo and a frontier trading post. Inquire *here* at "Casa Grande"
about *walking tours* hikes or four-wheel drive tours of the old Pueblo turquoise
mines in the nearby hills.

4.   In the second paragraph, delete the text "From Albuquerque, the tour begins at", and key **The last stop on the Trail is**

5.   Move the second paragraph to the end of the document as the last paragraph.

6.   Move the paragraph that begins "From Santa Fe" to follow the first paragraph.

7.   Move the paragraph that begins "Further along" to follow the second paragraph.

8.   Move the paragraph that begins "As you pass" to follow the third paragraph.

9.   Add the heading **THE TURQUOISE TRAIL** to the document using bold, all-capital letters. Insert two blank lines after the heading, and change the top margin of the document to 2 inches.

10.   Spell-check the document, adding words to the Southwest dictionary, if necessary.

11. Save the document as *[your three-letter identifier]*8-3.doc.

12. Print the document.

13. Close the document and exit Word (unless you will be doing the following exercise immediately).

Exercise 8.4: Challenge Yourself

Open the file 8-4 doc. Copy the headings "<u>Departing From</u>" and "<u>Rate</u>" to the adjacent two columns. Select the text for airfares, from "<u>Departing From</u>" through "$294-399". Change the 2-inch tab to 2.5 inches, and add a .5-inch left-aligned tab stop. Press the **Tab** key at the beginning of each line, from "<u>Departing From</u>" through "Arkansas".

Move all the columnar text to the end of the document. Insert one blank line between the end of the itinerary and the start of the columnar text.

Press **Enter** twice at the end of the airfare text, and then key the following text. Choose tab stops that allow proper spacing between columns and proper alignment:

<u>Land Rates Per Person*</u>

	<u>Twin</u>	<u>Single</u>	<u>Triple</u>	<u>Child</u>
May	$1079	$1549	$1049	$579
July 1-May 30	$1179	$1649	$1149	$679
Rest of Year	$1129	$1589	$1089	$629

*All meals are included.

In Day 4 of the itinerary, delete the last two sentences. Move the last sentence from Day 5 to the end of Day 4. In Day 1, delete the words "the many wonders of this city" from the third sentence. Copy this same sentence to the end of the Day 5 itinerary, and to the Day 7 itinerary, before the sentence that begins "Later in the afternoon".

Format each line of text that begins "Day" with a bullet and a .25-inch hanging indent. Change line spacing for all of the itinerary, from "Itinerary" to "Colorado", to 6 points after paragraphs.

Change the first line of the document to bold, all capitals. Remove the italics from "Itinerary", and make the word bold and underlined.

Spell-check the document. Add words to the Southwest dictionary, if necessary. Save the document as *[your three-letter identifier]*8-4.doc and print it. Close the document and exit Word.

Working with Multiple Document Windows

There are often occasions for working with more than one part of a document at a time. This occurs, for example, when you need to move text from one part of a long document to another part. There are also occasions when you want to use different documents at the same time—for example, to copy or move text from one document to another.

You can, of course, continually scroll back and forth throughout long documents, or open and close files every time you need them. But Word offers much easier ways to perform these tasks. You can open multiple windows of the same document or of different documents. Working with multiple windows can make it much more convenient to find and edit text.

Splitting a Document into Panes

One way to view two parts of a document at once is to split the document into *panes*. Panes are horizontal windows that each contain a portion of the document with which you are working.

There are two ways to split a window:

- Choose Split from the Window menu.

- Use the split box at the top of the vertical scroll bar.

When you choose Split from the Window menu, Word displays a *split bar*, and the pointer becomes a two-headed arrow positioned over the split bar. Use the mouse to position the bar, and then press **Enter** to insert the split. To remove the split bar, press the **Esc** key.

Pane
A portion of a document that is displayed onscreen in a horizontal window.

Split bar
A horizontal bar that can be moved to split a document window.

Window menu

To split a document using the Window menu:

1. Start Word, if necessary.

2. Open the file 2-3.doc.

3. Choose Split from the Window menu.

   The split bar appears with the split pointer—a two-headed arrow separated by two horizontal lines. See Figure 9-1 on page 166.

4. Use the mouse to move the split bar after the second paragraph, and then press **Enter**.

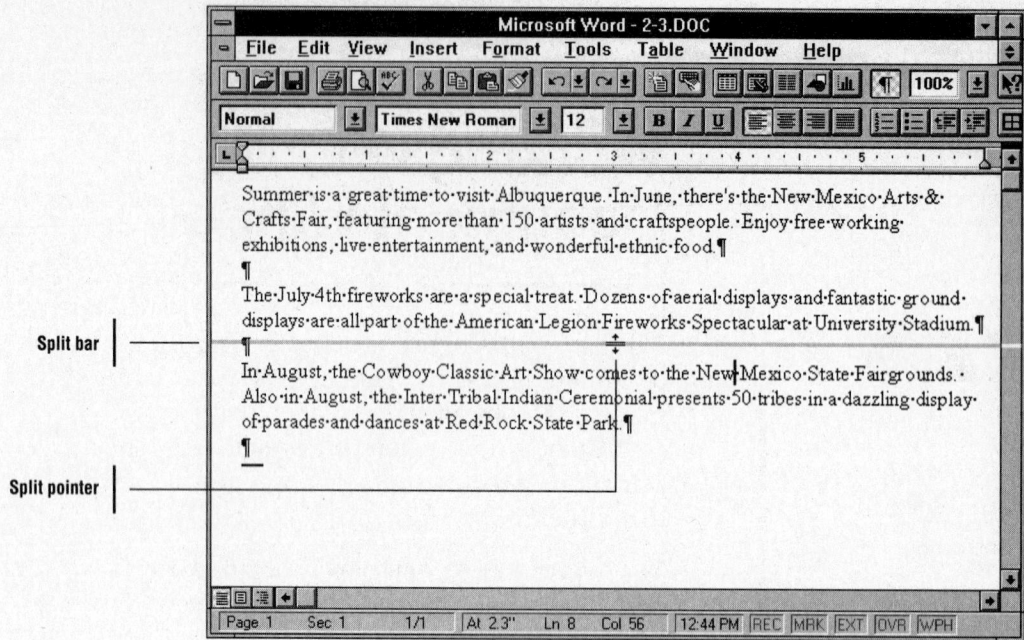

Figure 9-1
Using the split bar

Word splits the window into two panes that offer two views of the same document. You can scroll independently in each pane.

You can also split your document into two panes using the *split box*, which is the small, black rectangle at the top of the vertical scroll bar on the right side of the Word screen. When the mouse is pointing to the split box, Word displays the split pointer. Double-click to split the window into two equal panes, or drag the pointer to where you want to split the window.

To split a document window using the split box:

1. Open the file 9-0a.doc.

2. Move the mouse to the split box above the vertical scroll bar. Notice that the pointer changes to the split pointer. Double-click.

Word splits the document window into two equal panes.

Moving Between Panes

Once you have created a second pane, there are two ways to move between the panes:

- Move the insertion point into the pane and click.

- Press the **F6** key to switch between panes.

Each time you move to a pane, it becomes the active pane in which changes can be made.

Split box

The small, black rectangle at the top of the vertical scroll bar which is used to split a document window into two panes.

Split pointer on the split box

Each pane of a split document has its own scroll bars. Use them to locate the area of each file you wish to view rapidly. Each pane also has its own ruler. This lets you see and adjust the margins and tab settings for different parts of the document. Note that you can only split a document into two panes.

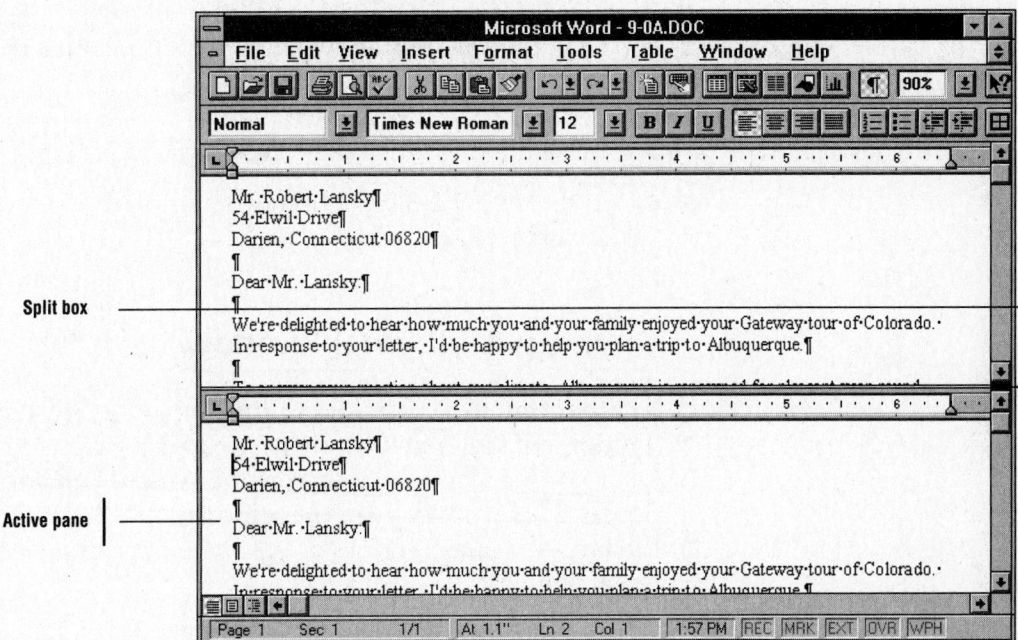

Figure 9-2
Document 9-0A.DOC split into two panes

Editing Panes

When you edit the contents of either pane, the changes become part of the overall document. For example, if you make changes in one pane, and then scroll to the same location in the other pane, the changes appear there as well.

To edit a pane:

1. In document 9-0A.DOC (which is now split into two panes), move the insertion point to the second pane, if it is not already there.

2. Click the up arrow on the scroll bar in the second pane to scroll to the top of the document.

3. Change the address to "55 Main Street".

    Notice that the change is also made in the first pane.

Closing Panes

When you are finished working with one section of a split document, it is easy to remove the split, which closes the panes. The quickest way is to double-click the split box, which is now located at the split position on the vertical scroll bar. You can also use the mouse to drag the split box off the document window.

To close panes:

1.   Move the mouse pointer to the split box.

2.   Drag the split box above the top of the scroll bar.

      The document is once again displayed in one window.

3.   Close the document 9-0A.DOC without saving the changes.

4.   In document 2-3.DOC, remove the split by double-clicking the split box.

Opening Additional Windows of a Document

Another way to work with multiple windows is to open additional windows of the same document. To open a new window for a document, choose New Window from the Window menu. Each new window you open is a copy of the same file, and has a number after the filename (such as ":2" or ":3"), so you can keep track of the additional windows.

To open an additional window:

Window menu

1.   With document 2-3.DOC open, choose New Window from the Window menu.

      Word opens a new window for document 2-3.DOC named 2-3.DOC:2, signifying the second open copy of the document. As in the split window examples described above, changes made in one copy of the document appear in the other copy or copies automatically. To work on one of the open windows as a separate document, you can rename it using the Save As command and then make the changes independent of the other copies.

Note: The Close command closes all windows that contain the active document.

2.   Choose Close from the File menu.

      Word closes both copies of the document.

Viewing More Than One Document at Once

You have viewed two copies of the same document on the screen. The next step is to view two different documents on the screen at once. This technique makes it easy and convenient to compare different files or to cut and paste information between them.

Normally, when you open two files, the second one appears full-screen, and the first one is no longer visible. To view the first document, you can choose the filename from a list of open documents in the Window menu. Once both files are open, you can view them both at one time by choosing Arrange All from the Window menu.

To open two files and view them both at one time:

1. Open the file 9-0b.doc.

2. Reopen the file 2-3.doc.

3. Choose the document you opened first, 9-0B.DOC, from the Window menu.

4. Choose Arrange All from the Window menu.

    Word displays both documents at the same time, dividing the screen into two equally sized windows.

Figure 9-3
Viewing two documents at once

Adjusting the Size of Document Windows

The Arrange All command allows you to view all open documents at once. When viewing several open documents, you can move, close, or change the size of the document windows. (See "Appendix E: Basic Windows Skills" to review the basic techniques for moving and sizing.)

To practice adjusting the size of windows:

1. With both documents displayed at once, click in document 2-3.DOC to make it the active window.

2. Point to the right border of the window.

   The pointer becomes a sizing pointer with a two-headed arrow.

3. Hold down the mouse button, and drag the window border to the left, until the window covers only the bottom, left quarter of the screen.

Sizing pointer

Figure 9-4
Adjusting the size of windows

4. Click in 9-0B.DOC to make it the active window.

5. Move the pointer to the top, left corner of the window, and drag the window corner to the right, until the window covers only the top, right quarter of the screen.

6. Choose Arrange All from the Window menu to resize the documents equally.

Note: Sizing a window by its corner will adjust both the height and length. Sizing a window by its border (top, bottom, right, or left) will adjust the height or width.

Two Views of a Table

Opening additional windows of a document and viewing them simultaneously is particularly helpful when editing a table. Suppose you want to view the first column of a table while entering information in the last column, but the table is too wide to view as a whole. You could open an additional window of the document and use the Arrange All command on the Window menu to view both windows at the same time. Since Word arranges the windows horizontally, you could resize the windows so they appear side by side vertically. Remember, any changes made in one window of any document are made in other open windows of the same document, so you could switch freely between the windows to edit the text.

Minimizing and Maximizing Document Windows

Minimize   Maximize

Document sizing buttons

After arranging or sizing windows, you can restore a document window to full size by clicking its Maximize button.

In addition, if several windows are open and arranged, but you only want to display two or three, click the Minimize button on the windows you do not want to see. When you minimize a window, it becomes an icon in the lower left corner of the application window. The icon may not be visible if it is hidden behind another window. To restore the icon to a document window, double-click the icon. You may have to size or move a document window to access the icon, or you can press **Shift+F6** to cycle through the active document windows.

To minimize and maximize document windows:

1. With 9-0B.DOC the active window, click the document's Maximize button.

    Word displays the document in full-screen size.

2. Choose Arrange All from the Window menu to display both documents again.

3. Click the Minimize button for the document 9-0B.DOC.

    Document 2-3.DOC becomes the active window, and document 9-0B.DOC is reduced to an icon.

9-0B.DOC

Document minimized to an icon

4. Drag the active window up by its title bar to show the icon under it.

5. Double-click the 9-0B.DOC icon.

6. Drag the top window down, or choose Arrange All from the Windows menu to display both windows.

Opening and Saving Multiple Documents

In Word, there are shortcuts for opening and saving several documents at one time. The Save All command, which is discussed in Lesson 2, allows you to save all the documents you have opened and any other files you may have created (such as templates or macros, which are discussed in later lessons). The Find File feature allows you to open several files at once, instead of opening files individually from the Standard toolbar or the File menu.

To save multiple documents using the Save All command:

1. At the top of the document 9-0B.DOC, key **9-0B.doc**

2. Move to the top of the document 2-3.DOC and key **2-3.doc**

3. Choose Save All from the File menu.

4. Close the documents.

The Find File command, which is available from the File menu, displays a detailed list of the files on your disk. It also allows you to view each file before opening it. To open several files at once, click the first file to choose it, hold down the **Ctrl** key, and click the additional files you want to open. When all files to be opened are chosen, click Open.

Figure 9-5
The Find File dialog box

To open multiple documents using the Find File command:

1. Choose Find File from the File menu.

   The Find File dialog box displays a list of the files in your current drive and directory. The first file in the list is highlighted and displayed in the content box.

Note: If your current drive is not displayed in the Find File dialog box, click the Search button. From the Location drop-down list, choose the correct drive, and then click OK.

2. Scroll down to choose the file 2-3.doc. Then hold down the **Ctrl** key, and click 9-0b.doc and 9-0c.doc.

3. Click Open to open all three files.

4. Choose Arrange All from the Window menu to view all three opened files.

Moving and Copying Text Among Multiple Windows

One of the most common reasons to use multiple windows is to edit text from one document to another. The Cut, Copy, and Paste commands work much the same with multiple windows as with individual windows, except you must make sure you are in the correct active window when you paste text.

You can also move and copy text among multiple windows using drag-and-drop editing. To do this, make sure you have properly sized the document windows, so the text to be dragged and the destination for the text are visible.

When working with multiple small windows, you may occasionally want to maximize the current window to full size and then minimize it when you are finished working with it.

To combine your editing skills with the multiple document techniques discussed in this lesson:

1. If it is not already activated, click in 2-3.DOC to activate the window. Delete the text "2-3.doc". Activate 9-0B.DOC, and delete the text "9-0b.doc".

2. Choose Save All from the File menu to save the corrections to these two documents.

3. Activate 9-0C.DOC. Select the first paragraph, and then click the Cut button on the Standard toolbar.

4. Activate 9-0B.DOC. Enlarge the window by moving the pointer to the top of the active title bar. When the pointer becomes a two-headed arrow, drag it up until the border is just below the title bar above it.

5. Move the insertion point to the end of the document, double space, and click the Paste button.

6. Activate 9-0C.DOC again. Close the window by double-clicking the document Control-menu box. Do not save the change.

7. Move the 2-3.DOC window up to the top of the screen.

8. In the 9-0B.DOC window, insert one blank line after the last paragraph.

9. In the 2-3.DOC window, select the first paragraph, which begins with "Summer", and drag it into the next window, at the end of document 9-0B.DOC.

10. Activate 2-3.DOC. Maximize the window by clicking its Maximize button in the upper, right corner of the window.

11. Select the rest of the text in 2-3.DOC, starting with the second paragraph (remember the shortcut: move the pointer in the selection bar, hold down the **Ctrl** key, and click the left mouse button). Copy the text to the Clipboard, and then close the document without saving it.

12. Paste the text at the bottom of 9-0B.DOC.

13. Make sure there is one blank line between paragraphs and no extraneous paragraph marks at the end of the document.

14. Spell-check the document.

15. Save the document as *[your three-letter identifier]*9-0.doc.

Double-click
to close

Document Control-menu
box

16. Print the document.

17. Close the documents and exit Word (unless you will be doing the following exercises immediately).

Key Terms

Pane   Split box

Split bar

Exercises

Exercise 9.1

1. Start Word, if necessary.

2. Open the file 4-3.doc.

3. Split 4-3.doc into two panes by double-clicking the split box.

4. In the lower pane, scroll to the paragraph that begins "For corporate clients". In the second sentence, change "provide" to "provides".

5. Activate the first pane. Scroll to the end of paragraph 5 to observe the correction.

6. Remove the split by double-clicking the split box.

7. Open the file 9-1.doc.

8. Choose Arrange All from the Window menu.

9. Activate 4-3.DOC, and copy paragraphs 2–4 (from "The hotel has 400" through "facsimile machines.") to the Clipboard.

10. Activate 9-1.DOC, and maximize the window.

11. Double space at the end of the document, and then paste the text from the Clipboard.

12. Check the memo formatting. Add another blank line after the "SUBJECT:" line, and add your reference initials.

13. Spell-check 9-1.DOC.

14. Save the document as *[your three-letter identifier]*9-1.doc.

15. Print the document.

16. Close 4-3.DOC without saving the changes. Then close *[your three-letter identifier]*9-1.DOC and exit Word (unless you will be doing the following exercises immediately).

Exercise 9.2

1. Start Word, if necessary.

2. Use the Find File command to open the files 9-2a.doc and 9-2b.doc:

   A. Choose Find File from the File menu.

   B. Scroll down to choose 9-2a.doc.

   C. Hold the **Ctrl** key and choose 9-2b.doc.

3. Choose Arrange All from the Window menu to view both files.

4. Adjust the 9-2B.DOC window so that it is slightly larger than the other window.

5. In the 9-2B.DOC window, scroll so that the fourth paragraph, which begins "Our local area", is visible.

6. In 9-2A.DOC, scroll to the second paragraph of the letter, which begins "We can set up".

7. Use drag-and-drop editing to copy the paragraph from one window to the other:

   A. Select the fourth paragraph (including the paragraph mark it) in the 9-2B.DOC window.

   B. Hold down the **Ctrl** key, and drag the paragraph to just before "We can set up" in 9-2A.DOC.

8. In 9-2B.DOC, copy paragraphs 6 and 7 (from "Our naturalist" through "for sightseeing.") to document 9-2A.DOC. Insert the text after the paragraph previously copied.

9. Make sure one blank line is inserted between paragraphs.

10. Close 9-2B.DOC without saving by double-clicking the document Control-menu box.

11. Maximize 9-2A.DOC, and then spell-check the document.

12. Add your reference initials to the document.

13. Save the document as *[your three-letter identifier]*9-2.doc and print it.

14. Close the document and exit Word (unless you will be doing the following exercises immediately).

Exercise 9.3

1. Start Word, if necessary.

2. Create a new document, and key the text in Figure 9-6, including the corrections. Format it as a standard business memo with 1-inch left and right margins. Insert the date as a field code.

Figure 9-6

Memo to Susan Allen from Nina Chavez

Subject is Phoenix Convention car rentals

Regarding car rentals for the Phoenix Convention next month, please advise clients of the following rates and upgrade charges. Car rentals are available for the entire stay and for additional days. All rental agreements for this trip offer unlimited mileage.

Remember to advise clients who pay with a ^major^ credit card that they need not buy the rental insurance.

3. Save the document as *[your three-letter identifier]*9-3.doc.

4. Use Find File to open the files 6-0.doc and 3-1.doc.

5. Arrange all three documents on the screen. From document window 3-1.DOC, copy the text from "Car Rental Classes and Rates" to "is $90." Paste it into 9-3.DOC as a separate paragraph after the text "for additional days."

6. From 6-0.DOC, copy the text that begins "Car rental upgrades are available" and the table following it. Paste it into *[your three-letter identifier]*9-3.DOC after the text inserted in the last step (which begins "Car Rental Classes").

7. Make sure one blank line is inserted before and after each of the above insertions.

8. From 3-1.DOC, copy the last two sentences in the last paragraph (from "One-way" to "guaranteed."). Paste them into *[your three-letter identifier]*9-3.DOC as a new paragraph after the sentence that begins "All rental agreements". Make sure one blank line appears after the insertion.

9. Close document windows 6-0.DOC and 3-1.DOC, and maximize *[your three-letter identifier]*9-3.DOC.

10. Delete the text "Car Rental Classes and Rates:" and the paragraph marks following it. Change the "I" of "In the" to lowercase, and then key before it:

    As to rates,

11. Make sure the text from "As to" to "is $90." is one paragraph.

12. In the columnar text, from "Category" to "24", clear the tabs, and set 2-, 3-, 4-, 5-, and 6-inch centered tabs.

13. Spell-check the document. Add names to the custom dictionary, if necessary.

14. Save the document and print it.

15. Close the document and exit Word (unless you will be doing the following exercise immediately).

Exercise 9.4 Challenge Yourself

Use Find File to open the files 9-4.doc and 7-0.doc. Arrange both files on the screen.

Format 9-4.DOC as a standard business memo, using 1-inch left and right margins. Insert the date as a field code. Key the following sentence at the end of the paragraph that begins "In reference to":

Hotel classifications can be described as follows:

Double space after this sentence, and set a 1.5-inch left-aligned tab stop. Key the text in Figure 9-7 that appears at the end of this exercise. Include the corrections.

After the last paragraph, which begins "Hotel classifications", double space and key:

A note about deposits and cancellations:

From 7-0.DOC, copy the paragraph under "Deposits/Cancellations". Paste the paragraph beneath the text you just keyed in 9-4.DOC, inserting one blank line above it. Indent the new text, from "A note about" to "by the supplier." by .5 inches on the left and right. Add a shadow border around the text.

Spell-check the document. Then copy the text with the border to a new document. Save the document as *[your three-letter identifier]*9-4a.doc and print it.

Save 9-4.DOC as *[your three-letter identifier]*9-4b.doc and print it. Close the documents and exit Word.

Figure 9-7

Classification	*Description* (underline)	
Tourist/Budget	limited amenities, functional accommodations	˄ *lowest prices*
Moderate	simple and comfortable, for the cost-conscious	
First Class	high-quality, offering a *wide* variety of ~~and~~ services	
Deluxe	outstanding accommodations, for the discriminating	
Luxury	the world's finest, offering the highest standard of services	

Find and Replace

When creating documents, especially long documents, you often need to review or change text. In Word, you can do this quickly and accurately using the Find and Replace commands.

The Find command locates all occurrences of specified text and formatting in a document. The Replace command finds the text and formatting and replaces it with a specified alternative.

Finding Text

With Word's Find (and Replace) command, you can locate whole words, parts of words, phrases, a sequence of characters, or special characters. Formatting, such as capitalization and character attributes, can also be specified as an option in the search. In addition, you can specify search criteria so that, for instance, you can find words that begin and end with certain letters but have different letters between them. You also can search for different spelling variations of the same word.

You can search the entire document, or you can specify the direction of the search from the insertion point (either up or down), and you can cancel the search at any time. To start a search, choose Find from the Edit menu to open the Find dialog box.

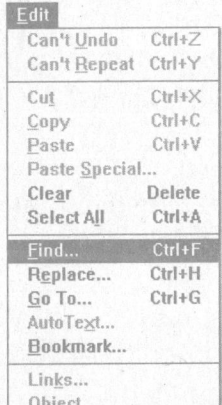

Edit menu

To use the Find command:

1. Start Word, if necessary.

2. Open the file 10-0.doc.

3. Choose Find from the Edit menu.

4. In the Find What text box, key **travel**

5. If necessary, choose All from the Search drop-down list box to search the entire document. See Figure 10-1 on page 180.

6. Click Find Next.

   Word searches the document and finds "Travel" in the first paragraph after the salutation.

7. Click Find Next.

   Word scrolls to the second paragraph and finds "Travel".

Note: To see more of the document text during a search, drag the dialog box by its title bar to the bottom, right corner of the screen.

Figure 10-1
The Find dialog box

8. Continue clicking Find Next until you reach the end of the document.

    Word finds several occurrences of "travel" in uppercase and lowercase, as a whole word and as part of the words "travelers" and "traveler".

9. Click OK in the dialog box that says Word has finished searching the document, and then click Cancel.

Matching the Case

To locate only words with certain letters in uppercase or lowercase, choose the Match Case option in the Find dialog box. This changes the search pattern. For example, if you choose this option and ask Word to find "Agency", it only searches for that word with the initial letter uppercase, and it will not find "agency" in all lowercase letters.

To find words with the matching case:

1. Move the insertion point to the left of "Chavez" in the closing, and choose Find from the Edit menu.

2. Key **Travel** in the Find What text box.

3. Click the Match Case check box to select it, and choose Up from the Search drop-down list box.

4. Click Find Next to begin the search.

5. Continue clicking Find Next until Word reaches the beginning of the document.

    Word finds "Travel", skipping over "travel", "traveler", and "travelers".

6. Click No in the dialog box that asks if you want to continue searching at the end, and then click Cancel.

    Notice how the position of the insertion point when you start the search and the search direction you choose affect the dialog box that ends the process. When Word searches through the entire document, the dialog box tells you that Word has finished searching the document, and the insertion point returns to its original position. When you search from a point other than the top or the bottom of the document, and you choose Up or Down as your search direction, Word asks if you want to continue the search. If you choose not to continue, the insertion point remains at the last occurrence found.

Finding Whole Words Only

Another way to narrow the search is to choose the Find Whole Words Only option. Word locates only separate words and not characters embedded in other words. For example, if you choose this option and ask Word to find "tour", it only searches for this word and not variations of it, such as "toured", "touring", or "detour".

To find whole words only and edit the document:

Note: If you want to find text that you searched for previously, you can click the down arrow next to the Find What text box and choose the text from your last four entries.

1. Move the insertion point to the beginning of the first paragraph, and choose Find from the Edit menu.

2. Key **travel** in the Find What text box. Click the Find Whole Words Only check box to select it, click the Match Case check box to deselect it, and choose Down from the Search drop-down list box.

3. Click Find Next to begin the search.

4. Continue clicking Find Next until Word reaches the end of the document.

    Word finds "Travel" and "travel", skipping over "traveler" and "travelers". After Word searches through the end of the document, a dialog box asks if you want to continue searching from the beginning.

5. Click No, and then click Cancel.

Using Pattern Matching

When using the Find command, a more advanced search method is the Use Pattern Matching option, which allows you to search for text strings. For example, if you want to search for all three-letter words that begin with "m", end with "t", and have an unspecified letter in the middle, you can search for "m?t", which will find "mat" and "met.

To use pattern matching:

1. Move the insertion point to the beginning of the document, and choose Find from the Edit menu.

2. Key **ca?** in the Find What text box. Make sure the option Use Pattern Matching is selected, and choose All from the Search drop-down list box.

3. Click Find Next.

    Word finds the "cat" in "location" in the third paragraph.

4. Click Find Next.

    Word finds the "cal" in "local" in the fifth paragraph.

5. Continue clicking Find Next until you reach the end of the document.

    Word finds "ca" and a third letter in "car", "cases", "can", and "care".

6. Click OK in the dialog box that says Word has finished searching the document, and then click Cancel.

There are several operators to perform advanced searches from the Find dialog box. You can key these operators in the Find What text box, or you can choose them from the Special drop-down list box (if Use Pattern Matching is selected).

Table 10-1: Operators for Advanced Searches

To Find	Operator	Example
Any single character	?	Key **m?t** to find "mat" and "met".
Any string of characters	*	Key **m*d** to find "mad", "maid", and "moved".
One of the specified characters	[ ]	Key **m[ae]n** to find "man" and "men".
Any single character in a range	[-]	Key **[r-t]ail** to find "rail", "sail", and "tail".
Any single character except the characters inside the brackets	[!]	Key **f[!a]rm** to find "firm" and "form", but not "farm". Key **l[!ou]ck** to find "lack" and "lick", but not "lock" or "luck".
Any single character except characters in the range inside the brackets	[!-]	Key **l[!a-m]ck** to find "lock" and "luck", but not "lack" or "lick".
An exact number of occurrences of the previous character or expression	{}	Key **me{2}t** to find "meet", but not "met".
At least a certain number of occurrences of the previous character or expression	{,}	Key **me{1,}t** to find "met" and "meet".
A range of occurrences of the previous character or expression	{,}	Key **20{1,3}** to find "20", "200", and "2000".
One or more occurrences of the previous character or expression	@	Key **lo@t** to find "lot" and "loot".
The beginning of a word	<( )	Key **<(count)** to find "counting" and "country", but not "encounter".
The end of a word	>( )	Key **(out)>** to find "out" and "clout", but not "outer".

Using Sounds Like

To find a word that is spelled several different ways in the text, or to find a word of which you are unsure of the spelling, you can use the Sounds Like option.

To use sounds like and edit text:

1. Move the insertion point to the beginning of the document, and choose Find from the Edit menu.

2. Key **traveler** in the Find What text box. Make sure the option Sounds Like is selected, and choose Down from the Search drop-down list box.

3. Click Find Next.

    Word finds "Travel" in the first paragraph, because "Travel" is close to "traveler".

4. Continue clicking Find Next until Word reaches "travellers" in the third paragraph.

5. Click Cancel to stop the search, and delete the second "l" in "travellers".

    To continue the search while staying in the document, use **Shift+F4**, the keyboard alternative to Find Next. Word continues to search through the document, allowing you to edit or move on to the next occurrence easily.

6. Continue to press **Shift+F4** until you reach the end of the document, changing every occurrence of "traveller" to "traveler". Click No when asked if you want to continue searching at the beginning.

7. Save the edited document as *[your three-letter identifier]*10-0.doc.

Finding Formatted Text

You can also search for text that is formatted. For instance, you can search for a particular word or phrase that is italicized, or you can search for all instances of bold text. You can also search for text that has been indented or that has had a particular style applied to it.

To find formatted text:

1. Move the insertion point to the beginning of the document, and choose Find from the Edit menu.

2. Key **Duke City** in the Find What text box. Click the Sounds Like check box to deselect it, if necessary.

3. Click the Format button, and then choose Font.

4. Choose Italic from the Font Style list box and click OK.

    Italic appears in the Format section of the Find dialog box.

Format options

5. Click Find Next.

   Word finds *"Duke City"*.

6. Click Cancel.

Finding and Replacing Text

The Replace command is a two-part procedure. It searches for the specified text or formatting and replaces it with the specified alternative. You can replace all instances of text or formatting in a document at once, or you can find and confirm each replacement. For example, an author can write an entire book using a character named William and then change the name to Ivan throughout the book with one keyboard command, or the author can choose to find and confirm each replacement of the name.

If you change your mind about making a replacement, press the **Esc** key or choose Cancel before making the replacement. If you change your mind after making the replacement, use the Undo command.

To use the Replace command, choose Replace from the Edit menu to open the Replace dialog box. Then specify the text, and choose the desired options.

Matching the Case

The Replace command, like the Find command, can search for only words that match the case you specify. The Match Case option narrows down the search, thereby speeding up the Find and Replace process.

To replace text with the matching case only:

1. With the file *[your three-letter identifier]*10-0.doc still open, open the original file 10-0.doc.

2. With the insertion point at the beginning of the document, choose Replace from the Edit menu.

3. Key **Travel Agency** in the Find What text box, and click the No Formatting button to remove Italic from the Format box, if necessary. See Figure 10-2 on page 185.

4. Press the **Tab** key to move to the Replace With text box, and then key **Travel**

5. Check Match Case, choose All from the Search drop-down list, and then click Find Next.

6. Click Replace at the first occurrence.

   Word changes "Travel Agency" to "Travel" and finds the next occurrence of "Travel Agency", skipping over any instances of "travel agency" in all lowercase.

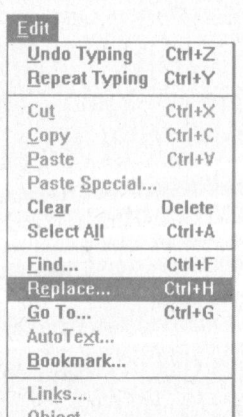

Edit menu

Note: To move from one text box to another within a dialog box, press the **Tab** key. This automatically highlights the text in the text box. Remember, pressing **Enter** will execute the dialog box command.

Note: If the dialog box covers a word you are replacing, use the down arrow on the vertical scroll bar to move the text into view.

Figure 10-2
The Replace dialog box

7. Continue to click Replace as Word finds each instance of "Travel Agency", until Word reaches the end of the document.

8. Click OK when Word has finished searching, and then click Close to return to the document.

Replacing Whole Words Only

The Replace command, like the Find command, can search for whole words only.

To replace whole words:

1. With the insertion point at the beginning of the document, choose Replace from the Edit menu.

2. Key **agency** in the Find What text box, and key **company** in the Replace With text box.

3. Make sure the Find Whole Words Only check box is checked and the Match Case check box is unchecked. Click Find Next.

4. Click Replace, and then click Close.

Using Pattern Matching and Sounds Like

Note: Find Next is similar to the Ignore option in spelling check. It moves to the next occurrence of the text without replacing the text. Remember to click Replace to make the edit.

As with the Find command, the Replace command also offers the Use Pattern Matching and Sounds Like options. These options are particularly useful if you want to replace several similar words or phrases with a single word or phrase, or if you are unsure of the spelling of the word or phrase you wish to replace.

Replacing All

The Replace dialog box offers the option to replace all occurrences of text or formatting in a document without confirmation. Word does this quickly and easily, according to the options chosen.

Practice using the Replace All option to change the name of the agency:

1. Move the insertion point to top of the document.

2. Choose Replace from the Edit menu.

3. Key **Duke City** in the Find What text box. Key **Albuquerque** in the Replace With text box. Uncheck all special options, if necessary, and choose All from the Search drop-down list.

4. Click Replace All.

    A dialog box appears, indicating the number of changes that have been made in the document.

5. Click OK, and then click close to view the document.

    The agency name is changed throughout the document.

Deleting Text with Replace

Earlier in the lesson, the Find command was used with the **Delete** key to delete text. The Replace command can be used to delete text automatically. Replace can find and delete text with confirmation using the Find Next button or without confirmation using the Replace All option.

To use Replace to delete text:

1. Position the insertion point at the top of the document, and choose Replace from the Edit menu.

2. In the Find What text box, key **Travel**, and press the **Spacebar** once. You cannot see a space character, but the position of the insertion point after the text indicates the space.

3. In the Replace With text box, delete the text, if necessary. Make sure the Match Case box is checked.

4. Click Replace All, click OK, and then click Close to view the document.

    The word "Travel" and the space following it are deleted from the agency name throughout the document. Note that "Travel" followed by a punctuation mark was not deleted. Note also that Replace All resulted in the deletion of the word "Travel" from the title "Travel Counselor" at the end of the letter. To avoid this, you would use the Replace command with confirmation instead of Replace All.

Undoing Replacements

If you change your mind after replacing text or formatting, there are two ways to undo the changes:

Undo button

- Choose the Undo command immediately after making the change. If you used Replace All, all changes are reversed. If you used Find Next, only the last change is reversed.

- Close the document without saving the changes. You can only use this method if you saved the document before using the Replace command.

To undo the replace and restore the document to its original form:

1. Click the Undo button on the Standard toolbar.

   Word undoes the change. If you performed any other action after the replace, and Word cannot undo the change, move on to step 2.

2. Close the document without saving changes.

   All previous changes made to the document are not saved.

3. Open the file 10-0.doc again.

   The document is displayed in its original form.

Using the Clipboard

If the text that you want to find or use as a replacement is already keyed in a document, you can use the Clipboard to avoid rekeying. There are three ways to do this:

- Copy the text to the Clipboard, and then press either **Shift+Insert** or **Ctrl+V** to paste the contents of the Clipboard into either the Find What or Replace With text box. You can paste up to 255 characters with this method.

- If the text to be pasted is more than 255 characters, copy it to the Clipboard, click the Special button, and choose Clipboard Contents from the drop-down list.

- Key **^c** (the special character for Clipboard Contents).

To replace text using the Clipboard:

1. Make [*your three-letter identifier*]10-0.DOC the active document window.

2. In the second paragraph after the salutation, delete "New Mexico" at the end of the first sentence, and key **the Southwest**

3. Copy the keyed text to the Clipboard, and then move the insertion point to the beginning of the next paragraph.

4. Choose Replace from the Edit menu.

5. Key **New Mexico** in the Find What text box.

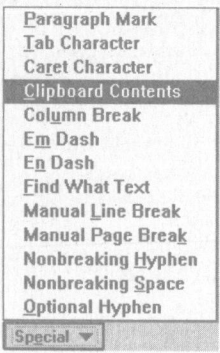

Paragraph Mark
Tab Character
Caret Character
Clipboard Contents
Column Break
Em Dash
En Dash
Find What Text
Manual Line Break
Manual Page Break
Nonbreaking Hyphen
Nonbreaking Space
Optional Hyphen

Special ▼

Special character options

6. Press the **Tab** key to move to the Replace With text box, click the Special button, and choose Clipboard Contents from the Special drop-down list. (In this case, you could also have pressed **Shift+Insert**, because the text contained on the Clipboard is less than 255 characters.)

7. Choose Down from the Search drop-down list.

8. Click Find Next to view the next occurrence of "New Mexico" and confirm the replacement of text. Click Replace until Word reaches the end of the document.

9. Click No to end the search, and then click Close.

Special Characters

The Find and Replace features can search for characters other than ordinary text. To do this, click the Special button, and choose an option from the Special drop-down list. For example, to remove blank lines in a document, you can search for two consecutive paragraph marks and replace them with a single paragraph mark. In addition to choosing these special characters from the Special drop-down list, you can also key the special codes that represent them into the Find What or Replace with dialog box. The special codes are listed in Table 10-2.

When searching for or replacing special characters, be sure they are displayed in the document. Click the Show/Hide ¶ button on the Standard toolbar, or choose Options from the Tools menu, and choose the View setting All under Nonprinting Characters.

Table 10-2: Find and Replace Special Characters	
Find or Replace	Special Character Code
Paragraph mark (¶)	**^p** Must be lowercase.
Tab character ()	**^t** Must be lowercase.
Any character	**?** Example: Key **?ffect** to find "affect" and "effect". Use with Find command only.
Any digit	**#** Example: Key **1#** to find "11", "12", etc. Use with Find command only.
Any letter	**$**
Caret character (^)	**^^**
Em dash	**^+**

Continued on next page

Table 10-2—Continued	
Find or Replace	**Special Character Code**
En dash	^=
Line break	^l Also called "newline character"
Manual page break	^m Must be lowercase.
Nonbreaking hyphen	^~
Nonbreaking space	^s Must be lowercase.
Optional hyphen	^- If you specify search text without optional hyphens, Word finds all matching text, including text containing optional hyphens. However, if you specify optional hyphens in the search text, Word finds only words having optional hyphens in the same position. For example, keying **cancel^-lation** finds only "cancel-lation".
Section break	^b Must be lowercase.
White space	^w Represents any number and combination of spaces, including nonbreaking spaces and tabs. Use with Find command only.
Clipboard contents	^c Use with Replace command to replace search text with Clipboard contents. Use for replacement text that is more than 255 characters.

For more information about special characters, see "special characters" in the Help menu.

To find and replace using special characters:

1. Position the insertion point at the top of *[your three-letter identifier]*10-0.doc, and then choose Replace from the Edit menu.

2. To delete the extra lines between paragraphs in the letter, key **^p^p^p** in the Find What text box. This instructs Word to look for three consecutive paragraph marks.

3. In the Replace What text box, key **^p^p**, and click Find Next.

    Word finds the extra lines of space before the address.

4. Click Find Next until Word locates the extra paragraph mark after the salutation. Click Replace.

5. Continue to click Replace for each of the extra paragraph marks up to "Sincerely," and then click Close to return to the document.

Figure 10-3
Using the Replace command for special characters

Finding and Replacing Formatting

In addition to finding and replacing text, Word can search for and replace both character and paragraph formatting.

Character formatting includes the options offered in the Font dialog box, such as Font Style and Underline. For example, you can search for bold text in a document and replace it with italics, or you can search for ordinary text and make it bold.

Paragraph formatting includes the options offered in the Paragraph dialog box, such as Alignment, Indents, and Spacing. For example, you can search for a 1-inch left indent and replace it with a .5-inch first-line indent.

Character or paragraph formatting can be specified by clicking the Format button in the Find or Replace dialog boxes and then choosing either Font or Paragraph. Formatting can also be specified by using keyboard shortcuts, such as **Ctrl+B** for bold.

Note: Some of the formatting features shown in the dialog boxes, such as Style in the Font drop-down list and Font in the Font dialog box, are discussed in future lessons.

Table 10-3: Find and Replace Formatting Guidelines	
Guideline	Procedure
Find specific text with specific formatting	Key search text in the Find What text box, and then specify its formatting by choosing Font or Paragraph from the Format drop-down list or by using a keyboard shortcut (for example, **Ctrl+B** for bold).
Find specific formatting	Delete any text in the Find What text box. Clear any existing formatting, and then specify formatting by choosing Font or Paragraph from the Format drop-down list or by using a keyboard shortcut.
Replace specific text but not its formatting	Key the search text in the Find What text box. Click the No Formatting button to clear any existing formatting. Key the replacement text in the Replace With text box, and clear any existing formatting.
Replace specific text and its formatting	Key the search text in the Find What text box and specify formatting. Key the replacement text in the Replace With text box and specify formatting.
Replace only formatting of specific text	Key the search text in the Find What text box and specify its formatting (you may only have to specify the formatting in some cases). Key the same text in the Replace With text box, and then specify formatting.
Replace only formatting	Delete any text in the Find What text box, and then specify formatting. Delete any text in the Replace What text box, and then specify the replacement formatting.

Character Formatting

When you choose Font from the Format drop-down list in the Find or Replace dialog box, Word opens a dialog box that is identical to the Font dialog box. However, all the text boxes are empty, and all the check boxes are filled with gray. When you leave a text box empty or a check box gray, Word ignores this character format in a search. To choose a format, click a drop-down arrow and choose an option, or click a check box. To remove a format, delete the text in the text box, or double-click a check box to clear it. See Figure 10-4 on page 192.

Character formatting can also be specified in a search with keyboard shortcuts. When specifying character formatting to find or replace, be sure the insertion point is in the appropriate text box before clicking the Format button or using a keyboard command.

Searching For Space Characters

A simple and helpful use of both Find and Replace is to look for extraneous space characters. It is not always easy to spot two consecutive space characters, especially in a long document, until after you print the document. Also, if you have clicked the Show/Hide ¶ button and are working on a document without viewing the special characters, it is very difficult to see where you may have inserted more than one space character.

To search for extra space characters in your document, you can use either the Find or Replace command. Using the Find command, you can choose White Space from the Special drop-down list, or you can key **^w** in the Find What text box. The characters "^w" represent white space, which can be space characters, tab characters, or nonbreaking spaces.

To search exclusively for space characters, use the **Spacebar**. For example, in the Find dialog box, place the insertion point in the Find What text box, and then press the **Spacebar** twice. You will not see any space characters in the text box, but the position of the insertion point will move over two spaces, indicating that you have entered the spaces. When you click Find Next, Word will search for two consecutive space characters.

The quickest way to eliminate two consecutive space characters in a document is to use the Replace command. In the Find What text box, press the **Spacebar** twice. In the Replace With text box, press the **Spacebar** once. Then click Replace All, and all occurrences of two consecutive space characters will be replaced with one space character.

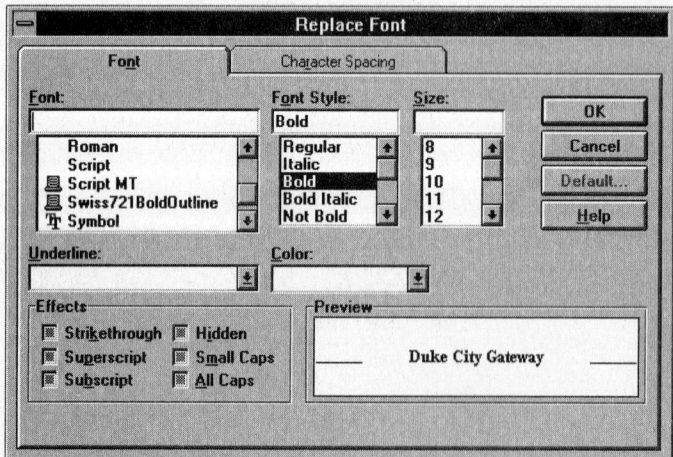

Figure 10-4
The Replace Font dialog box

To find and replace character formatting:

1. In *[your three-letter identifier]*10-0.doc, position the insertion point at the top of the document.

2. Choose Replace from the Edit menu.

3. Key **Duke City Gateway** in the Find What text box. Delete the text in the Replace With text box.

4. Click the Format button, and choose Font from the Format drop-down list. Choose Bold from the Font Style list box and click OK.

5. In the Replace dialog box, click Replace All. Click OK, and then click Close.

   "Duke City Gateway" is replaced with bold character formatting.

6. Choose Replace from the Edit menu again.

7. With the Find What text highlighted, click the Format button, and choose Font from the Format drop-down list. Choose Bold from the Font Style list box and click OK.

8. Move the insertion point to the Replace With text box, and click the No Formatting button to clear any existing formatting. Press **Ctrl+I** (the keyboard shortcut for italic text), and then press **Ctrl+B** (the keyboard shortcut for bold text) twice, so that "Not Bold" appears in the Format box.

9. Click Replace All, click OK, and then click Close.

   Word replaces the bold formatting with italics.

Figure 10-5
Replacing character formatting and text

Paragraph Formatting

To specify paragraph formatting in a search, choose Paragraph from the Format drop-down list in the Find or Replace dialog box. Word opens a dialog box that is identical to the Paragraph dialog box.

You can also specify paragraph formatting with keyboard commands. When specifying paragraph formatting to find or replace, be sure the insertion point is in the appropriate text box before clicking the Format button or using a keyboard command.

To find and replace paragraph formatting:

1. In *[your three-letter identifier]*10-0.doc, position the insertion point at the end of the salutation. Choose Replace from the Edit menu to begin the process of setting a first-line indent for paragraphs 2-8 after the salutation.

2. In the Find What text box, key **^p^p**. Click the No Formatting button to clear the existing formatting.

3. In the Replace With text box, key **^p^p**. Click the No Formatting button, and then choose Paragraph from the Format drop-down list.

4. Under Indentation, choose First Line from the Special drop-down list to set a .5-inch first-line indent, and then click OK.

Figure 10-6
The Replace Paragraph dialog box

5. Click Find Next. Click Find Next two more times, until Word highlights the paragraph marks after "Europe." Click Replace to format this paragraph. Remember, the paragraph mark at the end of a paragraph is what determines the paragraph's formatting.

6. Click Replace for the next seven paragraphs, through the paragraph ending "without a fee."

7. Close the dialog box to view the document.

8. Position the insertion point at the top of the document. Choose Replace from the Edit menu to replace the first-line indent with left and right indents.

9. In the Find What text box, delete the text. Choose Paragraph from the Format drop-down list, and then choose First Line from the Special drop-down list to search for this indent. Click OK.

10. In the Replace With text box, delete the text, and click the No Formatting button. Choose Paragraph from the Format drop-down list, and then set .25-inch left and right indents and choose (none) from the Special drop-down list. Click OK.

Figure 10-7
Replacing paragraph formatting

11. Click Replace All, click OK, and then close the dialog box to view the document.

    The first-line-indent formatting is replaced with a left and right indent, as specified.

12. Spell-check the document.

13. Save and print the document.

14. Close *[your three-letter identifier]*10-0.doc. Close 10-0.doc without saving changes. Exit Word (unless you will be doing the following exercises immediately).

Table 10-4: Keyboard Shortcuts for Find and Replace	
Keyboard Shortcut	Action
Shift+F4	Repeat Find or Replace
Shift+Insert	Paste Clipboard text into Find or Replace text box
Ctrl+V	Paste Clipboard text into Find or Replace text box

Exercises

Exercise 10.1

1. Start Word, if necessary.

2. Open the file 10-1.doc.

3. Change "Bike-a-Thon" to "Bike-In" using the Find command:

   A. Position the insertion point at the beginning of the document, and then choose Find from the Edit menu.

   B. Key **Bike-a-Thon** in the Find What text box. Click the No Formatting button to clear any formatting, if necessary. Choose Down from the Search drop-down list, and then click Find Next.

   C. At the first occurrence of the search text, click Cancel.

   D. Edit the text to "Bike-In".

   E. Press **Shift+F4** to repeat the search, and then repeat the edit. Continue to do this through the end of the document.

4. Change the name "Rick's Cycle Shop" to "Rick's Bike Shop" using the Replace command:

   A. Move the insertion point to the beginning of the document. Then choose Replace from the Edit menu.

   B. Key **Cycle** in the Find What text box, and key **Bike** in the Replace With text box.

   C. Click the No Formatting button, if necessary, and then click the Match Case and Find Whole Words Only check boxes to select them.

   D. Click Find Next. Click Replace. Repeat through the end of the document, and then return to the document.

5. Change "Bike-In" back to "Bike-a-Thon" and format the text in bold using the Replace command:

   A. Position the insertion point at the beginning of the document, and then choose Replace from the Edit menu.

   B. Key **Bike-In** in the Find What text box.

   C. Key **Bike-a-Thon** in the Replace With text box.

   D. Click the Format button, and then choose Font. Choose Bold from the Font Style list box, and then click OK.

   E. Click Replace All. Click OK, and then click Close to return to the document.

6. Spell-check the document.

7. Save the document as *[your three-letter identifier]*10-1.doc.

8. Print the document.

9. Close the document and exit Word (unless you will be doing the following exercises immediately).

Exercise 10.2

1. Start Word, if necessary.

2. Open the file 10-2.doc.

3. Use the Replace command to delete all tabs:

    A. With the insertion point at the beginning of the document, choose Replace from the Edit menu.

    B. Key ^t in the Find What text box. Clear any existing formatting.

    C. Delete any text in the Replace With text box, and clear any existing formatting.

    D. Click Replace All, click OK, and then click Close to return to the document.

4. Click the Undo button on the Standard toolbar to undo the replacement.

5. Change all the line spacing to 1.5 lines using the Replace command:

    A. With the insertion point at the beginning of the document, choose Replace from the Edit menu.

    B. Clear the text in the Find What text box. Clear any existing formatting, and then choose Paragraph from the Format drop-down list.

    C. Choose Single from the Line Spacing drop-down list and click OK.

    D. Go to the Replace With text box, clear any existing text and formatting, and then choose Paragraph from the Format drop-down list. Choose 1.5 Lines from the Line Spacing drop-down list and click OK.

    E. Click Replace All. Click OK, and then click Close.

6. Change the text "am" to " a.m.", with a space character before "a.m.", using the Replace command:

    A. With the insertion point at the beginning of the document, choose Replace from the Edit menu.

    B. Clear the formatting in the Find What text box. Make sure Find Whole Words Only is clear and Match Case is checked, and then key **am**

    C. Go to the Replace With text box, and clear the formatting. Press the **Spacebar** once, and then key **a.m.**

    D. Click Replace All. Click OK, and then click Close.

7. Change the name "Southwest" to "Southwest Airlines" using the Replace command with the Clipboard:

   A. From the text "America West Airlines" in the second line of the table, copy the word "Airlines".

   B. Move the insertion point to the beginning of the document, and then choose Replace from the Edit menu.

   C. In the Find What text box, delete the text and key **Southwest**

   D. In the Replace With text box, delete the text, and then key **Southwest ^c** (the "^c" is the text in the Clipboard), inserting a space character between "Southwest" and "^c".

   E. Click Replace All. Click OK, and then click Close.

8. Spell-check the document. Add any names to the Southwest dictionary, if necessary.

9. Change the heading to all capitals, and add another blank line under it. Change the top margin to 2 inches.

10. Save the document as *[your three-letter identifier]*10-2.doc.

11. Print the document.

12. Close the document and exit Word (unless you will be doing the following exercises immediately).

Exercise 10.3

1. Start Word, if necessary.

2. Open the file 7-0.doc.

3. Revise the paragraph under the heading "Record Keeping" as shown in Figure 10-8.

Figure 10-8

Use the computer to keep

[All correspondence between group participants and you ~~should be kept~~ up-to-date ~~in the computer~~. Each group is named and ~~kept~~ *stored* as its own database, so you always have access to all the active participants. There is a master list for each group that ~~should be~~ *is* (constantly) updated to reflect any change*s* in name, itinerary, accommodations, options bought, money paid, and so forth. This way, you can ~~tell~~ *see the status of the group plans* at a glance ~~where you are in finalizing the details~~ Valerie keeps a hard copy of all these records in her master file. *The computer files are stored on the network, in the directory C:\TRAVEL\GROUP*

---

4. Scroll to the paragraph beginning "July 1". Key the text **By no later than** before "July".

5. Copy the text just keyed and the space character after it to the beginning of the next four paragraphs.

6. Use the Replace command to replace all occurrences of "group travel" with "group tours". Make sure to correct any case changes that may occur with the replacement.

7. Add a .5-inch (default) tab to the beginning of each line of the list on page 2 that starts with "Airline tickets".

8. Use the Replace command to change the formatting of all underlined text to bold and italics. (Remember, you can press **Ctrl+U** twice or choose None from the Underline drop-down list for no underline.)

9. Replace "August" with "September" and "July" with "August" throughout the document.

10. On page 2, use the Replace command to delete the tab characters you inserted in the list and change the alignment to centered.

11. Delete the text at the bottom of the second page from "For more information" through "IATA".

12. Add your reference initials to the document, and then spell-check the document.

13. Save the document as *[your three-letter identifier]*10-3.doc.

14. Print the document.

15. Close the document and exit Word (unless you will be doing the following exercise immediately).

Exercise 10.4: Challenge Yourself

Open the file 10-4.doc. Format the lists that begin "The Great Sphinx" and "Hawaii" with .5-inch left indents.

In the second paragraph, delete "Our" and key **Duke City Gateway's**. Copy the keyed text to the Clipboard. Use the Replace command to replace uppercase and lowercase "our" with the Clipboard contents throughout the document. Confirm each replacement, and do not use the replacement text for "our own Southwest" or in the last paragraph.

Use the Replace command to replace "tours" with "expeditions", except when the word occurs in "special-interest tours". Use the Replace command to replace the text that has a .5-inch left indent with a 1-inch left indent, 1.5 line spacing, and italics.

Add a heading to the document by keying the following in bold, all-capital letters:

Interesting Tours For Travelers with Interests

Add a box around the heading using the thinnest double line. Adjust the right border to 5 inches on the ruler, and then center the text in the box.

Grammar-check and spell-check the document. Save the document as *[your three-letter identifier]*10-4.doc and print it. Close the document and exit Word.

A Press Release and a Schedule of Events

Background

Duke City Gateway Travel Agency is sponsoring the grand-opening events for Albuquerque's newest hotel, the Red River Hotel. The large hotel features two restaurants, sports facilities, and professional meeting facilities.

Events are scheduled for the entire grand-opening day. Duke City Gateway employees will promote the grand opening of the Red River Hotel and will be present at the grand-opening ceremonies to host events and entertain visitors.

Business Purpose

Create a press release announcing the grand opening of the Red River Hotel. Then, create a schedule of events for the grand-opening day.

Procedures

1. Start Word, if necessary.

2. Open the file p3-1.doc.

3. Below "FOR IMMEDIATE RELEASE", press **Enter** twice, and then key the text shown in Figure 10-9. Use double-spacing for all the keyed text.

4. Change the left and right margins to 1 inch.

5. Indent the paragraphs following "FOR IMMEDIATE RELEASE" .25 inches from the left and right margins.

6. Center the heading ("Grand Opening at the Red River Hotel") and make it bold.

7. Open the file p3-1a.doc.

8. Arrange the documents so that both are visible.

9. From document P3-1A.DOC, copy the text in the third paragraph, which begins "The Red River has" and ends with "sauna." Paste the text in document P3-1.DOC after the text "and weddings." in the last paragraph.

10. From document P3-1A.DOC, copy the sentence in the sixth paragraph, which begins "For corporate clients". Paste the text in document P3-1.DOC in the last paragraph after the sentence ending "sauna."

11. From document P3-1A.DOC, copy the sentence in the last paragraph, which begins "The Red River Hotel is conveniently". Paste the text as a separate and final paragraph in document P3-1.DOC.

12. At the end of document P3-1.DOC, key # # # and center it (this signifies the end of the press release).

13. Spell-check document P3-1.DOC.

14. Make any changes you feel would improve the appearance of the document, then save it as *[your three-letter identifier]*p3-1.doc and print it.

15. Close the documents, then open the file p3-2.doc.

16. Center the first two lines on the page and make them bold.

17. Switch the text after 11:00 a.m., which begins "Grand Tour", with the text after 12:00 p.m., which begins "Albuquerque".

18. After the last entry on the schedule of events, press **Enter** twice, then key:

    The new Red River Hotel has just been completed. The hotel has

19. Open the file *[your three-letter identifier]*p3-1.doc, and arrange the documents in the window.

20. From document P3-1.DOC, copy the text from "a heated indoor pool" to "banquet facilities." Paste the text in document P3-2.DOC after "The hotel has".

21. Close *[your three-letter identifier]*P3-1.DOC.

22. Key this sentence at the end of the paragraph:

    The Red River Hotel is conveniently located off I-40 on University.

23. Indent the paragraph .5 inches from the left and right margins.

24. Replace the italic character formatting of the times ("8:30 a.m.", etc.) with bold character formatting.

25. Make any changes you feel will improve the appearance of the document.

26. Spell-check the document, then save it document as *[your three-letter identifier]*p3-2.doc.

27. Print the document, and then close it and exit Word.

> ## Tips and Hints
>
> - Double-space the paragraphs in a press release to make the text easier to read.
>
> - Include a release date, contact name, and phone number on all press releases, so publishers know when to print the story and who to contact with questions about the press release.
>
> - Include three number signs (# # #) on the last page of the press release to indicate the end of the press release.
>
> - Include statements made by people involved in the event in your press release to make them more interesting.
>
> - Include a heading in your press release that captures the main idea of the information in the press release.

Figure 10-9

Grand Opening of the Red River Hotel

Duke City Gateway Travel, New Mexico's leading full-service travel agency, in conjunction with Red River, Inc., announces the grand opening of the Albuquerque Red River Hotel on Saturday, May 22. The schedule of events for the day includes a ribbon-cutting ceremony, a celebrity luncheon, and an evening jazz concert.

"We extend an open invitation to tourists, as well as to all members of the Albuquerque community, to attend the grand opening of Albuquerque's Red River Hotel," said Duke City Gateway's manager, Susan Allen. Duke City Gateway employees will be available all day to provide information and assistance.

The new Red River Hotel caters to tourists, corporate clients, and weddings.

Module 4

Page Formatting

Controlling Page and Section Breaks

Objectives

- Control soft and hard page breaks.

- Control widows and orphans.

- Insert section breaks.

- Format sections.

- Vertically align sections.

- Adjust the view of a document.

- Use the Go To command.

Soft page break
A page break automatically placed by Word, which is continually adjusted to reflect changes in the document.

Note: Remember, to locate a specific point in a document, you can also use the Find feature to move to a specific word or phrase.

In Word, text flows automatically from the end of one page to the next, just as text wraps automatically from the end of one line to the next. This lesson focuses on the techniques for controlling and customizing this process, particularly in long documents.

Sections, which were introduced in Lesson 5, are a common feature of long documents and have a significant impact on pagination. This lesson describes the use and management of sections in greater detail.

Soft and Hard Page Breaks

As you work on a document, Word is constantly calculating the amount of space available on the page. Page length is determined by the size of the paper and the top and bottom margin settings. For example, using standard-size paper and default margins, page length is nine inches. When a document exceeds this size, either through continuous keying, pasting of text, or changes in formatting, Word creates a *soft page break*. This is an automatic page break that is continually adjusted as text is added or deleted. It appears as a horizontal dotted line on the screen.

To observe the automatic adjustment of a soft page break:

1. Start Word, if necessary.

2. Open the file 11-0.doc.

3. Scroll to the bottom of page 3.

   Notice the soft page break separating the heading "Calling Home?" from the paragraph below it.

4. In the paragraph above the heading, which begins "In Western Europe", move the insertion point to the left of "We recommend" in the eighth line, and press **Enter** twice to start a new paragraph.

   Notice the adjustment of the soft page break. See Figure 11-1 on page 208.

A soft page break cannot be deleted. It can only be moved by adding or deleting text on a page, as demonstrated; by changing the document's margins; or by changing paragraph formatting.

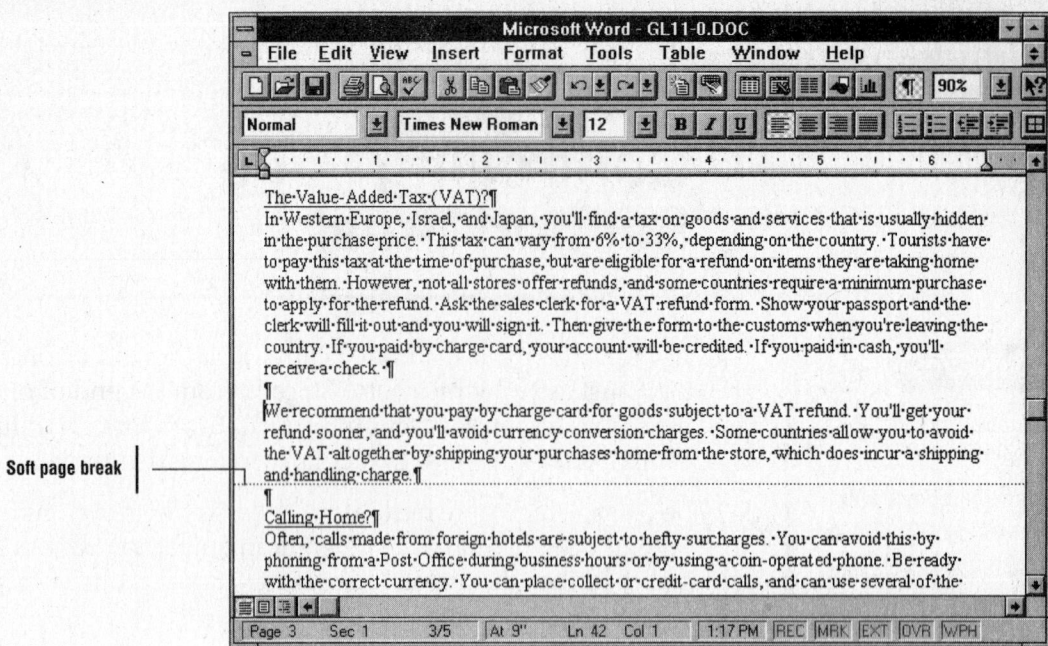

Soft page break

Figure 11-1
Moving a soft page break

Hard page break

A page break that is inserted manually and does not move, regardless of changes in the document.

You can control where a page breaks by inserting a *hard page break* manually. A hard page break does not move as the document is changed, and it can only be adjusted by you.

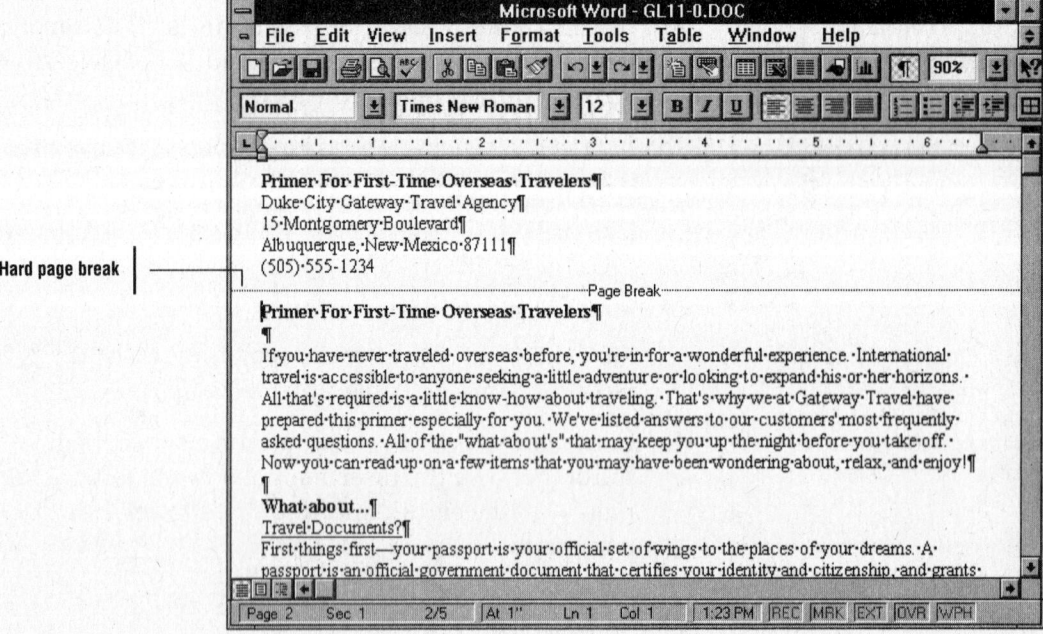

Hard page break

Figure 11-2
A hard page break

There are many reasons to insert a hard page break. You may want to start a new section, or your document may contain text that you do not want Word to break between two pages, such as a table. A hard page break appears on the screen as a dotted line with the words "Page Break".

There are two ways to insert a hard page break:

- Choose Break from the Insert menu.

- Use the keyboard command **Ctrl+Enter**.

To insert hard page breaks using both methods:

1. Move the insertion point to the bottom of page 2, to the beginning of the paragraph that starts "If you're torn".

2. Choose Break from the Insert menu.

   Word displays the Break dialog box.

Figure 11-3
The Break dialog box

3. Make sure Page Break is selected and click OK.

   Word inserts a hard page break, so that the paragraph is not separated between two pages. Pagination is adjusted in the document from this point forward.

4. Move through the document to the middle of page 4, and place the insertion point to the left of the text that begins "For specific information".

Note: When moving through long documents, remember the keyboard shortcuts: **Ctrl+Up** or **Down Arrow** to move up or down one paragraph, the **PgUp** or **PgDn** key to move up or down one window, and **Ctrl+Home** or **Ctrl+End** to move to the beginning or end of a document.

---

5. Press **Ctrl+Enter**.

   Word inserts a hard page break.

Insert
Break...
Page Numbers...
Annotation
Date and Time...
Field...
Symbol...
Form Field...

Footnote...
Caption...
Cross-reference...
Index and Tables...

File...
Frame
Picture...
Object...
Database...

Insert menu

There are three ways to remove a hard page break:

- Select it, or position the insertion point in the page break line, and then press the **Delete** key.

- Move the insertion point to the end of the text preceding the page break, and press the **Delete** key.

- Move the insertion point to the beginning of the text following the page break, and press the **Backspace** key.

To remove the last page break inserted:

1. Position the I-beam over the page break and click.

2. Press the **Delete** key.

3. Click the Undo button to restore the page break. Move the insertion point to the left of "For specific information", and then press the **Backspace** key.

   This method assures that only the page break is deleted.

Widows and Orphans

In traditional typing, and with many word processors, it is common for a single line of text to appear by itself at the top or bottom of a page. When a line of text appears by itself at the top of a page, it is called a *widow*. If it appears at the bottom of a page, it is called an *orphan*. Unless each page in a document must have the exact same number of lines, it is best to avoid widows and orphans. They distract the reader and detract from the cohesiveness of a document.

Word automatically checks a document to prevent widows and orphans. It moves an orphan forward to the next page and moves a widow back to the previous page. Widow/Orphan Control (no widows or orphans) is Word's default setting.

To make sure this setting is selected, choose Paragraph from the Format menu, and click the Text Flow tab. Check the Widow/Orphan Control check box. If you do not want to prevent all widows and orphans, clear the check box. See Figure 11-4 on page 211.

Controlling Page Breaks

In addition to Widow/Orphan control, the Text Flow tab in the Paragraph dialog box offers additional pagination options to control soft page breaks. These options are available by choosing Paragraph from the Format menu or choosing Paragraph from the shortcut menu.

- Page Break Before

  To print a specific paragraph at the top of a page, such as a chapter heading, place the insertion point in the paragraph, and then choose this option.

Widow
A line that appears by itself at the top of a page of text.

Orphan
A line that appears by itself at the bottom of a page of text.

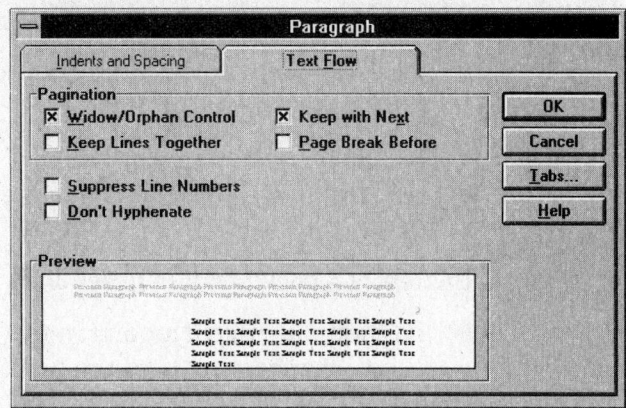

Figure 11-4

Text Flow options in the Paragraph dialog box

- Keep With Next

    To keep two paragraphs together on a page, place the insertion point in the paragraph you want to keep with the next paragraph, and then choose this option.

- Keep Lines Together

    To prevent a page break between lines of text in a paragraph, select the lines of text you want to keep together, and then choose this option.

When you choose any of these three options, Word displays a black, nonprinting square to the left of the paragraph (if nonprinting characters are displayed).

To make sure a paragraph starts at the top of a page, you can insert a hard page break immediately before it or use Page Break Before in the Paragraph dialog box as follows:

1. Close 11-0.doc without saving the changes, and then reopen the file by choosing the filename from the bottom of the File menu.

2. Move the insertion point to page 4, and place it in the paragraph that begins "For specific information".

3. Choose Paragraph from the Format menu, and click the Text Flow tab.

4. Click the Page Break Before check box, and then click OK.

    Word moves the soft page break, so that the paragraph starts at the top of page 5, and displays a black square to the left of the paragraph.

To keep two paragraphs together:

1. Move to the bottom of page 3, and place the insertion point in the heading "Calling Home?".

Black, nonprinting square

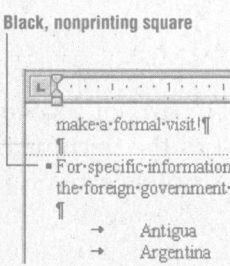

Using the Page Break Before option

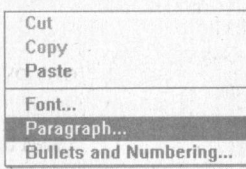

Shortcut menu

2. Choose Paragraph from the shortcut menu.

3. Click the Keep With Next check box, and then click OK.

   Word moves the page break to above the heading, keeping the two paragraphs together (remember, the heading is a paragraph, as is the text following it). The paragraph is marked with a black square.

To prevent a page break between lines of text in a paragraph:

1. Position the insertion point in the paragraph at the bottom of page 2 that begins "If you're torn".

2. Choose Paragraph from the Format menu.

3. Click the Keep Lines Together check box, and then click OK.

   The soft page break moves above the paragraph to keep the lines of text together.

Soft page break

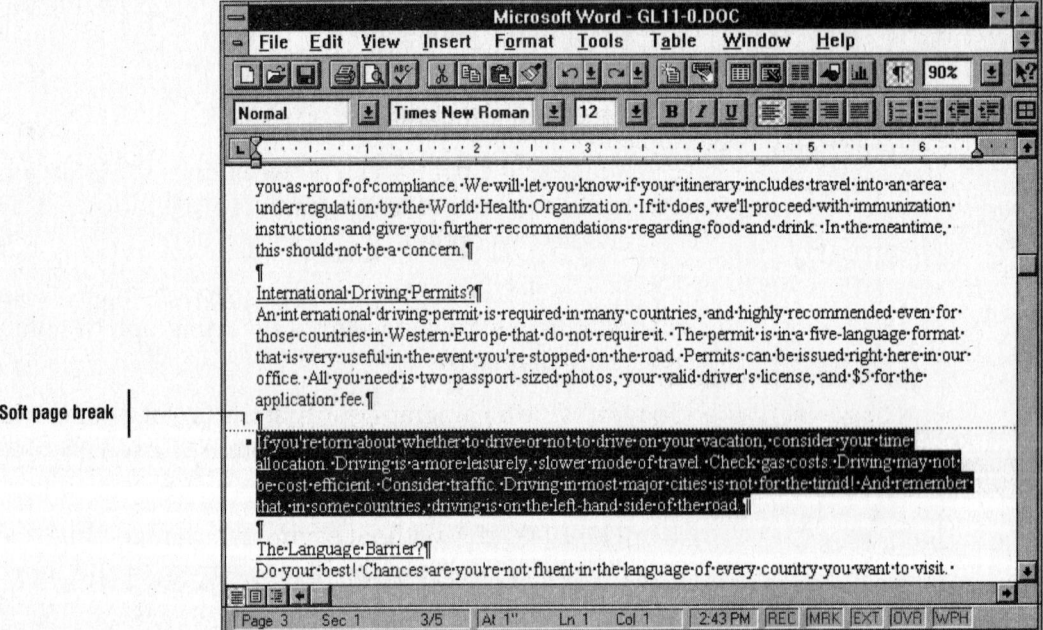

Figure 11-5
Using the Keep Lines Together pagination option

Controlling Section Breaks

As discussed in Lesson 5, section breaks separate parts of a document that have different formatting from the rest of the document. For example, changing the left and right margins of selected text results in a separate section that is marked by section breaks. This section starts on a new page, which affects the pagination in the document.

You can control the placement of section breaks in a document by specifying the type of section break. For example, a section break can be continuous—it can follow the preceding text without starting on a new page—or a section break can start on an even- or odd-numbered page.

Inserting Section Breaks

There are two ways to insert section breaks. You can format a part of a document differently, such as changing its margins, to create a separate section with section breaks, or you can select a point in a document where you want to start a new section, choose Break from the Insert menu, and specify the type of section break.

The Break dialog box, which you used earlier to insert page breaks, offers four options for section breaks:

- Next Page

    The section starts on a new page. This is the default setting when inserting section breaks.

- Continuous

    The section follows the text before it without a page break.

- Even Page

    The section starts on the next even-numbered page. If the section break falls on an even-numbered page, Word leaves the next odd-numbered page blank.

- Odd Page

    The section starts on the next odd-numbered page. If the section break falls on an odd-numbered page, Word leaves the next even-numbered page blank.

The Even Page and Odd Page options are useful for reports in which chapters must begin on either odd-numbered or even-numbered pages.

Removing a section break is similar to removing a page break. However, the section break, like the paragraph mark, stores whatever formatting you may have applied to the section. If you remove a section break, you delete the formatting for the section that precedes the section break. For example, if you have a two-section document, and you delete the section break at the end of section 1, the document becomes one section with the formatting of section 2. Use the Undo command to restore a section break that was deleted accidentally.

To insert section breaks using the Break dialog box:

1. Place the insertion point to the left of the paragraph at the top of page 5 that begins "For specific information".

2. Choose Paragraph from the shortcut menu, clear the Page Break Before check box, and click OK.

    Word removes the page break.

3. Choose Break from the Insert menu. Under Section Breaks, choose Continuous and click OK.

    Word begins a new section on the same page, from the position of the insertion point. Click above and below the section mark, and notice the page and section numbering on the status bar.

Figure 11-6
Inserting a continuous section break

4. Place the insertion point to the left of "For specific information" again, and press the **Backspace** key. (You can also place the insertion point at the section break or select it, and then press the **Delete** key.)

    Word removes the section break.

5. With the insertion point in the same place, choose Break from the Insert menu again. Select Next Page, and then click OK.

    Word begins a new section on the next page. Click above and below the section mark, and observe the page and section numbering on the status bar.

To insert section breaks by changing the formatting of text:

1. On page 2, select the text from the heading "**What About...**" through the fourth paragraph under it, which ends "just ask."

2. Choose Page Setup from the File menu.

3. Set the left and right margins to 1.5 inches. In Apply To, choose Selected Text, and then click OK.

    Word creates a separate section bordered on the top and bottom with section breaks. The section appears on its own page. Click above and below the section marks, and observe the page numbering on the status bar.

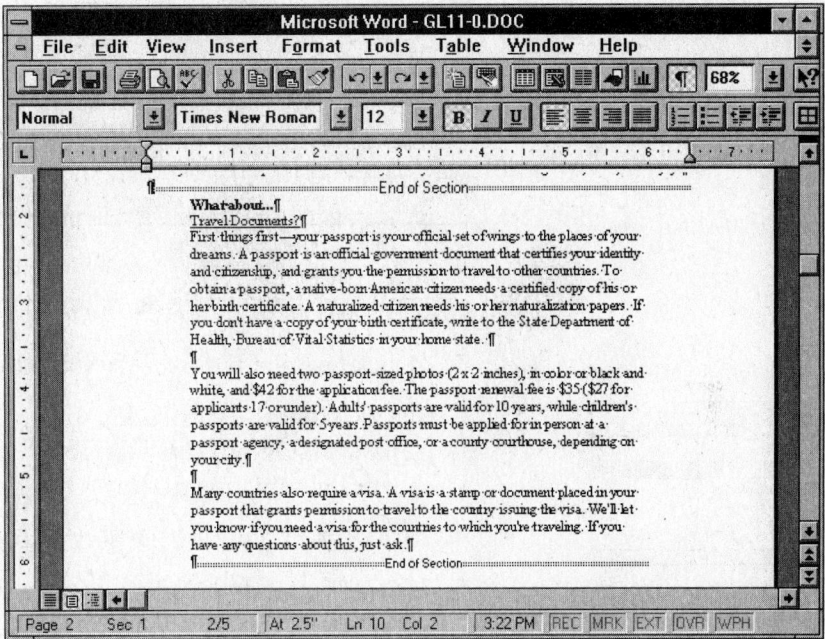

Figure 11-7
Section breaks at the top and bottom of the new section, as shown in page layout view

The document now contains two new sections: one that has a specified type of section break but the same formatting, and one that has different formatting but an unspecified type of section break.

Section Formatting

Once you have created a new section, you can change its formatting, or specify a different type of section break. For example, you can change a Next Page section break to a Continuous section break or apply new margin settings. To change the formatting of a section, choose Page Setup from the File menu, and then click the appropriate tab.

To apply formatting to sections:

1. Place the insertion point in section 2, at the beginning of the paragraph that starts "**What About**...".

    Notice that, although there is a section break above this section, the status bar indicates page 2, section 2, and page 2 of

5 pages. This shows that the section is a continuous section break, which does not start on a new page.

2. Choose Page Setup from the File menu, and click the Layout tab.

Figure 11-8
Layout options in the Page Setup dialog box

3. Click to open the Section Start drop-down list.

   Notice that the same section-break options available in the Break dialog box are available here (with the addition of New Column, which is discussed in Lesson 19).

4. Make no changes to the section break, and click the Margins tab.

5. Set 1.25-inch left and right margins. Make sure This Section appears in the Apply To box, and then click OK.

   Word applies the formatting to the section.

Types of section breaks

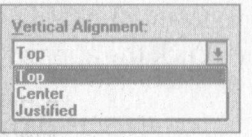

Vertical alignment options in the Page Setup dialog box

Vertical Alignment of Sections

Another way to format the way a section appears in a document is to specify the vertical alignment of the section on the page. For example, you can align a title page so that the text is centered between the top and bottom margins, or you can justify the alignment of the section so that the text extends from the top to the bottom margin. (This is similar in principle to the way Word justifies text between the left and right margins.)

To specify the vertical alignment of a section, choose Page Setup from the File menu, click the Layout tab, and then select one of the following alignment options:

• Top
  Aligns the top line of the page with the top margin. This is the default setting.

• Center
  Aligns the page between the top and bottom margins.

- Justified
  Aligns the top line of the page with the top margin and the bottom line with the bottom margin, with equal spacing between the lines of text.

To change the vertical alignment of a section:

1. Move the insertion point to the last section of the document.

2. Choose Page Setup from the File menu, and click the Layout tab.

3. Click the arrow to open the Vertical Alignment drop-down list, choose Center, and then click OK.

4. Click the Print Preview button on the Standard toolbar to view the section.

   The page is centered between the top and bottom margins.

5. Click Close to return to normal view.

Checking Pagination in Print Preview and Page Layout View

Use print preview or page layout view to check the pages of a document after you have applied page breaks, section breaks, or section formatting. Viewing the pages of a document in relation to each other may give ideas for improvement before printing. Remember, in page layout view, you can edit a document and change its page, paragraph, or character formatting.

Section breaks appear in page layout view the same as they appear in normal view. The actual section break is not visible in print preview. Page breaks are not indicated in page layout view or print preview by dotted lines, but by the actual page layout of each page as it will look when printed.

When viewing a multi-page document in page layout view, use the Page Forward and Page Back buttons to scroll up or down one page at a time. See Figure 11-9 on page 218.

Once in page layout view, you can use the Zoom Control box on the Standard toolbar to see whole pages. From the Zoom Control drop-down list, choose Whole Page to make each page fully visible, or choose Two Pages to see two pages at once, as in print preview. To change back to regular page layout view, choose Page Width.

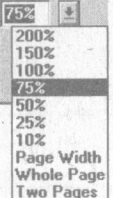

Page layout Zoom options on the Standard toolbar

Note: See Lesson 14 for more information about the Zoom command.

Start of a new page

Continuous section break

Page Layout view

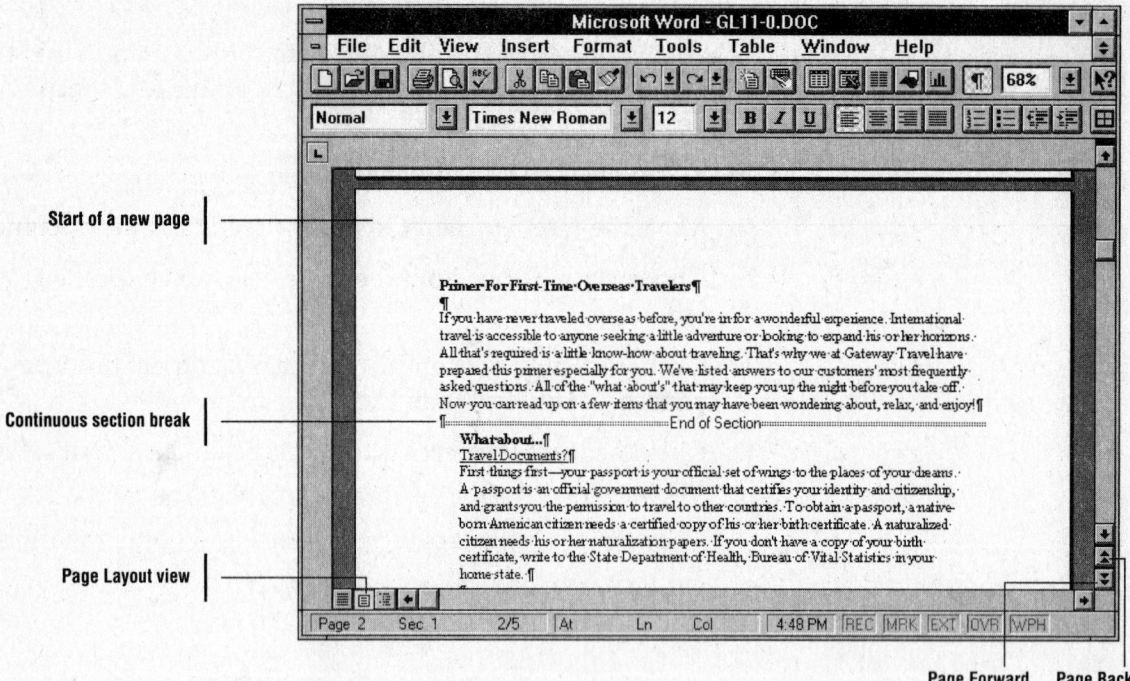

Page Forward   Page Back

Figure 11-9
Checking pagination in page layout view

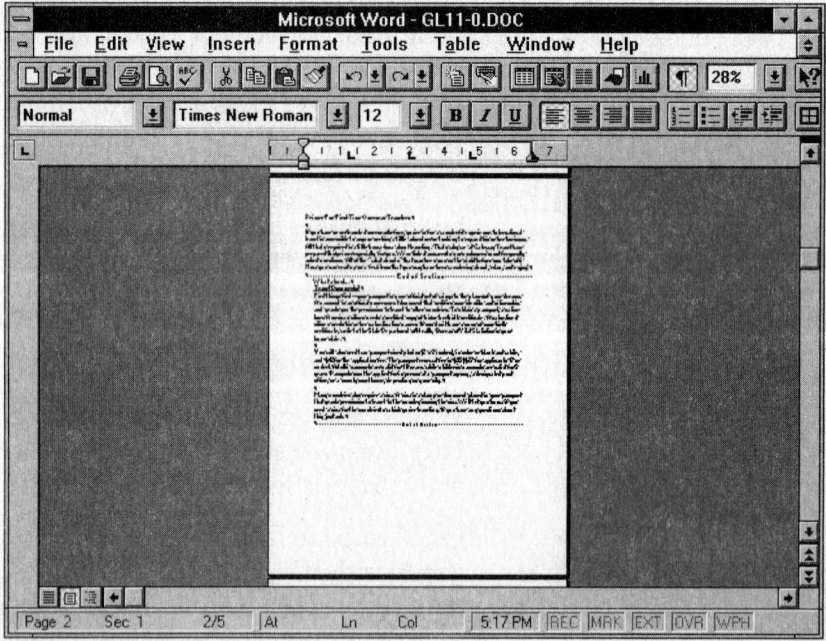

Figure 11-10
Viewing the whole page in page layout view

To check pagination and page layout by changing the view of a document:

1. Click the Page Layout View button above the status bar.

The document appears in page layout view, with section breaks and other formatting visible.

2. On the vertical scroll bar, click the Page Back button to scroll to the beginning of the document (or press **Ctrl+Home**).

3. Click the arrow to the right of the Zoom Control box on the Standard toolbar, and then choose Whole Page from the Zoom Control drop-down list.

   The full page is visible in page layout view

4. Scroll to the last page, and then choose Page Width from the Zoom Control drop-down list.

5. Choose Two Pages from the Zoom Control drop-down list.

   The document is reduced to display two pages at once.

6. Scroll back to the beginning of the document.

7. Click the Normal View button, and then switch to print preview.

8. Scroll to the last page of the document, and then choose Page Setup from the File menu (while still in print preview).

9. Click the Layout tab, if necessary, and change the vertical alignment to justified for this last section. Click OK.

   Word justifies the last page of the document (section 4) so that the text extends from the top to the bottom margin.

10. Click Close to return to normal view.

Using the Go To Command

Word offers several ways to move through a document quickly. The Find command, the scroll bar, and keyboard shortcuts are all methods discussed so far. Another method, the Go To command, lets you move to a specific line, page, or section of a document.

To use the Go To command, choose Go To from the Edit menu, press the **F5** key, or press **Ctrl+G**. Word opens the Go To dialog box, in which you can enter the appropriate instruction.

Figure 11-11
The Go To dialog box

The Go To dialog box offers the following options:

- Go to What
  Choose the type of location to which you want to move from this list. In addition to Page, Section, and Line, you can also choose Field, Graphic, and Table from this box.

- Enter
  This part of the dialog box corresponds to the item in the Go to What box. For example, if Page is chosen, then this part will be called Enter Page Number, and you key the page number to which you want to move. You can also key a plus sign (+) or a minus sign (-) before the number, and Word will count forward from the current location. For example, with Page chosen, key **+2**, and Word will move the insertion point two pages down in the document. Or, to move a specified distance through the document, key a number followed by the percent sign. For example, key **50%** to move to the middle of the document.

- Go To/Next
  When you have specified a location, click the Go To button. If the Enter box is empty, click the Next button to move ahead by whatever item is in the Go to What list box. For example, choose Section, and then click the Next button to move to the next section in the document.

- Previous
  Click this button to move back by whatever item is in the Go to What list box.

To use the Go To command:

1. With the insertion point in the last page of the document, choose Go To from the Edit menu.

2. With Page in the Go to What list box, key **1** in the Enter Page Number text box, click Go To, and then click Close.

   The insertion point moves to page 1.

3. Press **F5**. In the text box, key **s3l4**, press **Enter**, and then click Close. (You can also press the **Esc** key to close the Go To dialog box.)

   Section 3 is displayed, and the insertion point is at line 4.

4. Spell-check the document.

5. Save the document as *[your three-letter identifier]*11-0.doc.

6. Print the document.

7. Close the document and exit Word (unless you will be doing the following exercises immediately).

Note: You can also use the Enter area to enter an exact location with a corresponding prefix. For example, key **l50**, and Word will move to line 50 in the document. Key **p3**, and Word will move to page 3 of the document. Key **s2**, and Word will move to section 2 of the document. Key **s3p2l12**, and Word will move to section 3, page 2, line 12 of the document. You can key these specific locations without changing the Go to What item.

Note: Unlike scrolling, the Go To command moves the insertion point to the specified location.

Double-Clicking to Open Dialog Boxes

A quick way to open the Go To dialog box is to move the pointer to the left side of the status bar (for example, anywhere between "Page 1" and Col 1") and double-click. Double-clicking various parts of the Word screen opens different dialog boxes. To review the other double-clicking shortcuts:

- Double-click a tab marker or the lower border of the horizontal ruler to open the Tabs dialog box.

- Double-click an indent marker on the horizontal ruler to open the Paragraph dialog box.

- Double-click in either the left or right margin area of the horizontal ruler to open the Page Setup dialog box. (This is easiest in page layout view.)

- Double-click a section break to open the Page Setup dialog box (Layout tab).

- Double-click to the right of "REC" on the status bar to open the Record Macro dialog box. Macros are taught in Lesson 22.

Table 11-1: Keyboard Shortcuts for Controlling Page and Section Breaks

Keyboard Shortcut	Action
Ctrl+Enter	Insert hard page break
F5 or **Ctrl+G**	Open the Go To dialog box

Key Terms

Hard page break   Soft page break

Orphan   Widow

Exercises

Exercise 11.1

1. Start Word, if necessary.

2. Open the file 5-4.doc.

3. Move the columnar text from "<u>Airfares</u>" through "*All meals are included." to the end of the document. Make sure there are two blank lines between the first two lines of text on page 1.

4. Center the title on the first line of page 1 (which begins "New Mexico and Colorado"), and make it bold and all capitals.

5. Use the keyboard shortcut to insert a hard page break at "Day 7":

    A. Move the insertion point to the left of the text.

    B. Press **Ctrl+Enter**.

6. Insert a section break at "Airfares", so that the text starts on a new page:

    A. Move the insertion point to the left of the text.

    B. Choose Break from the Insert menu.

    C. Choose Next Page, and then click OK.

7. Use the Go To command to move the insertion point to the top of page 2:

    A. Press the **F5** key.

    B. Key **p2** in the text box, click Go To (or press **Enter**), and then click Close.

8. Press the **Backspace** key to delete the page break.

9. Move the soft page break to keep "Day 7" with the next paragraph:

    A. With the insertion point at "Day 7", choose Paragraph from the Format menu, and click the Text Flow tab.

    B. Under Pagination, check Keep with Next and click OK.

10. Center section 2 (which begins "Airfares") both vertically and horizontally:

    A. Place the insertion point in section 2.

    B. Choose Page Setup from the File menu, and click the Layout tab.

    C. Choose Center in the Vertical Alignment box.

    D. Click the Margins tab, and then increase the left margin to 1.75 inches.

    E. Click OK.

11. Select the text in section 2, and change the line spacing to 1.5 lines.

12. Select the text in section 1 from "*Itinerary*" through "and Colorado" (at the end of Day 9), and change the paragraph spacing to 6 pt after paragraphs.

13. View the pages of the document in print preview.

14. Spell-check the document.

15. Save the document as *[your three-letter identifier]*11-1.doc.

16. Print the document.

17. Close the document and exit Word (unless you will be doing the following exercises immediately).

Exercise 11.2

1. Start Word, if necessary.

2. Open the file 11-2.doc.

3. Use the Page Setup dialog box to format the paragraph that begins with "The Fountaines" and the two paragraphs after it with 1.25-inch left and right margins. Be sure to apply the formatting to the selected text only.

4. Change the section breaks to continuous section breaks:

   A. Place the insertion point in section 2, choose Page Setup from the File menu, and click the Layout tab.

   B. Make sure Continuous appears in the Section Start box, and then click OK.

   C. Place the insertion point in section 3. Open the same dialog box and choose Continuous. Click OK.

5. View the document in print preview.

6. View the document in page-layout view, and use the Zoom Control box on the Standard toolbar:

   A. Click the Page Layout View button.

   B. Choose Whole Page from the Zoom Control drop-down list.

   C. Choose Page Width from the Zoom Control drop-down list.

   D. Click the Normal View button to return to normal view.

7. Spell-check the document.

8. Add your reference initials and an enclosure notation to the document.

9. Save the document as *[your three-letter identifier]*11-2.doc.

10. Print the document.

11. Close the document and exit Word (unless you will be doing the following exercises immediately).

Exercise 11.3

1. Start Word, if necessary.

2. Open the file 11-3.doc.

3. Format the letter as a standard business letter from Ed Micali, Sales Representative. Insert the date as a field code. Include your reference initials and an enclosure notation. Keep the 1.25-inch left and right margins, and remember to allow a 2-inch top margin for page 1 of the letter.

4. On page 2, after the paragraph that begins "These dates are", key Figure 11-12 as a new paragraph, including the corrections.

Figure 11-12

Just a reminder⊙

[All U. S. citizens traveling to the Bahamas must carry proof of

                                    or a birth certificate
citizenship͓ such as a passport[. A driver's license is not considered

proof of citizenship, but you will need it for your rental car. Your

                                        and can seat (comfortably six people⊙
rental car, by the way, offers unlimited mileage?͓

---

5. At the bottom of page 1, use the Keep With Next pagination option for the text "Monday, September 3".

6. Using the Paragraph dialog box, format all the itinerary text (from "Saturday, August 25" through "at 4:10PM") with a .25-inch left and right indent.

7. Start a Next Page section break at "Monday, September 3", and then format section 2 with a 1-inch top margin.

8. Delete the paragraph mark just above the section break, if it is creating a soft return (and a blank page).

9. Underline the itinerary datelines, and view the document in print preview.

10. Switch back to Normal view, and replace "AM" with "a.m." and "PM" with "p.m.". Be sure to include a space before "a.m." and "p.m." in the Replace With text box. Delete any extra periods in sentences ending with "a.m." or "p.m.".

11. At the beginning of page 2, before the text "Monday, September 3" key the following three-line continuation page header:

    Mr. Michael Carver
    Page 2
    [today's date]

12. Make sure the header is not underlined or indented. Insert two blank lines after the date.

13. Spell-check the document.

14. Save the document as *[your three-letter identifier]*11-3.doc.

15. Print the document.

16. Close the document and exit Word (unless you will be doing the following exercise immediately).

Exercise 11.4: Challenge Yourself

Open the file 11-4.doc. Format the text from "**$1 Equals**" to "$1.37" with a 3-inch left margin. Change the line spacing for the text to 1.5 lines. Make both of the resulting section breaks continuous.

In the paragraph that begins "If you're wondering", change the end of the sentence to read "the cities listed on the following page." Move the last paragraph, which begins "The European Travel", so that it follows this paragraph.

Insert a section break at "**European Weather in June**", so that the text starts on the next page. For the text under this heading, change the tab settings to 3- and 4.5-inch centered tabs. Indent the text 1 inch from the left margin. Then change the line spacing for the text to double-spaced. Vertically align this section, so that it is centered between the top and bottom margins.

Use the Replace command to replace "June" with "July" in the document. Use the Go To command to go to Section 4, line 10. Change "80" to "85".

Spell-check the document, adding any foreign words to the world dictionary. Save the document as *[your three-letter identifier]*11-4.doc and print it. Close the document and exit Word.

Introduction to Page Numbers, Headers, and Footers

Background repagination
The automatic process of updating page breaks and page numbers that occurs after editing a document.

Header
Text that appears in the top margin of a page throughout a section or document.

Footer
Text that appears in the bottom margin of a page throughout a section or document.

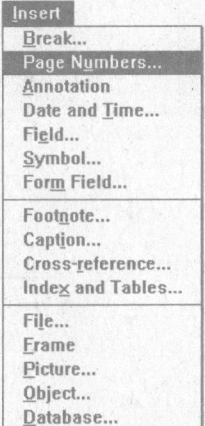

Insert menu

Numbering pages is a useful feature in Word that is applicable to all types of documents, particularly long documents. Word can automatically number the pages in a document and then update the numbering as the document is edited or formatted.

This lesson focuses on the many ways to apply and customize page numbering. It also introduces headers and footers, which are integral in the page-numbering process.

Page Numbers, Headers, and Footers

The pages of a document are always numbered as you work in Word—the status bar serves as a constant indicator of page and section numbers. Every time text or sections are added, deleted, or formatted, Word adjusts page breaks and page numbers. This is called *background repagination*. It is an automatic process that occurs when you pause while working on a document.

Page numbers do not appear on a printed document, unless you specify that they do. Page numbers can appear either in the top or the bottom margin of a page. The text in the top margin of a page is called a *header*; text in the bottom margin of a page is called a *footer*.

Headers and footers are not visible when a document is in normal view. They can only be seen in page layout view, in print preview, or on the printed page.

This lesson focuses on page numbers as headers or footers. Lesson 13: "Advanced Headers and Footers" discusses the use of other identifying information, such as a date or a document title, in headers and footers.

Adding Page Numbers

There are two ways to add page numbers to a document:

• Choose the Page Numbers command from the Insert menu

• Choose the Header and Footer command from the View menu

The Page Numbers command is used for basic page numbering. With this command, a single page number prints on all pages, or you

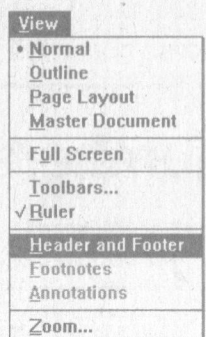

View menu

can begin page numbering with number 2 on page 2 for documents in which you want the first page to have no number.

The Header and Footer command is used for viewing, editing, and adding page numbers. It is also used for variations in page numbering, such as adding the word "Page" before the number.

Using the Page Numbers Command

When you choose the Page Numbers command from the Insert menu, Word displays the Page Numbers dialog box, from which you can choose the following options:

- Position
  Page numbers can appear at the top of the page as a header or at the bottom of the page as a footer. The default setting is the bottom of the page.

- Alignment
  Page numbers can be aligned with the left or right margin, or centered between the margins. The default setting is right-aligned.

- Show Number on First Page
  The default is to begin numbering on page 1. To begin on page 2, clear this check box.

- Format
  Pages can be sequenced with Arabic numerals (for example, 1, 2, 3), letters, or Roman numerals. The default setting is Arabic numerals.

The Preview box in the Page Numbers dialog box indicates the position and alignment of the number.

Figure 12-1
The Page Numbers dialog box

Using the Page Numbers command, you can apply page numbers with the default settings or choose other options.

To apply page numbers using the default settings:

1. Open the file 12-0.doc.

2. With the insertion point at the top of the document, choose Page Numbers from the Insert menu.

Word displays the Page Numbers dialog box. Notice the default settings Bottom of Page (Footer) and Right alignment are chosen.

3. Click Format.

The default numbering format is selected.

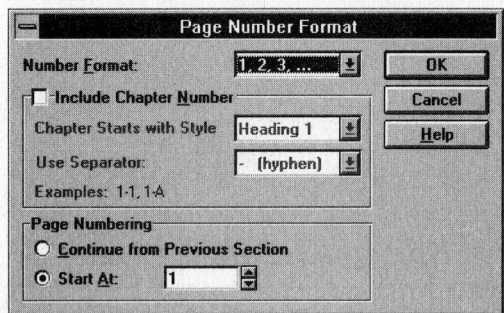

Figure 12-2
The Page Number Format dialog box

Note: The Page Number Format dialog box also lets you include chapter numbers with page numbers. For example, you can divide a long document in chapters by using a specific chapter heading style, and then have Word include the chapter number with the page number, such as 1-1 (chapter 1, page 1). Styles are discussed in Lesson 20.

4. Click OK in the Page Number Format dialog box, and then click OK in the Page Numbers dialog box.

5. Switch to print preview, and scroll through the document.

The numbers appear on the bottom right of each page, within the 1-inch bottom margin. Specifically, the page number is positioned .5 inches from the edge of the page. This is the default position for any header or footer.

6. Click the magnifying pointer on one of the numbers in the bottom right to view the number, if necessary.

7. Close print preview, and then close the document without saving the changes.

To apply page numbers by choosing different options:

1. Open the file 12-0.doc again.

Note: Remember, the fastest way to open a file that was recently opened is to choose the filename from the bottom of the File menu.

2. Choose Page Numbers from the Insert menu.

3. Choose Top of Page (Header) and Center alignment.

The Preview box shows the number placement.

4. Click the Show Number on First Page check box to clear it.

Page-number formats

5. Click Format, and then choose the last Roman numeral option from the Number Format drop-down list box.

6. Click OK in both dialog boxes to return to the document.

7. Switch to page layout view, and scroll through the document.

   The numbers for pages 2 and 3 are in Roman numerals and are centered at the top of the page. They appear within the 1-inch top margin, .5 inches from the edge. No number appears on page 1.

8. Switch back to normal view, and then close the document without saving the changes.

Using the Header and Footer Command

When you apply page numbers by choosing Header and Footer from the View menu, the document screen changes in several ways. Word switches to page layout view, moves the insertion point into the header area, and displays the Header and Footer toolbar. The header area appears as a dotted rectangle. With the insertion point in this area, use the preset tab settings to left-align, center, or right-align the page number. Then click the Page Numbers button on the Header and Footer toolbar. To move between the header and footer area, click the Switch Between Header and Footer button. The Header and Footer toolbar is discussed in more detail in Lesson 13.

Figure 12-3

Using the Header and Footer command to insert page numbers

To apply page numbers using the Header and Footer command:

1. Open the file 12-0.doc again.

2. Choose Header and Footer from the View menu.

   The document appears in page layout view with the Header and Footer toolbar. The insertion point is in the header area.

3. Press the **Tab** key to move to the preset center tab.

4. Key **Page**, and press the **Spacebar**. Then click the Page Numbers button.

5. Click the first button on the Header and Footer toolbar to switch to the footer area.

6. Click the Close button.

   The screen returns to normal view.

7. Switch to print preview to view the page numbers.

8. Close the document without saving changes.

Varying Page Numbers

In addition to choosing different options for the position and format of page numbers and choosing whether or not to number page 1, you vary page numbering in the following ways:

- Change the start of page numbering (for example, print "2" on page 1).

- Delay the start of page numbering (for example, print "1" on page 2).

- Change the format of page numbers among sections (for example, number one section of a document with Roman numerals, and the rest of the document with Arabic numerals).

Page Numbers and Section Breaks

Section breaks have an impact on page numbering. If a document has several sections, you can use the Header and Footer command to either number all the pages with the same format or number different sections with different formats. To use the same format to number all the pages, it is easiest to add the page numbers before adding the section breaks. Then Word adjusts the pagination each time you insert a section break. To vary page numbering within a document, it is sometimes necessary to add section breaks.

Remember, when choosing a continuous section break from the Break dialog box, the text does not start on a new page. When you choose Next Page, the text does.

Changing the Starting-Page Number

Word normally starts numbering a document on page 1. However, you can change numbering so that it starts on another page. For example, in a report such as the document 12-0.doc, you may want to insert an introductory page and change the numbering to start with page 2.

To change the starting-page number within a section, choose Page Numbers from the Insert menu and click Format. In the Start At box, key or choose a new starting-page number, and then click OK.

To change the starting-page number in a document:

1. Open the file 12-0.doc again.

2. Choose Page Numbers from the Insert menu.

3. Choose the Top of Page position, keep the Right alignment setting, and click Format.

4. Change the number in the Start At box to 2 and click OK.

5. Click OK to return to the document.

6. Switch to print preview, and scroll through the pages.

    Numbering begins on page 1 with number 2.

7. Click Close to exit print preview, and then close the document without saving it.

Number 2 on page 1 of the document

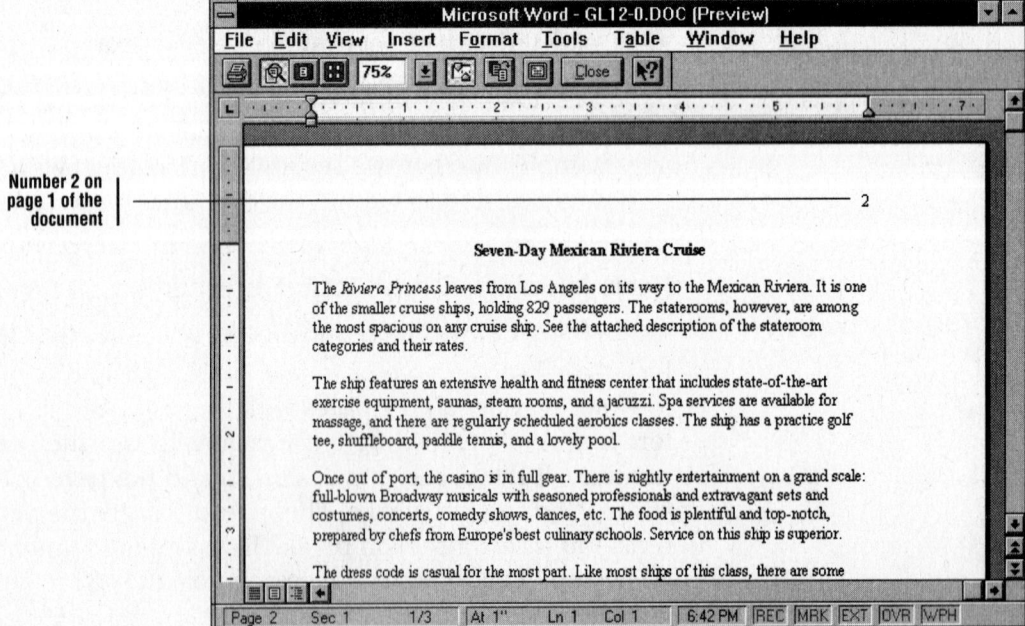

Figure 12-4

Viewing the starting-page number in print preview

Delaying the Start of Page Numbering

If a document has a title page or other introductory material, you may want to delay the start of page numbering in the document.

To delay the start of page numbering, first be sure the document is in normal view. Insert a section break where page numbering is to begin. (Remember, choose Next Page to start the section on a new page.)

Same As Previous button

With the insertion point in the new section, choose Header and Footer from the View menu. Click the Same As Previous button on the Header and Footer toolbar. This disconnects the headers and footers in the current section from the previous section. Then choose Page Numbers from the Insert menu, and choose the options you want. Word will apply the page numbering to the current section and to the sections following it.

The Same As Previous button is turned on by default. That means that all sections in a document will have the same header or footer. To change headers or footers from section to section, or to delay a header or footer, click the Same As Previous button to turn this option off.

To delay the start of page numbering in a document:

1. Open the file 12-0.doc again.

2. Create a title page by keying the following text at the beginning of the document (use the existing bold and centered formatting):

    **Seven-Day Mexican Riviera Cruise
    on the Riviera Princess
    Duke City Gateway Travel Agency
    (505) 555-1234**

3. After the keyed text, insert a section break. Be sure to choose Next Page from the Break dialog box.

    A new section is added at the beginning of the document.

4. To begin numbering in section 2, position the insertion point in the section, and choose Header and Footer from the View menu.

    Word displays the header area for section 2. The Same as Previous button is selected, indicating a link between the section headers. See Figure 12-5 on page 234.

5. Click the Same as Previous button to unlink the header between sections 1 and 2.

6. Press the **Tab** key twice to the right-aligned tab setting.

7. Key **Page**, press the **Spacebar**, and then click the Page Numbers button. Click Close.

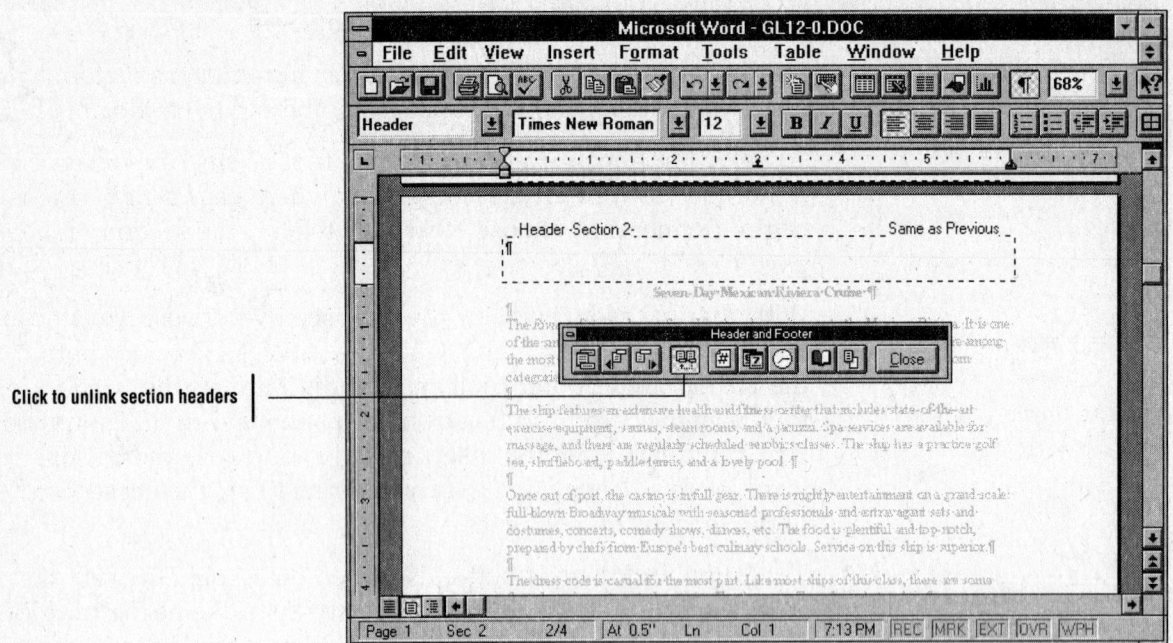

Click to unlink section headers

Figure 12-5
The header area for section 2

8. Switch to print preview, and scroll to the beginning of the document.

   Notice that there is no numbering on the title page (the new section 1) and that page numbering starts on page 1, section 2.

9. Save the document as *[your three-letter identifier]*12-0.doc.

Changing the Page-Number Format

In long documents with different sections, you can format one section differently than another. For example, you can start the introductory pages of a document with Roman numerals and continue with Arabic numerals for the rest of the document.

To do this, place the insertion point in the section you want to number and format differently. Choose Page Numbers from the Insert menu, and click the Format button. Choose the format you want from the Number Format box, and click OK in both dialog boxes.

To change the starting-page number and format:

1. In the document *[your three-letter identifier]*12-0.doc, place the insertion point in the first section.

2. Choose Page Numbers from the Insert menu.

3. Choose the header position and center alignment, and then click Format.

4. From the Number Format drop-down list, choose the lowercase Roman-numeral format. Make sure the Start At box reads "i" and click OK.

5. Click OK to return to the document.

6. Switch to print preview, and scroll through the document.

    Lowercase Roman numeral i is printed on page 1, section 1. Arabic numeral 1 appears on page 1, section 2.

To undo the special formatting of a section, use the Header and Footer command to open the header or footer area of a document and click the Save as Previous button. This changes the formatting to that of the section before it. You can also place the insertion point in the section, choose Page Numbers from the Insert menu, and choose the desired formatting.

Removing Page Numbers

Page numbers can be removed from an individual section or from the entire document. With the document in normal view, place the insertion point in the section from which you want to remove page numbers. Choose Header and Footer from the View menu. In the header or footer area, select the page number, then press the **Backspace** key or the **Delete** key. Word will remove the page numbers from the document or from the current section (if you have broken the link between headers or footers in different sections).

To remove page numbers from a document:

1. With the document in normal view, place the insertion point at the beginning of the document.

2. Choose Header and Footer from the View menu.

3. In the header area, select the page number for section 1, and press the **Delete** key.

4. While still in page layout view, scroll to the next page of the document (use the buttons on the vertical scroll bar to scroll one page at a time).

    Notice the page number is still in this section.

5. Scroll back to section 1.

Click to scroll to previous or next page

Scroll buttons in page layout view

6. With the insertion point in the section-1 header, click the Switch Between Header and Footer button on the Header and Footer toolbar.

7. In the footer area for section 1, click the Page Numbers button on the Header and Footer toolbar.

8. Scroll through the pages of the document.

    Page numbers have been applied to the footer of the document. Notice the page formatting matches the formatting previously chosen for each section.

9. Scroll back to section 1, and delete the page number in the footer.

10. Scroll to the next section.

    All the footer page numbers are deleted.

11. Click the Close button on the Header and Footer toolbar.

12. Save the document and print it.

13. Close the document and exit Word (unless you will be doing the following exercises immediately).

Removing Page Numbers in Page Layout View

You can remove page numbers in page layout view without first choosing the Header and Footer command from the View menu. To do this, switch to page layout view, and then scroll to the section and to the area of the section (header or footer) from which you want to delete page numbers. Move the pointer in the header or footer area and double-click. This activates the header or footer area and opens the Header and Footer toolbar. Then select the number and delete it as you normally would.

Remember, if you have kept headers and footers linked between sections in a document with multiple sections, all page numbering is removed when you delete a number from one section.

Troubleshooting

There are several factors that can affect page numbering in Word.

- As mentioned, in a document with multiple sections, page numbers will not appear throughout the document unless the insertion point is in the first section when applying the numbering.

- If you want a section to start with a new number or different formatting, be sure the section does not begin with a continuous section break.

- If you have renumbered a section in a different format, and the section following it does not reflect the original formatting, click Continue From Previous Section in the Page Number Format dialog box for that section. Word then renumbers that section from where the previous section ended.

- Page numbers can only be seen in print preview or page layout view. The status bar, which is visible in normal and page layout views, shows important information for page numbering, particularly for documents where the starting-page number has been changed.

  The first number indicates the position of the insertion point and the page number that will be printed on the page, if you have so specified. This number reflects any numbering changes made to the section or document. Whatever number format you have chosen will be reflected here. The second number is the section number. After that, Word displays two numbers: The first number represents the actual number of pages through to the insertion point, and the second number represents the total number of pages in the document.

Figure 12-6
The status bar showing a different first page

Key Terms

Background repagination   Header

Footer

Exercises

Exercise 12.1

1. Start Word, if necessary.

2. Open the file 7-2.doc.

3. Change the left and right margins to 1.5 inches. On page 2, insert a section break, so the paragraph that begins "Group travel is" starts on the next page.

4. Use the Page Numbers command to add page numbers to the bottom center of the page:

   A. Move the insertion point to the top of the document.

   B. Choose Page Numbers from the Insert menu.

   C. Keep the default position (footer), and choose Center under Alignment.

   D. Make sure the Show Number on First Page box is checked, and then click OK.

5. Switch to print preview to view the page numbers.

6. Change the page numbering, so that all numbers are preceded with the word "Page":

    A. With the insertion point at the top of the document, choose Header and Footer from the View menu.

    B. Click the Switch Between Header and Footer button to move to the footer area.

    C. Place the insertion point to the left of the page number, key **Page**, and press the **Spacebar**. Then click Close.

7. Switch to page layout view to view the page numbers.

8. Return to normal view, and then spell-check the document.

9. Save the document as *[your three-letter identifier]*12-1.doc.

10. Print the document.

11. Close the document and exit Word (unless you will be doing the following exercises immediately).

Exercise 12.2

1. Start Word, if necessary.

2. Open the file 11-0.doc.

3. Delay page numbering to the second page, so that number 1 prints on page 2 as a right-aligned header:

    A. Delete the page break at the top of page 2, and add a section break that starts on the next page.

    B. With the insertion point in the new section, choose Header and Footer from the View menu.

    C. Click the Same as Previous button to unlink the headers in sections 1 and 2.

    D. Press the **Tab** key until the insertion point is right-aligned.

    E. Click the Page Numbers button, and then click Close.

4. Go to page 3, and insert a section break at the paragraph "For specific information", so the text begins on a new page.

5. Remove the header from section 3:

    A. Place the insertion point in the section, and then choose Header and Footer from the View menu.

    B. Click the Same as Previous button to unlink the sections.

    C. In the Header area, select the number, and press the **Delete** key.

    D. Click Close.

6. Switch to print preview, scroll through each page of the document, and then return to normal view.

7. Start page numbering for section 3 with Roman numerals, centered on the page as a footer:

   A. With the insertion point in section 3, choose Header and Footer from the View menu.

   B. Click the Switch Between Header and Footer button.

   C. Click the Same as Previous button to unlink the footers between sections.

   D. Choose Page Numbers from the Insert menu. Choose Center alignment, and click the Format button.

   E. Choose uppercase Roman numerals from the Number Format drop-down list box. Click OK.

   F. Click OK to close the Page Numbers dialog box, and then close the Header and Footer toolbar.

8. View the pages of the document in page-layout view. Make sure no heading appears at the end of a page, separated from the text that follows it.

9. Return to normal view, and then spell-check the document.

10. Save the document as *[your three-letter identifier]*12-2.doc.

11. Print the document.

12. Close the document and exit Word (unless you will be doing the following exercises immediately).

Exercise 12.3

1. Start Word, if necessary.

2. Open the file 12-3.doc.

3. After the title page, delete the hard page break, and insert a section break that starts on the next page.

4. On page 1 of section 2, start numbering with 1. Center the number as a footer.

5. On page 2 of section 2, insert a hard page break at the bold heading "**Category, Location, and Rates**".

6. On page 4 of section 2, before the text "**Around-the-Clock Meals**", key the first paragraph that appears in Figure 12-7. Include the corrections. Edit the paragraph that begins "**Around-the-Clock Meals**", as shown in the second paragraph of the figure.

Figure 12-7

> non = stop serving of food. In addition to the regular
> three=meal=a=day schedule, you'll find announcements
> of midday snack times, afternoon tea times, and

Around the World Cuisine Cruise ship chefs are often specialists in cuisine from around the world. Depending upon where you are traveling, and the whim of the chef, cruises typically feature food *with* of regional *themes* ~~origin~~. For example, one night may be Italian Night ‒ serving up pastas, pizzas, and veal scallopini. Another night may be French Night, with escargot, duck al'orange, and an endless assortment of French pastries. A Mexican buffet may offer a savory spread of tacos, and tamales *^and fajitas*.

Around-the-Clock Meals Cruise ships are famous for ~~the many other meals that make up the day, from midday snacks to~~ midnight gourmet buffets. These meals are open seating and are served in different parts of the ship, including poolside or on one of the decks.

7. On page 6 of section 2, adjust the soft page break to keep the heading "**Ship Terminology**" with the text that follows it.

8. On page 8 of section 2, insert a section break at the heading "**Sample Cruise Itineraries**" that starts a new page. Adjust soft page breaks so that no lines of an itinerary are divided between two pages. (Use the paragraph pagination option Page Break Before.)

9. Renumber section 3, starting with page 1, using lowercase Roman numerals. Keep the same position (centered footer).

10. For all the cruise-itinerary text in section 3, change the tab to 1.5 inches.

11. Go to page 1, section 1, and vertically center the title-page text. Center each line of text between the right and left margins.

12. View the document in print preview to check the page numbering and formatting.

13. Spell-check the document. Do not spell-check the itineraries in the last section.

14. Save the document as *[your three-letter identifier]*12-3.doc.

15. Print the document.

16. Close the document and exit Word (unless you will be doing the following exercise immediately).

Exercise 12.4: Challenge Yourself

Open the file 12-4.doc. After the title page, delete the hard page break, and insert a section break that starts the text after it on the next page. Assume that another title page will be added, and begin numbering section 2 with "Page 3", including the word "Page". Use a right-aligned header.

Use the Replace command to replace all occurrences of two consecutive blank lines (three paragraph marks) with one blank line between paragraphs. Scroll through the document to make sure there is a blank line below every bold heading.

On page 8, in the text following the bold heading **"Sample Itinerary—The Great Southwest"**, left-align all the text following the day numbers at 1.75 inches. Repeat this formatting to the sample itineraries for **"The California Coast"**, **"London/Paris"**, **"The Western Caribbean"**, **"Cruise and Disney Vacation"**, and the itinerary under the heading **"Senior Citizen Travel"**. Make that itinerary heading bold.

On page 8, begin a new section on a new page from the heading **"Duke City Gateway Travel Itineraries"**. Number the pages in the section with lowercase letters, starting with "a". Use a centered footer, and delete the existing header.

Go to the beginning of section 2, which starts **"Introduction"**, and change numbering to start with "Page 1".

Center the text on the title page vertically and horizontally. Change the date field to a format that includes the day of the month. There should be no page number on this page.

Switch to page layout view to check the page numbers. Move any soft page breaks that separate a heading from the paragraph following it or that separate lines of an itinerary. (Insert a hard page break, or choose a pagination option.)

Spell-check the document. Then save the document as *[your three-letter identifier]*12-4.doc and print it. Close the document and exit Word.

Advanced Headers and Footers

Lesson 12 introduced the use of headers and footers for page numbers. This lesson focuses on the different kinds of descriptive information headers and footers can contain, such as the date, document title, and author's name. It also explains the many ways header and footer text can be formatted and positioned on the printed page.

Objectives

- Add headers and footers.
- Insert fields in headers and footers.
- Edit header and footer text.
- Apply formatting to header and footer text.
- Change the position of headers and footers.
- Create odd and even headers and footers.

Uses for Headers and Footers

Headers and footers are commonly used in documents to show such information as:

- Name of the document, section, or chapter

- Page or chapter numbers

- Date and/or time the document was created or revised

- Name of the author

- Graphic, such as a company logo

- Draft or revision number

The descriptive text in headers and footers can appear in many different combinations. For example, the second page of a business letter typically contains a header with the name of the addressee, the page number, and the date. A report may contain a footer with the report name and a header with the page number and chapter name. A newsletter may contain a header with the title and logo on the first page and a footer with the title and page number on the pages that follow.

In addition to having a different header or footer on the first page of a document, you can use a different header or footer on odd and even pages. Facing pages, which are the left and right pages in a bound document (see Lesson 5: "Changing Margins and Formatting Paragraphs"), can also have different headers and footers. These are discussed later in the lesson.

Figure 13-1
Examples of headers and footers

Adding Headers and Footers

When adding headers and footers, Word provides several options to customize and automate the process.

The Header and Footer Toolbar

The Header and Footer toolbar is the first step in understanding the basic elements of headers and footers. As explained in the previous lesson, when you choose Header and Footer from the View menu, Word moves the insertion point into the header area, which is surrounded by a dashed line, and opens the Header and Footer toolbar.

Figure 13-2
The Header and Footer toolbar

The buttons on the Header and Footer toolbar offer a variety of options:

• Switch Between Header and Footer
  Click to move to the header or footer area.

• Show Previous
  Click to move to the header or footer of the previous section.

- Show Next
  Click to move to the header or footer of the next section.

- Same as Previous
  Click to link or unlink the header or footer in one section to the header or footer in the previous section. If this button is depressed, the headers or footers between the two sections will be the same. If the button is not depressed, you can create a different header or footer for each section.

- Page Numbers
  Click to insert the page number.

- Date
  Click to insert the current date.

- Time
  Click to insert the current time.

- Page Setup
  Click to switch to the Layout tab in the Page Setup dialog box.

- Show/Hide Document Text
  Click to display or hide the document text.

Different First Page

To create a different first page, such as for a document's title page, you can create a separate section for the first page, as was done in the previous lesson, or you can choose the Different First Page option under the Layout tab in the Page Setup dialog box.

Figure 13-3

Header and footer options in the Page Setup dialog box

To add a different first page to a document:

1. Open the file 11-0.doc.

2. Choose Header and Footer from the View menu.

    Word displays the header area and opens the Header and Footer toolbar.

3. Click the Page Setup button on the Header and Footer toolbar.

4. Click Different First Page to select it and click OK.

   Word displays the first-page header area for page 1.

5. Click the Show Next button on the Header and Footer toolbar.

   Notice that this header area is just called "Header". Different text can be entered into each of these headers.

6. Click the Show Previous button, and then key **Duke City Gateway Travel Agency** in the first-page header at the left margin.

Figure 13-4
Creating a different first-page header

If you check Different First Page and key no text in the first-page header area, Word prints no header on the first page. Use this option when you want a header (or footer) on all pages of a document except the first page.

Page Number, Date, and Time Fields

In the previous lesson, the Page Numbers button was used to insert page numbers in a header. In this lesson, the Date and Time buttons are also used. The page number, date, and time are all entered as fields.

The page-number field is automatically updated whenever you repaginate a document. The date and time fields are automatically updated whenever you preview or print a document.

Note: There may be occasions when you do not want the date or time to be automatically updated. For example, you may want to print an earlier draft of a document, showing the date and time it was originally created. To instruct Word not to update the date and time, select the text containing this information in the header or footer area, and then press **Ctrl+F11**. To have Word begin updating this information again, press **Ctrl+Shift+F11**.

To add a header with the date, time, and page number:

1. Click the Show Next button on the Header and Footer toolbar.

2. Key **Page**, press the **Spacebar**, and then click the Page Numbers button.

   Notice that Word inserts the number 2.

3. Press **Enter**, and then click the Date button. Insert two spaces, and then click the Time button.

4. Click the Show Previous button to compare the document header with the first-page header.

5. Close the Header and Footer toolbar.

6. Save the document as *[your three-letter identifier]*13-0.doc.

Figure 13-5

A header showing the page number, date, and time

Additional Information Fields

Additional fields can be added to a document's header or footer, such as the author's name, the filename, the title of the document, the chapter number, and the total number of pages. You can key this information into a header or footer; however, the benefit of entering it as a field is that the information contained is updated automatically as you edit the document.

Information such as the filename and the number of pages is saved automatically with a document. However, information such as the author's name and the document title must be entered in

248   LESSON 13

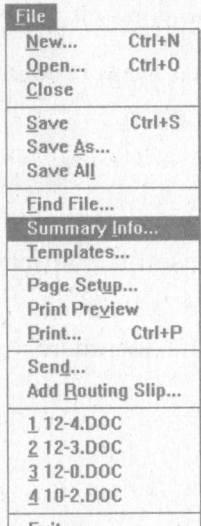

File menu

the Summary Info dialog box. If the Summary Info dialog box does not appear when you save a file, you can open it and add information to it by choosing Summary Info from the File menu.

To add a field to a header or footer, position the insertion point where you want the field to appear in the header or footer area, and then press **Ctrl+F9** to insert field characters ({}). Key one of the field codes in Table 13-1 between the field characters. To view the results, press **Alt+F9** or choose Toggle Field Codes from the shortcut menu. To update a field at any time, press the **F9** key or choose Update Field from the shortcut menu.

Table 13-1: Field Codes	
Key Field Code	To Insert
author	Author's name
title	Title of document
filename	Filename of document
numpages	Total number of pages in document

Another way to insert a field is to use the Field command, which is available from the Insert menu. This command allows you to insert many types of fields, most of which are discussed in later lessons.

To add additional fields to a header:

1. With *[your three-letter identifier]*13-0.DOC still open, choose Summary Info from the File menu.

2. Key your name in the Author box. In the Title box, key **Primer for First-Time Overseas Travelers** (if necessary).

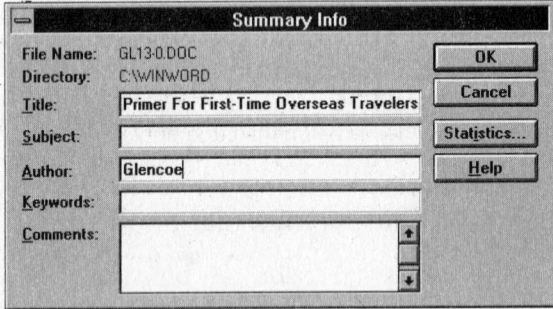

Figure 13-6
Entering information in the Summary Info dialog box

3. Click Statistics.

The filename and the number of pages, among many other statistics, are indicated.

4. Click Close, and then click OK to return to the document.

5. Place the insertion point in page 2, and then choose Header and Footer from the View menu.

6. In the header area, insert a space after "Page 2", and then key **of**

7. Insert a space, and then press **Ctrl+F9**.

   Word inserts field characters and places the insertion point between them. All the fields in the header appear as field codes.

8. Key **numpages**, and then press **Alt+F9** to turn off field codes (or choose Toggle Field Codes from the shortcut menu).

   The numpages field result is not yet visible, until you update the field.

9. Without moving the insertion point, click the right mouse button, and choose Update Field from the shortcut menu.

   Word inserts the document's total number of pages, so the header reads "Page 2 of 5". This total page number is updated as pagination in the document changes.

10. Press the **Tab** key to move the insertion point to the 6-inch right-aligned tab after "Page 2 of 5", and choose Field from the Insert menu.

    Word displays the Field dialog box.

Shortcut menu

Figure 13-7
The Field dialog box

11. From the Categories box, choose Document Information. From the Field Names box, scroll down and choose Title. Click OK.

    Word inserts the document title in the header, as entered in the Summary Info dialog box.

Header

Page 2 of 5 → → Primer For First-Time Overseas Travelers¶
May 23, 1994 10:38 AM¶

Primer For First-Time Overseas Travelers¶
¶

Figure 13-8
The new header with field information

Editing and Formatting Headers and Footers

In Word, header and footer text can be edited and formatted the same way you edit and format regular text in a document. This offers extensive flexibility in the appearance of headers and footers.

Character and Paragraph Formatting

Header and footer text can be selected and formatted using the Bold, Italic, or Underline buttons on the Formatting toolbar, or you can choose from any of the options in the Font dialog box.

Similarly, you can format header and footer text by setting tabs, margins, and indents or by changing alignment and line spacing. Apply paragraph formatting by using the ruler, the Formatting toolbar, or the Paragraph dialog box.

To format header or footer text:

Note: Fields are identified in Word with a gray highlight. For example, when you click a date field, it appears with a gray highlight to show it is a field. However, to select field text, you must either drag the I-beam over the text, or double-click at the beginning of the field text. The text then appears with a black highlight.

1. Select the document title in the header on page 2, and then click the Italic button on the Formatting toolbar.

    Word applies the formatting to the title.

2. With the insertion point in the first line of the header, drag the 6-inch right-aligned tab marker off the ruler.

    The text left-aligns with the first default setting after the 3-inch preset tab.

    Remember, when you open a header or footer, the ruler changes to the header or footer ruler, with a 3-inch centered tab and a 6-inch right-aligned tab. These tabs settings can, of course, be changed or deleted.

3. Click the Undo button to restore the original setting.

4. To change the line spacing, select both lines of the header text. (Move the pointer into the selection bar area to select both lines.)

5. Choose Paragraph from the Format menu, and click the Indents and Spacing tab. Under Line Spacing, choose Exactly. Then click OK.

    Word applies the new line spacing, which reduces the space between the two lines of text.

Header ruler

Header text with character and paragraph formatting

Figure 13-9
Formatting the header text

6. Close the header, and return to normal view.

    Notice that the ruler changes back to the document ruler once the header is closed.

Editing and Deleting Text

Header and footer text can be edited and deleted the same way you edit and delete regular text in a document. In addition, you can cut, copy, or paste text. As with the editing of regular document text, the Undo command can be used immediately after an edit if you change your mind.

As explained in earlier lessons, formatting instructions are contained in the paragraph mark. When you delete text in the header or footer area, the paragraph mark may still contain the formatting for the deleted text, such as alignment or character formatting. To clear formatting from the paragraph mark in the header or footer area, select the paragraph mark and press **Ctrl+Q**.

Working in Page Layout View

Not only can you view headers and footers in page layout view, but you can edit and format them, as well. Page layout view is the view that Word switches to when it opens the header or footer area.

When working on a document in page layout view, scroll to the header or footer text. Double-click the text, and Word opens the header or footer area (and the Header and Footer toolbar) for any changes you may wish to make. Remember, changes made to a header or footer on one page are reflected in all pages within the section.

To edit header or footer text in page layout view:

1. With *[your three-letter identifier]*13-0.DOC still open, switch to page layout view.

2. Scroll to the header on page 2 of the document.

3. Double-click the header text.

   Word moves the insertion point into the header area and opens the Header and Footer toolbar.

4. Copy the document title in the header to the Clipboard.

5. Click the Show Previous button to view the first-page header. Move the insertion point to the right of the company name in the header, and then press the **Tab** key twice.

6. Paste the Clipboard text in the header. Then move the right-aligned tab marker on the ruler to 6.25 inches.

7. Click Close to move out of the header area and return to page layout view.

8. Click within the document text on page 2, under the header.

   Notice that the ruler switches from the header ruler back to the document text ruler.

Header text

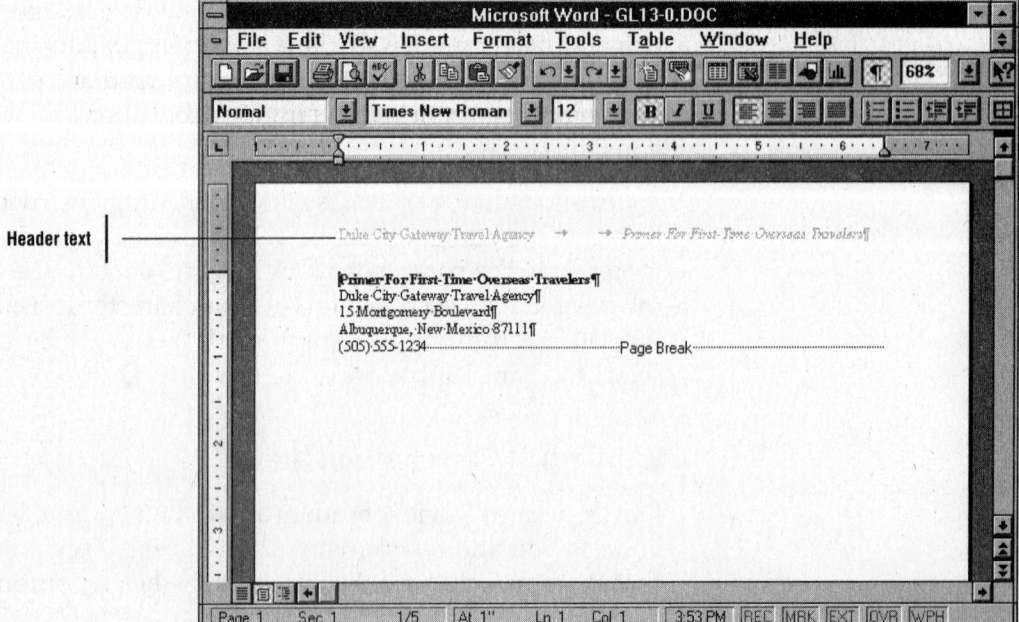

Figure 13-10
Viewing a header in page layout view

Changing the Date and Time Format

You can change the date and time format in a header as easily as you can change it in regular text. Time and date formats are discussed in Lesson 5.

After inserting the time or date field in a header or footer, select the field, and choose Time and Date from the Insert menu. In the dialog box, choose the preferred format and click OK. Word replaces the format throughout the section or document where the header or footer field appears. Instead of using the Date or Time buttons on the Header and Footer toolbar, you can insert the preferred date format directly from the Time and Date dialog box or from the Field dialog box.

To change the date format:

1. With the document still in page layout view, double-click the header text on page 2 to open the header area for editing.

2. Double-click at the beginning of the date field to select it, and then choose Date and Time from the Insert menu. Choose the first date format and click OK.

    Word replaces the formatting on each header with the date field.

3. Click the Page Forward button on the vertical scroll bar to see the change reflected on page 3.

Positioning of Headers and Footers

Earlier, the discussion about paragraph formatting explained how you can align, tab, or indent header and footer text. These are all methods of changing the horizontal position of headers and footers. You can also change the vertical position of headers and footers by increasing or decreasing the distance between the header or footer and the edge of the page, or between the header or footer and the document text.

Figure 13-11

Variables in header or footer position

Default header and footer settings

Settings in the Page Setup dialog box

Remember, when you create a header or a footer, Word positions the text .5 inches from the top edge of the page. This is the default setting that appears automatically when you open the Page Setup dialog box.

There are three ways to change the vertical position of headers and footers:

- Specify the header or footer distance from the edge of the page in the Page Setup dialog box

- Adjust the distance between the header or footer and the document text using the vertical ruler

- Insert blank lines above or below the header or footer in the header or footer area

To specify the vertical position using the Page Setup dialog box:

1. Switch to normal view, and then choose Page Setup from the File menu. Click the Margins tab, if necessary.

   The dialog box displays the .5-inch header and footer default positions.

2. Change the header position to .3 inches and click OK.

3. Switch to page layout view. Look at the headers on page 1 and page 2.

   The header text appears closer to the edge of the page and farther from the document text.

To adjust the distance between a header or footer and the document text using the vertical ruler, first open the header or footer area you wish to adjust. With the area open, point to either the top or bottom margin boundary on the vertical ruler. When the mouse changes to a double-headed arrow, drag the top margin boundary up or down to add or reduce space between the document text and the header. Drag the bottom margin boundary up or down to add or reduce space between the document text and the footer.

To adjust the position of a header using the vertical ruler:

1. Move to the header on page 1, and double-click the header text.

2. With the insertion point in the header area and the document now in page layout view, move the pointer to the top margin boundary of the document (the bottom of the white area on the vertical ruler). See Figure 13-12 on page 255.

3. When the pointer becomes a double-headed arrow, hold down the **Alt** key, and drag the margin boundary down to 1 inch on the ruler.

   The space between the header and the document text is increased.

4. Click the Show Next button to view the header on page 2.

   The space is increased throughout the pages of the document.

Note: Remember, when you hold down the **Alt** key, the ruler displays the actual measurements of the margin or text area.

Figure 13-12
Adjusting the space between a header and document text

Note: Remember that this document has no section breaks; therefore, a formatting change, such as a repositioned header, applies to every page.

5. Close the Header and Footer toolbar to return to normal view, and then save the document.

Another way to change the position of headers or footers is to insert blank lines in the header or footer area. For example, you can position a header or footer lower on the page by inserting blank lines before the header or footer text. Similarly, to increase the amount of space between a header and the document text, insert blank lines below the header text.

Continuation-Page Headings for Letters and Memos

Letters and memos of more than one page should follow a specific format, according to *The Gregg Reference Manual*. This format consists of a header beginning on page 2 that is 1 inch from the edge of the page. Two blank lines must separate the header and the continuation text.

Word's default header margin of .5 inches is used by many word-processing programs and may be accepted by some businesses.

Remember that the first page of a letter or memo is formatted with a 2-inch top margin. Therefore, you may need to use a section break to adjust the margins of your continuation pages.

However, if you use a 3-line continuation-page heading, you will not need to use a section break. You can use the existing 2-inch top margin and set the header margin to 1 inch. This allows the proper amount of space between the header and the continuation text.

(Note: There are 6 lines of text to an inch, unless you change the size of your text.)

See Appendices B and C for examples of the 3-line continuation-page heading.

Varying Headers and Footers

In addition to having a different header or footer on the first page and different page numbers between sections, Word offers additional ways to vary headers and footers within a document.

Odd and Even Pages

To vary header and footer text within a document or section, you can print different headers and footers on odd and even pages. For example, you can display the document title on odd pages and the author's name on even pages. This is a way of including a variety of identifying text without printing it all on each page.

To create different headers or footers for odd and even pages, choose Header and Footer from the View menu. Click the Page Setup button, and click the Layout tab, if necessary. Under Headers and Footers, click the Different Odd and Even check box, and then click OK. In the header or footer area, click the Show Previous or Show Next button to move to an even header or footer, and enter the desired text. Click the Show Next button to move to an odd header or footer, and enter the desired text. By creating a header or footer on one even page and on one odd page, all pages of the document will contain the alternating headers or footers (providing the document is one section and the headers and footers are linked).

To create different footers for odd and even pages:

1. Choose Header and Footer from the View menu (or double-click the Footer text in page layout view).

2. Click the first button on the Header and Footer toolbar to switch to the document footer.

3. Click the Page Setup button, and click the Layout tab, if necessary.

4. To create different odd and even footers starting with page 2, click the check box for Different Odd And Even, and make sure Different First Page is checked. Click OK.

5. Move to the even-page footer on page 2. See Figure 13-13 on page 257.

6. Key *Duke City Gateway Travel Agency* in italics.

7. Click the Show Next button.

    Word displays the odd page footer for page 3.

8. Key **Presented by**, and press the **Spacebar** once.

9. Choose Field from the Insert menu. Choose the field name Author from the Document Information category, and then click OK.

Figure 13-13
Creating different odd and even page footers

Word inserts your name, as entered earlier in the Summary Info dialog box.

10. Click the Page Forward button on the vertical scroll bar to view the different odd and even footers through the end of the document.

Facing Pages

As mentioned earlier, facing pages—also called mirrored pages—are the left and right pages in a bound document. Typically, the left page (the even-numbered page) and the right page (the odd-numbered page) have different headers or footers that are positioned on the outside edge of the page. For example, a left page may contain a header with the page number and document title, aligned to the left. The right page may contain a header with the page number and chapter title, aligned to the right.

Figure 13-14
Headers on facing pages

See Lesson 5 for a full description of facing pages, mirror margins, and gutter margins. To format a document with facing pages and different headers or footers, first choose Mirror Margins, and set a gutter in the Page Setup dialog box (under the Margins tab). Apply the options to the whole document or a particular section. Then open the odd and even header or footer areas and enter or edit the text.

To vary headers and footers on facing pages:

1. Change to normal view. Delete the hard page break at the beginning of page 2, and insert an Even Page section break.

    This will set up the document as if it were a small bound booklet, with page 2 printed on the reverse of page 1.

2. Center the text on page 1 vertically and horizontally.

3. With the insertion point in section 1, choose Page Setup from the File menu. Click the Margins tab, if necessary.

4. Click the Mirror Margins check box. Set a .25-inch gutter. Apply this to the whole document, and then click OK.

5. Choose Header and Footer from the View menu.

6. Delete the text in the header on page 1 of section 1.

7. Click the Show Next button to move to the header on page 2 of section 2.

8. Click the Page Setup button, and clear the Different First Page check box for this section. Make sure the Different Odd and Even check box is checked. Click OK.

9. Move to the odd-page header on page 3 of section 2.

10. Delete the line with the date and time fields. Delete one of the tabs before the document title to center-align the text at the 3-inch tab setting. Then insert a tab after the document title, and move the page numbering so it is right-aligned at the 6-inch tab setting.

11. Copy the odd-page header to the Clipboard.

12. Click the Show Previous button to move to the even-page header.

13. In the even-page header, create the mirror image of the odd header: Paste the text from the Clipboard in the header area, and then move the page numbering to the left margin.

14. Open the even-page footer. Make sure it is left-aligned like the even-page header.

15. Open the odd-page footer. Press the **Tab** key twice to right-align the text, and then close the footer area.

16. Switch to print preview to view the pages.

17. Spell-check the document.

18. Save the document, and then print it.

19. Close the document and exit Word (unless you will be doing the following exercises immediately).

Table 13-2: Keyboard Shortcuts for Headers and Footers	
Keyboard Shortcut	Action
Ctrl+F11	Turn off update for date and time fields
Ctrl+Shift+F11	Update date and time fields
Ctrl+F9	Insert field characters
Alt+F9	Turn on and off field-code display
F9	Update a field within field characters
Ctrl+Q	Clear formatting in a header or footer area

Exercises

Exercise 13.1

1. Start Word, if necessary.

2. Open the file 13-1.doc.

3. Format the document as a standard business letter from Nina Chavez, Travel Counselor, with your reference initials. Use the existing left and right margins, set the top margin to 2 inches, and insert the date as a field code.

4. Create a standard business-letter heading:

   A. Choose Header and Footer from the View menu.

   B. Click the Page Setup button. In the dialog box, check Different First Page and click OK.

   C. With the insertion point aligned to the left in the header area of page 2, key **Mr. Richard Ramirez**

   D. Press **Enter**, and then key *Waterhouse Investment Group* in italics.

   E. Press **Enter**, key **Page**, insert a space, and then click the Page Numbers button.

   F. Press **Enter**. Choose Date and Time from the Insert menu. Choose the fourth format and click OK.

5. Edit the header text:

   A. Select the header text *"Waterhouse Investment Group"*.

  B. Delete the text.

  C. Close the header area.

6. Change the vertical position of the header from the edge of the page:

  A. Choose Page Setup from the File menu.

  B. Set the header to 1 inch from the edge. Click OK.

7. Check the distance between the header and the document text:

  A. Switch to page layout view, and double-click the header text on page 2.

  B. Press **Enter** twice after the date.

  C. Move the pointer to the top margin boundary on the vertical ruler (the boundary between the bottom of the header and the top of the letter text).

  D. Hold down the **Alt** key and the left mouse button. Adjust the margin boundary so that it is just under the second paragraph mark in the header (1 inch on the ruler).

8. Spell-check the document.

9. Save the document as *[your three-letter identifier]*13-1.doc.

10. Print the document.

11. Close the document and exit Word (unless you will be doing the following exercises immediately).

Exercise 13.2

1. Start Word, if necessary.

2. Open the file 7-2.doc.

3. Insert a Next Page section break at the top of the document.

4. Above the section break, key a cover memo to Frank Youngblood from Susan Allen with today's date. For the subject, key:

  Excerpt from *How to Succeed in the Travel-Agency Business*

5. Key the following body text of the memo:

  The book, *How to Succeed in the Travel-Agency Business,* **published by Gateway Travel, contains a section about group travel that should interest you. Please distribute to the staff.**

6. Choose Summary Info from the File menu, and key **How to Succeed in the Travel-Agency Business** in the title box. Close the dialog box.

7. Format section 2 with different odd and even headers:

   A. Place the insertion point after the section break, and then choose Header and Footer from the View menu.

   B. Click the Page Setup button, click the Different Odd And Even and Different First Page check box, and then click OK.

8. Click the Show Next button to move to the odd-page header on page 3.

9. Insert the document title on the first line as a field:

   A. With the insertion point aligned to the left in the odd-page header, choose Field from the Insert menu.

   B. From the Document Information category, choose Title, and then click OK.

   C. Italicize the title.

10. Press **Enter**. Key **Page** (do not use italics), press the **Spacebar**, and then click the Page Number button. On a new line, click the Date button.

11. Open the even-page header.

12. On the first line, key **Duke City Gateway Travel**, and insert the page and date beneath it as in the odd header.

13. Change the horizontal position of the odd-header text:

    A. Click the Show Next button.

    B. Press the **Tab** key twice before each line in the header to right-align the text.

14. Make sure the entire document has a 2-inch top margin, and change the headers to appear 1 inch from the edge of the page.

15. View the document in print preview.

16. Spell-check the document.

17. Save the document as *[your three-letter identifier]*13-2.doc.

18. Print the document.

19. Close the document and exit Word (unless you will be doing the following exercises immediately).

Exercise 13.3

1. Start Word, if necessary.

2. Open the files 13-3.doc and 13-3a.doc.

3. Format 13-3.doc as a business letter from Doris Simms, Sales Representative. Insert today's date as a field. Set the right and left margins to 1 inch. Address the letter to:

Ms. Rachel Wolinsky
32 Tramway Boulevard
Albuquerque, NM 87123

4. After the paragraph that begins "The club location", start a new paragraph by keying:

   For a vacation that is less "beach-like," consider a special-interest tour:

5. Switch to the 13-3A.DOC window. Copy paragraphs 4-8, and paste them below the text you just keyed in document 13-3.doc.

6. Format the copied paragraphs with bullets and a .25-inch hanging indent.

7. Create a three-line header that prints on page 2 and is 1 inch from the edge.

8. With the header area still open and the document in page layout view, change the page setup to a 2-inch top margin and 1.25-inch left and right margins.

9. Make sure the date format used at the beginning of the letter and in the header is of the format "May 1, 1995".

10. Switch to print preview to view the document.

11. Spell-check the document.

12. Save the document as *[your three-letter identifier]*13-3.doc.

13. Print the document.

14. Close both documents and exit Word (unless you will be doing the following exercise immediately).

Exercise 13.4: Challenge Yourself

Open the file 12-3.doc. Format the title page as a separate section. Edit the title page as shown in Figure 13-15, which appears at the end of this exercise. Insert a blank line after the document title. Insert three blank lines before the agency name. On the middle blank line, insert the date as a field, using the format "May 1, 1995". Center the title-page text horizontally and vertically.

At the top of section 2, change the title to "**A GUIDE TO CRUISE TRAVEL**". Then number the document with a centered footer, starting with "2" on page 2, section 2.

Scroll through the document, and insert Next Page section breaks before the subheadings "**The Layout of the Ship**", "**Special Services/Additional Charges**", "**Ship Terminology**", and "**Types of Cruises**".

Add a left-aligned header, beginning with section 3, with the text "A Guide to Cruise Travel". (Hint: Unlink the section-3 header from the section-2 header.)

Working in page layout view, move to the document text in section 3, and key the heading *Life On Board* in bold italics above "**The Layout of the Ship**". Insert a blank line between the two headings. Then copy the text you keyed, and paste it in the header. Use the right-aligned tab stop.

Go to section 4, and key the heading *Important Information* in bold italics above "**Special Services/Additional Charges**". Insert a blank line between the two headings. Then unlink the section-4 header from the section-3 header and copy the text to the header using the right-aligned tab stop.

Following the same steps, add the heading "*Glossary*" above "**Ship Terminology**" in section 5 and in the section-5 header. Add the heading "*Cruises for Everyone*" above "**Types of Cruises**" in section 6 and in the section-6 header.

View the document in print preview. Make sure all pages are numbered consecutively from 2 to 13, and that page breaks do not occur within itineraries or just after headings. Then change the top margin for the entire document to 1.25 inches.

Save the document as *[your three-letter identifier]*13-4.doc and print it. Close the document and exit Word.

Figure 13-15

A GUIDE TO

Primer For First-Time Cruise Travelers   *Proposed by Frank Murillo*
                                              International Travel Counselor

Duke City Gateway Travel Agency

15 Montgomery Boulevard

Albuquerque, NM 87111

(505) 555-1234

A Brochure

Background

One of the biggest tourist events of the year in Albuquerque is the October International Balloon Fiesta with nine days of special events. For this event, Duke City Gateway offers its customers special vacation packages. To inform customers of the International Balloon Fiesta and the special vacation package, Duke City Gateway publishes a brochure.

Business Purpose

Create a brochure to promote Albuquerque's International Balloon Fiesta and Duke City Gateway's vacation package. The brochure will be three pages long, consisting of a title page and two pages of information.

Procedures

1. Open the file p4-1.doc.

2. Create a title page for the document as a separate section. On the new page, key:

   **Duke City Gateway Travel Agency's
   International Balloon Fiesta Vacation Packages
   Albuquerque, New Mexico**

3. Make the text bold, and center it horizontally and vertically. Change line spacing on this page to 1.5 lines.

4. On the first page of section 2, key **International Balloon Fiesta** in bold at the top of the page, and press **Enter** twice.

5. At the insertion point, insert the file 2-2.doc. To do this, choose File from the Insert menu, choose 2-2.doc from the File Name list, and then click OK.

6. Combine the new text and the paragraph that begins "Also available" into one paragraph. (If necessary, select the combined paragraph, open the Font dialog box, and choose Times New Roman, 12 points.)

7. Make the headings, "The Vacation Packages", "Restrictions", and "Other Arrangements" bold.

8. Add a shadow box border to the text from "Vacation Package: $699" to the first instance of "launching grounds".

9. Add the same border to the text from "Weekend Getaway" to the next instance of "launching grounds".

10. At the end of the document, press **Enter** twice, and key the bold heading **Coupons**

11. Press **Enter** twice and key:

    50% Off One Hot-Air-Balloon Ride

    Insert a line break (press **Shift+Enter**), and then key:

    This coupon entitles you to 50% off one hot-air-balloon ride from BALLOONS INC. Regular balloon ride rates are $35-$50 per hour.

12. Press **Enter** twice and key:

    FREE BREAKFAST

    Insert a line break, and then key:

    This coupon entitles you to one free breakfast with the purchase of one breakfast at the Ranch Resort.

13. Press **Enter** twice and key:

    20% Off Native American Craft Purchase

    Insert a line break, and then key:

    This coupon entitles you to 20% off the purchase of any item in the crafts displays at the launching grounds during the International Balloon Fiesta.

14. Add a double-line box border to each of the paragraphs to create three coupons. Center the text in each coupon, and change the line spacing to 1.5 lines.

15. Insert a page break before the heading "Restrictions".

16. Change the left and right margins in section 2 to 1.5 inches and the top margin to 2 inches.

17. Add a centered header to section 2 with the following text:

    Albuquerque International Balloon Fiesta

18. Add page numbers to section 2 using a footer. Start the page numbering at 1. Use center alignment, and include the word "Page" before the number.

19. Spell-check the document.

20. Make any changes you feel will improve the appearance of the document.

21. Save the document as *[your three-letter identifier]*p4-1.doc and print it.

22. Close the document and exit Word.

Tips and Hints

- Divide your documents into sections when you want to create separate headers and footers for different pages.

- Vary the position of the headers and footers in your document. For example, center a header on the page instead of leaving it flush with the left margin.

- Use the Page Numbers command to number the pages in your documents.

- Use print preview to view the sections and the positions of headers and footers in the document before you print it.

Module 5

Printing

Printing Options

Objectives

- Set up a printer.
- Use the Print Preview toolbar.
- Edit in print preview.
- Choose options in the Print dialog box.
- Cancel printing.
- Troubleshoot printing problems.

Printer-driver software
Software that instructs a computer about the printing capabilities of a printer.

Word offers many printing options to meet your printing needs. For example, the Print command does more than just print a document. You can use it to print selected text, a range of pages, or a document's summary information. This lesson reviews the printing process, from setup, to preview, to printing. Lesson 15 describes some of Word's special printing features.

Printer Setup

In order to print, you need to prepare both the printer and the computer. The printer must be loaded with paper and a toner cartridge or printer ribbon. The computer must be connected to the printer and loaded with *printer-driver software*. Printer-driver software tells the computer about the printing capabilities of the printer you are using. The printer-driver software for your printer was loaded when you installed Microsoft Windows.

The printer you choose in the Print Setup dialog box affects how Word will display and print a document. Therefore, choose the printer before you begin formatting a document. Only printers whose printer-driver software has been installed with Microsoft Windows will appear in the Print Setup dialog box.

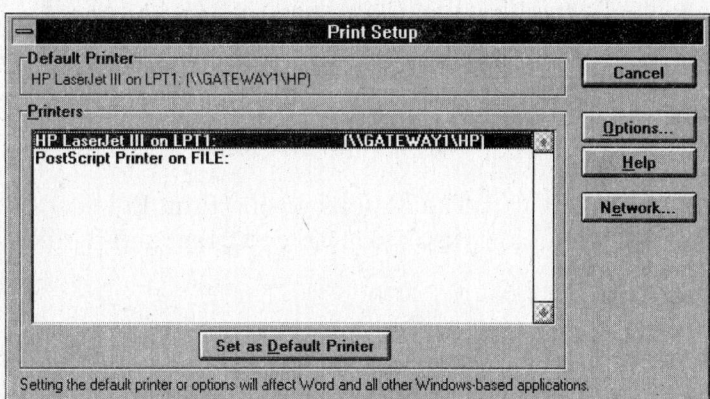

Figure 14-1
The Print Setup dialog box

To choose a printer from the Print setup dialog box:

1. Start Word, if necessary.

2. Choose Print from the File menu, and then click the Printer button.

Word displays the Print Setup dialog box. The printer you are using should appear in the dialog box.

3. Click Cancel, and then click OK to close both dialog boxes.

Previewing

It is always a good idea to preview the pages of a document before printing. Previewing a document in print preview or page layout view saves time and prevents wasting paper.

Using Print Preview

Print preview allows you to view a scaled-down version of a document. You can preview one page or several pages at a time. The pages appear complete with all the page elements. Use print preview to view the document as it will look when printed and to make any final adjustments.

To view a document in print preview:

1. Open the file 12-0.doc.

Print Preview button

2. Click the Print Preview button.

Unless you make changes in print preview, Word displays one page of the document, and the pointer is a magnifying glass.

Figure 14-2
The Print Preview toolbar

The buttons on the Print Preview toolbar allow you to change the display of the document and perform specific actions:

• Print

When you click this button, the Print dialog box appears, so you can print directly from print preview.

• Magnifier

When this button is depressed (as it is by default), you can use the magnifying glass pointer to magnify an area of the document by clicking the area. Once an area is magnified, you can click the Magnifier button to restore the I-beam pointer, which you can use to edit the document in print preview.

- One Page

    Click this button to display one page at a time.

- Multiple Pages

    Click this button to display two or more pages at a time. To do this, click the button, and then drag the pointer over the grid to choose the configuration of pages, or click within the grid to specify the number of pages. For example, click the second page in the top row to view two pages.

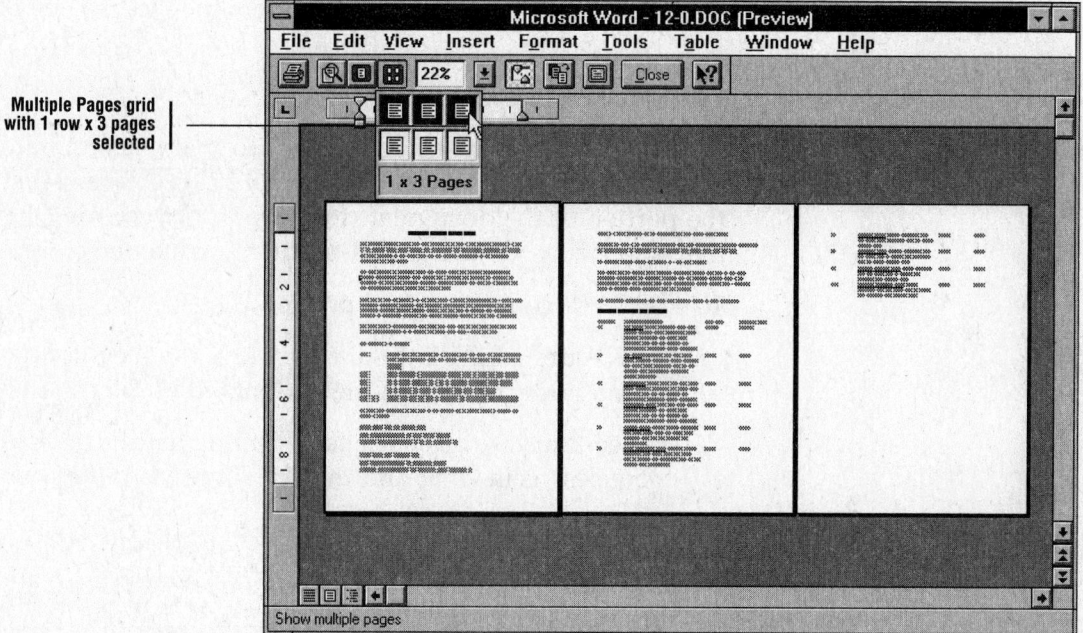

Multiple Pages grid with 1 row x 3 pages selected

Figure 14-3
Displaying multiple pages in print preview

- Zoom Control box

    Click the down arrow, and then choose a magnification to reduce or enlarge the page or pages displayed.

- View Ruler

    Click this button to show or hide the print preview ruler.

- Shrink to Fit

    Use this button to shrink a two-page document to fit on one page when the second page contains only a few lines of text.

- Full Screen

    Click this button to hide all elements of the print preview screen except the displayed page or pages and the Print Preview toolbar.

To exit print preview, you can click the Close button on the Print Preview toolbar or click the Normal View button in the bottom left of the screen.

To change the view of the document in print preview:

1. Click the Multiple Pages button on the Print Preview toolbar.

2. Drag the pointer over the grid to select the 1 x 3 configuration.

3. Release the pointer.

    Word displays all three pages in print preview.

4. Click the One Page button to restore the view to one page.

Editing in Print Preview

Editing in print preview allows you to make last-minute changes before printing a document. To edit in print preview, first magnify the portion of the document you wish to correct, and then change the magnifying pointer to an I-beam and make the corrections.

To edit the document in print preview:

1. Make sure page 1 is displayed. Move the magnifying glass pointer over the text in the bottom left of the page and click.

2. If necessary, scroll so the text "Sailing dates from Los Angeles" is in view, and then click the Magnifier button.

    The pointer becomes an I-beam.

3. Edit the off-peak season dates to November 1, 15, and 29.

4. Scroll to the top of the page, and select the text *"Riviera Princess"* in the first paragraph under the heading.

5. Press **Ctrl+B** to apply the bold attribute to the text.

6. Click the Magnifier button, and then click within the document to view the whole page again.

7. Click the Shrink to Fit button.

    Word reduces the document from 3 pages to 2, as indicated in the status bar. See Figure 14-4 on page 273.

8. Click the View Ruler button to make more room to view the document, and then use the Multiple Pages button to change the view to 2 pages (drag the pointer over the first two pages in the grid).

9. Click the Print button.

10. Close print preview, and then close the document without saving changes.

Shrink to Fit button

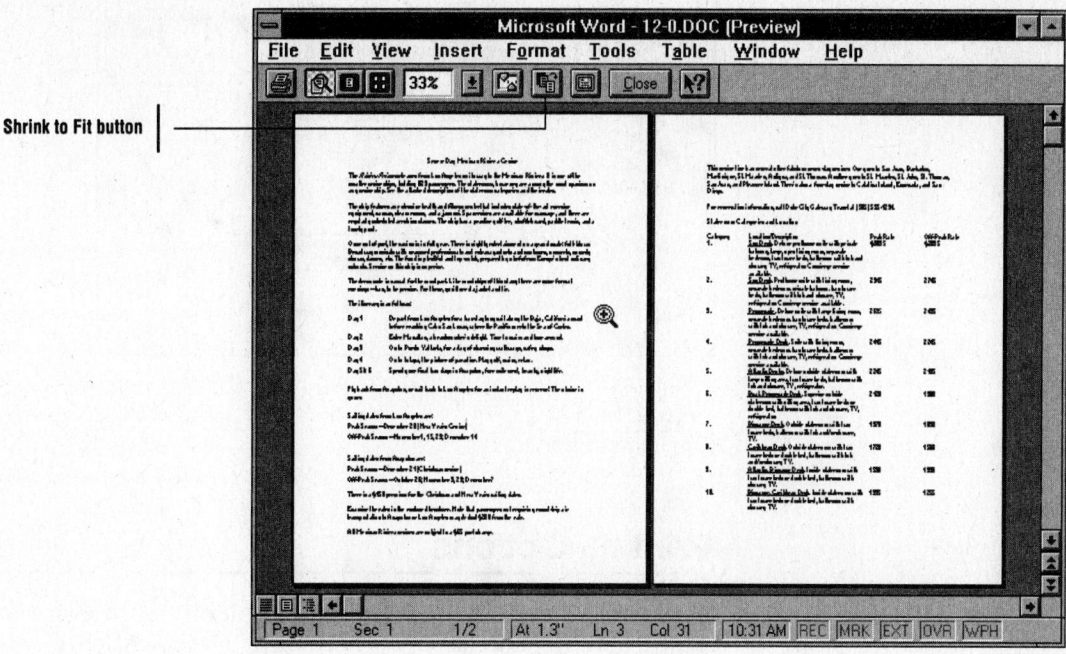

Figure 14-4
The Shrink to Fit option fits the document on 2 pages

The Zoom Command

The Zoom Control box, which is available on the Standard toolbar and the Print Preview toolbar, allows you to change the magnification of a document. The Zoom command, which is available from the View menu, is another way to customize the view of a document. Use the Zoom command to change the display to the size most convenient to your editing and viewing needs.

To use the Zoom command, choose Zoom from the View menu. In the Zoom dialog box, choose from three different levels of magnification: 200%, 100%, or 75%. (200% displays the document at twice its size, and 100% displays it at its normal size.) You can also specify a percent in the text box. Choose Page Width to restore the view to fit within the margins. If the document is in page layout view, the Whole Page and Many Page option buttons are available. To view more than two pages, click the monitor icon, and drag the pointer to choose the number of pages you want (as you would with the Multiple Pages button in print preview).

After choosing a magnification or reduction in the Zoom dialog box, the Preview box displays approximately how text will look with the chosen options. It also displays the font and font size. After making your choices, click OK. Word displays the document page to your specification. Each new window you open is displayed with the magnification level last specified. This display size has no effect on the printed document.

Figure 14-5
The Zoom dialog box

Printing Options

When you choose Print from the File menu, Word displays the Print dialog box. The options you choose in it affect how the document is printed and what portion of the document is printed. For example, you can print only the current page on which you are working, or only specified text. By default, when you click OK in the Print dialog box, Word prints the entire document that is currently open and displayed in the active window.

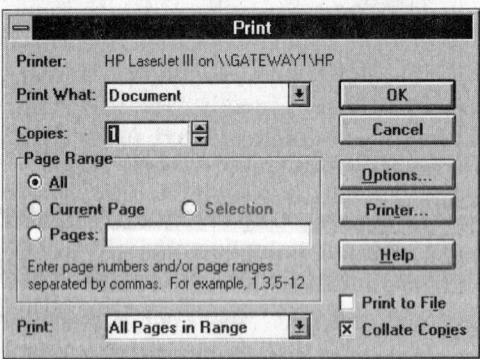

Figure 14-6
The Print dialog box

Print button

When you print a document by clicking the Print button on the Standard toolbar, Word prints the entire current document in the active window. The Print dialog box does not appear; therefore, you cannot choose any options for printing. Use the Print button only when you want to print the entire document.

Printing the Current Page

After you preview a document, you may decide to print only the current page to see how it looks or to proofread it. The current page is the page that contains the insertion point.

To print the current page:

1.   Open the file 12-0.doc again.

2.   On page 2, insert a hard page break before the heading **"Stateroom Categories and Location"**.

3.   With the insertion point in page 3, choose Print from the File menu. Click the Current Page option button, and click OK.

     Word prints the current page only.

Printing a Range of Pages

To print a range of pages:

1.   Choose Print from the File menu.

2.   Key **1-2** in the Pages text box and click OK.

     Word prints pages 1 through 2.

When specifying pages to print, it does not matter where the insertion point is in the document. For example, if the insertion point is in page 3, and you want to print page 1, you can key **1** in the Pages text box to print only page 1.

Printing Noncontiguous Pages

You can use the Print dialog box to print a group of pages that are not part of a contiguous range. To print noncontiguous pages, key the page numbers separated by commas. For example, to print pages 1, 4, and 6, key **1,4,6** in the Pages text box. To print pages 1 and 4 through 6, key **1,4-6** in the text box.

Printing Selected Text

Word allows you to print only selected text, such as a paragraph or a table within a document. When you select specific text to be printed, Word ignores any automatic (soft) page breaks and prints the beginning of the selected text at the top of the paper. When text is selected to print, the Selection option button is available in the Print dialog box.

To print only selected text:

1.   At the end of page 1, select the text from "Sailing dates from Acapulco" through "$200 from the rate." Notice that the selection spans a soft page break.

2.   Choose Print from the File menu.

3.   Click the Selection option button, and click OK.

Word prints the selected text only.

Printing Multiple Copies

In the workplace, you often may need to print more than one copy
of a document. Word offers the option to print multiple copies. Before choosing this option, decide whether or not you want Word to
collate the documents while printing. The Collate Copies check box
is checked by default. This means Word will print one complete copy
of a document before printing the second copy. If this option is not
checked, Word will print all the copies of each page of the document
one at a time, and you will have to collate the pages manually.

To print more than one copy:

1.   Choose Print from the File menu.

2.   Key **2** in the Copies text box.

3.   Key **1** in the Pages text box.

4.   Click OK.

Word prints two copies of page 1.

Printing to a File

In the Print dialog box, the Print to File option allows you to send a
document to a file or to a floppy disk instead of to the printer. This
enables you to prepare a version of the document for printing that is
transferable to another program or to a computer that does not have
Word installed. The Print to File option translates the instructions for
your Word-formatted document into instructions that another computer and printer can read to produce your document exactly as you
created it.

For example, suppose you create a document on your computer and
then wish to print it from another computer that is connected to a
better printer. You could make a regular copy of the file and bring
the file copy to the other computer. However, if the computer does
not have Word or is not configured the same way your computer is,
line and page breaks may differ, producing a different version of the
document. If you use the Print to File option, Word copies to a file or
floppy disk the computer code for the document, which can be interpreted by the other computer.

To print a document to a file, you must first choose the printer on
which you will print the file from the Print Setup dialog box. Click
the Set As Default Printer button, and then click Close. Check the
Print to File check box, and click OK. Word opens the Print to File
dialog box. In the Output File Name box, key a filename that is

different than your document's name, and then click OK. The file created using this method has the extension .prn (unless you key a different filename extension).

Figure 14-7
The Print to File dialog box

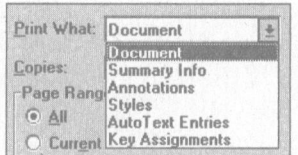

Options in the Print
dialog box

Printing Summary Information

The Print dialog box offers several options for printing information other than the contents of a document. For example, you can print the summary information that has been entered for a new document. Other material related to a document, such as annotations and styles (which are discussed in future lessons), may also be printed. These items can be printed with the document or separately.

To print only the summary information for the document:

1. First, save the open document as *[your three-letter identi-fier]*14-0.doc.

2. Enter summary information for the document by choosing Summary Info from the File menu. If you have not already done so, key your name as the author. The title should be entered already. For the subject, key **Cruise**. In the Comments box, key **3 pages including itinerary and stateroom categories**. Then click OK.

3. Choose Print from the File menu.

4. In the Print What box, choose Summary Info from the drop-down list box. Click OK.

   Word prints the summary information.

To print the summary information with the document, click the Options button in the Print dialog box. Word displays the Options dialog box for print settings. In the Include with Document box, click the Summary Info check box. Then click OK in the dialog box. Remember, a setting changed in an Options dialog box remains in effect until you reset the option.

Figure 14-8
Print settings in the Options dialog box

More Print Options in the Options Dialog Box

The Options dialog box for print settings offers five additional printing choices:

Note: You can also display the Options dialog box for print settings by choosing Options from the Tools menu and then clicking the Print tab.

- Draft Output

  When checked, a document is printed in draft form, which means the typeface will not be as distinct, and the pages will print faster. Graphics are not printed with this setting.

- Reverse Printing order

  When checked, a document begins printing with the last page and ends with the first.

- Update Fields

  When checked, Word updates the fields in the document before the document is printed.

- Update Links

  When checked, Word updates any linked information in the document before the document is printed.

- Background Printing

  When checked, Word allows you to continue working while a document is being printed. Background printing on is the default setting.

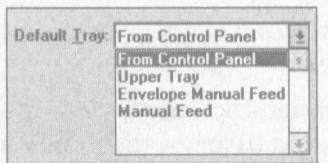

Printer tray options

You can also use the Options dialog box to specify the tray your printer will use to print a document.

Canceling Printing

In some instances, you may decide not to print a document after you have chosen the Print command. For example, you may notice that there is no paper in the printer after sending a document to the printer, or you have sent a long document to the printer before realizing you wanted to add a header.

If background printing is on, double-click the printer icon on the status bar to cancel printing, or open the Print dialog box, and click the Stop Print button.

If background printing is off, you can cancel printing by pressing the **Esc** key.

Note: If the document you have sent to print is short and your computer is fast, you may not be able to intercept the Print command.

To cancel a print job:

1. First choose Options from the Tools menu to see if Background Printing is on. Click the Print tab, and click the Background Printing check box to switch it on, if necessary. Click OK.

2. Click the Print button on the Standard toolbar.

3. Double-click the printer icon on the status bar immediately.

    The print job is canceled.

Double-click to
cancel printing

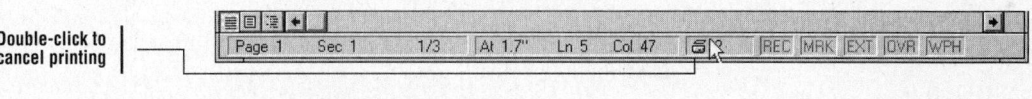

Figure 14-9
The status bar showing the printer icon

4. Save the document.

5. Close the document and exit Word (unless you will be doing the following exercises immediately).

Troubleshooting

To print from Word, the computer, the printer, and Windows software must all be set up correctly. Printing problems can often be resolved simply. If a printer does not print, first check to make sure that:

*   The printer is plugged in to an electrical outlet, and cables connecting the printer to the computer are firmly in place.

*   The printer has paper and a print ribbon or cartridge.

*   The printer is on-line (some printers have an on-line button you must press).

- The correct printer and printer settings are chosen in the Print Setup dialog box, and the printer is connected to the correct port (for example, LPT1 or LPT2).

If a printer prints text you did not want it to print, check to make sure that:

- You have chosen the correct page, range of pages, text, or other printing option.

- The printer can print the formatting you have included in the document. You may need to reformat the document for the printer.

- The fonts you are using match those available in the printer.

- The printer-driver software may be corrupted. You may need to reinstall the printer-driver software.

Key Term

Printer-driver software

Exercises

Exercise 14.1

1. Start Word, if necessary.

2. Open the file 7-0.doc.

3. Switch to print preview, and view both pages of the document:

   A. Click the Multiple Pages button.

   B. Drag the pointer over the first two pages of the grid.

4. Close print preview. In normal view, delete the text "Record Keeping", "Deposits/Cancellations", and the paragraphs under these headings. Delete the text at the end of the document, from "For more detailed information" through the end.

5. Switch back to print preview, and change the top margin to 2 inches.

6. Edit the document in print preview:

   A. Move the magnifying glass pointer over the memo heading and click.

   B. Click the Magnifier button to restore the I-beam pointer.

   C. Change the name after "FROM:" to your name.

   D. Select and delete the text under "Deadlines", up to "July 1".

E.   Use the keyboard shortcut **Ctrl+I** to make "July 1" italic. Repeat this formatting for the next four dates.

F.   Click the Magnifier button, and then click the document to view both pages.

7.   Click the Shrink to Fit button to fit the memo on one page.

8.   Click the View Ruler button to view the ruler, if necessary.

9.   Click the One Page button to center the document.

10. While still in print preview, use the File menu to save the document as *[your three-letter identifier]*14-1.doc, and then print the document.

11. Close print preview.

12. Close the document and exit Word (unless you will be doing the following exercises immediately).

Exercise 14.2

1.   Start Word, if necessary.

2.   Open the file 12-4.doc.

3.   Print the title page of the document:

A.   With the insertion point in page 1, choose Print from the File menu.

B.   Choose Current Page (or key **1** in the Pages text box) and click OK.

4.   Print noncontiguous pages 2, 10, 11, and 12:

A.   Choose Print from the File menu.

B.   In the Pages text box, key **2,10-12**

C.   Click OK.

5.   Cancel printing immediately by double-clicking the printer icon on the status bar (or by pressing the **Esc** key if background printing is off).

6.   Print a selection of the document:

A.   Go to page 10, and select the travel itinerary that begins **"Sample Itinerary — The Western Caribbean"**.

B.   Choose Print from the File menu.

C.   Choose Selection and click OK.

7.   Create summary information for the document and print it:

A.   Choose Summary Info from the File menu. For the document title, key **Your Gateway to the World**. For the subject, key **Introduction to Agency**. For the author, key

Susan Allen, agency owner/president. In the Comments box, key **12-page report including agency locations and itineraries**. Click OK.

    B.   Choose Print from the File menu.

    C.   Open the Print What box, choose Summary Info, and click OK.

8.   Spell-check the document, and save it as *[your three-letter identifier]*14-2.doc.

9.   Close the document and exit Word (unless you will be doing the following exercises immediately).

Exercise 14.3

1.   Start Word, if necessary.

2.   Open the file 14-3.doc.

3.   Format the document as a business letter with a 2-inch top margin and the date entered as a field. Add your reference initials to the letter.

4.   On page 1, delete the paragraph that begins "For local area residents" and the paragraph under it. (Delete the blank line under the second paragraph, as well.)

5.   Switch to print preview, and view both pages of the document at once.

6.   In print preview, edit the paragraph on page 2 that begins "Our staff of 12", as shown in Figure 14-10 below.

Figure 14-10

The 15 members of our staff

~~Our staff of 12~~ all have expertise in different areas of the travel business. You will be dealing primarily with me and with ~~the agency's~~ ~~manager, Frank Youngblood. Should you need to make overseas travel~~ ~~arrangements for yourself, your staff, or your family,~~ Frank Murillo will help you. ~~He is~~ the agency's international counselor. You *also* will be speaking *with* ~~on the phone to~~ Valerie Grier, our secretary/office manager, and most probably to our bookkeeper, Darrell Jackson. We're all here to ensure that your travel needs are *handled* ~~taken care of~~ efficiently.

---

7. Scroll up to the paragraph that begins "As an added service". Delete the paragraph, along with the paragraph under it and any extra blank lines.

8. View both pages of the document again, and then shrink the document to fit on one page.

9. Switch to normal view to spell-check the document.

10. Save the document as *[your three-letter identifier]*14-3.doc.

11. Print the document.

12. Close the document and exit Word (unless you will be doing the following exercise immediately).

Exercise 14.4: Challenge Yourself

Open the file 12-3.doc. First, create summary information for the document, including the document title, your name as author, and the comments: **11-page report for first-time cruise travelers, created by Duke City Gateway**.

Go to page 8, and insert a Next Page section break before the heading "**Sample Cruise Itineraries**". Number the pages in section 2 with a footer in which the document title appears left-aligned as a field and the page number is right-aligned. Begin numbering with page 1, and italicize the document title.

Use the Print dialog box to print section 2, and then print the summary information for the document. Go to page 7, and print two copies of the text from the heading "**Ship Terminology**" to "raise the anchor".

Save the document as *[your three-letter identifier]*14-4.doc. Close the document and exit Word.

Special Printing Features

Objectives

- Change paper size.
- Change page orientation.
- Print envelopes.
- Print a mailing label.

Word offers special printing features that allow you to print on different-sized paper and to change the orientation of text on a page. Another printing feature in Word is the ability to print envelopes and mailing labels. It is important to consider these special printing features before you begin formatting a document.

Printing Size and Orientation Options

There are times when you may want to print on different-sized paper, such as legal paper. You may want to change the orientation of the page and print horizontally between the top and bottom margins. The options for changing paper size and page orientation appear in the Page Setup dialog box. Choose Page Setup from the File menu, and then click the Paper Size tab.

Figure 15-1

Size and orientation options in the Page Setup dialog box

You can change the paper size and page orientation for the entire document or for sections of the document. In the same way that you change margins in the Page Setup dialog box, use the Apply To drop-down list box to choose:

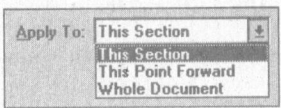

Options in the Apply To list box

- Whole Document

- This Point Forward

If the document has more than one section, or if text is selected, the list box will include additional options, such as This Section or Selected Text.

If a document has only one section, the changes will affect the whole document. If a document has more than one section, choose the section to which the change should be applied, or apply the change from the insertion point forward. Word automatically inserts section breaks when you apply the changes to selected text or from the insertion point forward.

Changing Paper Size

When you open a new document, the default paper size is 8½" x 11". The Paper Size drop-down list box in the Page Setup dialog box presents options for changing paper size. Depending upon the capabilities of the printer chosen in the Print Setup dialog box, you can change the paper size from the standard 8½" x 11". For example, if you need to print a document on a longer sheet of paper, choose Legal from the Paper Size list box. Legal-paper size is 8½" x 14". The width and height of the paper appears in the Width and Height boxes below the Paper Size list box. The values in these boxes change automatically when you choose a new paper size.

To change the paper size:

1. Start Word, if necessary.

2. Open a new document.

3. Choose Page Setup from the File menu, and click the Paper Size tab.

4. From the Paper Size drop-down list box, choose Legal.

5. View the change in the Preview box and click OK.

If you decide to change the paper size but do not find the size you need, you can change the values in the Width and Height boxes to create a custom paper size. When you enter values in the Width and Height boxes, "Custom Size" appears in the Paper Size list box.

To create a custom page:

1. Choose Page Setup from the File menu.

2. Key **9** in the Width box.

3. Key **12** in the Height box.

4. View the change in the Preview box, and then click OK.

5. Close the document without saving it.

Changing Page Orientation

In Word, you can choose between two page-orientation settings: Portrait and Landscape. A *portrait* page is taller than it is wide. For example, an 8½" x 11" portrait page is 8½ inches wide and 11 inches tall. This is the default in new Word documents. A *landscape* page

Paper-size options

Portrait

Landscape

Portrait page and
landscape page

Orientation options in
Page Setup

Note: When changing page
orientation, it is important to
keep in mind the formatting
of the original document.
Formatting can be greatly
affected by a change in
page orientation.

is wider than it is tall. When you change an 8½" x 11" page from portrait to landscape it becomes 11" x 8½", or 11 inches wide and 8½ inches tall. You can apply page-orientation changes to sections of a document or to the entire document.

To change page orientation:

1. Open the file 15-0.doc.

    The document is a letter with an attachment.

2. Move the insertion point to section 2, the attachment. Switch to print preview, and then click the One Page button, if necessary, to view section 2 only.

    The page appears in portrait style, 8½" x 11".

3. While still in print preview, choose Page Setup from the File menu. Click the Paper Size tab, if necessary.

    Notice that you can choose Page Setup options from print preview.

4. In the Orientation box, click the Landscape option button.

    View the page in the Preview box.

5. Click OK.

    The document appears in landscape style, 11" x 8½".

6. Return to normal view. Scroll between the two sections, and notice the margin changes on the ruler and in the document window.

7. Print page 2 of the document.

Changing the Paper Source

Frequently, businesses use different paper sources for different types of documents. For example, when using a laser printer, there may be one paper tray with legal paper and one with standard 8½" x 11" paper. In addition, different trays may contain different types of business stationery. One may contain letterhead stationery, and another may contain memo stationery.

The paper sources you choose in Word depend on the printer you have chosen in the Print Setup dialog box. A laser printer can use either paper trays or manual feed. You can use these in combination. For example, print the first page of a document on letterhead paper that is manually fed, and then print the remaining pages from a paper tray. Dot-matrix printers usually do not have paper trays. Instead, they have paper loaded into a tractor.

To access the Paper Source options, choose Page Setup from the File menu, and click the Paper Source tab. Then choose the appropriate paper source. Make sure you have loaded the chosen paper source before printing.

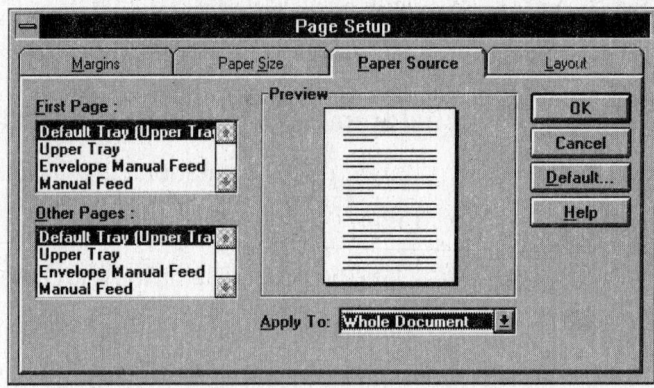

Figure 15-2
Paper Source options in Page Setup

Printing Envelopes

Instead of using a typewriter, you can create and print envelopes in Word. To do this, choose Envelopes and Labels from the Tools menu, and click the Envelopes tab in the dialog box.

Envelopes tab

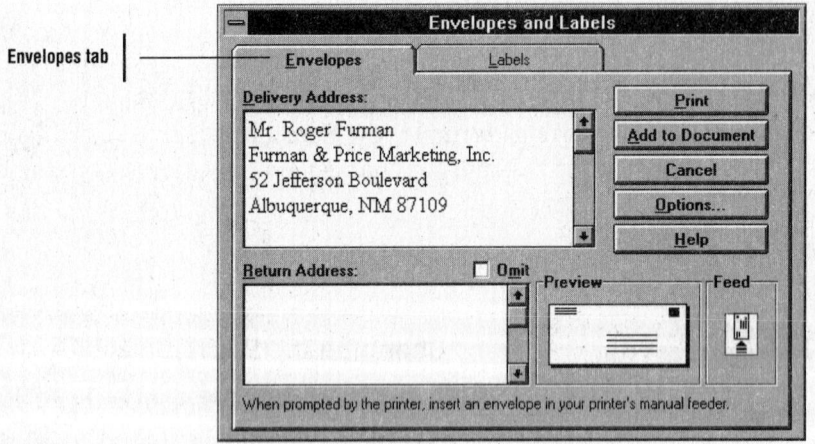

Figure 15-3
The Envelopes and Labels dialog box

To create and print an envelope, the Envelopes and Labels dialog box offers the following options:

- Delivery Address

   This is the mailing address for the document. You may not need to key the address, if it is already keyed in the document. Word searches the document for the short lines that look like an address and automatically inserts them in the Delivery Address box. You can also first select the address and then open the dialog box. Word inserts the selected text in the Delivery Address box. Text in this box can be edited, if necessary.

- Return Address

  You can enter information in the Return Address box. Or, if you are using an envelope with a preprinted return address, check the Omit Return Address box. When you enter or change an address in the Return Address box, Word asks if you want the new address to be the default return address. If you click Yes, the new return address will appear automatically each time you create an envelope. The return address can always be edited as needed.

- Preview

  The Preview box shows how the envelope will look when printed.

- Feed

  The Feed box shows how to place the envelope in the printer tray. This is the feeding method accepted by your printer.

- Print

  The Print button prints an envelope immediately and separately from the document. When you click the Print button, Word prints the envelope but does not save it.

- Add To Document

  This option saves the envelope by adding the address information to the beginning of the document as a new section (Page 0, Section 1). Word prints the envelope when you print the document.

To print an envelope:

1. Position the insertion point in section 1 of the document, and then choose Envelopes and Labels from the Tools menu.

   Word locates and inserts the address from the document in the Delivery Address box.

2. Make sure Omit Return Address is not checked, and then key in the Return Address box:

   Duke City Gateway Travel Agency
   15 Montgomery Boulevard
   Albuquerque, NM 87111

3. Prepare the printer with a standard business-size envelope, and then click Print.

   Word asks if you want to save the new return address as the default mailing address.

4. Click No, so the return address is not saved.

   Word prints the envelope.

Note: Although the feeding method is predetermined by your printer, you may have occasion to change the printer tray or position of the envelope in the tray. If necessary, click the Options button, and choose the Printing Options tab. Change the desired settings, and then print the envelope.

Tools menu

To add an envelope to a document for future printing:

1. Choose Envelopes and Labels from the Tools menu.

2. Key the return address again:

    Duke City Gateway Travel Agency
    15 Montgomery Boulevard
    Albuquerque, NM 87111

3. Click Add to Document. (Do not save the return address as the default mailing address.)

    Word adds the mailing address and return address to the top of the document.

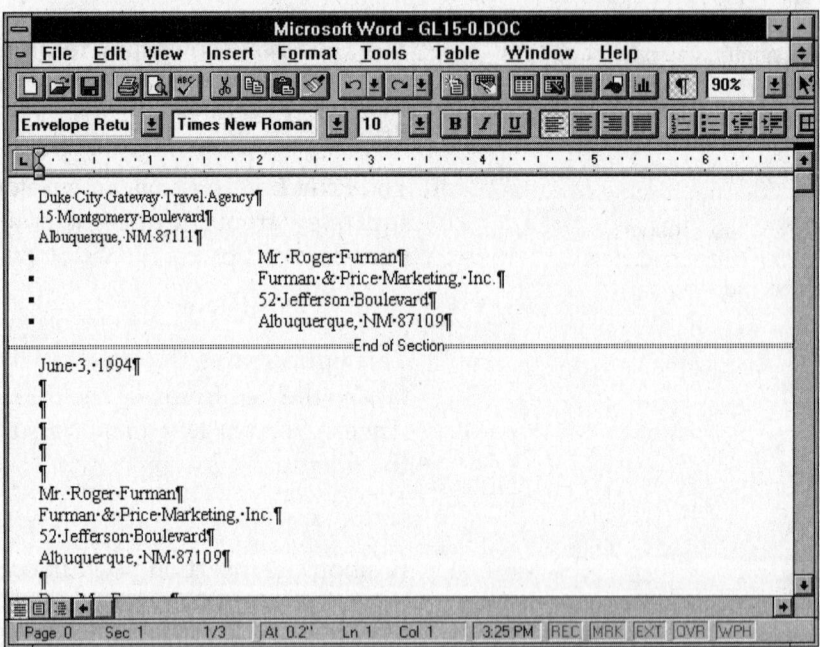

Figure 15-4
The envelope added to the document

4. Save the document as *[your three-letter identifier]*15-0.doc.

When you are ready to print the letter and the envelope, feed an envelope in the printer, and then use the Print command. Word will print the envelope first, and then the letter.

Word provides additional options for envelopes, such as the ability to change the envelope size, change the character formatting of the envelope text, or print bar codes on the envelope. To access the Envelope Options dialog box, click the Options button in the Envelopes and Labels dialog box or the icons in the Preview box or Feed box, and then click the Envelope Options tab.

Figure 15-5
The Envelope Options dialog box

Standard business envelope

Envelope Size

The default envelope size is Size 10, which is a standard business envelope. To print a different-sized envelope, choose another size from the Envelope Size list box, or choose Custom Size from the Envelope Size list box. You can then key a specific height and width for the envelope you want to use.

Printing Codes

If an envelope is to be mailed in the United States, you can print codes on it that can be read by the U.S. Postal Service for automated handling. These codes can reduce mailing costs and speed mail delivery.

Two types of codes can be printed on envelopes (if your printer can produce graphics):

FIM code identifies the front of the envelope

POSTNET bar code identifies the ZIP code

Envelope with printed codes

- The POSTNET (Postal Numeric Encoding Technique) bar code, which is a machine-readable code for the ZIP code of the delivery point.

- The FIM (Facing Identification Mark), which is used on courtesy reply mail to identify the front of an envelope. This is usually used by companies that provide return envelopes for bill paying.

Formatting and Positioning Text

The Envelope Options dialog box allows you to change the formatting of the return address and the delivery address by changing the size, font, or character attributes of the text. For example, you can make the return address smaller or make the delivery address bold. In addition, you can change the distance of the return address or delivery address from the left edge and the top edge of the envelope.

If the envelope is added to the document, the envelope text can easily be formatted in normal or page layout view before printing, and the address positions can be changed in page layout view or print preview.

To choose envelope options before printing an envelope:

1. Choose Envelopes and Labels from the Tools menu. Since the return address was not saved as the default return address, key it again.

2. Click the Options button, and then click the Envelope Options tab, if necessary.

3. Check the Delivery Point Bar Code check box to apply the POSTNET bar code.

   Note the change in the Preview box.

4. Click the Font button under Delivery Address.

5. Choose Bold, and then click OK.

6. Under Return Address, adjust the From Top measurement to .5" by clicking the up arrow four times.

7. Click OK in the Envelope Options dialog box, and then click Change Document in the Envelopes and Labels dialog box.

   This changes the existing envelope that was added to the document.

8. View the document in print preview.

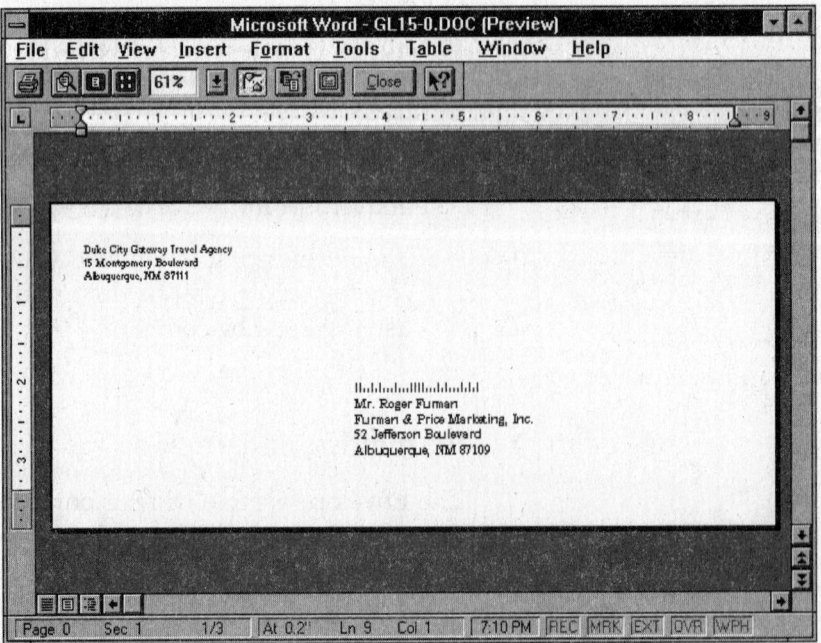

Figure 15-6
The envelope in print preview

9. Prepare the printer for a standard business envelope.

10. Print just the revised envelope. To do this, choose Print from the File menu, and key **s1** (remember, section 1 is the envelope) in the Pages text box. Click OK.

11. Save the document.

Printing Mailing Labels

Mailing labels are generally on sheets of 8½" x 11" paper. Word allows you to print one label on a sheet or print the same address on the entire sheet. This is helpful for mailing addresses that are used frequently. You can also choose to print the delivery address or the return address, specify the type of label product, and specify the height and width of a label. Labels can be created in Word for a variety of uses, such as file folders or diskettes.

To create labels, choose Envelopes and Labels from the Tools menu, and click the Labels tab.

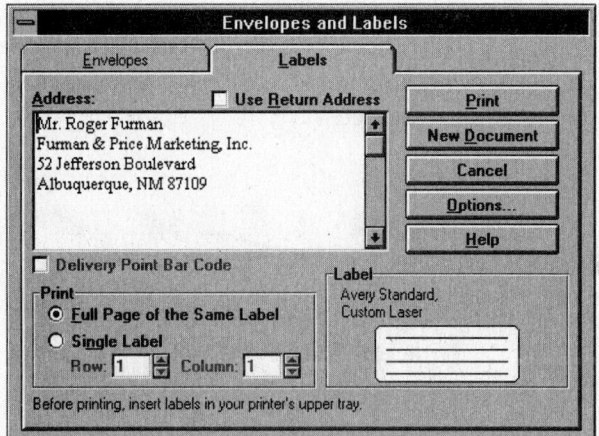

Figure 15-7

The Labels tab in the Envelopes and Labels dialog box

The Labels tab offers the following options:

- Address
  This is the delivery address. Word searches the document for this address, as it does when creating envelopes. You can also first select the address and then open the dialog box, or you can key any address in the Address box.

- Use Return Address
  Click this check box to print the return address instead of the delivery address. To print the return address, click the check box, and then key the return address.

- Delivery Point Bar Code
  As with envelopes, you can also add the POSTNET code to
  labels by clicking this check box.

- Full Page of the Same Label
  This option button allows you to print the same address on the
  entire sheet of labels.

- Single Label
  Use this option to print a single label. If necessary, specify the
  position of the label on the sheet. Word assumes you are
  beginning with a new sheet and with the label in row 1,
  column 1.

- Print
  The Print button prints the label immediately, without saving it.

Note: Labels are saved in table form. Tables are discussed in detail in Lesson 18.

- New Document
  The New Document button saves the label or sheet of labels in
  a new Word document for future use.

- Options
  Click the Options button (or click the label in the Label box) to
  choose another type of label. Word opens the Label Options
  dialog box, from which you can specify a label by product
  number. You can also click the Details button in this dialog
  box to specify the exact height and width of a particular label,
  if necessary.

Figure 15-8

The Label Options dialog box

To print a single mailing label:

1. With the insertion point still in *[your three-letter identi-fier]*15-0.doc, choose Envelopes and Labels from the Tools menu.

2. Click the Labels tab.

   Word locates the delivery address, as it does when creating an envelope. If there is more than one address in a document, you can select the text before opening the dialog box. You can also key any address or data in the Address box.

3. In the Print box, click the Single Label option button. Keep the default label position (row 1, column 1), unless your instructor directs you to do otherwise.

The label type is indicated in the Label box.

4. Click the Options button.

Word opens the Label Options dialog box.

5. Scroll through the Product Number list to view the different label options. Choose a different label type if your instructor directs you to do so.

6. Click OK in the Label Options dialog box.

7. Insert a sheet of labels into the printer, and then click Print in the Envelopes and Labels dialog box.

Word prints the delivery address on the specified label.

8. Save *[your three-letter identifier]*15-0.doc, close it, and exit Word (unless you will be doing the following exercises immediately).

Key Terms

Landscape   Portrait

Exercises

Exercise 15.1

1. Start Word, if necessary.

2. Open the file 15-1.doc.

3. Change the page orientation, and customize the paper size:

   A. Choose Page Setup from the File menu.

   B. Click the Paper Size tab.

   C. Click Landscape in the Orientation box.

   D. Set the width to 5 inches and the height to 3 inches.

4. Click the Margins tab, and set the top and bottom margins to .5 inches.

5. Click the Layout tab, and center the text vertically. Click OK.

6. View the document in print preview.

7. Change the paper size back to regular letter size:

    A. Choose Page Setup from the File menu.

    B. Choose Letter 8½ x 11 in from the Paper Size list box. Keep the landscape setting, and then click OK.

8. Change the line spacing to 1.5 lines.

9. Save the document as *[your three-letter identifier]*15-1.doc and print it.

10. Close the document and exit Word (unless you will be doing the following exercises immediately).

Exercise 15.2

1. Start Word, if necessary.

2. Open the file 15-2.doc.

3. Create an envelope for the first address, Golden Gateway Travel, and save it with the document:

    A. Select the text from the agency name through the ZIP code.

    B. Choose Envelopes and Labels from the Tools menu.

    C. Click the Envelopes tab.

    D. In the Return Address box, key:

        Windy City Gateway Travel
        305 Madison Street
        Chicago, IL 60607

    E. Click Options, and clear the postal-code check boxes, if necessary.

    F. Click the Add to Document button. Do not save the return address as the new default.

4. View the document in print preview.

5. Print the envelope:

    A. Feed an envelope in the printer.

    B. Choose Print from the File menu.

    C. In the Pages text box, key **s1** and click OK.

6. Create a mailing label for Golden Gate Travel:

    A. With the same address selected in the document, choose Envelopes and Labels from the Tools menu.

    B. Click the Labels tab.

    C. Click the Single Label option.

    D. Click Print.

7. Save the document as *[your three-letter identifier]*15-2.doc.

8. Close the document and exit Word (unless you will be doing the following exercises immediately).

Exercise 15.3

1. Start Word, if necessary.

2. Open the file 15-3.doc.

3. Print an envelope separate from the document to the first person on the list, Maria Cordova. As a return address, key:

    Duke City Gateway Travel Agency
    15 Montgomery Boulevard
    Albuquerque, NM 87111

4. Add an envelope to the document. Use Duke City Gateway, as listed above, as the return address. Add the POSTNET bar code. Address the envelope to:

    Big Apple Gateway Travel
    620 Fifth Avenue
    Rockefeller Center
    New York, NY 10022

5. Save the document as *[your three-letter identifier]*15-3.doc.

6. Print the envelope saved with the document.

7. Print another envelope separate from the document to the last participants on the list, Richard and Linda Elliot. Use no return address.

8. Close the document and exit Word (unless you will be doing the following exercise immediately).

Exercise 15.4: Challenge Yourself

Open the file 15-4.doc, and format the document as a standard business letter. Include your reference initials and an enclosure notation.

As a separate section after the letter, key the text in Figure 15-9, which appears at the end of this exercise. Use a 3-inch, left-aligned tab setting for the second column.

Change the orientation of section 2 to landscape. Move the tab setting of the second column, so that it is left-aligned at the center of the page. View the document in print preview, and then change the left and right margins for section 1 to 1.25 inches and the left margin for section 2 to 2 inches.

Spell-check the document, and save it as *[your three-letter identifier]*15-4.doc. Print the document, and then print a mailing label to the addressee on the letter. Use the same address to print an envelope with the POSTNET bar code and no return address. Close the document and exit Word.

Figure 15-9

Forward the Big Apple photos to the following New York "Night on the Town" participants:

Joseph Anaya   Cathy Peterson
3883 Cerillos Road   98 Sequoia Road
Santa Fe, NM 87501   Albuquerque, NM 87120

Charles Neira   Richard and Linda Elliott
87 Green Lake Road   8 Castillo Avenue
Rio Rancho, NM 87048   Belen, NM 87002

A Memo and an Invitation

Background

Duke City Gateway's manager, Susan Allen, is sending a memo to her staff announcing the grand opening of the new Red River Hotel in Albuquerque. Since she sent out a press release about the grand-opening ceremonies, Susan wants to make sure her employees are well informed about the hotel, in case they receive telephone inquiries about the event from the public. Also, although the grand opening is open to the public, Susan is sending out invitations to important members of the Albuquerque community to make sure they are properly invited to the grand opening of the hotel.

Business Purpose

Create a memo to the staff announcing the grand opening of the Red River Hotel and Duke City Gateway's role in the ceremonies. Then create an invitation to send to important members of the Albuquerque community. The invitation will be cut and folded when it is finished.

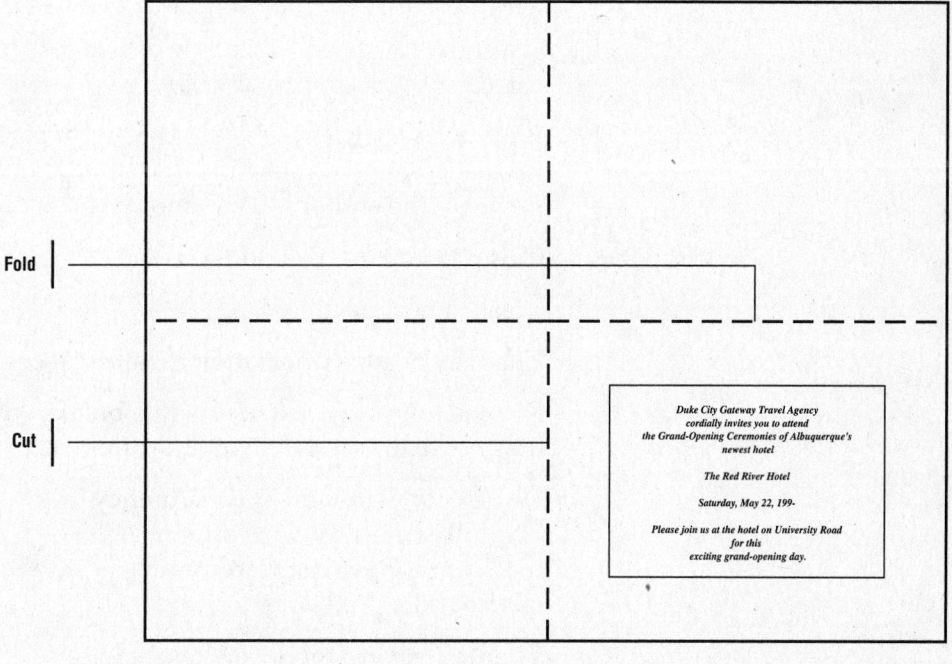

Figure 15-10
Diagram for invitation

Procedures

1. Open the files p5-1.doc and 4-3.doc.

2. Copy the last paragraph in 4-3.doc to the end of p5-1.doc as a new paragraph.

3. Close document 4-3.doc.

4. Make sure the memo has the appropriate top margin settings for each page, and then key a two-line continuation header for page 2:

   Red River Hotel
   Page

   Add the page number.

5. Adjust the left and right margins to 1.5 inches in print preview.

6. Spell-check the document.

7. Save the document as *[your three-letter identifier]*p5-1.doc.

8. Print two copies of pages 1 and 2.

9. Close the document.

10. Open the file p5-2.doc.

11. Select the text from "Schedule of Events " to the last event listed (the jazz concert at 9:00).

12. Print two copies of the selected text. Prepare the printouts for distribution by attaching one copy of the schedule of events to the end of each memo.

13. Close document p5-2.doc.

14. Create a new document.

15. Change the page orientation to landscape.

16. Key the following text, using line breaks within paragraphs. Make sure to insert a blank line after each paragraph:

    Duke City Gateway Travel Agency
    cordially invites you to attend
    the Grand-Opening Ceremonies of Albuquerque's
    newest hotel

    The Red River Hotel

    Saturday, May 22, 199-

Please join us at the hotel on University Road
for this
exciting grand-opening day.

17. Center the text, and make it bold and italic.

18. Add a thick, shadow border around the text.

19. View the document in print preview.

20. In print preview, adjust the margins so that the box is positioned at the bottom right of the page (allowing the top half to be folded over to create an invitation). See Figure 15-10.

21. Print one copy of the invitation.

22. Add the following summary information to the document:

    Title: **Invitation**

    Subject: **The Red River Hotel Opening**

    Author: *[your three-letter identifier]*

23. Print the summary information.

24. Add a custom return envelope to the document to mail back the invitations. Use Duke City Gateway Travel Agency's address (15 Montgomery Boulevard, Albuquerque, NM 87111) as the delivery address, and make the text italic. Customize the envelope size to 6.5 inches wide and 5 inches high. Include both types of postal codes on the envelope.

25. View the document in print preview, and make any changes you feel will improve the appearance of the document.

26. Save the document as *[your three-letter identifier]*p5-2.doc.

27. Close the document and exit Word.

Tips and Hints

- Use the Zoom Control box on the Standard toolbar to change your view of the page. You can view the page at its actual width or magnify the page.

- View multiple pages of a document in print preview. Switch to viewing one page to see a larger view.

- While changing margins in print preview, open the Page Setup dialog box to check your margin settings or make them more precise.

Advanced Character Formatting

Fonts and Type Sizes

Objectives

• Change fonts.

• Change type sizes.

• Change space between characters.

This lesson introduces you to Word features that allow you to specify type designs and type sizes for the documents you create and edit. It also shows you how to control the spacing between characters. Character attributes such as bold and italic were first introduced in Lesson 3. Lesson 16 now explores additional tools for calling attention to text and making it easy to read.

What Are Fonts and Type Sizes?

A font is a type design applied to an entire set of characters, including all the letters of the alphabet, numerals, punctuation marks, and other symbols, such as # and @.

Figure 16-1

Examples of fonts

As the figure shows, a font can be plain, like Helvetica, or more ornate, like Times New Roman. Fonts can also differ in their proportions, so that letters in some fonts appear short and wide, while letters in other fonts appear tall and thin.

Each font is available in a variety of type sizes, which are measured in *points*. There are 72 points to an inch. In other words, a point is $\frac{1}{72}$ of an inch.

Fonts and type sizes are character attributes. You can use any font or type size with text in combination with any other character attributes. For example, you can use any style of underlining for text in any font and type size.

Point

A measure of type size, with 72 points equaling one inch.

305

Figure 16-2
Examples of different point sizes

Note: The fonts and type sizes you can use with Word depend on the printer and whether it has font cartridges. They also depend on the software installed with the computer system. For example, Windows version 3.1 includes some fonts that do not come with earlier versions. A system may also have other software installed that provides additional fonts. Fonts such as Courier, Modern, Script, and Times New Roman are generally available with Word and Windows 3.1.

Figure 16-3
Some available Word fonts

The current template determines the default font and type size. The template most frequently used, the Normal template, uses Times New Roman 10-point type. Templates are discussed in more detail in Lesson 21.

You can use the Formatting toolbar or the Font dialog box to change the font and type size for any new or selected text. Keyboard shortcuts are also available for changing type sizes.

Changing Fonts and Type Sizes with the Formatting Toolbar

Choosing fonts and type sizes from the Formatting toolbar is generally faster than choosing them from the Font dialog box. Using the

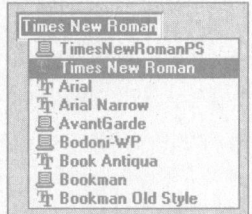

Font drop-down list box on the Formatting toolbar

Points drop-down list box on the Formatting toolbar

Formatting toolbar to change type size is even faster than using a keyboard shortcut.

The Font box on the Formatting toolbar shows the current font. Click the arrow to the right of it to display a drop-down list box of the fonts from which to choose.

The Points box shows the point size of the current type. Click the arrow to the right of it to display a drop-down list box of the type sizes available for the specified font.

To specify a font for new text using the Formatting toolbar, click the insertion point where you want the font to begin appearing. Then choose a font from the Font drop-down list box. The font name you choose appears in the Font box on the Formatting toolbar.

To change the font of existing text using the Formatting toolbar, select the text you want to change. Then choose the font you want from the Font drop-down list box. The new font name appears in the Font box on the Formatting toolbar, and the selected text appears in that font.

The same procedures apply to specifying a type size. For new text, choose a type size from the Points drop-down list box, and then begin keying text in the new type size. The new type size is reflected on the Formatting toolbar. For existing text, select the text, and then choose a type size from the Points drop-down list box. The selected text then appears in that type size.

To specify fonts and type sizes for new text using the Formatting toolbar:

1. Start Word, if necessary.

2. Open a new document.

3. Click the arrow to the right of the Font box on the Formatting toolbar, and then choose Century Schoolbook from the Font drop-down list box.

Note: If the fonts specified in the lesson are not available, ask your instructor for the name of a comparable font.

The Font drop-down list box closes, and the font name appears in the Font box on the Formatting toolbar.

4. Click the arrow to the right of the Points box on the Formatting toolbar. Then choose 24 from the Points drop-down list box.

The Points drop-down list box closes, and the number 24 appears in the Points box on the Formatting toolbar.

5. Key the title **Primer for First-Time Overseas Travelers**, and press **Enter** three times.

6. Choose Helvetica from the Font drop-down list box.

7. Choose 14 from the Points drop-down list box.

8. Key the following text:

    Duke City Gateway Travel Agency
    15 Montgomery Boulevard
    Albuquerque, NM 87111
    (505) 555-1234

9. Close the document without saving.

To change the font and type size of existing text using the Formatting toolbar:

1. Open the file 11-0.doc.

2. Select the title of the report on page 1, which begins "Primer For".

3. Choose 20 from the Points drop-down list box.

    The text appears in 20-point Times New Roman type.

4. Press **Enter** three times after the title, and then select the rest of the text on the title page.

5. Choose Arial from the Font drop-down list box. Then choose 14 from the Points drop-down list box.

    The selected text appears in 14-point Arial type.

6. Delete the hard page break before the title on page 2, and insert a Next Page section break, so that the title page is a separate section.

7. Center the text vertically and horizontally on the title page.

Choosing Fonts and Type Sizes from the Font Dialog Box

Fonts and type sizes are character attributes that can be chosen from the Font dialog box along with other character attributes. To open the Font dialog box, choose Font from the Format menu.

In the Font dialog box, the Font box shows the current font, and the Points box shows the point size of the current type. The list boxes below the Font box and the Points box show the available options. See Figure 16-4 on page 309.

The Preview box shows how text looks with the font, type size, and other character attributes specified. The appearance of the text in the Preview box changes whenever you change the font, type size, or other attributes. This lets you experiment with different fonts and type sizes before you click OK to specify a character format.

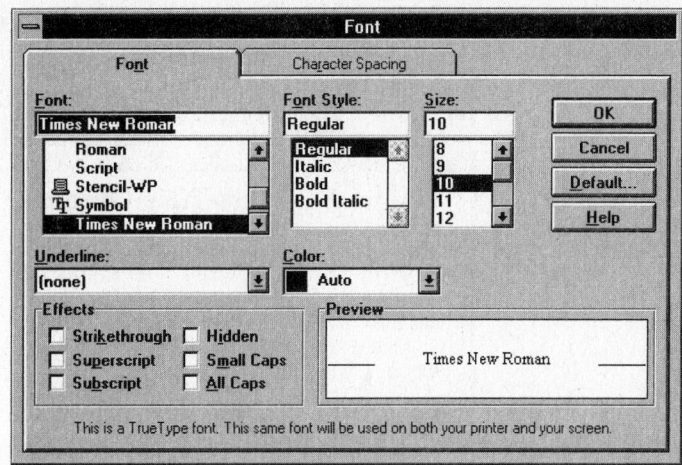

Figure 16-4
The Font dialog box

To change the font or type size for new text using the Font dialog box, position the insertion point where you want the new text to begin. Choose Font from the Format menu. Then choose a font from the Font list box or a type size from the Points list box. Click OK to close the dialog box and begin keying text.

To change the font or type size of existing text using the Font dialog box, select the text, open the Font dialog box, and then choose a font or type size from the list boxes.

To specify the font and type size for new text using the Font dialog box:

1. On page 1, section 1, place the insertion point after the phone number, and press **Enter** three times.

2. Choose Font from the Format menu.

3. In the Font dialog box, choose Italic from the Font Style list box.

4. Choose Times New Roman from the Font list box. Then choose 10 from the Points list box.

   The text appears in the Preview box in 10-point Times New Roman italics.

5. Click OK to close the Font dialog box, and then key:

   Southwestern U.S. Division, Gateway International Travel, Inc.

   The text appears with the specified character attributes. See Figure 16-5 on page 310.

To change the font and type size of existing text using the Font dialog box:

1. Select the heading "**What about . . .**" on page 1, section 2.

2. Choose Font from the Format menu.

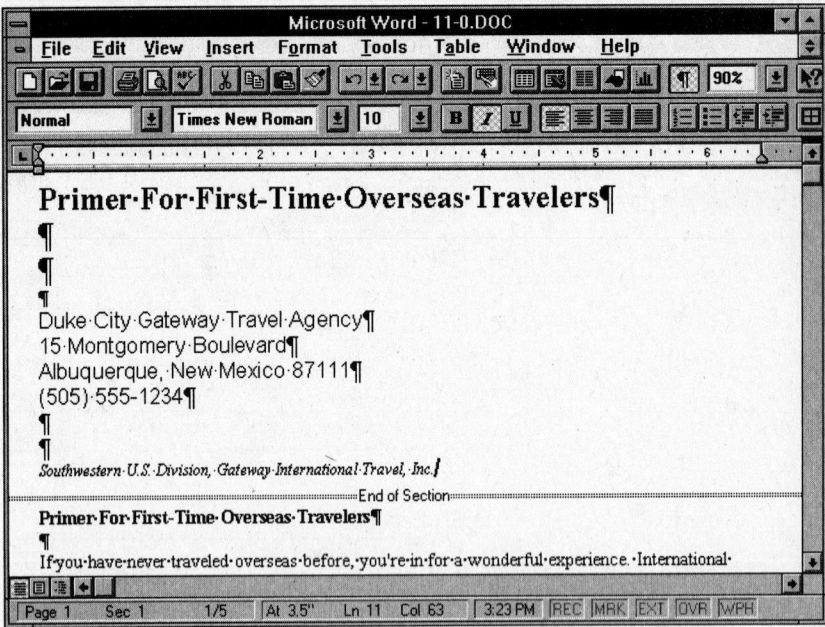

Figure 16-5
The document with different fonts and type sizes

3. In the Font dialog box, choose Century Schoolbook from the Font list box. Choose 14 from the Points list box.

   The text in the Preview box appears in 14-point Century Schoolbook type.

4. Click OK to close the Font dialog box.

   The selected text appears with the specified character attributes.

Using Unlisted Fonts

In Word, you can use fonts in a document that are not listed in the Font box. For example, you may want to format a document in a font that your printer does not have, but that another printer does. You can create the document in that font, and then print the document from the workstation that makes that font available.

To use a font that is not available on your printer, simply key the name of the font in the Font box. Word chooses a screen font that is closest in appearance to the font, so you can approximate the look of the document.

For example, suppose you want to use the font Helvetica, and it is not listed in the Font list box. Delete the text in the Font box and key **Helvetica**. You can then print the document in Helvetica from a computer with a printer that has the font.

This technique can also be used to create a document in a special font that will be sent to a print shop for typesetting.

Using Keyboard Shortcuts to Change Type Sizes

In addition to the Formatting toolbar and the Font dialog box, you can use keyboard shortcuts to change the type size of new or existing text.

The keyboard shortcut for increasing to the next available type size is **Ctrl+Shift+>**. The keyboard shortcut for decreasing to the next available type size is **Ctrl+Shift+<**. To use either of these keyboard shortcuts for existing text, select the text, and then use the shortcut. Each time you use the keyboard shortcut, you change the text to the next available type size. To use the shortcuts for new text, position the insertion point, use the shortcut, and then key the new text.

To change type sizes for existing text using the keyboard shortcuts:

1. Select the italicized line of text on page 1, section 1.

2. Press **Ctrl+Shift+>** twice.

   The number in the Points box on the Formatting toolbar increases from 10 to 12, and the selected text appears in 12-point type.

3. Select the first line of text on page 1, section 1 (the title).

4. Press **Ctrl+Shift+<** once.

   The number in the Points box changes from 20 to 18 (the next smallest Times New Roman type size), and the selected text appears in 18-point type.

To specify type sizes for new text using keyboard shortcuts:

1. Move the insertion point to section 2, choose Header and Footer from the View menu, and switch to the footer area.

2. In the footer area, center the paragraph mark, and then press **Ctrl+Shift+<** twice.

   The number in the Points box for the footer decreases from 12 to 10.

3. Key the following text:

   Duke City Gateway Travel - Your Gateway to the World

   The footer text appears in 10-point Times New Roman type.

4. Close the footer, and then switch to page-layout view.

5. Double-click in the footer area to open it, select the footer text, and then press **Ctrl+Shift+>** once.

   The footer text increases to 11 points.

6. Close the footer area, and switch back to normal view.

Character Spacing

In Word, you can adjust the spacing between characters in a document. You may want to do this to make text more readable or to create special effects. For example, if you are creating overhead transparencies for a presentation, you may want to adjust the character spacing to make the text more readable on a projection screen.

Changing Character Spacing

Use the Font dialog box to change character spacing. Click the Character Spacing tab in the Font dialog box to choose normal, expanded, or condensed spacing between characters. You can also click the up or down arrow in the By box to increase or decrease spacing in quarter-point increments.

The Preview box shows how text looks with the spacing and other character attributes that are specified. This allows you to experiment with different character-spacing options before you click OK to specify a character format.

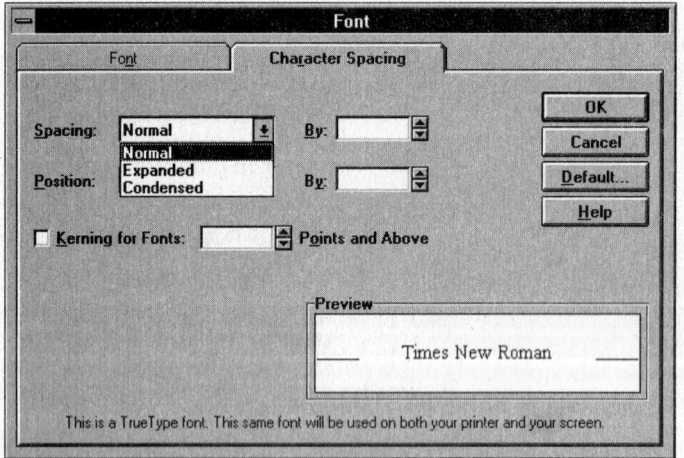

Figure 16-6
Choosing character spacing options in the Font dialog box

Expanded spacing provides more than the normal amount of space between characters. The Word default for expanded spacing provides 1 additional point of space between characters.

Condensed spacing provides less than the normal amount of space between characters. The Word default for condensed spacing provides 1 point less than the normal amount of space between characters. See Figure 16-7 on page 313.

You can use any of these methods to adjust character spacing:

* Choose an option from the Spacing drop-down list box. When you use this method to choose expanded or condensed

Normal | —— Duke City Gateway

Condensed by 1.5 points | —— Duke City Gateway

Expanded by 3 points | —— Duke City Gateway

Figure 16-7
Expanded, condensed, and normal character spacing

spacing, the Word default for that spacing option appears in the By box in the Spacing box.

- Choose an option from the Spacing drop-down list box. Then specify the number of points by which you want to increase or decrease spacing by keying the number in the By box.

- Click the up or down arrow in the By box to increase or decrease the spacing in $\frac{1}{10}$-point increments. Each time you click an arrow, the spacing increases or decreases by .10 points.

Kerning
Changes the spacing between specific pairs of letters to improve the appearance of text.

- Click the Kerning for Fonts check box. *Kerning* slightly changes the spacing between certain pairs of letters to improve the overall appearance of text. Kerning can be used only with proportionally spaced TrueType fonts or similar fonts that are larger than a certain minimum size.

Figure 16-8
Choosing Expanded spacing

Character spacing can only be adjusted in increments of .10 points. For example, if you key **2.75** in the By text box for additional spacing, you will only adjust the spacing by 2.7 points. If you attempt to change the spacing by increments other than .10 points, Word automatically rounds the number you key to the nearest .10 points.

To create new text with expanded or condensed spacing, move the insertion point to where you want the new text to begin. Choose Font from the Format menu, and then choose Expanded or Condensed from the Spacing drop-down list box in the Font dialog box.

To change Word's default for condensed spacing, click the down arrow in the By box once for each .10-point space reduction you want. To change Word's default for expanded spacing, click the up arrow in the By box once for each .10-point space increase you want. Click OK, and then key the new text.

To change the spacing of existing text to normal spacing or to Word's default for expanded or condensed spacing, select the text. In the Font dialog box, choose an option from the Spacing drop-down list box.

To change the spacing of existing text without using Word's default for expanded or condensed text, select the text. In the Font dialog box, click the down arrow in the By box to decrease the spacing between characters, or click the up arrow to increase the spacing. Remember, each click changes the spacing by $\frac{1}{10}$ of a point.

To change character spacing for new text:

1. Move the insertion point to the beginning of the second line of text on page 1, section 1, which shows the travel agency's name.

2. Choose Font from the Format menu, and click the Character Spacing tab, if necessary.

3. In the Font dialog box, choose Expanded from the Spacing drop-down list box.

   The number 1 appears in the By box, because 1 point of extra space between characters is the default for expanded spacing. The text in the Preview box appears with 1 point more space than normal between its characters.

4. Click OK to close the Font dialog box. Key **Compliments of:** and press **Enter** twice.

   The text appears with 1 point of extra spacing between characters.

5. Move the insertion point to section 2, and then choose Header and Footer from the View menu. Scroll down to the footer area.

6. Select the footer text, and then choose Font from the Format menu.

7. Choose Condensed from the Spacing drop-down list box.

   The number 1 appears in the By box, because 1 point less than the normal amount of space between characters is the default for condensed spacing. The text in the Preview box appears with 1 point less space than normal between its characters.

8. Click the up arrow in the By box three times.

The number in the By box changes from 1 to 0.7, and the text in the sample box appears with .7 points less space than normal between its characters.

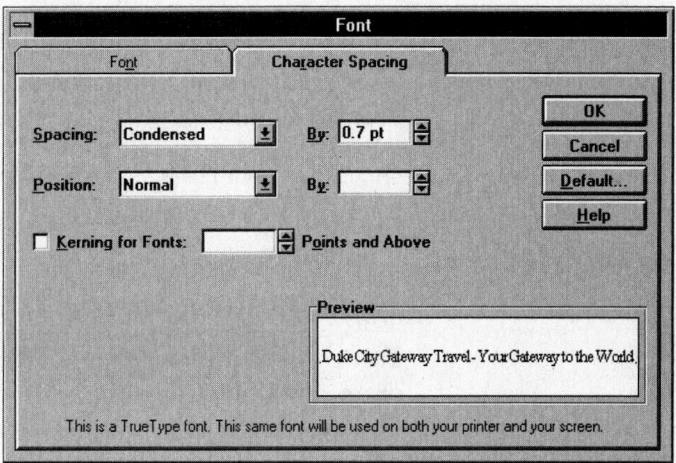

Figure 16-9
Adjusting condensed spacing

9. Click OK to close the Font dialog box, and then close the Header and Footer toolbar.

10. Save the document as *[your three-letter identifier]*16-0.doc.

11. Select the first two pages of the document and print the selection.

12. Close *[your three-letter identifier]*16-0.doc and exit Word (unless you will be doing the following exercises immediately).

Table 16-1: Keyboard Shortcuts for Changing Type Size	
Keyboard Shortcut	Action
Ctrl+Shift+>	Increase text size to next available size
Ctrl+Shift+<	Decrease text size to next available size

Key Terms

Kerning

Point

Exercises

Exercise 16.1

1. Start Word, if necessary.

2. Open the file 16-1.doc.

3. With the insertion point at the top of the document, use the Formatting toolbar to change the font to Helvetica or Arial:

   A. Click the arrow to the right of the Font box.

   B. Choose Helvetica or Arial from the Font drop-down list box.

4. Key the following paragraph:

   Traveling alone? Want to visit the Mayan ruins of Mexico, or go hot-air ballooning in the south of France? Join one of Duke City Gateway's special-interest tours, and meet others who share your hobby.

5. Press **Enter** twice. Change the character spacing of the paragraph you keyed to Word's default for expanded spacing:

   A. Select the paragraph.

   B. Choose Font from the Format menu.

   C. Click the Character Spacing tab, and choose Expanded from the Spacing drop-down list box. Click OK.

6. Change the formatting of the paragraph you keyed to 14-point bold, centered text, with a single-line box border.

7. Move the insertion point to the end of the document and press **Enter**.

8. Use the Formatting toolbar to change the font to Helvetica or Arial.

9. Use the Formatting toolbar to change the type size to 16 points:

   A. Click the arrow to the right of the Points box.

   B. Choose 16 from the Points drop-down list box.

10. Key the following paragraph:

    Call Gateway, and talk with one of our travel agents. Chances are, we'll be able to organize a trip with other single travelers who share your special interest.

11. Center the paragraph you just keyed, and change the top margin of the document to 1.5 inches.

12. Spell-check the document.

13. Save the document as *[your three-letter identifier]*16-1.doc.

14. Print the document.

15. Close the document and exit Word (unless you will be doing the following exercises immediately).

Exercise 16.2

1. Start Word, if necessary.

2. Open the file 16-2.doc.

3. Use the Font dialog box to change the entire document to the Arial font:

    A. Select the entire document.

    B. Choose Font from the Format menu.

    C. Click the Font tab, and choose Arial from the Font list box.

    D. Click OK to close the dialog box.

4. Change the character spacing for the seven indented lines (the Gateway locations) to Word's default condensed spacing:

    A. Select the seven indented lines.

    B. Choose Font from the Format menu.

    C. Click the Character Spacing tab, and choose Condensed from the Spacing drop-down list box.

    D. Click OK to close the dialog box.

5. Add the bold and italic attributes to the selected text.

6. Move the insertion point to the end of the document and press **Enter**.

7. Press **Ctrl+Shift+>** once to change the type size to 14 points.

8. Change the character spacing to condensed, with 0.7 points less space than normal between characters:

    A. Choose Font from the Format menu.

    B. Choose Condensed from the Spacing drop-down list box.

    C. In the By box, click the up arrow until the setting is 0.7 pt.

    D. Click OK to close the dialog box.

9. Key the following text:

    Other Gateway locations include offices in Boston, Atlanta, Washington, D.C., and Honolulu.

10. Add another blank line after the first line of the document, and then change the font of the first line to 20-point bold text.

11. Change the page orientation to landscape, center the text vertically, and change the left and right margins to 2 inches.

12. Spell-check the document, and save it as *[your three-letter identifier]*16-2.doc.

13. View the document in print preview, and then print it.

14. Close the document and exit Word (unless you will be doing the following exercises immediately).

Exercise 16.3

1. Start Word, if necessary.

2. Create a new document.

3. Change the font and type size to 24-point Century Schoolbook, and then key **Weekend in New York**

4. Press **Enter** twice, and then key the first line of Figure 16-10 using 12-point Arial type.

Figure 16-10

Luxury Accommodations and a Broadway Show

Join us for a "Night on the Town Weekend" including tickets to a great

show∧ *

Phantom of the Opera

Les Miserables

Grand Hotel ∧ *Cats*

From $550 ∧ **

Duke City Gateway Travel

15 Montgomery Boulevard
Albuquerque, ∧ *NM 87111*

555-1234
∧ * *One show per weekend, based on availability*
** *Includes air and hotel, based on double occupancy*

5. Press **Enter** twice. Using the same font and font size, key the next line (from "Join" through "show*").

6. Press **Enter** twice, and then key the next three lines in 14-point type, with character spacing that is 2 points more than normal. Do not insert a blank line between the lines of text.

7. Press **Enter** twice, and then key the next line in 12-point Arial, with normal character spacing.

8. Press **Enter** twice, and use the same font and font size to key the agency name, address, and phone number.

9. Press **Enter** twice, and then key the last two lines in 12-point Century Schoolbook.

10. Make the first line of the document bold, and then use the keyboard shortcut to decrease its type size by two points.

11. Center the document horizontally and vertically.

12. Spell-check the document.

13. Save the document as *[your three-letter identifier]*16-3.doc and print it.

14. Close the document and exit Word (unless you will be doing the following exercise immediately).

Exercise 16.4

Open the file 16-4.doc. Change the first line to 36-point Brush Script bold. Change the type size for the two lines beginning "Location" and "Date" to 14 points.

Above the paragraph that begins "Guests are", key the following as a separate paragraph in 12-point Times New Roman bold italic: **(All facilities and services will be available to the counselors at no cost.)** Change the character spacing for this text to 1.2 points of expanded spacing.

Format the text from "Location:" to "Mountain Top Restaurant" as two tabbed columns, with a right-aligned 1.25-inch tab before "Location:", "Date:", "Schedule:", and the times, and a left-aligned 1.75-inch tab before the rest of the text. Replace all line-break characters with paragraph marks. Change line spacing from "Location:" to "Mountain Top Restaurant" to 12 points after each paragraph. Key **p.m.** to the right of each time under "9:30 a.m." (for lines such as "10:15-12:15", key **p.m.** only after "12:15").

Center the first and last lines of the document, and apply a box border around the entire document. Center the document vertically. Spell-check the document, view it in print preview, and then save it as *[your three-letter identifier]*16-4.doc. Print the document, and then close it and exit Word.

Symbols, Special Characters, and Attributes

Objectives

- Understand special character and attribute options.
- Apply special character attributes to text.
- Insert special characters in a document.

This lesson shows how to use characters that do not appear on the keyboard in a document. It also introduces additional character attributes that are used for more advanced work with documents. For example, the strikethrough option allows you to call attention to text, and the hidden-text option allows you to create notes to yourself that do not appear when you print a document. This lesson also shows you how to enhance documents with double underlining, color, and other special character attributes.

Special Character Attributes

Character attributes, as discussed earlier, are options you can apply to characters to make them stand out from normal text. The basic optional character attributes are bold, italic, underlining, and all capitals.

In addition to these basic options, Word enables you to use these special character attributes:

- Double underline
- Words-only underline
- Dotted underline
- Color
- Strikethrough
- Superscript
- Subscript
- Hidden text
- Small capitals
- All capitals

You can use either key combinations (see the Keyboard Shortcuts table at the end of this lesson) or the Font dialog box to specify these special character attributes.

Double Underlining

Double underlining is just like single underlining, which was introduced in Lesson 3, except that the underlined text has two lines under it instead of one.

<u>This is an example of double-underlined text</u>.

Words-Only Underlining

When you apply the Single and Double Underline options, Word underlines spaces as well as letters, numbers, words, and punctuation. Use the Words Only option when you want single underlining only for characters you key, not for the spaces between them.

<u>This</u> <u>is</u> <u>an</u> <u>example</u> <u>of</u> <u>words-only</u> <u>underlining</u>.

Dotted Underlining

Unlike the other underlining options, which use a solid line or lines, the Dotted Underline option inserts a dashed line under the text.

This is an example of dotted underlining.

Color

You can format characters so that they appear on the screen in color. This enables you to use color for emphasizing text in documents that will be distributed electronically and read on the screen rather than on paper. You can also print the characters in color if the computer system uses a color printer.

Strikethrough

Strikethrough
An optional character attribute that causes a horizontal line to appear through the characters.

When you apply the *strikethrough* option to text, a horizontal line appears through the text.

~~This is an example of strikethrough text.~~

Many people use strikethrough to suggest that text be deleted. For example, if you think your manager should delete a word from a report he or she has asked you to review, you can select the word and apply the strikethrough option to it.

Superscript

Superscript
An optional character attribute that causes text to appear slightly above the other text on the same line.

Use the *superscript* option when you want characters to appear slightly higher than the other characters on the same line.

In this example, the word ^{keyboard} appears in superscript.

You may need to use superscript for trademark symbols or for asterisks or other characters that are used to call attention to notes.

Superscript is also used for exponents in math formulas and for some symbols in scientific formulas.

Subscript

Subscript
An optional character attribute that causes text to appear slightly below the other text on the same line.

Use the *subscript* option when you want characters to appear slightly lower than the other characters on the same line.

In this example, the word $_{keyboard}$ appears in subscript.

Subscript is useful for symbols or numbers in scientific formulas.

Hidden Text

Hidden text
Text that does not appear in the printed version of a document and that only appears on the screen if Word's hidden text option is turned on.

Hidden text does not appear in print, and it only appears on the screen if Word's view options are set to display hidden text. When you are keying or editing a draft of a document, you might want to use hidden text for notes to yourself or to others working on the draft.

Small Capitals

When you apply the small-capitals attribute to text, the text appears in small, all-capital letters. If you turn on the small-capitals option in many fonts, including Times New Roman and Helvetica, you can press the **Shift** key or the **Caps Lock** key to key regular capital letters.

THIS IS AN EXAMPLE OF SMALL CAPITALS IN THE HELVETICA FONT.

Notice that the capitals beginning the sentence and the font name are larger than the other capitals.

In a few fonts, all characters in small capitals appear exactly the same as characters in regular capitals.

All Capitals

When you apply the all-capitals attribute to text, the text appears in all-capital letters. This is the same as pressing the **Shift** key or the **Caps Lock** key to key in all capitals.

THIS IS AN EXAMPLE OF TEXT IN ALL CAPITALS.

Applying Special Character Attributes

There are two ways to apply special character attributes to new or existing text in a document:

- By choosing the attribute from the Font dialog box
- By using a keyboard shortcut for the special attribute

While the keyboard shortcut is the faster method, the Font dialog box allows you to see the attribute before you choose it.

Using the Font Dialog Box to Apply Special Attributes

To use the Font dialog box to apply special character attributes, choose Font from the Format menu. The Effects group in the Font dialog box contains check boxes for special character attributes, including Strikethrough, Hidden, and Small Caps. It also contains check boxes for Superscript and Subscript, which will reduce the size of text and position it a set distance above or below the *baseline* (the imaginary line upon which characters sit). To position the text a customized distance from the baseline, click the Character Spacing tab, and choose a distance from the By text box to the right of the Position text box.

Baseline
The imaginary line upon which characters sit.

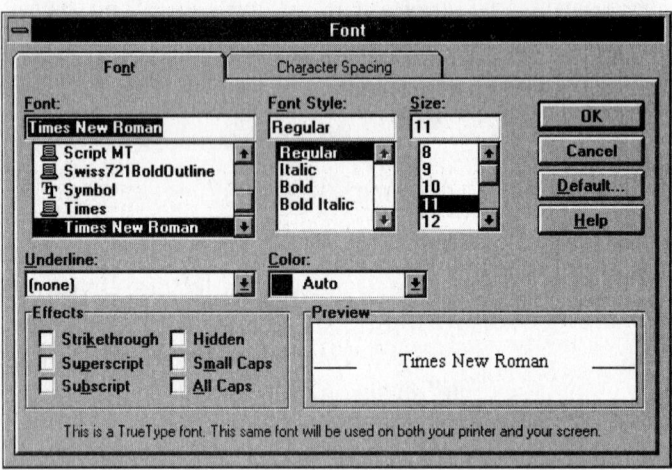

Figure 17-1
The Font dialog box

The Font dialog box also contains the Underline drop-down list box, which you can use to choose an underlining style. This lesson discusses the Words Only, Double, and Dotted options.

Use the Color drop-down list box to change the color in which the text appears.

The Sample box shows how text looks with the color, superscript or subscript options, and other character attributes that you specified. This lets you experiment with different colors, superscript or subscript options, and other attributes before you click OK to apply a character format.

To use the Font dialog box to apply special attributes:

1. Start Word, if necessary.

2. Open the file 17-0.doc. Be sure that Word is set to display hidden text. (Choose Options from the Tools menu, click the View tab to display view options, and then check the Hidden Text check box in the Nonprinting Characters option group.)

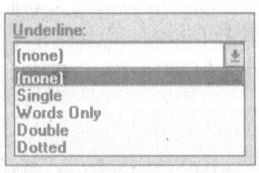

Underline options

Note: If the option All is checked in the Nonprinting Characters group, all the nonprinting characters listed above it will be displayed, including hidden text.

3. Select the "2" in "H20" at the end of the paragraph that begins "It was an unusually", and then choose Font from the Format menu to open the Font dialog box.

4. Click the Subscript checkbox to check it.

5. Click the Character Spacing tab. Choose Lowered from the Position box. Next to the Position by, click the down arrow to the right of the By box to change the subscript depth to 2 pt. Click OK.

6. Position the insertion point at the end of the paragraph that begins "The winners", press **Enter** twice, and key the following text as three tabbed columns that are left-aligned at 1.5, 3.25, and 5 inches:

Award	Name	Age
First Place	Jimmy Ferrini	22
Second Place	Fred Begey	31
Third Place	Juanita Hidalgo	29
Oldest Pedaler	Rick Lopez	48
Youngest Pedaler	Lucinda Parks	13

7. Apply the bold attribute to the first line keyed. Then select all the columnar text, and choose Font from the Format menu.

8. Click the Font tab, if necessary, check the Hidden check box in the Effects option group, and then click OK.

The selected text appears with dots under each line to indicate that it is hidden.

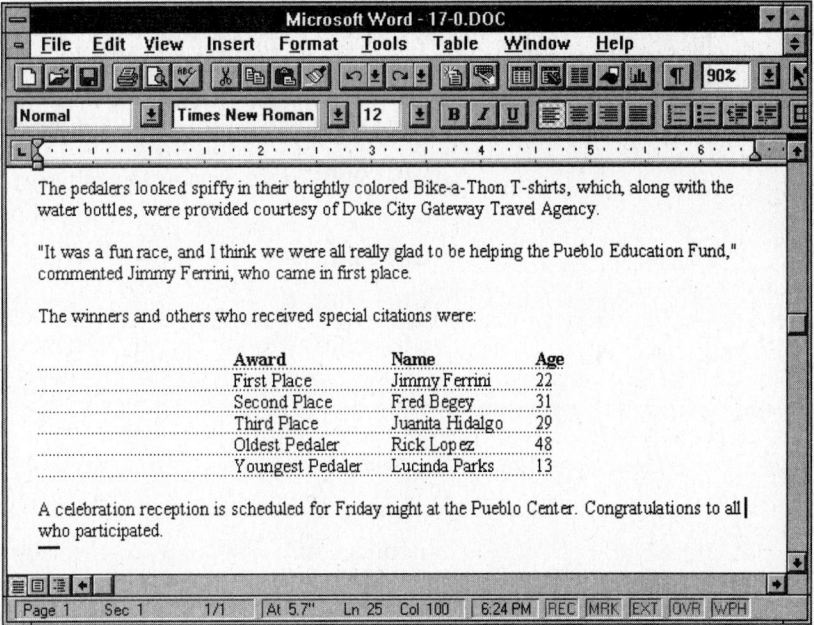

Figure 17-2
The document with hidden text

Note: Remember, by
unchecking the All option,
all nonprinting characters
disappear from the screen.

9. Turn off the Hidden Text option in the Options dialog box. If All was checked, uncheck it. Click OK.

   When the Options dialog box closes, the hidden text does not appear in the document.

Using Keyboard Shortcuts to Apply Special Attributes

You can use keyboard shortcuts to switch on or off most special character attributes. Using keyboard shortcuts to apply special attributes to new or existing text is generally faster than using the Font dialog box. However, when you use keyboard shortcuts for superscript or subscript text, you must use the default depth or height for the characters.

To use keyboard shortcuts to apply special character attributes:

1. Go to the beginning of the document. Press **Ctrl+Shift+K** to turn on the small-capitals option, key **Press Release Copy**, and press **Enter** twice.

   The text appears in small capitals.

2. Select the heading you just keyed, and press **Ctrl+Shift+D**.

   The selected text appears with double underlining.

PRESS RELEASE COPY

Small capitals and double
underlining

3. In the Options dialog box for viewing options, restore the All option under Nonprinting Characters.

Table 17-1: Keyboard Shortcuts for Special Character Attributes	
Keyboard Shortcut	Action
Ctrl+Shift+W	Turn on or off the words-only underline
Ctrl+Shift+D	Turn on or off double underlining
Ctrl+Shift+=	Turn on or off superscript
Ctrl+=	Turn on or off subscript
Ctrl+Shift+H	Turn on or off hidden text
Ctrl+Shift+K	Turn on or off small capitals
Ctrl+Shift+A	Turn on or off all capitals

What Are Symbols and Special Characters?

Special character
A character that does
not appear on a stan-
dard keyboard.

The fonts you use with Word have *special characters*, which are characters that do not appear on the keyboard. Special characters include letters, accent marks, punctuation marks, and other symbols from non-English alphabets, as well as many symbols used in English. For example, in Spanish, a question begins with an upside-down question

Note: Depending on the printer driver, some Word users may have the font ZapfDingbats instead of Wingdings. Both fonts consist entirely of special characters.

mark. This punctuation mark does not appear on most keyboards, but many fonts include it as a special character.

One of the fonts you can use with Word, which is called Wingdings, consists entirely of special characters, many of which are actually simple drawings. Another font, called Symbol, contains characters that are often used in technical documents. (Some of the characters in the Symbol font resemble those on the keyboard, but most are not used in everyday English documents.)

You can use special characters to enhance documents. For instance, the keyboard includes only one pair of double quotation marks ("), which are straight. Most of the time, you can use this character to open a quotation as well as to close it. Strictly speaking, however, the quotation marks that open a quote should be curled in one direction ("), and those that close a quote should curl in the opposite direction ("). If you are working on a document that requires these curled quotation marks, you can either insert them as special characters or use AutoCorrect to have Word insert them automatically.

Similarly, the only symbol on the keyboard that you can use for a dash is the hyphen (-). In some documents, however, it is important to distinguish between the *en dash*, which is about the same width as a hyphen, and the somewhat wider *em dash* (—). The em dash can be used in sentences where you would normally insert two dashes. Insert either en dashes or em dashes as special characters.

En dash
A special character that produces a dash about the width of a hyphen.

Em dash
A special character that produces a dash somewhat wider than a hyphen.

Inserting Symbols and Special Characters

There are three ways to insert symbols and special characters in documents:

- Using the Symbol command

- Using either pre-assigned keyboard shortcuts or keyboard shortcuts that you assign to insert the special characters manually

- Using the numeric keypad to insert the special characters manually

Using the Symbol Command to Insert Special Characters

You can use the Symbol command to insert special characters in the text you are keying. Choose Symbol from the Insert menu to display the Symbol dialog box.

The Symbol dialog box contains a Font drop-down list box that you can use to choose a font. It also contains a grid that includes all the characters available in the font you choose. Depending on the font, this grid might include characters that appear on the keyboard as well as special characters.

Insert
Break...
Page Numbers...
Annotation
Date and Time...
Field...
Symbol...
Form Field...

Footnote...
Caption...
Cross-reference...
Index and Tables...

File...
Frame
Picture...
Object...
Database...

Insert menu

Figure 17-3
The Symbol dialog box with Symbol font

Use the Font drop-down list box in the Symbol dialog box to choose the font that includes the symbols you want to insert. You can choose either the font you are currently using for normal text or fonts that contain mostly special characters.

The grid shows all the characters available in the chosen font. Some of the characters in the grid might appear too small for you to see them clearly. You can see an enlarged view of any character by clicking on it once with the left mouse button.

After you insert a special character, the only way to change its font is to select just the special character and then choose a different font for it. If you select the paragraph that contains the special character and then choose a different font for the paragraph, the font changes for the other text in the paragraph but not for the special character. However, the point size of the special character will change along with any other text you choose, and attributes such as bold, underline, or subscript that are applied to a selected block of text will be applied to any special characters in that block of text.

To choose a special character from the Symbol dialog box, position the insertion point where you want the special character to appear, and choose Symbol from the Insert menu to display the Symbol dialog box. Click the Symbols tab, if necessary, choose the font from the Font list box that contains the symbol you want to use, and double-click the symbol, or click the character once and click OK. You can also click the Special Characters tab and choose a symbol from the Character drop-down list box, which is a list of special characters that are used frequently.

To insert special characters using the Symbol dialog box:

1. Select " degrees" (including the space before it) in the first line of the paragraph that begins "It was an unusually".

2. Choose Symbol from the Insert menu.

   The Symbol dialog box appears.

3. Click the arrow to the right of the Font list box to display the Font drop-down list box, and then choose Symbol.

   The characters from the Symbol font appear in the grid.

4. Move the pointer to the degree sign (°), which is in the third row from the bottom of the grid, in the 5th box from the left.

5. Click the left mouse button.

   The box containing the degree sign appears enlarged. Remember, you can use this feature to be sure a special character is the one you want before you choose it.

6. Click Insert, and then click Close

   The dialog box closes, and the degree symbol appears in place of the text you selected in the document.

7. Click the insertion point immediately after the name "Trekker" in the paragraph that begins "It was an unusually".

8. Display the Symbol dialog box again with the Symbol font.

9. Double-click the trademark symbol (™) in the bottom row of the grid, in the 1st box from the left, and then click Close.

   The dialog box closes, and the trademark symbol appears in the document.

10. Move the insertion point immediately before the word "oldster" in the paragraph that begins "Special citations".

11. Choose Symbol from the Insert menu, and click the Special Characters tab.

12. Scroll down, and click Single Opening Quote. Click Insert, and then click Close.

13. Position the insertion point immediately after the word "oldster", and open the Symbol dialog box again.

14. Scroll down, and double-click Single Closing Quote. Then click Close.

15. Save the document as *[your three-letter identifier]*17-0.doc.

Using Keyboard Shortcuts to Insert Special Characters

Many of the symbols available from the Special Characters tab and some of the symbols available in the normal text font have been assigned shortcut keys, so that you can insert them into a document quickly.

To insert special characters using shortcut keys:

1. In the paragraph that begins "It was an unusually", select the text "--".

2. Press **Ctrl+Alt+-** (the minus sign on the numeric keypad).

   This is the keyboard shortcut for an em dash.

Using the Numeric Keypad to Insert Special Characters

If you know the code number for a special character, you can use the numeric keypad to insert the character in a document manually.

When using this method to insert a special character, press the **Alt** key and the character's code number, starting with zero. For example, in the Symbol font, character number 169 is a solid valentine shape (♥). With Symbol as the current font, you can turn on the numeric keypad and then press **Alt+0169** to insert this special character. (Remember, press the **Num Lock** key to turn the numeric keypad on or off.)

If you use this method to insert a symbol and then change the font for the text that contains it, the font for the symbol also changes. For example, if you use the keyboard shortcut **Alt+0169** when the current font is Symbol, the valentine heart appears. If you then change the text's font to Courier New, the copyright sign (©) replaces the symbol, because the copyright sign is character code number 169 in the Courier New font. Therefore, you should not use keyboard shortcuts to insert special characters if the font is likely to change and you do not want the characters to change at that time.

To insert special characters using the numeric keypad:

1. Open the file *[your three-letter identifier]*17-0.doc.

2. Select the em dash after the word "day" in the paragraph that begins "It was an unusually".

3. If necessary, turn on the numeric keypad (press the **Num Lock** key).

4. Press **Alt+0151**.

    An em dash is inserted.

5. Select the quotation marks at the beginning of the paragraph that begins "It was a fun".

6. Press **Alt+0147**.

    Curled open quotation marks are inserted.

7. Select the quotation marks at the end of the same quote, and then press **Alt+0148**.

    Curled closed quotation marks are inserted.

8. Save the document, and then print it.

9. Close the document and exit Word (unless you will be doing the following exercises immediately).

Table 17-2: Sample Characters and Code Numbers in the Symbol Font							
£	163	←	172	•	183	™	212
¥	165	↑	173	≠	185	√	214
ƒ	166	→	174	≡	186	⇔	219
♣	167	↓	175	≈	187	⇐	220
♦	168	°	176	…	188	⇑	221
♥	169	±	177	∅	198	⇒	222
♠	170	"	178	®	210	⇓	223
↔	171	≥	179	©	211	◊	224

Character Map

Character Map icon

Note: To find out the code numbers of additional characters not included in the table, minimize the Word window, and double-click the Character Map icon in the Windows Accessories group. Choose a font from the Character Map dialog box. When you click a character, its code number appears in the bottom, right corner of the dialog box.

Table 17-3: Keyboard Shortcuts for Special Characters and Attributes	
Keyboard Shortcut	Action
Ctrl+Shift+W	Turn on or off the words-only underline
Ctrl+Shift+D	Turn on or off double underlining
Ctrl+Shift+=	Turn on or off superscript
Ctrl+=	Turn on or off subscript
Ctrl+Shift+H	Turn on or off hidden text
Ctrl+Shift+K	Turn on or off small capitals
Ctrl+Shift+A	Turn on or off all capitals
Ctrl+Alt+-	Insert an em dash
Ctrl+`+"	Insert opening quotation marks
Ctrl+'+"	Insert closing quotation marks

Key Terms

Baseline

Em dash

En dash

Hidden text

Special character

Strikethrough

Subscript

Superscript

Exercises

Exercise 17.1

1. Start Word, if necessary.

2. Open the file 17-1.doc.

3. At the end of the paragraph that begins "B. Baggage Delay", apply the strikethrough attribute to the text "other than your residence":

    A. Select the text, and then choose Font from the Format menu.

    B. In the Font dialog box, check the Strikethrough checkbox in the Effects options group, and then click OK.

4. Apply the strikethrough attribute to the word "Terms" (excluding the colon) in the next paragraph.

5. With the insertion point after the strikethrough text and before the colon, change the text color to blue:

    A. Open the Font dialog box.

    B. Choose Blue from the Color drop-down list box.

    C. Uncheck Strikethrough, and click OK.

    D. Key **Conditions**

6. In the same paragraph, change the short dashes to em dashes using the keyboard shortcut:

    A. Select the short dashes after "authorities".

    B. Press the **Num Lock** key to turn on the numeric keypad, if necessary.

    C. Press **Ctrl+Alt+-** (the minus key on the numeric keypad).

    D. Substitute an em dash for the short dashes after "management" (use the Repeat command, the **F4** key).

7. Use the keyboard shortcut to apply double underlining to the title of the document:

    A. Select the title.

    B. Press **Ctrl+Shift+D**.

8. Use the keyboard shortcut to apply small capitals to the phrase "A. Baggage Loss or Damage:":

    A. Select the text.

    B. Press **Ctrl+Shift+K**.

9. Repeat this formatting for the text "B. Baggage Delay" in the next paragraph.

10. Spell-check the document, and save it as *[your three-letter identifier]*17-1.doc.

11. Print the document.

12. Close the document and exit Word (unless you will be doing the following exercises immediately).

Exercise 17.2

1. Start Word, if necessary.

2. Open the file 17-2.doc.

3. Change the format of the heading "July 199-" on both pages of the document so that it appears in bold, 16-point small capitals, with no underline.

4. Apply the double-underline attributes to each date label, starting with "Monday **5**".

5. Insert a stamped envelope symbol at the beginning of the line under "Tuesday **6**":

   A. Move the insertion point to the left of the tab character under "Tuesday **6**", and then choose Symbol from the Insert menu.

   B. In the Symbols dialog box, choose Wingdings from the Font drop-down list box.

   C. Move the pointer to the 12th box from the left in the top line of the grid. Click the left mouse button to view an enlargement of the symbol.

   D. Double-click the symbol to insert it in the document, and then click Close.

6. Insert a telephone symbol under "Thursday **8**", to the left of the tab character. Use the Wingdings font. The telephone symbol is in the 9th box from the left in the top row of the grid.

7. Insert an airplane symbol at the beginning of the first line under "Friday **9**" using the Wingdings font. The airplane symbol is the 7th box from the right in the 2nd row of the grid.

8. Press the **Tab** key, turn off the bold attribute, and then key **6:50 a.m., SWA flight 210 to Dallas**

9. Insert a right-pointing arrow symbol from the Symbol font at the beginning of the next line.

10. Press the **Tab** key, and then key **11:30 a.m., Bill Parret, SGC, Inc.**

11. Spell-check the document, and save it as *[your three-letter identifier]*17-2.doc.

12. Print the document.

13. Close the document and exit Word (unless you will be doing the following exercises immediately).

Exercise 17.3

1. Start Word, if necessary.

2. Open the file 17-3.doc.

3. Format the document as a business memo to Ed Micali from Frank Murillo. The subject is: The London/Paris Trip. Insert the date as a field.

4. In the third line below the memo heading, change "1 pound" to "£1", using the currency symbol for the pound from the normal text font.

5. On the next line, change "1/2" to the special character "½" from the normal text font.

6. In the next line, change "5 pounds" to "£5", using the pound symbol again from the normal text font.

7. In the line after "In Paris:", change "5 francs" to "5*f*" using the franc symbol from the normal text font.

8. In the next line, replace the word "francs" and the space that precedes it with the franc symbol by keying **Alt+0131**.

9. In the next line, replace "francs" and the space that precedes it with the franc symbol.

10. Spell-check the document, and then add your reference initials.

11. Save the document as *[your three-letter identifier]*17-3.doc and print it.

12. Close the document and exit Word (unless you will be doing the following exercise immediately).

Exercise 17.4: Challenge Yourself

Create a new document using 12-point type. Key the text in the figure that appears at the end of this exercise, including the corrections. Use single-spacing. Where extra line spacing is indicated in the figure (for example, after "Year-End Report"), insert an extra blank line.

Right-align the numerical text after "Sales" and "Expenses" at a 2.5-inch right tab setting. Change the first two lines to bold small capitals, and change the third, fifth, and seventh lines of text to small capitals. Change the fourth, sixth, and eighth lines of text to hidden text.

In each of the two lines that start with "Sales", replace the "+" with the hollow up arrow (⇑) from the Symbol font. In each of the two lines that start with "Expenses", replace the "-" with the hollow down arrow (⇓) from the Symbol font. Make sure there is a space character after and a tab character before the arrow symbols.

From the third line of text to the end of the document, change the spacing to 1.5 lines after each paragraph. Add an extra blank line under "Year-End Report", and then change the top margin of the document to 2 inches.

Spell-check the document, save it as *[your three-letter identifier]* 17-4.doc, and print it. Close the document and exit Word.

Figure 17-4

Duke City Gateway Travel

Year-End Report

Total Travel Sales

(insert year-end sales figures here)

Operating Expenses

(insert expense chart here)

Income

(show figures and calculate difference here)

Difference Between 1993 and 1994

Sales   + 24%

Expenses   - 3%

Difference Between 1992 and 1994

Sales   + 29%

Expenses   - 10%

An Advertisement

Background

Each year, the Albuquerque Chamber of Commerce asks Duke City Gateway to submit an advertisement for publication in the annual Albuquerque Vacation Guide. The Albuquerque Vacation Guide is distributed to local hotels, restaurants, travel agencies, and tourist information centers. It is also sent to people who request information directly from the Chamber of Commerce.

This year, Duke City Gateway is submitting an advertisement that highlights its special-interest tours.

Business Purpose

Create an advertisement for Duke City Gateway to submit to the Albuquerque Chamber of Commerce for the Albuquerque Vacation Guide.

The ad is in landscape orientation. It lists the special-interest tours and creates an interesting format for them.

Procedures

1. Create a new document.

2. Change the page orientation to landscape, change the left and right margins to 1.75 inches, and change the page layout to vertically centered alignment.

3. Key the text shown in Figure 17-5, which appears at the end of this project.

4. Use the Formatting toolbar to change the headline, which begins "Make Your Next Vacation", to:

   Font: Helvetica
   Size: 26 point
   Font Style: Bold
   Alignment: Center

5. Use the keyboard shortcut to reduce the point size of the headline to 24 point.

6. Use the Formatting toolbar to change the next sentence, which begins "Duke City Gateway Travel Agency", to:

   Font: Palatino (or a similar font, such as Times New Roman)
   Size: 12 point

7. Use the Font dialog box to change the tour names to:

   Font: Palatino (or Times New Roman)
   Size: 18 point
   Font Style: Bold
   Character spacing: Condensed

8. Press **Shift+Enter** after "Naturalist", center-align the tour names, and change the line spacing before and after the paragraph to 6pt.

9. Use the Font dialog box to change the paragraph beginning with "Travelers of all" to:

   Font: Helvetica
   Size: 14 point

10. Center the paragraph, and then add a 2¼-point, single-line box border and 20% shading to it.

11. Use the Font dialog box to change the paragraph that begins "Duke City Gateway Travel Agency will organize" to:

    Font: Palatino (or Times New Roman)
    Size: 12 point

12. Change the remaining lines of text, which are "Duke City Gateway Travel Agency" and "Your Gateway to the World", to:

    Font: Palatino (or Times New Roman)
    Size: 16 point
    Font Style: Bold, Small Caps
    Character Spacing: Expanded 1pt
    Alignment: Center

13. Use the Borders toolbar to insert a bottom border under "Duke City Gateway Travel Agency". Use a ¾ pt line.

14. Use the Insert menu to insert the ♦ (diamond) symbol between each tour name (use the Symbol font), and leave one blank space on each side of the symbol.

15. Insert a Registered Trademark (®) symbol after "Your Gateway to the World".

16. Use the keyboard to make the symbol superscript.

17. Add another blank line after the title, and then make any changes you feel would improve the appearance of the document.

18. Spell-check the document, and save it as *[your three letter identifier]*p6-1.doc.

19. Print the document.

20. Close the document and exit Word.

Tips and Hints

• Since advertisements in many publications are competing for the readers' attention, use an interesting headline. To make a headline interesting, ask the reader a question, or announce news about a product or service.

• Readers must be able to understand the message in an advertisement; therefore, keep the copy in your advertisements short and readable.

• In addition to an attention-grabbing headline, the visual elements in an advertisement are important. Use borders, symbols, and different character styles to add interest.

• The purpose of an advertisement is to sell something to a consumer. For this reason, it is important to target the advertisement for a specific audience and to make sure the advertisement is placed in an appropriate publication.

Figure 17-5

Make Your Next Vacation An Adventure!

Duke City Gateway Travel Agency offers local and international special-interest tours for the adventurous traveler, including:

Architecture Archaeological Photography Cycling Naturalist Safari
Bird-watching Hiking Camping Food and Wine Music

Travelers of all ages seek out special-interest tours, and there's a
tour to suit every interest. Whether it's food and wine, sports, ar-
chaeology, bird-watching, or music, Duke City Gateway Travel has a
tour for you.

Duke City Gateway Travel will organize any special-interest tour for
you. For 25 years, our customers have relied on us for all their
travel needs. Duke City Gateway Travel is one of a network of travel
agencies, with 50 offices worldwide. We are a full-service travel
agency with a highly qualified and dedicated staff, and we do not
charge fees for our services. For further information, please call us
weekdays from 9 a.m. to 5 p.m. at (505) 555-1234.

Duke City Gateway Travel Agency

Your Gateway to the World

Tables and Columns

Working with Tables

Table
A grid of columns and rows that contains information.

Cell
The intersection of a column and a row in a table.

Very often, information is easier to read in table format than in paragraph format. Lesson 6 explains how to create simple tables using tabs. This lesson describes Word's powerful table feature and the flexibility it offers in creating and editing tables.

What Are Tables?

A *table* is a grid of rows and columns that contains information in the form of text or pictures. Columns are vertical, and rows are horizontal. Columns and rows intersect to form *cells*.

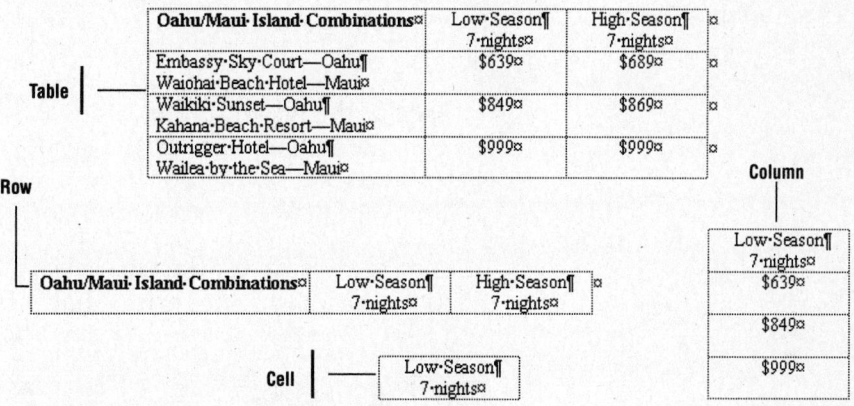

Figure 18-1
Columns, rows, and cells in a table

After creating a table, you can insert text or pictures in the cells. You can then add, delete, and change the sizes of cells, rows, and columns. When first creating a table, format it to accommodate the text you want to insert. After the table is created, you can experiment to find the most satisfactory widths for columns and heights for rows.

Creating Tables for New Text

There are two ways to create a table:

- Use the Table menu.

- Use the Insert Table button on the Standard toolbar.

Using the Table Menu to Create Tables

When you choose Insert Table from the Table menu, Word displays the Insert Table dialog box.

Figure 18-2
The Insert Table dialog box

To specify the number of columns in the table, key the number in the Number of Columns text box, or click the up or down arrow to the right of the box.

To specify the number of rows in the table, key the number in the Number of Rows text box, or click the up or down arrow to the right of the box.

To specify the width of the columns, key the number of inches per column in the Column Width text box, or click the up or down arrow to the right of the box. If the word "Auto" is chosen, Word will set the column width automatically.

To specify a format for the table, click the AutoFormat button. Word displays the Table AutoFormat dialog box.

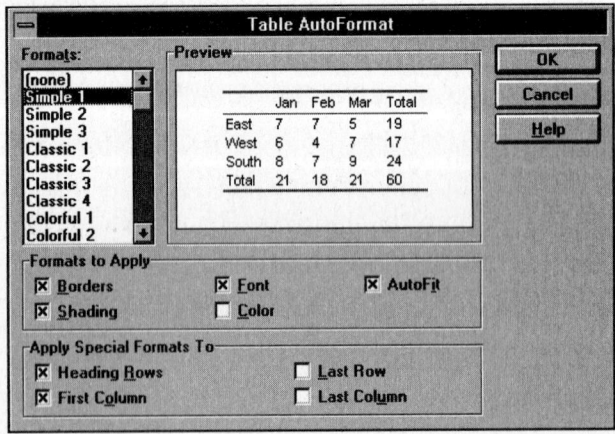

Figure 18-3
The Table AutoFormat dialog box

You can choose a predefined format from the Formats list box. The predefined formats change depending on what you choose for the Formats to Apply option and the Apply Special Formats To option. The Preview area shows you how the table will look.

To create both the layout and format of the table automatically, click the Wizard button. Word displays the Table Wizard dialog box. The Table Wizard is covered later in this lesson.

Gridlines
Lines that mark the boundaries of cells in a table.

You can display tables with or without *gridlines*, which are lines that mark the boundaries of the cells. Turn the gridlines option on or off from the Table menu. The default is gridlines on.

To use the Table menu to create a table:

1. Start Word, if necessary.

2. Create a new document using the Normal template.

3. Open the Table menu, and make sure Gridlines is checked.

4. Choose Insert Table from the Table menu to display the Insert Table dialog box.

5. Key **3** in the Number of Columns text box.

6. Key **13** in the Number of Rows text box.

7. Choose Auto in the Column Width box, if necessary.

   Word will adjust the column widths automatically. You can also indicate a specific column width by keying the column width in inches in the Column Width text box.

8. Click AutoFormat to display the Table AutoFormat dialog box.

9. Choose Classic 4 from the Formats list box, and then click OK to close the dialog box.

10. Click OK to close the Insert Table dialog box.

    The table appears, with gridlines showing cells arranged in 3 columns and 13 rows. The insertion point is in the first cell. Markers indicating the right margin of each column appear on the ruler.

11. Choose Gridlines from the Table menu to turn off the gridlines option.

    The space for the table remains in the document, but the gridlines do not.

12. Close the document without saving it.

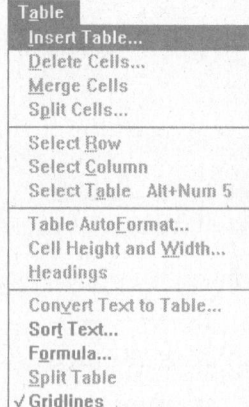

Table menu

Using the Toolbar to Create Tables

Instead of using the Table menu to create a table, you can use the Insert Table button on the Standard toolbar.

When you click the Insert Table button, a grid appears below the button. When the grid first appears, it contains five columns and four rows. You can, however, move the pointer beyond the grid's right margin to specify more columns or below its bottom margin to create more rows. To specify the number of columns and rows for

Insert Table button

Insert Table button with grid

6 x 3 Table

Specifying the number of rows and columns

the table, hold down the left mouse button, and move the pointer to highlight rows and columns.

When you move the pointer to highlight rows and columns, the dimensions of the table appear below the grid. For example, if you highlight six rows and three columns, "6 x 3 Table" appears below the grid. "Cancel" appears below the grid if no rows or columns are chosen.

To use the Standard toolbar to create tables:

1. Create a new document, and change the font to 12 point.

2. Open the Table menu, and make sure Gridlines is checked.

3. Click the Insert Table button on the Standard toolbar to display the table grid.

4. Position the pointer in the upper left cell of the grid.

5. Drag the pointer through six rows and three columns of the grid to create a 6 by 3 table, and then release the mouse button.

   The gridlines for the table appear, and the insertion point is in the first cell.

Keying and Editing Text in Tables

Keying and editing text in a cell in a table is much the same as working with text in paragraphs. Position the insertion point in the cell, and then key text or edit it using the **Insert**, **Delete**, or **Enter** keys. Keep in mind that **Enter** creates a new paragraph within a cell; it does not move the insertion point to the next cell.

To move the insertion point within a table, use the Arrow keys as you would with text outside tables. You can also use the following keyboard shortcuts to move from one cell to another:

Table 18-1: Shortcuts for Moving Between Cells	
To Move To	Press
Next cell	**Tab**
Previous cell	**Shift+Tab**
First cell in the current row	**Alt+Home**
Last cell in the current row	**Alt+End**
Top cell in the current column	**Alt+PgUp**
Last cell in the current column	**Alt+PgDn**

To key and edit text in a table:

1. In the first cell of the first row, key **$ Equals:**

2. Press the **Down Arrow** key to move the insertion point to the first cell in the next row. Key **Britain**

3. Press the **Tab** key to go to the next cell, and then key **pound**

4. Press the **Tab** key to go to the next cell, and then key **0.52**

5. Key the following lines of text in the remaining rows of the table, inserting each word or number in a different cell:

France	**franc**	**5.32**
Germany	**mark**	**1.51**
Greece	**drachma**	**177**
Italy	**lira**	**1,137**

Remember, press the **Tab** key to move to the next cell, and press **Shift+Tab** to move to the previous cell. Do not press **Enter**, because that will create a new paragraph within a cell.

6. Press **Alt+Home** to move to the first cell in the last row.

7. Press **Shift+Tab** to move to the third cell in the previous row. Change the text to "179".

8. Change the text in the cell beneath it to "1,137.00".

9. Go to the first cell in the first column (press **Alt+Home**, then **Alt+PgUp**). After "$", key **1**

Selecting Cells, Rows, and Columns

There are several ways to select the contents of cells, rows, and columns. Once selected, you can delete, copy, or move the contents. You can also change the format of the contents.

End-of-Cell and End-of-Row Markers

End-of-cell marker
A character within each cell in a table that indicates the end of that cell's contents.

End-of-row marker
A character to the right of the gridline for each row in a table that indicates the end of that row.

To help you select the contents within cells and rows, an *end-of-cell marker* (¤) indicates the end of each cell in a table, and a similar *end-of-row marker* (¤) indicates the end of each row in a table. (The character representing the end-of-cell and end-of-row markers may be different on your screen.)

The end-of-cell markers appear at the end of the contents in each cell. The end-of-row markers appear to the right of the gridline of each row.

End-of-cell   End-of-row
marker   marker

¤	¤
0.52¤	¤
5.32¤	¤
1.51¤	¤
179¤	¤
1,137.00¤	¤

Table markers

Note: The end-of-cell and end-of-row markers appear when Word's view options are set to display all nonprinting characters or paragraph marks. To display the end-of-cell and end-of-row markers, choose Options from the Tools menu. From the View tab, check the All check box under Nonprinting Characters.

Selection Bars

Lesson 2 explains how to use the selection bar to select a line or paragraph. In a table, each cell, row, and column has its own selection bar.

A *cell selection bar* is the unmarked area between a cell's left gridline and the left margin of the cell's text. A *row selection bar* is the area outside the left edge of the table. Actually, it is the same as the selection bar for the document. A *column selection bar* is an unmarked horizontal bar above the top border of the table. The pointer becomes a small, solid arrow when it is in the column selection bar.

Cell selection bar
The unmarked area between a cell's left gridline and the left margin of the cell's text used to select that cell and its contents.

Row selection bar
The area outside the left edge of a table used to select a row in that table.

Column selection bar
The unmarked horizontal bar above the top border of a table used to select a column in that table.

Figure 18-4
Pointing at the selection bar to select a cell, row, and column

Selecting Cells

You can select just the text or graphics within a cell, or you can select the entire cell, including its contents and end-of-cell marker. There are three ways to select a cell:

• Click the cell's selection bar.

  The contents and end-of-cell marker are highlighted.

• Drag the mouse pointer over the cell's contents.

  Only the cell's contents, not the end-of-cell marker, are highlighted.

• Press the **Tab** key to move to a cell.

  Only the cell's contents, not the end-of-cell marker, are highlighted.

To select cells:

1. If necessary, modify the view settings to display the end-of-cell markers.

2. Click the cell selection bar for the second cell in the second row.

   The entire cell, including the contents and end-of-cell marker, is highlighted.

3. Move the pointer so that it is over the "5" in "5.32" in the third cell in the third row. The pointer becomes an insertion point. Drag the insertion point over the text and the end-of-cell marker. Then release the mouse button.

   The cell's contents, but not the end-of-cell marker, are highlighted.

4. Press the **Tab** key twice to go to the second cell in the fourth row.

   Word highlights the text in the cell, but not the end-of-cell marker.

Selecting Rows

You can use any of these methods to select a row:

- Click the selection bar to the left of the row.

- Double-click the selection bar of any cell in the row.

- Position the insertion point anywhere in the row, and then choose Select Row from the Table menu.

- Position the insertion point at the beginning of the row, and then drag it to the end of the row.

- Drag the pointer down the selection bar to select several consecutive rows.

To select rows:

1. Click the selection bar to the left of the first row.

2. Double-click the selection bar for the second cell in the second row.

3. Position the insertion point anywhere in the word "mark" in the fourth row.

4. Choose Select Row from the Table menu.

5. Position the pointer in the selection bar outside the left edge of the row that begins "Greece", and then drag the pointer down to select that row and the next row.

Selecting Columns

Use any of these methods to select a column:

- Click the selection bar above the column.

- Position the insertion point in the first cell of the column, and drag it to the last cell.

- Position the insertion point in the column, press the **Alt** key, and click the left mouse button.

- Position the insertion point anywhere in the column, and choose Select Column from the Table menu.

- Drag the pointer across the column selection bar above the columns to select several consecutive columns.

To select columns:

1. Click the selection bar above the first column.

2. Position the insertion point in the first cell of the second column, and drag it to the last cell in the column.

3. Position the insertion point in the second column, and choose Select Column from the Table menu.

4. Position the pointer in the selection bar above the second column, and drag it to the third column.

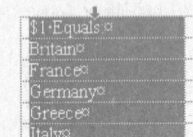

Selecting the first column

Selecting an Entire Table

There are two ways to select an entire table:

- Position the insertion point anywhere in the table, and choose Select Table from the Table menu.

- Position the insertion point anywhere in the table, and press **Alt+5** on the numeric keypad.

To select a table:

1. Position the insertion point anywhere in the table.

2. Choose Select Table from the Table menu.

3. Click the pointer anywhere in the table to deselect it.

4. Turn off Num Lock, if necessary, and then press **Alt+5** on the numeric keypad.

5. Click the pointer anywhere in the table to deselect it.

Note: Num Lock should be turned off before pressing **Alt+5** on the numeric keypad.

Editing Table Structures

In addition to editing the text and graphics in tables, you can edit the structure of tables. For example, you can add, delete, move, and copy rows, columns, and cells. You can also merge and split cells, change a table's position, and change a table's column spacing, column width, and row height.

Inserting Cells, Rows, and Columns

To add cells to a table, select the cells where you want to add new cells, and then choose Insert Cells from the Table menu (or click the Insert Cells button on the Standard toolbar). Word adds new cells to the left of or above the selected cells, depending on whether you click the Shift Cells Right or Shift Cells Down option button in the Insert Cells dialog box. Be sure to select the same number of cells you want to add.

Figure 18-5
The Insert Cells dialog box

To add a row to the end of a table, position the insertion point in the last cell of the table, and press the **Tab** key. You can also position the insertion point at the beginning of the first line below the table, and choose Insert Rows from the Table menu (or click the Insert Rows button on the Standard toolbar) to open the Insert Rows dialog box.

Figure 18-6
The Insert Rows dialog box

To add rows above existing rows, select the number of existing rows you want to add, including the end-of-row marker for each of the rows. Choose Insert Rows from the Table menu.

To add columns to the left of existing columns, select the number of existing columns you want to add. Choose Insert Columns from the Table menu, or click the Insert Columns button on the Standard toolbar.

To add columns to the right of the table, position the insertion point to the right of the table's first row, outside the gridline, and select the end-of-row markers for the table. Choose Insert Column from the Table menu, or click the Insert Columns button.

To add cells, columns, and rows to a table:

1. Move the insertion point to the beginning of the first cell in the second row, and drag it to the end of the second cell in the third row. Release the mouse button.

    The first two cells in the second and third rows are highlighted (from "Britain" through "franc").

2. Choose Insert Cells from the Table menu to display the Insert Cells dialog box, and then click Shift Cells Down. Click OK.

    The first two cells in the second and third rows move down to make room for four new cells. The cells in the third column do not shift down.

3. Select the row under "$1 Equals", and then click the Insert Rows button (the former Insert Table button).

    A new row appears above the selected row.

4. Select the second column, and then choose Insert Columns from the Table menu.

    A new column appears to the left of the column you selected.

5. Move the insertion point to the cell in the table's bottom right corner, and then press the **Tab** key.

    A new row appears, with the insertion point in its first cell.

6. Select the end-of-row marker of the table's first row.

7. Choose Insert Cells from the Table menu, and then click Insert Entire Column. Click OK.

    A fifth column appears at the right of the table.

8. Move the insertion point to the left of the paragraph mark below the table, and then choose Insert Rows from the Table menu.

9. In the Insert Rows dialog box, key **2** in the Number of Rows text box, and then click OK.

    Two new rows appear at the bottom of the table.

Deleting Cells, Rows, and Columns

You can delete cells, rows, and columns from a table by selecting them and then deleting them. You can also delete the contents of a table by highlighting the table and pressing the **Delete** key. The **Delete** key only deletes what is within the table, not the table's cells, rows, or columns.

When you delete cells, you also have to choose an option from the Delete Cells dialog box for adjusting the positions of the remaining cells. The options are to shift the remaining cells up or left or to delete an entire row or column.

Figure 18-7
The Delete Cells dialog box

To delete cells, rows, and columns:

1. Select the last row of the table, which contains no text, and then choose Delete Rows from the Table menu.

    Word deletes the row.

2. Select the first three cells in the third and fourth rows. Choose Delete Cells from the Table menu.

3. In the Delete Cells dialog box, click Shift Cells Up, and then click OK.

4. Select the second column, and then choose Delete Columns from the Table menu.

    Word removes the selected column.

Moving and Copying Cells, Rows, and Columns

You can move and copy cells and their contents to other cells using the same methods for moving and copying text presented in Lesson 8.

Note: It is a good idea to save your table before you begin to cut and copy text.

To move or copy cells, select them, including their contents and end-of-cell markers, copy or cut them, and then paste them elsewhere in the table. Be aware, however, that pasting cells into a table will replace entire cells, possibly overwriting contents you want to keep. A safe way to copy or move contents to new cells is first to use the Insert Cells command to add empty cells, and then to paste the cut or copied cells into the empty cells.

To move and copy cells, rows, and columns:

1. Save the document as *[your three-letter identifier]*18-0a.doc.

2. Select the row that begins "Britain", drag it to the empty row above it, and release the mouse button.

3. Select the row that begins "France", but not its end-of-row marker, and click the Cut button.

    The text is deleted from the cells. If you had selected the end-of-row marker, the entire row would have been deleted.

4. Move the insertion point to the row under "Britain", and choose Paste Cells from the Edit menu. (Make sure the current cell is not selected.)

Note: If you paste text to a position on the table where there is not enough room for all the cells, Word adds additional columns or rows to accommodate the text.

5. Select all the cells with numerical text in the third column, and then click the Copy button.

6. Move the insertion point to the cell in the second row of the last column. Click the Paste button.

7. Select and delete the third column.

8. Select all the columnar text from "Britain" to "1,137.00", and click the Cut button.

9. Move the insertion point to the first cell in the third row, and paste the text. Delete the remaining blank rows.

Merging and Splitting Cells

You can merge several cells into one row to create a single cell. For example, you might want to merge the cells in a row that contains a heading, so that the heading spans several rows. You can also merge cells in more than one row at once.

When you merge cells, Word substitutes a paragraph mark for each end-of-cell marker. After you merge cells, you can split them if you have not deleted the paragraph marks.

To merge and split cells:

1. Select all the cells in the first row of the table, and then choose Merge Cells from the Table menu.

   The heading "$1 Equals:" appears in a single cell that spans all three columns of the table. The heading is converted to a paragraph, and paragraph marks appear where the cells have been merged.

2. Select the cells that contain "Britain" and "pound", and then choose Merge Cells from the Table menu.

   The selected cells are merged to create one cell.

3. With the same cell selected, choose Split Cells from the Table menu.

   Word displays the Split Cells dialog box. You can split the selection back into the original number of cells or more.

4. Make sure the number of columns is 2, and then click OK.

   The cells are restored to two separate cells.

Positioning Tables

In general, if a table appears on a page with text, position the table by centering it horizontally. If a table appears on a page by itself, center it horizontally and vertically. To position tables horizontally, use the Cell Height and Width dialog box.

Figure 18-8
The Cell Height and Width dialog box

To position the table:

1. Select the table, and then choose Cell Height and Width from the Table menu.

2. Click the Row tab, if necessary.

3. Click the Center option button under Alignment and click OK.

    The table is centered between the left and right margins.

To position a table vertically, choose Page Setup from the File menu, click the Layout tab, and choose Center from the Vertical Alignment drop-down list box.

Changing Table Dimensions

In a table, you can change the width of the columns and the height of the rows. When you change the width of a column, the width of all columns to the right are adjusted in proportion to their original width, and the size of the table does not change. You can also change the width of a single cell. To do this, key the dimensions of column and cell widths and of row heights in inches.

To change the width of columns and height of rows in the table:

1. Select the entire table, and then choose Cell Height and Width from the Table menu.

2. Click the Column tab, and key **2** in the Width of Columns text box.

3. Key **.5** in the Space Between Columns text box and click OK.

    The width of each column decreases to 2 inches, and the spacing between the columns' contents and gridlines increases to ½ inch.

4. Select all but the first row of the table, and then choose Cell Height and Width from the Table menu.

5. Click the Row tab. Set the Height of Rows 2–6 to At Least, and set the measurement to 24 points (pt). Click OK.

The height of each row increases to at least 24 points, which is two lines.

To change the width of a cell:

1. Select the cell that contains "Greece". Position the pointer on the gridline to the right of the cell.

    The pointer changes to a two-headed horizontal arrow.

2. Drag the gridline to the right about 1 inch. Release the mouse button.

    The width of the single cell changes.

3. Click the Undo button to restore the cell's original width.

Use these shortcuts to change the width of a column:

Pointer as two-headed arrow

Dragging the guideline to resize a column

*   To change the width of a column, position the pointer on the gridline to the right of the column you want to resize. The mouse pointer changes to a two-headed horizontal arrow. Drag the gridline to the desired width, and release the mouse button.

*   To change the column width and the width of the next column to the right (so that the column to the right is not adjusted in proportion to its original width), position the pointer on the gridline to the right of the column you want to resize. The mouse pointer changes to a double-headed horizontal arrow. Hold down the **Shift** key as you drag the gridline to the desired width. Release the **Shift** key and the mouse button.

*   To change the column width and make all columns to the right equal, position the pointer on the gridline to the right of the column you want to resize. The mouse pointer changes to a double-headed horizontal arrow. Hold down the **Ctrl** key as you drag the gridline to the desired width. Release the **Ctrl** key and the mouse button.

Column marker

Ruler

*   To change the column width using the ruler, drag the small square column marker from the ruler above the column's right gridline to a new position in the ruler. Release the mouse button.

Formatting Cell Contents

Format characters and paragraphs in cells within tables the same way you format text outside of tables. For example, you can center column headings in a table and make them bold. You can also add tabs within a cell by pressing **Ctrl+Tab**.

To format text in a cell:

1. Select the cell in the top row of the table.

2. Click the Bold and the Center buttons on the Formatting toolbar.

    The text appears centered and bold.

Using Borders and Shading with Tables

Like other text, tables can have borders and shading. You can apply borders and shading to a single cell, a group of cells, or an entire table.

To apply borders and shading to a table:

1. Select the first cell again, and choose Borders and Shading from the Format menu.

2. In the Cell Borders and Shading dialog box, click the Borders tab, if necessary.

3. Click Box in the Preset options group.

    If you select a table or a group of cells, choose the Box or Shadow Preset option. If you select one cell, choose Box.

4. Click the 2¼-point line in the Style box. Then click the Shading tab.

5. Choose 20% from the Shading list box and click OK.

6. Deselect the row.

    The row appears with a box border and shading.

7. Save the document.

Using Table Wizard and Table AutoFormat

The Table Wizard gives you a fast and easy way to create a table, complete with layout and format. Choose Insert Table from the Table menu, and then click the Wizard button. The Table Wizard prompts you for information and automatically creates the table you specify.

To use the Table Wizard to create a new table with layout and format options:

1. Create a new document, and choose Insert Table from the Table menu to display the Insert Table dialog box.

2. Click the Wizard button to open the Table Wizard dialog box. See Figure 18-9 on page 358.

3. Choose Style 4, and click the Next button.

    The Table Wizard asks how many columns you want.

4. Specify 5 columns, and then click the Next button.

    The Table Wizard asks about column headings.

5. Choose Repeat headings and Left align, and then click the Next button.

    The Table Wizard asks you to specify row headings.

Figure 18-9
The Table Wizard dialog box

6. Choose Quarters for the row headings, and then click the Next button.

7. In the next dialog box, choose Center for the row-heading alignment, and click the Next button.

   The next dialog box asks you to specify the content of the table cells.

8. Choose Numbers: aligned on decimal, and then click the Next button.

9. Choose Portrait for the page orientation, and then click the Next button.

   The last Table Wizard dialog box asks if you want to display Help after the table is created.

10. Choose No, click the Finish button, and then click OK to close the Table AutoFormat dialog box.

    Word displays the completed table in the layout and format you specified.

11. In the first row, merge both cells to make one single cell, and then key the following text in the table:

    3-Year Revenue (in millions)

Quarters	1992	1993	1994	Total
Q 1	37.4	42.8	40.8	
Q 2	33.1	39.1	39.0	
Q 3	33.0	39.0	37.5	
Q 4	38.7	41.6	39.2	

12. Save the new document as *[your three-letter identifier]*18-0b.doc.

The Table AutoFormat command on the Table menu lets you apply predefined layout and format options to an existing table automatically.

To use the Table AutoFormat command for an existing table:

1. Switch to *[your three-letter identifier]*18-0a.doc.

2. Position the insertion point anywhere in the table, and choose Table AutoFormat from the Table menu.

   Word displays the Table AutoFormat dialog box.

AutoFormat "Simple 3"

3. Choose the Simple 3 format from the Formats list box.

4. Choose Borders, Shading, Font, and Autofit in the Formats To Apply box.

   Word will apply these parts of the predefined format to the table.

5. Choose Heading Rows in the Apply Special Format To box.

   Word will apply these special parts of the predefined format to the table.

6. Click OK to complete the table formatting and display the formatted table.

7. Save the document.

Converting Tables into Text

You can convert a table or selected rows in a table to paragraphs of text using the Convert Table To Text dialog box. The converted text can be separated with paragraph marks, commas, or tabs.

Figure 18-10
The Convert Table To Text dialog box

To convert text from a table:

1. Switch to the document with the revenue table. Select the last four rows of the table, and choose Convert Table to Text from the Table menu.

2. In the Convert Table To Text dialog box, choose the Tabs option to separate the text for different cells with tabs. Click OK.

   The text appears outside the table, with tab character marks between the words on each line and a paragraph mark at the end of each line.

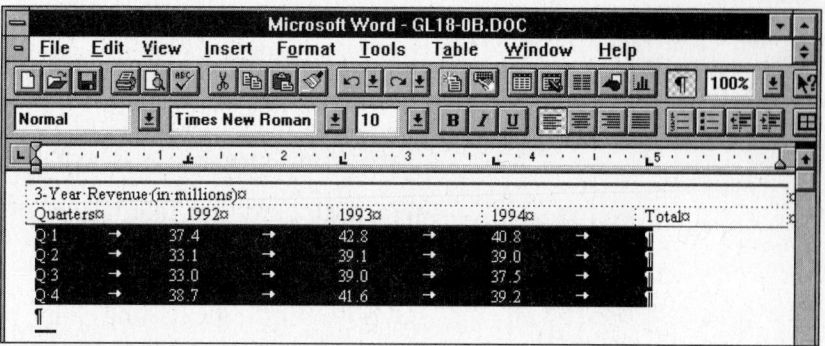

Figure 18-11
Converting a table to text

Converting Text into Tables

You also can convert existing text to a table. This procedure can be faster than creating a table and keying text in it.

To add converted text to an existing table, you may need to adjust the size and format of the new cells to make them conform with the rest of the table.

To convert text to a table:

1. Select the four lines of text under the table, and then choose Convert Text to Table from the Table menu.

    Word displays the Convert Text to Table dialog box.

2. Make sure the column setting is 5 and the row setting is 4, and then click OK.

    The text appears in a table, with each paragraph in a separate row and each tabbed item in a separate column.

3. Save the document.

Performing Calculations in a Table

You can add, subtract, multiply, and divide in a table, as well as calculate averages, percentages, and minimum and maximum values.

To add the contents of a row or column of cells, position the insertion point in the last cell of the row or column, and then choose Formula from the Table menu. Verify that the expressions in the Formula box are the ones you want for your operation, and then click OK.

When you add the contents of a row or column, the last cell does not need to be empty. If the cell is not empty, you can either add the result to the cell or replace what is in the cell with the result by selecting the cell before you perform the operation.

To perform different calculations, specify the cells to be used. As in a spreadsheet, the cells are referenced by letter (column) and number (row), starting with A1 for the first column and row, A2 for the first column and second row, B1 for the second column and first row, and so on.

You can perform simple calculations by keying the cell reference with the sign for adding, subtracting, multiplying, or dividing. For example, you can key **a2+b3** to add those cells or **a2/b3** to divide those cells.

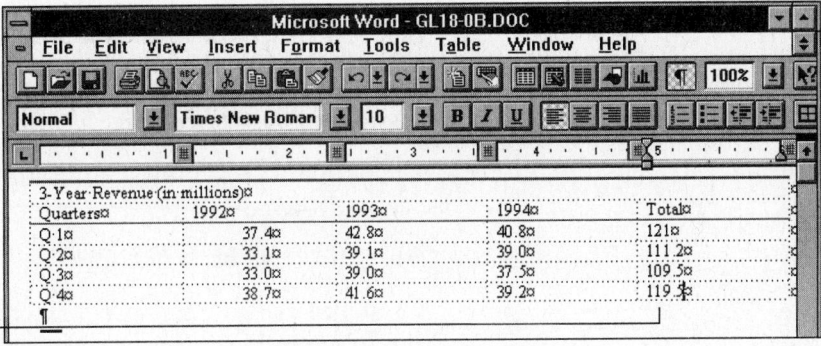

Word calculates totals

Figure 18-12

Performing calculations in a table

To add a row or column of numbers in a table:

1. In the revenue table, position the insertion point in the first cell under "Total".

2. Choose Formula from the Table menu.

    Based on the table content, Word presents the Formula dialog box with the appropriate formula for the operation. If the insertion point is in the last cell of a column of numbers, for instance, the =SUM(ABOVE) formula is presented. If the insertion point is in the last cell of a row, the =SUM(LEFT) formula is presented, as it is here.

3. Click OK to perform the operation.

    Word adds all the numerical text in the row, excluding the text in the first cell, "Q 1".

4. Move the insertion point to the next cell in the column, and choose Repeat Formula from the Insert menu.

5. Use the Repeat Formula command for the next two cells in the column.

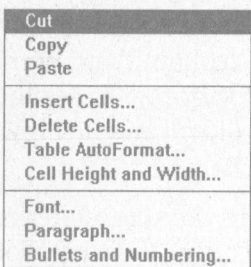

Shortcut menu

The Shortcut Menu

You can use the shortcut menu to perform common table functions quickly, such as inserting and deleting cells or rows or opening the Table AutoFormat dialog box. To display the shortcut menu, click the right mouse button with the insertion point inside the table.

To use the shortcut menu:

1. Select the revenue table.

2. Click the right mouse button, and choose Table AutoFormat from the shortcut menu.

3. Choose the Grid 3 format and click OK.

4. Select the top row of the table, and make the text bold and centered.

5. Switch to *[your three-letter identifier]*18-0a.doc.

6. Click the Borders button, and add a 1½-point top border to the second row.

7. Save and print both documents.

8. Close the documents and exit Word (unless you will be doing the following exercises immediately).

Splitting A Table

With a long table, you can split the table and add explanatory text between the parts. This makes the explanatory text stand out from the table, so it can be easily read.

Position the insertion point in the row that will be the first row of the new part. Choose Split Table from the Table menu. Word inserts a paragraph mark formatted in the normal style between the table parts. You can apply your own formatting to make the text stand out. You still have a single table that you can reference as such, but you also have separate parts that are visually distinctive, with explanatory text that can be easily read.

Table 18-2: Keyboard Shortcuts for Working with Tables	
Keyboard Shortcut	Action
Ctrl+Tab	Insert a tab within a cell
Alt+5 (numeric keypad)	Select table

Key Terms

Cell   End-of-row marker

Cell selection bar   Gridlines

Column selection bar   Row selection bar

End-of-cell marker   Table

Exercises

Exercise 18.1

1. Start Word, if necessary.

2. Create a new document using the normal template.

3. Make sure all nonprinting characters are displayed and the Gridlines option is checked.

4. Create a table with three rows and seven columns using the Table menu:

   A. Choose Insert Table from the Table menu.

   B. Key **7** in the Number of Columns text box.

   C. Key **3** in the Number of Rows text box. Click OK.

5. Key the first line of text in Figure 18-13. Key each column heading in a separate cell:

   A. Key **From** in the first cell.

   B. Press the **Tab** key to move to the next cell and key **To**

   C. Press the **Tab** key, and then key the next word in the first line. Continue in this manner until you have keyed all the column headings.

Figure 18-13

From	To	Airline	Flight	Date	Depart	Arrive
Phoenix	Albuquerque	Southwest	664	6/24	7:20AM	8:20AM
Albuquerque	Phoenix	America West	557	6/27	9:50AM	11:05AM

6. Key the second and third lines of Figure 18-13 in the second and third rows of the table, keying each entry in a separate cell. (In some cells, the text you key will wrap to a second line.)

7. Select the first row of the table by clicking the selection bar to the left of the row, and then click the Bold button.

8. Apply a border and shading to the selected row:

   A. Choose Borders and Shading from the Format menu, and click the Borders tab, if necessary.

   B. Choose Box in the Preset options group.

   B. Choose the 3-point line in the line Styles box.

   D. Click the Shading tab, and then choose 20% from the Shading list box. Click OK to close the dialog box.

9. Change the width of the first three columns to 1.2 inches:

   A. Select the columns by positioning the pointer in the selection bar above the first column and dragging it to the third column.

   B. Choose Cell Height and Width from the Table menu, and click the Column tab, if necessary.

   C. Key **1.2** in the Width of Columns text box and click OK.

10. Change the spacing between the columns to .2 inches, and change the row height of the columns:

    A. Select the entire table by positioning the insertion point anywhere in the table and choosing Select Table from the Table menu.

    B. Choose Cell Height and Width from the Table menu.

    C. Click the Column tab, if necessary, and key **.2** in the Space Between Columns text box.

    D. Click the Row tab, set the row height to At Least 48 point, and click OK.

11. Center the text in all the cells:

    A. Select the entire table, if necessary.

    B. Choose Paragraph from the Format menu.

    C. Choose Centered from the Alignment drop-down list box. Click OK.

12. Change the page orientation to landscape.

13. Center the table horizontally:

    A. Select the entire table.

    B. Choose Cell Height and Width from the Table menu.

    C. Click Center in the Alignment box. Click OK.

14. View the document in print preview, and then spell-check the document.

15. Save the document as *[your three-letter identifier]*18-1.doc and print it.

16. Close the document and exit Word (unless you will be doing the following exercises immediately).

Exercise 18.2

1. Start Word, if necessary.

2. Open the file 18-2.doc.

3. Make sure all nonprinting characters are displayed and the Gridlines option is checked.

4. Convert the five paragraphs beginning with "Day 1" to a table:

    A. Select the five paragraphs.

    B. Choose Convert Text to Table from the Table menu.

    C. Set Number of Columns to 1, set Column Width to 3 inches, and choose Paragraphs for Separate Text At.

5. Add a second column at the right of the table:

    A. Move the insertion point outside the right gridline.

    B. Choose Select Column from the Table menu.

    C. Choose Insert Columns from the Table menu.

6. Move the text, except "Day 1", in the first cell of the first row to the second cell in the first row.

7. Move the text, except "Day 2", in the first cell of the second row to the second cell in the second row.

8. Move the text, except "Day 3", in the first cell of the third row to the second cell in the third row.

9. Move the text, except "Day 4", in the first cell of the fourth row to the second cell in the fourth row.

10. Move the text, except "Day 5 & 6", in the first cell of the fifth row to the second cell in the fifth row.

11. Change the width of the first column to 1 inch without changing the width of the table:

    A.   Position the pointer to the right of the gridline of the first column. When the pointer becomes a two-headed arrow, hold down the **Shift** key.

    B.   Drag the gridline to the 1-inch mark on the ruler, and release the **Shift** key.

12.   Change the row height for the entire table:

    A.   Select the entire table, and then choose Cell Height and Width from the Table menu.

    B.   Click the Row tab, if necessary.

    C.   Set the row height to At Least 36 point and click OK.

13.   Add a row to the top of the table:

    A.   Select the first row.

    B.   Choose Insert Rows from the Table menu.

14.   Move the document heading into the second cell of the first row.

15.   Merge the cells in the first row:

    A.   Select both cells.

    B.   Choose Merge Cells from the Table menu.

16.   Change the heading to 12-point bold small capitals and center-align it.

17.   Align the table within the margins:

    A.   Select the entire table, and then choose Cell Height and Width from the Table menu.

    B.   Click the Row tab, if necessary.

    C.   Click Center alignment and click OK.

18.   Spell-check the document.

19.   Save the document as *[your three-letter identifier]*18-2.doc and print it.

20.   Close the document and exit Word (unless you will be doing the following exercises immediately).

Exercise 18.3

1.   Start Word, if necessary.

2.   Create a new document using the Normal template. Change the left and right margins to .5 inches and the top margin to 2 inches.

3.   Create a table with five rows and seven columns, and then key the text in Figure 18-14.

Figure 18-14

	Monday	Tuesday	Wednesday	Thursday	Friday	Sat./Sun.
J				1	2	3/4
U	5	6	7	8	9	10/11 Santa Fe
N	12	13	14	15	16	17/18
E	19	20	21	22	23	24/25

4. Add a sixth row to the table. Then key **26, 27, 28, 29,** and **30** in the second, third, fourth, fifth, and sixth cells of the last row, respectively.

5. Change the type size for the first column to 40 points.

6. Put a 3-point box border around the first column, and apply 20% shading.

7. Change the column width of the first column to .6. Change the column width of the second to seventh columns to 1.2.

8. Change the weekday headings in the top row to 16-point bold italics.

9. Change the row height for the first row to exactly 24 point.

10. Key **RSVP for Red Rock Ranch Trip** in the cell for June 6, beginning on the line below the date.

11. Key **Mail travel documents for Vegas** in the cell for June 1, beginning on the line below the date.

12. Key **Noon visit with regional managers** in the cell for June 19, beginning on the line below the date.

13. Key **Staff meeting** below the date in the cells for June 16 and June 30.

14. Change the row height for the second through sixth rows to exactly 72 pt.

15. Apply a 3-point grid border to the document, from the second to seventh columns.

16. Spell-check the document.

17. Save the document as *[your three-letter identifier]*18-3.doc and print it.

19. Close the document and exit Word (unless you will be doing the following exercise immediately).

Exercise 18.4: Challenge Yourself

Use the Calendar Wizard to create a monthly calendar. (To locate the Calendar Wizard, choose New from the File menu). Create the calendar in landscape orientation using the Banner style. Start the calendar at the current month for a three-month period.

View the calendar in print preview, and then save it as *[your three-letter identifier]*18-4.doc. Print the calendar, and then close it and exit Word.

Working with Columns

Objectives

- Create multiple-column layouts.

- Create and edit text in columns.

- Format text in columns.

- Change column width and spacing.

- Control column breaks.

A three-column layout

In Lesson 18, you created columns of text using the table feature. This lesson shows you how to arrange text in newspaper-style columns. Columns make a document more attractive and easier to read. They break up a page, add white space, and present information in shorter lines.

What Are Columns?

Text arranged in columns resembles text in newspapers and magazines. Text flows continuously from the top to the bottom of one column, then to the top of the next column.

You can arrange text in any number of columns. In addition, by creating more than one section, one document can have different text arranged in different numbers of columns. For example, a document can have one section with a standard one-column layout and another section with a three-column layout. A document can have up to 100 columns.

One-column section

Three-column section

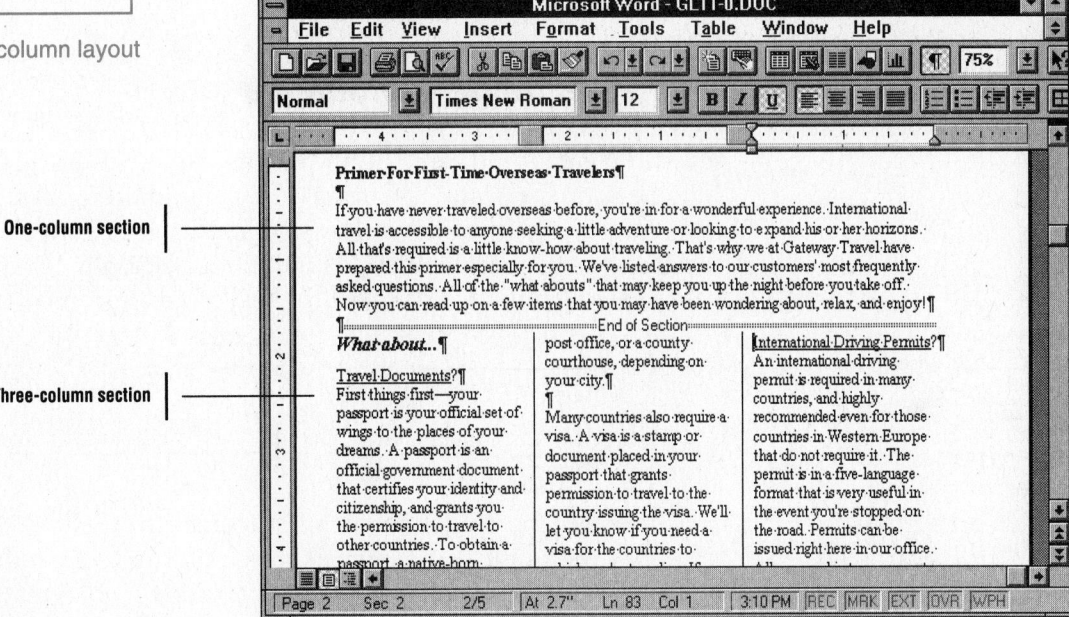

Figure 19-1

A one- and three-column layout in page layout view

When working with columns, use page layout view to see the columns as they are arranged on the page. In normal view, the text in a multiple-column layout appears on the screen as a single, continuous, narrow column. Another way to see how columns are arranged on a page is to use print preview.

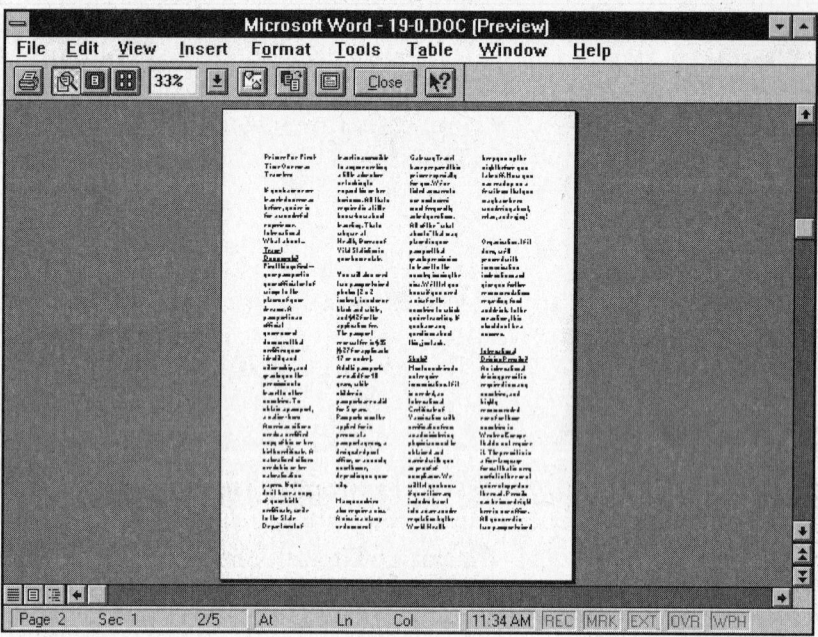

Figure 19-2
A four-column layout in print preview

Creating Multiple-Column Layouts

You can create multiple-column layouts using either the Columns dialog box or the Columns button on the Standard toolbar. In either case, before beginning to work with columns, switch to page layout view, if necessary, and either position the insertion point where you want to set up columns or select the text to arrange in columns.

Using the Columns Dialog Box to Set up Columns

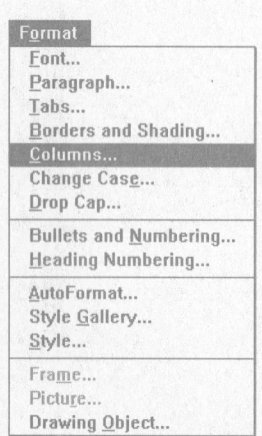

Format menu

To display the Columns dialog box for setting up columns, choose Columns from the Format menu.

Choose one of the predefined column formats from the Presets box, or specify the number of columns in the Number of Columns text box. Click the Equal Column Width check box if you want Word to make the width of the columns the same with equal spacing between them automatically. When you choose this option, you can adjust the Width and Spacing settings for Column #1, and Word automatically adjusts the remaining columns equally.

If you do not choose the Equal Column Width option, you can scroll to the column number and manually adjust the Width and Spacing settings for each individual column. Specify the column width in the Width box and the amount of space between columns in the Spacing box.

To print a vertical line between columns, check the Line Between check box. To start a new column, such as to place a heading at the top of a column, check the Start New Column check box.

The Preview box within the Columns dialog box shows how the column layout appears on the page.

Figure 19-3
The Columns dialog box

You can apply the layout to selected text, or you can apply the columns layout to the whole document or to all text following the insertion point by clicking the arrows to the right of the Apply To drop-down list box.

To use the Columns dialog box to set up columns:

1. Start Word, if necessary.

2. Open the file 11-0.doc.

3. Switch to page layout view.

4. Move the insertion point to the beginning of the heading **"What about..."** on page 2 of the document.

5. Choose Columns from the Format menu to display the Columns dialog box.

6. Key **3** in the Number of Columns text box.

    The Preview box shows three columns.

7. Check the Equal Column Width check box, if necessary.

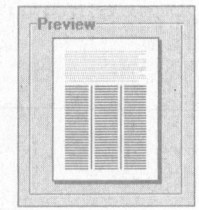

Column layout in the
Preview box

Using the Columns button

8. Key **.25** in the Spacing text box for Column # 1.

9. Check the Line Between check box.

10. Choose This Point Forward from the Apply To drop-down list box.

The Preview box reflects the options specified.

11. Click OK.

The document appears with the text arranged in three columns starting at the insertion point.

12. Switch to print preview.

The print-preview screen shows columns and the lines between columns as they appear in the printed document.

13. Click Close to return to page layout view.

Using the Toolbar to Set up Columns

Use the Columns button on the Standard toolbar to set up columns for the section in which the insertion point is positioned. If the document does not contain section breaks, Word applies the column layout to the entire document.

When you click the Columns button, a box appears below the button that allows you to choose the number of columns. Move the pointer across to choose the number of columns desired.

When using the Columns button to set up columns, Word applies the default settings for column width, lines between columns, and starting a new column. To change these settings, use the Columns dialog box.

To set up columns using the Columns button:

1. While still in page layout view, go to page 4 of document 11-0.doc. Move the insertion point to the beginning of the paragraph which starts "For specific information".

2. Choose Break from the Insert menu, and insert a Continuous Section Break.

3. Click the Columns button on the Standard toolbar.

4. Drag the pointer across one column in the columns box, and then release the mouse button.

The text beginning with "For specific information" appears as a single column. (Remember, the tabbed columns are part of the original document's formatting.)

5. Press **Enter** twice to insert two blank lines between the sections.

Creating and Editing Text in Columns

Keying new text and editing existing text in multiple-column layouts is the same as keying and editing text in standard one-column layouts. Moving the insertion point through a multiple-column layout, however, is different from moving it through a standard layout:

- Press the **Right Arrow** key at the end of any column to move the insertion point to the top of the next column.

- Press the **Left Arrow** key at the top of any column to move the insertion point to the bottom of the previous column.

- Press the **Down Arrow** key at the end of a column to move the insertion point from the bottom line of the column to the first line of the same column on the next page. If the document has a footer or the page contains blank lines between the end of the text and the page break, press the **Down Arrow** key more than once.

To enter and edit text in columns:

1. Click the Page Back button twice to scroll up two pages. In the paragraph above "The Language Barrier?" in the third column, move the insertion point before the text "Check gas costs."

2. Key the following:

   Driving is an excellent way to tour an area—providing you are not in a hurry. It allows you to explore freely and to mingle with local people at your own pace.

3. Move the insertion point to the end of the third column, and press the **Right Arrow** key.

   The insertion point moves to the first column at the top of the next page.

4. Press the **Left Arrow** key to return to the last column of the previous page.

5. Move the insertion point to the end of the first column (before the space) on the same page, and then press the **Right Arrow** key.

   The insertion point moves to the top of the next column.

Formatting Text in Columns

You create and change font and paragraph formats for text in columns the same way you format text in standard layouts. Use either the Font or Paragraph dialog box or the Formatting toolbar.

To format text in columns:

1. Just below the section break on page 2, select the text "**What about...**".

2. Use the Paragraph dialog box (choose Paragraph from the Format menu) to change spacing to 18 points after the paragraph.

3. Use the Font dialog box (choose Font from the Format menu, and click the Font tab, if necessary) to change the character format to 14-point bold italics.

4. Select the text "Travel Documents?" and the first line of the paragraph below it. Click the Justify button on the Formatting toolbar to justify the text.

5. Click the Undo button on the Standard toolbar.

6. Save the document as *[your three-letter identifier]*19-0.doc.

Changing Column Width and Spacing

After setting up columns, you can change their width as well as the spacing between them. Column width and spacing are interrelated: If you narrow the space between columns without changing the number of columns, the columns widen. If you narrow the columns themselves, the space between the columns widens. Use either the ruler or the Columns dialog box to change column width and spacing.

Using the Ruler to Change Column Width and Spacing

Using the ruler to change column width and spacing is generally faster than using the Columns dialog box. In page layout view, drag a column marker on the horizontal ruler.

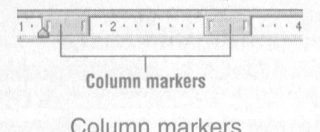

Column markers

When you adjust columns of equal width, the width of all columns changes equally. The text flow in all the columns changes to accommodate the new column width.

When you adjust columns of unequal width, only the width of the columns you adjust changes. The text flow in the adjusted column changes.

To use the ruler to change column width and spacing:

1. Turn on the ruler, if necessary. (Choose Ruler from the View menu.)

2. Go to page 3 of the document. With the insertion point in the first column, drag the right column marker .5 inches to the left on the ruler, and then release the mouse button.

Note: You can hold down the **Alt** key while adjusting column widths to see an exact measurement display.

Adjusting column marker

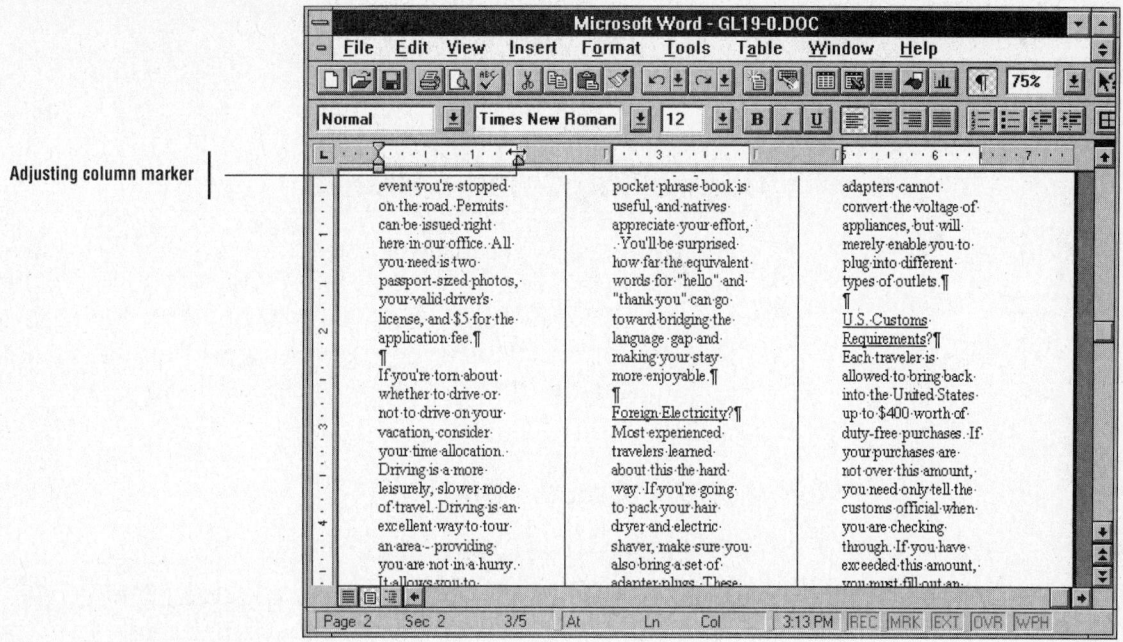

Figure 19-4
Using column markers to adjust columns of equal width

Word applies the narrower column width to all three columns in the section. The narrow width results in wider spacing between the columns. The change in column width and spacing changes the page breaks.

3. Click the Undo button to restore the original width.

Using the Columns Dialog Box to Change Column Width and Spacing

When using the Columns dialog box to change column width and spacing, the default measurement is inches. To specify column spacing in centimeters, key a number followed by a space, and then key **cm**. For example, to set the column spacing at .8 inch, key **.8** or **.8"**. To set the column spacing at 1.2 centimeters, key **1.2 cm**

To change column widths and spacing using the Columns dialog box:

1. With the insertion point still in the three-column section, choose Columns from the Format menu to display the Columns dialog box.

   The dialog box shows that each column is 2 inches wide, with .25 inches spacing between columns.

2. Set the Spacing for Column 1 to .4" and press the **Tab** key.

   Word changes the settings for all three columns to 1.9 inches wide, because the Equal Column Width check box is checked.

3. Click OK.

The columns are narrowed, and the page breaks are once again adjusted.

Controlling Column Breaks

When you set up columns for existing text or key new text in a multiple-column layout, Word breaks the columns at the end of the page or section. However, you can insert a column break manually, so that the columns end wherever you want. You can also balance the length of columns to give them a more even appearance.

Inserting Column Breaks

There are three ways to insert a column break:

- Move the insertion point to where you want to insert the column break. Choose Break from the Insert menu. In the Break dialog box, click the Column Break option button in the Insert group.

Figure 19-5
The Break dialog box

Note: You can also use the Paragraph dialog box to control column breaks. For example, if a column break separates a paragraph from its heading, select the heading, choose Paragraph from the Format menu, click the Text Flow tab, and choose the Keep With Next pagination option. To review these options, see "Controlling Page Breaks" in Lesson 11.

- Move the insertion point to where you want to insert the column break. Choose Columns from the Format menu. In the Columns dialog box, check the Start New Column check box, and then choose This Point Forward from the Apply To drop-down list box.

- Move the insertion point to where you want to insert the column break, and press **Ctrl+Shift+Enter**.

To delete a column break, move the insertion point to where you want to delete the break, and then press the **Backspace** key. You can also use the Undo command to delete a column break immediately after inserting it.

Balancing the Length of Columns

Column lengths are often unequal at the ends of sections or pages. However, you can balance the columns to make them even.

Figure 19-6
Columns of unequal and equal length

To balance columns, move the insertion point to the end of the page or section, choose Break from the Insert menu, and choose a Section Break option:

- Choose Next Page if the columns continue on the next page.

- Choose Continuous if the columns do not continue beyond this page.

- Choose Even Page if the columns continue on the next even-numbered page.

- Choose Odd Page if the columns continue on the next odd-numbered page.

To adjust column breaks:

1. At the end of the three-column section, delete the paragraph mark after "make a formal visit!" and all the text following it, up to but not including the last paragraph mark after "Paraguay".

   Section 2 is one column again.

2. With the insertion point in section 2, click the Columns button, and choose three columns.

   Notice the uneven columns on the last page.

3. Move the insertion point to the start of the heading "<u>The American Embassy</u>?" in the first column on the last page.

4. Choose Columns from the Format menu. Check Start New Column, and choose This Point Forward from the Apply To drop-down list box. Click OK.

   The heading is moved to the top of the next column.

5. Click the Undo button.

6. Move the insertion point to the end of the text, after "formal visit!".

7. Choose Break from the Insert menu. Under Section Break, choose Continuous. Click OK.

   Word balances the last page into three columns of equal length.

8. Switch to print preview to view the document.

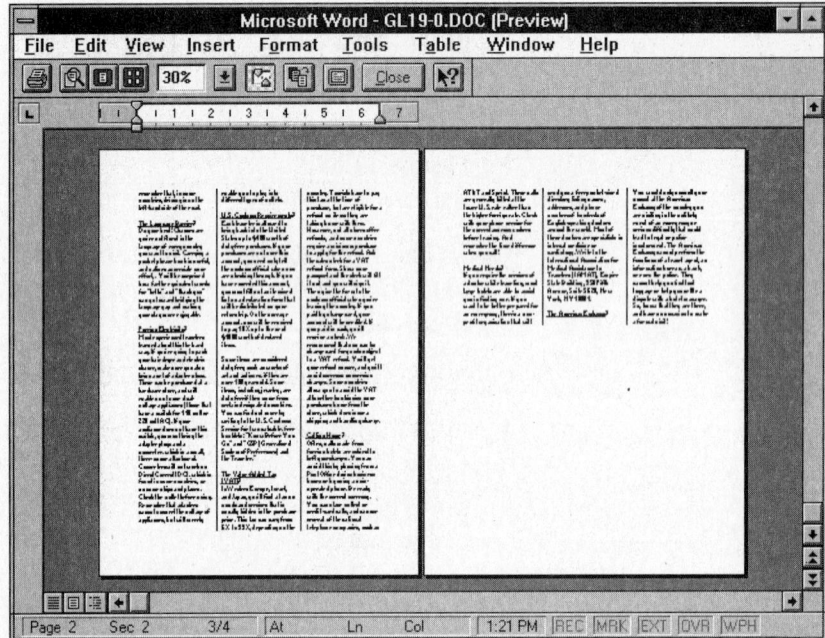

Figure 19-7
The last page with balanced columns in print preview

9. Return to page layout view, scroll through the document, and delete any extra paragraph marks that may occur at the top of the columns in section 2.

10. Spell-check the document.

11. Save the document.

12. Print section 2 of the document.

13. Close the document and exit Word (unless you will be doing the following exercises immediately).

Table 19-1: Keyboard Shortcut for Working with Columns	
Keyboard Shortcut	Action
Ctrl+Shift+Enter	Insert column break

One-Column Heading in a Multiple-Column Layout

If a multiple-column section has a title that you would like to appear as one column across the width of the page, you can do so by inserting a continuous section break before and after the title.

For example, section 1 of a document has three columns. Section 2 also has three columns, and you want the title of section 2 to span across the page as one column in 16-point type. To do this, insert a continuous section break after section 1. This balances the columns of section 1. Then format the new section as one column, and key the title. Make sure a continuous section break follows the title and precedes the next section, which will be set as three columns.

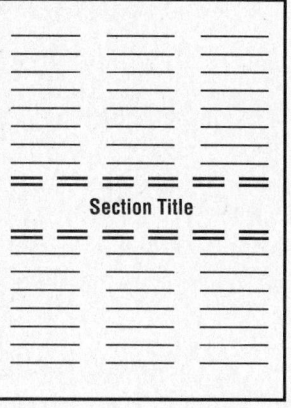

Figure 19-8

Page showing section title between columned sections

Exercises

Exercise 19.1

1. Start Word, if necessary.

2. Open the file 19-1.doc.

3. Create a three-column layout for the list of countries:

    A. Choose Page Layout from the View menu.

    B. Move the insertion point to the beginning of the word "Antigua".

    C. Choose Columns from the Format menu to display the Columns dialog box.

    D. Key **3** in the Number of Columns text box. Key **1** in the Spacing for Column #1 text box.

    E. Choose This Point Forward from the Apply To drop-down list box. Click OK.

4. Adjust the columns to three columns of equal length:

    A. Move the insertion point to the end of the columnar text.

    B. Choose Break from the Insert menu.

    C. In the Break dialog box, choose a Continuous Section Break and click OK.

5. At the top of the document, key in all capitals the heading **TOURIST OFFICES IN THE UNITED STATES**, followed by two blank lines.

6. Center the heading, and change it to 14-point bold.

7. Change the top margin to 2 inches.

8. Spell-check the document, and save it as *[your three-letter identifier]*19-1.doc.

9. Print the document.

10. Close the document and exit Word (unless you will be doing the following exercises immediately).

Exercise 19.2

1. Start Word, if necessary.

2. Open the files 15-2.doc and 12-4.doc.

3. Copy the second heading on the second page of document 12-4.DOC ("**Gateway Travel—Your Gateway to the World**") and the paragraph that follows it.

4. Paste the selected text at the beginning of document 15-2.DOC, and insert two blank lines between the text you just pasted and the heading "**Gateway Travel Offices**".

5. Delete the hard page break before "Ontario Gateway Travel", and then insert a continuous section break after the heading "**Gateway Travel Offices**".

6. Use the Columns button to set up a three-column layout for the list of travel offices:

    A. Switch to page layout view. With the insertion point in section 2, click the Columns button on the Standard toolbar.

    B. Drag the pointer across three columns in the column grid, and then release the mouse button.

7. Change the spacing between columns to .25 inches:

    A. Choose Columns from the Format menu.

    B. Set the Spacing for Column #1 to .25 inches. Click OK.

8. Move the insertion point to the beginning of the first travel-office listing, and then key:

Duke City Gateway Travel
15 Montgomery Boulevard
Albuquerque, NM 87111
Tel. (505) 555-1234
FAX (505) 555-1244

9. Insert a blank line before the next listing.

10. Insert a column break at the start of the listing for "New England Gateway Travel" in the first column:

   A. Move the insertion point to the start of the listing.

   B. Press **Ctrl+Shift+Enter**.

11. Insert a column break at the start of the listing for "Ontario Gateway Travel" using the Break dialog box.

12. Change the heading "**Gateway Travel—Your Gateway to the World**" to all capitals and 14-point bold italics. Center the heading, and add another blank line under it.

13. Add a blank line under the heading "**Gateway Travel Offices**", and center the heading.

14. Change the top margin to 1.5 inches.

15. Spell-check the document, and save it as *[your three-letter identifier]*19-2.doc.

16. Print the document.

17. Close the documents and exit Word (unless you will be doing the following exercises immediately).

Exercise 19.3

1. Start Word, if necessary.

2. Open the file 5-0.doc.

3. Change the page orientation to landscape.

4. Use the Standard toolbar to set up a two-column layout for the whole document, and then switch to page layout view.

5. At the top of the first column, key the heading:

New Mexico/Santa Fe Sightseeing: The Turquoise Trail Scenic and Historic Area

6. Insert two blank lines between the text you keyed and the next paragraph.

7. At the end of the document, insert a blank line, and then key the text in Figure 19-9, including the corrections.

Figure 19-9

tour of
No| New Mexico ~~tour~~ is complete without a visit to one of the 18 timeless

Pueblos. ~~If you~~ circle off Route 14 going toward interstate 25, ~~you can~~

and
|visit the Santo Domingo Pueblo. The pueblo was settled about 700 years

          today
ago and| is the home of 3,500 Native Americans. Don't miss Trader Fred's

world famous| trading post.| *for its rugs, jewelry, and crafts for over 100 years.*

8. Change the heading to 24-point italic.

9. Change the space between columns to 1 inch.

10. At the start of the text under the heading, insert a continuous section break.

11. Format the heading section as one column.

12. In the heading, delete the colon, and start the heading text from *"The Turquoise Trail"* on a new line. Change the text in the new line to small capitals, and center both lines of the heading.

13. Balance the length of the columns in section 2 using the Break dialog box.

14. Switch to print preview to view the document.

15. Spell-check the document.

16. Save the document as *[your three-letter identifier]*19-3.doc.

17. Print the document.

18. Close the document and exit Word (unless you will be doing the following exercise immediately).

Exercise 19.4: Challenge Yourself

Open the file 19-4.doc, and insert a continuous section break at the top of the document. Above the section break, key:

Big Turnout for the Bike-a-Thon

Switch to page layout view, and then format the second section with a three-column layout.

Change the type size and the font of the heading in section 1 to 24-point bold Arial. Then insert a blank line after the heading. Change the font in section 2 to Arial.

Format all the paragraphs under the heading with a .25-inch first-line indent. Change the space between the columns to .4 inches with a line between the columns.

Switch to print preview, and change the top margin to 2 inches, the bottom margin to 2.25 inches, and the left and right margins to 1.25 inches. Switch back to page layout view. In section 2, delete the blank lines between paragraphs, and then change the spacing to 6 points after paragraphs.

Insert a continuous section break at the end of the text in the last column to balance the columns.

Spell-check the document, save it as *[your three-letter identifier]* 19-4.doc, and print it. Close the document and exit Word.

A Newsletter

Background

Each season, Duke City Gateway publishes a newsletter to send to all of the agency's customers. The newsletter includes feature articles about the Southwest and information about weather, special vacation packages, and upcoming events.

The newsletter is prepared by all members of the agency and is edited by Frank Youngblood. Frank is also responsible for having the newsletter printed and distributed.

Business Purpose

Create a newsletter for the spring season.

Procedures

1. Open the file p7-1.doc.

2. Insert a continuous section break after the heading "The Duke City Traveler".

3. Format section 2 as two columns with .5 inches of space between the columns and a line between the columns.

4. Make the heading "Southwest Spotlight: The Turquoise Trail" bold, and change the type size to 14 point.

5. Make the heading "New Mexico: Spring Weather" 14 point bold.

6. Convert the text that includes the months and temperatures to a table.

7. Add a grid border to the table, and right-align the text.

8. Insert a page break after the table. On the next line, insert a continuous section break after the page break, and change the page to 1 column.

9. At the top of the section, key **Cruising**

10. Make the heading bold, centered, 24-point, and small caps.

11. Add a ¾ point box border to the heading that is 4 points from the text. Add a blank line after the box border.

12. On the same page, move the insertion point to the end of the paragraph that ends "discount prices we are offering:". Press **Enter** twice, and insert a table with 3 columns and 6 rows.

13. Key the following headings in the first row, and make them bold:

    First column: **Cruise Line**
    Second column: **Cruise Length**
    Third column: **Price**

14. Complete the table by keying the following information (leave one row blank, and begin keying in the third row):

Majesty	**5 days/4 nights**	**$1,150**
Chilton	**8 days/7 nights**	**$2,100**
Seaward	**4 days/3 nights**	**$1,000**
Navigator	**8 days/7 nights**	**$1,800**

15. Change the width of column 1 to 1.25 inches, column 2 to 1.5 inches, and column 3 to .75 inches.

16. Center the table horizontally on the page.

17. Insert a row of cells above the first row in the table.

18. Merge the cells, and change the row height to 36 points.

19. Key **Caribbean** in the cell.

20. Make the heading bold, center, small caps, and 14-point.

21. After this table, press **Enter** three times, and insert another table that has 4 columns and 6 rows.

22. Key in bold the following headings for the columns:

    Cruise Line   Cruise Type   Cruise Length   Price

23. Complete the table by keying the following information (leave one row blank, and begin keying in the third row):

Tropical	**South American**	**8 days/7 nights**	**$3,300**
Vacation	**Mexican**	**5 days/4 nights**	**$1,880**
Northern	**Alaska**	**12 days/11 nights**	**$4,300**
Exotica	**Hawaiian**	**11 days/10 nights**	**$3,999**

24. Change the width of column 1 to 1.25 inches and column 4 to .75 inches.

25. Center the table horizontally on the page.

26. Add a new row of cells above the first row.

27. Merge the cells, and change the row height to 36 points.

28. Key **Exotic** in bold, centered, 14-point small caps.

29. Move the insertion point to the end of the next paragraph, which ends "insider's view of the ships", press **Enter** once, and insert a page break.

30. Key **Spring Events** in bold, centered, 24-point small caps.

31. Add a ¾ point box border that is 4 points from the text.

32. Insert 4 lines of space after the heading, and then insert a continuous section break.

33. Change the new section into 3 columns with .5 space between the columns, and put lines between the columns.

34. Insert column breaks before "May" and "June". Delete any paragraph marks at the beginning of a column.

35. After the last entry in column 3, insert a continuous section break, and change the page to 1 column.

36. Allow three blank lines after the column break, and then key:

    Duke City Gateway Travel Agency
    15 Montgomery Boulevard
    Albuquerque, New Mexico 87110
    (505) 555-1234

37. Center the text, and make sure it is 14 points and single spaced.

38. Make any changes you feel will improve the appearance of the document.

39. Spell check the document, save it as *[your three-letter identifier]*p7-1.doc, and print it.

40. Close the document and exit Word.

Tips and Hints

- Add grid borders to tables to separate the rows and columns and give the table an organized appearance. By adding a blank row after the table heading, you can create a space before the table text.

- Try hyphenating text in columns to give it a less ragged appearance.

- Use multiple-column layouts in your newsletters to make them more interesting.

- Use an informal tone in the articles for your newsletter to make the reader feel comfortable.

Module 8

Styles, Templates and Macros

Styles

Word provides a time-saving feature, called styles, for formatting documents. Styles allow you to set paragraph- and character-formatting instructions for a whole paragraph or a small amount of selected text, save the instructions, and apply them to other text in a document.

Objectives

- Create styles.
- Apply styles.
- Redefine and rename styles.
- Delete styles.
- Save styles.
- Use style sheets.

Paragraph style
A set of paragraph- and character-formatting instructions that you name and use to format whole paragraphs in a Word document.

Character style
A set of character-formatting instructions that you name and use to format individual words or small amounts of text within a paragraph.

Normal style
The standard, default paragraph style that is applied automatically to new paragraphs in a document.

What Are Styles?

Word allows you to create two types of styles—paragraph styles and character styles.

Paragraph styles are paragraph- and character-formatting instructions that you specify to be applied to an entire paragraph or selected paragraphs. *Character styles* contain character-formatting instructions only and can be applied to small amounts of selected text within a paragraph that you wish to emphasize. You can specify font, type size, paragraph spacing, alignment, and other types of formatting. You can then assign a name to the set of formatting specifications and use the name to apply the same formatting to any other text or paragraphs in a document. A document can contain several different styles. For example, you can create one style for headings, another style for body text, and a third style to emphasize individual words.

Word includes standard styles in each new document you open. These include the body-text paragraph style, called *Normal*, three heading styles, and styles for headers and footers. Text you key in a new Word document is automatically formatted with the Normal style. All standard styles are based on the formatting of the Normal style. For example, if the font of the Normal style is Times New Roman, header and footer styles are the same font.

There are many good reasons to include styles in a document:

- Styles save time in formatting.
- Styles help give a document a consistent look.
- Styles are easy to create and use.

What Are Style Sheets?

Style sheet
A list of the styles found in a Word document.

In every document, Word keeps a list of style names and their formatting specifications. This collection of style information is called a *style sheet*. The style sheet lists the standard styles and the styles you

391

Style drop-down list box

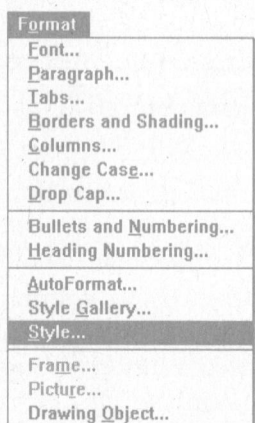

Format menu

have created for a document. You can view the styles in the style sheet using the Style drop-down list box on the Formatting toolbar. In the list box, paragraph styles are shown in bold text, and character styles are shown in normal text. The style for the paragraph containing the insertion point appears in the Style text box. You can also view the styles and the formatting instructions for the styles using the Style command on the Format menu.

To view the styles in the Style drop-down list box on the Formatting toolbar:

1. Open the file 20-0.doc.

2. Click the down arrow to the right of the word Normal on the Formatting toolbar.

    Word displays the standard paragraph and character styles and the styles created for the document.

3. Click outside the box to close it.

To view the styles and style specifications using the Style command on the Format menu:

1. Move the insertion point to the beginning of the document.

2. Choose Style on the Format menu.

    The style Normal is highlighted and checkmarked in the Styles list box on the left side of the dialog box.

3. View the formatting instructions for the style in the Description box, at the bottom center. Then click Cancel.

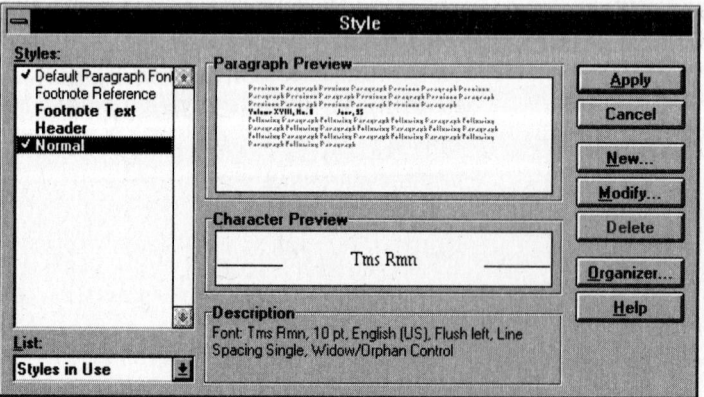

Figure 20-1
The Style dialog box

The style sheet is stored along with the document. It is not separate from the document, and you cannot remove the style sheet from a document. However, you can make changes to the style sheet by modifying the styles in your document. You can create, delete, rename, or redefine the styles in the style sheet.

Using AutoFormat and the Style Gallery

Word's AutoFormat feature allows you to format a document quickly and automatically. When you use AutoFormat, Word assigns a paragraph style to each paragraph in your document, using heading styles and body text styles where appropriate. Once AutoFormat has applied the styles, you can change the look of your document using the Style Gallery. The Style Gallery will change the features of each style that AutoFormat inserted in your document.

To format a document automatically:

1. Choose AutoFormat from the Format menu.

2. Click OK to verify that you want to proceed with AutoFormat.

   A dialog box opens offering choices to accept, reject, or review changes. You also can choose to open the Style Gallery from this dialog box.

Figure 20-2
You can either accept or reject the changes made by AutoFormat.

3. Click the Accept button.

4. Scroll through the document and notice the changes made.

   Word assigns styles based on the document's structure; for example, short lines are treated as headings. The following sections of this lesson show you how to make changes to styles.

5. On the Formatting toolbar, click the down arrow next to the Style box to open the Style drop-down list box.

   Notice the new styles added to the list.

6. Click outside the list box to close it.

The Style Gallery can be used to modify the look of a document after it has been formatted using AutoFormat. The style gallery will change the format attributes of the styles already assigned to the document by AutoFormat. See Figure 20-3 on page 394.

To use the Style Gallery:

1. Choose Style Gallery from the Format menu.

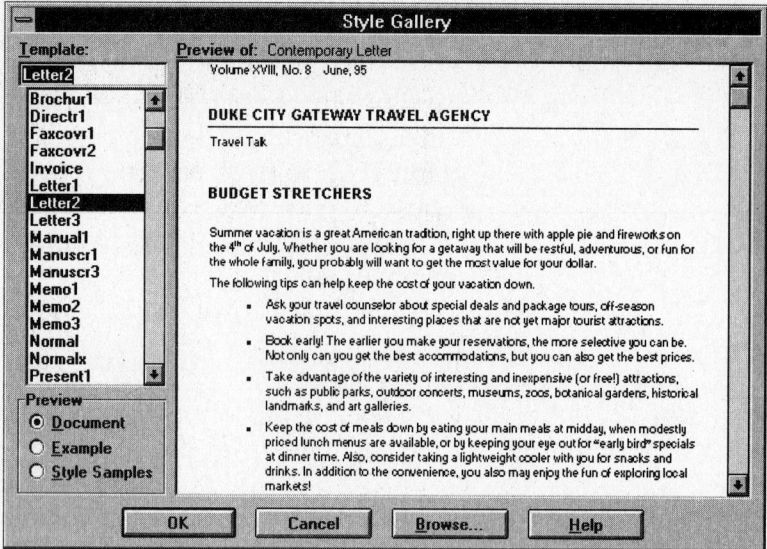

Figure 20-3
The Style Gallery dialog box

The Style Gallery dialog box fills the screen, displaying a sample of formatted text and a list of templates.

2. Choose Memo1 from the Template list box.

    The formatting of the sample text changes.

3. Choose Present1.

    The text is enlarged, suitable for overhead transparencies.

4. Choose Letter2 and click OK.

    Scroll through the document, and notice the formatting changes.

5. Open the Style drop-down list box on the Formatting toolbar, and scroll through the list.

    There are many new styles on the list.

6. Close the document without saving it.

Creating and Naming Paragraph Styles

Creating paragraph styles is as easy as formatting a paragraph. To create a style, you select a paragraph that you have already formatted and then give the format a name. The style will include all the formatting instructions that you have applied to the selected paragraph.

Style name
A name given to a style to identify it.

To identify styles, you give them *style names*. Style names may have up to 253 characters and can include any characters except the Backslash (\), braces, ({or}), or semicolon (;). Each new style name must be different from the other style names already in the document. You can create and name styles using either the Formatting toolbar or the Styles command from the Format menu.

To create and name a paragraph style using the Formatting toolbar:

1. Reopen the file 20-0.doc.

2. Select the heading "**BUDGET STRETCHERS**".

3. Change the text to 18-point Times New Roman bold.

4. Select the word "Normal" that is showing in the Style box on the Formatting toolbar.

5. Key **Headline** and press **Enter**.

   You have created and named the paragraph style "Headline."

To create and name a style using the Style command:

1. Select the paragraph beneath "**BUDGET STRETCHERS**".

2. Choose Style from Format menu.

3. Click the New button.

   The New Style dialog box opens.

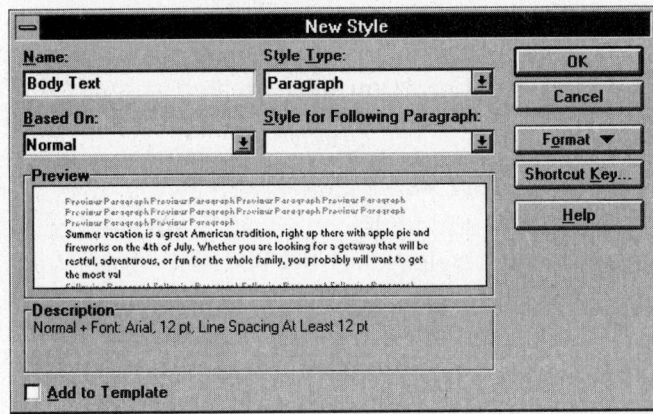

Figure 20-4
The New Style dialog box

4. Key **Body** in the Name text box.

5. Click the Format button, and then choose Font.

6. In the Font dialog box, choose Times New Roman from the Font list box and 14 from the Size list box. Click OK.

   Notice the change in the Description box.

7. Click OK.

8. Click the Apply button.

   You have created and named the style "Body" using the Style command.

Creating and Naming Character Styles

When creating character styles, you must use the Style dialog box. You cannot create character styles by selecting formatted text.

To create and name a character style:

1. Choose Style from the Format menu.

2. Click the New button.

3. Key **Emphasis** in the Name box.

4. Choose Character from the Style Type drop-down list box, to the right of the Name box.

5. Click the Format button, and then choose Font.

6. From the Font dialog box, choose Times New Roman, Single underline, and Italic.

7. Click OK to close the Font dialog box, and then click OK again to close the New Style dialog box.

8. Click Close to close the Style dialog box.

Applying Styles

Note: To apply a style to a paragraph, you can simply place the insertion point in the paragraph without selecting the text. Remember, this is also true for applying paragraph formatting to a paragraph.

Once you have created a style, you can apply it to any text in a document. To apply a paragraph style, first select the paragraph or paragraphs you want to format, and then either click the style name in the Style drop-down list box on the Formatting toolbar or use the Style command from the Format menu. To apply a character style, select the text to be formatted, and then choose a character style using the Formatting toolbar or the Style dialog box. Paragraph styles are displayed on the list box in boldface, and character styles are displayed in normal text. Paragraph styles always format an entire paragraph, even when only a part of the paragraph is selected, but character styles format only the text that is selected.

To apply a character style using the Formatting toolbar:

1. Select the text "special deals" in the first bulleted paragraph.

2. Choose Emphasis from the Style drop-down list on the Formatting toolbar.

    The selected text is now displayed as Times New Roman, italics and underlined.

To apply a paragraph style using the Formatting toolbar:

1. Position the insertion point in the text "Volume XVIII, No. 8" at the top of the document.

2. Choose Heading 1 from the Style drop-down list box.

    The style Heading 1 is applied to the text.

To apply a style using the Style command:

1. Position the insertion point in the text "HOME ON THE RANGE" at the bottom of the first page.

2. Choose Style from the Format menu.

3. Choose Headline from the Styles list box.

    Notice the formatting instructions of the style Headline in the Description box.

4. Click the Apply button.

    The style Headline is applied to the text.

When applying a style several times in one document, you can use the Repeat command. For example, after you have applied a style, select the next paragraph to which you want to apply that style (or place the insertion point in the paragraph). Then press the **F4** key to apply the style's formatting.

To reapply a style using the Repeat command:

1. Position the insertion point in the heading "CIBOLA NATIONAL FOREST" at the top of page 2.

2. Press the **F4** key.

Redefining and Renaming Styles

Once you have created and named a style, you can redefine the style by changing its formatting instructions. When you redefine a style, the changes you make will affect each paragraph that has that style. For example, if you applied a style to all the headings in your document, and you redefine the style, all the headings will be changed. You can also redefine any of the standard styles that are available in Word documents. To redefine a style, you can use the Formatting toolbar or the Style command on the Format menu.

To redefine a style using the Formatting toolbar:

1. Select the heading "HOME ON THE RANGE".

2. Change the text to 14-point italic.

3. Choose the style name Headline from the Style drop-down list box.

    The Reapply Style dialog box appears. You can choose to redefine the style or return the text to the style's original format.

4. Click OK to redefine the style.

    The redefined style is reflected in all uses of the style. Notice the change in "CIBOLA NATIONAL FOREST".

When you redefine a style using the Style dialog box, you click the Modify button, click the Format button, and choose a formatting command from the Format drop-down list.

Figure 20-5

The Format drop-down list in the Modify Style dialog box

To redefine a style using the Style command on the Format menu:

1. Position the insertion point in the text "Volume XVIII, No. 8" at the beginning of the document.

2. Choose Style from the Format menu.

3. Click the Modify button.

4. Click the Format button, and then choose Font.

5. In the drop-down list box for Underline, choose None.

6. Click OK to close the Font dialog box, and then click OK again to close the Modify dialog box.

7. Click Close to close the Style dialog box.

You can also rename any style that you have created. However, you cannot rename Word's standard styles. To rename a style, use the Style command on the Format menu.

To rename a style:

1. Choose Style from the Format menu.

2. Choose Headline from the Styles list box.

3. Click the Modify button.

4. Key **First Head** in the Name text box.

5. Click OK.

    The style First Head appears in the Styles list box, and Headline is no longer on the list.

6. Close the Style dialog box.

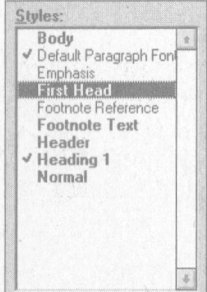

"First Head" appears on the Styles list box.

Deleting Styles

You can delete styles that you no longer need from the style sheet by using the Delete option in the Style dialog box. When you delete a style from the style sheet, any paragraph that contained the formatting for the style returns to the Normal style. Word does not allow you to delete the standard styles from the style sheet.

To delete a style:

1. Choose Style from the Format menu.

2. Choose Body from the Styles list box.

3. Click the Delete button.

4. Click Yes when prompted to verify the deletion, and then click Close.

   The Body style is deleted, and the paragraph returns to the Normal style.

Saving Styles

Word saves the styles you create for a document when you save the document. A style that is created and saved with a document is available for use only with that document. The next lesson explains how to save styles in templates, so they can be used on other documents.

Using Styles and Style Sheets

Formatting a document with styles improves the appearance and consistency of the document. When you organize a document using styles and style sheets, you save time and create an attractive, readable document. You can use options available in the Style dialog box to make formatting with styles easier. These options include the Style for Following Paragraph option and the Based On option.

The Style for Following Paragraph Option

The Style for Following Paragraph option helps you to automate the formatting of your document. You can apply a style to a paragraph and specify what style is to follow immediately after the paragraph. For example, you can create a style for a heading and specify a body text style for the next paragraph. Then, after keying the heading text, press **Enter**, and Word automatically changes the next paragraph to the body text style.

To specify a style as a next style, you first create and name the style, if it is not already available.

To specify a style as a next style:

1. Choose Style from the Format menu, and then click the New button.

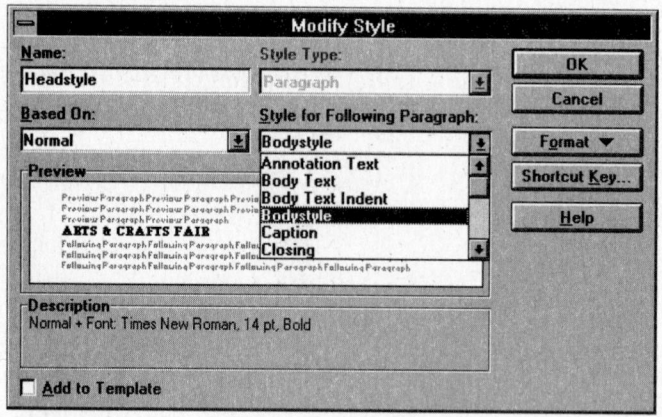

Figure 20-6

Choosing a style for the following paragraph

2. Key **Bodystyle** in the Name text box.

3. Click the Format button and choose Font.

4. Choose 12-point Times New Roman. Click OK.

    The new style attributes appear in the Description box.

5. Click OK again, and then click Close.

6. Near the bottom of the first page, change the text "ARTS & CRAFTS FAIR" to 14-point Times New Roman bold.

7. In the Style drop-down list box, key **Headstyle** and press **Enter**.

8. Choose Style from the Format menu.

    Notice that Headstyle is chosen in the Styles list box.

9. Click the Modify button.

10. In the Style for Following Paragraph drop-down list box, choose Bodystyle.

11. Click OK, and then click Close.

12. Move the insertion point to the end of "**ARTS & CRAFTS FAIR**" and press **Enter**.

    Bodystyle is indicated as the style for the next paragraph.

13. Key the following text:

    June 20-22
    10 a.m. - 6 p.m.
    State Fair Grounds

Note: When keying a telephone number, remember
to use a nonbreaking
space after the area code
and a nonbreaking hyphen
after the first three digits
to prevent a line break
within the number.

**For more information, contact the Albuquerque
Convention and Visitors Bureau at (303) 555-3696.**

The text is in Bodystyle: 12-point Times New Roman.

The Based On Option

The Based On option helps you format a document consistently. This
feature is useful in long documents with many styles that have similar formatting instructions. You can base the different styles in a
document on one base style that may include specific character or
paragraph formatting. For example, the standard styles that are
available with each new Word document are all based on the Normal
style. As explained earlier, if you modify the Normal style by changing the font, the fonts of the other standard styles are changed automatically to match the Normal style.

You can quickly reformat long documents by specifying one style as
the base style for the headings and one style as the base style for the
body text. For example, you can format a document with several different heading styles that are all based on one heading style and several different body-text styles based on one body-text style. Then, if
you decide to change the formatting of the headings or the body
text, you can easily change all the styles just by changing the two
base styles. Before you can create styles based on a base style, you
must create the base style.

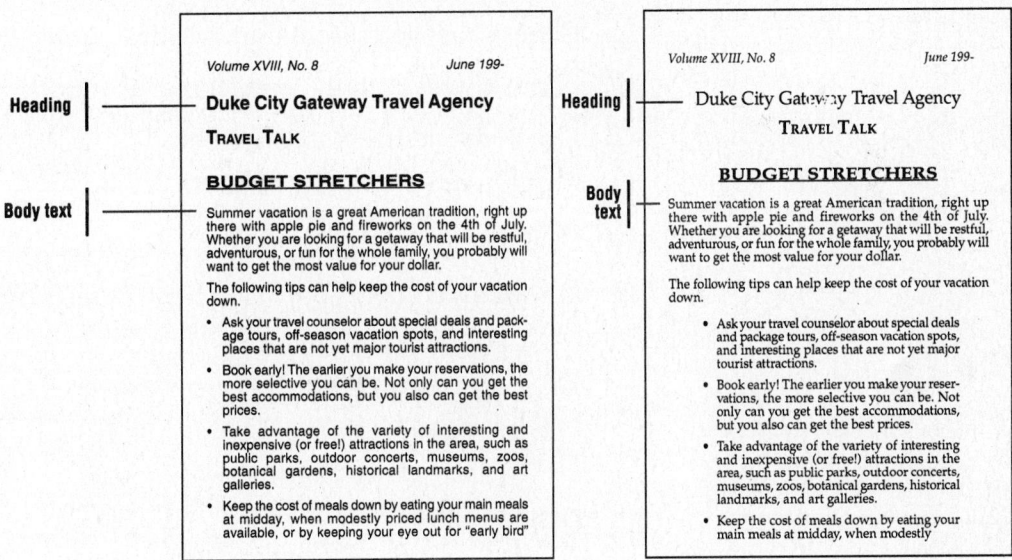

Figure 20-7
Using different base styles for headings and body text

To create a base style:

1. Select the text near the bottom of page 2 from "Travel Talk" to
    "Franchise".

2. Change the font to Times New Roman.

3. In the Style drop-down list box, key the name **Basebody** and press **Enter**.

To create other styles based on the base style:

1. Select the text in the next paragraph from "Editorial/ Advertising Office" to "87111".

2. Choose Basebody from the Style drop-down list box.

3. Choose Style from the Format menu, and then click New.

4. In the Name text box, key **Body2**

5. Click the Format button, and then choose Font.

6. Choose Italic, and then click OK.

   Notice the formatting instructions of the style in the Description box.

7. In the Based On list box, make sure Basebody is chosen, and then click OK.

8. Click the Apply button.

   Word applies the new style to the selected paragraph. The new style is based on the Basebody style.

9. Select the text from "President" through "Valerie Grier".

10. Choose Basebody from the Style drop-down list box.

11. Choose Style from the Format menu, and then click New.

12. Key **Body3** in the Name text box.

13. Click the Format button, and then choose Font.

14. Change the size to 10 and click OK.

15. In the Based On list box, make sure Basebody is chosen, and then click OK.

16. Click the Apply button.

   The paragraph is formatted in the Body3 style and is based on Basebody.

17. Deselect the text.

To make formatting changes to the base style:

1. Choose Style from the Format menu.

2. Choose Basebody from the Styles list box.

3. Click the Modify button.

4. Click the Format button, and then choose Font.

5. In the Font box, choose Courier New and click OK.

   Notice the change in the Description box.

6. Click OK, and then click Close.

   The Basebody style changes, along with the Body2 and Body3 styles.

Tips for Using Styles and Style Sheets

Word gives you options that make working with styles easier. You can:

- Print a document's styles

- Display the style area

- Create keyboard shortcuts for styles

Print a document's styles to view a list of all the styles used in the document, along with their formatting instructions.

Figure 20-8

The Styles option on the Print What drop-down list

To print the style sheet:

1. Choose Print from the File menu.

2. In the Print What drop-down list, choose Styles, and then click OK.

   Word prints the styles for your active document.

You can display the style area in a document. When you display the style area, the style names applied to the paragraphs in the document appear in the left margin.

To display the style area:

1. Choose Options from the Tools menu.

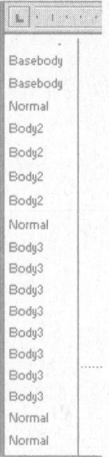

Style area

2. Under Category, click View, if necessary.

3. In the Style Area Width box, inside the Window box, key **0.6**

4. Click OK.

    The style area appears in the left margin.

Word allows you to assign shortcut keys to apply styles. Using a shortcut key, you can quickly apply a style without using the Formatting toolbar or Style command. When you create a shortcut key for a style, you usually include the **Ctrl** key, the **Shift** key, or the **Alt** key and a letter as part of the shortcut.

To assign a shortcut key to a style:

1. Choose Style from the Format menu.

2. In the Styles list box, choose Basebody.

3. Click the Modify button, and then click the Shortcut Key button.

    The Customize Keyboard dialog box opens.

4. In the Press New Shortcut Key box, press **Alt+B**.

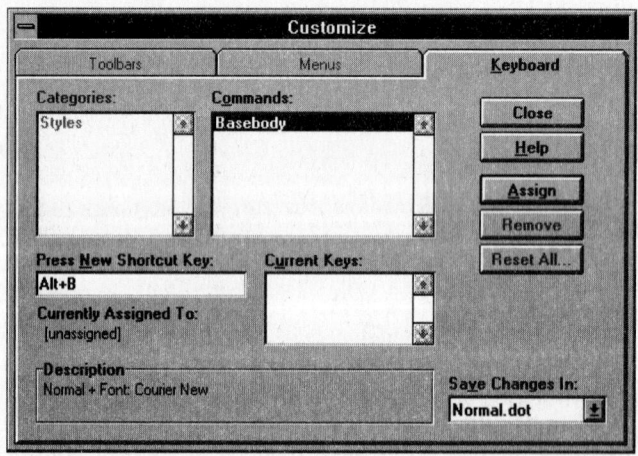

Figure 20-9
The Keyboard tab in the Customize dialog box

5. Click the Assign button, and then click Close.

6. Click OK to close the Modify Style dialog box, and then click Close to close the Style dialog box.

7. Select the paragraph on page 2 that begins "Come to Paella".

8. Press **Alt+B**.

    The style Basebody is applied to the text.

Using Another Document's Style Sheet

In Word, you can apply styles from one document to another using the Organizer option on the Style dialog box. For example, suppose you have two similar documents. In Document A, you have updated the styles to reflect different formatting. Instead of making the same changes to the styles in Document B, you can copy Document A's styles to Document B.

When you copy styles, all styles with the same name are updated with the new style's formatting. For example, Documents A and B both have a style called Heading 1. When you copy styles from Document A to Document B, the text in Document B with the style Heading 1 will take on the formatting from the Document A style. Style names that are not the same are added to the new document's list of styles.

To copy a style from one document to another: Open the Style dialog box, and then click the Organizer button. In the Organizer dialog box, click the Close File button on the left side. Then, when it changes to the Open File button, click it again, and choose the file that contains the styles you want to copy. On the right side of the dialog box, open the document to which the styles will be copied. On the left list of styles, choose all the styles to be copied, and then click the Copy button. Close the dialog box.

Using Styles Supplied with Word

Note: There are also styles that only appear when needed, such as styles for creating a table of contents or index. To view all the standard styles, choose Style from the Format menu, and then choose All Styles from the List drop-down list box in the lower left corner.

As mentioned earlier, Word provides you with standard styles in each new document. The standard styles that appear in the Styles drop-down list box are: Normal, Heading 1, Heading 2, Heading 3, and Default Paragraph Font. You can view these styles on the Formatting toolbar.

When you begin keying text in a new document, the text appears in the Normal style. When you press **Enter**, the new paragraphs are also in the Normal style. You can apply Word's other standard styles to the text as needed. Select the text to which you want to apply the style, and then choose the style name from the Style drop-down list box on the Formatting toolbar.

Standard styles also have the following shortcut keys: Normal, **Ctrl+Shift+N**; Heading 1, **Alt+Ctrl+1**: Heading 2, **Alt+Ctrl+2**; Heading 3, **Alt+Ctrl+3**.

To apply standard styles to text:

1. On page 1, select the Heading "Duke City Gateway Travel Agency".

2. From the Style drop-down list box, choose Heading 1.

3. Select the heading "Travel Talk".

4. From the Style drop-down list box, choose Heading 3.

    The standard styles are applied to the text.

5. Choose Options from the Tools menu to restore the style-name area width to 0.

6. Spell-check the document, and save it as *[your three-letter identifier]*20-0.doc.

7. Print the document.

    Notice that the different formatting of the different styles gives the document an inconsistent look. A document like this can, however, serve as a sample sheet from which to select preferred, printed formats.

8. Close the document and exit Word (unless you will be doing the following exercises immediately).

If Word's standard styles are not suitable for a document, you can redefine the formatting instructions of the standard styles. Remember, all the standard styles are based on the Normal style.

Table 20-1: Keyboard Shortcuts for Styles	
Keyboard Shortcut	Action
Ctrl+Shift+N	Apply Normal style
Alt+Ctrl+1	Apply Heading 1
Alt+Ctrl+2	Apply Heading 2
Alt+Ctrl+3	Apply Heading 3

Key Terms

Character style   Style name

Normal style   Style sheet

Paragraph style

Exercises

Exercise 20.1

1. Start Word, if necessary.

2. Open the file 20-1.doc.

3. Change the format of the first line of text, beginning with "Family", to 24-point Arial bold. Center the text.

4. Create a style for the text using the Formatting toolbar:

   A. Select the style name shown in the Style box on the Formatting toolbar.

   B. Key **Headline1**

   C. Press **Enter**.

5. Select the second line of text, beginning with "Transportation". Center the text.

6. Create a style using the Style command:

   A. Choose Style from the Format menu.

   B. Click the New button.

   C. In the Name box, key **Headline2**

   D. Click the Format button, and then choose Font.

   E. In the Font dialog box, choose 18-point Arial Italic and click OK.

   F. Click OK to close the New Style dialog box. Then click the Apply button.

7. On a new line after the phone number, key:

   Gateway Travel—Your Gateway To The World

8. Apply the Headline2 style to the new sentence:

   A. Select the text you keyed.

   B. Choose Headline2 from the Style drop-down list box on the Formatting toolbar.

9. Center the unstyled text.

10. Format the document with double-line spacing, and then center the document vertically.

11. Spell-check the document.

12. Save the document as *[your three-letter identifier]*20-1.doc.

13. Print the document.

14. Close the document and exit Word (unless you will be doing the following exercises immediately).

Exercise 20.2

1. Start Word, if necessary.

2. Open the file 15-3.doc.

3. Create a style for the first line of text:

A. Select the text, and then choose Style from the Format menu.

B. Click the New button.

C. In the Name box, key **HeadCenter**

D. Click the Format button, and then choose Font.

E. Choose 24-point Times New Roman and click OK.

F. Click the Format button again and choose Paragraph.

G. Click the Indents and Spacing tab, choose Center Alignment, and then click OK.

H. Click OK again to close the New Style dialog box, and then click the Apply button.

4. Create a style for the names and addresses:

A. Change the first name and address to 12-point Times New Roman italic.

B. In the Style Name list box on the Formatting toolbar, key **Address** and press **Enter**.

5. Select all the text in the table, and then choose Address from the Style drop-down list box to apply the style.

6. Delete the HeadCenter style from the style sheet:

A. Choose Style from the Format menu.

B. In the Styles list box, choose HeadCenter.

C. Click the Delete button. Click Yes to confirm the deletion.

D. Click Close.

7. Change the style Address from italic to bold:

A. Choose Style from the Format menu.

B. Choose Address from the Styles list box.

C. Click the Modify button.

D. Click the Format button, and then choose Font.

E. Click Bold in the Font Style list box and click OK.

F. Click OK again, and then click Close.

8. Change the type size of the text above the table to 16 point.

9. Spell-check the document, and save it as *[your three-letter identifier]*20-2.doc.

10. Print the document.

11. Close the document and exit Word (unless you will be doing the following exercises immediately).

Exercise 20.3

1. Start Word, if necessary.

2. Open the file 20-3.doc.

3. At the beginning of the document, key the text in Figure 20-10. Include the corrections.

Figure 20-10

Ms. Joan Piazza

WeatherTech Industries

42 Las Galinas Boulevard

Albuquerque, NM 87111

Dear Joan:

Regarding the sales incentive trip to the Caribbean for your account executives, I have researched accommodations ~~that meet your specifications~~ To cut down on cost, you may want to plan the trip so that you avoid paying peak=season rates.

The following list of Paradise Island hotels indicates each hotel's peak season:

---

4. Format the document as a business letter with today's date, from Nina Chavez, Travel Counselor. Use a three-line continuation header on page 2.

5. Display the style area so that it appears in the first .5 inches of the document screen.

6. Apply the standard style, Heading 1, to "Crown Beach Resort".

7. Apply the style Heading 2 to the dates "2/2-4/15".

8. Apply Heading 1 to the next hotel name.

9. Use the Repeat command to repeat the style formatting for the next three hotel names.

10. Apply Heading 2 to the date "3/23-3/31", and then use the Repeat command to repeat the style formatting for the next three dates.

11. Change the View option to remove the style area display.

12. Spell-check the document.

13. Save the document as *[your three-letter identifier]*20-3.doc.

14. Print the document and the styles for the document.

15. Close the document and exit Word (unless you will be doing the following exercise immediately).

Exercise 20.4: Challenge Yourself

Open the file 20-4.doc. Format the document as a memo from Doris Simms with the subject "Museum Update". Insert the date as a field, and change the left and right margins to 1.25 inches.

Create a style called "Text" based on the Normal style, with the italic attribute.

Insert the text **The Albuquerque Museum** as a separate paragraph above "National Atomic Museum". Format the text you just keyed in 14-point Times New Roman bold, and then use the formatted text to create a style called "Headstyle". Define the shortcut **Alt+Shift+H** for this style. Specify the style Text as the next style following the style Headstyle.

With the insertion point to the right of "The Albuquerque Museum", press **Enter**. Then key the following text in the next style:

For more information, call Elinor Roberts at 555-6787.

Press **Enter** twice, and then key **Pueblo Cultural Center**. Apply the Headstyle style to the text just keyed, press **Enter**, and key the following text in the next style:

For more information, call Marilyn Swift at 555-2344.

Use the Formatting toolbar to apply the style Headstyle to "National Atomic Museum". Apply the style Text to the next line, which begins "For more information".

Use the keyboard shortcut for Headstyle for the next museum name. Move to the end of the line, press **Enter**, and then key the following text in the next style:

For more information, call Jose Diaz at 555-4777.

Spell-check the document. Save the document as *[your three-letter identifier]*20-4.doc and print it. Print the document and the style sheet for the document. Close the document and exit Word.

Templates, Wizards, and AutoText

Objectives

- Use Word templates and wizards.
- Create new templates.
- Modify templates.
- Work with AutoText entries.
- Use the Spike.

Template
A file that contains the formatting information, styles, and sometimes text for a particular type of document.

Wizard
A template that contains sophisticated macros to automate document creation.

If you often create the same types of documents, such as memos or letters, or repeat the same text, such as standard salutations and closings, you will benefit from three of Word's timesaving features: templates, wizards, and AutoText. These features allow you to store document-formatting information and text so that you can use them again and again. They can increase your productivity with Word.

What Are Templates and Wizards?

A *template* is a file that contains the formatting information, styles, and sometimes text for a particular type of document. The purpose of the template is to provide a reusable model for all documents of the same type. You can use the template to speed up the creation of new documents. For example, you can create a letter template that contains the correct formatting, styles, and standard text for a business letter. Then you can use this template as a model for new business letters you create. By using the template, you avoid recreating the same formatting, styles, and text for each new letter.

A *wizard* is a sophisticated template that allows you to choose formatting options and prompts for text entries to be included in the resulting document. Wizards can format letters, memos, and reports quickly.

In Word, the default template file is NORMAL.DOT. New documents you create in Word contain all the formatting features that are assigned to the NORMAL.DOT template, such as the default font, type size, margins, and page orientation. When you save and name the new document, all the formatting information and text in the NORMAL.DOT template is transferred to the new document, but the original template file is not changed. It remains intact and can be reused to create future documents.

The NORMAL.DOT template is different from all other templates, because it stores some items that are available globally. That means that they can be used in every new document, regardless of the template you choose to use with the document. These global items are discussed later in this lesson and in Lesson 22.

The following features may be included in templates and wizards:

411

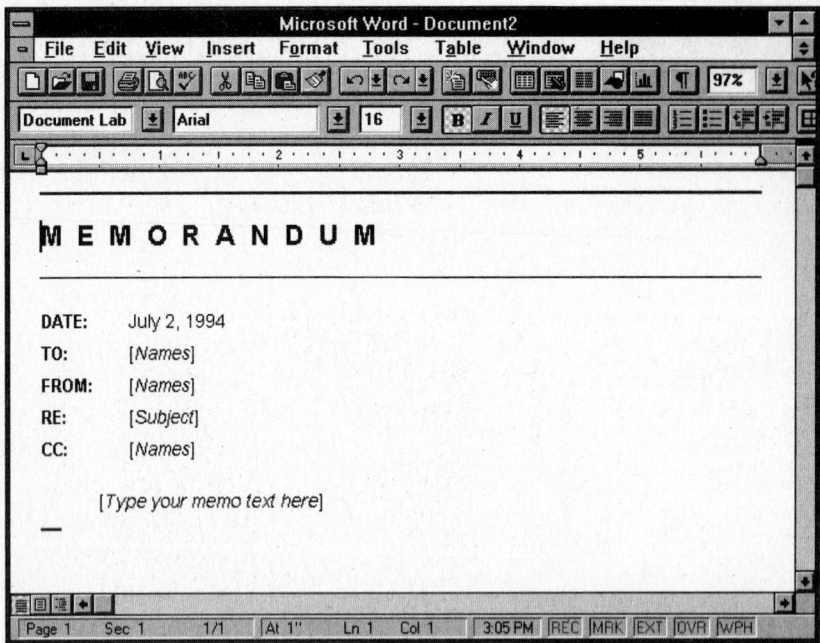

Figure 21-1
An example of a template for a business memo

- Formatting features, such as margins, columns, and page orientation for the entire document or sections of the document

- Standard text that is repeated in all documents of the same type, such as a company name and address in a letter template

- Character and paragraph formatting that are saved in styles

- Macros (automated procedures) and AutoText entries. The *AutoText* feature allows you to store frequently used text and graphics, so that they can be inserted into a document whenever needed with just a few keystrokes.

AutoText
A Word feature that allows you to store frequently used text and graphics that can be easily retrieved to be inserted in a document when needed.

Using Word Templates and Wizards to Create New Documents

Each time you create a new document, you can choose a template or a wizard for the document. When you choose New from the File menu, the New dialog box opens, displaying the Template list box. This box lists the different templates and wizards that are available for you to choose. By default, every new Word document that you open is based on the NORMAL.DOT template. To open a new document that is based on a template other than NORMAL.DOT, choose a template or wizard name from the Template list box and click OK. A new document that contains a copy of the chosen template opens automatically. The original template remains intact for future use. If you choose a wizard, a series of dialog boxes will open, allowing you

Note: The template and wizard names that appear in the Template list box include all of the Word-supplied templates and any templates that you have created. For template names to appear in the Template list box, they must be stored in the same directory as the Word program.

to make choices about formatting and possibly asking you to key text to be placed in the document. A document formatted by a wizard also contains a copy of a template.

Word supplies you with a number of useful templates and wizards that you can use to create new documents. Many of these are for standard business documents, such as letters, memos, articles, business proposals, and reports.

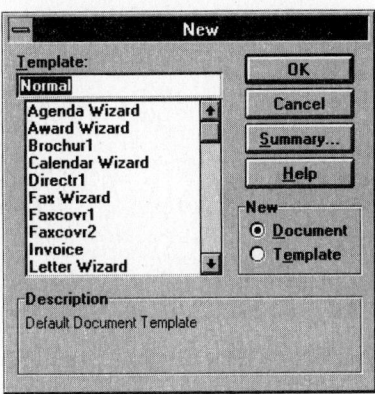

Figure 21-2
Templates and wizards listed in the New dialog box

Table 21-1: Template and Wizard Names and Descriptions	
Name	Description
Agenda Wizard	Creates an organized agenda for a meeting
Fax Wizard	Creates a fax cover sheet in one of three styles
Letter Wizard	Creates a business or personal letter, including sample wording
Letter1	Provides the framework for a classic-style business letter
Manual1	Provides the framework for creating training manuals or booklets
Memo Wizard	Formats a memo in one of three styles and inserts To, From, Date, and CC in the appropriate places
Present1	Provides the framework for creating overhead transparencies
Report2	Provides the framework for creating a business report in the contemporary style
Resume Wizard	Helps you create one of three styles of attractive resumes
Thesis	Provides the framework for creating a term paper or thesis

Templates and wizards have advanced features that automate the procedures for creating documents. They include:

- Dialog boxes

  When you create a document with a wizard, dialog boxes appear asking you to fill in certain information that will appear in the document, such as names and addresses.

- Predefined styles

  Each Word template includes a style sheet containing styles for different formatting instructions.

- Specialized commands

  Some Word templates or wizards may include commands that help you accomplish specific tasks. These commands are listed at the bottom of the dialog box.

To use the Memo Wizard:

1. Start Word, if necessary.

2. Choose New from the File menu.

3. In the Template list box, choose Memo Wizard and click OK.

   The Memo Wizard dialog box appears.

4. Read the dialog box information, and then click the Next button to accept the default.

5. Follow the instructions on the screen, pressing the Next button to get to the next step.

6. When the last dialog box appears, click the Finish button.

   The memo appears, indicating where to key the appropriate information.

7. Close the document without saving your changes.

Figure 21-3
A Memo Wizard dialog box

Creating New Templates

In Word, you can create templates for different types of documents. This is a very useful feature, because it allows you to set up your own standard formats for documents that are keyed frequently. For some types of documents, the process of creating a new template is easier than the process of modifying a Word template.

There are three ways to create a new template:

- You can create a blank template file using the default template and define the formatting information, styles, and text according to your own specifications.

- You can open an existing template, modify it, and save it with a new name.

- You can open an existing document, modify it, and save it as a new template.

Note: When you create a new template, Word automatically gives the template the extension .DOT. By default, all saved template files are stored in the Word program directory.

Modifying templates is discussed later in this lesson. However, even when you create a new template, as in the following procedure, you are actually using the NORMAL.DOT template as a starting point. You modify the template's formatting features and then save the resulting template with a new name.

You can insert a date field code in a template, so that the date is inserted automatically when you create a new document and is updated each time the document is printed. Sometimes, it is necessary to insert a date that does not change after the document is completed. You can use the SaveDate field code or the CreateDate field code for this purpose. The SaveDate code is updated each time a document is saved. The CreateDate code reflects the date the document was first created, and never changes.

To create a new template:

1. Select New from the File menu.

2. Choose the Template option.

   By choosing the Template option, you are indicating that you want to create a template, not a document.

3. Click OK.

   A new template file opens. Note that the title is Template1.

4. Choose Page Setup from the File menu, and set the margins for a standard, block-style business letter: Set a 2-inch top margin and 1-inch bottom, left, and right margins. (To review business-letter format, see Appendix B.)

5. Create a style named "Bodytext" that is 11-point Times New Roman for the text of the letter. Apply the Bodytext style to the paragraph mark at the top of the document.

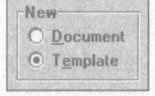

Creating a new template

6. To insert the CreateDate field code, choose Field from the Insert menu, and choose Date and Time from the Categories list box, and then choose CreateDate from the Field Names list box.

7. To format the date, click the Options button in the Field dialog box.

8. Choose the fifth format in the Date Time Formats list box, click the Add to Field button, and then click OK.

9. Click OK again to close the Field dialog box.

10. Press **Enter** six times.

11. Key the inside address and the salutation:

    Mr. Roger Furman
    Furman & Price Marketing, Inc.
    52 Jefferson Boulevard
    Albuquerque, NM 87109

    Dear Mr. Furman:

12. On the third line after the salutation, key the closing:

    Sincerely,

    Nina Chavez
    Travel Counselor

    vg

    There should be three blank lines between "Sincerely," and the letter writer's name and one blank line between the title and the typist's initials. See Figure 21-4 on page 417.

13. Choose Save As from the File menu.

    The Save As dialog box appears with a list of template files in the File Name list box.

14. Key the appropriate path and the filename **letter.dot**. For example, key **a:\letter.dot**

15. Click OK (or press **Enter**), and then close the template.

    The template is stored on the document diskette. Because this template is not stored in the Word program directory, its name will not appear in the Use Template box, but you will be able to use it later in the lesson.

You can also create a template by modifying an existing document and then saving it as a template.

To create a new template by modifying an existing document:

1. Choose New from the File menu.

2. Click the Template button.

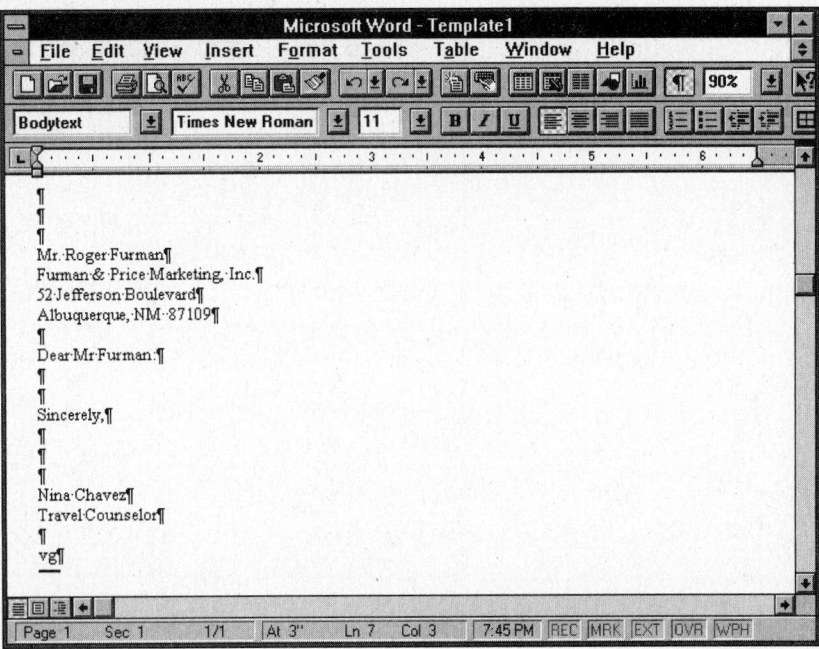

Figure 21-4
The new letter template

3. In the Template text box, key the appropriate path and the filename **21-0a.doc**, which you will use as a basis for the template. If your document diskette is in the a: drive, key **a:\21-0a.doc** and click OK.

   The document opens as a template file.

4. Format as a standard business memo: Set a 2-inch top margin and 1-inch bottom, left, and right margins. Set a 1-inch left-aligned tab.

5. Insert three blank lines at the top of the document, and then move to the first line. Key the memo heading, inserting one tab after each colon and double-spacing between each line:

   MEMO TO:

   FROM:

   DATE: *[insert CreateDate field code]*

   SUBJECT:

6. Delete the text below the heading from "I know you wanted" through the end of the document.

7. Change the Normal style to 12-point Times New Roman.

   You now have a memo format into which you can key future memos.

8. Press **Alt+F9** to see the CreateDate field code, and then press **Alt+F9** again to return the display to date text.

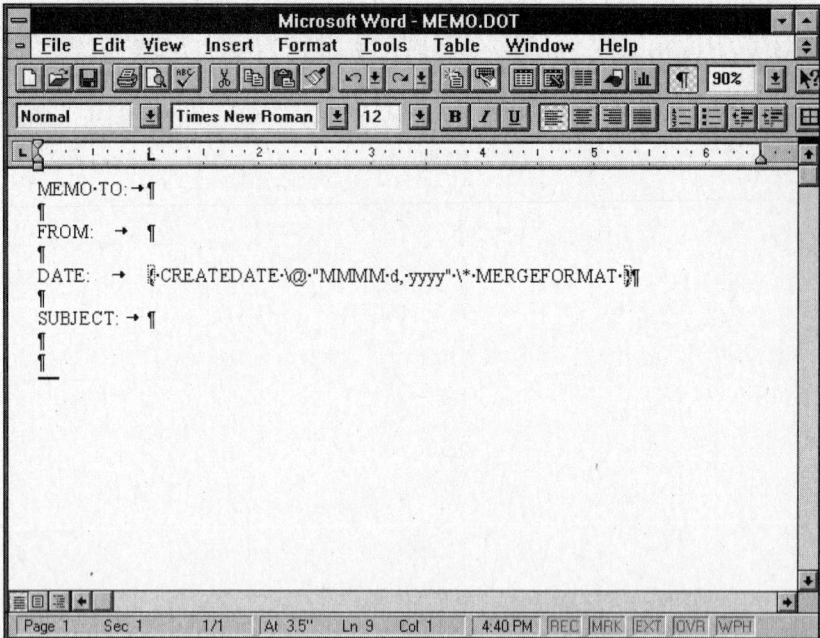

Figure 21-5
The template with CreateDate field code displayed

9.   Choose Save As from the File menu.

The Save As dialog box appears.

Note: The procedure for creating a new template from an existing template is discussed in this lesson under "Modifying Templates."

10.   Key the appropriate path and the filename **memo.dot**. For example, key **a:\memo.dot**. Click OK.

11.   Close the template.

Attaching Templates to Documents

Attach
Assign a template to an existing document.

Remember that all existing documents have templates, either the NORMAL.DOT template or another template that you assigned when you created the document. You can change the template assigned to an existing document. When you change to a different template, you *attach* the new template to the document. The main reason that you might want to attach a template to a document is to take advantage of the macros, AutoText entries, and other automated features of the template. For instance, you might have a report document that is largely unformatted and a report template with a macro that automates formatting that would be applicable to the document. By attaching the report template to the document, you can use the features of the template to format the report document quickly. You use the Template option on the File menu to attach a template to a document.

When you attach a template to an existing document, standard text and page formatting is not transferred to the document. The text content of the document remains unchanged. You do, however, have the option of transferring the template styles. If you choose to transfer the styles, template styles will override document styles that have the same style name. Document styles with names that do not match the template names will remain unchanged. Template styles with names that do not match the document styles will be added to the document's style sheet.

Modifying Templates

Once you create a template, Word allows you to change its formatting and redefine its styles. The easiest way to modify a template is to open the original template and make changes to it. A second way to modify a template is to copy a style sheet from another template or document into it. You can also create a modified version of a template and save it with a different filename. This allows you to save multiple templates of the same basic type but with variations in formatting and text.

Modifying Formatting

The changes you make to the formatting or text in a template will affect any future documents that are based on the template. These changes do not affect documents that were created from the template before you modified it.

To modify a template's formatting:

1. Choose Open from the File menu.

2. Choose Document Templates in the List Files of Type drop-down list box.

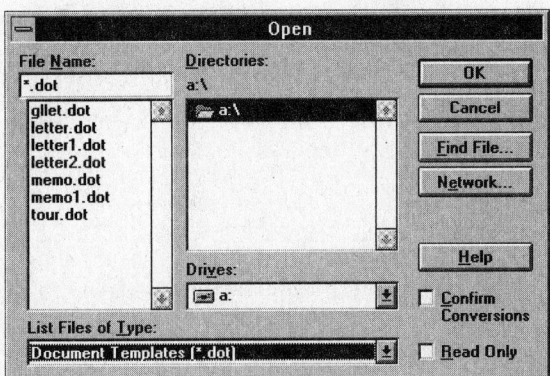

Figure 21-6

Choosing a document template from the Open dialog box

3. Choose the file letter.dot from your student disk and click OK.

4. Change the Bodytext style to 12-point Arial.

5. Change the letter format from a block to a standard modified-block format by left-aligning the date and closing with the center of the page. (Refer to Appendix B.)

6. On the first inside address line, replace "Mr. Roger Furman" with "Name". Then replace the three-line address with "Address".

7. On the Salutation line, delete "Mr. Furman", so that the line reads "Dear :".

8. In the closing, replace "Nina Chavez" with "Sender" and "Travel Counselor" with "Title".

9. Replace the typist's initials "vg" with "initials".

10. Choose Save from the File menu.

    The template is saved with the changes. The earlier version of the template has been overwritten by the new version.

11. Close the template.

Note: To keep both the block and modified-block letter templates, you would use the Save As command rather than the Save command. Then you would key a different filename for the modified-block template.

Copying Styles

You can modify the styles in a template in either of two ways. One way is to open the template and change the style definitions, as you did in the previous procedure. The second way is to copy styles from another document or template into the current template. Copying styles from one document into another or from one template into another is essentially the same procedure: Open the Style dialog box, and then click the Organizer button.

Figure 21-7
The Organizer dialog box

The Organizer dialog box has two list boxes. Under each list box is a Close File button that changes to an Open File button when clicked. Choose either a document or a template file to be displayed in each list box. The list boxes show all the styles in the opened files. You can copy a style from one file to the other by clicking on the style to be copied and then clicking the Copy button.

When copying styles, remember these rules:

- When styles are copied from one document or template to another, the styles being copied replace styles with the same style names in the other document or template.

- Styles that are copied to a template or document are added to the document's style sheet if the copied style names do not match any of the style names already in the document.

- Style names are case-sensitive—if you copy a style named "HEAD" (all uppercase letters) into a template or document that contains a style named "head" (all lowercase letters), the style "HEAD" will be added to the style sheet and will not replace the style "head".

To copy styles from one template to another:

1. Open the template memo.dot that you saved on your document diskette.

2. Open the Style drop-down list box on the Formatting toolbar to view the current styles.

3. Choose Style from the Format menu.

4. Click the Organizer button.

5. Click the Styles tab in the Organizer dialog box, if necessary.

6. Click the Close File button on the right side of the dialog box. (Be sure to choose Close File and not Close.)

    The button caption changes to Open File.

7. Click the Open File button, locate the template files in the winword\template directory, and choose the filename MEMO2.DOT. Click OK.

8. Choose Body Text from the MEMO2.DOT list box on the right side of the dialog box, and then click the Copy button.

9. Scroll down in the MEMO2.DOT list box and choose Normal.

10. Click the Copy button, and then click Yes to confirm the overwrite.

11. Click Close.

    The styles you chose from the MEMO2.DOT template have been copied to the MEMO.DOT template. The Normal style in the MEMO.DOT template has been replaced by the Normal style from MEMO2.DOT. Notice that the text has changed from Times New Roman 12 pt to Arial 11 pt.

12. Open the Styles drop-down list box on the Formatting toolbar to see the new style names.

13. Close the template without saving the newly copied styles.

What Is AutoText?

The purpose of AutoText is to store text and graphics items that you use frequently. By storing these items as AutoText entries, you avoid the need to rekey text or import graphics each time you want to use them.

Text and graphics stored as AutoText are easy to retrieve for use in your documents. Some of the items you might store include names and addresses, company logos, and standard text.

Like styles, AutoText can be stored in any template. If it is stored in the NORMAL.DOT template, it is available for all documents. If it is stored in a different template, it is available only when that template is in effect. If you click the AutoText tab on the Organizer dialog box, you can copy AutoText from one template to another in the same manner as styles are copied.

Creating AutoText Entries

AutoText button

It is very easy to add AutoText entries. Select the text or graphic you want to add, and then open the AutoText dialog box. You can open the AutoText dialog box by either choosing AutoText from the Edit menu or clicking the AutoText button on the Standard toolbar. The Name text box displays the beginning characters of the selected text. In most cases, you will change the name to a brief, easy-to-type description. For example, you might use the characters "FYI" to describe the text "For your information". When you want to use the AutoText entry, key **FYI** and then click the AutoText button, or press the shortcut key **F3**.

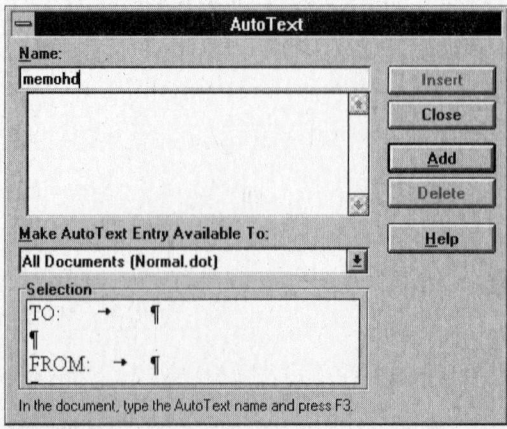

Figure 21-8

The AutoText dialog box

To create an AutoText entry:

1. Choose Open from the File menu. If necessary, choose Word Documents from the List Files of Type list box. Open the file 21-0b.doc.

2. Choose Templates from the File menu.

3. In the Document Template text box, key **a:\memo.dot** (or **b:\memo.dot** if you are using the b: drive).

4. Click the check box for Automatically Update Document Styles.

5. Click OK.

6. Delete the text to the right of each tab character in the memo heading, so that only MEMO TO:, FROM:, DATE:, and SUBJECT: remain. (Do not delete the tab character or the paragraph mark on each line.)

7. Select the four lines of text in the memo heading and the two blank lines after "SUBJECT:".

8. Choose AutoText from the Edit menu (or click the AutoText button).

9. In the Name text box, key **memohd**

10. Open the Make AutoText Entry Available To list box, and choose Documents Based on Memo.dot.

    By choosing Memo.dot, the AutoText can be used only in documents based on the MEMO.DOT template.

11. Click the Add button.

    You have created an AutoText entry that contains the text for the memo heading.

12. Save the document as *[your three-letter identifier]*21-0b.doc.

    A question box appears, asking if you want to save changes to the document template.

13. Click Yes.

    Saving the changes to the document template saves the AutoText entries for future use.

14. Close the document.

Inserting AutoText Entries

You can retrieve AutoText entries and insert them into documents using the AutoText command from the Edit menu, the AutoText button on the Standard toolbar, or the **F3** shortcut key. When you insert an AutoText entry using the AutoText command from the Edit menu, Word offers two options:

Edit	
Can't Undo	Ctrl+Z
Repeat New Default	Ctrl+Y
Cut	Ctrl+X
Copy	Ctrl+C
Paste	Ctrl+V
Paste Special...	
Clear	Delete
Select All	Ctrl+A
Find...	Ctrl+F
Replace...	Ctrl+H
Go To...	Ctrl+G
AutoText...	
Bookmark...	
Links...	
Object	

Edit menu

- You can insert the AutoText entry with its own formatting by choosing the Formatted Text option.

- You can insert the AutoText entry as plain text that will be changed to match the formatting of the text surrounding it by choosing the Plain Text option.

The shortcut key, **F3**, is a faster way to insert AutoText entries. However, to use the shortcut key, you must know the name of the AutoText entry you want to insert. Also, the entry will retain its original formatting. When you know the name of an AutoText entry, you can insert it by positioning the insertion point where you want the entry to appear in the document, keying its AutoText name, and pressing the **F3** key. The entry appears automatically at the insertion-point location.

To insert an AutoText entry using the Edit menu:

1. Open the file 21-0c.doc.

2. Choose Templates from the File menu.

3. In the Document Template text box, key **a:\memo.dot** (or **b:\memo.dot** if you are using the b: drive).

4. Click the Automatically Update Document Styles check box, and then click OK.

5. Position the insertion point at the beginning of the text in the document (before "I know you").

6. Choose AutoText from the Edit menu.

7. Choose the name memohd, and then click Insert.

   The AutoText entry is inserted at the beginning of the document. See Figure 21-9 on page 425.

To insert an AutoText entry using a shortcut key:

1. Create an AutoText entry named "zyte" that contains the phrase "the oak HilphanZyte coffee table" by selecting the phrase in the text, opening the AutoText dialog box, and keying **zyte** as the AutoText name. After you key the name, click the Add button.

2. After the text "March 21." at the end of the first paragraph, press **Enter** twice and key:

   Both Indira and I think that it is worth holding out for

3. Press the **Spacebar** once after "for" and key **zyte**

4. Press the **F3** key.

   You have used the shortcut key to insert the AutoText entry named zyte into the text.

5. If necessary, delete the space at the end of the AutoText entry you just inserted, and then add a period.

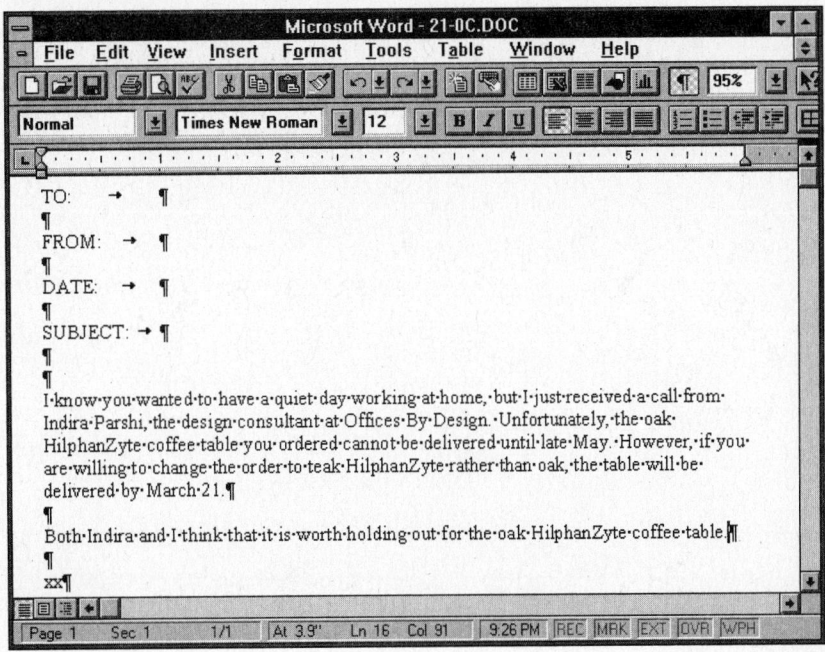

Figure 21-9
Inserting an AutoText entry

Saving a Table as an AutoText Entry

In addition to storing a phrase or a document opening (or closing), you can also store a table as an AutoText entry. For example, you may find that, in a particular business situation, you often use a specific table in your documents. The table may have specially formatted rows, columns, cell widths, and column headings. Instead of recreating the same table over and over, you can create it once and store it as an AutoText entry.

After creating the table, select it, and choose AutoText from the Edit menu. Give the table an AutoText name, and then click the Add button. To retrieve the table, select it from the AutoText dialog box, or key the AutoText name, and press the **F3** key (or click the AutoText button on the Standard toolbar). You can always modify the table by adding rows or columns or by changing the table headings, if necessary.

Revising AutoText Entries

Word allows you to edit AutoText entries by redefining an existing AutoText entry, renaming an entry, or deleting an entry.

Redefining an AutoText Entry

To redefine an existing AutoText entry, insert the AutoText entry into a document, edit the AutoText text, and redefine the AutoText entry using the AutoText dialog box.

To redefine an AutoText entry:

1. In the sentence that begins "Unfortunately," in the first paragraph, insert a space between the "n" and the "Z" in "HilphanZyte".

2. Select "the oak Hilphan Zyte coffee table" in the same sentence.

3. Choose AutoText from the Edit menu.

4. Choose the AutoText name zyte.

5. Click the Add button.

    A question box appears asking if you want to redefine the AutoText entry.

6. Click Yes to redefine the AutoText entry.

Renaming an AutoText Entry

To rename an existing AutoText entry, use the AutoText command on the Edit menu.

To rename an AutoText entry:

1. Select the AutoText text "the oak Hilphan Zyte coffee table" again.

2. Choose AutoText from the Edit menu.

3. Choose the AutoText name zyte.

4. Click the Delete button. Then key **Hilphan** in the Name text box.

5. Click the Add button.

    The AutoText name is changed from "zyte" to "Hilphan".

Figure 21-10
Renaming an AutoText entry

Deleting AutoText Entries

To delete an AutoText entry, use the AutoText command on the Edit menu.

To delete an AutoText entry:

1. Choose AutoText from the Edit menu.

2. Choose the AutoText name Hilphan.

3. Click the Delete button.

   The AutoText name Hilphan is deleted. Notice that the existing occurrences of the AutoText entry in the document are not deleted.

4. Click Close.

Printing AutoText Entries

Printing AutoText entries is similar to printing a style sheet. To print a document or template's AutoText entries, choose the Print command from the File menu, and choose AutoText Entries from the Print What drop-down list box. When you print the AutoText entries, Word prints out an alphabetical list of the AutoText names and text entries.

Using the Spike

Spike
An AutoText entry used to store multiple pieces of information.

The *Spike* is a special AutoText entry that you can use to store multiple pieces of information for use in documents. You can collect text or graphics from different parts of a document, store them in the Spike, and insert the collection in one location in the document. The Spike is different from the Clipboard in two ways. When you use the Clipboard, text is temporarily stored and then replaced when you cut or copy another item. When you use the Spike, you can cut and store several items at once. Also, the Clipboard lets you copy items as well as cut them. With the Spike, you can only cut them.

Before using the Spike to store text, delete the AutoText name Spike, if it exists, to clear any text that may remain from a previous Spike.

To store text in the Spike:

1. Open the AutoText dialog box, and delete Spike if it exists.

2. Select the first sentence of the memo, which begins "I know you".

3. Press the Spike key, **Ctrl+F3**.

   The sentence is deleted from its current location and stored in the Spike.

4. Select the first sentence in the next paragraph, which begins "Both Indira and I".

5. Press **Ctrl+F3**.

   The second sentence is stored in the Spike along with the first sentence.

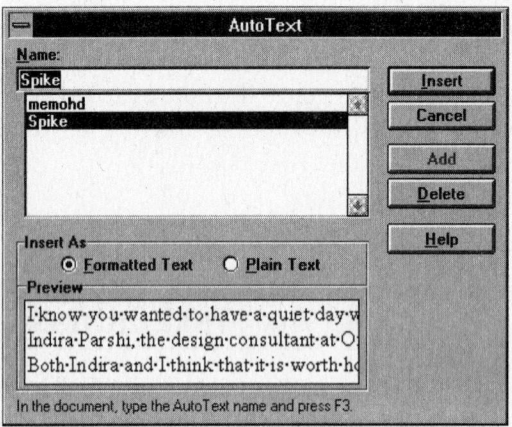

Figure 21-11

The Spike is added to the AutoText Name list box.

To insert the contents of the Spike:

1. Move the insertion point to the blank line after the first paragraph.

2. Key **spike**

3. Press the **F3** key.

   The contents of the Spike are inserted at the insertion point.

Note: To insert the contents of the Spike into text and delete them from the Spike at the same time, press the Unspike key, **Ctrl+Shift+F3**.

4. Make sure the contents of the Spike you just inserted are one paragraph. Delete any extra paragraph marks before the initials at the end of the document (there should be only two paragraph marks).

5. Delete the Spike entry from the AutoText dialog box to delete the Spike's contents.

6. Spell-check the document (change "Hilphan Zyte" to two words throughout), and save it as *[your three-letter identifier]*21-0c.doc.

7. Click Yes in the dialog box to save the changes you have made to the document template.

8. Print the document.

9. Close all open files and exit Word (unless you will be doing the following exercises immediately).

Table 21-2: Keyboard Shortcuts	
Keyboard Shortcut	Action
[AutoText name]+**F3**	Insert an AutoText entry
Ctrl+F3	Store selected text in the Spike
Spike+F3	Insert contents of the Spike
Ctrl+Shift+F3	Insert contents of the Spike, and then empty the Spike
Alt+F9	Toggle field code display on and off

Key Terms

Attach	Template
AutoText	Wizard
Spike	

Exercises

Exercise 21.1

1. Start Word, if necessary.

2. Create a document based on one of Word's press-release templates:

   A. Choose New from the File menu.

   B. In the Template list box, choose Presrel2. Click OK.

   C. Select the text "[Company Name]", and key **Duke City Gateway Travel Agency**

   D. Select the street address, and key **15 Montgomery Boulevard**

   E. Select the next line, which begins "[city", and key **Albuquerque, New Mexico 87111**

   F. Continue selecting bracketed text and replacing with the following:

[Title]	**25th Anniversary Celebration for Duke City Gateway Travel**
[Subtitle]	None (delete the subtitle line and the paragraph mark after it)
[Name]	**Doris Simms**

[Company]	**Duke City Gateway Travel**
[Phone Number]	**(505) 555 1234**
[City]	**Albuquerque**

3. Enter the body text of the press release by selecting "[*Type information here*]" and keying Figure 21-12. Press **Enter** twice to start a new paragraph.

Figure 21-12

This month, Duke City Gateway Travel Agency celebrates its 25th year in the travel business. The agency, located in downtown Albuquerque on Montgomery Boulevard, has been at the same location for all of its 25 years. It has served over 50,000 area residents, business travelers, and visitors to New Mexico.

"Each year is more exciting than the previous year. We're always so pleased to share our enthusiasm for the southwest with our customers," says the agency's owner, Susan Allen.

To mark the agency's 25th anniversary, a celebration will be held at the new Red River Hotel this Sunday at noon. Join Duke City Gateway's staff for a poolside champagne toast. Please call for reservations.

4. Store "Doris Simms" as an AutoText entry:

   A. At the beginning of the document, select the name "Doris Simms" (do not select the newline character).

   B. Choose AutoText from the Edit menu.

   C. Key **contact** in the Name box.

   D. Click Add.

5. Move the insertion point before "for reservations." in the last paragraph. Key **contact**, press the **Spacebar**, and then press the **F3** key.

6. Delete the AutoText entry:

   A. Choose AutoText from the Edit menu.

   B. Choose contact, and then click Delete.

   C. Click Close.

7. In the title text, insert a line break before "for". Change the body of the document to single spacing, if necessary.

8. Spell-check the document.

9. Save the document as *[your three-letter identifier]*21-1.doc. Do not save changes to the template.

10. Print the document.

11. Close the document and exit Word (unless you will be doing the following exercises immediately).

Exercise 21.2

1. Start Word, if necessary.

2. Open an existing Word template and modify it:

    A. Choose New from the File menu.

    B. Choose Letter1 from the Template list box.

    C. Click the Template option in the New option box. Then click OK.

3. Using the Page Setup command on the File menu, change all the margins to 1 inch.

4. Using the Style command on the Format menu, change the type size of the Normal style to 12 point.

5. Position the insertion point at the beginning of the line that starts "[Recipient", and press **Enter** four times to move the inside address down to the 3-inch position.

6. Replace the text in the first three lines as follows:

    [*Company Name*] **Duke City Gateway Travel**

    [*Street Address*]   **15 Montgomery Boulevard**

    [*City...Code*]   **Albuquerque, NM 87111**

7. Select the street address and the city lines. Use the Paragraph dialog box to clear the 3-inch right indent (change it to 0).

8. Set a 3.25 inch tab to left-align all three lines of the return address and the date.

9. Set a 3.25 inch tab to left-align the closing, from "Sincerely," to "[*Your position*]".

10. Spell-check the template.

11. Save the template as *[your three-letter identifier]*let1.dot, preceded by the appropriate drive.

12. Print the template.

13. Close the template and exit Word (unless you will be doing the following exercises immediately).

Exercise 21.3

1. Start Word, if necessary.

2. Create a new template using NORMAL.DOT as a base.

3. Format the template with 1-inch top, bottom, left, and right margins.

4. At the top of the page, key **Duke City Gateway Travel Agency**

5. Create an AutoText entry for "Duke City Gateway" called DCG. Store the AutoText entry in documents based on the new template (Template1 or Template2).

6. Move to the end of the line. Press **Enter** twice, and then key the following text on three lines, using line breaks as shown:

   Revised Statement of Travel Agency
   Responsibilities and Tour Conditions
   Effective May 15, 199-

7. Press **Enter**. Center all the text, and change the formatting to 14-point bold. Apply a shadow-box border around it.

8. Save the template as tour.dot (including the appropriate path), and then close the template.

9. Create a new document based on the TOUR.DOT template.

10. Move the insertion point to the paragraph mark below the box, press **Enter** twice, and key Figure 21-13. Include the corrections. Each time "DCG" appears in the figure, use the keyboard shortcut to insert the DCG AutoText entry.

Figure 21-13

Anyone reserving a DCG tour accepts the condition that DCG ~~has~~ *reserves* the exclusive right to cancel or change tour hotels, itineraries, and other tour features if ~~it~~ *DCG* deems *it* necessary to do so.

DCG asks *that* all customers who need special assistance ~~to~~ be accompanied by an adult. In addition please notify DCG in advance about your special needs. *Lack of such prior notification could cause delays or inconveniences.*

Itineraries may be subject to change due to weather, traffic, mechanical, and any other circumstances that prevent DCG from operating under conditions ~~that are normal~~. The published days and times of ~~our~~ *DCG* itineraries are as accurate as possible.

11. Change the line spacing for the inserted text to 1.5 lines and the point size to 12.

12. Add the last sentence in the document, which begins "The published", to the Spike.

13. Add the next-to-the-last sentence, which begins "Itineraries", to the Spike.

14. Move the insertion point after "do so." in the first paragraph, and press **Enter** twice. Then insert and empty the contents of the Spike.

15. Adjust spacing and punctuation where necessary.

16. Spell-check the document, save it as *[your three-letter identifier]*21-3.doc, and print it.

17. Close the document and exit Word (unless you will be doing the following exercise immediately).

Exercise 21.4: Challenge Yourself

Create a document based on the template *[your three-letter identifier]*let1.dot, created in Exercise 21.2.

Select the text "[*Type the body of your letter here*]", and key in its place Figure 21-14. Start a new paragraph where each paragraph mark is indicated.

Figure 21-14

```
Thank you for calling Duke City Gateway Travel Agency. ¶ I have enclosed
the travel brochures you requested, as well as your itinerary and
tickets. ¶Please feel free to call us with any questions you may have.
¶Have a wonderful trip. ¶We look forward to serving you again.
```

Change the paragraph spacing for the keyed text to 0 pts after paragraphs. Store the first paragraph, which begins "Thank you", as an AutoText entry called A1. Store it in the template. Store the second paragraph as AutoText entry A2. Store it in the template. Do the same for the next three paragraphs, storing them as A3, A4, and A5 respectively.

Spell-check the document, and save it as *[your three-letter identifier]*21-4a.doc. Save the changes to the template.

Open a new document based on the same template. In the new document, key the following name and address where indicated:

Mr. William Welden
5022 Alice Avenue
Albuquerque, NM 87110

For the body of the letter, use the AutoText paragraphs A2 and A4. Make sure there is one blank line between the two paragraphs and before "Sincerely". The letter is from Tom Carey, Travel Counselor. Use your initials at the bottom. Key **3** for the number of enclosures, and delete the cc line. Change the left and right margins to 1.5 inches and the top margin to 2 inches.

Spell-check the document, save it as *[your three-letter identifier]*21-4b.doc, and print it.

Create another letter using the same template. The letter is from Frank Murillo, Travel Counselor, and addressed to:

Ms. Amy Bailey
P.O. Box 301
Corrales, NM 87048

For the body of the letter, use AutoText paragraphs A1, A2, A3, and A4. Combine paragraphs A1, A2, and A3. Enter your initials, key **2** for the number of enclosures, and delete the CC: line. Change the left and right margins to 1.5 inches and the top margin to 2 inches.

Spell-check the document, save it as *[your three-letter identifier]* 21-4c.doc, and print it. Close the documents and exit Word.

Macros

Objectives

- Create macros.
- Run macros.
- Assign macros.
- Modify macros.
- Use Word's supplied macros.

Macro
An automated procedure consisting of a sequence of word-processing tasks.

The Word macro feature allows you to perform repetitive tasks involving command sequences and keystrokes quickly. With this feature, you can save a sequence of tasks as a single command. Then you can execute one command to perform the entire sequence automatically.

What Is a Macro?

A *macro* is an automated procedure consisting of a sequence of word-processing tasks. A macro can include menu commands, formatting options, keystrokes, and dialog-box selections. For example, you can create a macro that automatically opens a template or document that you use frequently. A macro cannot record mouse movements that position the insertion point or select text, so you must substitute keyboard equivalents for selecting text or repositioning the insertion point.

Storage Options for Macros

The storage options for macros are similar to those available for styles and AutoText. Macros can be stored globally in the NORMAL.DOT template or in a particular document template. You store general-purpose macros in the NORMAL.DOT template, so that you can use them with all documents. You store a macro in a document template when the macro has a special purpose that relates to that particular template.

To store macros in a template other than the NORMAL.DOT template, you attach a different template to the document and store the macros in that template. For macros to be stored in a document template, that template must be the active template.

To attach a template to a document:

1. Start Word, if necessary.
2. Open the file 22-0.doc.
3. Choose Templates from the File menu.
4. Click the Attach button.

435

Figure 22-1
The Attach Template dialog box

5. In the Drives drop-down list box, choose the drive where your student disk files are stored (for example, the a: drive).

6. In the List Files of Type drop-down list box, choose Document Templates (*.dot).

7. In the File Name list box, choose memo1.dot.

8. Click OK to close the Attach Template dialog box.

9. Click OK again to close the Templates and Add-ins dialog box.

    Now, the file 22-0.doc is attached to the template MEMO1.DOT on your student disk. When you record a macro, you will be able to store it either in the MEMO1.DOT template or globally in the NORMAL.DOT template.

10. Save the file as *[your three-letter identifier]*22-0.doc, but do not close it.

Creating Macros

There are two ways to create a macro. One way is to write it from scratch using a programming language called WordBasic. Experienced programmers can use WordBasic to automate complex operations. The second way is to record a sequence of word-processing tasks and give it a *macro name* by which the sequence can be retrieved. Macros created this way are called *recorded macros*. To record macros, use the Record Macro dialog box.

The Record Macro dialog box contains the Record Macro Name box, where you can key a brief name for the macro. If you do not key a name in this box, Word will automatically name the macro Macro1. If you then record other macros without naming them, Word will name them Macro2, Macro3, and so on. Macro names can be up to

Macro name
A name given to a recorded sequence by which the sequence can be retrieved.

Recorded macros
Macros created by recording and naming a sequence of tasks.

Macro Record floating
toolbar

Note: You can record a
macro even if you do not
have any documents open
on the screen. You can
choose Macro from the
File menu to record a
macro without opening a
document. This allows you
to record the steps to
open a document.

36 characters long with no spaces, commas, or periods. They must
begin with a letter.

You can also key a brief description of the macro in the Description
box. The Assign Macro To box lets you assign a keyboard shortcut
to run the macro or assign the macro to a toolbar or menu. Assigning macros is described later in this lesson.

As you record a macro, the Macro Record floating toolbar and the
recorder mouse pointer appear. Also, REC appears in the status bar
at the bottom of the window. When recording a macro, you must use
the keyboard to select text or move the insertion point. If you try to
do it with the recorder mouse pointer, you will hear a beep to remind
you that you cannot use the mouse to manipulate text. However, you
can use the mouse to choose commands from a menu, to choose
options from a dialog box, or to click buttons on a toolbar.

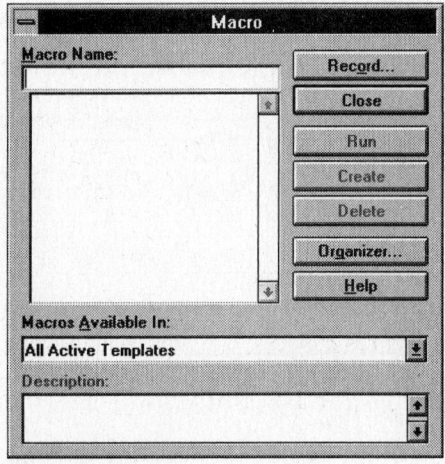

Figure 22-2
The Macro dialog box

To create a macro that saves and closes a document:

1. Choose Macro from the Tools menu.

2. Click the Record button.

    The Record Macro dialog box appears.

3. In the Record Macro Name text box, key **SaveAndClose**

4. In the Make Macro Available To list box, choose Documents
    Based On memo1.dot.

5. In the Description box, key **Saves and closes a document.** See
    Figure 22-3 on page 438.

6. Click OK to close the Record Macro dialog box.

    Notice that the Macro Record floating toolbar appears, and the
    mouse pointer has a recorder graphic attached to it.

Recorder mouse pointer

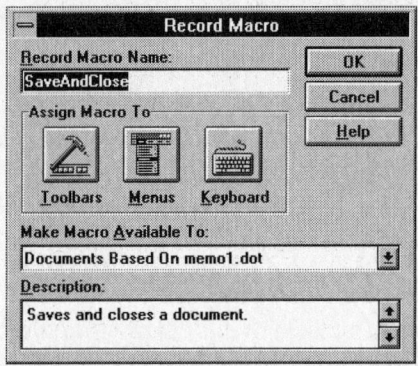

Figure 22-3
The Record Macro dialog box

7. To record the steps for saving and closing the file, choose Save from the File menu, and then choose Close from the File menu.

    When you choose Close, a confirmation box will warn you that you are still recording a macro.

Figure 22-4
Click the Yes button to confirm the file closing.

8. Click the Yes button.

    The document closes, but the Record Macro toolbar is still displayed.

9. Click the Stop button on the Record Macro toolbar to end the recording and complete the macro.

    You have recorded a macro for saving and closing a document. It will be saved in the MEMO1.DOT template.

Running Macros with the Macro Command

To execute the steps you record in a macro, you run the macro. When you run a macro, Word automatically executes the macro commands that you recorded, in the sequence that you recorded them. Word gives you several methods for running macros:

*   Using the Macro command from the Tools menu

*   Pressing the shortcut key for the macro

*   Choosing the macro name from a menu

*   Clicking the macro's button on a toolbar

You can use the Macro command to run any macro you have recorded and named. To use a shortcut key, the macro must be assigned to a shortcut key combination. To use a menu or a toolbar, the macro must be assigned to a menu or a toolbar. Assigning macros is discussed later in this lesson.

To run a macro using the Macro command:

1. Open the file *[your three-letter identifier]*22-0.doc.

2. At the right of each heading item, key and align the corresponding information at the 1-inch tab setting:

   Nina Chavez and Tom Carey
   Susan Allen
   March 20, 1995
   Travel Tips for Senior Citizens

3. Add your reference initials to the bottom of the memo.

4. Choose Macro from the Tools menu.

5. Choose All Active Templates from the Macros Available In box, if necessary.

6. Click SaveAndClose.

7. Click the Run button. If a dialog box opens, click Yes to save the changes.

   The macro runs, and the changes to the memo are saved. Then the memo is closed.

Assigning Macros to Shortcut Keys

Word allows you to assign a macro to a shortcut key when you record the macro or after the macro has been recorded. When you assign a macro to a shortcut key, you can use any combination of the **Alt, Ctrl,** or **Shift** keys along with a letter, number, or function key from **F2** to **F12**. When you enter the key in the Shortcut Key text box, Word tells you if that key is currently assigned by listing its macro name. If the key is not assigned, the box lists it as unassigned. You can use any key that is not currently assigned to another function.

To assign a macro to a shortcut key when recording the macro:

1. Open the file *[your three-letter identifier]*22-0.doc again.

2. After "Memo To:", delete the names, key **Distribution**, and then move the insertion point to the end of the document.

3. Choose Macro from the Tools menu.

4. Click the Record button.

5. In the Record Macro Name text box, key **Distribution**

Keyboard button in the
Record Macro dialog box

Note: When recording a
macro, you must use key-
board commands to edit
or format text. You cannot
use the mouse. If you key
incorrect text, use the
Backspace key.

6. Choose Documents Based On memo1.dot from the Make Macro Available To list box.

7. In the Description text box, key **Duke City Gateway staff**

8. Click the Keyboard button in the Assign Macro To box.

 The Customize dialog box opens.

9. In the Press New Shortcut Key text box, press **Alt+D**.

 Notice that **Alt+D** is currently unassigned.

10. If necessary, choose Memo1.dot from the Save Changes In list box, in the lower right corner of the dialog box.

11. Click Assign, and then click Close.

 The Macro Record toolbar and the record mouse pointer appear.

12. With the insertion point at the end of the document (after your reference initials), press **Enter** twice.

13. Press **Ctrl+U** to turn on underlining, and then key **Distribution**. Press **Ctrl+U** to turn underlining off, and then key a colon.

14. Press **Enter** twice, and then key:

 **T. Carey
 N. Chavez
 E. Micali
 F. Murillo
 D. Simms
 F. Youngblood**

15. Click the Stop button on the Record Macro toolbar.

 You have recorded a memo distribution list and assigned it the shortcut key combination **Alt+D**.

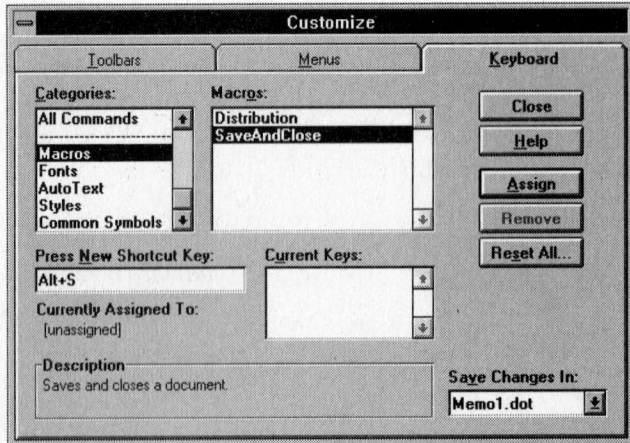

Figure 22-5
Assigning a shortcut key

To assign a macro to a shortcut key after it has been recorded:

1. Choose Customize from the Tools menu, and click the Keyboard tab, if necessary.

2. Choose Memo1.dot from the Save Changes In list box in the lower right corner of the dialog box.

3. Choose Macros from the bottom of the Categories list box.

4. Choose SaveAndClose from the Macros list box.

5. In the Press New Shortcut Key text box, press **Alt+S**.

6. Click the Assign button, and then click Close.

   The SaveAndClose macro is now assigned to the shortcut key combination **Alt+S**.

Assigning Macros to a Menu or Toolbar

You can also assign a macro to a menu or toolbar. When you assign a macro to a menu, you add the macro name to the menu where it will be available for you to choose it with the mouse. When you assign a macro to a toolbar, Word inserts a new button to represent the macro in an empty space on the designated toolbar.

To assign a macro to a menu:

1. Choose Customize from the Tools menu, and then click the Menus tab.

2. In the lower right corner of the dialog box, choose Memo1.dot.

3. Choose Macros at the bottom of the Categories list box.

4. Choose SaveAndClose from the Macros list box.

5. In the Change What Menu list box, choose &File.

6. In the Name on Menu text box, change "&SaveAndClose" to "SaveAn&dClose".

   The character to the right of the ampersand is underlined in the File drop-down menu. Because "S" is already underlined in the Save command, an unused letter, "d", is chosen in this case.

7. Click the Add button, and then click Close.

   The SaveAndClose macro is added to the File menu. It will be available in the current template only, because it has not been saved globally in the NORMAL.DOT template.

8. Click the File menu.

   The macro name SaveAndClose appears at the bottom of the menu. The keyboard shortcut for the macro also appears in the menu.

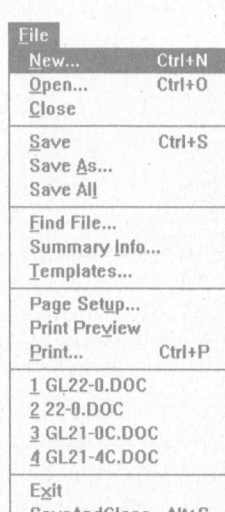

SaveAndClose at the bottom of the File menu

To assign a macro to the Standard toolbar:

1. Choose customize from the Tools menu, and then click the Toolbars tab.

2. Choose Memo1.dot from the Save Changes In list box.

3. Choose Macros from the Categories list box.

4. In the Macros list box, choose Distribution, and drag it to position it between the Spelling and Cut buttons on the Standard toolbar.

   A blank button appears on the Standard toolbar, and the Custom Button dialog box opens.

5. Click the fifth button in the fourth row in the Custom Button dialog box.

Figure 22-6
The Custom Button dialog box

6. Click the Assign button, and then click Close.

   A new button appears on the Standard toolbar, between the Spelling button and the Cut button.

7. Move the mouse pointer to the new button.

   Distribution appears in the yellow Tooltips box. The new Distribution button is saved with the MEMO1.DOT template. It will appear on the Standard toolbar only when the MEMO1.DOT template is attached to the current document.

New button for the
Distribution macro

Running Assigned Macros

Once you have assigned macros to shortcut keys, menus, or a toolbar, you no longer need to use the Macro command to run them. Assigned macros are extremely efficient to use, because they are so easy to run.

To run a macro using the shortcut key:

1. Delete the distribution list and the paragraph mark above it from the bottom of the memo.

2. With the insertion point at the end of the memo (to the right of your reference initials), press **Alt+D**.

   The macro is executed, and the distribution list appears at the end of the document.

To run a macro using a menu:

1. Delete the distribution list and the paragraph mark above it.

2. Choose SaveAndClose from the bottom of the File menu.

   The document is saved and closed.

3. Click Yes to save changes to the template if additional dialog boxes appear.

To run a macro using the Standard toolbar:

1. Open the file *[your three-letter identifier]*22-0.doc.

2. Position the insertion point at the end of the document.

3. Click the Distribution button that you inserted on the Standard toolbar.

   The macro is executed, and the distribution list appears in the document.

Making a Customized Template Available Globally

In Word, the NORMAL.DOT template is always available for use, no matter what other template may be attached to a document. Any AutoText, macros, and styles saved in the NORMAL.DOT template are always available.

But what happens if you attach a custom template, but need to use macros stored in a different custom template? You can make any template a global template so its macros, AutoText, and styles will be available to all documents, along with NORMAL.DOT.

To make a template available globally, do the following:

• Choose Templates from the File menu.

• In the Templates and Add-ins dialog box, click the Add button.

• Change to the drive and directory where the template is stored, choose it from the File Name list box, and click OK.

The template name will appear in the Global Templates and Add-ins list box in the Templates and Add-ins dialog box. You may put as many templates as you need on the list. Each item on the list has a check box. If the check box is checked, that template is available globally. To make it unavailable, uncheck it. To remove an item from the list, highlight it, and then click the Remove button.

Modifying Macros

In Word, you can modify macros by editing, replacing, and renaming them. You can also change the description of the macro or delete the macro using the Macro command from the Tools menu.

To rename a macro and change the macro's description:

1. Choose Macro from the Tools menu.

2. Choose the macro name Distribution from the Macro Name list box.

3. Select the text in the Description box, and key **List of travel counselors**

4. Click the Organizer button.

5. Click the Macros tab, if necessary, and then click the Rename button.

6. In the New Name box, change the name to "DistributionList" and click OK.

    The name of the macro changes from Distribution to DistributionList.

Figure 22-7
Renaming a macro

7. Click Close to close the Organizer dialog box, and then click Yes to save changes to memo1.dot.

8. Move the mouse pointer onto the Distribution button, between the Spelling and Cut buttons.

    The label in the yellow Tooltips box is DistributionList.

9. Use the SaveAndClose command on the File menu to close the document.

10. Click Yes to save changes to the document template.

Although it is easy to rerecord a short macro when you make a mistake, it is more convenient to edit macros that contain many commands or large amounts of text. Extensive editing or replacing of commands within a macro requires knowledge of the programming language WordBasic, which is beyond the scope of this lesson. You can, however, edit errors made when keying text, if you are careful not to alter other parts of the macro.

To edit a macro, choose the macro name from the Macro dialog box, and then choose Edit. The macro editing window opens, displaying the macro commands translated into the WordBasic programming language. Text that was keyed while recording the macro is displayed in quotes. Although it requires a knowledge of WordBasic to edit commands correctly, you can safely edit text contained in quotes just as you would in a normal document, as long as the quotes are not deleted.

As you study the commands, you will see that their functions are sometimes intuitive. For example, InsertPara is inserted each time you insert a blank line when recording. If you inserted too many blank lines, you can delete one or more of the InsertPara commands. If you need to insert a blank line, you can copy and paste one of the InsertPara commands already in the macro.

When you have completed the editing of the macro, save and close it the same way that you close a document.

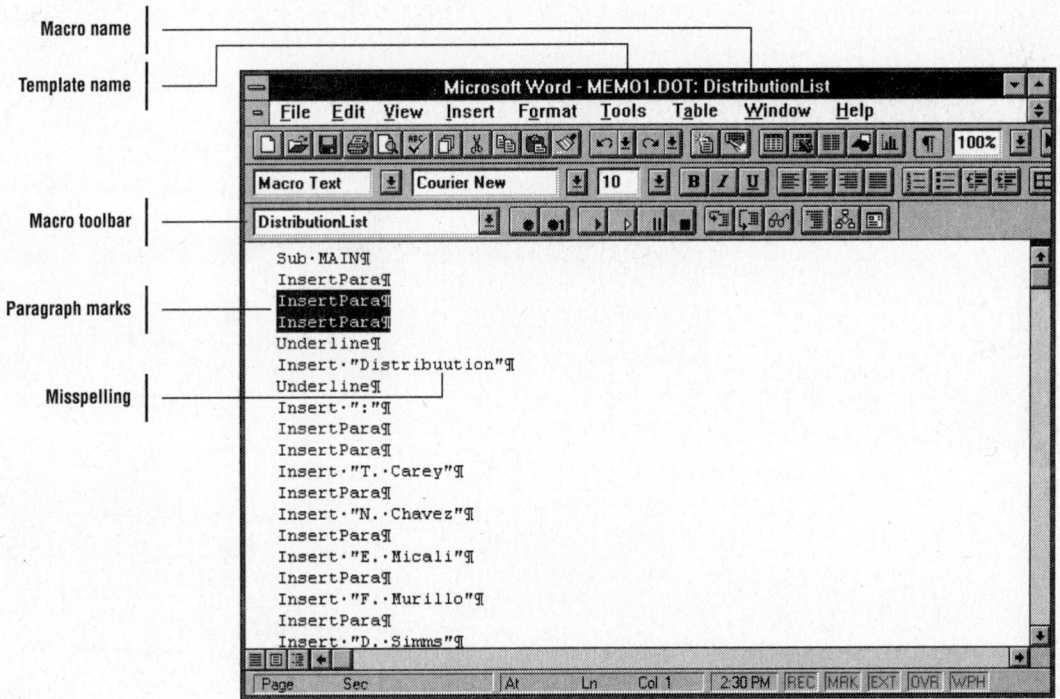

Figure 22-8
The macro editing window

Using Macros Supplied with Word

Word supplies four templates in the macro subdirectory under the winword directory that contain several macros you may find useful. For example, the LAYOUT.DOT template contains macros to increase and decrease font size. The macro examples supplied by

Word also serve as good examples for those interested in learning how to use WordBasic to create programmed macros. You can use the Organizer dialog box to copy macros from the Word-supplied templates to a custom template that you create, such as the MEMO1.DOT template used in this lesson.

To copy macros from the LAYOUT.DOT template:

1. Open the file *[your three-letter identifier]*22-0.doc.

2. Choose Macro from the Tools menu, and then click the Organizer button.

3. Click the Macros tab, if necessary.

4. In the Organizer dialog box, click the Close File button on the right side of the dialog box to close the Normal.dot template.

5. Click the Open File button.

6. Follow your instructor's directions to change to the winword directory, and then choose the macros directory.

7. In the File Name list box, choose layout.dot, and then click OK.

   The Organizer dialog box reappears, with the LAYOUT.DOT macros listed in the right list box.

Figure 22-9
Copying macros

8. Choose DecreaseFont from the LAYOUT.DOT list box, and then click the Copy button.

   DecreaseFont appears in the MEMO1.DOT list box.

9. Choose IncreaseFont from the LAYOUT.DOT list box, and then click the Copy button.

   Two macros have been copied to the memo1.dot template.

10. Click the Close button.

11. Click Yes to save changes to MEMO1.DOT.

To assign shortcut keys to the new macros in MEMO1.DOT:

1. Choose Customize from the Tools menu.

2. Click the Keyboard tab.

3. Choose Memo1.dot from the Save Changes In drop-down list box.

4. Choose Macros from the Categories list box.

5. Choose DecreaseFont from the Macros list box.

6. In the Press New Shortcut Key text box, press **Alt+<** (**Alt+Shift**+comma).

7. Click the Assign button.

8. Choose IncreaseFont from the Macros list box.

9. In the Press New Shortcut Key box, press **Alt+>** (**Alt+Shift**+period).

10. Click the Assign button.

11. Click the Close button.

To use the new macros in memo1.dot:

1. Select "Travel Tips for Senior Citizens" in the first paragraph of the memo.

2. Press **Alt+>** three times.

   The selected text size has increased.

3. Press **Alt+<** twice.

   The selected text size has decreased.

4. Save the document and the template.

5. Print the document.

6. Close the document and exit Word (unless you will be doing the following exercises immediately).

Saving Macros

When you record macros while working in an open document, Word does not save the macros in your document automatically. The macros are saved in the template attached to the document or to the NORMAL.DOT template. In order to save the macros, save the document, and then choose Yes when prompted to save the template.

Key Terms

Macro   Recorded macros

Macro name

Exercises

Exercise 22.1

1. Start Word, if necessary.

2. Create a new template.

3. Change the top margin to 2 inches.

4. At the top of the page, key **TRAVEL SURVEY RESULTS** in all capitals.

5. Press **Enter** twice and key:

   A SUMMARY OF THE ANNUAL CUSTOMER SURVEY ON VACATION TRAVEL PREFERENCES

6. Press **Enter** and key:

   By Doris Simms, Sales Representative

7. Center all the text, and change the font to 12-point Times New Roman. Make this the bodytext style.

8. Record a macro to activate the header area:

   A. Choose Macro from the Tools menu, and then click the Record button.

   B. Key **Header** in the Record Macro Name text box.

   C. In the Make Macro Available To list box, choose Documents Based On Template1 (or whatever the current template number is).

   D. In the description box, key **Activates the header area**

   E. Click the Keyboard button.

   F. In the Press New Shortcut Key text box, press **Alt+H**.

   G. Click the Assign button, and then click Close.

   H. Choose Header/Footer from the View menu.

9. Click the Stop button on the Macro Record toolbar.

10. Click Close on the Header and Footer toolbar.

11. Record a macro for activating the footer area. Name the macro "Footer", assign it the shortcut key **Alt+F**, give it the description "Activates the footer area", and store it in the template. Choose Header/Footer from the View menu, and then click the Switch Between Header and Footer button on the Header and Footer toolbar.

12. Stop recording the macro, and close the footer area.

13. Record a macro for inserting the current date:

    A. Move the insertion point after "Representative", and press **Enter** twice.

    B. Choose Macro from the Tools menu, and then click the Record button.

    C. Name the macro Date, make it available to documents based on Template1, give it the description "Inserts current date", and assign it the shortcut key **Alt+D**.

    D. Choose Date and Time from the Insert menu. Choose the fourth format and click OK.

    E. Stop the Recorder.

    F. Delete the date and the paragraph mark above it from the template.

14. Save the template as report.dot, and include the appropriate drive (for example, save it as a:\report.dot if you are using the a: drive).

15. Close the template.

16. Create a new document based on the report.dot template.

17. Press **Enter** twice after "Representative", and run the Date macro by pressing **Alt+D.**

18. Press **Alt+H** to run the Header macro, and key **Duke City Gateway Travel Report** in 10-point Times New Roman. Right-align the text in the header area.

19. Close the header.

20. Press **Alt+F** to run the Footer macro, and insert a page number in the footer.

21. Center the page number, and close the footer.

22. Press **Enter** twice after the date, and left-align the last paragraph mark. Key Figure 22-10 in single-spaced format with one blank line between paragraphs.

Figure 22-10

At the end of each year, the sales representatives of Duke City Gateway Travel ask 100 of the agency's best customers questions about vacation travel preferences. We poll travelers to find out their favorite regions to visit, the transportation they prefer, and the time of year they prefer to travel.

This year, we discovered that the favorite place to visit in the United States is California. Travelers like to fly to California and then rent a car and drive along the coast from San Diego to San Francisco and then head northeast to Lake Tahoe.

The seasons preferred for vacation travel in the United States are spring and summer. In the winter, vacationers usually fly south to Florida or the Caribbean to find sunshine, and some head north for snow skiing.

23. Spell-check the document.

24. Save the document as *[your three-letter identifier]*22-1.doc.

25. Print the document.

26. Close the document and exit Word (unless you will be doing the following exercises immediately).

Exercise 22.2

1. Start Word, if necessary.

2. Create a new template.

3. Format the page setup for a standard block-style business letter.

4. Record a macro for inserting the opening of the letter:

   A. Choose Macro from the Tools menu, and then click the Record button.

   B. Name the macro "Opening".

   C. Make the macro available to documents based on the current template.

   D. In the description box, key **Letter opening**

E. At the top of the page, insert the Create date field, choosing standard formatting. Press **Enter** six times and key:

**Mrs. Jean Anderson
115 Central Avenue
Albuquerque, NM 87110**

F. Press **Enter** twice, and key **Dear Mrs. Anderson:**

G. Click the Stop button on the Macro Record toolbar.

5. Press **Enter** twice after "Mrs. Anderson:", and record a macro for the closing of the letter:

A. Choose Macro from the Tools menu, and then click the Record button.

B. Name the macro "Closing", describe it as "Letter closing", and make it available to documents created with the current template.

C. Key **Sincerely**, press **Enter** four times, and then key:

**Nina Chavez
Travel Counselor**

D. Press **Enter** twice, and then key your reference initials.

E. Click the Stop button on the Macro Record toolbar.

6. Delete all of the text from the template, and save the template as newlet.dot with the appropriate drive (for example, a:\newlet.dot). Close the template.

7. Open a new document based on the NEWLET.DOT template.

8. Assign the macros to shortcut keys:

A. Choose Customize from the Tools menu, and click the Keyboard tab.

B. In the Save Changes In list box, choose Newlet.dot.

C. In the Categories list box, choose Macros.

D. In the Macros list box, choose Closing, and then assign the shortcut key **Alt+C**.

E. Assign the shortcut key **Alt+O** to the macro Opening.

9. With the insertion point at the top of the page, run the Opening macro.

10. Press **Enter** twice after "Mrs. Anderson", and key Figure 22-11. Include the corrections. Use single spacing for the text and double spacing between paragraphs.

Figure 22-11

I am writing on behalf of Duke City Gateway Travel to thank you for participating in our year end customer survey. We appreciate the time and energy you spent helping us.

We will use the results of the survey to develop *new and* exciting vacation packages for you to enjoy.

Once again, thanks for thinking of Duke City Gateway Travel as your primary travel planner. *We look forward to seeing you soon.*

11. Press **Enter** twice after "seeing you soon.", and run the closing macro.

12. Rename the Opening macro to LetterOpen:

   A. Choose Macro from the Tools menu, and click the Organizer button.

   B. Choose Opening from the list box.

   C. Click the Rename button.

   D. Key **LetterOpen** and click OK.

13. Follow the same procedures to rename the Closing macro to LetterClosing.

14. Close the Organizer dialog box, and click Yes to save the changes to NEWLET.DOT.

15. Spell-check the document.

16. Change the left and right margins to 1.5 inches and the font size to 12 point.

17. Save the document as *[your three-letter identifier]*22-2.doc.

18. Print the document.

19. Close the document and exit Word (unless you will be doing the following exercises immediately).

Exercise 22.3

1. Start Word, if necessary.

2. Create a new template.

3. At the top of the page, key the following as a two line heading:

   TRAVEL SURVEY RESULTS
   Types of Vacations Taken by 100 Duke City Gateway
   Customers

4. Center the text, and change it to 14-point Times New Roman.

5. Insert two blank lines, and then left-align the last paragraph mark.

6. Begin recording a macro named Table5x2. Assign the keyboard shortcut **Alt+T**, and make the macro available to documents based on the current template. Create a table that is five rows by two columns. Make the columns 2 inches wide, and center the table between the page margins.

7. With the macro recorder still on, key **Type of Vacation** in the first row of the first column. Press the **Tab** key. In the first row of the second column, key **Percentage**

8. Key the following text in rows two through five of the first column, using the **Tab** key and Arrow keys to move from cell to cell:

   Cruise
   Package Tour
   Special Interest
   Outdoor Adventure

9. Add a grid border to the table, and stop the macro recorder.

10. Delete the table, and save the template as trip.dot with the appropriate drive (for example, a:\trip.dot).

11. Close the template.

12. Open a new document based on the trip.dot template.

13. Move to the second line after the heading, and left-align the paragraph mark, if necessary.

14. Use the keyboard shortcut to run the Table5x2 macro.

15. Complete the table by keying the following values in rows two through five of the second column:

    19
    29
    40
    12

16. Center the text in the table, and change the top margin of the document to 2 inches.

17. Spell-check the document.

18. Save the document as *[your three-letter identifier]*22-3.doc.

19. Print the document.

20. Close the document and exit Word (unless you will be doing the following exercise immediately).

Exercise 22.4: Challenge Yourself

Create a template for a letterhead with the following information:

Duke City Gateway Travel Agency
15 Montgomery Boulevard
Albuquerque, NM 87111
Phone: (505) 555-1234
FAX: (505) 555-1244

Center the text, change the font to 12-point Arial, and move the insertion point to the last line of the letterhead. Begin recording a macro called CUST, and make it available to documents based on the current template. Assign the shortcut key **Alt+C**.

Insert three blank lines after the letterhead. In bold, centered, capital letters, key **CUSTOMER INFORMATION SHEET**. Turn off the bold attribute, insert three more blank lines, and left-align the last paragraph mark.

Key Figure 22-12, which appears at the end of this exercise. To enter the text with the fill-in lines, as shown, first select the paragraph mark, and open the Paragraph dialog box. Change line spacing to 24 points after, and set a 6-inch right-aligned tab with the underscore leader (choose 4 in the Leader options box in the Tab dialog box). Key **DATE:**, and then press the **Tab** key to insert the line. Press **Enter**, key **CUSTOMER:**, and press the **Tab** key again. At the end of the line, press **Enter** and the **Tab** key to insert a full line. Continue in this manner through the end of the figure.

Stop recording the macro. Delete all the text and lines from the first line after the letterhead to the end of the document. Save the template as ltrhd.dot with the appropriate drive and close it.

Create a new document using the ltrhd.dot template. Move to the end of the document, and run the CUST macro.

Spell-check the document, and save it as *[your three-letter identifier]* 22-4.doc. Print the document, close it, and exit Word.

Figure 22-12

DATE: _____

CUSTOMER: _____

TELEPHONE NUMBER: _____

FAX NUMBER: _____

NUMBER IN PARTY: _____

PREFERENCES: _____

_____

_____

_____

A Travel Update

Background

Each month, Duke City Gateway publishes a travel update to send to all of the agency's customers. This update includes information about special events, weather, and travel notes in the United States.

A few members of the Duke City Gateway staff prepare The North American Travel Update, and Frank Youngblood is responsible for distributing and printing the update.

Business Purpose

Create the May issue of the North American Travel Update.

Procedures

1. Create a new document, and change the left and right margins to 1 inch.

2. Key **North American Travel Update**

3. Press **Enter** twice, and key **Duke City Gateway Travel Agency**

4. Move the insertion point after "Agency", and insert a right tab at the 6-inch mark.

5. Press the **Tab** key, and key **May 1995** at the tab stop, and then press **Enter** three times.

6. Make the following changes to the first line of text:

   Font Size: 22 point

   Style: bold, centered

   Border: shadow

7. Select the text from "Duke City" to "May 1995", and make the following changes to the text:

   Font Size: 10 point

   Style: bold, italic

   Border: single-line box

8. Move to the end of the document, choose the Normal style, and key **May Events**

9. Select "May Events". Create and apply a style named UpdateHead for the text, including the following formatting in the style:

   Font Size: 16 point

   Style: bold, all caps, centered

   Space After: 24 points

10. Press **Enter** after "May Events", choose the Normal style, and key **Boston, Massachusetts**

11. Insert a left tab at the 3-inch mark, press the **Tab** key, and key **May 13-15**

12. Select the text from "Boston" to "15". Create and apply a style named CityName, including the following formatting:

    Font: Arial

    Font Size: 12 point

    Style: bold

    Line Spacing: single

    Tab: 3-inch left aligned

13. Create a Next Style to follow CityName. Call the new style Indentedpara, and include the following formatting:

    Font: Arial

    Font Size: 12 point

    Hanging Indent: at the 3-inch mark

14. Press **Enter** after "15", press the **Tab** key, and key **Annual Chowder Festival: Sample Boston's best clam, corn, and seafood chowders**

15. Press **Enter** after "chowders", and insert a page break.

16. Key **May Weather**, and then apply the UpdateHead style to the text.

17. Below the heading, change to the Normal style, and insert a table that has three columns and nine rows. Center the table horizontally.

18. Make the first column 1.5 inches wide and the last two columns 1 inch wide. Add a grid border to the table.

19. Across the first row, key **City** in the first column, **High** in the second column, and **Low** in the third column. Center these column heads.

20. Fill in the rows of the first column by keying:

    Atlanta

    Chicago

    Los Angeles

    New Orleans

    New York

    Orlando

    Seattle

    Washington, D.C.

21. Select the table, and then create and apply a style named Table, including the following formatting:

    Font: Arial

    Font Size: 12 point

    Style: regular

    Line Spacing: single

    Alignment: left

22. Center the column heads, and make them bold.

23. After the table, press **Enter** twice, key **Travel Notes**, and apply the UpdateHead style to the text.

24. After the heading, start a new paragraph. Change to left alignment, choose the Normal style, and then create a style for the paragraph named List with the following formatting (if the style name List already exists, use the name List1):

    Font: Times New Roman

    Font Size: 12 point

    Line Spacing: single

25. Start a new paragraph with the Normal style, and key in 12-point bold:

Duke City Gateway Travel Agency
15 Montgomery Boulevard
Albuquerque, New Mexico 87111
(505) 555-1234

26. Center the text, and make it bold.

27. Save the document as a template, and name it *[your three-letter identifier]*p8-1.dot.

28. Close the template, and then create a new document based on the template.

29. After the Boston, Massachusetts, paragraphs, key the following information:

New York, New York **May 29**
The New York Marathon

Cape May, New Jersey **May 7-9**
Victorian Fair: Victorian house tours, lawn parties, and arts and crafts

New Orleans, Louisiana **May 10-15**
Jazz Festival: Join the country's greatest jazz musicians for a week of jamming.

Tampa, Florida **May 20-22**
Strawberry Festival: Enjoy the spring harvest of the nation's best strawberries.

St. Louis, Missouri **May 5**
Annual May Day Parade down Main Street

Flint, Michigan **May 19-22**
The Greene's Nursery Annual Tulip Festival

Houston, Texas **May 28-29**
The Annual Amateur Rodeo and Western Show

San Diego, California **May 24-29**
Pacific Regatta: Watch hundreds of sailboats decorate the Pacific in this week-long regatta.

30. Apply the CityName style to the city names and dates. The Indentedpara style should automatically be applied to the descriptions.

31. On page 2, key the following temperatures in the table, and center the figures in the columns:

High	Low
79	60
65	50
72	52
83	68
69	52
88	66
64	50
75	54

32. Start a new paragraph after the table, and record a macro for drawing a single line under the paragraph. Give the macro the shortcut key **Alt+L**.

33. After the heading "TRAVEL NOTES", press **Enter,** choose the List style, and key:

Amtrak is now offering special rates on their cross-country rail packages. You can buy a rail pass with unlimited stops across the continental United States for one low price. Contact your travel counselor at Duke City Gateway for more details.

If you are planning a road trip for your next vacation, consider joining AAA road service. Not only does this service come to your rescue if your car breaks down, it also offers you free maps and great discounts on hotels.

The next time you are seeking ways to come up with a great gift idea for that special person, think travel. You can purchase travel gift certificates for dinners, travel agency services, airline tickets, hotel accommodations, and tours. Contact your travel counselor at Duke City Gateway for more details.

34. Select the text you keyed, and click the Bullets button on the Formatting toolbar.

35. Use the shortcut key **Alt+L** to insert a line before "Duke City Gateway Travel Agency". Leave one blank line above and below the line.

36. Make any changes you feel will improve the appearance of the document.

37. Spell-check the document, and save it as *[your three letter identifier]*p8-1.doc.

38. Print the document.

39. Close the document and exit Word.

Tips and Hints

- Create AutoText entries for words you will use frequently in your document.

- For longer documents, create styles for the headings and body text in the document, and remember to use the Next Style and Based On Style options.

- Use macros to automate some of the tasks you perform frequently while working in your document. Assign the macros shortcut keys or assign them to a menu or toolbar for easy access to the command.

- Create templates for everyday business documents, such as memos, letters, reports, and newsletters. The formatting you include in a template will help you save time producing new documents.

Module 9

Merging and Sorting

Mail Merging

Mail merging
A process of combining two documents during printing.

Main document
The document that contains the standard text that will appear in each copy of the printed document.

Data source
The document that contains the variable information, such as names, addresses, and other data, that is inserted into the main document when printed.

Record
In a data source, a set of related information, such as name, street, city, state, and ZIP code, for one person or business.

Businesses often want to send the same letter to several people on a mailing list. To do this, they could key the main body of the letter, include the name and address of the first person on the list, and then create several more letters containing the names and addresses of the other people on the list. Although this method works, it is time consuming and difficult to update when the mailing-list information changes. Fortunately, Word offers a much faster alternative called mail merging. *Mail merging* is a process by which Word inserts variable information from one document, such as names and addresses, into another, standard document for printing. Word automatically prints individual versions of the standard document with the variable information that you specify. The mail-merge feature can be used to create documents such as form letters and mailing labels.

Mail-Merge Basics

Two documents are needed in order to use the mail-merge feature: the main document and the data source. The *main document* is the document that contains the standard text that will appear in each copy of the printed document. The *data source* is the document that contains the variable information, such as names, addresses, and other data, that is inserted into the main document when printed. When executing the mail-merge command, Word inserts the variable information from the data source into specified locations in the main document. The mail-merge process involves:

• Creating a main document

• Planning and creating a data source and attaching it to the main document

• Specifying where the variable information will be inserted in the main document

• Merging the main document with the data source to print the documents

A data source contains the variable information that will be inserted into the main document. The data source consists of records. *Records* are sets of related information (such as the name, address, and salutation for one person) that are inserted into a merged document. Each record is made up of fields. Fields and their uses were introduced in Lesson 5. Fields are the individual pieces of information in a record. For example, a form letter may contain related information, such as the company name, contact name, address, and salutation. In the data source, the company name, contact name, address, and salutation are four different fields. All these fields together make up a record.

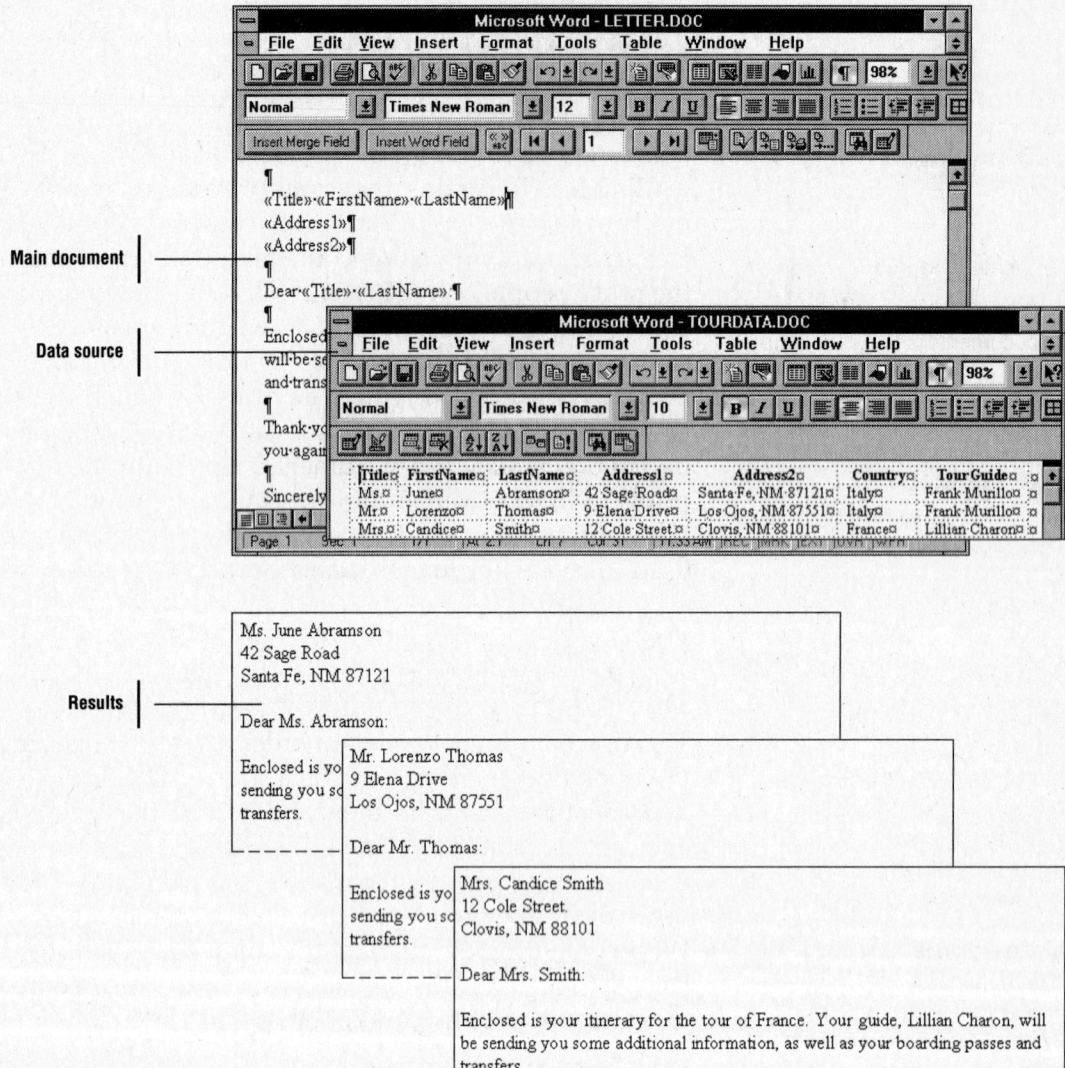

Figure 23-1
Mail merging a main document and a data source

Field name
Unique name given to a field in the data source.

Each field is identified in the data source with a unique name called a *field name*. In order to merge the information in the data source with the main document, insert the field names into the main document where you want the information to appear. When Word merges the main document and the data source, it replaces the field names with the actual data. See Figure 23-2 on page 467.

Planning a Data Source

Before creating a data source for a main document, it is important to consider the information that is to be included in the data source. Decide on the fields and the field names for the fields that you want

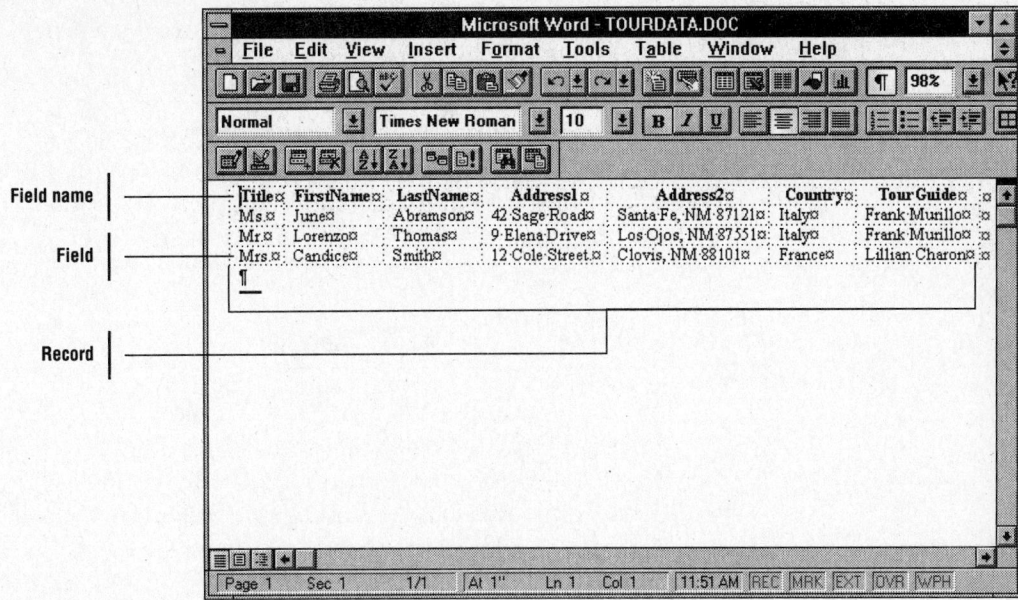

Figure 23-2
Records in a data source

to include in the records of your data source before creating it. For example, when creating a form letter, decide how much information needs to be included in each record. Most form letters include the title, name, street, city, state, and ZIP code of the person to whom the letter is being sent. Also consider:

- What type of information will be included in each record?

  Records may include information such as names, addresses, titles, salutations, and complimentary closings. Each record in a data source must have the same number of fields, but, if a field is not needed for a certain record, it can be left blank. For example, you can fill in a name field, but leave a title field blank.

- Will the data source be sorted?

  A data source can be sorted by the information in a field. Therefore, include information by which the data source could be sorted in separate fields. For example, in order to sort by city, state, or ZIP code, this information must be included in separate fields.

- Will the information in a field be used more than once?

  For example, a person's name could be entered in a letter in more than one place. The name appears in an address, in a salutation, and possibly in the body of the letter. In this situation, create separate fields in the data source for each form of the name. For example, create separate fields for the elements in the name: the title (Mr., Ms.), the first name, and the last name.

- How many fields will the data source contain?

  The maximum number of fields in a data source is 31.

- Include constant information, such as punctuation marks, in the main document. For example, if a comma is to appear after a complimentary closing, include the comma in the main document and not in the data source.

Beginning a Mail Merge

The automatic mail-merge feature in Word will lead you step-by-step through the mail-merge process. First, you will create a document. Next, you will create your data source, in which you will determine your field names and key in the variable information that will be inserted into your main document when you perform the mail merge. Then, you will complete your main document and merge the variable data into it.

To begin a mail merge:

1. Start Word, if necessary, and create a new document. Change the font size to 12 point and the top margin to 2 inches.

   This will be the main document.

2. Choose Mail Merge from the Tools menu.

The Mail Merge Helper dialog box appears.

Tools menu

Figure 23-3

The Mail Merge Helper dialog box

3. Click the Create button under Main Document, and choose Form Letters.

4. In the dialog box, click the Active Window button to use the document window you opened as your main document.

Now you are ready to go on to step 2, creating the data source.

Creating the Data Source

The data source is the variable information you will insert into your main document. For a form letter, you will have a record for each person or company to whom you are sending the form letter. For each record, you will enter specific information based upon the fields you choose to use in your letter. The names of the fields are entered into the header row.

To create the data source:

1. Click the Get Data button under Data Source, and choose Create Data Source.

    The Create Data Source dialog box opens, from which you will create the header row. The Field Names in Header Row list is a list of commonly used field names, in the order they are most likely to be entered as a record. You will delete the fields names you will not be using, and you will add the field names you need that are not in the list already.

Figure 23-4
The Create Data Source dialog box

2. Key **Street** in the Field Name box, and click the Add Field Name button.

3. Click the Move up arrow to move the Street field name up the list, between the LastName and JobTitle field names.

4. Choose JobTitle from the Field Names in Header Row list, and click the Remove Field Name button.

    The Company field name is highlighted.

5. Click the Remove Field Name button to delete Company from the Field Names in Header Row list.

6. Following the same steps, use the Remove Field Name button to remove the fields Address1, Address2, Country, HomePhone, and WorkPhone from the Field Names in Header Row list.

7. Click OK.

Word opens the Save Data Source dialog box.

Note: Instead of using Word's automatic mail-merge feature, you could create data sources manually and manually attach the data source to a main document. Create a data source manually by keying in each record as a separate paragraph and separating each field within the record with tabs or commas.

8. Key **1data** as the name for the data source document, and save the data source on the drive containing your student disk. Click OK.

9. In the dialog box that opens, click Edit Data Source to begin creating records for your merge.

The Data Form dialog box appears.

Figure 23-5
The Data Form dialog box

Once the field names have been entered in the data source, and the data source has been named, Word displays the Data Form dialog box. In the Data Form dialog box, each field name is followed by a text box, in which you can insert the information for that field. To move down to the next text box in the Data Source dialog box, press the **Tab** key. To move up to the previous text box in the Data Source dialog box, press **Shift+Tab**.

To complete the data source for the form letter:

1. With the insertion point in the Title text box, key **Mr.** and press the **Tab** key.

2. Continue to key the following information in the appropriate text boxes, pressing the **Tab** key after each one:

Note: ZIP Code is indicated in the data source as PostalCode.

FirstName: **Arthur**
LastName: **Peters**
Street: **32 Red Sky Road**
City: **Albuquerque**
State: **NM**
ZIP Code: **87111**

3.   Click the Add New button.

The record you keyed is added to the data-source document 1data.doc, and the text boxes in the Data Form dialog box are cleared.

4.   Key the following information in the appropriate field text boxes, clicking the Add New button after you complete each record:

Title:	**Ms.**
FirstName:	**Merita**
LastName:	**Loy-Jones**
Street:	**310 Lucia St.**
City:	**Albuquerque**
State:	**NM**
ZIP:	**87121**

Title:	**Mr.**
FirstName:	**Benjamin**
LastName:	**Barnes**
Street:	**9854 Reigor Lane**
City:	**Albuquerque**
State:	**NM**
ZIP:	**87109**

Title:	**Mrs.**
FirstName:	**Toni**
LastName:	**Abadini**
Street:	**1209 Lombard Road**
City:	**Bosque Farms**
State:	**NM**
ZIP:	**87068**

The data source is complete.

5.   Click OK.

The Data Form dialog box closes, and the main document appears. The main document, thus far, is blank.

The Mail Merge Toolbar

When you return to the main document after creating the data source, the Mail Merge toolbar appears beneath the Standard toolbar in the document window. The Mail Merge toolbar automates and simplifies some of Word's mail-merge features.

Figure 23-6
The Mail Merge toolbar

The Mail Merge toolbar displays the following buttons:

- Insert Merge Field

  This button allows you to insert the merge fields that you created in the data source into the main document. This tells Word where to insert the variable information from the data source into the main document.

- Insert Word Field

  This button allows you to insert special fields into the main document, such as ASK and FILLIN fields, which are discussed later in this lesson.

- Edit Data Source

  This button allows you to make changes to the fields and records in the data source.

- Check for Errors

  This button checks the data source and main document for errors before printing.

- Merge to Document

  This button merges the copies of the main document to a file rather than printing each document.

- Merge to Printer

  This button sends the merged documents to the printer.

Completing the Main Document

Your next step is to complete the main document. This document will contain all the text that will be the same for each mail-merge document, in addition to merge fields to indicate where variable information is to be inserted in the document during the mail merge.

Creating the main document is like creating any other Word document. To create the main document, key the standard text that you want to appear in each copy of the document that is merged. If necessary, include styles or paragraph formatting in the main document. When you reach the portion of the document in which you wish to have variable information, insert a merge field for that information using the Insert Merge Field button.

When you mail-merge the main document and the data source, the information from the data source that corresponds to a merge field will replace that merge field in the main document. The field names from the data file can be inserted into any location in the main document. A field name can be inserted into the main document as many times as it is needed. Also, the main document does not have to include all the fields from the record in the data source.

To create the main document with merge fields:

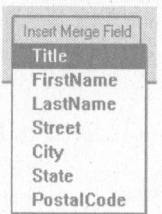

Insert Merge Field options

1. With the insertion point at the beginning of the document, insert today's date as a field from the Insert menu.

2. Press **Enter** six times, and then click the Insert Merge Field button on the Mail Merge toolbar.

3. Choose Title from the Insert Merge Field drop-down list.

4. Press the **Spacebar** once, click the Insert Merge Field button, and choose FirstName from the Insert Merge Field drop-down list.

5. Press the **Spacebar** once, click the Insert Merge Field button, and choose LastName.

6. Press **Enter**, click the Insert Merge Field button, and choose Street.

7. Press **Enter**, click the Insert Merge Field button, and choose City.

8. Key **,** (the comma), and press the **Spacebar**.

9. Click the Insert Merge Field button, choose State, press the **Spacebar**, click the Insert Merge Field button again, and choose PostalCode.

10. Press **Enter** twice and key **Dear**

11. Press the **Spacebar**, click the Insert Merge Field button, choose FirstName, and key **:** (the colon).

12. Press **Enter** twice, and key the following information, pressing **Enter** twice at the end of each paragraph:

    Enclosed are your airline tickets and the itinerary for your trip to Israel and Egypt. Please call me if you have any questions or concerns.

    I am sure you and your family will have a great time. Bon voyage!

13. Key **Sincerely,**

14. Press **Enter** five times, key **Travel Counselor**, press **Enter** twice, key your reference initials, and then key **Enclosure** on the next line.

15. Save the main document as *[your three-letter identifier]* 23-0a.doc and print it.

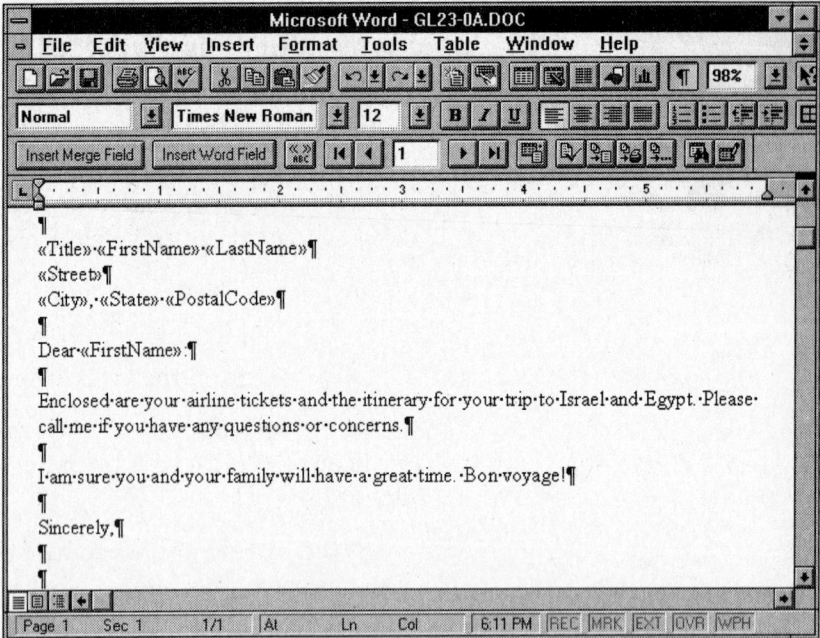

Figure 23-7
Merge fields inserted in the main document

Inserting Special Fields in the Main Document

Certain fields that do not appear in the data-source file can be inserted into the main document using the Insert Word Field button. The options in the Insert Word Field drop-down list are special options for inserting different types of fields, such as Ask and Fill-in fields, in the main document. Use one of the special fields to insert variable information in your document that you have not defined in the data source. When a special field, such as a Fill-in field, is inserted in a main document, and the document is mail merged, Word will prompt you for additional information in order to complete the merge. For example, insert a Fill-in field in the main document in place of a billing amount, and key in the prompt "Enter amount owed". Then, when the documents are mail merged, you will be prompted with "Enter amount owed". Key the amount owed in the dialog box, and it will appear in the merged copy of the main document.

To insert a Fill-in field:

1. Position the insertion point before the paragraph mark above "Travel Counselor".

2. Click the Insert Word Field button, and choose Fill-in from the Insert Word Field drop-down list.

    The Insert Word Field: Fill-in dialog box appears.

3. In the Prompt text box, key **Enter the Travel Counselor's name** and click OK.

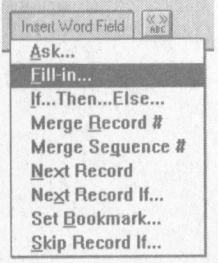

Insert Word Field options

The dialog box that will appear during the mail merge appears.

4. Click OK.

You will fill in the travel counselor's name at the prompt each time you mail merge.

You can view the field codes in the main document. To do this, use the shortcut menu or the View tab in the Options dialog box.

To view the field codes:

1. Select the entire document, click the right mouse button, and choose Toggle Field Codes from the shortcut menu.

Notice the change throughout the document.

2. With the document still selected, choose Toggle Field codes again from the shortcut menu.

Field codes are turned off.

Figure 23-8

Viewing field codes in the main document

Editing the Data Source

Edit Data Source button

Use the Edit Data Source button on the Mail Merge toolbar to make changes to the data source attached to the main document. When you click the Edit Data Source button, the data source appears. You can make changes to the text in the data-file records. Edit the text in the data source just as you edit any other text in a Word document.

After editing the data-source document, you may wish to view it. To do this, click the View Source button in the Data Form dialog box. Once the data-form table is displayed, you can change the table column widths or print the table.

First   Previous   Next   Last
Record   Record   Record   Record

Record text box

To edit the data source:

1. Click the Edit Data Source button on the Mail Merge toolbar.

2. Click the Next Record button to the right of the Record text box, so that "2" appears in the text box, and the second record is displayed in the dialog box.

3. In the Street field, delete "St." and key **Street**

4. To view the data-source document, click View Source.

    The document is displayed in table form.

Note: Adjusting the column widths of the data-source table has no effect on the final merged document.

5. Adjust the column widths, so that the text in each cell appears on one line.

6. Click the Edit Data Source button again, and then click OK.

Mail Merging

Once the merge fields are inserted into the main document, the data source and the main document can be mail merged. Start the process using the Mail Merge command from the Tools menu or the Merge to Printer button on the Mail Merge toolbar.

The Mail Merge Command

Choose Mail Merge from the Tools menu to open the Mail Merge Helper dialog box. The buttons in this dialog box allow you to make editing changes to the main document, to remove all files attached to the main document, to attach a data source to a main document, and to merge the data source with the main document. Click the Merge button in the Mail Merge Setup dialog box to start the mail merge.

To mail merge using the menu command:

1. Spell-check the document.

2. Choose Mail Merge from the Tools menu.

3. Click the Merge button under Merge the Data with the Document.

    The Merge dialog box appears. See Figure 23-9 on page 477.

The Merge dialog box presents merging options in the Merge To drop-down list, the Records to Be Merged box, and the When Merging Records box. The following options appear in the Merge To drop-down list:

Figure 23-9
The Merge dialog box

- New Document

  This option creates a new file with the merged documents in separate sections. This option is good for checking the merge before printing the documents on paper.

- Printer

  This options sends the merged documents to the active printer for printing.

- Electronic Mail

  This option sends the merged documents to the electronic-mail address or fax number you specify after clicking the Setup button.

The Records to Be Merged box in the Merge dialog box presents the following options:

- All

  This option prints all merged documents.

- From: and To:

  This option allows the user to choose a range of records to use for mail merging.

The When Merging Records box gives you the following options:

- Don't print blank lines when the data fields are empty.

  This is the default option. When this option is checked, Word does not print the blank lines that are caused by empty fields.

- Print blank lines when the data fields are empty.

  When this option is checked, the blank lines that are caused by empty fields are printed.

To mail merge using the Merge dialog box:

1. With the Merge dialog box open, choose New Document from the Merge To drop-down list.

2.   In the Records to Be Merged box, click All, if necessary, and then click Merge.

     A box appears, prompting you to enter the travel counselor's name.

3.   Key **Frank Murillo** and click OK each time you are prompted to enter the counselor's name.

     Word merges the records from the data source with the main document. "Form Letters1" appears in the title bar until you name the document.

4.   Scroll through the pages of the document, and notice the merged fields. Each letter is separated by a section break.

5.   Save the merged document as *[your three-letter identifer]*23-0b.doc.

The Mail Merge Buttons

Merge to New Document   Merge to Printer

Mail Merge buttons

The buttons on the Mail Merge toolbar also provide options for mail merging. The first merge button is the Merge to New Document button, which creates a new document with the merged documents. The second merge button is the Merge to Printer button, which sends the merged documents to the active printer.

To mail merge the document using the buttons on the Mail Merge toolbar:

1.   Switch to the main document, *[your three-letter identifier]* 23-0a.doc.

2.   Click the Merge to Printer button on the Mail Merge toolbar.

3.   In the Print dialog box, click OK.

4.   Key the travel counselor's name **Frank Murillo** (if necessary) and click OK each time you are prompted to do so.

5.   Close the documents, save the changes, and exit Word (unless you will be doing the following exercises immediately).

Using the Same Data Source with More Than One Document

Word's mail-merge feature is flexible. It allows you to attach the same data source to more than one main document. This comes in handy for mailing two or three documents to all the names or companies contained in one data source. For example, you could create a data source with different company names and addresses and then create two main documents, such as a form letter and an invitation. First, attach the data source to the form letter, and mail merge the documents. Then attach the same data source to the invitation, and mail merge the documents.

Key Terms

Data source   Mail merging

Field name   Record

Main document

Exercises

Exercise 23.1

1. Start Word, if necessary.

2. Create a new document based on the Memo1 template.

3. Choose Mail Merge from the Tools menu.

4. Click the Create button to create the main document, choose Form Letters, and click the Active Window button.

5. Click the Get Data button, and choose Create Data Source.

6. Create your header row:

   A. Remove all the field names currently in the Field Names in Header Row list.

   B. Key **DateSent** in the Field Name box, and click the Add Field Name button.

   C. Key **FullName** in the Field Name box, and click the Add Field Name button.

   D. Key **Leaves** in the Field Name box, and click the Add Field Name button.

   E. Key **Returns** in the Field Name box, and click the Add Field Name button. Click OK.

7. Save the data source as 23-1data.doc on the drive containing your student disk.

8. Click the Edit Data Source button, and complete the data source by keying in the following information in the proper fields (remember, press the **Tab** key to move to each new field, and click the Add New button at the end of each record):

DateSent	FullName	Leaves	Returns
March 6, 199-	Frank Youngblood	March 29	April 6
March 30, 199-	Ed Micali	April 16	April 27
April 28, 199-	Susan Allen	May 9	May 14
May 4, 199-	Mark Bloom	May 18	May 27

9. Click OK to return to the main document.

10. Address the memo to the Staff from Valerie Grier. The subject of the memo is Schedule. Delete the "CC:" line, and insert another blank line after the "RE:" line.

11. Insert a merge field after DATE:

    A. Delete the date field after "DATE:".

    B. Click the Insert Merge Field button and choose DateSent.

12. Key the following paragraph as the body of your memo, and insert merge fields in the noted places using the Insert Merge Field button (include one space before and one space after the merge fields, where necessary):

    Please be advised that (insert merge field for FullName) **will be out of the office from** (insert merge field for Leaves) **through** (insert merge field for Returns). **All calls should be directed to Susan Allen or me.**

13. Press **Enter** twice, and add your reference initials to the document.

14. Change the top margin to 2 inches.

15. Spell-check the document.

16. Save the document as *[your three-letter identifier]*23-1.doc.

17. Mail merge the data source and the main document:

    A. Choose Mail Merge from the Tools menu.

    B. Click the Merge button, choose Printer from the Merge To drop-down list, and click Merge.

    C. Click OK in the Print dialog box.

18. Close the documents, save the changes, and exit Word (unless you will be doing the following exercises immediately).

Exercise 23.2

1. Start Word, if necessary.

2. Create a new document based on the normal template.

3. Choose Mail Merge from the Tools menu.

4. Click the Create button to create the main document, choose Form Letters, and click the Active Window button.

5. Create your data source:

    A. Click the Get Data button, and choose Create Data Source.

    B. Create the following header row:

Rep
Contact
Title
Company
Commit

C. Click OK, and save the data source as 23-2data.doc.

D. Click the Edit Data Source button, and complete the data source by entering the following information in the appropriate fields:

Rep:	**Doris Simms**
Contact:	**October 29, 199-**
Title:	**Ethel Lewis, President**
Company:	**Congregational Sisterhood of Albuquerque**
Commit:	**No commitment was made by Lewis at this time.**
Rep:	**Doris Simms**
Contact:	**October 30, 199-**
Title:	**Mark Hunter, V.P. of Marketing**
Company:	**Taos Hotels**
Commit:	**Hunter will speak with Taos MIS and accounting divisions.**

6. Return to the main document and key:

Duke City Gateway Travel Agency
15 Montgomery Boulevard
Albuquerque, NM 87111

7. Press **Enter** three times, and then complete the Call Report by keying the following information, pressing **Enter** twice after each line:

CALL REPORT
Date:
Sales Representative:
Date of Contact:
Name and Title of Contact:
Company/Organization:
Commitment:

8. Set a 2.5-inch left-aligned tab for the text from "Date:" to "Commitment:". Then insert a tab character after each colon.

9. Insert the merge fields in the Call Report at the 2.5-inch tab setting:

A. Move the insertion point to the 2.5-inch tab setting after "Sales Representative:". Insert the Rep field.

B. Insert the Contact field after "Date of Contact:".

C. Insert the Title field after "Name and Title of Contact:".

   D. Insert the Company field after "Company/Organization:".

   E. Insert the Commit field after "Commitment:".

10. Insert a Fill-in field for the date:

   A. Move the insertion point to the tab setting after "Date:", click the Insert Word Field button, and choose Fill-in from the drop-down list.

   B. Key **Enter today's date** in the Prompt text box and click OK.

   C. Click OK.

11. Change the first three lines (the agency name and address) to 12-point bold text.

12. Spell-check the document, and save it as *[your three-letter identifier]*23-2a.doc.

13. Mail merge the main document and the data source to a new document:

   A. Choose Mail Merge from the Tools menu.

   B. Click the Merge button.

   C. Choose New Document from the Merge To drop-down list and click Merge.

   D. Key the current date at each prompt.

14. Return to the main document, and mail merge the document using the buttons on the Mail Merge toolbar:

   A. Click the Merge to Printer button on the Mail Merge toolbar.

   B. Click OK in the Print dialog box.

   C. Key the date at the prompts.

15. Print one record:

   A. Choose Mail Merge from the Tools menu.

   B. Click the Merge button.

   C. Choose Printer from the Merge To drop-down list.

   D. Click From in the Records to Be Merged box, and key **1** in the From box and **1** in the To box. Click Merge.

   E. Click OK in the Print dialog box.

   F. Key the date at the prompt.

16. Save the merged document file (Form Letters1) as *[your three-letter identifier]*23-2b.doc.

17. Close the documents and exit Word (unless you will be doing the following exercises immediately).

Exercise 23.3

1. Start Word, if necessary.

2. Open the file 23-3.doc, and use it as your main document for a mail merge.

3. Create a data source for the document with the following fields:

   Date
   Name
   Title
   Dept
   Company
   Address1
   CityStateZip
   To

4. Save the data source as 23-3data.doc.

5. Complete the data source by keying the information shown in Figure 23-10. (For the field CityStateZip, key the text as you would have it appear in the letter, with a comma and space after the city, and a space after the state.)

Figure 23-10

```
August 8, 199-

Mr. Paul I. Soper

Vice President

Human Resources

Suri Friedman Designs

8034 Menaul Rd.

Albuquerque, NM 87110

Paul


August 10, 199-

Mr. Aaron J. Hankly

Director

Personnel Department

Lasting Image Associates

4902 Silver Ave., Suite 230

Albuquerque, NM 87108

Mr. Hankly
```

August 9, 199–

Dr. Erica Singleton

Vice President

Human Resources

The Saddler Marketing Network

2034 Wyoming Boulevard NE

Albuquerque, NM 87112

Dr. Singleton

6. Return to the main document, and insert the Date merge field in place of the word "Date" in the document.

7. Starting at the sixth paragraph mark below the date, insert the merge fields Name, Title, Dept, Company, Address1, and CityStateZip on separate lines.

8. Insert a blank line above "Dear :", and then insert the To merge field before the colon.

9. Replace the underlining in the first paragraph (which begins "I know how") and the third paragraph (which begins "I would enjoy") of the letter with the Company merge field.

10. Check the documents for errors using the Check for Errors button on the Mail Merge toolbar. (Choose the option for simulating a mail merge.)

11. Check that the correct margins are set for the letter, and add your reference initials.

12. Spell-check the document, and save it as *[your three-letter identifier]*23-3.doc.

13. Mail merge the documents to the printer.

14. Save and close the documents, and then exit Word (unless you will be doing the following exercise immediately).

Exercise 23.4: Challenge Yourself

Open the file 23-4.doc, and format the heading (beginning with "Duke City" and including the address and telephone and fax numbers) as bold, centered text with a double-line box border. Under the heading, format the word "Invoice" in 14-point all caps and center it.

Convert the text from "Date:" to "Total Due:" to a one-column table. Change the column width to 2 inches, and then add a second column that is 4 inches wide. Add a grid border to the table. Change the row height to at least 36 pt. In the second column, to the right of "Date:", insert the date as a field. Choose the fourth format.

Save the main document as *[your three-letter identifier]*23-4a.doc, and use it as your main document for a mail merge.

Create a data source with the information in Figure 23-11, which appears at the end of this exercise. For the header row, use the field names **AcctNo**, **InvNo**, **Name**, **Address1** (for the street address), **Address2** (for the city, state, and ZIP code), **TktNo**, and **Total**. Save the document file as 23-4data.doc.

Insert the merge fields into the second column of the main document, and use the button on the Mail Merge toolbar to check the documents for errors. Use the button on the Mail Merge toolbar to merge the main document and the data source to a new document.

Save the merged document as *[your three-letter identifier]*23-4b.doc. Print the main document and the merged document. Save and close all documents and exit Word.

Figure 23-11

```
Account Number: 2037L

Invoice: 797411

Name: Nicole R. Sanchez

Address:    798 Armden Drive

            Chama, NM 87520

Ticket Number: 33679085

Total Due: $598.00


Account Number: 2943L

Invoice: 1856429

Name: Emery Ellis

Address:    2720 San Pedro Dr.

            Albuquerque, NM 87110

Ticket Number: 8731108

Total Due: $875.00


Account Number: 1243S

Invoice: 617831
```

Name: Sara O'Neill

Address: 83 Montgomery Boulevard

            Albuquerque, NM 87111

Ticket Number: 2289408

Total Due: $458.00

Sorting

Sorting
The process of reordering text, either alphanumerically, numerically, or by date.

Word's sorting feature is helpful in organizing documents. Use sorting to rearrange paragraphs, tabbed lists, or tables.

What is Sorting?

Sorting is the process of reordering text, either alphanumerically (by number and then by letter), numerically (by number), or by date. When you need to organize text according to one of the three sorting options, the sorting feature makes the process easy. To sort specific text, select a portion of the document before sorting, so that Word sorts only that text. Otherwise, Word sorts the entire document.

Sorting Order and Sorting Options

Word's sorting feature operates according to several rules to determine the placement of the text it sorts. The first is ascending and descending order. Ascending order is smallest to largest, such as 0-9 or A-Z. Descending order is largest to smallest, such as 9-0 or Z-A. Choose Ascending or Descending from the Sort By box in the Sort or Sort Text dialog box, which you access by choosing Sort or Sort Text from the Table menu.

The other rules of sorting relate to the type of sort chosen. The choices in the Type box in the Sort or Sort Text dialog box are Text, Number, and Date. Word orders text differently depending on the option chosen.

Figure 24-1
The Sort Text dialog box

487

- Text

  This option is the default type. Word sorts by numbers first and then by letters. When the data is a combination of letters, numbers, and special characters, Word follows these rules when sorting data alphanumerically:

  Text that starts with punctuation marks, such as !, ", $, and &, is placed before all other text, followed by text that begins with numbers. Text that begins with letters is placed last.

  Text that begins with uppercase letters is placed before text that begins with lowercase letters.

  If more than one text item or row in a table begins with the same character, Word sorts based on the next character in the text or row.

  A letter that contains an added mark, such as an accent, is sorted after the same letter without the mark, and before the next letter in the alphabet.

- Number

  This option sorts by number. Word recognizes the value of positive and negative numbers and places negative numbers before positive numbers in ascending sorts and positive numbers before negative numbers in descending sorts.

- Date

  This option sorts by date. In order for Word to recognize data as a date, it must be in one of the following formats:

  Month-Year (January-95)

  Month/Day/Year (1/31/95)

  Month-Day-Year (1-31-95)

  Day-Month-Year (31-1-95)

  Month Day, Year (January 31, 1995)

  Month/Day/Year Time (1/31/95 1:00 p.m.)

  The sorting order Word chooses when sorting dates depends on the date format used. For example, if you use the Month-Year format and ascending sort order, Word will sort January-95 before February-95. If you choose the Month/Day/Year format, and ascending order, Word will sort 1/2/95 before 1/12/95.

- Sort By

  From this drop-down list box, you can choose the form of text you wish to sort (for example, paragraphs or columns).

- Separate Fields At (in the Sort Options dialog box)

  To sort a multiple-column selection, choose the character (either a comma or a tab) that separates the columns.

- A check box for Sort Column Only (in the Sort Options dialog box)

  When checked, Word will sort only the selected column.

- A check box for Case Sensitive (in the Sort Options dialog box)

  When checked, Word will sort a capitalized word before the same word in lowercase.

Figure 24-2
The Sort Options dialog box

When to Sort

The sorting feature has many useful applications. For example, you can:

- Sort alphabetically or alphanumerically to organize an index or glossary
- Sort numerically to reorder the numerical information in a tabular report
- Sort numerically to organize a data-source file by ZIP code
- Sort by date to organize a data-source file containing date fields chronologically
- Sort numerically to organize numbered headings in an outline

It is also a good idea to sort only after you have saved the document.

Undoing a Sort

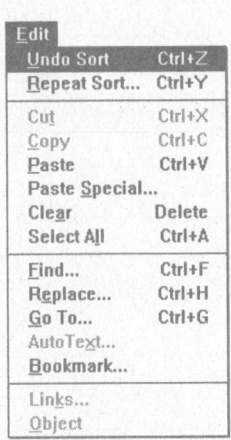

Edit menu

If necessary, you can undo a sort by choosing Undo Sort from the Edit menu. It is important to remember that you must undo the sort immediately after you sort by executing the Undo Sort command before you make any other changes to the document.

Sorting Paragraphs

Word sorts paragraphs based on the first character in the paragraph. You can sort all the paragraphs in a document or just selected paragraphs. If you do not select specific paragraphs to sort, Word will select the entire document automatically when you choose the Sort Text command from the Table menu. The paragraphs selected to sort can be any length.

To sort paragraphs in a specific order, number paragraphs before you sort. For example, in a document with five paragraphs that you want to rearrange by putting the fourth paragraph first and the fifth paragraph second, key the appropriate number before each paragraph, and then sort the paragraphs numerically. After the sort is complete, delete the numbers. In some cases, you may find it more efficient simply to cut and paste paragraphs to rearrange the order.

To sort paragraphs:

1. Start Word, if necessary.

2. Open the file 12-3.doc.

3. On page 2, select the paragraph that begins "**Decks**" and the two paragraphs below it (through "and strolling.").

4. Choose Sort Text from the Table menu.

5. Choose Text from the Type drop-down list and Ascending in the Sort By box, if necessary. Then click OK.

    Word sorts the paragraphs alphabetically. The paragraph marks that were between the paragraphs appear at the beginning of the selection, because Word sorts empty paragraph marks before text paragraphs.

6. Select the three sorted paragraphs (without the extra paragraph marks above the text), and choose Sort Text from the Table menu.

7. Choose Descending in the Sort By box. Click OK.

    Word sorts the paragraphs in descending alphabetical order.

8. Click the Undo button.

    The ascending alphabetical sort is restored.

9. Readjust the line spacing by inserting blank lines between the sorted paragraphs and deleting the extra paragraph marks above the first paragraph.

10. Save the document as *[your three-letter identifier]*24-0.doc.

Just as you sort paragraphs that contain more than one line, you can also sort paragraphs that contain only one line, such as items in a list. Suppose a document contains a list of the products a company sells,

Table

Insert Table...
Delete Cells...
Merge Cells
Split Cells...

Select Row
Select Column
Select Table   Alt+Num 5

Table AutoFormat...
Cell Height and Width...
Headings

Convert Text to Table...

Sort Text...

Formula...
Split Table
✓ Gridlines

Table menu

but the list is not organized. Use the Sort Text command to alphabetize the list of products.

To sort a list containing one-line paragraphs:

1. Go to page 5. In the paragraph under "**Dress Code**", delete the text from "bathing suits" through "is important." Insert a colon after "including".

2. Press **Enter**, and then key the following list:
   Sandals
   Bathing suit
   Bathing cap
   Jeans
   Exercise wear
   Shorts
   T-shirts
   Sun dresses

3. Select the list, and choose Sort Text from the Table menu.

4. Choose Text from the Type drop-down list and Descending in the Sort By box.

5. Click the Options button, check the Case Sensitive check box, and click OK.

   Word recognizes uppercase letters and sorts them before lowercase letters when the Case Sensitive box is checked.

6. Click OK.

   The list is alphabetized in descending order.

7. Select the list again, and then choose Sort Text from the Table menu.

8. Choose Ascending and click OK.

   The list is alphabetized in ascending order.

Sorting Lists Created with Tabs

If you have created a table using tabbed columns, Word can sort the text based on one of the tabbed lists. Word also can sort only one of the tabbed lists without sorting the rest of the text. By specifying Tab as the separator in the Sort Options dialog box, Word will recognize the tabbed text as columns. You can then identify the specific tabbed column by number in the Sort By box.

To sort the lists within tabbed text:

1. Under "**Tipping**" on page 6, select the tabbed text that begins with "Cabin steward" and ends with the second "At your discretion".

2. Choose Sort Text from the Table menu.

3. Choose Ascending and Text, if necessary. Click the Options button, and choose Tabs in the Separate Fields At box. Click OK.

4. Choose Field 1 from the Sort By drop-down list and click OK.

   The text is sorted alphanumerically and in ascending order by Field 1, which Word recognizes as the first column.

5. Select the text again, and choose Sort Text from the Table menu.

6. Choose Field 2 from the Sort By drop-down list and click OK.

   Word sorts the text alphanumerically and in ascending order by Field 2, the second tabbed column. Remember, alphanumeric sorting places numeric text first.

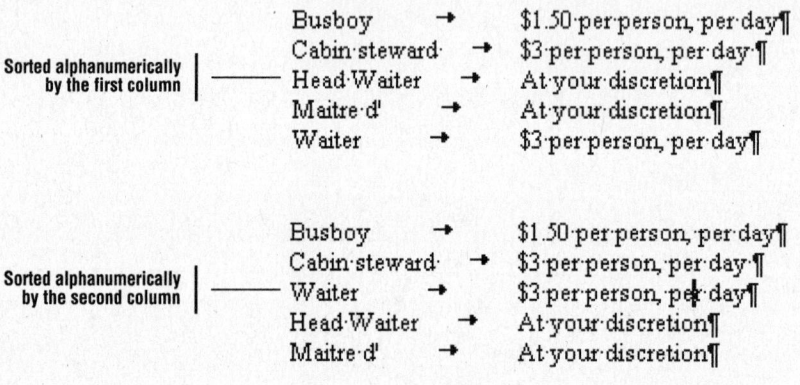

Figure 24-3
Tabbed text sorted two different ways

Sorting a Table

Note: It may not be appropriate to sort just one column of a table, if the cells of the column correspond to the cells in an adjacent column.

Any table created using Word's Table feature can be sorted. The process of sorting a table is similar to that of sorting a list created with tabs. Word sorts the rows in a table based on the column you select. When sorting tables, you can sort the whole table based on the first column of cells, the whole table based on another column of cells, or one column of the table without changing the whole table. Word sorts the table or column by the first character in each cell.

To sort a table:

1. Go to the table on page 3, under "Stateroom Categories and Location".

   The first column under "Category" is a numbered list. If you sort a numbered list, Word will renumber the list. In this procedure, you first need to convert the list to regular text, so the numbers can be reordered.

2. Select the first column, excluding the column heading in the first row, and delete the numbered list by clicking the Numbering button on the Formatting toolbar.

3. Key the same numbers as regular text, from 1 to 10, and then right-align the numbers.

4. Select the table, excluding the first row with the column headings.

5. Choose Sort from the Table menu.

6. Choose Ascending and Text, if necessary.

7. In the Sort By drop-down list, choose Column 2 and click OK.

   The table is sorted alphabetically by the second column (the Location/Description column).

8. Select the table again, excluding the first row with the column headings.

9. Choose Sort from the Table menu.

10. Choose Ascending, and choose Number from the Type drop-down list. Choose Column 3 from the Sort By drop-down list and click OK.

   The table is sorted in ascending numeric order by the third column (the Peak Rate column).

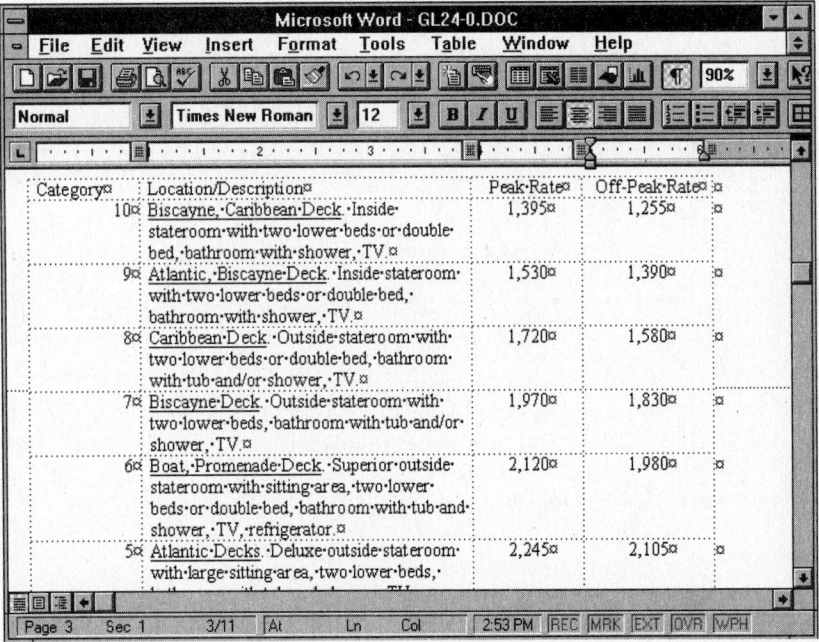

Figure 24-4
The table sorted by peak rates in ascending numeric order

11. Delete the dollar signs from the figures in the last row of the table.

12. Print pages 2 though 6 of the document.

13. Save the document, and then close it and exit Word (unless you will be doing the following exercises immediately).

Sorting Data-Source Files

Data-source files attached to a main document can be sorted before they are merged. The sort feature is useful for sorting a data-source file by information such as ZIP code, state, or invoice number. You sort the table in the data-source file in the same way as you sort a table created with Word's table feature. For example, to sort a data-source file by ZIP code, select the table (excluding the record header). Then, using the Sort dialog box, indicate the column number of the ZIP codes in the Sort By box. Click OK to apply the sorting.

Key Term

Sorting

Exercises

Exercise 24.1

1. Start Word, if necessary.

2. Open the file 24-1.doc.

3. Sort the text alphabetically in descending order:

   A. Position the insertion point in the table, and choose Sort from the Table menu.

   B. Choose Descending.

   C. Choose Text from the Type drop-down list.

   D. Make sure Column 1 is chosen in the Sort By box and click OK.

4. Undo the sort by choosing Undo Sort from the Edit menu.

5. Sort the list alphabetically in ascending order:

   A. Position the insertion point in the table.

   B. Choose Sort from the Table menu.

   C. Choose Ascending.

   D. In the Type drop-down list, choose Text, if necessary.

E. Make sure Column 1 is chosen in the Sort By box and click OK.

6. Select the table, and convert it to text (remember, choose Convert Table to Text from the Table menu, and then use paragraph marks to separate the text).

7. Change the sorted text to a two-column layout, so it can fit on one page.

8. Center the heading, and make it 14 points.

9. Save the document as *[your three-letter identifier]*24-1.doc.

10. Print the document.

11. Close the document and exit Word (unless you will be doing the following exercises immediately).

Exercise 24.2

1. Start Word, if necessary.

2. Open the file 24-2.doc.

3. Sort the tabbed list alphabetically:

A. Select the text from "Harmony Desk" to "279.99".

B. Choose Sort Text from the Table menu.

C. Choose Ascending.

D. In the Type drop-down list, choose Text.

E. Click Options, choose Tabs in the Separate Fields At box, and click OK.

F. Click OK.

4. Sort the tabbed list numerically based on the second column:

A. With the tabbed list still selected, choose Sort Text from the Table menu.

B. Choose Number from the Type drop-down list.

C. Choose Field 2 from the Sort By drop-down list and click OK.

D. Move the dollar sign up to the first figure in the list, and then align it with the dollar signs below it (insert seven space characters before the first dollar sign, or align all three dollar signs at a tab stop just before the 3-inch mark).

5. Position the insertion point after the last paragraph. Press **Enter** twice, and key the text in Figure 24-5. Single-space the list (from "desk chairs" through "two-drawer file cabinets"). Double-space before and after the list.

Figure 24-5

Last week, I took an inventory of our office furniture. We have:

desk chairs

desks

chairs with armrests

desk lamps

couches

bookshelves

four-drawer filing cabinets

two-drawer filing cabinets

With the exception of one of the couches (the one in Tom's office) and two of the chairs with armrests, all the furniture is in excellent condition.

6. Sort the list alphabetically:

   A. Select the list (from "desk chairs" to "two-drawer file cabinets").

   B. Choose Sort Text from the Table menu.

   C. Choose Ascending.

   D. Choose Text from the Type drop-down list.

   E. Make sure Paragraphs appears in the Sort By box and click OK.

7. Key the following numbers before the items of office furniture:

   7 bookshelves
   23 chairs with armrests
   4 couches
   13 desk chairs
   9 desk lamps
   11 desks
   9 four-drawer file cabinets
   11 two-drawer file cabinets

8. Sort the list numerically in descending order:

   A. Select the list.

   B. Choose Sort Text from the Table menu.

C. Choose Descending.

D. Choose Number from the Type drop-down list and click OK.

9. Spell-check the document.

10. Add your reference initials to the document.

11. Save the document as *[your three-letter identifier]*24-2.doc.

12. Print the document.

13. Close the document and exit Word (unless you will be doing the following exercises immediately).

Exercise 24.3

1. Start Word, if necessary.

2. Create a new document based on the Memo1 template.

3. In the heading, address the memo to Tom Carey from Susan Allen. Key **Sales Promotion Mailing List** as the subject, and delete the "CC:" line.

4. Format the paragraph spacing of the memo text line (where you begin keying the memo body text) to 0 pt after.

5. With the insertion point at the beginning of the memo text line, press **Enter** once, and then key the text in Figure 24-6. Include the corrections. Single-space the list of names. Double-space before and after the list of names.

Figure 24-6

Please add the following customers to our sales promotion letter mailing list. These are some of our best customers and we do not want to leave them out of our *future mailings* next mailing

Piestrup, Rhoda

Pienkowski, Cornelius

Besser, Susan G.

Stauber, Henrietta *s*

Elchsbind, Risa

Jorgenson, Lynette

6. Open the file 24-3.doc. Copy the entire document, except for "Tom:", and paste it below the last name in the memo.

7. Change the font of the entire memo (excluding "Memorandum" to Arial 12 point.

8. Spell-check the memo, and save it as *[your three-letter identifier]*24-3.doc.

9. Sort the first list of names in the memo alphabetically in descending order.

10. Sort the second list of names and dates by date in descending order.

11. Add your reference initials to the document.

12. Save the document again and print it.

13. Close the documents and exit Word (unless you will be doing the following exercise immediately).

Exercise 24.4: Challenge Yourself

Open the file 24-4.doc, and change line spacing for the entire document to 1.5 lines. Below the heading, change the four lines of text, from "TOUR OPERATOR" through "Sales Increase", to 16-point type. At the end of each of these four lines, insert a colon, and then insert a tab character that is right-aligned at 4 inches. For all the text in the document below these four lines, set a 3-inch, right-aligned tab. Make sure all the numerical text aligns at this tab stop.

Create a data source for the document, named 24-4data.doc, as follows:

TourOp	Sales93	Sales92	Increase
All Aboard	90,569	72,664	17,905
Horizons	98,513	93,979	4,534
Travel USA	99,364	87,886	11,478
American Dream	65,634	57,933	7,701

View the data source, and then sort it alphabetically in ascending order by the first column. Widen the first column, so all the text appears on one line.

In the main document, insert the corresponding mail-merge fields at the top of the document where you have inserted the tab characters (beginning to the right of "TOUR OPERATOR"). Save the main document as *[your three-letter identifier]*24-4a.doc. Print just the main document.

Mail merge the main document and the data source to a new document. Spell-check the new merged document, and save it as *[your three-letter identifier]*24-4b.doc.

On page 1 of the merged document, sort the list under "DAY TRIPS" alphabetically in ascending order by the first column. On page 2 of the merged document, sort the same list numerically in ascending order by the second column. On page 3 of the merged document, sort the same list numerically in descending order by the second column.

Print the merged document. Close the documents, saving the changes, and exit Word.

A Letter

Background

Duke City Gateway needs to send a letter to announce new golf-vacation packages.

Since the letter will be sent to more than one customer, Tom Carey has suggested that the letter be formatted in a mail-merge file, so he can create one copy of the letter and address it to several people.

Business Purpose

Create a letter and a data source. Then mail merge the letter to send to several customers.

Procedures

1. Open a new document, and use it as your main document for a mail merge.

2. Create a data source, using the following information as the header row:

   Title FirstName LastName Address1 City State PostalCode

3. Save the data source as p9data.doc.

4. Key the following information in the data source:

   Title: **Ms.**

   FirstName: **Maria**

   LastName: **Cordova**

   Address1: **15 Washington Avenue**

   City: **Santa Fe**

   State: **NM**

   PostalCode: **87501**

5. Complete the data file by keying the information from Figure 24-7, which appears at the end of this project.

6. Format the main document as a block-style letter. Use 1-inch left and right margins and a 2-inch top margin. Insert the date as a field.

7. At the point where you would key the name and address, insert the Title merge field, followed by the FirstName and LastName merge fields (leave one space between each of the fields).

8. Press **Enter**, and insert the Address1 merge field.

9. Press **Enter**, and insert the City merge field followed by a comma and a space, the State merge field, and the PostalCode merge field (leave one space between each field).

10. Press **Enter** twice, key **Dear** followed by a space, insert the FirstName merge field, and then key **:** (the colon).

11. Continue the letter by keying the following two paragraphs:

    As a valued customer of Duke City Gateway Travel Agency, we are offering you special low rates on our new golf-vacation packages. The National Golf Association has just released its ratings of the best golf resorts in the United States, and we have arranged vacation packages with top resorts in different regions of the country.

    The following is a listing by region of our exclusive golf-vacation packages at the top-rated United States golf courses:

12. Insert a table with three columns and eight rows. Make the first column 1.5 inches wide, the second column 2 inches wide, and the last column 1 inch wide.

13. Center the table horizontally.

14. To complete the table, key the following information in single-spaced format:

Location	Resort	Price
New England	Farmington Resort	$399
South	Plantation Resort	$459
Florida	Palm Grove Resort	$499
Southwest	Red River Resort	$699
California	Orange Grove Resort	$699
Midwest	Plainfield Resort	$599
Northwest	Rocky Hill Resort	$399

15. Select the third column of the table, and then center the text.

16. Below the table, key the following information in single-spaced format:

   All of the golf-vacation packages include:

   Per-person double-occupancy accommodations for three nights

   Breakfast and dinner

   Unlimited use of golf course and driving range for four days

   Round-trip airfare

   Airport shuttle

17. Rearrange the list of golf-package items to create a more logical order: Move "Round-trip airfare" to the top of the list, and move "Airport shuttle" into second place. Then format the items as a bulleted list.

18. Complete the letter by keying the following two closing paragraphs:

   Personal golf lessons are available at each resort at an additional cost. Lessons are conducted by the hour, and range from $45-$100 per hour, depending on the professional level of the instructor.

   If you would like to see for yourself how beautiful these courses really are, come in and visit our office. We will gladly show you our exclusive videos on each of these resorts. To take advantage of these special introductory prices on our new golf-vacation packages, contact me, Tom Carey, at (505) 555-1234.

19. Key **Sincerely** at the end of the letter, which is from Tom Carey, Travel Counselor. Include your reference initials.

20. Sort the golf courses in the table alphabetically by location. Underline the headings in the top row of the table.

21. Use the Shrink to Fit option in print preview to fit the letter on one page.

22. Spell-check the main document.

23. Save the main document as *[your three letter identifier]* p9-1.doc and print it.

24. Mail-merge the documents to a new document, and then name the merge document *[your three-letter identifier]* p9-2.doc.

25. Scroll through the pages of the new document. (You may have to remove a space before the address name in the last letter.) Print the merged document.

26. Save the changes, close the documents, and exit Word.

Tips and Hints

- Print your letters on company letterhead to give them a professional appearance.

- Review any items in lists or tables, and sort them into logical order.

- Include the appropriate courtesy title as a merge field.

- Once a data source has been created, it can be attached to other main documents. Therefore, if you need to send a new letter to the same names and addresses of the last letter sent, just create a new main document, and attach the old data source to the new letter.

Figure 24-7

Mr. Joseph Anaya
3883 Cerillos Road
Santa Fe, NM 87501

Ms. Sheila Friedman
P.O. Box 88
Grants, NM 87020

Mr. Charles Neira
87 Green Lake Road
Rio Rancho, NM 87048

Mr. Don Liu
4 Squaw Road
Albuquerque, NM 87120

Mrs. Cathy Petersen
98 Sequoia Road
Albuquerque, NM 87120

Ms. Mary Snow
801 Ranchitos Road
Albuquerque, NM 87107

Ms. Florence Lechtner
54 Indian School Road
Albuquerque, NM 87110

Mr. Donald Gagliano
45 Carson Drive
Los Lunas, NM 87021

Richard and Linda Elliott *(leave title field blank)*
8 Castillo Avenue
Belen, NM 87002

Module 10

Graphics

Working with Graphics

Objectives

- Insert graphics.
- Select graphics.
- Scale and crop graphics.
- Add borders to graphics.
- Move graphics.
- Delete graphics.
- Use the Drawing toolbar.

Pictures
Graphic images in Word documents.

Graphic file format
Defines the graphic's type, such as paint-type or draw-type.

To add interest to Word documents, place graphics in them. Graphics help attract attention to a document by guiding the reader's eye to specific locations on the page. Graphics include lines, borders, and images. In Word, graphic images are referred to as *pictures*.

Lesson 10 described how to add lines and borders to documents. This lesson describes the different ways to add graphics to Word documents and the ways to manipulate those graphics.

About Graphic File Formats

Graphic images from other applications can be inserted in Word documents. In order for Word to accept a graphic image from another application, it must be stored in a graphic file format that Word recognizes. The *graphic file format* defines the type of graphic. There are a few general categories of graphic file formats. These include:

- Paint-type graphics

  A *paint-type graphic* is a graphic that is stored as a pattern of electronic dots that are arranged to create an image. Paint-type graphics are created in programs such as PC Paintbrush.

- Draw-type graphics

  A *draw-type graphic* is a graphic that is stored as a combination of lines and shapes. Draw-type graphics are also known as *object-oriented graphics*.

- TIFF

  TIFF, short for tagged image file format, is a standard type of graphic file format that is widely available in many graphics programs. Graphics stored in the TIFF file format are similar to paint-type graphics, because they are made up of dots.

- EPS

  EPS, short for Encapsulated PostScript, is a draw-type graphic that has been saved using the PostScript page-description language.

Each type of graphic file format has a different file extension. A file extension is a three-character code added to the end of the file name. For example, when you save a Word document, the extension is

.DOC, and, when you save a Word template, the extension is .DOT. When graphic images are saved in the TIFF graphic file format, their file extension is .TIF. Other commonly used file extensions for graphics files are:

- .PCX for PC Paintbrush

- .EPS for Encapsulated PostScript

- .BMP for Windows Bitmaps

- .WMF for Windows Metafile Format

- .CGM for Computer Graphics Metafile

Before you can insert a graphic from another application into a Word document, your computer must have the appropriate graphic import filters installed. A *graphic import filter* is a software program that allows Word to recognize the graphic's file format and file extension.

Graphic import filter
A software program that allows Word to recognize graphics from other applications.

Note: All of the available graphic import filters should have been installed with Word.

The Word Clipart Subdirectory

Note: Depending on how Word was installed, clip art may also be found in a subdirectory of c:\msoffice.

A Clipart subdirectory is installed with Word. This subdirectory is found in the c:\winword directory. The Clipart subdirectory contains numerous draw-type graphics that can be inserted into Word documents. The following is a list of the names and descriptions of some of the graphic files available in the Clipart subdirectory:

Table 25-1: Graphic Files in the Clipart Subdirectory

Name	Description
3darrow1.wmf	Three-dimensional arrows
artist.wmf	An artist at an easel
buttrfly.wmf	A color butterfly
capitol.wmf	The capitol building in Washington, D.C.
coins.wmf	Stacks of coins
crowd.wmf	A crowd of people
helicptr.wmf	A helicopter
jazz.wmf	A collage of musical instruments
nosmoke.wmf	The no-smoking symbol

Inserting Graphics

You can insert graphics in Word documents using the Picture command from the Insert menu or the Clipboard. Graphics are inserted at the insertion point in a document.

The Picture Command

Use the Picture command to insert graphic images from other applications into a Word document. When you choose Picture from the Insert menu, the Insert Picture dialog box appears. This dialog box lists the graphic files available to insert in Word documents.

To insert a graphic file using the Picture command:

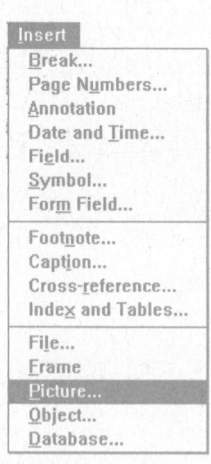

Insert menu

1. Start Word, if necessary.

2. Open the file 25-0.doc.

3. Position the insertion point before the fifth paragraph (which begins "For more information:").

4. Choose Picture from the Insert menu.

5. From the c:\winword\clipart directory, choose the filename 1stplace.wmf.

6. Check the Preview Picture check box, if necessary.

    The picture appears in the Preview box.

Figure 25-1

The Insert Picture dialog box

Note: The Link to File check box in the Picture dialog box allows you to link the graphic in the Word document to its original graphic file. Then, if you change the original graphic in another application, the graphic in the Word document is updated automatically.

7. Click OK.

    The picture is inserted in the document at the insertion point.

8. Press **Enter** to move the text "For more information:" to the next line.

Inserting Graphics Using the Clipboard

Using the Clipboard, you can copy a graphic from another Windows program and insert it into your Word document. To do this, copy a graphic image from another Windows application, such as PC Paintbrush, to the Clipboard. Close that application (the graphic remains on the Clipboard), and open the Word document. Then paste the graphic in the Word document. You can also use the Clipboard to copy a graphic image from one Word document to another.

To insert a graphic image using the Clipboard:

1. Click the picture.

    Handles appear around the picture, indicating that it is selected.

2. Click the Copy button on the Standard toolbar.

    The picture is stored in the Clipboard.

3. Save the document as *[your three-letter identifier]*25-0.doc, and then close the document.

4. Create a new document.

5. Click the Paste button on the Standard toolbar.

    The picture is inserted in the new document.

6. Close the new document without saving it.

Selecting a graphic to copy it

Selecting Graphics

Just as you selected a graphic to copy it, you must also select a graphic to manipulate it in the document. Click the mouse on a graphic to select it. When a graphic is selected, a border appears around it. Inside the border lines are eight small, square handles, called *sizing handles*, that you can use to resize the graphic.

To deselect a graphic, click another area of the page. To select a graphic with text, use the mouse to drag the I-beam over the graphic and the text. When you select a graphic and text together, the entire selection is highlighted.

To practice selecting and deselecting a graphic:

1. Open the file *[your three-letter identifier]*25-0.doc.

2. Click the picture to select it.

    A border appears with eight sizing handles inside the border.

3. Move the insertion point after the phone number at the end of the document to deselect the graphic.

    The border and sizing handles around the graphic disappear.

Sizing handles
The small, square handles inside the border lines of a selected graphic that are used for resizing.

Selecting a graphic to resize it

A picture and text selected

4. Drag the I-beam over the picture and the four lines of text below it.

The picture and the text are both highlighted.

5. Click the mouse to deselect the picture and text.

Viewing Graphics

In order to view a graphic in its exact location in a document, it is a good idea to switch to page layout view. Once in page layout view, graphics can be scaled, cropped, and moved easily.

In a long document that contains a few graphics, it is a good idea to turn on Picture Placeholders. When Picture Placeholders is turned on, boxes appear in place of the graphics in a document. This feature helps speed up scrolling through a long document and keying new text in a document. To turn on Picture Placeholders, choose Options from the Tools menu. Click the View tab, and then click Picture Placeholders in the Show box to select it.

Scaling and Cropping Graphics

Scale
To resize a graphic image.

Pictures in Word documents can be scaled or cropped. When you *scale* a graphic, you are reducing or enlarging the size of the image. Scale a graphic by first selecting the graphic and then dragging one of its sizing handles. Drag the handle in to reduce the size of the graphic or out to enlarge the graphic.

Proportional scaling
Scaling a graphic using a corner sizing handle to maintain the original proportions.

To scale a graphic proportionally, drag one of the four corner sizing handles in or out. With *proportional scaling*, you are resizing the graphic but maintaining its relative height and width (its original proportions). If you scale a graphic by dragging one of the top, bottom, or side sizing handles, the graphic's original proportions are distorted as its size changes.

Note: When a graphic is scaled, the status bar shows the percentage by which the graphic is reduced or enlarged.

Top handle resizes disproportionally

Corner handle resizes proportionally

Figure 25-2
A picture scaled proportionally and disproportionally

To scale a picture:

1. Click the picture to select it.

2. Move the pointer to the sizing handle in the bottom right corner.

3. Drag the sizing handle toward the center of the picture to reduce the size of the picture proportionally. As you are dragging, notice the scaling proportions changing on the status bar.

4. Drag the same sizing handle out to the right, and extend the picture all the way to the right margin (about 210% on the status bar).

You can also crop a picture. When you *crop* a picture, you are hiding parts of the image. The parts of the image that are cropped do not appear on the screen or print, but these parts are not eliminated.

To crop a picture proportionally, hold down the **Shift** key, and drag one of the four corner sizing handles. A corner sizing handle will crop a graphic from two sides. For example, if you move the pointer to the bottom right corner of the graphic, press the **Shift** key, and drag the sizing handle, the right and bottom sides of the graphic will be cropped proportionally. If you drag the sizing handle in the top left corner of the graphic, the top and left sides will be cropped proportionally.

To crop a picture from the top, bottom, or side only, hold down the **Shift** key, and drag the appropriate sizing handle.

Crop
To hide parts of a graphic image so that they do not appear on the screen or print.

Sizing handle for cropping graphics

Corner sizing handle crops bottom and right side

Bottom sizing handle crops bottom only

Figure 25-3
Different ways to crop a picture

To crop a picture:

1. Select the picture.

2. Hold down the **Shift** key as you drag the bottom sizing handle up toward the middle of the picture.

3. Release the mouse button and the **Shift** key.

Note: The Undo command can be used to undo the last sizing action, or you can use the Undo button's drop-down list to undo the last several sizing actions.

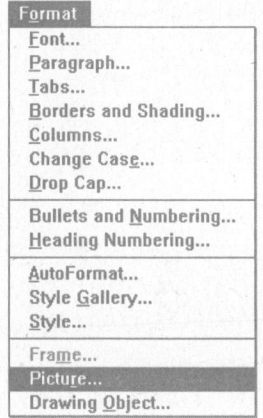

Format menu

Because Word remembers the original image, a scaled or cropped graphic can be restored to its original size. To restore a graphic to its original size, choose Picture from the Format menu, and click the Reset button. Or, press the **Ctrl** key, and double-click the graphic.

To restore a scaled graphic to its original size:

1. Select the picture.

2. Choose Picture from the Format menu.

   Word displays the Picture dialog box.

3. Click the Reset button, and then click OK.

Figure 25-4
The Picture dialog box

The Picture dialog box can also be used to crop or scale graphics. Select the graphic, open the dialog box, and then enter the desired measurements in the text boxes.

Adding Borders to Graphics

Note: A shadow box border can only be chosen from the Borders tab in the Borders and Shading dialog box, and not from the Borders toolbar.

Picture with a shadow border

To enhance the appearance of the graphics in a Word document, add borders around the graphics. Adding borders to graphics is similar to adding borders to paragraphs. To add a border to a graphic, select the graphic, and choose Borders and Shading from the Format menu. Click the Borders tab, and then choose the type of border and line style, or click the Borders button on the Formatting toolbar, and then choose a border and line style from the Borders toolbar.

To add a border to a picture:

1. Select the picture.

2. Choose Borders and Shading from the Format menu.

3. Click the Borders tab, if necessary.

4. Choose the Shadow box border and click OK.

   A shadow border is added to the picture.

Moving Graphics

Once a graphic is inserted in a Word document, it can be moved to a new location. Moving graphics in Word is similar to moving text. To move a graphic, you can use one of these methods:

- Select the graphic, and then use the Cut and Paste commands.

- Select the graphic, and press the **F2** key. Then move the insertion point to the new location and press **Enter**.

- Select the graphic, and drag it to a new location.

To move a picture:

1. Select the picture.

2. Press the **F2** key.

3. Move the insertion point to the end of the document.

4. Press **Enter**.

   The picture is moved to the new location.

Note: Once a picture is moved to the desired location, you can also align it using the alignment buttons on the Formatting toolbar. Positioning pictures is discussed in more detail in the next lesson.

Deleting a Graphic

To delete a graphic permanently from a Word document, select it and press the **Backspace** key, or select it and choose Cut from the Edit menu to place it on the Clipboard.

To delete a picture:

1. Select the picture at the end of the document.

2. Press the **Backspace** key.

   The picture is deleted from the document.

3. Click the Undo button to restore the picture.

The Drawing Toolbar

Drawing button on the Standard toolbar

When you click the Drawing button on the Standard toolbar, Word displays the Drawing toolbar, which offers many special drawing features to enhance documents. For example, you can use the Drawing toolbar to draw objects such as squares, rectangles, and polygons; to create a text box; or to add a callout to an illustration. Once a drawing object is created, it can be modified in a number of ways. For example, you can change the color or thickness of a drawing object or rotate an object. A series of objects can be grouped as one drawing object, which can then be moved or resized. You must first select a drawing object to modify it. A drawing object is selected like any graphic, by clicking it.

Figure 25-5

The Drawing toolbar

When the Drawing toolbar is open, Word switches to page layout view.

To use the Drawing toolbar:

1. Scroll to the bicycle at the top of the document.

    The bicycle drawing is a series of lines and shapes that have been grouped by selecting each individual object and clicking the Group button on the Drawing toolbar.

2. Click the Drawing button on the Standard toolbar.

    Word switches to page layout view as it opens the Drawing toolbar.

3. If necessary, drag the Drawing toolbar to a position above the ruler.

4. Click the bicycle drawing to select it.

    The drawing can now be sized or moved.

5. Double-click the drawing.

    Word opens a separate picture window for the drawing. The drawing can now be modified in other ways using the Drawing toolbar.

6. Move the arrow pointer to a line in the drawing, and click to select the drawing.

7. Click the Line Style button on the Drawing toolbar, and then click the third line from the top of the Line Style drop-down box.

    The drawing appears with a thicker line.

8. Click the Line Color button, and then click the blue color.

    The lines change from black to blue. See Figure 25-6 on page 516.

9. Click the Close Picture button on the Picture toolbar to return to the document.

    The modified drawing appears in the document.

Line Style button

Line style options

Click to close picture
window and return to
the document

Selected picture

Figure 25-6
Modifying a picture created with the Drawing toolbar

10. Click the drawing again to select it (click only once), and then use the Borders and Shading command to apply a thin box border to the drawing.

11. Scroll to the picture at the end of the document.

12. Click the Callout button on the Drawing toolbar.

    The pointer changes to a crosshair.

13. Move the pointer to the middle of the right border of the picture, click the left mouse button, and drag the line about one inch to the right.

14. Release the mouse button.

    A box appears with the insertion point in it.

15. Key **Prizes awarded courtesy of Rick's Cycle Shop**

16. Click outside the callout box.

    The callout appears next to the picture. The callout text can be selected and formatted. You can also use the ruler to change the margin boundary for the callout text.

17. Click the Drawing button to remove the Drawing toolbar.

18. View the document in print preview.

19. Save the document, and then print it.

20. Close the document and exit Word (unless you will be doing the following exercises immediately).

Note: Callouts are visible in page layout view and print preview, but not in normal view.

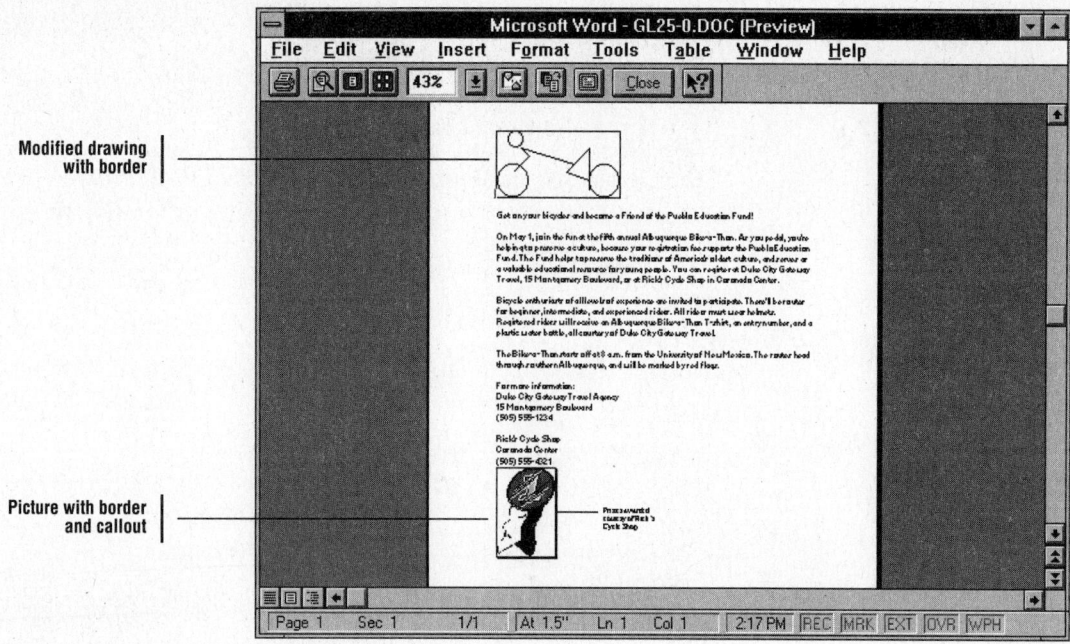

Modified drawing
with border

Picture with border
and callout

Figure 25-7
The document in print preview

Key Terms

Crop	Paint-type graphic
Draw-type graphic	Pictures
EPS	Proportional scaling
Graphic file format	Scale
Graphic import filter	Sizing handles
Object-oriented graphic	TIFF

Exercises

Exercise 25.1

1. Start Word, if necessary.

2. Open the file 25-1.doc.

3. Move the insertion point below the heading "Duke City Travel", and insert a picture:

    A. Choose Picture from the Insert menu.

    B. Select the filename jet.wmf from the c:\winword\clipart directory, and then click OK.

4. Move the picture:

    A. Click the picture to select it.

    B. Press the **F2** key.

    C. Move the insertion point above the heading "Duke City Gateway", and press **Enter** to insert the picture.

5. Scale the picture:

    A. Click the picture to select it.

    B. Drag the sizing handle in the bottom right corner to the right margin.

6. Restore the picture:

    A. Select the picture.

    B. Hold down the **Ctrl** key and double-click.

7. Click outside the picture to deselect it. Then change the type size of the text, from the heading ("Duke City Gateway") through "Friendly Service", to 28 point.

8. Insert a blank line before "Duke City Gateway".

9. Select the entire document, including the picture, and click the Center button on the Formatting toolbar.

10. Add a border to the picture:

    A. Select the picture.

    B. Choose Borders and Shading from the Format menu.

    C. Choose a box with a 1½ pt line and click OK.

11. View the document in print preview.

12. Save the document as *[your three-letter identifier]*25-1.doc and print it.

13. Close the document and exit Word (unless you will be doing the following exercises immediately).

Exercise 25.2

1. Start Word, if necessary.

2. Open the file 25-2.doc.

3. Change the type size for all the text to 24 point.

4. Move the insertion point to the left of "Turn off" in the third line, and insert the picture chekmark.wmf from the c:\winword\clipart directory.

5. Scale the picture:

    A. Select the picture.

    B. Drag the sizing handle in the bottom right corner toward the center of the picture, to 90% on the status bar.

6. Crop the picture:

    A. Select the picture.

    B. Hold down the **Shift** key as you drag the top sizing handle down to .25" on the status bar. Then release the mouse button and the **Shift** key.

7. Copy the picture to the Clipboard:

    A. Select the picture.

    B. Click the Copy button on the Standard toolbar.

8. Move the insertion point to the left of "Turn on" in the next sentence. Press **Enter**, and then paste the picture from the Clipboard.

9. Repeat step 8 for the next three sentences in the document.

10. Press **Enter** twice before "Thank you!".

11. At the top of the document, insert a blank line after "Reminder:".

12. View the document in print preview.

13. Save the document as *[your three-letter identifier]*25-2.doc and print it.

14. Close the document and exit Word (unless you will be doing the following exercises immediately).

Exercise 25.3

1. Start Word, if necessary.

2. Open the template letter1g.dot to modify it (or open one of Word's letter templates, and adapt it to the style described in Appendix B).

3. Change the top margin to 1 inch.

4. Above the date, insert the graphic letterhd.bmp from your student disk.

5. Insert 2 blank lines between the graphic and the date line.

6. Proportionally scale the letterhead to 5.5 inches wide.

7. Save the template as dukehd.dot on your student disk.

8. Close the template, and then open a new document based on the template.

9. Insert the date as a field, and address the letter to:

Mr. Robert Lambright
145 E. 15 Street
New York, NY 10003

10. For the body text, key the text in Figure 25-8, including the corrections. When you key "Ojo Caliente Hot Springs" in the first paragraph, create an AutoText entry for it called "Ojo". This entry is meant to be used automatically where "(Ojo)" is indicated in the figure.

Figure 25-8

In response to our conversation last week, I found a spa that meets your location and services specifications. *for* It is called Ojo Caliente Hot Springs, and it opened just two months ago. ¶ *{Ojo}* It *it* is located 100 miles from Albuquerque International Airport, and is only one hour from Santa Fe. It is surrounded by rugged mountains and desert, and has three different springs on the grounds. Services include massage, fitness training, and nutritional counseling. The enclosed brochure outlines all services and rates.

{Ojo}
~~The spa~~ has 25 rooms in the main building and 5 private cottages. The restaurant serves top-notch Southwestern food & *which is delicious and low in calories*.

Feel free to call with any questions you may have.

---

11. The letter is from Tom Carey, Travel Counselor. Key your reference initials at the bottom and an enclosure notation below them.

12. Delete the AutoText entry "Ojo".

13. Spell-check the document.

14. Save the document as *[your three-letter identifier]*25-3.doc and print it.

15. Close the document and exit Word (unless you will be doing the following exercise immediately).

Exercise 25.4: Challenge Yourself

Open the file 25-4.doc. Display the Drawing toolbar, and use the Line button to add a few new rays to the sun drawing. Use the Fill Color button to fill the circle portion of the drawing with yellow.

Change the style for the heading text to Heading 1. Change the line spacing in the text below the heading to double-spacing.

Above "Day 1", insert the picture tropics.eps from your student disk. Proportionally scale the picture so that it extends to the right margin. Move the picture to the end of the document. Insert a blank line above the picture, and then restore it to its original size.

Center-align the heading and the tropics picture, and then view the document in print preview. Save the document as *[your three-letter identifier]*25-4.doc and print it. Close the document and exit Word.

Positioning Graphics and Text

Objectives

- Add frames to text, pictures, and tables.
- Move and size frames.
- Flow text around frames.
- Align frames.
- Remove frames.
- Add captions to frames.
- Use WordArt.

Frames
Special enclosures that you add to paragraphs, pictures, or tables to position them on a page.

Normally, paragraphs, pictures, and tables are displayed in a document one after another. In Word, these items can be positioned anywhere on the page using a feature called frames.

What Are Frames?

Frames are rectangular enclosures that can be added to paragraphs, pictures, tables, or any other item inserted in a document. Frames allow you to position these items in a specific location on the page. For example, you can use a frame to position a heading in the margin of a page or to position a picture within a paragraph.

Viewing Frames

In order to view frames in their actual location, switch to page layout view. Frames appear in normal view, but they are not shown in their actual position on the page, and you cannot move them.

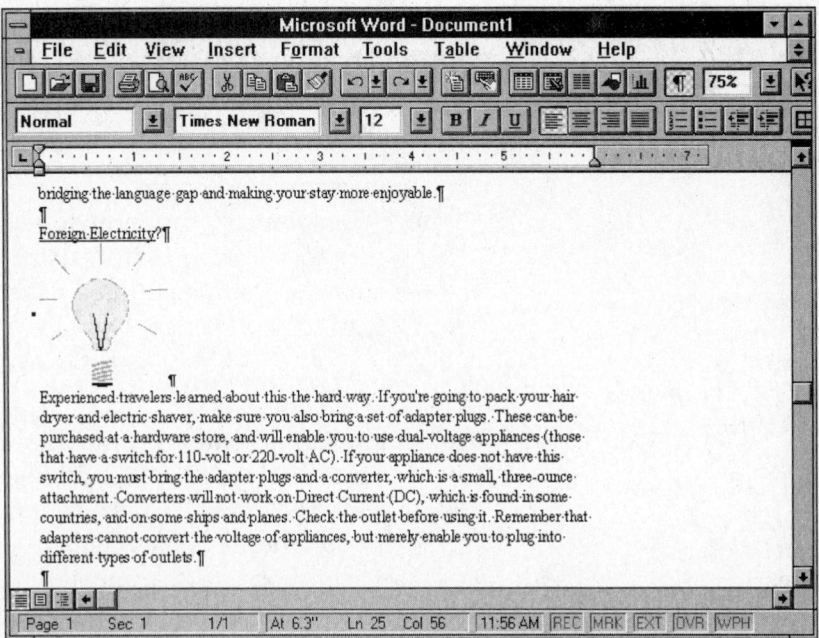

Figure 26-1
A framed picture in normal view

523

Figure 26-2
A framed picture in page layout view

Adding Frames

Before you can position a paragraph, picture, or table freely, you must add a frame to it in page layout view. If you are not in page layout view, and you try to add a frame, Word will prompt you with a dialog box that asks if you want to switch to page layout view. Click Yes, and then add the frame. Add frames to paragraphs, pictures, or tables by selecting the item to frame and choosing Frame from the Insert menu.

Note: When you apply a frame to text, Word adds a single-line, box border to the frame automatically. If necessary, this border can be removed from the frame, or the line style of the border can be changed.

You can insert an empty frame into a document to hold a position for text, a graphic, or a table. By inserting empty frames, you can create placeholders for items, such as graphics and tables, that you import from other applications. A *placeholder* is an empty frame that reserves a location in a document for text, graphics, or a table. To add an empty frame to a document, choose Frame from the Insert menu.

A frame is always anchored to the nearest paragraph. When you add a frame, an anchor appears next to it to indicate this. The anchor is a nonprinting character.

Placeholder
An empty frame inserted into a document to reserve a place for text, graphics, or a table.

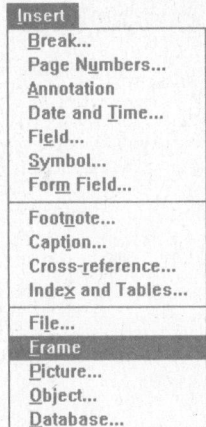

Insert menu

To add a frame to a paragraph:

1. Start Word, if necessary.

2. Open the file 26-0.doc.

3. On page 1, select the heading "Primer For First-Time Overseas Travelers".

4. Choose Frame from the Insert menu.

5. Click Yes in the dialog box to change to page layout view.

    A frame is added to the paragraph. The frame appears as a shaded border, and is accompanied by an anchor to show that the frame is anchored to the paragraph.

6. Click outside the frame to deselect it.

    Notice that Word applied a border to the frame automatically.

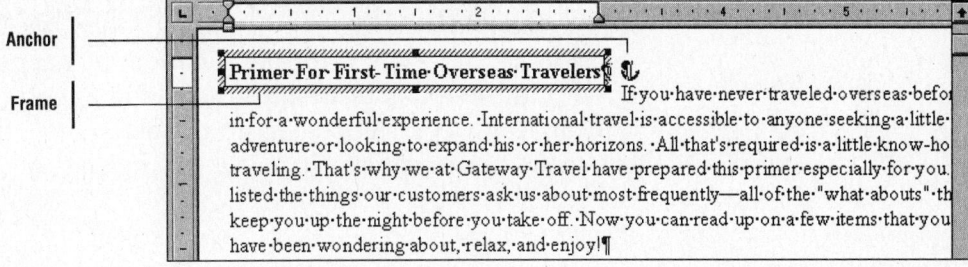

Anchor

Frame

Figure 26-3
A frame added to text

To add a frame to a picture:

1. After the first paragraph on page 1, which ends with "enjoy!", press **Enter**, and insert the clip-art file jet.wmf.

2. Click the picture to select it.

3. Choose Frame from the Insert menu.

    A frame is added to the picture. Notice the effect the frame has on the text following it. Notice also that Word does not apply a border to the framed picture automatically, as it does to framed text.

To insert an empty frame:

1. On the next page, move the insertion point to the left of the paragraph that begins "If you're torn".

2. Choose Frame from the Insert menu.

    The pointer changes to a crosshair.

3. Click before "If", and drag to the right to insert a frame. Using the ruler as your guide, release the mouse button when the frame is about 3 inches wide.

Note: When you apply a frame, the text following it is affected. This aspect of frames, known as text wrapping, is discussed later in the lesson.

An empty frame is inserted to the left of the paragraph. The frame has a border applied to it.

Figure 26-4
An empty frame inserted in the document

4. Switch to print preview to view the frames and the borders. Then return to page layout view.

Frames can be added to headers and footers in a Word document. When you add a frame to a header or footer, the frame's contents print on the pages where the header and footer appear. For example, use a frame to add a picture to a header or a footer, and the picture will appear with the header and footer when the document is printed. You manipulate frames in the headers and footers of your document using page layout view.

Figure 26-5
A framed picture in the document footer

Selecting Frames

Before manipulating the frames in Word documents, you must be able to select the frames. There are two ways to select a frame. To select a frame when the insertion point is not in the frame, click anywhere inside the frame. To select a frame when the insertion point is inside the frame, click any side of the frame. When the sizing handles appear inside the frame, the frame is selected.

To select a frame:

1. Move the insertion point to page 1, to the framed picture of the jet.

2. Click inside the frame to select it.

    The frame's sizing handles appear.

Selected frame

Sizing and Moving Frames

Two different mouse pointers are available when working with frames: the two-headed arrow and the four-headed arrow. The pointer is a four-headed arrow when it is within a frame or along the sides of a frame. It changes to a two-headed arrow when it is positioned over one of the sizing handles.

Sizing a frame is similar to sizing a picture. Select the frame, and then position the pointer on one of the sizing handles. When the pointer becomes a two-headed arrow, drag the sizing handle to reduce or enlarge the size of the frame.

To resize a frame:

1. Make sure the framed picture is still selected.

2. Move the pointer to the bottom right sizing handle.

3. When the pointer changes to a diagonal two-headed arrow, drag the sizing handle in to about 76% on the status bar.

    The framed picture is reduced to about 2 inches wide.

When the pointer changes to a four-headed arrow, you can move the frame. To move a frame, hold down the left mouse button, and drag the frame to the desired position.

To move and resize a frame:

1. Select the frame around the heading at the top of the page.

    The sizing handles appear.

2. Move the mouse pointer so that it points to the frame (use the tip of the arrow pointer).

3. When the four-headed arrow appears, drag the frame straight across to the right side of the page, so that the frame begins at about the 3-inch mark on the ruler.

4. Move the pointer over the right sizing handle on the right side of the frame.

5. When the pointer changes to a horizontal, double-headed arrow, drag the side of the frame about ½ inch to the right margin.

    The frame is resized.

6. With the frame selected, use the Center button on the Formatting toolbar to center the text within the frame.

7. Select the framed jet.

8. Move the pointer within the frame.

9. When the four-headed arrow appears, drag the frame straight across to the right side of the page, so that the right side of the

frame aligns with the framed text above it and the right margin.

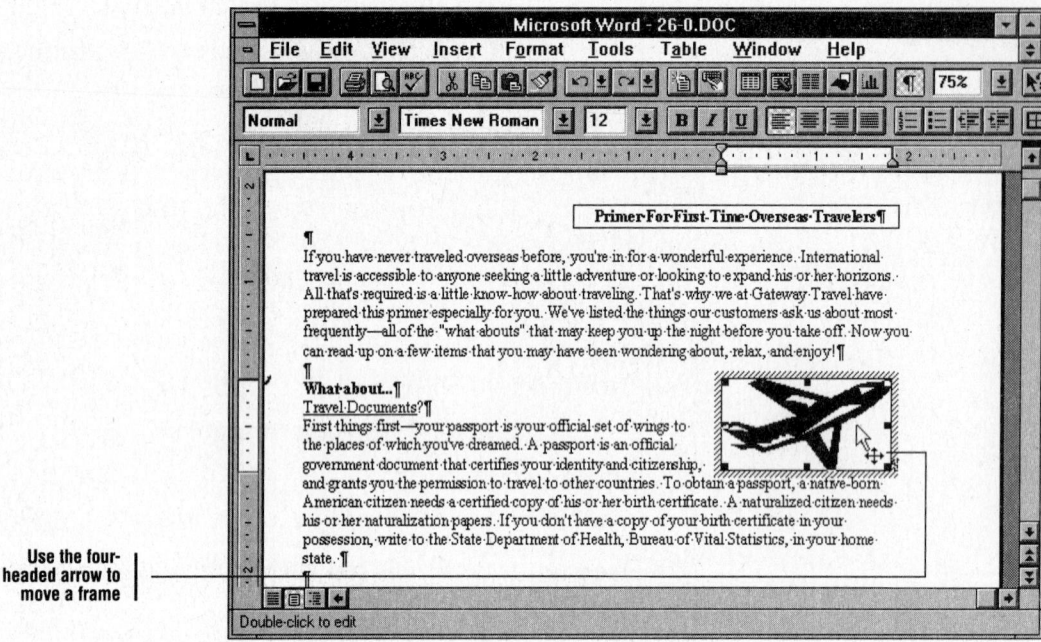

Use the four-headed arrow to move a frame

Figure 26-6
Resized and repositioned frames

Options in the Frame Dialog Box

The options in the Frame dialog box allow you to manipulate the frames in a document. For example, you can flow text around a frame, change the size of a frame, align a frame horizontally or vertically, move frames with text, and remove frames. To open the Frame dialog box, choose Frame from the Format menu.

Figure 26-7
The Frame dialog box

Flowing Text Around a Frame

The text-wrapping options appear in the Frame dialog box. The default text-wrapping option is Around. This option wraps text around all sides of the frame. If the text-wrapping option is changed to None, the text will not wrap around the frame, but the text will appear above and below the frame.

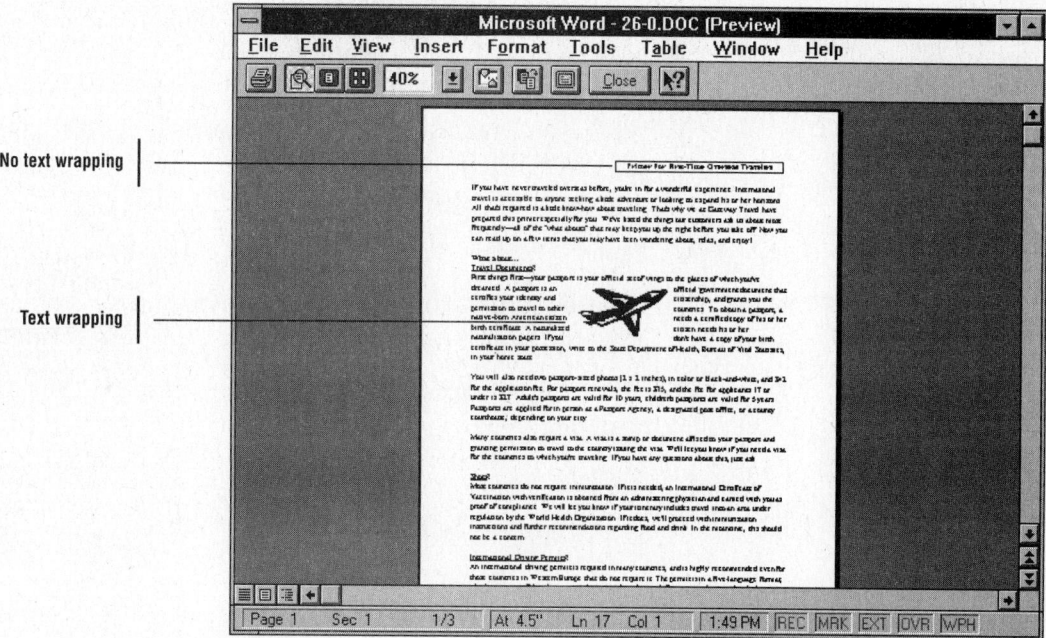

No text wrapping

Text wrapping

Figure 26-8

Using text-wrapping options for frames

To change text-wrapping options:

1. Select the frame around the heading at the top of the document.

2. Choose Frame from the Format menu.

3. Under Text Wrapping, choose None. Click OK.

   The text below the heading no longer wraps around the frame.

4. Click the jet picture to select the frame, and then choose Frame from the Format menu.

5. Change the Around option in the Text Wrapping box to None and click OK.

   The text that begins "**What about...**" no longer wraps around the frame.

6. Click the Undo button to restore the frame.

7. Using the four-headed arrow, drag the frame down and to the left, so that it is in the middle of the paragraph below "Travel Documents?".

   The text flows around the framed picture.

Note: You can leave space between a frame and the text around which it is wrapped. To specify the distance between the frame and the text wrapped around it, key a measurement in the Distance From Text box under Horizontal or Vertical in the Frame dialog box.

Changing the Size of Frames

In addition to sizing frames by dragging the sizing handles, you can change the size of frames by entering values in the Frame dialog box. Change the width and height of the frame by keying values in the Width and Height text boxes.

There are two options to consider when setting the width in the Frame dialog box:

Width settings

- Auto

  When selected, the width of the frame will be adjusted automatically if the item inside the frame is increased or decreased.

- Exactly

  Use this setting to specify a fixed width for a frame. The frame stays the same size when you adjust the item inside the frame.

The following are options to consider when setting the height in the Frame dialog box:

Height settings

- Auto

  The height of the frame stays the same as the item inside the frame.

- At Least

  Use this setting to specify a minimum height by which Word can increase the frame if you enlarge the item inside the frame.

- Exactly

  Use this setting to specify a fixed height for the frame. The height will not change if you change the size of the item inside the frame.

To change the frame size using the Frame dialog box:

1. Select the frame around the jet picture.

2. Choose Frame from the Format menu.

3. Under Size, set the Width to Exactly, and key **2** in the At box.

4. Click OK.

    The width of the frame increases to exactly 2 inches.

Aligning Frames

The options for horizontal and vertical placement in the Frame dialog box allow you to position frames in exact locations on the page and to specify the distance the frame is to be placed from other text. Use these options to specify a location for the frame or a point of reference on the page. For example, you can align a frame with the right margin, using the right margin as the point of reference. To do this,

Horizontal settings to
align a frame

select the frame, and choose Frame from the Format menu. Under Horizontal, choose Right from the Position drop-down list box and Margin from the Relative To drop-down list box.

Additional options for horizontal positioning from the Position drop-down list box are: Left, Right, Center, Inside, and Outside. Frames are aligned relative to the reference point that is chosen in the Relative To box. You can choose Margin, Page, or Column as the point of reference for the frame. If you choose Center in the Position box and Page in the Relative To box, the frame will be centered horizontally on the page. Use the Inside and Outside options when aligning frames in documents that contain facing pages.

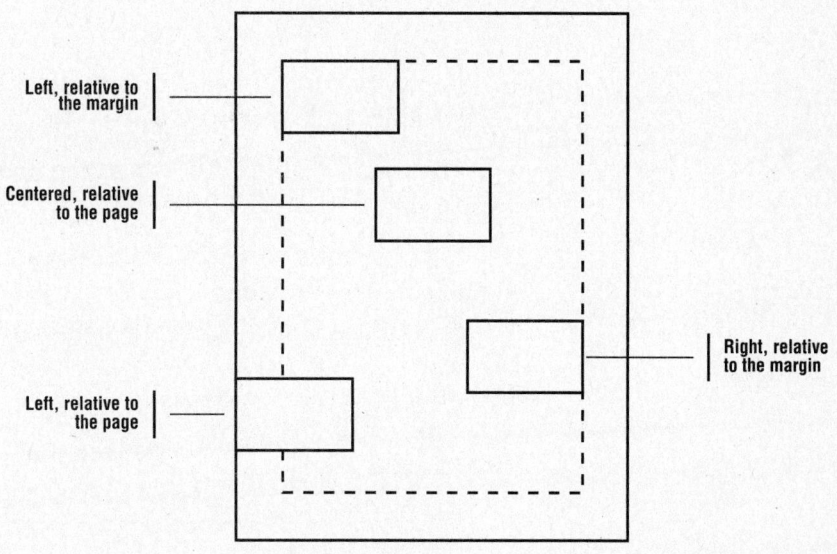

Figure 26-9

Examples of horizontally aligned frames in a one-column layout

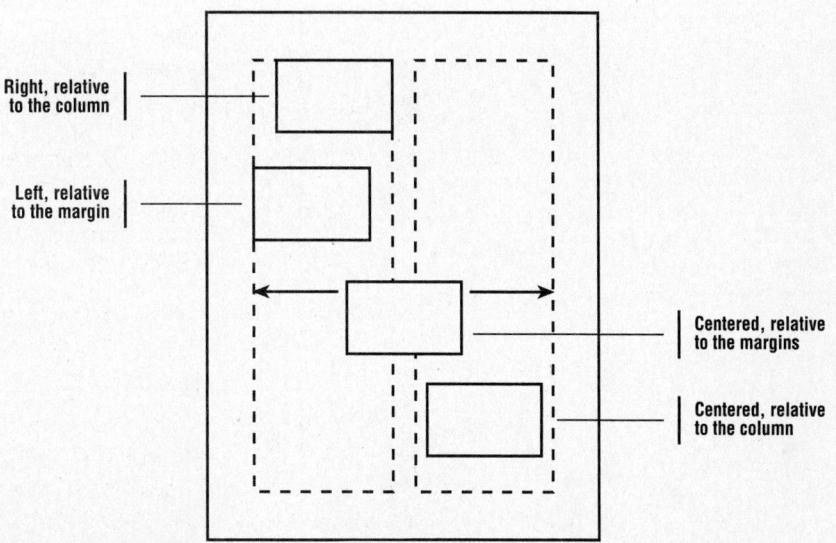

Figure 26-10

Examples of horizontally aligned frames in a two-column layout

To align a frame horizontally:

1. On page 2, position the insertion point to the left of the paragraph mark inside the empty frame.

2. Insert the picture blusedan.wmf from the winword\clipart directory.

3. Select the frame, and then choose Frame from the Format menu.

4. Under Horizontal, choose Right from the Position drop-down list box and Margin from the Relative To drop-down list box. Click OK.

   The frame is aligned at the right margin.

5. Repeat steps 3 and 4, this time choosing Center from the Position drop-down list box.

   The frame is aligned between the margins, and the text wraps around both sides of the frame.

Vertical settings to align a frame

The options in the Vertical box are similar to the options in the Horizontal box. You can align frames vertically between the top and bottom margins on the page by choosing Top, Center, or Bottom from the Position drop-down list box. Choose Margin, Page, or Paragraph from the Relative To drop-down list box. For example, to center a frame vertically between the top and bottom margins, choose Center from the Position box and Margin from the Relative To box.

Figure 26-11
Examples of vertically aligned frames

To align a frame vertically:

1. On page 1, select the framed picture of the jet.

2. Choose Frame from the Format menu.

3. Under Vertical, choose Center from the Position drop-down list box and Margin from the Relative To list box. Click OK.

The picture is centered between the top and bottom margins.

The Move with Text Option

The Move with Text option in the Frame dialog box is used to keep a frame next to the paragraph it is near. For example, if you frame headings for your paragraphs and align the headings with the left margin, check the Move with Text check box to keep each heading next to the corresponding paragraph. Framed headings move along with the paragraphs if the paragraphs are repositioned.

Removing Frames

You can remove a frame without deleting the contents inside the frame, or you can delete a frame and its contents. To remove a frame without deleting its contents, select the frame, choose Frame from the Format menu, and click Remove Frame. The contents of the frame then become part of the regular text. To delete the frame and the contents inside the frame, select the frame, and press the **Backspace** key.

To remove a frame without deleting the contents of the frame:

1. Select the frame around the heading on page 1.

2. Choose Frame from the Format menu.

3. Click the Remove Frame button.

The frame and the border are deleted.

Adding Captions

After adding a frame to a picture, you can add a caption to the frame that will stay with the picture when it or other items on the page are moved. Before adding a caption to a framed picture, select the picture, and make sure that the Height and Width boxes in the Frame dialog box are set to Auto. Then press **Enter**, and key a caption at the paragraph mark to accompany the picture. You can format the caption just as you format any other text in Word. The caption you create becomes part of the frame and will move along with the frame.

To add a caption to a frame:

1. On page 2, insert a hard page break before the heading "The Value-Added Tax (VAT)?", so that it begins on a new page.

2. Move the insertion point below the heading, before the text that begins "In Western Europe". Then insert the picture coins.wmf from the winword\clipart directory.

3. Apply a frame to the picture.

4. With the picture selected, press **Enter**. At the paragraph mark inserted below the picture, key the following in italics, without pressing the **Enter** key:

The VAT tax is often refundable.

The captioned text wraps within the width of the frame and becomes part of the framed picture.

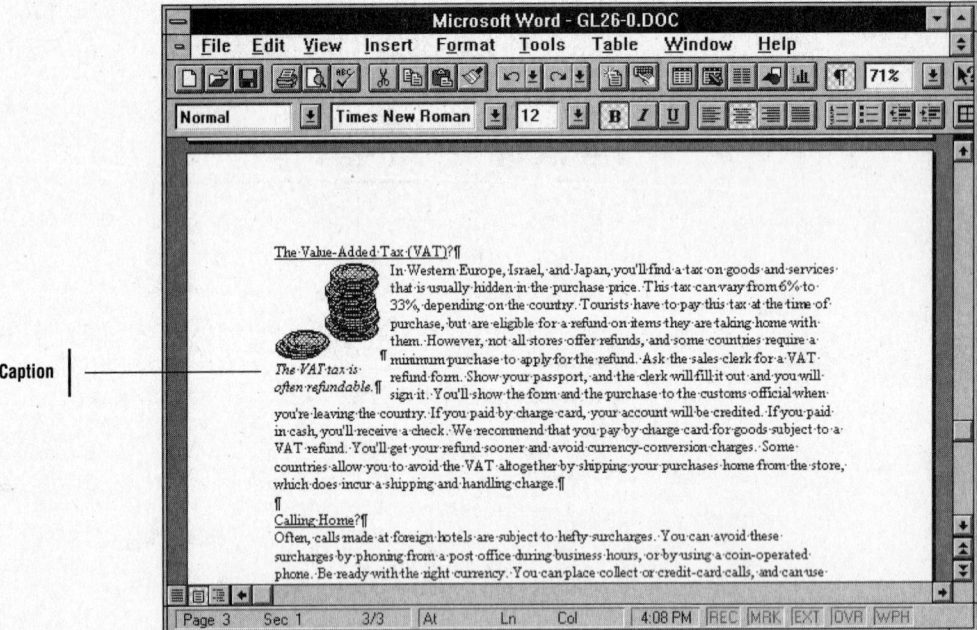

Figure 26-12
A framed picture with a caption

Using WordArt

Create special text effects in your Word documents using Microsoft WordArt. WordArt is a supplementary application of Word that uses *object linking and embedding (OLE)*. OLE allows you to create an object, such as a graphic, in another Microsoft application and then embed the object in a Word document. Once the object is part of the document, you can edit it from within Word.

An example of OLE is an embedded Excel worksheet in a Word document. If you double-click the worksheet within the document, you can access Excel to edit the worksheet without exiting Word.

The WordArt application lets you create a graphic object out of text. To open WordArt within a Word document, place the insertion point where you want to add the special text object, and then choose

Object linking and embedding (OLE)
A Microsoft utility that enables you to include an object from another application in Word and edit the object within Word.

Object from the Insert menu. Click the Create New tab, choose Microsoft WordArt 2.0 from the Object Type list box, and click OK.

Figure 26-13
The Object dialog box

WordArt opens within the document, complete with a special toolbar, text-entry box, and menu. Key the text you want to format in the text-entry box, choose the special-effect options from the WordArt menu and toolbar, and then click the Word document window. This closes WordArt. To edit the text object and reopen WordArt, double-click the object.

To create special effects using WordArt:

1. Left-align the heading at the top of page 1, and then move the insertion point to a blank line above the heading.

2. Choose Object from the Insert menu.

3. Choose Microsoft WordArt 2.0 from the Object Type list box and click OK.

   WordArt opens within the document. The WordArt menu bar, toolbar, and text-entry box appear on the screen. See Figure 26-14 on page 536.

4. In the text box at the top of the page, key the following two lines of text, keying the first line in all capitals:

   DUKE CITY GATEWAY
   Your Gateway to the World

5. On the WordArt toolbar, click the arrow to the right of "Plain Text" to choose a line and shape.

6. Choose the first shape in the third row (Arch Up).

   The text you keyed takes on the chosen shape.

Different fonts and special effects in WordArt

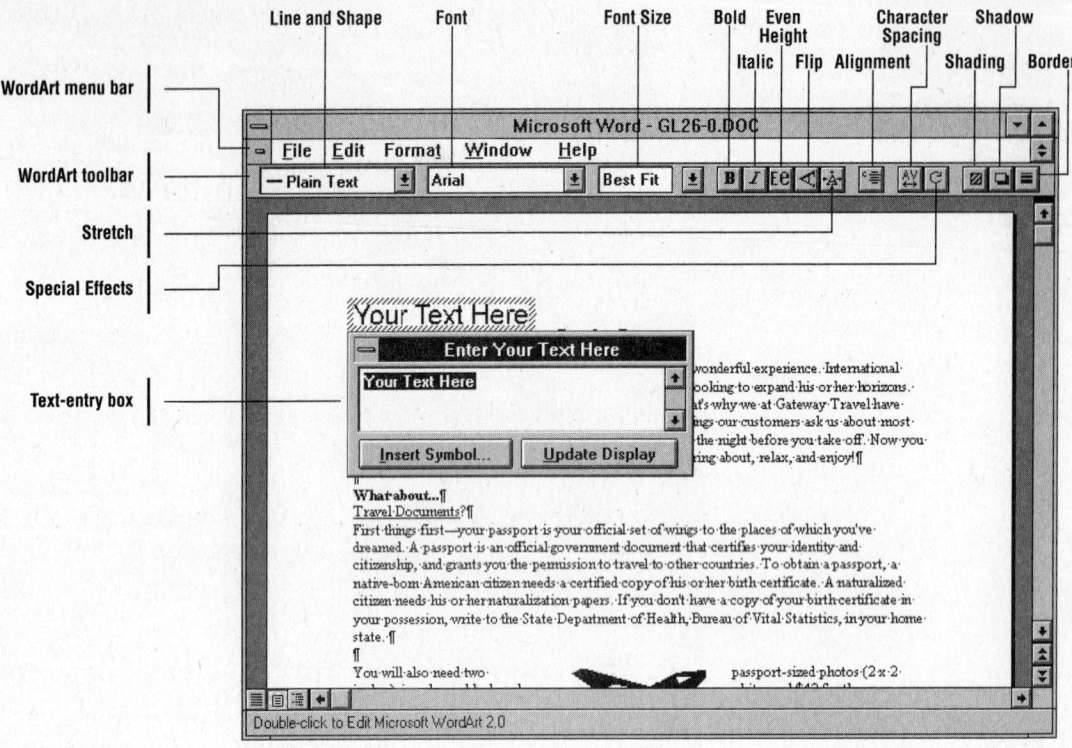

Figure 26-14
Opening WordArt within the Word document

7. Open the Font drop-down list and choose Impact.

8. Open the Font Size drop-down list, and choose 20 to enlarge the font.

9. Click the Shadow button, and choose one of the shadow styles in the top row.

10. Click outside the WordArt text.

The WordArt application closes, and the regular menu bar and toolbars appear.

Shortcut Menu for Graphics

Shortcut menus are available in Word for a variety of commands related to graphic objects. For example, if you click on a picture with the right mouse button, you can choose Frame Picture from the shortcut menu to add a frame instantly. If you click a framed picture with the right mouse button, the command Format Frame is available from the shortcut menu. In addition, you can choose Caption from the shortcut menu, which opens a dialog box to add a caption to the framed picture. The shortcut menu for a WordArt object allows you to add or format a frame. It also allows you to open the WordArt dialog box.

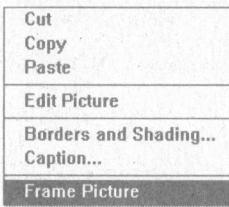

Shortcut menu

To frame the object designed in WordArt using the shortcut menu:

1. Use the right mouse button to click the WordArt design.

2. Choose Frame Picture from the shortcut menu.

    The design is framed, and the document text wraps around it.

3. Apply a 1½ pt box border to the framed design.

4. Switch to print preview to view the document.

5. Adjust page breaks, if necessary, for more attractive placement of headings.

6. Save the document as *[your three-letter identifier]*26-0.doc.

7. Print the document.

8. Close the document and exit Word (unless you will be doing the following exercises immediately).

Using the WordArt Dialog Box

When you double-click a WordArt object, this opens up the WordArt application, which includes the WordArt toolbar. Another way to edit a WordArt object is to click the object with the right mouse button, and then choose Open WordArt from the shortcut menu. This command opens the WordArt dialog box.

The WordArt dialog box contains all the elements normally seen in the WordArt application window, but they are all contained within the dialog box. As you choose the WordArt options, the changes appear in a Preview box. When you are finished editing the object, click OK. Word closes the dialog box and returns you to the document, which reflects the changes.

Key Terms

Frames

Object Linking and Embedding (OLE)

Placeholder

Exercises

Exercise 26.1

1. Start Word, if necessary.

2. Open the file 7-2.doc.

3. At the top of the page, insert two blank lines. Move the insertion point to the first blank line, and key the following heading in bold, uppercase letters:

   TIPS FOR SUCCESS IN THE TRAVEL-AGENCY BUSINESS

4. Press **Enter**, and add a frame to the heading:

   A. Select the heading.

   B. Choose Frame from the Insert menu.

   C. Click Yes in the dialog box that asks if you want to switch to page layout view.

5. Align the frame in the center of the page:

   A. Select the frame.

   B. Choose Frame from the Format menu.

   C. Under Horizontal, choose Center from the Position box and Page from the Relative To box.

   D. Under Text Wrapping, choose None. Click OK.

6. Select the frame, and change the border to a double-line style.

7. Move the insertion point to the paragraph mark under the framed heading, and insert the picture mapmen.wmf from the winword\clipart directory.

8. Add a frame to the picture.

9. Move the framed picture, so that it is centered within the margins:

   A. Select the picture.

   B. Choose Frame from the Format menu.

   C. Under Horizontal, choose Center from the Position box and Margin from the Relative To box.

   D. Under Vertical, choose Center from the Position box and Margin from the Relative To box. Click OK.

10. Spell-check the document.

11. Save the document as *[your three-letter identifier]*26-1.doc.

12. Print the first page of the document.

13. Close the document and exit Word (unless you will be doing the following exercises immediately).

Exercise 26.2

1. Start Word, if necessary.

2. Open the file 13-3a.doc, and switch to page layout view.

3. Change line spacing for the document to 1.5 lines.

4. At the top of the page, insert a blank line above the text, and key the following heading in bold, 18-point type:

   A Tour for Everyone

5. Add a frame to the heading.

6. Resize the frame slightly by dragging its right border out about .5 inches, and then center the text within the frame.

7. Change the border of the frame to a shadow border.

8. Insert a continuous section break above the paragraph that begins "We can arrange".

9. Format the text in the second section as two columns.

10. After the second paragraph in the first column, insert the picture continen.wmf from the winword\clipart directory.

11. Frame the picture using the shortcut menu.

12. Move the framed picture:

    A. Select the framed picture.

    B. Drag the frame to the right, until it covers some of the text in the second column and appears centered horizontally between the left and right margins.

13. Add a caption to the framed picture:

    A. Select the framed picture.

    B. Press **Enter**.

    C. At the paragraph mark, key the following text in 10-point bold text:

       Call Duke City Gateway Travel today for the tour to suit your special interest.

    D. Select the caption text, and change the line spacing for it to single.

14. Add a box border to the picture.

15. Add a box border to the outer frame that includes the picture and the caption.

16. Switch to print preview to view the document.

17. If the document does not fit on one page, delete the extra paragraph mark between paragraphs in section 2, and format the spacing for this text to 6 pt after paragraphs.

18. Spell-check the document.

19. Save the document as *[your three-letter identifier]*26-2.doc and print it.

20. Close the document and exit Word (unless you will be doing the following exercises immediately).

Exercise 26.3

1. Start Word, if necessary.

2. Open the file 20-0.doc.

3. Above the text "Summer vacation is", insert a continuous section break. Then format section 2 as two columns.

4. In page layout view, move the insertion point to the blank line after the paragraph that begins "Summer vacation is". Then insert the picture money.wmf from the winword\clipart directory.

5. Apply a frame to the picture.

6. Scale the picture by dragging the right sizing handle toward the right margin, until the status bar indicates 130%.

7. Center the picture horizontally using the Frame dialog box. Use the margins as a reference point. Change the vertical distance from text to .1.

8. Delete the heading "**BUDGET STRETCHERS**". With the insertion point in the heading's place, open Microsoft WordArt.

9. Key **Budget Stretching** in the text-entry box.

10. From the Line and Shape drop-down list on the WordArt toolbar, choose the shape Deflate (in the fifth row, second column). Close WordArt.

11. In the upper right corner, move the date to just under the volume number.

12. Frame the WordArt text, and then move it to the upper right corner of the document, aligned with the top and right margins.

13. Resize the WordArt text by dragging the left sizing handle out by 1.5 inches.

14. Double-click the WordArt text to edit it, and then click the Stretch button (three buttons to the right of the Italic button) on the WordArt toolbar. Close WordArt.

15. Apply a box border to the WordArt design.

16. To the left of the design, change the text "Travel Talk" to bold, 26-point small capitals. Change the type size of the three lines of text above "Travel Talk" to 10 point.

17. In the second column on the first page, below the phone number "555-1234", insert an empty frame that extends to the right and bottom margins.

18. On page 2 in the second column, format the text from "Published Monthly by" through "87111" in 10-point type and center it. Then move the text into the empty frame on page 1.

19. Within the frame you just filled, delete the third-to-last line of text (the agency's name). Resize the frame to fit the text, if necessary.

20. Delete the text on the second page, and then spell-check the document.

21. Save the document as *[your three-letter identifier]*26-3.doc and print it.

22. Close the document and exit Word (unless you will be doing the following exercise immediately).

Exercise 26.4: Challenge Yourself

Open the file 26-4.doc. Format the title page as a separate section. Number the pages in the second section, using a right-aligned header in the style of "Page 2". Create a footer for the second section. Key **Duke City Gateway Travel**, left-aligned. On the same line, key **Your Gateway to the World**, right-aligned.

Under the text in the footer, insert the picture star.wmf from the winword\clipart directory. Scale the picture to 25% of its original size, and then apply a frame to the picture. Drag the framed picture to the center of the footer line of text. To make sure the framed picture is centered horizontally, open the Frame dialog box, and choose the center horizontal position relative to the margin.

On page 2 of the document, at the paragraph mark above the paragraph that begins "Get to know us", insert the picture goldshak.eps from your student disk. Apply a frame to the picture, and then scale the framed picture to 75% of its original size. Drag the picture to the right side of the page, aligned with the right margin.

Apply a gridline border and a frame to the table on page 2. Center the table relative to the page, with no text wrapping.

On page 3, place the insertion point before the paragraph that begins "In addition to our expertise", and insert the picture wm&bcas2.wmf from the winword\clipart directory. Scale the picture to 50% of its original size, and then add a frame to it.

Remove the tab before the heading "**Corporate Travel**". Under this heading, unindent the text that wraps alongside the framed picture. At the end of the paragraph under "**Corporate Travel**" (after "put the plans through."), insert the picture speaker.wmf from the winword\clipart directory. Frame the picture, and then drag it to the right side of the page, so that the right side of the frame aligns with the right margin, and the top of the frame is just below the heading **"Corporate Travel"**.

On the title page of the document, center the text, and apply a frame to it. Center the frame vertically, relative to the page. Delete the border from the frame.

Save the document as *[your three-letter identifier]*26-4.doc, and then print pages 1-3. Close the document and exit Word.

Working with Forms

In Word, you can create a wide variety of customized forms for business documents, such as fax cover sheets, job applications, and questionnaires. Create your own forms by using Word's table feature and then enhance the appearance of the form using borders and shading, or use one of Word's templates for common business forms.

Objectives

- Create forms using tables.
- Add borders and shading to forms.
- Create blank lines in forms.
- Add check boxes.
- Work with on-line forms.

Forms

Forms can be either printed or on-line. *Printed forms* are forms that are printed out, then filled in later by hand. Examples of printed forms are job applications and questionnaires. *On-line forms* are forms that appear on the computer screen and are filled in using the computer. On-line forms often are used for company personnel records and invoices. You use the same Word features to create both printed and on-line forms, but there are a few special exceptions for creating on-line forms that are discussed later in this lesson.

Printed form

A form that is printed out and filled in by hand.

On-line form

A form that is filled in using the computer.

Figure 27-1

An example of a printed form

Using Tables to Create Forms

Text in a form is organized in the same way as text in a table, with rows and columns adjacent to each other. Forms also may contain blank lines for information to be filled in. After you create a table to use as a form, add interest to the table by using borders or shading in the cells or paragraphs of the table. Create a table using the Table button on the Standard toolbar or using the Insert Table command from the Table menu.

DATE¶		TIME¶		¤
¤		¤		
ROOM·NO.¶		AUTHORIZATION¤		¤
¤				
CHECK-IN·DATE¶		CODE¤		¤
¤				
CHECK-OUT·DATE¶		AMOUNT¤		¤
¤				

Figure 27-2
An example of a table used in a form

To create a table to use as a form:

1. Start Word, if necessary.

2. Create a new document. Change the font size for the document to 12 point.

3. Select Insert Table from the Table menu.

4. In the dialog box, key **1** for the number of columns and **15** for the number of rows. Click OK.

    A table with one column and 15 rows is inserted into the document. The table's rows extend from the left to the right margin.

5. Increase the height of the table's rows to three lines (36 points) by selecting the table, choosing Cell Height and Width from the Table menu, clicking the Row tab, and keying **36** in the At box for rows. Click OK.

6. Select the first two rows of the table, and switch to page layout view (use Page Width magnification).

7. Using the ruler, drag the right table column marker to the left about 1 inch, and then drag the left table column marker to the right about 1 inch.

    The first two rows are resized and centered above the other rows.

8. Move the insertion point to the first row, and key **Duke City Gateway Travel Agency** in bold, 14-point type.

9. In the second row, key **INCOMING TELEPHONE INQUIRY** in bold, 16-point, uppercase letters.

10. Center the text in the rows, and change the typeface to Arial.

Formatting Forms

Use other Word features to enhance the appearance of the table when creating the form. Format the form by adding borders or shading to the text or cells in the table. Use tab leaders to create blank lines to be filled in, and create check boxes.

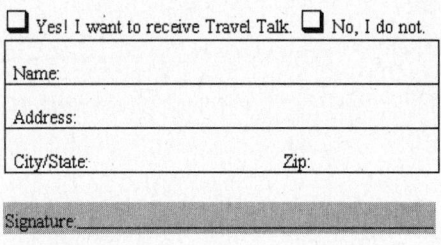

Figure 27-3
A form that incorporates different Word features

Adding Borders and Shading

Use the Borders toolbar or the Borders and Shading command to separate the different parts of the form or to emphasize one part of the form. Add borders or shading to selected paragraphs or cells in a table. Borders around table cells appear as a continuous grid, and borders around paragraphs appear as separate boxes. To apply a border or shading to a cell, make sure you select the cell and the end-of-cell marker. If you do not select the end-of-cell marker, Word will place a border or shading around the paragraph in the cell.

To apply a border and shading to the table:

1. Select the first two cells in the table that contain the keyed text, and click the Borders button on the Formatting toolbar.

2. From the Borders toolbar, choose the 1½ pt double-line style, and then click the Outside Border button.

3. Choose the ¾ pt single line, and then click the Inside Border button.

4. Select the first cell (which contains the agency name), and apply 10% shading from the Shading drop-down list.

Borders button

Note: You can also create a custom border for a paragraph or a cell (such as a border along the top, bottom, left, or right edge only) by clicking the corresponding boundaries of the paragraph or cell on the Borders toolbar.

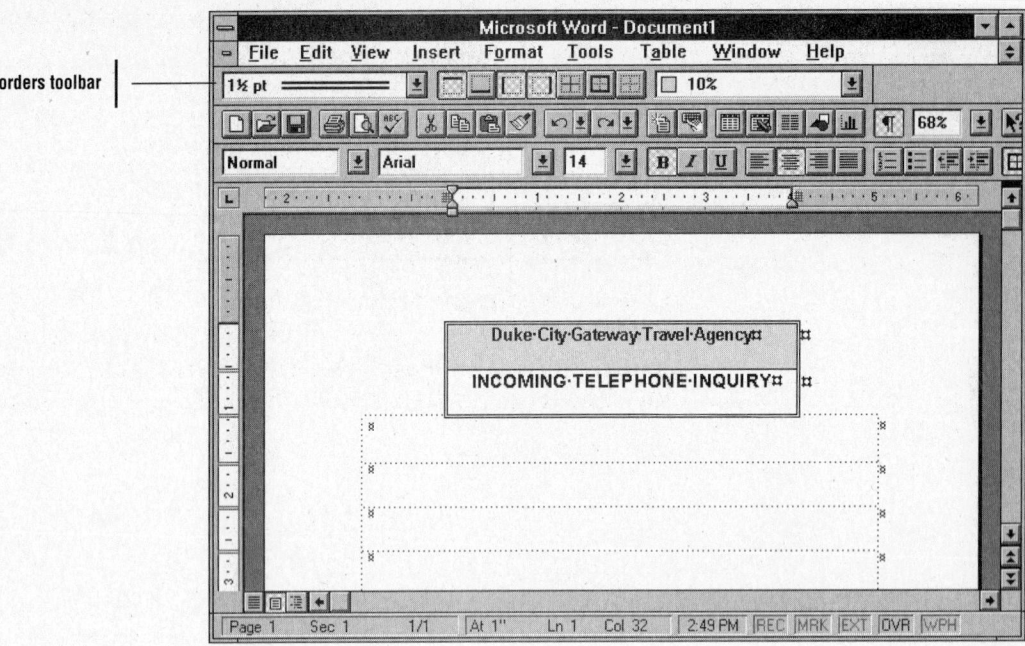

Borders toolbar

Figure 27-4
Formatting a table to create a form

Creating Blank Lines to Be Filled in

A typical printed form contains solid lines that are used as blank lines to be filled in. The lines usually follow a question that requires an answer or other text that requests information. For example, a job application contains blank lines for the applicant to fill in work experience. The best way to add horizontal lines to printed forms is to use tabs and leaders.

To create horizontal lines using tab leaders:

1. Position the insertion point in the third row. Press **Enter** twice to move the insertion point to the bottom of the row and key **To:**

2. In the fourth row, press **Enter** twice to move to the bottom of the row and key **From:**

3. In the fifth row, press **Enter** twice to move to the bottom of the row, and key **Date and Time:**

4. In the sixth row, press **Enter** twice to move to the bottom of the row and key **Company:**

5. In the seventh row, press **Enter** twice to move to the bottom of the row, and key **Phone Number:**

6. In the eighth row, press **Enter** twice to move to the bottom of the row and key **Message:**

7. Select rows 3 through 13, and choose Tabs from the Format menu.

8. In the Tab Stop Position box, key **5.5**. Choose the Right Alignment option button and the fourth solid-line leader. Click OK.

Figure 27-5
The Tabs dialog box

9. Move the insertion point to the right of "To:", and press **Ctrl+Tab**.

   A solid line is inserted from the insertion point to the right tab stop.

10. Repeat this procedure to insert a solid-line leader after the text in rows 4 through 8.

11. In the ninth row (below "Message:"), press **Enter** twice, and press **Ctrl+Tab** to insert a solid-line leader.

12. Repeat this procedure in rows 10 through 13.

   Six blank lines are available in the form to fill in the message.

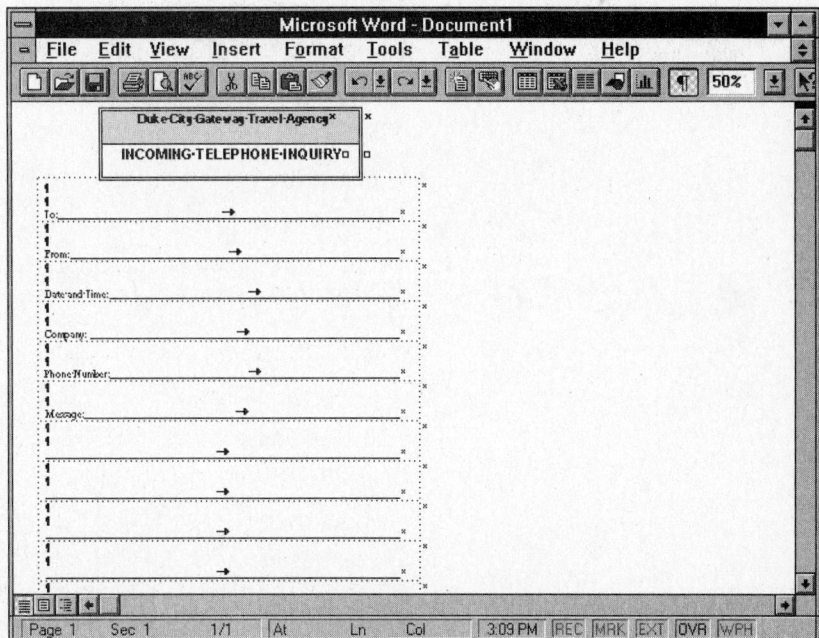

Figure 27-6
The table with blank lines (shown at 50% magnification)

Adding Check Boxes

Check boxes make filling out forms easier. For instance, you might place two check boxes after a question that requires a yes or no response. You can add a check box to a form by inserting a box symbol or by creating the check box with the Drawing toolbar.

When you add a check box by inserting a symbol, you can choose from a variety of box styles available with the font. For example, fonts such as Symbols and Wingdings contain check boxes, and Wingdings contains both plain and shaded boxes and circles. Remember, to insert a symbol, choose Symbol from the Insert menu, and then choose the desired character. Once you have inserted the check box, you can enlarge it by changing the font size.

To create a check box using the Drawing toolbar, first place the insertion point in the document where you want the shape to appear. Then click the Drawing button on the Standard toolbar.

Drawing button

The Rectangle drawing button on the Drawing toolbar can be used to create a square (by holding down the **Shift** key and then dragging) or a rectangle. The Oval button can be used to create a circle (by holding down the **Shift** key and then dragging) or an oval.

To add a check box to a form:

1. Position the insertion point in the last row of the table.

2. Choose Symbol from the Insert menu.

3. Click the Symbols tab, if necessary, and then choose Wingdings from the Font drop-down list. (If Wingdings is not available, choose the Symbol font).

4. Choose one of the box characters in the third row. (Click each one to see what they look like.)

Choosing a box character

5. Click the Insert button (or double-click the character), and then click Close.

   The box is inserted in the row.

6. After the box, press the **Spacebar** twice, and key **Will call again**

7. Clear any existing tabs, and set 2.5-inch and 4-inch left-aligned tab stops.

8. Select the check box, and copy it to the Clipboard.

9. Press **Ctrl+Tab** after "Will call again", paste the check box, press the **Spacebar** twice, and then key **Please call**

10. Press **Ctrl+Tab**, paste another check box, press the **Spacebar** twice, and then key **Returned your call**

    You have inserted three check boxes.

11. Select the first check box, and change the font to 22 pt.

12. Repeat the formatting for the next two check boxes.

Figure 27-7
The last row of the table with check boxes

Adjusting Spacing in Forms

There are many ways to adjust the space between items in a form. You can adjust the horizontal space by moving tab stops or by expanding the width of columns or cells. You can adjust the vertical space by adding or removing space before and after paragraphs or by changing the height of rows. You can also frame items and then adjust their positions on the page.

To adjust the spacing in a form:

1. In the last row, adjust the tab stops to space the second and third check boxes more evenly, if necessary.

2. Change the height of the next-to-last row to 24 pt.

3. In the third row (which contains the text "To:"), move the insertion point to the top paragraph mark.

4. Choose Split Table from the Table menu.

   The top two rows are split from the rest of the form to provide more space.

5. To enhance the form, position the insertion point after "Inquiry" in the second row, and press the **Spacebar** once. Then insert the Wingdings symbol of the telephone (in the first row, ninth box of the grid).

6. Use the Borders toolbar to apply a 2¼ pt outside border to the form (the lower table).

7. View the document in print preview, and save it as *[your three-letter identifier]*27-0a.doc.

8. Print the document, and then close it.

Working with On-Line Forms

On-line forms are created differently from printed forms. To create an on-line form, first create a new template. When the form is complete, you save the template. This allows you to create the form once and then open a new copy of it for each form you want to fill in.

Form field

An area in an on-line form where the user fills in information.

While creating the on-line form, instead of inserting your own check boxes or blank lines, you insert form fields. *Form fields* are the areas where the user fills in information. There are three types of form fields: text fields, check box fields, and drop-down fields.

To insert a form field, position the insertion point where you want the information to appear, and then choose Form Field from the Insert menu. In the Form Field dialog box, choose the type of form field. You can also open the Forms toolbar and use the appropriate buttons to insert the desired type of form field.

After creating an on-line form, it must be protected from any changes except for the information entered in the form fields. To protect the document, choose Protect Document from the Tools menu, or click the Protect Form button on the Forms toolbar. Protecting the form activates the form fields and allows the user to move only between form fields.

Click to open Forms toolbar

Figure 27-8
The Form Field dialog box

To create an on-line form:

1. Create a new template, and key the following heading:

    Duke City Gateway Travel Agency
    15 Montgomery Boulevard
    Albuquerque, NM 87111
    Telephone: (303) 555-1234
    Fax: (303) 555-4532

2. Center the heading, change the font size to 14 point, and make the first line bold.

3. After the last line in the heading, left-align the insertion point, press **Enter** three times, and change the font to 12 point. Then key **Account Number:**

4. Set left-aligned tab stops at 1.5", 3", and 4.5".

5. Move the insertion point to the right of "Account Number:", press the **Tab** key twice, and then key **Travel Counselor:**

6. Press **Enter** twice, and key **Date:**

7. Press **Enter** twice, and key **SOLD TO:**

8. Press the **Tab** key twice, and key **SENT TO:**

9. Press **Enter** twice, and insert a table with seven columns and three rows.

10. Key these seven column heads across the top row:

    Airline   FL/CL   Date   From   To   Leave   Arrive

11. Move the insertion point below the table, press **Enter** twice, and key **Senior Citizen Discount?**

12. Move the insertion point to the right of the first tab character after "Account Number:", and choose Form Field from the Insert menu.

    Word displays the Form Field dialog box.

13. Click the Show Toolbar button.

    Word displays the Forms toolbar.

Insert menu

Figure 27-9

The Forms toolbar

14. Click the Text Form Field button.

    Word inserts a shaded area that serves as the location for the account number. As with any shaded field area, the shading does not appear in the printed document.

15. Move to the right of "Travel Counselor:", press the **Tab** key, and then click the Drop-Down Form Field button.

16. Click the Form Field Options button, and key **Tom Carey** in the Drop-Down Item text box.

17. Click the Add button, key **Nina Chavez**, and then click OK.

    The first name keyed in the text box appears in the field area. However, a user who opens a document using this template can choose the appropriate name from the drop-down list.

18. After "Date:", press the **Tab** key, and insert the date as a field using the format 1/1/95.

19. After "SOLD TO:" and "SENT TO:", insert a text form field. Make sure there is a tab character before each field.

20. Position the insertion point after "Discount?" in the last line of the form, and click the Check Box Form Field button.

   A check box is inserted next to the text.

21. To enhance the form, make the first row of the table bold, apply a blue grid border to the table, and add 50% light-gray shading to the first row.

22. Click the Protect Form button on the Forms toolbar.

23. Save the template as *[your three-letter identifier]*form.dot, preceded by the appropriate drive, if necessary.

24. Close the template and the Forms toolbar.

Once the template is saved, you can use it to open new copies of the on-line form. You can open a copy of the template and fill in the needed information. To enter data in a form field and move to the next field, press **Enter** or the **Tab** key. To move to a previous form field, press **Shift+Tab**.

To use an on-line form:

1. Open a new file based on the on-line template. (Remember, to open a new file based on a template, choose New from the File menu. Identify the template in the Template box, including the path, if necessary. In the New box, make sure Document is chosen.)

   The template is opened as a new document.

2. Key the account number **194-1000** and press **Enter**.

   The next form field is activated, and an arrow appears next to the name to open the drop-down list.

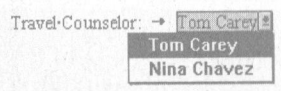

Drop-down form field

3. Click the arrow, choose the name Nina Chavez, and press **Enter**.

4. Key **Roger Furman** in the "SOLD TO:" field, and key **Business address** in the "SENT TO:" field.

5. In the check box field, key **x** to check it. (To clear a check box field, press the **Spacebar**.) See Figure 27-10 on page 553.

6. Save the document as *[your three-letter identifier]*27-0b.doc and print it.

7. Close the document and exit Word (unless you will be doing the following exercises immediately).

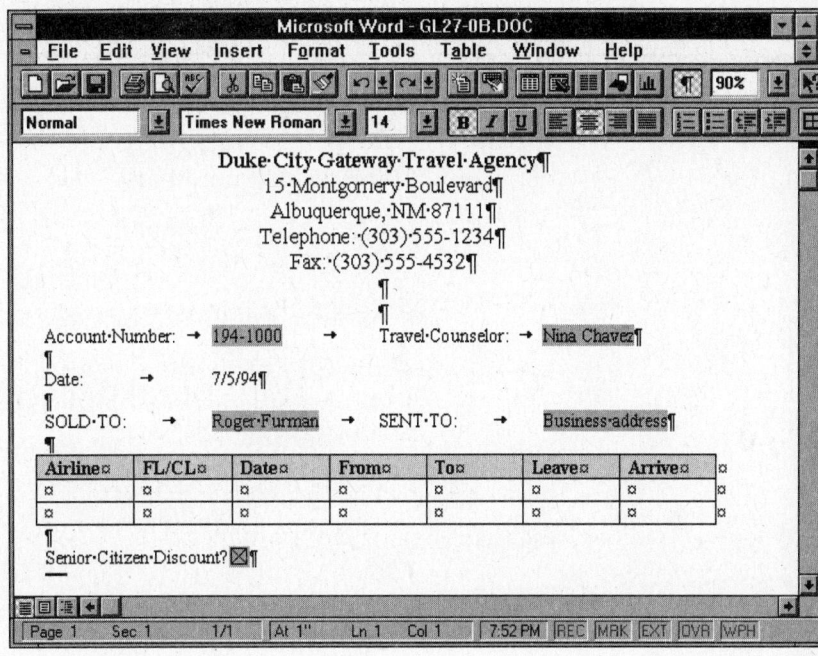

Figure 27-10
On-line form with field information entered

Using Macros in On-line Forms

On-line forms can include macros that can update form fields, validate data, or perform other tasks. Form fields can contain two types of macros: entry macros and exit macros. An entry macro is one that runs when a certain field is activated. An exit macro runs after you enter information in the field. For example, an on-line form can contain a form field for an account number. An entry macro can be assigned to this field that displays database information from which a user can choose an account number.

To assign a macro to a form field, double-click the form field to open the Options dialog box for the field. Under Run Macro On, choose the macro you want to run in either the Entry box or the Exit box. Macros used in form fields must be created and saved with the form template.

Key Terms

Form field

On-line form

Printed form

Exercises

Exercise 27.1

1. Start Word, if necessary.

2. Create a new document.

3. Create a fax cover sheet. Start by keying the following heading at the top of the page, using the Arial font:

   Duke City Gateway Travel Agency
   15 Montgomery Boulevard
   Albuquerque, NM 87111

4. Center the text. Then format the first line in 14-point bold type, with a shadow border and 1.25-inch left and right indents.

5. Press **Enter** twice after the ZIP code, and then key **Facsimile Cover Sheet** in 18-point bold type.

6. Press **Enter** twice, left-align the paragraph mark, and insert a table with 1 column and 13 rows.

7. Change the row height in the table to 36 points. (Select the table, choose Cell Height and Width from the Table menu, and set the At box to 36 pt).

8. Key **FROM:** in the first row, and then insert a solid-line leader to be used as a blank line:

   A. Select the entire table, and choose Tabs from the Format menu.

   B. Key **6** in the Tab Stop Position box.

   C. Click the Right Alignment option button.

   D. Choose the solid-line leader pattern and click OK.

   E. Position the insertion point after "FROM:", and press **Ctrl+Tab**.

9. In the second row, key **TELEPHONE NUMBER:** and press **Ctrl+Tab**.

10. In the third row, key **FAX NUMBER:** and press **Ctrl+Tab**.

11. Using the same procedure of keying text and pressing **Ctrl+Tab**, key the following text in the fourth through tenth rows:

    DATE:
    TO:
    COMPANY:
    TELEPHONE NUMBER:

FAX NUMBER:
TOTAL NUMBER OF PAGES (including cover sheet):
COMMENTS:

12. In the remaining rows, press **Ctrl+Tab** to insert solid-line leaders.

13. Adjust the space in the fourth row to 48 points.

14. Add another row at the end of the table. Insert a solid-line leader in the row.

15. Change the page layout so the text is centered vertically.

16. Spell-check the document.

17. Save the document as *[your three-letter identifier]*27-1.doc and print it.

18. Close the document and exit Word (unless you will be doing the following exercises immediately).

Exercise 27.2

1. Start Word, if necessary.

2. Open the file 27-2.doc.

3. Center the first three lines of text (from "Duke City" through the fax number), and make them bold.

4. Position the insertion point at the second paragraph mark below the paragraph that begins "Thank you". Then insert a table with 2 columns and 11 rows.

5. In the first row, key **ITEM** in the first cell and **RATING (1-10)** in the second cell.

6. Center the text in the first row, and make it bold.

7. Key the following items in the rows under "ITEM" (key each item in a separate row):

    Hotel Accommodations
    Meals
    Transportation
    Itinerary
    Knowledge Level of Tour Guide
    Helpfulness of Tour Guide
    Evening Events
    Allocation of Free Time
    Personal Service
    Luggage Delivery

8. Center all the text just keyed. Then add a grid border to the entire table and 25% blue shading to the first row.

9. Change the row height of rows 2 through 11 to 18 points. Make the first column 4 inches wide and the second column 2 inches wide.

10. To the right of the text "Additional Comments:", insert a solid-line leader that is right-aligned at 6.5 inches (remember to clear any existing tab stops). Using the same tab setting, insert four solid-line leaders below the text.

11. After the question "Would you take another Duke City Gateway tour?", insert check boxes for "Yes" and "No":

    A. Move the insertion point before "Yes", and choose Symbol from the Insert menu.

    B. From the Wingdings font, choose the box in the fifth row.

    C. Click Insert, and then click Close.

    D. Select the box, and change the font size to 16 points.

    E. Copy the box, and then paste it before "No".

12. To the right of the text "Why or why not?", insert a solid-line leader that is right-aligned at 6.5 inches. Using the same tab setting, insert two solid-line leaders under the text.

13. Change the paragraph formatting for "Additional Comments:" and the blank lines below it to 1.5 lines. Do the same for the text "Why or why not?" and the blank lines below it.

14. Spell-check the document.

15. Save the document as *[your three-letter identifier]*27-2.doc and print it.

16. Close the document and exit Word (unless you will be doing the following exercises immediately).

Exercise 27.3

1. Start Word, if necessary.

2. Open the file 27-3.doc.

3. Apply the bold attribute to the first line of text (the agency name).

4. Under "Client Profile", insert a shadow border around the text from "Name:" through "Business Fax:".

5. After each colon in the box, insert a solid-line leader that is right-aligned at 6 inches.

6. Below the box, press **Enter** twice, and insert a table with one column and ten rows.

7. In the first three rows of the table, set a right-aligned, 6-inch tab setting.

8. In the first row, key **Frequent Flyer Accounts:**, and then insert a solid-line leader after the text and in the next two rows.

9. In rows four and five, key the text in Figure 27-11. Use left-aligned tab stops at 2", 3.5", and 5" for the last three columns and a 14-point box character.

Figure 27-11

Preferred Seating:	☐Aisle	☐Center	☐Window
Special Meal Requests:	☐Low Calorie	☐Vegetarian	☐Seafood

---

10. In the sixth row, key **Notes:**, and then format rows six through ten with 6-inch, solid-line leaders.

11. Spell-check the document.

12. Save the document as *[your three-letter identifier]*27-3.doc and print it.

13. Close the document and exit Word (unless you will be doing the following exercise immediately).

Exercise 27.4: Challenge Yourself

Create a new template to create an on-line form. Insert a table with one column and seven rows. In the first row, key the following text as two lines in 14-point bold:

**Duke City Gateway Travel Agency
CALL REPORT**

Center the text, and add a double-line box border and 20% blue shading to the row. Change the row height of the second through seventh rows to 36 points, and add a grid border to the rows.

In rows two through seven, use 12-point normal type to insert the headings that appear in Figure 27-12, which is at the end of this exercise (include "Type of Contact", "Telephone", and "Meeting" in the same row). Insert form fields after the headings: Use a drop-down form field after "Sales Rep" that contains the two names listed and your name, use check box form fields after "Telephone" and "Meeting", and use text form fields for the rest of the headings. (Do not insert a form field to the right of "Type of Contact".) Left-align the first four form fields at a 2-inch tab stop. Left-align the last three form fields at a 1-inch tab stop.

Protect the template, and then save it as *[your three-letter identifier]* 27-4.dot. Close the template, and create a new document based on the template. In the first form field, enter today's date. Choose your name from the drop-down field. For contact, key **Julia Barnet, District Manager**. For company, key **Desert Electronics, Inc.** Check Telephone, and then key the following summary:

Interested in corporate travel for six account executives. May need to secure conference facility. Sent information. Will call back next week to arrange meeting for presentation.

Save the document as *[your three-letter identifier]*27-4.doc and print it. Close the document and exit Word.

Figure 27-12

Date: _____

Sales Rep: { *Valerie Grier*
            Frank Youngblood
            Your name

Contact: _____

Company/Organization: _____

Type of Contact:

Telephone ☐

Meeting ☐

Summary: _____

An Invoice

Background

Duke City Gateway sends invoices to its customers for their travel expenses. The agency has decided to discontinue using their old invoices and to design a completely new form.

The new form will be a printed form that contains tables in the design. It will include the invoice number, date, customer address, travel description, and prices.

Business Purpose

Create an invoice for Duke City Gateway to use to bill its customers.

Procedures

1. Create a new template.

2. At the top of the page, insert the picture jet.wmf from the winword\clipart directory.

3. With the insertion point to the right of the picture, open WordArt. In the text entry box, key:

   Duke City Gateway Travel Agency
   15 Montgomery Boulevard
   Albuquerque, NM 87111

4. Use the WordArt toolbar to change the font to Impact and the size to 16 point. Keep the Plain style.

5. Close WordArt, frame the WordArt object, and then move it so that it aligns with the top and right margins.

6. Below the picture and ClipArt text, insert a blank line, and then key **INVOICE** in 16-point bold Arial uppercase letters.

7. Press **Enter** twice, and key **Invoice Number:**. On the same line, set a 1.5-inch left-aligned tab (for the invoice number) and a 4-inch left-aligned tab (for the date). Press the **Tab** key twice and key **Date:**. Change the type size to 12-point normal (not bold) for the whole line.

8. Press **Enter** twice, and key **Invoice To:**

9. Press the **Enter** key once after "To:", and insert a table with one column and three rows. Change the column width to 3 inches, and then center the table between the left and right margins. This table is for the name and address of the customer.

10. Below the table, press **Enter** twice, and insert another table with two columns and seven rows. Make the first column 4.5 inches wide and the second column 1.5 inches wide.

11. In the table just created, change the row height of the first row to 24 points. Add a single-line border and 20% shading to the first row. Add a grid border to the remaining rows.

12. In the first row, key **Travel Description** in the first cell and **Price** in the second cell. Center the text, and make it 14-point bold.

13. Change the row height of the second through fourth rows to 36 points.

14. In the first cell of the fifth row, key **NET TOTAL:**. Make the text bold and right-aligned.

15. In the first cell of the sixth row, key **+ 6% Sales Tax:**. Right-align the text.

16. In the first cell of the seventh row, key **TOTAL DUE:**. Make the text bold and right-aligned.

17. Below the table, insert a blank line, and then insert another table with two columns and two rows. Make the first column 4.5 inches wide and the second column 1.5 inches wide.

18. Add a single-line grid border to the table.

19. In the first cell, key:

    Keep the above invoice for your records, and please submit this stub with your payment in full (check or credit card) to Duke City Gateway Travel Agency within ten days.

20. In the second row, key the following text, pressing **Enter** after each line:

    Please charge my credit card:
    VISA
    MasterCard
    American Express
    Card Number:
    Expiration Date: Signature:

21. Insert a 16-point check-box symbol before "Please charge my credit card", "VISA", "MasterCard", and "American Express".

22. After "Card Number", insert a solid-line leader (set a tab stop at 4 inches).

23. After "Expiration date", insert a solid-line leader (set a tab stop at 2.5 inches). Insert a solid-line leader after "Signature:", and then insert a blank line within the cell under "Signature:" and the leader.

24. In the first row of the second column, key **Amount Due:**

25. In the second row of the second column, key **Amount Enclosed:**

26. Using the Drawing toolbar, insert a rectangle below "Amount Enclosed".

27. Spell-check the template, and then save it as *[your three letter identifier]*p10-1.dot.

28. Create a new document based on the template.

29. After "Invoice Number", key **1001**

30. After "Date", press the **Tab** key, and then enter the current date.

31. In the 3-row table under "Invoice To:", key:

    Ms. Cathy Petersen
    98 Sequoia Road
    Albuquerque, NM 87120

32. In the second table, key the information shown below in the appropriate cells:

Travel Description	Price
Round-trip Airfare: **Albuquerque, NM to London, England** **Departure 1/1** **Return 1/14**	**$759.98**
Hotel Accommodations at the Savoy **from 1/1 to 1/14**	**$1,850.00**
Car Rental for 14 days	**$449.00**
Net Total:	**$3,058.98**
6% Sales Tax:	**$183.54**
Total Due:	**$3,242.52**

33. Right-align the prices in the "Price" column.

34. In the third table, key **$3,242.52** below "Amount Due".

35. Make any changes you feel will improve the appearance of the document.

36. Save the document as *[your three letter identifier]*p10-1.doc and print it.

37. Close the document and exit Word.

Tips and Hints

- Always create a form as a template, so you only have to create the design once.

- Use bold text, check boxes, borders, and shading to accent certain parts of the form.

- When creating an invoice, make sure to include the word "invoice" on the document. This helps avoid confusion when the customer receives the document.

- Use horizontal and vertical lines, such as a grid border, to organize the text in a form.

Module 11

File Management

Lesson

28: Word File Management

Word File Management

Objectives

- Use Find File to perform a search.

- Specify search criteria.

- Change Find File view options.

- Sort the Find File list.

- Perform file maintenance tasks using Find File.

- Use revision marks.

Previous lessons showed how to open files, close files, and print files using commands from the File menu in Word. This lesson shows how to perform the same file-maintenance tasks and others using the Find File command, which was introduced briefly in Lesson 9. The Find File command is a powerful file-management tool. It allows you to locate, sort, open, print, copy, and delete files. Using Find File, you can also view the contents of a file without opening it or view other information about the file, such as its subject, author, or keywords.

The Find File Dialog Box

To perform file-maintenance tasks using the Find File command, choose Find File from the File menu. The Find File dialog box opens.

File menu

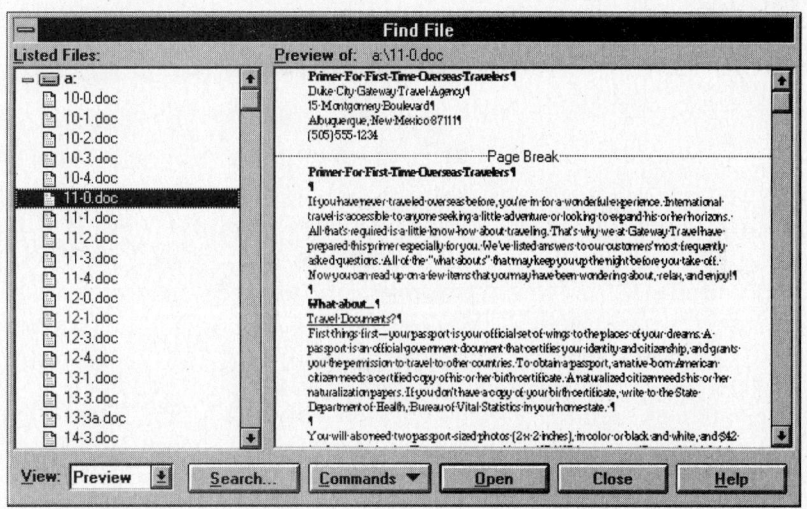

Figure 28-1
The Find File dialog box

The Find File dialog box contains:

- The Listed Files box

  The Listed Files box lists the files that Word locates. With Word's default settings for finding files, the list shows all the filenames with the .doc extension in the directory that contains Word's program files, but you can change the settings to locate different files. When you click a filename to choose it, the filename is highlighted in the list.

- The Preview box

  If the file you choose from the Listed File box contains a Word document or one in another format that Word can interpret, Word displays the contents of the file in the Preview box.

- The View drop-down list box

  Instead of previewing documents in the Find File dialog box, use the View drop-down list box to display other information about the listed files.

- Dialog box buttons

  Use the buttons at the bottom of the Find File dialog box to search for files, open files, or issue a variety of file-maintenance commands, such as sorting the listed files, copying files, or deleting files.

To display the Find File dialog box:

1. Start Word, if necessary.

2. Choose Find File from the File menu.

   The Find File dialog box opens and files are displayed according the the last Find File options specified.

Note: You also can display the Find File dialog box by choosing Open from the File menu and clicking the Find File button in the Open dialog box.

Performing a Search

Suppose you have saved hundreds of files on the computer's hard drive or on floppy disks, and you want to locate all files created on a specific date. Using the Search button in the Find File dialog box, you can choose specific drives or directories on which to search for all the files created on that date. Word creates a list of files that match your specifications. These specifications are called *search criteria*. Word's default search criteria produce a list of all files with the .doc file extension in the current Word directory.

Search criteria
Specifications that tell Word which files to locate in a search.

When it completes a search, Word displays the files it finds in alphabetical order by filename in the Find File dialog box. The Find File dialog box also shows the path or the drives and directories that it searched.

Specifying Search Criteria

The Search dialog box and the Advanced Search dialog box allow you to specify search criteria to locate files. To open the Search dialog box, click the Search button in the Find File dialog box, or click the Find File button in the Open dialog box. This opens the Search dialog box automatically. See Figure 28-2 on page 567.

The Search dialog box allows you to begin the search process by choosing from the following options:

Figure 28-2
The Search dialog box

Note: To search for more than one filename or extension, separate each item with a semicolon. For example, key *.doc;*.dot to find documents with either filename extension.

- File Name

  In the File Name text box, you can specify a filename for a document you want to locate or choose a filename extension from the File Name drop-down list to locate all files with that extension. To specify a filename, key it directly in the text box. You can use a question mark (?) for one unknown character or an asterisk (*) for more than one unknown character. For example, if you key **ab?.doc**, Word would locate all files with the .doc filename extension and with three-character filenames that start with "ab". If you key **abc*.***, Word searches for all files that begin with "abc" and have any filename extension.

- Location

  In the Location text box, you can key a drive and include a directory, or you can choose a drive from the Location drop-down list.

  If you want to include all the subdirectories in the specified directory, click the Include Subdirectories check box. After performing a search, if the list of files in the Find File dialog box still does not contain the file you want to locate, click the Search button, check the Rebuild File List check box, and repeat the search.

- Clear

  The Clear button clears all previously specified information in the Search dialog box.

- Advanced Search

  The Advanced Search button opens a dialog box that allows you to choose additional search criteria, such as a specific directory, document creation dates, or summary information.

Saving Searches

Once you have specified search criteria, you can name it and save it for future use. To save search criteria, first choose all the desired search options in the Search and Advanced Search dialog boxes. In the Search dialog box, click the Save Search As button. Key a name for the saved search criteria, and click OK. The name can then be chosen from the Saved Searches drop-down list box at a future date.

To delete a saved search from the Saved Searches drop-down list, choose the name, and then click the Delete Search button.

Once you choose the search criteria in the Search dialog box, you can click OK to start the search. Word closes the Search dialog box, locates the files that meet the search criteria, and lists their filenames in the Find File dialog box.

To specify search criteria:

1. Click the Search button in the Find File dialog box.

2. Click Clear to delete any previously entered search criteria.

3. Choose a: from the Location drop-down list box (or choose the appropriate drive for your student disk).

4. In the File Name box, key **18-?.doc** and click OK.

    The Search dialog box closes, and the Find File dialog box lists only four-character filenames on the specified drive that begin with "18-" and have the .doc extension.

5. Click the Search button to reopen the Search dialog box.

6. From the File Name drop-down list, choose Document Template (*.dot) and click OK.

    Word locates all the template files on the disk.

7. Click Close to close Find File.

Note: To use this procedure to search for a single file, key the exact filename in the File Name text box in the Search dialog box.

Advanced Search Criteria

When you click the Advanced Search button in the Search dialog box, the Advanced Search dialog box allows you to choose from the following options:

*   Location

    Like the Search dialog box, the Location tab in the Advanced Search dialog box allows you to specify a filename, a filename extension, and a location (drive and directory). It also allows you to add several locations. For example, you can specify that Word search through three different directories to find the filename or type of file for which you are looking.

Figure 28-3
The Location tab in the Advanced Search dialog box

- Summary

  The Summary tab allows you to choose search criteria based on document summary information. For example, you can search through document summary information by title, author, keywords, and subject.

  In addition, you can use the Containing Text box to search for specific text contained in the file you want to find. For example, if you key **insurance** in the Containing Text box, Word will search the specified location for all files that contain the word "insurance". Check the Match Case check box to locate files that contain the word with the exact capitalization as keyed. The Containing Text box also allows you to use pattern matching and special operators to specify approximate text criteria.

Note: Pattern matching and special operators are discussed in Lesson 10: "Find and Replace". See page 181.

Figure 28-4
Summary search options in the Advanced Search dialog box

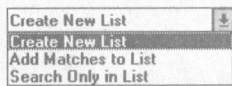

Search options

With each new advanced search, Word will create a new list. If you want to add the new search criteria to the current list of files in the Find File dialog box, choose Add Matches to List from the Options drop-down list. If you want the new search criteria to be applied only to the current list of files, choose Search Only in List from the Options drop-down list.

- Timestamp

    Use this tab to search for the date a file was created or last saved. For example, to search for files saved within a certain range of dates, key a From and a To date under Last Saved. You can also key the name of the person who saved or created the document. The dates keyed must be in the month/day/year format (1/31/95).

Figure 28-5
The Timestamp tab in the Advanced Search dialog box

To perform an advanced search:

1. Choose Find File from the File menu to open the Find File dialog box.

2. Click the Search button to open the Search dialog box.

3. In the File Name text box, change the *.dot extension to *.doc (or choose it from the File Name drop-down list box).

4. Click Advanced Search. Click the Location tab, if necessary, and check that the correct location is indicated.

5. Click the Summary tab. Key **cruise** in the Containing Text box. Leave the Match Case check box clear, and make sure Create New List is chosen.

6. Click OK in the Advanced Search dialog box and in the Search dialog box.

    Word searches through your disk for all documents that contain the word "cruise". When Word finishes building the new list, the files are listed in the Find File dialog box. If you were looking for a specific document with this word, you could view each document in the Preview box until you found it.

Viewing Information about Files

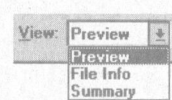

View options

By default, the Find File dialog box displays the contents of files in the Preview box. However, you can view files in Find File differently by choosing two other options:

- File Info

  This view option lists all the files in the Find File dialog box by filename, title, size, author, and last saved date.

- Summary

  This view option displays the summary information of a chosen file.

Figure 28-6
Viewing a file by its summary information

Note: If you have not entered a title for a document in the Summary Info dialog box, Word automatically uses the first few words of the document as the title. To add summary information to a file while still in Find File, choose the file from the list, click the Commands button, and then choose Summary from the pop-up list. Word displays the Summary Info dialog box for the file, to which you can add information.

To change file-viewing options:

1. In the Listed Files list box, click the filename 12-0.doc.

   The file is displayed in the Preview box.

2. Choose Summary from the View drop-down list.

   Summary information for the file is displayed.

Sorting the File List

By default, Word lists files in Find File alphanumerically by filename, but you have the option of listing the files differently. You can sort and list them by their authors' names, their creation dates, the names of the people who last saved them, the dates they were last saved, or their sizes (smallest to largest).

Figure 28-7
File-sorting options in the Options dialog box

To sort the list of files:

1. Click the Commands button in the Find File dialog box, and choose Sorting from the pop-up list.

2. In the Sort Files By box, choose Size and click OK.

   The files are listed in order of size rather than in alphanumeric order. To verify this, click the last filename in the list and notice its size in the Summary box.

File Maintenance

When you locate files with the Find File dialog box, you can perform file-maintenance tasks, such as opening, printing, copying, and deleting the files. The Find File dialog box can save you time by allowing you to perform these tasks on several files at once. For example, you can choose several files and then click the Open button to open all of them (as shown in Lesson 9). To choose more than one file, hold down the **Ctrl** key as you click each filename.

Opening Files

The Find File dialog box provides two options for opening files. After choosing a file or a group of files from the Find File list, you can:

- Click the Open button. This closes Find File and opens the file or group of files.

- Choose Open Read Only from the Commands pop-up list. This closes Find File and opens the file so you can read it but not edit it.

To open files using the Find File dialog box:

1. Click a filename in the Listed Files box of the Find File dialog box.

2. Hold down the **Ctrl** key, and then click another filename.

3. Click the Open button.

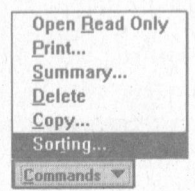

Command options in
Find File

Word opens the files.

4. Close both files.

Copying Files

From the Find File dialog box, you can make copies of files and add the copies to a different directory or to a new directory.

To copy files in Find File:

1. Open the Find File dialog box.

2. Click the filename 12-0.doc in the list of files.

3. Click the Commands button and choose Copy.

The Copy dialog box appears.

Figure 28-8
The Copy dialog box

4. Choose a: (or the appropriate drive for your student disk) from the Drives drop-down list box.

5. Click the New button to create a new directory.

Word displays the Create Directory dialog box.

6. Key **test** as the directory name and click OK.

The new directory appears in the Copy dialog box and is included in the path.

7. Click OK.

The file is copied to the new directory.

Printing Files

You can print files directly from the Find File dialog box. To print a file, choose its filename, click the Commands button, and choose Print. Then click OK in the Print dialog box.

To print a file:

1. Be sure your printer is turned on.

2.   Change the Find File view to Preview.

3.   With the files still sorted by size, click the first filename in the list (the smallest file).

4.   Click the Commands button and choose Print.

     The Print dialog box appears.

5.   Click OK.

     Word prints the file and closes Find File.

Deleting Files

You can use the Find File dialog box to delete files that you no longer need. To delete a file, choose its filename from the list, and then choose Delete from the Commands pop-up list. To prevent you from deleting files by mistake, Word asks you to verify the Delete command before it actually deletes the files.

To delete a file:

1.   Open the Find File dialog box.

2.   Click the Search button. In the Location text box, key the directory **test** to the right of the drive (for example, change the location to a:\test).

3.   Click OK.

     Word locates the file you copied into the new directory.

4.   Choose Delete from the Commands pop-up list.

     Word asks if you want to delete the file.

5.   Click Yes.

     Word deletes the file from the new directory. No files appear in the Find File dialog box.

6.   Click the Search button, and then click Clear.

7.   Click Close in the Search dialog box and in the Find File dialog box.

     All previous searches are cleared. The next time you open Find File, Word will display the Search dialog box instead of the Find File dialog box with previous search criteria.

Using Revision Marks

Revision marks
Marks that Word adds to a document to indicate changes you have made in its text.

Word offers a useful editing feature called revision marks. *Revision marks* are marks that Word adds to a document to indicate changes you have made in its text. For example, suppose you want to delete a sentence from a memo, but you want to check the change with your supervisor before you actually make it. After showing your work to your supervisor, you can use Word's Accept All command to save the memo with your changes, or you can use the Reject All command to save the memo without deleting the marked sentence.

When you turn on revision marking, Word applies these revision marks:

- Strikethrough text

  Any text you delete is displayed as strikethrough text (text that has a horizontal line running through the characters). Strikethrough text was first introduced in Lesson 17: "Symbols, Special Characters, and Attributes".

- Underlined text

  Any new text keyed is displayed with a single underline.

- Revision bar

  A *revision bar* is a vertical line that appears in the margin next to the text you revise. The default placement for revision bars is on the outside margin. This means that Word places revision bars in the left margin on even pages and in the right margin on odd pages.

Revision mark defaults can be changed to suit your preferences. For example, you can use different character formatting to mark new text, such as bold, italic, or another text color. You also have the option of not marking new text.

Note: When making revisions, the default color for strikethrough and underlined text is blue (for both the lines and the characters).

Revision bar
A vertical bar in the left or right margin that indicates where text has been revised.

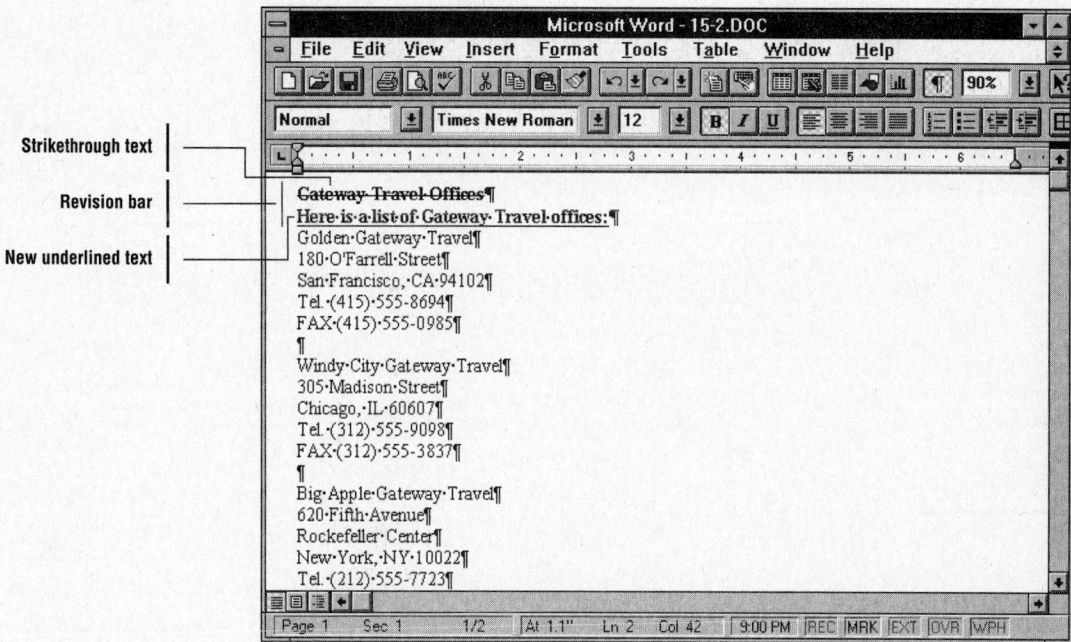

Figure 28-9
Text with revision marks

To add revision marks to a document, choose Revisions from the Tools menu. In the Revisions dialog box, check the Mark Revisions

While Editing check box. This turns on revision marking. Click Options to change the default attributes for old text, new text, and the revision bar, if desired. To turn off revision marking, choose Revisions from the Tools menu, and uncheck the Mark Revisions While Editing check box.

Figure 28-10
The Revisions dialog box

To use revision marks:

1. Open the file 15-2.doc.

2. Choose Revisions from the Tools menu.

   Word opens the Revisions dialog box.

3. Check the Mark Revisions While Editing check box.

4. Click the Options button.

   Notice the default settings of Underline for new text, Strikethrough for old text, and Outside Border to indicate the position of the revision bar.

5. Click OK in both dialog boxes.

6. Select the text "**Gateway Travel Offices**".

7. Press the **Backspace** key to delete the selected text.

   Word changes the text to strikethrough characters.

8. Deselect the text. Move the insertion point to the blank line below the strikethrough text and key:

   Here is a list of Gateway Travel offices:

   The new text appears underlined. A revision bar appears to the left of the old and new text. (In page layout view and in the printed document, the revision bar on an odd page will appear in the right margin.)

You can review the document once it has been marked for revisions and then decide if you wish to accept or reject the revisions. If you accept the revisions, Word deletes the strikethrough text, removes the underlining from the new text, and removes the revision bars. If you do not want to make the revisions, you can reject them and restore the original document.

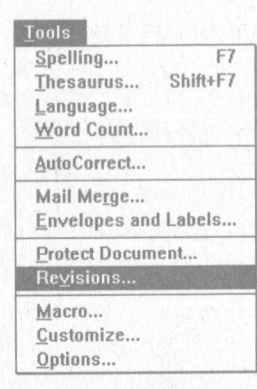

Tools menu

To accept or reject revisions, use the Accept All or Reject All button in the Revisions dialog box. You can select text and then accept or reject the revisions for the selected text. If you do not select text before clicking the Accept All or Reject All button, Word accepts or rejects the revisions in the entire document.

To undo revision marks:

1. Choose Revisions from the Tools menu to display the Revisions dialog box.

2. Click the Reject All button.

    Word asks if you want to reject all revisions.

3. Click Yes, and then click OK in the Revisions dialog box.

    The document appears without the revisions you made.

4. Close the document without saving changes and exit Word.

Key Terms

Revision bar   Search criteria

Revision marks

Appendices

Proofreaders' Marks

PROOFREADERS' MARK	DRAFT	FINAL COPY
ss Single-space	ss ⌈ I have heard ⌊ he is leaving	I have heard he is leaving
ds Double-space	ds ⌈ When will you ⌊ have a decision?	When will you have a decision?
+1ℓ# → Insert 1 line space	<u>Percent of Change</u> +1ℓ# → 16.25	<u>Percent of Change</u> 16.25
−1ℓ# → Delete (remove) 1 line space	Northeastern −1ℓ# → regional sales	Northeastern regional sales
⌣ Delete space	to gether	together
# Insert space	It may be	It may not be
↗ Move as shown	it is (not) true	it is true
∿ Transpose	belei̇vable is it so	believable it is so
◯ Spell out	②years ago 16 Elm St.	two years ago 16 Elm Street
∧ Insert a word	How much it?	How much is it?
ℓ OR — Delete a word	it may not be true	it may be true
∧ OR ⅄ Insert a letter	temperture	temperature
ℓ OR ⊖ Delete a letter and close up	commitṁent to buṅy	commitment to buy
⌒ Add on to a word	a real good day	a really good day
♈ OR / Change a letter	this supercedes	this supersedes
⌄ OR — Change a word	and if you won't	but if you can't
...... Stet (don't delete)	I was very glad	I was very glad
/ Make letter lowercase	Federal Government	federal government

PROOFREADERS' MARK	DRAFT	FINAL COPY
⹀ Capitalize	Janet L. greyston	Janet L. Greyston
⌄ Raise above the line	in her new book⁕	in her new book*
⌃ Drop below the line	H2S04	H_2SO_4
⊙ Insert a period	Mr‸Henry Grenada	Mr. Henry Grenada
⋀ Insert a comma	a large‸old house	a large, old house
⌵ Insert an apostrophe	my childrens car	my children's car
⌵ Insert quotation marks	he wants a loan	he wants a "loan"
= Insert a hyphen	a first‗rate job	a first-rate job
	ask the coowner	ask the co-owner
‑‑ OR ⊥/M Insert a dash or change a hyphen to a dash	Success‸at last! Here it is‸cash!	Success—at last! Here it is—cash!
___ Insert underscore	an issue of Time	an issue of <u>Time</u>
___ Delete underscore	a <u>very</u> long day	a very long day
(ital) ___ Set in italic	(ital) The New York Times	*The New York Times*
(bf) ～～ Set in boldface	(bf) the Enter key	the **Enter** key
(rom) ___ Set in roman	(rom) the *most* likely	the most likely
{ } Insert parentheses	left today (May 3)	left today (May 3)
¶ Start a new paragraph	ridiculous! If that is so	ridiculous! If that is so
2] Indent 2 spaces	Net investment in 2]tangible assets	Net investment in tangible assets
⊐ Move to the right	$38,367,000 ⊐	$38,367,000
⊏ Move to the left	⊏ Anyone can win!	Anyone can win!
= Align horizontally	Bob Mueller TO	TO: Bob Mueller
‖ Align vertically	‖ Jon Peters ‖ Ellen March	Jon Peters Ellen March

Standard Forms for Business Letters

Two frequently used formats for business letters are the Block Style and the Modified Block Style. Individual businesses and offices usually have a style preference.

Block Style

In the Block Style, text begins at the left margin. Nothing is indented except for quotations, tables, and other displayed material. (See page 584 for an example of the Block Style using paper with a letterhead.)

Modified-Block Style

In the Modified-Block Style, all text begins at the left margin except for the return address (if there is one), the date line, the complimentary closing, and the writer's identification, all of which begin at the center. A variation of the Modified Block Style indents the first line of each paragraph five spaces. (See page 585 for an example of the Modified Block Style using paper without a letterhead.)

Using Paper with a Letterhead

The first page of a business letter typically is written on paper with a letterhead. The letterhead usually consists of at least the following components: the company's name, its street address, its city, state, and ZIP code. Most letterheads indicate the area code and telephone number. Some letterheads also contain a graphic element (such as a logo) and a facsimile (fax) number.

Most large businesses have printed letterhead paper. However, with the increasing sophistication of word-processing programs, many businesses have also developed letterhead files that can be added to a letter and provide a professional-looking letterhead on a laser printer.

When not using a letterhead, a return address is required. A return address is also used when writing a personal-business letter (that is,

(Continued on page 586)

Business Letter—Block Style

Letterhead: The company's name and address, along with other information (such as a telephone number).

Date Line: The date (month, day, and year) on which the letter is typed; starts at the left on the third line below the letterhead or 2 inches from the top of the page.

Inside Address: The name and address of the person to whom you are writing.

Salutation: An opening greeting, such as "Dear Ms. Morales:".

Message: The text of the letter; all paragraphs are typed single-spaced with no indentions; leave one blank line between paragraphs.

Complimentary Closing: A parting phrase, such as "Sincerely," or "Sincerely yours", starts at the left.

Writer's Identification: The signer's name and title.

Reference Initials: The initials of the typist and sometimes those of the writer as well.

Enclosure Notation: A reminder that the letter is accompanied by an enclosure.

Copy Notation: The names of those who will receive copies of this letter.

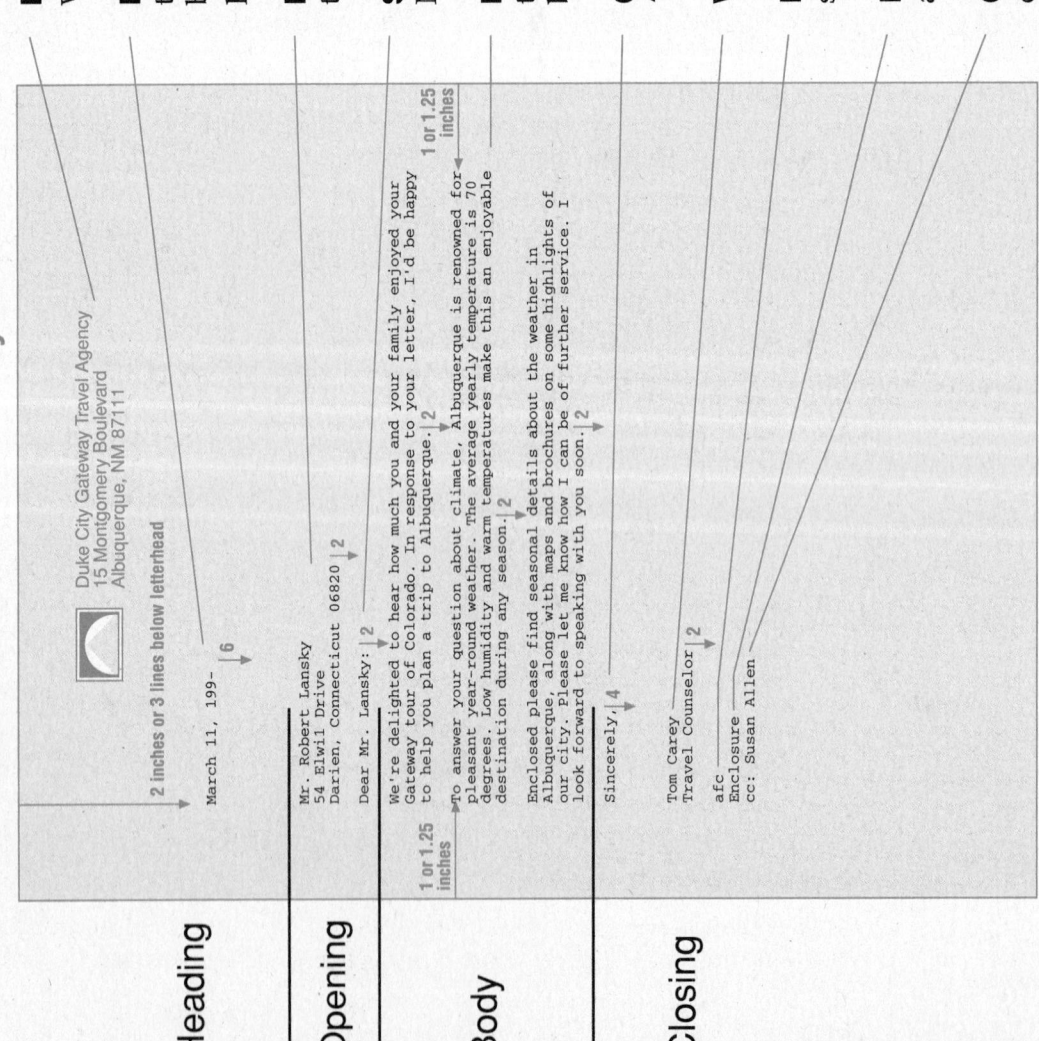

Heading

Opening

Body

Closing

2 inches or 3 lines below letterhead

Duke City Gateway Travel Agency
15 Montgomery Boulevard
Albuquerque, NM 87111

March 11, 199-

Mr. Robert Lansky
54 Elwil Drive
Darien, Connecticut 06820

Dear Mr. Lansky:

1 or 1.25 inches

We're delighted to hear how much you and your family enjoyed your Gateway tour of Colorado. In response to your letter, I'd be happy to help you plan a trip to Albuquerque.

1 or 1.25 inches

To answer your question about climate, Albuquerque is renowned for pleasant year-round weather. The average yearly temperature is 70 degrees. Low humidity and warm temperatures make this an enjoyable destination during any season.

Enclosed please find seasonal details about the weather in Albuquerque, along with maps and brochures on some highlights of our city. Please let me know how I can be of further service. I look forward to speaking with you soon.

Sincerely,

Tom Carey
Travel Counselor

afc
Enclosure
cc: Susan Allen

Business Letter—Modified-Block Style

Return Address: When not using letterhead paper, a return address is needed. A return address consists of the company's name and address. In a personal letter, the company's name is optional.

Date Line: The date (month, day, and year) on which the letter is typed; starts at center on the third line below the letterhead or 2 inches from the top of the page.

Inside Address: The name and address of the person to whom you are writing.

Salutation: An opening greeting, such as "Dear Ms. Morales:".

Message: The text of the letter; all paragraphs are typed single-spaced with no indentions; leave one blank line between paragraphs.

Complimentary Closing: A parting phrase, such as "Sincerely", or "Sincerely yours", starts at center.

Writer's Identification: The signer's name and title.

Reference Initials: The initials of the typist and sometimes those of the writer as well.

Enclosure Notation: A reminder that the letter is accompanied by an enclosure.

Delivery Notation: An indication that the letter has been sent in a special way.

Copy Notation: The names of those who will receive copies of this letter.

Heading

Opening

Body

Closing

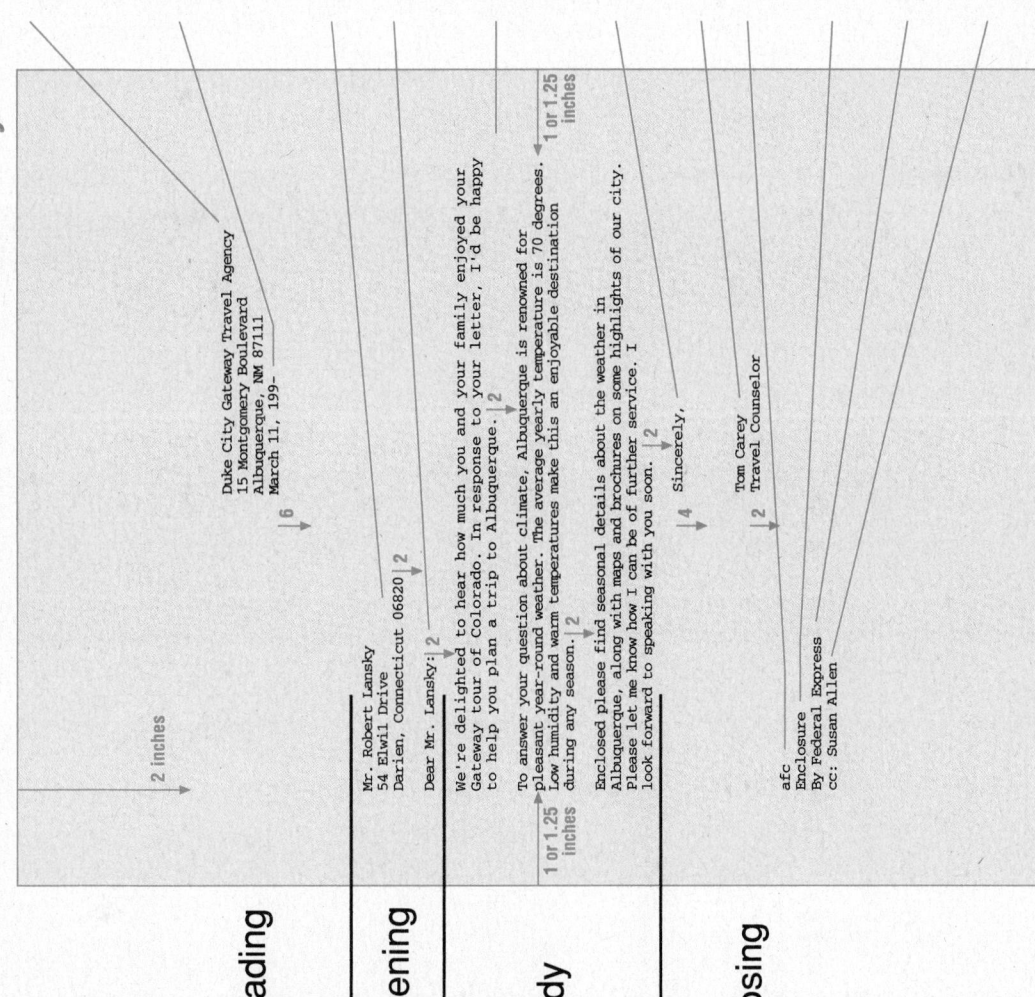

2 inches

Duke City Gateway Travel Agency
15 Montgomery Boulevard
Albuquerque, NM 87111
March 11, 199-
↓6

1 or 1.25 inches

Mr. Robert Lansky
54 Elwil Drive
Darien, Connecticut 06820 ↓2

Dear Mr. Lansky: ↓2

We're delighted to hear how much you and your family enjoyed your Gateway tour of Colorado. In response to your letter, I'd be happy to help you plan a trip to Albuquerque. ↓2

To answer your question about climate, Albuquerque is renowned for pleasant year-round weather. The average yearly temperature is 70 degrees. Low humidity and warm temperatures make this an enjoyable destination during any season. ↓2

Enclosed please find seasonal details about the weather in Albuquerque, along with maps and brochures on some highlights of our city. Please let me know how I can be of further service. I look forward to speaking with you soon. ↓2

Sincerely, ↓4

Tom Carey ↓2
Travel Counselor

afc
Enclosure
By Federal Express
cc: Susan Allen

1 or 1.25 inches

(Continued from page 583)

a letter you write as an individual, unrelated to business). The return address usually consists of your street address; your city, state, and ZIP code; your phone number (if appropriate); and the date. A business letter using a return address often includes the business name as well.

Continuation Pages

For letters that are two or more pages, use plain paper without letterhead for the continuation pages. Insert a header on the continuation pages that consists of the name of the addressee, the page number, and the date, using either of the following styles:

```
Mr. Steven Alvarez
Page 2
June 1, 199-
```

```
Mr. Steven Alvarez        2        June 1, 199-
```

Place the header 1 inch from the edge of the page. Insert two blank lines between the header and the continuation text.

Note: When creating business letters, *The Gregg Reference Manual* standard is 1 or 1.25 inches for left and right margins and 1 inch from the top edge for continuation page headers. Word default settings are 1.25 inches for left and right margins and .5 inches from the top edge for headers.

Standard Form for a Memorandum

Many businesses use preprinted memorandum forms that standardize the key information required by the business. When a business does not use a preprinted memo form, you can use paper with a letterhead or, if the company does not use a letterhead, you can use plain paper.

There isn't a single correct form for memos typed on letterhead or plain paper. However, the memo form shown on page 588 illustrates the elements of a good memo: "Memo To," "From," "Date," and "Subject".

For memos that are two or more pages, insert a header on the continuation pages that consists of the name of the addressee, the page number, and the date, using either of the following styles:

```
Ms. Susan Allen
Page 2
November 15, 199-
```

```
Ms. Susan Allen        2        November 15, 199-
```

Place the header 1 inch from the edge of the page. Insert two blank lines between the header and the continuation text.

Note: When creating business memos, *The Gregg Reference Manual* standard is 1 or 1.25 inches for left and right margins and 1 inch from the top edge for continuation page headers. Word default settings are 1.25 inches for left and right margins and .5 inches from the top edge for headers.

---

2 inches

1 inch

MEMO TO: Susan Allen |2

PROM: Tom Carey |2

DATE: November 15, 199- |2

SUBJECT: The Red River Hotel in Albuquerque |3

1 or 1.25 inches

The new Red River Hotel in Albuquerque has just been completed. It's the perfect place to stay for taking in all the local sights, or as a stopover to other New Mexico destinations. The hotel has extended very attractive discounts to all Gateway travel agencies, which we can extend to our customers. |2

1 or 1.25 inches

The hotel has 400 rooms, which are spacious and tastefully furnished. Each room is equipped with individual climate controls, direct-dial telephones, a color TV, a dressing room, and a heat lamp. Some two- and three-room suites are also available. |2

The hotel has two restaurants-one offering American food and the other offering some of the best New Mexican food available. It has an elegant lounge with live Mariachi music nightly. |2

The Red River has two heated pools, one indoor and the other outdoor. It also has full health-club facilities, including ten racquetball courts, five tennis courts, nautilus equipment, computerized treadmills, a steam room, and a sauna. Spa services, such as massages and facials, can be scheduled, as well as the services of a personal weight trainer. |2

                                        SA |2

afc

Standard Form for a Business Envelope

Many businesses use envelopes with preprinted return addresses for all correspondence. When the envelope contains a preprinted return address, you can key the name of the writer so that it prints above the preprinted return address. (However, some printers are not able to print a name that is too close to the edge of the envelope. In these cases, you will have to use a typewriter, insert the name by hand, or omit the name altogether.)

Preprinted Return Address

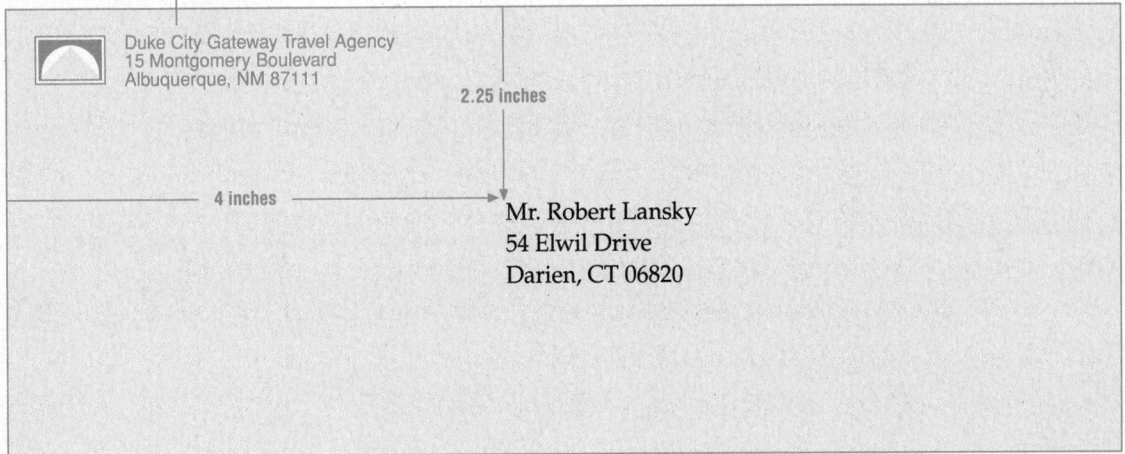

Duke City Gateway Travel Agency
15 Montgomery Boulevard
Albuquerque, NM 87111

2.25 inches

4 inches

Mr. Robert Lansky
54 Elwil Drive
Darien, CT 06820

For envelopes without a preprinted address, key the return address in the upper left corner, about .5 inches from the left and top edges.

If you wish to key a notation, such as "Confidential", it should begin on the third line below the return address. Underline the notation, and left-align it with the return address.

Note: When addressing business envelopes, *The Gregg Reference Manual* standard for the address is 4 inches from the left and 14 lines (about 2⅓ inches) from the top; the standard for the return address is .5 inches from the left and top edges. Word default settings for the address are 4 inches from the left and 2.25 inches from the top. Word default settings for the return address are .4 inches from the left edge and .25 inches from the top edge. However, these settings may vary slightly from printer to printer.

Basic Windows Skills

Many programs today use a program called Microsoft Windows (or Windows, for short). Windows is an operating environment for IBM and IBM-compatible computers. It supplements the computer's operating system, known as DOS (Disk Operating System), by adding a graphical screen display. Word for Windows, WordPerfect for Windows, PageMaker, Excel, and many other programs need Windows to operate.

Window
A rectangular area on the computer screen with borders that separate it from the rest of the screen.

In computer terms, a *window* is a rectangular area on the computer screen with borders that separate it from the rest of the screen. When you open a file in Windows, a window appears on the computer screen with the contents of the file inside it. When you close the file, the window disappears.

Window ─────

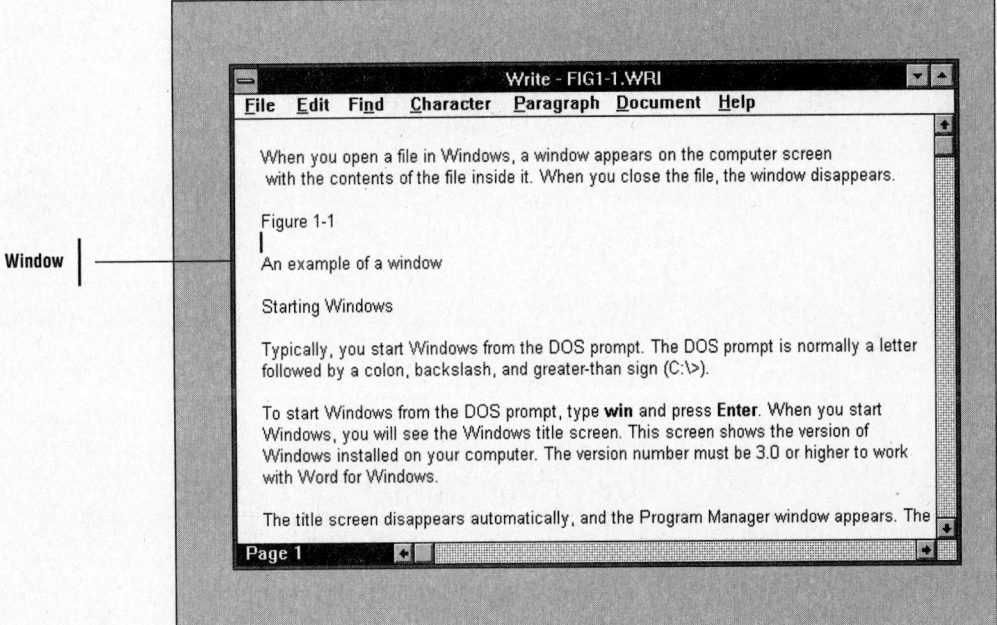

Figure E-1
An example of a window

Starting Windows

Typically, you start Windows from the DOS prompt. The DOS prompt is normally a letter followed by a colon, backslash, and greater-than sign (C:\>).

591

Note: Your computer may
require different startup
instructions. If it does, your
instructor will provide them.

To start Windows from the DOS prompt, type **win** and press **Enter**. When you start Windows, you will see the Windows title screen. This screen shows the version of Windows installed on your computer. The version number must be 3.0 or higher to work with most current Windows-based programs.

The title screen disappears automatically, and the Program Manager window appears. The Program Manager window shows you, at a glance, the program groups on your hard disk.

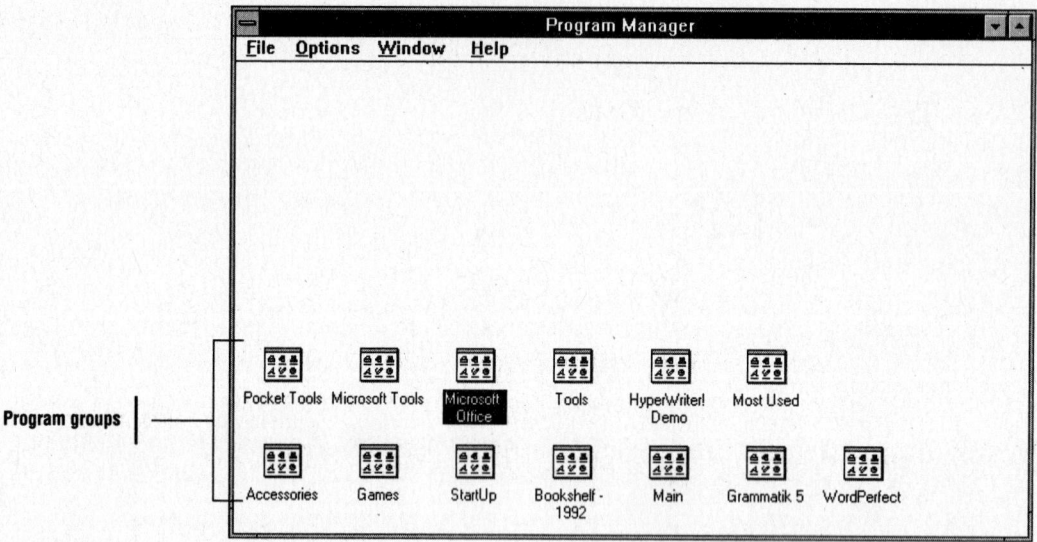

Program groups

Figure E-2
The Program Manager window

Think of the Program Manager window as a program organizer. From this window, you can quickly locate and start the programs on your computer.

Using the Mouse

Mouse pad
A small mat on which a
mouse may be rolled.

Pointer
A small symbol on the
screen that shows the po-
sition of the mouse.

To operate Windows and most Windows-based programs, you use a mouse. You roll the mouse on a small mat called a *mouse pad* (or on any flat surface, if you do not have a mouse pad). On one type of mouse, a rubber ball on the bottom of the mouse translates your movements to the computer. A *pointer*, a small symbol on the computer screen, shows your onscreen location as you move the mouse.

To select items on the computer screen using a mouse, you press a mouse button. Your mouse may have two or three buttons. Whenever you are told to "click" or "double-click" the mouse button, use the left button. In cases where you should use the right button, you will be told to do so.

Note: A trackball, which looks like an upside-down mouse, is sometimes used in place of a mouse. It provides the same functions as the mouse.

There are four ways to operate the mouse:

- Point

  When you *point*, you move the mouse until the on-screen pointer is on top of an item on the computer screen.

- Click

  When you *click*, you press the mouse button and then quickly release it.

- Double-click

  When you *double-click*, you quickly press and release the mouse button twice.

- Drag

  When you *drag*, you point to an object, hold down the mouse button, and move the mouse to a new position. Then you release the mouse button.

Practicing with the Mouse

Note: If you do not see a moving, arrow-shaped pointer on the computer screen, try moving the mouse farther to the left, right, toward you, or away from you until you see the pointer. Then pick up the mouse so the rubber ball underneath it does not touch the mouse pad or desktop. Move the mouse back to the center of the mouse pad, and put it down. The position of the pointer on the computer screen does not change until the ball under the mouse once again touches a flat surface.

In Windows (and in most Windows-based programs) there are often several ways to accomplish the same task. For example, you will learn three ways to close a window in the following practice session.

1. Place your hand over the mouse in a comfortable position with a finger on the left button, but do not press the button.

2. Move the mouse around on its mouse pad, and watch the computer screen. Look for a moving, arrow-shaped pointer.

3. Move the mouse toward you, away from you, to the left, and to the right, and watch the corresponding movements of the pointer on the computer screen.

4. Use the pointer to point to the word "File." To do this, move the mouse until the tip of the arrow is on top of File.

Pointer over word "File"

5. Move the mouse to the right, and stop when the pointer is on the word "Help."

6. Click (press and release) the left mouse button.

   A menu appears on the screen.

7. Point to the empty area to the right of the menu and click.

   The menu disappears.

8. Point to the program group symbol above the word "Main" and double-click (quickly press and release the mouse button twice).

   The Main window opens on the screen.

9. Point to the small square box at the upper left of the window.

Figure E-3
Your screen may look different from this screen, depending on the programs installed.

10. Point to the word "Close" and click.

    The window disappears.

11. Point to the Main program group again and click once.

    A menu appears above the program group.

12. Point to the word "Restore" and click.

    The Main window reopens.

13. Point to the small, square box in the upper left corner of the Main window and double-click.

    The window closes.

14. Again, point to the Main program group and click once.

    The menu again appears above the symbol.

15. Point to the empty area to the right of the menu and click.

The menu disappears.

16. This time, point to the word "File" at the top of the screen and click.

A menu appears below File.

17. Point to the word "Open" and click.

The Main windows reopens.

18. Close the window again by double-clicking the small, square box in the upper left corner of the Main window.

Icons

Icons

Small pictures or symbols on the computer screen representing programs or tools.

Program Manager icon

One feature that makes Windows and programs that work with Windows different from most other computer programs is their use of *icons*. Icons are small pictures or symbols on the computer screen. The symbol above the words "Program Manager" is an example of an icon.

Icons are used to represent many items on the computer screen, such as program groups, individual programs, and tools you use within programs. By getting to know the icons, you will be able to locate and choose the program groups, programs, and tools you need quickly.

To choose the Accessories icon in the Program Manager window:

1. Point to the icon above Accessories.

2. Click the left mouse button once.

A menu appears above the icon. If the word "Accessories" was not already shown with a dark background, the background changes now. That is how you know the icon has been chosen.

3. To choose the Main icon, point to the icon, and click the mouse button once.

The menu above the Accessories icon disappears. The word "Accessories" returns to a light background, indicating that it is no longer chosen. The word "Main" is shown on a dark background, indicating that the Main icon has now been chosen. A menu appears above the icon.

4. Point to an empty area in the window, and click the mouse button once.

The menu disappears; however, the Main icon is still chosen.

Parts of a Window

All windows contain several basic elements. The Program Manager window is a good example of a typical window.

Figure E-4
The Program Manager window

The common window elements are:

• Window borders

  The *window borders* are the boundary lines surrounding the window.

• Window corners

  The *window corners* are at the four corners of the window border. They are used to adjust the size of the window.

• Title bar

  The *title bar* is the shaded bar at the top of the window that displays the name of the window.

• Control-menu box

  The *Control-menu box* is the box in the upper left corner of the window. Clicking this box displays the Control menu, which contains options for manipulating windows.

- Minimize button

  The *Minimize button* is the box in the upper right corner containing a down arrow. Clicking this button shrinks the window to its icon.

- Maximize button

  The *Maximize button* is the box in the upper right corner containing an up arrow. Clicking this button enlarges the window to fill the entire screen.

- Menu bar

  The *menu bar* is the area under the title bar that displays the words File, Options, Window, and Help.

- Workspace

  The *workspace* is the area in the window that displays the contents of the window.

- Desktop

  The *desktop* is the area of the computer screen outside the window borders.

Types of Windows

As you work in Windows, you will notice that some windows have menu bars and some do not.

Application window
A window that contains a running application and has a menu bar.

An *application window* has a menu bar. For example, the Program Manager is an application window. The windows for Word, WordPerfect, PageMaker, and Excel are also application windows.

Application windows can contain subordinate windows. These windows do not contain menu bars. They appear in the workspace of an application window. They may contain documents, programs, groups of programs, files, or tools. More than one of these subordinate windows can be open in an application window at one time.

The following example shows two document windows (the Main window and the Accessories window) open in the Program Manager window at one time. See Figure E-5 on page 598.

Active window
The window currently in use on the computer screen.

When more than one window is open on the computer screen, only one of the windows is in use, or the *active window*. The active window appears in front of all other windows. On some computer screens, its title bar appears in a different color from the other windows. In the above example, the Main window is active.

Document
window

Application
window

Figure E-5
Two document windows open in an application window

Minimizing/Maximizing Windows

The Minimize and Maximize buttons in the upper right corner of a window let you change the window's size quickly. The Maximize button (with the up arrow in it) enlarges a window to fill the entire computer screen. This feature is particularly useful when you have a window open in another window. You can use the Maximize button to improve your ability to see what is in the window. Once you have maximized a window, the Maximize button for that window changes to the *Restore button* containing a double arrow. Clicking the Restore button returns the window to its original size.

The Minimize button (with the down arrow in it) reduces the window to its icon, which typically appears in the lower left corner of the screen. See Figure E-6 on page 599.

To maximize a window:

1. Point to the Maximize button in the upper right corner of the Program Manager window.

2. Click the left mouse button.

To restore a window to its original size:

1. Point to the Restore button in the window.

2. Click the left mouse button.

To minimize a window:

1. Point to the Minimize button in the window.

2. Click the left mouse button once.

Restore button
The box at the right of the title bar containing a double arrow that appears after maximizing a window and returns the window to its original size.

Restore button

Note: When you use the Maximize button in a window located within another window, the second window grows to the size of the original window. It will not fill the entire screen, unless the original window already does.

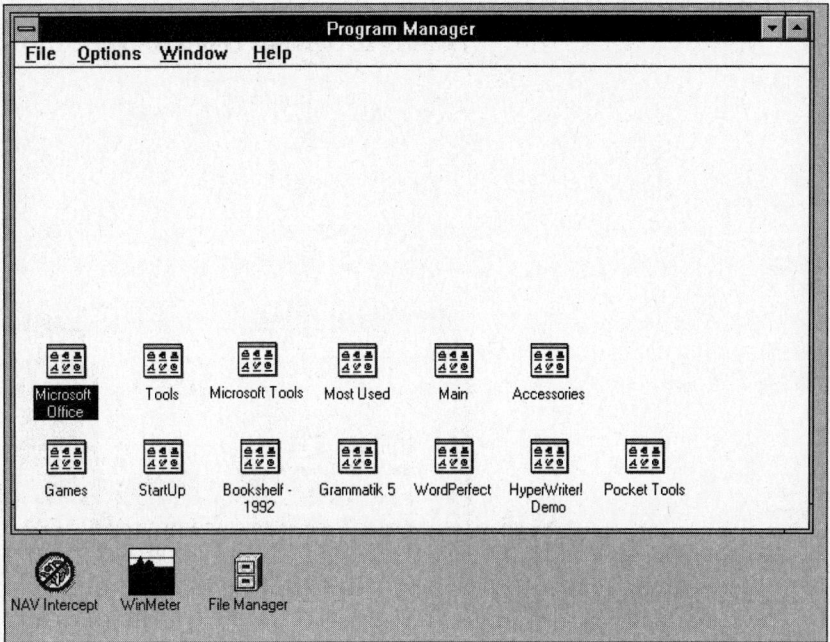

Figure E-6
A screen showing minimized windows

To restore a window to its original size:

1. Point to the window's icon.

2. Double-click the left mouse button. (After the first click, you may see a menu flash on the screen above the icon. This disappears when the window is restored after your second click.)

Moving Between Windows

When two or more windows are open simultaneously, you can only work in the active window. To work in another window, you must first make it active.

To move to a window and make it active:

1. Double-click the Main icon to open the Main window.

   When you open the Main window, it becomes the active window.

2. Double-click the Accessories icon to open the Accessories window.

   When you open the Accessories window, it moves in front of the Main window and becomes the active window.

3. Point to the Main window, and click the left mouse button.

   The Main window moves in front of the Accessories window and becomes active.

Note: If you move a larger window in front of a smaller one, you will not be able to point to the smaller window when you want to make it active. Instead, you can use the Minimize button in the current active window to reduce the larger window to its icon. Then you will be able to see the smaller window.

Rearranging Windows

When working with several open windows, some windows are hidden behind others. You can rearrange windows, so that a part of each one is visible.

You can layer each window within the Program Manager workspace so that you can see each window's title bar. These are *cascading windows*.

Cascading windows
Open windows that are arranged in layers with the title bar of each window visible.

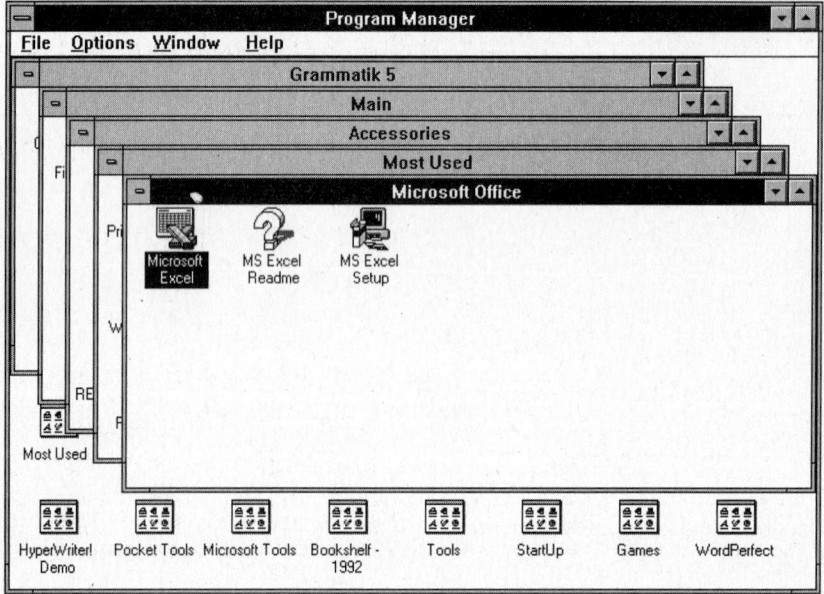

Figure E-7
Cascading windows within the Program Manager window

You can also arrange the windows so that they appear side by side within the Program Manager workspace. These are *tiled windows*.

Tiled windows
Open windows that are resized and arranged side by side on the screen.

Note: Tiled windows are arranged in smaller sizes. Therefore, not all icons may be visible within a tiled window.

Figure E-8
Tiled windows within the Program Manager window

Both options are chosen from the Window menu.

To rearrange windows:

1. Double-click the Games icon (or any other program group), so that there are three open windows.

2. Point to Window in the menu bar, and click the left mouse button.

3. Point to Cascade, and click the left mouse button.

    The three windows are layered with their title bars showing.

4. Click the title bar of the middle window.

    The middle window moves to the front and becomes the active window.

5. Point to Window in the menu bar, and click the left mouse button.

6. Point to Tile, and click the left mouse button.

    The three windows are displayed side by side within the Program Manager window.

7. Double-click any one of the icons that appear below the tiled windows.

    A new window overlaps one of the tiled windows and becomes the active window.

8. Point to Window in the menu bar, and click the left mouse button.

9. Point to Tile, and click the left mouse button.

    Now all four windows are tiled within the Program Manager window.

10. Click the Minimize button in each of the tiled windows.

    Each tiled window becomes an icon again.

Note: When you open an additional window after choosing the cascade or tile option, the window overlaps the rearranged windows. If you want the new windows to be part of the cascading or tiled windows, you must choose the option again.

Using Menus

While you do not need to understand all aspects of Windows to operate a Windows-based program successfully, you will find a basic knowledge of Windows features helpful. Because Windows-based programs are built on the structure of the Windows environment, you will be able to transfer much of what you learn about Windows to any Windows-based program. So, learning Windows will make learning virtually any Windows-based program much easier.

To conserve space in Windows, many available program features, or options, are kept in menus that you access from the menu bar. Windows has five menus, containing lists of options.

- File menu

  The File menu contains file-management options, such as Move, Copy, and Delete. It also contains the Exit Windows option for exiting the program.

- Options menu

  The Options menu contains options for arranging and sizing icons.

- Window menu

  The Window menu contains options for arranging windows and icons. It also lists the available windows and allows access to them.

- Help menu

  The Help menu contains options for accessing the Windows Help features.

Control-menu box

- Control menu

  This menu appears when you click the Control-menu box located to the left of the title bar. The Control menu contains options for changing the size and location of windows. All applications that work with Windows have a similar Control menu.

When a menu is closed, you see only its name in the menu bar. When a menu is open, you can view and choose menu options.

Figure E-9

On this screen, the File menu is open.

The menus are called *pull-down* or *drop-down menus* to describe the two ways you can open them.

The two ways to open menus and choose options are:

- By clicking the name of the menu in the menu bar. When you do this, the menu drops down, and the menu options appear. Then you can click the name of the option you want.

- By clicking the menu name and dragging the mouse to pull down the menu. When the menu is open, you can drag to the option you want and release the mouse button to choose it.

More About Menu Options

When you drag the pointer on top of a menu option, the name changes to light type on a dark background. This is called *highlighting*. The option that is highlighted when you release the mouse button is chosen.

Some menu options are only available at certain points in the program. When they are not available, they appear gray in the menu, and you are not able to choose them.

Some menu options are followed by three dots. These dots let you know that a dialog box appears if you choose that option. (Dialog boxes are discussed below.)

To the right of some menu options, you will notice keys (such as the **F7** key or the **Del** key) or a combination of keys (such as **Shift+F4** or **Ctrl+Esc**). These are keyboard commands that allow you to choose menu options using the keyboard. To use a combination of keys, hold down the first key, press the second key, then release both keys.

A triangle (▶) at the right side of a menu command indicates that the command leads to a *cascading menu*, which lists additional options that are available.

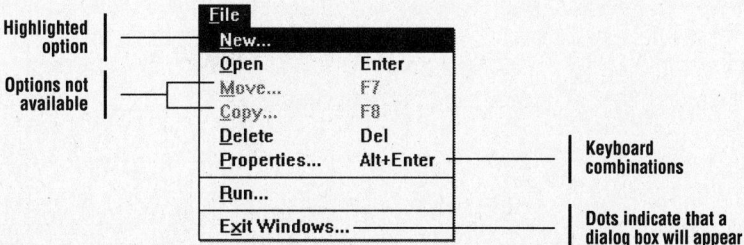

Figure E-10
Menus provide immediate information about options.

Introduction to Dialog Boxes

Dialog box
A box that displays a question or presents options and asks you to respond.

A good portion of your interaction with Windows-based programs will involve the use of *dialog boxes*. A dialog box displays a question or presents options and asks you to respond. It gives you a choice in how you want to proceed at certain points in the program.

Figure E-11
The Delete dialog box

Dialog boxes usually contain some or all of these items:

* Title

  The title is the name of the dialog box.

* Command buttons

  Command buttons are small rectangles, sometimes with rounded corners. You click a command button to choose an option.

  Some command buttons contain a word followed by three dots. When you click this type of command button, another dialog box appears offering you additional choices. Another type of command button contains a double chevron (»). Clicking this type of button causes another portion of the current dialog box to appear.

* List boxes

Drop-down list box
A list box that contains additional choices that appear when an arrow on the right side of the list box is clicked.

  List boxes contain a list of available choices. An arrow in a square box to the right of the list box indicates a *drop-down list box*. Clicking the box with the down arrow causes a list of available choices to appear. Clicking it again causes it to disappear.

* Text boxes

  Text boxes are rectangles in which you can type information.

* Option buttons

  Option buttons are small circles that indicate a list of mutually exclusive items. You can choose only one item from the list at a time. To change your choice, click a different button. The chosen option button contains a black dot.

- Check boxes

  Check boxes are small boxes offering you the chance to switch an option off or on. An **X** in the box indicates a yes response.

  To change the response in a check box, click the box.

Figure E-12
Often, you will use one dialog box to make several choices.

Choosing Dialog Box Options

The method you use to respond to options in a dialog box depends on the information in the box. The simplest dialog boxes have two buttons, representing a yes or no decision. More complex dialog boxes may require you to choose from among several buttons, type a choice in a text box, and make a choice from a list box.

Most dialog boxes use OK to represent a yes decision and Cancel to represent a no decision. In dialog boxes containing several options, clicking OK saves the options you have chosen, while clicking Cancel closes the dialog box without saving your choices.

To choose dialog box options using command buttons, click the button representing the choice you prefer. The procedure to exit Windows, for example, requires you to respond to a dialog box by clicking the appropriate button.

1. Click File in the menu bar of the Program Manager window.

2. Click Exit Windows in the File menu.

    The Exit Windows dialog box appears. Notice that this dialog box contains an OK and a Cancel command button.

3. Click the Cancel command button to close the dialog box and remain in Windows.

Moving Windows

You can move windows to new locations on the desktop using the mouse to create whatever desktop arrangement you like.

To move a window:

1. Point to the tile bar of the Program Manager window, and hold down the mouse button.

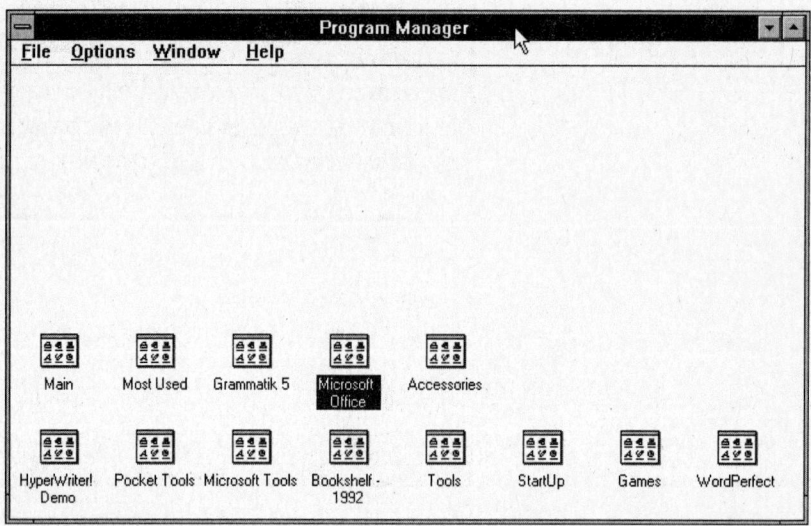

Figure E-13
Point to the title bar, and drag the window.

2. Drag the window to a new location on the desktop.

3. Release the mouse button.

Moving Items Within a Window

Items within a window, such as icons, dialog boxes, and other windows, are movable. You can arrange them any way you like. When windows or dialog boxes overlap inside a window, you can move them to see areas they are covering.

To move a window or a dialog box within a window:

1. Double-click the Accessories icon.

2. Point to the title bar of the Accessories window, and hold down the mouse button.

3. Drag the window to a new location while continuing to hold down the mouse button.

4. Release the mouse button.

5. Close the Accessories window.

Note: Some dialog boxes cannot be moved. You cannot move a window or dialog box outside the window it is in. If you need to see an area behind a window or dialog box and cannot move it out of the way, you can enlarge the original window using the Maximize button and then move it.

Note: If the Main icon is hidden by the another window, move the window to the left or right until you see the Main icon.

To move an icon:

1. Point to the Main icon.

2. Drag the icon to a new location while continuing to hold down the mouse button.

3. Release the mouse button.

Changing the Size of Windows

You can control the size of windows. You can use the Minimize, Maximize, and Restore buttons to adjust a window from the size of its icon to the size of the entire computer screen. But what if you want to make a window a particular size? Windows lets you use the mouse to adjust a window to any size.

To change the size of a window with the mouse:

1. Point to the right border of the Program Manager.

    The pointer changes to a double-headed arrow.

Double-headed arrows to change the size of windows horizontally, vertically, and diagonally.

2. With the pointer still shaped like a double-headed arrow, hold down the mouse button, and drag the window border toward the center of the window, until the window is about 2 inches wide.

Figure E-14

This window has been made narrow using the mouse.

3. Release the mouse button.

4. Now, point to the bottom window border.

    The pointer changes to a double-headed arrow.

5. With the pointer still shaped like a double-headed arrow, hold
    down the mouse button, and drag the window border up until
    the window is about 2 inches tall.

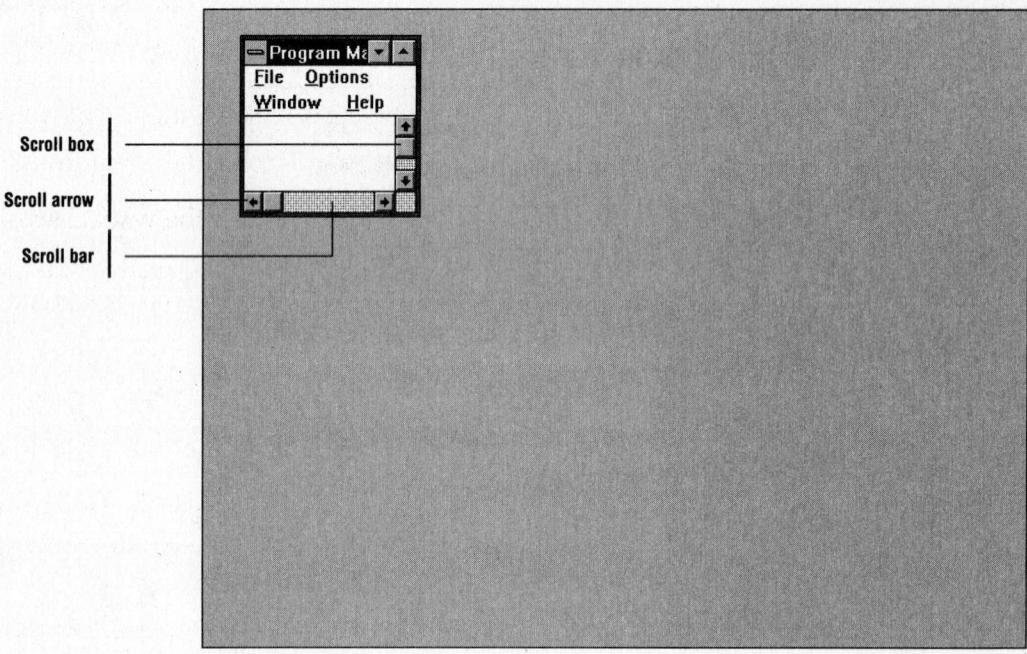

Figure E-15
Scroll bars appear as you reduce the size of the window.

6. Point to the bottom right corner of the reduced window.

    The pointer changes to a diagonal double-headed arrow,
    which lets you move two adjoining sides at the same time.

7. Hold down the mouse button, and drag outward until the
    window is slightly wider and taller, but not to its original size.

Using the Scroll Bars

Scroll bar
Bars appearing at the right
and bottom edges when
the contents of the window
are not entirely visible.

Scroll box
The box in a scroll bar that
represents your approxi-
mate position in the window.

With the window reduced from its original size, you can no longer
see the icons at the bottom of the window. To allow you to view the
hidden areas of the window, *scroll bars* appear along the right and
bottom edges. The scroll bars let you scroll up, down, left, and right
inside the window. The scroll bars represent the total area of the window both visible and hidden. The *scroll box* represents your approximate position in the window. (If the scroll bar is very short, a scroll
box does not appear on it.)

•   To move a short distance, click one of the *scroll arrows*.

Scroll arrow
The arrow at either end of
the scroll bar that, when
clicked, causes the work-
space to move a short distance in the opposite
direction of the arrow.

- To move a longer distance, click the scroll bar above or below the scroll box on the vertical scroll bar, and to the left or right of the scroll box on the horizontal scroll bar.

- To scroll continuously, point to one of the scroll arrows, and hold down the mouse button.

- To scroll to a particular position in the window, drag the scroll box to that position. Scroll bars represent the total area of the window, and the scroll box represents your position in the window. So, for example, if the scroll box is at the top of the vertical scroll bar, you are viewing the top of the window.

Practice using the scroll bars:

1. Point to the down scroll arrow of the vertical scroll bar.

2. Click the mouse button a few times, and watch the workspace shift until the bottom portion of the window containing the icons appears.

3. Point to the right scroll arrow of the horizontal scroll bar.

4. Click the mouse button once, and watch the screen.

   The workspace shifts a small distance to the right.

5. Point to the scroll bar to the right of the scroll box on the horizontal scroll bar, and click.

   The workspace shifts a greater distance to the right.

6. Point to the scroll box in the horizontal scroll bar, and drag the box left or right along the scroll bar. Then release the mouse button.

   The workspace shifts.

Note: The icons will re-main at the top of the win-dow and may be outside the workspace.

7. Click the lower right corner of the window, and drag outward to return the window to its approximate original size.

Choosing a Printer

Before you print from a Windows-based program, you should make sure that Windows and the program are set to print to the same printer. Otherwise, you may run into trouble when you try to print. If your computer is currently connected to a printer, someone has probably set up Windows for that printer already. However, we will review the steps to choose a printer, so you can check to make sure your printer is correctly identified in Windows.

Control Panel
A Windows application
with controls for adjusting
the screen and mouse and
for choosing the printer.

To choose a printer, you need to use the *Control Panel*. The Control Panel contains controls for adjusting the screen and mouse and for choosing the printer.

To access the Control Panel:

Note: You may have to scroll in the window to locate the Main icon.

1. In the Program Manager window, double-click the Main icon.

   The Main window opens.

2. Double-click the Control Panel icon.

   The Control Panel opens.

3. Double-click the Printers icon.

   The Printers dialog box opens. In the box labeled "Installed Printers" is a list of printers that can be installed on your computer. The printer currently in use is highlighted.

Figure E-16
Printers dialog box

4. If the highlighted printer is correct, you only need to click the Cancel button. If you need to choose a different printer, click the name of the printer. Click the Set As Default Printer button, and then click the Close button.

   If your printer does not appear in the Installed Printers list, it has not been installed on your computer. To install the printer, click the Add button, and choose the printer from the list that appears. Then click the Install button. You will not be able to install a printer unless the software required to run it, known as the *printer driver*, is also installed on your computer.

Printer driver
Software required to install a printer that controls how a computer and printer interact.

5. When you are finished, close the Control Panel, and arrange the icons in the Program Manager window (by clicking the Arrange Icons option in the Window menu).

Starting Applications from Within Windows

Applications
Computer programs used to do a particular kind of work, such as word processing.

Applications are programs you use to do your work, such as word-processing programs or desktop publishing programs. Windows-based applications use the Windows environment to provide their basic structure. Programs that are not based on Windows do not use Windows to provide their structure; however, you can start either type of application from within Windows.

To start an application from within Windows:

1. Turn on your computer and start Windows.

2. Double-click the icon in the Program Manager window that contains the program you want to open.

    The window for your program group opens.

3. Double-click an application icon.

    The application starts.

Exiting Applications

When you have finished working with an application, you exit the application and return to Windows. You usually have three options for exiting.

To exit a Windows application, you could:

*   Double-click the window's Control-menu box.

*   Click the Control-menu box, and then click Close on the Control menu.

*   Click File on the application's menu bar, and then click the Exit option in the File menu (not all applications have menu bars).

When you exit an application, a dialog box may appear asking you if you really want to exit the application. (The exact language will vary slightly from application to application.)

Exit your application:

1. Use any method described above to exit your application.

2. If a dialog box appears, indicate that you want to exit the application.

Asking for Help

If you get in trouble while you are using Windows, you can probably find the solution to your problem right on the computer screen. The Windows Help feature gives you immediate access to onscreen information about the program and how it works. This feature is often the fastest way to get assistance when you have a problem. One way to ask for Help is to use the **F1** key.

To use the **F1** key to ask for Help:

1. Press the **F1** key.

    The Help window appears. It contains information that relates to your current location in Windows.

2. Close the Help window.

The Help Menu

Another way to use the Help available in Windows is the Help menu. When you choose a Help menu option, a Help window opens.

To choose an option from the Help menu:

1. Click Help on the menu bar in the Program Manager window.

Figure E-17
The Help menu

2. Choose Contents from the Help menu to view the Help window.

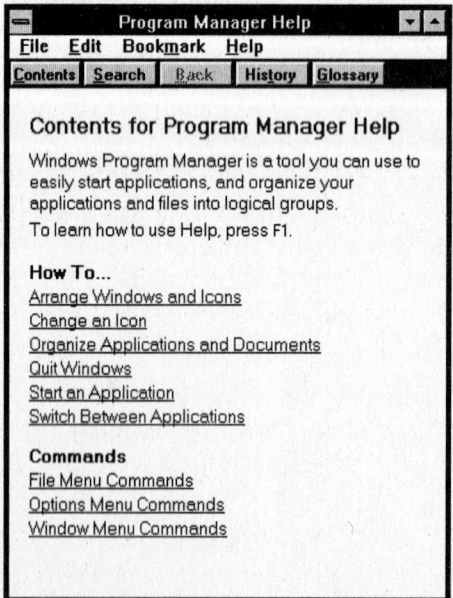

Figure E-18
A Help window

The Help Window

The Help window looks different from other windows you have seen in Windows. It has a menu bar with buttons underneath. You will use the menus and buttons to move from one Help screen to another. As you move to different screens, they appear in the Help window.

Practice using the Help window:

Note: As you move the pointer, it changes to a hand with a pointing finger.

1. Click the first How to topic, <u>Arrange Windows and Icons</u>.

    A Help window appears explaining how to arrange windows and icons. Notice that "title bar" in the first paragraph is highlighted.

2. Click the highlighted "title bar."

    When you click highlighted words, a definition of the word pops up in a box in the window.

3. Click again.

    The box disappears.

4. Click the Back button.

    This button takes you back to the previous Help topic.

5. Click the History button.

    A list of the Help topics you have viewed in this session appears.

6. Click the Search button.

    A Search dialog box appears. You can search for the topics that appear in the list in this dialog box, or you can type a word about which you want to request Help.

7. Click the Cancel button in the dialog box to close the Search dialog box. (You will search for Help in the next section.)

8. Click the Glossary button.

    An alphabetic listing of the terms used in Windows Help appears.

    You can choose words from the glossary list, and a definition for the term will appear. Click anywhere to remove the definition.

9. Close the glossary window.

10. Close the Help window.

The File menu contains a Print Topic option that lets you print the onscreen information about a topic on your printer. The other menus in the Help window provide advanced Help features, which you probably will not use very often, if at all. (For example, you can use the Annotate option in the Edit menu to make your own notations part of Help.)

Searching for Help

When you know the topic you would like to locate, you can let Windows find it for you:

1. Click Help on the menu bar in the Program Manager window.

2. Choose Search for Help on from the Help menu.

   The Search dialog box appears.

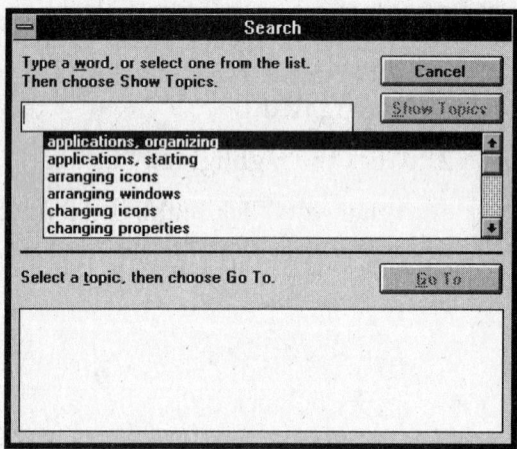

Figure E-19
The Search dialog box

3. Use the scroll bar to the right of the list of topics in the dialog box to find the topic "applications, starting" in the list.

4. Click "applications, starting" to choose it.

5. Click the Show Topics button in the Search dialog box.

   A list of topics appears in the box at the bottom of the dialog box. Each of these topics leads you to information related to starting an application.

6. Click "Starting an Application from a Group."

7. Click the Go To button.

   Information about the topic appears in the Help window.

8. After you have read the Help topic, close the Help window by double-clicking the Control-menu box.

Exiting Windows

When you have finished working in Windows, you should exit the program and return to the DOS prompt.

To exit Windows:

1. Point to File in the menu bar of the Program Manager window, and click the left mouse button.

2. Point to Exit Windows in the menu that appears, and click the left mouse button.

    A box appears, prompting you to confirm that you would like to end the Windows session.

3. Point to OK, and click the left mouse button.

    You are returned to the DOS prompt.

The number following the definition of a glossary term indicates the Lesson in which the term is first used.

Attach To assign a template to an existing document. (21)

AutoText A Word feature that allows you to store frequently used text and graphics that can be easily retrieved to be inserted in a document when needed. (21)

Background repagination The automatic process of updating page breaks and page numbers that occurs after editing a document. (12)

Baseline The imaginary line upon which characters sit. (17)

Border A line or box applied to paragraphs or sections in a document. (7)

Bullet A character (•) that precedes a paragraph in a bulleted list. (7)

Bulleted list A hanging indent, in which lines of text are preceded by bullet characters. (7)

Cell selection bar The unmarked area between a cell's left gridline and the left margin of the cell's text used to select that cell and its contents. (18)

Cell The intersection of a column and a row in a table. (18)

Character attribute A formatting option, such as bold or italic, that determines the appearance of text. (3)

Character format The combined character attributes of text. (3)

Character style A set of character-formatting instructions that you name and use to format individual words or small amounts of text within a paragraph. (20)

Clipboard A temporary storage area used to hold text that is cut or copied. (8)

Column selection bar The unmarked horizontal bar above the top border of a table used to select a column in that table. (18)

Crop To hide parts of a graphic image so that they do not appear on the screen or print. (25)

Custom tab A tab that is set to replace default tab settings. (6)

Data source The document that contains the variable information, such as names, addresses, and other data, that is inserted into the main document when printed. (23)

Default settings Settings predefined by Word if the user does not specify settings. (1)

Drag-and-drop editing A method of editing that allows you to move or copy text by dragging, without cutting, copying, or pasting. (8)

Draw-type graphic A graphic stored as a combination of lines and shapes. Also known as an *object-oriented graphic*. (25)

EPS A draw-type graphic format, stands for Encapsulated Postscript. (25)

Em dash A special character that produces a dash somewhat wider than a hyphen. (17)

En dash A special character that produces a dash about the width of a hyphen. (17)

End mark A short horizontal bar on the Word screen that indicates the end of the document. (1)

End-of-cell marker A character within each cell in a table that indicates the end of that cell's contents. (18)

End-of-row marker A character to the right of the gridline for each row in a table that indicates the end of that row. (18)

Field characters Brackets that show the beginning and end of a field. (5)

Field instructions Instructions in a field that tell Word how to perform the action. (5)

Field name Unique name given to a field in the data source. (23)

Field type The action the field is to perform in a document. (5)

Field A set of hidden codes in a Word document that tell Word where to insert specific text or graphics. (5)

File A document that has been created and then saved under a unique filename. (1)

Filename The unique name given to a document that is saved in Word. (1)

First-line indent An indent in which only the first line of a paragraph is indented from the left margin. (7)

Font A type design, such as Times New Roman or Courier. (3)

Footer Text that appears in the bottom margin of a page throughout a section or document. (12)

Form field An area in an on-line form where the user fills in information. (27)

Frames Special enclosures that you add to paragraphs, pictures, or tables to position them on a page. (26)

Graphic file format Defines the graphic's type, such as paint-type or draw-type. (25)

Graphic import filter A software program that allows Word to recognize graphics from other applications. (25)

Gridlines Lines that mark the boundaries of cells in a table. (18)

Gutter margin Extra space added to a margin to allow for binding. (5)

Hanging indent An indent in which the first line of a paragraph aligns at the left, and the remainder of the paragraph is indented from the left margin. (7)

Hard page break A page break that is inserted manually and does not move, regardless of changes in the document. (11)

Header Text that appears in the top margin of a page throughout a section or document. (12)

Hidden text Text that does not appear in the printed version of a document and that only appears on the screen if Word's hidden text option is turned on. (17)

Indent markers Markers that appear at the left and right margins on the ruler. (7)

Indent The distance between the sides of a paragraph and the margins. (7)

Insertion point A vertical blinking bar on the Word screen that indicates where an action will begin. (1)

Jump term A Help topic that is linked to other Help topics or to more information, usually identified by an underline and a color. (1)

Justified Text that is aligned with both the left and right margins by adjusting the spacing between words. (5)

Kerning Changes the spacing between specific pairs of letters to improve the appearance of text. (16)

Landscape A page-orientation setting in which the page is wider than it is tall. (15)

Leader Patterns of dots or dashes added to fill the tab spaces in a document. (6)

Left indent An indent that increases a paragraph's distance from the left margin. (7)

Line space The amount of vertical space used by characters in one line of text. (5)

Line-break character A symbol entered to start a new line within a paragraph. (2)

Macro name A name given to a recorded sequence by which the sequence can be retrieved. (22)

Macro An automated procedure consisting of a sequence of word-processing tasks. (22)

Mail merging A process of combining two documents during printing. (23)

Main document The document that contains the standard text that will appear in each copy of the printed document. (23)

Margins The distances between the text and the top, bottom, left, and right edges of the paper. (5)

Negative indent An indent that extends a paragraph into the left or right margin. (7)

Nonbreaking hyphen A hyphen in a hyphenated word that prevents the word from dividing at a line break. (5)

Nonbreaking space A space between two words, defined by a special character, that prevents Word from breaking a line between the two words. (2)

Nonprinting character A symbol for a tab, paragraph, or space that appears on the screen but not in the printed document. (2)

Normal style The standard, default paragraph style that is applied automatically to new paragraphs in a document. (20)

Numbered list A hanging indent, in which lines of text are preceded by sequential numbers or letters. (7)

Object linking and embedding OLE A Microsoft utility that enables you to include an object from another application in Word and edit the object within Word. (26)

Object-type graphic A graphic stored as a combination of lines and shapes. Also known as an *draw-oriented graphic*. (25)

On-line form A form that is filled in using the computer. (27)

Optional hyphen A hyphen that shows where a word should be divided if the word falls at the end of a line. (5)

Orphan A line that appears by itself at the bottom of a page of text. (11)

Paint-type graphic A graphic stored as a pattern of electronic dots that are arranged to created an image. (25)

Pane A portion of a document that is displayed onscreen in a horizontal window. (9)

Paragraph mark The symbol on the Word screen inserted each time you press Enter to indicate a new paragraph or start a new line. (1)

Paragraph style A set of paragraph- and character-formatting instructions that you name and use to format whole paragraphs in a Word document. (20)

Pictures Graphic images in Word documents. (25)

Placeholder An empty frame inserted into a document to reserve a place for text, graphics, or a table. (26)

Point A measure of type size, with 72 points equaling one inch. (16)

Portrait A page-orientation setting in which the page is taller than it is wide. (15)

Positive indent Any indent that occurs within the left and right margins. (7)

Printed form A form that is printed out and filled in by hand. (27)

Printer-driver software Software that instructs a computer about the printing capabilities of a printer. (14)

Proportional scaling Scaling a graphic using a corner sizing handle to maintain the original proportions. (25)

Ragged The uneven edge of text that is not aligned with a margin. (5)

Record In a data source, a set of related information, such as name, street, city, state, and ZIP code, for one person or business. (23)

Recorded macros Macros created by recording and naming a sequence of tasks. (22)

Revision bar A vertical bar in the left or right margin that indicates where text has been revised. (28)

Revision marks Marks that Word adds to a document to indicate changes you have made in its text. (28)

Right indent An indent that increases a paragraph's distance from the right margin. (7)

Row selection bar The area outside the left edge of a table used to select a row in that table. (18)

Scale To resize a graphic image. (25)

Search criteria Specifications that tell Word which files to locate in a search. (28)

Section breaks The double-dotted lines that appear on the screen to indicate the beginning and end of a section. (5)

Section A portion of a document that has its own formatting. (5)

Selection bar An unmarked area at the left edge of a document window, used to select text with the mouse. (2)

Selection The selected portion of a document (or the whole document), which appears highlighted on the screen. (2)

Sizing handles The small, square handles inside the border lines of a selected graphic that are used for resizing. (25)

Soft page break A page break automatically placed by Word, which is continually adjusted to reflect changes in the document. (11)

Sorting The process of reordering text, either alphanumerically, numerically, or by date. (24)

Special character A character that does not appear on a standard keyboard. (17)

Spike An AutoText entry used to store multiple pieces of information. (21)

Split bar A horizontal bar that can be moved to split a document window. (9)

Split box The small, black rectangle at the top of the vertical scroll bar which is used to split a document window into two panes. (9)

Strikethrough An optional character attribute that causes a horizontal line to appear through the characters. (17)

Style name A name given to a style to identify it. (20)

Style sheet A list of the styles found in a Word document. (20)

Subscript An optional character attribute that causes text to appear slightly below the other text on the same line. (17)

Superscript An optional character attribute that causes text to appear slightly above the other text on the same line. (17)

TIFF A standard graphic format, stands for tagged image file format. (25)

Tab marker A symbol on the horizontal ruler that indicates a custom tab setting. (6)

Tab stop The stopping point of a tab. (6)

Tab A set amount of space that is used to align text in a document. (6)

Table A grid of columns and rows that contains information. (18)

Template A file that contains the formatting information, styles, and sometimes text for a particular type of document. (21)

Widow A line that appears by itself at the top of a page of text. (11)

Wizard A template that contains sophisticated macros to automate document creation. (21)

Wordwrap The automatic placement of text on the next line. (1)

KEYBOARD SHORTCUTS

Introductory Word Skills

Ctrl+F12 or **Ctrl+O**	Open
Ctrl+N	New document
Ctrl+F4	Close document
Alt+F4	Exit Word
Shift+F12 or **Ctrl+S**	Save
F12	Save As
Ctrl+F2	Print Preview
Ctrl+P	Print
F1	Open Help
Shift+F1	Open context-sensitive Help
F4	Repeat last action
Ctrl+Z	Undo
F5 or **Ctrl+G**	Go to
Shift+F5	Go back
Shift+F10	Display shortcut menu

Moving the Insertion Point

Ctrl+Left Arrow	One word to left
Ctrl+Right Arrow	One word to right
Home	Beginning of line
End	End of line
Ctrl+Up Arrow	One paragraph up
Ctrl+Down Arrow	One paragraph down
Page Up	One window up
Page Down	One window down
Ctrl+Home	Beginning of document
Ctrl+End	End of document

Selecting Text

Shift+Right or **Left Arrow**	One character to right or left
Ctrl+Shift+Left Arrow	To start of word
Ctrl+Shift+Right Arrow	To end of word
Shift+End	To end of line
Shift+Home	To start of line
Shift+Up or **Down Arrow**	One line up or down
Ctrl+Shift+Up Arrow	To start of paragraph
Ctrl+Shift+Down Arrow	To end of paragraph
Shift+Page Up	One screen up
Shift+Page Down	One screen down
Ctrl+Shift+Home	To start of document
Ctrl+Shift+End	To end of document
Ctrl+A	Select all

Character Formatting

Ctrl+B	Turn on or off bold
Ctrl+I	Turn on or off italic
Ctrl+U	Turn on or off underline
Ctrl+Shift+D	Turn on or off double underline
Ctrl+Shift+W	Turn on or off words-only underline
Ctrl+Shift+A	Turn on or off all capitals
Shift+F3	Change case of characters
Ctrl+Spacebar	Remove character formatting
Ctrl+Shift+=	Turn on or off superscript
Ctrl+=	Turn on or off subscript
Ctrl+Shift+H	Turn on or off hidden text
Ctrl+Shift+K	Turn on or off small capitals
Ctrl+Shift+>	Increase text size
Ctrl+Shift+<	Decrease text size

Deleting, Copying, and Pasting

Ctrl+Backspace	Delete one word to left
Ctrl+Del	Delete one word to right
Ctrl+X	Cut text
Ctrl+C	Copy text
Ctrl+V	Paste text
Ctrl+Shift+C	Copy formats
Ctrl+Shift+V	Paste formats

Find and Replace

Ctrl+F	Find
Ctrl+H	Replace
Shift+F4	Repeat Find or Replace
Shift+Insert	Paste Clipboard contents into text box

Paragraph Formatting

Ctrl+L	Left-align
Ctrl+E	Center
Ctrl+R	Right-align
Ctrl+J	Justify
Ctrl+1	Single-space
Ctrl+2	Double-space
Ctrl+5	One-and-one half space
Ctrl+M	Indent from left margin
Ctrl+Shift+M	Decrease indent
Ctrl+T	Set hanging indent
Ctrl+Shift+T	Decrease hanging indent
Ctrl+Q	Remove paragraph formatting

Writing Tools

F7	Start spelling check
Shift+F7	Start thesaurus
Ctrl+- (hyphen)	Optional hyphen
Ctrl+Shift+- (hyphen)	Nonbreaking hyphen
Ctrl+Shift+Spacebar	Nonbreaking space

Line, Page, and Column Breaks

Shift+Enter	Insert line break
Ctrl+Enter	Insert hard page break
Ctrl+Shift+Enter	Insert column break

Tables

Tab	Move to next cell
Shift+Tab	Move to previous cell
Alt+Home	Move to first cell in current row
Alt+End	Move to last cell in current row
Alt+PgUp	Move to first cell in current column
Alt+PgDn	Move to last cell in current column
Alt+Shift+PgDn	Select column
Ctrl+Tab	Insert tab within cell
Alt+5 (numeric keypad)	Select table

Fields

F9	Update field
Ctrl+F9	Insert blank field
Alt+F9	Turn on and off field codes
Ctrl+F11	Lock fields
Ctrl+Shift+F11	Unlock fields
F11	Go to next field
Shift+F11	Go to previous field

Styles

Ctrl+K	Start AutoFormat
Ctrl+Shift+N	Apply Normal style
Alt+Ctrl+1	Apply Heading 1
Alt+Ctrl+2	Apply Heading 2
Alt+Ctrl+3	Apply Heading 3

AutoText and the Spike

[AutoText entry]+**F3**	Insert AutoText entry
Ctrl+F3	Store selected text in Spike
spike+**F3**	Insert contents of Spike
Ctrl+Shift+F3	Insert and empty contents of Spike